NEUROBIOLOGY OF MENTAL ILLNESS

NEUROBIOLOGY OF MENTAL ILLNESS

FOURTH EDITION

EDITED BY

Dennis S. Charney, MD

ANNE AND JOEL EHRENKRANZ, DEAN,
ICAHN SCHOOL OF MEDICINE AT MOUNT SINAI
EXECUTIVE VICE PRESIDENT FOR ACADEMIC AFFAIRS,
THE MOUNT SINAI MEDICAL CENTER
PROFESSOR, DEPARTMENTS OF PSYCHIATRY,
NEUROSCIENCE, AND
PHARMACOLOGY & SYSTEMS THERAPEUTICS
NEW YORK, NY

Pamela Sklar, MD, PhD

PROFESSOR, DEPARTMENTS OF PSYCHIATRY,
NEUROSCIENCE, AND GENETICS AND GENOMIC
SCIENCES
CHIEF, DIVISION OF PSYCHIATRIC GENOMICS
ICAHN SCHOOL OF MEDICINE AT MOUNT SINAI
NEW YORK, NY

Joseph D. Buxbaum, PhD

G. HAROLD AND LEILA Y. MATHERS PROFESSOR,
DEPARTMENTS OF PSYCHIATRY, NEUROSCIENCE, AND
GENETICS AND GENOMIC SCIENCES
CHIEF, DIVISION OF NEURODEVELOPMENTAL
DISORDERS
DIRECTOR, SEAVER AUTISM CENTER
ICAHN SCHOOL OF MEDICINE AT MOUNT SINAI
NEW YORK, NY

Eric J. Nestler, MD, PhD

NASH FAMILY PROFESSOR,
DEPARTMENTS OF NEUROSCIENCE, PSYCHIATRY,
AND PHARMACOLOGY & SYSTEMS THERAPEUTICS
CHAIR, DEPARTMENT OF NEUROSCIENCE
DIRECTOR, THE FRIEDMAN BRAIN INSTITUTE
ICAHN SCHOOL OF MEDICINE AT MOUNT SINAI
NEW YORK, NY

SECTION EDITORS

Eric J. Nestler, MD, PhD
Karl Deisseroth, MD, PhD
Pamela Sklar, MD, PhD
Helen S. Mayberg, MD
Kerry J. Ressler, MD, PhD

Antonello Bonci, MD
Nora D. Volkow, MD
David M. Holtzman, MD
Joseph D. Buxbaum, PhD
Dennis S. Charney, MD

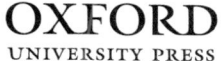
OXFORD
UNIVERSITY PRESS

OXFORD
UNIVERSITY PRESS

Oxford University Press is a department of the University of Oxford.
It furthers the University's objective of excellence in research, scholarship,
and education by publishing worldwide.

Oxford   New York
Auckland   Cape Town   Dar es Salaam   Hong Kong   Karachi
Kuala Lumpur   Madrid   Melbourne   Mexico City   Nairobi
New Delhi   Shanghai   Taipei   Toronto

With offices in
Argentina   Austria   Brazil   Chile   Czech Republic   France   Greece
Guatemala   Hungary   Italy   Japan   Poland   Portugal   Singapore
South Korea   Switzerland   Thailand   Turkey   Ukraine   Vietnam

Oxford is a registered trade mark of Oxford University Press
in the UK and certain other countries.

Published in the United States of America by
Oxford University Press
198 Madison Avenue, New York, NY 10016

Library of Congress Cataloging-in-Publication Data
Neurobiology of mental illness / edited by Dennis S. Charney . . . [et al.]. — 4th ed.
       p. ; cm.
Includes bibliographical references and index.
ISBN 978–0–19–993495–9 (hardcover : alk. paper); 978-0-19-939846-1 (paperback : alk. paper)
I. Charney, Dennis S.
[DNLM: 1. Mental Disorders—etiology.   2. Mental Disorders—physiopathology.   3. Mental Disorders—therapy.   4. Neurobiology. WM 140]
616.8—dc23
2012538316

This material is not intended to be, and should not be considered, a substitute for medical or other professional advice. Treatment for the conditions
described in this material is highly dependent on the individual circumstances. And, while this material is designed to offer accurate information
with respect to the subject matter covered and to be current as of the time it was written, research and knowledge about medical and health issues is
constantly evolving and dose schedules for medications are being revised continually, with new side effects recognized and accounted for regularly.
Readers must therefore always check the product information and clinical procedures with the most up-to-date published product information and
data sheets provided by the manufacturers and the most recent codes of conduct and safety regulations. The publisher and the authors make no
representations or warranties to readers, express or implied, as to the accuracy or completeness of this material. Without limiting the foregoing, the
publisher and the authors make no representations or warranties as to the accuracy or efficacy of the drug dosages mentioned in the material. The
authors and the publisher do not accept, and expressly disclaim, any responsibility for any liability, loss, or risk that may be claimed or incurred as a
consequence of the use and/or application of any of the contents of this material.

9 8 7 6 5 4 3 2 1

Printed in the United States of America
on acid-free paper

CONTENTS

SECTION IX

SPECIAL TOPIC AREAS   1065

Dennis S. Charney

PREFACE

These are exciting yet frustrating times for psychiatry. Our knowledge of basic brain function continues to increase at an accelerating pace as the tools of biology—from genetics and epigenetics to detailed exploration of brain circuits in animals and humans—become ever more powerful and penetrating. Yet this explosion of knowledge of the brain has not been translated into fundamental advances in our understanding of the pathophysiology of most major psychiatric syndromes, the diagnosis of these syndromes based on their underlying biological mechanisms, or the treatment and prevention of mental illness.

Why has there been such a divide between our basic knowledge and clinical advances? First and foremost, the brain has proved to be far more complicated than ever imagined a generation ago, and the disorders of the brain that manifest primarily in behavioral abnormalities (i.e., mental illness) are far more complicated too in terms of their genetic causes and the associated abnormalities at the epigenetic, cellular, and circuit levels. We have also learned that effective translation will not occur automatically or organically and will require a far more concerted effort than mounted thus far to link findings in basic neurobiology and genetics to the human syndromes. The good news is that leaders at the National Institutes of Health, academia, and industry recognize the need for such collaborations, with many exciting ventures now underway or planned to meet the challenges ahead.

We have completely revamped the fourth edition of *Neurobiology of Mental Illness* to address these challenging yet promising times. We have recruited two new book editors to add depth and breadth of expertise, and have engaged a team of all new section editors, each of whom represents a leader in his or her fields. Accordingly, new authors have been enlisted for a majority of the chapters that now comprise this book, with many new chapters added and old ones removed to reflect progress in the field. The result is a thoroughly updated view of the state of psychiatry, both its basic underpinnings and clinical evidence, with a view toward advances that can be expected in the coming years and the methodology that will bring us there.

As before, Section I provides an overview of basic neuroscience that is relevant to clinical psychiatry and expanding its foundations. Molecular neurobiology and molecular genetics are emphasized in the context of brain development, neuropharmacology, neuronal function, and neural networks and plasticity, with an eye on their contribution to complex behaviors.

Section II reviews the methods used to examine the biological basis of mental illness in animal models and in humans. This part has been expanded to reflect critically important technical advances in complex genetics (including powerful sequencing technologies and related bioinformatics), epigenetics, stem cell biology, optogenetics, cognitive neuroscience, and brain imaging. We believe that this range of exciting methodologies offer unique opportunities for the translation of preclinical and clinical research into badly needed breakthroughs in our therapeutic toolkit.

The remaining parts of the book cover the neurobiology and genetics of major psychiatric disorders: psychoses (including bipolar disorder), mood disorders, anxiety disorders, substance abuse disorders, dementias, disorders of childhood onset, and special topic areas. Each of these parts has been augmented in several different areas as a reflection of research progress. The last section, on special topics, includes chapters that address diagnostic schemes for mental illness. The release of our new edition coincides with the publication of DSM-5 (*Diagnostic and Statistical Manual-5*) by the American Psychiatric Association. Unfortunately, the diagnostic classification system utilized by DSM-5 remains limited by necessity, because it is still based primarily on phenomenology rather than etiology and pathophysiology. Alternative perspectives on diagnosis, for example, RDoC (research domain criteria), are therefore also presented. We predict that the research advances reviewed in our textbook will ultimately lead to diagnostic systems in which genetic and neurobiological abnormalities have a primary role.

This edition of *Neurobiology of Mental Illness* reflects the continuing reintegration of psychiatry into the mainstream of biomedical science. The research tools that are transforming other branches of medicine—epidemiology, genetics, epigenetics, molecular and cell biology, imaging, and medicinal chemistry—will also one day transform psychiatry. It is our hope that, like us, the reader is optimistic that the progress in genetics and in molecular, cellular, and systems neuroscience described in this textbook will eventually break new ground in the diagnosis, treatment, and prevention of disabling psychiatric disorders.

The Editors

CONTRIBUTORS

Jane B. Acri, PhD
Division of Pharmacotherapies and Medical Consequences
    of Drug Abuse
National Institute on Drug Abuse
National Institutes of Heath
Bethesda, MD

Susanne E. Ahmari, MD, PhD
Department of Psychiatry
New York State Psychiatric Institute
College of Physicians and Surgeons at Columbia University
New York, NY

Schahram Akbarian, MD, PhD
Departments of Psychiatry and Neuroscience; and
Friedman Brain Institute
Icahn School of Medicine at Mount Sinai
New York, NY

Gail A. Alvares
Brain & Mind Research Institute
The University of Sydney
Sydney, Australia

Alan Anticevic, PhD
Department of Psychiatry
Yale University School of Medicine; and
NIAAA Center for Translational Neuroscience of Alcoholism
New Haven, CT

Tracy L. Bale, PhD
Department of Psychiatry
Perelman School of Medicine
University of Pennsylvania
Philadelphia, PA

Deanna M. Barch, PhD
Departments of Psychology, Psychiatry and Radiology
Washington University School of Medicine
St. Louis, MO

Tami D. Benton, MD
Department of Child and Adolescent Psychiatry and
    Behavioral Science
Perelman School of Medicine at the University of Pennsylvania
Philadelphia, PA

Steven M. Berman, PhD
Department of Psychiatry and Biobehavioral Sciences
David Geffen School of Medicine-UCLA
Los Angeles, CA

Joseph Biederman, MD
Department of Psychiatry
Massachusetts General Hospital; and
Harvard Medical School
Boston, MA

R. James R. Blair, PhD
Unit of Affective Cognitive Neuroscience
Department of Health and Human Services
National Institute of Mental Health
National Institutes of Health
Bethesda, MD

Michael H. Bloch, MD
Yale Child Study Center and Department
    of Psychiatry
Yale University School of Medicine
New Haven, CT

Luke Bloy, PhD
Department of Radiology
Children's Hospital of Philadelphia
Philadelphia, PA

Joshua Blume, MD
Department of Psychiatry
Perelman School of Medicine at the University of
    Pennsylvania
Philadelphia, PA

Antonello Bonci, MD
Synaptic Plasticity Section
Intramural Research Program of the National Institute
    on Drug Abuse
Baltimore, MD

James B. Brewer, MD, PhD
Departments of Radiology and Neurosciences
University of California, San Diego
San Diego, CA

Katherine E. Burdick , PhD
Department of Psychiatry; and
Friedman Brain Institute
Icahn School of Medicine at Mount Sinai
New York, NY

Jeffrey Burns, MD
Department of Neurology
Kansas University Medical Center
Kansas City, KS

Joseph D. Buxbaum, PhD
Departments of Psychiatry, Neuroscience, and Genetic and
    Genomic Sciences; and
Friedman Brain Institute
Icahn School of Medicine at Mount Sinai
New York, NY

Christopher K. Cain, PhD
Center for Neural Science
New York University
New York, NY

William A. Carlezon, Jr., PhD
Departments of Psychiatry and Neuroscience
Harvard Medical School
Mclean Hospital
Belmont, MA

B.J. Casey, PhD
Sackler Institute for Developmental Psychobiology
Weill Medical College of Cornell University
New York, NY

Kristina Caudle, PhD
Sackler Institute for Developmental Psychobiology
Weill Medical College of Cornell University
New York, NY

Linda Chang, MD
Department of Medicine
John A. Burns School of Medicine, University of Hawai'i
Honolulu, HI

Dennis S. Charney, MD
Departments of Psychiatry, Neuroscience, and
    Pharmacology & Systems Therapeutics; and
Friedman Brain Institute
Icahn School of Medicine at Mount Sinai
New York, NY

Kimberly M. Christian, PhD
Institute for Cell Engineering
Departments of Neurology and Neuroscience
Johns Hopkins School of Medicine
Baltimore, MD

Helena Chang Chui, MD
Department of Neurology
Keck Medical Center of USC
Los Angeles, CA

Chiara Cirelli, MD, PhD
Department of Psychiatry
University of Wisconsin-Madison School
    of Medicine
Madison, WI

Christine C. Cloak, PhD
Department of Medicine
John A. Burns School of Medicine, University of Hawai'i
Honolulu, HI

Claire D. Craft
Department of Psychiatry
University of North Carolina School of Medicine
Chapel Hill, NC

Paul Crits-Christoph, PhD
Department of Psychiatry
Perelman School of Medicine at the University of Pennsylvania
Philadelphia, PA

Jeffrey Cummings, MD, ScD
Cleveland Clinic Lou Ruvo Center for Brain Health
Las Vegas, NV

Allison A. Curley, PhD
Department of Psychiatry
University of Pittsburgh School of Medicine
Pittsburgh, PA

Bruce N. Cuthbert, PhD
National Institute of Mental Health
National Institutes of Health
Bethesda, MD

Mark J. Daly, PhD
Analytic and Translational Genetics Unit
Massachusetts General Hospital, Boston, MA; and
Broad Institute of MIT and Harvard
Cambridge, MA

Karl Deisseroth, MD, PhD
Departments of Bioengineering and Psychiatry and
    Behavioral Sciences
Howard Hughes Medical Institute
Stanford University
Palo Alto, CA

Ariel Y. Deutch, PhD
Department of Psychiatry
Vanderbilt University School of Medicine
Nashville, TN

Mara Dierssen, MD, PhD
Cellular and Systems Neurobiology
Systems Biology Program
Center for Genomic Regulation
Barcelona, Spain

Ralph J. DiLeone, PhD
Department of Psychiatry
Yale University School of Medicine
New Haven, CT

Erin C. Dowd
Department of Psychology; and Neuroscience Program
Washington University School of Medicine
St. Louis, MO

Amanda Downey
Eating and Weight Disorders Program
Ichan School of Medicine at Mount Sinai
New York, NY

Wayne C. Drevets, MD
The Laureate Institute for Brain Research; and
Johnson & Johnson, Inc.
Tulsa, OK

Benoit Dubé, MD
Department of Psychiatry
Perelman School of Medicine at the University of
    Pennsylvania
Philadelphia, PA

Ronald S. Duman, PhD
Departments of Psychiatry and Pharmacology
Yale University School of Medicine
New Haven, CT

Amit Etkin, MD, PhD
Veterans Affairs Palo Alto Healthcare System; and
Sierra Pacific Mental Illness, Research, Education, and
    Clinical Center (MIRECC)
Department of Psychiatry and Behavioral Sciences
Stanford University School of Medicine
Stanford, CA

Christopher J. Evans, PhD
Brain Research Institute
David Geffen School of Medicine-UCLA
Los Angeles, CA

Dwight L. Evans, MD
Department of Psychiatry
Perelman School of Medicine at the University of
    Pennsylvania
Philadelphia, PA

Anne M. Fagan, PhD
Department of Neurology
Washington University School of Medicine
St. Louis, MO

Stephen V. Faraone, PhD
Department of Psychiatry
SUNY Upstate Medical University
Syracuse, NY

Jan Fawcett, MD
Department of Psychiatry
University of New Mexico School of Medicine
Albuquerque, NM

Adriana Feder, MD
Department of Psychiatry; and
Friedman Brain Institute
Icahn School of Medicine at Mount Sinai
New York, NY

Lief E. Fenno
Howard Hughes Medical Institute
Stanford University
Palo Alto, CA

Maura A. Furey, PhD
Section on Neuroimaging in Mood and Anxiety Disorders
National Institute of Mental Health
Bethesda, MD

James E. Galvin, MD, MPH
Comprehensive Center on Brain Aging; and
Department of Neurology
New York University Langone Medical Center
New York, NY

Mark S. George, MD
Departments of Psychiatry, Radiology, and Neurology
Medical University of South Carolina
Charleston, SC

Michael D. Geschwind, MD, PhD
Institute for Neurodegenerative Diseases
Department of Neurology
University of California, San Francisco Medical Center
San Francisco, CA

Jean-Antoine Girault, MD, PhD
Department of Neuroscience
Institut du Fer-à-Moulin
Paris, France

David Goldman, MD
Laboratory of Neurogenetics
National Institute on Alcohol Abuse and Alcoholism
National Institutes of Health
Rockville, MD

Madeleine S. Goodkind, PhD
Veterans Affairs Palo Alto Healthcare System; and
Sierra Pacific Mental Illness, Research, Education, and
    Clinical Center (MIRECC)
Department of Psychiatry and Behavioral Sciences
Stanford University School of Medicine
Stanford, CA

Ki A. Goosens, PhD
Department of Brain and Cognitive Sciences
Massachusetts Institute of Technology
Cambridge, MA

Bronwyn M. Graham, PhD
Athinoula A. Martinos Center for Biomedical Engineering
Harvard University School of Medicine
Cambridge, MA

Seth G. N. Grant, BSc (Medicine), MB, BS, FRSE
Centre for Clinical Brain Sciences
The University of Edinburgh
Edinburgh, UK

Paul Greengard, PhD
Laboratory of Molecular and Cellular Neuroscience
The Rockefeller University
New York, NY

Dorothy E. Grice, MD
Department of Psychiatry; and
Friedman Brain Institute
Icahn School of Medicine at Mount Sinai
New York, NY

Pamela C. Griesler, PhD
Department of Psychiatry
College of Physicians and Surgeons at
Columbia University
New York State Psychiatric Institute
New York, NY

Joshua D. Grill, PhD
Mary S. Easton Center for Alzheimer's Disease Research
David Geffen School of Medicine-UCLA
Los Angeles, CA

David Grodberg, MD
Department of Psychiatry; and
Friedman Brain Institute
Icahn School of Medicine at Mount Sinai
New York, NY

Adam J. Guastella, PhD
Brain & Mind Research Institute
The University of Sydney
Sydney, Australia

Raquel E. Gur, MD, PhD
Department of Psychiatry
Perelman School of Medicine
University of Pennsylvania
Philadelphia, PA

Fiorella Gurrieri, MD
Istituto di Genetica Medica
Università Cattolica del Sacro Cuore
Rome, Italy

Anett Gyurak, PhD
Veterans Affairs Palo Alto Healthcare System; and
Sierra Pacific Mental Illness, Research, Education, and
Clinical Center (MIRECC)
Department of Psychiatry and Behavioral Sciences
Stanford University School of Medicine
Stanford, CA

Brant Hager, MD
Department of Psychiatry
University of New Mexico School of Medicine
Albuquerque, NM

Stephen J. Haggarty, PhD
Department of Neurology
Massachusetts General Hospital
Boston, MA

Margaret Haglund, MD
Department of Psychiatry
David Geffen School of Medicine-UCLA
Los Angeles, CA

Shannon M. Hamilton, PhD
Department of Molecular and Human Genetics
Baylor College of Medicine
Houston, TX

Jason Hassenstab, PhD
Department of Neurology
Washington University School of Medicine
St. Louis, MO

Stephan Heckers, MD
Department of Psychiatry
Vanderbilt University School of Medicine
Nashville, TN

Jaimie M. Henderson, MD
Department of Neurosurgery
Stanford University School of Medicine
Palo Alto, CA

John M. Hettema, MD, PhD
Department of Psychiatry
Virginia Institute for Psychiatric and Behavioral Genetics
Virginia Commonwealth University
Richmond, VA

Thomas B. Hildebrandt, PhD
Department of Psychiatry; and
Friedman Brain Institute
Icahn School of Medicine at Mount Sinai
New York, NY

Georgia E. Hodes, PhD
Fishberg Department of Neuroscience; and
Friedman Brain Institute
Icahn School of Medicine at Mount Sinai
New York, NY

John L. Holt, PhD
Department of Medicine
John A. Burns School of Medicine, University of Hawai'i
Honolulu, HI

David M. Holtzman, MD
Department of Neurology
Washington University School of Medicine
St. Louis, MO

Mei-Chen Hu, PhD
Department of Psychiatry
College of Physicians and Surgeons at Columbia University
New York, NY

Steven E. Hyman, MD
Stanley Center for Psychiatric Research
Broad Institute of Harvard University and MIT
Cambridge, MA

Thomas R. Insel, MD
National Institute of Mental Health
National Institutes of Health
Bethesda, MD

Dan V. Iosifescu, MD
Departments of Psychiatry and Neuroscience; and
Friedman Brain Institute
Icahn School of Medicine at Mount Sinai
New York, NY

Elena I. Ivleva, MD, PhD
Department of Psychiatry
UT Southwestern Medical Center
Dallas, TX

J. David Jentsch, PhD
Department of Psychology
University of California, Los Angeles
Los Angeles, CA

Yan Jiang, PhD
Departments of Psychiatry and Neuroscience; and
Friedman Brain Institute,
Icahn School of Medicine at Mount Sinai
New York, NY

Keith A. Johnson, MD
Departments of Radiology and Neurology
Massachusetts General Hospital and Harvard Medical
    School; and
Centre for Alzheimer Research and Treatment
Department of Neurology
Brigham and Women's Hospital and Harvard Medical School
Boston, MA

Tanja Jovanovic, PhD
Department of Psychiatry and Behavioral Sciences
Emory University School of Medicine
Atlanta, GA

Peter W. Kalivas, PhD
Department of Neurosciences
Medical University of South Carolina
Charleston, SC

Denise B. Kandel, PhD
Department of Psychiatry
College of Physicians and Surgeons, and
Department of Sociomedical Sciences
Mailman School of Public Health Columbia University; and
New York State Psychiatric Institute
New York, NY

Stella Karantzoulis, PhD
Comprehensive Center on Brain Aging; and
Department of Neurology
New York University Langone Medical Center
New York, NY

Walter E. Kaufmann, MD
Department of Neurology
Boston Children's Hospital
Harvard Medical School
Boston, MA

Orion P. Keifer, Jr.
Department of Psychiatry and Behavioral Sciences
Emory University School of Medicine
Atlanta, GA

Brigitte L. Kieffer, PhD
Institute of Genetics and Molecular
    and Cellular Biology
Université Louis Pasteur
Strasbourg, Alsace, France

Meghan E. Keough, PhD
Department of Psychiatry and Behavioral Science
University of Washington at Harborview Medical Center
Seattle, WA

George Kirov, MRCPsych, PhD
MRC Centre for Neuropsychiatric Genetics
    and Genomics
Department of Psychological Medicine and Neurology
School of Medicine
Cardiff University
Wales, UK

Alexander Kolevzon, MD
Departments of Psychiatry and Pediatrics; and
Friedman Brain Institute
Icahn School of Medicine at Mount Sinai
New York, NY

Elisa E. Konofagou, PhD
Departments of Biomedical Engineering
    and Radiology
The Fu Foundation School of Engineering and Applied
    Science
Columbia University
New York, NY

Saïd Kourrich, PhD
Synaptic Plasticity Section
Intramural Research Program of the National Institute on
    Drug Abuse
Baltimore, MD

K. Ranga Rama Krishnan, MD
Neuroscience & Behavioral Disorders Program
Duke-NUS Graduate School
Singapore

David J. Kupfer, MD
Departments of Psychiatry Neuroscience and Clinical &
    Translational Science
University of Pittsburgh Schools of the
    Health Sciences
Pittsburgh, PA

Ester J. Kwon, PhD
Department of Brain and Cognitive Sciences
Massachusetts Institute of Technology
Cambridge, MA

Evelyn K. Lambe, PhD
Departments of Physiology, Obstetrics and Gynecology,
  and Psychiatry
University of Toronto
Toronto, Canada

Joseph E. LeDoux, PhD
Center for Neural Science
New York University
New York, NY

Francis S. Lee, MD, PhD
Department of Psychiatry
Weill Medical College of Cornell University
New York, NY

Kelly Lei
Department of Psychology and Program in Neuroscience
Florida State University
Tallahassee, FL

Douglas F. Levinson, MD
Department of Psychiatry and Behavioral Sciences
Stanford University School of Medicine
Stanford, CA

David A. Lewis, MD
Department of Psychiatry
University of Pittsburgh School of Medicine
Pittsburgh, PA

Peiying Liu, PhD
Departments of Psychiatry and Radiology
UT Southwestern Medical Center
Dallas, TX

Edythe D. London, PhD
Departments of Molecular & Medical Pharmacology and
  Psychiatry and Biobehavioral Sciences
Center for Addictive Behaviors
Semel Institute for Neuroscience and Human Behavior
David Geffen School of Medicine-UCLA
Los Angeles, CA

Rafael Maldonado, MD, PhD
Department of Pharmacology
Universitat Pompeu Fabra
Barcelona, Spain

Hanzhang Lu, PhD
Departments of Psychiatry and Radiology
UT Southwestern Medical Center
Dallas, TX

Dolores Malaspina, MD
Department of Psychiatry
New York University School of Medicine
New York, NY

Salvador Martínez, MD, PhD
Instituto de Neurociencias
UMH-CSIC
San Juan, Alicante, Spain

Daniel C. Mathews, MD
Experimental Therapeutics & Pathophysiology Branch
National Institute of Mental Health
Bethesda, MD

Helen S. Mayberg, MD
Departments of Psychiatry and Neurology
Emory University School of Medicine
Atlanta, GA

Bryan E. McGill, MD, PhD
Department of Neurology
Washington University School of Medicine
St. Louis, MO

Heather C. Mefford, MD, PhD
Department of Pediatrics
University of Washington School of Medicine
Seattle, WA

Julie W. Messinger
Department of Psychiatry
New York University School of Medicine
New York, NY

Mohammed R. Milad, PhD
Department of Psychiatry
Massachusetts General Hospital; and
Harvard University School of Medicine
Cambridge, MA

Bruce Miller, MD
Department of Neurology
University of California, San Francisco School of Medicine
San Francisco, CA

Guo-li Ming, MD, PhD
Institute for Cell Engineering
Departments of Neurology and Neuroscience
Johns Hopkins School of Medicine
Baltimore, MD

Amanda C. Mitchell, PhD
Departments of Psychiatry and Neuroscience; and
Friedman Brain Institute
Icahn School of Medicine at Mount Sinai
New York, NY

Hanns Möhler, PhD
Institute of Pharmacology and Toxicology
University of Zurich and Swiss Institute of Technology
Zurich, Switzerland

Lisa M. Monteggia, PhD
Department of Psychiatry
UT Southwestern Medical Center
Dallas, TX

Dave Morgan, PhD
Byrd Alzheimer's Institute
Department of Molecular Pharmacology and Physiology
Morsani College of Medicine
University of South Florida
Tampa, FL

John C. Morris, MD
Department of Neurology
Washington University School of Medicine
St. Louis, MO

Anne-Marie Mouly, PhD
Department of Sensory Neurosciences,
    Behavior, Cognition
Centre de Recherche en Neurosciences de Lyon
Lyon, France

Karen E. Murray
Department of Psychiatry and Behavioral Sciences
Emory University School of Medicine
Atlanta, GA

James W. Murrough, MD
Departments of Psychiatry and Neuroscience; and
Friedman Brain Institute
Icahn School of Medicine at Mount Sinai
New York, NY

Georges Naasan, MD
Department of Neurology
University of California, San Francisco School of Medicine
San Francisco, CA

Benjamin M. Neale, PhD
Analytic and Translational Genetics Unit
Massachusetts General Hospital; and
Stanley Center for Psychiatric Research
Broad Institute of MIT and Harvard
Cambridge, MA

Giovanni Neri, MD
Istituto di Genetica Medica
Università Cattolica del Sacro Cuore
Rome, Italy

Eric J. Nestler, MD, PhD
Fishberg Department of Neuroscience; and
Friedman Brain Institute
Icahn School of Medicine at Mount Sinai
New York, NY

Judith A. Neugroschl, MD
Department of Psychiatry; and
Friedman Brain Institute
Icahn School of Medicine at Mount Sinai
New York, NY

Antonia S. New, MD
Department of Psychiatry; and
Friedman Brain Institute
Icahn School of Medicine at Mount Sinai
New York, NY

Seth Davin Norrholm, PhD
Department of Psychiatry and Behavioral Sciences
Emory University School of Medicine
Atlanta, GA

Michael C. O'Donovan, PhD, FRCPsych
MRC Centre for Neuropsychiatric Genetics
    and Genomics
Department of Psychological Medicine
    and Neurology
School of Medicine
Cardiff University
Wales, UK

Dost Öngür, MD, PhD
Department of Psychiatry
Mclean Hospital; and
Harvard University School of Medicine
Belmont, MA

Takeshi Otowa, MD, PhD
Department of Neuropsychiatry
Graduate School of Medicine
University of Tokyo
Tokyo, Japan

Michael J. Owen, PhD, FRCPsych
MRC Centre for Neuropsychiatric Genetics
    and Genomics
Department of Psychological Medicine and Neurology
School of Medicine
Cardiff University
Wales, UK

Vani Pariyadath, PhD
Neuroimaging Research Branch
National Institute on Drug Abuse
National Institutes of Health
Baltimore, MD

Siobhan S. Pattwell, PhD
Sackler Institute for Developmental Psychobiology
Weill Medical College of Cornell University
New York, NY

Martin P. Paulus, MD
Department of Psychiatry
University of California, San Diego
San Diego, CA

Richard Paylor, PhD
Department of Molecular and Human Genetics
Baylor College of Medicine
Houston, TX

Javier A. Perez, PhD
Department of Psychiatry
Virginia Institute for Psychiatric and Behavioral Genetics
Virginia Commonwealth University
Richmond, VA

M. Mercedes Perez-Rodriguez, MD, PhD
Department of Psychiatry; and
Friedman Brain Institute
Icahn School of Medicine at Mount Sinai
New York, NY

Roy Perlis, MD
Department of Psychiatry
Massachusetts General Hospital
Boston, MA

Cyril J. Peter, PhD
Departments of Psychiatry and Neuroscience; and
Friedman Brain Institute
Icahn School of Medicine at Mount Sinai
New York, NY

Christopher Pittenger, MD, PhD
Departments of Psychiatry and Psychology
    and Yale Child Study Center
Yale University School of Medicine
New Haven, CT

Mikhail V. Pletnikov, MD, PhD
Departments of Psychiatry and Behavioral Sciences,
    Neuroscience and
Molecular and Comparative Pathobiology
Johns Hopkins University School of Medicine
Baltimore, MD

Joseph L. Price, PhD
Department of Anatomy and Neurobiology
Washington University School of Medicine
St. Louis, MO

Shaun M. Purcell, PhD
Department of Psychiatry; and
Friedman Brain Institute
Icahn School of Medicine at Mount Sinai
New York, NY

Kathryn J. Reissner, PhD
Department of Psychology; and
UNC Neuroscience Center UNC Chapel Hill
Chapel Hill, NC

Kerry J. Ressler, MD, PhD
Department of Psychiatry and Behavioral Sciences
Emory University School of Medicine
Atlanta, GA

Roxann Roberson-Nay, PhD
Department of Psychiatry
Virginia Institute for Psychiatric and Behavioral Genetics
Virginia Commonwealth University
Richmond, VA

Timothy P. L. Roberts, PhD
Department of Radiology
Perelman School of Medicine at University of
    Pennsylvania; and
Children's Hospital of Philadelphia
Philadelphia, PA

Chelsea L. Robertson
Center for Addictive Behaviors
Semel Institute for Neuroscience and Human Behavior
David Geffen School of Medicine-UCLA
Los Angeles, CA

Elise B. Robinson, ScD
Analytic and Translational Genetics Unit
Massachusetts General Hospital
Boston, MA; and
Broad Institute of MIT and Harvard
Cambridge, MA

Christopher A. Ross, MD, PhD
Departments of Psychiatry and Behavioral Sciences,
    Neuroscience, Neurology and Pharmacology
Johns Hopkins University School of Medicine
Baltimore, MD

Robert H. Roth, PhD
Departments of Psychiatry and Pharmacology
Yale University School of Medicine
New Haven, CT

Peter P. Roy-Byrne, MD
Department of Psychiatry and Behavioral Science
University of Washington at Harborview Medical Center
Seattle, WA

John L. R. Rubenstein, MD, PhD
Department of Psychiatry
University of California, San Francisco School of Medicine
San Francisco, CA

David R. Rubinow, MD
Department of Psychiatry
University of North Carolina, School of Medicine
Chapel Hill, NC

Scott J. Russo, PhD
Fishberg Department of Neuroscience; and
Friedman Brain Institute
Icahn School of Medicine at Mount Sinai
New York, NY

Mary Sano, PhD
Department of Psychiatry; and
Friedman Brain Institute
Icahn School of Medicine at Mount Sinai
New York, NY

Eric E. Schadt, PhD
Department of Genetics and Genomic Sciences
Icahn School of Medicine at Mount Sinai
New York, NY

Peter J. Schmidt, MD
Behavioral Endocrinology Branch
National Institute of Mental Health
Bethesda, MD

Susan K. Schultz, MD
Department of Psychiatry
University of Iowa Carver School of Medicine
Iowa City, IA

Charles E. Schwartz, PhD
JC Self Research Institute
Greenwood Genetic Center
Greenwood, SC

Jorge Sepulcre, MD, PhD
Department of Radiology
Massachusetts General Hospital and
  Harvard Medical School; and
Athinioula A. Martinos Center for Biomedical Imaging
Charlestown, MA

Larry J. Siever, MD
Department of Psychiatry; and
Friedman Brain Institute
Icahn School of Medicine at Mount Sinai
New York, NY; and
Department of Psychiatry
Bronx VA Medical Center
Bronx, NY

H. Blair Simpson, MD, PhD
Department of Psychiatry
New York State Psychiatric Institute
College of Physicians and Surgeons at Columbia University
New York, NY

Pamela Sklar, MD, PhD
Departments of Psychiatry, Neuroscience, and Genetic
  and Genomic Sciences; and
Friedman Brain Institute
Icahn School of Medicine at Mount Sinai
New York, NY

Phil Skolnick, PhD, DSc
Division of Pharmacotherapies and Medical
  Consequences of Drug Abuse
National Institute on Drug Abuse
National Institutes of Heath
Bethesda, MD

Adam S. Smith
Department of Psychology and Program in Neuroscience
Florida State University
Tallahassee, FL

Lianne Morris Smith, MD
Department of Psychiatry
New York University School of Medicine
New York, NY

Takahiro Soda, MD, PhD
Department of Brain and Cognitive Sciences
Massachusetts Institute of Technology
Cambridge, MA

Hongjun Song, PhD
Institute for Cell Engineering
Departments of Neurology and Neuroscience
Johns Hopkins School of Medicine
Baltimore, MD

Steven M. Southwick, MD
Department of Psychiatry
Yale University School of Medicine
New Haven, CT

Matthew W. State, MD, PhD
Department of Psychiatry and Langley Porter Psychiatric
  Institute
University of California, San Francisco
San Francisco, CA

Elliot A. Stein, PhD
Neuroimaging Research Branch
National Institute on Drug Abuse
National Institutes of Health
Baltimore, MD

Murray B. Stein, MD, MPH
Departments of Psychiatry and Family and Preventive
  Medicine
University of California, San Diego
San Diego, CA

Gregory M. Sullivan, MD
Department of Psychiatry
New York State Psychiatric Institute
College of Physicians and Surgeons at
  Columbia University
New York, NY

Regina M. Sullivan, PhD
Department of Child and Adolescent Psychiatry
NYU Child Study Center; and
Nathan S. Kline Institute for Psychiatric Research
New York, NY

Yvette F. Taché, PhD
Brain Research Institute
David Geffen School of Medicine-UCLA
Los Angeles, CA

Carol A. Tamminga, MD
Department of Psychiatry
UT Southwestern Medical Center
Dallas, TX

Rudolph E. Tanzi, PhD
Department of Neurology
Massachusetts General Hospital
Harvard Medical School
Boston, MA

John J. Taylor
Department of Psychiatry
Medical University of South Carolina
Charleston, SC

Alexia M. Thomas, PhD
Department of Molecular and Human Genetics
Baylor College of Medicine
Houston, TX

Giulio Tononi, MD, PhD
Department of Psychiatry
University of Wisconsin-Madison
  School of Medicine
Madison, WI

Li-Huei Tsai, PhD
Department of Brain and Cognitive Sciences
Massachusetts Institute of Technology
Cambridge, MA

Anita Van Zwieten
Brain & Mind Research Institute
The University of Sydney
Sydney, Australia

Surabi Veeraragavan, PhD
Department of Molecular and Human Genetics
Baylor College of Medicine
Houston, TX

Ragini Verma, PhD
Center for Biomedical Image Computing and Analytics
Department of Radiology
Perelman School of Medicine at University of Pennsylvania
Philadelphia, PA

Nora D. Volkow, MD
National Institute on Drug Abuse
National Institutes of Health
Bethesda, MD

A. Ting Wang, PhD
Departments of Psychiatry and Neuroscience; and
Friedman Brain Institute
Icahn School of Medicine at Mount Sinai
New York, NY

Zuoxin Wang, PhD
Department of Psychology
Florida State University
Tallahassee, FL

Joel C. Watts, PhD
Institute for Neurodegenerative Diseases
Department of Neurology
University of California, San Francisco
    Medical Center
San Francisco, CA

Kyle Williams, MD
Yale Child Study Center and Department of Psychiatry
Yale University School of Medicine
New Haven, CT

Neil Woodward, MD, PhD
Department of Psychiatry
Vanderbilt University School of Medicine
Nashville, TN

Gang Wu
Department of Psychiatry; and
Friedman Brain Institute
Icahn School of Medicine at Mount Sinai
New York, NY

Yihong Yang, PhD
National Institute on Drug Abuse
Baltimore, MD

Carlos A. Zarate Jr., MD
Experimental Therapeutics & Pathophysiology Branch
National Institute of Mental Health
Bethesda, MD

Huda Y. Zoghbi, MD
Department of Molecular and Human Genetics
Baylor College of Medicine
Houston, TX

SECTION I | INTRODUCTION TO BASIC NEUROSCIENCE

ERIC J. NESTLER

The first part of this book provides an overview of basic neuroscience and molecular biology. Each chapter represents an enormous body of material that could itself be the subject of an entire textbook. Accordingly, these chapters are not intended to be comprehensive reviews, but rather concise summaries of the fields that lay the foundation of basic biological principles required for the clinical material that is the main focus of the book.

Chapter 1 provides an overview of brain development. There is increasing evidence that certain neuropsychiatric disorders may involve abnormalities in the formation of the nervous system. Although the details of such abnormalities remain poorly understood, the chapter provides insights into the cellular and molecular processes that may be involved and the ways in which such processes can be influenced by genetic and external factors.

Chapter 2 describes the neurochemical organization of the brain. It summarizes the diverse types of molecules that neurons in the brain use as neurotransmitters and neurotrophic factors, and how these molecules are synthesized and metabolized. The chapter also presents the array of receptor proteins through which these molecules regulate target neuron functioning and the reuptake proteins that generally terminate the neurotransmitter signal. Today a large majority of all drugs used to treat psychiatric disorders, as well as most drugs of abuse, still have as their initial targets proteins involved directly in neurotransmitter function.

Chapter 3 summarizes the electrophysiological basis of neuronal function. Ultimately, brain function is mediated by interactions between nerve cells, and the readout of such interactions is an alteration in the electrical properties of the cells. Moreover, recent human genetic studies have identified variations in the genes that encode specific ion channels that are associated with various forms of mental illness, further demonstrating the importance of understanding the basis of neuronal excitability. The chapter reviews the several types of recording techniques that are commonly used to measure neuronal activity and then presents the many types of ion channels and receptors that control a neuron's electrophysiological responses.

Chapter 4 covers postreceptor intracellular messenger cascades through which neurotransmitters and neurotrophic factors, and their receptors, produce their diverse physiological effects. A major advance over the past generation of research has been an appreciation of the complex webs of intracellular signaling pathways that control every aspect of a neuron's functioning, from neurotransmitter signaling to cell shape and motility to gene expression. Although only a small number of medications used in psychiatry today have as their initial target intracellular signaling proteins, it is likely that drug development efforts will look increasingly to such proteins for the discovery of novel medications with fundamentally new mechanisms of action.

Chapter 5 describes prominent mechanisms of neural plasticity, that is, ways in which neurons adapt over time in response to environmental perturbations. It is this capacity for adaptation (or maladaptation) that makes it possible for the brain not only to learn and think but also to get sick. The chapter focuses on the several different ways in which experience alters the function of specific synapses (synaptic plasticity), including long-term potentiation and depression, as well as the inherent excitability of nerve cells (whole cell or homeostatic plasticity), along with the ever-increasing knowledge of their underlying molecular mechanisms.

Chapter 6 provides an overview of the genetic basis of the nervous system. The chapter covers the structure of DNA and chromatin in the nucleus, how genes encode messenger RNAs and proteins, and the mechanisms (e.g., alternative splicing and posttranslational processing) by which numerous proteins can be generated from individual genes. The chapter also describes how this process of gene expression is under dynamic regulation throughout the adult life of an organism via the regulation of transcription factors and other nuclear proteins, and how such mechanisms contribute in important ways to long-lived neural plasticity.

Chapter 7 covers epigenetic mechanisms in psychiatry. Epigenetic regulation in neurons describes a process in which the activity of a particular gene is controlled by the structure of chromatin in that gene's proximity. Recent work has demonstrated the dynamic nature of chromatin remodeling in the nervous system and its importance for the normal development of the nervous system as well as the brain's capacity to adapt over time to environmental challenges. Abnormalities in chromatin remodeling have also been implicated in a growing number of neurological and psychiatric disorders.

A great deal has been written recently about the need for translational research in psychiatry. Yet we all know how uniquely difficult translational research is in our field. This is due to several factors, including the unique complexity of the brain, the lack of ready access to the brains of our patients, and the complexity of psychiatric disorders with respect to etiology and pathophysiology. As a result, it is currently difficult, if not impossible, to relate most of the material covered in this first part of the book to studies of the clinical disorders. How does one study, for example, the transcription factor *cyclic adenosine monophosphate response element binding protein* (CREB) or changes in dendritic spine density, implicated in animal models of several psychiatric conditions, in living patients? We view this difficulty, though very real today, as a time-limited obstacle. As advances in human genetics and brain imaging progress, it will become possible to analyze diverse neurotransmitter and neurotrophic factor systems, intracellular signaling proteins, and even gene expression and chromatin profiles in our patients and ultimately within discrete brain regions implicated in disease pathophysiology. Such methodologies will complete psychiatry's transformation into a field of modern molecular medicine.

1 | OVERVIEW OF BRAIN DEVELOPMENT

JOHN L. R. RUBENSTEIN

There is increasing evidence that abnormalities in the development of the brain either predispose or directly cause some psychiatric disorders. Although it is not surprising that childhood disorders, such as autism, are caused by neurodevelopmental abnormalities, disorders that display their most characteristic symptoms during or after adolescence may be influenced by developmental abnormalities. For instance, several lines of evidence suggest that schizophrenia is a neurodevelopment disorder. Thus, there is a compelling rationale for behavioral scientists and clinicians to understand the basic mechanisms that regulate assembly of the brain, as this information may be critical in understanding the etiology and perhaps the prevention and treatment of major psychiatric disorders.

This chapter highlights many of the major processes involved in brain development, including: induction of the central nervous system (CNS), patterning of the primordia of major brain regions, proliferation of neuroepithelial cells, differentiation and migration of immature neurons and glia, formation of axon tracts and synapses, and the establishment and plasticity of neuronal networks. Although much of the information described in this chapter is based on studies in non-primate mammals, it is likely that these findings are pertinent to developing human brain. For a comprehensive resource on neural development see the series edited by Rubenstein and Rakic (2013).

INDUCTION AND PATTERNING OF THE EMBRYONIC CNS

Early CNS development involves an ordered sequence of inductive processes that begin with the formation of the neural plate followed by a hierarchical series of fate specification steps that lead to regionally distinct developmental programs (Hoch et al., 2009). Inductive processes generally involve two tissues; one is the target of induction and the other, called the *organizer*, produces the molecular signals that carry out the induction. The node is the first organizer, and regulates inductions during gastrulation. These molecular signals, which generally are proteins, induce in the target tissues a new pattern of gene expression that dictates their subsequent developmental program.

Development of the CNS begins during gastrulation by a process called *neural induction*. Proteins produced by organizer tissues cause the embryonic ectoderm to differentiate into a neural fate. This process involves activation of receptor tyrosine kinases, perhaps through fibroblast growth factors (FGFs), and inhibition of transforming growth factor-β (TGF-β) signaling through the noggin and chordin proteins that bind to bone morphogenetic proteins (BMPs) (Stern, 2006). In addition, inhibition of wingless (WNT) signaling is required, at least in some species (Stern, 2006). Induction of the neural ectoderm generates the neural plate, which will give rise to the entire CNS (Fig. 1.1); its lateral edges produce neurogenic placodes (for the olfactory epithelium and inner ear) and the neural crest, which gives rise to most of the peripheral nervous system (PNS) and contributes to the head skeleton.

Beginning during neural induction, inductive processes subdivide the neural plate into molecularly distinct domains that are the primordia of the major subdivisions of the CNS. One can distinguish three types of inductive processes during CNS regionalization: (1) anterior-posterior or A-P, (2) mediolateral or M-L, and (3) local. The A-P regionalization subdivides the neural plate into transverse domains. The principal transverse subdivisions of the brain are the prosencephalon (forebrain), mesencephalon (midbrain), and rhombencephalon (hindbrain) (Fig. 1.2). Further refinements of A-P regionalization subdivide the rhombencephalon into segment-like domains called *neuromeres* (*rhombomeres*). Part of the forebrain may also have neuromeric subdivisions called *prosomeres*. The inductive mechanisms underlying A-P regionalization are poorly understood but probably include vertical inductions (from underlying tissues) from mesoderm and endoderm, and planar inductions (from substances that transmit their effects in the plane of the neural plate), perhaps from the node.

The M-L regionalization produces distinct tissues that are longitudinally aligned along the long (A-P) axis of the CNS (Fig. 1.1). Medial inductions are regulated by substances produced by the axial mesodermal organizers: the notochord and prechordal plate. These organizers are midline structures that lie underneath the middle of the neural plate and produce substances, such as sonic hedgehog, that induce the medial neural plate to form the primordia of the floor plate and basal plate (see Fig. 1.1). Lateral inductions are mediated by substances such as TGF-β proteins (that include the BMPs), which are produced along the rim of the neural plate by the non-neural ectoderm. Lateral inductions participate in the development of the neural crest, roof plate, and alar plate (see Fig. 1.1).

The combination of A-P and M-L patterning generates a checkerboard organization of brain subdivisions (Fig. 1.2), each of which expresses a distinct combination of regulatory genes. Superimposed on this pattern are the local inductive

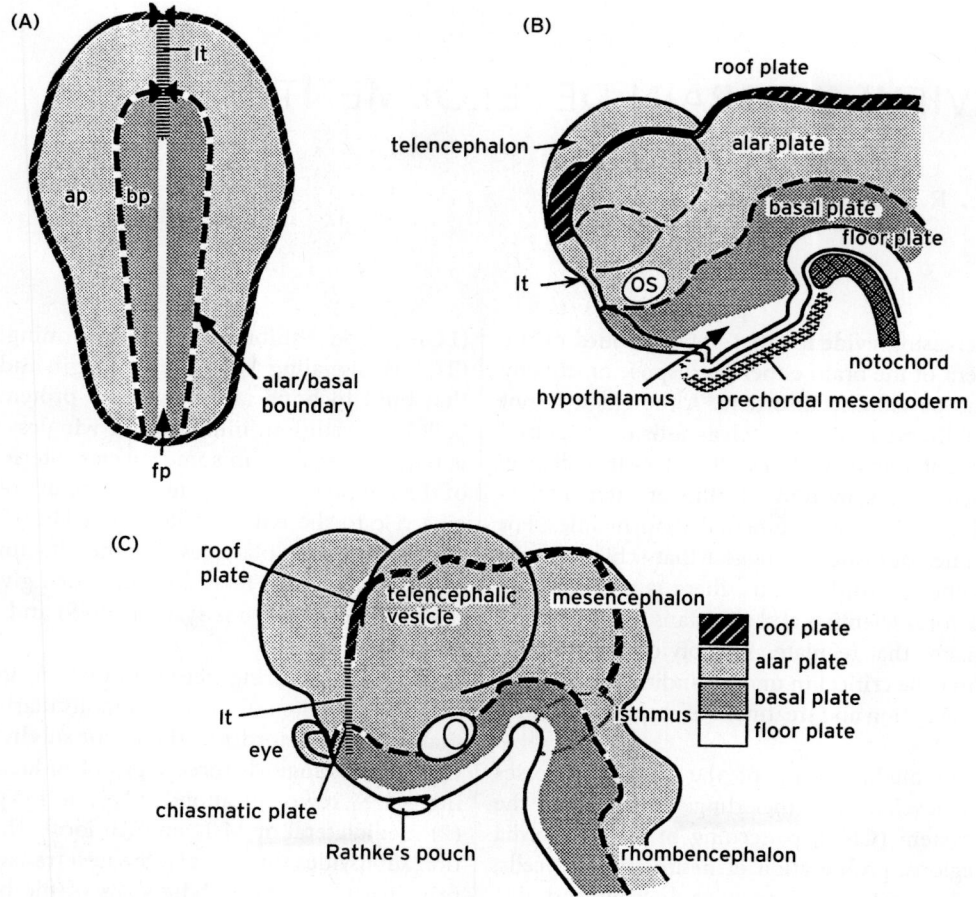

Figure 1.1 Schemas of the longitudinal organization of the brain (Shimamura et al., 1995). (A) Model of the longitudinal domains of the neural plate, including the primordia of the floor plate (fp), basal plate (bp), alar plate (ap), and roof plate (most lateral domain). (B) Medial view of the neural tube. (C) Rostrolateral view of the neural tube. lt: lamina terminalis; os: optic stalk.

signals that are essential for the formation of the vesicles that evaginate from the brain such as the telencephalon, eyes, and posterior pituitary. Evidence suggests that signals originating from ectodermal tissues (lens placode, anterior neural ridge, and anterior pituitary, respectively) adjacent to these structures produce signals that induce their formation.

Although the process of regionalization subdivides the neural plate into the primordia of the major brain regions, the process of morphogenesis transforms the shape of the neural plate into a tube that additionally has flexures and evaginations. Note that the folding of the neural plate into the neural tube converts the lateromedial dimension of the neural plate into the dorsoventral (D-V) dimension of the neural tube (Fig. 1.1).

A cross section through the D-V axis of the neural tube transects its four primary longitudinal subdivisions (Fig. 1.3). From ventral to dorsal these longitudinal columns are the floor, basal, alar, and roof plates. Each of these longitudinal columns may extend along the entire A-P axis of the CNS and contribute to distinct functional elements of the nervous system. The basal plate is the primordia for the motor neurons. The alar plate is the primordia for the secondary sensory neurons. The floor plate has several functions that are required during development. Like the notochord, the floor plate produces

sonic hedgehog and is believed to serve as a secondary ventral (medial) organizer where it also, in combination with chemotropic molecules such as netrins, guides the growth of axon tracts (Kolodkin and Tessier-Lavigne, 2011). Most of the roof plate forms the non-neuronal dorsal midline, which in some regions gives rise to specialized structures such as the choroid plexus and the pineal gland. The roof plate is marked by its high expression of BMPs and WNTs.

The regionalization process continues after neurulation (neural tube formation) to further subdivide large primordial regions into their constituent domains. These aspects of regionalization are probably carried out by planar inductive mechanisms via organizers that are within the neural tube. For example, secondary D-V patterning can be regulated by the floor plate (see the next section), whereas secondary A-P patterning can be regulated by the isthmus. The isthmus is a region between the mid- and hindbrain that produces inductive substances such as FGFs and WNT that regulate development of the midbrain and cerebellum. Primary cilia, an appendage on most cells, detects extracellular signals including sonic hedgehog and WNT. Mutations affecting cilia function are implicated in neurodevelopmental disorders affecting patterning and function of the brain (Louvi and Grove, 2011).

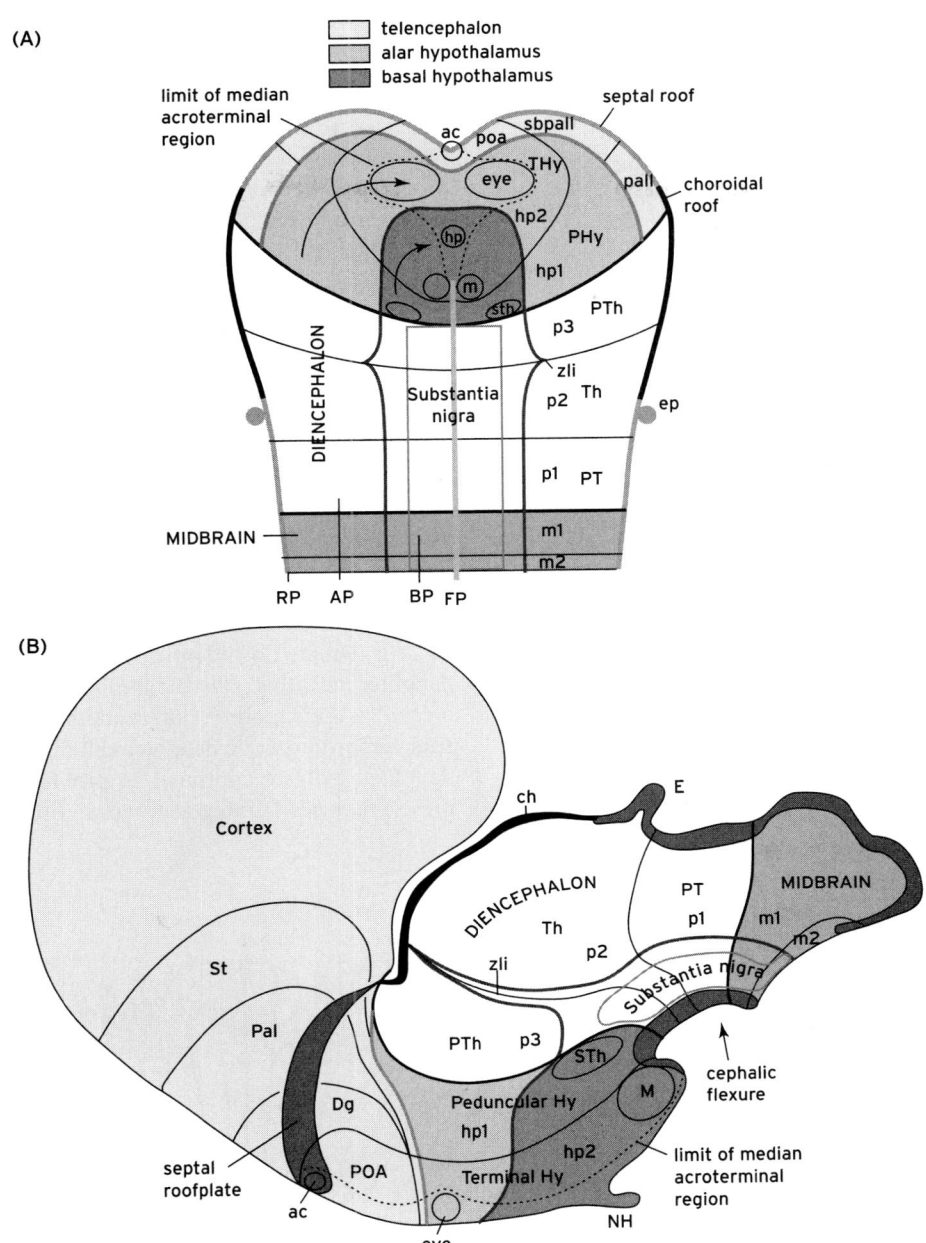

Figure 1.2 *Schemas of the organization of the rostral neural plate and neural tube (modified from Puelles et al., 2011). Looking down at a flattened neural plate (A). Transverse subdivisions from caudal-to-rostral include the midbrain, diencephalon (three prosomeres, p1, p2, and p3), and secondary prosencephalon, which includes the basal hypothalamus, alar hypothalamus, and telencephalon. Longitudinal domains: floor plate (fp), basal plate (bp), alar plate (ap), and roof plate (rp). Medial view of a mid-sagittally dissected neural tube (B). Subdivisions of the telencephalon include the cortex (including the hippocampus), striatum (St), pallidum (Pal), diagonal band/nucleus basalis (Dg), and preoptic area (POA). The hypothalamus (Hy) is postulated to have two transverse subdivisions (terminal and peduncular; hp2 and hp1), whose basal plates include the mammillary body (M), subthalamic nucleus (STh), and the midline neurohypophysis (NH; posterior pituitary). The alar plate of the diencephalon constitutes component of the thalamus, including the prethalamus (PTh), the thalamus proper (Th) and the pretectum (PT). Diencephalic basal plate components include the substantia nigra, which extends through the midbrain. The roof components of the forebrain include the epiphysis (E, ep), choroid plexus (ch), and the septal roof plate, where telencephalic commissures cross the midline, including the anterior commissure (ac).*

HISTOGENESIS OF BRAIN REGIONS: PROLIFERATION, CELL FATE DETERMINATION, MIGRATION, AND DIFFERENTIATION

The process of regionalization subdivides the CNS into the primordia of its major structures (e.g., cerebral cortex, striatum, thalamus, cerebellum) and initiates within these primordia their genetic programs of histogenesis that regulate cell fate determination, proliferation, differentiation, and migration (for more extensive reviews of this subject, see Kriegstein and Alvarez-Buylla, 2009; Marin and Rubenstein, 2001). These processes take place in specific zones within the wall of the neural tube (Fig. 1.4). Proliferation occurs in the ventricular

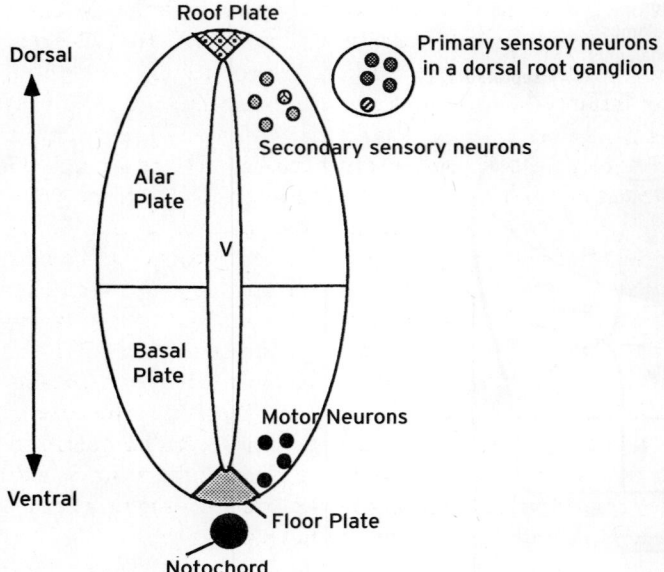

Figure 1.3 *Schematic cross section of the dorsoventral (D-V) organization of the spinal cord. The floor plate is induced by the notochord; together they produce the sonic hedgehog protein, which patterns the basal plate of the spinal cord, including the motor neurons. Neural crest cells originate from the dorsal-most part of the spinal cord and generate the primary sensory neurons of the spinal ganglia. Secondary sensory neurons are produced in the alar plate. V, ventricle.*

zone (VZ) and subventricular zone (SVZ), which line the inner surface of the neural tube, and are adjacent to the ventricular cavity. VZ progenitors, known as radial glia progenitors (RG) give rise to secondary (or intermediate) progenitors (IP), whose cell bodies generally reside in the SVZ. VZ and SVZ progenitors can both generate neurons and glia (astrocytes and oligodendrocytes). Newborn immature neurons produced in the progenitor zones migrate into the overlying mantle zone; in the case of the cerebral cortex, the mantle zone is called the cortical plate (Fig. 1.4a). In the developing human cerebral cortex, the progenitor domains are expanded compared to simpler mammals, such as rodents, and include an outer subventricular zone that has a large number of outer radial glial and intermediate progenitors (oRG and oIP) (Fig. 1.4b).

VZ progenitors are the most undifferentiated and mitotically active progenitors. Each brain region has a distinct proliferation program that regulates the rate of cell division, the number of times VZ cells divide, and the character of the cell division. Cell division can be symmetrical, producing daughter cells that are identical or asymmetrical, producing daughter cells that are non-identical. Symmetrical divisions produce daughter cells that, like their mother, continue to proliferate or, unlike their mother, differentiate or die. Asymmetric division can produce one daughter cell that differentiates and one daughter cell that continues to proliferate. The regulation of these processes is integral to controlling how many cells are

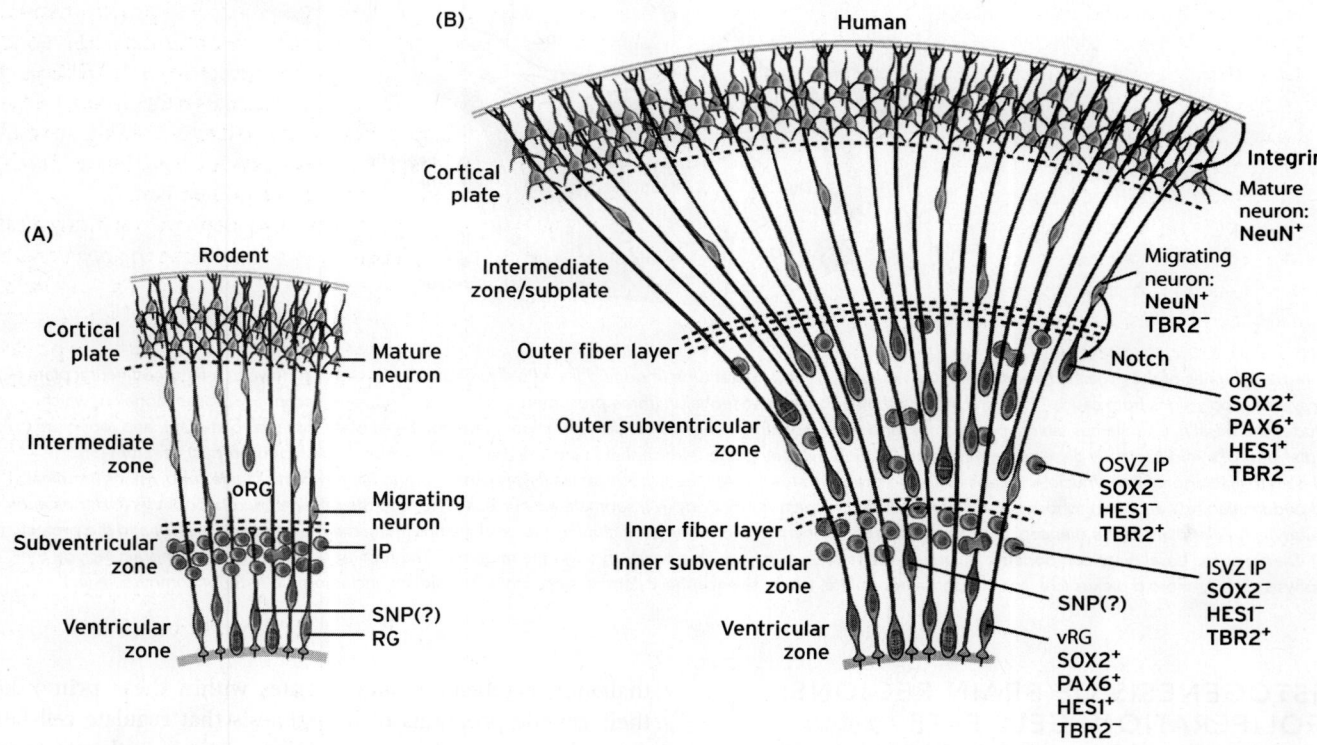

Figure 1.4 *Organization of progenitor and migration zones in the developing neocortex of rodents (A) and humans (B). (Taken with permission from Lui et al., 2011). Laminar divisions include the ventricular zone (VZ), subventricular zone (SVZ; inner and outer), intermediate zone (IZ), inner and outer fiber layers, subplate, and cortical plate. Transcription factors that are expressed in specific types of progenitors are listed: HES1, NeuN, PAX6, SOX1, TBR2. IP, intermediate progenitors; ISVZ, inner SVZ; oRG, outer radial glia progenitors; oSVZ, SNP, short neural precursor; outer SVZ progenitors; RG, radial glia progenitors; vRG, ventricular zone radial glia progenitors.*

produced in each region and when these cells are made. For example, the expansion of the cerebral cortex in primates may relate to increased numbers of symmetrical divisions of neuron-producing progenitors in the cortical SVZ (Liu et al., 2011).

There are many types of cells that make up the CNS; the two basic classes are neurons and glia (Lemke, 2001; Rowitch and Kriegstein, 2010). There are two general types of neurons: projection neurons, whose axons migrate to distant territories, and local circuit neurons (interneurons), whose axons ramify nearby. Within these general categories, there are distinct types of projection and local circuit neurons that differ by neurochemistry, firing characteristics, and connectivity (Wonders and Anderson, 2006). There are two types of CNS-derived glia, astrocytes and oligodendrocytes, whereas the other major glial type, the microglia, is mesodermally derived (Colognato and French-Constant, 2004). Astrocytes regulate the local chemical milieu and appear to regulate synapse formation and elimination (Eroglu and Barres, 2010). Oligodendrocytes produce the myelin sheaths that surround many axons; these sheaths function as insulators that increase the velocity of action potentials. Microglia are related to macrophages and subserve a phagocytic role to remove dead cells from the CNS.

Different types of neurons are generated at distinct D-V positions in the CNS. For instance, within the spinal cord, motor neurons are generated by ventral progenitors, whereas sensory neurons are generated by dorsal progenitors (Dessaud et al., 2008). Likewise, in the telencephalon, ventral progenitors produce neurons of the basal ganglia, whereas dorsal progenitors produce cortical neurons (Hebert and Fishell, 2008). This arrangement is the result of the D-V patterning mechanisms described earlier in this chapter. Although patterning of the nervous system produces separate primordia of major brain regions (e.g., cerebral cortex and basal ganglia), cell migration processes "mix" certain cell types between these primordia (see following paragraphs).

The mechanisms underlying cell fate decisions in the nervous system involve molecules within the cells (intrinsic signals controlled by proteins such as transcription factors; see Chapter 6) as well as molecules outside of the cells (extrinsic signals controlled by proteins such as growth/differentiation factors and their receptors). These proteins have integral roles in regulating whether a cell continues to divide, whether it undergoes symmetrical or asymmetrical division, whether the daughter cells go on to differentiate, and what type of cell they will become.

Notch signaling is an example of extrinsic control of differentiation and is mediated by *Notch* receptors and their ligands (e.g., Delta) (Justice and Jan, 2002). Activation of *Notch* by its ligand biases a cell not to differentiate into a neuron; thus neurogenesis requires inhibition of *Notch* signaling. *Notch* signaling controls the rate and timing of neuron production. Furthermore, high levels of *Notch* signaling biases progenitors toward an astrocytic fate. *Notch* signaling activates a cascade of molecular switches that culminates in the induction of transcription factors that change gene expression in the differentiating cell (Bertrand et al., 2002).

Although *Notch* signaling largely operates through basic helix-loop-helix transcription factors, many other types of transcription factors have central roles in brain development. These include *Homeobox*, *Sox*, *T-box*, *Winged-Helix*, and *HMG*-box families. Each family consists of subfamilies; for instance, key homeobox genes include *Arx*, *Dlx*, *Emx*, *Lhx*, *Nkx*, *Otx*, *Pax*, and *POU*, which control such processes as regional fate, cell type identity, neuronal maturation, and cell migration (Briscoe et al., 2000; Wilson and Rubenstein, 2000).

Once neurons are generated, the next step in their differentiation program is their migration to the appropriate destination (Ayala et al., 2007). Each brain region has a specific migration program. In cortical structures (e.g., cerebral cortex and superior colliculus) migrations are orchestrated to form layered or laminar structures. In most subcortical regions migrations form nuclear structures. There are two general types of migration: radial and tangential. Radial migration is movement perpendicular to the plane of the ventricle and toward the pial surface; tangential migration is movement parallel to the plane of the ventricle and pial surface.

Radial migration involves the interaction between the elongated processes of radial glial (RG) cells and the migrating immature neurons (Fig. 1.4). The immature neurons migrate through the subventricular and intermediate zones (Fig. 1.4) to specified locations within the wall of the neural tube where they disengage from the radial glial cell and continue to differentiate. Historically, an important molecule regulating this process was identified through analysis of the *reeler* mutant mouse (Rice and Curran, 2001). In the cerebral cortex of *reeler* mice, later-born neurons fail to migrate past their earlier-born siblings, leading to partial inversion of the usual inside-out lamination. The *reeler* gene encodes a secreted protein named *reelin* that can promote dissociation of neuroblasts from radial glia. Two low-density lipoprotein receptors (VLDLR and ApoER2) are receptors for reelin. Humans with *reelin* mutations can have neuropsychiatric disorders including mental retardation and epilepsy; changes in reelin function or levels may be associated with schizophrenia and autism.

Nervous system development also depends on tangential migration. This has long been known to occur in the cerebellum and in the rostral migratory stream (RMS) of the olfactory bulb, where adult neurogenesis is best characterized. In addition, most GABAergic local circuit neurons of the telencephalon are generated in the basal ganglia primordia and then tangentially migrate to the cerebral cortex and hippocampus (Marin and Rubenstein, 2001). This process results in mixing of gamma-aminobutyric acid (GABA)ergic neurons from the basal ganglia anlage with glutamatergic projection neurons of the cerebral cortex. GABAergic neurons are required for inhibitory regulation of excitatory transmission. Guidance cues for tangentially migrating interneurons include neuregulin1 (a schizophrenia risk gene), the CXCL12 cytokine, and semaphorins (Marin et al., 2001; Flames et al., 2004; Wang et al., 2011).

Progress has also been made in identifying genes that control cytoskeletal processes that are essential for migration. Several of these genes were first identified as causing neuronal migration defects in humans, including *Lisencephaly-1*, *Doublecortin*, and *Filamin* (Mochida and Walsh, 2004).

The time when a neuron is born (newborn neurons are not mitotically active and migrate away from the VZ) has an important influence on its fate (the type of neuron it becomes and its location within the brain). For instance, in the cerebral cortex there are seven layers: layers 1, 2, 3, 4, 5, 6, and the subplate. Layer 1 is the most superficial, and the subplate is closest to the VZ. In the cerebral cortex, cells that are born first populate the deepest layers; this produces the so-called inside-out pattern of histogenesis. Each layer has distinct functions. For instance, the subplate is believed to provide signals that direct the incoming thalamic axons to their appropriate cortical target zone; layers 5 and 6 contain neurons that project out of the cortex; neurons in layer 4 receive input from the thalamus; neurons in layers 2 and 3 have intracortical projections; reelin-secreting layer 1 neurons participate in regulating cortical histogenesis by modulating the radial migration process (Tissir and Goffinet, 2003).

WIRING OF THE BRAIN: FORMATION OF AXON PATHWAYS AND SYNAPSES

As the immature neurons and glia migrate from the proliferative zone to the differentiation zone (the mantle), they elaborate more complex cellular structures. Neurons extend several thin processes away from their cell body; these include multiple dendrites and a single axon. Perhaps the most distinctive feature of the nervous system is how axon processes navigate long distances to find their targets (Charron and Tessier-Lavigne, 2005; Guan and Rao, 2003). The growing tip of the axon is called the *growth cone*. This dynamic structure extends filopodia that explore their environment, searching for cues that either attract or repel them.

Molecules and their receptors have been identified that are chemoattractants or repellents for growing axons. These can function as long-range or as local signals. Some local signals are found on the surface of glial cells that serve as guideposts for the axons. The earliest axon pathways that develop create a scaffold for later-arriving axons. Through a process called *fasciculation*, later-arriving axons can adhere to axons that are already in an axon pathway. Molecules on the surface of the axons, some of which are related to immunoglobulins, can regulate selective fasciculation to generate axon bundles with common properties. When an axon has reached its target, a process called *defasciculation* enables the axon to separate from the axon bundle.

As axons grow and navigate, their plasma membrane contains guidance receptors that recognize molecules expressed by neighboring cells (Charron and Tessier-Lavigne, 2005; Guan and Rao, 2003). Guidance processes operate as growth cones grow along specific pathways. Important pathways that connect the left and right side of the CNS are midline structures (commissures), such as the optic chiasm and corpus callosum. Activation of guidance receptors determines whether an axon grows toward or away from a target cell. At least four conserved families of guidance molecules have been identified. The semaphorins comprise a 20-member family of soluble and membrane-bound molecules that elicit repulsive signals through two receptor families, neuropilins and plexins. The slit family of proteins consists of three members in mammals

and acts through Robo receptors in commissural axons to prevent these axons from recrossing the midline. Whereas the slits and semaphorins are repulsive, members of the netrin family can be repulsive or attractive for a growth cone, depending on the types of receptors expressed by the axon (receptor complexes containing either the colorectal cancer [DCC] or the neogenin protein lead to attraction; UNC-5-related protein leads to repulsion). Members of the ephrin family of ligands are membrane-bound and interact with two families of receptors, EphA and EphB (Kullander and Klein, 2002). EphrinB ligands, when bound to EphB receptors, are capable of bidirectional signaling whereby the cytoplasmic domain of the Ephrin ligand transmits a phosphorylation signal. In addition to regulating axon pathfinding, semaphorins, slits, netrins, and ephrins control neuronal migrations.

Upon reaching its target, the growth cone is further modified as it forms a part of the synapse (Sanes and Lichtman, 2001). Reciprocal signals between the growth cone and the postsynaptic target cell induce the production of molecules and membranous specializations found in synapses (Benson et al., 2001). Presynaptic cells produce synaptic vesicles filled with neurotransmitters, and the postsynaptic cells form dendrites with specialized domains containing neurotransmitter receptors (Jan and Jan, 2001). There is evidence that defects in synapse development and maintenance underlie some forms of autism (Walsh et al., 2008). Proteins of the neurexin/neuroligin families are of particular interest, as they are critical in dictating the types of synapses that form, and mutations in this class of genes are associated with a variety of neuropsychiatric disorders (Peñagarikano et al., 2011; Sudhof, 2008). Assembly and function of the synapse requires proteins such as Shank3, mutations of which can cause autism and schizophrenia (Herbert, 2011). Transduction of synaptic activity depends on ion channels; defects of these can contribute to autism susceptibility as in CACNA1C mutations, which recently have been characterized in induced pluripotential stem cells (iPSCs) from Timothy syndrome patients (Pasca et al., 2011).

In the 1950s, nerve growth factor (NGF) was discovered, the first of four so-called neurotrophins that provide signals that control such processes as neuronal survival and synapse strength (Huang and Reichardt, 2001). By the end of the 1980s the neurotrophic hypothesis was firmly entrenched, and it suggested that postsynaptic cells are responsible for releasing neurotrophins that the presynaptic neuronal process was attracted to via its expression of a so-called Trk receptor. The amount of neurotrophin released by a given cell determined whether a cell reached a given target and formed a synapse or otherwise was destined for "programmed death." The mechanisms underlying programmed cell death, or apoptosis, have recently been elucidated (Kuan et al., 2000).

The biochemical nature of apoptosis was first discovered by studying the nematode *Caenorhabditis elegans*. A genetic analysis identified a cascade of proteases, known as *caspases*, that control programmed cell death in all animals. Subsequently, mitochondrial-associated proteins have also emerged as important regulators of apoptosis including the Bcl-2 family, APAF, and cytochrome C. Apoptosis is recognized as a fundamental process that, together with progenitor cell proliferation, controls neuronal numbers during development. Presently, researchers are investigating whether some neurodegenerative disorders may be the result of aberrant apoptosis or neurotrophin signaling and whether neurotrophins or apoptosis inhibitors can be used clinically to treat neurodegenerative abnormalities.

The wiring of complex CNS systems requires the connection of multiple cell types that are located in different positions. The wiring diagram of the visual system is an instructive example of this process. The neural retina contains primary sensory receptor neurons (rods and cones), interneurons (e.g., amacrine, bipolar, and horizontal cells), glia (Müller cells), and projection neurons called *retinal ganglion cells*. The retinal ganglion cells extend axons that must make several choices on the path to their targets. First, they exit the eye through the optic nerve and confront the optic chiasmatic plate, a structure at the front of the hypothalamus. Axons from the temporal retina do not cross at the chiasm, whereas axons from the nasal retina do cross. Intrinsic signals that distinguish nasal and temporal cells (e.g., the brain factor-1 and -2 transcription factors) permit the growing axons to sort themselves out to follow the correct pathway. There appear to be signals that the axons detect in the chiasmatic plate that direct the axon traffic. Upon exiting the chiasm, the optic axons grow posteriorly toward their two main targets: the thalamus and the superior colliculus. The optic tracts grow along the surface of the hypothalamic mantle zone, passing many nuclei, until they reach the thalamus. Branches perpendicular to the trajectory of the optic tracts grow out from the axons. These branches then specifically enter the visual centers of the thalamus, principally the lateral geniculate nucleus (LGN), where they form synapses with the LGN neurons. Before describing the LGN in greater detail, it is important to point out that some optic axons continue to grow more posteriorly into the midbrain, where they form branches into the superior colliculus (or optic tectum). Here, the optic axons synapse in specific locations; axons from the temporal retina synapse in the anterior tectum, whereas axons from the nasal retina synapse in the posterior tectum. Molecules that may regulate this retinotopic map on the optic tectum are membrane-bound Eph-type receptors (found on the axons) and their membrane-bound protein ligands (found on the target cells). The Eph proteins probably make up part of the molecular system that orchestrates the precise mapping of axonal projections onto the target tissues in all CNS regions.

In the LGN, the optic axons also form a retinotopic map. In higher mammals, the LGN is a laminar structure; each layer in the adult is connected with only one eye. However, during development, axons from both eyes have processes that extend into many LGN layers. Experimental evidence suggests that neuronal activity is required for the sorting-out process that eliminates branches in some layers and strengthens the synapses in others. Neuronal activity–dependent processes and critical periods have an essential role in many steps that refine the patterns of connections in the CNS; these are addressed further below.

The projection neurons in the LGN send axons anteriorly into the telencephalon, where they traverse the striatum in the internal capsule and enter their target: the cerebral neocortex. The thalamocortical fibers enter the cortex while neurogenesis is still actively occurring and grow into a layer called the *intermediate zone* that is interposed between the proliferative (VZ and SVZ) and mantle (cortical plate) zones (Fig. 1.4). The thalamocortical fibers' next task is to innervate the correct region of the neocortex. The neocortex is subdivided into functionally distinct areas, each with a distinctive set of inputs. The LGN axons must innervate the primary visual cortex. Evidence suggests that some of the positional information that regulates this process is found in a transient layer of cortical neurons called the *subplate cells*. These are among the first cortical neurons to differentiate, and they are located in the deepest layer of the cortical plate, adjacent to the intermediate zone. The axons from different thalamic nuclei form transient synapses with the subplate cells in distinct cortical domains. The LGN fibers grow to a caudal position in the cortex, which will become the primary visual cortex. There the LGN axons form synapses with the subplate cells and wait in this location until the cerebral cortex has further matured. Then the LGN fibers leave the subplate, grow into the cortex, and form synapses with neurons in layer 4. After the axons leave the subplate, most of these cells die, leaving no trace of this important step in neurodevelopment.

Initially, inputs from both eyes converge within the same areas in layer 4 of the primary visual cortex. Then the axons from each eye segregate into distinct alternating domains called the *ocular dominance columns*. Evidence suggests that formation of these columns requires neuronal activity and that correlated activity from subregions of each eye plays a role in this process (see Katz and Shatz, 1996, for a review of this subject). Because ocular dominance formation occurs in utero, the neuronal activity is not induced by visual experience but is probably regulated by intrinsic neuronal discharges within the retina.

As the thalamocortical circuit is maturing, local connections between cortical layers 1–6 form a columnar intracortical circuit that is the basic unit of cortical function. Each region of visual space is represented in these cortical columns, and the ensemble of these columns becomes the primary visual cortex. Through processes that are beyond the scope of this chapter, the primary visual cortex regulates the development of secondary visual centers that are concerned with more complex aspects of processing and integrating visual information. These areas project to cortical association areas that integrate visual and other information, which then influences motor output areas of the cortex. Forming and refining of these more complex intracortical circuits continues into postnatal life. These postnatal aspects of CNS development are greatly influenced by visual experience.

POSTNATAL DEVELOPMENTAL PROCESSES

Many aspects of neuronal development continue throughout life, especially the elaboration and refinement of neuronal connections that are required to generate sensory maps, neural circuit assemblies that mediate sensory-motor integration and responses, and higher order cognitive and emotional representations. There is evidence that experiential activity-dependent processes are essential for the postnatal spatial assembly of the sensory map in the olfactory cortex (Franks et al., 2011), and therefore may underlie the assembly of higher order circuits. Furthermore, in adult animals, when peripheral sensory inputs are eliminated, such as through amputation of a finger, the cortical regions that previously received input from the removed finger now receive sensory inputs from the adjacent fingers. This alteration in the neocortical somatosensory map appears to result from changes in the sizes and shapes of axonal processes and the distribution of synapses. Thus, the synaptic connectivity of the adult cortex is capable of reorganization.

In addition to the ability of neuronal processes to continue to grow and change in shape in postnatal animals, there are at least two brain regions that postnatally produce neurons and glia. For instance, in rodents the SVZ of the lateral ventricles produces interneurons of the olfactory bulb, and the hippocampal subgranular zone continues to make new granular neurons; it is important to note that there may be less postnatal neurogenesis in the human olfactory bulb as the rostral migratory stream appears to disappear in infancy (Sanai et al., 2011). Adult neurogenesis in the hippocampal dentate gyrus is reduced by stress and may be important for spatial memory as well as aspects of antidepressant response (Perera et al., 2007).

Gliogenesis is also active postnatally. Oligodendrocytes continue to myelinate axons postnatally; some circuits are not fully myelinated until young adulthood. The degree of myelination is a critical determinant of action potential velocity, and therefore can have important consequences for circuit function. Furthermore, oligodendrocytes and astrocytes are essential for neuronal and synaptic integrity (Nave, 2010).

The neonatal brain is exposed to diverse sensory information; these experience-driven processes gain salience in neural circuit development and function. Experience-based learning involves alterations in the number and distribution of synapses, and molecular changes in synapses alter the strength of synaptic signaling. Processes such as *long-term potentiation* and *long-term depression* are regulated in part by changes in the numbers and types of neurotransmitter receptors (see Chapter 5).

For some types of experience-dependent learning there are limited time windows (*critical periods*) during which major changes to the brain's wiring diagram is plastic. For instance, early in postnatal development the primary visual cortex loses its ability to form eye-specific subdomains following closure of the critical period (Hensch, 2005). Closure of the critical period is regulated at least in part by the maturation of GABAergic cortical interneurons. These neurons are essential for creating the proper *excitation/inhibition balance* that is optimal for signal detection and for restraining uncontrolled excitation; defects in the development/function of cortical interneurons can cause epilepsy (Cobos et al., 2005), and are postulated to contribute to autism and schizophrenia (Rubenstein and Merzenich, 2003; Marin, 2012). For instance, neuregulin/ErbB4 signaling in GABAergic cortical interneurons regulates their ability to receive excitatory synapses and to form inhibitory synapses (Marin, 2012). Defects in synaptic development and function may underlie a substantial fraction of neuropsychiatric disorders. Indeed, single gene disorders that contribute to autism appear to largely encode proteins that affect the synapse (Walsh et al., 2008). In addition, mechanisms that globally control the transcriptional state of a cell through modulating the *epigenome* (chromatin state and covalent modifications to DNA) are implicated in psychiatric disorders. For instance, the MeCP2 protein binds methylated DNA; MeCP2 mutations cause Rett syndrome (autism spectrum disorder), in part through reducing GABAergic signaling (Chao et al., 2010). Of note, MeCP2 is part of the genomic machinery regulating how a neuron responds to incoming activity (Cohen and Greenberg, 2008).

PERSPECTIVE

There has been tremendous progress in understanding the mechanisms governing development of the brain. These insights now form the foundation for interpreting genomic modifications that are associated with neuropsychiatric disease risk, and with environmental perturbations that alter specific developmental processes. The convergence of these efforts promises further progress in elucidating etiology, identifying individuals at risk, and discovering modalities for prevention and therapy (through molecular and experiential interventions).

DISCLOSURE

Dr. Rubenstein has no conflicts of interest to disclose. He is funded by Nina Ireland, the Simons Foundation, Weston Havens Foundation, C.U.R.E. (Citizens United for Research in Epilepsy), CIRM (California Institute for Regenerative Medicine), NINDS R01 NS34661, NIMH R01 MH081880, and NIMH R37 MH049428.

REFERENCES

Alvarez-Buylla, A., Garcia-Verdugo, J.M., et al. (2001). A unified hypothesis on the lineage of neural stem cells. *Nat. Rev. Neurosci.* 2:287–293.

Ayala, R., Shu, T., et al. (2007). Trekking across the brain: the journey of neuronal migration. *Cell* 128:29–43.

Benson, D.L., Colman, D.R., et al. (2001). Molecules, maps and synapse specificity. *Nat. Rev. Neurosci.* 2:899–909.

Bertrand, N., Castro, D.S., et al. (2002). Proneural genes and the specification of neural cell types. *Nat. Rev. Neurosci.* 7:517–530.

Briscoe, J., Pierani, A., et al. (2000). A homeodomain protein code specifies progenitor cell identity and neuronal fate in the ventral neural tube. *Cell* 101:435–445.

Chao, H.T., Chen, H., et al. (2010). Dysfunction in GABA signalling mediates autism-like stereotypies and Rett syndrome phenotypes. *Nature* 468(7321):263–269.

Charron, F., and Tessier-Lavigne, M. (2005). Novel brain wiring functions for classical morphogens: a role as graded positional cues in axon guidance. *Development* 132:2251–2262.

Cobos, I., Calcagnotto, M.E., et al. (2005). Mice lacking Dlx1 show subtype-specific loss of interneurons, reduced inhibition and epilepsy. *Nat. Neurosci.* 8(8):1059–1068.

Cohen, S., and Greenberg, M.E. (2008). Communication between the synapse and the nucleus in neuronal development, plasticity, and disease. *Annu. Rev. Cell Dev. Biol.* 24:183–209.

Colognato, H., and French-Constant, C. (2004). Mechanisms of glial development. *Curr. Opin. Neurobiol.* 14:37–44.

Dessaud, E., McMahon, A.P., et al. (2008). Pattern formation in the vertebrate neural tube: a sonic hedgehog morphogen-regulated transcriptional network. *Development* 135(15):2489–2503.

Eroglu, C., and Barres, B.A. (2010). Regulation of synaptic connectivity by glia. *Nature* 468(7321):223–231.

Flames, N., Long, J.E., et al. (2004). Short- and long-range attraction of cortical GABAergic interneurons by neuregulin-1. *Neuron* 44(2):251–261.

Franks, K.M., Russo, M.J, et al. (2011). Recurrent circuitry dynamically shapes the activation of piriform cortex. *Neuron* 72(1):49–56.

Gaiano, N., and Fishell, G. (2002). The role of notch in promoting glial and neural stem cell fates. *Annu. Rev. Neurosci.* 25:471–490.

Gleeson, J.G., and Walsh, C.A. (2000). Neuronal migration disorders: from genetic diseases to developmental mechanisms. *Trends Neurosci.* 23:352–359.

Greer, J.M., and Capecchi, M.R. (2002). Hoxb8 is required for normal grooming behavior in mice. *Neuron* 33:23–34.

Guan, K.L., and Rao, Y. (2003). Signalling mechanisms mediating neuronal responses to guidance cues. *Nat. Rev. Neurosci.* 4(12):941–956.

Harrison, P.J., and Law, A.J. (2006). Neuregulin 1 and schizophrenia: genetics, gene expression, and neurobiology. *Biol. Psychiatry* 60(2):131–140.

Hébert, J.M., and Fishell, G. (2008). The genetics of early telencephalon patterning: some assembly required. *Nat. Rev. Neurosci.* 9(9):678–685.

Hensch, T.K. (2005). Critical period plasticity in local cortical circuits. *Nat. Rev. Neurosci.* 6(11):877–888.

Herbert, M.R. (2011). SHANK3, the synapse, and autism. *N. Engl. J. Med.* 365(2):173–175.

Hoch, R.V., Rubenstein, J.L.R., et al.. (2009). Genes and signaling events that establish regional patterning of the mammalian forebrain. *Semin. Cell Dev. Biol.* 20(4):378–378.

Huang, E.J., and Reichardt, L.F. (2001). Neurotrophins: roles in neuronal development and function. *Annu. Rev. Neurosci.* 24:677–736.

Jan, Y.N., and Jan, L.Y. (2001). Dendrites. *Genes Dev.* 15:2627–2641.

Justice, N.J., and Jan, Y.N. (2002). Variations on the Notch pathway in neural development. *Curr. Opin. Neurobiol.* 2:64–70.

Katz, L.C., and Shatz, C.J. (1996). Synaptic activity and the construction of cortical circuits. *Science* 274:1133–1138.

Kolodkin, A.L., and Tessier-Lavigne, M. (2011). Mechanisms and molecules of neuronal wiring: a primer. *Cold Spring Harb Perspect Biol.* 3(6):a001727.

Kriegstein, A., and Alvarez-Buylla, A. (2009). The glial nature of embryonic and adult neural stem cells. *Annu. Rev. Neurosci.* 32:149–184.

Kuan, C.Y., Roth, K.A., et al. (2000). Mechanisms of programmed cell death in the developing brain. *Trends Neurosci.* 23:291–297.

Kullander, K., and Klein, R. (2002). Mechanisms and functions of Eph and ephrin signalling. *Nat. Rev. Mol. Cell Biol.* 7:475–486.

Lemke, G. (2001). Glial control of neuronal development. *Annu. Rev. Neurosci.* 24:87–105.

Louvi, A., and Grove, E.A. (2011). Cilia in the CNS: the quiet organelle claims center stage. *Neuron.* 69(6):1046–1060.

Lui, J.H., Hansen, DV., et al. (2011). Development and evolution of the human neocortex. *Cell* 146(1):18–36.

Marín, O. (2012). Interneuron dysfunction in psychiatric disorders. *Nat. Rev. Neurosci.* 13(2):107–120.

Marin, O., and Rubenstein, J.L.R. (2001). A long remarkable journey: tangential migration in the telencephalon. *Nat. Rev. Neurosci.* 2:780–790.

Marín, O., Yaron, A., et al. (2001). Sorting of striatal and cortical interneurons regulated by semaphorin-neuropilin interactions. *Science* 293(5531):872–875.

Mochida, G.H., and Walsh, C.A. (2004). Genetic basis of developmental malformations of the cerebral cortex. *Arch. Neurol.* 61:637–640.

Nave, K.A. (2010). Myelination and support of axonal integrity by glia. *Nature* 468(7321):244–252.

Paşca, S.P., Portmann, T., et al. (2011). Using iPSC-derived neurons to uncover cellular phenotypes associated with Timothy syndrome. *Nat. Med.* 17(12):1657–1662.

Peñagarikano, O., Abrahams, B.S., et al. (2011). Absence of CNTNAP2 leads to epilepsy, neuronal migration abnormalities, and core autism-related deficits. *Cell* 147(1):235–246.

Perera, T.D., Coplan, J.D., et al.. (2007). Antidepressant-induced neurogenesis in the hippocampus of adult nonhuman primates. *J. Neurosci.* 27:4894–4901.

Puelles, L., Martinez-de-la-Torre, M., et al. (2011). The hypothalamus. In: Watson, C., Paxinos, G, and Puelles, L., eds. The Mouse Nervous System. Amsterdam: Academic Press, pp. 221–312.

Rakic, P. (1995). A small step for the cell, a giant leap for mankind: a hypothesis of neocortical expansion during evolution. *Trends Neurosci.* 18:383–388.

Rice, D.S., and Curran, T. (2001). Role of the reelin signaling pathway in central nervous system development. *Annu. Rev. Neurosci.* 24:1005–1039.

Rowitch, D.H., and Kriegstein, A.R. (2010). Developmental genetics of vertebrate glial-cell specification. *Nature* 468(7321):214–222.

Rubenstein, J.L., and Merzenich, M.M. (2003). Model of autism: increased ratio of excitation/inhibition in key neural systems. *Genes Brain Behav.* 2(5):255–267.

Rubenstein, J.L.R., and Puelles, L. (2003). Development of the nervous system. In: Epstein, C.J., Erikson, R.P., and Wynshaw-Boris, A., eds. Inborn Errors of Development. New York: Oxford University Press, pp. 75–88.

Rubenstein, J.L.R., and Rakic, P. (2013). Comprehensive Developmental Neuroscience. Oxford, UK: Academic Press.

Sanai, N., Nguyen, T., et al. (2011). Corridors of migrating neurons in the human brain and their decline during infancy. *Nature* 478(7369):382–386.

Sanes, J.R., and Lichtman, J.W. (2001). Development, induction, assembly, maturation and maintenance of a postsynaptic apparatus. *Nat. Rev. Neurosci.* 2:791–805.

Shimamura, K., Hartigan, D.J., et al. (1995). Longitudinal organization of the anterior neural plate and neural tube. *Development* 121:3923–3933.

Stern, C.D. (2006). Neural induction: 10 years on since the "default model." *Curr. Opin. Cell Biol.* 18(6):692–697.

Südhof, T.C. (2008). Neuroligins and neurexins link synaptic function to cognitive disease. *Nature* 455(7215):903–911.

Tissir, F., and Goffinet, A.M. (2003). Reelin and brain development. *Nat. Rev. Neurosci.* 4:496–505.

Walsh, C.A., Morrow, E.M., et al. (2008). Autism and brain development. *Cell* 135(3):396–400.

Wang, Y., Li, G., Stanco, A., et al. (2011). CXCR4 and CXCR7 have distinct functions in regulating interneuron migration. *Neuron* 69(1):61–76.

Wilson, S.W., and Rubenstein, J.L.R. (2000). Induction and dorsoventral patterning of the telencephalon. *Neuron* 28:641–651.

Wonders, C.P., and Anderson, S.A. (2006). The origin and specification of cortical interneurons. *Nat. Rev. Neurosci.* 7:687–696.

2 | NEUROCHEMICAL SYSTEMS IN THE CENTRAL NERVOUS SYSTEM

ARIEL Y. DEUTCH AND ROBERT H. ROTH

It has been more than a century since the introduction of the neuron doctrine by Santiago Ramon y Cajal marked the beginning of the modern neuroscience and positioned the neuron as the individual unit of the brain (see Valenstein, 2005). It has taken most of the subsequent century for investigators to begin to address how these individual neurons communicate. Although battles on the nature of the primary mode of communication, electrical or chemical, raged for more than 50 years after Cajal received the Nobel Prize in 1906, by the middle of the 20th century there was widespread acceptance that chemical signals were the primary means of interaction between two neurons. The "classic" view of transmission of signals between neurons was that transmitter molecules synthesized by the presynaptic neurons are released into the synaptic cleft when the neuronal membrane is depolarized, with the transmitter subsequently binding to specific postsynaptic receptors that are coupled to intracellular second messengers.

Although many thought the defining principles of neural transmission were worked out by the beginning of the 21st century, the past decade has been as scientifically tumultuous as any of the previous 100 years, with several findings challenging certain long-held and cherished beliefs about neurotransmitters.

WHAT DEFINES A NEUROTRANSMITTER?

Several criteria have been established that define a *neurotransmitter* (Iversen et al., 2008). These include the following: (*1*) a neurotransmitter should be synthesized in the neuron from which it is released; (*2*) the substance released from neurons should be present in a chemically or pharmacologically identifiable form: it should be capable of being measured and identified; (*3*) exogenous application of the neurotransmitter in physiologically relevant concentrations should elicit changes in the postsynaptic neuron that mimic the effects of stimulation of the presynaptic neuron; (*4*) the actions of a neurotransmitter should act on specific neuronal receptors and should therefore be blocked by administration of specific antagonists; and (*5*) there should be appropriate active mechanisms to terminate the actions of the neurotransmitter.

These criteria are based largely on studies of acetylcholine (ACh), the first neurotransmitter identified. The experimental steps required to advance a transmitter role for ACh were relatively simple because ACh is the transmitter at the neuromuscular junction. The ability to expose and maintain preparations of the neuromuscular junction, a peripheral site, permitted electrophysiological and biochemical studies of synaptic transmission. Physiological studies revealed fast excitatory responses of muscle fibers in response to stimulation of the nerve innervating the muscle, similar to the effects of ACh. Moreover, miniature end-plate potentials were observed, which Fatt and Katz (1952) demonstrated to be due to the "leakage" of the contents of individual ACh-containing vesicles from the presynaptic terminal. In contrast, overt depolarization is due to an increased number of quanta released over a set period of time. Finally, studies of the neuromuscular junction and another peripheral site, the superior cervical ganglion, allowed detailed analyses of the enzymatic inactivation of ACh. These studies of ACh established the standard to which subsequent studies of neurotransmitters would be held.

Many of the rules that were uncovered in studies of ACh apply to other transmitters. For example, the concept of the quantal nature of neurotransmission is central to current ideas of transmitter release. However, in the past generation, our ideas about the defining characteristics and functions of neurotransmitters have been expanded by the discovery of a number of chemical messengers that do not meet the criteria established for classical transmitters, but which clearly convey information from one neuron to another.

FUNCTIONAL ASPECTS OF MULTIPLE NEUROTRANSMITTERS

There are dozens if not hundreds of molecules that function as chemical messengers between neurons. Why do we need so many neurotransmitters? When transmitters were first being characterized it appeared that simple excitatory or inhibitory transmission would suffice, thus requiring two or at most a few transmitters. However, we now appreciate the complexity and nuance of interneuronal communication.

There are several factors that may contribute to the need for multiple chemical messengers (Deutch and Roth, 2012). The simplest explanation is that many axons terminate on a single postsynaptic neuron, which must be able to distinguish between these multiple inputs. Although multiple inputs terminate on different parts of the postsynaptic neuron (such as the soma or dendrite), many of these inputs are so closely positioned that inputs using the same transmitter cannot be discrimanated. Multiple transmitters allow the postsynaptic cell to distinguish differences in inputs by chemically coding the information, with the receptive neurons having distinct receptors and intracellular signaling pathways. This system also permits modulation of transmitter actions, changing a simple excitatory-inhibitory mode of communication to a situation where a single input determines the response of the neuron to a subsequent input.

A second reason for multiple transmitters may be related to the number of chemical messengers found in a single neuron. Thirty years ago, it was commonly thought that each neuron had but a single neurotransmitter; it is now clear that most if not all neurons have two or more chemical messengers (Deutch and Bean, 1995). Multiple transmitters in a single neuron permit the information transmitted by a neuron to a postsynaptic target to be encoded by different chemical messengers for different functional states. For example, the firing rates of a neuron differ over time, ranging from relatively slow firing rates to rapid bursts of firing. It may therefore be useful for a neuron to encode a high-frequency discharge by one transmitter and a lower-frequency discharge by another transmitter. Similarly, differences in firing pattern convey different information; for example, classical and peptide transmitters are differentially released by different patterns of discharge.

A third reason for multiple transmitters is that different types of transmitters are depleted at different rates. Classical transmitters are synthesized in the nerve terminal by enzymatic processing of a precursor; this process allows these transmitters to be released over extended periods of time while simultaneously being replenished at the terminal. In contrast, peptide transmitters are synthesized in the cell body and transported over long distances to the axon terminal. Peptides can therefore be depleted by repetitive firing of neurons before new stores of the peptide are synthesized and transported to the nerve terminal for use.

Yet another reason for multiple transmitters is that transmitters are released from different parts of a neuron. The prototypic site of release is the axon terminal. However, transmitters are also released from dendrites and can also be released from varicosities of an axon, not just the axon terminal. These different sites of release may be occupied by different transmitters.

The types of spatial arrangements between neurons may dictate yet another reason for multiple transmitters. We generally consider synapses to be the structural specializations for intercellular communication. However, transmitters may also be released from non-junctional appositions between two neurons. Multiple transmitters may allow the postsynaptic cell to distinguish between transmitters released from non-junctional appositions and areas of synaptic specializations.

A final factor that may contribute to the need for multiple transmitters is that postsynaptic responses to transmitters occur over different time periods. Such temporal differences allow the postsynaptic cell to respond in a manner that takes into account antecedent activity in the presynaptic neuron. Thus, one transmitter can set the stage for the response of a particular cell to subsequent stimuli, which can occur on the order of seconds, or even minutes.

So many substances are now commonly accepted as neurotransmitters that one cannot discuss them all, much less new transmitter candidates. We will therefore review in some detail the principles of neurotransmission for one group of classical neurotransmitters. A representative peptide transmitter is then discussed, emphasizing similarities and differences between neuropeptide and classical transmitters. Finally, we briefly touch on unconventional transmitters, a growing group that includes such unexpected members as soluble gases (e.g., nitric oxide and carbon monoxide).

CLASSICAL TRANSMITTERS

Classical is a relative term in science, and particularly in neuroscience. Despite the use of the adjective, some of the classical neurotransmitters were unknown 50 years ago. Nonetheless, there is a wealth of information concerning virtually every step in the biosynthetic and catabolic processes of the classical transmitters. One characteristic of classical transmitters is that the final synthesis of classical transmitters occurs in the axon terminal: precursors of the transmitter are transported from the cell body to the axon (or, in some cases dendrite), where the transmitter is released to influence a follower cell. Another defining characteristic of classical transmitters is that they (or their metabolic products) are accumulated by the presynaptic cell via an active process; there is no energy-dependent, high affinity reuptake process for non-classical transmitters.

The catecholamines are a group of three related classical transmitters that are synthesized in certain central neurons, as well as the peripheral nervous system, where they can have hormonal functions. Because of the involvement of the catecholamines in several neuropsychiatric disorders, ranging from schizophrenia and depression to Parkinson's disease and dystonias, these transmitters have been the focus of extensive investigation. A detailed description of the life cycle of catecholamine transmitters provides an excellent example of the various steps involved in intercellular communication by classical transmitters.

CATECHOLAMINES

Catecholamines are organic compounds with a catechol nucleus (a benzene ring with two adjacent hydroxyl substitutions) and an amine group (Fig. 2.1). The term *catecholamine* is used more loosely to describe dopamine (DA; dihydroxyphenylethylamine) and its metabolic products norepinephrine and epinephrine. These three transmitters are generated by successive enzymatic modification of the amino acid *tyrosine*, each step requiring a different enzyme. The three catecholamines are found as transmitters in distinct dopamine-, norepinephrine-, and

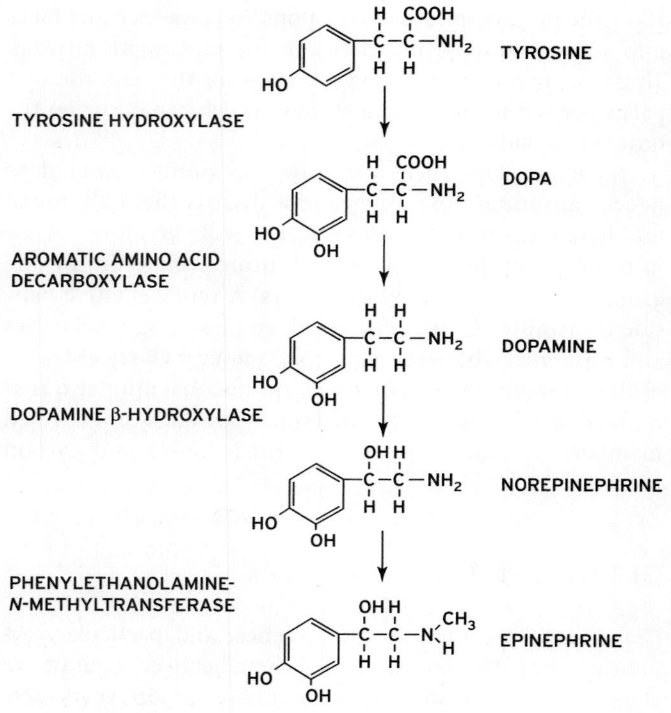

Figure 2.1 Synthetic pathway for catecholamines. From Hyman and Nestler (1993) from *The Molecular Foundations of Psychiatry,* (Copyright ©1993). American Psychiatric Publishing.

epinephrine-containing neurons because the biosynthetic enzymes that sequentially form these transmitters are localized to different cells.

CATECHOLAMINE SYNTHESIS

The amino acids *phenylalanine* and *tyrosine* are present in high concentration in plasma and the brain and are precursors for catecholamine synthesis. Under most conditions the starting point of catecholamine synthesis in the brain is tyrosine, which is derived from dietary phenylalanine by the hepatic enzyme *phenylalanine hydroxylase.* Decreased levels of this enzyme cause phenylketonuria, a disorder that if untreated (in part by limiting dietary intake of foods containing phenylalanine) results in severe intellectual deficits.

The amino acid *tyrosine* is accumulated by catecholamine neurons and then hydroxylated by the enzyme *tyrosine hydroxylase* (TH) to 3,4-dihydroxyphenylalanine (L-DOPA); this intermediary is immediately metabolized to DA by L-aromatic amino acid decarboxylase (AADC). In dopamine (DA)-containing neurons, this is the final synthetic step. However, neurons that use norepinephrine (NE) or epinephrine as transmitters also contain the enzyme *dopamine-β-hydroxylase* (DBH), which acts on DA to yield NE. Finally, brainstem neurons that use epinephrine as a transmitter, and adrenal medullary cells that release epinephrine, contain phenylethanolamine-*N*-methyltransferase (PNMT), which is responsible for the formation of epinephrine from norepinephrine (Fig. 2.1).

The entry of tyrosine into the brain occurs through a large neutral amino acid transporter; tyrosine competes with other large neutral amino acids at this transporter. Under normal conditions, brain levels of tyrosine are high enough to saturate TH, and thus changes in precursor availability do not affect catecholamine synthesis. As a result, TH is considered the rate-limiting step in catecholamine synthesis. There are, however, certain exceptions to this rule, including in poorly controlled diabetes, in which the size of the large neutral amino acid pool is altered.

Tyrosine Hydroxylase

A single TH gene in humans gives rise to four TH messenger ribonucleic acids (mRNAs) through alternative splicing. In most non-human primates, two mRNA species are present; in rodents there is but a single transcript. The functional significance of multiple transcripts is unknown, although it has been speculated that there may be subtle differences in enzyme activity of the different protein species.

The amount of TH protein and the activity of the enzyme determine overall TH function. Enzyme activity is dependent on phosphorylation of the enzyme at four distinct serine residues by different protein kinases. This provides remarkably specific control over TH activity. In addition to regulation of the enzyme by phosphorylation, TH activity can be regulated by end product (e.g., dopamine) inhibition. Catecholamines inhibit the activity of TH through competition for tetrahydrobiopterin, a required cofactor for TH. Levels of reduced tetrahydrobiopterin are not saturated under basal conditions and thus play an important role in regulating TH activity. This is best illustrated by DOPA-responsive dystonia, which is due to mutations in the gene encoding GTP-cyclohydrolase I, the rate-limiting enzyme in the synthesis of tetrahydrobiopterin (Segawa, 2011).

The two means by which catecholamine neurons can cope with an increased demand for synthesis are by inducing TH protein or by activating existing enzyme (through phosphorylation). The degree to which catecholamine synthesis depends on *de novo* synthesis of enzyme protein or changes in enzymatic activity differs in various catecholamine neurons. Noradrenergic neurons of the locus coeruleus, a brainstem nucleus that is the source of much of the forebrain NE innervation, respond to increased demands for synthesis primarily by increasing TH gene expression, ultimately leading to an increase in TH protein levels. In contrast, in midbrain DA neurons changes in TH mRNA levels are rarely seen, with regulation of synthesis in these DA cells primarily determined by changes in the activity of TH through posttranslational processes (phosphorylation).

L-Aromatic Amino Acid Decarboxylase (AADC)

The product of tyrosine hydroxylation is L-DOPA, which is immediately decarboxylated to generate DA. This step requires the enzyme AADC (also referred to as *DOPA decarboxylase*). AADC has low substrate specificity: because the enzyme decarboxylates tryptophan as well as tyrosine, it is a key step in the synthesis of serotonin and catecholamines. The activity of AADC is so high that L-DOPA is almost instantaneously converted to DA.

A single AADC gene encodes multiple transcripts that are differentially expressed in the central nervous system

(CNS) and peripheral tissues. L-aromatic amino acid decarboxylase mRNA is enriched in both catecholamine- and indoleamine-containing neurons in the CNS but is also found at low levels in other cell types.

Dopamine poorly penetrates the poor blood-brain barrier. In contrast, the DA precursor L-DOPA readily enters the brain and has therefore become the mainstay of the treatment of Parkinson's disease, the proximate cause of which is striatal DA insufficiency. Administration of L-DOPA to parkinsonian patients quickly increases brain DA levels and improves motor deficits.

Dopamine-β-Hydroxylase (DBH)

Noradrenergic and adrenergic neurons, but not dopaminergic neurons, contain DBH, the enzyme that converts DA to norepinephrine. In noradrenergic neurons this is the final step of catecholamine synthesis. Two different human DBH mRNAs are generated from a single gene.

Dopamine-β-hydroxylase has relatively poor substrate specificity and can oxidize in vitro almost any phenylethylamine to its corresponding phenylethanolamine. Thus, in addition to the oxidation of DA to form NE, DBH promotes the conversion of tyramine to octopamine and α-methyldopamine to α-methylnorepinephrine. This lack of substrate specificity has been exploited in the laboratory: several structurally analogous compounds can replace NE and function as "false transmitters," providing useful experimental tools. Contrary to the usual situation in which TH is the rate-limiting step in catecholamine synthesis, when the activity of locus coeruleus noradrenergic neurons is increased, DBH is thought to be saturated and becomes the rate-limiting step. DBH is localized to the vesicle, separating NE and its precursor dopamine into a vesicular, transmitter pool of NE and a cytosolic, non-transmitter pool for DA in noradrenergic neurons. If vesicular DBH is saturated, the result will be an accumulation of DA in the vesicle; when the vesicular contents are released by depolarization, both DA and NE are released. In this manner the noradrenergic vesicle becomes a Trojan horse for dopamine.

Phenylethanolamine-N-Methyltransferase (PNMT)

This enzyme methylates NE to form epinephrine. Central epinephrine neurons are located in two groups of brainstem cells; high levels of PNMT are also present in the adrenal medulla. PNMT has relatively poor substrate specificity and will transfer methyl groups to the nitrogen atom on a variety of β-hydroxylated amines. Nonspecific N-methyltransferases are also found in the lung and will methylate many indoleamines. The high levels of PNMT in the adrenal gland, coupled with relatively easy experimental access to the adrenal, have led to an extensive characterization of the enzyme in this gland, where enzyme activity and expression are tightly regulated by glucocorticoids and nerve growth factor.

Trace Amines and Trace Amine Receptors

A number of amines that are derived from catecholamine metabolism have been identified in the brain, including tyramine, octopamine, and β-phenythylamine. As their name indicates, these compounds are present in trace amounts relative to the classical catecholamines, and a number of different receptors for which trace amines have high affinities have been identified (Sotnikova et al., 2009). These receptors are expressed in brain and gut and may in part be responsible for certain side effects of treatments with therapeutic drugs, such as certain monoamine oxidase inhibitors (see following), and may contribute to some actions of psychoactive drugs such as amphetamine and lysergic acid diethylamide (LSD), which are agonists at a trace amine receptor.

STORAGE OF CATECHOLAMINES: SYNAPTIC VESICLES AND VESICULAR TRANSPORTERS

Catecholamine transmitters are stored in small vesicles located near the synapse and poised for fusion with the neuronal membrane and subsequent exocytosis. In addition to serving as a storage depot for catecholamines, vesicles sequester catecholamines from cytosolic enzymes and from some toxins that enter the neuron.

The accumulation of catecholamines by vesicles depends on a vesicular monoamine transporter (VMAT). Two VMAT genes have been cloned: one is in the adrenal medulla, and the other, designated VMAT2, is found in catecholamine and serotonin neurons of the CNS. VMAT2 broadly accumulates monoamines, including catecholamines and indoleamines such as serotonin.

The VMATs are targets of some psychotropic drugs. Reserpine, a blocker of VMAT, has been used for decades to treat hypertension and psychosis. Studies of reserpine shed light on how this drug can reduce psychotic symptoms (by decreasing DA accumulation into vesicles and thereby decreasing DA availability) and hypertension (by disrupting catecholamine synthesis in the adrenal medulla and thereby decreasing circulating catecholamine levels).

REGULATION OF CATECHOLAMINE SYNTHESIS AND RELEASE BY AUTORECEPTORS

We have discussed how catecholamines are synthesized and some of the regulatory features that govern synthesis of these transmitters. Another way in which the synthesis of catecholamines can be regulated is by the catecholamine released from the neuron. Once released, the transmitter (e.g., dopamine) interacts with a receptor located on the catecholamine axon that binds the transmitter (e.g., a dopamine D_2 receptor). This nerve terminal "autoreceptor" is part of a feedback loop that maintains synaptic dopamine within a homeostatic range. This feedback can be a negative feedback, in which the released transmitter shuts down further transmitter release; drugs that are antagonists of the autoreceptor can promote transmitter release. There are several types of autoreceptors. In addition to autoreceptors that regulate transmitter release, there are autoreceptors that govern transmitter synthesis, and still another type that controls the firing rate of the neuron. The precise cellular distribution of these autoreceptors is linked to their function. For example, release- and synthesis-modulating autoreceptors are found on axon terminals of catecholamine neurons, while impulse-modulating autoreceptors that regulate the firing rate of catecholamine neurons are localized to somatodendritic regions of the neuron. All three types of dopamine autoreceptors are thought to be D_2 receptors, one of the five types of dopamine receptors; this suggests that these D_2 receptors are coupled to different intracellular transduction cascades.

Release-modulating autoreceptors are found on all dopamine neurons, but synthesis-modulating autoreceptors are not. For example, both midbrain dopamine neurons that innervate the prefrontal cortex and certain hypothalamic dopamine neurons lack functional synthesis-modulating autoreceptors. Similarly, impulse-modulating autoreceptors are present on most but not all dopamine neurons. Such differences in the localization of autoreceptors to different types of neurons are thought to confer regional specificity on the function of dopamine neurons.

Autoreceptors for norepinephrine are also well characterized. Among these are noradrenergic autoreceptors that regulate release of NE, which are important targets for drugs used to treat cardiovascular and neuropsychiatric disorders. Norepinephrine autoreceptors in the brain are α_2-adrenergic receptors, the activation of which serves to inhibit norepinephrine release. In contrast, autoreceptors on peripheral nerves are β-adrenergic receptors and facilitate norepinephrine release.

INACTIVATION OF RELEASED CATECHOLAMINE NEUROTRANSMITTERS

Continuous (as opposed to discrete pulsatile) release of a transmitter does not provide target neurons with appropriate information about the dynamic state of the presynaptic neuron. Accordingly, there is a need for mechanisms to inactivate the released transmitter. The importance of this process can be easily appreciated by considering the consequences of unrestrained stimulation of channel-forming receptors through which calcium enters neurons: if intracellular Ca^{2+} levels increase too much, excitotoxic cell death results.

There are several specific mechanisms for terminating transmitter actions. Diffusion from the synapse is the most simple. However, in addition to being a slow mode of inactivation, diffusion is a poor means for terminating transmitter action because functional receptors are often present on the axon as well as in the immediate synaptic region The primary mode of inactivation appears to be uptake of the released transmitter by a plasma membrane-associated transporter protein. Because these transporters are typically located on cells that release the transmitter, inactivation by means of transporter-mediated reuptake is efficient and often allows for recycling of the transmitter or metabolites to lower energy demands on the neuron. A second way for transmitter actions to be terminated is by catabolic enzymes located either extra- or intracellularly.

Enzymatic Inactivation of Catecholamines

Two enzymes sequentially metabolize catecholamines. Monoamine oxidases (MAO) deaminate catecholamines to yield aldehyde derivatives; these are further catabolized by dehydrogenases and reductases. Catechol-O-methyltransferase (COMT) methylates the meta-hydroxy group on catechols, and these methylated intermediaries are further oxidized by MAO. Enzymatic inactivation, particularly by COMT, is the primary mode of terminating the actions of catecholamines circulating in the blood. In the brain, termination of catecholamine actions by reuptake mechanisms appears to be more important. Nevertheless, drugs that target the enzymatic inactivation of catecholamines have been very useful therapeutic strategies for several disorders, including depression.

Two MAO genes have been cloned, and two isoforms of the enzyme can be distinguished by substrate specificity. Both isoforms are present in the CNS and peripheral tissues. MAO_A displays high affinities for NE and serotonin, whereas MAO_B has a higher affinity for β-phenylethylamines. Drugs that inhibit MAO_A (*clorgyline, tranylcypromine*) are effective antidepressant drugs. However, these agents have serious side effects, including the development of hypertensive crisis: patients treated with MAO_A inhibitors who eat foods high in tyramine content (e.g., aged cheeses and Chianti, a particularly appetizing combination) do not effectively metabolize tyramine, which releases catecholamines from nerve endings and thereby dangerously increases blood pressure. These adverse effects associated with MAO_A inhibitors may be mediated in part by interactions with trace amine receptors.

Deprenyl is a specific inhibitor of MAO_B and is sometimes used in the treatment of Parkinson's disease (PD). The use of deprenyl in PD springs from studies of the neurotoxin 1-methyl-4-phenyl-1,2,3,6-tetrahydropyridine (MPTP), which causes a Parkinson's Disease (PD)-like syndrome. The tetrahydropyridine MPTP itself is not toxic, but its metabolite MPP^+, which is generated by the actions of MAO_B, is highly toxic. Because the MAO_B inhibitor deprenyl blocks the formation of MPP^+ from MPTP, pretreatment with deprenyl prevents MPTP-induced parkinsonism. This finding led to the suggestion that an environmental toxin similar to MPTP might cause parkinsonism, and studies of deprenyl in newly diagnosed PD patients ensued. Although initial analyses suggested that deprenyl slowed disease progression, subsequent analyses failed to sustain the early enthusiasm. It is now clear that deprenyl does not slow progression but may offer some symptomatic relief. This probably occurs by increasing DA levels secondary to the inhibition of MAO_B-mediated catabolism of DA. In addition, small amounts of amphetamine and methamphetamine, potent DA releasers, are generated by the metabolism of deprenyl and may contribute to symptomatic improvement in parkinsonian symptoms.

Catecholamine Reuptake: Membrane Transporter

The reuptake of transmitters released into the extracellular space via specific cell membrane proteins is thought to be the major mode of inactivation of classical transmitters. The accumulation of transmitters in the presynaptic neuron also permits intracellular degradative enzymes to act and further contribute to transmitter inactivation, particularly if the transmitter is not rapidly accumulated by vesicles.

Neuronal reuptake of catecholamines and other classical transmitters has several characteristics: the process is energy dependent, saturable, involves Na^+ co-transport, and requires extracellular Cl^- (Kristensen et al., 2011). It is worthwhile to note that transporters can operate bidirectionally and under certain conditions may paradoxically transport in the "wrong" direction, thereby "releasing" a transmitter.

Catecholamine transporters are found in catecholamine but not other neurons. There appears to be some catecholamine uptake by glial cells, but this is not a high-affinity reuptake process and the functional significance of this process remains obscure. However, there are high-affinity transporters for amino acid transmitters (such as γ-aminobutyric acid [GABA] and glutamate) that are localized to astrocytes and play a major role in regulating extracellular levels of these amino acid transmitters.

In mammals, two different catecholamine transporters, the dopamine (DAT) and norepinephrine (NET) transporters, have been identified. An amphibian epinephrine transporter has been cloned, but a mammalian homolog of this gene has not been identified. DAT and NET share significant sequence homology, and both exhibit relatively poor substrate specificity. In fact, NET has a higher affinity for DA than for NE.

Anatomical studies have revealed that DAT and NET are restricted to dopamine- and norepinephrine-containing cells, respectively. However, DAT is not present in measurable levels in all dopamine neurons. For example, the hypothalamic tuberoinfundibular neurons that release dopamine into the pituitary portal blood supply do not express detectable levels of DAT mRNA or protein. Because DA released from these neurons is rapidly carried away in the vasculature, there is probably no need for inactivation of DA by reuptake into tuberoinfundibular neurons.

Immunohistochemical studies have revealed that under basal conditions, DAT and other transmitter transporters are localized to the extrasynaptic region of the axon terminal (Pickel et al., 2002), suggesting that the transporter may be important in clearing DA that has diffused from the synaptic region. When one considers that DA receptors are also found adjacent to the synapse rather than at the synaptic junction (Pickel et al., 2002), extrasynaptic (so-called paracrine or volume) transmission may be of greater importance than previously realized for catecholamine transmission (Wickens and Arbuthnott, 2005).

Just as there is a tight process of regulation over enzyme activity, there are regulatory controls for neurotransmitter transporters. Chronic administration of catecholamine reuptake inhibitors decreases the number of transporter sites, consistent with a decrease in gene expression. In addition, the activity of catecholamine transporters appears to be regulated acutely by several mechanisms (Zahniser and Doolen, 2001). The recognition that transporter expression is dynamically regulated has broad implications for *in vivo* imaging studies of transporters (such as studies of DAT in PD) because drug treatments that patients receive may alter the apparent density of the transporter.

Studies of DAT knockout mice have revealed that a broad array of DA neuron functions is disrupted by loss of the transporter (Sotnikova et al., 2006). It is therefore not surprising that transporters are key targets of psychoactive drugs. Cocaine increases extracellular monoamine levels by blocking the transporters for DA, NE, and serotonin. The tricyclic antidepressants potently inhibit NE and serotonin reuptake, with significantly weaker effects on dopamine, and are one of the major means of treating certain types of depression. The newer serotonin-selective reuptake blockers, such as fluoxetine, are now the most widely prescribed antidepressant medications.

ANATOMY OF CATECHOLAMINE NEURONS

Neurons expressing dopamine, norepinephrine, and epinephrine are found in a wide variety of species, although there are some major differences in the anatomical organization of these neurons between species. For example, midbrain DA neurons are present in all vertebrates except bony fish (*teleosts*), and dopaminergic cells (although few in number) are present in flies and worms. There are some differences in the anatomy of the catecholaminergic neurons between primate and lower mammalian species, but these differences are mainly quantitative rather than qualitative, and the general organization of the catecholamine systems of primates and lower mammalian species is quite similar.

Dopamine neurons in the ventral midbrain cells project to several forebrain sites, including the striatum, limbic sites such as the amygdala, septum, and hippocampus, and to certain cortical sites (Fig. 2.2). The cortical DA innervation in primates is much broader than is seen in rodents. In addition to the midbrain DA neurons, several clusters of DA neurons are found in the diencephalon, including hypothalamic cells with long axons that innervate the spinal cord as well as intra-hypothalamic projections. Still another set of DA neurons is found in the olfactory bulb. The reader is referred to the review by Morelli and Bentivoglio (2005) for a more comprehensive discussion of the anatomy of DA neurons.

Norepinephrine-containing cells are located in the medulla and pons (Fig. 2.3). In the rostral pons, a small but important group of cells is found in the nucleus locus coeruleus. These neurons give rise to most of the noradrenergic innervation of

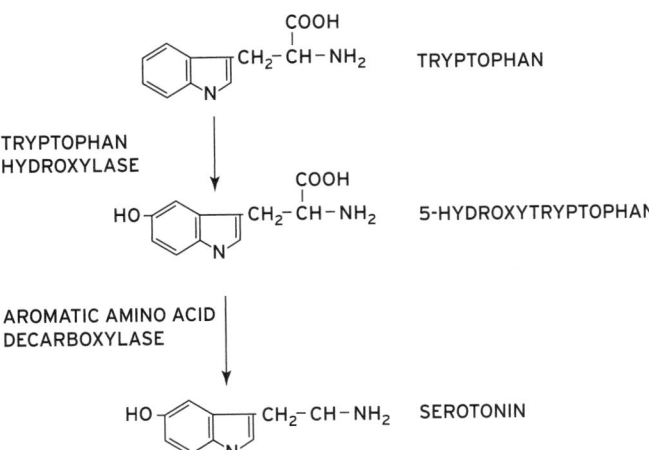

Figure 2.2 Dopaminergic projection systems in the brain. The major dopaminergic nuclei in the brain are the substantia nigra pars compacta (hatched), containing dopamine neurons that project to the striatum (also hatched); the ventral tegmental area (fine stipple), shown projecting to the frontal and cingulate cortex, nucleus accumbens, and other limbic structures (fine stipple); and the arcuate nucleus of the hypothalamus (coarse stipple), which provides a dopaminergic innervation of the pituitary. From Hyman and Nestler (1993) reprinted with permission from The Molecular Foundations of Psychiatry, (Copyright ©1993). American Psychiatric Publishing.

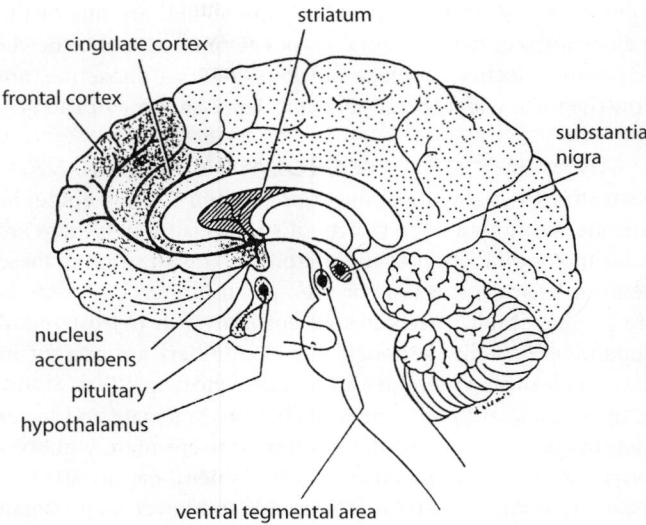

Figure 2.3 *Noradrenergic projection systems in the brain. Shown are the major noradrenergic nuclei of the brain, the locus coeruleus (hatched) and the lateral tegmental nuclei (fine stipple). Epinephrine-containing nuclei are shown in black. The projections from the locus coeruleus (as described in the text) are markedly simplified. Projections from the other noradrenergic nuclei are not shown. From Hyman and Nestler (1993) permission from The Molecular Foundations of Psychiatry, (Copyright ©1993). American Psychiatric Publishing.*

the forebrain, as well as of the brainstem and spinal cord. Other pontine and lower brainstem noradrenergic cells innervate certain nuclei in the hypothalamus and thalamus, and limbic areas such as the amygdala, septum, and hippocampus.

Epinephrine-containing cells are found in two nuclei in the medulla and provide descending projections as well as sending efferents to the pons that regulates the activity of the locus coeruleus NE-containing cells.

SEROTONIN

The major processes that regulate catecholamine synthesis and degradation are shared by all classical transmitters, including serotonin. Nonetheless, there are some relatively minor differences among the classical transmitters. The following discussion focuses on the differences between serotonin and catecholamine neurotransmitters.

SYNTHESIS OF SEROTONIN

The synthesis of serotonin (5-hydroxytryptamine) follows the basic scheme laid out for catecholamine transmitters: the uptake of a precursor amino acid (tryptophan) into a neuron, the sequential enzymatic formation of serotonin from tryptophan, the accumulation of serotonin by VMAT2 into vesicles, and, following release of the transmitter, inactivation by active reuptake of extracellular serotonin.

The precursor amino acid *tryptophan* enters the CNS via the large neutral amino acid transporter, where it competes with other amino acids (including phenylalanine and tyrosine). In serotonergic neurons, tryptophan is a substrate for tryptophan hydroxylase, which results in the formation of 5-hydroxytryptophan (5-HTP), the immediate serotonin precursor (Fig. 2.4). Tryptophan hydroxylase is not saturated, and

thus peripheral (including dietary) sources of tryptophan have a major influence on central serotonin synthesis.

There are two forms of tryptophan hydroxylase, one peripheral (TPH1) and the other central (TPH2). Situations requiring increased synthesis of serotonin are dealt with mainly by increasing the activity of the enzyme through phosphorylation; some long-term changes in demand may lead to increases in tryptophan hydroxylase gene expression.

5-Hydroxytryptophan is metabolized to serotonin by L-aromatic amino acid decarboxylase, the same enzyme that converts L-DOPA to dopamine. The serotonin formed can be metabolized to an acidic metabolite by MAO.

Although one usually thinks of serotonin as the end point of tryptophan pathways in the brain, there are two important exceptions to this rule. In the pineal gland serotonin is metabolized by serotonin-*N*-acetyltransferase to yield *N*-acetylserotonin, to which a methyl group is then added to form the hormone *melatonin*. Throughout the brain there is also a kynurenic acid shunt from tryptophan metabolism that results in the formation of several compounds, including quinolinic acid and kynurenic acid. Quinolinic acid is a potent agonist at *N*-methyl-D-aspartame (NMDA)-type glutamate receptors and causes seizures and neurotoxicity. In contrast, kynurenine is an NMDA antagonist. It has been suggested that the ratio of the two tryptophan derivatives may be of significance in conditions such as stroke, where cell death is mediated in part by NMDA receptors, as well as in schizophrenia (Wonodi and Schwarcz, 2010).

STORAGE AND REGULATION OF SEROTONIN RELEASE AND SYNTHESIS

Serotonin, like other classical transmitters, is stored intraneuronally in vesicles. The accumulation of 5-HT by vesicles depends on VMAT2, which also transports the catecholamines into vesicles. The other regulatory features of serotonin are essentially the same as seen in catecholamine transmitters, including the presence of serotonin autoreceptors that regulate serotonin release and synthesis, acting through functionally distinct somatodendritic and terminal autoreceptors. One

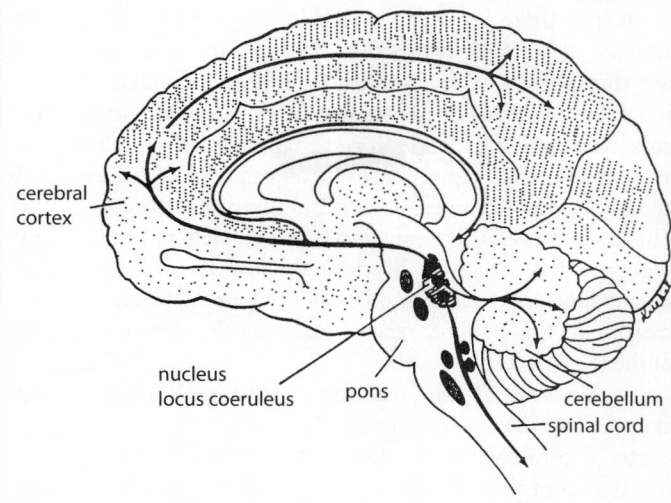

Figure 2.4 *Synthetic pathway for serotonin. From Hyman and Nestler (1993) reprinted with permission from The Molecular Foundations of Psychiatry, (Copyright ©1993). American Psychiatric Publishing.*

difference between serotonin and catecholamine neurons is that serotonin synthesis is not regulated by end-product inhibition *in vivo*. The release- and impulse-modulating autoreceptors in serotonin neurons are 5-HT$_1$ receptors. The 5-HT$_{1A}$ receptor is an autoreceptor present on the somatodendritic region of the serotonin neurons, whereas the 5-HT$_{1B}$ receptor is an autoreceptor located on serotonin nerve terminals. In addition, the 5-HT$_{1A}$ receptor is also found on some non-serotonergic neurons. Changes in the number and coupling of 5-HT$_1$ receptors in response to chronic treatment with serotonin-selective reuptake inhibitor antidepressants is thought to be critical to the therapeutic actions of these drugs.

INACTIVATION OF RELEASED SEROTONIN

Reuptake of released serotonin by the serotonin transporter (SERT) is the major means of terminating serotonin's actions. The serotonin transporter belongs to the same molecular family as the catecholamine membrane transporters and has the same requirements for action. The SERT is also the target for the most commonly used antidepressants, the serotonin-selective reuptake inhibitors (Thompson et al., 2011). Like the catecholamines, serotonin can be inactivated enzymatically by MAO.

ANATOMY OF SEROTONIN-CONTAINING NEURONS

There are a number of distinct groups of serotonin neurons, most of which are located on the midline of the pons and medulla. (see Fig. 2.5). Pontine serotonin cells in the dorsal and median raphe nuclei are the major source of diencephalic and telencephalic sites; cells in the medulla provide important descending serotonin projections to the spinal cord.

AMINO ACID TRANSMITTERS

The excitatory and inhibitor amino acid transmitters glutamate and γ-aminobutyric acid (GABA) are the most abundant transmitters in the brain. The cell bodies of monoamine neurons

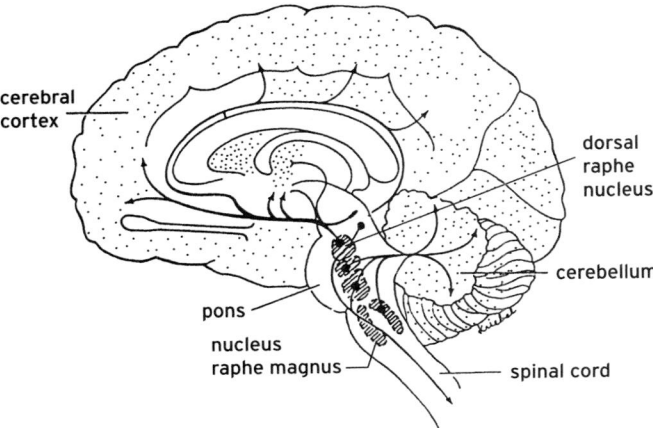

Figure 2.5 *Serotonergic projection systems in the brain. The major serotonergic nuclei in the brain are the brainstem raphe nuclei (hatched). The nuclei are shown slightly enlarged, and their diffuse projections (as described in the text) are markedly simplified. From Hyman and Nestler (1993) reprinted with permission from The Molecular Foundations of Psychiatry, (Copyright ©1993). American Psychiatric Publishing.*

are discretely localized in the brain, but glutamatergic and GABAergic neurons are found in virtually all areas of the brain. Although there are some significant differences between amino acid and monoamine transmitters, most of the major principles discussed in the section on catecholamine transmitters are applicable to amino acid transmitters. The amino acid transmitters are derived from intermediary glucose metabolism. The dual roles of GABA and glutamate as transmitters and metabolic intermediaries requires a means of segregating the transmitter and metabolic pools (Hassel and Dingledine, 2012; Olsen and Li, 2012). The other major difference between amino acid and monoamine transmitters is that the former are inactivated by uptake of the released transmitter through high-affinity transporters located on glial cells as well as by transporters found on neurons. This discussion focuses on those aspects of amino acid transmitters that differ from monoamine transmitters, as enumerated in the preceding. Although glycine is also an inhibitory transmitter, particularly in the spinal cord, GABA is discussed as the representative example of the inhibitory amino acid transmitter. Similarly, glutamate is discussed as the major excitatory transmitter, although other excitatory amino acids, including aspartate and sulfur-containing amino acids such as homocysteic acid, are also thought to be neurotransmitters.

AMINO ACID TRANSMITTER SYNTHESIS AND VESICULAR STORAGE

γ-aminobutyric acid is derived from glucose metabolism, with α-ketoglutarate from the Krebs (tricarboxylic acid) cycle being transaminated to glutamate by GABA α-oxoglutarate transaminase (GABA-T). The key step for the generation of the transmitter pool of GABA is the action of the enzyme *glutamic acid decarboxylase* (GAD), which converts glutamate to GABA. Glutamic acid decarboxylase is essentially restricted to neurons that use GABA as a transmitter and thus serves as a marker for GABAergic neurons.

Two isoforms of GAD are encoded by two different genes. The two GAD species (designated GAD$_{65}$ and GAD$_{67}$ on the basis of their mass) have somewhat different intracellular distributions and are differently regulated. Glutamic acid decarboxylase requires a pyridoxal phosphate cofactor for activity. The lower-mass enzyme, GAD$_{65}$, has a high affinity for the cofactor, but GAD$_{67}$ does not. The high affinity of GAD$_{65}$ for cofactor provides a way in which enzyme activity can be quickly and efficiently regulated. However, GAD$_{67}$ activity is not as readily regulated, although the amount of enzyme can be regulated at the transcriptional level.

The biosynthetic enzyme GAD is a cytosolic protein. However, GABA-T, which synthesizes the GABA precursor glutamate from α-ketoglutarate, is a mitochondrial enzyme. Thus, there appears to be a metabolic pool of GABA that is mitochondrial. The process by which glutamate destined for the transmitter pool is exported from the mitochondria is not fully understood.

Glutamate is the immediate precursor of the inhibitory transmitter GABA, but is also a major excitatory transmitter in different neurons. Neurons must therefore have some mechanisms to prevent GABA neurons from using glutamate as a transmitter. Glutamic acid decarboxylase is not found in neurons that use glutamate as a transmitter, thus ensuring that GABAergic neurons use GABA but not glutamate as a transmitter. Moreover, vesicular transporters for GABA are localized exclusively to GABAergic neurons. In contrast to the monoamine vesicular transporters, which use a pH gradient to transport monoamines into the cell, the vesicular GABA transporter uses electrochemical and pH gradients to drive transport.

Similarly, in glutamatergic neurons one of several vesicular glutamate transporters (VGluTs) allows glutamate to be stored in vesicles for use as a transmitter (El Mestikawy et al., 2011). The VGluTs are used as markers of glutamatergic neurons. Despite these means of separating the transmitter pools of glutamate and GABA, and the general utility in having excitatory and inhibitory transmitters being found in different neurons, there are some examples of co-localization of excitatory and inhibitory amino acid transmitters in single neurons (Zander et al., 2010).

Glutamate can also be formed directly from glutamine, which is synthesized in glial cells. The glutamine that is formed in glia can be transported out of the glia and into nerve terminals and then locally converted by glutaminase into glutamate. Thus, glial cells may in part regulate glutamate synthesis, as well as determine extracellular levels of glutamate by means of membrane-associated transporters. This underscores the complex functions of glia, which are now recognized to play several critical roles in brain function in addition to the support role previously envisioned (Halassa and Haydon, 2010; Panatier et al., 2011), including key roles in neurotransmission.

REGULATION OF AMINO ACID TRANSMITTER RELEASE BY AUTORECEPTORS

Autoreceptor-mediated regulation of GABA neurons occurs through $GABA_B$ receptors, which in contrast to postsynaptic ionotropic $GABA_A$ receptors are coupled to G proteins. $GABA_B$ receptors are also found on non-GABA cells, where they may regulate the release of glutamate and other transmitters. The release of glutamate from nerve terminals is also subject to autoreceptor regulation, a function subserved by G protein–coupled metabotropic glutamate receptors (mGluR). Three groups of mGluR receptors that include eight different receptors have been identified (Niswender and Conn, 2010); group II mGluRs are release-modulating autoreceptors. In addition to the well-characterized release-modulating mGluRs, electrophysiological studies have suggested the presence of a glutamate impulse–modulating autoreceptor. Various mGluRs are a target for the development of new drug treatments for a variety of neuropsychiatric disorders, including schizophrenia, Parkinson's disease, PTSD, and Fragile X syndrome.

INACTIVATION OF RELEASED GABA AND GLUTAMATE

The uptake of released GABA and glutamate is the primary means of terminating the actions of these transmitters. High-affinity GABA and glutamate uptake into both neurons and astrocytes occurs, the latter distinguishing these transmitters from the monoamines, which are not accumulated by high-affinity glial transporters.

In contrast to monoamine transporters, which include a single transporter for each of the monoamines (albeit with low substrate specificity), at least three transporters accumulate GABA (Kanner, 2006); other transporters present in the brain, such as a betaine transporter, can also accumulate GABA. The three types of membrane GABA transporters (GATs) do not readily correspond to different GAT isoforms in glia and neurons.

Glial and neuronal expression of membrane glutamate transporters also occurs, with at least four membrane glutamate transporters defined. These transporters display high affinities for glutamate, but differ in their affinities for other amino acids. Two glutamate transporters are primarily expressed in glia, with a third glutamate transporter being predominantly neuronal.

ANATOMY OF AMINO ACID TRANSMITTERS

GABA- and glutamate-containing neuronal elements can be found in almost every area of the brain. Nonetheless, certain discrete projections for excitatory and inhibitory neurons have been identified. For example, inhibitory GABAergic cells are usually local circuit neurons. However, some GABA neurons are projection neurons; among these are cells that project from the basal forebrain to the cortex and striatal GABAergic neurons that innervate the globus pallidus and substantia nigra. Among the many glutamatergic neurons are the pyramidal cells of the cortex, as well as a variety of long-axoned projection neurons in subcortical sites.

DIVERSITY OF AMINO ACID TRANSMITTERS

More so than other classical transmitters, GABA and glutamate as transmitters are marked by a complexity and diversity of function. There are multiple membrane transporters for GABA and glutamate, and multiple vesicular glutamate transporters. GABA and glutamate play transmitter and metabolic roles in neurons. There are a diverse group of receptors for GABA and glutamate, including ionotropic and metabotropic receptors. GABA and glutamate involve more than just neurons but critically bring into play glial cells.

We have focused this brief discussion on GABA and glutamate as amino acid transmitters, but there are other amino acids that are also transmitters or have been proposed to be neurotransmitters; these include, glycine, aspartate, and sulfur-containing amino acids. Among the most surprising of the amino acids transmitter candidates are D-amino acids (Wolosker et al., 2008). Conventional wisdom has held that L-enantiomers but not D-enantiomers of amino acids are active; D-amino acids were relegated to their functions in bacteria and invertebrates. However, D-serine and D-aspartame are present in relatively high concentrations in the human brain. D-serine is heterogeneously distributed, with the highest concentrations in regions with a high density of NADA glutamate receptors. An enzyme, *serine racemase*, which converts L-serine to D-serine, has been found in glia but not neurons, suggesting that glia may synthesize and release D-serine. However, classical considerations of transmitters hold that neurons but not glia communicate via release of transmitters. This conundrum has been resolved by noting that certain types of glia express α-amino-3-hydroxy-5-methyl-4-isoxa solepropionic acid (AMPA)-type glutamate receptors and respond to glutamate stimulation by releasing D-serine onto NADA-receptor-bearing neurons. Thus, in this case, glia serve as intermediate functional links between two neurons, and D-amino acids may be neurotransmitters, albeit unconventional ones (see following sections).

PEPTIDE TRANSMITTERS

Peptides, once viewed as pretenders to the royalty of neurotransmitters, have become firmly established as neurotransmitters over the past 30 years. The notion of peptide transmitters initially met with resistance because peptides did not meet some of the criteria developed for classical transmitters; some of these missing steps were subsequently shown to be due to methodological issues, including sensitivity of assay techniques.

There are two major differences between classical and peptide transmitters. The first is the intraneuronal site(s) of synthesis of the transmitter. Synthetic enzymes for classical transmitters are present in axon terminals as well as cell body regions, allowing a rapid response to increased demand for transmitter release from axon terminals. In contrast, peptide transmitters are typically synthesized in the cell body but not in axons. As such, increased demand for the peptide transmitter requires *de novo* protein synthesis and transport of the peptide to the terminal. The second major difference is that peptides are inactivated almost exclusively by enzymatic means; there are no high-affinity transporters that accumulate neuropeptides. Despite the failure of peptide transmitters to meet all of the classical criteria for transmitters, neuropeptides clearly convey information between neurons. Such information is not simply generalized information about the milieu, but is temporally and spatially coded information. Table 2.1 lists some of the many peptide transmitters in the brain.

The general principles of the peptide transmitters are discussed next. The discussion focuses on specific examples drawn from one widely distributed peptide, *neurotensin*.

SYNTHESIS AND STORAGE OF PEPTIDE TRANSMITTERS

Classical transmitters are typically synthesized by enzymatic processing of precursor(s) in the vicinity of the release site, usually the axon terminal. In contrast, peptide transmitters are formed from a prohormone precursor that is transcribed and translated in the cell body of the neuron, where it is then incorporated into vesicles. Thus, most peptide transmitters are formed from a single precursor from which active peptides are cleaved, in contrast to the successive enzymatic modifications of a precursor amino acid that give rise to most classical transmitters.

The general process can be easily understood by examining the case of the peptide transmitter neurotensin (NT). A large (170 amino acid) prohormone precursor of NT and a related

TABLE 2.1. Examples of peptide transmitters

Opioid and related peptides
Dynorphin
Endorphin
Enkephalins
Nociceptin (orphanin FQ)
Gut-brain peptides[a]
Cholecystokinin (CCK)
Gastrin
Secretin
Somatostatin
Vasoactive intestinal polypeptide (VIP)
Tachykinin peptides
Substance K
Substance P
Neuromedin N
Pituitary peptides[b]
Adrenal corticotropic hormone (ACTH)
Melanocyte stimulating hormone (MSH)
Oxytocin
Vasopressin
Hypothalamic releasing factors[c]
Corticotropin releasing hormone (CRH)
Growth hormone releasing factor (GHRF)
Luteinizing hormone releasing hormone (LHRH)
Thyrotropin releasing hormone (TRH)
Others
Angiotensin
Calcitonin gene-related peptide (CGRP)
Cocaine- and amphetamine-related transcript (CART)
Melanocyte concentration hormone (MCH)
Neurotensin
Hypocretin/Orexin

[a] Peptides first found in the gut and later shown to serve as neurotransmitters in the brain.
[b] Peptides first discovered as pituitary hormones and later shown to serve as neurotransmitters in the brain.
[c] Peptides first discovered for their role as hypothalamic-release hormones and later shown to serve as neurotransmitters in the brain.

peptide, *neuromedin N* (NMN), are encoded by a single gene that is transcribed to yield two mRNAs. The two transcripts are present in equal abundance in most brain areas. Different molar ratios of NT and NMN are found in some tissues because of differential processing of the prohormone.

Classical neurotransmitters are usually packaged in small (<50 nm) synaptic vesicles, while neuropeptide transmitters are localized to large (<100 nm) dense-core vesicles. Peptides are often released at higher neuronal firing rates than classical transmitters. The mechanisms that govern the different processes responsible for vesicular release of peptides and classical transmitters is still being untangled (Bean et al., 1995), and may be cell type-specific (Ramamoorthy et al., 2011)

RELEASE OF PEPTIDES

Depolarization-elicited release of peptides from dense-core vesicular stores is calcium-dependent. The amount of peptide transmitter that is released varies as a function of the firing rate and firing pattern of the neuron. For example, studies of neurons that use both DA and NT as transmitters have found that higher firing frequencies are required to elicit release of the peptide. The temporal pattern of impulses arriving at the nerve terminal also determines release characteristics: the release of many peptides is most prominent under conditions of burst firing, where neurons fire in very rapid succession followed by a quiescent period (Bean et al., 1995).

INACTIVATION OF PEPTIDE TRANSMITTERS

Peptides are inactivated enzymatically: there do not appear to be conventional transporters that accumulate released peptides. The enzymes that metabolize peptides are specific for certain dipeptide sites along the peptide chain. Thus, the same enzymes can catabolize any peptide with the requisite dipeptide linkages. An example is a metallo-endopeptidase that inactivates the small opioid transmitters called *enkephalins*. Although this enzyme is often called *enkephalinase*, it also participates in the enzymatic processing of other peptides, including NT. Because the enzymes cleave and inactivate peptides work at sites across many peptides, most peptides have several major peptidases involved in the catabolism of the peptide. Three endopeptidases enzymatically inactivate NT. Enkephalinase cleaves NT at two sites, Pro10-Tyr11 and Tyr11-Ile12, to yield a decapeptide. Another peptidase acts at the Arg8-Arg9 site, and the third at the same Pro10-Tyr11 site as enkephalinase. Such processing can give rise to multiple metabolic products of the parent peptide.

The enzymatic inactivation of classical transmitters results in products that are not active at the transmitter's receptors. However, this is not necessarily the case for peptide transmitters, in which the products of enzymatic breakdown may retain activity at the receptor site. Indeed, some peptide fragments that are generated by the actions of peptidases may have a higher affinity for the peptide's receptor than the parent molecule.

NEWER PEPTIDE TRANSMITTERS

No additions have been made to the list of classical transmitters for some time, although new receptors for these transmitters have been discovered at a rapid rate. In contrast to the stable number of classical transmitters, the number of peptide transmitters continues to grow. The increased number of peptide transmitters is due in part to molecular biological strategies aimed at identifying novel genes. Many peptides have been identified in this manner, and of these, a considerable number have subsequently been shown to be neuroactive and meet criteria for a transmitter. One recent example stands out. Two groups simultaneously identified a novel gene encoding a prohormone that gave rise to two isoforms of a peptide, designated *hypocretin* (de Lecea et al., 1998) or *orexin* (Sakurai et al., 1998). These peptides are expressed only in a small number of lateral hypothalamic neurons. Despite the small number of hypocretin/orexin neurons, these cells send axons to cover almost the entire brain. Two G protein–coupled hypocretin/orexin receptors are widely but differentially distributed in the brain. One of the most interesting aspects of these cells is that among the functions ascribed to them is arousal (Boutrel et al., 2010). Degeneration of hypocretin/orexin neurons in humans is the cause of narcolepsy, a disorder marked by excessive daytime sleepiness, while in narcoleptic dogs there is a mutation in one of the hypocretin/orexin receptors. Since the discovery of the hypocretins/orexins, it has become apparent that this transmitter is critically involved in attention and cognition, reward and motivated behavior, and feeding behavior and metabolism.

UNCONVENTIONAL TRANSMITTERS

Technical approaches limit advances in any scientific endeavor, including neuroscience. For example, prior to the development of radioimmunoassays, it was difficult to detect peptides in the brain, and hence peptides were not considered serious transmitter candidates. The development of contemporary analytical methods, which are capable of reliably measuring substances at attomole levels, has opened the door to the identification of many new neurotransmitters.

The criteria necessary for establishment of a neuroactive substance as a neurotransmitter may need to be reconsidered. We previously discussed the idea that a very simple definition of *neurotransmitter* would be a neuroactive substance that allows information to flow from one neuron to another (Deutch and Roth, 2012). This definition avoids the issues of glial contribution to the milieu of the neuron, despite the fact that glia may convey important information and play an active role in the CNS (Halassa and Haydon, 2010). One problem with this definition is that it does not specify either the temporal or spatial characteristics of a transmitter, and thus could denote as a neurotransmitter a hormone, which typically acts over an extended time course across relatively large distances. Nor does this definition cover roles for transmitters that are only now starting to be uncovered, such as soluble gases and neurotrophic factors. And D-serine, which we already discussed, can hardly be considered conventional, being synthesized in glia and posing as an intermediate between pre- and postsynaptic neurons, with even the synapse almost seeming to be an outdated concept.

In view of our inability to arrive at a satisfactory definition for transmitters, we suggest the term "unconventional transmitters." Because the unconventional may soon become conventional, it is likely that our choice of terms will bring only temporary relief.

NITRIC OXIDE AND GAS NEUROTRANSMITTERS

Nitric oxide (NO) is perhaps best known as an air pollutant and would not immediately come to mind as a neurotransmitter candidate. Indeed, it is difficult to envision gases as neurotransmitters because a gas cannot be conventionally stored by neurons or released in an impulse-dependent manner. Nitric oxide is not stored and thus does not meet one of the key criteria for a neurotransmitter. Other gases, including carbon monoxide and hydrogen sulfide, also appear to have a transmitter function (Mustafa et al., 2009). Because NO is not stored in cells, it cannot be released by exocytosis. Nitric oxide also lacks an active process to terminate its action, and its "receptor" is the intracellular signaling protein guanylyl cyclase. Finally, NO appears to regulate the function of presynaptic terminals. As one lists these characteristics of NO, it becomes obvious that "unconventional" is a very conservative modifier to "transmitter" in the case of NO. Despite some hesitancy to embrace fully NO as a neurotransmitter, there are now ample data on the processes that control the synthesis, "release," and termination of action of NO to consider gases as transmitters (Mustafa et al., 2009).

There is only one step in the synthesis of NO: the conversion of L-arginine by the enzyme nitric oxide synthase (NOS) to yield NO and citrulline. Three forms of NOS have been identified. *Macrophage-inducible NOS* (iNOS) is present in microglia, *endothelial NOS* (eNOS) is found in cells that line blood vessels, and *neuronal NOS* (nNOS) is indeed neuronal. All three NOS isoforms can be regulated, despite the use of the adjective *inducible* only for iNOS. Among the regulatory processes are phosphorylation (which decreases NOS activity) and hormonal control. In addition, levels of NOS can be modified by direct inhalation of NO as a feedback mechanism.

Nitric oxide is an uncharged molecule that diffuses freely across cell membranes. This allows NO to play a role in interneuronal communication. For example, NO may pass from one cell through an adjacent cell to influence a third neuron, which is not even a next-door neighbor of—much less synaptically coupled with—the original neuron. Indeed, recent data suggest that NO may act primarily as a retrograde messenger, modifying transmitter release and metabolism from presynaptic terminals. This situation has been most thoroughly explored in the hippocampus, where NADA-evoked NO release from pyramidal neurons increases glutamate release from presynaptic elements and may thereby influence long-term potentiation (and, by extension, learning and memory). Although one would suspect that a transmitter that acts by diffusion could not phasically regulate other cells, neuronal stimulation elicits NO release and therefore suggests phasic signaling capacity.

There is no active mechanism to terminate the effects of NO. However, the half-life of NO is only about 30 seconds, and thus this spontaneous decay to nitrite limits the duration of action of NO. In addition, NO can react with iron-containing compounds, such as hemoglobin, which effectively terminate the actions of NO.

ENDOCANNABINOIDS AND RETROGRADE NEUROTRANSMISSION

Marijuana has been used as a recreational drug and a therapeutic agent for thousands of years and remains a popular but largely illicit drug in the United States. The name *marijuana* is derived from the Mexican word *maraguanquo*, meaning "intoxicating plant." The behavioral effects of marijuana vary widely across individuals, with some becoming giddy and euphoric, while others become sedated and depressed. Use of the drug may lead to distortion of sensory perceptions and time. Potential adverse effects following acute administration include impairment of short-term memory and impaired motor coordination and tracking during the performance of certain tasks such as driving. The psychoactive properties of marijuana suggest that there is a specific brain receptor for the drug. The cannabinoid receptor (CB_1) was cloned and it was demonstrated that this receptor and a related CB_2 receptor are G protein–coupled receptors, present in both the brain and other tissues. Both receptors are coupled to $G_{i/o}$ and inhibit adenylyl cyclase. Initially it was thought that the CB_1 receptor is neuronal and CB_2 receptors are localized to peripheral sites. It is now clear that although CB_1 is the major cannabinoid receptor in brain, it is also found in the periphery, and there are CB_2 sites in brain.

The identification of cannabinoid receptors in turn led to the search for endogenous cannabinoid molecules (endocannabinoids, ECs). Progress has been rapid, and there is now a reasonably good understanding of the endogenous cannabinoid transmitters.

Endocannabinoids represent the first lipid transmitters. Because they are lipids they easily diffuse across membranes, and thus cannot be stored in vesicles. Instead, they are synthesized and released when needed from membrane-localized lipid precursors. Two major ECs have been identified, N-arachidonoylethanolamide (anandamide) and 2-arachidonoylglycerol (2-AG). The EC synthetic pathways and the mechanisms through which ECs can be released on demand are fairly well characterized (Alger and Kim, 2011). The synthesis of 2-AG is fairly well characterized, and involves an increase in intracellular calcium stimulating phospholipase C to subsequently yield diacylglycerol, which is a substrate for a lipase that converts DAG to 2-AG. The synthesis of anandamide is more complex, with alternative pathways leading to its formation. The inactivation of ECs involves three proteins. 2-AG is primarily metabolized by monoacylglycerol lipase (MGL), while anandamide is metabolized by fatty acid hydrolase (FAAH). There is also an energy- and sodium-dependent anandamide transporter that inactivates anandamide.

Endocannabinoids appear to act primarily as retrograde messengers at synapses. Upon appropriate stimulation of neurons that result in intracellular changes (such as increase in intracellular calcium), ECs are "released" from membranes and interact with cannabinoid receptors on the presynaptic axon; the CB1 receptor is present on both excitatory (glutamatergic) and inhibitory (GABAergic) axons. The interaction of ECs with CB1 presynaptic receptors modulates subsequent release of the amino acid transmitter from the presynaptic axons. This EC retrograde signaling is intimately involved in specific forms of short- and long-term synaptic plasticity that subserve learning and memory (Chevaleyre et al., 2006).

In light of the psychoactive properties of cannabis, there is considerable interest in potential therapeutic actions of drugs that alter EC synthesis or inactivation. Because recreational marijuana use is often accompanied by "the munchies," there have been trials of CB_1 antagonists in obesity; potential side effects essentially halted this line of drug development. CB antagonists have also been suggested to be of value in reducing cigarette smoking.

It has been widely speculated that cannabinoid receptors or ECs may be dysregulated in certain psychiatric disorders, particularly schizophrenia. Several indirect lines of evidence are consistent with a possible role of endogenous cannabinoids in the pathophysiology of schizophrenia. Early marijuana use is associated with an increased risk for a schizophrenic psychosis. Chronic marijuana use has been associated with cognitive deficits that progressively worsen with continued drug use and resemble to some degree the cognitive deficits of schizophrenia, and elevated cerebrospinal fluid levels of anandamide have been reported in patients with schizophrenia. There is an increase in the density of CB_1 receptors in the dorsolateral prefrontal cortex of patients with schizophrenia. Although some of these findings await independent verification, studies in laboratory animals are consistent with THC-induced cognitive deficits and transmitter changes. In particular, chronic administration of THC causes a decrease in DA turnover and ACh release in the prefrontal cortex that persists upon discontinuation of the drug treatment; during this drug-free period, attention and short-term memory deficits are present.

Both ECs and NO are retrograde signaling transmitters; there are other examples of retrograde messengers discussed next. It is not, in retrospect, surprising that there is both anterograde and retrograde transmission. We have already discussed certain mechanisms that permit the presynaptic axon to regulate its synthesis and release of transmitters (autoreceptors, end-product inhibition of synthesis). Retrograde signaling of information to modulate presynaptic release adds still another component to the tightly regulated orchestra of controls that homeostatically regulate neurotransmission.

NEUROTROPHIC FACTORS

Another group of molecules that appears to have retrograde neurotransmitter functions is the neurotrophins or growth factors. This diverse group of proteins is critical for the survival and differentiation of neurons (Huang and Reichardt, 2001). There are many different classes of neurotrophic factors, and within each class several members can be identified (Table 2.2). Although there are differences in the effects of members of a

TABLE 2.2. Examples of neurotrophic factors in brain

Neurotrophins
Brain-derived neurotrophic factor (BDNF)
Nerve growth factor (NGF)
Neurotrophin-3 (NT-3)
Neurotrophin-4 (NT-4)
Glial-derived neurotrophic factor (GDNF) family[a]
GDNF
Neurturin
Persephin
Tumor growth factor-β (TGFβ) family
TGFβ1–3
Bone morphogenic proteins (BMPs)
Myostatin
Sonic hedgehog
Insulin family
Insulin
Insulin-like growth factor-I (IGF-I)
Insulin-like growth factor-II (IGF-II)
Fibroblast growth factor (FGF) family
FGF (acidic)
FGF (basic)
Epidermal growth factor (EGF) family
ACh-receptor-inducing activity (ARIA)
Amphiregulin
EGF
Heregulin
TGF[a]
Cytokines[b]
Ciliary neurotrophic factor (CIF), leukemia inhibitory factor (LIF), cardiotrophin, interleukin-6 (IL-6) (gp 130-linked receptor)
Granulocyte colony stimulating factor (G-CSF) (G-CSF receptor)
IL-2, IL-4, others (CD132 receptor)
IL-3, IL-5, others (CDw131 receptor)
Leptin (OB-receptor)

[a] This family of neurotrophic factors interacts with the Ret signaling pathway (see Chapter 4).
[b] Cytokines are categorized according to the receptor with which they interact; all couple ultimately to the JAK-STAT signaling pathway (see Chapter 4).

given class of growth factors, and differences in the receptors through which these growth factors exert their effects, there are broad similarities in the basic principles concerning synthesis, release, and termination of action of these growth factors (Huang and Reichardt, 2001).

Neurotrophic factors are unconventional in several ways, including their synthesis and release characteristics. In addition, the target neurons of the neurotrophic factors are often presynaptic to the cell in which the factor is found, consistent with neurotrophic factors providing trophic support for developing axons.

Current appreciation of the synthesis and regulation of neurotrophic factors has been gained primarily through molecular biology studies. Neurotrophic factors are often translated from multiple mRNAs. An example is brain-derived neurotrophic factor (BDNF), which contains five different exons that encode BDNF protein. Four of the five exons are controlled by separate promoters, the alternative use of which generates eight different BDNF mRNAs. Yet there appears to be only one mature BDNF protein! Because the different promotors are regulated through different means, an intricate cascade of events leads to mature BDNF production, with different transcripts varying in stability and yielding different amounts of protein.

Our knowledge of the posttranslational processing of neurotrophic factors is relatively poor compared to that of peptide transmitters. Perhaps the best-known situation is that of nerve growth factor (NGF), where the mature protein is cleaved from a prohormone, somewhat analogous to the situation seen in peptides. However, the NGF prohormone is quite different from neuropeptide prohormones: three subunits of the prohormone are present, one of which is catalytic and cleaves the prohormone to generate NGF. An interesting twist in the synthesis of neurotrophins is the necessity for dimerization of neurotrophins to form active species. It was originally thought that neurotrophins were exclusively present as homodimers *in vivo*, in contrast to *in vitro* studies that indicated heterodimer assembly. However, recent data suggest that heterodimers of BDNF and NGF can be formed in mammalian cells *in vivo*.

Neurotrophins and other proteins are secreted or released from neurons through two different pathways. The constitutive pathway for secretion is not driven by extracellular stimulation and is used to secrete membrane components, viral proteins, and extracellular matrix molecules; in other words, the constitutive pathway is not the pathway generally associated with neurotransmitters. Yet neurotrophic factors have typically been considered to be secreted by the constitutive pathway, in contrast to the release of more conventional classical and peptide transmitters (e.g., those shown in Table 2.1) through the regulated pathway. Prohormones have an N-terminal signal sequence, which targets the protein to the endoplasmic reticulum and then to the Golgi network, from where it is ultimately packaged into vesicles. Because many neurotrophic factors lack a signal sequence, the idea that growth factors are secreted by the constitutive pathway occurred by default. However, specific antibodies used for immunohistochemical studies have suggested that BDNF is present in chromogranin-containing secretory granules and thus can be secreted through the regulated pathway as well as the constitutive pathway.

The pathway through which neurotrophic factors are secreted is critical because of the question whether the release can be evoked by neuronal depolarization. It appears that under basal conditions BDNF and NGF are constitutively released from somatodendritic regions of the neuron, but that depolarization leads to regulated release, although it is unclear if this release is calcium-dependent.

Among the functions subserved by neurotrophic factors are those commonly ascribed to growth factors, including involvement in development, differentiation, and survival of neurons. However, there are other more "transmitter"-like functions. Neurotrophic factor expression and release from neurons, like transmitter expression and release, are regulated by afferent signals. For example, NGF and BDNF expression are increased by the excitatory transmitter glutamate and decreased by the inhibitory transmitter GABA. In addition, the regulation of BDNF by events such as seizures is regionally, spatially, and temporally distinct, with seizures leading to BDNF induction in different types of hippocampal neurons and with specific patterns of promotor activation.

Finally, a transmitter role for neurotrophic factors is suggested by their ability to regulate other neurons. Neurotrophic factors activate receptor proteins on target cells, which then initiate complex cascades of intracellular signaling pathways leading to their diverse biological effects. These effects include not only the more traditional growth factor responses but also the same types of changes that are seen in response to classical transmitters, such as regulation of ion channels (albeit on a different time scale). This underscores the notion that neurotrophic factors can serve as transmitters, just as more conventional transmitters (e.g., monoamines) can exert some trophic effects on target cells.

NEUROTRANSMITTERS AND THEIR EVOLVING ROLES

Our views of what constitutes a neurotransmitter are constantly changing. We have moved from being limited to classical transmitters such as acetylcholine to accepting peptides as transmitters, and have grown comfortable with gases and lipids, which are neither stored nor actively released. Having considered these changes in our views of neurotransmitters, it is not surprising to learn that interneuronal communication may be only one of multiple roles played by transmitters. For example, mRNAs that encode enzymes involved in transmitter synthesis, such as the ACh-synthesizing enzyme *choline acetyltransferase*, are found in lymphocytes. The ACh-inactivating enzyme *acetylcholinesterase* is also expressed in lymphocytes, as are certain acetylcholine receptors. The expression of these markers of transmitter systems is not restricted to lymphocytes but is seen across different tissues: choline acetyltransferase is even found in spermatazoa! When one considers that so many different aspects of acetylcholine synthesis and action are found in blood cells, it is reasonable to speculate that changes in these factors in peripheral cells may in some cases reflect central changes in these transmitters in neuropsychiatric disorders. This tantalizing notion has been repeatedly explored, but no simple peripheral biomarker of central neuropsychiatric disorders has yet emerged from these studies.

There is inevitably strong resistance to change in scientific thinking, as Kuhn so compelling argued. Just as inevitably, our conventional wisdom changes and gives rise to new dogma. The consideration of interneuronal messengers such as NO and the endocannabinoids as neurotransmitters is indicative that we have entered a new era with a growing degree of (new) dogmatism. However, our most cherished beliefs will be challenged soon by new data, which will cause us to revise (and ultimately overthrow) our current views. This should not be a cause for alarm, bur perhaps celebration. As we have advanced in our understanding of the nature of neurotransmitters, so have we discovered new potential targets for the treatment of psychiatric disorders. While our current pharmacological treatment approaches will soon seem appallingly crude and ineffective, this can only emerge through an appreciation of transmitters and their receptor partners, as well as other near and distant relatives such as transporters and transduction mechanisms.

DISCLOSURES

Dr. Deutch serves on an Advisory Board for Eli Lilly and Co. He receives grant support from the National Institutes of Health. He is the chair of the Clinical and Scientific Advisory Board of the National Parkinson Foundation and a member of the Scientific Council of the Brain & Behavior Research Foundation. To the best of his knowledge he has no conflicts of interest, financial or otherwise, with regard to the subject matter of the chapter.

Dr. Roth receives grant support from the National Institutes of Health. To the best of his knowledge he has no conflicts of interest, financial or otherwise, with regard to the subject matter of the chapter.

REFERENCES

Alger, B.E., and Kim, J. (2011). Supply and demand for endocannabinoids. *Trends Neurosci.* 34:304–315.

Bean, A.J., Zhang, X., et al. (1995). Peptide secretion: what do we know? *FASEB J.* 8:630–638.

Boutrel, B., Cannella, N., et al. (2010). The role of hypocretin in driving arousal and goal-oriented behaviors. *Brain Res.* 1314:103–111.

Chevaleyre, V., Takahashi, K.A., et al. (2006). Endocannabinoid-mediated synaptic plasticity in the CNS. *Ann. Rev. Neurosci.* 29:37–76.

de Lecea, L., Kilduff, T.S., et al. (1998). The hypocretins: hypothalamus-specific peptides with neuroexcitatory activity. *Proc. Natl. Acad. Sci. USA* 95:322–327.

Deutch, A.Y., and Bean, A.J. (1995). Colocalization in dopamine neurons. In: Bloom, F.E., and Kupfer, D.J., eds. Psychopharmacology: The Fourth Generation of Progress. New York: Raven Press, pp. 197–206.

Deutch, A.Y., and Roth, R.H. (2012). Neurotransmitters. In: Squire, L., Bloom, F.E., Berg, D., du Lac, S., Ghosh, A., and Spitzer, N. C., eds. Fundamental Neuroscience, 4th Edition. San Francisco: Academic Press, pp. 117–138.

El Mestikawy, S., Wallén-Mackenzie, A., et al. (2011). From glutamate co-release to vesicular synergy: vesicular glutamate transporters. *Nat. Rev. Neurosci.* 12:204–216.

Fatt, P., and Katz, B. (1952). Spontaneous subthreshold activity at motor nerve endings. *J. Physiol. (Lond.).* 117:109–128.

Halassa, M.M., and Haydon, P.G. (2010). Integrated brain circuits: astrocytic networks modulate neuronal activity and behavior. *Annu. Rev. Physiol.* 72:335–355.

Hassel, B., and Dingledine. R. (2012). Glutamate and GABA receptors. In: Brady, S.R., Siegel, G.J., Albers, R.W., and Price, D.L., eds. Basic Neurochemistry, 8th Edition. Amsterdam: Academic Press, pp. 342–366.

Huang, E.J., and Reichardt, L.F. (2001). Neurotrophins: roles in neuronal development and function. *Annu. Rev. Neurosci.* 24:677–736.

Hyman, S.E., and Nestler, E.J. (1993). The Molecular Foundations of Psychiatry. Washington, DC: American Psychiatric Press.

Iversen, L., Iversen, S., et al. (2008). Introduction to Neuropsychopharmacology. New York: Oxford University Press.

Kanner, B.I. (2006). Structure and function of sodium-coupled GABA and glutamate transporters. *J. Membr. Biol.* 213:89–100.

Kristensen, A.S., Andersen, J., et al. (2011). SLC6 neurotransmitter transporters: structure, function, and regulation. *Pharmacol. Rev.* 63:585–640.

Morelli, M., and Bentivoglio, M. (2005). The organization and circuits of mesencephalic dopaminergic neurons and the distribution of dopamine receptors in the brain. In: Dunnett, S.B., Bentivoglio, M., Bjorklund, A., and Hokfelt, T., eds. Dopamine: Handbook of Chemical Neuroanatomy, vol. 21. Amsterdam: Elsevier, pp. 1–107.

Mustafa, A.K., Gadalla, M.M., et al. (2009). Signaling by gasotransmitters. *Sci. Signal.* 2:re2.

Niswender, C.M., and Conn, P.J. (2010). Metabotropic glutamate receptors: physiology, pharmacology, and disease. *Annu. Rev. Pharmacol. Toxicol.* 50:295–322.

Olsen, R.W., and Li, G.D. (2012). GABA. In: Brady, S.R., Siegel, G.J., Albers, R.W., and Price, D.L., eds. Basic Neurochemistry, 8th Edition. Amsterdam: Academic Press, pp. 367–376.

Panatier A., Vallée, J., et al. (2011). Astrocytes are endogenous regulators of basal transmission at central synapses. *Cell* 146:785–798.

Pickel, V.M., Garzón, M., and et al. (2002). Electron microscopic immunolabeling of transporters and receptors identifies transmitter-specific functional sites envisioned in Cajal's neuron. *Prog. Brain Res.* 136:145–155.

Ramamoorthy, P., Wang, Q., et al. (2011). Cell type-dependent trafficking of neuropeptide Y-containing dense core granules in CNS neurons. *J. Neurosci.* 31:14783–14788.

Sakurai, T., Amemiya, A., et al. (1998). Orexins and orexin receptors: a family of hypothalamic neuropeptides and G protein–coupled receptors that regulate feeding behavior. *Cell* 92:573–585.

Segawa, M. (2011). Dopa-responsive dystonia. *Handb. Clin. Neurol.* 100:539–557.

Sotnikova, T.D., Beaulieu, J.M., et al. (2006). Molecular biology, pharmacology and functional role of the plasma membrane dopamine transporter. *CNS Neurol. Disord. Drug. Targets* 5:45–56.

Sotnikova, T.D., Caron, M.G., et al. (2009). Trace amine-associated receptors emerging therapeutic targets. *Mol. Pharmacol.* 76:229–235.

Thompson, B.J., Jessen, B., et al. (2011). Transgenic elimination of high-affinity antidepressant and cocaine sensitivity in the presynaptic serotonin transporter. *Proc. Natl. Acad. Sci. USA* 108:3785–3790.

Valenstein, E.S. (2005). The War of the Soups and the Sparks. New York: Columbia University Press.

Wickens, J.R., and Arbuthnott, G.W. (2005). Structural and functional interactions in the striatum at the receptor level. In: Dunnett, S.B., Bentivoglio, M., Bjorklund, A., and Hokfelt, T., eds. Handbook of Chemical Neuroanatomy: Vol. 21. *Dopamine.* Amsterdam: Elsevier, pp. 199–239.

Wolosker, H., Dumin, E., Balan, L., and Foltyn, V.N. (2008). D-amino acids in the brain: D-serine in neurotransmission and neurodegeneration. *FEBS J.* 275:3514–3526.

Wonodi, I., and Schwarcz, R. (2010). Cortical kynurenine pathway metabolism: a novel target for cognitive enhancement in schizophrenia. *Schizophr. Bull.* 36:211–218.

Zahniser N.R., and Doolen S. (2001). Chronic and acute regulation of Na+/Cl-dependent neurotransmitter transporters: drugs, substrates, presynaptic receptors, and signaling systems. *Pharmacol. Ther.* 92:21–55.

Zander, J.F., Münster-Wandowski, A., et al. (2010). Synaptic and vesicular coexistence of VGLUT and VGAT in selected excitatory and inhibitory synapses. *J. Neurosci.* 30:7634–7645.

3 | PRINCIPLES OF ELECTROPHYSIOLOGY

EVELYN K. LAMBE

Neurons communicate with each other through electrochemical signaling. Their electrical state is vital to their ability to respond to stimuli and to release neurotransmitters, the chemical signal that is the main form of communication between neurons. Although we have understood for a long time how neurons send signals, we are only beginning to understand how this signaling in different brain regions is affected by prior activity and by the presence of neuromodulators.

Electrophysiologists examine how neurons communicate with each other and how different conditions (genetic variability, stress, pharmacological manipulations) affect this signaling. *Electrophysiology* as a subject covers a broad range of techniques, but all give access to a higher level of resolution than most brain-imaging methods. To understand the meaning of electrophysiological data, it is critical to understand how neurons work and to know about the typical electrophysiological methods. This chapter begins with a review of neuronal physiology, discusses the typical tools electrophysiologists use, and then gives examples of how electrophysiological approaches are relevant to understanding the neurobiology and treatment of mental illness.

HOW NEURONS WORK

Neurons are encased in phospholipid membranes in which proteins are embedded. The proteins of greatest relevance to electrophysiology are *ion channels* and *receptors*. The latter group falls into two types that are discussed in detail later in this chapter: receptors that are ligand-gated ion channels and receptors that couple to G proteins. The membrane is impermeable to charged particles unless they travel passively through ion channels or are actively moved by another group of proteins called *ion pumps*. Together, ion pumps and ion channels lead to the creation of concentration and electrical gradients across the membrane. We now discuss mechanisms by which these gradients are created and how they serve the neuron's ability to communicate.

RESTING POTENTIAL

To understand the baseline or resting condition of a neuron, one must appreciate how ions are distributed. The solution surrounding neurons, called *extracellular fluid*, is essentially like seawater. There is a high level of sodium ions and a low level of potassium ions in this external solution. Neurons spend a lot of energy pumping sodium ions out of, and potassium ions into, their intracellular space. As depicted in Figure 3.1, neurons thus have low internal sodium ion and high internal potassium ion concentrations. In addition to these positively charged sodium and potassium ions, neurons also contain negatively charged ions, most of which are membrane-impermeable anions (abbreviated as A^- on figures) such as sulfate ions. At rest, the membrane is permeable to potassium ions because of "leak" potassium channels; by contrast, there is very low permeability to sodium ions.

The array of channels that are open at a given time determines the membrane potential. Since the sodium-potassium pump has raised the internal potassium ion concentration above that found in the extracellular solution, potassium ions flow down their concentration gradient, leaving the cell through the leak potassium channels. As illustrated in Figure 3.2, this potassium ion movement leads to a local buildup of positive charge on the outside of the cell membrane near the potassium channels, and a local buildup of negative charge on the inside of the membrane. This electrical gradient opposes the concentration gradient. Rather than flowing through their ion channel from a place of high concentration to one of low concentration, the intracellular potassium ions are attracted to the buildup of negatively charged ions on the inside of the membrane and repelled by the local buildup of positively charged ions on the outside. So, the net flow of potassium ions stops. This steady state is called the *equilibrium potential* for potassium ions, or the *reversal potential* if determined experimentally. Since neurons have many more leak channels for potassium than for other ions, the equilibrium potential for potassium contributes disproportionately to the neuronal *resting potential*. The word *potential* refers to the difference in charge. At rest, the neuron is hyperpolarized; the inside of the membrane is more negative than the outside of the membrane. While the leak potassium channels are integral to setting a hyperpolarized resting potential, the exact resting potential is a function of the permeability of that neuron to potassium, sodium, and chloride ions. A typical membrane potential for a cortical pyramidal neuron at rest is −75 mV.

It is important to remember that this resting state is a dynamic process. Ion channels that are open have ions flowing through all the time; at rest, there is only no net flow. Under most conditions, the flow of ions through ion channels has negligible effects (less than 0.01%) on the total concentrations of ions inside and outside the cell. The energy-driven pumps are the main players at setting the intracellular concentration of ions, and the volume of extracellular fluid can be presumed

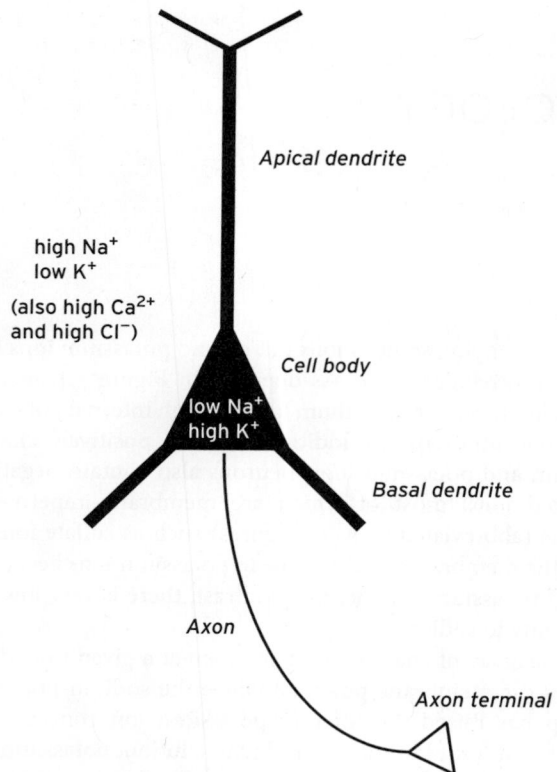

high Na⁺
low K⁺

(also high Ca²⁺
and high Cl⁻)

Apical dendrite

Cell body

low Na⁺
high K⁺

Basal dendrite

Axon

Axon terminal

Figure 3.1 *Schematic of a neuron showing concentration differences for various ions across the cellular membrane. The cytoplasm of the neuron is high in potassium ions (K⁺) and low in sodium ions (Na⁺), whereas the extracellular solution is high in sodium ions and low in potassium ions. Chloride (Cl⁻) and calcium (Ca²⁺) ions also occur at higher concentrations in the extracellular space compared to the intracellular space. Neurons receive inputs to their dendrites and send out information in the form of action potentials through their axons.*

to be infinite compared to that of the neuron. The ion channels lead to charge separations across the membrane, as illustrated in part C of Figure 3.2.

Calcium is another positively charged ion that is found at a higher concentration in the extracellular fluid than in the cytoplasm (mostly because the neuron spends energy sequestering calcium in intracellular storage compartments). At rest, the cell membrane has very low permeability to calcium ions. Calcium can enter the neuron through a variety of channels, some opened by neurotransmitters (these particular channels are usually also permeable to other cations such as sodium and potassium) and some opened by changes in membrane potential. Calcium ions are very important for many aspects of neuronal signaling and are discussed further in the next two sections.

HOW NEURONS COMMUNICATE: SPIKES

The negative resting potential, together with the concentration gradient of sodium across the cell membrane, allows the neuron the ability to communicate rapidly. At the resting potential, sodium ions don't have open ion channels to travel through because channels that are permeable to sodium are either ligand gated (e.g., by glutamate) or are voltage gated (i.e., the neuron has to become less negative before these channels

will open). Activation of glutamate receptors opens channels that allow sodium and calcium to flow along their concentration gradients into the cell, which makes the neuron less negative transiently—known as an *excitatory postsynaptic potential* or *EPSP*. If a given cell is sufficiently depolarized by the summation of several EPSPs arriving close together in time, the voltage-gated sodium channels will open. This level of depolarization is called *threshold* because once a few voltage-gated sodium channels open, sodium ions rush in down their concentration gradient, leading to more depolarization, which opens more voltage-gated sodium channels, and so on. Threshold is

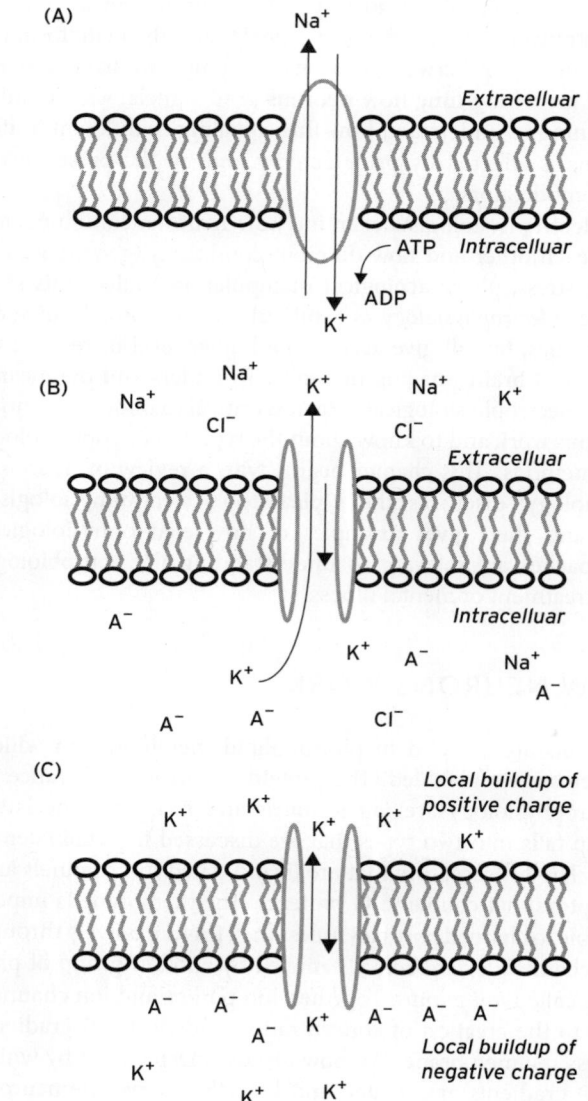

Figure 3.2 *Schematic of a portion of the phospholipid membrane. (A) Depiction of the sodium-potassium pump. This protein uses energy to create concentration gradients by pumping sodium ions (Na⁺) out of the neuron and potassium ions (K⁺) into the neuron. (B) The leak potassium channels are open at rest. Through these channels, potassium diffuses out of the neuron along its concentration gradient. This diffusion creates a local electrical gradient that opposes the concentration gradient. (C) A schematic of the separation of charge across the membrane created by diffusion through leak potassium channels. This separation of charge contributes to the resting potential, in which the inside of the cell membrane is more negative than the outside.*

thus the start of a positive-feedback "all-or-nothing process" that is called the *action potential*, as illustrated in Figure 3.3.

In an action potential, sodium rushes in through voltage-gated sodium channels, and this makes the membrane go from being negative relative to the local extracellular environment to being positive (remember: this is about local changes in electrical charge, not major changes in total intracellular or extracellular ion concentrations). As the cell membrane becomes more positive, however, two changes happen that tend to restore the neuron to its resting potential. First, voltage-gated potassium channels begin to open. The outward flow of potassium ions down their concentration gradient tends to bring the membrane potential to a more negative level. Second, voltage-gated sodium channels begin to inactivate. When they are inactivated, they are open but blocked. For this block to be relieved and the channels to close, the membrane potential must again become hyperpolarized. So with a hyperpolarizing force and the loss of the depolarizing force, the cell membrane becomes even more negative than the resting potential (calcium-activated potassium channels play an important role in this phenomenon called *afterhyperpolarization*, also shown in Fig. 3.3) and then returns to the resting potential as the voltage-gated potassium channels slowly close.

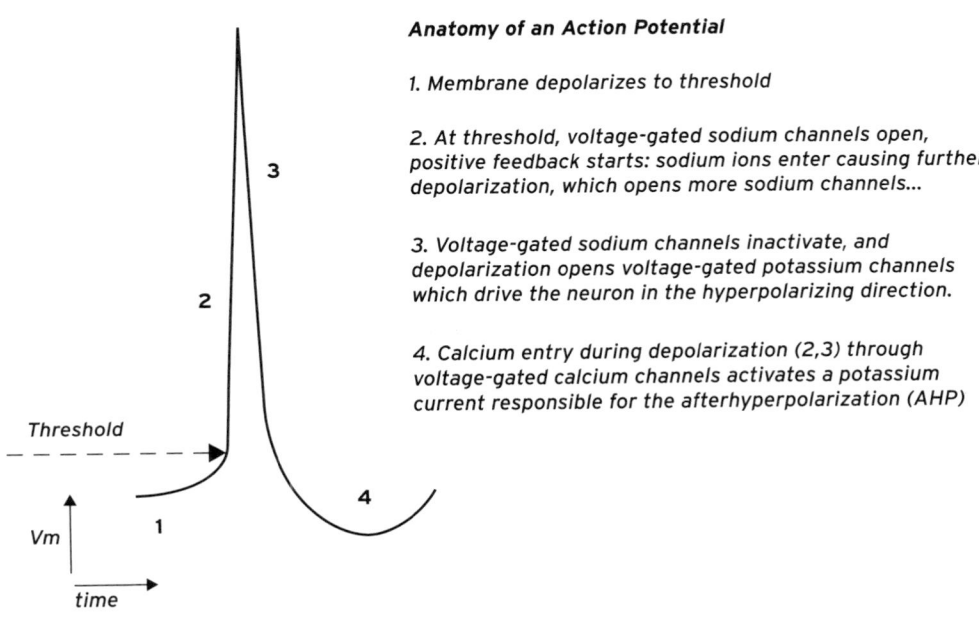

Anatomy of an Action Potential

1. Membrane depolarizes to threshold

2. At threshold, voltage-gated sodium channels open, positive feedback starts: sodium ions enter causing further depolarization, which opens more sodium channels...

3. Voltage-gated sodium channels inactivate, and depolarization opens voltage-gated potassium channels which drive the neuron in the hyperpolarizing direction.

4. Calcium entry during depolarization (2,3) through voltage-gated calcium channels activates a potassium current responsible for the afterhyperpolarization (AHP)

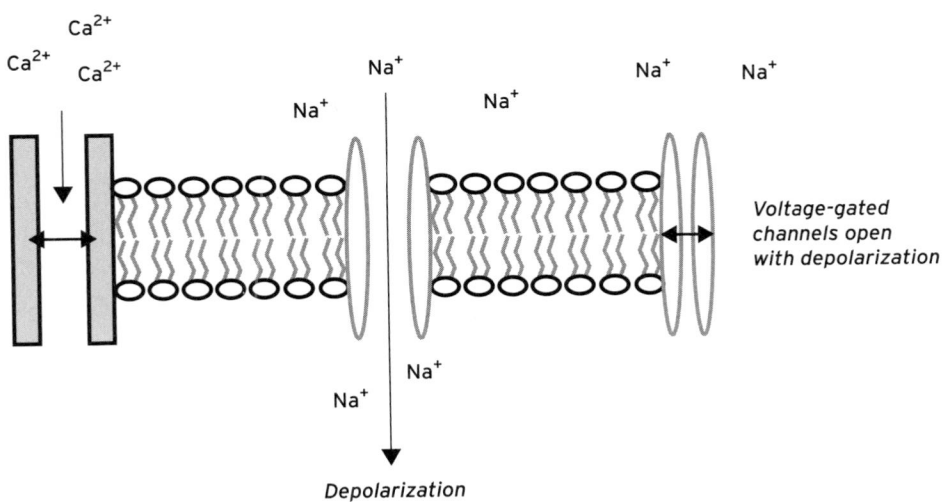

Voltage-gated channels open with depolarization

Figure 3.3 Action potentials are all-or-nothing events. When the membrane is depolarized to the threshold point, either by inputs from other neurons or through intrinsic mechanisms, voltage-gated sodium channels open, letting sodium ions (Na⁺) flow down their concentration gradient into the cell, further depolarizing the cell and opening more voltage-gated sodium channels. This depolarization also opens voltage-gated calcium channels and voltage-gated potassium channels. The latter are important for repolarizing the membrane potential. There is often an afterhyperpolarization, where the neuron overshoots its typical resting potential, as a result of additional potassium channel activation beyond the usual complement of leak potassium channels. Calcium ions (Ca²⁺), which entered while the neuron was depolarized, can contribute to the afterhyperpolarization by activating yet another set of potassium channels.

Voltage-gated sodium channel activation and inactivation explain much about how action potentials are generated and travel. Summation of several depolarizations or EPSPs arriving close together in time is usually required to trigger an action potential. A spike then depolarizes the entire neuron as the wave of depolarization opens more and more voltage-gated sodium channels. The axon, the output branch of the neuron, has evolved to enable particularly fast conduction. This thin branch is coated in myelin, which is similar in principle to the insulation that is used to increase the efficiency of electrical wires. Because the wave of depolarization is not substantially decreased between the gaps in myelin, it essentially "jumps" between the gaps or nodes (which have clusters of voltage-gated sodium channels). The action potential keeps traveling along neuronal structures toward their ends because sodium channel inactivation prevents sodium influx in a portion of the cell where the spike has already passed through. This phenomenon also limits how closely together spikes can be fired; this is known as the *refractory period*.

RELEASE OF NEUROTRANSMITTER

When the action potential reaches the end of the axon, it reaches a structure specialized for chemical transmission. Axon terminals have vesicles of neurotransmitter that are docked and ready to be released. Most axon terminals are the presynaptic structure of a synapse. Figure 3.4 shows a glutamatergic synapse. *Synapses* are an anatomical specialization for chemical neurotransmission, involving a presynaptic portion that releases the neurotransmitter and a postsynaptic portion that has a high density of relevant receptors and ion channels. The trigger for release of neurotransmitter is the influx of calcium through voltage-gated calcium channels in the axon terminal. Although there are such channels in many parts of the neuron, only in the axon terminal does calcium influx trigger neurotransmitter release. Once released, the neurotransmitter diffuses across the synapse to receptors on the postsynaptic cell. For example, if the transmitter is glutamate, it brings about an EPSP in the postsynaptic cell, as previously described.

EFFECT OF NEUROTRANSMITTERS ON POSTSYNAPTIC NEURONS: FAST, IONOTROPIC RECEPTORS

The major way neurons communicate with each other is through chemical transmission, by releasing neurotransmitters from their axon terminals onto the dendrites of target neurons where they bind to specialized receptors. It is important to appreciate how the resting potential of a given cell is affected by the neurons that communicate with it. When an excitatory neuron sends a signal down its axon to the postsynaptic neuron, it can excite the cell (make it less negative). When an inhibitory

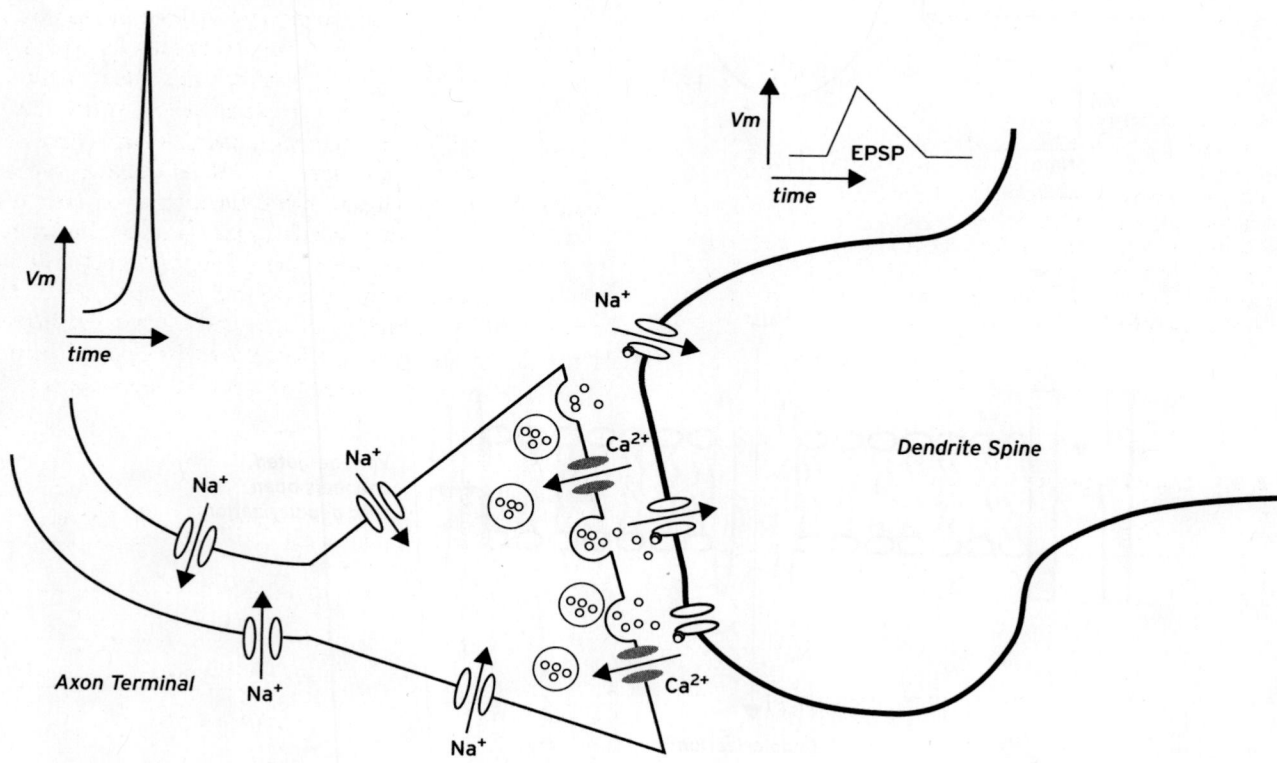

Figure 3.4 *When an action potential reaches the end of an axon, the flood of calcium ions (Ca^{2+}) into the terminal through voltage-gated calcium channels results in the fusion of vesicles with the cell membrane and the release of neurotransmitter. Molecules of neurotransmitter diffuse across the synaptic cleft and bind to receptors on the postsynaptic membrane. The binding of the neurotransmitter glutamate to AMPA receptors opens these ligand-gated ion channels to allow sodium (Na^+) and potassium (K^+) to pass through. This mixed cation current (mainly sodium ions diffusing into the neuron) is depolarizing and results in an excitatory postsynaptic potential (EPSP). If this EPSP depolarizes the postsynaptic neuron to threshold, perhaps through summation with another EPSP close together in time and space, it could cause an action potential in this postsynaptic neuron.*

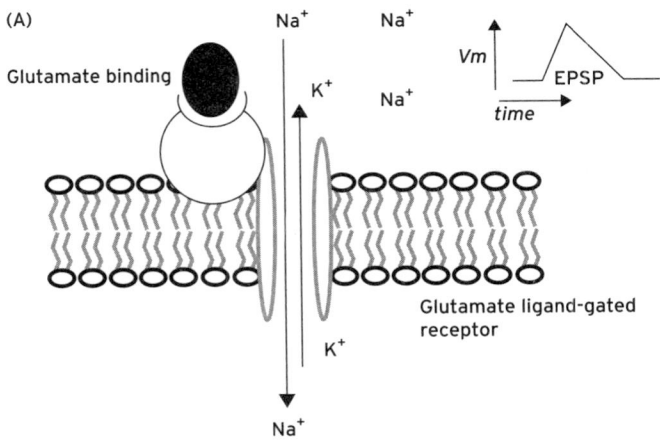

(A)

Glutamate binding

Glutamate ligand-gated receptor

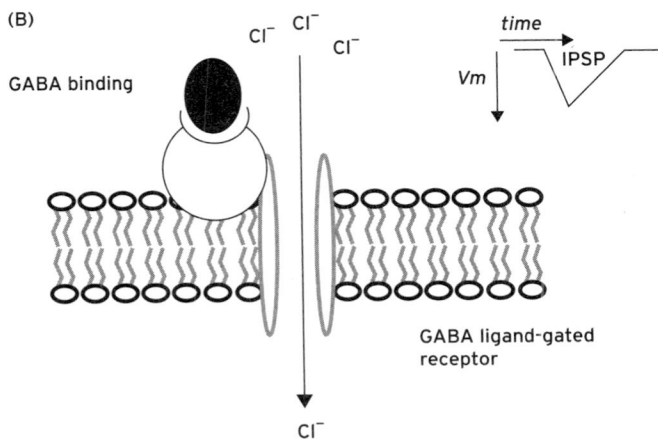

(B)

GABA binding

GABA ligand-gated receptor

Figure 3.5 Schematic of postsynaptic effects. (A) If glutamate is released and binds to postsynaptic α-amino-3-hydroxy-5-methyl-4-isoxasolepropionic (AMPA) receptors, it will open and allow a mixed cation current to depolarize the neuron, producing a subthreshold wave of depolarization called an excitatory postsynaptic potential (EPSP). (B) By contrast, if γ-aminobutyric acid (GABA) binds to a postsynaptic GABA$_A$ receptor, it will open to allow chloride ions (Cl$^-$) to flow down their concentration gradient into the cell. This current hyperpolarizes the neuron in a wave of negative potential called an inhibitory postsynaptic potential (IPSP).

cell sends a signal to this neuron, it can inhibit the cell (make it more negative). In both cases, this is accomplished by neurotransmitters binding to a receptor that is directly coupled to an ion channel (referred to as fast neurotransmission). The two major fast neurotransmitters are *glutamate* and *γ-aminobutyric acid* (GABA). Neurons are typically excited by glutamate binding and inhibited by GABA binding. As shown in Figure 3.5, activation of glutamate receptors creates an EPSP by opening channels that allow sodium and calcium ions to flow along their concentration gradients into the cell, which makes the neuron less negative transiently. By contrast, GABA binding opens a channel that allows negatively charged chloride ions to flow along their concentration gradient into the neuron, which makes it more negative transiently—known as an *inhibitory postsynaptic potential* (IPSP). Waves of potential spread passively along dendrites. If many inputs to a neuron are active within a narrow time window, these waves summate (or cancel in the case of concurrent excitatory and inhibitory potentials). In the special case when several excitatory neurons release glutamate onto a neuron nearly simultaneously, the EPSPs or waves of positive potential can raise the membrane potential to the level that can open voltage-gated sodium channels and trigger an action potential.

The ligand-gated channels represent the most direct form of coupling between a receptor and effector where both components are part of the same protein complex. This group of channels is described further in Table 3.1. Binding of the agonist results in a conformational change of the channel protein complex, resulting in a rapid and marked increase in the permeability of the channel to the ion or ions for which it is selective. For example, when glutamate binds to an α-amino-3-hydroxy-5-methyl-4-isoxasolepropionic acid (AMPA) receptor as shown in Figure 3.5, it opens a channel that is permeable to sodium and potassium ions (as well as calcium ions to a limited degree). Some ligand-gated channels also have a component of voltage gating. For example, glutamate is an agonist for the *N*-methyl-D-aspartate (NMDA) receptor as well; however, glutamate binding alone will not open the NMDA channel at hyperpolarized voltages. When the membrane is hyperpolarized, a magnesium ion blocks the channel from the extracellular side. The membrane must be depolarized to free

TABLE 3.1. Ligand-gated ion channels

NEUROTRANSMITTER	RECEPTOR SUBTYPE	ION CHANNEL PERMEABILITY	PHYSIOLOGICAL RESPONSE
Acetylcholine	Nicotinic	Na$^+$, K$^+$, Ca^{2+}	Fast excitation
Glutamate	AMPA	Na+, K$^+$ (Ca^{2+})	Fast excitation
	Kainite	Na+, K$^+$ (Ca^{2+})	Fast excitation
	NMDA	Na$^+$, K$^+$, Ca^{2+}	Slow excitation
Glycine	GlyRα/β	Cl$^-$	Fast inhibition
GABA	GABA$_A$	Cl$^-$	Fast inhibition
Serotonin	5-HT$_3$	Na$^+$, K$^+$, Ca^{2+}	Fast excitation

AMPA: α-amino-3-hydroxy-5-methyl-4-isoxasoleproptonic acid; GABA: γ-aminobutyric acid; NMDA: *N*-methyl-D-aspartate.

the magnesium ion and allow sodium, potassium, and calcium ions to pass through the NMDA channel into the neuron. In essence, this means that presynaptic axons must release sufficient glutamate onto the neuron not only to bind to NMDA receptors but also to depolarize that region of the cell (through activation of AMPA receptors and influx of sodium). So the NMDA receptor is thought to act as a coincidence detector, and its permeability to calcium ions allows for long-term changes in the cell through mobilization of second messenger systems.

EFFECT OF NEUROTRANSMITTERS ON POSTSYNAPTIC NEURONS: G PROTEIN-COUPLED RECEPTORS

In addition to glutamate and GABA, there are many other transmitters. So far, we have only discussed ligand-gated channels also known as *ionotropic receptors* (those where the receptor directly opens an ion channel). However, there are also *metabotropic receptors*. The latter can affect cellular processes quickly or over a longer time period through activation of second messenger systems. Glutamate, GABA, serotonin, and acetylcholine have both ionotropic and metabotropic receptors. Other neurotransmitters, such as dopamine and norepinephrine, appear to have only metabotropic receptors. In fact, most neurotransmitter receptors found in the brain are not an intrinsic component of ion channels but are coupled to ion channels through *G proteins* whose functional properties are intimately related to their ability to bind guanosine-5′ triphosphate (GTP). These metabotropic receptors can up- or downregulate the excitability of neurons in the short term and over a longer time period. Many examples of metabotropic G protein–coupled receptors in the brain and their functional effects are described Table 3.2.

G proteins are heterotrimers of α, β, and γ subunits, with the α subunit determining which of several major classes the G protein belongs and allowing us to predict its direct and indirect effects on ion channels. The direct effects involve interactions of the G protein subunits with ion channels. For example, the $\beta\gamma$ subunits of activated $G\alpha_i$ proteins dissociate and activate the inwardly rectifying potassium channels (Kir3 or GIRKs), ion channels that inhibit or hyperpolarize neurons. The indirect effects of G protein–coupled receptors, by contrast, affect ion channels through involving the modulation of second messenger cascades. The specific type of second messenger depends on the type of G protein α subunit. In this regard, the three major types of G proteins are $G\alpha_s$ (which stimulates the production of the second messenger, cyclic adenosine monophosphate [cAMP]), $G\alpha_i/G\alpha_o$ (which inhibit the production of the second messenger cAMP), and $G\alpha_q$ (which stimulates the second messenger phosphoinositol pathway). Table 3.2 identifies the second messenger cascades modulated by many G protein–coupled receptors in the brain. Such cascades can additionally have long-term effects on neuronal physiology through covalent modification of ion channels, as well as through changes in gene expression of receptors and channels. Through these indirect mechanisms, G proteins can modulate the fast, ionotropic transmission described in Table 3.1 and the previous section.

THE BASIC TOOLS OF THE ELECTROPHYSIOLOGIST

Electrophysiology is the study of the electrical properties of neurons, and the investigation of how these properties change under different conditions. Such recordings can be performed *in vivo*, in brain slice, or in isolated cells (either from dissociated brain slices or primary culture of neurons or another cell type). Each of these types of recordings has benefits and limitations in terms of the types of questions that can be addressed.

In vivo electrophysiologists record neuronal activity in certain regions of the brain to answer the question of how small groups of neurons respond during the performance of a task or when another brain area is stimulated. Data about individual neurons are extracted mathematically from the recordings of electrical activity at the place where the electrode was positioned. These experiments are extremely difficult logistically and are limited in terms of controlling different variables.

Questions about local circuitry can be better explored with slice physiology. This technique relies on the fact that it is possible under special conditions to keep a slice of brain alive and healthy for many hours. The investigator records from individual neurons and can examine how this neuron's electrical activity is affected by different conditions. Yet here too, there can be logistical difficulties accounting for so many variables.

Some investigators want to understand how one type of ion channel behaves under different conditions. To answer this sort of question, there are electrophysiologists who record from a small section of membrane from either a neuron or a cell from a line that has been molecularly altered such that it contains one channel or receptor of interest.

The brain is so complicated that any one level of electrophysiology will not answer all our questions. But the interplay of answers from labs using different techniques gives us unparalleled information about how neurons communicate with each other.

IN VIVO RECORDING

The spiking activity of individual neurons can be studied *in vivo* with extracellular recording via a microelectrode in the brain. This form of recording is referred to as *extracellular* because the electrode picks up signals from outside a cell. Recording in awake animals, termed *chronic unit recording*, allows for correlations between neuronal activity and behavioral state. If the animal is doing a task, patterns of neuronal activity correlated with correct performance can be contrasted with activity correlated with making a mistake. Patterns of activity can be correlated with broader behavioral states such as the different stages of sleep. Chronic unit recording is also performed sometimes in people with intractable epilepsy to better localize seizure foci before surgery. Extracellular recording is generally used to measure changes in firing activity. Some investigators will apply small quantities of a drug that affects a certain type of receptor, to see how either stimulating or blocking this receptor will change the firing pattern of a neuron or group of neurons. This is known as *microiontophoresis*.

TABLE 3.2. G Protein–coupled receptors

NEUROTRANSMITTER	RECEPTOR SUBTYPE	G PROTEIN	SECOND MESSENGER	ION CHANNEL	PHYSIOLOGICAL RESPONSE
Acetylcholine	M_1, M_5	G_q/G_{11}	⇑ IP_3 & DAG	⇓ K^+ currents	excitation
	M_2, M_3, M_4	G_i/G_o	⇓ cAMP	⇑ Kir3[a], ⇓ Ca^{2+}	inhibition
Cholecystokinin	CCK_1, CCK_2	G_q/G_{11}	⇑ IP_3 & DAG		excitation
Dopamine	D_1, D_5	G_s/G_{olf}	⇑ cAMP		variable
	D_2, D_3, D_4	G_i/G_o	⇓ cAMP	⇑ Kir3, ⇓ Ca^{2+}	inhibition
GABA	$GABA_B$	G_i/G_o	⇓ cAMP	⇑ Kir3, ⇓ Ca^{2+}	inhibition
Glutamate	mGlu group 1	G_q/G_{11}	⇑ IP_3 & DAG	⇓ K^+ currents	excitation
	mGlu groups 2 & 3	G_i/G_o	⇓ cAMP	⇑ Kir3, ⇓ Ca^{2+}	inhibition
Hypocretin/Orexin	Hcrt1, Hcrt2	G_q/G_{11}	⇑ IP_3 & DAG	⇓ K^+ currents, ⇑ cationic	excitation
Neuropeptide Y	Y_1, Y_2, Y_4, Y_5	G_i/G_o	⇓ cAMP	⇑ Kir3, ⇓ Ca^{2+}	inhibition
Norepinephrine	α_1	G_q/G_{11}	⇑ IP_3 & DAG	⇓ K^+ currents	excitation
	α_2	G_i/G_o	⇓ cAMP	⇑ Kir3, ⇓ Ca^{2+}	inhibition
	β_1, β_2	G_s	⇑ cAMP		variable
Opiate	μ, δ, κ	G_i/G_o	⇓ cAMP	⇑ Kir3, ⇓ Ca^{2+}	inhibition
Serotonin (5-HT)	$5\text{-}HT_1$ family	G_i/G_o	⇓ cAMP	⇑ Kir3, ⇓ Ca^{2+}	inhibition
	$5\text{-}HT_2$ family	G_q/G_{11}	⇑ IP_3 & DAG	⇑ K^+ currents	excitation
	$5\text{-}HT_{5A}$	G_i		⇑ Kir3	inhibition
	$5\text{-}HT_{4,6,7}$	G_s	⇑ cAMP		variable
Somatostatin	SST_{1-5}	G_i/G_o	⇓ cAMP	⇑ Kir3, ⇓ Ca^{2+}	inhibition
Tachykinins	NK_{1-3}	G_q/G_{11}	⇑ IP_3 & DAG	⇓ K^+ currents, ⇑ cationic	excitation
VIP	VIP_1, VIP_2	G_s	⇑ cAMP	⇑ cationic	excitation

[a] Kir3 is also known as GIRK (G protein–activated inwardly rectifying potassium current).
cAMP: cyclic adenosine monophosphate; DAG: diacylglycerol; GABA: γ-aminobutyric acid; 5HT: 5-hydroxytryptamine; IP_3: inositol triphosphate; VIP: vasoactive intestinal peptide.

Neurons can be further studied *in vivo* with multiphoton imaging. The longer wavelengths of light used for this imaging can penetrate deeply into thick, scattering brain tissue. As a result, multiphoton microscopy can be used to visualize fluorescent molecules hundreds of microns deep in the cortex. Usually the fluorescent dyes or calcium indicators have been infused with a pipette or were genetically expressed. Transgenic animals expressing green fluorescent protein (GFP) in a Golgi-like pattern in a population of neurons can be used to assess developmental or environmental changes in dendritic branches and spines.

SLICE RECORDING

Recording from individual neurons in brain slice is used to measure changes in membrane potential affected by the behavior of different ion channels. The slice is kept alive in a chamber under conditions that mimic those in vivo as closely as possible. The state of the art is to use an infrared camera that allows the visualization of the neurons in the slice so the experimenter can select a healthy neuron and guide the pipette up to the selected neuron under carefully controlled conditions, as illustrated in Figure 3.6. When the pipette is brought into contact with the neuron, a small amount of suction is applied. This induces the formation of a strong seal between the glass of the pipette and the cell membrane. At this point, further suction is applied and the small patch of membrane is opened. The pipette then has complete physical and electrical access to the neuron; this is known as *whole-cell patch recording*.

Slice physiologists can then look at changes in membrane potential or firing in response to certain treatments, such as application of a drug in the bath or more locally through

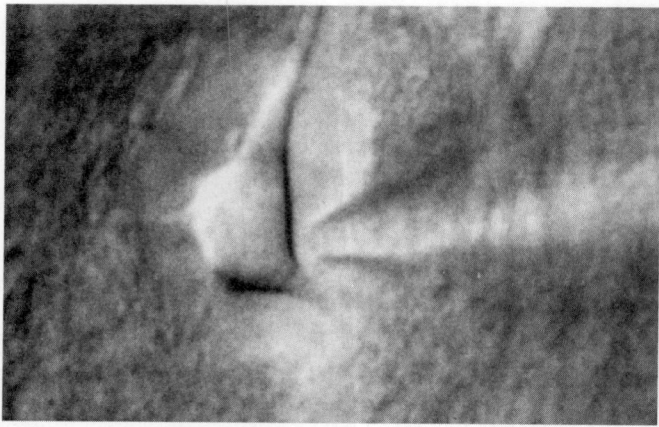

Figure 3.6 *Visualization of a pyramidal neuron in a slice of cerebral cortex using infrared-differential interference contrast optics. The pipette, shown to the right, will be brought into contact with the neuron. After formation of a gigaohm seal, a small amount of suction will be applied to allow recording in the whole-cell configuration.*

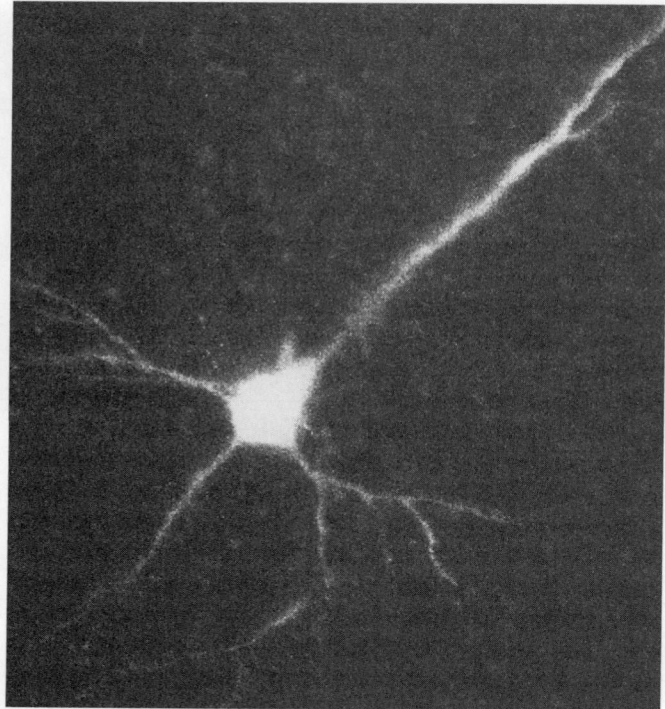

Figure 3.7 *A cortical pyramidal neuron previously filled with a fluorescent indicator through whole cell patch clamp. The membrane reseals after the patch pipette is pulled away.*

another pipette. When reading about slice physiology experiments, it is interesting to note whether the recordings were made in current clamp or voltage clamp. In the former, either depolarizing or hyperpolarizing current is injected and the effect on the membrane potential is assessed. This is similar to mimicking the effects of synaptic input. In voltage clamp, by contrast, the experimenter controls the membrane potential and measures the amount of current needed to maintain this "holding" potential. This is particularly useful for assessing the effects of some treatment on different voltage-gated ion channels because membrane potential is the key variable for this type of channel gating. Synaptic potentials are best measured in voltage clamp (they are measured as opposing currents needed to hold the membrane at the set potential) because they are relatively small and brief events that would be obscured by capacitive transients.

The complete physical access permitted in whole-cell recording allows the neuron to be filled with a fluorescent dye so that it can be visualized as shown in Figure 3.7. There are indicators available that change their level of fluorescence depending on the concentration of calcium. These calcium indicators allow us to "watch" the effects of calcium channels being opened by an action potential as it back-propagates through the dendritic arbor. The wave of depolarization opens voltage-gated calcium channels, increasing the concentration of calcium in spines and dendrites as shown in Figure 3.8.

BEYOND SLICE

There are many reasons why experimenters would like to reduce the complexity of the preparation they record in. For example, they might want to minimize inputs to the neuron they record from, to record from a small piece of membrane, or to record from a cell that has been genetically altered. Various possibilities for simplifying the system exist. These include mechanically dissociating a slice, creating a primary culture of the slice (though it is not possible to have neurons replicate themselves the way

other cell types will under cell culture conditions, it is feasible to create conditions where neurons from a brain slice will live for weeks rather than the hours they usually survive under typical slice conditions), or working with "neuronal-like" cell lines (cells originally from a tumor that will replicate themselves). The last are frequently transformed genetically so that they express certain receptors or ion channels that an electrophysiologist wishes to further characterize. For example, transfecting a cell line with different subunits of a particular channel in varying proportions permits one to investigate the kinetic properties of channels with different combinations of subunits. One way one could approach this question would be with single channel recording. Generally, one patches onto a cell, much the same way one would patch onto a neuron in slice. Then the electrode is pulled away. Depending on the technique, this can enable one to record from a small piece of membrane in several possible configurations. The single-channel approach allows the detailed examination of the kinetics of channel gating by different modulators and, in combination with genetically altered amino acids in channel subunits, the ability to understand which amino acids are critical for ion permeability through the pore or which endow vulnerability to various ion channel toxins.

ION CHANNELS AND MENTAL ILLNESS

Mental illness is a compelling example of a subtle dysfunction of neuronal communication that has dramatic consequences for how a person perceives and responds to the world. Our understanding of what triggers and perpetuates these illnesses is still in its infancy. We are only beginning to understand the genetic causes of specific mental illness and how these affect ion channels and brain physiology. Much of the brain functions normally, but certain processes unique to each mental illness go awry. Human imaging studies that assess brain activity levels suggest that the balance between excitation and inhibition in particular regions of the brain is abnormal in these disorders. For example, people with major depression have abnormally elevated activity in a specific brain region of the prefrontal cortex, the subcallosal cingulate gyrus, as well as in the amygdala (Hamani et al., 2011; Drevets et al., 2008). Interestingly, there is unexpectedly high comorbidity between major depression and seizure disorders (Kanner et al., 2008), which is consistent with altered excitation and inhibition in the brain in psychiatric disorders.

Recent studies have linked mental illnesses with genetic variability in the function of specific ion channels. For example, a single nucleotide polymorphism in the coding region of a nicotinic receptor subunit, CHRNA5, results in reduced function of the channel (Bierut et al., 2008; Kuryatov et al., 2011) and is strongly associated with increased vulnerability to nicotine addiction (Bierut et al., 2010). Rodent studies suggest that the reduction of the nicotinic receptor nonselective cation current resulting from this polymorphism will have behavioral consequences including a loss of sensitivity to the adverse effects of the drug nicotine (Tuesta et al., 2011) and a decrease in attentional performance (Bailey et al., 2010. Interestingly, this variation in the CHRNA5 gene has been found in half of people with schizophrenia (Hong et al., 2011), a group of people with a high prevalence of nicotine addiction (Myles et al., 2012) and deficits in attention (Hahn et al., 2012).

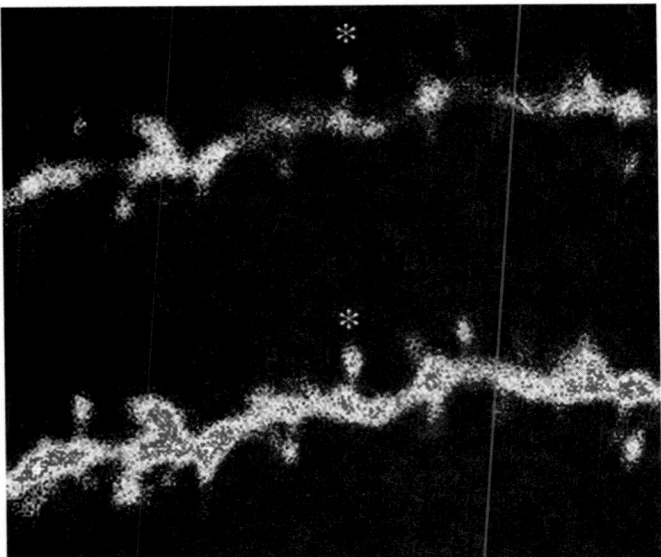

Figure 3.8 Multiphoton images of spines on a dendritic branch. The fluophore is Oregon Green BAPTA-1, a calcium indicator that becomes more intensely fluorescent when the level of calcium in the neuron increases. The upper image is this portion of the branch under baseline conditions of slice physiology. The lower image shows when the neuron is induced to fire repeated action potentials with injection of positive current. Action potentials open voltage-gated calcium channels along the dendrites and in the spines. One spine is marked by an asterisk to facilitate comparisons between low and high conditions of calcium influx. The influx of calcium raises the intensity of the indicator.

Genetic variants can affect the *expression levels* of the protein encoded by the gene. For example, polymorphisms in noncoding regions of the gene *NRG1* are associated with schizophrenia (Harrison and Law, 2006) and act in a gene-dose dependent manner to increase levels of the protein neuregulin 1 (Law et al., 2006), which interferes with the upregulation of NMDA glutamate receptor signaling (Pitcher et al., 2011). In essence, the genetic difference acts to reduce NMDA receptor mediated nonselective cation currents. Eliciting NMDA hypofunction pharmacologically, by comparison, is well known to provoke psychosis in otherwise healthy adults (see section on Psychotomimetics).

Genetic variation in a voltage-gated calcium channel gene, *CACNA1C*, has recently been found to be overrepresented in patients with several different mental illnesses, including patients with schizophrenia, bipolar disorder, and major depression (Bhat et al., 2012). It appears that at least one of the risk-associated single nucleotide polymorphisms increases the expression (Bigos et al., 2010) of this CaV1.2 channel that mediates an L-type or "long-lasting" calcium current. These channels open when the neuron is depolarized during a train of action potentials and allow calcium ions to rush down their concentration gradient into the neuron. This elevation in intracellular calcium ions is critical for changes in intracellular pathway activity, gene transcription, and synaptic plasticity (Bhat et al., 2012). Several studies have linked the polymorphisms in this particular calcium channel to widespread changes in the activation of brain networks necessary for executive function (Bhat et al., 2012).

ELECTROPHYSIOLOGY OF PSYCHOTROPIC DRUG ACTION

In the treatment of psychiatric illnesses such as depression and schizophrenia, certain drugs have been shown to be able to ameliorate some of the symptoms, although often with serious side effects. Most medicines for psychiatric illness have been found serendipitously and not by design. Despite understanding certain properties of these drugs (e.g., their acute ability to block a certain type of receptor), we do not fully appreciate how these properties change activity of brain systems over time in terms of bringing about improved function and in terms of causing side effects. In this section, several classes of psychoactive drugs are explored from the perspective of basic electrophysiology. In each case, a brief example is given of how we have come to better understand the initial or chronic action of such drugs using electrophysiological techniques. Because it is not feasible to study the neurophysiology of mental illness directly, where relevant, we also briefly describe possible animal models that may be helpful in the study of neuronal physiology relevant to mental illness.

ANXIOLYTICS

Several drugs to relieve anxiety—such as benzodiazepines, barbiturates, and even alcohol—work by enhancing inhibitory neurotransmission through the GABA system. They are the rare psychoactive drugs in which the acute action is also the therapeutic one; their therapeutic effects are directly correlated to the current blood level of the drug in the person taking it. Anxiolytics work by potentiating the $GABA_A$ receptor. As described in a previous section, the $GABA_A$ receptor is an ionotropic receptor that opens a chloride channel, tending to make the neuron less excitable, partly through hyperpolarization, and therefore less likely to be brought to spike threshold by an excitatory stimulus.

Benzodiazepines bind to a site on the $GABA_A$ receptor that increases the probability that GABA binding will open the chloride channel. They increase the chance that chloride can flow down its concentration gradient and hyperpolarize the neuron. In short, benzodiazepines potentiate the effect of synaptically released GABA. Barbiturates take this action one step further by increasing the duration of individual channel openings. Because GABA is the major inhibitory neurotransmitter in the brain, the anticonvulsant and sleep-inducing properties of these drugs are not surprising. Side effects such as withdrawal insomnia and withdrawal convulsions can be serious. Currently, dose level and metabolic clearance of the drug are the variables that are manipulated to try to maximize the therapeutic effect while minimizing side effects.

It is not well understood which regions of the brain are particularly involved in the antianxiety action of these drugs. Yet it appears that $GABA_A$ receptors are actually a heterogeneous population made up of different combinations of subunits. Certain combinations appear to be limited to regions of the brain, such as the amygdala and the limbic circuit, that are particularly involved in generating anxiety disorders. This may allow for the modification of the drugs to create compounds affecting the GABA system that are able to discriminate between anxiolytic, anticonvulsant, and sleep-inducing effects.

Another approach to anxiety disorders is through manipulating neuromodulatory systems such as serotonin or norepinephrine. One reason to focus on these systems is not necessarily because they are thought to be involved in the etiology of the illness, but because they are more limited in their actions. They modulate glutamate and GABA transmission, which means through neuromodulators one can manipulate glutamate and GABA transmission indirectly. Such indirect manipulation has less potential for extreme side effects (precipitating seizures or unconsciousness) than drugs that affect the glutamate or GABA systems directly.

PSYCHOTOMIMETICS

Psychotomimetics or hallucinogens are not used to treat mental illness; in fact, they can exacerbate schizophrenia and other types of psychosis. However, they give us an interesting window into the neurobiology of hallucinations and sensory perturbations. The effects of hallucinogens on an array of complex integrative processes such as cognition, perception, and mood suggest the involvement of the cerebral cortex. There are two major classes of psychotomimetics: psychedelics and NMDA antagonists. Both have been considered relevant animal models of psychosis.

The psychotomimetic effect of psychedelic hallucinogens depends on their stimulation of serotonin 5-HT_{2A} receptors. Slice physiology experiments in cerebral cortex have shown that selective stimulation of 5-HT_{2A} receptors decreases the threshold for recurrent network activity and enhances its duration far beyond that normally seen (Lambe and Aghajanian, 2007; Benekareddy et al., 2010). This effect of selective 5-HT_{2A} stimulation in cortex might be responsible for the sensory perturbations that people experience after taking psychedelic hallucinogens. Network activity has been suggested to provide a "context" in which information is interpreted and decisions are made. It has been hypothesized that aberrations in the modulation of network activity may account for the perceptual and cognitive abnormalities in schizophrenia. Normal modulation of network activity may work to enhance cortical efficiency by changing the signal-to-noise ratio.

The results of brain imaging studies by Vollenweider and colleagues tend to support this hypothesis (Vollenweider and Geyer, 2001; Vollenweider et al., 1997). They show that psilocybin, another 5-HT_{2A} receptor agonist, tends to activate the frontal cortex, and this activation correlates with the onset of sensory perturbations. Serotonin, the endogenous agonist of this receptor, does not cause this phenomenon. Most likely, this is due to its opposing actions through other receptors, such as the 5-HT_{1A} receptor. Whereas the 5-HT_{2A} receptor tends to inactivate potassium conductances and make neurons more excitable, 5-HT_{1A} receptor tends to activate potassium currents and make neurons less excitable. These opposing actions appear to have ramifications for psychoactive drugs such as the selective serotonin reuptake inhibitors (SSRIs) that tend to increase serotonin at synapses in the brain.

NMDA antagonists such as phencyclidine (PCP) and ketamine are dissociative anesthetics. In short, at high concentrations they are anesthetic and at lower concentrations they produce psychosis in adults (these psychiatric side effects do not occur in children, and ketamine is routinely used in pediatric anesthesia). Phencyclidine intoxication causes effects in otherwise healthy people that mimic positive and negative symptoms of schizophrenia, and it exacerbates psychotic symptoms in people with schizophrenia. Phencyclidine and ketamine are known to act as noncompetitive antagonists of the NMDA receptor, a subtype of glutamate receptor discussed previously. These antagonists bind to the open pore NMDA receptors and block the flow of cations through the channels. However, they do not block the AMPA subtype of glutamate receptors. It appears that blocking glutamate transmission through NMDA receptors increases glutamate release and excessively stimulates AMPA receptors in certain regions of the brain, including the prefrontal cortex. Although this increased stimulation of glutamate receptors in prefrontal cortex appears to differ from that induced by psychedelic hallucinogens, suppressing excessive glutamate release ameliorates many of the adverse behavioral effects in both cases.

ANTIDEPRESSANTS

The most commonly prescribed antidepressants, the SSRIs, increase serotonin in the brain by blocking the mechanism that actively removes serotonin from synapse. Over a period of chronic administration, this tends to desensitize the autoreceptors on serotonergic neurons, such that the feedback mechanism that normally limits the release of serotonin requires much higher levels of serotonin to be activated. It has been suggested that one possible explanation why some people may be vulnerable to developing depression is that their 5-HT_{1A} autoreceptors might be hypersensitive, which would tend to clamp down on the release of serotonin into the cortex. The time lag required for desensitization of the autoreceptors might explain why a therapeutic improvement is not observed until 2–3 weeks after onset of drug treatment. Single-cell recordings suggest that repeated daily administration of antidepressants enhances the effects of 5-HT in the forebrain with a time course that parallels the therapeutic effects of antidepressants (Mongeau et al., 1997).

Low doses of NMDA antagonists have rapid antidepressant effects (Berman et al., 2000). Recent electrophysiological work suggests the cellular mechanism involves a rapid upregulation of dendritic spines in prefrontal cortex (Li et al., 2010). This morphological change is opposite of the changes elicited by chronic stress and is compromised in transgenic mice with the human coding polymorphism (Val66Met) that results in a reduction of depolarization-induced BDNF release (Liu et al., 2012).

Stress can be used to produce animal models of depression. Preclinical and clinical studies have demonstrated that stress and depression result in cell atrophy and loss in limbic and cortical brain regions (Duman and Monteggia, 2006). These effects can be reversed with such diverse antidepressant treatments as SSRIs, electroconvulsive shock, and exercise. Interestingly, a number of gene products that mediate neurotrophin and growth factor signaling are reduced in depressed patients and in stressed animals. Antidepressant treatments, by contrast, elevate the expression of multiple genes involved in neurotrophin signaling pathways. Together, these findings implicate neurotrophic factors in the etiology and treatment of depression. Some electrophysiology studies of the neurotrophic hypothesis of depression have examined the properties of new neurons generated in the dentate through adult neurogenesis (van Praag et al., 2002) and their contributions to synaptic plasticity in the hippocampus (Ge et al., 2007). Other electrophysiology studies have used transgenic mice with alterations of neurotrophic factors or receptors to assess the effects of long-term changes in these systems on brain physiology (Rios et al., 2006).

ANTIPSYCHOTICS

Like most psychoactive drugs, antipsychotic drugs were discovered serendipitously. Although chlorpromazine, the original antipsychotic, had actions at many receptors, its ability to act as an antagonist at the dopamine D_2 receptor turned out to be critical. Although there are many antipsychotic drugs today, almost every single one has some ability to downregulate the activation of D_2 receptors by endogenous dopamine, either by direct antagonism or by partial agonism (Kapur and Remington, 2001). Positron emission tomography (PET) imaging studies have used radiolabeled versions of these drugs

to assess the degree and length of binding. For the typical antipsychotic, reduction of "positive" symptoms (for example, *psychosis, hallucinations, delusions*) requires the antipsychotic drug to have bound to ~65% of D_2 receptors. However, there is a very narrow window of binding before motor side effects, called *extrapyramidal symptoms*, set in at binding higher than 70%. A major development in psychiatry has been the emergence of an antipsychotic drug, *clozapine*, that does not cause these motor side effects. It is often referred to as an atypical antipsychotic in contrast to previous "typical" antipsychotics such as chlorpromazine and haloperidol. Of perhaps even greater significance is the fact that clozapine, unlike typical antipsychotics, treats negative symptoms of schizophrenia (for example, *flat affect, anhedonia, withdrawal*).

The emergence of clozapine has focused more recent research on differences between typical antipsychotics and clozapine. The latter has a very complicated profile of action that includes effects at dopamine, norepinephrine, serotonin, acetylcholine, and histamine receptors. Clozapine is a significantly more potent 5-HT_{2A} antagonist and a significantly less potent D_2 antagonist compared to the typical antipsychotics. This pattern, together with the large body of work on the psychotomimetic effects of 5-HT_{2A} agonists, awakened interested in the therapeutic effects of a pure 5-HT_{2A} antagonist. However, this drug did not succeed in clinical trials. It may be clozapine's more moderate action at D_2 receptors, rather than its ability to block pure 5-HT_{2A} receptors, which is responsible for its ability to improve negative symptoms as well as its reduced propensity to induce motor side effects.

One hypothesis that has been proposed to explain the clinical efficacy of antipsychotic drugs relates to the "depolarization block" of midbrain dopamine neurons projecting to the prefrontal cortex (Bunney, 1992). The blockade of autoreceptors on dopaminergic neurons leads to chronic depolarization of these neurons, which prevents the relief from sodium channel inactivation. Electrophysiological experiments revealed that one difference between clozapine and typical antipsychotics is that chronic administration of clozapine results in depolarization block only of the midbrain dopaminergic cells that project to the medial prefrontal cortex, whereas chronic administration of typical antipsychotics results in depolarization block of the neostriatum as well as the medial prefrontal cortex. This former is thought to account for the extrapyramidal symptoms associated with typical antipsychotics.

There have been several animal models postulated for schizophrenia. The psychotomimetic drug model of the disease has proved informative about what types of neurotransmission are involved in acute psychosis. The amphetamine model has proved useful for understanding the paranoid state. However, given the evidence for neurodevelopmental abnormalities in schizophrenia, several groups of researchers have tried to model this illness in rodents through lesions early in development (Lipska and Weinberger, 2000). One such model, involving lesions to the ventral-hippocampus, has been shown to result in the postpubertal onset of dopaminergic abnormalities (Goto and O'Donnell, 2002; O'Donnell, 2012) similar to what is hypothesized to occur in schizophrenia. These animal models allow the *in vitro* and *in vivo* electrophysiological examination of how an early brain lesion alters interactions between the dopaminergic and glutamatergic systems in adulthood.

OVERVIEW AND FUTURE DIRECTIONS

This chapter explored how basic electrophysiology can be used to clarify how neurons communicate with each other and how different drugs affect this signaling. Appreciating how a neuron maintains its electrical state and its ability to release neurotransmitters onto other cells is critical to appreciating the many subtle ways that thought can be influenced by genetic variations in ion channels. Understanding the electrophysiological mechanisms by which neurotransmitter receptors can modulate the activity of neurons is essential to appreciate the immediate and long-term consequences of psychoactive drugs. Recent progress in the molecular genetics of psychiatric illness, together with the capacity to model relevant human single nucleotide polymorphisms in transgenic mice, promises to provide new opportunities for targeting electrophysiological studies toward uncovering the role of susceptibility genes in these illnesses.

DISCLOSURE

Dr. Lambe has no conflicts of interest to disclose. She is funded only by the Canadian Institutes of Health Research (Canada Research Chair and MOP 89825), the Province of Ontario (Early Researcher Award), and the National Science and Engineering Council (Discovery Grant).

REFERENCES

Bailey, C.D., De Biasi, M., et al. (2010). The nicotinic acetylcholine receptor alpha5 subunit plays a key role in attention circuitry and accuracy. *J. Neurosci.* 30(27):9241–9252.

Benekareddy, M., Goodfellow, N.M., et al. (2010). Enhanced function of prefrontal serotonin 5-HT(2) receptors in a rat model of psychiatric vulnerability. *J. Neurosci.* 30(36):12138–12150.

Berman, R.M., Cappiello, A., et al. (2000). Antidepressant effects of ketamine in depressed patients. *Biol. Psychiatry* 47(4):351–354.

Bhat, S., Dao, D.T., et al. (2012). CACNA1C (Ca(v)1.2) in the pathophysiology of psychiatric disease. *Prog. Neurobiol.* 99(1):1–14.

Bierut, L.J. (2010). Convergence of genetic findings for nicotine dependence and smoking related diseases with chromosome 15q24–25. *Trends Pharmacol. Sci.* 31(1):46–51.

Bierut, L.J., Stitzel, J.A., et al. (2008). Variants in nicotinic receptors and risk for nicotine dependence. *Am. J. Psychiatry* 165(9):1163–1171.

Bigos, K.L., Mattay, V.S., et al. (2010). Genetic variation in CACNA1C affects brain circuitries related to mental illness. *Arch. Gen. Psychiatry* 67(9):939–945.

Bunney, B.S. (1992). Clozapine: a hypothesised mechanism for its unique clinical profile. *Br. J. Psychiatry Suppl.* 17:17–21.

Drevets, W.C., Price, J.L., et al. (2008). Brain structural and functional abnormalities in mood disorders: implications for neurocircuitry models of depression. *Brain Struct. Funct.* 213(1–2):93–118.

Duman, R.S., and Monteggia, L.M. (2006). A neurotrophic model for stress-related mood disorders. *Biol. Psychiatry* 59(12):1116–1127.

Ge, S., Yang, C.H., et al. (2007). A critical period for enhanced synaptic plasticity in newly generated neurons of the adult brain. *Neuron* 54(4):559–566.

Goto, Y., and O'Donnell, P. (2002). Delayed mesolimbic system alteration in a developmental animal model of schizophrenia. *J. Neurosci.* 22(20):9070–9077.

Hahn, B., Robinson, B.M., et al. (2012). Visuospatial attention in schizophrenia: deficits in broad monitoring. *J. Abnorm. Psychol.* 121(1):119–128.

Hamani, C., Mayberg, H., et al. (2011). The subcallosal cingulate gyrus in the context of major depression. *Biol. Psychiatry* 69(4):301–308.

Harrison, P.J., and Law, A.J. (2006). Neuregulin 1 and schizophrenia: genetics, gene expression, and neurobiology. *Biol. Psychiatry* 60(2):132–140.

Hong, L.E., Yang, X., et al. (2011). A CHRNA5 allele related to nicotine addiction and schizophrenia. *Genes Brain Behav.* 10(5):530–535.

Kanner, A.M. (2008). Mood disorder and epilepsy: a neurobiologic perspective of their relationship. *Dialogues Clin. Neurosci.* 10(1):39–45.

Kapur, S., and Remington, G. (2001). Dopamine D(2) receptors and their role in atypical antipsychotic action: still necessary and may even be sufficient. *Biol. Psychiatry* 50(11):873–883.

Kuryatov, A., Berrettini, W., et al. (2011). Acetylcholine receptor (AChR) $\alpha 5$ subunit variant associated with risk for nicotine dependence and lung cancer reduces $(\alpha 4\beta 2)_2\alpha 5$ AChR function. *Mol. Pharmacol.* 79(1):119–125.

Lambe, E.K., and Aghajanian, G.K. (2007). Prefrontal cortical network activity: opposite effects of psychedelic hallucinogens and D1/D5 dopamine receptor activation. *Neuroscience* 145(3):900–910.

Law, A.J., Lipska, B.K., et al. (2006). Neuregulin 1 transcripts are differentially expressed in schizophrenia and regulated by 5' SNPs associated with the disease. *Proc. Natl. Acad. Sci. USA* 103(17):6747–6752.

Li, N., Lee, B., et al. (2010). mTOR-dependent synapse formation underlies the rapid antidepressant effects of NMDA antagonists. *Science* 329(5994):959–964.

Lipska, B.K., and Weinberger, D.R. (2000). To model a psychiatric disorder in animals: schizophrenia as a reality test. *Neuropsychopharmacology* 23(3):223–239.

Liu, R.J., Lee, F.S., et al. (2012). Brain-derived neurotrophic factor Val66Met allele impairs basal and ketamine-stimulated synaptogenesis in prefrontal cortex. *Biol. Psychiatry* 71(11):996–1005.

Mongeau, R., Blier, P., et al. (1997). The serotonergic and noradrenergic systems of the hippocampus: their interactions and the effects of antidepressant treatments. *Brain Res. Brain Res. Rev.* 23(3):145–195.

Myles, N., Newall, H.D., et al. (2012). Tobacco use before, at, and after first-episode psychosis: a systematic meta-analysis. *J. Clin. Psychiatry* 73(4):468–475.

O'Donnell, P. (2012). Cortical disinhibition in the neonatal ventral hippocampal lesion model of schizophrenia: new vistas on possible therapeutic approaches. *Pharmacol. Ther.* 133(1):19–25.

Pitcher, G.M., Kalia, L.V., et al. (2011). Schizophrenia susceptibility pathway neuregulin 1-ErbB4 suppresses Src upregulation of NMDA receptors. *Nat. Med.* 17(4):470–478.

Rios, M., Lambe, E.K., et al. (2006). Severe deficits in 5-HT2A-mediated neurotransmission in BDNF conditional mutant mice. *J. Neurobiol.* 66(4):408–420.

Tuesta, L.M., Fowler, C.D., et al. (2011). Recent advances in understanding nicotinic receptor signaling mechanisms that regulate drug self-administration behavior. *Biochem. Pharmacol.* 82(8):984–995.

van Praag, H., Schinder, A.F., et al. (2002). Functional neurogenesis in the adult hippocampus. *Nature*, 415(6875):1030–1034.

Vollenweider, F.X., and Geyer, M.A. (2001). A systems model of altered consciousness: integrating natural and drug-induced psychoses. *Brain. Res. Bull.* 56(5):495–507.

Vollenweider, F.X., Leenders, K.L., et al. (1997). Positron emission tomography and fluorodeoxyglucose studies of metabolic hyperfrontality and psychopathology in the psilocybin model of psychosis. *Neuropsychopharmacology* 16(5):357–372.

4 | PRINCIPLES OF SIGNAL TRANSDUCTION

JEAN-ANTOINE GIRAULT AND PAUL GREENGARD

SIGNAL TRANSDUCTION

All cells react to changes in their environment and to clues that may be important for their survival and/or function. This is true for unicellular as well as multicellular organisms. Unicellular organisms react to light, to chemical gradients of nutrients, and to specific molecules released by other cells from the same species. In multicellular organisms, the harmonious functioning of billions of cells, assembled in tissues as sophisticated as the human brain, requires a highly complex network of intercellular signaling involving molecules known as *hormones*, *neurotransmitters*, *cytokines*, *growth factors*, and so forth. Yet the molecular mechanisms by which these signals are perceived and interpreted by individual cells are quite similar to those used by much simpler unicellular beings. Indeed, work over the past years has demonstrated an amazing degree of conservation of many of these molecular mechanisms among brewer's yeast (*Saccharomyces cerevisiae*), nematode worms (*Caenorhabditis elegans*), fruit flies (*Drosophila melanogaster*), and mammals, including humans. In addition, specialized cells, such as the cones or the rods in the retina, or the olfactory epithelial cells, have retained the ability to perceive changes in the physical or chemical environment. These specialized cells translate information from the external world into changes in neuronal activity that can be communicated to the rest of the organism.

The term *signal transduction* is used to describe the cascades of biochemical reactions by which cells translate various extracellular signals into appropriate responses, whether the primary extracellular signal comes from other cells or from the external world. Signal transduction involves a number of key players and reactions that we examine successively. The initial reaction involves a "receptor," the protein that interacts with the extracellular signal and triggers its effects. Subsequently, a series of reactions of varying degrees of complexity ensues, resulting in a vast array of physiological responses. In many instances, the coupling between receptors and effector pathways requires an intermediate agent, a guanosine 5′-triphosphate (GTP) binding protein or *G protein*, which acts as a molecular switch, and the generation of a second messenger. Second messengers are small molecules that are generated within cells in response to extracellular signals (the latter correspond to "first messengers"). One particular class of signaling molecules comprises small molecules that can readily cross biological membranes and act as intercellular messengers and second messengers. Such molecules include fatty acids such as arachidonic acid, and the gas nitric oxide. The major covalent modification of proteins involved in signal transduction is phosphorylation. This modification has been shown to result in changes of innumerable biological properties of nerve cells, such as activation of biosynthetic enzymes, activation of transcription factors, regulation of the permeability of ion channels, regulation of neurotransmitter release, and alteration of the sensitivity to neurotransmitters.

GENERAL PROPERTIES OF SIGNAL TRANSDUCTION PATHWAYS

Signal transduction pathways have a number of important properties in common that are interesting to consider before describing these pathways in detail.

First, many signaling cascades have a tremendous capability of signal amplification. This explains why, in some instances, cells are able to detect only a single photon—in the case of retina photoreceptor cells—or a few molecules in their environment. A second property is specificity. Cells are able to discriminate between a virtually unlimited number of extracellular molecules and to react to very few of them. Moreover, different signals acting on the same cells will have different effects. This is true in spite of the fact that receptor proteins belong to a limited number of classes and that many of the components of the signaling cascades are rather ubiquitous. Thus, during development, a characteristic set of genes, the products of which are involved in signal transduction, is selected in each cell type, providing it with the capability to react in an appropriate way to specific signals. A third important characteristic of signal transduction pathways is their pleiotropy. Thus, a single extracellular signal can generate multiple responses in the cell. For instance, a single neurotransmitter can trigger the opening of some ion channels and the closing of others, the activation of multiple enzymes, the modification of cytoskeletal organization, and the stimulation of the expression of specific genes.

Another property of signal transduction pathways is that they allow the integration of several simultaneous or successive signals. The cascades of reactions triggered by each signal interact with the others at many levels, sometimes reinforcing each other, sometimes canceling each other. As a result, the final output in terms of cellular response is a subtle combination of what would have been induced by each extracellular signal separately and may indeed be quite different from responses to individual signals. Some signals may, for instance, have little effect by themselves yet inhibit or potentiate considerably the response to other signals. In the nervous system this property is called *neuromodulation*. These properties of integration and transformation of multiple signaling pathways are often quite complex, and computer modeling is necessary to help predict their output.

Finally, the response to extracellular signals can have long-lasting effects on cells and modify their subsequent response to the same or other signals. One obvious example involves gene expression: One hormone, for instance, will induce the expression of a gene necessary for the response to a neurotransmitter. In fact, there are many different ways by which such long-lasting changes in cellular responses can be implemented. They represent the molecular basis for "cellular" learning and memory, a capacity that all cells possess to some extent. Thus at any given time the response of a cell to external signals depends on its previous history. Such mechanisms have a special importance in neurons in which they represent the cellular basis for synaptic plasticity, which is thought to underlie "psychological" learning and memory (Chapter 5).

THE IMPORTANCE OF ELUCIDATING SIGNAL TRANSDUCTION PATHWAYS

Deciphering the complex networks of reactions that constitute signal transduction pathways is important for understanding the physiology of cells and multicellular organisms, including the human brain. Moreover, such understanding is certainly critical for elucidating the mechanisms of diseases that are still elusive, and eventually treating them. It is easy to understand that dysfunctions of signal transduction pathways will have profound and deleterious consequences on the properties of cells. This point is well illustrated by the fact that cancers result from the dysfunction of signaling pathways that regulate cell growth and division. Similarly, many naturally occurring toxins exert their effects by interrupting or diverting normal intracellular signaling pathways. Recent work has identified mutations in genes which code for signaling proteins as the cause of mental retardation and syndromic autism spectrum disorders. It seems likely that, as our knowledge of signal transduction in neurons progresses, we will discover that alterations of signal transduction pathways play an important role in a number of neurological or psychiatric diseases. In addition, the multiple enzymes involved in these pathways represent potential targets for therapeutic drugs. Lithium is one example of a drug that is already used in psychiatry and is thought to exert its effect by acting on signal transduction mechanisms (see following). The study of complete genome sequences, including those of brewers' yeast (*Saccharomyces cerevisiae*), a plant (*Arabidopsis thaliana*), a round worm (*Caenorhabditis elegans*), fruit fly (*Drosophila melanogaster*), and human (*Homo sapiens*), allows an estimation of the number of genes devoted to signal transduction in various eukaryotic organisms (Table 4.1). Comparison of signaling networks in organisms of various complexities provides useful information about their organizing and functioning principles. Exhaustive identification of the components of such networks in humans pinpoints potential candidates for genetic alterations that may underlie

neurological or psychiatric disease, or more likely enhance the susceptibility to such diseases. It also provides novel targets for designing new pharmacological tools aimed at modifying specific signaling pathways either to correct natural deficits or to counteract the consequences of their alterations, regardless of the cause of these alterations.

RECEPTORS: HOW CELLS DETECT EXTRACELLULAR SIGNALS

Cells can detect chemical as well as physical signals from their environment. We concentrate on chemical signals that are the more relevant for understanding brain physiology. The first step in signal transduction is the interaction of the extracellular signaling molecule with a receptor. A receptor is a protein that is able to bind the signaling molecule with high affinity and specificity, and to trigger a biological response in reaction to this binding. Extracellular signaling molecules include neurotransmitters, hormones, growth factors, and related substances and can be divided into two broad categories: those that do not penetrate the cells and act at the level of the plasma membrane and those that readily penetrate the cells and act on intracellular targets. It should be emphasized that these two mechanisms of action are not always exclusive and that compounds such as steroid hormones appear to have membrane receptors in addition to their well-characterized intracellular receptors.

SIGNALS THAT ACT AT THE LEVEL OF THE PLASMA MEMBRANE

Receptors that have been characterized at the level of the plasma membrane can be divided into several classes depending on their organization and properties. Representatives of each of these classes of receptors are present in neurons, where they play diverse roles.

NEUROTRANSMITTER-GATED ION CHANNELS
Biological membranes are impermeable to small ions including Na^+, K^+, Ca^{2+}, and Cl^- (Chapter 3). The concentrations of these ions are very different in the intracellular and extracellular compartments, due to the existence of active transport mechanisms. Ion channels are proteins that form pores within the membranes and allow the selective flow of specific ions to which they are permeable. The magnitude and direction of ion flow depend on two forces: the concentration gradient and the electrical potential difference between the two sides of the membrane. Opening or closing of one class of channels allows or blocks flow of ions to which this class of channels is permeable. This, in turn, regulates the electrical potential across the membrane. At rest, the intracellular side of the membrane is electronegative as compared to the extracellular side (usually −60 to −80 mV).

The opening of several ion channels is directly regulated by neurotransmitters. Such channels are called *neurotransmitter-gated channels* or *ionotropic receptors* (Box 4.1). The neurotransmitter binds to the ion channel and triggers

TABLE 4.1. Estimated numbers of proteins involved in signal transduction

PROTEIN FAMILY	HUMAN	FLY	WORM	YEAST	MUSTARD WEED
Eukaryotic protein kinases*	575	319	437	121	1049
Ser/Thr and dual specificity protein kinases°	395	198	315	114	1102
Tyr protein kinases°	106	47	100	5	16
Ser/Thr protein phosphatases°	15	19	51	13	29
Tyr and dual specificity protein phosphatases*	112	35	108	12	21
Cyclic nucleotide phosphodiesterases°	25	8	6	1	0
G protein–coupled receptors*	569	97	358	0	16
G protein alpha°	27	10	22	2	5
G protein beta°	5	3	2	1	1
G protein gamma°	13	2	2	0	0
Ras superfamily°	141	64	62	26	86
SH2 domains	119*	39°	48°	1	3°
SH3 domains^	215*	75°	62*	27°	4°
Voltage-gated Ca²⁺ channels alpha subunits°	32	7	10	2	2
Caspases°	13	7	3	0	0
Nuclear hormone receptors°	59	25	183	1	4

The numbers of some proteins important for signal transduction are given for human (*Homo sapiens*), fly (*Drosophila melanogaster*), round worm (*Caenorhabditis elegans*), yeast (*Saccharomyces cerevisiae*), and mustard weed (*Arabidopsis thaliana*). Since the sequencing and analysis of the genomes of these organisms is not fully complete, these numbers represent only lower limits. Data are based on the publications by the International Human Genome Sequencing Consortium (Nature, 2001 409:860–921) indicated by an asterisk (*) and by Celera Genomics and associates (Science, 2001 291:1304–1351) indicated by °.

its opening by inducing a change in its conformation. Since no intermediate biochemical reaction is involved, the effects of neurotransmitters on ligand-gated channels are very fast. This type of receptor underlies most of the fast synaptic excitatory or inhibitory transmission in brain. In addition, the response of ionotropic receptors to neurotransmitters can be regulated by several extracellular or intracellular signals, providing a fine tuning of their properties (see the examples of glutamate *N*-methyl-D-aspartate [NMDA] receptor and γ-aminobutyric acid [GABA-A] receptor, Box 4.1). Such modulatory sites are targets for molecules of great pharmacological importance, including benzodiazepines and barbiturates, which increase the response to GABA (Box 4.1).

G PROTEIN–COUPLED RECEPTORS

A large number of receptors work in close association with heterotrimeric GTP-binding proteins or G proteins that are composed of three subunits (α, β, and γ; Box 4.2; see also Box 4.7). Although these receptors belong to several different gene families, they have a major structural feature in common,

which has been conserved throughout evolution: *the polypeptide chain of these receptors crosses the plasma membrane seven times.* Therefore, these receptors are called *7-transmembrane domain receptors* or *serpentine receptors*. When these receptors bind their specific ligand, they undergo a conformational change that has consequences for the associated G protein (Box 4.2), leading to the dissociation of a GTP-bound α subunit and β/γ complex, each of which is able to interact with various targets including ion channels and enzymes (Box 4.7). Interestingly, these G protein–coupled receptors (often referred to as GPCRs) are also involved in the detection of clues from the environment: receptors for odors, pheromones, and light belong to this category.

RECEPTORS THAT ARE THEMSELVES ENZYMES

Some receptors are transmembrane proteins that are composed of an extracellular domain that binds the extracellular signaling molecule, a single transmembrane domain, and an intracellular domain that possesses an enzymatic activity. Binding of

BOX 4.1 NEUROTRANSMITTER-GATED ION CHANNELS

The neurotransmitter receptors responsible for fast synaptic transmission are ligand-gated ion channels. They comprise several subunits arranged in such a way as to form a central pore through which ions can cross the plasma membrane. Binding of the neurotransmitter triggers the opening of this pore. Neurotransmitter-gated ion channels are specific for one or several ions, the nature of which is responsible for their excitatory or inhibitory effects.

Receptors for excitatory neurotransmitters such as acetylcholine (nicotinic subtype), or glutamate (subtypes named after chemicals not present in the brain but which activate them specifically, *alpha-amino-3-hydroxy-5-methyl-4-isoxazolepropionic acid* [AMPA] and *kainate*), let Na^+ ions flow into the neuron, and K^+ ions flow out [see (A)]. At resting potential, the Na^+ influx predominates and is responsible for the depolarizing, excitatory effects of these neurotransmitters. The open state of neurotransmitter-gated ion channels is usually unstable. They switch spontaneously to a desensitized state, in which the ion channel is closed, although the neurotransmitter is still bound with high affinity. Desensitization is thought to be a protective mechanism against overstimulation.

NMDA receptors are a subtype of glutamate receptors, named after their specific synthetic agonist (*N-methyl-D-aspartate*), that have a number of unique properties [see (B)]. First, glycine must also be bound to these receptors for them to open in response to glutamate. Second, at resting membrane potential, when NMDA receptors open, they are obstructed by Mg^{2+} ions. This block is relieved only when the membrane is depolarized simultaneously by another mechanism (e.g., stimulation of nearby glutamate receptors of the AMPA subtype). Finally, in addition to Na^+ and K^+, NMDA receptors are highly permeable to Ca^{2+}. The resulting Ca^{2+} influx is responsible for the role of NMDA receptors in synaptic plasticity and also for its deleterious, excitotoxic effects in pathological conditions.

Receptors for GABA [GABA-A subtype, see (C)] and glycine (not shown) are selectively permeable to Cl^- ions. In most instances, the resulting Cl^- influx is responsible for the inhibitory effects of these neurotransmitters. GABA-A receptors account for most of the inhibitory receptors in the central nervous system, whereas glycine receptors are restricted to the brainstem and spinal cord. GABA-A receptors are modulated by two classes of drugs that have important clinical applications. Benzodiazepines (e.g., diazepam) or barbiturates (e.g., phenobarbital), although they cannot open the GABA-A ion channel by themselves, increase the response to GABA. The existence and the nature of endogenous ligands for the benzodiazepine and barbiturate modulatory sites on GABA-A receptors are still a matter of dispute.

Other abbreviations: GABA: γ-aminobutyric acid.

Further reading: Benarroch, 2007; Cull-Candy et al., 2001; Dani and Bertrand, 2007; Derkach et al., 2007; Johnston, 2005; Mayer, 2005; Mohler et al., 2002; Nutt and Malizia, 2001; Paoletti, 2011; Traynelis et al., 2010.

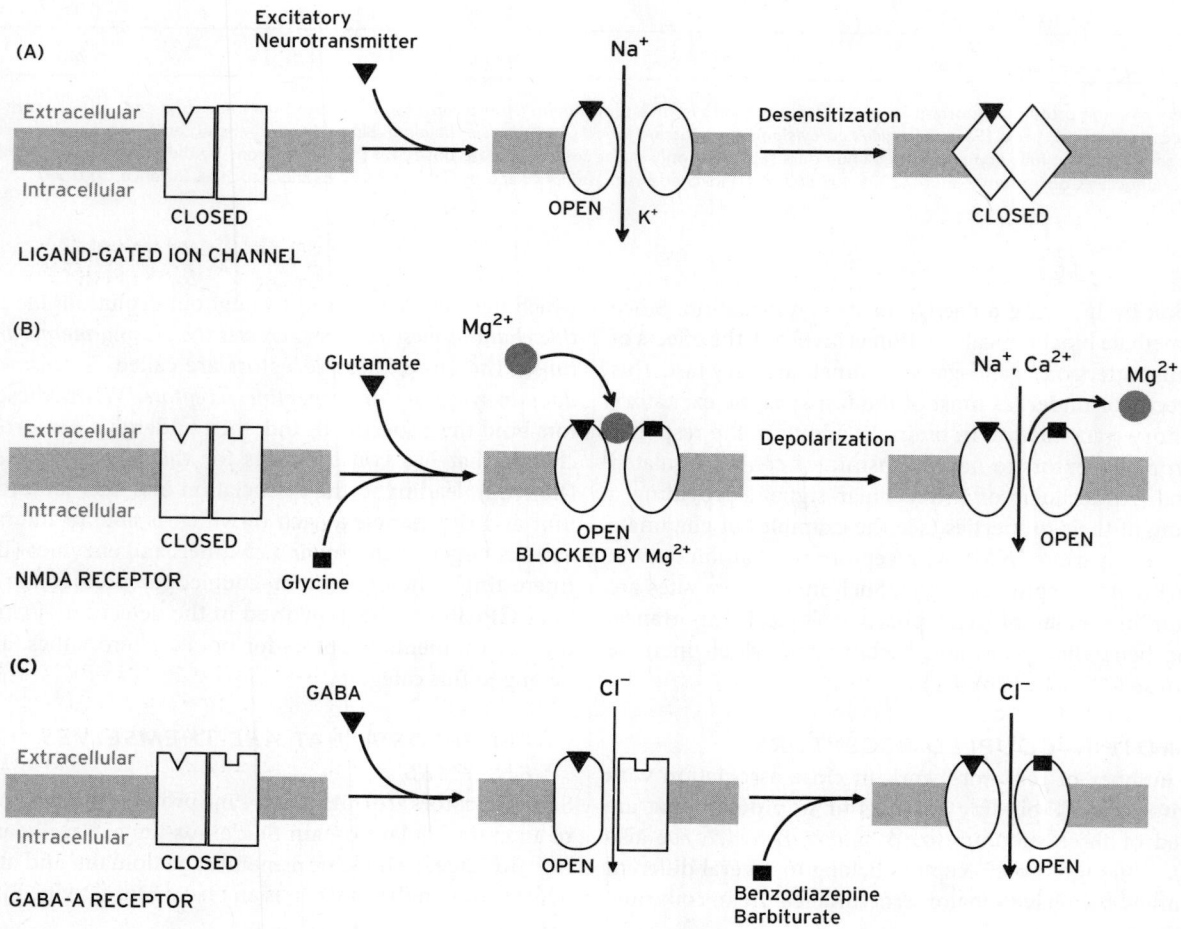

BOX 4.2 G PROTEIN–COUPLED RECEPTORS

A large number of neurotransmitter receptors belong to the category of seven transmembrane domain *G protein–coupled receptors* (GPCRs), which also includes receptors for hormones, light, odorants, pheromones, and Ca²⁺. These receptors are associated with heterotrimeric G proteins (see Box 4.7). Heterotrimeric G proteins comprise three subunits: α, β, and γ, which are not transmembrane proteins but are associated with the membrane by covalently bound fatty acid molecules. In the resting state, GDP is bound to the α subunit, which is closely attached to the β/γ complex. When the neurotransmitter binds to the receptor, the conformation of the receptor changes, inducing a change in the conformation of the α subunit, which expels GDP and replaces it by GTP. GTP-bound α subunit is no longer capable of interacting with the receptor or β/γ. Instead, GTP-bound α and β/γ diffuse away from each other and from the receptor, while still attached to the membrane, and interact with specific targets. After a short time GTP is hydrolyzed to GDP, and GDP-bound α reassociates with β/γ. At about the same time, the neurotransmitter leaves its receptor, which returns to its resting state and reassociates with α-GDP and β/γ.

There are several different types of α, β, and γ subunits, encoded by different genes. The nature of the α subunit that associates with a given receptor determines the actions that can be triggered by this receptor. β/γ subunits have their own effects on similar targets that can be in the same direction as that of their cognate α subunit, or, sometimes, in the opposite direction. β/γ subunits have additional specific properties, such as recruiting to the membrane a protein kinase (*G protein–coupled receptor kinase* or GRK), which phosphorylates the receptor and prevents its further interaction with G proteins. This represents an important mechanism of desensitization of G protein–coupled receptors.

Other abbreviations: G protein: guanine nucleotide binding protein; GDP: guanosine 5′-diphosphate; GTP: guanosine 5′-triphosphate; Pi: inorganic phosphate.

Further reading: Bockaert and Pin, 1999; DeWire et al., 2007; Gainetdinov et al., 2004; Kobilka, 2011; May et al., 2007; Moore et al., 2007; Rosenbaum et al., 2009.

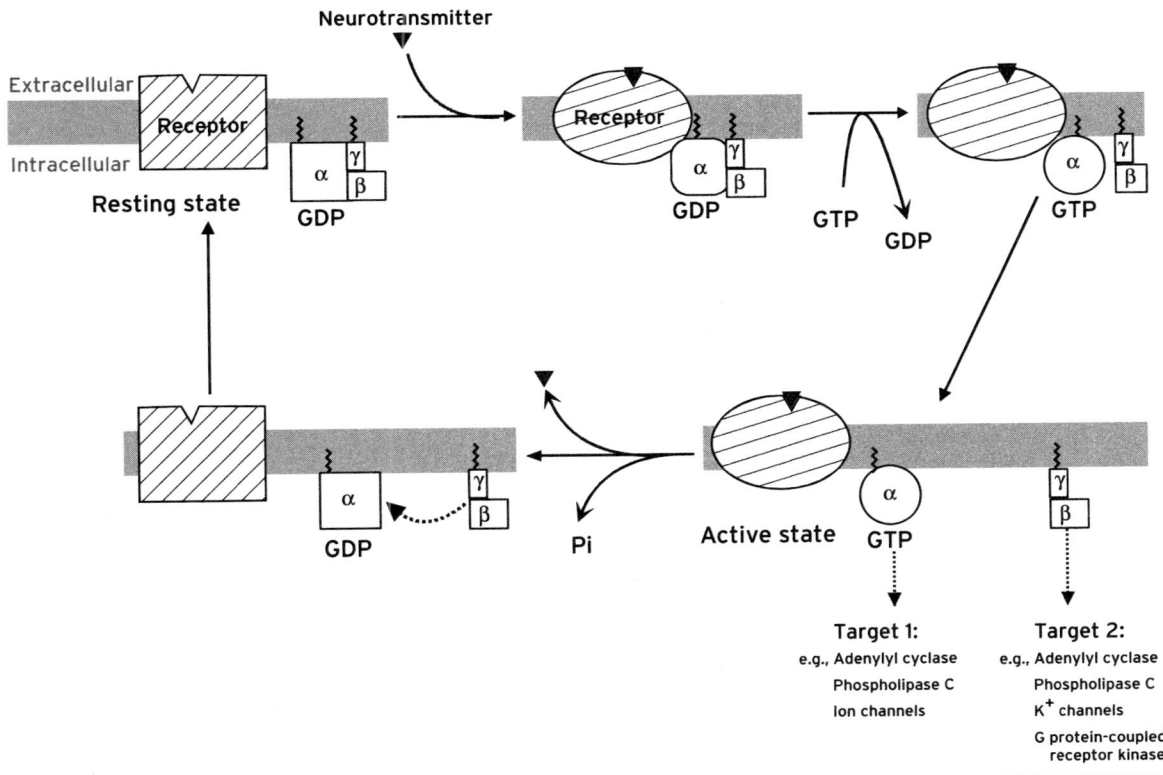

the ligand to the extracellular domain dramatically alters the activity of the intracellular enzymatic domain. This activation often results from the dimerization of the receptor.

The best-known receptors in this category are tyrosine kinase receptors for polypeptide growth factors, including nerve growth factor (NGF) and related neurotrophins (Box 4.3). Their ligands are polypeptides that are often soluble but can also be attached to the membrane of other cells. The intracellular domain of this type of receptor is a protein kinase, which is able to phosphorylate itself and other proteins on tyrosines (see Box 4.14). Phosphorylation on tyrosine triggers cascades of reactions that are detailed in Box 4.3. These reactions involve recruitment of specific proteins through domains such as the SH2 (Src-homology 2) domain that bind to their target peptide sequence only when the tyrosine it contains is phosphorylated (Box 4.4). Thus, a variety of intracellular

BOX 4.3 PROTEIN TYROSINE KINASE RECEPTORS

Receptors for many polypeptide growth factors, including nerve growth factor and related neurotrophins, are transmembrane tyrosine kinases. These receptors are composed of a single peptide chain whose extracellular domain can bind the growth factor, whereas the intracytoplasmic domain is a protein tyrosine kinase (see Box 4.14). In the absence of growth factor, the tyrosine kinase is inactive. In the presence of growth factor, two identical receptors interact with each other (*homodimerization*), and this results in the activation of the tyrosine kinase domains. They phosphorylate several tyrosine residues located in each other's sequence (*autophosphorylation*). Autophosphorylation on tyrosine provides docking sites for a number of proteins that possess SH2 domains (see Box 4.4), resulting in the phosphorylation-dependent clustering of several important proteins around the growth factor receptor. These proteins, many of which also become phosphorylated on tyrosine, include phospholipase C γ (PLCγ) that hydrolyzes phosphatidylinositol 4,5 bisphosphate into diacylglycerol and inositol 1,4,5 trisphosphate (IP$_3$, see Boxes 4.10 and 4.12),

phosphatidylinositol 3 kinase (PI3 kinase) that phosphorylates phosphatidylinositol at position 3 and activates its own signal transduction pathway (see Box 4.18), phosphotyrosine phosphatases (PTP), adaptor molecules, and others. Adaptor molecules are proteins that possess, in addition to an SH2 domain, SH3 domains (see Box 4.4). By these SH3 domains the adaptors are bound to proline-rich regions of guanine nucleotide exchange factors (GEFs; see Box 4.7). GEFs are enzymes that catalyze the exchange of GDP for GTP on small G proteins of the Ras family. Their recruitment to the membrane, mediated by the adaptor, brings them in contact with Ras, which they put in its GTP-bound, active form (see Boxes 4.7 and 4.8). The precise nature of the SH2-containing enzymes or adaptor molecules that are recruited varies from one growth factor receptor to another; however, the principles of signaling are the same in all cases.

Other abbreviations: G protein: guanine nucleotide binding protein; GDP: guanosine 5′-diphosphate; GTP: guanosine 5′-triphosphate; P: phosphate group; SH2: Src-homology domain 2; SH3: Src-homology domain 3.

Further reading: Kalb, 2005; Lemmon and Schlessinger, 2010; Papin et al., 2005; Schlessinger, 2002.

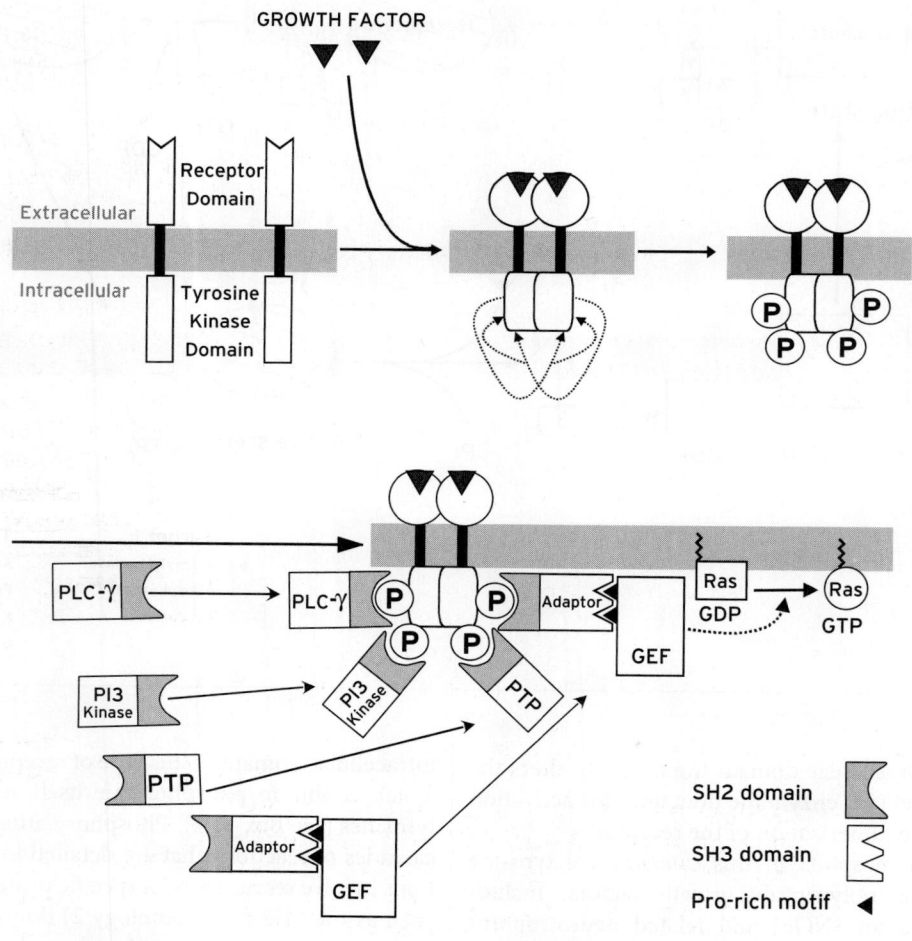

signaling pathways are activated (see following Boxes 4.8, 4.10, and 4.18).

A variation on the same theme is represented by receptors that do not possess an enzymatic activity by themselves but that associate with tyrosine kinases. For example, receptors for some neurotrophic factors, such as glial derived neurotrophic factor (GDNF), are extracellular proteins attached to the membrane by a lipid anchor (*glycosyl-phosphatidyl inositol*). Due to their localization, they cannot transduce the signal directly to the interior of the cell. They do it by virtue of their association to a transmembrane protein whose intracellular domain is a tyrosine kinase (c-Ret in the case of GDNF receptor). An important class of receptor comprises transmembrane proteins that have the capability to associate with intracytoplasmic tyrosine kinase. This class includes receptors for key messengers in the immune response (e.g., cytokines, interferon), hormones (e.g., growth hormone, prolactin, leptin), and polypeptides that have growth factor activity (e.g., erythropoietin, ciliary derived neurotrophic factor). The intracellular segment of these receptors binds a tyrosine kinase of the JAK family (*Janus kinase*; see Box 4.5). Other types of receptors, including the receptors for the antigen of lymphocytes, have a similar, although more complicated, organization. In this case the enzyme is a member of the Src family of tyrosine kinases. Similarly, integrins, which are receptors for extracellular matrix proteins, associate on their intracellular side with a tyrosine kinase called *FAK* (focal adhesion kinase).

Several other families of receptors are transmembrane proteins that possess other types of enzymatic activities. One group corresponds to receptors for transforming growth factor beta (TGFβ), activin, and inhibin, the intracellular domain of which possesses a protein serine/threonine kinase activity. Another group of receptors, including the receptor for atrial natriuretic factor (ANF), have an intracellular domain that is a guanylyl cyclase, an enzyme that generates the second messenger cyclic guanosine 3′,5′-monophosphate (cGMP). Other receptors, such as those for Fas and tumor necrosis factor α (TNFα), which are able to trigger programmed cell death (apoptosis), associate with various intracellular proteins that, among other things, activate proteolytic enzymes.

EXTRACELLULAR SIGNALS THAT PENETRATE CELLS

Most of the molecules that act on membrane receptors cannot cross the plasma membrane because of their charge, which makes them highly hydrophilic, or their size. However, some signaling molecules are readily able to cross the lipid bilayer of the plasma membrane because of their hydrophobic nature and/or their small size. These molecules include steroid hormones and the related vitamin D derivatives, thyroid hormones, and retinoic acid. Steroid hormones bind to intracellular receptors that, in addition to the hormone binding domain, contain a deoxyribonucleic acid (DNA) binding domain, and a domain capable of stimulating messenger ribonucleic acids (mRNA) transcription of specific genes (Box 4.6). In the absence of hormone, the receptor is in an inactive conformation, unable to enhance

BOX 4.4 SH2 AND SH3 DOMAINS

SH2 (Src-homology domain 2) and SH3 (Src-homology domain 3) were first identified in the cytoplasmic tyrosine kinase Src. They have now been recognized in a large number of proteins, many of which are involved in signal transduction.

SH2 domains bind to peptide sequences within proteins that contain a phosphorylated tyrosine. In the absence of phosphorylation, there is no binding. In addition, SH2 domains recognize a few amino acids located on the carboxy-terminal side of the phosphorylated tyrosine, thus providing specificity to this type of interaction: each SH2 domain binds preferentially to specific protein regions phosphorylated on tyrosine.

SH3 domains bind to proline-rich regions that adopt a characteristic conformation. Each SH3 domain reacts preferentially with particular proline-rich sequences, providing specificity to this type of interaction. SH3-mediated interactions are constitutive and do not depend on phosphorylation. In fact, SH3 and proline-rich regions are one example of a large number of pairs of protein domains that are able to interact with each other with high affinity and specificity. These protein–protein interactions are important in signal transduction and in other neuronal functions, such as the clustering of receptors at the postsynaptic sites.

Other abbreviations: P: phosphate group; Tyr: tyrosine.

Further reading: Kuriyan and Cowburn, 1997; Pawson and Scott, 1997; Pawson, 2004; Schlessinger and Lemmon, 2003.

(A) SH2 DOMAINS

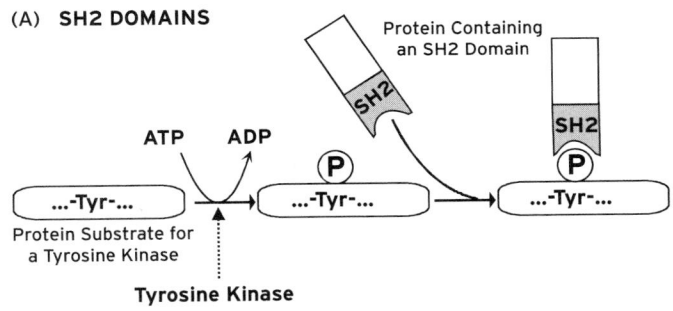

(B) SH3 DOMAINS

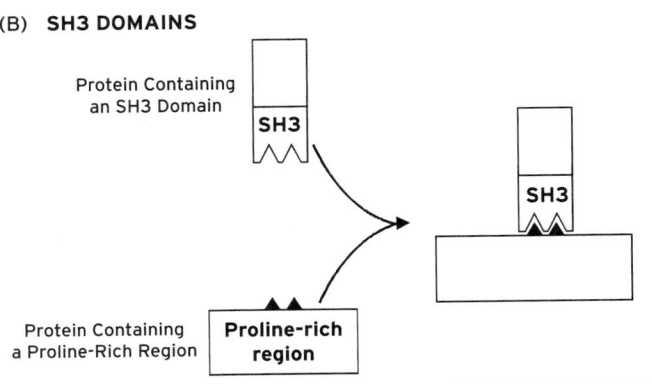

BOX 4.5 JAK-STAT-COUPLED RECEPTORS

A large number of receptors for polypeptide messengers (e.g., *cytokines, interferon, growth hormone, prolactin, leptin, erythropoietin, ciliary derived neurotrophic factor*) utilize a tyrosine phosphorylation signaling mechanism. In contrast to the growth factor receptors depicted in Box 4.3, the cytoplasmic domain of these receptors does not possess tyrosine kinase activity. However, this domain is associated with a cytoplasmic tyrosine kinase belonging to the JAK subfamily (these kinases have two tyrosine kinase domains, only one of which is catalytically active, and are called *Janus tyrosine kinase* after the two-faced Roman god). When the receptor binds its ligand, it dimerizes and becomes phosphorylated by the associated JAK tyrosine kinases. Remarkably, activation of this class of receptor can regulate gene expression via a single family of intermediary proteins called *STAT* (signal transducer and activator of transcription). One important consequence of the phosphorylation of the receptor is the recruitment of STAT, which possesses an SH2 domain (Box 4.4). When STAT molecules are bound to the phosphorylated receptor by their SH2 domain, they become phosphorylated by the JAKs. This allows a switch in the interaction of the SH2 domain of the two molecules of STAT that, instead of binding to the receptor, bind to each other. The resulting dimer detaches from the receptor and enters the nucleus, where it binds to the promoter region of specific genes and, in combination with several other proteins, induces their transcription (Chapter 6).

Other abbreviations: P: phosphate group; SH2: Src-homology domain 2.

Further reading: Imada and Leonard, 2000; O'Shea et al., 2005; Seidel et al., 2000; Yamaoka et al., 2004.

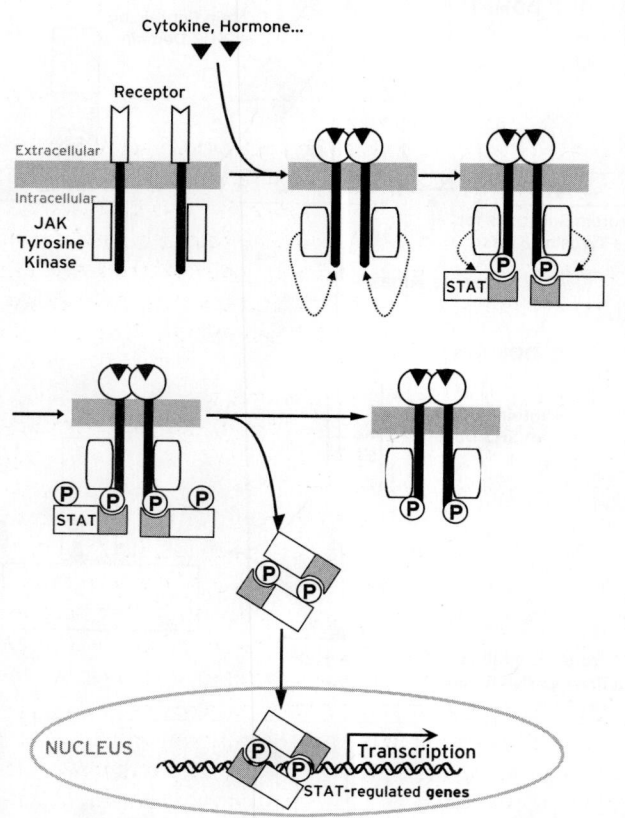

transcription, and, usually, sequestered in the cytoplasm. In the presence of steroid hormone, the receptor switches to an active form, which translocates to the nucleus, where it binds to the promoter region of specific genes and activates their transcription. Retinoic acid and thyroid hormones have similar modes of action.

G PROTEINS: MOLECULAR SWITCHES IN SIGNAL TRANSDUCTION

G proteins are proteins that possess a specific domain capable of binding GTP or guanosine 5′-diphosphate (GDP). In general, the GDP-bound form is inactive and the GTP-bound form is active (Box 4.7). G proteins act as molecular switches that can be turned on by replacement of GDP by GTP, or turned off by hydrolysis of GTP to GDP. They belong to two classes: small G proteins that contain little more than the GDP/GTP binding domain, and large heterotrimeric G proteins in which the GDP/GTP interacting subunit α is associated with two other subunits, β and γ (Box 4.7). Small G proteins are involved in many cellular functions (see Table 4.2 in Box 4.7). The role of the small G protein *Ras* in triggering a cascade of phosphorylation reactions in response to growth factors' action on receptor tyrosine kinases is depicted in Box 4.8. Heterotrimeric G proteins are important in the action of seven transmembrane domain receptors (Box 4.2) and are also coupled to multiple effectors (Box 4.7).

SECOND MESSENGERS

CYCLIC NUCLEOTIDES

Cyclic adenosine 3′-5′-monophosphate (cAMP) was the initial second messenger to be identified. It is generated by a class of enzymes called *adenylyl cyclases* that form cAMP using adenosine 5′-triphosphate (ATP) as a precursor. The major action of cAMP is to activate the protein kinase called *cAMP-dependent protein kinase*. The metabolism and actions of cAMP are detailed in Box 4.9. cGMP is also a second messenger. It is formed by guanylyl cyclases that belong to two groups: as mentioned earlier, some are transmembrane receptors for polypeptides such as ANF; others are soluble enzymes activated by nitric oxide (see the following Box 4.13). cGMP has several targets in mammalian cells, one of which is cGMP-dependent protein kinase.

PHOSPHOLIPID METABOLITES

In addition to their importance in the structure of membranes, phospholipids are precursors for many signaling molecules. The structures of some glycerophospholipids are depicted in Box 4.10. These phospholipids generate signaling molecules under the control of different classes of phospholipases, each of which cleaves the precursor at a specific position (Box 4.10). In addition to glycerophospholipids, other membrane lipids such as sphingomyelin have been found to be involved in

BOX 4.6 RECEPTORS FOR STEROID HORMONES

In contrast to other intercellular messengers such as neurotransmitters, peptide hormones, or growth factors, steroid hormones are capable of readily penetrating the target cells. This is due to their lipophilic nature that allows them to cross the plasma membrane. The glucocorticoid receptor (GR) is a protein located in the cytoplasm, where it is sequestered by association with several proteins, including one called *heat shock protein 90* (HSP90). When the GR has bound cortisol, it undergoes a conformational change that releases it from the associated proteins. The hormone-bound receptor then diffuses into the nucleus, where, as a dimer, it binds to specific DNA sequences in the promoter region of glucocorticoid-responsive genes. The hormone-bound receptor stimulates the transcription of these genes. Other steroid hormones have similar mechanisms of action, except that in some instances their receptor is always located within the nucleus but becomes capable of activating transcription only in the presence of the hormone. Thyroid hormones, vitamin D metabolites, and retinoic acid (a compound important for the regulation of development) have similar mechanisms of action.

Further reading: Dilworth and Chambon, 2001; Mark et al., 2006; Weatherman et al., 1999.

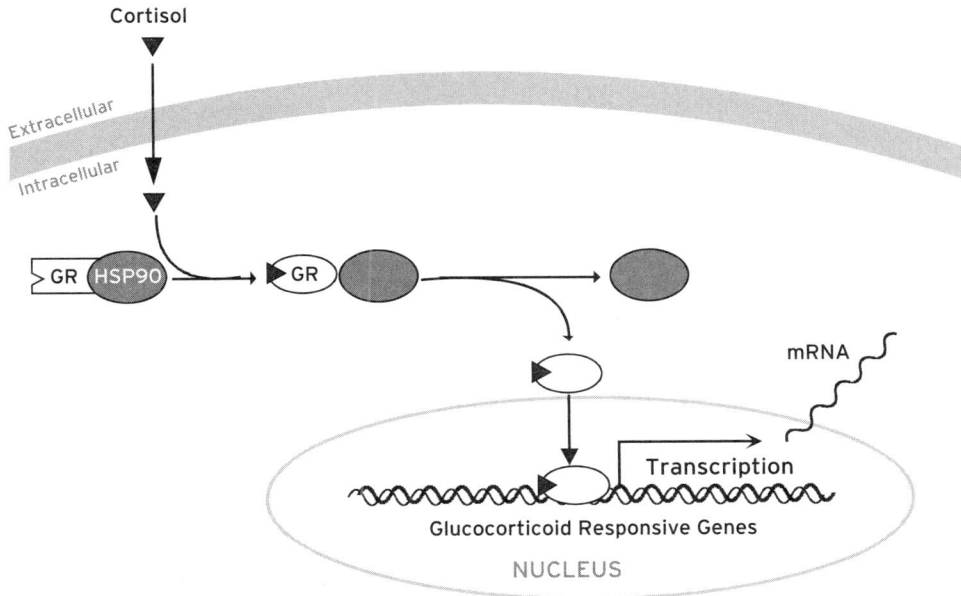

signal transduction. A breakdown product of sphingomyelin, ceramide, may play a role of second messenger. It should be noted that breakdown of membrane phospholipids does not only generate metabolites that contain fatty acids and are relatively hydrophobic, but also water-soluble molecules that are second messengers. An important molecule in that category is inositol-trisphosphate (IP3), a second messenger released from a membrane phospholipid (phosphatidylinositol-4,5bisphosphate) following the action of phospholipase C (PLC, Boxes 4.10 and 4.11). IP3 triggers the release of Ca^{2+} from intracellular stores (see Box 4.12).

CA²⁺

Normal concentrations of Ca^{2+} in the cytosol are very low, due to the impermeability of membranes to this ion and the efficiency of the mechanisms of extrusion (Box 4.12). Ca^{2+} can flow into the cytosol either from the outside through neurotransmitter- or voltage-operated Ca^{2+} channels, or from internal stores (i.e., the endoplasmic reticulum) through Ca^{2+} channels called *inositol-trisphosphate* (IP_3) receptors and *ryanodine receptors* (see Box 4.12). Ca^{2+} has many biological effects that are brought about by its binding to a number of enzymes and their subsequent activation (see Table 4.3 in Box 4.12). Ca^{2+} binds directly to some of these enzymes that contain specific Ca^{2+}- binding domains. In many cases, however, Ca^{2+} interacts first with a small protein, *calmodulin*. The Ca^{2+}/calmodulin complex binds to many proteins, including signaling enzymes, and alters their properties. An important class of such enzymes is the Ca^{2+}/calmodulin-dependent protein kinases.

Depolarization of neurons triggers the opening of voltage-gated Ca^{2+} channels, leading to an increase in intracellular Ca^{2+}. In nerve terminals, this is the signal responsible for neurotransmitter release. Ca^{2+} influx also provides a mechanism by which nerve cell stimuli, such as the action potential, can be transduced into biochemical signals important for the regulation of neurotransmitter synthesis, gene expression, and many other responses in neurons. Ca^{2+} is an essential trigger of the biochemical reactions that result in long-term depression and long-term potentiation of synaptic efficacy. These forms of synaptic plasticity are thought to be important cellular bases of learning and memory. In addition to its paramount role in neuronal physiology, Ca^{2+} is a key player in the induction of neuronal death in pathological circumstances. For instance,

BOX 4.7 G PROTEINS

G proteins can bind GDP or GTP. They act as molecular switches that are active in the GTP-bound form and inactive in the GDP-bound form. Although G proteins are not transmembrane proteins, they are attached to the membrane by various lipid molecules covalently bound to the protein and inserted into the membrane. Examples of G proteins are listed in Table 4.2.

Small G proteins are simple molecular switches. In the resting state they are bound to GDP and are inactive. The exchange of GDP for GTP is catalyzed by a guanine nucleotide exchange factor (GEF). In the case of Ras, the GEF is brought into play by its adaptor-mediated attachment to phosphorylated growth factor receptors (Box 4.3). In its GTP-bound form, Ras is active and triggers a cascade of phosphorylation reactions (Box 4.8). The inactivation of Ras requires a specific type of protein, called *GAP* (GTPase activating protein). GAP allows Ras to hydrolyze GTP and to return to the inactive, GDP-bound state.

Although the principle of their function is similar to that of small G proteins, large G proteins are more complicated. These heterotrimeric G proteins are composed of three subunits (α, β, and γ). The α subunit is the one that binds GDP and GTP. The exchange of GDP for GTP is triggered by seven transmembrane domain receptors, when they are bound to their ligand, a neurotransmitter or hormone (Box 4.2). Then, α-GTP and β/γ can diffuse freely at the level of the membrane and act on various targets (Box 4.2). The α subunit has the ability to hydrolyze GTP and to return spontaneously to the inactive GDP-bound form, behaving as a time device. Alpha subunits are the targets of bacterial toxins: α_s is irreversibly activated by cholera toxin, whereas α_i and α_o are irreversibly inhibited by the toxin of *Bordetella pertussis*, the agent of whooping cough.

(A) **Small G proteins**

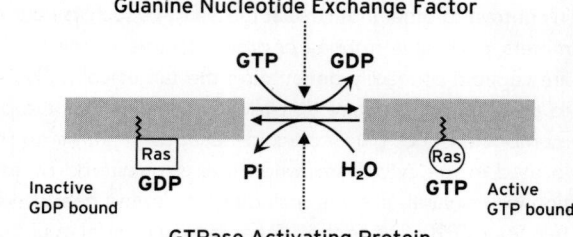

(B) **Heterotrimeric G proteins**

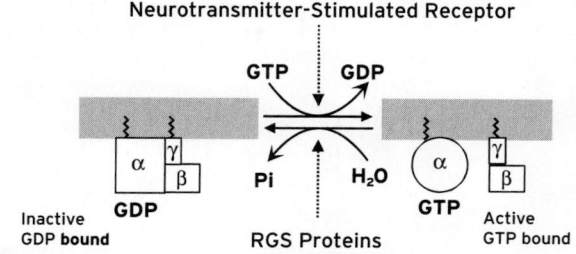

Recently, GAPs for some α subunits have been identified. They are called *RGS* (regulator of G protein signaling) and facilitate the return to the inactive GDP-bound form of the G protein.

Other abbreviations: G protein: guanine nucleotide binding protein; GDP: guanosine 5'-diphosphate; GTP: guanosine 5'-triphosphate; Pi: inorganic phosphate.

Further reading: Bourne, 1995, 1997; Jaffe and Hall, 2005; Koelle, 2006; Luttrell, 2006; Steyaert and Kobilka, 2011.

TABLE 4.2. Examples of GTP-binding proteins

GTP-BINDING PROTEIN CLASS	NAME	FUNCTION
Small G proteins	Ras	Responds to growth factors, activates Raf/MAP kinase pathway
	Rho	Regulates actin filaments
	Rab	Regulates vesicle trafficking, including synaptic vesicles
Heterotrimeric G proteins		
α subunit (binds GTP)	α_S, α_{Olf}	Activate adenylyl cyclase
	α_i	Inhibits adenylyl cyclase, activates K$^+$ channels
	α_t	Stimulates cGMP phosphodiesterase (retina)
	$\alpha_q, \alpha_{11, 14-16}$	Stimulate phospholipase C
	α_O	Inhibits Ca^{2+} channels
	$\alpha_{12, 13}$	Activate Na$^+$/H$^+$ exchanger
β/γ (does not bind GTP directly, but associates to α subunits)	$\beta_{1-5}, \gamma_{1-8}$	Activate or inhibit adenylyl cyclase and phospholipase C, activate K$^+$ channels, MAP kinase pathway, recruit β-adrenoceptor kinase

CGMP: cyclic guanosine 3'-5'-monophosphate; GTP: guanosine 5'-triphosphate; MAP kinase: mitogen-activated protein kinase.

Stimulation of growth factor receptors results in the conversion of Ras to its active GTP-bound form (Boxes 4.3 and 4.7). Ras exerts its effects by triggering a protein kinase cascade that results, among other things, in the increased transcription of specific genes. The first step is the recruitment to the membrane, by Ras-GTP, of a protein kinase called *Raf*, which, thus, becomes activated (there are several isoforms of Raf: A-Raf-1, B-Raf, and cRaf-1). Raf phosphorylates a second protein kinase called *MEK* (MAP kinase/ERK kinase). Phosphorylation of MEK activates it, making it capable of phosphorylating ERK (extracellular signal-regulated kinase) also called *MAP kinase* (mitogen-activated protein kinase). MEK is an unusual protein kinase that is able to phosphorylate ERK on threonine and tyrosine residues. This double phosphorylation activates ERK

that can phosphorylate cytoplasmic substrates such as phospholipase A2 (Box 4.10) or enter the nucleus. In the nucleus, ERK phosphorylates transcription factors, including Elk-1, a component of the ternary complex factor, thus increasing the transcription of specific genes. This cascade of biochemical reactions is important in the regulation of cell growth and differentiation. In fact, it represents one example of a highly conserved set of kinase cascades that are involved in signal transduction in all eukaryotic cells. For example, two other pathways leading to the activation of MAPKs termed *JNK* and *p38-MAPK* are organized in a very similar manner.

Other abbreviations: ERK: extracellular signal regulated kinase; GTP: guanosine 5'-triphosphate; JNK: *c-Jun N*-terminal kinase; P: phosphate group.

Further reading: Girault et al., 2007; Lu et al., 2006; Shalin et al., 2006; Zebisch et al., 2007.

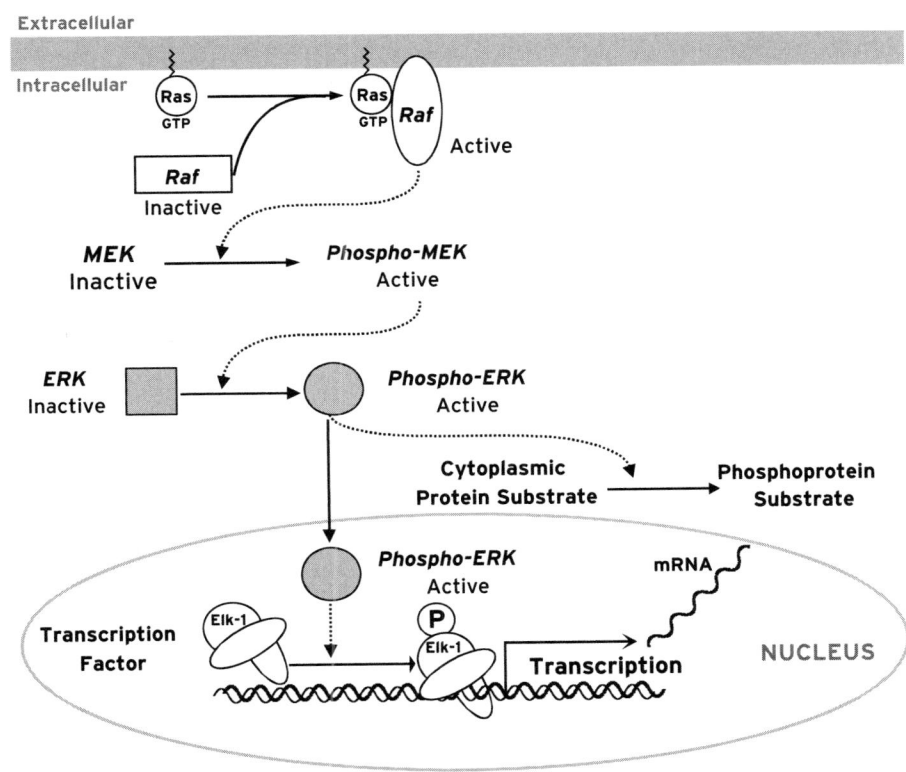

during hypoxia extracellular glutamate levels increase, leading to an abnormal stimulation of glutamate NMDA receptors. This, in combination with the partial depolarization of neuronal membranes and impairment of Ca^{2+} extrusion mechanisms (due to an energy deficiency), leads to a prolonged increase in cytosolic Ca^{2+} concentrations. Ca^{2+} triggers several cascades of reactions that can lead to neuronal death. Such reactions are the subject of intense investigations, with the hope that their pharmacological inhibition will improve survival and recovery in stroke and other neurological diseases.

DIFFUSIBLE MOLECULES ACTING AS INTERCELLULAR AND INTRACELLULAR MESSENGERS

ARACHIDONIC ACID AND ITS METABOLITES

Arachidonic acid is a 20-carbon fatty acid with four double bonds. It is released from precursor phospholipids by phospholipase A2 (Box 4.10). It can act in the cells in which it has been produced, for instance, by stimulating protein kinase C. Arachidonic acid can also diffuse to neighboring cells or nerve terminals and act as a local intercellular messenger. In addition,

BOX 4.9 cAMP

Cyclic adenosine 3'-5'-monophosphate (cAMP) is formed from ATP by a class of transmembrane enzymes, *adenylyl cyclases*. Adenylyl cyclases are activated by two related subtypes of α subunits of heterotrimeric G proteins: α_s (stimulatory) and α_{olf} (olfactory, which is found in olfactory epithelium and some brain neurons such as striatal neurons). Adenylyl cyclases are inhibited by α_i (inhibitory). In addition, some adenylyl cyclases can be stimulated or inhibited by β/γ subunits of heterotrimeric G proteins, or Ca^{2+} combined with calmodulin. cAMP is inactivated by hydrolysis into AMP by phosphodiesterases, a family of enzymes that are inhibited by theophylline and related methylxanthines. cAMP has very few targets in vertebrates, including a cAMP-gated ion channel that is most prominently found in olfactory neurons, cAMP-regulated guanine nucleotide exchange factors (GEF; see Box 4.7), and the cAMP-dependent protein kinase that is present in all cells. cAMP-dependent protein kinase is a tetramer composed of two catalytic subunits and two regulatory subunits (only one of each is shown on the figure). When cAMP binds to the regulatory subunits (two molecules of cAMP bind to each regulatory subunit), they dissociate from the catalytic subunits that, once free, are active as protein kinases. The catalytic subunit phosphorylates numerous specific substrates including ion channels, receptors, and enzymes synthesizing neurotransmitters. In addition, the catalytic subunit can enter the nucleus, where it phosphorylates transcription factors. One well-characterized transcription factor phosphorylated in response to cAMP is CREB (cAMP-response element binding protein). CREB forms a dimer that binds to a specific DNA sequence in the promoter region of cAMP-responsive genes, called *CRE* (cyclic AMP-response element). However, CREB is unable to promote transcription when it is not phosphorylated, whereas phospho-CREB strongly stimulates transcription. Genes regulated by CREB include immediate early genes *c-Fos* and *c-Jun* (Box 4.16). It should be noted that CREB is also activated by Ca2+/calmodulin dependent protein kinases and by protein kinases downstream from MAP kinases (see Table 4.3, Box 4.11).

Other abbreviations: ATP: adenosine 5'-triphosphate.

Further reading: Arnsten et al., 2005; Michel and Scott, 2002; Smith et al., 1999.

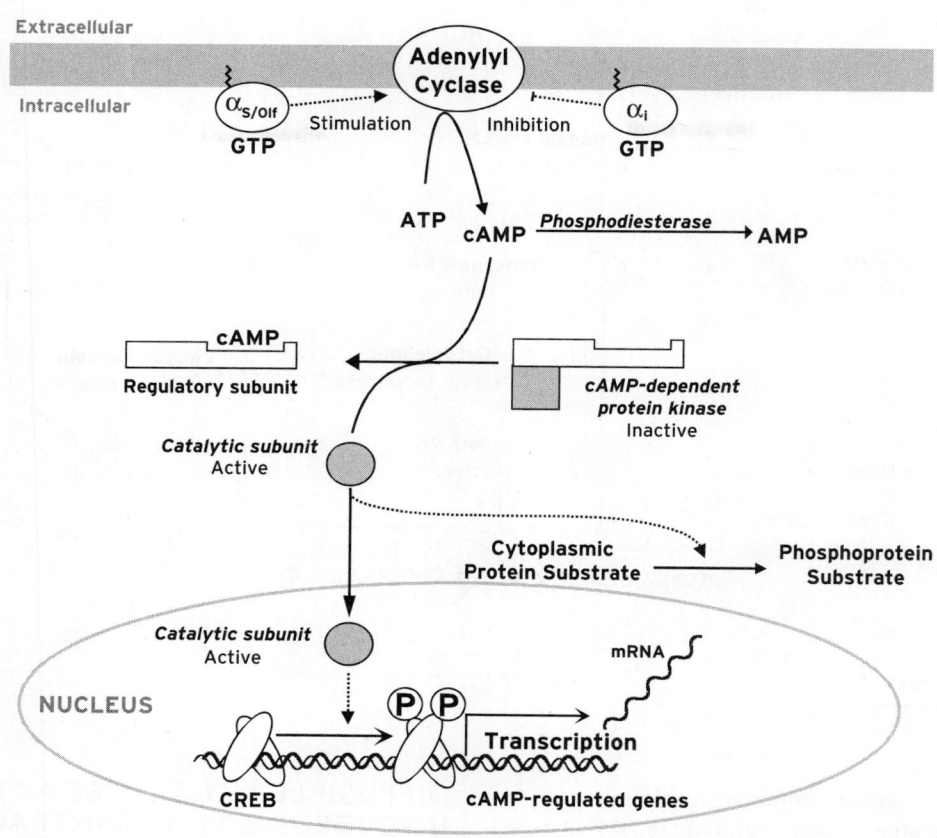

it is a precursor for a large family of signaling molecules called *eicosanoids* (*eicosi* is the Greek radical for 20, referring to the length of the carbon chain). Such molecules include prostaglandins, thromboxanes, and hydroperoxymetabolites. A particular class of interesting derivatives of arachidonic acid is composed of endogenous ligands for brain cannabinoid receptors, referred to as *endocannabinoids*. Cannabinoid receptors are the targets of Δ9-tetrahydrocannabinol, the main active substance in cannabis (hashish and marijuana). Endocannabinoids include arachidonoylethanolamine, also called *anandamide* (from *ananda*, the Sanskrit word for "bliss"), and 2-arachidonoylglycerol, which are released from specific phospholipid precursors in a

The basic backbone of major phospholipids is made up of glycerol that is esterified on positions 1 and 2 by fatty acids and on position 3 by a phosphate group, forming phosphatidic acid. The two fatty acids are inserted into the membrane to which they attach the phospholipid. A water-soluble molecule is linked to the phosphate, giving rise to various types of phospholipids such as phosphatidyl-choline, phosphatidyl-ethanolamine, or phosphatidyl-inositol. Enzymes called *phospholipases* are capable of hydrolyzing specific chemical bonds within these phospholipids, as indicated by solid arrows in the figure.

Phospholipase A2 (PLA2) releases the fatty acid located in position 2 of the glycerol backbone. PLA2 acts preferentially on phosphatidyl-choline or phosphatidyl-ethanolamine, in which the fatty acid in position 2 is arachidonic acid, releasing a lysophospholipid and free arachidonic acid. Arachidonic acid is moderately hydrophobic and can diffuse within the cell in which it has been formed, or to neighboring cells. It has several intrinsic biological activities by itself and is also a precursor for many active molecules called *eicosanoids*, including prostaglandins, thromboxanes, and hydroperoxymetabolites. PLA2 is activated by many extracellular signals including neurotransmitters, although the mechanism of its regulation is still incompletely understood.

Phospholipase C (PLC) hydrolyzes the bond between the phosphate group and the glycerol backbone. PLC acts preferentially on phosphatidylinositol 4,5 bisphosphate and generates diacylglycerol and inositol 1,4,5 trisphosphate (IP_3; see Box 4.11). Diacylglycerol stays in the membrane and participates in the activation of protein kinase C. IP_3 is very water-soluble and diffuses in the cytosol. It binds to a receptor located on the endoplasmic reticulum and triggers the release of Ca^{2+} from internal stores (Box 4.11). Among many other actions, Ca^{2+} participates in the activation of protein kinase C. PLC is activated by many neurotransmitters that act on G protein–coupled, seven transmembrane domain receptors. PLC is stimulated by α_q-GTP and α_{11}-GTP as well as by some β/γ complexes (Boxes 4.2 and 4.7).

Phospholipase D (PLD) acts preferentially on phosphatidylcholine and hydrolyzes the bond between the phosphate group and the water-soluble molecule that esterifies it. Thus, it releases phosphatidic acid and choline. It is not known if choline has a role in signal transduction. On the other hand, phosphatidic acid stimulates protein kinase C subtypes. Although PLD is activated by several extracellular signals, including neurotransmitters, the mechanism of its activation is still incompletely understood.

Other abbreviations: G protein: guanine nucleotide binding protein.

Further reading: Cockcroft, 2006; Farooqui et al., 2006.

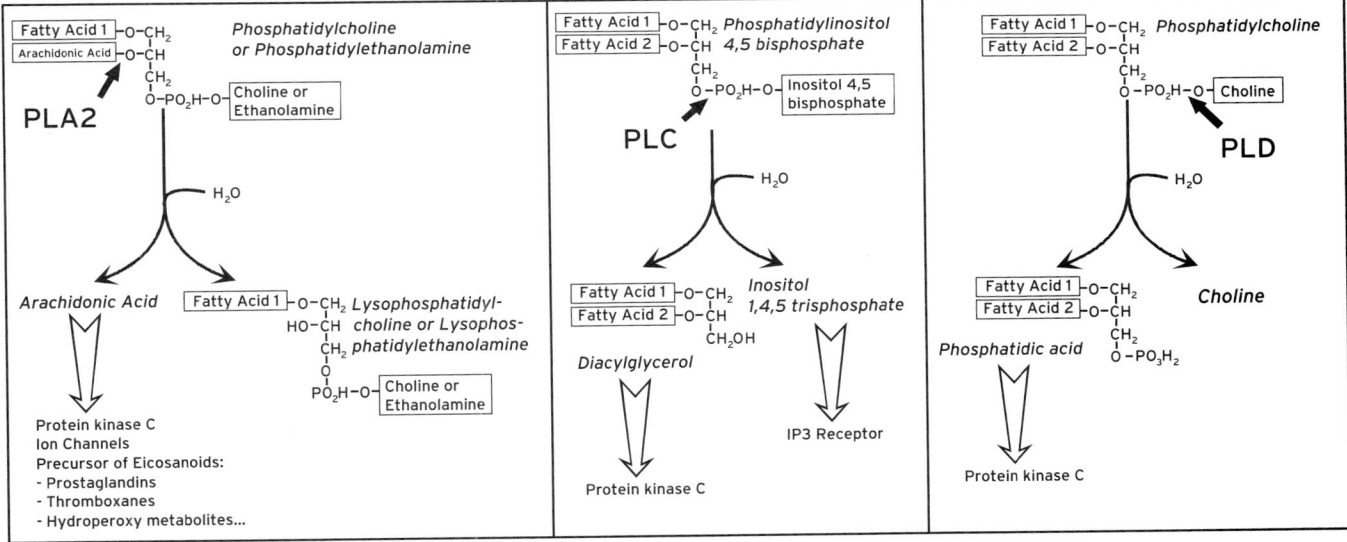

Ca^{2+}-dependent manner. Endocannabinoids, which do not easily cross cell membranes, are intercellular messengers, rather than second messengers, and are implicated in important aspects of neuromodulation, such as retrograde signaling from postsynaptic to presynaptic sites.

NITRIC OXIDE

Nitric oxide (NO) is a gas molecule that has important biological functions. On the one hand, it is a highly reactive chemical species that is used by macrophages to destroy exogenous substances. On the other hand, it is a chemical messenger, which can diffuse freely, over a short range, through cellular membranes. Nitric oxide was originally discovered as a vasodilator substance generated by endothelial cells that acts on smooth muscle cells of blood vessels. In neurons, *NO synthase*, the enzyme that generates NO, is activated by Ca^{2+} (Box 4.13). A well-characterized effect of NO is to increase cGMP by activation of soluble guanylyl cyclase. Because of its diffusible nature, NO is a retrograde messenger in the nervous system, diffusing

BOX 4.11 INOSITOL-TRISPHOSPHATE

Inositol 1,4,5 trisphosphate (IP_3) is an important second messenger. It is generated by the enzyme phospholipase C (PLC) that hydrolyzes a membrane phospholipid, *phosphatidylinositol 4,5 bisphosphate* (see Box 4.10). PLC is activated by neurotransmitters that act on G protein–coupled, seven transmembrane domain receptors (Box 4.2). PLC generates diacylglycerol and IP_3. IP_3 is very water soluble and diffuses in the cytosol. It binds to a receptor located on the endoplasmic reticulum and thereby triggers the release of Ca^{2+} from internal stores (see Box 4.12). Inositol 1,4,5 trisphosphate is inactivated by several phosphoinositol phosphatases that remove successively the phosphate molecules from the inositol backbone. These phosphatases can act in various sequences, not necessarily that depicted in the figure. The phosphatase that removes the phosphate in position 1 of the inositol backbone is inhibited by lithium (Li^+). Inositol can be reincorporated into membrane phospholipids by its coupling to an activated form of diacylglycerol (CDP-diacylglycerol) and phosphorylated on positions 4 and 5 by specific kinases to regenerate phosphatidylinositol 4,5 bisphosphate (broken arrow in the figure). Chronic treatment with lithium may decrease the amount of inositol that can be incorporated into neuronal phospholipids and thus dampen the effects of neurotransmitters that activate PLC. This property of lithium may participate in its mood stabilizing effects.

Other abbreviations: CDP: cytosine 5'-diphosphate; G protein: guanine nucleotide binding protein; Pi: inorganic phosphate.

Further reading: Berridge et al., 2000; Berridge, 2009; Collin et al., 2005; Iino, 2007; Pietrobon, 2005; Stutzmann and Mattson, 2011.

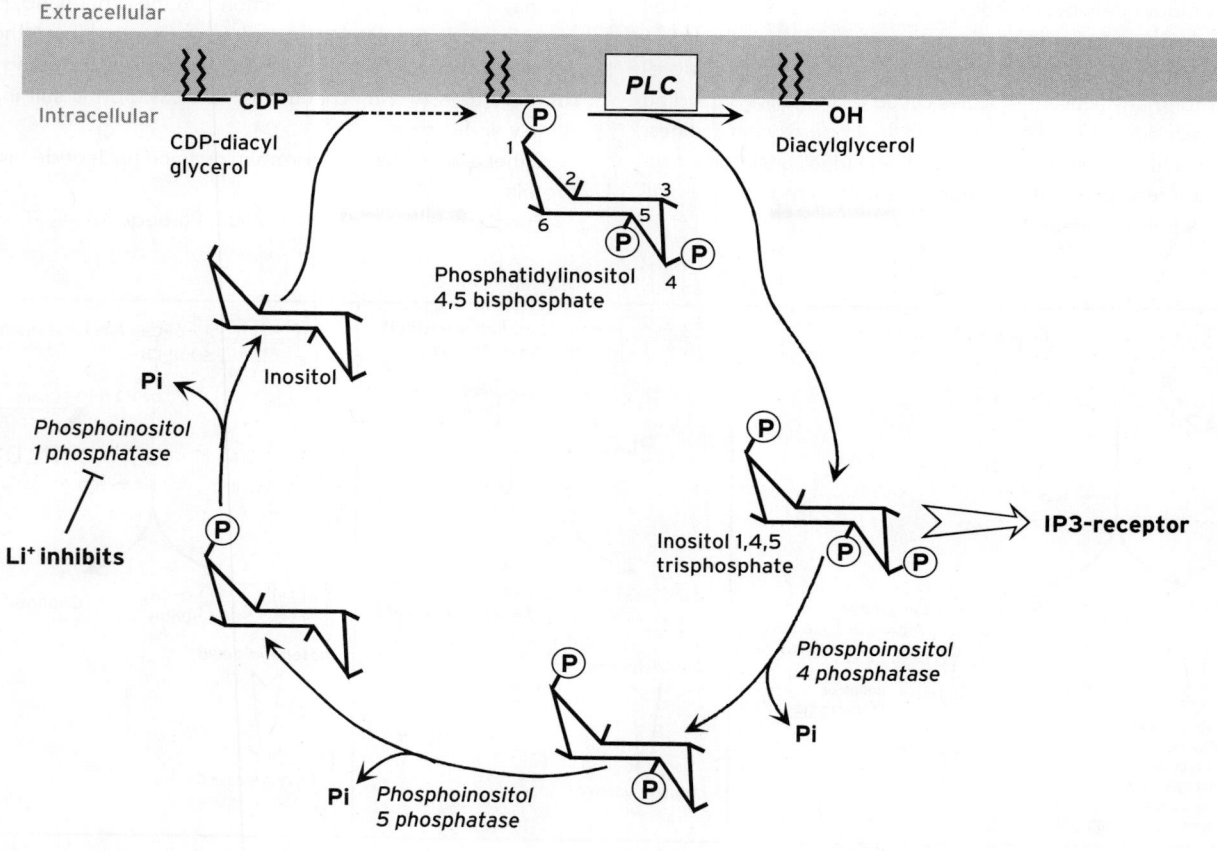

from the postsynaptic to the presynaptic side of synapses, and thus plays a role in synaptic plasticity (Chapter 5).

PROTEIN PHOSPHORYLATION

Protein phosphorylation is a reversible covalent chemical modification of proteins that plays a central role in signal transduction (Box 4.14). The vast majority of known signal transduction pathways involve the activation of one or several protein kinases, the enzymes that phosphorylate substrate proteins (see examples of protein kinases in Table 4.4 in Box 4.14). In most instances, it is by altering the state of phosphorylation of key intracellular proteins that intercellular messengers including neurotransmitters, hormones, growth factors, and others ultimately exert most of their effects. The amino acids whose side chains are phosphorylated in the context of signal transduction in multicellular animals (metazoans) are predominantly *serine*, *threonine*, and *tyrosine*. Most protein kinases belong to a very large and ancient gene family. They include serine/threonine kinases, tyrosine kinases, and a few dual specificity protein kinases (Table 4.1).

BOX 4.12 Ca²⁺

Ca²⁺ is a divalent cation whose concentrations are relatively high in the extracellular space (around 1.2 mM) and more than 10,000 times lower within the cytosol (around 100 nM). Some intracellular organelles, however, namely *mitochondria* and *endoplasmic reticulum*, contain high concentrations of Ca²⁺. In resting conditions the plasma membrane is impermeable to Ca²⁺. Ca²⁺ can penetrate neurons through specific channels, which include voltage-gated Ca²⁺ channels (VGCC) and glutamate receptors of the NMDA subtype. When these channels are open, in response to depolarization in the case of VGCC or in the presence of glutamate in the case of *N*-methyl-D-aspartate (NMDA) receptor (see Box 4.1), Ca²⁺ flows readily into the cytosol following its concentration gradient and the electrical potential. Ca²⁺ can also be released into the cytosol from internal stores that are mostly located in the endoplasmic reticulum. Two types of Ca²⁺ channels are responsible for the release of Ca²⁺ from internal stores. One is the inositol 1,4,5 trisphosphate (IP₃) receptor whose opening is triggered by IP₃, a second messenger generated by phospholipase C (Boxes 4.10 and 4.11). The other is the ryanodine receptor, named after *ryanodine*, a drug that triggers its opening, although it is not a physiological ligand. In fact, opening of ryanodine receptors is elicited by Ca²⁺ itself by a mechanism called *Ca²⁺-induced Ca²⁺ release*, which can give rise to propagation of waves of Ca²⁺ release along the endoplasmic reticulum. In the cytosol, Ca²⁺ is mostly bound to specific binding proteins. Some of them appear to play a role primarily as buffering proteins, preventing excessive rises in cytosolic free Ca²⁺. Other proteins are the actual targets of Ca²⁺, which account for its potent biological effects. Among the best characterized targets are calmodulin and calmodulin-related proteins. When they are bound to Ca²⁺, calmodulin and the related proteins undergo a conformational change that enables them

TABLE 4.3. Examples of target proteins for cytosolic free Ca²⁺

Ca²⁺-BINDING DOMAIN	TARGET PROTEIN	FUNCTION
Calmodulin	Ca²⁺/calmodulin kinases I, II, IV	Protein kinases that increase phosphorylation of multiple proteins
	Elongation factor 2 (EF2) kinase	Protein kinase that phosphorylates EF2 and inhibits protein synthesis
	Calcineurin (Phosphatase 2B)	Protein phosphatase that decreases phosphorylation of specific proteins
	Adenylyl cyclase	Increases cAMP
	Phosphodiesterase	Decreases cAMP
	NO synthase	Triggers NO production
Calmodulin-like	Calpains	Proteases that cut specific proteins
C2 domains	Protein kinase C	Increases phosphorylation of multiple proteins
	Phospholipase A2	Releases arachidonic acid
	Synaptotagmin	Regulates neurotransmitter release

to interact with, and activate, a number of enzymes (Table 4.3). Ca²⁺ can also bind to another type of protein domain called *C2* that is found in several different proteins (Table 4.3). Free Ca²⁺ in the cytosol is maintained at very low levels by several

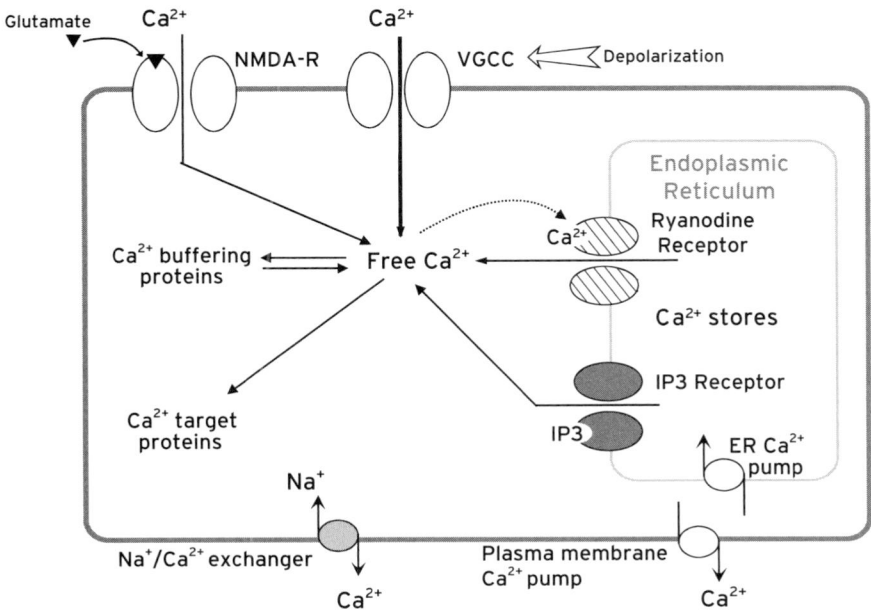

(continued)

BOX 4.12 *CONTINUED*

highly active processes, which include Ca^{2+} pumps and Ca^{2+} exchangers. Ca^{2+} pumps have a high affinity but a low capacity for Ca^{2+} and are used for fine-tuning Ca^{2+} levels. They are located on the plasma membrane and the membrane of the endoplasmic reticulum, and their energy is provided by ATP hydrolysis. Na^+/Ca^{2+} exchangers, whose driving force is provided by the Na^+ gradient, have a large capacity, but a low affinity for Ca^{2+}.

Other abbreviations: C2: second constant domain within protein kinase C sequence; cAMP: cyclic adenosine 3'-5'-monophosphate; ER: endoplasmic reticulum; NMDA-R: *N*-methyl-D-aspartate subtype of glutamate receptor.

Further reading: Berridge et al., 2000; Berridge, 2009; Collin et al., 2005; Mikoshiba and Hattori, 2000; Pietrobon, 2005.

BOX 4.13 NITRIC OXIDE

Nitric oxide (NO) is a gas that is highly diffusible and chemically reactive. In the nervous system it is used as a locally active intra- or intercellular messenger. The enzyme responsible for the formation of NO is NO synthase (NOS). It is activated by Ca^{2+} associated to calmodulin. In neurons, opening of glutamate receptors of the *N*-methyl-D-aspartate (NMDA) subtype is a major source of Ca^{2+} influx (Box 4.1) that can lead to the activation of NOS. NOS is a complex enzyme that uses molecular oxygen, O_2, to generate NO by transforming arginine into citrulline. NO can cross membranes readily and diffuse to neighboring cells or nerve endings. Thus, the rest of the cascade depicted in the figure can take place in a cell different from that in which NO was generated, as symbolized by the dotted pair of lines in the figure. A major target of NO is soluble guanylyl cyclase. This enzyme is activated by NO and uses guanosine 5'-triphosphate (GTP) to form cyclic guanosine 3',5'- monophosphate (cGMP), a second messenger that remains within the cell in which it is produced. cGMP exerts its effects by activating several enzymes, one of which is cGMP-dependent protein kinase. Phosphorylation of specific proteins by cGMP-dependent protein kinase accounts for some of the physiological effects of NO.

Other abbreviations: GC: guanylyl cyclase; NMDA-R: *N*-methyl-D-aspartate subtype of glutamate receptor; PKG: cGMP-dependent protein kinase.

Further reading: Iino, 2006; Snyder et al., 1998.

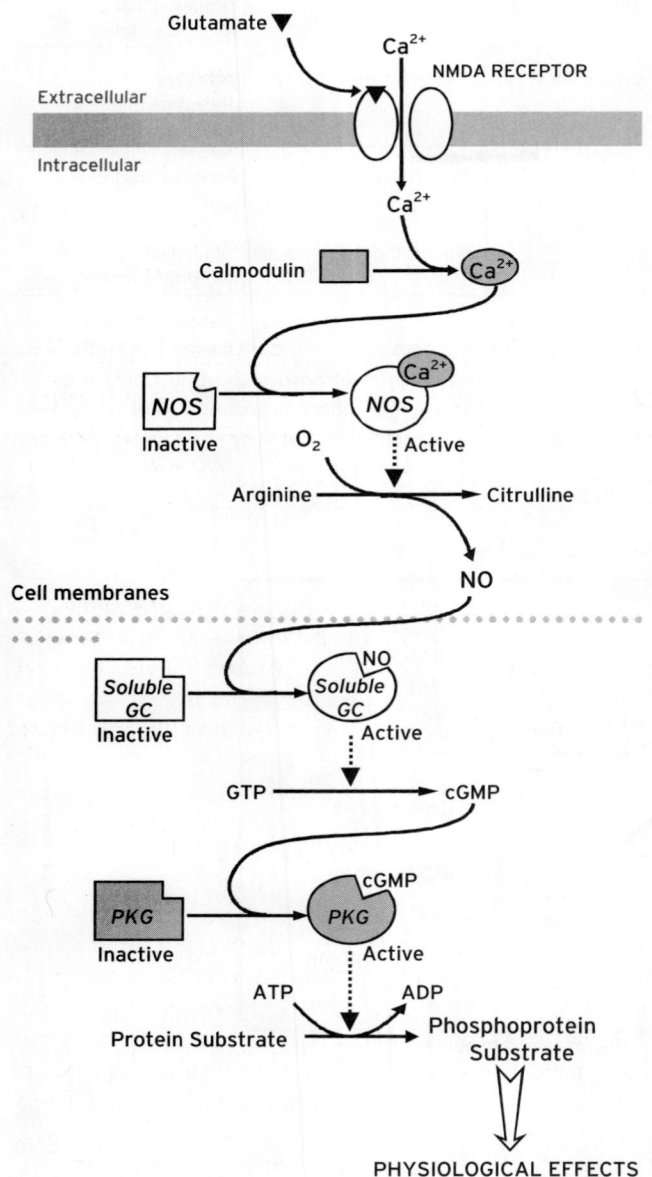

The presence of a bulky and negatively charged phosphate group on the side chain of these amino acids can change dramatically the properties of the protein, leading to the activation or inhibition of enzymes, opening or closing of ion channels, modulation of neurotransmitter receptors, activation of transcription factors, and so forth (examples of neuronal proteins regulated by phosphorylation are listed in Table 4.6 in Box 4.14). Thus, phosphorylation reactions play an effector role when the substrate proteins are critical components for the behavior of cells (see Box 4.14). In addition, protein phosphorylation is involved in cascades of signal transduction in two other ways. First, phosphorylation of amino acid residues can promote the recruitment of proteins important for signal transduction, as exemplified by interaction of protein regions phosphorylated on tyrosine with Src-homology-2 (SH2) domains (Boxes 4.3–4.5). Second, many signaling pathways involve protein kinase cascades in which a first kinase activates a second kinase, which activates a third one, and so on. Functions of such kinase cascades (see Box 4.8 for an example and also Box 4.18) are to provide amplification and, in some cases, to turn graded inputs into switch-like all-or-none responses (bistable systems).

The state of phosphorylation of a protein is determined by its relative rates of phosphorylation and dephosphorylation. The enzymes that remove phosphate groups from proteins are called *phosphoprotein phosphatases* (Box 4.14, Table 4.5) and

BOX 4.14 PROTEIN PHOSPHORYLATION

Phosphorylation is carried out by protein kinases, which, in the presence of Mg^{2+}, transfer a phosphoryl group from ATP to serine, threonine, or tyrosine residues. Because these kinases often recognize the amino acid sequence surrounding the serine, threonine, or tyrosine to be phosphorylated, protein kinases have a high degree of substrate specificity. Protein kinases form a very large group of related enzymes, each of which has its own localization, regulation, and substrate specificity (Table 4.4). Some protein kinases are either receptors for extracellular signals (Box 4.3) or are associated with such receptors (Box 4.5). Several protein kinases are activated directly by second messengers and account for most of the effects of these second messengers. These include cAMP- and cGMP-dependent protein kinases (Boxes 4.9 and 4.13), protein kinases activated by Ca^{2+} associated to calmodulin (Box 4.11), and protein kinase C, which is activated by Ca^{2+}, diacylglycerol, and/or several other lipid derivatives (Box 4.10). Some protein kinases are themselves regulated by phosphorylation and participate in kinase cascades (see Box 4.8).

The reverse reaction, the removal of the phosphate group, is catalyzed by phosphoprotein phosphatases. This class of enzymes, if not quite as large as that of protein kinases, includes many members belonging to several gene families (Table 4.5). Different types of phosphatases are responsible for the removal of phosphate groups from serine and threonine side chains and from tyrosine side chains. A very large number of important neuronal proteins are regulated by phosphorylation/dephosphorylation (Table 4.6).

Other abbreviations: ATP: adenosine 5'-triphosphate; cAMP: cyclic adenosine 3'-5'-monophosphate; cGMP: cyclic guanosine 3'-5'-monophosphate.

Further reading: Greengard, 2001; Johnson and Hunter, 2005; Mansuy and Shenolikar, 2006; Papin et al., 2005.

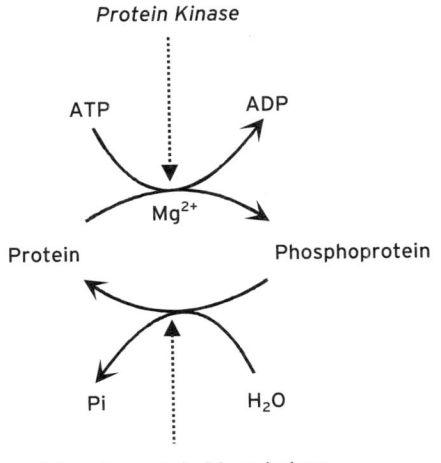

TABLE 4.4. Examples of protein kinases

PHOSPHORYLATED AMINO ACID	ACTIVATION MECHANISM	PROTEIN KINASE
Serine and/or threonine	cAMP	cAMP-dependent protein kinase
	cGMP	cGMP-dependent protein kinase
	Ca^{2+}-calmodulin	Ca^{2+}/calmodulin kinases I, II,IV
		Elongation factor 2 kinase
	Ca^{2+}, DAG, arachidonic acid	Protein kinase C
	Interaction with Ras-GTP	Raf
	Recruitment to the membrane by phosphoinositides	Akt (or PKB)
	Phosphorylation	MAP kinases (ERK, JNK, p38-MAP kinase)
	Phosphorylation, dephosphorylation, cyclin binding	Cyclin-dependent kinases
	Extracellular ligand binding	Receptors for TGFβ, activin, inhibin, etc.
Tyrosine	Extracellular ligand binding	Receptors for insulin or growth factors
	Interaction with a receptor	JAK, Src family kinases
Threonine and tyrosine	Phosphorylation	MAP kinase (or MEK)

may be as important in signal transduction as protein kinases. The regulation of protein phosphatases is, in general, not as well understood as that of protein kinases. There are nevertheless well-documented examples of protein phosphatases whose activity is regulated by neurotransmitters, as illustrated in Box 4.15.

SIGNALING BY PROTEOLYSIS

In contrast to non-covalent protein–protein interactions and to protein phosphorylation, which are reversible, proteolysis is irreversible. In addition to its obvious role in the degradation of proteins, proteolysis is involved in intracellular signaling cascades. For example, signals that lead to programmed cell death, or *apoptosis*, activate a set of proteases, the *caspases*. Caspases activate each other in an ordered manner by limited proteolysis and also contribute directly to cell death by cleaving a number of cellular proteins (Box 4.16).

TABLE 4.5. Classification of phosphoprotein phosphatases*

TARGET PHOSPHO-AMINO ACID	PROPERTIES	CLASSICAL NAME	NEW NAME
Phosphoserine and/or phosphothreonine	Sensitive to specific protein inhibitors (phospho-inhibitor 1, phospho-DARPP-32, inhibitor 2)	Phosphatase 1	PPP1
	Insensitive to these inhibitors		
	Insensitive to divalent cations	Phosphatase 2A	PPP2
	Activated by Ca^{2+}	Phosphatase 2B (Calcineurin)	PPP3
	Requires Mg^{2+}	Phosphatase 2C	PPM
Phosphotyrosine	Transmembrane "receptor-like" proteins	RPTP	
	Cytoplasmic proteins (usually possess targeting domains)	PTP	
Dual specificity: phosphoserine and/or phosphothreonine and/or phosphotyrosine		Phosphatases acting on MAP kinase or cyclin-dependent kinases	

*Several other Ser/Thr protein phosphatases have been identified, including PP4 and PP6, which are close to PP2A, and PP5 and PPP7. A new nomenclature has been proposed that takes into account the sequence similarities of the catalytic domain. PPP, phosphoprotein phosphatase, PPM, protein phosphatases dependent from Mg^{2+} or Mn^{2+}.

TABLE 4.6. Examples of neuronal proteins regulated by phosphorylation/dephosphorylation

REGULATED PROTEIN	PROTEIN KINASE	EFFECT
Ion channels		
Ca^{2+} (L type)	cAMP-dependent	Increases Ca^{2+} permeability
K^+ (Kv1.2, 1.3)	Tyrosine kinase	Closes the channel
Na^+	PKC, cAMP-dependent	Decreases Na^+ permeability
Neurotransmitter-gated ion channels		
Glutamate (AMPA-subtype)	cAMP-dependent	Increases response
Glutamate (NMDA-subtype)	PKC, tyrosine kinase	Increases response
GABA-A	Tyrosine kinase	Increases response
G protein-coupled receptors		
β-adrenoceptor	β-adrenoceptor kinase	Desensitization, recruitment of partners
Neurotransmitter synthesizing enzymes		
Tyrosine hydroxylase	cAMP-, Ca^{2+}/calmodulin-dependent, MAP kinase	Increases catecholamine synthesis
Tryptophan hydroxylase	Ca^{2+}/calmodulin-dependent	Increases serotonin synthesis
Synaptic vesicle proteins		
Synapsins	Ca^{2+}/calmodulin-dependent	Facilitates neurotransmitter release
Transcription factors		
CREB	cAMP-dependent, kinases activated by MAP kinases	Increases transcription

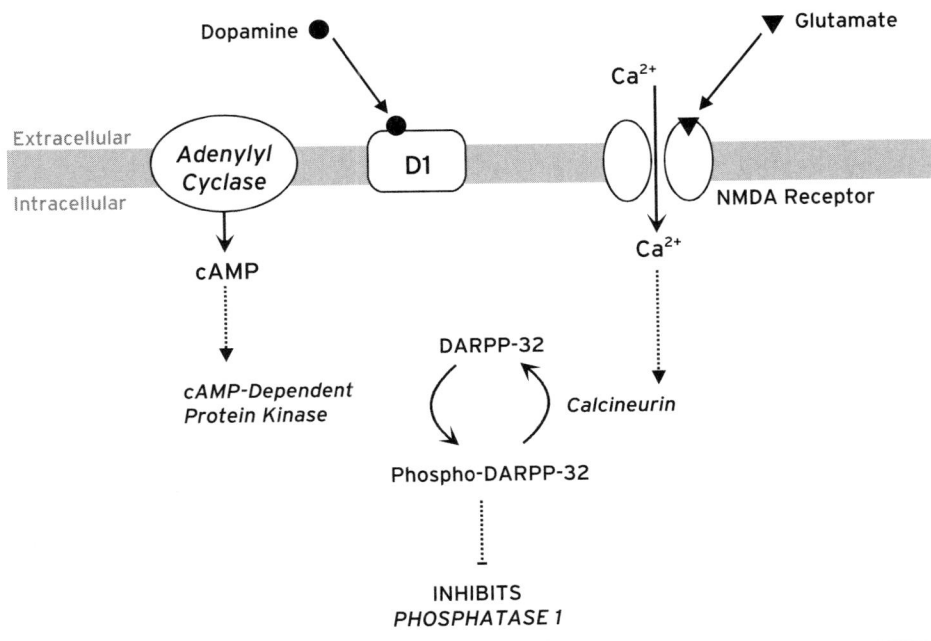

Other types of intracellular proteases can play a role in signaling, outside of the context of cell death. For example, calpains are proteases activated by increased levels of cytosolic free Ca^{2+} (Table 4.3 in Box 4.11). One important system for the degradation of cellular proteins is a large multiprotein complex called *proteasome*. Proteins are targeted to the proteasome by conjugation to a small polypeptide termed *ubiquitin*, under the action of specific enzymes and cofactors. The ubiquitin "tag" triggers the degradation of improperly folded proteins but also has a role in signaling (Box 4.16). Thus, recently several pathways of regulated proteolysis of specific proteins have been identified as important components of signal transduction not only for programmed cell death, but also during development as well as in the mature nervous system. Moreover, abnormal regulation of proteolysis is likely to be a key aspect in pathological conditions such as Alzheimer's disease.

REGULATION OF GENE EXPRESSION

Regulation of gene expression is an important target of signal transduction in neurons, as in other cells. Because of its long-lasting effects, it is important in mediating the actions of neurotrophins, as well as in learning and memory (Chapter 5). Signaling pathways involving growth factor receptors and the mitogen-activated protein (MAP) kinase cascade (Boxes 4.3 and 4.8), JAK-STAT associated receptors (Box 4.5), steroid hormones (Box 4.6), cAMP (Box 4.9), and proteolysis (Box 4.16) lead to changes in gene expression. Other pathways involving Ca^{2+}/calmodulin-activated protein kinases, or protein kinase C also exert profound effects on gene expression, via similar mechanisms. In fact, the promoter region of regulated genes often contains several consensus DNA sequences capable of interacting with specific transcription factors (see Chapter 6). The overall rate of transcription of

BOX 4.16 SIGNALING BY PROTEOLYSIS

In contrast to phosphorylation, which is reversible, proteolysis is irreversible. Nevertheless it is an important component of several signaling pathways. All cells can undergo a programmed cell death or apoptosis, which is a way to control precisely cell numbers during development and to eliminate abnormal cells. Excessive apoptosis is also a mechanism underlying many neurological diseases. A specific group of evolutionarily conserved proteases are termed *caspases* because they contain a cysteine residue in their active site and cleave their substrates in the vicinity of aspartate residues. Caspases are the final common pathway of apoptosis [see (A)]. Caspases exist as inactive precursors, the procaspases that become active following limited proteolysis. Upstream caspases are activated by autocleavage following interaction with specific factors in response to various signals. For example, procaspase-8 is activated by ligation of "death receptors" such as Fas and the p75 neurotrophin receptor, while procaspase-9 is activated by the release of proapoptotic factors from mitochondria. Once in their active form, these caspases cleave and activate effector caspases, such as caspase-3, which contribute to cell death by cutting multiple cellular proteins. Degradation of proteins by the proteasome is important for the elimination of abnormal or improperly folded proteins. It is also involved in some signaling pathways. Proteins are targeted for degradation in the proteasome by the attachment to their lysine side chains of one or several polypeptides called *ubiquitin*. For example, this mechanism is important for the activation of the transcription factor NFκB (*nuclear factorκB*, named because of its role in the regulation of κ immunoglobulin light chains in B lymphocytes) [see (B)]. NFκB plays a role in many biological responses ranging from early development to inflammation. NFκB is a dimer of two subunits maintained in an inactive state in the cytoplasm by interaction with an inhibitor protein termed *IκB*. Activation of NFκB in response to stimulation of various receptors involves its dissociation from IκB, triggered by phosphorylation. IκB is then ubiquitinated and degraded by the proteasome, allowing NFκB to translocate to the nucleus and activate transcription of multiple genes, some of which may have antiapoptotic effects.

Other abbreviation: TNFα: tumor necrosis factor alpha.

Further reading: Baud and Karin, 2001; Jiang and Wang, 2004; Yan and Shi, 2005; Patrick, 2006.

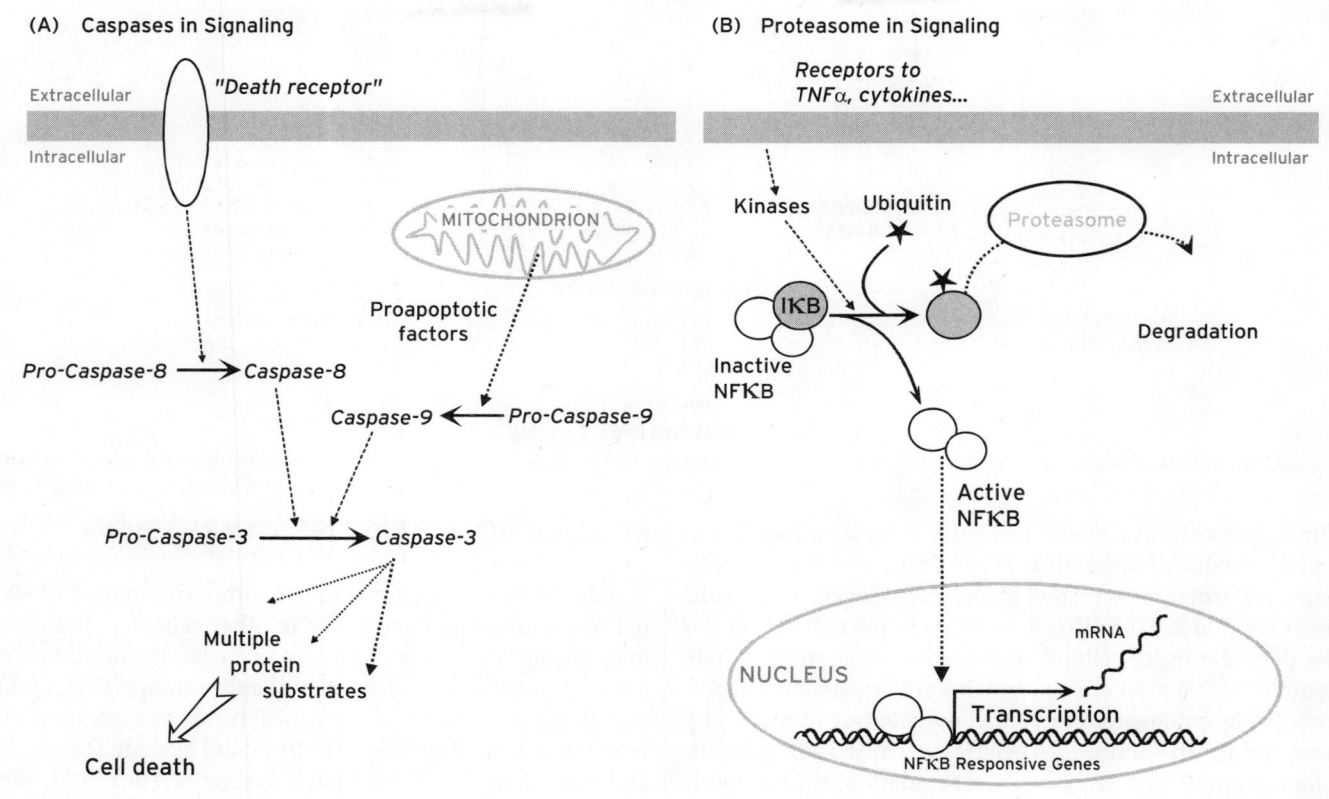

(A) Caspases in Signaling

(B) Proteasome in Signaling

such genes depends on the interaction between various transcription factors and the housekeeping proteins involved in mRNA synthesis. The nuclear localization, DNA-binding, and activity of transcription factors can be modulated by phosphorylation. In addition, signaling pathways regulate histones, which are basic proteins associated to DNA to form the chromatin, thereby facilitating or preventing the accessibility and transcription of specific genes. These regulations

BOX 4.17 IMMEDIATE EARLY GENES

The transcription of genes encoding certain transcription factors, such as c-Fos and c-Jun depicted here, is readily regulated by extracellular signals that act by various signal transduction pathways involving cAMP, Ca²⁺, or phosphorylation cascades (see Boxes 4.9, 4.12, and 4.8, respectively). The levels of c-Fos and c-Jun are very low in basal conditions, but their transcription increases dramatically and transiently in many neurons within minutes following various extracellular signals or depolarization. The increased transcription of these genes is the consequence of the phosphorylation of transcription factors that are already present in the cell under an inactive form, and which are activated by phosphorylation (examples of such factors are Elk-1, see Box 4.8, and cAMP-responsive element binding protein [CREB], see Box 4.9). Such genes are called *immediate early genes*, and stimulation of their transcription does not require protein synthesis to occur. When c-Fos and c-Jun messenger ribonucleic acids (mRNAs) are translated into proteins, these proteins dimerize and form an active transcription factor that binds to specific DNA sequences in the promoter region of other genes and stimulates their transcription. Transcription of these latter genes occurs several hours after the initial stimuli and is prevented by protein synthesis inhibitors that block the synthesis of c-Fos and c-Jun proteins (Chapter 6).

Other abbreviations: cAMP: cyclic adenosine 3′-5′-monophosphate.

Further reading: Girault et al., 2007; Guzowski et al., 2005; Hyman et al., 2006.

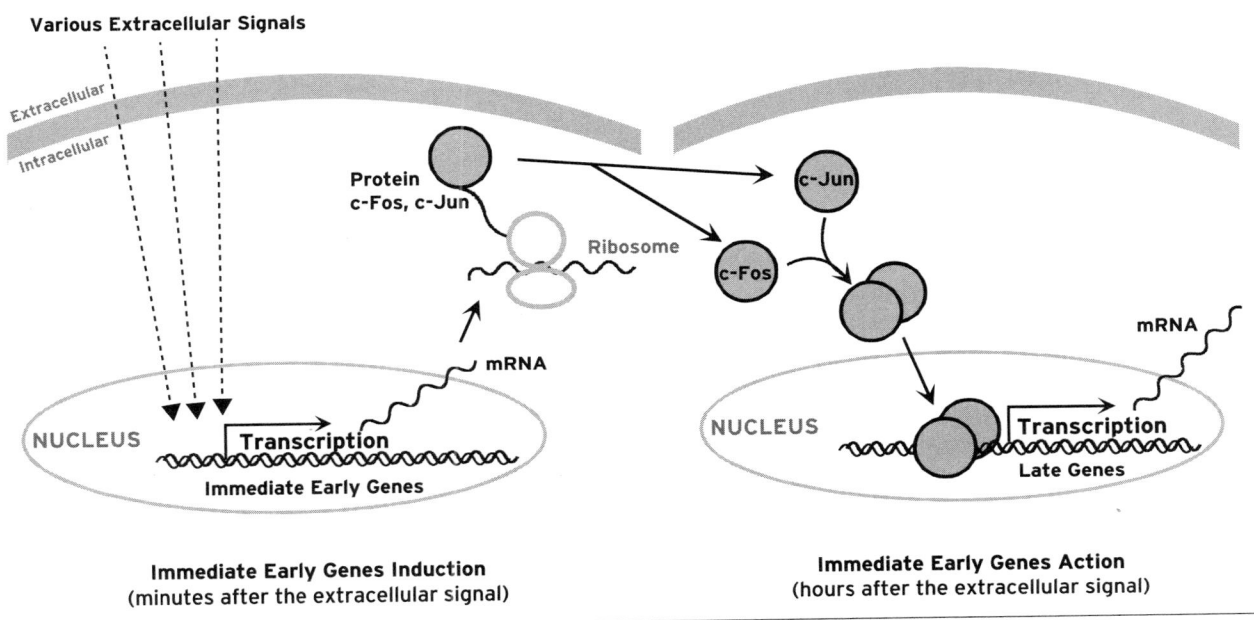

Various Extracellular Signals

Extracellular

Intracellular

Protein
c-Fos, c-Jun

Ribosome

c-Jun

c-Fos

mRNA

mRNA

NUCLEUS

Transcription

Immediate Early Genes

NUCLEUS

Transcription

Late Genes

Immediate Early Genes Induction
(minutes after the extracellular signal)

Immediate Early Genes Action
(hours after the extracellular signal)

include different types of modification of histones such as phosphorylation, methylation, and acetylation. Thus, several signal transduction pathways can converge to modulate precisely the levels of gene expression. Some transcription factors are present at low levels in basal conditions but can be rapidly induced in response to extracellular signals. These transcription factors belong to the class of immediate early genes, which include *c-Fos* and *c-Jun* and are useful markers of neuronal activity (Box 4.17).

TERMINATION OF SIGNALS

Intuitively, for cells to adapt swiftly to changes in their environment or incoming signals, it seems critical that they be able to stop rapidly the responses they started, pretty much as driving a car requires both an accelerator and a brake. This may be appropriate either when the external signal itself is off, or when the signal is too intense or too prolonged, so that excessive responding could become deleterious. In fact, most reactions of signal transduction are reversible and cells have developed highly sophisticated ways to control the duration and intensity of their responses. Most receptors go through several types of inactivation that prevent excessive stimulation. Many ligand-gated ion channels undergo desensitization. This means that in the presence of the neurotransmitter the receptor switches spontaneously into a closed (i.e., inactive) conformation, which is usually rather stable and corresponds to a state of high affinity for the neurotransmitter (see Box 4.1). G protein–coupled receptors also undergo desensitization and down-regulation (removal of the receptor from the cell surface by endocytosis), a process that involves phosphorylation of the receptor. Many G protein-coupled receptors are regulated by phosphorylation by a specific class of protein kinases (*G protein–coupled receptor kinases*, GRKs) that act specifically on the active, neurotransmitter-bound form of the receptor. Phosphorylation of the receptor by GRKs decreases or blocks its ability to interact with G proteins and facilitates

BOX 4.18 PI3 KINASE Akt mTOR PATHWAY

The importance of this pathway was initially identified in the context of insulin actions and control of glucose metabolism and cell growth. Further studies have shown its paramount importance in many cell functions and recently in brain development, function, and diseases. The initial step is the activation of PI3 kinase (PI3K), which is a lipid kinase that phosphorylates phosphatidyl-inositol-4,5 bisphosphate (PIP2, for the class I PI3 kinase depicted here) on the position 3 of the inositol moiety to form phosphatidyl-inositol-3,4,5 trisphosphate (PIP3). There are several classes of PI3 kinases that can be activated by receptor tyrosine kinases in response to growth factors (Box 4.3) or by some G protein–coupled receptors (Box 4.2). The dephosphorylation of PIP3 is catalyzed by PTEN (phosphatase and tensin homolog).

When PIP3 is formed at the inner face of the plasma membrane it recruits proteins that have domains that recognize specifically this phospholipid, such as the pleckstrin-homology (PH) domain. Akt (also termed PKB) and 3-phosphoinositide-dependent protein kinase 1(PDK-1) are two related protein kinases that have a PH domain [see (B)]. PDK-1 phosphorylates and activates Akt, which, in turn, phosphorylates and regulates many proteins including the tuberous sclerosis complex proteins 1 and 2 (TSC1/2). The TSC1/2 heteromer is a GTPase-activating protein for the small G protein Rheb (Box 4.7). Rheb, when it is bound to GTP, activates the mTOR complex 1 (mTORC1, comprising mTOR and Raptor). mTOR is a protein kinase and was identified as the mammalian target of rapamycin (hence its name), a potent immunosuppressor

which acts by inhibiting the protein kinase activity of mTORC1. This complex cascade of reactions explains how PI3 kinase and Akt can activate mTORC1 by preventing the action of TSC1/2, which has an inhibitory role through its action on Rheb. mTOR can also associate to a protein termed Rictor to form mTOR complex 2 (mTORC2). The regulation of this complex is less well understood than that of mTORC1, but it plays an important role in the pathway by phosphorylating and activating Akt.

mTORC1 has several substrates including the eIF4E-binding protein (4EBP). 4EBP normally inhibits the action of eukaryotic initiation factor 4E (eIF4E) an essential element for protein translation initiation. Phosphorylation of 4EBP by mTORC1 relieves its inhibitory effect and favors protein translation. Another substrate of mTORC1 is the S6 kinase, which phosphorylates the ribosomal protein S6, further contributing to protein synthesis regulation. In summary this pathway stimulates cell growth through increase in protein translation. Recent work has also shown its implication in synaptic plasticity.

Interestingly, several genes coding for proteins of this pathway, including PTEN, TSC1, and TSC2, are mutated in human conditions associated with epilepsy, mental disability, and autism spectrum disorder. Such mutations appear to result in constitutive activation of this pathway and the possible therapeutic effects of rapamycin are currently being investigated.

The arrows with a pointed head indicate activation, whereas those with a bar indicate an inhibition. The circled P on the arrow indicates that the activation or the inhibition is mediated by phosphorylation.

Further reading: Crino, 2011; Richter and Klann, 2009; Vanhaesebroeck et al., 2010.

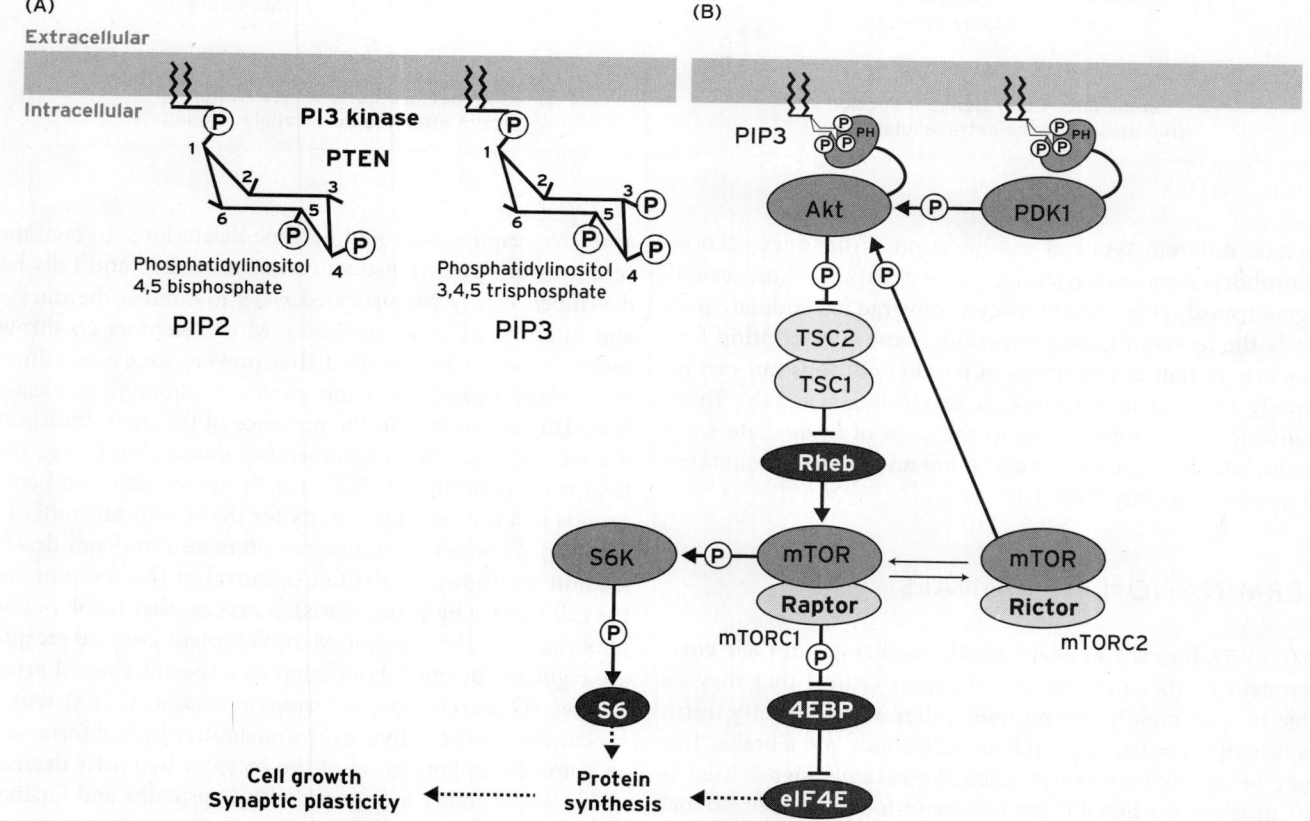

(A)

(B)

its endocytosis. Indeed, most receptors, including G protein–coupled receptors, as well as tyrosine kinase receptors and many others, are subjected to endocytosis when they are activated by their cognate ligand. Internalization of the receptor may lead to its degradation or to its recycling to the membrane. In fact, regulation of the number of receptors present at the membrane, by adjustment of their endocytosis and exocytosis rates, appears to be an important mechanism by which cells alter their sensitivity to external signals. For example, regulation of the number of glutamate receptors in the postsynaptic membrane is an important aspect of synaptic plasticity.

G proteins have built-in inactivating mechanisms: spontaneous or induced GTP hydrolysis leads to the inactivation of the G protein (see Box 4.7). The importance of this mechanism is underlined by the dramatic consequences of its blockade. Cholera toxin–induced blockade of GTP hydrolysis by $G\alpha_S$ in the intestinal epithelium is responsible for a potentially lethal water loss, while mutations that hamper the GTPase activity of Ras are potently oncogenic. Second messengers themselves are rapidly degraded by specific enzymes. Phosphodiesterases transform cAMP and cGMP into inactive AMP and GMP, respectively (see Box 4.9). Inositol phosphates are dephosphorylated by specific phosphatases (see Box 4.11). Free cytosolic Ca^{2+} is buffered by binding proteins and rapidly eliminated by various pumps and exchangers either to the outside of the cell or into intracellular stores (see Box 4.12). These various mechanisms can be important pharmacological targets. For example, lithium inhibits phospho-inositol-phosphatases, while inhibitors of cGMP phosphodiesterase have attracted a lot of public attention for their effects on sexual performance through vasodilation.

Protein phosphorylation reactions are also reversible, due to the presence of protein phosphatases (see Box 4.14), and the tightly regulated activity of these enzymes is an integral part of signaling mechanisms (see Box 4.15). It is worth mentioning that in many cases signaling pathways appear to be active to some degree even in the absence of extracellular signals, but that inactivation mechanisms (e.g., GTPases, phosphodiesterases, or phosphatases) counteract this spontaneous activity. What the extracellular signal does is to tilt the balance by enhancing the rate of activation and/or decreasing the rate of inactivation of the signaling. Although this permanent bustle of signaling pathways may, at first sight, appear costly for the cell, it may be advantageous by providing the capability to react very rapidly to extracellular signals.

PSYCHOPHARMACOLOGIC AGENTS AND SIGNAL TRANSDUCTION

Most of the therapeutic agents used at present in psychiatry act at the level of synaptic transmission by altering either the reuptake of neurotransmitters into presynaptic terminals, their degradation, or their action on target nerve cells. Benzodiazepines are potent modulators of GABA-A receptors. Most antipsychotic agents (neuroleptics) are antagonists at dopamine receptors. Most antidepressants are inhibitors of the plasma membrane transporters for norepinephrine and/or serotonin. Other drugs have intracellular targets such as the monoamine oxidase inhibitor class of antidepressants, which inhibit an enzyme that degrades catecholamines and serotonin. In contrast to agents that act at the level of neurotransmitters, lithium is thought to exert its mood-stabilizing effects in part by dampening phosphatidylinositol turnover. It provides an example of a psychotherapeutic agent that appears to act directly at the level of a signal transduction pathway. Recent work has identified other signaling pathways as potential additional targets for lithium, including the protein kinase *glycogen-synthase kinase-3*. Although few psychotherapeutic drugs used at present act directly on signaling mechanisms, several compounds have already proven their usefulness in other fields of medicine, including cancer treatment and immunosuppression. It is safe to predict that due to the intense research in this field, new classes of drugs with interesting applications in psychiatry will be developed. An example of drug under investigation is rapamycin, initially discovered as an immunosuppressant, which blocks the protein kinase mammalian target of rapamycin (mTOR, Box 4.18). mTOR is an effector of the PI3 kinase/Akt pathway, which controls cell survival, cell growth, and synaptic plasticity. Genetic alterations of this pathway are involved in a large variety of diseases, some of which alter brain development and function.

The antipsychotic effects of neuroleptics, as well as the therapeutic effects of antidepressants, take several days to appear, whereas their actions on receptors, transporters, or enzymes are immediate. This discrepancy indicates that many biochemical steps are probably involved between the primary targets of these drugs and the biological changes responsible for their clinically useful effects. These steps may include signal transduction pathways, which have started to be studied only very recently. It is likely that elucidation of such signaling pathways will be required to explain the therapeutic effects of neuroleptics and antidepressants and will be helpful in the design of new and more rapid active treatments. Likewise the signaling pathways underlying learning and memory at the cellular level are being deciphered at a rapid pace. Recent work has shown that abnormal incentive learning plays an important role in drug addiction (see Chapters 45 and 46), and possibly in other psychiatric diseases. The understanding of intracellular signaling pathways involved in the action of drugs of abuse is progressing rapidly and sheds light on the molecular basis of this frequent condition.

CONCLUSIONS

Signal transduction pathways form a complex network of biochemical reactions that allow cells to translate changes in their environment into appropriate responses. In spite of their complexity, these pathways have been highly conserved during evolution, and neurons use the same types of signaling cascades as other cells. In neurons, they are important for the modulation of the fast reactions involved in neuronal activity. They also provide the basis for the reactions that lead to neuronal growth and synapses formation and plasticity, and thus for the development of the nervous system, as well as for learning and memory. It is likely that, in the near future, environmental or genetic alterations of signal transduction pathway components will be found to be important in some psychiatric diseases. The understanding of these pathways is just at its beginning. To date, a few compounds acting on signal transduction mechanisms have already found clinical application. Moreover, this is an area of intense research, and it is likely that an increasing number of psychotherapeutic agents will be discovered that act by altering signal transduction mechanisms.

DISCLOSURES

Dr. Girault has no conflicts of interest to disclose. His salary is paid by Inserm (a public national research institute) and work in his laboratory is funded by French (*Agence Nationale de la Recherche*) and European (Framework Program 7, European Research Council) grants.

Dr. Greengard receives grant support from the National Institutes of Health and the U.S. Department of Defense. He has no conflicts of interest with regard to the subject matter of the chapter.

REFERENCES

Arnsten, A.F., Ramos, B.P., et al. (2005). Protein kinase A as a therapeutic target for memory disorders: rationale and challenges. *Trends Mol. Med.* 11:121–128.

Baud, V., and Karin, M. (2001). Signal transduction by tumor necrosis factor and its relatives. *Trends Cell Biol.* 11:372–377.

Benarroch, E.E. (2007). GABAA receptor heterogeneity, function, and implications for epilepsy. *Neurology* 68:612–614.

Berridge, M.J. (2009). Inositol trisphosphate and calcium signalling mechanisms. *Biochim. Biophys. Acta* 1793:933–940.

Berridge, M.J., Lipp, P., et al. (2000). The versatility and universality of calcium signalling. *Nat. Rev. Mol. Cell Biol.* 1:11–21.

Bockaert, J., and Pin, J.P. (1999). Molecular tinkering of G protein-coupled receptors: an evolutionary success. *EMBO J.* 18:1723–1729.

Bourne, H.R. (1995). GTPases: a family of molecular switches and clocks. *Philos. Trans. R. Soc. Lond. B Biol. Sci.* 349:283–289.

Bourne, H.R. (1997). How receptors talk to trimeric G proteins. *Curr. Opin. Cell Biol.* 9:134–142.

Cockcroft, S. (2006). The latest phospholipase C, PLCeta, is implicated in neuronal function. *Trends Biochem. Sci.* 31:4–7.

Collin, T., Marty, A., et al. (2005). Presynaptic calcium stores and synaptic transmission. *Curr. Opin. Neurobiol.* 15:275–281.

Crino, P.B. (2011). mTOR: A pathogenic signaling pathway in developmental brain malformations. *Trends Mol. Med.* 17:734–742.

Cull-Candy, S., Brickley, S., et al. (2001). NMDA receptor subunits: diversity, development and disease. *Curr. Opin. Neurobiol.* 11:327–335.

Dani, J.A., and Bertrand, D. (2007). Nicotinic acetylcholine receptors and nicotinic cholinergic mechanisms of the central nervous system. *Annu. Rev. Pharmacol. Toxicol.* 47:699–729.

Derkach, V.A., Oh, M.C., et al. (2007). Regulatory mechanisms of AMPA receptors in synaptic plasticity. *Nat. Rev. Neurosci.* 8:101–113.

DeWire, S.M., Ahn, S., et al. (2007). Beta-arrestins and cell signaling. *Annu. Rev. Physiol.* 69:483–510.

Dilworth, F.J., and Chambon, P. (2001). Nuclear receptors coordinate the activities of chromatin remodeling complexes and coactivators to facilitate initiation of transcription. *Oncogene* 20:3047–3054.

Farooqui, A.A., Ong, W.Y., et al. (2006). Inhibitors of brain phospholipase A2 activity: their neuropharmacological effects and therapeutic importance for the treatment of neurologic disorders. *Pharmacol. Rev.* 58:591–620.

Gainetdinov, R.R., Premont, R.T., et al. (2004). Desensitization of G protein-coupled receptors and neuronal functions. *Annu. Rev. Neurosci.* 27:107–144.

Girault, J.A., and Greengard, P. (2004). The neurobiology of dopamine signaling. *Arch. Neurol.* 61:641–644.

Girault, J.A., Valjent, E., et al. (2007). ERK2: a logical AND gate critical for drug-induced plasticity? *Curr. Opin. Pharmacol.* 7:77–85.

Greengard, P. (2001). The neurobiology of slow synaptic transmission. *Science* 294:1024–1030.

Guzowski, J.F., Timlin, J.A., et al. (2005). Mapping behaviorally relevant neural circuits with immediate-early gene expression. *Curr. Opin. Neurobiol.* 15:599–606.

Hyman, S.E., Malenka, R.C., et al. (2006). Neural mechanisms of addiction: the role of reward-related learning and memory. *Annu. Rev. Neurosci.* 29:565–598.

Iino, M. (2006). Ca²⁺-dependent inositol 1,4,5-trisphosphate and nitric oxide signaling in cerebellar neurons. *J. Pharmacol. Sci.* 100:538–544.

Iino, M. (2007). Regulation of cell functions by Ca2+ oscillation. *Adv. Exp. Med. Biol.* 592:305–312.

Imada, K., and Leonard, W.J. (2000). The Jak-STAT pathway. *Mol. Immunol.* 37:1–11.

Jaffe, A.B., and Hall, A. (2005). Rho GTPases: biochemistry and biology. *Annu. Rev. Cell Dev. Biol.* 21:247–269.

Jiang, X., and Wang, X. (2004). Cytochrome C-mediated apoptosis. *Annu. Rev. Biochem.* 73:87–106.

Johnston, G.A. (2005). GABA(A). receptor channel pharmacology. *Curr. Pharm. Des.* 11:1867–1885.

Johnson, S.A., and Hunter, T. (2005). Kinomics: methods for deciphering the kinome. *Nat. Methods* 2:17–25.

Kalb, R. (2005). The protean actions of neurotrophins and their receptors on the life and death of neurons. *Trends Neurosci.* 28:5–11.

Kobilka, B.K. (2011). Structural insights into adrenergic receptor function and pharmacology. *Trends Pharmacol. Sci.* 32:213–218.

Koelle, M.R. (2006). Heterotrimeric G protein signaling: Getting inside the cell. *Cell* 126:25–27.

Kuriyan, J., and Cowburn, D. (1997). Modular peptide recognition domains in eukaryotic signaling. *Annu. Rev. Biophys. Biomol. Struct.* 26:259–288.

Lemmon, M.A., and Schlessinger, J. (2010). Cell signaling by receptor tyrosine kinases. *Cell* 141:1117–1134.

Lu, L., Koya, E., et al. (2006). Role of ERK in cocaine addiction. *Trends Neurosci.* 29:695–703.

Luttrell, L.M. (2006). Transmembrane signaling by G protein-coupled receptors. *Methods Mol. Biol.* 332:3–49.

Mansuy, I.M., and Shenolikar, S. (2006). Protein serine/threonine phosphatases in neuronal plasticity and disorders of learning and memory. *Trends Neurosci.* 29:679–686.

Mark, M., Ghyselinck, N.B., et al. (2006). Function of retinoid nuclear receptors: lessons from genetic and pharmacological dissections of the retinoic acid signaling pathway during mouse embryogenesis. *Annu. Rev. Pharmacol. Toxicol.* 46:451–480.

May, L.T., Leach, K., et al. (2007). Allosteric modulation of G protein-coupled receptors. *Annu. Rev. Pharmacol. Toxicol.* 47:1–51.

Mayer, M.L. (2005). Glutamate receptor ion channels. *Curr. Opin. Neurobiol.* 15:282–288.

Michel, J.J., and Scott, J.D. (2002). Akap mediated signal transduction. *Annu. Rev. Pharmacol. Toxicol.* 42:235–257.

Mikoshiba, K., and Hattori, M. (2000). IP3 receptor-operated calcium entry. *Sci. STKE* 2000(51):PE1.

Mohler, H., Fritschy, J.M., et al. (2002). A new benzodiazepine pharmacology. *J. Pharmacol. Exp. Ther.* 300:2–8.

Moore, C.A., Milano, S.K., et al. (2007). Regulation of receptor trafficking by GRKs and arrestins. *Annu. Rev. Physiol.* 69:451–482.

Nairn, A.C., Svenningsson, P., et al. (2004). The role of DARPP-32 in the actions of drugs of abuse. *Neuropharmacology* 47 Suppl 1:14–23.

Nutt, D.J., and Malizia, A.L. (2001). New insights into the role of the GABA(A)-benzodiazepine receptor in psychiatric disorder. *Br. J. Psychiatry* 179:390–396.

O'Shea, J.J., Park, H., et al. (2005). New strategies for immunosuppression: interfering with cytokines by targeting the Jak/Stat pathway. *Curr. Opin. Rheumatol.* 17:305–311.

Paoletti, P. (2011). Molecular basis of NMDA receptor functional diversity. *Eur. J. Neurosci.* 33:1351–1365.

Papin, J.A., Hunter, T., et al. (2005). Reconstruction of cellular signalling networks and analysis of their properties. *Nat. Rev. Mol. Cell Biol.* 6:99–111.

Patrick, G.N. (2006). Synapse formation and plasticity: recent insights from the perspective of the ubiquitin proteasome system. *Curr. Opin. Neurobiol.* 16:90–94.

Pawson, T. (2004). Specificity in signal transduction: from phosphotyrosine-SH2 domain interactions to complex cellular systems. *Cell* 116:191–203.

Pawson, T., and Scott, J.D. (1997). Signaling through scaffold, anchoring, and adaptor proteins. *Science* 278:2075–2080.

Pietrobon, D. (2005). Function and dysfunction of synaptic calcium channels: insights from mouse models. *Curr. Opin. Neurobiol.* 15:257–265.

Richter, J.D., and Klann, E. (2009). Making synaptic plasticity and memory last: mechanisms of translational regulation. *Genes Dev.* 23:1–11.

Rosenbaum, D.M., Rasmussen, S.G., et al. (2009). The structure and function of G-protein-coupled receptors. *Nature* 459:356–363.

Schlessinger J. (2002). Ligand-induced, receptor-mediated dimerization and activation of EGF receptor. *Cell 110:*669–672.

Schlessinger, J., and Lemmon, M.A. (2003). SH2 and PTB domains in tyrosine kinase signaling. *Sci. STKE* 2003(191):RE12.

Seidel, H.M., Lamb, P., et al. (2000). Pharmaceutical intervention in the JAK/STAT signaling pathway. *Oncogene* 19:2645–2656.

Shalin, S.C., Egli, R., et al. (2006). Signal transduction mechanisms in memory disorders. *Prog. Brain Res.* 157:25–41.

Smith, C.M., Radzio-Andzelm, E., et al. (1999). The catalytic subunit of cAMP-dependent protein kinase: prototype for an extended network of communication. *Prog. Biophys. Mol. Biol.* 71:313–341.

Snyder, S.H., Jaffrey, S.R., et al. (1998). Nitric oxide and carbon monoxide: parallel roles as neural messengers. *Brain Res. Rev.* 26:167–175.

Steyaert, J., and Kobilka, B.K. (2011). Nanobody stabilization of G protein-coupled receptor conformational states. *Curr. Opin. Struct. Biol.* 21:567–572.

Stutzmann, G.E., and Mattson, M.P. (2011). Endoplasmic reticulum Ca(2+). handling in excitable cells in health and disease. *Pharmacol. Rev.* 63:700–727.

Svenningsson, P., Nishi, A., et al. (2004). DARPP-32: an integrator of neurotransmission. *Annu. Rev. Pharmacol. Toxicol.* 44:269–296.

Traynelis, S.F., Wollmuth, L.P., et al. (2010). Glutamate receptor ion channels: structure, regulation, and function. *Pharmacol. Rev.* 62:405–496.

Vanhaesebroeck, B., Guillermet-Guibert, J., et al. (2010). The emerging mechanisms of isoform-specific PI3K signalling. *Nat. Rev. Mol. Cell. Biol.* 11:329–341.

Weatherman, R.V., Fletterick, R.J., et al. (1999). Nuclear-receptor ligands and ligand-binding domains. *Annu. Rev. Biochem.* 68:559–581.

Yamaoka, K., Saharinen, P., et al. (2004). The Janus kinases (Jaks). *Genome Biol.* 5:253.

Yan, N., and Shi, Y. (2005). Mechanisms of apoptosis through structural biology. *Annu. Rev. Cell Dev. Biol.* 21:35–56.

Yger, M., and Girault, J.A. (2011). DARPP-32, Jack of all trades...master of which? *Front. Behav. Neurosci.* 5:1–14.

Zebisch, A., Czernilofsky, A.P., et al. (2007). Signaling through RAS-RAF-MEK-ERK: from basics to bedside. *Curr. Med. Chem.* 14:601–623.

5 | SYNAPTIC AND NEURAL PLASTICITY

SAÏD KOURRICH AND ANTONELLO BONCI

Brain function is generated by an extraordinarily complex yet organized neuronal network where information transmission is orchestrated by elementary cellular mechanisms. Ultimately, the firing patterns of neurons code information within the brain, and the frequency and variation of the firing patterns determine the nature of this information. Information transmission within the brain involves complex and subtle variations in neuronal activity. In particular, electrical signals in the brain are constantly modulated and are heavily influenced by excitatory (glutamate) and inhibitory (gamma-aminobutyric acid, GABA) inputs. These, in turn, are translated into excitatory and inhibitory postsynaptic potentials (EPSPs and IPSPs, respectively), which eventually give rise to action potentials. When triggered, an action potential travels from the somatodendritic compartment along an axon to its presynaptic terminal. Here, it triggers the release of neurotransmitters, which are molecules that transmit information chemically by binding to their specific postsynaptic receptors on adjacent neurons. A persistent change in any of these events will affect information coding and impact underlying cognitive or sensory processes. Potassium (K^+), sodium (Na^+), and calcium (Ca^{2+}) voltage-gated channels all participate in the generation and conduction of action potentials. Because voltage-gated ion channels are heterogeneously distributed throughout neurons (Lujan, 2010), their functional states alter various aspects of neuronal transmission, including action potential generation, neurotransmitter release, and postsynaptic receptor sensitivity. Indeed, synaptic and intrinsic excitability are constantly working in concert to shape global neuronal excitability and control information transmission within the nervous system.

This chapter will provide basic descriptions of the principal forms of activity- and experience-dependent plasticity that can persistently affect neuronal transmission. The first part will present the synaptic factors that determine how well pre- and postsynaptic sides of neurons communicate, that is, *synaptic plasticity*. The second part will describe lasting changes in intrinsic factors that control action potential generation and conduction, that is, *intrinsic plasticity*. The third part will discuss the capacity of a neuron to regulate its function to reach stability based on changes in its environment, that is, *homeostatic plasticity*. Research on this form of plasticity is still in its infancy. Examples will be used to describe how experience, such as learning or exposure to drugs of abuse, can persistently affect each segment of information transmission. We will show that although some of these changes may be adaptive, others become deleterious and lead to neurological and psychiatric disorders.

SYNAPTIC PLASTICITY
BRIEF HISTORY AND BASIC FEATURES

Neuronal plasticity, a concept that emerged at the end of the 19th century with Santiago Ramon y Cajal and others (Berlucchi and Buchtel, 2009), describes the processes by which neurons or synapses change their internal parameters in response to experience. However, it has only been in the mid-20th century that this concept has been seriously considered to underlie higher cognitive functions such as learning and memory (Hebb, 1949). Indeed, Hebb was the first to pose a specific theoretical process by which neuronal plasticity might occur. He postulated that *"when an axon of cell A is near enough to excite B and repeatedly or persistently takes part in firing it, some growth process or metabolic change takes place in one or both cells such that A's efficiency, as one of the cells firing B, is increased"* (Hebb, 1949: p. 62). In other words, he proposed that the synchronous firing of two neurons, A and B, leads to enduring changes in synaptic efficacy, or how efficiently neurons communicate with each other, and that this synaptic efficacy is the cellular basis for encoding and storing information. Over the last few decades, his theory prompted an intense search for the cellular mechanisms mediating specific behaviors and higher cognitive functions. This search was greatly influenced by the techniques of electrophysiology, a major technical advancement in neural science made around the same time, which allows the recording of neuronal electrical activity.

The idea that long-lasting increases in synaptic transmission could occur in living animals was confirmed in 1973 (Bliss and Lomo, 1973). In their experiment, performed in anesthetized rabbits, Bliss and Lomo applied a repetitive stimulation to the perforant path input to the hippocampus and recorded excitatory postsynaptic potentials generated by the first neuronal relay, dentate granule cells. The authors observed an increased excitatory synaptic transmission that lasted from minutes to hours and named it long-term potentiation (LTP). The discovery of LTP was exciting not just because neuronal transmission persisted but also because it was discovered in the hippocampus, a structure known to be critical for learning and memory. To this day, one of the major questions investigated in this research is whether cellular mechanisms of LTP underlie formation of memories. Despite being most frequently studied in the rat hippocampus, LTP has also been demonstrated *in vitro* and *in vivo* in many other species and regions of the central nervous system, suggesting that perhaps persistent increase in synaptic efficacy is a physiological mechanism used by the brain to store specific information that is later used for behavioral adaptability in the larger sense.

The features that make LTP attractive as a model for information storage reside in its fundamental properties. In addition to its *persistence*, as mentioned previously, LTP develops only if the firing of a presynaptic neuron is followed by the firing of a postsynaptic neuron; or when multiple inputs weakly stimulate the same synapse to depolarize a cell enough to reach the level of LTP induction, a property called *associativity* or *cooperativity*. Furthermore, changes at one synapse, via a synaptic tagging mechanism, do not spread to other synapses, which is a feature that makes LTP *input-specific*. Because the number of synapses in the brain is estimated to a quadrillion, input specificity is one the most appealing properties of LTP, as it provides a means to store endless amounts of specific information. For these reasons, increased synaptic transmission has become a model for studying how behavioral experience, such as learning, induces long-term changes in synaptic transmission, and reciprocally how long-term changes in synaptic transmission affect learning capabilities.

As much as LTP is a long-lasting increase in synaptic transmission, it has its counterpart, long-term depression (LTD), which is a long-lasting decrease in synaptic transmission, a phenomenon first discovered in the cerebellum (Ito and Kano, 1982). Whereas high-frequency stimulation is needed to induce LTP, LTD is triggered following low-frequency stimulation.

PHASES OF LTP

LTP is composed of several distinct phases, including (*1*) a first phase, referred to as short-term plasticity (STP); (*2*) an early phase, referred to as E-LTP; and (*3*) a late phase, referred to as L-LTP. Although STP and E-LTP can sometimes share common cellular mechanisms, each of these components is associated with specific changes in synaptic function.

In brief, STP is a form of potentiation that decays in the order of minutes shortly after the post-tetanic potentiation (PTP). STP is characterized by its presynaptic locus and its resistance to protein kinase inhibitors (Lauri et al., 2007). In particular, changes in presynaptic function are usually associated with changes in the probability of neurotransmitter release (P_r), namely, glutamate at excitatory synapses and GABA at inhibitory synapses, and are the likelihood of vesicle fusion and transmitter release occurring at a presynaptic terminal in response to an action potential. The parameters that determine the changes in P_r during STP are not well understood. However, prominent candidates for the mechanism include the size of the readily releasable vesicle pool and the SNAREs machinery for neurotransmitter exocytosis, whose function directly depends on the presynaptic Ca^{2+} concentration. Early-LTP, developing while STP decays, lasts for a few hours. Although both E-LTP and STP are characterized by changes in presynaptic function, E-LTP is sensitive to several kinase inhibitors, but is resistant to protein synthesis inhibitors. The third phase, L-LTP, is thought to last for days and requires protein synthesis (Lauri et al., 2007).

CELLULAR MECHANISMS

As mentioned, LTP is a phenomenon that exhibits critical characteristics that make it an ideal model for the physiological mechanisms of learning and memory. A well-studied form of LTP is Hebbian LTP, a form of plasticity that is induced following Hebbian rules of associativity, namely, LTP develops only if the firing of a presynaptic neuron is followed by the firing of a postsynaptic neuron. In other words, two events have to co-occur to trigger the induction mechanism. This form of LTP has been best characterized in the CA1 field of hippocampus, and as such the cellular mechanisms described in this section are from studies performed in CA1, except when mentioned (Fig. 5.1A). The NMDA receptor, which is a glutamate receptor, has the characteristic of a coincidence detector, meaning it needs two events to occur simultaneously to respond. First, glutamate must bind to the postsynaptic receptor, which means that the presynaptic neuron has been excited and released glutamate. Second, the postsynaptic neuron must be partially depolarized in order to remove the Mg^{2+} block that normally prevents Ca^{2+} from flowing through the NMDAR. This means that the postsynaptic neuron receives glutamate when it is still depolarized due to recent activity. Such a physiological state happens either when high-frequency stimulation is used (*cooperativity*) or when the postsynaptic neuron is significantly excited to send action potentials from the axon hillock back to the dendrite, a phenomenon called back-propagation (*associativity*) (see section paragraph "At the Dendritic Level" in the section "Intrinsic Plasticity"). When these two events occur together, they allow for a large influx of Ca^{2+} into the postsynaptic neuron, which triggers action potentials and a cascade of events in the postsynaptic neuron that induces LTP. Ca^{2+} will trigger activation of Ca^{2+}-dependent protein kinases that are necessary for LTP maintenance (CaMK, PKC, PKA, and tyrosine protein kinase fyn). Ca^{2+}/calmodulin-dependent protein kinase II (CaMKII), which is an enriched forebrain enzyme, is the best characterized of these kinases. CaMKII has the capacity to autophosphorylate in the presence of increased Ca^{2+} concentrations, and will phosphorylate synaptic AMPARs to increase their functions and/or promote their trafficking from intracellular compartments to the plasma membrane, which helps maintain increased synaptic strength (Lisman et al., 2012). For long-lasting maintenance of LTP, *de novo* AMPARs are also added to the synapses via transcriptional events. Increased postsynaptic Ca^{2+} influx activates adenylate cyclase, and through the metabolism of ATP, cAMP is produced, which activates cAMP kinase and allows its translocation into the nucleus. Cyclic AMP kinase phosphorylates the nuclear transcription factor CREB (cAMP-responsive element binding protein), which triggers the expression of new AMPAR subunits to be inserted at the synaptic membrane (Benito and Barco, 2010). Additionally, CREB-dependent gene expressions also lead to the synthesis of proteins that participate in making structural changes. Lastly, through an unknown mechanism, the postsynaptic neuron releases a retrograde messenger (nitric oxide) that can act on presynaptic protein kinases to enhance neurotransmitter release (Fig. 5.1A).

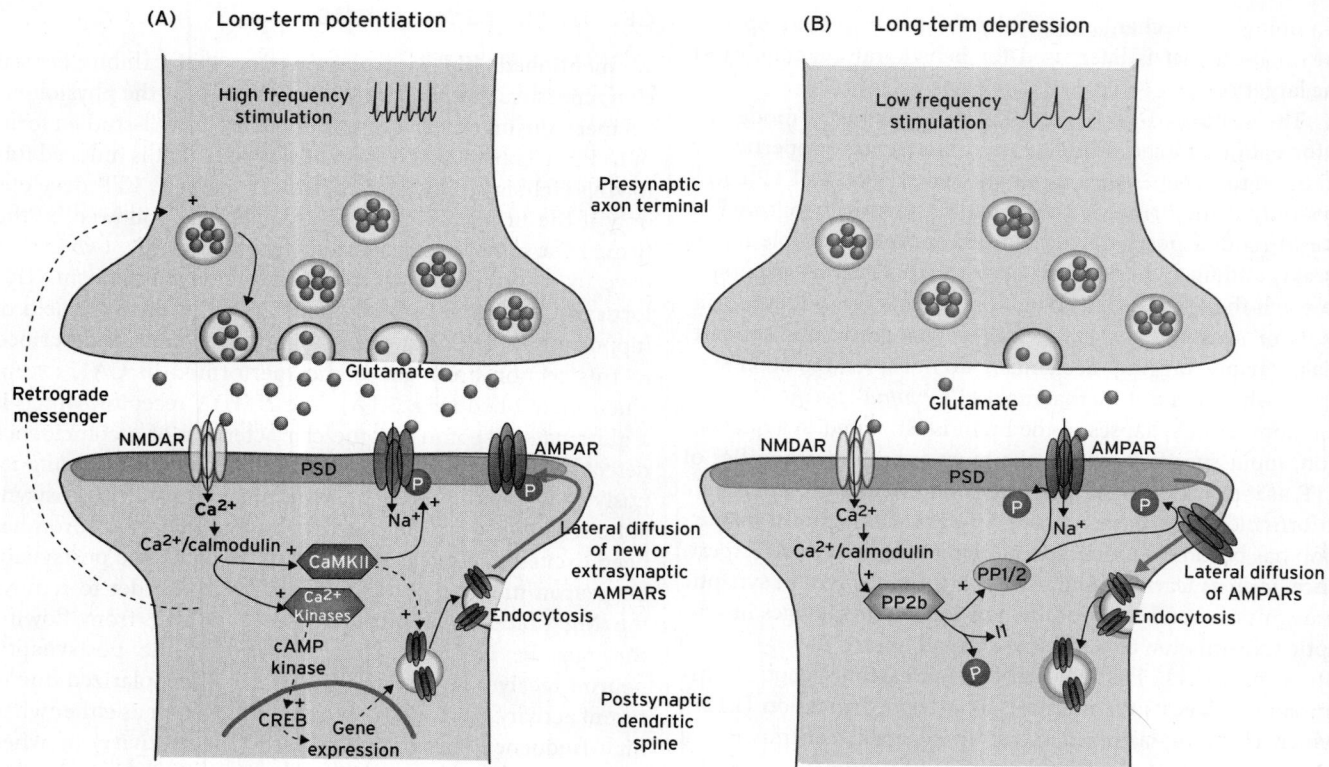

(A) Long-term potentiation

High frequency stimulation

Presynaptic axon terminal

Retrograde messenger

Glutamate

NMDAR

PSD

AMPAR

Ca²⁺

Na⁺

Ca²⁺/calmodulin +

CaMKII

Ca²⁺ Kinases

Lateral diffusion of new or extrasynaptic AMPARs

Endocytosis

cAMP kinase

CREB

Gene expression

Postsynaptic dendritic spine

(B) Long-term depression

Low frequency stimulation

Glutamate

NMDAR

PSD

AMPAR

Ca²⁺

Na⁺

Ca²⁺/calmodulin

PP1/2

PP2b

I1

Lateral diffusion of AMPARs

Endocytosis

Figure 5.1 *Possible cellular mechanisms involved in LTP and LTD in the CA1 field of hippocampus. (A) An intense and brief stimulation (e.g., high frequency stimulation, HFS) induces the release of enough glutamate to trigger a strong activation of AMPARs. Through influx of Na⁺ and efflux of K⁺, AMPARs activation depolarizes the postsynaptic membrane, which frees NMDARs from Mg²⁺ block (not represented). In turn, besides moderate influx of Na⁺ and efflux of K⁺, NMDARs conduct a strong influx of Ca²⁺. Together with NMDARs, voltage-gated Ca²⁺ channels (VGCCs) may also contribute to intracellular rise of Ca²⁺ (not represented), which would trigger activation of several Ca²⁺-dependent protein kinases (CaMKII, PKC, PKA and the tyrosine protein kinase Fyn). Through a phosphorylation mechanism, the active autophosphorylated form of CaMKII increases AMPARs function and trafficking of cytoplasmic inactive AMPARs to the postsynaptic density (PSD), a specialized region of the postsynaptic membrane that is dense in proteins and directly opposed to the presynaptic zone, the site of neurotransmitters release. For LTP maintenance, increased intracellular Ca²⁺ may also activate adenylate cyclase, which through cAMP kinase-dependent phosphorylation pathway activates the nuclear transcription factors CREB (cAMP-responsive element binding). In turn, CREB triggers expression of new AMPARs and other proteins that participate in structural changes. New and cytoplasmic AMPARs are integrated at the synaptic membrane through exocytosis and lateral diffusion from extrasynaptic membrane to the PSD, a mechanism that involves transmembrane AMPA receptor regulatory proteins (TARPs) and various scaffolding proteins (e.g., MAGUKs). The postsynaptic neuron may also release retrograde messengers (e.g., nitric oxide) that act on presynaptic protein kinases and thereby enhance neurotransmitter release. (B) A low-frequency stimulation (LFS) induces a weaker AMPARs-dependent depolarization, which leads to a moderate NMDAR-dependent increase in intracellular Ca²⁺. Similar to LTP, Ca²⁺ binds to calmodulin; however in this case, Ca²⁺/calmodulin activates the protein phosphatase calcineurin (also called PP2b). In turn, calcineurin dephosphorylates inhibitor 1, which was maintaining PP1 and/or PP2 inactive. PP1 and/or PP2 dephosphorylate synaptic AMPARs, which triggers lateral diffusion and a clathrin-dependent endocytosis for endosomal degradation. For clarity, other contributors to synaptic plasticity, including VGCCs and metabotropic glutamate receptors, are not represented. Dashed arrows indicate either cellular mechanisms that are still unknown or mechanisms that require multiple steps.*

LTD, which is the opposite of LTP, also requires postsynaptic Ca²⁺ influx through NMDAR activation (Fig. 5.1B). In contrast to LTP induction, which requires strong Ca²⁺ influx, LTD is induced by a low frequency stimulation that yields moderate levels of intracellular Ca²⁺, which also bind to calmodulin to form a complex. However, in the case of LTD, the complex activates Ca²⁺-calmodulin-dependent phosphatase calcineurin (also named PP2b), which triggers a dephosphorylation cascade. By inhibiting inhibitor 1, calcineurin activates protein phosphatase 1 and/or phosphatase 2 (PP1/2). Dephosphorylation of AMPARs by PP1/2 triggers a clathrin-dependent endocytosis of receptors, which results in decreased synaptic efficacy (Fig. 5.1B). Interestingly, PP1/2 also targets the active autophosphorylated form of CaMKII. By dephosphorylating CaMKII, PP1/2 facilitates LTD and may also prevent further LTP from occurring (Collingridge et al., 2010).

Although these processes appear simple, the cellular mechanisms through which LTP and LTD occur following neuronal activity are still heavily researched. For example, while intracellular domains of AMPARs are important for plasticity, it is not yet clear whether activity directly targets the AMPARs themselves. Recent scientific studies have shown that there is a new type of regulatory proteins for AMPARs, the TARPS (transmembrane AMPA receptor regulatory proteins). These auxiliary subunits, closely working with several other types of scaffolding proteins (e.g., membrane-associated guanylate kinases, MAGUKs), are involved in trafficking, synaptic targeting, gating, and pharmacological behaviors of AMPARs (Jackson and Nicoll, 2011). Furthermore, LTP and LTD can be elicited in various brain nuclei and subregions, and each may express differences in induction's of cellular mechanisms.

One of the most striking and unexpected mechanisms is that some forms of LTP and LTD are NMDAR-independent. For example, LTP at the mossy fiber pathway-CA3 relay in the hippocampus is presynaptic and NMDAR-independent, a phenomenon that can also apply to LTD. In this case, the source of Ca^{2+} originates from voltage-gated Ca^{2+} channels and the Ca^{2+} release from intracellular stores that are triggered by the activation of metabotropic glutamate or other metabotropic receptors (Collingridge et al., 2010). At the presynaptic terminal, Ca^{2+} influx, via activation of a cAMP–dependent pathway, promotes glutamate release.

EXPERIENCE-DEPENDENT SYNAPTIC PLASTICITY

SYNAPTIC PLASTICITY IN LEARNING AND MEMORY

Physiologically, LTP exhibits two key properties that support its role in memory formation. The first is its persistence over time, and the second is that LTP develops only if the firing of the presynaptic neuron is followed by the firing of the postsynaptic neuron, that is, the co-occurrence requirement discussed earlier. The requirement for the postsynaptic neuron to be partially depolarized when glutamate binds to receptors is an extremely important characteristic of LTP because it permits neural networks to learn associations. Importantly, LTP can be elicited by low levels of stimulation that mimic physiologically relevant neural activity.

Behaviorally, conditioning tasks can produce LTP-like changes in the hippocampus, and many drugs that influence learning and memory have parallel effects on LTP. Additionally, mutant mice that display little hippocampal LTP have difficulty learning the Barnes circular maze, a task that tests spatial memory (Mayford et al., 1996). In contrast, Joe Z. Tsien's laboratory generated a transgenic mouse that overexpresses the NR2B subunit in the forebrain (Tang et al., 1999). NR2B is an NMDAR subunit that permits a larger influx of Ca^{2+} into the cell. Since NMDAR is a coincidence detector, an increase in NMDAR function should increase the capability of a neuron to detect coincidences and potentially improve learning mechanisms. They found that NR2B-overexpressing mice showed greater LTP associated with improved memory (Tang et al., 1999). Although there is a consensus linking LTP in the hippocampus to learning and memory processes, investigations are still ongoing (Lynch, 2004).

SYNAPTIC PLASTICITY IN NEUROLOGICAL DISORDERS

There is increasing evidence that neurological disorders, including Alzheimer's disease (Spires-Jones and Knafo, 2012) and substance abuse disorders are associated with persistent changes in synaptic strength (Bowers et al., 2010). In this section, we will provide a brief review of the functional evidence linking changes in AMPAR-mediated transmission with substance abuse disorders. A thorough chapter, "Cellular and Molecular Mechanisms of Addiction," is provided by Dr. Peter Kalivas (Chapter 52).

Studies have mainly focused on two brain areas of the mesolimbic reward circuit, the ventral tegmental area (VTA) and the nucleus accumbens (NAc). In the VTA, the ability of drugs of abuse to produce synaptic plasticity was first demonstrated using a single experimenter-administered cocaine injection. Remarkably, subsequent studies have shown that a single injection of a variety of abused drugs (e.g., cocaine, morphine, nicotine), but not non-abused drugs (fluoxetine or carbamazepine), leads to the potentiation of glutamatergic synapses in VTA dopamine (DA) neurons. This potentiation is mediated by a transient increase in AMPAR-mediated synaptic response (5 days), but is no longer potentiated 10 days after the cocaine injection. Furthermore, cocaine-induced LTP in the VTA was associated with an increase in the proportion of GluR1-containing, GluR2-lacking AMPARs—receptors that exhibit a Ca^{2+} permeability. Regardless of the number of injections, LTP in VTA stayed transient. Because associative learning mechanisms may play a vital role in the development of addiction, changes in synaptic plasticity in VTA DA neurons should also be examined using voluntary cocaine self-administration models. In stark contrast to the consequences of passive cocaine administration, cocaine self-administration enhanced AMPAR-mediated responses in VTA DA neurons for at least 3 months of abstinence. Importantly, self-administration of natural rewards also induced LTP in VTA DA neurons, but this potentiation was transient, lasting for up to 7 days. These findings suggest that learning in relation to natural rewards has much shorter lasting effects on VTA function than does drug self-administration (Bowers et al., 2010).

In the NAc, changes after single or repeated exposure to a drug of abuse are different from those seen in the VTA. As in the VTA, repeated exposure to drugs of abuse can strongly modulate NAc excitatory synaptic transmission. Glutamatergic plasticity has been examined primarily after repeated cocaine exposure, either passively through experimenter administration or actively through self-administration. Interestingly, little or no change in synaptic transmission has been observed in the NAc shell during early withdrawal after repeated drug exposure. However, studies generally agree that repeated passive or active drug exposure and protracted abstinence are associated with increased NAc AMPAR signaling, although there are likely to be differences in the type of AMPAR function that is altered (Bowers et al., 2010).

INTRINSIC PLASTICITY

DEFINITION AND BASIC FEATURES

Intrinsic plasticity is the plasticity of non-synaptic factors that control neuronal excitability. These factors directly affect the probability that a neuron will fire an action potential in response to excitatory inputs. Conceptually, these factors can be any elements located on the soma, dendrites, or axon, that is, remote from the synapse, which passively or actively modulate membrane excitability. However, the study of intrinsic plasticity is still in its infancy and concerns mainly short- and long-term changes in voltage-gated ion channels. These channels are the "building blocks" that shape action potentials, and are also the same "building blocks" that shape firing patterns. Voltage-gated ion channels (Na^+, Ca^{2+}, and K^+) are ubiquitous transmembrane proteins mediating ionic exchange between extra- and intracellular compartments and are coded by hundreds of genes. Combined with alternative splicing and heteromeric assembly within subfamilies, they provide neurons with tremendous possibilities and a remarkable ability for fine-tuning intrinsic excitability. However, the K+ channels, which tend to hyperpolarize neurons, are exceptionally more complex in their role and structures when compared to other voltage-gated conductances (Hille, 2001). This diversity of K+ channels likely illustrates their role in regulating neuronal excitability both tonically and in response to intra- or extracellular stimuli in order to provide appropriate behaviors in specific contexts. This complexity in role is reflected in their subcellular localizations (somatic, dendritic, axonal, or synaptic) and additional auxiliary subunits that regulate their functions. Questions about how experience, for example, learning or exposure to drug of abuse, alters neuronal intrinsic excitability and how these changes relate to behaviors remain unanswered in the field of intrinsic plasticity, and the cellular mechanisms underlying these changes are currently under investigation.

A LOOK AT INTRINSIC PLASTICITY AT THE SUBCELLULAR LEVEL

AT THE DENDRITIC LEVEL

Dendrites express various types of voltage-gated ion channels, and many of these channels are not expressed uniformly throughout the dendrite. This feature provides the dendrite with a unique capability to regulate signal integration. Depending on the strength of the synaptic input, either an EPSP or a dendritic spike is generated. These electrical events are then either dampened and fade away, or increased and generate somatic action potentials. The direction of the effect depends on the population and types of voltage-gated ion channels expressed along the dendrite. For example, a decrease in dendritic K+ currents may boost dendritic excitability and allow excitatory inputs generated at the synapse to travel to the soma, which results in the generation of action potentials. In the classical view, these action potentials will travel along the axon and trigger neurotransmitter release at the axon terminal. However, action potentials can also travel back to the dendritic tree, a phenomenon known as back-propagation. Back-propagation is strongly influenced by the electrical properties of dendrites, where voltage-gated Na+ channels boost back-propagating action potentials while K+ channels (e.g., Kv4.2 subtype) determine their amplitudes and widths (Shah et al., 2010). At the functional level, back-propagating action potentials provide the additional level of depolarization needed for the synapses to trigger the cellular mechanisms necessary to induce some forms of associative synaptic plasticity (Shah et al., 2010) (see also section paragraph "Cellular Mechanisms" in section "Synaptic Plasticity"). In other words, they provide a feedback signal informing the synapses about the output state of the neuron, and the time window in which this occurs determines the direction of synaptic changes. For example, a significantly strong output that arrives shortly after a synaptic input will set the synapse at a permissive state that allows the induction of associative synaptic potentiation. If the constraints imposed by the time window are not met, LTD is favored. It should be noted, however, that the rules for such phenomena have been updated recently (Caporale and Dan, 2008). It appears that the distribution and types of specific Na+ and K+ channels expressed along the dendrite play a critical role in the induction of associative synaptic plasticity. Conversely, induction of associative synaptic plasticity triggers a decrease in A-type K+ currents mediated by internalization of Kv4.2 channels (Shah et al., 2010), an event that could enhance subsequent synaptic potentials. This illustrates how intrinsic and synaptic excitability work together to shape global neuronal excitability and determine the direction of future changes in synaptic transmission (Fig. 5.2).

AT THE AXOSOMATIC LEVEL

After propagating along the dendrites and soma, excitatory and inhibitory inputs are summed and generate an action potential at the axon hillock if the depolarization level reaches the action potential threshold. A change in axosomatic excitability will then have dramatic effects on the throughput of all the synapses that contact that neuron. Voltage-gated Na+ channels are highly expressed on the soma and are a major determinant of action potential threshold, and changes in their function or density affect the generation of action potentials. For example, in dorsal root ganglion neurons, in addition to the downregulation of A-type K+ and T-type Ca2+ currents, an increase in voltage-gated Na+ currents decreases the action potential threshold—an effect that is associated with chronic inflammatory pain. Together, enduring changes in these currents contribute to long-lasting dorsal root ganglion hyperexcitability that is thought to mediate chronic hyperalgesia (Beck and Yaari, 2008) (Fig. 5.2).

AT THE AXON INITIAL SEGMENT (AIS) LEVEL

Immediately distal to the axon hillock, the AIS is the subcellular region with the highest density of Na+ channels, a feature that provides it with the lowest action potential threshold. At the AIS, variations in neuronal activity can induce changes in ion channel functions (Na+ and K+) and/or a shift in AIS position and length. For example, in cultured hippocampal neurons, a long-term increase in neuronal activity shifts the AIS more distally, which returns to its original position when activity renormalizes. On the other hand, a persistent decrease in activity increases the length of the AIS. Because the composition and density of Na+ channels at the AIS did not change, this alteration reflected a true change in AIS structure. Physiologically, increased activity that moves the AIS distally is associated with decreased intrinsic excitability. Decreased activity, for example, in the case of auditory deprivation, is associated with more Na+ channels that occupy a longer AIS, which translates into increased intrinsic excitability by lowering action potential threshold (Grubb et al., 2011). Such activity-dependent changes set the AIS as a site where homeostatic adaptation can occur. Dynamic changes in its structure and position may be a homeostatic response, which provide the neuron with the remarkable capability to readjust its action potential discharge in response to chronic increases or decreases in neuronal activity (see also next section, "Homeostatic Plasticity").

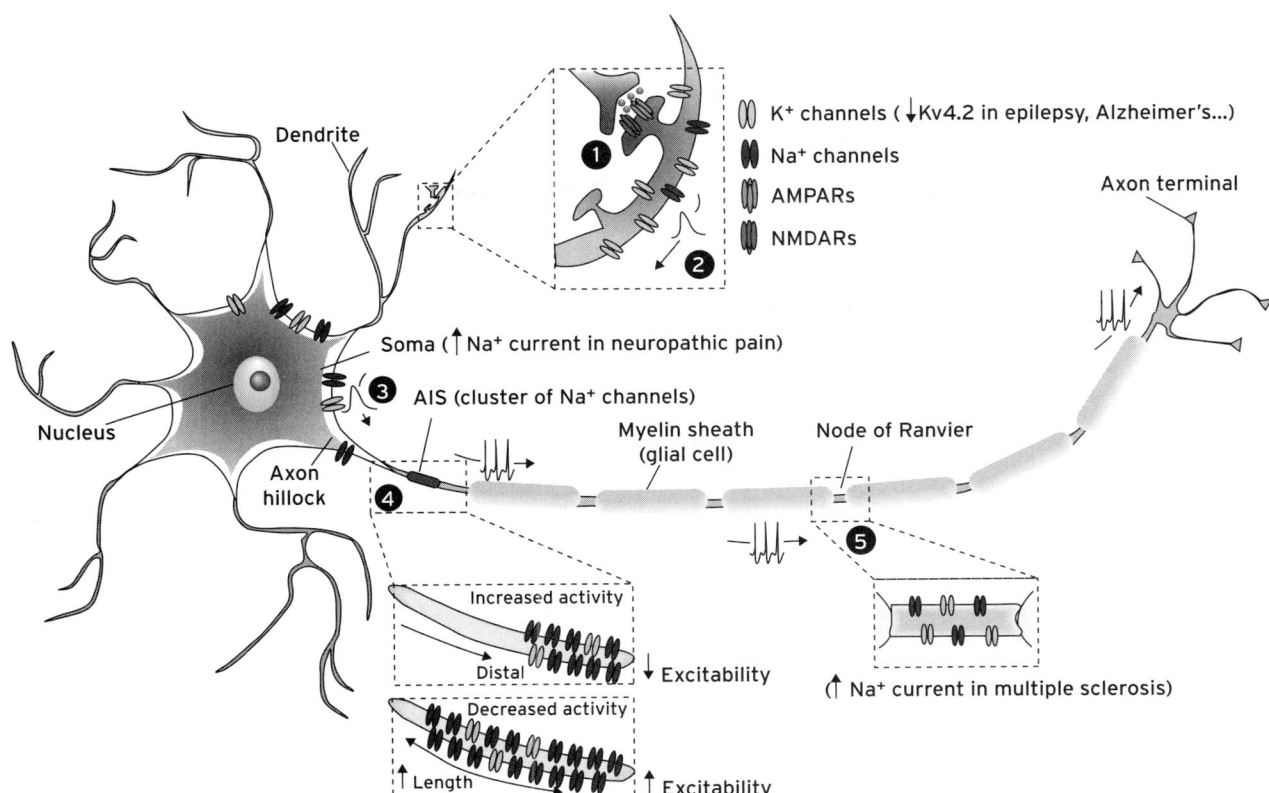

Figure 5.2 *Schematic depicting the different subcellular compartments of a neuron and examples of reported changes in factors that influence intrinsic excitability. When a neuron receives a signal through presynaptic neurotransmitter release (1), it travels through successive subcellular compartments before it can transmit the information to the next neuron. In particular, at the synaptic level (1) the signal generates an excitatory postsynaptic potential (EPSP) that travels along the dendrite (2) and the soma (3) before reaching the axon hillock and the axon initial segment (AIS) (4), structures that are rich in voltage-gated Na^+ channels. At this step, if an EPSP is strong enough to depolarize the membrane to action potential threshold, then action potentials are generated. In myelinated neurons, action potentials will travel in a saltatory conduction mode from one node of Ranvier (5) (interruption in myelin sheath) to the next, until they reach the axon terminal, where they will trigger neurotransmitter release. At each of these steps, which can undergo activity- and/or experience-dependent intrinsic plasticity, the signal is modulated by voltage-gated ion channels (Na^+, K^+, and Ca^{2+}). The physiological and behavioral consequences of these changes are diverse.*

As much as changes in neuronal activity alter AIS function and structure, mutational changes in proteins that are specifically expressed at the AIS can disrupt its proper function and engender neurological disorders. Although little is known about AIS-related disorders, it appears that disruption of AIS excitability may be a potential mechanism for febrile seizures. Mutation in *SCN1B*, a gene that codes for the auxiliary Na^+ channels subunit β1 found at the AIS, causes a common form of childhood epilepsy. Mutation in this gene tends to hyperpolarize the action potential threshold by lowering Na^+ channel voltage activation, which increases sensitivity to temperature-triggered seizures (Grubb et al., 2011) (Fig. 5.2).

AT THE AXONAL LEVEL

Once an action potential is triggered, it travels along the axon to the presynaptic terminal where it triggers release of neurotransmitters. Among other factors, action potential conduction is strongly influenced by myelin, an insulating sheath wrap made up of glial cells. At regular intervals, called the nodes of Ranvier, this sheath is interrupted, which allows the generation of electrical activity. This allows the action potential to propagate in a saltatory fashion, which is quicker and uses less energy. Nodes of Ranvier express a specific set of voltage-gated K^+ and Na^+ ion channels. Alterations in channel function will affect the proper conduction of the signal. However, in some cases, alterations can be beneficial. For example, in the early stages of multiple sclerosis, a demyelinating disease that has debilitating consequences, increases in the expression of Na^+ channels actually compensate for a decrease in action potential propagation induced by loss of myelin (Mantegazza et al., 2010) (Fig. 5.2).

MOLECULAR SUBSTRATES AND MECHANISMS

Ion channels can be modulated through their numbers and functional kinetics. While their numbers often involve either internalization in the case of decreases, or translational processes in the case of increases, mechanisms that lead to changes in their activation kinetics are more complex. The most well known and best described modes of functional modulation of ion channels are the phosphorylation/dephosphorylation mechanisms (Barros et al., 2012). Like many other proteins, ion channels are the substrates of kinases, such as serine/threonine and tyrosine kinases, and phosphatases. Site-specific phosphorylations at the cytoplasmic domains, either at the N- or the C-terminal of the pore-forming α-subunits, have various consequences for channel function, including regulation of current amplitudes and kinetics (Barros et al., 2012). Such modulations contribute to both short- and long-term regulations of ion influx and thus affect the electrical properties of membranes. Several phosphorylated residues located at the N-terminal are targets for regulating the gating properties of voltage-gated K⁺ channels. Phosphorylations at this site alter the most studied channel inactivation mode, the so-called ball-and-chain or N-type inactivation (fast-inactivation), which consists of an occlusion of the internal mouth of the channel pore by a protein localized at the amino(N)-terminal. For example, PKC-dependent phosphorylation of the Kv3.4 N-terminal slows down or eliminates N-type inactivation, which accelerates repolarization and shortens action potential duration (Barros et al., 2012; Ritter et al., 2012). Kv3.4 is a member of the fast-inactivating A-type K⁺ currents and is expressed in nociceptive dorsal root ganglion neurons. Slowing down or eliminating N-type inactivation of Kv3.4 is hypothesized to be involved in the transition from acute to chronic pain. Other mechanisms of regulations also exist. For example, in chronic epilepsy, dendritic decreases in Kv4.2-mediated A-type K⁺ currents can occur via various signaling pathways that can either change the functions of existing channels through kinase-dependent phosphorylation (PKA/PKC/MAPK) or decrease their availability at the membrane through a clathrin-dependent internalization or a transcriptional downregulation. Interestingly, another mode of regulation that may contribute to declining cognitive functions observed in Alzheimer's disease is the direct block of the Kv4.2 channel by β amyloid, a protein produced by the sequential cleavage of the amyloid precursor protein by secretases (Beck and Yaari, 2008).

EXPERIENCE-DEPENDENT INTRINSIC PLASTICITY

Although the functional and behavioral consequences of persistent changes in intrinsic excitability remain elusive, several hypotheses have been raised. The role of some of the forms of experience-dependent intrinsic plasticity discussed next is to actually render the neural system resistant or predisposed to undergoing future plastic changes, a phenomenon called metaplasticity (Abraham and Bear, 1996).

INTRINSIC PLASTICITY IN LEARNING AND MEMORY

Although synaptic plasticity is widely assumed to mediate learning and memory, a number of studies show that learning experience can modify excitability, implying that the regulation of intrinsic ion channels may contribute to learning and memory processes, and in some cases actually correlates with learning performance (Disterhoft and Oh, 2006; Zhang and Linden, 2003). Since K⁺ currents are highly involved in the fine-tuning of neuronal intrinsic excitability, studies often report functional changes in this ion channel family. Results from multidisciplinary approaches, including genetic manipulations, pharmacological tools, and electrophysiological measurements, seem to indicate that specific K⁺ channels and/or currents are involved in forming specific types of memories

and participating in specific stages of learning depending on their anatomical and subcellular localization and biophysical properties. The first results that showed changes in intrinsic excitability during learning and memory experience were from studies on invertebrates. For example, Cowan and Siegel (1986) observed that a specific deleterious mutation in the *Shaker* gene (coding for a subset of voltage-dependent K⁺ channels) attenuated the acquisition and short-term memory in a classical olfactory conditioning in *Drosophila* (Cowan and Siegel, 1986). Later, experience-dependent changes in K⁺ conductances during memory processes were reported in several other learning paradigms in both invertebrates and vertebrates (Zhang and Linden, 2003). However, because such adaptations may encode or underlie various phenomena, it has been difficult to relate them to specific behavioral of physiological functions. Here, we will briefly cite the most prominent hypotheses.

(1) Savings
Savings is the capability of a system, even after the performance has declined to basal level, to learn faster when retrained on the same or similar tasks. For example, *in vivo* intracellular recordings in cat sensorimotor cortex following an associative conditioning task revealed an increase in spiking capability that persisted even after the conditioning was extinguished, which suggests that this form of cellular memory is not coding the memory of the conditioning itself. Interestingly, subsequent conditionings, similar to the previous and new ones, were acquired faster (Zhang and Linden, 2003). Hypothetically, increased cellular excitability can represent a form of memory that primes the brain for new learning, a phenomenon called *savings*.

(2) Permissive Role
In this case, learning-induced changes in intrinsic excitability disappear when learning is still strong, which suggests again that such changes are not a part of the engram itself. For example, Disterhoft and colleagues measured increased intrinsic excitability in pyramidal hippocampal neurons, characterized by a reduction of action potential afterhyperpolarization (AHP) during a learning task in rabbits. Reduced AHP occurred before a behavioral response was acquired and was no longer present when animals, still showing a strong behavioral response, were tested a few weeks later. Disterhoft and colleagues hypothesized that because increases in pyramidal hippocampal neurons' intrinsic excitability precede acquisition of behavioral responses, they might have a permissive function in memory. In other words, increased neuronal excitability may render the hippocampus hyperexcitable and predispose the neural network to generate long-term neuronal change, for example, LTP, which will *in fine* constitute the memory trace. This hypothesis is supported by the fact that reduced AHP occurs before efficient learning and that AHP reductions are directly correlated with enhanced learning capability (Disterhoft and Oh, 2006) (See also earlier section paragraph "At the Dendritic Level".)

(3) Rule Learning and/or Learning Set
As defined by Harry F. Harlow in 1949, learning set is "*the learning how to learn efficiently in the situations the animal*

frequently encounters" (Harlow, 1949: p. 51). An interesting experimental example of this was provided by Barkai and his colleagues (Saar and Barkai, 2009), who showed that rats that have learned to discriminate a pair of odors for a reward exhibited an increased neuronal intrinsic excitability in the piriform (olfactory) cortex. The rats could discriminate subsequent new pairs of odors in fewer trials, but only when the new pair was presented soon (1–3 days) after the first pair, that is, when the increased piriform intrinsic excitability was still present. If this delay was extended to 5–7 days, when changes in intrinsic excitability had disappeared, the rats failed to acquire the task as quickly and took the same time as untrained animals. In summary, recordings in the piriform cortex had an increased neuronal intrinsic excitability, which decayed with a similar time course as the learning capabilities (Saar and Barkai, 2009). This is in stark contrast with the concept of "savings," where changes in intrinsic excitability outlast the performance in the conditioning task. Here, the capability for faster learning occurs only when increased intrinsic excitability is still present.

INTRINSIC PLASTICITY IN NEUROLOGICAL DISORDERS

Although plasticity of intrinsic excitability can be beneficial, as in the case of learning and memory, it is also emerging as a maladaptive alteration with potentially deleterious outcomes that can lead to neurological disorders. Most of the advancements investigating the role of intrinsic plasticity in CNS disorders have come from studies on epilepsy and neuropathic pain (Beck and Yaari, 2008). For example, it is hypothesized that chronic epilepsy is caused by an increase in hippocampal neuron dendritic excitability. In particular, a single episode of status epilepticus leads to a decrease in A-type voltage-gated K^+ currents, a major regulator of dendritic excitability (Hille, 2001). Whether this phenomenon contributes to the reoccurrence of epileptic seizures is still under investigation. Other disorders have also been associated with decreased dendritic A-type K^+ currents, including traumatic brain injury (TBI) (Lei et al., 2012), an event that can lead to cognitive deficits, and Alzheimer's disease (Zou et al., 2011). It has only been recently that lasting changes in the function of voltage-gated channels in specific regions of the brain have been linked to various neurological disorders, including chronic stress (Krishnan et al., 2007), affective disorders, and schizophrenia (Roberts, 2006).

Plasticity of intrinsic excitability following experience of drugs of abuse was reported in the early 1970s; however, in the past 10 years this field has drawn increasing attention. One of its critical aims is to understand how chronic experience with drugs of abuse leads to persistent changes in intrinsic excitability, and how these changes relate to the behavioral phenotypes that characterize addiction. In this regard, perhaps the first evidence was provided by George K. Aghajanian's laboratory (Nestler et al., 1999), where the authors showed that acute *in vitro* or *in vivo* morphine application decreases action potential firing in the locus coeruleus (LC), the major noradrenergic nucleus in the brain. In contrast, repeated *in vivo* morphine renormalized firing rates toward control levels. Interestingly, naltrexone application, an opioid receptor antagonist that is used in alcohol and opioid dependence, increased firing only in morphine-treated animals—an effect that is dependent on K^+ channels and is tightly correlated with withdrawal symptoms, including irritability and wet dog shakes. This set of intriguing data likely represents the first demonstration of *in vivo* neuronal homeostatic adaptation, where chronic morphine exposure triggered a non-synaptic increase in LC neurons' excitability to counteract morphine-induced decreased firing rate. Along the same line, exposure to psychostimulant drugs modulates ionic currents as well, including Na^+, Ca^{2+}, and K^+. These changes, where K^+ current modulation plays a primary role, translate into transient or persistent firing adaptations. For example, chronic exposure to cocaine or amphetamine leads to a persistent firing rate depression in the shell subregion of the nucleus accumbens (NAc) (Kourrich and Thomas, 2009), a brain region involved in motivation and reward (Kelley, 2004). Although the causal relationship between NAc neurons' firing capability and addiction-related behaviors is still under investigation, a recent study has demonstrated that NAc firing rate depression enhances behavioral sensitization to cocaine (Kourrich et al., 2012), a behavioral phenotype thought to reflect increased rewarding properties of cocaine that may contribute to the development of addictive processes (Robinson and Berridge, 2008).

Finally, alcohol has also been shown to modulate the firing rate in the NAc. Although the first study to investigate the changes in neuronal intrinsic properties following chronic alcohol drinking was performed in 1984 (Durand and Carlen, 1984), it has only been recently that these changes have been attributed to a specific ion channel, the small conductance Ca^{2+}-activated K^+ channel (SK) (Hopf et al., 2010), a strong regulator of repetitive firing. Chronic alcohol consumption induces a long-lasting reduction of SK3 subtype expression, which enhances the firing rate in the core subregion of the NAc. Interestingly, *in vivo* activation of SK3 reduced motivation for alcohol seeking behaviors (Hopf et al., 2010).

HOMEOSTATIC PLASTICITY

DEFINITION AND BRIEF HISTORY

In the second half of the 19th century, Claude Bernard first defined homeostasis as the capacity for a system to regulate its function according to changes in its environment to reach stability. At the neuronal level, homeostasis has been proposed as a means for the brain to reach stability upon destabilization of the neural circuit activity. In this way, a neuron can adjust its excitability to compensate for perturbations in activity, a process that can requires hours to days (Turrigiano and Nelson, 2004). These types of compensations in activity level can affect both intrinsic and synaptic factors that control global neuronal excitability.

Perhaps the first *in vivo* demonstration to show that neurons are capable of compensation for chronic suppression of activity were suggested by a series of articles published between 1970 and 1990 from George K. Aghajanian's laboratory (see section paragraph "Intrinsic Plasticity in Neurological Disorders") (Nestler et al., 1999); however, it is after 1990 that similar phenomena started to be revealed *in vitro*. In particular, Ramakers et al. (1990) demonstrated that chronic activity blockade produces a rebound in hyperexcitability in central neuronal networks *in vitro* (Ramakers et al., 1990), a phenomenon that also occurs in isolated lobster stomatogastric ganglion neurons (Turrigiano et al., 1994), which suggests that neurons regulate their conductances to maintain stable activity patterns and that the intrinsic properties of a neuron depend on its recent history of activation. Later studies demonstrated that neurons could also modulate their synaptic functions by increasing or decreasing AMPAR function in response to chronic alteration in activity (O'Brien et al., 1998; Turrigiano et al., 1998). These studies raised a number of critical questions. For instance, does homeostatic adaptation require changes in the network, that is, pre- and postsynaptic, or are these changes cell-autonomous? Also, what are the sensors and monitors of cell activity that initiate

compensatory changes, and what are the cellular mechanisms that are triggered by chronic changes in activity? This section will provide a brief description of the different types (Fig. 5.3) of homeostatic plasticity as well as descriptions of the monitors of cellular activity, and the known basic cellular mechanisms involved in neuronal homeostatic plasticity (Fig. 5.4).

DIVERSITY IN HOMEOSTATIC PLASTICITY

CELL-AUTONOMOUS

As defined by Turrigiano and Nelson (2004: p. 103), cell-autonomous plasticity is "*the plasticity in the properties of an individual neuron resulting from changes in its own activity, independent of the activity of other neurons in the network*" (Fig. 5.3A). Two seminal studies addressed this possibility. In the first, synaptic activity was blocked and the postsynaptic neuron chemically depolarized (Leslie et al., 2001). In the second, the neuron was hyperpolarized via a transfection of Kir2.1, an inward-rectifier K+ channel involved in maintaining hyperpolarized membrane

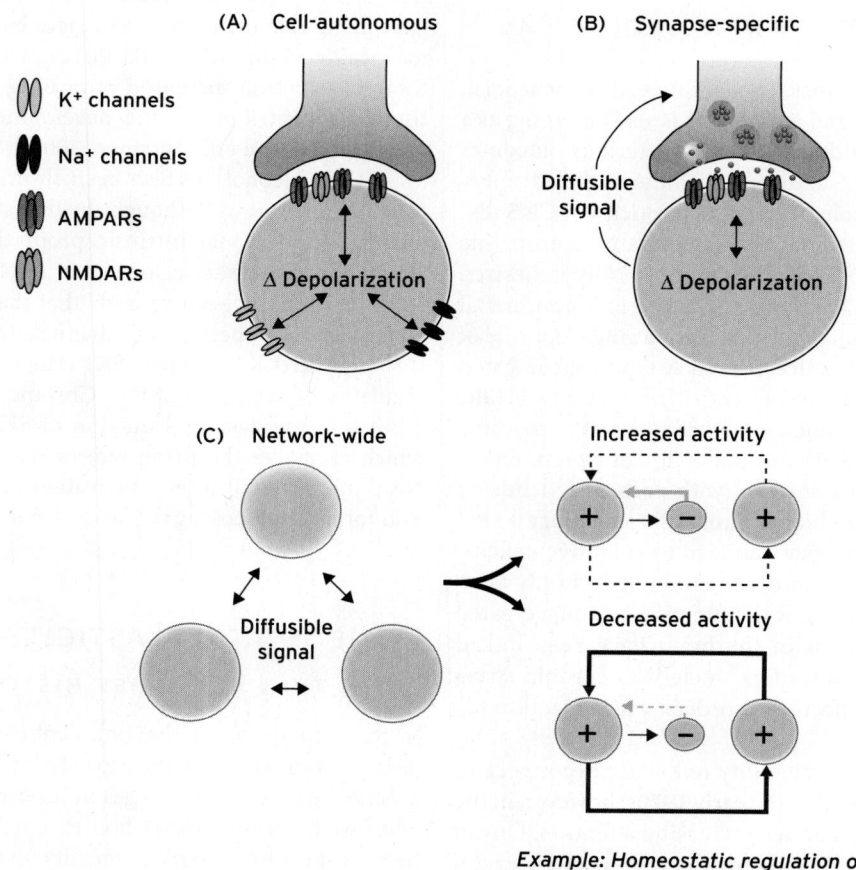

Figure 5.3 *Diagrams representing three models of homeostatic neuroadaptations. All modes are supposed to be triggered by variations in postsynaptic depolarization, likely through changes in intracellular Ca²⁺ concentrations. (A) Cell-autonomous homeostasis is when a neuron can sense, integrate, and correct its own neuronal activity to a set value without requiring external factors. (B) Synapse-specific homeostasis is when, at a specific synapse, local signaling regulates pre- and/or postsynaptic excitability. This may involve a retrograde diffusible signal(s) from the post- to presynaptic side to regulate neurotransmitter release. (C) Network-wide homeostasis is when a network of neighboring cells adjusts neural network excitability through a diffusible activity signal. The diffusible signal can act on both the neighboring cells and the neuron itself (not represented) and can either increase or decrease neuronal excitability depending on neuronal types. As an example, homeostatic regulation of excitation-inhibition balance may involve diffusion of brain-derived neurotrophin (BDNF), which can differentially regulate excitability of excitatory versus inhibitory neurons. When activity is increased, the diffusible signal can trigger cellular mechanisms that weaken excitatory transmission (Dotted line) and enhance inhibitory transmission (Solid gray line). If activity is decreased, the opposite mechanism occurs.*

potentials (Burrone et al., 2002). In both cases, the neuron compensated for its changes in neuronal activity by either decreasing (Leslie et al., 2001) or increasing synaptic input, which restored neuronal activity to control levels. Interestingly, Leslie et al. (2001) found that these changes were independent of fast excitatory and inhibitory synaptic transmission (AMPAR, NMDAR, and GABAR), action potential generation, and activity-dependent release of brain-derived neurotrophic factor (BDNF). These findings suggest that neurons can sense an average level of activity and compensate for it in an autonomous fashion (Turrigiano, 2008). Later studies established unequivocal evidence for cell-autonomous mechanisms and particularly the capacity for a neuron to adjust its synaptic input following changes in its somatic, but not dendritic or synaptic, intrinsic properties (Goold and Nicoll, 2010; Ibata et al., 2008).

SYNAPSE-SPECIFIC

In the synapse-specific model, chronic changes in neuronal activity involve synaptic signaling that will trigger compensatory changes in pre- and/or postsynaptic function, such as changes in presynaptic release probability, quantal size, and the number of postsynaptic glutamate receptors (Turrigiano, 2007) (Fig. 5.3B).

Synapse-specific homeostatic plasticity was originally found in the invertebrate *Drosophila*, where muscle membrane hyperpolarization through overexpression of Kir2.1 triggered presynaptic adaptations in order to compensate for impaired muscle excitability. This compensatory mechanism occurs rapidly and is characterized by increased glutamate release (quantal content) without a change in quantal size. Because changes occurred only on the presynaptic side, it suggests the

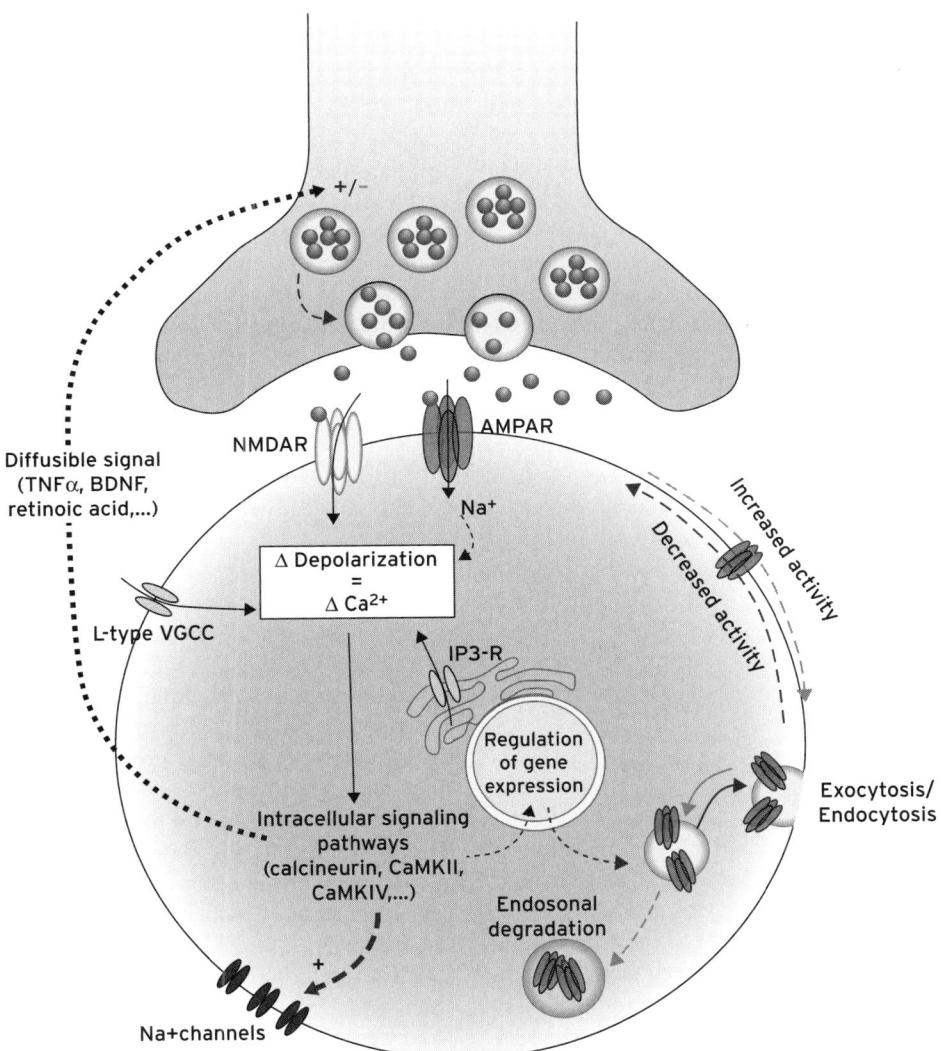

Figure 5.4 Diagram representing a summary of cellular mechanisms that have been shown to be involved in homeostatic plasticity. After sensing its depolarization level (intracellular Ca^{2+}), a neuron can trigger a variety of mechanisms that aim to readjust neuronal excitability to a set value. Via AMPARs activation the neuron depolarizes and allows activation of NMDARs and VGCCs, which directly increases intracellular Ca^{2+} concentration. Ca^{2+}-dependent pathways may also lead to the activation of IP3 receptors and further influence intracellular Ca^{2+} concentration. Intracellular Ca^{2+} can then recruit various intracellular signaling pathways, including CaMKII-, CaMKIV- and calcineurin-dependent pathways, which in turn, likely through phosphorylation/dephosphorylation mechanisms adjust postsynaptic levels of a variety of targets (Na^+ channels, K^+ channels, AMPARs, etc.). Additionally, the postsynaptic neuron may also, through mechanisms that are still unclear, release diffusible activity signals (BDNF, Tumor necrosis factor alpha TNFα, retinoic acid, etc.) that can act presynaptically to regulate neurotransmitter release. In dark gray are examples of mechanisms that are regulated when activity is decreased, and in light gray, when activity is increased.

involvement of a trans-synaptic signaling cascade. Although the signaling mechanism remains elusive, presynaptic homeostasis following postsynaptic changes in activity also occurs at central synapses (Turrigiano, 2007). Though not discussed here, synaptic homeostasis can also involve changes in postsynaptic glutamate receptors with no perceptible changes in presynaptic function (Turrigiano, 2008).

NETWORK-WIDE

Network-wide homeostasis occurs when neurons regulate their synaptic function following changes in network activity. This homeostatic adaptation involves a diffusible signal that is sensed by neurons in the network that triggers changes in their synaptic activity to restore normal neural network activity (Fig. 5.3C). For example, in cultured cortical networks, interneurons decrease their inhibitory inputs to pyramidal neurons when pyramidal neuronal activity is decreased. Specifically, when a pyramidal neuron firing rate is decreased, its capability to release BDNF is decreased as well. Decreased levels of BDNF translate into increased excitatory transmission between pyramidal neurons. Importantly, neighboring interneurons can sense the decreased BDNF and decrease their inhibitory inputs onto pyramidal neurons to restore the firing capability for the neurons in the network (Turrigiano and Nelson, 2004). The mechanism by which decreased BDNF triggers opposite synaptic adaptations in pyramidal neurons versus interneurons is not yet known.

The regulation of synaptic transmission in cortical networks is a critical mechanism that preserves an adequate balance of excitation and inhibition (Fig. 5.3C), and a disruption in the balance of excitation to inhibition can have dramatic consequences. For example, this type of disruption is one of the leading hypotheses to explain some forms of autism where an imbalance occurs in the form of an increased ratio of excitation/inhibition in various systems, including mnemonic, social, sensory, and emotional systems (Rippon et al., 2007; Rubenstein and Merzenich, 2003). Disruption in excitation-inhibition balance has also been reported in neurological disorders as diverse as epilepsy (Fritschy, 2008), schizophrenia (Kehrer et al., 2008), and mental retardation (Eichler and Meier, 2008).

MOLECULAR SUBSTRATES

Homeostatic mechanisms are triggered by perturbations in the level of neuronal activity. However, the means through which a neuron detects variations in its activity are still unclear. Because the level of depolarization directly influences intracellular Ca^{2+} concentration, a prerequisite for many activity-dependent enzymes to function, intracellular Ca^{2+} level has become a prominent candidate for monitoring cellular activity. Ca^{2+} levels are influenced by Ca^{2+} influx through neurotransmitter receptors, voltage-gated Ca^{2+} channels, and Ca^{2+} release from intracellular stores, each of which potentially provides a temporal and spatial readout of cellular activity (Davis and Bezprozvanny, 2001). Once the neuron senses changes in its activity, it activates molecular effectors to execute compensatory changes, likely through Ca^{2+}-calmodulin protein kinases-activated pathways (Fig. 5.4).

A subject of a long series of studies, CaMKII is a Ca^{2+} sensor that is sensitive to the oscillations in the intracellular concentration of Ca^{2+}, a critical feature that encodes information (De Koninck and Schulman, 1998). A unique characteristic of this kinase is its autophosphorylation ability, through which it produces an "autonomous" form that is constitutively active well beyond the activating stimulus. This characteristic allows the kinase to remember previous activity and influences subsequent response to stimuli (Lisman et al., 2012). A facet of CaMKII that makes it an attractive executor for homeostatic adaptations resides in its capability to modulate a variety of targets, including synaptic strength, intrinsic excitability, and gene expression (Lisman et al., 2012; Maier, 2011). Intriguingly, α and β isoforms forming the CaMKII holoenzyme are not only differentially sensitive to Ca^{2+} concentration, but also differentially affect synaptic functions (Thiagarajan et al., 2002). Taken together, these characteristics make CaMKII an ideal monitor and effector that can trigger intracellular signaling to correct chronic variations in neuronal activity. In addition to CaMKII, two recent studies have revealed a critical role for CaMKIV, another type of calmodulin-dependent kinase, in cell-autonomous regulation of synaptic transmission (Goold and Nicoll, 2010; Ibata et al., 2008). Specifically, decreased neuronal activity triggers increased synaptic strength, a mechanism mediated through a drop in somatic Ca^{2+} concentration and reduced activation of CaMKIV (Ibata et al., 2008). The opposite phenomenon was later reported by Goold and Nicoll (2010) where neuronal activity was increased, further supporting a role for CaMKIV in bidirectional regulation of neuronal homeostasis.

CONCLUSION

This chapter succinctly described some fundamental types of neural plasticity. Generally speaking, plasticity is a ubiquitous phenomenon that occurs in various subcellular compartments, where each regulates specific aspects of neuronal communication. Subcellular compartments can engage in a variety of cellular mechanisms targeting voltage- and/or ligand-gated ion channels to change persistently their functions upon exposure to various types of experiences, including learning and exposure to drugs of abuse. For the purpose of brevity, we did not describe structural plasticity in this chapter, which is another type of neural plasticity that is also very important (Bosch and Hayashi, 2011). Combined with the discovery of unequivocal evidence for adult neurogenesis (Lledo et al., 2006), it demonstrates that neurons not only change their functions, but also their shapes and numbers. Now, new challenges for researchers include achieving a better understanding of how diverse types of plasticity occur as well as elucidating their functional relevance and how they relate to changes in behaviors. Moreover, because multiple types of plasticity can coexist in a neural network or even in the same neuron, we need to better understand how they interact with one another to shape neural activity and lead to adaptive or maladaptive behaviors that are observed in neurological and psychiatric disorders.

DISCLOSURES

Dr. Kourrich and Dr. Bonci have no conflicts of interests to disclose. This work was supported by the Intramural Research Program at the National Institute on Drug Abuse.

REFERENCES

Abraham, W.C., and Bear, M.F. (1996). Metaplasticity: the plasticity of synaptic plasticity. *Trends Neurosci.* 19:126–130.

Barros, F., Dominguez, P., et al. (2012). Cytoplasmic domains and voltage-dependent potassium channel gating. *Front. Pharmacol.* 3:49.

Beck, H., and Yaari, Y. (2008). Plasticity of intrinsic neuronal properties in CNS disorders. *Nat. Rev. Neurosci.* 9:357–369.

Benito, E., and Barco, A. (2010). CREB's control of intrinsic and synaptic plasticity: implications for CREB-dependent memory models. *Trends Neurosci.* 33:230–240.

Berlucchi, G., and Buchtel, H.A. (2009). Neuronal plasticity: historical roots and evolution of meaning. *Exp. Brain Res.* 192:307–319.

Bliss, T.V., and Lomo, T. (1973). Long-lasting potentiation of synaptic transmission in the dentate area of the anaesthetized rabbit following stimulation of the perforant path. *J. Physiol.* 232:331–356.

Bosch, M., and Hayashi, Y. (2011). Structural plasticity of dendritic spines. *Curr. Opin. Neurobiol.* 22:383–388.

Bowers, M.S., Chen, B.T., et al. (2010). AMPA receptor synaptic plasticity induced by psychostimulants: the past, present, and therapeutic future. *Neuron* 67:11–24.

Burrone, J., O'Byrne, M., et al. (2002). Multiple forms of synaptic plasticity triggered by selective suppression of activity in individual neurons. *Nature* 420:414–418.

Caporale, N., and Dan, Y. (2008). Spike timing-dependent plasticity: a Hebbian learning rule. *Annu. Rev. Neurosci.* 31:25–46.

Collingridge, G.L., Peineau, S., et al. (2010). Long-term depression in the CNS. *Nat. Rev. Neurosci.* 11:459–473.

Cowan, T.M., and Siegel, R.W. (1986). Drosophila mutations that alter ionic conduction disrupt acquisition and retention of a conditioned odor avoidance response. *J. Neurogenet.* 3:187–201.

Davis, G.W., and Bezprozvanny, I. (2001). Maintaining the stability of neural function: a homeostatic hypothesis. *Annu. Rev. Physiol.* 63:847–869.

De Koninck, P., and Schulman, H. (1998). Sensitivity of CaM kinase II to the frequency of Ca^{2+} oscillations. *Science* 279:227–230.

Disterhoft, J.F., and Oh, M.M. (2006). Learning, aging and intrinsic neuronal plasticity. *Trends Neurosci.* 29:587–599.

Durand, D., and Carlen, P.L. (1984). Decreased neuronal inhibition in vitro after long-term administration of ethanol. *Science* 224:1359–1361.

Eichler, S.A., and Meier, J.C. (2008). E-I balance and human diseases—from molecules to networking. *Front. Mol. Neurosci.* 1:2.

Fritschy, J.M. (2008). Epilepsy, E/I Balance and GABA(A) Receptor Plasticity. *Front. Mol. Neurosci.* 1:5.

Goold, C.P., and Nicoll, R.A. (2010). Single-cell optogenetic excitation drives homeostatic synaptic depression. *Neuron* 68:512–528.

Grubb, M.S., Shu, Y., et al. (2011). Short- and long-term plasticity at the axon initial segment. *J. Neurosci.* 31:16049–16055.

Harlow, H.F. (1949). The formation of learning sets. *Psychol. Rev.* 56:51–65.

Hebb, D.O. (1949). Organization of Behavior. New York: Wiley.

Hille, B. (2001). Ion Channels of Excitable Membranes, 3rd Edition. Sunderland, MA: Sinauer Associates.

Hopf, F.W., Bowers, M.S., et al. (2010). Reduced nucleus accumbens SK channel activity enhances alcohol seeking during abstinence. *Neuron* 65:682–694.

Ibata, K., Sun, Q., et al. (2008). Rapid synaptic scaling induced by changes in postsynaptic firing. *Neuron* 57:819–826.

Ito, M., and Kano, M. (1982). Long-lasting depression of parallel fiber-Purkinje cell transmission induced by conjunctive stimulation of parallel fibers and climbing fibers in the cerebellar cortex. *Neurosci. Lett.* 33:253–258.

Jackson, A.C., and Nicoll, R.A. (2011). The expanding social network of ionotropic glutamate receptors: TARPs and other transmembrane auxiliary subunits. *Neuron* 70:178–199.

Kehrer, C., Maziashvili, N., et al. (2008). Altered excitatory-inhibitory balance in the NMDA-hypofunction model of schizophrenia. *Front. Mol. Neurosci.* 1:6.

Kelley, A.E. (2004). Ventral striatal control of appetitive motivation: role in ingestive behavior and reward-related learning. *Neurosci. Biobehav. Rev.* 27:765–776.

Kourrich, S., Klug, J.R., et al. (2012). AMPAR-independent effect of striatal alphaCaMKII promotes the sensitization of cocaine reward. *J. Neurosci.* 32:6578–6586.

Kourrich, S., and Thomas, M.J. (2009). Similar neurons, opposite adaptations: psychostimulant experience differentially alters firing properties in accumbens core versus shell. *J. Neurosci.* 29:12275–12283.

Krishnan, V., Han, M.H., et al. (2007). Molecular adaptations underlying susceptibility and resistance to social defeat in brain reward regions. *Cell* 131:391–404.

Lauri, S.E., Palmer, M., et al. (2007). Presynaptic mechanisms involved in the expression of STP and LTP at CA1 synapses in the hippocampus. *Neuropharmacology* 52:1–11.

Lei, Z., Deng, P., et al. (2012). Alterations of A-type potassium channels in hippocampal neurons after traumatic brain injury. *J. Neurotrauma* 29:235–245.

Leslie, K.R., Nelson, S.B., et al. (2001). Postsynaptic depolarization scales quantal amplitude in cortical pyramidal neurons. *J. Neurosci.* 21:RC170.

Lisman, J., Yasuda, R., et al. (2012). Mechanisms of CaMKII action in long-term potentiation. *Nat. Rev. Neurosci.* 13:169–182.

Lledo, P.M., Alonso, M., et al. (2006). Adult neurogenesis and functional plasticity in neuronal circuits. *Nat. Rev. Neurosci.* 7:179–193.

Lujan, R. (2010). Organisation of potassium channels on the neuronal surface. *J. Chem. Neuroanat.* 40:1–20.

Lynch, M.A. (2004). Long-term potentiation and memory. *Physiol. Rev.* 84:87–136.

Maier, L.S. (2011). CaMKII regulation of voltage-gated sodium channels and cell excitability. *Heart Rhythm* 8:474–477.

Mantegazza, M., Curia, G., et al. (2010). Voltage-gated sodium channels as therapeutic targets in epilepsy and other neurological disorders. *Lancet Neurol.* 9:413–424.

Mayford, M., Bach, M.E., et al. (1996). Control of memory formation through regulated expression of a CaMKII transgene. *Science* 274, 1678–1683.

Nestler, E.J., Alreja, M., et al. (1999). Molecular control of locus coeruleus neurotransmission. *Biol. Psychiatry* 46:1131–1139.

O'Brien, R.J., Kamboj, S., et al. (1998). Activity-dependent modulation of synaptic AMPA receptor accumulation. *Neuron* 21:1067–1078.

Ramakers, G.J., Corner, M.A., et al. (1990). Development in the absence of spontaneous bioelectric activity results in increased stereotyped burst firing in cultures of dissociated cerebral cortex. *Exp. Brain Res.* 79:157–166.

Rippon, G., Brock, J., et al. (2007). Disordered connectivity in the autistic brain: challenges for the "new psychophysiology." *Int. J. Psychophysiol.* 63:164–172.

Ritter, D.M., Ho, C., et al. (2012). Modulation of Kv3.4 channel N-type inactivation by protein kinase C shapes the action potential in dorsal root ganglion neurons. *J. Physiol.* 590:145–161.

Roberts, E. (2006). GABAergic malfunction in the limbic system resulting from an aboriginal genetic defect in voltage-gated Na+-channel SCN5A is proposed to give rise to susceptibility to schizophrenia. *Adv. Pharmacol.* 54:119–145.

Robinson, T.E., and Berridge, K.C. (2008). Review. The incentive sensitization theory of addiction: some current issues. *Philos. Trans. R. Soc. Lond. B Biol. Sci.* 363:3137–3146.

Rubenstein, J.L., and Merzenich, M.M. (2003). Model of autism: increased ratio of excitation/inhibition in key neural systems. *Genes Brain Behav.* 2:255–267.

Saar, D., and Barkai, E. (2009). Long-lasting maintenance of learning-induced enhanced neuronal excitability: mechanisms and functional significance. *Mol. Neurobiol.* 39:171–177.

Shah, M.M., Hammond, R.S., et al. (2010). Dendritic ion channel trafficking and plasticity. *Trends Neurosci.* 33:307–316.

Spires-Jones, T., and Knafo, S. (2012). Spines, plasticity, and cognition in Alzheimer's model mice. *Neural. Plast.* 2012, Article ID 319836.

Tang, Y.P., Shimizu, E., et al. (1999). Genetic enhancement of learning and memory in mice. *Nature* 401:63–69.

Thiagarajan, T.C., Piedras-Renteria, E.S., et al. (2002). alpha- and betaCaMKII. Inverse regulation by neuronal activity and opposing effects on synaptic strength. *Neuron* 36:1103–1114.

Turrigiano, G. (2007). Homeostatic signaling: the positive side of negative feedback. *Curr. Opin. Neurobiol.* 17:318–324.

Turrigiano, G., Abbott, L.F., et al. (1994). Activity-dependent changes in the intrinsic properties of cultured neurons. *Science* 264:974–977.

Turrigiano, G.G. (2008). The self-tuning neuron: synaptic scaling of excitatory synapses. *Cell* 135:422–435.

Turrigiano, G.G., Leslie, K.R., et al. (1998). Activity-dependent scaling of quantal amplitude in neocortical neurons. *Nature* 391:892–896.

Turrigiano, G.G., and Nelson, S.B. (2004). Homeostatic plasticity in the developing nervous system. *Nat. Rev. Neurosci.* 5:97–107.

Zhang, W., and Linden, D.J. (2003). The other side of the engram: experience-driven changes in neuronal intrinsic excitability. *Nat. Rev. Neurosci.* 4:885–900.

Zou, X., Coyle, D., et al. (2011). Beta-amyloid induced changes in A-type K(+) current can alter hippocampo-septal network dynamics. *J. Comput. Neurosci.* 32:465–477.

6 | PRINCIPLES OF MOLECULAR BIOLOGY

STEVEN E. HYMAN AND ERIC J. NESTLER

Advances in molecular biology and in understanding the genetics of complex human phenotypes have opened a new world of possibilities for research on mental disorders and their treatment. However, because the syndromes with which psychiatry is ultimately charged are expressed at the level of behavior, molecular and genetic work must be complemented by ongoing research in the more integrative aspects of neuroscience and behavioral science described elsewhere in this textbook. Thus, for example, the pathophysiology of mental disorders depends on the complex interaction of genetic (bottom-up) factors and environmental (top-down) factors affecting the development and subsequent function of the brain. Many scientific disciplines must contribute to that understanding.

Despite substantial evidence that genes and environment are inseparable partners in brain development and plasticity—and therefore in the formation of personalities, talents, and all other aspects of behavior, including vulnerability to mental illness and very likely responsiveness to treatments for mental illness—simplistic versions of the nature–nurture debate never seem to disappear. It is true that from the time a one-cell embryo is formed from the fusion of sperm and egg, the genetic endowment of that individual is fixed. An important focus of current research, however, is to find out precisely what that means with respect to behavioral traits. It is now becoming increasingly clear that behavioral phenotypes, including vulnerability to serious mental disorders such as schizophrenia, bipolar disorder, depression, and autism, result from the interaction of multiple (perhaps hundreds of) genes, very likely acting at different times during brain development in interaction with the environment. An important goal of psychiatric research is therefore to understand how genetic information is read out during development and how the brain changes as a result of stochastic or random processes during development, as well as in response to experience of the sensory world and other environmental inputs, such as drugs, infections, and injuries.

The goal of this chapter is to describe the fundamental molecular processes by which information is encoded in the genome and how this information is expressed within an environmental context. We describe what genes are, how they function, and how their expression is regulated by signals from outside the cell. This chapter shows that the control of gene expression by extracellular signals is a critical arena for gene–environment interactions relevant to psychiatry (Hyman and Nestler, 1993). Chapter 7 builds on this foundation by describing *epigenetic* regulation in psychiatry, namely, how stable changes in the structure of *chromatin* (the combination of DNA and proteins that comprise the nucleus) at particular genes—and hence in the behaviors those genes regulate—can be produced without changes in the genetic code itself.

NUCLEIC ACIDS

Deoxyribonucleic acid (DNA) contains the genetic blueprints of cells, that is, the information to produce ribonucleic acid (RNA) and proteins, which in turn create the fundamental structural and functional properties of our cells. The latest estimate is that the human genome contains approximately 25,000 genes, which use about 1.5% of ~3,000,000,000 base pairs of DNA. Deoxyribonucleic acid exists as a double helix, each strand of which is an unbranched chain built out of small building blocks called *nucleotide bases*. DNA and RNA are synthesized from four types of nucleotide bases. The four nucleotides that make up DNA are the *purines, adenine* (A) and *guanine* (G), and the *pyrimidines, cytosine* (C) and *thymine* (T), each containing a deoxyribose sugar group. In RNA the pyrimidine *uracil* (U) takes the place of thymine, and the sugar group is ribose instead of deoxyribose. Individual nucleotides are joined into strands of DNA or RNA via the phosphate groups that form a phosphodiester linkage.

The alternating deoxyribose sugar and phosphate groups that connect the bases of each DNA strand form a "sugar-phosphate backbone" on the outside of the double helix with the bases arrayed on the inside of the double helix (Fig. 6.1). In DNA, the nucleotide base A is paired with (or is complementary to) T on the opposite strand, and G is paired with C. In RNA, U, which is structurally similar to T, is also complementary to A. The rules of base pairing observed in DNA result from the fact that only complementary pairs of nucleotides form a maximum number of stabilizing hydrogen bonds. Any other arrangement of bases destabilizes the structure of the DNA. A critical property of a linear polymer such as DNA (or RNA) is that it can serve as a template for the synthesis of other macromolecules. The principle of complementary base pairing provides the mechanism by which information can be transferred. An enzyme, a DNA polymerase in the case of DNA replication, or RNA polymerase in the case of transcription of DNA into RNA, can proceed down a template strand of DNA, adding a nucleotide base complementary to the base on the template strand as it forms a new strand of nucleic acid (Fig. 6.1).

Although the actual enzymatic steps involved in the replication of DNA are quite complex, the overall principles are

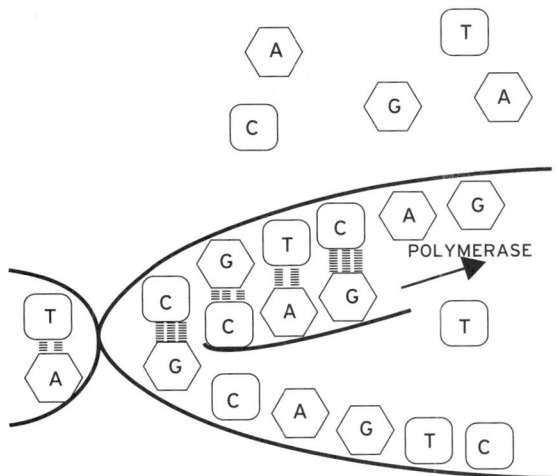

Figure 6.1 *Schematic of complementary base pairing of deoxyribonucleic acid (DNA). Two complementary strands of DNA hybridize with one another to form a double helix. The sugar-phosphate backbones of the two strands are found on the outside of the double helix; the bases are found on the inside. Formation of a DNA double helix is stabilized when hydrogen bonds form between complementary bases of the two strands. Two hydrogen bonds form when A is across from T; three hydrogen bonds form when G is across from C. Other appositions of bases are destabilizing and do not occur. A strand of DNA can serve as a template for a second strand of nucleic acid (DNA or ribonucleic acid [RNA]). A polymerase enzyme assembles individual nucleotides into a new strand using the first strand as a template. The sequence of the new strand is therefore determined by the template, permitting the transfer of information across generations. Complementary base pairing is also the fundamental principle in the synthesis of RNA from DNA and in many experimental situations in which it is desirable to detect the presence of a specific DNA or RNA strand.*

simple. Replication begins with separation of the two complementary DNA strands in a local region. Each strand then serves as a template for a new DNA molecule by the sequential polymerization of nucleotides. Eventually the replication process generates two complete DNA double helices, each identical in sequence to the original. Replication of DNA is said to be semiconservative because each daughter DNA molecule contains one of the original parental strands plus one newly synthesized strand. Transcription of DNA into RNA is conceptually similar except that only one DNA strand serves as a template and, when synthesis of the RNA is complete, it is released and the DNA strands can reanneal into their stable double-helical structure.

INFORMATION FLOWS FROM DNA TO RNA TO PROTEIN

DNA carries information in its linear sequence of nucleotides. Although the linear polynucleotide structure of DNA is well suited for the stable storage of information and for self-replication, its chemical simplicity and its relatively rigid helical structure limit its biological functions. Thus, the information contained within DNA must be read out to yield RNA and proteins. Like DNA, RNA is chemically quite simple (i.e., composed of four nucleotides), but because it is

a flexible single strand, free to fold into numerous conformations, it is functionally more versatile than DNA.

Messenger RNA (mRNA) functions as an intermediate between the sequence of DNA that comprises the transcribed regions of genes and the sequence of proteins. Not all RNA serve as mRNA, however. Other RNAs function in varied roles in cells. Ribosomes, the organelles on which proteins are synthesized, are constructed out of complexes of several types of ribosomal RNA (rRNAs) with proteins. Transfer RNAs (tRNAs) transport specific amino acids to the ribosomes for incorporation into proteins during the process in which mRNA is translated into protein. More recently, scientists have characterized several other types of non-coding RNAs, categorized as long or short based on their length. These non-coding RNAs are considered a form of epigenetic regulation and are discussed in greater detail in Chapter 7. Briefly, long non-coding RNAs, generally characterized as >200 nucleotides in length, regulate chromatin structure and gene expression (Taft et al., 2010). The most prevalent short non-coding RNAs, termed microRNAs (miRNAs), bind to specific mRNAs and inhibit their translation and/or promote their degradation (Bartel, 2009; Vo et al., 2010). The discovery of miRNAs has been translated into a powerful tool called *RNA interference* or *RNAi*, which uses small hairpin RNAs (shRNAs), which are cleaved into small inhibitory RNAs, to experimentally suppress expression of a targeted mRNA and protein.

Like DNA, mRNA carries information encoded in its linear sequence of nucleotides. DNA and mRNA specify amino acid building blocks for proteins in linear stretches of three nucleotides. Proteins consist of unbranched chains of amino acid building blocks. An amino acid is a small molecule that contains an amino group (NH_2) and a carboxylic acid or carboxy group (COOH) plus a variable side chain. The side chains used by the 20 common amino acids differ markedly in size, shape, hydrophobicity, and charge. Amino acids are linked to each other by peptide bonds that join the amino group of one amino acid to the carboxy group of another amino acid.

Within the portion of an mRNA that is translatable into a protein, each successive group of three nucleotide bases (called a *codon*) specifies either one amino acid or termination of the protein chain. The rules specifying the correspondence between a codon and an amino acid are called the *genetic code*. Because RNA is a linear polymer of 4 nucleotides, there are 4^3 or 64 possible codons but only 20 amino acids. As a result, although each codon specifies only a single amino acid, most amino acids are specified by more than one codon. The genetic code is therefore said to be degenerate. With only a few minor exceptions, the code has been conserved across evolution. The codons in an mRNA molecule do not interact directly with the amino acids they specify; the translation of mRNA into protein depends on the presence of tRNAs that serve as adapter molecules that recognize a specific codon and the corresponding amino acid (Fig. 6.2).

The ribosome is a structure composed of proteins and structural rRNAs; these organelles provide a structure on which tRNAs can interact (via their anticodons) with the codons of an mRNA in sequential order. The ribosome finds a specific start site on the mRNA that sets the reading frame and then moves

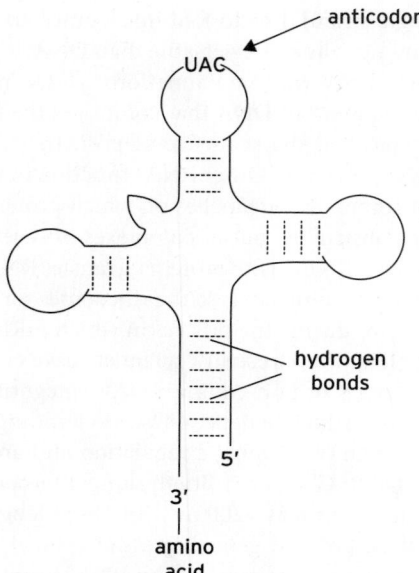

Figure 6.2 *Transfer RNA (tRNA): Transfer RNA (tRNA) is a single strand of RNA that folds on itself through the apposition of complementary base pairs and the subsequent formation of hydrogen bonds, indicated by the dashed lines in the figure. One of the loops formed contains the anticodon, the sequence of three nucleotides on the tRNA that binds to the complementary codon on a messenger RNA molecule. For the anticodon AGA shown in the figure, the corresponding codon on the mRNA would be UCU. The free end of the tRNA binds to a specific amino acid. Each tRNA, with a given anticodon, binds only one type of amino acid determined by the genetic code. In the case shown in the figure, the amino acid bound would be serine. From Hyman and Nestler (1993) reprinted with permission from The Molecular Foundations of Psychiatry, (Copyright ©1993). American Psychiatric Publishing.*

along the mRNA molecule progressively, translating the nucleotide sequence one codon at a time, using tRNAs to add amino acids to the growing end of the polypeptide chain (Fig. 6.3).

Over the past decade, it has become clear that a small number of mRNAs, along with associated protein translation machinery, are transported to dendrites of neurons, where they mediate rapid changes in protein synthesis in response to synaptic activity (Wang et al., 2010). This transport is mediated by the presence of specific sequences in the 3'-untranslated region

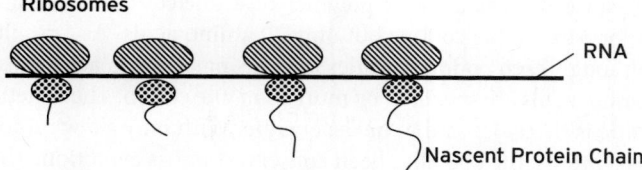

Figure 6.3 *Protein translation. Ribosomal subunits bind together on mature messenger ribonucleic acids (mRNAs) to form actively translating ribosomes. The ribosome begins adding amino acids when it reaches a "start codon" on the mRNA and processes down the mRNA, one codon at a time, adding the appropriate amino acid as it is delivered by a transfer RNA (tRNA). When a "stop codon" is reached, the ribosome releases the polypeptide chain and dissociates from the mRNA. Each mRNA that is being actively translated has multiple ribosomes moving sequentially down its length, forming a polyribosome complex. From Hyman and Nestler (1993) reprinted with permission from The Molecular Foundations of Psychiatry, (Copyright ©1993). American Psychiatric Publishing.*

of certain mRNAs, which are targeted by RNA-binding proteins to form RNA granules for transport. Fragile X mental retardation protein (FMRP) is an example of one of these RNA-binding proteins, which plays an important role in controlling dendritic protein synthesis. Loss of FMRP expression causes Fragile X mental retardation syndrome (see Chapter 7).

In contrast with nucleic acids, which are constructed of four bases that are chemically similar, proteins are constructed out of 20 very different amino acids. By incorporating so many different types of amino acids, each with its chemically diverse side chains, proteins have extraordinary functional versatility, unlike DNA or RNA. The specific properties of proteins depend not only on the linear sequence of their amino acid building blocks (*primary structure*), but also on the tendency of certain combinations of amino acids to form intrinsic structural motifs (*secondary structures*, for example, α helices or β sheets) and by their folded three-dimensional characteristics (*tertiary structure*). In addition, proteins form stable interactions (*complexes*) with other proteins (*quaternary structure*). In such cases, the individual polypeptide chains are called *subunits*. The folding of proteins, and the interactions of proteins with each other and with other molecules such as nucleic acids, is highly regulated by chemical modifications of the protein, most often of particular side chains. For example, one ubiquitous mechanism of regulation of protein function is by the covalent addition of a phosphate group (by specific enzymes called *protein kinases*) to the hydroxyl groups found in serine, threonine, or tyrosine side chains (Chapters 4 and 5). Cells may contain tens of thousands of distinct proteins, each with unique structural and functional properties, including neurotransmitter receptors, neuropeptides, ion channels, enzymes, and a very large number of other types of proteins.

GENES AND CHROMOSOMES

As a first approximation, genes were initially defined as stretches of DNA that encode a single protein or a single functional RNA, such as an rRNA or a tRNA. This rule breaks down quickly, however, because there are mechanisms, such as *alternative splicing* of the primary RNA transcript into different mRNAs, that may intervene between a given gene and a finished protein. Moreover, individual protein precursors may be cleaved into numerous functionally active peptides. As a result of these and other processes, many individual genes actually encode multiple proteins, although we still do not know what fraction of all genes function in this manner.

Genes are arrayed on extremely long chains of DNA called *chromosomes*. Eukaryotic chromosomes contain not only genes, but also large amounts of intergenic DNA. Indeed, within the human genome, the ~25,000 genes take up perhaps only 3% of chromosomal DNA. Moreover, genes are not distributed equally along the chromosomes but are often found in clusters. Some chromosomes are "gene rich" and others are relatively "gene poor." Within intergenic regions there is a great deal of DNA with unique sequences of unknown function, as well as long stretches of tandemly repeated sequences known as *satellite DNA*. Included within these regions are *retrotransposons*, such as LINE-1 (long interspersed nuclear element-1) repeats, which are transcribed by RNA polymerase and encode several enzymes including reverse transcriptase (an enzyme that synthesizes a strand of DNA from RNA). The resulting DNA strands can then incorporate into the genome, where they can disrupt normal gene expression. An interesting line of current research is to understand the role of LINE-1 and related retrotransposons as a novel mechanism controlling neural gene expression (see Chapter 7).

The chromosomes of eukaryotic cells are so long (~2 meters if stretched out linearly) that they would not fit in the nucleus in their extended form. Thus, stretches of the DNA that are not being actively transcribed are tightly packed into a conformation described as a coiled coil, which permits the chromosomes to fit within the nucleus. To create packed conformations, lengths of DNA are coiled around structural and regulatory proteins, of which the most important are the histones. These structures are termed *nucleosomes*. Regions of DNA that are being actively transcribed into RNA may be greater than 1000-fold more extended than regions that are transcriptionally quiescent. The unwinding of tightly packed nucleosomes, which enables their expression, is mediated by highly complex modifications of histones and many other nuclear proteins, which are discussed in detail in Chapter 7 (Borrelli et al., 2008).

GENE EXPRESSION

As described in the preceding paragraphs, proteins are not synthesized directly from the DNA that encodes them, but in two sequential processes, *transcription of DNA into mRNA*, which occurs in the nucleus, and *translation of the mRNA into protein* according to the rules of the genetic code, which occurs in the cytoplasm. Transcription of protein-coding genes can be divided into three major steps. First, the enzyme primarily involved in

RNA synthesis, *RNA polymerase*, must interact with the gene at an appropriate transcription start site and begin transcribing (*initiation*). Second, the RNA polymerase must successfully transcribe an appropriate length of RNA (*elongation*). Third, transcription of the RNA must terminate appropriately. The resulting RNA is then posttranscriptionally processed. It receives a stretch of adenines, a poly-(A) tail, which makes it more stable in the cell. This process of polyadenylation is dynamically regulated and can exert a powerful influence on expression of the resulting mRNAs (Proudfoot, 2011). It is also spliced to remove internal sequences (*introns*) that are not appropriate for translation into protein in that particular cell. The spliced "exportable" sequences (*exons*) exit the nucleus to be translated into protein in the cytoplasm (Fig. 6.4). Alternative splicing vastly increases the number of protein products produced by the cell, with certain genes, for example, the neurexins, generating hundreds of splice variants (Padgett, 2012).

TRANSCRIPTIONAL CONTROL

We have now reviewed the flow of information from gene to protein. Every step along the way is regulated, but the major control point in reading out the information contained within the genome is transcription initiation. Indeed, this is the step at which environmental signals often exert powerful regulatory control on gene expression, during development and in mature cells. How does this come about?

In addition to encoding information that ultimately directs the synthesis of proteins, genes contain regulatory information. Every cell in our bodies contains all of our genes in its nucleus, but not every gene is active in every cell. Our cells differ—indeed, their identity is defined—by the fact that each type of cell in the body expresses only a subset of the entire

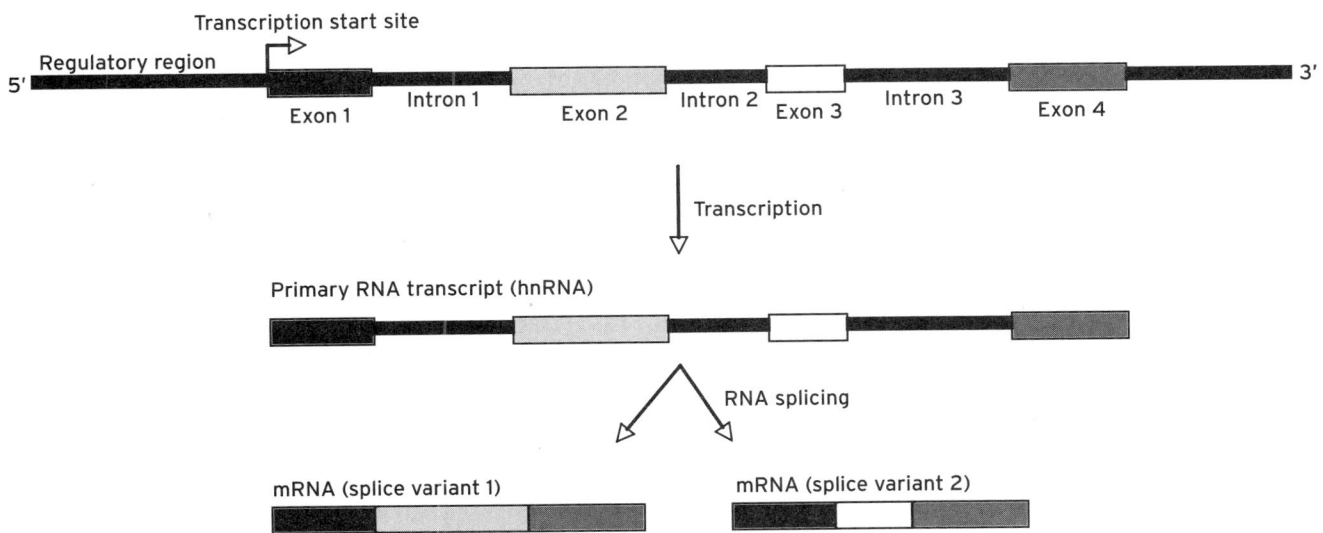

Figure 6.4 *RNA splicing. Horizontal black lines represent deoxyribonucleic acid (DNA) regulatory regions and introns. Black, gray, and white rectangles represent exons. The region to the left of the first exon is the 5' regulatory region of the gene, but cis-regulatory elements are also found in introns and sometimes downstream of the last exon. The primary transcript, also known as heterogeneous ribonucleic acid (hnRNA), contains exons and introns and gives rise, in the case shown, to two alternatively spliced messenger ribonucleic acids (mRNAs): one containing exons 1, 2, and 4, and one containing exons 1, 3, and 4. These splice variants, after export from the nucleus and translation in the cytoplasm, give rise to distinct proteins.*

complement of genes. In any given cell, some genes are "on," being read out to make mRNA and hence proteins, and the rest are silent. Thus, for example, in the red blood cell precursors of the bone marrow, the genes that encode globins, proteins that are the critical building blocks of hemoglobin, are actively making globin-encoding mRNA. In our midbrains, a subset of cells are making a protein called *tyrosine hydroxylase*, the rate-limiting enzyme for the synthesis of catecholamines, like dopamine and norepinephrine. It would not be adaptive for these cells to synthesize large amounts of hemoglobin, just as red blood cell precursors need not use energy to synthesize tyrosine hydroxylase. The processes by which certain genes are "silenced" in a tissue-specific manner during development are now increasingly understood at the chromatin or epigenetic level (Chapter 7).

Regulatory sequences within genes work by virtue of their ability to bind specific proteins. Certain regulatory sequences specify the beginnings and ends of segments of DNA that can be transcribed into RNA. Other regulatory sequences determine in what cell types and under what circumstances their gene can be read out. DNA sequences that subserve such control functions are often called *cis-regulatory elements* (Fig. 6.5). The term *cis* refers to the fact that the relevant regulatory sequences are physically linked, on the DNA, to the region being controlled, which is usually a segment of DNA that can be transcribed into RNA. The proteins that bind to cis elements have been described as *trans-acting* factors because they may be encoded anywhere in the genome rather than on the same stretch of DNA that they regulate. Those proteins that are involved in specifying whether, and under what circumstances, a gene will be transcribed are more generally known as *transcription factors*. Many transcription factors bind DNA directly; others interact only indirectly via protein–protein interactions with factors that bind DNA.

Those cis-regulatory elements that specify the site within a gene at which transcription starts, and on which the complex of proteins that forms the basal transcription apparatus is assembled, are called the *basal* or *core promoter*. The core promoters

for many protein-encoding genes consist of a sequence motif rich in the nucleotides A and T, called the *TATA box*. The TATA box is generally located ~30 nucleotides upstream of the actual site at which transcription of DNA into RNA is initiated. In the nervous system, however, numerous genes do not contain identifiable TATA boxes, which means that their transcription start sites are defined differently. In eukaryotes, transcription of protein-coding genes is carried out by the enzyme RNA polymerase II, which does not directly contact DNA but interacts with the complex of proteins that assembles at the TATA box or distinct transcription start site (Fig. 6.5).

SEQUENCE-SPECIFIC TRANSCRIPTION FACTORS INTERACT WITH THE BASAL TRANSCRIPTION APPARATUS TO PRODUCE SIGNIFICANT LEVELS OF TRANSCRIPTION

The basal transcription complex assembled at the TATA box or other transcription start site is only sufficient to initiate low levels of transcription of DNA into RNA. To achieve significant levels of gene expression, the basal transcription complex requires help from additional transcription factors that recognize and bind to cis-regulatory elements found elsewhere within the gene. Cis-elements that exert control near the core promoter itself have been called *promoter elements*, and those that act at a distance—often several hundred to more than 1,000 nucleotide base pairs away—have been called *enhancer elements*, but the commonly made distinction between promoter and enhancer elements is artificial. Both are composed of small "modular" sequences of DNA (generally 7–12 base pairs in length), each of which is a specific binding site for one or more transcription factors. Multiple cis-regulatory elements arrayed throughout the control regions of a gene, and the proteins they bind, act in combinatorial fashion to give each gene its distinct patterns of expression and regulation.

Transcription factors that are tethered to DNA by binding cis-elements are often described as sequence-specific transcription factors. Most such proteins have a modular structure composed of physically separate domains: a domain that recognizes and binds a specific DNA sequence, an activation domain that interacts with the basal transcription complex to activate or inhibit it, and a multimerization domain that permits the formation of homo- and heteromultimers with other transcription factors (Fig. 6.5). Many transcription factors are active only as dimers or higher order complexes. Within transcription factor dimers, whether homodimers or heterodimers, it is common for both partners to contribute jointly to the DNA binding domain and the activation domain. Sequence-specific transcription factors may contact the basal transcription complex directly; in many cases, they interact through the mediation of adapter proteins. In either case, transcription factors that bind cis-regulatory elements at a distance from the core promoter can interact with the basal transcription apparatus because the DNA forms loops that bring distant regions in contact with each other (Fig. 6.6A and B). Once bound to DNA, transcription factors serve as scaffolds for the recruitment of many types of activator or repressor proteins that serve to

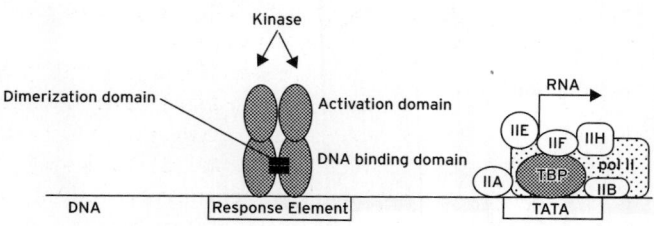

Figure 6.5 *Cis- and trans-regulation. The figure shows two cis-regulatory elements (open rectangles) along the stretch of deoxyribonucleic acid (DNA) (thin line). The element to the left represents a response element that serves as a binding site for a hypothetical transcription factor that binds as a homodimer. The other is the thymine adenine thymine adenine (TATA) element, shown binding the TATA binding protein (TBP). Multiple general transcription factors and ribonucleic acid (RNA) polymerase II (pol II) associate with TBP. This basal transcription apparatus recruits RNA polymerase II into the complex and also forms the substrate for interactions with activator proteins, such as those binding to the activator elements shown. The transcription factor shown binding to the response element is a substrate for a protein kinase that phosphorylates its activation domain (see text).*

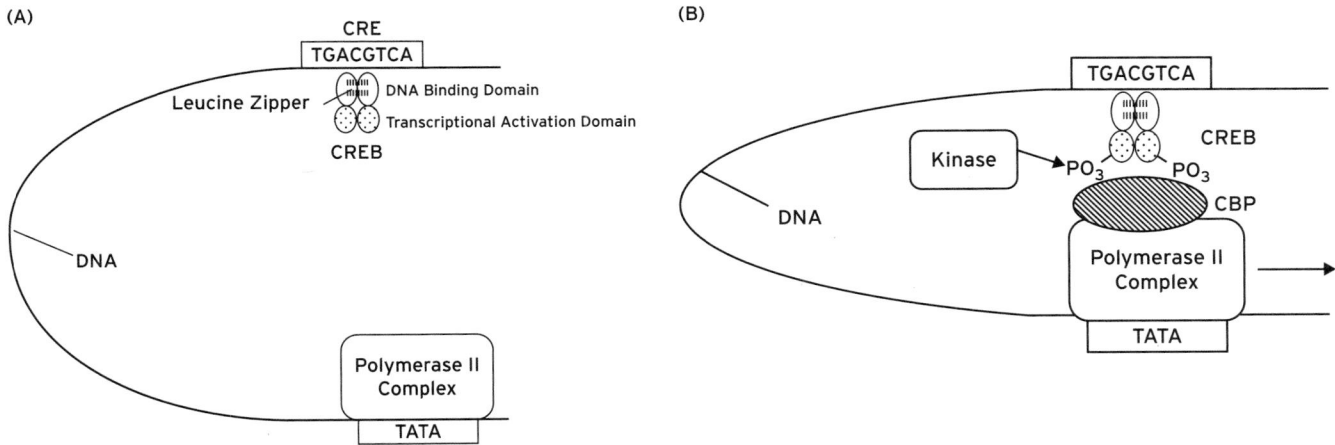

Figure 6.6 *Looping of deoxyribonucleic acid (DNA) permits activator (or repressor) proteins binding at a distance to interact with the basal transcription apparatus. In the figure, the basal transcription apparatus is shown as a single box bound at the thymine adenine thymine adenine (TATA) element. The activator protein, cyclic adenosine monophosphate (cAMP)-response element binding protein (CREB), is shown bound as a homodimer to its cognate cis-regulatory element, the cAMP-response element (CRE), at a distance from the TATA element (panels A and B). Upon phosphorylation, many activators such as CREB are able to recruit adapter proteins that mediate between the activator and the basal transcription apparatus. An adapter protein that binds phosphorylated CREB is called CREB binding protein (CBP), a form of histone acetyltransferase (HAT) that acetylates nearby histones to facilitate gene transcription (see Chapter 7). With the recruitment of the adapter, a mature transcription complex forms that permits the synthesis of ribonucleic acid (RNA) by RNA polymerase II (panel B).*

epigenetically activate or repress gene expression, respectively (see Chapter 7).

REGULATION OF GENE EXPRESSION BY EXTRACELLULAR SIGNALS

All regulation of gene expression by extracellular signals requires a mechanism that carries a signal from the cell membrane to the nucleus. In many cases, intracellular signaling molecules, such as protein kinases, serve this function. This is illustrated by CREB (cAMP response element binding protein), which mediates many of the effects of the cyclic adenosine monophosphate (cAMP) system, and other intracellular pathways, on gene expression (Altarejos and Montminy, 2011). CREB is bound under basal cellular conditions to its cognate cis-regulatory element (the cyclic AMP-response element, or CRE). Stimuli that increase levels of cAMP activate cAMP-dependent protein kinase (PKA), which results in liberation of the kinase's catalytic subunits (Chapter 4). A portion of the free catalytic subunit then enters the nucleus, where it phosphorylates CREB, permitting it to activate transcription. Similarly, stimuli that activate other intracellular signaling cascades (e.g., Ca^{2+} or extracellular signal-regulated kinase [ERK] pathways) lead to the activation of other protein kinases, which also phosphorylate and activate CREB.

In other cases, a transcription factor, itself activated at the cell membrane or in the cytoplasm, then translocates to the nucleus. This is illustrated by the transcription factor NF-κB (nuclear factor κB), which is involved, among other things, in the activation of genes involved in inflammatory responses but also implicated in diverse neural phenomena (Hayden and Ghosh, 2012). Under basal conditions, NF-κB is retained in the cytoplasm by its inhibitory binding protein (IκB); this interaction masks a protein sequence within the NF-κB molecule that serves as a nuclear localization signal. Phosphorylation of IκB

by IκB-kinase (IκK) leads to dissociation of NF-κB, which permits it to enter the nucleus, where it binds to its response elements; IκB is then digested within the cytoplasm.

The preceding discussion highlights that the critical nuclear translocation step can involve the transcription factor itself or another signaling molecule. Either mechanism can activate a third scenario: Some transcription factors are expressed only at very low levels when cells are in their unstimulated state. Their genes contain response elements that lead to their synthesis when cells are activated. Thus, gene expression may occur in cascades, with the stimulation of preexisting transcription factors leading to the expression of genes encoding (among many other genes) additional transcription factors, which can then stimulate yet other genes. Activation of genes by preexisting transcription factors occurs more rapidly than activation of genes by factors that must be synthesized *de novo*. Thus, not surprisingly, different neurotransmitters, drugs, and other stimuli may activate gene expression with widely varying time courses ranging from minutes to many hours.

Many transcription factors are members of families, presumably related by evolution, with related structures and functions. In the following section we illustrate the function of representative families of transcription factors, which serve as instructive examples of the diverse mechanisms governing the regulation of transcription in the nervous system.

THE CREB FAMILY OF TRANSCRIPTION FACTORS

CREB was the first-discovered and best-characterized member of a family of related proteins that bind to a particular DNA sequence termed the *CRE*, as mentioned (Altarejos and Montminy, 2011). The family is composed of CREB, the ATFs (activating transcription factors), and the CREMs (cAMP-response element modulators). CREB itself plays a major role in mediating the effects of cAMP and Ca^{2+} and of those neurotransmitters that act through cAMP or Ca^{2+}, on gene expression. A large number of genes contain CREs, including the gene encoding the transcription factor c-Fos and the genes encoding tyrosine hydroxylase, BDNF (brain-derived neurotrophic factor), and several neuropeptides, such as proenkephalin, prodynorphin, somatostatin, and VIP (vasoactive intestinal polypeptide). Members of the CREB/ATF family bind to CREs as dimers. The dimerization domain used by the CREB/ATF proteins and several other families of transcription factors is called a *leucine zipper*, an alpha helical motif in which every seventh residue is a leucine. The proteins form a coil in which electrostatic interactions stabilize dimer formation.

The methods used to characterize CREs, and indeed all cis-regulatory elements, involve deleting them, or mutating them more subtly, and then reintroducing them into eukaryotic cells in culture by transfection. When a critical base in a DNA regulatory element is mutated, it weakens or destroys the binding site for the relevant transcription factor. If the protein can no longer bind, the gene can no longer be activated by the physiological stimulus under investigation, such as cAMP. By comparing response element sequences that have been investigated by mutagenesis within many genes, an idealized consensus sequence can be derived. The consensus nucleotide sequence of the CRE is TGACGTCA, with the nucleotides CGTCA absolutely required.

The consensus CRE sequence illustrates an important principle, the palindromic nature of many transcription factor binding sites. In the sequence TGACGTCA, it can be readily observed that the sequence on the two complementary strands, which run in opposite directions, is identical. Many cis-regulatory elements are perfect or approximate palindromes permitting binding of transcription factors in the form of dimers, where each member of the dimer recognizes one of the half-sites.

The primary mechanism by which CREB is regulated is through its phosphorylation on a single serine residue (Ser133) by any of several protein kinases, including PKA, Ca^{2+}/calmodulin-dependent protein kinase IV (CaMKIV), and several kinases in the ERK cascade (see Chapter 4). CREB is constitutively synthesized so that it exists in neurons under basal conditions, although its expression can be regulated under certain circumstances, such as in response to psychotropic drug treatments. Nonphosphorylated CREB is localized to the nucleus, where it is bound to its response elements without considerable transcriptional activity (Fig. 6.6A). Phosphorylation of CREB activates its transcriptional activity by permitting CREB to interact with CBP (Fig. 6.6B). As noted in the preceding, CBP is called an *adapter protein* because it intervenes between a sequence-specific transcription factor CREB and the basal transcription apparatus, thus activating transcription. Despite its name, CBP provides this adapter function for several regulated transcription factors in addition to CREB family proteins.

The mechanism by which neurotransmitters that increase cAMP levels regulate gene expression via CREB is straightforward. Neurotransmitter-receptor stimulation increases levels of cAMP and of activated PKA. Activated PKA (that is,

free catalytic subunits of the enzyme) is then translocated into the nucleus, where it phosphorylates and activates CREB. Phosphorylation of CREB, in turn, serves to activate the expression of genes that contain CREB bound to their promoter regions. Similar mechanisms operate for neurotransmitters (or nerve impulses) that activate CREB via stimulation of cellular Ca^{2+} signals and for neurotrophic factors that activate CREB via stimulation of ERK cascades.

The convergence of multiple signaling pathways on CREB may be very significant for the function of the nervous system. For example, associative memory appears to result from the integration of multiple signals that converge on target neurons, integration that could be achieved in part via CREB phosphorylation. Indeed, experiments performed by numerous laboratories on multiple species from *Drosophila* to rats, in which CREB was inactivated by different experimental methods, yield organisms with deficits in long-term memory, while increases in CREB function produce animals with enhanced memory (e.g., Josselyn, 2010; Barco and Marie, 2011). CREB has also been implicated in many additional psychiatric phenomena including drug addiction and depression (Blendy, 2006; Cao et al., 2010; Carlezon et al., 2005).

CREB illustrates yet another important principle of transcriptional regulation. As described the preceding section, CREB is a member of a larger family of related proteins. The ATFs and CREMs (distinct CREM products are generated from a single CREM gene via alternative splicing) bind CREs as dimers; many can dimerize with CREB itself. Activating transcription factor-1 (ATF1) appears to be very similar to CREB; it can be activated by the cAMP and Ca^{2+} pathways. Many of the other ATF proteins and CREM isoforms appear to activate transcription; however, certain CREMs, such as one called *ICER* (inducible cAMP repressor), act to repress it. Inhibitory CREM isoforms lack a glutamine-rich transcriptional activation domain found in CREB. Thus, certain CREB–CREM heterodimers might bind CREs but fail to activate transcription. Some inhibitory CREMs (e.g., ICER) are induced by CREB itself but with a delayed time course. In this way, these proteins may help terminate genes that had been activated by a CREB signal. Work in recent years has begun to demonstrate the involvement of ATFs and CREMs in an individual's adaptations to numerous environmental stimuli, such as stress and drugs of abuse (e.g., Green et al., 2008).

THE AP-1 FAMILY OF TRANSCRIPTION FACTORS

Another group of transcription factors that plays a central role in the regulation of neural gene expression by extracellular signals is the AP-1 proteins (Morgan and Curran, 1995). The name *AP-1* was originally applied to a transcriptional activity, then called *Activator Protein-1*, that was subsequently found to be composed of multiple proteins that bind as heterodimers (and a few as homodimers) to the DNA sequence TGACTCA, the AP-1 sequence. AP-1 proteins are divided into two groups, the *Fos* and *Jun* families. Like the CREB/ATF family, AP-1 proteins dimerize via a leucine zipper. The consensus AP-1 sequence is a heptamer, which forms a palindrome flanking a central C or G. The AP-1 sequence differs from the CRE sequence by only a single base. Yet this one base difference strongly biases protein binding away from CREB (which requires an intact CGTCA motif) to the AP-1 family of proteins and means that, under most circumstances, this sequence will not confer cAMP responsiveness on a gene. Instead, AP-1 sequences tend to confer responsiveness to growth factor–stimulated signaling pathways such as the ERK pathways and to the protein kinase C pathway. Indeed, the AP-1 sequence was historically described as a TPA-response element (TRE) because the phorbol ester *12-O-tetradecanoyl-phorbol-13-acetate* (TPA), which activates protein kinase C, strongly induces gene expression via AP-1 proteins. It is a staggering illustration of the specificity of cellular regulation that a single base change (from a CRE to an AP-1 site) in a gene thousands of bases long can result in such a profound change in gene regulation.

AP-1 proteins generally bind DNA as heterodimers composed of one member each of the Fos and Jun families. The Fos family includes c-Fos, Fra-1 (Fos-related antigen-1), Fra-2, and FosB (which gives rise to full-length FosB plus a truncated splice variant termed ΔFosB). The Jun family includes c-Jun, JunB, and JunD. Heterodimers form between members of the Fos and Jun families via the leucine zipper. The potential complexity of transcriptional regulation is greater still because some AP-1 proteins can heterodimerize via the leucine zipper with members of the CREB–ATF family (e.g., ATF2 with c-Jun).

Jun proteins, in particular JunD, are expressed constitutively at appreciable levels in neural cells. In contrast, all Fos proteins are expressed at low or even undetectable levels under basal conditions, but with stimulation, can be induced to high levels of expression. Thus, unlike genes that are regulated by constitutively expressed transcription factors such as CREB, genes that are regulated by c-Fos/c-Jun heterodimers require new transcription and translation of these AP-1 proteins.

GENES ENCODING FOS AND JUN FAMILY PROTEINS ARE OFTEN TERMED IMMEDIATE EARLY GENES

Genes, such as the c-Fos gene itself, that are activated rapidly (within minutes), transiently, and without requiring new protein synthesis are frequently referred to as *cellular immediate early genes* (IEGs) (Morgan and Curran, 1995) (see Chapter 4). Genes that are induced or repressed more slowly (over hours), and are dependent on new protein synthesis, may be described as *late response genes*. The term *IEG* was initially applied to describe viral genes that are activated immediately upon infection of eukaryotic cells by commandeering host cell transcription factors for their expression. Viral IEGs generally encode transcription factors needed to activate viral late gene expression. This terminology has been extended to cellular (i.e., nonviral) genes with varying success. The terminology is problematic because there are many cellular genes induced independently of protein synthesis, but with a time course intermediately between those of classical IEGs and late response genes. In fact, some genes may be regulated with different time courses or requirements for protein synthesis in response to different extracellular signals. Moreover,

it must be recalled that many cellular genes regulated as IEGs encode proteins that are not transcription factors (e.g., prodynorphin or BDNF). Despite these caveats, the concept of IEG-encoded transcription factors in the nervous system has been useful heuristically. Because of their rapid induction from low basal levels in response to neuronal depolarization (the critical signal being Ca^{2+} entry) and to second messenger and growth factor pathways, several IEGs have been used as cellular markers of neural activation, permitting novel approaches to functional neuroanatomy. This includes not only the Fos and Jun families of transcription factors, but also Zif268 (also called *Egr1*), which belongs to a distinct family of transcription factors that binds to its own response elements. Examples of the use of c-Fos as a marker of neuronal activation include induction of c-Fos in dorsal horn of the spinal cord by nociceptive stimuli, in motor and sensory thalamus by stimulation of sensory cortex, in supraoptic/paraventricular nuclei by water deprivation, and in numerous brain regions by acute and chronic opiate and cocaine administration, as well as in response to a number of other psychotropic drug treatments.

THE COMPOSITION OF AP-1 COMPLEXES CHANGES OVER TIME

Following acute stimulation of cells, different members of the Fos family are induced with varying time courses of expression, which leads to a progression of distinct AP-1 protein complexes over time (Nestler, 2008). It is believed that these changes produce varying patterns of expression of AP-1-regulated genes, thereby permitting neurons to adapt to the pattern of stimulation to which they are being subjected.

Under resting conditions, c-Fos mRNA and protein are barely detectable in most neurons; however, c-Fos gene expression can be induced dramatically in response to a variety of stimuli. As just one example, experimental induction of a grand mal seizure causes marked increases in levels of c-Fos mRNA in the rat brain within 30 minutes and induces substantial levels of c-Fos protein within 2 hours. c-Fos is highly unstable and is degraded back to low, basal levels within 4–6 hours. Administration of cocaine or amphetamine causes a similar pattern of c-Fos expression in the striatum. In either of these stimulus paradigms, other Fos-like proteins are also induced, but with a longer temporal latency than c-Fos; their peak levels of expression lag behind c-Fos by approximately 1 hour. Moreover, expression of these proteins persists a bit longer than that of c-Fos but still returns to basal levels within 8–12 hours.

With repeated stimulation, however, the c-Fos gene, and to a lesser extent the genes for other Fos-like proteins, become refractory to further activation (i.e., their expression becomes desensitized). However, in most systems, isoforms of ΔFosB continue to be expressed (Nestler, 2008). These isoforms exhibit very long half-lives in brain (1–2 weeks). As a result, ΔFosB accumulates in specific neurons in response to repeated perturbations and persists long after cessation of these perturbations (Fig. 6.7). Such stable accumulation of ΔFosB, which is responsible for desensitizing expression of c-Fos, has been shown to play an important role in mediating the long-term effects of drugs of abuse and several other treatments on the nervous system.

THE c-Fos GENE IS ACTIVATED BY MULTIPLE SIGNALING PATHWAYS

The precise intracellular mechanisms by which extracellular stimuli induce c-Fos expression are now well understood (Fig. 6.8). Stimuli that depolarize neurons (e.g., seizure activity, glutamate) induce c-Fos through a Ca^{2+}-dependent mechanism that involves the phosphorylation, by CaMKIV, of a CREB protein that is already present in the cell and bound to CREs in the c-Fos gene. Neurotransmitters that activate the cAMP pathway in target neurons phosphorylate CREB on the same amino acid residue via PKA. Phosphorylation of CREB, as outlined in the previous section, activates its transcriptional activity and leads to increased c-Fos expression.

The c-Fos gene can also be induced by the ERK pathway, which is activated by many types of growth factors, via at least two distinct mechanisms, which may operate to different extents in different cell types. One mechanism, discussed in the preceding description of CREB, involves the phosphorylation of CREB by ribosomal S6 kinase (RSK) directly downstream of ERK. A second mechanism involves the phosphorylation and activation, also by ERK, of a different transcription factor termed *Elk-1* (E twenty-six [ETS]-like transcription factor 1). Elk-1 binds, along with still another transcription factor, serum response factor (SRF), to the serum response element (SRE) within the c-Fos gene. A third mechanism mediates c-Fos induction by cytokines via activation of the JAK (Janus kinase)-STAT (signal transducers and activators of transcription) pathway. The c-Fos gene contains a response element called the SIE (SIF [sis-inducible factor]-inducible element), which binds and is activated by STAT transcription factors. Cytokine regulation of JAK-STAT signaling is described in greater detail in what follows.

The activation of IEG products such as c-Fos in response to a large number of stimuli raises the question of how specificity of response is achieved. First, specificity is partly achieved by the particular neural circuitry involved; that is, c-Fos and the other proteins are induced only along those particular neural pathways activated in response to the stimulus. Second, specificity is achieved by specialization within neuronal cell types. For example, in particular cell types not every gene that contains an appropriate binding site (e.g., an AP-1 site) to which c-Fos can bind is in a chromatin configuration that permits access to c-Fos-containing complexes (Chapter 7). Third, individual transcription factors generally cannot act alone to induce or repress the expression of a given gene. Multiple types of transcription factors, binding to distinct regulatory elements within a gene's promoter region, must often act in concert to produce significant effects on gene expression.

Fourth, as alluded to the above-described point, protein products of many IEGs including c-Fos can bind DNA with high affinity only after binding to other transcription factors to form heterodimers. Such interactions are well exemplified by c-Fos and c-Jun. By itself, c-Fos is unable to bind DNA with high affinity. c-Jun homodimers can bind DNA but do so with relatively low affinity. However, c-Fos/c-Jun heterodimers bind to the AP-1 site with high affinity to regulate transcription. In contrast, heterodimers of c-Fos and JunB appear to be relatively inactive. Due to the existence of numerous members of the Fos and Jun families, complex regulatory schemes can readily be imagined by which a great deal of specificity in regulating cellular genes can be attained.

Although the primary mechanism by which Fos family members are regulated appears to be at the level of their transcription, the proteins are also regulated by phosphorylation. This is best illustrated by c-Fos itself, which is heavily phosphorylated on several closely spaced serine residues in the C-terminal region of the protein by PKA and CaMKs and by protein kinase C. c-Fos phosphorylation appears to be a critical regulatory mechanism for the protein: The difference between normal c-Fos (cellular Fos) and its viral counterpart v-Fos (which is oncogenic) is a frame-shift mutation that deletes the serine residues from the viral protein. It has been suggested that phosphorylation of c-Fos triggers the protein's ability to suppress its own transcription, thereby providing key regulatory feedback control of the expression of this transcription factor. Another example is the phosphorylation of Jun proteins by Jun-kinases (JNKs). Jun-kinases are activated by cellular forms of stress and, like ERK, are considered to be part of the MAP (mitogen-activated protein)-kinase family (see Chapter 4). The resulting phosphorylation of Jun transcription factors is thought to be an important part of a cell's adaptation to stress.

REGULATION OF GENE EXPRESSION BY CYTOKINES AND NONRECEPTOR PROTEIN TYROSINE KINASES

Cytokines subserve a wide array of functions within and outside of the nervous system (Chapters 1 and 2). Such cytokines include leukemia inhibitory factor (LIF), ciliary neurotrophic factor (CNTF), and interleukin-6 (IL-6), to name just a few. Recall from Chapter 4 that each of these cytokines produces its biological effects through activation of the gp130 class of plasma membrane receptor and the subsequent activation of the JAK-STAT pathway, noted earlier (Horvath, 2000; Ihle, 2001). The crucial feeding peptide, *leptin*, also acts via a JAK-STAT linked receptor.

The gp130-linked receptors for these cytokines and related signals do not contain protein kinase domains. Rather, the cytoplasmic portions of the receptors interact with nonreceptor protein tyrosine kinases of the JAK family, which include JAK1, JAK2, and Tyk2. Cytokine receptors show some specificity for the types of JAKs activated in a given cell type. Signal transduction to the nucleus involves the tyrosine phosphorylation, by the JAKs, of one or more of a family of transcription factor proteins called *STATs*. Upon phosphorylation, STAT proteins translocate to the nucleus, where they bind appropriate cytokine response elements present in target genes. The transcriptional activity of STAT proteins can be illustrated by regulation of c-Fos, as depicted in Fig. 6.8. Analogous mechanisms are involved in mediating the ability of cytokines to regulate many neural genes, including those for VIP and several other neuropeptides.

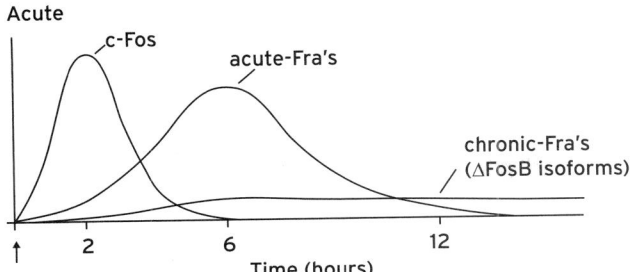

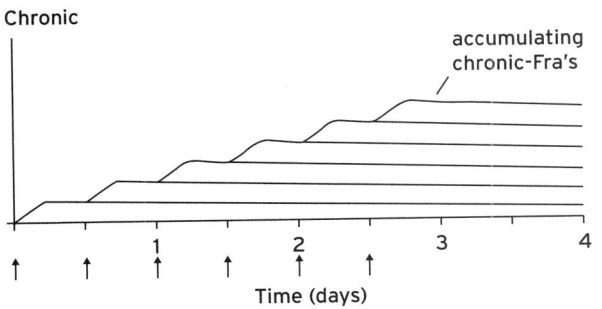

Figure 6.7 *Scheme for the gradual accumulation of ΔFosB versus the rapid and transient induction of c-Fos and several other Fos family proteins in the brain. (Top) Several waves of Fos family proteins are induced by many acute stimuli in neurons. c-Fos is induced rapidly and degraded within several hours of the acute stimulus, whereas others (FosB, ΔFosB, FRA-1 [Fos-related antigen-1], FRA-2) are induced somewhat later and persist somewhat longer than c-Fos. In contrast, ΔFosB is induced (although at low levels) following a single acute stimulus but persists in brain with a half-life of 1–2 weeks due to its unique stability. In a complex with Jun family proteins, these waves of Fos family proteins form AP-1 binding complexes with shifting composition over time. (Bottom) With repeated (e.g., twice daily) stimulation, each acute stimulus induces a low level of ΔFosB. This is indicated by the lower set of overlapping lines, which indicate ΔFosB induced by each acute stimulus. The result is a gradual increase in the total levels of ΔFosB with repeated stimuli during a course of chronic treatment. This is indicated by the increasing stepped line in the graph. The increasing levels of ΔFosB with repeated stimulation result in the gradual induction of a long-lasting AP-1 complex, which underlies persisting forms of neural plasticity in the brain. Adapted from Nestler (2008).*

Wnt SIGNALING CASCADES AND THE REGULATION OF GENE EXPRESSION

Wnt (Wingless) is a secreted protein that activates a seven-transmembrane receptor, termed Frizzled (Fzd) (Inestrosa and

Arenas, 2010). (Many of the names given to proteins in this pathway are based on morphological phenotypes seen upon deletion of homologous genes in *Drosophila*.) Wnt activation of Fzd leads to the activation of Disheveled (Dvl) by promoting its polymerization. The primary downstream signaling mechanism of activated Dvl is termed the "canonical" pathway (Fig. 6.9), where Dvl polymerization triggers its binding to Axin, which in turn triggers the AKT (a serine/threonine kinase)–mediated phosphorylation and *inhibition* of GSK3β (glycogen synthase kinase-3β). GSK3β phosphorylates several downstream targets, including β-catenin, which functions as a transcription factor (Inestrosa and Arenas, 2010). GSK3β phosphorylation of β-catenin promotes β-catenin's *degradation*; hence, Wnt-Dvl, by inhibiting GSK3β, activates β-catenin–mediated transcription. Dvl polymerization also triggers the activation of Rac1, a small GTPase, which promotes the translocation of β-catenin to the nucleus. β-Catenin is a required cofactor for the transcription factors TCF (T cell transcription factor) and LEF (lymphoid enhancer factor). TCF/LEF binds to TCF/LEF response elements (also known as WREs or Wnt response elements) present in numerous genes to regulate gene expression. The Wnt-Dvl-GSK3β-β-catenin signaling cascade has been implicated in numerous neuropsychiatric syndromes and is the target for several types of psychotropic drugs, in particular, mood stabilizers such as lithium (e.g., Li and Jope, 2010; Wilkinson et al., 2011). There is thus keen interest in identifying the target genes of this cascade in limbic brain regions that mediate these clinically important behavioral effects.

STEROID HORMONE RECEPTORS ARE LIGAND-ACTIVATED TRANSCRIPTION FACTORS

The differentiation of many cell types in the brain is established by exposure to steroids. For example, exposure to estrogen or testosterone during critical developmental periods results in sexually dimorphic development of certain nuclei. The steroid hormone receptor superfamily (also called the *nuclear receptor superfamily*) includes the receptors for lipid-soluble molecules that diffuse readily across cell membranes, such as glucocorticoids, gonadal steroids, mineralocorticoids, retinoids, thyroid

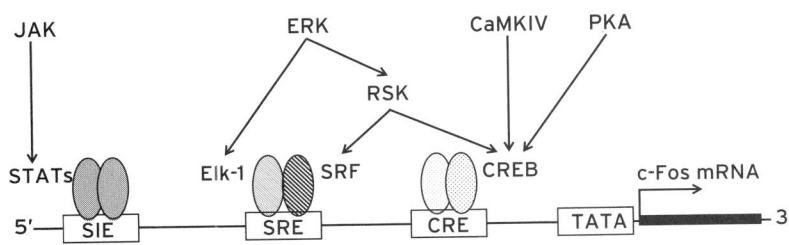

Figure 6.8 *Regulation of c-Fos gene transcription. A cAMP response element (CRE) binds cAMP response element binding protein CREB, a serum response element (SRE) binds serum response factor (SRF) plus another transcription factor termed Elk-1 (E twenty-six [ETS]-like transcription factor 1) or ternary complex factor (TCF), and a SIF (sis-inducible factor)-inducible element (SIE) binds signal transducers and activators of transcription (STAT proteins). These three elements represent a small number of all known transcription factor–binding sites in the c-Fos gene. Proteins that bind at these sites are constitutively present in cells and are activated by phosphorylation. CREB can be activated by protein kinase A, Ca²⁺/calmodulin-dependent protein kinases (CaMKs), or ribosomal S6 kinases (RSKs); Elk-1 can be activated by extracellular signal-regulated kinases (ERKs); and STATs can be activated by Janus kinases (JAKs). Because the activation of c-Fos by any of multiple signaling pathways requires only signal-induced phosphorylation rather than new protein synthesis, it can be triggered rapidly by a wide array of stimuli.*

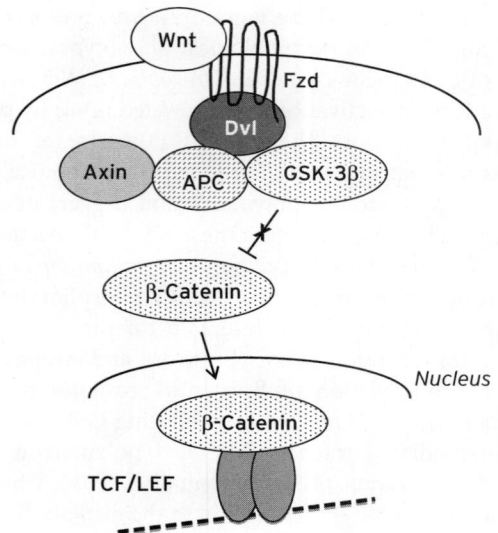

Figure 6.9 *Regulation of gene expression by Wnt (Wingless) signaling cascades. Wnt activates the Frizzled (Fzd) receptor, which through Disheveled (Dvl) binds a complex composed of adenomatous polyposis coli (APC), Axin, glycogen synthase kinase-3β (GSK-3β), and other proteins. This leads to the phosphorylation and inhibition of GSK-3β and to the stabilization and accumulation of β-catenin, which then translocates to the nucleus (a process facilitated by Dvl), where it binds to TCF (T cell transcription factor) and LEF (lymphoid enhancer factor) transcription factors to regulate expression of specific genes. A growing number of neural genes have been recognized in recent years as targets for Wnt signaling.*

hormone, vitamin D, and cholesterol-related steroids (Chawla et al., 2001). They act on their receptors within the cell cytoplasm, in marked distinction to the other types of intercellular signals described that act on plasma membrane receptors (see Chapter 4). Another unique feature of the nuclear receptor superfamily is that their receptors are actually transcription factors. Like other transcription factors described, the steroid hormone receptors are modular in nature. Each has a transcriptional activation domain at its amino terminus, a DNA binding domain, and a hormone binding domain at its carboxy terminus. The DNA binding domains recognize different types of steroid hormone response elements within the regulatory regions of genes. The DNA binding domains of the steroid hormone receptors are described as zinc finger domains, a cysteine-rich motif that contains a zinc ion. This motif is used by many other transcription factors (so-called zinc finger proteins), but by few factors that are regulated by extracellular signals.

Once bound by hormone, activated steroid hormone receptors translocate into the nucleus, where they bind to their cognate response elements. Such binding then increases or decreases the rate at which these target genes are transcribed, depending on the precise nature and DNA sequence context of the element. Steroid hormone receptors can therefore be considered ligand-activated transcription factors. In recent years, steroid hormone receptors have been shown to regulate the transcription of genes that do not contain steroid response elements by forming protein-protein interactions with other transcription factors, for example, AP-1 and CREB proteins. This discovery reveals highly complex regulatory mechanisms by which steroid hormones control gene expression (Biddie et al., 2011).

Although the primary mechanism by which the transcriptional activity of steroid hormone receptors is regulated is through their ligand binding and consequent nuclear translocation, the receptors are also regulated *in vivo* at transcriptional and posttranslational levels. The total amount of the receptors expressed in specific target tissues can be altered by numerous types of environment stimuli. For instance, levels of expression of the glucocorticoid receptor are under highly dynamic regulation within several limbic brain regions in response to chronic stress, and can mediate life-long changes in stress vulnerability (Zhang and Meaney, 2010).

DISCLOSURES

Dr. Nestler serves on the scientific advisory boards of PsychoGenics, Inc., Merck Research Laboratories, and Berg Pharma. He also is an ad hoc consultant for Johnson & Johnson.

Dr. Hyman serves on the Novartis Science Board and has advised Astra-Zeneca within the last year. Both advisory roles focus on early stage drug discovery. His research is funded by the Stanley Foundation.

REFERENCES

Altarejos, J.Y., and Montminy, M. (2011). CREB and CRTC co-activators: sensors for hormonal and metabolic signals. *Nat. Rev. Mol. Cell Biol.* 12:141–151.

Barco, A., and Marie, H. (2011). Genetic approaches to investigate the role of CREB in neuronal plasticity and memory. *Mol. Neurobiol.* 44:330–349.

Bartel, D.P. (2009). MicroRNAs: target recognition and regulatory functions. *Cell* 136:215–233.

Biddie, S.C., John, S., et al. (2011). Transcription factor AP1 potentiates chromatin accessibility and glucocorticoid receptor binding. *Mol. Cell* 43:145–155.

Blendy, J.A. (2006). The role of CREB in depression and antidepressant treatment. *Biol. Psychiatry* 59:1144–1150.

Borrelli, E., Nestler, E.J., et al. (2008). Decoding the epigenetic language of neuronal plasticity. *Neuron* 60:961–974.

Carlezon, W.A., Jr., Duman, R.S., et al. (2005). The many faces of CREB. *Trends Neurosci.* 28:436–445.

Cao, J.-L., Vialou, V.F., et al. (2010). Essential role of the cAMP-CREB pathway in opiate-induced homeostatic adaptations of locus coeruleus neurons. *Proc. Natl. Acad. Sci. USA* 107:17011–17016.

Chawla, A., Repa, J.J., et al. (2001). Nuclear receptors and lipid physiology: opening the X-files. *Science* 294:1866–1870.

Green, T.A., Alibhai, I.N., et al. (2008). Induction of activating transcription factors ATF2, ATF3, and ATF4 in the nucleus accumbens and their regulation of emotional behavior. *J. Neurosci.* 28:2025–2032.

Hayden, M.S., and Ghosh, S. (2012). NF-κB, the first quarter century: remarkable progress and outstanding questions. *Genes Dev.* 26:203–234.

Horvath, C.M. (2000). STAT proteins and transcriptional responses to extracellular signals. *Trends Biochem. Sci.* 25:496–502.

Hyman, S.E., and Nestler, E. (1993). The Molecular Foundations of Psychiatry. Washington, DC: American Psychiatric Association.

Ihle, J.N. (2001). The Stat family in cytokine signaling. *Curr. Opin. Cell Biol.* 13:211–217.

Inestrosa, N.C., and Arenas, E. (2010). Emerging roles of Wnts in the adult nervous system. *Nat. Rev. Neurosci.* 11:77–86.

Josselyn, S.A. (2010). Continuing the search for the engram: examining the mechanism of fear memories. *J. Psychiatry Neurosci.* 35:221–228.

Li, X., and Jope, R.S. (2010). Is glycogen synthase kinase-3 a central modulator in mood regulation? *Neuropsychopharmacology* 35:2143–2154.

Morgan, J.I., and Curran, T. (1995). Immediate-early genes: ten years on. *Trends Neurosci.* 18:66–77.

Nestler, E.J. (2008). Transcriptional mechanisms of addiction: role of delta-FosB. *Philos. Trans. R. Soc. Lond. B Biol. Sci.* 363:3245–3255.

Padgett, R.A. (2012). New connections between splicing and human disease. *Trends Genet.* 28:147–154.

Proudfoot, N.J. (2011). Ending the message: poly(A) signals then and now. *Genes Dev.* 25:1770–1782.

Taft, R.J., Pang, K.C., et al. (2010). Non-coding RNAs: regulators of disease. *J. Pathol.* 220:126–139.

Vo, N.K., Cambronne, X.A., et al. (2010). MicroRNA pathways in neural development and plasticity. *Curr. Opin. Neurobiol.* 20:457–465.

Wang, D.O., Martin, K.C., et al. (2010). Spatially restricting gene expression by local translation at synapses. *Trends Neurosci.* 33:173–182.

Wilkinson, M.B., Dias, C., et al. (2011). A novel role of the WNT-Dishevelled-GSK3β signaling cascade in the mouse nucleus accumbens in a social defeat model of depression. *J. Neurosci.* 31:9084–9092.

Zhang, T.Y., and Meaney, M.J. (2010). Epigenetics and the environmental regulation of the genome and its function. *Annu. Rev. Psychol.* 61:439–466.

7 | EPIGENETICS OF PSYCHIATRIC DISEASES

BRYAN E. MCGILL AND HUDA Y. ZOGHBI

Coined by Conrad Waddington in 1946, the term *epigenetic* was originally used to describe the effect of gene-environment interactions on the expression of particular phenotypes. Today, the same word commonly refers to stable changes in gene expression that occur without altering the underlying deoxyribonucleic acid (DNA) sequence. Epigenetic changes are characterized by being mitotically stable, meaning that they can be faithfully inherited through generations of somatic cell division. Furthermore, epigenetic changes result in stable phenotypic alterations for the organism. In recent years, a number of molecular pathways have been identified that mediate the establishment, maintenance, and interpretation of the epigenetic code (Goldberg et al., 2007). In this chapter, we provide a brief primer on the epigenetic mechanisms that are currently known to exist in humans: DNA methylation, covalent histone modification, chromatin remodeling by polycomb-group (PcG) and trithorax-group (trxG) proteins, ribonucleic acid (RNA) interference, and imprinting. Following that, we discuss examples whereby errors in these processes contribute to the pathogenesis of psychiatric diseases, using examples culled from research using *in vitro* systems, animal models, and humans where applicable.

MECHANISMS OF EPIGENETICS

DNA METHYLATION AND METHYL-CpG-BINDING PROTEINS

In humans (and other mammals), the cytosine base in DNA can be covalently modified at the carbon-5 position of its ring structure by the addition of a methyl group. The modified bases, designated 5-methylcytosines, are found primarily in symmetric CpG dinucleotide pairs. A minority of CpG pairs is found scattered throughout the genome. In large part, these are methylated, and they are involved in establishing a transcriptionally repressive environment. The majority of CpG dinucleotides are located in so-called CpG islands, which primarily occur in the promoters of protein-encoding genes. The remainder of CpG islands occupy sites within genes that identify alternative transcriptional initiation sites. Similar to the effect of methylation on cytosine in isolated CpG pairs, methylation of cytosines in CpG islands suppresses downstream transcription and silences local genes (Defossez and Stancheva, 2011; Illingworth and Bird, 2009; Suzuki and Bird, 2008).

In mammals, a class of proteins known as DNA methyltransferases (DNMTs) mediates DNA methylation. This family of proteins includes five polypeptides: DNMT1, DNMT2, DNMT3a, DNMT3b, and DNMT3L (Goll and Bestor, 2005). DNMT1, the first of this family to be identified, was originally distinguished by a preference for hemimethylated DNA compared with unmethylated DNA (Yoder et al., 1997). Given that methylated DNA is replicated semiconservatively, this resulted in the description of DNMT1 as a "maintenance DNA methyltransferase," as it was inferred that DNMT1 would faithfully curate the methylation pattern of DNA from parent to offspring during cell division. Subsequent data identified a *de novo* DNA methyltransferase function of DNMT1 and noted that under some conditions DNMT1 methylates hemimethylated and umethylated DNA with equal efficiency, making the relative contribution of this enzyme to maintenance and *de novo* DNA methylation less clear (Svedružić, 2011). In any case, DNMT1 activity is critical to normal development, as evidenced by the embryonic lethal phenotype of *Dnmt1* knockout mice (Li et al., 1992).

DNMT3a and DNMT3b are *de novo* methyltransferases and methylate hemimethylated or unmethylated DNA without preference. DNMT3a and DNMT3b also methylate cytosine in CpA and CpT dinucleotides in addition to cytosine in CpG dinucleotides. Mice lacking DNMT3a die within a month of birth, and mice lacking DNMT3b die *in utero*. Human mutations in the DNMT3b gene are notable for causing ICF (immunodeficiency-centromeric instability-facial anomalies) syndrome, a neurodevelopmental disorder characterized by intellectual disability (Chédin, 2011).

DNMT3L and DNMT2 bear structural similarities to the other DNA methyltransferase proteins, but they lack the ability to methylate DNA. DNMT3L interacts with DNMT3a and DNMT3b and is necessary for appropriate methylation of imprinted genes. The phenotype of DNMT3L null mice illustrate the relevance of this function, as both males and females of this strain are viable but sterile (Chédin, 2011). DNMT2 has a protein domain that is structurally identical to the catalytic core of the bacterial methyltransferase enzyme *HhaI*, but it appears to have little or no DNA methyltransferase activity under laboratory conditions. It methylates transfer RNA (tRNA). DNMT2 knockout mice have no apparent phenotypic abnormalities (Schaefer and Lyko, 2010).

Besides playing a role in normal development, DNA methylation is critical to the function of terminally differentiated neurons. Mice deficient for both *Dnmt1* and *Dnmt3a* in neurons perform poorly compared with control animals in behavioral assessments of long-term memory, and they have impaired long-term potentiation, an electrophysiologic

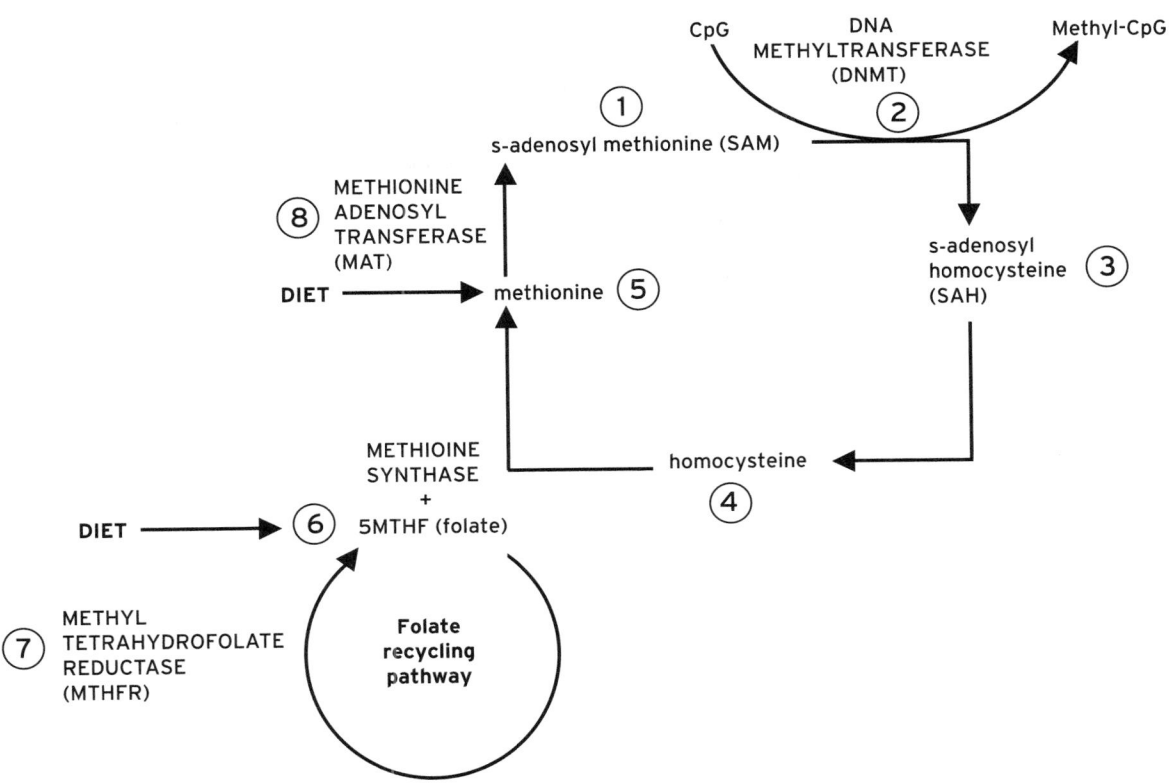

Figure 7.1 *Biochemical pathways link dietary folic acid and methionine to DNA methylation. (1) S-adenosyl methionine (SAM) provides the methyl group that (2) DNA methyltransferase (DNMT) uses to methylate CpG dinucleotides in DNA. When SAM donates its methyl group to DNMT, it is converted to S-adenosylhomocysteine (SAH) (3). Then, SAH is converted to homocysteine (4). Homocysteine is converted to methionine (5) by methionine synthase in a reaction that consumes 5-methyltetrahydrofolate (5MTHF), the major circulating form of the nutrient folic acid (6). Folate is regenerated in a series of enzymatic reactions, the last of which is carried out by methylene tetrahydrofolatereductase (MTHFR) (7). SAM is generated from the methionine by the enzyme methionine adenosyltransferase (MAT) (8). Food is the ultimate source of methionine and folic acid.*

correlate of long-term memory. These same mice have reduced levels of DNA methylation upstream of genes important for neural activity and synaptic plasticity, and this correlates with increased gene expression, at least for the immediate early gene *Stat1* (Feng, Zhou, et al., 2010). Further illustrating this point, pharmacologic inhibition of DNMT1 function has been shown to impair long-term recall of conditioned fear memory (Miller and Sweatt, 2007). These findings suggest that DNMTs regulate expression of genes critical to learning and memory, both during development and in adult animals (Day and Sweatt, 2011).

DNA methyltransferases obtain the methyl group used to methylate DNA from the methyl donor *S*-adenosylmethionine (SAM) (Fig. 7.1). SAM is produced from methionine by the enzyme methionine adenosyl transferase. DNA methylation depletes the available pool of SAM and generates the metabolite S-adenosyl-homocysteine, which is converted to homocysteine. The ultimate source of methionine, the precursor of SAM, is the diet. However, methionine can also be regenerated from homocysteine by the enzyme methionine synthase. This reaction requires the methyl donor 5-methyl tetrahydrofolate (5MTHF), the major circulating form of the nutrient folic acid (folate). As with methionine, dietary intake is the ultimate source of folate. In this way, levels of DNA methylation are closely linked to the nutritional status of the organism (Muskiet and Kemperman, 2006).

DNA methylation regulates gene expression via at least two mechanisms (Fig. 7.2). First, methyl-CpGs directly interfere with the binding of some transcription factors (Watt and Molloy, 1988). Second, DNA methylation regulates gene expression via the methyl-CpG-directed recruitment of methylated DNA binding proteins that bind methylated DNA and act as scaffolds to recruit protein complexes that primarily repress, and in some cases activate, gene transcription (Defossez and Stancheva, 2011).

The first family of methylated DNA binding proteins is characterized by the presence of a conserved methyl-CpG-binding domain (MBD), and includes the proteins MeCP2, MBD1, MBD2, and MBD4. MBD1 and MBD2 participate in gene silencing; MBD4 has DNA glycosylase activity and helps repair DNA damage (Defossez and Stancheva, 2011). MeCP2, the first member of this family to be purified (Lewis et al., 1992), binds methylated CpGs in proximity to a run of at least four adenine or thymine nucleotides. Once bound, MeCP2 recruits a variety of corepressor complexes, including one containing Sin3a and the histone deacetylases HDAC1 and HDAC2. In addition, MeCP2 recruits histone methyltransferases, DNA methyltransferases, and transcriptional activators like ATP-dependent chromatin remodeling proteins and the transcription factor CREB1 (Chahrour et al., 2008; Chahrour and Zoghbi, 2007). MBD3, MBD5, and MBD6 proteins exist as well,

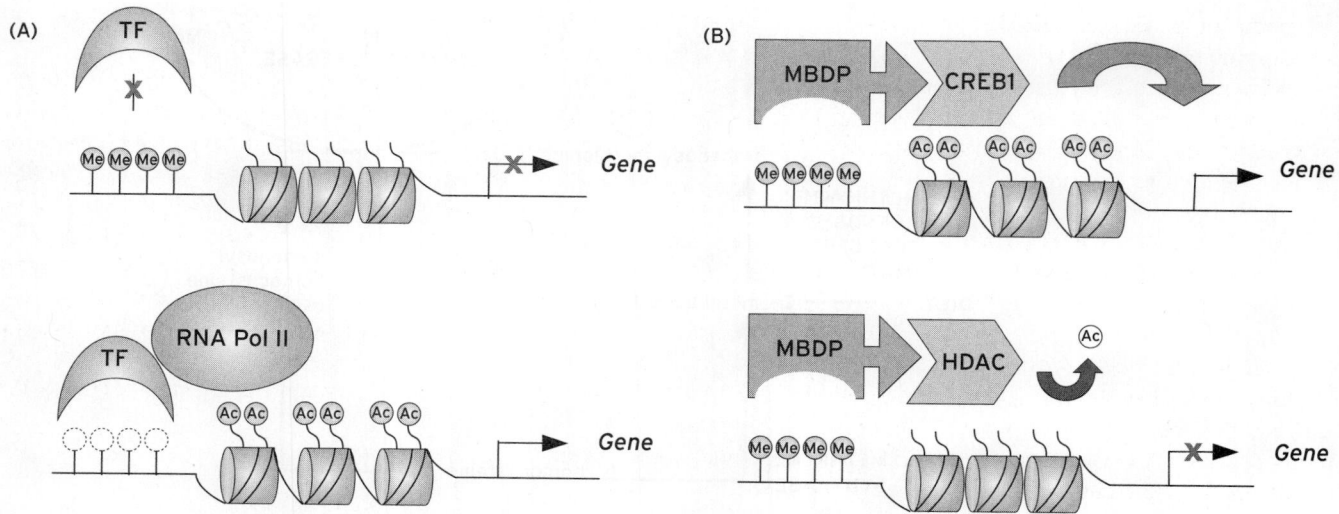

Figure 7.2 *Mechanisms of epigenetic gene regulation by DNA methylation. (A) DNA methylation may cause gene repression by interfering with transcription factor binding. The transcription factor binds unmethylated DNA, recruits RNA polymerase II (RNA pol II), and the target gene is transcribed. (B) Alternatively, DNA methylation may attract methyl-CpG binding proteins (here labeled MBDP). In turn, methyl-CpG binding proteins recruit coactivators, such as CREB1, or corepressors, such as histone deacetylases (HDACs). In this figure, the DNA strand is represented by a dark gray line, nucleosomes are represented by gray cylinders, histone tails are represented by squiggly lines, and histone modifications (here, acetylation) are represented by circles atop the squiggly lines. DNA methylation of CpG sites is represented by shaded lollipops. The absence of DNA methylation is represented by dotted lollipops.*

but they lack functional MBD domains and do not bind methylated DNA (Defossez and Stancheva, 2011).

The second family of methylated DNA binding proteins includes Kaiso and the Kaiso-like proteins ZBTB4 and ZBTB38. These proteins are zinc finger transcription factors that preferentially bind a specific DNA sequence called a Kaiso binding site (KBS), which is characterized by a central TpG dinucleotide. TpG shares structural similarity with methyl-CpG, and in fact Kaiso and its relatives bind methyl-CpG with equal affinity to the canonical KBS (Defossez and Stancheva, 2011).

UHRF1 (also known as ICBP90) and UHRF2 comprise the third and final family of methylated DNA binding proteins. These proteins bind methylated DNA via an SRA (*SET and Ring finger Associated*) protein domain. UHRF1 also interacts with histone proteins and has enzymatic activity, functioning as a ubiquitin E3 ligase. UHRF2 was identified by virtue of its close structural similarity to UHRF1, but other than its interaction with methylated DNA little is known about its function (Defossez and Stancheva, 2011).

Although much is known about the proteins that methylate DNA and interpret DNA methylation, far less is understood about DNA demethylation. Numerous studies have pointed to the occurrence of DNA demethylation during both embryonic development as well as during gametogenesis (Feng, Jacobsen, et al., 2010), although some have refuted this (Li and O'Neill, 2012). Two methods of DNA demethylation exist: active and passive demethylation. Passive DNA demethylation is accomplished by preventing DNMT1 from interacting with replicating DNA. Because duplication of DNA methylation patterns occurs in a semiconservative manner, each successive round of DNA replication further dilutes the original complement of methylated cytosines, resulting in demethylation. Therefore, passive demethylation is dependent on DNA replication,

which occurs only during cell division during development (Morgan et al., 2005).

Active demethylation requires neither DNA replication nor cell division, and is therefore accessible to mature neurons, unlike passive demethylation. In mammals, there is evidence to support three ways by which demethylation occurs in postmitotic cells. The first and simplest process uses a 5'-methyl-cytosine DNA glycosylase and the base excision repair pathway, normally a DNA damage repair mechanism, to demethylate 5-methyl cytosines. First, a 5'-methyl-cytosine DNA glycosylase cleaves the covalent link between the 5meC and the deoxyribose sugar. Then, an endonuclease removes the deoxyribose sugar. Finally, a DNA polymerase and a DNA ligase insert an unmethylated cytosine into the same spot (Zhu, 2009). In mammals, MBD4 has DNA glycosylase activity at guanine/thymine nucleotide mismatches, at least *in vitro* (Zhu, 2000). In mammalian cell lines, the non-enzymatic protein Gadd45a promotes DNA demethylation in a process that requires both XPB, a DNA helicase, and XPG, a DNA 3' endonuclease (Barreto et al., 2007). Although intriguing, a subsequent study in cells did not find proof of Gadd45a involvement in DNA demethylation (Jin et al., 2008). However, *in vivo* studies in mice found evidence of activity-dependent upregulation of *Gadd45b* expression in the dentate gyrus, a domain of the hippocampus important in learning and memory formation. In response to electrical stimulation of the brain, Gadd45b localized to the *Bdnf* regulatory region IX and the *Fgf1* promoter and decreased methylation was observed at these sites. The same gene regulatory regions remained methylated in *Gadd45b* knockout mice in response to the same stimulus (Ma et al., 2009). Thus, although the components of this demethylation pathway remain unknown, evidence is accumulating that DNA demethylation occurs in mammals.

Another proposed mechanism of DNA demethylation begins with deamination of 5-methyl cytosine to generate thymine. Then, a glycosylase that recognizes guanine/thymine DNA base mismatches removes the thymine base. Finally, just as with the first mechanism described in the preceding, an endonuclease removes the deoxyribose sugar, and a DNA polymerase and a DNA ligase together insert an unmethylated cytosine into the same spot (Zhu, 2009). *In vitro*, the mammalian proteins Dnmt3a and Dnmt3b demonstrate 5-methyl cytosine deaminase activity. In an experimental system in cell culture, estradiol treatment leads to demethylation of the *pS2* gene promoter and subsequent *pS2* transcription. Prior to demethylation, Dnmt3a and Dnmt3b bind the *pS2* promoter in association with the DNA glycosylase TDG and base excision repair proteins. Pharmacological inhibition of Dnmt3a and Dnmt3b blocks *pS2* demethylation, suggesting that these proteins are responsible for demethylation of the *pS2* promoter (Métivier et al., 2008). Further studies will be needed to confirm these findings and determine whether or not they apply to whole organisms as well.

A third mechanism of demethylation involves initial chemical conversion of 5-methyl cytosine to 5-hydroxymethyl cytosine. This is followed by deamination of 5-hydroxymethyl cytosine to thymine, and subsequent replacement of thymine with unmethylated cytosine using base excision repair. In mammals, the Tet1 protein performs the initial hydroxylation step, and Apobec1 deaminates 5-hydroxymethyl cytosine. Initially worked out in cell culture, there is evidence that this pathway also exists in mouse brain, where interference with either Tet1 or Apobec1 expression blocks electrical stimulation-induced demethylation at the *Bdnf* regulatory region IX and the *Fgf1* promoter (Guo et al., 2011).

COVALENT HISTONE MODIFICATION

Nuclear DNA is organized into a three-dimensional molecular structure known as chromatin. The most basic form of chromatin is the nucleosome, which is composed of DNA wrapped around a complex of eight histone proteins, including two copies each of protein H2A, H2B, H3, and H4. Nucleosomes are separated from one another by short stretches of naked DNA, and the alternating sequence of nucleosome-naked DNA-nucleosome forms a filament with a "beads on a string" appearance called a 10nm fiber. The 10nm fiber represents an open chromatin configuration known as euchromatin, and it is this configuration that allows for active gene transcription. The 10nm fiber coils further in a solenoid pattern to form a 30nm fiber, and most DNA maintains this degree of compaction during interphase. Compacted, transcriptionally inactive chromatin is known as heterochromatin. During cell division the 30nm fiber condenses further to generate the chromosome complement of every human cell (Ruthenburg et al., 2007; Fussner et al., 2011).

It is evident that chromatin configuration (i.e., open or closed, euchromatin or heterochromatin) determines the complement of active genes in the cell nucleus, and that manipulating chromatin compaction alters the cohort of expressed genes. Covalent chemical modification of histone proteins represents one method of controlling chromatin configuration. Research over the last two decades has identified histone modification

as a major mechanism of transmitting and maintaining epigenetic information (Strahl and Allis, 2000).

Histone proteins are primarily modified on their N-terminal tails, which jut out from the globular nucleosome core like spokes on a wheel. Numerous chemical modifications have been identified on the amino acids that form these tails, including methylation, acetylation, phosphorylation, gylcosylation, formylation, hydroxylation, and crotonylation (Tan et al., 2011). Additionally, the small proteins ubiquitin and SUMO can be covalently attached to various histones, leading to histone ubiquitylation and SUMOylation, respectively. These modifications change chromatin structure, and thereby gene expression, via multiple mechanisms (Fig. 7.3). First, covalent modifications change the

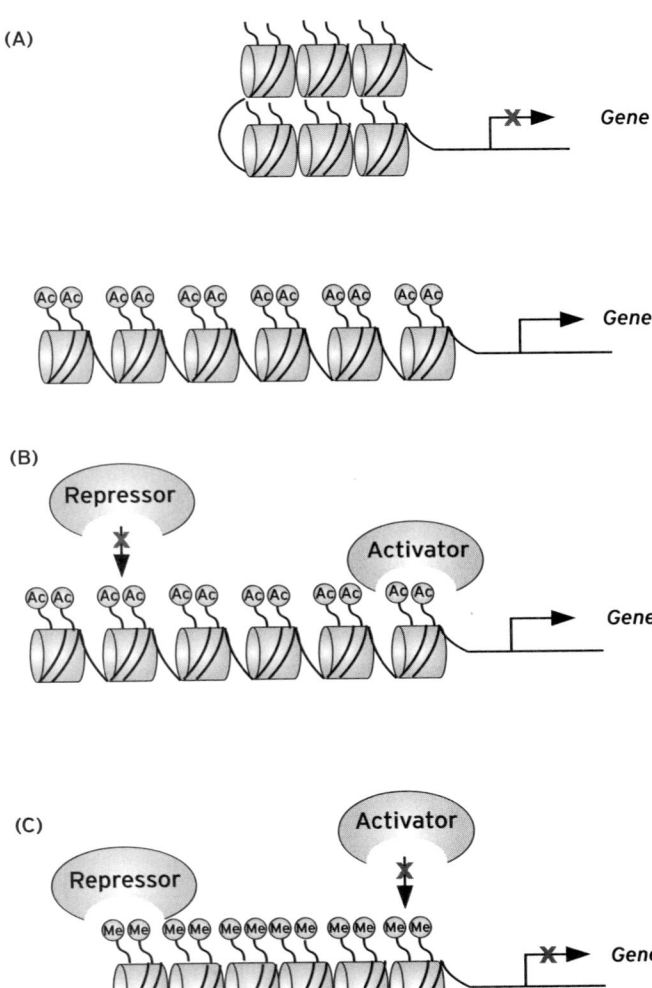

Figure 7.3 *Mechanisms of epigenetic gene regulation by covalent histone modification. (A) Covalent histone modification may directly alter chromatin compaction by altering the affinity of histone proteins for one another or for DNA. (B) Alternatively, modifications may attract transcriptional activators that recognize particular chemical moieties or repel transcriptional repressors that ordinarily bind histones in the absence of a particular modification. (C) Other modifications may have the opposite effects on transcriptional activators and repressors. In this figure, the deoxyribonucleic acid (DNA) strand is represented by a dark gray line, nucleosomes are represented by gray cylinders, histone tails are represented by squiggly lines, and histone modifications [here, acetylation in (B) and methylation in (C)] are represented by circles atop the squiggly lines.*

electrostatic charge of specific amino acids. For example, lysine residues are positively charged, and histone lysine acetylation removes that charge. The net effect of numerous such chemical modifications is enough to change chromatin structure on a larger scale both by affecting individual nucleosome interactions with DNA in *cis* and nucleosome-nucleosome interactions in *trans*. Second, posttranslational covalent modifications to histone proteins changes the molecular topology of nucleosomes such that they may attract or interfere with the binding of various chromatin-modifying enzymes, transcriptional coactivators, and transcriptional corepressors to DNA. In this way, the combination of histone modifications at a particular locus can determine cell specific gene transcription (Ruthenburg et al., 2007).

Of the various chemical modifications to histone tail amino acid residues, methylation and acetylation are the most well understood. Histone methylation occurs on the basic amino acid residues lysine (K), arginine (R), and histidine (H). Lysine can be mono-, di-, or trimethylated on a single residue, whereas arginine can be mono- or dimethylated, and histidine accommodates only monomethylation. Enzymes that methylate lysines include SET domain containing proteins and DOT1-like proteins. Arginines are methylated by protein arginine methyltransferases, or PRMTs. Histidine methyltransferases remain undiscovered. Lysine demethylases include the amine oxidases and the jumonji domain containing iron-dependent dioxygenases. There are no known arginine or histidine demethylases. Various protein domains recognize each individual histone methylation mark, and the effects of individual marks can have dramatically different effects on chromatin conformation and gene expression. For example, histone H3 lysine 4 trimethylation (H3K4me3) is a mark of active chromatin, whereas histone H3 lysine 27 trimethylation (H3K27me3) is a mark of inactive chromatin. Combinatorial effects are also possible. As a case in point, the combination of H3K4me3 and H3K27me3 results in activated chromatin (Greer and Shi, 2012) .

Histone acetylation, which occurs on lysine (K) residues, is also well characterized. In general, histone acetylation is associated with an open chromatin conformation and correlates with transcriptionally active genes. Histones are acetylated by enzymes called histone acetyltransferases (HATs), which are recruited to chromatin by transcriptional activators. Some HATs are also able to directly bind chromatin on their own. Acetylation neutralizes the positive charge of lysine residues, decreasing the affinity of histone proteins for the negatively charged DNA double helix and opening the chromatin structure. Acetylation also provides a binding surface for specialized proteins that mediate the effects of this histone modification, including proteins that promote open chromatin conformation, such as the SWI/SNF family of proteins. These proteins recognize acetylated lysines with protein domains called bromodomains, which allow binding of the modified residues (Choi and Howe, 2009).

In contrast to acetylation, histone deacetylation generally promotes a closed chromatin conformation and repression of gene transcription. Deacetylation is carried out by histone deacetylases (HDACs), and exposes positively charged lysine residues on histones, which are then free to interact with the negatively charged DNA strand. Just as histone acetylation recruits proteins that open chromatin and promote gene transcription, histone deacetylation attracts proteins that promote a repressed chromatin state. Proteins containing SANT (*SWI3*, *ADA2*, *N*-CoR, and *TFIIB*) domains recognize deacetylated lysines on histone proteins and recruit HDACs to help maintain gene repression (Shahbazian and Grunstein, 2007).

An important exception to the rule that histone deacetylation correlates with gene repression is the case of histone H4 lysine 16 (H4K16). Deacetylation of this residue correlates with gene activation when it occurs in euchromatic regions of DNA. This finding suggests that other individual acetylated residues may have specific effects on gene expression, and represents an active area of research for scientists interested in histone modification (Shahbazian and Grunstein, 2007).

In addition to the role of histone tails in the control of gene expression, other mechanisms exist whereby histones may modulate the epigenetic transfer of information. For example, splice variants of each of the core histone proteins exist, some of which can be modified at alternative sites. Inclusion of another histone protein not part of the nucleosome, HP1, allows further condensation of chromatin into a more heterochromatic state by linking nucleosomes to one another (Zeng et al., 2010).

CHROMATIN REMODELING BY POLYCOMB- AND TRITHORAX-GROUP PROTEINS

Another mechanism of epigenetic gene regulation involves the manipulation of higher order chromatin structure by polycomb-group (PcG) and trithorax-group (trxG) proteins. Both groups of proteins were initially discovered in the fruit fly, *Drosophila melanogaster*, where they organize development along the anterior-posterior axis by regulating the expression of so-called homeotic genes. PcG and trxG proteins regulate gene expression in mammals as well, particularly at imprinted loci, making them relevant to epigenetic processes occurring in humans (Schuettengruber et al., 2007).

In general, PcG proteins repress gene expression by combining to form one of two multimember protein complexes, PRC1 and PRC2. PRC1 is composed of the mammalian homologs of four core proteins found in *D. melanogaster*: Polycomb, Polyhomeotic, Posterior sex combs, and Sex combs extra. Polycomb has a chromodomain that binds trimethylated histone H3 at lysine 27 (H3K27me3); Sex combs extra ubiquitylates histone H2A, and Posterior sex combs is a cofactor for the ubiquitin ligase function of Sex combs extra (Simon and Kingston, 2009). The repressive function of Polyhomeotic depends on its ability to self-associate and form polymerized chains of Polyhomeotic protein (Robinson et al., 2012a). The mechanism by which PRC1 represses gene transcription is not known. One hypothesis proposes that PRC1 blocks transcription by interfering with the disassembly and reassembly of nucleosomes that is required for transcriptional elongation. Another hypothesis proposes that PRC1-induced ubiquitylation of histone proteins blocks transcription by interfering with RNA polymerase movement along the DNA strand (Simon and Kingston, 2009).

Like PRC1, PRC2 is composed of four core subunits, the mammalian homologs of the *D. melanogaster* proteins Enhancer of Zeste, Suppressor of Zeste, Extra Sex Combs, and nucleosome remodeling factor 55 (NURF55). Enhancer of Zeste is a SET-domain containing histone methyltranferase that carries out the primary repressive function of PRC2 by trimethylating histone H3 at lysine 27 (H3K27me3). The other core proteins allow PRC2 to bind histones and stimulate its histone methyltransferase function (Simon and Kingston, 2009).

Similar to PcG proteins, trxG proteins form multi-subunit protein complexes of their own that fall into two categories: histone modifying complexes and ATP-dependent chromatin remodeling complexes. The former category includes COMPASS, COMPASS-like, TAC1, and ASH1. These complexes stimulate gene transcription by trimethylating histone H3 at lysine 4 (H3K4me3), and acetylating histone H4 at lysine 16 (H4K16ac) and acetylating histone H3 at lysine 27 (H3K27ac). The latter category includes SWI/SNF, ISWI, and CHD1, CHD2, CHD3, CHD4, CHD6, CHD7, and CHD8. These complexes expend ATP energy to alter chromatin structure in one of three ways: by disrupting DNA-nucleosome interactions, by repositioning nucleosomes along the chromatin fiber, and by ejecting or exchanging entire nucleosomes (Schuettengruber et al., 2011).

RNA INTERFERENCE

RNA interference (RNAi) is an epigenetic mechanism that is mediated by the production of various types of non-coding RNA (ncRNA). ncRNA species include micro RNA (miRNA), Piwi-interacting RNA (piRNA), long non-coding RNA (lncRNA), and the small RNA subspecies called small interfering RNA (siRNA), small nucleolar RNA (snoRNA), and repeat-associated siRNA (rasiRNA). Experimental evidence is accumulating for other varieties of ncRNA, and it is likely that further subtypes will be delineated in the future. The various forms of ncRNA are differentiated from one another by their sizes and cellular functions. miRNAs, the best described among the ncRNAs, are 23-nucleotide-long RNA species transcribed from DNA by RNA polymerase II. Initially present in the nucleus as a hairpin structure, miRNAs in mammals are processed by the enzyme Drosha and exported to the cytoplasm by the RAN-GTPase exportin 5. Once there, miRNAs are further processed by a protein called Dicer. The mature miRNA is incorporated into the RNA-induced silencing complex (RISC), the key component of which is the protein Argonaute. RISC separates the two strands of the miRNA and uses the so-called guide strand to target specific mRNA sequences. These mRNA targets may be degraded by the RNAse H, or "slicer," activity of the Argonaute component of RISC. Alternatively, RISC can suppress mRNA translation and shunt the mRNA to other endogenous cytoplasmic RNA degradation pathways (Fig. 7.4). A similar mechanism is utilized by siRNA small RNAs. Targets of this pathway include genes that encode key members of other epigenetic signaling pathways, including the DNA methyltransferases DNMT1, DNMT3a, and DNMT3b, and EZH2, a histone methyltransferase and component of the

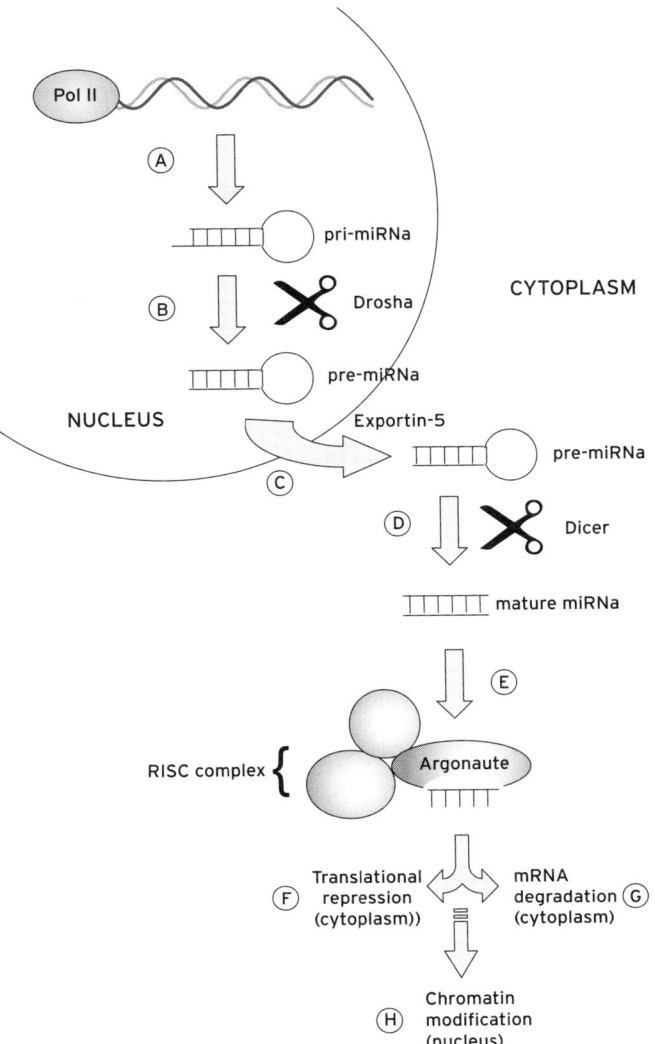

Figure 7.4 *The RNA interference pathway. pri-miRNA, the initial miRNA precursor, is transcribed from palindromic DNA sequences by RNA polymerase II (A). pri-miRNAs are trimmed by the enzyme Drosha in the nucleus (B) to make pre-miRNs and exported to the cytoplasm by Exportin-5 (C). There, pre-miRNA is further processed by Dicer to mature miRNA (D). miRNA is cleaved into its complementary strands and the guide strand is loaded into the RISC protein complex, the major component of which is the protein Argonaute (E). miRNA can suppress translation by sequestering mRNA (F) or targeting it for degradation (G). Alternatively, miRNA can return to the nucleus, where it regulates transcription and chromatin formation via mechanisms that are still being investigated (H).*

polycomb complex PRC2 (Cam, 2010; Costa, 2010; Wiklund et al., 2010).

In addition to directing mRNA degradation, ncRNA regulates the establishment of heterochromatin. This occurs when an ncRNA associates with the RNA-induced transcriptional suppressor (RITS) complex in the nucleus. The ncRNA is used to target promoter RNA (pRNA), which is RNA transcribed from the promoter region of a gene. This leads to the recruitment of histone methyltransferases that methylate local chromatin, particularly at histone H3 lysine 9 (H3K9), which in turn attracts histone deacetylases. The combination of histone methylation at H3K9 and deacetylation produces a closed chromatin structure that suppresses gene transcription (Wiklund et al., 2010).

IMPRINTING

The term *imprinting* describes an epigenetic phenomenon in which a gene is expressed differentially (often monoallelically) in a parent-of-origin-specific manner. Approximately 131 imprinted genes have been identified at the time of this writing (July 2012). Most imprinted genes occur in clusters throughout the genome and frequently occur in close association with CpG islands. The functions of imprinted genes are tightly linked to specific developmental and somatic processes, including neural activity, energy use and metabolism, the development of specific tissues, and intrauterine growth.

At least three mechanisms exist to regulate imprinted gene expression. The first and best characterized mechanism is illustrated by the *Igf2* gene (Fig. 7.5A). *Igf2* is normally repressed on the maternal chromosome, which instead expresses the *H19* non-coding RNA (ncRNA). The maternal chromosome contains an imprinting control region (ICR) upstream of the *H19* gene. The ICR remains unmethylated on the maternal chromosome and binds the CTCF protein and the cohesin protein complex. This protein-DNA interaction denies the *Igf2* gene access to its enhancer sequence and suppresses *Igf2* expression on the maternal chromosome. Instead, *H19* is expressed. Meanwhile, on the paternal chromosome, cytosines in the ICR are methylated, which impairs CTCF and cohesin binding. This allows access to the *Igf2* enhancer, which activates *Igf2* expression. In this context, *H19* is suppressed.

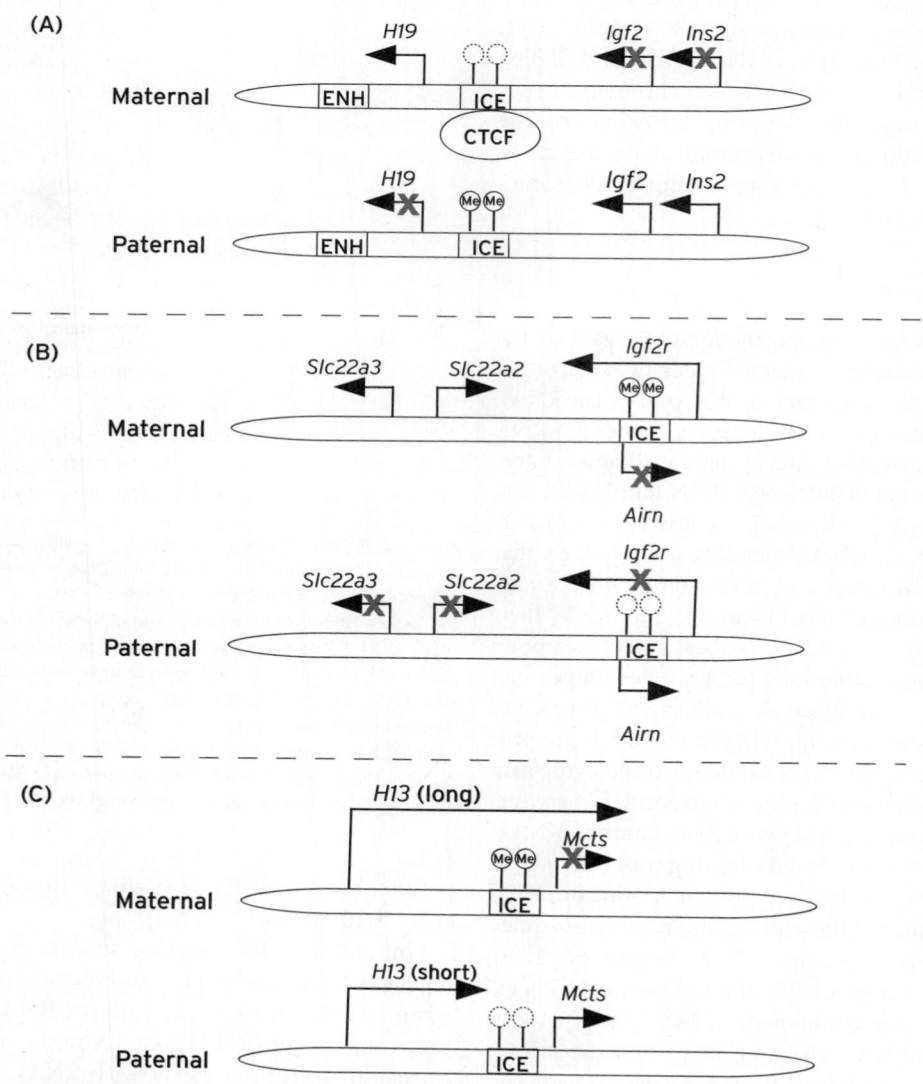

Figure 7.5 *Mechanisms of imprinting. There are three general mechanisms by which genes are imprinted. (A) In the first model, DNA methylation at the imprinting control region (ICR) regulates binding of a protein like CTCF. The presence or absence of the protein dictates which imprinted genes are expressed. (B) In the second model, DNA methylation at the ICR controls expression of an antisense transcript, like Airn. When expressed, the antisense transcript interferes with transcription of the sense transcript from the same allele, leading to differential expression of the target gene. (C) In the third model, DNA methylation at the ICR controls polyadenylation site choice, leading to expression of a short or long form of a gene. In this figure, DNA methylation of CpG sites is represented by shaded lollipops (see text for details).*

The second mechanism of imprinted gene regulation is exemplified by the *Igf2r* gene (Fig. 7.5B). *Igf2r* contains an intronic CpG island within its sequence that functions as an ICR. On the maternal chromosome, this CpG island is methylated, and the *Igf2r* gene is expressed. On the paternal chromosome, the CpG island is unmethylated. The unmethylated sequence functions as a promoter for the *Airn* gene, which is transcribed antisense to the *Igf2r* gene. *Airn* encodes an ncRNA, which suppresses *Igf2r* expression via a mechanism that is still being investigated.

The *H13* gene provides an example of the third mechanism of imprinted gene regulation (Fig. 7.5C). *H13* has multiple alternative polyadenlyation sites separated by an ICR that serves as the promoter for the *Mcts* gene. On the maternal allele the ICR is methylated, which blocks expression of *Mcts* and allows a long, functional form of the *H13* gene to be transcribed. On the paternal allele, the ICR is unmethylated and *Mcts* is expressed. In the presence of *Mcts* expression the *H13* gene is transcribed using an alternative polyadenylation site that yields a truncated, inactive form of the *H13* transcript (Barlow, 2011; Bartolomei and Ferguson-Smith, 2011; Koerner and Barlow, 2010).

NEUROPSYCHIATRIC DISORDERS ASSOCIATED WITH EPIGENETIC DEFECTS

ADDICTION

Epigenetic mechanisms of gene regulation have proven to be fundamental to the development of addictive behaviors in preclinical animal models. To date, most data collected have focused on the effects of cocaine on epigenetic gene regulation. Cocaine treatment leads to increased histone H3 and H4 acetylation, a mark of gene activation, at immediate early genes that are activated by the drug, including *cFos*, *Bdnf*, and *Cdk5* (Kumar et al., 2005). This effect is mediated by both cocaine-induced recruitment of the histone acetyltransferase, CREB binding protein (CBP) (Levine et al., 2005), and cocaine-induced inhibition of the histone deacetylase, HDAC5 (Renthal et al., 2007). Genes encoding the histone deacetylases Sirt1 and Sirt2 are among those that are transcriptionally activated by cocaine, and may be responsible for sustaining the transcriptional response to the drug (Renthal et al., 2009). Supporting this concept, genetic and pharmacologic manipulations of HATs and HDACs predictably alter the behavioral response to cocaine in animals. For example, mice heterozygous for a *Creb1* null mutation (predicted to decrease histone acetylation) have reduced acetylation at *cFos*, reduced *cFos* expression, and reduced locomotor activity in response to cocaine (Levine et al., 2005). Likewise, viral mediated enhancement of HDAC expression (also predicted to decrease histone acetylation) in mice impairs cocaine induced place preference, a behavioral model for addiction in humans (Kumar et al., 2005). Conversely, small molecule inhibitors of HDAC enzymatic activity enhance *cFos* expression and the behavioral response to cocaine (Kumar et al., 2005).

Histone acetylation also underlies the effects of other drugs of abuse, such as nicotine. Chronic nicotine treatment of mice leads to hyperacetylation of histone proteins and increased *FosB* expression. In addition to mediating the rewarding effects of drugs of abuse, histone acetylation may also play a role in priming the users of one drug to the addictive effects of another. For example, chronic use of nicotine prior to treatment with cocaine enhanced *FosB* expression more than cocaine alone without prior nicotine treatment. This effect was mediated by a nicotine-induced reduction in HDAC activity, and a similar effect was achieved using a small-molecule inhibitor of HDACs. Epidemiologic analysis indicates that humans who used cocaine and who concurrently smoked cigarettes had a higher incidence of cocaine dependence, suggesting that similar epigenetic mechanisms operate in humans and are responsible for regulating complex addictive behaviors (Levine et al., 2011).

In addition to histone acetylation, histone methylation has been implicated in addiction. Chronic cocaine use causes genome-wide reduction in histone H3 lysine 9 trimethylation (H3K9me3), a histone modification associated with gene silencing and heterochromatin formation, in nucleus accumbens. This leads to de-repression of intergenic regions of DNA and activation of retrotransposons (Maze et al., 2011). Similar analysis of histone H3 lysine 9 dimethylation (H3K9me2) and histone H3 lysine 27 dimethylation (H3K27me2), both repressive marks, found that repeated cocaine treatment led to increased methylation at these sites at nearly 900 genes, as compared with a reduction in methylation at these sites in fewer than one third as many genes (Renthal et al., 2009). Together, these findings indicate that repeated cocaine use both dampens gene expression and transcriptionally activates genes at the same time, reinforcing the concept that epigenetic changes in response to environmental stimuli are exceedingly complex, even in isolated brain regions and even in response to well-defined stimuli. As with histone acetylation, it is possible to interfere with the effects of cocaine by manipulating histone methylation. For example, cocaine downregulates the G9a histone methyltransferase, and genetic upregulation of *G9a* expression reduces behavioral sensitivity to the drug (Maze et al., 2010). This suggests that treatments targeting epigenetic systems may be powerful tools in the fight against addiction.

DNA methylation also plays a role in mediating the addictive properties of cocaine. Cocaine decreases global DNA methylation in the prefrontal cortex of mammals. This may be mediated by *Dnmt3b*, the expression of which is downregulated following cocaine treatment. Dietary supplementation with methionine, a methyl donor, rescues *Dnmt3b* expression and abolishes conditioned place preference, a model of addictive behavior in animals (Tian et al., 2012). Likewise, cocaine downregulates *Dnmt3a* expression in the nucleus accumbens, and methionine supplementation and *Dnmt3a* overexpression there abolish addictive behaviors in mice (LaPlant et al., 2010). These results are particularly exciting because they suggest that simple dietary modification with methionine supplementation can interfere with the addictive effects of cocaine.

RNA interference by non-coding RNA (ncRNA) also regulates addictive behaviors. This has been most convincingly demonstrated for the ncRNA, miR-212, which is transcribed in the dorsal striatum of animals under conditions of unfettered access to cocaine. Surprisingly, miR-212 appears to protect against the effects of chronic cocaine use, as siRNA knockdown of miR-212 increased cocaine intake and enhanced its addictive properties in mice, whereas miR-212 upregulation protected against these effects (Hollander et al., 2010). Interestingly, miR-212 is negatively regulated by MeCP2, thereby implicating yet another epigenetic marker in the process of addiction (Im et al., 2010) . Thus, even though the crucial histone modifications, ncRNA transcripts, and methylated sites vary between addictive substances examined and even between brain regions for the same substance, it is clear that epigenetic systems are crucial to establishing and maintaining an animal's sensitivity to drugs of abuse.

DEPRESSION

The genetics of affective disorders, including major depressive disorder, have proven to be relatively intractable to traditional forward genetic analyses. Studies of monozygotic twins, which find a 50% discordance rate for major depressive disorder (MDD), suggest that a major reason for the failure of forward genetics to solve MDD is that it is less heritable by traditional Mendelian genetics. This seems to agree with clinical experience, which suggests that susceptibility to MDD is based on complex gene x environment interactions. Epigenetic mechanisms are thus attractive to researchers interested in the biological basis of MDD as they provide a mechanism whereby environmental perturbations can lead to gene expression changes, which in turn affect behavioral phenotypes (Sun et al., 2012). The last few years have seen an explosion of preclinical data evaluating epigenetic mechanisms of depressive behaviors in animals, as outlined in the following paragraphs.

Both covalent modifications of histone proteins and DNA methylation have been tied to depression. In the setting of chronic stress, increased DNA methylation occurs at multiple Bdnf promoters, and the transcripts from these promoters are downregulated. The antidepressant imipramine abrogates this effect. Imipramine also increases histone acetylation at the same Bdnf promoters that are silenced by DNA methylation in the setting of chronic stress, and this hyper-acetylation is accompanied by increased Bdnf expression. Remarkably, genetic upregulation of histone deacetylases, which reverses the effect of imipramine on histone acetylation, is sufficient to block the antidepressant effect of this drug (Tsankova et al., 2006).

Similar to the effect of chronic stress on Bdnf, chronic stress also silences Gdnf expression in BALB mice, which are susceptible to depressive behavior in the setting of chronic stress. Following stress, BALB mice have increased DNA methylation upstream of Gdnf at a CpG site that is bound by a protein complex including MeCP2 and HDAC2. Predictably, these mice have decreased acetylation at histone H3 at the Gdnf locus. Imipramine blocks these effects of stress, leading to reduced CpG methylation, reduced MeCP2 and HDAC2 recruitment, and increased histone H3 acetylation at Gdnf. Imipramine-treated BALB mice have increased Gdnf expression and less depressive behaviors than their untreated counterparts. In contrast, B6 mice, a stress-resistant strain, recruit MeCP2 complexed with CREB, a transcriptional activator, to the same methyl-CpG site upstream of Gdnf in response to chronic stress. B6 mice have increased histone H3 acetylation at Gdnf and increased Gdnf expression in response to stress (Uchida et al., 2011). This suggests that subtle alterations in the epigenetic control of gene expression may underlie individual differences in the behavioral response to stress, and that successful therapeutic interventions may hinge on reversing maladaptive epigenetic changes.

Broad, unbiased evaluation of histone modifications have also yielded insight into the epigenetic response to stress. For instance, both social defeat stress and social isolation stress affect histone methylation similarly by increasing dimethylation at histone H3 lysine 27 (H3K27me2) and at lysine 9 (H3K9me2) in the nucleus accumbens. Both modifications enhance transcriptional repression. Nearly three quarters of the genes repressed under both paradigms overlap, supplying evidence that different stressors activate epigenetic programs that are largely identical (Wilkinson et al., 2009). However, acute and chronic stress affect histone modifications differently. In the hippocampus, acute stress increases the overall level of trimethylation at histone H3 lysine 9 (H3K9me3), whereas chronic stress decreases H3K9me3 (Hunter et al., 2009). Remote effects of stress on histone modifications are possible as well; histone H3 acetylation initially decreases one hour after the last session of chronic stress, only to significantly increase by 10 days afterward. Decreased expression of HDAC2 occurs concurrently with increases in histone acetylation in mice exposed to chronic stress. Postmortem samples from humans with depression also demonstrate decreased HDAC2 and increased histone acetylation, indicating that epigenetic responses to stress may be similar across species (Covington et al., 2009).

In addition to providing new avenues for understanding the molecules that mediate depression, the study of epigenetic mechanisms has led to a greater understanding of the biological basis for the effects of antidepressants. For example, fluoxetine prevents reductions in global histone acetylation in hippocampus in response to chronic stress, such that levels of histone acetylation in stressed animals exposed to fluoxetine closely resemble those of unstressed animals (Hunter et al., 2009). Imipramine reverses the effects of social defeat stress on dimethylation at histone H3 lysine 9 and histone H3 lysine 27 in the nucleus accumbens. The histone methylation pattern observed after imipramine treatment overlaps considerably with the histone methylation pattern observed in stress-resilient mice, again emphasizing that different methods of overcoming stress appear to utilize similar epigenetic programs (Wilkinson et al., 2009).

The fact that traditional antidepressants alter histone acetylation and methylation has led to investigation of new drugs that directly interfere with the enzymatic mediators of these histone modifications. MS-275, an inhibitor of HDACs, has potent antidepressant properties in multiple behavioral settings in preclinical animal models (Covington et al., 2009; 2011), and it has a similar effect on gene expression patterns as fluoxetine (Covington et al., 2009). SAHA, another HDAC inhibitor, also works as an antidepressant in preclinical animal models (Covington et al., 2009). Further study of compounds like these may lead to improved therapies for mood disorders.

Besides histone modification, DNA methylation plays a role in depression by controlling the neuroendocrine response to stress. Specifically, it regulates the expression of key components of the limbic-hypothalamic-pituitary-adrenal (LHPA) axis, which is activated in states of depression and anxiety. This was first demonstrated in a series of experiments examining the methylation status of the *Nr3c1* gene, which encodes the glucocorticoid receptor. Rat pups raised in a highly nurturing environment had decreased DNA methylation of *Nr3c1*. The reduced methylation status of this gene was accompanied by increased glucocorticoid receptor expression, leading to increased feedback inhibition on the LHPA axis, which relies on glucocorticoid-glucocorticoid receptor interaction to inactivate it after exposure to a stressor. Rat pups raised in a poorly nurturing environment experienced the reverse effect, methylating their *Nr3c1* gene, downregulating *Nr3c1* expression, and hyperactivating their LHPA axis with exposure to subsequent stressors (Weaver et al., 2004). Intriguingly, an investigation of the methylation status of the human glucocorticoid receptor gene (*NR3C1*) in postmortem samples from human suicides found increased methylation of the gene and decreased glucocorticoid receptor expression in suicides with a history of child abuse, as compared with suicides without such experience, suggesting that a similar mechanism may underlie the human LHPA response to stress (McGowan et al., 2009).

DNA methylation also plays a key role in regulating the expression of the corticotropin releasing hormone gene, which encodes CRH, a neuropeptide released by the paraventricular nucleus of the hypothalamus in response to stress. At baseline the promoter region of the *Crh* gene is methylated in mice, but it is demethylated in mice susceptible to the effects of chronic social defeat stress, a model of human depression, whereas mice resistant to the effects of this stressor maintain *Crh* methylation. Predictably, *Crh* expression is increased in the susceptible mice. Increased *Crh* expression in these mice is associated with increased expression of the *Gadd45b* gene, which encodes a demethylating enzyme, and decreased expression of the *Dnmt3b* gene, which encodes a DNA methyltransferase, in the hypothalamus, suggesting that changes in *Crh* methylation status occur in concert with exposure to environmental stressors such as the social defeat paradigm utilized in these experiments (Elliott et al., 2010). Changes in *Crh* methylation appear to be a common response to a variety of chronic stressors, as similar results have been observed in rodents exposed to maternal deprivation and chronic variable stress. Moreover, DNA methylation at this locus is persistent, suggesting that it provides a long-term memory of the experience within the animal's brain (Chen et al., 2012; Sterrenburg et al., 2011).

Just as the LHPA axis is induced by alterations made to DNA methylation, there is evidence that these changes are reversible. For example, *Crh* demethylation in response to stress was attenuated by the antidepressant imipramine in one animal model (Elliott et al., 2010). Treatment with the methyl-donor methionine reversed the effects of remote maternal deprivation stress on *Nr3c1* gene expression in adult animals, suggesting that changes in DNA methylation, far from being permanent, are amenable to interventions made throughout an animal's lifetime (Weaver et al., 2005).

SCHIZOPHRENIA

Interest in epigenetics as a source of pathology in schizophrenia stems from observations in the early part of the 20th century suggesting a link between diet and the development of schizophrenia. First, children born to women who became pregnant during famines in China and the Netherlands were found to be at higher risk for developing schizophrenia later in life (St. Clair et al., 2005; Susser et al., 1996). These children were also at higher risk for the development of neural tube defects, which other studies have linked to folic acid deficiency. Thus, it has been hypothesized that low serum folate levels during pregnancy also contribute to an increased risk for developing schizophrenia (Susser et al., 1996).

As described in the preceding, folic acid provides a dietary source of methyl groups that can be used to methylate DNA. Thus, one reason why gestational folate status may be an important risk factor for the development of schizophrenia could be that DNA methylation patterns are initially established during pregnancy in humans (Morgan et al., 2005). Malnutrition leading to folic acid deficiency may interfere with the establishment of a normal pattern of DNA methylation during prenatal development, or so some have argued. In support of this, studies in rodents demonstrate that altering the amount of folic acid available to pregnant dams affects the degree of DNA methylation that is observed in their pups (Waterland, 2006).

In light of this argument, numerous attempts have been made to link DNA methylation to the pathogenesis of schizophrenia, but these have met only limited degrees of success. With respect to DNA methylation, initial candidate gene approaches identified methylation changes correlating with disease (schizophrenia) state for the genes *RELN*, *COMT*, and *SOX10*. However, the findings related to *RELN* and *COMT* were not replicated in independent experiments, and further studies have not reevaluated the *SOX10* gene (Akbarian, 2010). A single study examining methylation changes in CpG islands upstream of 50 candidate genes for schizophrenia failed to identify any consistent differences in DNA methylation between samples from patients with schizophrenia and controls (Siegmund et al., 2007). To date, only one unbiased screen of DNA methylation in schizophrenia has been performed. This experiment succeeded in identifying approximately 100 loci that were differentially methylated between schizophrenics and controls in prefrontal cortex. Bioinformatic analysis of the genes identified indicated that they tended to cluster in functional categories thought to be relevant to schizophrenia, including GABAergic signaling. However, follow-up validation of gene expression changes identified in the initial screen verified only 5 of 12 (40%) of the candidate genes that were tested, suggesting that these results must be interpreted cautiously (Mill et al., 2008).

Histone modifications have also been examined in schizophrenia. Akbarian et al. (2005) examined covalent histone modifications in postmortem prefrontal cortex tissue from schizophrenics and found evidence of increased levels of histone H3 arginine 17 methylation in a subgroup of patients with schizophrenia with reduced metabolic gene expression. Another subgroup, this one with increased expression of the ornithine aminotransferase (*OAT*) gene, was found to have increased levels of histone H3 serine 10 phosphorylation and histone H3 lysine 17 acetylation. Meanwhile, Huang et al. found a correlation between reduced *GAD1* gene expression and decreased trimethylation at histone H3 lysine 4 (H3K4me3), a mark for open chromatin, in postmortem samples from women with schizophrenia, but not from men (Huang et al., 2007). Further study will be required to determine whether these results are reproducible. In addition, the significance of abnormal histone modification to the pathogenesis of schizophrenia remains to be determined.

Expression profiling of micro-RNAs from postmortem brain tissue from schizophrenics and case controls has implicated a list of 14 different miRNAs in the pathogenesis of the disease. However, with the exception of miR-132, which was identified in two studies by separate researchers, there has been no independent validation of the other targets. miR-132 is attractive to scientists since it targets transcripts encoding BDNF and NMDA receptor subunits (Mellios and Sur, 2012). More recently, a consortium of scientists reported the results of a large genome-wide association study (GWAS) that found evidence of linkage to an SNP within the miR-137 transcript. Although it is a single report, the strength of the data is related to the large cohort of samples analyzed (over 20,000) and the finding that four of the seven other loci identified are predicted targets of miR-137 (Ripke et al., 2011).

RETT SYNDROME

Evidence for the role of epigenetic processes in psychiatric disease also comes from genetic disorders with prominent psychiatric phenotypes. Some of these disorders are caused by mutations in genes encoding components of epigenetic systems (Table 7.1). For example, mutations in *MECP2*, the X-linked gene that encodes the methyl-DNA binding protein MECP2, cause Rett syndrome (RTT) (Amir et al., 1999). The clinical features of Rett syndrome are silent during the first 6 to 18 months of life, at which point children undergo a period of developmental regression and lose milestones they had previously attained, especially language. Children with RTT develop microcephaly, growth restriction, hypotonia, and ataxia. Features of autonomic nervous system dysfunction appear, including abnormal breathing patterns (hyperventilation and apnea are common), and vasomotor instability. Movement disorders are characteristic. As young children, patients with RTT have upper extremity stereotypies, such as hand wringing. Later in life, spasticity, dystonia, and parkinsonian features appear. Behavioral features also figure prominently in RTT. Autistic features, including minimal to absent language skills, repetitive behaviors, and social withdrawal, are a core component of the RTT phenotype. Low mood, inconsolable crying, anxiety, and periodic screaming in fits of apparent terror are observed in RTT as well (Chahrour and Zoghbi, 2007; Samaco and Neul, 2011).

Besides RTT, mutations in *MECP2* cause a host of other neuropsychiatric phenotypes. For example, some *MECP2* mutations cause autism alone. Other *MECP2* mutations, particularly in the 3' UTR of the gene, have been linked to juvenile onset schizophrenia, psychosis, alcoholism, phobia, and attention-deficit/hyperactivity disorder (ADHD) (Cohen et al., 2002; Shibayama et al., 2004). The A140V *MECP2* mutation causes the PPM-X syndrome, which is characterized by intellectual disability, manic-depressive psychosis, pyramidal tract signs, parkinsonism, and macroorchidism (Klauck et al., 2002). *MECP2* duplication causes a unique syndrome, which in part is characterized by autistic features and mood disorder (Van Esch, 2012).

The phenotypic variability associated with mutations in *MECP2* is in part due to its physical location on the X chromosome, which makes it subject to X chromosome inactivation (XCI). Thus women who carry two X chromosomes may

TABLE 7.1. Syndromes with prominent neuropsychiatric phenotypes that are linked to mutations in genes regulating epigenetic processes

DISEASE	GENE(S)	NEUROPSYCHIATRIC PHENOTYPE(S)
Rett syndrome	*MECP2*	Anxiety, autism, childhood-onset schizophrenia
Rubinstein-Taybi syndrome	*CREBBP, EP300*	Hyperactivity, mood lability, obsessive behaviors, autistic features
α-thalassemia/mental retardation syndrome, X-linked	*ATRX*	Autistic features, mood lability, emotional outbursts, self-injurious and obsessive behaviors
Angelman syndrome	*UBE3A*	Autistic features
Prader-Willi syndrome	Unknown. Linked to paternally expressed genes at 15q11-q13	Autistic features
Fragile X syndrome	*FMR1*	Autistic features, attention deficit/hyperactivity
Kabuki syndrome	*MLL2, KDM6A*	Autistic features, aggressive/oppositional behavior, hyperactive/impulsive behavior, anxiety, and obsessions

manifest partial features of RTT depending on XCI patterns. Favorable XCI, which occurs when a majority of cells express the wild type (WT) *MECP2* allele instead of the mutated *MECP2* allele, accounts for the partial neuropsychiatric phenotypes in females. Males with severe *MECP2* mutations suffer from early lethality because they have only one X chromosome. However, males with mild *MECP2* mutations may develop less severe disease manifesting as a neuropsychiatric disorder compatible with life (Chahrour and Zoghbi, 2007).

How mutations in *MECP2* cause RTT has been an area of active investigation for more than a decade now. Mouse models of RTT have contributed a great deal to this effort. Both the complete absence of MeCP2 and the replacement of endogenous MeCP2 with a truncated, mutant protein recapitulate the features of RTT in mice (Chen et al., 2001; Guy et al., 2001; Shahbazian et al., 2002). Neuron-specific *Mecp2* knockout mice, which lack MECP2 throughout the brain, are indistinguishable from animals that lack MECP2 throughout their entire body (Chen et al., 2001; Gemelli et al., 2006). Mice have also been generated that lack MECP2 specifically in forebrain neurons, aminergic neurons, hypothalamic neurons, and astrocytes (Ballas et al., 2009; Chao et al., 2010; Fyffe et al., 2008; Gemelli et al., 2006; Maezawa et al., 2009; Samaco et al., 2009). These animals display varying degrees of pathology and recapitulate one or more aspects of the RTT phenotype. Deletion of *MeCP2* in adult mice also causes RTT, indicating a lifelong need for the MeCP2 protein to maintain normal brain function (McGraw et al., 2011). Importantly, expressing wild type MECP2 in animals lacking a copy of the gene (MECP2 "null" animals) rescues the RTT phenotype (Guy et al., 2007; Robinson et al., 2012b), and expression of MeCP2 in either astrocytes or in microglia prolongs breathing, motor function, and survival (Derecki et al., 2012; Lioy et al., 2011) suggesting that therapeutic approaches when discovered might hold some promise for treating the disease in the future (Samaco and Neul, 2011).

Currently our understanding of the mechanism by which *MECP2* mutation produces the RTT phenotype is limited and incomplete. Initially, researchers focused on identifying the genes regulated by MeCP2, theorizing that a complete description of this complement of genes would readily explain aspects of the RTT phenotype. The *Bdnf* gene, encoding the neuropeptide brain-derived neurotrophic factor (BDNF), is one such MeCP2 target gene. Reduction of endogenous *Bdnf* levels via genetic engineering exacerbates the phenotype of *Mecp2* null mice, whereas genetic overexpression of *Bdnf* extends the life span of *Mecp2* null mice (Chang et al., 2006), and drugs that enhance BDNF levels improve synaptic function in neurons (Ogier et al., 2007) and improve disease symptoms in mice (Tropea et al., 2009).

Another MECP2 target is *Crh*, the gene encoding corticotropin releasing hormone (CRH). Released in response to stress, CRH elicits anxiety-like behavior in animals and induces the release of adrenal corticosteroids (cortisol in humans, corticosterone in mice). Mice expressing a truncated version of MECP2 have enhanced *Crh* expression and increased anxiety-like behavior (McGill et al., 2006). Disruption of *Crh* signaling via genetic downregulation of *Crh* expression or pharmacologic blockade of CRH signaling was sufficient to reverse anxiety-like behavior in *MECP2* transgenic mice. Thus *Crh*, like *Bdnf*, is a MECP2 target gene that can be modified to ameliorate RTT phenotypes (Samaco et al., 2012).

Classically, MECP2 has been thought of as a transcriptional repressor, binding specific promoters and recruiting corepressor proteins to shut down gene expression. However, recent data have challenged this view. For example, genome-wide expression profiling studies have revealed that many genes are downregulated in absence of MeCP2 and upregulated when it is overexpressed. In fact, more genes are activated by MeCP2 than are repressed, at least in the hypothalamus (Chahrour et al., 2008; Yasui et al., 2007). Perhaps more surprisingly, MeCP2 is present in neurons at concentrations akin to those of histone proteins, and binds chromatin every two nucleosomes. In the absence of MeCP2, more histone protein H1 is bound to chromatin, suggesting that one of MeCP2's roles is to function as a chromatin remodeling protein (Skene et al., 2010).

Finally, evidence is accumulating in favor of a role for MECP2 in activity dependent gene regulation and experience-dependent synaptic plasticity. Some of this evidence comes from studies of addiction in rodents (see "Addiction" section in this chapter). Neuronal activity has been shown to elicit MECP2 phosphorylation, and early experiments suggested that this posttranslational modification changed the affinity of MECP2 for DNA at specific sites, including the *Bdnf* promoter (Chen et al., 2003; Martinowich et al., 2003). However, a more recent genome-wide evaluation of MeCP2 binding sites did not replicate this finding (Cohen et al., 2011). One view is that MeCP2 phosphorylation changes local chromatin structure, although this remains untested. Mice genetically engineered to express a phosphorylation deficient form of MeCP2 display different phenotypes depending on the mutated sites. Mutation of S421A causes lack of habituation to familiar objects and mice, and seems to render mice less able to distinguish between the novel and the familiar (Cohen et al., 2011). In contrast, mutations of S421A/S424A lead to several phenotypes reminiscent of the features observed in mice that overexpress MeCP2 (Li et al., 2011).

ANGELMAN SYNDROME AND PRADER-WILLI SYNDROME

Imprinting errors at chromosome 15q11-q13 cause two childhood neurological disorders, Angelman syndrome (AS) and Prader-Willi syndrome (PWS). Angelman syndrome is characterized by a constellation of features including intellectual disability, epilepsy, and ataxia. Patients with AS have unique behavioral features that set them apart from other neurodevelopmental disorders. They display frequent outbursts of laughter, sometimes out of context. They appear happy, and often smile. They have some autistic features, most prominently poor or absent language and stereotypic hand-flapping movements, but unlike children with autism, they are sociable and many enjoy interacting with others. Additional behavioral features include poor sleep, restlessness, short attention span, and hyperactivity (Mabb et al., 2011; Williams, 2010).

AS is caused by failure to express the maternal allele of the gene *UBE3A*. For the vast majority of patients with AS (75%), this is a result of a maternally inherited deletion of the 15q11-q13 region that includes the *UBE3A* gene. Other patients (15%) inherit a more conventional missense or nonsense mutation that renders the maternal copy of the *UBE3A* gene nonfunctional. Fewer patients (7%) have paternal uniparental disomy and inherit both copies of *UBE3A* from their fathers. Finally, a minority of patients with AS (3%) inherit a microdeletion that eliminates the maternal copy of the AS imprinting control region (ICR), which causes the maternally inherited allele to function as a paternally inherited allele (Mabb et al., 2011) (Fig. 7.6).

Intense research has focused on uncovering the molecular mechanisms that govern imprinting at chromosome 15q11-q13, the site crucial to the development of AS and PWS. The locus containing the *UBE3A* gene can be transcribed in the forward direction, which produces the UBE3A protein, and in the reverse direction, which produces a non-coding antisense transcript, *UBE3A-ATS*. DNA methylation at the AS ICR on the maternal allele blocks transcription of *UBE3A-ATS*. As a result, *UBE3A* is transcribed without interference. However, DNA methylation is lacking on the AS ICR of the paternal allele. As a result the *UBE3A-ATS* transcript is produced, which blocks expression of the *UBE3A* gene from that allele (Mabb et al., 2011). Recent studies using genetic manipulations in mice suggest that *Ube3a-ATS* is an atypical non-polyadenylated RNA Polymerase II transcript that represses *Ube3a* on the paternal allele (Meng et al., 2012).

The phenotype of PWS differs significantly from AS. Infants with PWS typically come to clinical attention because of hypotonia, poor suck, and resultant failure to gain weight. Later in childhood, children with PWS develop hyperphagia and are at risk to develop morbid obesity if access to food is not carefully controlled. Hypogonadism is another characteristic feature of PWS, and both males and females may have small genitalia.

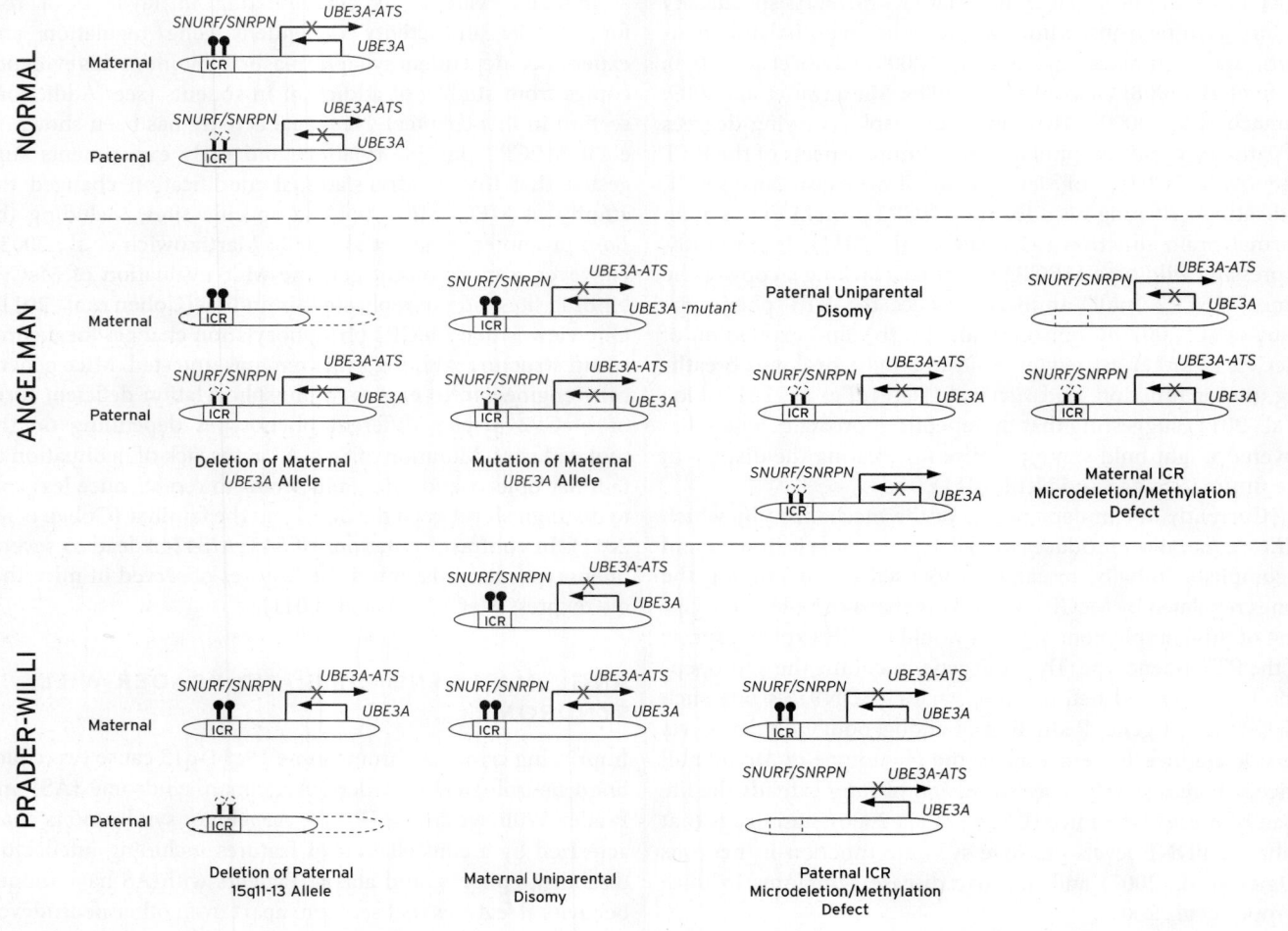

Figure 7.6 *Causes of Angelman syndrome and Prader-Willi syndrome. Angelman syndrome (AS) and Prader-Willi syndrome (PWS) are caused by mutations and imprinting errors at chromosome 15q11-q13. Normally, UBE3A is expressed from the maternal chromosome, while a group of genes, including SNURF-SNRPN, are expressed from the paternal chromosome. The 3' terminus of the SNURF-SNRPN gene cluster contains UBE3A-ATS, an antisense transcript that transcriptionally silences UBE3A. Expression of UBE3A-ATS, SNURF-SNRPN, and the other paternally expressed genes is regulated by the differential methylation of the AS imprinting control region (not shown) and the PWS imprinting control region (labeled as "ICR" in the figure). Differential methylation of the AS-ICR occurs transiently during embryonic development and is not shown here. DNA methylation at the PWS-ICR is represented by shaded lollipops, whereas unmethylated DNA at this site is indicated by dotted lollipops. AS is caused by mutations and epimutations that result in decreased expression of the maternal copy of UBE3A or the function of its protein product, UBE3A. PWS is caused by mutations and epimutations that disrupt the expression of paternally imprinted genes in the SNURF-SNRPN gene cluster at chromosome 15q11-q13 (see text for more details).*

Endocrine dysfunction is common, and central deficiencies of growth hormone, adrenal hormones, and thyroid hormone may coexist. Intellectual disability in the moderate to severe range occurs as a rule for PWS. Behavioral features of the syndrome include autism, present in 20% of patients, psychosis, present in 10%–20% of adult patients with PWS, hyperactivity, and compulsive behaviors (Cassidy et al., 2012; Whittington and Holland, 2010).

In contrast to AS, the most common cause of PWS (65%–75%) is deletion of the paternal allele containing the 15q11-q13 region. Another 20%–30% of PWS cases are caused by maternal uniparental disomy for this chromosomal region. A minority of cases (1%–3%) are due to microdeletions of the paternal copy of the PWS imprinting control region (ICR) or defects in DNA methylation at this site (Buiting, 2010). The PWS ICR is located just upstream of the *SNURF-SNRPN* gene and is contiguous with a CpG island located within the proximal 5' portion of this gene. On the paternal allele of the 15q11-q13 region, the PWS ICR is unmethylated, whereas it is methylated on the maternal allele. Again, this leads to *UBE3A-ATS* transcription and blockade of *UBE3A* expression. In addition to *UBE3A-ATS*, the unmethylated PWS ICR on the paternal allele permits expression of a number of other genes that are not expressed from the maternal allele. These include the genes *MKRN3*, *MAGEL2*, *NECDIN*, *C15orf2*, *SNURF-SNRPN*, and multiple genes encoding small nucleolar RNAs (snoRNAs). Rare patients with deletions of one of these snoRNA genes, *SNORD116*, display most features of PWS, suggesting that this gene plays a major role in the PWS phenotype. However, the exact contribution of other genes in this cluster remains to be determined (Buiting, 2010; Cassidy et al., 2012).

FRAGILE X SYNDROME

Fragile X syndrome (FXS) is the most common cause of X-linked intellectual disability (ID) and the second most common cause of ID overall after Trisomy 21. In addition to ID, features of FXS include dysmorphic features such as elongated faces, enlarged ears, a prominent jaw, and macroorchidism. Psychiatric features figure prominently in the FXS phenotype and include autistic spectrum disorders (autism and pervasive developmental disorder), which are present in a third of people with FXS. The vast majority (90%–95%) of people with FXS have symptoms of inattentiveness and hyperactivity. Anxiety may be crippling in FXS, and emotional lability can lead to aggressive outbursts and stereotyped behaviors (Tranfaglia, 2011).

FXS is caused by expansion of a cytosine-guanine-guanine (CGG) nucleotide triplet repeat in the 5' untranslated region of the *FMR1* gene, located within the gene's first exon. Normal alleles of *FMR1* contain less than 45 repeats, whereas the presence of more than 200 repeats causes FXS. Alleles containing 55–200 repeats are termed "premutations," and are prone to spontaneous expansion in subsequent generations. Premutation alleles cause an adult onset progressive neurodegenerative disease, Fragile X associated tremor ataxia syndrome (FXTAS), further discussion of which is outside the scope of this chapter (Penagarikano et al., 2007).

Disease-causing *FMR1* alleles are hypermethylated within the triplet repeat and also within a CpG island located in the *FMR1* promoter. The hypermethylated, disease-causing alleles are transcriptionally silenced and fail to express the *FMR1* product, the fragile X mental retardation protein (FMRP). In addition to the direct effects of DNA methylation on silencing *FMR1*, local changes in covalent histone modifications have been identified at the expanded *FMR1* allele. Histone H3 and H4 acetylation is reduced, and trimethylated histone H3 lysine 9 and trimethylated histone H3 lysine 27 is increased at the disease-causing allele, whereas the normal, unexpanded allele has the opposite histone marks. This indicates that in addition to DNA methylation, local chromatin modifications at the expanded allele contributes to *FMR1* silencing by maintaining a condensed and transcriptionally restrictive structure (Penagarikano et al., 2007). Additionally, the 5' UTR of *FMR1* is transcribed in both sense and antisense directions, which makes it conceivable that it generates double stranded RNA capable of activating the RNA-induced transcriptional silencing (RITS) pathway. Thus, some investigators have put forward the hypothesis that RNA interference may play a role in *FMR1* silencing. However, this remains unproven (Kumari and Usdin, 2009).

KABUKI SYNDROME

Kabuki syndrome is a neurodevelopmental disorder with characteristic dysmorphologic features, including high arched eyebrows, elongated palpebral fissures, everted lower eyelids, large, prominent ears, a depressed nasal tip, various skeletal abnormalities, and fetal fingertip pads. Approximately 85% of patients with Kabuki syndrome have developmental delay and intellectual disability. In addition, autistic features are prominent in a subset of patients with Kabuki syndrome, and some patients have other psychiatric features, including aggressive/oppositional behavior, hyperactive/impulsive behavior, anxiety, and obsessions (Adam and Hudgins, 2005; Ho and Eaves, 1997). Recently, Kabuki syndrome was linked to epigenetic phenomena when the gene *MLL2* was identified as the cause of 56%–76% of cases. *MLL2* encodes a histone lysine methyltransferase and functions as a trithorax-group protein, preferentially mediating trimethyl modification of histone H3 lysine 4 (Ng et al., 2010). Further studies of Kabuki patients lacking *MLL2* mutation identified mutations in *KDM6A*, a gene encoding an MLL2 interacting protein, as causative of some cases of Kabuki syndrome. Like MLL2, KDM6A is a trithorax-group protein. It functions as a histone demethylase that removes mono-, di-, and trimethylation marks from histone H3 lysine 27 residues, thereby activating gene transcription. KDM6A also interacts with the SWI/SNF protein, Brg1, and participates in repositioning nucleosomes to change chromatin structure (Lederer et al., 2012). At this time it is not known whether or not there is a mechanistic link between *MLL2*, *KDM6A*, and the neuropsychiatric features of Kabuki syndrome.

RUBINSTEIN-TAYBI SYNDROME (RSTS)

Errors in covalent histone modification also have been linked to the pathogenesis of Rubinstein-Taybi syndrome (abbreviated

RSTS). Patients with RSTS have characteristic facial features including microcephaly, down-slanted palpebral fissures, a beaked nose, micrognathia, a high-arched palate, and dental anomalies. Broad thumbs and great toes also help identify people with RSTS. Intellectual disability is a prominent feature of RSTS, and other neuropsychiatric pathology including hyperactivity, mood lability, obsessive-compulsive behaviors, and autistic features also occur frequently in RSTS (Roelfsema and Peters, 2007; Verhoeven et al., 2010).

Mutations in the gene *CREBBP*, encoding cAMP-response element binding (CREB) binding protein (CBP) account for about 60% of RSTS cases, and mutations in a related gene, *EP300*, encoding the E1A binding protein p300, account for another 3% of RSTS cases. The cause of the remaining 45% of cases is unknown but could be due to further genetic heterogeneity, somatic mosaicism for mutations in *CREBBP* and *EP300*, or mutations in distant regulatory regions of *CREBBP* and *EP300*. Both CBP and p300 are histone acetyltransferases, and mutations that disrupt the acetyltransferase domain of CBP are sufficient to cause RSTS, illustrating the relevance of histone acetylation to human health (Roelfsema and Peters, 2007) .

A variety of genetically engineered mouse models of RSTS have been produced, including *Crebbp* knockouts, forebrain specific *Crebbp* knockouts, and transgenic mice overexpressing an inactive form of *Crebbp*. All of these animals have impaired long-term memory, a cardinal feature of RSTS. Molecular analysis indicates that these mice have reduced histone acetylation and altered expression of immediate early genes in the hippocampus, a brain region crucial to the consolidation of long-term memories. Importantly, histone deacetylase inhibitors reverse the memory phenotype, even in adult mice, suggesting that elements of the RSTS phenotype may be overcome by treatments that modulate the same epigenetic system that is dysregulated by disease-causing mutations in *CREBBP* and *EP300*. Further investigations focusing on how disrupted histone acetylation accounts for the behavioral features of RSTS will provide an avenue to discover how alteration of epigenetic processes causes psychiatric disease (Roelfsema and Peters, 2007; Valor et al., 2011).

X-LINKED ALPHA THALASSEMIA MENTAL RETARDATION SYNDROME (ATRX)

X-linked alpha thalassemia mental retardation syndrome (ATRX) is a rare disorder with characteristic physical features including short nose, anteverted nares and epicanthal folds, microcephaly, hypotonia, and abnormal genitalia. Some patients develop alpha thalassemia. Patients with ATRX have moderate to severe intellectual disability with prominent language impairment. The behavioral phenotype of ATRX includes autistic features, rapid mood swings from manic to depressive states, and repetitive activity (Gibbons, 2006).

ATRX is caused by mutations in the *ATRX* gene, which encodes a SWI/SNF family helicase/ATPase. The ATRX protein contains a domain with homology to DNMT3 that permits DNA binding and a domain that permits binding to trimethylated histone H3 lysine 9. ATRX interacts with other proteins that are key epigenetic regulators, including MeCP2.

Recently, a macromolecular protein complex containing ATRX, MeCP2, and other proteins was found to regulate the expression of imprinted genes in the brain. *ATRX* loss of function disrupted expression of these imprinted genes. For one of these genes, *H19*, inappropriate overexpression was associated with increased acetylation at histone H3 and H4 and decreased trimethylation at histone H4 lysine 20 and histone H3 lysine 9, changes associated with a more open chromatin configuration (Kernohan et al., 2010). In addition to gene expression changes, *ATRX* loss of function also leads to the loss of forebrain neurons in mice. As with the other neurodevelopmental disorders described, research has yet to bridge the gap between the dysregulation of epigenetic gene expression and the neuropsychiatric phenotype of ATRX (Gibbons, 2006).

CONCLUSION

Although epigenetics as a field of study is young, the discipline of psychiatric epigenetics can genuinely be described as in its infancy. Fundamental questions regarding the exact role of epigenetic processes in the development and pathogenesis of psychiatric disease remain unanswered. How are global and local patterns of epigenetic modification different in patients with psychiatric diseases as compared to the general population? Are epigenomic changes the cause or the consequence of psychiatric disease? Are any psychiatric diseases epigenetically inherited? Do environmental effects on the epigenome contribute to the development of psychiatric disease? Can treatments that modify epigenetic marks be used to successfully treat psychiatric conditions successfully? Although there are many unknowns, one thing is certain: As our understanding of the basic mechanisms controlling the establishment, maintenance, interpretation, and modification of the epigenetic code increases, so too will our ability to apply this knowledge to answer these and other questions.

DISCLOSURES

Dr. Zoghbi serves on the advisory board of the Mcknight Neuroscience fund and is a senior editor for *eLife*. She receives compensation from both. She is also member of the jury for the Vilcek Prize, Gruber Genetics Prize, and Janssen Prize (and receives compensation), and for the Lasker Prize (no compensation). She receives grant support from HHMI, NIH, IRSF, and RSRT. Dr. Zoghbi holds a patent for MECP2 Rett testing.

Dr. McGill has no conflicts of interest to disclose.

REFERENCES

Adam, M.P., and Hudgins, L. (2005). Kabuki syndrome: a review. *Clin. Genet.* 67:209–219.

Akbarian, S. (2010). The molecular pathology of schizophrenia—focus on histone and DNA modifications. *Brain Res. Bull.* 83:103–107.

Akbarian, S., Ruehl, M.G., et al. (2005). Chromatin alterations associated with down-regulated metabolic gene expression in the prefrontal cortex of subjects with schizophrenia. *Arch. Gen. Psychiatry* 62:829–840.

Amir, R.E., Van den Veyver, I.B., et al. (1999). Rett syndrome is caused by mutations in X-linked MECP2, encoding methyl-CpG-binding protein 2. *Nat. Genet.* 23:185–188.

Ballas, N., Lioy, D.T., et al. (2009). Non-cell autonomous influence of MeCP2-deficient glia on neuronal dendritic morphology. *Nat. Neurosci.* 12:311–317.

Barlow, D.P. (2011). Genomic imprinting: a mammalian epigenetic discovery model. *Annu. Rev. Genet.* 45:379–403.

Barreto, G., Schäfer, A., et al. (2007). Gadd45a promotes epigenetic gene activation by repair-mediated DNA demethylation. *Nature* 445:671–675.

Bartolomei, M.S., and Ferguson-Smith, A.C. (2011). Mammalian genomic imprinting. In Sassone-Corsi, P., Fuller, M.T., and Braun, R., eds. Germ Cells: A Subject Collection from Cold Spring Harbor Perspectives in Biology. Cold Spring Harb Perspect. Biol. 3. Cold Spring Harbor, NY: Cold Spring Harbor Laboratory Press, pp. 167–184.

Buiting, K. (2010). Prader-Willi syndrome and Angelman syndrome. *Am. J. Med. Genet. C Semin. Med. Genet.* 154C:365–376.

Cam, H.P. (2010). Roles of RNAi in chromatin regulation and epigenetic inheritance. *Epigenomics* 2:613–626.

Cassidy, S.B., Schwartz, S., et al. (2012). Prader-Willi syndrome. *Genet. Med.* 14:10–26.

Chahrour, M., Jung, S.Y., et al. (2008). MeCP2, a key contributor to neurological disease, activates and represses transcription. *Science* 320:1224–1229.

Chahrour, M., and Zoghbi, H.Y. (2007). The story of Rett syndrome: from clinic to neurobiology. *Neuron* 56:422–437.

Chang, Q., Khare, G., et al. (2006). The disease progression of Mecp2 mutant mice is affected by the level of BDNF expression. *Neuron* 49:341–348.

Chao, H.-T., Chen, H., et al. (2010). Dysfunction in GABA signalling mediates autism-like stereotypies and Rett syndrome phenotypes. *Nature* 468:263–269.

Chédin, F. (2011). The DNMT3 family of mammalian de novo DNA methyltransferases. *Prog. Mol. Biol. Transl. Sci.* 101:255–285.

Chen, J., Evans, A.N., et al. (2012). Maternal deprivation in rats is associated with corticotrophin-releasing hormone (CRH) promoter hypomethylation and enhances CRH transcriptional responses to stress in adulthood. *J. Neuroendocrinol.* 24:1055–1064.

Chen, R.Z., Akbarian, S., et al. (2001). Deficiency of methyl-CpG binding protein-2 in CNS neurons results in a Rett-like phenotype in mice. *Nat. Genet.* 27:327–331.

Chen, W.G., Chang, Q., et al. (2003). Derepression of BDNF transcription involves calcium-dependent phosphorylation of MeCP2. *Science* 302:885–889.

Choi, J.K., and Howe, L.J. (2009). Histone acetylation: truth of consequences? *Biochem. Cell Biol.* 87:139–150.

Cohen, D., Lazar, G., et al. (2002). MECP2 mutation in a boy with language disorder and schizophrenia. *Am. J. Psychiatry* 159:148–149.

Cohen, S., Gabel, H.W., et al. (2011). Genome-wide activity-dependent MeCP2 phosphorylation regulates nervous system development and function. *Neuron* 72:72–85.

Costa, F.F. (2010). Non-coding RNAs: meet thy masters. *Bioessays* 32:599–608.

Covington, H.E., 3rd, Maze, I., et al. (2009). Antidepressant actions of histone deacetylase inhibitors. *J. Neurosci.* 29:11451–11460.

Covington, H.E., 3rd, Vialou, V.F., et al. (2011). Hippocampal-dependent antidepressant-like activity of histone deacetylase inhibition. *Neurosci. Lett.* 493:122–126.

Day, J.J., and Sweatt, J.D. (2010). DNA methylation and memory formation. *Nat. Neurosci.* 13:1319–1323.

Day, J.J., and Sweatt, J.D. (2011). Epigenetic mechanisms in cognition. *Neuron* 70:813–829.

Defossez, P.-A., and Stancheva, I. (2011). Biological functions of methyl-CpG-binding proteins. *Prog. Mol. Biol. Transl. Sci.* 101:377–398.

Derecki, N.C., Cronk, J.C., et al. (2012). Wild-type microglia arrest pathology in a mouse model of Rett syndrome. *Nature* 484:105–109.

Elliott, E., Ezra-Nevo, G., et al. (2010). Resilience to social stress coincides with functional DNA methylation of the Crf gene in adult mice. *Nat. Neurosci.* 13:1351–1353.

Feng, J., Zhou, Y., et al. (2010). Dnmt1 and Dnmt3a maintain DNA methylation and regulate synaptic function in adult forebrain neurons. *Nat. Neurosci.* 13:423–430.

Feng, S., Jacobsen, S.E., et al. (2010). Epigenetic reprogramming in plant and animal development. *Science* 330:622–627.

Fussner, E., Ching, R.W., et al. (2011). Living without 30nm chromatin fibers. *Trends Biochem. Sci.* 36:1–6.

Fyffe, S.L., Neul, J.L., et al. (2008). Deletion of Mecp2 in Sim1-expressing neurons reveals a critical role for MeCP2 in feeding behavior, aggression, and the response to stress. *Neuron* 59:947–958.

Gemelli, T., Berton, O., et al. (2006). Postnatal loss of methyl-CpG binding protein 2 in the forebrain is sufficient to mediate behavioral aspects of Rett syndrome in mice. *Biol. Psychiatry* 59:468–476.

Gibbons, R. (2006). Alpha thalassaemia-mental retardation, X linked. *Orphane. J. Rare Dis.* 1:15.

Goldberg, A.D., Allis, C.D., et al. (2007). Epigenetics: a landscape takes shape. *Cell* 128:635–638.

Goll, M.G., and Bestor, T.H. (2005). Eukaryotic cytosin methyltransferases. *Annu. Rev. Biochem.* 74:481–514.

Greer, E.L., and Shi, Y. (2012). Histone methylation: a dynamic mark in health, disease and inheritance. *Nat. Rev. Genet.* 13:343–357.

Guo, J.U., Su, Y., et al. (2011). Hydroxylation of 5-methylcytosine by TET1 promotes active DNA demethylation in the adult brain. *Cell* 145:423–434.

Guy, J., Gan, J., et al. (2007). Reversal of neurological defects in a mouse model of Rett syndrome. *Science* 315:1143–1147.

Guy, J., Hendrich, B., et al. (2001). A mouse Mecp2-null mutation causes neurological symptoms that mimic Rett syndrome. *Nat. Genet.* 27:322–326.

Ho, H.H., and Eaves, L.C. (1997). Kabuki make-up (Niikawa-Kuroki) syndrome: cognitive abilities and autistic features. *Dev. Med. Child Neurol.* 39:487–490.

Hollander, J.A., Im, H.-I., et al. (2010). Striatal microRNA controls cocaine intake through CREB signalling. *Nature* 466:197–202.

Huang, H.-S., Matevossian, A., et al. (2007). Prefrontal dysfunction in schizophrenia involves mixed-lineage leukemia 1-regulated histone methylation at GABAergic gene promoters. *J. Neurosci.* 27:11254–11262.

Hunter, R.G., McCarthy, K.J., et al. (2009). Regulation of hippocampal H3 histone methylation by acute and chronic stress. *Proc. Natl. Acad. Sci. USA* 106:20912–20917.

Illingworth, R.S., and Bird, A.P. (2009). CpG islands—"a rough guide." *FEBS Lett.* 583:1713–1720.

Im, H.-I., Hollander, J.A., et al. (2010). MeCP2 controls BDNF expression and cocaine intake through homeostatic interactions with microRNA-212. *Nat. Neurosci.* 13:1120–1127.

Jin, S.-G., Guo, C., et al. (2008). GADD45A does not promote DNA demethylation. *PLoS Genet.* 4:e1000013.

Kernohan, K.D., Jiang, Y., et al. (2010). ATRX partners with cohesin and MeCP2 and contributes to developmental silencing of imprinted genes in the brain. *Dev. Cell* 18:191–202.

Klauck, S.M., Lindsay, S., et al. (2002). A mutation hot spot for nonspecific X-linked mental retardation in the MECP2 gene causes the PPM-X syndrome. *Am. J. Hum. Genet.* 70:1034–1037.

Koerner, M.V., and Barlow, D.P. (2010). Genomic imprinting—an epigenetic gene-regulatory model. *Curr. Opin. Genet. Dev.* 20:164–170.

Kumar, A., Choi, K.-H., et al. (2005). Chromatin remodeling is a key mechanism underlying cocaine-induced plasticity in striatum. *Neuron* 48:303–314.

Kumari, D., and Usdin, K. (2009). Chromatin remodeling in the noncoding repeat expansion diseases. *J. Biol. Chem.* 284:7413–7417.

LaPlant, Q., Vialou, V., et al. (2010). Dnmt3a regulates emotional behavior and spine plasticity in the nucleus accumbens. *Nat. Neurosci.* 13:1137–1143.

Lederer, D., Grisart, B., et al. (2012). Deletion of KDM6A, a histone demethylase interacting with MLL2, in three patients with Kabuki syndrome. *Am. J. Hum. Genet.* 90:119–124.

Levine, A.A., Guan, Z., et al. (2005). CREB-binding protein controls response to cocaine by acetylating histones at the fosB promoter in the mouse striatum. *Proc. Natl. Acad. Sci. USA* 102:19186–19191.

Levine, A., Huang, Y., et al. (2011). Molecular mechanism for a gateway drug: epigenetic changes initiated by nicotine prime gene expression by cocaine. *Sci. Transl. Med.* 3:107ra109.

Lewis, J.D., Meehan, R.R., et al. (1992). Purification, sequence, and cellular localization of a novel chromosomal protein that binds to methylated DNA. *Cell* 69:905–914.

Li, E., Bestor, T.H., et al. (1992). Targeted mutation of the DNA methyltransferase gene results in embryonic lethality. *Cell* 69:915–926.

Li, H., Zhong, X., et al. (2011). Loss of activity-induced phosphorylation of MeCP2 enhances synaptogenesis, LTP and spatial memory. *Nat. Neurosci.* 14:1001–1008.

Li, Y., and O'Neill, C. (2012). Persistence of cytosine methylation of DNA following fertilisation in the mouse. *PLoS ONE* 7:e30687.

Lioy, D.T., Garg, S.K., et al. (2011). A role for glia in the progression of Rett's syndrome. *Nature* 475:497–500.

Ma, D.K., Jang, M.-H., et al. (2009). Neuronal activity-induced Gadd45b promotes epigenetic DNA demethylation and adult neurogenesis. *Science* 323:1074–1077.

Mabb, A.M., Judson, M.C., et al. (2011). Angelman syndrome: insights into genomic imprinting and neurodevelopmental phenotypes. *Trends Neurosci.* 34:293–303.

Maezawa, I., Swanberg, S., et al. (2009). Rett syndrome astrocytes are abnormal and spread MeCP2 deficiency through gap junctions. *J. Neurosci.* 29:5051–5061.

Martinowich, K., Hattori, D., et al. (2003). DNA methylation-related chromatin remodeling in activity-dependent BDNF gene regulation. *Science* 302:890–893.

Maze, I., Covington, H.E., 3rd, et al. (2010). Essential role of the histone methyltransferase G9a in cocaine-induced plasticity. *Science* 327:213–216.

Maze, I., Feng, J., et al. (2011). Cocaine dynamically regulates heterochromatin and repetitive element unsilencing in nucleus accumbens. *Proc. Natl. Acad. Sci. USA* 108:3035–3040.

McGill, B.E., Bundle, S.F., et al. (2006). Enhanced anxiety and stress-induced corticosterone release are associated with increased Crh expression in a mouse model of Rett syndrome. *Proc. Natl. Acad. Sci. USA* 103:18267–18272.

McGowan, P.O., Sasaki, A., et al. (2009). Epigenetic regulation of the glucocorticoid receptor in human brain associates with childhood abuse. *Nat. Neurosci.* 12:342–348.

McGraw, C.M., Samaco, R.C., et al. (2011). Adult neural function requires MeCP2. *Science* 333:186.

Mellios, N., and Sur, M. (2012). The emerging role of microRNAs in schizophrenia and autism spectrum disorders. *Front. Psychiatry* 3:39.

Meng, L., Person, R.E., et al. (2012). Ube3a-ATS is an atypical RNA polymerase II transcript that represses the paternal expression of Ube3a. *Hum. Mol. Genet.* 21:3001–3012.

Métivier, R., Gallais, R., et al. (2008). Cyclical DNA methylation of a transcriptionally active promoter. *Nature* 452:45–50.

Mill, J., Tang, T., et al. (2008). Epigenomic profiling reveals DNA-methylation changes associated with major psychosis. *Am. J. Hum. Genet.* 82:696–711.

Miller, C.A., and Sweatt, J.D. (2007). Covalent modification of DNA regulates memory formation. *Neuron* 53:857–869.

Morgan, H.D., Santos, F., et al. (2005). Epigenetic reprogramming in mammals. *Hum. Mol. Genet.* 14(Spec No 1):R47–R58.

Muskiet, F.A.J., and Kemperman, R.F.J. (2006). Folate and long-chain polyunsaturated fatty acids in psychiatric disease. *J. Nutr. Biochem.* 17:717–727.

Ng, S.B., Bigham, A.W., et al. (2010). Exome sequencing identifies MLL2 mutations as a cause of Kabuki syndrome. *Nat. Genet.* 42:790–793.

Ogier, M., Wang, H., et al. (2007). Brain-derived neurotrophic factor expression and respiratory function improve after ampakine treatment in a mouse model of Rett syndrome. *J. Neurosci.* 27:10912–10917.

Penagarikano, O., Mulle, J.G., et al. (2007). The pathophysiology of Fragile X syndrome. *Annu. Rev. Genomics Hum. Genet.* 8:109–129.

Renthal, W., Kumar, A., et al. (2009). Genome-wide analysis of chromatin regulation by cocaine reveals a role for sirtuins. *Neuron* 62:335–348.

Renthal, W., Maze, I., et al. (2007). Histone deacetylase 5 epigenetically controls behavioral adaptations to chronic emotional stimuli. *Neuron* 56:517–529.

Ripke, S., Sanders, A.R., et al. (2011). Genome-wide association study identifies five new schizophrenia loci. *Nat. Genet.* 43:969–976.

Robinson, A.K., Leal, B.Z., et al. (2012a). The growth-suppressive function of the polycomb group protein polyhomeotic is mediated by polymerization of its sterile alpha motif (SAM) domain. *J. Biol. Chem.* 287:8702–8713.

Robinson, L., Guy, J., et al. (2012b). Morphological and functional reversal of phenotypes in a mouse model of Rett syndrome. *Brain* 135:2699–2710.

Roelfsema, J.H., and Peters, D.J.M. (2007). Rubinstein-Taybi syndrome: clinical and molecular overview. *Exp. Rev. Mol. Med.* 9:1–16.

Ruthenburg, A.J., Li, H., et al. (2007). Multivalent engagement of chromatin modifications by linked binding modules. *Nat. Rev. Mol. Cell Biol.* 8:983–994.

Samaco, R.C., Mandel-Brehm, C., et al. (2009). Loss of MeCP2 in aminergic neurons causes cell-autonomous defects in neurotransmitter synthesis and specific behavioral abnormalities. *Proc. Natl. Acad. Sci. USA* 106:21966–21971.

Samaco, R.C., Mandel-Brehm, C., (2012). Crh and Oprm1 mediate anxiety-related behavior and social approach in a mouse model of MECP2 duplication syndrome. *Nat. Genet.* 44:206–211.

Samaco, R.C., and Neul, J.L. (2011). Complexities of Rett syndrome and MeCP2. *J. Neurosci.* 31:7951–7959.

Schaefer, M., and Lyko, F. (2010). Solving the Dnmt2 enigma. *Chromosoma* 119:35–40.

Schuettengruber, B., Chourrout, D., et al. (2007). Genome regulation by polycomb and trithorax proteins. *Cell* 128:735–745.

Schuettengruber, B., Martinez, A.-M., et al. (2011). Trithorax group proteins: switching genes on and keeping them active. *Nat. Rev. Mol. Cell Biol.* 12:799–814.

Shahbazian, M.D., and Grunstein, M. (2007). Functions of site-specific histone acetylation and deacetylation. *Annu. Rev. Biochem.* 76:75–100.

Shahbazian, M., Young, J., et al. (2002). Mice with truncated MeCP2 recapitulate many Rett syndrome features and display hyperacetylation of histone H3. *Neuron* 35:243–254.

Shibayama, A., Cook, E.H., Jr., et al. (2004). MECP2 structural and 3'-UTR variants in schizophrenia, autism and other psychiatric diseases: a possible association with autism. *Am. J. Med. Genet. B Neuropsychiatr. Genet.* 128B:50–53.

Siegmund, K.D., Connor, C.M., et al. (2007). DNA methylation in the human cerebral cortex is dynamically regulated throughout the life span and involves differentiated neurons. *PLoS ONE* 2:e895.

Simon, J.A., and Kingston, R.E. (2009). Mechanisms of polycomb gene silencing: knowns and unknowns. *Nat. Rev. Mol. Cell Biol.* 10:697–708.

Skene, P.J., Illingworth, R.S., et al. (2010). Neuronal MeCP2 is expressed at near histone-octamer levels and globally alters the chromatin state. *Mol. Cell* 37:457–468.

St. Clair, D., Xu, M., et al. (2005). Rates of adult schizophrenia following prenatal exposure to the Chinese famine of 1959–1961. *JAMA* 294:557–562.

Sterrenburg, L., Gaszner, B., et al. (2011). Chronic stress induces sex-specific alterations in methylation and expression of corticotropin-releasing factor gene in the rat. *PLoS ONE* 6:e28128.

Strahl, B.D., and Allis, C.D. (2000). The language of covalent histone modifications. *Nature* 403:41–45.

Sun, H., Kennedy, P.J., et al. (2012). Epigenetics of the depressed brain: role of histone acetylation and methylation. *Neuropsychopharmacology* 38:124–137.

Susser, E., Neugebauer, R., et al. (1996). Schizophrenia after prenatal famine: further evidence. *Arch. Gen. Psychiatry* 53:25–31.

Suzuki, M.M., and Bird, A. (2008). DNA methylation landscapes: provocative insights from epigenomics. *Nat. Rev. Genet.* 9:465–476.

Svedružić, Ž.M. (2011). Dnmt1 structure and function. *Prog. Mol. Biol. Transl. Sci.* 101:221–254.

Tan, M., Luo, H., et al. (2011). Identification of 67 histone marks and histone lysine crotonylation as a new type of histone modification. *Cell* 146:1016–1028.

Tian, W., Zhao, M., et al. (2012). Reversal of cocaine-conditioned place preference through methyl supplementation in mice: altering global DNA methylation in the prefrontal cortex. *PLoS ONE* 7:e33435.

Tranfaglia, M.R. (2011). The psychiatric presentation of Fragile X: evolution of the diagnosis and treatment of the psychiatric comorbidities of Fragile X syndrome. *Dev. Neurosci.* 33:337–348.

Tropea, D., Giacometti, E., et al. (2009). Partial reversal of Rett syndrome-like symptoms in MeCP2 mutant mice. *Proc. Natl. Acad. Sci. USA* 106:2029–2034.

Tsankova, N.M., Berton, O., et al. (2006). Sustained hippocampal chromatin regulation in a mouse model of depression and antidepressant action. *Nat. Neurosci.* 9:519–525.

Uchida, S., Hara, K., et al. (2011). Epigenetic status of Gdnf in the ventral striatum determines susceptibility and adaptation to daily stressful events. *Neuron* 69:359–372.

Valor, L.M., Pulopulos, M.M., et al. (2011). Ablation of CBP in forebrain principal neurons causes modest memory and transcriptional defects and a dramatic reduction of histone acetylation but does not affect cell viability. *J. Neurosci.* 31:1652–1663.

Van Esch, H. (2012). MECP2 duplication syndrome. *Mol. Syndromol.* 2:128–136.

Verhoeven, W.M.A., Tuinier, S., et al. (2010). Psychiatric profile in Rubinstein-Taybi syndrome: a review and case report. *Psychopathology* 43:63–68.

Waterland, R.A. (2006). Assessing the effects of high methionine intake on DNA methylation. *J. Nutr.* 136:1706S–1710S.

Watt, F., and Molloy, P.L. (1988). Cytosine methylation prevents binding to DNA of a HeLa cell transcription factor required for optimal expression of the adenovirus major late promoter. *Genes Dev.* 2:1136–1143.

Weaver, I.C.G., Cervoni, N., et al. (2004). Epigenetic programming by maternal behavior. *Nat. Neurosci.* 7:847–854.

Weaver, I.C.G., Champagne, F.A., et al. (2005). Reversal of maternal programming of stress responses in adult offspring through methyl supplementation: altering epigenetic marking later in life. *J. Neurosci.* 25:11045–11054.

Whittington, J., and Holland, A. (2010). Neurobehavioral phenotype in Prader-Willi syndrome. *Am. J. Med. Genet. C Semin. Med. Genet.* 154C:438–447.

Wiklund, E.D., Kjems, J., et al. (2010). Epigenetic architecture and miRNA: reciprocal regulators. *Epigenomics* 2:823–840.

Wilkinson, M.B., Xiao, G., et al. (2009). Imipramine treatment and resiliency exhibit similar chromatin regulation in the mouse nucleus accumbens in depression models. *J. Neurosci.* 29:7820–7832.

Williams, C.A. (2010). The behavioral phenotype of the Angelman syndrome. *Am. J. Med. Genet. C Semin. Med. Genet.* 154C:432–437.

Yasui, D.H., Peddada, S., et al. (2007). Integrated epigenomic analyses of neuronal MeCP2 reveal a role for long-range interaction with active genes. *Proc. Natl. Acad. Sci. USA* 104:19416–19421.

Yoder, J.A., Soman, N.S., et al. (1997). DNA (cytosine-5)-methyltransferases in mouse cells and tissues: studies with a mechanism-based probe. *J. Mol. Biol.* 270:385–395.

Zeng, W., Ball, A.R., Jr., et al. (2010). HP1: heterochromatin binding proteins working the genome. *Epigenetics* 5:287–292.

Zhu, B., Zheng, Y., et al. (2000). 5- Methylcytosine DNA glycosylase activity is also present in the human MBD4 (G/T mismatch glycosylase) and in a related avian sequence. *Nucleic Acids Res.* 28:4157–4165.

Zhu, J.-K. (2009). Active DNA demethylation mediated by DNA glycosylases. *Annu. Rev. Genet.* 43:143–166.

SECTION II | NEW METHODS AND NEW TECHNOLOGIES FOR PRECLINICAL AND CLINICAL NEUROBIOLOGY

KARL DEISSEROTH

The mammalian brain is extraordinarily difficult to study. Whether in the clinical or the preclinical realm, investigators focusing on psychiatric disease not only lack fundamental understanding of the key pathophysiological processes but also lack understanding of the normal function of the relevant circuits (or even knowledge of which are the relevant circuits). This challenge is due in large part to technological limitations linked to the complexity and inaccessibility of the circuitry, and for this reason the future of mental illness research depends upon the development and application of new technologies for studying brain function. Collected here in this volume are chapters from leading developers and pioneers of new neuroscience technologies relevant to mental illness.

In Chapter 8 transgenic tools and animal models of mental illness are addressed. Recent exciting progress not only in accelerating mouse genetic targeting, but also in advancing the genetic tractability of rats, has been and will continue to be crucial for delivering causal understanding of the impact of specific genetic modifications or manipulations. Of course, even technologically novel genetic methods do not stand alone but, rather, require smooth integration with physiology, pharmacology, behavior, and more recently, viral engineering and transduction methods. Together these genetic manipulation approaches show great promise for advancing our understanding of the mechanisms and physiology underlying brain function in health and in psychiatric disease-related states.

In Chapter 9 the influence of stem cell technology is discussed in opening up a new landscape for investigating the processes underlying both normal human brain development and developmental pathogenesis of psychiatric disease-related states. It is now possible to generate renewable sources of human neurons from normal or disease-impaired individuals, via (among other methods) cellular reprogramming, thereby defining a novel translational bridge between animal studies and human disease. Such research will not replace but, rather, complement traditional animal models, while at the same time representing a paradigm shift in our investigation of neural substrates of mental disorders.

In Chapter 10 optogenetic technologies are addressed; optogenetics is defined as the combination of genetic and optical methods to achieve gain- or loss-of-function of temporally defined events in specific cells embedded within intact living tissue or organisms, usually via introduction of microbial opsin genes that confer to cells both light detection capability and specific effector function. This approach has now been used to control neuronal activity in a wide range of animals, resulting in insights into fundamental aspects of circuit function, as well as circuit dysfunction and treatment in pathological states. Here we review the current state of optogenetics for neuroscience and psychiatry, and address the rapidly evolving challenges and future opportunities.

In Chapter 11 applications of focused ultrasound are reviewed, which may help address the fact that current treatments of neuropsychiatric disease are limited by the lack of noninvasive, reversible, and regionally selective brain-directed drug delivery methods (in large part because of the blood–brain barrier or BBB). Focused ultrasound (FUS) has been found to provide the capability of noninvasively, locally, and transiently opening the BBB in the context of central nervous system diseases. Remaining challenges that are discussed in the chapter include (1) safety and efficacy tradeoffs, (2) mechanism, (3) quantitative measures of BBB change properties, and (4) practical aspects of application for both small (rodent) and large (nonhuman primate) animals.

Chapter 12 reviews some of the advances made in genetic technologies and their application to large-scale gene-mapping efforts in neuropsychiatric disease. From genome-wide association studies to whole-exome sequencing, the sheer amount of data recently generated is unparalleled. Studies of both common and rare variation in diseases such as schizophrenia, bipolar disorder, and autism are now yielding convergent and robust findings, although the high degree of genetic complexity of these diseases (particularly in terms of the number of genes implicated) has also been made evident.

In Chapter 13 the epigenome is explored—as defined by DNA methylation, posttranslational histone modifications, and other regulators of genome organization and function. In the context of psychiatric disorders, these aspects of genetic control have all become increasingly relevant and widely studied. Related therapeutic options—largely based on preclinical studies in rodents—are also addressed, with linkages forged to human brain biology and the pharmacology of mental illness.

In Chapter 14 novel genetic modeling approaches are reviewed that may enable therapeutic predictions and inform decision making. These approaches will range from deciding on genes to probe experimentally, to defining the best treatment for an individual given detailed molecular, genetic, and other personal data. It will be crucial to infer causality and maintain rigorous quantitative methodology with high-dimensional, large-scale data structures, as large and complex as those encountered by climatology and astrophysics. A new breed of mental health researchers with a new set of tools and styles of thinking are coming to the field, with transformative possibilities emerging.

Chapter 15 reviews neuroimaging modalities that can reflect and inform different aspects of brain anatomy and physiology. Key to the research potential of neuroimaging is noninvasiveness, with clear advantages for global and unperturbative observation as well as speedy clinical translation of applications for insight, diagnosis, and treatment. This chapter focuses on key emerging methodologies that may exert substantive impact on mental illness research in the near future.

Finally, Chapter 16 provides an overview of the ways in which brain imaging modalities may interact with, and guide, brain stimulation. These interactions can arise from structural or functional scans on a subject later used to guide offline treatment planning in terms of stimulation site choice. Key caveats, limitations, and opportunities are reviewed. Additionally, scans can be used to track effects of brain stimulation. In a key distinction, such feedback can be processed and analyzed offline or, alternatively, in real time as the brain is being stimulated, employing modalities such as positron emission tomography (PET), single-photon emission computed tomography (SPECT), and functional magnetic resonance imaging (fMRI). This is an exciting avenue of research that provides potential for insight into the global and individualized causal physiology underlying mental illness.

Together, the chapters in this section endeavor to review the principles and possibilities linked to a range of exciting new methodologies for brain research. While translational approaches are emphasized, it is anticipated that basic scientists will also find this compendium helpful as a resource and guide. Technological limitations and opportunities linked to the complexity of the mammalian central nervous system will continue to define the frontiers of neuroscience research for decades to come.

8 | TRANSGENIC TOOLS AND ANIMAL MODELS OF MENTAL ILLNESS

LISA M. MONTEGGIA, WILLIAM A. CARLEZON, JR., AND
RALPH J. DILEONE

INTRODUCTION

Genetics researchers often utilize the study of mutants to better understand the function of genes. For many decades, the field used mutation analysis to identify important genes. However, the completion of the genome project and the development of high-throughput genomic techniques have made it possible to rapidly evaluate expression of hundreds of genes. These approaches can be used on populations of RNA or protein from specific tissue sources or cell types, and have resulted in a massive influx of gene regulatory data. While expression changes under different conditions may suggest a function, it is necessary to conduct more traditional genetic analysis in model organisms to define gene function. This conversion of extensive genomic data to *functional* genomic understanding is multidisciplinary and has implications for many fields, including psychiatry.

Mutant analysis in model systems has helped to define and elucidate signal transduction pathways and transcriptional hierarchies. While yeast, flies, and worms have helped define basic genetic pathways, the use of mice as the representative organism of complex mammalian systems has become increasing popular. The mouse is particularly relevant in neuroscience and psychiatry, where the development of effective models is dependent on complex mammalian brain circuitry and behavior. Although the current technology will be emphasized here, the infrastructure established over decades of work made the modern techniques both possible and more powerful.

The extensive history of mouse studies has enabled large-scale efforts to understand gene function. A consortium of mutagenesis centers has generated novel mouse mutants that will likely provide new insights into the pathophysiology of neurobiological and psychiatric disorders. However, modern mouse research also takes advantage of transgenics and targeted gene knockouts, where specific genes are added or removed from the mouse genome. This "reverse genetic" strategy (from a cloned gene to mutant animal) has redefined experimental possibilities and has dominated the landscape of mouse genetics for the last 20 years. As new genes are implicated in a biological process, it is possible to directly assess their relevance in a complete animal system. The reverse genetic approach is increasingly needed since the completion of the genome project has shown that a large number of genes cannot be placed into a functional category from their primary sequence information.

This chapter focuses on how genetic animal models are relevant for advancing our understanding of psychiatric disorders. The creation of genetically modified animal models has led to our ability to study the contribution of individual genes and their products in the brain. These genetic models have also complemented and extended our understanding of heuristic and pharmacological models of psychiatric diseases. We will discuss conventional approaches to generating transgenic mice, in which a gene of interest is added to the animal, and knockout mice, in which a gene of interest is disrupted or inactivated. We will also address technologies such as viral-mediated gene transfer that allow for spatial and temporal control over gene function. The use of these technical advances has elevated the use of the rat, another well-studied model in neurobiology and behavioral studies, as a genetic model. Finally, many of these transgenic techniques, especially viral-mediated gene transfer, are being used with a powerful new system, called optogenetics, whereby specific sets of neurons are controlled with pulses of light. Optogenetics depends upon expression of light-activated ion channels, or pumps, to elicit action potential firing or to suppress activity in neurons. Transgenic resources have thus become more important in the field, since they allow for control of specific neurons with light (Tye and Deisseroth, 2012).

TRANSGENIC MICE

Transgenic mice are created by adding DNA directly to the genome (Box 8.1). As the first efficient approach to taking previously isolated genes and evaluating possible functions *in vivo*, this technique revolutionized mouse genetics by allowing for direct tests of gene function in an entire animal system. Transgenic experiments are often used to: (*1*) overexpress a gene at high levels, (*2*) misexpress a gene in the wrong place or at the wrong time, (*3*) express a mutant or modified form or a gene, or (*4*) study gene regulation via reporter gene constructs. Gene overexpression can yield important information of the dosage sensitivity of the gene product while misexpression experiments can indicate whether or not a gene will cause defects when abnormally expressed. Expression of certain mutant forms can also be used to reduce the function of the endogenous gene ("dominant negative").

Transgenic mouse lines can be made and established rapidly. Transgenic mice are generated via nuclear microinjection of cloned DNA into fertilized mouse eggs. The DNA construct usually inserts into a single random site of the genome as multiple copies (usually between 5 and 50). Since this transgene integration often occurs at the one- or two-cell stage, the transgenic founder mouse contains the transgenes in most cell types and can pass the transgene directly to progeny. Expression is then mediated by regulatory elements contained within the original construct (Box 8.1). However, transgene expression is usually influenced by DNA sequences surrounding the insertion site,

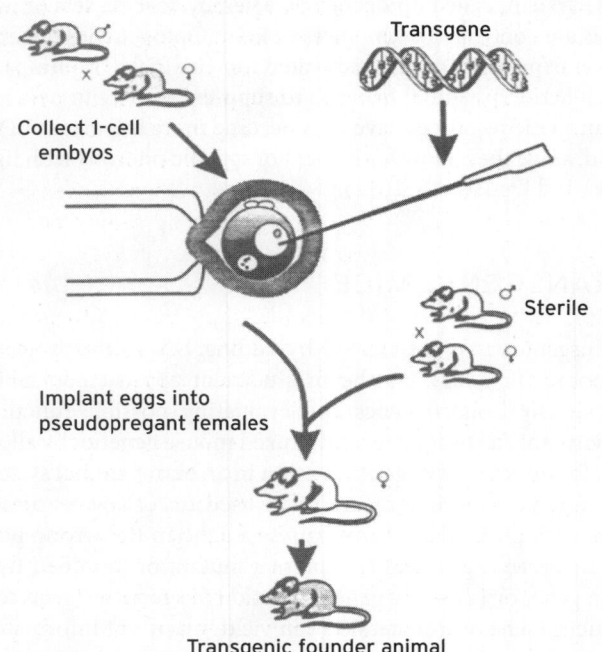
which necessitates the creation and characterization of multiple founder mice to find lines with the desired expression patterns. This concern is mitigated by use of larger pieces of DNA as described next.

LARGE-CLONE TRANSGENICS AND DISEASE MODELS

Traditional transgenics are made with relatively small DNA constructs (3–25 kilobases) that can be generated through standard cloning techniques. While sufficient for many experiments, the complexity of gene regulation, and the large size of mammalian genes, often demands the use of larger fragments of DNA to effectively model gene regulation and disease states. Large-clone transgenics are made using bacterial artificial chromosomes (BACs) and yeast artificial chromosomes (YACs) (Heintz, 2001). BACs are large circular DNA plasmids that allow long stretches of DNA to be cloned and propagated in bacteria. BACs can be used to successfully propagate up to 300 kilobases (300,000 base pairs [bp]) of mammalian DNA in bacteria while YACs can propagate over 1,000 kilobases (1,000,000 base pairs) of mammalian DNA in yeast, allowing for transgenics to be made with entire genes and surrounding genomic regulatory sequences. Large-clone transgenics have been used to effectively model diseases that are caused by mutations in large genes. The accurate expression of the mutant form is likely to yield models that most closely mimic the human pathology. For example, YACs containing the entire human Huntingtin protein have been used to model Huntington's disease (Hodgson et al., 1999). The YACs were modified to express the glutamine repeats that are found in individuals with the disease. Mice transgenic for these constructs developed the cellular, physiological, and behavioral characteristics similar to human Huntington's patients, including selective striatal neurodegeneration. Transgenic approaches have also been useful in delineating the role of the amyloid precursor protein (APP) in Alzheimer's disease (Box 8.2).

Large-clone transgenics have also used to determine the significance of gene dosage effects on behavior and disease states. For example, DNA around the Down syndrome candidate region was introduced via large-clone transgenics and mice were screened for learning abnormalities. This led to identification of the minibrain-related gene, *Dyrk-1*, as a candidate gene for Down syndrome (Smith et al., 1997). The large size of most mammalian genes necessitates the large-clone approach for these studies.

BAC TRANSGENICS AS REPORTER GENES

Another powerful application of large-scale clones has been the generation of reporter lines that express readily detectable marker proteins, such as green fluorescent protein (GFP). By using BACs surrounding specific genes, a series of mouse lines have been generated that allow researchers to detect, study, and isolate specific neuron populations that are otherwise difficult to detect (Heintz, 2004). These BAC reporter mice have been used to distinguish direct and indirect output neurons within the striatum, allowing for definitive characterization

Alzheimer's disease (AD) is a neurodegenerative disease characterized by a gradual decline in cognition and memory over a period of years. The neuropathology of AD is marked by the presence of extracellular senile plaques and intracellular neurofibrillary tangles. While the debate over the causative factor for AD remains controversial, growing evidence suggests plaques are required for the development of AD. Plaques are generated by accumulation of a 42–amino acid amyloid ß protein (Aß), which is derived from the amyloid precursor protein (APP). Genetic studies have identified mutations in the *APP* gene and in the presenilin genes (*PS1* and *PS2*) in familial forms of AD. Disorders that lead to the oversecretion of APP result in Alzheimer's disease–like syndromes.

Transgenic mice overexpressing APP and presenilin mutations have been used to model AD. The first successful attempt, using a platelet-derived growth factor promoter to drive expression of a familial APP mutation, resulted in mice with elevated levels of APP as well as increased amyloid deposits (Games et al., 1995; Masliah, 1996). More recently, transgenics have been generated that link the elevated APP to learning and memory deficits (Hsiao, 1996; Moran et al., 1995). Transgenic mice coexpressing the wild-type human *APP* gene and various PS1 mutations exhibited high levels of Aß in the brain, suggesting the PS1 mutations may influence Aß production and contribute to the pathology of the disease (Citron et al., 1997). This model has recently been used to test the effectiveness of immunomodulatory therapy (Janus et al., 2000; Morgan et al., 2000). The ability of transgenic mice to model aspects of AD represents a major advancement toward understanding the pathophysiology of this disease

Specific behaviors, such as certain paradigms in addiction, have been better studied in rat models, and transgenic rats have been used in recent work. For example, use of rats transgenic for a reporter gene that is activated in neurons (*cFos-lacZ*) allowed researchers to isolate and study neurons that are activated after exposure to cocaine, or a context associated with cocaine (Koya et al., 2009). Other investigators have generated rat lines that allow genetic or optogenetic manipulation of dopamine or acetylcholine neurons (Witten et al., 2011).

CONVENTIONAL KNOCKOUT MICE

Transgenic mice created via microinjection allow for efficient gain-of-function analysis or expression of exogenous molecules. Although this approach is powerful and can be used to model a subset of diseases, there was still a need to test the necessity of gene products via loss-of-function analysis. The goal of removing genes in a directed fashion motivated a number of approaches to modify the endogenous genes within the mouse genome. Ultimately, the knockout strategy depended upon modifying the genome of embryonic stem (ES) cell lines and subsequently generating a mouse from the modified cell lines.

Early research on cell lines derived from early embryos and embryonic carcinomas indicated that these lines could retain totipotency, or the ability to give rise to all differentiated cell types of the mouse. Cells derived from the inner cell mass of a mouse blastula were used to establish the first embryonic stem cell lines. Importantly, ES cell lines could be cultured and frozen, and they allowed recombination to occur between introduced DNA and homologous sequences in the cellular genome (Fig. 8.1). However, the rates of recombination that occur in ES cells are very low compared with random insertion events. To select for the rare recombination event, a "positive-negative" strategy was developed to select for inserts into the desired (homologous) position, while selecting against random insertions (Mansour et al., 1988). After a single copy (maternal or paternal) of the gene was modified, the cells were expanded and introduced into a developing mouse embryo. The cells became incorporated into the developing embryo, and the resulting founder mouse was a mosaic of wild-type cells and mutant cells. This founder must be bred to confirm the presence of the transgene in the progeny. Finally, progeny were mated to generate mice that were missing both copies of the gene (homozygous mutants).

Knockouts originally used a replacement strategy to exchange an endogenous gene with a neomycin-resistant gene cassette (PGK-neo^r). Later generation knockouts took advantage of the recombination event to replace the original gene with a reporter gene or a mutated version of an original gene. These "knock-in" studies yielded powerful data on gene expression and gene redundancy and are now standard practice in current gene analysis. This strategy could be used to misexpress a gene as with transgenic microinjections. Although more time-consuming than traditional transgenic approaches, no knowledge of regulatory elements is required since placing the

of different electrophysiological properties in these important neurons (Kreitzer and Malenka, 2007). Likewise, these same BACs can be used to express proteins, such as Cre recombinase, that allow investigators to target genetic manipulations to specific neuronal types. These Cre driver lines are critical in conditional knockout and transgenic mice, which are discussed in more detail later in the chapter.

RAT TRANSGENIC MODELS

While less common, transgenic rats have been made and are powerful tools for assessing physiology or behavior that is better characterized in rat models. For example, a transgenic model of Huntington's disease was generated in rats to allow for longitudinal imaging studies in a larger brain (von Hörsten et al., 2003). Working memory deficits have been characterized in transgenic rats overexpressing the adenosine receptor (A$_{2A}$) in the rat brain (Giménez-Llort et al., 2007). In addition, transgenic reporter rats have been generated for the study of circadian rhythms (Yamazaki et al., 2000). As the generation of transgenic rats becomes more efficient, including application of large-clone techniques, rat reporter and disease models will become more common and more powerful for behavioral and psychiatric research.

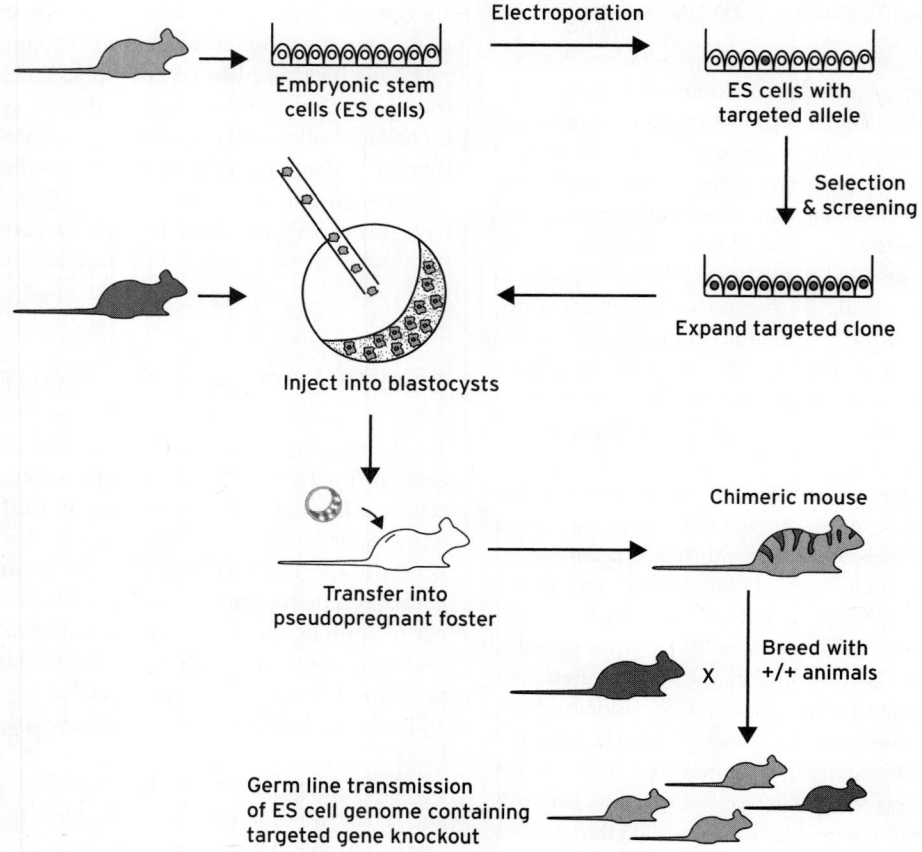

Electroporation

Embryonic stem
cells (ES cells)

ES cells with
targeted allele

Selection
& screening

Expand targeted clone

Inject into blastocysts

Transfer into
pseudopregnant foster

Chimeric mouse

Breed with
+/+ animals

X

Germ line transmission
of ES cell genome containing
targeted gene knockout

Figure 8.1 Knockout mouse production. Adapted from Joyner A. (2000). *Gene Targeting: A Practical Approach*. New York: Oxford University Press.

new gene into the same position of the genome should ensure correct expression.

KNOCKOUT DISEASE MODELS

Many human neurological and psychiatric diseases are likely to be due to loss of gene function that cannot be readily modeled with transgenics. For example, a subset of dominant human mutations is caused by loss of function of only one gene copy. This is known as *haplo-insufficiency* and is best modeled by evaluating heterozygote mice that are missing only one copy of a gene. This is particularly relevant and best studied in cancer models, where heterozygote mutant mice are more prone to tumor formation due to somatic loss of the normal copy. However, it is also possible that a loss of a single copy of a gene is sufficient to recapitulate aspects of psychiatric diseases in animal models. Recently, it was found that animals missing only one copy of the *Reeler* gene displayed gene expression changes as well as dendritic defects similar to those found in postmortem tissue from schizophrenic patients (Liu et al., 2001). It may be useful to conduct more widespread and thorough behavioral testing on heterozygous mice to evaluate the effects of reduced gene expression on behavior.

Like transgenic mice, knockout mice can be used to target specific genes in order to test a hypothesis or model a disease state. Box 8.3 and Table 8.1 highlight results obtained from knockout studies on molecules related to the dopamine system, which have clearly helped to elucidate the specific role of receptors, enzymes, and proteins. Knockouts have also been useful in testing the specificity and effects of pharmacological agents. By completely removing a receptor, for example, knockout mice can be screened for the effects of various drugs. For example, mice missing the 5-HT$_{2C}$ receptor have a paradoxical locomotor increase in response to the nonselective serotonin agonist *m*-chlorophenylpiparazine, which normally induces a locomotor decrease (Heisler and Tecott, 2000). It was subsequently discovered that the agonist was acting on 5-HT$_{1B}$ receptors in the absence of 5-HT$_{2C}$, revealing the dependence of drug response on the genetic constitution of the individual.

While genetic knockout studies have traditionally focused on the use of mice, the completion of the rat genome project (Gibbs et al., 2004), and the extensive history and use of rats in studying behavior and modeling psychiatric disease, has motivated efforts for generating rat knockouts. There are mutagenesis strategies being used to systematically generate a large set of rat knockouts (Smits et al., 2006). This will undoubtedly lead to more use of rat knockouts for modeling behavior and psychiatric disease.

LIMITATIONS OF KNOCKOUT MICE

Early studies with knockout mice produced many surprises while also exposing a number of limitations. A drawback of knockout mice is that there can be functional redundancy of many gene products, leading to a lack of an appreciated phenotype.

BOX 8.3 KNOCKOUTS AND THE DOPAMINERGIC SYSTEM

Dopamine (DA) plays an important role in Parkinson's disease, drug addiction, and schizophrenia among other neuropsychiatric diseases. However, the role of individual components of the dopaminergic system in these disorders remains unknown. The ability to knock out specific genes involved in DA synthesis, release, signaling, and reuptake allows for a comparison of specific genetic alterations with pharmacological models of these disorders.

Dopamine (DA) is synthesized from tyrosine by tyrosine hydroxylase (TH) in the nerve cell cytoplasm and then loaded onto vesicles by vesicular monoamine transporters (VMATs). Once dopamine is released from the synapse, it can (1) activate either presynaptic (D2) or postsynaptic (D1–D5) dopamine receptors, (2) be degraded by catechol-O-methyl transferase (COMT) or monoamine oxidase (MAO), or (3) be taken up by a plasma membrane transporter (DAT).

Mice that lack TH die at birth, implicating catecholamines in fetal development (Zhou et al., 1995). The loss of VMAT disrupts the ability of dopamine to be loaded in the synaptic vesicles and results in mice that die shortly after birth (Takahashi et al., 1997; Wang et al., 1997). In contrast, knockouts of all of the dopamine receptor genes (D1–D5) are viable with mild alterations in locomotor activity (Accili et al., 1996; Baik et al., 1995; Clifford et al., 1998; Dulawa et al., 1999; Holmes et al., 2001; Kelly et al., 1998; Rubinstein et al., 1997; Xu et al., 1994, 1997). The loss of the DA degradative enzymes does not produce alterations in locomotor activity but does result in increased aggression and reactivity to stress (Gogos et al., 1998; Shih et al., 1999). The DAT knockouts have high extracellular DA concentration and display alterations in various behavioral abnormalities, including deficits in spatial cognitive function and sensorimotor gating (Giros et al., 1996; Jones et al., 1998). These knockouts of the dopaminergic system allow for a comparison of specific genetic alterations with pharmacological models of psychiatric and neurological disorders and may contribute to new therapeutic approaches in drug discovery.

TABLE 8.1. Knockouts and the dopaminergic system

KNOCKOUT MICE	PHENOTYPES
Tyrosine hydroxylase (TH)	Lethal (Zhou and Palmiter, 1995)
VMAT2	Lethal (Takahashi et al., 1997; Wang et al., 1997)
D1 DA receptor	Hyperactivity, spatial learning deficit (Clifford et al., 1998; Xu et al., 1994)
D2 DA receptor	Hypoactive, some dysfunction of prepulse inhibition (PPI) sensorimotor gating (Baik et al., 1995; Kelly et al., 1998)
D3 DA receptor	Hyperactive (Accili et al., 1996; Xu et al., 1997)
D4 DA receptor	Hypoactive (Dulawa et al., 1999; Rubinstein et al., 1997)
D5 DA receptor	Normal (Holmes et al., 2001)
COMT	Normal activity; increased aggression, impairment of emotional reactivity (Gogos et al., 1998)
MAO-A	Normal activity; increased aggression, more reactive to stress (for review, see Shih et al., 1999)
MAO-B	Normal activity; more reactive to stress (for review, see Shih et al., 1999)
DAT	Hyperactive, deficits in PPI sensorimotor gating and spatial cognitive impairments (Giros et al., 1996; Jones et al., 1998)

Nevertheless, the use of knockout mice can also produce valuable information regarding the particular gene of interest as long as caveats of the model are appreciated. Recent genetic studies have identified several mutations, copy number variations, and other alterations associated with neuropsychiatric disorders with several reports focused in particular on autism and schizophrenia. The generation of animal models that mimic these abnormalities can have a strong impact on treatment advance, as they will enable detailed examination of neuronal circuit abnormalities derived from these genetic malformations. However, it is important to note that modeling complex genetic modifications in mice is difficult. For instance, alterations in methylation patterns, large gene deletions, or even single nucleotide polymorphisms may have distinct effects depending on the species in question. Moreover, chromosomal abnormalities such as those associated with Down syndrome are hard to replicate in mice. Nevertheless, these attempts will likely yield novel insight as

long as they are well-executed studies done in a well-controlled manner by avoiding overinterpretation of the model.

Another limitation in studying constitutive knockout mice is the occurrence of lethality that can occur if a critical gene is deleted. Since developmental biologists did most of the early work, the early terminal phenotypes that were often observed were of interest. However, early lethality precludes studies of gene function in adult animals demanding use of conditional mutagenesis strategies that are outlined in the next section. Combining knockouts and transgenics can be used to overcome this limitation. For example, by generating a tyrosine hydroxylase (TH) knockout mouse that has been genetically engineered to express the TH gene only in noradrenergic cells, it is possible to generate a mouse that is missing dopamine and yet creates normal norepinephrine (Zhou and Palmiter, 1995). These dopamine-deficient mice survive until birth, indicating that the fetal lethality of constitutive tyrosine hydroxylase knockout mice was caused by the lack of norepinephrine. These mice can be kept alive via daily injections of L-DOPA and have been used extensively to better evaluate the function of dopamine in locomotion, nest building, and feeding. While this strategy was used successfully, it is not always possible to develop effective rescue experiments. More recent work has established strategies for better control of transgenic and knockout effects.

CONDITIONAL CONTROL OF GENE EXPRESSION

The ideal system to control gene expression would be a "genetic switch" that can be operated at will to turn genes on or off. Newer transgenic models are taking advantage of these inducible systems to clearly define the relationship between the transgene expression and the phenotype. In these models, the transgenic expression is regulated temporally by administration of an exogenous agent. Most approaches involve the use of a binary system, or two-gene system, in which one transgene controls the expression of a second. Binary systems that control gene expression can be classified into two groups: (*1*) transcriptional transactivator systems, to overexpress a gene of interest, and (*2*) site-specific recombination systems, to knock out a gene of interest (Fig. 8.2).

TRANSCRIPTIONAL TRANSACTIVATOR SYSTEMS

There are many different types of transcriptional transactivator systems; here we focus on the most commonly used system, the tetracycline gene regulation system (Gossen and Bujard, 1992). In this system, the first transgene encodes the tetracycline transactivator (tTA) under the control of enhancer sequences that dictate expression patterns. The second transgene encodes the gene of interest to be overexpressed under the control of a tetracycline responsive promoter (TetOp) (Fig. 8.2A). In this system, tTA binds to TetOp and results in transcription on the gene of interest unless tetracycline (or, doxycycline, a

tetracycline analogue that can cross the blood–brain barrier) is present. Tetracycline interferes with the ability of tTA to bind to TetOp and drive expression of the gene of interest and is referred to as the "tet-off" system. Thus, mice remain treated with doxycycline until the time the researcher wants to study the overexpression of the gene. This is an inducible system because the gene of interest is controlled by the presence or absence of doxycycline. It is also a cell-targeted system, since the transgene of interest will only be expressed in those cells that express tTA, which is controlled by the choice of promoter in the first transgene construct.

INDUCIBLE TRANSGENICS AND DISEASE MODELS

The tetracycline gene regulation system has been used to successfully overexpress genes in the central nervous system. The first published report overexpressed the calcium-calmodulin-dependent protein kinase II (CaMKII) selectively within the hippocampus of adult mice (Mayford et al., 1996). The resulting mice had cellular phenotypes including impaired functioning of place cells as well as decrements in long-term potentiation within the hippocampus. These mice also had a decrement in spatial learning, which is thought to be a hippocampal-dependent task. These findings suggest that CaMKII in an important step in cellular and behavioral forms of plasticity and highlight the functional importance of the gene in the hippocampus.

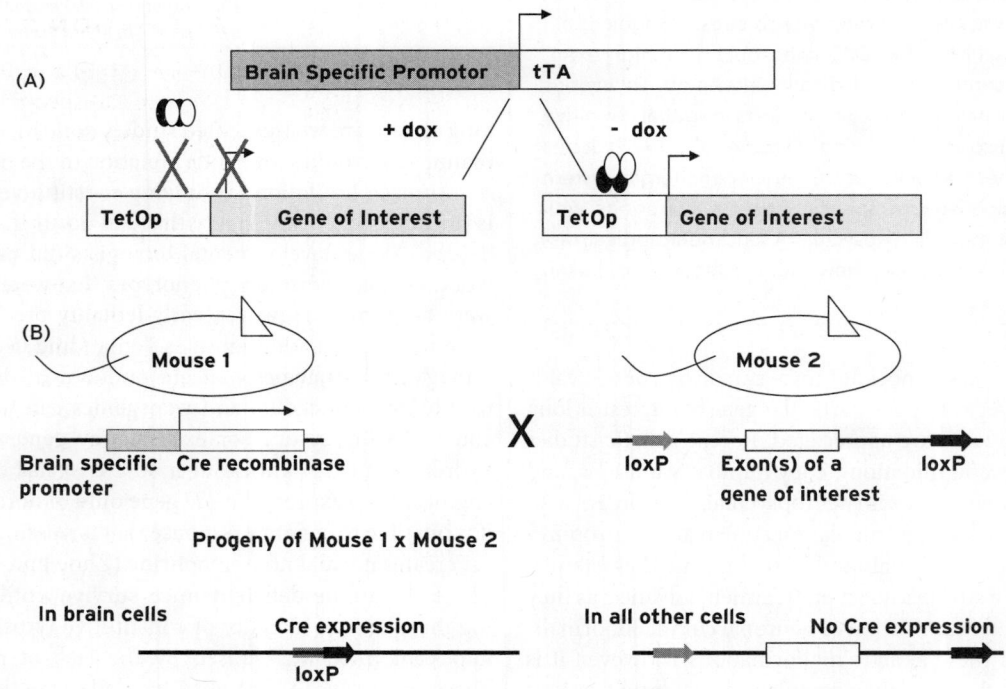

Figure 8.2 *Binary systems for gene induction and removal. A, Schematic of the tetracycline transactivator system for the generation of double transgenic animals. In this system, a brain-specific promoter drives expression of the tetracycline transactivator (tTA) gene selectively to the brain. In the presence of doxycycline (dox), a tetracycline analogue, tTA cannot bind to its promoter (TetOp), and the gene of interest is not expressed. In the absence of dox, tTA binds to TetOp and results in transcription of the gene of interest selectively to the brain. B, Schematic of the Cre/loxP system for conditional knockouts: Genetic techniques are used to express Cre recombinase under the control of a brain-specific promoter. A second construct contains loxP sites flanking a critical region of the gene to be knocked out. The two lines of mice are crossed, and resulting bigenic mice show a loss of the gene of interest, which occurs at the time of development and selectively in those cells in the brain in which the brain-specific promoter is active. The gene of interest is expressed at wild-type levels in cells not expressing Cre recombinase.*

Other studies have direct implications for better understanding of brain disease. For example, Yamamoto et al. (2000) found that the neuropathology and motor dysfunction caused by overexpression of huntingtin were reversible by simply turning off the transgene. This has important mechanistic implications that are relevant to the development of effective therapeutics. In contrast, the inducible transgenic strategy has been used to show that 5-HT$_{1A}$ serotonin receptor function is required during development, and not in the adult, to produce normal anxiety responses in mice (Gross et al., 2002). Another use of inducible transgenic technology is to mimic molecular changes that may be seen in psychiatric disease states as exemplified in Box 8.4.

There are many advantages of the tetracycline gene-regulated system, including the reversibility of the system and the ability to target it to a specific cell type with the use of a cell type–specific enhancer/promoter. There are, however, also limitations to the system. First, the dynamics of gene induction is relatively slow (hours to days) since this system requires the mice to be removed from doxycycline to induce expression of the target gene of interest. Second, transgene expression can be influenced by the position that it has inserted into the genome and not just by the promoter that is driving its expression. While these concerns are of importance, the tetracycline gene-regulated system is still being used with remarkable

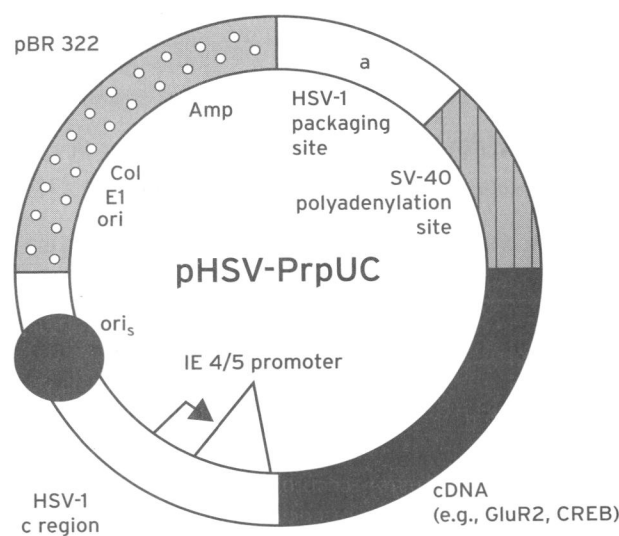

Figure 8.3 *The amplicon (plasmid-based) vector HSV-PrpUC, into which foreign cDNA (e.g., that encoding GluR2, cAMP-responsive element binding protein [CREB]) is subcloned. The viral backbone contains minimal wild-type viral genes and relies upon specially engineered cell lines for propagation and helper virus to produce the proteins needed for packaging.*

success to study the function of genes in the adult nervous system. These inducible transgenic systems are of particular use in psychiatry, where minor developmental disturbances could have subtle, but persistent repercussions.

SITE-SPECIFIC RECOMBINATION SYSTEMS

One way to target a genetic deletion in a regionally and temporally dependent manner is with site-specific recombination. Site-specific recombinases are enzymes that catalyze recombination between specific DNA sites. The Cre recombinase from P1 bacteriophage is the most widely used enzyme. Cre recognizes a 34-bp site (loxP, or locus of recombination) to catalyze recombination. If two loxP sites are placed in the same orientation on a piece of DNA, the region between the two sites will be excised by the recombinase (Nagy, 2000).

Recombinase sites are not normally found in the mammalian genome. The recombinase sites are inserted into the genome of ES cells by homologous recombination such that the sites flank an exon (or exons) of a gene of interest. The gene with flanking recombinase sites is referred to as a "floxed" gene. The recombinase sites should be placed in the genome so as not to interfere with the expression or function of the gene of interest before the recombination event. A selection strategy is employed to identify those ES cells containing the floxed gene in a similar manner to that used to generate a conventional knockout (see Fig. 8.1). The resulting floxed mice still have the functional endogenous gene because the Cre recombinase has not yet been introduced into the system. To obtain a knockout of the targeted gene, the floxed mouse is bred to a second mouse in which a regional or cell type–specific transcriptional promoter controls Cre recombinase expression (Fig. 8.2B). These mice are referred to as "conditional" knockouts, since the knockout occurs only in certain regions and is dependent on Cre recombinase expression

BOX 8.4 OVEREXPRESSION OF ΔFosB AND THE LINK TO DRUG ABUSE

Chronic exposure to many drugs of abuse (e.g., cocaine, amphetamine, morphine, and nicotine) results in the accumulation of the transcription factor ΔFosB in the striatum. ΔFosB is a protein that, once induced, persists for a very long time in the brain. The striatum regions are important for mediating many behavioral aspects of addiction. The molecular mechanisms that are responsible for the long-term induction of ΔFosB in the striatum may represent one biological basis underlying the transition from a nonaddicted to an addicted state.

The tetracycline gene-regulated system has been used to successfully overexpress the transcription factor ΔFosB to the striatum region of the brain (Chen et al., 1998). The resulting mice were more responsive to the rewarding effects of cocaine (Kelz et al., 1999). The use of additional genomic technologies (i.e., viral-mediated gene transfer) has provided evidence that ΔFosB-associated upregulation of GluR2 (an AMPA glutamate receptor) causes, at least in part, the increases in sensitivity to cocaine (Kelz et al., 1999) and other types of rewards (Todtenkopf et al., 2006) (See Fig. 8.3). Interestingly, in a parallel set of experiments with the tetracycline gene-regulated system, mice were generated that overexpress a dominant-negative inhibitor of ΔFosB in the striatum, and these mice were less responsive to cocaine (Peakman et al., 2003). These findings demonstrate a direct role for ΔFosB in the rewarding properties of cocaine and may suggest a role for this molecule in promoting a switch from casual drug use to addiction. By limiting overexpression of ΔFosB in adult mice, this molecular phenotype is mimicked without the potential developmental effects that might have been caused by more traditional transgenic analysis.

(Box 8.5). This approach has proved quite useful in the development of adult knockout mice where the traditional knockout of the gene is fatal and has moved us closer to understanding the function of specific genes (in the brain) and modeling human genetic diseases. Alternatively, viral vectors (see the following) expressing Cre recombinase can be used to ablate expression of floxed genes at various times during development or to selectively delete a gene of interest in a particular brain region. The use of a viral-mediated approach is often used when there is not a specific regional or cell type–specific transcriptional promotor that would target the brain region of interest and thus turn Cre recombinase on in the appropriate site. The viral-mediated approach can circumvent this problem but relies on a surgical approach for each animal to inject the viral vector into the selected region of interest.

BOX 8.5 CRE-DRIVEN LINES CAN INFLUENCE THE PHENOTYPE OF THE CONDITIONAL KNOCKOUT

Recently, conditional knockouts of neurotrophin 3 (NT-3) were generated to study the role of this growth factor in adult brain. Traditional knockouts of NT-3 die shortly after birth. Two independent groups have generated conditional NT-3 knockouts in which the loss of NT-3 is restricted to the brain and the conditional NT-3 knockouts survive into adulthood. The first group generated conditional NT-3 knockouts by crossing floxed NT-3 mice with animals expressing Cre recombinase under the control of the neural-specific promoter, synapsin 1 (Ma et al., 1999). The conditional knockouts had an ablation of NT-3 in many regions of the brain, including the hippocampus. These conditional knockouts were examined in several parameters of synaptic transmission and displayed no difference between wild-type controls, suggesting that NT-3 does not play a role in synaptic transmission and some forms of hippocampal-dependent learning. The second group used the neural-specific nestin promoter to drive Cre expression in floxed NT-3 mice (Akbarian et al., 2001). These nestin-Cre expressing mice caused a more widespread pattern of NT-3 loss in the brain than the synapsin I–Cre expressing mice. In contrast to the synapsin-Cre results, the nestin-Cre NT-3 conditional knockouts established a role for this growth factor in modulating noradrenergic function and opiate withdrawal in the brain.

The conditional knockouts generated by the two different groups resulted in progeny with different patterns of NT-3 loss in the brain and different reported phenotypes. This example illustrates the importance of using different Cre-driven expression lines to elucidate "gene–function" relationships in conditional knockouts. However, there are many important limitations with the currently available Cre-driven expression lines. First, there are not many enhancer and promoter sequences that are successful in expressing Cre recombinase specifically to the brain, let alone to particular regions or cell types. Second, many of these promoters do not express the Cre recombinase in the predicted locations. One approach is to identify better regulatory sequences to drive recombinase expression. Alternatively, knocking the recombinase directly into a known genetic locus by homologous recombination may allow for better control of its expression.

The first successful attempt of a conditional brain-specific gene knockout was the ionotropic glutamate receptor N-methyl-D-aspartate (NMDAR1) gene. The NMDAR1 gene is an obligatory subunit of NMDA receptors. A floxed NMDAR1 mouse was crossed with a transgenic line expressing Cre under the control of the calcium-calmodulin-dependent kinase II (CaMKII) promoter. The CaMKII promoter turns on Cre recombinase in specific regions of the brain without any peripheral expression. The resulting mice displayed a relatively selective knockout of NMDAR1 in the hippocampus that resulted in an impairment in hippocampal long-term potentiation and spatial memory. These cellular and behavioral phenotypes provided support for the view that endogenous NMDAR1 is important in hippocampal-dependent tasks (McHugh et al., 1996; Shimizu et al., 2000; Tsien et al., 1996a, b).

CONDITIONAL KNOCKOUTS AND DISEASE MODELS

Conditional knockouts have also been used to model aspects of Rett syndrome (RTT), a childhood neurological disorder that occurs almost exclusively in females. An exciting recent discovery has been the identification of the gene responsible for RTT (Amir et al., 1999). The majority of Rett syndrome is caused by mutations in the methyl-CpG-binding protein (MeCP2) gene located on the X chromosome (Wan et al., 1999). The MeCP2 gene encodes a protein that binds to methylated DNA. Original attempts to knock out the MeCP2 gene by traditional knockout approaches resulted in early lethality of the mice. Conditional knockout techniques resulted in the generation of viable mice that have a neurological phenotype similar to human RTT (Chen et al., 2001; Guy et al., 2001). Behavioral characterization of the conditional MeCP2 knockout mice showed that the loss of this gene in broad forebrain regions was sufficient to mediate behavioral aspects of the disorder and starts to provide a framework of the brain regions that may be important in mediating some of these behavioral components of the disease (Gemelli et al., 2006). A mouse model that recapitulates aspects of a human disorder is a major advancement in studying this disease and may provide a model in which pharmacological agents can be tested for prevention or possible reversal of the behavioral phenotypes. In an important extension of this work, recent work demonstrated that reintroduction of MeCP2 in adult MeCP2 constitutive knockout mice rescues the disease phenotype supporting an acute rather than a developmental role for MeCP2 in neuronal function (Guy et al., 2007). In addition, in another set of experiments the deletion of MeCP2 in distinct age windows uncovered a divergent requirement for MeCP2 at distinct developmental stages (Cheval et al., 2012). Overall, these studies on MeCP2 provide a road map on how to take advantage of the conditional expression/deletion mouse model to recapitulate disease phenotype in a developmentally specific manner.

Conditional knockouts are also showing great promise in elucidating the genetics of synaptic vesicle function. Synaptic vesicles influence neurotransmitter release and thus play important roles in mediating synaptic transmission. There are a vast number of synaptic vesicle proteins, of which the majority have been knocked out by traditional genetic approaches.

Traditional knockouts have provided support for the role of many of these proteins in neurotransmitter release, but their functional redundancy and lack of regional specificity make it difficult to assess their role in individual neurotransmitter systems. This limitation is particularly important in diseases that are thought to be due to imbalances of particular neurotransmitter systems such as schizophrenia that may be due to an elevated dopaminergic and reduced glutaminergic transmission. The ability to target a knockout to a particular brain region in delineating the role of these particular proteins to specific neurotransmitter systems may contribute to our of understanding particular molecular mechanisms of psychiatric illnesses (Fernandez-Chacón and Sudhof, 1999).

VIRAL-MEDIATED GENE TRANSFER

Another strategy for genetic intervention in the brain is to engineer viral vectors that carry a specific gene (or coding sequence) of interest. These constructs can then be microinjected directly into discrete brain regions. This technique exploits the natural ability of viruses to deliver genetic material to cells. When delivered to the brain, these vectors cause infected cells to express (or, in the case of endogenous genes, overexpress) transferred genes (transgenes) or sequences. Vectors can be used to increase the expression of endogenous genes, mutated genes (e.g., encoding dominant-negative proteins), or siRNA. As such, viral-mediated gene transfer complements the use of mutant (knockout or transgenic) mice in neuropsychiatric research and is particularly useful when the goal is to manipulate expression of a single gene (1) in a specific brain region (2) at a specific time (3) in animals that developed normally.

There are several types of viruses that can be adapted for use as viral vectors, including those based on herpes simplex virus (HSV-1), adenovirus (AV), adeno-associated virus (AAV), lentivirus (LV), and more recently, canine adenovirus (CAV). Considering that each type of vector has unique advantages and disadvantages (see Carlezon et al., 2000b; Neve et al., 2005), the selection of the most appropriate viral backbone depends upon the goals of the experiment. For example, HSV (Fig. 8.3) is an excellent vector when targeting neurons because it is naturally neurotropic and it accommodates relatively large foreign cDNA sequences, but it is associated with a short duration (~5 days) of transgene expression. AV, on the other hand, is associated with a longer duration of transgene expression (months), but it is not selective for neurons and can elicit immune responses in the host. AAV elicits less of an immune response, but it can accommodate only small foreign cDNA sequences, thereby restricting the genes that can be transferred. LV vectors—which belong to the same class of viruses as the human immunodeficiency virus (HIV)—integrate into the host DNA and cause permanent increases in transgene expression but are often associated with biosafety concerns. CAV is of interest because it is neurogenic and retrogradely transported (Soudais et al., 2001) and thus can be used to express or ablate genes within specific neuronal pathways.

Generally, viral vectors are replication deficient: they transfer the gene (or sequence) of interest into cells, but they lack the genes that enable the wild-type virus to replicate or cause a destructive (lytic) infection. Currently, there are two types of replication-deficient vectors. *Genomic* vectors can be conceptualized as "gutted" viruses; the starting point is a competent virus from which harmful (lytic) genes have been removed, and to which the foreign cDNA has been added (for review, see Fink et al., 1996). Conversely, *amplicon* vectors (see Fig. 8.3) can be conceptualized as "modular" viruses; the starting point is a plasmid (amplicon) carrying the exogenous gene, to which minimal viral sequences are added that allow it to be packaged into virus particles with the aid of a helper virus and specialized cell lines (for review, see Carlezon et al., 2000b; Neve et al., 2005).

Typically in neuropsychiatric research, small quantities of viral vectors (for a rat or mouse, 1–2 µl) are microinjected directly into discrete brain regions during stereotaxic surgery. Following a period of time that allows transgene expression to increase (or to increase and then wane), the consequences of increased transgene expression are evaluated in biochemical or behavioral assays. For a viral vector to have utility for this type of research (or ultimately, for gene therapy), the consequences of increased transgene expression must be detectable against the damage caused by the delivery procedure and any cytopathic effects of the viral vector (Fig. 8.4). Theoretically, it is possible to engineer viral vectors that express any biological entity with a known sequence. For example, vectors have been used that encode enzymes (e.g., TH, Cre recombinase), transcription factors (e.g., CREB, NAC-1), receptors (e.g., dopamine D1), receptor subunits (e.g., GluRs), growth-associated proteins (e.g., GAP43), microRNAs (miRs; e.g., miR-212), and reporter proteins (β-galactosidase, green fluorescent protein). Moreover, vectors encoding antisense sequences, dominant-negative mutations (assuming that they exist), or siRNA for any of these entities can be engineered. There are some practical limitations, including the size of the foreign cDNA and the ease with which it can be subcloned into the viral backbone. The larger the cDNA construct, the less efficient the amplification will be during replication, which leads to less favorable amplicon-to-helper virus ratios and lower titers of the vector (see Carlezon et al., 2000b). Assuming that the sequence of the construct is known, the cDNA itself is available, and that no untoward complications are encountered during subcloning, new HSV vectors can be engineered and generated usually within a period of several weeks, and sometimes within days.

EARLY APPLICATIONS OF VIRAL-MEDIATED GENE TRANSFER

During et al. (1994) performed one of the first *in vivo* applications of viral-mediated gene transfer. The goal in this study was to use the vectors as gene therapy to elicit behavioral recovery in an animal model of Parkinson's disease. In this model, rats were given unilateral, intrastriatal microinjections of the neurotoxin 6-hydroxydopamine (6-OHDA) to deplete local concentrations of dopamine. Viral-mediated gene transfer (by stereotaxic microinjections of vector) was then used to convert

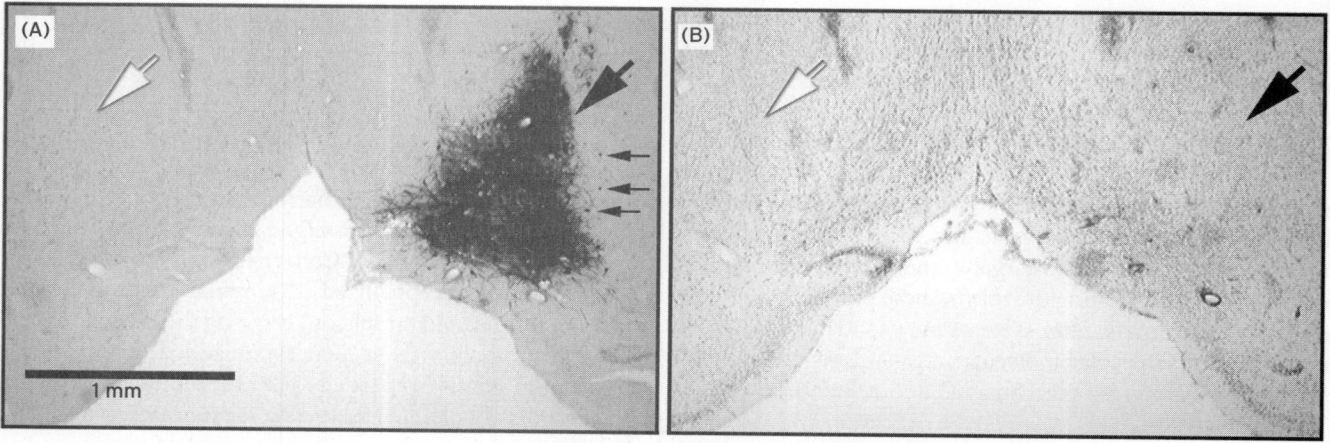

Figure 8.4 Histological examination of nucleus accumbens (NAc) tissue 3 days after gene transfer. A, Large solid arrow: brain site at which the viral vector HSV-LacZ was microinjected. This vector encodes the reporter protein Escherichia coli β-galactosidase, which causes a dark blue reaction product in the presence of substrate. Small solid arrows: individual cells expressing β-galactosidase. Open arrow: noninjected NAc. B, An adjacent, Nissl-stained slice from the same brain, showing minimal evidence of toxicity or damage despite strong transgene expression. Damage produces gliosis and darker Nissl staining.

the endogenous cells of the striatum (primarily GABAergic medium spiny neurons) into L-dopa-producing cells by delivering the gene for TH, the rate-limiting enzyme in the synthesis of dopamine. Hypothetically, increased expression of TH would lead to restored striatal dopamine levels and recovery of function. During et al. (1994) reported significant increases in the expression of TH within the striatum accompanied by partial behavioral recovery after viral-mediated gene transfer and concluded that TH gene therapy was effective in this model. Although other investigators (Isacson, 1995) who used the same viral vector preparations in their studies proposed alternative explanations for the behavioral data of During et al. (1994), this early work highlighted the theoretical potential of viral-mediated gene transfer to facilitate recovery from neurodegenerative processes and, more generally, the use of viral vectors to study how gene expression in discrete brain regions can influence behavior.

More recently, viral-mediated gene transfer has been used to study complex motivational states associated with neuropsychiatric disorders such as addiction and depression. The use of viral vectors is particularly well suited to the study of addiction because exposure to drugs of abuse causes many changes in gene expression within the brain (Nestler, 2005). Since viral vectors offer the capability to study individual changes in gene expression in discrete brain regions, it is possible to mimic certain aspects of the drug-exposed state without ever administering the drugs themselves. For example, repeated exposure to drugs of abuse can cause increases in sensitivity ("sensitization") to the rewarding effects of drugs (Lett, 1989; Piazza et al., 1990), a phenomenon that may contribute to the addiction process (Robinson and Berridge, 2001). Because the dopamine projection from the ventral tegmental area (VTA) of the midbrain to the nucleus accumbens (NAc) of the basal forebrain has been implicated in the habit-forming (rewarding) effects of virtually all abused drugs, many studies on the molecular basis of addiction have focused on this circuitry. Repeated intermittent exposure to morphine or cocaine can increase expression of the AMPA (glutamate) receptor subunit GluR1 within the

VTA and NAc (Churchill et al., 1999; Fitzgerald et al., 1996). To directly test the hypothesis that these drug-induced molecular adaptations *cause* drug-induced behavioral adaptations (including sensitization), viral vectors were used to elevate GluR1 levels within the VTA of rats not exposed previously to drugs. Rats with viral-mediated elevations in GluR1 expression within anterior portions of the VTA showed dramatic increases in sensitivity to the rewarding effects of morphine (Carlezon et al., 1997, 2000a). These data suggest that the behavioral consequences of repeated exposure to morphine are mimicked by gene transfer of GluR1 into the VTA, and support a causal relation between previously disparate drug-induced molecular and behavioral adaptations. Remarkably, elevated expression of GluR1 in the NAc appears to have the opposite effect—reduced sensitivity to reward (Todtenkopf et al., 2006)—highlighting the fact that altered expression of any given gene cannot be assumed to have uniform functional consequences from brain region to brain region (Carlezon et al., 2005).

Hints about the genes and intracellular mechanisms involved in depressive disorders have also evolved from this type of addiction research. Exposure to drugs of abuse increases the function of the transcription factor CREB (cAMP-responsive element binding protein) in striatal regions, including the NAc (Cole et al., 1995; Turgeon et al., 1997). CREB regulates the expression of many genes (Shaywitz and Greenberg, 1999), including that for dynorphin (Hurd et al., 1992), an opioid peptide implicated in dysphoric (aversive) states (Pfeiffer et al., 1986). Viral vector-mediated elevations of CREB in the NAc of rats make low doses of cocaine aversive, and higher doses of cocaine less rewarding (Carlezon et al., 1998). In addition to producing these signs of anhedonia—a hallmark symptom of depression characterized by a diminished ability to experience rewarding stimuli as rewarding—elevations of CREB in the NAc also produce other symptoms of depression in animal models (Pliakas et al., 2001). Antagonists of brain receptors for dynorphin (κ-opioid receptors) eliminate the signs of aversion and depression (Carlezon et al., 1998; Mague et al., 2003; Pliakas et al., 2001), suggesting that CREB-mediated induction of dynorphin contributes directly to these complex behavioral states. Other investigators have used viral vectors to express miRs or "anti-miRs," identifying novel intracellular mechanisms involved in regulation of CREB function and motivated behavior (Hollander et al., 2010).

Together, these types of "biobehavioral" studies demonstrate how viral-mediated gene transfer offers a unique methodology with which to examine how alterations in a single, localized gene product can lead to changes in behaviors that reflect complex motivational states. Moreover, they may help to identify intracellular pathways and alterations in gene expression that are potential targets for new generations of pharmacotherapies for addiction, depression, and possibly other neuropsychiatric disorders (see Box 8.6).

BOX 8.6 COMPLEMENTARY GENOMIC STRATEGIES TO STUDY ΔFosB AND GluR2

As described in Box 8.4, mice engineered to overexpress ΔFosB in the ventral striatum (NAc) are more sensitive to the stimulant and rewarding effects of cocaine (Kelz et al., 1999). Presumably, the proximal cause of heightened drug sensitivity is not increased expression of ΔFosB per se, but rather, increased expression of a target gene (or genes) regulated by this long-lasting transcription factor. Protein immunoblotting studies revealed that the ΔFosB-overexpressing mice also had large increases in GluR2 expression in the NAc, raising the possibility that local alterations in the expression of this AMPA receptor subunit contribute to increased drug sensitivity. To test the hypothesis that elevated GluR2 expression in the NAc is sufficient to cause increased sensitivity to the rewarding effects of cocaine, rats were given stereotaxic microinjections of an HSV vector encoding GluR2 (HSV-GluR2) into this brain region. Rats that received this manipulation showed dramatic increases in sensitivity to the rewarding effects of cocaine in place conditioning studies, mimicking the effects of increased expression of ΔFosB in mice (Kelz et al., 1999). They also showed heightened sensitivity to the rewarding effects of electrical stimulation of the medial forebrain bundle (Todtenkopf et al., 2006). These findings provide strong evidence that the increases in cocaine reward seen in ΔFosB transgenic mice are attributable, at least in part, to elevated expression of GluR2 in the NAc.

The use of additional viral vector constructs provided strong evidence that elevated expression of GluR2 in the NAc increases cocaine reward because of effects on calcium (Ca^{2+}) permeability of neurons within this region. There are numerous possible explanations for how local alterations in Ca^{2+} flux might influence drug reward, considering the role of Ca^{2+} in cellular functions including membrane depolarization, neurotransmitter release, signal transduction, and plasticity (Malinow and Malenka, 2002; Zucker, 1999). Regardless, the combined use of complementary genomic techniques allowed the testing of complex working hypotheses and led not only to the elucidation of drug reward mechanisms, but also to the identification of potential targets for new generations of medications for addiction.

OTHER DEVELOPMENTS IN VIRAL-MEDIATED GENE TRANSFER

TRANSGENE TAGGING

A general improvement to gene transfer methods has been the incorporation of "tags" onto the transgene product to facilitate its detection in the brain, and to differentiate between endogenous gene expression and viral-mediated transgene expression. One increasingly popular and powerful strategy is to incorporate the gene for the green fluorescent protein into the vectors. Coexpression of GFP enables researchers to visually detect cells infected by the vector against a background of endogenous gene expression. There are numerous engineering strategies that can be used to tag vector-infected cells (see Neve et al., 2005). The advantages of tagging proteins are obvious: for example, in cases where viral-mediated elevations in transgene expression have been found to have biobehavioral significance (e.g., GluR2 in the nucleus accumbens), electrophysiologists can visually identify infected neurons for study. An added advantage of the GFP tag is the ability to track the subcellular location of the transgene product, which may increase interest in the use of viral vectors for anatomical studies. Additionally, any of several nonfluorescent tags can be fused to the transgene product because they are not expressed in the brain endogenously, including -HA (hemaglutinen), -FLAG (Asp-Tyr-Lys-Asp-Asp-Asp-Asp-Lys), and -myc (an epitope of the avian myelocytomatosis oncogene). This type of work comes with an important caveat, however: it is imperative to demonstrate that the addition of the tag directly to the transgene product does not affect the native function of the protein.

NEURONAL SPECIFICITY AND DURATION OF EXPRESSION

Current limitations of many viral vectors include their lack of selectivity for neuronal subtypes (e.g., neurotransmitter-specific) and the transient nature of their effects. Reportedly, substitution of a viral transgene promoter with a neuronal promoter can solve both of these limitations. For example, HSV vectors that contain a fragment of the TH promoter cause increased transgene expression selectively in TH-positive (e.g., dopaminergic) neurons, and the expression has been observed for months after infection (Jin et al., 1996). However, the size of neuronal promoters can make packaging less efficient, thereby causing significant reductions in viral titers. Similar techniques have been utilized to restrict LV-mediated transgene expression to neurons (Jakobsson et al., 2006). While AAV can express products for extended periods of time, there is a stricter limit to how many base pairs of DNA the virus can carry.

These challenges have been overcome by combining transgenics and viral approaches to achieve specificity in neuronal expression. By combining transgenic mice that express Cre recombinase in specific neurons, with Cre-dependent viral vectors, expression is achieved in restricted types of cells (e.g., Cardin et al., 2010). This approach has been used extensively with optogenetics, where activated inhibition of specific types of neurons is highly desirable.

DEACTIVATION AND ACTIVATION OF GENES

One intriguing possibility is to use viral vectors in conjunction with other genomic technologies, such as mutant (knockout) mice. A current limitation of knockout mice (inducible knock-outs notwithstanding) is that they lack the gene under study for their entire lives, raising the possibility of developmental adaptations that may complicate interpretation of results (Gingrich and Hen, 2000). However, the use of viral vectors that express the DNA-splicing enzyme Cre recombinase can eliminate this limitation. The general strategy is to engineer mutant mice such that the gene (or genes) to be knocked out is flanked by loxP sites ("floxed"), molecular targets for Cre recombinase (Nagy, 2000). Microinjection of a vector expressing Cre recombinase can then cut and fuse the DNA at the loxP sites, permanently knocking out the gene flanked by the sites. This approach enables regional and temporal selectivity to the genetic manipulation—two current limitations of mutant mouse technology, and two current advantages of viral-mediated gene transfer. Viral vector–induced excision of floxed genes has been used to demonstrate that expression of brain-derived neurotrophic factor (BDNF) in the mesolimbic system plays an essential role in stress-induced development of depressive-like behaviors (Berton et al., 2006) and self-administration of and relapse to drugs of abuse (Graham et al., 2007). Expression of Cre in CAV may offer unique opportunities to dissect complex circuitry: as one example, infusion of CAV-Cre into the nucleus accumbens would allow retrograde expression or ablation of genes specifically within ventral tegmental area (VTA) dopamine neurons that project to this region, while sparing VTA dopamine neurons that project to other areas (e.g., frontal cortex). Viral vectors have also been utilized together with siRNA to achieve gene knockdown with spatial and temporal specificity (Hommel et al., 2003). This approach has also applied to generate conditional knockdown rats with gene loss restricted to the midbrain region (Hommel et al., 2006). The use of viral vectors to deliver siRNA is not trivial, however, and often requires additional engineering of the viral backbone and siRNA oligonucleotide (Sandy et al., 2005; Saydam et al., 2005).

It may also be possible to design viral vectors that cause transgene expression that is subject to pharmacological regulation. For example, a vector has been created that expresses an RU486 (mifepristone)-inducible transactivator (Oligino et al., 1998). Transgenes under control of this transactivator are expressed only in the presence of RU486. Similarly, inducible LV vectors have been created that contain promoter elements that render transgene expression sensitive to doxycycline (Markusic et al., 2005). This strategy is analogous to the use of inducible promoters to regulate gene expression in mutant mice, which dramatically improves the temporal resolution of altered gene expression and facilitates the identification of causal relations between altered gene expression and altered behavior.

LIMITATIONS OF VIRAL-MEDIATED GENE TRANSFER

As an *in vivo* technique for neuropsychiatry research, viral-mediated gene transfer has two main limitations. First, the vectors must be injected directly into the brain region of interest. This involves anesthesia, stereotaxic microinjections, damage to brain regions dorsal to the injection sites from the injection track, damage to the injection sites themselves from the hydraulic pressure of the microinjection, and several days recovery time for the animal. The size and shape of the targeted brain region can make the microinjection procedure difficult or prevent certain regions from being targeted with specificity. Many of these limitations are similar to those encountered with other brain manipulations (e.g., lesions), and their severity is often associated with the skill and experience of the researchers performing the *in vivo* procedures. Historically, cytotoxic effects of the viral vectors themselves or from an immune response from the host are also concerns, although improvements in vector engineering and purification (see Carlezon et al., 2000b) have greatly diminished their severity. The second limitation is that, in general, the vectors do not target specific types of cells. Whereas vectors such as HSV, AAV, and CAV target neurons, others such as AV and LV are not naturally selective for neurons or glia. More importantly, none of the current vectors can selectively target specific types of neurons (e.g., dynorphin-containing GABAergic medium spiny neurons). As previously noted, however, the use of Cre-dependent viruses in transgenic Cre driver lines has made neuronal specificity easier to achieve. As with any technique, these limitations of viral-mediated gene transfer must be weighed against its advantages and potential.

THE FUTURE OF VIRAL-MEDIATED GENE TRANSFER

Gene therapy is an obvious medical application for viral vectors. The use of viral vectors to transfer therapeutic genes or siRNA to treat neurological conditions (e.g., brain tumors) shows great promise (Saydam et al., 2005). However, gene therapy for neuropsychiatric disorders must overcome several technological challenges before it can become a reality (Neve et al., 2005). As previously emphasized, the ability to control the efficacy of the vectors will continue to be a critical consideration. In the past, most vectors have utilized strong or "promiscuous" promoters that tend to drive gene expression beyond physiological levels, raising the possibility of unwanted—and possibly detrimental—effects on cell function. An improved ability to target specific cell types while tightly regulating the timing and strength of gene expression will open up a wealth of opportunities for clinical applications. There are also conceptual hurdles. Aside from the fact that it seems unlikely that any neuropsychiatric disorder is due to alterations in a single gene, the brain is not particularly accessible or hospitable to genetic intervention. In addition, neuropsychiatric disorders such as schizophrenia may have their origins in molecular processes that occur transiently in small subsets of cells at very specific times during development. Once established, these molecular misadaptations may be difficult or impossible to correct with delayed interventions. Thus, while viral-mediated gene transfer is presently well suited for brain research in animals, a substantial amount of work is needed before it can be determined whether it has practical applications in evolving fields of molecular medicine.

DISCLOSURES

Dr. Carlezon discloses that he has a U.S. patent (assignee: McLean Hospital) covering the use of kappa-opioid antagonists for the treatment of depressive disorders.

Drs. Monteggia and Dileone declare no competing financial interests.

REFERENCES

Accili, D., Fishburn, C.S., et al. (1996). A targeted mutation of the D3 dopamine receptor gene is associated with hyperactivity in mice. *Proc. Natl. Acad. Sci. USA* 93:1945–1949.

Akbarian, S., Bates, B., et al. (2001). Neurotrophin-3 modulates noradrenergic neuron function and opiate withdrawal. *Mol. Psychiatry* 6:593–604.

Amir, R.E., Van den Veyver, I.B., et al. (1999). Rett syndrome is caused by mutations in X-linked MECP2, encoding methyl-CpG-binding protein 2. *Nat. Genet.* 23:185–188.

Baik, J.H., Picetti, R., et al. (1995). Parkinsonian-like locomotor impairment in mice lacking dopamine D2 receptors. *Nature* 377:424–428.

Berton, O., McClung, C.A., et al. (2006). Essential role of BDNF in the mesolimbic dopamine pathway in social defeat stress. *Science* 311: 864–868.

Cardin, J.A., Carlén, M., et al. (2010). Targeted optogenetic stimulation and recording of neurons *in vivo* using cell-type-specific expression of Channelrhodopsin-2. *Nat. Protoc.* 5: 247–254.

Carlezon, W.A., Jr., Boundy, V.A., et al. (1997). Sensitization to morphine induced by viral-mediated gene transfer. *Science* 277: 812–814.

Carlezon, W.A., Jr., Duman, R.S., et al. (2005). The many faces of CREB. *Trends Neurosci.* 28: 436–445.

Carlezon, W.A., Jr., Haile, C.N., et al. (2000a). Distinct sites of opiate reward and aversion within the midbrain identified by a herpes simplex virus vector expressing GluR1. *J. Neurosci.* 20: RC62.

Carlezon, W.A., Jr., Nestler, E.J., et al. (2000b). Herpes simplex virus-mediated gene transfer as a tool for neuropsychiatric research. *Crit. Rev. Neurobiol.* 14:47–67.

Carlezon, W.A., Jr., Thome, J., et al. (1998). Regulation of cocaine reward by CREB. *Science* 282:2272–2275.

Chen, J., Kelz, M.B., et al. (1998). Transgenic animals with inducible, targeted gene expression in brain. *Mol. Pharmacol.* 54:495–503.

Chen, R.Z., Akbarian, S., et al. (2001). Deficiency of methyl-CpG binding protein-2 in CNS neurons results in a Rett-like phenotype in mice. *Nat. Genet.* 27:327–331.

Cheval, H., Guy, J., et al. (2012). Postnatal inactivation reveals enhanced requirement for MeCP2 at distinct age windows. *Hum. Mol. Genet.* 21:3806–3814.

Churchill, L., Swanson, C.J., et al. (1999). Repeated cocaine alters glutamate receptor subunit levels in the nucleus accumbens and ventral tegmental area of rats that develop behavioral sensitization. *J. Neurochem.* 72: 2397–2403.

Citron, M., Westaway, D., et al. (1997). Mutant presenilins of Alzheimer's disease increase production of 42-residue amyloid beta-protein in both transfected cells and transgenic mice. *Nat. Med.* 3:67–72.

Clifford, J.J., Tighe, O., et al. (1998). Topographical evaluation of the phenotype of spontaneous behaviour in mice with targeted gene deletion of the D1A dopamine receptor: paradoxical elevation of grooming syntax. *Neuropharmacology* 37:1595–1602.

Cole, R.L., Konradi, C., et al. (1995). Neuronal adaptation to amphetamine and dopamine: molecular mechanisms of prodynorphin gene regulation in rat striatum. *Neuron* 14: 813–823.

Dulawa, S.C., Grandy, D.K., et al. (1999). Dopamine D4 receptor-knockout mice exhibit reduced exploration of novel stimuli. *J. Neurosci.* 19:9550–9556.

During, M.J., Naegele, J.R., et al. (1994). Long-term behavioral recovery in Parkinsonian rats by an HSV vector expressing tyrosine hydroxylase. *Science* 266:1399–1403.

Fernandez-Chacón, R., Sudhof, T.C. (1999). Genetics of synaptic vesicle function: toward the complete functional anatomy of an organelle. *Annu. Rev. Physiol.* 61:753–776.

Fink, D.J., DeLuca, N.A., et al. (1996). Gene transfer to neurons using herpes simplex virus-based vectors. *Annu. Rev. Neurosci.* 19:265–287.

Fitzgerald, L.W., Ortiz, J., et al. (1996). Drugs of abuse and stress increase the expression of GluR1 and NMDAR1 glutamate receptor subunits in the rat ventral tegmental area: common adaptations among cross-sensitizing agents. *J. Neurosci.* 16:274–282.

Games, D., Adams, D., et al. (1995). Alzheimer-type neuropathology in transgenic mice overexpressing V717F beta-amyloid precursor protein. *Nature* 373:523–527.

Gemelli, T., Berton, O., et al. (2006). Postnatal loss of MeCP2 in the forebrain is sufficient to mediate behavioral aspects of Rett Syndrome in mice. *Biol. Psychiatry.* 59(5):468–476.

Gibbs, R.A., Weinstock, G.M., et al. (2004). Rat Genome Sequence Project Consortium. Genome sequence of the Brown Norway rat yields insights into mammalian evolution. *Nature* 428:493–521.

Giménez-Llort, L., Schiffmann, S.N., et al. (2007). Working memory deficits in transgenic rats overexpressing human adenosine A2A receptors in the brain. *Neurobiol. Learn. Mem.* 87:42–56.

Gingrich, J.A., and Hen, R. (2000). The broken mouse: the role of development, plasticity and environment in the interpretation of phenotypic changes in knockout mice. *Curr. Opin. Neurobiol.* 10:146–152.

Giros, B., Jaber, M., et al. (1996). Hyperlocomotion and indifference to cocaine and amphetamine in mice lacking the dopamine transporter. *Nature* 379:606–612.

Gogos, J.A., Morgan, M., et al. (1998). Catechol-O-methyltransferase-deficient mice exhibit sexually dimorphic changes in catecholamine levels and behavior. *Proc. Natl. Acad. Sci. USA* 95:9991–9996.

Gossen, M., and Bujard, H. (1992). Tight control of gene expression in mammalian cells by tetracycline-responsive promoters. *Proc. Natl. Acad. Sci. USA* 89:5547–5551.

Graham, D.L., Edwards, S., et al. (2007). Dynamic BDNF activity in nucleus accumbens with cocaine use increases self-administration and relapse. *Nat. Neurosci.* 10:1029–1037.

Gross, C., Zhuang, X., et al. (2002). Serotonin1A receptor acts during development to establish normal anxiety-like behaviour in the adult. *Nature* 416(6879):396–400.

Gurney, M.E., Pu, H., et al. (1994). Motor neuron degeneration in mice that express a human Cu,Zn superoxide dismutase mutation. *Science* 264(5166):1772–1775.

Guy, J., Gan, J., et al. (2007). Reversal of neurological defects in a mouse model of Rett syndrome. *Science* 315:1143–1147.

Guy, J., Hendrich, B., et al. (2001). A mouse Mecp2-null mutation causes neurological symptoms that mimic Rett syndrome. *Nat. Genet.* 27:322–326.

Heintz, N. (2001). BAC to the future: the use of bac transgenic mice for neuroscience research. *Nat. Rev. Neurosci.* 2(12):861–870.

Heintz, H. (2004). Gene expression nervous system atlas (GENSAT). *Nat. Neurosci.* 7:483.

Heintz, N., and Zoghbi, H.Y. (2000). Insights from mouse models into the molecular basis of neurodegeneration. *Annu. Rev. Physiol.* 62:779–802.

Heisler, L.K., and Tecott, L.H. (2000). A paradoxical locomotor response in serotonin 5-HT(2C) receptor mutant mice. *J. Neurosci.* 20(8):RC71.

Hodgson, J.G., Agopyan, N., et al. (1999). A YAC mouse model for Huntington's disease with full-length mutant huntingtin, cytoplasmic toxicity, and selective striatal neurodegeneration. *Neuron* 23(1):181–192.

Hollander, J.A., Im, H.-I., et al. (2010). Striatal microRNA controls cocaine intake through regulation of CREB signaling. *Nature* 466:197–202.

Holmes, A., Hollon, T.R., et al. (2001). Behavioral characterization of dopamine D5 receptor null mutant mice. *Behav. Neurosci.* 115:1129–1144.

Hommel, J.D., Sears, R.M., et al. (2003). Local gene knockdown in the brain using viral-mediated RNA interference. *Nat. Med.* 9:1539–1544.

Hommel, J.D., Trinko, R., et al. (2006). Leptin receptor signaling in midbrain dopamine neurons regulates feeding. *Neuron* 51:801–810.

Hsiao, K., Chapman, P., et al. (1996). Correlative memory deficits, Abeta elevation, and amyloid plaques in transgenic mice. *Science* 274:99–102.

Hurd, Y.L., Brown, E.E., et al. (1992). Cocaine self-administration differentially alters mRNA expression of striatal peptides. *Brain Res. Mol. Brain Res.* 13:165–170.

Isacson, O. (1995). Behavioral effects and gene delivery in a rat model of Parkinson's disease. *Science* 269:856–857.

Jakobsson, J., Nielsen, T.T., et al. (2006). Efficient transduction of neurons using Ross River glycoprotein-pseudotyped lentiviral vectors. *Gene Ther.* 13:966–973.

Janus, C., Pearson, J., et al. (2000). A beta peptide immunization reduces behavioural impairment and plaques in a model of Alzheimer's disease. *Nature* Dec 21–28;408(6815):979–982.

Jin, B.K., Belloni, M., et al. (1996). Prolonged *in vivo* gene expression by a tyrosine hydroxylase promoter in a defective herpes simplex virus amplicon vector. *Hum. Gene Ther.* 7:2015–2024.

Jones, S.R., Gainetdinov, R.R., et al. (1998). Profound neuronal plasticity in response to inactivation of the dopamine transporter. *Proc. Natl. Acad. Sci. USA* 95:4029–4034.

Kelly, M.A., Rubinstein, M., et al. (1998). Locomotor activity in D2 dopamine receptor-deficient mice is determined by gene dosage, genetic background, and developmental adaptations. *J. Neurosci.* 18:3470–3479.

Kelz, M.B., Chen, J., et al. (1999). Expression of the transcription factor delta-FosB in the brain controls sensitivity to cocaine. *Nature* 401:272–276.

Koya, E., Golden, S.A., et al. (2009). Targeted disruption of cocaine-activated nucleus accumbens neurons prevents context-specific sensitization. *Nat. Neurosci.* 12:1069–1073.

Kreitzer, A.C., and Malenka, R.C. (2007). Endocannabinoid-mediated rescue of striatal LTD and motor defects in Parkinson's disease models. *Nature* 445:643–647.

Lett, B.T. (1989). Repeated exposures intensify rather than diminish the rewarding effects of amphetamine, morphine, and cocaine. *Psychopharmacology* 98:357–362.

Liu, W.S., Pesold, C., et al. (2001). Down-regulation of dendritic spine and glutamic acid decarboxylase 67 expressions in the reelin haploinsufficient heterozygous reeler mouse. *Proc. Natl. Acad. Sci. USA* 98(6):3477–3482.

Ma, L., Reis, G., et al. (1999). Neuronal NT-3 is not required for synaptic transmission or long-term potentiation in area CA1 of the adult rat hippocampus. *Learn. Mem.* 6:267–275.

Mague, S.D., Pliakas, A.M., et al. (2003). Antidepressant-like effects of k-opioid receptor antagonists in the forced swim test in rats. *J. Pharmacol. Exp. Ther.* 305:323–330.

Malinow, R., and Malenka, R.C. (2002). AMPA receptor trafficking and synaptic plasticity. *Annu. Rev. Neurosci.* 25:103–125.

Mansour, S.L., Thomas, K.R., et al. (1988). Disruption of the proto-oncogene int-2 in mouse embryo-derived stem cells: a general strategy for targeting mutations to non-selectable genes. *Nature* 336(6197):348–352.

Markusic, D., Oude-Elferink, R., et al. (2005). Comparison of single regulated lentiviral vectors with rtTA expression driven by an autoregulatory loop or a constitutive promoter. *Nucleic Acids Res.* 33:e63.

Masliah, E., Sisk, A., et al. (1996). Comparison of neurodegenerative pathology in transgenic mice overexpressing V717F beta-amyloid precursor protein and Alzheimer's disease. *J. Neurosci.* 16:5795–5811.

Mayford, M., Bach, M.E., et al. (1996). Control of memory formation through regulated expression of a CaMKII transgene. *Science* 274:1678–1683.

McHugh, T.J., Blum, K.I., et al. (1996). Impaired hippocampal representation of space in CA1-specific NMDAR1 knockout mice. *Cell* 87:1339–1349.

Moran, P.M., Higgins, L.S., et al. (1995). Age-related learning deficits in transgenic mice expressing the 751-amino acid isoform of human beta-amyloid precursor protein. *Proc. Natl. Acad. Sci. USA* 92:5341–5345.

Morgan, D., Diamond, D.M., et al. (2000). A beta peptide vaccination prevents memory loss in an animal model of Alzheimer's disease. *Nature* 408(6815):982–985.

Nagy, A. (2000). Cre recombinase: the universal reagent for genome tailoring. *Genesis* 26:99–109.

Nestler, E.J. (2005). Is there a common molecular pathway for addiction? *Nat. Neurosci.* 8:1445–1449.

Neve, R.L., Neve, K.A., et al. (2005). Use of herpes virus vectors to study brain function. *BioTechniques* 39:381–391.

Oligino, T., Poliani, P.L., et al. (1998). Drug inducible transgene expression in brain using a herpes simplex virus vector. *Gene. Ther.* 5:491–496.

Peakman, M.-C., Colby, C., et al. (2003). Inducible, brain-region specific expression of a dominant negative mutant of c-Jun in transgenic mice decreases sensitivity to cocaine. *Brain. Res.* 970:73–86.

Pfeiffer, A., Brantl, V., et al. (1986). Psychotomimesis mediated by kappa opiate receptors. *Science* 233:774–776.

Piazza, P.V., Deminiere, J.M., et al. (1990). Stress- and pharmacologically-induced behavioral sensitization increases vulnerability to acquisition of amphetamine self-administration. *Brain. Res.* 514:22–26.

Pliakas, A.M., Carlson, R., et al. (2001). Altered responsiveness to cocaine and increased immobility in the forced swim test associated with elevated cAMP response element binding protein expression in nucleus accumbens. *J. Neurosci.* 21:7397–7403.

Robinson, T.E., Berridge, K.C. (2001). Incentive-sensitization and addiction. *Addiction* 96:103–114.

Rubinstein, M., Phillips, T.J., et al. (1997). Mice lacking dopamine D4 receptors are supersensitive to ethanol, cocaine, and methamphetamine. *Cell* 90:991–1001.

Sandy, P., Ventura, A., et al. (2005). Mammalian RNAi: a practical guide. *Biotechniques* 39:1–10.

Saydam, O., Glauser, D.L., et al. (2005). Herpes Simplex virus 1 amplicon vector-mediated siRNA targeting epidermal growth factor receptor inhibits growth of human glioma cells *in vivo*. *Mol. Ther.* 12: 803–812.

Shaywitz, A.J., and Greenberg, M.E. (1999). CREB: a stimulus-induced transcription factor activated by a diverse array of extracellular signals. *Annu. Rev. Biochem.* 68:821–861.

Shih, J.C., Chen, K., et al. (1999). Monoamine oxidase: from genes to behavior. *Annu. Rev. Neurosci.* 22:197–217.

Shimizu, E., Tang, Y.P., et al. (2000). NMDA receptor-dependent synaptic reinforcement as a crucial process for memory consolidation. *Science* 290:1170–1174.

Smith, D.J., Stevens, M.E., et al. (1997). Functional screening of 2 Mb of human chromosome 21q22.2 in transgenic mice implicates minibrain in learning defects associated with Down syndrome. *Nat. Genet.* 16(1):28–36.

Smits, B.M., Mudde, J.B., et al. (2006). Generation of gene knockouts and mutant models in the laboratory rat by ENU-driven target-selected mutagenesis. *Pharmacogenet. Genom.* 16:159–169.

Soudais, C., Laplace-Builhe, C., et al. (2001). Preferential transduction of neurons by canine adenovirus vectors and their efficient retrograde transport *in vivo*. *FASEB J* 15:2283–2285.

Takahashi, N., Miner, L.L., et al. (1997). VMAT2 knockout mice: heterozygotes display reduced amphetamine- conditioned reward, enhanced amphetamine locomotion, and enhanced MPTP toxicity. *Proc. Natl. Acad. Sci. USA* 94:9938–9943.

Todtenkopf, M.S., Parsegian, A., et al. (2006). Brain reward regulated by glutamate receptor subunits in the nucleus accumbens shell. *J. Neurosci.* 26:11665–11669.

Tsien, J.Z., Chen, D.F., et al. (1996a). Subregion- and cell type-restricted gene knockout in mouse brain. *Cell* 87:1317–1326.

Tsien, J.Z., Huerta, P.T., et al. (1996b). The essential role of hippocampal CA1 NMDA receptor-dependent synaptic plasticity in spatial memory. *Cell* 87:1327–1338.

Turgeon, S.M., Pollack, A.E., et al. (1997). Enhanced CREB phosphorylation and changes in c-Fos and FRA expression in striatum accompany amphetamine sensitization. *Brain. Res.* 749:120–126.

Tye, K.M., and Deisseroth, K. (2012). Optogenetic investigation of neural circuits underlying brain disease in animal models. *Nat. Rev. Neurosci.* 13:251–266.

von Hörsten, S., Schmitt, I., et al. (2003). Transgenic rat model of Huntington's disease. *Hum. Mol. Gen.* 12:617–624.

Wan, M., Lee, S.S., et al. (1999). Rett syndrome and beyond: recurrent spontaneous and familial MECP2 mutations at CpG hotspots. *Am. J. Hum. Genet.* 65:1520–1529.

Wang, Y.M., Gainetdinov, R.R., et al. (1997). Knockout of the vesicular monoamine transporter 2 gene results in neonatal death and supersensitivity to cocaine and amphetamine. *Neuron* 19:1285–1296.

Witten, I.B., Steinberg, E.E., et al. (2011). Recombinase-driver rat lines: tools, techniques, and optogenetic application to dopamine-mediated reinforcement. *Neuron* 72:721–733.

Xu, M., Koeltzow, T.E., et al. (1997). Dopamine D3 receptor mutant mice exhibit increased behavioral sensitivity to concurrent stimulation of D1 and D2 receptors. *Neuron* 19:837–848.

Xu, M., Moratalla, R., et al. (1994). Dopamine D1 receptor mutant mice are deficient in striatal expression of dynorphin and in dopamine-mediated behavioral responses. *Cell* 79:729–742.

Yamamoto, A., Lucas, J.J., et al. (2000). Reversal of neuropathology and motor dysfunction in a conditional model of Huntington's disease. *Cell* 101(1):57–66.

Yamazaki, S., Numano, R., et al. (2000). Resetting central and peripheral circadian oscillators in transgenic mice. *Science* 288:682–685.

Zhou, Q.Y., Palmiter, R.D. (1995). Dopamine-deficient mice are severely hypoactive, adipsic, and aphagic. *Cell* 83:1197–1209.

Zucker, R.S. (1999). Calcium- and activity-dependent synaptic plasticity. *Curr. Opin. Neurobiol.* 9:305–313.

9 | APPLICATION OF STEM CELLS TO UNDERSTANDING PSYCHIATRIC DISORDERS

KIMBERLY M. CHRISTIAN, HONGJUN SONG, AND GUO-LI MING

ABBREVIATIONS

αSMA, alpha smooth muscle actin; AD, Alzheimer's disease; AFP, alpha-fetoprotein; APP, amyloid-β precursor protein; Ascl1, achaete-scute homolog 1; ASD, autism spectrum disorder; BAC, bacterial artificial chromosome; BDNF, brain-derived neurotrophic factor; CACNA1C, calcium channel, voltage-dependent, L type, alpha 1C subunit; CNS, central nervous system; CREB, cAMP response element-binding; cyclic AMP, 3′-5′-cyclic adenosine monophosphate; DISC1, disrupted-in-schizophrenia 1; ESC, embryonic stem cell; FD, familial dysautonomia; Fez1, fasciculation and elongation protein zeta-1; FXS, fragile X syndrome; GABA, gamma-aminobutyric acid; GSK3β, glycogen synthase kinase 3 beta; HD, Huntington's disease; hESC, human embryonic stem cell; IKBKAP, I-k-B kinase complex–associated protein; iPSC, induced pluripotent stem cell; Klf4, Kruppel-like factor 4; LRRK2, leucine-rich repeat kinase 2; me3H3K27, trimethylated histone 3 lysine 27; MECP2, methyl-CpG-binding protein 2; Myt1l, myelin transcription factor 1-like; Ndel1, nuclear distribution protein nudE-like 1; Oct4, octamer-binding protein 4; PD, Parkinson's disease; PINK1, PTEN-induced putative kinase 1; PNS, peripheral nervous system; PSD95, postsynaptic density-95 kDa; RTT, Rett syndrome; Sox2, SRY-box-containing gene 2; SZ, schizophrenia; TH, tyrosine hydroxylase; TS, Timothy syndrome; Tuj1, class III beta-tubulin; ZFN, zinc finger nuclease

INTRODUCTION

How can the material substance of our brain become organized into a state that disturbs our very sense of self? What is the neural basis of hallucinatory or delusional perceptual experience that is dissociated from external triggers? And how do persistently maladaptive responses to stimuli manifest in the neural circuitry? Some of the most profound questions with respect to mental illness have been prohibitively difficult to address because of our limited ability to probe the human brain—to observe its development and deconstruct its systems into component parts. To circumvent this constraint, researchers have employed a variety of investigative approaches to make specific predictions about the processes underlying normal and pathological neural function in humans. Animal models have served as a viable and essential proxy for investigating mechanisms underlying clinically relevant pathophysiology in humans.

Conservation of gene function and pharmacological isomorphism provide correlative evidence to validate the use of these animals to model features of neurological disease. In patients, functional imaging, EEG (electroencephalography) and MEG (magnetoencephalography), genetic association studies, and postmortem analyses of brain tissue have all generated substantial and critical information regarding the pathology associated with psychiatric disorders. However, the molecular-, cellular-, and circuitry-level dynamics in the human brain that generate the symptomatology have been elusive because the system itself is not generally amenable to invasive studies.

The advent of stem cell technology has the potential to radically alter our investigative approach by opening a new window into the processes underlying human brain development and pathogenesis. Stem cells exhibit two hallmark properties, namely, unlimited self-renewal and the capacity to differentiate into different cell types (Gage, 2000). By harnessing the potential of stem cells to undergo unlimited self-renewal and specific differentiation, we are now able to generate a renewable source of living human neurons to study under controlled experimental conditions. This provides us with an exciting opportunity to expose human neural components to rigorous investigation and establish a translational bridge between animal studies and the diagnosis and treatment of disease. Although the human brain as a holistic system is still largely inaccessible to direct manipulation, investigating elemental units of neuronal communication and function may lead to a deeper understanding of the cellular mechanics that contribute to systemic dysregulation. Stem cell research will not supplant animal models or noninvasive studies of patients, but is a vital complement to these approaches and heralds a paradigm shift in our investigation of the neural substrates of mental disorders.

Cellular reprogramming is a method designed to convert differentiated somatic cells into different states, such as pluripotent stem cells, neural stem cells, or neurons, via forced expression of specific transcription factors. The prospective utility of cellular reprogramming for reducing the burden of neurological disease derives from two overarching goals—the ability to generate specific cell types to replace neural populations damaged by injury or disease and the generation of a renewable source of genetically tractable human neurons and glial cells to study the mechanisms underlying pathological development. The field is progressing at a rapid pace, and the number of reports using cellular reprogramming to investigate the mechanistic basis of neuropsychiatric disorders will likely increase exponentially in the near future. At this nascent stage, the most striking advances in human reprogramming technology are driven by disease-specific questions as researchers begin to work on transforming some of the most vexing issues in the investigation of the human central nervous system into tractable research problems. Whether the focus is on identifying unknown etiology, engineering genetic rescue, or discovering a novel therapeutic compound, investigators are being challenged to find innovative solutions to unique problems, and the approaches they develop may be generalized to other domains. As the field matures, the cross-pollination of ideas from diverse research programs should facilitate generation of target cell populations and efficacious methods to characterize and rescue relevant phenotypes. In this chapter, we first introduce different types of stem cells used to investigate psychiatric disorders, then highlight some novel approaches in the field of cellular reprogramming and examples that use stem cells to understand psychiatric disorders, and conclude with discussion of some of the central challenges in the field. Because there are currently only a few published studies using patient-derived reprogrammed nerve cells to investigate cellular dysregulation in psychiatric disorders, we will include a discussion of prominent findings from other neurological diseases to illustrate salient issues that are applicable to all efforts to exploit the potential of cellular reprogramming (Table 9.1). Interested readers can consult other detailed review articles (Brennand et al., 2012; Dolmetsch and Geschwind, 2011; Vaccarino et al., 2011).

STEM CELLS FROM DIFFERENT SOURCES

EMBRYONIC STEM CELLS

Stem cells are defined by two essential characteristics—the capacity for self-renewal and the ability to generate multiple cell types (Gage, 2000). Although stem cells exist in many adult tissues, the number is limited, and fate choices are often constrained to a few cell types. Embryonic stem cells (ESCs) can be maintained in culture indefinitely and exhibit no restriction on fate specification. Early attempts to generate multiple neuronal subtypes to study in culture began with efforts to direct differentiation of mouse ESCs. Significant progress has been made in recent years to develop protocols to differentiate ESCs into different types of neurons in the CNS and PNS as well as glial cells (Gottlieb, 2002).

Human embryonic stem cell (hESC) lines derived from human blastocysts were first characterized in 1998 and exhibited the essential properties of self-renewal and pluripotency observed in mouse ESC lines (Thomson et al., 1998). The creation of these early hESC lines was invaluable to the study of early human development and offered the first real possibility of generating a renewable source of diverse cell types in the human nervous system. However, the ethical issues surrounding the acquisition of source material for hESCs has constrained the development of additional lines, which may limit applicability to a genetically diverse population.

INDUCED PLURIPOTENT STEM CELLS

One of the most significant technological advances in stem cell biology was the seminal study by Takahashi and Yamanaka demonstrating that both embryonic and adult fibroblasts of mice could be reprogrammed to a state of pluripotency through the retroviral-mediated introduction of four transcription factors—Oct3/4, Sox2, c-MYC, and Klf4 (Takahashi and Yamanaka, 2006). These induced pluripotent stem cells (iPSCs) exhibited all the classic hallmarks of stem cells, including self-renewal and the capability of differentiating into cells from all three embryonic germ layers. Critically, it was soon shown that this strategy was also effective for reprogramming of human fibroblasts and many other somatic cell types into pluripotent iPSCs (Park et al., 2008; Takahashi et al., 2007; Yu et al., 2007). Perhaps the most salient and exciting aspect of this technology is that differentiated cells arising from iPSCs retain the genetic information of the fibroblast donor, thus providing a renewable, genetically tractable resource for different types of human cells. This cardinal feature has a profound impact for investigating human disease in that it allows direct observation of neurons and glial cells that have a clinically relevant genetic profile. Efforts to validate pluripotency and stability of iPSC lines have converged on an array of standard assays to demonstrate fundamental properties of stem cells and similarity to ESCs (Fig. 9.1). Depending on the method of reprogramming, it may be necessary to show the silencing of viral-mediated introduction of transgenes. Karyotyping is typically performed to ensure that there are no gross chromosomal abnormalities. iPSC colonies should be positive for typical pluripotency markers, including Nanog, SSEA3, SSEA4, TRA-1-60, TRA-1-181, TRA-2-49, Sox2, OCT4, and alkaline phosphatase (Fig. 9.1A–C). Competency to generate all three embryonic germ layers can be demonstrated through expression of layer-specific markers for ectoderm (e.g., Tuj1), mesoderm (e.g., αSMA), and endoderm (e.g., AFP), following differentiation (Fig. 9.1D–F). Finally, the current in vivo benchmark for pluripotency is the teratoma assay in which undifferentiated iPSCs are intramuscularly injected into immunodeficient mice to induce formation of tumors that include all three germ layers. Once pluripotency has been achieved, the resultant iPSCs can be induced to differentiate toward specific lineages, including neural progenitors (Fig. 9.1G), which give rise to immature neurons (Fig. 9.1H), and finally, mature neurons expressing synaptic markers (Fig. 9.1H).

DIRECT PROGRAMMING INTO NEURONS OR NEURAL STEM CELLS

In the first iterations of cellular reprogramming, fibroblasts were converted to a state of pluripotency through the introduction of transcription factors delivered via a retrovirus (Takahashi and Yamanaka, 2006). Subsequently, additional induction methods were developed that were able to confer pluripotency while minimizing risk associated with viral-mediated transgene insertion. Although newer methods have minimized or eliminated the risk of residual expression of transgenes, the transient induction of pluripotency required for iPSC generation

TABLE 9.1. Patient-specific iPSC Studies of neurological disorders

DISEASE	MUTATION	REPROGRAMMING METHOD	DIFFERENTIATION	PHENOTYPE	RESCUE	REFERENCE
AD	APP duplication in two patients (APP^{Dp}); no identified mutations in two sporadic AD patients (sAD)	Retrovirus (Oct3/4, Sox2, Klf4, c-Myc)	Glutamatergic, GABAergic, and cholinergic neurons	Increased amyloid-β, p-tau, and aGSK-3β expression in both APP^{Dp} lines and one of two sAD lines	Partial rescue of amyloid-β, p-tau, and aGSK-3β expression with γ and β-secretase inhibitors	Israel et al. (2012)
AD	Three sporadic AD patients, three familial AD patients with mutations in either PSEN1 or PSEN2	Direct conversion to neurons via lentivirus (Ascl1, Brn2, Myt1l, Oligo2, Zic1)	Glutamatergic forebrain neurons	Familial AD-iPSCs show increased expression of Aβ; dysregulated processing of amyloid precursor protein	WT PSEN1 expression rescues	Qiang et al. (2011)
FD	IKBKAP point mutation	Lentivirus (Oct3/4, Sox2, Klf4, c-Myc)	CNS and PNS precursors	Limited tissue-specific splicing; reduction in ASCL1 expression	Kinetin rescue of splicing and autonomic neuron generation	Lee et al. (2009)
FXS	FMR1 CGG repeat expansions (one mosaic patient, two with >600 repeats)	Retrovirus (Oct3/4, Sox2, Klf4, c-Myc)	Neurons, glia	Neuronal differentiation, process morphology	—	Sheridan et al. (2011)
FXS	FMR1 premutation –30, 94 CGG repeat	Retrovirus (Oct3/4, Sox2, Klf4, c-Myc)	Neurons	Reduced neurite length, synaptic puncta, PSD-95	—	Liu et al. (2012)
HD	HTT CAG expansion repeat mutations (50 CAG; 109 CAG)	Integration-free episomes	Neurons, astrocytes	CAG-repeat-associated presence of cytoplasmic vacuoles in astroyctes	—	Juopperi et al. (2012)
HD	HTT CAG expansion repeat mutations (72)	—	DAARP32 neurons	Cell death, mitochondrial bioenergetics, elevated stress response	BAC homologous recombination gene editing to reduce repeat length rescued mitochondrial and cell death vulnerability	An et al. (2012)
HD	HTT CAG expansion repeat mutations (60, 180)	Lentivirus (Oct4, Sox2, Klf4, cMyc, Nanog, Lin28)	DAARP32 neurons	Cell death, BDNF sensitivity, cytoskeleton, adhesion, cell energetics	—	HD iPSC Consortium (2012)
PD	LRRK2 dominant missense mutation	Retrovirus (Oct3/4, Sox2, Klf4)	Midbrain dopaminergic neurons	Differential gene expression; increased α-synuclein expression, increased susceptibility to H_2O_2, 6-OHDA, and MG-132	—	Nguyen et al. (2011)
PD	PINK1 nonsense or missense mutations	Retrovirus (Oct3/4, Sox2, Klf4, c-Myc)	Dopaminergic neurons	Impaired stress-induced translocation of Parkin to mitochondria; increased PGC-1α and mtDNA following depolarization	Overexpression of WT PINK1 restored translocation capacity and prevented PGC-1α increase	Seibler et al. (2011)

(continued)

TABLE 9.1. (Continued)

DISEASE	MUTATION	REPROGRAMMING METHOD	DIFFERENTIATION	PHENOTYPE	RESCUE	REFERENCE
PD	α synuclein point mutation	Tetracycline-inducible lentivirus (Oct3/4, Sox2, Klf4, c-Myc)	Dopaminergic neurons	—	ZFN gene editing; repair of point mutation in patient iPSCs; introduction of point mutation in hESCs	Soldner et al. (2011)
PD	PINK1, LRRK2	Retrovirus (Oct3/4, Sox2, Klf4, c-Myc)	Neurons	Mitochondrial dysfunction	Rescue via coenzyme Q$_{10}$, rapamycin, or the LRRK2 kinase inhibitor GW5074	Cooper et al. (2012)
PD	Parkin mutations	Lentivirus (Oct3/4, Sox2, Klf4, c-Myc, Nanog)	Midbrain dopaminergic neurons	Increased oxidative stress, spontaneous DA release, decreased DA uptake	Overexpression of WT-parkin rescued all phenotypes	Jiang et al. (2012)
RTT	*MeCP2* missense, nonsense, and frameshift mutations	Retrovirus (Oct3/4, Sox2, Klf4, c-Myc)	GABAergic and glutamatergic neurons	Reduced soma size, number of spines, glutamatergic synapses; altered Ca^{2+} transients, sEPSCs, sIPSCs	IGF1—partial increase in synapse number; gentamycin—restored MeCP2 expression in nonsense mutation	Marchetto et al. (2010)
RTT	MeCP2-null mutation	Retrovirus (Oct3/4, Sox2, Klf4, c-Myc)	Neurons	Soma size reduction	—	Cheung et al. (2011)
RTT	Domain-specific mutations (MBD, TRD, CTD)	Retrovirus (Oct3/4, Sox2, Klf4, c-Myc)	Neurons, glia	Decreased neuronal differentiation	—	Kim et al. (2011b)
SZ	4bp deletion in *DISC1*- frameshift	Integration-free episomes	—	—	—	Chiang et al. (2011)
SZ	Not known	Tetracycline-inducible lentivirus (Oct3/4, Sox2, Klf4, c-Myc)	Glutamatergic, GABAergic, and dopaminergic neurons	Decreased neuronal connectivity, increased *NRG1* expression	Loxapine rescue of neuronal connectivity deficits, *NRG1* expression	Brennand et al. (2011)
TS	*CACNA1C* point mutation	Retrovirus (Oct3/4, Sox2, Klf4, c-Myc)	Layer-specific cortical neurons	Differential gene expression; TH expression	—	Pasca et al. (2011)

ABBREVIATIONS: RTT, Rett syndrome; FD, familial dysautonomia; TS, Timothy syndrome; FXS, fragile X syndrome; HD, Huntington's disease; SZ, schizophrenia; PD, Parkinson's disease; AD, Alzheimer's disease; TH, tyrosine hydroxylase; DA, dopamine; MAO-A, monoamine oxidase A; MAO-B, monoamine oxidase-B; ZFN, zinc finger nuclease; mtDNA, mitochondrial DNA; MBD, methyl-CpG binding domain; TRD, transcriptional repression domain; CTD, carboxyl terminal domain.

is still time consuming and labor intensive and poses a risk for tumor formation during transplantation. To address many of these issues, a rapidly evolving technology is the direct conversion of somatic cells to neuronal lineages (Chambers and Studer, 2011). An early study demonstrating the possibility of direct programming described direct conversion of murine adult somatic cells to functional neurons using a set of three neural-lineage-specific transcription factors, Ascl1, Brn2, and Myt1l (Vierbuchen et al., 2010), a strategy that subsequently proved effective for human fibroblast conversion as well (Pang et al., 2011). Independent laboratories used a partially overlapping set of transcription factors in combination with specific microRNAs, such as miRNA-9 and miRNA-124, to achieve similar results (Ambasudhan et al., 2011; Yoo et al., 2011).

Nevertheless, direct programming of somatic cells to neurons has its own set of potential pitfalls and experimental

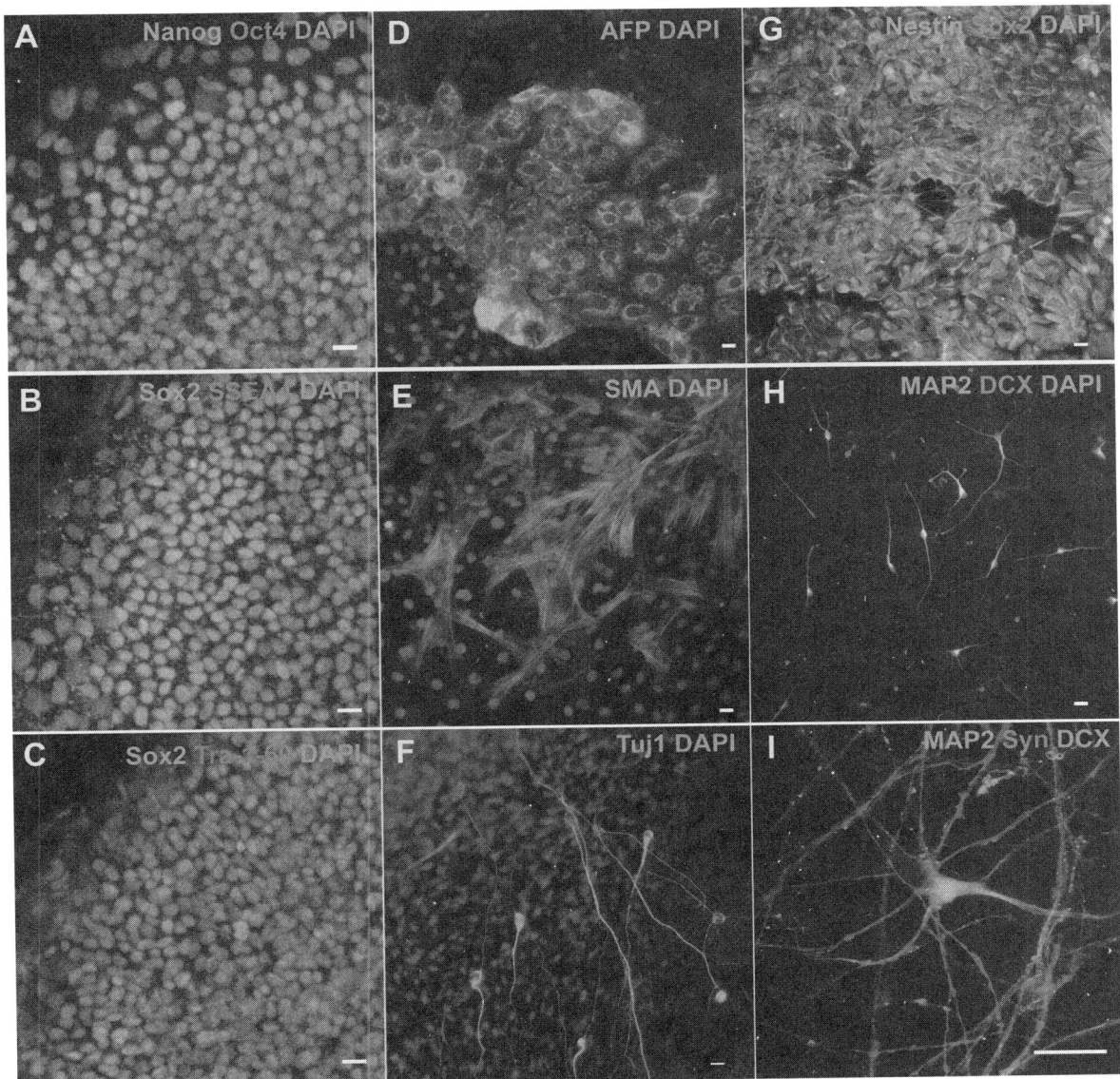

Figure 9.1 *Generation of neurons from human iPSCs. (A–C) Confocal images of iPSC colonies expressing pluripotency markers: (A) Nanog (green), Oct4 (red), DAPI (blue); (B) Sox2 (green), SSEA4 (red), DAPI (blue); (C) Sox2 (green), Tra-1–60 (red), DAPI (blue). (D–F) In vitro differentiation into three embryonic germ layers revealed by immunostaining for markers of α-fetoprotein (endoderm) (D), α smooth muscle actin (mesoderm) (E), and Tuj1 (ectoderm) (F). (G–I) Neuronal differentiation: (G) Neural progenitors cells 7 d after neural induction stained for Nestin (green), Sox2 (red), and DAPI (blue); (H) immature neurons 7 d after differentiation, stained for MAP2 (green), DCX (red), and DAPI (blue); (I) 4 week-old neurons stained for MAP2 (green), DCX (blue), and synapsin (red). Scale bar = 20 μm. (See color insert).*

challenges. While expedient, the process of direct conversion to neurons requires a large pool of source material and allows for the possibility of population-level variability. In addition, neurons generated as a result of direct programming exhibited little proliferative potential and limited ability for stable expansion. More recently, methods have been developed to generate multipotent neural stem cells and neural progenitors (Han et al., 2012; Kim et al., 2011a; Lujan et al., 2012; Thier et al., 2012). One approach relied on a slight modification of traditional methods for reprogramming by limiting the duration of Oct4 expression (Thier et al., 2012). The rationale of this approach was that sustained expression of the remaining transcription factors (Sox2, Klf4, and c-Myc) would create a selective pressure for neural-lineage induction while restricting

Oct4 expression to the first 5 days of reprogramming would limit the induction of pluripotency. As a result the induced neural stem cells were capable of differentiation into all three neural cell types—neurons, astrocytes, and oligodendrocytes—and, critically, this differentiation capacity remained stable over long-term expansion of more than 50 passages. A markedly different approach was used by two independent groups, which achieved generation of stable and expandable neural progenitor and stem cell pools in the absence of Oct4 (Han et al., 2012; Lujan et al., 2012). Interestingly, each group relied on a unique set of transcription factors in which Sox2 was the only common element, further supporting an integral role of Sox2 in neural induction. Sox2 has now been demonstrated to be capable of converting both mouse and human fibroblasts to multipotent neural stem cells through single-factor conversion (Ring et al., 2012).

ENDOGENOUS NEURAL STEM CELLS

Although it was long believed to be devoid of postnatal proliferation, the adult central nervous system was shown to be capable of *de novo* cellular production in a pivotal series of studies in the 1960s, which were largely overlooked for the next several decades (Altman and Das, 1965). In the intervening years, it was conclusively demonstrated that two primary areas of the mature brain do exhibit ongoing neurogenesis throughout life in most species, including humans, and that specialized populations of neural stem cells occur endogenously in the mature mammalian brain (Gage, 2000). The subventricular zone gives rise to immature neurons that traverse the rostral migratory stream to populate the olfactory bulb. And in the hippocampus, neural stem cells in the subgranular zone are the source of newborn granule cells in the dentate gyrus. Because the hippocampus is an integrative site that supports many forms of learning and memory, much effort has been devoted to understanding the role of this site-specific generation of a select population of neurons (Aimone et al., 2011). Intriguingly, adult neurogenesis has been implicated in affective disorders, with the most striking evidence arising from a correlation between levels of neurogenesis and the efficacy of antidepressants in animal models (Samuels and Hen, 2011). These data suggest that adult neurogenesis may play an active role in mediating emotional behavior. Many mental disorders are associated with reduced hippocampal volume and correlate with decreased levels of neurogenesis in animal models, suggesting that depressed levels of cell proliferation may play a role in hippocampal atrophy and cognitive impairments, although there are limited data to demonstrate a casual influence of neurogenesis levels on disease etiology. Adult neurogenesis can also play a significant role as a model system to explore basic principles of how newborn neurons are integrated in the mature brain, which will be critical to the development therapeutic cell replacement strategies (Christian et al., 2010). While mechanistic investigations of this phenomenon are limited to animal models, it provides a viable *in vivo* model that can be used to complement *in vitro* studies of human neurons. Furthermore, the presence of a robust neurogenic niche in the adult rodent brain provides a unique opportunity for transplantation studies of human neural stem cells to examine their development, maturation, and integration (Juopperi et al., 2012).

MODELING NEUROLOGICAL DISORDERS USING STEM CELLS

MONOGENIC DISEASES

Initially, the most approachable diseases to investigate mechanistically are those associated with highly or completely penetrant single gene mutations. This genetic determinism reduces complexity and narrows the investigative focus for characterization of the relevant pathology. To date, the most significant breakthroughs in terms of identifying potential strategies to reverse or prevent phenotypic disturbances have come from the study of monogenic diseases. Starting from a functional evaluation of a circumscribed genetic domain, two general approaches are being developed that show considerable promise in being able to rescue cellular phenotypes observed during the differentiation of neurons from patient-specific iPSCs—biochemical rescue and targeted gene editing (Fig. 9.2).

In diseases with a predominant psychiatric impact, there are few examples of monogenic diseases, but there is a subset of autism spectrum disorders (ASD) for which a causative genetic locus has been identified. Rett syndrome, Timothy syndrome, and fragile X syndrome are all associated with mutations in single genes and will be instructive in developing technologies for genetically mediated rescue or screening for biochemical compounds to ameliorate or reverse cellular phenotypes.

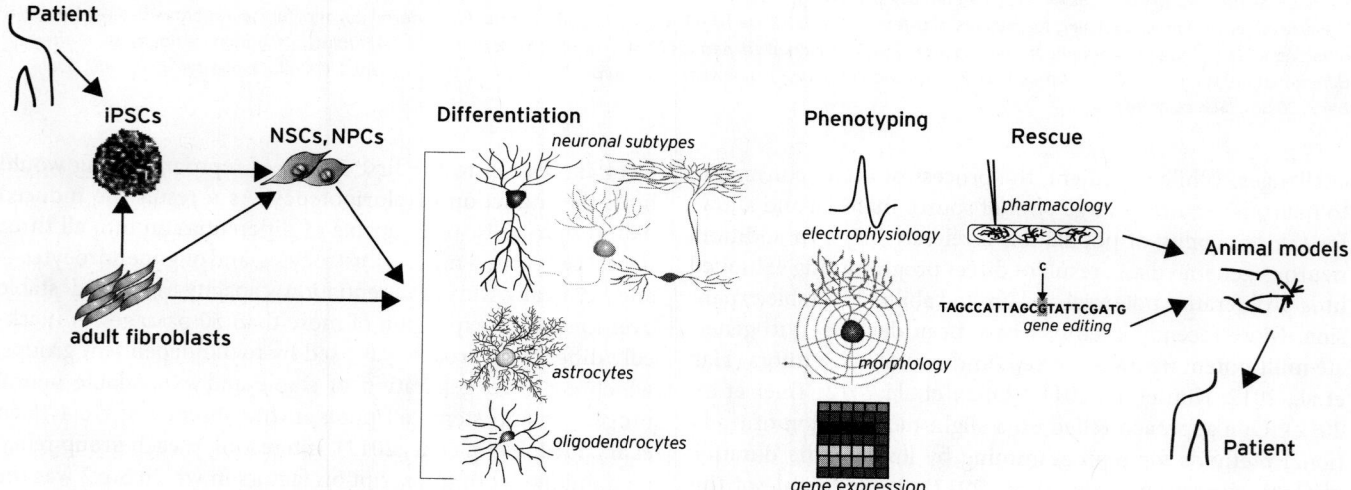

Figure 9.2 *Flowchart for application of cellular reprogramming to neurological disorders. Schematic representing process from acquisition of fibroblasts from patients, reprogramming to iPSCs or directly to neural lineages, phenotypic screening of cellular properties, identification of strategies to rescue phenotypes, validation in animal models, and ultimately, the development of novel therapeutic strategies that can be tested in clinical trials.*

RETT SYNDROME

Capitalizing on the opportunity to investigate a monogenic ASD developmental disorder marked by both cognitive and motor impairments, several laboratories have generated and begun to characterize neurons derived from Rett syndrome (RTT) patients. Caused by a mutation in the X-linked gene, methyl-CpG-binding protein 2 (MeCP2), symptoms of RTT emerge in females around 6–18 months of age, following a period of unremarkable and grossly normal development (Chahrour and Zoghbi, 2007). At the age of onset, developmental processes slow and often regress, resulting in decelerated head growth, movement stereotypy, and severe impairments of verbal and communicative skills. The first characterization of RTT patient–derived neurons revealed several morphological and electrophysiological phenotypes, including altered soma size, spine density, synapse number, calcium signaling, and evoked activity, compared with neurons derived from disease-free subjects (Marchetto et al., 2010). Partial rescue of the decrease in synapse number in RTT neurons was achieved through application of the nonspecific growth factor, IGF1, an effect previously observed in a mouse model of RTT (Tropea et al., 2009). Because the majority of causative MECP2 variants are nonsense mutations, the authors then explored the possibility of using a pharmacological approach to impair ribosomal proofreading and allow read-through of the premature stop codon to restore MECP2 expression. Low-dose application of the antibiotic gentamicin was able to enhance MECP2 expression and showed a similar effect as IGF1 in increasing synapse number. Using two fundamentally different mechanisms for pharmacological rescue of phenotypes, this study demonstrated that at least some facets of cellular dysregulation could be reversed in human neurons. It is somewhat surprising that the enhanced MECP2 expression did not rescue more of the morphological and electrophysiological deficits since it had been previously shown in a mouse model of RTT that introduction of MECP2 could reverse behavioral deficits in adult mice (Guy et al., 2007). However, many parameters remain to be explored to determine the temporal requirements for pharmacological treatment in the restoration of cellular function. Following this initial study, independent laboratories confirmed several of the cellular phenotypes (Cheung et al., 2011; Kim et al., 2011b).

One procedural complication in the evaluation of female iPSC lines is the ability to accurately characterize the status of X-inactivation in clonal progeny, an issue that has been central to the investigation of RTT patient iPSCs. Initially, it was reported that reactivation of the silenced X chromosome occurred during reprogramming, resulting in a differentiated population of human neurons that exhibited random X-inactivation based on variable expression of an epigenetic silencing marker, trimethylated histone 3 lysine 27 (me3H3K27), and the loss of Xist RNA, a noncoding transcript involved in silencing the inactive X chromosome (Marchetto et al., 2010). Other studies, however, found that iPSCs retained the allelic X-inactivation from the founder somatic cell, which was transcriptionally maintained, despite the emergent loss of Xist over extended passaging of the iPSCs (Ananiev et al., 2011; Cheung et al., 2011; Tchieu et al., 2010). Still others have shown that reprogramming does not alter X-inactivation status from the parent cell but that late-passage iPSCs can lose both Xist RNA and me3H3K27 markers, which is believed to signal transcriptional derepression of the inactive X chromosome (Mekhoubad et al., 2012). Yet another group suggested that neither reprogramming of a mosaic culture of fibroblasts nor extensive passaging of fibroblasts results in activation of both X chromosomes, but that there is an intrinsic bias toward a dominant X chromosome and that cells in which the unfavored X chromosome is active are more resistant to proliferation, potentially as a result of shortened telomeres (Pomp et al., 2011). Finally, a systematic study of cell culture conditions showed that spontaneous X reactivation during reprogramming does occur rarely but that the frequency is heavily influenced by feeder conditions (Tomoda et al., 2012). Collectively, the preponderance of current evidence suggests that, unlike reprogramming of murine cells, human cells do not typically undergo transient reactivation of both X chromosomes and that transcriptional assays may be more sensitive than Xist or me3H3K27 in detecting the presence of X-inactivation. Further, allelic skewing toward a dominant X-chromosome may impact the reprogramming, proliferative, and differentiation capacity of female iPSCs.

TIMOTHY SYNDROME

Caused by a single-point mutation in the CACNA1C gene, Timothy syndrome (TS) is a rare disorder that has a pervasive impact on the developing central nervous system and leads to autism or ASD, in conjunction with other deficits including cardiac arrhythmia and intermittent hypoglycemia. Because most TS patients meet the diagnostic criteria for ASD, this disease provides a useful entry point to investigate cellular phenotypes associated with a psychiatric disease with limited genetic complexity (Splawski et al., 2004). CACNA1C encodes the α_1 subunit of the L-type calcium channel, $Ca_V1.2$, and the missense mutation responsible for TS impairs voltage-dependent channel inactivation. To identify the functional impact of the single point mutation on human neurons, iPSCs from TS patients were generated and compared with neurons derived from control subjects without the disease (Pasca et al., 2011). Consistent with the proposed role of the point mutation in regulating $Ca_V1.2$ inactivation kinetics, action potentials recorded from TS neurons exhibited a broader profile, and there was an elevated increase in intracellular calcium following depolarization. This change in intracellular calcium had consequent effects on Ca^{2+}-mediated activity-dependent gene expression through the CREB pathway as evidenced by whole-genome expression profiles. Downstream targets of CREB include tyrosine hydroxylase (TH), the rate-limiting enzyme necessary for dopamine and norepinephrine production. In TS-derived neurons, baseline TH levels were higher, and in contrast to control neurons, there was no downregulation of TH following prolonged depolarization.

The differentiation protocol used in this study was designed to promote the generation of cortical neurons. One of the most striking phenotypes observed in the population-level analysis of TS-derived neurons was a propensity for differentiation into upper-layer cortical neurons. This finding suggests a new investigative target for postmortem studies to determine whether patients have an imbalance in the composition of cortical neurons. A bias toward upper-layer neurons would effectively increase the proportion of neurons projecting to subcortical regions at the expense of callosal projections and could significantly alter signaling pathways among distributed neural systems. Finally, in an attempt to define the specificity of the mutation and role of the L-type calcium channels in the observed pathology, application of roscovitine, which increases inactivation of this channel subtype, was highly effective in ameliorating expression of TH in differentiated neurons. L-type calcium channels have been independently associated with other psychiatric disorders, including bipolar disorder and schizophrenia (Green et al., 2010; Nyegaard et al., 2010), and these results suggest a potential strategy to reduce abnormal expression of TH via enhanced channel inactivation.

FRAGILE X SYNDROME

Fragile X syndrome (FXS) is a genetically mediated ASD and the most common form of inherited intellectual disability. Caused by an expansion of a CGG repeat (>200 repeats) in the X chromosome–linked fragile X mental retardation gene 1 (FMR1) gene, the extent of cognitive deficits can range from mild to severe. The first published report of human iPSCs from FXS patients compared FXS-iPSC lines from three unrelated males with a clinical diagnosis of FXS and CGG repeat length in the full mutation range (Sheridan et al., 2011). Retroviral-mediated reprogramming resulted in several iPSC lines in which the CGG repeat length differed slightly from the donor fibroblast, but it was uncertain whether this change reflected an undetected mosaicism in the fibroblast population or was a consequence of the reprogramming itself. Initial characterization of the patient lines compared with unaffected control lines revealed no significant difference in the capacity to differentiate to a neuronal lineage but a distinct morphological phenotype in the neural progenitor cells in the form of shorter length and decreased complexity of neural processes. A subsequent study focused on premutation CGG repeat length and generated iPSCs from a female with both a normal repeat length (30) and a premutation repeat length (94) on separate X chromosome alleles (Liu et al., 2012). Functional characterization of differentiated neurons revealed several phenotypes, including decreased neurite length, decreased expression of the synaptic marker, PSD-95, elevated spontaneous calcium transients, and heightened responses to glutamate, while repeat length appeared stable throughout reprogramming and differentiation. Together, these studies provide initial evidence of morphological and synaptic abnormalities that are consistent between FXS patients and a carrier of a premutation length CGG repeat sequence and suggest the existence of a graded phenotype associated with repeat-level regulation of FMR1 expression.

FAMILIAL DYSAUTONOMIA

One of the first studies to rely on hypothesis-driven investigation of neurological disease mechanisms using cellular reprogramming focused on familial dysautonomia, a rare and lethal disease most commonly arising from a point mutation in the I-k-B kinase complex–associated protein (IKBKAP) gene (Lee et al., 2009). This mutation causes splicing defects and tissue-specific expression of the IKAP protein and a progressive loss of sensory and autonomic neurons, but it is unknown at what point during development these neurons become vulnerable to degeneration. Fibroblasts from FD patients and control subjects were obtained and used to generate viable iPSC lines. After targeting differentiation to five tissues spanning all three embryonic germ layers, the authors identified lower absolute levels of wild-type IKAP expression in neural crest precursors, the lineage most affected in FD. Transcriptome analysis of purified FD neural crest precursors revealed decreased transcripts of genes that regulate neurogenesis and differentiation compared with controls, which was reflected in a relative decrease of FD neural crest precursors to differentiate into neurons. Migration deficits were also observed in the neural crest precursors derived from patient iPSCs. All of these data suggest that at least some of the phenotypes associated with FD could result from early defects in neuronal development, as opposed to degeneration of a well-developed peripheral nervous system. Previous studies using lymphocytes from patients had identified the plant cytokinin, kinetin, as a bioactive compound capable of reducing expression of mutant IKBKAP. Acute application of kinetin to neural crest precursors increased the ratio of normal to mutant transcript of IKBKAP. Chronic application of kinetin beginning prior to differentiation reduced the deficits in neurogenic gene expression and increase in markers of peripheral neurons, although no rescue of migratory defects was observed. Although FD is not a predominantly psychiatric disorder, this early study was instrumental in illustrating the potential of using patient-derived iPSCs for initial screening of cellular phenotypes and the evaluation of candidate compounds for biochemically mediated rescue. In addition, it demonstrates how recapitulation of developmental processes can pinpoint the time of pathological onset and disambiguate between neurodevelopmental and neurodegenerative effects.

PARKINSON'S DISEASE

Parkinson's disease (PD) is a late-onset progressive neurodegenerative disorder that affects dopaminergic neurons in the substantia nigra of the basal ganglia. Primary symptoms of PD involve impairments in motor control and postural stability, although cognitive impairments and psychological disturbances are often associated with the disease. Several genetic loci have been associated with the rare cases of familial PD, including mutations in α-synuclein, LRRK2, PTEN-induced putative kinase 1 (PINK1), parkin, and DJ-1 (Martin et al., 2011). Risk for sporadic PD may be partially mediated by variation in these and other unidentified genes in combination with environmental risk factors that have yet to be fully understood. Although early studies showed successful generation of iPSCs from patients with sporadic forms of PD, more recent studies have focused on patients with a single known mutation in an attempt to isolate specific genetic influences on cellular pathology and establish a baseline from which to investigate functional dysregulation. These studies targeting monogenic influences have revealed several characteristic phenotypes in differentiated dopaminergic or tyrosine hydroxylase–positive neurons. The G2019S missense mutation in the *LRRK2* gene, associated with both familial and sporadic PD cases, resulted in the increased expression α-synuclein, the protein that aggregates to form Lewy bodies, a signature of PD and other degenerative diseases (Nguyen et al., 2011). Also, in support of previous animal and cellular models, differentiated dopaminergic neurons from these LRRK2-mutated patient iPSCs showed a modest upregulation of select oxidative stress genes in basal conditions and enhanced vulnerability to neurotoxins and hydrogen peroxide–induced cell death. Investigation of a different genetic locus, the PINK1 mutation, revealed deficits in depolarization-induced translocation of Parkin to mitochondria, which was restored through lentiviral-mediated expression of wild-type PINK1 in the mutant iPSC lines (Seibler et al., 2011). Because Parkin is believed to act in a PINK1-dependent manner to degrade dysfunctional mitochondria, levels of mitochondrial DNA were quantified and shown to be higher in the mutant dopaminergic neurons, although increased levels of a mitochondrial biogenic protein were also observed, raising the possibility of enhanced mitochondrial production in the mutant neurons. In a separate study, direct investigation of Parkin mutations (affecting exons 3 and 5) did not reveal any differences in expression levels of mitochondrial DNA or α-synuclein (Jiang et al., 2012). However, mutant neurons showed increased spontaneous release of dopamine and decreased dopamine uptake due to misfolding of dopamine transporter proteins that impacted dopamine binding sites. Hypersensitivity to dopamine-induced oxidative stress was also observed in the patient-derived neurons, likely a result of the compromised Parkin-regulated expression of monamine oxidases A and B in mutant neurons.

Several of these initial studies to characterize the cellular phenotypes of disease-relevant mutations in PD-associated genes used expression of wild-type protein to effectively rescue deficits, suggesting the genetic specificity of the observed phenotypes. More recently, investigators have begun to explore alternative means of reversing cellular pathology through pharmacology. In a comprehensive study of several iPSC lines derived from patients with either a PINK1 or one of two known LRRK2 mutations, treatment of differentiated neural cells with the antioxidant coenzyme Q_{10} reduced vulnerability to low-dose exposure to the chemical toxins valinomycin and concanamycin A as measured by cellular release of lactate dehydrogenase (Cooper et al., 2012). Interestingly, the sensitivity to chemical stressors was enhanced in the derived neural cells when compared directly with the fibroblasts, suggesting that the observed pathology was selective to cell types that are more functionally similar to the affected neuronal populations in the patients.

In one of the first studies to employ targeted gene editing in the investigation of neurological disease, Soldner et al. took a counterbalanced approach to generate several isogenic iPSC lines that differed in two point mutations in the α-synuclein gene associated with familial PD (Soldner et al., 2011). The distinct advantage of this approach is the virtual elimination of genetic variability that is introduced when comparing patient iPSCs with "control" iPSCs derived from disease-free individuals, who differ not only in disease status but genetic background. In complementary sets of experiments, the authors repaired the point mutations in patient-derived iPSCs to generate isogenic lines with either mutant or wild-type α-synuclein expression and introduced the point mutations to hESCs to express the mutant form of α-synuclein. The strategy used for the targeted manipulation of the base pair changes was a zinc finger nuclease (ZFN) gene-editing technique that employs a combination of DNA-binding domains specific to the target sequence with a generic cleavage domain. Nuclease-mediated introduction of double-strand breaks in the DNA are then repaired through either nonhomologous end joining or homology-directed repair end joining. Use of this strategy requires additional assays to verify the absence of off-target cleavage sites and genomic alterations. Although neuronal phenotypes in the edited iPSCs were not extensively characterized, this study provided an important proof of principle that selective gene editing is feasible, and this technique will be instrumental in identifying the specific role of restricted genetic variation in monogenic diseases.

HUNTINGTON'S DISEASE

Huntington's disease (HD) is another late-onset neurodegenerative disorder that initially impacts medium spiny neurons in the striatum, progresses to involve other brain regions, and induces pervasive motoric and cognitive impairments. HD is caused by an autosomal dominant mutation in the Huntingtin gene characterized by excessive polyglutamine (CAG) repeats, the number of which strongly correlates with the age of onset. In a collaborative study published by the Huntington's Disease iPSC Consortium, a total of 14 iPSC lines from HD patients and controls were extensively characterized. Interestingly, the CAG repeat length appeared to exhibit a graded phenotypic profile in only a subset of assays, including a measure of calcium homeostasis (The HD iPSC Consortium, 2012). In a separate study, gene editing through the use of bacterial artificial chromosome (BAC)-based homologous recombination was successful in reducing the number of CAG repeats in HD patient iPSCs (An et al., 2012), resulting in two corrected iPSC lines with 21 and 20 repeats, below the pathological threshold (36 CAG repeats). Strikingly, the genetic correction was able to protect neural stem cells against cell death following withdrawal of growth factors, restored levels of brain-derived neurotrophic factor (BDNF), and enhanced mitochondrial function. In one of the few studies to evaluate glial phenotypes in relation to neurological disease, astrocytic differentiation of HD iPSCs revealed distinct vacuoles in the somatic cytoplasm of cells derived from two genetically related HD patients, which was more pronounced in astrocytes generated from the patient with a longer CAG repeat length and early-onset HD (Juopperi et al., 2012). Initial characterization showed indistinguishable properties between patient and control iPSC-derived neurons. Interestingly, HD neural progenitors transplanted to the neurogenic subventricular of the adult mouse brain were capable of generating immature neurons that migrate along the endogenous rostral migratory stream and differentiate into mature neurons in the olfactory bulb. *In vivo* transplantation of neural precursors was later shown to result in successful differentiation of GABAergic neurons and modest functional recovery in rats subjected to unilateral striatal lesions (Jeon et al., 2012). In vivo neuronal pathology following transplantation of patient-derived neural progenitors was only observed at remote time points. This observation suggests the possibility that latent phenotypes may emerge after an extended period of development and integration *in vivo* and, importantly, that the rodent brain may serve as viable model to evaluate age-dependent factors regulating neural pathology.

POLYGENIC DISEASES

For most psychiatric disorders, there is no single identified genetic cause. These complex polygenic diseases, which are known to include schizophrenia, affective disorders, and the vast majority of ASDs, are instead associated with several hundred "risk" genes that may increase the probability of disease onset to variable degrees but alone are not causally sufficient to induce the disease (Eichler et al., 2010). Because these genes confer only susceptibility, there are several other factors that can modify the net risk for a given individual. Any number of combinations of environmental influences, epigenetic mechanisms, and genetic interactions could enhance susceptibility for disease. Disentangling the individual contributions of each factor to the pathophysiology is extremely challenging. Using iPSCs to address this issue should proceed in a systematic fashion starting from known parameters. If the donor material is obtained from patients, the one certainty is that the genetic background is at least permissive for the disease state. Building upon that knowledge, it is then feasible to explore the impact of additional influences on cellular integrity.

SCHIZOPHRENIA

One such strategy was recently employed in a phenotypic screen of iPSCs derived from unrelated patients with sporadic schizophrenia (SZ) who had no identified genetic link (Brennand et al., 2011). This study was among the first to characterize the functional properties of human neurons from patients with a psychiatric disease and describes a comprehensive battery of assays designed to reveal pathological disturbances predicted to be relevant for SZ. Several prominent cellular phenotypes were identified, including a deficit in cellular connectivity among differentiated neurons, which was partially rescued through application of the antipsychotic drug loxapine. Markers of synaptic function, including PSD95 and glutamate receptor expression, were diminished in the patient-derived iPSCs but functional synaptic transmission appeared largely intact. In order to investigate changes in gene expression shared among lines derived from different patients, the authors analyzed RNA expression profiles and identified a subset of genes related to the cyclic AMP- and WNT-signaling pathways that were common to all SZ-iPSC lines. Strikingly, only 25% of the genes that were differentially regulated in the SZ-iPSCs had been previously identified as putative risk genes, and many of these genes are involved in signaling pathways not previously associated with SZ.

These results illustrate both the potential utility of patient-derived iPSCs to identify novel gene interactions in complex genetic disorders and the constraints imposed by the technical challenges of generating multiple iPSC lines on a large enough scale to validate the role of these interactions in cellular phenotypes in diverse patient populations. Importantly, however, this study effectively demonstrates how a genetically complex disease can be probed mechanistically through patient-specific iPSCs and lead to the identification of novel cellular targets of pathology.

Although schizophrenia is a genetically complex disease, several genes have emerged as prominent risk factors. Originally identified at the breakpoint of a balanced (1;11) (q42;q14) chromosome translocation in a large Scottish family, mutations in DISC1 have been shown to segregate with schizophrenia, schizoaffective disorders, and major depression in several studies (Porteous et al., 2011). Genetic mouse models have been developed to manipulate DISC1 expression, and several phenotypes have been identified in behavioral assays such as prepulse inhibition, latent inhibition, working memory, and sociability that are reminiscent of symptoms in SZ patients (Johnstone et al., 2011). However, similar to the heterogeneity observed in the clinical profile of patients and family members with DISC1 mutations, the behavioral deficits observed in the rodent models also varied across studies using different strategies to disrupt DISC1 expression. Recently, an episomal-vector-based approach was used for integration-free reprogramming of fibroblasts from several family members who harbor a 4 bp mutation in the *DISC1* gene (Chiang et al., 2011). In this family, the DISC1 mutation is associated with increased risk for schizophrenia, schizoaffective disorder, and major depression (Sachs et al., 2005). Reprogramming efficiency and differentiation capacity were similar to control iPSCs in the initial characterization assays. Together, these two studies, focused on generation of iPSCs from schizophrenia patients, represent complementary strategies to identify relevant pathology and etiological factors. Data generated from both approaches may eventual converge on a common set of developmental mechanisms that are vulnerable to dysregulation in individuals at risk for SZ.

ALZHEIMER'S DISEASE

Another strategy to begin to resolve the ambiguity in the etiology of diseases not fully explained by heritable mutations was described in a recent study that directly compared iPSCs from familial and sporadic Alzheimer's disease (AD) patients (Israel et al., 2012). A late-stage neurodegenerative disease, AD induces widespread cellular pathology in both cortical and subcortical regions and is associated with the presence of neurofibrillary tangles and amyloid plaques identified in postmortem analyses. Familial forms of AD can result from a duplication in the amyloid-β precursor protein gene (*APP*). In this study, patient-derived iPSCs were generated from two patients with familial AD and two patients with sporadic AD. Interestingly, neurons generated from one of the sporadic AD patients showed a phenotypic similarity along a number of dimensions with both lines generated from the familial AD patient. All three lines exhibited increased levels of amyloid-β and phosphorylated tau, suggesting a mechanistic link between plaque and tangle formation. Strikingly, the line from the second sporadic AD patient exhibited none of these phenotypes and thus indicated the possibility of categorical discrimination of patients with sporadic AD based on a phenotypic profile. However, it remains an outstanding question whether the difference in cellular phenotypes from these two sporadic AD patients results from distinct mechanisms or instead a variable latency in the development of phenotypes in neurons differentiated from reprogrammed cells.

In relatively late-onset diseases such as AD and even SZ, a critical question is the nature and duration of the prodromal period. At what point is cellular or systems-level pathology discernible? And is there a critical window, before the onset of deterministic pathological development, when successful intervention is possible? This is a particularly salient issue with respect to newly differentiated human neurons as cellular pathology may not be present in cells that have not been sufficiently challenged by exogenous or endogenous demands. Although we are fully capturing the static genetic background of patients, culturing derived human neurons in a dish cannot recapitulate the dynamic conditions of a mature human brain, either in terms of acute environmental demands or the trajectory of its past history. It is an open and important question how the developmental timeline in cultured human neurons maps onto the endogenous state of *in vivo* neuronal development. In this respect, one of the potential advantages of direct programming to neurons or neural stem cells is that differentiated neurons may, in fact, retain age-specific features of the donor material (Saha and Jaenisch, 2009), while differentiation of iPSCs may most closely recapitulate embryonic development due to a complete resetting of the cellular clock. Although a comparison between iPSCs and direct induction of neurons from fibroblasts of a single patient has yet to be tested in a late-onset disease model, direct conversion of skin fibroblasts from sporadic and familial AD patients was recently reported (Qiang et al., 2011). Familial AD-induced neurons revealed deficits in the processing of the amyloid precursor protein and increased production of amyloid-β, caused by a dominant mutation in the *Presenilin-1* gene, characteristic features associated with AD pathology. It remains to be seen whether direct conversion will have any advantage in modeling age-dependent disease mechanisms, but this is a rapidly developing area of research and one of the many strategies being pursued to optimize cellular reprogramming.

MODELING PSYCHIATRIC DISORDERS IN NONHUMAN ANIMALS

Moving forward, reprogramming technology should be integrated with *in vivo* animal experimentation to build dynamic models of disease etiology and a platform to evaluate the efficacy of proposed treatment. To maximize the potential of stem cells to inform our understanding of disease mechanisms, we should work to apply knowledge gained from cellular analyses toward a systems-level inquiry of how pathology in neural components can affect global brain function. And conversely, we will need to identify how to engineer targeted rescue of disease phenotypes, while leaving normally functioning systems intact. Nonhuman animal models will be vital to this effort and can provide a means to evaluate basic properties of neural stem cells and progenitors in the mature brain.

IN VIVO TRANSPLANTATION

One of the most often discussed benefits of patient-specific cellular reprogramming is the potential for cellular replacement with minimal risk of immune rejection. Undoubtedly, this holds great promise for any number of human diseases that affect tissues with relatively homogenous cellular distribution and function. For disorders of the central nervous system, however, the vast heterogeneity of cell type and widespread anatomical distribution of deeply integrated functional systems may preclude the straightforward replacement of affected neural populations. For many predominantly psychiatric diseases, we do not yet know the extent of the causally relevant pathology, nor do we have a strategy for directing integration of exogenous populations to distributed loci within the brain.

But *in vivo* transplantation of derived human neurons in animal models is an important step in the full characterization of neuronal function. The ability of stem cells and progenitors to differentiate and integrate in situ not only will be critical for cell engineering in therapeutic applications but also will provide another level of analysis to identify disease-relevant phenotypes. By introducing patient-specific neural precursors to the developing or mature brains of rodents or nonhuman primates, we may be able to observe latent phenotypes that were not readily apparent in cell culture conditions. Further, we will be able to expose transplanted neurons to physiological stressors in an intact animal model to investigate the impact of environmental conditions on genetically mediated disease risk. To date, several studies have provided proof of principle to demonstrate that transplanted neural stem cells and progenitors are capable of differentiation into mature neurons with signature properties of effective synaptic signaling and targeting. In a stroke model, neuroepithelial-like stem cells derived from adult human iPSCs were transplanted to either the cortex or striatum and the grafted cells differentiated into several neuronal subtypes including GABAergic interneurons and projection neurons (Oki et al., 2012). Neural precursors from HD patient iPSCs have also been successfully grafted into adult mice and rat brains, and initial characterizations showed immunohistological evidence of mature neurons (Jeon et al., 2012; Juopperi et al., 2012).

ENDOGENOUS NEUROGENESIS AS A MODEL SYSTEM

In addition to providing a host system to interrogate *in vivo* functionality of human neurons, nonhuman animals also provide an empirically tractable system in which to explore the basic properties of endogenous neurogenesis. Because adult neurogenesis mirrors embryonic neurodevelopment on a dilated timescale, it is more amenable to systematic investigation of intracellular and niche signaling pathways. As an *in vivo* cellular model, adult neurogenesis has been effectively used to explore neurodevelopmental mechanisms of psychiatric disease. This model has been most extensively characterized with respect to the schizophrenia risk gene, *DISC1*. Accruing evidence implicates *DISC1* in a wide range of neurodevelopmental processes. During embryonic neuronal development, knockdown of *DISC1* can lead to premature exit from cell cycle and early differentiation, reducing the proliferative capacity of neural progenitors (Mao et al., 2009) and disorganization of dendritic arbors in the developing cerebral cortex (Kamiya et al., 2005). In adult hippocampal neurogenesis, *DISC1* interacts with several binding partners to regulate several aspects of neuronal development. Effects on proliferation of neural progenitors are mediated through the GSk3β-signaling pathway (Mao et al., 2009). Interaction with KIAA1212/Girdin impacts several morphological phenotypes, including soma size, primary dendrite formation, dendritic length, and migration patterns (Enomoto et al., 2009; Kim et al., 2009). Direct interactions of DISC1 with NDEL1 and FEZ1 each lead to a complementary, nonoverlapping subset of phenotypes (Duan et al., 2007; Kang et al., 2011). Globally, *DISC1* acts as a negative regulator of neuronal and dendritic development during the temporally extended time course of adult neurogenesis. Knockdown of *DISC1* in proliferating cells results in the acceleration and overshoot of neuronal development *in vivo*, an effect that is at least partially mediated by concomitant levels of GABAergic signaling (Kim et al., 2012). Systematic investigation of the *DISC1*-signaling pathways during adult neurogenesis provides important mechanistic information about the potential role of this gene in risk for disease pathology that can subsequently be probed in human neurons derived from patients and "at-risk" family members. Further, it is possible to identify novel synergistic or epistatic genetic interactions within a single signal transduction pathway that may begin to explain the variable penetrance of many risk genes and "missing heritability" observed in many genome-wide association studies (Eichler et al., 2010).

CHALLENGES FOR MODELING PSYCHIATRIC DISORDERS

Tremendous progress has been made in the effort to generate renewable sources of human neurons for mechanistic investigation of psychiatric disease, but many significant challenges remain. With the publication of each new study, the field evolves, and new information emerges about critical variables that may influence effective reprogramming, neuronal generation, and the variability in iPSCs, all of which could impact the investigation of disease-specific and patient-invariant phenotypes necessary for the development of widely applicable therapeutic approaches.

During embryonic development, epigenetic mechanisms constrain and direct cell fate, transforming totipotent stem cells into lineage-specific progenitors and, ultimately, terminally differentiated cell types. A goal of cellular reprogramming is to erase the epigenetic signature of the source tissue, creating a cellular tabula rasa from which researchers can direct fate specification to the desired cell type. However, several studies have shown that iPSCs can retain DNA methylation signatures similar to the tissue of fibroblast origin, indicating incomplete reprogramming (Plath and Lowry, 2011). ESCs remain the standard against which iPSCs are measured to evaluate pluripotency and unbiased potential for differentiation. Characterizing the extent of residual genetic and epigenetic somatic memory in iPSCs remains an ongoing challenge, but efforts are being made to directly compare those generated from different somatic tissues and across independent laboratories to isolate sources of variability (Boulting et al., 2011).

While differentiation capacity may be largely impacted by the extent of reprogramming, the optimization of specific protocols to direct targeted differentiation is also still very much a work in progress. Researchers are just beginning to refine differentiation protocols to enrich specific cell populations and have demonstrated successful generation of GABAergic, glutamatergic, dopaminergic, and layer-specific cortical neurons as well as astrocytes and oligodendrocytes (Hansen et al., 2011). However, many of these studies have only been able to bias differentiation toward the desired fate, resulting in a mixed population that could still require an additional step to isolate homogenous populations for studies of cell-autonomous phenotypes. But in the investigation of psychiatric disease, identification of genetically mediated, cell-autonomous pathology should be countered by an equally vigorous attempt to understand dysfunction within integrated neural networks. One approach will be to pursue *in vivo* transplantation strategies, but another would be to develop small-scale models of neuronal interactions *in vitro*. By modeling features of endogenous cell distributions in a given brain region, it may be possible to isolate discrete signaling defects between specific neural subtypes and begin to approximate physiological conditions.

Certainly, this represents one of the most significant challenges looking forward—how to ask the right questions so that we can observe signatures of neuronal dysfunction *in vitro* that may be relevant to disease etiology. Newly differentiated human neurons *in vitro* exist in an environment that is temporally and spatially distinct from the system we are trying to understand. Many of the specific phenotypes observed thus far in patient-derived iPSCs are remarkably congruent with data from animal models or postmortem studies and support current working hypotheses. However, many of the patient-derived neurons exhibit minimal or unexpected phenotpyes when compared with controls. But our current methodological tools may not have the resolution and sensitivity to detect all the environmental influences on cellular function, which properties are specific to neurons in a dish versus neurons in a brain, and how the history and age of the neuron affects its function. In addition to the procedural challenges facing all researchers invested in cellular reprogramming, investigators of psychiatric disorders are additionally challenged in using *de novo* human neurons to investigate a biological system that can store and retrieve information for decades, a system in which function is often measured by the capacity for both constitutive plasticity and long-term memory.

CONCLUSION

Both conceptually and empirically, there is a huge chasm between traditional animal models of psychiatric illness and the limited range of information we have been able to garner from studies of patients and postmortem analysis of human brains. Cellular reprogramming has enabled us to partially fill this gap by establishing a new intermediate level of investigation. Physicians often lament that for many neuropsychiatric disorders, their only option is to treat the symptoms of disease, as opposed to its underlying cause. Stem cell technology has the potential to transform this palliative approach to one in which novel therapies are generated from rational design based on causal mechanisms. It remains to be seen whether this field will live up to its promise and whether some of the most troubling issues can be resolved in order to enable revolutionary new therapies for patients. Also uncertain is the extent to which fundamental principles that evolve from a focus on the most prominent psychiatric disorders, namely, affective disorders, schizophrenia, and ASD, can be successfully applied to other disorders such as compulsive and dissociative disorders. In principle, generalization is possible, but for many of these less well-studied disorders, there is a paucity of data on putative risk genes, postmortem analyses, and validated behavioral correlates in animals, all of which are critical to the generation of testable hypotheses using patient-derived human neurons.

But what is appealing about the use of iPSCs and investigations of patient-specific human neurons is the possibility to redefine diagnostic criteria of disease based on a mechanistic understanding of the features underlying relevant pathology. Identification of etiological factors can inform the discussion over whether a categorical or dimensional approach to the diagnosis and treatment of patients is most efficacious. What has been missing in this debate over the years is a mechanistic understanding of symptomatology that may transcend traditional boundaries of behavioral categorization. And it is likely that the granularity of analysis will change the more we understand the mechanisms. For example, positive and negative symptoms of schizophrenia may have different neural substrates, but the negative symptoms may be mechanistically similar to features of depressive disorders. Stem cell researchers should build upon this diagnostic framework to test discrete hypotheses regarding neural structure and function while adopting an agnostic stance toward the possibility of shared mechanisms among categorically distinct diseases.

De novo generation of human neurons that are isogenic to patients reflects a remarkable achievement and a putative turning point in our attempt to understand human neurological diseases. But mental illness is humbling in its complexity, and we are a long way from being able to answer the questions posed at the outset of this chapter. Nor can we expect that iPSCs will provide the consummate solution. We will not be able to delineate the phenomenology of mental illness by investigating neurons in a dish. Psychiatric disorders are often characterized by complex deficits such an impairment in exerting volitional control over behavior, the persistence of aberrant sensory processing, or maladaptive responses to external demands. We cannot expect that investigations of dissociated human neurons will be able to provide a comprehensive explanation for what is ultimately an embodied phenomenon, and it is a mistake to presume that a cell-based reductionist strategy will be able to capture all the relevant features of psychiatric disease. Our brains are composed of neurons and glia and a rich milieu of chemical neurotransmitters and modulators. What cellular reprogramming has given us is a means to examine the building blocks of the human brain to search for patient-invariant phenotypes and molecular mechanisms associated with complex diseases. For the first time, we can generate and manipulate human neurons that have confirmed disease-relevant genetic profiles. While the majority of psychiatric diseases may not be immediately amenable to cell-replacement strategies, there is a wealth of information to be gleaned from an understanding of the basic mechanisms. The promise of this technology is nearly boundless, and it is our sincere hope that the excitement, innovation, and productivity expressed by researchers thus far will continue to grow and contribute to a better understanding of how dysfunction of neural components and processes can lead to some of the most devastating ailments. Most importantly, we may learn how to reverse or prevent dysfunction to alleviate the suffering of people who have limited information about why or how their symptoms emerge. A better mechanistic understanding of mental illness will not only enable the development of new therapeutic approaches but will also help affirm that these diseases are the consequence of specific neural pathology and dysregulation of discrete neural processes.

DISCLOSURES

Dr. Christian has no conflicts of interest to disclose and receives funding from the Brain & Behavior Research Foundation.

Dr. Song is a consultant for Roche and receives funding from NIH and the Simons Foundation Research Initiative.

Dr. Ming has no conflicts of interest to disclose and receives funding from NIH, Maryland Stem Cell Research Fund, and the Brain & Behavior Research Foundation.

REFERENCES

Aimone, J.B., Deng, W., et al. (2011). Resolving new memories: a critical look at the dentate gyrus, adult neurogenesis, and pattern separation. *Neuron* 70:589–596.

Altman, J., and Das, G.D. (1965). Autoradiographic and histological evidence of postnatal hippocampal neurogenesis in rats. *J. Comp. Neurol.* 124:319–335.

Ambasudhan, R., Talantova, M., et al. (2011). Direct reprogramming of adult human fibroblasts to functional neurons under defined conditions. *Cell Stem Cell* 9:113–118.

An, M.C., Zhang, N., et al. (2012). Genetic correction of Huntington's disease phenotypes in induced pluripotent stem cells. *Cell Stem Cell* 11:253–263.

Ananiev, G., Williams, E.C., et al. (2011). Isogenic pairs of wild type and mutant induced pluripotent stem cell (iPSC) lines from Rett syndrome patients as *in vitro* disease model. *PLoS One* 6, e25255.

Boulting, G.L., Kiskinis, E., et al. (2011). A functionally characterized test set of human induced pluripotent stem cells. *Nat. Biotechnol.* 29:279–286.

Brennand, K.J., Simone, A., et al. (2011). Modelling schizophrenia using human induced pluripotent stem cells. *Nature* 473:221–225.

Brennand, K.J., Simone, A., et al. (2012). Modeling psychiatric disorders at the cellular and network levels. *Mol. Psychiatry* 17:1239–1253.

Chahrour, M., and Zoghbi, H.Y. (2007). The story of Rett syndrome: from clinic to neurobiology. *Neuron* 56:422–437.

Chambers, S.M., and Studer, L. (2011). Cell fate plug and play: direct reprogramming and induced pluripotency. *Cell* 145:827–830.

Cheung, A.Y., Horvath, L.M., et al. (2011). Isolation of MECP2-null Rett Syndrome patient hiPS cells and isogenic controls through X-chromosome inactivation. *Hum. Mol. Genet.* 20:2103–2115.

Chiang, C.H., Su, Y., et al. (2011). Integration-free induced pluripotent stem cells derived from schizophrenia patients with a DISC1 mutation. *Mol. Psychiatry* 16:358–360.

Christian, K., Song, H., et al. (2010). Adult neurogenesis as a cellular model to study schizophrenia. *Cell Cycle* 9:636–637.

Cooper, O., Seo, H., et al. (2012). Pharmacological rescue of mitochondrial deficits in iPSC-derived neural cells from patients with familial Parkinson's disease. *Sci. Transl. Med.* 4:141–190.

Dolmetsch, R., and Geschwind, D.H. (2011). The human brain in a dish: the promise of iPSC-derived neurons. *Cell* 145:831–834.

Duan, X., Chang, J.H., et al. (2007). Disrupted-In-Schizophrenia 1 regulates integration of newly generated neurons in the adult brain. *Cell* 130:1146–1158.

Eichler, E.E., Flint, J., et al. (2010). Missing heritability and strategies for finding the underlying causes of complex disease. *Nat. Rev. Genet.* 11:446–450.

Enomoto, A., Asai, N., et al. (2009). Roles of disrupted-in-schizophrenia 1-interacting protein girdin in postnatal development of the dentate gyrus. *Neuron* 63:774–787.

Gage, F.H. (2000). Mammalian neural stem cells. *Science* 287:1433–1438.

Gottlieb, D.I. (2002). Large-scale sources of neural stem cells. *Annu. Rev. Neurosci.* 25:381–407.

Green, E.K., Grozeva, D., et al. (2010). The bipolar disorder risk allele at CACNA1C also confers risk of recurrent major depression and of schizophrenia. *Mol. Psychiatry* 15:1016–1022.

Guy, J., Gan, J., et al. (2007). Reversal of neurological defects in a mouse model of Rett syndrome. *Science* 315:1143–1147.

Han, D.W., Tapia, N., et al. (2012). Direct reprogramming of fibroblasts into neural stem cells by defined factors. *Cell Stem Cell* 10:465–472.

Hansen, D.V., Rubenstein, J.L., et al. (2011). Deriving excitatory neurons of the neocortex from pluripotent stem cells. *Neuron* 70:645–660.

The HD iPSC Consortium. (2012). Induced pluripotent stem cells from patients with Huntington's disease show CAG-repeat-expansion-associated phenotypes. *Cell Stem Cell* 11:264–278.

Israel, M.A., Yuan, S.H., et al. (2012). Probing sporadic and familial Alzheimer's disease using induced pluripotent stem cells. *Nature* 482:216–220.

Jeon, I., Lee, N., et al. (2012). Neuronal properties, *in vivo* effects and pathology of a Huntington's disease patient-derived induced pluripotent stem cells. *Stem Cells* 30:2054–2062.

Jiang, H., Ren, Y., et al. (2012). Parkin controls dopamine utilization in human midbrain dopaminergic neurons derived from induced pluripotent stem cells. *Nat. Commun.* 3:668.

Johnstone, M., Thomson, P.A., et al. (2011). DISC1 in schizophrenia: genetic mouse models and human genomic imaging. *Schizophr. Bull.* 37:14–20.

Juopperi, T.A., Kim, W.R., et al. (2012). Astrocytes generated from patient induced pluripotent stem cells recapitulate features of Huntington's disease patient cells. *Mol. Brain* 5:17.

Kamiya, A., Kubo, K., et al. (2005). A schizophrenia-associated mutation of DISC1 perturbs cerebral cortex development. *Nat. Cell Biol.* 7:1167–1178.

Kang, E., Burdick, K.E., et al. (2011). Interaction between FEZ1 and DISC1 in regulation of neuronal development and risk for schizophrenia. *Neuron* 72:559–571.

Kim, J., Efe, J.A., et al. (2011a). Direct reprogramming of mouse fibroblasts to neural progenitors. *Proc. Natl. Acad. Sci. USA* 108:7838–7843.

Kim, J.Y., Duan, X., et al. (2009). DISC1 regulates new neuron development in the adult brain via modulation of AKT-mTOR signaling through KIAA1212. *Neuron* 63:761–773.

Kim, J.Y., Liu, C.Y., et al. (2012). Interplay between DISC1 and GABA signaling regulates neurogenesis in mice and risk for schizophrenia. *Cell* 148:1051–1064.

Kim, K.Y., Hysolli, E., et al. (2011b). Neuronal maturation defect in induced pluripotent stem cells from patients with Rett syndrome. *Proc. Natl. Acad. Sci. USA* 108:14169–14174.

Lee, G., Papapetrou, E.P., et al. (2009). Modelling pathogenesis and treatment of familial dysautonomia using patient-specific iPSCs. *Nature* 461:402–406.

Liu, J., Koscielska, K.A., et al. (2012). Signaling defects in iPSC-derived fragile X premutation neurons. *Hum. Mol. Genet.* 21:3795–3805.

Lujan, E., Chanda, S., et al. (2012). Direct conversion of mouse fibroblasts to self-renewing, tripotent neural precursor cells. *Proc. Natl. Acad. Sci. USA* 109:2527–2532.

Mao, Y., Ge, X., et al. (2009). Disrupted in schizophrenia 1 regulates neuronal progenitor proliferation via modulation of GSK3beta/beta-catenin signaling. *Cell* 136:1017–1031.

Marchetto, M.C., Carromeu, C., et al. (2010). A model for neural development and treatment of Rett syndrome using human induced pluripotent stem cells. *Cell* 143:527–539.

Martin, I., Dawson, V.L., et al. (2011). Recent advances in the genetics of Parkinson's disease. *Annu. Rev. Genomics Hum. Genet.* 12:301–325.

Mekhoubad, S., Bock, C., et al. (2012). Erosion of dosage compensation impacts human iPSC disease modeling. *Cell Stem Cell* 10:595–609.

Nguyen, H.N., Byers, B., et al. (2011). LRRK2 mutant iPSC-derived DA neurons demonstrate increased susceptibility to oxidative stress. *Cell Stem Cell* 8:267–280.

Nyegaard, M., Demontis, D., et al. (2010). CACNA1C (rs1006737) is associated with schizophrenia. *Mol. Psychiatry* 15:119–121.

Oki, K., Tatarishvili, J., et al. (2012). Human-induced pluripotent stem cells form functional neurons and improve recovery after grafting in stroke-damaged brain. *Stem Cells* 30:1120–1133.

Pang, Z.P., Yang, N., et al. (2011). Induction of human neuronal cells by defined transcription factors. *Nature* 476:220–223.

Park, I.H., Zhao, R., et al. (2008). Reprogramming of human somatic cells to pluripotency with defined factors. *Nature* 451:141–146.

Pasca, S.P., Portmann, T., et al. (2011). Using iPSC-derived neurons to uncover cellular phenotypes associated with Timothy syndrome. *Nat. Med.* 17:1657–1662.

Plath, K., and Lowry, W.E. (2011). Progress in understanding reprogramming to the induced pluripotent state. *Nat Rev Genet* 12:253–265.

Pomp, O., Dreesen, O., et al. (2011). Unexpected X chromosome skewing during culture and reprogramming of human somatic cells can be alleviated by exogenous telomerase. *Cell Stem Cell* 9:156–165.

Porteous, D.J., Millar, J.K., et al. (2011). DISC1 at 10: connecting psychiatric genetics and neuroscience. *Trends Mol. Med.* 17:699–706.

Qiang, L., Fujita, R., et al. (2011). Directed conversion of Alzheimer's disease patient skin fibroblasts into functional neurons. *Cell* 146:359–371.

Ring, K.L., Tong, L.M., et al. (2012). Direct reprogramming of mouse and human fibroblasts into multipotent neural stem cells with a single factor. *Cell Stem Cell* 11:100–109.

Sachs, N.A., Sawa, A., et al. (2005). A frameshift mutation in Disrupted in Schizophrenia 1 in an American family with schizophrenia and schizoaffective disorder. *Mol. Psychiatry* 10:758–764.

Saha, K., and Jaenisch, R. (2009). Technical challenges in using human induced pluripotent stem cells to model disease. *Cell Stem Cell* 5:584–595.

Samuels, B.A., and Hen, R. (2011). Neurogenesis and affective disorders. *Eur. J. Neurosci.* 33:1152–1159.

Seibler, P., Graziotto, J., et al. (2011). Mitochondrial Parkin recruitment is impaired in neurons derived from mutant PINK1 induced pluripotent stem cells. *J. Neurosci.* 31:5970–5976.

Sheridan, S.D., Theriault, K.M., et al. (2011). Epigenetic characterization of the FMR1 gene and aberrant neurodevelopment in human induced pluripotent stem cell models of fragile X syndrome. *PLoS One* 6, e26203.

Soldner, F., Laganiere, J., et al. (2011). Generation of isogenic pluripotent stem cells differing exclusively at two early onset Parkinson point mutations. *Cell* 146:318–331.

Splawski, I., Timothy, K.W., et al. (2004). Ca(V)1.2 calcium channel dysfunction causes a multisystem disorder including arrhythmia and autism. *Cell* 119:19–31.

Takahashi, K., Tanabe, K., et al. (2007). Induction of pluripotent stem cells from adult human fibroblasts by defined factors. *Cell* 131:861–872.

Takahashi, K., and Yamanaka, S. (2006). Induction of pluripotent stem cells from mouse embryonic and adult fibroblast cultures by defined factors. *Cell* 126:663–676.

Tchieu, J., Kuoy, E., et al. (2010). Female human iPSCs retain an inactive X chromosome. *Cell Stem Cell* 7:329–342.

Thier, M., Worsdorfer, P., et al. (2012). Direct conversion of fibroblasts into stably expandable neural stem cells. *Cell Stem Cell* 10:473–479.

Thomson, J.A., Itskovitz-Eldor, J., et al. (1998). Embryonic stem cell lines derived from human blastocysts. *Science* 282:1145–1147.

Tomoda, K., Takahashi, K., et al. (2012). Derivation conditions impact x-inactivation status in female human induced pluripotent stem cells. *Cell Stem Cell* 11:91–99.

Tropea, D., Giacometti, E., et al. (2009). Partial reversal of Rett Syndrome-like symptoms in MeCP2 mutant mice. *Proc. Natl. Acad. Sci. USA* 106:2029–2034.

Vaccarino, F.M., Stevens, H.E., et al. (2011). Induced pluripotent stem cells: a new tool to confront the challenge of neuropsychiatric disorders. *Neuropharmacology* 60:1355–1363.

Vierbuchen, T., Ostermeier, A., et al. (2010). Direct conversion of fibroblasts to functional neurons by defined factors. *Nature* 463:1035–1041.

Yoo, A.S., Sun, A.X., et al. (2011). MicroRNA-mediated conversion of human fibroblasts to neurons. *Nature* 476:228–231.

Yu, J., Vodyanik, M.A., et al. (2007). Induced pluripotent stem cell lines derived from human somatic cells. *Science* 318:1917–1920.

10 | OPTOGENETIC TECHNOLOGIES FOR PSYCHIATRIC DISEASE RESEARCH: CURRENT STATUS AND CHALLENGES

LIEF E. FENNO AND KARL DEISSEROTH

INTRODUCTION

Studying intact systems with simultaneous local precision and global scope is a fundamental challenge in biology. This familiar tradeoff leads to important conceptual and experimental difficulties in psychiatric disease research and, indeed, throughout the study of complex biological systems. Part of a solution may arise from the technology of optogenetics: the combination of genetic and optical methods to achieve gain- or loss-of-function of temporally defined events in specific cells embedded within intact living tissue or organisms (Deisseroth, 2010; Deisseroth et al., 2006, 2011, 2012; Fenno et al., 2011; Scanziani and Häuser, 2009). Such precise causal control within the functioning intact system can be achieved via introduction of genes that confer to cells both light detection capability and specific effector function. For example, microbial opsin genes can be expressed in mammalian neurons to mediate millisecond precision and reliable elicitation or inhibition of action potential firing in response to light pulses, while hybrid opsin receptor proteins called optoXRs can recruit defined biochemical signaling pathways in response to light (Fig. 10.1; recent primers on this methodology have been published [Yizhar et al., 2011a; Zhang et al., 2011]).

This approach has now been used to control neuronal activity in a wide range of animals, resulting in insights into fundamental aspects of circuit function, as well as circuit dysfunction and treatment in pathological states (Deisseroth, 2012; Tye et al., 2012). Here we review the current state of optogenetics for neuroscience and psychiatry and address the evolving challenges and future opportunities. Despite both rapid growth and wide scope of applications, fundamental challenges remain to be addressed.

BACKGROUND: CURRENT FUNCTIONALITY OF TOOLS

Diverse and elegant mechanisms have evolved to enable organisms to harvest light for survival functions. For example, opsin genes encode 7-transmembrane (TM) proteins that (when bound to the small organic chromophore all-*trans* retinal) constitute light-sensitive rhodopsins, which are found across all kingdoms of life (Fenno et al., 2011). Many prokaryotes employ these proteins to control proton gradients and to maintain membrane potential and ionic homeostasis, and many motile microorganisms have evolved opsin-based photoreceptors to modulate flagellar motors and thereby direct phototaxis toward environments with optimal light intensities for photosynthesis. Owing to their structural simplicity (both light-sensing and effector domains are encoded within a single gene) and fast kinetics, microbial opsins can be treated as precise and modular photosensitization components for introduction into non–light sensitive cells to enable rapid optical control of specific cellular processes. For example, channelrhodopsins (Fig. 10.1, left) such as ChR2 induce nonselective cationic photocurrents in response to illumination, resulting in a net depolarization and spike firing in neurons, first demonstrated in 2005 (Boyden et al., 2005). Halorhodopsins (Fig. 10.1, middle; NpHR) conduct chloride, and bacteriorhodopsin and related opsins conduct protons (not shown) in response to illumination, both hyperpolarizing neurons (Chow et al., 2010; Zhang et al., 2007, 2011) reviewed in Mattis et al., 2012; Yizhar et al., 2011a). Many other nonopsin classes of naturally occurring protein have been explored as well, including flavin chromophore-utilizing light-activated adenylyl cyclases, as well as artificially engineered systems in which light sensation modules become physically linked to effector modules (Airan et al., 2009; Gulyani et al., 2012; Möglich and Moffat, 2007; Stierl et al., 2011; Wu et al., 2009).

The relatively small number of initial genomically identified opsins has now been dwarfed by an ever-increasing portfolio of derivatives designed to manipulate peak wavelength, current magnitude, and inactivation time constant (τ_{off}). τ_{off} is an intrinsic property that describes the time taken for an opsin to spontaneously relax from the conducting state to the nonconducting state after the cessation of light. The τ_{off} of ChR2 is ~12 ms whereas (e.g.) that of the mutant ChR2-H134R is approximately doubled (Mattis et al., 2012; Fig. 10.2); this property in part determines the maximum frequency at which a neuron may produce precisely timed light-initiated action potentials (Gunaydin et al., 2010; Mattis et al., 2012). Indeed, an opportunity was seen to speed up optogenetic control function by modulating τ_{off}; destabilizing the open state of the channel could lead to a more rapid spontaneous reversion to the nonconducting state of ChR2 following light cessation, thereby increasing the frequency ceiling for driving

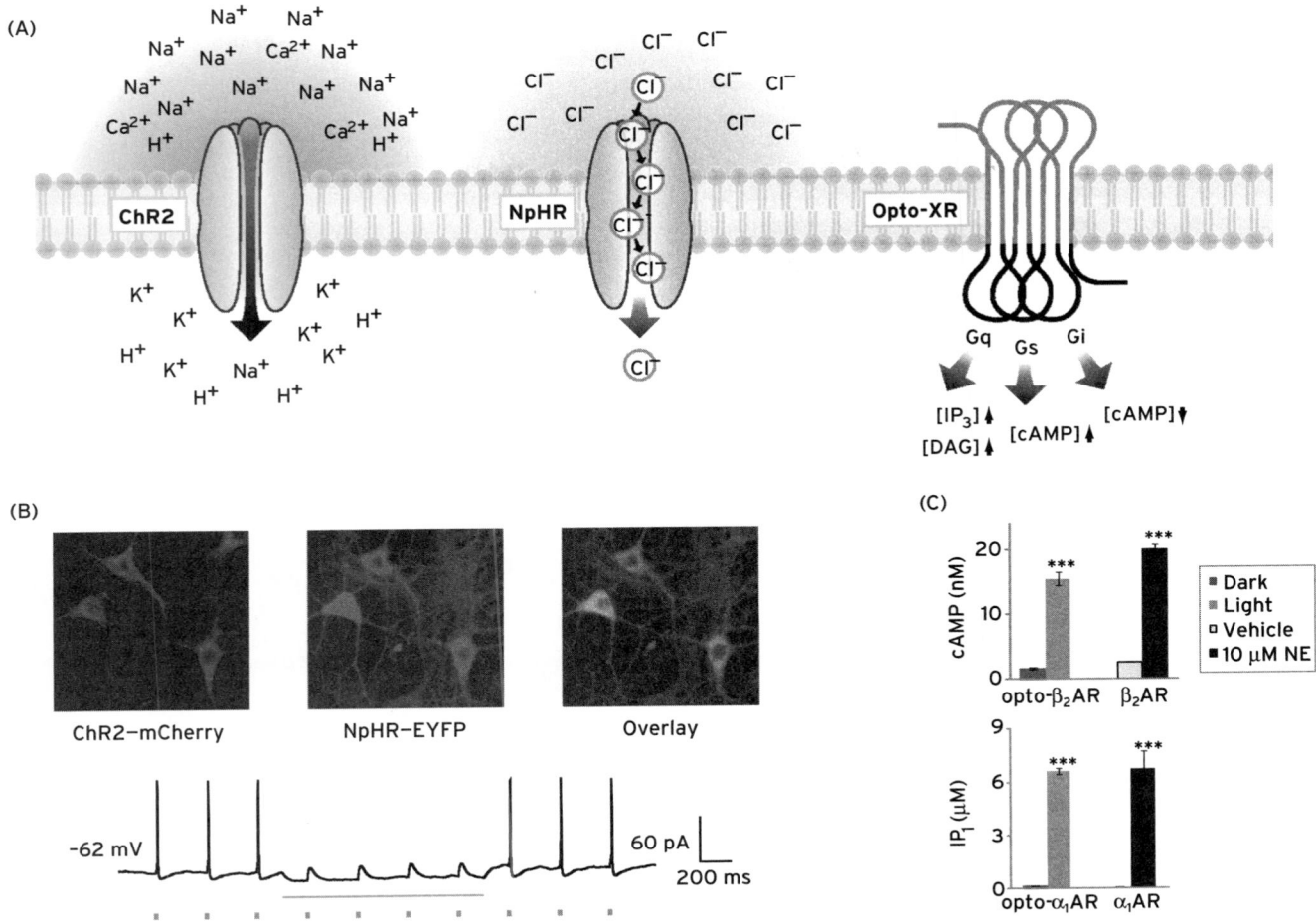

Figure 10.1 Optogenetic tool families. (A) Channelrhodopsins (left), such as ChR2, induce nonselective cationic photocurrents in response to illumination, resulting in a net depolarization and spike firing in neurons. Halorhodopsins (middle; NpHR) conduct chloride, and bacteriorhodopsin and related opsins conduct protons (not shown) in response to illumination, both hyperpolarizing neurons. The optoXRs (right) are chimeric proteins that elicit biochemical signal cascades in response to illumination. The specific biochemical cascade is determined by the source of the intracellular loops. (B) Whole-cell patch clamp response of a neuron expressing both ChR2 and NpHR. Pulses of dark gray light activate ChR2 and induce sufficient depolarizing photocurrent to produce action potentials whereas dark gray light induces an inward chloride current that hyperpolarizes the neuron and prevents firing. (C) Response of HEK cells expressing optoβ2 or native β2 adrenergic receptor (top), or optoα1 or native α1 adrenergic receptor (bottom). Production of downstream biochemical effectors is similar in magnitude from optical stimulation of optoXRs (left) and agonist-induced response in native receptors (right). (Panel A adapted from Fenno et al., 2011; panel B adapted from Zhang et al., 2007; panel C adapted from Airan et al., 2009.)

neurons—an especially important consideration for some classes of fast-spiking inhibitory interneurons, including those expressing parvalbumin (PV). By applying observations in the bacteriorhodopsin literature to ChR2 based on the high degree of homology among Type I rhodopsins, it was found that shifting a single amino acid residue was sufficient to approximately halve the τ_{off} (ChETA; Gunaydin et al., 2010; Mattis et al., 2012), thereby increasing the top high-fidelity frequency to at least 200 Hz and increasing overall performance. A separate creative approach to creating a channelrhodopsin with a rapid τ_{off} arose from chimeras of ChR1 and ChR2 (ChEF/ChIEF) (Lin et al., 2009; Mattis et al., 2012) (Fig. 10.2).

Opsins optimized for rapid closure and high-frequency stimulation are complemented by ChR2 variants designed to induce prolonged depolarization after light cessation. The engineering approach to design these proteins also took advantage of homology between ChR2 and BR to produce variants

that stabilize, as opposed to destabilize, the active retinal conformer. These "step function opsins" (SFO) allow precise induction and inactivation of a depolarizing current "step" into the population of neurons, the duration of which is dependent upon the particular mutation (C128S: 100s, Berndt et al., 2008; D156A: 6.9 min, Bamann et al., 2008; C128S/D156A: 29 min [stabilized step function opsins/SSFOs], Yizhar et al., 2011b) (Fig. 10.2). As these are derivatives of ChR2, they are activated by blue (470 nm) light. This depolarizing step can then be terminated with yellow light (590 nm), which drives the opsin to its resting state. In the case of SSFO, the most stable of the SFOs, the depolarization step occurs without crossing the sodium channel activation threshold, which has the useful effect of modestly sensitizing a population of neurons to incoming excitatory input.

One additional benefit of an extended τ_{off} is that the cell expressing the protein may effectively act as a photon

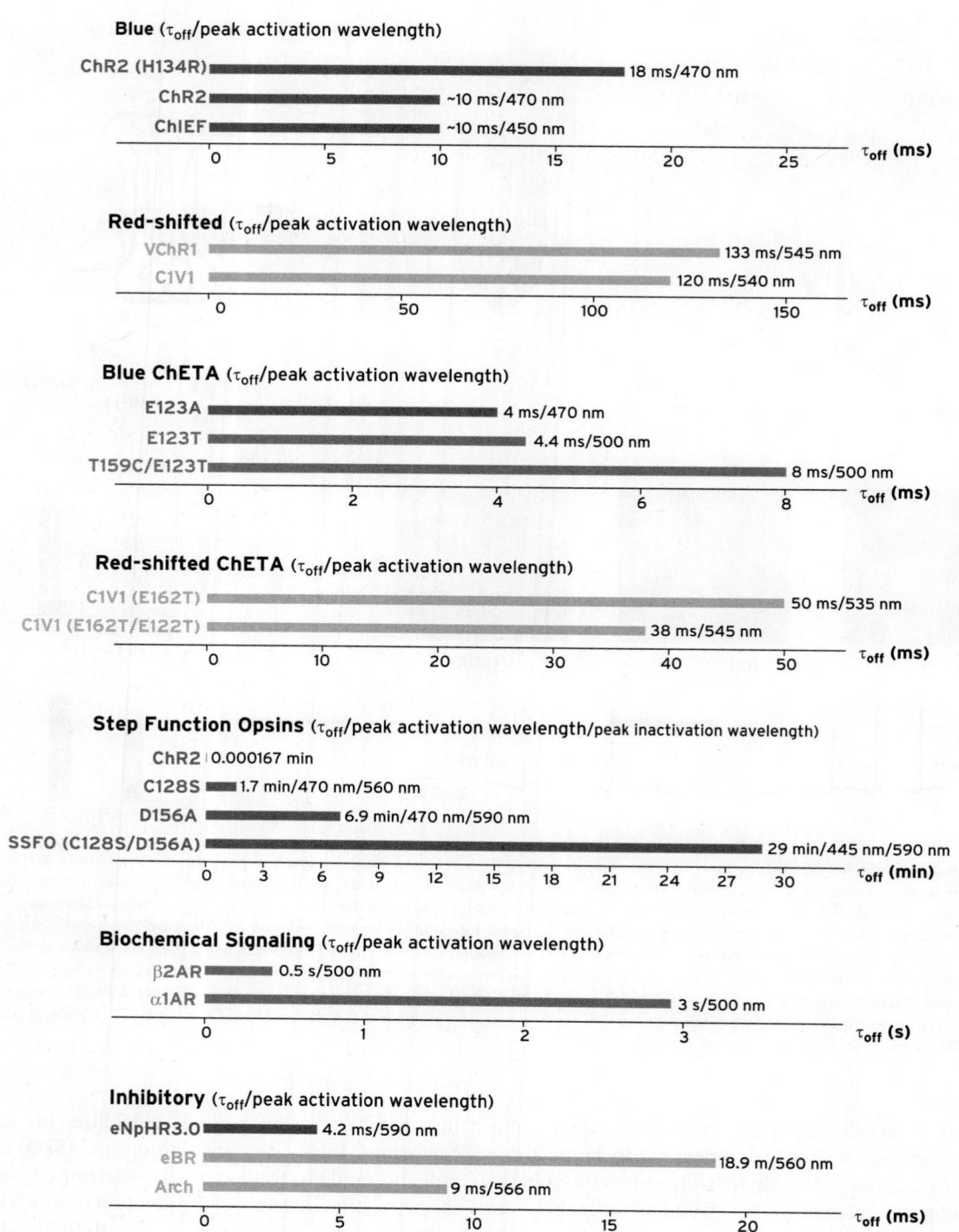

Figure 10.2 Properties of optogenetic tools. Deactivation time constants. (τ_{off}) and activation/inactivation wavelengths are illustrated for comparison purposes and as a look-up table. ChR2 is grouped with step function opsins for scale purposes. Decay kinetics were measured where precise published values were not available. Values from room temperature except for optoXRs (37°C). (Adapted from Fenno et al., 2011.)

integrator: in the case of SSFO, once a channel has been activated, it remains open for a period approximately 150,000 times longer than native ChR2 (Yizhar et al., 2011b). The implication of cellular photon integration is that the total number of photons needed to induce a maximal photocurrent in the cell may be spread over a longer period of time (in contrast to stimulation parameters of ChR2 that require a high density of photons in order to activate enough channels to move the neuron

beyond action potential threshold). In the context of behavioral neuroscience, this property has been exploited to allow for extracerebral light delivery, obviating the need to implant fiber optic light delivery devices into animals for behavioral trials at depths of at least 2.8 mm (Yizhar et al., 2011b).

A second dimension into which considerable engineering resources have been invested is "red-shifting" the maximum excitation wavelength of channelrhodopsins. A tool that is sufficiently red activated might be able to be modulated independently of ChR2, thus allowing for the manipulation of multiple, independent populations of neurons within the same space (Yizhar et al., 2011b; Zhang et al., 2008). While both VChR1 and the recently described MChR1 are significantly red shifted relative to ChR2, VChR1 does not produce sufficient photocurrents to reliably drive suprathreshold events in neural populations, and the function of MChR1 in neurons has yet to be described (although data from other heterologous systems suggests that its currents will be similar in magnitude to VChR1; Govorunova et al., 2011). The most potent red-shifted channelrhodopsins currently available are not derived from any one organism but are chimaeras between ChR1 and VChR1 (C1V1); resulting currents are significantly larger than ChR2 (Mattis et al., 2012; Yizhar et al., 2011b), and action potentials may be elicited by even 630 nm red light (Yizhar et al., 2011b). In a recent series of experiments, C1V1 was shown to independently modulate cell bodies and terminals in the same tissue as neurons expressing ChR2 (experiments conducted in brain slice, in anesthetized ("optrode") recordings *in vivo*, and in awake, behaving animals (Yizhar et al., 2011b). Independent modulation of multiple populations is of immediate utility in understanding the dynamics of circuits and, indeed, has been used to examine independent inputs into thalamus as well as the interplay between pyramidal neurons and parvalbumin-expressing, fast-spiking interneurons in medial prefrontal cortex (mPFC; Yizhar et al., 2011b).

In summary, the explosion of channelrhodopsins, mutational variants, and chimaeras since the original introduction of ChRs into neurons in 2005 has included the engineering of tools differently specialized for increased photocurrent, for driving action potentials at high frequencies, for depolarizing neurons for extended periods in the absence of direct action potential generation, and for combinatorial control via red-shifting of excitation wavelength. However, while using channelrhodopsins to control the excitability of a population of neurons with fine temporal resolution allows neuroscientists to ask if the activity of a genetically and/or anatomically specified population of neurons is sufficient to cause a given outcome, the reverse side of this experimental coin is to ask if the activity of these elements is necessary for the outcome. To obtain direct evidence of necessity, a tool is required that is able to silence the activity of a targeted population of neurons while leaving others unaffected. The light-activated halorhodopsin (HR) is an electrogenic pump producing inward chloride flux that can hyperpolarize and thereby inhibit neurons (e.g., the HR from *Natronomonas pharaonis*, or NpHR; reviewed in Zhang et al., 2011). Optogenetic function of proton efflux pumps that can hyperpolarize neurons have since also been described (reviewed in Mattis et al., 2012; Zhang et al., 2011). Local environmental acidification can result from proton efflux; the consequence to neighboring neurons will require further investigation.

In addition to optically modulated mediators of neuronal membrane potential, a class of tools for optical control of biochemical signaling cascades (the optoXRs) now exist for temporally precise manipulation of G-Protein Coupled Receptor (GPCR) signaling cascades (Fig. 10.1). These chimeric proteins are composed of the light-sensing extracellular domain of the Type II mammalian rhodopsin and the intracellular domain of a given GPCR, for instance, α1 and β2 adrenergic receptors (G_q- and G_s-coupled, respectively; Airan et al., 2009; Kim et al., 2005), and 5-HT1a ($G_{i/o}$-coupled; Oh et al., 2010), and activate native signaling pathways in response to light. These receptors are activated by 500-nm light and are useful for control of biochemical signaling both *in vivo* (Airan et al., 2009) and *in vitro* (Airan et al., 2009; Kim et al, 2005; Oh et al., 2010).

As these examples show, the experimental potential of optogenetics has triggered a surge of genome prospecting and molecular engineering to expand the repertoire of tools and generate new functionality, in turn catalyzing further mechanistic studies of microbial proteins. High-resolution crystal structures are now available for all the major opsin classes (e.g., Kolbe et al., 2000), including most recently channelrhodopsin (ChR; Kato et al., 2012); this information has been of enormous value, not only for enhancing understanding of microbial opsin-based channels, but also for guiding optogenetics in the generation of variants with novel function related to spectrum, selectivity, and kinetics. The high-resolution, crystal-structural insights have also been used to help guide the assembly of light-sensitive modules together with effector modules into artificial proteins, thereby creating parallel information streams capable of carrying optogenetic control signals for modulation purposes (Gulyani et al., 2012; Möglich and Moffat, 2007).

CURRENT NEUROSCIENCE APPLICATIONS AND DISEASE MODELS

This diversity of optogenetic tool function will be important for making significant headway in our understanding both of normal brain function and of dysfunctional processes in neuropsychiatric disease (e.g., many disease states may relate to impaired interaction of multiple distinct cell- or projection types, pointing to the experimental value of achieving multiple-color excitation and multiple-color inhibition optogenetically within the same living mammalian brain) (Deisseroth, 2012; Tye et al., 2012). Indeed, recent years have already seen a swiftly growing wave of applications of optogenetics to questions in neuropsychiatric disease, with the deployment of millisecond precision optical excitation or inhibition of specific circuit elements within behaving mammals. Overall this line of work is very timely at the societal level; psychiatric disease represents the leading cause of disability worldwide, but major pharmaceutical companies are withdrawing from developing new treatments, and many are shutting down psychiatry programs—a situation with major medical, social, and economic implications. Reasons cited include the lack of neural circuit-level understanding of symptom states, which impairs identification of final common pathways for treatment and hobbles development of predictive animal models. Identification of simplifying hypotheses and unifying theories by optogenetic or other means is one of the most pressing needs and exciting avenues of research into neurological and psychiatric disease.

Optogenetic technology now exists in a special relationship with psychiatry because one of the unique and most versatile features of optogenetics (modulation of defined neural projections by fiberoptic-based "projection-targeting," in which cells are transduced with opsin in region A but illumination is delivered in region B where only a subset of the expressing cells from A send axonal projections; (Fig. 10.3; Gradinaru et al, 2007, 2009, 2010; Petreanu et al., 2007; Stuber et al., 2011; Tye et al., 2011; Yizhar et al., 2011a) is well aligned with what may be a core feature of psychiatric disease (altered function along pathways of neural communication). The fiberoptic neural interface not only allows this selective recruitment of cells defined by projection target, but also overcomes the depth limitations caused by light scattering, and allowed access to (and optogenetic control of) any brain region even in freely moving mammals. This device debuted in 2007 (Aravanis et al., 2007) and was first applied that year (Adamantidis et al., 2007) to address questions relevant to narcolepsy and sleep–wake transitions. Specific activity patterns were played into hypocretin neurons (genetically targeted by use of a cell type–specific promoter that was functional in an injected opsin-bearing viral vector) in the lateral hypothalamus in freely moving mice; certain patterns but not others were found to favor sleep–wake transitions, providing the first causal understanding of specific activity patterns in well-defined cells underlying mammalian behaviors.

Memory deficits (notably in working memory but also in aspects of long-term episodic or declarative memory) are seen in autism and schizophrenia but more prominently in cognitive impairment and dementia. The persistence of episodic memories is also highly relevant to posttraumatic stress disorder (PTSD) and other anxiety disorders, in which the memory can be a contextual fear memory. Recent work using optogenetics has now found that long-term contextual fear memories surprisingly involve both hippocampus and neocortex, even in the remote phase (Goshen et al., 2011); this work may help inform our understanding of PTSD and attempts to ameliorate the debilitating consequences of this disease. Other optogenetics-based studies have explored diverse aspects of fear memory formation and expression in amygdala, hippocampus, neocortex, and other neural circuits, in freely moving mammals (Ciocchi et al., 2010; Haubensak et al., 2010; Liu et al., 2012). Optogenetic methods have also been used to probe unconditioned anxiety, and a specific intra-amygdala pathway has been optogenetically resolved that appears to bidirectionally set anxiety expression level in real time as mammals behave (Tye et al., 2011).

An even more versatile cell type–targeting approach involves mouse Cre-driver lines in which the enzyme Cre-recombinase is expressed across generations as a transgene, only in targeted cells. Cre-dependent viruses are constructed and injected that will therefore express opsin only in the targeted (Cre-expressing) cells. This technique led to the first control of specific recombinase-targeted populations in freely moving mice (Tsai et al., 2009) via selective opsin expression in tyrosine hydroxylase–expressing (dopaminergic) neurons in the ventral tegmental area, to probe reward and conditioning. Cre targeting was also (in separate studies) used to control the cholinergic cells of the nucleus accumbens to identify a role for these neurons in cocaine conditioning (Witten et al., 2010), and to modulate the intriguing parvalbumin or fast-spiking inhibitory neurons (Sohal et al., 2009); prior pioneering work had shown that the parvalbumin neurons are altered in schizophrenia and had long been suggested to be involved in modulating certain kinds of brain rhythmicity such as gamma oscillations, which are also known to be abnormal in schizophrenia. Optogenetic studies were able to define a causal role of these neurons in the modulation of gamma oscillations, which in turn were found to modulate information flow within neocortical circuitry (Sohal et al., 2009).

Altered gamma oscillations are also seen in autism, another disorder (like schizophrenia) in which information processing and social function deficits are seen, although with a markedly different quality. A long-standing hypothesis in the field had been that elevated excitation–inhibition imbalance could give rise to social dysfunction of the kind seen in autism, but the physiology (unlike the genetics) had been difficult to test in a causal fashion. Optogenetic interventions were able to directly and causally implicate excitation–inhibition balance changes in setting up abnormal social function as well as giving rise to abnormal information processing and gamma oscillations (Yizhar et al., 2011b) of the kind seen in autism and schizophrenia.

While the above neocortical interventions did not discriminate among neocortical layers, it is presumed that pyramidal neurons of different layers play different roles in the circuit. To address this caveat, multiple studies have described the introduction of optogenetic tools using *in utero* electroporation (IUE), and IUE takes advantage of distinct temporal windows during which the pyramidal neurons of different cortical layers are born. With knowledge of when the neurons of a layer are produced, one may introduce an expression construct with a given optogenetic tool to target only that layer. This has been used with success in rodents (Adesnik and Scanziani, 2010; Gradinaru et al., 2007; Petreanu et al., 2009) to analyze the contribution of layer-specific pyramidal populations to neocortical information processing. Similar to transgenic mouse lines, constructs electroporated *in utero* are expressed at birth, allowing for acute slice preparation of young animals. One drawback of this strategy is lower expression level of the opsin, possibly due to reduced expression construct copy number.

IUE-introduced ChR2, in a recent study from Adesnik and Scanziani (2010), was integral to a description of the role of excitatory/inhibitory (E/I) interactions in layer-specific communication between and across cortical columns. Their approach to examining cortical circuitry involved introduction of ChR2 into layer 2/3 as well as use of a stimulating light ramp that increased in intensity over time. Driving excitation in layer 2/3 pyramidal neurons in this way with ChR2 was sufficient to induce gamma-band oscillations in nonexpressing cells from both inhibitory and excitatory classes, assessed by patch clamp. Using a simultaneous four-cell patch clamp, this group found that transmission of ChR2-driven excitation and inhibition across layers (vertically) in cortex was clearest from layer 2/3 to 5, and less so to 4 or 6.

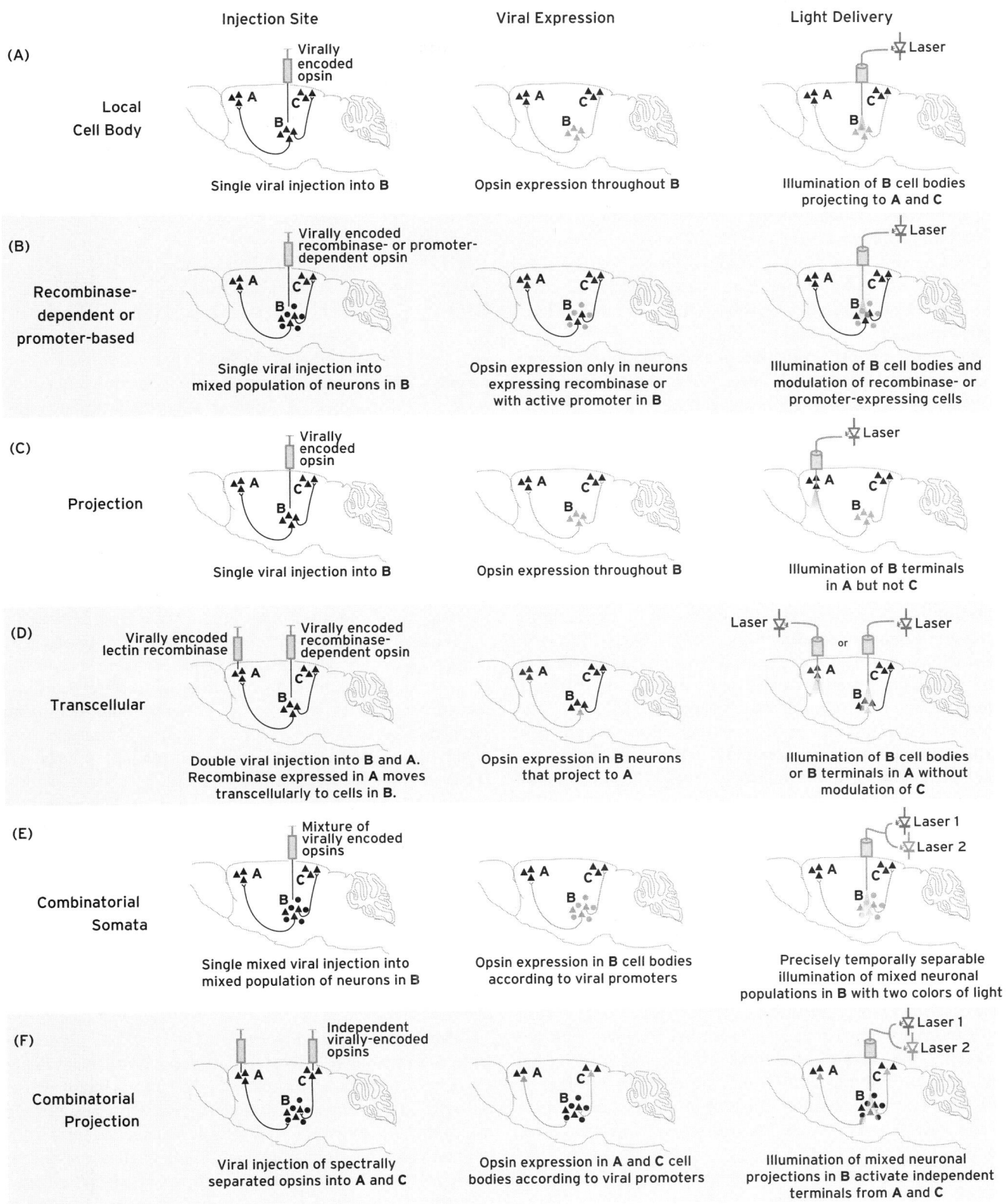

Figure 10.3 In vivo optogenetic targeting strategies. (A) Viral targeting of a neuron population based on promoter specificity followed by stimulation of the same area as the injection. (B) Viral targeting of a neuron population based on expression of Cre-recombinase followed by stimulation of the same area as the viral injection. (C) Viral targeting of a neuron population followed by stimulation of a downstream target region; note that this will likely be a subset of the total population of neurons expressing opsin. (D) Dual viral targeting of a downstream population with lectin-recombinase (e.g., WGA-CRE) and upstream injection of cre-dependent DIO virus followed by stimulation of either the somata or axons of opsin-expressing population. (E) Injection of multiple opsins expressed in separate populations within the same space based on promoter or recombinase-mediated specificity followed by multiwavelength stimulation at the somata. (F) Trans-synaptic or retrograde targeting of axons in two separate locations followed by central multiwavelength stimulation location to differentially modulate somata of neurons based on their projections. (Adapted from Yizhar et al., 2011.)

Additionally, checks and balances involving inhibition and excitation were found to be operative when spatially distinct subsets of cells expressing ChR2 were stimulated. Strikingly, when single cells in layer 2/3 were stimulated with current injection, photostimulation of nearby layer 2/3 cortical columns decreased induced spiking activity of the patched cell. In contrast, cells in layer 5 induced to spike with current injection saw a significant increase in firing rate during layer 2/3 photostimulation, which was reduced by lateral 2/3 excitation. In combination, it was found that layer 2/3 cells compete with layer 2/3 neighbors to drive cortical output via layer 5. These experiments utilized optogenetics to ask questions that could not be answered with other available neuroscience tools lacking this spatial and temporal specificity.

A distinct direct examination of the excitation/inhibition ratio imbalance in neocortex developed and employed novel ChR variants, including the "stabilized step function opsin" modified to remain in the activated state for >30 min after the introduction of blue light (but still inactivated using yellow light) (Yizhar et al., 2011a, b). Like other SFOs, the photocurrent generated by SSFO is subthreshold and thus does not directly generate action potentials by driving a neuron above threshold. Yizhar et al. combined the novel opsin variants and viral delivery to manipulate E/I cortical balance through expression of SSFO in either pyramidal neurons (via the specific promoter CaMKIIα to increase E) or in parvalbumin expressing inhibitory interneurons (using a DIO-SSFO virus in combination with PV::Cre transgenic mouse to increase I). It was found that baseline gamma-band activity was increased in response to E/I elevation, even in freely moving mice (Yizhar et al., 2011b); moreover, both social behaviors and episodic learning (but not anxiety, locomotion, or novel object exploration) were nearly abolished in response to E/I elevation but not reduction (Yizhar et al., 2011b).

Further investigation in slice to examine potential mechanisms underlying this deficit revealed that information processing by pyramidal neurons became saturated at a much lower input frequency during SSFO activation of pyramidal neurons, whereas activation of PV neurons decreased the gain of the transfer curve, but without changing the slope; indeed, E/I balance elevation but not reduction was found to actually reduce information throughput in neocortical pyramidal neurons, assessed in bits per second (Yizhar et al., 2011b). Last, combinatorial optogenetics (discussed below) was employed to examine the effect of simultaneously increasing excitation and inhibition (with a resultant E/I more similar to baseline than during manipulation of either E or I in isolation); partial restoration of social function was observed (Yizhar et al., 2011b).

In summary, the expanding optogenetic toolbox is beginning to pay dividends in addressing mysteries and challenges in psychiatric disease research that have long been out of reach (including in the above studies and many others, e.g., Abbott et al., 2009; Busskamp and Roska, 2011; Covington et al., 2010; Ivanova and Pan, 2009; Lobo et al., 2010; Paz et al., 2011; Tan et al., 2008, 2012; Tonnesen et al., 2009). Optogenetic work has even begun to provide clues to treatment mechanisms and refinement; for example, in the case of the deep brain stimulation (DBS) mechanism, optogenetic studies have suggested that the likely direct initial target of DBS (at least in the case of Parkinson's disease) is not local cell bodies but afferent axons to the region (in this case, to the subthalamic nucleus), which may arise from globally distributed brain regions (Gradinaru et al., 2009). However, major areas of optogenetic tool advancement are nevertheless required in the future, as detailed next.

UNSOLVED PROBLEMS AND OPEN QUESTIONS: TECHNOLOGY FROM CELL BIOLOGY, OPTICS, AND BEHAVIOR

One group of technological challenges to be addressed in optogenetics lies within the natural domain of mammalian biology. First, the development of improved subcellular trafficking will be important. Membrane trafficking strategies have improved the expression of opsins at the membrane (Gradinaru et al., 2008, 2010; Zhao et al., 2008), but further exploration in this area may produce targeting strategies that allow selective opsin expression in subcellular compartments such as dendrites, soma, or axon terminals. Indeed, while efforts have been made in this regard, achieving truly robust (near 100%) exclusion of heterologously expressed optogenetic proteins from axons would prevent undesired optical drive of axons of passage during illumination of an opsin-expressing brain region. While the expression of opsins in axons is one of the most useful features of this approach in allowing "projection targeting"–based recruitment of cells defined only by selective illumination and projection pattern, this effect also confounds certain kinds of functional mapping procedures that employ optogenetics (Petreanu et al., 2009).

Second, it would be valuable to develop a robust and versatile optical (nonpharmacological) strategy to (when desired) prevent the propagation of optogenetically elicited action potentials in the antidromic direction or along axon collaterals during projection-targeting experiments. Again, sometimes this antidromic drive is desired, but in other cases it is not (wherein the experimenter seeks to allow generalizable selective excitation only of spatially defined projections, and wishes to not take advantage of the existing capability to recruit cells defined by projection).

Third, improved high-speed volumetric (3D) light delivery strategies with single-cell resolution would be of great value, so that populations of cells even within intact mammalian brain tissue could be recruited optogenetically with any required extent of synchrony or asynchrony. Optogenetics applications *in vivo* to questions in mammalian circuit dynamics and behavior have typically involved synchronous optogenetic control of entire genetically targeted cell populations over millimeter scale spatial domains, for example, in studies of sleep–wake transitions, Parkinsonian circuitry, gamma rhythms, feeding behavior, olfaction, aggression, and memory consolidation. Yet methods for guiding spatial delivery of light excitation itself in 3D volumes could allow much improved precision and complexity in optogenetic modulation, taking the next step beyond the single-photon, guided-light strategies which have already been used in mammalian tissue for applications such as refined optogenetic circuit mapping and dissection of anxiety circuitry (Tye et al., 2011). Improved optogenetic two-photon illumination theoretically could provide a distinct means to manipulate single or multiple genetically and spatially targeted cells with high temporal resolution over sustained intervals and within intact tissue volumes, in order to delineate and define components that work in concert to generate circuit dynamics or behavior.

Fourth, it would be immensely valuable to develop methods to rapidly and efficiently extract brainwide wiring (connectomic) patterns, or at least projection patterns, from optogenetically driven cells that had been shown to have a known and quantified impact on behavior in the very same animal (Deisseroth, 2012).

Fifth, robust extension of optogenetic tool-targeting strategies to non–genetically tractable species or cell types will be enormously helpful. The generation of Cre-driver rats has been important (Witten et al., 2011), and projection targeting provides an independent step forward. But improved intersectional targeting strategies will also be crucial since few relevant cell types can be specified by only a single descriptor such as cell body location, projection target, or activity of one promoter/enhancer region. Design and validation of opsin-carrying viruses that depend on multiple recombinases (e.g., with Boolean AND or other logical gates) will be essential, and improved methods to selectively *exclude* optogenetic tool expression in cells with a given genetic identity will also be useful. Finally, true retrograde and anterograde wiring-based strategies (i.e., targeting cells that project to a particular region, or cells that receive projections from a particular region) would greatly enhance the flexibility of optogenetic control, both in mice and in other species; such strategies exist but are not always robust or well tolerated.

Sixth, it would be of great value to rapidly and efficiently extract the brainwide elicited-activity patterns arising from optogenetic control of a targeted population. This can be achieved to some extent with ofMRI (optogenetic functional magnetic resonance imaging; Lee et al., 2010), an optogenetic method that enables unbiased global assessment of the neural circuits upstream and downstream of focal stimulation. However, fMRI methods in general suffer from poor spatial and temporal resolution. Whether the optimal method to obtain brainwide activity records in freely moving animals would be through activity imaging compatible with optogenetics, or with deposition of some recoverable permanent activity trace (Deisseroth, 2012) in the cellular population of interest (since light-based imaging methods encounter fundamental limitations of resolution arising from scattering in mammalian brain tissue), remains to be seen. In general, improved integration of optogenetic control with readouts will be important—whether behavioral, electrophysiological (e.g., Anikeeva et al., 2011), or imaging. Moreover, closing the loop so that neural activity or behavioral readouts can feed back and control the inputs played in via optogenetics will be of great interest—as will the development of computational methods to begin "reverse engineering" the studied circuitry by identifying the underlying transformations of information carried out in the tissue.

Addressing the above technological challenges, all squarely in the domain of modern neuroscience, will help provide experimental leverage that may lead to key insights into neural circuit function and dysfunction that would be difficult or impossible to establish by other means.

UNSOLVED PROBLEMS AND OPEN QUESTIONS: GENOMICS AND BIOPHYSICS

Another group of technological challenges to be addressed in optogenetics falls more into the natural domain of microbial biologists and biophysicists (although, of course, many laboratories and investigators span the mammalian and the microbial realms).

First, the ongoing identification of additional genomically identified tools (via searching databases, broad-based sequencing efforts, and ecological genome mining) will profoundly improve our ability to perturb and understand biological systems. Many thousands of new opsin genes alone, to say nothing of other classes of light-sensitive modules, will be accessible in this way. For example, even though known opsins already span most of the visual spectrum and a very broad kinetics space (Fenno et al., 2011; Yizhar et al., 2011), it is very likely that new kinds of light sensitivity, kinetic properties, and even ion selectivity will emerge. One important goal is moving into the infrared, which will achieve (1) deeper light penetration at a given irradiance value, (2) reduced scattering for improved resolution, and (3) provision of an additional control channel; infrared actuation has already been achieved for certain non-opsin-based optogenetic approaches but possibly pushes against certain physics-based limitations for retinal-based photoreceptors.

Second, engineering of these known or new tools for a narrowed (as well as shifted) action spectrum would enable more clean separation of control channels. For example, engineering of blue-shifted hyperpolarizing opsins with narrower activation wavelength spectra could ultimately allow for enhanced combinatorial neuronal inhibition experiments within scattering mammalian tissues. While action spectrum peaks for existing tools span the visible spectrum and beyond, the broad shoulders of relevant action spectra may prevent use of more than two or three channels of control at once, unless spectra can be narrowed. Such efforts might involve mutations that prevent access of the photocycle to specific states or intermediates that have shifted absorbance properties. This class of opsin engineering will be facilitated by structure-based insights into the photocycle; to understand the ChR photocycle in more detail, further structural studies beyond the current closed-state structure (Kato et al., 2012), including of open and intermediate photocycle states, are clearly needed. These efforts may also lead to the generation of mutants with novel kinetic properties.

Third, engineering the light sensors of optogenetics for higher quantum efficiency, greater light sensitivity, and/or increased current elicited per optogenetic-protein molecule, would be of substantial value in allowing the use of lower irradiances for targeting a given tissue volume or depth, which may be important in minimizing photodamage, heating, or power use/deposition constraints. While for opsins many orders-of-magnitude-increased light sensitivity can be achieved with the bistable or step-function approach, this comes at a kinetic cost (slowing down the deactivation after light-off; Berndt et al., 2009).

Fourth, developing an electrically inhibitory optogenetic channel (rather than a pump) would be of immense value. Current hyperpolarizing tools are all pumps rather than channels and therefore do not provide shunting or input resistance changes (and also can only move one ion per photon); as a result these optogenetic tools are not nearly as effective as the channels or native inhibitory receptors, especially in projection-targeting experiments wherein the goal is to intercept action potentials in axons. Achieving this goal would also rapidly enable the generation of a hyperpolarizing SFO or bistable optogenetic tool that would allow sustained inhibition of neurons without requiring constant illumination. New structural knowledge of the ChR cation-conducting pathway (Kato et al., 2012) and pore vestibules may facilitate construction of ChR variants with potassium selectivity for this purpose, as well as improved photocurrents, light sensitivity, and kinetic properties.

Fifth, "dead" optogenetic tool mutants with expression and targeting properties comparable to active tools, but with no light-induced effector function, would be useful as controls. Currently, controls for optogenetic experiments often include XFP-expressing organisms or viruses, but this approach may not fully account for potential side effects of expressing the optogenetic tools themselves on parameters such as membrane capacitance and endogenous protein trafficking. Again, knowledge of pore structure (and pump mechanisms) may facilitate the generation of such tools.

Sixth, in addition to light-sensitive pumps and channels, continued expansion of optically recruited biochemical signaling will be important, with increasing attention to strategies for modular and easily programmable pathway recruitment, improved specificity, expanded spectral responsivity bands, and adaptation to additional classes of native chromophores (such as flavins, biliverdins, and the like). The optoXR family of light-activated 7TM neurotransmitter/neuromodulator receptors will see addition of novel tools based on chimeras between vertebrate rhodopsins and both well-known and orphan GPCRs. And light-sensitive domains are being added to an increasing number of receptor and even intracellular signaling proteins, so that optogenetics will expand to occupy the full breadth of cell signaling, far beyond the study of neural activity.

CONCLUSION

In summary, continued investigation from the microbial and biophysical side into ecological diversity, high-resolution structures, photocycle properties, and functional phylogenetics of light-sensitive protein modules will enable the discovery and engineering of new and improved classes of optogenetic control. Moreover, investigation from the neuroscience side into targeting, trafficking, selective spatiotemporal properties of illumination, precise circuit element recruitment, and diverse compatible readout engineering will fundamentally advance the scope and precision of resulting insights into complex, intact biological systems. Existing methods represent only the tip of the iceberg in terms of what could be ultimately achieved for neuroscience and neuropsychiatry disease research, in maximally enabling the principled design and application of optogenetics.

DISCLOSURES

Dr. Fenno has no conflicts of interest to disclose.

Dr. Deisseroth has disclosed his optogenetic research findings to the Stanford Office of Technology Licensing, which has filed patent applications for the possible use of the findings and methods in identifying new treatments for neuropsychiatric disease; Dr. Deisseroth is also co-founder and scientific advisor to a company, Circuit Therapeutics, which employs related methods to develop new treatments for neuropsychiatric disease. All materials, methods and reagents remain freely available for academic and non-profit research in perpetuity through the Deisseroth optogenetics website (http://www.optogenetics.org).

REFERENCES

Abbott, S.B., Stornetta, R.L., et al. (2009). Photostimulation of retrotrapezoid nucleus phox2b-expressing neurons *in vivo* produces long-lasting activation of breathing in rats. *J. Neurosci.* 29(18):5806–5819.

Adamantidis, A.R., Zhang, F., et al. (2007). Neural substrates of awakening probed with optogenetic control of hypocretin neurons. *Nature* 450(7168):420–424.

Adesnik, H., and Scanziani, M. (2010). Lateral competition for cortical space by layer-specific horizontal circuits. *Nature* 464(7292):1155–1160.

Airan, R.D., Thompson, K.R., et al. (2009). Temporally precise *in vivo* control of intracellular signalling. *Nature* 458:1025–1029.

Anikeeva, P., Andalman, A.S., et al. (2011). Optetrode: a multichannel readout for optogenetic control in freely moving mice. *Nat. Neurosci.* 15:163–170.

Aravanis, A.M., Wang, L.P., et al. (2007). An optical neural interface: *in vivo* control of rodent motor cortex with integrated fiberoptic and optogenetic technology. *J. Neural. Eng.* 4(3):S143–156.

Bamann, C., Kirsch, T., et al. (2008). Spectral characteristics of the photocycle of channelrhodopsin-2 and its implication for channel function. *J. Mol. Biol.* 375:686–694.

Berndt, A., Yizhar, O., et al. (2009). Bi-stable neural state switches. *Nat. Neurosci.* 12:229–234.

Boyden, E.S., Zhang, F., et al. (2005). Millisecond-timescale, genetically targeted optical control of neural activity. *Nat. Neurosci.* 8:1263–1268.

Busskamp, V., and Roska, B. (2011). Optogenetic approaches to restoring visual function in retinitis pigmentosa. *Curr. Opin. Neurobiol.* 21(6):942–946.

Chow, B.Y., Han, X., et al. (2010). High performance genetically targetable optical neural silencing by light-driven proton pumps. *Nature* 463:98–102.

Ciocchi, S., Herry, C., et al. (2010). Encoding of conditioned fear in central amygdala inhibitory circuits. *Nature* 468:277–282.

Covington, H.E., III, Lobo, M.K., et al. (2010). Antidepressant effect of optogenetic stimulation of the medial prefrontal cortex. *J. Neurosci.* 30(48):16082–16090.

Deisseroth, K. (2010). Optogenetics: controlling the brain with light. *Sci. Am.* 303(5):48–55.

Deisseroth, K. (2011). Optogenetics. *Nat. Methods* 8:26–29.

Deisseroth, K. (2012). Optogenetics and psychiatry: applications, challenges, and opportunities. *Biol. Psychiatry* 71:1030–1032.

Deisseroth, K., Feng, G., et al. (2006). Next-generation optical technologies for illuminating genetically targeted brain circuits. *J. Neurosci.* 26:10380–10386.

Fenno, L., Yizhar, O., et al. (2011). The development and application of optogenetics. *Annu. Rev. Neurosci.* 34:389–412.

Goshen, I., Brodsky, M., et al. (2011). Dynamics of retrieval strategies for remote memories. *Cell* 147:678–689.

Govorunova, E.G., Spudich, E.N., et al. (2011). New channelrhodopsin with a red-shifted spectrum and rapid kinetics from Mesostigma viride. *MBio.* 2(3):e00115–e11.

Gradinaru, V., Mogri, M., et al. (2009). Optical deconstruction of parkinsonian neural circuitry. *Science* 324:354–359.

Gradinaru, V., Thompson, K.R., et al. (2007). Targeting and readout strategies for fast optical neural control *in vitro* and *in vivo*. *J. Neurosci.* 27:14231–14238.

Gradinaru, V., Thompson, K.R., et al. (2008). eNpHR: a Natronomonas halorhodopsin enhanced for optogenetic applications. *Brain Cell Biol.* 36:129–139.

Gradinaru, V., Zhang, F., et al. (2010). Molecular and cellular approaches for diversifying and extending optogenetics. *Cell* 141:154–165.

Gulyani, A., Vitriol, E., et al. (2012). A biosensor generated via high-throughput screening quantifies cell edge Src dynamics. *Nat. Chem. Biol.* 8(8):737.

Gunaydin, L.A., Yizhar, O., et al. (2010). Ultrafast optogenetic control. *Nat. Neurosci.* 13:387–392.

Haubensak, W., Kunwar, P.S., et al. (2010). Genetic dissection of an amygdala microcircuit that gates conditioned fear. Nature 468:270–276.

Ivanova, E., and Pan, Z.H. (2009). Evaluation of the adeno-associated virus mediated long-term expression of channelrhodopsin-2 in the mouse retina. *Mol. Vis.* 15:1680–1689.

Kato, H., Zhang, F., et al. (2012). Crystal structure of the channelrhodopsin light-gated cation channel. Nature 482:369–374.

Kim, J.M., Hwa, J., et al. (2005). Light-driven activation of beta 2-adrenergic receptor signaling by a chimeric rhodopsin containing the beta 2-adrenergic receptor cytoplasmic loops. *Biochemistry* 44:2284–2292.

Kolbe, M., Besir, H., et al. (2000). Structure of the light-driven chloride pump halorhodopsin at 1.8 A resolution. *Science* 288:1390–1396.

Lee, J.H., Durand, R., et al. (2010). Global and local fMRI signals driven by neurons defined optogenetically by type and wiring. *Nature* 465(7299):788–792.

Lin, J.Y., Lin, M.Z., et al. (2009). Characterization of engineered channelrhodopsin variants with improved properties and kinetics. *Biophys. J.* 96:1803–1814.

Liu, X., Ramirez, S., et al. (2012). Optogenetic stimulation of a hippocampal engram activates fear memory recall. *Nature* 484:381–385.

Lobo, M.K., Covington, H.E., III, et al. (2010). Cell type-specific loss of BDNF signaling mimics optogenetic control of cocaine reward. *Science* 330(6002):385–390.

Mattis, J., Tye, K.M., et al. (2012). Principles for applying optogenetic tools derived from direct comparative analysis of microbial opsins. *Nat. Methods* 9:159–172.

Möglich, A., and Moffat, K. (2007). Structural basis for light-dependent signaling in the dimeric LOV domain of the photosensor YtvA. *J. Mol. Biol.* 373(1):112–126.

Oh, E., Maejima, T., et al. (2010). Substitution of 5-HT1A receptor signaling by a light-activated G protein-coupled receptor. *J. Biol. Chem.* 285:30825–30836.

Paz, J.T., Bryant, A.S., et al. (2011). A new mode of corticothalamic transmission revealed in the Gria4(−/−) model of absence epilepsy. *Nat. Neurosci.* 14(9):1167–1173.

Petreanu, L., Huber, D., et al. (2007). Channelrhodopsin-2-assisted circuit mapping of long-range callosal projections. *Nat. Neurosci.* 10(5):663–668.

Petreanu, L., Mao, T., et al. (2009). The subcellular organization of neocortical excitatory connections. *Nature* 457(7233):1142–1145.

Scanziani, M., and Häuser, M. (2009). Electrophysiology in the age of light. *Nature* 461(7266):930–939.

Sohal, V.S., Zhang, F., et al. (2009). Parvalbumin neurons and gamma rhythms enhance cortical circuit performance. *Nature* 459(7247):698–702.

Stierl, M., Stumpf, P., et al. (2011). Light modulation of cellular cAMP by a small bacterial photoactivated adenylyl cyclase, bPAC, of the soil bacterium Beggiatoa. *J. Biol. Chem.* 286:1181–1188.

Stuber, G.D., Sparta, D.R., et al. (2011). Excitatory transmission from the amygdala to nucleus accumbens facilitates reward seeking. *Nature* 475(7356):377–380.

Tan, K.R., Yvon, C., et al. (2012). GABA neurons of the VTA drive conditioned place aversion. *Neuron* 73:1173–1183.

Tan, W., Janczewski, W.A., et al. (2008). Silencing preBotzinger complex somatostatin-expressing neurons induces persistent apnea in awake rat. *Nat. Neurosci.* 11(5):538–540.

Tonnesen, J., Sorensen, A.T., et al. (2009). Optogenetic control of epileptiform activity. *Proc. Natl. Acad. Sci. USA* 106(29):12162–12167.

Tsai, H.C., Zhang, F., et al. (2009). Phasic firing in dopaminergic neurons is sufficient for behavioral conditioning. *Science* 324(5930):1080–1084.

Tye, K.M., and Deisseroth, K. (2012). Optogenetic investigation of neural circuits underlying brain disease in animal models. *Nat. Rev. Neurosci.* 13:251–266.

Tye, K.M., Prakash, R., et al. (2011). Amygdala circuitry mediating reversible and bidirectional control of anxiety. *Nature* 471:358–362.

Witten, I.B., Lin, S.C., et al. (2010). Cholinergic interneurons control local circuit activity and cocaine conditioning. *Science* 330:1677–1681.

Witten, I.B., Steinberg, E.E., et al. (2011). Recombinase-driver rat lines: tools, techniques, and optogenetic application to dopamine-mediated reinforcement. Neuron 72:721–733.

Wu, Y.I., Frey, D., et al. (2009). A genetically encoded photoactivatable Rac controls the motility of living cells. *Nature* 461(7260):104–108.

Yizhar, O., Fenno, L.E., et al. (2011a). Optogenetics in neural systems. Neuron 71:9–34.

Yizhar, O., Fenno, L.E., et al. (2011b). Neocortical excitation/inhibition balance in information processing and social dysfunction. *Nature* 477:171–178.

Zhang, F., Vierock, J., et al. (2011). The microbial opsin family of optogenetic tools. *Cell* 147:1446–1457.

Zhang, F., Wang, L.P., et al. (2007). Multimodal fast optical interrogation of neural circuitry. *Nature* 446:633–639.

Zhao, S., Cunha, C., et al. (2008). Improved expression of halorhodopsin for light-induced silencing of neuronal activity. *Brain Cell Biol.* 36(1–4):141–154.

11 | BLOOD–BRAIN BARRIER OPENING AND DRUG DELIVERY USING FOCUSED ULTRASOUND AND MICROBUBBLES

ELISA E. KONOFAGOU

INTRODUCTION

Current treatments of neurological and neurodegenerative diseases are limited due to the lack of a truly noninvasive, transient, and regionally selective brain drug delivery method (Pardridge, 2005). The brain is particularly difficult to deliver drugs to because of the blood–brain barrier (BBB). The impermeability of the BBB is due to tight junctions connecting adjacent endothelial cells and highly regulatory transport systems of the endothelial cell membranes (Abbott et al., 2006). The main function of the BBB is ion and volume regulation in order to ensure conditions necessary for proper synaptic and axonal signaling (Stewart and Tuor, 1994). However, the same impermeability properties that keep the brain healthy are the reason for the difficulties in its efficient pharmacological treatment. The BBB prevents most neurologically active drugs from entering the brain, and, as a result, has been determined as the rate-limiting factor in brain drug delivery (Pardridge, 2005). Until a solution to the trans-BBB delivery problem is found, treatments of neurological diseases will remain impeded.

BBB PHYSIOLOGY: STRUCTURE AND FUNCTION

The BBB is a specialized substructure of the vascular system, consisting of endothelial cells connected together by tight junctions. The luminal and abluminal membranes line the inner wall of the vessel and act as the permeability barrier. The combination of tight junctions and these two membranes characterizes the BBB as having low permeability to large and ionic substances. However, certain molecules such as glucose and amino acids are exceptions because they are actively transported. It has also been shown that lymphocytes can traverse the BBB by going through temporarily opened tight junctions of the endothelial walls. The astrocytes have been proven to offer a protective mechanism of the neurons to any mechanical effect (Abbott et al., 2006).

BBB AND NEUROTHERAPEUTICS

Several neurological disorders remain intractable to treatment by therapeutic agents because of the BBB, the brain's natural defense. By acting as a permeability barrier, the BBB impedes entry from blood to the brain of virtually all molecules with higher than 400 Da of molecular weight, thus rendering many potent neurologically active substances and drugs ineffective simply because they cannot be delivered to where they are needed. As a result, traversing the BBB remains the rate-limiting factor in brain drug delivery development (Pardridge, 2005, 2006).

FOCUSED ULTRASOUND

Focused ultrasound (FUS) utilizes the same concept of acoustic wave propagation as the more widely known diagnostic ultrasound applications. However, instead of acquiring and displaying echoes generated at several tissue interfaces for imaging, FUS employs concave transducers that usually have a single geometric focus, at which most of the power is delivered during sonication in order to induce mechanical effects, thermal effects, or both. Note that the more widely used "high-intensity focused ultrasound (HIFU)" name of the method is not used here for BBB opening since the intensities used are low, that is, on the level of what is used in diagnostic ultrasound.

BBB OPENING USING FUS AND MICROBUBBLES

Blood–brain barrier opening induced by ultrasound at or near ablation intensities was first observed while accompanied by neuronal damage (Bakay et al., 1956; Ballantine et al., 1960; Patrick et al., 1990; Vykhodtseva et al., 1995). After reducing the acoustic intensity and duty cycle (the time the power is on relative to the time the power is off), BBB opening was still observed, but without the macroscopic damage detected as lesions (Mesiwala et al., 2002). With the addition of intravenously (IV) injected microbubbles prior to sonication, BBB opening was determined to be transient (Hynynen et al., 2001) in the presence of Optison™ (Optison™; Mallinckrodt Inc., St. Louis, MO), which are albumin-coated, octafluoropropane-filled microbubbles of 3–4.5 μm in diameter and are usually used to enhance blood vessels on clinical ultrasound images through opacification. The BBB opening procedure could also be monitored with MRI and MR contrast agents (Hynynen et al., 2001). This showed the potential of opening the BBB without damaging parenchymal cells, such as neurons. Further investigation entailed study of this phenomenon with Optison™ to search for a difference in threshold of BBB opening and neuronal damage and understand the mechanism of the opening in rabbits, with (Hynynen et al., 2003; McDannold et al., 2004; Sheikov et al., 2004) or without (Hynynen et al., 2005) a craniotomy. The advantage of having microbubbles present in the blood supply is that it allows for the reduction of the ultrasound intensity, the containment of most of the disruption within the vasculature, and the reduction of the likelihood of irreversible neuronal damage (Choi et al., 2005, 2006, 2007a, 2007b; Hynynen et al., 2003, 2005, 2006; McDannold et al., 2004, 2005, 2006; Sheikov et al., 2004, 2006). Although there are many indications that damage can be contained to minimal hemorrhage (Hynynen et al., 2006), the complete safety profile remains to be assessed. In addition, indications to various mechanisms such as the dilation of vessels, temporary ischemia, mechanically induced opening of the tight junctions, and the activation of various transport mechanisms have been reported (Mesiwala et al., 2002; Sheikov et al., 2004, 2006).

Our group has demonstrated feasibility of BBB opening through intact skull and skin and successful imaging of the BBB opening in the area of the hippocampus at submillimeter imaging resolution using a 9.4T MR scanner in both wild-type (Choi et al., 2005, 2007a, 2007b; Konofagou et al., 2009) and Alzheimer's mice (Choi et al., 2008). Our group also concentrates on a specific brain region (e.g., the hippocampus), which is key in neurodegenerative disease, such as Alzheimer's, and can be successfully and reproducibly targeted (Konofagou and Choi, 2008). Delivery of molecules of up to 2,000 kDa in molecular weight was also demonstrated (Choi et al., 2010). Preliminary histology indicated no structural damage in the area of the hippocampus (Baseri et al., 2010). Finally, it is important to note that the microbubbles used for BBB opening have been approved by the Food and Drug Administration (FDA) for human use in contrast echocardiography, for example, for the detection of myocardial infarction (Kaufmann et al., 2007). It is equally important to specify that the pressure amplitudes used for BBB opening are of similar range to ultrasound diagnostic levels (<1.5–2 MPa) and, therefore, assumed safe for human use (Christensen, 1988) while the pulse duration is by orders of magnitude longer.

MICROBUBBLES IN CONTRAST ULTRASOUND AND ASSOCIATED BIOEFFECTS

Currently, in the United States, microbubbles are only FDA approved for echocardiography in patients with suboptimal images of the cardiac chambers. However, microbubbles have shown promise for imaging myocardial perfusion using intermittent contrast destruction pulses. Therefore, most *in vivo* bioeffects studies have focused on the heart (Miller, 2007). For a given frequency, separate pressure thresholds exist for microbubble destruction and the onset of bioeffects (Chen et al., 2002; Li et al., 2003, 2004). Safe cardiac perfusion imaging would then be done with the microbubble clearance pulse being between these thresholds. Extravascular drug delivery to the brain would then be performed near the threshold for transient opening, but well below the conditions for permanent damage. Human doses for commercially available microbubbles used in contrast echocardiography could provide a useful benchmark for therapy trials. However, the human dose for imaging purposes varies widely (Table 11.1). A typical dose ranges between 6 and 12 × 107 microbubbles per kg (60–120 microbubbles per mg). Mean diameters are given, but detailed information of the polydispersed size distributions is lacking. Thus, the effects of microbubble size and concentration on safety are difficult to decouple from previous studies using these commercial agents. Our ability to generate and isolate microbubbles of distinct and narrow size distributions with well-defined concentrations will allow us to probe these effects in the proposed study.

Several studies have shown an increase in bioeffects with increasing microbubble dose. For Definity and Optison, increases in rat cardiomyocyte cell death and premature heartbeats and microvessel leakage were found after exposure to ultrasound, also called sonication (Li et al., 2003; Miller et al., 2005). Similar dose–response relationships have been observed for BBB opening (Kaps et al., 2001; Yang et al., 2007). Miller et al. (2005) compared insonation of Optison, Definity, and Imagent in the rat heart and found that microvascular effects were similar when expressed as the number of microbubbles injected. They concluded that shell type and encapsulated gas have little effect on bioeffects. Given the polydispersed size distribution of the different formulations, however, the effects

TABLE 11.1. Clinically used contrast agents and their specifications

FORMULATION (MANUFACTURER)	SHELL/GAS	CONCENTRATION (ml⁻¹)	MEAN DIAMETER (μm)	GAS VOLUME FRACTION[a]	DOSE (ml/kg)
Optison (GE Healthcare)	Albumin/C_3F_8	8×10^8	3.0–4.5	1.1%–3.8%	0.006–0.1[b]
Definity (Bristol-Myers Squibb)	Lipid/C_3F_8	1.2×10^{10}	1.1–3.3	0.8%–23%	0.01–0.02[c]
Sonovue (Bracco)	Lipid/SF_6	2×10^8	2.5	0.2%	0.003–0.3[c]

[a]Determined from concentration and mean diameter.
[b]Data obtained from Optison package insert.
[c]Data from NIH Molecular Imaging and Contrast Agent Database (MIDAC).

of size are difficult to glean from that study. However, little is known about the effects of microbubble size on bioeffects. Christiansen et al. (2003) found that intra-arterial injection was more effective than intravenous injection for gene transfection through sonoporation. This result was attributed to the difference in microbubble sizes delivered to the insonified region. Several biophysical studies have shown remarkable size dependence for microbubble oscillation and destruction (Borden et al., 2005; Chomas et al., 2001).

CLINICAL RELEVANCE OF BBB DISRUPTION

NEURODEGENERATIVE DISEASE

Over 4 million U.S. men and women suffer from Alzheimer's disease: 1 million from Parkinson's disease, 350,000 from multiple sclerosis, and 20,000 from ALS (amyotrophic lateral sclerosis). Worldwide, these four diseases account for more than 20 million patients. Although great progress has been made in recent years toward the understanding of neurodegenerative diseases like Alzheimer's, Parkinson's, multiple sclerosis, ALS, and others, few effective treatments and no cures are currently available. Aging greatly increases the risk of neurodegenerative disease, and the average age of Americans is steadily increasing. Today, over 35 million Americans are over the age of 65. Within the next 30 years, this number is likely to double, putting more and more people at increased risk of neurodegenerative disease. Alzheimer's disease, which has emerged as one of the most common brain disorders, begins in the hippocampal formation and gradually spreads to the remaining brain at its most advanced stages, and it is characterized partly by deposition of amyloid plaques in the brain tissue but also in the blood vessels themselves (Iadecola, 2004). For the purpose of this study, we will focus on the treatment of Alzheimer's disease through the FUS-induced BBB opening, and therefore, the targeted region in the brain will be the hippocampus.

DRUG DELIVERY IN NEURODEGENERATIVE DISEASE

Over the past decade, numerous small- and large-molecule products have been developed for treatment of neurodegenerative diseases with mixed success. When administered systemically *in vivo*, the BBB inhibits their delivery to the regions affected by those diseases. A review of the Comprehensive Medicinal Chemistry database indicates that only 5% of the more than 7,000 small-molecule drugs treat the central nervous system (CNS) (Pardridge, 2006). With these, only four CNS disorders can be treated: depression, schizophrenia, epilepsy, and chronic pain (Ghose et al., 1999; Lipinski, 2000). Despite the availability of pharmacological agents, potentially devastating CNS disorders and age-related neurodegenerative diseases, such as Alzheimer's disease, Parkinson's disease, Huntington's disease, multiple sclerosis, and amythrophic lateral sclerosis, remain undertreated mainly because of the impermeability of the BBB (Pardridge, 2005, 2006). The goal of this proposal is thus to optimize the FUS method and elucidate its mechanism in order to ultimately deliver therapeutics to the brain and significantly facilitate treatment of currently intractable and devastating neurodegenerative diseases.

A successful drug delivery system requires transient, localized, and noninvasive targeting of a specific tissue region. None of the current techniques clinically used, or currently under research, address these issues within the scope of the treatment of neurodegenerative diseases. As a result, the present situation in neurotherapeutics enjoys few successful treatments for most CNS disorders. Some of those routes of administration are listed in Table 11.2. Several pharmaceutical companies use the technique known as "lipidization," which is the addition of lipid groups to the polar ends of molecules to increase the permeability of the agent (Fischer et al., 1998). However, the effect is not localized as the permeability of the drug increases not only in the targeted region, but also over the entire brain and body. There can thus be a limit to the amount absorbed before the side effects become deleterious (Fischer et al., 1998).

TABLE 11.2. Techniques shown to induce trans-BBB transport or BBB disruption

METHOD	DESCRIPTION	PROBLEMS	NONINVASIVE?	LOCALIZED?
Lipidization	"Lipidizes" the drug. Allows uptake in the BBB.	Increases penetration across *all* biological membranes.	Yes	No
Transcranial brain drug delivery (Fig. 11.2)	Neurosurgically based drug delivery method. Diffusion-based method.	Invasive. Diffusion reduces the initial concentration by 90% when traveling only 0.5 mm.	No	Yes
Solvent/adjuvant-mediated BBB disruption	Solvent and adjuvants disrupt the BBB using dilation, contraction, and other methods.	Disrupts the BBB in all of the brain. Potentially toxic.	Yes	No
Delivery through endogenous transporters	Uses endogenous transporters to traverse the BBB.	Requires medicinal chemistry to modify drugs and knowledge of the endogenous transporters.	Yes	No
Ultrasound	Focused ultrasound (FUS) with microbubbles	Possible irreversible damage may be induced.	Yes	Yes

A second set of techniques under study are neurosurgically based drug delivery methods, which involve the invasive implantation of drugs into a region by a needle (Blasberg et al., 1975; Fung et al., 1996). The drug spreads through diffusion and is localized to the targeted region, but diffusion does not allow for molecules to travel far from their point of release. In addition to this, invasive procedures traverse untargeted brain tissue, causing unnecessary damage. As a result, effective drugs have recently been shelved after reports of adverse effects. Other techniques utilize solvents mixed with drugs or adjuvants (pharmacological agents) attached to drugs to disrupt the BBB through dilation and contraction of the blood vessels [Pardridge, 2005, 2006, 2007]). However, this disruption is not localized within the brain, and the solvents and adjuvants used are potentially toxic. This technique may constitute a delivery method specific to the brain, but it requires special attention to each type of drug molecule and a specific transport system resulting in a time-consuming and costly process while still not being completely localized to the targeted region. FUS in combination with microbubbles constitutes thus the only truly transient, localized, and noninvasive technique for opening the BBB. Due to these unique advantages over other existent techniques (Table 11.2), FUS may facilitate the delivery of already developed pharmacological agents and could significantly impact how devastating CNS diseases are treated.

However, despite the fact that FUS is currently the only technique that can open the BBB locally and noninvasively, several key aspects of this phenomenon remain unexplored. A clear correlation of BBB opening with microbubbles has been shown (Choi et al., 2005; Hynynen et al., 2001; McDannold et al., 2004). Although the presence of microbubbles allows for a reduction in the necessary acoustic pressure for BBB opening, it also allows for the possibility of disrupting the microbubble through inertial cavitation (Leighton, 1994; Neppiras, 1980; Pardridge, 2007). The resulting effects not only can open the tight junctions but also could induce irreversible damage to the blood vessels and their surrounding cells (Baseri et al., 2010). Recent studies have indicated that BBB opening may occur without necessarily incurring inertial cavitation, without (Hynynen et al., 2003) or with (McDannold et al., 2006) craniotomy. However, it is not clear how the different types of mechanical effects lead to BBB opening and how the role of the microbubble can be optimized. Given the strong coupling of microbubble size and concentration to the response to sonication, a mechanistic study to BBB opening by contrast-assisted focused ultrasound must include these parameters. Control over both ultrasound and microbubble parameters is essential for the proper optimization and understanding of the FUS technique. However, to our knowledge no study to date has included a thorough investigation of both of these components.

FUS-FACILITATED BBB OPENING IN DRUG DELIVERY FOR TREATMENT OF NEURODEGENERATIVE DISEASE

Realizing the strong premise of this technique for facilitation of drug delivery to specific brain regions, we showed that the BBB can be opened reliably and reproducibly in the hippocampal region in mice (Choi et al., 2005, 2006, 2007a, 2007b, 2007c, 2008, 2009, 2010; Konofagou et al., 2008, 2009). By developing a better understanding of the underlying physical parameters that are responsible for the opening of the BBB, namely, the ultrasound and microbubble parameters, we will be in a position to fully exploit this methodology and to do so safely. The feasibility of the technique at optimized ultrasound and microbubble parameters for reversible BBB opening, as determined in vivo, has been tested on wild-type mice as a first step to identify the potential of this technique in the treatment of neurodegenerative diseases (Choi et al., 2008). The MR imaging methods developed allow for high sensitivity, high spatial resolution, and high temporal resolution. The latter is achieved through the slow diffusion of intraperitoneally injected gadolinium. The added potential of combining this ultrasound technique with any therapeutic agent may renew possibilities in potentially employing available pharmacological agents, whose development has currently been abandoned because of poor BBB penetration. This may thus result in the novel and effective treatment of several potentially devastating neurological and neurodegenerative diseases. As previously indicated, we will concentrate on the feasibility of noninvasive and localized treatment of Alzheimer's disease by specifically targeting the hippocampus. However, the FUS technique can, in principle, be combined and applied in the case of any neurological disease. Therefore, findings of this study may impact not only treatment of a specific disease but also the entire field of brain diseases. In summary, FUS stands to make a very important impact in the brain drug delivery, and the proposed study aims at its optimization through understanding of the type of interaction between the microbubble, the tissue, and the FUS beam.

DRUG DELIVERY THROUGH THE OPENED BBB

The delivery of many large agents using focused ultrasound and microbubbles has been demonstrated in previous studies by our group and others: MRI contrast agents such as Omniscan (573 Da) (Choi et al., 2007b) and Magnevist® (938 Da) (Choi et al., 2007), Evans Blue (Kinoshita et al., 2006), Trypan Blue (Raymond et al., 2008), Herceptin (148 kDa) (Kinoshita et al., 2006), horseradish peroxidase (40 kDa) (Sheikov et al., 2008), doxorubicin (544 Da) (Treat et al., 2007), multisized Dextran (Choi et al., 2010), and rabbit anti-Aβ antibodies (Raymond et al., 2008). Despite the promise shown by the delivery of such a variety of compounds, several questions about the effectiveness of the delivery remain. In particular, it is still not known whether therapeutic molecules can cross through the BBB opening into the intracellular neuronal space so that they can trigger the required downstream effects for neuronal regeneration.

METHODS FOR INDUCING AND ASSESSING BBB OPENING

FUS AND MICROBUBBLES

The experimental setup is shown in Figure 11.1. The FUS transducer (center frequency: 1.5 MHz; focal depth: 60 mm;

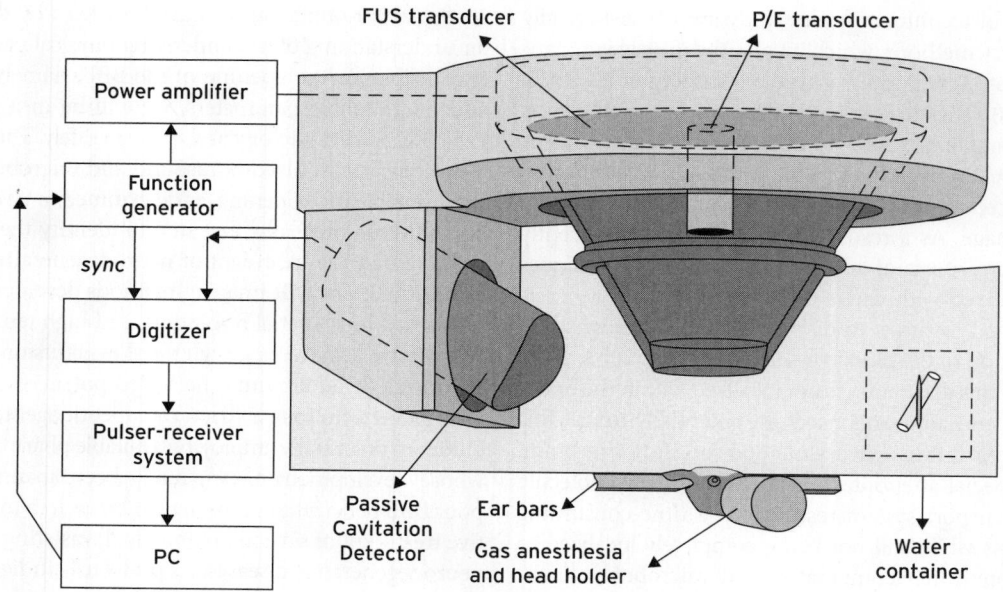

FUS transducer   P/E transducer

Power amplifier

Function generator

sync

Digitizer

Pulser-receiver system

PC

Passive Cavitation Detector

Ear bars

Gas anesthesia and head holder

Water container

Figure 11.1 *Block diagram and illustration of the experimental setup. The PCD was positioned at 60° relative to the longitudinal axis of the FUS beam. The overlap between the focal regions of PCD and FUS occurring inside the murine brain is illustrated in the inset.*

outer radius: 30 mm; inner radius: 11.2 mm, model cdc7411–3, Imasonic, Besançon, France) is used to perform sonication immediately following bubble administration. The transducer is driven by a function generator (Agilent Technologies, Palo Alto, CA) through a 50-dB power amplifier (ENI Inc., Rochester, NY). A cone filled with degassed and distilled water is attached to the transducer system. The transducer is attached to a computer-controlled positioner (Velmex Inc., Bloomfield, NY). The PCD, a 5-cm cylindrically focused broadband hydrophone (Sonic Concepts, Bothell, WA), with a cylindrical focal region (height 19 mm, diameter 3.64 mm) is placed at 60° from the longitudinal axis of the FUS beam. The PCD and the FUS transducer are confocally aligned. The acoustic emissions from the microbubbles are captured with the PCD and collected using a digitizer (model 14200, Gage Applied Technologies, Inc., Lachine, QC, Canada) through a 20 dB amplifier (model 5800, Olympus NDT, Waltham, MA). Microbubbles (Definity®: mean diameter range: 1.1–3.3 μm, Lantheus Medical Imaging, MA, or lipid-shelled microbubbles manufactured in-house and size isolated using differential centrifugation [57]) are activated and used within 24 hr after activation. Following activation, a 1:20 dilution solution is prepared using 1× phosphate-buffered saline (PBS) and slowly injected into the tail vein (1 μl per gram of mouse body weight). Both transducers use pulsed-wave FUS (burst rate: 10 Hz; burst duration: 20 ms; duty cycle: 20%) in two 30-s sonication intervals with a 30-s intermittent delay. Peak-rarefactional acoustic pressures of 0.15, 0.30, 0.45, and 0.60 MPa are typically used as they have been shown to provide the best tradeoff between safety and BBB opening (Baseri et al., 2010). One side of the hippocampus in the horizontal orientation is sonicated in each mouse. Acoustic parameters other than the pressure have also been studied with respect to their role in BBB disruption. One of those is the pulse length (Choi et al., 2011). In that study, mouse brains were pulse sonicated

(center frequency: 1.5 MHz, peak-negative pressure: 0.3 MPa, pulse length [PL]: 2.3 μs, pulse repetition frequency [PRF]: 6.25, 25, 100 kHz) continuously or with a burst length of 1,000 pulses (burst repetition frequency [BRF]: 0.1, 1, 2, or 5 Hz) through the intact scalp and skull for 11 min. One minute after the start of sonication, fluorescence-tagged dextran (60 μg/g, molecular weight: 3 kDa) and Definity® microbubbles (0.05 μl/g) were intravenously injected. After 20 min of circulation, the mice were transcardially perfused, and the brains were sectioned and imaged using fluorescence microscopy. In order to determine the microbubble size dependence, mice have been injected intravenously with lipid-shelled bubbles of either 1–2, 4–5, or 6–8 μm in diameter while the concentration was 10^7 numbers/mL (Choi et al., 2009).

CONFIRMATION OF BBB OPENING BY MAGNETIC RESONANCE IMAGING

A vertical-bore 9.4 T MR system (Buker Biospin, Billerica, MA) was used to confirm the blood–brain barrier opening in the murine hippocampus. Each mouse was anesthetized using 1%–2% of isoflurane gas and was positioned inside a single resonator. The respiration rate was monitored throughout the procedure using a monitoring or gating system (SA Instruments Inc., Stony Brook, NY). Prior to introducing the mouse into the scanner, intraperitoneal (IP) catheterization was performed. Two different protocols were used for MR imaging. The first protocol was a three-dimensional (3D), T1-weighted SNAP gradient echo pulse sequence, which acquired horizontal images using TR/TE = 20/4 ms, a flip angle of 25°, NEX of 5, a total acquisition time of 6 min and 49 s, a matrix size of 256 × 256 × 16 pixels and a field of view (FOV) of 1.92 × 1.92 × 0.5 cm³, resulting in a resolution of 75 × 75 × 312.5 μm³. The second protocol was a 3D T2*-weighted GEFC gradient echo pulse sequence, which acquired horizontal images using TR/TE = 20/5.2 ms, a flip angle of 10°, NEX of 8, a total acquisition time of 8 min and 12 s, a matrix size of 256 × 192 × 16 pixels, and a FOV of 2.25 × 1.69 × 0.7 cm³, resulting in a resolution of 88 × 88 × 437.5 μm³. Both protocols were applied approximately 30 min after IP injection of 0.30 ml of gadodiamide (590 Da, Omniscan˙, GE Healthcare, Princeton, NJ), which allowed sufficient time for the gadodiamide to diffuse into the sonicated region.

ACOUSTIC EMISSION SIGNAL ACQUISITION AND ANALYSIS

The acoustic emission signals acquired by the PCD are sampled at 25 MHz to accommodate the highest memory limit of the digitizer involved in each case. A customized spectrogram function (30 cycles, i.e., 20 μs, Chebyshev window; 95% overlap; 4096-point FFT) in MATLAB˙ (2007b, Mathworks, Natick, MA) is used to generate a time–frequency map, which provided the spectral amplitude in time. The spectrogram can then clearly indicate how the frequency content of a signal changes over time. Therefore, the onset of the broadband response and its duration could be clearly demonstrated on the spectrogram.

The acoustic emissions are quantified *in vivo*. A high-pass, Chebyshev type 1, filter with a cutoff of 4 MHz was first applied to the acquired PCD signal. The acoustic emission collected by the focused hydrophone was used in the quantification of the ICD; the harmonic (nf, $n = 1, 2, \ldots, 6$), subharmonic ($f/2$) and ultraharmonics ($nf/2$, $n = 3, 5, 7, 9$) frequencies produced by stable cavitation (Farny et al., 2009) were filtered out by excluding 300-kHz bandwidths around each harmonic and 100-kHz bandwidths around each sub- and ultraharmonic frequency. These bandwidths were designed to filter for the broadband response and to ensure that the stable cavitation response was not included in the ICD calculation. The root mean square (RMS) of the spectral amplitude (V_{RMS}) could then be obtained from the spectrogram after filtering. To maximize the broadband response compared to the sonication without microbubbles, only the first 50 μs of sonication were considered in the ICD calculation, which was performed by integrating the V_{RMS} variation within an interval of 0.75 μs (i.e., calculating the area below the V_{RMS} curve between 0.095 ms and 0.145 ms). In order to remove the effect of the skull in the ICD calculation, the V_{RMS} in the case without microbubbles was also calculated and was subtracted from the results with the microbubbles to obtain the net bubble response. A Student's t-test was used to determine whether the ICD was statistically different between different pressure amplitudes. A p-value of $p < 0.05$ was considered to denote a significant difference in all comparisons.

ACOUSTIC PARAMETER DEPENDENCE AND MECHANISM OF BBB OPENING

The BBB opening pressure threshold is identified to fall between 0.30 and 0.45 MPa in the case of the 1-to-2-μm bubbles and between 0.15 and 0.30 MPa in the 4- to 5- and 6- to 8-μm cases

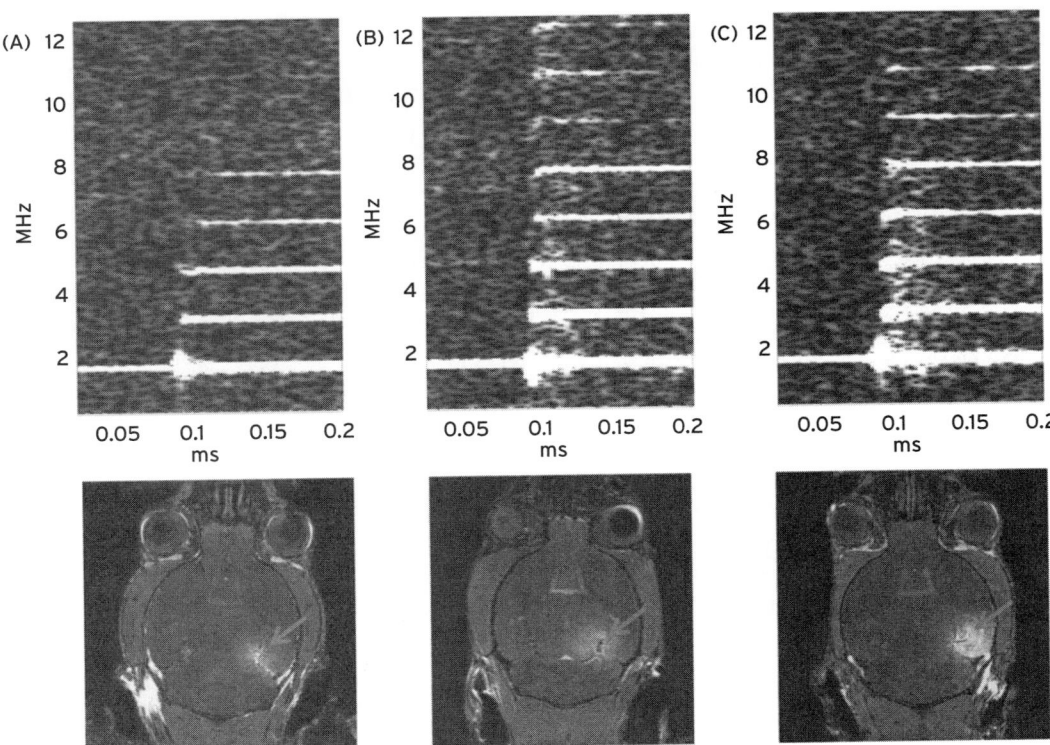

Figure 11.2 *Spectrogram during the first 0.2 ms sonication. Broadband acoustic emissions were detected at (B) 0.45 MPa and (C) 0.60 MPa but not at (A) 0.30 MPa. Corresponding MRI images confirm that the blood–brain barrier could be opened at 0.30 MPa, that is, without inertial cavitation [60,64]. The arrows indicate the location of BBB opening.*

(Choi et al., 2009; Tung et al., 2010). At every acoustic pressure, both the region of contrast enhancement in the MRI imaging and the amplitude of broadband emissions increased with the bubble diameter. The IC threshold is found to be bubble independent and to lie between 0.30 and 0.45 MPa for all bubble sizes (Fig. 11.2). In fluorescence imaging, the PL of 2.3 μs was found to be sufficient for BBB opening and Dextran delivery (Choi et al., 2011).

MOLECULAR DELIVERY THROUGH THE BBB OPENING

A molecular delivery study (Choi et al., 2007c, 2010) indicated that the range of molecular size for trans-BBB delivery spreads to well beyond the 574 Da (Gadolinium; Fig. 11.2) to 67 kDa (Albumin; Fig. 11.3[v]) and 2,000 kDa (Dextrans; Fig. 11.3[iii]). As expected, at 2,000 kDa (or, ~20 nm), the fluorescent region is the smallest (since the molecule is the largest and thus diffusion the slowest) and mostly outside of the hippocampus. Therefore, FUS-induced BBB opening was shown feasible for noninvasive, local, and transient opening of the BBB for drug delivery of agents of several tens of kDa, providing thus the opportunity of delivering available pharmacological agents to specific brain regions for treatment of neurological disease.

SAFETY AND REVERSIBILITY OF BBB OPENING

In order to determine the safety window of the FUS technique, through histological and immunohistological techniques (Baseri et al., 2010), we have identified the safe operating parameters of ultrasound exposure for neurons, astrocytes, and endothelial cells (Fig. 11.4). In summary, BBB opening starts occurring at around 0.2–0.3 MPa rarefactional pressure amplitude and beyond. At pressures under 0.6 MPa (Fig. 11.4[i]), no extravasation of red blood cells (RBC) or neuronal damage was observed in the regions of the hippocampus exhibiting the most pronounced BBB opening. Beyond 0.6 MPa (Fig. 11.4[ii]), RBC extravasation was detected, and beyond 0.9 MPa neuronal damage was observed. These preliminary findings suggest that there is overlap between the feasibility and safety windows within the pressure range of 0.3–0.6 MPa; that is, the BBB can be opened throughout the entire hippocampus without endothelial or neuronal damage at those pressures (Fig. 11.4; Baseri et al., 2010; Konofagou and Choi, 2008). FUS-induced BBB opening was reported to close within 72 hours in rabbits (Hynynen et al., 2001). The blood-brain barrier closure occurs within the first 24 hours after BBB opening at low pressures and within 2–3 days at higher pressures and monodispersed bubbles (Samiotaki et al., 2012).

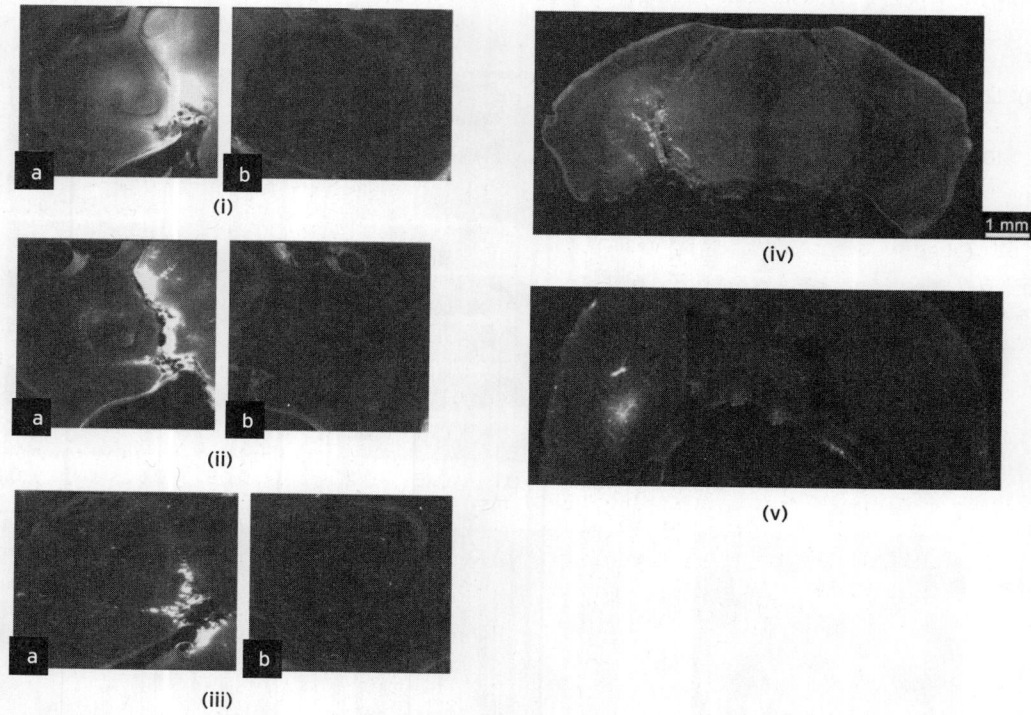

Figure 11.3 *Study of the molecular size through the bbb opening using dextrans and fluorescence imaging. Horizontal slice of Dextran of molecular weight equal to (i) 3, (ii) 70, and (iii) 2000 kDa on the (a) left (targeted) and (b) right (not targeted) hippocampus; (iv) coronal slice of the entire brain at 70 kDa Dextran showing the fluorescent left hippocampus (crescent shaped); (v) fluorescent albumin (67 kDa) permeated in the putamen through the opened BBB.*

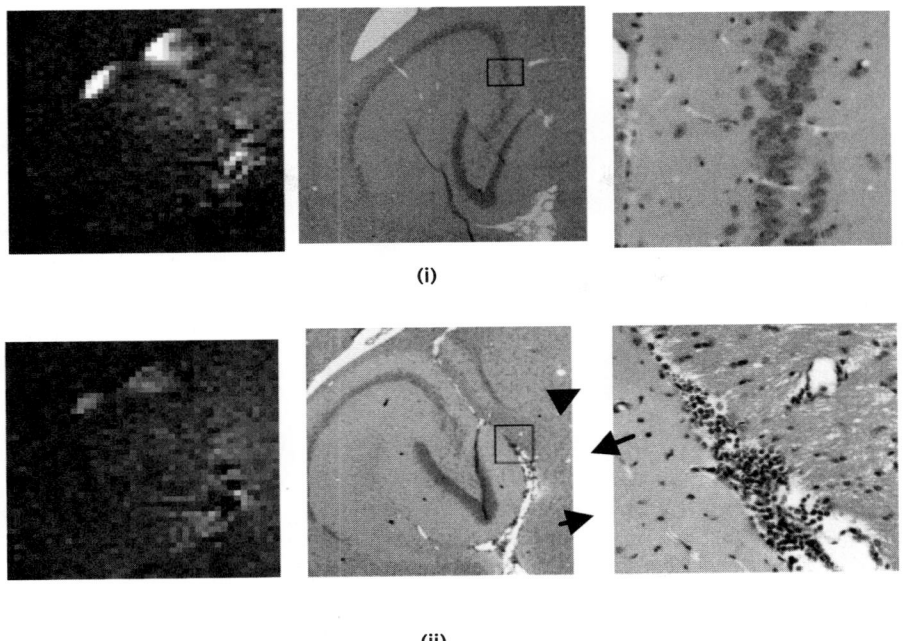

(i)

(ii)

Figure 11.4 *Comparison between MRI (left) and histology (center [1×] and right [200×] near the region of most enhanced BBB opening according to the MRI) after FUS-induced BBB opening on the left hippocampus at (i) 0.45 and (ii) 0.75 MPa peak rarefactional pressure. It shows that at lower pressures (i) the endothelial and neurons are intact while at higher pressures (ii) there is extravasation of red blood cells (indicated by arrowhead) and neuronal death (indicated by arrow). This indicates the safety window of the FUS technique in BBB opening.*

PROPERTIES OF BBB OPENING

Dynamic contrast-enhanced (DCE) MRI has been performed before and after the intraperitoneal injection of gadodiamide over 60 min (Vlachos et al., 2010). The general kinetic model (GKM) and reference region model (RRM) were used to estimate the permeability in the entire brain (Vlachos et al., 2010). At 0.3 MPa and 4- to-5-μm bubbles (Feshitan et al., 2009), the permeability were found to equal 0.02 ± 0.0123 min^{-1} and increase by at least 100 times in the region of BBB opening compared with the control side (Fig. 11.5). Cavitation (Fig. 11.2) and permeability (Fig. 11.5) findings demonstrated that the inertial cavitation threshold is independent of the bubble size while both the ICD and MR amplitude increased at larger bubble sizes, also indicating a correlation between the cavitation and permeability increase (Tung et al., 2010). The fact that the permeability increased with the pressure and microbubble size indicated that the BBB opening occurs at multiple sites within the capillary tree and that the BBB opening is larger with larger microbubbles, most likely due to the larger area of contact between the bubble and the capillary wall.

BBB OPENING IN LARGE ANIMALS

A 500-kHz FUS transducer was used transcranially in Macaca Mulatta monkeys (Marquet et al., 2011). This transducer was mounted on a stereotaxic frame, enabling treatment planning using the brain atlas. *In vivo* experiments were conducted in six monkeys (30 sonications) using Definity or 4–5 μm,

custom-made, lipid-shelled microbubbles. The BBB opening was confirmed using T1-weighted, spoiled gradient pulse-echo MR sequence at 3 T and gadodiamide IV injection. Damage was assessed using a T2 sequence with the same system. To obtain the BBB closing time line, the T1-weighted MR sequence was repeated along with gadodiamide IV injection over 4 days. MR images were registered to a monkey brain atlas allowing targeting quality assessment. Postprocessing was performed on combined pre- and postcontrast agent T1 images to quantify BBB disruption at the targeted regions, that is, caudate, hippocampus (Fig. 11.6), and visual cortex.

The blood-brain barrier opening was achieved in six different animals using peak negative pressures ranging from 0.2 to 0.6 MPa. No damage was detected at pressures below 0.45 MPa. The actual BBB-opened location was found to be in very good agreement with the targeted one under close to normal incidence angles with the absolute targeting error being less than 1 mm laterally and less than 4 mm axially. The maximum opening-volume-to-target overlap was 85% with an average of 52% depending on the brain region targeted (Deffieux and Konofagou, 2010; Marquet et al., 2011). Initial findings on the closing time line showed that the BBB was fully restored within 2 days after treatment.

THERAPEUTIC DELIVERY THROUGH THE BBB OPENING

Neurotrophic delivery to the brain has been proven essential in reversing the neuronal degeneration process but so far has been hindered by the blood–brain barrier. In a recent study

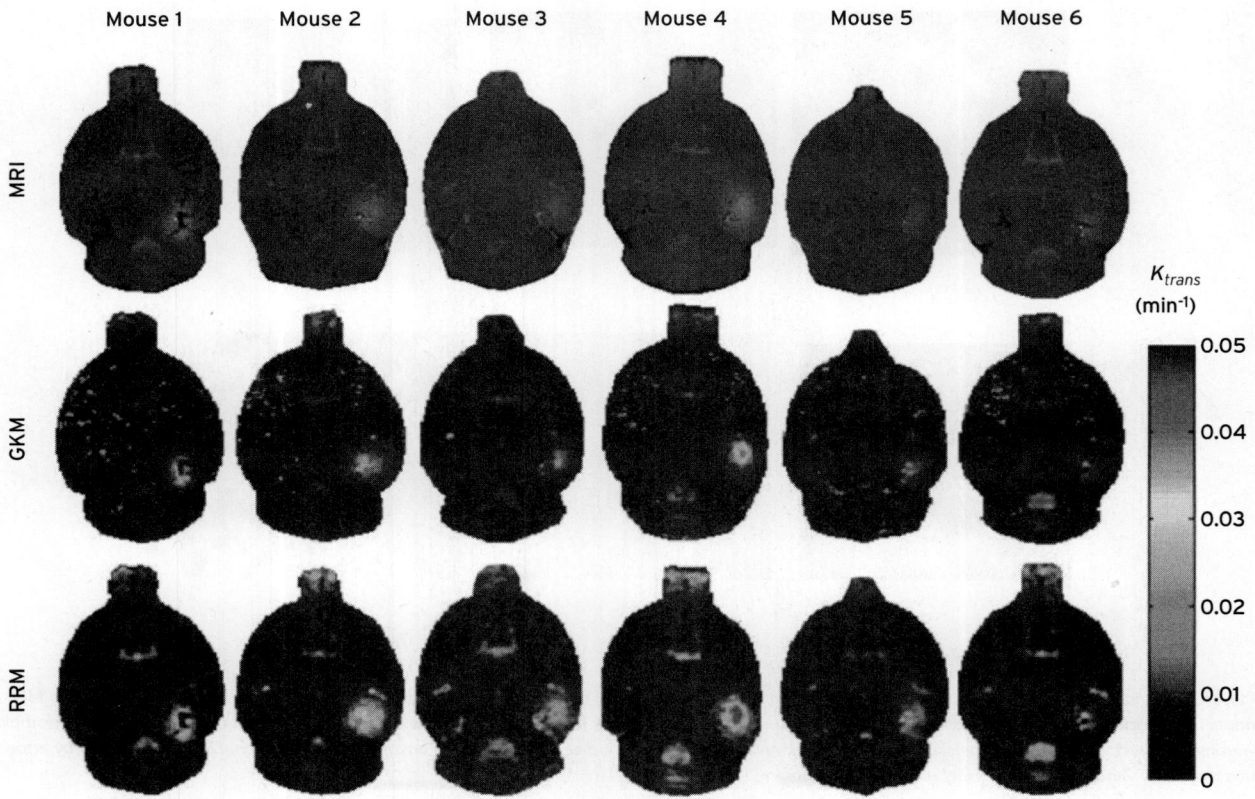

Figure 11.5 *T1 images (first row) and their corresponding permeability maps generated from GKM (second row) and RRM (third row) for all mice. The transverse slice with maximum T1 signal enhancement is selected. The Ktrans values are indicated in the color bar. The maps have been superimposed over the corresponding DCE-MR images. In the case of Mouse 1, the last acquired DCE-MR image is presented instead of a regular T1[61]. (See color insert).*

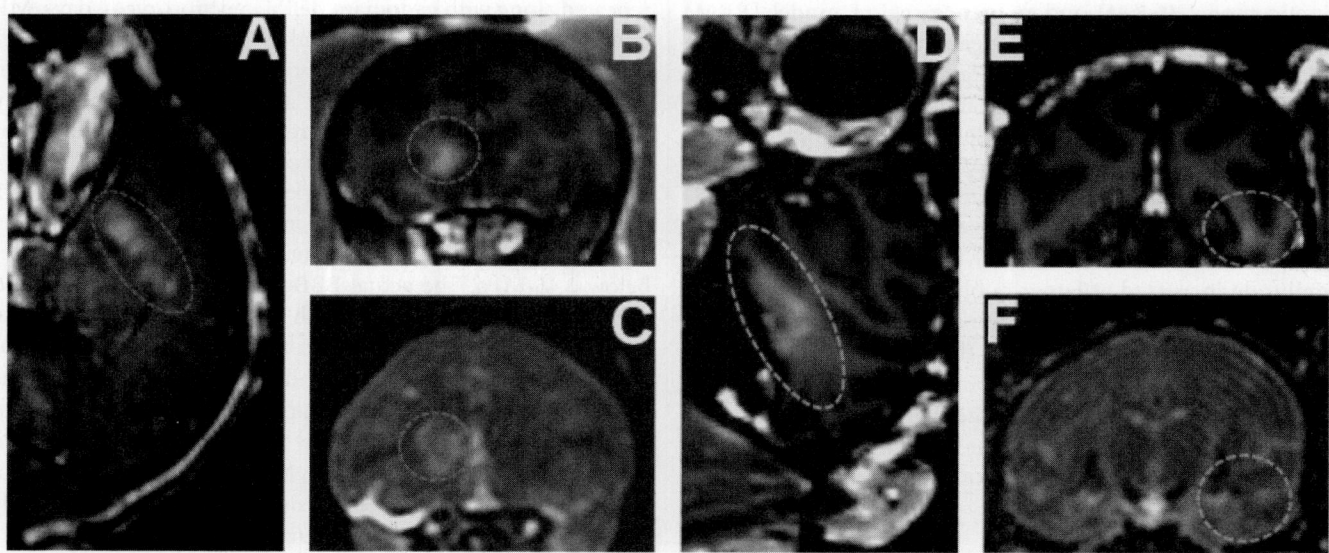

Figure 11.6 *In vivo BBB opening in monkeys. (A, C) BBB opening experiment targeting the caudate using custom-made microbubbles and applying 0.6 MPa (dashed line shows region of interest). (D, F) BBB opening experiment targeting hippocampus using Definity® microbubbles and applying 0.6 MPa (dashed line shows region of interest). (A, B, D, E) 3D Spoiled Gradient-Echo (SPGR) T1-weighted sequence was applied after intravenous (IV) injection of gadodiamide 1 hr after sonication. (A, D) Sagittal slices at the region of interest. (B, E) Corresponding coronal slices. (C, F) 3D T2-weighted sequence. An edema was visible using custom-made microbubbles while no damage was detected using Definity® microbubbles.*

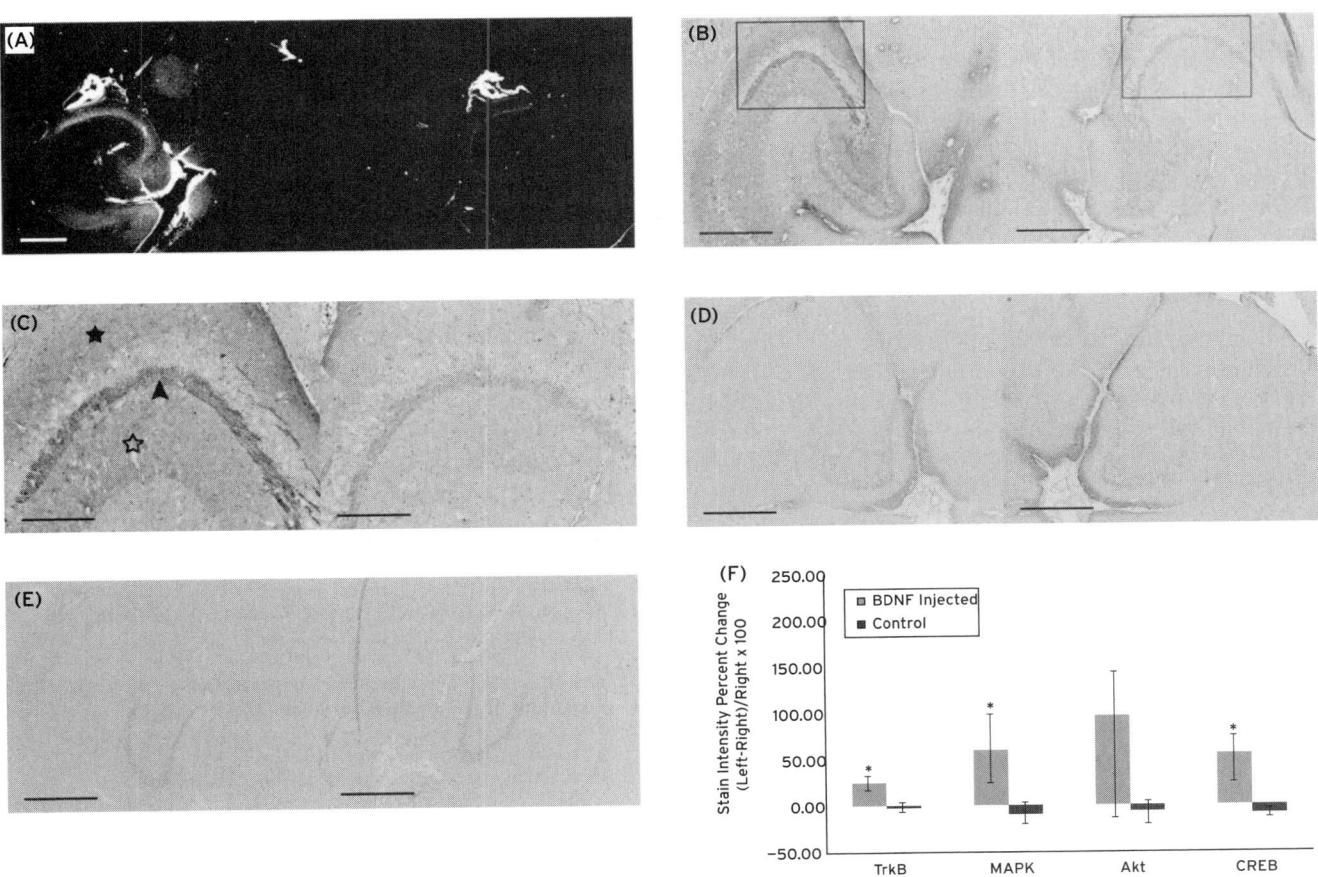

Figure 11.7 (A) Fluorescent image of a 100-micron frozen brain section from a mouse that was sacrificed 20 min after sonication. The sonicated hippocampus (left) shows much higher fluorescent intensity than the unsonicated hippocampus (right), depicting blood–brain barrier opening and the extravasation of fluorescent-tagged (Alexa Fluor 594) BDNF in the sonicated region; (B) a 5-micron frozen section from the same mouse was immunohistochemically stained using a primary antibody against phosphorylated MAPK (pMAPK). Consistent with the fluorescent image in (A), the intensity of DAB staining is much greater in the left sonicated hippocampus compared with the right control; the black box shows the enlarged area in (C), where immunoreactivity to pMAPK is shown in mossy fiber terminals (arrowhead), suprapyramidal CA3 dendrites (black star), and the axons of the Schaffer collateral system (hollow star). (D) Immunohistochemical staining of a 5-micron frozen section from a mouse that was sacrificed 3 min after sonication; the same primary antibody against pMAPK was used. No difference in DAB intensity is observed between the sonicated and the control hippocampus. (E) Negative control for the same mouse in (A); no primary antibody (against pMAPK) was added to this 5-micron frozen section during the staining procedure. All magnifications are 40× and scale bars are 500 μm except for (C), which is 100× and 200 μm, respectively. In (F), immunohistology stain intensity analysis shows percentage change between the left (FUS) and the right (no FUS) sides of the mice brains. A significant difference ($p < 0.05$, N = 3; depicted by asterisks) was found between the BDNF-administered animal group and the control (no BDNF) animal group for the TrkB, MAPK, and CREB antibodies. Bars represent mean ± standard deviation.

by our group, not only was it shown that the brain-derived neurotrophic factor (BDNF) can cross the ultrasound-induced BBB opening but also that it can trigger signaling pathways in the pyramidal neurons of mice in vivo from the membrane to the nucleus (Fig. 11.7) (Baseri et al., 2012). This opens entirely new avenues in the brain drug delivery where focused ultrasound in conjunction with microbubbles can generate downstream effects at the cellular and molecular level and thus increase the drug's efficacy and potency in controlling or reversing the disease.

SUMMARY

The studies described this chapter demonstrate that FUS in conjunction with microbubbles was hereby shown to effectively and reproducibly open the blood–brain barrier transcranially in vivo with its recovery occurring within the first 24 hours. The permeability of the FUS-opened BBB was shown to increase by at least two orders of magnitude, indicating facilitation of drug delivery through FUS. Molecules of a wide range of sizes were capable of traversing the opened BBB without any associated structural damage. A dependence of the BBB permeability on the pressure and the microbubble size indicated that multiple sites of BBB opening within the ultrasound beam occur simultaneously while each BBB opening site increases with the microbubble size. Finally, a new pulse sequence was designed that showed feasibility at very short pulse lengths, and transcranial BBB opening in larger animals, such as nonhuman primates and humans, was shown feasible in simulations and ex vivo experiments as well as in vivo primate monkeys (Fig. 11.6) (Marquet et al., 2011; Tung et al., 2011).

The preclinical studies described point to the considerable progress that has been made in understanding the characteristics of the BBB as well as the safety and efficacy of delivering small molecules into the brain parenchyma using focused ultrasound with microbubbles. Studies are ongoing in order to ensure successful clinical translation in the near future.

DISCLOSURE

Dr. Konofagou has no conflicts of interest to disclose. The research in the chapter was supported by NIH R01 EB009041, NIH R21 EY018505, NSF CAREER 064471, the Kinetics Foundation, and the Kavli Institute.

REFERENCES

Abbott, N.J., Ronnback, L., et al. (2006). Astrocyte-endothelial interactions at the blood-brain barrier. *Nat. Rev. Neurosci.* 7:41–53.

Bakay, L.,H. Ballantine, T., Jr., et al. (1956). Ultrasonically produced changes in the blood-brain barrier. *AMA Arch. Neurol. Psychiatry* 76:457–467.

Ballantine, H.T., Jr., Bell, E., et al. (1960). Progress and problems in the neurological applications of focused ultrasound. *J. Neurosurg.* 17:858–876.

Baseri, B., Choi, J.J., et al. (2012). Activation of signaling pathways following localized delivery of systemically administered neurotrophic factors across the blood–brain barrier using focused ultrasound and microbubbles. *Phys. Med. Biol.* 57:N65–N81.

Baseri, B., Choi, J.J., et al. (2010). Safety assessment of blood-brain barrier opening using focused ultrasound and definity microbubbles: a short-term study. *Ultras. Med. Biol.* 36(9):1445–1459.

Blasberg, R., Patlak, C., et al. (1975). Intrathecal chemotherapy brain tissue profiles after ventriculocisternal perfusion. *J. Pharmacol. Exp. Ther.* 195:73–83.

Borden, M., Kruse, D., et al. (2005). Influence of lipid shell physicochemical properties on ultrasound-induced microbubble destruction. *IEEE. Trans. Ultrason. Ferroelect. Freq. Contr.* 52:1992–2002.

Chen, S., Kroll, M.H., et al. (2002). Bioeffects of myocardial contrast microbubble destruction by echocardiography. *Echocardiography* 19:495–500.

Choi, J.J., Feshitan, J.A., et al. (2009). The dependence of the ultrasound-induced blood-brain barrier opening characteristics on microbubble size *in vivo*. In: Ebbini, E., ed. *8th International Symposium on Therapeutic Ultrasound*, AIP Conference Proceedings. Minneapolis, MN, pp. 58–62.

Choi, J.J., Pernot, M., et al. (2007a). Spatio-temporal analysis of molecular delivery through the blood-brain barrier using focused ultrasound. *Phys. Med. Biol.* 52:5509–5530.

Choi, J.J., Pernot, M., et al. (2005). Feasibility of transcranial, localized drug-delivery in the brain of Alzheimer's-model mice using focused ultrasound. In: IEEE Ultrasonics Symposium, 2005, pp. 988–991.

Choi, J.J., Pernot, M., et al. (2006). Noninvasive blood-brain barrier opening in live mice. *AIP Conf. Proc.* 829:271–275.

Choi, J.J., Pernot, M., et al. (2007b). Noninvasive, transcranial and localized opening of the blood-brain barrier using focused ultrasound in mice. *Ultrasound Med. Biol.* 33:95–104.

Choi, J., Selert, K., et al. (2011). Noninvasive and localized neuronal delivery using short ultrasonic pulses and microbubbles. *Proc. Natl. Acad. Sci. USA* 108(40):16539–16544.

Choi, J.J., Small, S.A., et al. (2006). Optimization of blood-brain barrier opening in mice using focused ultrasound. In: *IEEE Ultrasonics Symposium, 2006*, pp. 540–543.

Choi, J.J., Wang, S., et al. (2008). Noninvasive and transient blood-brain barrier opening in the hippocampus of Alzheimer's double transgenic mice using focused ultrasound. *Ultrason. Imaging* 30:189–200.

Choi, J.J., Wang, S., et al. (2007c). Molecular delivery and microbubble dependence study of the FUS-induced blood-brain barrier opening *in vivo*. In: *Ultrasonics Symposium, 2007 IEEE International Ultrasound Symposium Proceedings*, pp. 1192–1195.

Choi, J.J., Wang, S., et al. (2010). Molecules of various pharmacologically-relevant sizes can cross the ultrasound-induced blood-brain barrier opening *in vivo*. *Ultrasound Med. Biol.* 36(1):58–67.

Christensen, D.A. (1988). *Ultrasonic Bioinstrumentation*. New York: John Wiley.

Christiansen, J., French, B.A., et al. (2003). Targeted tissue transfection with ultrasound destruction of plasmid-bearing cationic microbubbles. *Ultrasound. Med. Biol.* 29:1759–1767.

Chomas, J.E., Dayton, P., et al. (2001). Threshold of fragmentation for ultrasonic contrast agents. *J. Biomed. Opt.* 6:141–150.

Deffieux, T.A., and Konofagou, E.E. (2010).Numerical study and experimental validation of a simple transcranial focused ultrasound system applied to blood-brain barrier opening. *IEEE-UFFC Trans.* 57(12):2637–265,.

Farny, C.H., Holt, R.G., et al. (2009). Temporal and spatial detection of HIFU-induced inertial and hot-vapor cavitation with a diagnostic ultrasound system. *Ultrasound Med. Biol.* 35:603–615.

Feshitan, J.A., Chen, C.C., et al. (2009). Microbubble size isolation by differential centrifugation. *J. Colloid. Interface Sci.* 329:316–324.

Fischer, H., Gottschlich, R., et al. (1998). Blood-brain barrier permeation: molecular parameters governing passive diffusion. *J. Membr. Biol.* 165:201–211.

Fung, L., Shin, M., et al. (1996). Chemotherapeutic drugs released from polymers distribution of 1,3-bis(2-chloroethyl)-1-nitrosourea in the rat brain. *Pharm. Res.* 13:671–682.

Ghose, A., Viswanadhan, V.N., et al. (1999). A knowledge-based approach in designing combinatorial or medicinal chemistry libraries for drug discovery. 1. A qualitative and quantitative characterization of known drug databases. *J. Comb. Chem.* 1:55–68.

Hynynen, K., McDannold, N., et al. (2001). Noninvasive MR imaging-guided focal opening of the blood-brain barrier in rabbits. *Radiology* 220:640–646.

Hynynen, K., McDannold, N., et al. (2003). Non-invasive opening of BBB by focused ultrasound. *Acta Neurochir. Suppl.* 86:555–558.

Hynynen, K., McDannold, N., et al. (2006). Focal disruption of the blood-brain barrier due to 260-kHz ultrasound bursts: a method for molecular imaging and targeted drug delivery. *J. Neurosurg.* 105:445–454.

Hynynen, K., McDannold, N., et al. (2005). Local and reversible blood-brain barrier disruption by noninvasive focused ultrasound at frequencies suitable for trans-skull sonications. *NeuroImage* 24:12–20.

Iadecola, C. (2004). Neurovascular regulation in the normal brain and in Alzheimer's disease. *Nat. Rev. Neurosci.* 5:347–360.

Kaps, M., Seidel, G., et al. (2001). Pharmacokinetics of echocontrast agent infusion in a dog model. *J. Neuroimaging* 11:298–302.

Kaufmann, B.A., Wei, K., et al. (2007). Contrast echocardiography. *Curr. Probl. Cardiol.* 32:51–96.

Kinoshita, M., McDannold, N., et al. (2006). Noninvasive localized delivery of Herceptin to the mouse brain by MRI-guided focused ultrasound-induced blood-brain barrier disruption. *Proc. Natl. Acad. Sci. USA* 103:11719–11723, Aug 1.

Konofagou, E. and Choi, J.J. (2008). Ultrasound-induced treatment of neurodegenerative diseases across the blood-brain barrier. In Al-Jumaily, A., and Alizad, A. eds. *Biomedical Applications of Vibration and Acoustics in Therapy, Bioeffects and Modelling*. New York: ASME Press, pp. 63–80.

Konofagou, E.E., Choi, J., et al. (2009). Characterization and optimization of trans-blood-brain barrier diffusion *in vivo*. In: Ebbini, E. ed. *8th International Symposium on Therapeutic Ultrasound*, AIP Conference Proceedings. Minneapolis, MN, pp. 418–422.

Leighton, T. (1994). *The Acoustic Bubble*, 1st Edition. London: Academic.

Li, P., Armstrong, W.F., et al. (2004). Impact of myocardial contrast echocardiography on vascular permeability: comparison of three different contrast agents. *Ultrasound Med. Biol.* 30:83–91.

Li, P., Cao, L.Q., et al. (2003). Impact of myocardial contrast echocardiography on vascular permeability: an *in vivo* dose response study of delivery mode, pressure amplitude and contrast dose. *Ultrasound Med. Biol.* 29:1341–1349.

Lipinski, C. (2000). Drug-like properties and the causes of poor solubility and poor permeability. *J. Pharmacol. Toxicol. Methods* 44:235–249.

Marquet, F., Tung, Y.-S., et al. (2011). Noninvasive, transient and selective blood-brain barrier opening in non-human primates *in vivo*. *PLoS ONE*, 6(7):e22598.

McDannold, N., King, R.L., et al. (2004). MRI monitoring of heating produced by ultrasound absorption in the skull: *in vivo* study in pigs. *Magn. Reson. Med.* 51:1061–1065.

McDannold, N., Vykhodtseva, N., et al. (2006). Targeted disruption of the blood-brain barrier with focused ultrasound: association with cavitation activity. *Phys. Med. Biol.* 51:793–807.

McDannold, N., Vykhodtseva, N., et al. (2005). MRI-guided targeted blood-brain barrier disruption with focused ultrasound: histological findings in rabbits. *Ultrasound Med. Biol.* 31:1527–1537.

Mesiwala, A.H., Farrell, L., et al. (2002). High-intensity focused ultrasound selectively disrupts the blood-brain barrier *in vivo*. *Ultrasound Med. Biol.* 28:389–400.

Miller, D.L. (2007). Overview of experimental studies of biological effects of medical ultrasound caused by gas body activation and inertial cavitation. *Prog. Biophys. Mol. Bio.* 93:314–330.

Miller, D., Li, P., et al. (2005). Influence of contrast agent dose and ultrasound exposure on cardiomyocyte injury induced by myocardial contrast echocardiography in rats. *Radiology* 237:137–143.

Neppiras, E.A. (1980). Acoustic cavitation. *Phys. Rep.* 61:159–251.

Pardridge, W.M. (2005). The blood-brain barrier: bottleneck in brain drug development. in *NeuroRx* 2:3–14.

Pardridge, W.M. (2006). Molecular Trojan horses for blood-brain barrier drug delivery. *Disc. Med.* 6:4.

Pardridge, W.M. (2007). Drug targeting to the brain. *Pharm. Res.* 24:1733–1744.

Patrick, J.T., Nolting, M.N., et al. (1990). Ultrasound and the blood-brain barrier. *Adv. Exp. Med. Biol.* 267:369–381.

Raymond, S.B., Treat, L.H., et al. (2008). Ultrasound enhanced delivery of molecular imaging and therapeutic agents in Alzheimer's disease mouse models. *PLoS ONE* 3:e2175.

Samiotaki, M., Vlachos, F., et al. (2012). A quantitative pressure and microbubble-size dependence study of focused ultrasound-induced blood-brain barrier opening reversibility *in vivo* using MRI. *Magn. Reson. Med.* vol. 67(3):769–777.

Sheikov, N., McDannold, N., et al. (2006). Brain arterioles show more active vesicular transport of blood-borne tracer molecules than capillaries and venules after focused ultrasound-evoked opening of the blood-brain barrier. *Ultrasound Med. Biol.* 32:1399–1409.

Sheikov, N., McDannold, N., et al. (2008). Effect of focused ultrasound applied with an ultrasound contrast agent on the tight junctional integrity of the brain microvascular endothelium. *Ultrasound Med. Biol.* 34(7):1093–1104.

Sheikov, N., McDannold, N., et al. (2004). Cellular mechanisms of the blood-brain barrier opening induced by ultrasound in presence of microbubbles. *Ultrasound Med. Biol.* 30:979–989.

Stewart, P.A., and Tuor, U.I. (1994). Blood-eye barriers in the rat: correlation of ultrastructure with function. *J. Comp. Neurol.* 340:566–576.

Treat, L.H., McDannold, N., et al. (2007). Targeted delivery of doxorubicin to the rat brain at therapeutic levels using MRI-guided focused ultrasound. *Int. J. Cancer* 121:901–907.

Tung, Y.-S., Vlachos, F., et al. (2011). The mechanism of the interaction between focused ultrasound and microbubbles in blood-brain barrier opening in mice. *J. Acous. Soc. Amer.* 108(40), 130(5):3059–3067.

Tung, Y., Vlachos, F., et al. (2010). In vivo transcranial cavitation threshold detection during ultrasound-induced blood-brain barrier opening. *Phys. Med. Biol.*, 55(20):6141–6155.

Vlachos, F., Tung, Y.S., et al. (2010). Permeability assessment of the focused ultrasound-induced blood-brain barrier opening using dynamic contrast-enhanced MRI. *Phys. Med. Biol.* 55:5451–5466.

Vykhodtseva, N.I., Hynynen, K., et al. (1995). Histologic effects of high intensity pulsed ultrasound exposure with subharmonic emission in rabbit brain *in vivo*. *Ultrasound Med. Biol.* 21:969–979.

Yang, F.Y., Fu, W.M., et al. (2007). Quantitative evaluation of focused ultrasound with a contrast agent on blood-brain barrier disruption. *Ultrasound Med. Biol.* 33:1421–1427.

12 | GENETIC METHODOLOGIES AND APPLICATIONS

SHAUN M. PURCELL

The past decade has witnessed tremendous advances in the molecular technologies and data-analytic methods at our disposal for studying the genetic bases of complex diseases and traits. These advances have enabled the creation of comprehensive catalogs of different forms of human genetic variation, as well as large-scale studies focused on specific diseases or traits. In this chapter, we outline the general principles behind some of these advances and discuss their application to studying complex traits, with a focus on neuropsychiatric disease in particular.

MOTIVATIONS FOR MAPPING THE GENETIC BASIS OF DISEASE

Genetic epidemiology is fundamentally concerned with relating *genotype* (i.e., variation between individuals' genomes) to *phenotype* (i.e., the presence or absence of a disease, or measure of a trait such as height or cholesterol level) (Altshuler et al., 2008). There are a number of relatively distinct motivations for this work, which can be conceived of both in terms of proximal and distal goals of the research. Recently, there has been a great deal of focus on identifying specific *alleles* (variable forms of a *locus*, which is a gene or region) that "explain the heritability" as a primary benchmark and major goal of genetic studies, as discussed later. For many downstream applications, however, perhaps an equally important, but distinct, proximal goal of genetics is to point to the genes and/or gene networks that are causally associated with disease.

Following from these proximal goals (identifying the specific alleles that explain heritability and identifying the relevant genes and pathways) there are several distinct, more distal goals or applications, the success of which will depend on different aspects of the genetic discoveries made. In theory, understanding the genetics of a disease could be used for risk prediction, either at the population level or within families (following the model of genetic counseling for Mendelian disease); for prediction of disease course, severity, or drug response in affected individuals; to identify targets for drug discovery research; to inform on the relationships and comorbidities between different diseases; or even to provide a framework for causal inference around environmental effects (Smith and Ebrahim, 2003). More generally, advances in understanding disease genetics will ultimately, but undoubtedly, provide fundamental insights into human biology, development, and evolution. However, the ease with which genetics will achieve success in these various applications relates to different aspects of the unknown, underlying *genetic architecture* of any particular disease or trait.

The question of the genetic architecture of common disease has been a central one: it relates to the types of approaches that will work best to map genes, as well as to what we can expect to learn from genetic studies in the near future. For a heritable disease, genetic architecture describes *how many* independent genetic effects contribute to risk, at the level of both the population and the specific individual; it also describes the typical *frequency* and *effect size* of these variants; *how they combine* to produce a phenotype (e.g., additively or interactively) and the extent to which multiple genetic risk factors for a disease coalesce into a smaller number of distinct *biological pathways or networks*. Other aspects of genetic architecture include the *mode of inheritance* (e.g., recessive effects), the presence of positive, negative, or balancing *selection* acting on risk variants, the extent to which genetic effects are shared (or contribute to different disease rates) *across populations*, the extent to which variants influence multiple outcomes through *pleiotropy* (one gene having multiple downstream effects), and the extent to which genetic effects are moderated by environmental exposures (*gene–environment interaction*).

The success of risk prediction, for example, in the general population will be crucially dependent on the proportion of variance explained by detected variants, which is a function of both the frequency and penetrance (a measure of effect size that equals the chance that a carrier develops disease) of risk alleles. By learning which specific alleles (the particular variants of genes) increase or decrease risk or type or course of disease, one can in theory predict an individual's risk or provide tailored medical treatment to patients based on their genotype. In practice, truly personalized genomic medicine is still only a long-term goal in most instances, rather than a current or imminent reality, although this is likely to be an area of great progress over the coming decade.

However, inasmuch as the distal goals relate to identifying *loci*, to point to potential drug targets, for example, the extent to which detected variants account for heritability might not be critically relevant: for instance, there are multiple examples of genetic studies that have pointed to weak genetic effects in genes that are already known targets of existing, successful therapies. Thus, genetic studies have a parallel set of aims that are almost orthogonal to the goal of explaining variability in a population, involving the identification of the *networks of genes* implicated in disease. Here the aim is to use this information to point to the biological mechanisms involved in disease pathogenesis.

CLASSICAL GENETIC EPIDEMIOLOGY: FROM FAMILY STUDIES, SEGREGATION, AND LINKAGE ANALYSIS, TO LINKAGE DISEQUILIBRIUM MAPPING

Classical genetic epidemiology posed a series of increasingly specific questions: For a particular disease or trait, are there genetic influences? Is the genetic basis simple or complex? Where are those genes located? Which specific forms of the gene cause disease? The tools to answer these questions were, respectively, family and twin studies, segregation analysis, linkage analysis, and association analysis. Twin and family studies are used primarily to estimate the heritability of a trait (the extent to which variation in outcome is due to variation in genes) by contrasting the phenotypic similarity of relatives of differing genetic similarity. More recently, twin and family study designs have also proved useful in molecular studies of genetic and epigenetic variation (van Dongen et al., 2012). One notable family study of schizophrenia and bipolar disorder involved tens of thousands of patients from Sweden and showed clear evidence for a shared genetic basis common to both disorders (Lichtenstein et al., 2009). Looking at a range of first-degree relative classes, such studies estimate the probandwise concordance rate (the probability an individual develops disease given they have an affected relative of a particular type) and the familial relative risk (λ), which for a given class of relative, is the concordance rate divided by the population prevalence of disease. Both approaches ask how much more likely an individual is to develop disease if he or she has an affected relative. Estimates of λ for MZ twins, full siblings, parent–offspring pairs, and half-siblings track strongly with the extent of genetic similarity in those pairs, indicative of a considerable genetic basis for these diseases. This and other studies put the heritability of schizophrenia to be very high, with estimates from 60% to 80%, for example.

Segregation analysis considers the broader pattern of disease within larger pedigrees. For Mendelian disease, segregation analysis can estimate whether there is likely to be a single disease allele in each family, and if so, its mode of inheritance. For complex diseases that are caused by multiple genes and environmental influences, segregation analysis is typically uninformative (beyond demonstrating above-chance levels of familial clustering). Linkage analysis also uses pedigrees to identify specific (but very broad) chromosomal loci that cosegregate with disease in a particular family. Linkage analysis primarily gained popularity after the introduction of molecular marker maps in the 1980s. For example, by genotyping 300–400 "microsatellite" markers (short tandem repeats of variable length between individuals), one can infer the pattern of gene flow in a family (specifically, of shared chromosomal regions coinherited from a single ancestor and so identical-by-descent, IBD) and then search for chromosomal positions at which the profile of IBD maximally correlates with the coinheritance pattern of the phenotype. Linkage analysis proved spectacularly useful in mapping Mendelian disease genes of major effect: rare mutations that almost always lead to correspondingly rare diseases. In contrast, for complex, common diseases, linkage analysis has yielded very few durable results (for neuropsychiatric disease, one notable exception is the DISC1 locus).

This is, in large part, because linkage analysis has low power to detect variants of only modest effect. The general failure of linkage analysis (given that it has, in fact, been widely applied for many diseases, including schizophrenia) can be taken to indicate that the genetic architecture of most common diseases is unlikely to be well characterized as primarily consisting of a small number of "hotspot" regions: that is, genes or loci at which a sizeable proportion of cases carry a highly or even moderately penetrant risk variant.

Association analysis (or linkage disequilibrium mapping) has replaced linkage analysis as the workhorse of genetic epidemiology over the past decade. Association analysis is conceptually straightforward: typically in populations of unrelated individuals, association analysis simply looks for specific variants (alleles) that are significantly more frequent in people with the disease compared with those without. Compared with linkage analysis, this approach is more powerful to detect variants of smaller effect (Risch and Merikangas, 1996).

To more concretely contrast the effect sizes expected for a "major gene" disorder versus a complex, common disease, consider that for a rare disease, say, affecting 1 in 10,000 individuals, a major gene effect may increase risk more than 10,000-fold: for example, if baseline risk in noncarriers of the gene is 0.00003, then the penetrance (risk of disease given genotype) would be 30% or more. In this scenario, even though the gene is not completely Mendelian (deterministic in its effect), a very large proportion (more than one third) of carriers will develop the disease, and conversely, a very large proportion of all affected individuals will carry that particular disease allele (again, more than one third). In comparison, for a common disease with a population prevalence of 1 in 100 individuals, for common alleles researchers expect realistic effect sizes along the lines of, at most, a 1.2-fold, rather than 10,000-fold, increase in risk. If this risk allele has a population frequency of, say, 40%, it implies that carriers have ~1.2% risk of developing disease and we would expect to see the allele in ~44% of cases compared with ~40% of unaffected individuals. This relatively small difference means that the variant is harder to detect statistically. (It also means that this allele, by itself, will have very little predictive utility: i.e., knowing an individual's genotype at this locus would only marginally improve one's ability to predict, above chance, whether or not the individual will develop disease. Of course, for a heritable disease, we would expect many such loci to contribute to disease risk that could be informative if analyzed collectively.)

Historically, the principal limitation in applying association analysis broadly was that, unlike linkage analysis in which only a relatively modest number of molecular markers provide a genome-wide survey of gene flow within families (because very large chunks of chromosome are shared between closely related individuals), testing a specific marker for association only queries a tiny proportion of the total extent of variability that exists genome-wide. This arises from the properties of linkage disequilibrium in human populations, as described later. Thus, hundreds of thousands of markers would be needed to cover the whole genome, and the sufficiently high-throughput genotyping methods needed to achieve this have only come into existence more recently. In practice, for a long time this meant that association analysis was limited to testing a small number of variants in a small number of *candidate genes*. Candidates were usually selected on the basis of prior knowledge, or assumptions, about the pathophysiology of disease. In neuropsychiatric genetics, despite a considerable body of work, studies of candidate genes largely failed to lead to broadly reproducible results. There are multiple reasons to explain this state of affairs (reviewed by Kim et al., 2011). Perhaps most obviously, many of the original hypotheses about the disease may have been incorrect, or at least fundamentally incomplete descriptions of a much more complex process. For a number of diseases such as Type II diabetes and Crohns' disease, the biology pointed to by recent, robust genetic findings from genome-wide association studies (see following) has often been at odds with the prior assumptions about what would be genetically important. This is, of course, a good thing from the perspective of genetic studies, in that we wish for genetics to be a source of novel insights and hypotheses—that is, to tell us something new. Typically the error rates of candidates genes studies would also have been high: false positives (Type I errors in hypothesis testing) are hard to control, given varying degrees of multiple testing, and false negatives (Type II errors) are likely as sample sizes used for most candidate gene studies were typically very small by today's standards. In schizophrenia, as of 2011, 732 autosomal genes had been tested by 1,374 hypothesis-driven candidate gene studies, although most genes were investigated in only one (61%) or two (16%) studies (Kim et al., 2011). Typically no replication was attempted, or it was underpowered, or the statistical evidence was, at best, hard to reconcile from the literature (e.g., when different markers in the same gene were tested across different studies, or when

replication was claimed but the direction of effect for the same marker differed between studies). Furthermore, genetic variation in the candidate genes tested was typically only very poorly captured, even for common variation, often with only one or two markers being genotyped per gene.

EXPANDING KNOWLEDGE OF THE HUMAN GENOME

Reference maps and databases have been critical in many areas of genomics: from the human genome reference sequence itself, to maps of coding and other functional elements in the sequence. Equally important for disease and population genetics has been the more recent construction of maps, or catalogs, of observed *variation* within and between different human populations. The two most notable efforts are the International HapMap project (International HapMap Consortium, 2007) and, more recently, the 1000 Genomes project (1000 Genomes Consortium, 2010). The HapMap project employed large-scale genotyping to type almost 4 million known single-nucleotide polymorphisms (SNPs) in 270 individuals of African, Asian, and European ancestry. As well as generating lists of technically validated polymorphic sites along with estimates of allele frequencies in multiple populations, a central aim was to characterize and describe the patterns of correlation between nearby variants, referred to as *linkage disequilibrium* (LD). As illustrated in Figure 12.1, two or more alleles at nearby sites are said to be in LD if they co-occur more than expected by chance, that is, than if they were inherited independently of

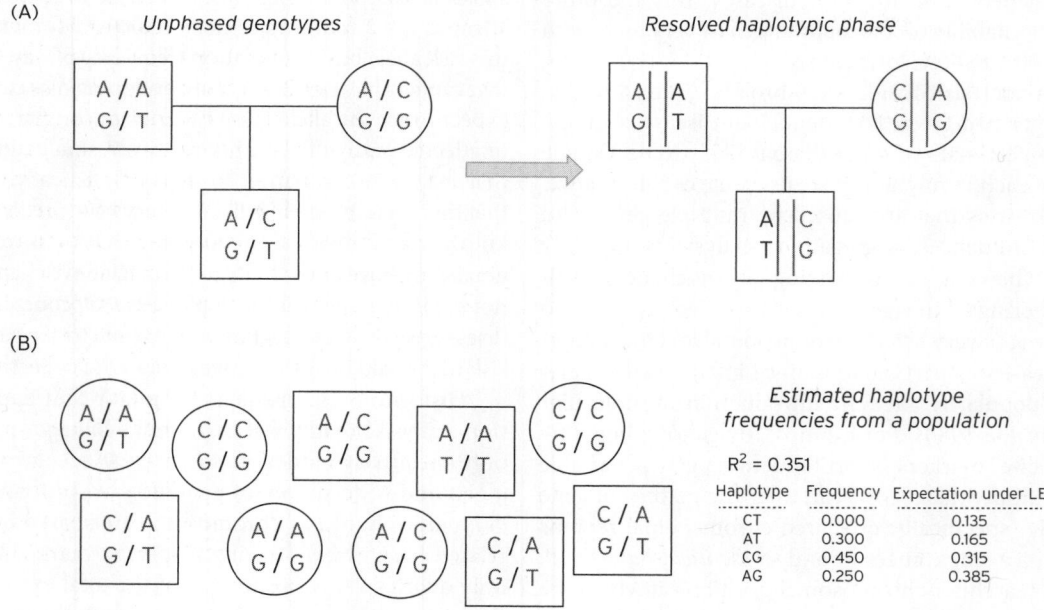

Figure 12.1 *Linkage disequilibrium and haplotype phasing. (A) Using family information can often resolve phase unambiguously. Here a trio is genotyped for two biallelic SNPs: for the first site, A or C alleles (top genotype in all plots); for the second site, G or T alleles (bottom genotype in all plots) in this example. From inspection, the mother necessarily transmits the CG haplotype, implying that the offspring carries AT and CG haplotypes, rather than AG and CT haplotypes. (B) In the absence of family data, it is still possible to estimate haplotype frequencies from genotypes at SNPs in linkage equilibrium. In this toy, illustrative example, the EM algorithm would conclude that the CT haplotype does not exist in this population based on this very small sample of 10, meaning that the two SNPs are in LD (here R² is estimated at 0.351). Individuals would be assigned a combination of AT, CG, and AG haplotypes only, which will be consistent with their SNP genotypes.*

each other. In reality, *haplotypes* (collections of alleles on the same physical stretch of chromosome) are the primary unit of inheritance, not individual alleles. Two alleles on the same haplotype will tend to be either both cotransmitted from parent to offspring, or will both be untransmitted, thereby inducing a correlation between the alleles at the population level. The further away two sites physically reside on the chromosome, the more likely that they will be separated by a meiotic *recombination event*. Thus, LD between any two sites tends to "break down," or be attenuated, over distance. This property can be used to localize genes, in that it implies that two sites that are in LD are also likely to be physically colocated on the same stretch of chromosome. This is the principle behind linkage disequilibrium mapping.

Obtaining genotype data on an individual for two nearby heterozygous sites does not directly reveal the underlying haplotypes carried by that individual, although in families the haplotype can often be inferred straightforwardly. For example, if the individual carries an *A/C* (heterozygous) genotype for the first site and *G/T* for the second, there are two possible haplotypic configurations: that the *AG* haplotype was inherited from one parent, and therefore *CT* from the second, or that *AT* was inherited from the first and *CG* from the second. The process of resolving which configuration is more likely is called *phasing*. As in the Figure 12.1, phase is often unambiguous when one studies multiple members of the same family. Alternatively, statistical approaches (based on algorithms such as expectation maximization [EM] or Markov Chain Monte Carlo [MCMC] and population genetic models) can be used to resolve phase in samples of unrelated individuals, by considering the observed correlation between sites and treating the unknown phase information statistically in terms of a missing-data problem (Browning and Browning, 2012). In some situations it is also possible to use sequencing to type haplotypes directly, using molecular rather than statistical means, sequencing along the same physical stretch of chromosome.

The actual structure and extent of LD in humans reflects both demographic factors and the history of the population studied, as well as biological properties of the genome, influencing the rate of recombination at particular sites. The typical structure and extent of LD is of critical importance to the implementation of association analysis as applied to large genomic regions. Fundamentally, association mapping (or *linkage disequilibrium* mapping, as previously noted) relies on the fact that by testing a particular variant, one is implicitly testing a host of nearby variants, for which the genotyped markers act as proxies, or *tags*.

The HapMap project provides a comprehensive empirical description of the typical profiles of LD in the populations studied. To a first approximation, patterns of LD can be well characterized by "haplotype blocks," meaning that there are regions of the genome (very variable in size, but often on the order of 10 to 100 kb) in which there is very high LD, meaning that only a small subset of all possible haplotypes (combinations of alleles in that region) are observed in the population. For example, considering 10 SNPs, each with two alleles, there are $2^{10} = 1024$ possible haplotypes, although under very strong LD we may observe only two or three of these at appreciable population frequencies. These "blocks" are separated by "recombination hotspots"—places in the genome with a historically higher rate of recombination, which acts to reduce LD by separating alleles on the recombinant haplotype. The results from the HapMap helped inform the design of experiments that aimed to intelligently select the smallest possible set of markers necessary to capture, or tag, most of the known common variation in a region. In the 10-SNP example, it may only be necessary to genotype 1 or 2 SNPs for example, without significant loss of information compared with genotyping all 10.

A common measure of LD in association studies is R^2, where a value of 0 indicates no LD (two sites are statistically independent) and 1 indicates that one marker is effectively a perfect proxy for the second. An intermediate value, say of 0.8, indicates that one marker captures 80% of the information one would obtain if using one marker as a proxy for the other, instead of directly genotyping the second marker. If the untyped marker is a causal risk factor for disease, then one may still expect to observe a statistical signal of association (e.g., based on a simple comparison of case and control allele frequencies) at the genotyped marker, albeit one that is attenuated due to incomplete LD. (In fact, to retain equivalent power to detect association at the marker, in this case one would require $1/R^2 = 1/0.8$ or 125% of the sample size compared with typing the causal marker directly). By estimating the average extent of LD, analyses of HapMap data showed that one could expect to capture the majority of common (typically defined as above 5% marker allele frequency) variation in European and Asian populations at a reasonable level of certainty (e.g., $R^2 > 0.8$) by genotyping on the order of 500,000 SNPs genome-wide. This paved the way for the first genome-wide association studies (GWASs), which began typing 100,000–300,000 markers using newly developed, standardized commercial microarrays, soon establishing 500,000–1,000,000 SNPs as routine (Carlson et al., 2004). As described later, association analysis of these datasets has driven many genetic discoveries in the past decade.

Superseding the tagging approach in many respects, the more general approach of *imputation* leverages the actual HapMap sample data itself to fill in data that are "missing" in a GWAS but present in the HapMap, relying on LD information implicit in the HapMap across all SNPs. Imputation allows researchers to probabilistically assign genotypes for all common HapMap SNPs (over 2 million in the European samples), even if only 500,000 have been directly genotyped in the study, by taking advantage of the redundancy due to LD. One of the major applications of imputation is to facilitate the comparison and aggregation of studies that use different GWAS arrays, by mapping everything to the common set of HapMap SNPs. This also obviates many of the practical difficulties that plagued candidate gene studies, in which different markers were typed in different studies.

The HapMap and GWAS in general are largely focused on assaying only common genetic variation: typically sites at which at least 5% of chromosomes carry an "alternate" allele compared with the reference sequence. The vast majority of variants that have population frequencies below 1% will not be present in the HapMap or on standard microarrays and so will be effectively invisible to GWAS approaches. A major push in recent years has been to leverage advances in so-called *next-generation sequencing* (NGS) technologies to build catalogs of lower frequency variation. This technology employs massively parallel approaches to sequence many millions of small fragments of DNA, generating very large numbers of short reads (around 100 bases) that can be mapped back to the reference sequence and variant sites called in an individual. The 1000 Genomes Project (*www.1000genomes.org/*) has used this technology to sequence the entire genomes of over 1,000 individuals, in order to create maps of known low-frequency variants and reference panels for imputation. Combining publicly available 1000 Genomes data with standard GWAS data, one can reliable impute over 10,000,000 polymorphic sites, many of which are of low frequency (under 1%) and many of which represent potentially functional polymorphisms (e.g., nonsynonymous allelic substitutions in genes, or short insertions and deletions that could shift the reading frame of a gene). To measure very rare mutations that are specific to a family or a particular ancestral group that is not represented in the 1000 Genomes data, it will still be necessary to sequence samples directly. But given current cost constraints, the 1000 Genomes data afford a new lease of life for existing GWAS samples. In addition to utility in imputing a good deal of low-frequency variation, these data may be particularly helpful in ascribing a putative function to associated regions or haplotypes, as a consequence of the near-complete ascertainment of all commonly variable sites.

Another type of genomic map that has recently been completed, and that will likely play a critical part in both the analysis and interpretation of many genetic studies of disease, is the ENCODE project (Encyclopedia of DNA Elements; http://www.genome.gov/10005107). This project aimed to map all functional elements in the human genome sequence beyond protein-coding genes: for example, regions (that may often be cell- and tissue specific) related to factors such as chromatin structure, methylation, histone modification, sequence-specific transcription factors, and RNA-binding proteins. As many association signals from GWAS fall outside of known protein coding genes, a more comprehensive annotation and understanding of the full sequence will be important in translating statistical signal into biological knowledge (Degner et al., 2012).

GENOME-WIDE ASSOCIATION STUDIES

In many respects, the development of reliable, cost-effective, high-throughput genotyping technologies, using microarrays that can simultaneously assay hundreds of thousands of single-nucleotide polymorphisms, has addressed all the basic limitations inherent in the early application of association (or linkage disequilibrium) mapping. Because almost all of the common variation in the genome can be assayed, genetic studies have become fundamentally data-driven enterprises and do not need to rely on prior hypotheses being correct. Order-of-magnitude, cheaper, per-genotype costs have enabled a large amount of genetic data to be amassed; the use of standardized microarrays (combined with imputation analysis) has also facilitated pooling of data across studies to achieve larger samples through meta-analysis, and therefore greater power,

which is vitally important in complex trait genetics (Lohmueller et al., 2003). At the same time, the large multiple-testing burden inherent in genome-wide scans has forced investigators to address the issue of false positive rates early and head on in the context of GWAS. Based on empirical and theoretical considerations, most investigators now require a p-value of less than 5×10^{-8} for an association to be declared *genome-wide significant*. In a well-controlled study, findings that reach this stringent threshold have been shown to have a very high probability of replicating in subsequent studies. Finally, GWAS studies generally do a more comprehensive job at capturing common variation in a given gene compared with early candidate-based studies using older genotyping technologies, including capturing the vast amount of variation in intergenic regions).

APPLICATIONS OF GENOME-WIDE ASSOCIATION MAPPING AND ANALYTIC ISSUES

Genome-wide association studies have been very widely adopted for a large number of diseases. One of the pioneering studies was of seven diseases and a shared control sample, the Wellcome Trust Case Control Consortium (2007). The U.S. National Human Genome Research Institute (NHGRI) maintains a catalog (www.genome.gov/GWAStudies) of published associations from GWAS for a diverse range of diseases and traits. To date, over 1,600 associations have been published, all meeting the strict threshold of genome-wide significance (Figure 12.2).

There is a great deal of evidence to suggest that for most common diseases these genome-wide findings represent the tip of the iceberg of true common variant associations. In many cases, including for neuropsychiatric disease, there are multiple lines of evidence that point to an abundance of true signals below the formal threshold for genome-wide significance. When looking at many replicated genome-wide significant results, the statistical power to detect a variant of that frequency and reported effect size is typically low, even acknowledging that they may be inflated by the so-called "winner's curse" effect (that means that effect sizes for variants that are detected at very strict significance thresholds will tend to be larger than their true value, reflecting the fact that they may have needed "the luck of the draw" from sampling variation to push them over the bar). This implies either that the investigator was extremely lucky (managing to detect one particular true positive despite very low power to do so) or, perhaps more parsimoniously, that there must be a (much) larger reservoir of similar effects truly existing, from which this study sampled a particular subset, in proportion to the statistical power. More directly, one can take sets of independent subthreshold associations (e.g., SNPs with p-values between 1×10^{-4} and 5×10^{-8}) and ask whether more than expected are nominally significant in an independent sample (e.g., at $P < 0.01$ or $P < 0.05$), or show effects in a consistent direction (above 50% correspondence of risk versus protective effects expected by chance alone, often referred to as a "sign test"). For many diseases, such analyses strongly support the presence of many subthreshold true associations. Furthermore, approaches such

TABLE 12.1. Sample sizes required (case/control pairs for a 1% disease) under different genetic models

CAUSAL ALLELE		GENOTYPED MARKER		REQUIRED SAMPLE SIZE OF 80% POWER	
MAF	GRR	MAF	R^2	$\alpha = 0.05$	$\alpha = 5 \times 10^{-8}$
0.40	1.2	(Directly typed causal allele)		949	4,792
0.40	1.2	0.50	0.67	1,400	7,064
0.40	1.2	0.10	0.17	5,880	29,668
0.01	3.0	(Directly typed causal allele)		410	2,070
0.01	3.0	0.50	0.01	21,213	107,030
0.01	3.0	0.10	0.09	2,533	12,780

Contrasting power under two particular scenarios, involving a common and a low-frequency variant. Power calculated using the Genetic Power Calculator (http://pngu.mgh.harvard.edu/purcell/gpc/) and shows the number of case/control pairs required to achieve 80% power (i.e., an 80% chance of correctly rejecting the null hypothesis when the SNP truly has an effect) for two significant thresholds: a nominal 0.05, and genome-wide significant 5×10^{-8}. (These α values represent the chance of a false-positive test result.) The two causal scenarios are not intended to be directly comparable; rather, the numbers presented are meant to show the impact of requiring a strict significance threshold on required sample size, and the impact of incomplete LD (by genotyping a marker instead of directly genotyping the causal variant) under the two scenarios. Aside from the fact that, in general, large sample sizes are required for these types of effects, we see in particular that if the marker has a frequency very different from the causal variant, the R^2, which is always set at the highest possible value given the two allele frequencies, it will be necessarily low, and therefore, power will be power, and the sample size required to achieve 80% will be high. The first scenario represents the type of SNP we may expect to find in a GWAS; the second scenario represents (perhaps an optimistically large) effect as one might hope to see in exome sequencing or an exome array study.

as *gene set–enrichment analysis* applied to lists of subthreshold associations can be used to indicate whether the genes implicated appear to be a random selection of all genes, as would be expected if the associated regions were, in fact, selected purely by chance, as opposed to preferentially belonging to certain known pathways, or clustering in networks, beyond chance expectation—that is consistent with a nontrivial proportion of the associations being true positives. For example, Lango Allen et al. (2010) reported hundreds of variants influencing human height clustered in functionally related pathways. Evidence for a substantial number of likely true subthreshold associations for a given disease can be taken to indicate that larger sample sizes will yield genome-wide significant associations, as more true positives are pushed over the threshold.

Other studies have taken more direct approaches to address the idea of *highly polygenic* disease architectures (i.e., involving hundreds or thousands of distinct genetic loci). In particular, analyses of common variants in GWAS data for various highly heritable phenotypes, including height (Yang et al., 2010) and schizophrenia (International Schizophrenia Consortium, 2009), have indicated that a sizeable proportion of the total heritability may be due to the combined action of extremely modest effects across many loci (many of which may never be expected to rise to the level of genome-wide significance even in very large samples). Under such models it is likely unrealistic to ever expect a complete genetic model of a disease, although it is important to note that very high polygenicity (in which the power to unambiguously detect any one of a large number of loci is very low) does not by itself preclude progress toward the broader goals of genetic studies, namely, the identification of critical biological pathways and networks, and even individual risk prediction and personalized therapies.

Table 12.1 gives concrete numbers for the sample sizes required under different genetic models, for both common

and rare variants of varying effect sizes. Given the large sample sizes indicated in Table 12.1 for the type of variant that characterizes most "GWAS hits," *meta-analysis* (or combined, *mega-analysis*) has played an increasingly important role in genetic disease studies, in which consortia of consortia pool results or raw genotype data to collectively achieve greater power to detect variants of small effect.

Although it has become clear that Type II errors (false negatives) are the primary hurdle in GWAS (low power to detect small effects), there has been considerable attention to the issue of Type I errors (false positives). At the dawn of the GWAS era, many researchers were reasonably concerned that the massive multiple testing, as well as the scope for bias to arise from technical artifact or epidemiological confounding, would lead to hopelessly inflated false-positive signals. Given that most GWAS studies have been population based (utilizing samples of unrelated cases and controls) as opposed to family based, one concern was that *population stratification* might give rise to false positives, if cases and controls are not well matched for ancestry, given that different populations systematically vary in allele frequency at many sites across the genome, for reasons unrelated to the disease being studied. In contrast, association analyses that adopt a family-based approach (e.g., the *transmission disequilibrium test*, or TDT, which tests for overtransmission of a specific allele from heterozygous parents to affected offspring) implicitly guard against such confounding effects (e.g., by contrasting transmitted versus untransmitted alleles from within the same parent, in the case of the TDT). In practice, the presence of genome-wide genotypic data allows one to empirically assess the presence of heterogeneity in ancestry in a sample of individuals (Rosenberg et al., 2002), and to correct it statistically in tests of association (using approaches such as principal components analysis). Although most GWASs have been conducted in populations of European

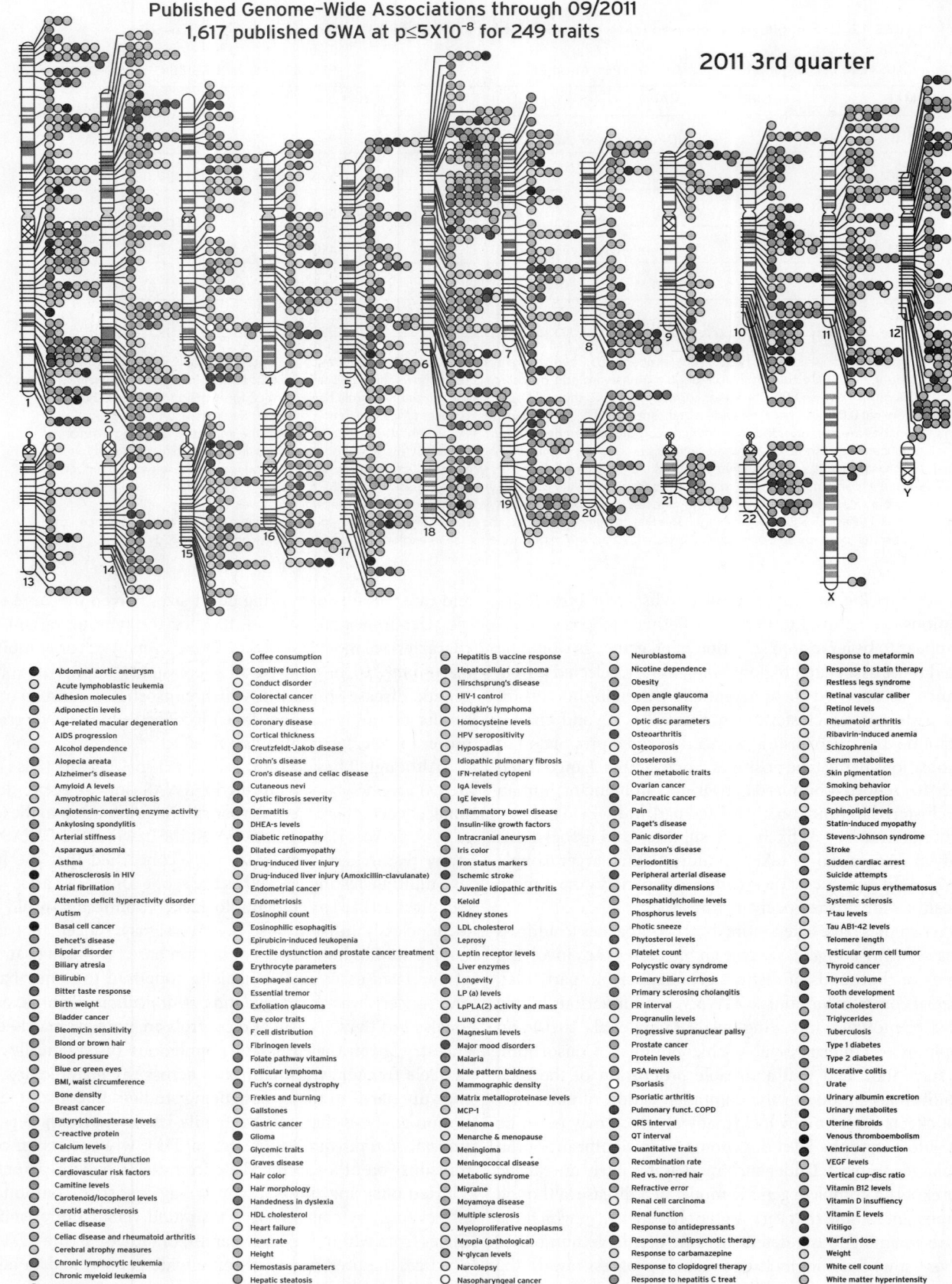

Figure 12.2 *The National Human Genome Research Institute GWAS catalog. A list of published GWAS associations published up until 9/2011 (www.genome.gov/ GWAStudies). Shaded circles indicate different classes of phenotype, enumerated in text that follows. The shaded-coded key does a rather poor job at indicating which associations are mapped genomically, but perhaps more importantly, the legend does convey the breadth of phenotypes for which successful GWAS have been performed. Many of these discovered loci were completely novel.*

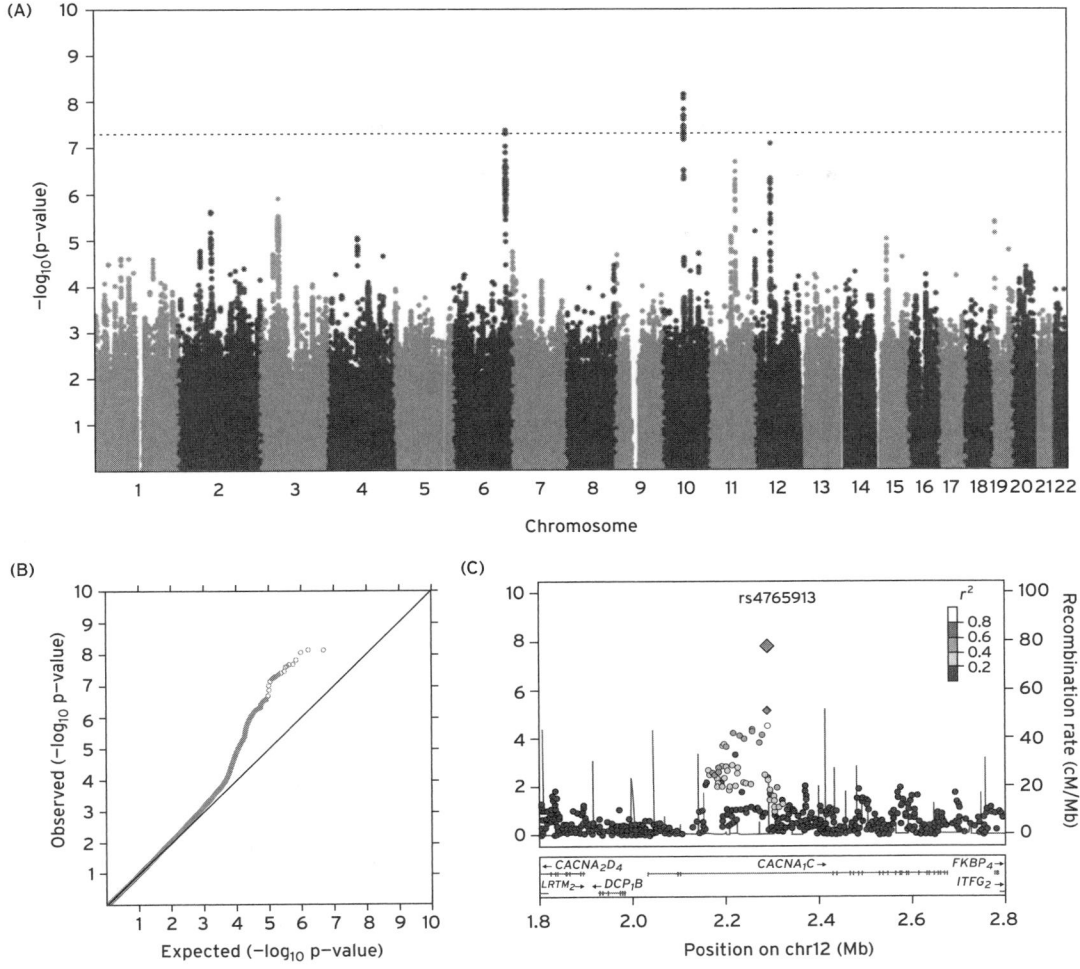

Figure 12.3 *Reporting GWAS results: Q-Q, Manhattan, and "regional" plots. These figures are taken from the Psychiatric Genomics Consortium Bipolar Disorder Working Group's Nature Genetics 2011 report of a mega-analysis of bipolar disorder GWAS data. (A) A so-called "Manhattan plot," in which individual SNP association statistics are ordered along the x-axis; the p-value is plotted on a –log10(P) scale, so values over 7.3 represent genome-wide significance. (B) The same data are shown in a Q–Q plot (quantile–quantile), which plots the observed statistic (–log10(P)) in rank order against the expected value under the global null hypothesis of no association. Points along the diagonal are therefore consistent with chance. The plots can show evidence of systematic bias (if the entire line grossly departs from the diagonal) or signal that is more likely to be true (if only the top portion of the data does, indicating there are more nominally significant hits than would be expected by chance). (C) A third commonly used plot when reporting GWAS results is a "region" plot. This shows the association statistics in a particular region as well as gives information on the LD (R^2) between markers.(Psychiatric GWAS Consortium Bipolar Disorder Working Group, 2011)..*

decent, there is potentially a lot to be learned from application to a more diverse range of populations, and new analytic challenges, for example, in highly admixed populations (Rosenberg et al., 2010). Quality control procedures play an important role in GWAS—for example, testing for deviations from *Hardy-Weinberg equilibrium*, or detecting SNPs with particularly high rates of failed genotyping. GWAS can still be prone to false positives from technical bias or other types of analytic error, simply by virtue of the large number of tests performed: this concern is in large part addressed by placing a strong emphasis on the need to seek *replication* in independent samples of any putative strong signals.

Although one in theory can approach the analysis of genotype–phenotype relations using GWAS data in a number of ways, in practice most of the substantive findings (as represented in the NHGRI catalog) come from simple, sequential tests of one SNP (either imputed or directly genotyped) at a

time. Typically, a technique such as logistic or linear regression is employed, assuming a purely additive dosage model at each site. Simpler alternatives include Armitage trend test or Fisher's exact test; more complex alternatives include nonparametric regression models, linear mixed models, and Bayesian approaches—in broad terms though, it is not obvious that the precise choice of statistical machinery employed would have impacted the substantive conclusions drawn to date.

Subsequent chapters summarize the results to date of GWAS and other types of genetic studies, for a range of neuropsychiatric diseases. There have been fewer, if any, cases of "low-hanging fruit" to emerge from common variant studies of diseases such as schizophrenia and bipolar disorder, compared with other common diseases such as Crohn's disease or Type I diabetes. Nonetheless, numerous genome-wide significant hits have emerged for both disorders, and, as noted, consideration of subthreshold results would strongly suggest that more are to be expected with larger sample sizes. Indeed, several large meta-analyses are currently underway: the analysis of common variation in neuropsychiatric disease is very much a work in progress, but one that appears to have found a steady footing from which to move forward.

THE FREQUENCY SPECTRUM OF DISEASE ALLELES: MODELS OF RARE AND COMMON VARIATION

Almost by definition, most genetic variation is attributable to common polymorphism in the human genome. For this reason, along with the fact that common SNPs in any one population constitute a relatively limited and easily assayable universe, common variation was an obvious first target for large-scale, genome-wide genetic studies, in the form of SNP-based GWASs. It has, of course, long been recognized that common SNPs are by no means the only class of variation a geneticist may wish to study. Particularly in the context of disease, one can reasonably argue (supported by observations in rare, Mendelian disease) that larger types of variant— those impacting more than just a single, usually intergenic, nucleotide—might also be more likely to have a strong impact on disease risk. *Structural variants* are one such class, involving the deletion, duplication, inversion, or translocation of potentially millions of nucleotides. Similarly, evolutionary arguments can be used to suggest that alleles of *high penetrance* are unlikely to be very common, assuming the disease has had a continued, negative impact on fitness over many generations, and so would have been selected against. The hypothesis that *rare variants* may primarily underlie common disease risk, in the same way they do for rare disease, expresses this logic (Cirulli and Goldstein, 2010).

For schizophrenia, examples of very rare structural variants that are strong risk alleles were identified over two decades ago, using the classical techniques of cytogenetics and linkage mapping in extended pedigrees. For example, a 1.5–3 Mb microdeletion at 22q11.2 leads to velo-cardio-facial syndrome (VCFS), a phenotypically heterogeneous syndrome, which displays an approximately 30% probability of leading to schizophrenia. Because the deletion occurs at 1 in ~4,000 live births, this variant is expected to contribute to risk in ~1% of all schizophrenia patients.

A second example of a highly penetrant, rare structural variant is the balanced translocation between 1q42 and 11q14, segregating with major psychiatric disease in a single extended Scottish pedigree and mapped using linkage analysis. One of the translocations breakpoints was later shown to disrupt a particular gene, now known as *DISC1*, "disrupted in schizophrenia 1" (St. Clair et al., 1990). The success of mapping *DISC1* prompted a wave of functional studies to investigate its roles in neurodevelopment, although the precise mechanism by which the translocation acts to increase risk for major psychiatric illness in this family still eludes researchers. Whether or not that mechanism is ever fully understood, many would argue that the finding still provides a useful window into the larger, more complex pathways involved in the disease.

In its extreme form, the *multiple rare variant* model is taken to mean that although many rare disease variants may exist *in a population*, most affected individuals will carry only one, which was sufficient to cause their disease; similarly, most unaffected individuals would not be expected to carry any risk alleles. This model is in contrast to the polygenic common variant model, in which both affected and unaffected individuals would be expected to carry many risk alleles: under this model, cases simply carry more of them on average, as a consequence of the increased genetic burden leading to increased risk of disease. The extreme form of the multiple rare variant model essentially recasts a common disease as a collection of multiple, clinically indistinguishable diseases—that could in theory also be etiological CGH distinct in a fundamental manner, but that should often be amenable to the same family-based approaches that worked for Mendelian disease (i.e., if most affected families are, in fact, segregating a single, high-penetrance allele). In practice, extreme forms of the multiple–rare variant model are unlikely to be the general rule for any common disease (certainly if linkage analysis has been adequately performed in appropriately sized pedigree collections, this model can already be ruled out).

Perhaps a better default or working model for most common diseases should instead be that multiple variants of varying effect sizes are likely to exist anywhere across the frequency spectrum (Gibson, 2012; Owen et al., 2010). For diseases with childhood or early-adult onset at least, we would expect selection to constrain alleles of larger effect to lower population frequencies. Although the exact relationship between frequency and effect sizes arising from the action of selection will be hard to predict generally, it is safe to conclude that common variants of very large effect are unlikely to exist; otherwise, all combinations of variant will likely occur, in proportion to the frequency spectrum of neutral variation. What may make some diseases, including neuropsychiatric disease, particularly challenging from a genetic perspective, is likely to be the sheer number of loci in the genome that, if perturbed by either a rare or common variant, can increase risk for disease. This challenge will be equally pertinent for various study designs, from sequencing to GWAS.

STUDIES OF RARE STRUCTURAL VARIATION: COPY NUMBER VARIANTS AND NEUROPSYCHIATRIC DISEASE

Structural variants, such as the 22q11.2 deletion previously described, have a well-established role in a range of rare disease phenotypes as well as genomic alterations that occur in cancers (Mills et al., 2011; Wain et al., 2009). Technologies such as array-CGH (comparative genomic hybridization) are now routinely used in prenatal screening as well as research settings, replacing traditional karyotype techniques for detecting unbalanced chromosomal changes. Rare copy number variants (CNVs, deletions or duplications of genetic material) ranging from 100 kb or less to multiple megabases can also be called from analysis of the same SNP microarrays used in GWAS studies: this fortuitous fact has meant that relatively large GWAS samples have been able to be assayed for changes in copy number variation. For autism and schizophrenia (International Schizophrenia Consortium, 2008; Sebat et al., 2007), such events clearly play an important role. Several studies have found, in particular, an increased rate of *de novo* CNVs in both autism and schizophrenia patients: such events will effectively be uncensored with respect to natural selection. The increased rate of *de novo* mutation in schizophrenia patients is also consistent with epidemiological observations of increased paternal age (as the probability of a germ line mutation in the father is known to increase with his age also).

Approximately a dozen specific loci have been mapped with high statistical confidence, being likely to harbor CNVs that increase risk for disease (Sullivan et al., 2012). Such events are typically large (often impacting dozens of genes), rare in the general population (with a frequency under 1/1000), and are estimated to increase risk for disease by up to 10-fold or more. Interestingly, the same CNVs have been shown to increase risk both for autism and schizophrenia as well as other neurodevelopmental and behavioral disorders. In addition, autism and schizophrenia patients show a modest but significant increased burden of rare CNVs across their genomes, again consistent with the high polygenicity of neuropsychiatric disease. For other neuropsychiatric diseases, the role of CNVs is either less pronounced or no relationship has yet been clearly established.

NEXT-GENERATION SEQUENCING TECHNOLOGIES AND MEDICAL SEQUENCING

The advent of next-generation sequencing, as well as driving large genomics projects such the 1000 Genomes, has been widely and largely very successfully applied to a host of rare, Mendelian diseases over the past few years. One of the most common applications of NGS to date has been *whole-exome sequencing* (Bamshad et al., 2011). Here targeted approaches allow investigators to first greatly enrich the pool of DNA fragments to be sequenced for particular regions of interest: in the case of whole-exome sequencing, this involves "capturing" the ~1% of the genome that is known to contain exons of protein-coding genes. This relatively small fraction of the genome can then be sequenced at high depth (i.e., with 20 or more reads spanning most targeted bases) to ensure high sensitivity to detect if not all then at least the vast majority of variant (nonreference) sites present in an individual's exome. In comparison with sequencing the whole genome, exome sequencing is still considerably cheaper per unit, although *per base* sequenced, it is less cost effective. In practice, though, sequence data on the exome is typically more valuable in the sense that any one variant has a higher prior likelihood of being functional, and that one can more readily ascribe and interpret that function in terms of its impact on the resulting gene product, and what else is known about that gene (e.g., where it is expressed, what other disorders are associated with mutations in that gene, what other proteins interact with the protein coded by that gene). Perhaps the main drawback with

exome sequencing is the expanding definition of what is practically implied by "the exome": other interesting regions such as regulatory regions near genes, rare transcripts, and noncoding RNAs are typically not captured comprehensively, and this fact alone may for many motivate the move to whole-genome sequencing. The amount of data generated by whole-genome sequencing is orders-of-magnitude larger than for the exome, and so computational challenges in analyzing and even storing the data become major concerns for large studies.

A typical exome-sequencing experiment on one individual currently targets around 200,000 genomic intervals, each usually corresponding to one exon of a protein-coding gene, around 150 bases in length, targeting around 20,000 RefSeq genes and spanning around 30 Mb of genomic sequence. In a high-depth sequencing study, each targeted base is often covered, on average, by as many as 50 to 100 "short reads." These reads are typically 70–100 bases in length, often physically paired such that any two reads are expected to fall at nearby genomic locations. Variants are discovered by aligning these reads to the reference sequence and looking for differences: this is a technically involved and potentially error-prone procedure, although the informatics for this have improved markedly in the past few years, in no small part driven by large projects such as the 1000 Genomes. From a whole-genome sequencing study, one expects to find something on the order of 3 to 4 million variant sites; from whole-exome sequencing, this figure is typically in the range of 15,000–20,000 (depending on experimental details as well as the ancestry of the sampled individual).

When sequencing more than a few individuals, a very large proportion of all sites discovered will be "singletons"— variants observed in only one of the sequenced samples, and most of these will be novel, in the sense that they will not have been previously identified and deposited in databases such as dbSNP (http://www.ncbi.nlm.nih.gov/projects/SNP/), which currently contains around 50 million known variants. This fact alone clearly poses challenges for the analysis of sequence data to map risk alleles for disease. In practice, the rarity of individual variants means that researchers employ a range of methods to statistically aggregate multiple mutations across a particular gene and collectively test them for association with a disease, in so-called *gene-based* rare-variant analysis. Although large studies of thousands of patients and controls are underway, across a range of diseases, unambiguous discoveries are yet to emerge from these studies. For common, complex traits, exome sequencing will be much more challenging than for Mendelian disorders, and very large sample sizes may well be required, as is the case for studies of common variation (Kiezun et al., 2012).

Because genotyping technology is still cheaper and more accurate than sequencing, a number of groups have recently collaborated to create an *exome array* (http://genome.sph. umich.edu/wiki/Exome_Chip_Design): that is, a standard SNP microarray using the same technology deployed for GWAS, but that primarily contains approximately 200,000 low-frequency mutations that are *nonsynonymous* (alter the protein's amino-acid sequence) and observed in at least two studies (and so represent variants that are segregating in populations at low frequencies, perhaps 0.1%, as opposed to truly "private" mutations that may be specific to single families and may never be seen again). Because this array is far cheaper than exome sequencing on a per individual basis, it can be applied rapidly to very large samples. Comprehensive results from these studies are not yet available, although by the end of 2013, we should have a very clear sense of whether this particular slice of the frequency spectrum of nonsynonymous SNPs plays a major role for many diseases, or goes toward explaining the heritability not directly accounted for by the top results of GWASs.

Other applications of sequencing to map rare variants for common diseases are using families rather than standard case control, population-based designs. Families can have a number of advantages: ascertaining families with an unusually high "density" of affected individuals for a given disease increases the probability that a rare highly penetrant variant is present in that family. One can, in principle, use IBD information from linkage analysis to prioritize specific regions of the genome for sequencing or analysis. One can use family information to resolve haplotype phase and to impute sequence data across family members (as related individuals, by definition, represent different combinations of the same smaller set of "founder" chromosomes). One disadvantage is that for many adult-onset diseases it is far harder to collect intact family collections in large numbers.

Additionally, one can use families to detect new, or *de novo*, mutations. In neuropsychiatric disease, and particularly autism and schizophrenia, the hypothesis that *de novo* mutation may play a significant role in disease risk is attractive to many researchers and is supported by the epidemiological observation that affected individuals tend to have older fathers (which is, in turn, known to correlate within increased germ line mutation that will be transmitted to offspring). A number of exome-sequencing studies using *trios* (affected offspring and two parents) have been published for these two diseases. The results to date are interesting and do point to nonrandom networks of genes that are enriched for highly deleterious mutations in patients. At the same time, it does not appear to be the case that a sizeable proportion of affected individuals carry a *de novo* mutation that is likely to be the sole cause of their disease; furthermore, relatively few genes have emerged that are observed to be recurrently hit by *de novos* across these studies beyond the level expected by chance—again speaking to the very high polygenicity of these diseases. The genes and mutations in specific patients that do emerge from this approach may well be particularly interesting to study, however, in that

(because *de novo* mutations are effectively uncensored with respect to natural selection) they could in theory display a very high penetrance. Such "large-effect" alleles could in many cases be preferable mutations to follow up in functional studies, for example, using IPS cells or animal models.

Figure 12.4 illustrates some of the different genetic designs and technologies currently available for relating DNA variation to phenotype, in relation to the part of the allelic frequency spectrum they are designed to probe. Ultimately, it is likely that approaches that look for convergence of genetic signals across these different studies may be fruitful (Nejentsev et al., 2009).

INTEGRATIVE ANALYSES OF GENETIC NETWORKS AND PATHWAYS

Future progress in complex traits genetics is likely to rely on two factors, no matter what particular type of genetic study is adopted: *(1)* increasingly large sample collections and *(2)* integrative modeling approaches that not only consider genetic information from different studies as illustrated in Figure 12.4, but also consider multiple genetic signals in their broader context (Raychaudhuri, 2011). This includes intersection of multilocus genotype data with functional information, from gene expression studies, from protein–protein interaction networks, or from other curated gene sets and pathways. Jointly modeling the impact of risk variants on intermediate phenotypes or *endophenotypes* (Gottesman and Gould, 2003), for example, from brain imaging studies, and a fuller analysis of *pleiotropic* effects, where the same variant influences multiple (and potentially seemingly unconnected) disorders or traits (Cotsapas et al., 2011; Craddock et al., 2009), are both likely to be powerful approaches moving forward, particularly when seeded by solid knowledge of multiple associated loci from the primary genetics studies.

ALTERNATIVE GENETIC MODELS

The majority of genetic studies assume simple, additive models of effect, whether the variant is common or rare. On one hand this is typically a simplifying assumption of convenience made during analysis, although in practice it is often likely to be a reasonable one. Although there is little empirical evidence for *nonadditive* effects being a generally important component of

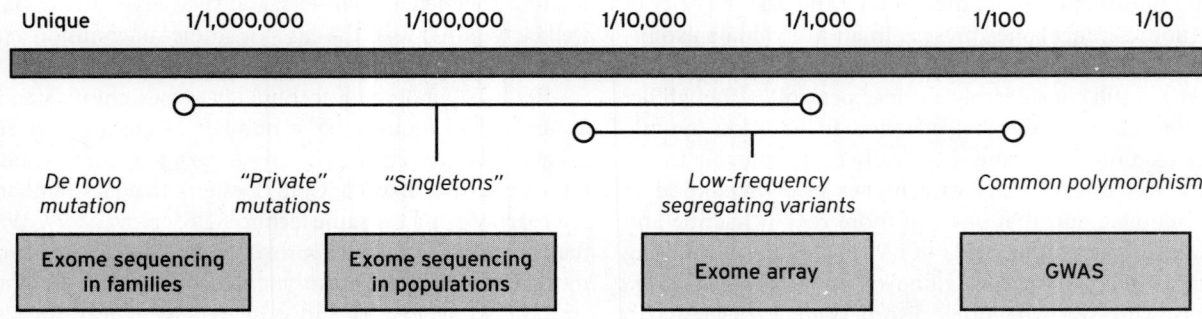

Figure 12.4 *Summary of genetic study types targeting different intervals of the allelic frequency spectrum. The values along the horizontal bar indicate the minor allele frequency that is targeted by different genetic technologies, from common variation to sequencing for newly arising mutation.*

the architecture of common disease, finding specific instances of such effects could be very informative. Examples of nonadditive effects include basic dominant/recessive (and compound heterozygote) models at a single locus and extended regions of homozygosity due to recent inbreeding unmasking rare recessive effects (Keller et al., 2012), interaction between genes (epistasis as reviewed by Cordell [2009]), and between genes and environments (Thomas, 2010), as well as sex-specific, imprinting, and parent-of-origin effects. Whether or not allowing for these more complex, potentially unbounded models will help to map disease genes is unclear, but in any case, intensive study of the growing number of genes already mapped by the additive models with respect to these alternate models (including pleiotropic effects on other phenotypes) has potential to be a great value.

SUMMARY

The tools available to the complex trait geneticist have evolved rapidly over the past decade. Consequently, psychiatric genetics has made considerable progress during the same time frame (Sullivan et al., 2012). Different genetic strategies, from studies of *de novo* variation in exome sequencing, large deletion and duplication copy number variants, and rare and low-frequency variants segregating in populations, to common polymorphisms are underway. It seems clear that all approaches will continue to bear fruit in the coming years, although the full promise of neuropsychiatric genetics is not yet achieved. In the (hopefully not too distant) future, the *interpretation* of multiple genetic associations in their biological context, rather than their initial discovery per se, will increasingly become the central challenge faced, but it will remain critically grounded on the initial gene discovery work going on today.

DISCLOSURE

Dr. Purcell has no conflicts of interests to disclose.

REFERENCES

Altshuler, D., Daly, M.J., et al. (2008). Genetic mapping in human disease. *Science* 322(5903):881–888. (PMID: 18988837)

Bamshad, M.J., Ng, S.B., et al. (2011). Exome sequencing as a tool for Mendelian disease gene discovery. *Nat. Rev. Genet.* 12(11):745–755.

Browning S.R., and Browning, B.L. (2012). Haplotype phasing: existing methods and new developments. *Nat. Rev. Genet.* 12:703–714.

Carlson, C.S., Eberle M.A., et al. (2004). Mapping complex disease loci in whole-genome association studies. *Nature* 429(6990):446–452. (PMID: 15164069)

Cirulli, E.T., and Goldstein, D.B. (2010). Uncovering the roles of rare variants in common disease through whole-genome sequencing. *Nat. Rev. Genet.* 11(6):415–425. (PMID: 20479773)

Cordell H.J. (2009). Detecting gene–gene interactions that underlie human diseases. *Nat. Rev. Genet.* 10:392–404.

Cotsapas C., Voight, B.F., et al. (2011). Pervasive sharing of genetic effects in autoimmune disease. *PLoS Genet.* 7(8) (PMID: 21852963)

Craddock, N., Kendler, K., et al. Cross-Disorder Phenotype Group of the Psychiatric GWAS Consortium. (2009). Dissecting the phenotype in genome-wide association studies of psychiatric illness. *Br. J. Psychiatry* 195(2):97–99.

Degner, J.F., Pai, A.A., et al. (2012). DNase I sensitivity QTLs are a major determinant of human expression variation. *Nature* 482(7385):390–394.

ENCODE Project Consortium. (2012). http://www.nature.com/encode/ Encyclopedia of DNA Elements. URL http://www.genome.gov/10005107

Genetic Power Calculator http://pngu.mgh.harvard.edu/purcell/gpc/

Gibson, G. (2012). Rare and common variants: twenty arguments. *Nat. Rev. Genet.* 13(2):135–145. (PMID: 22251874)

Gottesman I., and Gould, T. (2003). The endophenotype concept in psychiatry: etymology and strategic intentions. *Am. J. Psych.* 160(4):636–645. (PMID: 12668349)

International HapMap Consortium. (2007). A second generation human haplotype map of over 3.1 million SNPs. *Nature* 449:851–861.

International Schizophrenia Consortium. (2008). Rare chromosomal deletions and duplications increase risk of schizophrenia. *Nature* 455:237–241.

International Schizophrenia Consortium. (2009). Common polygenic variation contributes to risk of schizophrenia and bipolar disorder. *Nature* 460(7256):748–752. Epub 2009 Jul 1.

Keller M.C., Simonson, M.A., et al.; Schizophrenia Psychiatric Genome-Wide Association Study Consortium. (2012). Runs of homozygosity implicate autozygosity as a schizophrenia risk factor. *PLoS Genet.* 8(4):e1002656.. (PMID: 22511889)

Kiezun, A., Garimella K., et al. (2012). Exome sequencing and the genetic basis of complex traits. *Nat. Genet.* 44(6):623–630. (PMID: 22641211)

Kim, Y., Zerwas S., et al. (2011). Schizophrenia genetics: where next? *Schizophr. Bull.* 37(3):456–463.

Lango Allen H., Estrada, K., et al. (2010). Hundreds of variants clustered in genomic loci and biological pathways affect human height. *Nature* 467:832–838.

Lichtenstein, P., Yip, B.H., et al. (2009). Common genetic determinants of schizophrenia and bipolar disorder in Swedish families: a population-based study. *Lancet* 373(9659):234–239.

Lohmueller, K.E., Pearce, C.L., et al. (2003). Meta-analysis of genetic association studies supports a contribution of common variants to susceptibility to common disease. *Nat. Genet.* 33:177–182.

Mills, R.E., Walter, K., et al.; 1000 Genomes Project. (2011). Mapping copy number variation by population-scale genome sequencing. *Nature* 470(7332):59–65. (PMID: 21293372)

Nejentsev, S., Walker, N., et al. (2009). Rare variants of IFIH1, a gene implicated in antiviral responses, protect against type 1 diabetes. *Science* 324(5925):387–339. (PMID: 19264985)

NHGRI GWAS Catalog: A Catalog of Published Genome-Wide Association Studies. http://www.genome.gov/gwastudies/

Owen M.J., Craddock, N., et al.(2010). Suggestion of roles for both common and rare risk variants in genome-wide studies of schizophrenia. *Arch. Gen. Psychiatry* 67(7):667–673. (PMID: 20603448)

Psychiatric GWAS Consortium Bipolar Disorder Working Group. (2011). Large-scale genome-wide association analysis of bipolar disorder identifies a new susceptibility locus near ODZ4. *Nat. Genet.* 43(10):977–983.

Raychaudhuri S. (2011). Mapping rare and common causal alleles for complex human diseases. *Cell* 147(1):57–69. (PMID: 21962507)

Rosenberg, N.A., Huang, L., et al. (2010). Genome-wide association studies in diverse populations. *Nat. Rev. Genet.* 11(5):356–366. (PMID: 20395969)

Rosenberg, N.A., Pritchard J.K., et al. (2002). Genetic structure of human populations. *Science* 298(5602):2381–2385.

Risch, N., and Merikangas, K. (1996). The future of genetic studies of complex human diseases. *Science* 273(5281):1516–1517. (PMID: 8801636)

Sebat J., Lakshmi, B., et al. (2007). Strong association of *de novo* copy number mutations with autism. *Science* 316:445–449.

Smith G.D., and Ebrahim, S. (2003). "Mendelian randomization": can genetic epidemiology contribute to understanding environmental determinants of disease? *Int. J. Epidemiol.* 32(1):1–22.

St Clair, D., Blackwood D., et al. (1990). Association within a family of a balanced autosomal translocation with major mental illness. *Lancet.* 336(8706):13–16. (PMID 1973210)

Sullivan, P.F., Daly M.J., et al.(2012). Genetic architectures of psychiatric disorders: the emerging picture and its implications. *Nat. Rev. Genet.* 13(8):537–551. (PMID: 22777127)

Thomas, D. (2010). Gene-environment-wide association studies: emerging approaches. *Nat. Rev. Genet.* 11(4):259–272.

The 1000 Genomes Project Consortium. (2010). A map of human genome variation from population-scale sequencing. *Nature* 467(7319):1061–1073.

van Dongen J., Slagboom, P.E., et al. (2012). The continuing value of twin studies in the omics era. *Nat. Rev. Genet.* 13:640–653.

Wain L.V., Armour, J.A., et al. (2009). Genomic copy number variation, human health, and disease. *Lancet* 374(9686):340–350. (PMID: 19535135)

The Wellcome Trust Case Control Consortium. (2007). Genome-wide association study of 14,000 cases of seven common diseases and 3000 shared controls. *Nature* 447:661–678.

Yang J., Benyamin, B., et al. (2010). Common SNPs explain a large proportion of the heritability for human height. *Nat. Genet.* 42(7):565–569.

13 | THE BRAIN AND ITS EPIGENOME

AMANDA C. MITCHELL, YAN JIANG, CYRIL J. PETER,
KI A. GOOSENS, AND SCHAHRAM AKBARIAN

INTRODUCTION

Psychiatric disorders, including autism, mood and anxiety, or psychosis spectrum disorders, substance abuse, and addiction each lack a unifying molecular or cellular pathology, and most cases are believed to be of multifactorial etiology with numerous environmental and genetic components involved. This, taken together with the fact that laboratory animal models, including rats and mice, do not reflect the full complexities surrounding disorders of higher cognition and emotion (Nestler and Hyman, 2010), poses a formidable challenge to the quests of understanding the pathophysiology of disease and developing efficient therapies for the majority of patients. Consider that conventional psychopharmacology, including drugs targeting monoamine signaling, for example, dopaminergic, serotonergic, and noradrenergic pathways, elicits an insufficient therapeutic response in one half or less of patients diagnosed with schizophrenia and related illnesses (Lehman et al., 2004), or depression and anxiety (Krishnan and Nestler, 2010). Thus, it will be necessary to further explore the neurobiology and molecular pathology of mental disorders, in order to develop novel treatment strategies of higher efficacy.

One promising avenue of research that is moving center stage in basic and clinical neurosciences alike is epi- (Greek for "over," "above") genetics (Labrie et al., 2012). Not long ago *epigenetics* was mainly viewed through the prism of a single mark, DNA cytosine methylation, in the context of cell division related to, for example, embryonic development or cancer. This work might suggest that epigenetics bears little relevance for the postnatal and mature brain with its large proportion of postmitotic and differentiated cells. At least four independent lines of evidence fuel the current interest in neuroepigenetics, making it repeatedly a "hot topic" at recent annual conventions of neuroscientists and psychiatrists. First, based on human and animal brain studies, it is becoming increasingly clear that epigenetic markings, including DNA methylation and many types of histone modifications, remain "plastic" throughout all periods of development and aging, with ongoing dynamic regulation even in neurons and other differentiated cells. Changes in neuronal activity, learning, and memory, including the establishment of reward- and addiction-related behaviors, and numerous other paradigms all have been shown to be associated with DNA methylation and histone modification changes at specific genomic sequences in brain chromatin (Day and Sweatt, 2011; Robison and Nestler, 2011). These principal insights immediately propelled epigenetics into the forefront of brain research, as it provides a molecular system operating at the genome–environment intersect, and obviously is a topic of interest deeply rooted in the concepts of modern psychology and the behavioral sciences. Second, recent work has revealed that each of the causative mutations in a subset of monogenetic neurological disorders (including but not limited to Rubinstein-Taybi, Kleefstra, Rett, and other syndromes) disrupts the function of a protein involved in the regulation of chromatin structure and function (Haggarty and Tsai, 2011). These findings from clinical genetics indicated that the developing brain, indeed, is sensitive to dysregulation of the epigenetic machinery, and that some neurological conditions could arise from more widespread chromatin defects affecting the immature brain. Moreover, similar types of mutations were subsequently found in some cases with adult-onset psychosis or dementia, which implies that "chromatin disorders" encompass a much wider range of neuropsychiatric disease, contrasting the traditional view that they reflect "static" lesions confined to the developing nervous system (Jakocevski and Akbarian, 2012). Third, a subset of chromatin-modifying drugs—compounds with inhibitory activity directed against histone deacetylases are a well-known example—demonstrated a promising therapeutic potential in animal models for cognitive and emotional disease (Machado-Vieira et al., 2011), and even for neurodegenerative conditions (Fischer et al., 2010). Finally, even some of the most optimistic estimates on the role of protein-coding sequences as genetic risk factors for major psychiatric disease predict that only 25%–50% of sporadic cases of autism and schizophrenia carry disease-associated mutations altering protein sequence and function (O'Roak et al., 2011; Xu et al., 2011). Therefore, a subset of the remaining disease-associated variants are thought to involve regulatory and probably noncoding DNA, and by exploring the pattern and distribution of various epigenetic markings (which, in concert, define the functional architecture of chromatin, including open or silenced euchromatin, constitutive heterochromatin, etc.), one could expect to obtain important clues about the molecular pathology associated with the disease-related DNA variants (Houston et al., 2012). In the following, we will, after a concise introduction to the various markings and molecules that define a cell's epigenome, touch upon each of four points raised in the preceding, and then finish this chapter with a brief discussion about how epigenetic technologies and discoveries could have a lasting impact on our understanding of the neurobiology and heritability of mental disorders.

THE EPIGENOME—GENERAL PRINCIPLES

The elementary unit of chromatin is the nucleosome, or 146 bp of genomic DNA wrapped around an octamer of core histones, connected by linker DNA and linker histones. The collective set of covalent DNA and histone modifications and variant histones provides the major building blocks for the "epigenome," or the epigenetic landscapes that define the functional architecture of the genome, including its organization into many tens of thousands of transcriptional units, clusters of condensed chromatin, and other features that are differentially regulated in different cell types and developmental stages of the organism (Li and Reinberg, 2011; Rodriguez-Paredes and Esteller, 2011). An in-depth description of all epigenetic markings would be far beyond this review chapter, but multiple recent excellent reviews on this topic provide an excellent starting point for the reader interested to learn more about these topics (Ederveen et al., 2011; Kinney et al., 2011; Zhou et al., 2011). Here, we confine the discussion to a subset of the epigenetic markings repeatedly explored in the human and animal brain.

Common terminology used in chromatin studies includes (1) *nucleosomes*, comprised of a protein octamer of four small proteins, the *nucleosome core histones*, around which 146 bp of DNA is wrapped around. Transcription start sites are often defined by a nucleosome-free interval, probably for increased access of the transcriptional initiation complex and other regulators of gene expression. Arrays of nucleosomes,

connected by linker DNA and linker histones, comprise the 10-nm "beads-on-a-string" chromatin fiber; (2) *euchromatin* defines loose chromatin typically at sites of actively transcribed genes and units poised for transcription; (3) *heterochromatin* defines tightly packed nucleosomal arrays. Constitutive heterochromatin remains highly condensed in most interphase nuclei. Examples include pericentric and telomeric repeat DNA, the inactivated X chromosome ("Barr body") of female somatic cells, and other chromosomal structures often found in close proximity to the nuclear envelope and also around the nucleolus (see Fig. 13.1). Facultative heterochromatin includes silenced genes that upon differentiation or other stimuli could switch to a state of active transcription.

DNA (HYDROXY)-METHYLATION

Two related but functionally very different types of DNA modifications, methylation (m) and hydroxymethylation (hm) of cytosines in CpG dinucleotides, provide the bulk of the epigenetic modifications in vertebrate DNA (Kriaucionis and Heintz, 2009). There are additional types of DNA modifications, which are mostly chemical intermediates in the context of mC5 and hmC5 (cytosines methylated at the carbon 5 position) synthesis and breakdown (He et al., 2011; Ito et al., 2011). While the majority of DNA (hydroxy)-methylation is found at sites of CpG dinucleotides and, more generally, in the CpG-enriched sequences of the genome, a recent study in rat cerebral cortex

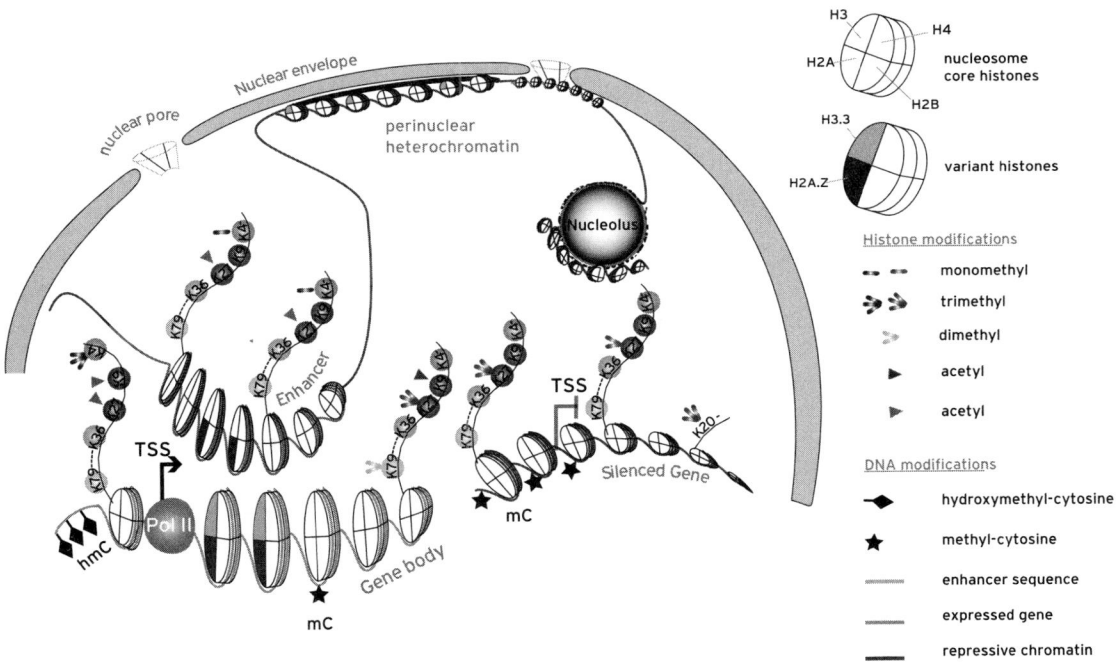

Figure 13.1 *The epigenome, from nucleus to nucleosome. Schematic illustration of a gene poised for transcription by polymerase II (Pol II) initiation complex, with nucleosome-free interval at transcription start site (TSS). Distal enhancer sequence which in looplike structure moves in close proximity to active gene. Marks a small subset of heterochromatic portions of the genome, including silenced gene and heterochromatic structures bordering the nuclear envelope and pore complex, and also the nucleolar periphery. A small subset of representative histone variants and histone H3 site-specific lysine (K) residues at N-terminal tail (K4, K9, K27, K36, K79) and H4K20 residue are shown as indicated, together with panel of mono- and trimethyl, or acetyl modifications that differentiate between active promoters, transcribed gene bodies, and repressive chromatin, as indicated. DNA cytosines that are hydroxymethylated at the C5 position are mostly found at active promoters, while methylated cytosines are positioned within body of actively transcribed genes and around repressed promoters and in constitutive heterochromatin.*

reported that the amount of mC5 found at nonCpG sites is far higher than previously assumed (Xie et al., 2012). The mC5 and hmC5 markings show a differential (but not mutually exclusive) pattern of genomic occupancy. The hmC5 mark is concentrated toward the 5′ end of genes and the proximal-most portion of transcriptional units, and broadly correlates with local gene expression levels (Jin et al., 2011; Song et al., 2011). On the other hand, less than 3% of mC5 markings are positioned around the 5′ end of genes (Maunakea et al., 2010). The classical concept on the transcriptional regulatory role of DNA methylation, which also has guided many brain-related studies, is that promoter-bound repressive chromatin remodeling complexes negatively regulate transcription (Sharma et al., 2005). There are many studies that report changes in promoter DNA methylation (mostly in conjunction with decreased gene expression) in preclinical models of psychosis, depression, and addiction, as well as in brain tissue in subjects diagnosed with one of these conditions. Interestingly, however, while the largest amount, or 97%, of mC5s are found in intra- and intergenic sequences and within DNA repeats (Maunakea et al., 2010), only few of these studies have explored brain DNA methylation changes at repeat DNA and other sequences outside of promoters.

The role of hmC5, however, in transcriptional regulation still remains controversial. Yi Zhang's group (Wu et al., 2011) performed genome-wide profile of 5hmC in both wild-type and Tet1-depleted mouse embryonic stem (ES) cells, and their data suggested that 5hmC is enriched at both gene bodies of actively transcribed genes and extended promoter regions of Polycomb-repressed developmental regulators. There is also evidence that besides TSSs, hmC5 is also enriched in enhancer region marked by H3K4me1 and H3K27ac in human embryonic stem cells (Stroud et al., 2011; Szulwach et al., 2011a). From a *Nature* paper published (Williams et al., 2011), it was reported that hmC5 was enriched by both TSSs and gene bodies, and its catalytic enzyme TET1 interacts with Sin3A corepressor complex and is involved in transcriptional repression of a significant portion of polycomb group target genes.

HISTONE MODIFICATIONS

The epigenetic regulation of chromatin by virtue of chemical histone modifications is even more complex than DNA methylation discussed previously, and it is now thought that there are far more than 100 amino acid residue-specific posttranslational modifications (PTMs) in a typical vertebrate cell (Tan et al., 2011), including mono (me1), di (me2)-, and tri (me3) methylation, acetylation, and crotonylation; polyADP-ribosylation and small protein (ubiquitin, SUMO) modification of specific lysine residues; and as arginine (R) methylation and "citrullination," serine (S) phosphorylation, tyrosine (T) hydroxylation, and several others (Kouzarides, 2007; Tan et al., 2011; Taverna et al., 2007). These site- and residue-specific PTMs are typically explored in the context of chromatin structure and function, with an epigenetic histone code (a combinatorial set of histone PTMs that differentiates between promoters, gene bodies, enhancer, and other regulatory sequences, condensed heterochromatin, and so on [Zhou et al., 2011]). For an overview on the principle (but by far not an exhaustive illustration of all molecular markings defining the epigenome), see Figure 13.1. It is important to emphasize that histone PTMs rarely occur in isolation, and instead multiple histone PTMs appear to be coregulated and, as a group, define the aforementioned chromatin states (Berger, 2007). Many active promoters, for example, are defined by high levels of histone H3 lysine 4 methylation and various histone lysine acetylation markings (Zhou et al., 2011). Furthermore, there is also evidence for a coordinated and sequential regulation; phosphorylation of histone H3 at the serine (S)10 position often serves as a trigger for subsequent acetylation of neighboring lysine residues H3K9 and H3K14 in the context of transcriptional activation, while at the same time blocking repression-associated methylation of H3K9 (Nowak and Corces, 2004).

HISTONE VARIANTS

In addition to the core histones H2A/H2B/H3/H4, histone variants such as H3.3, H2A.Z, and H2A.X exist (Fig. 13.1). The role of these variant histones, which differ from the canonical histone only at very few amino acid positions, is often discussed in the context of replication-independent expression and assembly (Woodcock, 2006), and several histone variants robustly affect nucleosome stability and compaction (Jin and Felsenfeld, 2007). One popular model postulates that during the process of gene expression, RNA polymerase and the transcriptional activation and elongator complexes destabilize nucleosomes, which in turn promotes nucleosome remodeling and variant histone incorporation, which then further potentiate or stabilize gene expression (Bintu et al., 2011; Sutcliffe et al., 2009).

THE EPIGENOME IS PACKAGED INTO HIGHER ORDER CHROMATIN STRUCTURES

Epigenetic decoration of nucleosomes, including the DNA and histone modifications, and histone variants described previously, in itself, would fall short to adequately describe the epigenome, or even the localized chromatin architecture at any given (genomic) locus. This is because nucleosomal organization leads to only a 7-fold increase in packaging density of the genetic material, as compared with naked DNA; however, the actual level of compaction in the vertebrate nucleus in interphase (which defines the nucleus during the time period a cell is not dividing, including postmitotic cells such as neurons) is about three orders of magnitude higher (Belmont, 2006). The chromosomal arrangements in the interphase nucleus are not random, however. Specifically, loci at sites of active gene expression are more likely to be clustered together and positioned toward a central position within the nucleus, while heterochromatin and silenced loci move more toward the nuclear periphery (Cremer and Cremer, 2001; Duan et al., 2010). Chromatin loopings, in particular, are among the most highly regulated "supranucleosomal" structures and are associated with transcriptional regulation, by, for example, positioning distal regulatory enhancer or silencer elements that—in the linear genome—are positioned potentially many hundred kilobases apart from a gene, to interact directly with that specific promoter (Gaszner and Felsenfeld, 2006; Wood et al., 2010). Despite the growing realization of the importance of these and other higher order chromatin structures for transcriptional regulation, this is an area where very little is known about regulation in the nervous system, let alone potential alterations in psychiatric disease. Until recently, there were only three studies in the literature that explored loop formations in brain tissue (Dhar et al., 2009; Horike et al., 2005; Jiang et al., 2010), with a few additional papers using the brain as negative control for their studies on the sensory epithelium of the nose (Lomvardas et al., 2006) or the hematopoietic system (Simonis et al., 2006). However, to date, nothing is known about chromatin loopings in human brain.

Three-dimensional chromatin architectures are commonly mapped using derivatives of chromosome conformation capture (3C). This technique was originally developed for simple eukaryote systems such as yeast (Dekker et al., 2002) but has been further advanced to include 4C, 5C, HiC, and ChIA-PET (Simonis et al., 2007), allowing the mapping of chromosomal architectures across many megabases, or in the case of HiC and ChIA-PET, even genome-wide. At its core, the technique explores physical interactions between DNA fragments separated by interspersed sequence (chromosome architecture in cis) or between sequences positioned in different chromosomes (interactions in trans). Cross-linked chromatin is digested with a specific restriction enzyme, religated and amplified using primer pairs for which forward and reverse primers match to different portions of the genomic locus of interest. It will be important to clarify in the nearby future whether the 3C technique and its derivatives are applicable to human postmortem brain tissue. If so, then the exploration of chromatin loopings in normal and diseased brain could potentially provide valuable insights about the chromosomal architectures surrounding any given locus, including potential aberrations in the context of disease-associated polymorphisms or DNA structural variants. Presently, the exploration of many regulatory sequences is simply not possible because they are, to put it simply, not "visible" in the linear genome sequence, because of their spatial separation from transcription start sites or annotated genes by many hundreds of kilobases, potentially. To highlight the potential use of chromosome conformation capture in the context of psychiatric disease, consider the example of the major histocompatibility complex (MHC) locus, which long has been implicated in psychiatric disease (Smeraldi et al., 1976), conferring significant genetic risk to schizophrenia and related disease as most recently shown in three large genome-wide association studies (GWASs) published jointly in 2009 (Purcell et al., 2009; Shi et al., 2009; Stefansson et al., 2009). These studies identified up to 45 disease-associated SNPs (single-nucleotide polymorphisms) in the 26–33 megabase region of the MHC loci on chromosome 6. Strikingly, 50% of these SNPs are not located near genes. In fact, the strongest SNP at rs13194053 ($p = 9.54 \times 10^{-9}$) is more than 29 kb away from its nearest gene, HIST1H2AH. A functional role for many intergenic regions would not be surprising since many intergenic regions alter expression of upstream and downstream genes (Kleinjan and van Heyningen, 2005), and the mechanistic workup of these SNPs will certainly require application of chromosome conformation capture and related technologies.

CHROMATIN MARKINGS REMAIN PLASTIC THROUGHOUT THE LIFE SPAN OF THE HUMAN BRAIN, WITH IMPLICATIONS FOR THE NEUROBIOLOGY OF PSYCHIATRIC DISEASE

DEVELOPMENTAL PLASTICITY OF BRAIN EPIGENOMES

Most or perhaps all epigenetic markings studied to date, including DNA methylation, are now thought to be reversible and subject to bidirectional regulation in somatic tissues including brain, and there is no a priori reason for the unidirectional accumulation of a specific epigenetic mark while the brain is maturing and aging (Cheung et al., 2010; Guo et al., 2011; Klose and Zhang, 2007; Loenarz and Schofield, 2011; Miller and Sweatt, 2007; Ooi and Bestor, 2008). Nonetheless, multiple lines of evidence suggest that there is substantial reorganization of chromatin structures during the course of postnatal development and aging. Human cerebral cortex, for example, shows complex and gene-specific changes in the amount of methyl-cytosine (mC5; cytosines are methylated at the carbon 5 position). There is a fast rise in mC5 at many promoters during the transition from peri- to postnatal ages that continues at a slower pace into old age in conjunction with subtle changes (mostly a decline) in expression of transcripts originating from these promoters (Hernandez et al., 2011; Numata et al., 2012; Siegmund et al., 2007). Such age-related epigenetic drifts could impact vulnerability to neurodegenerative disease. A fascinating example has been recently reported for the cerebellum of the mouse, where levels of the mC5 derivative, hydroxymethyl-cytosine 5hmC, increase by 10-fold from postnatal Week 1 to adulthood (Szulwach et al., 2011b). Notably, among the genes that are affected by increasing 5hmC amounts at their promoters during cerebellar maturation, pathways for aging-related neurodegenerative diseases and angiogenesis were overrepresented and included at least 15 genes linked to hereditary forms of spinocerebellar ataxia, a neurological syndrome defined by severe motor dysfunction with the degeneration of cerebellar Purkinje neurons and other systems (Szulwach et al., 2011b). Also, of relevance, ten-eleven translocation (TET) proteins are responsible for converting mC5 to hmC5, and the active domains of these proteins belong to the same dioxygenase superfamily as hypoxia-inducible factor (HIF), an oxygen sensor that has been ascribed with a key role in angiogenesis and oxidative stress responses (Szulwach et al., 2011b). It will be extremely interesting to explore whether oxidation and other stress factors in the cellular environment, via TET-mediated regulation of DNA methylation levels, could leave a lasting imprint on chromatin structures in neurons or glia.

Like the aforementioned dynamic changes in DNA methylation during the course of development and aging, the epigenetic landscapes of histone modifications also undergo substantial reorganization across the life span of the human brain. For example, histone methylation markings that differentiate between open and repressive chromatin surrounding NMDA receptor gene promoters show highly dynamic changes in cerebellar cortex during the transition from perinatal stages and infancy to adulthood (Stadler et al., 2005) that reflect, in part, development changes in levels of the corresponding gene transcripts (Akbarian et al., 1996). Furthermore, hundreds of loci undergo histone methylation changes in cortical neurons during the first few years of life (Cheung et al., 2010). The brains from mice that are prone to accelerated senescence (the SAMP8 line) and have learning and memory deficits show age-related drifts in histone PTMs: these epigenetic drifts are defined by a loss of the markings associated with active gene expression, such as histone H4 lysine 20 monomethyl (H4-K20me1) and H3-K36me3 (Fig. 13.1), in conjunction with a robust rise in the repressive mark, H3-K27me3 (Wang et al., 2010). The hippocampus of aged, 16-month-old wild-type mice shows deficits in acetylated histone H3-lysine 12 (H4K12) (Peleg et al., 2010), a histone PTM that is broadly correlated with the transcriptional elongation process (Hargreaves et al., 2009). In addition, drugs with histone deacetylase inhibitor (HDACi) activity induce upregulation of H4-K12ac dramatically and thereby could improve hippocampal-dependent learning and memory in aged mice (Peleg et al., 2010). It is possible that age-related drifts in brain epigenomes negatively affect neuronal (Fischer et al., 2010; Lu et al., 2004) and oligodendroglial (Copray et al., 2009) transcriptomes, thereby contributing to a decline in the signaling capacity of nerve cells, defects in axon myelination, and other molecular defects that have been linked to cognitive disorders of the adult brain, including those that like Alzheimer's disease are associated with neurodegeneration (Yankner et al., 2008) and others such as schizophrenia that are not accompanied by ongoing loss of nerve cells (Tang et al., 2009). Taken together, these findings leave little doubt that brain epigenomes are indeed subject to dynamic changes throughout all periods of maturation and aging, which may have important implications for the neurobiology of disease.

Posttraumatic stress disorder (PTSD) is probably a good example to illustrate how current concepts in epigenetics influence thoughts about pathophysiology of psychiatric disease. Obviously, from a heuristic perspective, it is very attractive to design working hypotheses that attribute a key role for epigenetic markings inside the nucleus of neurons and other brain cells subserving a memory function that, in response to an intense "environmental" influence (e.g., trauma), convey lasting alterations in a subject's emotional and physical health and resilience (Zovkic and Sweatt, 2012). Indeed, some recent studies in human subjects point to the promising potential of such types of working models. For example, a recent study on peripheral cells collected pre- and postdeployment from U.S. military service members identified global DNA methylation levels in repetitive DNA sequences, including LINE-1 and Alu repeat elements, as biomarkers that were significantly associated with resilience or, conversely, vulnerability to PTSD (Rusiecki et al., 2012). Similarly, studies in civilian/urban populations discovered that changes in blood DNA methylation signatures in PTSD subjects selectively affected cytokine and steroid signaling, immune defense, and inflammation-related genes, consistent with various lines of evidence implicating some degree of peripheral immune dysregulation in this disorder (Smith et al., 2011; Uddin et al., 2010). Based on the aforementioned studies in blood, one would predict that brain chromatin, too, is involved in the neurobiology of PTSD, and human postmortem brain shows distinct DNA and histone methylation changes in amygdala and hippocampus, ventral striatum, and other anatomical structures with a critical role for emotion, affect, and memory (Zovkic and Sweatt, 2012). Indeed, there is excessive methylation of the glucocorticoid receptor gene promoter NR3C1 and ribosomal DNA repeats in the hippocampus of adult suicide victims who also suffered childhood abuse (McGowan et al., 2008, 2009). Furthermore, the prefrontal cortex of suicide completers exhibits a shift from open to repressive chromatin-associated histone methylation for the TRKB neurotrophin high-affinity receptor, and for various genes regulating polyamine metabolism (Ernst et al., 2009; Fiori and Turecki, 2010). Furthermore, downregulated histone deacetylase 2 (HDAC2) expression in ventral striatum of subjects diagnosed with depression is thought to lead to an overall increase in histone H3 acetylation in this mesolimbic structure (Covington et al., 2009). In the aforementioned studies, many of these epigenetic changes are associated with decreased expression of the corresponding gene transcripts, which reaffirms the importance of epigenetic mechanisms and transcriptional regulation for the pathophysiology of psychiatric disease.

While postmortem brains of psychiatric disease cases are notoriously hampered by the fact that most subjects received psychoactive medication prior to death, some evidence from animal studies would suggest that at least a subset of the chromatin changes in diseased brain, as mentioned previously, are not mere epiphenomena due to medication or postmortem confounds such as tissue autolysis but, instead, closely associated with the disease process. To mention just two examples, the hippocampal glucocorticoid receptor gene Nr3c1 shows excessive methylation not only in patients (McGowan et al., 2009), but also in adults rats brought up with suboptimal maternal care ("low licking" versus "high licking" mothers) (Weaver et al., 2004), and chronic social defeat stress in mice and rats elicits histone acetylation changes in ventral striatum and hippocampus very similar to those encountered in depressed human subjects (Covington et al., 2009; Hollis et al., 2010).

MONOGENETIC ETIOLOGIES OF NEUROPYCHIATRIC DISEASE INCLUDES MUTATIONS IN PROTEINS INVOLVED IN READING, WRITING, OR ERASURE OF EPIGENETIC MARKINGS

There are many hundreds of genes that encode proteins that either write, erase, or read the molecular markings of the epigenome (Filippakopoulos et al., 2010; Janzen et al., 2010); however, we want to make the reader aware that some experts feel this type of terminology can be misleading, especially because the regulation of many epigenetic markings could turn out to be only a "cog" in the chromatin-remodeling machinery but not a key driver (Henikoff and Shilatifard, 2011). The genome encodes three DNA methyltransferases, *DNMT1*, *DNMT3a*, and *DNMT3b*, that establish and maintain DNA methylation markings, and in addition, there are complex DNA demethylation pathways involving mC5 hydroxylation and oxidation via ten-eleven translocation dioxygenases, or activation-induced deaminase (AID)/APOBEC-mediated deamination of mC5 or hmC5, followed by base excision repair-mediated replacement with (unmethylated) cytosine (Bhutani et al., 2011; Guo et al., 2011). Furthermore, the collective set of histone methyltransferases (KMTs) and demethylases (KDMs) together could easily account for >100 genes in a mammalian genome, suggestiong that the molecular framework to establish and erase histone methylation marks is likely to be extremely complex and probably differentially regulated across various cell types, or developmental stages, of the organism (Copeland et al., 2009; Rotili and Mai, 2011). Reader proteins, which bind to a specific epigenetic mark, are defined by their characteristic "reader module"; well-studied examples include the methyl-CpG binding domain (MBD) for mC5-DNA, the bromodomain for lysine acetylation, and "chromo," "Tudor," malignant brain tumor ("MBT")," "WD40repeat," plant homeodomain (PHD) finger domains targeting methylated lysines or arginines in a residue-specific manner (Taverna et al., 2007). For the "open-chromatin" mark histone H3-trimethyl-lysine 4 (H3K4me3), these include many components of the RNA polymerase II–associated transcriptional initiation complex, while other marks such as H3K9me3 are primarily targeted by transcriptional repressors and regulators of chromatin condensation (Vermeulen et al., 2010).

The collective set of reader, writer, and eraser proteins includes at least 15 genes that are associated with monogenetic forms of neurodevelopmental or adult-onset neuropsychiatric disease (Jakocevski and Akbarian, 2012). While an exhaustive discussion of these various neurodevelopmental syndromes would be beyond the scope of this book chapter, it is important to point out that while chromatin defects in the brain were until very recently considered static lesions of early development that occurred in the context of rare genetic syndromes, it is now clear that mutations and maladaptations of the epigenetic machinery cover a much wider continuum, including adult-onset neurodegenerative disease. For example, while hypomorphic (partial loss-of-function) mutations in the DNA methyltransferase *DNMT3B* were already known to cause a multiorgan syndrome—Immunodeficiency, Centromere Instability, Facial anomalies (ICF 1)—that includes mental retardation and defective brain development (Hansen et al., 1999; Okano et al., 1999), it was only recently discovered that select mutations in DNA methyltransferase–coding regions, including *DNMT1*, are responsible for some cases of hereditary sensory and autonomic neuropathy, type 1 (HSAN1) (Klein et al., 2011), a rare neurodegenerative condition characterized by various neuropathies and early-onset dementia in the third or fourth decade of life. In other pedigrees, DNMT1 mutations were linked to narcolepsy and late-onset deafness and cerebellar ataxia (Winkelmann et al., 2012). Likewise, structural variants in the X-linked gene *MECP2*, encoding the methyl-CpG-binding protein 2, not only

cause Rett syndrome (RTT), a disorder of early childhood with an incidence of 1 in 10,000 that is associated with cognitive deficits and a broad range of neurological symptoms (Amir et al., 1999; Chouery et al., 2011), but are also thought to be responsible for some cases of autism and schizophrenia with onset in childhood or adolescence (Piton et al., 2011). Furthermore, consider the DNA variants and mutations encompassing the *KMT1D* gene (9q34.3), encoding a histone H3-lysine 9 specific methyltransferase initially recognized as the causative gene responsible for a distinct neurodevelopmental and multiorgan syndome, the Kleefstra mental retardation syndrome (Kleefstra et al., 2009). Meanwhile, however, *KMT1D* mutations are also responsible for some cases with schizophrenia (Kirov et al., 2012), and various nonspecific psychiatric phenotypes and even neurodegenerative disease in the postadolescence period (Verhoeven et al., 2011).

Taken together, these findings leave little doubt that mutations that fall within the coding sequence or otherwise affect levels of expression of a select set of regulatory proteins involved in DNA or histone methylation could cause neuropsychiatric disease even after brain development has largely been completed, including some cases diagnosed with psychosis or early-onset dementia. One could speculate that *DNMT1*, *MECP2*, *KMT1D*, and other monogenetic causes of neuropsychiatric disease (Jakocevski and Akbarian, 2012) could then also play a wider role in the pathophysiology of autism, schizophrenia, and other illnesses, outside of what has been discussed—and among the overall population of psychiatric patients very rarely occurring—cases with mutations and deletions of these chromatin regulatory proteins. For example, a recent postmortem study on 16 cases on the autism spectrum, exploring genome-wide occupancies of histone H3-tri-methyl-lysine 4 (H3K4me3), a mark sharply upregulated at transcription start sites (see Fig. 13.1) in prefrontal neurons, reported an abnormally broad histone methylation profile ("spreading") at the 5′ end of many hundreds or thousands of genes for four of their cases, while the remaining twelve cases showed much more limited alterations at a few loci only (Shulha et al., 2012). While purely speculative at this point, it remains possible that these subsets of autism cases with an apparently more generalized abnormality in prefrontal histone methylation profiles are affected by defects in the pathways governing the writing, reading, or erasure of H3K4me3 and related markings. These may include pathways that are critical for the orderly activity of *KDM5C/SMCX/JARID1C*, the X-linked H3K4-specific histone demethylase that is also responsible for some cases of mental retardation, autism, and other neurodevelopmental disease, or the H3K4 methyltransferase MLL1 previously implicated in the neurobiology of schizophrenia (Adegbola et al., 2008; Akbarian and Huang, 2009; Huang et al., 2007; Iwase et al., 2007).

"EPIGENETIC DRUG" DEVELOPMENT IN PSYCHIATRY—READY FOR PRIME TIME?

While most major psychiatric disorders, including the broader range of autism, mood, or psychosis spectrum disorders, each lack a unifying neuropathology, the pathophysiology almost certainly involves dysregulated gene expression in cerebral cortex and other brain regions. Starting with the initial reports on gene expression changes in prefrontal cortex and hippocampus of subjects diagnosed with schizophrenia, a large number of postmortem brain studies have been published, collectively suggesting that distinct sets of gene transcripts are frequently, albeit never consistently, expressed at altered levels in at least a subset of psychiatric disease cases, when compared with control brain cohorts. Well-known examples, as they pertain to schizophrenia or mood disorder, involve transcripts for GABAergic inhibitory signaling, or myelination and other oligodendrocyte-specific function, and in some studies more generalized transcriptome changes compromising metabolic activities, as well as many markers of pre- and postsynaptic neurotransmission (Akbarian and Huang, 2006; Aston et al., 2004; Benes, 2010; Charych et al., 2009; Dracheva et al., 2004; Duncan et al., 2010; Guidotti et al., 2005; Hakak et al., 2001; Hashimoto et al., 2008; Katsel et al., 2005; Martins-de-Souza et al., 2009; Regenold et al., 2007; Sibille et al., 2009; Tkachev et al., 2003; Woo et al., 2008).

Therefore, drugs that interfere with chromatin-bound proteins involved in transcriptional regulation could be of interest both to preclinical researchers interested in modeling the aforementioned gene expression deficits in the animal, as well as to groups in academia or industry that are interested in exploring novel psychopharmacologic treatments. In this context, it is worth mentioning that sodium valproate, one of the most frequently prescribed drugs in neurology and psychiatry largely due to its anticonvulsive and mood-stabilizing properties, is a weak but broadly acting inhibitor of histone deacetylase enzymes (HDAC) (Guidotti et al., 2011). Histone acetylation is viewed as a facilitative signal for transcription, while HDAC cleaves off the acetyl groups from the histone lysine residues and is commonly associated with repressive chromatin remodeling (Sharma et al., 2006). Thus, HDAC inhibitors (HDACi) are thought to upregulate gene expression at some loci, by shifting the balance toward acetylation (of promoter-bound histones). For example, it has been suggested that valproate-induced histone hyperacetylation may exert some of its therapeutic effects via transcriptional upregulation at "GABAergic" and other neuronal genes (Guidotti et al., 2011). In animal experiments, histone deacetylase inhibitors improve learning and memory function in a variety of paradigms, including at advanced age and also in mice with mutation in Creb-binding protein, CBP (which is mutated in subjects with Rubinstein-Taybi syndrome). Other preclinical work strongly suggests that HDACi may exert therapeutic effects in depression and related psychiatric illnesses (Covington et al., 2009; Morris et al., 2010; Schroeder et al., 2007). Whether HDACi's would emerge in the future, indeed, as novel psychopharmacologic treatment options for the treatment of psychiatric disorders is not yet clear. However, it is the broad therapeutic potential of HDACi in the animal model, which goes far beyond the aforementioned psychiatric conditions and includes acute and chronic neurodegenerative disease including acute brain injury and stroke, as well as Parkinson's, Alzheimer's, and Lou Gehrig's (motor neuron) disease, and various triplet repeat disorders including Huntington's chorea and spinocerebellar ataxia (Baltan et al., 2011; Chuang et al., 2009; Fischer et al., 2010; Tsou et al., 2009).

Similar to the HDACi previously mentioned, there is some evidence for the therapeutic potential of drugs affecting histone methylation, but it remains unclear whether these findings would in the future bear fruit and lead to novel psychiatric treatment options. Of interest are small molecules such as BIX-01294, which inhibit a select set of histone methyltransferases (HMTs), including histone H3K9-specific HMT G9a/Glp (Kubicek et al., 2007). The H3K9 methylation mark, particularly the di- and trimethylated forms, are associated with repression and negative regulation of transcription, and consequently, expression of some genes in brains is increased after exposure to BIX-01294 (Kubicek et al., 2007). Behavioral changes after BIX-01294 have been reported as well, including increased reward and addiction behavior in the context of cocaine and other stimulant exposure (Maze et al., 2010). The drug's mechanism of action could, at least in part, involve the inhibition of G9a/Glp-mediated repressive chromatin remodeling at the promoters of Bdnf, Cdk5, Arc, and other genes, which then in turn could lead to increased spine density and synaptic connectivity (Maze et al., 2010). Like the histone-modifying drugs previously discussed, several structurally unrelated DNA methylation inhibitors, including cytidine analogues 5-azacytidine or compounds such as N-phthalyl-L-tryptophan/RG108, when administered directly into brain tissue of mice and rats, alter synaptic plasticity and hippocampal learning and memory and are thereby associated with powerful modulation of reward- and addiction-related behavior (Han et al., 2010; LaPlant et al., 2010; Levenson et al., 2006; Lubin et al., 2008; Miller et al., 2010; Miller and Sweatt, 2007). Whatever the underlying mechanism of action, we predict that, as in cancer treatment and other areas of medicine where presently worldwide hundreds of clinical trials involve epigenetic drug targets, in psychiatry, too, the therapeutic potential of chromatin-modifying drugs will soon be tested on a broader basis, given the plethora of promising findings that are currently emerging from preclinical and translational research.

EPIGENETICS AS A TOOL TO EXPLORE DISEASE-ASSOCIATED DNA STRUCTURAL VARIANTS AND POLYMORPHISMS OUTSIDE OF PROTEIN-CODING SEQUENCES

As already discussed, a significant portion of (psychiatric) disease-associated mutations and polymorphisms are thought to cause functional changes other than alterations in protein-coding sequence. This poses a potential challenge, as the functional role of the "normal" DNA sequence and the (disease-related) structural variants may be hard to discern by sequence analyses alone. To provide the reader with an illustrative example of the challenging tasks that lie ahead for psychiatric (epi)genetics, consider the example of the major histocompatibility complex locus, which long has been implicated in mental illness, conferring significant genetic risk for schizophrenia and related diseases as most recently shown in three large genome-wide association studies published jointly in 2009 (Purcell et al., 2009; Shi et al., 2009; Stefansson et al., 2009). Intergenic disease–associated SNPs identified in the MHC region of chromosome 6 may interact via proteins with functional regions of the genome. Indeed, when open chromatin-associated histone methylation markings, including the H3K4 tri- and mono-methyl mark, and the genomic occupancy pattern of the transcription factor (and potential barrier protein preventing the uncontrolled spread of heterochromatin), CTCF (CCCTC-binding factor), was profiled in neuronal chromatin from human prefrontal cortex and in peripheral cell lines, it became apparent that several schizophrenia-associated SNPs are highly enriched with one or several of these markings (Fig. 13.2). Because the H3K4 tri- and mono-methyl markings are often associated with transcriptional regulation, including promoter- and enhancer-like functions, one could speculate that the risk alleles are probably interfering with local transcription. While this is purely speculative at this point in time, the preceding example illustrates how the study of epigenetic markings bears the potential to provide important clues on the role of otherwise poorly characterized DNA sequences outside of coding regions.

Obviously, the study of chromatin structures could also provide important information for DNA sequences for which a functional role is already known, such as an annotated promoter. One of the best-known examples involves the fragile X mental retardation (*FMR1*) gene in fragile X mental retardation syndrome, where the abnormal expansion of a CGG codon from (normally) 5–40 repeats from 50 to over 200 triggers excessive promoter DNA methylation, effectively shutting down gene expression by silencing the surrounding chromatin (Oberle et al., 1991). This is true even for genes with a much

more subtle contribution to disease risk, such as *GAD1* encoding glutamic acid decarboxylase (67kDa) GABA synthesis enzyme, for which some halplotypes and polymorphisms, positioned within a few Kb from the GAD1 transcription start site, confer genetic risk for accelerated loss of frontal lobe gray matter (Addington et al., 2005; Straub et al., 2007) and, via epistatic interaction with catechol-o-methyltransferase (COMT) alleles, regulate synaptic dopamine and modulate overall GABA tissue levels in the prefrontal cortex (Marenco et al., 2010). The same genetic variants surrounding the *GAD1* promoter recently emerged as a major driver for the disease-related decline in *GAD67* transcript and the epigenetic decoration of the proximal *GAD1* promoter in subjects with schizoprenia, including the balance between "open" and "repressive" histone methylation markings histone H3 trimethyl-lysines, K4me3 and K27me3 (Huang et al., 2007). These findings, taken together, clearly illustrate the potential of epigenetic approaches to shed light on the functional impact of structural variants involving regulatory, noncoding DNA, both for rare mutations with high disease risk/penetrance (e.g., *FMR1* in fragile X) or for common variants that make only much smaller contribution to the overall disease risk (e.g., *GAD1* in schizophrenia).

SYNOPSIS AND OUTLOOK

"Neuroepigenetics" is a new discipline (Day and Sweatt, 2010) that presently takes center stage in the field of mental health research, mainly because: (*1*) Recent findings suggest that the epigenetic landscapes of the human brain remain "plastic" throughout all periods of brain development and aging, with ongoing dynamic regulation occurring even in neurons and other postmitotic constituents (Cheung et al., 2010; Hernandez et al., 2011; Numata et al., 2012; Siegmund et al., 2007). (*2*) The

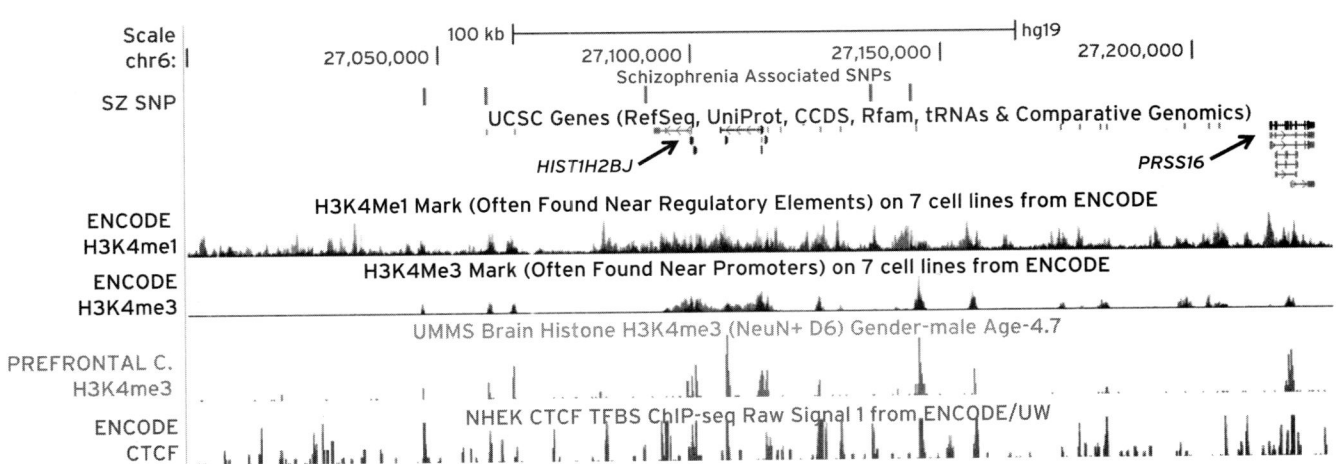

Figure 13.2 *Epigenetic profiles encompassing the MHC region on chromosome 6, which harbors strong linkage disequilibrium (r^2 = 0.52–0.77) of five schizophrenia single-nucleotide polymorphisms (SNPs) in the major histocompatibility complex (MHC) region (27,000,000–27,300,000) (Purcell et al., 2009; Stefansson et al., 2009). The most significant SNP rs6913660 is located greater than 50 kb from the nearest gene (HIST1H2BJ). The chr 6:27,000,000–27,300,000 region on the UCSC genome browser is shown with six tracks represented: (i) five schizophrenia-associated SNPs in linkage disequilibrium in the following order: rs6904071, rs926300, rs6913660, rs13219181, and rs1319453; (ii) UCSC genes; (iii) histone 3 lysine 4 monomethylation (H3K4me1) marks on seven cells from ENCODE; (iv) histone 3 lysine 4 trimethylation (H3K4me3) marks on seven cell lines from ENCODE; (v) H3K4me3 marks from prefrontal cortex neuron in a 4.7-year-old boy; and (vi) CTCF ChIP-seq data from the NHEK cell line. Notice that several schizophrenia-associated SNPs are found within H3K4me1, H3K4me3, and CTCF peak sequences, indicating possible physical interactions between these various chromatin fragments.*

range of neurological conditions due to a primary chromatin defect extends far beyond the early developmental period and may even include a subset of cases with adult-onset psychosis, or dementia and other neurodegenerative disease (Klein et al., 2011; Winkelmann et al., 2012). (3) Chromatin-modifying drugs could lead to novel treatments for neurological and psychiatric disease (Baltan et al., 2011; Chuang et al., 2009; Fischer et al., 2010; Peter and Akbarian, 2011; Tsou et al., 2009). (4) Exploration of chromatin structures could be expected to uncover, in a substantial portion of cases, the functional impact of disease-relevant mutations in regulatory and other sequences that are otherwise difficult to "capture" by DNA sequence analyses alone. Indeed, the important role of epigenetically regulated noncoding DNA was ascertained by recent bioinformatical studies showing that many noncoding DNA sequences are generally deficient of SNP and undergo a purifying selection (Tolstorukov et al., 2011).

Finally, it is worth mentioning that, based on next-generation sequencing of epigenetic markings in sperm, perhaps as much as 4% of the human genome could maintain nucleosomal organization and many types of epigenetic decoration when transmitted through the germline. This includes many loci considered of critical importance for early pre- and postimplantation development, imprinted gene clusters, microRNA clusters, homeobox (HOX) gene clusters, and the promoters of many stand-alone developmental transcription and signaling factors (Hammoud et al., 2010). These and related findings will most certainly further stimulate research aimed at uncovering evidence for epigenetic heritability of psychiatric disease, including depression, schizophrenia, and addiction, to name a few, which all have in common that for a majority of subjects no straightforward genetic risk architecture has been identified.

Without doubt, psychiatric epigenetics will remain a most productive area of research for many years to come.

DISCLOSURE

The authors declare no conflicts of interests to disclose.

Work conducted in the authors' laboratories is sponsored by the National Institutes of Health to S. A., the Brain Behavior Research Foundation to S. A., the NIMH (R01 MH084966 to K. A. G.), and the U.S. Army Research Laboratory and the U.S. Army Research Office (grant 58076-LS-DRP) to K. A. G.

REFERENCES

Addington, A.M., Gornick, M., et al. (2005). GAD1 (2q31.1), which encodes glutamic acid decarboxylase (GAD67), is associated with childhood-onset schizophrenia and cortical gray matter volume loss. *Mol. Psychiatry* 10:581–588.

Adegbola, A., Gao, H., et al. (2008). A novel mutation in JARID1C/SMCX in a patient with autism spectrum disorder (ASD). *Am. J. Med. Genet. A* 146A, 505–511.

Akbarian, S., and Huang, H.S. (2006). Molecular and cellular mechanisms of altered GAD1/GAD67 expression in schizophrenia and related disorders. *Brain. Res. Rev.* 52:293–304.

Akbarian, S., and Huang, H.S. (2009). Epigenetic regulation in human brain-focus on histone lysine methylation. *Biol. Psychiatry* 65:198–203.

Akbarian, S., Sucher, N.J., et al. (1996). Selective alterations in gene expression for NMDA receptor subunits in prefrontal cortex of schizophrenics. *J. Neurosci.* 16:19–30.

Amir, R.E., Van den Veyver, I.B., et al. (1999). Rett syndrome is caused by mutations in X-linked MECP2, encoding methyl-CpG-binding protein 2. *Nat. Genet.* 23:185–188.

Aston, C., Jiang, L., et al. (2004). Microarray analysis of postmortem temporal cortex from patients with schizophrenia. *J. Neurosci. Res.* 77:858–866.

Baltan, S., Murphy, S.P., et al. (2011). Histone deacetylase inhibitors preserve white matter structure and function during ischemia by conserving ATP and reducing excitotoxicity. *J. Neurosci.* 31:3990–3999.

Belmont, A.S. (2006). Mitotic chromosome structure and condensation. *Curr. Opin. Cell. Biol.* 18:632–638.

Benes, F.M. (2010). Amygdalocortical circuitry in schizophrenia: from circuits to molecules. *Neuropsychopharmacol.* 35:239–257.

Berger, S.L. (2007). The complex language of chromatin regulation during transcription. *Nature* 447:407–412.

Bhutani, N., Burns, D.M., et al. (2011). DNA demethylation dynamics. *Cell* 146:866–872.

Bintu, L., Kopaczynska, M., et al. (2011). The elongation rate of RNA polymerase determines the fate of transcribed nucleosomes. *Nat. Struct. Mol. Biol.* 18:1394–1399.

Charych, E.I., Liu, F., et al. (2009). GABA(A) receptors and their associated proteins: implications in the etiology and treatment of schizophrenia and related disorders. *Neuropharmacology* 57:481–495.

Cheung, I., Shulha, H.P., et al. (2010). Developmental regulation and individual differences of neuronal H3K4me3 epigenomes in the prefrontal cortex. *Proc. Natl. Acad. Sci. USA* 107:8824–8829.

Chouery, E., Ghoch, J.A., et al. (2011). A novel deletion in ZBTB24 in a Lebanese family with Immunodeficiency, Centromeric Instability, and Facial Anomalies Syndrome Type 2. *Clin. Genet.* 82:480–493.

Chuang, D.M., Leng, Y., et al. (2009). Multiple roles of HDAC inhibition in neurodegenerative conditions. *Trends Neurosci.* 32:591–601.

Copeland, R.A., Solomon, M.E., et al. (2009). Protein methyltransferases as a target class for drug discovery. *Nat. Rev. Drug Discov.* 8:724–732.

Copray, S., Huynh, J.L., et al. (2009). Epigenetic mechanisms facilitating oligodendrocyte development, maturation, and aging. *Glia* 57:1579–1587.

Covington, H.E., III, Maze, I., et al. (2009). Antidepressant actions of histone deacetylase inhibitors. *J. Neurosci.* 29:11451–11460.

Cremer, T., and Cremer, C. (2001). Chromosome territories, nuclear architecture and gene regulation in mammalian cells. *Nat. Rev. Genet.* 2:292–301.

Day, J.J., and Sweatt, J.D. (2010). DNA methylation and memory formation. *Nat. Neurosci.* 13:1319–1323.

Day, J.J., and Sweatt, J.D. (2011). Epigenetic mechanisms in cognition. *Neuron* 70:813–829.

Dekker, J., Rippe, K., et al. (2002). Capturing chromosome conformation. *Science* 295:1306–1311.

Dhar, S.S., Ongwijitwat, S., et al. (2009). Chromosome conformation capture of all 13 genomic loci in the transcriptional regulation of the multisubunit bigenomic cytochrome C oxidase in neurons. *J. Biol. Chem.* 284:18644–18650.

Dracheva, S., Elhakem, S.L., et al. (2004). GAD67 and GAD65 mRNA and protein expression in cerebrocortical regions of elderly patients with schizophrenia. *J. Neurosci. Res.* 76:581–592.

Duan, Z., Andronescu, M., et al. (2010). A three-dimensional model of the yeast genome. *Nature* 465:363–367.

Duncan, C.E., Webster, M.J., et al. (2010). Prefrontal GABA(A) receptor alpha-subunit expression in normal postnatal human development and schizophrenia. *J. Psychiatr. Res.* 44:673–681.

Ederveen, T.H., Mandemaker, I.K., et al. (2011). The human histone H3 complement anno 2011. *Biochim. Biophys. Acta* 1809:577–586.

Ernst, C., Chen, E.S., et al. (2009). Histone methylation and decreased expression of TrkB.T1 in orbital frontal cortex of suicide completers. *Mol. Psychiatry* 14:830–832.

Filippakopoulos, P., Qi, J., et al. (2010). Selective inhibition of BET bromodomains. *Nature* 468:1067–1073.

Fiori, L.M., and Turecki, G. (2010). Genetic and epigenetic influences on expression of spermine synthase and spermine oxidase in suicide completers. *Int. J. Neuropsychopharmacol.* 13:725–736.

Fischer, A., Sananbenesi, F., et al. (2010). Targeting the correct HDAC(s) to treat cognitive disorders. *Trends Pharmacol. Sci.* 31:605–617.

Gaszner, M., and Felsenfeld, G. (2006). Insulators: exploiting transcriptional and epigenetic mechanisms. *Nat. Rev. Genet.* 7:703–713.

Guidotti, A., Auta, J., et al. (2005). GABAergic dysfunction in schizophrenia: new treatment strategies on the horizon. *Psychopharmacol. (Berl)* 180:191–205.

Guidotti, A., Auta, J., et al. (2011). Epigenetic GABAergic targets in schizophrenia and bipolar disorder. *Neuropharmacology* 60:1007–1016.

Guo, J.U., Su, Y., et al. (2011). Hydroxylation of 5-methylcytosine by TET1 promotes active DNA demethylation in the adult brain. *Cell* 145:423–434.

Haggarty, S.J., and Tsai, L.H. (2011). Probing the role of HDACs and mechanisms of chromatin-mediated neuroplasticity. *Neurobiol. Learn. Mem.* 96:41–52.

Hakak, Y., Walker, J.R., et al. (2001). Genome-wide expression analysis reveals dysregulation of myelination-related genes in chronic schizophrenia. *Proc. Natl. Acad. Sci. USA* 98:4746–4751.

Hammoud, S.S., Purwar, J., et al. (2010). Alterations in sperm DNA methylation patterns at imprinted loci in two classes of infertility. *Fertil. Steril.* 94:1728–1733.

Han, J., Li, Y., et al. (2010). Effect of 5-aza-2-deoxycytidine microinjecting into hippocampus and prelimbic cortex on acquisition and retrieval of cocaine-induced place preference in C57BL/6 mice. *Eur. J. Pharmacol.* 642:93–98.

Hansen, R.S., Wijmenga, C., et al. (1999). The DNMT3B DNA methyltransferase gene is mutated in the ICF immunodeficiency syndrome. *Proc. Natl. Acad. Sci. USA* 96:14412–14417.

Hargreaves, D.C., Horng, T., et al. (2009). Control of inducible gene expression by signal-dependent transcriptional elongation. *Cell* 138:129–145.

Hashimoto, T., Bazmi, H.H., et al. (2008). Conserved regional patterns of GABA-related transcript expression in the neocortex of subjects with schizophrenia. *Am. J. Psychiatry* 165:479–489.

He, Y.F., Li, B. et al. (2011). Tet-mediated formation of 5-carboxylcytosine and its excision by TDG in mammalian DNA. *Science* 333:1303–1307.

Henikoff, S., and Shilatifard, A. (2011). Histone modification: cause or cog? *Trends Genet.* 27:389–396.

Hernandez, D.G., Nalls, M.A., et al. (2011). Distinct DNA methylation changes highly correlated with chronological age in the human brain. *Hum. Mol. Genet.* 20:1164–1172.

Hollis, F., Wang, H., et al. (2010). The effects of repeated social defeat on long-term depressive-like behavior and short-term histone modifications in the hippocampus in male Sprague-Dawley rats. *Psychopharmacol. (Berl)* 211:69–77.

Horike, S., Cai, S., et al. (2005). Loss of silent-chromatin looping and impaired imprinting of DLX5 in Rett syndrome. *Nat. Genet.* 37:31–40.

Houston, I., Peter, C.J., et al. (2012). Epigenetics in the human brain. *Neuropsychopharmacol.* 38:183–197.

Huang, H.S., Matevossian, A., et al. (2007). Prefrontal dysfunction in schizophrenia involves mixed-lineage leukemia 1-regulated histone methylation at GABAergic gene promoters. *J. Neurosci.* 27:11254–11262.

Ito, S., Shen, L., et al. (2011). Tet proteins can convert 5-methylcytosine to 5-formylcytosine and 5-carboxylcytosine. *Science* 333:1300–1303.

Iwase, S., Lan, F., et al. (2007). The X-linked mental retardation gene SMCX/JARID1C defines a family of histone H3 lysine 4 demethylases. *Cell* 128:1077–1088.

Jakocevski, M., and Akbarian, S. (2012). Epigenetic mechanisms in neurodevelopmental and neurodegenerative disease. *Nat. Med.* 18:1194–1204.

Janzen, W.P., Wigle, T.J., et al. (2010). Epigenetics: tools and technologies. *Drug Discov. Today Technol.* 7:e59–e65.

Jiang, Y., Jakovcevski, M., et al. (2010). Setdb1 histone methyltransferase regulates mood-related behaviors and expression of the NMDA receptor subunit NR2B. *J. Neurosci.* 30:7152–7167.

Jin, C., and Felsenfeld, G. (2007). Nucleosome stability mediated by histone variants H3.3 and H2A.Z. *Genes Dev.* 21:1519–1529.

Jin, S.G., Wu, X., Li, A.X., et al. (2011). Genomic mapping of 5-hydroxymethylcytosine in the human brain. *Nucleic Acids Res.* 39:5015–5024.

Katsel, P., Davis, K.L., et al. (2005). Variations in myelin and oligodendrocyte-related gene expression across multiple brain regions in schizophrenia: a gene ontology study. *Schizophr. Res.* 79:157–173.

Kinney, S.M., Chin, H.G., et al. (2011). Tissue-specific distribution and dynamic changes of 5-hydroxymethylcytosine in mammalian genomes. *J. Biol. Chem.* 286:24685–24693.

Kirov, G., Pocklington, A.J., et al. (2012). *De novo* CNV analysis implicates specific abnormalities of postsynaptic signalling complexes in the pathogenesis of schizophrenia. *Mol. Psychiatry* 17:142–153.

Kleefstra, T., van Zelst-Stams, W.A., et al. (2009). Further clinical and molecular delineation of the 9q subtelomeric deletion syndrome supports a major contribution of EHMT1 haploinsufficiency to the core phenotype. *J. Med. Genet.* 46:598–606.

Klein, C.J., Botuyan, M.V., et al. (2011). Mutations in DNMT1 cause hereditary sensory neuropathy with dementia and hearing loss. *Nat. Genet.* 43:595–600.

Kleinjan, D.A., and van Heyningen, V. (2005). Long-range control of gene expression: emerging mechanisms and disruption in disease. *Am. J. Hum. Genet.* 76:8–32.

Klose, R.J., and Zhang, Y. (2007). Regulation of histone methylation by demethylimination and demethylation. *Nat. Rev. Mol. Cell Biol.* 8:307–318.

Kouzarides, T. (2007). Chromatin modifications and their function. *Cell* 128:693–705.

Kriaucionis, S., and Heintz, N. (2009). The nuclear DNA base 5-hydroxymethylcytosine is present in Purkinje neurons and the brain. *Science* 324:929–930.

Krishnan, V., and Nestler, E.J. (2010). Linking molecules to mood: new insight into the biology of depression. *Am. J. Psychiatry* 167:1305–1320.

Kubicek, S., O'Sullivan, R.J., et al. (2007). Reversal of H3K9me2 by a small-molecule inhibitor for the G9a histone methyltransferase. *Mol. Cell* 25:473–481.

Labrie, V., Pai, S., et al. (2012). Epigenetics of major psychosis: progress, problems and perspectives. *Trends Genet.* 28:427–435.

LaPlant, Q., Vialou, V., et al. (2010). Dnmt3a regulates emotional behavior and spine plasticity in the nucleus accumbens. *Nat. Neurosci.* 13:1137–1143.

Lehman, A.F., Lieberman, J.A., et al. (2004). Practice guideline for the treatment of patients with schizophrenia, second edition. *Am. J. Psychiatry* 161:1–56.

Levenson, J.M., Roth, T.L., et al. (2006). Evidence that DNA (cytosine-5) methyltransferase regulates synaptic plasticity in the hippocampus. *J. Biol. Chem.* 281:15763–15773.

Li, G., and Reinberg, D. (2011). Chromatin higher-order structures and gene regulation. *Curr. Opin. Genet. Dev.* 21:175–186.

Loenarz, C., and Schofield, C.J. (2011). Physiological and biochemical aspects of hydroxylations and demethylations catalyzed by human 2-oxoglutarate oxygenases. *Trends Biochem. Sci.* 36:7–18.

Lomvardas, S., Barnea, G., et al. (2006). Interchromosomal interactions and olfactory receptor choice. *Cell* 126:403–413.

Lu, T., Pan, Y., et al. (2004). Gene regulation and DNA damage in the ageing human brain. *Nature* 429:883–891.

Lubin, F.D., Roth, T.L., et al. (2008). Epigenetic regulation of BDNF gene transcription in the consolidation of fear memory. *J. Neurosci.* 28:10576–10586.

Machado-Vieira, R., Ibrahim, L., et al. (2011). Histone deacetylases and mood disorders: epigenetic programming in gene-environment interactions. *CNS Neurosci. Ther.* 17:699–704.

Marenco, S., Savostyanova, A.A., et al. (2010). Genetic modulation of GABA levels in the anterior cingulate cortex by GAD1 and COMT. *Neuropsychopharmacol.* 35:1708–1717.

Martins-de-Souza, D., Gattaz, W.F., et al. (2009). Alterations in oligodendrocyte proteins, calcium homeostasis and new potential markers in schizophrenia anterior temporal lobe are revealed by shotgun proteome analysis. *J. Neural. Transm.* 116:275–289.

Maunakea, A.K., Nagarajan, R.P., et al. (2010). Conserved role of intragenic DNA methylation in regulating alternative promoters. *Nature* 466:253–257.

Maze, I., Covington, H.E., III, et al. (2010). Essential role of the histone methyltransferase G9a in cocaine-induced plasticity. *Science* 327:213–216.

McGowan, P.O., Sasaki, A., et al. (2008). Promoter-wide hypermethylation of the ribosomal RNA gene promoter in the suicide brain. *PLoS One* 3, e2085.

McGowan, P.O., Sasaki, A., et al. (2009). Epigenetic regulation of the glucocorticoid receptor in human brain associates with childhood abuse. *Nat. Neurosci.* 12:342–348.

Miller, C.A., Gavin, C.F., et al. (2010). Cortical DNA methylation maintains remote memory. *Nat. Neurosci.* 13:664–666.

Miller, C.A., and Sweatt, J.D. (2007). Covalent modification of DNA regulates memory formation. *Neuron* 53:857–869.

Morris, M.J., Karra, A.S., et al. (2010). Histone deacetylases govern cellular mechanisms underlying behavioral and synaptic plasticity in the developing and adult brain. *Behav. Pharmacol.* 21:409–419.

Nestler, E.J., and Hyman, S.E. (2010). Animal models of neuropsychiatric disorders. *Nat. Neurosci.* 13:1161–1169.

Nowak, S.J., and Corces, V.G. (2004). Phosphorylation of histone H3: a balancing act between chromosome condensation and transcriptional activation. *Trends Genet.* 20:214–220.

Numata, S., Ye, T., et al. (2012). DNA methylation signatures in development and aging of the human prefrontal cortex. *Am. J. Hum. Genet.* 90:260–272.

Oberle, I., Rousseau, F., et al. (1991). Instability of a 550-base pair DNA segment and abnormal methylation in fragile X syndrome. *Science* 252:1097–1102.

Okano, M., Bell, D.W., et al. (1999). DNA methyltransferases Dnmt3a and Dnmt3b are essential for *de novo* methylation and mammalian development. *Cell* 99:247–257.

Ooi, S.K., and Bestor, T.H. (2008). The colorful history of active DNA demethylation. *Cell* 133:1145–1148.

O'Roak, B.J., Deriziotis, P., et al. (2011). Exome sequencing in sporadic autism spectrum disorders identifies severe *de novo* mutations. *Nat. Genet.* 43:585–589.

Peleg, S., Sananbenesi, F., et al. (2010). Altered histone acetylation is associated with age-dependent memory impairment in mice. *Science* 328:753–756.

Peter, C.J., and Akbarian, S. (2011). Balancing histone methylation activities in psychiatric disorders. *Trends. Mol. Med.* 17:372–379.

Piton, A., Gauthier, J., et al. (2011). Systematic resequencing of X-chromosome synaptic genes in autism spectrum disorder and schizophrenia. *Mol. Psychiatry* 16:867–880.

Purcell, S.M., Wray, N.R., et al. (2009). Common polygenic variation contributes to risk of schizophrenia and bipolar disorder. *Nature* 460:748–752.

Regenold, W.T., Phatak, P., et al. (2007). Myelin staining of deep white matter in the dorsolateral prefrontal cortex in schizophrenia, bipolar disorder, and unipolar major depression. *Psychiatry Res.* 151:179–188.

Robison, A.J., and Nestler, E.J. (2011). Transcriptional and epigenetic mechanisms of addiction. *Nat. Rev. Neurosci.* 12:623–637.

Rodriguez-Paredes, M., and Esteller, M. (2011). Cancer epigenetics reaches mainstream oncology. *Nat. Med.* 17:330–339.

Rotili, D., and Mai, A. (2011). Targeting histone demethylases: a new avenue for the fight against cancer. *Genes and Cancer* 2:663–679.

Rusiecki, J.A., Chen, L., et al. (2012). DNA methylation in repetitive elements and post-traumatic stress disorder: a case-control study of US military service members. *Epigenomic.* 4:29–40.

Schroeder, F.A., Lin, C.L., et al. (2007). Antidepressant-like effects of the histone deacetylase inhibitor, sodium butyrate, in the mouse. *Biol. Psychiatry* 62:55–64.

Sharma, R.P., Grayson, D.R., et al. (2005). Chromatin, DNA methylation and neuron gene regulation—the purpose of the package. *J. Psychiatry Neurosci.* 30:257–263.

Sharma, R.P., Rosen, C., et al. (2006). Valproic acid and chromatin remodeling in schizophrenia and bipolar disorder: preliminary results from a clinical population. *Schizophr. Res.* 88:227–231.

Shi, J., Levinson, D.F., et al. (2009). Common variants on chromosome 6p22.1 are associated with schizophrenia. *Nature* 460:753–757.

Shulha, H.P., Cheung, I., et al. (2012). Epigenetic signatures of autism: trimethylated H3K4 landscapes in prefrontal neurons. *Arch. Gen. Psychiatry* 69:314–324.

Sibille, E., Wang, Y., et al. (2009). A molecular signature of depression in the amygdala. *Am. J. Psychiatry* 166:1011–1024.

Siegmund, K.D., Connor, C.M., et al. (2007). DNA methylation in the human cerebral cortex is dynamically regulated throughout the life span and involves differentiated neurons. *PLoS One* 2, e895.

Simonis, M., Klous, P., et al. (2006). Nuclear organization of active and inactive chromatin domains uncovered by chromosome conformation capture-on-chip (4C). *Nat. Genet.* 38:1348–1354.

Simonis, M., Kooren, J., et al. (2007). An evaluation of 3C-based methods to capture DNA interactions. *Nat. Methods* 4:895–901.

Smeraldi, E., Bellodi, L., et al. (1976). Further studies on the major histocompatibility complex as a genetic marker for schizophrenia. *Biol. Psychiatry* 11:655–661.

Smith, A.K., Conneely, K.N., et al. (2011). Differential immune system DNA methylation and cytokine regulation in post-traumatic stress disorder. *Am. J. Med. Genet. B Neuropsychiatr. Genet.* 156B:700–708.

Song, C.X., Szulwach, K.E., et al. (2011). Selective chemical labeling reveals the genome-wide distribution of 5-hydroxymethylcytosine. *Nat. Biotechnol.* 29:68–72.

Stadler, F., Kolb, G., et al. (2005). Histone methylation at gene promoters is associated with developmental regulation and region-specific expression of ionotropic and metabotropic glutamate receptors in human brain. *J. Neurochem.* 94:324–336.

Stefansson, H., Ophoff, R.A., et al. (2009). Common variants conferring risk of schizophrenia. *Nature* 460:744–747.

Straub, R.E., Lipska, B.K., et al. (2007). Allelic variation in GAD1 (GAD67) is associated with schizophrenia and influences cortical function and gene expression. *Mol. Psychiatry* 12:854–869.

Stroud, H., Feng, S., et al. (2011). 5-hydroxymethylcytosine is associated with enhancers and gene bodies in human embryonic stem cells. *Genome Biol.* 12:R54.

Sutcliffe, E.L., Parish, I.A., et al. (2009). Dynamic histone variant exchange accompanies gene induction in T cells. *Mol. Cell Biol.* 29:1972–1986.

Szulwach, K.E., Li, X., et al. (2011a). Integrating 5-hydroxymethylcytosine into the epigenomic landscape of human embryonic stem cells. *PLoS Genet.* 7:e1002154.

Szulwach, K.E., Li, X., et al. (2011b). 5-hmC-mediated epigenetic dynamics during postnatal neurodevelopment and aging. *Nat. Neurosci.* 14:1607–1616.

Tan, M., Luo, H., et al. (2011). Identification of 67 histone marks and histone lysine crotonylation as a new type of histone modification. *Cell* 146:1016–1028.

Tang, B., Chang, W.L., et al. (2009). Normal human aging and early-stage schizophrenia share common molecular profiles. *Aging Cell* 8:339–342.

Taverna, S.D., Li, H., et al. (2007). How chromatin-binding modules interpret histone modifications: lessons from professional pocket pickers. *Nat. Struct. Mol. Biol.* 14:1025–1040.

Tkachev, D., Mimmack, M.L., et al. (2003). Oligodendrocyte dysfunction in schizophrenia and bipolar disorder. *Lancet* 362:798–805.

Tolstorukov, M.Y., Volfovsky, N., et al. (2011). Impact of chromatin structure on sequence variability in the human genome. *Nat. Struct. Mol. Biol.* 18:510–515.

Tsou, A.Y., Friedman, L.S., et al. (2009). Pharmacotherapy for Friedreich ataxia. *CNS Drugs* 23:213–223.

Uddin, M., Aiello, A.E., et al. (2010). Epigenetic and immune function profiles associated with posttraumatic stress disorder. *Proc. Natl. Acad. Sci. USA* 107:9470–9475.

Verhoeven, W.M., Egger, J.I., et al. (2011). Kleefstra syndrome in three adult patients: further delineation of the behavioral and neurological phenotype shows aspects of a neurodegenerative course. *Am. J. Med. Genet. A* 155A:2409–2415.

Vermeulen, M., Eberl, H.C., et al. (2010). Quantitative interaction proteomics and genome-wide profiling of epigenetic histone marks and their readers. *Cell* 142:967–980.

Wang, C.M., Tsai, S.N., et al. (2010). Identification of histone methylation multiplicities patterns in the brain of senescence-accelerated prone mouse 8. *Biogerontology* 11:87–102.

Weaver, I.C., et al. (2004). Epigenetic programming by maternal behavior. *Nat. Neurosci.* 7:847–854.

Williams, K., Christensen, J., et al. (2011). TET1 and hydroxymethylcytosine in transcription and DNA methylation fidelity. *Nature* 473:343–348.

Winkelmann, J., Lin, L., et al. (2012). Mutations in DNMT1 cause autosomal dominant cerebellar ataxia, deafness and narcolepsy. *Hum. Mol. Genet.* 21:2205–2210.

Woo, T.U., Kim, A.M., et al. (2008). Disease-specific alterations in glutamatergic neurotransmission on inhibitory interneurons in the prefrontal cortex in schizophrenia. *Brain Res.* 1218:267–277.

Wood, A.J., Severson, A.F., et al. (2010). Condensin and cohesin complexity: the expanding repertoire of functions. *Nat. Rev. Genet.* 11:391–404.

Woodcock, C.L. (2006). Chromatin architecture. *Curr. Opin. Struct. Biol.* 16:213–220.

Wu, H., D'Alessio, A.C., et al. (2011). Genome-wide analysis of 5-hydroxymethylcytosine distribution reveals its dual function in transcriptional regulation in mouse embryonic stem cells. *Genes Dev.* 25:679–684.

Xie, W., Barr, C.L., et al. (2012). Base-resolution analyses of sequence and parent-of-origin dependent DNA methylation in the mouse genome. *Cell* 148:816–831.

Xu, B., Roos, J.L., et al. (2011). Exome sequencing supports a *de novo* mutational paradigm for schizophrenia. *Nat. Genet.* 43:864–868.

Yankner, B.A., Lu, T., et al. (2008). The aging brain. *Annu. Rev. Pathol.* 3:41–66.

Zhou, V.W., Goren, A., et al. (2011). Charting histone modifications and the functional organization of mammalian genomes. *Nat. Rev. Genet.* 12:7–18.

Zovkic, I.B., and Sweatt, J.D. (2012). Epigenetic mechanisms in learned fear: implications for PTSD. *Neuropsychopharmacology* 38:77–93.

14 | NETWORK METHODS FOR ELUCIDATING THE COMPLEXITY OF COMMON HUMAN DISEASES

ERIC E. SCHADT

INTRODUCTION

Our understanding of common human diseases and how best to treat them are hampered by the complexity of the human system in which they are manifested. Unlike simple Mendelian disorders in which highly expressive, highly penetrant mutations make it possible to identify the causal genes within families, segregating traits associated with the disorders (Mulvihill, 1999), common human diseases originate from a more complex interplay between constellations of changes in DNA (both rare and common variation) and a broad range of environmental factors like diet, age, sex, and exposure to environmental toxins.

With roughly 3 billion nucleotides making up the human genome, the number of nucleotide changes that can affect the activities of a moderate to large number of genes is effectively infinite with respect to our ability to experimentally determine the effects of combinations of such changes. Whereas the focus in years past regarding DNA variation and its association to disease had been focused on protein-coding sequences, given declarations of intergenic DNA being comprised mainly of "junk" (Smith et al., 1972), today we know that greater than 80% of the human genome is actively bound by proteins that regulate the expression of genes (Ecker et al., 2012), providing a vast array of knobs and switches to modulate not only the activity of genes, but also of whole gene networks. Therefore, leveraging naturally occurring DNA variation in human populations can be considered among the most attractive approaches to inferring the constellation of genes that affect disease risk. For most noncancer human diseases like Alzheimer's disease, autism, and schizophrenia, changes in DNA that correlate with changes in disease can be inferred as tagging or directly representing causal components of disease. In this way, the DNA variation directly elucidates disease etiology and so is extremely useful. Genome-wide association studies (GWAS) are now well proven to uncover genetic loci that affect disease risk or disease progression (Stranger et al., 2011).

The complex array of interacting factors does not influence the activity of single genes in isolation but, instead, affects entire network states that, in turn, increase or decrease the risk of disease or affect disease severity. In the context of common human diseases, the disease states can be considered as emergent properties of molecular networks (Chen et al., 2008), as opposed to responses to changes in a small number of genes driving core biological processes associated with the disease. Integrating large-scale, high-dimensional molecular and physiological data holds promise in not only defining the molecular networks that directly respond to genetic and environmental perturbations that associate with disease, but also in causally associating such networks with the physiological states associated with disease.

Of course, genetics is but one dimension in a big sea of data dimensions that we can now leverage to better understand human conditions such as psychiatric disorders. Models of disease that consider a greater diversity of data that inform on disease will necessarily deliver more accurate diagnoses. In fact, we are in the midst of a big data revolution that permeates nearly every aspect of our lives. Electronic devices that consume much of our attention on a daily basis enable rapid transactions among individuals on unprecedented scales, where all of the information involved in these daily transactions can be seamlessly stored in digital form, whether the transactions involve monitoring of activity levels using Fitbit-like devices, cell phone calls, text messages, credit card purchases, e-mail, or visits to the doctor's office in which all tests carried out are digitized and entered into your electronic medical record (Fig. 14.1). The digital universe more generally now far exceeds one zettabyte (i.e., 21 zeros or one billion terabytes—think 63 billion 16 gigabyte iPhones). Thus, our ability to store and access unimaginable scales of data has been revolutionized by technological innovations that are often observed to operate at super Moore's law rates.

The life and biomedical sciences have not stood on the sidelines of this revolution. There has been an incredible wave of new technologies in genomics—such as next-generation sequencing technologies (Eid et al., 2009), sophisticated imaging systems, and mass spectrometry-based flow cytometry (Bandura et al., 2009)—enabling data to be generated at very large scales. As a result we can monitor the expression of tens of thousands of protein- and noncoding genes simultaneously (Chen et al., 2008; Emilsson et al., 2008), score hundreds of thousands of SNPs (single-nucleotide polymorphisms) in individual samples (Sklar et al., 2011; Stranger et al., 2011), sequence entire human genomes now for less than $5,000 (Drmanac et al., 2012), and relate all of these data patterns to a great diversity of other biologically relevant information (clinical data, biochemical data, social networking data, etc.). Given technologies on the horizon like the IBM DNA transistor with theoretical sequencing limits in the hundreds of millions of

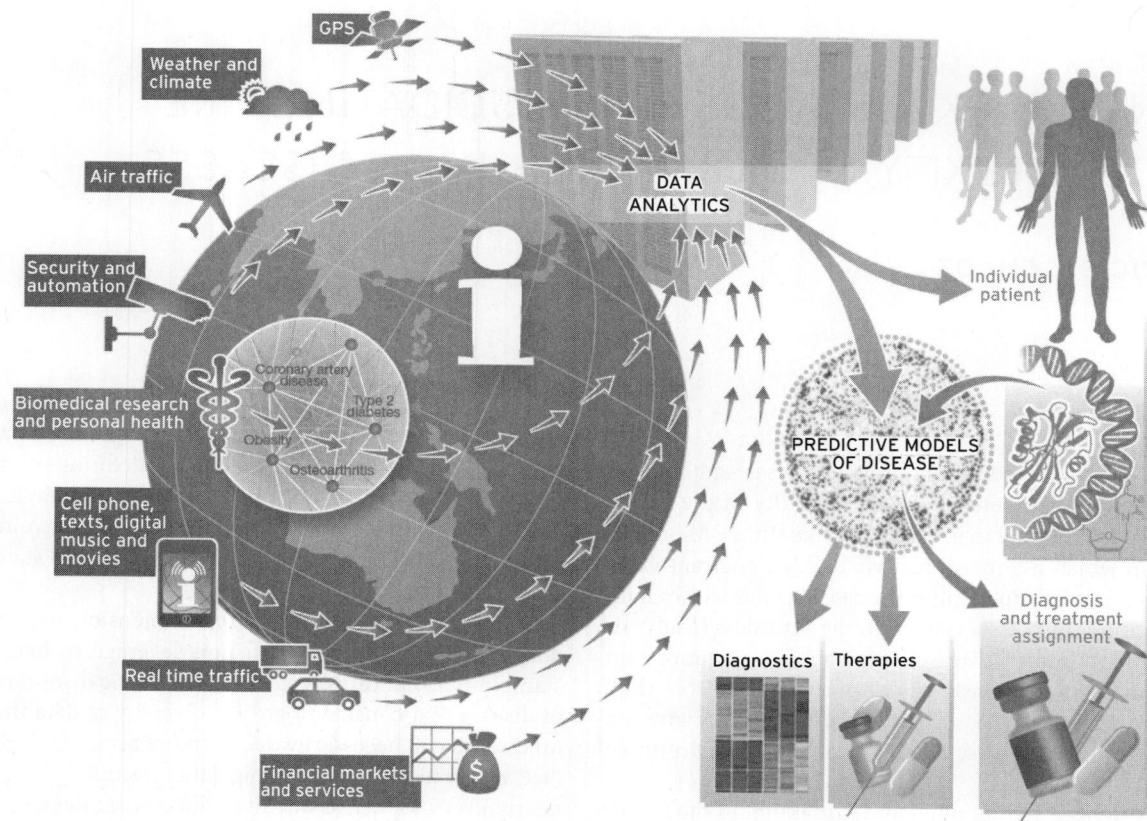

Figure 14.1 *Big data is all around us, enabled by technological advances in micro- and nanoelectronics, nano materials, interconnectivity provided by sophisticated telecommunication infrastructure, massive network-attached storage capabilities, and commodity-based high-performance computing infrastructures. The ability to store all credit card transactions, all cell phone traffic, all e-mail traffic, video from extensive networks of surveillance devices, and satellite and ground sensing data informing on all aspects of the weather and overall climate, and to now generate and store massive data informing on our personal health including whole-genome sequencing data and extensive imagining data, is driving a revolution in high-end data analytics to make sense of the big data, and drive more accurate descriptive and predictive models that inform decision making on every level, whether identifying the next big security threat or making the best diagnosis and treatment choice for a given patient.*

bases per second per transistor (imagine millions of these transistors packed together in a single handheld device) (Schadt et al., 2010), we would not be talking in the future about Google rolling through neighborhoods with Wi-Fi-sniffing equipment (Kravets, 2010), but rather, we'll be talking about DNA-sniffing equipment rolling through neighborhoods sequencing everything they encounter in real time and then pumping such data into big data clouds to link with all other available information in the digital universe.

If we want to achieve understanding from big data, organize it, compute on it, and build predictive models from it, then we must employ statistical reasoning beyond the more classic hypothesis testing of yesteryear. We have moved well beyond the idea that we can simply repeat experiments to validate findings generated in populations. In fact, while first instances of the central dogma of biology looked something like the simple graph depicted in Figure 14.2 (top), today, given that the complex interplay of multiple dimensions of data (DNA, RNA, protein, metabolite, cellular, physiologic, ecologic, and social structures more generally) demands a more holistic view be taken in which we embrace complexity in its entirety, the central dogma is evolving to look something more like the graph depicted in Figure 14.2 (bottom). Our emerging view

of complex biological systems is one of a dynamic, fluid system that is able to reconfigure itself as conditions demand (Barabasi and Oltvai, 2004; Han et al., 2004; Luscombe et al., 2004; Pinto et al., 2004; Zerhouni, 2003). Despite these transformative advances in technology and the need to embrace complexity, it remains difficult to assess where we are with respect to our understanding of living systems, relative to a complete comprehension of such systems. One of the primary difficulties in our making such an assessment is that the suite of research tools available to us seldom provides insights into aspects of the overall picture of the system that are not directly measured.

In this chapter I discuss a particular class of modeling approaches that integrate diverse types of data on broad scales, in ways that enable others to interpret their data in a more holistic, informative context, to derive predictions that inform decision making on multiple levels, whether deciding on the next set of genes to validate experimentally or the best treatment for a given individual, given detailed molecular and higher order data on their condition. Central to these models will be inferring causality among molecular traits and between molecular and higher order traits by leveraging DNA as a systematic source of perturbation. In contrast to the more

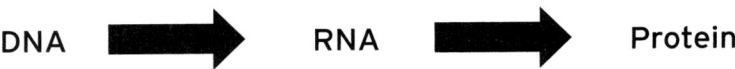

Original Central Dogma of Biology

DNA ➡ RNA ➡ Protein

___

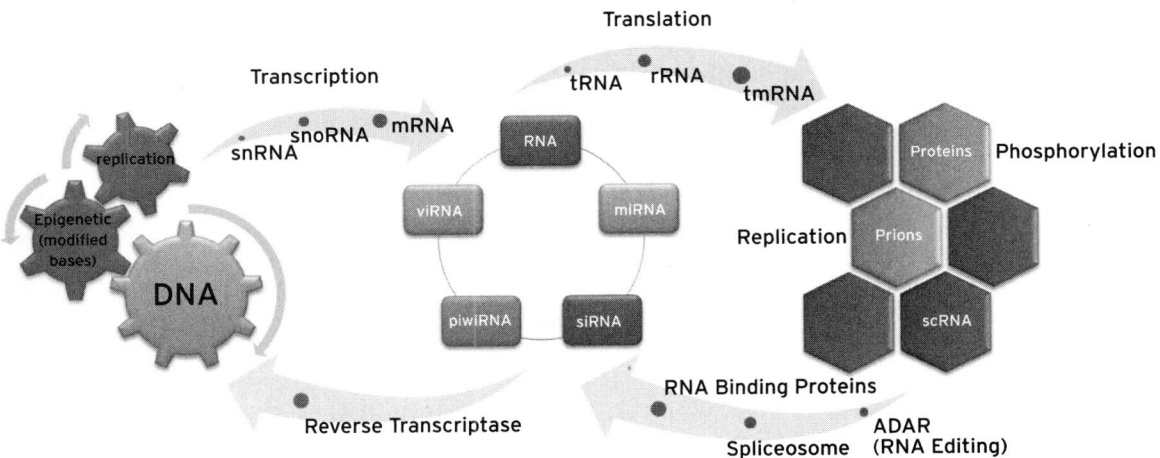

Evolving Central Dogma of Biology

Figure 14.2 *The evolving central dogma of biology. The upper panel represents the original central dogma of biology, a simple view driven by early observations with low-resolution tools that uncovered a central relationship between DNA, RNA, and proteins, namely, that RNA is transcribed from DNA, and RNA, in turn, is translated into proteins. New higher resolution technologies have enabled a far more complex view of the central dogma to emerge (bottom panel), with epigenetic changes to DNA that are transgenerational, leading to non-Mendelian patterns of inheritance, a complex array of RNA molecules such as microRNA, viRNA, piwiRNA, and siRNA that do not code for proteins but carry out complex regulatory functions, and sophisticated protein complexes involved in splicing, RNA editing, and RNA binding all feeding back on transcription, leading to a more network-oriented view of the central dogma.*

qualitative approaches biological researchers have employed in the past, getting the most from these new types of high-dimensional, large-scale data requires constructing more complex, predictive models from them, refining the ability of such models to assess disease risk, progression, and best treatment strategies, and ultimately translating these complex models into a clinical setting where doctors can employ them as tools to understand most optimally your current condition and how best to improve it. Such solutions require a robust engineering approach, where integrating the new breed of large-scale datasets streaming out of the biological sciences and constructing predictive models from them will require approaches more akin to those employed by physicists, climatologists, and other strongly quantitative disciplines that have mastered the collection and predictive modeling of high-dimensional data.

THE MANY MOVING PIECES OF BIOLOGICAL SYSTEMS: A MOVIE ANALOGY

Tools to interrogate biological systems in the past were crude and did not permit the more holistic querying of such systems at multiple scales. In fact, if we were to view the full suite of interacting parts in living systems, from the molecular on up to

the ecological levels, we would achieve a more complete understanding of the cellular-, organ-, and organism-level processes that underlie complex phenotypes such as disease, much in the same way we achieve understanding by watching a movie. The continuous flow of information in a movie enables our minds to exercise an array of priors that provide the appropriate context and that constrain the possible relationships (structures) not only within a given frame or scene, but also over the entire course of the movie. As our senses take in all of the streaming audio and visual information, our internal network reconstruction engine (centered at the brain) pieces the information together to represent highly complex and nonlinear relationships depicted in the movie, so that in the end we are able to achieve an understanding of what the movie intends to convey at a hierarchy of levels.

What if we were to view a movie as we have viewed biological systems in the past? What if instead of viewing a movie as a continuous stream of frames of coherent pixels and sound, we viewed single dimensions of these data, and we viewed them independently from one another? Understanding in this case would likely be difficult, if not impossible, to achieve. As an example, consider a 2-hour feature length film comprised of 216,000 frames (30 frames per second), where each frame is comprised of $1,280 \times 720$ pixels (roughly one million pixels). First, it is worth noting that the number of pixels of information, roughly 199 billion, represented in this film is quite large (if each pixel were represented by 32 bits, the film would comprise more than 6 terabytes of information). Suppose we decided to use the tools of reductionist biology to view the film, where instead of viewing the film as a rapid succession of frames of one million pixels each, we viewed a single frame in which the intensity value for each pixel across all 216,000 frames in the movie was averaged. This gross, aggregate average would provide very little, if any, information regarding the movie, not unlike our attempts to understand complex living systems by examining single snapshots of a subset of molecular traits in a single cell type and in a single context at a single point in time. Even if we viewed our movie as independent, one-dimensional slices through its frames, where each slice was viewed as pixel intensities across that one dimension changing over time (like a dynamic mass spectrometry trace), this view would provide significantly more information, but it would still be very difficult to understand the meaning of the movie by looking at all of the one-dimensional traces independently, unless more sophisticated mathematical algorithms were employed to link the information together.

Despite the complexity of biological systems, even at the cellular level, research in the context of large-scale, high-dimensional omics data has tended to focus on single data dimensions, whether constructing coexpression networks based on gene expression data, carrying out genome-wide association analyses based on DNA variation information, or constructing protein interaction networks based on protein–protein interaction data. While we achieve some understanding in this way, progress is limited because none of the dimensions on their own provide a complete enough context within which to interpret results fully. This type of limitation has become apparent in genome-wide association studies or whole-exome or genome-sequencing studies, where thousands of highly replicated loci have been identified and highly replicated as associated with disease, but our understanding of disease is still limited because the genetic loci do not necessarily inform on the gene affected, on how gene function is altered, or more generally, how the biological processes involving a given gene are altered at particular points of time or in particular contexts (Altshuler et al., 2008; Chen et al., 2008; Emilsson et al., 2008; Witte, 2010). It is apparent that if different biological data dimensions could be formally considered simultaneously, we would achieve a more complete understanding of biological systems (Chen et al., 2008; Emilsson et al., 2008; Hsu et al., 2010; Schadt et al., 2008; Zhong et al., 2010). (See the documentary film *The New Biology* at http://www.youtube.com/watch?v=sjTQD6E3lH4.)

To form a more complete understanding of complex human diseases like psychiatric disorders, we must not only evolve technologies to sample systems at ever higher rates and with ever greater breadth, but we must also innovate methods that consider many different dimensions of information to produce more descriptive models (movies) of the system. There are, of course, many different types of modeling approaches that have been and continue to be explored. Descriptive models quantify relationships among variables in data that can, in turn, enable classification of systems under study into different meaningful groups; whether stratifying disease populations into disease subtypes to assign patients to the most appropriate treatment, or categorizing customers by product preference, descriptive models are useful for classifying but cannot necessarily be used to predict how any given variable will respond to another at the individual level. For example, while patterns of gene expression such as those identified for breast cancer and now in play at companies like Genomic Health can very well distinguish good from poor prognoses (van 't Veer et al., 2002; van de Vijver et al., 2002), such models are not generally as useful for understanding how genes in patterns associated with disease are causally related or distinguishing key driver genes from passenger genes.

Predictive models, on the other hand, incorporate historic and current data to predict how one variable may respond to another in a particular context or predict response or future states of components of a system at the individual level. In the biological context, predictive models aim to accurately predict (*in silico*—using the model to run simulations on a computer) molecule expression–level changes, cell state dynamics, and phenotype transitions in response to specific perturbation events. For example, understanding how the constellation of genes identified for diseases like schizophrenia or autism (Neale et al., 2012; Ripke et al., 2011) are actually related to one another in probabilistic causal ways can lead to an understanding of how perturbing a given gene (say, for treatment) will impact the corresponding molecular networks and ultimately the pathophysiology of the diseases they impact. Key to constructing predictive models is elucidating causal relationships between traits of interest. Resolving causal relationships requires a systematic source of perturbation, and here I discuss the use of DNA variation as a systematic perturbation source to infer causal relationships among molecular traits and between molecular traits and higher order traits like disease (Chen et al., 2008; Emilsson et al., 2008; Mehrabian et al., 2005; Millstein et al., 2009; Schadt et al., 2005; Yang et al., 2009; Zhu et al., 2004; Zhu et al., 2012; Zhu et al., 2008).

CAUSALITY AS A STATISTICAL INFERENCE

In the life sciences, most researchers are accustomed to thinking about causality from the standpoint of physical interactions. In the molecular biology or biochemistry setting, when two molecular traits are indicated as causally related, we typically mean that one of the molecular entities (e.g., a small molecule compound) has been determined experimentally to physically interact with or to induce processes that directly affect the other molecular entity (e.g., the target protein of the small molecule) and consequently leads to a phenotypic change of interest (e.g., lower LDL cholesterol levels). In this case we have an understanding of the causal factors relevant to the activity of interest, so that careful experimental manipulation of these factors allows for the identification of genuine causal relationships. However, in the context of many thousands of variables related in unknown ways, the aim is to examine the behavior of those variables across populations in ways that facilitate statistically inferring causal relationships. For example, statistical associations between changes in DNA, changes in molecular phenotypes, and changes in higher order phenotypes like functional MRI readouts or disease can be examined for patterns of conditional dependency among the variables that allow directionality to be inferred among them. In this case we can employ indirect measures of processes that mediate changes in one trait conditional on another to make a statistically inferred causal link. This is not unlike the types of statistical inferences that are leveraged in other disciplines to make new discoveries. For example, less than 5% of known extrasolar planets have been directly observed, so that most are observed indirectly. One method for detecting planets that cannot be directly observed considers that when a planet is orbiting a star, the gravitational pull of the planet on the star will place the star into a subtle orbit, which from our vantage point will appear as the star moving closer to and further away from the Earth in a cyclical fashion. Such movement can be measured as displacements in the star's spectral lines due to the Doppler effect (Erskine et al., 2005), and so the presence of the planet acting on the star can be statistically inferred.

Similarly, consider genetic variants associated with, say, schizophrenia or autism (many such loci have now been identified; Elia et al., 2012; Glessner et al., 2009; Neale et al., 2012; Pinto et al., 2010; Ripke et al., 2011; Wang et al., 2009). Further, suppose the expression of some number of genes assayed in relevant regions of the brain relating to these disorders were also associated with these same genetic variants. By examining the changes in the levels of expression of these genes in response to changes in genotype at any of the genetic loci of interest, one can directly assess the extent to which these expression changes induced by the genetic loci well explain the degree of association between the locus genotypes and disease trait. In this way, just as the characteristic wobble of a star induced by an orbiting planet predicts the presence of the planet, the characteristic "wobble" of the expression levels of a gene and its association to the disease state predicts a causal path between the gene and disease state, as described in more detail later.

Critical to identifying causal relationships is distinguishing between correlation and causation. The old adage, "correlation does not imply causation," is familiar to most. This is among the first fallacies one learns about in beginning logic courses: *post hoc ergo propter hoc* (Latin for "after this, therefore because of this"). Measurements taken over time on independent variables can be correlated because trends reflected by such variables are coincidentally similar or changes in each variable are independently caused by a common source, in addition to being correlated as a result of a cause–effect relationship. It is also interesting to note that while correlation and causation are related, our intuitive notation that causation implies correlation is not always correct either. For example, suppose U and V are random variables with the same distribution and suppose $X = U + V$ and $Y = U - V$. In this case the covariance between X and Y [defined as $E(XY) - E(X)E(Y)$, where E represents the expectation function] is 0 and so the correlation is 0, even though there is a direct functional dependence between the

variables (Feller, 1967). Only when two variables are linearly dependent (which is often the case in research) is our intuitive notion of functional dependence implying perfect correlation correct.

Structure learning approaches that seek to infer causal relationships among correlated variables often employ conditional dependency arguments or mutual information measures to resolve causality by introducing a third correlated variable. By conditioning each of the variables on the third and examining the residual correlation between them in each case, a decision can be made as to the direction of the flow of information between the variables. However, this type of reasoning has generally failed to result in predictive causal inference because in the absence of systematic perturbations, the number of graphs that can be represented between just three traits is large (125 graphs representing directed and undirected relationships between three correlated variables are possible), and many of these possible relationships between the traits are not statistically distinguishable (Sieberts and Schadt, 2007). For example, if variables X, Y, and Z are observed in a population to be correlated (e.g., suppose X, Y, and Z represent the expression levels of three genes assayed in a given region of the brain in a population of individuals with schizophrenia) and the true relationship between the variables is $X \rightarrow Z \leftarrow Y$, this relationship cannot be statistically distinguished from $X \rightarrow Y \leftarrow Z$ and $Z \rightarrow X \leftarrow Y$, even though these relationships give rise to contradictory causal relationships.

To break this type of statistical symmetry, a source of perturbation is required. Classically in biology we have introduced artificial perturbations by knocking a gene out, overexpressing a gene, or chemically perturbing a given protein to assess the consequences on a given trait of interest. More recently, in the neurosciences, optogenetics methods have provided novel ways to perturb genes on the short time scales needed to elucidate the complexity of networks at play in neurons in living mammals (Boyden et al., 2005). If experimentally controlled artificial perturbations on a given gene cause a change in a trait of interest, then we infer a causal relationship between that gene and trait. However, DNA variation in the germline provides an excellent systematic perturbation source that can also be used to resolve causal relationships in biological systems. Because variations in DNA cause variations in RNA, proteins, metabolites, and subsequently, higher order phenotypes, this source of variation can be leveraged to infer causality. Unlike artificial perturbations such as gene knockouts, transgenics, or chemical or optogenetic perturbations that may induce artificial correlations that are not observed in more natural settings, naturally occurring genetic variation defines those perturbations that give rise to the broad array of phenotypic variations (such as disease and drug response) that we are precisely interested in elucidating. The past seven years has demonstrated that causal links between DNA variations and molecular and higher order phenotypes can provide information on causal relationships between those traits (Chen et al., 2007; Chen et al., 2008; Davey Smith and Ebrahim, 2003; Didelez and Sheehan, 2007; Emilsson et al., 2008; Kulp and Jagalur, 2006; Millstein et al., 2009; Schadt et al., 2005; Schadt et al., 2003; Yang et al., 2009; Zhu et al., 2004; Zhu et al., 2008). Causality in this instance can be inferred because there is random segregation of the chromosomes during gametogenesis, thus providing the appropriate randomization mechanism to protect against confounding, similar to what is achieved in randomized clinical trials by randomly assigning patients to treatments to test the causal effects of a drug of interest (Lawlor et al., 2008; Nitsch et al., 2006). However, quantifying the uncertainty in making such causal calls has been challenging. For example, causal effect estimates often considered in Mendelian randomization approaches can be confounded by pleiotropic effects and reverse causation, limiting the utility of such approaches for problems that involve the reconstruction of regulatory networks, in which pleiotropy is common and there may be little a priori information regarding the structure of the causal relationships between the traits of interest (Millstein et al., 2009).

Recently, though, formal statistical tests for inferring causal relationships between quantitative traits mediated by a common genetic locus have been developed (Millstein et al., 2009). To understand how such a test works, consider marker genotypes at a given DNA locus L that are correlated with a given molecular phenotype, G, and a higher order phenotype T (Fig. 14.3). The causal relationship G → T is implied if three conditions are satisfied under the assumption that L is sufficiently randomized: (1) L and G are associated, (2) L and T are associated, and (3) L is independent of T given G (i.e., L and T|G are not associated) (Chen et al., 2007). If a given locus L is independent of G given T (G|T), this is consistent with T being causal for G (T → G), and if L is associated with G|T, then this is consistent with G being causal for T (G → T). We can boil all of these observations down to four conditions from which a statistical test can be formed to test for causality: (1) L and T are associated, (2) L is associated with G|T, (3) G is associated with T|L, and (4) L is independent of T|G. Each of these conditions can be assessed with a corresponding statistical test. For example, if we assume the marker corresponding to locus L is biallelic, where L_1 and L_2 represent indicator variables for the

two alleles in a codominant coding scheme, then the four conditions can be tested in the parameters of the following three regression models:

$$T_i = \alpha_1 + \beta_1 L_{1i} + \beta_2 L_{2i} + \varepsilon_{1i} \tag{14.1}$$

$$G_i = \alpha_2 + \beta_3 T_i + \beta_4 L_{1i} + \beta_5 L_{2i} + \varepsilon_{2i} \tag{14.2}$$

$$T_i = \alpha_3 + \beta_6 G_i + \beta_7 L_{1i} + \beta_8 L_{2i} + \varepsilon_{3i}, \tag{14.3}$$

where G_i and T_i represent the gene and trait levels, respectively, for individual i in a population of interest, and the ε_{ij} represents independently distributed random noise variables with variance σ_j^2 (Chen et al., 2007). Given these models the four component tests of interest are:

$$H_0: \{\beta_1, \beta_2 = 0\}, \quad H_1: \{\beta_1, \beta_2\} \neq 0 \tag{14.4}$$

$$H_0: \{\beta_4, \beta_5 = 0\}, \quad H_1: \{\beta_4, \beta_5\} \neq 0 \tag{14.5}$$

$$H_0: \beta_6 = 0, \quad H_1: \beta_6 \neq 0 \tag{14.6}$$

$$H_0: \{\beta_7, \beta_8 \neq 0\}, \quad H_1: \{\beta_7, \beta_8\} = 0. \tag{14.7}$$

The four conditions of interest can be tested using standard F-tests for linear model coefficients (conditions 1–3) and a slightly more involved test for the last condition, given it is an equivalence testing problem (Millstein et al., 2009). Given these individual statistical tests on the different regression parameters, a causal inference test can then be carried out by testing the strength of the chain of mathematical conditions that collectively are consistent with causal mediation (i.e., the strength of the chain is only as strong as its weakest link, so that the intersection of the rejection regions of the component tests provides for the causality test we seek). For a series of statistical tests of size α_γ and rejection region R_γ, the "intersection union" test with rejection region equal to the intersection over all R_γ, is a level $\sup(\alpha_\gamma)$ test, so that the p-value for the causal inference test corresponds to the p-value for an intersection union test, or, simply, the supremum of the four p-values for the component tests (Chen et al., 2007). This test has been implemented as the CIT package in the R statistical programming language and is freely available.

Applications of this type of test can be applied to resolve the types of causal relationships depicted in Fig. 14.3. Application of these ideas in segregating mouse populations have led to the identification and validation of many genes causal for a number of metabolic traits, including obesity, diabetes, and heart disease. In one such population constructed between the B6 and DBA inbred strains of mouse, 111 F2 intercross animals were placed on a high-fat, atherogenic diet for 4 months at 12 months of age. All animals were genotyped using a genome-wide panel of markers, clinically characterized with respect to a number of metabolic traits, and the livers were expression profiled using a comprehensive gene expression microarray. Given the pattern of genetic association between the metabolic and gene expression traits, causal inference testing was carried

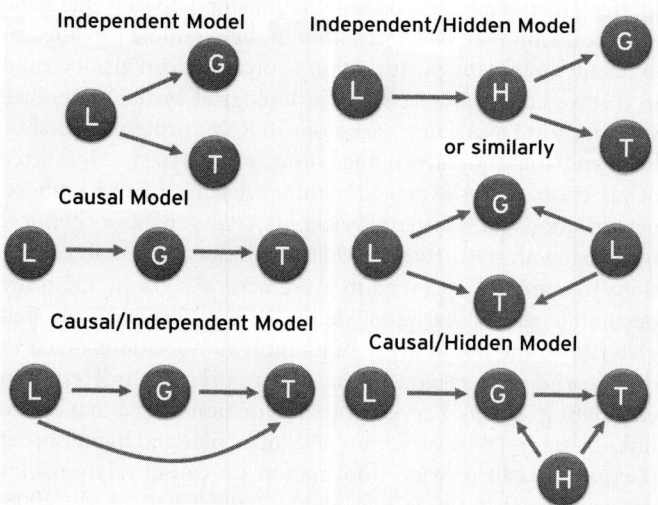

Figure 14.3 Given two traits G and T are correlated in a given population with changes in DNA at locus L, there are five basic causal models to consider in testing the hypothesis that variations in trait G cause variations in trait T. Here H denotes an unmeasured molecular or higher order trait.

out to identify the genes in this population best supported as causal of obesity-related traits (Schadt et al., 2003; Schadt et al., 2005). Of the top nine genes identified in this study supported as causal for obesity-related traits, eight of the genes were ultimately experimentally validated (Yang et al., 2009). The only gene that failed to validate was an X-linked gene that was lethal if completely knocked out and so represented a more complicated example for which the appropriate tools could not be constructed to validate.

Of course, this exact same type of reasoning can be used to causally relate imaging traits, DNA variation, and expression data to clinical phenotype data in the context of psychiatric disorders (Fig. 14.4). Consider associations identified between SNP genotypes and gene expression traits assayed in dorsal-lateral prefrontal cortex (DLPFC). Given the association of SNPs with expression in DLPFC, such SNPs are of interest for testing association to functional MRI (fMRI) traits. Given a set of SNPs in which there is an association between gene expression in DLFPC, fMRI, and schizophrenia status, we can statistically model whether the relationship between the traits is causal, reactive, or independent as described in the preceding (Fig. 14.4). This provides a causal statistical inference procedure applied to functional MRI

and disease trait data, using DNA variation as the systematic perturbation source that can address the pressing question of whether changes in neuroimaging traits are the result of schizophrenia or whether these changes lead to the schizophrenia phenotype.

FROM ASSESSING CAUSAL RELATIONSHIPS AMONG TRAIT PAIRS TO PREDICTIVE GENE NETWORKS

Leveraging DNA variation as a systematic perturbation source to resolve the causal relationships among traits is necessary but not sufficient for understanding the complexity of living systems. Cells are comprised of many tens of thousands of proteins, metabolites, RNA, and DNA, all interacting in complex ways. Complex biological systems are comprised of many different types of cells operating within and between many different types of tissues that make up different organ systems, all of which interact in complex ways to give rise to a vast array of phenotypes that manifest themselves in living systems. Modeling the extent of such relationships between molecular entities, between cells, and between organ systems is a daunting

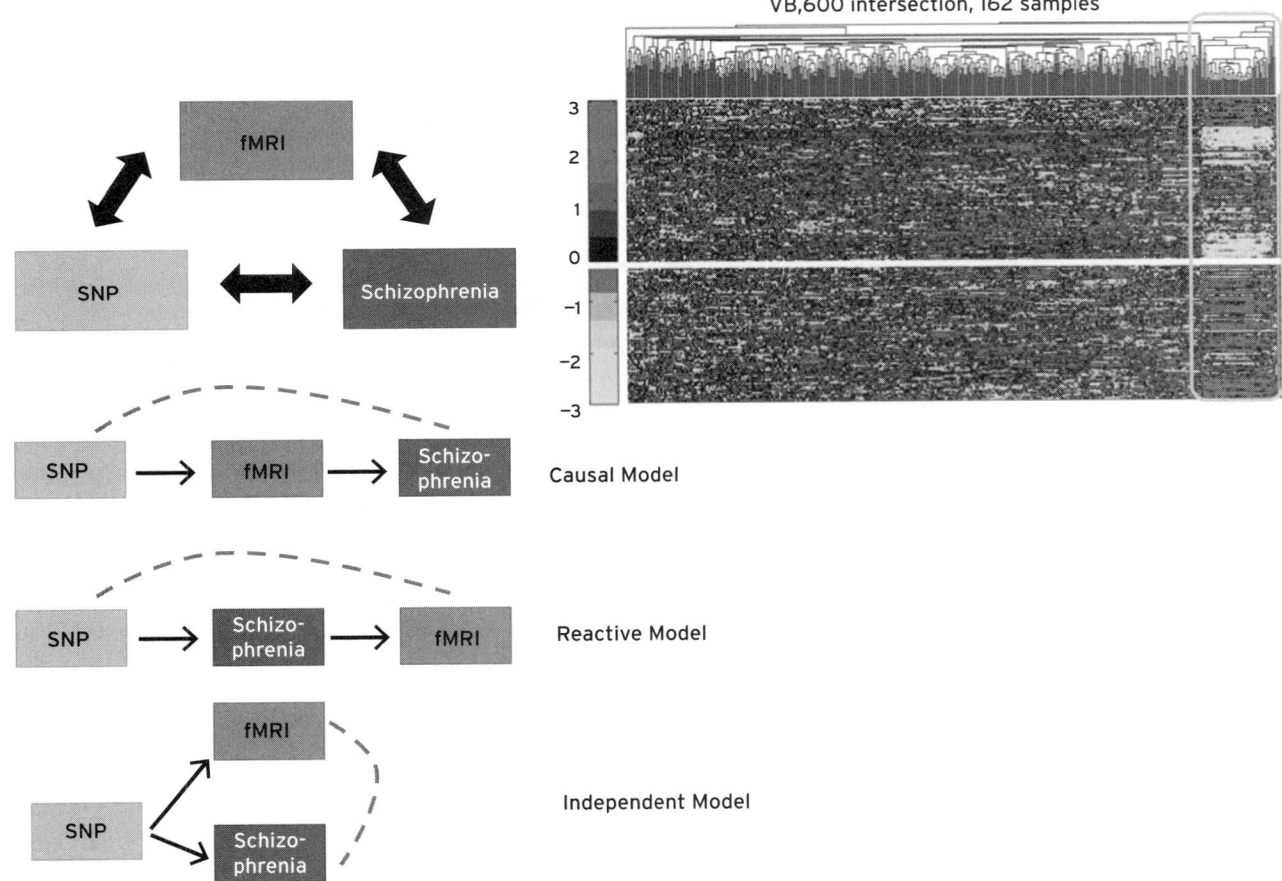

Figure 14.4 Inferring causal relationships between functional MRI traits and schizophrenia traits using SNPs that associate with the expression of genes in the dorsal-lateral prefrontal cortex as a perturbation source. The heat map represents a two-dimensional hierarchical clustering of functional MRI traits in which the highlighted cluster distinguishes schizophrenia cases from controls. Associations between functional MRI traits, gene expression, disease status, and SNP genotypes can be integrated to infer causal relationships between functional MRI traits and disease status.

task. Networks are a convenient framework for representing the relationships among these different variables. In the context of biological systems, a network can be viewed as a graphical model that represents relationships among DNA, RNA, protein, metabolite, and higher order phenotypes like disease state. In this way, networks provide a way to represent extremely large-scale and complex relationships among molecular and higher order phenotypes like disease in any given context.

BUILDING FROM THE BOTTOM UP OR TOP DOWN?

Two fundamental approaches to the reconstruction of molecular networks dominate computational biology today. The first is what is referred to as the bottom-up approach in which fundamental relationships between small sets of genes that may comprise a given pathway are established, thus providing the fundamental building blocks of higher order processes that are then constructed from the bottom up. This approach typically assumes that we have more complete knowledge regarding the fundamental topology (connectivity structure) of pathways, and given this knowledge, models are constructed that precisely detail how changes to any component of the pathway affect other components as well as the known functions carried out by the pathway (i.e., bottom-up approaches are hypothesis driven). The second approach is referred to as a top-down approach in which we take into account all data and our existing understanding of systems and construct a model that reflects whole system behavior and from there tease apart the fundamental components from the top down. This approach typically assumes that our understanding of how the network is actually wired is sufficiently incomplete, that our knowledge is sufficiently incomplete, and that we must objectively infer the relationships by considering large-scale, high-dimensional data that informs on all relationships of interest (i.e., top-down approaches are data driven).

Given our incomplete understanding of more general networks and pathways in living systems, in this chapter I focus on a top-down approach to reconstructing predictive networks, given that this type of structure learning from data is critical to derive hypotheses that cannot otherwise be efficiently proposed in the context of what is known (from the literature, pathway databases, or other such sources). However, top-down and bottom-up approaches are complementary to one another, although these approaches have largely been pursued as separate disciplines, with, interestingly, little crosstalk occurring between them. One of the future directions I discuss in the conclusion is the need to mathematically unify these two classes of predictive modeling to produce probabilistic causal networks that more maximally leverage all available data and knowledge.

In the context of integrating genetic, molecular profiling and higher order phenotypic data, biological networks are comprised of nodes that represent molecular entities that are observed to vary in a given population under study (e.g., DNA variations, RNA levels, protein states, or metabolite levels). Edges between the nodes represent relationships between the molecular entities, and these edges can either be directed, indicating a cause–effect relationship, or undirected, indicating an association or interaction. For example, a DNA node in the network representing a given locus that varies in a population of interest may be connected to a transcript abundance trait, indicating that changes at the particular DNA locus induce changes in the levels of the transcript. The potentially millions of such relationships represented in a network define the overall connectivity structure of the network, or what is otherwise known as the topology of the network. Any realistic network topology will be necessarily complicated and nonlinear from the standpoint of the more classic biochemical pathway diagrams represented in textbooks and pathway databases like KEGG (Kanehisa, 2002). The more classic pathway view represents molecular processes on an individual level, while networks represent global (population-level) metrics that describe variation between individuals in a population of interest, which, in turn, define coherent biological processes in the tissue or cells associated with the network. One way to manage the complexity of network structures that can obtain is to impost constraints on network structures to make them more computational tractable. For example, it is common when learning network structures to disallow loops or cycles in the network structure (otherwise known as the network topology, the connectivity structure of the network), in which cases we refer to the network as acyclic.

The neurosciences have a rich history of employing network-based approaches to understand the complexity of the human brain and the causes of psychiatric illnesses. Resources like the Allen Brain Atlas (http://www.alleninstitute.org) provide an anatomically comprehensive map of gene expression of the human brain that can facilitate network-based analyses (Hawrylycz et al., 2012). Others have employed techniques developed for constructing gene coexpression networks to construct interaction networks on fMRI data (Mumford et al., 2010), and others still have generated protein interaction networks to reflect features of the network architecture in brains of those with illnesses such as Huntington's disease (Shirasaki et al., 2012). Larger scale efforts have also been undertaken to integrate larger scale transcriptomic data in the context of diseases like autism to understand how changes in these networks may give rise to autism or reflect the types of pathways or biological processes involved in such a disease (Voineagu et al., 2011). These efforts are important not only for better understanding psychiatric diseases, but also for elucidating novel drug targets or biomarkers that better assess disease risk or severity. However, most of these current efforts do not lead to predictive models of disease but, rather, provide a descriptive framework within which to uncover associations between a myriad of molecular, cellular, imaging, and clinical traits and disease.

AN INTEGRATIVE GENOMICS APPROACH TO CONSTRUCTIVE PREDICTIVE NETWORK MODELS

Systematically integrating different types of data into probabilistic networks using Bayesian networks has been proposed and applied for the purpose of predicting protein–protein interactions (Jansen et al., 2003) and protein function (Lee et al., 2004). However, these Bayesian networks are still based on associations between nodes in the network as opposed to causal relationships. As previously discussed for the simple case of two traits, from these types of networks we cannot infer whether a specific perturbation will affect a complex disease trait. To make such predictions, we need networks capable of representing causal relationships. Probabilistic causal networks are one way to model from the top down such relationships, where causality again in this context reflects a probabilistic belief that one node in the network affects the behavior of another. Bayesian networks (Pearl, 1988) are one type of probabilistic causal network that provides a natural framework for integrating highly dissimilar types of data.

Bayesian networks are directed acyclic graphs in which the edges of the graph are defined by conditional probabilities that characterize the distribution of states of each node given the state of its parents (Pearl, 1988). The network topology defines a partitioned joint probability distribution over all nodes in a network, such that the probability distribution of states of a node depends only on the states of its parent nodes: formally, a joint probability distribution $p(X)$ on a set of nodes X can be decomposed as $p(X) = \Pi p(X^i | \mathrm{Pa}(X^i))$, where $\mathrm{Pa}(X^i)$ represents the parent set of X^i. The biological networks of interest we wish to construct are comprised of nodes that represent a quantitative trait such as the transcript abundance of a given gene or levels of a given metabolite. The conditional probabilities reflect not only relationships between genes, but also the stochastic nature of these relationships, as well as noise in the data used to reconstruct the network.

The aim in any network reconstruction such as this is to find the best model, the model that best reflects the relationships between all of the variables under consideration, given a set of data that informs on the variables of interest. In a probabilistic sense, we want to search the space of all possible networks (or models) for that network that gives the highest likelihood of occurring given the data. Bayes' formula allows us to determine the likelihood of a network model M given observed data D as a function of our prior belief that the model is correct and the probability of the observed data given the model is: $P(M|D) \sim P(D|M)P(M)$. The number of possible network structures grows superexponentially with the number of nodes, so an exhaustive search of all possible structures to find the one best supported by the data is not feasible, even for a relatively small number of nodes. A number of algorithms exist to find the optimal network without searching exhaustively, like Monte Carlo Markov Chain (MCMC) (Madigan and York, 1995) simulation. With the MCMC algorithm, optimal networks are constructed from a set of starting conditions. This algorithm is run thousands of times to identify different plausible networks, each time beginning with different starting conditions. These most plausible networks can then be combined to obtain a consensus network. For each of the reconstructions using the MCMC algorithm, the starting point is a null network. Small random changes are made to the network by flipping, adding, or deleting individual edges, ultimately accepting those changes that lead to an overall improvement in the fit of the network to the data. To assess whether a change improves the network model or not, information measures like the Bayesian Information Criterion (BIC) (Schwarz, 1978) are employed, which reduces overfitting by imposing a cost on the addition of new parameters. This is equivalent to imposing a lower prior probability $P(M)$ on models with larger numbers of parameters.

Even though edges in Bayesian networks are directed, we cannot in general infer causal relationships from the structure directly, just as I discussed in relation to the causal inference test. For a network with three nodes, X_1, X_2, and X_3, there are multiple groups of structures that are mathematically equivalent. For example, the three models, M1: $X_1 \rightarrow X_2, X_2 \rightarrow X_3$; M2: $X_2 \rightarrow X_1, X_2 \rightarrow X_3$; and M2: $X_2 \rightarrow X_1, X_3 \rightarrow X_2$, are all Markov equivalent, meaning that they all encode for the same conditional independence relationship: $X_1 \perp X_3 | X_2$, X_1, and X_3 are independent conditional on X_2. In addition, these models are mathematically equivalent:

$$\begin{aligned} p(X) = p(M1|D) &= p(X_2|X_1)p(X_1)p(X_3|X_2) \\ &= p(M2|D) = p(X_1|X_2)p(X_2)p(X_3|X_2) \\ &= p(M3|D) = p(X_2|X_3)p(X_3)p(X_1|X_2). \end{aligned}$$

Thus, from correlation data alone we cannot infer whether X_1 is causal for X_2 or vice versa from these types of structures. It is worth noting, however, that there is a class of structures, V-shape structures (e.g., Mv: $X_1 \rightarrow X_2, X_3 \rightarrow X_2$), that have no Markov-equivalent structure. In such cases it is not possible based on correlation data alone to infer causal relationships. Because there are more parameters to estimate in the Mv model than in the M1, M2, or M3 models, there is a large penalty in the Bayesian information criterion (BIC) score for the Mv model. Therefore, in practice, a large sample size is needed to differentiate the Mv model from the M1, M2, or M3 models.

INTEGRATING GENETIC DATA AS A STRUCTURE PRIOR TO ENHANCE CAUSAL INFERENCE IN THE BAYESIAN NETWORK RECONSTRUCTION PROCESS

In general, Bayesian networks can only be solved to Markov-equivalent structures, so it is often not possible to determine the causal direction of a link between two nodes even though Bayesian networks are directed graphs. However, the Bayesian network reconstruction algorithm can take advantage of genetic data to break the symmetry among nodes in the network that lead to Markov-equivalent structures, thereby providing a way to infer causal directions in the network in an unambiguous fashion (Zhu et al., 2004). The reconstruction algorithm can be modified to incorporate genetic data as prior evidence that two quantitative traits may be causally related based on a previously described causality test (Zhu et al., 2004). The genetic priors can be constructed from three basic sources. First, gene expression traits associated with DNA variants that are coincident with the gene's physical location (referred to as *cis-acting expression quantitative trait loci* or *cis eQTLs*) (Doss et al., 2005) are allowed to be parent nodes of genes with coincident trans eQTLs (the gene in this case does not physically reside at the genetic locus of interest), $p(cis \rightarrow trans) = 1$, but genes with trans eQTLs are not allowed to be parents of genes with cis eQTLs, $p(trans \rightarrow cis) = 0$. Second, after identifying all associations between different genetic loci and expression traits at some reasonable significance threshold, genes from this analysis with cis- or trans-eQTL can be tested individually for pleiotropic effects at each of their eQTLs to determine whether any other genes in the set are driven by common eQTLs (Jiang and Zeng, 1995; Lum et al., 2006). If such pleiotropic effects are detected, the corresponding gene pair and locus giving rise to the pleiotropic effect can then be used to infer a causal/reactive or independent relationship based on the causality test previously described. If an independent relationship is inferred, then the prior probability that gene A is a parent of gene B can be scaled as

$$p(A \rightarrow B) = 1 - \frac{\sum_i p(A \perp B|A,B,l_i)}{\sum_i 1},$$

where the sums are taken over all loci used to infer the relationship. If a causal or reactive relationship is inferred, then the prior probability is scaled as

$$p(A \rightarrow B) = \frac{2\sum_i p(A \rightarrow B|A,B,l_i)}{\sum_i p(A \rightarrow B|A,B,l_i) + p(B \rightarrow A|A,B,l_i)} p.$$

Finally, if the causal/reactive relationship between genes A and B cannot be determined from the first two sources, the complexity of the eQTL signature for each gene can be taken into consideration. Genes with a simpler, albeit stronger, eQTL signature (i.e., a small number of eQTL that explain the genetic variance component for the gene, with a significant proportion of the overall variance explained by the genetic effects) can be considered as more likely to be causal compared with genes with more complex and possibly weaker eQTL signatures (i.e., a larger number of eQTLs explaining the genetic variance component for the gene, with less of the overall variance explained by the genetic effects). The structure prior that gene A is a parent of gene B can then be taken to be

$$p(A \rightarrow B) = 2\frac{1 + n(B)}{2 + n(A) + n(B)},$$

where n(A) and n(B) are the number of eQTLs at some predetermined significance level for genes A and B, respectively.

INCORPORATING OTHER OMICS DATA AS NETWORK PRIORS IN THE BAYESIAN NETWORK RECONSTRUCTION PROCESS

Just as genetic data can be incorporated as a network prior in the Bayesian network reconstruction algorithm, so can other types of data like transcription factor binding site (TFBS) data, protein–protein interaction (PPI) data, and protein–small molecule interaction data. PPI data can be used to infer protein complexes to enhance the set of manually curated protein complexes (Guldener et al., 2006). PPI-inferred protein complexes can be combined with manually curated sets, and each protein complex can then be examined for common transcription factor binding sites at the corresponding genes. If some proportion of the genes in a protein complex (e.g., half) carry a given TFBS, then all genes in the complex can be included in the TFBS gene set as being under the control of the corresponding transcription factor.

Given that the scale-free property is a general property of biological networks (i.e., most nodes in the network are linked to a small number of nodes whereas a smaller number of nodes are linked to many nodes) (Albert et al., 2000), inferred and experimentally determined TFBS data can be incorporated into the network reconstruction process by constructing scale-free priors, in a manner similar to the scale-free priors others have constructed to integrate expression and genetic data (Lee et al., 2006). Given a transcription factor T, and a set of genes, G, that contain the binding site of T, the TF prior, p_{tf}, can be defined so that it is proportional to the number of expression traits correlated with the TF expression levels, for genes carrying the corresponding TFBS:

$$\log\left(p_{tf}\left(T \rightarrow g\right)\right) \alpha \log\left(\sum_{gi \in G} p_{qtl}\left(T \rightarrow g_i\right)\delta\right)$$

where $p_{qtl}(T \rightarrow g)$ is the prior for the QTL and $\delta = \begin{cases} 1, if\ corr(T,g_i) \geq r_{cutoff} \\ 0, if\ corr(T,g_i) < r_{cutoff} \end{cases}$. The correlation cutoff r_{cutoff} can be determined by permuting the data and then selecting the maximum correlation values in the permuted datasets (corresponding to some predetermined, reasonable false discovery rate). This form of the structure prior favors transcription factors that have a large number of correlated responding genes. From the set of priors computed from the inferred and experimentally determined TFBS set, only nonnegative priors should be used to reconstruct the Bayesian network. For those protein complexes that could not be integrated into the network reconstruction process using scale-free priors, uniform priors were used for pairs of genes in these complexes (i.e., $p_{pc}(g_i \rightarrow g_j) = p_{pc}(g_j \rightarrow g_i) = c$).

Small molecule–protein interactions can also be incorporated into the Bayesian network reconstruction process. Chemical reactions reflected in biochemical pathways and the associated catalyzing enzymes can be identified as metabolite–enzyme pairs from existing pathway databases like KEGG. These relationships can then be stored in an adjacency matrix in which a 1 in a cell represents a direct connection between the metabolite and the enzyme. The shortest distance $d_{m,e}$ from an enzyme e to a metabolite m can then calculated using the repeated matrix multiplication algorithm. The structure prior for the gene expression of an enzyme e affecting the metabolite concentration is related to their shortest distance $d_{m,e}$ as $p(m \rightarrow e) \alpha e^{-\lambda d_{m,e}}$. The shorter the distance, the stronger the prior.

ILLUSTRATING THE CONSTRUCTION OF PREDICTIVE BAYESIAN NETWORKS WITH AN EXAMPLE

To illustrate how different types of data can be integrated to construct predictive gene networks, we can consider a simple model system, yeast, that makes the point on how different pieces of molecular information can be brought together to infer causal networks. A yeast example in this instance is preferable to one involving psychiatric disorders given the latter would be complicated and the validations less straightforward than we can demonstrate in a simple model system. However, the procedures applied and steps indicated in the following would be essentially the same for any disease or system of interest, given that the Bayesian network reconstruction algorithm described is generally applicable to data collected in any population and for any phenotype of interest.

In our simple yeast system, consider the following two classes of data: (1) DNA variation, gene expression, and metabolite data measured in a previously described cross between laboratory (BY) and wild (RM) yeast strains (referred to here

as the BXR cross) for which DNA variation, RNA expression, and metabolite levels have been assessed (Brem and Kruglyak, 2005; Brem et al., 2002; Zhu et al., 2012), and (2) protein–DNA binding, protein–protein interaction, and metabolite–protein interaction data available from public data sources and generated independently of the BXR cross (referred to here as non-BXR data). The BXR yeast data are reflected as nodes in the network to be constructed, where edges in the network reflect statistically inferred causal relationships among the expression and metabolite traits. The non-BXR interaction data from public sources are used to derive the types of structure priors previously discussed on the network to both constrain the size of the search space in finding the best network and enhance the ability to infer causal relationships between the network nodes (Zhu et al., 2008).

To illustrate the steps in the type of Bayesian network reconstruction procedure previously described and detailed more formally (Zhu, Chen et al.) and to examine contributions from the different data types used to construct the network, I focus on genes and metabolites involved in the *de novo* biosynthesis of pyrimidine ribonucleotides (Fig. 14.5). For

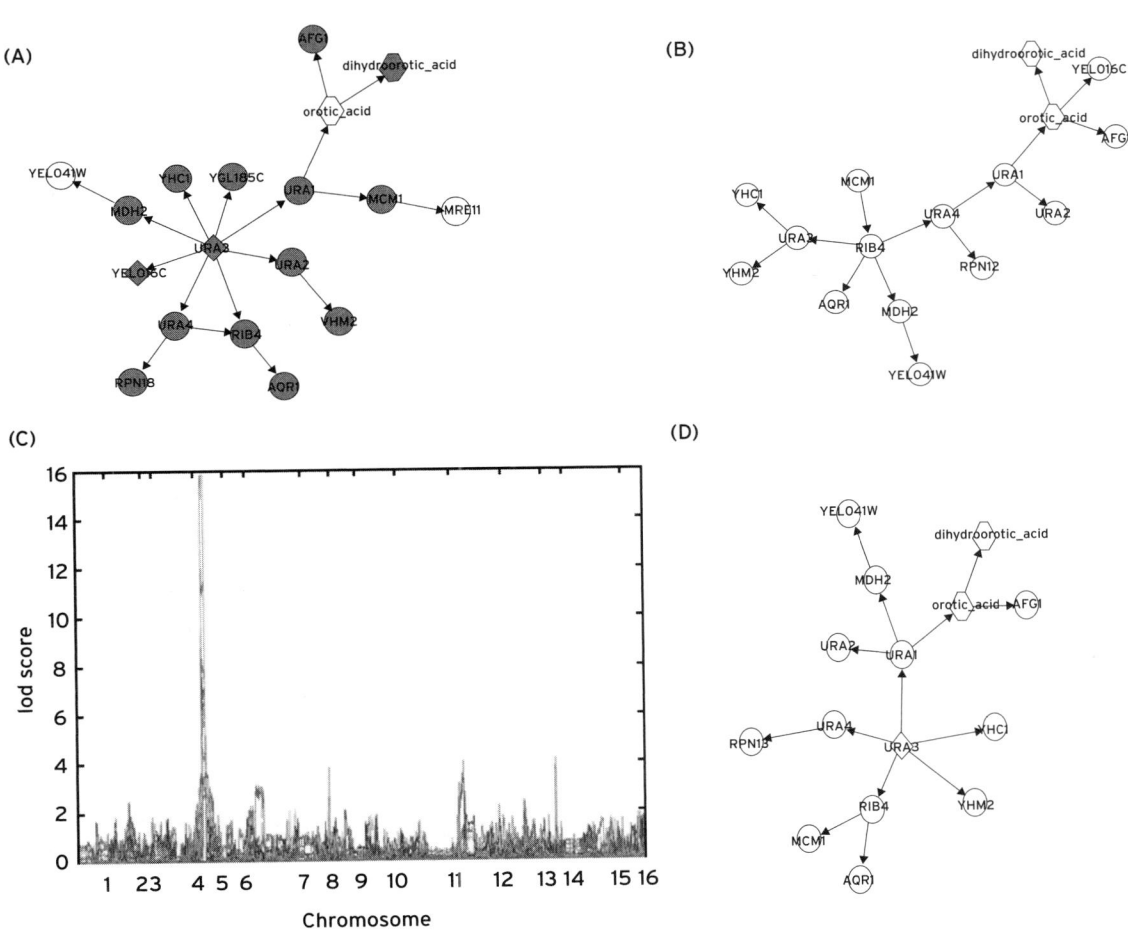

Figure 14.5 *Example yeast network. (A) Subnetwork identified in a previously constructed whole-genome yeast network in which URA3 was predicted as the causal regulator for genes and metabolites linked to a genetic locus on chromosome 5 coincident with the physical location of URA3. Gray nodes are genes or metabolites whose variations are linked to the chromosome 5 locus. Hexagon-shaped nodes represent metabolites, circular nodes represent genes, and diamond-shaped nodes represent genes with cis eQTLs. (B) Trait values of nodes compared with genotype data for the URA3 subnetwork. eQTLs and metQTLs are prominently featured as residing in the chromosome 5 URA3 locus. (C) Bayesian network reconstructed using only trait data. (D) Bayesian network reconstructed using trait data and priors derived from other types of data.*

simplicity I focus on the reconstruction of this smaller subset of genes, although the steps are similar if building a network from a more comprehensive set of genes. The subnetwork depicted in Figure 14.5a was identified from the full Bayesian network constructed from the BXR data (Zhu, Chen et al.). *URA3* in this network was predicted as a causal regulator of gene expression traits linked to the *URA3* locus. That is, using the full Bayesian network, in silico perturbations were carried out by simulating changes in each of the nodes and identifying those nodes that resulted in the most significant changes in other nodes in the network. As a result of this simulation, *URA3* was identified as the regulator modulating the most significant number of nodes in the subnetwork in a causal fashion (Fig. 14.5a). A deletion of *URA3* was engineered in the parental strain RM11–1a as a selectable marker, and segregation of this locus among the BXR progeny is the most likely cause for expression variation of uracil biosynthesis genes linked to this locus (Brem et al., 2002). Variations of two metabolites are also linked to this locus: dihydroorotic acid, which is converted to orotic acid by the enzyme Ura1p, and orotic acid itself, reflecting the functional consequence of transcriptional variation in genes involved in de novo pyrimidine base biosynthetic processes on metabolite levels. The causal relationships between *URA1*, orotic acid, and dihydroorotic acid as well as the subnetwork for genes linked to the *URA3* locus recapitulate the known pyrimidine base biosynthesis pathway (Zhu, Chen et al.). This subnetwork not only captures the coregulation of gene expression and metabolite abundance but also elucidates the mechanism of how genetic variation in *URA3* affects orotic acid and dihydroorotic acid levels.

Step 1: Identification of the URA3-centered de novo biosynthesis of pyrimidine ribonucleotides subnetwork. There are 18 nodes in the subnetwork shown in Figure 14.5a. These nodes are highly correlated with one another, with 68% of all pairwise relationships significant at the 0.01 significance level. The continuous gene expression data for these 18 genes can then be discretized into three states representing downregulated, no-change, and upregulated states, and then the mutual information of all pairs of nodes are calculated. In this case, 54% of all pairs are significant at $p < 0.01$ (the mutual information of the permutated data is calculated and fit into a normal distribution, which is then used to assess significance of the mutual information of the observed data). All 18 of the trait values corresponding to these nodes are significantly associated with the genotypes at the URA3 locus (Fig. 14.5c).

Step 2: Reconstructing networks using only expression and metabolite traits (excluding DNA variation data). The process of reconstructing networks using only trait data is straightforward. The trait data are input into a standard Bayesian network reconstruction program in which 1,000 network structures are generated from a Monte Carlo Markov Chain process using different random seed numbers (1,000 random seed numbers are generated by a

master process, then each slave process starts an MCMC process using one of the generated seed numbers). Once the 1,000 network structures have been generated, common features are extracted to derive a consensus network. With this construction, the consensus network may contain loops, which are prohibited in Bayesian networks. Therefore, to ensure the consensus network structure is a directed acyclic graph, the edges in the original consensus network are removed if and only if (1) the edge was involved in a loop, and (2) the edge was the most weakly supported of all edges making up the loop. The network resulting from this process is depicted in Figure 14.5b.

Step 3: Constructing priors using eQTL data. The network in Step 2 is constructed without considering any of the genetic data. Because eQTL data represent a systematic source of perturbation on the expression data, integrating these data has the potential to better resolve causal relationships. Toward this end, expression and genotype data in the BXR cross are compared to detect eQTLs. The gray nodes in Figure 14.5a indicate that nearly all of the nodes have QTLs linked to a single locus on chromosome 5. Expression traits that associate with a common eQTL are then subjected to a statistical test to infer causal relationships between the traits, as described. Among the nodes tested, URA3 and YEL016C have cis-acting eQTLs linked to the chromosome 5 locus. Nodes with cis-acting eQTLs are allowed to be causal parent nodes to nodes with trans-acting QTLs. However, nodes with trans-QTLs are not allowed to be causal parent nodes to nodes with cis-acting eQTLs.

Step 4: Constructing priors using KEGG data. The network constructed in Step 2 also does not consider known relationships among genes and metabolites as defined by canonical pathways. The relationships between enzymes and metabolites are well established in many cases. To incorporate this knowledge into the network reconstruction process, we construct priors using canonical pathway data in the following way. There are two metabolites in the *URA3* subnetwork. Their distances to each other and related enzymes are defined in the KEGG database. The structure prior for the gene expression of an enzyme *e* affecting a metabolite concentration is constructed using their shortest distance $d_{m,e}$ as $p(m \to e) \alpha e^{-\lambda d_{m,e}}$.

Step 5: Constructing networks using expression data, metabolite data, and the genetic and canonical pathway priors defined in Steps 3 and 4. The process of reconstructing networks using trait data and priors from other data types is similar to the reconstruction process applied to trait data only described in Step 2. In addition to trait data, priors derived from other data types are also input into the standard Bayesian network reconstruction process. The trait data of the 18 nodes and related priors are input into the network reconstruction process, and the resulting network is shown in Figure 14.5d. The root node of the Bayesian network is URA3, which is the gene with the cis-acting eQTL associated with other traits in the network.

Step 6: Comparing the networks constructed in Steps 2 and 5. The main difference between the networks depicted in Fig. 14.5b and 14.5d are the head nodes. In general, directed links in a Bayesian network do not necessarily represent causal relationships (Zhu et al., 2004). The network constructed from the trait data only reflects relationships not supported by the genetic perturbation data. The genetic relationships are well captured by the more integrated network described in Step 5. For example, the link RIB4 → URA3 depicted in Fig. 14.5b is opposite that identified in Fig. 14.5d. Because the genetic perturbation at the URA3 locus affects the expression activity of that gene in cis and the expression activity of the gene RIB4 in trans, the experimentally supported relationship is URA3 → RIB4. I note that the enzyme/ metabolite and metabolite/metabolite relationships are similar with or without the priors derived from the KEGG pathways.

All data and software used to construct the Bayesian networks for this example are available at http://www.mssm.edu/ research/institutes/genomics-institute/rimbanet.

ELUCIDATING THE COMPLEXITY OF HUMAN DISEASE: FROM THE METABOLIC TO THE PSYCHIATRIC

We have carried out studies using the modeling described in detail for the yeast cross, but in human and mouse population segregating a number of different diseases such as obesity, diabetes, and heart disease. For example, in a segregating mouse population in which an extensive suite of disease traits associated with metabolic syndrome were manifested, including obesity, diabetes, and atherosclerosis (Chen et al., 2008), we carried out the type of network analysis previously discussed using genetic data typed in all animals and gene expression data generated from the liver and adipose tissues of all animals in the population. With this approach we found that of the many functional units (subnetworks) identified in the networks that reflected core biological processes specific to the liver and adipose tissues, only a handful were strongly causally associated with the metabolic syndrome traits. One module (referred to here as the inflammatome module) in particular stood out not only because it was conserved across the liver and adipose tissues, between the sexes, and between species (Emilsson et al., 2008), but also because it was supported as strongly causal for nearly all of the metabolic traits scored in the cross (fat mass, weight, plasma glucose, insulin, and lipid levels, and aortic lesions) (Chen et al., 2008). Again, the causal relationship between the inflammatome module and the disease traits was established by leveraging the changes in DNA in this population that were simultaneously associated with disease and expression traits. The entire subnetwork was shown to be under the control of genomic loci associated with the metabolic traits, while the predictive network modeling

strongly indicated that the module was causal for the disease traits and was not simply reacting to or acting independently of these traits.

Of the more than 100 genes supported in the inflammatome module as causal for metabolic disease traits like obesity and diabetes, many genes like *Zfp90*, *Alox5*, *C3ar1*, and *Tgfbr2* had been previously identified and validated as causal for metabolic traits (Mehrabian et al., 2005; Schadt et al., 2005). In addition, three other genes were selected for validation because they were independently supported as causal for metabolic traits in other studies (*Lpl* and *Lactb*) or because they were supported as causal for such a wide variety of metabolic traits (*Ppm1l*) (Chen et al., 2008). Interestingly, the degree of connectivity in this causal metabolic subnetwork was extreme. Perturbations to genes in this module that were previously validated as causal for the metabolic traits caused expression changes in many other genes validated as causal for metabolic traits. For example, overexpression of *Zfp90* in mouse not only generated an expression response that was significantly overlapping with the causal metabolic module but also caused changes in other genes like *Pparg* known to have an impact on metabolic traits (Chen et al., 2008).

These same approaches can be applied to brain-related disorders, such as Alzheimer's disease. In fact, we recently more fully characterized the inflammatome module described earlier, linking it to 11 different diseases: atherosclerosis, obesity, diabetes, inflammatory pain, COPD (chronic obstructive pulmonary disease), asthma, fibrosis, stroke, neuropathic pain, sarcopenia, and inflammation (Wang et al., 2012). This same module can also be seen to be significantly enriched not only for genes that are differentially expressed in the brain between Alzheimer's and control subjects, but also for genes that are differentially expressed in different brain regions in both Alzheimer's and schizophrenia patients versus controls. That is, the intersection between the set of genes identified as differentially expressed in both Alzheimer's and schizophrenia patients (Horesh et al., 2011) is very significantly enriched for genes that are in the inflammatome module. Therefore, the extensive research carried out on the inflammatome module, the causal networks that have been constructed for this network, may hold clues regarding inflammation-related processes that are at play in brain-associated disorders such as Alzheimer's and schizophrenia.

CONCLUSION AND FUTURE DIRECTIONS

The generation of ever higher dimensional data (DNA sequencing, RNA sequencing, epigenomic profiling, proteomic profiling, metabolomic profiling, and so on) at ever higher scales demands sophisticated mathematical approaches to integrate these data in more holistic ways to uncover not only patterns of molecular, cellular, and higher order activities that underlie the biological processes that define physiological states of interest, but also causal relationships among molecular and cellular phenotypes and between these phenotypes and clinical traits like disease or drug response. Among the more successful frameworks for representing large-scale, high-dimensional data are networks. Here I have detailed one particular approach to reconstructing predictive network models of living systems that leverages DNA variation as a systematic variation source and Bayesian network reconstruction algorithms to take a top-down approach to modeling complex systems. Because state-of-the-art therapies in the future will be based on targeting combinations of genes (Schadt, 2009; Schadt, Friend et al., 2009), and for such applications not only is it important to infer the direction of each interaction (i.e., do you antagonize or activate a given target?), but also one must be able to predict the degree to which each gene should be knocked down or activated (in a quantitative sense), only by generating accurate predictive models of complex phenotypes can we most efficiently search for such combinations to pursue for experimental proof of concept.

The success of modeling complex systems in the future will depend on constructing networks that are predictive of complex behavior, not merely descriptive. In order to achieve these more predictive models in complex systems like humans, we must expand existing networks so that they reflect relationships between cell types and tissues, not just within a single cell type or tissue; capture a greater range of molecular phenotypes to enhance understanding of relevant functional units that define biological processes of interest; and improve modeling capabilities, ideally drawing on the expertise of other fields that have pioneered causality-type reasoning. The complex phenotype-associated molecular networks we can construct today are necessarily based on grossly incomplete sets of data. Even given the ability to assay DNA and RNA variation in whole populations in a comprehensive manner, the information is not complete, given rare variation, DNA variation other than SNP/co number, variation in noncoding RNA levels, and variation in the different isoforms of genes are far from being completely characterized in any sample, let alone in entire populations. Beyond DNA and RNA, measuring all protein-associated traits, interactions between proteins and DNA/RNA, metabolite levels, epigenetic changes, and other molecular entities important to the functioning of living systems are not yet possible with existing technologies. Further, the types of high-dimensional data we are able to routinely generate today in populations represent only a snapshot at a single time point, which may enable the identification of the functional units of the system under study and how these units relate to one another, but it does not enable a complete understanding of how the functional units are put together, the mechanistic underpinnings of the complex set of functions carried out by individual cells and by entire organs and whole systems comprised of multiple organs.

One of the future developments expected to be most impactful in this context is the unification of bottom-up and top-down modeling approaches that maximally leverage the strengths of each approach while minimizing the weaknesses. Integrating models derived from bottom-up approaches into top-down approaches is currently hampered by the fact that the existing approaches do not typically fully parameterize the network structure in ways that match the intrinsic quantitative nature of top-down approaches. In bottom up-approaches, the structural information detailing how different molecular entities are connected is typically derived from the literature or pathway databases, but such structural information is only qualitative, failing to define quantitatively how one node responds to another. On the other hand, in existing top-down approaches, unless a tremendous amount of training data are available to cover all of the categories represented in the conditional probability distribution (CPD) defining how nodes are connected in the network (such as with Bayesian network reconstruction approaches), it is not generally possible to accurately estimate the full set of parameters associated with the reconstructed network structure. Worse, carrying out parameter estimation on a network structure that is not correct can be misleading, given false-positive and false-negative predictions. In cases where heuristic searches are used to orient the edges in a given network structure, the end result is that model parameters have not been fitted accurately, given the network itself is not correct. Without proper parameterization of network structures from these conventional systems biology approaches, the networks serve only as descriptive models that are not generally capable of generating in silico predictions.

The limitations of bottom-up and top-down approaches can be addressed by devising bottom-up modeling approaches that deliver structures that can serve as prior information for top-down approaches, thereby providing a direct path for parameterizing bottom-up models in the context of a richer set of omics data and network architectures, while simultaneously reducing the size of the search space for top-down approaches. Such bottom-up approaches are beginning to emerge (Chang et al., 2011). By automatically parameterizing large networks given a particular network structure and corresponding interaction functions (e.g., activation or repression of gene activity) associated with all node pairs by either leveraging prior information or performing a heuristic search, bottom-up approaches will be capable of generating direct quantitative predictions that are compatible with top-down approaches. Central to the success of this approach is the observation that the complexity of the structure of biological networks leads to robust parameter estimates in a constrained parameter space (Blanchini and Franco, 2011; Wilhelm et al., 2004; Wu et al., 2009) and the fact that a statistical model's parameters are, in fact, constrained to a cubic space (e.g., the conditional probabilities that represent parameters in our modeling approach are constrained to fall between 0 and 1). This stands in contrast to current bottom-up modeling approaches like continuous ordinary differential equation (ODE) modeling in which the parameter space is generally unconstrained (infinitely large).

Current systems biology approaches relating to network learning and modeling have exclusively utilized a top-down (reverse-engineering) approach to learn network structure based on association scores (Carro et al., 2010; Fiedler et al., 2009; Margolin et al., 2006; Stuart et al., 2003; Zhu et al., 2008). Association scores are designed to uncover the best correlations between variables. Bayesian networks are among the most popular models for this purpose. In theory, it is known that learning the optimal (global maximum) Bayesian network structure from the data is a problem that cannot be solved in polynomial time (what is referred to as an NP-hard problem);

further, because many substructures that must be considered during the reconstruction process are from classes of structures that are equivalent (the Markov equivalence issue previously noted), the statistical scores for all of the structures in a given equivalence class are equal, so that completely contradictory causal relationships are indistinguishable from one another. The integration of bottom-up and top-down approaches in a more holistic mathematical framework has the potential to further address these issues, potentially enhancing the power to uncover true causal relationships.

DISCLOSURE

Dr. Schadt has no conflicts of interests to disclose.

REFERENCES

Albert, R., Jeong, H., et al. (2000). Error and attack tolerance of complex networks. *Nature* 406(6794):378–382.

Altshuler, D., Daly, M.J., et al. (2008). Genetic mapping in human disease. *Science* 322(5903):881–888.

Bandura, D.R., Baranov, V.I., et al. (2009). Mass cytometry: technique for real time single cell multitarget immunoassay based on inductively coupled plasma time-of-flight mass spectrometry. *Anal. Chem.* 81(16):6813–6822.

Barabasi, A.L., and Oltvai, Z.N. (2004). Network biology: understanding the cell's functional organization. *Nat. Rev. Genet.* 5(2):101–113.

Blanchini, F., and Franco, E. (2011). Structurally robust biological networks. *BMC Syst. Biol.* 5:74.

Boyden, E.S., Zhang, F., et al. (2005). Millisecond-timescale, genetically targeted optical control of neural activity. *Nat. Neurosci.* 8(9):1263–1268.

Brem, R.B., and Kruglyak, L. (2005). The landscape of genetic complexity across 5,700 gene expression traits in yeast. *Proc. Natl. Acad. Sci. USA* 102(5):1572–1577.

Brem, R.B., Yvert, G., et al. (2002). Genetic dissection of transcriptional regulation in budding yeast. *Science* 296(5568):752–755.

Carro, M.S., Lim, W.K., et al. (2010). The transcriptional network for mesenchymal transformation of brain tumours. *Nature* 463(7279):318–325.

Chang, R., Shoemaker, R., et al. (2011). Systematic search for recipes to generate induced pluripotent stem cells. *PLoS Comput. Biol.* 7(12):e1002300.

Chen, L.S., Emmert-Streib, F., et al. (2007). Harnessing naturally randomized transcription to infer regulatory relationships among genes. *Genome Biol.* 8(10):R219.

Chen, Y., Zhu, J., et al. (2008). Variations in DNA elucidate molecular networks that cause disease. *Nature* 452(7186):429–435.

Davey Smith, G., and Ebrahim, S. (2003). "Mendelian randomization": can genetic epidemiology contribute to understanding environmental determinants of disease? *Int. J. Epidemiol.* 32(1):1–22.

Didelez, V., and Sheehan, N. (2007). Mendelian randomization as an instrumental variable approach to causal inference. *Stat. Methods Med. Res.* 16(4):309–330.

Doss, S., Schadt, E.E., et al. (2005). Cis-acting expression quantitative trait loci in mice. *Genome Res.* 15(5):681–691.

Drmanac, R., Sparks, A.B., et al. (2012). Human genome sequencing using unchained base reads on self-assembling DNA nanoarrays. *Science* 327(5961):78–81.

Ecker, J.R., Bickmore, W.A., et al. (2012). Genomics: ENCODE explained. *Nature* 489(7414):52–55.

Eid, J., Fehr, A., et al. (2009). Real-time DNA sequencing from single polymerase molecules. *Science* 323(5910):133–138.

Elia, J., Glessner, J.T., et al. (2012). Genome-wide copy number variation study associates metabotropic glutamate receptor gene networks with attention deficit hyperactivity disorder. *Nat. Genet.* 44(1):78–84.

Emilsson, V., Thorleifsson, G., et al. (2008). Genetics of gene expression and its effect on disease. *Nature* 452(7186):423–428.

Erskine, D.J., Edelstein, J., et al. (2005). Externally dispersed interferometry for planetary studies. *Proc. SPIE* 5905: 249–260.

Feller, W. (1967). An Introduction to Probability Theory and Its Applications. New York: Wiley.

Fiedler, D., Braberg, H., et al. (2009). Functional organization of the S. cerevisiae phosphorylation network. *Cell* 136(5):952–963.

Glessner, J.T., Wang, K., et al. (2009). Autism genome-wide copy number variation reveals ubiquitin and neuronal genes. *Nature* 459(7246):569–573.

Guldener, U., Munsterkotter, M., et al. (2006). MPact: the MIPS protein interaction resource on yeast. *Nucleic Acids Res.* 34(Database issue):D436–D441.

Han, J.D., Bertin, N., et al. (2004). Evidence for dynamically organized modularity in the yeast protein-protein interaction network. *Nature* 430(6995):88–93.

Hawrylycz, M.J., Lein, E.S., et al. (2012). An anatomically comprehensive atlas of the adult human brain transcriptome. *Nature* 489(7416):391–399.

Horesh, Y., Katsel, P., et al. (2011). Gene expression signature is shared by patients with Alzheimer's disease and schizophrenia at the superior temporal gyrus. *Eur. J. Neurol.* 18(3):410–424.

Hsu, Y.H., Zillikens, M.C., et al. (2010). An integration of genome-wide association study and gene expression profiling to prioritize the discovery of novel susceptibility Loci for osteoporosis-related traits. *PLoS Genet.* 6(6):e1000977.

Jansen, R., Yu, H., et al. (2003). A Bayesian networks approach for predicting protein-protein interactions from genomic data. *Science* 302(5644):449–453.

Jiang, C., and Zeng, Z.B. (1995). Multiple trait analysis of genetic mapping for quantitative trait loci. *Genetics* 140(3):1111–1127.

Kanehisa, M. (2002). The KEGG database. *Novartis Found. Symp.* 247:91–101; discussion 101–103, 119–128, 244–152.

Kravets, D. (2010). Privacy in peril: lawyers, nations clamor for Google Wi-Fi data. *Wired, Wired Magazine* .

Kulp, D.C., and Jagalur, M. (2006). Causal inference of regulator-target pairs by gene mapping of expression phenotypes. *BMC Genomics* 7:125.

Lawlor, D.A., Harbord, R.M., et al. (2008). Mendelian randomization: using genes as instruments for making causal inferences in epidemiology. *Stat. Med.* 27(8):1133–1163.

Lee, I., Date, S.V., et al. (2004). A probabilistic functional network of yeast genes. *Science* 306(5701):1555–1558.

Lee, S.I., Pe'er, D., et al. (2006). Identifying regulatory mechanisms using individual variation reveals key role for chromatin modification. *Proc. Natl. Acad. Sci. USA* 103(38):14062–14067.

Lum, P.Y., Chen, Y., et al. (2006). Elucidating the murine brain transcriptional network in a segregating mouse population to identify core functional modules for obesity and diabetes. *J. Neurochem.* 97(Suppl 1):50–62.

Luscombe, N.M., Babu, M.M., et al. (2004). Genomic analysis of regulatory network dynamics reveals large topological changes. *Nature* 431(7006):308–312.

Madigan, D., and York, J. (1995). Bayesian graphical models for discrete data. *Int. Stat. Rev.* 63: 215–232.

Margolin, A.A., Wang, K., et al. (2006). Reverse engineering cellular networks. *Nat. Protoc.* 1(2):662–671.

Mehrabian, M., Allayee, H., et al. (2005). Integrating genotypic and expression data in a segregating mouse population to identify 5-lipoxygenase as a susceptibility gene for obesity and bone traits. *Nat. Genet.* 37(11):1224–1233.

Millstein, J., Zhang, B., et al. (2009). Disentangling molecular relationships with a causal inference test. *BMC Genet.* 10: 23.

Mulvihill, J.J. (1999). Catalog of Human Cancer Genes: McKusick's Mendelian Inheritance in Man for Clinical and Research Oncologists (onco-MIM). Baltimore: Johns Hopkins University Press.

Mumford, J.A., Horvath, S., et al. (2010). Detecting network modules in fMRI time series: a weighted network analysis approach. *NeuroImage* 52(3):1465–1476.

Neale, B.M., Kou, Y., et al. (2012). Patterns and rates of exonic *de novo* mutations in autism spectrum disorders. *Nature* 485(7397):242–245.

Nitsch, D., Molokhia, M., et al. (2006). Limits to causal inference based on Mendelian randomization: a comparison with randomized controlled trials. *Am. J. Epidemiol.* 163(5):397–403.

Pearl, J. (1988). Probabalistic Reasoning in Intelligent Systems: Networks of Plausible Inference. San Mateo, CA: Morgan Kaufmann Publishers.

Pinto, D., Pagnamenta, A.T., et al. (2010). Functional impact of global rare copy number variation in autism spectrum disorders. *Nature* 466(7304):368–372.

Pinto, S., Roseberry, A.G., et al. (2004). Rapid rewiring of arcuate nucleus feeding circuits by leptin. *Science* 304(5667):110–115.

Ripke, S., Sanders, A.R., et al. (2011). Genome-wide association study identifies five new schizophrenia loci. *Nat. Genet.* 43(10):969–976.

Schadt, E.E. (2009). Molecular networks as sensors and drivers of common human diseases. *Nature* 461(7261):218–223.

Schadt, E.E., Friend, S.H., et al. (2009). A network view of disease and compound screening. *Nat. Rev. Drug Discov.* 8(4):286–295.

Schadt, E.E., Lamb, J., et al. (2005). An integrative genomics approach to infer causal associations between gene expression and disease. *Nat. Genet.* 37(7):710–717.

Schadt, E.E., Molony, C., et al. (2008). Mapping the genetic architecture of gene expression in human liver. *PLoS Biol.* 6(5):e107.

Schadt, E.E., Monks, S.A., et al. (2003). Genetics of gene expression surveyed in maize, mouse and man. *Nature* 422(6929):297–302.

Schadt, E.E., Turner, S., et al. (2010). A window into third-generation sequencing. *Hum. Mol. Genet.* 19(R2):R227–R240.

Schwarz, G. (1978). Estimating the dimension of a model. *Ann. Stat.* 6(2):461–464.

Shirasaki, D.I., Greiner, E.R., et al. (2012). Network organization of the huntingtin proteomic interactome in mammalian brain. *Neuron* 75(1):41–57.

Sieberts, S.K., and Schadt, E.E. (2007). Moving toward a system genetics view of disease. *Mamm Genome* 18(6–7):389–401.

Sklar, P., Ripke, S., et al. (2011). Large-scale genome-wide association analysis of bipolar disorder identifies a new susceptibility locus near ODZ4. *Nat. Genet.* 43(10):977–983.

Smith, H.H., Brookhaven National Laboratory, et al. (1972). Evolution of Genetic Systems. New York: Gordon and Breach.

Stranger, B.E., Stahl, E.A., et al. (2011). Progress and promise of genome-wide association studies for human complex trait genetics. *Genetics* 187(2):367–383.

Stuart, J.M., Segal, E., et al. (2003). A gene-coexpression network for global discovery of conserved genetic modules. *Science* 302(5643):249–255.

van de Vijver, M.J., He, Y.D., et al. (2002). A gene-expression signature as a predictor of survival in breast cancer. *N. Engl. J. Med.* 347(25):1999–2009.

van 't Veer, L.J., Dai, H., et al. (2002). Gene expression profiling predicts clinical outcome of breast cancer. *Nature* 415(6871):530–536.

Voineagu, I., Wang, X., et al. (2011). Transcriptomic analysis of autistic brain reveals convergent molecular pathology. *Nature* 474(7351):380–384.

Wang, I.M., Zhang, B., et al. (2012). Systems analysis of eleven rodent disease models reveals an inflammatome signature and key drivers. *Mol Syst Biol.* 8:594.

Wang, K., Zhang, H., et al. (2009). Common genetic variants on 5p14.1 associate with autism spectrum disorders. *Nature* 459(7246):528–533.

Wilhelm, T., J. Behre, et al. (2004). Analysis of structural robustness of metabolic networks. *Syst. Biol. (Stevenage)* 1(1):114–120.

Witte, J.S. (2010). Genome-wide association studies and beyond. *Annu Rev. Public Health* 31: 9–20, 4 p following 20.

Wu, Y., Zhang, X., et al. (2009). Identification of a topological characteristic responsible for the biological robustness of regulatory networks. *PLoS Comput. Biol.* 5(7):e1000442.

Yang, X., Deignan, J.L., et al. (2009). Validation of candidate causal genes for obesity that affect shared metabolic pathways and networks. *Nat. Genet* 41(4):415–423.

Zerhouni, E. (2003). Medicine: the NIH roadmap. *Science* 302(5642):63–72.

Zhong, H., Beaulaurier, J., et al. (2010). Liver and adipose expression associated SNPs are enriched for association to type 2 diabetes. *PLoS Genet.* 6: e1000932.

Zhu, J., Chen, Y., et al. (2010). Characterizing dynamic changes in the human blood transcriptional network. *PLoS Comput. Biol.* 6(2):e1000671.

Zhu, J., Lum, P.Y., et al. (2004). An integrative genomics approach to the reconstruction of gene networks in segregating populations. *Cytogenet. Genome Res.* 105(2–4):363–374.

Zhu, J., Sova, P., et al. (2012). Stitching together multiple data dimensions reveals interacting metabolomic and transcriptomic networks that modulate cell regulation. *PLoS Biol.* 10(4):e1001301.

Zhu, J., Zhang, B., et al. (2008). Integrating large-scale functional genomic data to dissect the complexity of yeast regulatory networks. *Nat. Genet.* 40(7):854–861.

15 | BRAIN IMAGING METHODOLOGIES

HANZHANG LU, YIHONG YANG, AND PEIYING LIU

Neuroimaging is versatile in that it contains many submodalities that can reflect different aspects of brain anatomy, physiology, and function. Collectively, they provide a powerful toolbox for researchers and clinicians to better understand the neurobiology of the disease and improve diagnosis. The greatest advantage of neuroimaging is that most modalities can be performed noninvasively; thereby it represents the most direct means to "look" inside the brain in living humans. This chapter focuses on several emerging methodologies that are capable of making a major impact in mental illness in the coming years.

MEASUREMENT OF CEREBRAL PERFUSION USING MRI

Estimation of cerebral perfusion parameters provides a useful means to evaluate tissue integrity and viability (Alsop et al., 2000; de Crespigny et al., 1998; Harris et al., 1996; Loeber et al., 1999). It should be emphasized that the utility of cerebral perfusion measurement is not limited to diseases of vascular origin (e.g., stroke or vascular dementia), but many psychiatric and neurologic diseases may also benefit from perfusion measurement. The reason is that perfusion measures can provide an indirect index of neural activity in the brain parenchyma due to neurovascular coupling (Roy and Sherrington, 1890). That is, if the brain region has greater neural activity, the local perfusion tends to be greater, too (Kuschinsky, 1996). Over the past few years, several MRI techniques have been extensively tested for the purpose of perfusion measurement, and they can now be used to quantitatively study perfusion parameters, including cerebral blood flow (CBF), cerebral blood volume (CBV), and mean transit time (MTT).

Dynamic susceptibility contrast (DSC) MRI uses a Food and Drug Administration (FDA)-approved MR contrast reagent (namely, the *gadolinium complex of diethylenetriamine pentaacetic acid, Gd-DTPA*) administered intravenously and employs rapid image acquisitions (e.g., 1 image/second) to monitor the first passage of the reagent in the brain (Ostergaard et al., 1996b; Rosen et al., 1990). Unlike perfusion tracers used in positron emission tomography (PET), the Gd-DTPA reagent is a nondiffusable tracer and does not penetrate the blood–brain barrier (BBB). However, using a model that accounts for the input–output functions of the vasculature, it is still possible to estimate the perfusion parameters, including CBV, CBF, and MTT (Ostergaard et al., 1996a, 1996b). One important requirement to accurately determine perfusion using DSC MRI is the estimation of arterial input function (AIF), which describes the time course of the reagent concentration in the incoming arterial blood (Calamante et al., 2004; Rausch et al., 2000; van Osch et al., 2003). This is typically done by selecting pixels containing large arteries and using the averaged time course as the AIF (Cha et al., 2005; Law et al., 2004). If absolute quantification is not necessary, one can calculate the relative perfusion parameters by normalizing the values against the value in a region-of-interest (ROI), often the white matter.

A steady-state (SS) contrast MRI approach can also be used to evaluate cerebral perfusion, in this case only the CBV. This method acquires two MRI images before and after the contrast reagent injection and utilizes the fact that Gd-DTPA is an intravascular reagent and only occupies the vascular space (Kuppusamy et al., 1996; Lu et al., 2005; Moseley et al., 1992; Schwarzbauer et al., 1993). As a result, the difference signal is proportional to the CBV. Several variants of the technique are available, and their main differences reside in the use of different methods to normalize the signal, thereby converting the dimensionless MRI signal to physiologic values. Figure 15.1 shows a CBV map using the vascular-space-occupancy (VASO) approach, in which the normalization factor was obtained from a cerebrospinal fluid (CSF) region (Lu et al., 2005). In comparison with DSC MRI, the SS contrast MRI has the advantages that the model is relatively simple and does not require the knowledge of the AIF. In addition, the SS approach does not require rapid acquisitions; therefore, higher spatial resolution can be achieved and the image distortion is minimal. A pitfall is that this technique only estimates CBV (Lu et al., 2005), but not other parameters such as CBF, which is believed to be more useful in predicting tissue viability.

Cerebral blood flow can also be evaluated noninvasively using a technique called *arterial spin labeling* (ASL) MRI (Aslan et al., 2010; Dai et al., 2008; Detre et al., 1992; Detre and Alsop, 1999; Edelman et al., 1994; Golay et al., 1999; Kim, 1995; Kwong et al., 1995; Wong, 2007; Wu et al., 2007). The ASL pulse sequence starts with a radiofrequency (RF) pulse to magnetically label the incoming blood in the arterial vessels. Then, after a certain waiting period (1–2 seconds) to allow the blood to flow into the perfused tissue, an image is taken that contains signal from labeled blood and static tissue. In a second scan, the blood is not labeled, and similar waiting and acquisition schemes are undertaken. By subtracting one image from the other, the static tissue signal is canceled out, and the remaining difference image reflects the amount of labeled blood water that has flowed into the tissue, which can be used to calculate CBF. This technique can now measure a whole-brain CBF map

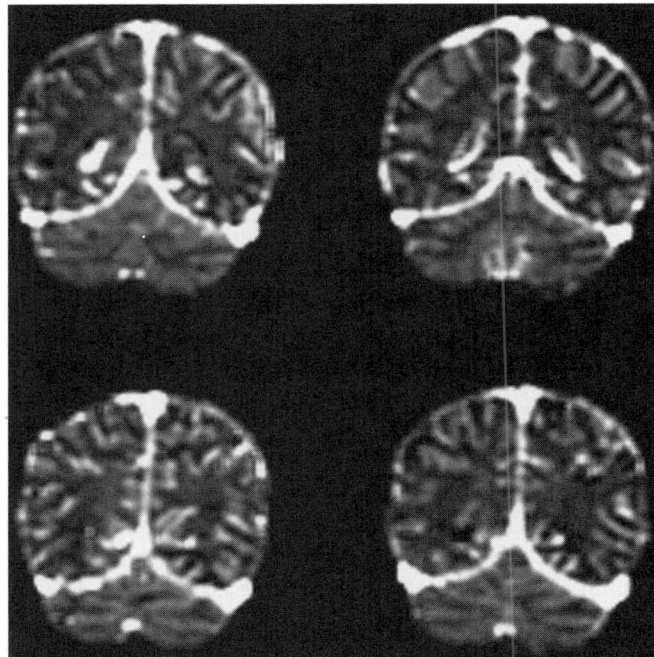

Figure 15.1 Absolute cerebral blood volume maps using VASO MRI. Imaging parameters: coronal slices, resolution 1.5 × 1.5 mm²; acquisition time was 5 minutes.

within 5 minutes on a standard clinical MRI scanner; thus, it can be easily included in an imaging session with relatively little added cost. Figure 15.2 shows a CBF map measured with a pseudocontinuous ASL method. The main advantage of the ASL technique is that the experimental procedure is noninvasive and straightforward. A pitfall is that the quantification is not trivial, and it involves several confounding factors, including arterial transit time and vessel signal contributions (Buxton et al., 1998; Calamante et al., 1996; Hendrikse et al., 2003; Liu et al., 2011; Yang et al., 2000).

ASSESSING BRAIN FUNCTIONS USING MRI

Neuronal activity in the brain is accompanied by an increased consumption of glucose and oxygen. In addition, there are pronounced changes in blood supply to the activated regions, characterized by increased CBF and CBV (Roy and Sherrington, 1890). The precise mechanism of this neurovascular coupling is not clear. But it is thought to be mediated by one or more factors related to metabolism and/or neurotransmitters (Iadecola, 2004). Regardless of the mechanism, it is important to note that the increase in blood supply overcompensates for the increase in oxygen metabolism. As a result, the blood oxygenation in the draining veins and the capillaries is actually more oxygenated during the stimulation period compared with the resting state. This forms the basis of blood oxygenation level–dependent (BOLD) functional magnetic resonance imaging (fMRI) signal (Kwong et al., 1992; Ogawa et al., 1992). The hemoglobin in erythrocytes has different MR properties during the oxygenated and deoxygenated states. Deoxygenated blood is paramagnetic, which reduces the transverse relaxation times (T2 and T2*) of the water signal (inside the blood compartment and outside the blood compartment), whereas oxygenated blood is not paramagnetic. As a result, the MR signal is directly correlated with the amount of deoxyhemoglobin in the voxel (Ogawa et al., 1993). The BOLD effect on T2* is more pronounced than that on T2. As a result, the T2* weighted gradient-echo echo-planar-imaging (EPI) sequence is the most widely used pulse sequence.

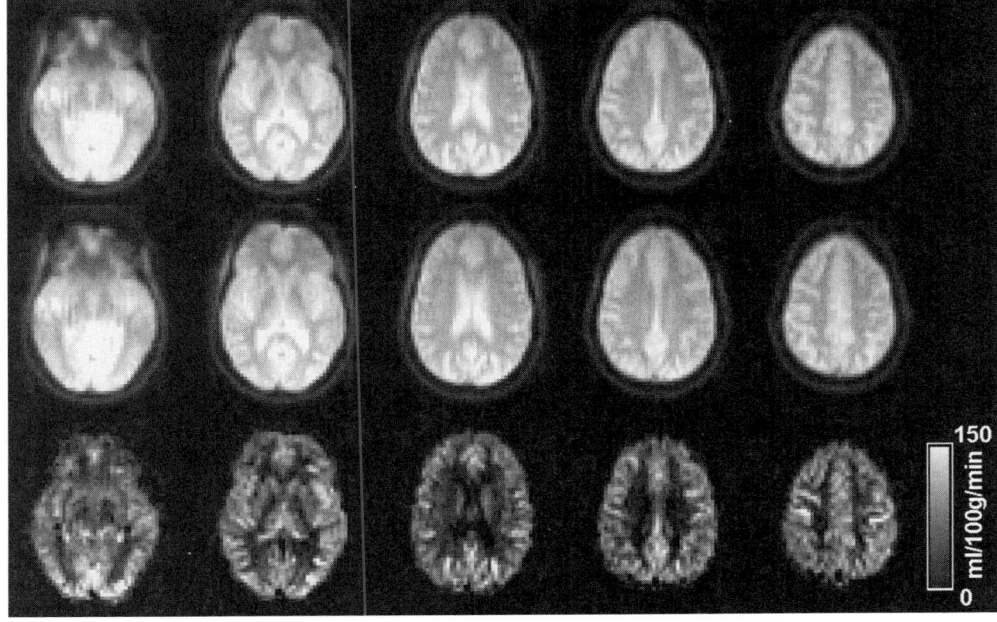

Figure 15.2 Absolute cerebral blood flow (CBF) maps using pseudocontinuous ASL MRI. The duration of the image acquisition was approximately 5 minutes and no contrast agent was used.

While evoked fMRI based on specific external stimuli has been used for more than two decades, there has been a recent surge in the use of BOLD MRI to study resting-state brain activity. We therefore focus our discussion on the resting state fMRI. Since the current analysis of the resting state data has primarily focused on the connection between two or more brain regions rather than individual regions, this technique is also known to as functional connectivity MRI (fcMRI).

Intrinsic brain activity can be investigated using spontaneous fluctuations in resting-state fMRI signals (Biswal et al., 1995). As illustrated in Figure 15.3, fMRI signals from the left and right primary sensorimotor cortices show highly synchronized fluctuations at rest, and "functional connectivity" maps based on the synchrony can be obtained by cross-correlation analysis using signal from a selected brain area as a "seed point" or reference. Brain connectivity maps in the absence of task performance have been reported to follow specific brain circuits, including sensorimotor, visual, auditory, and language-processing networks (Beckmann et al., 2005; Biswal et al., 1995; Cordes et al., 2000; Fox et al., 2005; Greicius et al., 2003; Lowe et al., 1998; Xiong et al., 1999). Among these observations, the existence of a brain network including posterior cingulate cortex (PCC) and medial prefrontal cortex (MPF) has been reported (Fox et al., 2005; Greicius et al., 2003). This finding supports previous suggestions that there is a functionally significant "default brain mode" in the resting state (Gusnard et al., 2001; Raichle et al., 2001). Because the brain expends a considerable amount of energy for neuronal-signaling

processes in the absence of a particular task (Shulman et al., 2004; Sibson et al., 1998), it is further argued that, in pursuit of better understanding of brain functions, observation of intrinsic brain activity may be at least as important as that of evoked activity (Gusnard et al., 2001; Raichle et al., 2001).

Various applications of resting-state fMRI to brain diseases have been demonstrated, including studies of Alzheimer's disease (Greicius et al., 2003; Li et al., 2002), schizophrenia (Liang et al., 2006), epilepsy (Waites et al., 2006), cocaine dependence (Li et al., 2000), and antidepressant effects (Anand et al., 2005). Using a cross-correlation-based analysis method, Li et al. (2002) quantified functional synchrony in the hippocampus of patients with Alzheimer's disease and demonstrated lower correlation of signals in patients with Alzheimer's disease compared with age-matched mild cognitive impairment (MCI) participants and healthy controls. Their study suggested that resting-state synchrony may be used as a quantitative marker for diagnosis and stage of Alzheimer's disease. Greicius et al. (2003) investigated the default brain mode activity in patients with Alzheimer's disease using independent component analysis (ICA). They found that patients with Alzheimer's disease showed decreased resting-state activity in the posterior cingulate and hippocampus, suggesting disrupted connectivity between these two brain regions, consistent with the posterior cingulated hypometabolism commonly found in previous PET studies of early Alzheimer's disease. These studies demonstrated the utility of resting-state functional connectivity in the study of neurological and neuropsychiatric disorders.

Advanced approaches for analyzing resting-state fMRI data, beyond the traditional seed-based and ICA methods, have been developed in recent years. Quantitative analysis of complex networks, based on graph theory, has been successfully exploited to study brain organizations (Bullmore and Sporns, 2009; Sporns et al., 2005). Graph theory analyzes "graphs" consisting of nodes (e.g., anatomical regions of the brain) and edges (e.g., functional connectivity strength) connecting the nodes. It has been shown that brain systems exhibit topological features of complex networks, including "small-world" characteristics (Watts and Strogatz, 1998), modular structures (Meunier et al., 2010), and highly connected hubs (Buckner et al., 2009). For example, a small-world network possesses both high clustering and short path lengths, resulting in efficient information transfer on both local and global scales. The human brain, like many other networks such as social network and electrical power grids, has small-world properties representing an optimal balance between integration and segregation between subunits. Network analysis methods have been demonstrated to be useful in identifying dynamic changes of brain networks associated with development (Fan et al., 2011), aging (Wu et al., 2012), and neuropsychiatric diseases (Yao et al., 2010).

Despite extensive applications of resting-state functional connectivity in basic and clinical studies, the underlying neural mechanisms of these synchronized fluctuations in resting-state fMRI signal remain obscure. Effort has been made in recent years to investigate whether these coherent fluctuations have a neural basis. Using an animal model, the mechanisms were first examined by combined electrophysiological recordings and fMRI scans in the resting rat brain

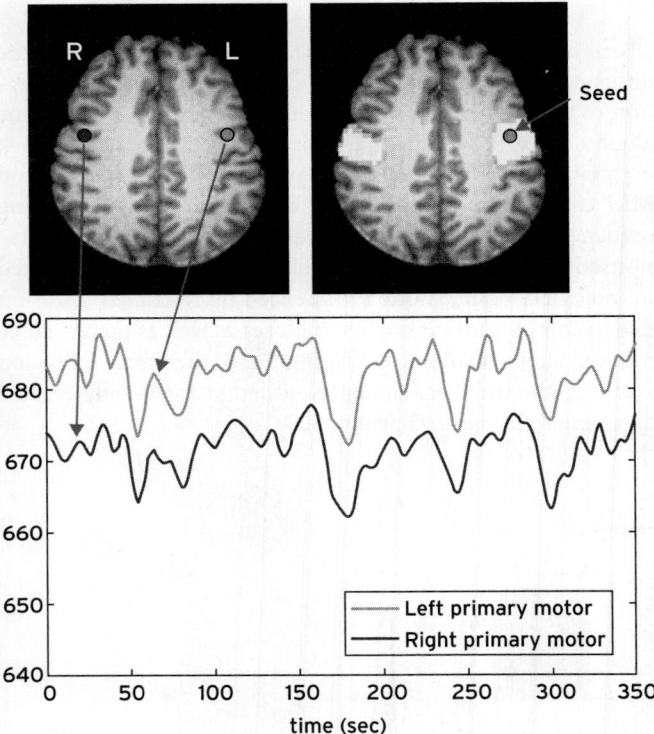

Figure 15.3 *Functional MRI signals at rest (bottom) from the left and right primary sensorimotor cortices (upper left), and functional connectivity map (upper right), obtained from cross-correlation analysis using the left sensorimotor cortex as a reference.*

(Lu et al., 2007). It was demonstrated that the interhemispheric γ-band power correlation and functional connectivity between the left and right somatosensory cortices were significantly greater than those between the somatosensory cortex and the visual cortex, and the electrophysiological and hemodynamic metrics were significantly and similarly modulated by anesthetic dose, suggesting a region-specific and anesthetic-induced state-dependent effect (Lu et al., 2007). The tight relationship between electrophysiological and resting fMRI signals was also demonstrated in human brains in patients with intractable epilepsy undergoing evaluation with surgically implanted grids of subdural electrodes (He et al., 2008). These studies provided an important bridge between the brain networks readily revealed by spontaneous BOLD signals and their underlying neurophysiology.

DIFFUSION-BASED MRI TECHNIQUES

Diffusion occurs as a result of random thermal motion of small particles such as water molecules in a given medium. The effects of molecular diffusion on MR signals have been studied since 1950s (Carr and Purcell, 1954; Hahn, 1950). A significant improvement of diffusion measurement using MR techniques was made in 1960s (Stejskal and Tanner, 1965) by utilizing magnetic gradient pulses to encode the phase dispersion caused by diffusion. Diffusion-weighted imaging (DWI) was developed in 1980s (Le Bihan et al., 1986) as an integration of MRI and diffusion-sensitive magnetic gradients. In ideal free diffusion, the diffusivity is uniform along all directions, or *isotropic*. However, a diffusion process in biological tissue, such as brain white matter, could be *anisotropic* because the diffusive molecules may experience direction-dependent restrictions due to specific arrangements of tissue structures. Diffusion tensor imaging (DTI) was developed in 1990s (Basser et al., 1994) as a tool to quantify the anisotropy of diffusion in biological tissue. An important advantage of DTI is that it provides rotation-invariant measurements, which means that the measurements are independent from participant positions, thus making longitudinal and group comparisons possible (Basser and Pierpaoli, 1996). In recent years, "beyond-tensor" imaging techniques (Tuch et al., 2003) have been proposed to overcome challenges encompassed in DTI, such as the handling of complex white matter structures. Tractography, a promising technique to delineate neuronal

pathways based on DTI or beyond-tensor techniques, has also been developed (Xue et al., 1999).

PRINCIPLES OF DIFFUSION MRI

For unrestricted diffusion in a three-dimensional space, the displacements of an ensemble of molecules can be described by the Einstein equation (Einstein, 1926)

$$\langle \mathbf{r}^2 \rangle = 6D\tau_D$$

where $<r^2>$ is the mean-squared displacement, τ_D is the diffusion time, and D is the diffusion coefficient. Fundamental principles of diffusion MRI can be illustrated by the traditional pulsed gradient experiment (Stejskal and Tanner, 1965) designed to measure the spin echo signal attenuation caused by phase dispersion of diffusive nuclear spins in the presence of diffusion-sensitive gradients. As illustrated in Figure 15.4, in a spin echo pulse sequence, a pair of identical gradients is placed on both sides of the 180-degree refocus RF pulse. For a static spin, the two gradients would result in phase shifts with the same magnitude but opposite signs, respectively, leading to cancellation of the phase change at the echo time. However, for a diffusive spin the gradients would produce a net phase shift, and phase dispersion in an ensemble of spins would cause signal attenuation at the echo time. The spin echo signal in the presence of diffusion gradients, $S(b)$, with respect to that in the absence of the gradients, $S(0)$, can be expressed as

$$S(b) = S(0)\exp(-bD)$$

where b is called "b-factor," a measure of the strength of the diffusion-weighting gradients, and is determined by the duration of the gradients δ, separation of the gradients Δ, and the amplitude of the gradient G. For the setting in Figure 15.4, $b = \gamma^2 G^2 \Delta^2 (\Delta - \delta/3)$, where γ is the gyromagnetic ratio. Diffusion MRI can be implemented by a combination of an imaging sequence with the diffusion-sensitive gradients to map diffusion coefficient in an object. Diffusion coefficient measured in biological tissue is often influenced by restricted diffusion due to complex microscopic structures as well as macroscopic motion such as blood perfusion, and therefore, diffusion strength measured in biological systems is generally termed *apparent diffusion coefficient* or ADC.

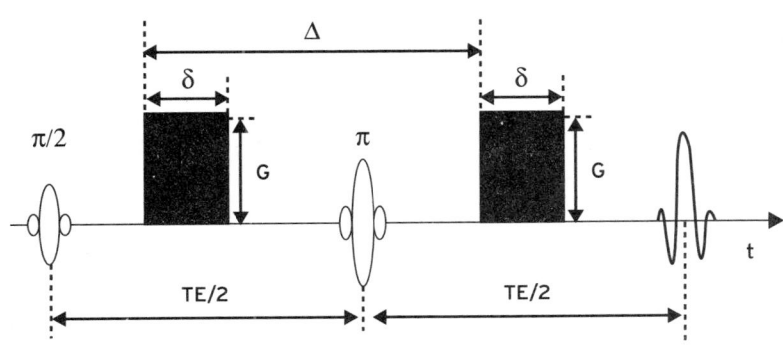

Figure 15.4 *Schematic diagram of the Stejskal-Tanner pulsed gradient diffusion experiment.*

DIFFUSION TENSOR IMAGING

Diffusion tensor imaging is a diffusion-imaging technique to characterize diffusion anisotropy (Basser et al., 1994). Molecular diffusion in biological tissue is often anisotropic due to varied restriction along different directions. For instance, water molecules in a white matter fiber fascicle typically diffuse faster along the fibers compared with those that cross the fibers. Diffusion in such an anisotropic medium needs to be described by multiple diffusion coefficients accounting for the direction dependence. In the formulation of DTI (Basser et al., 1994), the diffusion coefficient is no longer characterized by a scalar parameter D, but rather, by a 3×3 tensor D:

$$D = \begin{pmatrix} D_{XX} & D_{XY} & D_{XZ} \\ D_{YX} & D_{YY} & D_{YZ} \\ D_{ZX} & D_{ZY} & D_{ZZ} \end{pmatrix}$$

where $D_{ij}(i, j = x, y, z)$ denotes the cross-correlation of the diffusion coefficient between the i and j axis, and thus, D is always symmetric, that is, $D_{ij} = D_{ji}$. Similarly, a 3×3 matrix b is employed in DTI with elements b_{ij} representing the b-factor corresponding to the element D_{ij} in D. Thus, the diffusion-weighted signal attenuation can be expressed in the DTI formulation,

$$S(b) = S(0) \exp\left(-\sum_{i=X,Y,Z} \sum_{j=X,Y,Z} b_{ij} D_{ij} \right)$$

To determine the six independent elements in D, one needs to perform at least six diffusion-weighted measurements with the b matrices independent from each other. An additional experiment is also needed to provide a nondiffusion-weighted reference image. Therefore, a minimum of seven measurements is required to determine the diffusion tensor D. Recent studies have indicated that using more directions for diffusion encoding generally helps to improve the accuracy and/or the efficiency of the DTI technique, if these directions are appropriately optimized (Le Bihan et al., 2001).

Diffusion tensor can be analyzed based on the eigen-analysis theorem (Golub and Van Loan, 1996). Several rotation-invariant indices have been widely used to visualize and quantify diffusion tensor maps in biological applications. These include (Basser et al., 1994) the mean diffusivity (MD), the average diffusion strength in all directions

$$MD = \langle \mathbf{D} \rangle = \frac{\lambda_1 + \lambda_2 + \lambda_3}{3}$$

and the fractional anisotropy (FA), a *normalized* ($0 \leq FA < 1$) degree of the diffusion anisotropy

$$FA = \sqrt{\frac{3\left((\lambda_1 - \langle \mathbf{D} \rangle)^2 + (\lambda_2 - \langle \mathbf{D} \rangle)^2 + (\lambda_3 - \langle \mathbf{D} \rangle)^2 \right)}{2\left(\lambda_1^2 + \lambda_2^2 + \lambda_3^2 \right)}}$$

where λ_1, λ_2, and λ_3 are eigenvalues of the diffusion tensor. Figure 15.5 illustrates maps of MD and FA calculated from the diffusion tensor map acquired from a human brain. In general, the MD map shows high intensities in ventricles and gray matter, where the diffusion is relatively isotropic with higher strength. The FA map highlights the white matter tracts in the brain, where the diffusion is highly anisotropic. The primary eigenvector of the diffusion tensor is useful to indicate the orientation of the well-organized tissue, such as fiber boundless in white matter, and can be used to track neural pathways.

"BEYOND-TENSOR" DIFFUSION TECHNIQUES

Despite the success of DTI in a variety of applications, challenges exist in handling complex brain structures, in which diffusion patterns are far more complicated than a tensor model can deal with. For instance, DTI often fails to correctly describe diffusion patterns in brain areas with fiber crossings. In the case of multiple fiber components sharing a single voxel, the major eigenvector of the diffusion tensor could be substantially biased from the actual fiber orientation, resulting in misleading fiber tracing. This is fundamentally limited by the tensor model because the diffusion tensor is only a second-order approximation (in terms of mean square fitting) to the real three-dimensional diffusion process (Basser et al., 2000). "Beyond-tensor" diffusion techniques based on

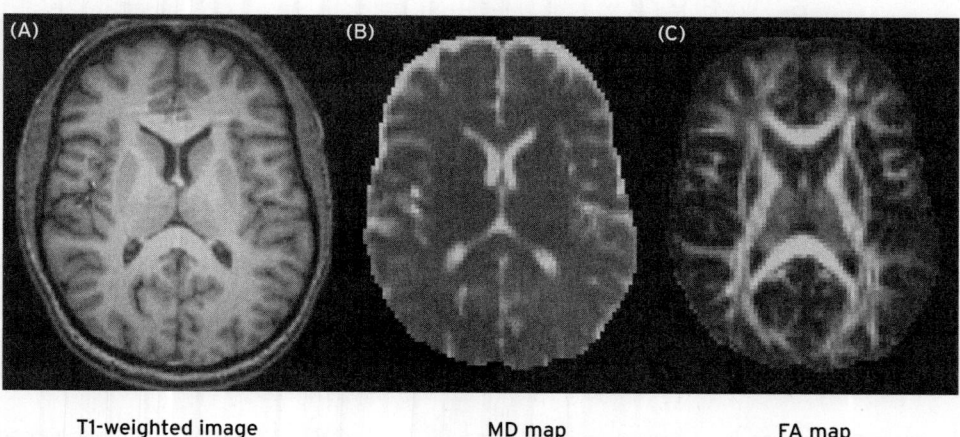

| T1-weighted image | MD map | FA map |

Figure 15.5 *T1-weighted image (A) and corresponding mean diffusivity (B) and fractional anisotropic (C) images of a brain section.*

higher order mathematical models, such as high angular resolution diffusion (HARD) and q-space imaging (QSI) have been proposed recently to overcome these difficulties (Frank, 2001; Jensen et al., 2005; Tuch et al., 2003; Zhan et al., 2004).

MAGNETIC RESONANCE SPECTROSCOPY

Magnetic resonance spectroscopy (MRS) is a noninvasive technique that can be used to investigate biochemistry of living systems. The first *in vivo* ^{31}P MRS experiment was conducted on a mouse head using a conventional spectrometer with a RF coil surrounding the entire head (Chance et al., 1978). Spectra of brain without contamination from other tissues were first obtained using a localization technique with a surface coil (Ackerman et al., 1980). In the past decades, MRS has evolved into a powerful tool for biological research and clinical diagnosis. Unlike MRI, which measures the signal from protons in water molecules, MRS usually detects the signal from compounds in much lower concentrations. Besides the most sensitive nuclear ^{1}H, MRS can also detect a range of nuclei including ^{31}P, ^{13}C, ^{19}F, ^{15}N, ^{23}Na, and ^{7}Li.

SPATIAL LOCALIZATION

The simplest way to obtain a localized spectrum is to use a surface coil, which produces a limited excitation volume close to the coil (Ackerman et al., 1980). The sensitivity distribution of the volume depends on the shape and orientation of the coil. For a single-loop coil, the selective volume is roughly a cylindrical region with a radius and length about the same as the coil radius. A disadvantage of using surface coils for localization is that the sensitivity is extremely inhomogeneous in the volume, which makes quantification of spectroscopic data difficult.

Single-volume spectroscopy techniques use shaped RF pulses along with field gradients to selectively excite the spins in a defined volume. The most commonly used approaches in this category are point resolved spectroscopy (PRESS) (Bottomley, 1984) and stimulated echo acquisition mode (STEAM) (Frahm et al., 1987). Similar to slice selection in imaging, these techniques select a volume using three slab-selective RF pulses in the presence of field gradients in three orthogonal directions. A spin echo or stimulated echo is formed by the signal from the intersection of the three selected slabs.

Spectroscopic imaging (SI) or chemical shift imaging (CSI) uses phase encoding and/or frequency encoding to obtain spatial and spectroscopic information (Brown et al., 1982; Lauterbur et al., 1975). Like imaging, this technique acquires spectroscopic data in a matrix of spatially resolved voxels, allowing for observation of spectra in multiple regions simultaneously.

^{1}H MRS

Proton MRS can reliably detect *N*-acetyl-aspartate (NAA), creatine (Cr)/phosphocreatine (PCr), choline (Cho)-containing compounds including phosphocholine (PC) and glycerophosphocholine (GPC), and *myo*-inositol (Ins) in the brain. At high field strengths (>7 T), glutamate (Glu), glutamine (Gln), and other metabolites can be resolved. A spectrum acquired from the cingulate of a rat brain at 9.4 T is illustrated in Figure 15.6.

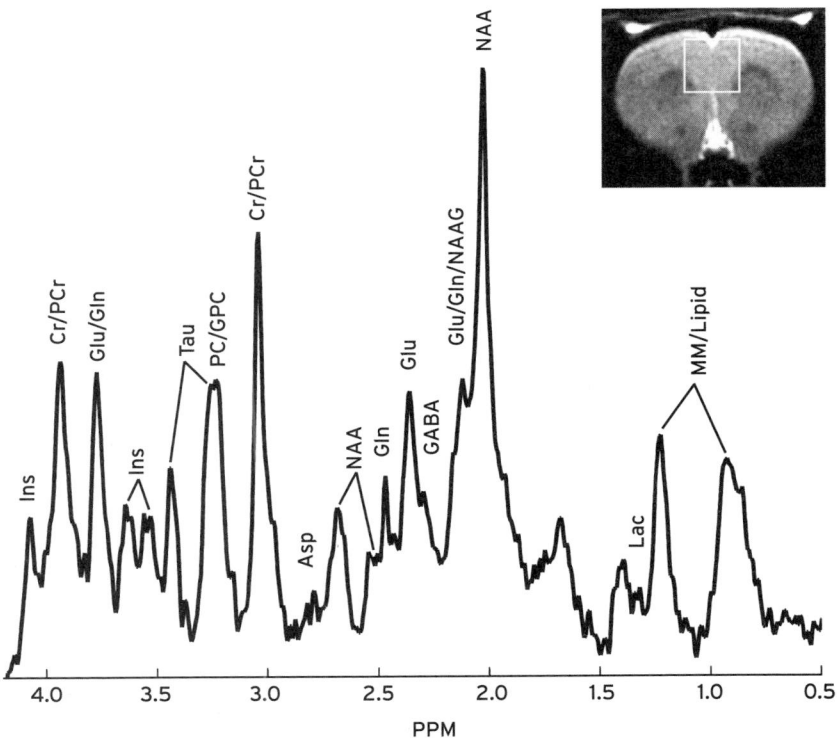

Figure 15.6 *A STEAM spectrum from the rat cingulate, volume size = 3 × 3 × 3 mm³, TR/TE/TM = 3000/9.1/10 ms, NEX = 300. Asp = aspartate, Cr = creatine, GABA = γ-aminobutyric acid, Gln = glutamine, GPC = glycerophosphocholine, Glu = glutamate, Lac = lactate, Ins = myo-inositol, NAA = N-acetyl-aspartate, NAAG = N-acetyl-asparty-glutamate, PC = phosphocholine, PCr = phosphocreatine, Tau = taurine, MM = macromolecules.*

Brain metabolites measured by ¹H MRS are involved in cellular metabolism, neurotransmission, and cell membrane synthesis, or serve as a marker specific to neurons or glia (de Graaf, 1998; Govindaraju et al., 2000). NAA is commonly believed to be a marker of mature neurons, and a reduction of NAA level in the brain is indicative of neuronal loss and/or dysfunction. The protons of an N-acetyl CH_3 group provide the most prominent singlet resonance at 2.02 ppm, which can be measured robustly. Cr and PCr are observed as a strong singlet resonance at 3.03 pm. The Cr/PCr level is relatively stable across the brain and is, therefore, often used as an internal concentration reference. This measure should be used with caution because reduced levels of Cr are observed in some pathological conditions, such as tumors and stroke. Cho is an important precursor of cell membrane synthesis, and increases of Cho indicate membrane damage to myelin or neuron. Cho, PC, and GPC give rise to a prominent singlet resonance at 3.20 ppm. Ins is believed to be a glial marker and an increase of Ins reflects gliosis. This compound has a prominent doublet of doublet centered at 3.52 ppm and a triplet at 3.61 ppm.

Glu is the major excitatory neurotransmitter in the central nervous system (CNS). Closely coupled to Glu, Gln is mostly located in glial cells as the end product of Glu catabolism and is a reservoir for Glu production in the neuron. γ-aminobutyric acid (GABA) is the major inhibitory neurotransmitter in CNS. These neurotransmitters play important roles in many neurological and psychiatric disorders, such as epilepsy, depression, and drug addiction. However, reliable detection and accurate quantification of Glu, Gln, or GABA *in vivo* remains challenging using proton ¹H MRS at low and middle magnetic field strengths (1.5–4.7 T), primarily due to spectral overlap of these compounds. Recently, new techniques such as echo time (TE)-averaged PRESS (Hurd et al., 2004) and STEAM with optimized timing parameters (Hu et al., 2007) have been developed to deal with this problem. An example of resolved Glu and Gln STEAM spectrum on the human brain with optimized TE and mixing time (TM) at 3 T is illustrated in Figure 15.7. Glu and Gln peaks at 2.35–2.45 ppm are well resolved and can be accurately quantified.

The three resonances of GABA at 1.89, 2.28, and 3.01 ppm are overlapped with the much stronger signals of NAA, Glu, and Cr, respectively. However, the resonance frequencies of GABA are affected by "J-coupling" while the overlapping singlet peaks of NAA and Cr are not. As such, editing spectroscopic techniques can separate the desired J-coupled compounds from the overlapping ones by manipulating their magnetizations (Mescher et al., 1998; Rothman et al., 1993). In the difference editing sequence, a selective 180° pulse is used to refocus the magnetization evolution due to J-coupling of the GABA-H4 spin (3.01 ppm). When editing pulses are turned ON/OFF in a two-step acquisition, the J-evolution of GABA-H4 is refocused/intact respectively, while the strong singlet resonance Cr at 3.03 ppm remains unchanged between the two scans. Difference of the two scans will eliminate the Cr resonance while preserving the GABA-H4 resonance at almost the same frequency. This spectral editing technique has been successfully implemented on 3T MR scanners recently and

has shown promise in assessing patients with neuropsychiatric disorders (Hasler et al., 2007).

SPECTRAL QUANTIFICATION

The goal of spectral quantification is to estimate metabolite concentrations from spectroscopic data. Although the area underneath a spectrum is directly proportional to the number of nuclei within the sensitive volume of the coil, it is not straightforward to achieve this goal. A number of factors have to be taken into account in quantifying spectroscopic data (Kauppinen and Williams, 1994).

Spectroscopic signal intensity is related to relaxation times and equilibrium magnetization. Magnetization recovers during a repetition time (TR) with longitudinal relaxation time (T_1) and decays during a TE with transverse relaxation time (T_2). Effects of T_1 and T_2 can be minimized using long TR and short TE. In many circumstances, however, knowledge of the relaxation times is needed to correct for these effects.

Spectral peak intensities can be affected by data acquisition and processing strategies as well as the existence of macromolecules in the sensitive volume. For instance, in chemical shift imaging using phase encoding for spatial localization (Brown et al., 1982), the early data points in the free induction decay (FID) are not collected, resulting in baseline and line shape distortions in the spectrum. Appropriate processing techniques are needed to estimate the missing data points and thus to correct for spectral distortions. Macromolecules contribute to a broad baseline in a spectrum, which has to be removed in data acquisition or processing. Techniques to extract signal intensities, such as LCModel (Provencher, 1993) and jMRUI (Naressi et al., 2001), have been developed and widely used for spectral quantification.

Metabolite concentrations can be presented as ratios, for example, relative to Cr, which is thought to be relatively stable in normal brains. Recent studies demonstrated that absolute quantification of metabolites has added value for unambiguous data interpretation (Jansen et al., 2006). However, extra calibration steps are required to achieve absolute quantification. Several strategies have been developed for this purpose, including internal endogenous marker, external reference, replace-and-match method, water signal reference, and principle of reciprocity (Jansen et al., 2006). Although absolute quantification requires more time and expertise, it can improve the diagnosis utility of MR spectroscopy.

MEASUREMENT OF CEREBRAL METABOLIC RATE OF OXYGEN

Cerebral metabolic rate of oxygen ($CMRO_2$) is a measure of energy consumption in the brain. Because aerobic metabolism is the primary form of energy production in the brain (Magistretti and Pellerin, 1999), $CMRO_2$ is an important index of tissue viability and brain function. Disrupted oxygen metabolism is associated with a number of pathophysiologic conditions such as Alzheimer's disease (Buckner et al., 2005; Ogawa et al., 1996), brain aging (Lu et al., 2011), multiple sclerosis

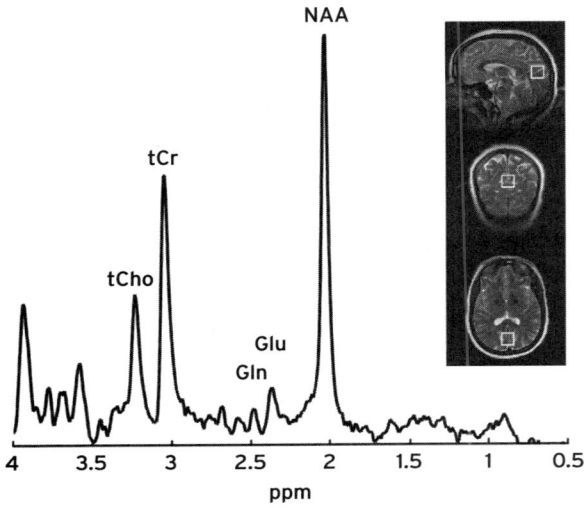

Figure 15.7 *A STEAM spectrum with optimized TE/TM (72/6 ms) in the medial occipitoparietal junction of the human brain (voxel size = 20 × 20 × 20 mm3). Glu and Gln peaks are well resolved at 2.35–2.45 ppm.*

(Ge et al., 2012; Sun et al., 1998), Parkinson's disease (Borghammer et al., 2008), diabetes (Sieber et al., 1993; Uchino et al., 2010), traumatic brain injury (Glenn et al., 2003), and normal pressure hydrocephalus (Walter et al., 2005). Traditionally, brain oxygen metabolism can only be measured with positron emission tomography (PET). Unfortunately, the measurement is only available in a limited number of institutions where an on-site cyclotron is available and, furthermore, technical limitations such as long scan duration, high cost, and high risk have prevented oxygen metabolism measurement from becoming a routine procedure. Recent advances in MRI technologies have provided an opportunity to fill this gap. Over the past few years, a number of emerging techniques have been developed and extensively tested to a point that it is now feasible to measure human brain metabolism using completely noninvasive procedures on a standard 3-Tesla scanner.

$CMRO_2$ can be measured by combining several noninvsive measures obtained from MRI and pulse oximetry (Xu et al., 2009). The theoretical basis of the method is the Fick principle (Kety and Schmidt, 1948):

$$CMRO_2 = CBF \cdot (Y_a - Y_v) \cdot C_a$$

A graphical illustration of this relationship is shown in Figure 15.8a. In brief, arterial vessels deliver blood that has an oxygenation level of Y_a, the flow rate of which is denoted by CBF. When the blood transits through capillary beds, a portion of the carried oxygen is extracted by brain tissue for its metabolism, the rate of which is denoted by $CMRO_2$. The portion that remains in the blood will determine the venous oxygenation, Y_v, and is drained through veins. C_a is the amount of oxygen molecules that a unit volume of blood can carry, assumed to be 897 μmol O_2/100 ml blood based on physiology literature (Guyton and Hall, 2005). Therefore, once CBF, Y_a, and Y_v are experimentally measured, $CMRO_2$ can be determined using the Fick principle.

In the preceding equation, Y_a can be easily measured with noninvasive pulse oximetry on a fingertip. Note that arterial oxygenation is identical throughout the body; thus, measurement made at a finger can be used for brain calculation. A number of MR techniques are available for quantitative measurements of CBF. For global CBF, one can use a phase contrast MRI applied on the feeding arteries of the brain (Fig. 15.8b) (Aslan et al., 2010; Bonekamp et al., 2011; Lu et al., 2011; Xu et al., 2009). For region-specific CBF, a noninvasive technique, arterial-spin-labeling (ASL), can be used (Aslan et al., 2010; Dai et al., 2008; Detre and Alsop, 1999; Edelman et al., 1994; Golay et al., 1999; Kim, 1995; Kwong et al., 1995; Liu et al., 2011; Wong, 2007; Wu et al., 2007). The most challenging component is the measurement of Y_v, which has seen a great deal of technical development over the past several years.

One of the MRI approaches to quantify global venous oxygenation is based on the relationship between blood T2 and oxygenation and was termed T2-relaxation-under-spin-tagging (TRUST) (Lu and Ge, 2008). The TRUST MRI technique applies the spin labeling principle on the venous side and acquires control and labeled images, the subtraction of which yields pure venous blood signal (Fig. 15.8c). T2 value of the pure venous blood is then determined using nonselective T2 preparation pulses, minimizing the effect of flow on T2 estimation (Lu and Ge, 2008; Lu et al., 2012). Despite the lack of spatial information, this approach has the advantage of being fast and reliable (Liu et al., 2012). Intrasession and intersession coefficient of variation (CoV) of this technique was 2.8% ± 1.3% and 5.9% ± 1.6%, respectively, suggesting a high reproducibility of this technique. This $CMRO_2$ technique has so far been applied in studies of cognitive aging, Alzheimer's disease (AD), cocaine addiction, and multiple sclerosis (MS) (Ge et al., 2012; Lu et al., 2011). Another promising T2-based MRI method, quantitative imaging of extraction of oxygen and tissue consumption (QUIXOTIC) (Bolar et al., 2011), aimed to measure regional oxygenation. This technique uses velocity-selective spin tagging to separate venular blood from arterial blood and static tissue (Bolar et al., 2011). In combination with ASL MRI technique, absolute $CMRO_2$ map can, in principle, be generated.

Venous oxygenation can also be measured using susceptibility differences between oxygenated and deoxygenated blood. It has been shown that blood oxygenation in major blood vessels can alter the magnetic susceptibility difference between intravascular blood and surrounding brain parenchyma (Fernandez-Seara et al., 2006; Haacke et al., 1997). This concept has been extended to measure venous oxygenation in smaller vessels, which, in combination with regional CBF measured by ASL technique, yields regional $CMRO_2$ values (Fan et al., 2012). The major limitation of the susceptibility-based approaches is that the veins being measured need be parallel to the main magnetic field. The angle between vessel geometry and main magnetic field will cause bias to the oxygenation measurements.

Alternatively, calibrated fMRI has been shown to provide quantitative measurement of $CMRO_2$ as well. This approach is based on a generalized calibrated MRI signal model (Bulte et al., 2012; Gauthier et al., 2011). By having the subjects undergo

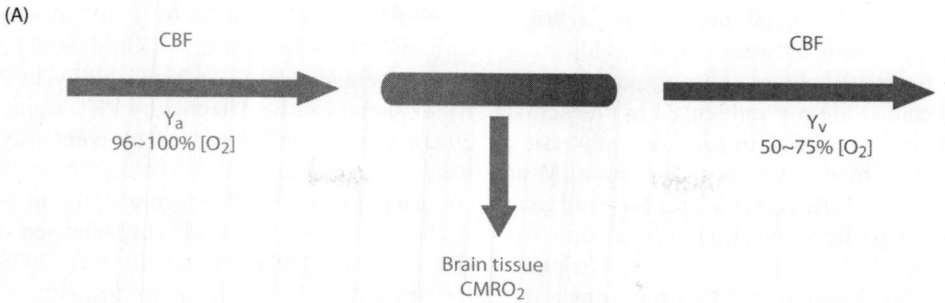

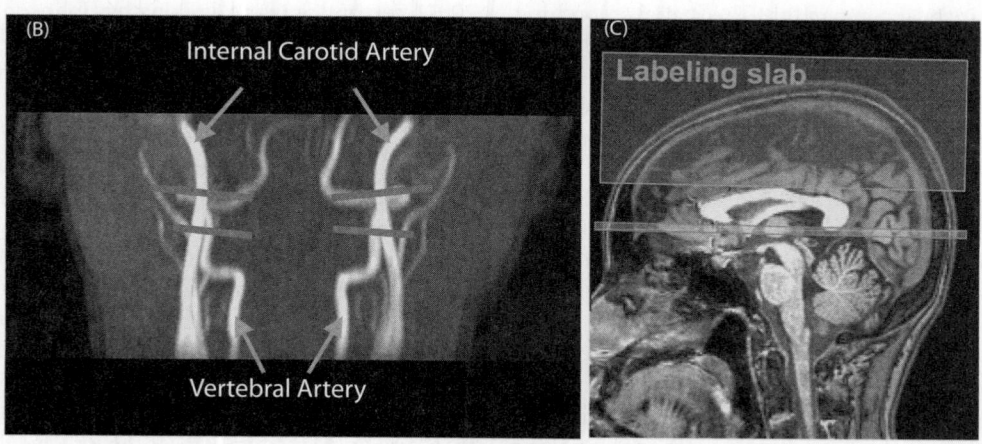

Figure 15.8 Illustration of cerebral metabolic rate of oxygen (CMRO₂) measurement using MRI techniques. (A) Relationship among physiologic parameters associated with oxygen demand and supply. (B) Slice locations of phase contrast MRI for the measurement of cerebral blood flow. Each of the imaging slices (gray horizontal) is placed at one of the four feeding arteries of the brain before they enter the skull. (C) Slice location of T2-relaxation-under-spin-tagging (TRUST) MRI for the measurement of venous oxygenation in superior sagittal sinus. Small rectangular slab—imaging slice. Large rectangular slab—labeling slab.

two physiologic challenges of hypercapnia and hyperoxia breathing, two forms of the signal equations can be obtained. Solving the two equations will provide parameters that can further yield CMRO₂ map (Gauthier and Hoge, 2012). A major limitation of the calibrated fMRI method is the complexity of experiment procedures, the subject burden to perform hypercapnia and hyperoxia breathing, and the large number of assumptions used in the model.

STRUCTURAL IMAGING USING MRI

With recent advances in high-field MR imaging technology and the development of parallel imaging acquisitions, structural MR images can be obtained with higher spatial resolutions and signal-to-noise ratio (SNR). Whole-brain images with a resolution of $1 \times 1 \times 1$ mm³ are now routinely acquired with scan durations of 4 to 8 minutes. This renders to MRI the capability of evaluating regional volumetric changes for various tissue types, such as gray matter, white matter, and CSF; this is especially useful for studies of psychiatric disorders because the involved brain regions may be relatively diffused and changes can be subtle. The typical MR pulse sequence used is called magnetization-prepared rapid acquisitions of gradient-echo (MPRAGE) (Mugler and Brookeman, 1991), and the resulting images are T1 weighted, with clear contrast

between gray and white matters. This technique is increasingly used to assess brain atrophy in longitudinal and cross-sectional studies. The MRI data can be analyzed using one of three different methods.

One method is to manually draw ROI on a slice-by-slice basis and to calculate the volume for each tissue type (Convit et al., 1997). The intersubject variability in head size can be corrected by dividing the ROI volume by the total intracranial volume. The advantage of such a method is that the procedure is relatively straightforward, and the results are less sensitive to SNR and image inhomogeneity. However, this approach is very time consuming, and the operators need to be well trained to produce consistent results. A less labor-intensive ROI approach is to use a semiautomatic procedure, in which a large ROI is selected based on simple landmarks; an algorithm is applied to segment the ROI into gray matter, white matter, and CSF; and the normalized tissue volume is used for atrophy comparison (Rusinek et al., 2003).

A second method is voxel-based morphometry (VBM). This processing strategy first uses spatial coregistration to normalize individual brains into the coordinates of a brain template (Ashburner and Friston, 2000; Rombouts et al., 2000; Wright et al., 1995), so that equivalent structures in different brains are roughly in the same location. Image segmentation is then performed to partition the normalized brain image into gray matter, white matter, and CSF. It is important to note

that, after the segmentation, the signal intensity in the original image is replaced by a value between 0 and 1, indicating the probability that the voxel belongs to gray matter, white matter, or CSF. These values are not influenced by the actual signal intensity in the raw MPRAGE image. This conversion from MRI signal to brain mask value is crucial in VBM as the scaling factor of the raw MRI signal is arbitrary and may be different for different participants. Therefore, a comparison of the signals in the MPRAGE image across participants is not meaningful. The next key step in VBM processing is the smoothing of the mask images. It is this step that creates the contrast between a normal brain and an atrophic brain, which can be used for statistical comparison. The spatial smoothing, in effect, allows the signal in a single voxel to reflect the concentration of the tissue in its surrounding areas. Therefore, a voxel in a thick gray matter layer will have a larger value than a voxel in a thin layer after smoothing, even though their values before smoothing were identical (e.g., both 1). In addition, the smoothing also reduces the effect of regional brain shape differences, which cannot be compensated for in the normalization step. Following smoothing, statistical comparison is performed on a voxel-by-voxel basis to detect the regions that show significant changes in tissue concentration. The advantage of the VBM method is that the processing steps are highly automated, and one can assess the atrophy for the entire brain easily. One disadvantage is that this processing requires the anatomical data to be of high quality, in terms of resolution and SNR, and data acquired using different MRI scanners or different imaging parameters may yield drastically different results.

A third method for analyzing structural images is deformation-based morphometry (Freeborough and Fox, 1998; Shen and Davatzikos, 2002). In this method, the brain image is transformed into the coordinates of a template brain or a baseline brain image. Then the information in the transformation matrix is used to determine whether the position of a particular brain structure is shifted or the shape has changed. Certain indices are often obtained from the transformation matrix (e.g., the Jacobian determinant), and they can be used for statistical analysis. The advantage of the deformation-based approach is that it does not use spatial smoothing to generate the volumetric information. On the other hand, the performance of this method would require the algorithm to be able to detect deformations at a very small scale.

AMYLOID IMAGING WITH POSITRON EMISSION TOMOGRAPHY

During the past decade, the neuroimaging community has seen the successful development of a few radiotracers for imaging of beta-amyloid (Aβ) (Jureus et al., 2010; Klunk et al., 2004; Koole et al., 2009; Zhang et al., 2005, 2007;), a hallmark protein in Alzheimer's disease (Hardy and Selkoe, 2002).

While a relatively large number of tracers have been reported to be capable of amyloid-specific imaging, two of them have made particularly large impact and are the foci of the discussion in this section.

Pittsburgh compound-B (PIB) is the most successful carbon-11-based radiotracer (Klunk et al., 2004). It is a benzothiazole agent that has high affinity to bind Aβ, and the tracer signal can be detected by PET scanners (Mathis et al., 2003). The PIB compound has been extensively tested in multisite studies (Klunk and Mathis, 2008). Validation studies comparing in vivo PIB imaging signal to postmortem tissue Aβ have also been reported, which showed strong correlations (Bacskai et al., 2007; Ikonomovic et al., 2008). Amyloid imaging using PIB has shown utility in many research areas such as Alzheimer's disease, mild cognitive impairment (Forsberg et al., 2008; Jack et al., 2008; Kemppainen et al., 2007; Pike et al., 2007), cerebral amyloid angiopathy (Johnson et al., 2007), cognitive aging (Aizenstein et al., 2008; Edison et al., 2007; Fotenos et al., 2008; Kemppainen et al., 2008; Mintun et al., 2006; Nelissen et al., 2007; Rodrigue et al., 2012), and Parkinson's disease (Johansson et al., 2008). Due to the large number of participants on whom PIB has been used and the extensive experience the field has gained on this tracer, it is now becoming a reference tracer that newly developed tracer is compared with (Klunk and Mathis, 2008). A limitation of PIB is that it is based on carbon-11 radioisotope, and the half-life of this agent is relatively short (~20 minutes). Therefore, in practice terms, the tracer would have to be generated on-site and be administered to the patient almost immediately. The equipment that is used to generate the carbon-11 radioisotope is called a cyclotron, and only less than 10% of the PET facilities in the United States have an on-site cyclotron. This requirement of PIB limits the use of this agent to the few medical centers and research institutions. Therefore, the impact of this agent so far has been mainly limited to the research realm.

The other tracer discussed in this section, Florbetapir, does not have this limitation. Florbetapir is based on fluorine-18 radioisotope, which has a half-life of about 110 minutes (Zhang et al., 2007). With this long half-life, it is feasible and practical for the agent to be synthesized at a centralized facility and then be shipped to various clinical and research PET facilities. This is a huge advantage in terms of practicality and scope of impact. On April 10, 2012, Florbetapir was approved by the U.S. Food and Drug Administration for use on adults who are being evaluated for Alzheimer's disease and other causes of cognitive decline. Therefore, the impact of amyloid imaging has evolved from research tools to clinical practice.

At present, the high costs associated with amyloid imaging remain to be the main obstacle to many researchers. It is estimated that the costs to obtain the amyloid imaging data are several times greater than that to collect the MRI data.

SUMMARY

It is clear that neuroimaging technologies will continue to contribute to our understanding of mental disorders and may emerge as a diagnostic tool and eventually be used for monitoring treatments. Many imaging biomarkers have already been proposed for the evaluation of diseases and to guide therapeutic procedures. Among neuroimaging modalities, MRI is a versatile technique in that it provides a variety of tools for in vivo

assessment of human brain, ranging from anatomical structure and neuronal functions to cerebral perfusion. Meanwhile, it is necessary to be cautious in interpreting and understanding MR data. Although MR images are often shown in high resolution and sometimes labeled in colors, investigators should always try to gain a full understanding of the results and be informed about potential uncertainties in the measurements and confounding factors in the quantification. PET imaging has the advantages of high specificity and sensitivity. With the development of new tracers, this imaging modality also has greater potentials in better understanding the neurobiology of mental illness.

DISCLOSURES

Dr. Lu has no conflicts of interest to disclose. He is funded by NIH R01 MH084021, NIH R01 NS067015, NIH R01 AG042753, R21 AG034318, and NIH R21 NS078656.

Dr. Yang has no conflicts of interest to disclose.

Dr. Liu has no conflicts of interest to disclose.

REFERENCES

Ackerman, J.J., Grove, T.H., et al. (1980). Mapping of metabolites in whole animals by 31P NMR using surface coils. *Nature* 283:167–170.

Aizenstein, H.J., Nebes, R.D., et al. (2008). Frequent amyloid deposition without significant cognitive impairment among the elderly. *Arch. Neurol.* 65:1509–1517.

Alsop, D.C., Detre, J.A., et al. (2000). Assessment of cerebral blood flow in Alzheimer's disease by spin-labeled magnetic resonance imaging. *Ann. Neurol.* 47:93–100.

Anand, A., Li, Y., et al. (2005). Antidepressant effect on connectivity of the mood-regulating circuit: an FMRI study. *Neuropsychopharmacol.* 30:1334–1344.

Ashburner, J., and Friston, K.J. (2000). Voxel-based morphometry—the methods. *NeuroImage* 11:805–821.

Aslan, S., Xu, F., et al. (2010). Estimation of labeling efficiency in pseudocontinuous arterial spin labeling. *Magn. Reson. Med.* 63:765–771.

Bacskai, B.J., Frosch, M.P., et al. (2007). Molecular imaging with Pittsburgh Compound B confirmed at autopsy: a case report. *Arch. Neurol.* 64:431–434.

Basser, P.J., Mattiello, J., et al. (1994). MR diffusion tensor spectroscopy and imaging. *Biophys. J.* 66:259–267.

Basser, P.J., Pajevic, S., et al. (2000). *In vivo* fiber tractography using DT-MRI data. *Magn. Reson. Med.* 44:625–632.

Basser, P.J., and Pierpaoli, C. (1996). Microstructural and physiological features of tissues elucidated by quantitative-diffusion-tensor MRI. *J. Magn. Reson. B* 111:209–219.

Beckmann, C.F., DeLuca, M., et al. (2005). Investigations into resting-state connectivity using independent component analysis. *Philos. Trans. R. Soc. Lond. B Biol. Sci.* 360:1001–1013.

Biswal, B., Yetkin, F.Z., et al. (1995). Functional connectivity in the motor cortex of resting human brain using echo-planar MRI. *Magn. Reson. Med.* 34:537–541.

Bolar, D.S., Rosen, B.R., et al. (2011). QUantitative Imaging of eXtraction of oxygen and TIssue consumption (QUIXOTIC). using venular-targeted velocity-selective spin labeling. *Magn. Reson. Med.* 66:1550–1562.

Bonekamp, D., Degaonkar, M., et al. (2011). Quantitative cerebral blood flow in dynamic susceptibility contrast MRI using total cerebral flow from phase contrast magnetic resonance angiography. *Magn. Reson. Med.* 66:57–66.

Borghammer, P., Vafaee, M., et al. (2008). Effect of memantine on CBF and CMRO2 in patients with early Parkinson's disease. *Acta Neurol. Scand.* 117:317–323.

Bottomley, P.A. (1984). Selective volume method for performing localized NMR spectroscopy. *U.S. Patent No.*: 4,480,228. Washington, DC: U.S. Patent and Trademark Office.

Brown, T.R., Kincaid, B.M., et al. (1982). NMR chemical shift imaging in three dimensions. *Proc. Natl. Acad. Sci. USA* 79:3523–3526.

Buckner, R.L., Sepulcre, J., et al. (2009). Cortical hubs revealed by intrinsic functional connectivity: mapping, assessment of stability, and relation to Alzheimer's disease. *J. Neurosci.* 29:1860–1873.

Buckner, R.L., Snyder, A.Z., et al. (2005). Molecular, structural, and functional characterization of Alzheimer's disease: evidence for a relationship between default activity, amyloid, and memory. *J. Neurosci.* 25:7709–7717.

Bullmore, E., and Sporns, O. (2009). Complex brain networks: graph theoretical analysis of structural and functional systems. *Nat. Rev. Neurosci.* 10:186–198.

Bulte, D.P., Kelly, M., et al. (2012). Quantitative measurement of cerebral physiology using respiratory-calibrated MRI. *NeuroImage* 60:582–591.

Buxton, R.B., Frank, L.R., et al. (1998). A general kinetic model for quantitative perfusion imaging with arterial spin labeling. *Magn. Reson. Med.* 40:383–396.

Calamante, F., Morup, M., et al. (2004). Defining a local arterial input function for perfusion MRI using independent component analysis. *Magn. Reson. Med.* 52:789–797.

Calamante, F., Williams, S.R., et al. (1996). A model for quantification of perfusion in pulsed labelling techniques. *NMR Biomed.* 9:79–83.

Carr, H.Y., and Purcell, E.M. (1954). Effects of diffusion on free precession in nuclear magnetic resonance experiments. *Phys. Rev.* 94:630–638.

Cha, S., Tihan, T., et al. (2005). Differentiation of low-grade oligodendrogliomas from low-grade astrocytomas by using quantitative blood-volume measurements derived from dynamic susceptibility contrast-enhanced MR imaging. *AJNR Am. J. Neuroradiol.* 26:266–273.

Chance, B., Nakase, Y., et al. (1978). Detection of 31P nuclear magnetic resonance signals in brain by *in vivo* and freeze-trapped assays. *Proc. Natl. Acad. Sci. USA* 75:4925–4929.

Convit, A., De Leon, M.J., et al. (1997). Specific hippocampal volume reductions in individuals at risk for Alzheimer's disease. *Neurobiol. Aging* 18:131–138.

Cordes, D., Haughton, V.M., et al. (2000). Mapping functionally related regions of brain with functional connectivity MR imaging. *AJNR Am. J. Neuroradiol.* 21:1636–1644.

Dai, W., Garcia, D., et al. (2008). Continuous flow-driven inversion for arterial spin labeling using pulsed radio frequency and gradient fields. *Magn. Reson. Med.* 60:1488–1497.

de Crespigny, A., Rother, J., et al. (1998). Magnetic resonance imaging assessment of cerebral hemodynamics during spreading depression in rats. *J. Cereb. Blood Flow Metab.* 18:1008–1017.

de Graaf, R.A. (1998). *In Vivo NMR Spectroscopy.* New York: Wiley.

Detre, J.A., and Alsop, D.C. (1999). Perfusion magnetic resonance imaging with continuous arterial spin labeling: methods and clinical applications in the central nervous system. *Eur. J. Radiol.* 30:115–124.

Detre, J.A., Leigh, J.S., et al. (1992). Perfusion imaging. *Magn. Reson. Med.* 23:37–45.

Edelman, R.R., Siewert, B., et al. (1994). Qualitative mapping of cerebral blood flow and functional localization with echo-planar MR imaging and signal targeting with alternating radio frequency. *Radiology* 192:513–520.

Edison, P., Archer, H.A., et al. (2007). Amyloid, hypometabolism, and cognition in Alzheimer disease: an [11C]PIB and [18F]FDG PET study. *Neurology* 68:501–508.

Einstein, A. (1926). *Investigations on the Theory of Brownian Motion.* New York: Dover.

Fan, A.P., Benner, T., et al. (2012). Phase-based regional oxygen metabolism (PROM). using MRI. *Magn. Reson. Med.* 67:669–678.

Fan, Y., Shi, F., et al. (2011). Brain anatomical networks in early human brain development. *NeuroImage* 54:1862–1871.

Fernandez-Seara, M.A., Techawiboonwong, A., et al. (2006). MR susceptometry for measuring global brain oxygen extraction. *Magn. Reson. Med.* 55:967–973.

Forsberg, A., Engler, H., et al. (2008). PET imaging of amyloid deposition in patients with mild cognitive impairment. *Neurobiol. Aging* 29:1456–1465.

Fotenos, A.F., Mintun, M.A., et al. (2008). Brain volume decline in aging: evidence for a relation between socioeconomic status, preclinical Alzheimer disease, and reserve. *Arch. Neurol.* 65:113–120.

Fox, M.D., Snyder, A.Z., et al. (2005). The human brain is intrinsically organized into dynamic, anticorrelated functional networks. *Proc. Natl. Acad. Sci. USA* 102:9673–9678.

Frahm, J., Merboldt, K.D., et al. (1987). Localized proton spectroscopy using stimulated echoes. *J. Magn. Reson.* 72:502–508.

Frank, L.R. (2001). Anisotropy in high angular resolution diffusion-weighted MRI. *Magn. Reson. Med.* 45:935–939.

Freeborough, P.A., and Fox, N.C. (1998). Modeling brain deformations in Alzheimer disease by fluid registration of serial 3D MR images. *J. Comput. Assist. Tomogr.* 22:838–843.

Gauthier, C.J., and Hoge, R.D. (2012). Magnetic resonance imaging of resting OEF and CMRO(2). using a generalized calibration model for hypercapnia and hyperoxia. *NeuroImage* 60:1212–1225.

Gauthier, C.J., Madjar, C., et al. (2011). Elimination of visually evoked BOLD responses during carbogen inhalation: implications for calibrated MRI. *NeuroImage* 54:1001–1011.

Ge, Y., Zhang, Z., et al. (2012). Characterizing brain oxygen metabolism in patients with multiple sclerosis with T2-relaxation-under-spin-tagging MRI. *J. Cereb. Blood Flow Metab.* 32:403–412.

Glenn, T.C., Kelly, D.F., et al. (2003). Energy dysfunction as a predictor of outcome after moderate or severe head injury: indices of oxygen, glucose, and lactate metabolism. *J. Cereb. Blood Flow Metab.* 23:1239–1250.

Golay, X., Stuber, M., et al. (1999). Transfer insensitive labeling technique (TILT): application to multislice functional perfusion imaging. *J. Magn. Reson. Imaging* 9:454–461.

Golub, G.H., and Van Loan, C.F. (1996). Matrix Computations. Baltimore: Johns Hopkins University Press.

Govindaraju, V., Young, K., et al. (2000). Proton NMR chemical shifts and coupling constants for brain metabolites. *NMR Biomed.* 13:129–153.

Greicius, M.D., Krasnow, B., et al. (2003). Functional connectivity in the resting brain: a network analysis of the default mode hypothesis. *Proc. Natl. Acad. Sci. USA* 100:253–258.

Gusnard, D.A., Raichle, M.E., et al. (2001). Searching for a baseline: functional imaging and the resting human brain. *Nat. Rev. Neurosci.* 2:685–694.

Guyton, A.C., and Hall, J.E. (2005). Respiration. In: Guyton, A.C., Hall, J.E., eds. Textbook of Medical Physiology. Philadelphia: Saunders/Elsevier, p. 506.

Haacke, E.M., Lai, S., et al. (1997). *In vivo* measurement of blood oxygen saturation using magnetic resonance imaging: a direct validation of the blood oxygen level-dependent concept in functional brain imaging. *Hum. Brain Mapp.* 5:341–346.

Hahn, E.L. (1950). Spin echo. *Phys. Rev.* 80:580–594.

Hardy, J., and Selkoe, D.J. (2002). The amyloid hypothesis of Alzheimer's disease: progress and problems on the road to therapeutics. *Science* 297:353–356.

Harris, G.J., Lewis, R.F., et al. (1996). Dynamic susceptibility contrast MRI of regional cerebral blood volume in Alzheimer's disease. *Am. J. Psychiatry* 153:721–724.

Hasler, G., van der Veen, J.W., et al. (2007). Reduced prefrontal glutamate/glutamine and gamma-aminobutyric acid levels in major depression determined using proton magnetic resonance spectroscopy. *Arch. Gen. Psychiatry* 64:193–200.

He, B.J., Snyder, A.Z., et al. (2008). Electrophysiological correlates of the brain's intrinsic large-scale functional architecture. *Proc. Natl. Acad. Sci. USA* 105:16039–16044.

Hendrikse, J., Lu, H., et al. (2003). Measurements of cerebral perfusion and arterial hemodynamics during visual stimulation using TURBO-TILT. *Magn. Reson. Med.* 50:429–433.

Hu, J., Yang, S., et al. (2007). Simultaneous detection of resolved glutamate, glutamine, and gamma-aminobutyric acid at 4 T. *J. Magn. Reson.* 185:204–213.

Hurd, R., Sailasuta, N., et al. (2004). Measurement of brain glutamate using TE-averaged PRESS at 3T. *Magn. Reson. Med.* 51:435–440.

Iadecola, C. (2004). Neurovascular regulation in the normal brain and in Alzheimer's disease. *Nat. Rev. Neurosci.* 5:347–360.

Ikonomovic, M.D., Klunk, W.E., et al. (2008). Post-mortem correlates of *in vivo* PiB-PET amyloid imaging in a typical case of Alzheimer's disease. *Brain* 131:1630–1645.

Jack, C.R., Jr., Lowe, V.J., et al. (2008). 11C PiB and structural MRI provide complementary information in imaging of Alzheimer's disease and amnestic mild cognitive impairment. *Brain* 131:665–680.

Jansen, J.F., Backes, W.H., et al. (2006). 1H MR spectroscopy of the brain: absolute quantification of metabolites. *Radiology* 240:318–332.

Jensen, J.H., Helpern, J.A., et al. (2005). Diffusional kurtosis imaging: the quantification of non-gaussian water diffusion by means of magnetic resonance imaging. *Magn. Reson. Med.* 53:1432–1440.

Johansson, A., Savitcheva, I., et al. (2008). [(11)C]-PIB imaging in patients with Parkinson's disease: preliminary results. *Parkinsonism Relat. Disord.* 14:345–347.

Johnson, K.A., Gregas, M., et al. (2007). Imaging of amyloid burden and distribution in cerebral amyloid angiopathy. *Ann. Neurol.* 62:229–234.

Jureus, A., Swahn, B.M., et al. (2010). Characterization of AZD4694, a novel fluorinated Abeta plaque neuroimaging PET radioligand. *J. Neurochem.* 114:784–794.

Kauppinen, R.A., and Williams, S.R. (1994). Nuclear magnetic resonance spectroscopy studies of the brain. *Prog. Neurobiol.* 44:87–118.

Kemppainen, N.M., Aalto, S., et al. (2007). PET amyloid ligand [11C]PIB uptake is increased in mild cognitive impairment. *Neurology* 68:1603–1606.

Kemppainen, N.M., Aalto, S., et al. (2008). Cognitive reserve hypothesis: Pittsburgh Compound B and fluorodeoxyglucose positron emission tomography in relation to education in mild Alzheimer's disease. *Ann. Neurol.* 63:112–118.

Kety, S.S., and Schmidt, C.F. (1948). The effects of altered arterial tensions of carbon dioxide and oxygen on cerebral blood flow and cerebral oxygen consumption of normal young men. *J. Clin. Invest.* 27:484–492.

Kim, S.G. (1995). Quantification of relative cerebral blood flow change by flow-sensitive alternating inversion recovery (FAIR) technique: application to functional mapping. *Magn. Reson. Med.* 34:293–301.

Klunk, W.E., Engler, H., et al. (2004). Imaging brain amyloid in Alzheimer's disease with Pittsburgh Compound-B. *Ann. Neurol.* 55:306–319.

Klunk, W.E., and Mathis, C.A. (2008). The future of amyloid-beta imaging: a tale of radionuclides and tracer proliferation. *Curr. Opin. Neurol.* 21:683–687.

Koole, M., Lewis, D.M., et al. (2009). Whole-body biodistribution and radiation dosimetry of 18F-GE067: a radioligand for *in vivo* brain amyloid imaging. *J. Nucl. Med.* 50:818–822.

Kuppusamy, K., Lin, W., et al. (1996). *In vivo* regional cerebral blood volume: quantitative assessment with 3D T1-weighted pre- and postcontrast MR imaging. *Radiology* 201:106–112.

Kuschinsky, W. (1996). Regulation of cerebral blood flow: an overview. In: Mraovitch, S., Sercombe, R., eds. Neurophysiological Basis of Cerebral Blood Flow Control: An Introduction. London: Johns Libbey, pp. 245–262.

Kwong, K.K., Belliveau, J.W., et al. (1992). Dynamic magnetic resonance imaging of human brain activity during primary sensory stimulation. *Proc. Natl. Acad. Sci. USA* 89:5675–5679.

Kwong, K.K., Chesler, D.A., et al. (1995). MR perfusion studies with T1-weighted echo planar imaging. *Magn. Reson. Med.* 34:878–887.

Lauterbur, P.C., Kramer, C.D., et al. (1975). Zeugmatographic high resolution nuclear magnetic resonance spectroscopy imaging of chemical inhomogeneity within macroscopic object. *J. Am. Chem. Soc.* 97:6866–6868.

Law, M., Yang, S., et al. (2004). Comparison of cerebral blood volume and vascular permeability from dynamic susceptibility contrast-enhanced perfusion MR imaging with glioma grade. *AJNR Am. J. Neuroradiol.* 25:746–755.

Le Bihan, D., Breton, E., et al. (1986). MR imaging of intravoxel incoherent motions: application to diffusion and perfusion in neurologic disorders. *Radiology* 161:401–407.

Le Bihan, D., Mangin, J.F., et al. (2001). Diffusion tensor imaging: concepts and applications. *J. Magn. Reson. Imaging* 13:534–546.

Li, S.J., Biswal, B., et al. (2000). Cocaine administration decreases functional connectivity in human primary visual and motor cortex as detected by functional MRI. *Magn. Reson. Med.* 43:45–51.

Li, S.J., Li, Z., et al. (2002). Alzheimer disease: evaluation of a functional MR imaging index as a marker. *Radiology* 225:253–259.

Liang, M., Zhou, Y., et al. (2006). Widespread functional disconnectivity in schizophrenia with resting-state functional magnetic resonance imaging. *NeuroReport* 17:209–213.

Liu, P., Uh, J., et al. (2011). Determination of spin compartment in arterial spin labeling MRI. *Magn. Reson. Med.* 65:120–127.

Liu, P., Xu, F., et al. (2012). Test-retest reproducibility of a rapid method to measure brain oxygen metabolism. *Magn. Reson. Med.*

Loeber, R.T., Sherwood, A.R., et al. (1999). Differences in cerebellar blood volume in schizophrenia and bipolar disorder. *Schizophr. Res.* 37:81–89.

Lowe, M.J., Mock, B.J., et al. (1998). Functional connectivity in single and multislice echoplanar imaging using resting-state fluctuations. *NeuroImage* 7:119–132.

Lu, H., and Ge, Y. (2008). Quantitative evaluation of oxygenation in venous vessels using T2-Relaxation-Under-Spin-Tagging MRI. *Magn. Reson. Med.* 60:357–363.

Lu, H., Law, M., et al. (2005). Novel approach to the measurement of absolute cerebral blood volume using vascular-space-occupancy magnetic resonance imaging. *Magn. Reson. Med.* 54:1403–1411.

Lu, H., Xu, F., et al. (2012). Calibration and validation of TRUST MRI for the estimation of cerebral blood oxygenation. *Magn. Reson. Med.* 67:42–49.

Lu, H., Xu, F., et al. (2011). Alterations in cerebral metabolic rate and blood supply across the adult lifespan. *Cereb. Cortex* 21:1426–1434.

Lu, H., Zuo, Y., et al. (2007). Synchronized delta oscillations correlate with the resting-state functional MRI signal. *Proc. Natl. Acad. Sci. USA* 104:18265–18269.

Magistretti, P.J., and Pellerin, L. (1999). Cellular mechanisms of brain energy metabolism and their relevance to functional brain imaging. *Philos. Trans. R. Soc. Lond. B Biol. Sci.* 354:1155–1163.

Mathis, C.A., Wang, Y., et al. (2003). Synthesis and evaluation of 11C-labeled 6-substituted 2-arylbenzothiazoles as amyloid imaging agents. *J. Med. Chem.* 46:2740–2754.

Mescher, M., Merkle, H., et al. (1998). Simultaneous *in vivo* spectral editing and water suppression. *NMR Biomed.* 11:266–272.

Meunier, D., Lambiotte, R., et al. (2010). Modular and hierarchically modular organization of brain networks. *Front. Neurosci.* 4:200.

Mintun, M.A., Larossa, G.N., et al. (2006). [11C]PIB in a nondemented population: potential antecedent marker of Alzheimer disease. *Neurology* 67:446–452.

Moseley, M.E., Chew, W.M., et al. (1992). Hypercarbia-induced changes in cerebral blood volume in the cat: a 1H MRI and intravascular contrast agent study. *Magn. Reson. Med.* 23:21–30.

Mugler, J.P., III, and Brookeman, J.R. (1991). Rapid three-dimensional T1-weighted MR imaging with the MP-RAGE sequence. *J. Magn. Reson. Imaging* 1: 561–567.

Naressi, A., Couturier, C., et al. (2001). Java-based graphical user interface for the MRUI quantitation package. *Magma* 12:141–152.

Nelissen, N., Vandenbulcke, M., et al. (2007). Abeta amyloid deposition in the language system and how the brain responds. *Brain* 130:2055–2069.

Ogawa, M., Fukuyama, H., et al. (1996). Altered energy metabolism in Alzheimer's disease. *J. Neurol. Sci.* 139:78–82.

Ogawa, S., Menon, R.S., et al. (1993). Functional brain mapping by blood oxygenation level-dependent contrast magnetic resonance imaging. A comparison of signal characteristics with a biophysical model. *Biophys. J.* 64:803–812.

Ogawa, S., Tank, D.W., et al. (1992). Intrinsic signal changes accompanying sensory stimulation: functional brain mapping with magnetic resonance imaging. *Proc. Natl. Acad. Sci. USA* 89:5951–5955.

Ostergaard, L., Sorensen, A.G., et al. (1996a). High resolution measurement of cerebral blood flow using intravascular tracer bolus passages. Part II: Experimental comparison and preliminary results. *Magn. Reson. Med.* 36:726–736.

Ostergaard, L., Weisskoff, R.M., et al. (1996b). High resolution measurement of cerebral blood flow using intravascular tracer bolus passages. Part I: Mathematical approach and statistical analysis. *Magn. Reson. Med.* 36:715–725.

Pike, K.E., Savage, G., et al. (2007). Beta-amyloid imaging and memory in non-demented individuals: evidence for preclinical Alzheimer's disease. *Brain* 130:2837–2844.

Provencher, S.W. (1993). Estimation of metabolite concentrations from localized *in vivo* proton NMR spectra. *Magn. Reson. Med.* 30:672–679.

Raichle, M.E., MacLeod, A.M., et al. (2001). A default mode of brain function. *Proc. Natl. Acad. Sci. USA* 98:676–682.

Rausch, M., Scheffler, K., et al. (2000). Analysis of input functions from different arterial branches with gamma variate functions and cluster analysis for quantitative blood volume measurements. *Magn. Reson. Imaging* 18:1235–1243.

Rodrigue, K.M., Kennedy, K.M., et al. (2012). Beta-amyloid burden in healthy aging: regional distribution and cognitive consequences. *Neurology* 78:387–395.

Rombouts, S.A., Barkhof, F., et al. (2000). Unbiased whole-brain analysis of gray matter loss in Alzheimer's disease. *Neurosci. Lett.* 285:231–233.

Rosen, B.R., Belliveau, J.W., et al. (1990). Perfusion imaging with NMR contrast agents. *Magn. Reson. Med.* 14:249–265.

Rothman, D.L., Petroff, O.A., et al. (1993). Localized 1H NMR measurements of gamma-aminobutyric acid in human brain *in vivo*. *Proc. Natl. Acad. Sci. USA* 90:5662–5666.

Roy, C.S., and Sherrington, C.S. (1890). On the regulation of the blood-supply of the brain. *J. Physiol.* 11:85–108.

Rusinek, H., De Santi, S., et al. (2003). Regional brain atrophy rate predicts future cognitive decline: 6-year longitudinal MR imaging study of normal aging. *Radiology* 229:691–696.

Schwarzbauer, C., Syha, J., et al. (1993). Quantification of regional blood volumes by rapid T1 mapping. *Magn. Reson. Med.* 29:709–712.

Shen, D., and Davatzikos, C. (2002). HAMMER: hierarchical attribute matching mechanism for elastic registration. *IEEE Trans. Med. Imaging* 21: 1421–1439.

Shulman, R.G., Rothman, D.L., et al. (2004). Energetic basis of brain activity: implications for neuroimaging. *Trends Neurosci.* 27:489–495.

Sibson, N.R., Dhankhar, A., et al. (1998). Stoichiometric coupling of brain glucose metabolism and glutamatergic neuronal activity. *Proc. Natl. Acad. Sci. USA* 95:316–321.

Sieber, F.E., Brown, P.R., et al. (1993). Cerebral blood flow and metabolism in dogs with chronic diabetes. *Anesthesiology* 79:1013–1021.

Sporns, O., Tononi, G., et al. (2005). The human connectome: a structural description of the human brain. *PLoS Comput. Biol.* 1: e42.

Stejskal, E.O., and Tanner, J.E. (1965). Spin diffusion measurement: spin echoes in the presence of a time-dependent field gradient. *J. Chem. Phys.* 42:288–292.

Sun, X., Tanaka, M., et al. (1998). Clinical significance of reduced cerebral metabolism in multiple sclerosis: a combined PET and MRI study. *Ann. Nucl. Med.* 12:89–94.

Tuch, D.S., Reese, T.G., et al. (2003). Diffusion MRI of complex neural architecture. *Neuron* 40:885–895.

Uchino, K., Lin, R., et al. (2010). Increased cerebral oxygen metabolism and ischemic stress in subjects with metabolic syndrome-associated risk factors: preliminary observations. *Transl. Stroke Res.* 1:178–183.

van Osch, M.J., Vonken, E.J., et al. (2003). Measuring the arterial input function with gradient echo sequences. *Magn. Reson. Med.* 49:1067–1076.

Waites, A.B., Briellmann, R.S., et al. (2006). Functional connectivity networks are disrupted in left temporal lobe epilepsy. *Ann. Neurol.* 59:335–343.

Walter, C., Hertel, F., et al. (2005). Alteration of cerebral perfusion in patients with idiopathic normal pressure hydrocephalus measured by 3D perfusion weighted magnetic resonance imaging. *J. Neurol.* 252:1465–1471.

Watts, D.J., and Strogatz, S.H. (1998). Collective dynamics of 'small-world' networks. *Nature* 393:440–442.

Wong, E.C. (2007). Vessel-encoded arterial spin-labeling using pseudocontinuous tagging. *Magn. Reson. Med.* 58:1086–1091.

Wright, I.C., McGuire, P.K., et al. (1995). A voxel-based method for the statistical analysis of gray and white matter density applied to schizophrenia. *NeuroImage* 2:244–252.

Wu, K., Taki, Y., et al. (2012). Age-related changes in topological organization of structural brain networks in healthy individuals. *Hum. Brain Mapp.* 33:552–568.

Wu, W.C., Fernandez-Seara, M., et al. (2007). A theoretical and experimental investigation of the tagging efficiency of pseudocontinuous arterial spin labeling. *Magn. Reson. Med.* 58:1020–1027.

Xiong, J., Parsons, L.M., et al. (1999). Interregional connectivity to primary motor cortex revealed using MRI resting state images. *Hum. Brain Mapp.* 8:151–156.

Xu, F., Ge, Y., et al. (2009). Noninvasive quantification of whole-brain cerebral metabolic rate of oxygen (CMRO$_2$). by MRI. *Magn. Reson. Med.* 62:141–148.

Xue, R., van Zijl, P.C., et al. (1999). *In vivo* three-dimensional reconstruction of rat brain axonal projections by diffusion tensor imaging. *Magn. Reson. Med.* 42:1123–1127.

Yang, Y., Engelien, W., et al. (2000). Transit time, trailing time, and cerebral blood flow during brain activation: measurement using multislice, pulsed spin-labeling perfusion imaging. *Magn. Reson. Med.* 44:680–685.

Yao, Z., Zhang, Y., et al. (2010). Abnormal cortical networks in mild cognitive impairment and Alzheimer's disease. *PLoS Comput. Biol.* 6: e1001006.

Zhan, W., Stein, E.A., et al. (2004). Mapping the orientation of intravoxel crossing fibers based on the phase information of diffusion circular spectrum. *NeuroImage* 23:1358–1369.

Zhang, W., Kung, M.P., et al. (2007). 18F-labeled styrylpyridines as PET agents for amyloid plaque imaging. *Nucl. Med. Biol.* 34:89–97.

Zhang, W., Oya, S., et al. (2005). F-18 stilbenes as PET imaging agents for detecting beta-amyloid plaques in the brain. *J. Med. Chem.* 48:5980–5988.

16 | IMAGE-GUIDED BRAIN STIMULATION

MARK S. GEORGE, JOSEPH J. TAYLOR, AND JAIMIE M. HENDERSON

GENERAL ISSUES IN BRAIN TARGETING IN PSYCHIATRY

This chapter builds on the prior chapter, which described the new methods for imaging the brain. With our ability to image the brain's structure or function, we now have more sophisticated models, or maps, of how the brain works in health and disease. Luckily, in concert with the advances in brain imaging, there has been a steady expansion of new techniques that can focally stimulate the brain either invasively or noninvasively (Higgins and George, 2008). These new brain stimulation or neuromodulation methods work hand in hand with brain-imaging methods in order to determine where to stimulate or to examine the effects of stimulation (Sackeim and George, 2008). This chapter provides an overview of the ways in which the brain stimulation methods interact with, and even inform, brain imaging (Siebner et al., 2009). In particular, we will discuss the techniques where imaging is used to guide or target the stimulation. Before discussing the individual brain stimulation methods, there are several overview points needed in order to understand this exciting new area.

KEY POINT #1

In combining brain stimulation and imaging, is the stimulation being done offline after the imaging (guided by structure or function), or offline before and after imaging using imaging to assess the effects of stimulation, or are the imaging and stimulation online and truly interleaved? Figure 16.1 highlights an important point in understanding how to classify or conceptualize the different ways of integrating brain stimulation and brain imaging (from Siebner et al., 2009). "Offline" means that the stimulation and imaging are occurring on different occasions. "Online" means that stimulation and imaging are occurring simultaneously. In the neurosurgical literature, "offline" scans are also referred to as historical scans, as opposed to "online" real-time or intraoperative scans.

Perhaps the most common method to use imaging information to inform brain stimulation is to perform either a structural or functional scan on a patient or subject and then to use the offline scan to determine where to place the stimulation at a later time point. As we will discuss, there are many different ways to use an offline image to guide brain stimulation, and it is important to know the advantages and limitations of "image-guided" stimulation.

A less common offline approach is to perform the scan to assess the effects of the brain stimulation approach. This can involve either a single scan after the stimulation, or a scan immediately before and then again after the stimulation, subtracting the two scans to determine the effect of the stimulation.

Finally, in some situations one can actually perform stimulation at the same time as the brain is being stimulated. This online stimulation allows one to visualize and understand the effects of stimulation. Currently this can be done with positron emission tomography (PET), single-photon emission computed tomography (SPECT), and functional magnetic resonance imaging (fMRI).

KEY POINT #2

When using scans to determine where to place the stimulation, it is important to remember that *there are differences between brain structure and function, and the two do not necessarily overlap.* Certain scans such as conventional computerized tomography (CT) or T1 MRI image the structure of the brain—its size and shape. Other scans reveal information about the function of the brain. These include images of blood flow (such as flow SPECT, oxygen [O15] PET, or the very common blood oxygen level–dependent [BOLD] fMRI technique) or metabolism (fluorodeoxyglucose [FDG] PET). It is important to realize that structure is not the same thing as function, and vice versa. One can have a brain region that appears normal structurally, but a small lacunar stroke at a distant location can make the function of broad areas of cortex change drastically. Similarly, one can have a vastly abnormal structural scan, say, congenital hemiatrophy, but with normal behavior and grossly normal brain function. It is thus important to understand which type of imaging information is present in a scan. Most commonly, areas of functional activation are overlaid onto a structural scan to allow more precise localization of function. Figure 16.2 depicts examples of different forms of imaging that can be used to guide or evaluate the brain stimulation methods.

KEY POINT #3

In the case of cortical stimulation, *it can be difficult to identify homologous cortical structural sites across different individuals, in part due to morphological differences and varying gyral morphology.* Identification of highly conserved areas such as the motor strip and primary visual cortical regions is relatively straightforward with high-field MR imaging. However, gyral morphology varies greatly across individuals. About one third of humans have only two prefrontal gyri, and thus, they do not

(A) "Online" approach: concurrent TMS and neuroimaging

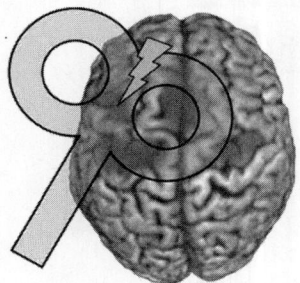

(B) "Offline" approach: neuroimaging before TMS

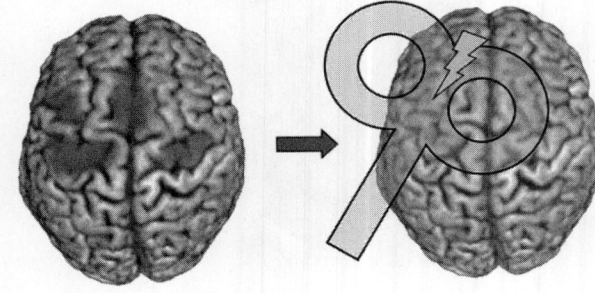

(C) "Offline" approach: TMS before neuroimaging

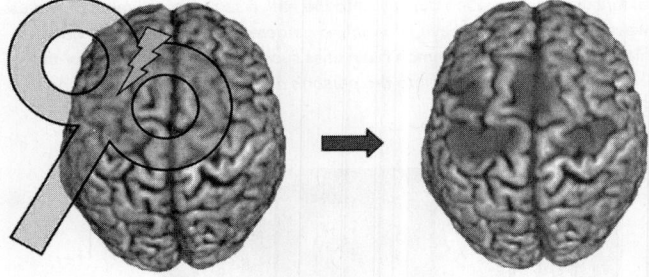

Figure 16.1 Different ways to combine imaging and stimulation. Image A shows the situation where the stimulation (in this case TMS) is being performed simultaneously with the imaging study. This is called "online" or real-time imaging. Image B shows the more common example where the information gathered in a separate scanning session, either structural or functional information, or both, is then used to position or target the location of the brain stimulation tool. This is called "offline imaging." Image C shows another example of offline imaging where imaging is done after the stimulation, in order to understand the effects of the stimulation. (Reprinted with permission from Siebner et al. 2009.)

by definition have a middle frontal gyrus. Even identical twins have widely varying gyral patterns (White et al., 2002). Thus, it may be difficult to guide brain stimulation methods to cortical regions based solely on a structural scan. For a full discussion of these issues (see Brett et al., 2002).

KEY POINT #4

Finally, *should targeting of functional areas be performed using a single scan from a single individual, or using pooled group means from many scans mapped onto an individual's anatomy?* On top of the variation in cortical structure, there is another problem where the functional location of a task varies as well across individuals. For example, the brain region that a given

individual uses to solve cognitive tasks can vary widely. In part the common practice of pooling group activation studies into a common group image, and then displaying that on a structural scan in a common brain space, may have led the field to "overphrenologize" with respect to the cortical location, within individuals, that works to create a behavior. An example of this between-individual variation can be seen in Figure 16.3. Cigarette smokers were shown smoking-related cues while they were in an MRI scanner (Hanlon et al., 2012). Commonly these BOLD fMRI individual results would be averaged, and the results would be presented in a group image with one large area of mean activation. This would lead some to think that stimulation over the location in any given individual of the mean activation might actually influence craving. However, in Figure 16.2 we identified the actual peak locations for each individual. One can easily see the large variety of prefrontal brain regions used in this task. Thus, it may be that for certain behaviors we should do within-individual functional scanning in order to make sure that the stimulation method is in the correct location for that individual. There may be some locations that will stimulate a certain majority of individuals. There are additional concerns about the repeatability of the fMRI activation maps over time within individuals (Johnson et al., 2004), especially after they have learned or practiced a task.

With these guiding principles discussed or at least outlined, it is now worthwhile to examine exactly how the different brain stimulation methods have been combined with neuroimaging tools.

ISSUES FOR SPECIFIC BRAIN STIMULATION METHODOLOGIES

We will start with the least invasive of the brain stimulation methods, transcranial direct current stimulation (tDCS) and then proceed in terms of level of invasiveness, ending with deep brain stimulation (DBS). For each of these methods, we will discuss studies with offline scanning used to target or direct the device, then summarize studies with offline scanning illuminating what effect the device has on functional imaging scans, and finally discuss true online scanning.

TRANSCRANIAL DIRECT CURRENT STIMULATION

DESCRIPTION

tDCS involves placing two electrodes on the scalp and passing a small (usually 12 V) direct current between them. This remarkably simple technology has been around for over 100 years but has recently undergone a renaissance (Higgins and George, 2008). As current passes through the brain, it attempts to exit under the anode, causing the underlying cortex to become increasingly active (Nitsche et al., 2008). The opposite is true of the cathode. Areas under the cathode are largely inhibited in their function. If tDCS is applied to the scalp (and thus underneath to the brain), there is no immediately observable behavior change. In contrast to direct electrical stimulation, deep brain stimulation, or even transcranial magnetic stimulation (TMS), from the standpoint of changed external behavior,

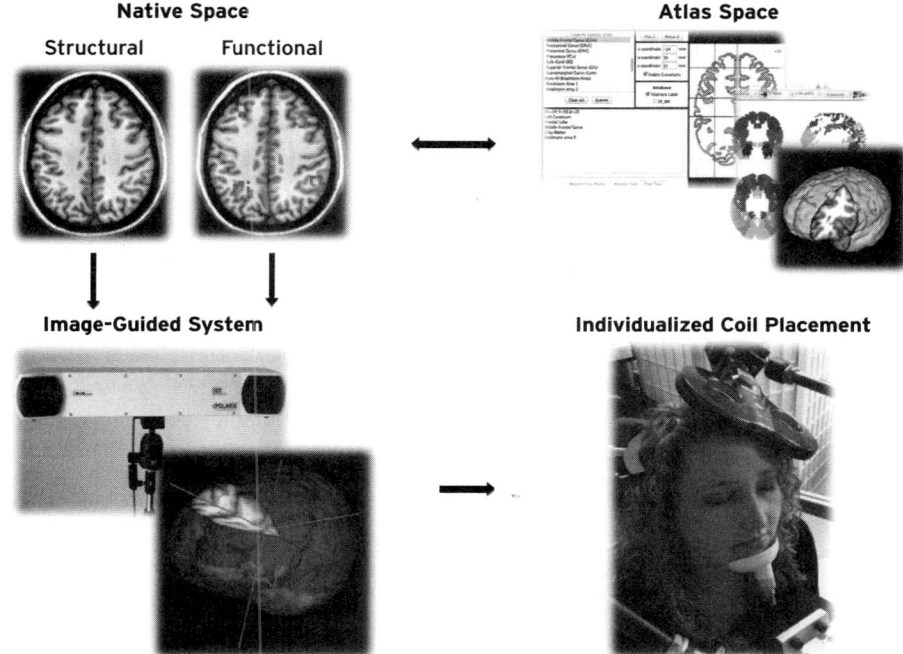

Figure 16.2 *These are different ways that one can go from an image to targeting the stimulation method. At the far left is a structural scan. Commercial systems can then directly position the stimulation method over the skull in order to accurately stimulate the intended region. Because this image remains in the person's native space, there is little distortion and high fidelity. One can also overlay individual functional information directly onto the native space structural scan and use this to position the stimulation tool accurately for that person. Not uncommonly, however, researchers will have information gathered from multiple individuals. Because everyone's head varies in size, researchers then stereotactically normalize this information into a common brain atlas such as the Talairach atlas or the MNI atlas. In order to stimulate within an individual, this group information must be reverse transformed back into the person's native space and overlaid on their structural scan. This can then be targeted for brain stimulation using frameless stereotactic systems.*

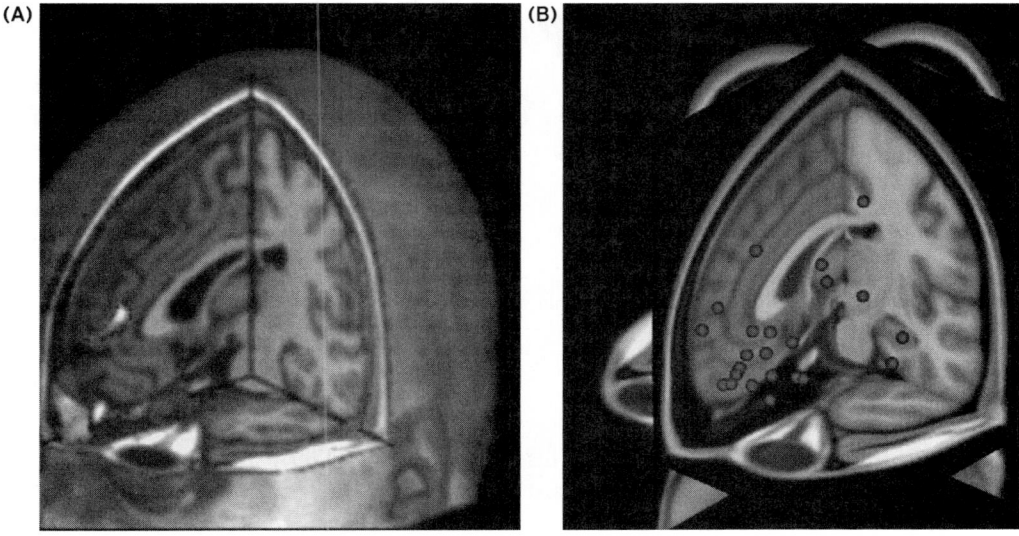

Figure 16.3 *This figure illustrates the problem of between-individual variability in the functional location of various higher-order tasks. Much of the imaging literature consists of images like panel A on the left. This is the group mean area of activation for cigarette smokers who have been shown pictures of cigarettes. It is an area that is activated when they crave. It represents the mean, however. The panel to the right depicts each individual subject's major area of activation during the task. The image on the right is thus the raw data that creates the image on the left. If you were to stimulate the region in the left panel, many of the patients might not have a change in their craving, because their functional circuit varies widely from the group mean (seen on the scatter image to the right). This problem lies at the heart of how to use imaging to guide the brain stimulation treatments in a variety of disorders. (Reprinted with permission from Hanlon et al., 2012.)*

nothing much happens during tDCS exposure. However, depending on the task being performed, and the region, tDCS can consistently either augment or subtly inhibit the activity within that brain region and thus influence performance and behaviors that rely on that brain region. Thus, tDCS is not really a brain stimulation method (stimulation here meaning directly causing neurons to depolarize due to an external stimulation) and is more of a neuromodulator (meaning that it changes the natural firing rates of a brain region). Some conceptualize the energy of tDCS like the effects of a catalyst on a chemical reaction. The presence of anodal tDCS requires less energy for the brain region to do its function (Molaee-Ardekani et al., in press; Nitsche et al., 2007, 2008; Pena-Gomez et al., 2011; Stagg et al., 2011).

In general the pads are large, 2 × 2 cm sponges soaked in saline. These are secured on the head with straps. One group has developed a novel ring architecture that can provide more focal cortical stimulation, with the cathodes externally surrounding a central anode (Datta et al., 2008). However, even with this advance, tDCS is the most spatially crude of the current brain stimulation tools.

COMPUTER MODELS
Because of its simple design, with an MRI scan of a subject one can then model the likely flow of the tDCS current with different electrodes. This type of modeling was initially performed with time-intensive massive computers. Newer advances have reduced the time needed for these modeled maps.

OFFLINE TARGETING FOR PLACEMENT
Some investigators are using MRI image–generated maps to adjust the tDCS sponges in order to make sure current is flowing in the intended brain regions (see Datta et al., 2011; Turkeltaub et al., 2011)

OFFLINE IMAGING OF THE EFFECTS
Some of the most interesting imaging studies of tDCS have involved using MR spectroscopy to measure GABA or glutamate after subjects have received a standard tDCS dose. Excitatory (anodal) tDCS causes locally reduced GABA while inhibitory (cathodal) stimulation causes reduced glutamatergic neuronal activity with a highly correlated reduction in GABA (Stagg et al., 2009).

ONLINE INTERLEAVED SCANNING
There have not been many studies using tDCS during scanning, in part due to technical issues of artifacts, although there is one commercially available system (Pena-Gomez et al., 2011).

TRANSCRANIAL MAGNETIC STIMULATION

DESCRIPTION
Transcranial magnetic stimulation (TMS) allows for focal brain stimulation noninvasively from outside of the skull. An external electromagnet is pulsed and creates a powerful (1–3 T) magnetic field that passes unimpeded through the skull. When the magnetic field encounters neurons, it creates a charge in them and causes depolarization. Because the magnetic field declines exponentially with distance from the coil, most TMS coils are only able to stimulate the superficial areas of the cortex. There is ongoing debate about how to design coils that can penetrate deeper into the brain. Most researchers agree that there is a depth/focality tradeoff, meaning that the deeper in the brain one penetrates with TMS, the less focal one can be (Deng et al., 2012; Peterchev et al., 2011).

A single TMS pulse over the motor area can produce a twitch or movement in the contralateral body. The electrical dose needed within the electromagnet to cause a thumb twitch (called the motor threshold [MT]) varies considerably across individuals but is remarkably constant within an individual over time. Early MRI structural studies found that about 60% of the between-individual variance in MT is accounted for by the distance from the skull to cortex (Kozel et al., 2000; McConnell et al., 2001). It is harder to determine how much TMS energy is needed to stimulate other "behaviorally silent" brain regions outside of the motor strip. In early MRI work with elderly subjects, we determined that 120% of the MT would likely result in a prefrontal dose of TMS sufficient to excite the prefrontal cortex, and thus 120% MT is commonly used in TMS depression treatment (Nahas et al., 2004).

COMPUTER MODELS
The Deng study cited earlier is the most extensive series of computer models to date of TMS. In early work in the field, researchers were able to actually use the MRI scanner to image the magnetic field distortions caused by the TMS coil (Bohning et al., 1997).

OFFLINE TARGETING FOR PLACEMENT
There are now several commercial systems available that allow a researcher or clinician to match ("register") a structural MRI scan of a patient to the location of the TMS coil on the head surface, enabling real-time guidance of the TMS coil for a research study or treatment session. One of these systems (Nexstim, Helsinki, Finland) has been FDA (U.S. Food and Drug Administration) approved for presurgical mapping of the motor areas, allowing for safer resective surgery. The fidelity of this system is less than 7 mm difference from direct cortical stimulation. That is, the area actually stimulated by the TMS coil is within 7 mm of where the system indicates it to be on the scan, as confirmed with intraoperative direct electrical stimulation. This system also has a graphical interface that "knows" the field strength of the TMS coil, and then calculates based on the subject's gyral orientation and can render an approximation of the induced electrical field generated by the TMS coil held over the scalp in a certain orientation.

While the technology exists to guide TMS to specific cortical regions, the neuroscience question of where to stimulate for a specific behavior is much more complicated. As discussed earlier, there are within-individual variations in the location, between-session changes due to plasticity or learning, and the fundamental problem that complex behaviors often depend on the coordinated activity of a network of regions.

This issue can be illustrated in the current controversy about where to stimulate with figure 8 TMS coils in order to treat depression. The early TMS clinical studies used a crude system called the "5 cm rule" to find the prefrontal cortex location for stimulating. One of us (M.S.G.) developed this with other researchers in the early 1990s by consulting the Talairach atlas and reasoning that 5 cm anterior and in a parasagittal line from the motor thumb area would place the coil in the center of the prefrontal cortex (Brodman areas 9, 46). Thus, after finding the scalp location that best produced contralateral thumb twitching (which was needed in order to determine the motor threshold and determine the person's dose), one could then put a cloth ruler on the scalp, find the prefrontal location, and proceed with treatment, without having to obtain an MRI and use formal image guidance. Unfortunately, this system did not take into account variations in head size or the location of motor cortex, and it likely results in 30% of patients being treated in the supplementary motor area, and not prefrontal cortex (Herwig et al., 2001). Thus, the field has now moved to systems using 6 cm, or based on the flexible EEG 10/20 system (Beam et al., 2009). An early analysis of imaging studies done in depression studies using the 5 cm rule found that more remitters received stimulation in anterior and more lateral locations (Herbsman et al., 2009) (see Fig. 16.4). A recent large study of the NIH OPT-TMS trial found that with the 5 cm rule, about 30% of patients needed the coil to be moved forward in order to be over prefrontal cortex. Even with this nudge forward, 7 patients still had stimulation in premotor areas. None of these 7 patients remitted from their depression with TMS, suggesting but not proving that they were stimulated in the wrong location (Johnson et al., 2012).

Would personalized scanning be helpful in using TMS as a treatment for depression? This is an area where much more research is needed. A key issue is what task one would use to activate the intended treatment location. Affective regulation of response to pictures is one candidate that some researchers are exploring.

OFFLINE IMAGING OF THE EFFECTS

There have been many offline studies of the effects of TMS. It seems fairly clear that 10–20 minutes of treatment with high frequency TMS (10–20 Hz) causes increased activity (flow or metabolism) in local and connected regions in the brain. In contrast, 20 minutes of treatment with 1 Hz stimulation can cause the brain to temporarily decrease activity (Speer et al., 2000). These early PET studies mirrored the effects seen with TMS over the motor cortex measured electrophysiologically, and they are one of the cornerstones of knowledge about how to use TMS to temporarily excite or inhibit regional brain activity.

Additionally, important offline TMS studies include MRI scans performed before and after a course of treatment, showing no pathological changes in the brain as a function of treatment (Nahas et al., 2000). Finally, Baeken et al. (2011) performed PET scanning with a serotonin ligand before and after a course of daily left-prefrontal TMS. Successful rTMS treatment correlated positively with 5-HT(2A) receptor binding in the DLPFC bilaterally and correlated negatively with right-hippocampal 5-HT(2A) receptor uptake values. This type of imaging study reminds readers that the brain stimulation methods are really tools to change focal pharmacology (Baeken et al., 2011).

ONLINE INTERLEAVED SCANNING— COMBINING TMS WITH IMAGING

TMS can be performed inside the PET camera, producing truly interleaved online images of the local and distributed effects of the TMS pulse (Fox et al., 1997). Although there was initial controversy about the effect of the TMS pulse on the PET cameras, this has largely been resolved.

TMS can also be performed within an MRI scanner. This was initially thought to be impossible and unsafe, due to interactions between the TMS magnetic field and the MRI scanner's field. There are some restrictions on what can be done (only figure 8 coils, biphasic pulses, etc.); however, truly interleaved TMS fMRI is possible (Bohning et al., 1999, 2000). These early imaging studies were important as they allowed researchers to determine the full brain effect of a TMS pulse. It appears that a TMS pulse results in brain metabolic changes that are similar in magnitude and extent to normal brain activity that results in a thought or produces a movement. Figure 16.5 shows the ways that interleaved TMS-fMRI can be used to precisely stimulate the appropriate region of the brain, and then, using the MRI scanner, to monitor the effects of the stimulation.

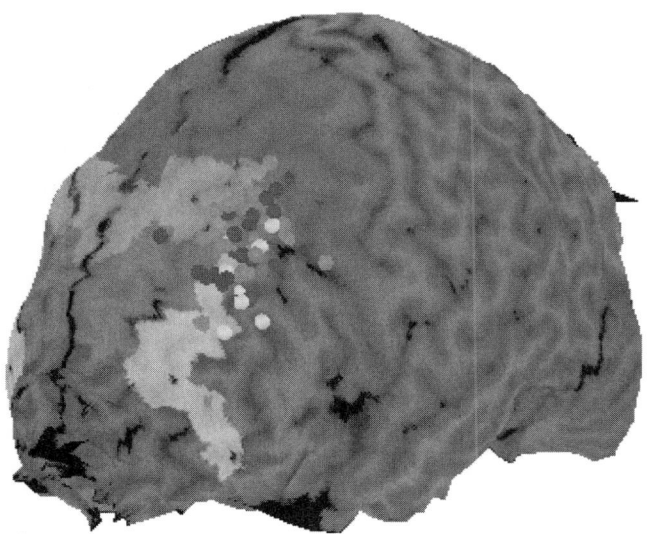

Figure 16.4 *This figure illustrates the need for better positioning of the TMS coil for treating depression. David Avery and colleagues gathered structural MRI scans in all depressed patients being treated in double-blind trial of TMS for depression. The scalp location was determined using the rigid 5 cm rule, where the coil was placed 5 cm anterior from the best location for stimulating the thumb. Note the spread of the location when the data are all presented in a common atlas space. About one third of the patients were treated in supplementary motor areas (dark gray shaded areas). Patients who received placebo are in dark gray shaded circles. There were no placebo remitters. Patients who received active TMS are in light gray shaded circles, with active remitters in white shaded circles. The actively treated patients who remitted, on average, were treated at a location more anterior and more lateral than those who did not remit. This has led to adjustments in the way TMS coils are placed for treatment, with most methods now resulting in treatment more anterior and lateral than in early studies. (Reprinted with permission from Herbsman et al., 2009.)*

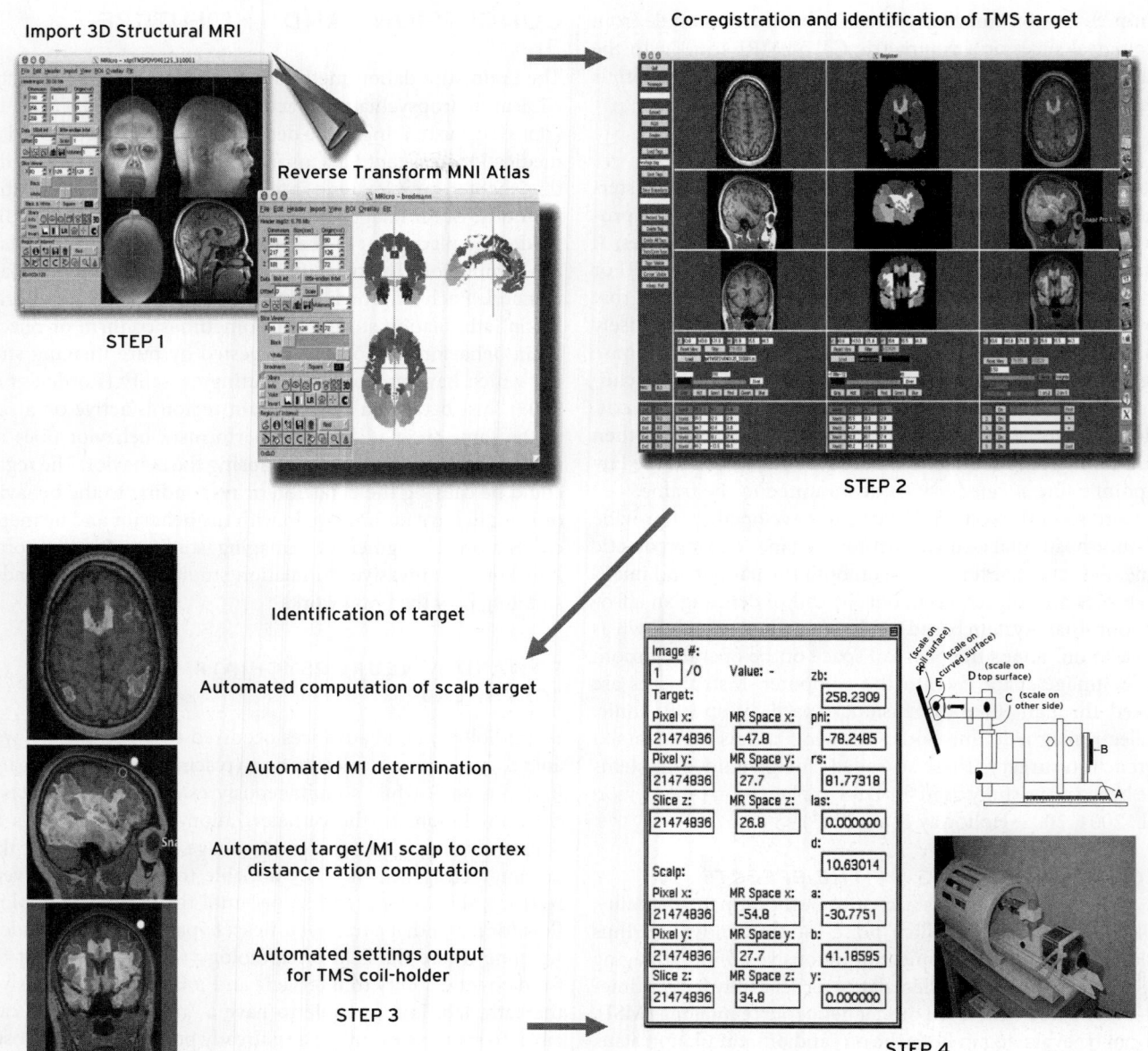

Figure 16.5 *This image depicts how one can precisely position the TMS coil for accurate online stimulation within the scanner. Essentially, the person's native-space MRI scan is seeded with the data that describe the different Brodman areas. One can then determine on the person's scan, with the Brodman information loaded onto it, where to stimulate. These coordinates are then entered into a program that will calculate where on the scalp to position the coil, and that will then enter the correct adjustments to be made into the TMS coil holder. We call this "point and shoot." This approach has been reduced to a robot for PET studies. It is difficult, though not impossible, to build robots that work within the MRI suite that might do the same thing.*

DBS

DESCRIPTION

Deep brain stimulation involves implanting electrodes into subcortical structures for the treatment of neurological and psychiatric disorders. It has been used in various forms since the 1950s, although it has only been since the late 1980s that chronically implanted systems have been widely available (Hariz et al., 2010). A linear array of electrodes (known as a "lead") is implanted into the target site using stereotactic surgical technique, and attached to an implantable pulse generator that provides continuous or intermittent pulsed electrical stimuli. Using an external programmer, the stimulation frequency, pulse width, and amplitude can all be dynamically adjusted. DBS is approved by the FDA for the treatment of Parkinson's disease and tremor and is currently under investigation for use in the treatment of psychiatric disorders (Greenberg et al., 2008; Lozano et al., 2012).

COMPUTER MODELS

Stereotactic technique (from the Greek "στερεός," meaning "solid," and "τακτική," meaning "ability in disposition") is a method for introducing a therapeutic intervention to a particular three-dimensional location within the body, or more frequently, the brain. It involves correlating a target chosen

from preoperative image modality (either an atlas made from histological slices or a volumetric CT or MRI scan) with the analogous location in the target organ of interest. DBS is thus an inherently image-guided therapy.

OFFLINE TARGETING FOR PLACEMENT
DBS electrodes are most commonly introduced using a stereotactic frame, which mounts to the patient's head and provides mechanical adjustments in three orthogonal planes. A system of rods or markers, which can be imaged with MRI or CT (known as "fiducials"), provides a reference system that allows any point within the cranial volume to be precisely defined in three-dimensional space with reference to the base ring of the stereotactic frame. Once this target point is chosen, specialized software generates the settings for each axis, which are then entered into the frame. A burr hole is then made through the skull, and the lead is introduced to the target point using a trajectory guide mounted to the frame.

More recently, systems have been developed that provide real-time positional feedback without reliance on a stereotactic frame. Fiducial markers visible on both the patient and imaging studies are still required, but instead of defining an absolute coordinate system based on the frame, a process known as "registration" aligns the physical space of the operating room to the "image space" within the computer. Instruments are tracked through three-dimensional space by optical, sonic, or electromagnetic methods, allowing a less constrained approach to surgery. These so-called "image-guided" systems have been successfully used for DBS implantation (Henderson et al., 2004, 2005; Holloway et al., 2005).

OFFLINE IMAGING OF THE EFFECTS
DBS is commonly used as a continuous treatment modality, unlike rTMS or tDCS, which pulse intermittently, and thus could be thought of as being continuously "online." Imaging modalities such as PET collect data over relatively longer timescales compared with fMRI or magnetic source imaging (MSI), and can be evaluated in both the on- and off-stimulation state. Many such studies have been carried out in patients undergoing DBS for various indications (Ballanger et al., 2009). PET has been successfully used to image the effects of DBS in the treatment of depression, showing normalization of prefrontal metabolic changes similar to those seen during other effective treatments (Mayberg et al., 2005).

ONLINE INTERLEAVED SCANNING
Since DBS systems consist of electrically conducting wires and electronic pulse generators, the introduction of strong magnetic fields such as those used for MRI scanning could induce current or heating. Patients with implanted DBS systems might thus be at risk for serious complications (Henderson et al., 2005), potentially limiting the use of functional MRI. Despite these concerns, several investigators have used fMRI to evaluate the effects of DBS in patients with movement disorders and chronic pain (Jech et al., 2001; Rezai et al., 1999; Stefurak et al., 2003). fMRI has thus far not been performed in patients undergoing DBS for the treatment of psychiatric disorders.

CONCLUSIONS AND THE FUTURE

The brain stimulation methods are now making an impact in clinical neuropsychiatric practice, with prefrontal TMS FDA approved for treating acute depression, and DBS approved for medication-resistant Parkinson's disease. We have reviewed in this chapter how imaging informs the use of the stimulation methods. Brain images can either provide the road map that guides the placement of the stimulator or assess the effects of the stimulation. The two—imaging and stimulation—go hand in hand. Each improves the other. "Knockout or temporary lesion" stimulation studies can sometimes confirm or reject a brain behavior relationship suggested by pure imaging studies, which have problems attributing causality (Rorden et al., 2008). Just because a certain brain region is active on a scan at the same time as someone performs a behavior does not mean that that brain region is causing the behavior. The region could be causing the behavior, or responding to the behavior, or it could have nothing to do with the behavior and be merely correlational. Augmenting imaging studies with temporary knockout noninvasive stimulation studies can help in understanding how the brain works.

TOWARD A NEUROPSYCHIATRIC "CATH. LAB?"

In cardiology, rapid advances occurred when physicians were able to perform an intervention (placing a stent or expanding an artery) while simultaneously examining the effects of the stimulation. In the catheterization lab, cardiologists are constantly using fluoroscopy to image the heart while they are interacting with it. They are able to diagnose, intervene, reimage, reintervene, and so on, until they achieve full blood flow (or deem that a full open-heart bypass surgery is needed). Imagine where the field of cardiology would be without this fundamental ability to intervene and image simultaneously in the cath. lab. Is it possible to have a "neuropsychiatric cath. lab"? To a simple extent, this is already possible, and neurosurgeons or interventional neuroradiologists do investigate aneurysms and strokes in a catheter lab environment. But problems with blood flow are not the main issue in many neuropsychiatric diseases that are not caused by acute problems with blood flow. Rather, the problem is one of abnormal or pathological activity of a circuit or system (e.g., the fear circuitry in anxiety disorders, mood regulation circuitry in depression, motor movement in Parkinson's disease, craving circuits in the addictions). Imagine having an imaging tool (like BOLD fMRI) that could quickly assess circuit behavior within an individual, and the psychiatrist or neurologist can then stimulate within the scanner in a manner that will produce long-term potentiation (LTP)–like or long-term depression (LTD)–like changes that would alter the function of the circuit. One could then immediately reimage the activity of the circuit with real-time output (Johnson et al., 2012) and continue to intervene until the circuit behaved normally. The studies reviewed in this chapter demonstrate that for some issues the field is not far from creating such an environment. However, in other areas, there is much work to be done before such a dream could be realized.

Only more research will tell us if combined imaging/stimulation approaches might eventually treat some, many, or most psychiatric diseases.

DISCLOSURES

Dr. George has no equity ownership in any device or pharmaceutical company.

He does occasionally consult with industry, although he has not accepted consulting fees from anyone who manufactures a TMS device, because of his role in NIH and DOD/VA studies evaluating this technology. His total industry-related compensation per year is less than 10% of his total university salary.

Current or Recent (within past two years)
Pharmaceutical Companies
None
Imaging and Stimulation Device Companies
Brainsonix (TMS): Consultant (unpaid)
Brainsway (TMS): Consultant (unpaid), Research Grant
Cephos (fMRI deception): Consultant (unpaid), MUSC owns patent rights
Mecta (ECT): Consultant (unpaid), Research Grant
Neuronetics (TMS): Consultant (unpaid), company donated equipment for OPT-TMS trial, VA antisuicide study
Cervel/ NeoStim (TMS): Consultant (unpaid), Research Grant
NeoSync (TMS): Consultant (unpaid), Research Grant
PureTech Ventures (tDCS, others): Consultant
Publishing Firms
American Psychiatric Press: Two recent books
Elsevier Press: Journal Editor
Lippincott: One recent book and a second edition
Wiley: One recent book
MUSC has filed eight patents or invention disclosures in my name regarding brain imaging and stimulation.

Mr. Taylor has no conflicts of interest to disclose. He is funded by NIDA (1F30DA033748-01).

Dr. Henderson serves on the Advisory Board of Nevro Corp. (stock options) and Circuit Therapeutics (stock options). He has also served in a consulting role for Proteus Biomedical (stock options). Stanford University receives support from Medtronic, Inc. for education of a trainee in Stereotactic and Functional Neurosurgery, which Dr. Henderson directs.

REFERENCES

Baeken, C., De Raedt, R., et al. (2011). The impact of HF-rTMS treatment on serotonin(2A) receptors in unipolar melancholic depression. *Brain Stimul.* 4:104–111.

Ballanger, B., Jahanshahi, M., et al. (2009). PET functional imaging of deep brain stimulation in movement disorders and psychiatry. *J. Cereb. Blood. Flow. Metab.* 29:1743–1754.

Beam, W., Borckardt, J.J., et al. (2009). An efficient and accurate new method for locating the F3 position for prefrontal TMS applications. *Brain Stimul.* 2:50–54.

Bohning, D.E., Pecheny, A.P., et al. (1997). Mapping transcranial magnetic stimulation (TMS) fields *in vivo* with MRI. *NeuroReport* 8:2535–2538.

Bohning, D.E., Shastri, A., et al. (1999). A combined TMS/fMRI study of intensity-dependent TMS over motor cortex. *Biol. Psychiatry* 45:385–394.

Bohning, D.E., Shastri, A., et al. (2000). Motor cortex brain activity induced by 1-Hz transcranial magnetic stimulation is similar in location and level to that for volitional movement. *Invest. Radiol.* 35:676–683.

Brett, M., Johnsrude, I.S., et al. (2002). The problem of functional localization in the human brain. *Nat. Rev. Neurosci.* 3:243–249.

Datta, A., Baker, J.M., et al. (2011). Individualized model predicts brain current flow during transcranial direct-current stimulation treatment in responsive stroke patient. *Brain Stimul.* 4:169–174.

Datta, A., Elwassif, M., et al. (2008). A system and device for focal transcranial direct current stimulation using concentric ring electrode configurations. *Brain Stimul.* 1:318.

Deng, Z.D., Lisanby, S.H., et al. (2012). Electric field depth-focality tradeoff in transcranial magnetic stimulation: simulation comparison of 50 coil designs. *Brain Stimul.* [Epub ahead of print.]

Fox, P., Ingham, R., et al. (1997). Imaging human intra-cerebral connectivity by PET during TMS. *NeuroReport* 8:2787–2791.

Greenberg, B.D., Gabriels, L.A., et al. (2008). Deep brain stimulation of the ventral internal capsule/ventral striatum for obsessive-compulsive disorder: worldwide experience. *Mol. Psychiatry* 15(1):64–79.

Hanlon, C.A., Jones, E.M., et al. (2012). Individual variability in the locus of prefrontal craving for nicotine: implications for brain stimulation studies and treatments. *Drug Alcohol. Depend.*

Hariz, M.I., Blomstedt, P., et al. (2010). Deep brain stimulation between 1947 and 1987: the untold story. *Neurosurg. Focus* 29.

Henderson, J.M., Holloway, K.L., et al. (2004). The application accuracy of a skull-mounted trajectory guide system for image-guided functional neurosurgery. *Comput. Aided Surg.* 9:155–160.

Henderson, J.M., Tkach, J., et al. (2005). Permanent neurological deficit related to magnetic resonance imaging in a patient with implanted deep brain stimulation electrodes for Parkinson's disease: case report. *Neurosurgery* 57:E1063; discussion E1063.

Herbsman, T., Avery, D., et al. (2009). More lateral and anterior prefrontal coil location is associated with better repetitive transcranial magnetic stimulation antidepressant response. *Biol. Psychiatry* 66:509–515.

Herwig, U., Padberg, F., et al. (2001). Transcranial magnetic stimulation in therapy studies: examination of the reliability of "standard" coil positioning by neuronavigation. *Biol. Psychiatry* 50(1):58–61.

Higgins, E.S., and George, M.S. (2008). Brain Stimulation Therapies for Clinicians. Washington, DC: American Psychiatric Press.

Holloway, K.L., Gaede, S.E., et al. (2005). Frameless stereotaxy using bone fiducial markers for deep brain stimulation. *J. Neurosurg.* 103:404–413.

Jech, R., Urgosik, D., et al. (2001). Functional magnetic resonance imaging during deep brain stimulation: a pilot study in four patients with Parkinson's disease. *Mov. Disord.* 16:1126–1132.

Johnson, K.A., Baig, M., et al. (2012). Prefrontal rTMS for treating depression: location and intensity results from the OPT-TMS multi-site clinical trial. *Brain Stimul.*

Johnson, K.A., Hartwell, K., et al. (2012). Intermittent "real-time" fMRI feedback is superior to continuous presentation for a motor imagery task: a pilot study. *J. Neuroimaging* 22:58–66.

Johnson, K.A., Mu, Q., et al. (2004). Repeatability of within-individual blood oxygen level-dependent functional magnetic resonance imaging maps of a working memory task for transcranial magnetic stimulation targeting. *Neuroscience Imaging* 1:95–111.

Kozel, F.A., Nahas, Z., et al. (2000). How coil-cortex distance relates to age, motor threshold, and antidepressant response to repetitive transcranial magnetic stimulation. *J. Neuropsychiatry Clin. Neurosci.* 12:376–384.

Lozano, A.M., Giacobbe, P., et al. (2012). A multicenter pilot study of subcallosal cingulate area deep brain stimulation for treatment-resistant depression. *J. Neurosurg.* 116:315–322.

Mayberg, H.S., Lozano, A.M., et al. (2005). Deep brain stimulation for treatment-resistant depression. *Neuron* 45:651–660.

McConnell, K.A., Nahas, Z., et al. (2001). The transcranial magnetic stimulation motor threshold depends on the distance from coil to underlying cortex: a replication in healthy adults comparing two methods of assessing the distance to cortex. *Biol. Psychiatry* 49:454–459.

Molaee-Ardekani, B., Marquez-Ruiz, J., et al. (2013). Effects of transcranial Direct Current Stimulation (tDCS) on cortical activity: a computational modeling study. *Brain Stimul.*

Nahas, Z., Debrux, C., et al. (2000). Lack of significant changes on magnetic resonance scans before and after 2 weeks of daily left prefrontal repetitive transcranial magnetic stimulation for depression. *J. ECT* 16:380–390.

Nahas, Z., Li, X., et al. (2004). Safety and benefits of distance-adjusted prefrontal transcranial magnetic stimulation in depressed patients 55–75 years of age: a pilot study. *Depress. Anxiety* 19:249–256.

Nitsche, M.A., Cohen, L.G., et al. (2008). Transcranial direct current stimulation: state of the art 2008. *Brain Stimul.* 1:206–223.

Nitsche, M.A., Doemkes, S., et al. (2007). Shaping the effects of transcranial direct current stimulation of the human motor cortex. *J. Neurophysiol.* 97:3109–3117.

Pena-Gomez, C., Sala-Lonch, R., et al. (2011). Modulation of large-scale brain networks by transcranial direct current stimulation evidenced by resting-state functional MRI. *Brain Stimul.* 5:252–263.

Peterchev, A.V., Wagner, T.A., et al. (2011). Fundamentals of transcranial electric and magnetic stimulation dose: definition, selection, and reporting practices. *Brain Stimul.* 5:435–453.

Rezai, A.R., Lozano, A.M., et al. (1999). Thalamic stimulation and functional magnetic resonance imaging: localization of cortical and subcortical activation with implanted electrodes. Technical note. *J. Neurosurg.* 90:583–590.

Rorden, C., Davis, B., et al. (2008). Broca's area is crucial for visual discrimination of speech but not non-speech oral movements. *Brain Stimul.* 1:383–385.

Sackeim, H.A., and George, M.S. (2008). Brain Stimulation—basic, translational and clinical research in neuromodulation: why a new journal? *Brain Stimul.* 1:4–6

Siebner, H.R., Bergmann, T.O., et al. (2009). Consensus paper: Combining TMS with neuroimaging. *Brain Stimul.* 2:58–80.

Speer, A.M., Kimbrell, T.A., et al. (2000). Opposite effects of high and low frequency rTMS on regional brain activity in depressed patients. *Biol. Psychiatry* 48:1133–1141.

Stagg, C.J., Best, J.G., et al. (2009). Polarity-sensitive modulation of cortical neurotransmitters by transcranial stimulation. *J. Neurosci.* 29:5202–5206.

Stagg, C.J., Jayaram, G., et al. (2011). Polarity and timing-dependent effects of transcranial direct current stimulation in explicit motor learning. *Neuropsychologia* 49:800–804.

Stefurak, T., Mikulis, D., et al. (2003). Deep brain stimulation for Parkinson's disease dissociates mood and motor circuits: a functional MRI case study. *Mov. Disord.* 18:1508–1516.

Turkeltaub, P.E., Benson, J., et al. (2011). Left lateralizing transcranial direct current stimulation improves reading efficiency. *Brain Stimul.* 5:201–207.

White, T., Andreasen, N.C., et al. (2002). Brain volumes and surface morphology in monozygotic twins. *Cereb. Cortex* 12:486–493.

SECTION III | PSYCHOTIC DISORDERS

PAMELA SKLAR

Psychotic disorders disturb particularly human aspects of perception and cognition. The overall burden of suffering for patients, family, and society are huge, and these disorders have seemingly proven refractory to the best neurobiological and genetic experimental strategies. We remain without fundamental clarity regarding many key issues that could lead to improved diagnosis and treatment. There is now cause for optimism. In the last decade we have moved from knowing nothing about the types and number of genetic loci involved in these diseases to having a substantial understanding of rare and common variants that increase disease risk. The purpose of this section is to discuss the current state of research and understanding in nosology, genetics, genomics, biology, imaging, cognition, and pharmacology of psychotic disorders. Organizationally, the first five chapters cover the basic science and phenomenology of psychosis, the subsequent three chapters delve into animal and cellular models, and the final chapters address theoretical models and clinical aspects of psychosis and the neurobiology of bipolar disorder.

In Chapter 17, Morris Smith, Meissinger, and Malaspina discuss the historical evolution of the term "psychosis" and its prototypical disorder, schizophrenia, as well as its relationship to other mental illnesses with prominent psychotic symptoms such as bipolar disorder and schizoaffective disorder. They explain the development of current diagnostic schema, criteria, and reliability, as found in the American Psychiatric Association's *Diagnostic and Statistical Manual of Mental Disorders* (DSM) and the *International Statistical Classification of Diseases and Related Health Problems* (ICD). Importantly, since the current nosology is phenomenological and symptom-based, they discuss directions for the future and ways in which genetics and neurobiology are likely to drive a more refined understanding of the disease categories.

In Chapter 18, Sklar covers the current status of the genetics of psychotic disorders, in particular schizophrenia and bipolar disorder. While both disorders have been repeatedly demonstrated to be familial, until recently they have proven unyielding to standard genetic tools. This has dramatically changed over the last half decade, and several aspects of the underlying architecture—the type and number of genetic changes that lead to liability—are now well established. This chapter explores the role of structural variation and common and rare single nucleotide variation. The overall focus is on understanding that the genetics of these disorders is highly complex, being both polygenic and multifactorial, with the strong prediction that psychotic disorder genetics will be ultimately defined through future research.

In Chapter 19, genomic syndromes in psychotic disorder are discussed by Kirov, O'Donovan, and Owen. One of the most fertile areas of genetic discovery over the last five years has been identifying structural lesions, copy number variants (CNVs), in the genome that predispose individuals to schizophrenia, bipolar disorder, and autism. These lesions generally have strong effects, harbor many genes, and result in multiple phenotypes; the current understanding of the most robustly associated CNVs are reviewed. However, understanding the role of these lesions is a rapidly changing area that will be influenced by neurobiology, clinical studies, and integration with other types of genomic data.

In Chapter 20, the applications of neuroimaging techniques to study the brain in schizophrenia are explored. Heckers, Woodward, and Ongur synthesize a vast literature that includes computed tomography (CT), single photon emission computed tomography (SPECT), positron emission tomography (PET), magnetic resonance imaging (MRI) of a variety of types, magnetic resonance imaging spectroscopy (MRS), and diffusion tensor imaging (DTI). Consistent observations regarding brain volume, connectivity, chemistry, and activation during psychosis have been observed and replicated, but the future lies in the exciting possibilities for deriving diagnostic markers by connecting neuroimaging with neurobiology, genetics, and clinical treatment.

In Chapter 21, Anticevic, Dowd, and Barch focus not on the psychotic symptoms such as delusions and hallucinations, but on abnormalities in cognitive functions that are responsible for some of the most debilitating aspects of schizophrenia and bipolar disorder. Over the years many direct tests of cognitive processing abnormalities in patients and controls have been made. Critical observations regarding working memory deficits in both its encoding and maintenance phase are leading to a deeper understanding of this aspect of schizophrenia. The direct connections that can be made through the use of functional neuroimaging are described and point to the involvement of the dorsolateral prefrontal cortex. In addition, dysfunction within reward and motivation systems are reviewed. Finally, exciting potential links with underlying biology and circuitry, particularly as they relate to the balance of excitatory and inhibitory signaling are drawn that should ultimately unravel the circuit changes responsible for symptom production and disease.

In Chapter 22, Pletnikov and Ross discuss the progress and limitations of using mouse models in studying psychotic disorders. The current generation of models is based largely on environmental exposures, drug-induced behaviors that

correlated with pharmacological developments, or lesion studies, and mimic aspects of the phenotype, but not the underlying pathophysiology convincingly. However, there is great hope for the future in applying the mature and advanced transgenic tools and animal models to newly emerging, validated loci from genetic and genomic studies.

In Chapter 23, Curley and Lewis explore the cellular details of inhibitory neurotransmission, its role in the synchronized firing of cells and networks, and the strong connections with schizophrenia. They discuss the elegant studies that have led to understanding the basic structure of inhibitory neurons, their subtypes, transmitters, contacts, and organization, as well as the mechanisms used for controlling and timing the activity of large numbers of cortical pyramidal cells. Numerous intriguing observations regarding GABA signaling as well as interneuron abnormalities and upstream NMDA-receptor signaling that have been observed in patients with schizophrenia emphasize the importance of inhibitory signaling in the pathology of schizophrenia.

In Chapter 24, exploration of cellular aspects of brain function continues with a focus on synaptic physiology. In this chapter, Grant focuses attention on the billions of contacts through which nerve cells communicate. Understanding the neurotransmitter receptors, ion channels, and membrane proteins that are in play at the synapse, as well as disruptions in rare neurological and developmental disorders, is likely to point to common pathways that will also be relevant to schizophrenia and other psychotic disorders.

In Chapter 25, Kwon, Soda, and Tsai discuss the developmental theory of schizophrenia. They particularly focus on a series of developmental factors that have not been discussed elsewhere in this section including the environment, the role of myelin development, and pathways that are critical to neuronal development and neuronal migration.

In Chapter 26, Gur follows up the neurodevelopmental focus of the previous chapter with a clinical discussion of the proneness to psychosis. Identifying individuals with early symptoms that represent a "psychosis risk syndrome" is being helped forward through following neurobehavioral outcomes such as cognition in high-risk patients. This approach is complemented by detailed imaging measures investigating aspects of brain physiology, and increasingly, brain circuitry. These studies are frequently longitudinal, and the early work has largely been focused on, and will be discussed in relationship to, prodromal schizophrenia.

In Chapter 27, Tamminga and Ivleva review the neurochemical models of these illnesses. The evidence for and against the long-standing theories, including dopamine hyperfunction, glutamatergic hypofunctions, and altered inhibitory neurotransmission, are elucidated. The relation of these theories to treatment modalities is made clear, as well as a review of the current status of molecular targets for both the positive psychotic symptoms and cognitive dysfunction.

In Chapter 28, Burdick, Haggarty, and Perlis review the neurobiology of bipolar disorder. While there are genetic loci that overlap between schizophrenia and bipolar disorder, there are substantial differences between the two syndromes as well. In this chapter, the particular aspects of the clinical syndrome and neurobiology that appear more distinct from schizophrenia are covered, including evidence for involvement of circadian systems, mitochondrial function, and epigenetics.

17 | DIAGNOSIS OF THE PSYCHOSES

LIANNE MORRIS SMITH, JULIE W. MESSINGER, AND DOLORES MALASPINA

INTRODUCTION

Despite the currently accepted practice of separating textbook discussions of the non-affective ("schizophrenia-spectrum") psychoses from the affective psychoses, this chapter considers both illnesses. The schizophrenia spectrum disorders (specifically, schizophrenia and schizoaffective disorder) were combined with bipolar disorder in this section because the diagnostic boundary between the non-affective and affective psychoses is an active topic of debate. This debate, initially sparked in the 19th century by observations of clinical contrasts between *dementia praecox* (now denoted schizophrenia) and manic-depressive insanity, continues to be fueled by mounting scientific evidence of overlap and dissimilarities in the epidemiology, genetics, neuroanatomy, and neuropsychiatry between and within the categories (for review, see Crow, 1995, and Moller, 2003). In order to provide the reader with a broad appreciation of the theories underlying the diagnostic grouping and separation of the categories, their clinical characteristics (as typified by schizophrenia and bipolar disorder) will be reviewed both individually and jointly. The clinical entity of schizoaffective disorder will also be a primary topic of discussion as it represents a bridging of the affective and non-affective psychoses. The scope of this section will be limited to schizophrenia, schizoaffective disorder, and bipolar disorder to allow greater depth of discussion, as most studies of psychosis have focused on these illnesses with relatively less data on other psychotic disorders (e.g., brief psychotic disorder, schizophreniform disorder, and delusional disorder).

THE CONCEPT OF PSYCHOSIS

Psychosis, a mental state characterized by impaired reality testing, is manifested by a constellation of symptoms that have been eloquently described since the age of Hippocrates (c. 460 B.C.– c. 370 B.C.). Schizophrenia is the best known of the psychotic disorders, and many of the classic symptoms of psychosis were originally described in patients that would today be diagnosed as having schizophrenia. Eugen Bleuler (1857–1939), the Swiss psychiatrist who coined the term *schizophrenia* (from the Greek *skhizein* "to split" and *phren* "mind"), summarized the schisms in behavior, thought, and emotion that he observed in patients with schizophrenia which are now mnemonically known as "the four As": affect, associations (particularly the loose associations characteristic of a thought disorder), autism, and ambivalence. Kurt Schneider (1887–1967), a German

psychiatrist, later compiled a core group of "hallmark" disturbances of behavior and thought, termed *first rank symptoms* (FRSs) including delusions and hallucinations, which he emphasized were not meant to be diagnostic of schizophrenia but a useful guide in identifying the disorder. Schneider additionally described a list of *second rank symptoms* that were also intended as an aide in the particular diagnosis of schizophrenia versus other psychotic disorders. One of the most popular systems for categorizing symptoms of schizophrenia is the positive/negative grouping. The British neurologist John Hughlings Jackson (1835–1911) provided one of the earliest and the most extensive applications of the positive and negative symptom model to psychosis (a model he initially developed in the context of evolutionary theory). Jackson hypothesized that the brain is organized into strata of higher (more civilized) and lower (more primitive) layers. He proposed that delusions and hallucinations, the positive symptoms of psychosis, were "release" phenomena seen when impaired higher cortical regulators allowed emergence of unchecked activity from lower cerebral levels. Negative symptoms (e.g., affective blunting and avolition) were "dissolution" phenomena reflecting loss of functioning in higher centers. Multiple subsequent studies, using statistical techniques such as factor analysis, have found that the symptoms of schizophrenia, the classic disease of psychosis, do not fit into two disparate categories. Andreasen et al. (1995), for example, found that the symptoms of schizophrenia fell into three natural categories; they separate into psychotic and disorganized dimensions, and negative symptoms.

Although schizophrenia is considered the classic psychotic disorder and is the source of many of the original descriptions of psychosis, it was recognized as early as the 19th century that psychosis manifests across a broad range of other non-schizophrenic mental conditions including, most prominently, the affective disorders. It was also evident that the symptomatology presented by different patients with schizophrenia is a highly heterogeneous combination of the aforementioned positive and negative symptoms. This observation led to the concept of "the group of schizophrenias." Emil Kraepelin's (1856–1926) dichotomous distinction between dementia praecox and manic-depressive insanity (modern-day schizophrenia and bipolar disorder, respectively), which he primarily differentiated by differences in episodicity of symptoms and the long-term outcome, was one of the earliest attempts to categorize mental illnesses based on observable behavioral phenomena, which practice continues to the current day.

Phenomenology, a philosophical school founded by Austrian mathematician Edmund Husserl (1859–1938), was

formally applied to psychopathology, including the psychoses, by the German psychiatrist and philosopher Karl Jaspers (1883–1969) (Burgy, 2008). Jaspers's phenomenology focused on detailing descriptive accounts of a patient's current subjective experiences heavily based on his/her self-report (unlike Kraepelin, he deemphasized longitudinal course), and emphasized the form of symptoms rather than content (e.g., the experience of visual hallucinations rather than the actual visions) in the diagnosis of a mental illness. In the more modern, Anglophone interpretation, phenomenology refers to diagnosis based on the observation of externally observable phenomena (Burgy, 2008), with a less strict emphasis on the subjective experience of the patient.

The nosology, or diagnostic categorization, of psychotic disorders has been and continues to be heavily based on phenomenological (behavioral) descriptions of signs and symptoms, with considerably less focus on etiology. An area of particularly heated debate in psychiatric nosology is the distinction between the functional psychoses, schizophrenia and bipolar disorder, which can both present with severe psychosis. Despite the propensity for psychosis in both types of disorders, schizophrenia has been considered a primary psychotic disorder with minimal fluctuations in affective symptoms. By contrast, psychosis for those with affective illnesses (bipolar disorder and depression) is considered to be a secondary phenomenon (reviewed in Ivleva et al., 2008). However, the clinical distinction between "primary" psychosis and psychotic affective illness is often diagnostically unclear, as evidenced by the eventual designation of the nosologic category of schizoaffective psychosis in 1933 by Jacob Kasanin. Although Kraepelin's dichotomy holds in the formal diagnostic literature, the validity of this distinction has been in question since the 1890s. Recent studies demonstrating the evidence for significant overlap in genetic liability for affective disorders and schizophrenia is discussed in chapter 18.

Another significant hindrance to clarity and reliability in the nosology of psychosis was an initial lack of a common language to describe mental illnesses. The widespread embrace of Freudian psychoanalytic theory in the early- to mid-20th century, which may have had the greatest impact in the United States, considerably shifted the goal of work with patients from nosology and diagnosis via the detailed observation of behaviors to the identification and exploration of intrapsychic conflicts (Andreasen, 2007). The landmark United States–United Kingdom Study (Zubin and Gurland, 1977) provided a needed and striking illustration of the heterogeneity in diagnostic practices between regions that resulted from inconsistent definition and utilization of specific diagnostic criteria. The study found that while there were similar total admissions rates for mental disorders in the United Kingdom and United States, there was a fourfold higher first admission rate for schizophrenia compared to affective psychosis in the United States versus the United Kingdom. The authors attributed this disparity to the "free-wheeling psychiatric interviews" and prevailing "psychiatric culture" of symptom interpretation in each country. Furthermore, they found that the United States and United Kingdom schizophrenia-affective psychosis diagnostic ratios converged significantly when clinicians used a structured clinical interview which combined the Present State Examination (Wing et al., 1974) and the Psychiatric Status Schedule (Spitzer et al., 1970). Zubin and Gurland's study served to highlight the improved reliability of standardized diagnoses based on operational criteria. It also underscored the underlying similarities between the affective psychoses and schizophrenia related psychosis.

THE DIAGNOSIS OF PSYCHOTIC DISORDERS BY THE FEIGHNER CRITERIA AND THE RESEARCH DIAGNOSTIC CRITERIA

Despite the American Psychiatric Association's first *Diagnostic and Statistical Manual of Mental Disorders* (DSM-I), published in 1952, and second version (DSM-II) released in 1968, there remained significant concern in the scientific and clinical communities that the DSM and other standard glossaries of the time did not contain explicit criteria for psychiatric diagnoses that distinguished schizophrenia, schizoaffective disorder, and affective psychoses. The inconsistency and unreliability in diagnosis that was exemplified in the United States–United Kingdom study (Zubin and Gurland, 1977) remained despite the new environment of rekindled interest in nosology and the movement toward standardization. These circumstances led to the publication of the Feighner Criteria (Feighner et al., 1972), developed by a group of researchers based at the Washington University School of Medicine in St. Louis, Missouri. The Feighner Criteria provided diagnostic criteria for 15 mental illnesses, based on the most current evidence (clinical description, follow-up studies, and family investigations) at the time. Of particular interest to our topic, of course, was the categorization of the functional psychoses. In the Feighner system, mania was classified along with depression under the Primary Affective Disorders, while schizophrenia formed its own separate group, in accordance with Kraepelin's dichotomy. Schizophrenia was marked by chronicity of delusions, hallucinations, or a thought disorder, lasting at least six months, with evidence of a fixed deterioration of psychosocial functioning (see Table 17.1A). There was relatively little detail provided on positive, negative, and disorganized symptoms, in contrast to later glossaries. Additionally, the criteria did not mention bipolar disorder, although mania (see Table 17.1B) was described with a requirement of at least two weeks duration of classic mood and behavioral symptoms, and a listing of exclusion criteria (including no prior episodes of schizophrenic illness). Schizoaffective disorder was also not included although in clinical practice it was considered under the category Undiagnosed Psychiatric Illness. The authors acknowledged the omission of several categories of illness that were coded in the DSM-II based on insufficient clinical data for diagnostic validation (Feighner et al., 1972).

Following the publication of the Feighner Criteria, the Research Diagnostic Criteria (RDC; Spitzer et al., 1978) were developed as a collaborative project of investigators from the Washington University School of Medicine and the New York State Psychiatric Institute. The RDC, published just ahead of the release of the *Diagnostic and Statistical Manual of Mental*

TABLE 17.1A. Feighner criteria for diagnosis of schizophrenia

For a diagnosis of schizophrenia, A through C are required.

A. Both of the following are necessary:
   (1) A chronic illness with at least 6 months of symptoms prior to the index evaluation without return to the premorbid level of psychosocial adjustment
   (2) Absence of a period of depressive or manic symptoms sufficient to qualify for affective disorder or probable affective disorder
B. The patient must have had at least one of the following:
   (1) Delusions or hallucinations without significant perplexity or disorientation associated with them
   (2) Verbal production that makes communication difficult because of a lack of logical or understandable organization (In the presence of muteness the diagnostic decision must be deferred.)
C. At least three of the following manifestations must be present for a diagnosis of "definite" schizophrenia, and two for a diagnosis for "probable" schizophrenia:
   (1) Single
   (2) Poor premorbid social adjustment or work history
   (3) Family history of schizophrenia
   (4) Absence of alcoholism or drug use within one year of onset of psychosis
   (5) Onset of illness before age 40

TABLE 17.1B. Feighner criteria for diagnosis of mania

For a diagnosis of mania, A through C are required.

A. Euphoria or irritability
B. At least three of the following symptom categories must also be present:
   (1) Hyperactivity (includes motor, social, and sexual activities)
   (2) Push of speech (pressure to keep talking)
   (3) Flight of ideas (racing thoughts)
   (4) Grandiosity (may be delusional)
   (5) Decreased sleep
   (6) Distractibility
C. A psychiatric illness lasting at least 2 weeks with no preexisting psychiatric conditions such as schizophrenia, anxiety neurosis, phobic neurosis, obsessive compulsive neurosis, hysteria, alcoholism, drug dependency, antisocial personality, homosexuality and other sexual deviations, mental retardation, or organic brain syndrome

Disorders III (DSM III; American Psychiatric Association, 1980), were "developed to enable research investigators to apply a consistent set of criteria for the description or selection of samples of subjects with functional psychiatric illnesses" (Spitzer et al., 1978: p. 773). They were initially developed as a National Institutes of Mental Health (NIMH)-sponsored collaborative project on the psychobiology of depressive disorders. However, they were adopted by a variety of other research groups and also had a significant impact on clinical work since several of the definitions, criteria, and semistructured interviews stemming from the study were utilized in DSM-III. The RDC, which was partially an elaboration of Feighner's Criteria, defined 25 major diagnostic categories and significantly expanded psychosis diagnoses. The definition of schizophrenia was modified and subcategories were delineated (see Tables 17.2A and 17.2B). Of note, the Feighner Criteria minimum duration of six months was reduced

TABLE 17.2A. Research diagnostic criteria (RDC) for schizophrenia, schizoaffective disorder, and bipolar disorder

SCHIZOPHRENIA
Course:
   Acute-subacute-subchronic-chronic
Subtypes:
   Paranoid
   Disorganized
   Catatonic
   Mixed (undifferentiated)
   Residual
SCHIZOAFFECTIVE DISORDER-MANIC OR DEPRESSED
Course:
   Acute-chronic
Subtypes:
   Mainly schizophrenia
   Mainly affective
BIPOLAR AFFECTIVE DISORDER
MANIC DISORDER
HYPOMANIC DISORDER
BIPOLAR WITH MANIA
BIPOLAR WITH HYPOMANIA

TABLE 17.2B. The research diagnostic criteria (RDC) for schizophrenia

A through C are required for the period of illness being considered.

A. During an active phase of the illness (may or may not now be present), at least two of the following are required for definite and one for probable:
   (1) Thought broadcasting, insertion, or withdrawal
   (2) Delusions of being controlled (or influenced), other bizarre delusions, or multiple delusions
   (3) Somatic, grandiose, religious, nihilistic, or other delusions without persecutory or jealous content lasting at least 1 week
   (4) Delusions of any type if accompanied by hallucinations of any type for at least 1 week
   (5) Auditory hallucinations in which either a voice keeps up a running commentary on the patient's behavior or thoughts as they occur or two or more voices conversing with each other
   (6) Nonaffective verbal hallucinations spoken to the patient
   (7) Hallucinations of any type throughout the day for several days or intermittently for at least 1 month
   (8) Definite instances of marked formal thought disorder accompanied by either blunted or inappropriate affect, delusions or hallucinations of any type, or grossly disorganized behavior
B. Signs of the illness lasted at least 2 weeks from the onset of a noticeable change in the patient's usual condition (current signs of the illness may not now meet criterion A and may be the residual symptoms only, such as extreme social withdrawal, blunted or inappropriate affect, mild formal thought disorder, or unusual thoughts or perceptual experiences).
C. At no time during the active period of illness being considered (delusions, hallucinations, marked formal thought disorder, bizarre behavior, etc.) did the patient meet full criteria for either probable or definite manic or depressive syndrome to such a degree that it was a prominent part of the illness.

(Spitzer et al., [1978] from Neurobiology of Mental Illness, 3rd Edition)

to two weeks in order to exclude the brief reactive psychoses and to include non-chronic cases. To exclude borderline and paranoid states, the "A criteria" symptoms were expanded to better reflect Schneider's (1959) first rank symptoms. Schizophrenia was also

subtyped according to temporality of symptoms (acute-chronic) and phenomenology of the episode (paranoid, disorganized, catatonic, mixed/undifferentiated, residual). Schizoaffective disorder (SAD) was newly included but as its own category of illness, given its unclear relationship to schizophrenia. Schizoaffective disorder was separated into manic and depressive subtypes in the RDC, with further qualifiers of temporality (acute-chronic) and phenomenologic characteristics (mainly schizophrenic versus mainly affective). The authors were not reticent in declaring the limitations of their diagnosis of SAD, stating:

> There is no consensus on how to diagnose this condition, or even whether or not it represents a variant of affective disorder, schizophrenia, or a separate condition…we define this class symptomatically, requiring some temporal overlap of both the active signs of schizophrenia and the full depressive or manic syndrome.
>
> (SPITZER et al., 1978: p. 776)

They also hypothesized that the acute form of SAD may be a form of atypical mood disorder, whereas the chronic form may be more related to schizophrenia.

The RDC also expanded the number of categories addressing bipolarity, with the inclusion of Manic Disorder and Bipolar Depression with Mania (Bipolar I). They note that Manic Disorder might be the more appropriate diagnosis for some "excited" patients formerly diagnosed with paranoid schizophrenia, and provide exclusion criteria to delineate it from SAD, manic type. Hypomanic Disorder and Bipolar Depression with Hypomania (Bipolar II) were also newly included but with the caveat that hypomania excludes psychotic features.

THE DIAGNOSIS OF PSYCHOTIC DISORDERS IN DSM-IV AND ICD-10

The fourth edition of the DSM (DSM-IV) was published in 1994, with a subsequent text revision (DSM-IV-TR) released in 2000. The DSM-5 is scheduled for publication in 2013, and with minimal alterations will replace DSM-IV-TR as the primary reference used for the diagnosis of psychiatric disorders in the United States. To the extent that it is possible, more harmony was sought between the DSM-5 and the 10th edition of the *International Statistical Classification of Diseases and Related Health Problems* (ICD-10; World Health Organization, 1992b), which is more commonly used in other countries. Both systems of diagnosis provide a categorical classification of mental disorders based on sets of defined phenomenological criteria. The definitions of schizophrenia, schizoaffective disorder, and bipolar disorder according to the DSM-IV-TR and ICD-10 are defined and contrasted later in this section.

In the DSM-IV-TR, schizophrenia is grouped under Schizophrenia and Other Psychotic Disorders. The diagnosis of schizophrenia requires the presence of at least two characteristic positive and negative signs and symptoms ("A" criteria) for a significant period over a 1-month interval (or less if successfully treated). No "A" criterion symptom is considered pathognomonic for schizophrenia, other than bizarre delusions

(the authors acknowledge that bizarreness can be challenging to judge) or auditory hallucinations involving running commentary or two voices conversing. The positive symptoms include delusions and hallucinations, as well as disorganized thoughts and behavior; three main negative symptoms (affective flattening, alogia, avolition) are specified, with other negative symptoms listed under Associated Features and Disorders. The B criterion specifies the need for significant impairment in psychosocial functioning. Criterion C specifies that the total duration of the behavioral change must be present for at least 6 months, and may include prodromal or residual periods when only negative symptoms are expressed or positive symptoms are seen in an attenuated form. Criteria D, E, and F are exclusion criteria, requiring rule-out of schizoaffective and mood disorders, substance-induced or causative medical conditions, and pervasive developmental disorders. The subtypes of schizophrenia (paranoid, disorganized, catatonic, undifferentiated, residual) are discontinued in the DSM-5.

In the ICD-10, schizophrenia is described under the category Schizophrenia, Schizotypal, and Delusional Disorders. Similar to the DSM-IV, the ICD-10 lists signs and symptoms, including classic Schneiderian first-rank and second-rank phenomena. The ICD-10 provides a more considerably detailed list of phenomena (see Table 17.3); for example, "persistent hallucinations in any modality, when occurring every day for at least 1 month, when accompanied by delusions (which may be fleeting or half-formed) without clear affective content, or when accompanied by persistent overvalued ideas" can be compared to the DSM's simply listed requirements for "delusions" or "hallucinations." The ICD-10 requires at least one item from a list of four symptoms, or two items from a second list of symptoms, which includes negative symptoms. The former list is akin to the DSM-IV specification that the presence of either bizarre delusions or voices dialoguing or providing running commentary alone is, with appropriate satisfaction of the Criteria B–F, diagnostic of schizophrenia. The most significant difference between the DSM and the ICD-10 is in the duration criteria. ICD-10 requires a one-month period of active symptoms, while DSM requires a one-month duration of active symptoms in the context of at least six months of the behavioral disturbance. Individuals with an overall duration of behavioral disturbance lasting between one and six months would meet criteria for a diagnosis of schizophreniform disorder in the DSM, whereas they would meet criteria for schizophrenia in the ICD-10.

In the DSM, schizoaffective disorder is listed under Schizophrenia and Other Psychotic Disorders. Schizoaffective disorder is defined as a chronic, uninterrupted illness in which mood (manic, mixed, or depressive) episodes overlap for a substantial portion of time with the active or residual symptoms of schizophrenia. It is divided into manic and depressive types, which require a history of a manic/mixed or exclusively depressive episodes, respectively. Criterion A specifies that the phase in which the mood and psychotic symptoms coincide must involve the full symptomatic and temporal criteria for the active phase symptoms of schizophrenia (see Criterion A for schizophrenia) and for the particular mood episode. The illness must also include at least a two-week period of positive psychotic symptoms (delusions or hallucinations) in the

TABLE 17.3. ICD-10 Diagnosis of schizophrenia, schizoaffective disorder, and bipolar disorder

SCHIZOPHRENIA

G1. Either at least one of the syndromes, symptoms and signs listed under (1), or at least two of the symptoms and signs listed under (2), should be present for most of the time during an episode of psychotic illness lasting for at least one month (or at some time during most of the days).
   (1) At least one of the following:
      a) Thought echo, thought insertion or withdrawal, or thought broadcasting
      b) Delusions of control, influence, or passivity, clearly referred to body or limb movements or specific thoughts, actions, or sensations; delusional perception
      c) Hallucinatory voices giving a running commentary on the patient's behavior, or discussing him between themselves, or other types of hallucinatory voices coming from some part of the body
      d) Persistent delusions of other kinds that are culturally inappropriate and completely impossible (e.g. being able to control the weather, or being in communication with aliens from another world)
   (2) or at least two of the following:
      a) Persistent hallucinations in any modality, when occurring every day for at least one month, when accompanied by delusions (which may be fleeting or half-formed) without clear affective content, or when accompanied by persistent over-valued ideas
      b) Neologisms, breaks, or interpolations in the train of thought, resulting in incoherence or irrelevant speech
      c) Catatonic behavior, such as excitement, posturing, or waxy flexibility, negativism, mutism, and stupor
      d) "Negative" symptoms such as marked apathy, paucity of speech, and blunting or incongruity of emotional responses (it must be clear that these are not due to depression or to neuroleptic medication)
G2. Most commonly used exclusion criteria: If the patient also meets criteria for manic episode or depressive episode, the criteria listed under G1.1 and G1.2 must have been met before the disturbance of mood developed
G3. The disorder is not attributable to organic brain disease (in the sense of F0), or to alcohol- or drug-related intoxication, dependence, or withdrawal
Comments: In evaluating the presence of the these abnormal subjective experiences and behavior, special care should be taken to avoid false-positive assessments, especially where culturally or sub-culturally influenced modes of expression and behavior, or a subnormal level of intelligence, are involved.

TYPES

Paranoid, Hebephrenic, Catatonic, Undifferentiated, Post-schizophrenic depression, Residual schizophrenia, Simple schizophrenia

SCHIZOAFFECTIVE DISORDER

Note: This diagnosis depends upon an approximate "balance" between the number, severity, and duration of the schizophrenic and affective symptoms.
G1. The disorder meets the criteria of one of the affective disorders of moderate or severe degree, as specified for each sub-type.
G2. Symptoms from at least one of the symptom groups listed in the following, clearly present for most of the time during a period of at least two weeks (these groups are almost the same as for schizophrenia):
   (1) Thought echo, thought insertion or withdrawal, thought broadcasting
   (2) Delusions of control, influence, or passivity, clearly referred to body or limb movements or specific thoughts, actions, or sensations
   (3) Hallucinatory voices giving a running commentary on the patient's behavior, or discussing him between themselves; or other types of hallucinatory voices coming from some part of the body
   (4) Persistent delusions of other kinds that are culturally inappropriate and completely impossible, but not merely grandiose or persecutory, e.g. has visited other worlds; can control the clouds by breathing in and out; can communicate with plants or animals without speaking, etc.
   (5) Grossly irrelevant or incoherent speech, or frequent use of neologisms
   (6) The intermittent but frequent appearance of some forms of catatonic behavior, such as posturing, waxy flexibility, and negativism
G3. Criteria G1 and G2 must be met within the same episode of the disorder, and concurrently for at least some time of the episode. Symptoms from both criteria G1 and G2 must be prominent in the clinical picture.
G4. Most commonly used exclusion criteria: the disorder is not attributable to organic brain disease, or to psychoactive substance-related intoxication, dependence or withdrawal.

TYPES

Schizoaffective disorder, manic type
Schizoaffective disorder, depressive type
Schizoaffective disorder, mixed type
Other schizoaffective disorders
Schizoaffective disorder, unspecified

MANIA WITH PSYCHOTIC SYMPTOMS

A. The episode meets the criteria for mania without psychotic symptoms with exception of criterion C.
B. The episode does not simultaneously meet the criteria for schizophrenia (F20) or schizo-affective disorder, manic type (F25.0).
C. Delusions or hallucinations are present, other than those listed as typical schizophrenic in G1.1b, c, and d (i.e. delusions other than those that are completely impossible or culturally inappropriate, and hallucinations that are not in the third person or giving a running commentary). The commonest examples are those with grandiose, self-referential, erotic, or persecutory content.
D. Most commonly used exclusion criteria: the episode is not attributable to psychoactive substance use (F1) or any organic mental disorder, in the sense of F0.

(Continued)

TABLE 17.3. (*Continued*)

A fifth character may be used to specify whether the hallucinations or delusions are congruent or incongruent with the mood:
Mania with mood congruent psychotic symptoms (such as grandiose delusions or voices telling the subject that he has superhuman powers)
Mania with mood incongruent psychotic symptoms (such as voices speaking to the subject about affectively neutral topics, or delusions of reference or persecution)

ICD-10 SUBTYPES OF SCHIZOPHRENIA, SCHIZOAFFECTIVE DISORDER, AND BIPOLAR DISORDER

F20 SCHIZOPHRENIA

F20.0 Paranoid schizophrenia
F20.1 Hebephrenic schizophrenia
F20.2 Catatonic schizophrenia
F20.3 Undifferentiated schizophrenia
F20.4 Post-schizophrenic depression
F20.5 Residual schizophrenia
F20.6 Simple schizophrenia
F20.8 Other schizophrenia
F20.9 Schizophrenia, unspecified
A fifth character may be used to classify course:
– Continuous
– Episodic with progressive deficit
– Episodic with stable deficit
– Episodic remittent
– Incomplete remission
– Complete remission
– Other
– Course uncertain, period of observation too short

F25 SCHIZOAFFECTIVE DISORDER

F25.0 Schizoaffective disorder, manic type
F25.1 Schizoaffective disorder, depressive type
F25.2 Schizoaffective disorder, mixed type
F25.8 Other schizoaffective disorders
F25.9 Schizoaffective disorder, unspecified
A fifth criteria may be used to classify the following subtypes:
– Concurrent affective and schizophrenic symptoms only
– Concurrent affective and schizophrenic symptoms, plus persistence of the schizophrenic symptoms beyond the duration of the affective symptoms

F31 BIPOLAR AFFECTIVE DISORDER

F31.0 Bipolar affective disorder, current episode hypomanic
F31.1 Bipolar affective disorder, current episode manic without psychotic symptoms
F31.2 Bipolar affective disorder, current episode manic with psychotic symptoms
– With mood-congruent psychotic symptoms
– With mood-incongruent psychotic symptoms
F31.3 Bipolar affective disorder, current episode mild or moderate depression
– Without somatic syndrome
– With somatic syndrome
F31.4 Bipolar affective disorder, current episode severe depression without psychotic symptoms
F31.5 Bipolar affective disorder, current episode severe depression with psychotic symptoms
– With mood-congruent psychotic symptoms
– With mood-incongruent psychotic symptoms
F31.6 Bipolar affective disorder, current episode mixed
F31.7 Bipolar affective disorder, currently in remission
F31.8 Other bipolar affective disorders
F31.9 Bipolar affective disorder, unspecified

(From the World Health Organization, 1993, used with permission)

absence of mood symptoms. This latter specification primarily serves to differentiate schizoaffective disorder from mood disorders with psychotic features. Criterion C specifies that the mood symptoms must have been present for a "substantial portion" of the illness as determined by "clinical judgment." In the DSM-5, the "substantial portion" of mood disturbance necessary for schizoaffective diagnosis is greater than 50% from the illness onset. Criterion D excludes symptoms due to the direct effects of a substance or medical condition.

Similarly, schizoaffective disorder is classified under the Psychotic Disorders section of the ICD-10. The ICD-10 criteria are similar to those of DSM-IV-TR as they both require positive and/or negative symptoms and affective symptoms for diagnosis, and specify manic, mixed, and depressive types.

However, the requirement for a temporal dissociation of symptom types is specified differently. According to the ICD-10 diagnostic guidelines, "a diagnosis of schizoaffective disorder should be made only when both definite schizophrenic and definite affective symptoms are prominent simultaneously, or within a few days of each other, within the same episode of illness" (World Health Organization, 1992a: p. 90). This contrasts with the relatively specific DSM requirement for at least two weeks of psychotic symptoms in the absence of affective symptoms. Consequently, there would be some cases (without the required temporal dissociation of symptoms) classified as schizoaffective disorder by the ICD-10 and a psychotic mood disorder by the DSM (Jager et al., 2011).

Bipolar Disorder is categorized under the Mood Disorders section of the DSM-IV. The category of Bipolar Disorder includes Bipolar I Disorder, Bipolar II Disorder, Cyclothymia, and Bipolar Disorder Not Otherwise Specified. The focus here will be on bipolar disorder I, as it is the category that is most consistently associated with psychotic features, with half of bipolar disorder cases experiencing psychosis and/or thought disorder. A diagnosis of bipolar I disorder requires a history of at least one episode of mania or, more commonly, a history of recurrent mood disturbances meeting criteria for at least one episode of mania with additional episodes of mixed features, hypomania, or major depression. There are six different criteria sets that specify the nature of the most recent episode, which include Single Manic Episode, Most Recent Episode Hypomanic, Most Recent Episode Manic, Most Recent Episode Mixed, Most Recent Episode Depressed, and Most Recent Episode Unspecified. The remainder of the bipolar I disorder criteria sets apply to individuals who have had recurrent episodes of mania or mania and depression. A characteristic of bipolar disorder that usually differentiates it from the schizophrenia spectrum disorders is its episodic nature with symptom-free intervals associated with a significant improvement in psychosocial function; this contrasts with the classically more chronic course of schizophrenia and schizoaffective disorder, which is usually associated with a greater impairment in and poor prognosis for psychosocial function.

In the ICD-10, bipolar I disorder is similarly categorized as a Mood (Affective) Disorder. The congruence between the DSM-IV and ICD-10 diagnoses of bipolar I disorder is relatively good compared to the diagnostic congruence for schizophrenia and schizoaffective disorder. For example, Cheniaux et al. (2009) found congruence levels (as measured by Cohen's kappa values) between the DSM-IV and ICD-10 diagnoses of bipolar disorder of 0.83 compared to lower scores in schizophrenia (0.61) and schizoaffective disorder (0.37). Both classification systems require a history of episodic disturbances in mood and activity levels, including at least one episode of mania. However the ICD-10 requires a history of at least two mood episodes, at least one of which is manic, for a diagnosis of Bipolar Affective Disorder. This contrasts with the DSM-IV in which a single manic episode qualifies for a diagnosis of Bipolar I Disorder, Single Manic Episode. The ICD-10 acknowledges this discordance, stating that a single episode of mania is "distinguished from bipolar and other multiple episode disorders because substantial proportions of patients have only one episode of illness" (World Health Organization, 1992a: p. 94).

CHANGES IN THE DSM-5

As described previously, no particular psychotic symptom or single illness feature can be used to distinguish who will receive a diagnosis of a bipolar or other psychotic affective disorder versus a schizophrenia-related psychosis; of course this process presumes that medical, substance-related, and other exclusionary causes of psychosis have been ruled out. The diagnostic categorizations of "the psychoses" in the DSM-5 will entail the clinician's determination of the relative duration and overlap of any manic and/or depressive episodes as they occurred with psychotic symptoms. The duration will extend from the estimated onset of the disorder to the time of the current diagnosis and not just consider the current episode, as was often practiced in previous considerations of the schizoaffective diagnosis. For individuals meeting the A criterion of schizophrenia and continually having mood symptoms that meet the criteria for affective syndromes, or where the affective symptoms are successfully treated, the appropriate diagnosis will be a psychotic mood disorder. By contrast, if the bipolar or depressive syndrome accompanies less than 50% of the entire illness duration of psychosis, the DSM-5 criteria will specify a schizophrenia diagnosis. Schizoaffective disorder is reserved for cases who have at least 2 weeks of non-affective psychosis meeting the A criteria for schizophrenia; they must also have had concurrent affective syndromes for more than 50% of their illness course. In DSM-IV, schizophrenia and schizoaffective disorder were distinguished by the imprecise clinical determination of whether or not the symptoms meeting criteria for a mood episode were present "for a substantial part of the overall duration of both the active and residual period of the illness" (American Psychiatric Association, 2000: p. 323). The concept of "substantial" was so variably interpreted that the reliability of a schizoaffective diagnosis was quite poor. Schizophrenia quite commonly includes mood features, which do not necessarily change the appropriate diagnosis to schizoaffective disorder in DSM-5.

Notably, the implicit acceptance of the overlap of bipolar and schizophrenia conditions is not disputed in the DSM-5, but the convention of separating the chapters on bipolar disorder and schizophrenia is consistent with the decision to make only conservative changes to the DSM-5. The need to improve diagnostic reliability for schizophrenia, schizoaffective disorder, and psychotic affective conditions will contribute to the evolution of evidence-based studies by improving the reliability for categorical diagnoses, such as the 50% determination. The overlap of bipolar and schizophrenia conditions is certainly evident in the frequent longitudinal instability of an individual's diagnosis, which commonly shifts among schizophrenia, bipolar or other affective psychosis, and schizophrenia. These common shifts in diagnosis for a patient, between affective and schizophrenia diagnostic categories, puzzle both patients and clinicians, but neither treatment nor prognosis is altered by these designations. It is expected that the most appropriate diagnosis will shift over time, but that the cross-sectional assessments by different clinicians will be more reliable and fewer schizophrenia cases should be misdiagnosed as having schizoaffective disorder based on the DSM-5 criteria requiring

that an affective syndrome is present for more than 50% of the entire illness for a schizoaffective diagnosis.

Other possible approaches to addressing the substantial overlap of bipolar disorder and schizophrenia for the DSM-5 were suggested. On one hand, subdivisions of a psychotic illness into separate epochs of psychosis related to schizophrenia, bipolar disorder, major depressive psychosis, and substance-induced psychosis are appealing to some groups, but have a weak evidence base. On the other hand, quantifying the different symptom domains of all severe mental disorders by dimensional metrics is very compelling; that is, providing separate ratings for psychosis, mania, depression, cognitive limitations, avolition and diminished emotional expression, anxiety, and other dimensions depending on the disorders at a specific time point. These domain scores could shift over time with treatment, brain development, and symptom evolution, but would provide an anchor for description and intervention at specific time points, rather than the constrained longitudinal categorical diagnoses. Again, there is an insufficient database to support this large departure from current practice in the DSM-5.

Other changes in the schizophrenia chapter of the DSM-5 include an elevation of the catatonia concept, such that the condition may stand on its own or accompany a host of other conditions; the consideration of a period of attenuated psychotic symptoms in the appendix, as a route to better understand the adolescent and young adult transitions to psychotic disorders; and limiting the negative symptoms to those that can be observed rather than inferred, namely, avolition/asociality, and diminished emotional expression rather than anhedonia and other negative symptom constructs. The essential "A criteria" for schizophrenia will include two (or more) of the following, each present for a significant portion of time during a one-month period (or less if successfully treated). At least one of these should include 1, 2, or 3: (1) delusions; (2) hallucinations; (3) disorganized speech; (4) grossly abnormal psychomotor behavior, including catatonia; (5) negative symptoms, for example, diminished emotional expression or avolition. The special consideration for bizarre delusions is discontinued in the DSM-5. The "B criteria" specify deterioration in function, or failure to achieve expected levels for those with earlier onset; the "C criteria" set the disturbance duration of at least 6 months (or less if successfully treated), including periods of prodromal or residual symptoms. Durations less than a month indicate brief psychotic disorder and 1 month to up to 6 months are noted as schizophreniform disorder, which may have good or bad prognostic signs of likelihood to become a chronic condition. Changes to the bipolar disorder section in the DSM-5 are notable for the new inclusion of increased energy/activity as a core symptom of Manic Episodes and Hypomanic Episodes.

THE MAJOR RATING SCALES FOR PSYCHIATRIC DIAGNOSIS

Distinguishing between different psychotic illnesses in a reliable way is often challenging for clinicians and researchers. Numerous structured and semistructured diagnostic interviews have been developed to provide standardized ways for clinicians to collect the information necessary to make a differential diagnosis, thus increasing reliability across clinician diagnoses. The most common of these interviews are the Structured Clinical Interview for DSM Disorders (SCID; Spitzer et al., 1992), the Diagnostic Interview for Genetic Studies (DIGS; Nurnberger et al., 1994), and the Schedule for Affective Disorders and Schizophrenia (SADS; Endicott and Spitzer, 1978), all of which have demonstrated reliability (Keller et al., 1981; Lobbestael et al., 2011; Nurnberger et al., 1994).

While these interviews all provide structured questions and prompts aimed at gathering the same basic data (e.g., identifying information, developmental history, psychiatric history, medical history, and current symptomatology), the interviews differ in the diagnostic criteria to which the information corresponds. For example, the SCID was initially developed based on DSM-III criteria and had to be revised following the publication of the DSM-IV in 2000. Similarly the SADS was developed based on the Research Diagnostic Criteria (RDC). As a result the SCID most directly corresponds to DSM criteria and the SADS most directly corresponds to the RDC criteria, which may present a challenge for clinicians who want to apply the information obtained from these interviews to a different set of diagnostic criteria. An advantage that the DIGS has over the other two interviews is that the questions and prompts were written to collect information that allows clinicians to make diagnoses based on multiple diagnostic criteria. The OPerational CRITeria (OPCRIT; Craddock et al., 1996), which is embedded in the DIGS, is a checklist of criteria from all of the major diagnostic classification systems that can be entered into computerized software, which then allows for the generation of diagnoses across the major diagnostic systems. This system allows for easy, standardized, and reliable comparison of diagnosis across multiple diagnostic systems and has demonstrated good to excellent agreement with multiple clinician consensus diagnoses.

RESEARCH DOMAIN CRITERIA: THE FUTURE OF PSYCHIATRIC DIAGNOSIS

Given the overlap of phenomenology, genes, neurobiology, risk factors, and course between the bipolar and schizophrenia-related disorders, it is clear that the categorical diagnoses are not optimal. Nonetheless these are standard instruments for diagnosis, insurance, utilization reports, clinical trials, and even for the Federal Drug Association (FDA). Their use in research, however, may have stymied our progress in discerning the etiology and finding optimal interventions for individual illness features, which can be called "domains" of behavior. The RDoC is a strategy proposed by the National Institute of Mental Health to find a synergy between behavioral analysis and neuroscience that can serve to deconstruct the current and former categorical mental illnesses into their component specific observable behaviors for research. These domains of psychopathology will cut across disorders and will even be identified, to a variable extent, in people who do not meet criteria for any psychiatric diagnosis (www.nimh.nih.gov). The RDoC considers that

a disruption in behavior may be driven by changes in one or more genes that impact a specific neurocircuitry. The major constructs encompassing the domain will encompass motivation, cognition, and social behavior in the first iteration of the RDoC. The specific domains will include Negative Valence Systems (i.e., systems for aversive motivation), Positive Valence Systems, Cognitive Systems, Systems for Social Processes, and Arousal/Regulatory Systems. Each domain is expected to be definable by different classes of variables reflecting neurobiological and clinical approaches; including neurochemistry, cellular systems, neurocircuitry, behavioral tasks, and self-reports. It is furthermore expected, given the lifelong development and remodeling of the brain, that many or most behaviors and their underlying neurobiology will be developmentally modified, as observed for most symptom phenomena in psychiatric patients. RDoC will not immediately be a useful clinical tool, but it will gather the knowledge that is essential for the clinical diagnostic schemes of the future.

CONCLUSION

Over the past century the concept of psychosis has shifted from a unitary model, in which psychosis was considered a single illness, to the current model, in which it is recognized that psychosis manifests across a broad range of separate psychiatric disorders. Current diagnostic criteria (DSM-IV and ICD-10) are largely consistent with Kraepelin's dichotomy and the Feighner Criteria in making a distinction between primary psychotic illnesses (e.g., schizophrenia) and the functional/affective psychoses. Recognition of overlap between these two categories is seen in schizoaffective disorder, a diagnosis given to individuals who simultaneously meet criterion A for schizophrenia and criteria for an affective episode for "a substantial part of the overall duration of both the active and residual period of the illness" (American Psychiatric Association, 2000: p. 323). The diagnostic criteria for schizoaffective disorder are refined with the publication of the DSM-5 to clarify vague wording and increase diagnostic reliability, such that the diagnosis will be reserved for individuals who meet criterion A for schizophrenia and meet criteria for an affective episode for more than 50% of their illness course. Still, there remains great overlap between phenomenology, genes, neurobiology, and risk factors across all psychotic disorders. New behavioral domain approaches to psychopathology research, such as the NIMH's RDoC initiative, will provide approaches to assessment that are not bound by diagnostic categories, which may help further clarify these diagnostic categories over time.

DISCLOSURES

The chapter authors have no conflicts of interest to disclose.

REFERENCES

American Psychiatric Association. (1952). Diagnostic and Statistical Manual of Mental Disorders, 1st Edition. Washington, DC: Author.

American Psychiatric Association. (1968). Diagnostic and Statistical Manual of Mental Disorders, 2nd Edition. Washington, DC: Author.

American Psychiatric Association. (1980). Diagnostic and Statistical Manual of Mental Disorders, 3rd Edition. Washington, DC: Author.

American Psychiatric Association. (1994). Diagnostic and Statistical Manual of Mental Disorders, 4th Edition. Washington, DC: Author.

American Psychiatric Association. (2000). Diagnostic and Statistical Manual of Mental Disorders, 4th Edition, Text Revision. Washington, DC: Author.

Andreasen, N.C., Arndt, S., et al. (1995). Symptoms of schizophrenia: methods, meanings, and mechanisms. *Arch. Gen. Psychiatry* 52:341–351.

Andreasen, N.C. (2007). DSM and the death of phenomenology in America: an example of unintended consequences. *Schizophr. Bull.* 33:108–112.

Burgy, M. (2008). The concept of psychosis: historical and phenomenological aspects. *Schizophr. Bull.* 34:1200–1210.

Cheniaux, E., Landeira-Fernandez, J., et al. (2009). The diagnoses of schizophrenia, schizoaffective disorder, bipolar disorder and unipolar depression: interrater reliability and congruence between DSM-IV and ICD-10. *Psychopathology* 42:293–298.

Craddock, M., Asherson, M.P., et al. (1996). Concurrent validity of the OPCRIT diagnostic system: comparison of OPCRIT diagnoses with consensus best-estimate lifetime diagnoses. *Br. J. Psychiatry* 169:58–63,

Crow, T.J. (1995). A continuum of psychosis, one human gene, and not much else—the case for homogeneity. *Schizophr. Res.* 17(2):135–145.

Endicott, J., and Spitzer, R.L. (1978). A diagnostic interview: the schedule for affective disorders and schizophrenia. *Arch. Gen. Psychiatry* 35:837–844.

Feighner, J.P., Robins, E., et al.(1972) Diagnostic criteria for use in psychiatric research. *Arch. Gen. Psychiatry* 26:57–63.

Ivleva, E., Thaker, G., et al. (2008). Comparing genes and phenomenology in the major psychoses: schizophrenia and bipolar 1 disorder. *Schizophr. Bull.* 34:734–742.

Jager, M., Haack, S., et al. (2011). Schizoaffective disorder—an ongoing challenge for psychiatric nosology. *Eur. Psychiatry* 26:159–165.

Kasanin, J. (1933). The acute schizoaffective psychoses. *Am. J. Psych.* 90:97–126.

Keller, M.B., Lavori, P.W., et al. (1981). Test-retest reliability of assessing psychiatrically ill patients in a multi-center design. *J. Psychiat. Res.* 16:213–227.

Lobbestael, J., Leurgans, M. et al. (2011). Inter-rater reliability of the Structured Clinical Interview for DSM-IV Axis I Disorders (SCID I) and Axis II Disorders (SCID II). *Clin. Psychol. Psychother.* 18:75–79.

Moller, H.J. (2003). Bipolar disorder and schizophrenia: distinct illnesses or a continuum? *J. Clin. Psychiatry* 64(Suppl 6):23–27.

National Institute of Mental Health Research Domain Criteria (RDoC). *National Institute of Mental Health.* www.nimh.nih.gov/research-funding/rdoc/nimh-research-domain-criteria-rdoc.shtml. Accessed July 2012.

Nurnberger, J.I., Blehar, M.C., et al. (1994). Diagnostic interview for genetic studies: rationale, unique features, and training. *Arch. Gen. Psychiatry* 51:849–859.

Schneider, K. (1959). Clinical Psychopathology. New York: Grune & Stratton.

Spitzer, R.L., Endicott, J., et al. (1970). The psychiatric status schedule: a technique for evaluating psychopathology and impairment in role functioning. *Arch. Gen. Psychiatry* 23:41–55.

Spitzer, R.L., Endicott, J., et al. (1978). Research diagnostic criteria: rationale and reliability. *Arch. Gen. Psychiatry* 35:773–782.

Spitzer, R.L., Williams, J.B., et al. (1992). The structured clinical interview for DSM-III-R (SCID). I: History, rationale, and description. *Arch. Gen. Psychiatry* 49:624–629.

Wing, J.K., Cooper, J.E., et al. (1974). Present State Examination. London: Cambridge University Press.

World Health Organization. (1992a). Classification of Mental and Behavioural Disorders, Clinical Descriptions and Diagnostic Guidelines. Geneva: Author.

World Health Organization. (1992b). International Statistical Classification of Diseases and Related Health Problems (ICD-10), Tenth Revision. Volumes 1–3. Geneva: Author.

Zubin, J., and Gurland, B.J. (1977). The United States–United Kingdom project on diagnosis of the mental disorders. *Ann. NY Acad. Sci.* 285:676–686.

18 | GENETICS OF SCHIZOPHRENIA AND BIPOLAR DISORDER

PAMELA SKLAR

INTRODUCTION

This chapter provides an overview of the genetics of schizophrenia and bipolar disorder. Over the last 100 years or so genetic studies have included the epidemiology of families and twins, traditional genetic linkage and positional cloning in pedigrees, and candidate gene association studies. The evolution of genetic information rapidly expanded as we entered the genomic era with important new insights from genome-wide microarray and sequencing studies.

We can expect this expansion in genetic knowledge to continue and likely escalate. This chapter will cover information supporting several basic ideas. First, that there is strong and consistent evidence that both disorders are genetic. Second, neither disorder is caused by a *single* abnormal gene. Third, biological candidate genes and traditional linkage studies proved inadequate to identify genetic causes for reasons that are now largely understood. Fourth, copy number variation plays an important role in schizophrenia. Fifth, genome-wide association studies have identified multiple significant loci for schizophrenia and bipolar disorder. Sixth, next generation sequencing studies are beginning to catalog rare variants and their potential role in schizophrenia and bipolar disorder. Finally, integration of all of the various sources of genetic risk information will be difficult and will require interdisciplinary work and new biological strategies.

GENETIC EPIDEMIOLOGY

Schizophrenia and bipolar disorder are both strongly familial. It is only over the last ~120 years that they have been investigated as separate, distinct disorders. This distinction, based on clinical observations and symptoms, was codified by Emil Kraepelin in the late 1890s. As highlighted in Chapter 20, many clinical and phenotypic aspects of the diseases have long been known to overlap. Genetic, imaging, and some cognitive observations have increasingly converged, and thus bipolar disorder genetics will be discussed along with schizophrenia, rather than among the mood disorders.

Recent systematic re-review of extant literature confirms that the lifetime risk of schizophrenia is approximately 1% and that there is evidence for a modest variation in prevalence when investigated by latitude (McGrath et al., 2008). The incidence is elevated in migrants over native-born individuals (4.6-fold). Several recent studies of schizophrenia using Scandinavian hospital registers suggest the prevalence may be somewhat lower (Lichtenstein et al., 2009). Estimating the lifetime risk of bipolar disorder is more difficult as diagnostic schemes have changed significantly over the last 100 years particularly with the formulation of bipolar II disorder in DSM-III-R in 1987. Subsequent changes have tended to broaden the diagnostic scope and the larger spectrum of symptoms has increased the overall prevalence. However, discussing the accuracy and potential impacts of these diagnostic changes is beyond the scope of this chapter (Yutzy et al., 2012). Recent population-based studies in the United States find roughly a 1% lifetime prevalence for bipolar I disorder (Merikangas et al., 2007), with some differences between countries (Merikangas et al., 2011). Prevalence of bipolar II disorder was estimated at 1.1 (Merikangas et al., 2007). Most genetic studies focus on bipolar I disorder only or bipolar I disorder and bipolar II disorder.

FAMILY AND TWIN STUDIES IN SCHIZOPHRENIA

As described in Chapter 12, the first step in gene mapping is to establish whether a trait or disease has a genetic liability, typically undertaken through family and twin studies. The first family study of schizophrenia was carried out almost one hundred years ago by Ernst Rudin. Even though his work predated the development of modern statistical methods for analyzing these data, he was able to appreciate that schizophrenia ran in families, although not in a manner consistent with Mendel's laws. Since then the rates of transmission in hundreds of families have been studied with consistent results. In fact, even application of modern statistical methods to Rudin's original data confirm these observations (Kendler and Zerbin-Rudin, 1996). The relative risk for first-degree relatives (λ) of an individual with schizophrenia is ~10. This has recently been confirmed and extended in a large Swedish population registry-based study of 32,536 individuals with schizophrenia and their family members. The size of this study allowed for examination of a wider variety of familial relationships and again the familial relative risks for parents, siblings, and children were 8.6–10.3 (Lichtenstein et al., 2006). Further investigation using twin studies supports underlying genetic factors for the observed familial clustering. The concordance rate (the likelihood that the second twin will develop the disorder once the first is diagnosed) between genetically identical monozygotic twins is high (41%–65%) and substantially lower for dizygotic twins (0%–28%) (Cardno and Gottesman, 2000). A meta-analysis of 12 twin studies derived a heritability estimate of 81% (Sullivan et al., 2003). Heritability estimates based on Swedish and Danish registry data were somewhat lower (67%) and may represent diagnostic differences in the newer

studies. However, the larger registry based studies are likely to be more broadly representative of the types of samples that are used in the genome-wide studies discussed below (Wray and Gottesman, 2012).

It is frequently stated that most patients with schizophrenia do not have affected relatives and are thus "sporadic" in nature. However, Yang and colleagues have demonstrated that a low rate of affected relatives would be expected with a disease that is uncommon (1% prevalence), highly heritable, and highly polygenetic with risk mediated by many common variants of small effects (Yang et al., 2010). Thus, the lack of close relatives alone is insufficient to support an exclusively sporadic, or non-inherited component to the etiology of schizophrenia.

FAMILY AND TWIN STUDIES IN BIPOLAR DISORDER

Early family studies of bipolar disorder did not distinguish individuals with depressive episodes only, or what is now classified as major depressive disorder, from individuals with depressive episodes as well as manic episodes, what is now classified as bipolar disorder. More recent studies have done so, and the most recent have further included separate analyses of bipolar II disorder. In the modern studies that included control populations and that used a population risk of 1%–2%, the relative risk for first-degree relatives (λ) of bipolar patients is approximately 7–10 (Barnett and Smoller, 2009). Family studies of bipolar II disorder are indeterminate. This is likely because bipolar II disorder symptomatically resembles both major depression and bipolar I disorder and may be genetically related to one, or both. Complicating this is a lower interrater reliability for the diagnosis of bipolar II disorder as well as the small samples sizes available (Smoller and Finn, 2003). Family studies also point to familial enrichment of several other phenotypes that may prove useful in refining genetic studies once genes and loci have been identified. These include observing evidence for familial clustering of early age-of-onset, mania versus depression on first onset, mood episode frequency, psychosis, lithium-responsiveness, rapid-cycling, and panic disorder (Barnett and Smoller, 2009). Like schizophrenia, twin studies of bipolar disorder support a genetic underpinning to the family study results. The most recent studies find the concordance rate for monozygotic twins is higher (0.5–0.6) than for dizygotic twins (0.39–0.43) resulting in heritability estimates of 79%–93% (Kendler et al., 1995; McGuffin et al., 2003; Kieseppa et al., 2004).

EPIDEMIOLOGICAL OVERLAP BETWEEN SCHIZOPHRENIA AND BIPOLAR DISORDER

For the traditional linkage studies that will be described below, families with the clearest inheritance of either schizophrenia or bipolar disorder, but not both, were sought. Supporting this focus were two family studies from the early 1990s that indicated there was no genetic overlap in families (Kendler et al., 1993; Maier et al., 1993). However, two more recent studies have suggested that this was not a settled issue. Researchers found increased risks of affective disorder in the families of schizophrenia patients (Mortensen et al., 2003), and one found the reverse (Maier et al., 2002). Several small twin studies came to similar contradictory conclusions. However, in 2009 a very large population-based study was reported that was able to take advantage of the quality of information in the Swedish Hospital Discharge Registry to more definitively answer the question of the familial relationships (Lichtenstein et al., 2009). Analyzing data on over 35,000 patients with schizophrenia, 40,000 patients with bipolar disorder, and their family members, they were able to calculate the relative risk for a wide variety of family and adoptive relationships. Table 18.1 displays these results. For schizophrenia probands, the relative risk of schizophrenia was highest for first-degree relatives, but the relative risk of developing bipolar disorder was also elevated, although not as high. The reverse applied to bipolar disorder probands, where they had increased risks of both bipolar disorder and schizophrenia in their first-degree relatives. In fact, there was sufficient power in this study to look at a variety of adoptive relationships confirming earlier studies that adopted away children with a biologic parent with schizophrenic or bipolar are at increased risk of developing the same disease as their biological parent.

The nature of the genetic relationship between schizophrenia and bipolar disorder is also highlighted by patients with schizoaffective disorder, often referred to as a schizophrenia spectrum disorder. Patients with the manic/bipolar subtype meet diagnostic criteria for both schizophrenia and bipolar disorder, while those with the depressed subtype meet criteria for schizophrenia and major depressive disorder. Some work suggests increased familial risk of bipolar disorder and schizophrenia for each subtype, respectively. However, not all family and twin studies concur. Molecular genetic overlap that will be discussed below reinvigorates the discussion and may provide additional data to improve nosology (Craddock et al., 2009; Hamshere et al., 2009).

ENVIRONMENTAL AND NON-INHERITED GENETIC FACTORS

Several non-genetic risk factors for schizophrenia have been reproducibly identified and have been reviewed (Brown, 2011). The most well documented of these include obstetrical complications, urban birth, season of birth, famine while *in utero*, migration, prenatal infections, and cannabis use. Advancing paternal age has also been shown to be associated with increased risk of schizophrenia (Miller et al., 2011). Patients with schizophrenia have decreased reproductive fitness as measured by reduced fecundity measured as a fertility ratio in comparison to siblings, particularly in males (23% vs. 47% in females), that is not offset by increased fecundity in siblings (Power et al., 2012). This implies that negative selection is at work, and that there is a supply of new mutations that are occurring that are contributing to the risk of schizophrenia. In a whole genome sequencing study in Iceland, paternal age was estimated to explain most of the increased *de novo* mutation rate observed (Kong et al., 2012), providing

TABLE 18.1. Recurrence risks for schizophrenia and bipolar disorder. [Used with permission from: Lichtenstein, *Lancet* (2009) 373:17–23.]

RELATION TO PROBAND		RISK FOR SCHIZOPHRENIA WHEN PROBAND HAS SCHIZOPHRENIA		RISK FOR BIPOLAR DISORDER WHEN PROBAND HAS BIPOLAR DISORDER		RISK FOR SCHIZOPHRENIA WHEN PROBAND HAS BIPOLAR DISORDER		RISK FOR BIPOLAR DISORDER WHEN PROBAND HAS SCHIZOPHRENIA	
		RR	95% CL	RR	95% CL	RR	95% CL	RR	95% CL
BIOLOGICAL RELATIONSHIP									
Parent	offspring	9.9	8.5–11.6	6.4	5.9–7.1	2.4	2.1–2.6	5.2	4.4–6.2
Sibling	Sibling	9.0	8.1–9.9	7.9	7.1–8.8	3.9	3.4–4.4	3.7	3.2–4.2
Sibling	Maternal half-sibling	3.6	2.3–5.5	4.5	2.7–7.4	1.4	0.7–2.6	1.2	0.6–2.4
Sibling	Paternal half-sibling	2.7	1.9–3.8	2.4	1.4–4.1	1.6	1.0–2.7	2.2	1.3–3.8
ADOPTIVE RELATIONSHIP									
Biological parent	Adopted away offspring*	13.7	6.1–30.8	4.3	2.0–9.5	4.5	1.8–10.9	6.0	2.3–15.2
Sibling	Adopted away biological sibling	7.6	0.7–87.8	–	–	3.9	0.2–63.3	5.0	0.3–79.9
Adoptive parent	Adoptee	–	–	1.3	0.5–3.6	1.5	0.7–3.5	–	–
Sibling	Non-biological sibling	1.3	0.1–15.1	–	–	–	–	2.0	0.1–37.8

R = relative risk. *Adopted children whose biological parents have disease.

a potential molecular correlate. There are fewer studies investigating environmental factors in bipolar disorder. However, there is some evidence of effects on risk of seasonality of birth, advanced paternal age, and stressful life events (Alloy et al., 2005; Frans et al., 2008; Disanto et al., 2012), environmental factors that overlap those observed in schizophrenia and major depressive disorder.

EARLY GENETIC STUDIES/TRADITIONAL GENETIC METHODS

LINKAGE ANALYSES

The genetic observations described above led to searches for the responsible genes. As genome-wide markers became available in the 1980s, they were used for linkage studies in families with schizophrenia or bipolar disorder. As was discussed in Chapter 12, linkage analysis follows the transmission of disease and particular genetic markers in families to identify chromosomal segments for closer follow-up and has primarily been successful in diseases caused by mutations with large effect sizes in a single or small number of genes. Many linkage studies of both disorders have been performed. The overall conclusion that can be drawn is that no genomic loci are likely to harbor large effect genes that account for a substantial portion of genetic liability. Even a meta-analysis of 32 independent linkage studies using data from 7,413 schizophrenia cases in 3,255 pedigrees was not able to identify

significant chromosomal regions linked to schizophrenia at above the chance level (Ng et al., 2009). While the overall number of linkage studies in bipolar disorder is more modest, the overall observation was the same in the meta-analysis of 18 studies of 2,437 bipolar cases in 592 pedigrees (Segurado et al., 2003). This was recently extended using a linkage panel of 6,000 single nucleotide markers to achieve more complete linkage information across the genome in 2,782 bipolar disorder cases without producing significant results (Badner et al., 2012). Phenotypic heterogeneity and diagnostic inaccuracy have often been postulated as a primary explanation for lack of clear success in linkage studies. However, similar diagnostic methods and patient samples were used in the genome-wide association studies (GWAS) of common variants and rare copy number variants with strikingly different results that will be described below. Furthermore, it is often argued that there are some suggestive regions that overlap in several studies and might contain loci, however the most likely explanation for the overlap is random chance resulting from the large number of studies performed and the relative lack of fine scale genomic resolution of linkage analysis.

Despite this, positional cloning, the process whereby specific genes are identified within a linkage peak, has been carried in some linkage regions, particularly on chromosomes 8p12 and 6p22.3. In those regions, two candidate genes were of particular focus, neuregulin1 (*NRG1*) and dysbindin (*DTNBP1*), respectively. Disrupted in Schizophrenia 1 (*DISC1*), is a gene interrupted by a balanced chromosomal translocation between chromosomes 1 and 11 (t(1;11) (q42;q14)), that segregates in

a single Scottish family with schizophrenia, bipolar disorder, and major depression. No other families with translocations, or other segregating structural abnormalities in *DISC1* have been found. Numerous association studies have focused on this gene in both schizophrenia and bipolar disorder with inconsistent results. A meta-analysis of data from 11,626 cases and 15,237 controls did not find evidence for association for any of the 1,241 SNPs in DISC1 that were tested (Mathieson et al., 2012). In addition, studies have generally not found an excess of rare variants at this locus. Despite the paucity of evidence for a major role in genetic risk of schizophrenia, there have been many interesting biological studies of this gene that will be described in later chapters.

CANDIDATE GENES STUDIES OF SCHIZOPHRENIA AND BIPOLAR DISORDER

Hundreds of candidate gene association studies have been performed over the last decade. Most were defined as candidates based on biological theories from pharmacological observations or secondary to abnormalities observed in postmortem human brain tissue from patients. Taken as a whole, the results of these studies are inconsistent and may represent poor candidate choices because of our fundamental lack of understanding of the underlying biology and/or poor gene coverage and/or small sample sizes. Numerous detailed publications review the status of the most frequently studied of these genes, and a list of them is maintained by the schizophrenia research forum (see http://www.szgene.org). It is of note that initial results from GWAS do not find the prior biological candidate genes enriched among significant or nearly significant loci (Collins et al., 2012). The most extensively investigated are covered in other chapters of this section. Candidate genes in bipolar disorder have focused on *BDNF*, circadian genes, phosphinositide signaling, and Wnt/GSK3beta signaling (Martinowich et al., 2009). As with schizophrenia, initial results from GWAS do not find the prior biological candidates enriched among significant or nearly significant loci (Seifuddin et al., 2012).

COPY NUMBER VARIATION

Copy number variants (CNVs) are deletions or duplications of genetic material and can range from several base pairs (often called "indels") to 100,000s to millions of bases. The risk of developing schizophrenia is markedly elevated in the presence of certain CNVs (Table 18.2). A large body of work reviewed in detail elsewhere (Malhotra and Sebat, 2012) has defined

TABLE 18.2. Disease-associated copy number variants

LOCUS (CHROMOSOME LOCATION MB HG18)	TYPE OF CNV	RELATIVE RISK	NUMBER OF GENES (APPROXIMATE)	RATE IN SCZ CASES/ RATE IN CONTROLS	SCZ (OTHER POTENTIALLY ASSOCIATED DISEASE PHENOTYPES)[b]
1q21.1 (144.9–146.3)	Deletion	9.2[a]	12	0.18/0.02	SCZ (ID, epilepsy, ASD)
2p16.3 (*NRXN1*)	Exonic deletions	7.5–8.97[a]	1		SCZ (ID, epilepsy, ASD, ADHD)
3q29 (197.4–198.8)	Deletion	49.5[a]	21	0.097/0.002	SCZ (ID, ASD, BD)
7q36.3 (158.4–158.8)	Duplication	3.2[b]	2 (*VIPR2*)	0.19/0.06	SCZ (ASD)
15q11.2 (20.2–20.8)	Deletion	2.2[a]	8	0.57/0.27	SCZ (ID, epilepsy)
15q13.3 (28.7–30.3)	Deletion	8.3[a]	8	0.19/0.023	SCZ (ID, epilepsy, ASD)
16p13.1 (15.0–16.2)	Duplication	2.1[a]	8	0.28/0.13	SCZ (ID, ADHD)
16p11.2 (29.5–30.2)	Duplication	9.8[a]	26	0.3/0.031	SCZ (ID, epilepsy, ASD, ADHD, BD)
17p12 (14.0–15.4)	Deletion	5.9[a]	5	0.16/0.026	SCZ (hereditary neuropathy with pressure palsies)
17q12 (31.8–33.3)	Deletion	18.4[a]	17	0.06/0.0003	SCZ (ID, ASD)
22q11.2 (17.4–19.8)	Deletion	44-infinity[a]	30	0.31/0	SCZ (LD, ASD)

[a]Based on (Grozeva, Conrad, et al., 2012) which included enhanced control population; [b]based on (Malhotra and Sebat, 2012); ASD-autism spectrum disorder, ID-intellectual disability or developmental disability, BD-bipolar disorder

the following principles of the CNVs associated with schizophrenia from studying over 10,000 samples initially using array-comparative genomic hybridization and subsequently SNP microarrays.

- Genome-wide rates of large (>100 kb), rare (<1%) CNVs are elevated.

- Rates of *de novo* CNVs are elevated.

- CNVs generally contain many genes and confer large relative risks (2.1–49.5)

- SCZ associated CNVs are often found in multiple additional disease phenotypes including most commonly ASD, LD, and epilepsy.

- Specific genomic locations are recurrent sites of these CNVs (see Table 18.2)

- CNVs are enriched in neuronal functions particularly those that are involved in synaptic activity and neurodevelopmental processes. Additional support for proteins enriched in synaptic signaling has been found in recent work on *de novo* CNVs.

Characteristics of the individual loci, genes, and phenotypic overlaps are discussed in Chapter 19.

The role of CNVs in bipolar disorder has been less well studied and remains somewhat controversial, with some studies findings increased rates and others not (Malhotra and Sebat, 2012; Olsen et al., 2011). Overall, the association of rare CNVs is less prominent, and only one specific CNV (3q29) is reported with an effect size > 5 for bipolar disorder, although a study of 185 proband-parent trios found a rate of *de novo* CNVs that was 4.8-fold higher then controls and similar to what was observed in schizophrenia (Malhotra et al., 2011).

GENOME-WIDE ASSOCIATION STUDIES

Development of the technology for simultaneously genotyping hundreds of thousands of SNPs as well as the positional information regarding the sites of almost all common SNPs has allowed for progressively more informative GWAS studies. These studies have the advantage of being unbiased with respect to prior biologically driven theories, but of course have well-known limitations. The theoretical underpinnings of GWAS have been discussed in an earlier chapter, and the specific implications for psychiatric disease covered in several excellent reviews (PGC, 2009; Sullivan et al., 2012).

SCHIZOPHRENIA

There are now >10 published GWAS studies of European samples (Table 18.3) (Lencz et al., 2007; O'Donovan et al., 2008; Sullivan et al., 2008; Need et al., 2009; Purcell et al., 2009; Shi et al., 2009; Stefansson et al., 2009; Athanasiu et al., 2010; Schizophrenia Psychiatric Genome-Wide Association

Study (GWAS) Consortium, 2011; Shi et al., 2011; Steinberg et al., 2011; Bergen et al., 2012; Hamshere et al., 2012; Rietschel et al., 2012). Other studies have included African American and Japanese samples, but sample sizes remain small at present. A large sample has been reported by the Psychiatric Genomics Consortium (PGC). This consortium was formed in 2007, recognizing that individual studies that utilized only several thousand individuals would be underpowered and that sharing of data and rapid meta-analysis would significantly accelerate the gene discovery process. An international group of scientists from over 60 institutions and 19 countries continues to work together and timely updates will be provided on their website (https://pgc.unc.edu/). An overlapping group of European scientists from seven European institutions work together as part of the SGENE consortium (http://www.sgene.eu/).

A stringent and well-accepted criteria for genome-wide significance takes into account the total number of independent SNPs tested (approximately 1 million) and thus should be equal to or below 5×10^{-8} (Pe'er et al., 2008). If we assume that most common variant loci have modest effect sizes (<1.5-fold), then the power to detect loci using stringent thresholds that adjust for the total genome-wide testing burden is low. Thus, while many groups began by using their own samples, they rapidly proceeded to replication of the best loci through collaboration with additional groups. This can easily be appreciated by reviewing Table 18.3, noting that most of the primary or stage 1 samples did not detect associated loci, but that following either replication/stage 2 or large meta-analysis (e.g., PGC or SGENE) several loci were convincingly associated.

Since linkage disequilibrium varies across the genome, the associated regions vary in size; some contain multiple genes, some one, or even none. Table 18.4 contains genome-wide significant findings as of November 2012. The most significant individual marker is listed along with the nearest gene, the study in which it was first reported, and the study in which it has been reported in the largest overall sample size. The first regions were identified in a series of studies published in 2008 and 2009. O'Donovan and colleagues first reported a locus *ZNF804A*, a transcription factor of unknown function (O'Donovan et al., 2008). This was followed by three studies published simultaneously that analyzed over 3,000 cases each. These studies reported an association across the large region of the major histocompatibility complex (MHC) on chromosome 6. Two additional regions, each of which pointed to specific genes, were reported by the SGENE consortium, transcription factor 4, *TCF4*, and neurogranin, *NRGN* (Stefansson et al., 2009). The largest study, undertaken by the Schizophrenia Psychiatric Genome-Wide Association Study Consortium, assembled and directly analyzed genotype data from 17 individual samples for a total of 8,394 cases and 12,462 in the primary analysis. Overall, five new loci were detected (1p21.3, 2q32.3, 8p23.2, 8q21.3, and 10q24.32). A graphical representation of the data is displayed in Figure 18.1. In the replication study of the 81 most associated SNPs, a strongly positive deviation from expectation in the number of results detected in the same direction as

TABLE 18.3. Studies reporting full GWAS in schizophrenia in european samples

| PUBLICATION | YEAR | PRIMARY OR STAGE 1 | | GWS STAGE1 | REPLICATION OR STAGE 2[a] | | GWS STAGE 2 |
		CASES	CONTROLS		CASES	CONTROLS	
Lencz	2007	178	144	–	–	–	NA
O'Donovan	2008	479	2,937	–	7,308	12,834	+
Sullivan	2008	417	411	–	–	–	NA
ISC	2009	3,322	3,587	+	8,008	19,077	+
Shi	2009	2,681	2,653	–	8,008	19,077	+
Stefansson	2009	2,663	13,498	–	12,945	34,591	+
Need	2009	871	869	–	1,460	12,995	–
Athanasiu	2010	201	307	–	2,864	14,087	–
SCZ-PGC	2011	9,394	12,462	+	8,442	21,397	+
Shi Y[b]	2011	3,750	6,468	–	4,383	4,539	+
Steinberg[c]	2011	–	–	NA	18,206	42,536	+
Rietschel	2011	1,169	3,714	–	3,738	7,802	+
Bergen	2012	1,507	2,093	–	11,271	14,601	+
Hamshere	2012	–	–	NA	2,640	2,878	+

[a]Replication and Stage 2 samples often tested only a subset of the most associated SNPs in the larger sample. [b]Large Chinese sample; [c]enlarged sample based on Stefansson, 2009, only subset of SNPs tested in primary study; GWS = genome-wide significant

the original effect (but not independently genome-wide significant) was found. This means that sample sizes are insufficient and that as they grow additional associated loci will be found. The PGC is completing meta-analysis of case and control samples that is 2–3 times larger than those previously reported. The expectation, based on simulations that compare the rates of identification of additional loci in other genetically complex traits such as height, is that there will be a dramatic increase in genome-wide significant loci. Thus, the loci listed in Table 18.4 are provisional. Ultimately this list may also contain some of the prior biological candidate genes, albeit with effects sizes that are more modest than those originally observed.

It is important to note that the relative risk conferred by each individual variant listed in the table is small and thus, even in aggregate, contributes a negligible amount to the overall heritability. Rather than jump to the conclusion that the genetic causes of schizophrenia must be either rare, or *de novo* as many authors have, the International Schizophrenia Consortium tested whether there were many variants, even thousands of variants, each contributing a very small amount to the overall liability of developing schizophrenia. Individually, none of these variants was able to generate a signal, but taken in groups of 10s or 1000s of SNPs they were able to predict aggregate risk of having schizophrenia in independent samples (Fig. 18.2). The Consortium developed score profiles from groups of SNPs that were below a variety of more and more

relaxed *P* value thresholds. This was done in order to be able to include SNPs with very small effect sizes. Using the derived profiles and applying them to independent schizophrenia samples, they found that for all the thresholds tested, they were highly significantly associated, as a group, in the independent schizophrenia samples, but critically, not in a wide variety of other non-psychiatric genetic diseases like Crohn's disease and diabetes. These results cannot be explained by rare variants alone, or by other artifacts such as population stratification, and thus indicate there are meaningful contributions from many common variants to the overall liability to schizophrenia. These results have subsequently been replicated in several larger samples. A recent study estimated the proportion of variation in the susceptibility to schizophrenia that had been explained by GWAS SNPs was ~25%–30% using some of the largest GWAS studies (Lee, DeCandia, et al., 2012). A highly polygenic model suggests that genetically influenced individual differences across domains of brain development and function may form a diathesis for major psychiatric illness, perhaps as multiple growth and metabolic pathways influence human height.

While GWAS does not identify specific functional variants and genes, several interesting observations have already emerged from this early work. The MHC is an exceedingly gene-rich region, including both HLA genes as well as a family of histones, an olfactory receptor cluster, and a number of brain-related genes. To complicate matters, the MHC is a

TABLE 18.4. Disease associated susceptibility variants by GWAS for schizophrenia and bipolar disorder

CANDIDATE OR NEAREST GENE (CHROMOSOME LOCATION)	ASSOCIATED VARIANT	RELATIVE RISK[a]	FREQUENCY OF RISK ALLELE	P VALUE[b]	ASSOCIATED DISEASE PHENOTYPE	FIRST REPORTED; LARGEST SAMPLE
MIR137 (1p21.3)	rs1625579	1.12	0.8	1.6×10^{-11}	SCZ	SCZ-PGC
SDCCAG8 (1q43)	rs6703335	1.12	NA	4.2×10^{-8}	SCZ	Hamshere
VRK2 (2p15.1)	rs2312147	1.09	0.61	1.9×10^{-9}	SCZ	Steinberg
ZNF804A (2q32.1)	rs1344706	1.11	0.33	4.1×10^{-13} (BD and SCZ) 2.5×10^{-11} (SCZ)	SCZ and BD[c]; SCZ alone	O'Donovan; Williams
PCGEM1 (2q32.3)	rs17662626	1.2	0.91	4.7×10^{-8}	SCZ	SCZ-PGC
ITIH3-ITIH4 (3p21.1)	rs2239547	1.11	0.74	3.6×10^{-10}	SCZ alone and combined with BD	Hamshere
Extended MHC region (6p21.3–22–1)	Many	1.13–1.36	0.78–0.92	1.7×10^{-11}	SCZ	ISC; Steinberg
CSMD1 (8p23.2)	rs10503253	1.11	0.19	1.5×10^{-8}	SCZ	SCZ-PGC
LSM1 (8p11.2)	rs16887244	0.83	0.32	1.3×10^{-10}	SCZ	Shi Y
MMP16 (8q21.3)	rs7004633	1.1	0.18	2.8×10^{-8}	SCZ	SCZ-PGC
ANK3 (10q21.2)	rs10994359	1.22	0.69	2.4×10^{-8}	BD; SCZ and BD combined	Ferreira
CNNM2 (10q24.32)	rs7914558	1.08	0.59	1.8×10^{-9}	SCZ	SCZ-PGC
NT5C2 (10q24.33)	rs11191580	1.15	0.91	1.1×10^{-8}	SCZ	SCZ-PGC
AMBRA1 (11p11.2)	rs11819869	1.25	0.19	3.9×10^{-9}	SCZ	Rietchel
ODZ4 (11q14.1)	rs12576775	1.14	xx	4.4×10^{-8}	BD	PGC-BD
NRGN (11q24.2)	rs12807809	1.12	0.83	2.8×10^{-9}	SCZ	Stefansson; Steinberg
CACNA1C (12p13.33)	rs4765905	1.14	0.35	1.5×10^{-8}	BD; SCZ alone and combined with BD	Ferreira; SCZ-PGC
TCF4 (18q21.2)	rs9960767	1.2	0.056	4.2×10^{-9}	SCZ	Stefansson; Steinberg
CCDC68 (18q21.2)	rs12966547	1.09	0.58	2.6×10^{-10}	SCZ	SCZ-PGC
NCAN (19p13.1)	rs1064395	1.17	0.20	2.1×10^{-9}	BD	Cichon

[a] Relative risk in largest sample presented. In most cases SNPs are in LD with additional potentially functional variants; [b] P value in largest sample presented; [c] SCZ and BD analyzed together as a single phenotype.

multi-megabase region of unusually extensive linkage disequilibrium and gene density, making it impossible to attribute the association signal to particular genes, or to a particular HLA haplogroup. One of the strongest new associations is over 100 kb from the nearest protein-coding gene, but is within the transcript for *MIR137*. Prior work has identified a role for miR137 in several important areas of brain development including neurogenesis and neuronal maturation. While there is an additional gene, dihydrophyrimidine dehydrogenase (*DPYD*), in which rare *de novo* functional mutations were found in two schizophrenia patients (Xu et al., 2012), the connection between *MIR137* is strengthened by the observation that four schizophrenia associated genes at the genome-wide significant level are *MIR137* targets. Of course, both may be contributing to the phenotype. In general, one reasonable, although not proven, hypothesis is that associated loci will fall into meaningful biologic pathways with explanatory power for the disease. Many methods have been developed for this (e.g., ALIGATOR: Holmans et al., 2009; INRICH: Lee, O'Dushlaine, et al., 2012; DAPPLE: Rossin et al., 2011; and GRAIL: Raychaudhuri et al., 2009), and there are a wide variety of databases with curated gene sets (e.g., Gene Ontology-GO: http://www.geneontology.

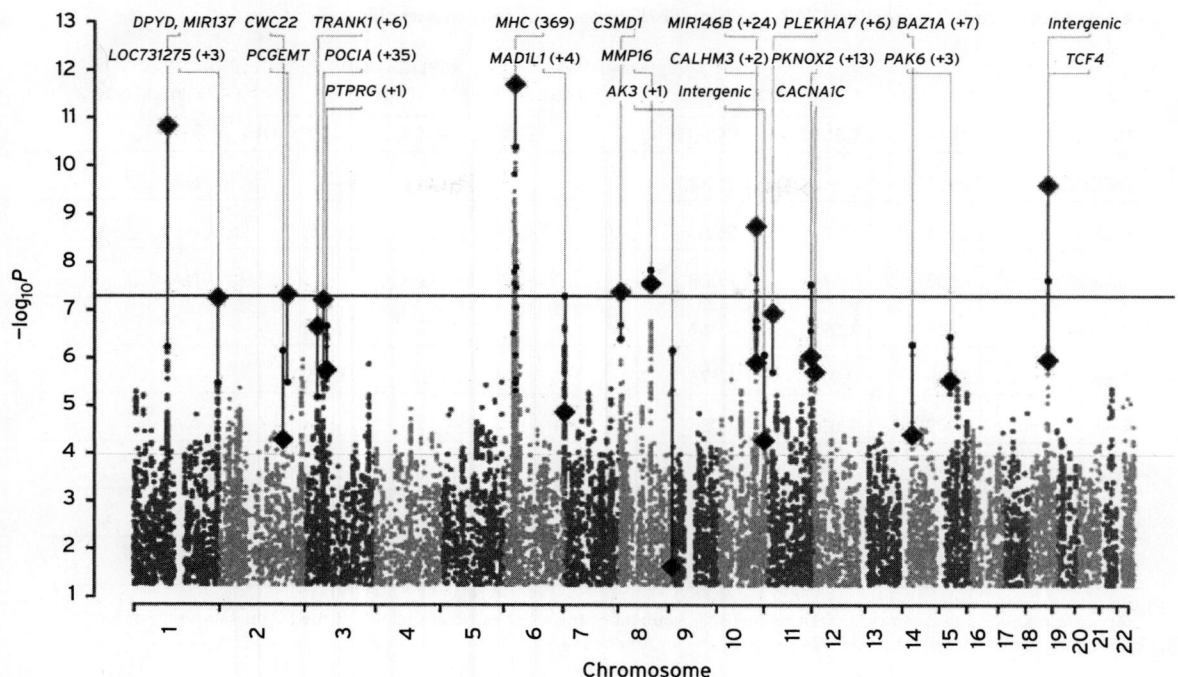

Figure 18.1 Manhattan plot adapted from Schizophrenia Psychiatric Genome-Wide Association Study (GWAS) Consortium, 2011. Each point represents either a directly genotyped or imputed SNP. SNPs are plotted on the x-axis starting from the p arm of chromosome 1 to chromosome 22. The y-axis displays the statistical significance as the $-\log_{10}P$ value of the association results for each SNP. For the stage 1 results, 16 regions with one or more SNP achieving $P < 10^{-6}$ are highlighted and labeled with the name of the nearest gene. SNPs selected for stage 2 replication are highlighted, with the resulting combined P value after replication (i.e., after incorporation of stage 2 results) indicated by the large diamonds. Diamonds above highlighting indicate SNPs that were more significantly associated after replication, and diamonds below highlighting indicate SNPs that were less significantly associated after replication. P values below 0.05 are not shown adapted from Ripke et al., 2011 (Consortium 2011).

org/; Kyoto Encyclopedia of Genes and Genome-KEGG: http://www.genome.jp/kegg/). However, currently these databases are likely underrepresented in human brain pathways, just those that should be most useful for schizophrenia studies. Furthermore, consensus has not been achieved on proper thresholds for statistical significance for these studies given the wide variety of methods, and numbers and types of genes and pathways that may be analyzed. Application of these methods to GWAS data have not yet identified consistent and replicable loci, most likely because the overall number of input loci has been too small to have adequate power.

Ultimately, developing etiological validation of genetic observations is important, and one method is through testing their effects on gene expression. Microarray based gene expression studies using postmortem tissue from schizophrenia patients have identified regional brain abnormalities, as well as abnormalities in several biological processes such as synaptic transmission, inhibitory neurotransmission, and myelination (Horvath et al., 2011). Furthermore, sequence dependent gene expression abnormalities have been reported in a variety of the biological candidate genes or those that emerged from earlier linkage studies such as *NRG1*, *DISC1*, and *DTNBP1*. As discussed earlier, there is no evidence for a predominant role in genetic liability for these genes. However, systematic surveys of the presence of common and rare human variation on protein coding genes and gene expression found that the genome contains a surprising number of functional alleles that profoundly alter gene expression (Kang et al., 2011; MacArthur et al.,

2012). The role of the gene expression changes in the etiology of schizophrenia will require understanding whether genes or pathways with statistically compelling risk associations are among this group. As a first step in this direction, several groups have investigated whether associated loci are enriched for expression quantitative trait loci (eQTLs). Using gene expression microarray data from 163 control postmortem brain samples, polygenic schizophrenia risk alleles derived from large-scale GWAS were statistically enriched for cis-eQTLs (Richards et al., 2011). Gene expression data from several developmental and spatial transcriptional atlases of the human brain have recently been made available (NCBI Gene Expression Omnibus GSE25219 and GSE30272). Comprehensive next generation sequencing surveys are also in progress for human postmortem samples from hundreds of schizophrenia patients. Integration of these resources and other complex datatypes that are emerging from the Encyclopedia of DNA Elements (ENCODE) project with DNA variation will enable an understanding of the biological role of disease associated variation.

BIPOLAR DISORDER

There are also ~10 published studies of GWAS genotyped Europeans. Table 18.5 lists GWAS studies of bipolar disorder, many of which included both types 1 and 2. As in schizophrenia, it is in the largest studies or the replication and stage 2 samples that genome-wide significant loci were identified. A particular difficulty in the early bipolar disorder GWAS

TABLE 18.5. Studies reporting GWAS in bipolar disorder in european samples

| PUBLICATION | YEAR | PRIMARY OR STAGE 1 | | GWS STAGE 1 | REPLICATION OR STAGE 2[a] | | GWS STAGE 2 |
		CASES	CONTROLS		CASES	CONTROLS	
WTCCC	2007	1,868	2,938	–	–	–	NA
Baum[b]	2008	461	563	–	772	876	+
Sklar	2008	1,461	2,008	–	–	–	NA
Ferreira	2009	1,098	1,267	–	4,387	6,209	+
Scott	2009	2,076	1,676	–	3,683	14,507	–
Smith[c]	2009	1,003	1,033	–	–	–	NA
PGC-BD	2011	7,481	9250	+	11,974	51,792	+
Cichon	2011	682	1300	–	8,441	35,362	+
Hamshere	2012	–	–		2,504	2,878	+

[a]Replication and Stage 2 samples often tested only a subset of the most associated SNPs in the larger sample. [b]Pooled genotyping only. [c]Study included GWAS in 345 African American cases. NA-not applicable.

literature occurred because many of the samples used partially overlapping case and controls. The first small study that used pooled genotyping, reported a genome-wide significant association to *DGKH* that has subsequently not been replicated in the larger studies that followed (Baum et al., 2008). Subsequently, Ferreira and colleagues (Ferreira et al., 2008) identified the region of *ANK3* (encoding ankyrin 3) and *CACNA1C* (encoding the alpha subunit of the L-type calcium channel) and those from a third reported an association to *NCAN* (encoding neurocan) (Cichon et al., 2011), while other studies did not report genome-wide significant loci (Scott et al., 2009; Sklar et al., 2008; Smith et al., 2009, 2011). The PGC Bipolar Disorder Working Group reported results from the largest study to date (Psychiatric GWAS Consortium Bipolar Disorder Working Group, 2011). Genotype data were assembled from 11 samples and a combined analysis of 16,731 samples and 46,912 replication samples identified two genome-wide significant loci, *CACNA1C* and a new locus, *ODZ4* (encoding a human homolog of the *Drosophila* pair-rule gene *ten-m* (*odz4*)). Of note, strong association (but not genome-wide significant) was reported by Scott in 2009 in the region of *NEK4-ITIH1-ITIH3* on chromosome 3; this region was recently shown to be genome-wide significant in follow-up studies of schizophrenia, and has a replication *P* value below 0.05 for bipolar disorder in an independent sample (Hamshere et al., 2012).

As we discussed for schizophrenia, there is strong evidence that increasing the sample sizes for bipolar disorder will make it possible to identify additional loci. In the replication portion of the PGC-BD study, 34 of the most associated SNPs were tested in an additional 4,496 cases and 42,422 controls. Of those tested, 31 of the 34 SNPs had a signal in the same direction of effect as the original—highly unlikely to have occurred by chance ($P = 3.8 \times 10^{-7}$). However, not all loci were independently replicated—in particular, two significant loci

in the stage 1 samples, *ANK3* and *SYNE1*. These results may represent the "winner's curse" with smaller real effects sizes and larger samples needed for replication or with false positive associations. This will become clearer as data from additional samples becomes available.

The PGC-BD group also provided direct evidence for a polygenic component in bipolar disorder. Performing the same score profile analysis, but starting with bipolar disorder samples to define the score, they showed a highly statistically significant enrichment of putatively associated bipolar disorder score profile alleles across a wide variety of *P* value thresholds. These data are consistent with the presence of many common susceptibility variants of relatively weak effects.

Pathway analysis in the PGC-BD sample showed significant enrichment in the GO category of voltage-gated calcium channel activity (GO:0015270) in an analysis that controlled for many of the potential biases caused by not accounting for SNP density, gene density, and gene size. Three calcium channel subunits were included in this category, *CACNA1C*, *CACNA1D* and *CACNB3*. The first two encode the major L-type alpha subunits found in the brain, consistent with prior literature regarding the role of ion channels in bipolar disorder, the mood stabilizing effects of ion channel modulating drugs, and the specific treatment literature suggesting direct efficacy of L-type calcium channels blockers in the treatment of bipolar disorder (Casamassima et al., 2010). *ODZ4*, located on chromosome 11, encodes a member of a family of cell surface proteins, the teneurins. These genes are likely involved in cell surface signaling and neuronal pathfinding. *NCAN* is an extracellular matrix glycoprotein that is brain expressed. Ncan$^{-/-}$ mice show abnormalities in a variety of behavioral paradigms, some of which are often used as models of mania, such as increased exploratory behavior and increased amphetamine-induced hyperactivity (Miro et al., 2012). *ANK3* codes for a multifunctional protein, which forms a critical component of the

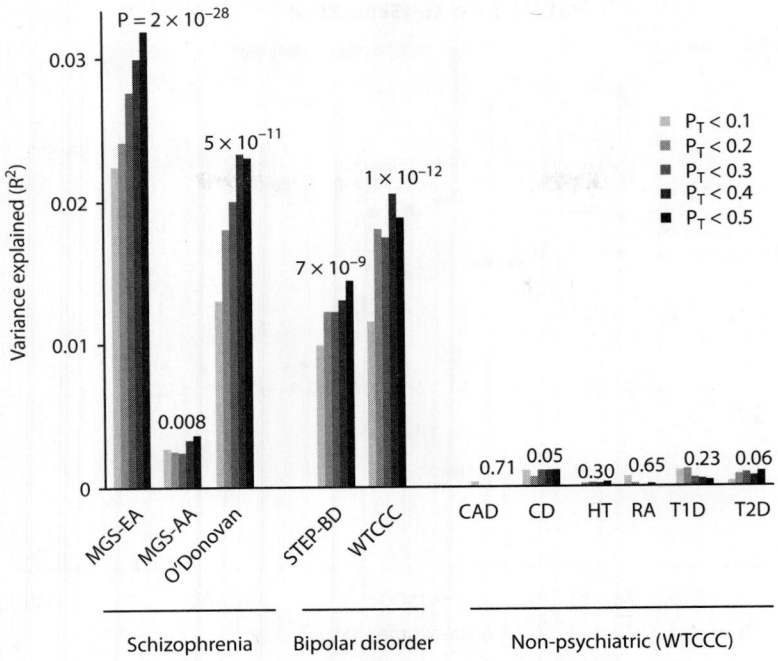

Figure 18.2 *Variance explained in the target samples on the basis of score profiles derived in the entire ISC for five significance thresholds (P Value$_{Threshold}$ < 0.1, 0.2, 0.3, 0.4, and 0.5, plotted left to right in each study). The y-axis indicates Nagelkerke's pseudo R²; the number above each set of bars is the P value for the P Value$_{Threshold}$ < 0.5 target sample analysis. CAD, coronary artery disease; CD, Crohn's disease; HT, hypertension; RA, rheumatoid arthritis; T1D, type I diabetes; T2D, type II diabetes. Used with permission from Purcell, Wray (2009).*

axon initial segment and of nodes of Ranvier with described functions in the developmental and physiological regulation of neural activity including the assembly of voltage-gated sodium channels. As in schizophrenia, enrichment of cis e-QTL were found when testing the top ~1,000 SNPs in novel human cerebellar postmortem brain tissue (P < 0.001).

Phenotypic aspects, such as clinical symptom dimensions, of the categorical disease diagnosis are beginning to emerge. These have included negative mood delusions, mood incongruent psychotic symptoms, suicidality, and temperament, and while some have reported signals that just achieve genome-wide significance, they need to be interpreted with caution (Goes et al., 2012; Greenwood et al., 2012; Meier et al., 2012; Willour et al., 2012). These studies are necessarily smaller in size and thus confronted with low statistical power and problems from the lack of replication samples, since detailed phenotyping is not widely available.

GWAS OVERLAP BETWEEN SCHIZOPHRENIA AND BIPOLAR DISORDER

Overlap in both specific genetic vulnerability loci as well as an overlap in polygenic background has been observed. Large-scale GWAS have found strengthened signals that are also genome-wide significant when combining results from schizophrenia and bipolar disorder for *ZNF804A*, *ITIH3-ITIH4*, *ANK3*, and *CACNA1C*. In Fig. 18.2, the score profile that was defined using a schizophrenia case-control sample was also able to statistically significantly discriminate between bipolar disorder cases and controls in two independent bipolar disorder samples. This is a strong demonstration

that there is a large molecular overlap in vulnerability alleles for the two disorders. The strength of these observations differs from earlier indications from linkage and candidate gene studies because of the sample sizes, statistical significance, and replication status of the results. Graphical representations of genes and regions of interest from GWAS results have been made publicly available through the easy to use program RICOPILI (http://www.broadinstitute.org/mpg/ricopili/). It is hoped that this will facilitate translation of genetic findings into neurobiological and clinical follow-up by interested scientists. Examples of loci in schizophrenia and bipolar disorder are shown in Fig. 18.3.

LARGE-SCALE SEQUENCING STUDIES

Several observations imply that cataloging rare single nucleotide variants (SNVs) enriched in patients is important. As with the CNVs discussed earlier, advanced paternal age is associated with increased risk of schizophrenia (age 45–49 relative risk = 1.24; >50 = 1.79) suggesting a role for *de novo* mutations. We know, conclusively, that rare large structural mutations, many of which are *de novo* or relatively new in the population, such as that deletions of hundreds of kilobases, have a large effect on the SCZ risk. In addition, work described previously from the genome-wide studies of common variants strongly supports a threshold liability model, which by definition will include inherited variants on the rare end of the spectrum. Integrating between and across multiple sources of variation will be a large-scale challenge for the future. Already several studies are pointing to hints from new and segregating

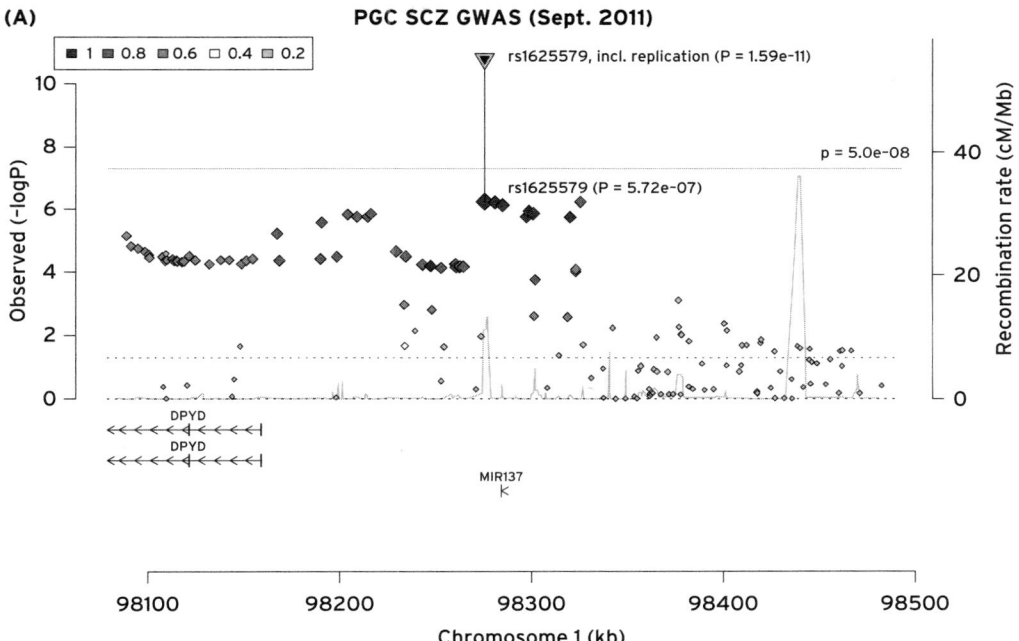

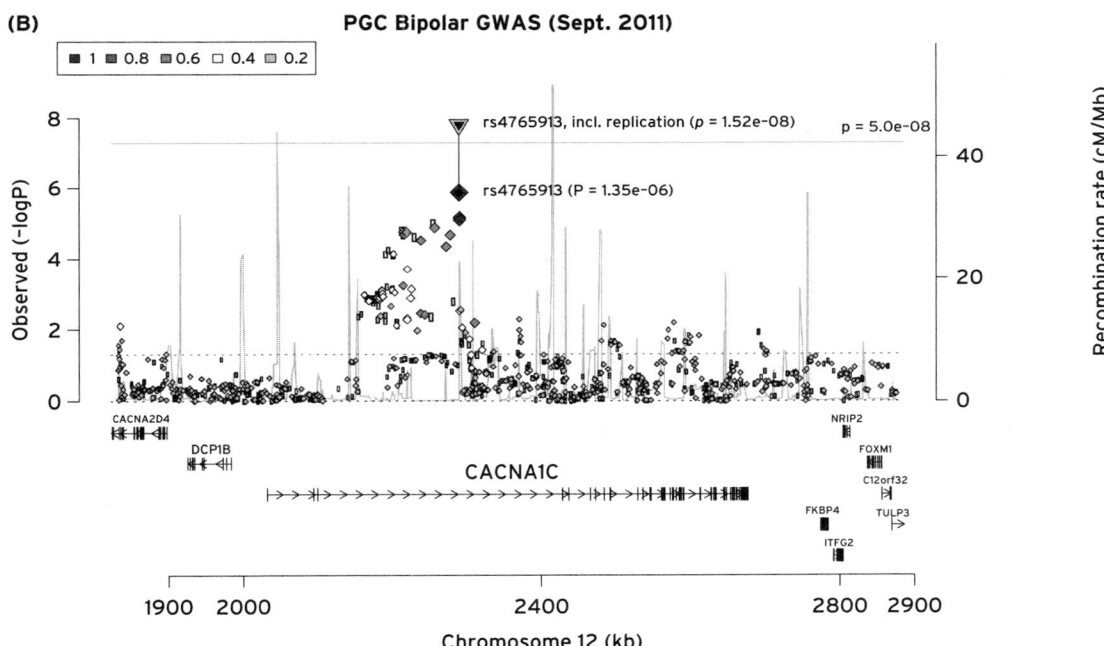

Figure 18.3 *Representative regional plots in schizophrenia and bipolar disorder. (A) Top association signal in schizophrenia on chromosome 1 in PGC-SCZ; (B) Top association signal in bipolar disorder on chromosome 12 in PGC-BD. Each point represents either a directly genotyped or imputed SNP. SNPs are plotted on the x-axis starting surrounding the gene or SNP of interest 5′ to 3′. The y-axis displays the statistical significance as the $-\log_{10}P$ value of the association results for each SNP. Genes are indicated and exons marked with vertical lines. The horizontal line at 5×10^{-3} marks the genome-wide significance threshold. Linkage disequilibrium (r^2) with most significant SNP is indicated as shading of each SNP according to the legend in the upper left of each graphic. Graphic produced by Ricopili.*

variants, that will require replication in large samples. The field is in its infancy, but similar to GWAS studies it can be broken into genome-wide, candidate, and single gene studies.

Prior to the availability of high-throughput sequencing machines, identifying mutations or rarer variants could only be accomplished by sequencing single or modest numbers of genes, usually based on biologically driven hypotheses (Table 18.6). As part of the Synapse-to-Disease Project, the coding regions of 401 genes found in the synapse, with ~30% located on the X chromosome, were sequenced in 143 schizophrenia samples and 285 population controls (Wing et al., 1990). Following confirmation as new mutations, by sequencing

TABLE 18.6. *De novo* variants observed in schizophrenia sequencing studies

REFERENCE	SAMPLES	CONTROLS	GENES OR REGIONS SEQUENCED	RATE OF EXONIC SCZ *DE NOVO* SNVS	RATE OF EXONIC CONTROL *DE NOVO* SNVS	NUMBER OF SCZ *DE NOVO* SNVS	NUMBER OF CONTROL *DE NOVO* SNVS	MS/NS CASES
Awadalla et al., 2010	143 SCZ probands	185	401 synapse-expressed genes[a]	NA	NA	8	1	2/2
Girard, et al., 2011	14 SCZ proband/parent trios	–	Exome	1.88	NA	15	NA	11/4
Need, et al., 2012		–	Exome	1.88	NA	15	NA	11/4
Xu et al., 2012[b]	146 Afrikaner & 85 US SCZ proband/parent trios	34	Exome	0.65	0.50	29	17	121/6
Frank et al., 2011	503	538	10 Glutamate genes-exons[c]					
Ayoub et al., 2012	450	605	*GRM1* exons only					
Sullivan et al., 2012	727	733	10 candidate genes-exons[d]					

[a]Only 39 genes found to have *de novo* variants in cases were sequenced in the controls. [b]*GRM1, DLG1, GRIN2A, GRIN1, DLG4, GRIN2B, DLG2–1, DLG2–4, DLG3, GRIA1, GRIA2* [c]*COMT, DAOA, DISC1, DRD3, DTNBP1, HTR2A, NRG1, SLC6A3, SLC6A4.* [d]includes samples presented in Xu, et al. (Xu, Roos, et al., 2011). Note that several studies of the DISC1 used a pooled DNA sequencing strategy and single gene sequencing studies in fewer then 100 cases are not included in this table. Ms-missense, Ns-nonsense.

both parents, they found 8 *de novo* changes in patients, and 1 in the controls. Amino acid altering mutations were found in several genes previously highlighted in autism or in structural variant pathways including *SHANK3, NRXN1, GRIN2B,* and *KIF7.* The coding regions of 10 genes selected to have some biological and genetic evidence (predating genome-wide association studies) for a role in schizophrenia were sequenced in 727 cases and 733 controls (Crowley et al., 2012). In this study genotyping follow-up of 92 variants, including all rare, novel nonsense, missense, or splice site variants in an independent sample of 2,191 cases and 2,659 controls. Although the replication sample was only modestly powered, no evidence was found suggesting that these genes are enriched for rare coding variation for either the individual variants, or when the variants from a single gene were analyzed together. This is in line with the results from common genomic variants as discussed above for biologically chosen candidate genes. Of note, *DISC1* was included and did not show evidence for an association with rare variants.

Four exome sequencing studies have been reported using next generation, high-throughput technology, and many more will emerge (Table 18.6). Two studies investigated whether there is an increased rate of *de novo* mutations by sequencing the coding regions (exome sequencing) using hybrid capture followed by next generation sequencing, and both used filtering strategies to arrive at a small set of novel mutations for validation (Girard et al., 2011; Xu et al., 2012). In the first study of 14 schizophrenia probands and both parents, 15 *de novo* mutations were found in 8 of the probands, with a notable

number of them being nonsense mutations. An initial small study by Xu et al. reporting 53 cases was followed in 2012 with a larger study of 231 SCZ trios (Xu et al., 2012). In the larger study, the point mutation rate of the exome sequence tested did not differ between cases and controls, but there were differences in the rate and ratios of specific types of mutations, some of which could have a larger functional potential. The missense to silent ratio was elevated 4.84-fold over controls, and no nonsense or canonical splice site mutations were observed in controls. Caution in interpreting these early results is indicated. Recent work from the larger scale studies of *in silico* predicted loss of function mutations indicate that not all nonsense and consensus splice site mutations are functional (MacArthur et al., 2012). Of note, however, only 50% of the patients carried even one potentially functional SNV. Even more surprising was that observation of lack of the same gene being affected by recurrent *de novo* mutations across studies. Only a single gene, dihydropyrimidine dehydrogenase (*DPYD*) contained more than one highly likely functional mutation. The hope that mutations would fall easily into pathways or recur repeatedly in a specific subset of genes is not likely.

In a population-based study, exome and whole genome sequencing of 166 cases of schizophrenia and 307 controls (Need et al., 2012) was followed by genotyping of ~5,000 of the best candidates in additional unrelated cases (*n* = 2,617) and controls (1,800). No individual SNV was significant, given the low power of the primary sample for rare variation. However, even in the follow-up sample no variants were significant. This

study indicates that there may not be very many moderately rare variants (1%–5%) of large effects (>2-fold). Similarly, three candidate genes studies did not find differences between cases and controls in the number of rare variants observed.

Taken together these very early results suggest that rare variation, like common variation, will play a role in liability, but effect sizes may be smaller than hoped and the number of variants larger then hoped, and thus considerably larger sample sizes will be needed to evaluate this. To date no genome-wide deep sequencing studies have been published, however, at the time of writing this chapter, several large studies are in progress whose results will enrich the understanding of the overall architecture.

NEAR FUTURE NEEDS

In the last decade, we have moved from knowing nothing about the types and number of genetic loci involved in these diseases to having a substantial understanding of rare and common variants that increase disease risk, and the path forward is clear for further, future locus identification. Many types of variants of weak effects will be involved, and thus large samples will be necessary regardless of whether common or rare loci are sought. What has not advanced as rapidly is the translation of these findings into biological experimentation. In this respect we are no worse off than with many Mendelian diseases, where the gene cloning is not followed rapidly by insights into pathophysiology and novel treatments (Huntington's disease and Cystic Fibrosis are two examples). For schizophrenia and bipolar disorder, this is in large part because the number and type of loci is much greater than ever anticipated, and because our long history of powerful reductionist science is well developed to study single genes rather than pathways and circuits. However, the large size of the risk gene pool should ultimately allow for more shots on goal as we consider choosing targets for novel drug development.

Many areas of investigation in the near term should prove fruitful in improving our ability to detect causal pathways and relatively more important genes. For common and rare variants, the initial genetic identification generally does not lead to an obvious functionally testable hypothesis regarding the relationship with disease. In the case of common SNPs they may be intergenic, or only related to the functional SNP; in the case of SNVs, the identified variants may have no obvious function, or may be in a seemingly irrelevant gene. In particular, strategies that seek to integrate genetic data with the wealth of biological information publicly available through the Encyclopedia of DNA Elements (ENCODE) and Roadmap to Epigenomics projects, databases of protein interactions, biological pathways, and gene expression will be able to increase the signal to noise ratio. For example, intersecting between different types of genetic variants by evaluating the burden of rare variants in loci identified in CNVs and/or de novo SNVs is likely to improve the detection of consistent underlying pathways. Similarly, integrating genotype data with RNA expression and neuroimaging should likewise be helpful and be employed to build predictive models. Any models derived from this work will need to be experimentally validated, and here there is great hope that human stem cells—induced human pluripotent stem cells derived from patients, that recapitulate the human genetic background—can be differentiated into the tissue of interest, and manipulated experimentally, and this will prove a powerful intermediate for developing and testing pathophysiological understanding (Brennand and Gage, 2012).

Finally, the studies reviewed in this chapter have focused on European samples because those have the largest sample sizes and thus have had the greatest power. These studies need to be extended to additional ethnic groups to begin to elucidate both the shared loci as well as those that are specific.

SUMMARY

This chapter has reviewed strong and convincing genetic evidence that indicates a contribution of many DNA changes to the risk of becoming ill. For schizophrenia, there are large contributions of rare copy number variants and common single nucleotide variants, with an overall highly polygenic genetic architecture. There is a role for rare single nucleotide variation as well as de novo genetic variation being pointed to in new sequencing studies, but their overall contribution to risk is less clear. For bipolar disorder, the role of copy number variation appears to be much less pronounced. Specific common single nucleotide polymorphisms are associated, there is evidence for polygenicity, but as yet no deep sequencing surveys have been published. Several intriguing biological pathways are suggested by these genetic findings related to microRNAs and calcium channel signaling. Several surprises have emerged from the genetic data that indicate there is significantly more molecular overlap in copy number variants between autism and schizophrenia, and in common variants between schizophrenia and bipolar disorder. Translating these results into biological and etiological understanding has not yet advanced, and will likely only do so when experimental methods are developed than can address the large numbers of genes and variants within them that, along with environmental and stochastic effects, result in the development of disease for a particular person.

DISCLOSURE

Dr. Sklar is on the Board of Directors of Catalytic, Inc.

REFERENCES

Alloy, L.B., Abramson, L.Y., et al. (2005). The psychosocial context of bipolar disorder: environmental, cognitive, and developmental risk factors. *Clin. Psychol. Rev.* 25(8):1043–1075.

Athanasiu, L., Mattingsdal, M., et al. (2010). Gene variants associated with schizophrenia in a Norwegian genome-wide study are replicated in a large European cohort. *J. Psychiatr. Res.* 44(12):748–753.

Badner, J.A., Koller, D., et al. (2012). Genome-wide linkage analysis of 972 bipolar pedigrees using single-nucleotide polymorphisms. *Mol. Psychiatry* 17(8):818–826.

Barnett, J.H., and Smoller, J.W. (2009). The genetics of bipolar disorder. *Neuroscience* 164(1):331–343.

Baum, A.E., Akula, N., et al. (2008). A genome-wide association study implicates diacylglycerol kinase eta (DGKH) and several other genes in the etiology of bipolar disorder. *Mol. Psychiatry* 13(2):197–207.

Bergen, S.E., O'Dushlaine, C.T., et al. (2012). Genome-wide association study in a Swedish population yields support for greater CNV and MHC involvement in schizophrenia compared with bipolar disorder. *Mol. Psychiatry* 17(9):880–886.

Brennand, K.J., and Gage, F.H. (2012). Modeling psychiatric disorders through reprogramming. *Dis. Model Mech.* 5(1):26–32.

Brown, A.S. (2011). The environment and susceptibility to schizophrenia. *Prog. Neurobiol.* 93(1):23–58.

Cardno, A.G., and Gottesman, I.I. (2000). Twin studies of schizophrenia: from bow-and-arrow concordances to Star Wars Mx and functional genomics. *Am. J. Med. Genet.* 97(1):12–17.

Casamassima, F., Hay, A.C., et al. (2010). L-type calcium channels and psychiatric disorders: a brief review. *Am. J. Med. Genet. B Neuropsychiatr. Genet.* 153B(8):1373–1390.

Cichon, S., Muhleisen, T.W., et al. (2011). Genome-wide association study identifies genetic variation in neurocan as a susceptibility factor for bipolar disorder. *Am. J. Hum. Genet.* 88(3):372–381.

Collins, A.L., Kim, Y., et al. (2012). Hypothesis-driven candidate genes for schizophrenia compared to genome-wide association results. *Psychol. Med.* 42(3):607–616.

Craddock, N., O'Donovan, M.C., et al. (2009). Psychosis genetics: modeling the relationship between schizophrenia, bipolar disorder, and mixed (or "schizoaffective") psychoses. *Schizophr. Bull.* 35(3):482–490.

Crowley, J.J., Hilliard, C.E., et al. (2012). Deep resequencing and association analysis of schizophrenia candidate genes. *Mol. Psychiatry.* [Epub ahead of print.]

Disanto, G., Morahan, J.M., et al. (2012). Seasonal distribution of psychiatric births in England. *PLoS One* 7(4):e34866.

Ferreira, M.A., O'Donovan, M.C., et al. (2008). Collaborative genome-wide association analysis supports a role for ANK3 and CACNA1C in bipolar disorder. *Nat. Genet.* 40(9):1056–1058.

Frans, E.M., Sandin, S., et al. (2008). Advancing paternal age and bipolar disorder. *Arch. Gen. Psychiatry.* 65(9):1034–1040.

Girard, S.L., Gauthier, J., et al. (2011). Increased exonic de novo mutation rate in individuals with schizophrenia. *Nat. Genet.* 43(9):860–863.

Goes, F.S., Hamshere, M.L., et al. (2012). Genome-wide association of mood-incongruent psychotic bipolar disorder. *Transl. Psychiatry.* 2:e180.

Greenwood, T.A., Akiskal, H.S., et al. (2012). Genome-wide association study of temperament in bipolar disorder reveals significant associations with three novel loci. *Biol. Psychiatry* 72(4):303–310.

Grozeva, D., Conrad, D.F., et al. (2012). Independent estimation of the frequency of rare CNVs in the UK population confirms their role in schizophrenia. *Schizophr. Res.* 135(1–3):1–7.

Hamshere, M.L., Green, E.K., et al. (2009). Genetic utility of broadly defined bipolar schizoaffective disorder as a diagnostic concept. *Br. J. Psychiatry* 195(1):23–29.

Hamshere, M.L., Walters, J.T., et al. (2012). Genome-wide significant associations in schizophrenia to ITIH3/4, CACNA1C and SDCCAG8, and extensive replication of associations reported by the Schizophrenia PGC. *Mol. Psychiatry.* [Epub ahead of print.]

Holmans, P., Green, E.K., et al. (2009). Gene ontology analysis of GWA study data sets provides insights into the biology of bipolar disorder. *Am. J. Hum. Genet.* 85(1):13–24.

Horvath, S., Janka, Z., et al. (2011). Analyzing schizophrenia by DNA microarrays. *Biol. Psychiatry* 69(2):157–162.

Kang, H.J., Kawasawa, Y.I., et al. (2011). Spatio-temporal transcriptome of the human brain. *Nature* 478(7370):483–489.

Kendler, K.S., McGuire, M., et al. (1993). The Roscommon Family Study. IV. Affective illness, anxiety disorders, and alcoholism in relatives. *Arch. Gen. Psychiatry* 50(12):952–960.

Kendler, K.S., Pedersen, N.L., et al. (1995). A pilot Swedish twin study of affective illness including hospital- and population-ascertained subsamples: results of model fitting. *Behav. Genet.* 25(3):217–232.

Kendler, K.S., and Zerbin-Rudin, E. (1996). Abstract and review of "Studien Uber Vererbung und Entstehung Geistiger Storungen. I. Zur Vererbung und Neuentstehung der Dementia praecox" (Studies on the inheritance and origin of mental illness: I. To the problem of the inheritance and primary origin of dementia praecox). 1916. *Am. J. Med. Genet.* 67(4):338–342.

Kieseppa, T., Partonen, T., et al. (2004). High concordance of bipolar I disorder in a nationwide sample of twins. *Am. J. Psychiatry* 161(10):1814–1821.

Kong, A., Frigge, M.L., et al. (2012). Rate of de novo mutations and the importance of father's age to disease risk. *Nature* 488(7412):471–475.

Lee, P.H., O'Dushlaine, C., et al. (2012). INRICH: interval-based enrichment analysis for genome-wide association studies. *Bioinformatics* 28(13):1797–1799.

Lee, S.H., DeCandia, T.R., et al. (2012). Estimating the proportion of variation in susceptibility to schizophrenia captured by common SNPs. *Nat. Genet.* 44(3):247–250.

Lencz, T., Lambert, C., et al. (2007). Runs of homozygosity reveal highly penetrant recessive loci in schizophrenia. *Proc. Natl. Acad. Sci. USA* 104(50):19942–19947.

Lichtenstein, P., Bjork, C., et al. (2006). Recurrence risks for schizophrenia in a Swedish national cohort. *Psychol. Med.* 36(10):1417–1425.

Lichtenstein, P., Yip, B.H., et al. (2009). Common genetic determinants of schizophrenia and bipolar disorder in Swedish families: a population-based study. *Lancet* 373(9659):234–239.

MacArthur, D.G., Balasubramanian, S., et al. (2012). A systematic survey of loss-of-function variants in human protein-coding genes. *Science* 335(6070):823–828.

Maier, W., Lichtermann, D., et al. (1993). Continuity and discontinuity of affective disorders and schizophrenia. Results of a controlled family study. *Arch. Gen. Psychiatry* 50(11):871–883.

Maier, W., Lichtermann, D., et al. (2002). The dichotomy of schizophrenia and affective disorders in extended pedigrees. *Schizophr. Res.* 57(2–3):259–266.

Malhotra, D., McCarthy, S., et al. (2011). High frequencies of de novo CNVs in bipolar disorder and schizophrenia. *Neuron* 72(6):951–963.

Malhotra, D., and Sebat, J. (2012). CNVs: harbingers of a rare variant revolution in psychiatric genetics. *Cell* 148(6):1223–1241.

Martinowich, K., Schloesser, R.J., et al. (2009). Bipolar disorder: from genes to behavior pathways. *J. Clin. Invest.* 119(4):726–736.

Mathieson, I., Munafo, M.R., et al. (2012). Meta-analysis indicates that common variants at the DISC1 locus are not associated with schizophrenia. *Mol. Psychiatry* 17(6):634–641.

McGrath, J., Saha, S., et al. (2008). Schizophrenia: a concise overview of incidence, prevalence, and mortality. *Epidemiol. Rev.* 30:67–76.

McGuffin, P., Rijsdijk, F., et al. (2003). The heritability of bipolar affective disorder and the genetic relationship to unipolar depression. *Arch. Gen. Psychiatry* 60(5):497–502.

Meier, S., Mattheisen, M., et al. (2012). Genome-wide significant association between a "negative mood delusions" dimension in bipolar disorder and genetic variation on chromosome 3q26.1. *Transl. Psychiatry* 2: e165.

Merikangas, K.R., Akiskal, H.S., et al. (2007). Lifetime and 12-month prevalence of bipolar spectrum disorder in the National Comorbidity Survey replication. *Arch. Gen. Psychiatry* 64(5):543–552.

Merikangas, K.R., Jin, R., et al. (2011). Prevalence and correlates of bipolar spectrum disorder in the world mental health survey initiative. *Arch. Gen. Psychiatry* 68(3):241–251.

Miller, B., Messias, E., et al. (2011). Meta-analysis of paternal age and schizophrenia risk in male versus female offspring. *Schizophr. Bull.* 37(5):1039–1047.

Miro, X., Meier, S., et al. (2012). Studies in humans and mice implicate neurocan in the etiology of mania. *Am. J. Psychiatry* 169(9):982–990.

Mortensen, P.B., Pedersen, C.B., et al. (2003). Individual and familial risk factors for bipolar affective disorders in Denmark. *Arch. Gen. Psychiatry* 60(12):1209–1215.

Need, A.C., Ge, D., et al. (2009). A genome-wide investigation of SNPs and CNVs in schizophrenia. *PLoS Genet.* 5(2):e1000373.

Need, A.C., McEvoy, J.P., et al. (2012). Exome sequencing followed by large-scale genotyping suggests a limited role for moderately rare risk factors of strong effect in schizophrenia. *Am. J. Hum. Genet.* 91(2):303–312.

Ng, M.Y., Levinson, D.F., et al. (2009). Meta-analysis of 32 genome-wide linkage studies of schizophrenia. *Mol. Psychiatry* 14(8):774–785.

O'Donovan, M.C., Craddock, N., et al. (2008). Identification of loci associated with schizophrenia by genome-wide association and follow-up. *Nat. Genet.* 40(9):1053–1055.

Olsen, L., Hansen, T., et al. (2011). Copy number variations in affective disorders and meta-analysis. *Psychiatr. Genet.* 21(6):319–322.

Pe'er, I., Yelensky, R., et al. (2008). Estimation of the multiple testing burden for genomewide association studies of nearly all common variants. *Genet. Epidemiol.* 32(4):381–385.

PGC (2009). A framework for interpreting genome-wide association studies of psychiatric disorders. *Mol. Psychiatry* 14(1):10–17.

Power, R.A., Kyaga, S., et al. (2012). Fecundity of patients with schizophrenia, autism, bipolar disorder, depression, anorexia nervosa, or substance abuse vs their unaffected siblings. *Arch. Gen. Psychiatry* 1–8. [Epub ahead of print.]

Psychiatric GWAS Consortium Bipolar Disorder Working Group (2011). Large-scale genome-wide association analysis of bipolar disorder identifi es a new susceptibility locus near ODZ4. *Nat. Genet.* 43(10):977–983.

Purcell, S.M., Wray, N.R., et al. (2009). Common polygenic variation contributes to risk of schizophrenia and bipolar disorder. *Nature* 460(7256):748–752.

Raychaudhuri, S., Plenge, R.M., et al. (2009). Identifying relationships among genomic disease regions: predicting genes at pathogenic SNP associations and rare deletions. *PLoS Genet.* 5(6):e1000534.

Richards, A.L., Jones, L., et al. (2012). Schizophrenia susceptibility alleles are enriched for alleles that affect gene expression in adult human brain. *Mol. Psychiatry* 17(2):193–201.

Rietschel, M., Mattheisen, M., et al. (2012). Association between genetic variation in a region on chromosome 11 and schizophrenia in large samples from Europe. *Mol. Psychiatry* 17(9):906–917.

Rossin, E.J., Lage, K., et al. (2011). Proteins encoded in genomic regions associated with immune-mediated disease physically interact and suggest underlying biology. *PLoS Genet.* 7(1):e1001273.

Schizophrenia Psychiatric Genome-Wide Association Study (GWAS) Consortium. (2011). Genome-wide association study identifies five new schizophrenia loci. *Nat. Genet.* 43(10):969–976.

Scott, L.J., Muglia, P., et al. (2009). Genome-wide association and meta-analysis of bipolar disorder in individuals of European ancestry. *Proc. Natl. Acad. Sci. USA* 106(18):7501–7506.

Segurado, R., Detera-Wadleigh, S.D., et al. (2003). Genome scan meta-analysis of schizophrenia and bipolar disorder, part III: Bipolar disorder. *Am. J. Hum. Genet.* 73(1):49–62.

Seifuddin, F., Mahon, P.B., et al. (2012). Meta-analysis of genetic association studies on bipolar disorder. *Am. J. Med. Genet. B Neuropsychiatr. Genet.* 159B(5):508–518.

Shi, J., Levinson, D.F., et al. (2009). Common variants on chromosome 6p22.1 are associated with schizophrenia. *Nature* 460(7256):753–757.

Shi, Y., Li, Z., et al. (2011). Common variants on 8p12 and 1q24.2 confer risk of schizophrenia. *Nat. Genet.* 43(12):1224–1227.

Sklar, P., Smoller, J.W., et al. (2008). Whole-genome association study of bipolar disorder. *Mol. Psychiatry* 13(6):558–569.

Smith, E.N., Bloss, C.S., et al. (2009). Genome-wide association study of bipolar disorder in European American and African American individuals. *Mol. Psychiatry* 14(8):755–763.

Smith, E.N., Koller, D.L., et al. (2011). Genome-wide association of bipolar disorder suggests an enrichment of replicable associations in regions near genes. *PLoS Genet.* 7(6):e1002134.

Smoller, J.W., and Finn, C.T. (2003). Family, twin, and adoption studies of bipolar disorder. *Am. J. Med. Genet. C Semin. Med. Genet.* 123(1):48–58.

Stefansson, H., Ophoff, R.A., et al. (2009). Common variants conferring risk of schizophrenia. *Nature* 460(7256):744–747.

Steinberg, S., de Jong, S., et al. (2011). Common variants at VRK2 and TCF4 conferring risk of schizophrenia. *Hum. Mol. Genet.* 20(20):):4076–4081.

Sullivan, P.F., Daly, M.J., et al. (2012). Genetic architectures of psychiatric disorders: the emerging picture and its implications. *Nat. Rev. Genet.* 13(8): 537–551.

Sullivan, P.F., Kendler, K.S., et al. (2003). Schizophrenia as a complex trait: evidence from a meta-analysis of twin studies. *Arch. Gen. Psychiatry* 60(12):1187–1192.

Sullivan, P.F., Lin, D., et al. (2008). Genomewide association for schizophrenia in the CATIE study: results of stage 1. *Mol. Psychiatry* 13(6):570–584.

Willour, V.L., Seifuddin, F., et al. (2012). A genome-wide association study of attempted suicide. *Mol. Psychiatry* 17(4):433–444.

Wing, J.K., Babor, T., et al. (1990). SCAN. Schedules for Clinical Assessment in Neuropsychiatry. *Arch. Gen. Psychiatry* 47(6):589–593.

Wray, N.R., and Gottesman, I.I. (2012). Using summary data from the Danish national registers to estimate heritabilities for schizophrenia, bipolar disorder, and major depressive disorder. *Front. Genet.* 3:118.

Xu, B., Ionita-Laza, I., et al. (2012). *De novo* gene mutations highlight patterns of genetic and neural complexity in schizophrenia. *Nat. Genet.* 44(12):1365–1369.

Xu, B., Roos, J.L., et al. (2011). Exome sequencing supports a *de novo* mutational paradigm for schizophrenia. *Nat. Genet.* 43(9):864–868.

Yang, J., Visscher, P.M., et al. (2010). Sporadic cases are the norm for complex disease. *Eur. J. Hum. Genet.* 18(9):1039–1043.

Yutzy, S.H., Woofter, C.R., et al. (2012). The increasing frequency of mania and bipolar disorder: causes and potential negative impacts. *J. Nerv. Ment. Dis.* 200(5):380–387.

19 | GENOMIC SYNDROMES IN SCHIZOPHRENIA

Overlapping Phenotypes

GEORGE KIROV, MICHAEL C. O'DONOVAN, AND MICHAEL J. OWEN

ABBREVIATIONS

CNV   copy number variant
DD   developmental delay
CM   congenital malformations
ASD   autism spectrum disorders
SCZ   schizophrenia
ADHD   attention-deficit hyperactivity disorder
LCR   low copy repeat
NAHR   non-allelic homologous recombination

BACKGROUND

Chromosomes can be impacted by events that result in the duplication, deletion, or inversion of segments of DNA as well as other more complex rearrangements. When the affected segments are relatively large (several million bases of DNA), they can often be seen by light microscopy, a process known as karyotyping. Smaller rearrangements are only detectable by molecular genetic techniques, for example fluorescence in situ hybridization (FISH). Using these approaches, a number of rare causes of severe forms of developmental delay (DD) have been identified that involve whole chromosomes (e.g., Down's syndrome) or relatively large segments of chromosomes (e.g., Prader-Willi/Angelman syndrome, Smith-Magenis syndrome, and the 1p36 deletion syndrome). In schizophrenia (SCZ), these low resolution approaches made two striking findings. Thus carriers of the 2.3Mb deletion of 22q11.2 that causes the DiGeorge/Velo-Cardio-Facial syndrome (VCFS) have been shown to be at very high risk of the disorder (Murphy et al., 1999), and so were members of a single large pedigree who carry a balanced translocation involving chromosomes 1 and 11, the translocation breakpoint on chromosome 1 intersecting the eponymously named Disrupted in Schizophrenia gene (*DISC1*). However, with the introduction of technology with better resolution, including comparative genomic hybridization (CGH), high density genotyping microarrays, and more recently, whole genome sequencing, it is now possible to undertake genome-wide screens for much smaller deletions and duplications, with the resolution offered by sequencing being at the single nucleotide level.

Chromosomal deletions and duplications above 1,000 bases in size have been called DNA copy number variants (CNVs). Some CNVs are common and are not thought to play a major role in human disease. Others are rare, and, while many may be non-pathogenic, a subset of these cause uncommon phenotypes known as genomic disorders (Lupski, 1998, 2009), the name arising from the fact that the disorders are caused via changes to genome structure rather than sequence, and that the genome architecture incites an instability of the genome. The alterations in the genome can occur through recombination between highly homologous stretches of DNA, known as low copy repeats (LCRs), that is, non-allelic homologous recombination (NAHR, Stankiewicz and Lupski, 2002), although other mechanisms have been recognized since (Lupski, 2009). There is now compelling evidence that CNVs also play a role in common disorders, among which SCZ is a prime example.

SCZ is a chronic mental disorder with a lifetime risk of ~1% and a strong genetic component, indicated by heritability estimates of 60–80% and a ~10-fold elevated recurrence risk in first-degree relatives (Gottesman, 1991; Lichtenstein et al., 2009) (see Chapter 18, Pamela Sklar). Despite the evidence for a strong genetic component, until recently there had been very few confirmed genetic susceptibility factors. This picture changed with the publication of a number of genome-wide SNP and CNV studies based on large samples of cases and controls.

Here we summarize the findings for loci for which we consider the evidence of involvement in SCZ as virtually indisputable. Such evidence arises mainly from strong statistical support, replication in independent studies (Table 19.1), and evidence that they are pathogenic for other neurodevelopmental disorders. We will also summarize the evidence for involvement of these loci in other disorders.

THE MAJOR SOURCES OF EVIDENCE CONSIDERED IN THIS REVIEW

The main primary sources of data we consider in this review come from the largest studies on SCZ. The ISC study (ISC, 2008) investigated 3,391 cases and 3,181 controls from six European populations, genotyped with Affymetrix 5.0 or 6.0 arrays. The authors filtered out loci that were common in the sample (>1%) and CNVs <100 kb in size, as they are less reliable for calling. Another team, Stefansson et al. (2008), started off by identifying *de novo* occurring CNVs in the Icelandic population, and then examined their frequencies in a total of 4,718 cases and 41,199 controls from nine European countries and China. Kirov et al.

(2009) examined 471 cases and 2,792 controls who took part in the Wellcome Trust Case Control Consortium study (WTCCC) study and were genotyped with the early version Affymetrix 500K arrays. A large collaborative study on European and African Americans was published by Levinson et al. (2011). It analyzed 3,945 subjects with SCZ or schizoaffective disorder and 3,611 comparison subjects. We also use the main papers that implicated several specific loci: Mulle et al. (2010) for deletions at 3q29; ISC (2008) and Stefansson et al. (2008) for deletions at 15q11.2 and 15q13.3; Kirov et al. (2009) for deletions at *NRXN1*; Moreno-de-Luca et al. (2010) for deletions at 17q12; Ingason et al. (2011a) for duplications at 16p13.1; Ingason et al. (2011b) for maternal duplications at the PWS region on 15q11.2-q13.1; and McCarthy et al. (2009) for duplications at 16p11.2. We have taken care to exclude any overlapping samples. Data on additional ~10,000 controls from the UK population was published by Grozeva et al. (2012), and that paper will be used extensively, as it also summarizes the findings in these loci.

Every CNV that has been robustly implicated in SCZ (Table 19.1) has also been evaluated in large datasets of subjects referred for genetic testing because they had intellectual disability, DD, congenital malformations (CM), or autism spectrum disorders (ASD). Two very large non-overlapping datasets on such patients were reported recently. Girirajan et al. (2012) reported on a sample of 32,587 cases with DD/CM/ASD, and Kaminsky et al. (2011) reported results gathered by a large consortium of cytogenetic laboratories on another very large sample of 15,749 subjects. Combined with the availability of data from other large studies of candidate CNVs in specific disorders, those data permit a reasonable estimation of the frequencies in other neurodevelopmental disorders of what are extremely rare events. A caveat is that these samples comprise a heterogeneous mixture of conditions ascertained through referral for genetic testing, and consequently, the data on each disorder of potential interest (e.g., ASD or DD) may be limited. However, a large proportion of these cases were known to suffer from intellectual disability, DD, and/or ASD, and evidence for the involvement of most of the loci has also come from smaller datasets recruited specifically for the presence of ASD, so we regard the estimates in Table 19.1 as giving a good approximation of the true rates in both DD and ASD.

REVIEW OF INDIVIDUAL CNV LOCI

All coordinates in this chapter are according to the genome build NCBI36/hg18.

DELETIONS AT 1q21.1 (144,9–146,3 Mb)

Deletions at 1q21.1 were independently implicated in SCZ by the first large-scale genome-wide CNV studies of the disorder (ISC, 2008; Stefansson et al., 2008). In a recent review of the published data (Grozeva et al., 2012), we identified 20 reported deletions among over 11,000 cases compared with 11 deletions in almost 60,000 controls. These rates differ highly significantly between the groups (P = 2.9×10^{-9}) and correspond to an odds ratio (OR) of 9.2 for the deletion. Shortly after the findings in SCZ, deletions at this locus were reported to be enriched among a heterogeneous group of individuals who had been referred for genetic testing (Brunetti-Pierri et al., 2008; Mefford et al., 2008). Among the variable phenotypes in carriers, most consistently present were autism, heart defects, and cataracts. Of particular interest, the deletion was also associated with microcephaly, while the reciprocal duplication was associated with macrocephaly. Intriguingly, the region contains the HYDIN2 gene, a paralog of *HYDIN*. Since disruption of *Hydin* causes hydrocephalus in mouse, this has led to speculation that the head size phenotype might be related to altered copy number state of *HYDIN2* (Brunetti-Pierri et al., 2008; Mefford et al., 2008), although it is unclear that *HYDIN2* is translated and it is currently annotated as a pseudogene.

The studies by Girirajan et al. (2012) and Kaminsky et al. (2011) found the deletion at very similar rates of 0.31% and 0.35% respectively, in large samples of people referred to diagnostic laboratories because of DD, intellectual disability, ASD, and various CM. The combined rate of the deletion among such subjects is 0.32%, which is higher than the 0.18% found in SCZ. It is not yet possible to conclude whether this rate is statistically higher in DD/ASD, as the above cohorts included other (non-neurodevelopmental) phenotypes where this CNV has also been specifically implicated, such as congenital heart disease. An excess of duplications in SCZ cases has also been suggested by Levinson et al. (2011). Such an increase in SCZ looks even more likely, as the rate of these duplications is also increased in cases with DD/ASD/CM in the series of Girirajan et al. (2012) and Kaminsky et al. (2011).

DELETIONS IN *NRXN1*

NRXN1 encodes neurexin 1, which is one of a family of presynaptic transmembrane proteins that bind with postsynaptic proteins called neuroligins. They are the only cell adhesion molecules known to be specific to synapses, where they mediate essential interactions between pre- and postsynaptic structures (Südhof, 2008). *NRXN1* has been shown to have a vital role in the formation, maintenance, and release of neurotransmitters at synapses. In the first published study to implicate CNVs in *NRXN1* in SCZ, we and colleagues found a deletion that spanned the promoter and the first exon of the gene which was transmitted to two affected siblings (Kirov et al., 2008). While the statistical evidence that this deletion was disease relevant was weak, the observation in our study of a case with a *de novo* CNV spanning *APBA2* (coding for a protein known to interact with neurexin 1) provided some circumstantial support. Subsequently a strong body of evidence has emerged for the involvement in SCZ of exonic deletions at *NRXN1*, as reviewed by Kirov et al. (2009).

Unlike the other CNVs discussed in this chapter, those affecting *NRXN1* are not flanked by LCRs and therefore deletions at this locus come in various sizes and disrupt different parts of the gene. Currently, and as first noted by Rujescu et al. (2008), compelling evidence (P = 3.7×10^{-6}) for the involvement of CNVs at *NRXN1* concerns specifically exon spanning deletions which have a substantial effect on risk (OR = 7.44; 95% CI = 3.2–17.2) (Kirov et al., 2009). Duplications affecting *NRXN1* are surprisingly rare and have not been associated with diseases.

TABLE 19.1. CNV loci that can be regarded as increasing risk to develop SCZ. The numbers of carriers and the total number of subjects in each study are presented (nn/nn). The sources used to derive the figures are abbreviated with just the names of the first authors and are listed in the references as follows: Grozeva et al. (2012); Girirajan et al. (2012); Kaminsky et al. (2011); Kirov et al. (2009); Ching et al. (2010); Glessner et al. (2009); Ballif et al. (2008); Burnside et al. (2011); de Kovel et al. (2010); Ingason et al. (2011b); Levinson et al. (2011); Dibbens et al. (2009); Nagamani et al. (2011); Williams et al. (2010); Kuang et al. (2011); McCarthy et al. (2009); Rees et al. (2011); Schaaf CP et al. (2012). Genomic coordinates are according to NCBI36/hg18

LOCUS	CONTROLS FREQUENCY	SCZ FREQUENCY	DD/CM/ASD FREQUENCY	OTHER PHENOTYPES
1q21.1 Del 144,9–146,3 Mb	0.02% (Grozeva) 11/57,580	0.18% (Grozeva) 20/11,392	0.31% (Girirajan) 100/32,587 0.35% (Kaminsky) 55/15,749	Congenital heart disease, Microcephaly
2p16.3 **NRXN1** 50,01–51,11 Mb Exonic del	0.02% (Kirov) 9/42,054	0.16% (Kirov) 14/8,798	0.34% (Ching) 12/3,540 0.21% (Schaaf) 17/8,051	ASD: 0.36% (Glessner) 8/2,195
3q29 Del 197,4–198,8 Mb	0.002% (Grozeva) 1/51,200	0.097% (Grozeva) 9/9,323	0.095% (Ballif) 14/14,698 0.061% (Girirajan) 20/32,587 0.057% (Kaminsky) 9/15,749	Microcephaly
15q11.2 Del 20,3–20,8 Mb	0.27% (Grozeva) 160/60,367	0.57% (Grozeva) 68/11,863	0.4% (Burnside) 69/17,000 0.71% (Girirajan) 166/23,380	Epilepsy: 1% (de Kovel) 12/1,234
15q11.2-q13.1 dup (PWS region) 21,2–26,2 Mb	0.007% (Ingason) 3/41,370	0.05% (Ingason) 4/7,582	0.25% (Girirajan) 82/32,587 0.22% (Kaminsky) 35/15,749	ASD: 0.68% (Glessner) 15/2,195
15q13.3 Del 29–30,3 Mb	0.023% (Grozeva) 13/51,151	0.19% (Levinson) 21/10,866	0.26% (Girirajan) 85/32,587 0.29% (Kaminsky) 46/15,749	Epilepsy: 0.98% (de Kovel; Dibbens) 16/1,639
16p13.1 Dup 15.0–16.2 Mb	0.13% (Grozeva) 63/47,854	0.28% (Grozeva) 20/7,075	0.4% (Nagamani) 56/14,000 0.3% (Girirajan) 98/32,587 0.29% (Kaminsky) 45/15,749	ADHD: 0.84% (Williams) 10/1,191 Aortic dissection: 1.1% (Kuang) 13/1,232
16p11.2 Dup 29,5–30,1 Mb	0.031% (Grozeva) 12/38,665	0.3% (McCarthy) 26/8,590	0.25% (Girirajan) 83/32,587 0.25% (Kaminsky) 39/15,749	ASD: 0.45% (Rees) 17/3,746 Microcephaly
17q12 Del 31,8–33,3 Mb	0.003% (Grozeva) 2/58,188	0.06% (Moreno-De-Luca) 4/6,340	0.08% (Girirajan) 26/32,587 0.11% (Kaminsky) 18/15,749	Renal cysts, Diabetes
22q11.21 Del 17,4–19,8 Mb	0% (Grozeva) 0/55,620	0.31% (Levinson) 35/11,400	0.54% (Girirajan) 175/32,587 0.59% (Kaminsky) 93/15,749	Congenital heart disease, many others

Two large studies on DD/ASD/congenital anomalies/epilepsy found deletions in *NRXN1* at higher rates than in controls: Schaaf et al. (2012) found 17 carriers of exonic CNV among 8,051 individuals, and reported that 93% of the patients with exonic deletions manifested DD or intellectual disability, 56% had ASDs, and 59% had infantile hypotonia, while congenital malformations and dysmorphic features appeared only infrequently. Probands with epilepsy were also highly overrepresented among the carriers, at 53%, and ADHD was found in 41%. Ching et al. (2010) reported a similar rate of 12/3,540 exonic deletions among another cohort of probands with similar phenotypes. The combined rate of these two studies (29/11,591) is 0.25%, slightly higher than the 0.16% found in SCZ. Deletions in *NRXN1* have also been found in cases recruited specifically for the presence of ASD (Glessner et al., 2009), again at the somewhat higher rate of 0.36%, compared to SCZ (Table 19.1). Here the sample sizes are smaller than those for SCZ, and so the estimate of the prevalence in ASD is less exact to allow a conclusion as to whether these CNVs are more specific for SCZ or ASD.

DELETIONS AT 3q29 (197,4–198,8 Mb)

These deletions span 21 genes and, after anecdotal observations in some studies, were reported to be associated with SCZ by Mulle et al. (2010). The finding was confirmed by Levinson et al. (2011). In a synthesis of the data (Grozeva et al., 2012), deletions were shown to have been found in about 1 in 1,000 cases, a rate 50 times higher than in controls, a highly significant increase ($P = 4.2 \times 10^{-7}$, OR = 49.5, 95% CI = 6.9–2168). Three large studies reported on the rate of this deletion in other neurodevelopmental disorders (Table 19.1). Ballif et al. (2008) reported the highest rate of 14/14,698 cases affected with CM/mental retardation. The deletion was found in 20 cases out of 32,587 people affected with DD/CM/ASD in the Girirajan et al. (2012) series, and in 9 among the 15,749 subjects of the Kaminsky et al. (2011) series. This gives a total frequency of 0.068% (43/63,034) among such disorders, slightly lower than the 0.097% found among SCZ cases. The near absence of this deletion among controls (a single observation so far in >50,000 controls) suggests a high pathogenicity. This is reflected by the very high selection coefficient of 0.81 estimated for this locus (discussed later in the section "Mutation Rates and Selection Coefficients").

DELETIONS AT 15q11.2 (BP1-BP2, 20,3–20,8 Mb)

There are five documented LCRs near the centromere of chromosome 15 that can instigate NAHR and give rise to CNVs. These LCRs have been called breakpoints (BP) and in the literature are designated BP1 to BP5. Several CNVs arising between different BPs in this region have been implicated in SCZ and other neurodevelopmental disorders. Deletions at 15q11.2 are the most centromeric of these CNV loci and involve the region between BP1 and BP2. The first report that deletions at this locus are risk factors for SCZ came from the work of Stefansson et al. (2008). CNVs at this locus are the most common of those discussed in this review, indeed in the study of the ISC, they surpassed the threshold for exclusion (>1% for deletion and duplication combined) and as a

result, this locus was not considered in that initial report (ISC, 2008). We have recently summarized the results of all published large studies (Grozeva et al., 2012): deletions have been reported in 68 out of 11,863 cases (0.57%) and in 160 of 60,367 controls (0.27%), Fisher Exact Test P = 5.7×10^{-7}.

Despite the very low p-value, this locus confers only a modest OR for SCZ of 2.2 (95% CI = 1.6 to 2.9). Additional support for the pathogenic role for this deletion in human disease has come from work on other neurodevelopmental disorders. Burnside et al. (2011) found 69 cases with deletions here among 17,000 subjects referred for genetic testing, a rate of 0.4%. Phenotypes in carriers of the 15q11.2 deletion included autism, DD, motor and language delays, and behavioral problems. Girirajan et al. (2012) found a somewhat higher rate in their study, CNV deletions occurring here in 0.71% of their sample. Together, these two studies report the deletion in 235 out of 40,380 subjects affected with unexplained DD/intellectual disability/physical anomalies/ASD, a rate of 0.58%. This is almost identical to the rate reported in SCZ (0.57%), and twice that in controls.

High rates of this deletion have also been reported in subjects with epilepsy: De Kovel et al. (2010) found a rate of 1% among 1,234 patients with idiopathic generalized epilepsy. The sample size here is too small to accept this estimate of frequency as accurate, and the main finding in epilepsy remains to be replicated.

The chromosomal segment between BP1 and BP2 contains four highly conserved genes that are expressed in the brain: *TUBGCP5*, *NIPA1*, *NIPA2*, and *CYFIP1*. *CYFIP1* is a gene encoding a postsynaptic protein involved in regulating postsynaptic sensitivity at glutamatergic NMDAR receptors. As reported in their study of *de novo* and case-control CNVs (Kirov et al., 2012) genes that encode such proteins are enriched among CNVs found in those with SCZ, suggesting the hypothesis that *CYFIP1* may be the gene relevant to the disorder at this locus. Details on the role of the postsynaptic density complex in SCZ, and of the involvement of CNVs containing genes that code for proteins embedded within that complex, are presented in Chapter 24 (Seth Grant).

DUPLICATIONS AT 15q11.2-q13.1 (BP2-BP3, 21,2–26,2 Mb)

This 4Mb region is known as the Prader-Willi/Angelman syndrome critical region (PWS/AS). Due to differential methylation of paternal and maternal chromosomes in this region, a phenomenon known as imprinting, some genes are only expressed from the maternally transmitted chromosome, others from the paternally transmitted one. Accordingly, CNVs at this locus functionally impact on different genes depending on the transmitting parent, and as a result, the phenotype also differs by parent of origin. Deletions of the paternal chromosome cause PWS, while deletions of the maternal chromosome cause AS. Duplications of this region are also involved in human disease; indeed they have been claimed to be one of the most common causes of autism (Glessner et al., 2009), where the majority are maternally derived.

It is of note that PWS patients who have maternal uniparental disomy (lacking the paternal chromosome but having inherited two maternal copies) have high rates of psychosis, usually of a

schizoaffective or cycloid type (Verhoeven et al., 1998), whereas those with the usual PWS (lacking the paternal chromosome, but having only a single maternal chromosome in this locus) do not. This suggests that excess expression of a gene in this region (normally expressed only on maternal chromosomes) might contribute to psychosis. Compatible with this, Ingason et al. (2011b) reported four duplications of this region of maternal origin among 7,582 patients affected with SCZ. The rate of this maternal duplication in SCZ is approximately 0.05%, which is more than five times higher than the rate in controls but is much lower than in autism (0.68%). Coupled with the high rate of psychosis in PWS patients with maternal uniparental disomy, it seems very likely this duplication is involved in psychotic disorders.

DELETIONS AT 15q13.3 (BP4-BP5, 29–30,3 Mb)

This 1.3Mb deletion was independently implicated as a risk factor for SCZ in both of the first large CNV studies of the disorder (ISC, 2008; Stefansson et al., 2008). The rate of the deletion in those with SCZ is 0.19% (21/10,887), about 10 times higher than that of controls, $P = 2.7 \times 10^{-9}$, OR = 8.3 (95% CI = 4–18.2) (Grozeva et al., 2012).

Similar to the other CNVs discussed here, this deletion can present with a range of phenotypes. Thus, the overall rate of 0.28% in DD/CM/ASD is similar, and possibly higher to that of SCZ, with similar rates reported in the two largest studies: Girirajan et al. (2012) found 85 deletions in 32,587 subjects referred for DD/CM/ASD, and Kaminsky et al. (2011) found 46/15,749 in their series. Ben-Shachar et al. (2009) pointed out the incomplete penetrance and highly variable expressivity associated with this deletion in a series of 14 children with the deletion, who had been identified from a series of 8,200 individuals referred to medical genetics for diagnostic testing. Phenotypes in the children carrying this CNV included DD, mental retardation, ASD, speech delay, aggressiveness, and attention-deficit hyperactivity disorder (ADHD). Deletions were observed in several phenotypically normal parents and siblings, confirming its incomplete penetrance.

This deletion is also highly likely to be pathogenic for epilepsy. Two studies of generalized idiopathic epilepsy reported a rate of about 1% in patients (combined results of the two studies): 16/1,639 patients (de Kovel et al., 2010; Dibbens et al., 2009). Epilepsy also appears to be more common than expected among carriers of the deletion who also suffer with mental retardation (Sharp et al., 2008). Overall, this CNV seems to be most highly enriched in those with epilepsy than it is for other developmental phenotypes, although as before, a caveat is that sample sizes used in the epilepsy studies are more than an order of magnitude smaller than those for SCZ and DD/CA. It is also of note that very few of the SCZ patients who had this deletion had documented epilepsy.

DUPLICATIONS AT 16p13.1 (15.0–16.2 Mb)

The pathogenicity of this CNV locus was first suggested by Ullmann et al. (2007), who found duplications in four male patients with severe autism. Ingason et al. (2011a) subsequently reported a threefold increase in the rate of this duplication in

4,345 cases with SCZ, which is in line with, although slightly larger than, what we find in a review of the literature in which we reported a prevalence of 0.28% (20/7,075) in cases compared with 0.13% in controls (63/47,854) in controls, $p = 0.005$, OR = 2.1 (95% CI = 1.2–3.6).

Following the pattern of the other CNVs, increased rates of this duplication have been reported in other disorders. Williams et al. (2010) found an increased rate of 0.84% in ADHD. The rates reported in DD/CM/ASD are similar to those in SCZ (Table 19.1): 0.29% among 15,749 subjects in the study by Kaminsky et al. (2011), 0.3% among 32,587 subjects in the study by Girirajan et al. (2012), and 0.40% among 14,000 subjects in the study by Nagamani et al. (2011). Phenotypic manifestations in the three studies listed above included behavioral abnormalities, cognitive impairment, congenital heart defects, and skeletal defects. Another phenotype is aortic dissection, with a carrier rate of ~1% (Kuang et al., 2011), although given the size of the sample, this study is underpowered for accurate estimation of frequency and requires replication.

The reciprocal deletion has not been confidently implicated in SCZ yet, although a non-significant trend was reported in the Ingason et al. (2011a) study, where deletions were present in 0.12% of cases and 0.04% of controls (P > 0.05). The deletion appears to also confer high risk for DD and ASD. Thus, in the study by Girirajan et al. (2012), deletions at 16p13.1 were found in 0.14% of the 32,587 subjects. Intriguingly, very high rates of this deletion have been reported in people with epilepsy, with one study (Heinzen et al., 2010) reporting a 0.6% rate (23/3,812).

DUPLICATIONS AT 16p11.2 (29,5–30,1 Mb)

This gene-rich duplication (24 genes) was first implicated as a risk factor for autism, where it is regarded as one of the most frequent chromosomal abnormalities (e.g., Glessner et al., 2009; Sanders et al., 2011), with a rate of 0.45% (reviewed in Rees et al., 2011). A meta-analysis of studies on SCZ (McCarthy et al., 2009) also found a highly increased rate of duplications at this locus in SCZ: 0.3% (26/8,590), while the latest estimate of the control rate is 0.031 (12/38,665), an almost 10-fold increase in SCZ: OR = 9.8, 95% CI = 4.8–21.3, $P = 1.8 \times 10^{-11}$ (Grozeva et al., 2012). This CNV is also present at high rates in DD/CM: Girirajan et al. (2012) and Kaminsky et al. (2011) found it in a total of 122 out of 48,446 subjects referred for genetic testing, a rate (0.25%) similar to but somewhat lower than in ASD and SCZ. Carriers were typically microcephalic, a phenotype that through studies of zebra fish and of mouse, appears to be attributable to dosage of KCTD13 (Golzio et al., 2012). KCTD13 encodes polymerase delta-interacting protein 1, which has been speculated to have a role in cell cycle during neurogenesis, although it is not clear yet from human studies that this gene per se is involved in SCZ.

The rate of the reciprocal deletion is markedly increased in DD/CM: Girirajan et al. (2012) found it among 125/32,587 cases (0.38%) and Kaminsky et al. (2011) in a similar rate of 67/15,749 (0.43%) a more than 10-fold increase over the 0.03% in controls (McCarthy et al., 2009). However, as yet there is no evidence that the prevalence of this deletion is increased in people affected with SCZ (McCarthy et al. 2009).

DELETIONS AT 17q12 (31,8–33,3 Mb)

Deletions of 1.5Mb at this region have been implicated in SCZ (Moreno-De-Luca et al., 2010), and in autism/neurocognitive impairment (Loirat et al., 2010; Moreno-De-Luca et al., 2010). This CNV can also present with various medical conditions including macrocephaly, genitourinary tract anomalies such as renal cysts, recurrent infections, and diabetes (Moreno-De-Luca et al., 2010; Nagamani et al., 2010). The rate among individuals referred for genetic testing in the combined datasets of Girirajan et al. (2012) and Kaminsky et al. (2011) is 0.09% (44/48,336), an approximately 30-fold increase compared to controls, where it has been detected in only two out of 58,188 controls (0.003%). As this CNV is very rare, and has not been tested in sufficiently large cohorts of SCZ, the evidence for its involvement in SCZ is still modest and requires further evaluation, it having been reported so far in only 4/6,340 cases (0.06%) a rate that is still about 20-fold higher than in controls, $p = 0.001$, OR = 18.4 (95% CI = 2.6–203).

DELETIONS AT 22q11.2 (17,4–19,8 Mb)

This was the first CNV of established pathogenicity in psychosis, for which it still confers the highest known elevation in risk of any molecular lesion. It has been extensively reviewed in the literature (e.g., Murphy et al., 1999). Small studies have reported substantial variation in prevalence in the disorder, but the best estimate is 0.31% (35/11,400) (Levinson et al., 2011), compared with zero observations among 55,620 controls. Around 80% of cases are due to *de novo* mutations (reviewed by Rees et al., 2011). Around 30% of carriers develop psychosis, but despite this incomplete penetrance, the deletion carriers are not found in control populations, probably because they can also develop cardiac anomalies, mild mental retardation, or other behavioral abnormalities, leading to their exclusion from control populations. About 40% of carriers have mild mental retardation, and the mean IQ is in the range of 70–80. Around 30% of deletion carriers have ASD. The rate among referrals for genetic testing for DD/CM/ASD is 0.55% in the combined datasets of Girirajan et al. (2012) and Kaminsky et al. (2011), with virtually identical rates between the two studies: 175/32,587 (0.54%) and 93/15,749 (0.59%) respectively. This is approximately twice the rate found in SCZ.

Despite intensive investigation over more than a decade, and a number of intriguing candidates, the gene(s) within this CNV relevant to psychosis have not been unequivocally established. The role of the reciprocal duplication is much less clear, with increased rates reported in DD/ASD/CM (Girirajan et al., 2012; Kaminsky et al., 2011), but not in SCZ.

COMPARISON BETWEEN RECIPROCAL DELETIONS AND DUPLICATIONS OF THE REGIONS

As can be seen from Table 19.1, the specific deletion or duplicated CNVs that have been implicated in SCZ have also been implicated in DD and or ASD. However, whereas most of the reciprocal CNVs in Table 19.1 have also been implicated in DD and/or ASD, there are to date no instances where both deletion

and duplication at a given locus have been confidently confirmed to increase risk of SCZ. This could be due to lack of power of these studies, and indeed increased risk for duplications at 1q21.1 and deletions at 16p13.1 has been suggested and awaits replication (Ingason et al., 2011a; Levinson et al., 2011). Of the three duplications listed in Table 19.1, the reciprocal deletions at 15q11.2-q13.1 are known to cause Prader-Willi or Angelman syndromes (depending on parental origin), while deletions at 16p11.2 and 16p13.1 are found at high rates in DD/ASD. The same applies to rearrangements at 7q11.23, where deletions cause Williams Beuren syndrome, while duplications have been implicated in SCZ (Kirov et al., 2012) and are known to cause ASD (Sanders et al., 2011). Similarly the reciprocal duplications of the deleted loci from Table 19.1 (except for 1q21.1) have not yet been implicated as increasing risk for SCZ, although many have been found at increased rates in the Girirajan et al. (2012) and Kaminsky et al. (2011) series with DD/CM (e.g., duplications at 1q21.1, 3q29, 15q13.3, 17q12, 22q11.2). The absence of association at most of the reciprocal loci could be due to lack of power in the SCZ studies, but could also reflect a degree of specificity in the role of CNVs in SCZ and DD/ASD.

Figure 19.1 (based on Table 19.1) shows the frequencies of each CNV at SCZ implicated loci in SCZ, DD/CM/ASD, and controls. At several of the loci (1q21.1, *NRXN1*, 15q13.3, duplications at the PWS/AS region and deletions at the VCFS region on 22q11.2), the CNV frequencies are substantially higher in DD/CM/ASD compared with SCZ, but at none is the frequency markedly higher in SCZ than in DD/CM/ASD. We have not attempted a formal statistical analysis of these comparisons given the data have been generated and analyzed with very different methods and platforms. Nevertheless, it appears that with some exceptions the SCZ-associated CNVs are either similar in frequency or are even more common in DD/ASD than in SCZ.

At present, it is premature to do direct comparisons between SCZ and samples ascertained specifically for studies of ASD (as opposed to general referral for molecular genetics testing), as those studies are still too small to allow confident comparisons. However, tentatively, the available data suggest a more prominent role in autism than in SCZ for maternally inherited duplications of the PWS/AS region (0.68%), deletions at *NRXN1* (0.36%), and possibly duplications at 16p11.2 (0.45%), but larger studies of ASD (without CM/DD) are required to resolve this question.

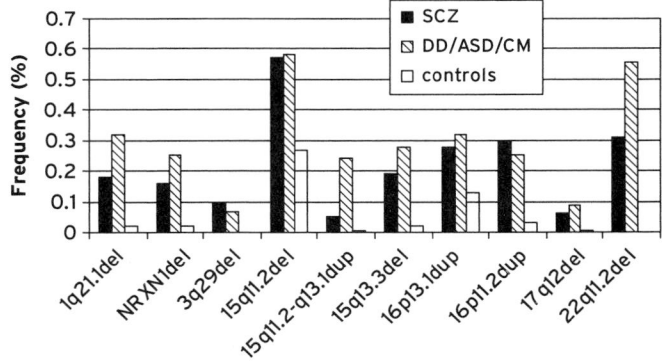

Figure 19.1 Comparison of the rates of the reviewed CNVs in SCZ, DD/ASD/CM, and controls.

As highlighted in the previous sections, several CNVs result in increased risk to develop DD/CM/ASD, but not SCZ, but the converse is not true. If we accept that SCZ represents a milder phenotype based on later age at onset and less impaired cognition, this may suggest that those that do not cause SCZ have higher pathogenicity. In support of this hypothesis, we would note that there are many other CNV loci that we do not discuss in this chapter, that cause severe DD, intellectual deficit, and some recognized syndromes, for example 1p36 syndrome, Sotos or Smith-Magenis syndrome. These CNVs are not known to include SCZ as a phenotype, although the identification of such CNVs in a proband with SCZ or ASD should raise the question of causality.

There was an expectation that these CNVs will also increase risk to develop bipolar affective disorder, as the two disorders share genetic factors (Lichtenstein et al., 2009). Several studies failed to find such links and the overall rate of large and rare CNVs in bipolar disorder was found to be similar to that among controls (e.g., Grozeva et al., 2010). However, the rate of de novo CNVs is increased in bipolar patients compared to controls, at 4.3%, which is nearly as high as the rates reported in SCZ (Malhotra et al., 2011), indicating that certain CNVs also increase risk to develop this disorder. This might apply especially to large duplications (Malhotra et al., 2011), such as the duplication at 16p11.2 (McCarthy et al., 2009).

MUTATION RATES AND SELECTION COEFFICIENTS

SCZ is associated with substantially reduced fecundity, estimated at less than half compared to healthy controls. As a result, genetic variants that confer high risk to SCZ might be expected to be subject to strong negative selection and therefore be eventually excluded from the population. If the prevalence of SCZ is stable in the population, and the evidence suggests it is, or at least it has not decreased to the current rate from a much higher level, it is a reasonable first proposition that the high penetrance variants that are excluded by selection should be replenished by new (de novo) mutations (though other explanations are also possible). In the case of CNVs, studies of proband parent trios (reviewed by Rees et al., 2012) have shown that this is indeed true. An early study (Xu et al., 2008) found that a de novo CNV occurred in 10% of individuals with SCZ who had no family history of SCZ in a close family member, but the rate of de novo CNV occurrence in SCZ has dropped somewhat as sample sizes have enlarged. Thus, recent estimates are in the order of around 5% compared with a rate in controls of around 1% or 2% (summarized by Kirov et al., 2012). The de novo CNVs were also much larger than those found to be transmitted, another indication that they are under selection pressure (otherwise their properties would be similar to those of CNVs that are neutral and segregating in the population at large). Moreover, that the observed de novos represent a replenishing of schizophrenia risk CNVs is supported by the fact that a large number of the 34 de novo CNVs we reported (Kirov et al., 2012) were either in some of the confirmed SCZ loci discussed in this chapter, or in loci for which there is a high index of suspicion for their involvement

in SCZ, such as the duplication at the WBS region and the DLG2 gene.

Assuming that the prevalence of a CNV is stable in the general population, it is possible to estimate the strength of the selection pressure acting against it. As discussed previously, if a CNV is under selection pressure, then its prevalence will decline in each generation unless new de novo CNVs occur at a rate equal to that at which they are removed as a result of reduced fecundity of carriers. The selection pressure or selection coefficient (s) against a CNV approximates to the proportion of CNVs at a locus that are the direct result of de novo events in a representative sample of the population: ($s = [N$ de novo]/[N total]). It is also possible to estimate the average number of people that will carry a de novo CNV before it is eliminated from the population. This is called pervasiveness and is estimated as $1/s$ (see Rees et al., 2012). In Table 19.2 we present estimates of selection pressure and pervasiveness. All the loci from Table 19.1 are under a strong selection pressure of between 0.11 and 0.81, and are expected each be carried by between 1.2 (for the more pathogenic 17q12 and 22q11.2 deletions) and 9.1 people (for the more common 15q11.2 deletion and 16p13.1 duplication) before they are eliminated from the general population. In other words all these CNVs confer risk to disorders that markedly reduce fecundity or survival and if the frequency in the population is stable, must have high mutation rates. Their mutation rates are indeed high, estimated between 1.7×10^{-5} and 1.4×10^{-4} (Rees et al., 2011). Thus, between 1 in 7,000 newborns (for 15q11.2 deletion) and 1 in 58,000 newborns (for 17q12 deletion) will have a new mutation at each of the loci listed in Table 19.1.

CONCLUSIONS

The recent CNV studies have changed the landscape of SCZ genetics. There are now at least 10 confirmed loci that cause substantial increases in the risk to develop the disorder, and we expect that the list will grow once larger samples are tested, as many CNVs are so rare that tens of thousands of patients need to be genotyped for a confident statistical conclusion to be reached. These studies have shown a rather unexpected overlap with the genetic causes of DD and ASD, with all of the implicated large CNVs conferring increased risk to develop these disorders. For several of the CNVs, the carriers appear even more likely to develop these earlier onset disorders (DD/ASD/intellectual disability), and one could speculate that other genetic or environmental factors protect carriers from developing a disorder during early childhood, but instead they develop SCZ in later life. The penetrance for developing any disorder is incomplete, and it would be fascinating if any protective factors are identified. These large CNVs cause a reduction in fecundity in their carriers, and would be eliminated from the population very quickly, if it were not for their high mutation rates. The main cause for the increased mutation rate at these loci is the abundance of LCRs in the human genome, that causes instability, mostly via NAHR events.

The presence of clearly identified genetic changes that increase risk to develop SCZ raises the question whether

TABLE 19.2. Selection coefficients for associated SCZ CNV loci. Del = deletion, Dup = duplication. Selection coefficients (s) are updated from those estimated by Rees et al. (2011) with data from the recent large paper by Girirajan et al. (2012). The second column presents the numbers of *de novo* mutations in each locus out of the total number (*de novo* + transmitted) reported in studies that systematically ascertained the rates of *de novos* in these loci. Pervasiveness refers to the average number of people who will carry the mutation before it is eliminated from the general population.

CNV LOCUS	N(*DE NOVO*)/ N(TOTAL)	SELECTION COEFFICIENT S (*DE NOVO* RATIO)	PERVASIVENESS (1/S)
1q21.1 del	22/76	0.29	3.4
NRXN1 exonic del	7/32	0.22	4.5
3q29 del	17/21	0.81	1.2
15q11.2 del	7/64	0.11	9.1
15q13.3 del	20/69	0.29	3.4
15q11.2-q13.1 dup	17/34	0.50	2.0
16p13.1 dup	7/63	0.11	9.1
16p11.2 dup	19/66	0.29	3.4
17q12 del	12/16	0.75	1.3
22q11.2 del	482/601	0.80	1.3

subjects with this disorder should undergo genetic testing and counseling, if requested. This is now routine practice in children with unexplained DD/ASD, and could easily be applied to patients suffering with SCZ. The yield is likely to be much lower than among subjects with DD/ASD/CM, as only about 2–3% of SCZ sufferers are likely to carry a known pathogenic CNV. It will be up to the genetics community and patients to discuss whether such testing will be beneficial and cost-effective for the treatment and counseling of sufferers and their families.

DISCLOSURES

The authors have not disclosed any conflicts of interest.

REFERENCES

Ballif, B.C., et al. (2008). Expanding the clinical phenotype of the 3q29 microdeletion syndrome and characterization of the reciprocal microduplication. *Mol. Cytogenet.* 1:8.

Ben-Shachar, S., Lanpher, B., et al. (2009). Microdeletion 15q13.3: a locus with incomplete penetrance for autism, mental retardation, and psychiatric disorders. *J. Med. Genet.* 46:382–388.

Burnside, R., Pasion, R., et al. (2011). Microdeletion/microduplication of proximal 15q11.2 between BP1 and BP2: a susceptibility region for neurological dysfunction including developmental and language delay. *Hum. Genet.* 130:517–528.

Brunetti-Pierri, N., Berg, J.S., et al. (2008). Recurrent reciprocal 1q21.1 deletions and duplications associated with microcephaly or macrocephaly and developmental and behavioral abnormalities. *Nat. Genet.* 40:1466–1471.

Ching, M.S., Shen, Y., et al. (2010). Children's Hospital Boston Genotype Phenotype Study Group. Deletions of NRXN1 (neurexin-1) predispose to a wide spectrum of developmental disorders. *Am. J. Med. Genet. B Neuropsychiatr. Genet.* 153B:937–947.

de Kovel, C.G., Trucks, H., et al. (2010). Recurrent microdeletions at 15q11.2 and 16p13.11 predispose to idiopathic generalized epilepsies. *Brain* 133(Pt 1):23–32.

Dibbens, L.M., Mullen, S., et al.; EPICURE Consortium. (2009). Familial and sporadic 15q13.3 microdeletions in idiopathic generalized epilepsy: precedent for disorders with complex inheritance. *Hum. Mol. Genet.* 18:3626–3631.

Girirajan, S., Rosenfeld, J.A., et al. (2012). Phenotypic heterogeneity of genomic disorders and rare copy-number variants. *N. Engl. J Med.* 367:1321–1331.

Glessner, J.T., Wang, K., et al. (2009). Autism genome-wide copy number variation reveals ubiquitin and neuronal genes. *Nature* 459:569–573.

Golzio, C., Willer, J., et al. (2012). KCTD13 is a major driver of mirrored neuroanatomical phenotypes of the 16p11.2 copy number variant. *Nature* 485:363–367.

Gottesman, I.I. (1991). *Schizophrenia Genesis: The Origins of Madness.* New York: Henry Holt.

Grozeva, D., Kirov, G., et al.; Wellcome Trust Case Control Consortium. (2010). Rare copy number variants: a point of rarity in genetic risk for bipolar disorder and schizophrenia. *Arch. Gen. Psychiatry* 67:318–327.

Grozeva, D., Conrad, D.F., et al.; Wellcome Trust Case Control Consortium. (2012). Independent estimation of the frequency of rare CNVs in the UK population confirms their role in schizophrenia. *Schizophr. Res.* 135:1–7.

Heinzen E.L., Radtke R.A., et al.(2010) Rare deletions at 16p13.11 predispose to a diverse spectrum of sporadic epilepsy syndromes. *Am. J. Hum. Genet.* 86:707–718.

Ingason A., Rujescu D., et al. (2011a). Copy number variations of chromosome 16p13.1 region associated with schizophrenia. *Mol. Psychiatry.* 16:17–25.

Ingason A., Kirov G., et al. (2011b). Maternally derived microduplications at 15q11-q13: implication of imprinted genes in psychotic illness. *Am. J. Psychiatry* 168:408–417.

International Schizophrenia Consortium. (2008). Rare chromosomal deletions and duplications increase risk of schizophrenia. *Nature* 455:237–241.

Kaminsky, E.B., Kaul, V., et al. (2011). An evidence-based approach to establish the functional and clinical significance of copy number variants in intellectual and developmental disabilities. *Genet. Med.* 13:777–784.

Kirov, G., Grozeva, D., et al.; International Schizophrenia Consortium; the Wellcome Trust Case Control Consortium. (2009). Support for the involvement of large CNVs in the pathogenesis of schizophrenia. *Hum. Mol. Genet.* 18:1497–1503.

Kirov, G., Gumus, D., et al. (2008). Comparative genome hybridization suggests a role for NRXN1 and APBA2 in schizophrenia. *Hum. Mol. Genet.* 17:458–465.

Kirov, G., Pocklington, A.J., et al. (2012). *De novo* CNV analysis implicates specific abnormalities of postsynaptic signalling complexes in the pathogenesis of schizophrenia. *Mol. Psychiatry* 17:142–153.

Kirov, G., Rujescu, D., et al. (2009). Neurexin 1 (NRXN1) deletions in schizophrenia. *Schizophr. Bull.* 35:851–854.

Kuang, S.Q., Guo, D.C., et al.; GenTAC Investigators. (2011). Recurrent chromosome 16p13.1 duplications are a risk factor for aortic dissections. *PLoS. Genet.* 7(6):e1002118.

Levinson, D.F., Duan, J., et al. (2011). Copy number variants in schizophrenia: confirmation of five previous findings and new evidence for 3q29 microdeletions and VIPR2 duplications. *Am. J. Psychiatry.* 168:302–316.

Lichtenstein, P., Yip, B.H., et al. (2009). Common genetic determinants of schizophrenia and bipolar disorder in Swedish families: a population-based study. *Lancet.* 373:234–239.

Loirat, C., Bellanne-Chantelot, C., et al. (2010). Autism in three patients with cystic or hyperechogenic kidneys and chromosome 17q12 deletion. *Nephrol. Dial. Transplant.* 25:3430–3433.

Lupski, J.R. (1998). Genomic disorders: structural features of the genome can lead to DNA rearrangements and human disease traits. *Trends. Genet.* 14:417–422.

Lupski, J.R. (2009). Genomic disorders ten years on. *Genome. Med.* 1:42.

McCarthy, S.E., Makarov, V., et al. (2009). Microduplications of 16p11.2 are associated with schizophrenia. *Nat. Genet.* 41:1223–1227.

Malhotra, D., McCarthy, S., et al. (2011). High frequencies of *de novo* CNVs in bipolar disorder and schizophrenia. *Neuron* 72:951–963.

Mefford, H.C., Sharp, A.J., et al. (2008). Recurrent rearrangements of chromosome 1q21.1 and variable pediatric phenotypes. *N. Engl. J. Med.* 359:1685–1699.

Moreno-De-Luca, D., Mulle, J.G., et al. (2010). Deletion 17q12 is a recurrent copy number variant that confers high risk of autism and schizophrenia. *Am. J. Hum. Genet.* 87:618–630.

Mulle, J.G., Dodd, A.F., et al. (2010). Microdeletions of 3q29 confer high risk for schizophrenia. *Am. J. Hum. Genet.* 87:229–236.

Murphy, K.C., Jones, L.A., et al. (1999). High rates of schizophrenia in adults with velo-cardio-facial syndrome. *Arch. Gen. Psychiatry* 56:940–945.

Nagamani, S.C., Erez, A, et al. (2010). Clinical spectrum associated with recurrent genomic rearrangements in chromosome 17q12. *Eur. J. Hum. Genet.* 18:278–284.

Nagamani, S.C.S., Erez, A., et al. (2011). Phenotypic manifestations of copy number variation in chromosome 16p13.11 *Eur. J. Hum. Genet.* 19:280–286.

Rees, E., Moskvina, V., et al. (2011). *De novo* rates and selection of schizophrenia-associated copy number variants. *Biol. Psychiatry* 70:1109–1114.

Rees, E., Kirov, G., et al. (2012). *De novo* mutation in schizophrenia. *Schizophr. Bull.* 38:377–381.

Rujescu, D., Ingason, A., et al. (2011). Multiple recurrent *de novo* CNVs, including duplications of the 7q11.23 Williams syndrome region, are strongly associated with autism. *Neuron* 70:863–885.

Schaaf, C.P., Boone, P.M., et al. (2012). Phenotypic spectrum and genotype-phenotype correlations of NRXN1 exon deletions. *Eur. J. Hum. Genet.* 20:1240–1247.

Sharp, A.J., Mefford, H.C., et al. (2008). A recurrent 15q13.3 microdeletion syndrome associated with mental retardation and seizures. *Nat. Genet.* 40:322–328.

Stankiewicz, P., and Lupski, J.R. (2002). Genome architecture, rearrangements and genomic disorders. *Trends. Genet.* 18:74–82.

Stefansson, H., Rujescu, D., et al. (2008). Large recurrent microdeletions associated with schizophrenia. *Nature.* 455:232–236.

Südhof, T.C. (2008). Neuroligins and neurexins link synaptic function to cognitive disease. *Nature* 455:903–911.

Verhoeven, W.M., Curfs, L.M., et al. (1998). Prader-Willi syndrome and cycloid psychoses. *J. Intellect. Disabil. Res.* 42(Pt 6):455–462.

Ullmann, R., Turner, G., et al. (2007). Array CGH identifies reciprocal 16p13.1 duplications and deletions that predispose to autism and/or mental retardation. *Hum. Mutat.* 28:674–682.

Williams, N.M., Zaharieva, I., et al. (2010). Rare chromosomal deletions and duplications in attention-deficit hyperactivity disorder: a genome-wide analysis. *Lancet* 376:1401–1408.

Xu, B., Roos, J.L., et al. (2008). Strong association of *de novo* copy number mutations with sporadic schizophrenia. *Nat. Genet.* 40:880–885.

20 | NEUROIMAGING OF PSYCHOTIC DISORDERS

STEPHAN HECKERS, NEIL WOODWARD, AND DOST ÖNGÜR

STUDYING THE BRAIN TO UNDERSTAND PSYCHOSIS

Neuroimaging studies of brain structure and function have significantly advanced our understanding of psychotic disorders. They transformed psychosis research at a very basic level—by capturing the elusive pathology with brain images (Johnstone et al., 1976). At a time when few psychiatrists were neuroscientists, this was crucial for redefining psychotic disorders as brain disorders. Neuroimaging of psychotic disorders began in the 1970s with computed tomography (CT) studies of brain structure, followed by single photon emission computed tomography (SPECT) and positron emission tomography (PET) studies of blood flow, glucose metabolism, and receptor chemistry. It culminated in the application of several magnetic resonance imaging (MRI)–based techniques, including structural MRI, functional MRI (fMRI), MR spectroscopy (MRS), and diffusion tensor imaging (DTI). The widespread use of MR machines in academic medical centers has liberated a new generation of researchers from the constraints of postmortem research and the limitations of inferring brain abnormalities through neurochemical effects in plasma or urine.

Despite tremendous progress, the neuroimaging of psychotic disorders remains heavily influenced by Emil Kraepelin's concept of psychotic disorders. He introduced the dichotomy of nonaffective and affective psychoses at the end of the 19th century and asserted that schizophrenia is caused by a cellular pathology of the cerebral cortex, leading to marked cognitive deficits, whereas bipolar disorder is not. He also began the neuroscientific study of psychotic disorders, using two very different approaches: he conducted psychological experiments in patients and he encouraged the pathological exploration of their brains after death. Encouraged by early successes, anatomists and pathologists dominated the field of schizophrenia research in the first half of the 20th century. They described mainly qualitative abnormalities in the cellular organization of the cerebral cortex and the thalamus. However, by the 1950s, they concluded that the neuropathology was elusive and that they were not able to diagnose schizophrenia in the laboratory. Similarly, the efforts of experimental psychologists did not lead to diagnostic tests that could assist clinicians in the management of psychotic patients.

Two discoveries reinvigorated the neuroscientific study of psychotic disorders. The serendipitous discovery of neuroleptic/antipsychotic drugs raised important questions about their mechanism at the level of cells and circuits. The subsequent discovery of the neurotransmitter dopamine and its role in mediating the effect of neuroleptic/antipsychotic drugs helped focus the research on a small group of neurons in the midbrain and their diffuse projections to the cortex and subcortical regions. This led to the prominence of neurochemical models for the explanation of schizophrenia, first the dopamine model in the 1960s and then the glutamate model in the 1980s.

Many themes of the neuroimaging research reviewed here overlap with those in postmortem research (see Chapter 23) and cognitive neuroscience research (see Chapter 21). However, the ability to study brain structure and function repeatedly and to correlate it with cognitive and clinical outcomes are unique strengths of neuroimaging studies and will ensure a prominent position of this research methodology in the study of psychotic disorders. Here we provide an overview of the neuroimaging studies of psychotic disorders (mainly schizophrenia and schizoaffective disorder). We will focus on meta-analyses and comprehensive reviews, but will include some seminal studies that have shaped our current understanding of psychotic disorders.

THE GOALS OF NEUROIMAGING IN THE STUDY OF PSYCHOTIC DISORDERS

First and foremost, we look toward neuroimaging to establish illness markers that can distinguish a clinically defined group of patients (e.g., schizophrenia) from healthy controls and from other patient groups (e.g., mood disorder). The ideal outcome is a test that can assist the clinician in the diagnosis and management of the psychotic patient.

Second, we expect that neuroimaging will aid in the understanding of the psychosis phenotype. This includes explanations of abnormal mental states, such as delusions and hallucinations, and of the prominent deficits in the realm of attention, memory, language, and thought.

Third, neuroimaging methods need to improve our neural models of psychotic disorders, including the prominent anatomical models of prefrontal cortex and medial temporal lobe pathology and the neurotransmitter models of dopamine, glutamate, and GABA dysfunction.

Finally, neuroimaging can build a bridge to the genetic mechanisms of the disease. This can be explored by studying monozygotic and dizygotic twins, by studying nonaffected relatives of psychotic patients, or by studying the association of risk genes with neuroimaging markers.

Our review is organized according to these four goals of neuroimaging in the study of psychotic disorders. It is important to note that these goals are not necessarily aligned with each other and that relatively specialized communities of researchers have emerged to pursue these studies. Even the same result, for example, abnormal hippocampal structure and function, may be interpreted in largely non-overlapping contexts. For example, one researcher may want to develop it as a diagnostic marker in the early stages of psychosis, whereas another might explore the same finding as an indication of abnormal GABAergic or glutamatergic function in schizophrenia. Yet another setting for the same finding is to study the neural consequences of potential risk alleles such as DISC1 or BDNF. The same scenario holds true for abnormalities of the prefrontal cortex, the thalamus, the cerebellum, or the basal ganglia. The relative merits of these goals are rarely considered, and the neuroimaging community has yet to define shared goals in order to make progress in schizophrenia research.

ESTABLISHING MARKERS OF DISEASE

The vast majority of structural and functional neuroimaging studies compare a group of psychotic patients, at one time point, with a group of healthy control subjects. This cross-sectional approach is modeled after the use of neuroimaging in clinical radiology, where the image of a single patient is contrasted with the standard of a healthy person. Some studies have compared two different groups of patients (e.g., schizophrenia versus bipolar disorder) in order to explore shared or distinct features of psychopathology. So far, few researchers have taken advantage of the unique strength of neuroimaging methods to follow patients over time. This is due in large part to the challenges of a longitudinal study design. In addition, there are several pitfalls when disambiguating illness effects from treatment effects. However, it is likely that the longitudinal study design will ultimately secure a prominent position of neuroimaging in the scientific study and clinical management of psychotic patients.

CROSS-SECTIONAL STUDY OF BRAIN STRUCTURE

There are two main approaches to quantifying brain structure: manual tracing and automated methods. The initial studies of brain structure in schizophrenia used the manual approach to quantify the volume of a specific region-of-interest (ROI). The earliest of these studies employed computed tomography and focused on measuring the size of the ventricles (Johnstone et al., 1976). The subsequent development of MRI afforded substantially better spatial resolution of brain tissue types, that is, gray matter, white matter, and cerebrospinal fluid (CSF), which prompted a large number of volumetric studies. Qualitative and quantitative reviews of structural MRI studies using manual tracing methods confirmed the earlier finding of ventricular enlargement. They also concluded that schizophrenia is associated with reductions in whole brain volume, particularly gray matter volumes of the medial temporal lobe (including hippocampus and amygdala), the superior temporal gyrus, the frontal and parietal lobes, and several subcortical regions (including the basal ganglia, thalamus, and cerebellum) (Shenton et al., 2001). With better image resolution of more recent studies, this general pattern has not changed substantially (Shenton et al., 2010). While consistent across studies, the magnitude of these changes is subtle, generally falling within the range of 5–10% for specific structures and <5% for whole brain and total gray matter volumes (Wright et al., 2000).

Three regions of interest, the superior temporal gyrus (STG), the thalamus, and the hippocampus, have been studied extensively. Thirty-five out of 46 (76%) studies reported a significant difference in STG volume (mainly reduction) and 18 out of 30 studies reported correlations of STG volume with the severity of auditory hallucinations or thought disorder (Sun et al., 2009). Thirteen studies reported volume reduction of both left and right thalamus in both first-episode patients (six studies) and chronic patients (seven studies), with Cohen's d effect sizes ranging from −0.32 to −0.48 (Adriano et al., 2010). Finally, 13 studies of first-episode patients and 22 studies of chronic patients provided compelling evidence for smaller left and right hippocampal volumes in schizophrenia, with Cohen's d effect sizes ranging from −0.56 to −0.65 (Adriano et al., 2012). Taken together, there is compelling evidence for localized gray matter volume changes in schizophrenia.

Advances in computing power and computational anatomy spurred the development and application of automated methods for investigating structural brain changes in schizophrenia. In addition to the obvious advantage of being less laborious, compared to manual tracing approaches, automated methods can quantify multiple brain structures, examine changes at higher resolution—for example, down to the voxel-wise level in the case of voxel-based morphometry (VBM), and quantify aspects of cerebral morphology that are difficult to measure, such as cortical thickness.

Three meta-analyses of VBM studies used the activation likelihood estimation (ALE) method to review the current evidence of gray matter (Fornito et al., 2009; Glahn et al., 2008) and white matter (Di et al., 2009) abnormalities in schizophrenia. The ALE method tests for the likelihood that, across the studies under review, spheres around specific brain coordinates differ between groups. A more recent study (Bora et al., 2011) used the signed differential mapping (SDM) method, which includes not only positive changes as in the ALE method, but also negative results for the estimation of group differences. The results of these recent meta-analyses largely confirm the previous ROI-based studies, with two exceptions. First, medial temporal lobe abnormalities are not as prominent in meta-analyses of the VBM studies. This is possibly due to the lower sensitivity of the ALE and SDM methods to the complex anatomy in a relatively circumscribed region (Bora et al., 2011). Second, several brain regions, which had not been implicated by the ROI studies, emerged from the VBM studies. In large part this is due to a more difficult delineation of cortical regions, resulting in fewer studies. This is particularly striking for the insula, for which an ALE-based meta-analysis (Glahn et al., 2008) and an SDM-based meta-analysis (Bora et al., 2011) provided the initial evidence. This has now been confirmed by a third meta-analysis (Shepherd, Matheson, et al., 2012), which localized the changes

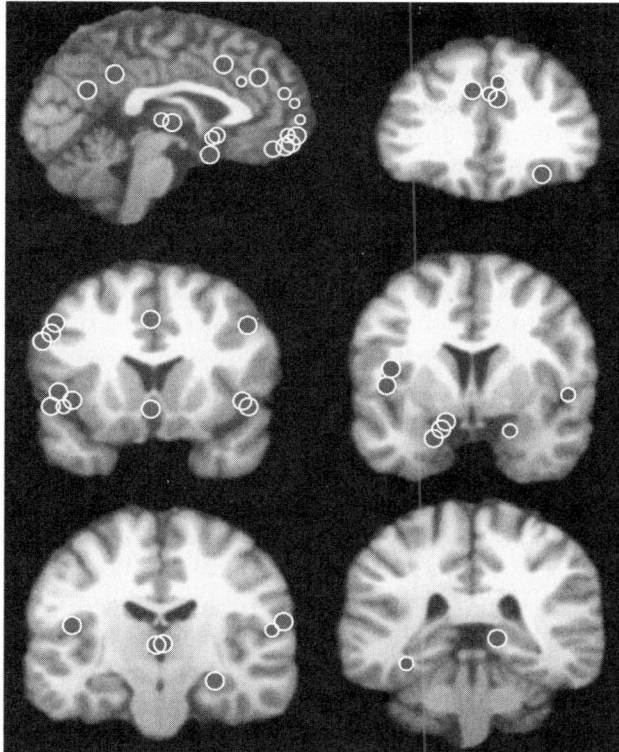

Figure 20.1 *Reduced grey matter density in chronic schizophrenia. Dots indicate the spatial proximity of foci identified across multiple voxel-based meta-analyses, with coronal slices progressively posterior from left to right. Reproduced from: Shepherd, A. M., K. R. Laurens, et al. (2012). "Systematic meta-review and quality assessment of the structural brain alterations in schizophrenia." Neuroscience and Biobehavioral Reviews with permission from Elsevier.*

to the anterior insula (connected to limbic cortex) in both first-episode and chronic patients.

Two recent meta-analyses using the ALE method examined the specificity of the changes observed in schizophrenia compared to bipolar disorder. Both reviews concluded that there is considerable overlap in gray matter volume reduction in schizophrenia and bipolar disorder, with both involving gray matter loss in the anterior cingulate/medial prefrontal cortex, lateral prefrontal cortex, and bilateral insula. However, the extent of gray matter volume loss is greater in schizophrenia and includes additional areas, such as the thalamus and temporal lobe (Ellison-Wright and Bullmore, 2010; Yu et al., 2010).

A comprehensive summary of both ROI and VBM studies of structural brain alterations in schizophrenia concluded that we now have evidence for gray matter reductions of anterior cingulate, frontal (particularly medial and inferior) and temporal lobes, hippocampus/amygdala, thalamus, and insula that may be magnified over time (Shepherd et al., 2012a) (Fig. 20.1).

CROSS-SECTIONAL STUDY OF BRAIN FUNCTION

Cognition is markedly impaired in schizophrenia, with relatively greater deficits in episodic memory, executive cognitive abilities, such as problem solving and working memory,

and processing speed (see Chapter 21). Not surprisingly, the bulk of functional imaging investigations in schizophrenia have focused on elucidating the neural correlates of cognitive impairment, as opposed to clinical symptoms, such as delusions and hallucinations. The advent of functional neuroimaging, beginning with PET in the 1980s then fMRI in the early 1990s, opened new avenues of research into the neural basis of cognitive impairment in schizophrenia. Early PET studies revealed abnormal activity in the prefrontal cortex, often consisting of reduced activation compared to control subjects during performance of executive cognitive tasks (Weinberger et al., 1986a). The non-invasive nature of fMRI coupled with widespread availability, relative to PET imaging, resulted in a rapid increase of functional neuroimaging studies of cognition in schizophrenia. Meta-analyses and qualitative reviews of this literature have revealed several consistent findings (Glahn et al., 2005; Minzenberg et al., 2009; Ragland et al., 2009; Goghari et al., 2010; Niendam et al., 2012; Whalley et al., 2012).

In line with earlier PET studies, schizophrenia patients often demonstrate reduced activation of the dorsolateral PFC during performance of executive cognitive tasks (Glahn et al., 2005; Minzenberg et al., 2009). However, reduced brain activity extends beyond the PFC to include rostral anterior cingulate cortex, thalamus, and inferior/posterior parietal cortex. In addition, increased rather than decreased PFC activity in schizophrenia is observed in several regions, including the midline cortical areas, premotor cortex, and ventrolateral PFC (Glahn et al., 2005; Minzenberg et al., 2009). This more complex pattern of localized increases and decreases of PFC activity during performance of executive cognitive tasks has led to models that go beyond the simple notion of hypofrontality in schizophrenia. On the one hand, the alterations are more consistent with a pattern of dysregulation and decreased efficiency, rather than a simple loss of cortical activity. On the other hand, a distributed network of frontal, subcortical, and posterior brain regions is engaged during the performance of executive cognitive tasks, and the PFC is one of several abnormal nodes in a dysregulated network in schizophrenia.

Reduced activation of the prefrontal cortex, especially the dorsolateral PFC, is also observed during episodic memory (Achim and Lepage, 2005; Ragland et al., 2009). Episodic memory (the ability to encode and retrieve the details of events) and relational memory (the ability to remember not just single items but also their relationships) are significantly impaired in schizophrenia, and it is therefore not surprising that neuroimaging studies have explored the neural basis of this deficit. In addition to the abnormalities of dorsolateral PFC during memory performance, several studies have also reported an abnormal recruitment of the hippocampus and the closely connected parahippocampal cortex. This pattern has been interpreted as an abnormal corticohippocampal network or an abnormal connectivity within the hippocampal formation (Heckers and Konradi, 2010).

PARSING HETEROGENEITY

While neuroimaging studies have supported Kraepelin's assertion that psychotic disorders have a neural basis, they have

also revealed significant heterogeneity. This is apparent in two metrics of the available meta-analyses: the low to medium effect sizes of the group differences and the significant results when measuring the inconsistency between study results. In other words, neuroimaging studies do not have to answer the question "Is the brain abnormal in psychotic disorders?" since the evidence is strongly affirmative. Instead, we now need to turn to the question "Which patient has what abnormality?" in order to parse the still considerable heterogeneity of psychotic disorders. This line of research may proceed along the well-established path of studying diagnostic categories. But neuroimaging methods are very well suited to complement this with an alternative approach. It takes dimensions of psychopathology, cognition, or neural systems as a starting point in order to uncover mechanisms that are not expected to confirm the existing nosology of psychotic disorders. Such cross-cutting dimensions can enrich the diagnostic classification and can provide new avenues to study the mechanism of psychotic disorders, with the hope to develop markers for the development or testing of new treatments.

Neuroimaging findings have not matured yet as validators of the various psychotic disorder diagnoses and will not be included as biological markers in the revision of the *Diagnostic and Statistical Manual of Mental Disorders* (DSM-5). It is likely that traditional dichotomies such as schizophrenia/healthy control or schizophrenia/bipolar disorder are not sufficient to overcome the low validity and limited clinical utility of neuroimaging methods. However, the ability to correlate brain structure and function with the clinical features of psychotic disorders is one of the strengths of neuroimaging and deserves more attention.

Liddle and colleagues characterized 30 chronic outpatients with schizophrenia, who had a stable pattern of psychotic symptoms, using factor analysis (Liddle et al., 1992). The symptoms were grouped into three syndromes, namely, prominent positive symptoms (reality distortion), prominent negative symptoms (psychomotor poverty), or prominent thought disorder (disorganization). Each of the three patterns was associated with altered perfusion at different loci, including increased medial temporal lobe blood flow in the reality distortion syndrome and decreased prefrontal cortex blood flow in the psychomotor poverty and disorganization syndromes. A similar approach was pursued by VBM studies, which revealed distinct patterns of gray matter density in the three syndromes, with a shared pattern of prefrontal and perisylvian alterations (Nenadic et al., 2012).

Several neuroimaging studies have explored the neural correlates of the negative syndrome or schizophrenia patients with persistent negative symptoms (Hovington and Lepage, 2012). This subgroup constitutes approximately 15–20% of all schizophrenia patients. They show more pronounced reductions of cortical gray matter, more widespread deficits of prefrontal and temporal recruitment during the performance of cognitive tasks, and more significant impairments of several cognitive abilities, especially memory. This group of patients deserves further attention in neuroimaging studies, especially in the early stages of the disease, when treatment effects are less likely to obscure the effects of prominent negative symptoms.

Patients with schizophrenia have also been contrasted with other psychotic patients, for example, schizoaffective disorder and psychotic bipolar disorder patients. A recent review of these studies concluded that medial temporal lobe changes differentiated bipolar patients from patients with schizophrenia, but that alterations in the prefrontal cortex were less discriminating (Whalley et al., 2012). This line of research challenges Kraepelin's schizophrenia/bipolar dichotomy in two ways. First, it is now clear that bipolar disorder is as much a brain disorder as is schizophrenia, while Kraepelin did not consider bipolar disorder worthy of study in the laboratory or the morgue. More importantly, patients with psychotic bipolar disorder share many of the clinical features of schizophrenia, but may differ with regard to disease onset, progression, and outcome, resulting in different treatments. This allows neuroimaging researchers to disentangle the shared mechanisms of clinical features (e.g., hallucinations, delusions) from the more fundamental mechanisms of the disease. They also allow, to some degree, the study of a major confound in neuroimaging studies of psychotic disorders, namely, pharmacological treatment.

EFFECTS OF ILLNESS AND TREATMENT

Most abnormalities of brain structure and function are described initially in chronic, treated patients, and researchers are then moving to studies of patients in the early stages of the illness, if possible with no or little exposure to current treatments whenever possible.

While many studies of early psychosis confirmed the findings in chronic patients, they typically detect less significant or less widespread changes. For example, a meta-analysis comparing studies of chronic patients to first-episode schizophrenia concluded that many of the structural brain changes observed in chronic patients are present at first episode, including gray matter loss in bilateral insula, left uncus/amygdala, anterior cingulate, and thalamus (Ellison-Wright et al., 2008). For more detail see Chapter 26.

LONGITUDINAL STUDIES

The unique strength of neuroimaging studies is the ability to follow patients over time to study brain abnormalities at all stages of the illness and even predating the illness (high-risk state and prodrome). This puts neuroimaging in the unique position to study the neural mechanisms of course, outcome, and response to treatment. While longitudinal studies are superior to cross-sectional studies, simply by design, they are challenging and are confounded by the effect of treatment and different genetic and environmental backgrounds.

A review of longitudinal studies in chronic schizophrenia (follow-up duration ranging from 1 to 10 years) reported reductions in frontal lobe and thalamus volume and less consistent reductions of whole brain and temporal lobe, particularly STG, volumes. No progressive differences were reported in the hippocampus or cerebellum (Hulshoff Pol and Kahn, 2008). A meta-analysis of ventricular volume change found compelling evidence for increased lateral ventricular volume

over time, in both first-episode and chronic patients (Kempton et al., 2010).

A recent meta-analysis confirmed these earlier findings, reporting a significant change over time for whole brain gray matter, frontal lobe gray matter, and left caudate. No progressive changes were reported in temporal, parietal, or occipital lobe gray matter, hippocampus, amygdala, or cerebellum over a range of 1 to 10 years (Olabi et al., 2011). Interestingly, illness duration before baseline was negatively associated with the effect size in the hippocampus, implying that the magnitude of this volume difference changes as the disease progresses. The consequences of progressive changes in brain structure in schizophrenia remain unclear, but may be associated with poorer outcome, worse negative symptoms, and greater cognitive impairment. It is unclear whether bipolar disorder is associated with similar changes in brain structure over time, as relatively few studies have been carried out (Schneider et al., 2012).

HIGH-RISK STUDIES

Complementing the longitudinal studies of psychotic patients are studies of subjects who are not psychotic, but are at high risk to develop a psychotic disorder. Such cohorts can be defined by a high familial loading for psychotic disorders, that is, at least one or more than one (multiplex) first-degree relative with a psychotic disorder. An alternative recruitment strategy is the detailed characterization of basis symptoms of psychosis or brief, limited, and intermittent psychotic symptoms that do no cross the threshold for a categorical diagnosis. Such studies are time-consuming and require considerable effort in recruitment and follow-up. Recent meta-analyses have reviewed this still young branch of neuroimaging research (Fusar-Poli et al., 2011; Smieskova et al., 2010). They indicate that gray matter volume reductions in temporoparietal, bilateral prefrontal, and limbic cortices are a marker of increased risk for psychosis. In addition, gray matter reductions in superior temporal and inferior frontal areas are associated with later transition to psychosis (Fusar-Poli et al., 2011). These structural studies are complemented by a smaller number of fMRI, PET, and MRS studies, which also point to abnormalities in frontal and temporolimbic brain regions (Smieskova et al., 2010). In contrast to structural imaging studies of the early and chronic stages of schizophrenia, high-risk studies have repeatedly shown an increase in whole brain and gray matter volumes. This somewhat counterintuitive finding has been interpreted as an indication of dynamic brain changes at the time of transition into psychosis and deserves further study.

STATISTICAL CONSIDERATIONS

The vast majority of the neuroimaging studies reviewed here have set out to identify a structural or functional brain abnormality that can separate a group of patients from a healthy control group or a different group of patients. It is important to briefly review several issues of study design and inference testing, including representativeness of the study sample, strength of the statistical effect, and the sensitivity and specificity of the findings.

Most relevant is the feasibility and clinical utility of the study design. Do the research studies recruit a representative sample of patients from the larger population? While this seems possible for structural imaging studies, it is unlikely for functional studies, which require the active participation of study subjects. It is particularly challenging if the neural function under study (e.g., working memory) is impaired in the patients, but the design of the study asks for matched performance in order to draw stronger inferences about neural mechanisms. This often excludes a large number of patients who cannot perform adequately during the test.

The effect size of most neuroimaging findings in psychotic disorders is less than 0.5, and very few are above 1.0. A recent meta-analysis of structural neuroimaging studies using ROI methods (excluding VBM studies) of several psychiatric disorders concluded that the significance of the group differences has been inflated (Ioannidis, 2011). In short, the number of positive results was too large to be true: the number of positive results was almost double than what would have been expected based on power calculations for the included samples. The excess significance may be due to unpublished negative results or due to selective exploratory analyses (Ioannidis, 2011). The more recent meta-analyses of VBM studies also add a word of caution, as they consistently show a high degree of inconsistency between study results. Taken together, we need to remain cautious about the strength of the statistical inferences.

Finally, even if a difference of brain structure or function is significant, it is not clear whether such a marker is sensitive and specific enough to classify an individual patient accurately. This has been explored in several studies using structural MR datasets. For example, a study of 36 patients with recent-onset psychosis and 36 healthy control subjects showed significantly lower gray matter density in the patients, and a machine learning algorithm was able to correctly classify patients with 86% accuracy (Sun et al., 2009). A similar accuracy was reported in a study of high-risk subjects (Koutsouleris et al., 2009). For now, a skilled clinical interview remains the most efficient and cost-effective diagnostic tool. However, these are encouraging first studies of pattern classification of imaging data in the diagnosis of psychotic disorder patients.

UNDERSTANDING THE PHENOTYPE

So far we have reviewed neuroimaging as a tool to establish disease markers. The non-invasive methods of MR imaging have also attracted the interest of researchers who study the phenomenology of psychosis and are interested in the mechanisms of abnormal mental states, irrespective of categorical diagnoses and their impact on disease management. In essence, they employ neuroimaging to study core questions of psychiatric phenomenology and psychopathology, such as "How does the brain hallucinate?"

Most neuroimaging studies of hallucinations have focused on auditory verbal hallucinations, the most prevalent form of hallucinations in schizophrenia (Allen et al., 2012; Jardri

et al., 2011; Palaniyappan et al., 2012). The initial studies simply compared patients with a history of frequent hallucinations and those who reported a low level of hallucinatory experiences. More recently, ratings for the severity of hallucinations were correlated with brain structure and function (Palaniyappan et al., 2012). These studies have confirmed a hypothesis that can be traced back to postmortem studies 100 years ago: patients with a prominent history of auditory hallucinations have a smaller superior temporal gyrus. In addition to the structural abnormalities of the STG, there is also evidence for structural abnormalities of the insula, anterior and posterior cingulate cortex, inferior frontal gyrus, thalamus, cerebellum, and precuneus. Finally, data are emerging that link auditory hallucinations to abnormalities of brain chemistry, including increased levels of glutamine (Allen et al., 2012).

Few neuroimaging studies have explored patients during the experience of psychotic symptoms (symptom-capture studies). For example, a patient is studied during the experience of auditory hallucinations, and brain activity is then compared to periods when the hallucinations are not present (Dierks et al., 1999). In addition to the unique challenges of this study design (e.g., infrequent events, reliance on the subject to indicate the experience of the symptom), the studies cannot resolve whether the functional brain abnormalities are primary or secondary to the event of interest. For example, is the activation of the primary auditory cortex the origin of the voices or is the association cortex recruiting the primary auditory cortex during the experience of hearing voices? Despite these caveats, the few symptom-capture studies have provided compelling evidence for an abnormal activation in a bilateral neural network, including Broca's area, anterior insula, precentral gyrus, frontal operculum, middle and superior temporal gyri, inferior parietal lobule, and hippocampus/parahippocampal region (Jardri et al., 2011) (Fig. 20.2). This indicates that the experience of auditory verbal hallucinations involves increased activity in areas involved in speech generation and perception as well as verbal memory.

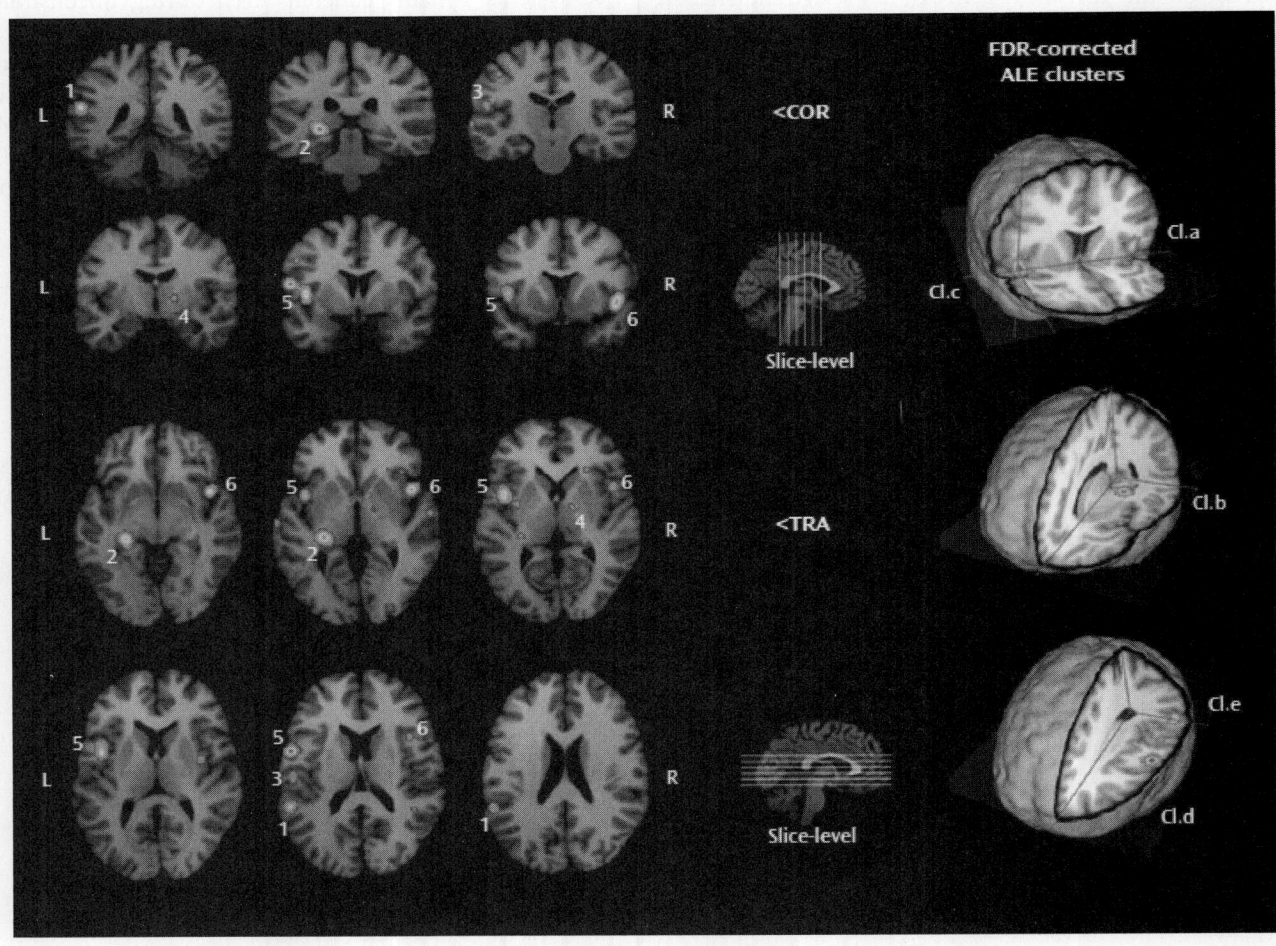

Figure 20.2 *Functional brain activity associated with auditory verbal hallucinations in schizophrenia. The first three columns depict the activation likelihood estimation (ALE) results on coronal (COR) views (upper panel) as well as on transverse (TRA) views (lower panel) of the brain anatomy. The fourth column depicts slice levels shown on sagittal views. The fifth column shows clusters (Cl.a to Cl.e) of consistent activity among patients with schizophrenia spectrum disorders experiencing auditory verbal hallucinations. Reproduced from: Jardri, R., A. Pouchet, et al. (2011). "Cortical activations during auditory verbal hallucinations in schizophrenia: a coordinate-based meta-analysis." The American Journal of Psychiatry 168(1): 73–81; used with permission. (See color insert).*

There are several other phenomena of psychosis that deserve further study using neuroimaging methods: What brain changes characterize catatonia, with its characteristic periods of mutism and stupor? What happens in the brain of a patient who is unable to think and speak coherently? What is at the core of the fractured self? While these questions remain intriguing, developing the proper experimental approaches to capture such phenomena is a challenge.

STUDYING THE NEURAL MECHANISMS

Over the last 100 years, several leitmotifs have captured the attention of neuroscientists who explored the neural basis of psychotic disorders. Here we focus on network models and neurochemistry changes observed in schizophrenia measured using MRS.

NETWORK MODELS OF SCHIZOPHRENIA

The idea that the pathology of schizophrenia involves abnormalities in brain connectivity (i.e., dysconnectivity) can be traced back to the turn of the 20th century (Gage and Hickok, 2005). Dysconnectivity models of schizophrenia received relatively little attention at the time and remained largely ignored for much of the 20th century. The advent of structural neuroimaging, which provided clear evidence that multiple brain regions are affected in schizophrenia, combined with advances in our understanding of the large-scale functional organization

of the human brain, reinvigorated interest in network models of schizophrenia.

Two important advances in functional imaging contributed to the renaissance of dysconnectivity theories of schizophrenia. The first is the development and increased use of network-based approaches to analyzing functional imaging data. In contrast to standard functional imaging methods that focus on detecting differences in brain activity between behavioral conditions (i.e., activations), network-based approaches examine statistical dependencies in activity across brain regions. The most common of these methods, functional connectivity, quantifies correlations between brain regions. Usually this is accomplished by selecting a brain region, called a "seed," and calculating its correlation with other brain areas. Brain regions that demonstrate correlated activity over time are said to be functionally connected. The second key development is the emergence of resting-state fMRI. As its name implies, no task is performed during the scanning session; subjects are instructed to rest quietly for several minutes. Application of functional connectivity methods to resting-state fMRI data has revealed that activity in several canonical brain networks corresponding to sensory, motor, and cognitive systems remains coherent even during unconstrained mental activity (see Fig. 20.3) (Zhang and Raichle, 2010). The correspondence between resting-state networks and known anatomical connections, along with their striking resemblance to activation patterns observed with task-based fMRI, support the validity of resting-state fMRI (Honey et al., 2009; Smith et al., 2009). Combined, these two developments have

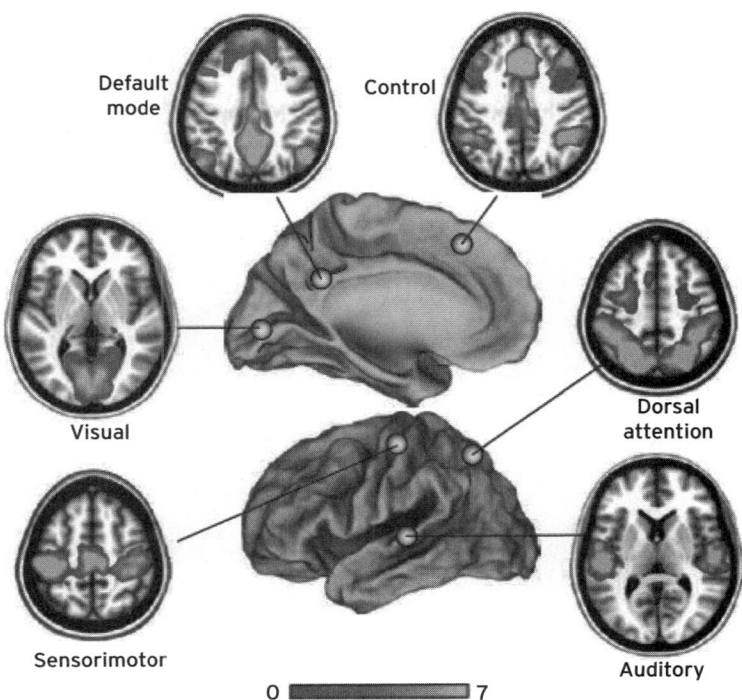

Figure 20.3 Intrinsic neuronal activity of the brain. Correlation of neuronal activity between a seed region (each circle) and the rest of the brain reveals six major networks: visual, sensorimotor, auditory, default mode, dorsal attention, and executive control. The scale numbered 0–7 indicates relative correlation strength. Reproduced from: Zhang, D. and M. E. Raichle (2010). "Disease and the brain's dark energy." Nat.Rev.Neurol. 6(1): 15–28 with permission from Nature Publications Group. (See color insert).

created novel opportunities to test dysconnectivity theories of schizophrenia.

Several network models of schizophrenia have been proposed. Cortical models integrate the deficits in executive cognitive functioning with frontal cortical gray matter loss and alterations in dorsolateral prefrontal cortex (PFC) microcircuitry. Others link the deficits in episodic memory to hippocampal volume loss and abnormalities of intrinsic or extrinsic hippocampal connectivity. The final set of network models focuses on cortical-subcortical networks. These models are supported by evidence of structural changes in cortex, striatum, thalamus, and cerebellum; alterations in dopamine signaling, and, more recently, animal studies showing that focal disturbances in subcortical structures recapitulates many of the key cognitive and neurotransmitter changes observed in schizophrenia. We review neuroimaging support for each of these network models of schizophrenia. Particular attention is paid to studies that applied network-based analytic approaches to functional imaging data.

ALTERATIONS IN PREFRONTAL CORTEX NETWORKS IN SCHIZOPHRENIA

Executive cognitive functions that rely on the integrity of the PFC, including working memory, initiation, planning, and cognitive flexibility, are impaired in schizophrenia (Heinrichs and Zakzanis, 1998). Not surprisingly, the initial functional imaging investigations of schizophrenia patients attributed executive cognitive impairment to PFC dysfunction (Weinberger, Berman et al., 1986b). Postmortem studies showing reduced dendritic spines, fewer axon terminals, and smaller soma volumes of pyramidal cells, in the context of normal number of neurons, along with a variety of changes in cortical GABA interneurons provides a possible mechanistic explanation for the structural and functional changes in the PFC (Lewis, 2012).

The PFC, however, is densely connected to other cortical areas, particularly the posterior parietal cortex, temporal lobe, and subcortical brain structures, and damage to or dysfunction of these regions can also produce impairments in executive cognitive functions (Fuster, 2008). Functional neuroimaging has confirmed that, in addition to the PFC, the posterior parietal cortex, and rostral/dorsal anterior cingulate cortex are consistently activated by a variety of executive cognitive tasks (Niendam et al., 2012). The combination of traditional lesion studies and functional neuroimaging has led to the idea that a "superordinate" fronto-cingulo-parietal network (FCPN) underlies executive cognitive functioning (Niendam et al., 2012).

There is considerable evidence of activation differences during performance of executive cognitive tasks in schizophrenia. A recent meta-analysis of 41 imaging studies concluded that reduced neural activity in schizophrenia extends beyond the PFC to include additional regions of the FCPN, including the rostral/dorsal anterior cingulate and inferior/posterior parietal cortex (Minzenberg et al., 2009). Dysconnectivity within the FCPN, and PFC more generally, during task performance has been confirmed by functional connectivity analyses. The general picture to emerge from these investigations is that connectivity of the PFC is reduced in schizophrenia, and that PFC connectivity with parietal and temporal lobe regions is especially affected (Pettersson-Yeo et al., 2011). PFC dysconnectivity has also been consistently observed in resting-state studies. As with task-based imaging, these studies have shown reduced connectivity within the PFC and between dorsolateral PFC and parietal cortex (Cole et al., 2011; Woodward et al., 2011; Zhou et al., 2007). Importantly, PFC dysconnectivity is present in both first-episode and chronic patients, unaffected relatives of patients, and even individuals at high risk for developing schizophrenia (Pettersson-Yeo et al., 2011). Combined, the evidence strongly suggests that functional connectivity of the PFC, particularly the dorsolateral PFC, is altered in schizophrenia and that the abnormality is a fundamental component of the illness that transcends cognitive state and illness stage.

HIPPOCAMPAL NETWORK DYSFUNCTION

Smaller hippocampal volume was the initial evidence for an involvement of the hippocampus in schizophrenia. This finding is now firmly established, and postmortem as well as animal studies have supported several models of hippocampal dysfunction in schizophrenia (Heckers and Konradi, 2010).

For example, one model proposes that the reciprocal connections of the hippocampus and the multimodal association cortex are perturbed in schizophrenia and that this leads to the well-known deficits of abnormal episodic and relational memory. Functional neuroimaging studies have supported this hypothesis with evidence for an impaired recruitment during memory encoding and retrieval (Heckers and Konradi, 2010). But it remains unclear whether hippocampal or cortical nodes in this network drive the memory dysfunction. It is also not clear when these changes occur, since first episode and at-risk subjects already show hippocampal alterations, and whether the changes are amenable to treatment.

Several competing models propose that only some aspects of the hippocampus are abnormal in schizophrenia, leading to a specific rather than general pathology. This includes proposed changes of anterior but not posterior hippocampal regions, of the CA 2/3 but not the CA1 sector and of interneurons but not glutamatergic cells (Lisman et al., 2008; Heckers and Konradi, 2010). Some of these hypotheses are supported by postmortem and animal studies and can now be studied with neuroimaging studies. For example, high-resolution (7T) imaging can resolve the regions and sectors of the human hippocampus. Similarly, studies of cerebral blood flow and blood volume can provide an index of tonic activity of the hippocampus and can test for GABAergic and glutamatergic dysfunction in schizophrenia (Small et al., 2011).

CORTICAL-SUBCORTICAL NETWORK DYSFUNCTION

Cortical projections to striatum and cortex are arranged topographically in several segregated networks, linking different cortical areas to specific subregions of the striatum and thalamus. This arrangement raises the possibility that schizophrenia may involve selective dysfunction

of cortical-subcortical circuits or, alternatively, widespread disruption by a focal abnormality within a zone of convergence, such as the thalamus. Indeed, reduced thalamic volume loss is a consistent structural neuroimaging finding (Adriano et al., 2010), and a variety of striatal and thalamic abnormalities have been reported in postmortem studies, although postmortem findings tend to be less consistent than volumetric changes observed on MRI (Dorph-Petersen and Lewis, 2011).

The "cognitive dysmetria" hypothesis posits that the diverse array of symptoms associated with schizophrenia are the consequence of a core defect in coordinated information processing related to disruption of networks linking cortex, thalamus, and cerebellum (Andreasen et al., 1999). This hypothesis was prompted by a series of PET functional imaging investigations that repeatedly found reduced activity in the cortex, thalamus, and cerebellum during performance of cognitive tasks (Andreasen et al., 1999). Reduced activity in the frontal cortex and thalamus, especially mediodorsal nucleus, continues to be a robust finding in fMRI investigations (Minzenberg et al., 2009). Alterations in thalamocortical connectivity, especially between the PFC and mediodorsal thalamus, and in cortico-cerebellar connectivity have also been observed in several resting-state studies (Collin et al., 2011; Skudlarski et al., 2010; Welsh et al., 2010; Woodward et al., 2012).

Cortico-striatal models of schizophrenia emerged from PET investigations of glucose metabolism and dopamine receptor function (Buchsbaum and Hazlett, 1998; Honey et al., 2009; Meyer-Lindenberg et al., 2002). In addition, reduced activation of the striatum is commonly observed in fMRI studies of executive function (Minzenberg et al., 2009). However, the effects of antipsychotic medications on the function and structure of the striatum poses interpretational challenges (Buchsbaum and Hazlett, 1998; Brandt and Bonelli, 2008). It is noteworthy in this regard that unaffected relatives of schizophrenia patients show altered striatal activity, which suggests that at least some of the functional abnormalities detected in patients are not a consequence of antipsychotic treatment (Vink et al., 2006). As with other network models tested using functional imaging, it is unclear where the primary point of pathology resides, as dysfunction in any node could lead to pathological changes in the network. Interestingly, multimodal imaging investigations in both schizophrenia patients and prodromal subjects have found that abnormal functional activation of the prefrontal cortex is associated with elevated striatal dopamine signaling (Fusar-Poli et al., 2010; Meyer-Lindenberg et al., 2002).

NEUROCHEMICAL SYSTEMS

In addition to brain structure and activity, neuroimaging methods can also be used to study brain chemistry. One such method is magnetic resonance spectroscopy (MRS), a non-invasive MRI approach that can easily be implemented on routine scanners. Signal from several nuclei can be detected using MRS, but the ones most useful for brain research are proton (^{1}H)MRS and phosphorus (^{31}P)MRS. These approaches provide information on brain chemicals relevant to various aspects of neurotransmission and brain metabolism. The utility of MRS has historically been limited by poor spatial and temporal resolution and by technical non-uniformity across research centers. The typical MRS dataset is acquired over several minutes from voxels that are several centimeters in each dimension. Nevertheless, recent advances in MRS data acquisition and analysis techniques coupled with the greater availability of higher field strength magnets has generated new opportunities for obtaining insight into neurochemical abnormalities in psychotic disorders from smaller brain regions with shorter duration scans.

Many current theories regarding the pathophysiology of psychotic disorders in general and schizophrenia in particular implicate abnormalities in glutamatergic and GABAergic neurotransmission (Lisman et al., 2008). Since glutamate (Glu) and GABA are the principal excitatory and inhibitory neurotransmitters in the brain, these abnormalities have major implications for brain function in schizophrenia. ^{1}H MRS provides the ability to assess concentrations of Glu, GABA, and other related brain metabolites such as glutamine (Gln), the principal metabolite of Glu at the synapse. Due to technical limitations, most publications on glutamate-related metabolites in schizophrenia have reported a composite measure termed Glx. Glx contains contributions from Glu, Gln, GABA, and aspartate. As a result, Glx is best considered a general index of multiple glutamate-related metabolites but provides no information on individual ones. Recent advances have allowed the resolution of signals coming from Glu, Gln, and GABA. Glu and Gln play roles in intermediary metabolism in addition to their functions in neurotransmission. Therefore, brain levels of these metabolites cannot be interpreted solely in the context of synaptic activity. However, since Glu released into the synapse is converted to Gln in glial cells, the relative concentrations of Gln and Glu may provide information more closely related to neurotransmission than the concentration of either molecule alone (Yuksel and Ongur, 2010) (Fig. 20.4). GABA levels in the brain parenchyma are thought to be more closely related to neurotransmission since GABA does not play a prominent role in intermediary metabolism.

A recent meta-analysis of 28 published ^{1}H MRS studies concluded that medial PFC Glu levels were reduced and Gln levels elevated in schizophrenia (Marsman et al., 2013). In addition, age-by-group analyses revealed that Glu and Gln concentrations decreased at a faster rate with age in patients with schizophrenia than in healthy controls. With the caveat that brain concentrations of Glu and Gln can be affected by metabolic processes unrelated to neurotransmission, this pattern of findings has been tentatively interpreted as evidence for a two-step abnormality in schizophrenia: during the first episode of psychosis there may be elevations in Glu neurotransmission leading to depletion of Glu and buildup of its metabolite Gln; with chronic disease there is an impoverishment of the entire Glu neurotransmission machinery, leading to lower than normal levels of both Glu and Gln. In addition to emerging from a meta-analysis, this pattern has also been found in an elegant longitudinal study in a single patient cohort (Theberge et al., 2007). In addition to dynamic Glu and Gln changes in the PFC and thalamus, Theberge and colleagues also reported that the

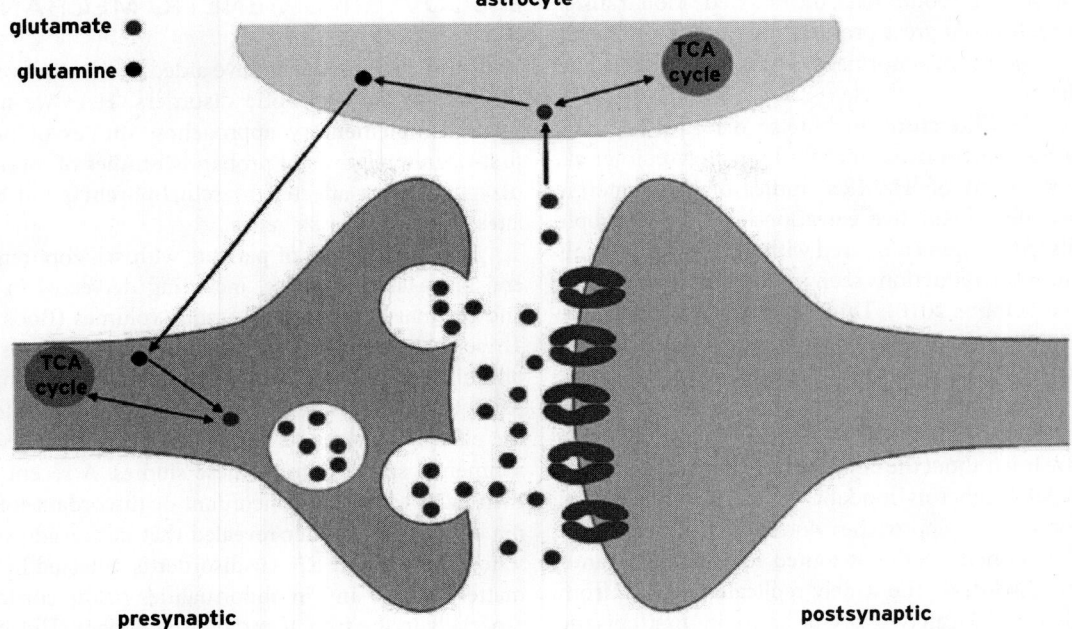

Figure 20.4 *Schematic representation of glutamate-glutamine (Glu-Gln) cycling at the synapse. Glu is synthesized from TCA cycle metabolites or from Gln, packaged into synaptic vesicles and released into the synaptic cleft. After interacting with postsynaptic receptors, the actions of Glu are terminated by uptake into adjacent glial cells (red profiles), where it is converted to Gln. Gln then diffuses back to neurons to complete the cycle.*

glutamate ●

glutamine ●

astrocyte

TCA cycle

TCA cycle

presynaptic

postsynaptic

change in Gln seen during the transition from first episode to chronic illness correlated with gray matter losses in temporal and parietal cortices in the same patients during the same period.

Although the relationship of GABA level abnormalities to neurotransmission would be more straightforward to interpret than those of Glu and Gln, ¹H MRS studies of GABA have reported conflicting findings in schizophrenia. Using similar GABA-dedicated MRS acquisition techniques, some studies (including one with first-episode patients) have reported GABA reductions in this condition (Goto et al., 2009; Yoon et al., 2010), while others (including one with unmedicated patients) have reported elevations (Ongur et al., 2010; Kegeles et al., 2012). Demographic and clinical patient differences or other variables may explain the discrepancy. But it appears unlikely that there is a substantial and sustained abnormality in parenchymal GABA levels in schizophrenia, since that would already be detected across all studies. Instead, there seems to be a decoupling between brain GABA levels and the well-documented abnormalities in GABAergic neurotransmission in schizophrenia.

NEURONAL HEALTH AND BIOENERGETICS

In addition to neurochemical systems, MRS studies also provide information on a range of metabolites related to neuronal health as well as energy production and utilization in the brain *in vivo*. The three most prominent and most easily quantifiable metabolites in the ¹H spectrum from the human brain are *N*-acetylaspartate (NAA), creatine (Cr), and choline (Cho). NAA is an amino acid found almost exclusively and in high concentrations (around 10 mM) in neurons. Its precise functions are not well understood

but a large experimental and clinical literature has identified NAA concentrations as a marker for neuronal integrity and health (Lyoo and Renshaw, 2002). The Cr signal arises from Cr as well as its phosphorylated counterpart phosphocreatine (PCr), which functions as a high-energy phosphate store for cellular energy needs. Similarly, the Cho signal arises from several choline-including metabolites mostly related to cell membrane metabolism (with a minor contribution from acetylcholine).

The literature contains multiple well-done ¹H MRS studies quantifying NAA, Cr, and Cho in the neocortex, hippocampus, and white matter in schizophrenia. The most consistent finding across these studies, confirmed in a meta-analysis, is a reduction in NAA in all brain regions (Steen et al., 2005). This pattern is widely interpreted as reflecting abnormalities in neuronal integrity and health in schizophrenia, although NAA measures per se cannot determine whether there are reductions in neuron number. Some, but not all, of these studies have also reported reductions in Cr, which may indicate a bioenergetic abnormality in schizophrenia.

³¹P MRS is a related technique that provides information on phosphate-containing metabolites in the brain. Some studies have reported abnormalities in phosphomonoesters (PME) and phosphodiesters (PDE) in schizophrenia using this approach (Keshavan et al., 1993). Due to the role PMEs and PDEs play in cell membrane turnover, these findings were often interpreted as suggesting an impoverishment of dendritic remodeling and synaptic pruning. More recently, new ³¹P MRS techniques are making it possible to obtain dynamic measures of brain bioenergetics *in vivo*. These approaches rely on the principle of magnetization transfer to calculate reaction rate constants for the creatine kinase (CK) and ATP synthase reactions noninvasively in the human brain (Du et al., 2012). Although in early stages of

application to psychiatric conditions, the magnetization transfer ^{31}P MRS approach holds great promise for examining bioenergetic and mitochondrial abnormalities in schizophrenia and bipolar disorder.

So far, the MRS literature on bipolar disorder is small. Reductions in NAA are a consistent finding (Bertolino et al., 2003). A recent review of ^{1}H MRS studies of glutamatergic metabolites revealed distinctive elevations in Glx in people with bipolar disorder when compared with healthy individuals and in contrast to the reductions seen in major depressive disorder (Yuksel and Ongur, 2010). This would suggest an increase in the overall pool of glutamate-related metabolites in bipolar disorder. In addition, there may be systematic variation in the Gln/Glu ratio across the depressive/euthymic/manic phases of the illness (Yuksel and Ongur, 2010).

What can we learn about the neurobiology of psychosis from MRS studies? Although this modality is less well-developed compared to other MRI approaches due to its inherently low resolution, it has nonetheless contributed to our understanding of psychotic disorders. The widely replicated finding from ^{1}H MRS studies of elevated Gln/Glu ratio in first-episode schizophrenia followed by a reduction in Glx in chronic illness is a good example. This pattern of findings suggests a dynamic process of inappropriately elevated glutamatergic neurotransmission followed by an impoverishment in this process.

It is intriguing to consider the future of MRS in the study of psychotic disorders. The advent of higher magnetic field MRI scanners aids MRS through increased signal to noise ratio and better spectral dispersion, which allows separation of metabolite signals. In fact, higher field strengths benefit MRS more so than other MRI approaches. Thus, widespread availability of ultra-high field (4 Tesla and higher) magnets will help MRS at least partially overcome its key shortcoming of poor temporal and spatial resolution. MRS data collection from millimeter voxels using shorter acquisition times is leading to whole-brain data collection—a technique termed chemical shift imaging. Collection of MRS data in parallel with fMRI and DTI will provide converging evidence of abnormalities in glutamatergic or GABAergic neurotransmission or neuronal metabolism and allow investigators to gain deeper insights into pathophysiology (for some early examples, see Falkenberg et al., 2012; Northoff et al., 2007). In addition, better MRS data acquisition hardware and software have improved our ability to non-invasively measure brain processes of great interest to psychiatric neuroscience (such as neurotransmission and bioenergetics) in the past decade. Some possible directions include improved quantification of lactate (related to energetic abnormalities), glutathione (the brain's principal antioxidant), and N-acetylaspartylglutamate (NAAG-a neuromodulator); the promise of quantifying markers of neural stem cells in the human brain *in vivo* (Manganas et al., 2007); and the use of diffusion MRS and T1 and T2 relaxation characteristics to quantify the brain's microenvironment.

It has been said that "MRS is a technique of the future and always will be." The inherent poor sensitivity of the MRS signal has hampered the development of this field in psychiatric research, but the technique holds promise for studies of neurochemical processes in psychotic disorder patients.

DISCOVERING GENETIC MECHANISMS

Neuroimaging methods have aided in the discovery of genetic risk factors for psychotic disorders. Here we briefly review three complementary approaches: studies of non-psychotic first-degree relatives of probands, studies of monozygotic and dizygotic twins affected by schizophrenia, and neural correlates of psychosis risk genes.

Family members of patients with schizophrenia show several brain abnormalities, including decreases in whole brain and (primarily left) hippocampus volumes (Boos et al., 2007). These changes are similar to those seen in patients with schizophrenia and parallel the findings of memory impairments in patients and relatives. However, it is not possible to disentangle the effects of risk genes (such as DISC 1 or BDNF) and environmental stressors from these studies. A recent study of 158 twin pairs who were concordant or discordant for schizophrenia or bipolar disorder revealed that increased genetic risk for schizophrenia and bipolar disorder is reflected in loss of white matter volume and in abnormalities of the cortical thickness, especially in the frontal and temporal lobes (Hulshoff Pol et al., 2012). In addition, a direct comparison of monozygotic twins discordant for schizophrenia revealed that, above and beyond the shared genetic risk, the affected twin showed reduced gray matter volume in prefrontal, cingulate, and superior temporal cortex (Borgwardt et al., 2010).

More recently, neuroimaging studies have revealed some of the neural mechanisms of putative schizophrenia risk genes from early candidate gene association studies (Meyer-Lindenberg, 2010). For example, allelic variants in the gene neuregulin 1 have been associated with smaller hippocampal volume and larger ventricular volumes. Similarly, the gene *DISC1*, originally identified in a large Scottish pedigree with multiple individuals affected by schizophrenia and bipolar disorder, has been associated with reduced hippocampal gray matter and increased hippocampal-PFC connectivity (Meyer-Lindenberg, 2010). These are two examples for the role of neuroimaging in the exploration of the allelic effects of schizophrenia risk genes.

SUMMARY

Neuroimaging studies have restored Kraepelin's optimism that we will find the neural mechanisms of psychotic disorders. What is needed now is a dimensional assessment of psychopathology that allows neuroimaging researchers to go beyond the classic categories of psychotic disorders and reveal the mechanisms of genes and environmental risk factors leading to psychosis. The unique strengths of neuroimaging, namely, the repeated assessment of patients (especially in the early stages of the illness) and the ability to correlate brain imaging data with clinical and treatment variables, will ensure a prominent position for this research domain in the study of psychotic disorders.

DISCLOSURES

Dr. Heckers is a member of the DSM-5 work group on Psychotic Disorders. He has no other conflicts to disclose.

Dr. Woodward has no conflicts of interest to disclose. He has received support from NIMH and NARSAD. Grant Support: NIMH (1R21MH096177-01A1) and National Alliance for Research on Schizophrenia and Depression (NARSAD) Young Investigator Award.

Dr. Ongur's research is funded by NIMH and Shervert Frazier Research Institute at McLean Hospital, and he is PI on a research contract with Rules Based Medicine Inc. (a for-profit entity), he teaches a CME course for New England Educational Institute (not-for-profit), and he draws income as Associate Editor for the journal *Archives of General Psychiatry*.

REFERENCES

Achim, A.M., and Lepage, M. (2005). Episodic memory-related activation in schizophrenia: meta-analysis. *Br. J. Psychiatry* 187:500–509.

Adriano, F., Caltagirone, C., et al. (2012). Hippocampal volume reduction in first-episode and chronic schizophrenia: a review and meta-analysis. *Neuroscientist* 18(2):180–200.

Adriano, F., Spoletini, I., et al. (2010). Updated meta-analyses reveal thalamus volume reduction in patients with first-episode and chronic schizophrenia. *Schizophr. Res.* 123(1):1–14.

Allen, P., Modinos, G., et al. (2012). Neuroimaging auditory hallucinations in schizophrenia: from neuroanatomy to neurochemistry and beyond. *Schizophr. Bull.* 38(4):695–703.

Andreasen, N.C., Nopoulos, P., et al. (1999). Defining the phenotype of schizophrenia: cognitive dysmetria and its neural mechanisms. *Biol. Psychiatry* 46(7):908–920.

Bertolino, A., Frye, M., et al. (2003). Neuronal pathology in the hippocampal area of patients with bipolar disorder: a study with proton magnetic resonance spectroscopic imaging. *Biol. Psychiatry* 53(10):906–913.

Boos, H.B., Aleman, A., et al. (2007). Brain volumes in relatives of patients with schizophrenia: a meta-analysis. *Arch. Gen. Psychiatry* 64(3):297–304.

Bora, E., Fornito, A., et al. (2011). Neuroanatomical abnormalities in schizophrenia: a multimodal voxelwise meta-analysis and meta-regression analysis. *Schizophr. Res.* 127(1–3):46–57.

Borgwardt, S.J., Picchioni, M.M., et al. (2010). Regional gray matter volume in monozygotic twins concordant and discordant for schizophrenia. *Biol. Psychiatry* 67(10):956–964.

Brandt, G.N., and Bonelli, R.M. (2008). Structural neuroimaging of the basal ganglia in schizophrenic patients: a review. *Wien. Med. Wochenschr.* 158(3–4):84–90.

Buchsbaum, M.S., and Hazlett, E.A. (1998). Positron emission tomography studies of abnormal glucose metabolism in schizophrenia. *Schizophr. Bull.* 24(3):343–364.

Cole, M.W., Anticevic, A., et al. (2011). Variable global dysconnectivity and individual differences in schizophrenia. *Biol. Psychiatry* 70(1):43–50.

Collin, G., Hulshoff Pol, H.E., et al. (2011). Impaired cerebellar functional connectivity in schizophrenia patients and their healthy siblings. *Front. Psychiatry* 2:73.

Di, X., Chan, R.C., et al. (2009). White matter reduction in patients with schizophrenia as revealed by voxel-based morphometry: an activation likelihood estimation meta-analysis. *Prog. Neuropsychopharmacol. Biol. Psychiatry* 33(8):1390–1394.

Dierks, T., Linden, D.E., et al. (1999). Activation of Heschl's gyrus during auditory hallucinations. *Neuron* 22(3):615–621.

Dorph-Petersen, K.A., and Lewis, D.A. (2011). Stereological approaches to identifying neuropathology in psychosis. *Biol. Psychiatry* 69(2):113–126.

Du, F., Cooper, A., et al. (2012). Creatine kinase and ATP synthase reaction rates in human frontal lobe measured by (31)P magnetization transfer spectroscopy at 4T. *Magn. Reson. Imaging.*

Ellison-Wright, I., and Bullmore, E. (2010). Anatomy of bipolar disorder and schizophrenia: a meta-analysis. *Schizophr. Res.* 117(1):1–12.

Ellison-Wright, I., Glahn, D.C., et al. (2008). The anatomy of first-episode and chronic schizophrenia: an anatomical likelihood estimation meta-analysis. *Am. J. Psychiatry* 165(8):1015–1023.

Falkenberg, L.E., Westerhausen, R., et al. (2012). Resting-state glutamate level in the anterior cingulate predicts blood-oxygen level-dependent response to cognitive control. *Proc. Natl. Acad. Sci. USA* 109(13):5069–5073.

Fornito, A., Yucel, M., et al. (2009). Mapping grey matter reductions in schizophrenia: an anatomical likelihood estimation analysis of voxel-based morphometry studies. *Schizophr. Res.* 108(1–3):104–113.

Fusar-Poli, P., Borgwardt, S., et al. (2011). Neuroanatomy of vulnerability to psychosis: a voxel-based meta-analysis. *Neurosci. Biobehav. Rev.* 35(5):1175–1185.

Fusar-Poli, P., Howes, O.D., et al. (2010). Abnormal frontostriatal interactions in people with prodromal signs of psychosis: a multimodal imaging study. *Arch. Gen. Psychiatry* 67(7):683–691.

Fuster, J.M. (2008). *The Prefrontal Cortex.* London, Amsterdam, Burlington, San Diego: Elsevier.

Gage, N., and Hickok, G. (2005). Multiregional cell assemblies, temporal binding and the representation of conceptual knowledge in cortex: a modern theory by a "classical" neurologist, Carl Wernicke. *Cortex* 41(6):823–832.

Glahn, D.C., Laird, A.R., et al. (2008). Meta-analysis of gray matter anomalies in schizophrenia: application of anatomic likelihood estimation and network analysis. *Biol. Psychiatry* 64(9):774–781.

Glahn, D.C., Ragland, J.D., et al. (2005). Beyond hypofrontality: a quantitative meta-analysis of functional neuroimaging studies of working memory in schizophrenia. *Hum. Brain Mapp.* 25(1):60–69.

Goghari, V.M., Sponheim, S.R., et al. (2010). The functional neuroanatomy of symptom dimensions in schizophrenia: a qualitative and quantitative review of a persistent question. *Neurosci. Biobehav. Rev.* 34(3):468–486.

Goto, N., Yoshimura, R., et al. (2009). Reduction of brain gamma-aminobutyric acid (GABA) concentrations in early-stage schizophrenia patients: 3T Proton MRS study. *Schizophr. Res.* 112(1–3):192–193.

Heckers, S., and Konradi, C. (2010). Hippocampal pathology in schizophrenia. In: N.R. Swerdlow, ed. *Current Topics in Behavioral Neurosciences: Behavioral Neurobiology of Schizophrenia and Its Treatment.* New York: Springer, pp. 529–553.

Heinrichs, RW., and Zakzanis, K.K. (1998). Neurocognitive deficit in schizophrenia: a quantitative review of the evidence. *Neuropsychology* 12(3):426–445.

Honey, C.J., Sporns, O., et al. (2009). Predicting human resting-state functional connectivity from structural connectivity. *Proc. Natl. Acad. Sci. USA* 106(6):2035–2040.

Hovington, C.L., and Lepage, M. (2012). Neurocognition and neuroimaging of persistent negative symptoms of schizophrenia. *Exp. Rev. Neurother.* 12(1):53–69.

Hulshoff Pol, H.E., and Kahn, R.S. (2008). What happens after the first episode?: a review of progressive brain changes in chronically ill patients with schizophrenia. *Schizophr. Bull.* 34(2):354–366.

Hulshoff Pol, H.E., van Baal, G.C., et al. (2012). Overlapping and segregating structural brain abnormalities in twins with schizophrenia or bipolar disorder. *Arch. Gen. Psychiatry* 69(4):349–359.

Ioannidis, J.P. (2011). Excess significance bias in the literature on brain volume abnormalities. *Arch. Gen. Psychiatry* 68(8):773–780.

Jardri, R., Pouchet, A., et al. (2011). Cortical activations during auditory verbal hallucinations in schizophrenia: a coordinate-based meta-analysis. *Am. J. Psychiatry* 168(1):73–81.

Johnstone, E.C., Crow, T.J., et al. (1976). Cerebral ventricle size and cognitive impairment in chronic schizophrenia. *Lancet* 2: 924–926.

Kegeles, L.S., Mao, X., et al. (2012). Elevated prefrontal cortex gamma-aminobutyric acid and glutamate-glutamine levels in schizophrenia measured *in vivo* with proton magnetic resonance spectroscopy. *Arch. Gen. Psychiatry* 69(5):449–459.

Kempton, M.J., Stahl, D., et al. (2010). Progressive lateral ventricular enlargement in schizophrenia: a meta-analysis of longitudinal MRI studies. *Schizophr. Res.* 120(1–3):54–62.

Keshavan, M.S., Sanders, R.D., et al. (1993). Frontal lobe metabolism and cerebral morphology in schizophrenia: 31P MRS and MRI studies. *Schizophr. Res.* 10(3):241–246.

Koutsouleris, N., Meisenzahl, E.M., et al. (2009). Use of neuroanatomical pattern classification to identify subjects in at-risk mental states of psychosis and predict disease transition. *Arch. Gen. Psychiatry* 66(7):700–712.

Lewis, D.A. (2012). Cortical circuit dysfunction and cognitive deficits in schizophrenia—implications for preemptive interventions. *Eur. J. Neurosci.* 35(12):1871–1878.

Liddle, P.F., Friston, K.J., et al. (1992). Patterns of cerebral blood flow in schizophrenia. *Br. J. Psychiatry* 160: 179–186.

Lisman, J.E., Coyle, J.T., et al. (2008). Circuit-based framework for understanding neurotransmitter and risk gene interactions in schizophrenia. *Trends Neurosci.* 31(5):234–242.

Lyoo, I.K., and Renshaw, P.F. (2002). Magnetic resonance spectroscopy: current and future applications in psychiatric research. *Biol. Psychiatry* 51(3):195–207.

Manganas, L.N., Zhang, X., et al. (2007). Magnetic resonance spectroscopy identifies neural progenitor cells in the live human brain. *Science* 318(5852):980–985.

Marsman, A., van den Heuvel, M.P., et al. (2013). Glutamate in schizophrenia: a focused review and meta-analysis of 1H-MRS studies. *Schizophr. Bull.* 39(1):120–129.

Meyer-Lindenberg, A. (2010). From maps to mechanisms through neuroimaging of schizophrenia. *Nature* 468(7321):194–202.

Meyer-Lindenberg, A., Miletich, R.S., et al. (2002). Reduced prefrontal activity predicts exaggerated striatal dopaminergic function in schizophrenia. *Nat. Neurosci.* 5(3):267–271.

Minzenberg, M.J., Laird, A.R., et al. (2009). Meta-analysis of 41 functional neuroimaging studies of executive function in schizophrenia. *Arch. Gen. Psychiatry* 66(8):811–822.

Nenadic, I., Gaser, C., et al. (2012). Heterogeneity of brain structural variation and the structural imaging endophenotypes in schizophrenia. *Neuropsychobiology* 66(1):44–49.

Niendam, T.A., Laird, A.R., et al. (2012). Meta-analytic evidence for a superordinate cognitive control network subserving diverse executive functions. *Cogn. Affect. Behav. Neurosci.* 12(2):241–268.

Northoff, G., Walter, M., et al. (2007). GABA concentrations in the human anterior cingulate cortex predict negative BOLD responses in fMRI. *Nat. Neurosci.* 10(12):1515–1517.

Olabi, B., Ellison-Wright, I., et al. (2011). Are there progressive brain changes in schizophrenia? A meta-analysis of structural magnetic resonance imaging studies. *Biol. Psychiatry* 70(1):88–96.

Ongur, D., Prescot, A.P., et al. (2010). Elevated gamma-aminobutyric acid levels in chronic schizophrenia. *Biol. Psychiatry* 68(7):667–670.

Palaniyappan, L., Balain, V., et al. (2012). Structural correlates of auditory hallucinations in schizophrenia: a meta-analysis. *Schizophr. Res.* 137(1–3):169–173.

Pettersson-Yeo, W., Allen, P., et al. (2011). Dysconnectivity in schizophrenia: where are we now? *Neurosci. Biobehav. Rev.* 35(5):1110–1124.

Ragland, J.D., Laird, A.R., et al. (2009). Prefrontal activation deficits during episodic memory in schizophrenia. *Am. J. Psychiatry* 166(8):863–874.

Schneider, M.R., DelBello, M.P., et al. (2012). Neuroprogression in bipolar disorder. *Bipolar Disord.* 14(4):356–374.

Shenton, M.E., Dickey, C.C., et al. (2001). A review of MRI findings in schizophrenia. *Schizophr. Res.* 49(1–2):1–52.

Shenton, M.E., Whitford, T.J., et al. (2010). Structural neuroimaging in schizophrenia: from methods to insights to treatments. *Dialogues Clin. Neurosci.* 12(3):317–332.

Shepherd, A.M., Laurens, K.R., et al. (2012a). Systematic meta-review and quality assessment of the structural brain alterations in schizophrenia. *Neurosci. Biobehav. Rev.* 36(4):1342–13456.

Shepherd, A.M., Matheson, S.L., et al. (2012b). Systematic meta-analysis of insula volume in schizophrenia. *Biol. Psychiatry* 72(9):775–784.

Skudlarski, P., Jagannathan, K., et al. (2010). Brain connectivity is not only lower but different in schizophrenia: a combined anatomical and functional approach. *Biol. Psychiatry* 68(1):61–69.

Small, S.A., Schobel, S.A., et al. (2011). A pathophysiological framework of hippocampal dysfunction in ageing and disease. *Nat. Rev. Neurosci.* 12(10):585–601.

Smieskova, R., Fusar-Poli, P., et al. (2010). Neuroimaging predictors of transition to psychosis—a systematic review and meta-analysis. *Neurosci. Biobehav. Rev.* 34(8):1207–1222.

Smith, S.M., Fox, P.T., et al. (2009). Correspondence of the brain's functional architecture during activation and rest. *Proc. Natl. Acad. Sci. USA* 106(31):13040–13045.

Steen, R.G., Hamer, R.M., et al. (2005). Measurement of brain metabolites by ^{1}H magnetic resonance spectroscopy in patients with schizophrenia: a systematic review and meta-analysis. *Neuropsychopharmacology* 30(11):1949–1962.

Sun, D., van Erp, T.G., et al. (2009). Elucidating a magnetic resonance imaging-based neuroanatomic biomarker for psychosis: classification analysis using probabilistic brain atlas and machine learning algorithms. *Biol. Psychiatry* 66(11):1055–1060.

Sun, J., Maller, J.J., et al. (2009). Superior temporal gyrus volume change in schizophrenia: a review on region of interest volumetric studies. *Brain Research Reviews* 61(1):14–32.

Theberge, J., Williamson, K.E., et al. (2007). Longitudinal grey-matter and glutamatergic losses in first-episode schizophrenia. *Br. J. Psychiatry* 191: 325–334.

Vink, M., Ramsey, N.F., et al. (2006). Striatal dysfunction in schizophrenia and unaffected relatives. *Biol. Psychiatry* 60(1):32–39.

Weinberger, D., Berman, K., et al. (1986a). Physiologic dysfunction of dorsolateral prefrontal cortex in schizophrenia: I. Regional cerebral blood flow evidence. *Arch. Gen. Psychiatry* 43:114–125.

Weinberger, D.R., Berman, K.F., et al. (1986b). Physiologic dysfunction of dorsolateral prefrontal cortex in schizophrenia. I. Regional cerebral blood flow evidence. *Arch. Gen. Psychiatry* 43(2):114–124.

Welsh, R.C., Chen, A.C., et al. (2010). Low-frequency BOLD fluctuations demonstrate altered thalamocortical connectivity in schizophrenia. *Schizophr. Bull.* 36(4):713–722.

Whalley, H.C., Papmeyer, M., et al. (2012). Review of functional magnetic resonance imaging studies comparing bipolar disorder and schizophrenia. *Bipolar Disord.* 14(4):411–431.

Woodward, N.D., Karbasforoushan, H., et al. (2012). Thalamocortical dysconnectivity in schizophrenia. *Am. J. Psychiatry* 169(10):1092–1099.

Woodward, N.D., Rogers, B., et al. (2011). Functional resting-state networks are differentially affected in schizophrenia. *Schizophr. Res.* 130(1–3):86–93.

Wright, I.C., Rabe-Hesketh, S., et al. (2000). Meta-analysis of regional brain volumes in schizophrenia. *Am. J. Psychiatry* 157(1):16–25.

Yoon, J.H., Maddock, R.J., et al. (2010). GABA concentration is reduced in visual cortex in schizophrenia and correlates with orientation-specific surround suppression. *J. Neurosci.* 30(10):3777–3781.

Yu, K., Cheung, C., et al. (2010). Are bipolar disorder and schizophrenia neuroanatomically distinct? An anatomical likelihood meta-analysis. *Front. Hum. Neurosci.* 4:189.

Yuksel, C., and Ongur, D. (2010). Magnetic resonance spectroscopy studies of glutamate-related abnormalities in mood disorders. *Biol. Psychiatry* 68(9):785–794.

Zhang, D., and Raichle, M.E. (2010). Disease and the brain's dark energy. *Nat. Rev. Neurol.* 6(1):15–28.

Zhou, Y., Liang, M., et al. (2007). Functional dysconnectivity of the dorsolateral prefrontal cortex in first-episode schizophrenia using resting-state fMRI. *Neurosci. Lett.* 417(3):297–302.

21 | COGNITIVE AND MOTIVATIONAL NEUROSCIENCE OF PSYCHOTIC DISORDERS

ALAN ANTICEVIC, ERIN C. DOWD, AND DEANNA M. BARCH

OVERVIEW

Typically, when we think of the core symptoms of psychotic disorders such as schizophrenia, we think of people who hear voices, see visions, and have false beliefs about reality (i.e., delusions). However, clinicians have long recognized that abnormalities in cognitive function and motivated behavior are a key component of psychosis, and of schizophrenia in particular. As such, the last three decades have witnessed a relative explosion of research on cognition in schizophrenia, much of it couched within the framework of understanding the cognitive neuroscience of schizophrenia and the neural correlates of cognitive deficits. This emphasis on cognition in schizophrenia is in part due to the growing body of research suggesting that cognitive dysfunction in this illness is a substantial source of disability and loss of functional capacity for patients (Nuechterlein et al., 2011). This work is complemented by an additional recent focus on understanding the psychological and neurobiological impairments leading to deficits in motivation and goal-directed behavior in schizophrenia (Barch and Dowd, 2010; Gold et al., 2008; Kring and Moran, 2008), raising critical and important questions about the potential interactions between motivational and cognitive impairments in schizophrenia, and their influence on function, course, and outcome in this illness.

The challenge we face in understanding the cognitive and motivational neuroscience of schizophrenia is that individuals with this illness appear to exhibit deficits in a diverse array of domains (Mesholam-Gately et al., 2009). It is of course possible that this seemingly diverse array of impairments reflects dissociable deficits, each with its own psychological and neural pathophysiology. However, such an explanation does little to help us move forward in our conceptualization of the final common pathway leading to cognitive or motivational dysfunction in this illness, or in other psychotic disorders. Instead, we and others have argued that a common mechanism contributing to cognitive impairments across a range of domains in schizophrenia may arise due to an inability to actively represent goal information in working memory (WM) as needed to guide behavior, and that this deficit reflects profound impairments in the function of the dorsolateral prefrontal cortex (DLPFC) and its interactions with other brain regions such as parietal cortex, thalamus, and striatum, as well as altered function of neurotransmitter systems such as dopamine (DA), γ-aminobutyric acid (GABA), and glutamate. Importantly, in recent years, this hypothesis postulating a "core" deficit in goal representation has been expanded to integrate work on emotion, reward processing, and motivational impairments in schizophrenia. Specifically, we postulate that these deficits may reflect, at least in part, impairments in the ability to actively maintain and utilize internal representations of emotional experiences, previous rewards, and motivational goals in order to drive current and future behavior in a way that would normally allow individuals to obtain desired outcomes. In the sections that follow, we provide a discussion of the evidence for such impairment in schizophrenia, how it manifests in domains typically referred to as executive control, WM, and episodic memory, and how it may help us understand impairments in reward processing and motivation in schizophrenia. We conclude with a brief discussion of emerging evidence of cortical microcircuit pathophysiology in schizophrenia and how it may relate to cognitive and motivational deficits in this population.

CONTEXT PROCESSING AND PROACTIVE CONTROL IN SCHIZOPHRENIA

CONTEXT PROCESSING

In previous work based in part on computational modeling, Cohen and colleagues put forth the hypothesis that DA activity in DLPFC was responsible for the processing of context, and that a disturbance in this mechanism could be responsible for a range of cognitive deficits in schizophrenia (Braver et al., 1999; Cohen and Servan-Schreiber, 1992). Here, context refers to prior task-relevant information that is represented in such a form that it can bias selection of the appropriate behavioral response. Because context representations are maintained on-line, in an active state, they are continually accessible and available to influence processing in the service of ongoing goals. Consequently, context can be viewed as the subset of representations within WM that govern how other representations are used. One important insight that emerged from this work was that a single deficit in one aspect of executive control could contribute to deficits in cognitive domains often treated as independent. As such, this theory argued that deficits in WM, attention, and inhibition in schizophrenia can all be understood in terms of a broader deficit in context-processing (Braver et al., 1999; Cohen et al., 1999; Cohen and Servan-Schreiber, 1992). When a task involves competing, task-irrelevant processes (as in the Stroop task), context representations serve to inhibit such

task-irrelevant processes by providing top-down support for task-relevant processes. When a task involves a delay between a cue and a later contingent response, context representation involves maintaining task-relevant information against the interfering and cumulative effects of noise over time. Further, in both inhibition and WM conditions, context representations serve an attentional function by selecting task-relevant information for processing over other potentially competing sources of information (Miller and Cohen, 2001). Thus, the context hypothesis was used to explain why patients with schizophrenia demonstrate deficits on several tasks thought to tap WM, as well as deficits on other executive control tasks that may not involve a high WM load (e.g., Stroop); in other words, patients show deficits on tasks in which context information needs to be determined and maintained, even if this context information constitutes a low WM load (Barch et al., 2003; Cohen et al., 1999). Numerous studies have provided support for these hypotheses concerning context-processing deficits in schizophrenia (for a review, see Barch and Braver, 2007), as well as evidence for impairments in individuals at risk for schizophrenia (e.g., MacDonald et al., 2005; Snitz et al., 2006), suggesting that such deficits may be associated with liability to schizophrenia as well as manifest illness.

PROACTIVE AND REACTIVE CONTROL IN SCHIZOPHRENIA

In more recent years, context processing in cognition has been reconceptualized more broadly as the function of proactive cognitive control (Braver, 2012; Edwards et al., 2010). This conceptualization builds on earlier ideas of context processing to argue for flexible mechanisms of cognitive control that allow humans to deal with the diversity of challenges that we face in everyday life. In this theory, termed dual mechanisms of control (Braver, 2012; Edwards et al., 2010), a distinction is made between proactive and reactive modes of cognitive control. The proactive control model can be thought of as a form of "early selection," in which goal-relevant information is actively maintained in a sustained or anticipatory manner, before the occurrence of cognitively demanding events. This allows for optimal biasing of attention, perception, and action systems in a goal-driven manner. In this case, goals refer to the information one needs to accomplish a particular task or the intended outcome of a series of actions or mental operations. In real life, such goal information may include the main points one wishes to communicate in a conversation, or the need to organize a shopping trip so that one can make sure to get everything that is needed. In contrast, in the reactive mode, attentional control is recruited as a "late correction" mechanism that is mobilized only when needed, such as after a high-interference event is detected (e.g., an unexpected distracting stimulus is encountered and there is a need to retrieve the topic of conversation). Thus, proactive control relies on the *anticipation* and prevention of interference before it occurs, whereas reactive control relies on the *detection* and resolution of interference after its onset.

This theory postulates that proactive control depends on actively representing information in lateral prefrontal cortex (PFC), and that the updating and maintenance of such information relies on precise inputs from neurotransmitter systems such as DA into PFC. However, as discussed in the following, it is clear that other neurotransmitter mechanisms such as GABA and glutamate are critical for active maintenance of information in PFC, and that deficits in N-methyl-D-aspartate (NMDA) receptor function may underlie impaired delay-related activity during WM in schizophrenia (e.g., Krystal et al., 2003; Wang et al., 2008). As outlined in detail in Braver (2012), proactive and reactive control functions are not mutually exclusive, and some balance between the two modes is necessary to successfully meet most ongoing cognitive demands. However, Braver (2012) has argued that the two control modes can be distinguished based on their temporal characteristics (e.g., *when* they are engaged in the course of cognitive processing) and the requirement to actively maintain control representations over time for proactive control. Further, Braver has suggested that there may be biases to favor one processing mode over the other, which may be dependent on task demands (e.g., high conflict situations may push toward a proactive control mode), as well as on individual differences in factors such as WM capacity, fluid intelligence, and even personality traits such as reward sensitivity. Proactive control may also be particularly vulnerable to disruption, given that it is resource demanding and dependent on temporally precise active maintenance mechanisms. Thus, populations characterized by disordered PFC function (such as schizophrenia) may rely more heavily on reactive control, as it may be more robust in the face of such dysfunction (Edwards et al., 2010). Consistent with this hypothesis, there is ample evidence for an association between impairments in DLPFC activity and deficits of proactive control in schizophrenia (e.g., Minzenberg et al., 2009) as well as those at risk for the development of schizophrenia (e.g., MacDonald et al., 2009). Further, there is growing evidence for a critical role of impaired connectivity between the DLPFC and other cognitive control related brain regions (e.g., Anticevic et al., 2013, Repovs et al., 2011; Yoon et al., 2008), positive impacts of DA enhancement on cognitive control in psychosis (e.g., Barch, 2005), and intriguing evidence for GABAergically mediated (Lewis and González-Burgos, 2008) impairment in neural oscillations that may support representations in DLPFC (e.g., Cho et al., 2006).

WORKING MEMORY IN SCHIZOPHRENIA

COGNITIVE NEUROSCIENCE MODELS OF WORKING MEMORY

Although a good deal of work has been devoted to understanding cognitive control deficits in schizophrenia, perhaps the greatest amount of cognitive neuroscience research in schizophrenia has been focused on WM since the seminal writings of Patricia Goldman-Rakic (Goldman-Rakic, 1995). There is a huge body of evidence to suggest that individuals with schizophrenia show deficits in WM (e.g., Forbes et al., 2009; Lee and Park, 2005). However, WM is a complex construct with many subprocesses. As such, we need to move beyond simply saying that individuals with schizophrenia

experience WM deficits, toward understanding what specific aspects of WM are impaired in this illness and how they may relate to shared deficits in context processing. To do so, it is important to discuss some of the leading cognitive neuroscience models of WM as they provide conceptual leverage on findings in schizophrenia by anchoring our understanding in findings in healthy adults. WM traditionally refers to temporary storage and manipulating information "on-line," typically in the service of some goal (Baddeley, 2000). According to one prominent cognitive model, WM is thought to be comprised of a central executive resource system, and two slave subsidiary systems: the phonological loop and the visuospatial sketchpad—i.e., WM is conceptualized as a multistore process relying on distinct subcomponents. This cognitive model was later updated to include a fourth component: the episodic buffer (Baddeley, 2000). Alternatively, rather than dividing the WM process into "cognitive" modules, one can consider WM to consist of distinct stages in time. In that sense, the WM process can be roughly subdivided into three distinct temporal components (Jonides et al., 2008): (1) encoding of novel information and forming an internal representation, (2) active maintenance of this information over some period (i.e., refreshing the memory trace, which is aligned with the function of two slave subsystems), and (3) manipulation of maintained information in the service of some goal (i.e., the central executive).

BEHAVIORAL FINDINGS ON WORKING MEMORY IN SCHIZOPHRENIA

There is robust evidence suggesting that individuals with schizophrenia display deficits in WM (e.g., Forbes et al., 2009; Lee and Park, 2005). These deficits are present in both medicated and unmedicated patients, the first-degree relatives of individuals with schizophrenia, and individuals with schizotypal personality, suggesting that WM is a critical abnormality manifesting across the schizophrenia spectrum. There is relatively little evidence that such WM deficits can be unambiguously attributed to dysfunction in either the verbal or visual-spatial buffer systems, as individuals with schizophrenia exhibit abnormalities on WM tasks with many different material types, with relatively little evidence for selective deficits for one material type over another (Lee and Park, 2005; Forbes et al., 2009). This has led to the suggestion that WM deficits in schizophrenia might primarily reflect deficits in the central executive, or the active maintenance and manipulation of information over time, an interpretation consistent with a central role for deficits in the proactive control of behavior. Such a modality non-specific deficit in the ability to maintain and manipulate information over time would also be consistent with emerging hypotheses detailing synaptic-level pathophysiology in schizophrenia (Marin, 2012), which is not likely to selectively disrupt verbal vs. non-verbal cortical circuits (discussed in what follows).

However, it is also important to consider the temporal aspects of WM function, and the distinction between encoding and maintenance, which rely on distinct neural dynamics. An influential meta-analysis suggested that the degree of WM impairment in schizophrenia is fairly constant even when extending the maintenance period (Lee and Park, 2005), such that the effect sizes of WM impairment across studies did not change as a function of the delay period used. This may imply that breakdowns in WM may be occurring as early as the encoding stage—i.e., when internal representations are still forming. In turn, such deficits in the initial generation of representations could impact the stability of such representations and the ability to accurately maintain them over time. Consistent with this hypothesis, studies examining encoding deficits have demonstrated that patients with schizophrenia exhibit short-term memory deficits even in the absence of a delay (e.g., Tek et al., 2002) and when allowed only a fixed duration to encode. However, such "encoding" deficits can be minimized if individuals with schizophrenia are given a longer period of time to process the information, suggesting that such deficits may reflect "speed of processing" rather than fundamental deficits in the ability to encode information into WM (e.g., Badcock et al., 2008). Nevertheless, speed-of-processing reductions at encoding may still be interpreted as an "encoding" deficit in that a reduction in the speed with which the information can be robustly encoded will degrade the quality of internal representations. At the same time, a number of studies have provided evidence for deficits in the ability to maintain information across time in schizophrenia, even after controlling for encoding differences (e.g., Badcock et al., 2008; Tek et al., 2002). One issue that still needs to be fully resolved in the context of WM tasks, especially those involving a match versus non-match decision, is to what extent group differences are exacerbated by tasks involving more complex "probe" decisions, which are difficult for patients given their slow processing speed and/or decision-making difficulties and may contribute to poor performance without reflecting deficits in working memory per se. In that sense, simple continuous report WM tasks (Badcock et al., 2008), similar to those used in non-human primate work (Funahashi et al., 1989), may prove better equipped for careful characterization of encoding versus delay deficits (as they circumvent match/non-match decisions).

Taken together, the existing evidence base suggests that there are abnormalities evident across both encoding and maintenance phases of WM in schizophrenia. The encoding deficits may be due to increases in time necessary to rapidly form an accurate internal representation (e.g., Badcock et al., 2008), while the deficits in the maintenance of information are consistent impairments in the central executive aspects of WM and impairments in the ability to proactively represent information necessary to guide behavior. Further, behavioral WM studies in schizophrenia argue that deficits exist not only in the maintenance mechanisms but also in the ability to resist external sources of interference and that these abnormalities are present in both visuospatial and verbal domains. Such impairments are consistent with a role for a fundamental impairment in the ability to represent and maintain representation in WM that can be used to guide goal directed behavior, and with an in impairment in the ability to use proactive cognitive control mechanisms in order to regulate behavior.

PREFRONTAL RECRUITMENT DURING WORKING MEMORY IN SCHIZOPHRENIA

Building on the behavioral evidence of WM deficits, there is a growing functional neuroimaging literature demonstrating the presence of brain abnormalities associated with WM dysfunction in schizophrenia. The majority of findings suggest that regions comprising the dorsal frontal-parietal network are affected in patients and may be contributing to WM abnormalities. Specifically, reductions in DLPFC (Brodmann's Area 9/46) activations have been documented while patients perform WM tasks, suggesting that patients exhibit task-related "hypofrontality" (Barch et al., 2001; Callicott et al., 1998). These findings have also been confirmed through quantitative meta-analytic studies (Glahn et al., 2005; Van Snellenberg et al., 2006). Such DLPFC deficits are present even in medication naïve individuals (Barch et al., 2001), and are also present, albeit to a lesser extent, in the first-degree relatives of individuals with schizophrenia (e.g., MacDonald et al., 2009), suggesting a potential role as an endophenotypic marker.

However, there have been discrepant findings with regard to over- or underrecruitment of DLPFC regions during WM (Callicott et al., 2003). A number of findings have suggested that WM capacity in healthy subjects may be dependent on level of recruitment of DLPFC, which is thought to operate according to an inverted "U" model of WM capacity (Goldman-Rakic et al., 2000). In other words, the model suggests that with increasing WM demands there is a concomitant parametric DLPFC signal increase. However, as WM load demands reach and exceed capacity limitations, DLPFC signals begin to drop, presumably due to information load exceeding available computational resources (Goldman-Rakic et al., 2000). In line with this hypothesis, recent evidence suggests that patients with schizophrenia may exhibit a shifted inverted U function, such that capacity limitations are reached faster (i.e., with lower WM load levels), which may result in over- or underrecruitment when compared to healthy controls depending on level of WM load at which the groups are compared (Johnson et al., 2006). In other words, at low difficulty levels patients may find performance more effortful and may have to recruit more PFC resources than healthy controls to accomplish the same task, leading to findings of "hyperactivity" in PFC cortex. Consistent with this model, a meta-analysis by Van Snellenberg and colleagues demonstrated that the magnitude of WM performance differences between patients and healthy controls was positively correlated with the magnitude of activation differences in dorsal-lateral prefrontal regions (Van Snellenberg et al., 2006).

THE TEMPORAL DYNAMICS OF PREFRONTAL ACTIVATION DURING WORKING MEMORY IN SCHIZOPHRENIA

The previous discussion focused on the general involvement of PFC, specifically the DLPFC, in WM. However, one can also consider the ways in which cognitive mechanisms involved in proactive control and the active representation of information may influence the magnitude and timing of brain activation in WM. A failure to use proactive control would suggest that patients might show reduced activity during encoding and/or maintenance in lateral PFC regions if they fail to effectively encode or maintain information over the delay in preparation for responding. There are several studies showing evidence consistent with such an alteration in activity in DLPFC during encoding (e.g., Anticevic et al., 2013; Edwards et al., 2010; Johnson et al., 2006) and/or maintenance (Anticevic et al., 2013; Driesen et al., 2008; Edwards et al., 2010). This impairment in encoding and maintenance of information may shift individuals with schizophrenia into a greater reliance on more *reactive* modes of processing. In other words, when a response is needed, patients may need to engage additional computational mechanisms to retrieve the memoranda, potentially resulting in *increased* activation in brain regions associated with memory retrieval or response selection. Consistent with this hypothesis, studies that have specifically examined retrieval-related activity have found evidence for *increased* activation among individuals with schizophrenia in either the same or different regions that showed reduced encoding/maintenance related activation (Johnson et al., 2006; Edwards et al., 2010). Future work may determine whether such increased retrieval signals are accompanied by increases in functional connectivity in a distributed retrieval-associated network, and importantly, whether such "compensatory" signal increases and/or connectivity changes are predictive of better performance in patients.

ALTERED DEFAULT MODE PROCESSING DURING WORKING MEMORY IN SCHIZOPHRENIA

The preceding discussion focused on the role of the DLPFC in WM and the importance of impaired DLPFC function to understanding impairments in WM and proactive control in schizophrenia. However, there is also a growing literature suggesting that WM deficits in schizophrenia may be associated with failures to "deactivate" regions overlapping with what is termed the default mode network (DMN) (e.g., Anticevic et al., 2013; Metzak et al., 2012; Whitfield-Gabrieli et al., 2009; although see Mannell Franco et al., 2010, for how cognitive load may modulate this effect). The DMN is a network of brain regions including the medial anterior PFC and the posterior cingulate that normally show reduced activity during cognitively demanding externally oriented mental processing in healthy individuals. DMN activation has been hypothesized to be associated with self-referential and spontaneous cognition (Raichle and Snyder, 2007). It is now widely accepted, based on evidence from both task-based and connectivity findings, that in healthy adults there exists an inverse/anticorrelated relationship between these distributed neural systems purportedly supporting these different aspects of cognition (Fox et al., 2005). In fact, our previous work in healthy adults has demonstrated that the degree of DMN suppression is directly related to accurate WM performance (e.g., Anticevic et al., 2010). The combination of altered DLPFC activity (frequently reduced) and a failure to suppress DMN regions in schizophrenia suggests that there

may be a malfunction in reciprocal communication between brain networks involved in active task engagement and passive mental states or attention to internal representations. Related to this point, the preceding sections discussed interference resolution as a critical component of WM function and that there is clear evidence for breakdowns in filtering of interfering signals during WM maintenance in schizophrenia. In that sense, one can conceptualize the lack of DMN suppression in individuals with schizophrenia as possibly contributing additional sources of unwanted signals during WM. In other words, if there is a breakdown of such distributed regional suppression during WM in patients, superfluous activation of regions involved in passive mentation may contribute an additional source of "noise" during WM and render the ongoing task representations more susceptible to interference. Therefore, these findings raise the possibility that DMN suppression deficits may compromise signal processing in cortical networks by rendering network function "noisy" or inefficient, given that a lowered DMN signal is thought to reflect the suppression of cognitive operations carried out by the DMN (e.g., Raichle and Snyder, 2007). However, as of yet, the direction and causality of the relationship between altered DMN activity and impaired DLPC function during WM in schizophrenia have not been established. Put differently, we do not yet know whether a failure to suppress DMN activity is simply a by-product of a failure to engage frontoparietal control nodes to an appropriate extent to support WM and proactive cognitive control, or whether there is an independent deficit in DMN processing or connectivity with the DLPFC such that an inability to suppress DMN interferes with DLPFC function and processing. Additional research is needed to arbitrate between these differing possibilities and to better understand the complex causal dynamics as well as synergistic contributions of the DMN to cognitive impairment in schizophrenia.

SUMMARY OF WORKING MEMORY FINDINGS IN SCHIZOPHRENIA

In summary, both behavioral and functional neuroimaging evidence points to WM abnormalities in schizophrenia, which extend across both the encoding and maintenance phases and which are consistent with deficits in the ability to generate and maintain internal representations that can be used to guide behavior in a proactive fashion. These deficits are also associated with abnormalities in the function of brain regions such as the DLPFC and the DMN, as well as with connectivity in a distributed cortical circuit that includes frontoparietal, striatal, and thalamic interactions. Such deficits may involve not only abnormalities in sustaining activation across a delay, but also breakdowns in interference resolution from incoming distraction.

EPISODIC MEMORY

COGNITIVE NEUROSCIENCE MODELS OF EPISODIC MEMORY

As with efforts to understand the nature of WM deficits in schizophrenia, it is useful to briefly review the cognitive neuroscience literature on the processing and brain regions involved

in episodic memory (EM) as a means to organize the research pertaining to EM deficits in schizophrenia. A key place to start is work on the specific role that the hippocampal formation plays in EM. A common theme in theories regarding the role of the hippocampal formation in EM is the idea that it is critical for the rapid binding of novel configurations of information (e.g., Cohen and Eichenbaum, 2001; Squire, 1987). Consistent with this hypothesis, a number of human neuroimaging studies have shown activation of the hippocampus during the encoding or retrieval of novel relational information (e.g., Wendelken and Bunge, 2010), and work in amnestic patients emphasizes the importance of hippocampal structures in relational processing (e.g., Bowles et al., 2010). Moreover, a number of functional neuroimaging studies in healthy humans have demonstrated that enhanced hippocampal/parahippocampal activity at the time of encoding predicts subsequent successful retrieval of that information (e.g., Brewer et al., 1998; Wagner et al., 1998). In addition, work with depth electrodes implanted in humans undergoing epilepsy surgery has also demonstrated that hippocampal activity at the time of encoding predicted subsequent memory for verbal stimuli (Cameron et al., 2001). Although more recent models of EM also suggest differential roles for hippocampal versus perirhinal regions of the medial temporal lobes in encoding of item versus relational memory (Davachi, 2006), there is a still a strong consensus on the importance of the hippocampus for relational encoding of a range of information types.

The field has also garnered information about the important contribution made by PFC structures to EM. Damage to the prefrontal cortex can lead to EM deficits, among other cognitive impairments (e.g., Janowsky et al., 1989). Such findings have contributed to the hypothesis that PFC damage alters EM by impairing strategic contributions to memory formation and retrieval (e.g., Janowsky et al., 1989). For example, studies have shown activation of ventral PFC regions such as Brodmann's areas 45 and 47 when participants are asked to process verbal information using semantic elaboration strategies (e.g., Wagner et al., 1998) that promote subsequent memory. For a recent meta-analysis, see (Spaniol et al., 2009). Further, there is recent work suggesting that DLPFC may contribute specifically to successful relational memory formation and retrieval (e.g., Blumenfeld et al., 2011).

EPISODIC MEMORY IMPAIRMENTS IN SCHIZOPHRENIA

As described in the preceding, most theories of hippocampal function posit a key role in binding together novel configurations of information. One way to examine whether individuals with schizophrenia have binding deficits is to determine if they are more impaired on memory for associative information (e.g., the association of previously unrelated words or items) as compared to memory for individual items. To address this question, Achim and Lepage conducted a meta-analysis comparing performance on associative and item memory tests in individuals with schizophrenia, and concluded that there was evidence for a 20% greater impairment in associative as compared to item memory in individuals with schizophrenia

(Achim and Lepage, 2003). However, a number of the associative memory studies included in this meta-analysis were tests of source memory rather than associations of novel pairs of items, and the human neuropsychological and imaging literatures suggest that PFC function may make an important contribution to source memory (Mitchell and Johnson, 2009). In addition, few of the studies that have compared item and associative memory have dealt with the ubiquitous problems of discriminating power. Associative memory tests are often more difficult than item memory tests. Greater task difficulty by itself does not necessarily indicate higher discriminating power, but it does raise the question of whether a pattern of greater impairment on associative versus item memory is truly indicative of a selective deficit in binding of novel information. More recently, clinical researchers have begun to use tasks derived from the animal literature on hippocampal function, such as the transitive interference test, which measures the ability to learn the relationships among hierarchically arranged stimulus pairs, as well as the transitive patterning test, in which individuals have to learn about relationships between items for correct selection. Individuals with schizophrenia are impaired on critical conditions of these tasks requiring relational processing, but not on conditions that require simpler associative reinforcement mappings (e.g., Heckers et al., 2004). Other work has used eye-movement measures of relational memory, shown to be impaired in patients with hippocampal lesions (e.g., Hannula and Ranganath, 2009), to identify relational memory impairments in schizophrenia (e.g., Hannula et al., 2010). There is also work indicating impairments in both item and relational retrieval for information that was relationally encoded in schizophrenia (Ragland et al., 2012b). Still other work has provided evidence for greater deficits in recollection than familiarity in schizophrenia, which have also been interpreted as reflecting relational memory impairments (e.g., van Erp et al., 2008).

Many researchers have taken this body of work to suggest that EM impairments in schizophrenia reflect medial temporal lobe deficits, with a specific focus on the hippocampus (e.g., Heckers and Konradi, 2010). However, the findings in healthy individuals about the role of the PFC cortex in EM raise the possibility that at least some EM impairments among individuals with schizophrenia also reflect deficits in PFC mediated cognitive functions that contribute to successful memory encoding and retrieval, including strategic mechanisms that may facilitate memory formation. Consistent with this hypothesis, a number of studies suggest that individuals with schizophrenia are impaired in their ability to generate effective mnemonic strategies. However, when provided with strategies that promote successful episodic encoding, individuals with schizophrenia are typically able to benefit as much as controls from these strategies and can even show intact item recognition when provided with support for effective encoding (for review, see Barch, 2005). Further, a meta-analysis of brain activity alterations during EM performance in schizophrenia showed consistent evidence for reduced activation in both ventrolateral and DLPFC, but did not find consistent evidence for altered hippocampal activity (Ragland et al., 2009). Recent work on relational memory encoding

and retrieval has shown evidence for impaired DLPFC function associated with impaired relational memory function in schizophrenia (Ragland et al., 2012a), though other recent work has also implicated hippocampal function (e.g., Hanlon et al., 2011). These findings do suggest a need to also take into account a role for PFC mediated cognitive functions as well as hippocampally mediated processes in understanding the source and nature of EM deficits in schizophrenia. Further, the findings on strategic changes in schizophrenia and the role of DLPFC in EM suggests that examining the role of executive control deficits and effective encoding manipulations may be a fruitful avenue for future research on enhancing EM in schizophrenia.

Prior to transitioning to motivational deficits in schizophrenia an important final point relates to heterogeneity of cognitive deficits and the possibility of their occurrence across diagnostic categories. The chapter's focus is on schizophrenia, but cognitive deficits are also observed in other neuropsychiatric conditions that may share behavioral and genetic features with schizophrenia. One example is bipolar illness. Evidence suggests that psychotic symptoms occur in 50–70% of individuals with bipolar disorder (Dunayevich and Keck, 2000; Goodwin and Jamison, 1990) and psychosis aggregates within families of bipolar patients (Potash et al., 2001). One possibility is that comorbid psychosis symptoms in bipolar illness represent a more severe form of the illness associated with worse prognosis (Bellivier et al., 2001; Coryell et al., 2001; but see Keck et al., 2003) and poorer cognitive performance (Glahn et al., 2007) as well as abnormalities in brain structure (Strasser et al., 2005) and function (Pearlson et al., 1995) that may be observed in schizophrenia and associated with cognitive deficits. Therefore, it will be vital to carefully establish to what extent observed cognitive and associated neural disturbances scale, not only as a function of schizophrenia heterogeneity, but also whether cognitive deficits manifest across diagnoses with shared risk. In the concluding section we highlight such need for future studies to investigate endophenotypic markers that may underlie shared versus dissociable disturbances along the psychosis spectrum. Perhaps one way to investigate neural correlates of cognitive (or emotional) disturbances that may scale along the schizophrenia spectrum or co-occur in bipolar illness is to capitalize on the dimensional approach articulated by NIMH Research Domain Criteria (RDoC) initiative (Cuthbert and Insel, 2010; Keshavan et al., 2011; Potash, 2006). One hypothesis suggests that these seemingly separate illnesses represent different endpoint phenomenological expressions of a similar underlying problem at a neural circuit level (Keshavan et al., 2011; Potash, 2006). Emerging reports using novel connectivity approaches in schizophrenia (Cole et al., 2011) and bipolar illness with psychosis history (Anticevic et al., 2012a) indeed raise the intriguing possibility that there may be shared neural (and consequently behavioral) disturbances across the two conditions, which may extend to cognitive deficits. Thus, future work should quantify prefrontal function that may relate to illness severity and comorbidity of psychosis across diagnoses. We return to these issues in the concluding remarks.

Next, we turn to additional disturbances in schizophrenia that extend beyond cognitive deficits.

GOAL REPRESENTATIONS AND MOTIVATIONAL DEFICITS IN SCHIZOPHRENIA

The preceding discussion focused on "cold" cognitive impairments in proactive control, WM, and EM in schizophrenia. These domains have received massive research attention in the schizophrenia literature, which is quite logical given the evidence for their importance in understanding function and outcome, their presence across the spectrum of psychosis, and their links to genetic risk for the development of psychosis. However, a variety of emotional and motivational impairments have also long been clinically documented in patients (Barch and Smith, 2008; Gold et al., 2008; Meehl, 1962), and there has been resurgence of interest in understanding the psychological and neural bases of what are often referred to as "negative symptoms" in schizophrenia. These aspects of schizophrenia pathology include constructs such as asociality (disengagement from others), avolition (a reduction in the motivation to initiate or persist in goal-directed behavior), and anhedonia (a reduction in the ability to experience pleasure). This resurgence of interest in negative symptoms in schizophrenia has been driven by at least two factors. The first factor is the realization that addressing the pervasive cognitive impairment present in schizophrenia may not be enough to fully understand and remediate the functional impairments that can make life so difficult for individuals with this disorder. In other words, we may also need to understand how cognitive impairments interact with reward and emotional processing systems in a way that leads to profound abnormalities in goal-driven behaviors. A second factor, paralleling the aforementioned developments in cognitive neuroscience, is that major advances have occurred in the field of affective neuroscience that provide a theoretical and empirical foundation on which to draw in order to identify candidate psychological and neural mechanisms that drive interactions between cognitive function, reward, and motivation (e.g., Wallis 2007). Here we would like to propose that there may be some common mechanisms that drive impairments in cognition and motivated behavior (e.g., anhedonia/amotivation) in schizophrenia—specifically the ability to use representations about motivational salient incentives or rewards to generate and represent goal-directed action plans necessary to achieve those incentives or rewards. This perspective builds on our previously articulated goal and the hope for the field; namely, to understand several complex and seemingly distinct behavioral manifestations in schizophrenia via parsimonious final common mechanistic pathways (Yizhar et al., 2011).

In order to understand the basis for this argument, it is important to overview the psychological processes and neural systems thought to support linking experienced or anticipated rewards and/or incentives with the action plans that need to be generated and maintained in order to obtain these rewards. The literature on the neural bases of reward and motivation is large and complex. However, one can organize this literature by focusing on four major components to the translation of appetitive or reward information into behavioral responses (Berridge et al., 2009; Schultz, 2007; Wallis, 2007) (see Fig. 21.1). While this conceptualization is clearly an oversimplification, it provides a useful set of organizing principles in approaching the study of which contributors to goal-directed behavior are impaired in schizophrenia. The first component *hedonics or liking* (Fig. 21.1a) reflects the ability to "enjoy" the stimulus or event that may provide pleasure or reward. It had traditionally been thought that the neurotransmitter dopamine (DA) was the primary substrate of liking (Berridge, 2004), but more recent research has shown that experimental depletion of DA does not reduce liking when it can be measured by facial expression and/or subjective reports (Berridge et al., 2009). Instead, hedonic responses (at least to primary sensory stimuli) seem to be mediated by activation of the opioid and GABAergic systems in the nucleus accumbens shell and its projections to the ventral pallidum, as well as in the orbital frontal cortex (OFC) (e.g., Berridge et al., 2009).

A second component *reward prediction and wanting* (Fig. 21.1b) is mediated by the midbrain DA system, particularly the projections to ventral and dorsal striatum (Schultz, 2007; Berridge et al., 2009). Many DA neurons in the substantia nigra and ventral tegmental area respond to stimuli that *predict* reward, as well as to the rewarding stimuli themselves, with the degree of response depending on reward predictability. These types of DA/striatal responses have been captured by temporal difference models that simulate learning about stimuli that predict rewards (e.g., Montague et al., 1996). These mechanisms are also thought to underlie basic aspects of reinforcement learning that may occur without conscious awareness (e.g., Frank et al., 2004). A prominent, though slightly different theory, emphasizes the role of the DA-learning process in transferring incentive salience from the reward itself to reward-predicting cues, thus imbuing these cues with motivational properties themselves (e.g., a "wanting" response; Berridge et al., 2009).

A third component is *cost-benefit analysis*, or the ability to integrate information from different sources to derive and update the value of potentially rewarding outcomes. One aspect, thought to be mediated in part by orbitofrontal cortex (OFC) (e.g., Padoa-Schioppa and Cai, 2011), is the ability to represent value information (Fig. 21.1c), which takes into account not only the hedonic properties of a stimulus, but also the internal state of the organism (e.g., value of juice when thirsty versus not), the delay before the reward occurs, the available reward options (e.g., juice versus wine after a hard day), and the changing contingencies associated with a stimulus (a previously rewarded response is now punished) (e.g., Dias et al., 1996). Some researchers have described the OFC as being involved in "working memory for value," or the ability to maintain, update, and integrate different sources of information about value over a short period of time (e.g., Frank and Claus, 2006). Human functional neuroimaging studies also highlight activation of OFC under conditions requiring value representations (e.g., O'Doherty, 2007), particularly those in which response contingencies need to be updated, such as

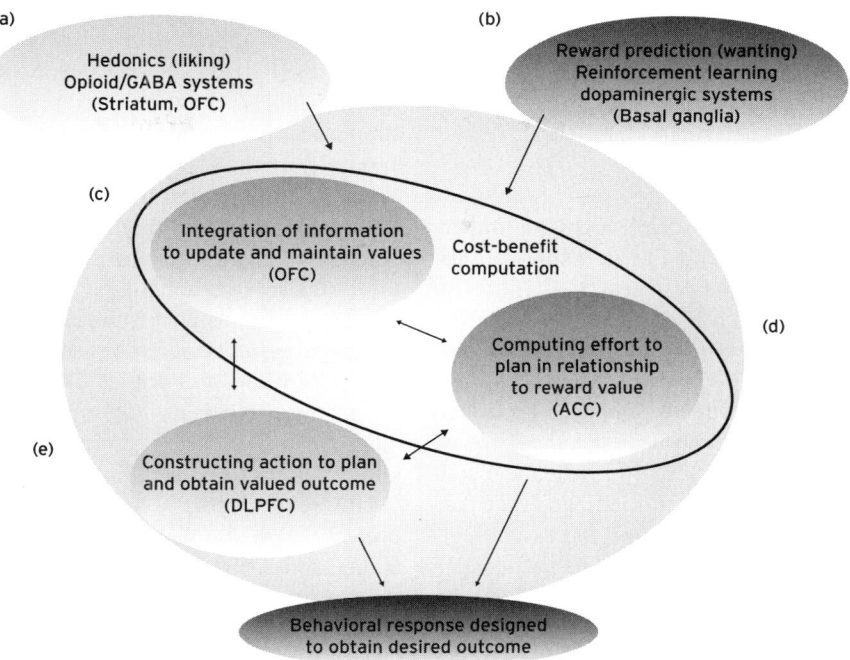

Integration of neuropathology at the level of phenomenology and symptoms

(a) Hedonics (liking) Opioid/GABA systems (Striatum, OFC)

(b) Reward prediction (wanting) Reinforcement learning dopaminergic systems (Basal ganglia)

(c) Integration of information to update and maintain values (OFC)

Cost-benefit computation

(d) Computing effort to plan in relationship to reward value (ACC)

(e) Constructing action to plan and obtain valued outcome (DLPFC)

Behavioral response designed to obtain desired outcome

Figure 21.1 Integration of neuropathology at the level of phenomenology and symptoms—goal representations and motivational deficits in schizophrenia. (Figure adapted from Barch and Dowd, 2010.) This figure outlines a conceptual overview of several processes thought to be involved in translating reward information into goal-directed behaviors, which may be compromised in schizophrenia.

reversal learning (e.g., Cools et al., 2007). In addition, humans with OFC lesions can show reversal learning impairments (e.g., Fellows and Farah, 2005).

Another aspect of representing value information is *effort computation* (Fig. 21.1d), that is, determining the cost of engaging in whatever actions it will take to obtain that outcome. For example, you may really want to eat some ice cream, and may perceive eating ice cream as rewarding, but you may not want to extend the effort to go to the store to get the ice cream. Some research suggests that the dorsal anterior cingulate cortex (ACC) may be important for evaluating the effort associated with different action plans, with contributions from DA input from nucleus accumbens and related forebrain circuitry (e.g., Salamone et al., 2007). For example, research has shown that ACC lesions, as well as depletions of accumbens DA, lead animals to choose low effort but low reward options over higher reward, but higher effort options (e.g., Rushworth et al., 2007; Salamone et al., 2007).

A fourth component is the ability to *generate and execute goal-directed action plans necessary to achieve the valued outcome* (Fig. 21.1e), a function closely aligned with the concept of proactive control. A number of researchers have discussed the role of the lateral PFC in relation to this component in the context of reward and motivation (in particular DLPFC) (Braver et al., 1999; Miller and Cohen, 2001; Wallis, 2007), a function that is consistent with a number of other lines of research and theory, including: (*1*) the role of the DLPFC in top-down control of cognitive processing; (*2*) models suggesting that the DLPFC provides a bias signal that helps to facilitate goal-directed behavior (Miller and Cohen, 2001); (*3*) evidence

for impaired action planning following lateral PFC lesions (e.g., Zalla et al., 2001); and (*4*) evidence that increases in DLFPC activity mediate "motivated" cognitive control enhancements that occur with the provision of incentives in both animals (e.g., Sakagami and Watanabe, 2007) and humans (e.g., Jimura et al., 2010). In other words, intact DLPFC function may be necessary to translate information about value into goal representations and to maintain such information so that is can be implemented as action plans to achieve the desired outcome.

HEDONICS AND LIKING IN SCHIZOPHRENIA

Numerous studies have emphasized that individuals with schizophrenia and controls show similar patterns of valence and arousal (e.g., liking) in their self-reported emotional responses to affect-eliciting stimuli (for reviews, see Kring and Moran, 2008; Cohen and Minor, 2010). The neuroimaging studies examining striatal responses to the receipt of monetary rewards in schizophrenia have also shown a consistent pattern of intact responses. Specifically, these studies have found robust ventral striatal responses to the receipt of money (e.g., Simon et al., 2009; Dowd and Barch, 2012). Interestingly, Simon and colleagues found that the magnitude of the reward receipt response in the ventral striatum was inversely associated with severity of depression, but not with anhedonia (Simon et al., 2009). Schlagenhauf and colleagues did not find group differences in the response to rewards in the ventral striatum, though they did not clearly see intact responses in patients, and there were reduced striatal responses to loss-avoidance among the individuals with schizophrenia (Schlagenhauf et al., 2009).

However, while striatal responses to reward receipt seem to be largely intact in schizophrenia, some of these studies did report abnormal cortical responses to reward receipt (Schlagenhauf et al., 2009; Walter et al., 2010; Waltz et al., 2010). A more mixed picture has arisen from functional neuroimaging studies that have examined brain responses to other types of pleasurable stimuli in schizophrenia (e.g., Crespo-Facorro et al., 2001; Dowd and Barch, 2010; Grimm et al., 2012; Paradiso et al., 2003; Plailly et al., 2006; Waltz et al., 2009).

In sum, the self-report literature provides relatively consistent evidence for intact self-reports of "liking" in schizophrenia, though there is evidence that greater self-reports of anhedonia or negative symptom ratings are associated with less "liking" (e.g., Dowd and Barch, 2010). In addition, the functional neuroimaging literature on the receipt of monetary rewards shows consistent evidence for intact receipt responses. However, the functional neuroimaging literature on responses to other types of rewarding stimuli provides a more confusing picture, with some evidence for reduced insular responses, and mixed evidence for altered striatal responses. Further, those studies that have examined individual differences in negative symptoms do suggest an important relationship between the magnitude of striatal responses to rewarding or pleasurable stimuli and anhedonia among individuals with schizophrenia (Waltz et al., 2009; Dowd and Barch, 2010).

REWARD PREDICTION AND WANTING IN SCHIZOPHRENIA

In schizophrenia, there is robust evidence for altered DA and basal ganglia function (e.g., Fusar-Poli and Meyer-Lindenberg, 2013; Howes et al., 2012). As such, it is surprising that a relatively large number of studies have suggested intact reinforcement learning in schizophrenia using a range of tasks in which learning is either relatively easy or relatively implicit (e.g., Heerey et al., 2008; Waltz et al., 2007), though with some exceptions (e.g., Pantelis et al., 1999). However, when the paradigms become more difficult and require the explicit use of representations about stimulus-reward contingencies, individuals with schizophrenia show more consistent evidence of impaired reinforcement learning (e.g., Gold et al., 2012; Waltz et al., 2007; Yilmaz et al., 2012). Interestingly, there are hints that these impairments may be greater when individuals with schizophrenia must learn from reward versus from punishment (Cheng et al., 2012; Gold et al., 2012; Waltz et al., 2007). Although such deficits could reflect impaired basal ganglia-mediated reinforcement learning mechanisms, they may also reflect impairments in more explicit and rapid on-line learning mechanisms that may be mediated by OFC and/or DLPFC, as hypothesized by Gold and colleagues (Gold et al., 2008) and discussed in what follows.

In the neuroimaging literature, studies of reward prediction (wanting) have primarily used paradigms that directly examine neural responses to reward-predicting cues, sometimes following conditioning trials and sometimes through explicit instruction, such as in the monetary incentive delay (MID) task. A number of studies have reported reduced ventral striatum activity to cues predicting reward in schizophrenia in the MID. These results have been found in unmedicated individuals with schizophrenia (e.g., Nielsen et al., 2012a), as well as in individuals taking typical antipsychotics, but not in individuals treated with atypicals (e.g., Simon et al., 2009), nor in prodromal individuals (Juckel et al., 2012). Kirsch also found reduced ventral striatal responses to reward cues in individuals with schizophrenia taking typicals compared to atypicals (Kirsch et al., 2007), and Nielsen et al. (2012b) found reduced ventral striatal responses to anticipation cues in antipsychotic-naive patients with schizophrenia, which improved following treatment with amisulpride. Importantly, a number of these studies also showed a relationship between negative symptom severity and deficits in anticipatory ventral striatal activity. Juckel and colleagues showed that the severity of negative symptoms predicted the reduction in ventral striatal responses in unmedicated and typically medicated patients. In addition, Simon and colleagues showed that the magnitude of this response was inversely correlated with apathy ratings, and Waltz showed a relationship between negative symptom severity and ventral striatal activation during anticipated gains (Waltz et al., 2010). We have also studied reward prediction using a Pavlovian task, and found a relationship between reduced striatal response to reward-predictive cues and greater anhedonia among individuals with schizophrenia (Dowd and Barch, 2012).

A number of studies have also examined prediction error responses—an increase in striatal (presumably dopaminergic) responses to unexpected rewards and a decrease in striatal responses when predicted rewards do not occur. Murray found evidence for reduced prediction error responses to rewards among schizophrenia spectrum patients in bilateral midbrain and right ventral striatum, coupled with enhanced prediction error responses to neutral stimuli (Murray et al., 2008). Somewhat consistent with this finding, Morris found reduced prediction error responses in the striatum in schizophrenia, as well as enhanced responses for unsurprising reward stimuli that were not expected to elicit prediction errors (Morris et al., 2012). Gradin found reduced prediction error responses in the caudate, but increased activation associated with expected reward value in the ventral striatum (Gradin et al., 2011). Waltz and colleagues examined positive and negative prediction error responses in a passive paradigm that required participants to learn about the timing of a potential reward (Waltz et al., 2009). These researchers found evidence for reduced positive prediction error responses in a range of regions that included the striatum (dorsal and ventral) as well as insula, but relatively intact negative prediction errors in these same regions. Interestingly, Waltz et al. did find that the magnitude of prediction errors in basal ganglia among patients was negatively correlated with avolition scores. In more recent work, Walter et al. (2010) found intact prediction error responses in the striatum for both positive and negative prediction errors, though this was a relatively low negative symptom sample.

To summarize, the literature on reinforcement learning and reward prediction in schizophrenia suggests relatively intact learning on simple reinforcement learning paradigms, though this may reflect a ceiling. On more difficult tasks, there is more consistent evidence for impaired performance,

though in terms of absolute levels of performance rather than in learning rates. The open question in regard to this literature is the degree to which these impairments reflect differences in striatum-influenced learning mechanisms that may be more implicit, versus explicit learning mechanisms that may be more cortically mediated. Consistent with the hypothesis that some of these reinforcement learning impairments may reflect striatal mechanisms, a growing number of studies in the imaging literature suggest reduced ventral striatal reward prediction/"wanting" responses in unmedicated and typically medicated individuals with schizophrenia (though not in those taking atypical antipsychotics) and evidence for reduced positive prediction errors. However, not all studies have found impaired striatal responses to reward prediction cues or to prediction error, and there is also evidence that the magnitude of these striatal impairments may be related to the severity of negative symptoms, again pointing to the importance of examining individual difference relationships among individuals with schizophrenia. Further, a number of studies have also found altered activation in frontal regions during reward prediction or reinforcement learning, suggesting a potentially important role for cortically mediated mechanisms.

VALUE COMPUTATIONS AND OFC FUNCTION IN SCHIZOPHRENIA

There are two experimental paradigms that have been frequently used as probes of lateral and medial OFC function: probabilistic reversal learning and the Iowa gambling task. Both tasks require individuals to integrate information about rewards and punishments across trials, and to use such information to update value representations appropriately. Several studies suggest impaired reversal learning in schizophrenia (e.g., Waltz and Gold, 2007), though a few studies using the ID-ED task did not find simple reversal learning deficits in schizophrenia (e.g., Jazbec et al., 2007). These reversal-learning impairments are present even when individuals with schizophrenia and controls are matched on initial acquisition performance (Weiler et al., 2009). The literature on the Iowa gambling task in schizophrenia also provides evidence for impairment (e.g., Kim et al., 2009), again with some exceptions (e.g., Turnbull et al., 2006). There is also evidence for structural and functional changes in OFC in schizophrenia (e.g., Pantelis et al., 2003; Plailly et al., 2006), though such changes have not been directly related to reversal learning or Iowa gambling task performance. There is also reasonable evidence for olfactory functioning deficits in schizophrenia (e.g., Kamath et al., 2013), which could be related to OFC function (given that olfactory cortex is located in OFC) (Moberg and Turetsky, 2003), although it is not clear whether olfactory functions rely on the same OFC regions that support value computations. In sum, there is good evidence from the behavioral literature for deficits in tasks thought to reflect OFC function in schizophrenia, but no direct evidence of impaired OFC function in relationship to deficits in value computation, as one might find in imaging studies of probabilistic reversal learning (Cools et al., 2002).

EFFORT COMPUTATIONS AND ACC FUNCTION IN SCHIZOPHRENIA

To our knowledge, there is no work directly addressing effort computations in schizophrenia. Several studies suggest that individuals with schizophrenia show reduced error-related ACC responses (e.g., Polli et al., 2008), as well as reduced post-error slowing (e.g., Kerns et al., 2005). However, there is also evidence that patients with schizophrenia can show normal error correction performance even in the context of reduced ACC responses to errors (e.g., Polli et al., 2006) and that the relationship between the magnitude of the error-related negativity (ERN) and error-related behaviors is intact in schizophrenia (Morris et al., 2006). Thus, there is some reason to believe that conflict monitoring, error processing, and ACC function may be altered in individuals with schizophrenia, though more work is needed to address whether these reflect the same mechanisms supporting effort computations.

GOAL-DIRECTED ACTION AND DLPFC FUNCTION IN SCHIZOPHRENIA

As previously reviewed, there is strong evidence from a variety of sources for impairments in goal representation, proactive control, and DLPFC function in schizophrenia. Thus, an important question is whether some of the motivational impairments observed in schizophrenia reflect, at least in part, problems in translating reward information into goal representations that can be used and maintained in DLPFC to guide goal-directed behavior. One means of examining this issue is to determine how motivational incentives impact cognitive performance, potentially via modulation of DLPFC activity. Several studies suggest that individuals with schizophrenia are not able to improve their performance on cognitive tasks when offered monetary incentives (e.g., Hellman et al., 1998); while an equal number suggest at least some evidence for improvement with reward (e.g., Rassovsky et al., 2005), though the studies showing improvements have not used executive control tasks. There is also work on the use of token economies in schizophrenia that suggests functioning can be improved through an explicit reward system, though token economies provide a number of "external" supports for maintaining reward-related information that could compensate for deficits in the ability to translate reward information into action plans. However, to date, there are no fMRI studies examining whether or not incentives modulate DLPFC activity during cognitive control or WM tasks in schizophrenia.

Recent elegant work by Ursu and colleagues provides some data at least indirectly consistent with the presence of deficits in the ability to maintain emotionally relevant information in schizophrenia (Ursu et al., 2011). In the scanner, Ursu and colleagues presented participants with affective or neutral pictures for a brief period followed by a delay interval during which subjects "maintained" the affective state. Following the delay, all participants provided ratings of their emotional experience of the previously presented stimulus. Interestingly, during the initial stimulus presentation phase (i.e., while the physical stimulus was presented on screen), patients and healthy

comparison subjects showed little difference in neural activity, as revealed by a direct contrast. In fact, both groups activated a distributed network of regions previously associated with processing affective stimuli, including the visual cortex, insula, thalamus, midbrain structures, and other regions. However, when required to "maintain" the affective content over the delay, individuals with schizophrenia exhibited marked reductions in signal across regions previously linked to cognitive control (e.g., DLPFC). The lack of maintenance signals correlated with negative symptom severity in their sample. It is important to note that Ursu and colleagues found an association with negative and not positive stimuli, which somewhat limits the generalizability of their findings to discussion of reward and motivation. Nevertheless, this general pattern of reduced PFC signal in the context of maintaining affective information is in correspondence with a body of evidence showing that schizophrenia is associated with reduced DLPFC signals during cognitive control and WM tasks described in the preceding, and is consistent with the hypothesis that individuals with schizophrenia may have difficulty representing information about rewards and incentives that can be used to drive goal directed behavior (Heerey and Gold, 2007).

SUMMARY OF REWARD AND MOTIVATIONAL NEUROSCIENCE IN SCHIZOPHRENIA

Taken together, the results of the current literature review are generally consistent with the interpretation that hedonics are relatively intact in schizophrenia. In contrast, the literature increasingly suggests that there may be a deficit in putatively DA mediated reward learning and/or reward prediction functions. Such findings suggest that impairment in striatal reward prediction mechanisms may influence "wanting" in schizophrenia in a way that reduces the ability of individuals with schizophrenia to use anticipated rewards to drive motivated behavior. Although there is ample evidence for impaired DLPFC function and action planning in schizophrenia, there is little work directly examining the influence of rewards on the ability to modulate these mechanisms in schizophrenia. However, the literature on DLPFC mediated cognitive impairments in schizophrenia, and the recent work by Ursu (Ursu et al., 2011) suggests some potentially intriguing interactions between reward predictions and proactive control in contributing to motivational impairments in schizophrenia. To illustrate, consider the following scenario: An individual with schizophrenia may report that they enjoy chocolate chip cookies, but may not be able to engage in the behaviors necessary to obtain or make more chocolate chip cookies (Barch and Dowd, 2010; Kring and Moran, 2008). Planning, purchasing, preparing, or baking the cookies requires ongoing maintenance of contextual or cue information that should trigger associations about the food's rewarding properties, which will ultimately guide the volitional pursuits over time that may lead to such a reward (in this case intake of appetitive food). An intact reward valuation and prediction system is necessary for this set of behaviors to take place, and deficits in these functions in schizophrenia may reduce the ability of appetitive food cues to drive behavior. However, these functions also depend on the intact ability to maintain appetitive cues or context over time—a process that may be reliant on WM and proactive cognitive control, which are compromised in schizophrenia (Barch and Dowd, 2010). Thus, deficits in reward prediction and learning may be exacerbated by the inability to actively maintain rewarding information in WM, which may extend beyond simple appetitive stimuli to more abstract rewards. What is needed next is research that directly tests the ability to use and maintain internal representations of reward information to modulate behavior and brain function in schizophrenia, along with work that characterizes links between deficits in this ability and everyday function in this illness.

The previous discussion reviews the potential mechanisms of impairment in schizophrenia as potentially dissociable psychological and neural systems that may make independent contributions to impairments in goal directed behavior in schizophrenia. However, it is also possible that there are impairments in several of these functions and systems that reflect one or multiple common mechanisms. One potential common denominator that could lead to impairments in each of the functions (outside of hedonics) is altered DA function in both subcortical and cortical regions (e.g., Fusar-Poli and Meyer-Lindenberg, 2013; Howes et al., 2012). Almost all of the functions described earlier are heavily reliant on intact DA function, which has widespread influences on both cognitive and motivational systems. Thus, should future research indicate that many or all of the processes involved in translating reward into goal directed action are impaired in schizophrenia, it may suggest a role for a core deficit in DA function that modulates multiple components of the system as one parsimonious explanation. However, it is also possible that ongoing research will provide evidence for selective impairments or differential involvement of neurotransmitter systems in individual components of the system (e.g., GABA or glutamate to DLPFC deficits), providing important clues as to pathways for intervention. Further, antipsychotic medications that block DA receptors have the potential to impact these cognitive and motivational systems at several stages, and addressing potential medication confounds will therefore be critical to future work in this field. While practical and ethical constraints make controlled examination of medication effects difficult, there are several strategies that, when combined, may yield a fuller picture of how reward-related functions are affected by medications in this population. The reward prediction literature has begun to tackle these questions by examining unmedicated patients and comparing results between different medication types. Other approaches could include: examining genetically related, medication-naïve populations such as first-degree relatives and schizotypal personality disorder patients; delaying a dose of medication in order to perform within-subjects comparisons at high and low D2R blockade, and/or performing PET and fMRI studies in the same sample to gain information about individual levels of DA synthesis, availability, or receptor distribution to directly link DA function to behavior and brain responses associated with proactive control and motivation. Finally, due to well-known system-level DA and glutamate interactions (Coyle, 2006) it will be critical for future studies to fully disambiguate whether DA dysregulation, even

if functionally important for the aforementioned deficits, is the proximal cause of these deficits or a downstream abnormality of other neurotransmitter and microcircuit alterations (Lewis et al., 2012). Such complex multilevel integration, from synaptic mechanism to system-wide effects of interacting neurotransmitter abnormalities, will be vital to mechanistically understand emerging behavioral pathology in schizophrenia.

UNDERSTANDING AFFECTIVE AND COGNITIVE DEFICITS IN SCHIZOPHRENIA ACROSS LEVELS OF ANALYSES

Thus far we have discussed the complex cognitive and motivational processes affected in schizophrenia from the perspective of psychological processing as well as the brain regions and broadly defined neural and neurotransmitter systems that may support these processes. This is the level of analysis most commonly examined using cognitive neuroscience approaches, and the levels for which the most data exist about impairment in schizophrenia level, mainly due to the functional resolution of non-level human neuroimaging. Indeed, such approaches have honed our search for mechanisms involved in these behavioral deficits. However, such cognitive neuroscience approaches when used in isolation have more difficulty identifying underlying cellular mechanisms (in humans, and therefore patients suffering from mental illness, at least). Such a cellular and molecular level of understanding is crucial to identify effective pharmacological therapies that directly translate from an understanding of the impaired mechanisms leading to abnormal cognitive and motivational process. We believe it will be critical to close the existing gaps in our understanding of emotion and cognition in schizophrenia across levels of explanation: from synaptic signaling at the microcircuit level, to system-level disruptions and ultimately abnormal behavior. We acknowledge that a comprehensive review of the neurobiology and neurochemical alterations in schizophrenia is beyond the scope of the present chapter (see prior reviews for excellent treatments of this topic (e.g., Krystal et al., 2003; Lewis et al., 2012; Marin, 2012; Moghaddam and Javitt, 2012). However, we briefly highlight how evolving cellular-level hypotheses of microcircuit disruptions offer a possible foundation for understanding higher-order emergent neural system and behavioral deficits in schizophrenia that demand mechanistic explanations.

As discussed in this chapter, the clinical cognitive and motivational neuroscience approach to schizophrenia has identified region-level abnormalities in both function and anatomy across areas such as DLPFC, hippocampus, amygdala, thalamus, and striatum (Fig. 21.2). Regions such as DLPFC, striatum, amygdala, and thalamus comprise a set of cortical-subcortical networks and loops, which function in concert and are influenced by multiple neuromodulatory signaling pathways (Fig. 21.2). Indeed, as reviewed previously, disruptions in numerous interacting neurotransmitter systems, including DA, GABA, and glutamate have been implicated in schizophrenia (e.g., Krystal et al., 2003; Lewis et al., 2012). For example, there is mounting evidence for DA alterations in the striatum of patients with schizophrenia that result in hyperactivity (e.g.,

(a) Micro-circuit level disturbances in cortical function

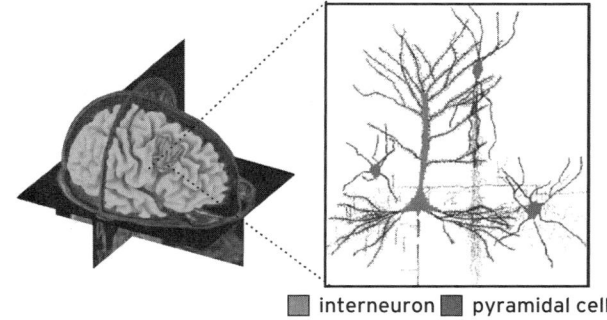

⬛ interneuron ⬛ pyramidal cell

(b) Cortical-striatal-limbic circuit disruption in schizophrenia

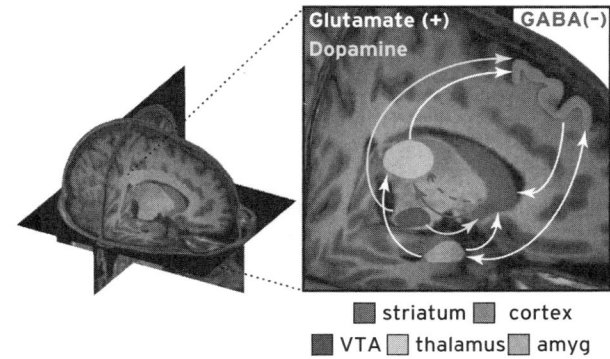

⬛ striatum ⬛ cortex
⬛ VTA ⬛ thalamus ⬛ amyg

Figure 21.2 Conceptual illustration of neural circuitry across levels of computation that may be involved in affective and cognitive disturbances in schizophrenia. The figure highlights how, in order to explain deficits at the phenomenological/behavioral level, we need to bridge observations across multiple levels of analysis in schizophrenia. (a) At the regional level there is clear evidence for both structural and functional abnormalities in cortical and striatal/thalamic circuits in schizophrenia (Bora et al., 2011; Shepherd et al., 2012). Based on emerging findings from basic animal (e.g., Yizhar et al., 2011; Lewis et al., 2012), postmortem (e.g., Lewis et al., 2012), and pharmacological studies (Krystal et al., 2003), there is an increasing understanding of microcircuit abnormalities that may be at play in schizophrenia, contributing to regional abnormalities (Marin, 2012). One possibility is that that abnormalities in the balance of excitation/inhibition in cortical microcircuitry (E/I balance) contribute to downstream system-level disturbances that encompass distributed circuits and neurotransmitter systems. One leading hypothesis postulates an imbalance between cortical excitation and inhibition between pyramidal cells and interneurons, producing a state of "disinhibition," which may in turn affect regional and neural system-level function in schizophrenia (Yizhar et al., 2011). (b) Less is known about how some of these regional deficits and microcircuit alterations manifest in possible system-level disruptions in functional loops between prefrontal, striatal, limbic, and thalamic nodes in schizophrenia (Lisman, 2012). Deficits in these interacting functional systems need to be considered when interpreting abnormalities between affective and cognitive operations in schizophrenia. Furthermore, there is known interplay between interacting neurotransmitter systems in cortico-striatal-thalamic loops that may be compromised in schizophrenia (e.g., Coyle, 2006). Considering effects across all of these levels will be critical to mechanistically understand complex schizophrenia phenomenology.

Fusar-Poli and Meyer-Lindenberg, 2013; Howes et al., 2012). Patients also present with reduced (in particular hypostimulation of D1 receptors in PFC; Abi-Dargham et al., 2002). Patients may also exhibit disruptions in glutameric signaling at the NMDA receptor (Krystal et al., 2003), as well as disruptions in

GABA synthesis and signaling from interneurons onto pyramidal cells (e.g., Lewis et al., 2012) (Fig. 21.2b). As noted, there is still an ongoing debate as to which one of these disruptions may be the proximal cause of downstream symptoms (Coyle, 2006), but given that disruptions across interactive neurotransmitter systems are likely to contribute to dysfunction across the illness course (Marsman et al., 2013), considering these complex interactions will be vital as we move toward a more complete understanding of this illness.

One way to organize these multiple, interactive dysfunctions across levels of analysis is to consider how they may be impacted by pathology at the level of cortical microcircuitry (Fig. 21.2) (Lewis et al., 2012; Marin, 2012). That is, perhaps if we were to start from cellular-level hypotheses of disrupted cortical computations in schizophrenia, we may ultimately be able to better understand complex dynamics that emerge at higher levels of observation. Here we need to consider that optimal cortical function depends on the balanced interaction of pyramidal excitatory (glutamatergic) and inhibitory (GABAergic) neurons (Shadlen and Newsome, 1994) (i.e., excitation/inhibition balance—E/I balance). Disruptions of this E/I balance can have drastic behavioral consequences, with implications for a number of neuropsychiatric conditions (Marin, 2012; Yizhar et al., 2011). In schizophrenia specifically there may be a functional deficit in the interaction between excitatory and inhibitory cortical neurons (e.g., Lewis et al., 2012; Marin, 2012). This may arise from a disruption in cortical inhibition stemming perhaps from reduced inhibitory drive via GABA interneurons onto pyramidal cells and ultimately resulting in *disinhibition* of pyramidal cells (Lewis et al., 2012; Marin, 2012). One finding consistent with this possibility is that postmortem studies of patients with schizophrenia consistently show reduced levels of the mRNA for the 67-kilodalton isoform of glutamic acid decarboxylase (GAD67, encoded by *GAD1*), a key factor in optimal GABA levels, in the DLPFC (for review see Lewis et al., 2012). Importantly, it is well documented that GABAergic interneurons function by exerting lateral inhibition and synchronizing persistent firing of pyramidal cells in DLPFC (Rao et al., 2000), thus providing one potential mechanism for the tuning of representations across cortex. That is, lateral inhibition might enhance the processing and maintenance of salient information relative to less behaviorally relevant representations. Disruptions of this balance between pyramidal and GABA interneurons may be one crucial pathophysiological mechanism operating in schizophrenia, relevant to the patterns of neural and behavioral responses that we discuss presently.

At present, it is unknown how these cellular disruptions in E/I balance may manifest at the level of neural systems and ultimately diverse psychological processes compromised in this illness (Yizhar et al., 2011). The challenge facing the field is to close this gap and understand the pathways that lead to such disruptions, which will potentially allow for future hypothesis-driven compensations aimed at ameliorating such circuit abnormalities. There are multiple paths forward that can help close this gap:

1. One approach is to start at the level of cells and make predictions regarding the higher levels of analysis. A way to accomplish this goal could involve computational modeling, particularly models that are rooted in neurophysiologic data and that build on assumptions based on molecular and systems neuroscience (e.g., Wang, 2010). We have, as proof-of-principle, applied this framework in the context of WM (Anticevic et al., 2012b), but more work will be needed to extend such tools to other psychological constructs and processes.

2. Another approach is to test hypotheses regarding neural dysfunction in schizophrenia via pharmacological manipulations in healthy adults (Corlett et al., 2007). This is accomplished through perturbations of the underlying circuitry thought to be compromised in individuals suffering from the illness, via relatively well understood neurochemical mechanisms. In turn, such manipulations may reveal clues regarding specific links between disruptions in neurotransmitter systems, which can be connected to system-level deficits and ultimately behavior.

3. Continued development of more sophisticated animal models of the neural pathology that may be present in this illness that are well linked to both intermediate and behavioral phenotypic markers should also be pursued (Yizhar et al., 2011). For instance, primate physiology experiments of WM, in combination with targeted neurochemical and optogenetic manipulations (Tye and Diesseroth, 2012), provide this framework (e.g., Arnsten and Rubia, 2012).

4. As articulated by the Research Domain Criteria (RDoC) initiative (Insel and Cuthbert, 2009), examining behavioral deficits and alterations in the underlying neural systems transdiagnostically (Anticevic et al., 2012b) and via continuous measures of symptom severity could provide further clues about common versus unique mechanisms that may co-occur in schizophrenia and other severe neuropsychiatric illnesses such as bipolar disorder.

5. Lastly, large-scale imaging genomic studies as well as detailed spatial and temporal genetic transcriptomics approaches (e.g., Kang et al., 2011) could hone our search for genes that influence cortical development, that may ultimately disrupt the cortical microcircuitry detailed in the preceding.

We argue that these and other complementary neuroscientific approaches will be critical to close our vast explanatory gaps in clinical neuroscience of schizophrenia.

CONCLUDING REMARKS AND FUTURE DIRECTIONS

In this chapter, we have reviewed the extensive evidence that individuals with schizophrenia experience deficits in the active representation of information necessary to guide behavior, a critical aspect of proactive control and WM function (see Fig. 21.3). Further, we have also reviewed evidence that WM

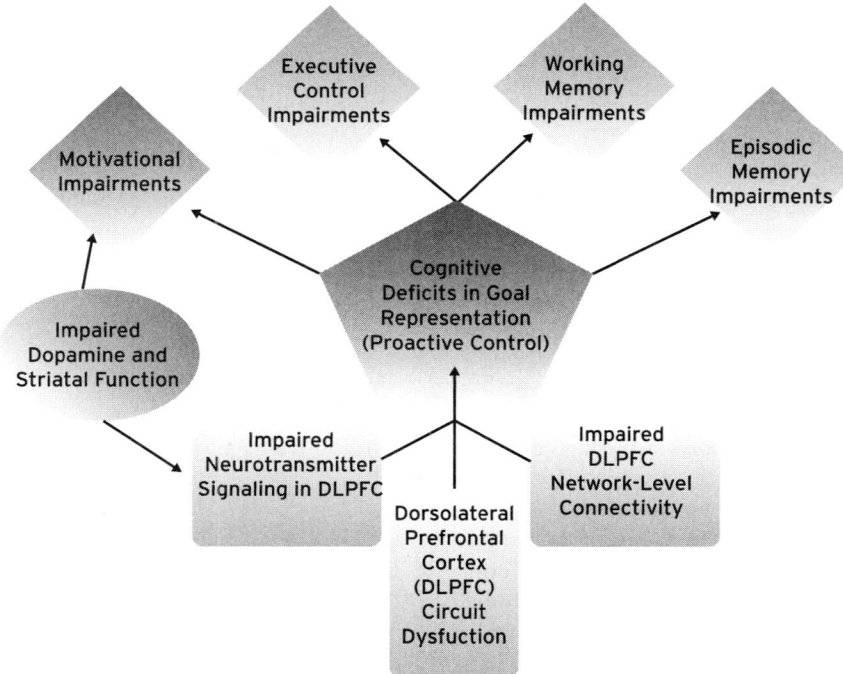

Figure 21.3 Goal representation, cognition, and motivation in schizophrenia. The figure highlights the complex multilevel interactions that need to be considered in the context of cognitive and motivational deficits in schizophrenia. For instance, regional deficits in prefrontal nodes such as DLPFC (bottom boxes) arising from multiple factors—namely disrupted local neurotransmission (e.g. GABA, dopamine, and glutamate), deficits in microcircuit computations, as well as network-level connectivity disturbances in key cortical nodes. Such regional abnormalities may be exacerbated by neurotransmitter disturbance in downstream circuits, such as dopamine signaling in striatum (oval), which also impact on motivational problems in schizophrenia (left diamond). Such region and system-level disturbances may converge on a "core" cognitive deficit in goal and context representation (center polygon), which is ultimately measurable via neurocognitive behavioral tests. Importantly, such a "core" deficit may impact various complex cognitive operations that rely and tap into similar circuits (top diamonds).

deficits in schizophrenia are associated with disturbances in a distributed cortical frontoparietal, striatal, and thalamic circuit, though impairments in DLPFC function may play a particularly key role. Such impairments may involve not only abnormalities in sustaining activation across a delay, but also breakdowns in interference resolution from incoming distraction. We have also discussed evidence suggesting that individuals with schizophrenia have deficits in episodic memory function that involve impairments in relational integration and retrieval. These deficits in relational processing of components of episodic memory appear to reflect impairments in both binding processes supported by the hippocampus and the types of beneficial encoding strategies supported by regions of PFC. Importantly, we have also suggested that impairments in DLPFC-mediated active maintenance of information may contribute to deficits in motivated behavior in schizophrenia, by interfering with the ability to use and/or maintain representations of rewards, incentives, or other affective information necessary to generate action plans needed to obtain positive outcomes. Although we realize that this is an oversimplification, as outlined in Figure 21.3, we have found it useful to conceptualize the common mechanisms that may be contributing to deficits across cognitive domains and which may link cognitive and motivational deficits. We have proposed proactive control and DLPFC dysfunction as one common mechanism,

as well as the possible contribution of impaired DA function along other interactive neurotransmitter systems. Other researchers will have suggestions about different types of common mechanisms; what we wish to emphasize here is the utility of a more unified account of the diversity of impairments in schizophrenia as a means to move forward our understanding of pathophysiology and treatment options.

There are several other important directions for future work in the cognitive and motivational neuroscience of schizophrenia. The first direction is to link this work back to genetics, risk for psychosis, and endophenotypic markers, so we can better understand the causal pathways leading to deficits in cognitive and motivational processes in psychosis, and their potential synergistic interactions. There is already a good deal of evidence that a variety of cognitive deficits present in schizophrenia may be associated with genetic risk for psychosis, as they are present in the first-degree relatives of individuals with schizophrenia who do not manifest psychotic symptoms. There is also some work beginning to link the severity of such impairment, at the neural and/or behavioral level with particular genetic risk factors. The second is closely aligned with the goals of the recently developed and aforementioned RDoC initiative, the aim of which is to redefine the structure of psychopathology based on known neural systems and neurobiological mechanisms. Deficits in the types and profiles of cognitive and motivational

processes described in this chapter are not limited to schizophrenia, and at least some are present (albeit sometimes in an attenuated form) across the spectrum of psychotic disorders (e.g., psychosis NOS, schizotypal personality disorder; e.g., Barch et al., 2003; Barch et al., 2004) and across the traditional divisions between affective and non-affective psychoses (e.g., Depp et al., 2007; Reichenberg et al., 2009). Such findings raise the possibility that there are common mechanisms that lead to cognitive dysfunction across psychotic disorders, a hypothesis that is consistent with a growing emphasis on identifying core neural systems that contribute to impairments that cut across traditional diagnostic boundaries (Insel, 2010). As such, much more research is needed that directly compares cognitive and motivational deficits across typical diagnostic boundaries, with a particular focus on understanding whether similar deficits at the behavioral level are linked to similar deficits at the neural level and with an emphasis on linking such impairments to specific psychopathological processes (e.g., anhedonia) or function. While there is clearly a need for continued research effort, we find that the field of schizophrenia research is at a truly exciting juncture where ever-expanding neuroimaging technologies, translational findings, computational modeling techniques, and genetic approaches provide true potential for hypothesis-driven rational treatment development based on understanding of disease mechanisms.

DISCLOSURES

Dr. Anticevic is funded by National Alliance for Research on Schizophrenia and Depression (NARSAD).

Dr. Dowd does not have any conflicts of interest to disclose.

Dr. Barch has been funded by National Institute of Mental Health (NIMH), National Alliance for Research on Schizophrenia and Depression (NARSAD), and National Institute on Aging (NIA), has received research grants from Allon and Novartis, and has consulted for Pfizer.

REFERENCES

Abi-Dargham, A., Mawlawi, O., et al. (2002). Prefrontal dopamine D1 receptors and working memory in schizophrenia. *J. Neurosci.* 22(9):3708–3719.

Achim, A.M., and Lepage, M. (2003). Is associative recognition more impaired than item recognition memory in schizophrenia?: a meta-analysis. *Brain Cogn.* 53:121–124.

Anticevic, A., Brumbaugh, M.S., et al. (2012a). Global prefrontal and fronto-amygdala dysconnectivity in bipolar I disorder with psychosis history. *Biol. Psychiatry* [Epub ahead of print].

Anticevic, A., Gancsos M., et al. (2012b). NMDA receptor function in large-scale anti-correlated neural systems with implications for cognition and schizophrenia. *Proc. Natl. Acad. Sci. USA* 109(41):16720–16725.

Anticevic, A., Repovs, G., et al. (2010). When less is more: TPJ and default network deactivation during encoding predicts working memory performance. *NeuroImage* 49:2638–2648.

Anticevic, A., Repovs, G., et al. (2012c). A broken filter: prefrontal functional connectivity abnormalities in schizophrenia during working memory interference. *Schizophr. Res.* 141(1):8–14.

Anticevic, A., Repovs, G., et al. (2013). Working memory encoding and maintenance deficits in schizophrenia: neural evidence for activation and deactivation abnormalities. *Schizophr. Bull.* 39(1):168–178.

Arnsten, A.F., and Rubia, K. (2012). Neurobiological circuits regulating attention, cognitive control, motivation, and emotion: disruptions in neurodevelopmental psychiatric disorders. *J. Am. Acad. Child Adolesc. Psychiatry* 51(4):356–367.

Badcock, J.C., Badcock, D.R., et al. (2008). Examining encoding imprecision in spatial working memory in schizophrenia. *Schizophr. Res.* 100(1–3):144–152.

Baddeley, A.D. (2000). The episodic buffer: A new component of working memory? *Trends Cogn. Sci.* 4:417–423.

Barch, D.M. (2005). The cognitive neuroscience of schizophrenia. In: T. Cannon and S. Mineka, eds. Annual Review of Clinical Psychology. Washington, D.C: American Psychological Association, vol. 1, pp. 321–353.

Barch, D.M., and Braver, T.S. (2007). Cognitive control in schizophrenia: Psychological and neural mechanisms. In: R.W. Engle, G. Sedek, U. von Hecker, and A.M. McIntosh, eds. Cognitive Limitations in Aging and Psychopathology. Cambridge: Cambridge University Press, pp. 122–159.

Barch, D.M., Carter, C.S., et al. (2001). Selective deficits in prefrontal cortex regions in medication naive schizophrenia patients. *Arch. Gen. Psychiatry* 50:280–288.

Barch, D.M., Carter, C.S., et al. (2003). Context processing deficit in schizophrenia: diagnostic specificity, 4-week course, and relationships to clinical symptoms. *Journal of Abnormal Psychology* 112:132–143.

Barch, D.M., Carter, C.S., et al. (2004). Factors influencing Stroop performance in schizophrenia. *Neuropsychology* 18(3):477–484.

Barch, D.M., and Dowd, E.C. (2010). Goal representations and motivational drive in schizophrenia: the role of prefrontal-striatal interactions. *Schizophr. Bull.* 36(5):919–934.

Barch, D.M., and Smith, E. (2008). The cognitive neuroscience of working memory: relevance to CNTRICS and schizophrenia. *Biol. Psychiatry* 64(1):11–17.

Bellivier, F., Golmard, J.L., et al. (2001). Admixture analysis of age at onset in bipolar I affective disorder. *Arch. Gen. Psychiatry* 58(5):510–512.

Berridge, K.C. (2004). Motivation concepts in behavioral neuroscience. *Phys. Behav.* 81(2):179–209.

Berridge, K.C., Robinson, T.E., et al. (2009). Dissecting components of reward: "liking," "wanting," and learning. *Curr. Opin. Pharmacol.* 9(1):65–73.

Blumenfeld, R.S., Parks, C.M., et al. (2011). Putting the pieces together: the role of dorsolateral prefrontal cortex in relational memory encoding. *J. Cogn. Neurosci.* 23(1):257–265.

Bora, E., Fornito, A., et al. (2011). Neuroanatomical abnormalities in schizophrenia: a multimodal voxelwise meta-analysis and meta-regression analysis. *Schizophr. Res.* 127(1–3):46–57.

Bowles, B., Crupi, C., et al. (2010). Double dissociation of selective recollection and familiarity impairments following two different surgical treatments for temporal-lobe epilepsy. *Neuropsychologia* 48(9):2640–2647.

Braver, T.S. (2012). The variable nature of cognitive control: a dual mechanisms framework. *Trends Cogn. Sci.* 16(2):106–113.

Braver, T.S., Barch, D.M., et al. (1999). Cognition and control in schizophrenia: A computational model of dopamine and prefrontal function. *Biol. Psychiatry* 46:312–328.

Brewer, J., Zhao, Z.H., et al. (1998). Parahippocampal and frontal responses to single events predict whether those events are remembered or forgotten. *Science* 281:1185–1187.

Callicott, J.H., Mattay, V.S., et al. (2003). Complexity of prefrontal cortical dysfunction in schizophrenia: more than up or down. *Am. J. Psychiatry* 160(12):2209–2215.

Callicott, JH., Ramsey, N.F., et al. (1998). Functional magnetic resonance imaging brain mapping in psychiatry: methodological issues illustrated in a study of working memory in schizophrenia. *Neuropsychopharmacology* 18(3):186–196.

Cameron, K.A., Yashar, S., et al. (2001). Human hippocampal neurons predict how well word pairs will be remembered. *Neuron* 30(1):289–298.

Cheng, G.L., Tang, J.C., et al. (2012). Schizophrenia and risk-taking: impaired reward but preserved punishment processing. *Schizophr. Res.* 136(1–3):122–127.

Cho, R.Y., Konecky, R.O., et al. (2006). Impairments in frontal cortical gamma synchrony and cognitive control in schizophrenia. *Proc. Natl. Acad. Sci. USA* 103(52):19878–19883.

Cohen, A.S., and Minor, K.S. (2010). Emotional experience in patients with schizophrenia revisited: meta-analysis of laboratory studies. *Schizophr. Bull.* 36(1):143–150.

Cohen, J.D., Barch, D.M., et al. (1999). Context-processing deficits in schizophrenia: converging evidence from three theoretically motivated cognitive tasks. *Journal of Abnormal Psychology* 108:120–133.

Cohen, J.D., and Servan-Schreiber, D. (1992). Context, cortex and dopamine: a connectionist approach to behavior and biology in schizophrenia. *Psychol. Rev.* 99(1):45–77.

Cohen, N.J., and Eichenbaum, H. (2001). From Conditioning to Conscious Recollection. New York: Oxford University Press.

Cole, M.W., Anticevic, A., et al. (2011). Variable global dysconnectivity and individual differences in schizophrenia. *Biol. Psychiatry* 70(1):43–50.

Cools, R., Clark, L., et al. (2002). Defining the neural mechanisms of probabilistic reversal learning using event-related functional magnetic resonance imaging. *J. Neurosci.* 22(11):4563–4567.

Cools, R., Lewis, S.J., et al. (2007). L-DOPA disrupts activity in the nucleus accumbens during reversal learning in Parkinson's disease. *Neuropsychopharmacology* 32(1):180–189.

Corlett, P.R., Honey, G.D., et al. (2007). From prediction error to psychosis: ketamine as a pharmacological model of delusions. *J. Psychopharmacol.* 21(3):238–252.

Coryell, W., Leon, A.C., et al. (2001). The significance of psychotic features in manic episodes: a report from the NIMH collaborative study. *J. Affect. Disord.* 67(1–3):79–88.

Coyle, J.T. (2006). Glutamate and schizophrenia: beyond the dopamine hypothesis. *Cell. Mol. Neurobiol.* 26(4–6):365–384.

Crespo-Facorro, B., Paradiso, S., et al. (2001). Neural mechanisms of anhedonia in schizophrenia: a PET study of response to unpleasant and pleasant odors. *JAMA* 286(4):427–435.

Cuthbert, B.N., and Insel, T.R. (2010). Toward new approaches to psychotic disorders: the NIMH Research Domain Criteria project. *Schizophr. Bull.* 36(6):1061–1062.

Davachi, L. (2006). Item, context and relational episodic encoding in humans. *Curr. Opin. Neurobiol.* 16(6):693–700.

Depp, C.A., Moore, D.J., et al. (2007). Neurocognitive impairment in middle-aged and older adults with bipolar disorder: comparison to schizophrenia and normal comparison subjects. *J. Affect. Disord.* 101(1–3):201–209.

Dias, R., Robbins, T.W., et al. (1996). Dissociation in prefrontal cortex of affective and attentional shifts. *Nature* 380: 69–72.

Dowd, E.C., and Barch, D.M. (2010). Anhedonia and emotional experience in schizophrenia: neural and behavioral indicators. *Biol. Psychiatry* 67(10):902–911.

Dowd, E.C., and Barch, D.M. (2012). Pavlovian reward prediction and receipt in schizophrenia: relationship to anhedonia. *PLoS ONE* 7(5):e35622.

Driesen, N.R., Leung, H.C., et al. (2008). Impairment of working memory maintenance and response in schizophrenia: functional magnetic resonance imaging evidence. *Biol. Psychiatry* 64(12):1026–1034.

Dunayevich, E., and Keck, P.E., Jr. (2000). Prevalence and description of psychotic features in bipolar mania. *Curr. Psychiatry Rep.* 2(4):286–290.

Edwards, B.G., Barch, D.M., et al. (2010). Improving prefrontal cortex function in schizophrenia through focused training of cognitive control. *Front. Hum. Neurosci.* 4:32.

Fellows, L.K., and Farah, M.J. (2005). Different underlying impairments in decision-making following ventromedial and dorsolateral frontal lobe damage in humans. *Cereb. Cortex* 15(1):58–63.

Forbes, N.F., Carrick, L.A., et al. (2009). Working memory in schizophrenia: a meta-analysis. *Psychol. Med.* 39(6):889–905.

Fox, M.D., Snyder, A.Z., et al. (2005). The human brain is intrinsically organized into dynamic, anticorrelated functional networks. *Proc. Natl. Acad. Sci. USA* 102(27):9673–9678.

Frank, M.J., and Claus, E.D. (2006). Anatomy of a decision: striato-orbitofrontal interactions in reinforcement learning, decision making, and reversal. *Psychol. Rev.* 113(2):300–326.

Frank, M.J., Seeberger, L.C., et al. (2004). By carrot or by stick: cognitive reinforcement learning in parkinsonism. *Science* 306(5703):1940–1943.

Funahashi, S., Bruce, C.J., et al. (1989). Mnemonic coding of visual space in the monkey's dorsolateral prefrontal cortex. *J. Neurophysiol.* 61(2):331–349.

Fusar-Poli, P., and Meyer-Lindenberg, A. (2013). Striatal presynaptic dopamine in schizophrenia, Part I: meta-analysis of dopamine active transporter (DAT) density. *Schizophr. Bull.* 39(1):22–32.

Glahn, D.C., Bearden, CE., et al. (2007). The neurocognitive signature of psychotic bipolar disorder. *Biol. Psychiatry* 62(8):910–916.

Glahn, D.C., Ragland, J.D., et al. (2005). Beyond hypofrontality: a quantitative meta-analysis of functional neuroimaging studies of working memory in schizophrenia. *Hum. Brain Mapp.* 25(1):60–69.

Gold, J.M., Waltz, J.A., et al. (2012). Negative symptoms and the failure to represent the expected reward value of actions: behavioral and computational modeling evidence. *Arch. Gen. Psychiatry* 69(2):129–138.

Gold, J.M., Waltz, J.A., et al. (2008). Reward processing in schizophrenia: a deficit in the representation of value. *Schizophr. Bull.* 34(5):835–847.

Goldman-Rakic, P.S. (1995). Cellular basis of working memory. *Neuron* 14:477–485.

Goldman-Rakic, P.S., Muly, E.C., et al. (2000). D1 receptors in prefrontal cells and circuits. *Brain Res. Rev.* 31: 295–301.

Goodwin, F.K., and Jamison, K.R. (1990). Manic Depressive Illness. New York: Oxford University Press.

Gradin, V.B., Kumar, P., et al. (2011). Expected value and prediction error abnormalities in depression and schizophrenia. *Brain* 134(Pt 6):1751–1764.

Grimm, O., Vollstadt-Klein, S., et al. (2012). Reduced striatal activation during reward anticipation due to appetite-provoking cues in chronic schizophrenia: a fMRI study. *Schizophr. Res.* 134(2–3):151–157.

Hanlon, F.M., Houck, J.M., et al. (2011). Bilateral hippocampal dysfunction in schizophrenia. *NeuroImage* 58(4):1158–1168.

Hannula, D.E., and Ranganath, C. (2009). The eyes have it: hippocampal activity predicts expression of memory in eye movements. *Neuron* 63(5):592–599.

Hannula, D.E., Ranganath, C., et al. (2010). Use of eye movement monitoring to examine item and relational memory in schizophrenia. *Biol. Psychiatry* 68(7):610–616.

Heckers, S., and Konradi, C. (2010). Hippocampal pathology in schizophrenia. *Curr. Top. Behav. Neurosci.* 4:529–553.

Heckers, S., Zalesak, M., et al. (2004). Hippocampal activation during transitive inference in humans. *Hippocampus* 14(2):153–162.

Heerey, E.A., Bell-Warren, K.R., et al. (2008). Decision-making impairments in the context of intact reward sensitivity in schizophrenia. *Biol. Psychiatry* 64(1):62–69.

Heerey, E.A., and Gold, J.M. (2007). Patients with schizophrenia demonstrate dissociation between affective experience and motivated behavior. *J. Abnorm. Psychol.* 116: 268–278.

Hellman, S.G., Kern, R.S., et al. (1998). Monetary reinforcement and Wisconsin Card Sorting performance in schizophrenia: why show me the money? *Schizophr. Res.* 34(1–2):67–75.

Howes, O.D., Kambeitz, J., et al. (2012). The nature of dopamine dysfunction in schizophrenia and what this means for treatment: meta-analysis of imaging studies. *Arch. Gen. Psychiatry.*

Insel, T.R. (2010). Rethinking schizophrenia. *Nature* 468(7321):187–193.

Insel, T.R., and Cuthbert, B. N. (2009). Endophenotypes: bridging genomic complexity and disorder heterogeneity. *Biol. Psychiatry* 66(11):988–989.

Janowsky, J.S., Shimamura, A.P., et al. (1989). Cognitive impairment following frontal lobe damage and its relevance to human amnesia. *Behav. Neurosci.* 103(3):548–560.

Jazbec, S., Pantelis, C., et al. (2007). Intra-dimensional/extra-dimensional set-shifting performance in schizophrenia: impact of distractors. *Schizophr. Res.* 89(1–3):339–349.

Jimura, K., Locke, H.S., et al. (2010). Prefrontal cortex mediation of cognitive enhancement in rewarding motivational contexts. *Proc. Natl. Acad. Sci. USA* 107(19):8871–8876.

Johnson, M.R., Morris, N.A., et al. (2006). A functional magnetic resonance imaging study of working memory abnormalities in schizophrenia. *Biol. Psychiatry* 60(1):11–21.

Jonides, J., Lewis, R.L., et al. (2008). The mind and brain of short-term memory. *Annu. Rev. Psychol.* 59:193–224.

Juckel, G., Friedel, E., et al. (2012). Ventral striatal activation during reward processing in subjects with ultra-high risk for schizophrenia. *Neuropsychobiology* 66(1):50–56.

Kamath, V., Moberg, P.J., et al. (2013). Odor hedonic capacity and anhedonia in schizophrenia and unaffected first-degree relatives of schizophrenia Patients. *Schizophr. Bull.* 39(1):59–67.

Kang, H.J., Kawasawa, Y.I., et al. (2011). Spatio-temporal transcriptome of the human brain. *Nature* 478:483–489.

Keck, P.E., Jr., McElroy, S.L., et al. (2003). Psychosis in bipolar disorder: phenomenology and impact on morbidity and course of illness. *Comp. Psychiatry* 44(4):263–269.

Kerns, J.G., Cohen, J.D., et al. (2005). Decreased conflict- and error-related activity in the anterior cingulate cortex in subjects with schizophrenia. *Am. J. Psychiatry* 162(10):1833–1839.

Keshavan, M.S., Morris, D.W., et al. (2011). A dimensional approach to the psychosis spectrum between bipolar disorder and schizophrenia: the Schizo-Bipolar Scale. *Schizophr. Res.* 133(1–3):250–254.

Kim, YT., Lee, K.U., et al. (2009). Deficit in decision-making in chronic, stable schizophrenia: from a reward and punishment perspective. *Psychiatry Investig.* 6(1):26–33.

Kirsch, P., Ronshausen, S., et al. (2007). The influence of antipsychotic treatment on brain reward system reactivity in schizophrenia patients. *Pharmacopsychiatry* 40(5):196–198.

Kring, A.M., and Moran, E.K. (2008). Emotional response deficits in schizophrenia: insights from affective science. *Schizophr. Bull.* 34(5):819–834.

Krystal, J.H., D'Souza, D.C., et al. (2003). NMDA receptor antagonist effects, cortical glutamatergic function, and schizophrenia: toward a paradigm shift in medication development. *Psychopharmacol. (Berl.).* 169(3–4):215–233.

Lee, J., and Park, S. (2005). Working memory impairments in schizophrenia: a meta-analysis. *J. Abnorm. Psychol.* 114(4):599–611.

Lewis, D.A., Curley, A.A., et al. (2012). Cortical parvalbumin interneurons and cognitive dysfunction in schizophrenia. *Trends Neurosci.* 35(1):57–67.

Lewis, D.A., and González-Burgos, G. (2008). Neuroplasticity of neocortical circuits in schizophrenia. *Neuropsychopharmacology* 33(1):141–165.

Lisman, J. (2012). Excitation, inhibition, local oscillations, or large-scale loops: what causes the symptoms of schizophrenia? *Curr. Opin. Neurobiol.* 22(3):537–544.

MacDonald, A.W., 3rd, Goghari, V.M., et al. (2005). A convergent-divergent approach to context processing, general intellectual functioning, and the genetic liability to schizophrenia. *Neuropsychology* 19(6):814–821.

MacDonald, A.W., 3rd, Thermenos, H.W., et al. (2009). Imaging genetic liability to schizophrenia: systematic review of FMRI studies of patients' nonpsychotic relatives. *Schizophr. Bull.* 35(6):1142–1162.

Mannell, M.V., Franco, A.R., et al. (2010). Resting state and task-induced deactivation: a methodological comparison in patients with schizophrenia and healthy controls. *Hum. Brain Mapp.* 31(3):424–437.

Marin, O. (2012). Interneuron dysfunction in psychiatric disorders. *Nat. Rev. Neurosci.* 13(2):107–120.

Marsman, A., van den Heuvel, M.P., et al. (2013). Glutamate in schizophrenia: a focused review and meta-analysis of 1H-MRS studies. *Schizophr. Bull.* 39(1):120–129.

Meehl, P.E. (1962). Schizotaxia, schizotypy, schizophrenia. *Am. Psychologist* 17: 827–838.

Mesholam-Gately, R.I., Giuliano, A.J., et al. (2009). Neurocognition in first-episode schizophrenia: a meta-analytic review. *Neuropsychology* 23(3):315–336.

Metzak, P.D., Riley, J.D., et al. (2012). Decreased efficiency of task-positive and task-negative networks during working memory in schizophrenia. *Schizophr. Bull.* 38(4):803–813.

Miller, E.K., and Cohen, J.D. (2001). An integrative theory of prefrontal cortex function. *Annu. Rev. Neurosci.* 24:167–202.

Minzenberg, M.J., Laird, A.R., et al. (2009). Meta-analysis of 41 functional neuroimaging studies of executive function in schizophrenia. *Arch. Gen. Psychiatry* 66(8):811–822.

Mitchell, K.J., and Johnson, M.K. (2009). Source monitoring 15 years later: what have we learned from fMRI about the neural mechanisms of source memory? *Psychol. Bull.* 135(4):638–677.

Moberg, P.J., and Turetsky, B.I. (2003). Scent of a disorder: olfactory functioning in schizophrenia. *Curr. Psychiatry Rep.* 5(4):311–319.

Moghaddam, B., and Javitt, D. (2012). From revolution to evolution: the glutamate hypothesis of schizophrenia and its implication for treatment. *Neuropsychopharmacology* 37(1):4–15.

Montague, P.R., Dayan, P., et al. (1996). A framework for mesencephalic dopamine systems based on predictive Hebbian learning. *J. Neurosci.* 16:1936–1947.

Morris, R.W., Vercammen, A., et al. (2012). Disambiguating ventral striatum fMRI-related BOLD signal during reward prediction in schizophrenia. *Molecular Psychiatry* 17(3):235, 280–239.

Morris, S.E., Yee, C.M., et al. (2006). Electrophysiological analysis of error monitoring in schizophrenia. *J. Abnorm. Psychol.* 115(2):239–250.

Murray, G.K., Corlett, P.R., et al. (2008). Substantia nigra/ventral tegmental reward prediction error disruption in psychosis. *Mol. Psychiatry* 13(3):239, 267–276.

Nielsen, M.O., Rostrup, E., et al. (2012a). Alterations of the brain reward system in antipsychotic naïve schizophrenia patients. *Biol. Psychiatry* 71(10):898–905.

Nielsen, M.O., Rostrup, E., et al. (2012b). Improvement of brain reward abnormalities by antipsychotic monotherapy in schizophrenia. *Arch. Gen. Psychiatry* 12:1–10.

Nuechterlein, K.H., Subotnik, K.L., et al. (2011). Neurocognitive predictors of work outcome in recent-onset schizophrenia. *Schizophr. Bull.* 37(suppl 2):S33–S40.

O'Doherty J.P. (2007). Lights, Camembert, Action! The role of human orbitofrontal cortex in encoding stimuli, rewards and choices. *Ann. NY Acad. Sci.* 1121:254–272.

Padoa-Schioppa, C., and Cai, X. (2011). The orbitofrontal cortex and the computation of subjective value: consolidated concepts and new perspectives. *Ann. NY Acad. Sci.* 1239:130–137.

Pantelis, C., Barber, F.Z., et al. (1999). Comparison of set-shifting ability in patients with chronic schizophrenia and frontal lobe damage. *Schizophr. Res.* 37(3):251–270.

Pantelis, C., Velakoulis, D., et al. (2003). Neuroanatomical abnormalities before and after onset of psychosis: a cross-sectional and longitudinal MRI comparison. *Lancet* 361(9354):281–288.

Paradiso, S., Andreasen, N.C., et al. (2003). Emotions in unmedicated patients with schizophrenia during evaluation with positron emission tomography. *Am. J. Psychiatry* 160(10):1775–1783.

Pearlson, G.D., Wong, D.F., et al. (1995). *In vivo* D2 dopamine receptor density in psychotic and nonpsychotic patients with bipolar disorder. *Arch. Gen. Psychiatry* 52(6):471–477.

Plailly, J., d'Amato, T. et al. (2006). Left temporo-limbic and orbital dysfunction in schizophrenia during odor familiarity and hedonicity judgments. *NeuroImage* 29(1):302–313.

Polli, F.E., Barton, J.J., et al. (2006). Schizophrenia patients show intact immediate error-related performance adjustments on an antisaccade task. *Schizophr. Res.* 82(2–3):191–201.

Polli, F.E., Barton, J.J., et al. (2008). Reduced error-related activation in two anterior cingulate circuits is related to impaired performance in schizophrenia. *Brain* 131(Pt 4):971–986.

Potash, J.B. (2006). Carving chaos: genetics and the classification of mood and psychotic syndromes. *Harv. Rev. Psychiatry* 14(2):47–63.

Potash, J.B., Willour, V.L., et al. (2001). The familial aggregation of psychotic symptoms in bipolar disorder pedigrees. *Am. J. Psychiatry* 158:1258–1264.

Ragland, J.D., Laird, A.R., et al. (2009). Prefrontal activation deficits during episodic memory in schizophrenia. *Am. J. Psychiatry* 166(8):863–874.

Ragland, J.D., Blumenfeld, R.S., et al. (2012a). Neural correlates of relational and item-specific encoding during working and long-term memory in schizophrenia. *NeuroImage* 59(2):1719–1726.

Ragland, J.D., Ranganath, C., et al. (2012b). Relational and item-specific encoding (RISE): task development and psychometric characteristics. *Schizophr. Bull.* 38(1):114–124.

Raichle, M.E., and Snyder, A.Z. (2007). A default mode of brain function: a brief history of an evolving idea. *Neuroimage* 37(4):1083–1090; discussion 1097–1089.

Rao, S.G., Williams, G.V., et al. (2000). Destruction and creation of spatial tuning by disinhibition: GABA(A) blockade of prefrontal cortical neurons engaged by working memory. *J. Neurosci.* 20(1):485–494.

Rassovsky, Y., Green, M.F., et al. (2005). Modulation of attention during visual masking in schizophrenia. *Am. J. Psychiatry* 162(8):1533–1535.

Reichenberg, A., Harvey, P.D., et al. (2009). Neuropsychological function and dysfunction in schizophrenia and psychotic affective disorders. *Schizophr. Bull.* 35(5):1022–1029.

Repovs, G., Csernansky, J.G., et al. (2011). Brain network connectivity in individuals with schizophrenia and their siblings. *Biol. Psychiatry* 15(69):967–973.

Rushworth, M.F., Behrens, T.E., et al. (2007). Contrasting roles for cingulate and orbitofrontal cortex in decisions and social behaviour. *Trends Cogn. Sci.* 11(4):168–176.

Sakagami, M., and Watanabe, M. (2007). Integration of cognitive and motivational information in the primate lateral prefrontal cortex. *Ann. NY Acad. Sci.* 1104:89–107.

Salamone, J.D., Correa, M., et al. (2007). Effort-related functions of nucleus accumbens dopamine and associated forebrain circuits. *Psychopharmacol. (Berl.).* 191(3):461–482.

Schlagenhauf, F., Sterzer, P., et al. (2009). Reward feedback alterations in unmedicated schizophrenia patients: relevance for delusions. *Biol. Psychiatry* 65(12):1032–1039.

Schultz, W. (2007). Multiple dopamine functions at different time courses. *Annu. Rev. Neurosci.* 30:259–288.

Shadlen, M.N., and Newsome, W.T. (1994). Noise, neural codes and cortical organization. *Curr. Opin. Neurobiol.* 4:569–579.

Shepherd, A.M., Laurens, K.R., et al. (2012). Systematic meta-review and quality assessment of the structural brain alterations in schizophrenia. *Neurosci. Biobehav. Rev.* 36(4):1342–1356.

Simon, J.J., Biller, A., et al. (2009). Neural correlates of reward processing in schizophrenia—relationship to apathy and depression. *Schizophr. Res.*

Snitz, B.E., Macdonald, A.W., 3rd, et al. (2006). Cognitive deficits in unaffected first-degree relatives of schizophrenia patients: a meta-analytic review of putative endophenotypes. *Schizophr. Bull.* 32(1):179–194.

Spaniol, J., Davidson, P.S., et al. (2009). Event-related fMRI studies of episodic encoding and retrieval: meta-analyses using activation likelihood estimation. *Neuropsychologia* 47(8–9):1765–1779.

Squire, L.R. (1987). Memory and Brain. New York: Oxford University Press.

Strasser, H.C., Lilyestrom, J., et al. (2005). Hippocampal and ventricular volumes in psychotic and nonpsychotic bipolar patients compared with schizophrenia patients and community control subjects: a pilot study. *Biol. Psychiatry* 57(6):633–639.

Tek, C., Gold, J., et al. (2002). Visual perceptual and working memory impairments in schizophrenia. *Arch. Gen. Psychiatry* 59(2):146–153.

Turnbull, O.H., Evans, C.E., et al. (2006). A novel set-shifting modification of the Iowa gambling task: flexible emotion-based learning in schizophrenia. *Neuropsychology* 20(3):290–298.

Tye, K.M., and Diesseroth, K. (2012). Optogenetic investigation of neural circuits underlying brain disease in animal models. *Nat. Rev. Neurosci.* 13(4):251–266.

Ursu, S., Kring, A.M., et al. (2011). Prefrontal cortical deficits and impaired cognition-emotion interactions in schizophrenia. *Am. J. Psychiatry* 168(3):276–285.

van Erp, T.G., Lesh, T.A., et al. (2008). Remember and know judgments during recognition in chronic schizophrenia. *Schizophr. Res.* 100(1–3):181–190.

Van Snellenberg, J.X., Torres, I.J., et al. (2006). Functional neuroimaging of working memory in schizophrenia: task performance as a moderating variable. *Neuropsychology* 20:497–510.

Wagner, A.D., Schacter, D., et al. (1998). Building memories: remembering and forgetting of verbal experiences as predicted by brain activity. *Science* 281(5380):1188–1191.

Wallis, J.D. (2007). Orbitofrontal cortex and its contribution to decision-making. *Annu. Rev. Neurosci.* 30:31–56.

Walter, H., Heckers, S., et al. (2010). Further evidence for aberrant prefrontal salience coding in schizophrenia. *Front. Behav. Neurosci.* 3:62.

Waltz, J.A., and J. M. Gold (2007). Probabilistic reversal learning impairments in schizophrenia: further evidence of orbitofrontal dysfunction. *Schizophr. Res.* 93(1–3):296–303.

Waltz, J.A., Frank, M.J., et al. (2007). Selective reinforcement learning deficits in schizophrenia support predictions from computational models of striatal-cortical dysfunction. *Biol. Psychiatry* 62(7):756–764.

Waltz, J.A., Schweitzer, J.B., et al. (2009). Patients with schizophrenia have a reduced neural response to both unpredictable and predictable primary reinforcers. *Neuropsychopharmacology* 34(6):1567–1577.

Waltz, J.A., Schweitzer, J.B., et al. (2010). Abnormal responses to monetary outcomes in cortex, but not in the basal ganglia, in schizophrenia. *Neuropsychopharmacology* 35(12):2427–2439.

Wang, H., Stradtman, G.G., et al. (2008). A specialized NMDA receptor function in layer 5 recurrent microcircuitry of the adult rat prefrontal cortex. *Proc. Natl. Acad. Sci. USA* 105(43):16791–16796.

Wang, X.-J. (2010). Neurophysiological and computational principles of cortical rhythms in cognition. *Phys. Rev.* 90(3):1195–1268.

Weiler, J.A., Bellebaum, C., et al. (2009). Impairment of probabilistic reward-based learning in schizophrenia. *Neuropsychology* 23(5):571–580.

Wendelken, C., and Bunge, S.A. (2010). Transitive inference: distinct contributions of rostrolateral prefrontal cortex and the hippocampus. *J. Cogn. Neurosci.* 22(5):837–847.

Whitfield-Gabrieli, S., Thermenos, H., et al. (2009). Hyperactivity and hyperconnectivity of the default network in schizophrenia and in first-degree relatives of persons with schizophrenia. *Proc. Natl. Acad. Sci. USA* 106(4):1279–1284.

Yilmaz, A., Simsek, F., et al. (2012). Reduced reward-related probability learning in schizophrenia patients. *Neuropsychiatr. Dis. Treat.* 8:27–34.

Yizhar, O., Fenno, L.E., et al. (2011). Neocortical excitation/inhibition balance in information processing and social dysfunction. *Nature* 477(7363):171–178.

Yoon, J.H., Tamir, D., et al. (2008). Multivariate pattern analysis of functional magnetic resonance imaging data reveals deficits in distributed representations in schizophrenia. *Biol. Psychiatry* 64(12):1035–1041.

Zalla, T., Plassiart, C., et al. (2001). Action planning in a virtual context after prefrontal cortex damage. *Neuropsychologia* 39(8):759–770.

22 | MOUSE MODELS OF SCHIZOPHRENIA AND BIPOLAR DISORDER

MIKHAIL V. PLETNIKOV AND CHRISTOPHER A. ROSS

INTRODUCTION

Animal models are experimental systems that are developed to study particular aspects of a disease, as no model can accurately reflect all features of the disease. Modeling of human neuropsychiatric disorders in animals is especially challenging (Nestler and Hyman, 2010).

An example of both the opportunities and difficulties of mouse model research is seen with Huntington's disease (HD). HD is a single gene disorder whose genetics and neurobiology are relatively well understood (Ross and Tabrizi, 2011). The clinical symptoms of human HD include pathognomonic involuntary and voluntary movement disorders, cognitive decline, and emotional changes, with inexorable progression to death. These are accompanied by selective neuronal degeneration in the striatum and other brain regions. The disease is caused by a single mutation, a CAG repeat expansion at the *Huntingtin* locus. There have been over a dozen attempts to model this disease in mice (Crook and Housman, 2011). These models had some outstanding successes. For instance, the characteristic intranuclear inclusions containing aggregated Huntingtin protein were first discovered in the mouse model, and this discovery enabled their identification in humans. The mice generally do have some motor and cognitive abnormalities, and in some cases there is a progressive phenotype ending in early death. However, most of the models do not have the massive striatal neurodegeneration seen in the human disease. Most of the models do not have the involuntary movement disorder. Many of the models have weight gain instead of the progressive weight loss seen in most HD cases. Thus, it is important to keep in mind that even in a disorder that should be relatively straightforward, the mouse models have both strengths and weaknesses, and demand careful and cautious interpretation.

During the last three decades multiple animal models of schizophrenia and bipolar disorder have been generated, based on environmental exposures, drug-induced behaviors, or lesions. We might categorize different kinds of animal models in terms of their relationship to the cognate human diseases.

Phenotypic models attempt to model aspects of the phenotype of the disease, often picking behaviors that are reliably measured in animals, such as motor activity, acoustic startle responses, or various kinds of learning. These may or may not reproduce the pathophysiology of the human disorder, but may be useful for pharmacology.

Pathophysiological models attempt to mimic some key aspect of the biology, though not necessarily the etiology of the human disorders. For instance, since abnormal neurodevelopment is increasingly seen as central to schizophrenia, perturbations of brain development (Lu, 2011) may model some aspects of the biology of the disorder. It is important to interpret developmental mouse models in the context of emerging knowledge of the circuitry of psychiatric disorders (Lewis and Sweet, 2009; Ross et al., 2006), including cortical and subcortical circuits. Much attention has been given to modeling alterations in dopamine signaling; however this may be more relevant to antipsychotic pharmacology than to human disease pathogenesis.

Finally, etiologic models have the potential to match most closely the human disorders. Presumably, the pathophysiology should also be congruent if the etiology is congruent. Etiologic models could be either environmental or genetic. However, while environmental factors, including pharmacologic exposure, clearly contribute to psychiatric disorders, the exact factors and their time course, are not yet well defined, and so it is difficult to model them. Therefore, taking into account the strong evidence for genetic contributions to the development of schizophrenia and bipolar disorder, genetic models may be the most specific way to attempt to match the human neurobiology, and hopefully model pathogenesis and, ideally, response to treatment.

In this review we will mention some of the non-genetic models, but focus on genetic mouse models, evaluate their advantages and limitations, and comment on potential new prospects for the field. We will focus on single gene alterations and attempts to model copy number variation. For most genetic contributors to human psychiatric disorder, the pathophysiologic mechanisms are poorly understood. For instance, genetic variation could lead to overall loss of function, gain of function, misregulation of gene expression and function, or other more complex changes. Until specific causative mutations are identified, models will have to depend on hypotheses about gain or loss of function or other alterations.

NON-GENETIC MODELS

PHARMACOLOGICAL MODELS

One approach to animal models of schizophrenia and bipolar disorders is based on use of pharmacological challenges. These models are mainly relatively acute phenotypic models, though exposure to psychostimulants, cannabis, PCP, and other drugs may contribute to susceptibility to human psychiatric disorders. In addition, these pharmacologic models may be able to mimic the behavioral effects of treatments used in clinic (pharmacological isomorphism) and to predict pharmacological effects of experimental compounds to become future therapeutics (predictive validity) (Matthysse, 1986).

Among pharmacological animal models of schizophrenia, phencyclidine (PCP)- or amphetamine-induced hyperactivity are most popular. Similarly, amphetamine-induced hyperactivity has been widely used to model mania (Berggren et al., 1978; Davies et al., 1974; Gould et al., 2001; Kato et al., 2007), although lithium does not seem to attenuate amphetamine-induced changes in healthy volunteers (Silverstone, 1998). The major caveat of drug-induced hyperactivity models is that hyperactivity is one of a broad set of symptoms of several psychiatric diseases, including schizophrenia, attention-deficit hyperactivity disorder, and bipolar disorder (Young, 2011). Since pharmacological treatments of schizophrenia and bipolar disorder are largely symptom-based or palliative, animal models that mimic behavioral responses to drugs are less likely to provide insights into the pathogenic mechanisms of disease and more likely to illuminate behavior pharmacology (Elenbroek and Cools, 1995).

BEHAVIORAL OR SYMPTOM-ORIENTED MODELS

Another approach to animal models of schizophrenia and bipolar disorder mimics behavioral abnormalities of the disease. Critically, in addition to evaluation of how accurate modeled animal behaviors reflect human symptoms, animal models of face validity are also scrutinized in pharmacological studies to evaluate if an altered behavior is responsive to treatments also used in clinical settings. For example, disrupted prepulse inhibition (PPI) of the acoustic startle and abnormal social interaction mimic impaired sensorimotor gating and social withdrawal observed in schizophrenia patients and can be improved by typical and atypical antipsychotics). Symptoms of mania that can be modeled in animals include increased activity, irritability, reduced need for sleep (or other changes in sleep patterns), aggressive behavior, sexual drive, distractibility, and risk-taking behavior, all of which are commonly observed in human mania (Einat, 2006). Models of the depressive phase of bipolar disorder usually utilize models validated in the context of depression research (see the chapter on models of depression), such as models of anhedonia, sleep disorder, poor hygiene, and changes in appetite or weight (Cryan and Holmes, 2005).

However, key positive and negative symptoms of schizophrenia or mood swings in bipolar disorder cannot be fully reproduced in animals. Even when schizophrenia-like alterations such as hyperactivity or social behavior deficit are modeled, it is unclear whether they arise from the same pathological processes, since hyperactivity can be induced by a great variety of drugs and manipulations irrelevant to the etiology and neuropathology of schizophrenia or bipolar disorder (Ridley and Baker, 1982).

PATHOGENIC NON-GENETIC MODELS

An additional approach to animal models involves attempts to reproduce pathogenic processes underlying the disease. These models are based on the concept that behavioral deficits in humans are due to disturbances in the brain functioning that could be modeled in animals (Elenbroek, 1995). Abnormal neurodevelopment is believed to be an important factor leading to behavioral deficits (Jaaro-Peled et al., 2010). Thus, animal models of abnormal brain and behavior development are likely to be most informative for our understanding of the neurobiology of schizophrenia and bipolar disorder (Insel, 2010; Kamiya et al., 2012).

During the last three decades several animal models of schizophrenia have been generated based on environmental exposures and lesions in developing and adult rodents (Lipska and Weinberger, 1993, 1995). The similar approaches have been utilized for neurodevelopmental models of bipolar disorder. For example, the exposure of the animals to early social isolation or early postnatal lesions in amygdala may produce the symptoms resembling aspects of mania, such as increased locomotor activity and enhanced sensitivity to the locomotor-activating effects of amphetamine (Swerdlow, 2001). In the context of recent reports on using transcranial magnetic stimulation as a treatment for depression, use of electrically or chemically induced kindling to study the development of new episodes in bipolar disorder is also of an interest (Kalynchuk, 2000). Still, all these non-genetic pathogenic animal models do not really address the etiology of the diseases and will unlikely advance uncovering new therapeutic targets.

GENETIC MOUSE MODELS OF SCHIZOPHRENIA

Genetic models have the potential to model both etiology and pathogenesis. Recent genetic studies are finally yielding replicable genetic loci for the human disorder. Most mouse work to date has relied on genes identified in linkage studies, which may contribute risk in small families though not necessarily in the entire population. However in other disorders, genes identified in small families have often turned out later to be relevant to the population at large. Since psychiatric genetics is still in a relatively early stage, it is difficult now to know which genes will confer the greatest amount of risk in different populations. Furthermore, alterations of genes whose gene products are involved in pathogenic pathways may be very useful even if the gene altered does not turn out to contribute a large amount of risk in human populations. In the future, likely more models will be available from loci confirmed in large GWAS or sequencing studies. For now, much of the work is on genes identified in smaller studies.

MODELS BASED ON GENES FROM GENOME-WIDE ASSOCIATION STUDIES

Most of the candidate genes studied to date emerged from relatively small linkage or association studies, and have not been seen in genome-wide association studies, so their relevance to schizophrenia in the population is uncertain (Sklar et al., 2008). Genome-wide association studies offer an unbiased assessment of variation across the entire genome, with the ability to identify specific disease variants (Bergen et al., 2012; Lee et al., 2012). A recent list of the risk genes associated with schizophrenia at genome-wide significance level includes zinc finger binding protein 804A (ZNF804A), the major histocompatibility (MHC) region on chromosome 6, neurogranin (NRGN), and transcription factor 4 (TCF4) (e.g., Lee et al., 2012). In addition, Ripke and colleagues have identified the microRNA MIR137 and its targets (Ripke et al., 2011). Generating animal models with the risk variants and characterizing molecular, cellular, behavioral, and other processes will help to link these genes to disease mechanisms. However, animal model research in this field is only starting. Here, we review a few experimental studies available in the literature to date (fall of 2012).

MHC

The most replicated schizophrenia GWAS association is the MHC locus, though multiple genes involved in immunity, neurodevelopment, synaptic plasticity, and other processes present a challenge for linking specific genes in this region to pathophysiology (Corriveau et al., 1998; Huh et al., 2000;). Many MHC mouse studies focus on species-specific recognition as a part of mating behavior (Hurst, 2009). A few investigations have been performed to address roles for this locus in other behaviors. For example, it has been reported that mice deficient for both H2-K(b) and H2-D(b)(K(b)D(b−/−)) have a lower threshold for induction of long-term depression (LTD) at parallel fiber to Purkinje cells synapses and improvement in acquisition and retention of a Rotarod behavioral task. These results suggest a role for classical MHCI molecules in synaptic plasticity and motor learning (McConnell et al., 2009). Unlike wild-type animals, mice lacking both β-2-microglobulin and transporter associated with antigen processing (β2M−/−TAP−/−) showed a greater hypothalamic pituitary adrenal activation to saline injection, while lipopolysaccharide-induced cytokine expression in the hypothalamus was similar in β2M−/−TAP−/− and wild type mice, suggesting that class I MHC plays a role in stress reactivity (Sankar et al., 2012).

An interesting approach to the behavioral effects of the MHC locus is to compare behaviors between MHC-congenic strains of mice or rats, which are genetically identical to each other except for the locus. Spatial learning and memory in male and female mice of two MHC-congenic strains (C57BL/6J and B6-H-2K) in two versions of the Hebb-Williams maze were evaluated. In the food-reward paradigm, males required fewer sessions to learn than females, but there were no strain differences in acquisition. The B6-H-2K mice reached the goal box faster than the C57BL/6J mice. In the water-escape paradigm, the C57BL/6J mice required more sessions than the B6-H-2K mice during acquisition. Thus, these two strains are comparable

in cognitive ability but still show differences in performance in the Hebb-Williams maze (Stanford et al., 2003).

TCF4

A putative role of the basic helix-loop-helix (bHLH) transcription factor TCF4 in the adult brain has been evaluated in transgenic mice that moderately overexpress TCF4 in the postnatal brain. TCF4 transgenic mice display profound deficits in contextual and cue-dependent fear conditioning and sensorimotor gating. Molecular analyses revealed the dynamic circadian deregulation of neuronal bHLH factors in the adult hippocampus. This study describes the first animal model relating to TCF4, and suggests that this transcriptional factor contributes to cognitive processing (Brzózka et al., 2010).

MODELS BASED ON COPY NUMBER VARIATION

Recent studies have implicated structural variations in the genome (copy number variations) in schizophrenia (Malhotra and Sebat, 2012). A 22q11 deletion has long been known to lead to 25-fold increase in the risk for schizophrenia (Murphy et al., 1999), though it is uncertain to what extent this corresponds to other forms of the disease. 22q11.2 deletion syndrome, DiGeorge syndrome (DGS), or velo-cardio-facial syndrome (VCFS) is associated with craniofacial and cardiovascular abnormalities, immunodeficiency, hypocalcemia, short stature, and cognitive dysfunctions (Karayiorgou et al., 2010). The orthologous region of the human 22q11.2 locus is located on mouse chromosome 16 with a high degree of conservation within the 22q11.2 region (Drew, 2011). Both long-range deletion models and single gene knockout (KO) preparations have been described. Here, we only briefly review mouse models related to the deletion. Comprehensive recent reviews of this topic are available elsewhere (e.g., Karayiorgou et al., 2010).

Two of the long-range deletion models—the Df(16)A−/− model (Stark, 2008) and the LgDel/- model (Merscher et al., 2001)—lack the entire 1.5 Mb region on one chromosome, most closely modeling the human 22q11.2 deletion. These models have been reported to display impaired working memory and prepulse inhibition (PPI) of the acoustic startle, similar to the phenotypes of individuals with the 22q11.2 deletion syndrome (Paylor, 2006; Stark, 2008).

Among single gene KO mouse models involving the region of the deletion, PRODH is a promising candidate gene (Li, 2008) that encodes a mitochondrial enzyme to metabolize L-proline, a putative neuromodulator of Glu and GABA neurotransmission. Genetic variants in this gene have been associated with hyperprolinemia type 1 and schizophrenia (Harrison and Weinberger, 2005). Mutant mice with reduced PRODH enzymatic activity show abnormal associative conditioning (Gogos et al., 1999; Paterlini et al., 2005). These mutant mice were reported to have increased levels of COMT, possibly as a compensation for enhanced DA signaling in prefrontal cortex (PFC). Blockade of COMT in PRODH KO mice impairs learning in T-maze task (Paterlini et al., 2005). These results suggest an epistatic interaction between COMT and PRODH (Kvajo et al., 2011), consistent with a similar interaction reported for patients with 22q11.2 deletion (Raux, 2007). A growing

appreciation of the fact that a large number of schizophrenia cases result from copy number variations provides the good rationale for the development of models based on chromosomal engineering and other advanced techniques to manipulate sizable segments of DNA (Nomura and Takumi, 2012).

MODELS BASED ON GENES FROM LINKAGE STUDIES

Genetic models of candidate genes emerging from early linkage studies have been also generated, including dysbindin, neuregulin 1, and Disrupted-in-Schziophrenia-1 (DISC1), which have attracted the most attention and are described here in greater detail. It is notable that most candidate genes that have been studied to date have not been well supported by GWAS studies (Collins et al., 2012). These include COMT, dopamine receptors, neuregulin, dystrophin, BDNF, and other genes. It is possible that genes that do not have a signal in GWAS studies may still be important in familial or other subtypes of the disorder.

DYSBINDIN

Dystrobrevin-binding protein 1, or dysbindin, encoded by the DTNBP1 gene and discovered through screening for binding partners of α-dystrobrevin (Benson et al., 2001) is a part of the dystrophin-associated protein complex (DPC) and of the biogenesis of lysosome-related organelles complex 1 (BLOC-1) (Nazarian et al., 2006). The dysbindin locus was first identified in an Irish study (Straub et al., 2002), and some research has supported relevance of this gene to schizophrenia, including haplotypes of the gene linked to the negative symptoms, or cognitive functioning in healthy people (Talbot, 2009). Postmortem studies also found reduced expression of the gene and protein in the hippocampus and PFC (Talbot, 2009; Weickert, 2008), where decreased expression of the protein can affect synaptic neurotransmission (Iizuka et al., 2007) and synaptic stability.

The role for dysbindin in vivo has been mainly evaluated using mice with spontaneous deletion in the Dtnbp1gene, leading to loss of dysbindin in "sandy" mice of DBA/2J strain (Li et al., 2003; Talbot, 2009). Sandy mice model type VII Hermansky-Pudlak syndrome, which is characterized by oculocutaneous albinism, prolonged bleeding, and pulmonary fibrosis. Earlier studies suggested that dysbindin can be involved in regulation of exocytosis and vesicle biogenesis in neurons and detected diminished levels of snapin (a SNAP25-binding protein) in sandy mice that may partially explain alteration in neurotransmission and behaviors (Chen et al., 2008; Feng et al., 2008). Nagai et al. (2010) observed decreased KCl-evoked DA release in prefrontal cortex, in line with attenuated behavioral sensitization after repeated methamphetamine. In addition, lower expression of dysbindin was associated with decreased NMDA-evoked currents in PFC neurons and decreased NR1 expression that correlated with spatial working memory performance (Karlsgodt et al., 2011). Parvalbumin (PV)-positive neurons were reported to be affected in these mutant mice as well, including impaired inhibition and decreased PV cell immunoreactivity, suggesting a link between this candidate gene and the auditory endophenotypes (Carlson et al., 2011).

These endophenotypic studies were further extended in a recent MRI analysis that found the structural volume deficits in cortical regions, subiculum and dentate gyrus, and the striatum were found in mutant mice (Lutkenhoff et al., 2012).

The molecular and neuronal abnormalities in sandy mice may underlie the behavioral phenotypes, including deficits in social interaction, long-term memory, novel object recognition, and working memory (Feng et al., 2008; Jentsch et al., 2009). Moreover, the most recent reports have described interaction of dysbindin with another candidate gene, Disrupted-in-Schizophrenia-1 (DISC1), suggesting overlapping intracellular signaling pathways for these two important proteins (Camargo et al., 2007; Ottis et al., 2011).

NEUREGULIN 1

Neuregulin 1 (NRG1) and its receptors, ErbB2 and ErbB4, appeared in linkage studies (Stefansson et al., 2002), though again, not yet in genome-wide association studies. Thus, while there has been a large amount of interesting neurobiology brought forward to date, it is not yet clear how relevant it will be to human disease.

Neuregulin-1, also known as heregulin, acetylcholine receptor inducing activity (ARIA), glial growth factor (GGF), or sensory and motor neuron derived factor (SMDF), is encoded by the NRG1 gene located on chromosome 8p13 (Law et al., 2006). Chromosome 8p, mainly the region around 8p21.1–22, has been implicated as a locus harboring one or more susceptibility genes by several linkage studies (Goes FS et al., 2008). Association of this gene with schizophrenia has been replicated, although some contradictions exist (Chen et al., 2006; Harrison and Law, 2006). The SNPs associated with schizophrenia were positioned either before exon 1 or in the introns, and no functional mutations have been identified (Gogos et al., 1999; Mei and Xiong, 2008). Polymorphisms in the intronic regions of this gene are associated with variation in cognitive functions in healthy individuals (Silberberg, 2006; Roussos et al., 2012) and may alter NRG1 expression. Both upregulation and downregulation in expression of mRNA or protein in postmortem brain samples have been reported (Hashimoto et al., 2004; Law et al., 2006; Chong et al., 2008).

NRG1 has been implicated in neuronal migration, synaptogenesis, gliogenesis, neuron-glia interplay, myelin formation, and synaptic neurotransmission (Harrison, 2006). Recently, one of the NRG-1 isoforms has been found to be predominantly expressed prenatally, suggesting a role in neurodevelopment (Tan, 2007). Alternative splicing of NRG1 results in at least 15 isoforms that all contain an extracellular epidermal growth factor (EGF)-like domain, which is sufficient for NRG1 biological activity, and the transmembrane (TM) domain that is common to most NRG1 isoforms (Mei, 2008). Deletion of Nrg1 and its receptor, ErbB4, are lethal, and mice die before birth (Meyer and Birchmeier, 1995). Thus, most studies have been performed using either heterozygous mice or Nrg1 hypomorphic mice that have mutations in the different domains of the gene.

Meyer and Birchmeier generated mice with targeted deletion of the EGF-like domain (NRG1-EGF+/−) by fusing exon 6 of the neuregulin gene to β-galactosidase, which results in

partial deletion of the EGF-like domain of all three major types of Nrg1 (Meyer and Birchmeier, 1995). These mice exhibited elevated activity in open field, improved rotorod performance, and a better performance in T-maze spontaneous alternation task that may be explained by hyperactivity (Gerlai et al., 2000) that can be partially reversed with clozapine (Stefansson et al., 2002). Nrg1 mutant mice also exhibit improved habituation to a new environment, and impairment in PPI after pharmacological challenge with psychostimulants (Duffy et al., 2008).

An NRG-1 KO mouse model that lacks the transmembrane domain was also generated. Heterozygous (HET) mice have no gross alterations in the appearance but display increased activity and deficient PPI reversible by clozapine (Karl, 2007). Mice have no abnormalities in spatial learning but are aggressive (O'Tuathaigh et al., 2007). Compared to wild-type mice, Nrg1+/− mice display increased locomotor activity at 12–16 weeks of age, but not at 6 months. John Waddington and his associates evaluated Nrg1 "knockouts" for four topographies of orofacial movement, both spontaneously and under challenge with the D(1)-like dopamine receptor agonist, SKF 83959. They report that mutants exhibit increased spontaneous and induced incisor chattering, vertical jaw movements, and tongue protrusions. The level of horizontal jaw movements was elevated, while that of tongue protrusions was decreased in mutants, suggesting that Nrg1 may be involved in the regulation of orofacial dyskinesia (Tomiyama, 2012). Deletion of Nrg1 also leads to reduced thermal pain but does not alter the antinociceptive effects of tetrahydrocannabinol (THC) (Walsh, 2010). Another behavioral pharmacology study assessed the effects of MK-801 and phencylclidine (PCP) in these mice. Nrg1 male mutants display attenuated responses to the effects of acute PCP, while subchronic treatment with MK-801 and PCP comparably affect social behaviors in WT and KO mice. The total ventricular and olfactory bulb volumes were found decreased in mutants, but there were no group differences in levels of N-acetylaspartate, glutamate, or GABA (O'Tuathaigh et al., 2010).

The behavior of mice heterozygous for a mutation in neuregulin-1's immunoglobulin (Ig)-like domain (Ig-Nrg-1 mice) was also assessed. These mutants demonstrate clozapine suppression of open-field and running wheel activity and impaired latent inhibition. Unlike other Nrg-1 mutants, Ig-Nrg-1 mice are not hyperactive, suggesting a distinct contribution of this domain to behavioral phenotypes (Rimer et al., 2005). The relatively mild phenotypes of Nrg1 HET mutants might be a result of functional compensation by Nrg2 and/or Nrg3.

A loss-of-function mouse model for type III Nrg1 was also generated. Type III NRG1 is transcribed by a different promoter and is expressed in mPFC, ventral hippocampus, and ventral subiculum. Adult type III Nrg1 HET mice have enlarged lateral ventricles and decreased dendritic spine density on pyramidal neurons. These brain abnormalities were associated with impaired spatial alternation and PPI rescued by chronic nicotine treatment. This model demonstrates a role of type III Nrg1 signaling in the neural circuits involved in sensorimotor gating and short-term memory (Chen et al., 2008).

Several studies evaluated the effects of increased Nrg1 expression using transgenic approaches. Overexpressing Nrg1 in all tissues increased locomotor activity, decreased fear conditioning, and abnormal social behaviors (Kato et al., 2010). Transgenic Nrg1 mice were found to have more parvalbumin-positive neurons and elevated levels of myelination markers in PFC (Kato et al., 2010).

NRG1 acts by stimulating a family of single-transmembrane receptor tyrosine kinases called ErbB proteins (Mei and Xiong, 2008). ErbB proteins have homology with the EGF receptor (EGFR, also known as ErbB1). ErbB4 is the only autonomous NRG1-specific ErbB that can both interact with the ligand and become activated by it as a tyrosine kinase. NRG1 signaling is mediated by heterodimers of ErbB2–ErbB3, ErbB2–ErbB4 and ErbB3–ErbB4 and by the homodimer ErbB4–ErbB4. Consistently, ErbB2 and ErbB3 mutant mice, whose strain origin was identical to that of heregulin mutants, showed no sign of the behavioral alterations (Gerlai et al., 2000). In contrast, ErbB4 heterozygous mice are hyperactive (Stefansson et al., 2002).

In order to study the role for the Nrg1 receptor in progenitor cells, a conditional KO model was generated using mice that express Cre under the nestin promoter. KO mice survived into adulthood and showed no behavioral deficits in locomotion. KO mice also display reduced grip strength compared to WT mice, while HET mice showed an intermediate phenotype. However, HET KO showed abnormalities in Morris water maze learning and memory task relative to WT (Golub et al., 2004).

Selective deletion of ErbB4 in PV-positive neurons prevented NRG1 from promoting activity-dependent GABA release to inhibit the activity of pyramidal neurons. These mutant mice showed hyperactivity, impaired contextual and working memory, and disrupted PPI. Some of these phenotypes were ameliorated by acute treatment with a low dose of diazepam, consistent with impaired GABA neurotransmission. These results indicate that NRG1 regulates the activity of pyramidal neurons by promoting GABA release from PV-positive interneurons, identifying a critical function of NRG1 in balancing brain activity (Wen et al., 2010).

DISRUPTED-IN-SCHZIOPHRENIA-1 (DISC1)

The Disrupted-in-Schizophrenia-1 (DISC1) gene was discovered in a large Scottish family in which a balanced chromosomal translocation [t(1;11)] segregates with schizophrenia, bipolar disease, major depression, and anxiety disorders (St Clair et al., 1990). The translocation t(1;11) (q42;q14) disrupts two genes named Disrupted in Schizophrenia 1 and 2 (DISC1 and DISC2). In contrast to DISC1, the function of DISC2 that encodes a noncoding RNA antisense to DISC1 is unclear. The existence of a clear, identifiable mutation has put DISC1 in a unique position in schizophrenia research (Chubb et al., 2008; Millar et al., 2001).

DISC1 is located within a chromosomal region that has been reported to harbor susceptibility genes for psychiatric illness in several populations (Ekelund et al., 2001; Hennah, 2005; Hennah et al., 2009). Several studies have also reported that healthy subjects and patients with schizophrenia carrying DISC1 variants have alterations in gray matter volume of the hippocampus and PFC (Callicott et al., 2005; Cannon et al., 2005), deficient memory and attention (Cannon et al., 2005; Hennah, 2005), and hippocampal or PFC activation (Callicott et al., 2005). Still, there are also negative reports for linkage to

the *DISC1* locus), SNP associations (Lim, 2009; Sanders, 2008; Wood, 2007), and the rearrangements within the *DISC1* locus. Furthermore there is little support for the DISC1 locus in large association studies to date.

DISC1 protein likely acts as a scaffold protein, with multiple motifs mediating binding to several proteins (Camargo, 2007). DISC1 is expressed in adult rat heart, liver, kidney, brain, and thymus. Brain expression of DISC1 encompasses the hippocampal dentate gyrus, cerebral cortex, hypothalamus, amygdala, cerebellum, and olfactory bulbs (as reviewed in Chubb et al., 2008; Mackie et al., 2007).

RNAi knockdown of Disc1 in the embryonic cortex affects migration, produces mispositioning of neurons (Kamiya et al., 2005), decreases proliferation, and alters neuronal distribution in the developing cortex and adult hippocampus (Mao et al., 2009). In contrast, Disc1 knockdown in proliferating neurons in the mature dentate gyrus enhances migration, growth of dendrites and axons, and maturation of granule neurons. In addition, transient knockdown of DISC1 in the pre- and perinatal stages in pyramidal neurons of PFC leads to altered dopaminergic maturation and resultant behavioral abnormalities in adult mice (Niwa et al., 2010).

DISC1 mouse models have been instrumental in uncovering the mechanisms whereby this protein and its partners contribute to neurodevelopment with relevance to the pathogenesis of schizophrenia.

Risk Allele Model

Drs. Gogos and Karayiorgou have developed a Disc1 mouse model based on the 129 mouse strain, in which a spontaneous 25-bp deletion in exon 6 induces a frame shift in the open reading frame, resulting in 13 novel amino acids, followed by a premature stop codon in exon 7. This strain was modified by homologous recombination to have a termination codon in exon 8 and a premature polyadenylation site in intron 8 to produce a truncated transcript (Koike et al., 2006). Western blot analysis of brain extracts from mutant mice demonstrated the absence of two major Disc1 isoforms and the expression of short N-terminal isoforms (Koike et al., 2006). After backcrossing to the C57B6/j background, these mice show impaired working memory and no alterations in locomotion or PPI. Subsequent studies have found that mutants have disorganized newly born and mature neurons of the dentate gyrus and altered short-term plasticity. Recently, defects in axonal targeting and changes in short-term (Kvajo et al., 2008) plasticity at the mossy fiber/CA3 circuit have been presented for this mouse model as well as elevated levels of cAMP (Kvajo et al., 2011). Thus a natural polymorphism in Disc1 gene may be responsible for the neural and behavioral abnormalities reminiscent of schizophrenia.

Disc1 KO Mice

Generation of Disc1 knockout mice, lacking exons 2 and 3, has been recently reported (Kuroda et al., 2011). Mutant mice have no gross brain or behavior abnormalities but exhibit elevated anxiety and impulsivity (Kuroda et al., 2011). As expression of short transcripts in these KO mice is still observed, a mouse model with deletion of the entire genetic locus is needed to better decipher the function of *DISC1*.

ENU-Induced Model

Two mouse models based on mutations in the mouse Disc1 gene as a result of *N*-nitroso-*N*-ethylurea (ENU) mutagenesis were also described (Clapcote et al., 2007). Two novel missense mutations lead to Q31L and L100P amino acid exchanges in the exon 2, respectively. Notably, these mouse models are characterized by distinct phenotypes. 31L mice display increased immobility in forced swim test (FST), decreased sociability and social novelty, and decreased sucrose consumption, L100P mutants demonstrate increased locomotor activity, decreased PPI, decreased LI, and decreased performance in T-maze were found in L100P mutant mice. These models demonstrate that polymorphisms in Disc1 gene can produce variable behavioral alterations, consistent with distinct aspects of psychiatric disorders. Unfortunately, further study of some of the DISC1 models has not clearly substantiated some of the initially reported behavioral phenotypes (Shoji et al., 2012).

An analysis of the brain abnormalities in Disc1 mutants found a reduced neuronal number, decreased neurogenesis, and altered neuronal distribution and shorter dendrites and decreased surface area and spine density in cortical neurons of Disc1 L100P mutant mice (Lee et al., 2011). Genetic variations in DISC1 can influence interaction between PDE4, GSK-3, and DISC1 (Lipina et al., 2012).

The chromosomal translocation affects the C-terminal of the three major isoforms (Millar et al., 2001). Possible outcomes of the translocation in the *DISC1* gene include haploinsufficiency or the production of a mutant truncated DISC1 protein. Expression of truncated human DISC1 in neuronal PC12 rat cells or mouse brain affects interacting partners via dominant-negative mechanisms, leading to altered levels and distribution of endogenous Disc1 (Kamiya et al., 2005; Pletnikov et al., 2008). In this context, studying effects of mutant DISC1 on neurodevelopment can provide valuable mechanistic insights into the pathogenesis of schizophrenia.

Constitutive Overexpression of Mutant DISC1

A transgenic mouse model with constitutive expression of mutant human DISC1 was developed (Hikida et al., 2007). Transgenic mice express mutant human DISC1 under regulation of the CAMKII promoter in forebrain neurons and exhibit elevated novelty-induced activity, impaired PPI, and more immobility in FST. Mutant mice also have decreased numbers of PV-positive neurons in the cortex and a transient enlargement of the lateral ventricles, demonstrating that forebrain neuronal expression of mutant human DISC1 can produce subtle neurobehavioral alterations resembling aspects of major psychiatric diseases (Hikida et al., 2007).

A *BAC-transgenic mouse model* with expression of C-terminus truncated mouse Disc1 under the endogenous Disc1 promoter was also described (Shen et al., 2008). These mice have thinning of the cortex, enlarged lateral ventricles, corpus callosum agenesis, impaired LI, and greater immobility in FST.

Inducible C-Fragment DISC1 Model

Silva and Cannon's groups have introduced a DISC1 model in which the putative "translocated" C-terminus fragment

of DISC1 is expressed under regulation of the CAMKII promoter in forebrain neurons in an inducible manner (Li et al., 2007). Remarkably, early postnatal but not adult expression of the fragment produces impaired performance in a DNMP task, attenuated social interaction, and a shorter latency to immobilization in FST. These behavioral changes were accompanied by reduced dendritic complexity and decreased basal synaptic transmission in the hippocampus. This inducible model was the first to demonstrate that early postnatal perturbation in Disc1 can lead to neurobehavioral changes, consistent with the neurodevelopmental hypothesis of schizophrenia.

Inducible Mutant Human DISC1 Model

A different mouse model of inducible expression of mutant human DISC1 in forebrain neurons was generated using the Tet-off system (Pletnikov et al., 2008). In this model, expression of mutant DISC1 is regulated by the CAMKII promoter and can be regulated with doxycycline. Expression of mutant DISC1 was described to produce no gross developmental defects but was associated with increased spontaneous locomotor activity in male but not female mice, decreased social interaction in male mice, enhanced aggressive behavior and poorer memory in Morris water maze task in female mice. In addition, expression of mutant DISC1 led to lateral ventricle enlargement in adult mice and reduced dendritic arborization in primary cortical neurons and decreased expression of a synaptic protein, SNAP-25, consistent with human postmortem studies that show decreased dendritic length and dendritic arborization in frontal cortical areas (Harrison, 1999).

To evaluate the roles of DISC1 at various stages of neurodevelopment, the effects of mutant DISC1 were examined during prenatal and/or postnatal periods. Regardless of timing of expression, decreased levels of cortical dopamine (DA) and fewer parvalbumin-positive neurons in the cortex were found in mutant mice. Combined prenatal and postnatal expression produced increased aggression and enhanced response to psychostimulants in male mice along with increased linear density of dendritic spines on neurons of the dentate gyrus of the hippocampus, and lower levels of endogenous DISC1 and LIS1. Selective prenatal expression was associated with smaller brain volume, whereas postnatal expression gave rise to decreased social behavior in male mice and depression-like responses in female mice as well as enlarged lateral ventricles and decreased DA content in the hippocampus of female mice, and decreased level of endogenous DISC1. Mutant DISC1 affects methamphetamine-induced sensitization and conditioned place preference: a comorbidity model (Pogorelov et al., 2012). The diverse changes in mutant DISC1 mice are reminiscent of findings in major mental diseases.

DISC1 models may be as relevant to bipolar disorder and psychotic depression as to schizophrenia.

MOUSE MODELS OF BIPOLAR DISORDER

The human genetics of bipolar disorder is perhaps less well established compared to that of schizophrenia. However, a number of genes have emerged from GWAS studies (Welcome Trust Case Control Consortium, 2007; Sklar et al., 2008; Craddock and Sklar, 2009; Lichtenstein et al., 2009; Schulze et al., 2009; Green et al., 2010; Curtis et al., 2011; Psychiatric GWAS Consortium Bipolar Disorder Working Group 2011; Sullivan et al 2012), and the hope is that as the power of these studies increases, additional candidate genes will be forthcoming. Furthermore, the increasing sophistication of genetic analyses is making it possible to suggest possible pathways (Pandey et al., 2012), including Wnt signaling circadian rhythm pathways, cadherin signaling pathway, axonal guidance, and neuroactive ligand-receptor interactions.

One of the notable themes emerging from current psychiatric genetics is the overlap between schizophrenia and bipolar disorder as well as the overlap between schizophrenia and autism. We hypothesize that risk for schizophrenia is more related to neurodevelopmental brain changes, whereas risk for bipolar disorder may be more related to neuronal signaling and plasticity.

CACNA1C

Voltage-gated calcium channels have emerged from these studies as strong genetic candidates, with overlap for both schizophrenic and bipolar disorder. There is extensive knowledge of the biology of voltage-gated calcium channels, which will not be repeated in detail here. They are critical for neuronal-membrane-excitability regulated entry of calcium into cells, and are involved in regulation of many signaling pathways and activity related to gene transcription (Bhat et al., 2012). Intriguingly inhibitors of voltage-gated calcium channels have been used in treating bipolar disorder with some mixed success.

Mouse model studies related to voltage-gated calcium channels are just beginning to address issues of behavior related to psychiatric disorders. For instance, voltage-gated calcium channel CACNA1C haploinsufficiency was associated with decreased exploratory behavior, diminished response to amphetamine, and altered behavior in the forced swim and tail suspension tests with sex-specific differences (Dao et al., 2010). These studies though raise the issue of what mouse model is likely to be most appropriate given the human genetics. There is some genetic evidence that the genetic variation at the L-type calcium channel may be a partial gain of function. Thus, mouse models of the disorder may be most appropriately established using transgenic overexpression or other comparable genetic modifications.

ANKYRIN-G

Another very intriguing genetic association in bipolar disorder is with the ANK3 locus, which codes for the ankyrin-G protein. This was found to be the strongest risk factor in one of the initial GWAS studies or is replicated more modestly or variably in subsequent GWAS studies, but has more recently emerged again as a leading candidate gene in population studies.

Ankyrin-G is an especially intriguing candidate as it has well-established roles in maintenance of the structure of the axon initial segment, and in maintenance of axodendritic polarity *in vivo* (Pan et al., 2006; Roussos et al., 2012; Sobotzik et al., 2009;

Zhou et al., 1998). Ankryin-G maintains voltage-gated sodium channels and potassium channels at the axon initial segment, and thus is critical for generation and regulation of the axon potential. It is also critical for axon potential transmission, since it is located at nodes of Ranvier as well. Intriguingly ankyrin-G also appears to be relevant for functional localization of dystrophin complexes (Ayalon et al., 2008), potentially suggesting the relationship between these two risk genes.

The genetic organization of the ankyrin gene locus is complex (Rueckert et al., 2012). Most of the bipolar disorder genetic variation at the ANK3 locus is in the promoter region, suggesting alterations of expression, though it is possible there are also alterations in splicing given the complex splice and promoter usage variation. Thus, for this gene again it is unclear what genetic manipulation may be most relevant to the human disorder; however, partial loss of function would appear to be a good candidate. There has been one knockout mouse model generated in which one of the isoforms has been deleted (Pan et al., 2006; Zhou et al., 1998). This isoform is highly expressed in cerebellum, so the animals have a significant degree of ataxia, making other behavioral tests difficult to interpret. Recent data suggest that these animals may have cognitive and emotional changes as well as motor changes. In addition, they have intriguing alterations in cerebellar circuitry. The loss of ankyrin-G expression in Purkinje cells leads to a redistribution of synaptic input onto Purkinje cells, presumably with profound alterations for neuronal connectivity in signaling. In addition, an ankyrin mouse model with knockout of most isoforms expressed in brain has recently been generated. A conditional knockout enables the deletion of ankyrin-G in the forebrain. Preliminary data suggest that this model may have hyperactivity and alterations in cognitive and emotional behavior consistent with some aspects of human psychiatric disorder.

NEUROCAN

Several studies have found strong associations between the Neurocan (NCAN) gene and bipolar disorder (e.g., Cichon et al., 2011). Neurocan is a component of the extracellular matrix in brain and CNS, expressed at highest levels around birth in the mouse, and may be involved with regulation of synaptic connectivity and plasticity.

A recent study (Miro et al., 2012) combined clinical analyses and mouse behavioral studies. Genotype/phenotype correlations were tested in patients with bipolar disorder, depression, and schizophrenia. Instead of using DSM4 diagnoses, the clinical features were factor-analyzed. In the combined patient sample, the NCAN risk allele was significantly associated with the "mania" factor, in particular "overactivity." A mouse with genetic deletion of neurocan was available (Zhou et al., 2001), and had no gross developmental abnormalities, though altered synaptic transmission and plasticity had been observed. Behavior of the NCAN KO mice was then studied in more detail (Miro et al., 2012). The NCAN KO mice were hyperactive and showed more frequent "risk-taking" behaviors, less "depression-like" conduct, greater amphetamine hypersensitivity, and increased saccharin preference. These behavioral changes were ameliorated by lithium treatment.

DIACYLGLYCEROL KINASE

A locus that has recently been identified in relation to bipolar disorder is the diacylglycerol kinase DGK locus. Behavioral tests using DGK beta knockout mice showed hyperactivity reduced anxiety and reduced "depression"-like behaviors. These behaviors were attenuated by the administration of lithium. These mice also showed impairment in GSK3 beta signaling (Kakefuda et al., 2010). Taken together these data suggest that DGK beta knockout mice have some behavioral abnormalities that could be relevant to human psychiatric disorders, and these mice merit further study.

ODZ4

Recent GWAS studies have identified the ODZ4 or teneurin-4. Relatively little attention has been paid to this gene to date. A mouse mutation designated furue has some behavioral changes and substantial alterations in myelination of small diameter axons and differentiation of oligodendrocytes. Given that white matter changes have been detected in human psychiatric disorders, this model may also merit further study.

OTHER GENES AND PATHWAYS

There is some support for the role of circadian-rhythm-related genes in risk for affective disorder, though perhaps more for depression than bipolar disorder (Kennaway, 2010), and of course sleep and circadian rhythm disturbances are notable in human affective disorder. Several different mouse models of alterations of clock genes have been reported with changes in anxiety, exploratory behavior, activity, and cognitive behavior as well as alterations in circadian periodicity (Arey and McClung, 2012; Keers et al., 2012; Kozikoski et al., 2011; McClung, 2011). Pharmacologic data and some studies of gamma oscillations suggest possible translation to human psychiatric disorder (Dzirasa et al., 2011).

The beta-catenin pathway has recently emerged in genetic studies and also has pharmacologic data to support it. Interestingly, overexpression of beta catenin results in behavioral changes including alterations in the forced swim test and alterations in drug response (Gould et al., 2007).

Other studies have modeled pathways that may be relevant to psychiatric disorders such as the GSK3 beta pathway (Ackermann et al., 2010). Polymorphisms in DISC1 have also been reported to disrupt Wnt and GSK3 beta signaling (Singh et al., 2011).

It has been claimed that a mouse strain termed "Madison" shows behavioral changes reminiscent of mania. Gene expression array changes and drug responses may also be comparable to the human disorder; however, it is unclear if there is any genetic convergence with human genetic risk factors (Saul et al., 2012; Scotti et al., 2011).

As noted above, numerous studies have implicated glutamate signaling, and some studies have suggested that glutamate receptors are relevant for bipolar disorder (Knight et al., 2011). A number of studies of glutamate receptor mouse models have been generated. A detailed consideration of these

studies is beyond the scope of this current chapter, since the genetic correlation is not clear. There is an extensive literature on dopamine transporter knockout mice. These have dramatic hyperactivity and other behavioral changes reminiscent of affective disorder. However, the relationship to the human genetics is still unclear.

FUTURE DEVELOPMENTS

Psychiatric genetics is still in its infancy, with replicable risk loci just beginning to be identified. Functional genomics studies, including better mouse models, will have greater opportunities when mutations with clear effects on gene transcription, splicing, translation, and regulation are identified. Even the knowledge of whether genetic variation leads broadly to loss or gain of function will be helpful, though either can lead to failure of neuronal homeostasis (Ramocki and Zoghbi, 2008). Although the current models have advanced our understanding of the neurobiology of schizophrenia and bipolar disorder, there are still many issues that need to be addressed in the future research.

The methodologies to manipulate the mouse genome at different levels of its organization are constantly improving (see Chapter 8). Simple knockout and transgenic technologies produce artificial systems with the deletion of one or both copies of a gene, or with its overexpression. New models with point mutations in coding sequence or mutations in regulatory elements will better reflect the complex molecular processes implicated in schizophrenia or bipolar disorder (Chen, 2006). The use of zinc finger nucleases and transcription activator-like effector nucleases to manipulate the genome (Cheng et al., 2012) may provide additional options. Inducible and conditional systems allow the alteration to be expressed in a time-dependent and specially controlled fashion.

A drawback of current mouse models is related to the fact that schizophrenia and bipolar disorder are polygenic diseases, and current techniques alter the genome one gene at a time. Combining multiple genetic mutations in a single model could be more informative. Attempts to model neuropsychiatric disorders based on gene expression changes (Lin et al., 2012) may be very difficult to interpret, but targeting several susceptibility genes that belong to different signaling pathways may be a promising direction. Once single gene models are well characterized, it may be possible to perform genetic crosses or other attempts to model polygenic inheritance.

Alternatively it may be possible to make single manipulations at key regulatory positions with pleomorphic effects.

An important aspect of the complex etiology of schizophrenia and bipolar disorder is a contribution of environmental factors (Brown, 2010; van Os et al., 2008). Combining both genetic and environmental risk factors by exposing genetically altered mice to adverse environments at different times across

TABLE 22.1. Behavioral tests used in animal models of schizophrenia (adapted from Nestler and Hyman 2010, used with permission)

TEST	MEASURES	STRENGTHS	WEAKNESSES
Stimulant-induced hyperactivity	Locomotion and stereotypy	Translational potential as can be observed in humans Quantifiable and objectively assessed Easily performed	Acute challenges with drugs do not reflect the pathogenesis Use for testing antipsychotics is based on circularity
Habituation and prepulse inhibition (PPI) of the acoustic startle Latent inhibition	Sensorimotor gating Attention, impulsivity	Translational potential as can be observed in humans Quantifiable and objectively assessed	Weak specificity as PPI and latent inhibition impairment can be observed in several neurological and psychiatric conditions
Social interaction tests relevant to schizophrenia – 3-chamber test – Male-male dyadic interaction in open field – Intruder-resident test – Social approach-avoidance – Social play	Non-aggressive and aggressive species-specific social behaviors, including following, sniffing, crawl-over and crawl-under; attacking, biting, tail-rattling, play activity in juveniles	Easily performed	Face validity is unclear The brain mechanisms may be species-specific (olfaction in mice vs. vision and language in humans) Difficult to automate Not specific to schizophrenia
Progressive ratio schedule procedures to evaluate motivation (avolition?)	Operant tasks to assess relationship between increase in reward and response demands	Translational potential as can be observed in humans Quantifiable and objectively assessed	Not specific to schizophrenia Levels of motivation can vary across animals, while perseveration in response may reflect enhanced impulsivity Require substantial expertise
Cognitive paradigms	Various measures of attention, different types of learning and memory	Several validated tests Can be measured objectively Strong translational potential	Time consuming Easily influenced by environmental conditions Requires substantial behavioral expertise

TABLE 22.2. Behavioral tests used in animal models of mood disorders (Adapted from Nestler and Hyman 2010, used with permission)

TEST	MEASURES	STRENGTHS	WEAKNESSES
Behavioral "despair" – Forced swim – Tail suspension – Learned helplessness	Antidepressant effects	Easily performed	Unclear relation to depressive states Sensitive to a limited set of antidepressants
Anhedonia – Sucrose preference – Sexual behavior	Preference for positive (i.e., pleasurable) stimuli	Face validity Can be objectively measured Do not require sophisticated equipment	Not specific to mood disorders Time consuming
Novelty-suppressed feeding	Latency to feeding and time of food consumption in open field	Easily performed Objective assessment Sensitivity to chronic antidepressant administration	Can be associated with anxiety rather than depression
Social defeat paradigm	Long-term inhibition of social interaction	Objective assessment Sensitivity to chronic antidepressant administration	Can be associated with anxiety as well Time consuming
Maternal deprivation	Stress calls by pups (ultrasonic vocalization)	Objective assessment Easily performed	Not specific to mood disorders Easily influenced changes in test conditions
Elevated plus maze	Risk-taking behavior measures such as forward stretches, head down turns	Easily performed	Require some experience to detect these behaviors Also associated with anxiety
Sleep deprivation-induced behavioral changes	Home cage activity Weight monitoring Eating and drinking monitoring	Easily performed Objective	Require home cage activity monitoring equipment Time consuming Difficult to control the individual effects of deprivation

the life span of the mouse could better reflect the complexity of the pathogenesis of these diseases. Although still in infancy, the initial gene-environment interaction studies have already revealed some issues important for future research. For example, combining an environmental challenge with a genetic mutation in the susceptibility gene can produce both protective and pathogenic effects, depending on the type of adverse environment and the time of interaction. Combinations of genetic and environmental factors can also result in new phenotypes previously unseen in unchallenged mutant mice or wild-type mice exposed the environmental insult (Abazyan et al., 2010; Behan et al., 2012; O'Tuathaigh et al., 2010). Given that simple laboratory environmental changes could be responsible for appreciable variations in the mouse behavior (Crabbe et al., 1999), one needs to be extremely cautious in interpretations of the changes produced in genetic mouse models due to environmental factors.

Behavior readouts have limitations (see Tables 22.1 and 22.2 and Box 22.1). Many of the behavioral tests currently in use were developed for pharmacological studies. As new genetic and environmental models are developed, there should be an iterative process of developing and refining behavioral tests. Brain imaging, electrophysiology, or other endophenotypes are likely to provide additional information, which may be more translatable to the human diseases.

Most studies to date have focused on neuronal functions of susceptibility genes. However, many of the candidate genes are also expressed by glial cells (Iijima et al., 2009). Manipulation of expression in non-neuronal cells may be important. For example, a recent study has provided the first evidence for interaction between DISC1 and serine racemase in astrocytes, connecting DISC1 and D-serine/NMDA receptor hypofunction (Ma, 2012).

Thus, genetic mouse models will continue to be important tools for psychiatric research. They have been illuminating the functions of candidate genes in neurodevelopment and are stimulating a search for future pathogenic treatments. The approach of using factor analysis of human clinical phenotypic features, association with genetic risk loci, and then in turn correlating with phenotypes of mice with alterations at the same loci (e.g., Miro et al., 2012) is intriguing. More sophisticated and advanced genetic manipulations in combination with better understanding of the human clinical phenotypes will be needed to refine the present models to make them more relevant to human psychiatric diseases.

DISCLOSURES

Dr. Pletnikov has no conflicts of interest to disclose. He is funded by NIH only. Grant Support: NIH (P50MH084018 and 5R01MH083728–04).

Dr. Ross has no conflicts of interest to disclose.

We propose the following considerations for future animal models of schizophrenia and bipolar disorder:

CONSTRUCT VALIDITY

- Construct validity based on human genetic studies
  - Manipulation at a locus identified in human population genetic (e.g., GWAS or sequencing) studies
  - Manipulation using a specific causative point or deletion mutation
  - Copy number variation models
- Construct validity based on human environmental studies
  - Human environmental stressors such as prenatal immune activation
- Construct validity based on interaction of genetic and environmental factors

FACE VALIDITY

- Behavioral features
  - For schizophrenia
    - Behavioral and social changes (social withdrawal, anhedonia)
    - Cognitive deficits (working memory)
  - For affective disorder
    - Mania-like alterations, such as hyperactivity and hypersexuality, risk-taking behavior, and impulsivity
    - Depression-like behaviors
    - Altered circadian rhythms, sleep disorders
- Endophenotypes
  - Structural brain change including lateral ventricle enlargement
  - Functional and chemical brain changes (e.g., fMRI, micro-PET, MRS)
  - Electrophysiological changes such as reduced N100, mismatch negativity (MMN), changed theta and gamma oscillation
  - Histological changes such as
    - Interneuron and synaptic pathology
    - Abnormal neurogenesis
    - Molecular and cell signaling changes

PHARMACOLOGICAL VALIDITY FOR EXISTING MEDICATIONS

- Antipsychotics for schizophrenia models
- Lithium and valproate for bipolar models
- Antidepressant for depression models

PREDICTION OF NEW FEATURES THAT ARE SUBSEQUENTLY VALIDATED IN HUMAN

- Novel endophenotypes
- Novel neuropathology
- Novel pharmacological targets

REFERENCES

Abazyan, B., Nomura, J., et al. (2010). Prenatal interaction of mutant DISC1 and immune activation produces adult psychopathology. *Biol. Psychiatry*, 68(12):1172–1181.

Ackermann, T.F., Kempe, D.S., et al. (2010). Hyperactivity and enhanced curiosity of mice expressing PKB/SGK-resistant glycogen synthase kinase-3 (GSK-3). *Cell. Physiol. Biochem.* 25(6):775–786.

Arey, R., and McClung, C.A. (2012). An inhibitor of casein kinase 1ε/δ partially normalizes the manic-like behaviors of the ClockΔ19 mouse. *Behav. Pharmacol.* 23(4):392–396.

Ayalon, G., Davis, J.Q., et al. (2008). An ankyrin-based mechanism for functional organization of dystrophin and dystroglycan. *Cell* 135:1189–1200.

Behan, A.T., Hryniewiecka, M., et al. (2012). Chronic adolescent exposure to delta-9-tetrahydrocannabinol in COMT mutant mice: impact on indices of dopaminergic, endocannabinoid and GABAergic pathways. *Neuropsychopharmacology* 37(7):1773–1783.

Benson, M.A., Newey, S.E., et al. (2001). Dysbindin, a novel coiled-coil-containing protein that interacts with the dystrobrevins in muscle and brain. *J. Biol. Chem.* 276(26):24232–24241.

Bergen, S.E., and Petryshen, T.L. (2012). Genome-wide association studies of schizophrenia: does bigger lead to better results? *Curr Opin Psychiatry*, 25(2):76–82.

Berggren, U., Tallstedt, L., et al. (1978). The effect of lithium on amphetamine-induced locomotor stimulation. *Psychopharmacol. (Berl.).* 59:41–45.

Bhat, S., Dao, D.T., et al. (2012). CACNA1C (Ca(v)1.2) in the pathophysiology of psychiatric disease. *Prog. Neurobiol.* 99 (1):1–14.

Brown, A.S., and Derkits, E.J. (2010). Prenatal infection and schizophrenia: a review of epidemiologic and translational studies. *Am J. Psychiatry* 167(3):261–280.

Brzózka, M.M., Radyushkin, K., et al. (2010). Cognitive and sensorimotor gating impairments in transgenic mice overexpressing the schizophrenia susceptibility gene Tcf4 in the brain. *Biol. Psychiatry* 68(1):33–40.

Callicott, J.H., Straub, R.E., et al. (2005). Variation in DISC1 affects hippocampal structure and function and increases risk for schizophrenia. *Proc. Natl. Acad. Sci. USA* 102(24):8627–8632.

Camargo, L.M., Collura, V., et al. (2007). Disrupted in Schizophrenia 1 Interactome: evidence for the close connectivity of risk genes and a potential synaptic basis for schizophrenia. *Mol. Psychiatry* 12(1):74–86.

Cannon, T.D., Hennah, W., et al. (2005). Association of DISC1/TRAX haplotypes with schizophrenia, reduced prefrontal gray matter, and impaired short- and long-term memory. *Arch. Gen. Psychiatry* 62(11):1205–1213.

Carlson, G.C., Talbot, K., et al. (2011). Dysbindin-1 mutant mice implicate reduced fast-phasic inhibition as a final common disease mechanism in schizophrenia. *Proc. Natl. Acad. Sci. USA* 108(43):E962–E970.

Chen, Y.-J.J., Johnson, M.A., et al. (2008). Type III neuregulin-1 is required for normal sensorimotor gating, memory-related behaviors, and corticostriatal circuit components. *J. Neuroscience*, 28(27):6872–6883.

Chen, J., Lipska, B.K., et al. (2006). Genetic mouse models of schizophrenia: from hypothesis-based to susceptibility gene-based models. *Biol. Psychiatry* 59(12):1180–1188.

Cheng, L.T., Sun, L.T., et al. (2012). Genome editing in induced pluripotent stem cells. *Genes Cells* 17(6):431–438. Epub 2012 Apr 4. Review. PubMed PMID: 22487259.

Chong, V.Z., Thompson, M., et al. (2008). Elevated neuregulin-1 and ErbB4 protein in the prefrontal cortex of schizophrenic patients. *Schizophr. Res.* 100(1–3):270–280.

Chubb, J.E., Bradshaw, N.J., et al. (2008). The DISC locus in psychiatric illness. *Mol. Psychiatry* 13(1):36–64.

Cichon, S., Mühleisen, T.W., et al. (2011). Genome-wide association study identifies genetic variation in neurocan as a susceptibility factor for bipolar disorder. *Am. J. Hum. Genet.* 88(3):372–381.

Clapcote, S.J., Lipina, T.V., et al. (2007). Behavioral phenotypes of Disc1 missense mutations in mice. *Neuron* 54(3):387–402.

Collins, A.L., Kim, Y., et al.; International Schizophrenia Consortium. (2012). Hypothesis-driven candidate genes for schizophrenia compared to genome-wide association results. *Psychol. Med.* 42(3):607–616.

Corriveau, R.A., Huh, G.S., et al. (1998). Regulation of class I MHC gene expression in the developing and mature CNS by neural activity. *Neuron* 21(3):505–520.

Crabbe, J.C., Wahlsten, D., et al. (1999). Genetics of mouse behavior: interactions with laboratory environment. *Science*, 284(5420):1670–1672.

Craddock, N., and Sklar, P. (2009). Genetics of bipolar disorder: successful start to a long journey. *Trends Genet.* 25(2):99–105.

Crook, Z.R., and Housman, D. (2011). Huntington's disease: can mice lead the way to treatment? *Neuron*, 69(3):423–435. Review. Erratum in: *Neuron* 69(5):1038. PubMed PMID: 21315254.

Cryan, J.F., and Slattery, D.A. (2007). Animal models of mood disorders: recent developments. *Curr. Opin. Psychiatry* 20(1):1–7.

Curtis, D., Vine, A.E., et al. (2011). Case-case genome-wide association analysis shows markers differentially associated with schizophrenia and bipolar disorder and implicates calcium channel genes. *Psychiatr. Genet.* 21(1):1–4.

Dao, D.T., Mahon, P.B., et al. (2010). Mood disorder susceptibility gene CACNA1C modifies mood-related behaviors in mice and interacts with sex to influence behavior in mice and diagnosis in humans. *Biol. Psychiatry* 68(9):801–810.

Davies, J. A., Jackson, B., et al. (1974). The effect of amantadine, L-dopa, (plus)-amphetamine and apomorphine on the acquisition of the conditioned avoidance response. *Neuropharmacol.* 13:199–204.

Drew, L.J., Stark, K.L., et al. (2011). Evidence for altered hippocampal function in a mouse model of the human 22q11.2 microdeletion. *Mol. Cell Neurosci.* 47:293–305.

Duffy, L., Cappas, E., et al. (2008). Behavioral profile of a heterozygous mutant mouse model for EGF-like domain neuregulin 1. *Behav. Neurosci.* 122(4):748–759.

Dzirasa, K., McGarity, D.L., et al. (2011). Impaired limbic gamma oscillatory synchrony during anxiety-related behavior in a genetic mouse model of bipolar mania. *J. Neurosci.* 31(17):6449–6456.

Einat, H. (2006). Modelling facets of mania–new directions related to the notion of endophenotypes. *J. Psychopharmacol.* 20:714–722.

Ekelund, J., Hovatta, I., et al. (2001). Chromosome 1 loci in Finnish schizophrenia families. *Hum. Mol. Genet.* 10(15):1611–1617.

Elenbroek, B., and Cools, A.R. (1995). Animal models of psychotic disturbances. In: J.A., Den Boer, H.G.M., Westenberg, and H.M., van Praag, eds. Advances in the Neurobiology of Schizophrenia. New York: Wiley, pp. 89–109.

Feng, Y.-Q., Zhou, Z.-Y., et al. (2008). Dysbindin deficiency in sandy mice causes reduction of snapin and displays behaviors related to schizophrenia. *Schizophr. Res.*, 106(2–3):218–228.

Gerlai, R., Pisacane, P., et al. (2000). Heregulin, but not ErbB2 or ErbB3, heterozygous mutant mice exhibit hyperactivity in multiple behavioral tasks. *Behav. Brain Res.* 109(2):219–227. Retrieved from http://www.ncbi.nlm.nih.gov/pubmed/10762692

Goes F.S., Sanders L.L., Potash J.B. The genetics of psychotic bipolar disorder. *Curr Psychiatry Rep.* 2008 Apr;10(2):178–89.

Gogos, J.A., Santha, M., et al. (1999). The gene encoding proline dehydrogenase modulates sensorimotor gating in mice. *Nat. Genet.* 21(4):434–439.

Golub, M.S., Germann, S.L., et al. (2004). Behavioral characteristics of a nervous system-specific erbB4 knock-out mouse *Behav. Brain Res.* 153(1):159–170.

Gould, T.D., and Einat, H. (2007). Animal models of bipolar disorder and mood stabilizer efficacy: a critical need for improvement. *Neurosci. Biobehav. Rev.* 31(6):825–831.

Gould, T.D., Einat, H., et al. (2007). Beta-catenin overexpression in the mouse brain phenocopies lithium-sensitive behaviors. *Neuropsychopharmacology* 32(10):2173–2183.

Gould, T.J., Keith, R.A., et al. (2001). Differential sensitivity to lithium's reversal of amphetamine-induced open-field activity in two inbred strains of mice. *Behav. Brain Res.* 118:95–105.

Green, E.K., Grozeva, D., et al. (2010). The bipolar disorder risk allele at CACNA1C also confers risk of recurrent major depression and of schizophrenia. *Mol. Psychiatry* 15(10):1016–1022.

Green, E.K., Hamshere, M., et al. (2012). Replication of bipolar disorder susceptibility alleles and identification of two novel genome-wide significant associations in a new bipolar disorder case-control sample. *Mol. Psychiatry.*

Harrison, P.J. (1999). The neuropathology of schizophrenia. A critical review of the data and their interpretation. *Brain* 122(Pt 4):593–624.

Harrison, P.J., and Weinberger, D.R. (2005). Schizophrenia genes, gene expression, and neuropathology: on the matter of their convergence. *Mol. Psychiatry* 10(1):40–68; image 5.

Harrison, P.J, and Law, A.J. (2006). Neuregulin 1 and schizophrenia: genetics, gene expression, and neurobiology. *Biol. Psychiatry* 60(2):132–140.

Hashimoto, R., Straub, R.E., et al. (2004). Expression analysis of neuregulin-1 in the dorsolateral prefrontal cortex in schizophrenia. *Mol. Psychiatry* 9(3):299–307.

Hennah, W., Thomson, P., et al. (2009). DISC1 association, heterogeneity and interplay in schizophrenia and bipolar disorder. *Mol. Psychiatry* 14(9):865–873.

Hennah, W., Tuulio-Henriksson, A., et al. (2005). A haplotype within the DISC1 gene is associated with visual memory functions in families with a high density of schizophrenia. *Mol. Psychiatry* 10(12):1097–1103.

Hikida, T., Jaaro-Peled, H., et al. (2007). Dominant-negative DISC1 transgenic mice display schizophrenia-associated phenotypes detected by measures translatable to humans. *Proc. Natl. Acad. Sci. USA* 104(36):14501–14506.

Huh, G.S., Boulanger, L.M., et al. (2000). Functional requirement for class I MHC in CNS development and plasticity. *Science* 290(5499):2155–2159.

Hurst, J.L. (2009). Female recognition and assessment of males through scent. *Behav. Brain Res.* 200(2):295–303.

Iijima, S., Masaki, H., et al. (2009). Immunohistochemical detection of dysbindin at the astroglial endfeet around the capillaries of mouse brain. *J. Mol. Histol.* 40(2):117–121.

Iizuka, Y., Sei, Y., et al. (2007). Evidence that the BLOC-1 protein dysbindin modulates dopamine D2 receptor internalization and signaling but not D1 internalization. *J. Neurosci.* 27(45):12390–12395.

Insel, T.R. (2010). Rethinking schizophrenia. *Nature* 468(7321):187–193.

Jaaro-Peled, H., Ayhan, Y., et al. (2010). Review of pathological hallmarks of schizophrenia: comparison of genetic models with patients and nongenetic models. *Schizophr. Bull.* 36(2):301–313.

Jentsch, J.D., Trantham-Davidson, H., et al. (2009). Dysbindin modulates prefrontal cortical glutamatergic circuits and working memory function in mice. *Neuropsychopharmacol.* 34(12):2601–2608.

Kakefuda, K.H., Oyagi, A., et al. (2010). Diacylglycerol kinase β knockout mice exhibit lithium-sensitive behavioral abnormalities. *PLoS One* 5(10):e13447.

Kalynchuk, L.E. (2000). Long-term amygdala kindling in rats as a model for the study of interictal emotionality in temporal lobe epilepsy. *Neurosci. Biobehav. Rev.* 24:691–704.

Kamiya, A., Kubo, K., et al. (2005). A schizophrenia-associated mutation of DISC1 perturbs cerebral cortex development. *Nat. Cell Biol.* 7(12):1167–1178.

Kamiya, A., Sedlak, T.W., et al. (2012). DISC1 Pathway in brain development: exploring therapeutic targets for major psychiatric disorders. *Front. Psychiatry* 3:25.

Karayiorgou, M., Simon, T.J., et al. (2010). 22q11.2 microdeletions: linking DNA structural variation to brain dysfunction and schizophrenia. *Nat. Rev. Neurosci.* 11(6):402–416.

Karl, T., Duffy, L., et al. (2007). Altered motor activity, exploration and anxiety in heterozygous neuregulin 1 mutant mice: implications for understanding schizophrenia. *Genes Brain Behav.* 6(7):677–687.

Karlsgodt, K.H., Robleto, K., et al. (2011). Reduced dysbindin expression mediates N-methyl-D-aspartate receptor hypofunction and impaired working memory performance. *Biol. Psychiatry* 69(1):28–34.

Kato, T., Kasai, A., et al. (2010). Phenotypic characterization of transgenic mice overexpressing neuregulin-1. *PloS One* 5(12):e14185.

Kato, T., Kubota, M., et al. (2007). Animal models of bipolar disorder. *Neurosci. Biobehav. Rev.* 31(6):832–842.

Keers, R., Pedroso, I., et al. (2012). Reduced anxiety and depression-like behaviours in the circadian period mutant mouse afterhours. *PLoS One* 7(6):e38263.

Kennaway, D.J. (2010). Clock genes at the heart of depression. *J. Psychopharmacol.* 24(2):5–14.

Knight, H.M., Walker, R., et al. (2011). GRIK4/KA1 protein expression in human brain and correlation with bipolar disorder risk variant status. *Am. J. Med. Genet. B Neuropsychiatr. Genet.* 159B(1):21–29.

Koike, H., Arguello, P.A., et al. (2006). Disc1 is mutated in the 129S6/SvEv strain and modulates working memory in mice. *Proc. Natl. Acad. Sci. USA* 103(10):3693–3697.

Kozikowski, A.P., Gunosewoyo, H., et al. (2011). Identification of a glycogen synthase kinase-3β inhibitor that attenuates hyperactivity in CLOCK mutant mice. *Chem. Med. Chem.* 6(9):1593–1602.

Kuroda, K., Yamada, S., et al. (2011). Behavioral alterations associated with targeted disruption of exons 2 and 3 of the Disc1 gene in the mouse. *Hum. Mol. Genet.* 20(23):4666–4683.

Kvajo, M., McKellar, H., et al. (2008). A mutation in mouse Disc1 that models a schizophrenia risk allele leads to specific alterations in neuronal architecture and cognition. *Proc. Natl. Acad. Sci. USA* 105(19):7076–7081.

Kvajo, M., McKellar, H., et al. (2011). Altered axonal targeting and short-term plasticity in the hippocampus of Disc1 mutant mice. *Proc. Natl. Acad. Sci. USA* 108(49):E1349–E1358.

Law, A.J., Lipska, B.K., et al. (2006). Neuregulin 1 transcripts are differentially expressed in schizophrenia and regulated by 5' SNPs associated with the disease. *Proc. Natl. Acad. Sci. USA* 103(17):6747–6752.

Lee, F.H.F., Fadel, M.P., et al. (2011). Disc1 point mutations in mice affect development of the cerebral cortex. *J. Neurosci.* 31(9):3197–3206.

Lee, K.W., Woon, P.S., et al. (2012). Genome wide association studies (GWAS) and copy number variation (CNV) studies of the major psychoses: what have we learnt? *Neurosci. Biobehav. Rev.* 36(1):556–571.

Leussis, M.P, Berry-Scott, E.M., et al. (2012). The ANK3 bipolar disorder gene regulates psychiatric-related behaviors that are modulated by lithium and stress. *Biol. Psychiatry*.

Leussis, M.P., Madison, J.M., et al. (2012). Ankyrin 3: genetic association with bipolar disorder and relevance to disease pathophysiology. *Biol. Mood Anxiety Disord*. 2(1):18.

Lewis, D.A., and Sweet, R.A. (2009). Schizophrenia from a neural circuitry perspective: advancing toward rational pharmacological therapies. *J. Clin. Invest*. 119(4):706–716. Epub 2009 Apr 1. Review. PubMed PMID: 19339762; PubMed Central PMCID: PMC2662560.

Li, W., Zhang, Q., et al. (2003). Hermansky-Pudlak syndrome type 7 (HPS-7) results from mutant dysbindin, a member of the biogenesis of lysosome-related organelles complex 1 (BLOC-1). *Nat. Genet*. 35(1):84–89.

Li, W., Zhou, Y., et al. (2007). Specific developmental disruption of Disrupted-in-Schizophrenia-1 function results in schizophrenia-related phenotypes in mice. *Proc. Natl. Acad. Sci. USA* 104(46):18280–18285.

Li, T., Ma, X., et al. (2008). PRODH gene is associated with executive function in schizophrenic families. *Am. J. Med. Genet. B Neuropsychiatr. Genet*. 147B, 654–657.

Lichtenstein, P., Yip, B.H., et al. (2009). Common genetic determinants of schizophrenia and bipolar disorder in Swedish families: a population-based study. *Lancet* 373(9659):234–239.

Lim, S. M., Kim, et al. (2009). Association study of DISC1 in Korean population with autism spectrum disorders. *Psychiatric Genet*. 19(3):160.

Lin, C.Y., Sawa, A., et al. (2012). Better understanding of mechanisms of schizophrenia and bipolar disorder: from human gene expression profiles to mouse models. *Neurobiol. Dis*. 45(1):48–56.

Lipina, T.V., Wang, M., et al. (2012). Synergistic interactions between PDE4B and GSK-3: DISC1 mutant mice. *Neuropharmacol*. 62(3):1252–1262.

Lipska, B.K., and Weinberger, D.R. (1993). Delayed effects of neonatal hippocampal damage on haloperidol-induced catalepsy and apomorphine-induced stereotypic behaviors in the rat. *Brain Res. Dev. Brain Res*. 75(2):213–222.

Lipska, B.K., and Weinberger, D.R. (1995). Genetic variation in vulnerability to the behavioral effects of neonatal hippocampal damage in rats. *Proc. Natl. Acad. Sci. USA* 92(19):8906–8910.

Lu, L., Mamiya, T., et al. (2011). Genetic animal models of schizophrenia related with the hypothesis of abnormal neurodevelopment. *Biol. Pharm. Bull*. 34(9):1358–1363.

Lutkenhoff, E., Karlsgodt, K.H., et al. (2012). Structural and functional neuroimaging phenotypes in dysbindin mutant mice. *NeuroImage* 62(1):120–129.

Ma, T.M., Abazyan, S., et al. (2012). Pathogenic disruption of DISC1-serine racemase binding elicits schizophrenia-like behavior via D-serine depletion. *Mol. Psychiatry*.

Mackie, S., Millar, J.K., et al. (2007). Role of DISC1 in neural development and schizophrenia. *Curr. Opin. Neurobiol*. 17(1):95–102.

Malhotra, D, and Sebat, J. (2012). CNVs: harbingers of a rare variant revolution in psychiatric genetics. *Cell* 148(6):1223–1241.

Mao, Y., Ge, X., et al. (2009). Disrupted in schizophrenia 1 regulates neuronal progenitor proliferation via modulation of GSK3beta/beta-catenin signaling. *Cell* 136(6):1017–1031.

Matthysse, S. (1986). Animal models in psychiatric research. *Prog. Brain Res*. 5:1–25.

McConnell, M.J., Huang, Y.H., et al. (2009). H2-K(b) and H2-D(b) regulate cerebellar long-term depression and limit motor learning. *Proc. Natl. Acad. Sci. USA* 106(16):6784–6789.

McClung, C.A. (2011). Circadian rhythms and mood regulation: insights from pre-clinical models. *Eur. Neuropsychopharmacol*. 21(4):S683–S693.

Mei, L., and Xiong, W.-C. (2008). Neuregulin 1 in neural development, synaptic plasticity and schizophrenia. *Nat. Rev. Neurosci*. 9(6):437–452.

Merscher, S., Funke, B., et al. (2001). TBX1 is responsible for cardiovascular defects in velo-cardio-facial/DiGeorge syndrome. *Cell* 104(4):619–629.

Meyer, D., and Birchmeier, C. (1995). Multiple essential functions of neuregulin in development. *Nature* 378(6555):386–390.

Millar, J.K., Christie, S., et al. (2001). Genomic structure and localisation within a linkage hotspot of Disrupted In Schizophrenia 1, a gene disrupted by a translocation segregating with schizophrenia. *Mol. Psychiatry* 6(2):173–178.

Miró, X., Meier, S., et al. (2012). Studies in humans and mice implicate neurocan in the etiology of mania. *Am J. Psychiatry* 169(9):982–990.

Murphy, K.C., Jones, L.A., et al. (1999). High rates of schizophrenia in adults with velo-cardio-facial syndrome. *Arch. Gen. Psychiatry* 56(10):940–945.

Nagai, T., Kitahara, Y., et al. (2010). Dysfunction of dopamine release in the prefrontal cortex of dysbindin deficient sandy mice: an *in vivo* microdialysis study. *Neurosci. Lett*. 470(2):134–138.

Nazarian, R., Starcevic, M., et al. (2006). Reinvestigation of the dysbindin subunit of BLOC-1 (biogenesis of lysosome-related organelles complex-1) as a dystrobrevin-binding protein. *Biochem. J*. 395(3):587–598.

Nestler, E.J., and Hyman, S.E. (2010). Animal models of neuropsychiatric disorders. *Nat. Neurosci*. 13(10):1161–1169.

Niwa, M., Kamiya, A., et al. (2010). Knockdown of DISC1 by *in utero* gene transfer disturbs postnatal dopaminergic maturation in the frontal cortex and leads to adult behavioral deficits. *Neuron* 65(4):480–489.

Nomura, J., and Takumi, T. (2012). Animal models of psychiatric disorders that reflect human copy number variation. *Neural Plast*. 2012:589524.

Ottis, P., Bader, V., et al. (2011). Convergence of two independent mental disease genes on the protein level: recruitment of dysbindin to cell-invasive Disrupted-in-Schizophrenia 1 aggresomes. *Biol. Psychiatry* 70(7):604–610.

O'Tuathaigh, C.M.P., Babovic, D., et al. (2007). Phenotypic characterization of spatial cognition and social behavior in mice with "knockout" of the schizophrenia risk gene neuregulin 1. *Neurosci*. 147(1):18–27.

O'Tuathaigh, C.M.P., Harte, M., et al. (2010). Schizophrenia-related endophenotypes in heterozygous neuregulin-1 "knockout" mice. *Eur. J. Neurosci*. 31(2):349–358.

O'Tuathaigh, C.M., Hryniewiecka, M., et al. (2010). Chronic adolescent exposure to Δ-9-tetrahydrocannabinol in COMT mutant mice: impact on psychosis-related and other phenotypes. *Neuropsychopharmacology* 35(11):2262–2273.

Pan, Z., Kao, T., et al. (2006). A common ankyrin-G-based mechanism retains KCNQ and Nav channels at electrically active domains of the axon. *J. Neurosci*. 26(10):2599–2613.

Pandey, A., Davis, N.A., et al. (2012). Epistasis network centrality analysis yields pathway replication across two GWAS cohorts for bipolar disorder. *Transl. Psychiatry* 2:e154.

Paterlini, M., Zakharenko, S.S., et al. (2005). Transcriptional and behavioral interaction between 22q11.2 orthologs modulates schizophrenia-related phenotypes in mice. *Nat. Neurosci*. 8(11):1586–1594.

Paylor, R., Glaser, B., et al. (2006). Tbx1 haploinsufficiency is linked to behavioral disorders in mice and humans: implications for 22q11 deletion syndrome. *Proc. Natl. Acad. Sci. USA* 103:7729–7734.

Pletnikov, M.V., Ayhan, Y., et al. (2008). Inducible expression of mutant human DISC1 in mice is associated with brain and behavioral abnormalities reminiscent of schizophrenia. *Mol. Psychiatry* 13(2):173–186:115.

Pogorelov, V.M., Nomura, J., et al. (2012). Mutant DISC1 affects methamphetamine-induced sensitization and conditioned place preference: a comorbidity model. *Neuropharmacol*. 62(3):1242–1251.

Psychiatric GWAS Consortium Bipolar Disorder Working Group. (2011). Large-scale genome-wide association analysis of bipolar disorder identifies a new susceptibility locus near ODZ4. *Nat. Genet*. 43(10):977–983. Erratum in: *Nat. Genet*. 2012 Sep;44(9):1072.

Raux, G., Bumsel, E., et al. (2007). Involvement of hyperprolinemia in cognitive and psychiatric features of the 22q11 deletion syndrome. *Hum. Mol. Genet*. 16:83–91.

Ridley, R., and Baker, H.F. (1982). Stereotypy in monkeys and humans. *Psychol. Med*. 12:61–72.

Rimer, M., Barrett, D.W., et al. (2005). Neuregulin-1 immunoglobulin-like domain mutant mice: clozapine sensitivity and impaired latent inhibition. *Neuroreport* 16(3):271–275.

Ripke, S., Sanders, A.R., et al. Schizophrenia Psychiatric Genome-Wide Association Study (GWAS) Consortium. (2011).Genome-wide association study identifies five new schizophrenia loci. *Nat. Genet*. 43(10):969–976.

Ross, C.A, Margolis, R.L., et al. (2006). Neurobiology of schizophrenia. *Neuron* 52(1):139–153.

Ross, C.A., and Tabrizi, S.J. (2011). Huntington's disease: from molecular pathogenesis to clinical treatment. *Lancet Neurol*. 10(1):83–98.

Roussos, P., Katsel, P., et al. (2012). Molecular and genetic evidence for abnormalities in the nodes of Ranvier in schizophrenia. *Arch. Gen. Psychiatry* 69(1):7–15.

Rueckert, E.H., Barker D., Ruderfer D., Bergen S.E., O'Dushlaine C., Luce C.J., Sheridan S.D., Theriault K.M., Chambert K., Moran J., Purcell S.M., Madison J.M., Haggarty S.J., Sklar P. (2012). Cis-acting regulation of brain-specific ANK3 gene expression by a genetic variant associated with bipolar disorder. *Mol. Psychiatry*. [Epub ahead of print] PubMed PMID: 22850628.

Sankar, A., MacKenzie, R.N. (2012). Loss of class I MHC function alters behavior and stress reactivity. *J. Neuroimmunol*. 244(1–2):8–15.

Sanders, A. R., Duan, J., et al. (2008). No significant association of 14 candidate genes with schizophrenia in a large European ancestry sample: implications for psychiatric genetics. *Am. J. Psychiatry* 165(4):497–506.

Saul, M.C., Gessay, G.M., et al. (2012). A new mouse model for mania shares genetic correlates with human bipolar disorder. *PLoS One* 7(6):e38128.

Schulze, T.G., Detera-Wadleigh, S.D., et al. (2009). Two variants in ankyrin 3 (ANK3) are independent genetic risk factors for bipolar disorder. *Mol. Psychiatry* 14(5):487–491.

Scotti, M.A., Lee, G., et al. (2011). Behavioral and pharmacological assessment of a potential new mouse model for mania. *Physiol. Behav.* 103(3–4):376–383.

Shen, S., Lang, B., et al. (2008). Schizophrenia-related neural and behavioral phenotypes in transgenic mice expressing truncated Disc1. *J. Neurosci.* 28(43):10893–10904.

Shoji, H., Toyama, K., et al. (2012). Comprehensive behavioral analysis of ENU-induced DISC1-Q31L and -L100P mutant mice. *BMC Res. Notes* 5:108.

Silberberg, G., Darvasi, A., et al. (2006). The involvement of ErbB4 with schizophrenia: association and expression studies. *Am. J. Med. Genet. B Neuropsychiatr. Genet.* 141B(2):142–148.

Silverstone, P.H., Pukhovsky, A., et al. (1998). Lithium does not attenuate the effects of D-amphetamine in healthy volunteers. *Psychiatry Res.* 79:219–226.

Singh, K.K., De Rienzo, G., et al. (2011). Common DISC1 polymorphisms disrupt Wnt/GSK3β signaling and brain development. *Neuron* 72(4):545–558.

Sklar, P., Smoller, J.W., et al. (2008). Whole-genome association study of bipolar disorder. *Mol. Psychiatry* 13(6):558–569.

Sobotzik J.M., Sie J.M., Politi C., Del Turco D., Bennett V., Deller T., Schultz C. (2009). AnkyrinG is required to maintain axo-dendritic polarity in vivo. *Proc. Natl. Acad. Sci. U S A.* 106(41):17564–17569. Epub 2009 Sep 24. PubMed PMID: 19805144; PubMed Central PMCID: PMC2765162

Stark, K.L., Xu, B., et al. (2008) Altered brain microRNA biogenesis contributes to phenotypic deficits in a 22q11-deletion mouse model. *Nat. Genet.* 40:751–760.

St Clair, D., Blackwood, D., et al. (1990). Association within a family of a balanced autosomal translocation with major mental illness. *Lancet* 336(8706):13–16.

Stanford, L., and Brown, R.E. (2003). MHC-congenic mice (C57BL/6J and B6-H-2K) show differences in speed but not accuracy in learning the Hebb-Williams Maze. *Behav. Brain Res.* 144(1–2):187–197.

Stefansson, H., Sigurdsson, E., et al. (2002). Neuregulin 1 and susceptibility to schizophrenia. *Am. J. Hum. Genet.* 71(4):877–892.

Straub, R.E., Jiang, Y., et al. (2002). Genetic variation in the 6p22.3 gene DTNBP1, the human ortholog of the mouse dysbindin gene, is associated with schizophrenia. *Am. J. Hum. Genet.* 71(2):337–348.

Sullivan, P.F., Daly, M.J., et al. (2012). Genetic architectures of psychiatric disorders: the emerging picture and its implications. *Nat. Rev. Genet.* 13(8):537–551. Review.

Swerdlow, N.R., Halim, N., et al. (2001). Lesion size and amphetamine hyperlocomotion after neonatal ventral hippocampal lesions: more is less. *Brain Res. Bull.* 55:71–77.

Talbot, K. (2009). The sandy (sdy) mouse: a dysbindin-1 mutant relevant to schizophrenia research. *Prog. Brain Res.* 179:87–94.

Tan, W., Wang, Y., et al. (2007). Molecular cloning of a brain-specific, developmentally regulated neuregulin 1 (NRG1) isoform and identification of a functional promoter variant associated with schizophrenia. *J. Biol. Chem.* 282(33):24343–24351.

Tomiyama, K., O'Tuathaigh, C.M., et al. (2009). Phenotype of spontaneous orofacial dyskinesia in neuregulin-1 'knockout' mice. *Prog. Neuropsychopharmacol. Biol. Psychiatry* 33(2):330–333.

van den Buuse, M., Wischhof, L., et al. (2009). Neuregulin 1 hypomorphic mutant mice: enhanced baseline locomotor activity but normal psychotropic drug-induced hyperlocomotion and prepulse inhibition regulation. *Int. J. Neuropsychopharmacol.* 12(10):1383–1393.

van Os, J., Rutten, B.P., et al. (2008). Gene-environment interactions in schizophrenia: review of epidemiological findings and future directions. *Schizophr. Bull.* 34(6):1066–1082.

Walsh, J., Tighe, O., et al. (2010). Disruption of thermal nociceptive behaviour in mice mutant for the schizophrenia-associated genes NRG1, COMT and DISC1. *Brain Res.* 1348:114–119.

Weickert, C.S., Straub, R.E., et al. (2004). Human dysbindin (DTNBP1) gene expression in normal brain and in schizophrenic prefrontal cortex and midbrain. *Arch. Gen. Psychiatry* 61(6):544–555.

Weickert, C. S., Rothmond, D. A., et al. (2008). Reduced DTNBP1 (dysbindin-1) mRNA in the hippocampal formation of schizophrenia patients. *Schizophr. Res.* 98(1–3):105–110.

Wellcome Trust Case Control Consortium. (2007). Genome-wide association study of 14,000 cases of seven common diseases and 3,000 shared controls. *Nature* 447(7145):661–678.

Wen, L., Lu, Y.-S., et al. (2010). Neuregulin 1 regulates pyramidal neuron activity via ErbB4 in parvalbumin-positive interneurons. *Proc. Natl. Acad. Sci. USA* 107(3):1211–1216.

Wood, L. S., Pickering, E. H., et al. (2007). Significant support for DAO as a schizophrenia susceptibility locus: examination of five genes putatively associated with schizophrenia. *Biol. Psychiatry*, 61(10):1195–1199.

Young, J.W., Henry, B.L., et al. (2011). Predictive animal models of mania: hits, misses and future directions. *Br. J. Pharmacol.* 164(4):1263–1284.

Zhou, D., Lambert, S., et al. (1998). Ankyrin$_G$ is required for clustering of voltage-gated Na channels at axon initial segments and for normal action potential firing. *J. Cell Biol.* 143(5):1295–1304.

Zhou X.H., Brakebusch C., Matthies H., Oohashi T., Hirsch E., Moser M., Krug M., Seidenbecher C.I., Boeckers T.M., Rauch U., Buettner R., Gundelfinger E.D., Fässler R. (2001). Neurocan is dispensable for brain development. *Mol Cell Biol.* 21(17):5970–5978.

23 | CORTICAL GABA NEURONS IN SCHIZOPHRENIA

ALLISON A. CURLEY AND DAVID A. LEWIS

Cognitive impairments are a core feature of schizophrenia and the best predictor of functional outcome; however, current pharmacotherapies offer only limited cognitive improvement. Therefore, knowledge of the abnormalities in brain circuitry that give rise to the cognitive abnormalities is critical for developing new treatments. Higher order cognitive processes, such as working memory, the ability to transiently retain and manipulate a limited amount of information in order to guide thought or behavior, are strongly associated with neural network oscillations, the synchronized firing of large assemblies of cells, that are dependent on signaling via the inhibitory neurotransmitter γ-aminobutyric acid (GABA) (Bartos and Elgueta, 2012). The cells that synthesize and release GABA, appropriately termed GABA neurons (or interneurons), exhibit a variety of abnormalities in schizophrenia. Thus, alterations in GABA neurons are thought to, at least in part, underlie the cognitive deficits of schizophrenia. Consequently, in this chapter we provide: (1) an introduction to interneurons and their role in cognition, (2) a description of the GABAergic alterations found in schizophrenia, (3) a review of potential mechanisms underlying these alterations, and (4) a discussion of the consequences of impaired GABA signaling. The prefrontal cortex (PFC) is a brain area especially critical for cognition, and where interneurons have been most extensively studied in schizophrenia, and thus we concentrate on this region here.

INTRODUCTION TO INTERNEURONS

SUBTYPES OF GABA NEURONS

Excitatory pyramidal cells comprise 75–80% of the neurons in the primate neocortex, and the remaining 20–25% are GABA neurons. In contrast to pyramidal cells that mainly send their axons over long distances, interneurons primarily project locally. GABA neurons in the cerebral cortex can be divided into different subclasses based on their electrophysiological, molecular, and anatomical properties (Ascoli et al., 2008) (Fig. 23.1). Electrophysiologically, interneurons are classified as fast-spiking (FS) or non-fast-spiking (non-FS), based on their firing patterns in response to depolarization above spiking threshold. FS cells exhibit a nearly constant interval between spikes. In contrast, non-FS cells typically show an adapting firing pattern, such that the interspike interval increases with stimulus duration. Interneuron subpopulations can also be distinguished by the molecular markers they express. With a few exceptions, the calcium binding proteins parvalbumin (PV),

calbindin (CB), and calretinin (CR) are found in distinct cell types. FS cells contain PV (hereafter referred to as PV neurons), do not contain any neuropeptides, and give rise to axons that target the perisomatic region, the cell body and proximal dendrites, of pyramidal cells. PV neurons comprise ~25% GABA neurons in the primate PFC (but a much larger proportion of GABA neurons in rodent cortex), and PV-positive cell bodies and axon terminals are present in the highest density in layers deep 3–4. PV cells are divided into two main classes: (1) basket (PV_b) cells, whose axons target the soma, proximal dendrites, and spines of pyramidal cells, and (2) chandelier (PV_ch) cells, whose axon terminals form distinctive vertical arrays termed cartridges that exclusively target the axon initial segment (AIS) of pyramidal cells.

Non-FS cells are more heterogeneous and include a number of distinct subpopulations (Fig. 23.1). One subpopulation contains the neuropeptide cholecystokinin (CCK). A subset of these cells also contains CR, and a separate subset expresses the cannabinoid 1 receptor (CB1R). The latter are known as CCK basket (CCK_b) cells. All CCK_b cells target the perisomatic region of pyramidal cells, and in the primate neocortex, CCK-immunoreactive cell bodies are principally localized to layers 2-superficial 3, and their axon terminals are present mainly in layers 2, 4, and 6. A second subtype of non-FS cells expresses CB and the neuropeptide somatostatin (SST), and furnishes axons that synapse onto the distal dendrites of pyramidal cells. SST cells are present in all layers of the cortex, as well as the underlying white matter. A third subtype contains CR, is found primarily in layers 1 and 2, and provides axon terminals that mainly innervate pyramidal neuron dendrites and other interneurons.

GABA SYNTHESIS

GABA is synthesized by the 67 kiloDalton and 65 kiloDalton isoforms of glutamic acid decarboxylase (GAD67 and GAD65, respectively) which decarboxylate glutamate to produce GABA (Fig. 23.2). GAD65 and GAD67 are encoded by separate genes (GAD1 and GAD2, respectively) on different chromosomes, and undergo different posttranslational modifications (Akbarian and Huang, 2006). Many, but not all, GABA neurons appear to contain both isoforms. GAD67 is distributed throughout the neuron, whereas GAD65 is primarily located in axon terminals. The activity of both enzymes is regulated by their cofactor pyridoxal 5'-phosphate, which activates or inactivates the enzyme when it is bound and released, respectively. GAD67 is saturated with cofactor and therefore largely exists in the active form, while

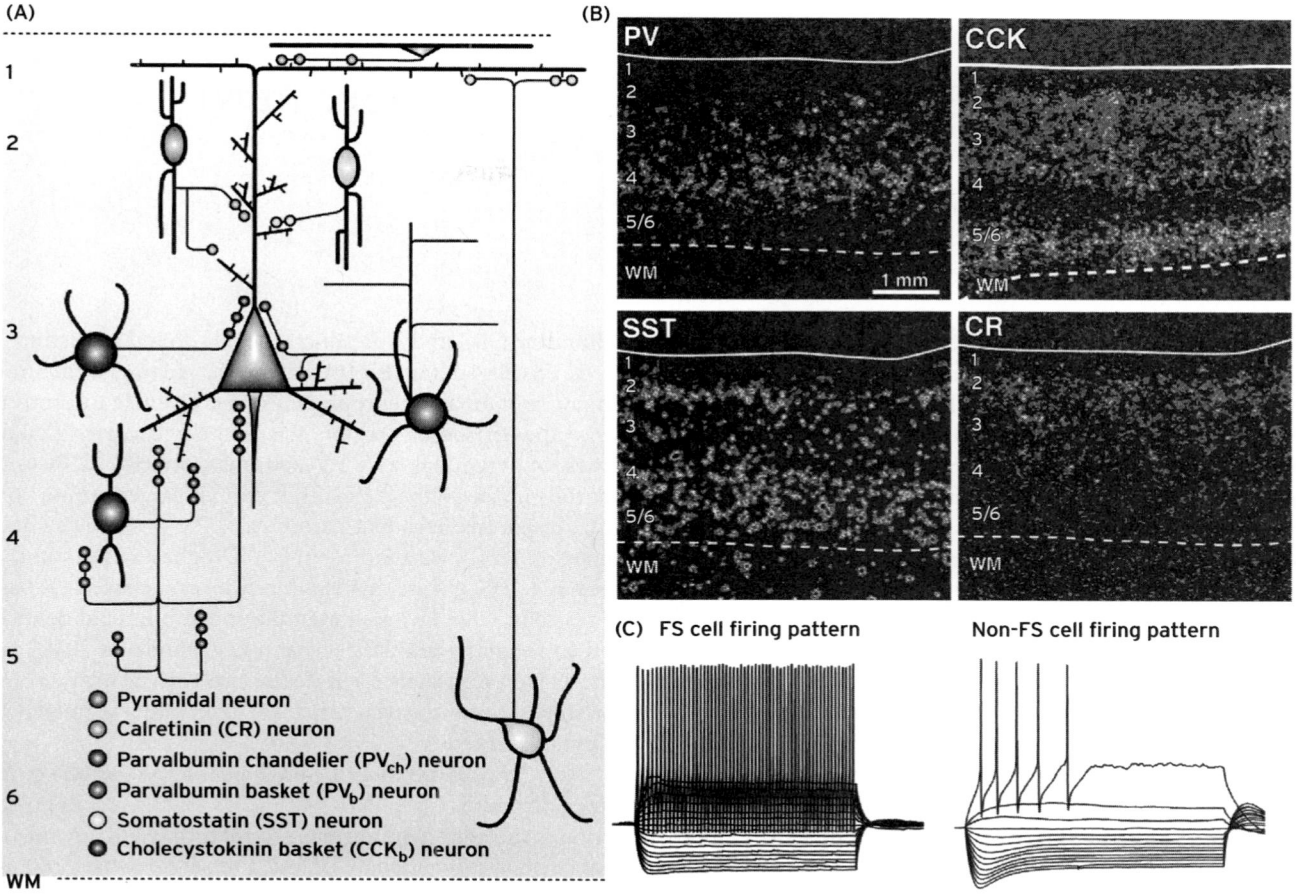

(A)

1
2
3
4
5
6

WM

○ Pyramidal neuron
○ Calretinin (CR) neuron
○ Parvalbumin chandelier (PV$_{ch}$) neuron
○ Parvalbumin basket (PV$_b$) neuron
○ Somatostatin (SST) neuron
○ Cholecystokinin basket (CCK$_b$) neuron

(B)

PV | CCK
SST | CR

1 mm

(C) FS cell firing pattern | **Non-FS cell firing pattern**

Figure 23.1 *Diversity of cortical GABA neurons. GABAergic interneurons can be classified based on morphological (A), molecular (B), and electrophysiological (C) properties. Some interneurons express the calcium binding proteins parvalbumin (PV) or calretinin (CR), whereas others contain the neuropeptides somatostatin (SST) or cholecystokinin (CCK). (A) PV and CCK neurons target the perisomatic region of pyramidal cells, while SST and CR neurons target pyramidal neuron dendrites. PV neurons can be divided into chandelier (PV$_{ch}$) and basket (PV$_b$) cells based on their morphology. The axon terminals of PV$_{ch}$ cells exclusively target the pyramidal cell axon initial segment, while the terminals of PV$_b$ cells synapse onto the soma and proximal dendrites. (B) The different interneuron subtypes are distributed distinctively across the layers of the cortex, as evidenced by the different expression patterns of their mRNAs. (C) PV cells exhibit a fast spiking (FS) firing pattern, characterized by a high firing frequency and constant interval between action potentials, while the remaining subclasses are classified as non-FS cells that fire at a lower frequency and exhibit progressively increasing intervals between action potentials. (Image adapted from Gonzalez-Burgos et al. Am J Psychiatry (2007) 164 (1):12; and Hashimoto et al. Mol Psychiatry (2008) 13:147–161.) (See color insert.)*

GAD65 is mostly inactive (with low levels of cofactor binding). Thus, the activity of GAD67 is principally regulated by expression and appears to be responsible for the majority of cortical GABA synthesis, producing up to 90% of the GABA in mouse brain. In contrast, GAD65 seems to be mainly active during conditions of high synaptic demand (Patel et al., 2006).

GABA RECEPTORS

Released GABA exerts its effects through binding to the two major types of GABA receptors—GABA$_A$ and GABA$_B$ receptors (Fig. 23.2). The ionotropic GABA$_A$ receptor is composed of 5 subunits that form a central ion pore, with the most common composition being two α, two β, and one γ subunit. The subunit composition of GABA$_A$ receptors determines important functional and pharmacological properties, such as the kinetics of the postsynaptic signal decay (Gonzalez-Burgos et al., 2011). Activation of these receptors results in an increased chloride conductance, with the direction of ion flow being

determined by the intracellular chloride concentration resulting from the activity of the chloride transporters NKCC1 and KCC2, that bring chloride into and out of the cell, respectively. In the majority of cases, chloride flows inward through GABA$_A$ receptors and hyperpolarizes the membrane, producing the classic inhibitory postsynaptic response (Fig. 23.2).

GABA$_B$ receptors form heterodimers, each composed of a GABA$_{B1}$ and GABA$_{B2}$ subunit, and both subunits are required to produce a functional receptor. Activation of metabotropic GABA$_B$ receptors stimulates the opening of potassium channels and closing of calcium channels via G proteins, resulting in hyperpolarization. GABA$_B$ receptors are located both pre- and postsynaptically.

ROLE OF GABA NEURONS IN NETWORK OSCILLATIONS AND COGNITION

A single interneuron not only makes multiple contacts onto a pyramidal cell, but also contacts many different pyramidal

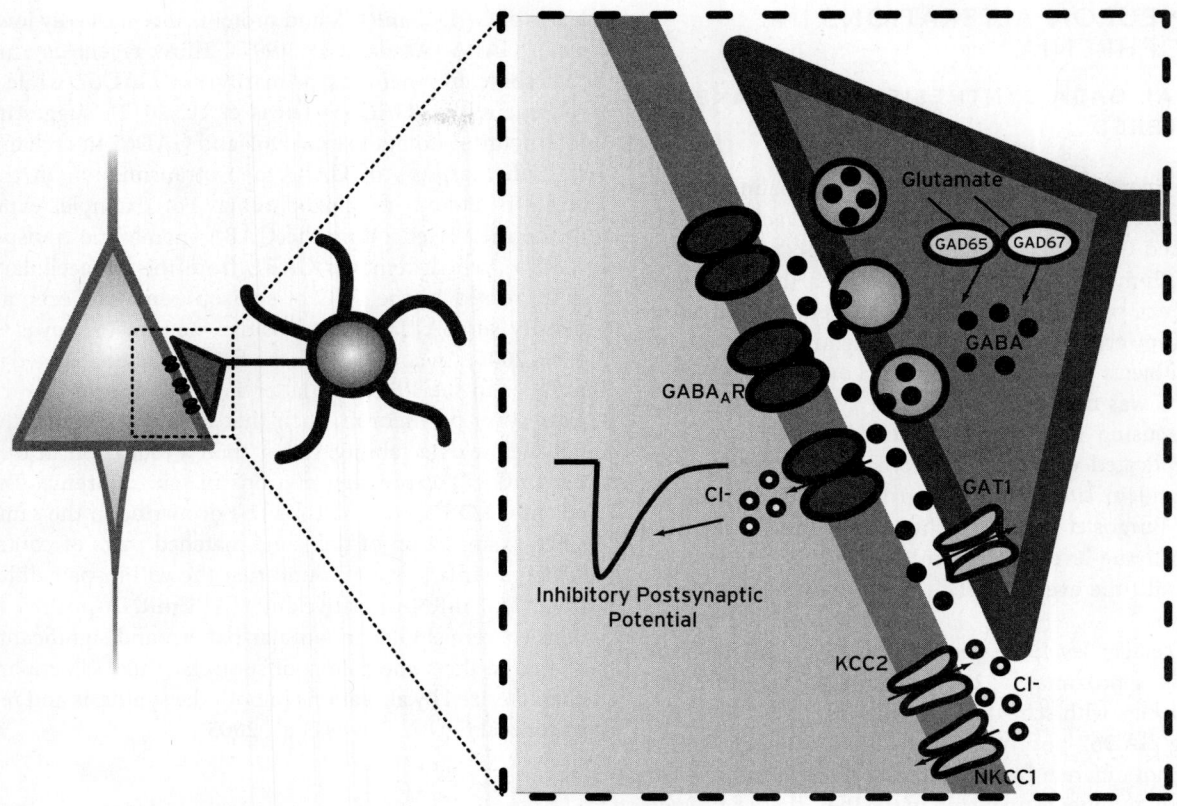

Figure 23.2 Basics of ionotropic GABA neurotransmission. GABA is synthesized from glutamate by the enzyme GAD67 or GAD65. After release from synaptic vesicles into the synaptic cleft, GABA binds to postsynaptic GABA$_A$ receptors. GABA$_A$ receptor activation stimulates the opening of chloride channels. The direction and magnitude of the chloride current produced by GABA$_A$ receptor activation is regulated by the transporters NKCC1 and KCC2, which uptake and extrude chloride, respectively. In the majority of cases, chloride flows inward and hyperpolarizes the membrane, producing the classic inhibitory postsynaptic potential. GABA membrane transporter 1 (GAT1) removes GABA from the synaptic cleft, thereby regulating the concentration of GABA that reaches postsynaptic receptors.

cells (Gonzalez-Burgos and Lewis, 2008). This places interneurons in a position to exert strong inhibitory control over large numbers of pyramidal cells, so that the firing of a single interneuron transiently silences many pyramidal cells. When the pyramidal cells are then released from inhibition, they fire in concert. This inhibitory mechanism of controlling and timing the activity of large numbers of pyramidal cells by interneurons is crucial for proper cortical function. It maintains neural activity within a functional range, preventing the runaway cortical activity of seizures, and exerts an important influence on the timing of neural activity. In addition, the synchronized firing of networks of interconnected interneurons and pyramidal cells produces rhythmic oscillations of different frequencies.

Different subtypes of GABA neurons appear to play distinct roles in the generation of oscillations of different frequencies (Klausberger and Somogyi, 2008). PV$_b$ neurons are known to be crucial in the generation of γ oscillations, the synchronized activity of networks of pyramidal neurons at 30–80 Hz (Gonzalez-Burgos et al., 2010). For example, although the activity of multiple interneuron subtypes is associated with γ oscillations, they are most tightly coupled to the firing of PV$_b$ neurons. Moreover, recent evidence using optogenetic

techniques has demonstrated that suppression and activation of PV neurons suppresses and generates, respectively, γ activity *in vivo*, indicating that PV neurons are both necessary and sufficient for the generation of γ oscillations (Sohal et al., 2009). The GABA$_A$ α1-containing receptors that predominate at PV$_b$ cell synapses exhibit a fast decay of the inhibitory synaptic potential (IPSP) that is consistent with the firing rate of γ oscillations (Gonzalez-Burgos and Lewis, 2008). In contrast, CCK$_b$ neurons are the interneuron subtype that is most strongly coupled to the slower θ oscillations (4–7 Hz) (Klausberger and Somogyi, 2008). In addition, the GABA$_A$ α2-containing receptors that are prominent at CCK$_b$ synapses onto pyramidal cells in rodents exhibit a slower IPSP decay, consistent with θ oscillations.

PFC θ and γ oscillations are associated with higher order cognitive processes such as working memory (Curley and Lewis, 2012). For example, θ and γ band activity is induced during the delay period of working memory tasks, and the power of θ and γ synchrony increases in proportion to working memory load. In addition, injection of a GABA$_A$ receptor antagonist into the PFC disrupts working memory performance in monkeys (Lewis et al., 2005). Thus, CCK$_b$-and PV$_b$-mediated θ and γ oscillations, respectively, are crucial to normal cognitive function.

INTERNEURON ALTERATIONS IN SCHIZOPHRENIA

CORTICAL GABA SYNTHESIS AND UPTAKE ARE ALTERED

The first evidence of altered cortical GABA signaling in schizophrenia came from early findings of decreased activity of GAD and reduced GABA release and uptake in postmortem tissue samples (Blum and Mann, 2002). However, the most consistent evidence supporting altered GABA neurotransmission is reports of lower levels of the mRNA encoding GAD67 in the PFC of subjects with schizophrenia. Lower GAD67 mRNA in the PFC was first demonstrated in 1995 by Akbarian and colleagues using in situ hybridization, and has since been widely replicated using DNA microarray, quantitative PCR (qPCR), and in situ hybridization (Blum and Mann, 2002; Gonzalez-Burgos et al., 2010). Thus far, 10 studies have found deficits in tissue-level GAD67 mRNA in the PFC in schizophrenia, with the average deficit ranging in magnitude from 12% to 68%.

On a cellular level, the density of GAD67 mRNA-positive neurons is approximately 25–35% lower across PFC layers 1–5 of subjects with schizophrenia (Lewis et al., 2005). In the remaining GAD67-positive neurons, the expression level per neuron is not different from that of comparison subjects. Since total neuron number is unaltered in the PFC, these data suggest that GABA neurons are not missing in schizophrenia, but that the majority express normal levels of GAD67 mRNA and a subset express levels so low as to not be detectable.

Although a GAD67 mRNA deficit in the PFC has been widely and consistently reported, knowledge of protein levels is of particular importance given that mRNA and protein levels are not necessarily correlated, since a number of factors regulate transcription and translation (Blum and Mann, 2002). For example, pharmacological manipulation of GABA levels is associated with changes in GAD67 protein but not mRNA. However, similar to the mRNA deficit, levels of GAD67 protein are also lower in the PFC in schizophrenia, and in the largest study to date, the magnitudes of the tissue-level reductions in mRNA and protein (15% and 10%, respectively) were similar (Curley et al., 2011).

In contrast to the reductions in GAD67, the mRNA and protein levels of GAD65 have been reported to be unchanged or only slightly reduced in the PFC in schizophrenia (Lewis et al., 2012). Moreover, the density of GAD65-immunoreactive (-IR) terminals is also unaltered. Thus, schizophrenia is characterized by a preferential deficit of GAD67, but not of GAD65, in the PFC. Given that GAD67 mediates the majority of GABA synthesis in the cortex, lower GAD67 in schizophrenia is thought to result in a reduction of cortical GABA levels that significantly impairs synaptic transmission and inhibition of postsynaptic targets.

Although it is possible that compensatory increases in GAD65 may normalize GABA levels in the illness, this scenario is unlikely for a number of reasons. First, as described earlier, most reports of GAD65 levels in schizophrenia have found no alteration. Second, GAD67 knockout mice exhibit normal levels of GAD65 mRNA and protein, and markedly lower levels of GABA (Asada et al., 1997). Third, recent data indicate that some interneurons primarily use GAD67 while others rely mainly on GAD65 (Lewis et al., 2012), suggesting that interneurons do not use GAD65 and GAD67 interchangeably.

Other aspects of GABA neurotransmission in the PFC are also altered in schizophrenia. For example, expression of the mRNA encoding the GABA membrane transporter 1 (GAT1), which removes GABA from the extracellular space, is decreased in the PFC of schizophrenia subjects, and the density of GAT1 mRNA-positive neurons is lower (Lewis et al., 2005). In concert with the findings of unchanged neuron number in the PFC, this latter finding suggests lower GAT1 expression per neuron, such that in some neurons the level falls below detectability, rather than a reduction in the number of GAT1-expressing neurons in schizophrenia. The deficits in GAD67 and GAT1 may be occurring in the same cells, since examination of the same matched pairs of control and schizophrenia subjects found that the within-pair differences in GAD67 mRNA-positive and GAT1 mRNA-positive neuron density were similar in laminar pattern and significantly correlated in the same cohort of subjects. Thus, schizophrenia is characterized by alterations in both the synthesis and reuptake of cortical GABA (Lewis et al., 2005).

PARVALBUMIN NEURONS ARE PARTICULARLY AFFECTED IN SCHIZOPHRENIA

Given that different subtypes of interneurons possess distinct electrical, molecular, and anatomical properties, the functional outcome of impaired GABA neurotransmission in schizophrenia depends on the subpopulation(s) of neurons affected. PV cells are one subtype of GABA neuron that is known to contain lower GAD67 mRNA in schizophrenia (Lewis et al., 2012). Dual label in situ hybridization has shown that approximately 50% of PV mRNA-positive neurons lack detectable levels of GAD67. In addition, PV mRNA levels are significantly decreased, and laminar analyses have revealed that this reduction occurs principally in layers 3 and 4, layers where lower GAD67 mRNA is also present.

However, in contrast to GAD67 mRNA, although the expression of PV mRNA per neuron is decreased, neither the density of neurons with detectable levels of PV mRNA nor the density of PV-immunoreactive neurons is altered in schizophrenia (Lewis et al., 2012). Although some studies have reported a lower density of PV-immunoreactive neurons in schizophrenia, these results may have been confounded by a reduced sensitivity for PV immunoreactivity resulting from the tissue processing method utilized. Moreover, the lower density of PV-immunoreactive neurons was reported in layers 3–5, where the largest decrement in PV mRNA is found. Thus, levels of PV protein are likely to have fallen below detectability in conditions of reduced sensitivity, and thus the reported findings likely do not reflect lower PV neuron number, but rather an inability to visualize all of the neurons that are present (Stan and Lewis, 2012). In addition, in matched pairs of schizophrenia and control subjects, the within-subject pair difference in

PV mRNA expression per neuron was positively correlated with the difference in density of GAD67 mRNA-positive neurons, suggesting that GAD67 is dramatically lower in a subpopulation of neurons that contain lower, but still detectable, levels of PV mRNA (Lewis et al., 2005).

CONVERGENT EVIDENCE POINTS TO WEAKER INHIBITION FROM PV BASKET CELLS

A recent study demonstrated that the axon terminals of PV_b cells exhibit an approximately 50% reduction in GAD67 protein (Lewis et al., 2012). In addition to lower GABA synthesis, several lines of evidence suggest that PV_b cells exhibit other presynaptic alterations that result in weaker inhibition onto pyramidal cells in the PFC of subjects with schizophrenia (Lewis et al., 2012) (Fig. 23.3). First, mRNA and protein levels

of μ opioid receptors are increased in the PFC of subjects with schizophrenia. Perisomatic μ opioid receptors, which are localized to PV_b cells, hyperpolarize the cell body through the activation of inwardly rectifying potassium channels, making the cell less likely to fire, and μ opioid receptors localized to axon terminals lead to the suppression of vesicular GABA release. Therefore, the greater complement of μ opioid receptors in schizophrenia could contribute to increased suppression of GABA release and result in deficient PV_b cell output (Lewis et al., 2012).

On the postsynaptic side of the PV_b-pyramidal cell synapse, additional alterations are present that may further lower the PV_b-mediated inhibition of pyramidal neurons (Fig. 23.3). First, PV_b-pyramidal neuron synapses are populated by α1-containing $GABA_A$ receptors, and lower α1 mRNA has been demonstrated in schizophrenia PFC by several studies

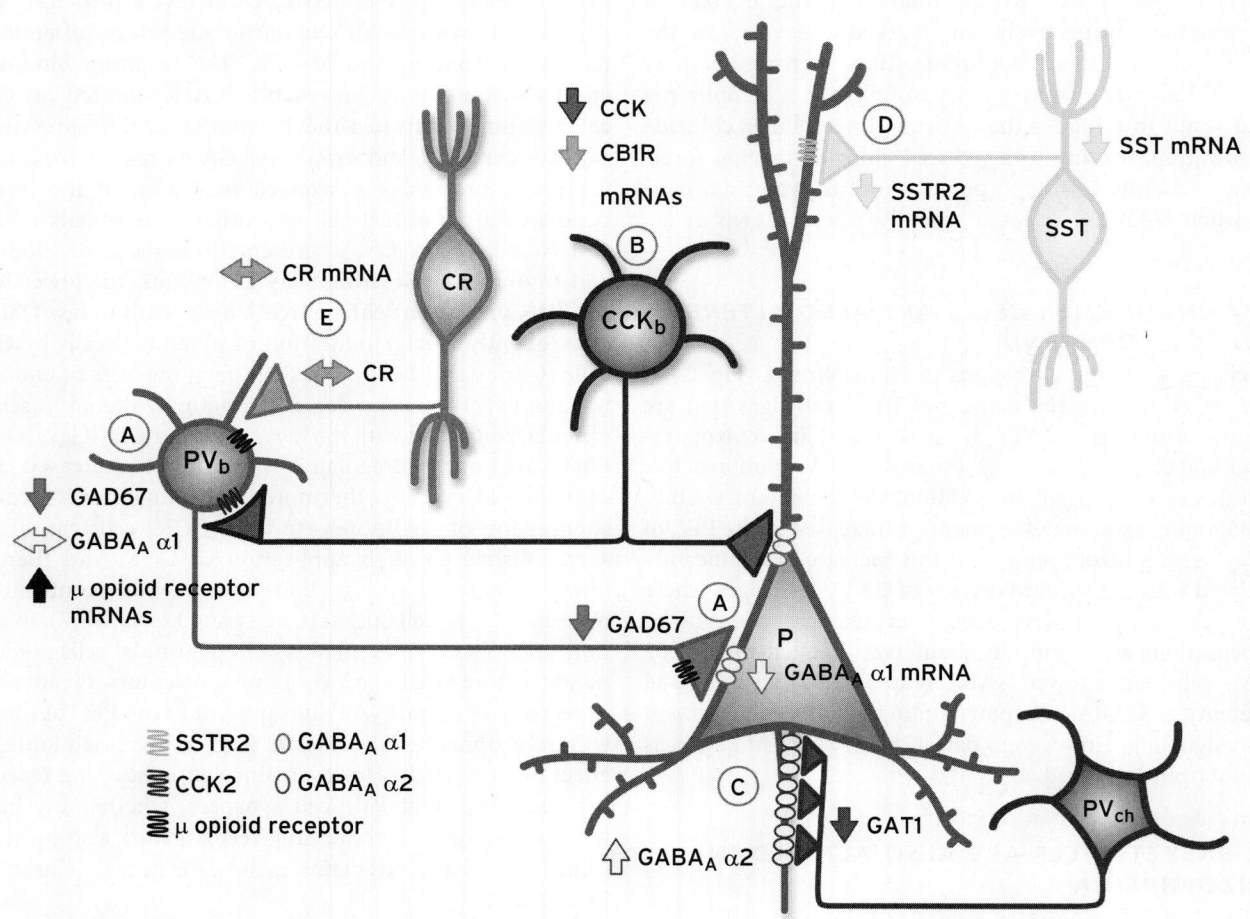

Figure 23.3 Schematic summary of alterations in neuronal circuitry in the PFC of subjects with schizophrenia. (A) The perisomatic inhibition of pyramidal (P) neurons by parvalbumin basket (PV_b) cells is lower due to (1) lower GAD67 mRNA and protein, and therefore less GABA synthesis; (2) higher levels of μ opioid receptor expression in PV_b cells that reduces their activity and suppresses GABA release; (3) reduced expression of cholecystokinin (CCK) mRNA, which stimulates the activity of, and GABA release from, PV_b cells; and (4) less mRNA for, and presumably fewer, postsynaptic $GABA_A$ α1 receptors in pyramidal neurons. (B) The perisomatic inhibition of pyramidal neurons by cholecystokinin-expressing basket (CCK_b) cells is enhanced due to lower levels of CCK and cannabinoid 1 receptor (CB1R) mRNAs that reduce depolarization-induced suppression of inhibition (DSI). Levels of GAD67 in CCK_b cells are unknown, but are thought to be very low, relative to PV cells, in the healthy state. (C) PV-expressing chandelier (PV_{ch}) cells have decreased GABA membrane transporter 1 (GAT1) protein in their axon terminals and increased postsynaptic $GABA_A$ α2-containing receptors at pyramidal neuron axon initial segments. The levels of GAD67 protein in PV_{ch} cells in schizophrenia are not known. (D) Somatostatin (SST)-containing cells contain lower mRNA levels of SST, and expression of its receptor, SSTR2, is also lower. Levels of GAD67 in SST cells have not been measured. (E) Calretinin (CR)-containing cells are thought to be unaffected, since levels of CR mRNA and protein are unchanged. GAD67 levels in CR cells are unknown. (See color insert.)

(Lewis et al., 2012). In addition, mRNA levels of the β2 and γ2 subunits, which coassemble with the α1 subunit, are also lower in schizophrenia. The lower levels of α1 and β2 are most prominent in layers 3–4, exhibiting the same laminar pattern as the PV mRNA deficit. Furthermore, in PFC layer 3, α1 mRNA levels are significantly reduced by 40% in pyramidal cells, but unchanged in interneurons. These data suggest that the number of GABA$_A$ receptors postsynaptic to PV$_b$ cell inputs is selectively lower in pyramidal cells, contributing to weaker PV$_b$ inhibition of pyramidal cells in schizophrenia (Lewis et al., 2012).

Finally, inhibitory inputs onto pyramidal cells may be less hyperpolarizing in schizophrenia. The chloride transporters NKCC1 and KCC2 partially control the driving force of chloride entry into pyramidal neurons, thereby determining the strength of the postsynaptic response to GABA. The mRNA levels of two phosphatases, OSXR1 and WNK3, which phosphorylate NKCC1 and KCC2, increasing and decreasing their function, respectively, are markedly elevated in the PFC of subjects with schizophrenia. Thus, increased activity of NKCC1 and decreased activity of KCC2 in schizophrenia would result in a higher than normal intracellular chloride concentration, leading to a reduced chloride driving force, and subsequently less hyperpolarization of pyramidal neurons when GABA is released from PV$_b$ cells (Lewis et al., 2012).

PV CHANDELIER CELLS ARE ALSO ALTERED IN SCHIZOPHRENIA

PV$_{ch}$ cells also exhibit alterations in schizophrenia (Fig. 23.3) (Lewis et al., 2012). The density of PV$_{ch}$ cartridges that are immunoreactive for GAT1 is 40% lower in schizophrenia, although the density of other GAT1-immunoreactive structures is unchanged. In addition, the density of GABA$_A$ α2-containing axon initial segments is increased in the PFC of subjects with schizophrenia, and this increase is significantly correlated with the reduced density of GAT1 cartridges. These reciprocal alterations have been interpreted as coordinated compensations attempting to counteract a deficit in GAD67 in PV$_{ch}$ cells, since lower GABA reuptake and an increased probability of GABA$_A$ receptor binding would both augment GABA signaling. However, to date, GAD67 levels in PV$_{ch}$ cells have not been measured.

CCK BASKET CELLS ARE ALSO ALTERED IN SCHIZOPHRENIA

Abnormalities in PV neurons alone may not account for the lower GAD67 mRNA and protein levels observed in schizophrenia. In addition to the reductions in layers 3–4 in the PFC, lower levels of GAD67 mRNA have also been observed in layers 1, 2, and 5, where relatively few PV-expressing GABA neurons are located and where PV mRNA expression is unaltered in schizophrenia (Lewis et al., 2005). These findings suggest that other subsets of interneurons residing outside layers 3–4 may also exhibit reductions in GAD67. One candidate population is CCK$_b$ cells, whose cell bodies are principally localized to layers 2-superficial 3 (Fig. 23.3). Lower levels of CCK and

CB1R mRNAs, and lower CB1R protein levels, are present in the PFC of schizophrenia subjects. Furthermore, in matched pairs of schizophrenia and control subjects, the within-subject pair difference in GAD67 mRNA levels was positively correlated with differences in both CCK and CB1 mRNAs, suggesting that the GAD67 mRNA deficit in layers 2–3 is present in CCK$_b$ cells. However, GAD67 levels have not yet been directly assessed in CCK$_b$ cells in schizophrenia. A recent finding that CB1R-expressing axon terminals in monkey PFC tissue have very low levels of GAD67 protein suggests that CCK$_b$ cells may rely mainly on GAD65 for GABA synthesis. Consistent with this hypothesis, nearly all CCK-expressing, but only a few PV-expressing, cells in mouse neocortex express GAD65. Thus, CCK$_b$ cells may not contain lower GAD67 in schizophrenia (Curley and Lewis, 2012).

CCK$_b$ cells are known to participate in a process termed depolarization-induced suppression of inhibition (DSI). In this phenomenon, elevated calcium levels produced from depolarization stimulate the retrograde release of endocannabinoids from pyramidal cells. The resulting binding of endocannabinoids to presynaptic CB1Rs located on CCK$_b$ cell terminals activates the receptors, inhibits presynaptic calcium channels, and suppresses GABA release from CCK$_b$ terminals, producing a reduced inhibition of the original depolarized pyramidal cell and other nearby cells (Wilson and Nicoll, 2002). DSI is present throughout development and into adulthood in monkey PFC. Thus, the lower levels of CB1R present in schizophrenia may result in less DSI and consequently greater inhibition of pyramidal cells by CCK$_b$ cells (Curley and Lewis, 2012). In fact, markers of endocannabinoid synthesis and degradation are unaltered in schizophrenia, consistent with the idea that lower CB1R levels in the illness are not downregulated in response to increased endocannabinoid levels. Furthermore, endocannabinoid-mediated suppression of GABA release from CCK$_b$ cells can also be accomplished through application of CCK, and therefore lower CCK levels in schizophrenia may also contribute to increased CCK$_b$ cell output (Curley and Lewis, 2012). In addition, since CCK$_b$ cell synapses onto pyramidal cells predominantly feature GABA$_A$ α2-containing receptors, the increased expression of α2 mRNA that is present in the PFC of subjects with schizophrenia is consistent with an increased inhibitory effect of CCK$_b$ cells. However, since α2-containing receptors are also present at PV$_{ch}$ cell synapses, whether the higher levels of GABA$_A$ α2-containing receptors are also present at CCK$_b$ cell synapses remains to be determined (Curley and Lewis, 2012).

Alternatively, if GAD67 is lower in CCK$_b$ cells in schizophrenia, reduced CCK and CB1R levels may represent a compensation designed to increase GABA neurotransmission. Consistent with this idea, germ-line reductions of GAD67 in mouse PFC are associated with lower CB1R levels, and the alterations in GAD67 and CB1R are positively correlated, similar to schizophrenia. However, since GAD67 protein levels are normally very low in CCK$_b$ axon terminals from monkey PFC, germ-line reductions in GAD67 may lower CB1R levels by acting at the circuit level rather than within CCK$_b$ cells (Curley and Lewis, 2012).

SST NEURONS ARE ALSO AFFECTED IN SCHIZOPHRENIA

A fourth population of interneurons that exhibit alterations in schizophrenia is cells expressing SST (Fig. 23.3). Lower SST mRNA is present in the PFC of subjects with schizophrenia (Fung et al., 2010), and the reductions are significantly correlated with the deficit observed in GAD67 mRNA in the same subject cohort. Lower levels of somatostatin receptor 2 mRNA are also present in the PFC of subjects with schizophrenia (Beneyto et al., 2012). However, GAD67 levels in SST cells have not been directly examined in schizophrenia, and thus the nature of their involvement in the disease pathology is currently unclear.

CALRETININ CELLS DO NOT SEEM TO BE ALTERED IN SCHIZOPHRENIA

The ~40–50% of interneurons that express CR in the primate PFC do not appear to be affected in schizophrenia (Fig. 23.3). CR mRNA, CR-immunoreactive neurons, and CR-immunoreactive axon terminals are all unaltered in the illness (Lewis et al., 2005). In contrast to PV_b, PV_{ch}, CCK_b, and SST cells, CR cells primarily target other GABA neurons, and thus the fact that these cells seem to be spared in schizophrenia is suggestive of a selective deficit in the inhibition of pyramidal cells, but not of interneurons, in the illness.

ALTERATIONS IN GABA NEURONS ARE FOUND IN OTHER BRAIN REGIONS

An important question that arises from the findings of GABA neuron abnormalities in the PFC is whether these changes are specific to this brain region or are also present in other cortical areas. In fact, reductions in GAD67 mRNA have been reported (although not yet replicated in every location) in the primary motor, primary visual, anterior cingulate, and orbitofrontal cortices, as well as the superior temporal gyrus and hippocampus (Gonzalez-Burgos et al., 2010; Thompson Ray et al., 2011). In addition, other markers of GABA neurotransmission, including PV, GAT1, SST, and $GABA_A$ α1, are lower across multiple cortical regions in schizophrenia, with similar magnitudes of reduction observed across brain regions for each transcript (Lewis et al., 2012). Lower $GABA_B$ receptor immunoreactivity has been reported in the hippocampus, entorhinal cortex, and inferior temporal cortex of subjects with schizophrenia (Mizukami et al., 2002). Importantly, similar to the PFC, CR and GAD65 mRNA are unaltered across multiple cortical regions (Lewis et al., 2012; although axon terminal GAD65 protein levels are lower in primary auditory cortex, see Moyer et al., 2012). Thus, the changes observed in the PFC do not appear to be specific to this brain region, and similar GABA neuron alterations are likely to be present in a variety of cortical regions.

IN VIVO MEASUREMENT OF GABA LEVELS HAS YIELDED INCONSISTENT RESULTS

Despite an abundance of postmortem data suggesting reduced GABA synthesis and alterations in other aspects of GABA neurotransmission in the illness, in vivo measurements of cortical GABA using proton magnetic resonance spectroscopy have yielded conflicting results, with decreased, increased, and unchanged levels reported in different cortical regions (Kegeles et al., 2012; Maddock and Buonocore, 2012). Thus, it is currently unknown whether impaired GABA synthesis is accompanied by lower GABA levels in schizophrenia. Further complicating the issue, magnetic resonance spectroscopy studies assess total tissue levels of GABA, not those associated with synapses, and therefore the relationship between these studies and GABAergic neurotransmission in schizophrenia remains unclear.

ALTERATIONS IN GABA NEURONS ARE DUE TO THE DISEASE PROCESS OF SCHIZOPHRENIA

An important consideration is whether the alterations in markers of GABA neurotransmission described earlier are specific to the disease process of schizophrenia, or represent a consequence of illness chronicity, treatment, or comorbid diagnoses (Lewis et al., 2005). In general, studies in animals exposed to medications used in the treatment of schizophrenia, and the comparison of subjects with schizophrenia on or off such medications at the time of death, suggest that altered GABA-related gene expression in schizophrenia is not attributable to medication effects. Similarly, alcohol use does not seem to affect GAD67, PV, or GAT1 mRNA levels (Lewis et al., 2005), and nicotine and cannabis use also do not account for the lower GAD67 mRNA levels in schizophrenia (Curley et al., 2011).

Furthermore, since GAD67 expression is activity-dependent (Akbarian and Huang, 2006), lower expression might just index the less stimulating social, occupational, and intellectual environment associated with illness chronicity. However, a recent study found no association between GAD67 mRNA expression and age-corrected length of illness (Curley et al., 2011). In addition, the same study found no association between predictors of illness severity or measures of functional outcome and GAD67 mRNA levels.

Another important consideration is whether the observations in schizophrenia are specific to the illness, or are shared among other psychiatric diseases such as bipolar disorder (BPD) and major depressive disorder (MDD). Current evidence suggests that all three disorders do share some common GABAergic alterations, although they are also characterized by differences in their pattern of alterations, and by substantial heterogeneity in findings across studies. For example, lower GAD67 has also been found in BPD and MDD (Guidotti et al., 2000; Thompson Ray et al., 2011), and lower PV has been reported in BPD (Torrey et al., 2005) but not MDD (Beasley et al., 2002; Rajkowska et al., 2007). In contrast, another recent study in the PFC found lower SST levels in MDD and reduced PV in BPD, but no change in GAD67, GAD65, or CR mRNA expression in either illness (Sibille et al., 2011). In addition, microarray studies that examined the expression patterns of large groups of genes have found alterations in a number of GABA-related genes in MDD and BPD (Kato et al., 2007; Klempan et al., 2009). Thus, while these major psychiatric illnesses do seem to be characterized by alterations in GABA

neurons, the exact degree of overlap between illnesses remains to be determined.

MECHANISMS UNDERLYING ALTERATIONS IN GABA NEUROTRANSMISSION IN SCHIZOPHRENIA

A thorough interpretation of the GABA neurotransmission deficit in schizophrenia requires knowledge of the underlying mechanism(s). Since lower GAD67 is the most robust finding in postmortem tissue, here we consider some of the candidate mechanisms for this reduction.

ALLELIC VARIATION IN GAD1

GAD1, the gene that encodes GAD67, is located on chromosome 2q31 (Akbarian and Huang, 2006). Single nucleotide polymorphisms (SNPs) in GAD1 have been implicated in the risk for adult- and childhood-onset schizophrenia (Marenco et al., 2010), and have also been associated with GAD67 mRNA levels (Straub et al., 2007), indicating that alterations in the gene may underlie lower GAD67 mRNA levels in schizophrenia. Existing data suggest several possible mechanisms by which these allelic variants may alter GAD67 mRNA levels. For example, although no risk SNPs are located within the coding region of GAD1 (Akbarian and Huang, 2006), one located in the promoter region is associated with altered transcription factor binding, which may lead to impaired promoter function (Zhao et al., 2007). In addition, epigenetic mechanisms, which control gene activity without altering DNA sequence, may also contribute. Methylation of certain lysine residues on nuclear histone proteins, around which DNA is wound, result in shifts between active and repressed transcription (Tsankova et al., 2007). In female schizophrenia subjects, GAD1 risk SNPs are associated with lower PFC GAD67 mRNA and a shift from active to repressed histone methylation (Huang et al., 2007), providing a potential mechanism through which allelic variation may lower GAD67 mRNA levels. However, this mechanism may be specific to females, and thus the exact role of epigenetic mechanisms in GAD1 transcription requires further study.

Despite this evidence, low penetrance, small effect sizes, and a lack of concordance between studies regarding the specific SNPs involved suggest that allelic variation in the GAD1 gene likely plays only a minor role as a causative factor underlying lower GAD67 in schizophrenia (Insel, 2010). Further confusing the issue, schizophrenia GAD1 risk alleles have recently been associated with *increased* GABA levels in healthy subjects (Marenco et al., 2010), and therefore the exact role of GAD1 risk alleles in the pathogenesis of GAD67 deficits in schizophrenia remains to be determined.

REDUCED SIGNALING THROUGH TRKB

In contrast to a primary genetic effect, lower GAD67 expression may be a consequence of an upstream mechanism. One such mechanism that could lead to a reduction in GAD67, as well as in PV and GAT1, in schizophrenia is reduced signaling through the TrkB receptor and its ligand brain-derived neurotrophic factor (BDNF) (Lewis et al., 2005). TrkB/BDNF signaling is crucial for interneuron development, especially in PV cells, which comprise the majority of TrkB-expressing interneurons. Treatment with BDNF *in vitro* upregulates GAD and promotes GABA release, and BDNF-overexpressing mice exhibit accelerated PV interneuron maturation (Balu and Coyle, 2011).

Both TrkB and BDNF mRNA and protein are lower in the PFC of subjects with schizophrenia (Balu and Coyle, 2011). In fact, in matched pairs of control and schizophrenia subjects, the within-pair differences in TrkB mRNA are positively correlated with those of both GAD67 and PV mRNAs. In addition, mice with a genetic knockdown of TrkB, but not BDNF, exhibit lower levels of GAD67 and PV mRNAs, suggesting that reduced signaling through the TrkB receptor may underlie lower levels of both mRNAs in schizophrenia. Furthermore, knockdown of TrkB produces a reduced density of GAD67 mRNA-positive cells, without a change in the mRNA levels per cell, similar to the pattern observed in schizophrenia. Although GAT1 expression has not been examined in these animals, it also appears to be modulated by the TrkB/BDNF signaling pathway. In hippocampal cells, inhibition of tyrosine kinases lowers GAT1 phosphorylation and GABA reuptake, while application of BDNF increases GAT1 function (Law et al., 2000).

NMDA HYPOFUNCTION IN PV NEURONS

Glutamate-mediated excitatory neurotransmission occurs through a variety of fast ionotropic receptors (NMDA, AMPA, and kainate), as well as the slower G protein-coupled metabotropic receptors. The NMDA receptor hypofunction hypothesis of schizophrenia originated from the observation that NMDA receptor antagonists recapitulate many clinical features of schizophrenia. Although attempts to document alterations in the level of NMDA receptor subunits in schizophrenia have been mixed, the hypothesis has been strengthened by findings that several schizophrenia risk genes, such as neuregulin 1 and ErbB4, affect NMDA receptor signaling, and by preclinical and clinical studies demonstrating that NMDA receptor enhancement ameliorates disease symptoms (Gonzalez-Burgos and Lewis, 2012).

Interneurons are known to depend on NMDA-mediated excitation, and thus lower glutamatergic drive onto GABA neurons may result in subsequent reductions in markers of inhibitory neurotransmission (Lewis and Moghaddam, 2006). The vast majority (80–90%) of PV neurons express NR1 receptors (Huntley et al., 1994; González-Albo et al., 2001), and so PV neurons are thought to be particularly affected by lower NMDA receptor signaling. In fact, NMDA receptor antagonists lower GAD67, PV, and GAT1 mRNAs (Behrens and Sejnowski, 2009; Bullock et al., 2009). In addition, reduced levels of GAD67 and PV protein are observed in mice with a selective knockout of the NR1 receptor on ~50% of cortical and hippocampal interneurons, presumably mostly PV neurons, during early postnatal development (Gonzalez-Burgos and Lewis, 2012).

CONSEQUENCE OF REDUCED EXCITATION

GAD67 is activity-dependent (Akbarian and Huang, 2006), and reductions in excitatory signaling have been shown to produce many of the same alterations in inhibitory function observed in schizophrenia. For example, monocular deprivation of the lateral geniculate nucleus of the thalamus results in lower GAD67 mRNA in the primary visual cortex of primates. Thus, one hypothesis is that the reduced excitatory activity in schizophrenia is an "upstream" pathology that produces a compensatory downregulation of inhibitory activity, in an attempt to maintain the balance of excitatory and inhibitory activity (E/I balance) needed for proper cortical functioning. E/I balance is important to prevent both runaway excitatory activity (too much excitation) and a dying out of cortical activity (too much inhibition). Thus, reduced excitatory activity of pyramidal cells may result in a compensatory downregulation of inhibitory activity onto these neurons, as evidenced by the multiple different types of reductions in effectors of GABA neurotransmission (Lewis et al., 2012).

In fact, a number of alterations are present in excitatory pyramidal cells in schizophrenia (Glausier and Lewis, 2012). First, there is a significant reduction in the density of dendritic spines, a finding that is most pronounced in layer 3. In addition, although the total number of pyramidal neurons is unchanged in the PFC, somal size is significantly lower, and neuropil and dendritic tree size are reduced. In conjunction with these morphological alterations, certain molecules that regulate spine formation and maintenance are also altered in schizophrenia. For example, mRNA levels of the Rho GTPase cell division cycle 42 (Cdc42), which promotes spine formation, are lower in the PFC of subjects with schizophrenia, and the decrease in Cdc42 mRNA is significantly correlated with the reduction in layer 3 spine density. The inhibition of Cdc42 effector protein 3 (Cdc42EP3) by Cdc42 is thought to enable synaptic potentiation, and mRNA levels of Cdc42EP3 are increased in schizophrenia. Thus, the combination of lower Cdc42 and higher Cdc42EP3 levels may contribute to the spine loss observed in schizophrenia (Glausier and Lewis, 2012).

CONSEQUENCES OF ALTERATIONS IN GABA NEURONS IN SCHIZOPHRENIA: NETWORK OSCILLATIONS AND WORKING MEMORY

As previously reviewed, schizophrenia is associated with alterations in a variety of interneuron subtypes. The abnormalities in two of these cell types, PV_b and CCK_b cells, are particularly interesting in light of their role in neural network oscillations associated with cognition, and here we consider the consequences of alterations in these cells in schizophrenia. Lower levels of CCK and CB1R in CCK_b cells are hypothesized to strengthen the inhibition of postsynaptic pyramidal cells. On the other hand, lower levels of GAD67 and increased levels of μ opioid receptors in PV_b cells are thought to weaken the inhibition of postsynaptic pyramidal cells. In addition, PV_b cells receive input from CCK_b cells, and application of CCK can activate PV neurons (Krook-Magnuson et al., 2012); thus, lower

CCK in schizophrenia may also contribute to weaker PV_b cell activity. Lower levels of $GABA_A$ α1-containing receptors and a reduced chloride driving force in pyramidal neurons may also decrease the strength of hyperpolarizing inputs from PV_b cells and exacerbate this reduction in inhibition. Thus, a convergence of evidence suggests that the relative strengths of pyramidal cell inhibition from CCK_b and PV_b cells are increased and decreased, respectively, in schizophrenia (Curley and Lewis, 2012).

An important determinant of the functional consequences of these alterations is whether the disturbances in each cell type affect the same pyramidal neurons (Curley and Lewis, 2012). Although CCK mRNA levels in schizophrenia have not been examined in a laminar fashion, CB1R immunoreactivity is significantly lower in layers deep 3–4 and 6. The density of PV-immunoreactive axon terminals is also lower in layers deep 3–4, suggesting that the alterations in both PV_b and CCK_b terminals are present in the middle cortical layers, despite the locations of their cell bodies in different layers. On the other hand, recent data suggest that all pyramidal neurons receive PV_b cell inputs, whereas only some receive CCK_b inputs and show DSI (Krook-Magnuson et al., 2012), which may indicate that, while all pyramidal cells are affected by impaired inhibition from PV_b cells, only some are affected by alterations in CCK_b cell inputs. However, whether the affected PV_b and CCK_b cells target the same pyramidal neurons in schizophrenia remains to be determined (Curley and Lewis, 2012).

CCK_b and PV_b cells play an important role in the θ and γ oscillations, respectively (Klausberger and Somogyi, 2008), that underlie working memory function. Although in healthy subjects the amplitude of θ and γ oscillations increases in proportion to working memory load, subjects with schizophrenia exhibit impairments in θ and γ band power and working memory performance. Thus, changes in the inhibitory output from CCK_b and PV_b cells, and the resulting shift in their relative control of pyramidal cells, could disrupt normal network functioning and θ and γ band power. Moreover, since θ and γ oscillations are coupled during memory tasks, a disturbance in one frequency may result in corresponding deficits in the other frequency. Thus, alterations in the perisomatic inhibition of PFC pyramidal neurons by CCK_b and PV_b neurons are a plausible mechanism underlying θ and γ oscillation deficits and cognitive impairments in schizophrenia (Curley and Lewis, 2012).

CONCLUSIONS

Schizophrenia is characterized by a number of cortical interneuron alterations. Abnormalities are present in PV_b, PV_{ch}, CCK_b, and SST, but not CR cells, and occur in a number of cortical regions in addition to the PFC. These alterations appear to reflect the disease process of schizophrenia, as they are not a consequence of illness chronicity, treatment, or comorbid diagnoses. A number of plausible mechanisms could underlie the most robust finding, a reduction in GAD67 mRNA and protein, including allelic variation in GAD1, reduced signaling through the TrkB receptor, NMDA receptor hypofunction in PV neurons, or reduced excitation. The alterations in two cell types in particular, PV_b and CCK_b cells, are particularly

important given their roles in θ and γ oscillations, respectively, and provide a possible mechanism underlying the oscillation deficits and cognitive impairments of schizophrenia.

DISCLOSURES

Dr. Lewis currently receives grant/research support from Bristol-Myers Squibb and Pfizer. He is a consultant for Bristol-Myers Squibb and Concert.

Dr. Curley has no conflicts of interest to disclose.

REFERENCES

Akbarian, S., and Huang, H.S. (2006). Molecular and cellular mechanisms of altered GAD1/GAD67 expression in schizophrenia and related disorders. *Brain Res. Rev.* 52:293–304.

Asada, H., Kawamura, Y., et al. (1997). Cleft palate and decreased brain gamma-aminobutyric acid in mice lacking the 67-kDa isoform of glutamic acid decarboxylase. *Proc. Natl. Acad. Sci. USA.* 94:6496–6499.

Ascoli, G.A., Alonso-Nanclares, L., et al. (2008). Petilla terminology: nomenclature of features of GABAergic interneurons of the cerebral cortex. *Nat. Rev. Neurosci.* 9:557–568.

Balu, D.T., and Coyle, J.T. (2011). Neuroplasticity signaling pathways linked to the pathophysiology of schizophrenia. *Neurosci. Biobehav. Rev.* 35:848–870.

Bartos, M., and Elgueta, C. (2012). Functional characteristics of parvalbumin- and cholecystokinin-expressing basket cells. *J. Physiol.* 590:669–681.

Beasley, C.L., Zhang, Z.J., et al. (2002). Selective deficits in prefrontal cortical GABAergic neurons in schizophrenia defined by the presence of calcium-binding proteins. *Biol. Psychiatry* 52:708–715.

Behrens, M.M., and Sejnowski, T.J. (2009). Does schizophrenia arise from oxidative dysregulation of parvalbumin-interneurons in the developing cortex? *Neuropharmacol.* 57:193–200.

Beneyto, M., Morris, H.M., et al. (2012). Lamina- and cell-specific alterations in cortical somatostatin receptor 2 mRNA expression in schizophrenia. *Neuropharmacol.* 62:1598–1605.

Blum, B.P., and Mann, J.J. (2002). The GABAergic system in schizophrenia. *Int. J. Neuropsychopharmacol.* 5:159–179.

Bullock, W.M., Bolognani, F., et al. (2009). Schizophrenia-like GABAergic gene expression deficits in cerebellar Golgi cells from rats chronically exposed to low-dose phencyclidine. *Neurochem. Int.* 55:775–782.

Curley, A.A., Arion, D., et al. (2011). Cortical deficits of glutamic acid decarboxylase 67 expression in schizophrenia: clinical, protein, and cell type-specific features. *Am. J. Psychiatry* 168:921–929.

Curley A.A., and Lewis D.A. (2012). Cortical basket cell dysfunction in schizophrenia. *J. Physiol.* 590:715–724.

Fung, S.J., Webster M.J., et al. (2010). Expression of interneuron markers in the dorsolateral prefrontal cortex of the developing human and in schizophrenia. *Am. J. Psychiatry* 167:1479–1488.

Glausier, J.R., and Lewis D.A. (2012). Dendritic spine pathology in schizophrenia. *Neuroscience*.

González-Albo, M.C., Elston, G.N., et al. (2001). The human temporal cortex: characterization of neurons expressing nitric oxide synthase, neuropeptides and calcium-binding proteins, and their glutamate receptor subunit profiles. *Cereb. Cortex.* 11:1170–1181.

Gonzalez-Burgos, G., Fish, K.N., et al. (2011). GABA neuron alterations, cortical circuit dysfunction and cognitive deficits in schizophrenia. *Neural Plast.* 2011:723184.

Gonzalez-Burgos, G., Hashimoto, T., et al. (2010). Alterations of cortical GABA neurons and network oscillations in schizophrenia. *Curr. Psychiatry Rep.* 12:335–344.

Gonzalez-Burgos, G., and Lewis, D.A. (2008). GABA neurons and the mechanisms of network oscillations: implications for understanding cortical dysfunction in schizophrenia. *Schizophr. Bull.* 34:944–961.

Gonzalez-Burgos, G., and Lewis, D.A. (2012). NMDA receptor hypofunction, parvalbumin-positive neurons and cortical gamma oscillations in schizophrenia. *Schizophr. Bull.* 38:950–957.

Guidotti, A., Auta J., et al. (2000). Decrease in reelin and glutamic acid decarboxylase67 (GAD67) expression in schizophrenia and bipolar disorder: a postmortem brain study. *Arch. Gen. Psychiatry* 57:1061–1069.

Huang, H.S., Matevossian, A., et al. (2007). Prefrontal dysfunction in schizophrenia involves mixed-lineage leukemia 1-regulated histone methylation at GABAergic gene promoters. *J. Neurosci.* 27:11254–11262.

Huntley, G.W., Vickers, J.C., et al. (1994). Distribution and synaptic localization of immunocytochemically identified NMDA receptor subunit proteins in sensory-motor and visual cortices of monkey and human. *J. Neurosci.* 14:3603–3619.

Insel, T.R. (2010). Rethinking schizophrenia. *Nature* 468:187–193.

Kato, T., Kakiuchi, C., et al. (2007). Comprehensive gene expression analysis in bipolar disorder. *Can. J. Psychiatry* 52:763–771.

Kegeles, L.S., Mao X., et al. (2012). Elevated prefrontal cortex γ-aminobutyric acid and glutamate-glutamine levels in schizophrenia measured *in vivo* with proton magnetic resonance spectroscopy. *Arch. Gen. Psychiatry* 69:449–459.

Klausberger, T., and Somogyi, P. (2008). Neuronal diversity and temporal dynamics: the unity of hippocampal circuit operations. *Science* 321:53–57.

Klempan, T.A., Sequeira, A., et al. (2009). Altered expression of genes involved in ATP biosynthesis and GABAergic neurotransmission in the ventral prefrontal cortex of suicides with and without major depression. *Mol. Psychiatry* 14:175–189.

Krook-Magnuson, E., Varga, C., et al. (2012). New dimensions of interneuronal specialization unmasked by principal cell heterogeneity. *Trends. Neurosci.* 35:175–184.

Law, R.M., Stafford, A., et al. (2000). Functional regulation of gamma-aminobutyric acid transporters by direct tyrosine phosphorylation. *J. Biol. Chem.* 275:23986–23991.

Lewis, D.A., Curley, A.A., et al. (2012). Cortical parvalbumin interneurons and cognitive dysfunction in schizophrenia. *Trends Neurosci.* 35:57–67.

Lewis, D.A., Hashimoto, T., et al. (2005). Cortical inhibitory neurons and schizophrenia. *Nat. Rev. Neurosci.* 6:312–324.

Lewis, D.A., and Moghaddam, B. (2006). Cognitive dysfunction in schizophrenia: convergence of gamma-aminobutyric acid and glutamate alterations. *Arch. Neurol.* 63:1372–1376.

Maddock, R.J., and Buonocore, M.H. (2012). MR spectroscopic studies of the brain in psychiatric disorders. *Curr. Top. Behav. Neurosci.* 11:199–251.

Marenco, S., Savostyanova, A.A., et al. (2010). Genetic modulation of GABA levels in the anterior cingulate cortex by GAD1 and COMT. *Neuropsychopharmacol.* 35:1708–1717.

Mizukami, K., Ishikawa, M., et al. (2002). Immunohistochemical localization of GABAB receptor in the entorhinal cortex and inferior temporal cortex of schizophrenic brain. *Prog. Neuropsychopharmacol. Biol. Psychiatry* 26:393–396.

Moyer, C.E., Delevich, K.M., et al. (2012). Reduced glutamate decarboxylase 65 protein within primary auditory cortex inhibitory boutons in schizophrenia. *Biol. Psychiatry* 72:734–743.

Patel, A.B., de Graaf, R.A., et al. (2006). Evidence that GAD65 mediates increased GABA synthesis during intense neuronal activity *in vivo*. *J. Neurochem.* 97:385–396.

Rajkowska, G., O'Dwyer, G., et al. (2007). GABAergic neurons immunoreactive for calcium binding proteins are reduced in the prefrontal cortex in major depression. *Neuropsychopharmacology* 32:471–482.

Sibille, E., Morris, H.M., et al. (2011). GABA-related transcripts in the dorsolateral prefrontal cortex in mood disorders. *Int. J. Neuropsychopharmacol.* 14:721–734.

Sohal, V.S., Zhang, F., et al. (2009). Parvalbumin neurons and gamma rhythms enhance cortical circuit performance. *Nature* 459:698–702.

Stan, A., and Lewis, D.A. (2012). Altered cortical GABA neurotransmission in schizophrenia: insights into novel therapeutic strategies. *Curr. Pharm. Biotechnol.* 13:1557–1562.

Straub, R.E., Lipska, B.K., et al. (2007). Allelic variation in GAD1 (GAD67) is associated with schizophrenia and influences cortical function and gene expression. *Mol. Psychiatry* 12:854–869.

Thompson Ray, M., Weickert C.S., et al. (2011). Decreased BDNF, trkB-TK+ and GAD(67) mRNA expression in the hippocampus of individuals with schizophrenia and mood disorders. *J. Psychiatry. Neurosci.* 36:195–203.

Torrey, E.F., Barci, B.M., et al. (2005). Neurochemical markers for schizophrenia, bipolar disorder, and major depression in postmortem brains. *Biol. Psychiatry* 57:252–260.

Tsankova, N., Renthal, W., et al. (2007). Epigenetic regulation in psychiatric disorders. *Nat. Rev. Neurosci.* 8:355–367.

Wilson, R.I., and Nicoll, R.A. (2002). Endocannabinoid signaling in the brain. *Science* 296:678–682.

Zhao, X., Qin, S., et al. (2007). Systematic study of association of four GABAergic genes: glutamic acid decarboxylase 1 gene, glutamic acid decarboxylase 2 gene, GABA(B) receptor 1 gene and GABA(A) receptor subunit beta2 gene, with schizophrenia using a universal DNA microarray. *Schizophr. Res.* 93:374–384.

24 | SYNAPTIC DISEASE IN PSYCHIATRY

SETH G. N. GRANT

INTRODUCTION

Synapses are the junctions between nerve cells. A single neuron can have thousands of synapses, and the overall number in the human brain is estimated to be around a million billion (10^{15}). Pathology of synapses is known as "synaptopathy" and there are over 100 nervous system diseases caused by mutations disrupting synaptic proteins (Bayes et al., 2011). Single gene mutations have been described in over 200 synapse genes causing a wide variety of psychiatric, neurological, and developmental diseases. Synaptopathy is now recognized as a major cause of common and rare brain diseases.

The complete set of proteins found within synapses is known as the synapse proteome (Bayes and Grant, 2009). This is further divided into the presynaptic and postsynaptic proteomes, referring to the sets of proteins in the presynaptic terminal on the axon and the postsynaptic terminal on the dendrite (Fig. 24.1). The size of the synapse proteome is around 2,000 proteins, representing about 10% of the human genome.

The understanding of synaptopathy requires an appreciation of the basic organization of proteins within the synapse proteome. There is a need to understand the classes (or types) of proteins, how they are physically organized and assembled together, and in which parts of the brain they are expressed. These organizational principles aid in understanding why mutations in particular proteins produce particular phenotypes and diseases.

This chapter will introduce the reader to the molecular science of synaptic disease. The focus will be on the relationship between mutations and the proteins that are found in synapses, and how these mutations cause the phenotypes that comprise the clinical symptoms and signs of the diseases. The chapter will not provide exhaustive lists of gene mutations, as these are constantly being updated. The reader can find lists of synaptic proteome components and their disease mutations on the Genes to Cognition Website (www.genes2cognition.org/synaptopathy). The reader is directed toward specialist chapters for descriptions of the genetics of psychiatric disease and to general neuroscience textbooks for descriptions of the basic physiology and function of synapses.

BRIEF HISTORICAL PERSPECTIVES ON SYNAPTIC DISEASE IN THE PREMOLECULAR ERA

The great dispute between Cajal and Golgi, the two leading neuroanatomists of the 19th century, centered on whether the axons and dendrites of neurons were in continuity or physically separated (DeFelipe, 2010). The importance of this question echoes today because it is the molecular specialization of the contact made between the two separated nerve cells—the structure that Sherrington called the synapse—that is the key to the etiology of many brain diseases.

Until the arrival of electron microscopy in the mid-20th century, neuroanatomical observations of synapses were at the limit of light microscopic methods and discriminating the size and shape of different synapses was difficult. Although these methods revealed that some brain diseases, such as forms of intellectual disability, display morphological abnormalities in synapse structure, there was no systematic way for neuropathologists to use microscopy to classify synaptopathies and thereby determine how many diseases involve pathology at synapses.

Pharmacological studies were more successful in invoking the possibility that synapse disease was involved in psychiatric illness. Evidence such as changes in levels of neurotransmitters or the striking behavioral effects of drugs that modulate the levels or action of neurotransmitters led to the view that an imbalance of neurotransmitter function was either of primary etiological significance or a secondary manifestation of synapses adjusting to the primary disease process. The inability of either neuropharmacology or neuroanatomy to distinguish between the cause or effect has been an obstacle to understanding the relevance of changes in synapses in disease.

Another impediment to scientific advancement was the lack of systematic knowledge about the molecules that are found at synapses. As recently as the 1990s, there was only partial understanding of all the neurotransmitter receptors and even less known about the enzymes and structural proteins found in synapses. As a result of proteomic and genomic studies, there has been at least a 10-fold increase in the number of proteins discovered at the synapse. We now have comprehensive lists of all synaptic proteins and their gene sequences and thus the fundamental "parts list" of synapses (Bayes and Grant, 2009).

ORGANIZATION OF SYNAPSE PROTEOME

The synapse proteome is organized into a hierarchy of structures: genes and RNA encode individual proteins that are organized into macromolecular assemblies, and ultimately these assemblies are organized into the overall subcellular structure of the presynaptic and postsynaptic terminal (Fig. 24.1). The

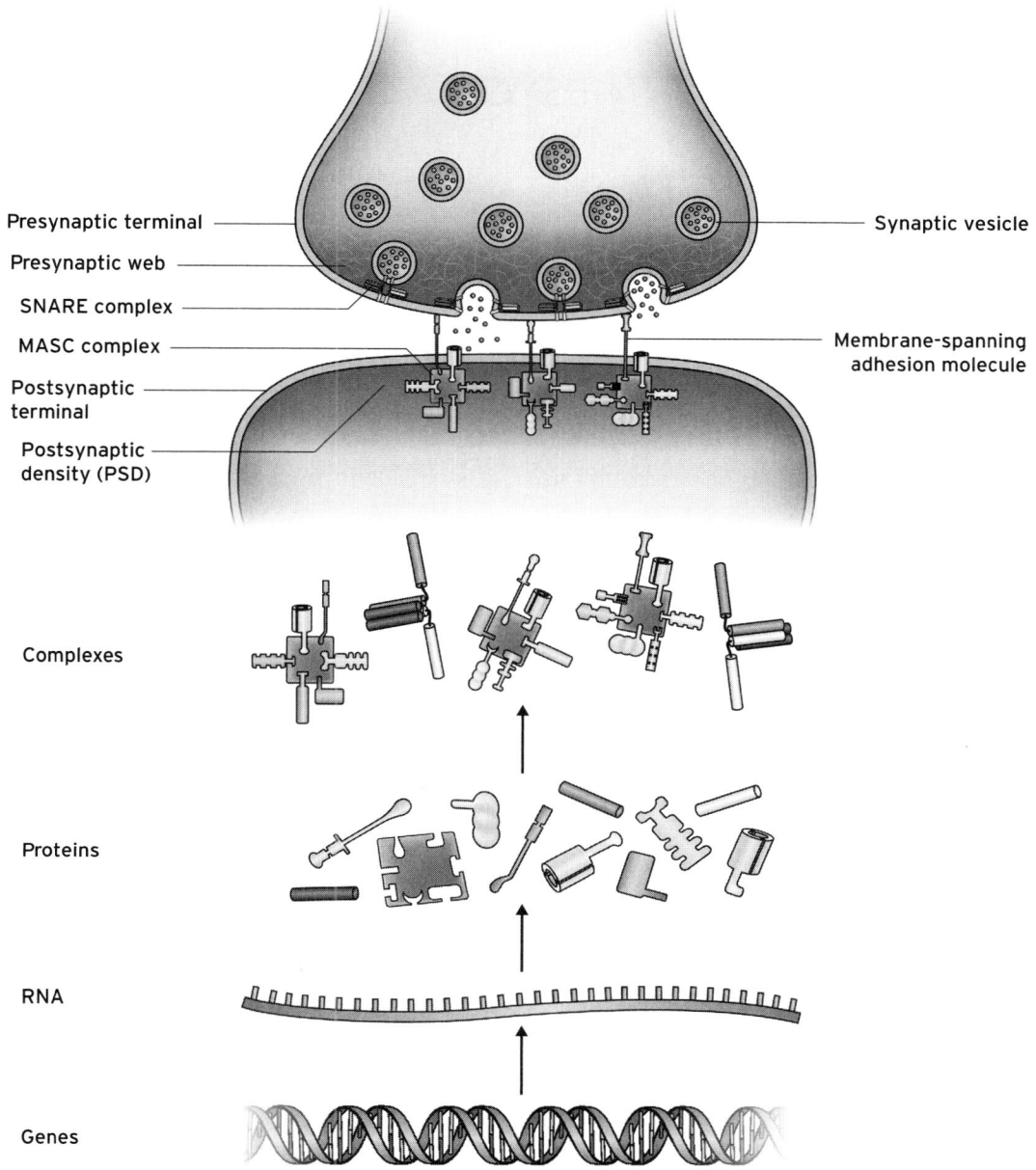

Presynaptic terminal

Presynaptic web

SNARE complex

MASC complex

Postsynaptic terminal

Postsynaptic density (PSD)

Synaptic vesicle

Membrane-spanning adhesion molecule

Complexes

Proteins

RNA

Genes

Figure 24.1 *The synapse proteome. A simplified molecular hierarchy linking genes to synapse structure emphasizing the importance of multiprotein complexes is shown. SNARE and MASC are two prototype complexes in the presynaptic and postsynaptic terminal respectively. The presynaptic web and postsynaptic density (shaded areas) are zones where the complexes are found and visible with electron microscopy. The presynaptic and postsynaptic terminals are interlinked by membrane spanning adhesion molecules that connect the protein assemblies within each neuron.*

subcellular structure of the synapse is visible with electron microscopy (EM), and landmark features of the presynaptic terminal are synaptic vesicles and an electron-dense region beneath the presynaptic membrane (referred to as the presynaptic web). Within the postsynaptic terminal the characteristic feature at the EM level is another electron-dense region described as the postsynaptic density (PSD). Within these microscopic features are specialized multiprotein complexes, each of which is an assembly of dozens of proteins in the MegaDalton size range like that of ribosomes (Husi and Grant, 2001). The presynaptic and postsynaptic terminals are interlinked by membrane spanning adhesion molecules that connect the protein assemblies within each neuron.

Synaptic disease results from the disruption in the proteins and structures in the hierarchy of the synapse proteome, and it is important to understand general principles of proteome organization and in particular the nature of its constituent multiprotein complexes. There are two prototype complexes at synapses: in the postsynaptic terminal the complexes known as MASC (MAGUK Associated Signaling Complexes) link neurotransmitter receptors and ion channels to intracellular signaling enzymes and adhesion proteins (Husi et al., 2000); and within the presynaptic terminal, synaptic vesicle release is mediated by the SNARE (Soluble NSF-Attachment protein REceptor) protein complexes (Sudhof and Rizo, 2011). MASC and SNARE complexes together are

responsible for organizing at least 15% of all the synapse proteome (over 300 proteins) and comparative genomic studies reveal they are some of the most highly conserved proteins in the brain (Bayes et al., 2011; Emes and Grant, 2011, 2012). MASCs are important in neurotransmitter receptor function and disease and will be described in greater detail to illustrate general principles of multiprotein complex structure and function.

Neurotransmitter receptors, ion channels, and other membrane proteins play the vital role of detecting the signals in the milieu surrounding the synapse, which are principally the dynamic fluctuations in the concentration of neurotransmitter released from the presynaptic terminal. Although neurotransmitter receptors are responsible for binding the ligand, it is now known that their regulation of intracellular biochemical events is mediated by the proteins that physically couple to the receptors (Komiyama et al., 2002; Migaud et al., 1998). A plethora of intracellular and other extracellular adhesion proteins are brought into proximity to the receptor through scaffold proteins (Fig. 24.2) (Fernandez et al., 2009). This clustering of signaling proteins into "particles" confers far more sophisticated signaling properties than an ion channel in isolation. Signaling complexes are widespread in eukaryotes and play a vital role in coordinating communication between cells of metazoans and in unicellular eukaryotes for detecting changes in the external environment (Good et al., 2011; Nourry et al., 2003).

The most widely studied example of a postsynaptic MASC is that formed between the glutamate receptors of the N-methyl-D-aspartate (NMDA) family and the scaffold protein Post Synaptic Density 95 (PSD95). PSD95 is a Membrane Associated Guanylate Kinase (MAGUK) family protein and known to interact with over 100 postsynaptic proteins (Fernandez et al., 2009; Husi et al., 2000). These include a variety of signaling, adhesion, and cytoskeletal proteins (Table 24.1). MASC is highly sensitive to the patterns of neuronal activity, which it senses by its neurotransmitter receptor components. The signals from the neurotransmitter receptors are transmitted to the cytoplasmic proteins in part through the influx of Ca^{2+}, which then binds to Ca^{2+}-sensitive proteins that are tethered to PSD95. These in turn catalyze intracellular signaling events such as kinase mediated phosphorylation regulating downstream biochemical pathways. For example, SynGAP is a Ras-GTPase activating protein that regulates the ERK/MAPKinase pathway and it is itself activated by Ca^{2+} influx through the NMDA receptor, which is also tethered to PSD95 (Komiyama et al., 2002). The enzymes in MASC thus engage and drive cell biological pathways that change the properties of the synapse, regulate local protein synthesis, and also transmit signals into the nucleus. It is important to emphasize that the signaling complexes can simultaneously orchestrate and coordinate multiple different downstream signaling pathways that form a network (Coba et al., 2009; Pocklington et al., 2006). Thus MASC is a signal detector and processor that monitors

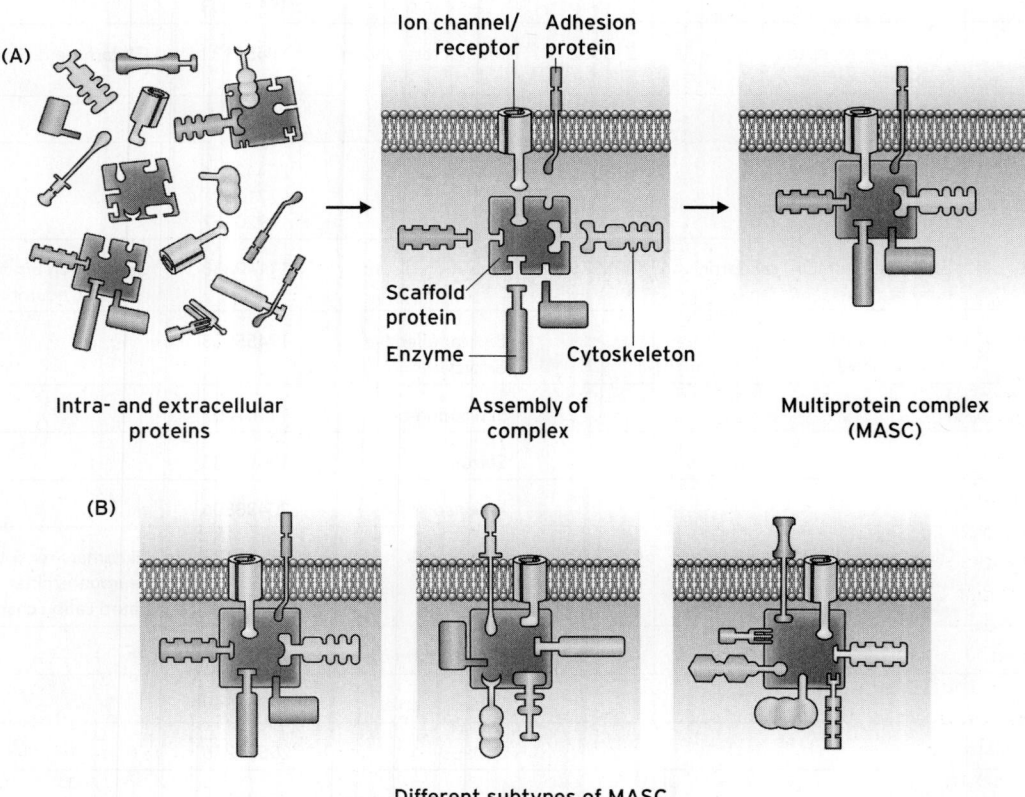

Figure 24.2 Composition of MAGUK associated signaling complexes. (A) Assembly of MASC requires scaffold proteins that bind to a variety of intracellular and extracellular proteins. (B) Different combinations of the binding proteins can assemble into different subtypes of MASC.

TABLE 24.1. Genes encoding proteins in MAGUK Associated Signaling Complexes (MASC) are involved in many neurological and psychiatric diseases. Diseases were annotated from the Genetic Association Database and by manual curation. Genes and Protein identifiers are shown (Gene Name, Entrez Gene ID, UniProt). Molecular Function curated from GO (Gene ontology) and Reference number from PubMed.

GENE NAME	ENTREZ GENE ID	PROTEIN NAME	UNIPROT ACC	DISEASE	REFERENCE	GO MOLECULAR FUNCTIONS
RECEPTOR/CHANNELS/TRANSPORTERS						
ATP1B1	481	Sodium/potassium-transporting ATPase subunit beta-	P05026	Rett syndrome	19455133	Sodium: potassium-exchanging ATPase activity
				Neurodegeneration	19455133	
CACNG2	10369	Voltage-dependent calcium channel gamma-2 subunit	Q9Y698	Bipolar disorder	19455133	Voltage-gated calcium channel activity
				Schizophrenia	18571626	
GRIA1	2890	Glutamate receptor 1, GluR-1	P42261	Schizophrenia	19455133	Glutamate receptor
				Alzheimer's	19455133	
				Epilepsy	19455133	
GRIA2	2891	Glutamate receptor 2, GluR-2	P42262	Schizophrenia	19455133 18163426	Glutamate receptor
				Epilepsy	19455133	
GRIA3	2892	GRIA3 protein	Q17R51	Schizophrenia	19736351 19455133	Glutamate receptor
				X-Mental retardation	19449417	
GRIA4	2893	GRIA4 protein	A6QL61	Schizophrenia	12497607 19125103	Glutamate receptor
GRIK2	2898	Glutamate receptor, ionotropic kainate 2	Q13002	Mental retardation	19455133	Glutamate receptor
				Schizophrenia	12467946	
				Autism	20442744 1771262 11920157	
GRIN1	2902	Glutamate [NMDA] receptor subunit zeta-1	Q05586	Attention disorder	11140838	Calcium ion binding, glutamate receptor, neurotransmitter binding
				Bipolar affective disorder	19455133	
				Schizophrenia	11109007	
				Seizure	19455133	
				Parkinson's	20438806	
GRIN2A	2903	Glutamate [NMDA] receptor subunit epsilon-1	Q12879	Alzheimer's	19455133	Glutamate receptor, neurotransmitter binding, voltage-gated cation channel activity
				Huntington's disease	15742215	
				Schizophrenia	12082569	
				Epilepsy	20890276	
				Mental retardation	20890276	
				Autism	19058789	

(Continued)

TABLE 24.1. (*Continued*)

GENE NAME	ENTREZ GENE ID	PROTEIN NAME	UNIPROT ACC	DISEASE	REFERENCE	GO MOLECULAR FUNCTIONS
GRIN2B	2904	Glutamate [NMDA] receptor subunit epsilon-2	Q13224	Schizophrenia	11317224	Glutamate receptor, neurotransmitter binding, voltage-gated cation channel activity
				Bipolar affective disorder	19005876	
				Huntington's disease	15742215	
				Mental retardation	2089027	
				Alzheimer's	11844890	
				Parkinson's	11844890	
KCNA1	3736	Potassium voltage-gated channel subfamily A member 1	Q09470	Episodic ataxia, type 1	19455133	Potassium ion transmembrane transporter activity
KCNJ10	3766	ATP-sensitive inward rectifier potassium channel 10	P78508	Schizophrenia	20933057	ATP binding, voltage-gated K+-channel
				Epilepsy	15725393	
				Seizure	15120748	
KCNJ4	3761	KCNJ4 protein	Q58F07	Schizophrenia	19455133	Inward rectifier potassium channel activity
VDAC1	7416	Recommended name: Voltage-dependent anion-selective channel protein 1 Short name = VDAC-1 Short name = hVDAC1 Alternative name(s): Outer mitochondrial membrane protein porin 1 Plasmalemmal porin Porin 31HL Porin 31HM	P21796	Alzheimer's	19455133	Porin activity, voltage-gated anion channel activity
				Schizophrenia	19455133	
				Narcolepsy	20677014	
				Bipolar affective disorder	19455133	
VDAC2	7417	Voltage-dependent anion-selective channel protein 2	P45880	Bipolar affective disorder	19455133	Nucleotide binding, porin activity, voltage-gated anion channel activity
				Alzheimer's disease	16385451	
ENZYME						
ACOT7	11332	Cytosolic acyl coenzyme A thioester hydrolase	O00154	Schizophrenia	19455133	Carboxylesterase activity, palmitoyl-CoA hydrolase activity
ATP5A1	498	ATP synthase subunit alpha, mitochondrial	P25705	Alzheimer's	19455133	ATP synthase activity
ATP5C1	509	ATP synthase subunit gamma, mitochondrial	P36542	Bipolar affective disorder	19455133	Hydrogen ion transporting ATP synthase activity, transmembrane transporter activity
CNP	1267	2',3'-cyclic-nucleotide 3'-phosphodiesterase	P09543	Schizophrenia	19455133	2',3'-cyclic-nucleotide 3'-phosphodiesterase activity

(*Continued*)

TABLE 24.1. (*Continued*)

GENE NAME	ENTREZ GENE ID	PROTEIN NAME	UNIPROT ACC	DISEASE	REFERENCE	GO MOLECULAR FUNCTIONS
ERBB4	2066	Receptor tyrosine-protein kinase erbB-4	Q15303	Schizophrenia	16249994	Cell surface receptor for neuregulins and EGF family members
GAPDH	2597	Glyceraldehyde-3-phosphate dehydrogenase	P04406	Alzheimer's	19455133, 15507493	ADP binding: glyceraldehyde-3-phosphate dehydrogenase (NAD+) (phosphorylating) activity Inferred from electronic annotation. Source: Inter Proglyceraldehyde-3-phosphate dehydrogenase (NAD+) (phosphorylating) activity Inferred from sequence or structural similarity. Source: UniProtKBpeptidyl-cysteine S-nitrosylase activity
GDA	9615	Guanine deaminase	Q9Y2T3	Schizophrenia	2047103	Guanine deaminase activity, zinc ion binding
MSRB2	22921	Methionine-R-sulfoxide reductase B2, mitochondrial	Q9Y3D2	Bipolar affective disorder	19455133	Protein-methionine-R-oxide reductase activity: sequence-specific DNA binding transcription factor activity Inferred from electronic annotation. Source: InterProprotein-methionine-R-oxide reductase activity Inferred from sequence or structural similarity PubMed 14699060. Source: HGNCsequence-specific DNA binding transcription factor activity Traceable author statement Ref.1. Source: ProtIınczinc ion binding
				Alzheimer's	16385451	
NLN	57486	Neurolysin, mitochondrial	Q9BYT8	*Impaired function*	22222624	Metal ion binding, metalloendopeptidase activity
PDHA1	5160	Recommended name: Pyruvate dehydrogenase E1 component subunit alpha, somatic form, mitochondrial EC= 1.2.4.1 Alternative name(s): PDHE1-A type I	P08559	Depression	19455133	*Pyruvate dehydrogenase (acetyl-transferring) activity*
PGK1	5230	Phosphoglycerate kinase 1		Parkinson's	19455133	Kinase, ATP bindingphosphoglycerate kinase activity transferase
				Mental retardation	19455133	
				Bipolar disorder	19455133	
PRDX1	5052	Peroxiredoxin-1	Q06830	Alzheimer's	19455133	Antioxidant, oxidoreductase, peroxidase
PRDX2	7001	Peroxiredoxin-2	P32119	Parkinson's	19455133	Antioxidant, oxidoreductase, peroxidase
				Frontotemporal lobar degeneration	2236042	

(*Continued*)

TABLE 24.1. (*Continued*)

GENE NAME	ENTREZ GENE ID	PROTEIN NAME	UNIPROT ACC	DISEASE	REFERENCE	GO MOLECULAR FUNCTIONS
				Schizophrenia	19165527	
				Alzheimer's	12650976	
TNIK	23043	TNIK protein	Q7Z4L4	Schizophrenia	19023125	Small GTPase regulator activity
DPYSL2	1808	Dihydropyrimidinase-related protein 2, DRP-2	Q16555	Alzheimer's	17683481	Dihydropyrimidinase activity, protein kinase binding
				Schizophrenia	16321170, 15858820, 16380905	
				Epilepsy	15672539	
				Down syndrome	11771764	
				Biploar disorder	16380905	
PROTEIN PHOSPHATASES						
PPP3CA		Serine/threonine-protein phosphatase 2B catalytic subunit alpha isoform	Q08209	Schizophrenia	19455133	Calcium ion binding, calmodulin-dependent protein phosphatase activity
				Parkinson's disease	18628988	
				Alzheimer's disease	20590401	
SER/THR KINASES						
CAMK2A	815	Calcium/calmodulin-dependent protein kinase type II subunit alpha	Q9UQM7	Bipolar disorder	19455133	ATP binding; calmodulin-dependent protein kinase activity; kinase activity
CAMK2B	816	Calcium/calmodulin-dependent protein kinase type II subunit beta	Q13554	Schizophrenia	19455133	ATP binding; calmodulin-dependent protein kinase activity
				Depression	19455133	
				Autism	19058789	
MAPK1	5594	Mitogen-activated protein kinase 1	P28482	Schizophrenia	19455133	MAP kinase activity: RNA polymerase II carboxy-terminal domain kinase activity Source: UniProtKB-KWDNA binding Inferred from electronic annotation. Source: UniProtKB-KWMAP kinase activity Traceable author statement PubMed 10706854. Source: ProtInc RNA polymerase II carboxy-terminal domain kinase activity
				Depression	19455133	
RELN	5649	Reelin	P78509	Autism	11317216	Protein serine/threonine/tyrosine kinase activity
				Schizophrenia	12082559	
				Alzheimer's disease	18599960	
				Bipolar Disorder	19691043	

(Continued)

TABLE 24.1. (*Continued*)

GENE NAME	ENTREZ GENE ID	PROTEIN NAME	UNIPROT ACC	DISEASE	REFERENCE	GO MOLECULAR FUNCTIONS
CYTOSKELETAL/STRUCTURAL/CELL ADHESION						
ADAM22	53616	Disintegrin and metalloproteinase domain-containing protein 22, ADAM 22	Q9P0K1	Epilepsy	19455133	Metalloendopeptidase activity; receptor activity; zinc ion binding;
CAPZA2	830	F-actin-capping protein subunit alpha-2	P47755	Mental retardation	19455133	Regulates the growth of the actin filaments at the barbed end.
LGI1	9211	Leucine-rich glioma-inactivated protein 1	O95970	Epilepsy	20659151	Protein binding
NEFL	4747	Recommended name: Neurofilament light polypeptide Short name = NF-L Alternative name(s): 68 kDa neurofilament protein Neurofilament triplet L protein	P07196	CMT1	19455133	Protein C-terminus binding, structural constituent of cytoskeleton
				Schizophrenia	19455133	
				Bipolar	19455133	
				CMT2	19455133	
				ALS	19455133	
				Parkinson's	12231460	
NRCAM	4897	Neuronal cell adhesion molecule	Q92823	Autism	17106428	Neuron-neuron adhesion and promotes directional signaling during axonal cone growth.
				Schizophrenia	19154219	
NRXN1	9378	NRXN1 protein	Q49A31	Autism	18490107	Acetylcholine receptor binding, calcium-dependent protein binding, cell adhesion molecule binding, neuroligin family protein binding
				Schizophrenia	18940311	
PLP1	5354	Myelin proteolipid protein	P60201	Pelizaeus–Merzbacher disease	2479017	Structural constituent of myelin sheath, structural molecule activity
				Depression40	19455133	
				Multiple sclerosis	9460711	
				Demyelinating disease	19455133	
				Spastic paraplegia	19455133	
				leukodystrophies	16416265	
Vesicular/trafficking/transport						
CLTC	1213	Recommended name: Clathrin heavy chain 1 Alternative name(s): Clathrin heavy chain on chromosome 17 Short name= CLH-17	Q00610	Mental retardation	19455133	Binding, structural molecule activity

(*Continued*)

TABLE 24.1. (*Continued*)

GENE NAME	ENTREZ GENE ID	PROTEIN NAME	UNIPROT ACC	DISEASE	REFERENCE	GO MOLECULAR FUNCTIONS
DEVELOPMENT						
CYFIP1	23191	Cytoplasmic FMR1-interacting protein 1	Q7L576	Prader-Willi syndrome	14508708	Actin filament binding; Rac GTPase binding
MAGUKs / Adaptors / Scaffolders						
PDZ-domain containing scaffolders						
DLG1	1739	Disks large homolog 1	Q12959	Schizophrenia	19455133, 18665322	Guanylate kinase activity, phosphoprotein phosphatase activity, potassium channel regulator activity
DLG2	1740	Disks large homolog 2	Q15700	Schizophrenia	19736351, 19455133	Guanylate kinase activity
				Parkinson's disease	17052657	
DLG3	1741	Disks large homolog 3	Q92796	Schizophrenia	19455133	Guanylate kinase activity
				Bipolar disorder	19455133	
				Depression	19455133	
				X-Mental retardation	19455133	
DLG4	1742	Disks large homolog 4	P78352	Schizophrenia	19455133, 20921115, 12950712	ADP-activated nucleotide receptor activity
				Bipolar disorder	19455133	
SHANK3	85358	SH3 and multiple ankyrin repeat domains protein 3, Shank3	Q9BYB0	Autism	22223503	GKAP/Homer scaffold activity; SH3 domain binding
				Schizophrenia type 15	20385823	
				Phelan-McDermid syndrome	21984749, 21984749	
TJP1	7082	Tight junction protein ZO-1	Q07157	Prader-Willi syndrome	8825647	Calmodulin binding, protein binding
non-PDZ-domain containing scaffolders						
DLGAP1	9229	Disks large-associated protein 1	O14490	Schizophrenia	19455133	Protein binding, postsynaptic scaffold in neuronal cells
YWHAE	7531	Recommended name: 14–3-3 protein epsilon Short name = 14–3-3E	P62258	Miller–Dieker lissencephaly	19455133	Histone deacetylase binding, phosphoprotein binding, protein binding protein domain specific binding
YWHAG	7532	14–3-3 protein gamma	P61981			Insulin-like growth factor receptor binding, protein binding, protein kinase C inhibitor activity, receptor tyrosine kinase binding
DTNBP1	84062	Dysbindin	Q96EV8	Schizophrenia	12474144	Protein binding, intracellular vesicle trafficking. Plays a role in synaptic vesicle trafficking and in neurotransmitter release
				Bipolar disorder	15820225	

(Continued)

TABLE 24.1. (*Continued*)

GENE NAME	ENTREZ GENE ID	PROTEIN NAME	UNIPROT ACC	DISEASE	REFERENCE	GO MOLECULAR FUNCTIONS
DISC1	27185	Recommended name: Disrupted in schizophrenia 1 protein	Q9NRI5	Schizophrenia	15342131	Protein binding, developmental protein
				Asperger syndrome	17579608	
				Bipolar disorder	15838535	
				Alzheimer's disease	19118814	
				Amyotrophic lateral sclerosis	19451621	
				Depression	19548263	
TRANSCRIPTION AND TRANSLATION						
FMR1	2332	Fragile X mental retardation protein 1, FMRP, FMR-1	Q06787	Mental retardation	11415517	mRNA binding, inhibit translations
				Parkinson's disease	15929093	
				Mental disorder	15617547	
				X-Mental retardation	9415473	
EHMT1	79813	Histone-lysine *N*-methyltransferase, EHMT1	Q9H9B1	Schizophrenia	22083728	Chromatin regulator, methyltransferase
MECP2	4204	Methyl-CpG-binding protein 2	P51608	Angelman syndrome	11283202	Double-stranded methylated DNA binding, transcription corepressor activity
				Rett syndrome	15034579	
				Mental retardation syndromic X-linked type 13	10986043	
				Autism X-linked type 3	12770674	
TCF4	6925	Transcription factor 4		Pitt-Hopkins syndrome	17478476	Sequence-specific DNA binding RNA polymerase recruiting transcription factor activity
				Schizophrenia	10889556	
G-PROTEINS AND MODULATORS						
G-proteins						
GNAO1	2775	Guanine nucleotide-binding protein G(o) subunit alpha	P09471	Schizophrenia	19455133	Transducer, GTP binding/ activity, metal ion binding, signal transducer activity
Modulators						
SYNGAP1	8831	Ras GTPase-activating protein SynGAP	Q96PV0	Mental retardation autosomal dominant type 5	19196676	GTPase activation, phospholipid binding
				Autism	21237447	
NRG1	3084	Pro-neuregulin-1, membrane-bound isoform	Q02297	Schizophrenia	12478479	Direct ligand for ERBB3 and ERBB4 tyrosine kinase receptors
				Bipolar disorder	15939841	
				Autism	17519028	
				Bipolar disorder	18466879	

(Continued)

TABLE 24.1. (*Continued*)

GENE NAME	ENTREZ GENE ID	PROTEIN NAME	UNIPROT ACC	DISEASE	REFERENCE	GO MOLECULAR FUNCTIONS
SYNAPTIC VESICLES AND PROTEIN TRANSPORT						
Synaptic vesicle						
NSF	4905	Vesicle-fusing ATPase	P46459	Schizophrenia	19455133	ATP binding/ activity, metal ion binding
				Alzheimer's disease	15917099	
				Huntington's disease	15040808	
				Parkinson's disease	14570706	
RPH3A	22895	Rabphilin-3A	Q9Y2J0	Huntington's disease	17877635	Transporter activity, zinc ion binding
RYR2	6262	Ryanodine receptor 2	Q92736	Autism	21151189	Calcium ion binding, receptor activity, ryanodine-sensitive calcium-release channel activity, suramin binding
STX1a	6804	Recommended name: Syntaxin-1A Alternative name(s): Neuron-specific antigen HPC-1	Q16623	Alzheimer's	10891589	Calcium channel inhibitor activity
				Epilepsy	19557857	
				Migraine disorders	19368856	
				Schizophrenia	10924661, 1521946	
				Autism	21118708	
				CJD	10842016	
STXBP1	6812	Syntaxin-binding protein 1	P61764	Schizophrenia	19455133	SNARE binding, identical protein binding, syntaxin binding
				Epileptic encephalopathy	18469812	
Transporters						
SLC25A4	291	ADP/ATP translocase 1	P12235	Bipolar affective disorder	19455133	ATP:ADP antiporter activity, adenine transmembrane transporter activity
				Opthalmoplegia	12112115	

neuronal activity and organizes the functional state of the synapse and nerve cell.

Analysis of MASC from brain tissue has shown there is a very large number of proteins (100–300) and it is clear that these are not all found within a single physical complex. Rather, they are shared into different complexes or subtypes forming a family of MASCs (Fig. 24.2). Recent large-scale systematic studies examining the neuroanatomical distribution of gene expression reveal differences in the levels of synapse proteins in different parts of the mouse and human brain (Emes et al., 2008; Hawrylycz, 2012). From these data

it is evident that the various MASC subtypes are differentially distributed in the brain, with some components expressed in particular synapses and neurons and others in different locations (Fig. 24.2B) (Emes et al., 2008). The differential expression of MASC components has implications for disease because mutations in proteins will therefore not affect all synapses and neurons equally. While this is not well documented in humans, studies in genetically modified mice show that mutations that interfere with core MASC components, such as the MAGUK proteins that assemble the complexes, have pronounced electrophysiological and behavioral phenotypes

(Carlisle et al., 2008; Cuthbert et al., 2007; Migaud et al., 1998; Nithianantharajah et al., 2012).

In contrast to the signal transduction complexes formed by neurotransmitters, the complexes in the presynaptic terminal for neurotransmitter release have a mechanical role in catalyzing the fusion of the presynaptic membrane with synaptic vesicles (Sudhof and Rizo, 2011). Core proteins include the SNARE and SM (Sec1/Munc18-like) proteins. These proteins form a helical complex bringing the membranes together and are later dissociated by additional proteins (NSF, N-ethylmaleimide sensitive factor). Further interacting proteins including chaperones, synaptotagmin, Munc, and RIM proteins play key roles in tethering to Ca^{2+} channels (that permit Ca^{2+} entry following the arrival of the action potential) and triggering the SNARE proteins.

In addition to signaling complexes and synaptic vesicle complexes, there are also other types of complexes or assemblies at synapses. For example, the multiprotein complexes regulating the synthesis and turnover of proteins including ribosomes and proteasomes are present in the postsynaptic terminal (Haas and Broadie, 2008; Steward et al., 1996; Zalfa et al., 2006). Dysfunction in protein metabolism impacts on many different postsynaptic proteins and thereby produces general debilitating effects. For example, a genetic disorder of cognition involving dysregulation of protein synthesis is Fragile X syndrome. The gene encoding FMRP (Fragile X Mental Retardation Protein) regulates mRNA translation, and its disruption results in widespread changes in MASC and PSD proteins (Darnell et al., 2011). FMRP is also found within multiprotein complexes with CYFIP and other proteins (Schenck et al., 2001; Zalfa et al., 2006; Zalfa et al., 2007). Thus the overall organization and function within the postsynaptic terminal is carried out by sets of large multiprotein machines. The relevance of these complexes to disease will be highlighted in the following sections by studies showing that multiple mutations impact on these complexes.

SYNAPSE MUTATIONS CAUSE A WIDE RANGE OF DISEASES

The first global view of genetic disease burden on the human synapse proteome came from the systematic characterization of the postsynaptic proteome (Bayes et al., 2011). The study discovered a total of 1,461 PSD proteins from the neocortex, of which a "consensus set" of 748 were common to all samples and subjects. Each PSD gene was annotated to known monogenic diseases identified from the Online Mendelian Inheritance in Man (OMIM) database: 269 monogenic diseases were encoded by 199 genes from the total PSD, and 155 diseases were encoded from 110 genes in the consensus PSD, overall representing ~14% of PSD proteins. The number of disease relevant mutations is continuing to increase with new sequencing data. Diseases with primary symptoms in the nervous system represented ~50% of the total diseases in both PSD sets (133 diseases in total PSD and 82 in consensus PSD) and of all nervous system diseases, ~80% were central nervous system disorders.

Many of these diseases are rare single gene disorders, and others are more common diseases, such as epilepsy and mental retardation, which were caused by mutations in multiple PSD genes (Fig. 24.3). Classifications of human diseases rely on the *International Classification of Diseases*, now in its 10th revision (ICD10). ICD10 relies primarily on overall disease description and from the total of 22 ICD10 disease categories (chapters), PSD diseases mapped primarily to four chapters with most in *Diseases of the nervous system*, which includes neurological disorders: epilepsies, atrophies, paralytic, movement disorders, and neurodegenerative conditions including

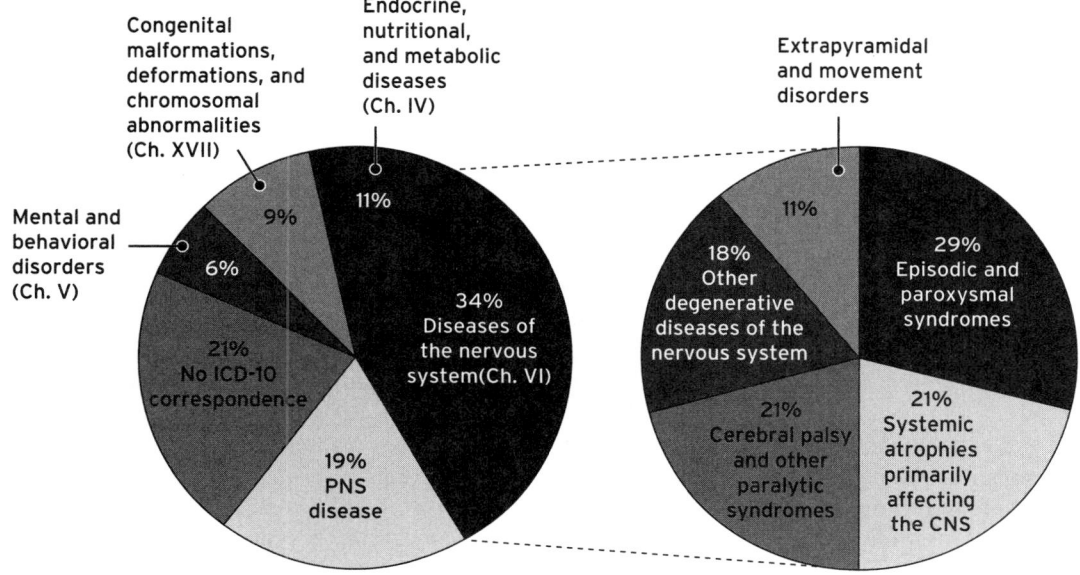

Figure 24.3 *Diseases of the human postsynaptic density. Over 130 brain diseases caused by mutations disrupt the human postsynaptic proteome and are here categorized according to the International Classification of Disease chapter system. The left chart shows the distribution into all disease categories with four chapters (IV-VII) representing those affecting the brain. Note that peripheral nervous system (PNS) is also affected. The right chart is an expansion of the disease subclassifications within Chapter VI. (Further details can be found in Bayes et al., 2011, from which this was adapted.)*

Alzheimer's and Parkinson's disease. Other major categories of human CNS disorders were also represented, including psychiatric, developmental, and metabolic diseases. The broad range of diseases caused by mutations disrupting the PSD show that neurological and psychiatric diseases have a common etiology in synaptopathy.

DISEASE MUTATIONS CONVERGE ON SYNAPTIC PROTEIN COMPLEXES

Schizophrenia and autism are two diseases that together afflict several percent of the population and produce lifelong problems in cognitive functioning. Large-scale genome-wide studies have excluded the possibility that all patients have a mutation in a single gene and the prevailing view is that each of these diseases arises from mutations in multiple different genes. The study of *de novo* copy number variation has recently become a powerful tool for identifying pathogenic mutations in diseases that have complex multigenic genetics. The essence of the approach is to compare the genome of patients with their normal parents and seek the *de novo* mutations that arose with the disease: these are more likely to be causal than (inherited) genetic variants found using other approaches (Vissers et al., 2010). In a study of hundreds of families with an affected offspring with schizophrenia, *de novo* mutations were identified in many genes, and it was found that there was a highly significant enrichment of mutations in synapse proteins, and in particular the MASC proteins in the PSD (Fig. 24.4) (Kirov et al., 2012).

The convergence of many mutations causing schizophrenia onto MASC strongly supports the view that these complexes are the level in the molecular hierarchy at which the disease and its phenotypes are regulated. In other words, the disease is caused by disruptions to a set of proteins that form MASC—the disease is a "postsynaptic complexopathy." Similar studies of autism *de novo* CNVs also reported mutations in these postsynaptic signaling complexes and the postsynaptic density (Levy et al., 2011; Pinto et al., 2010). Not only were the same complexes impacted by mutations in these diseases, but some of the same genes. Another similar study of attention-deficit hyperactivity disorder (Elia et al., 2011) and Tourette's syndrome (Fernandez et al., 2011) identified *de novo* mutations that also overlapped with these sets. Thus these genetic and proteomic data reveal that these diseases, which have similar clinical manifestations must have a common underlying etiology, and this etiology is in the disruption of the synaptic signaling complexes.

These examples have emphasized that different *single* gene mutations disrupting the complexes can result in disease in the individual patient. Another genetic mechanism relevant to the model of genetic convergence on multiprotein complexes is to have two or more weaker mutations in different proteins that together have an additive effect—a phenomenon known as epistasis. An example of this type of analysis on glutamate receptors and interacting MAGUK proteins was recently reported in a cohort of schizophrenia and bipolar disorder patients (Frank et al., 2011). Another genetic mechanism

whereby a "spectrum" of related phenotypes can arise is through different mutations (including deletions and duplications) in the same gene as exemplified in Charcot-Marie-Tooth disease (Shchelochkov et al., 2010). It is likely that all of these genetic mechanisms acting on the complexes will be a source of the spectrum of clinical disorders.

While there may be many important disease mutations impacting on synaptic signaling complexes these findings do not imply that other genes such as those encoding proteins in other complexes cannot also produce some of the same diseases and phenotypes. As noted earlier, FMRP when mutated results in the Fragile X syndrome, a relatively common cause of intellectual impairment with autism-like features. Another example would be mutations in transcription factors or genes that regulate transcription such as EHMT1 or MECP2 that could disrupt the expression of proteins in the synapse (Kirov et al., 2012). As a result of the rapid progress in genome sequencing, there are new mutations in psychiatric diseases being discovered each month. Biochemical characterization of the synaptic complexes that these genes regulate is expected to expand in coming years.

A GENETIC AND PROTEOMIC ARCHITECTURE OF BRAIN DISEASE PHENOTYPES

The following section aims to take the reader away from the use of the term "disease" to a more fundamental and reductionist descriptive approach of behavior phenotypes. There are two essential concepts to embrace. First, the clinical manifestation of a disease is a constellation or set of abnormal symptoms or signs. For example, Huntington's disease (HD) is a description of a set of motoric and cognitive impairments. Second, mutations produce phenotypes (because of the disruption of the proteins controlling that behavior or physiological function), and any mutation usually produces multiple phenotypes. The mutation in the Huntington gene that results in HD is an excellent example. Thus a simple hierarchy where diseases are on top and beneath them are the specific phenotypes and beneath these are the genes (and their mutations) can be constructed as shown in Fig. 24.5.

With available knowledge of gene mutations and their phenotypes a map of gene-phenotype-disease relationship can be constructed for any set of genes, such as the postsynaptic proteome (Bayes et al., 2011). This not only permits the identification of the sets of proteins directly relevant to a phenotype (and disease) but can be used to reveal other proteins that interact with them, which may be new disease candidates. Using the knowledge of the postsynaptic proteome all the known Mendelian diseases were cataloged from OMIM, and all the relevant phenotypes identified using the Human Phenotype Ontology (HPO) (Robinson and Mundlos, 2010), which is another catalog that systematically lists all the phenotypes for OMIM diseases. This showed that mutations in 80 PSD genes resulted in 115 human neural phenotypes. Since there are more phenotypes than genes, it is clear that some mutations produce multiple phenotypes. Conversely, many

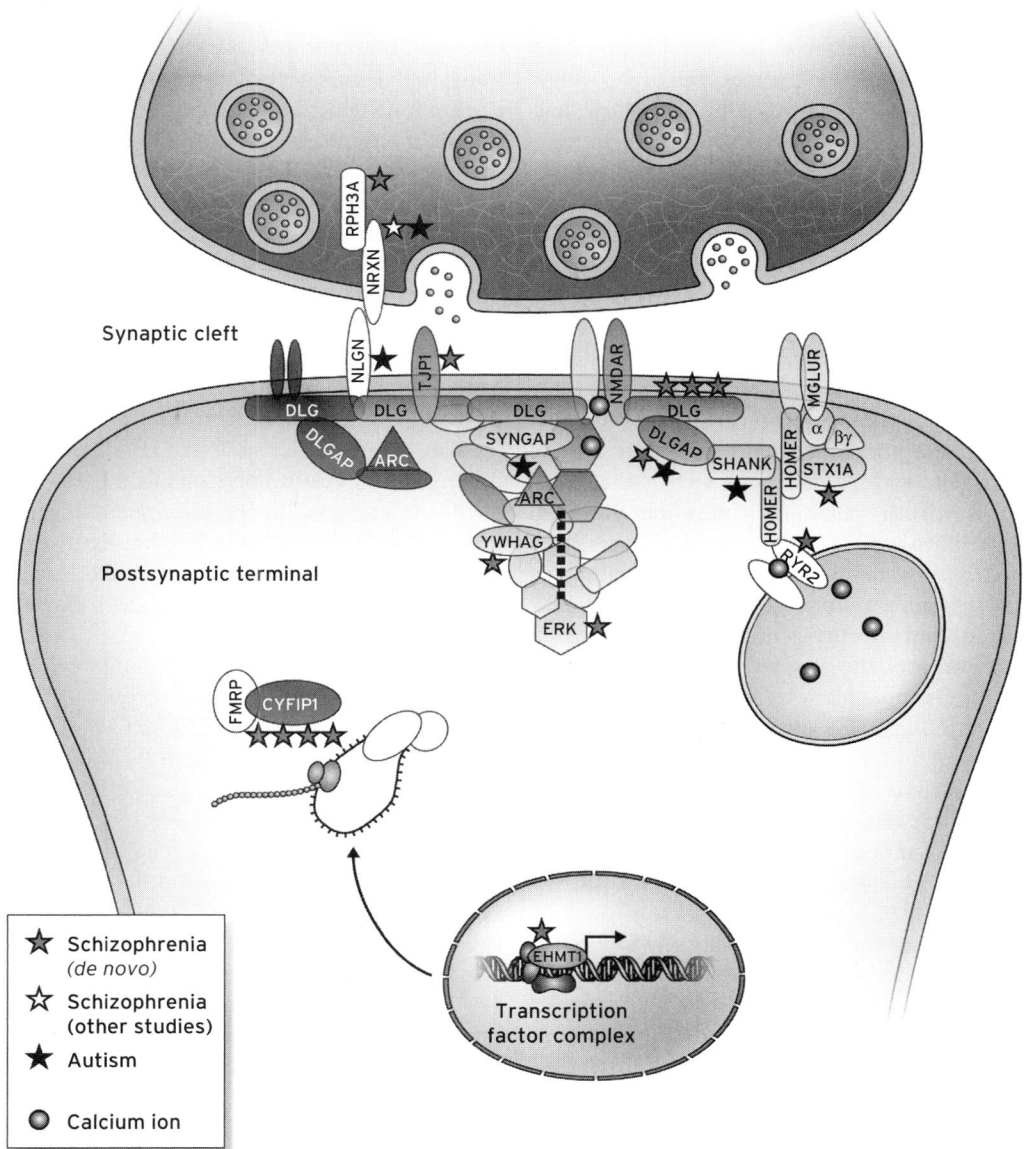

Figure 24.4 *Schizophrenia and autism mutations at the synapse. Schematic of the synapse proteome showing individual proteins and complexes impacted by mutations in schizophrenia and autism. From a study of de novo copy number variation in 662 schizophrenia proband-parent trios (Kirov et al., 2012) multiple mutations in MASC proteins were found (indicated by gray star). Other studies of schizophrenia and autism have identified mutations in the same sets of proteins (light and dark stars respectively) (See Table 24.1). These disease mutations also impact on presynaptic proteins including those linked to MASC across the synaptic cleft by the adhesion proteins. Within the postsynaptic terminal the complex formed by FMRP and CYFIP1 that controls protein translation is shown with mRNA. This complex is important in schizophrenia and autism (Fragile X Mental Retardation) for controlling synthesis of MASC and PSD proteins. Calcium ions are important in activating postsynaptic signaling proteins in the complexes and these flow into the cytoplasm from the synaptic cleft via the NMDA receptor and other membrane channels as well as from internal membrane-bound stores. The transcription factor complexes in the nucleus are also shown. Individual shapes are specific proteins and relevant names are included and correspond to Table 24.1.*

(over 100) phenotypes were caused by mutations in more than one PSD gene and some of these involved large subsets of genes. For example, 40 known mutations cause mental retardation, 29 cause seizures, and 20 cause spasticity. These kinds of studies were also performed in mice, where the genetic mutations are well controlled and the phenotypes accurately measured with similar results. For example, 57 postsynaptic gene mutations result in learning and memory phenotypes, 38 in emotion, and 21 in the phenotype of impaired social interaction.

This large-scale phenotype mapping shows that the symptoms and signs that are the diagnostic features of a disease will depend on which subset of PSD proteins is disrupted. For example, mutations affecting a "cognitive subset of proteins" will result in more cognitive symptoms, and mutations in a "motor subset" will present with more motor symptoms. This is shown in Fig. 24.5, where subnetworks of the postsynaptic proteome comprising interacting proteins control these different phenotypes. Because a protein may be in two phenotype networks, a single mutation can produce two phenotypes. Thus

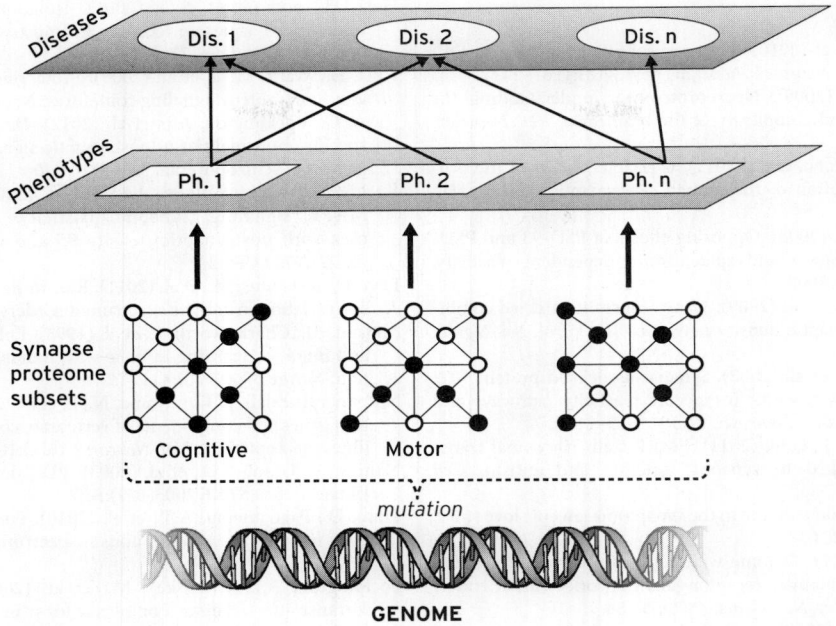

Figure 24.5 *Diseases are sets of phenotypes regulated by sets of proteins. Any single disease is defined by a set of clinical symptoms and signs or phenotypes. Proteins in complexes are interconnected (shown by synapse proteome subsets where each protein is a circle) and mutations in subsets of these proteins (shaded circles) cause specific phenotypes (e.g., cognitive or motor, as indicated). Mutations at the level of the genome produce the altered protein function within these proteins. This hierarchy aims to explain how multiple different gene mutations result in disease phenotypes through their convergent effect on specific subsets of proteins within the synapse proteome.*

the phenotype spectrum or constellation is dependent not only on the gene, but also on the interactions of its encoded protein with other synaptic proteins. These subsets also help explain why some phenotypes are common to multiple diseases. From this outline, it will be possible in future to develop a molecular categorization of PSD diseases mapping diseases and phenotypes onto protein complexes or networks of PSD proteins.

These studies of the genetic and proteomic architecture of the whole postsynaptic proteome also apply to sets of proteins found in physical complexes such as MASC, and reveal their role in the etiology of multiple diseases. As shown in Table 24.1 and Fig. 24.4, disruption of the different proteins in MASC results in a set of diseases. This indicates a common molecular etiology at the level of the multiprotein complexes for diseases that have heretofore been considered to be separate. This helps explain why these diseases are similar and in some instances very difficult to distinguish, as well as why the same gene mutation can be found in two diseases.

FUTURE PERSPECTIVES

The present era of psychiatry is one where genome sequencing is having a major impact by identifying DNA variants in disease. It is clear that genetic based diagnosis will be a major asset in the future, but alone will not be sufficient for classification of the disease. It will also be necessary to use new behavioral diagnostic approaches that go beyond interviews, such as the computerized touchscreen based methods of cognitive testing (Barnett et al., 2010; Nithianantharajah et al., 2012). Together

with genome sequencing, there will be a more definitive definition of both the underlying molecular mechanisms as well as phenotypic characteristics that may indicate degree or extent of disease progression. These types of measure will also be necessary to assess outcomes in clinical trials.

The identification of the phenotypes that comprise the disease (sometimes called endophenotypes) and their specific molecular basis will focus attention on new therapeutic targets. Targets that are within the subsets of proteins controlling a phenotype could be used to treat all the diseases that share that phenotype. Progress in this area will require more research toward understanding the organization of the sets of proteins into multiprotein complexes and new types of drug screening assays.

The recognition that synaptopathies are important in neurology and psychiatry and in pediatric disorders of the nervous system suggests that there are avenues for changing the structure of clinical training programs around synapses. Clinicians who are experts on synaptic diseases could cross the traditional boundaries between psychiatry and neurology. This would require training programs based on fundamental neuroscience of synapses together with a rigorous understanding of human genetics.

DISCLOSURE

Dr. Grant serves on the Board of Synome Ltd. and does not receive financial compensation or salary support for his participation. He receives grant support from the European Union and the Medical Research Council.

REFERENCES

Barnett, J.H., Robbins, T.W., et al. (2010). Assessing cognitive function in clinical trials of schizophrenia. *Neurosci. Biobehav. Rev.* 34(8):1161–1177.

Bayes, A., and Grant, S.G. (2009). Neuroproteomics: understanding the molecular organization and complexity of the brain. *Nat. Rev. Neurosci.* 10(9):635–646.

Bayes, A., van de Lagemaat, L.N., et al. (2011). Characterization of the proteome, diseases and evolution of the human postsynaptic density. *Nat. Neurosci.* 14(1):19–21.

Carlisle, H.J., Fink, A.E., et al. (2008). Opposing effects of PSD-93 and PSD-95 on long-term potentiation and spike timing-dependent plasticity. *J. Physiol.* 586(Pt 24):5885–5900.

Coba, M.P., Pocklington, A.J., et al. (2009). Neurotransmitters drive combinatorial multistate postsynaptic density networks. [*In Vitro*]. *Sci. Signal.* 2(68):ra19.

Cuthbert, P.C., Stanford, L.E., et al. (2007). Synapse-associated protein 102/dlgh3 couples the NMDA receptor to specific plasticity pathways and learning strategies. [*In Vitro*]. *J. Neurosci.* 27(10):2673–2682.

Darnell, J.C., Van Driesche, S.J., et al. (2011). FMRP stalls ribosomal translocation on mRNAs linked to synaptic function and autism. *Cell* 146(2):247–261.

DeFelipe, J. (2010). From the connectome to the synaptome: an epic love story. *Science* 330(6008):1198–1201.

Elia, J., Glessner, J.T., et al. (2011). Genome-wide copy number variation study associates metabotropic glutamate receptor gene networks with attention deficit hyperactivity disorder. *Nat. Genet.* 44(1):78–84.

Emes, R.D., and Grant, S.G. (2012). Evolution of synapse complexity and diversity. *Ann. Rev. Neurosci.* 35:111–131.

Emes, R.D., and Grant, S.G. (2011). The human postsynaptic density shares conserved elements with proteomes of unicellular eukaryotes and prokaryotes. *Front. Neurosci.* 5:44.

Emes, R.D., Pocklington, A.J., et al. (2008). Evolutionary expansion and anatomical specialization of synapse proteome complexity. *Nat. Neurosci.* 11(7):799–806.

Fernandez, E., Collins, M.O., et al. (2009). Targeted tandem affinity purification of PSD-95 recovers core postsynaptic complexes and schizophrenia susceptibility proteins. *Mol. Syst. Biol.* 5:269.

Fernandez, T.V., Sanders, S.J., et al. (2011). Rare copy number variants in Tourette syndrome disrupt genes in histaminergic pathways and overlap with autism. *Biol. Psychiatry* 71(5):392–402.

Frank, R.A., McRae, A.F., et al. (2011). Clustered coding variants in the glutamate receptor complexes of individuals with schizophrenia and bipolar disorder. *PloS One* 6(4):e19011.

Good, M.C., Zalatan, J.G., et al. (2011). Scaffold proteins: hubs for controlling the flow of cellular information. *Science* 332(6030):680–686.

Haas, K.F., and Broadie, K. (2008). Roles of ubiquitination at the synapse. *Biochim. Biophys. Acta* 1779(8):495–506.

Hawrylycz, M.J. (2012). An anatomically comprehensive atlas of the adult human brain transcriptome. *Nature* 489(7416):391–399.

Husi, H., and Grant, S.G. (2001). Isolation of 2000-kDa complexes of N-methyl-D-aspartate receptor and postsynaptic density 95 from mouse brain. *J. Neurochem.* 77(1):281–291.

Husi, H., Ward, M.A., et al. (2000). Proteomic analysis of NMDA receptor-adhesion protein signaling complexes. *Nat. Neurosci.* 3(7):661–669.

Kirov, G., Pocklington, A.J., et al. (2012). *De novo* CNV analysis implicates specific abnormalities of postsynaptic signalling complexes in the pathogenesis of schizophrenia. *Mol. Psychiatry* 17(2):142–153.

Komiyama, N.H., Watabe, A.M., et al. (2002). SynGAP regulates ERK/MAPK signaling, synaptic plasticity, and learning in the complex with postsynaptic density 95 and NMDA receptor. *J. Neurosci.* 22(22):9721–9732.

Levy, D., Ronemus, M., et al. (2011). Rare *de novo* and transmitted copy-number variation in autistic spectrum disorders. *Neuron* 70(5):886–897.

Migaud, M., Charlesworth, P., et al. (1998). Enhanced long-term potentiation and impaired learning in mice with mutant postsynaptic density-95 protein. *Nature* 396(6710):433–439.

Nithianantharajah, J., Komiyama, N.H., et al. (2013). Synaptic scaffold evolution generated components of vertebrate cognitive complexity and mental illness susceptibility. *Nat. Neurosci.* 16(1):16–24.

Nourry, C., Grant, S.G., et al. (2003). PDZ domain proteins: plug and play! [Review]. *Sci. STKE* 2003(179):RE7.

Pinto, D., Pagnamenta, A.T., et al. (2010). Functional impact of global rare copy number variation in autism spectrum disorders. *Nature* 466(7304):368–372.

Pocklington, A.J., Cumiskey, M., et al. (2006). The proteomes of neurotransmitter receptor complexes form modular networks with distributed functionality underlying plasticity and behaviour. *Mol. Syst. Biol.* 2:2006.0023.

Robinson, P.N., and Mundlos, S. (2010). The human phenotype ontology. [Review]. *Clin. Genet.* 77(6):525–534.

Schenck, A., Bardoni, B., et al. (2001). A highly conserved protein family interacting with the fragile X mental retardation protein (FMRP) and displaying selective interactions with FMRP-related proteins FXR1P and FXR2P. *Proc. Natl. Acad. Sci. USA* 98(15):8844–8849.

Shchelochkov, O.A., Cheung, S.W., et al. (2010). Genomic and clinical characteristics of microduplications in chromosome 17. [Review]. *Am. J. Med. Genet. Part A* 152A(5):1101–1110.

Steward, O., Falk, P.M., et al. (1996). Ultrastructural basis for gene expression at the synapse: synapse-associated polyribosome complexes. *J. Neurocytology* 25(12):717–734.

Sudhof, T.C., and Rizo, J. (2011). Synaptic vesicle exocytosis. *Cold Spring Harb Perspect. Biol.* 3(12).

Vissers, L.E., de Ligt, J., et al. (2010). A *de novo* paradigm for mental retardation. *Nat. Genet.* 42(12):1109–1112.

Zalfa, F., Achsel, T., et al. (2006). mRNPs, polysomes or granules: FMRP in neuronal protein synthesis. *Curr. Opin. Neurobiol.* 16(3):265–269.

Zalfa, F., Eleuteri, B., et al. (2007). A new function for the fragile X mental retardation protein in regulation of PSD-95 mRNA stability. *Nat. Neurosci.* 10(5):578–587.

25 | NEURODEVELOPMENT AND SCHIZOPHRENIA

ESTER J. KWON,* TAKAHIRO SODA,* AND LI-HUEI TSAI

INTRODUCTION

Schizophrenia affects approximately 1% of the world's population and is a major contributor to both years lost to disability and health care costs. Despite the significant impetus to understand the etiology of schizophrenia and to develop therapeutics to ease the burden of disease, progress has been limited. This may be due to the complexity of the underlying genetics as well as heterogeneity within and between psychiatric diagnoses. What is clear is that there is a genetic component to schizophrenia risk as well as environmental factors that are important for the manifestation of disease. At this point, the genetic causes of schizophrenia remain largely elusive except for highly penetrant but rare variants, which account only for a small fraction of schizophrenia cases. The most notable example is disrupted in schizophrenia-1 (DISC1), which was identified in a Scottish family with a near Mendelian inheritance of psychiatric diseases. Although rare variants are not the genetic cause of schizophrenia for the vast majority of cases, they may be instructive for the identification of underlying pathways that are dysregulated in schizophrenia.

A NEURODEVELOPMENTAL MODEL OF SCHIZOPHRENIA

A neurodevelopmental model of schizophrenia has been hypothesized by numerous researchers. This model postulates that some of the key aspects of brain development that normally occur both pre- and postnatally are not occurring correctly, either in time or space. Complex neural circuitry needs to form and be modulated by experience. Classically, proliferation, migration, arborization and myelination occur prenatally. Elaboration and refining of dendritic trees and synapses as well as myelination of the nervous system continues through the first two-decades of life. There are opportunities for genetic and environmental abnormalities and variation to profoundly influence the trajectories of all of these critical functional processes. Temporal correlation is noted between the prodromal aspects of schizophrenia, in particular abnormalities in cognition and in the neuroanatomic development of regions of the cerebral cortex. As reviewed in earlier chapters, there is some evidence suggesting that reduced interneuron activity may be involved. Some of the key evidence that developmental processes are awry and their potential causes is reviewed in the following and in the subsequent two chapters.

ENVIRONMENTAL EFFECTS DURING DEVELOPMENT

The 50% concordance of schizophrenia between monozygotic twins demonstrates that there is a clear genetic component to disease onset, and the incomplete concordance highlights that there are also other factors in play. Many epidemiological observations associated with increased risk of schizophrenia suggest exposures that might influence brain development. For a comprehensive review see Brown (2011).

Significant effort has been put into correlating pre- and perinatal disturbances to the development of schizophrenia. Numerous studies have linked phenomena such as maternal nutrition and infection, season of birth, and obstetrical complications to the manifestation of schizophrenia later in life (Lewis and Levitt, 2002). Studies of children born from mothers who were in early pregnancy during the Dutch Hunger winter have shown association with schizophrenia, as well as with depression and mood disorders, increasing the risk of schizophrenia approximately twofold. The association of famine with schizophrenia was also observed in the 1959–1961 Chinese famines in two separate regions, Liuzhou and Wuhu (Rapoport et al., 2012). Improvements in imaging technology and longitudinal studies with collection of tissue and blood samples will aid the understanding of how these factors contribute to schizophrenia onset in the future.

An example of association with an environmental factor that may be present during adolescence, and that has now been replicated in several carefully controlled studies is being in a minority group position. Studies examining association of schizophrenia with being in a minority group position show that development of psychosis is dependent on the proportion of their own ethnic group present in the area. Furthermore, the association is seen in first- and second-generation migrants and across several ethnic groups, indicating that it is not the ethnicity or migration itself that is causing the association. Other examples include growing up in an urban environment and experiencing developmental trauma (van Os et al., 2010). These three factors clearly have components of stress, although it is still not understood what types of stress and during which developmental times stresses occur that are related to the onset of psychosis. In addition to these environmental factors, there are also examples of more acute triggers that track with schizophrenia. A meta-analysis of people who have antibodies to toxoplasma gondii has found associations to schizophrenia that replicated previous findings, showing that toxoplasma gondii infection conferred an odds ratio of ~2.7 (Torrey et al., 2012).

* Authors contributed equally and are presented in alphabetical order.

The presence of antibodies indicated an infection up to the point of analysis, which was after onset of disease; work remains to be done pinpointing whether there is a time window of infection that is relevant for the development of psychosis. Another factor thought to be associated with the onset of psychosis is the use of cannabis. Although reverse causation is a concern when studying cannabis use, a meta-analysis of studies where baseline psychosis was a criterion for exclusion found that there was an increased risk of psychosis with cannabis use associated with an odds ratio of 1.4 (Moore et al., 2007).

Each of these associations implicate periods of stress, for example, nutritional, immunological, or social, in the onset of schizophrenia. These associated factors serve as proxies for what stimulus is really affecting the molecular basis of schizophrenia progression, which remains to be uncovered in future studies. Epigenetics (e.g., DNA methylation, histone acetylation, and noncoding RNA) has been shown to be able to have a strong influence in the case of maternal nutrition and the development of obesity and diabetes and may be important in the role of neurodevelopmental influences in schizophrenia (Bale et al., 2010).

NEUROPATHOLOGY ASSOCIATED WITH SCHIZOPHRENIA

The macroscopic phenotypes that have most predictably tracked with schizophrenia are ventricular enlargement and slight reductions in brain volume and weight as measured in whole brain imaging studies or in postmortem samples (Lawrie and Abukmeil, 1998). Other endophenotypes of schizophrenia include structural changes in various brain regions, changes in gray matter volume, cortical thickness, and neuronal integrity (Harrison and Weinberger, 2005).

Brain imaging studies of rare childhood onset schizophrenia cases (1/500 cases of schizophrenia), which are often similar to more severe outcomes of schizophrenia, provide an opportunity to understand how brain development may be perturbed in schizophrenia, and they are less likely to be influenced by environmental factors such as substance abuse, which is known to cause structural changes to the brain. Longitudinal studies were conducted starting in 1991 at the NIMH, where more than 100 child-onset schizophrenia patients and their siblings underwent brain imaging four–five times every two years. The average age of onset was 10 years, and there was an equal distribution between males and females (Gogtay et al., 2011). These studies show that phenotypes are preserved between child and adult onset schizophrenia, such as increased lateral ventricular sizes, and decreased overall gray matter, hippocampus, and amygdala volumes (Gogtay and Rapoport, 2008). In the course of normal development, gray matter volumes follow an inverted U-shape curve, where they increase throughout childhood and peak at puberty, whereas white matter volumes steadily increase into adulthood. The NIH longitudinal study showed that in child onset schizophrenia gray matter loss occurs throughout development and that white matter development is retarded when compared with control cases. These data support the concept that schizophrenia is a progressive disease with perturbations throughout neurodevelopment that lead up to its onset in early adulthood.

Another longitudinal study was conducted on ultra-high-risk schizophrenia candidates, as determined by their mental health state and family history of mental illness, in Melbourne, Australia (Gogtay et al., 2011). The candidates were on average 19 years of age and 40% developed schizophrenia within 12 months of the initiation of the study, allowing for the imaging of brains and discovery of perturbations during the period of onset between those candidates who developed psychosis and those who did not. They found that there was gray matter loss in the left medial and inferior temporal regions, the anterior cingulated cortex, and in the left orbitofrontal cortex in patients who developed psychosis, which was not seen in those who did not develop psychosis (Gogtay et al., 2011).

Although there is a decrease in brain volume, a significant change in number of neurons has not been observed. One hypothesis is that the decrease in volume is due to the loss of neuronal processes, such as axons, dendrites, and dendritic spines, referred to collectively as the neuropil. Analyses of postmortem brains have shown a marked decrease in dendritic spines in schizophrenic patients when compared with controls, especially in cortical pyramidal neurons (Garey, 2010). A diffusion-weighted magnetic resonance imaging technique called diffusion tensor imaging (DTI) is used to image fiber pathways and connection integrity of white matter in living subjects. In white matter, the flow of water is largely restricted to the tracts and therefore has directionality that can be used as a proxy for the integrity of the fibers.

Before the onset of the majority of schizophrenia cases in late adolescence/early adulthood, there are cognitive deficits that can be observed before diagnosis is made (Gold and Weinberger, 1995). Furthermore, these cognitive deficits are found in undiagnosed family members who have not been exposed to treatment, indicating that there is a genetic disposition for cognitive dysfunction that may be used as a hallmark of severity of disease. The most consistent finding resulting from functional magnetic resonance imaging (fMRI) studies in schizophrenic patients is changes in activity in the dorsolateral prefrontal cortex (DLPFC) during working memory tasks. Schizophrenic patients have decreased performance on working memory tasks, which is correlated with decreased activity in the DLPFC. One nuance is that for tasks in which schizophrenic patients have similar performance as control subjects, there is an increased activity in the DLPFC (Lewis et al., 2005). The impairment in working memory has led investigators to posit several hypotheses based on neurotransmitters and connectivity.

OLIGODENDROCYCTES, MYELIN, DEVELOPMENT, AND SCHIZOPHRENIA

White matter integrity is measured in DTI by fractional anisotrophy, which is representative of myelination and tract organization. Over the many DTI studies performed on schizophrenia cohorts, there are decreases in fractional anisotrophy measurements in white matter across many brain

regions, most consistently in the cingulate, corpus callosum, and frontal lobes (Thomason and Thompson, 2011). Moreover, in a study of prodromal ultra-high-risk psychosis candidates, there were decreases in fractional anisotrophy that preceded disease onset (Karlsgodt et al., 2009). In addition, there is a well-characterized reduction in expression of oligodendrocytes and myelin related genes in postmortem brain samples. Structural analyses in postmortem brain have also shown both a decreased density of oligodendrocytes and damaged myelin sheaths in schizophrenia cases compared to controls. Furthermore, a wide variety of candidate genes involved in oligodendrocyte development have found modest associations with increased risk of schizophrenia (see Takahashi et al., 2011, for review).

The temporal process of myelination is correlated with the developmental trajectory of schizophrenia. Myelination is incomplete at birth and develops gradually, with some cortical areas not being completed until adulthood. For example, regions expected to be of particular relevance to schizophrenia such as cortical and hippocampal pathways are not fully myelinated until adulthood. Diseases whose primary pathology is in white matter, such as the leukodystrophies, are often accompanied by psychosis, which suggests a shared altered basic role for myelination and oligodendrocytes. Furthermore, an appealing hypothesis is that oligodendrocyte and myelin dysfunction exerts its role in schizophrenia by altering key features of synaptic activity such as synaptic plasticity or the production of synchronous oscillating activities implicated in establishing aspects of cognition (Walterfang et al., 2011).

NEUROTRANSMITTERS AND ANTIPSYCHOTIC DRUGS

There are several theories associating dysfunction of neurotransmitter pathways and schizophrenia based on neuropharmacological studies, which include the GABA, NMDA, and dopamine theories. It is important to note that none of these are theories are exclusive, neither among themselves nor to the other theories presented, which will be discussed in a subsequent chapter.

Antipsychotic drugs used to treat schizophrenia are effective in mitigating the positive symptoms, such as hallucinations and delusions. The first widely used antipsychotic, chlorpromazine, blocks the dopamine D2 receptor. Derivative first- and second-generation antipsychotics by and large also target the dopamine D2 receptor. Though the D2 receptor has been generally established as the site of action for antipsychotics, the mechanism of action is less clear. There are several pathways downstream of the dopamine D2 receptor, and it is becoming apparent that the localization of dopamine D2 receptor interaction proteins, in addition to the location of the D2 receptor itself, may impact which downstream pathways become affected.

The D2 receptor acts as a classical G protein–coupled receptor, and has been associated with the $G\alpha i/o\ G\beta\gamma$ heterotrimeric G protein complex. Activation of this pathway is associated with the inhibition of downstream cAMP signaling. Coupling of these receptors to presynaptic K^+ channels has been shown to lead to the inhibition of neurotransmitter release. In addition, it has been reported that these receptors and D1/D2 heterooligomeric receptors activate downstream Ca^{2+} signaling via coupling to $GqG\beta\gamma$ and the activation of phospholipase C.

The D2 receptor has also been shown to activate another signaling pathway, the phosphatidylinositol (3,4,5)-triphosphate kinase (PI3K)/AKT/mammalian Target of Rapamycin (mTOR) pathway, a pathway that regulates the Wnt signaling cascade. The P13K/AKT/mTor pathway is also activated by another class of membrane-bound receptors, the receptor tyrosine kinases. In the baseline state, AKT is bound to phosphatidylinositol(3, 4)-bisphosphate (PIP2). Upon activation of a receptor tyrosine kinase or a G protein–coupled receptor, PI3K phosphorylates PIP2 to form PIP3. AKT bound to PIP3 is then phosphorylated by mTOR complex 2 (mTORC2), then phosphorylated by phosphinositide dependent kinase 1 (PDPK1). The phosphorylation by both kinases activates AKT to then phosphorylate its many downstream targets, including mTOR (implicated in autism), GSK3β (involved in the Wnt signaling cascade), BAD (a pro-apoptotic mitochondrial protein), and IκB kinase (IKK; regulator of NFκB mediated transcription).

The intersection of the AKT pathway with the pharmacology of psychiatric disorder treatment is notable. Dopamine D2 receptors have been shown to modulate AKT signaling by recruiting a signaling complex that results in the inactivation of AKT. Upon D2 receptor activation and phosphorylation by G protein–coupled receptor kinase (GRK), β-arrestin and protein phosphatase 2A (PP2A) are recruited to the cell membrane, where they interact with and dephosphorylate AKT. Antipsychotics, which are antagonists to the D2 receptor, block this signaling cascade and allow AKT to remain active (Freyberg et al., 2010).

Lithium, a treatment for bipolar disorder that can also be prescribed in conjunction with antipsychotics for the treatment of schizophrenia, is shown to lead to inhibition of glycogen synthase kinase β (GSK3β). It has been shown that lithium activates AKT to phosphorylate GSK3β, leading to GSK3β inhibition. Lithium has also been proposed to solubilize AKT from the β-arrestin/PP2A complex, which mediates portions of downstream D2 receptor signaling functions (Beaulieu, 2012). Thus, both antipsychotic and lithium treatments secondarily affect the Wnt pathway via affecting AKT activity.

RARE AND COMMON GENETIC VARIATION IN SCHIZOPHRENIA

Recent genetic evidence has found that *de novo* duplications and deletions of DNA, termed copy number variations (CNVs), increase the risk of schizophrenia. As noted in an earlier chapter, many of these CNVs have been associated with a wide variety of developmental phenotypes. One early CNV study found novel CNVs greater than 100 kilobases in schizophrenic patients and their families and found an increased number of CNVs in patients, with a disproportionate number in genes related to neurodevelopmental pathways (Walsh et al., 2008).

International collaborative efforts have resulted in findings from genome-wide association studies (GWASs) with cohorts on the scale of tens of thousands of control and schizophrenia cases (Ripke et al., 2011; Stefansson et al., 2009). While further GWAS findings are anticipated, even the early studies suggest that there may be some convergence of gene candidates involved in neurodevelopmental phenomena and synaptic processes. The haploinsufficiency of one identified gene identified as genome-wide significant by GWAS, *TCF4*, leads to Pitt-Hopkins mental retardation in humans (Brockschmidt et al., 2007) and is also involved in the specification of specific subsets of neural progenitors in the mouse (Flora et al., 2007). Another genome-wide significant GWAS identified gene, *CACNA1C*, encodes a subunit of an L-type calcium channel leading to the intriguing theory that there may be aberrant synaptic transmission underlying the brain activation changes observed in functional neuroimaging studies (Bigos et al., 2010). There is a major ongoing effort to understand the biology of schizophrenia GWAS candidates and whether they are dysregulated and/or dysfunctional in the context of human disease.

Collectively, gene candidates of schizophrenia identified by studying both CNVs and common risk SNPs are converging on pathways that regulate neurodevelopmental and synaptic phenomena. It is also important to note that there is emerging evidence of a shared set of risk factors between psychiatric disorders including schizophrenia and bipolar, as well as autism. There are also several recurrent CNVs that are common between schizophrenic and autistic patients, such as 1q21.1, 15q11.2, 15q13.3, 17q12 (Malhotra and Sebat, 2012; Mefford et al., 2008; Stefansson et al., 2008).

PATHWAYS

Based on the neuropharmacology and neuropathological findings, there have been several theories suggested to understand the etiology of schizophrenia including the GABA, dopamine, and glutamate hypotheses. Although each of these pathways is likely to contribute to and/or be resultant from schizophrenia pathology, none alone is sufficient to explain the onset of disease and the presence of the spectrum of symptoms displayed by schizophrenic patients. An alternative way of understanding the etiology of schizophrenia and disease-associated genetic loci is to examine their involvement in dysregulated biochemical pathways. One such study compared significant and non-significant SNPs from the International Schizophrenia Consortium to pathways described in the Kyoto Encyclopaedia of Genes and Genomes (O'Dushlaine et al., 2011). The only significantly associated pathway found was the cell-adhesion molecule pathway, which is important for synaptic formation and cell signaling. One caveat to this approach is that the functions of many genes identified in CNV and GWAS studies are yet unknown, and thus insights gained from these types of analyses are just emerging. It may therefore be more fruitful at this early stage of understanding schizophrenia genetics to specify genes that are unmistakably linked to disease and study

their function as a starting point to understand the context of common risk alleles that have lower effect sizes and occur in complex constellations.

As noted earlier, perturbation of neurodevelopmental processes in schizophrenia is a theory that is accumulating supporting evidence. There are pre- and perinatal environmental factors described in the preceding that are thought to associate with risk of schizophrenia as well as the changes in neuroanatomical structures and cognition observed before the manifestation of disease. There are also many gene candidates of neuropsychiatric disease that perturb biochemical pathways associated with neurogenesis and neuronal migration as well as spine morphogenesis, which are discussed in the following and are summarized in Table 25.1. The confluence of genetic and environmental factors on neurodevelopmental pathways is depicted in Figure 25.1.

EARLY DEVELOPMENT PATHWAYS

DISC1

DISC1 was identified in a Scottish pedigree in which it was disrupted by a balanced translocation, t(1:11)(q42.1;q14.3). The translocation segregated with psychiatric disorders such as schizophrenia, major depression, and bipolar disease with a combined OR 7.1. Mouse models expressing a transgene of human DISC1 recapitulating the Scottish translocation exhibit increased ventricle size, decreased gray matter volume, and changes in dendritic arborization in cortical and hippocampal neurons, mimicking the endophenotypes found in humans. Mouse models of DISC1 and their neuroanatomical, behavioral, and cellular phenotypes are summarized in the review by Jaaro-Peled (2009). The mice also exhibit behavioral abnormalities such as hyperactivity, increased immobility in the forced swim test, decreased sociability, and impaired working memory. Mouse models have also been demonstrated to have reduced embryonic and adult hippocampal neurogenesis. DISC1 is also implicated in proper integration of newborn neurons in the adult dentate gyrus.

DISC1 is a pleiotropic protein with numerous interaction partners affecting multiple biochemical signaling pathways that impact neuronal development and function. Some validated interacting partners for DISC1 include NDE1, NDEL1, LIS1, Kalirin-7, ATF4/5, GSK3β, and the PDE4 family of phosphodiesterases. The study of DISC1 is instructive since it is implicated in psychiatric disease and has a major role in early developmental phenomena and synaptic pathways.

WNT PATHWAY

The Wnt family consists of 19 secreted lipoproteins that act as morphogens and play important roles in the development and patterning of various limbs and organs. Wnts bind to their cell surface receptor, the Frizzled (Fz) family of seven transmembrane G protein–coupled receptors, of which 10 have been identified to date. The various Wnt and Fz proteins have

TABLE 25.1. Genetic loci, effect size, affected genes, and their known role in neuronal development. A select table highlighting the known risk loci with putative effects on genes affecting neuronal development

GENETIC ASSOCIATION	DISEASE[a]	OR[b]	CANDIDATE GENE	NEURODEVELOPMENTAL PHENOMENON	REFERENCES
CNV (3q29)	SCZ, ASD	49.5	DLG1	Wnt pathway	Mulle et al. (2010)
CNV (3q29)	SCZ, ASD	49.5	PAK2	Wnt pathway	Mulle et al. (2010), Zhou et al. (2011)
CNV (22q11.2)	SCZ, ASD	21	TBX1	Wnt pathway, Wnt transcription target	Hiramoto et al. (2011), Huh and Ornitz (2010), Paylor et al. (2006)
CNV (17q12)	ASD	18.4	ADA2A	Wnt pathway	Yang et al. (2008)
CNV (1q21.1)	SCZ, ASD, micro-/macrocephaly	9.2	BCL9	Wnt pathway	Malhotra and Sebat (2012), Mefford et al. (2008), Stefansson et al. (2008)
t(1:11)(q42.1;q14.3)	SCZ, MD, BP	7.1	DISC1	Wnt pathway, neurogenesis, neuronal migration, synaptic morphology	Brandon and Sawa (2011), Jaaro-Peled (2009), Mao et al. (2009), Ming and Song (2009)
rs10761482, rs10994359	BP, SCZ	1.15	ANK3	Wnt pathway, synaptic transmission	Orsulic et al. (1999), Ripke et al. (2011)
rare missense mutations	ASD	NA	CHD8	Wnt pathway	Neale et al. (2012), O'Roak et al. (2012)
mutations	SCZ	NA	ERBB4/NRG1	Wnt pathway, neuronal migration, synaptic morphology	Muraoka-Cook et al. (2009)
rs17512836	SCZ, microcephaly	1.15	TCF4	progenitor specification	Brockschmidt et al. (2007), Flora et al. (2007), Ripke et al. (2011), Stefansson et al. (2009)
CNV (16p13.1)	SCZ, ASD	9.8	NDE1	neuronal migration	Bradshaw et al. (2011), Ingason et al. (2011)
rs7004633	SCZ	1.11	MMP16	Wnt transcription target, neurite outgrowth	Lowy et al. (2006)
CNV (16p11.2)	SCZ, ASD	9.8	TAOK2	dendritic morphology	de Anda et al. (2012), McCarthy et al. (2009)
CNV (22q11.2)	SCZ, ASD	21	DCGR8	spine morphology	Karayiorgou et al. (2010)
GWAS, mutations	SCZ	2.07	KALRN	spine morphology	Brandon and Sawa (2011), Kushima et al. (2012), Ma et al. (2003), Ma et al. (2008a), Ma et al. (2008b)
rs1625579	SCZ	1.12	MIR137	spine morphology	Ripke et al. (2011), Smrt et al. (2010), Sun et al. (2011), Szulwach et al. (2010)
rs4765905	BP, SCZ	1.09	CACNA1C	synaptic transmission	Bigos et al. (2010), Ripke et al. (2011)
rs1807809	BP, SCZ	1.15	NRGN	synaptic transmission	Stefansson et al. (2009)

distinct and overlapping patterns throughout the body, which is thought to account for the variability of phenotypes that result upon loss of function, and multiple downstream pathways have been shown to be activated downstream of Wnt binding.

CANONICAL WNT SIGNALING

The canonical Wnt signaling pathway is defined by the involvement of the transcriptional coactivator β-catenin and the downstream signaling cascades that are associated with it. β-catenin is normally confined to the cell membrane as part of the adherens junctions complex in neuronal progenitors in the central nervous system. Upon Wnt ligand binding, Fz proteins bind to disheveled proteins (Dvl). In the absence of Wnt binding, Dvl is part of a destruction complex in conjunction with axis inhibitor (Axin), adenomatous polyposis coli (APC), casein kinase 1 alpha (CK1α), and GSK3β. This destruction complex binds and phosphorylates β-catenin at multiple sites, designating it for proteosomal degradation and preventing the accumulation of β-catenin in the absence of Wnt. In the presence of Wnt stimulation, Fz-associated Dvl polymerizes and binds Axin through DIX domains. Axin binding recruits

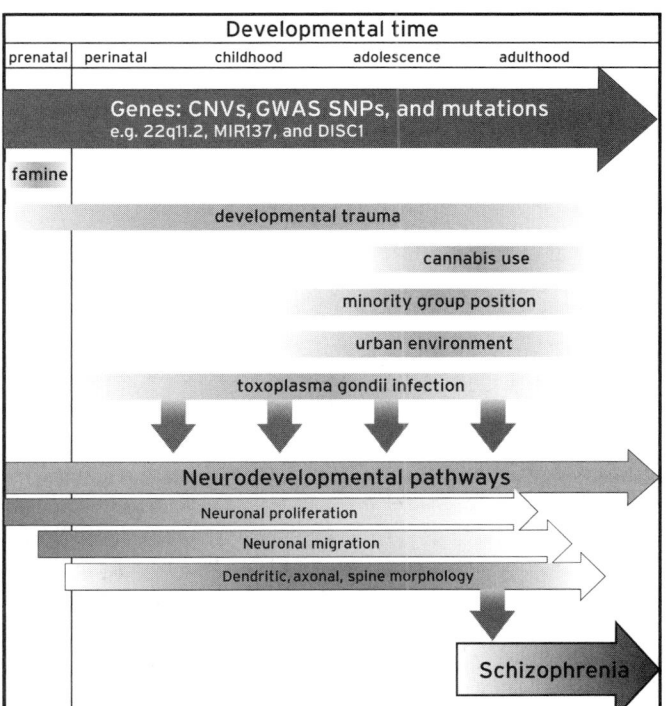

Figure 25.1 Factors that influence schizophrenia. Genes and environmental components affect neurodevelopmental pathways throughout life spans.

CK1α and GSK3β to the LRP5/6 complex, resulting in their phosphorylation and increased affinity for Axin. The interaction with LRP5/6 directly inhibits the phosphorylation of β-catenin by GSK3β, allowing for the cytosolic accumulation of β-catenin and its subsequent nuclear localization.

In the nucleus, β-catenin acts as a transcriptional co-activator of the T-cell factor and lymphoid enhancer-binding protein (TCF/LEF) transcription factors, which control the dynamics of the cell cycle partly via the regulation of cyclinD1. TCF/LEF has three identified domains: a high mobility group (HMG) box domain that is crucial for DNA interaction, a caspase activated deoxyribonuclease (CAD) domain necessary for binding to Groucho/TLE, and an N-terminal β-catenin binding domain. In the absence of nuclear β-catenin, the TCF/LEF occupying TCF/LEF DNA binding sites is bound to tetrameric Groucho/TLE, which recruits transcriptional repressors, such as histone deacetylases (HDACs), keeping the DNA in a condensed, repressed state. β-catenin directly competes with, and displaces Groucho/TLE (Daniels and Weis, 2005), and recruits general transcriptional activators such as the histone acetyltransferase CBP, the SWI/SNF complex protein Brg-1, and TATA- binding protein, as well as a more specific core complex consisting of Pygopus and Legless/BCL9 (Logan and Nusse, 2004). CBP acetylates histone residues in the promoter region, and the recruitment of Pygopus and Legless/BCL9 leads to the methylation of H3K9 residues by SET-1 methyltransferases, altering the chromatin structure from a condensed, transcriptionally repressed state to a more relaxed and open state, allowing for transcription (Fiedler et al., 2008). A comprehensive review of the Wnt signaling pathway in development can be found here (van Amerongen and Nusse, 2009).

ROLE OF THE CANONICAL WNT SIGNALING PATHWAY IN NEURONAL DEVELOPMENT

Numerous proteins within the canonical Wnt signaling pathway have been linked with neuronal development. GSK3 inactivation, achieved by a conditional knockout of both GSK3α and β resulted in a larger brain with an expansion of the progenitor pool with a concomitant reduction in the thickness of the cortex, indicating that GSK3 promotes progenitor proliferation while suppressing neuronal differentiation (Kim et al., 2009). Overexpression of stabilized β-catenin also results in mice with an increase in brain size, and an increased fraction of cells reentering the cell cycle, essentially phenocopy the GSK3 knockout phenotype, while mice with β-catenin mutations which selectively abolish its transactivation function have defects in forebrain development, accompanied by a decrease in the neuronal progenitor pool (Valenta et al., 2011), reiterating the crucial role of the proteins in the canonical Wnt pathway in the maintenance of the neuronal progenitor pool.

In summary, many factors crucial to the canonical Wnt pathway, as well as numerous interacting proteins with the pathway, have been shown to play crucial roles in neurogenesis, neuronal migration, axon/dendrite growth and morphology, and synaptic development. For a more extensive review of Wnt signaling and development, see Kim and Snider (2011).

DISC1 AND THE WNT SIGNALING PATHWAY

DISC1 has been shown to bind to and inhibit the activity of GSK3β, one of two forms of an enzyme that is known to lead to the phosphorylation of many downstream proteins that are crucial for the pathophysiology of many nervous system disorders. One GSK3β target is TAU, which forms aggregates in many nervous system disorders including Alzheimer's disease (TAU forms the neurofibrillary tangles that are used in the Braak and Braak postmortem staging of disease progress), Parkinson's disease, and tuberous sclerosis. Another GSK3β target is β-catenin, the crucial component of the canonical Wnt signaling pathway. DISC1 promotes the maintenance of the neuronal progenitor pool by inhibiting GSK3β, allowing cytoplasmic β-catenin to accumulate, and transduce canonical Wnt signaling. The loss of DISC1 leads to decreased neuronal progenitor proliferation by promoting early cell cycle exit in neurons (Mao et al., 2009; Ming and Song, 2009). DISC1 provides further evidence that the Wnt signaling pathway may be involved in both neurodevelopment and psychiatric disorders.

WNT PATHWAY AND PSYCHIATRIC DISEASE GENE CANDIDATES

Several players in the Wnt signaling pathways have been associated with psychiatric disease, in addition to DISC1 (Fig. 25.2). Glycosylation is a form of regulation of Wnt ligands and their receptors, and perturbations of glycosylation are known to affect their function, localization, and signaling. SNPs in genes that are involved in glycan synthesis (Kegg pathway: hsa01030) associate with schizophrenia (O'Dushlaine et al., 2011), which raises a possibility that a part of the phenotypes caused by perturbations in this molecular pathway act via disruption of

the Wnt pathway. Furthermore, several candidate genes, such as MMP16 and Tbx1, are transcriptionally regulated via Wnt activation of TCF/LEF transcription (Huh and Ornitz, 2010; Lowy et al., 2006). Mice hemizygous for Tbx1, located in the 22q11.2 microdeletion, display behavioral phenotypes that are associated with psychiatric disease (Hiramoto et al., 2011; Paylor et al., 2006).

Chromodomain helicase DNA binding protein 8 (CHD8), associated with autism in several exome sequencing studies (Neale et al., 2012; O'Roak et al., 2012), is also recruited to TCF/LEF sites along with β-catenin. CHD8 has been shown to counter the activating activity of β-catenin, by binding to β-catenin and also Histone1, and thus limiting the relaxation of chromatin. BCL9, mentioned earlier as a core component of the transcriptional complex mediating Wnt signaling, is one of the genes in the 1q21.1 recurrent CNV, in which microdeletions have been associated with schizophrenia and microcephaly, and microduplications associated with autism and macrocephaly. Furthermore, ADA2A, in the 17q12 microdeletion associated with autism, is known to be an acetyltransferase required for transcriptional activity and proliferative effects mediated by β-catenin (Yang et al., 2008).

Microdeletions of 3q29 have been associated with microencephaly, dysmorphology, and autistic features, and more recently schizophrenia (Mulle et al., 2010). Several genes in this locus have roles in the Wnt pathway. Discs, large homolog 1 (DLG1 or Sap97) is one of the binding partners of Fz and is known to signal downstream of Wnt binding by binding to APC, affecting cell proliferation. p21 protein (Cdc42/Rac)-activated kinase 2 (PAK2), also in the 3q29 CNV, also serves to phosphorylate and promote the nuclear localization of β-catenin (Zhou et al., 2011).

Neuregulin 1 and its receptor ErbB4, are other well-studied candidates found to have SNPs associated with schizophrenia and play roles in neuronal migration and synapse formation (Mei and Xiong, 2008). ErbB4 is a receptor tyrosine kinase, and its family members have been shown to activate cascades that phosphorylate and lead to the intracellular localization of β-catenin: overexpression of ErbB4 Cyt2 increased nuclear β-catenin and TCF-LEF transcriptional activity (Muraoka-Cook et al., 2009).

WNT SIGNALING AND CELL MORPHOLOGIES

Binding of Wnt to Fz leads to activation of pathways involved in planar cell polarity, acting through Dvl, activating RhoA and Ras-related C3 botulinum toxin substrate 1 Rac1 (Gao et al., 2011; Shafer et al., 2011). Rac1 activation then activates c-Jun N-terminal kinase (JNK) downstream of Wnt7b (Rosso et al., 2005). JNK activation has been shown to be crucial for the proper development of axons and dendrites (de Anda et al., 2012; Rosso et al., 2005), and to enhance or inhibit canonical Wnt activation, depending on the Wnt ligand (Billiard et al., 2005). Tao Kinase 2, in the 16p11.2 region, which has CNVs that associate with both autism and schizophrenia (deletion

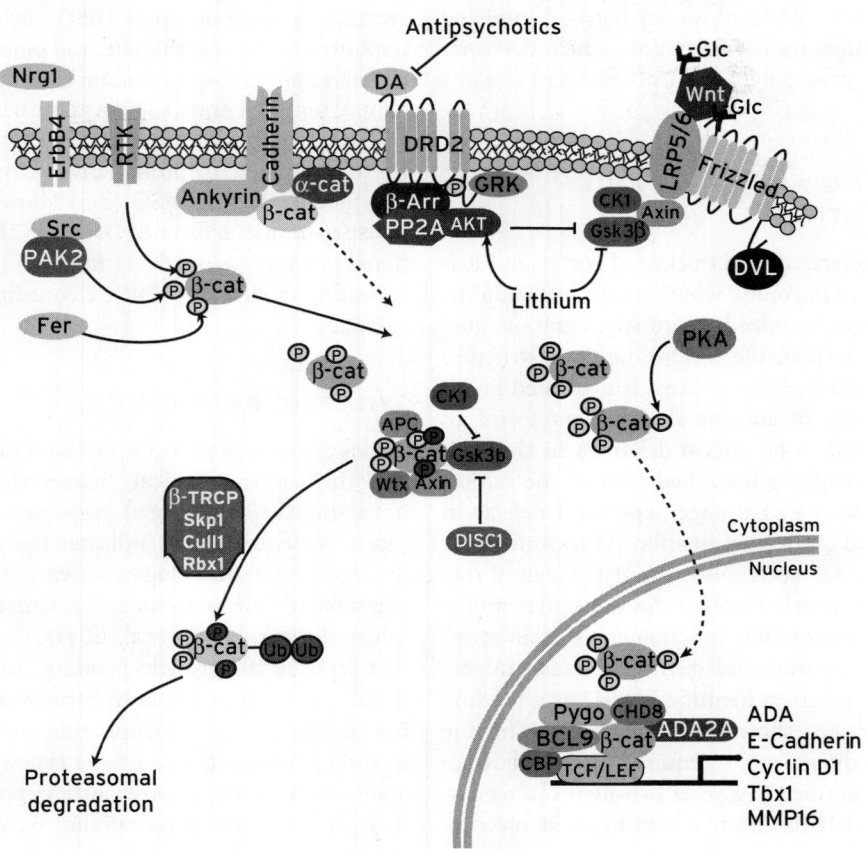

Figure 25.2 *Many genes associated with psychiatric disorders regulate or are regulated by the Wnt signaling pathway.*

and duplication, respectively), also plays a role in the activation of JNK and affects basal dendrite formation (de Anda et al., 2012; McCarthy et al., 2009).

The proteins in the canonical Wnt pathway also have an effect on postmitotic neurons independent of their effect on β-catenin. One of the alternative β-catenin independent pathways that is downstream of LRP5/6- Frizzled signaling depends on the inhibition of GSK3β. GSK3β is known to destabilize microtubules by phosphorylating microtubule proteins such as TAU, MAP1B, and MAP2. Inhibition of GSK3β stabilizes microtubules, promoting axon growth and growth cone remodeling. The phosphorylation of collapsin response mediator protein 2 (CRMP2) by GSK3 is crucial for neuronal polarity, and CRMP2 has been shown to be involved in determining axon/dendrite fate (Yoshimura et al., 2005). Knockdown of Axin results in the abolishment of axon formation in postmitotic neurons. APC, part of the destruction complex in Wnt signaling, also plays a role in neurite extension and neuronal migration. In this manner, the Wnt pathway is able to exert effects on neuronal morphology.

Binding of Wnt to Ryk has been shown to directly activate the Src pathway, similar to the activation of many other receptor tyrosine kinases. The activation of Src, in turn, has been shown to be crucial for axon guidance. Ryk has also been shown to interact directly to Fz8, as well as Dvl, and to potentiate the canonical Wnt signaling pathway, suggesting that the presence of Ryk in conjunction with Fz may either stabilize the Dvl-Fz interaction, or enhance Axin interaction with Fz (Lu et al., 2004). The convergence of neuropharmacological and genetic evidence makes the Wnt pathway(s), if not a promising target, at least a convenient framework within which the function of psychiatric risk gene polymorphisms and rare variants can be tested.

DISC1, ITS BINDING PARTNERS, AND NEURONAL MIGRATION

Lissencephaly is characterized by a thickened cortex and loss of the organized layers of the brain, which results in a smoothened brain. Because synchronized neuronal migration during embryogenesis is responsible for the laminar structure of the brain, it is thought that this process is disrupted in lissencephaly. The majority of autosomal dominant forms of lissencephaly were found to be due to deletions in chromosome 17, where gene mapping identified LIS1 as the critical gene. Mouse models show Lis1-dosage dependent defects in neuronal migration and cortical lamination (Hirotsune et al., 1998). The centrosome has been shown to play a central role in neuronal migration, which involves the molecular motor dynein. Lis1 regulates microtubule function and dynein activity, both of which are coordinated during neuronal migration. A yeast two-hybrid screen identified Ndel1 as a binding partner of Lis1. It has been shown that Ndel1 allows for the interaction of Lis1 and dynein and is required for dynein function. Ndel1 was also identified in a yeast two-hybrid screen to interact with Disc1. Ndel1 has been shown to be involved in neuronal migration, neuronal localization, and neurite and axon development (Kamiya et al., 2006). Disrupting DISC1/

Ndel1 interaction disrupts neurite outgrowth in PC12 cells (Pletnikov et al., 2007), and also prevents the colocalization of DISC1 and Lis1, which localizes with the dynein heavy chain, indicating that DISC1 plays an important role in the function of Ndel1/Lis1 complex by regulating its localization. In addition, Nde1 has also been associated with DISC1/Ndel1/Lis1 to regulate neuronal proliferation, migration, and neurite extension (Bradshaw et al., 2011) and is found in the 16p13.1 CNV (Ingason et al., 2011).

It has been shown that DISC1 also interacts with this complex via its interaction with DIX domain containing-1 (Dixdc1), the third mammalian gene discovered to contain a Disheveled-Axin (DIX) domain (Dixdc1). DISC1, Dixdc1, and Ndel1 form a tripartite interaction, and the presence of either DISC1 or DIXDC1 seems to be able to properly localize Ndel1, indicating that these two proteins may have redundant effects on neuronal migration (Singh et al., 2010). This also indicates that a partial loss of function of either of these two genes can be offset by the function of the other, potentially explaining why differences in the ability of DISC1 variants to bind to Ndel does not result in an appreciable difference in human disease burden.

A molecular switch between the Wnt signaling and neuronal migration function of DISC1 has been recently uncovered (Ishizuka et al., 2011). DISC1 was found to be a target of PKA-mediated phosphorylation, downstream of cAMP activation. The study identified two putative PKA mediated phosphorylation sites on DISC1, and discovered that one of the sites, at serine 710, is responsible for the differential localization and binding properties observed in neuronal progenitors versus migrating neurons. DISC1 in neuronal progenitors is unphosphorylated at this site, and binds to and inhibits GSK3β activity: upon phosphorylation at this site, DISC1 increases its affinity for BBS1 and localizes at the centrosome. Crucially, the authors demonstrated that the phospho-dead form of DISC1 (S710A) rescued the proliferative but not the migrational phenotype observed in DISC1 knockdown conditions, while the phospho-mimetic form of DISC1 (S710E) rescued the migrational phenotypes of DISC1 function (Ishizuka et al., 2011). It is becoming clear that DISC1 coordinates multiple signaling cascades.

SYNAPTIC PATHWAYS

Spines are the postsynaptic entity of most excitatory synapses, and their morphological characteristics are important for imparting their functional properties and plasticity. There is recent evidence that has indicated that dendrites and spines are dysregulated in neurological diseases that are accompanied by cognitive impairment, such as autism spectrum disorders and schizophrenia (Penzes et al., 2011). Dysregulation of pathways that regulate the growth, pruning, and maintenance of dendritic spines is a particularly intriguing hypothesis for explaining components of schizophrenia etiology, since the onset is in early adulthood, when there is active synaptic pruning. In addition, analysis of postmortem brain samples show that there is decreased spine number on cortical pyramidal neurons in schizophrenia patients compared to controls (Garey et al., 1998).

DISC1

Discussed earlier was the role of DISC1 in neurogenesis and migration in the developing brain. DISC1 is observed to be present at 40% of synapses in postmortem tissue and primary cultures, and enriched in the postsynaptic density after subcellular fractionation (Brandon and Sawa, 2011). In primary neuron culture, it has been shown that DISC1 knockdown leads to increases in spine size and decreases in spine density, which is also seen in various DISC1 mouse models. In addition to this, there are increases in mini excitatory postsynaptic current frequencies, and knockdown of GluN1 leads to decreases in DISC1 levels. Yeast two-hybrid screens with DISC1 found that its binding partners were enriched for synaptic proteins and proteins associated with NMDA-dependent signaling. It has been subsequently found that binding partners of DISC1 are important for the regulation of spine morphologies, and DISC1 is involved in their regulation.

KALIRIN

A binding partner of DISC1 identified was Kalirin, which is a Rac GTP nucleotide exchange factor. The KALRN gene encodes several isoforms, of which Kalirin-7 is the most abundant form in the rat. It contains a PDZ binding motif and interacts with several other proteins via their PDZ domain. Kalirin-7 is localized to postsynaptic densities of excitatory synapses, and Kalirin-7 clusters are generally positively stained with PSD-95, AMPA, and NMDA receptors in the rat brain (Ma et al., 2008b). Kalirin-7 is known to be crucial for spine morphogenesis and function. *In vitro* overexpression in hippocampal cultures causes increases in spine density, while shRNA-mediated knockdown causes the converse (Ma et al., 2003). KALRN$^{-/-}$ knockout mice have decreases in spine density and dendritic complexity and show impairments in long-term potentiation in the Schaeffer collateral, decreases in spontaneous excitatory postsynaptic currents, and deficits in several animal behaviors associated with schizophrenia (working memory, social interaction, and prepulse inhibition) (Ma et al., 2008a). It has been determined that in the basal state, DISC1 coordinates interaction between Kalirin-7 and PSD-95, which prevents Kalirin-7 activation of Rac1. Upon NMDA receptor activation, a fraction of Kalirin-7 dissociates from DISC1 is able to activate Rac1, whose constitutive activation is known to lead to decreases in spine size. In humans, there are decreased Kalirin mRNA levels in the DLPFC in schizophrenic postmortem brain tissue. In addition, Kalirin has been associated with schizophrenia in a Japanese GWAS and sequencing of its exons has identified rare mutations which also associate with schizophrenia (Brandon and Sawa, 2011; Kushima et al., 2012).

CHANNEL PROPERTIES AND SYNAPTIC TRANSMISSION

In a cross-analysis GWAS between schizophrenia and bipolar disease, ANK3 and CACNA1C were found to be reach genome-wide significance (Ripke et al., 2011). ANK3 encodes for ankyrin 3, a protein found in the axon initial segment which is important for clustering Ca^{++} and Na$^+$ channels into electrically active areas of the axon (Pan et al., 2006), while CACNA1C encodes a subunit for an L-type voltage-gated calcium channel. Interestingly, ankyrin 3 is also known to be a component of the cadherin complex, and disruption of the cadherin complex is known to lead to mislocation of β-catenin (Orsulic et al., 1999), suggesting it may have also have a role in regulating Wnt signaling. Neurogranin, implicated in bipolar disorder and schizophrenia (Stefansson et al., 2009), is a key regulator of the Ca^{2+} binding messenger protein calmodulin, limiting its activity by sequestration. Based on the association of these genes in both schizophrenia and bipolar disorder, channel properties and synaptic transmission may be a shared feature of these two diseases.

There are also intersections of calcium signaling and the Wnt pathway. Wnt activates the G proteins associated with Fz proteins to modulate downstream calcium signaling. The Fz proteins are coupled to the Gαi/o Gβγ heterotrimeric G protein complex (Katanaev et al., 2005), and Wnt binding to Fz liberates the Gβγ subunits to activate a calcium-dependent pathway that involves the activation of phospholipase C cascade. The perturbation of these signaling pathways can have consequences beyond this pathway, and can impact the canonical Wnt pathway as well.

MICRORNA PATHWAYS

microRNAs (miRNAs) have been identified as a new regulatory layer that guides synaptic morphologies and functions; they have activity dependent regulation and can have differential subcellular localization (Siegel et al., 2011). Some 30% of humans who have deletion of 22q11.2 develop schizophrenia. Children with this deletion have cognitive dysfunction and similar macroscopic changes to brain structure such as decreased total brain, gray matter, and white matter volumes. Mouse models of this deletion show increased prepulse inhibition and decreased hippocampal dependent learning (Karayiorgou et al., 2010). One intriguing candidate present in 22q11.2 is Dcgr8, a protein important in the miRNA processing machinery. Dcgr8 knockout mice have decreased primary dendrites and spines as well as a decrease in functional glutamatergic synapses.

The strongest association signal in a meta-analysis of a schizophrenia GWAS was found in the putative primary transcript of the microRNA-137 (miR-137) (Ripke et al., 2011). Moreover, four predicted targets of miR-137 reached genome-wide significance and were demonstrated to have sequence-specific downregulation by miR-137 (Kwon et al., 2011), indicating that GWASs may have identified a pathway dysregulated in schizophrenia. miR-137 has been demonstrated to play a role in the dendritic arborization and spine density of adult newborn neurons and on embryonic and adult neurogenesis, although with opposite effects between the two periods (Smrt et al., 2010; Sun et al., 2011; Szulwach et al., 2010). The differential action of miR-137 between embryonic and adult neurogenesis may hold clues to how schizophrenia onset may switch in early adulthood.

CONCLUSION

There is growing evidence that schizophrenia is a neurodevelopmental disorder. The disease progression of schizophrenia is well underway before manifestation; there is cognitive

impairment, decreased connectivity and organization of white matter tracts in DTI studies, and gross anatomical changes that can be detected before onset. Significant progress has been made in understanding the genetics of schizophrenia in the past five years, and there are many emerging lines of evidence networking existing theories of schizophrenia etiology with genes that contribute risk to schizophrenia. Among the various emerging gene candidates from GWAS and CNV studies, several are associated with neurodevelopmental pathways. It is also becoming evident that there are many intersections between neuropsychiatric disorders, such as schizophrenia, bipolar disorder, autism spectrum disorder, and major depressive disorder. Treating the genetics as an aggregate of causative genes with effect sizes, just as the diagnosis of many psychiatric disorders is an aggregate of symptoms with magnitudes, may be useful in parsing their complexity moving forward. At this stage of unraveling the genetics of psychiatric disorders, studying unambiguously associated genes to elucidate pathways that underlie disease may set the framework for appreciating the complexity of gene candidates identified by GWASs. It is also worth noting that these molecular pathways that are important during neurodevelopment are also active throughout adulthood, and that a single protein can have pleiotropic effects; persistent dysregulation/dysfunction of a protein can have lasting effects and affect different pathways depending on developmental time. As geneticists continue genome-wide sequencing studies, such as CNV studies, GWASs, exome sequencing, and whole genome sequencing, and basic biologists uncover functions of identified genes and the effect of the risk alleles on these functions, there is no doubt new discoveries about the etiology of psychiatric disorders will become apparent, and novel therapeutic targets will emerge. In the future, personalized medicine tailored to the unique genetic burden of individual patients may be used to prevent developmental abnormalities that later lead to increased susceptibility to schizophrenia.

DISCLOSURES

Dr. Kwon has no conflicts of interest to disclose. She is funded by a Simons postdoctoral fellowship.

Dr. Soda has no conflicts of interest to disclose. He was supported by award Number T32GM07753 from the National Institute of General Medical Sciences. The content is solely the responsibility of the authors and does not necessarily represent the official views of the National Institute of General Medical Sciences or the National Institutes of Health.

Dr. Tsai serves on the Scientific Advisory Board of Sirtris Pharmaceuticals, Inc. and is a consultant for Lilly UK. She receives grant support from the NIH, Howard Hughes Medical Institute, and the Simons Foundation.

REFERENCES

Bale, T.L., Baram, T.Z., et al. (2010). Early life programming and neurodevelopmental disorders. *Biol. Psychiatry* 68:314–319.

Beaulieu, J.M. (2012). A role for Akt and glycogen synthase kinase-3 as integrators of dopamine and serotonin neurotransmission in mental health. *J. Psychiatry Neurosci.* 37:7–16.

Bigos, K.L., Mattay, V.S., et al. (2010). Genetic variation in CACNA1C affects brain circuitries related to mental illness. *Arch. Gen. Psychiatry* 67:939–945.

Billiard, J., Way, D.S., et al. (2005). The orphan receptor tyrosine kinase Ror2 modulates canonical Wnt signaling in osteoblastic cells. *Mol. Endocrinol.* 19:90–101.

Bradshaw, N.J., Soares, D.C., et al. (2011). PKA phosphorylation of NDE1 is DISC1/PDE4 dependent and modulates its interaction with LIS1 and NDEL1. *J. Neurosci.* 31:9043–9054.

Brandon, N.J., and Sawa, A. (2011). Linking neurodevelopmental and synaptic theories of mental illness through DISC1. *Nat. Rev. Neurosci.* 12:707–722.

Brockschmidt, A., Todt, U., et al. (2007). Severe mental retardation with breathing abnormalities (Pitt-Hopkins syndrome) is caused by haploinsufficiency of the neuronal bHLH transcription factor TCF4. *Hum. Mol. Genet.* 16:1488–1494.

Brown, A.S. (2011). The environment and susceptibility to schizophrenia. *Prog. Neurobiol.* 93:23–58.

Daniels, D.L., and Weis, W.I. (2005). Beta-catenin directly displaces Groucho/TLE repressors from Tcf/Lef in Wnt-mediated transcription activation. *Nat. Struct. Mol. Biol.* 12:364–371.

de Anda, F.C., Rosario, A.L., et al. (2012). Autism spectrum disorder susceptibility gene TAOK2 affects basal dendrite formation in the neocortex. *Nat. Neurosci.* 15:1022–1031.

Fiedler, M., Sanchez-Barrena, M.J., et al. (2008). Decoding of methylated histone H3 tail by the Pygo-BCL9 Wnt signaling complex. *Mol. Cell.* 30:507–518.

Flora, A., Garcia, J.J., et al. (2007). The E-protein Tcf4 interacts with Math1 to regulate differentiation of a specific subset of neuronal progenitors. *Proc. Natl. Acad. Sci. USA* 104:15382–15387.

Freyberg, Z., Ferrando, S.J., et al. (2010). Roles of the Akt/GSK-3 and Wnt signaling pathways in schizophrenia and antipsychotic drug action. *Am. J. Psychiatry* 167:388–396.

Gao, B., Song, H., et al. (2011). Wnt signaling gradients establish planar cell polarity by inducing Vangl2 phosphorylation through Ror2. *Dev. Cell.* 20:163–176.

Garey, L. (2010). When cortical development goes wrong: schizophrenia as a neurodevelopmental disease of microcircuits. *J. Anat.* 217:324–333.

Garey, L.J., Ong, W.Y., et al. (1998). Reduced dendritic spine density on cerebral cortical pyramidal neurons in schizophrenia. *J. Neurol. Neurosurg. Psychiatry* 65:446–453.

Gogtay, N., and Rapoport, J.L. (2008). Childhood-onset schizophrenia: insights from neuroimaging studies. *J. Am. Acad. Child Adolesc. Psychiatry* 47:1120–1124.

Gogtay, N., Vyas, N.S., et al. (2011). Age of onset of schizophrenia: perspectives from structural neuroimaging studies. *Schizophr. Bull.* 37:504–513.

Gold, J.M., and Weinberger, D.R. (1995). Cognitive deficits and the neurobiology of schizophrenia. *Curr. Opin. Neurobiol.* 5:225–230.

Harrison, P.J., and Weinberger, D.R. (2005). Schizophrenia genes, gene expression, and neuropathology: on the matter of their convergence. *Mol. Psychiatry* 10:40–68; image 45.

Hiramoto, T., Kang, G., et al. (2011). Tbx1: identification of a 22q11.2 gene as a risk factor for autism spectrum disorder in a mouse model. *Hum. Mol. Genet.* 20:4775–4785.

Hirotsune, S., Fleck, M.W., et al. (1998). Graded reduction of Pafah1b1 (Lis1) activity results in neuronal migration defects and early embryonic lethality. *Nat. Genet.* 19:333–339.

Huh, S.H., and Ornitz, D.M. (2010). Beta-catenin deficiency causes DiGeorge syndrome-like phenotypes through regulation of Tbx1. *Development* 137:1137–1147.

Ingason, A., Rujescu, D., et al. (2011). Copy number variations of chromosome 16p13.1 region associated with schizophrenia. *Mol. Psychiatry* 16:17–25.

Ishizuka, K., Kamiya, A., et al. (2011). DISC1-dependent switch from progenitor proliferation to migration in the developing cortex. *Nature* 473:92–96.

Jaaro-Peled, H. (2009). Gene models of schizophrenia: DISC1 mouse models. *Prog. Brain. Res.* 179:75–86.

Rapoport, J.L., Giedd, J.N., and Gogtay N. (2012). Neurodevelopmental model of schizophrenia: update 2012. *Mol. Psych.* 17(12):1228–1238.

Kamiya, A., Tomoda, T., et al. (2006). DISC1-NDEL1/NUDEL protein interaction, an essential component for neurite outgrowth, is modulated by genetic variations of DISC1. *Hum. Mol. Genet.* 15:3313–3323.

Karayiorgou, M., Simon, T.J., et al. (2010). 22q11.2 microdeletions: linking DNA structural variation to brain dysfunction and schizophrenia. *Nat. Rev. Neurosci.* 11:402–416.

Karlsgodt, K.H., Niendam, T.A., et al. (2009). White matter integrity and prediction of social and role functioning in subjects at ultra-high risk for psychosis. *Biol. Psychiatry* 66:562–569.

Katanaev, V.L., Ponzielli, R., et al. (2005). Trimeric G protein-dependent frizzled signaling in Drosophila. *Cell* 120:111–122.

Kim, W.Y., and Snider, W.D. (2011). Functions of GSK-3 signaling in development of the nervous system. *Front. Mol. Neurosci.* 4:44.

Kim, W.Y., Wang, X., et al. (2009). GSK-3 is a master regulator of neural progenitor homeostasis. *Nat. Neurosci.* 12:1390–1397.

Kushima, I., Nakamura, Y., et al. (2012). Resequencing and association analysis of the KALRN and EPHB1 genes and their contribution to schizophrenia susceptibility. *Schizophr. Bull.* 38:552–560.

Kwon, E., Wang, W., et al. (2011). Validation of schizophrenia-associated genes CSMD1, C10orf26, CACNA1C and TCF4 as miR-137 targets. *Mol. Psychiatry.*

Lawrie, S.M., and Abukmeil, S.S. (1998). Brain abnormality in schizophrenia. A systematic and quantitative review of volumetric magnetic resonance imaging studies. *Br. J. Psychiatry* 172:110–120.

Lewis, D.A., Hashimoto, T., et al. (2005). Cortical inhibitory neurons and schizophrenia. *Nat. Rev. Neurosci.* 6:312–324.

Lewis, D.A., and Levitt, P. (2002). Schizophrenia as a disorder of neurodevelopment. *Annu. Rev. Neurosci.* 25:409–432.

Logan, C.Y., and Nusse, R. (2004). The Wnt signaling pathway in development and disease. *Annu. Rev. Cell. Dev. Biol.* 20:781–810.

Lowy, A.M., Clements, W.M., et al. (2006). Beta-catenin/Wnt signaling regulates expression of the membrane type 3 matrix metalloproteinase in gastric cancer. *Cancer. Res.* 66:4734–4741.

Lu, W., Yamamoto, V., et al. (2004). Mammalian Ryk is a Wnt coreceptor required for stimulation of neurite outgrowth. *Cell* 119:97–108.

Ma, X.M., Huang, J., et al. (2003). Kalirin, a multifunctional Rho guanine nucleotide exchange factor, is necessary for maintenance of hippocampal pyramidal neuron dendrites and dendritic spines. *J. Neurosci.* 23:10593–10603.

Ma, X.M., Kiraly, D.D., et al. (2008a). Kalirin-7 is required for synaptic structure and function. *J. Neurosci.* 28:12368–12382.

Ma, X.M., Wang, Y., et al. (2008b). Kalirin-7 is an essential component of both shaft and spine excitatory synapses in hippocampal interneurons. *J. Neurosci.* 28:711–724.

Malhotra, D., and Sebat, J. (2012). CNVs: harbingers of a rare variant revolution in psychiatric genetics. *Cell.* 148:1223–1241.

Mao, Y., Ge, X., et al. (2009). Disrupted in schizophrenia 1 regulates neuronal progenitor proliferation via modulation of GSK3beta/beta-catenin signaling. *Cell* 136:1017–1031.

McCarthy, S.E., Makarov, V., et al. (2009). Microduplications of 16p11.2 are associated with schizophrenia. *Nat. Genet.* 41:1223–1227.

Mefford, H.C., Sharp, A.J., et al. (2008). Recurrent rearrangements of chromosome 1q21.1 and variable pediatric phenotypes. *N. Engl. J. Med.* 359:1685–1699.

Mei, L., and Xiong, W.C. (2008). Neuregulin 1 in neural development, synaptic plasticity and schizophrenia. *Nat. Rev. Neurosci.* 9:437–452.

Ming, G.L., and Song, H. (2009). DISC1 partners with GSK3beta in neurogenesis. *Cell* 136:990–992.

Moore, T.H., Zammit, S., et al. (2007). Cannabis use and risk of psychotic or affective mental health outcomes: a systematic review. *Lancet* 370:319–328.

Mulle, J.G., Dodd, A.F., et al. (2010). Microdeletions of 3q29 confer high risk for schizophrenia. *Am. J. Hum. Genet.* 87:229–236.

Muraoka-Cook, R.S., Sandahl, M.A., et al. (2009). ErbB4 splice variants Cyt1 and Cyt2 differ by 16 amino acids and exert opposing effects on the mammary epithelium *in vivo. Mol. Cell. Biol.* 29:4935–4948.

Neale, B.M., Kou, Y., et al. (2012). Patterns and rates of exonic de novo mutations in autism spectrum disorders. *Nature* 485:242–245.

O'Dushlaine, C., Kenny, E., et al. (2011). Molecular pathways involved in neuronal cell adhesion and membrane scaffolding contribute to schizophrenia and bipolar disorder susceptibility. *Mol. Psychiatry* 16:286–292.

O'Roak, B.J., Vives, L., et al. (2012). Sporadic autism exomes reveal a highly interconnected protein network of de novo mutations. *Nature* 485:246–250.

Orsulic, S., Huber, O., et al. (1999). E-cadherin binding prevents beta-catenin nuclear localization and beta-catenin/LEF-1-mediated transactivation. *J. Cell. Sci.* 112 (Pt 8), 1237–1245.

Pan, Z., Kao, T., et al. (2006). A common ankyrin-G-based mechanism retains KCNQ and NaV channels at electrically active domains of the axon. *J. Neurosci.* 26:2599–2613.

Paylor, R., Glaser, B., et al. (2006). Tbx1 haploinsufficiency is linked to behavioral disorders in mice and humans: implications for 22q11 deletion syndrome. *Proc. Natl. Acad. Sci. USA* 103:7729–7734.

Penzes, P., Cahill, M.E., et al. (2011). Dendritic spine pathology in neuropsychiatric disorders. *Nat. Neurosci.* 14:285–293.

Pletnikov, M.V., Xu, Y., et al. (2007). PC12 cell model of inducible expression of mutant DISC1: new evidence for a dominant-negative mechanism of abnormal neuronal differentiation. *Neurosci. Res.* 58:234–244.

Rapoport, J.L., Giedd, J.N., and Gogtay, N. (2012). Neurodevelopmental model of schizophrenia: update 2012. *Mol. Psych.* 17(12):1228–1238.

Ripke, S., Sanders, A.R., et al. (2011). Genome-wide association study identifies five new schizophrenia loci. *Nat. Genet.* 43:969–976.

Rosso, S.B., Sussman, D., et al. (2005). Wnt signaling through Dishevelled, Rac and JNK regulates dendritic development. *Nat. Neurosci.* 8:34–42.

Shafer, B., Onishi, K., et al. (2011). Vangl2 promotes Wnt/planar cell polarity-like signaling by antagonizing Dvl1-mediated feedback inhibition in growth cone guidance. *Dev. Cell.* 20:177–191.

Siegel, G., Saba, R., et al. (2011). microRNAs in neurons: manifold regulatory roles at the synapse. *Curr. Opin. Genet. Dev.* 21:491–497.

Singh, K.K., Ge, X., et al. (2010). Dixdc1 is a critical regulator of DISC1 and embryonic cortical development. *Neuron* 67:33–48.

Smrt, R.D., Szulwach, K.E., et al. (2010). MicroRNA miR-137 regulates neuronal maturation by targeting ubiquitin ligase mind bomb-1. *Stem Cells* 28:1060–1070.

Stefansson, H., Ophoff, R.A., et al. (2009). Common variants conferring risk of schizophrenia. *Nature* 460:744–747.

Stefansson, H., Rujescu, D., et al. (2008). Large recurrent microdeletions associated with schizophrenia. *Nature* 455:232–236.

Sun, G., Ye, P., et al. (2011). miR-137 forms a regulatory loop with nuclear receptor TLX and LSD1 in neural stem cells. *Nat. Commun.* 2:529.

Szulwach, K.E., Li, X., et al. (2010). Cross talk between microRNA and epigenetic regulation in adult neurogenesis. *J. Cell. Biol.* 189: 127–141.

Takahashi, N., Sakurai, T., et al. (2011). Linking oligodendrocyte and myelin dysfunction to neurocircuitry abnormalities in schizophrenia. *Prog. Neurobiol.* 93:13–24.

Thomason, M.E., and Thompson, P.M. (2011). Diffusion imaging, white matter, and psychopathology. *Annu. Rev. Clin. Psychol.* 7:63–85.

Torrey, E.F., Bartko, J.J., et al. (2012). Toxoplasma gondii and other risk factors for schizophrenia: an update. *Schizophr. Bull.* 38:642–647.

Valenta, T., Gay, M., et al. (2011). Probing transcription-specific outputs of beta-catenin *in vivo. Genes. Dev.* 25:2631–2643.

van Amerongen, R., and Nusse, R. (2009). Towards an integrated view of Wnt signaling in development. *Development* 136:3205–3214.

van Os, J., Kenis, G., et al. (2010). The environment and schizophrenia. *Nature* 468:203–212.

Walterfang, M., Velakoulis, D., et al. (2011) Understanding aberrant white matter development in schizophrenia: an avenue for therapy? *Expert. Rev. Neurother.* 11:971–987

Walsh, T., McClellan, J.M., et al. (2008). Rare structural variants disrupt multiple genes in neurodevelopmental pathways in schizophrenia. *Science* 320:539–543.

Yang, M., Waterman, M.L., et al. (2008). hADA2a and hADA3 are required for acetylation, transcriptional activity and proliferative effects of beta-catenin. *Cancer. Biol. Ther.* 7:120–128.

Yoshimura, T., Kawano, Y., et al. (2005). GSK-3beta regulates phosphorylation of CRMP-2 and neuronal polarity. *Cell* 120:137–149.

Zhou, L., Ercolano, E., et al. (2011). Merlin-deficient human tumors show loss of contact inhibition and activation of Wnt/beta-catenin signaling linked to the PDGFR/Src and Rac/PAK pathways. *Neoplasia* 13:1101–1112.

26 | NEUROBIOLOGY OF MENTAL ILLNESS PSYCHOSIS PRONENESS

RAQUEL E. GUR

INTRODUCTION

Across medicine, early identification of disorders is recognized as important and at times critical for intervention. A prodrome is an early symptom or set of symptoms, which may be specific (e.g., aura before migraine) or non-specific (e.g., fever, malaise, decreased appetite in infectious illnesses), and is a precursor to a disease. Early detection creates the potential for intervention at a stage where it could disrupt the pathological process or help manage the disorder and ameliorate its course.

The application of the prodrome concept to schizophrenia builds on clinical lore where a prolonged period of two to three years is common before the emergence of psychotic symptoms that meet *Diagnostic and Statistical Manual* (DSM) criteria for schizophrenia or spectrum psychotic disorders. This period is associated with sub-threshold symptoms and some functional decline. A rapidly growing literature since the mid-1990s has examined the clinical course of individuals with prodromal presentation and gauged conversion rates to schizophrenia. Based on the literature and considering potential implications, the DSM-5 work group has examined how "psychosis risk syndrome" or "attenuated psychotic symptoms syndrome," terms applied to define the prodromal phase of schizophrenia, should be incorporated into the next diagnostic manual (Carpenter and van Os, 2011). As this debate unfolds, it is critical to evaluate systematically concomitant neurobiological processes that can be examined prospectively to elucidate the pathophysiology of vulnerability to psychosis. Complementally, such work can identify markers of resilience by studying those at risk who do not proceed to a more severe form of the syndrome.

Methodological advances in neuroscience have enabled us to probe brain function in schizophrenia. Because it is a neurodevelopmental disorder, understanding the pathophysiology of schizophrenia is central to establishing the neurobiology pertinent to the continuum of psychosis. The study of at risk individuals with quantitative phenotypic measures of brain and behavior can address fundamental questions regarding the presence of abnormalities at an early phase of presentation and their relation to outcome. Importantly, such measures can be integrated with genomics to elucidate underlying mechanisms of vulnerability and resilience. Therefore, this framework of research can help behavioral neuroscience join the genomic effort underway toward precision medicine.

This chapter will summarize current literature on the prodromal state as examined with neurobehavioral and neuroimaging methods. Findings will be integrated considering the NIMH Research Domain Criteria (RDoC) initiative (http://www.nimh.nih.gov).

NEUROBEHAVIOR

Behavioral performance that can be linked to brain function has been examined in neurocognitive measures. More recently, social cognition measures have been included in evaluating those at clinical risk for psychosis, commonly integrating cognitive and social psychology paradigms. A small literature has focused on olfaction.

NEUROCOGNITION

Impaired cognition is prominent in schizophrenia and is associated with disrupted functioning. Whether cognitive deficits are progressive or stable has been debated. Examination of first-episode patients, before initiation of treatment with antipsychotic medications, and their longitudinal follow-up made it possible to determine that the neurocognitive profile in first-episode patients resembles that evident in individuals with schizophrenia with a more chronic course of illness. The pattern of deficits in the executive and memory domains implicates frontotemporal dysfunction. The extension of neurocognitive assessment with tests applied in schizophrenia research to individuals with attenuated psychotic symptoms has been commonly applied in prodromal investigations. Some inconsistencies are noted as studies vary in ascertainment, assessment instruments, tests applied, and the information provided on potential moderators, such as substance use. Previous reviews of this growing literature have been qualitative. Two recent quantitative meta-analyses highlight the emerging findings reported in multiple studies in the literature (Fusar-Poli et al., 2012b; Giuliano et al., 2012).

Giuliano and colleagues (2012) conducted a meta-analysis of fourteen studies that met specified inclusion criteria, published until February 2011, which examined the psychosis risk syndrome. A sample of 1,215 individuals at risk for psychosis was compared to 851 healthy controls on neurocognitive domains derived from multiple tests that are frequently examined in schizophrenia. Tests included measures of general cognitive abilities, language functions, episodic memory, attention, visuospatial abilities, and working memory. Overall,

small to medium effect sizes of neurocognitive impairment were noted in the psychosis risk group, with significant deficits in 9 of the 10 domains examined. The motor skills domain was the only one that did not differ between the groups. Longitudinal follow-up in seven of the studies showed that those in the psychosis risk group, who transitioned to psychosis at follow-up, had medium to large neurocognitive deficits at baseline compared to healthy controls, except for motor speed (Addington et al., 2008; Brewer et al., 2003, 2005; Chung et al., 2008; Dickinson and Gold, 2008; Gschwandtner et al., 2006; Hawkins et al., 2004; Miyake et al., 2000; Pflueger et al., 2007; Pinkham et al., 2007; Reichenberg et al., 2010; Seidman et al., 2010; Smith et al., 2006; Szoke et al., 2008). Given the small samples, the limited period of follow-up, subjects' attrition, and potential treatment effects, the longitudinal results are preliminary and limited.

Fusar-Poli et al. (2012b) have also focused their meta-analysis on cognitive functioning in individuals who were at clinical high risk for psychosis. They examined 19 studies published before January 2011. Specified and carefully delineated inclusion criteria were applied, and only 19 studies of the 78 studies screened were included (Addington et al., 2008; An et al., 2010; Brewer et al., 2005; Broome et al., 2007; Chung et al., 2008; Frommann et al., 2011; Green et al., 2012; Ilonen et al., 2010; Korver et al., 2010; Koutsouleris et al., 2012; Lindgren et al., 2010; Magaud et al., 2010; Pflueger et al., 2007; Seidman et al., 2010; Silverstein et al., 2006; Simon et al., 2007; Szily and Keri, 2009; van Rijn et al., 2011; Woodberry et al., 2010). The sample consisted of 1,188 clinical risk participants and 1,029 controls. Diffuse deficits across several neurocognitive domains were evident in the clinical risk group. Impairments in general intelligence, executive functions, attention, working memory, verbal fluency, verbal and spatial memory, and social cognition characterized the clinical risk group. Processing speed did not distinguish between the groups. Transition to psychosis was examined in 7 studies, with mean longitudinal follow-up of 19 months (Becker et al., 2010; Brewer et al., 2005; Koutsouleris et al., 2012; Pukrop et al., 2007; Riecher-Rossler et al., 2009; Seidman et al., 2010; Woodberry et al, 2010). The group of converters had lower general intelligence at baseline, and more impaired performance in verbal fluency, verbal and visual memory, and working memory, compared to those who did not develop psychosis at follow-up.

To examine the regional distribution of neurocognitive deficits implicated by the test results, we have entered the z-scores of the prodromal group into the "behavioral imaging" algorithm (Gur et al., 1990). This algorithm uses z-scores from neuropsychological tests to create a three-dimensional representation of brain regions that are likely impaired based on the pattern of deficits. We entered the results from the meta-analyses and averaged both when the same measures were included in both analyses (see Table in Fig. 26.1). The algorithm generates three views (Fig. 26.1) of brain cortex, identifying regions of impaired functioning in individuals at clinical risk. As can be seen, the abnormalities seem more pronounced in the left than the right hemisphere, especially in the juncture of frontal, temporal, and parietal lobes.

SOCIAL COGNITION

Relative to the large number of studies that investigated neurocognition in clinical risk groups, as highlighted in the meta-analyses previously summarized, a handful of studies examined processes that relate to the perception, interpretation, and response to other people's behavior. As social cognition is a later addition to studies in schizophrenia and the clinical risk studies are an extension of these efforts, more work is necessary.

Giuliano and colleagues' (2012) qualitative part of the review of the psychosis risk syndrome presents data on social cognition that is insufficiently represented in the literature for quantitative meta-analysis. Three studies are included, and while deficits in emotion processing and theory of mind tasks are noted, the results are too preliminary to be conclusive (Addington et al., 2008; Chung et al., 2008; Pinkham et al., 2007). Fusar-Poli et al. (2012b) meta-analysis noted a significant impairment in 255 clinical risk participants compared to 235 controls in six studies that included measures of the social cognition domain (Addington et al., 2008; An et al., 2010; Chung et al., 2008; Green et al., 2012; Szily and Keri, 2009; van Rijn et al., 2011). While these preliminary studies are encouraging, and ultimately may yield insights into negative symptoms, this effort is in its initial stages.

OLFACTION

The Giuliano et al. review (2012) mentions only two studies on olfactory identification in the psychosis risk syndrome, with medium mean effect size. Similarly, only two studies (Brewer et al., 2003) examined the transition to schizophrenia spectrum disorders at follow-up. These are preliminary data not yet suitable for meta-analysis, and further research is required.

Thus, the pattern of neurobehavioral performance in individuals at clinical risk for psychosis shows diffuse deficits in multiple domains, similar to those evident in first-episode and more chronic patients with schizophrenia. Specifically, deficits in verbal memory and working memory implicating left frontotemporal dysfunction have been extensively documented in schizophrenia. While longitudinal studies are limited, the literature suggests that those individuals who transition to schizophrenia spectrum disorders manifest neurocognitive deficits already at baseline to a greater extent than those who do not transition. This buttresses the importance of examining schizophrenia related disorders neurodevelopmentally and in integration with neuroimaging.

NEUROIMAGING

The application of neuroimaging methodology to the study of schizophrenia, including first-episode presentation, has enabled the examination of brain structure and function and demonstrated key aberrations in the syndrome (Fusar-Poli et al., 2012c). The extension of this line of research to the investigation of vulnerability to psychosis can provide important information on brain changes associated with the emerging psychotic process. Magnetic resonance imaging

Test	Measure	Fusar-Poli 2012	Giuliano 2012	Combined
WAIS-R	Digit Span	-0.39	-0.4	-0.395
	Block Design	-0.2	-0.4	-0.3
	Digit Symbol	-0.35	-0.52	-0.435
WMS-R	Logical Memory I	-0.25	-0.49	-0.37
	Visual Repro I (RCFT Imm)	-0.39	NA	-0.39
	Visual Repro II (RCFT Delayed)		-0.16	-0.16
CVLT	Trials 1-5	-0.47	-0.68	-0.575
RAVLT	Sum 1-5	-0.37	-0.47	-0.42
	WCST Total Perseverative Resp	-0.25	-0.36	-0.305
Stroop	Color	NA	-0.25	-0.25
	Color Word	NA	-0.09	-0.09
Finger Tap	RH + LH	-0.09	-0.22	-0.155
Trail Making	A Seconds	-0.34	-0.41	-0.375
	B Seconds	-0.39	-0.47	-0.43
CPT	Vigilance (Total Correct)	-0.35	-0.4	-0.375
CFL	FAS Total Unique	-0.27	-0.48	-0.375
Animal Naming	Total Unique	-0.45	-0.66	-0.555
WRAT-R2	Reading	NA	-0.35	-0.35

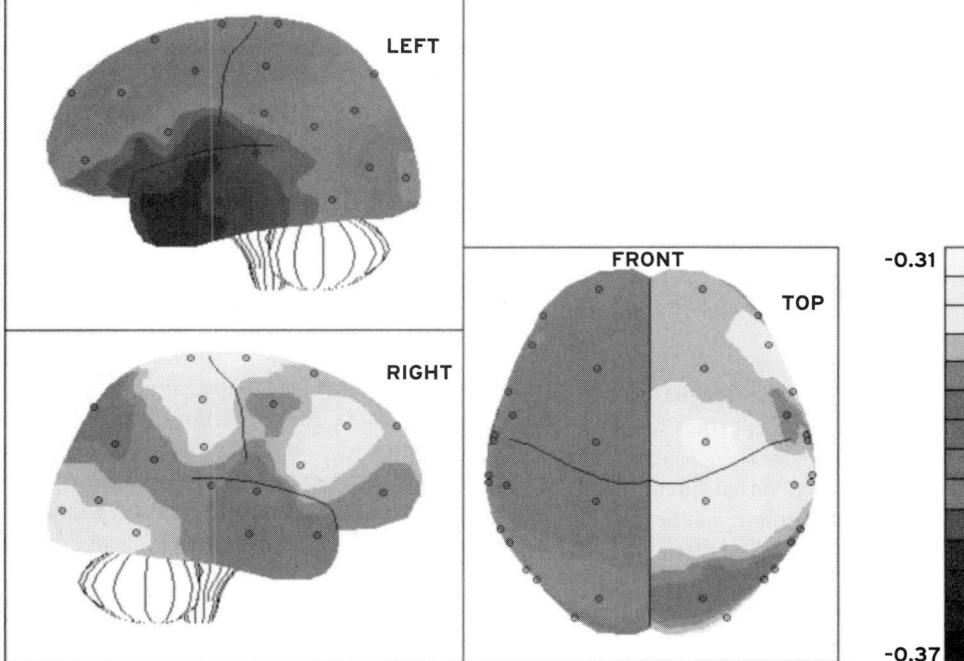

Figure 26.1 *Behavioral Image displays of left hemisphere, right hemisphere, and top view. Values are based on the meta-analyses of tests examined and summarized in the table. The color scale indicates effect sizes of psychosis prone individuals relative to healthy controls. (See color insert).*

(MRI) enables evaluation of brain structure, gray matter and white matter volumes, connectivity, and activity in response to neurobehavioral probes. As the techniques for image acquisition and processing advance rapidly, more refined assessment of brain integrity is feasible.

STRUCTURAL MRI

Detailed morphometric measures can be obtained in individual and group data that provide gray matter, white matter, and CSF whole brain and regional volumes. Parameters commonly scrutinized are highlighted in Figure 26.2.

Structural MRI measures have been tested as endophenotypes in several studies of first-degree family members who are at genetic risk for schizophrenia. Family members show

a similar pattern but diminished extent compared to that observed in probands, with increased ventricular volume and decreased gray matter volume. The literature on clinical risk for psychosis, recently reviewed (Fusar-Poli et al., 2012a), is relatively limited in size of samples and extent of follow-up.

A meta-analysis of voxel-based morphometry studies compared psychosis risk and first-episode schizophrenia patients to healthy controls (Fusar-Poli et al., 2012c). Fourteen studies met specified selection criteria and included participants who were never treated with antipsychotic medications. There were 198 individuals at risk for psychosis compared to 254 healthy controls, and 206 first-episode patients compared to 202 controls. Image acquisition in most studies was on a 1.5 Tesla scanner. Gray matter volume reduction was evident in several regions including the right temporal, limbic prefrontal cortex

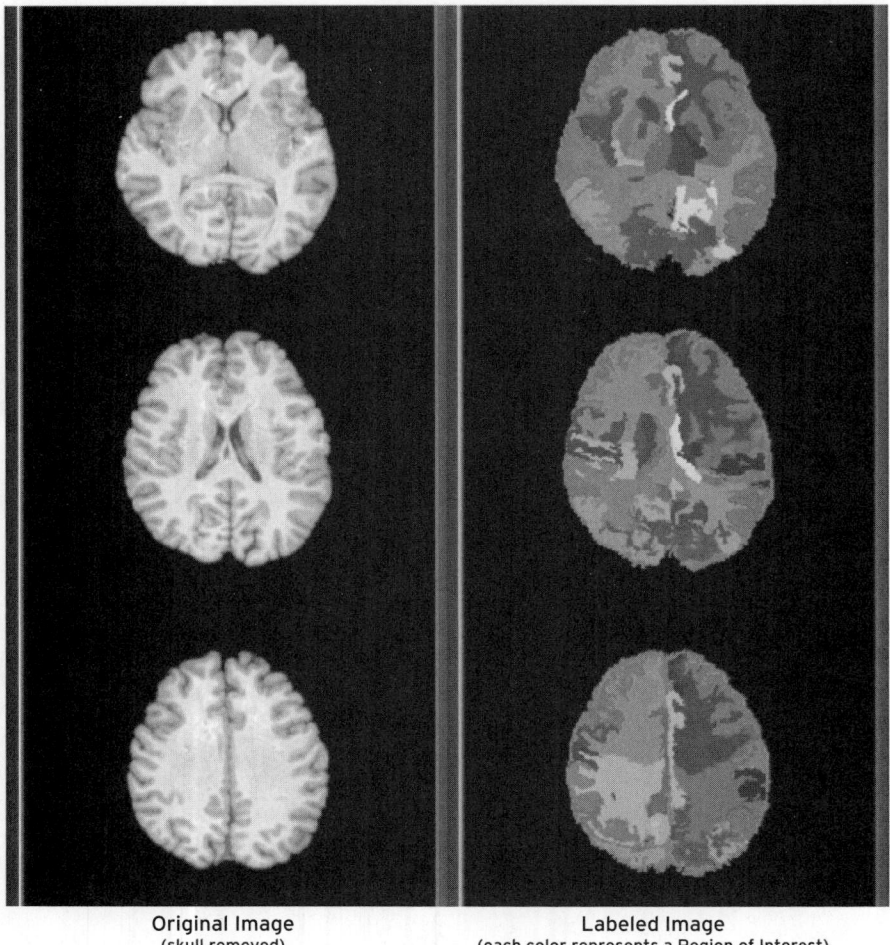

Original Image
(skull removed)

Labeled Image
(each color represents a Region of Interest)

Figure 26.2 *MRI template-warping for parcellating regions of interest. A template in which regions are labeled and demarcated is warped into an individual's MRI recording the extent of changes required. As a result, axial slices such as seen on the left are labeled as seen on the right column. Regional volumes can then be calculated for quantitative analysis allowing, for example, comparison between psychosis prone and healthy participants. (See color insert).*

in the clinical risk group, and in the temporal insular cortex and cerebellum in the first-episode group. Notably, the onset of psychosis was associated with decreased gray matter volume in temporal, anterior cingulate, cerebellar, and insular regions. In one study, greater severity of psychotic symptoms was related to right superior temporal lobe gyrus volume decrease. These regions have been implicated in multiple studies of schizophrenia and subserve functions that are aberrant in schizophrenia and relate to cognition and emotion processing.

It is notable that while the neuroanatomic studies, when reporting lateralized effects, suggest greater structural abnormalities in the right hemisphere, the neurocognitive studies suggest greater left hemispheric dysfunction. This seeming discrepancy may reflect the lack of emphasis on laterality in neuroimaging studies, which typically examine data on a voxelwise basis within a hemisphere. It could also reflect greater sensitivity of neuropsychological tests to left hemispheric dysfunction. On the other hand, cognitive deficits could reflect compensatory activation, and if these effects are validated in future studies they could thus suggest avenues for remediation.

There are multiple methodological limitations entailed in MRI meta-analytic approaches, and the studies are mostly cross-sectional and include participants who did not transition to psychosis. However, the results suggest that brain regions that show volume reduction in schizophrenia also show abnormalities in those at risk for psychosis (Fusar-Poli et al., 2012c). Larger samples in a longitudinal design will be important to advance the understanding of underlying neuroanatomical differences between groups. White matter changes have also been reported in schizophrenia, early in the course of illness, as well as in individuals at risk for psychosis (Carletti et al., 2012; Fusar-Poli et al., 2011a).

DIFFUSION TENSOR IMAGING

Diffusion tensor imaging (DTI) quantifies restricted water diffusivity in white matter, enabling non-invasive detection of subtle white matter abnormalities and facilitating the understanding of complex large-scale brain networks. Figure 26.3 illustrates measures obtained in DTI.

Abnormalities in DTI have been reported in schizophrenia, both in chronic patients and in first-episode presentation (Peters et al., 2009), with reduced white matter integrity in frontotemporal tracts. The literature on psychosis risk is limited to several

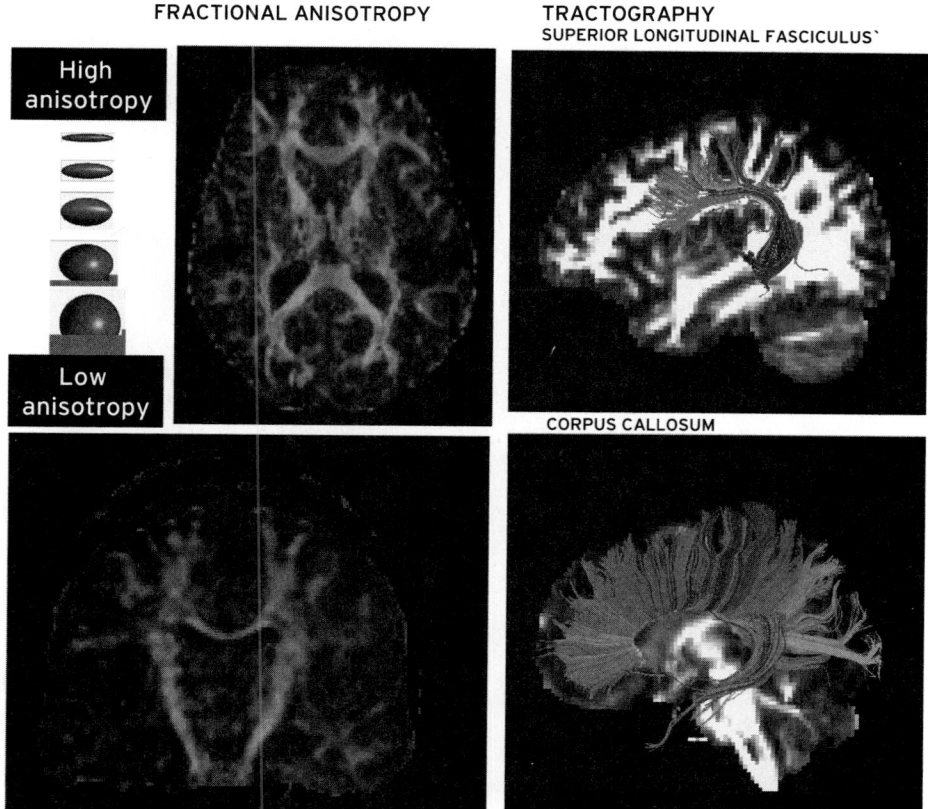

High anisotropy

Low anisotropy

CORPUS CALLOSUM

Figure 26.3 Diffusion tensor imaging (DTI) illustrates fractional anisotropy (left) and tractography (right). Fractional anisotropy reveals white matter architecture while tractography depicts the integrity of fiber tracts. (See color insert).

cross-sectional studies, with differing findings including reduced fractional anisotropy in frontal lobe (Bloemen et al., 2010) or in the superior longitudinal fasciculus (Borgwardt et al., 2011). A longitudinal study (Carletti et al., 2012) compared three groups: individuals at risk for psychosis ($n = 32$) healthy controls ($n = 32$), and first-episode schizophrenia ($n = 15$). The psychosis risk and control participants were rescanned on a 1.5 Tesla after 28 months. At baseline, the first-episode group had decreased fractional anisotropy and increased diffusivity relative to controls, and the psychosis risk group was intermediate between the other two groups. At follow-up, further reduction in fractional anisotropy was evident in left frontal region only in those psychosis risk individuals ($n = 8$) who transitioned to psychosis. This suggests that progressive changes occur at disease onset, which has been reported before for gray matter (Borgwardt et al., 2007; Smeiskova et al., 2010). Again, however, the available data are meager and must be considered very preliminary.

fMRI

Functional MRI has been applied to individuals at risk for psychosis, commonly in small samples with neurobehavioral probes that have shown differences between schizophrenia patients and controls. Neurobehavioral domains examined include working memory, using the n-back paradigm. Overall, psychosis risk groups show decreased activation in the blood oxygenation level-dependent (BOLD) response in dorsolateral and medial prefrontal regions (Fusar-Poli et al., 2012c). The pattern of activity is similar to that seen early in the course of schizophrenia, but less pronounced abnormalities are observed. To evaluate activation changes with disease progression, longitudinal designs are necessary. Such designs have been applied in several fMRI studies, reviewed by Smieskova and colleagues (2010). This small literature suggests that individuals who transition to psychosis differ from those who do not, with the latter group showing normalization. Thus, the application of fMRI holds promise as a tool that may facilitate elucidation of the underlying pathophysiology of the psychotic process (Fig. 26.4).

CONNECTIVITY

The resting BOLD signal in fMRI paradigms can provide a measure of connectivity, reflecting "cross-talk" integration among brain regions. It examines the time-series correlations among brain regions, indicating which regions show synchronized activation. Aberrations in schizophrenia in frontotemporal connectivity have been reported and have also been seen in those at clinical risk (Crossley et al., 2009). This literature too is at its infancy.

NEUROTRANSMITTERS

Several neurotransmitters that have been related to the pathophysiology of schizophrenia have been examined in those at psychosis risk. Dopamine dysregulation has been linked to

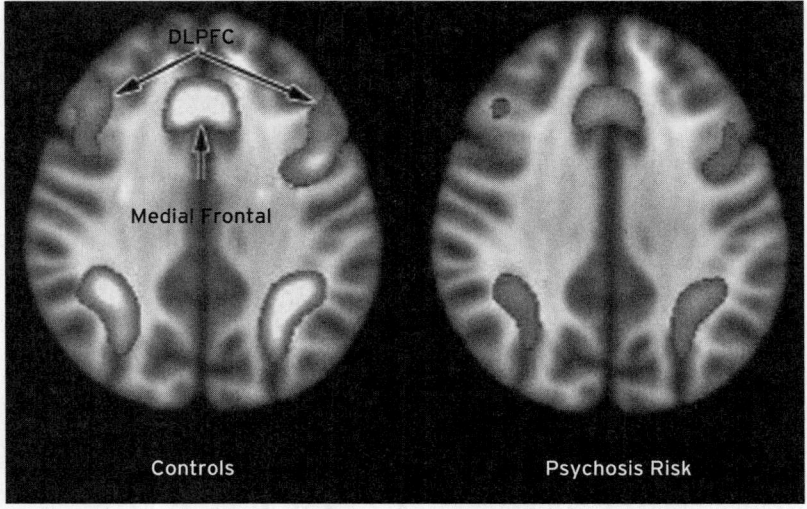

Figure 26.4 *Functional MRI (fMRI) BOLD activation in response to a working memory task. A normal pattern of activation (left) and reduced activity in clinical risk for psychosis (right) illustrates the pattern observed in studies applying the n-back paradigm.*

psychosis, and positron emission tomography (PET) studies have shown increased dopamine striatal activity in schizophrenia (Fusar-Poli and Meyer-Lindenberg, 2013; Howes et al., 2009). Striatal 6-fluoro-L-dopa F18-dopa was also elevated in psychosis risk individuals and related to symptom severity (Tibbo et al., 2004).

Glutamate has also been implicated in the pathophysiology of schizophrenia and studies have examined individuals at genetic risk for psychosis using magnetic resonance spectroscopy (MRS). Increased glutamine/glutamate ratio in medial frontal cortex was reported in adolescents at genetic risk (Tibbo et al., 2004). In a study integrating fMRI and MRS, 24 psychosis risk individuals were compared to 17 healthy controls (Fusar-Poli et al., 2011c). BOLD response to a verbal fluency task showed that the psychosis risk group had greater bilateral activation than controls in midfrontal gyrus. Glutamate levels in the thalamus were lower in psychosis prone individuals. Furthermore, the pattern of correlations with activation suggests that prefrontal, hippocampal, and temporal functioning are related to thalamic glutamate levels and differentiate those at risk from controls.

ELECTROPHYSIOLOGY

As in schizophrenia research, the investigation of brain function has included several studies that have examined brain activity with electrophysiological measures. For example, P300 amplitude was reported to be smaller in a group of 100 clinical risk individuals, early or late in the prodromal state, compared to 40 healthy controls (Frommann et al., 2008). The findings were interpreted as suggesting that selective left temporoparietal amplitude deficits could be a trait abnormality, while deficits at sagittal midline electrodes may relate to changes that underlie the emergence of psychotic symptoms.

A study integrating P300 and volumetric MRI measures (Fusar-Poli et al., 2011b) examined 39 psychosis risk individuals and 41 healthy controls. P300 at intake was lower, and gray matter was reduced in several regions including the right superior frontal gyrus, left medial frontal gyrus, left inferior frontal gyrus, right orbital gyrus, and right supramarginal gyrus in the psychosis risk group. The longitudinal design made it possible to follow a subgroup, with some subjects transitioning to psychosis. Progressive gray matter alterations in prefrontal and subcortical areas were noted in the psychosis risk group, but no significant changes in P300 amplitude over time were observed.

CHALLENGES AND PROMISES

Advancing the neurobiology of schizophrenia is extremely challenging and requires converging multidisciplinary team science approaches. The bar is even higher when attempting to do what we need to in order to elucidate mechanisms that underlie the pathophysiology early in the course of emerging psychosis. Before turning to the scientific challenges and promises, the context of the debate is important to consider.

Medicine is undergoing a paradigm shift in which "Big Science" is applied to multiple biomarkers in order to permit early identification and targeted interventions that aim at biological processes rather than symptoms. Unfortunately, psychiatry is at risk to stay at the sidelines of the move toward such precision medicine not just because of the complexity of behavior and its organ, the brain, but also because of societal attitudes. Unlike other medical disorders, the burden of stigma and the consequences of false early identification of individuals who may not transition to psychosis weigh heavily when discussing the inclusion of clinical risk in DSM-5. Yet, a shift in research paradigms as envisioned by RDoC provides an opportunity to bypass the stigma by obtaining dimensional data on behavior without emphasis on categorical diagnostic classification. Such a framework can be well integrated into large-scale genomic studies and afford the data essential for addressing fundamental basic and clinical questions that can

fill existing gaps in understanding. Such systematic efforts will help answer questions currently enigmatic or with limited data reflecting an early phase of investigation.

The heterogeneity in clinical features and variability in brain behavior measures necessitate large samples and longitudinal follow-up. Large longitudinal samples are also essential for integration of quantitative phenotypic neurobiological data with genomics. Such efforts are required for progress in advancing the understanding of neurodevelopmental trajectories that underlie the continuum of psychosis.

Several methodological challenges merit consideration and discussion. Some uniformity and standardization in the approach to these issues could ultimately lead to consensus in the next stages of this undertaking.

Ascertainment. The population captured in clinical risk studies is based on help-seeking youths. Some sites develop a referral network that may include community mental health providers, schools, and advertisement in the community at large. Is the pattern of presentation related to the method of ascertainment? Demographics? How does the presentation of help-seekers differ from population-based studies? To enable generalizability and sensitivity of measures, consistent information should be provided, even in the form of supplemental data in journal articles.

Comorbidity. There is inconsistency in the literature in reporting comorbid conditions, such as substance use, despite an extensive literature of psychosis in the context of substance use, such as cannabis. Similarly, the role of environmental stressors that can facilitate or curtail the emergence of psychosis needs attention.

Diagnostic instruments. Several instruments have been applied to assess sub-threshold psychotic symptoms. Adopting a common instrument will be helpful in standardization, and research groups can add other instruments to address further questions. Such standardization will help establish common training across research sites and facilitate clinical training of professionals as the field moves forward. There is also a need to focus on negative symptoms early in the course of psychosis, as the clinical presentation is at times mistakenly diagnosed as depression.

Neurobehavioral measures. Core domains should be included in future studies to enable comparison across samples and pulling data together systematically. Easy access to behavioral measurement procedures is necessary to enable data gathering across diverse settings beyond academic sites.

Neuroimaging measures. For more complex brain indices, such as those obtained in neuroimaging and electrophysiology, further considerations on data acquisition and processing are required. In such studies it is crucial to standardize data analytic approaches, and increasingly multimodal neuroimaging is feasible and could help propel the field. Structural, functional, and connectivity data can now be obtained in single sessions, and longitudinal follow-up is feasible. Importantly, the neuroimaging data need to be integrated with clinical and neurocognitive data.

Sample size. The large volume of data generated in neuroimaging studies underscores the need for large samples. Even larger samples are needed if the aim is to integrate neuroimaging data with genomics. The typical concluding paragraph in neuroimaging papers, which states that "larger samples are required" should become limited.

When genomics is running forward and bioinformatics is keeping up, we have unprecedented opportunities with available and developing technologies to attempt to answer questions that are crucial and critical for early intervention. Such knowledge may help pave the way for novel approaches to ameliorate the impact of illness and enable vulnerable individuals to get back on track as much as possible. Concerns over medicating the young and perhaps those not bound to schizophrenia spectrum disorders is understandable. However, this valid concern should not become a paralyzing fear. As the field is adopting behavioral interventions that show promise, as well as discovering natural substances that can help modulate the disease process, it is up to us to be vigilant as health professionals and do no harm. By educating the public, and free of conflict of interest, we can be in a position to impart knowledge gained, admit our ignorance, and strive to obtain the best data possible in the service of those who need it.

As we gain better understanding of the neurodevelopmental trajectories associated with "deep phenotyping" of brain behavior quantitative measures, and have data on adequately powered samples, we will be in a position to evaluate the degree and extent of departure from the normative growth curve. Implications of symptoms, their duration, persistence, intensification, and impact on functioning can be monitored. Such efforts will lead to better understanding of variability in presentation, vulnerability, resilience, and early intervention.

DISCLOSURE

Dr. Gur has no conflicts of interest to disclose.

REFERENCES

Addington, J., Penn, D., et al. (2008). Facial affect recognition in individuals at clinical high risk for psychosis. *Br. J. Psychiatry* 192:67–68.

An, S.K., Kang, J.I., et al. (2010). Attribution bias in ultra-high risk for psychosis and first-episode schizophrenia. *Schizophr. Res.* 118:54–61.

Becker, H.E., Nieman, D.H., et al. (2010). Neurocognitive functioning before and after the first psychotic episode: does psychosis result in cognitive deterioration? *Psychol. Med.* 40:1599–1606.

Bloemen, O.J., de Koning, M.B., et al. (2010). White-matter markers for psychosis in a prospective ultra-high-risk cohort. *Psychol. Med.* 40:1297–1304.

Borgwardt, S., McGuire, P.K., et al. (2011). Gray matters! Mapping the transition to psychosis. *Schizophr. Res.* 133:63–67.

Borgwardt, S.J., Riecher-Rossler, A., et al. (2007). Regional gray matter volume abnormalities in the at-risk mental state. *Biol. Psychiatry* 61:1148–1156.

Brewer, W.J., Francey, S.M., et al. (2005). Memory impairments identified in people at ultra-high risk for psychosis who later develop first-episode psychosis. *Am. J. Psychiatry* 162:71–78.

Brewer, W.J., Wood, S.J., et al. (2003). Impairment of olfactory identification ability in individuals at ultra-high risk for psychosis who later develop schizophrenia. *Am. J. Psychiatry* 160:1790–1794.

Broome, M.R., Johns, L.C., et al. (2007). Delusion formation and reasoning biases in those at clinical high risk for psychosis. *Br. J. Psychiatry Suppl.* 51:38–42.

Carletti, F., Woolley, J.B., et al. (2012). Alterations in white matter evident before the onset of psychosis. *Schizophr. Bull.* 38:1170–1179.

Carpenter, W.T., and van Os J. (2011). Should attenuated psychosis syndrome be a DSM-5 diagnosis? *Am. J. Psychiatry* 168:460–463.

Chung, Y.S., Kang, D.H., et al. (2008). Deficit of theory of mind in individuals at ultra-high-risk for schizophrenia. *Schizophr. Res.* 99:111–118.

Crossley, N.A., Mechelli, A., et al. (2009). Superior temporal lobe dysfunction and fronto-temporal dysconnectivity in subjects at risk of psychosis and in first-episode psychosis. *Hum. Brain. Mapp.* 30:4129–4137.

Dickinson, D., Gold, J.M. (2008). Less unique variance than meets the eye: overlap among traditional neuropsychological dimensions in schizophrenia. *Schizophr. Bull.* 34:423–434.

Frommann I., Brinkmeyer, J., et al. (2008). Auditory P300 in individuals clinically at risk for psychosis. *Int. J. Psychophysiol.* 70:192–205.

Frommann, I., Pukrop, R., et al. (2011). Neuropsychological profiles in different at-risk states of psychosis: executive control impairment in the early—and additional memory dysfunction in the late—prodromal state. *Schizophr. Bull.* 37:861–873.

Fusar-Poli, P., Bonoldi, I., et al. (2012a). Predicting psychosis: meta-analysis of transition outcomes in individuals at high clinical risk. *Arch. Gen. Psychiatry* 69:220–229.

Fusar-Poli, P., Borgwardt, S., et al. (2011a). Neuroanatomical correlates of vulnerability to psychosis: a voxel-based meta-analysis. *Neurosci. Biobehav. Rev.* 35:1175–1185.

Fusar-Poli, P., Crossley, N., et al. (2011b). Gray matter alterations relted to P300 abnormalities in subjects at high risk for psychosis: longitudinal MRI-EEG study. *NeuroImage.* 55:320–328.

Fusar-Poli, P., Deste, G., et al. (2012b). Cognitive functioning in prodromal psychosis: a meta-analysis. *Arch. Gen. Psychiatry* 69:562–571.

Fusar-Poli, P., McGuire, P., et al. (2012c). Mapping prodromal psychosis: a critical review of neuroimaging studies. *Eur. Psychiatry* 27:181–191.

Fusar-Poli, P., Meyer-Lindenberg A. (2013). Striatal presynaptic dopamine in schizophrenia, part II: meta-analysis of [18F]/[11C] DOPA PET studies. *Schizophr. Bull.* 39:33–42.

Fusar-Poli, P., Stone, J.M., et al. (2011c). Thalamic glutamate levels as a predictor of cortical response during executive functioning in subjects at high risk for psychosis. *Arch. Gen. Psychiatry* 68:881–890.

Giuliano, A.J., Li, H., et al. (2012). Neurocognition in the psychosis risk syndrome: a quantitative and qualitative review. *Curr. Pharm. Des.* 18:399–415.

Green, M.F., Bearden, C.E., et al. (2012). Social cognition in schizophrenia: Part 1. Performance across phase of illness. *Schizophr. Bull.* 38:854–864.

Gschwandtner, U., Pfluger, M., et al. (2006). Fine motor function and neuropsychological deficits in individuals at risk for schizophrenia. *Eur. Arch. Psychiatry Clin. Neurosci.* 256:201–206.

Gur, R.C., Saykin, A.J., et al. (1990). "Behavioral imaging": III. Inter-rater agreement and reliability of weightings. *Neuropsychiatr. Neuropsychol. Behav. Neurol.* 3:113–124.

Hawkins, K.A., Addington, J., et al. (2004). Neuropsychological status of subjects at high risk for a first episode of psychosis. *Schizophr. Res.* 67:115–122.

Howes, O., Montgomery, A., et al. (2009). Elevated striatal dopamine function linked to prodromal signs of schizophrenia. *Arch. Gen. Psychiatry* 66:13–20.

Ilonen, T., Heinimaa, M., et al. (2010). Differentiating adolescents at clinical high risk for psychosis from psychotic and non-psychotic patients with the Rorschach. *Psychiatry Res.* 179:151–156.

Korver, N., Nieman, D.H., et al. (2010). Symptomatology and neuropsychological functioning in cannabis using subjects at ultra-high risk for developing psychosis and healthy controls. *Aust. N.Z. J. Psychiatry* 44:230–236.

Koutsouleris, N., Davatzikos, C., et al. (2012). Early recognition and disease prediction in the at-risk mental states for psychosis using neurocognitive pattern classification. *Schizophr. Bull.* 38:1200–1215.

Lindgren, M., Manninen, M., et al. (2010). The relationship between psychotic-clike symptoms and neurocognitive performance in a general adolescent psychiatric sample. *Schizophr. Res.* 123:77–85.

Magaud, E., Kebir, O., et al. (2010). Altered semantic but not phonological verbal fluency in young help-seeking individuals with ultra high risk of psychosis. *Schizophr. Res.* 123:53–58.

Miyake, A., Friedman, N.P., et al. (2000). The unity and diversity of executive functions and their contributions to complex "Frontal Lobe" tasks: a latent variable analysis. *Cogn. Psychol.* 40:49–100.

Peters, B.D., de Haan, L., et al. (2009). Recent-onset schizophrenia and adolescent cannabis use: MRI evidence for structural hyperconnectivity? *Psychopharmacol. Bull.* 42:75–88.

Pflueger, M.O., Gschwandtner, U., et al. (2007). Neuropsychological deficits in individuals with an at risk mental state for psychosis—working memory as a potential trait marker. *Schizophr. Res.* 97:14–24.

Pinkham, A.E., Penn, D.L., et al. (2007). Emotion perception and social skill over the course of psychosis: a comparison of individuals "at-risk" for psychosis and individuals with early and chronic schizophrenia spectrum illness. *Cogn. Neuropsychiatry* 12:198–212.

Pukrop, R., Ruhrmann, S., et al. (2007). Neurocognitive indicators for a conversion to psychosis: comparison of patients in a potentially initial prodromal state who did or did not convert to a psychosis. *Schizophr. Res.* 92:116–125.

Reichenberg, A., Caspi, A., et al. (2010). Static and dynamic cognitive deficits in childhood preceding adult schizophrenia: a 30-year study. *Am. J. Psychiatry* 167:160–169.

Riecher-Rossler, A., Pflueger, M.O., et al. (2009). Efficacy of using cognitive status in predicting psychosis: a 7-year follow-up. *Biol. Psychiatry* 66:1023–1030.

Seidman, L.J., Giuliano, A.J., et al. (2010). Neuropsychology of the prodrome to psychosis in the NAPLS Consortium: relationship to family history and conversion to psychosis. *Arch. Gen. Psychiatry* 67:578–588.

Silverstein, S., Uhlhaas, P.J., et al. (2006). Perceptual organization in first episode schizophrenia and ultra-high-risk states. *Schizophr. Res.* 83:41–52.

Simon, A.E., Cattapan-Ludewig, K., et al. (2007). Cognitive functioning in the schizophrenia prodrome. *Schizophr. Bull.* 33:761–771.

Smieskova, R., Fusar-Poli, P., et al. (2010). Neuroimaging predictors of transition to psychosis: a systematic review and meta-analysis. *Neurosci. Biobehav. Rev.* 38:1207–1222.

Smith, C.W., Park, S., et al. (2006). Spatial working memory deficits in adolescents at clinical high risk for schizophrenia. *Schizophr. Res.* 81:211–215.

Szily, E., and Keri, S. (2009). Anomalous subjective experience and psychosis risk in young depressed patients. *Psychopathology* 42:229–235.

Szoke, A., Trandafir, A., et al. (2008). Longitudinal studies of cognition in schizophrenia: metaanalysis. *Br. J. Psychiatry* 192:248–257.

Tibbo, P., Hanstock, C., et al. (2004). 3T proton MRS investigation of glutamate and glutamine in adolescents at high genetic risk for schizophrenia. *Am. J. Psychiatry* 161:1116–1118.

van Rijn, S., Aleman, A., et al. (2011). Misattribution of facial expressions of emotion in adolescents at increased risk of psychosis: the role of inhibitory control. *Psychol. Med.* 41:499–508.

Woodberry, K.A., Seidman, L.J., et al. (2010). Neuropsychological profiles in individuals at clinical high risk for psychosis: relationship to psychosis and intelligence. *Schizophr. Res.* 123:188–198.

27 | PSYCHOTIC DISORDERS: NEUROCHEMISTRY AND PHARMACOTHERAPY

CAROL A. TAMMINGA AND ELENA I. IVLEVA

PSYCHOSIS AS AN INDEPENDENT CLINICAL PHENOTYPE

Psychosis is a symptom dimension that appears in multiple brain disorders, most commonly in psychiatric disorders, but occasionally in neurological and other medical diagnoses. Psychotic symptoms include hallucinations, delusions, and thought disorder, as well as thought and behavioral disorganization. These symptoms are experienced by psychotic individuals as actual cognitive or sensory experiences and involve all sensory modalities (auditory, visual, olfactory, gustatory, and tactile). Several first-person accounts written by brilliant and self-perceptive individuals with psychosis record the nature of psychosis and show that there is a profound loss of reality testing around psychotic experiences. John Nash describes the nature of his delusion:

> These ideas just keep coming into my head. I can't prevent it. (I) believe that there is a conspiracy among military leaders to take over the world, and that (I) am in charge of the takeover. (I) secretly feel that I am the left foot of God. And that God is walking on the earth. (Nasar, 1998)

Elyn Saks details her experience of psychotic "disorientation":

> Consciousness gradually loses its coherence. The "me" becomes a haze...reality breaks up like a bad radio signal. There is no longer a sturdy vantage point from which to look out, take things in, assess what's happening. No core lens through which to see the world, to make judgments and comprehend risk. Random moments of time follow one another. Sights, sounds, thoughts, and feelings don't go together. No organizing principle takes successive moments in time and puts them together in a coherent way from which sense can be made. And it's all taking place in slow motion. (Saks, 2007).

The clinical manifestations of psychosis as just described, with hallucinations, delusions, thought disorder, and disorganization, are a disturbance of cognition, not a global loss of cognitive capacity as distinct from dementing illnesses. Indeed, psychosis can be thought of as a "gain-of-function" symptom, with increased associational productions, which generate bizarre perceptual experiences, thoughts, and memories with psychotic content; this is in contrast to dementias, which are "loss-of-function" cognitive disorders. Because the psychotic experiences appear entirely real to the person suffering them, it is easy for the individuals to act on the commands, the psychotic perceptions, or delusional thinking; this can result in bizarre, illogical, or aggressive behavior. Psychosis is a broadly expressed symptom set across diagnoses and thus could be an intermediate phenotype, perhaps a symptom dimension representing a final common pathway of cerebral dysfunction (including limbic cortex, we will argue). It is easy to presume that this symptom set has its own common and distinctive anatomy and pathophysiology, as well as molecular targets and treatments, although this has yet to be fully demonstrated (Fig. 27.1).

Psychotic symptoms in psychiatric diagnosis are highly sensitive to antipsychotic drugs, drugs that block dopamine D2 receptors or diminish dopamine mediated transmission, with limited evidence that serotonin antagonists (MDL100907), muscarinic agonists (xanomiline, Shekhar et al., 2008), or glutamate agonists (LY2140023) (Kinon and Gomez, 2012) can have an effect, albeit partial. It is often debated whether the behavioral state of psychosis can be modeled in a laboratory animal, with the difficulty being the ability to detect symptoms with the actual object dependent on language (behavioral state of psychosis). However, measurable behaviors that have been associated with psychotic human behavior, like altered pre-pulse inhibition (PPI), declarative memory dysfunction (e.g., fear conditioning correlates), and alterations in intentional bias, and the use of human psychotomimetic drugs can be used to represent psychosis, as putative human correlates of psychosis (Yanagi et al., 2012).

In psychotic diseases, as discussed in several of the earlier chapters, psychosis is not the only symptom set that causes dysfunction. In schizophrenia, which is generally considered to be the most persistent and severe of the psychotic disorders, patients suffer from cognitive dysfunction, negative symptoms, mood symptoms, and anxiety, in addition to psychosis. In psychotic bipolar disorder, it is not only psychosis, but also mood instability with mania, depression, and mixed states, as well as cognitive dysfunction that characterize persons with that diagnosis. The coexisting symptom dimensions (like cognitive dysfunction or negative symptoms) are not treated by antipsychotic drugs; they have their own disease course, with symptom-onset characteristically occurring before the psychosis and their distinctive life course. For these reasons many clinical scientists, exemplified by the NIMH *Measurement and Treatment Research to Improve Cognition in Schizophrenia* (MATRICS) group (Marder and Fenton, 2004), proposed

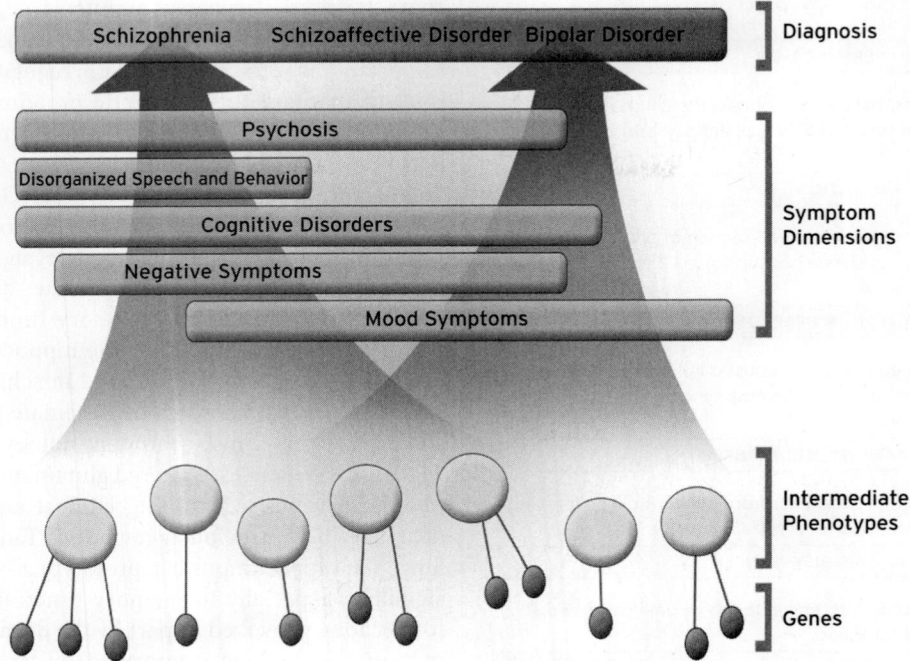

Figure 27.1 *The genes, intermediate phenotypes, and symptom dimensions that characterize the categorical diseases that we diagnose have been shown to overlap extensively. Therefore, to deconvolve the biology, we need to focus on disease dimensions and their underlying intermediate phenotypes, which will more directly relate to the genes underlying psychiatric conditions. (Previously published in Ivleva E.I., Tamminga C. 2009. Psychosis as a defining dimension in schizophrenia. In: Sadock, B.J., Sadock, V.A., and Ruiz, P. [Eds.], Kaplan & Sadock's Comprehensive Textbook of Psychiatry, 9th edition. Vol. 1. Philadelphia, PA: Lippincott Williams & Wilkins, schizophrenia. In: Sadock, B. Chapter 12.16, pp. 1594–1605.)*

formulating these entities as independent symptom dimensions, each with their own anatomy, molecular determinants, and pharmacology, hence likely to have their own treatments.

Thus, disease dimensions have become the therapeutic target of experimental therapeutics today.

MOLECULAR MECHANISMS OF PSYCHOSIS: MODELS OF THE ILLNESSES

DOPAMINE HYPERFUNCTION

Dopamine hyperfunction was the first molecular hypothesis of schizophrenia (Table 27.1). The only effective treatments discovered so far for psychosis are medications that reduce dopamine-mediated transmission in brain. Their action was identified serendipitously early in 1950 by Delay and Denniker, who used chlorpromazine initially as merely a sedative agent, but were alert enough to notice its selective antipsychotic activity. The use of chlorpromazine spread around the world very quickly for the treatment of psychosis, especially schizophrenia due to extremely high medical need. The identification of the dopaminergic mechanism of chlorpromazine was detected pharmacologically within the next decade by Carlsson and Lindquist (Carlsson and Lindquist, 1963), as dopamine receptor antagonism. Moreover, the subsequent design and development of dopamine receptor antagonists and now of partial dopamine agonists have confirmed the therapeutic action of this family of drugs on psychosis. So, it is well established that drugs which block dopamine receptors in brain improve

psychosis. It was an easy step from this body of knowledge to the idea that schizophrenia itself, and psychosis in particular, are diseases whose mechanisms involve a hyperfunction of the dopamine system. For the last half-century, clinical scientists have examined the "dopamine hypothesis of schizophrenia" using schizophrenia brain tissue, cerebrospinal fluid (CSF), blood, transformed cells, human brain imaging, and anything else available to demonstrate evidence of dopamine hyperactivity. Sadly, these studies as a group have not been able to verify the dopamine hypothesis of schizophrenia (Kendler and Schaffner, 2011). There is no replicable increase in dopamine receptor number, except that associated with chronic antipsychotic use; there is no consistent evidence of altered dopamine metabolites or proteins associated with dopamine signaling in schizophrenia brain tissue; although there is some evidence of increased dopamine release gathered through displacement imaging, this is not a feature unique to schizophrenia. Kendler et al. reviewed this area exhaustively and asked why the hypothesis was not falsified faster, a question important to experimental therapeutics (Kendler and Schaffner, 2011). At the present time, while the hypothesis is often quoted, it is not relied on within the field for the discovery of disease mechanism or for drug development. However, antipsychotic drugs are still identified by their antidopaminergic action, and there is no reconsideration of the well-substantiated observation that dopamine antagonism improves psychotic symptoms. To resurrect the usefulness of the "dopamine hypothesis of schizophrenia" in the field, a new and clear aspect of dopamine pharmacology will have to be identified as altered in schizophrenia.

TABLE 27.1. Molecular models of psychosis

DOPAMINE SIGNALING HYPERFUNCTION
First molecular hypothesis, based on pharmacological data. Postulates have not been confirmed. Yet, all antipsychotic drugs are antidopaminergic.
GLUTAMATE SIGNALING REDUCTION
Based first on the potent psychotomimetic action of phencyclidine. Considerable biochemical evidence has supported this model. There may be regional effects.
GABA SIGNALING REDUCTION IN PREFRONTAL CORTEX
Fast-spiking GABA interneurons show reduced inhibition; may be especially relevant for loss of cortical gamma synchrony and cognitive dysfunction in PFC.
ALTERED CNS NEUROPLASTICITY MECHANISMS
Psychosis could represent the loss of appropriate controls on learning and memory plasticity mechanisms. A still speculative idea.
MODELS BASED ON PSYCHOSIS RISK GENES
These models are interesting but remain tentative until psychosis genetics becomes fully established.
PSYCHOTOMIMETIC DRUG MODELS
These are the classical psychosis models. They have been highly useful for drug development but cannot be used to inform pathophysiology.

GLUTAMATE AND EXCITATORY TRANSMISSION

In the meantime, proteins in the glutamate system have been shown to be altered in schizophrenia tissue, and pharmacological blockade of NMDA glutamate receptors in normal people has been shown to mimic symptoms of schizophrenia, generating the idea that glutamatergic action is reduced in schizophrenia. Pharmacology of the NMDA receptor suggests that a reduction in glutamate signaling at this receptor can mimic some of the psychotic symptoms of schizophrenia (Tamminga, 1999), as well as its cognitive symptoms in normal human volunteers (Krystal et al., 1994a). Molecular alterations in glutamate-related proteins are documented in postmortem tissue and CSF, changes that could impair signaling at this receptor (Gao et al., 2000; Tamminga, 1999; Tsai et al., 1995). Therefore, molecular targets within the NMDA receptor complex have become interesting targets for drug development in both psychosis and cognition (Table 27.1).

Glutamate signaling impinges most neurons in the brain and supports activity-dependent signaling, neuronal growth, and synaptic plasticity (Benarroch, 2011; Lynch and Guttmann, 2001; Nikam and Kornberg, 2001). The glutamate system is regionally diverse and complex, with multiple interacting receptors, modulating co-transmitters, and multiple postsynaptic intracellular signaling systems. Presynaptic, postsynaptic, and astrocytic mechanisms all contribute to overall excitatory signaling and to unique plasticity mechanisms that are involved with glutamatergic transmission (Lee et al., 2010; Shepherd and Huganir, 2007; Song and Huganir, 2002); these compartments are all candidate systems for pathology in glutamate-related brain diseases. Regional

characteristics of synapse architecture, local circuitry, and specialized postsynaptic signaling mechanisms, suggest that important aspects of glutamate regulation are local. The roles of many of these synaptic proteins were discussed in Chapter 25. Even within regions, functional specialization occurs on a microcircuit level with the same glutamatergic architecture serving distinct functions (Greer and Greenberg, 2008). It is already known that the hippocampus and its surrounding cortex features glutamate signaling to a greater extent than other neocortical tissue, a characteristic that underlies its learning and memory functions (Franzek and Beckmann, 1996). Moreover, the hippocampus is one of the brain regions functionally altered in schizophrenia, suggesting the potential relevance of glutamate transmission in this structure to psychosis pathophysiology (Tamminga et al., 2010). The evidence for altered glutamate signaling in schizophrenic psychosis, including clinical and pharmacological, data, have been previously reviewed (Tamminga et al., 2010). Since the hippocampus is a prototypical excitatory organ, its signaling, especially in memory function, has been studied for decades, provoked in part by the dramatic demonstration of its essential role in memory by the case of Henry Moliason (HM) (Rempel-Clower et al., 1996). Thus there exists a rich understanding around the role of glutamate and excitatory transmission in declarative memory. There exists evidence and plausible models that psychosis is due to reduced glutamatergic transmission at the NMDA-sensitive receptor and several hypotheses have been proposed to account for this (Olney and Farber, 1995; Tsai and Coyle, 2002). While no definitive mechanisms have yet been demonstrated, the idea that psychosis in schizophrenia may involve inadequate glutamatergic transmission at the NMDA receptor is widely acknowledged and remains plausible. In addition, evidence implicates the hippocampus, in particular in psychosis, involving its unique cortical anatomy and its subfield-specific functions (Tamminga et al., 2010)

GABA AND INHIBITORY TRANSMISSION

As detailed in Chapter 24, considerable evidence implicates alterations in GABAergic transmission in the manifestations of schizophrenia, based on very early and simple ideas of neocortical function, dependent on controlled excitation extensively modulated by GABA-mediated inhibition. Modern postmortem research has shown cell-specific GABA reductions in neocortex, most precisely worked out in prefrontal cortex (PFC) (Krystal et al., 1994b). In PFC schizophrenia tissue, reduced concentrations of GAD67, one of the synthetic enzymes for GABA, occur and are especially prominent in CCK- and parvalbumin-containing inhibitory interneurons. Upregulated postsynaptic GABA receptors have been found (Krystal et al., 1994b), which have been interpreted to reflect reduced synaptic levels of GABA in the specific synapses in PFC. Speculations have connected this GABA reduction with PFC regional cerebral activation reductions, with reduced cognitive function possibly mediated by the loss of gamma synchrony already associated with schizophrenia. Some (Wang et al., 2011) but not all (Kegeles et al., 2000) data implicate GABA reduction

in other areas of PFC and in hippocampus, leaving the role of GABA in hippocampal function less clear.

LEARNING AND MEMORY PLASTICITY DYSFUNCTION

Observations drawn from *in vivo* imaging studies in schizophrenia (which show *increased* perfusion in the hippocampus; Heckers et al., 1998; Medoff et al., 2001; Schobel et al., 2009) and from postmortem schizophrenia tissue studies (which show *decreased* GluN1 expression in hippocampal subfields, especially dentate gyrus [DG]; Deicken et al., 1999; Gao et al., 2000) converge to suggest that homeostatic plasticity mechanisms might be altered in the hippocampus in patients (Eichenbaum, 2000; McClelland et al., 1995; Preston and Wagner, 2007). We have proposed a speculative and testable model of psychosis, based on evidence of altered hippocampal learning and memory, and suggest that altered glutamate-mediated functions in hippocampal subfields are involved in psychotic and deficient declarative memory manifestations of schizophrenia (Tamminga et al., 2010).

It is the functional effect secondary to this reduced glutamate signaling in DG in CA3 that could be of interest for psychosis. DG projects to CA3 in the mossy fiber pathway, a link within the trisynaptic circuit. We suspect that this decrease in activity-dependent signaling from DG sensitizes its target tissue (CA3) to incoming stimuli and generates a lower LTP threshold and increased cellular sensitivity; this could generate higher levels of neuronal activity in CA3, to be projected onto CA1. We suggest that this results in an increase in synaptic strength in CA3, accompanied by increased associational memory function. The ability of homeostatic plasticity phenomena to support this kind of model is included in data generated in the Malenka, Bear, and Malinow laboratories, among others (Tamminga et al., 2010). It is a speculation that increases in CA3 associational function could generate false associations, some with psychotic content, which could then get laid down in memory as psychotic thoughts and memories. This idea is consistent with the reduction in glutamate signaling in DG (indicated by a decrease in GluR1 protein), as well as the increase in hippocampal perfusion that we detect with rCBF measures (Tamminga et al., 2010) and the finding that BDNF is increased regionally in CA3 in schizophrenia tissue (Ghose et al., 2006). Dysfunction of associational memory with changes localized to CA3 would lead to the assumption that occasional and fleeting mistakes in CA3 could be responsible for the psychosis-like phenomena in normal and in "prodromal" individuals. Persistent and high increases in CA3 activity could stimulate psychosis thinking and generate manifestations that would resemble schizophrenia.

GENETIC ASSOCIATIONS AS MODELS

Modern genetic outcomes have contributed to the realization that schizophrenia and psychosis are complex genetic illnesses. Whereas there was early evidence for specific risk genes, the problems with replication and power soon suggested that many genes generate risk for schizophrenia and psychosis. Recent genome-wide association studies suggest that there may be more than 1,000 risk genes, each of small effect, for psychosis syndromes (Wellcome Trust Case Control Consortium, 2007). Although the majority of the candidate genes were first implicated in schizophrenia, recent reports have suggested an overlap in genetic susceptibility across the traditional diagnostic categories. GWAS, candidate genes, family, and twin genetic studies all indicate overlap across diagnostic categories, as outlined in Chapter 19. This implicates the potential for common genetic risk across the whole psychosis spectrum. It also suggests that simpler behaviors, like intermediate phenotypes for psychosis, may be useful in genotyping to develop a more precise understanding of the basis of psychotic illness (Fig. 27.1). Understanding the genes associated with intermediate phenotypes of psychosis will surely inform genetic mouse models for psychosis, as soon as the relationship between genes and intermediate phenotypes becomes clarified.

ANIMAL MODELS OF PSYCHOSIS

Animal models of human brain diseases, which are stringently based on disease features having strong construct validity, are critical for testing disease pathophysiology and novel treatment development (Young et al., 2009, 2010). However, because the mechanistic basis of schizophrenia remains obscure, our ability to develop verified animal models has been critically challenged (Nestler and Hyman, 2010). Current preclinical models of schizophrenia are primitive and mechanistically speculative, with no forward vision of how to verify the models; there is often insufficient indication that these models are related to disease pathophysiology in human constructs. Nonetheless, developments in the conceptualization of complex diseases like schizophrenia will allow more kinds of animal models to be relevant and their verification more direct (Hyman and Fenton, 2003).

The *Schizophrenia Research Forum* lists 87 putative rodent models for aspects of schizophrenia. These models can be organized into three main categories and model not only psychosis in schizophrenia but also cognitive dysfunction and negative symptoms, all dimensions of illness in schizophrenia. These animal models are based on psychotomimetic drug stimulation, early adversity and lesion models, and schizophrenia risk gene models.

Psychotomimetic agents include amphetamine, phencyclidine and their congeners. These are drugs that cause psychosis in humans, often including schizophrenia-like symptoms, and tend to exacerbate the psychotic manifestations in schizophrenia. It has been assumed that an understanding of the mechanism(s) of these psychosis-inducing actions might contribute to our fundamental understanding of psychosis, although this has not yet been the case. Psychotomimetic drugs have been administered to animals both for psychosis pathophysiology studies and in order to model pharmacological antagonist approaches as treatments.

The approach of introducing environmental adversity to animals early in development to model schizophrenia grew out of observations and epidemiological data showing that early

childhood adversity, including prenatal, perinatal, and developmental adverse events, predispose individuals to schizophrenia in adulthood (Akbarian, 2010; Brown, 2011). How these childhood adversities predispose individuals to develop illness in adulthood is not known but could be associated with epigenetic alterations that develop in childhood to pose risks during adulthood. The idea that early changes in brain structure or function, or in epigenetic signaling, contribute to an adult onset illness has been a generative concept in the field of schizophrenia pathophysiology.

Closest to a study of disease mechanism has been the study of genetically modified animals at schizophrenia-risk loci. These animal models are reviewed in Chapter 9, and provide critical evidence of specific molecular lesions which can be associated with illness. It is unfortunate that these risk genes are not strong enough to be comprehensive, but will become increasingly useful as the molecular bases of psychosis is defined.

ESTABLISHED AND EXPERIMENTAL PSYCHOSIS TREATMENTS

HISTORY OF ANTIPSYCHOTIC DRUG DEVELOPMENT

Discovery of the antipsychotic action of chlorpromazine in the mid-1950s identified the first therapeutic agent for schizophrenia and it happened serendipitously. Its selective antipsychotic properties were noticed with its first application, and its use spread around the world within a few years, signaling the overwhelming medical need for psychosis treatments. In the decade following this clinical discovery, not only was the probable mechanism of antipsychotic drug action articulated as monoamine (especially dopamine) receptor blockade (Carlsson and Lindquist, 1963) but also many additional antipsychotic compounds were generated, based on the clear molecular target being the dopamine receptor. These dopamine antagonists have formed the exclusive effective, but incomplete, antipsychotic armamentarium for psychiatrists throughout the past half-century. Each of the traditional and newer antipsychotics is associated with a distinctive side effect profile but with the same primary antipsychotic effects (Davis, 1969).

TRADITIONAL ANTIPSYCHOTIC DRUGS

There are many primary and review papers in this area (Gallego et al., 2012; Leucht et al., 2012), allowing the emphasis here to highlight the trajectory of drug development and special features important to the clinical use of antipsychotic drugs.

Chlorpromazine, after its serendipitous discovery, was evaluated in the early 1950s in multicenter trials (Davis, 1969). The trials inevitably included drug-naïve individuals, because this was the first effective drug for psychosis. Patient response was brisk and extensive; improvement occurred incrementally over several weeks. Remarkable reductions of 80% or more in psychotic symptoms were reported, including resolution of hallucinations, delusions, and thought disorder. The drug

was broadly applied and the development of additional compounds strongly encouraged because of the long awaited efficacy of a drug treatment for florid psychosis. Side effects of chlorpromazine include parkinsonism and akathisia, and also hypotension, sedation, and amenorrhea. Hepatotoxicity and electrocardiographic changes were less frequent but more serious side effects. Tardive dyskinesia occurred as well. Today the use of chlorpromazine has gradually diminished, based mostly on its sedative and cardiovascular side effects, and still significant parkinsonism.

Haloperidol was introduced in the late 1950s, and until recently, was the most widely prescribed antipsychotic for schizophrenia and psychosis in general. Its potent antipsychotic action with little sedation, despite acute chronic motor side effects, sustained its widespread recommendation as an antipsychotic. It remains to be seen if new drugs will offer side-effect advantages over haloperidol to increase compliance and reduce relapse sufficiently to balance their increased cost. The pharmacology of haloperidol is broadly documented because the drug is often used as the prototypical control antipsychotic for animal and human studies. Functional imaging studies of humans have addressed the question of where in the brain haloperidol exerts its actions, relating its extensive pharmacology to its clinical actions. In this regard it is interesting to note that haloperidol increases neuronal activity throughout the basal ganglia, in both dorsal and ventral regions, and in the thalamus, while it decreases neuronal activity in the PFC and in the anterior cingulate cortex (ACC) (Holcomb et al., 1996). We presume that activations in dorsal basal ganglia relate to motor side effects, while functional alterations in PFC and ACC may underlie therapeutic actions, although this interpretation is still speculative. The antipsychotic efficacy of haloperidol was initially established in controlled clinical trials in the early 1960s (Davis, 1969). But it was not until recently that a dose-response study was conducted across the apparent dose-sensitive range for haloperidol, showing a highly potent action without a linear relationship between dose and antipsychotic action (Zimbroff et al., 1997). Haloperidol produced significant parkinsonism and akathisia across all doses used, even at the lowest dose tested (4 mg/day).

Clozapine is an antipsychotic drug, which, although it has led the "new drug" era, is not itself new. Clozapine has a uniquely superior antipsychotic action, demonstrated in treatment-resistant individuals and in partial treatment responders (Kane et al., 1988). While it is the only superior antipsychotic, the molecular mechanism(s) associated with this action are unknown, although often suggested to be associated with its broad but low affinity for many monoamine receptors; its pharmacology is consistent with these characteristics (Coward, 1992). Clozapine has several active metabolites, two abundant examples of which are norclozapine and desmethylclozapine. Clozapine's neurochemical profile showing reduced dopamine receptor occupancy in striatum and increased serotonin receptor occupancy in cortex (Farde et al., 1992) is characteristic of the second generation of antipsychotics (Kapur et al., 1999). Functional imaging results are consistent with those for haloperidol, although the striatal activations are only in limited ventral regions, not broadly throughout the

basal ganglia, compared with extensive actions by haloperidol (Lahti et al., 2002). Moreover, clozapine differs from haloperidol in that it increases neuronal activity in the ACC and PFC, areas that are important to core cognitive functions like attention and working memory. Acute motor side effects are not often seen with clozapine including parkinsonism and akathisia. In addition, clozapine appears by all estimates to have an extremely low (if any) incidence of tardive dyskinesia. With respect to other side effects, however, clozapine is at the top of the list. It causes agranulocytosis with an incidence of 0.5–1%, a condition which has a 3–15% mortality. The risk for agranulocytosis is highest in the second and third months after beginning treatment; risk is reduced after the first six months and remains flat and relatively low after the first twelve treatment months of treatment. In addition, the drug can induce seizures, increase heart rate, and stimulate cardiac arrhythmias. The drug causes substantial weight gain, and alters carbohydrate metabolism while it affects plasma lipids, a symptom complex called the metabolic syndrome (Allison et al., 1999; Henderson et al., 2000; Wirshing et al., 1999). It also causes other less medically significant, but bothersome side effects like sedation and drooling. It is surprising that, with this serious side effect profile, clozapine is used at all; however, the value of its added benefit in psychosis weighs successfully against all of these side effects, particularly for the seriously ill schizophrenic person.

One of the active metabolites of clozapine is *N-desmethylclozapine* (NDMC); it has similar pharmacological properties to clozapine with the exception of demonstrating M_1/M_5 agonist actions instead of the M_1/M_5 antagonist actions of clozapine (Burstein et al., 2005; Weiner et al., 2004). This distinction suggests that NDMC will have an improved action on cognitive dysfunction in schizophrenia along with the superior clozapine-like antipsychotic action. Indirect evidence supports this prediction with the observation that among clozapine treated patients, a linear correlation exists between cognitive performance and the ratio of NDMC/clozapine (Davies et al., 2005).

SECOND-GENERATION ANTIPSYCHOTIC DRUGS

Risperidone is a benzisoxazol derivative with high affinity for the $5HT_{2A}$ and D_2 receptors. Its *in-vitro* affinity for serotonin $5HT_{2A}$ is 20 times higher than for dopamine D_2 receptors. Risperidone efficacy has been evaluated in schizophrenia across a broad dose range (2–16 mg/day) in several large multicenter trials showing a reduction in positive and negative symptoms; positive symptoms responded to risperidone in a similar fashion as to haloperidol; negative symptom response may be greater (Marder and Meibach, 1994). A risperidone dose of 3–6 mg/day produces the most desired outcome in the usual patients (Love et al., 1999). Risperidone has been extensively used as an antipsychotic in the elderly, in part because of its favorable motor side effect profile with limited sedation. A long-acting injectable preparation of risperidone is available, made up of active medication encapsulated in a Medisorb polymer, generating microspheres. After a single injection of a recommended dose of 25–50 mg, the microspheres will generate a slow and steady release of risperidone

between three and seven weeks after injection. Steady state plasma levels occur after four injections. Clinical actions begin three weeks after the injection and will extend 4–6 weeks after that. This long-acting risperidone has shown full antipsychotic efficacy in several large multicenter clinical trials. Its primary actions and side effects are similar to the parent drug. Its recommended dose is 25 mg every two weeks, with an increase to 37.5 mg or 50 mg where necessary. This is the first long-acting preparation of any second-generation drug and has the potential to improve medication compliance in persons with psychosis. Motor side effects are relatively low with risperidone at doses below 4 mg/day. At doses above 10 mg/day, parkinsonism and akathisia are similar to haloperidol. Hyperprolactinemia is common and frank galactorrhea regularly seen with risperidone. Weight gain occurs, but to a mild degree. The metabolic syndrome, although apparent with risperidone, is not as frequent as with clozapine or olanzapine (Allison et al., 1999).

Olanzapine is a structural congener of clozapine and has many of the same pharmacologic characteristics as clozapine, with significant exceptions in side effects (i.e., no agranulocytosis) and in efficacy (*i.e.* equal, but not superior efficacy). Olanzapine efficacy was established based on four large placebo- and haloperidol-controlled multicenter registration trials (Tamminga and Kane, 1997; Tollefson et al., 1997b). Consistently, olanzapine showed a clear antipsychotic response in actively psychotic schizophrenic patients, significantly greater than placebo and equivalent to haloperidol on positive symptoms. There was a suggestion that olanzapine could be more effective for negative symptoms than haloperidol (Tollefson et al., 1997a). Motor side effects with olanzapine treatment are remarkably diminished compared to traditional drugs. Whereas at high doses, mild akathisia can be seen, anticholinergic drug use for motor side effects is low. Weight gain can be substantial. Metabolic syndrome with abnormal carbohydrate metabolism, frank diabetes, and elevated plasma lipid measures is reported, thus increasing metabolic and cardiovascular burden (Bettinger et al., 2000; Osser et al., 1999). No blood dyscrasias are associated with olanzapine use, a side effect closely evaluated because of the structural similarity between olanzapine and clozapine.

The other second-generation antipsychotic drugs include *quetiapine ziprasidone, and aripiprazole*. Each of the second-generation drugs has demonstrated antipsychotic activity and moderate, if any, motor side effects. Quetiapine is distinguished by its sleep action (prolongs sleep without inducing it) and it is often administered before bed but it still retains the metabolic side effects of clozapine-like drugs. Ziprasidone and aripiprazole both have low levels of metabolic side effects and are antipsychotic drugs that avoid gross weight gain. Additional drugs with antipsychotic activity have continued to be marketed, including lurazidone (Kane, 2011), asenipine (Potkin, 2011), paliperidone (Richelson, 2010), and iloperidone (Weiden, 2012), and others are under development. All of the new drug actions include antidopaminergic activity, so success at novel drug development for psychosis outside of the dopaminergic modulation class has not achieved full success. It remains unclear why the effective pharmacotherapy of psychosis is so focused.

GLUTAMATERGIC DRUGS

Drugs that block the NMDA receptor generate robust psychotic manifestations in normal people, as well as psychosis exacerbation in patients, and generate psychotic-like behaviors in animals. Moreover, analysis of human tissue from schizophrenia cases shows alterations in NMDA receptor and signaling proteins. Therefore, glutamate enhancers, especially those acting at the NMDA receptor, have been put forward as rational hypothetical antipsychotics. In 2006, when Schoeppe et al. reported the efficacy of LY2140023, an agonist at the mGluR2/3 metabotropic receptor which is thought to augment glutamate release through a presynaptic mechanism, there was considerable excitement (Kinon and Gomez, 2012). However, the promise has not been born out, and public summaries of two follow-up studies have both been negative. Several additional glutamatergic drugs are still in development, both as stand-alone antipsychotics and as co-treatments with standard drugs for cognitive dysfunction (Kinon, 2011). Results from additional glutamate enhancing strategies will inform this area further as they become available. It is widely speculated that these drugs may act effectively in subgroups of individuals with glutamate-mediated lesions accounting for their psychosis.

MUSCARINIC AGONISTS

An interesting antipsychotic candidate, xanomiline, was originally developed as a cognition-enhancing drug for Alzheimer's disease, and now has shown surprising effects in a single-site schizophrenia trial (Shekhar et al., 2008). Xanomiline showed both a significant (although not large) antipsychotic action in schizophrenia as well as an advantage for cognition. Whether or not these manifestations can be demonstrated in a large multisite trial is an unanswered question. Cholinesterase inhibitors are not effective antipsychotic agents but have a much lower potency as cholinergic drugs than direct-acting cholinergic agonists. There are additional cholinergic agents available to test (Sellin et al., 2008) and considerable activity in the development of allosteric modulators of selected muscarinic receptors subtypes. It may be possible within the next few years to follow up on this original clever finding.

COGNITIVE DYSFUNCTION IN PSYCHOSIS AND EXPERIMENTAL TREATMENTS

Cognitive dysfunction in schizophrenia is often associated with poor psychosocial outcome, correlating significantly with aspects of poor psychosocial outcomes, therefore effective treatment is important (Green, 1996). This motivated the NIMH to open up the area of cognition treatments in schizophrenia, in part by spearheading the NIMH Measurement and Treatment Research to Improve Cognition in Schizophrenia (MATRICS) project (Marder and Fenton, 2004). The literature supports the presence of several, but not all, cognitive dimensions as abnormal in schizophrenia, including "speed of processing," "attention and vigilance," "working memory," "verbal learning and memory," "visual learning and memory," "reasoning and problem solving," and "social cognition." Animal research suggests that each cognitive domain could be distinctive in its anatomy, pharmacology, and likely in its molecular treatment. Many studies are ongoing to identify treatments for cognitive dysfunction.

MOLECULAR TARGETS FOR COGNITION IN SCHIZOPHRENIA

No treatments currently exist for cognitive dysfunction in psychosis. No human targets are apparent, and no understanding of the molecular basis exists. However, abundant animal literature exists to support interest in several different molecular targets in schizophrenia.

The role of the hippocampal alpha-7 nicotinic receptor in sensory gating and attention, and its alteration in schizophrenia provide the basis for strategies augmenting alpha-7 nicotinic signaling in schizophrenia (Martin et al., 2004). In addition, the delineation of selective deficits in GABA receptor subunits within subpopulations of GABA-containing neurons in the prefrontal cortex have led to the strategy of augmenting GABA signaling in prefrontal cortex pharmacologically (Lewis et al., 2004). These strategies are currently being tested in humans with pharmacologic probes.

With non-human primate models of working memory, Goldman-Rakic elegantly established the importance of D_1 dopamine signaling for working memory, a key area of cognition dysfunction in schizophrenia. Diverse experiments suggest that dopamine signaling at the D_1 receptor could be insufficient in persons with schizophrenia (Akil et al., 2003; Karlsson et al., 2002; Okubo et al., 1997; Potkin et al., 2003; Selemon et al., 1995). In animals, D_1 but not D_2 antagonists disrupt working memory and D_1 agonists promote cognition (Goldman-Rakic et al., 2004). Therefore, the augmentation of D_1 signaling in schizophrenia is one of the most viable approaches for improving cognition, especially for augmenting working memory.

Serotonin, as a neurotransmitter, uses different CNS receptors for its signaling pathways. Evidence supports a role for the 5-HT1a, 5-HT2a, 5-HT4, and 5-HT6 receptor systems as potential targets for schizophrenia cognition (Roth et al., 2004). The 5-HT1a receptors are located in regions of brain that subserve learning and memory, including the hippocampus and neocortex. Considerable animal evidence suggests that 5-HT1a active drugs could be cognitively enhancing in humans; clinical evidence also supports this idea, but without being clear if it is a 5-HT1a partial agonist or a 5-HT1a full antagonist that would have the best cognition-enhancing action (Roth et al., 2004). Modest, but indirect evidence, supports the role of the 5-HT2, 5-HT4, and 5-HT6 receptors in cognition enhancement. Studies are currently being carried out in humans with cognitive disorders testing candidates from each of these families.

Additional data (mostly preclinical) exist to support several other molecular targets for cognitive enhancements in schizophrenia, including the muscarinic cholinergic receptors (Friedman, 2004), the metabotropic glutamate receptor (Moghaddam, 2004), and adrenergic receptors (Arnsten, 2004).

It is an era of discovery for schizophrenia therapeutics (Insel, 2012). The possibility that multiple, dimension-specific co-treatments could be necessary for full response in the illness will be tested.

DISCLOSURES

Dr. Tamminga has the following conflict of interest, disclosures, and financial support. To my knowledge, all of my possible conflicts of interest and those of my coauthors, financial or otherwise, including direct or indirect financial or personal relationships, interests, and affiliations, whether or not directly related to the subject of the chapter, are listed here.

- American Psychiatric Association—Deputy Editor >$10,000

- Astellas—Ad Hoc Consultant <$10,000

- The Brain & Behavior Foundation—Council Member; Unpaid Volunteer

- Eli Lilly Pharmaceuticals—Ad Hoc Consultant <$10,000

- International Congress on Schizophrenia Research—Organizer; Unpaid volunteer

- Intra-cellular Therapies—Advisory Board, Drug Development <$10,000

- Institute of Medicine—Council Member; Unpaid Volunteer

- Lundbeck, Inc—Ad Hoc Consultant <$10,000

- NAMI—Council Member; Unpaid Volunteer

- National Institute of Medicine—Council Member <$10,000

- PureTech Ventures—Ad Hoc Consultant <$10,000

Dr. Ivleva has no conflicts of interest to disclose. She is funded by NIMH & BBRF/NARSAD only. Grant Support: NIMH (1 R01 MH077851–01A1, PI: Tamminga, Role: co-investigator), BBRF/NARSAD (17801, Role: PI).

REFERENCES

Akbarian, S. (2010). Epigenetics of schizophrenia. Curr. Top. Behav. Neurosci. 4:611–628.

Akil, M., Kolachana, B.S., et al. (2003). Catechol-O-methyltransferase genotype and dopamine regulation in the human brain. J. Neurosci. 23:2008–2013.

Allison, D.B., Mentore, J.L., et al. (1999). Antipsychotic-induced weight gain: a comprehensive research synthesis. Am. J. Psychiatry 156:1686–1696.

Arnsten, A.F.T. (2004). Adrenergic targets for the treatment of cognitive deficits in schizophrenia. Psychopharmacology 174:25–31.

Benarroch, E.E. (2011). NMDA receptors: recent insights and clinical correlations. Neurology 76:1750–1757.

Bettinger, T.L., Mendelson, et al. (2000). Olanzapine-induced glucose dysregulation. Ann. Pharmacother. 34:865–867.

Brown, A.S. (2011). The environment and susceptibility to schizophrenia. Prog. Neurobiol. 93:23–58.

Burstein, E.S., Ma, J.N., et al. (2005). Intrinsic efficacy of antipsychotics at human D2, D3, and D4 dopamine receptors: identification of the clozapine metabolite N-desmethylclozapine as a D2/D3 partial agonist. J. Pharmacol. Exp. Ther. 315:1278–1287.

Carlsson, A., and Lindquist, L. (1963). Effect of chlorpromazine or haloperidol on formation of 3-methoxytyramine and normetanephrine in mouse brain. Acta Pharmacol. Toxicol. 20:140–145.

Coward, D.M. (1992). General pharmacology of clozapine. [Review] [56 refs]. Br. J. Psychiatry Suppl. 17:5–11.

Davies, M.A., Compton-Toth, B.A., et al. (2005). The highly efficacious actions of N-desmethylclozapine at muscarinic receptors are unique and not a common property of either typical or atypical antipsychotic drugs: is M1 agonism a pre-requisite for mimicking clozapine's actions? Psychopharmacology 178:451–460.

Davis, J.M. (1969). Review of antipsychotic drug literature. In: Klein, D.F., and Davis, J.M., eds. Diagnosis and Drug Treatment of Psychiatric Disorders. Baltimore: Williams and Wilkins, pp. 52–138.

Deicken, R.F., Pegues, M., et al. (1999). Reduced hippocampal N-acetylaspartate without volume loss in schizophrenia. Schizophr. Res. 37:217–223.

Eichenbaum, H. (2000). A cortical-hippocampal system for declarative memory. Neuroscience 1:41–50.

Farde, L., Nordstrom, A.L., et al. (1992). Positron emission tomographic analysis of central D1 and D2 dopamine receptor occupancy in patients treated with classical neuroleptics and clozapine. Relation to extrapyramidal side effects. Arch. Gen. Psychiatry 49:538–544.

Franzek, E., Beckmann, H. (1996). [Genetic heterogeneity of schizophrenia. Results of a systematic twin study]. Nervenarzt. 67:583–594.

Friedman, J.I. (2004). Cholinergic targets for cognitive enhancement in schizophrenia: focus on cholinesterase inhibitors and muscarinic agonists. Psychopharmacology 174(1):45–53.

Gallego, J.A., Bonetti, J., et al. (2012). Prevalence and correlates of antipsychotic polypharmacy: a systematic review and meta-regression of global and regional trends from the (1970)s to (2009). Schizophr. Res. 138:18–28.

Gao, X.M., Sakai, K., et al. (2000). Ionotropic glutamate receptors and expression of N-methyl-D-aspartate receptor subunits in subregions of human hippocampus: effects of schizophrenia. Am. J. Psychiatry 157:1141–1149.

Ghose, S., Chin, R., et al. (2006). Distinct gene expression correlations in schizophrenia between NR1 and GAD67 in the anterior hippocampus. Abstract, Society for Neuroscience.

Goldman-Rakic, P.S., Castner, S.A., et al. (2004). Targeting the dopamine D1 receptor in schizophrenia: insights for cognitive dysfunction. Psychopharmacology 174(1):3–16.

Green, M.F. (1996). What are the functional consequences of neurocognitive deficits in schizophrenia? Am. J. Psychiatry 153:321–330.

Greer, P.L., and Greenberg, M.E. (2008). From synapse to nucleus: calcium-dependent gene transcription in the control of synapse development and function. Neuron 59:846–860.

Heckers, S., Rauch, S.L., et al. (1998). Impaired recruitment of the hippocampus during conscious recollection in schizophrenia. Nature 1:318–323.

Henderson, D.C., Cagliero, E., et al. (2000). Clozapine, diabetes mellitus, weight gain, and lipid abnormalities: A five-year naturalistic study. Am. J. Psychiatry 157:975–981.

Holcomb, H.H., Cascella, N.G., et al. (1996). Functional sites of neuroleptic drug action in the human brain: PET/FDG studies with and without haloperidol. Am. J. Psychiatry 153:41–49.

Hyman, S.E., and Fenton, W.S. (2003). Medicine: what are the right targets for psychopharmacology? Science 299:350–351.

Insel, T.R. (2012). Next-generation treatments for mental disorders. Sci. Transl. Med. 4:155ps19.

Kane, J., Honigfeld, G., et al. (1988). Clozapine for the treatment-resistant schizophrenic. A double-blind comparison with chlorpromazine. Arch. Gen. Psychiatry 45:789–796.

Kane, J.M. (2011). Lurasidone: a clinical overview. J. Clin. Psychiatry 72(Suppl 1):24–28.

Kapur, S., Zipursky, R.B., et al. (1999). Clinical and theoretical implications of 5-HT2 and D2 receptor occupancy of clozapine, risperidone, and olanzapine in schizophrenia. Am. J. Psychiatry 156:286–293.

Karlsson, P., Farde, L., et al. (2002). PET study of D(1) dopamine receptor binding in neuroleptic-naive patients with schizophrenia. Am. J. Psychiatry 159:761–767.

Kegeles, L.S., Shungu, D.C., et al. (2000). Hippocampal pathology in schizophrenia: magnetic resonance imaging and spectroscopy studies. Psychiatry Research 98:163–175.

Kendler, K.S., Schaffner, K.F. (2011). The dopamine hypothesis of schizophrenia: an historical and philosophical analysis. Philos. Psychiatry Psychol. 18:41–63.

Kinon, B. (2011). A long-term, phase 2, safety study of LY(2140)023 monohydrate vs atypical antipsychotic standard of care in schizophrenia. *Schizophr. Bull.* 37:311.

Kinon, B.J., and Gomez, J.C. (2012). Clinical development of pomaglumetad methionil: A non-dopaminergic treatment for schizophrenia. *Neuropharmacol.* 66:82–86.

Krystal, J.H., Karper, L.P., et al. (1994a). Subanesthetic effects of the noncompetitive NMDA antagonist, ketamine, in humans: psychotomimetic, perceptual, cognitive, and neuroendocrine responses. *Arch. Gen. Psychiatry* 51:199–214.

Krystal, J.H., Karper, L.P., et al. (1994b). Subanesthetic effects of the noncompetitive NMDA antagonist, ketamine, in humans. Psychotomimetic, perceptual, cognitive, and neuroendocrine responses. *Arch. Gen. Psychiatry* 51:199–214.

Lahti, A.C., Holcomb, H.H., et al. (2002). Functional effects of antipsychotic drugs: comparing clozapine with haloperidol. *Biol. Psychiatry* 53(7):601–608.

Lee, M.C., Yasuda, R., et al. (2010). Metaplasticity at single glutamatergic synapses. *Neuron* 66:859–870.

Leucht, S., Tardy, M., et al. (2012). Maintenance treatment with antipsychotic drugs for schizophrenia. *Cochrane Database Syst. Rev.* 5:CD(0080)16.

Lewis, D.A., Volk, D.W., et al. (2004). Selective alterations in prefrontal cortical GABA neurotransmission in schizophrenia: a novel target for the treatment of working memory dysfunction. *Psychopharmacology* 174:143–150.

Love, R.C., Conley, R.R., et al. (1999). A dose-outcome analysis of risperidone. *J. Clin. Psychiatry* 60:771–775.

Lynch, D.R., Guttmann, R.P. (2001). NMDA receptor pharmacology: perspectives from molecular biology. *Curr. Drug Targ.* 2:215–231.

Marder, S.R., Meibach, R.C. (1994). Risperidone in the treatment of schizophrenia. *Am. J. Psychiatry* 151:825–835.

Marder, S.R., Fenton, W. (2004). Measurement and treatment research to improve cognition in schizophrenia: NIMH MATRICS initiative to support the development of agents for improving cognition in schizophrenia. *Schizophr. Res.* 72:5–9.

Martin, L.F., Kem, W.R., et al. (2004). Alpha-7 nicotinic receptor agonists: potential new candidates for the treatment of schizophrenia. *Psychopharmacology* 174:54–64.

McClelland, J.L., McNaughton, B.L., et al. (1995). Why there are complementary learning systems in the hippocampus and neocortex: insights from the successes and failures of connectionist models of learning and memory. *Psychology Rev.* 102:419–457.

Medoff, D.R., Holcomb, H.H., et al. (2001). Probing the human hippocampus using rCBF: contrasts in schizophrenia. *Hippocampus* 543–550.

Moghaddam, B. (2004). Targeting metabotropic glutamate receptors for treatment of the cognitive symptoms of schizophrenia. *Psychopharmacology* 174:39–44.

Nasar, S. (1998). A Beautiful Mind: A Biography of John Forbes Nash, Jr., Winner of the Nobel Prize in Economics, 1994. New York: Simon & Schuster.

Nestler, E.J., and Hyman, S.E. (2010). Animal models of neuropsychiatric disorders. *Nat. Neurosci.* 13:1161–1169.

Nikam, S.S., and Kornberg, B.E. (2001). AMPA receptor antagonists. *Curr. Med. Chem.* 8:155–170.

Okubo, Y., Suhara, T., et al. (1997). Decreased prefrontal dopamine D1 receptors in schizophrenia revealed by PET. *Nature* 385:634–636.

Olney, J.W., and Farber, N.B. (1995). Glutamate receptor dysfunction and schizophrenia. *Arch. Gen. Psychiatry* 52:998–1007.

Osser, D.N., Najarian, D.M., et al. (1999). Olanzapine increases weight and serum triglyceride levels. *J. Clin. Psychiatry* 60:767–770.

Potkin, S.G. (2011). Asenapine: a clinical overview. *J. Clin. Psychiatry* 72(Suppl 1):14–18.

Potkin, S.G., Saha, A., et al. (2003). Aripiprazole, an antipsychotic with a novel mechanism of action and risperidone vs placebo in patients with schizophrenia and schizoaffective disorder. *Arch. Gen. Psychiatry* 60:681–690.

Preston, A.R., and Wagner, A.D. (2007). The medial temporal lobe and memory. In: Kesner, R.P. and Martinez, J.L., eds. Neurobiology of Learning and Memory. Burlington, MA: Elsevier, pp. 305–337.

Rempel-Clower, N.L., Zola, S.M., et al. (1996). Three cases of enduring memory impairment after bilateral damage limited to the hippocampal formation. *J. Neurosci.* 16:5233–5255.

Richelson, E. (2010). New antipsychotic drugs: how do their receptor-binding profiles compare? *J. Clin. Psychiatry* 71:1243–1244.

Roth, B.L., Hanizavareh, S.M., et al. (2004). Serotonin receptors represent highly favorable molecular targets for cognitive enhancement in schizophrenia and other disorders. *Psychopharmacology* 174:17–24.

Saks, E.R. (2007). The Center Cannot Hold: My Journey through Madness. New York: Hyperion.

Schobel, S.A., Lewandowski, N.M., et al. (2009). Differential targeting of the CA1 subfield of the hippocampal formation by schizophrenia and related psychotic disorders. *Arch. Gen. Psychiatry* 66:938–946.

Selemon, L.D., Rajkowska, G., et al. (1995). Abnormally high neuronal density in the schizophrenic cortex: a morphometric analysis of prefrontal area 9 and occipital area 17. *Arch. Gen. Psychiatry* 52:805–818.

Sellin, A.K., Shad, M., et al. (2008). Muscarinic agonists for the treatment of cognition in schizophrenia. *Cent. Nerv. Syst. Spect.* 13:985–996.

Shekhar, A., Potter, W.Z., et al. (2008). Selective muscarinic receptor agonist xanomeline as a novel treatment approach for schizophrenia. *Am. J. Psychiatry* 16:1033–1039.

Shepherd, J.D., and Huganir, R.L. (2007). The cell biology of synaptic plasticity: AMPA receptor trafficking. *Annu. Rev. Cell Dev. Biol.* 23:613–643.

Song, I., and Huganir, R.L. (2002). Regulation of AMPA receptors during synaptic plasticity. *Trends Neurosci.* 25:578–588.

Tamminga, C. (1999). Glutamatergic aspects of schizophrenia. *Br. J. Psychiatry Suppl.* 37:12–15.

Tamminga, C.A., and Kane, J.M. (1997). Olanzapine (Zyprexa): characteristics of a new antipsychotic. *Exp. Opin. Investig. Drugs* 6:1743–1752.

Tamminga, C.A., Stan, A.D., et al. (2010). The hippocampal formation in schizophrenia. *Am. J. Psychiatry* 167:1178–1193.

Tollefson, G.D., Beasley, C.M., Jr., et al. (1997a). Olanzapine versus haloperidol in the treatment of schizophrenia and schizoaffective and schizophreniform disorders: results of an international collaborative trial. *Am. J. Psychiatry* 154:457–465.

Tollefson, G.D., Tran, P.V., et al. (1997b). Olanzapine versus risperidone in the treatment of psychosis. *Schizophr. Res.* 24:191–192.

Tsai, G., and Coyle, J.T. (2002). Glutamatergic mechanisms in schizophrenia. *Annu. Rev. Pharmacol. Toxicol.* 42:165–179.

Tsai, G., Passani, L.A., et al. (1995). Abnormal excitatory neurotransmitter metabolism in schizophrenic brains. *Arch. Gen. Psychiatry* 52:829–836.

Wang, A.Y., Lohmann, K.M., et al. (2011). Bipolar disorder type 1 and schizophrenia are accompanied by decreased density of parvalbumin- and somatostatin-positive interneurons in the parahippocampal region. *Acta Neuropathol.* 122:615–626.

Weiden, P.J. (2012). Iloperidone for the treatment of schizophrenia: an updated clinical review. *Clin. Schizophr. Relat. Psychosis* 6:34–44.

Weiner, D.M., Meltzer, H.Y., et al. (2004). The role of M1 muscarinic receptor agonism of N-desmethylclozapine in the unique clinical effects of clozapine. *Psychopharmacology* 177:207–216.

Wellcome Trust Case Control Consortium. (2007). Genome-wide association study of 14,000 cases of seven common diseases and 3,000 shared controls. *Nature* 447:661–678.

Wirshing, D.A., Wirshing, W.C., et al. (1999). Novel antipsychotics: comparison of weight gain liabilities. *J. Clin. Psychiatry* 60:358–363.

Yanagi, M., Southcott, S., et al. (2012). Animal models of schizophrenia emphasizing construct validity. *Prog. Mol. Biol. Transl. Sci.* 105:411–444.

Young, J.W., Powell, S.B., et al. (2009). Using the MATRICS to guide development of a preclinical cognitive test battery for research in schizophrenia. *Pharmacol. Thera.* 122:150–202.

Young, J.W., Zhou, X., et al. (2010). Animal models of schizophrenia. *Curr. Top. Behav. Neurosci.* 4:391–433.

Zimbroff, D.L., Kane, J.M., et al. (1997). Controlled, dose-response study of sertindole and haloperidol in the treatment of schizophrenia. Sertindole Study Group. *Am. J. Psychiatry* 154:782–791.

28 | THE NEUROBIOLOGY OF BIPOLAR DISORDER

KATHERINE E. BURDICK, STEPHEN J. HAGGARTY, AND ROY PERLIS

INTRODUCTION

Efforts to understand the fundamental neurobiology of bipolar disorder, as with other psychiatric illnesses, have been hindered by the inability to directly access the primary organ of interest in living patients, as well as a lack of valid cellular and animal models of disease. As a result, the majority of data to date comes either from postmortem studies, from peripheral cells, and from investigations of the effects of known therapeutic agents in bipolar disorder, particularly lithium. New technologies are emerging that may inform these studies; these include new kinds of cellular models (Brennand et al., 2011; Sheridan et al., 2011), including models that will be informed by the genetic studies described elsewhere (Chapter 19), as well as new ways of characterizing those models. As such, any summary of relevant neurobiology is undoubtedly incomplete and likely to have a short half-life.

The genetics of bipolar disorder were extensively covered in an earlier chapter in view of substantial overlaps with schizophrenia. However, topics that are relatively more specific to bipolar disorder are the focus of the current chapter. Several areas will be covered. First, the temporal development of bipolar disorder from high-risk to prodromal to first-episode symptoms will be discussed. Second, evidence that bipolar disorder has well-documented, measurable cognitive abnormalities, in contrast with older views, is explored. Third, the disruption in circadian biology in bipolar disorder patients is discussed. Fourth, we describe the current, existing model systems that have implicated a number of signaling pathways, processes, and animal models that are likely to be relevant to bipolar disorder itself and/or therapeutic mechanisms. These include circadian abnormalities, epigenetic processes including histone modification, Wnt/GSK3 signaling, other modulators of neuroplasticity, and mitochondrial function. The evidence for each of these is summarized in the following.

HIGH-RISK STUDIES IN BIPOLAR DISORDER

As discussed in Chapter 19, the heritability of bipolar disorder is high, and substantial evidence indicates that the illness runs in families. Specifically, first-degree relatives of patients with bipolar illness are at about a 10-fold increased risk of developing bipolar disorder as compared with individuals who do not have a family history. These data suggest that one useful approach to understanding the risk factors associated with bipolar disorder, as well as the longitudinal development of the illness, is to study high-risk offspring of bipolar parents. Unlike studies focused on prodromal or chronic patient cohorts, high-risk offspring samples are not as likely to be confounded by existing symptoms, medications, and other comorbid conditions such as substance use disorders.

Children with at least one parent who is diagnosed with bipolar disorder are at a fourfold increased risk of developing a mood disorder over their lifetime (Lapalme et al., 1997). The rate of diagnosis of bipolar disorder in high-risk offspring ranges broadly from 3% to 50% but is consistently higher than in the general population (1–2%) (Kessler et al., 2005). Most high-risk studies are limited by very small sample sizes and are descriptive in nature, making it difficult to identify specific risk factors for conversion to the full-blown illness. Very few studies have systematically assessed clinical or environmental risk factors; however, certain personality traits such as behavioral disinhibition are more commonly seen in high-risk offspring than in those without enhanced risk (Hirshfeld-Becker et al., 2006) and significant negative life events during childhood increase the likelihood of developing a subsequent mood disorder (Hillegers et al., 2004). There is also some evidence that high-risk children and adolescents have neurocognitive impairments across several domains including processing speed, working memory, executive functions, and response inhibition (Salvadore et al., 2008), but these deficits are milder than those noted in first-episode and more chronic patients with bipolar disorder and are rather nonspecific.

Neurobiological risk factors for bipolar disorder have also been identified in high-risk offspring including stress-vulnerability associated with hypothalamic-pituitary-adrenal (HPA)-axis dysfunction and increased inflammatory/immune response; however, again data are limited by small cohorts. Most studies assessing biomarkers in offspring of bipolar parents include individuals who are themselves diagnosed with either depression or another psychiatric disorder, confounding the interpretation of these findings. Nevertheless, early evidence indicates subtle abnormalities in HPA-axis functioning in high-risk offspring such as elevated salivary cortisol levels upon waking when compared with children with no family history (Ellenbogen et al., 2004). Likewise, at least one study has identified markers of an activated immune system in offspring of bipolar parents prior to the development of overt affective symptoms as evidenced by altered expression in genes that are involved in the inflammatory process (Padmos et al., 2008).

Despite the increased risk for illness that is associated with being born to a bipolar parent, most offspring do not go on

to develop bipolar disorder, making high-risk studies time-consuming and expensive with inherently small sample sizes. Other approaches have been implemented to increase the likelihood of studying individuals who will develop the full-blown illness, including studies focusing on the clinical prodrome and the early phase of the illness.

THE PRODROME

The bipolar prodrome constitutes a period of disturbance characterized by distinct features/symptoms that lead up to the onset of the full-blown disorder. The schizophrenia prodrome has been well characterized and has been researched for decades, yielding significant findings that point toward clinical and cognitive predictors as was discussed in Chapter 27. Large consortia have been formed, such as the North American Prodrome Longitudinal Study (NAPLS; Addington et al., 2007), in order to collect sample sizes that are sufficient for obtaining maximal predictive power. However, the field of bipolar disorder has yet to firmly establish the presence of a prodrome or to identify clear, replicated clinical/cognitive predictors for the disorder. Data from retrospective studies suggest that there are attenuated forms of symptoms seen in the disorder as well as less specific psychiatric features that precede the onset of the illness; however, there are very few prospective studies confirming these findings.

CLINICAL PREDICTORS

According to retrospective reports, between 45% and 96% of bipolar disorder patients reported prodromal symptoms at least one month prior to the full onset of bipolar disorder (Correll et al., 2007; Conus et al., 2010). Depressive symptoms are typically reported as the first prodromal signs, however some manic symptoms were also reported, including sleep disturbance/decreased need for sleep and increased energy/activity. Psychotic symptoms have also been identified as a prodromal symptom (Jackson et al., 2003), although they tend to occur later in the prodrome and have low specificity.

Prospective accounts of prodromal symptoms support mood lability (Angst et al., 2003) and attenuated positive symptoms as putative prodromal symptoms in bipolar disorder (Thompson et al., 2003). Data indicating attenuated positive symptoms as prodromal to bipolar disorder are limited by the fact that most of these samples were being collected in the context of a schizophrenia high-risk study; therefore, those who went on to develop bipolar disorder may not be representative of the general at-risk population. During the prodromal phase, these patients presented with similar clinical and neurocognitive profiles compared to individuals who ultimately developed a schizophrenia spectrum disorder.

COGNITIVE PREDICTORS

Global and specific neurocognitive impairments are prominent during the prodrome for schizophrenia (Davidson et al., 1999). In contrast, global measures of cognitive function, such as IQ, do not appear to be viable cognitive predictors of bipolar disorder. Most studies agree that there is no significant IQ deficit in individuals before they develop bipolar disorder (Meyer et al., 2004; Reichenberg et al., 2002; Zammit et al., 2004) if they are at high risk for the disorder based on family history (Frangou et al., 2005), or if they are in the early stages of the disorder (Hill et al., 2009; Zanelli et al., 2010). There is even some evidence to suggest that an *increased* IQ may be predictive of bipolar disorder (MacCabe et al., 2010). This is in stark contrast with the schizophrenia literature, which consistently finds IQ deficits in those at increased risk and in the early stages of the disorder.

Although global measures are not useful in predicting impending onset of bipolar disorder, some specific neurocognitive domains, such as declarative memory and executive function, remain promising. Deficits in these domains have been reported in unaffected siblings (Christensen et al., 2006), in offspring from bipolar parents (Klimes-Dougan et al., 2006; Maziade et al., 2009), and in first-episode patients (Hill et al., 2009; Zanelli et al., 2010), and are consistent with deficits reported in chronic patients with bipolar disorder. Cognitive deficits in memory and executive function are noted during acute episodes, as well as during euthymic periods (Martinez-Aran et al., 2004). In fact, convergent and meta-analytic data suggest that verbal memory, in particular, may be the most valuable cognitive phenotype for bipolar disorder (Glahn et al., 2004).

FIRST EPISODE

The onset of bipolar disorder is marked by the first affective episode of either polarity; however, the diagnosis itself is not made until the first manic episode occurs. In up to 2/3 of cases, the first episode of mania is preceded by a major depressive episode (Daban et al., 2006) but most studies of first-episode bipolar disorder focus on patients who are experiencing their first hospitalization or their first mania.

Given the relative preservation of premorbid functioning in bipolar disorder, the period surrounding the first mania is of particular importance. At the time of first episode, frank symptoms of psychosis present in approximately 60% of subjects; neurocognitive deficits are significant, and functional abilities are disrupted. Onset of first episode typically occurs during adolescence; however, many patients will have been suffering undiagnosed, or misdiagnosed, for months or even years prior to initial treatment (Weller et al., 1995). With adequate treatment, first-episode bipolar subjects show relatively high rates of remission from mania within six months, ranging from 80% to 100% in most studies; however, relapse rates within the first year are also high (35–52%). Moreover, syndromic recovery rates, defined by no longer meeting DSM criteria for an acute episode, are considerably higher than symptomatic recovery rates, suggesting a persistent clinical course marked by subsyndromal symptoms in most patients (Tohen et al., 1992). Of particular concern are the consistently replicated findings of social, occupational, and general functional recovery rates falling far below remission rates (Conus et al., 2006; Tohen et al., 2003).

Neurocognitive functioning at the time of first episode also tends to decline significantly as compared with premorbid functioning; although the deficits are generally less severe than those noted in first episode schizophrenia samples (Hill et al., 2009). Overall there is substantial evidence documenting poor outcomes in first-episode bipolar disorder. Certain illness features such as earlier age at onset and comorbid drug and alcohol abuse (McGorry et al., 1996) can exacerbate these poor outcomes and should be the focus of future early intervention efforts.

CIRCADIAN ABNORMALITIES

It has long been understood that changes in sleep, daytime activity, and energy levels are cardinal features of acute mania and depression, with more recent data suggesting that these symptoms may represent trait-related risk factors for BPD (Plante and Winkelman, 2008). Changes in the sleep-wake cycle and other circadian rhythms represent core features of bipolar disorder, with sleep abnormalities reported in ~90% of patients during acute episodes. Even when euthymic, many BPD patients continue to demonstrate circadian disruptions, including diminished sleep efficiency and lower daytime activity levels. These trait-like circadian disruptions are of particular clinical relevance as changes in sleep are highly predictive of impending affective instability, and BPD patients with poor sleep quality report diminished quality of life (Gruber et al., 2009).

The exact nature of the circadian abnormality in BPD is unknown; theories posit a potential uncoupling of the biological clock from external variables that entrain circadian rhythms (e.g., light) versus the desynchronization of the sleep-wake cycle such that it falls out of phase with other biological rhythms (Dallaspezia and Benedetti, 2009). Euthymic BPD patients are commonly characterized by an "eveningness" chronotype, such that their time-to-sleep preference is phase-shifted to a later than average hour, one that is not typically aligned with the 24-hour light-dark cycle (Plante and Winkelman, 2008). Harvey et al. reported that 70% of remitted BPD patients had diminished sleep efficiency and decreased daytime activity levels (Harvey et al., 2005). More recently, Ritter et al. found that patients with BPD demonstrated increased sleep latency compared to healthy controls as determined by actigraphy. In addition, patients with BPD self-reported a persistent pattern of increased insomnia and hypersomnia, as well as sensitivity to shifts in circadian rhythm (Ritter et al., 2012). Interestingly, participants at increased risk for BPD reported a similar pattern, suggesting that circadian abnormalities may represent a core illness feature that precedes the onset of frank mood episodes.

Along these lines, a decreased *need* for sleep (the ability to maintain energy without adequate sleep) has been shown to be present prior to the illness onset and during the prodrome (Skjelstad et al., 2010). Unaffected offspring of BPD patients demonstrate disrupted sleep and activity levels versus healthy subjects without a family history (Ankers and Jones, 2009), suggesting that circadian abnormalities may be a genetically

mediated, central feature of the disorder. In order to provide support for this hypothesis, molecular genetic studies have tested candidate genes that are known to regulate circadian functions (e.g., *CLOCK, PERIOD*) for association to BPD (Dallaspezia and Benedetti, 2009). Some evidence for modest level of association has been found. For example, a *CLOCK* gene polymorphism was found to be nominally associated with moderate features of the illness such as diurnal preference (Katzenberg et al., 1998), levels of evening activity, and delayed sleep onset in BPD (Benedetti et al., 2007). In general, studies of circadian genes are limited by (*1*) the small sample sizes available in which relevant phenotypes can be tested, and thus (*2*) the lack of appropriate replication samples, which are critical to establish valid genetic association. Information on circadian abnormalities is not routinely available in samples that have been used in genome-wide association studies. Thus the data are intriguing, but extensive further studies will be necessary to ensure relevance to the etiology of bipolar disorder.

The nature of the circadian abnormality in BPD is not known; however, a recent review by Dallaspezia and Benedetti (2009) described two related hypotheses: (*1*) patients with BPD have a biological clock that is detached from environmental variables that act to regulate circadian rhythms; and/or (*2*) the normal sleep-wake cycle in BPD is not in phase with other biological rhythms (e.g., melatonin release). As noted, data in BPD support a high rate of an "eveningness" chronotype, a preference for later bedtimes/wake-times, and for carrying out mental and physical activity in the evening as opposed to the morning (Giglio et al., 2010). Eveningness is associated with a circadian phase delay, a shift in the normal temperature reduction and melatonin secretion that triggers onset of the circadian-based sleep cycle, as well as waking times that are misaligned to circadian phase (Duffy et al., 1999). Such circadian desynchronization results in elevated melatonin, a sleep-promoting hormone, early in the day thereby impairing wakefulness and vigilance (Benca et al., 2009). Importantly, these data suggest that impaired sleep quality in BPD is associated with reduced quality of life. Animal models of circadian abnormalities are discussed in what follows.

EPIGENETICS

Epigenetic mechanisms, including methylation of DNA and DNA-associated proteins, represent key means of regulating gene expression. Histone proteins "package" DNA in units called nucleosomes, and thereby regulate access of transcription factors and other proteins to that DNA. The nucleosomes are regulated by histone-modifying complexes and ATP-dependent remodeling complexes (Gardner et al., 2011; Racki and Narlikar, 2008), and these groups of proteins either modify histones directly or alter the position of nucleosomes, to influence the accessibility of DNA itself. Two groups of enzymes of particular importance to these epigenetic mechanisms are the histone acetyltransferases (HATs), which tend to alter chromatin in a manner that makes DNA more accessible for transcription, and the histone deacetylases, which tend to

have opposing effects and repress transcription (Berndsen and Denu, 2008; Selvi et al., 2010). Other enzymes modify DNA itself, primarily through addition or removal of methyl groups (Guo et al., 2011; Mikaelsson and Miller, 2011).

Evidence implicating histone deactylases (HDACs) in mood and psychotic disorders, including bipolar disorder, comes from two major sources: animal data in disease models, and known HDAC effects of existing therapeutics. Preliminary human studies also suggest some role for epigenetic effects in bipolar disorder.

ANIMAL MODELS: MEMORY AND STRESS RESPONSE

The link between epigenetics and psychiatric illness began with evidence that chromatin plays a key role in memory formation and in learning (Guan et al., 2002; Korzus et al., 2004; Levenson et al., 2004). Work in *Aplysia* from the Kandel lab demonstrated the effects of excitatory and inhibitory neurotransmitters on transcription were mediated by HATs and HDACs, respectively (Guan et al., 2002). Later work in mutant mice heterozygous for the specific HAT identified in that system, CREB-binding protein (CBP), indicated deficits in synaptic plasticity as well as long-term potentiation in hippocampus, which was associated with reduced histone acetylation. Notably, an inhibitor of HDACs was able to reduce both the molecular and cellular effects of reduced CBP function suggesting a potential novel approach to therapeutic development for cognitive disorders (Alarcon et al., 2004; Wood et al., 2005).

A particularly relevant form of memory for psychiatric disorders amenable to investigation in animal models is fear conditioning, in which a neutral stimulus is paired with a noxious stimulus resulting in anxiety and fear in the presence of what was previously a neutral stimulus. While anxiety is not a core feature of bipolar disorder, it is highly comorbid with a prevalence of 50% or more in clinical samples. Initial investigations found conditioned fear to be associated with acetylation of histone H3 in hippocampus; fear conditioning could be enhanced with administration of an HDAC inhibitor (Levenson et al., 2004). At a cellular level, administration of the HDAC inhibitor enhanced hippocampal long-term potentiation in area CA1. Subsequent investigations suggest that HDAC inhibitors may potentiate memory even in mouse models of neurodegeneration (Graff et al., 2012), and find consistent effects with modulation of HDAC function. In particular, increased expression of Hdac2 appears to suppress memory formation and reduce synapse number, while reduced Hdac2 expression has opposing effects (Guan et al., 2009).

Multiple pharmacologic treatments for mood disorders can modulate chromatin structure or DNA methylation. The monoamine oxidase inhibitor antidepressant tranylcypromine also acts as a direct inhibitor of lysine histone demethylase 1 (*LSD1*) (Lee et al., 2006). Antidepressants from other classes, including the tricyclic imipramine and the selective serotonin reuptake inhibitors (SSRI), indirectly inhibit DNA methyltransferase (*DNMT1*) in primary cortical culture (Zimmermann et al., 2012). Finally, the antimanic drug valproic acid is known to inhibit one class of HDACs (Phiel et al., 2001), including HDAC2 described in the preceding to play a key role in cognition.

Non-pharmacologic interventions have been shown to influence chromatin modification as well. In a rat study, electroconvulsive seizures (analogous to human electroconvulsive therapy) elicited increases in histone acetylation (Tsankova et al., 2004). Among the genes influenced by an increase in open chromatin was the promoter region of brain-derived neurotrophic factor (*Bdnf*), whose expression is known to be increased following electroconvulsive seizures. Additional chromatin changes were observed following chronic administration of electroconvulsive seizures.

Animal models of the stress response may also be important for understanding bipolar disorder. Stressful life events such as early adversity have been shown to increase risk for development of mood disorders, including bipolar disorder (Gilman et al., 2012; Horesh et al., 2011; Post et al., 2001), while acute stress may be associated with onset of mood episodes.

One of the most direct links between epigenetics and behavior comes from studies that demonstrated in rats that maternal behavior influenced histone acetylation as well as DNA methylation in offspring observed one week after and persisting at ninety days after birth (Weaver et al., 2004). Most notably, these offspring exhibited hyperactivity of the hypothalamic-pituitary-adrenal axis when exposed to acute restraint stress. Conversely, when pups were fostered by mothers exhibiting higher levels of grooming and licking behavior, these changes were reversed—an infusion of an HDAC inhibitor, trichostatin A, could also normalize stress response.

Importantly, the changes in histone acetylation may exhibit a complex kinetic relationship with stress response. For example, following a similar restraint stress paradigm (Hunter et al., 2009), some chromatin marks decreased while others increased at seven days, with opposing changes observed following twenty one days, which may represent an attempt to maintain homeostasis following acute stress exposure.

Additional animal models of stress response also support a role for epigenetic effects. For example, forced swim tests increase histone phosphorylation as well as other chromatin marks (Chandramohan et al., 2008), which can be blocked by antagonism of N-methyl-D-aspartate (NMDA) receptors or downstream signaling pathways. Similarly, chronic social defeat, in which mice are exposed to an aggressive male mouse for a brief period daily, yields increase in histone methylation in the defeated mouse up to one month after exposure (Tsankova et al., 2006). Work with this latter model has also yielded important insight into epigenetic mechanisms of antidepressant effect, discussed further in the following.

ANIMAL MODELS OF MOOD AND PSYCHOSIS

Epigenetic effects in animal models of mood and psychosis have been investigated in two main ways. First, initial studies have characterized changes in chromatin or DNA methylation among animals following exposure to specific stressors known to produce mood disorder-like phenotypes. Second, some

studies have directly examined the effects of perturbing function of HDACs or other enzymes important in chromatin modification and remodeling. An example of the former is studies in the mouse social defeat model, indicating increased histone methylation a month after stress exposure (Tsankova et al., 2006). Specific changes in nucleus accumbens were observed in histone methylation (Wilkinson et al., 2009).

Several studies investigated the perturbing effects of known HDAC inhibitors in mouse models. Results with a lower-potency HDAC inhibitor, sodium butyrate, have been inconsistent. One study suggested augmentation of fluoxetine effect in the tail suspension tests (Schroeder et al., 2007), and another showed antidepressant-like effects on both tail suspension and forced swim tests (Yamawaki et al., 2012). On the other hand, a 21-day treatment study using sodium butyrate failed to show change in forced swim test behavior, even though changes in histone acetylation were observed (Gundersen and Blendy, 2009). More potent HDAC inhibitors yielded consistent effects. In the forced swim test, a model of acute stress, the nonselective HDAC inhibitor SAHA diminishes depression-like behaviors (Uchida et al., 2011). A more selective HDAC inhibitor, MS275, can reverse depression-like effects in the mouse social defeat model (Covington et al., 2009). The antidepressant imipramine also reduces the depression phenotype in this model, and is associated with increase in other marks associated with the more active form of chromatin. In addition to the drug-induced manipulation of HDACs, mouse investigations that directly manipulate HDAC expression have yielded convergent results in certain cases. For example, increased expression of Hdac5 in mouse hippocampus, previously shown to be reduced by imipramine treatment, yielded prodepressant effects (Tsankova et al., 2006).

One of the most intriguing links between histone modification and bipolar disorder comes from investigations of the CLOCK gene (Doi et al., 2006), which itself codes for a histone acetyltransferase. This gene interacts with HDACs and other histone-modifying enzymes (Etchegaray et al., 2006; Katada and Sassone-Corsi, 2010; Nakahata et al., 2008) that may be involved in generating circadian rhythms. A direct role for CLOCK in interacting with a small network of genes including BMAL1, PER1–3, and CRY1 and 2 has been demonstrated to be central for generation of circadian rhythms (Brown et al., 2012). A dominant-negative mutation in CLOCK has been demonstrated to elicit mania-like increases in activity and disruption of sleep-wake cycle in mouse models (Roybal et al., 2007). Such phenotypic changes have high face validity given the prominence of disruption of circadian rhythms in many bipolar patients (Milhiet et al., 2011).

The dominant-negative mutation CLOCK mouse model (King et al., 1997) has also provided an opportunity to investigate the effects of known bipolar therapies. For example, chronic lithium treatment appears to normalize anxiety and depressive behaviors in these models (Roybal et al., 2007), while an inhibitor of GSK3β, a putative lithium target, reduces another mania-like phenotype in these mouse models, referred to as novelty-induced hyperactivity (Kozikowski et al., 2011). This last finding may provide an important link between investigation of histone modification and the GSK3β/Wnt pathway discussed in more detail in what follows.

Another mouse model of a manic-like phenotype likewise supports a role for epigenetic effects of known antimanic therapies. The HDAC inhibitor sodium butyrate, like valproic acid, reduces the hyperactivity induced by psychostimulants in mice (Arent et al., 2011; Kim et al., 2008). The mechanism of this effect has not been directly demonstrated, though other lines of evidence indicate that valproic acid, like certain antipsychotic treatments, does demonstrate epigenetic effects (Tremolizzo et al., 2005).

Psychosis is a prominent feature of bipolar disorder that may occur during both manic and depressive episodes and some antipsychotic medications have demonstrated efficacy in treating psychosis as well as preventing mania depression. Here too, antipsychotic mechanism of action has been linked to epigenetic effects. In mice, chronic administration of the antipsychotic clozapine yields increased expression of Hdac2 in frontal cortex, coupled with decreased expression of the metabotropic glutamate receptor 2 (mGluR2), a transcriptional target of Hdac2 (Kurita et al., 2012). Other atypical antipsychotics exerted similar effects, which were dependent on antagonism of serotonin receptor 2A. Conversely, injection of the HDAC inhibitor SAHA increased mGluR2 expression, and chronic SAHA administration prevented some psychotic-like phenotypes such as deficits in prepulse inhibition induced by an NMDA receptor antagonist, MK801.

HUMAN STUDIES

A small but expanding set of studies suggests that individuals with mood disorders may exhibit changes in chromatin. Such studies are challenging because chromatin modification is highly time-, experience-, and tissue-specific. Absent a way to directly measure chromatin modification *in vivo* without directly sampling brain tissue, these studies rely either on postmortem tissue or on peripheral cells such as lymphocytes.

A number of studies find mood disorders to be associated with changes in expression of chromatin-modifying enzymes, using either lymphocytes or postmortem brain tissue (Abe et al., 2011; Covington et al., 2011; Hobara et al., 2010; Iga et al., 2007). One comprehensive examination of 11 different HDACs in lymphocytes from mood disorder patients found multiple changes, some of which appeared to be state-dependent. That is, among individuals with major depressive disorder, HDAC2 and HDAC5 expression was reduced only during the depressive episodes, while individuals with BPD exhibited an increase in HDAC4 (Hobara et al., 2010). Conversely, BPD subjects demonstrated reduced expression of HDAC6 and HDAC8 regardless of mood state. While those changes appeared to be independent of medication treatment, work in postmortem brain samples from individuals with schizophrenia (Kurita et al., 2012) has suggested that chronic antipsychotic use increased expression of HDAC2.

Two studies have directly demonstrated modification in levels of acetylation for a particular histone, H3, among individuals with bipolar disorder. The first compared blood-derived

lymphocytes in BPD patients and healthy controls (Gavin et al., 2009); notably, H3 acetylation was increased in lymphocytes from valproate-treated patients (Sharma et al., 2006). A post-mortem brain study found consistent results among individuals with major depression, with H3 methylation levels reduced (Covington et al., 2011).

GLYCOGEN SYNTHASE KINASE 3 (GSK3) PATHWAY

Several lines of evidence implicate the Wnt/GSK3 pathway in the etiology of neuropsychiatric disorders. First, the Wnt pathway is known to play a crucial role in neurodevelopment. The peak age of emergence of both bipolar disorder and schizophrenia is known to correspond to critical periods in brain development (Chapter 26). Second, this pathway is targeted by pharmacological agents used to treat these disorders, most notably lithium (Gould and Manji, 2005; Klein and Melton, 1996). Finally, and most directly, the Wnt/GSK3 pathway has been implicated by the demonstration that at least two psychotic disorder liability genes influence this pathway: inhibition of GSK3 by the protein encoded by the schizophrenia-associated gene Disrupted-in-Schizophrenia 1 (*DISC1*) (Mao et al., 2009), and *TCF4*, which is a known target gene of β-catenin(David et al., 2010).

GSK3β has become a focus of investigation in bipolar disorder in large part because of its position as one target of lithium (Klein and Melton, 1996). In particular, the antidepressant properties of lithium preparations are thought at least in part to occur as a result of inhibition of GSK3β (Beaulieu et al., 2007; Beaulieu et al., 2004; Pan et al., 2011), although the downstream mechanisms remain poorly understood (Bachmann et al., 2005; Chen et al., 2000; Gould and Manji, 2002). At the cellular level, with inhibition of GSK3β by lithium (Beaulieu et al., 2008; Klein and Melton, 1996), the degradation of β-catenin is blocked, resulting in its accumulation in the cytoplasm and translocation to the nucleus, where it acts as an activator of transcription of TCF/LEF-dependent genes, such as *CCND1*, *AXIN2*, which can play a key role in cell cycle progression and neuroplasticity (Harris and Peifer, 2005).

NEUROGENESIS AND NEUROPLASTICITY

The discovery that neurogenesis occurs in adult brains, first in mouse and subsequently in human brains, prompted great excitement about the potential therapeutic implications. The observation of subtle abnormalities of histopathology, and in magnetic resonance spectroscopy studies, suggests that abnormalities in neuronal or glial proliferation or differentiation may contribute to the pathophysiology of bipolar disorder.

In particular, one postmortem study in mood disorder patients suggested a region-specific reduction in glial cell counts (Ongur et al., 1998), while another found normal glial density but reduction in neuronal size (Cotter et al.,

2005). Other studies fail to find any consistent differences in cytoarchitecture in bipolar disorder (Beasley et al., 2009). Complicating the interpretation of these studies are differences in region assessed, general methodology, and medication exposure. Taken together, however, at least some evidence exists for cellular abnormalities in bipolar disorder.

One possible indicator of synapse integrity *in vivo* is N-acetyl aspartate (NAA). Considered a marker of neuronal metabolism (see next section), NAA appears to increase along with synapse formation and reductions may be associated with axon dysfunction (Baslow, 2003). A recent review examined nearly 150 studies utilizing magnetic resonance spectroscopy in schizophrenia and bipolar disorder (Kraguljac et al., 2012). In those studies, among the most consistent findings were diminished levels of NAA in basal ganglia in individuals with bipolar disorder. A subset of studies have also found reductions in NAA in prefrontal cortex, including among children and adolescents diagnosed with bipolar disorder (Caetano et al., 2011). Notably, a recent study found reduced prefrontal NAA levels compared to controls in lithium-nonexposed bipolar patients, but normal levels in patients treated chronically with lithium (Hajek et al., 2012), consistent with a prior investigation of NAA and lithium in older adults (Forester et al., 2008), though another study did not observe such changes in adolescents (Patel et al., 2008).

Multiple studies have demonstrated that lithium promotes neurogenesis in adult rodent brain in hippocampus (Chen, et al., 2000; Hanson et al., 2011), an effect dependent on Wnt pathway integrity (Wexler et al., 2008). Anticonvulsants also demonstrate effects on neuronal proliferation and differentiation (Boku et al., 2011; Laeng et al., 2004). Studies in rodent models also suggest that lithium may oppose the antiproliferative effects of glucocorticoids, and further link lithium's proneurogenic effects to Wnt/GSK3β, discussed in the preceding (Boku et al., 2009).

Beyond neuronal proliferation and differentiation, bipolar disorder may impact maturation and remodeling of synapses, so-called neuroplasticity. Here again indirect evidence comes from lithium's effects in model systems. For example, lithium augments long-term potentiation in the rat dentate (Son et al., 2003). Convergent effects of lithium and valproate have been observed in postsynaptic density gene expression (Nanavati et al., 2011).

An interesting proof-of-principle of lithium's effects on synapse function comes from models of Fragile X syndrome, which exhibit synaptic dysfunction that includes increases in glutamate-dependent long-term depression in hippocampus. Chronic lithium treatment in the mouse model normalizes these deficits, suggesting yet another mechanism by which lithium impacts synapse formation and maintenance (Choi et al., 2011).

MITOCHONDRIAL DYSFUNCTION

Another hypothesis about the pathophysiology of bipolar disorder relates to abnormalities in mitochondrial function. Evidence for such abnormalities comes from multiple lines of

investigation, ranging from studies of peripheral lymphocytes to magnetic resonance imaging. Complicating the investigation of mitochondria is the breadth of effects associated with them: in addition to their centrality in cellular metabolism, they play key roles in buffering calcium and regulating cell death (apoptosis).

A small number of studies have investigated the role of mitochondrial function in producing depressive- or manic-like phenotypes. In one study, manipulation of the mitochondrial polymerase gene *POLG* produced disruption of circadian rhythms (Kasahara et al., 2006), effects that could be eliminated with lithium administration or electroconvulsive shock (Kasahara et al., 2008). From a therapeutic perspective, a mouse study of creatine supplementation, a putative enhancer of mitochondrial function, suggested an antidepressant-like response among female but not male rats (Allen et al., 2010).

In humans, some studies of peripheral cells suggest abnormalities both of mitochondrial structure and function. An investigation of fibroblasts and lymphoblastoid cell lines from patients with bipolar disorder found abnormal cellular location of mitochondria (Cataldo et al., 2010). Deprived of glucose, peripheral monocytes from bipolar patients failed to exhibit the upregulation in genes related to electron transport observed in healthy control subjects (Naydenov et al., 2007). Abnormalities in calcium buffering and homeostasis have also been observed in peripheral cells from bipolar patients. These include elevated basal levels of calcium and elevated calcium peaks after stimulation of peripheral blood cell lines (Dubovsky et al., 1992; Kato et al., 2003; Kusumi et al., 1992). *In vitro* studies suggest that lithium protects mitochondria exposed to excessive calcium (Shalbuyeva et al., 2007) and improves oxidative stress tolerance (Allagui et al., 2009).

Direct evidence that genetic abnormalities cause mitochondrial dysfunction in bipolar disorder is limited (Clay et al., 2011; Conus et al., 2006). Neither parent of origin studies nor single nucleotide association studies have arrived at consistent conclusions. These studies are technically difficult due to high levels of heteroplasmy as well as high levels of ancestral variation in mtDNA. Notably, however, the 22q11 deletion syndrome, or velo-cardio-facial syndrome, has been associated with both psychotic and manic-like presentations in up to one-third of patients (Baker and Vorstman, 2012). While they have received less attention than other candidates, the deleted locus includes multiple genes important in mitochondrial function (Maynard et al., 2008). Likewise, Mendelian mitochondrial disorders are sometimes associated with mood or psychotic symptoms (Anglin et al., 2012).

Human imaging studies also suggest the potential role for mitochondrial dysfunction in bipolar disorder; magnetic resonance spectroscopy (MRS), which allows direct imaging of ATP and phosphocreatine, has been particularly relevant here. Two early studies suggested changes in frontal lobe metabolism (Kato et al., 1993, 1998) in a state-dependent fashion; whether these represent cause or effect cannot be determined. In general, multiple investigators have suggested that a key aspect of pathophysiology in bipolar disorder is the shift of neuronal metabolism from oxidative phosphorylation to glycolysis (Kato and Kato, 2000; Stork and Renshaw, 2005). Consistent

with this hypothesis, an investigation of bipolar depression using proton-MRS found elevated lactate levels compared to healthy subjects.

Bipolar pharmacotherapies may moderate these abnormalities observed by MRS. One report found lithium-associated changes in an aggregate measure of glutamate, glutamine, and GABA (Friedman et al., 2004). A study of quetiapine in rapid-cycling bipolar disorder patients correlated clinical improvement in manic symptoms with reduction in lactate levels (Kim et al., 2007). Other mood disorder studies incorporating MRS have similarly suggested that efficacious depression treatments act in part by modulating brain metabolism (Iosifescu et al., 2008).

SUMMARY

The neurobiology of bipolar disorder is still in a phenomenological and descriptive phase. The temporal pattern of development of bipolar disorder includes high-risk, prodromal, and first-episode symptoms, but does not have either the prominent prodrome, or the cognitive abnormalities observed in schizophrenia. A disruption in circadian biology in bipolar disorder patients is a consistent finding, and several intriguing animal models are being investigated. There is substantial evidence for neurobiological abnormalities in aspects of epigenetic regulation of several pathways and in the mitochondria. As yet the progress in genetics largely has not converged with the existing neurobiological abnormalities and will be an important part of future research.

DISCLOSURES

Dr. Burdick has no conflicts of interest to disclose.

Dr. Haggarty has no conflicts of interest to disclose.

Over the past 12 months, Dr. Perlis received fees for consulting or scientific advisory board membership from Bristol Myers-Squibb, Genomind, Healthrageous, Proteus Biomedical, Pamlab, and RIDVentures. He received royalties/patent fees from UBC/Medco.

REFERENCES

Abe, N., Uchida, S., et al. (2011). Altered sirtuin deacetylase gene expression in patients with a mood disorder. *J. Psychiatr. Res.* 45(8):1106–1112.

Addington, J., Cadenhead, K.S., et al. (2007). North American Prodrome Longitudinal Study: a collaborative multisite approach to prodromal schizophrenia research. *Schizophr. Bull.* 33(3):665–672.

Alarcon, J.M., Malleret, G., et al. (2004). Chromatin acetylation, memory, and LTP are impaired in CBP+/- mice: a model for the cognitive deficit in Rubinstein-Taybi syndrome and its amelioration. *Neuron* 42(6):947–959.

Allagui, M.S., Nciri, R., et al. (2009). Long-term exposure to low lithium concentrations stimulates proliferation, modifies stress protein expression pattern and enhances resistance to oxidative stress in SH-SY5Y cells. *Neurochem. Res.* 34(3):453–462.

Allen, P.J., D'Anci, K.E., et al. (2010). Chronic creatine supplementation alters depression-like behavior in rodents in a sex-dependent manner. *Neuropsychopharmacology* 35(2):534–546.

Anglin, R.E., Garside, S.L., et al. (2012). The psychiatric manifestations of mitochondrial disorders: a case and review of the literature. *J. Clin.* 73(4):506–512.

Angst, J., Gamma, A., et al. (2003). Risk factors for the bipolar and depression spectra. *Acta Psychiatr. Scand. Suppl.* (418):15–19.

Ankers, D., and Jones, S.H. (2009). Objective assessment of circadian activity and sleep patterns in individuals at behavioural risk of hypomania. *J. Clin. Psychol.* 65(10):1071–1086.

Arent, C.O., Valvassori, S.S., et al. (2011). Neuroanatomical profile of antimaniac effects of histone deacetylases inhibitors. *Mol. Neurobiol.* 43(3):207–214.

Bachmann, R.F., Schloesser, R.J., et al. (2005). Mood stabilizers target cellular plasticity and resilience cascades: implications for the development of novel therapeutics. *Mol. Neurobiol.* 32(2):173–202.

Baker, K., and Vorstman, J.A. (2012). Is there a core neuropsychiatric phenotype in 22q11.2 deletion syndrome? *Curr. Opin. Neurol.* 25(2):131–137.

Baslow, M.H. (2003). N-acetylaspartate in the vertebrate brain: metabolism and function. *Neurochem. Res.* 28(6):941–953.

Beasley, C.L., Honavar, M., et al. (2009). Two-dimensional assessment of cytoarchitecture in the superior temporal white matter in schizophrenia, major depressive disorder and bipolar disorder. *Schizophren. Res.* 115(2–3):156–162.

Beaulieu, J.M., Gainetdinov, R.R., et al. (2007). The Akt-GSK-3 signaling cascade in the actions of dopamine. *Trends. Pharmacol. Sci.* 28(4):166–172.

Beaulieu, J.M., Marion, S., et al. (2008). A beta-arrestin 2 signaling complex mediates lithium action on behavior. *Cell* 132(1):125–136.

Beaulieu, J.M., Sotnikova, T.D., et al. (2004). Lithium antagonizes dopamine-dependent behaviors mediated by an AKT/glycogen synthase kinase 3 signaling cascade. *Proc. Natl. Acad. Sci. USA* 101(14):5099–5104.

Benca, R., Duncan, M.J., et al. (2009). Biological rhythms, higher brain function, and behavior: Gaps, opportunities, and challenges. *Brain Res. Rev.* 62(1):57–70.

Benedetti, F., Dallaspezia, S., et al. (2007). Actimetric evidence that CLOCK 3111 T/C SNP influences sleep and activity patterns in patients affected by bipolar depression. *Am. J. Med. Genet. B Neuropsychiatr. Genet.* 144B(5):631–635.

Berndsen, C.E., and Denu, J.M. (2008). Catalysis and substrate selection by histone/protein lysine acetyltransferases. *Curr. Opin. Struct. Biol.* 18(6):682–689.

Boku, S., Nakagawa, S., et al. (2009). Glucocorticoids and lithium reciprocally regulate the proliferation of adult dentate gyrus-derived neural precursor cells through GSK-3beta and beta-catenin/TCF pathway. *Neuropsychopharmacology* 34(3):805–815.

Boku, S., Nakagawa, S., et al. (2011). Effects of mood stabilizers on adult dentate gyrus-derived neural precursor cells. *Prog. Neuropsychopharmacol. Biol. Psychiatry* 35(1):111–117.

Brennand, K.J., Simone, A., et al. (2011). Modelling schizophrenia using human induced pluripotent stem cells. *Nature* 473(7346):221–225.

Brown, S.A., Kowalska, E., et al. (2012). (Re)inventing the circadian feedback loop. *Dev. Cell* 22(3):477–487.

Caetano, S.C., Olvera, R.L., et al. (2011). Lower N-acetyl-aspartate levels in prefrontal cortices in pediatric bipolar disorder: a (1)H magnetic resonance spectroscopy study. *J. Am. Acad. Child. Adolesc. Psychiatry* 50(1):85–94.

Cataldo, A.M., McPhie, D.L., et al. (2010). Abnormalities in mitochondrial structure in cells from patients with bipolar disorder. *Am. J. Pathol.* 177(2):575–585.

Chandramohan, Y., Droste, S.K., et al. (2008). The forced swimming-induced behavioural immobility response involves histone H3 phospho-acetylation and c-Fos induction in dentate gyrus granule neurons via activation of the N-methyl-D-aspartate/extracellular signal-regulated kinase/mitogen- and stress-activated kinase signalling pathway. *Eur. J. Neurosci.* 27(10):2701–2713.

Chen, G., Rajkowska, G., et al. (2000). Enhancement of hippocampal neurogenesis by lithium. *J. Neurochem.* 75(4):1729–1734.

Choi, C.H., Schoenfeld, B.P., et al. (2011). Pharmacological reversal of synaptic plasticity deficits in the mouse model of fragile X syndrome by group II mGluR antagonist or lithium treatment. *Brain Res.* 1380:106–119.

Christensen, M.V., Kyvik, K.O., et al. (2006). Cognitive function in unaffected twins discordant for affective disorder. *Psychol. Med.* 36(8):1119–1129.

Clay, H.B., Sillivan, S., et al. (2011). Mitochondrial dysfunction and pathology in bipolar disorder and schizophrenia. *Int. J. Dev. Neurosci.* 29(3):311–324.

Conus, P., Abdel-Baki, A., et al. (2010). Pre-morbid and outcome correlates of first episode mania with psychosis: is a distinction between schizoaffective and bipolar I disorder valid in the early phase of psychotic disorders? *J. Affect. Disord.* 126(1–2):88–95.

Conus, P., Berk, M., et al. (2006). Pharmacological treatment in the early phase of bipolar disorders: what stage are we at? *Aust. N. Z. J. Psychiatry* 40(3):199–207.

Correll, C.U., Penzner, J.B., et al. (2007). Early identification and high-risk strategies for bipolar disorder. *Bipolar. Disord.* 9(4):324–338.

Cotter, D., Hudson, L., et al. (2005). Evidence for orbitofrontal pathology in bipolar disorder and major depression, but not in schizophrenia. *Bipolar. Disord.* 7(4):358–369.

Covington, H.E., 3rd, Maze, I., et al. (2009). Antidepressant actions of histone deacetylase inhibitors. *J. Neurosci.* 29(37):11451–11460.

Covington, H.E., 3rd, Maze, I., et al. (2011). A role for repressive histone methylation in cocaine-induced vulnerability to stress. *Neuron* 71(4):656–670.

Daban, C., Martinez-Aran, A., et al. (2006). Specificity of cognitive deficits in bipolar disorder versus schizophrenia. A systematic review. *Psychother. Psychosom.* 75(2):72–84.

Dallaspezia, S., and Benedetti F. (2009). Melatonin, circadian rhythms, and the clock genes in bipolar disorder. *Curr. Psychiatry Rep.* 11(6):488–493.

David, M.D., Canti, C., et al. (2010). Wnt-3a and Wnt-3 differently stimulate proliferation and neurogenesis of spinal neural precursors and promote neurite outgrowth by canonical signaling. *J. Neurosci. Res.* 88(14):3011–3023.

Davidson, M., Reichenberg, A., et al. (1999). Behavioral and intellectual markers for schizophrenia in apparently healthy male adolescents. *Am. J. Psychiatry* 156(9):1328–1335.

Doi, M., Hirayama, J., et al. (2006). Circadian regulator CLOCK is a histone acetyltransferase. *Cell* 125(3):497–508.

Dubovsky, S.L., Murphy, J., et al. (1992). Abnormal intracellular calcium ion concentration in platelets and lymphocytes of bipolar patients. *Am. J. Psychiatry* 149(1):118–120.

Duffy, J.F., Dijk, D.J., et al. (1999). Relationship of endogenous circadian melatonin and temperature rhythms to self-reported preference for morning or evening activity in young and older people. *J. Investig. Med.* 47(3):141–150.

Ellenbogen, M.A., Hodgins, S., et al. (2004). High levels of cortisol among adolescent offspring of parents with bipolar disorder: a pilot study. *Psychoneuroendocrinology* 29(1):99–106.

Etchegaray, J.P., Yang, X., et al. (2006). The polycomb group protein EZH2 is required for mammalian circadian clock function. *J. Biol. Chem.* 281(30):21209–21215.

Forester, B.P., Finn, C.T., et al. (2008). Brain lithium, N-acetyl aspartate and myo-inositol levels in older adults with bipolar disorder treated with lithium: a lithium-7 and proton magnetic resonance spectroscopy study. *Bipolar Disord.* 10(6):691–700.

Frangou, S., Haldane, M., et al. (2005). Evidence for deficit in tasks of ventral, but not dorsal, prefrontal executive function as an endophenotypic marker for bipolar disorder. *Biol. Psychiatry* 58(10):838–839.

Friedman, S.D., Dager, S.R., et al. (2004). Lithium and valproic acid treatment effects on brain chemistry in bipolar disorder. *Biol. Psychiatry* 56(5):340–348.

Gardner, K.E., Allis, C.D., et al. (2011). Operating on chromatin, a colorful language where context matters. *J. Mol. Biol.* 409(1):36–46.

Gavin, D.P., Kartan, S., et al. (2009). Histone deacetylase inhibitors and candidate gene expression: an *in vivo* and *in vitro* approach to studying chromatin remodeling in a clinical population. *J. Psychiatr. Res.* 43(9):870–876.

Giglio, L.M., Magalhaes, P.V., et al. (2010). Circadian preference in bipolar disorder. *Sleep Breath.* 14(2):153–155.

Gilman, S.E., Dupuy, J.M., et al. (2012). Risks for the transition from major depressive disorder to bipolar disorder in the National Epidemiologic Survey on Alcohol and Related Conditions. *J. Clin. Psychiatry* 73(6):829–836.

Glahn, D.C., Bearden, C.E., et al. (2004). The feasibility of neuropsychological endophenotypes in the search for genes associated with bipolar affective disorder. *Bipolar Disord.* 6(3):171–182.

Gould, T.D., and Manji, H.K. (2002). The Wnt signaling pathway in bipolar disorder. *Neuroscientist* 8(5):497–511.

Gould, T.D., and Manji, H.K. (2005). Glycogen synthase kinase-3: a putative molecular target for lithium mimetic drugs. *Neuropsychopharmacology* 30(7):1223–1237.

Graff, J., Rei, D., et al. (2012). An epigenetic blockade of cognitive functions in the neurodegenerating brain. *Nature* 483(7388):222–226.

Gruber, J., Harvey, A.G., et al. (2009). Sleep functioning in relation to mood, function, and quality of life at entry to the Systematic Treatment Enhancement Program for Bipolar Disorder (STEP-BD). *J. Affect. Disord.* 114(1–3):41–49.

Guan, J.S., Haggarty, S.J., et al. (2009). HDAC2 negatively regulates memory formation and synaptic plasticity. *Nature* 459(7243):55–60.

Guan, Z., Giustetto, M., et al. (2002). Integration of long-term-memory-related synaptic plasticity involves bidirectional regulation of gene expression and chromatin structure. *Cell* 111(4):483–493.

Gundersen, B.B., and Blendy, J.A. (2009). Effects of the histone deacetylase inhibitor sodium butyrate in models of depression and anxiety. *Neuropharmacology* 57(1):67–74.

Guo, J.U., Su, Y., et al. (2011). Hydroxylation of 5-methylcytosine by TET1 promotes active DNA demethylation in the adult brain. *Cell* 145(3):423–434.

Hajek, T., Bauer, M., et al. (2012). Large positive effect of lithium on prefrontal cortex N-acetylaspartate in patients with bipolar disorder: 2-centre study. *J. Psychiatry Neurosci.* 37(3):185–192.

Hanson, N.D., Nemeroff, C.B., et al. (2011). Lithium, but not fluoxetine or the corticotropin-releasing factor receptor 1 receptor antagonist R121919, increases cell proliferation in the adult dentate gyrus. *J. Pharmacol. Exp. Ther.* 337(1):180–186.

Harris, T.J., and Peifer M. (2005). Decisions, decisions: beta-catenin chooses between adhesion and transcription. *Trends. Cell Biol.* 15(5):234–237.

Harvey, A.G., Schmidt, D.A., et al. (2005). Sleep-related functioning in euthymic patients with bipolar disorder, patients with insomnia, and subjects without sleep problems. *Am. J. Psychiatry* 162(1):50–57.

Hill, S.K., Reilly, J.L., et al. (2009). A comparison of neuropsychological dysfunction in first-episode psychosis patients with unipolar depression, bipolar disorder, and schizophrenia. *Schizophr. Res.* 113(2–3):167–175.

Hillegers, M.H., Burger, H., et al. (2004). Impact of stressful life events, familial loading and their interaction on the onset of mood disorders: study in a high-risk cohort of adolescent offspring of parents with bipolar disorder. *Br. J. Psychiatry* 185:97–101.

Hirshfeld-Becker, D.R., Biederman, J., et al. (2006). Psychopathology in the young offspring of parents with bipolar disorder: a controlled pilot study. *Psychiatry Res.* 145(2–3):155–167.

Hobara, T., Uchida, S., et al. (2010). Altered gene expression of histone deacetylases in mood disorder patients. *J. Psychiatr. Res.* 44(5):263–270.

Horesh, N., Apter, A., et al. (2011). Timing, quantity and quality of stressful life events in childhood and preceding the first episode of bipolar disorder. *J. Affect. Disord.* 134(1–3):434–437.

Hunter, R.G., McCarthy, K.J., et al. (2009). Regulation of hippocampal H3 histone methylation by acute and chronic stress. *Proc. Natl. Acad. Sci. USA* 106(49):20912–20917.

Iga, J., Ueno, S., et al. (2007). Altered HDAC5 and CREB mRNA expressions in the peripheral leukocytes of major depression. *Prog. Neuropsychopharmacol. Biol. Psychiatry* 31(3):628–632.

Iosifescu, D.V., Bolo, N.R., et al. (2008). Brain bioenergetics and response to triiodothyronine augmentation in major depressive disorder. *Biol. Psychiatry* 63(12):1127–1134.

Jackson, A., Cavanagh, J., et al. (2003). A systematic review of manic and depressive prodromes. *J. Affect. Disord.* 74(3):209–217.

Kasahara, T., Kubota, M., et al. (2006). Mice with neuron-specific accumulation of mitochondrial DNA mutations show mood disorder-like phenotypes. *Mol. Psychiatry* 11(6):577–593, 523.

Kasahara, T., Kubota, M., et al. (2008). A marked effect of electroconvulsive stimulation on behavioral aberration of mice with neuron-specific mitochondrial DNA defects. *PloS One* 3(3):e1877.

Katada, S., and Sassone-Corsi, P. (2010). The histone methyltransferase MLL1 permits the oscillation of circadian gene expression. *Nat. Struct. Mol. Biol.* 17(12):1414–1421.

Kato, T., Ishiwata, M., et al. (2003). Mechanisms of altered Ca2+ signalling in transformed lymphoblastoid cells from patients with bipolar disorder. *Int. J. Neuropsychopharmacol.* 6(4):379–389.

Kato, T., and Kato N. (2000). Mitochondrial dysfunction in bipolar disorder. *Bipolar. Disord.* 2(3 Pt 1):180–190.

Kato, T., Murashita, J., et al. (1998). Decreased brain intracellular pH measured by 31P-MRS in bipolar disorder: a confirmation in drug-free patients and correlation with white matter hyperintensity. *Eur. Arch. Psychiatry Clin. Neurosci.* 248(6):301–306.

Kato, T., Takahashi, S., et al. (1993). Alterations in brain phosphorous metabolism in bipolar disorder detected by *in vivo* 31P and 7Li magnetic resonance spectroscopy. *J. Affect. Disord.* 27(1):53–59.

Katzenberg, D., Young, T., et al. (1998). A CLOCK polymorphism associated with human diurnal preference. *Sleep* 21(6):569–576.

Kessler, R.C., Berglund, P., et al. (2005). Lifetime prevalence and age-of-onset distributions of DSM-IV disorders in the National Comorbidity Survey Replication. *Arch. Gen. Psychiatry* 62(6):593–602.

Kim, D.J., Lyoo, I.K., et al. (2007). Clinical response of quetiapine in rapid cycling manic bipolar patients and lactate level changes in proton magnetic resonance spectroscopy. *Prog. Neuropsychopharmacol. Biol. Psychiatry* 31(6):1182–1188.

Kim, W.Y., Kim, S., et al. (2008). Chronic microinjection of valproic acid into the nucleus accumbens attenuates amphetamine-induced locomotor activity. *Neurosci. Lett.* 432(1):54–57.

King, D.P., Zhao, Y., et al. (1997). Positional cloning of the mouse circadian clock gene. *Cell* 89(4):641–653.

Klein, P.S., and Melton, D.A. (1996). A molecular mechanism for the effect of lithium on development. *Proc. Natl. Acad. Sci. USA* 93(16):8455–8459.

Klimes-Dougan, B., Ronsaville, D., et al. (2006). Neuropsychological functioning in adolescent children of mothers with a history of bipolar or major depressive disorders. *Biol. Psychiatry* 60(9):957–965.

Korzus, E., Rosenfeld, M.G., et al. (2004). CBP histone acetyltransferase activity is a critical component of memory consolidation. *Neuron* 42(6):961–972.

Kozikowski, A.P., Gunosewoyo, H., et al. (2011). Identification of a glycogen synthase kinase-3beta inhibitor that attenuates hyperactivity in CLOCK mutant mice. *Chem. Med. Chem.* 6(9):1593–1602.

Kraguljac, N.V., Reid, M., et al. (2012). Neurometabolites in schizophrenia and bipolar disorder—a systematic review and meta-analysis. *Psychiatry Res.* 203(2–3):111–125.

Kurita, M., Holloway, T., et al. (2012). HDAC2 regulates atypical antipsychotic responses through the modulation of mGlu2 promoter activity. *Nat. Neurosci.* 15(9):1245–1254.

Kusumi, I., Koyama, T., et al. (1992). Thrombin-induced platelet calcium mobilization is enhanced in bipolar disorders. *Biol. Psychiatry* 32(8):731–734.

Laeng, P., Pitts, R.L., et al. (2004). The mood stabilizer valproic acid stimulates GABA neurogenesis from rat forebrain stem cells. *J. Neurochem.* 91(1):238–251.

Lapalme, M., Hodgins, S., et al. (1997). Children of parents with bipolar disorder: a metaanalysis of risk for mental disorders. *Can. J. Psychiatry* 42(6):623–631.

Lee, M.G., Wynder, C., et al. (2006). Histone H3 lysine 4 demethylation is a target of nonselective antidepressive medications. *Chem. Biol.* 13(6):563–567.

Levenson, J.M., O'Riordan, K.J., et al. (2004). Regulation of histone acetylation during memory formation in the hippocampus. *J. Biol. Chem.* 279(39):40545–40559.

MacCabe, J.H., Lambe, M.P., et al. (2010). Excellent school performance at age 16 and risk of adult bipolar disorder: national cohort study. *Br. J. Psychiatry* 196(2):109–115.

Mao, Y., Ge, X., et al. (2009). Disrupted in schizophrenia 1 regulates neuronal progenitor proliferation via modulation of GSK3beta/beta-catenin signaling. *Cell* 136(6):1017–1031.

Martinez-Aran, A., Vieta, E., et al. (2004). Cognitive function across manic or hypomanic, depressed, and euthymic states in bipolar disorder. *Am. J. Psychiatry* 161(2):262–270.

Maynard, T.M., Meechan, D.W., et al. (2008). Mitochondrial localization and function of a subset of 22q11 deletion syndrome candidate genes. *Mol. Cell Neurosci.* 39(3):439–451.

Maziade, M., Rouleau, N., et al. (2009). Shared neurocognitive dysfunctions in young offspring at extreme risk for schizophrenia or bipolar disorder in eastern quebec multigenerational families. *Schizophr. Bull.* 35(5):919–930.

McGorry, P.D., Edwards, J., et al. (1996). EPPIC: an evolving system of early detection and optimal management. *Schizophr. Bull.* 22(2):305–326.

Meyer, S.E., Carlson, G.A., et al. (2004). A prospective study of the association among impaired executive functioning, childhood attentional problems, and the development of bipolar disorder. *Dev. Psychopathol.* 16(2):461–476.

Mikaelsson, M.A., and Miller, C.A. (2011). DNA methylation: a transcriptional mechanism co-opted by the developed mammalian brain? *Epigenetics* 6(5):548–551.

Milhiet, V., Etain, B., et al. (2011). Circadian biomarkers, circadian genes and bipolar disorders. *J. Physiol. Paris.* 105(4–6):183–189.

Nakahata, Y., Kaluzova, M., et al. (2008). The NAD+-dependent deacetylase SIRT1 modulates CLOCK-mediated chromatin remodeling and circadian control. *Cell* 134(2):329–340.

Nanavati, D., Austin, D.R., et al. (2011). The effects of chronic treatment with mood stabilizers on the rat hippocampal post-synaptic density proteome. *J. Neurochem.* 119(3):617–629.

Naydenov, A.V., MacDonald, M.L., et al. (2007). Differences in lymphocyte electron transport gene expression levels between subjects with bipolar disorder and normal controls in response to glucose deprivation stress. *Arch. Gen. Psychiatry* 64(5):555–564.

Ongur, D., Drevets, W.C., et al. (1998). Glial reduction in the subgenual prefrontal cortex in mood disorders. *Proc. Natl. Acad. Sci. USA* 95(22):13290–13295.

Padmos, R.C., Hillegers, M.H., et al. (2008). A discriminating messenger RNA signature for bipolar disorder formed by an aberrant expression of inflammatory genes in monocytes. *Arch. Gen. Psychiatry* 65(4):395–407.

Pan, J.Q., Lewis, M.C., et al. (2011). AKT kinase activity is required for lithium to modulate mood-related behaviors in mice. *Neuropsychopharmacology* 36(7):1397–1411.

Patel, N.C., DelBello, M.P., et al. (2008). Temporal change in N-acetyl-aspartate concentrations in adolescents with bipolar depression treated with lithium. *J. Child. Adolesc. Psychopharmacol.* 18(2):132–139.

Phiel, C.J., Zhang, F., et al. (2001). Histone deacetylase is a direct target of valproic acid, a potent anticonvulsant, mood stabilizer, and teratogen. *J. Biol. Chem.* 276(39):36734–36741.

Plante, D.T., and Winkelman, J.W. (2008). Sleep disturbance in bipolar disorder: therapeutic implications. *Am. J. Psychiatry* 165(7):830–843.

Post, R.M., Leverich, G.S., et al. (2001). Developmental vulnerabilities to the onset and course of bipolar disorder. *Dev. Psychopathol.* 13(3):581–598.

Racki, L.R., and Narlikar, G.J. (2008). ATP-dependent chromatin remodeling enzymes: two heads are not better, just different. *Curr. Opin. Genet. Dev.* 18(2):137–144.

Reichenberg, A., Weiser, M., et al. (2002). A population-based cohort study of premorbid intellectual, language, and behavioral functioning in patients with schizophrenia, schizoaffective disorder, and nonpsychotic bipolar disorder. *Am. J. Psychiatry* 159(12):2027–2035.

Ritter, P.S., Marx, C., et al. (2012). The characteristics of sleep in patients with manifest bipolar disorder, subjects at high risk of developing the disease and healthy controls. *J. Neural. Transm.* 119(10):1173–1184.

Roybal, K., Theobold, D., et al. (2007). Mania-like behavior induced by disruption of CLOCK. *Proc. Natl. Acad. Sci. USA* 104(15):6406–6411.

Salvadore, G., Drevets, W.C., et al. (2008). Early intervention in bipolar disorder, part I: clinical and imaging findings. *Early. Interv. Psychiatry* 2(3):122–135.

Schroeder, F.A., Lin, C.L., et al. (2007). Antidepressant-like effects of the histone deacetylase inhibitor, sodium butyrate, in the mouse. *Biol. Psychiatry* 62(1):55–64.

Selvi, B.R., Cassel, J.C., et al. (2010). Tuning acetylation levels with HAT activators: therapeutic strategy in neurodegenerative diseases. *Biochim. Biophys. Acta.* 1799(10–12):840–853.

Shalbuyeva, N., Brustovetsky, T., et al. (2007). Lithium desensitizes brain mitochondria to calcium, antagonizes permeability transition, and diminishes cytochrome C release. *J. Biol. Chem.* 282(25):18057–18068.

Sharma, R.P., Rosen, C., et al. (2006). Valproic acid and chromatin remodeling in schizophrenia and bipolar disorder: preliminary results from a clinical population. *Schizophr. Res.* 88(1–3):227–231.

Sheridan, S.D., Theriault, K.M., et al. (2011). Epigenetic characterization of the FMR1 gene and aberrant neurodevelopment in human induced pluripotent stem cell models of fragile X syndrome. *PloS One* 6(10):e26203.

Skjelstad, D.V., Malt, U.F., et al. (2010). Symptoms and signs of the initial prodrome of bipolar disorder: a systematic review. *J. Affect. Disord.* 126(1–2):1–13.

Son, H., Yu, I.T., et al. (2003). Lithium enhances long-term potentiation independently of hippocampal neurogenesis in the rat dentate gyrus. *J. Neurochem.* 85(4):872–881.

Stork, C., and Renshaw, P.F. (2005). Mitochondrial dysfunction in bipolar disorder: evidence from magnetic resonance spectroscopy research. *Mol. Psychiatry* 10(10):900–919.

Thompson, K.N., Conus, P.O., et al. (2003). The initial prodrome to bipolar affective disorder: prospective case studies. *J. Affect. Disord.* 77(1):79–85.

Tohen, M., Ketter, T.A., et al. (2003). Olanzapine versus divalproex sodium for the treatment of acute mania and maintenance of remission: a 47-week study. *Am. J. Psychiatry* 160(7):1263–1271.

Tohen, M., Stoll, A.L., et al. (1992). The McLean First-Episode Psychosis Project: six-month recovery and recurrence outcome. *Schizophr. Bull.* 18(2):273–282.

Tremolizzo, L., Doueiri, M.S., et al. (2005). Valproate corrects the schizophrenia-like epigenetic behavioral modifications induced by methionine in mice. *Biol. Psychiatry* 57(5):500–509.

Tsankova, N.M., Berton, O., et al. (2006). Sustained hippocampal chromatin regulation in a mouse model of depression and antidepressant action. *Nat. Neurosci.* 9(4):519–525.

Tsankova, N.M., Kumar, A., et al. (2004). Histone modifications at gene promoter regions in rat hippocampus after acute and chronic electroconvulsive seizures. *J. Neurosci.* 24(24):5603–5610.

Uchida, S., Hara, K., et al. (2011). Epigenetic status of Gdnf in the ventral striatum determines susceptibility and adaptation to daily stressful events. *Neuron* 69(2):359–372.

Weaver, I.C., Cervoni, N., et al. (2004). Epigenetic programming by maternal behavior. *Nat. Neurosci.* 7(8):847–854.

Weller, E.B., Weller, R.A., et al. (1995). Bipolar disorder in children: misdiagnosis, underdiagnosis, and future directions. *J. Am. Acad. Child. Adolesc. Psychiatry* 34(6):709–714.

Wexler, E.M., Geschwind, D.H., et al. (2008). Lithium regulates adult hippocampal progenitor development through canonical Wnt pathway activation. *Mol. Psychiatry* 13(3):285–292.

Wilkinson, M.B., Xiao, G., et al. (2009). Imipramine treatment and resiliency exhibit similar chromatin regulation in the mouse nucleus accumbens in depression models. *J. Neurosci.* 29(24):7820–7832.

Wood, M.A., Kaplan, M.P., et al. (2005). Transgenic mice expressing a truncated form of CREB-binding protein (CBP) exhibit deficits in hippocampal synaptic plasticity and memory storage. *Learn. Mem.* 12(2):111–119.

Yamawaki, Y., Fuchikami, M., et al. (2012). Antidepressant-like effect of sodium butyrate (HDAC inhibitor) and its molecular mechanism of action in the rat hippocampus. *World J. Biol. Psychiatry* 13(6):458–467.

Zammit, S., Allebeck, P., et al. (2004). A longitudinal study of premorbid IQ Score and risk of developing schizophrenia, bipolar disorder, severe depression, and other nonaffective psychoses. *Arch. Gen. Psychiatry* 61(4):354–360.

Zanelli, J., Reichenberg, A., et al. (2010). Specific and generalized neuropsychological deficits: a comparison of patients with various first-episode psychosis presentations. *Am. J. Psychiatry* 167(1):78–85.

Zimmermann, N., Zschocke, J., et al. (2012). Antidepressants inhibit DNA methyltransferase 1 through reducing G9a levels. *Biochem. J.* 448(1):93–102.

SECTION IV | MOOD DISORDERS

HELEN S. MAYBERG

Depression is one of the most common of all psychiatric disorders and is a leading cause of disability worldwide. Current psychiatric tenets assume a core biological basis for this condition; however the disorder continues to be clinically defined by patient self-report, with treatments generally prescribed without consideration of etiology or pathophysiology. As presented in the following state-of-the-art chapters, there has been tremendous progress toward defining a comprehensive multidimensional neurobiology of mood disorders. The authors in this section provide critical perspective on recent basic, translational, and clinical research advances contributing to an evolving integrative understanding of illness risk and vulnerability, molecular and circuit pathophysiology, and novel diagnostic and treatment strategies.

The section opens with a comprehensive review by Fawcett and Hager of the history and changing nosology of depression diagnosis. This chapter provides broad perspective on the potential changes in the clinical research landscape anticipated by the introduction of DSM-5 (Chapter 29), as well as the need for improved clinical characterization of depression subtypes and syndromic dimensions to fully define mechanisms and develop and test novel treatments. Levinson next present an update on the genetics of depression, summarizing the challenges, limitations, and potential of various approaches including candidate gene studies, genomewide association studies, and evolving applications of sequencing and stem cell technologies (Chapter 30).

Hodes and Russo follow with a critique of the theoretical and practical applications of a wide range of genetic, developmental, and stress-based animal models currently in use to study depression. This chapter provides a comprehensive summary of behavioral endophenotypes and associated peripheral and central biomarkers and behavioral assays relevant to the human condition (Chapter 31).

Duman (Chapter 32) and Furey, Mathews, and Zarate (Chapter 33) offer complementary basic and clinical perspectives on molecular and cellular mechanisms contributing to depression pathogenesis and treatment response with a particular emphasis on their role in development and clinical testing of a new generation of rapid-acting antidepressant agents. Price and Drevets provide important anatomical context to such molecular and cellular findings in their comprehensive review of brain circuits implicated in depression and mood regulation covering basic anatomy, structural and functional neuroimaging, and postmortem pathological studies (Chapter 34).

Krishnan (Chapter 35) extends the discussion of the neuroanatomy of depression to a late-life perspective highlighting vascular pathophysiology and both postmortem and imaging studies of depression in the elderly. Rubinow, Schmidt, and Craft (Chapter 36) focus on the role of gonadal steroids and mood disorders with a comprehensive review of cellular mechanisms, clinical syndromes, and treatment mechanisms. Benton, Blume, Crits-Christoph, Dubeé, and Evans next provide an updated perspective on depression and medical illness (Chapter 37) emphasizing studies of cardiac disease, diabetes, HIV/AIDS, and cancer. The section concludes with comprehensive summary of depression treatments by Iosifescu, Murrough, and Charney (Chapter 38), presenting an overview of treatment efficacy, side effects, and mechanisms of action of the major classes of available interventions and discussing new research on predictive biomarkers and advances in novel treatment development.

Clearly, considerable progress has occurred since publication of the last edition. Judging from this set of comprehensive reviews, the field appears poised for disruptive new advances impacting diagnosis, evidence-based treatment development, and, ultimately, improved care of patients with this common and disabling disorder.

DISCLOSURE

Dr. Mayberg has a consulting agreement with St. Jude Medical Neuromodulation, which has licensed her intellectual property to develop SCC DBS for the treatment of severe depression (US 2005/0033379A1).

29 | THE DIAGNOSIS OF MOOD DISORDERS

JAN FAWCETT AND BRANT HAGER

Every established order tends to produce (to very different degrees and with very different means) the naturalization of its own arbitrariness....Schemes of thought and perception can produce the objectivity that they do produce by misrecognition of the limits of the cognition that they make possible, thereby founding immediate adherence ...to the world of tradition experienced as a "natural world" and "taken for granted." PIERRE BOURDIEU, in Wilson (1993)

INTRODUCTION

Sadness and distress are part of everyday life, as are elation, irritability, and associated fluctuations in energy, activity, enjoyment, and cognition. More severe, disabling mood traits and states, which today we conceptualize as mood disorders, have been described throughout recorded history. Ancient mood disorder diagnostic concepts served the early physician by identifying putative underlying mechanisms, guiding correspondingly appropriate treatment, and estimating patient prognosis. Modern mood disorder diagnostic concepts continue to aid the contemporary physician in similar ways. However, modern mood disorder diagnostic concepts serve many other masters, including research, public health, financial, and medico-legal endeavors.

In mental health clinical care, an optimally conceptualized categorical mood disorder diagnosis validly, accurately, reliably, and rapidly identifies an individual patient as belonging to one or more specific mood disorder diagnostic groups, and not belonging to others. For the clinician, such an optimal mood disorder diagnosis allows for rapid identification of disorder type, determination of caseness, diagnostic elimination of other conditions, concise formulation about putative underlying mechanisms, selection of optimally effective therapy, and prediction of course and prognosis.

In mental health research, an optimally conceptualized categorical mood disorder diagnosis validly, accurately, reliably, and efficiently defines a controlled, descriptively homogeneous mood disorder group for study. Making such an optimal diagnosis allows for statistically robust conclusions regarding mood disorder diagnosis-related natural history, correlations, and outcomes in response to treatment. Given the need for diagnostic homogeneity, an optimal research diagnosis values the elimination of false positives over the elimination of false negatives (Spitzer et al., 1978). Diagnostic false positives dilute the sameness of a research sample, and the exclusion of diagnostic false negatives may be mitigated by increased sample sizes. Ultimately, an optimal research diagnosis, subjected to rigorous study, may point to candidate disease mechanisms, and fruitful areas for possible intervention, control, and cure.

In addition, categorical mood disorder diagnoses also help to establish the fact that a given diagnosis is of public health significance, worthy of reimbursement for treatment, and appropriate for research funding. These latter three diagnostic purposes serve as a crucial bridge between clinical and research efforts, as the clinician's diagnostic task ultimately relies on payment for services, research into neurobiologic etiogenesis and treatments, and empirical data on diagnostic validity, accuracy, reliability, and outcomes.

As we shall see, however, current categorical diagnostic approaches to mood disorders, even ones as optimally conceptualized previously, pose problems for both clinical care and research. To explore this crucial issue, the following chapter will outline an early history of mood disorder diagnostic concepts, discuss the evolution of contemporary mood disorder diagnostic concepts up to the most current diagnostic systems, and finally address the myriad questions of how clinical description of mood disorders might be improved to further the usefulness of diagnosis for treatment and research.

What criteria are most valid and reliable for determining when sadness, distress, elation, irritability, and associated fluctuations in energy, activity, enjoyment, and cognition constitute a disorder, indicating altered pathophysiology, and requiring treatment? How might we improve mood disorder diagnosis to better advance our efforts to predict course and specific treatment response, understand underlying causes, and develop more effective treatments? This chapter will address these questions.

HISTORY

EARLY HISTORY OF MOOD DISORDER DIAGNOSIS

The earliest lineaments of psychiatry contain remarkable descriptors of pathological mood states and traits, and trace prescient contours of our current dilemmas in mood disorder diagnosis. Ancient physicians throughout Europe, the Middle East, South Asia, and East Asia, described sundry accounts

of what we might today call syndromes of depression, mania, psychosis, agitated excitement, anxiety, and adjustment reactions, among others (Horowitz and Wakefield, 2007; Maciocia, 2009; Sharma, 1994; Solomon, 2001). Hippocrates, writing in the 5th and 4th centuries B.C.E., illuminated several cases of melancholia, and distinguished between melancholia with and without external cause (Horowitz and Wakefield, 2007). Aristotle himself added the notion of melancholia as a temperament as well as an illness. Hippocrates also mentioned the maniacal affliction, and stated that both maniacal and melancholic diseases occur especially during spring (Hippocrates and Adams (Tr.), 2010: p. 135). Speculations about the relationship between melancholia and mania began to appear in the occidental literature circa 1st century B.C.E., and came to full fruition between the efforts of Aretaeus of Cappadocia, 2nd century C.E., and Alexander of Tralles, 6th century C.E. (Goodwin and Jamison, 2007).

Equally elaborative, yet seldom referenced in allopathic literature, are mood descriptors from Ayurvedic and Chinese medicine. The *Caraka Samhita*, a core Ayurvedic document with origins conservatively dated to the 7th century B.C.E., features a chapter on insanity, including syndromes of euphoric excitement, irritable agitation, and withdrawn despondency. The *Caraka Samhita* includes allowances for simultaneous occurrence of any combination of these three syndromes, and is replete with lists of prodromal symptoms, vivid syndromic descriptors, and references to humoral as well as exogenous mechanisms (Sharma, 1994). The *Rites of Zhou*, a 12th century B.C.E. Chinese non-medical text, mentions *Kuang*, the disease of irritable raving, and by the 2nd century B.C.E., Chinese medical texts, such as the *Spiritual Axis* and the *Classic of Difficulties*, linked irritable raving, both cyclically and mechanistically, to *Dian*, the disease of withdrawn, worried, unresponsive dullness (Maciocia, 2009). Other ancient Chinese medicine contributions, especially the *Essential Prescriptions of the Golden Chest*, circa 3rd century C.E., included additional syndromes of restless fatigue and agitated sadness (Maciocia, 2009).

Taken together, these first forays into mood diagnosis demonstrate an ostensible distillation of case-based observations, rooted firmly in humoral heuristics, without the apparent benefit of formal statistical empiricism.

The Middle Ages in Europe saw a period of supernatural etiologic speculation in medicine. Mood disorders, along with other forms of mental illness, took on the assumption and stigma of demonic possession and religious uncleanliness, whose care, cure, and punishment was the ken of the priesthood (Solomon, 2001). Later, the Renaissance, the Enlightenment, and the associated Scientific Revolution in Europe heralded a resurgence of classical, case-based psychiatric observations, with humoral explanations, dovetailed with sundry attempts at anatomical correlation (Goodwin and Jamison, 2007).

These ancient forays into mood disorder diagnosis established melancholia and mania as facts of human existence, posed questions about the relationships between them, and hypothesized about the mechanisms underlying such conditions. Furthermore, they delimited a spectrum of philosophic conceptualizations of, and reactions to, mood disorders, from the Greek protomedical model of mood disorders as diseases to be treated, to the Aristotelian notion of melancholia in particular as character to be valued, to the medieval notion of mood disorders as evil to be despised and eradicated. Such ontologic, epistemologic, nosologic, and ethical treatment issues pertaining to mood disorders persist to this day.

RECENT HISTORY OF MOOD DISORDER DIAGNOSIS

The contemporary era of empirical, medical model mood disorder diagnosis, based on systematic amassment of case-based observations without humoral assumptions, began in earnest in the 19th century C.E. In 1838 Jean Etienne Dominique Esquirol proposed the idea that the psychological faculty of mood could be disordered independently from the behavioral problems of melancholic underactivity and manic hyperactivity, laying groundwork for our current conceptions of mood rather than activity as central to mood disorder diagnosis (Healy, 2002: p. 15). In 1854, echoing Aretaeus of Cappadocia and Alexander of Tralles, Jean Pierre Falret and Jules Bailarger independently proposed that mania and depression represented manifestations of an underlying, unitary illness, which Falret termed *folie circulaire*, and Bailarger named *folie de double forme* (Healy, 2002: p. 16). In 1881 Emanuel Mendel defined hypomania as "that form of mania which typically shows itself only in the mild stages abortively, so to speak," and in 1882 Karl Kahlbaum published his observations of a milder, cyclic, manic-depressive illness, cyclothymia (Goodwin and Jamison, 2007: p. 7). Kahlbaum is also credited as first describing dysthymia, a state of chronic unhappiness lacking the full neurovegetative manifestations of melancholia, as well as first advocating the full, historical description of all of a psychiatric patient's signs and symptoms, in order to form diagnostic syndromes (Healy, 2002, pp. 19–20).

From the late 19th century into the first part of the 20th century, Emil Kraeplin arose as a major figure in descriptive psychiatry, melding disparate psychiatric diagnostic concepts into an overarching, comprehensive, and parsimonious classification scheme. Whereas Kraeplin did not invent nosological empiricism, he built creatively on the syndrome concept of Kahlbaum, and brought to bear a dedicated, systematic, and at the time unparalleled method of tracking and analyzing psychiatric signs and symptoms. Kraeplin leveraged detailed, longitudinal clinical observations to synthesize a unitary concept of manic-depressive illness, including the concept of mixed states, which resonates to this day in our current DSM and ICD classifications. Kraeplin's synthetic concepts allowed for better prediction of the course and prognosis of major mental illness, and sharper delimitation of mood from psychotic disorders (Goodwin and Jamison, 2007).

In contrast with Kraeplin, Bleuler, in 1924, proposed that mood (termed affective by Bleuler) and psychotic illnesses fell along a spectrum without a firm boundary, presaging the current concepts of schizoaffective disorder and recent findings into the extensive genetic overlap between bipolar disorder and schizophrenia (Goodwin and Jamison, 2007).

Since the late 19th and early 20th centuries—with the exception of the psychoanalytic and psychobiologic influences

in American psychiatry during the majority of the 20th century, as well as the constructivist-humanist critiques of the antipsychiatry movement—mood disorder diagnosis worldwide has largely taken on a stance valuing the medical model of descriptive empiricism over models with more rationalistic explanatory power (McHugh and Slavney, 1983). However, to this day mental health clinicians treating mood disorders continue to employ a plethora of useful rationalistic diagnostics, through the lenses of psychoanalytic, psychodynamic, cognitive-behavioral, and biopsychosocial formulations, as well as through the persistent clinical assumptions of the monoamine hypothesis and associated theories of biological etiogenesis (Beck, 2011; Driessen et al., 2009; Engel, 1977, 1980; Gabbard, 2005).

EVOLUTION OF THE DSM AND ICD

The *American Diagnostic and Statistical Manual* (DSM) traces its origins to two key predecessors, *The Statistical Manual for the Use of Institutions for the Insane*, and the *Nomenclature of Psychiatric Disorders and Reactions, War Department Technical Bulletin, Medical 203*.

The *Statistical Manual for the Use of Institutions for the Insane* was created in 1918 through collaboration between the Committee on Statistics of the American Medico-Psychological Association and the US Census Bureau (American Psychiatric Association, 1952; Grob, 1991). Prior to this time, the US Census Bureau had made successive attempts to keep count of patients with various disorders housed in state hospitals. The Bureau's accounting of mental illness, however, was of little clinical use to practicing psychiatrists. For example, in the 1840 US Census, the Bureau recorded only one category of mental illness: "idiocy/insanity" (American Psychiatric Association, 2000). By the 1880 US Census, the Bureau distinguished seven categories of mental illness: mania, melancholia, monomania, paresis, dementia, dipsomania, and epilepsy (American Psychiatric Association, 2000). The massive expansion of asylum psychiatry in the early 19th century appears to have driven this nosological enrichment, as alienists of the day observed progressively larger numbers of institutionalized patients, and discerned increasingly differentiated shades of madness and insanity (Healy, 2002). Such efforts at continual nosological improvement, in conjunction with increasing scientific and political interest in the social, demographic, and economic correlates of mental illness, culminated in the aforementioned *Statistical Manual for the Use of Institutions for the Insane*, including 22 principle categories (Grob, 1991). However, it was not until the events of World War II that psychiatric nosology in the United States became clinically useful, and its further evolution clinically driven.

In World War II, American psychiatry—influenced by psychobiologic and psychoanalytic thinking, in combination with barbiturate-aided abreactions—asserted its usefulness by mitigating the effects of psychiatric reactions among soldiers, thus ameliorating chronic disability and consequent attrition of fighting troops. During the war, the Army Medical Corps' psychiatric division, led by Brigadier General William C. Menninger, used the *Nomenclature of Psychiatric Disorders and Reactions, War Department Technical Bulletin, Medical 203*, as its primary diagnostic manual (Office of the Surgeon General, Army Service Forces, 1946). Medical 203 applied to inpatients as well as outpatients, and thus had broader clinical utility for both military and civilian psychiatric clinicians. With the exception of organic psychoses and character, intellectual, and paranoid disorders, Medical 203 conceptualized the majority of psychiatric disorders as reactions to the stresses of war, a conceptualization with clear situational pertinence and convincing rationale, traceable to both Pierre Janet and Adolf Meyer.

After World War II, the World Health Organization (WHO) began work on ICD-6, published in 1948. The release of ICD-6 represented a significant event in international psychiatric nosology. ICD-6 marked the first attempt by the WHO to attempt classification of causes of morbidity as well as mortality, including Section V, on mental, psychoanalytic, and personality disorders (Moriyama et al., 2011). Psychiatric classification in ICD-6 largely followed that used by the US military and related Veterans Administration system, and eventually by DSM-I (American Psychiatric Association, 1952).

As with the ICD-6, the concept of psychiatric disorders as reactions was incorporated into the DSM-I by the American Psychiatric Association in 1952 (American Psychiatric Association, 1952). In this way, DSM-I was influenced heavily by the psychobiologic work of Adolf Meyer, who taught that psychiatric disorders were reactions to various stresses at various phases of the life cycle. Similarly, DSM-I was also influenced strongly by psychoanalytic theories, which were pervasive at the time and originally incorporated into the language of Medical 203, leading some diagnoses to be defined in psychodynamic terms (Grob, 1991). In the Medical 203, affective (mood) disorder diagnoses included neurotic depressive reaction, manic-depressive reaction, psychotic depressive reaction, and melancholia, with related diagnostic categories of note including acute situational maladjustment, and cyclothymic personality. In DSM-I, a similar rubric obtained for mood disorder diagnoses, called affective reactions, which were also enriched by additional symptomatic descriptors to aid the diagnostician. DSM-I also further subdivided adjustment reactions into various time periods across the life span, and added a category for schizophrenic reaction, schizoaffective type.

DSM-II, appearing in 1968, retained Meyerian psychobiologic influences in the categories of psychotic depressive reaction and adjustment reactions subdivided across the lifespan. DSM-II also demonstrated increased psychoanalytic influences through the various categories of neuroses, including depressive neurosis. Cyclothymia remained as a personality disorder. However, DSM-II dropped the reaction designation for most mood disorders, and indeed divorced the occurrence of major mood disorders from their psychobiologic context. DSM-II stipulated that, regarding the major affective disorders, "The onset of the mood does not seem to be related directly to a precipitating life experience" (American Psychiatric Association, 1968, pp. 35–36). The major affective disorders in DSM-II included involutional melancholia, manic depressive illness (manic, depressed, and circular types), and other and unspecified major affective disorders. These reorganizations of DSM-II occurred in the overarching context of

nosologic synchronization with ICD-8 (American Psychiatric Association, 1965).

The WHO adopted ICD-9 in 1975. ICD-9 expanded the list of ICD mental disorder categories, and included narrative descriptions of disorders similar to that of DSM-II (American Psychiatric Association, 1980; Moryama et al., 2011). The related ICD-9-CM, or clinical modification, released in 1978, included more detailed coding procedures, for categorizing and tracking clinical morbidity. The DSM has continued to use the ICD-9-CM coding system since release of the DSM-III, discussed next.

DSM-III, published in 1980, embodied a major departure from prior DSM and ICD editions, by focusing on operationalized symptom criteria validated by family history and follow-up studies, tested for interrater reliability, and almost totally divorced from a priori etiologic designations. DSM-III arose almost entirely from Spitzer et al.'s (1978) Research Diagnostic Criteria, which in turn evolved directly from Feighner et al.'s (1972) diagnostic criteria (Feighner et al., 1972; Spitzer et al., 1978). DSM-III dropped the etiologically presumptive diagnoses of depressive neurosis, involutional melancholia, and psychotic depressive reaction from DSM II, although it retained synonymic mention of depressive neurosis under the new category of dysthymic disorder. DSM-III also reclassified adjustment disorders according to the type of emotional disturbance (depressed mood, anxious mood, or both), and/or disturbance of conduct.

The psychopharmacologic revolution, which burgeoned in the early 1950s and came to full fruition in the 1960s, informed the shift of DSM-III toward the medical model of diagnosis, and away from the psychobiologic and psychoanalytic stances of prior editions. The discovery and demonstration of empirical effectiveness of the neuroleptic chlorpromazine, the tricyclic antidepressant imipramine, the monoamine oxidase inhibitor isocarboxazid, and the mood stabilizer lithium carbonate served as potent stimuli for a disease-oriented approach to psychoses and mood disorders, and led to a paradigm shift that supported a proliferation of neurobiologic research into mood disorders.

Furthermore, the social, political, and economic climate of the 1960s and 1970s placed American psychiatry in a position necessitating justification of its services. The influence of the antipsychiatry movement, the failure of psychoanalysis to impact severe and persistent mental illness, and governmental budgetary tightening all exerted pressure on American psychiatry to identify itself as a useful and necessary specialty. Part of this justification included the effort to demarcate more sharply between normal and abnormal states, that is, defining those disorders requiring treatment and deserving reimbursement for care (Wilson, 1993). One unforeseen consequence of American psychiatry's need to justify its existence and funding through nosologic definition has been a tendency to pathologize as disordered what might otherwise be interpreted as normative human emotional experience (Healy, 1997; Horowitz and Wakefield, 2007).

Another important change in DSM-III comprised the shift from the diagnostic category of manic-depressive illness, which captured recurrent depression as well as mania, mixed states, and cyclic alterations between the three, to the diagnostic category of bipolar disorder, which required only the historical presence of mania for diagnosis, and the category of major depression, which required only the historical presence of one major depressive episode for diagnosis. As Goodwin and Jamison (2007) have pointed out, this shift prioritized the polarity of a mood disorder (bipolar versus unipolar) over the recurrence or longitudinal course of a mood disorder. In DSM-III, bipolar disorders were further subdivided according to the polarity of their current episode, and included an additional category of atypical bipolar disorder, which captured the disorder of hypomania in a person with a prior major depressive episode, later designated Bipolar II Disorder in DSM-IV. DSM-III furthermore reclassified cyclothymia as an affective disorder, rather than a personality disorder (American Psychiatric Association, 1980).

Lastly, DSM-III added prognostically informative specifiers to describe the current manic or major depressive disorder, and a category of Atypical Depression. Manic Episode specifiers included In Remission, With Psychotic Features (Mood-congruent vs. Mood-incongruent), and Without Psychotic Features. Major Depressive Episode specifiers included the preceding, plus With Melancholia and Without Melancholia. The category of Atypical Depression introduced a place where clinicians could diagnose clinically significant depressive symptoms that did not meet full criteria for a previously defined specific affective disorder (American Psychiatric Association, 1980).

DSM-III-R added some changes in 1987. Notably, in an attempt to define better caseness, the diagnosis of major mood episodes now required a change from prior level of functioning (for major depressive episode), or impairment in functioning (for manic episode) (American Psychiatric Association, 1987).

DSM-IV updated these changes in 1994, and made further revisions leading to DSM-IV-TR in 2000. DSM-IV was fashioned based on 150 literature reviews, including data-reanalyses, field trials comparing DSM-III, DSM-III-R, ICD-10, and proposed DSM-IV criteria (American Psychiatric Association, 1994). Proposed changes had to be supported by published empirical data. For example, in one DSM-IV mood disorders field trial, 91% of subjects, who presented with depressed mood plus two other depressive disorder symptoms, met the criteria for current or lifetime major depression or dysthymia, suggesting to the authors that additional categories for milder forms of depression were not needed to account for the vast majority of depressive morbidity (Keller et al., 1995). As a result, the categories of minor depressive disorder and recurrent brief depressive disorder did not rise to the level of independent diagnoses, but instead remained under the rubric of depressive disorder, not otherwise specified. In 2000, DSM-IV-TR was completed to correct factual errors in DSM-IV, and include relevant research data developed since 1994.

The release of ICD-10 in 1995 brought the ICD system up to date regarding operationalized psychiatric diagnostic criteria (World Health Organization, 1993). Although their coding differs, the diagnostic criteria for mood disorders in ICD-10 largely correspond to those of DSM-IV-TR, as outlined in the following.

CURRENT MOOD DISORDER DIAGNOSTIC SYSTEMS

Following the example of DSM-III and its progeny, current mood disorder diagnostic systems, including the DSM IV-TR and ICD-10 Diagnostic Criteria for Research, emphasize the recognition of discrete, non-overlapping syndromes, comprising various combinations of core, prototypal mood episodes. An abbreviated list of mood disorder diagnostic criteria from ICD-10 Diagnostic Criteria for Research may be found in Table 29.1. For comparison with current DSM mood disorder diagnostic criteria, the reader is directed to DSM-IV-TR (American Psychiatric Association, 2000), described in brief in the following text, and the imminent DSM-5, scheduled for release in May 2013.

The DSM-IV-TR chapter on mood disorders stresses the exclusion of medically induced conditions, substance-induced conditions, stress-induced conditions such as bereavement, other mood disorders, and symptomatically similar psychotic disorders. ICD-10 stipulates the exclusion of other mood disorders, and medically induced or substance-induced conditions. DSM-IV-TR requires the presence of clinically significant distress or impairment for mood disorder diagnosis, whereas ICD-10 does not. In both texts, bipolar syndromes assume hierarchical precedence over unipolar syndromes, and syndromes with higher symptom counts assume hierarchical precedence over syndromes with lower symptom counts. In DSM-IV-TR, a variety of prognostically informative specifiers add further characterization to the current mood episode, and to the overarching mood disorder. Both the DSM-IV-TR and the ICD-10 attempt to capture dimensionality in mood disorder diagnosis by identifying, for the current episode, polarity (manic, mixed, or depressed), severity (mild, moderate, or severe), and presence or absence of psychotic features (assumed to occur only during severe mood episodes, an assumption disentangled by the upcoming DSM-5). Dimensionality in diagnosis is also implied by a spectrum covering syndromes with fewer to greater symptom counts (dysthymic disorder, cyclothymic disorder, major depressive disorder, bipolar II disorder, bipolar I disorder).

The structure of both current nosologic systems relies on syndromic prototypology, with diagnoses based on the presence of one or more core stem criteria, and the addition of any combination of a defined number of associated criteria. This prototypal approach inherently results in diagnostic heterogeneity, with hundreds of possible combinations underlying a single clinical diagnosis. Another consequence of this prototypal approach is the assumption of symptomatic equivalence amongst the criteria. In DSM-IV-TR major depressive episode, for example, depressed mood and anhedonia assume equivalent and interchangeable importance as stem criteria, and the remaining seven symptoms/signs also carry equal diagnostic weight as associated criteria.

EPISODES

MAJOR DEPRESSIVE EPISODE

Depressed mood and/or anhedonia comprise the core stem criteria for DSM-IV-TR major depressive episode. Additional criteria for major depressive disorder in DSM-IV-TR include: weight loss/gain or appetite increase/decrease; insomnia or hypersomnia; psychomotor agitation or retardation; fatigue or loss of energy; feelings of worthlessness or inappropriate guilt; diminished ability to think or concentrate, or indecisiveness; and recurrent thoughts of death or recurrent suicidal ideation or suicide attempt or suicide plan. The DSM-IV-TR diagnosis of a major depressive episode requires the presence of at least one core stem criterion, plus four of the other listed depressive signs or symptoms, for at least two weeks. The DSM-IV-TR diagnosis of a major depressive episode furthermore stipulates that criteria are not currently met for a mixed episode, that depressive symptoms cause clinically significant distress or impairment, and that symptoms are not better accounted for by substance use, a general medical condition, or bereavement. ICD-10 criteria for a depressive episode echo most of the DSM-IV-TR criteria, with the exceptions that ICD-10 also recognizes diminished energy or increased fatigability as a core stem criterion, ICD-10 does not stipulate a bereavement exclusion, ICD-10 excludes patients who have ever met criteria for a lifetime hypomanic or manic episode, ICD-10 recognizes loss of confidence and self-esteem as an additional criterion, ICD-10 does not require clinically significant distress or impairment, and ICD-10 has a diagnostic threshold of four total symptoms instead of five. ICD-10 may thus pick up less severe depressive states than DSM-IV-TR.

MANIC EPISODE

In both DSM-IV-TR and ICD-10, core stem criteria for a manic episode include elevated, expansive, or irritable mood. Elevated or expansive mood carry more weight as core criteria, as their presence requires only three additional associated criteria to make the diagnosis, whereas irritable mood requires four. Additional criteria for manic episode in DSM-IV-TR include: inflated self-esteem or grandiosity; decreased need for sleep; flight or ideas or racing thoughts; distractibility, increase in goal directed activity or psychomotor agitation; and excessive involvement in pleasurable activities with high potential for painful consequences. The diagnosis requires syndromic duration of one week, or lesser duration if hospitalization is required. Again, DSM-IV-TR also requires clinically significant distress or impairment for diagnosis, whereas ICD-10 does not. DSM-IV-TR and ICD-10 also differ in some of their additional criteria for a manic episode. For example, ICD-10 recognizes as an additional criterion the loss of normal social inhibitions with resultant inappropriate behavior. ICD-10 also separates marked sexual energy or indiscretions from foolhardy or reckless behavior with a high degree of risk, whereas in DSM-IV-TR these phenomena are subsumed under one criterion.

MIXED EPISODE

The diagnosis of mixed episode in DSM-IV-TR requires the simultaneous presence of criteria for a major depressive episode and a manic episode. In ICD-10, a mixed episode is captured under the diagnosis of F38.0, mixed affective episode, and bipolar disorder current episode mixed. ICD-10 does not require the full depressive and manic syndromes to be present concurrently for a mixed episode diagnosis, but rather the

TABLE 29.1. ICD-10 mood disorders (World Health Organization, 1993)

F30–F39 MOOD [AFFECTIVE] DISORDERS

F30 MANIC EPISODE

F30.0 Hypomania

A. The mood is elevated or irritable to a degree that is definitely abnormal for the individual concerned and sustained for at least four consecutive days.

B. At least three of the following must be present, leading to some interference with personal functioning in daily living:

 (1) increased activity or physical restlessness;

 (2) increased talkativeness;

 (3) difficulty in concentration or distractibility;

 (4) decreased need for sleep;

 (5) increased sexual energy;

 (6) mild spending sprees, or other types of reckless or irresponsible behavior;

 (7) increased sociability or overfamiliarity.

C. The episode does not meet the criteria for mania (F30.1 and F30.2), bipolar affective disorder (F31.-), depressive episode (F32.-), cyclothymia (F34.0), or anorexia nervosa (F50.0).

D. Most commonly used exclusion criteria: the episode is not attributable to psychoactive substance use (F1) or any organic mental disorder, in the sense of F0.

F30.1 Mania without psychotic symptoms

A. A mood that is predominantly elevated, expansive, or irritable, and definitely abnormal for the individual concerned. This mood change must be prominent and sustained for at least a week (unless it is severe enough to require hospital admission).

B. At least three of the following must be present (four if the mood is merely irritable), leading to severe interference with personal functioning in daily living:

 (1) Increased activity or physical restlessness;

 (2) Increased talkativeness ("pressure of speech");

 (3) Flight of ideas or the subjective experience of thoughts racing;

 (4) Loss of normal social inhibitions resulting in behavior that is inappropriate to the circumstances;

 (5) Decreased need for sleep;

 (6) Inflated self-esteem or grandiosity;

 (7) Distractibility or constant changes in activity or plans;

 (8) Behavior that is foolhardy or reckless and whose risks the subject does not recognize, e.g., spending sprees, foolish enterprises, reckless driving;

 (9) Marked sexual energy or sexual indiscretions.

C. The absence of hallucinations or delusions, although perceptual disorders may occur (e.g., subjective hyperacusis, appreciation of colors as specially vivid, etc.).

D. Most commonly used exclusion criteria: the episode is not attributable to psychoactive substance use (F1) or any organic mental disorder, in the sense of F0.

F30.2 Mania with psychotic symptoms

A. The episode meets the criteria for mania without psychotic symptoms (F30.1) with exception of criterion C.

B. The episode does not simultaneously meet the criteria for schizophrenia (F20) or schizoaffective disorder, manic type (F25.0).

C. Delusions or hallucinations are present, other than those listed as typical schizophrenic in F20 G1.1b, c, and d (i.e., delusions other than those that are completely impossible or culturally inappropriate, and hallucinations that are not in the third person or giving a running commentary). The commonest examples are those with grandiose, self-referential, erotic, or persecutory content.

(Continued)

TABLE 29.1. (*Continued*)

F30–F39 MOOD [AFFECTIVE] DISORDERS

D. Most commonly used exclusion criteria: the episode is not attributable to psychoactive substance use (F1) or any organic mental disorder, in the sense of F0.

A fifth character may be used to specify whether the hallucinations or delusions are congruent or incongruent with the mood:

F30.20 mania with mood congruent psychotic symptoms (such as grandiose delusions or voices telling the subject that he has superhuman powers)

F30.21 mania with mood incongruent psychotic symptoms (such as voices speaking to the subject about affectively neutral topics, or delusions of reference or persecution)

F30.8 Other manic episodes

F30.9 Manic episode, unspecified

F31 BIPOLAR AFFECTIVE DISORDER

Note: Episodes are demarcated by a switch to an episode of opposite or mixed polarity or by a remission.

F31.0 Bipolar affective disorder, current episode hypomanic

A. The current episode meets the criteria for hypomania (F30.0).

B. There has been at least one other affective episode in the past, meeting the criteria for hypomanic or manic episode (F30.-), depressive episode (F32.-), or mixed affective episode (F38.00).

F31.1 Bipolar affective disorder, current episode manic without psychotic symptoms

A. The current episode meets the criteria for mania without psychotic symptoms (F30.1).

B. There has been at least one other affective episode in the past, meeting the criteria for hypomanic or manic episode (F30.-), depressive episode (F32.-), or mixed affective episode (F38.00).

F31.2 Bipolar affective disorder, current episode manic with psychotic symptoms

A. The current episode meets the criteria for mania with psychotic symptoms (F30.2).

B. There has been at least one other affective episode in the past, meeting the criteria for hypomanic or manic episode (F30.-), depressive episode (F32.-), or mixed affective episode (F38.00).

A fifth character may be used to specify whether the psychotic symptoms are congruent or incongruent with the mood:

F31.20 with mood-congruent psychotic symptoms

F31.21 with mood-incongruent psychotic symptoms

F31.3 Bipolar affective disorder, current episode moderate or mild depression

A. The current episode meets the criteria for a depressive episode of either mild (F32.0) or moderate severity (F32.1).

B. There has been at least one other affective episode in the past, meeting the criteria for hypomanic or manic episode (F30.-) or mixed affective episode (F38.00).

A fifth character may be used to specify the presence of the somatic syndrome as defined in F32, in the current episode of depression:

F31.30 without somatic syndrome

F31.31 with somatic syndrome

F31.4 Bipolar affective disorder, current episode severe depression without psychotic symptoms

A. The current episode meets the criteria for a severe depressive episode without psychotic symptoms (F32.2).

B. There has been at least one well-authenticated hypomanic or manic episode (F30.-) or mixed affective episode (F38.00) in the past.

F31.5 Bipolar affective disorder, current episode severe depression with psychotic symptoms

A. The current episode meets the criteria for a severe depressive episode with psychotic symptoms (F32.3).

B. There has been at least one well-authenticated hypomanic or manic episode (F30.-) or mixed affective episode (F38.00) in the past.

A fifth character may be used to specify whether the psychotic symptoms are congruent or incongruent with the mood.

F31.50 with mood-congruent psychotic symptoms

F31.51 with mood-incongruent psychotic symptoms

(*Continued*)

TABLE 29.1. (*Continued*)

F30–F39 MOOD [AFFECTIVE] DISORDERS

F31.6 Bipolar affective disorder, current episode mixed

A. The current episode is characterized by either a mixture or a rapid alternation (i.e., within a few hours) of hypomanic, manic, and depressive symptoms.

B. Both manic and depressive symptoms must be prominent most of the time during a period of at least 2 weeks.

C. There has been at least one well-authenticated hypomanic or manic episode (F30.-), depressive (F32.-) or mixed affective episode (F38.00) in the past.

F31.7 Bipolar affective disorder, currently in remission

A. The current state does not meet the criteria for depressive or manic episode in any severity, or for any other mood disorder in F3 (possibly because of treatment to reduce the risk of future episodes).

B. There has been at least one well-authenticated hypomanic or manic episode (F30.-) in the past and, in addition, at least one other affective episode (hypomanic or manic (F30.-), depressive (F32.-), or mixed (F38.00).

F31.8 Other bipolar affective disorders

F31.9 Bipolar affective disorders, unspecified

F32 DEPRESSIVE EPISODE

G1. The depressive episode should last for at least 2 weeks.

G2. There have been no hypomanic or manic symptoms sufficient to meet the criteria for hypomanic or manic episode (F30.-) at any time in the individual's life.

G3. Most commonly used exclusion clause: The episode is not attributable to psychoactive substance use (F10–F19) or to any organic mental disorder (in the sense of F00-F09).

SOMATIC SYNDROME

Some depressive symptoms are widely regarded as having special clinical significance and are here called "somatic." (Terms such as "biological," "vital," "melancholic," or "endogenomorphic" are used for this syndrome in other classifications.) A fifth character (as indicated in F31.3; F32.0 and F32.1; F33.0 and F33.1) may be used to specify the presence or absence of the somatic syndrome. To qualify for the somatic syndrome, four of the following symptoms should be present:

(1) marked loss of interest or pleasure in activities that are normally pleasurable;

(2) lack of emotional reactions to events or activities that normally produce an emotional response;

(3) waking in the morning 2 hours or more before the usual time;

(4) depression worse in the morning;

(5) objective evidence of marked psychomotor retardation or agitation (remarked on or reported by other people);

(6) marked loss of appetite;

(7) weight loss (5% or more of body weight in the past month);

(8) marked loss of libido.

In *The ICD-10 Classification of Mental and Behavioural Disorders: Clinical Descriptions and Diagnostic Guidelines*, the presence or absence of the somatic syndrome is not specified for severe depressive episode, since it is presumed to be present in most cases. For research purposes, however, it may be advisable to allow for the coding of the absence of the somatic syndrome in severe depressive episode.

F32.0 Mild depressive episode

A. The general criteria for depressive episode (F32) must be met.

B. At least two of the following three symptoms must be present:

(1) depressed mood to a degree that is definitely abnormal for the individual, present for most of the day and almost every day, largely uninfluenced by circumstances, and sustained for at least 2 weeks.

(2) loss of interest or pleasure in activities that are normally pleasurable;

(3) decreased energy or increased fatigability.

(*Continued*)

TABLE 29.1. *(Continued)*

F30–F39 MOOD [AFFECTIVE] DISORDERS

C. An additional symptom or symptoms from the following list should be present, to give a total of at least four:

    (1) loss of confidence and self-esteem;

    (2) unreasonable feelings of self-reproach or excessive and inappropriate guilt;

    (3) recurrent thoughts of death or suicide, or any suicidal behavior;

    (4) complaints or evidence of diminished ability to think or concentrate, such as indecisiveness or vacillation;

    (5) change in psychomotor activity, with agitation or retardation (either subjective or objective);

    (6) sleep disturbance of any type;

    (7) change in appetite (decrease or increase) with corresponding weight change

A fifth character may be used to specify the presence or absence of the "somatic syndrome" (as defined in F32):

F32.00 Without somatic syndrome

F32.01 With somatic syndrome

F32.1 Moderate depressive episode

A. The general criteria for depressive episode (F32) must be met.

B. At least two of the three symptoms listed for F32.0, criterion B, must be present.

C. Additional symptoms from F32.0, criterion C, must be present, to give a total of at least six.

A fifth character may be used to specify the presence or absence of the "somatic syndrome" as defined in F32:

F32.10 Without somatic syndrome

F32.11 With somatic syndrome

F32.2 Severe depressive episode without psychotic symptoms

Note: If important symptoms such as agitation or retardation are marked, the patient may be unwilling or unable to describe many symptoms in detail. An overall grading of severe episode may still be justified in such a case.

A. The general criteria for depressive episode (F32) must be met.

B. All three of the symptoms in criterion B, F32.0, must be present.

C. Additional symptoms from F32.0, criterion C, must be present, to give a total of at least eight.

D. There must be no hallucinations, delusions, or depressive stupor.

F32.3 Severe depressive episode with psychotic symptoms

A. The general criteria for depressive episode (F32) must be met.

B. The criteria for severe depressive episode without psychotic symptoms (F32.2) must be met with the exception of criterion D.

C. The criteria for schizophrenia (F20.-) or schizoaffective disorder, depressive type (F25.1) are not met.

D. Either of the following must be present:

    (1) delusions or hallucinations, other than those listed as typically schizophrenic in F20, criterion G1(1)b, c, and d (i.e., delusions other than those that are completely impossible or culturally inappropriate and hallucinations that are not in the third person or giving a running commentary); the most common examples are those with depressive, guilty, hypochondriacal, nihilistic, self-referential, or persecutory content;

    (2) depressive stupor.

A fifth character may be used to specify whether the psychotic symptoms are congruent or incongruent with mood:

F32.30 With mood-congruent psychotic symptoms (i.e., delusions of guilt, worthlessness, bodily disease, or impending disaster, derisive or condemnatory auditory hallucinations)

F32.31 With mood-incongruent psychotic symptoms (i.e., persecutory or self-referential delusions and hallucinations without an affective content)

(Continued)

TABLE 29.1. (*Continued*)

F30–F39 MOOD [AFFECTIVE] DISORDERS

F32.8 Other depressive episodes

Episodes should be included here that do not fit the descriptions given for depressive episodes in F32.0–F32.3, but for which the overall diagnostic impression indicates that they are depressive in nature. Examples include fluctuating mixtures of depressive symptoms (particularly those of the somatic syndrome) with non-diagnostic symptoms such as tension, worry, and distress, and mixtures of somatic depressive symptoms with persistent pain or fatigue not due to organic causes (as sometimes seen in general hospital services).

F32.9 Depressive episode, unspecified

F33 RECURRENT DEPRESSIVE DISORDER

G1. There has been at least one previous episode, mild (F32.0), moderate (F32.1), or severe (F32.2 or F32.3), lasting a minimum of 2 weeks and separated from the current episode by at least 2 months free from any significant mood symptoms.

G2. At no time in the past has there been an episode meeting the criteria for hypomanic or manic episode (F30.-).

G3. Most commonly used exclusion criteria: the episode is not attributable to psychoactive substance use (F1) or any organic mental disorder, in the sense of F0.

It is recommended to specify the predominant type of previous episodes (mild, moderate, severe, uncertain).

F33.0 Recurrent depressive disorder, current episode mild

A. The general criteria for recurrent depressive disorder (F33) are met.

B. The current episode meets the criteria for depressive episode, mild severity (F32.0).

A fifth character may be used to specify the presence of the somatic syndrome, as defined in F32, in the current episode:

F33.00 without somatic syndrome

F33.01 with somatic syndrome

F33.1 Recurrent depressive disorder, current episode moderate

A. The general criteria for recurrent depressive disorders (F33) are met.

B. The current episode meets the criteria for depressive episode, moderate severity (F32.1).

A fifth character may be used to specify the presence of the somatic syndrome, as defined in F32, in the current episode:

F33.10 without somatic syndrome

F33.11 with somatic syndrome

F33.2 Recurrent depressive disorder, current episode severe without psychotic symptoms

A. The general criteria for recurrent depressive disorders (F33) are met.

B. The current episode meets the criteria for severe depressive episode without psychotic symptoms (F32.2).

F33.3 Recurrent depressive disorder, current episode severe with psychotic symptoms

A. The general criteria for recurrent depressive disorders (F33) are met.

B. The current episode meets the criteria for severe depressive episode with psychotic symptoms (F32.3).

A fifth character may be used to specify whether the psychotic symptoms are congruent or incongruent with the mood:

F33.30 with mood congruent psychotic symptoms

F33.31 with mood incongruent psychotic symptoms

F33.4 Recurrent depressive disorder, currently in remission

A. The general criteria for recurrent depressive disorder (F33) have been met in the past.

B. The current state does not meet the criteria for a depressive episode (F32.-) of any severity, or for any other disorder in F3 (the patient may receive treatment to reduce the risk of further episodes).

F33.8 Other recurrent depressive disorders

F33.9 Recurrent depressive disorder, unspecified

(*Continued*)

TABLE 29.1. *(Continued)*

F30–F39 MOOD [AFFECTIVE] DISORDERS

F34 PERSISTENT MOOD [AFFECTIVE] DISORDERS

F34.0 Cyclothymia

A. A period of at least 2 years of instability of mood involving several periods of both depression and hypomania, with or without intervening periods of normal mood.

B. None of the manifestations of depression or hypomania during such a 2-year period should be sufficiently severe or long-lasting to meet criteria for manic episode or depressive episode (moderate or severe); however, manic or depressive episode(s) may have occurred before, or may develop after, such a period of persistent mood instability.

C. During at least some of the periods of depression at least three of the following should be present:

   (1) A reduction in energy or activity;

   (2) Insomnia;

   (3) Loss of self-confidence or feelings of inadequacy;

   (4) Difficulty concentrating;

   (5) Social withdrawal;

   (6) Loss of interest or enjoyment in sex and other pleasurable activities;

   (7) Less talkative than normal;

   (8) Pessimistic about the future or brooding over the past.

D. During at least some of the periods of mood elevation at least three of the following should be present:

   (1) Increased energy or activity;

   (2) Decreased need for sleep;

   (3) Inflated self-esteem;

   (4) Sharpened or unusually creative thinking;

   (5) More gregarious than normal;

   (6) More talkative or witty than normal;

   (7) Increased interest and involvement in sexual and other pleasurable activities;

   (8) Overoptimism or exaggeration of past achievements.

Note: If desired, specify whether onset is early (in late teenage or the twenties) or late (usually between age 30 to 50 subsequent to an affective episode).

F34.1 Dysthymia

A. A period of at least 2 years of constant or constantly recurring depressed mood. Intervening periods of normal mood rarely last for longer than a few weeks and there are no episodes of hypomania.

B. None, or very few, of the individual episodes of depression within such a 2-year period are severe enough, or last long enough, to meet the criteria for recurrent mild depressive disorder (F33.0).

C. During at least some of the periods of depression at least three of the following should be present:

   (1) A reduction in energy or activity;

   (2) Insomnia;

   (3) Loss of self-confidence or feelings of inadequacy;

   (4) Difficulty concentrating;

   (5) Often in tears;

   (6) Loss of interest or enjoyment in sex and other pleasurable activities;

(Continued)

TABLE 29.1. (Continued)

F30–F39 MOOD [AFFECTIVE] DISORDERS

(7) Feeling of hopelessness or despair;

(8) A perceived inability to cope with the routine responsibilities of everyday life;

(9) Pessimistic about the future or brooding over the past;

(10) Social withdrawal;

(11) Less talkative than normal.

Note: If desired, specify whether onset is early (in late teenage or the twenties) or late (usually between age 30 to 50 subsequent to an affective episode).

F34.8 Other persistent mood [affective] disorders

A residual category for persistent affective disorders that are not sufficiently severe or long-lasting to fulfill the criteria for cyclothymia (F34.0) or dysthymia (F34.1) but that are nevertheless clinically significant. Some types of depression previously called "neurotic" are included here, provided that they do not meet the criteria for either cyclothymia (F34.0) or dysthymia (F34.1) or for depressive episode of mild (F32.0) or moderate (F32.1) severity.

F34.9 Persistent mood [affective] disorder, unspecified

F38 OTHER MOOD [AFFECTIVE] DISORDERS

There are so many possible disorders that could be listed under F38 that no attempt has been made to specify criteria, except for mixed affective episode (F38.00). Investigators requiring criteria more exact than the Diagnostic Guidelines should construct them according to the requirements of their study.

F38.0 Other single mood [affective] disorders

F38.00 Mixed affective episode

A. The episode is characterized by either a mixture or a rapid alternation (i.e., within a few hours) of hypomanic, manic, and depressive symptoms.

B. Both manic and depressive symptoms must be prominent most of the time during a period of at least 2 weeks.

C. No previous hypomanic, depressive, or mixed episodes.

F38.1 Other recurrent mood [affective] disorders

F38.10 Recurrent brief depressive disorder

A. The disorder meets the symptomatic criteria of either mild (F32.0), moderate (F32.1), or severe depressive episode (F32.2)

B. The depressive episodes occur about once a month over the past year.

C. The individual episodes last less than 2 weeks (typically 2 to 3 days).

D. The episodes do not occur solely in relation to the menstrual cycle.

F38.8 Other specified mood [affective] disorders

This is a residual category for affective disorders that do not meet the criteria for any other categories F30-F38.

F39 Unspecified mood [affective] disorder

mixture or rapid alternation of manic and depressive *symptoms* for two weeks, with the number and intensity of symptoms not defined. As such, ICD-10 may pick up a wider variety of mixed states, including agitated depressive episodes or subsyndromal hypomanic states concurrent with depressive episodes.

HYPOMANIC EPISODE

In DSM-IV-TR, the diagnosis of hypomanic episode differs from that of manic episode only in required duration (minimum four days versus minimum one week), and degree of dysfunction (hypomanic episode defined as not severe enough to cause hospitalization or marked impairment). ICD-10 criteria for a hypomanic episode share the same duration requirements as

DSM-IV-TR, but require only three additional symptoms, regardless of whether the core mood is elevated or irritable. ICD-10 furthermore does not recognize expansive mood as a core criterion for a hypomanic episodes, yet recognizes some different additional criteria, such as increased sociability or overfamiliarity.

DISORDERS

MAJOR DEPRESSIVE DISORDER AND RECURRENT DEPRESSIVE DISORDER

The DSM-IV-TR diagnosis of major depressive disorder requires the presence of one or more major depressive episodes, and the exclusion of other mood disorders, concurrent psychotic disorders, or medically induced or substance-induced mood disorders. The diagnosis of ICD-10 recurrent depressive disorder requires at least two depressive episodes, and exclusion of medically induced or substance-induced mood disorders, whereas exclusion of bipolar mood disorders is already implied in the ICD-10 criteria for depressive episode.

BIPOLAR I AND II DISORDERS, AND BIPOLAR AFFECTIVE DISORDER

Bipolar I disorder in DSM-IV-TR requires the presence of at least one manic or mixed episode, although the current episode may be specified as hypomanic, manic, mixed, or depressed. Bipolar II disorder is defined as the presence of one or more major depressive episodes, and at least one episode of hypomania, without history of full mania or mixed episodes. For both bipolar I and II disorders, schizoaffective disorders and psychotic disorders must not better account for the disorder at hand. ICD-10 bipolar affective disorder stipulates the presence of a hypomanic, manic, mixed, or depressive episode, plus at least one other mood episode, which must be hypomanic or manic if the current episode is depressed. In this way, ICD-10 groups together the DSM-IV-TR diagnoses of bipolar I and II disorders.

DYSTHYMIC DISORDER AND CYCLOTHYMIA

Dysthymic disorder in DSM-IV-TR requires the presence of a predominantly depressed mood, plus two or more additional depressive symptoms, whose total does not meet or exceed the threshold for major depressive disorder, plus no more than two months of euthymia, during a period of at least two years. Additional criteria for dysthymic disorder in DSM-IV-TR include: poor appetite or overeating; insomnia or hypersomnia; low energy or fatigue; poor concentration or difficulty making decisions; and feelings of hopelessness. Major depressive episodes or other mood episodes may supervene after two years of the diagnosis of DSM-IV-TR dysthymic disorder. Of course, all the usual DSM-IV-TR mood disorder exclusionary criteria apply. ICD-10 defines dysthymia in largely the same way as DSM-IV-TR, although in addition to the stem core criterion of depressed mood, ICD-10 requires at least three additional depressive symptoms. ICD-10 also allows for the possibility of a full depressive episode during the initial diagnostic period of dysthymia, and recognizes a greater diversity of additional diagnostic criteria, such as tearfulness, loss of interest or enjoyment in pleasurable activities, perceived inability to cope, pessimism or brooding, social withdrawal, and diminished talkativeness.

DSM-IV-TR cyclothymia requires the presence of two years of alternating periods of hypomania and depressive symptoms not meeting criteria for major depressive episode, without more than two months of euthymia at any time during the disturbance. The patient must not have evidence of full mania, mixed states, or major depressive episodes for the first two years of the disorder, but may go on to develop full blown bipolar disorder after this time. The usual exclusion of other mood disorders, psychotic disorders, and medically induced as well as substance-induced disorders apply. ICD-10 defines cyclothymia in much the same fashion as DSM-IV-TR, although without the two-month limit on euthymic periods, and with specifically spelled-out symptom criteria for the periods of hypomania and depressive symptoms, including some unique hypomanic symptoms such as sharpened or unusually creative thinking, increased gregariousness, increased wittiness, and overoptimism or exaggeration of past achievements.

MEDICALLY INDUCED AND SUBSTANCE-INDUCED MOOD DISORDERS

Mood disturbances comprise common manifestations of many general medical conditions, substance use syndromes, and treatment with prescribed medical therapies. Medically ill patients require screening for and evidenced-based treatment of mood disorders (Evans et al., 2005), as do patients with substance use disorders, and patients undergoing known mood-altering medical therapies.

Clinically significant depressive symptoms have been reported in 14–43% of patients with HIV (Cysique et al., 2007; Gibbie et al., 2007), up to 85% of patients with Hepatitis C (Nelligan et al., 2008), 8–18% of patients with diabetes (Gendelman et al., 2009; Li et al., 2008), 20% of patients with COPD (Cleland et al., 2007), 50% of patients with asthma (Van Lieshout et al., 2009), 9–31% of patients after CVA (Brodaty et al., 2007), 14% of patients with CAD (Shanmugasegaram et al., 2012), 20% of patients after acute myocardial infarction (Thombs et al., 2006), 20–55% of patients with epilepsy (Kanner 2003), 19–61% of patients after TBI (Kim et al., 2007), 40–60% of patients with multiple sclerosis (Wallin et al., 2006), 30–50% of patients with Alzheimer's disease (Lee and Lyketsos, 2003), 22–29% of patients with cancer (Raison and Miller, 2003), 20–30% of patients with obesity (Stunkard et al., 2003), 30–54% of patients with chronic pain conditions (Campbell et al., 2003), and 4–75% of patients with idiopathic Parkinson's disease (McDonald et al., 2003). Depressive symptoms also feature prominently in patients with endocrine disturbances, including 57–80% of patients with Cushing's syndrome (Haskett, 1985; Kelly, 1996), 30% of patients with hyperthyroidism (Kathol and Delahunt, 1986), and frequently in hypothyroidism (Whybrow et al., 1969). Hyperparathyroidism, hypoparathyroidism, Addison's disease, B vitamin deficiencies, folic acid deficiency, malnutrition, electrolyte imbalances, acid-base disturbances, and uremia have also been associated with clinically significant depressive symptoms, among other neuropsychiatric disturbances (Harrison and Kopelman, 2009, pp. 617–688).

Depressive symptoms in HIV correlate with treatment non-adherence and decreased viral response (Sumari de-Boer et al., 2012; Tsai et al., 2013), and in hepatitis C correlate with treatment non-adherence (Liu et al., 2010). Depressive symptoms in type I diabetes associate with lower therapeutic adherence (Van Tilburg et al., 2001), increased risk of medical complications (de Groot et al., 2001), and increased mortality (Milano and Singer, 2007). Depressive symptoms after CVA correlate with poor functional recovery and higher mortality (Gothe et al., 2012). Depressive symptoms following myocardial infarction predict repeat MI and death (Barth et al., 2004; Glassman et al., 2002). A diagnosis of major depressive disorder in hospitalized elderly patients correlates with increased in-hospital mortality and length of inpatient care (Koenig et al., 1989). Depressive symptoms in cancer patients correlate with greater physical disability (Bukberg, 1984) and increased mortality (Brown et al., 2003). Furthermore, depressive symptoms in the context of many general medical disorders, such as hepatitis C undergoing interferon treatment (Kraus et al., 2008), HIV (Tsai et al., 2013), CVA (Hackett et al., 2008), and multiple sclerosis (Mohr et al., 2001) are responsive to treatment.

Clinically significant manic symptoms have been reported in 1% of post-CVA patients and 9% of post-TBI patients (Jorge et al., 1993), 2–12% of Huntington's disease patients (Mendez, 1994), 39% of patients with thyrotoxicosis (Brownlie et al., 2000), 27% of patients with Cushing's syndrome (Haskett, 1985), and 3–22% of patients with epilepsy (Robertson, 1992). Clinically significant manic symptoms have also been associated with CNS tumors; multiple sclerosis; complex partial seizures; viral, fungal, and Treponemal meningoencephalitides; Parkinson's disease; Wilson's disease; Cushing's disease; hyperthyroidism; B vitamin deficiencies,; and other general medical conditions (Krauthammer and Klerman, 1978; Levenson 2011: p. 227; Mendez, 2000).

In an effort to account for mood disturbances in the context of general medical conditions and substance use disorders: DSM-IV-TR and ICD-10 list diagnostic criteria for mood disorders due to general medical condition, and DSM-IV-TR in particular lists diagnostic criteria for substance-induced mood disorder.

DSM-IV-TR criteria for Mood Disorder due to a General Medical Condition stipulate the presence of prominent and persistent mood symptoms corresponding to the core stem criteria for Major Depressive Episode and/or Manic Episode, in addition to evidence that the disorder is a physiologic consequence of a general medical condition, not better accounted for by another mental disorder, not occurring exclusively during the course of delirium, and causing clinically significant distress or impairment. In contrast to the diagnoses of primary idiopathic mood disorders, the DSM-IV-TR diagnosis of Mood Disorder due to a General Medical Condition does not dictate a threshold number of symptoms; the presence of one stem criterion suffices for the diagnosis. DSM-IV-TR further specifies subtypes, including With Depressive Features, With Manic Features, With Mixed Features, and With Major Depressive-Like Episode. ICD-10 criteria for Mental Disorders due to Brain Damage and Dysfunction and to Physical Disease require objective evidence or history of a medical disorder known to cause cerebral dysfunction, a presumed temporal relationship between development of the medical condition and the mental disorder, recovery or improvement of mental disorder following recovery or improvement from the medical condition, absence of convincing evidence for alternative causation of the mental disorder, and full criteria for one of the primary mood disorders outlined later in ICD-10. The latter criterion makes ICD-10 criteria more stringent than DSM-IV-TR in diagnosing mood disorders due to general medical conditions. ICD-10 further defines subtypes of Organic Manic/Bipolar/Depressive/Mixed Affective Disorder. ICD-10 delineates between provisional and certain diagnoses of organic mood disorders, with certainty dictated by the presence of evidence of recovery or improvement of mental disorder following recovery or improvement from the medical condition.

Similarly, many substance intoxication and withdrawal syndromes include core mood disorder disturbances. For example, euphoria, increased sociability, excitement, inexhaustibility, rambling speech, insomnia, mood lability, agitation, irritability, dysphoria, aggression, heightened sexuality, restlessness, anxiety, depression, interpersonal sensitivity, appetite changes, fatigue, psychomotor retardation, hypersomnia, fatigue, and hallucinations may occur during intoxication or withdrawal from ethanol, amphetamines, cocaine, caffeine, cannabis, or hallucinogens (American Psychiatric Association, 2000). Furthermore, many drug therapies for general medical conditions have been associated with clinically significant depressive symptoms, including corticosteroids, interferon alpha, interleukin 2, GRH agonists, mefloquine, and propranolol (Patten and Barbui, 2004). Drug therapies for general medical conditions have also been associated with clinically significant manic symptoms, including dopaminergic agents, noradrenergic agents, serotonergic agents, corticosteroids, and anabolic steroids (Krauthammer and Klerman, 1978; Levenson, 2011: p. 227).

DSM IV-TR criteria for Substance-Induced Mood Disorder require the presence of prominent and persistent mood symptoms, corresponding to core stem criteria for Major Depressive Episode and/or Manic Episode, in addition to evidence that the mood symptoms are temporally (within one month) or etiologically linked to substance use, intoxication, or withdrawal, not better accounted for by another mood disorder, not occurring exclusively during the course of delirium, and causing clinically significant distress or impairment. DSM-IV-TR does not dictate a threshold number of additional mood symptoms for diagnosis. Subtypes include With Depressive Features, With Manic Features, and With Mixed Features. Specifiers include With Onset During Intoxication, and With Onset During Withdrawal. ICD-10 does not define specific criteria for substance-induced mood disorders.

OTHER MOOD DISORDERS

Other mood disorders in DSM-IV-TR are captured by diagnoses of depressive disorder NOS, bipolar disorder NOS, and mood disorder NOS. ICD-10 similarly accounts for several other mood disorders. DSM-IV-TR in particular allows that these diagnoses may be made when the clinician cannot determine whether the mood disorder is primary or due to a general medical condition.

SPECIFIERS

DSM IV-TR includes prognostically informative specifiers for major depressive, manic, mixed, and recurrent episodes. Episode specifiers include severity, psychotic features, partial or full remission, single or recurrent episodes, melancholic features (for MDE only), atypical features (for MDE and dysthymia only), catatonic features, postpartum onset, and chronicity (for MDE only). Specifiers for recurrent mood episodes include with or without full interepisode recovery, with seasonal pattern, or with rapid cycling. In ICD-10, specifiers for severity, psychotic features, and recurrence apply to depressive episodes singly or as part of bipolar or recurrent depressive disorders, and are implied for manic, mixed, or hypomanic episodes in the diagnosis of bipolar affective disorder. In the following are presented selected specifiers, with brief descriptions and clinical implications.

SEVERITY

Severity in DSM-IV-TR mood disorders is defined in two ways: total symptom counts above that required for diagnosis, and degree of impairment attributable to the disorder. ICD-10 defines the severity of depressive episodes in terms of total symptom counts, and defines hypomanic versus manic episodes in terms of symptom counts and degree of impairment.

A study by Lux et al. (2010) examined the coherence and validity of the DSM-IV definition of the severity of major depression in a sample of 1,015 Caucasian twins who met criteria for major depressive disorder in the year prior to the study interview. The authors operationalized three measures of severity, including criteria counts (the DSM-IV definition of severity), scaled severity of individual symptoms (which is not present in DSM-IV), and impairment of function in occupational, social, and relational domains (which is not present in the DSM-IV diagnostic criteria, but is reflected to some extent in the separate GAF rating on axis V). Validators of severity in the study included co-morbid psychiatric conditions, personality traits, characteristics of the index episode, prior history of depression, demographic characteristics at index episode, future episodes, and depressive episodes of the co-twin. The authors found that criteria count and severity of individual symptoms were each significantly associated with 14 validators, and that functional impairment was associated with 12 validators. No one measure of severity accounted for all validators, and each measure of severity appeared to tap into different sets of validators. The authors concluded that clinicians should probably use a combination of severity measures, including the severity of individual symptoms.

Severity can be attributed to other aspects of a mood disorder as well, including duration (chronic MDE is shown to respond more poorly to treatment), comorbid symptom severity [several studies have shown severe anxiety correlates with increased time spent in depression over decades, as well as higher risk for suicide], and comorbid substance abuse (predictive of poor long-term outcomes, and suicidal behavior) (Kim et al., 2011; Rush et al., 2012).

Severity in research studies of major mood disorders often takes the form of arbitrarily defined cutoffs on the more common mood disorder rating scales, such as the Hamilton Depression Rating Scale, Montgomery Asberg Depression Rating Scale, Young Mania Rating Scale, and so on.

Severity of depressive and manic episodes among patients with bipolar I and II disorders correlates longitudinally with degree of psychosocial dysfunction (Judd et al., 2005). In addition, severe depressive episodes in both major depressive disorder and bipolar disorder have been associated with treatment resistance (Mendlewicz et al., 2010; Souery et al., 2007). However, antidepressant trials in major depressive disorder tend to show larger effect sizes in more severely depressed populations (Fournier et al., 2010).

PSYCHOTIC FEATURES

DSM-IV-TR defines "with psychotic features" as the presence of delusions or hallucinations concurrent with the mood episode. DSM-IV-TR allows for both mood-congruent and mood-incongruent psychotic features. ICD-10 defines with psychotic features similarly, but excludes those delusions most typical of schizophrenia, such as bizarre delusions or voices with running commentary. In ICD-10, psychotic features in depressive, manic, or mixed episodes may also be mood-congruent or mood-incongruent. Neither DSM-IV-TR nor ICD-10 allows for psychotic features in mild or moderate depressive episodes or hypomania.

Baseline psychotic features in major depressive disorder tend to recur highly in subsequent major depressive episodes (Coryell et al., 1994). Psychotic features in major depressive disorder also appear to portend later onset of mania or hypomania (Fiedorowicz et al., 2011) Furthermore, psychotic features in mood disorders in general associate with worse prognosis. For example, over 10 years of follow-up, psychotic features in major depressive disorder portend longer duration of depressive episodes, shorter intervals between depressive episodes, and greater persistence of subthreshold mood symptoms (Coryell et al., 1996).

PARTIAL OR FULL REMISSION

DSM-IV-TR defines partial remission of a mood episode as having some symptoms of a mood episode, but not meeting full criteria, for at least two months. Full remission is defined as not demonstrating any symptoms of a mood episode for at least two months. ICD-10 defines remission in mood disorders as no longer meeting full criteria for an episode within the disorder, thus grouping together partial and full remission groups. ICD-10 does not define how long mood episode criteria need to be absent for remission.

In general, partial remission carries continued illness-related morbidity and risk of relapse. In major depressive disorder, for example, partial remission and other subthreshold depressive states are associated longitudinally with greater psychosocial impairment than full remission, with the gradient of impairment increasing with increasing numbers of depressive symptoms (Judd et al., 2000). This finding holds true with regard to subthreshold depressive states in bipolar I and II disorders as well (Judd et al., 2005).

SINGLE OR RECURRENT MAJOR DEPRESSIVE DISORDER

DSM-IV-TR defines recurrence in major depressive disorder as two or more major depressive episodes, as does ICD-10. As described in the text of the DSM-IV-TR, within major depressive disorder, a single major depressive episode has about a 60% change of recurrence, a second major depressive episode increases the risk of recurrence to about 70%, and a third major depressive episode increases recurrence risk to 90%. Although DSM-IV-TR and ICD-10 define recurrence in major depressive disorder as two or more major depressive episodes, highly recurrent major depressive disorders begin to behave more akin to bipolar disorder than major depressive disorder (Goodwin and Jamison, 2007). For example, highly recurrent major depressive disorder probands show family histories enriched with bipolar disorders, convert to frank bipolarity more often than single episode or lowly recurrent major depressive disorder probands, and may respond preferentially to treatments shown to be effective in bipolar disorders. For these reasons, the DSM-IV-TR and ICD-10 definitions of recurrence have been criticized for not delineating definitions for highly recurrent major depressive disorder.

MELANCHOLIC FEATURES

Melancholic features, including dense anhedonia, non-reactive mood, diurnal variation, and neurovegetative signs, are among the oldest described symptoms in psychiatry. DSM-IV-TR defines melancholic features as requiring either loss of pleasure or lack of reactivity to usually pleasurable stimuli, plus three or more additional criteria such as: distinct quality of depressed mood; depression worse in the morning; early morning awakening; marked psychomotor retardation or agitation; and excessive or inappropriate guilt. ICD-10 refers to melancholic features as the somatic syndrome, defined similarly to DSM-IV-TR but without drawing a distinction between core and stem criteria. ICD-10 also notes that many other monikers have accompanied this syndrome in other classification schemes.

Melancholic features in major depressive disorder associate with increased comorbidity of anxiety disorders, greater number of lifetime depressive episodes, more severe impairment, lower levels of neuroticism, and increased risk of major depressive disorder in both mono- and dizygotic co-twins (Kendler, 1997). Melancholic features in major depressive disorder, bipolar I disorder, and bipolar II disorder also correlate with treatment resistance (Mendlewicz et al., 2010; Souery et al., 2007).

ATYPICAL FEATURES

In contrast to the implications of the term, atypical features of depression are not unusual in mood disorders. Historically, the term "atypical depression" stemmed from the striking difference between the clinical appearance of such presentations and that of the more classical endogenous or melancholic depressive syndromes, as well as the differential response of a particular form of atypical depression to MAOI pharmacotherapy as demonstrated by a research group from Columbia University (Davidson, 2007). The DSM-IV-TR criteria for atypical features in depression, derived from the criteria described by the aforementioned Columbia University group, include the stem criterion of mood reactivity, plus at least two of the following additional criteria: increased appetite or weight gain; hypersomnia; leaden paralysis; and a long-standing pattern of extreme sensitivity to perceived interpersonal rejection, occurring most of the time over a two-week period. ICD-10 does not include an atypical features specifier for depressive disorders.

Earlier studies in atypical depression that showed a higher rate of response to MAOI medications than tricyclic antidepressants have been eclipsed by more recent studies showing that SSRI antidepressants such as fluoxetine are equally effective as MAOIs in atypical depression.

CATATONIC FEATURES

The DSM-IV-TR catatonic features specifier is applied when the clinical picture of a mood episode is characterized by marked psychomotor disturbance including two or more of the following: marked motoric immobility such as catalepsy or stupor; excessive motor activity; extreme negativism or mutism; peculiarities of motor movement such as posturing or stereotypies or mannerisms or grimacing; and echolalia or echopraxia. ICD-10 does not have a catatonic features specifier in its section on mood disorders.

A patient with catatonia requires careful supervision to avoid self-harm, or harm to others. Malnutrition, exhaustion, hyperpyrexia, or self-inflicted injury may occur. Catatonic states have been reported in up to 5–9% of psychiatric inpatients. Between 25 and 50% of cases of catatonia occur in mood disorders and 10–15% occur in schizophrenia (American Psychiatric Association, 2000). Catatonia also occurs in postpartum psychosis in 0.1–0.5% of women within weeks of delivery, although it can occur within hours (Strain et al., 2012). However, catatonia is not unique to psychiatric conditions, as it has also been associated with a plethora of general medical conditions. Lastly, as with all catatonic syndromes, catatonic features in mood disorders may respond preferentially to high dose benzodiazepine pharmacotherapy, and may require electroconvulsive therapy (ECT) for definitive treatment.

POSTPARTUM ONSET

The DSM-IV-TR postpartum specifier can be applied to a mood disorder if the onset is within 4 weeks after childbirth. Symptoms may include fluctuations in mood, mood lability, and preoccupation with infant well-being, which may range from overconcern to frank delusions. The presence of severe ruminations or delusional thoughts about the infant is associated with a significantly increased risk of harm to the infant. ICD-10 does not specify postpartum onset. Postpartum depression affects 10–15% of women within six months after delivery. It is important to distinguish postpartum mood episodes from the "baby blues" that affect up to 70% of women within 10 days of delivery (American Psychiatric Association, 2000; Strain, 2012).

CHRONIC MAJOR DEPRESSIVE EPISODE

DSM-IV-TR defines a chronic specifier for major depressive episode, whereas ICD-10 does not. Chronicity in DSM-IV-TR requires that full major depressive episode criteria have been met for at least the past two years. Chronicity in a major depressive episode confers a poorer prognosis. Chronic major depressive disorder in particular has been associated with greater baseline socioeconomic disadvantage, lower baseline quality of life, lower baseline social and occupational functioning, and higher baseline medical disease and anxiety disorder burden. Furthermore, after treatment with antidepressant pharmacotherapy, chronic depression demonstrates continued poorer functioning and greater anxiety, despite an adjusted treatment response rate statistically indistinguishable from non-chronic depression (Sung et al., 2012). Another report, from the STAR*D study, demonstrates that patients with chronic index episodes of major depressive disorder have lower and slower remission rates, as well as higher relapse rates, than patients with non-chronic index episodes (Rush et al., 2012). In addition, unlike in many studies of non-chronic major depressive disorder, in chronic major depressive disorder the addition of psychotherapy to pharmacotherapy does not appear consistently to provide short-term or long-term treatment benefits above pharmacotherapy alone, with the exception of small add-on effects on quality of life (von Wolff et al., 2012). CBASP (Cognitive Behavioral Analysis System of Psychotherapy) may represent one exception to these latter findings, as this form of psychotherapy has demonstrated add-on effects to pharmacotherapy in chronic major depressive disorder (Keller et al., 2000).

FULL INTEREPISODE RECOVERY

DSM-IV-TR defines full interepisode recovery as full remission attained between the two most recent mood episodes. Similar to partial versus full remission, full interepisode recovery portends better functionality.

SEASONAL PATTERN

In DSM-IV-TR, the seasonal pattern specifier describes a regular temporal occurrence of major depressive episodes in major depressive, bipolar I, or bipolar II disorders. Criteria require that both onset and remission of major depressive episodes occur at characteristic times of the year, that at least two major depressive episodes have occurred with this temporal seasonal pattern over the past two years, and that the number of major depressive episodes occurring during this temporal seasonal pattern outnumber the non-seasonal episodes. ICD-10 does not stipulate a seasonal pattern specifier in its mood disorders chapter. Seasonal major depressive episodes in major depressive disorder may respond to light therapy, although this therapy may also increase the rate of switching to hypomanic or manic episodes when used to treat seasonal depressive episodes in bipolar I or II disorder (American Psychiatric Association, 2000).

WITH RAPID CYCLING

The DSM-IV-TR rapid cycling specifier is applied to either bipolar I or bipolar II disorder diagnoses. The essential feature of the DSM-IV-TR definition of rapid-cycling bipolar disorder is the occurrence of four or more mood episodes during the previous year. ICD-10 does not account for a rapid cycling specifier. Rapid cycling occurs in 10–20% of individuals with bipolar disorder, and is much more commonly found in females, who comprise 70–90% of individuals with a rapid cycling pattern. These episodes are not linked to any particular phase of the menstrual cycle and are seen in both pre- and postmenopausal women (American Psychiatric Association, 2000). Induction of rapid cycling has been reported in association with maintenance tricyclic antidepressant use in five bipolar patients, despite concurrent treatment with lithium (Wehr and Goodwin, 1979). Successful treatment of rapid cycling bipolar disorder has been demonstrated using high dose levothyroxine, carbamazepine, and lamotrigine (Joyce, 1988; Stancer and Persad, 1982; Stromgren and Boller, 1985; Wang et al., 2010) .

MOOD DISORDERS IN LATE LIFE

Neither DSM-IV-TR nor ICD-10 outlines criteria for depressive or bipolar disorders in late life (typically defined as older than 60–65 years). However, some important biopsychosocial considerations and phenomenological differences bear mentioning. Normative aging may be associated with altered sleep patterns, diminished sleep quality, diminished energy, decreased cognitive performance, motoric slowing, and interpersonal losses associated with sadness and bereavement. Furthermore, older patients typically manifest more general medical conditions, including conditions themselves linked to clinically significant depressive and/or manic symptoms. Lastly, given the physiologic effects of aging on pharmacokinetics, in combination with frequent pharmacologic treatment of general medical and psychiatric conditions, late life patients may be at particular risk for exposure to mood-altering pharmacotherapy.

Onset of major depressive disorder after age 60 is common, accounting for up to 50% of major depressive disorder diagnoses in late life. Adults with onset of major depressive disorder after age 60 typically evidence a history of less personality dysfunction, and lower burden of psychiatric family history. Patients with major depressive disorder in late life may exhibit more prominent melancholic symptoms, and psychotic symptoms, including prominent delusions of persecution, incurable illness, guilt, and nihilism or non-existence (Blazer and Steffens, 2009: p. 286). Furthermore, patients with depressive disorders in late life may also exhibit cognitive disturbances suggestive of dementia, termed pseudodementia (Snowdon, 2011), which typically demonstrates slowed processing speed, dysexecutive problems, and memory retrieval deficits. With successful treatment of depressive illness, pseudodementia appears reversible in the short term, yet predictive of later onset primary dementia (Saez-Fonseca et al., 2007). Similar to findings that late life patients with major depressive disorder demonstrate less comorbid personality pathology than younger patients with major depressive disorder (Devanand et al., 2002), late life patients with dysthymia also differ from younger patients with dysthymia in that they exhibit less comorbid personality pathology (Devanand et al., 2000). Specifically, late life patients with dysthymia or major depressive disorder appear preferentially to demonstrate cluster C personality pathology, in contradistinction to the cluster B personality pathology preferentially common in younger patients with dysthymia or major depressive disorder.

Bipolar disorder in late life may exhibit less classic euphoric mania, and more mixed depressive and manic symptomatology, with agitated depression and dysphoric mania commonly seen (Shulman and Post, 1980; Spar et al., 1979). Delirious mania may also present in late life bipolar disorder, exhibiting symptoms of mania along with catatonic symptoms and disturbed cognition (Blazer and Steffens, 2009: p. 285).

SEPARATION FROM OTHER CONDITIONS, DIFFERENTIAL DIAGNOSIS, AND COMORBIDITY

As outlined previously, in both DSM-IV-TR and ICD-10, diagnosing a primary idiopathic mood disorder requires exclusion of other mood disorders, psychotic disorders, and medically induced or substance-induced disorders. Both systems leave it to the clinician's discernment to determine whether the apparent episode or disorder at hand is better accounted for by another condition. This diagnostic task is non-trivial, as many psychiatric disorders, general medical conditions, and substance use syndromes feature signs and symptoms that overlap significantly with mood disorders. For example, hypothyroidism and major depressive disorder both share possible symptoms of anergia, lassitude, impaired concentration and memory, weight gain, depressed mood, and dullness of expression. For the purposes of appropriate treatment planning, however, it remains clinically important to differentiate between primary idiopathic mood disorders, symptomatically overlapping psychiatric conditions, mood disorders due to general medical conditions, substance-induced mood disorders, and co-occurrence of primary and secondary disorders. A differential diagnosis list of possible medically induced and substance-induced mood disorders, as well as symptomatically overlapping psychiatric conditions, is listed in Table 29.2.

TABLE 29.2. General differential diagnosis for mood episodes and mood disorders

Substance-Induced Mood Disorder
Alcohol intoxication, withdrawal, abuse, or dependence
Sedative or hypnotic intoxication, withdrawal, abuse, or dependence
Stimulant intoxication, withdrawal, abuse, or dependence
Opioid intoxication, withdrawal, abuse, or dependence
Cannabis intoxication, withdrawal, abuse, or dependence
Anabolic steroid abuse or therapy
Corticosteroid therapy or withdrawal
Other immunomodulatory therapies
Chemotherapy for oncologic disease
HAART
Interferon therapy, e.g., in hepatitis C
Beta blockers
Malarial prophylaxis, especially with mefloquine
SSRIs, SNRIs, NRIs, TCAs, MAOIs
Stimulant therapy
Mood Disorder due to a General Medical Condition
Obstructive Sleep Apnea
Hyperthyroidism or Hypothyroidism

(Continued)

TABLE 29.2. *(Continued)*

Hyperparathyroidism or Hypoparathyroidism
Hyperpituitarism or Hypopituitarism
Hypercortisolemia or Hypocortisolemia
Hypotestosteronemia
Diabetes
Electrolyte Disturbances
Acid-Base Disturbances
Malnutrition
Vitamin Deficiency
Renal Failure
Hepatic Failure
Wilson's Disease
Malignancy
Brain Tumor or Metastasis
Systemic Effects of Peripheral Malignancy
Paraneoplastic Syndromes
Paraneoplastic Limbic Encephalitis
Coronary Artery Disease
Other Cardiovascular Disease
Anemia
Arrhythmias
Congestive Heart Failure
Valvular Heart Disease
Respiratory Illness
COPD
Asthma
Obstructive Sleep Apnea
Infectious Disease
HIV / AIDS
Viral Hepatitis
Osteomyelitis
Endocarditis
Mononucleosis
Lyme Disease
Opportunistic Infections

(Continued)

TABLE 29.2. (*Continued*)

Autoinflammatory Disease

Multiple Sclerosis

Systemic Lupus Erythematosis

Autoimmune Encephalitis

Cerebrovascular Disease

Cerebrovascular Accident

Vascular Dementia

Cerebrovascular Malformation

Parkinsonism

Idiopathic Parkinson's Disease

Antipsychotic-Induced Parkinsonism

Parkinson's Dementia

Dementia with Lewy Bodies

Progressive Supranuclear Palsy

Multisystem Atrophy

Huntington's Disease

Other Dementias

Dementia of Alzheimer's Type

Frontotemporal Dementia

Amyotrophic Lateral Sclerosis

Seizure Disorders

Ictal

Postictal

Interictal

Traumatic Brain Injury

Chronic Pain

Delirium

Catatonia due to General Medical Condition

Brief Psychotic Disorder, Schizophrenia, Schizophreniform Disorder, Schizophrenia, Delusional Disorder, or Psychotic Disorder NOS

Schizoaffective Disorder

Bipolar I or II Disorder

Major Depressive Disorder

Dysthymic or Cyclothymic Disorder

Adjustment Disorder

Bereavement

(Continued)

TABLE 29.2. (*Continued*)

Demoralization

Attention Deficit Hyperactivity Disorder

Posttraumatic Stress Disorder

Generalized Anxiety Disorder

Eating Disorders

Neurasthenia

Primary Sleep Disorder

Personality Disorders

In keeping with the broad differential diagnosis of mood disorder symptoms, psychiatric standards of care stipulate screening evaluations for general medical conditions and substance use syndromes that may mimic primary idiopathic mood disorders. History of present illness, past medical history, past psychiatric history, substance use history, current medications, family history, social history, developmental history, legal history, review of systems, and focused physical examination are indicated when evaluating patients with mood disorder symptoms. Cognitive screening examinations, such as the MMSE (Folstein et al., 1975) or MOCA (Nasreddine et al., 2005), are also indicated in the routine evaluation of mood disorders, especially so in older patients and patients with a known or suspected cognitive disorder. Routine and inexpensive screening tests in mood disorder diagnosis may include CBC, chemistry panel, liver function tests, TSH, free T4, B12, folic acid, thiamine, *T. pallidum* antibody, HCG, urine drug metabolite screen, and ECG. Further tests indicated by history and physical examination may include an HIV screen, infectious hepatitis panel, ESR, ANA, timed serum or salivary cortisol, free testosterone, prolactin, EEG, polysomnography, and MRI. Medical or neurological consultation is also warranted, whenever a general medical or neurologic condition is suspected.

Discerning the source of mood symptoms in the face of multiple likely etiologies requires recognition of several logical diagnostic possibilities. Given the presence of two mood-related conditions, A and B, diagnostic possibilities include:

1. An overarching unitary condition AB that has been erroneously, conceptually split

2. A and B represent related conditions arising from a shared root cause

3. Condition A causes condition B

4. Condition B causes condition A

5. Condition A is causally independent from but influences condition B

6. Condition B is causally independent from but influences condition A

7. Condition A and B are causally independent from each other, but mutually influence each other

8. Condition A and B are fully causally independent and do not influence each other.

These logical possibilities underscore the difficulty of diagnostic separation of mood disorders from other conditions, differential diagnosis, and comorbidity assessment. Stemming from these logical possibilities, several approaches obtain to diagnosing mood disorders in the context of known mood-altering medical conditions, substance use, and overlapping psychiatric conditions. These approaches may exist in pure, or combined, forms.

1. Inclusive approach: applies signs and symptoms that satisfy mood disorder diagnostic criteria, or normative cutoffs on depressive symptom screening instruments, without subtracting signs and symptoms that may be related to another condition. Threshold severity and number of total signs and symptoms required for diagnosis remain unchanged from those applied to primary mood disorder diagnosis. This approach maximizes sensitivity and reliability, but minimizes specificity. Examples include the assessment of depressive symptoms in general medical conditions using low cutoff scores on the PHQ-9 (Kroenke et al., 2001; Lamers et al., 2008; Stafford et al., 2007) or CES-D (Jones et al., 2005; Koenig et al., 1998; Weissman et al., 1977).

2. Exclusive approach: applies signs and symptoms that satisfy mood disorder diagnostic criteria, while subtracting signs and symptoms that may be related to other conditions. Threshold severity and number of total signs and symptoms required for diagnosis remain unchanged. An example of this approach may be found in Bukberg et al.'s (1984) assessment of depressive symptoms in hospitalized cancer patients. This approach encourages specificity at the expense of sensitivity.

3. Increased threshold approach: applies signs and symptoms that satisfy mood disorder diagnostic criteria, or signs and symptoms from depressive screening instruments, with or without subtracting signs and symptoms that may be related to other conditions. However, the threshold symptom severity, number of total signs and symptoms, or cutoff score required for diagnosis increase. Examples include the assessment of depressive symptoms in general medical conditions using high cutoff scores on the PHQ-9 (Justice et al., 2004; Williams et al., 2005) or CES-D (Hermanns et al., 2006). This approach also encourages specificity at the expense of sensitivity.

4. Symptom substitution approach: applies signs and symptoms that satisfy mood disorder diagnostic criteria, while subtracting signs and symptoms that may be related to a general medical condition or substance use. These subtracted signs and symptoms are replaced by other signs and symptoms intended to more closely capture mood symptoms, as opposed to general medical condition or other psychiatric disorder manifestations. Threshold severity and number of total signs and symptoms required for diagnosis may increase or remain the same. This approach, as exemplified in Endicott's (1984) examination of depression in patients with cancer, is also evident in the structure of numerous depressive screening instruments for use in patients with possibly confounding comorbid conditions, including the Hospital Anxiety and Depression Scale (Zigmond and Snaith, 1983), the Geriatric Depression Scale (Yesavage et al., 1982–1983), and the Calgary Scale for Depression in Schizophrenia (Addington et al., 1992). The various versions of the Beck Depression Inventory (Beck et al., 1961, 1996) also exemplify a symptom substitution approach, as they rely more heavily on mood and cognitive symptoms than neurovegetative symptoms. This approach also encourages specificity at the expense of sensitivity.

5. Etiologic approach: attempts to ascribe specific symptoms to their most likely underlying etiology, whether primary idiopathic, medical, or substance-induced, then arrives at a mood disorder diagnosis by applying only those symptoms attributable to the mood disorder. Both DSM-IV-TR and ICD-10 exemplify this approach to mood disorder diagnosis, which also encourages specificity at the expense of sensitivity.

In their classic paper on depression in 460 medically ill older adults, Koenig et al. (1997) outlined the prevalence of major and minor depressive disorders in this population according to inclusive, etiologic, exclusive-inclusive, exclusive-etiologic, substitutive-inclusive, or substitutive-etiologic approaches. The authors demonstrated that an inclusive approach resulted in the highest prevalence rates for major and minor depression, an exclusive-etiologic approach resulted in the lowest prevalence of major depression, and an etiologic approach resulted in the lowest prevalence of minor depression. The exclusive-etiologic approach identified the most severe and persistent major depressions. However, the authors also showed that known depression-associated characteristics (predictive validity) and associations with depression scale scores (convergent validity) did not vary remarkably. The authors concluded by suggesting that clinicians or researchers choose from the various diagnostic approaches based on the goals and purpose of the examination. For example, an epidemiologist studying depressive morbidity in a general medical condition may wish to utilize an inclusive approach in order to highlight the problem for public health attention, whereas a clinician working in a resource-limited setting may wish to use an exclusive-etiologic approach to identify those patients with the most severe depressive symptoms for treatment.

DIAGNOSTIC VALIDITY

In their landmark paper on diagnostic criteria for psychiatric research, Feighner et al. (1972) outlined five phases for establishing diagnostic validity in psychiatric illness: clinical description, laboratory studies, delimitation from other disorders, follow-up study, and family study.

Certainly, current mood disorder nosologies contain a wealth of clinical descriptors, and take pains to delimit specific mood disorders. Furthermore, family and twin studies have repeatedly demonstrated the heritable nature of all the major mood disorder syndromes, although specific genes appear to explain only small effects in the etiology of mood disorders. Patients with mood disorders also demonstrate a plethora of laboratory abnormalities, although none so sensitive or specific to point to a unified biological etiogenesis. This last fact points to the need further to define mood disorder subtypes, symptom components, and cross-syndromic dimensional constructs, which may serve better to elucidate candidate mechanisms for neurobiologic investigation.

In addition to the preceding problems with genetic and laboratory investigation, follow-up study also points to some weaknesses in the validity of current mood disorder diagnoses. DSM-IV-TR and ICD-10 emphasize cross-sectional diagnosis, causing problems with recall bias and diagnostic instability over time. For example, patients with prior hypomania show demonstrably poor recall of having had hypomania, and a non-trivial portion of patients diagnosed with major depressive disorder turn out rather to have bipolar disorder (Fiedorowicz et al., 2011; Goodwin and Jamison, 2007).

Furthermore, individual symptoms or signs within a given mood disorder diagnosis may vary in their individual validity. For example, a study by Lux et al. (2010) investigated a sample of 1,015 Caucasian twins using logistic regression analyses to compare the associations of individual symptom criteria, and two groups of criteria reflecting cognitive and neurovegetative symptoms, with a wide range of diagnostic validators including demographic factors, risk for future episodes in the co-twin, pattern of comorbidity, and personality traits. Cognitive symptoms included "depressed mood," "loss of interest," "worthlessness-guilt," and "suicidal ideation." Neurovegetative symptoms included "sleep," "appetite/weight," "psychomotor changes," and "fatigue." "Trouble concentrating" was excluded as a criterion. Interestingly, the investigators found that individual symptom criteria differed substantially in their associations with specific diagnostic validators, and that the cognitive criteria group generally produced stronger associations with diagnostic validators than did the neurovegetative criteria group. These results challenge the equivalence assumption inherent to the criteria for major depressive disorder, and suggest a degree of covert heterogeneity among these criteria, part of which is captured by the cognitive symptoms being more strongly associated with the most clinically relevant characteristics. They suggest that a detailed evaluation of DSM-IV major depressive episode criteria is overdue.

Recently the construct validity of major depression has been tested with item response theory analysis. Carragher et al. (2011) have shown that the current criteria for major depressive disorder performed well in defining a latent continuum for major depression. In general, the criteria fell along a range of depression severity, with death/suicidal thoughts, worthlessness/guilt, and psychomotor difficulties appearing along the severe end of the range, and concentration difficulties/indecision and sleep disturbance appearing along the middle to mild end of the range.

DIAGNOSTIC ACCURACY

The soft, syndromic, heterogeneous, and cross-sectional nature of current mood disorder diagnoses makes difficult the establishment of a gold standard reference. Structured diagnostic interviews, combined with medical record review and expert reassessment, appear to come closest to a gold standard approach to diagnosis in routine clinical research. Spitzer's (1983) "LEAD Standard"—L = Longitudinal evaluation of symptomatology, E = Evaluation by expert consensus, AD = All Data from multiple sources—captures the essence of such combined methods. Numerous studies have demonstrated that structured diagnostic interviews outperform routine clinical diagnosis, and that the addition of medical record review brings diagnostic accuracy close to that attained from use of all four LEAD sources (Basco et al., 2000; Miller et al., 2001). However, whereas such methods allow for the calculation of accuracy and reliability data, they do not take advantage of statistical methods such as latent class analysis, which may contribute to improved accuracy in the assessment of such markedly complex phenomena as mood disorder diagnosis (Faraone and Tsuang, 1994).

DIAGNOSTIC RELIABILITY

Field trials of mood disorder diagnoses from DSM-IV and ICD-10 reveal marked variability in interrater reliability. One DSM-IV mood disorders field trial, reported by Keller et al. (1995), included 524 adult patients, comprising approximately 100 patients from each of five US university medical center sites. The study selected patients based on complaint of depressed mood, plus the presence of at least two other DSM-III-R symptoms of major depression or dysthymia, with no minimum duration of symptoms required. The interrater reliability investigation protocol utilized videotaped interviews. In reported results, diagnoses of both major depression and dysthymia demonstrated good to excellent intrasite interrater reliability, and fair to good intersite interrater reliability. Six month test-retest interrater reliability was poor to fair for the diagnosis of major depression, and fair for the diagnosis of dysthymia.

In contrast, the ICD-10 field trial included 11,491 adult patients, unselected by any preconceived symptomatic threshold for inclusion. The ICD-10 field trial reported only intrasite reliability, between pairs of raters from 32 countries. The study reported good to excellent intrasite interrater reliability for overarching categories of manic episode, bipolar affective disorder, depressive episode, recurrent depressive disorder, and schizoaffective disorder. Subtypes of these overarching categories had fair to good intrasite interrater reliability, as had dysthymia and adjustment disorders. Mixed anxiety depressive disorder demonstrated very poor intrasite interrater reliability (Sartorius et al., 1995).

It is important to note that the former field trial included enriched clinical samples, thereby potentially inflating real-world clinical reliability, whereas the latter used unenriched convenience samples, more closely approximating usual clinical practice.

The search for laboratory anomalies associated with the major mood disorders has a long and convoluted history. For example, John Cade's discovery of the mood stabilizing properties of lithium occurred in the context of testing his hypothesis that excess urea in the urine of mentally ill patients signified a general marker of mental illness. In an animal model of this hypothesis, Cade used lithium urate to increase the amount of urea he could administer to his guinea pigs, and observed that lithium protected against the toxic effects of urea. Other lithium salts appeared to tranquilize the animals, and successful trials of lithium for manic agitation soon followed (Cade, 1949).

The era of modern, neohumoral mechanisms as etiologies and diagnostic tests, however, began in earnest with the monoamine and catecholamine hypotheses. Various authors investigated catecholamine metabolites as diagnostic tests for major depression, and later as tests for predicting response to tricyclic antidepressants. However, neither endeavor resulted in evidence supporting a diagnostic or predictive role for these markers.

Other investigators have examined the HPA axis, the hypothalamic-pituitary-thyroid axis, EEG abnormalities, neurotrophic factors, neuroimaging patterns, inflammatory markers, risk conferring genes, and second messenger system components in relation to mood disorders. While such investigations have contributed unquestionably to our understanding of aspects of mood disorder pathophysiology, none have resulted in diagnostic tests able to discern between disordered and non-disordered patients with enough accuracy to warrant clinical use. One recent attempt at compiling various inflammatory, neurotrophic, and neuroendocrine markers in the diagnosis of major depressive disorder, resulted in a reported sensitivity of 91.1%, specificity of 81.3%, positive predictive value of 79%, and negative predictive value of 92% (Papakostas, 2011). This effort represents a significant advance over prior attempts, but if used alone would still result in possibly harmful exposure to unnecessary antidepressant pharmacotherapy or psychotherapy for 21 out of 100 "positive" patients. Note also that the study used DSM-IV criteria, diagnosed via a structured clinical interview, as the comparative gold standard, suggesting that clinicians simply use these clinical procedures for diagnosis in the first place.

LIMITATIONS OF CURRENT CATEGORICAL DIAGNOSES

"With the publication of DSM-III, psychiatrists had an agreed-upon language for naming what they saw, yet this language did not explicitly engage the issue of the nature of the disorders it named."

MITCHELL WILSON (Wilson, 1993)

IMPORTANT PROGNOSTIC SPECIFIERS NOT INCLUDED IN DSM

TREATMENT RESISTANCE

Several authors have proposed that treatment resistance in major depressive disorder represents an independent and important prognostic feature. Systematic methods for assessing treatment resistance include the Maudsley Staging Method (MSM), the Antidepressant Treatment History Form (ATHF), the Massachusetts General Hospital Staging Model (MGH-s), the Thase Rush Staging Model (TRSM), and the European Staging Model (ESM) (Ruhe et al., 2012). In general, these models attempt to assess treatment resistance by scoring the number and adequacy of prior medication trials, the presence of augmentation trials, dose optimizations, and combination strategies, and the use of ECT. The MSM additionally includes measures of index episode duration and severity, which, as demonstrated in the specifiers section, have their own prognostic implications.

A recent review by Ruhe et al. (2012) illustrates the value of the treatment resistant depression concept. In a series of ECT studies, the highest scoring antidepressant trial on baseline ATHF correlated with higher relapse one year status post ECT (Sackeim et al., 1990), lower response to ECT (Prudic et al., 1996), and higher relapse on Li after effective ECT (Shapira et al., 1995). In addition, in outpatient MDD treatment, higher scores on the MGH-s, but not the TRSM, correlated retrospectively with absence of remission (Petersen et al., 2005). Lastly, Fedaku et al. (2009a, 2009b) demonstrated that total MSM score correlated with short-term failure to achieve remission, as well as long-term persistence of a depressive episode, and presence of a depressive episode over 50% of follow-up time. In contrast, total TRSM score correlated more weakly with short-term failure to achieve remission, and did not correlate with long-term outcomes (Fedaku et al., 2009b). Of the preceding treatment resistant depression models, only the ATHF has published interrater reliability data, with a reported intraclass correlation coefficient of 0.94. (Sackeim et al., 1990). Overall, treatment resistance in unipolar depressive disorders appears to have prognostic importance in predicting lack of treatment response, and delineation of treatment resistance may be a helpful diagnostic concept in developing future treatment studies in this therapeutically challenging subgroup.

ANXIETY

A recent review by Goldberg and Fawcett (2012) found that both anxiety diagnoses and anxiety symptoms occur frequently in both unipolar and bipolar depression, and that both anxiety diagnoses and severity of anxiety symptoms in unipolar and bipolar depression also correlate with poor treatment outcomes and higher risk for suicidal behavior and completed suicide.

Fava et al. (2008) reported from the STAR*D study, one of the largest major depressive disorder treatment outcome studies ever conducted, that severity of anxiety symptoms, as extracted from a subscale of the Hamilton Depression Scale, also predicted poor treatment outcomes in this sample.

As Coryell et al. (2012) note, "Many longitudinal studies of depressive disorders have associated comorbid anxiety with poorer outcomes as reflected in a lower likelihood of treatment response, longer times to recovery from index episodes and greater amounts of depressive morbidity over time." (Coryell et al., 2012: p. 210) Drawing from the NIMH Collaborative Depression Study sample, Coryell and colleagues further delineated this relationship by showing that severity of anxiety symptoms during an index depressive episode correlated with duration of future depressive episodes for both unipolar and bipolar depression (Coryell et al., 2012). Furthermore, baseline anxiety symptom severity predicted duration of future depressive episodes more strongly than did baseline depressive symptom severity, and the predictive power of baseline anxiety symptom severity outlasted that of baseline depressive symptom severity. In addition, the same group also demonstrated that severity of anxiety symptoms during an index bipolar depressive episode correlated with greater percentage of time spent in subsequent depressive episodes versus manic or hypomanic episodes (Coryell et al., 2009). Both of these findings showed dose-response relationships between baseline global anxiety symptom severity and outcomes—relationships that persisted over two decades of follow-up. In neither study did comorbid anxiety disorders at baseline correlate with outcomes at follow-up, indicating that anxiety symptom severity during depressive episodes represents an important prognostic feature inherent to mood disorder diagnosis.

SUBSYNDROMAL MIXED STATES

Cassano et al. (1999) have noted that a failure to recognize subthreshold expressions of mania has contributed to the under-diagnosis of bipolar disorder. More recent studies have shown a frequent occurrence of subthreshold manic symptoms in unipolar mood disorders that correlates with rates of switching to bipolar diagnoses over time. (Fiedorowicz et al., 2011)

TRAUMA HISTORY

Childhood sexual trauma is a risk factor for many mental disorders, including bulimia, alcohol dependence, other drug dependence, and mood disorders. Kendler et al. (2000) found that, of 1,411 adult female twins, 30.4% reported any childhood sexual abuse (CSA), and 8.4% reported childhood sexual intercourse. In turn, any CSA was associated with an increased risk (OR 1.93) for major depressive disorder in adulthood in this sample, and childhood sexual intercourse was associated with an even higher risk (OR 3.24) for major depressive disorder in adulthood. A case control study by Cong et al. (2011) similarly reported that any form of CSA was associated with an increased risk for recurrent major depressive disorder in adulthood, and that incrementally greater severity of CSA heightened this risk. Heim et al. (2010) also reported that a particularly strong link has been found between childhood trauma in general and the mood and anxiety disorders, and Sareen et al. (2012) found in an epidemiological study of Canadian Forces that adverse childhood experiences (ACE) increased the risk of mood and anxiety disorders among active military personnel. Furthermore, it has been reported that childhood abuse dramatically increases the risk for later suicide attempts. Studies of the stress of maternal separation in rats have yielded lasting changes in the HPA axis function, leading to theories that comparable early traumatic events in humans may increase the risk of various disorders, including mood and anxiety disorders, through similar biological mechanisms.

ARBITRARY SELECTION OF CORE CRITERIA

It is worthwhile to note that selection of the core criteria for many of our current psychiatric categorical diagnoses arose from arbitrary processes. For example, between the Feighner criteria and Research Diagnostic Criteria, researchers dropped the terms "fearful" and "worried" from the list of acceptable dysphoric moods, and elevated the "presence of a pervasive loss of interest or pleasure" as one of the core stem criteria (Spitzer et al., 1978). Spitzer et al. (1978) report that the former change occurred to avoid the inclusion of patients with only anxiety, a reasonable justification. However, given the preceding evidence on the importance of anxiety in depression, evidence whose roots were apparent at the time, why not list "fearful and worried" as an additional criterion? Furthermore, the elevation of anhedonia to a core stem criterion occurred based on "the clinical recognition that many patients with an obvious depressive syndrome do not acknowledge feeling depressed" (Spitzer et al., 1978). Fair enough, yet the authors cited no empirical evidence to support either change.

THRESHOLDS, CASENESS, AND DISCRIMINATIVE ABILITY

ARBITRARINESS OF THRESHOLDS AND FLUIDITY OF CASENESS

In an interesting historical account of the development of the Feighner criteria, Kendler et al. (2010) report that W. L. Cassidy, one of Feighner's main influences in constructing the diagnostic criteria for major depression, decided on his diagnostic threshold of 6 out of 10 criteria, because: "it sounded about right" (Kendler et al., 2010).

Furthermore, why is the duration of two weeks of symptoms a criterion for a major depressive episode? The early Feighner criteria, precursors of the Research Diagnostic Criteria that were in turn a model for DSM-III in 1980, used a one-month duration criterion. It is difficult to generate the data to justify any particular duration, but the problem of an overlap with "normal reactions of distress to an event" or "demoralization" still exists, as evidenced by current arguments for dropping or keeping the DSM-IV bereavement exclusion for the diagnosis of a major depressive episode. It is worth considering whether to define clinical depression as a binary state, or whether it should be considered on a severity continuum with a certain number of symptoms, severity of individual symptoms, chronicity, and impairment levels defining a spectrum for the syndrome.

RELATED CONDITIONS BLURRING WITH MOOD DISORDERS

Is there a difference between demoralization (learned hopelessness) and depression (Clarke and Kissane, 2002)? When does demoralization become clinical depression? Are these conditions more similar or different when it comes to treatment response? Could descriptive diagnoses be determined that would separate these conditions with respect to specific treatment response, are they on a severity dimension, or are they indistinguishable in terms of mechanism or treatment? Is there a point in the development of learned hopelessness or demoralization when a basic change takes place to establish major depression? Is that point defined by the inability to respond to positive input? Does demoralization become a clinical depression when an individual is no longer capable of responding to positive stimuli, that is, when the dopaminergic pleasure system is turned off (Treadway and Zald, 2011)? On one hand, maybe there is some other mechanism that leads to a qualitative change. On the other hand, maybe there is no discontinuous mechanism but simply a severity or coping mechanism spectrum that is quantitative, not qualitative. In order to determine this, we need the best possible system for behavioral classification. Even then this may not be a possible discrimination.

Maybe there are risk factors (e.g., negative affect) that can be discriminated behaviorally. Recently, in studying subjects of early abuse (before age 18) that were over 45 (allowing a characterization of their life trajectory), LaNoue et al. (2012) found that patients who scored high on the construct of negative affect (which has been shown to be a lifelong trait) were more likely to see their entire life as "ruined," in contrast to those who scored low on negative affect on the NEO Personality Inventory (McCrae, 1991). In contrast, patients with low negative affect were less likely to experience lasting impairment and recurrence of symptoms after experiencing early abuse. The patients with low negative affect were more likely to agree that childhood abuse ruined their childhood, but that it did not affect them in adulthood. Responses like "that was then, but this is now" and even "it made me stronger" were volunteered by these subjects, as opposed to "it ruined my childhood and my life" being a characteristic view expressed by high negative affect subjects. High negative affect or "neuroticism" has also been shown to predict recurrence in patients with major depression (Lanoue et al., 2012). Interestingly, despite the concept that neuroticism is a stable trait, SSRI treatment in depression may reduce levels of neuroticism, underscoring a potential mechanism for serotonergic antidepressant action (Tang et al., 2009).

A study by Kendler et al. (2001) showed moderate effects for genetic vulnerability (65% and 50% in females and males, respectively), as well as moderate effects for stress in the origin of depression. Caspi et al.'s (2003) findings demonstrating genetic moderation of life stress on the occurrence of depression point to tantalizing epigenetic methods of understanding vulnerability and resiliency, which may eventually aid in combined genetic-behavioral description of patients who are demoralized versus depressed.

Perhaps our understanding of mood disorder causes and treatments must be tempered not by either-or thinking, but by empirically based pluralism, as discussed by Kendler (2012).

FAILURE OF CURRENT DIAGNOSTIC SYSTEMS TO ELUCIDATE NEUROBIOLOGICAL MECHANISMS OR DEVELOP MORE EFFECTIVE TREATMENTS

The pharmacologic revolution of the 1960s led to a massive increase in neurobiological research starting with the measurement of metabolic and hormonal peripheral changes, to EEG sleep studies, to animal studies of functional brain changes associated with the recently successful antipsychotic and antidepressant medications. Family and twin studies attested to the familial transmission of various major disorders such as schizophrenia, bipolar disorder, and depressive disorders. Technology accelerated and in the late 1980s and

early 1990s molecular biology, genetics, and human brain imaging became possible, offering the promise of more basic understanding of brain function and the pathophysiology of mental disorders.

These technical advances have led to a great increase in knowledge about the complexities of all mental disorders, including mood disorders. As more progress has been attained, the basic understanding of the etiology of mood disorders and other mental disorders has remained elusive, with much work yet to be done.

One reason is the unfolding complexity leading to boxes inside of boxes in the psychobiology of the brain, and the recognition of complex interactions between genetics and environmental inputs, termed epigenetics, which has added a massive layer of complexity to our understanding of the interaction of our brains' gene expression with environmental circumstances. Another problem that has surfaced is the limitation of our current categorical system of diagnoses in mapping with both genetic and imaging findings.

PROPOSED SOLUTIONS: DIMENSIONAL CONSTRUCTS

SPECTRUM CONCEPTS LINKING SYNDROMES

As Cassano et al. (1999) point out, failure to recognize subthreshold symptoms of mania contributes to frequent underdiagnosis of bipolar disorder Reasons for the non-recognition of subthreshold bipolar symptoms include the relative lack of suffering compared with depressive symptoms, enhanced productivity, ego-syntonicity, and the assumption by clinicians that such symptoms represent the instability of affect associated with comorbid personality disorders. From the National Comorbidity Survey Replication, Angst et al. (2010) reported that 40% of patients with a diagnosis of major depressive disorder had subthreshold hypomanic symptoms. From the Collaborative Depression Study (CDS) Akiskal et al. (1995) found that, of 559 patients diagnosed with unipolar major depression and followed over 11 years, 8.6% converted to a diagnosis of Bipolar II Disorder, and 3.9% converted to a diagnosis of Bipolar I Disorder. A more recent publication from the CDS found that, of 142 patients diagnosed with Bipolar Disorder I or II, 76% had subsyndromal manic symptoms accompanying their depressive episodes (Judd et al., 2012). Overt irritability and psychomotor agitation were the most prominent symptoms (57% and 39% respectively), and the subsyndromal symptoms were associated with increased severity of depression. These findings show that depression is often on a spectrum with bipolar features. The recent literature showing evidence that response to antidepressants may be diminished in bipolar patients and may lead to more mood instability also stands as a reminder of the importance of distinguishing patients presenting with major depressive episodes that are on a bipolar spectrum (Fountoulakis et al., 2012; Phelps et al., 2008; Sidor and MacQueen, 2011). Given such findings, bipolar spectrum concepts have attempted to unify our understanding of the fluidity between unipolar disorders, bipolar disorders, and monomanic disorders, and, within each of these disorders, the fluidity between normal symptom expression, temperamental expression, and full disorder expression (Angst, 2007; Phelps et al., 2008).

BEHAVIORAL CONSTRUCTS DESCRIBING SYNDROME COMPONENTS

In the area of psychopharmacologic treatment, which stimulated our current era of psychobiologic, genetic, and imaging research, it has become clear that, while medications are approved by the Federal Drug Administration as efficacious for various diagnostic categories such as Major Depressive Disorder or Bipolar Disorder, these medications actually seem to address various "behavioral dimensions" that cross diagnostic categories.

Neither the DSM-IV-TR nor the ICD-10 encourages dimensional characterization of manic, mixed, or depressed episodes according to the relative severity of specific symptom components such as depressed mood, motor retardation, anxiety/agitation, insomnia, hostility/interpersonal sensitivity, anhedonia, or suicidality (Bagby et al., 2004; Katz et al., 2004). Katz et al. (2011) have argued for the regular measurement of specific symptom components in treatment studies. Symptom components of depressed mood, motor retardation, and hostility appear to respond differentially to distinct classes of pharmacotherapy. Such differential responses appear to arise early in the course of pharmacotherapy, and these early responses appear to predict later overall and sustained responses. Symptom components that cluster together in factor analytic studies, and show differential responses to treatment, may serve as candidate endophenotypes for further study.

For example, a study by Katz et al. (2004) showed that symptom components of major depression, identified by cluster analysis, not only include symptoms absent from the accepted DSM criteria, but also show different response times when treated with noradrenergic versus serotonergic medications. Another study, by Martinotti et al. (2012), demonstrated differential improvement of anhedonia in major depressive disorder using agomelatine versus venlafaxine XR, in the context of equivalent improvement of the overall syndrome.

Study of other behavioral components of depression such as anticipatory anhedonia, consummatory anhedonia, psychomotor slowing, anxiety-agitation, or angry impulsiveness, may yield specific targets for treatment, or reveal correlations with research domains such as genetic endophenotypes, brain circuit changes, epigenetic events like childhood abuse or adversity, or biomarkers such as HPA axis activation or changes in glucocorticoid receptor function.

The use of theoretically related clinical components, such as decisional anhedonia, anxiety severity, and impulsiveness with affective lability, may also come to prove more useful for understanding the clinical effect of various available or experimental medications (e.g., ketamine, pramipexole) with fairly well understood mechanisms of action. A categorical diagnosis supplemented by severity measures of various behavioral components of mood disorders may prove a valuable advance in clinical utility compared to categorical diagnoses alone. Studies by Katz et al. may prove a starting point for such efforts.

TOWARD FUTURE MODELS: DSM-5 AND RESEARCH DOMAIN CRITERIA

Current categorical diagnoses based on clinical consensus have failed to align with findings emerging from clinical science and genetics, which has slowed the development of new treatments targeted to underlying pathological mechanisms. As mentioned previously, it has been proposed that studying various measurable behavioral traits and dimensions, and looking for correlates with various domains such as genetics, electrical brain functions, or imaging studies, may produce more useful findings than looking for correlates of these domains using categorical diagnoses. Such proposals have led to the development of the Research Domain Criteria (RDoC) by the NIMH (Insel and Cuthbert, 2010).

Behavioral dimensions such as depression, anxiety, psychosis, impulsivity, irritability, agitation, emotional liability, anhedonia, blunting, and negative affect are all "targets" for psychotropic medication, various electronic treatments, and psychotherapies. Many of these symptom complexes occur across categorical diagnoses. For instance, various forms of psychosis occur across schizophrenia, mood disorders, dementias, drug addictions, and even borderline personality disorder. Impulsivity is seen as a behavioral trait across a similar range of disorders. The RDoC hope to leverage such cross-cutting behavioral dimensions in order to better understand the pathogenesis of mental illness, and develop the next generation of treatments.

Currently, DSM-5 is under development for release in 2013. Like DSM-IV-TR, DSM-5 has used literature reviews, results of field trials, review of proposed changes by a scientific review committee, and, where necessary, review of changes by a community public health review committee, as the basis for decisions about changes in diagnostic criteria, or the addition/deletion of diagnoses. In addition, DSM-5 has also used feedback from Internet postings of changes under consideration. DSM-5 has retained most of the diagnostic criteria of DSM-IV-TR, but has added a dimensional perspective to diagnoses in some areas such as mood disorders, psychotic disorders, and personality disorders, in order to address diagnostic overlap and increase the clinical information relevant for treatment planning. Evidence showing the existence of frequent mixed symptoms across mania, hypomania, and depression (depressive symptoms in the manias and manic or hypomanic symptoms in depression) has led to a mixed specifier in DSM-5, allowing the clinician to acknowledge the presence of a mood disorder spectrum in treatment planning. Building evidence for the importance of comorbid anxiety symptoms in the prognosis and treatment mood disorders has also led to the availability of an anxiety severity dimension across all mood disorder diagnoses in DSM-5. Finally, across all DSM-5 diagnoses, clinicians will be asked to record their assessment of the level of concern for suicide in individual patients. The suicide risk assessment will be based off of a list of risk factors for suicide, in combination with the clinician's own clinical judgment, and will be reflected in the clinician's treatment plan.

These changes in DSM-5 reflect recognition of the spectrum-like nature of psychiatric diagnoses, and the importance of individual symptom severity in psychiatric disorders, including mood disorders. Such changes may further lead to additional identification of symptom components in major depression, mania, and mixed states relevant to specific medication response prediction, as well as biological correlates and endophenotypes in research paradigms of etiologic mechanisms.

CONCLUSION

What we know today is mood disorders make up an indelible part of the human experience. Since antiquity, the diagnosis of mood disorders has evinced increasing levels of sophistication, in keeping with historical paradigms and scientific influences. Current mood disorder diagnostic classification schemes comprise a collection of atheoretical, prototypal, categorical, operationalized diagnostic criteria, which have modest clinical utility, and have led to intriguing neurobiologic hypotheses. Even so, we have come to expect more clinical and research utility from mood disorder diagnoses, in order to make further progress in understanding mood disorder mechanisms and developing the next generation of mood disorder treatments. After reviewing the development and current state of mood disorder diagnosis, it appears that empirical efforts to elucidate further behavioral components and dimensional constructs salient to mood disorders may help in advancing both treatment and neurobiologic research.

DISCLOSURES

Dr. Hager has no conflicts of interest to disclose.

Dr. Fawcett has not disclosed any conflicts of interest.

REFERENCES

Addington, D., Addington, J., et al. (1992). Reliability and validity of a depression rating scale for schizophrenics. *Schizophr. Res.* 6(3):201–208.

Akiskal, H.S., Maser, J.D., et al. (1995). Switching from "unipolar" to bipolar II: an 11-year prospective study of clinical and temperamental predictors in 559 patients. *Arch. Gen. Psychiatry* 52(2):114–123.

American Psychiatric Association. (1952). Diagnostic and Statistical Manual: Mental Disorders. Washington, DC: Author.

American Psychiatric Association. (1965). Diagnostic and Statistical Manual: Mental Disorders—with Special Supplement on Plans for Revision. Washington, D.C.: Author.

American Psychiatric Association. (1968). Diagnostic and Statistical Manual of Mental Disorders, 2nd Edition. Washington, DC: American Psychiatric Association.

American Psychiatric Association. (1980). Diagnostic and Statistical Manual of Mental Disorders, 3rd Edition. Washington, DC: Author.

American Psychiatric Association. (1987). Diagnostic and Statistical Manual of Mental Disorders, 3rd Edition, Revised. Washington, DC: Author.

American Psychiatric Association. (1994). Diagnostic and Statistical Manual of Mental Disorders, 4th Edition. Washington, DC: Author.

American Psychiatric Association. (2000). Diagnostic and Statistical Manual of Mental Disorders, 4th Edition, Text Revision (DSM-IV-TR). Arlington, VA: Author.

Angst, J. (2007). The bipolar spectrum. *Br. J. Psychiatry* 190:189–191.

Angst, J., Azorin, J.M., et al.; BRIDGE Study Group. (2011). Prevalence and characteristics of undiagnosed bipolar disorders in patients with a major depressive episodes: the Bridge study. *Arch. Gen. Psychiatry* 68(8):791–798.

Angst, J., Cui, L., et al. (2010). Major depressive disorder with subthreshold bipolarity in the National Comorbidity Survey Replication. *Am. J. Psychiatry* 167(10):1194–1201.

Bagby, R.M., Ryder, A.G., et al. (2004). The Hamilton Depression Rating Scale: has the gold standard become a lead weight? *Am. J. Psychiatry* 161(12):2163–2177.

Barth, J., Schumacher, M., et al. (2004). Depression as a risk factor for mortality in patients with coronary artery disease: a meta-analysis. *Psychosom. Med.* 66(6):802–813.

Basco, M.R., Bostic, J.Q., et al. (2000). Methods to improve diagnostic accuracy in a community mental health setting. *Am. J. Psychiatry* 157(10):1599–1605.

Beck, A.T., Steer, R.A., et al. (1996). Comparison of Beck Depression Inventories—IA and II in psychiatric outpatients. *J. Pers. Assess.* 67(3):588–597.

Beck, A.T., Ward, C.H., et al. (1961). An inventory for measuring depression. *Arch. Gen. Psychiatry* 4:561–571.

Beck, J.S. (2011). Cognitive Behavior Therapy: Basics and Beyond. New York: Guilford Press.

Blazer, D.G., and Steffens, D.C., eds. (2009). The American Psychiatric Publishing Textbook of Geriatric Psychiatry, 4th Edition. Arlington, VA: American Psychiatric Publishing.

Brodaty, H., Withall, A., et al. (2007). Rates of depression at 3 and 15 months poststroke and their relationship with cognitive decline: the Sydney Stroke Study. *Am. J. Geriatr. Psychiatry* 15(6):477–486.

Brown, K.W., Levy, A.R., et al. (2003). Psychological distress and cancer survival: a follow-up 10 years after diagnosis. *Psychosom. Med.* 65(4):636–643.

Brownlie, B.E., Rae, A.M., et al. (2000). Psychoses associated with thyrotoxicosis—"thyrotoxic psychosis": a report of 18 cases, with statistical analysis of incidence. *Eur. J. Endocrinol.* 142(5):438–444.

Bukberg, J., Penman, D., et al. (1984). Depression in hospitalized cancer patients. *Psychosom. Med.* 46(3):199–212.

Cade, J.F.J. (1949). Lithium salts in the treatment of psychotic excitement. *Med. J. Australia.* 36(10):349–351.

Campbell, L.C., Clauw, D.J., et al. (2003). Persistent pain and depression: a biopsychosocial perspective. *Biol. Psychiatry* 54(3):399–409.

Carragher, N., Mewton, L., et al. (2011). An item response analysis of the DSM-IV criteria for major depression: findings from the Australian National Survey of Mental Health and Wellbeing. *J. Affect. Disord.* 130(1–2):92–98.

Caspi, A., Sugden, K., et al. (2003). Influence of life stress on depression: moderation by a polymorphism in the 5-HTT gene. *Science* 301(5631):386–389.

Cassano, G.B., Dell'Osso, L., et al. (1999). The bipolar spectrum: a clinical reality in search of diagnostic criteria and an assessment methodology. *J. Affect. Disord.* 54(3):319–328.

Clarke, D.M., and Kissane, D.W. (2002). Demoralization: its phenomenology and importance. *Aust. N. Z. J. Psychiatry* 36(6):733–742.

Cleland, J.A., Lee, A.J., et al. (2007). Associations of depression and anxiety with gender, age, health-related quality of life and symptoms in primary care COPD patients. *Fam. Pract.* 24(3):217–223.

Cong. E., Li, Y., et al. (2011). Childhood sexual abuse and the risk for recurrent major depression in Chinese women. *Psychol. Med.* 11:1–9.

Coryell, W., Fiedorowicz, J.G., et al. (2012). Effects of anxiety on the long-term course of depressive disorders. *Br. J. Psychiatry* 200(3):210–215.

Coryell, W., Leon, A., et al. (1996). Importance of psychotic features to long-term course in major depressive disorder. *Am. J. Psychiatry* 153(4):483–489.

Coryell, W., Solomon, D.A., et al. (2009). Anxiety and outcome in bipolar disorder. *Am. J. Psychiatry* 166(11):1238–1243.

Coryell, W., Winokur, G., et al. (1994). The long-term stability of depressive subtypes. *Am. J. Psychiatry* 151(2):199–204.

Cysique, L.A., Deutsch, R., et al.; HNRC Group (2007). Incident major depression does not affect neuropsychological functioning in HIV-infected men. *J. Int. Neuropsychol. Soc.* 13(1):1–11.

Davidson, J.R. (2007). A history of the concept of atypical depression. *J. Clin. Psychiatry* 68(Suppl 3):10–15.

de Groot, M., Anderson, R., et al. (2001). Association of depression and diabetes complications: a meta-analysis. *Psychosom. Med.* 63(4):619–630.

Devanand, D.P. (2002). Comorbid psychiatric disorders in late life depression. *Biol. Psychiatry* 52(3):236–242.

Devanand, D.P., Turret, N., et al. (2000). Personality disorders in elderly patients with dysthymic disorder. *Am. J. Geriatr. Psychiatry* 8(3):188–195.

Driessen, E., Cuijpers, P., et al. (2009). The efficacy of short-term psychodynamic psychotherapy for depression: a meta-analysis. *Clin. Psych. Rev.* 30(1):25–36.

Endicott, J. (1984). Measurement of depression in patients with cancer. *Cancer* 53(10):2243–2249.

Engel, G.L. (1977). The need for a new medical model: a challenge for biomedicine. *Science* 196(4286):129–136.

Engel, G.L. (1980). The clinical application of the biopsychosocial model. *Am. J. Psychiatry* 137(5):535–544.

Evans, D.L., Charney, D.S., et al. (2005). Mood disorders in the medically ill: scientific review and recommendations. *Biol. Psychiatry* 58(3):175–189.

Faraone, S.V., and Tsuang, M.T. (1994). Measuring diagnostic accuracy in the absence of a "gold standard." *Am. J. Psychiatry* 151(5):650–657.

Fava, M., Rush, A.J., et al. (2008). Difference in treatment outcome in outpatients with anxious versus nonanxious depression: a STAR*D report. *Am. J. Psychiatry* 165(3):342–351.

Feighner, J.P., Robins, E., et al. (1972). Diagnostic criteria for use in psychiatric research. *Arch. Gen. Psychiatry* 26(1):57–63.

Fekadu, A., Wooderson, S., et al. (2009a). A multidimensional tool to quantify treatment resistance in depression: the Maudsley staging method. *J. Clin. Psychiatry* 70(2):177–184.

Fekadu, A., Wooderson, S., et al. (2009b). The Maudsley staging method for treatment-resistant depression: prediction of longer term outcome and persistence of symptoms. *J. Clin. Psychiatry* 70(7):952–957.

Fiedorowicz, J.G., Endicott, J., et al. (2011). Subthreshold hypomanic symptoms in progression from unipolar major depression to bipolar disorder. *Am. J. Psychiatry* 168(1):40–48.

Folstein, M.F., Folstein, S.E., et al. (1975). "Mini-mental state." A practical method for grading the cognitive state of patients for the clinician. *J. Psychiatr. Res.* 12(3):189–198.

Fountoulakis, K.N., Kasper, S., et al. (2012). Efficacy of pharmacotherapy in bipolar disorder: a report by the WPA section on pharmacopsychiatry. *Eur. Arch. Psychiatry Clin. Neurosci.* 262(Suppl 1):1–48.

Fournier, J.C., DeRubeis, R.J., et al. (2010). Antidepressant drug effects and depression severity: a patient-level meta-analysis. *JAMA* 303(1):47–53.

Gabbard, G.O. (2005). Psychodynamic Psychiatry in Clinical Practice. Arlington, VA: American Psychiatric Publishing.

Gendelman, N., Snell-Bergeon, J.K., et al. (2009). Prevalence and correlates of depression in individuals with and without type I diabetes. *Diabetes Care* 32(3):575–579.

Gibbie, T., Hay, M., et al. (2007). Depression, social support and adherence to highly active antiretroviral therapy in people living with HIV/AIDS. *Sex. Health* 4(4):227–232.

Glassman, A.H., O'Connor, C.M., et al.; Sertraline Antidepressant Heart Attack Randomized Trial (SADHEART) Group. (2002). *JAMA* 288(6):701–709.

Goldberg, D., and Fawcett, J. (2012). The importance of anxiety in both major depression and bipolar disorder. *Depress. Anxiety* 29(6):471–478.

Goodwin, F.K., and Jamison, K.R. (2007). Manic-Depressive Illness: Bipolar Disorders and Recurrent Depression. New York: Oxford.

Gothe, F., Enache, D., et al. (2012). Cerebrovascular diseases and depression: epidemiology, mechanisms and treatment. *Panminerva Med.* 54(3):161–170.

Grob, G.N. (1991). Origins of DSM-I: a study in appearance and reality. *Am. J. Psychiatry* 148(4):421–431.

Hackett, M.L., Anderson, C.S., et al. (2008). Interventions for treating depression after stroke. *Cochrane Databas. Syst. Rev.* 4:CD003437.

Harrison, N.A., and Kopelman, M.D. (2009). Endocrine diseases and metabolic disorders. In David, A.S., Fleminger, S., Kopelman, M.D., Lovestone, S., Mellers, J.D.C., eds. Lishman's Organic Psychiatry: A Textbook of Neuropsychiatry, 4th Edition. West Sussex: Wiley-Blackwell.

Haskett, R.F. (1985). Diagnostic categorization of psychiatric disturbance in Cushing's syndrome. *Am. J. Psychiatry* 142(8):911–916.

Healy, D. (1997). The Anti-Depressant Era. Cambridge, MA: Harvard University Press.

Healy, D. (2002). The Creation of Psychopharmacology. Cambridge, MA: Harvard University Press.

Heim, C., Shugart, M., et al. (2010). Neurobiological and psychiatric consequences of child abuse and neglect. *Dev. Psychobiol.* 52(7):671–690.

Hermanns, N., Kulzer, B., et al. (2006). How to screen for depression and emotional problems in patients with diabetes: comparison of screening characteristics of depression questionnaires, measurement of diabetes-specific emotional problems and standard clinical assessment. *Diabetologia* 49(3):469–477.

Hippocrates. (2010). Works of Hippocrates (F. Adams, Translator). MobileReference.

Horowitz, A.V., and Wakefield, J.C. (2007). The Loss of Sadness: How Psychiatry Transformed Normal Sorrow into Depressive Disorder. New York: Oxford.

Insel, T., and Cuthbert, B. (2010). Research domain criteria (RDoC): toward a new classification framework for research on mental disorders. *Am. J. Psychiatry* 167(7):748–751.

Jones, J.E., Hermann, B.P., et al. (2005). Screening for major depression in epilepsy with common self-report depression inventories. *Epilepsia* 46(5):731–735.

Jorge, R.E., Robinson, R.G., et al. (1993). Secondary mania following traumatic brain injury. *Am. J. Psychiatry* 150(6):916–921.

Joyce, P.R. (1988). Carbamazepine in rapid cycling bipolar affective disorder. *Int. Clin. Psychopharmacol.* 3(2):123–129.

Judd, L.L., Akiskal, H.S., et al. (2005). Psychosocial disability in the course of bipolar I and II disorders: a prospective, comparative, longitudinal study. *Arch. Gen. Psychiatry* 62(12):1322–1330.

Judd, L.L., Akiskal, H.S., et al. (2000). Psychosocial disability during the long-term course of unipolar major depressive disorder. *Arch. Gen. Psychiatry* 57(4):375–380.

Judd, L.L., Schettler, P.J., et al. (2012). Prevalence and clinical significance of subsyndromal manic symptoms, including irritability and psychomotor agitation, during bipolar major depressive episodes. *J. Affect. Disord.* 138(3):440–448.

Justice, A.C., McGinnis, K.A., et al.; Veterans Aging Cohort 5-Site Study Project Team. (2004). Psychiatric and neurocognitive disorders among HIV-positive and negative veterans in care: Veterans Aging Cohort Five-Site Study. *AIDS* 18(Suppl 1):S49–S59.

Kanner, A.M. (2003). Depression in epilepsy: prevalence, clinical semiology, pathogenic mechanisms, and treatment. *Biol. Psychiatry* 54(3):388–398.

Kathol, R.G., and Delahunt, J.W. (1986). The relationship of anxiety and depression to symptoms of hyperthyroidism using operational criteria. *Gen. Hosp. Psychiatry* 8(1):23–28.

Katz, M.M., Berman, N., et al. (2011). The componential approach enhances the effectiveness of 2-week trials for new antidepressants. *J. Clin. Psychopharmacol.* 31(2):253–254.

Katz, M.M., Tekell, J.L., et al. (2004). Onset and early behavioral effects of pharmacologically different antidepressants and placebo in depression. *Neuropsychopharmacology* 29(3):566–579.

Keller, M.B., Klein, D.N., et al. (1995). Results of the DSM-IV mood disorders field trial. *Am. J. Psychiatry* 152(6):843–849.

Keller, M.B., McCullough, J.P., et al. (2000). A comparison of nefazodone, the Cognitive Behavioral Analysis System of Psychotherapy, and their combination in for the treatment of chronic depression. *N. Eng. J. Med.* 342(20):1462–1470.

Kelly, W.F. (1996). Psychiatric aspects of Cushing's syndrome. *QJM* 89(7):543–551.

Kendler, K.S. (1997). The diagnostic validity of melancholic major depression in a population-based sample of female twins. *Arch. Gen. Psychiatry* 54(4):299–304.

Kendler, K.S. (2012). The dappled nature of causes of psychiatric illness: replacing the organic-functional/hardware-software dichotomy with empirically based pluralism. *Mol. Psychiatry* 17(4):377–388.

Kendler, K.S., Bulik, C.M., et al. (2000). Child sexual abuse and adult psychiatric and substance abuse disorders in women. *Arch. Gen. Psychiatry* 57:953–959.

Kendler, K.S., Gardner, C.O., et al. (2001). Genetic risk factors for major depression in men and women: similar or different heritabilities and same or partly distinct genes? *Psychol. Med.* 31(4):605–616.

Kendler, K.S., Munoz, R.A., et al. (2010). The development of the Feighner criteria: a historical perspective. *Am. J. Psychiatry* 167(2):134–142.

Kim, E., Lauterbach, E.C., et al.; ANPA Committee on Research. (2007) Neuropsychiatric complications of traumatic brain injury: a critical review of the literature (a report by the ANPA Committee on Research). *J. Neuropsychiatry Clin. Neurosci.* 19(2):106–127.

Kim, S.W., Stewart, R., et al. (2011). Relationship between a history of suicide attempt and treatment outcomes in patients with depression. *J. Clin. Psychopharmacol.* 31(4):449–456.

Koenig., H.G. (1998). Depression in hospitalized patients with congestive heart failure. *Gen. Hosp. Psychiatry* 20(1):29–43.

Koenig, H.G., George, L.K, et al. (1997). Depression in medically ill hospitalized older adults: prevalence, characteristics, and course of symptoms according to six diagnostic schemes. *Am. J. Psychiatry* 154(10):1376–1383.

Koenig, H.G., Shelp, F., et al. (1989). Survival and health care utilization in elderly medical inpatients with major depression. *J. Am. Geriatr. Soc.* 37(7):599–606.

Kraus, M.R., Schafer, A., et al. (2008). Therapy of interferon-induced depression in chronic hepatitis C with citalopram: a randomized, double-blind, placebo-controlled study. *Gut* 57(4):531–536.

Krauthammer, C., and Klerman, G. (1978). Secondary mania: mania associated with antecedent physical illness or drugs. *Arch. Gen. Psychiatry* 35(11):1333–1339.

Kroenke, K., Spitzer, R., et al. (2001). The PHQ-9: validity of a brief depression severity measure. *J. Gen. Intern. Med.* 16(9):606–613.

Lamers, F., Jonkers, C.C., et al. (2008). Summed score of the Patient Health Questionnaire-9 was a reliable and valid method for depression screening in chronically ill elderly patients. *J. Clin. Epidemiol.* 61(7):679–687.

Lanoue, M., Graeber, D.A., et al. (2012). Negative affect predicts adults' ratings of the current, but not childhood, impact of adverse childhood events. *Community Ment. Health.* E-pub (Mar 30).

Lee, H.B., and Lyketsos, C.G. (2003). Depression in Alzheimer's disease: heterogeneity and related issues. *Biol. Psychiatry* 54(3):353–362.

Levenson, J.L., Ed. (2011). The American Psychiatric Publishing Textbook of Psychosomatic Medicine: Psychiatric Care of the Medically Ill, 2nd Edition Arlington, VA: American Psychiatric Publishing.

Li, C., Ford, E.S., et al. (2008). Prevalence of depression among U.S. adults with diabetes: findings from the 2006 behavioral risk factor surveillance system. *Diabetes Care* 31(1):105–107.

Liu, S.S., Schneekloth, T.D., et al. (2010). Impact of depressive symptoms and their treatment on completing antiviral treatment in patients with chronic hepatitis C. *J. Clin. Gastroenterol.* 44(8):178–185.

Lux, V., Aggen, S.H., et al. (2010). The DSM-IV definition of severity of major depression: inter-relationship and validity. *Psychol. Med.* 40(10):1691–1701.

Maciocia, G. (2009). The Psyche in Chinese Medicine. New York: Churchill Livingstone.

Martinotti, G., Sepede, G., et al. (2012). Agomelatine versus venlafaxine XR in the treatment of anhedonia in major depressive disorder, a pilot study. *J. Clin. Psychopharmacology* 32(4):487–491.

McCrae, R.R. (1991). The five-factor model and its assessment in clinical settings. *J. Pers. Assess.* 57(3):399–314.

McDonald, W.M., Richard, I.H., et al. (2003). Prevalence, etiology, and treatment of depression in Parkinson's disease. *Biol. Psychiatry* 54(3):363–375.

McHugh, P.R., and Slavney, P.R. (1983). The Perspectives of Psychiatry. Baltimore: Johns Hopkins University Press.

Mendez, M.F. (1994). Huntington's disease: update and review of neuropsychiatric aspects. *Int. J. Psychiatry Med.* 24(3):189–208.

Mendez, M.F. (2000). Mania in neurologic disorders. *Curr. Psychiatry Rep.* 2(5):440–445.

Mendlewicz, J., Massat, I., et al. (2010). Identification of clinical factors associated with resistance to antidepressants in bipolar depression: results from an European multicentre study. *Int. Clin. Psychopharm.* 25(5):297–301.

Milano, A.F., and Singer, R.B. (2007). Mortality in co-morbidity (II)—excess death rates derived from a follow-up study on 10,025 subjects divided into 4 groups with or without depression and diabetes mellitus. *J. Insur. Med.* 39(9):160–166.

Miller, P.R., Dasher, R., et al. (2001). Inpatient diagnostic assessments: 1. Accuracy of structured vs. unstructured interviews. *Psychiatry Res.* 105(3):255–264.

Mohr, D.C., Boudewyn, A.C., et al. (2001). Comparative outcomes for individual cognitive-behavioral therapy, supportive-expressive group psychotherapy, and sertraline for the treatment of depression in multiple sclerosis. *J. Consult. Clin. Psychol.* 69(6):942–949.

Moriyama, I.M., Loy, R.M., et al. (2011). History of the Statistical Classification of Diseases and Causes of Death. Hyattsville, MD: National Center for Health Statistics.

Nasreddine, Z.S., Phillips, N.A., et al. (2005). The Montreal Cognitive Assessment, McCA: a brief screening tool for mild cognitive impairment. *J. Am. Geriatr. Soc.* 53(4):695–699.

Nelligan, J.A., Loftis, J.M., et al. (2008). Depression comorbidity and antidepressant use in veterans with chronic hepatitis C: results from a retrospective chart review. *J. Clin. Psychiatry* 69(5):810–816.

Office of the Surgeon General, Army Service Forces. (1946). Nomenclature of psychiatric disorders and reactions: War Department Technical Bulletin, Medical 203. *J. Clin. Psychol.* 2:289–296.

Patten, S.B., and Barbui, C. (2004). Drug-induced depression: a systematic review to inform clinical practice. *Psychother. Psychosom.* 73(4):207–215.

Papakostas, G.L., Shelton, R.C., et al. (2011, Dec. 13). Assessment of a multi-assay, serum-based biological diagnostic test for major depressive disorder: a pilot and replication study. *Mol. Psychiatry* 1–8.

Petersen, T., Papakostas, G.I., et al. (2005). Empirical testing of two models for staging antidepressant treatment resistance. *J. Clin. Psychopharmacol.* 25(4):336–341.

Phelps, J., Angst, J., et al. (2008). Validity and utility of bipolar spectrum models. *Bipolar Disord.* 10(1 Pt 2):179–193.

Prudic, J., Haskett, R.F., et al. (1996). Resistance to antidepressant medications and short-term clinical response to ECT. *Am. J. Psychiatry* 153(8):985–992.

Raison, C.L., and Miller, A.H. (2003). Depression in cancer: new developments regarding diagnosis and treatment. *Biol. Psychiatry* 54(3):283–294.

Robertson, M.M. (1992). Affect and mood in epilepsy: an overview with a focus on depression. *Acta. Neurol. Scand. Suppl.* 140:127–132.

Ruhe, H.G., van Rooijen, G., et al. (2012). Staging methods for treatment resistant depression. *J. Affect. Disord.* 137(1–3):35–45.

Rush, A.J., Wisniewski, S.R., et al. (2012). Is prior course of illness relevant to acute or longer-term outcomes in depressed out-patients? A START*D report. *Psychol. Med.* 42(6):1131–1149.

Sackeim, H.A., Prudic, J., et al. (1990). The impact of medication resistance and continuation pharmacotherapy on relapse following response to electroconvulsive therapy in major depression. *J. Clin. Psychopharmacol.* 10(2):96–104.

Saez-Fonseca, J.A., Lee, L., et al. (2007). Long-term outcome of depressive pseudodementia in the elderly. *J. Affect. Disord.* 101(1–3):123–129.

Sansone, R.A., and Sansone, L.A. (2010). Demoralization in patients with medical illness. *Psychiatry (Edgmont.)* 7(8):42–45.

Sareen, J., Henriksen, C.A., et al. (2012). Adverse childhood experiences in relation to mood and anxiety disorders in a population-based sample of active military personnel. *Psychol. Med.* 21:1–12.

Sartorius, N., Ustun, T.B., et al. (1995). Progress toward achieving a common language in psychiatry, II: results from the international field trials of the ICD-10 diagnostic criteria for research for mental and behavioral disorders. *Am. J. Psychiatry* 152(10):1427–1437.

Shanmugasegaram, S., Russel, K.L., et al. (2012). Gender and sex differences in prevalence of major depression in coronary artery disease patients: a meta-analysis. *Maturitas* 73(4):305–311.

Shapira, B., Gorfine, M., et al. (1995). A prospective study of lithium continuation therapy in depressed patients who have responded to electroconvulsive therapy. *Convuls. Ther.* 11(2):80–85.

Sharma, P. (1994). Caraka-Samhita. Delhi: Chaukhambha Orientalia.

Shulman, K., and Post, F. (1980). Bipolar affective disorder in old age. *Br. J. Psychiatry* 136:26–32.

Sidor, M.M., and MacQueen, G.M. (2011) Antidepressants for the acute treatment of bipolar depression: a systematic review and meta-analysis. *J. Clin. Psychiatry* 72(2):156–167.

Snowdon, J. (2011). Pseudodementia, a term for its time: the impact of Leslie Kiloh's 1961 paper. *Australas. Psychiatry* 19(5):391–397.

Solomon, A. (2001). The Noonday Demon. New York: Touchstone.

Souery, D., Oswald, P., et al. (2007). Clinical factors associated with treatment resistance in major depressive disorder: results from a European multicenter study. *J. Clin. Psychiatry* 68(7):1062–1070.

Spar, J.E., Ford, C.V., et al. (1979). Bipolar affective disorder in aged patients. *J. Clin. Psychiatry* 40(12):504–507.

Spitzer, R.L., Endicott, J., et al. (1978). Research Diagnostic Criteria: rationale and reliability. *Arch. Gen. Psychiatry* 35(6):773–782.

Stafford, L., Berk, M., et al. (2007). Validity of the Hospital Anxiety and Depression Scale and Patient Health Questionnarie-9 to screen for depression in patients with coronary artery disease. *Gen. Hosp. Psychiatry* 29(5):417–424.

Stancer, H.C., and Persad, E. (1982). Treatment for intractable rapid-cycling manic depressive disorder with levothyroxine: clinical observations. *Arch. Gen. Psychiatry* 39(3):311–312.

Strain, A.K., Meltzer-Brody, S., et al. (2012). Postpartum catatonia treated with electroconvulsive therapy: a case report. *Gen. Hosp. Psychiatry* 34(4):436–437.

Stromgren, L.S., and Boller, S. (1985). Carbamazepine in treatment and prophylaxis of manic-depressive disorder. *Psychiatr. Dev.* 3(4):349–367.

Stunkard, A.J., Faith, M.S., et al. (2003). Depression and obesity. *Biol. Psychiatry* 54(3):330–337.

Sumari-de Boer, I.M., Sprangers, M.A., et al. (2012). HIV stigma and depressive symptoms are related to adherence and virological response to antiretroviral treatment among immigrant and indigenous HIV infected patients. *AIDS Behav.* 16(6):1681–1689.

Sung, S.C., Haley, C.L., et al., for the CO-MED study team. (2012). The impact of chronic depression on acute and long-term outcomes in a randomized trial comparing selective serotonin reuptake inhibitor monotherapy versus each of 2 different antidepressant medication combinations. *J. Clin. Psychiatry* 73(7):967–976.

Tang, T.Z., DeRubeis, R.J., et al. (2009). Personality change during depression treatment: a placebo-controlled trial. *Arch. Gen. Psychiatry* 66(12):1322–1330.

Thombs, B.D., Bass, E.B., et al. (2006). Prevalence of depression in survivors of acute myocardial infarction. *J. Gen. Intern. Med.* 21(1):30–38.

Treadway, M, and Zald, D.H. (2011). Reconsidering anhedonia in depression: lessons learned from translational neuroscience. *Neurosci. Biobehav. Rev.* 35(3):537–555.

Tsai, A.C., Karasic, D.H., et al. (2013). Directly observed antidepressant medication treatment and HIV outcomes among homeless and marginally housed HIV-positive adults: a randomized controlled trial. *Am. J. Public. Health* 103(2):308–315.

Van Leishout, R.J., Bienenstock, J., et al. (2009). A review of candidate pathways underlying the association between asthma and major depressive disorder. *Psychosom. Med.* 71(2):187–195.

Van Tilburg, M.A., McCaskill, C.C., et al. (2001). *Psychosom. Med.* 63(4):551–555.

von Wolff, A., Holzel, L.P., et al. (2012). Combination of pharmacotherapy and psychotherapy in the treatment of chronic depression: a systematic review and meta-analysis. *BMC. Psychiatry* 12(1):61.

Wallin, M.T., Wilken, J.A., et al. (2006). Depression and multiple sclerosis: review of a lethal combination. *J. Rehabil. Res. Dev.* 43(1):45–62.

Wang, E., Gao, K., et al. (2010). Lamotrigine adjunctive therapy to lithium and divalproex in depressed patients with rapid cycling bipolar disorder and a recent substance abuse disorder: a 12-week, double-blind, placebo-controlled pilot study. *Psychopharmacol. Bull.* 43(4):5–21.

Wehr, T.A., and Goodwin, F.K. (1979). Rapid cycling in manic-depressives induced by tricyclic antidepressants. *Arch. Gen. Psychiatry* 36(5):555–559.

Weissman, M.M., Sholomskas, D., et al. (1977). Assessing depressive symptoms in five psychiatric populations: a validity study. *Am. J. Epidemiol.* 106(3):203–214.

Whybrow, P.C., Prange, A.J., Jr., et al. (1969). Mental changes accompanying thyroid gland dysfunction. A reappraisal using objective psychological measurement. *Arch. Gen. Psychiatry* 20(1):48–63.

Williams, L.S., Brizendine, E.J., et al. (2005). Performance of the PHQ-9 as a screening tool for depression after stroke. *Stroke* 36(3):635–638.

Wilson, M. (1993). DSM-III and the transformation of American psychiatry: a history. *Am. J. Psychiatry* 150(3):399–410.

World Health Organization. (1993). The ICD-10 Classification of Mental and Behavioural Disorders: Diagnostic criteria for research. Geneva: World Health Organization.

Yesavage, J.A., Brink, T.L., et al. (1982–1983). Development and validation of a geriatric depression screening scale: a preliminary report. *J. Psychiatr. Res.* 17(1):37–49.

Zigmond, A.S., and Snaith, R.P. (1983). The hospital anxiety and depression scale. *Acta Psychiatr. Scand.* 67(6):361–370.

30 | GENETICS OF DEPRESSION

DOUGLAS F. LEVINSON

Of the three major psychiatric disorders in adults—schizophrenia, bipolar disorder, and major depressive disorder—major depression has proven to be the most challenging for modern genetic methods. This is perhaps not surprising, given that major depression is the most common and the most influenced by non-genetic factors. Here we will review the progress that has been made with an emphasis on more recent findings, discuss the challenges that remain, and point to possible directions for future research.

DEFINING DEPRESSION FOR GENETIC STUDIES

Genetic researchers face the same problem that has vexed clinicians for centuries: how to classify the sad and painful mood states that are among the most important non-infectious causes of morbidity and disability throughout the world according to World Health Organization statistics. Most people experience periods of sadness in their lives, often in response to painful events. At the other extreme, the most disabling forms of "clinical depression" involve periods ranging from weeks to years or even decades when the individual is consumed by a mental state ("melancholia" in ancient terminology) that seems obviously abnormal even to a casual observer: feelings of sadness, desolation, and guilt; a painful absence of the slightest pleasure; suicidal impulses or acts; an inability to concentrate or make decisions (sometimes reaching a state of complete incapacitation); and a set of characteristic physical symptoms including disturbed sleep, appetite, energy, and movement (either agitated or slowed). Another approach (adopted by some molecular genetic studies) is to define continuous, normally distributed personality traits such as "neuroticism" (more descriptively labeled "negative emotionality"), an index of the degree to which someone experiences unpleasant mood states and anxiety in diverse situations throughout life.

Most modern genetic studies have focused on the category of major depressive disorder, which has remained essentially constant from the introduction of the Washington University or Feighner Criteria in 1972 through the DSM-IV criteria in 1994, as reviewed elsewhere (Maj, 2012). Previous criteria (such as DSM-II) had used categories such as "neurotic" and "reactive" depression, which mixed causal assumptions with vague descriptions of signs and symptoms. *Major depressive episodes*, by contrast, have been defined by a simple checklist of behaviors and experiences that could be readily observed and reported by most people: dysphoric mood state plus at least

four of eight additional criteria (five of eight in the Feighner and RDC versions) for two or more weeks, with impairment of function. *Major depressive disorder* is defined by depressive episodes without certain additional features: the diagnosis is bipolar type I disorder if manic episodes are observed (with or without depression); bipolar type II disorder if there are depressive episodes plus milder hypomanic episodes; and, if psychotic symptoms such as delusions or hallucinations are present well beyond the depressive episode, either schizoaffective disorder or schizophrenia (depending on the relative duration of mood and psychotic symptoms). These criteria for major depressive disorder have proven remarkably robust. The diagnosis can be made reasonably reliably on the basis of self-report or by interviews conducted in-person, by telephone, or with informants such as family members (family history); and it is predictive of increased risk of recurrent depression, response to antidepressant treatments compared with placebo, and increased risk of depression in relatives.

On the other hand, no clinician or researcher believes that these criteria define a single "illness." A large proportion of the population (12–20%) experiences at least one depressive episode (Hasin et al., 2005; Weissman et al., 1996). It is twice as frequent in females as in males, for reasons that remain unclear. There is great diversity in the severity, acute features, and lifelong course of depression across individuals. No major genetic effects or robust biological markers have been identified. Although clinicians tend to believe that some patients have particularly severe, disabling forms of depression, no objective subtyping method has ever been validated or widely accepted, either for categories or for continuous variables. Similarly, while there are potential "endophenotypes" (variables that may represent biological variation underlying the trait of interest, such as depression), such as imaging and gene expression assays, there is no variable that has been clearly shown to define a more heritable or homogeneous subtype of depression.

GENETIC EPIDEMIOLOGY OF MAJOR DEPRESSIVE DISORDER

Definitions of phenotypes for molecular genetic studies of depression have been informed by genetic epidemiological studies, that is, investigations of relatives (including the special case of twins) that attempt to tease out categories or continuous variables that are both familial and heritable, and to determine the extent to which they are related to each other.

These studies have arrived at a number of consistent conclusions, although there are also important unresolved issues. It is clear that major depression aggregates in families, and (based on twin and adoption studies) that this familial aggregation is likely to be due to genetic factors (Sullivan et al., 2000). These factors do not act in a simple Mendelian fashion (major dominant or recessive effects of single mutations) in any substantial number of cases, based on the pattern of depression in families and the failure to find large single pedigrees in which a mutation could be detected by linkage methods. Thus, major depression is considered a *complex trait*, with multiple DNA sequence variations likely to be combining to influence risk in many cases, with non-genetic factors interacting with genes or perhaps entirely causing depression in some cases.

Two parameters have been of great interest to genetic investigators in planning studies of complex traits: heritability, typically estimated from *twin studies*, and relative risk, based on *family studies*:

1. Heritability is the total proportion of the variance in the trait in a population that is due to genes. For a categorical trait such as a diagnosis, this is based on the proportions of identical (monozygotic, MZ) versus non-identical (dizygotic, DZ) twins of ill probands who are also ill. While in theory a higher MZ concordance could be due to non-genetic, for example, obstetric, factors, in practice this is rarely the case. There would be little point to molecular genetic studies of a trait without substantial heritability. The largest meta-analysis of twin studies of major depression estimated heritability at 0.37 (Sullivan et al., 2000). This estimate is driven by large population-based twin studies in which clinically less severe cases tend to predominate. Higher heritability estimates of 50–70% have been observed in a few small twin studies of more severe cases recruited from clinical settings (Kendler et al., 1995; McGuffin et al., 1996), and from a twin study in which unreliability of self-report was taken into account (by considering depression to be present if it was reported in at least one of two interviews) (Kendler, Neale et al., 1993). A more recent large registry-based study was consistent with the meta-analytic result, but estimated significantly higher heritability in women (0.42) than in men (0.29), a difference that had been considered controversial previously (Kendler et al., 2006). The large sample sizes required for current molecular genetic study designs have been attained in most cases by recruiting all individuals who have major depression criteria during at least one period in their life. But heritability of 37% is modest, which might explain why more significant genetic findings have been obtained for schizophrenia and bipolar disorder, with heritabilities of 70% or more. Ideally, larger twin and family studies of more clinically severe cases might be used to define subtypes with higher heritability, but such studies are difficult to carry out.

2. Relative risk (RR) is an odds ratio computed from the lifetime risks of disease in groups of (usually first-degree) relatives of ill versus control probands (the latter serving as an estimate for the general population, using the same diagnostic methods in both groups), as an estimate of the true ratio of these risks in the population. (Here, "relative" risk refers to the risk in group A vs. group B, rather than to the fact that "relatives" are being studied.) For major depression, the RR to first-degree relatives across studies is a little under three (Sullivan et al., 2000). Genetic researchers are actually interested in the increase in risk attributable to each specific genetic mutation or variation, because this determines the power to detect the effect with a given study design and sample size. For a complex disorder, it is not known in advance how many genetic loci are interacting to influence risk, or whether mutations with larger effects (which would be easier to find) might be present in some individuals. We now know that there is a close relationship between how harmful a DNA sequence variant is (i.e., its RR for a disease) and its frequency (the proportion of chromosomes in a population on which it is found) (Boyko et al., 2008). Family-based linkage methods are appropriate to search for rare variants with at least moderately large effects on risk (at least 5- or 10-fold increases) in one or a proportion of families (Levinson, 1993), while genome-wide association study (GWAS) methods use very large samples to search for more common variants whose individual effects have generally proven to be quite small (usually up to 10–15% increases in risk) (McCarthy et al., 2008). Our failure to observe clear linkage in single pedigrees suggests that loci with very large effects on depression risk either do not exist or are extremely rare. The absence of significant GWAS findings to date, despite sample sizes similar to those that have been successful in schizophrenia and bipolar disorder, suggests that the effects of individual loci are quite small and/or that etiologic heterogeneity is very high, perhaps with multiple genetic risk mechanisms and diversity in the importance of genetic and non-genetic factors in subsets of cases that cannot currently be differentiated.

PREDICTORS OF FAMILIAL RISK

Given these challenges, it would be helpful to be able to focus genetic studies on cases whose relatives are at the greatest risk of depression, suggesting a greater involvement of genetic factors and perhaps larger locus-specific effects. Substantial efforts have been made to identify characteristics of probands that predict familial risk (as a proxy for involvement of genetic factors), but the results remain controversial. Several proband characteristics have been reported by different investigators to have some predictive value: recurrent episodes (Sullivan et al., 2000), earlier age at onset (AO) (Levinson et al., 2003; Weissman et al., 1984), severity as indexed by the number of MDD criteria endorsed by each subject (Kendler et al., 2007), and depression in both the parental and grandparental generation, with anxiety being an early sign of risk (Grillon et al., 2005). A review of family studies of major depression (Sullivan et al., 2000) found that recurrent episodes in the proband were most consistently predictive of familial risk.

The present author has interpreted the available evidence as suggesting that the familial nature of depression cases in genetic studies might be increased by requiring at least two episodes (persisting beyond 18 years of age), with age at onset of a full depressive syndrome before the age of 30 and evidence of recurrent depression in a parent or sibling (Levinson et al., 2003), although younger age at onset also might introduce heterogeneity due to greater overlap with bipolar disorder and a greater role for childhood psychological trauma. But no very large epidemiological or family study has provided a reliable estimate of the RR to first-degree relatives of probands with both early onset and recurrence. There is one informative large population-based study of almost 14,000 adult twin pairs from the Swedish National Twin Registry (Kendler et al., 2007). Age at onset, recurrence, and number of endorsed criteria (as an index of severity) each predicted increased familial risk, but more modestly than would have been predicted by previous studies. However, RRs were not computed.

Investigators have also differed in their approaches to the relationship between depression and anxiety. In population-based twin studies, it has become clear that there is a substantial overlap in the genetic factors that predispose to major depression and to anxiety disorders, based on mathematical modeling of their co-occurrence in individuals and in MZ versus DZ twin pairs (Kendler et al., 2003). This close relationship is reflected in the fact that factor-analytic studies of questionnaire-based data on persisting personality traits always identify a major factor similar to what Eysenck termed "neuroticism" (McCrae and John, 1992), which is measured with questions about chronic tendencies to feel dysphoric and anxious, particularly in response to stress. Some genetic investigators have studied neuroticism (or similar dimensional scores) rather than clinical categories, or have defined phenotypes based either on depression-or-anxiety diagnoses or a composite score reflecting both depression and anxiety symptoms (see the following). However, most genetic studies have focused on major depression as a categorical diagnosis, and alternative definitions have not yet succeeded in producing more robust findings.

RELATIONSHIP OF MAJOR DEPRESSION TO BIPOLAR DISORDER AND SCHIZOPHRENIA

The relationship between major depression and bipolar disorder is complex and poorly understood. Clinically, most patients with bipolar-I disorders experience both major depressive and manic episodes (some experience only mania), while bipolar-II disorder is defined by recurrent depressive episodes plus hypomanic episodes. A review of the familial relationships among bipolar and unipolar disorders (Smoller and Finn, 2003) computed summary risks based on family studies (and few additional data have been published since then): the estimated lifetime risk of any bipolar disorder (I or II) was 8.7% in relatives of bipolar probands (mostly bipolar-I), 2.2% in relatives of major depression probands, and 0.7% in

relatives of controls; for major depression in relatives, estimated lifetime risks in the same groups were 14.1%, 17.9%, and 5.2% (although recent studies produced higher estimates for major depression in all groups). In almost all studies, the risk of major depression is similarly increased in relatives of bipolar-I and major depression probands, while the risk of bipolar disorders is increased approximately 10-fold in relatives of bipolar probands, but not significantly in relatives of major depression probands. Because the prevalence of major depression in the population is so much higher than that of bipolar disorders, the relatives of bipolar patients are much more likely to develop major depressive than bipolar disorders. Based on twin data, it has been estimated that bipolar and major depressive ("unipolar") disorders share some, but not most, of their genetic risk factors (Craddock and Forty, 2006), and this seems consistent with the family study data: genetic factors that underlie bipolar disorders also increase the risk of major depression, but it seems likely that only a minority of individuals with major depression have a substantially increased genetic risk of bipolar disorder.

The situation appears even more complex if one considers the distinction between bipolar-I and -II disorders. While few of the large family studies have considered these disorders separately with adequate groups of control relatives, it appears that in relatives of bipolar-II probands there may be a greater risk of bipolar-II than of bipolar-I disorder, that is, there may be some genetic differences between those two disorders (Smoller and Finn, 2003). This is of interest to major depression researchers, because while the severe manic episodes of bipolar-I disorder are starkly different from anything experienced by major depression patients, there is a continuum of clinical presentations among individuals with predominately depressive disorders ranging from those who have never experienced anything remotely resembling mania, to those who experience brief "subthreshold" periods that resemble hypomania, to those in whom clear-cut hypomania is a recurrent and significant problem (leading to a bipolar-II diagnosis). Those of us who treat patients with severe, recurrent mood disorders see many individuals in whom the degree of subtle "bipolarity" is difficult to judge. By contrast, large population-based depression studies typically use diagnostic methods that are not sensitive to bipolar symptoms (i.e., they are not asked about them at all, or screening is brief, or interviewers are not trained to explore these symptoms), and most of the depression cases observed in these studies seem to be milder and less complex than those in specialized clinical settings.

The issue is illustrated by our experiences in the Genetics of Recurrent Early-onset Depression (GenRED) study (Levinson et al., 2003, 2007; Shi et al., 2011). In the initial planning stages for the first phase of the project that recruited multiply affected families, several collaborators argued that a large proportion of individuals with recurrent, early-onset depression would prove to have bipolar-II disorder. We therefore expanded the hypomania section of the Diagnostic Interview for Genetic Studies, and stressed this area during interviewer training. During recruitment, potential probands with any clear episode of mania or hypomania were excluded, as were individuals with any sibling or parent in whom a bipolar disorder could not be ruled out with reasonable confidence by either direct interview or indirect family history data. This was not a population-based study—subjects were either volunteers responding to announcements about families with two or more depressed siblings, or were recruited from clinical settings—and severity was typically high. In the 680 families in the final family sample, 4% (47) of the 1,158 directly interviewed affected siblings received diagnoses of bipolar-II disorder, which is higher than the frequency in control relatives in available studies and similar to the frequency among relatives of bipolar-I or bipolar-II probands. Thus, while it was certainly not impossible (as some had feared) to collect a large sample of purely depressed probands and siblings, some degree of overlap with bipolar-II disorder is suggested by the data.

Many efforts have been made to identify clinical features to differentiate "true" major depression from depression that is more closely related to bipolar disorders, despite the absence of manic episodes. Investigators have looked at predictors of subsequent appearance of mania in depression patients (Beesdo et al., 2009; Zimmermann et al., 2009), differences between depressive features in unipolar versus bipolar patients (Blacker et al., 1996; Zimmermann et al., 2009), and subtyping of major depression cases in the families of bipolar probands. (Mitchell et al., 2011) Consistent empirical support is lacking for discrete subtypes. Two recent studies have taken fresh looks at this question. A longitudinal population-based study (Zimmermann et al., 2009) identified individuals with histories of depression with or without subthreshold manic symptoms. Those with such symptoms were more likely to have a family history of bipolar disorder and to develop mania during follow-up (7.2% vs. 1.7% in those with no manic symptoms). The study was unusual in that manic symptoms were carefully explored in subjects from a population-based design, and interestingly, over 40% of depression cases did report what the investigators interpreted as subtle manic symptoms, suggesting that the prevalence of manic symptoms in the population might have been underestimated previously. A study of the relatives of probands with bipolar disorders compared the features of depressive episodes in relatives with either unipolar depressive or bipolar disorders (Mitchell et al., 2011). The major depressive relatives could be clustered into two groups, one of which had features that were also more frequent in the bipolar depression relatives (such as psychomotor retardation and difficulty thinking). Findings like these might prove useful for subtyping subjects in genetic studies of mood disorders, with the caveat that it is difficult to rate subtle clinical features consistently in studies (such as the GWAS described later) in which thousands of subjects are evaluated at multiple sites.

Family studies have also demonstrated that relatives of probands with schizophrenia are at increased risk of major depression (Gershon et al., 1988; Maier et al., 1993). An increased risk of schizophrenia and of schizoaffective-depressed disorder has been reported in the relatives of probands with the psychotic form of major depression (depressive episode with psychotic features—usually delusional beliefs with themes consistent with depressive ideas—that remit with the depression), although not in the relatives of non-psychotic depressive probands (Kendler et al., 1993; Maier et al., 1993). Thus, molecular genetics investigators are currently using GWAS data to search for genetic associations that cut across diagnostic boundaries among mood and psychotic disorders, as discussed in the following.

ADVERSE LIFE EVENTS INCLUDING CHILDHOOD TRAUMA

It is now well established that individuals who experience more, and more severe, adverse (stressful) life events are at increased risk of depression (Nanni et al., 2012) and other psychiatric disorders (Nelson et al., 2002) during adulthood. Early separation from a parent is also a risk factor (Kendler et al., 2002). More severe abuse (e.g., sexual abuse with penetration) confers greater risk (Kendler et al., 2004). A recent meta-analysis of 16 epidemiological studies reported an odds ratio of 2.27 for increased risk of recurrent and persistent (long duration) major depression after childhood abuse, as well as an increased risk of non-response to depression treatment (OR = 1.43) in 10 studies (Nanni et al., 2012). There is evidence that early psychological trauma may have diverse neurobiological effects on the developing brain, including alterations of hypothalamic-pituitary axis function and structural and functional brain changes, which have been hypothesized to mediate the vulnerability to persistent adult psychopathology (McCrory et al., 2010). These findings raise the question of whether adverse events are an independent "cause" of depression and other disorders, or whether their effects interact with genotype.

This has been studied indirectly, using family history of depression as a proxy for genetic risk, in the same longitudinal population-based study previously discussed with regard to bipolar disorder (Zimmermann et al., 2008). During a 10-year follow-up period, individuals with histories of early separation or any of seven types of adverse events (including childhood abuse), had an increased risk of major depression (OR = 1.8). However, an interaction between adverse events and genetic liability was demonstrated: adverse events did not increase risk of depression in those with no family history; but in those with a family history, family history alone increased risk (OR = 1.6 vs. those with neither family history or adverse events), and adverse events conferred a further increase (OR = 1.6 vs. those with family history and no adverse events; OR = 2.5 vs. those with neither a family history or adverse events). Thus, it is possible that large genetic studies of depression cases with versus without adverse events such as childhood abuse could detect sequence variants that contribute to this interaction.

MOLECULAR GENETIC STUDIES: OVERVIEW

Three types of studies will be reviewed here.

(i) **Linkage** analysis was the first approach that permitted searching the genome in an unbiased fashion for genetic factors underlying a disease or trait. Linkage studies use hundreds or thousands of sequence variants scattered throughout the genome as markers to determine whether ill members in the same family tend to share the same marker alleles in specific locations, suggesting that an etiologic variant might exist somewhere in a broad region (tens of millions of nucleic acids). Several large and a few other small linkage studies of major depression have been reported, with several significant findings that have not yet been linked to specific genes. Linkage methods have been dramatically successful for Mendelian diseases, but usually not for complex diseases as noted previously.

(ii) The **GWAS** is a more recent, and potentially more powerful, method to search for associations between a disease and specific sequenced variants throughout the genome (McCarthy et al., 2008; Visscher et al., 2012). A GWAS interrogates only the more common single nucleotide polymorphisms (SNPs) in the genome (and other common variants, such as copy number polymorphisms, that might be nearby), taking advantage of the phenomenon of linkage disequilibrium (LD; correlation of SNPs within small chromosomal segments called LD blocks) to permit panels of between 500,000 and several million SNPs to detect associations to most of the common SNPs in the genome. GWAS methods have been extraordinarily successful in detecting associations for many common, complex diseases and traits, including schizophrenia (Ripke et al., 2011) and bipolar disorder (Sklar et al., 2011).

(iii) Most published molecular genetic studies of major depression have focused on **candidate genes**, and particularly on just a few polymorphisms that are known to have functional effects—for example, changes in expression of genes that influence neurotransmitters that are modulated by antidepressant drugs. Recently, many of these studies have been motivated by a model first suggested by Caspi and colleagues (Caspi et al., 2003), who reported that adverse life events interact with the "short" allele in the promoter region of SLC6A4, the gene that encodes the serotonin transporter protein that transports serotonin back into the presynaptic cell from the synapse, and which is blocked by many antidepressant drugs.

A fourth area of research involves study of genome-wide **gene expression** using microarray technology (and in the future, RNA sequencing methods). Both environmental and genetic factors influence gene expression, but if a "signature" of genes with increased or decreased expression could be identified in subsets of depression cases, the basis for the alterations could then be sought. These studies bear directly on the molecular pathology of depression (Chapter 33 of this volume) and will not be reviewed here. They do not yet intersect with research on specific genetic sequence variants as risk factors, but a convergence of these approaches is a goal of both fields of research.

LINKAGE STUDIES

The 10 genome-wide linkage studies of depression that have been reported to date are described in Table 30.1. As shown in the table, only two (Holmans; Breen) focus on the major depression phenotype and have sample sizes that might be considered reasonable for the study of complex traits (more than 500 families, more than 1,000 cases); two were primarily studies of alcohol (Nurnberger, Pergadia) or cocaine dependence (Yang), in which the analysis focused on the phenotype of a major depressive episode and/or dependence; and one (Schol-Gelok) defined depression on the basis of symptom scores or history of antidepressant treatment rather than assessment of major depression. Two of the studies were analyzed twice. Zubenko and colleagues reanalyzed their original linkage data to provide better empirical estimation of significance levels, but the sample, diagnoses, genotypes, and main findings were the same in both analyses. Two separate analyses have been published that used the same set of genotypes for a sample of Utah families ascertained through major depression probands—with many of the nuclear families forming distantly related clusters: once (Abkevich et al., 2003) with bipolar-I and -II relatives included as affected, and then (Camp et al., 2005) with only the recurrent early-onset major depression cases, and also with anxiety disorders considered as a related phenotype (analyses of depression-or-anxiety and of depression-and-anxiety). Overall, the three largest analyses (Camp, Holmans, Breen) required recurrent major depression, two also required early onset (Camp, Holmans), and the third had primarily early-onset probands (Breen).

Two of these larger studies reported findings that were significant after correction for genome-wide testing. The GenRED study (Levinson et al., 2007) reported significant linkage to recurrent early-onset major depression on chromosome 15q25–26, with a Kong-Cox lod score of 4.78 in 631 European-ancestry families after fine-mapping with SNPs (after scanning the genome with microsatellite markers). No other study has reported significant linkage in this region, although two other studies reported that the same region yielded one of their better linkage results (Breen et al., 2011b; Camp et al., 2005). The DENT study (Breen et al., 2011b) reported significant linkage to recurrent major depression on chromosome 3p25–26, with a lod score of 4.0 in 839 families using a dense microsatellite marker set. Significant linkage in the 3p25–26 region was also reported in a second, much smaller study (Pergadia et al., 2011) of 116 families originally selected from a population-based sample for heavy smoking, but which had two or more members with major depression. Another interesting region is on chromosome 8p (interestingly, the same region that has produced the best linkage findings in schizophrenia, although not reaching a genome-wide significant level across studies (Ng et al., 2009), and which has produced among the stronger (but not individually significant) findings in several depression linkage studies and also in studies of neuroticism and related traits (see the following).

The larger question is whether linkage findings will prove useful in elucidating the genetic susceptibility to depression. Investigators (including the present author) applied linkage

TABLE 30.1. Genome-wide linkage scans of depression and related phenotypes

FIRST AUTHOR (YEAR)*	FAMILIES	AFFECTED CASES	PHENOTYPE(S)	SIGNIFICANT OR SUGGESTIVE RESULTS
Nurnberger, 2001	262	839	Alcohol dependence + MD (235); MDD (94); Alcohol dependence (604)	Suggestive (1p31.1, AD, or MD) Suggestive (7q 150 cM, MD)
Zubenko, 2002 Maher, 2010	81	unclear	MDD-RE, MDD-R, "major" mood disorders, "all" mood disorders, "depressive spectrum" disorders. Sex as covariate.	Significant (2q33-35)
Utah study[a] Abkevich, 2003	110	1,107	MDD or BP-I or BP-II (probands MDD)	Significant (12q22-23.2)
Camp, 2005	87 (19–112)[b]	75–718[b]	MDD-RE; MDD-RE or anxiety disorder; MDD-RE plus anxiety disorder.	Suggestive (MDD-RE or anxiety—3p12-q12, 7p; MDD-RE and anxiety—18q21-22)
Holmans, 2007 Levinson, 2007	656	1,748	MDD-RE	Significant (15q25–26) Suggestive, sex effect (8p22-p21.3, 17p12)
Middeldorp, 2009	133	278	MDD (from samples selected for high depression/anxiety factor scores)	Suggestive (17q, 8p, 2q)
Ayub, 2008	1	63	MDD (mostly recurrent)	None
Schol-Gelok, 2010	45[c]	115	Elevated depression symptom scores or antidepressant medication	Significant (2p16.1-15)[d]
Breen, 2011	839	2,164	MDD-R; severe MDD-R; very severe MDD-R	Significant (3p25-26)
Yang, 2011	384 (AA) 355 (EA)	unclear	Cocaine dependence; MDD; both (~52%, 25%, and 23% of cases)	Significant (7q36.3 for CD+MDE in AA) Suggestive (multiple)
Pergadia, 2011	116	270	MDD (families selected for heavy smoking)	Significant (3p25-26)

"Significant" (5% probability of false positive result) and "suggestive" (expected < once per genome scan) results are noted, generally based on permutation tests. MDD-RE = recurrent, early-onset mdd (onset < age 25 in Zubenko et al; <31 in Holmans et al. (<41 for cases other than probands) and in Camp et al. MDD-R = recurrent MDD. MD = major depression ± comorbid alcohol or substance use. BP = bipolar. AA = African American. EA = European ancestry.

a. Abkevich et al. and Camp et al. drew their pedigrees from the same Utah sample. Abkevich et al. considered all MDD cases plus BP-I and BP-II as affected, and selected families with four or more such cases. Camp et al. considered MDD-RE cases (and/or, in alternative analyses, all DSM-IV anxiety disorders) as affected, excluded BP cases, and selected families with 3 or more MDD-RE cases.

b. 87 large families studied. P-values were corrected for multiple testing: for each of three diagnostic models, pedigrees were split for analysis by limiting the genealogies to 3, 4, 5, or 6 generations. The N of families and of affected cases varied with diagnostic model and genealogical rule.

c. Nuclear families that were distantly related within an isolated population (analyses were corrected for this relatedness).

d. Note that this study used a map of ~6,000 SNPs but did not mention any correction for the inflation of linkage scores that occurs when there is linkage disequilibrium between markers in a region.

* References: (Abkevich et al., 2003; Ayub et al., 2008; Breen et al., 2011b; Camp et al., 2005; Holmans et al., 2007; Levinson et al., 2007; Maher et al., 2010; Middeldorp et al., 2009; Nurnberger et al., 2001; Pergadia et al., 2011; Schol-Gelok et al., 2010; Yang et al., 2011; Zubenko et al., 2002)

methods to depression because they represented the only unbiased, genome-wide scanning method available before the availability of GWAS arrays and whole-genome sequencing. But we have learned a great deal more about the genome since then, and it is now more apparent that linkage studies are successful when the genetic architecture of a trait (the number, frequency, and effect sizes of the causative variants) has features that are not likely to be met by most complex disorders. Linkage studies of small samples are mostly likely to be successful when one or a very small number of mutations can individually cause a disease in a Mendelian (dominant or recessive) fashion, such that single large pedigrees, or a small sample of nuclear families or sibling pairs, can produce significant results. Such findings have never been observed for depression. Variants with smaller effect sizes can be detected, but only in much larger samples and only if they are carried by a substantial minority of cases. As an example of a genetic model that would result in reasonable power to detect linkage, if 30% of probands in a study carried a variant whose population frequency was 4%, and if carriers of that variant had a 35% risk of illness compared with 1.38% for non-carriers, then the population frequency of the disease would be 4%, the increase in risk to sibs in those families would be 3.5, and the increase in risk to siblings that would be observed in the population as a whole—due to that specific variant—would be 27%, which is the lower limit of the effect that can be reliably detected in 800–1,000 affected sibling pairs. The ratio of risks (penetrances) to carriers versus non-carriers (25) is comparable to the odds ratio for genotypic risk, but we now know that SNPs with population frequencies as high as 4% virtually never contribute to serious diseases with an OR of 25. Alternatively, there could be one gene in a linkage region (or, more likely, several risk genes in the same region) in which many different families in the population were carrying very rare variants with high penetrances—but one would expect that in this case there would be many large, multiply affected families in which significant linkage could be detected in each family separately, which is not the case.

Nevertheless, linkage studies do have some advantages over current GWAS methods. Whereas GWAS can only detect the (small) effects of common SNPs, linkage analysis in very large samples could detect the aggregate effects of many rare variants in a region, each with moderate effects on risk, thus prioritizing that region for further study. It is quite possible that all depression linkage findings are false positives. But there is another, more complex possibility. It is well known that when statistical effects are analyzed in samples that are underpowered (i.e., too small to reliably detect the actual effect sizes), the measured effect sizes in each sample will vary widely around the true value (Goring et al., 2001). Thus, excessively high estimates will be observed in some samples, and excessively low values in others. This is one version of the "winner's curse" effect—if one chooses the best test result out of many tests in an underpowered sample, the measured effect is likely to be a large overestimate, and will fail to "replicate" in other underpowered samples. With a sufficiently large sample, the true effect size will be estimated with statistical significance, and will replicate in a second sample of similar size. But if samples of 600–800 families cannot detect true effects reliably, then many thousands of families would be required, and funding for such a study is highly unlikely. Therefore we will not know whether any depression risk variants exist in the best depression linkage regions until whole-genome or targeted sequencing methods are applied to larger samples of cases and controls.

Note that there have also been genome-wide linkage studies of neuroticism as a continuous variable measured in population-based samples, and of harm avoidance, a related measure. A recent rank-based meta-analysis of eight neuroticism linkage scans with and without an additional three scans of anxiety disorders (Webb et al., 2012) reported that in the combined analysis, the top 12 "bins" (in 7 chromosomal regions), in aggregate, contained more highly ranked linkage scores than expected by chance (none of them overlapping with the best major depression findings), but no single region

achieved genome-wide-corrected significance in any of the analyses. Thus, linkage analyses of neuroticism have not been more successful than those of major depression, and the same issues previously discussed for depression would apply to linkage studies of a complex, normally distributed trait like neuroticism. A full discussion of neuroticism and related studies is beyond the scope of this chapter.

GENOME-WIDE ASSOCIATION STUDIES

GWAS DATA FOR MAJOR DEPRESSION

Eight Genome-Wide Association Studies (GWAS) analyses of major depression have been reported (Table 30.2), and others are in progress. The Psychiatric GWAS Consortium carried out a mega-analysis of these datasets (Major Depressive Disorder Working Group of the Psychiatric GWAS Consortium, 2012): in a collaborative effort, a central analysis team was provided with the original genotypes for each study, applied identical quality control procedures to each dataset, identified and eliminated any duplication of samples based on genotypes (i.e., when there was overlap in control samples, or occasionally when the same case was enrolled in more than one study), computed principal component scores reflecting ancestry differences, imputed genotypes for all un-typed SNPs in each sample from the HapMap 3 SNP set for a total of 1.2 million SNPs, and carried out association tests for each SNP with ancestry scores and study site as covariates. Then, additional investigators provided genotypes from 7 independent datasets for 554 SNPs with p < 0.001 in the initial (discovery) sample, and a meta-analysis of the discovery and replication data was completed. As shown in Table 30.2, the discovery sample included 9,240 cases and 9,519 controls, and the replication sample included 6,783 cases and 50,695 controls (with most of these latter controls from the Icelandic dataset, and thus only contributing to the analysis of that sample), for a total of 16,023 cases in the final analysis. (Note that for some studies, the dataset in the mega-analysis was different from its own publication, as described in the table legend, usually due either to dividing up the datasets differently based on ancestry and genotyping platform or to partitioning of control samples that were used in more than one study.)

There were no findings in this analysis that met the conventional genome-wide-corrected significance threshold (P < 5 × 10^{-8}). A series of planned secondary analyses was also carried out: separate analysis of females (N = 6,118) and males (N = 3,122) versus same-sex controls; of all controls versus cases with recurrent major depression (N = 6,743), recurrent major depression with onset before age 31 (N = 4,710), onset before the age of 13 (N = 774); and cases (N = 3,814) with high scores on a factor score representing "typical" physiological features of depression (weight loss and insomnia). Age of onset was also analyzed as a continuous trait, within cases. No significant findings were observed (correcting for genome-wide analysis but not for multiple analysis models) in these underpowered subsamples.

A different type of secondary analysis did produce a positive result. This approach tests whether the independent SNPs with the lowest P-values in one dataset (eliminating SNPs in LD with a more significant SNP) have the same direction of

TABLE 30.2. Genome-wide association studies of major depression

SAMPLE	COUNTRY	PUBLISHED STUDY			PGC ANALYSIS		REF
		TOTAL	CASES	CONTROLS	CASES	CONTROLS	
PGC MDD GWAS DISCOVERY SAMPLE							
GAIN	Netherlands	3,540	1,738	1,802	1,696	1,765	(Sullivan et al., 2009)
GenRED	US	2,656	1,020	1,636	1,030	1,253	(Shi et al., 2011)
GSK[a]	Germany	3,566	1,514	2,052	887	864	(Muglia et al., 2010)
MDD2000-QIMR	Australia	6,104	2,431	3,673	1,450	1,711	(Wray et al., 2012)
MPIP	Germany	719	353	366	376	537	(Ising et al., 2009)
RADIANT [b]	Germany	1,968	604	1,364	935	1,290	(Lewis et al., 2010; Rietschel et al., 2010)
RADIANT	UK	3,230	1,636	1,594	1,625	1,588	(Lewis et al., 2010)
STAR*D	US	2,857	1,221	1,636	1,241	511	(Shyn et al., 2011)
Totals					9,240	9,519	
PGC MDD REPLICATION SAMPLE (554 SNPS WITH P < 0.001 IN THE DISCOVERY SAMPLE)							
deCODE	Iceland				1,067	33,162	
GenPod/NEWMEDS	UK				477	5,462	(Lewis et al., 2011)
Harvard i2b2	US				460	442	
PsyCoLaus	Switzerland				1,303	1,491	(Firmann et al., 2008)
SHIP-LEGEND	Germany				313	1,493	(Volzke et al., 2011)
TwinGene	Sweden				1,861	7,701	
GenRED2/ DepGenesNetworks	US				1,302	944	
Totals					6,783	50,695	
PGC COMBINED MDD-BIPOLAR ANALYSIS (819 SNPS WITH P < 0.0001 IN EITHER DISCOVERY DATASET; WITH NO SUBJECT OVERLAP)							
PGC MDD					9,238	8,039	(Major Depressive Disorder Working Group of the Psychiatric GWAS Consortium, 2012)
PGC BIP					6,998	7,775	(Sklar et al., 2011)
Totals					16,236	15,814	

[a]The PsyCoLaus sample was included in the published GSK report, but not the PGC discovery sample; it was included as a replication sample.
[b]The Bonn/Mannheim sample and the German subsample of the RADIANT published report were combined for analysis in the PGC discovery analysis.

association in a second dataset (OR > 1 or OR < 1 for the same SNP allele), using a simple version of the sign test (one-sided) based on the binomial distribution: if none of the SNPs are associated with the disease, then the ORs in the first dataset are positive by chance, and in the second dataset, half of the directions should be consistent and half inconsistent. The assumption here is that, even if none of the SNPs are significant after genome-wide correction, some of them may in fact be contributing to disease risk in a polygenic fashion. If the true effect sizes are small, then the P-value in the first dataset represents an overestimate of the effect (i.e., winner's curse). So the only prediction one can make in the second dataset is that the ORs will be in the same direction. In the PGC depression analysis, for female cases and controls, the discovery and replication datasets had ORs in the same direction for the best discovery SNPs significant more than 50% of the time (P < 0.006). The analysis was not significant for the smaller subsample of males (P = 0.17) or for males and females combined (P = 0.05). This result suggests that some of the top SNPs contribute to disease risk, but that the study was underpowered to detect association with these SNPs at a significant level.

The failure to detect significant SNP associations stands in contrast to the PGC mega-analysis and replication analyses, using identical methods, of schizophrenia (Ripke et al.,

2011) and of bipolar disorder (Sklar et al., 2011), both of which detected strongly significant associations; and to the many GWAS analyses of non-psychiatric disorders that detected associations with similar sample sizes (see http://www.genome.gov/gwastudies/ for an up-to-date catalog of GWAS findings). A recent paper (Wray et al., 2012) discussed several ways to estimate the relative sample sizes needed to explain the same proportion of phenotypic variance in two diseases with different heritabilities and prevalences. The authors point out that GWAS has been most successful for disorders with high heritability and low prevalence (such as schizophrenia and bipolar disorder), rather than low heritability and high prevalence (such as depression). Depending on the method and the assumptions made about genetic architecture of the disease, they estimate that GWAS analysis of depression would require 2.4–5 times as many cases as a schizophrenia analysis to detect the same proportion of total variance; given that the PGC schizophrenia mega-analysis included approximately 10,000 cases, this would mean that 24,000–50,000 cases would be desirable for major depression. Or, if one assumes that hospitalized MDD (or some other definition of a clinical severe subtype) has a higher heritability and lower prevalence, perhaps only 1.8 times as many cases might be needed (18,000), but there were only 4,710 cases in the PGC secondary analysis of recurrent early-onset major depression, which tends to be clinically severe. Collecting such large samples would be very expensive. Some of us who study depression would argue that it would be worthwhile, given the fact that GWAS studies of other diseases have produced many pathophysiological clues and the high worldwide burden of disability from depression. But it is understandable that others in the scientific community might conclude otherwise, particularly during difficult economic times.

Copy number variants (chromosomal deletions and duplications) are also detected from GWAS array data. Three groups have reported on CNV analyses of major depression to date. A significant association was reported between major depression and duplications that spanned SLIT3, CCDC99, and DOCK2, observed in 5 of 1,693 cases (from the GAIN GWAS sample) versus 0 of 34,506 controls (Glessner et al., 2010). The finding has not yet been replicated. Another study reported four nominally significant CNV regions in 604 MDD patients and 1,643 controls, but the findings do not withstand correction for genome-wide testing of CNVs (Degenhardt et al., 2012). A third study, using GWAS data for 3,106 cases of recurrent depression versus 459 screened (for absence of lifetime major depression) and 5,619 unscreened controls, reported that cases had more rare, large deletion CNVs (those with a frequency of less than 1% in controls and length greater than 100,000 bp), with no difference for duplications (Rucker et al., 2011). Interestingly overall frequency of rare CNVs was highest in depression cases, intermediate in unscreened controls, and lowest in screened controls. They did not find any specific CNVs to be associated with depression. Larger CNV analyses of major depression will be needed.

CROSS-DISORDER FINDINGS

Another approach of great current interest is the use of GWAS data to detect associations that cut across current diagnostic boundaries, and to estimate the overall correlation in the SNP contributions to different disorders or traits. Two papers have investigated association to SNPs in the *CACNAC1* gene (encoding the α-1C subunit of the L-type voltage-gated calcium channel), which had previously been reported to be significantly associated with bipolar disorder in two overlapping datasets (the largest of which was the PGC bipolar mega-analysis) . The first analysis, of quite small GWAS samples, reported that the most significant SNP in the bipolar analyses was also nominally associated with major depression (P = 0.013) and with schizophrenia (P = 0.034), with similar ORs (1.15) as in the larger bipolar studies (Green et al., 2010). A second analysis, using over half of the data used in the PGC bipolar analysis plus the GAIN major depression dataset, reported significant association to a combined bipolar-major depression phenotype (Liu et al., 2011).

A second finding was reported in a combined analysis of the PGC major depression and bipolar disorder (BP-I) discovery datasets after eliminating any sample overlap (16,236 cases and 15,814 controls, Table 30.2), treating both disorders as a single phenotype. One significant finding was observed for multiple SNPs on chromosome 3p21.1 in a region containing many genes. Significant associations in this region were previously reported in a combined analysis of PGC bipolar and schizophrenia data (Sklar et al., 2011) and in a previous combined analysis of some of the same bipolar and major depression datasets included in the larger PGC analysis (McMahon et al., 2010). The PGC depression group suggested caution in interpreting this as a cross-disorder finding, given that the bipolar cases provided most of the evidence for association, with the depression replications samples not supporting the finding. The same point was made in a comment (Breen et al., 2011a) on the McMahon et al. combined analysis.

The sign test approach, discussed earlier for evaluating consistency between PGC depression discovery and replication samples, was also applied to the depression-bipolar analysis. There were 176 independent SNPs in this analysis (drawn from both the depression and bipolar analyses). Of the 100 SNPs that were the best bipolar findings, 65 had the same direction of effect in the depression analysis (P = 0.0018), whereas of the 76 best independent SNPs from the depression analysis, 46 had the same direction of effect in the bipolar analysis (P = 0.042). This suggests that at least some of the common SNPs that confer risk of bipolar disorder also confer some degree of risk to major depression.

The PGC Cross-Disorder Group is currently completing a comprehensive combined mega-analysis of GWAS data for depression, schizophrenia, bipolar disorder, autism, and attention deficit hyperactivity disorder, which should shed further light onto possible cross-disorder associations.

NEUROTICISM

GWAS analyses have also been carried out for personality questionnaires from population-based samples. In a meta-analysis of 15 samples (10 discovery and 5 replication) totaling 20,669 individuals with data for the NEO Five-Factor Inventory, which includes neuroticism (de Moor et al., 2012) no significant associations were detected for neuroticism.

Another approach to cross-dataset analysis did produce positive findings regarding the relationship between depression and neuroticism scores. Polygenic profile (score) analysis (Purcell et al., 2009) is based on the hypothesis that for many complex diseases, there are large numbers of risk-modifying SNPs, most with such small effect sizes that they will not produce statistically significant results with feasible sample sizes. To test this hypothesis, a genome-wide set of independent SNPs (i.e., pruned to eliminate LD among SNPs) is selected from a first ("training") dataset. For each SNP, the association test result (e.g., log of the OR for a specified test allele) in that dataset is adopted as a weighting factor. Then, for each SNP in the second ("test") dataset, the number of observed test alleles is multiplied by the weight, and the resulting scores are summed across all SNPs. If the polygenic risk factors in the two datasets are similar, then cases and controls will have significantly different scores. The test is generally repeated using larger and larger proportions of the SNPs, rank ordered by their P-values in the training dataset (e.g., the SNPs with the best 10%, 20%, 30%, etc., of P-values in the training dataset). The test has produced robustly significant results, for example, across virtually all pairs or combinations of schizophrenia GWAS datasets (Purcell et al., 2009; Ripke et al., 2011). In an analysis of a training dataset of GWAS data for personality traits in 13,835 subjects and separate test datasets for depression (3,839 GAIN subjects and 5,082 MD2000 subjects) and bipolar disorder (3,375 cases and 3,370 controls from the STEP-BD and Wellcome Trust samples), weights from the results for neuroticism scores in the training dataset differentiated depression cases and controls in analyses of five different "bins" of SNPs at $P < 0.05$. Weights based on the analysis of extraversion scores were significant at $P < 0.05$ for differentiating bipolar cases and controls. This is an intriguing result although the significance level is modest.

STUDIES OF CANDIDATE GENES AND POLYMORPHISMS

Historically, the term "candidate genes" has referred to genes that were selected for study because their biological function was considered potentially relevant to the pathophysiology of a disease. Because the biological mechanisms that contribute to depression risk are not known, most depression "candidate genes" have been nominated because of their potential relevance to the mechanisms of action of antidepressant drugs, particularly polymorphisms (SNPs but also insertion-deletion and variable-number-of-tandem-repeats [VNTRs]) with putative functional effects on gene expression. The vast majority of published studies of genetic factors in depression have analyzed one or a small number of such polymorphisms, usually in samples that are now considered vastly underpowered given the small effect sizes that were being reported.

ASSOCIATION TO MAJOR DEPRESSION

A comprehensive meta-analysis of these studies (Lopez-Leon et al., 2008) analyzed data from 129 studies of 20 polymorphisms in 18 genes that had been studied at least three times, and showed results for previous meta-analysis of polymorphisms in two genes for which no additional studies had appeared in the interim. Fifteen of these 20 genes were related to neurotransmitters or receptors involved in antidepressant actions. Fixed and random effects meta-analyses were carried out of counts for two alleles, of heterozygotes versus homozygotes, and contrasting the two homozygotes (although no correction was provided for these multiple tests). Nominally significant results (the 95% confidence interval for the OR did not include 1.0) were observed in one or more of these analyses for single polymorphisms in each of six genes: DRD4 (dopamine-4 receptor; 319 cases vs. 808 controls; allelic OR = 1.73; $P < 0.01$), APOE (apolipoprotein ε2,3,4 alleles; 827 cases vs. 1,616 controls; allelic OR = 0.51 for ε2 vs. ε3, n.s. for ε4 vs. ε3; $P < 0.001$); GNB3 (guanine nucleotide binding protein 3; 375 cases vs. 492 controls; allelic OR = 1.38, homozygote OR = 2.13; $P < 0.01$ for both effects); MTHFR (methylenetetrahydrofolate reductase; 875 cases vs. 3,859 controls; allelic OR = 1.20; $P < 0.01$); SCL6A3 (dopamine transporter; 151 cases vs. 272 controls; heterozygote test OR = 2.06; $P < 0.01$); and SLC6A4 (the 44 bp insertion/deletion polymorphism referred to as 5-HTTLPR, in the promoter of the serotonin transporter gene; 3,752 cases vs. 5,707 controls; allelic OR = 1.11; $P < 0.01$).

A larger meta-analysis was published in 2010 for the short and long alleles of the 5-HTTLPR indel, including 46 samples with at least 7,769 cases vs. 16,107 controls (this is the present author's count from the main table in the paper, but certain counts were not clear, so the totals are probably larger) (Clarke et al., 2009). This is by far the most frequently studied single polymorphism in psychiatric and psychological research. The OR estimate for allele counts (the number of s alleles) was 1.076 ($P = 0.001$), with the dominant model not significant (s/s or s/l > l/l) and the recessive model (s/s > s/l or l/l) yielding an OR = 1.16 ($P < 0.001$). In an unusually thoughtful discussion, these authors comment on many of the methodological issues that have plagued these candidate gene studies, including small sample sizes, variable and often unreliable genotyping methods, and diversity of many other aspects of study design as well as ancestral backgrounds. For this particular well-known polymorphism, the authors list several caveats that suggest the possibility of technical artifacts that might also explain the positive results: (1) the polymorphism is notoriously difficult to assay, and authors have usually not commented on what quality control procedures were implemented to ensure accuracy; (2) no association (OR = 0.96) was observed in the 5 studies that genotyped the third allele (a SNP in the long allele that was reported to make it functionally similar to a short allele, see the following); (3) in the 33 studies of European-ancestry samples, the evidence for association was marginal (OR = 1.06, confidence interval = 1.01–1.10, $P = 0.019$), thus the association was primarily driven by 7 East Asian samples; and the P-value for association was correlated with the short allele frequency in controls, which could suggest genotyping problems.

ADVERSE EVENTS AND 5-HTTLPR GENOTYPE

In 2003 Caspi and colleagues introduced what has become an influential approach for studying genotype-environment interactions (Caspi et al., 2003). The 5-HTTLPR (5-HTT [serotonin]-linked polymorphic region) insertion-deletion polymorphism just 5' to the promoter region of the serotonin transporter gene (now called SLC6A4) had been identified in 1996 (Heils et al., 1996). Within a region of GC-rich 21–23 bp repeat sequences, there was a common variant allele that contained a 44 bp deletion, thus designated as the "short" allele versus the more common "long" or intact allele. Several lines of evidence suggested that the short allele reduced transcription of the gene product. Because the serotonin transporter is the site of action of the commonly used type of antidepressant drugs (serotonin-specific reuptake inhibitors, which block the transporter site), the effect of genotypic variation at this polymorphic site had already been studied many times. Caspi and colleagues measured the number of short and long alleles carried by each of 847 individuals whose health and psychological development had been studied longitudinally from childhood to age 26. The data permitted rating of the subjects for two measures of life stress: number of stressful life events between age 21 and 26, and childhood maltreatment between the ages of 3 and 11. The outcome measures were major depressive symptoms (or alternatively, major depression diagnosis) in the year before the 26th birthday (for the analysis of life events), and occurrence of a major depressive diagnosis between 21 and 26 (for the child maltreatment analysis). Genotype did not significantly predict the overall outcome of depression, or either type of stress. However, the number of s alleles predicted (*1*) the slope of the increase in depression outcomes (symptoms or diagnosis) as the number of stressful life events increased; and (*2*) the increase in the probability of a major depressive episode in those with probable or severe maltreatment versus no maltreatment.

This finding has been controversial since its initial publication, but it has been an attractive model for many investigators, and has been applied to the study of many different groups of subjects in relation to diverse stressors. More has also been learned about the polymorphism itself. As noted previously, an SNP inside the long allele has been described (rs25531) whose rare G allele alters an AP2 transcription factor binding site and thus reportedly makes the resulting allele (termed L_G) functionally equivalent to the short allele (Hu et al., 2005). However, only a small minority of behavioral studies have genotyped this SNP. Additional SNPs in the region have also been studied, and it has been reported that other SNPs are associated with greater changes in transcription than the short/long variant (Martin et al., 2007), but these have also not been studied further. It has been noted that the most commonly used assay for the short-long alleles is prone to error due to bias toward calling of short alleles (Martin et al., 2007; Wray et al., 2009). Most behavioral studies have genotyped only the short/long polymorphism.

Because there have been both positive and negative findings in a diverse set of studies, meta-analyses are of particular interest. Here, too, the evidence is contradictory, with two recent analyses taking very different approaches and arriving at opposite conclusions. The first meta-analysis (Risch et al., 2009) selected 14 studies (with 14,250 participants, of whom 1,769 developed major depression) for a narrow test of one

version of the primary Caspi et al. finding: that the recent onset of categorical major depression could be predicted by an interaction between s/s, s/l and l/l genotype status and the number of recent life events (0, 1, 2, ≥3). They found that the number of events was predictive (as has been repeatedly shown including by Caspi et al.), but that neither genotype nor the interaction of genotype and life events predicted major depression onset. The main advantage of these authors' approach was in rigorously defining the requirements for inclusion of studies, so that the predictor and outcome measures were consistent with the original finding. The authors' more general interpretation of the result was that gene-environment interactions are rarely true findings in the absence of a main effect for genotype.

However, the analysis was criticized for excluding so many of the positive studies for various methodological differences. A second meta-analysis was thus carried out (Karg et al., 2011) that included 54 studies with 40,749 participants. They opted for an inclusive approach, considering diverse types of stressful events, with most studies being categorized for secondary analyses into three groups based on the type of stress: number of all stressful life events (N = 26,921), childhood trauma (N = 6,936), and specific medical conditions (N = 6,592). Thus, these authors opted for inclusiveness, tolerating differences in predictive measures and study design as long as the outcome could be analyzed in terms of consistency with the hypothesis that increased numbers of short alleles would be predictive of increased vulnerability to development of depression by either continuous or categorical outcome measures. The analysis of all studies strongly supported the hypothesis (P = 0.00002). Interestingly, the secondary analyses supported the hypothesis for childhood maltreatment (P = 0.00007) and specific medication conditions (P = 0.0004), but not for number of stressful life events (P = 0.03 without correcting for multiple tests), and the latter analysis was also sensitive to removal of many individual studies and to the use of self-report scales. So in one sense the two analyses were consistent (number of stressful events does not robustly interact with genotype in predicting depression), but the positive result in the larger meta-analysis for definable stressors like specific medical conditions suggests that the more general hypothesis could be true.

A CRITIQUE OF CANDIDATE GENE STUDIES

Psychiatric candidate gene studies have been fraught with problems from the perspective of investigators in the field of modern genomics (the study of all genes and their relationships to each other and to the environment):

1. Given the number of sequence variants in the genome and the lack of prior knowledge to formulate strong pathophysiological hypotheses about psychiatric disorders (until recently), the a priori probability of any one candidate polymorphism being associated with a given disorder is essentially zero, and thus false positives are likely to be very common (Sullivan et al., 2001). Combined with the typical practice of requiring only a nominal significance level for each separate study of a single polymorphism (P < 0.05), rather than correcting

for all tests performed for a particular outcome (as is done in genome-wide linkage and association studies), there is ample room for skepticism about the results of these studies.

2. Virtually all psychiatric candidate gene studies have investigated common polymorphisms which, as noted previously, are unlikely to have large effects (ORs for association). Yet, psychiatric and psychological researchers have persisted in studying them with samples that are vastly underpowered for detecting small effects.

3. Many of the initial positive findings for the "popular" candidate genes were reported at a time when genotyping assays had much higher error rates, and with much greater variability across labs in accuracy of genotyping, than is the case with current high-throughput genotyping arrays. Sen and Burmeister (2008) demonstrated empirically that psychiatric candidate gene studies have been prone to genotyping errors: they found that in 325 studies of 17 polymorphisms, deviation from Hardy–Weinberg equilibrium (the expected distribution of homozygous and heterozygous genotypes based on the frequencies of the alleles) was significantly correlated with the sample size. Genotyping error is by far the most likely explanation for this. This effect was observed separately for the many studies of 5-HTTLPR. This might not be critical if all investigators routinely balanced the order in which cases and controls were genotyped in each batch of assays, but frequently, case and control DNA specimens are obtained, stored, or even genotyped separately so that systematic differences can result from variation in error rates across batches of sample or across labs. For many years, genetics investigators were very resistant to performing duplicate assays to evaluate test genotyping error rates, although it is now routine.

4. Almost all published "candidate gene" studies are really studies of one or a few polymorphisms and ignore the gene as a unit of study. (The term "polymorphism" simply refers to a specific position in the genome where different chromosomes in a population have different DNA sequences. It arose when sequence variants were genotyped by methods that required the migration of processed DNA on gels, resulting in pictures of two or more horizontal bands that were due to radioactive or other labels attached to the variant sequences. Thus the "shapes" of the variants were different, hence "polymorphic.") The most widely studied polymorphisms in psychiatric genetics were selected because there was evidence that they resulted in different levels of expression of the gene. But the polymorphisms that have been frequently studied do not represent the only genetic determinants of expression levels of their genes, and comprehensive studies of variation in each gene have rarely been carried out. In one such example, it was shown that several SNPs in the serotonin transporter gene (SLC6A4, 5-HTT) were significantly associated with expression, some of them more strongly than 5-HTTLPR (Martin et al., 2007). Yet,

no other behavioral study of this gene has ever considered these other variants. Instead, behavioral researchers commonly refer to a study of, for example, the 5-HTTLPR polymorphism as a study of the "serotonin transporter gene," as if the genotype at this polymorphism is all one needs to know about the gene. Similarly, investigators write that "we studied the X, Y, and Z genes" when they studied one polymorphism in each gene.

We may be turning a corner in this area of research. Unbiased genome-wide studies are beginning to produce robust evidence for association of genes to disorders such as schizophrenia and bipolar disorder. Subsequent studies of gene expression, gene-gene, or gene-environment interactions, and biological and clinical effects of genotype can be carried out on the basis of a strong prior hypothesis, and study results are more likely to have biological relevance to pathophysiology. Also, with the advent of high-throughput sequencing methods, it is gradually becoming easier and cheaper (but still not routine in 2012) to carry out comprehensive studies of sequence variants in targeted regions or throughout the genome. It is to be hoped that the next generation of candidate gene studies will avoid the pitfalls that have been so common in the past.

CONCLUSIONS AND FUTURE DIRECTIONS

It has proven difficult to detect specific genetic associations for depression-related phenotypes. It is likely that this is due to modest heritability, high prevalence, and substantial heterogeneity of genetic and non-genetic factors without known clinical or biological markers to permit analysis of more homogeneous subgroups. Linkage studies have produced some promising findings, but common SNPs do not have sufficiently large effects on risk to explain these findings (and significant common SNP associations have not been observed in the best linkage regions), so large targeted or whole-genome sequencing studies will be needed to determine whether there are rare risk variants in these regions, or whether they are false positive results. GWAS analyses have not yet yielded significant results for single SNPs after genome-wide correction, and it seems likely that much larger GWAS samples would be required to accomplish this. There are additional studies in progress, most notably a study of 5,000 cases and 5,000 controls in China (Flint et al., 2012), but it is unclear whether a several-fold increase in total worldwide sample size will be available in the near future. There have been some promising results suggesting overlapping findings in major depression and bipolar disorder (i.e., that bipolar risk genes might increase risk of major depression in some individuals), and larger-scale cross-disorder analyses that will be available soon from the Psychiatric Genomics Consortium should provide new information about the degree of genetic overlap and about specific cross-disorder associations. Gene expression studies of postmortem brain specimens have produced promising results, but small samples and confounding factors remain problematic. Finally, in the present author's judgment, "candidate gene" studies of single polymorphisms have not been productive in elucidating the genetic basis of risk for depressive disorders, and have been prone to methodological and technical problems; and the much-studied hypothesis of gene-environment interactions involving stress and the 5-HTTLPR polymorphism remains controversial.

What can we expect in the near future? Advances in studies of depression have always been driven by new genetic technologies but also by improvements in clinical methods and study designs, and we will consider both here.

Larger GWAS analyses (i.e., association of common SNPs) will be forthcoming as large-scale genetic projects are completed, such as (to give examples from the United States) the Kaiser Permanente Research Program on Genes, Environment, and Health (Hoffmann et al., 2011) and the Million Veteran Program (http://www.research.va.gov/MVP/). One dilemma inherent to such projects is that they must rely on brief assessments and/or information from medical records, so that detailed clinical characterization is usually impossible. It is not yet known whether very large sample sizes will overcome the high degree of heterogeneity that is likely to result from this type of strategy. But it is clear that epidemiologists are beginning to think in creative new ways about studying larger population-based and clinical samples, and new sampling and data collection methods would be useful for depression research. Larger analyses of rare CNVs in depression samples will also emerge. Emerging findings of genetic associations that cut across current diagnostic boundaries could begin to shed light on genetic mechanisms in depression.

All of the developing technologies of modern genomics will be applied to depressive disorders as costs decline: genome-wide sequencing; targeted high-throughput sequencing (including exome sequencing, although regulatory sequences might be particularly critical in common complex disorders); RNA sequencing; and epigenetic assays. The first genome-wide epigenetic study of major depression was recently published (Sabunciyan et al., 2012). DNA methylation was studied in postmortem prefrontal cortex samples from 39 individuals with major depression histories and 26 controls, with a small follow-up sample. No replicable results were reported. Nevertheless, larger-scale studies using diverse epigenetic designs are likely to be attempted because of substantial evidence suggesting that epigenetic factors could be relevant to depression (Sun et al., 2012).

Because depression is such a common and modestly heritable disorder, it is possible that virtually all genetic risk factors have individually small effects. In this case, more powerful methods for analyzing the aggregate role of genetic pathways should provide useful, and it is to be expected that increasing knowledge about the functions of genes, coupled with advances in proteomic research, will lead to substantial progress. Research on animal models and pharmacological mechanisms could also provide critical clues. Studies of gene-environment interactions may also prove to be critical; this may depend on further improvement in epidemiological technologies for identifying and recruiting large relevant samples, for example, individuals with severe childhood abuse in whom genetic factors might be interacting in specific ways with the effects of trauma.

Studies of neurons generated from individuals with depression (and other disorders) using cell reprogramming technologies (Brennand and Gage, 2011; Pang et al., 2011) are likely to permit studying genetic, structural, and physiological changes in brain tissue in much larger samples, while circumventing the problems inherent in the use of postmortem tissue. The potential disadvantage is that these cells may not be entirely representative of cells in specific tissues that have fully developed functional connections with other brain regions. Further advances in the use of sequencing technologies to study immunological variation could also prove useful, given the putative role of inflammatory responses in depression.

Not to be overlooked is the continued importance of genetic epidemiological research. During a time of increasing criticism of categorical definitions of psychiatric disorders and of emerging genetic findings that cut across those boundaries, it may be useful to remember that the first breakthroughs in etiological research into the major adult disorders—namely, robust SNP association findings for schizophrenia (Ripke et al., 2011) and for bipolar disorder (Sklar et al., 2011), and high-penetrance CNV associations for schizophrenia (Levinson et al., 2011)—were discovered in cases that met criteria developed on the basis of careful dissection of twin and family study data. For depression, there is an even larger genetic epidemiological dataset, but there are many holes in our knowledge. Much of the existing data are from large-scale twin studies that necessarily have used abbreviated clinical assessments to achieve large sample size; they shed little light on such issues as differences between the mild forms of depression that are often observed in population-based studies and the disabling disorders observed in the clinic; the relationships among depressive, mild manic, and severe manic symptoms in the population; the extent to which clinically severe depressive and/or anxiety disorders might define less common and more heritable traits; and so on. New cross-disorder genetic findings will raise additional questions that might best be answered by careful genetic epidemiological studies of the distribution and co-occurrence of symptoms and syndromes that share genetic risk factors. Ultimately, technologies will be needed that permit more detailed phenotypic assessment of very large samples.

DISCLOSURE

Dr. Levinson has no conflicts of interest to disclose. He is funded by NIMH. Grant Support: NIH grants R01MH094740, MH096262, R01MH094421, and P50HG003389.

REFERENCES

Abkevich, V., Camp, N.J., et al. (2003). Predisposition locus for major depression at chromosome 12q22–12q23.2. Am. J. Hum. Genet. 73(6):1271–1281.

Ayub, M., Irfan, M., et al. (2008). Linkage analysis in a large family from Pakistan with depression and a high incidence of consanguineous marriages. Hum. Hered. 66(3):190–198.

Beesdo, K., Hofler, M., et al. (2009). Mood episodes and mood disorders: patterns of incidence and conversion in the first three decades of life. Bipolar Disord. 11(6):637–649.

Blacker, D., Faraone, S.V., et al. (1996). Unipolar relatives in bipolar pedigrees: a search for elusive indicators of underlying bipolarity. Am. J. Med. Genet. 67(5):445–454.

Boyko, A.R., Williamson, S.H., et al. (2008). Assessing the evolutionary impact of amino acid mutations in the human genome. PLoS. Genet. 4(5):e1000083.

Breen, G., Lewis, C.M., et al. (2011a). Replication of association of 3p21.1 with susceptibility to bipolar disorder but not major depression. *Nat. Genet.* 43(1):3–5.

Breen, G., Webb, B.T., et al. (2011b). A genome-wide significant linkage for severe depression on chromosome 3: the depression network study. *Am. J. Psychiatry* 168(8):840–847.

Brennand, K.J., and Gage, F.H. (2011). Concise review: the promise of human induced pluripotent stem cell-based studies of schizophrenia. *Stem Cells* 29(12):1915–1922.

Camp, N.J., Lowry, M.R., et al. (2005). Genome-wide linkage analyses of extended Utah pedigrees identifies loci that influence recurrent, early-onset major depression and anxiety disorders. *Am. J. Med. Genet. B Neuropsychiatr. Genet.* 135B(1):85–93.

Caspi, A., Sugden, K., et al. (2003). Influence of life stress on depression: moderation by a polymorphism in the 5-HTT gene. *Science.* 301(5631):386–389.

Clarke, M.C., Tanskanen, A., et al. (2009). Evidence for an interaction between familial liability and prenatal exposure to infection in the causation of schizophrenia. *Am. J. Psychiatry* 166(9):1025–1030.

Craddock, N., and Forty, L. (2006). Genetics of affective (mood) disorders. *Eur. J. Hum. Genet.* 14(6):660–668.

de Moor, M.H., Costa, P.T., et al. (2012). Meta-analysis of genome-wide association studies for personality. *Mol. Psychiatry* 17(3):337–349.

Degenhardt, F., Priebe, L., et al. (2012). Association between copy number variants in 16p11.2 and major depressive disorder in a German case-control sample. *Am. J. Med. Genet. B Neuropsychiatr. Genet.* 159B(3):263–273.

Firmann, M., Mayor, V., et al. (2008). The CoLaus study: a population-based study to investigate the epidemiology and genetic determinants of cardiovascular risk factors and metabolic syndrome. *BMC Cardiovasc. Disord.* 8:6.

Flint, J., Chen, Y., et al.; Converge Consortium. (2012). Epilogue: lessons from the CONVERGE study of major depressive disorder in China. *J. Affect. Disord.* 140(1):1–5.

Gershon, E.S., DeLisi, L.E., et al. (1988). A controlled family study of chronic psychoses. Schizophrenia and schizoaffective disorder. *Arch. Gen. Psychiatry* 45(4):328–336.

Glessner, J.T., Wang, K., et al. (2010). Duplication of the SLIT3 locus on 5q35.1 predisposes to major depressive disorder. *PLoS One* 5(12):e15463.

Goring, H.H., Terwilliger, J.D., et al. (2001). Large upward bias in estimation of locus-specific effects from genomewide scans. *Am. J. Hum. Genet.* 69(6):1357–1369.

Green, E.K., Grozeva, D., et al. (2010). The bipolar disorder risk allele at CACNA1C also confers risk of recurrent major depression and of schizophrenia. *Mol. Psychiatry* 15(10):1016–1022.

Grillon, C., Warner, V., et al. (2005). Families at high and low risk for depression: a three-generation startle study. *Biol. Psychiatry* 57(9):953–960.

Hasin, D.S., Goodwin, R.D., et al. (2005). Epidemiology of major depressive disorder: results from the National Epidemiologic Survey on Alcoholism and Related Conditions. *Arch. Gen. Psychiatry* 62(10):1097–1106.

Heils, A., Teufel, A., et al. (1996). Allelic variation of human serotonin transporter gene expression. *J. Neurochem.* 66(6):2621–2624.

Hoffmann, T.J., Kvale, M.N., et al. (2011). Next generation genome-wide association tool: design and coverage of a high-throughput European-optimized SNP array. *Genomics* 98(2):79–89.

Holmans, P., Weissman, M.M., et al. (2007). Genetics of recurrent early-onset major depression (GenRED): final genome scan report. *Am. J. Psychiatry* 164(2):248–258.

Hu, X., Oroszi, G., et al. (2005). An expanded evaluation of the relationship of four alleles to the level of response to alcohol and the alcoholism risk. *Alcohol. Clin. Exp. Res.* 29(1):8–16.

Ising, M., Lucae, S., et al. (2009). A genomewide association study points to multiple loci that predict antidepressant drug treatment outcome in depression. *Arch. Gen. Psychiatry* 66(9):966–975.

Karg, K., Burmeister, M., et al. (2011). The serotonin transporter promoter variant (5-HTTLPR):stress, and depression meta-analysis revisited: evidence of genetic moderation. *Arch. Gen. Psychiatry* 68(5):444–454.

Kendler, K.S., Gatz, M., et al. (2006). A Swedish national twin study of lifetime major depression. *Am. J. Psychiatry* 163(1):109–114.

Kendler, K.S., Gatz, M., et al. (2007). Clinical indices of familial depression in the Swedish Twin Registry. *Acta Psychiatr. Scand.* 115(3):214–220.

Kendler, K.S., Kuhn, J.W., et al. (2004). Childhood sexual abuse, stressful life events and risk for major depression in women. *Psychol. Med.* 34(8):1475–1482.

Kendler, K.S., McGuire, M., et al. (1993). The Roscommon Family Study. IV. Affective illness, anxiety disorders, and alcoholism in relatives. *Arch. Gen. Psychiatry* 50(12):952–960.

Kendler, K.S., Neale, M.C., et al. (1993). The lifetime history of major depression in women: reliability of diagnosis and heritability. *Arch. Gen. Psychiatry* 50(11):863–870.

Kendler, K.S., Pedersen, N.L., et al. (1995). A pilot Swedish twin study of affective illness including hospital- and population-ascertained subsamples: results of model fitting. *Behav. Genet.* 25(3):217–232.

Kendler, K.S., Prescott, C.A., et al. (2003). The structure of genetic and environmental risk factors for common psychiatric and substance use disorders in men and women. *Arch. Gen. Psychiatry* 60(9):929–937.

Levinson, D.F. (1993). Power to detect linkage with heterogeneity in samples of small nuclear families. *Am. J. Med. Genet.* 48(2):94–102.

Levinson, D.F., Duan, J., et al. (2011). Copy number variants in schizophrenia: confirmation of five previous findings and new evidence for 3q29 microdeletions and VIPR2 duplications. *Am. J. Psychiatry* 168(3):302–316.

Levinson, D.F., Evgrafov, O.V., et al. (2007). Genetics of recurrent early-onset major depression (GenRED): significant linkage on chromosome 15q25-q26 after fine mapping with single nucleotide polymorphism markers. *Am. J. Psychiatry* 164(2):259–264.

Levinson, D.F., Zubenko, G.S., et al. (2003). Genetics of recurrent early-onset depression (GenRED): design and preliminary clinical characteristics of a repository sample for genetic linkage studies. *Am. J. Med. Genet. B Neuropsychiatr. Genet.* 119B(1):118–130.

Lewis, C.M., Ng, M.Y., et al. (2010). Genome-wide association study of major recurrent depression in the U.K. population. *Am. J. Psychiatry* 167:949–957.

Lewis, G., Mulligan, J., et al. (2011). Polymorphism of the 5-HT transporter and response to antidepressants: randomised controlled trial. *Br. J. Psychiatry* 198(6):464–471.

Liu, Y., Blackwood, D.H., et al. (2011). Meta-analysis of genome-wide association data of bipolar disorder and major depressive disorder. *Mol. Psychiatry* 16(1):2–4.

Lopez-Leon, S., Janssens, A.C., et al. (2008). Meta-analyses of genetic studies on major depressive disorder. *Mol. Psychiatry* 13(8):772–785.

Maher, B.S., Hughes, H.B., 3rd, et al. (2010). Genetic linkage of region containing the CREB1 gene to depressive disorders in families with recurrent, early-onset, major depression: a re-analysis and confirmation of sex-specific effect. *Am. J. Med. Genet. B Neuropsychiatr. Genet.* 153B(1):10–16.

Maier, W., Lichtermann, D., et al. (1993). Continuity and discontinuity of affective disorders and schizophrenia. Results of a controlled family study. *Arch. Gen. Psychiatry* 50(11):871–883.

Maj, M. (2012). Development and validation of the current concept of major depression. *Psychopathology* 45(3):135–146.

Major Depressive Disorder Working Group of the Psychiatric GWAS Consortium. (2012). A mega-analysis of genome-wide association studies for major depressive disorder. *Mol.Psychiatry.* In press.

Martin, J., Cleak, J., et al. (2007). Mapping regulatory variants for the serotonin transporter gene based on allelic expression imbalance. *Mol. Psychiatry* 12(5):421–422.

McCarthy, M.I., Abecasis, G.R., et al. (2008). Genome-wide association studies for complex traits: consensus, uncertainty and challenges. *Nat. Rev. Genet.* 9(5):356–369.

McCrae, R.R., and John, O.P. (1992). An introduction to the five-factor model and its applications. *J. Pers.* 60(2):175–215.

McCrory, E., De Brito, S.A., et al. (2010). Research review: the neurobiology and genetics of maltreatment and adversity. *J. Child Psychol. Psychiatry* 51(10):1079–1095.

McGuffin, P., Katz, R., et al. (1996). A hospital-based twin register of the heritability of DSM-IV unipolar depression. *Arch. Gen. Psychiatry* 53(2):129–136.

McMahon, F.J., Akula, N., et al. (2010). Meta-analysis of genome-wide association data identifies a risk locus for major mood disorders on 3p21.1. *Nat. Genet.* 42(2):128–131.

Middeldorp, C.M., Sullivan, P.F., et al. (2009). Suggestive linkage on chromosome 2, 8, and 17 for lifetime major depression. *Am. J. Med. Genet. B Neuropsychiatr. Genet.* 150B(3):352–358.

Mitchell, P.B., Frankland, A., et al. (2011). Comparison of depressive episodes in bipolar disorder and in major depressive disorder within bipolar disorder pedigrees. *Br. J. Psychiatry* 199(4):303–309.

Muglia, P., Tozzi, F., et al. (2010). Genome-wide association study of recurrent major depressive disorder in two European case-control cohorts. *Mol. Psychiatry* 15(6):589–601.

Nanni, V., Uher, R., et al. (2012). Childhood maltreatment predicts unfavorable course of illness and treatment outcome in depression: a meta-analysis. *Am. J. Psychiatry* 169(2):141–151.

Nelson, E.C., Heath, A.C., et al. (2002). Association between self-reported childhood sexual abuse and adverse psychosocial outcomes: results from a twin study. *Arch. Gen. Psychiatry* 59(2):139–145.

Ng, M.Y., Levinson, D.F., et al. (2009). Meta-analysis of 32 genome-wide linkage studies of schizophrenia. *Mol. Psychiatry* 14(8):774–785.

Nurnberger, J.I., Jr., Foroud, T., et al. (2001). Evidence for a locus on chromosome 1 that influences vulnerability to alcoholism and affective disorder. *Am. J. Psychiatry* 158(5):718–724.

Pang, Z.P., Yang, N., et al. (2011). Induction of human neuronal cells by defined transcription factors. *Nature* 476(7359):220–223.

Pergadia, M.L., Glowinski, A.L., et al. (2011). A 3p26–3p25 genetic linkage finding for DSM-IV major depression in heavy smoking families. *Am. J. Psychiatry* 168(8):848–852.

Purcell, S.M., Wray, N.R., et al. (2009). Common polygenic variation contributes to risk of schizophrenia and bipolar disorder. *Nature* 460(7256):748–752.

Rietschel, M., Mattheisen, M., et al. (2010). Genome-wide association-, replication-, and neuroimaging study implicates HOMER1 in the etiology of major depression. *Biol. Psychiatry* 68(6):578–585.

Ripke, S., Sanders, A.R., et al. (2011). Genome-wide association study identifies five new schizophrenia loci. *Nat. Genet.* 43(10):969–976.

Risch, N., Herrell, R., et al. (2009). Interaction between the serotonin transporter gene (5-HTTLPR):stressful life events, and risk of depression: a meta-analysis. *JAMA* 301(23):2462–2471.

Rucker, J.J., Breen, G., et al. (2011). Genome-wide association analysis of copy number variation in recurrent depressive disorder. *Mol. Psychiatry.* In press.

Sabunciyan, S., Aryee, M.J., et al. (2012). Genome-wide DNA methylation scan in major depressive disorder. *PLoS One* 7(4):e34451.

Schol-Gelok, S., Janssens, A.C., et al. (2010). A genome-wide screen for depression in two independent Dutch populations. *Biol. Psychiatry* 68(2):187–196.

Sen, S., and Burmeister, M. (2008). Hardy-Weinberg analysis of a large set of published association studies reveals genotyping error and a deficit of heterozygotes across multiple loci. *Hum. Genomics* 3(1):36–52.

Shi, J., Potash, J.B., et al. (2011). Genome-wide association study of recurrent early-onset major depressive disorder. *Mol. Psychiatry* 16:193–201.

Shyn, S.I., Shi, J., et al. (2011). Novel loci for major depression identified by genome-wide association study of sequenced treatment alternatives to relieve depression and meta-analysis of three studies. *Mol. Psychiatry* 16(2):202–215.

Sklar, P., Ripke, S., et al. (2011). Large-scale genome-wide association analysis of bipolar disorder identifies a new susceptibility locus near ODZ4. *Nat. Genet.* 43(10):977–983.

Smoller, J.W., and Finn, C.T. (2003). Family, twin, and adoption studies of bipolar disorder. *Am. J. Med. Genet. C Semin. Med. Genet.* 123C(1):48–58.

Sullivan, P.F., de Geus, E.J., et al. (2009). Genome-wide association for major depressive disorder: a possible role for the presynaptic protein piccolo. *Mol. Psychiatry* 14(4):359–375.

Sullivan, P.F., Eaves, L.J., et al. (2001). Genetic case-control association studies in neuropsychiatry. *Arch. Gen. Psychiatry* 58(11):1015–1024.

Sullivan, P.F., Neale, M.C., et al. (2000). Genetic epidemiology of major depression: review and meta-analysis. *Am. J. Psychiatry* 157(10):1552–1562.

Sun, H., Kennedy, P.J., et al. (2012). Epigenetics of the depressed brain: role of histone acetylation and methylation. *Neuropsychopharmacology* 38(1):124–137.

Visscher, P.M., Brown, M.A., et al. (2012). Five years of GWAS discovery. *Am. J. Hum. Genet.* 90(1):7–24.

Volzke, H., Alte, D., et al. (2011). Cohort profile: the study of health in Pomerania. *Int. J. Epidemiol.* 40(2):294–307.

Webb, B.T., Guo, A.Y., et al. (2012). Meta-analyses of genome-wide linkage scans of anxiety-related phenotypes. *Eur. J. Hum. Genet.* 20(10):1078–1084.

Weissman, M.M., Bland, R.C., et al. (1996). Cross-national epidemiology of major depression and bipolar disorder. *JAMA* 276(4):293–299.

Weissman, M.M., Wickramaratne, P., et al. (1984). Onset of major depression in early adulthood. Increased familial loading and specificity. *Arch. Gen. Psychiatry* 41(12):1136–1143.

Wray, N.R., James, M.R., et al. (2009). Accurate, large-scale genotyping of 5HTTLPR and flanking single nucleotide polymorphisms in an association study of depression, anxiety, and personality measures. *Biol. Psychiatry* 66(5):468–476.

Wray, N.R., Pergadia, M.L., et al. (2012). Genome-wide association study of major depressive disorder: new results, meta-analysis, and lessons learned. *Mol. Psychiatry* 17(1):36–48.

Yang, B.Z., Han, S., et al. (2011). A genomewide linkage scan of cocaine dependence and major depressive episode in two populations. *Neuropsychopharmacology* 36(12):2422–2430.

Zimmermann, P., Bruckl, T., et al. (2008). The interplay of familial depression liability and adverse events in predicting the first onset of depression during a 10-year follow-up. *Biol. Psychiatry* 63(4):406–414.

Zimmermann, P., Bruckl, T., et al. (2009). Heterogeneity of DSM-IV major depressive disorder as a consequence of subthreshold bipolarity. *Arch. Gen. Psychiatry* 66(12):1341–1352.

Zubenko, G.S., Hughes, H.B., 3rd, et al. (2002). Genetic linkage of region containing the CREB1 gene to depressive disorders in women from families with recurrent, early-onset, major depression. *Am. J. Med. Genet.* 114(8):980–987.

31 | ANIMAL MODELS OF MOOD DISORDERS

GEORGIA E. HODES AND SCOTT J. RUSSO

WHY USE ANIMAL MODELS?

One of the first questions that arises when planning a research project is what approach to use. How do we accurately model a disease in a rodent to understand the human pathophysiology and gain insight into new treatments? This is increasingly challenging for psychiatric disorders where the human diagnosis is based largely on self-report. Nevertheless, ongoing efforts in neuroscience to develop valid rodent models focus on key behavioral domains that are conserved across species that accurately model symptoms of depressive disorders. While other animal models, including non-human primates, dogs, and even fish, are used to model depression-like behavior, the majority of research is currently being done in the rodent model, which will therefore be the primary focus of this chapter.

Given advances in technology one might question why we still need to model behavior in an animal. Aren't there computer programs available to model drug or genetic manipulations? The reality is that animal models are currently the key to understanding a multitude of diseases. While there are computer-generated programs such as "Sniffy the virtual rat" (http://www.wadsworth.com/psychology_d/special_features/sniffy.html) that model some aspects of operant conditioning, there is currently no substitute for *in vivo* research. At this point there is still too much that is unknown about how the brain and body work to accurately model drug action *in silico*, and thus, rodent studies are critical to determine drug safety before human trials. Adding additional complexity, even when animal models have been used for drug screening purposes, sometimes the findings do not translate to humans. For example a cortisol releasing factor-1 antagonist Pexacerfont recently underwent clinical trials for generalized anxiety disorder. Although the drug was effective in animal models of anxiety, in human trials, the drug was completely ineffective, underscoring the difficulty in treating human behavioral disorders (Coric et al., 2010). Until we have a better understanding of the underlying biology driving mood disorders, we need to depend on animal models to develop safe and effective treatments.

This chapter will focus on animal models of depression, although there is significant overlap between rodent models of mood and anxiety disorder making our discussion relevant to both disorders. We will discuss the behavioral domains tested to explore depression and discuss the benefits and drawbacks of each approach. We will examine models stemming from two basic approaches. The first uses behavioral manipulations (i.e., chronic stress) to induce depression-associated behavior in normal mice. The second uses breeding strategies to try and understand how naturalistic genetic variation can lead to a depression-like phenotype. These approaches and the symptoms of depression in humans that they model are presented in Table 31.1 and discussed throughout the chapter. Both of these approaches are valid and can inform us about the mechanisms of mood disorders and identify new compounds to treat them.

WHAT CONSTITUTES AN ANIMAL MODEL?

A relevant animal model is capable of reproducing one or more core symptoms of the disorder and should have face, construct, and predictive validity (Dalla et al., 2010). Face validity is the ability of the model to mimic the symptoms of the disorder. An example would be a model, like chronic mild stress (CMS) that results in decreased preference for a natural reward (i.e., sucrose water) (Willner, 2005). In this model, animals are exposed to alternating minor stressors for approximately two to four weeks. These stressors can include forced circadian shifts, tilted cages, physical restraint, or wet bedding (Willner, 2005), the main point being that the animal's environment is constantly changing in uncomfortable ways with no predictable pattern. This model has face validity because it induces anhedonia or the inability to experience pleasure, which is a core symptom of depression. Exposure to CMS reduces sucrose preference as well as decreasing the rewarding properties of intracranial self-stimulation (Dalla et al., 2010). Any model that measurably decreases the animal's engagement in these types of reward-related behaviors would have good face validity and be considered to model a core symptom of the disorder.

Construct validity evaluates the plausibility or rationale of the model to explain the human disorder. Construct validity is basically addressing the question, does the basis of the model make sense in light of what we know about the human disorder? An example of a model with good construct validity is the early life stress model (Plotsky et al., 2005), though it should be noted that all stress models have a degree of construct validity, since stress is a major precipitating factor in human depression. In this model, animals are separated from their mothers for three hours at a time from postnatal day (PND) 2 to PND 14. During that time they are kept warm but not held or stimulated. In adulthood, they display a number of measures of depression including altered hypothalamic-pituitary-adrenal axis (HPA) activity, increased addiction liability (Moffett et al., 2007), and decreased coping behavior when faced with a stressor (Gardner et al., 2005). Animals that are

TABLE 31.1. Diagnostic symptoms of depression and the behavioral measures used to model them in animals

DSM IV DEPRESSION SYMPTOM	BEHAVIORAL DOMAIN	ANIMAL MODEL
Depressed mood for majority of the day	Not measurable	No available model
Diminished interest or pleasure in most activities for majority of the day including social withdrawal	Decreased sucrose preference (Cryan and Mombereau, 2004) Shift in sensitivity to intracranial self stimulation (Cryan and Mombereau, 2004) Novelty-induced hypophagia (Dulawa and Hen, 2005) Social Interaction test (Krishnan et al., 2008)	CMS (Dalla et al., 2010; Krishnan et al., 2008) Olfactory bulbectomy (Cryan and Mombereau, 2004) Learned helplessness (Anisman and Matheson, 2005) Social defeat stress (Krishnan et al., 2007) Prenatal stress (Goel and Bale, 2009) FSL rats (Overstreet, 2012) WKY rats (Malkesman and Weller, 2009) Rouen helpless mice (El Yacoubi and Vaugeois, 2007)
Weight loss (when not dieting) or weight gain consisting of a change in more than 5% of body weight within a month, or decrease or increase in appetite nearly every day	Measure food intake (Dulawa and Hen, 2005) Weight (Neumann et al., 2011) Novelty-suppressed feeding (Dulawa and Hen, 2005)	CMS (Dallman et al., 2000), Social defeat (Krishnan et al., 2007) FSL rats (Neumann et al., 2011) WKY rats (Pare and Redei, 1993)
Increased or decreased sleeping every day	Shift in REM sleep patterns (Steiger and Kimura, 2010) Theta activity in hippocampus and amygdala (Kronfeld-Schor and Einat, 2012) Changes in body temperature or activity during sleep/wake cycle (Kronfeld-Schor and Einat, 2012)	CMS (Dalla et al., 2010; Kronfeld-Schor and Einat, 2012) Olfactory bulbectomy (Song and Leonard, 2005) Prenatal stress (Maccari et al., 2003; Steiger and Kimura, 2010) Social defeat stress (Kronfeld-Schor and Einat, 2012) FSL rats (Overstreet et al., 2005) WKY rats (Steiger and Kimura, 2010) Rouen helpless mice (Steiger and Kimura, 2010)
Observable psychomotor agitation or retardation. Psychomotor retardation includes decrease in ability to perform "self care," difficulties with day-to-day physical activities. Psychomotor agitation includes unintentional purposeless movements including activities resulting in self harm.	Exploration of a novel environment in the open field test (Cryan and Mombereau, 2004) Motor coordination using a Roto-rod test (Cryan and Mombereau, 2004) Grooming activity in the splash test Active or avoidance (Cryan and Mombereau, 2004) Social interaction test (Cryan and Mombereau, 2004)	CMS (Krishnan et al., 2008), Olfactory bulbectomy (Song and Leonard, 2005) Learned helplessness (Seligman et al., 1975) Early life stress (Gardner et al., 2005) Social defeat stress (Krishnan et al., 2007) WKY rats (Pare and Redei, 1993)
Fatigue or loss of energy	Swimming activity in forced swim test (Cryan and Mombereau, 2004) Immobility in the tail suspension test (Cryan and Mombereau, 2004) Running wheel activity (Cryan and Mombereau, 2004) Active avoidance	Learned helplessness (Seligman et al., 1975) Early life stress (Gardner et al., 2005) Prenatal stress (Weinstock, 2008) FSL rats (Dalla et al., 2010) WKY rats (Pare and Redei, 1993) Rouen helpless mice (El Yacoubi and Vaugeois, 2007)
Feelings of worthlessness, excessive or inappropriate guilt for the majority of the time period	Not measureable	No available model
Cognitive difficulties including indecisiveness	Eye blink conditioning Barnes maze (Mueller and Bale, 2007) Radial arm maze (Song and Leonard, 2005) Morris water maze (Song and Leonard, 2005)	Olfactory bulbectomy (Song and Leonard, 2005) Prenatal stress (Mueller and Bale, 2007; Weinstock, 2008)
Suicidal ideation and recurrent thoughts of death	Not measurable	No available model

only separated from their mothers for 15-minute intervals during the same time period show resiliency to stress on all of these domains (Plotsky et al., 2005). From the human literature, studies of orphans in Romania in the 1980s, showed that children who are not held or stimulated during early postnatal life can develop biological and emotional changes including depression, and cognitive deficits (Chugani et al., 2001). These studies support that the early life model of stress has good construct validity. From what we know about human depression, it makes sense that early life adversity can contribute to susceptibility to depression.

Predictive validity is the ability of known treatments to reverse the symptoms induced by the model. An example of a model of depression with good predictive validity is the repeated social defeat model (Krishnan et al., 2007). In this model the experimental mice are exposed each day to a novel aggressor and allowed to physically interact for 10 minutes. Animals are then separated with a perforated Plexiglas barrier that allows for sensory contact but no physical interaction. On the following day, animals are given a social interaction test that measures the time spent in the vicinity of a novel object and a novel animal. Animals that show susceptibility to the stressor will avoid the novel animal, a phenotype that is essentially permanent and only reversed by chronic, but not acute, treatment with antidepressants, including imipramine and fluoxetine (Berton et al., 2006). Importantly, these antidepressant treatments in humans also require chronic administration, thus providing excellent predictive validity. It should be noted that some models fulfill one or more of these criteria, however, ideally a model of depression will fulfill all three criteria. All of the models discussed in this section, chronic unpredictable stress, early life stress, and social defeat stress, have face, construct, and predictive validity.

Another set of criteria that have been used for determining the validity of a model are those proposed by McKinney and Bunny in the late 1960s (McKinney and Bunny, 1969). They proposed that a model should show similarity of symptoms or traits to the disorder being modeled, much like face validity. The model should also have an observable and objectively measurable behavioral change. Like predictive validity, the behavioral change should be sensitive to or reversible with known antidepressant agents, although as these known antidepressants have limited efficacy at best, they may not be the best determinants of a valid animal model for novel drug development. Finally, the model should be reproducible between investigators and laboratories. This is a key issue with some animal models of depression. For example some researchers have had difficulties in replicating the effects of chronic mild stress across laboratories (Cryan and Mombereau, 2004). A number of factors can contribute to difficulties in replicating behavioral effects, including strain of animal, age, sex, temperature differences, health of the animal colony, and so forth.

Lastly, a particularly important form of validity, not often used, involves the degree to which an animal model recapitulates the biological causes of depression in humans. This criterion has been termed pathological validity (Krishnan and Nestler, 2011) and is critical to future drug development efforts. To date, a number of peripheral biomarkers such as changes in release and feedback of cortisol, alterations in cytokine profiles, postmortem brain molecular changes, and structural and functional brain imaging changes have been identified in humans, some of which also been found in validated animal models. These are summarized in Table 31.2 and referred to throughout the chapter in the context of each model. At this time there is still too much unknown about the etiology of depression to develop bona fide models using clinically accepted diagnostic criteria to establish the pathological validity. However, it a good criterion to keep in mind as the field moves forward.

WHAT IS DEPRESSION AND HOW DO WE MODEL SYMPTOMS?

Depression is a debilitating disorder that currently affects 16.5% of people in United States within their lifetime and can affect up to 6.7% of the population in any given year (Kessler et al., 1993). Women are twice as likely as men to experience an episode of depression within their lifetime (Kessler et al., 1993). Depression is diagnosed based on a heterogeneous cluster of symptoms listed from the *Diagnostic and Statistical Manual of Mental Disorders* (DSM-IV). To meet criteria for depression a patient must report depressed mood or lack of interest plus four additional symptoms for two or more weeks. As shown in Table 31.1, the other symptoms include decreased interest and pleasure, weight or appetite change, changes in sleep patterns including either sleeping too much or too little, psychomotor agitation or retardation, fatigue, feelings of worthlessness or guilt, cognitive difficulties including decreases in ability to concentrate or feelings of indecisiveness, and recurrent thoughts of suicide or death (American Psychiatric Association, 2000). Because diagnosis of depression is dependent on expression of a group of symptoms rather than a biomarker-based test it leads to issues in modeling. Two individuals can exhibit very different clusters of symptoms and yet both are diagnosed with the same disorder. For example, patient A reports feelings of sadness accompanied by loss of appetite, insomnia, psychomotor agitation, and suicidal ideation. Patient B reports a lack of interest along with increased appetite and weight gain, hypersomnia, psychomotor retardation, and feelings of indecisiveness. While both patients would receive a diagnosis of major depression, their symptomology is completely different. Given this, animal models tend to focus on endophenotypes or behavioral domains that model these core symptoms rather than trying to fulfill the full criteria for depression diagnosis. In this way, animal models allow us to understand the brain circuits that control the endophenotypes, which may allow us to develop more selective therapeutics that treat the domain rather than the diverse cluster of symptoms that define depression. The next section will include a discussion of common measures used to examine the validity of these models for each depression-like phenotype.

ENDOPHENOTYPES OF DEPRESSION

Behavioral screens used to discern a depressive phenotype can be sorted into three core domains: appetitive tasks, measures of behavioral despair, and ethologically relevant behaviors, such as grooming and social interaction. In addition, researchers use physiological measures that are consistently altered in human subjects with depression, or have otherwise been validated in animal models of depression. These include, but are not limited to, peripheral endocrine, metabolic, and immune markers, along with cellular and structural changes identified through brain imaging. Each of these pathological markers will be discussed throughout the following sections in the context of animal models that exhibit pathological validity (summarized in Table 31.2).

TABLE 31.2. Behavioral and pathological validity of animal models of depression

ANIMAL MODEL	BEHAVIORAL DOMAIN	RODENT PERIPHERAL ALTERATIONS	RODENT STRUCTURAL ALTERATIONS
Olfactory bulbectomy	Increased open field exploration (Song and Leonard, 2005) Increased anhedonia (Cryan and Mombereau, 2004) Decreased spatial learning (Song and Leonard, 2005) Decreased avoidance learning (Song and Leonard, 2005)	Elevated basal CORT (Song and Leonard, 2005) Increased pro-inflammatory cytokines (Song and Leonard, 2005)	Increased cell death (Song and Leonard, 2005) Decreased volume of hippocampus (Song and Leonard, 2005) Decreased dendritic spines and synapses (Song and Leonard, 2005)
Chronic mild stress	Increased anhedonia (Dalla et al., 2010) Decreased grooming (Willner, 2005) Increased immobility in FST (Willner, 2005) Potentiation of learned helplessness (Willner, 2005)	Increased basal CORT (Dallman et al., 2000) Increased pro-inflammatory cytokines (Grippo et al., 2005) Development of metabolic disorder (Dallman et al., 2000)	Decreased neurogenesis (Kubera et al., 2011) Decreased dendritic spine density and shift in spine type (Michelsen et al., 2007)
Learned helplessness	Decreased active avoidance (Seligman et al., 1975)	Alterations in brain region specific cytokine protein levels (Lee et al., 2008)	Decreased neurogenesis (Malberg and Duman, 2003) Decreased synaptic proteins (Reines et al., 2008)
Prenatal stress	Increased immobility in FST and TST (Alonso et al., 1991; Goel and Bale, 2009) Increased anhedonia (Goel and Bale, 2009) Decreased spatial learning (Weinstock, 2008) and alterations in spatial navigation strategies (Mueller and Bale, 2007)	Increased basal CORT and alterations in negative feedback (Goel and Bale, 2009)	Decreased neurogenesis (Weinstock, 2008) Decreased dendritic spine density (Weinstock, 2008)
Early life stress	Increased immobility (Krishnan and Nestler, 2011) Increase in submissive postures during social defeat (Gardner et al., 2005) Decreased spatial learning (Krishnan and Nestler, 2011)	Exaggerated CORT response to stress (Plotsky et al., 2005) Down regulation of cytokine gene expression within the brain (Dimatelis et al., 2012)	Decreased neurogenesis (Mirescu et al., 2004)
Repeated social defeat stress	Increased social avoidance (Krishnan et al., 2007) Increased anhedonia (Krishnan et al., 2007) Increased anxiety behaviors (Krishnan et al., 2007)	Exaggerated CORT response to a second stressor (Krishnan et al., 2007) Increase in pro-inflammatory cytokines (Gomez-Lazaro et al., 2011) Altered metabolism (Krishnan et al., 2007)	Decreased neurogenesis (Lagace et al., 2010) Decreased dendritic spine density and shift in spine type (Christoffel et al., 2011)
FSL rats	Increased time immobile in FST (Overstreet, 2012) Decreased social interaction (Overstreet, 2012) Increased anhedonia (Overstreet et al., 2005)	Decreased CRF and ACTH (Overstreet et al., 2005) Low body weight (Overstreet et al., 2005) Basal reductions in pro-inflammatory cytokines (Overstreet et al., 2005) More prone to infection (Overstreet et al., 2005)	Increased neurogenesis (Husum et al., 2006)
Wistar Kyoto rats	Increased time immobile in FST (Pare and Redei, 1993) Decreased active avoidance (Pare and Redei, 1993) Increased anhedonia (Malkesman and Weller, 2009) Increased anxiety (Malkesman and Weller, 2009)	Increased basal CORT and CORT response to stress (Malkesman and Weller, 2009) Decreased HPA negative feedback to stress (Malkesman and Weller, 2009) More severe stress-induced ulcers (Pare and Redei, 1993) Low body weight (Malkesman and Weller, 2009)	Possible reduction in neurogenesis (Kronenberg et al., 2007) Possible decreased dendritic length (Falowski et al., 2011)
Rouen helpless mice	Increased immobility in FST and TST (Cryan and Mombereau, 2004) Increased anhedonia (El Yacoubi and Vaugeois, 2007)	Elevated basal levels of CORT (El Yacoubi and Vaugeois, 2007)	Not examined

BEHAVIORAL DOMAINS

APPETITIVE TASKS

Appetitive tasks generally measure the core symptom of depression, anhedonia, although some are also negatively affected by anxiety or cognitive deficits. A first-pass screen for anhedonia is done using sucrose preference tests, which consists of giving an animal a choice between a 1% sucrose solution and water. Although many derivations of the procedures have been published, access to a two-bottle choice for sucrose or water is given for an acute period of time (1–2 hours) (Dalla et al., 2010) or overnight (Krishnan et al., 2007). The researcher then measures how much sucrose is consumed versus the total amount of fluid consumed (both sucrose and water) and the percent sucrose preference is reported. While most animals greatly prefer the sucrose over water, a variety of stressors and genetic manipulations result in decreased sucrose preference (Cryan and Mombereau, 2004) while chronic treatment with classic antidepressants can reverse the effects of some chronic stressors on sucrose preference (Willner, 2005). One issue that arises when using this test to compare effects between the sexes is that females show a greater sucrose preference as baseline than males (Dalla et al., 2010). While sucrose preference tests are the most widely published measures of anhedonia, there are many other appetitive tasks that operate on similar principles. For example, sexual activity and the preference a male exhibits toward a sexually receptive female is considered to be a measure of natural reward preference (Willner, 2005). This measure also has validity given that depressed humans exhibit similar sexual dysfunction. The "gold standard" to measure reward function is intracranial self-stimulation (Carlezon and Chartoff, 2007). In this test, an electrode is implanted directly into the medial forebrain bundle, containing dense dopaminergic fibers emanating in the VTA, and the animals are allowed to press a lever to stimulate dopamine release. The more current necessary to invoke an operant response is thought to reflect reward thresholds and are significantly increased in stress disorders, meaning that they need greater activation of the circuitry to find things reinforcing.

Other appetitive tasks make use of food restriction or food rewards to measure a depression-like behavior. Novelty-suppressed feeding (NSF) is a task that measures the latency of an animal to eat in a novel environment. In this task, animals are food-restricted over night and then placed in a new environment the following day. One pellet of food is placed in the center of the novel space and the latency to approach and feed is measured (Dulawa and Hen, 2005). This was originally considered an anxiety test, however, evidence that latency to eat could be reversed or shortened by giving the animals chronic antidepressants led people to use the test as a measure of depression (Santarelli et al., 2003). In addition, a biological process in the hippocampus called neurogenesis, thought to control antidepressant efficacy, was shown to be necessary for the antidepressant effects on latency to feed in this task (Santarelli et al., 2003). A variation of this test is called novelty-induced hypophagia (NIH). The NIH test does not require food restriction. Instead animals are trained to eat a novel palatable substance in the home cage (Dulawa and Hen, 2005). Once the animal is reliably eating the substance, the latency to feed is measured

in a novel environment (Dulawa and Hen, 2005). While this again taps into aspects of anxiety/exploratory-based behavior, chronic, but not acute, treatment with antidepressants shortens the latency to eat in the novel environment.

BEHAVIORAL DESPAIR

A number of depression tests are considered measures of behavioral despair. These include the forced swim test (FST) (Fig. 31.1 A, B), tail suspension test (TST) (Fig. 31.1 C, D), and active avoidance tests. Behavioral despair tests can be thought to model feelings of sadness, psychomotor retardation, and fatigue. However, they are all confounded if the animal has a motor deficit and the active avoidance tasks are additionally confounded by cognitive deficits, since the animal has to learn how to escape or avoid a shock.

The FST was developed by Porsolt in the late 1970s. In this test, rats are placed in a cylinder containing 15 cm of room temperature water for 15 minutes. Twenty-four hours later they are again placed in the same cylinder and the amount of time the animal spends floating (immobile) is measured (Porsolt et al., 1978). The concept behind the test is that animals with higher levels of emotional despair would give up struggling sooner and remain immobile, thereby forgoing an attempt to escape the aversive environment. Importantly, the FST was the first animal model of depression that could be used as a rapid screening device for antidepressants, since tricyclics, MAOIs, and atypical antidepressants all decrease immobility on this test (Detke and Lucki, 1996). Variations of this test were later used to differentiate between different types of antidepressants. Drugs that engaged the norepinephrine (NE) system, such as tricyclic antidepressants, resulted in decreased immobility and increased climbing behavior. Drugs such as selective serotonin reuptake inhibitors (SSRIs) decreased immobility but also increased their swimming behavior (Detke and Lucki, 1996). An additional modification shortening the test to one day was then validated for use in mice and since has been used in a number of genetic mutant mice to screen for potential depression phenotypes (Krishnan and Nestler, 2011). The TST is essentially a variation of FST developed so that despair could be measured without the use of water. Removing the water element was thought to prevent hypothermia and increase repeatability (Steru et al., 1985) because water level and temperature can alter behavioral outcome. In this test mice are suspended by their tails for six minutes and the amount of time spent immobile is recorded as a behavioral measure of despair (Steru et al., 1985). The benefit of these types of tests is that they are rapid and allow for high throughput screening of new compounds. In addition, they are fairly accurate at detecting the efficacy of current antidepressants. However, they lack predictive validity in that acute antidepressants effectively decrease the time spent immobile in both the FST and TST even though chronic treatment is necessary to alleviate depression symptoms in humans. In general, these types of tests work well for determining antidepressant efficacy and screening potential new drugs based on the monoamine hypothesis, but their validity as a model for depression or use in testing novel mechanisms of action is highly questionable.

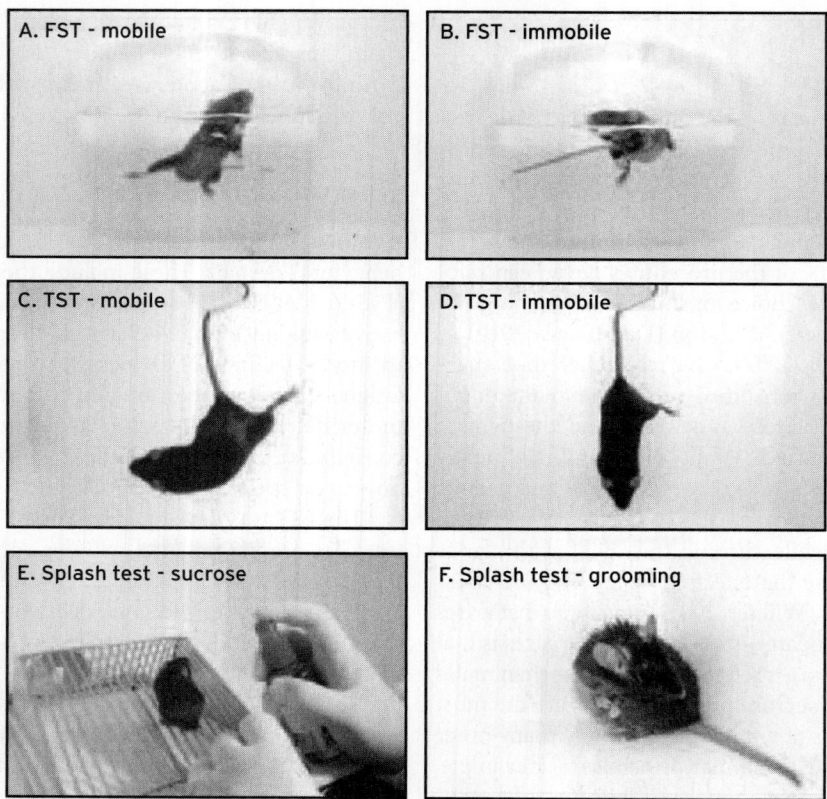

Figure 31.1 *Behavioral assays of depression-like behavior in mice. Common behavioral tests used to assay depression-associated behavior. (A) Time spent swimming in the forced swim test (FST) is considered an antidepressant measure, as SSRIs will increase engagement in this type of behavior. (B) The time spent floating or in an immobile posture is considered prodepressant, as stress manipulations increase this behavior. (C) Struggling behavior in the tail suspension test (TST) is considered an antidepressant measure, as antidepressants increase engagement in this activity. (D) The amount of time the animal spends immobile is considered a depression-like response, as stress based manipulations increase the amount of time spent immobile. (E) In the splash test, an animal is sprayed with a 10% sucrose solution to make their coats sticky. (F) The amount of time spent grooming is measured as an indicator of a depression-like state; animals that are stressed spend less time grooming and this can be reversed by chronic antidepressant treatment. (Photography credit: Christopher Wood.)*

Active escape avoidance is another commonly used measure of behavioral despair. In an active avoidance task animals are required to perform an operant behavior allowing them to escape an aversive environment. The operant response requirement can vary from simple (i.e., running through a doorway from one side of a cage to another) to complex (i.e., pushing a lever, turning a wheel, or poking their nose into a hole). Usually the stimulus that makes the environment aversive is a mild foot shock. A subset of animals that are stressed will fail to engage in active avoidance behavior (Krishnan and Nestler, 2011). This task has face validity and it is often used to test learned helplessness behavior, since animals experiencing repeated stress learn that they have no control over their environment and therefore don't attempt escape (Overmier and Seligman, 1967). Chronic treatment with antidepressants can reverse active avoidance deficits induced by the learned helplessness paradigm (Malberg and Duman, 2003), therefore the model has good predictive validity.

ETHOLOGICALLY RELEVANT BEHAVIORS

A number of behavioral tests for depression measure the degree to which ethologically relevant behaviors are altered. These are behaviors that the animal would normally engage in within their natural environment. Two examples of this type of test include social avoidance behavior (Fig. 31.3) and the splash test (Fig. 31.1 E, F). Social avoidance behavior is defined as the amount of time an animal spends in the presence of a novel animal versus a novel object. This test is used to model two core symptoms of depression: lack of interest or pleasure, since rodents are social organisms and find these interactions to be naturally rewarding, and psychomotor retardation, as we can measure the total distance traveled within the environment as well as the time spent near the target or in the corners. While a version of this test, often referred to as sociability test, is also used extensively to test features of autism and memory, in depression, it is commonly used as a behavioral endpoint following repeated social defeat stress (Fig. 31.2). During testing the experimental animal is placed in a novel environment with a novel object, consisting of a small wire mesh cage. The amount of time the animal spends within the interaction zone with a novel animal placed inside the mesh cage is measured. A ratio of the time spent in the interaction zone with the novel animal divided by the time spent in the same area without the novel mouse can be used to determine if an animal exhibits social avoidance. Under control conditions, most animals prefer the

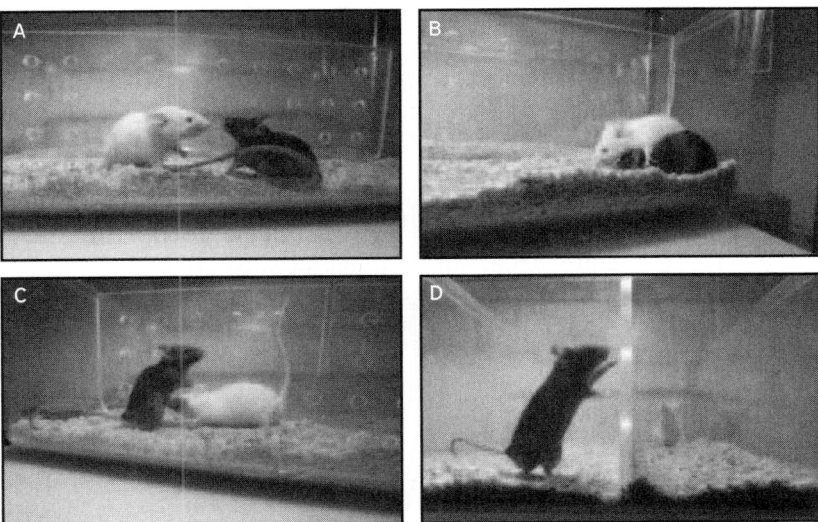

Figure 31.2 *Repeated Social Defeat Stress and Social Interaction Testing. Repeated social defeat stress is an animal model of depression with strong face, construct, and predictive validity. The experimental mouse is housed with a new aggressor every day for 10 days. (A) The smaller C57BL/6J mouse is given a 10-minute physical interaction with a larger CD-1 mouse that is screened to show aggression within his home cage. (B) CD-1 aggressor mouse is pinning the C57BL/6J mouse, one type of aggressive behavior. (C) The C57BL/6J mouse is displaying a submissive posture to the CD-1 mouse. (D) After the physical interaction, the C57BL/6J mouse is separated by a divider that allows for sensory, but not physical, stimulation for the next 24 hours. (Photography credit: Christopher Wood.)*

social target and increase their interaction time when the novel mouse is placed in the mesh cage. Conversely, susceptible mice avoid the novel animal and typically hide within the corners of the arena. This model has predictive, construct, and face validity, since chronic, but not acute, antidepressant treatment can reverse avoidance behavior in mice (Berton et al., 2006) and there is an extensive literature showing the contribution of repeated social subordination in the development of depressive disorders in humans (Gilbert, 2006). The model also has pathological validity; a number of biological targets have been identified in this model that are similarly changed in postmortem brain from humans with depression (Krishnan et al., 2007; Wilkinson et al., 2011).

Another ethologically relevant measure of a depressed state is a decrease in grooming behavior. All organisms including humans and rodents tend to decrease grooming when they are sick or stressed (Isingrini et al., 2010). These types of tests can be used to model lack of interest in normal activities of daily life, another core symptom of depression. Rodent studies such as the splash test score grooming intensity as a behavioral measure of an animal's psychological state. In this test animals are sprayed with a 10% sucrose solution that makes their coat sticky. The amount of time the animal spends grooming is then measured as an indicator of a depression-like state. This test has predictive and face validity since animals experiencing chronic stress will spend less time grooming, like depressed humans, and chronic, but not acute, antidepressants have been shown to reverse this effect (Isingrini et al., 2010). Together these endophenotypes give us multiple functional behavioral outputs that are relevant to depressive-like states in humans. It should be noted however, that each test focuses on aspects of core symptoms of depression and are most effective when used

as part of a larger test battery providing a powerful set of tools to explore the underlying biology of depression.

ANIMAL MODELS OF DEPRESSION

While there are no clinically accepted genetic or biological causes of depression in humans, it is clear that stress exposure increases depression onset and severity. Therefore, most models of depression utilize various environmental stressors to induce a depression-like behavioral phenotype and then study the underlying biological consequences of such stress on the key behavioral domains described earlier. Environmental models use "normal" animals and manipulate their environment through physical or psychological stress, surgical manipulation, or other methods to produce a depression-like phenotype. Examples of this type of stressor include early life stress, CMS, and olfactory bulbectomy. Genetic models make use of naturally occurring or trait-based selective breeding or gene knockout/transgenic technology to produce a depressive state. These studies can vary from examining natural strain differences in depression-associated behavior to conditional removal or overexpression of genes of interest, although the latter is beyond the scope of the current chapter and is discussed in detail in subsequent chapters. Recently, there has been increasing interest in epigenetic models of depression. These models examine the impact of environmental stressors on parent-offspring heritability of traits that are outside of genetic sequence differences. Alternatively they consider differences in the stress response not driven by genetic sequence differences. While epigenetics is clearly an important area of research, it is discussed in detail in subsequent chapters and is beyond the scope of the current discussion. The following section will discuss examples of a variety of these animal models of depression and discuss their validity within the context of the behavioral domains previously described.

OLFACTORY BULBECTOMY

The majority of these studies have been performed in rats, with only a small subset in mice (Cryan and Mombereau, 2004). In this model the olfactory bulbs are removed resulting in a variety of behavioral, cellular, neuroendocrine, and immune changes consistent with depression (Cryan and Mombereau, 2004). Animals that undergo olfactory bulbectomy are highly aggressive and hyperactive, including increased investigation of novel environments and increased nocturnal activity (Song and Leonard, 2005). They also show cognitive impairment similar to patients with depression. These cognitive impairments include decreased abilities to perform spatial learning tasks that engage the hippocampus, such as the radial arm maze and Morris water maze, along with deficits in active avoidance tasks (Song and Leonard, 2005). Olfactory bulbectomy results in anhedonia measured by decreased sucrose preference (Cryan and Mombereau, 2004) and reduced sexual activity (Song and Leonard, 2005). These deficits are due to the removal of the olfactory bulbs, as inducing anosmia by flushing zinc through the nasal cavities does not cause any significant depression phenotype (Song and Leonard, 2005). The removal of the olfactory bulbs also leads to cell death and degeneration in a number of areas implicated in depression in humans, including the hippocampus, amygdala, dorsal raphe, cortex, and locus coeruleus. Within the hippocampus there is a reduction in volume along with a decrease in the number of dendritic spines. These changes have also been reported in the piriform cortex (Song and Leonard, 2005) and the amygdala (Cryan and Mombereau, 2004). Chronic antidepressant treatment can reverse behavioral and structural changes (Song and Leonard, 2005). In addition, removal of the olfactory bulbs also induces changes similar to those seen in depressed humans within the immune system. These include increases in serum concentrations of the pro-inflammatory cytokine interleukin (IL)-1β and prostaglandin E$_2$ along with a decrease in circulating levels of the anti-inflammatory cytokine IL-10 (Song and Leonard, 2005). Olfactory bulbectomized animals also have elevated basal corticosterone (CORT) levels, the rodent homolog for the stress hormone cortisol in humans. While this model does not have good construct validity and only moderate face validity, it does have excellent predictive validity, as chronic antidepressant treatments consistently reverse the behavioral effects of olfactory bulbectomy (Cryan and Mombereau, 2004). The paradigm also has excellent reproducibility across labs. Interestingly, olfactory bulbectomy is one of the few models of depression that does not show sex differences in the behavioral measures. Both males and females show behavioral effects of olfactory bulbectomy in tests of locomotor activity, exploration of a novel environment, anxiety, and sucrose preference (Song and Leonard, 2005) making it a test of interest for those studying depression in females.

CHRONIC MILD STRESS

In the chronic mild stress (CMS) paradigm, sometimes referred to as chronic variable or unpredictable stress (CVS or CUS), animals are exposed to variable stressors for a length of time extending between 6 (LaPlant et al., 2009) and 28 days (Willner, 2005). The stressors are typically minimally invasive but are given in a varied and unpredictable order. Animals can be exposed to more than one stressor in a day and the stressors are administered during all phases of their light:dark cycle. Stressors include restraint, tail suspension, disruption of the light/dark cycle, cage tilt, food and/or water restriction, changing of cage mates, temperature reductions, exposure to soiled or wet bedding, and random foot-shocks (Willner, 2005). Animals exposed to CMS generally show anhedonic behaviors, such as decreased sucrose consumption, impairments in natural reward associations, and changes in responsiveness to intracranial self-stimulation (Dalla et al., 2010). Animals exposed to CMS display increased immobility in the FST (Willner, 2005) and are more likely to show decreased active avoidance if they are subsequently exposed to the learned helplessness paradigm described in the following section in this chapter (Willner, 2005). They also show deficits in grooming, sexual behavior, and immune function (Willner, 2005). Biological profiling shows that CMS can induce increases in circulating levels of the pro-inflammatory cytokines tumor necrosis factor (TNF) α and IL1β (Grippo et al., 2005) both in the brain and the body. Four weeks of CMS exposure also results in increased basal levels of CORT (Grippo et al., 2005) along with disruptions in circadian release of CORT leading to reduced peak levels and an elongation of the trough of the cycle (Dallman et al., 2000). This dysregulation of normal HPA feedback results in changes in the storage of calories and fat leading to the development of a metabolic syndrome (Dallman et al., 2000). CMS can reduce neurogenesis in rodents although this may be due to effects on cell survival rather than cell proliferation (Kubera et al., 2011). CMS can also alter spine density in the prefrontal cortex and hippocampus of rodents consistent with work in humans showing reduced volume of these structures by magnetic resonance imaging (MRI) (Michelsen et al., 2007). Importantly, many of these effects can be reversed with chronic, but not acute, antidepressant exposure, giving this model good predictive validity. Also, an abbreviated six-day variation of this model can induce depression-like behaviors in females, but not males, making it an ideal model for understanding biological differences in stress responses between males and females (LaPlant et al., 2009). The utility of CMS to understand the neurobiology of depression in both males and females makes it a very useful tool to test new compounds for the treatment of depression and possibly identify targets for individualized approaches to treatment in men and woman.

LEARNED HELPLESSNESS

The learned helplessness paradigm was developed in the late 1960s. In the original experiments, dogs were given a single session of multiple inescapable shocks and then presented with an active avoidance task (Overmier and Seligman, 1967). They were allowed to escape the shock by jumping over a barrier in a shuttle box. In control animals that were not exposed to a previous bout of inescapable shock, the animals quickly learned to escape the aversive environment. Dogs that had experienced a prior uncontrollable shock failed to learn to escape the shuttle box and would exhibit helpless behavior (i.e., dogs would lie down and whimper) (Seligman, 1972). This test was later adapted for use in rodents and is now considered to be a primary depression test. Adaptations of the protocol have included yoked controls, allowing the researcher to directly compare behavioral and biological effects of having control over shock termination. Here, both groups of animals are exposed to the shock before avoidance training but only one group can control the termination of the shock (Seligman et al., 1975). Animals that can terminate the stressor, usually by performing an operant task, learn to escape in a subsequent active avoidance task, whereas yoked animals receiving the same shock without control over termination show a much greater degree of helplessness behavior. Interestingly, there are individual differences in susceptibility to inescapable stress; a third of the animals exposed to inescapable shock display susceptibility and engage in helplessness behavior, whereas a majority of animals are resilient to the stress and still learn to escape (Russo et al., 2012). This suggests that there may be an epigenetic component, since many of these studies are performed in genetically identical inbred animals, though further studies are needed. The difference in susceptibility also highlights a degree of face validity to the model, since most humans are resilient in the face of stress and don't develop significant depression symptoms. The model also has good construct validity, as loss of control over one's environment is highly stressful and can contribute to onset of a depressive episode (Gilbert, 2006) and all classes of antidepressant reverse learned helplessness in adult male rats (Zazpe et al., 2007). The model has some pathological validity, since helpless rodents have decreased hippocampal synaptic proteins such as PSD 95 and synaptophysin, and decreased neurogenesis (Malberg and Duman, 2003), which are consistent with some of the structural changes observed by MRI in humans. Both behavioral and structural deficits can be reversed by chronic, but not acute, treatment with antidepressants (Malberg and Duman, 2003), indicating that the model has good predictive validity (Malberg and Duman, 2003; Reines et al., 2008). Helpless animals also show reductions in IL-2 levels in brain regions implicated in depression including the hippocampus and prefrontal cortex (Lee et al., 2008). In the periphery IL-2 is involved with T-cell development and the recognition of "self" within the immune system (Lee et al., 2008) and within the brain it has been demonstrated to control emotion associated behaviors (Lee et al., 2008). However, females do not have the same stress-related behavioral deficits in LH (Shors et al., 2007), nor do they exhibit any chronic stress-related decrease in neural plasticity (Shors et al., 2007). Therefore the utility of the test is limited, especially when studying females. Regardless, LH models important aspects of mood disorders, and therefore, warrants further mechanistic

studies to determine pathological validity across a wider array of biomarker targets.

DEVELOPMENTAL STRESSORS

Stress exposure during critical periods of development has been shown to produce long-lasting changes in depression and anxiety-like behavior (Russo et al., 2012). Prenatal stress paradigms involve exposing pregnant females to stress and examining the effects of this stress exposure on the adult offspring. The effects of prenatal stress depends in part on the critical prenatal period when the mother is exposed to the stressor (Goel and Bale, 2009; Weinstock, 2008). Any number of prenatal stressors, including CMS (Goel and Bale, 2009), restraint stress, foot shock, and swim stress have been used (Weinstock, 2008). Stress during the early prenatal period (PND 1–7) results in a depression-like phenotype in male but not female mice (Goel and Bale, 2009), as measured by increased immobility in the FST and TST. Male mice exposed to gestational stress at this time point also displayed decreased sucrose preference (Goel and Bale, 2009). Interestingly, during this period, stress leads to dysmasculinization, causing males to engage in female-like behavioral strategies in their exploration of the Barnes maze (Mueller and Bale, 2007). Physiological changes in HPA-axis sensitivity to stress have been shown. Male mice exhibit larger stress-induced increases in CORT along with alterations of gene expression involved with negative feedback of the HPA (Goel and Bale, 2009). Later gestational stress can lead to a more pronounced depression-like phenotype in females than males, although this depends heavily on the behavioral domain being studies (Weinstock, 2008). Restraint stress (PND 15- parturition) leads to greater immobility in the FST in females than males (Alonso et al., 1991). However, other studies have reported that late gestational restraint stress (PND 14–20) impacts cognitive abilities in males but not females (Weinstock, 2008). Both restraint stress and foot shock starting at PND 8 have been reported to decrease spatial learning in males (Weinstock, 2008). These mice also had reductions in dendritic spine densities within the hippocampus that were thought to be associated with the cognitive deficit (Weinstock, 2008). Other studies performed only in males have found late gestational restraint stress also leads to adult reductions in cell proliferation within the hippocampus (Weinstock, 2008). Like early gestational stress, late gestational stress leads to hypercortisolemia in adults along with dysregulation of HPA negative feedback (Weinstock, 2008). Late gestational restraint stress also leads to alterations in circadian rhythm and changes in REM sleep (Maccari et al., 2003). These alterations include increases in paradoxical and fragmented sleep along with a decrease in deep slow wave sleep (Maccari et al., 2003). This model has good predictive validity, since treatment of offspring exposed to late gestational stress with chronic antidepressants in adulthood can reverse behavioral effects in the FST and alter glucocorticoid receptor expression (Maccari et al., 2003).

Early life stress can also produce significant depression-like phenotypes (Russo et al., 2012). Most studies have used maternal separation during the early postnatal period followed by behavioral, hormonal, and molecular analysis of the separated offspring during adulthood (Plotsky and Meaney, 1993). Studies typically separate pups for either 15 or 180 minutes a day during the postnatal period. Offspring separated for 15 minutes a day did not differ from normal facility reared controls or else showed resilience to stress exposure later in life (Plotsky et al., 2005). This phenomenon is referred to as stress tolerance and may promote active coping strategies (Russo et al., 2012). Conversely, animals exposed to early life stress have displayed greater immobility, and decreased spatial learning (Krishnan and Nestler, 2011). Rats exposed to maternal separation and then put through a repeated social defeat paradigm in adulthood used a passive coping mechanism to the stressor and engaged in more submissive postures and behavior (Gardner et al., 2005). Other studies have demonstrated that early life stress can make animals more prone to self-administer alcohol and cocaine (Moffett et al., 2007). They also exhibit greatly exaggerated HPA responses to stress (Plotsky et al., 2005) and have decreased cell proliferation in hippocampus leading to a smaller overall volume (Mirescu et al., 2004). Interestingly, studies in rodents have demonstrated that most early life stress affects male, but not female, rodents in adulthood (Diehl et al., 2007). In general it is currently thought that male animals are more susceptible to most forms of early life stress than females (Goel and Bale, 2009), whereas females are more susceptible to stress after puberty (Dalla et al., 2010). More research is clearly needed to understand how stress susceptibility changes across

the life span in both sexes. In sum, early life stress models are excellent for understanding a host of biological and behavioral changes important in depression. They exhibit excellent face, construct, and predictive validity as well as a growing body of evidence that suggests the model has pathological validity.

REPEATED SOCIAL DEFEAT STRESS

Repeated social defeat stress (Fig. 31.2) can unmask behavioral differences in vulnerability to stress across a wide spectrum of behavioral domains. In this model, experimental mice are placed into the home cage of a novel larger aggressive mouse each day for 10 days (Krishnan et al., 2007). The larger mouse quickly establishes dominance through physical interaction for a brief five to ten minute period, and then a perforated Plexiglas divider is placed in the cage to physically separate the two animals, allowing them to experience continued sensory cues. At the end of 10 days, experimental mice are separated into resilient and susceptible populations based on their social interaction score (Fig. 31.3), described earlier in the behavioral domains section of this chapter. Susceptibility and resilience scores are calculated as a ratio of the time spent near the novel animal divided by the time spent near the novel object. Animals that prefer the novel animal are considered resilient and behave like control animals that have not been exposed to stress. Animals that avoid the novel animal and spend more time near the novel object are considered susceptible. Approximately two-thirds

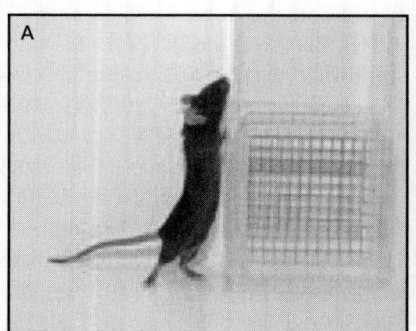
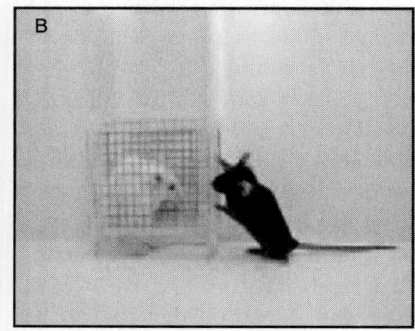
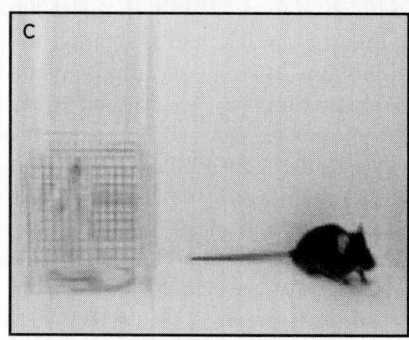

Figure 31.3 Social interaction testing. The social interaction test is used as a behavioral endpoint for stress-based manipulations such as repeated social defeat stress. In this test an animal is placed in a novel environment and allowed to interact with a novel object or a novel animal. (A) The time the mouse spends near a novel object is measured. (B) The amount of time spent interacting with the novel animal is measured. Control and resilient mice spend more time with the novel animal than the novel object. (C) The amount of time spent avoiding the novel animal is measured. Stress-susceptible mice will spend more time with the novel object than the novel animal. (Photography credit: Christopher Wood.)

of the mice exhibit social avoidance behavior and are considered susceptible, while the remaining one third do not show avoidance behavior and are considered resilient (Krishnan et al., 2007). Interestingly, both susceptible and resilient mice exhibit significant anxiety phenotypes, yet only susceptible mice show depression-like phenotypes measured by social avoidance, anhedonia, disruptions of the circadian system, and metabolic changes, including weight gain (Krishnan et al., 2007). The fact that only a subset of animals shows vulnerability to the effects of stress is again consistent with human responses to stress and provides construct validity. Some of the behavioral effects, including social avoidance and metabolic syndrome, can be reversed with chronic, but not acute, antidepressant treatment (Berton et al., 2006). Mechanistically, social defeat stress leads to a transient decrease in cell proliferation in both susceptible and resilient mice (Lagace et al., 2010), though reduced neurogenesis has been functionally implicated in resiliency, which may be somewhat counter to the reduced hippocampal volume identified in depression in humans (Lagace et al., 2010). Susceptibility to social defeat stress increases dendritic spine density on medium spiny neurons in the nucleus accumbens, a region critical for emotion and reward (Christoffel et al., 2011). These changes in spine profiles correlated with social avoidance behavior. Social defeat stress also increases circulating levels of pro-inflammatory cytokines in susceptible mice (Gomez-Lazaro et al., 2011). While social defeat is clearly a powerful model of depression exhibiting face, construct, and predictive validity, one of the major limitations of this type of stress is that it is difficult to test in female mice. Female mice do not normally attack each other, making it difficult to establish antagonistic interactions based on these dominance hierarchies. A few recent studies using a female rodent that is monogamous and territorial (California mouse; *Peromyscus californicus*) (Trainor et al., 2011) or nursing dams have effectively established social dominance in females (Shimamoto et al., 2011). Importantly, these studies have shown similar effects as males in measures such as anhedonia, drug addiction, and metabolic effects. However, more research is clearly necessary to determine whether the same molecular cascades and neural circuitry are affected in both sexes.

SELECTIVE BREEDING MODELS

While there are no known genetic causes of depression, there is clearly a strong familial linkage (Gilbert, 2006), suggesting that certain heritable complex genetic traits may predispose one to depression. For years, researchers have utilized selective breeding strategies to uncover the genetic basis of disease and, not surprisingly, there are a few lines, including the Flinder's sensitive line (FSL) and the Wistar-Kyoto (WKY) line, that show increased depression-associated phenotypes. Although the FSL was not originally investigated as a model of depression, it became clear that some of the neurochemical changes recapitulated alterations in humans with depression. The FSL rats were derived from Sprague–Dawley rats by selecting animals that were sensitive to cholinergic and anticholinergic compounds (Overstreet, 2012). It was later determined

that FSL rats show increased time spent immobile in the FST and decreased social interaction behavior (Overstreet, 2012). In addition, FSL rats are less motivated to work for a natural reward and have lower body weight and alteration in REM sleep (Overstreet et al., 2005). Interestingly, male FSL rats show greater behavioral deficits than females; females only show reductions in latency to immobility but not in time spent immobile (Dalla et al., 2011). The male response in the FST has been used to screen novel antidepressant compounds because they can be tested in concert with the Flinder's resistant line (FRL), which do not show the same behavioral deficits and are not responsive to acute antidepressant treatment. Interestingly, FSL rats are only responsive to chronic, antidepressant treatment, making this line particularly useful for its predictive validity. Pathological changes are also shown in the FSL rats. They have reductions in CRF and ACTH, similar to the subset of depressed subjects with hypocortisolemia and psychomotor retardation (Overstreet et al., 2005). The FSL rats also show abnormalities in immune function. There is a reduction in the number of natural killer cells in FSL rats, and they are more vulnerable to infection. However, FSL rats show basal reductions in pro-inflammatory cytokines such as IL-6 (Overstreet et al., 2005) that are normally elevated in the blood of subjects with depression (Dowlati et al., 2010). While FSL rats have increased cell proliferation in the dorsal hippocampus compared to the FRL line, during aging, they have a sharp decline in cell proliferation concurrent with a decrease in serotonergic enervation of the hippocampus thought to increase depression associated behavior (Husum et al., 2006). These findings warrant future investigation in that they may provide insight into the mechanisms of increased depression prevalence during aging. In general, the model shows good predictive validity in male animals. The face and pathological validity is mixed, as some symptoms do overlap with those of depression, whereas a number of biological measures do not. There is also a degree of construct validity, as humans with depression have abnormal sensitivity to cholinergic agents (Overstreet, 2012). Importantly, the model shows good reproducibility, at least in male rats, as multiple labs have found similar effects of antidepressants on the FST response (Dalla et al., 2011; Overstreet, 2012). However the fact that females show less depression behavior than males offers an important caveat, since females of most other rodent strains and women exhibit greater stress-induced depression-like behavior and higher depression prevalence, respectively (Dalla et al., 2010).

As mentioned previously, the WKY rats are also predisposed to greater depression behavior as a result of selective breeding. WKY rats were originally bred as a control for a hypertensive line (Malkesman and Weller, 2009). WKY rats compared to other strains show greater stress susceptibility, including increased immobility in the FST, decreased active avoidance when exposed to the learned helplessness paradigm, and increased vulnerability to stress-induced ulcers (Pare and Redei, 1993). Females show greater immobility than males in their response in the FST and also develop more severe ulcers, although this varies across the estrous cycle (Pare and Redei, 1993). In addition, WKY rats show greater anhedonia, anxiety-like behavior, and stress-induced weight loss compared with other strains

(Malkesman and Weller, 2009). This cluster of behavioral symptoms have led researchers to classify this as a model of comorbid depression and anxiety disorder (Malkesman and Weller, 2009). Mechanistically, WKY rats display dysregulation of the HPA axis including increased levels of CORT and ACTH along with an elongation of the elevation in CORT and a decrease in ACTH levels following an acute swim stress (Malkesman and Weller, 2009). Little is known about differences in brain plasticity, as most studies have compared the WKY rats to the spontaneously hypertensive strain, but these studies have shown that WKY rats have lower rates of cell proliferation and survival (Kronenberg et al., 2007). This strain has recently been used to explore the antidepressant and anxiolytic effects of novel antidepressant drugs acting on the kappa-opioid system (Carr et al., 2010). The model has good face and predictive validity, but lacks construct validity, as the basis for the susceptibility of WKY rats to stress is not yet understood. Reproducibility between laboratories is mixed because differences in breeding strategies by commercial breeders can lead to significant genetic drift (Overstreet, 2012).

In addition to selective breeding models in rat, Rouen helpless or "depressed" mice have been heavily used to study the mechanisms of depression and for novel antidepressant discovery. These mice were originally generated in 1995 by breeding CD-1 mice with high and low immobility scores in the TST (Cryan and Mombereau, 2004). Fourteen generations later these mice were shown to display increased immobility in the FST and TST, alterations in REM sleep, anhedonia, and elevated basal levels of CORT (El Yacoubi and Vaugeois, 2007). The helpless phenotype appears more often in females than males, making it a valid line for studying sex differences (Yacoubi et al., 2011). The model has good predictive validity as a number of classic antidepressants are able to reverse the behavioral effects in both sexes (El Yacoubi and Vaugeois, 2007). Reproducibility is also good, as multiple labs have identified similar behavioral phenotypes (Svenningsson et al., 2006). This model was used to first identify a functional role for P11 (Svenningsson et al., 2006), a protein that interacts with serotonin 1B receptors. P11 is decreased in helpless male and female mice, as well as in postmortem tissue from subjects with depression (El Yacoubi and Vaugeois, 2007; Svenningsson et al., 2006) and is proposed to be a potential novel target for the development of new antidepressants. The selective breeding strategy is one method of developing animal models of depression with pathological validity for discovering complex genetic variations that may underlie depression. However, there are some major drawbacks to selective breeding models. The generation of animals is time consuming and expensive, multiple overlapping genetic factors make it impossible to understand contributions of specific genes, and genetic drift occurring over time can affect the reproducibility of phenotypes (Overstreet, 2012; Yacoubi et al., 2011). Despite these factors, selective breeding may help to understand how these complex psychiatric phenotypes are maintained in a population and eventually, through the use of high-throughput genetic sequencing, we may even determine the complex genetic contributions driving depression susceptibility.

SUMMARY AND CONCLUSIONS

In this chapter we have discussed the validity of each major animal model of mood disorders currently being used to uncover novel mechanisms of psychiatric illness and to develop new therapeutics. These models range from those based on stress exposure to induce a depression-like phenotype in genetically identical mice to models that use selective breeding to examine the complex genetic contributions to depression between strains. Some of the models make use of acute or short-term stress exposure such as learned helplessness, whereas others depend on exposure to chronic stress, such as CMS and social defeat stress. All of the models discussed at least partially fulfill the criterion for face, construct, and predictive validity, which is critical to establishing animal models that accurately mimic the disease. However, as we have discussed throughout this chapter, we need to judge the validity of these animal models with greater stringency and incorporate new criteria, such as reproducibility across labs and pathological validity. Pathological validity is especially important and will lead to a greater understanding of the underlying biology of depression. Over time, this may help clinicians to develop diagnostic criteria based on these biological changes and move drug discovery efforts beyond monoamine-based antidepressants, which only lead to successful remission in approximately 40% of the population (Krishnan and Nestler, 2008). New, rapid onset treatments such as ketamine (Berman et al., 2000) are undergoing clinical trials and show promise, however, all currently approved antidepressants are based on serendipitous discovery and do not directly target the underlying pathology of mood disorders. Additionally, diagnosis is based largely on non-overlapping clusters of behavioral symptoms that are often shared across disorders, making it difficult to achieve specificity in diagnosis. Thus, we need to develop biomarkers and diagnostic tests for the core symptoms of depression, and diagnose and treat based on these factors. For this, the use of valid animal models is critical and we need to continually develop and expand on our models to cover an even greater range of behavioral deficits. Moreover, few basic drug discovery studies use female animals as experimental subjects (Beery and Zucker, 2010), despite the fact that in humans, there are twice as many women that suffer from depression as men (Kessler et al., 1993). While there are a few models that accurately reflect this sex difference in depression prevalence, many do not. Thus, we need to be cognizant of this limitation in validity and understand that there may be individual- or sex-based differences in our models that will impact our results. In summary, the field has made tremendous progress in developing animal models of mood disorders that, in some cases, have a high degree of validity in modeling human depression. By using a battery of tests to understand distinct behavioral domains we can gain a greater insight into the biology of depression behavior. Over time, we can use these animal models that mimic the pathophysiology of depression to develop biomarker diagnostic tests and eventually more effective treatments with fewer negative side effects.

ACKNOWLEDGMENTS

Preparation of this review was supported by grants from the National Institute of Mental Health: R01 MH090264 (SJR), and National Institute on Drug Abuse training grant 5TDA07135-28 (GEH).

DISCLOSURES

Dr. Russo has no conflicts of interest to disclose. His work is funded by a NIMH R01 MH090264 and J&J IMHRO Rising Star Award.

Dr. Hodes has no conflicts of interest to disclose. She is funded by NIDA (5TDA07135-28) and the Brain and Behavior Research foundations NARSAD Young Investigator award.

REFERENCES

Alonso, S.J., Arevalo, R., et al. (1991). Effects of maternal stress during pregnancy on forced swimming test behavior of the offspring. *Physiol. Behav.* 50(3):511–517.

American Psychiatric Association. (2000). Diagnostic and Statistical Manual of Mental Disorders: DSM-IV-TR, 4th Edition. Washington DC: Author.

Anisman, H., and Matheson, K. (2005). Stress, depression, and anhedonia: caveats concerning animal models. *Neurosci. Biobehav. Rev.* 29(4–5):525–546.

Beery, A.K., and Zucker, I. (2010). Sex bias in neuroscience and biomedical research. *Neurosci. Biobehav. Rev.* 35(3):565–572.

Berman, R.M., Cappiello, A., et al. (2000). Antidepressant effects of ketamine in depressed patients. *Biol. Psychiatry* 47(4):351–354.

Berton, O., McClung, C.A., et al. (2006). Essential role of BDNF in the mesolimbic dopamine pathway in social defeat stress. *Science* 311(5762):864–868.

Carlezon, W.A., Jr., and Chartoff, E.H. (2007). Intracranial self-stimulation (ICSS) in rodents to study the neurobiology of motivation. *Nat. Protoc.* 2(11):2987–2995.

Carr, G.V., Bangasser, D.A., et al. (2010). Antidepressant-like effects of kappa-opioid receptor antagonists in Wistar Kyoto rats. *Neuropsychopharmacology.* 35(3):752–763.

Christoffel, D.J., Golden, S.A., et al. (2011). IkappaB kinase regulates social defeat stress-induced synaptic and behavioral plasticity. *J. Neurosci.* 31(1):314–321.

Chugani, H.T., Behen, M.E., et al. (2001). Local brain functional activity following early deprivation: a study of postinstitutionalized Romanian orphans. *NeuroImage.* 14(6):1290–1301.

Coric, V., Feldman, H.H., et al. (2010). Multicenter, randomized, double-blind, active comparator and placebo-controlled trial of a corticotropin-releasing factor receptor-1 antagonist in generalized anxiety disorder. *Depress. Anxiety* 27(5):417–425.

Cryan, J.F., and Mombereau, C. (2004). In search of a depressed mouse: utility of models for studying depression-related behavior in genetically modified mice. *Mol. Psychiatry* 9(4):326–357.

Dalla, C., Pitychoutis, P.M., et al. (2010). Sex differences in animal models of depression and antidepressant response. *Basic Clin. Pharmacol. Toxicol.* 106(3):226–233.

Dalla, C., Pitychoutis, P.M., et al. (2011). Sex differences in response to stress and expression of depressive-like behaviours in the rat. *Curr. Top. Behav. Neurosci.* 8:97–118.

Dallman, M.F., Akana, S.F., et al. (2000). Bottomed out: metabolic significance of the circadian trough in glucocorticoid concentrations. *Int. J. Obes. Relat. Metab. Disord.* 24(Suppl 2):S40–S46.

Detke, M.J., and Lucki, I. (1996). Detection of serotonergic and noradrenergic antidepressants in the rat forced swimming test: the effects of water depth. *Behav. Brain. Res.* 73(1–2):43–46.

Diehl, L.A., Silveira, P.P., et al. (2007). Long lasting sex-specific effects upon behavior and S100b levels after maternal separation and exposure to a model of post-traumatic stress disorder in rats. *Brain. Res.* 1144:107–116.

Dimatelis, J.J., Pillay, N.S., et al. (2012). Early maternal separation leads to down-regulation of cytokine gene expression. *Metab. Brain. Dis.* 27(3):393–397.

Dowlati, Y., Herrmann, N., et al. (2010). A meta-analysis of cytokines in major depression. *Biol. Psychiatry* 67(5):446–457.

Dulawa, S.C., and Hen, R. (2005). Recent advances in animal models of chronic antidepressant effects: the novelty-induced hypophagia test. *Neurosci. Biobehav. Rev.* 29(4–5):771–783.

El Yacoubi, M., and Vaugeois, J.M. (2007). Genetic rodent models of depression. *Curr. Opin Pharmacol.* 7(1):3–7.

Falowski, S.M., Sharan, A., et al. (2011). An evaluation of neuroplasticity and behavior following deep brain stimulation of the nucleus accumbens in an animal model of depression. *Neurosurgery* 69(6):1281–1290.

Gardner, K.L., Thrivikraman, K.V., et al. (2005). Early life experience alters behavior during social defeat: focus on serotonergic systems. *Neuroscience* 136(1):181–191.

Gilbert, P. (2006). Evolution and depression: issues and implications. *Psychol. Med.* 36(3):287–297.

Goel, N., and Bale, T.L. (2009). Examining the intersection of sex and stress in modelling neuropsychiatric disorders. *J. Neuroendocrinol.* 21(4):415–420.

Gomez-Lazaro, E., Arregi, A., et al. (2011). Individual differences in chronically defeated male mice: behavioral, endocrine, immune, and neurotrophic changes as markers of vulnerability to the effects of stress. *Stress* 14(5):537–548.

Grippo, A.J., Francis, J., et al. (2005). Neuroendocrine and cytokine profile of chronic mild stress-induced anhedonia. *Physiol. Behav.* 84(5):697–706.

Husum, H., Aznar, S., et al. (2006). Exacerbated loss of cell survival, neuropeptide Y-immunoreactive (IR) cells, and serotonin-IR fiber lengths in the dorsal hippocampus of the aged Flinders sensitive line "depressed" rat: implications for the pathophysiology of depression? *J. Neurosci. Res.* 84(6):1292–1302.

Isingrini, E., Camus, V., et al. (2010). Association between repeated unpredictable chronic mild stress (UCMS) procedures with a high fat diet: a model of fluoxetine resistance in mice. *PLoS One* 5(4):e10404.

Kessler, R.C., McGonagle, K.A., et al. (1993). Sex and depression in the National Comorbidity Survey. I: Lifetime prevalence, chronicity and recurrence. *J. Affect. Disord.* 29(2–3):85–96.

Krishnan, V., Berton, O., et al. (2008). The use of animal models in psychiatric research and treatment. *Am. J. Psychiatry* 165(9):1109.

Krishnan, V., Han, M.H., et al. (2007). Molecular adaptations underlying susceptibility and resistance to social defeat in brain reward regions. *Cell* 131(2):391–404.

Krishnan, V., and Nestler, E.J. (2008). The molecular neurobiology of depression. *Nature* 455(7215):894–902.

Krishnan, V., and Nestler, E.J. (2011). Animal models of depression: molecular perspectives. *Curr. Top. Behav. Neurosci.* 7:121–147.

Kronenberg, G., Lippoldt, A., et al. (2007). Two genetic rat models of arterial hypertension show different mechanisms by which adult hippocampal neurogenesis is increased. *Dev. Neurosci.* 29(1–2):124–133.

Kronfeld-Schor, N., and Einat, H. (2012). Circadian rhythms and depression: human psychopathology and animal models. *Neuropharmacology* 62(1):101–114.

Kubera, M., Obuchowicz, E., et al. (2011). In animal models, psychosocial stress-induced (neuro)inflammation, apoptosis and reduced neurogenesis are associated to the onset of depression. *Prog. Neuropsychopharmacol. Biol. Psychiatry* 35(3):744–759.

Lagace, D.C., Donovan, M.H., et al. (2010). Adult hippocampal neurogenesis is functionally important for stress-induced social avoidance. *Proc. Natl. Acad. Sci. USA* 107(9):4436–4441.

LaPlant, Q., Chakravarty, S., et al. (2009). Role of nuclear factor kappaB in ovarian hormone-mediated stress hypersensitivity in female mice. *Biol. Psychiatry* 65(10):874–880.

Lee, Y.T., Wang, W.F., et al. (2008). Effects of escapable and inescapable stressors on behavior and interleukin-2 in the brain. *Neuroreport* 19(12):1243–1247.

Maccari, S., Darnaudery, M., et al. (2003). Prenatal stress and long-term consequences: implications of glucocorticoid hormones. *Neurosci. Biobehav. Rev.* 27(1–2):119–127.

Malberg, J.E., and Duman, R.S. (2003). Cell proliferation in adult hippocampus is decreased by inescapable stress: reversal by fluoxetine treatment. *Neuropsychopharmacology* 28(9):1562–1571.

Malkesman, O., and Weller, A. (2009). Two different putative genetic animal models of childhood depression—a review. *Prog. Neurobiol.* 88(3):153–169.

Mckinney, W.T., Jr., and Bunny, W.E., Jr. (1969). Animal model of depression. I. Review of evidence: implications for research. *Arch. Gen. Psychiatry* 21(2):240–248.

Michelsen, K.A., van den Hove, D.L., et al. (2007). Prenatal stress and subsequent exposure to chronic mild stress influence dendritic spine density and morphology in the rat medial prefrontal cortex. *BMC. Neurosci.* 8:107.

Mirescu, C., Peters, J.D., et al. (2004). Early life experience alters response of adult neurogenesis to stress. *Nat. Neurosci.* 7(8):841–846.

Moffett, M.C., Vicentic, A., et al. (2007). Maternal separation alters drug intake patterns in adulthood in rats. *Biochem. Pharmacol.* 73(3):321–330.

Mueller, B.R., and Bale, T.L. (2007). Early prenatal stress impact on coping strategies and learning performance is sex dependent. *Physiol. Behav.* 91(1):55–65.

Neumann, I.D., Wegener, G., et al. (2011). Animal models of depression and anxiety: what do they tell us about human condition? *Prog. Neuropsychopharmacol. Biol. Psychiatry* 35(6):1357–1375.

Overmier, J.B., and Seligman, M.E. (1967). Effects of inescapable shock upon subsequent escape and avoidance responding. *J. Comp. Physiol. Psychol.* 63(1):28–33.

Overstreet, D.H. (2012). Modeling depression in animal models. *Methods Mol. Biol.* 829:125–144.

Overstreet, D.H., Friedman, E., et al. (2005). The Flinders Sensitive Line rat: a selectively bred putative animal model of depression. *Neurosci. Biobehav. Rev.* 29(4–5):739–759.

Pare, W.P., and Redei, E. (1993). Sex differences and stress response of WKY rats. *Physiol. Behav.* 54(6):1179–1185.

Plotsky, P.M., and Meaney, M.J. (1993). Early, postnatal experience alters hypothalamic corticotropin-releasing factor (CRF) mRNA, median eminence CRF content and stress-induced release in adult rats. *Brain. Res. Mol. Brain. Res.* 18(3):195–200.

Plotsky, P.M., Thrivikraman, K.V., et al. (2005). Long-term consequences of neonatal rearing on central corticotropin-releasing factor systems in adult male rat offspring. *Neuropsychopharmacology* 30(12):2192–2204.

Porsolt, R.D., Anton, G., et al. (1978). Behavioural despair in rats: a new model sensitive to antidepressant treatments. *Eur. J. Pharmacol.* 47(4):379–391.

Reines, A., Cereseto, M., et al. (2008). Maintenance treatment with fluoxetine is necessary to sustain normal levels of synaptic markers in an experimental model of depression: correlation with behavioral response. *Neuropsychopharmacology* 33(8):1896–1908.

Russo, S.J., Murrough, J.A., et al. (2012). Neurobiology of resilience. *Nat. Neurosci.* 15(11):1475–1484.

Santarelli, L., Saxe, M., et al. (2003). Requirement of hippocampal neurogenesis for the behavioral effects of antidepressants. *Science* 301(5634):805–809.

Seligman, M.E. (1972). Learned helplessness. *Annu. Rev. Med.* 23 407–412.

Seligman, M.E., Rosellini, R.A., et al. (1975). Learned helplessness in the rat: time course, immunization, and reversibility. *J. Comp. Physiol. Psychol.* 88(2):542–547.

Shimamoto, A., Debold, J.F., et al. (2011). Blunted accumbal dopamine response to cocaine following chronic social stress in female rats: exploring a link between depression and drug abuse. *Psychopharmacology. (Berl.)* 218(1):271–279.

Shors, T.J., Mathew, J., et al. (2007). Neurogenesis and helplessness are mediated by controllability in males but not in females. *Biol. Psychiatry* 62(5):487–495.

Song, C., and Leonard, B.E. (2005). The olfactory bulbectomised rat as a model of depression. *Neurosci. Biobehav. Rev.* 29(4–5):627–647.

Steiger, A., and Kimura, M. (2010). Wake and sleep EEG provide biomarkers in depression. *J. Psychiatr. Res.* 44(4):242–252.

Steru, L., Chermat, R., et al. (1985). The tail suspension test: a new method for screening antidepressants in mice. *Psychopharmacology (Berl.)* 85(3):367–370.

Svenningsson, P., Chergui, K., et al. (2006). Alterations in 5-HT1B receptor function by p11 in depression-like states. *Science* 311(5757):77–80.

Trainor, B.C., Pride, M.C., et al. (2011). Sex differences in social interaction behavior following social defeat stress in the monogamous California mouse (Peromyscus californicus). *PLoS One* 6(2):e17405.

Weinstock, M. (2008). The long-term behavioural consequences of prenatal stress. *Neurosci. Biobehav. Rev.* 32(6):1073–1086.

Wilkinson, M.B., Dias, C., et al. (2011). A novel role of the WNT-Dishevelled-GSK3{beta} signaling cascade in the mouse nucleus accumbens in a social defeat model of depression. *J. Neurosci.* 31(25):9084–9092.

Willner, P. (2005). Chronic mild stress (CMS) revisited: consistency and behavioural-neurobiological concordance in the effects of CMS. *Neuropsychobiology* 52(2):90–110.

Yacoubi, M.E., Popa, D., et al. (2011). Genetic association between helpless trait and depression-related phenotypes: evidence from crossbreeding studies with H/Rouen and NH/Rouen mice. *Int. J. Neuropsychopharmacol.* 1–12.

Zazpe, A., Artaiz, I., et al. (2007). Reversal of learned helplessness by selective serotonin reuptake inhibitors in rats is not dependent on 5-HT availability. *Neuropharmacology* 52(3):975–984.

32 | MOLECULAR AND CELLULAR PATHOGENESIS OF DEPRESSION AND MECHANISMS FOR TREATMENT RESPONSE

RONALD S. DUMAN

INTRODUCTION

Major depressive disorder (MDD) is a debilitating illness that effects approximately 17% of the US population at some point in life, causing enormous economic burden and devastating personal suffering (Kessler, 2005). MDD is a heterogeneous illness characterized by impaired mood, low self-esteem, inability to experience pleasure (i.e., anhedonia), cognitive deficits, and altered eating and sleeping patterns. The available medications are only effective in approximately two-thirds of depressed patients, but can take months to years and still leaves one-third of patients untreated (Trivedi, 2006). The low rates of efficacy and lag time for treatment response are particularly problematic for a patient population at high risk for suicide.

Our inability to rapidly and successfully treat and ultimately cure MDD is due in large part to the lack of information on the underlying causes of this disorder. Early theories of depression and treatment response were centered on disruption of monoamine neurotransmitter systems, 5-hydroxytryptamine (5-HT) and norepinephrine (NE), but more recent studies have focused on dysregulation of the major amino acid neurotransmitters glutamate and γ-aminobutyric acid (GABA), and the role of disrupted neuroplasticity in depression. A delicate balance of glutamate and GABA, the major excitatory and inhibitory neurotransmitters, in key limbic and cortical circuits is required for control of emotion and mood. This balance is also critical for the function and health of neurons, which are controlled in part via activity dependent regulation of neurotrophic factors. Altered activity levels, either increases or decreases, over sustained periods of time can result in neuronal damage, atrophy and loss, contributing to cellular and behavioral abnormalities in depression.

Clinical brain imaging and postmortem studies provide evidence that MDD is associated with structural abnormalities, and preclinical work in rodent models of depression also demonstrate alterations of neurons and glia at the cellular level. Stress and other environmental factors, combined with genetic polymorphisms are thought to contribute to an individual's vulnerability or resilience to depression. This could also explain the heterogeneity of depressive disorders, as the combination of life exposure to stress/trauma and genetic makeup determine whether a particular person will develop MDD. Another limiting factor is that there are no validated biomarkers of depression or treatment response.

The recent discovery of a rapid-acting antidepressant ketamine that is effective in patients who have failed to respond to typical antidepressants represents a major advance for the treatment of depression. Research on the mechanisms underlying the actions of ketamine further highlight the importance of altered synaptic connections in depression and provide targets for development of a new generation of antidepressants. This chapter will discuss the neurotransmitter systems, cellular and structural changes, and the role of neurotrophic factors and inflammatory cytokines in the pathophysiology and treatment of depression. Work on the synaptogenic and behavioral actions of ketamine, as well as novel antidepressant targets will also be presented.

ALTERED NEUROTRANSMISSION AND NEUROPLASTICITY IN DEPRESSION

Many theories of depression have involved alterations of neurotransmitter systems in limbic and cortical brain regions that control emotion, mood, and cognition. Most notable are the early hypotheses that involved the monoamines 5-HT and NE, and more recently the amino acid neurotransmitters glutamate and GABA. A brief review of the role of these monoamines and amino acid neurotransmitter systems is provided in this review. Also discussed is one of the key processes for regulation of neurotransmission, neuroplasticity, which has been implicated in psychiatric illnesses including depression. There have been a number of neuropeptide systems implicated in the pathophysiology and/or treatment of depression, including corticotrophin releasing factor, neuropeptide Y, neurokinin/substance P, galanin, and others that will not be discussed here due to space limitations.

ALTERED MONOAMINE NEUROTRANSMITTER SYSTEMS

The first evidence-based neurobiological theories of MDD focused on dysregulation of the monoamine neurotransmitter systems. This included evidence that early drugs with antidepressant efficacy increased monoamine levels by blocking the reuptake or breakdown of these neurotransmitters. Agents that produced these kinds of effects included the tricyclic antidepressants, such as imipramine, a nonselective inhibitor of the 5-HT and NE transporters, as well as iproniazid and tranylcypromine, drugs that inhibit monoamine oxidase, the enzyme responsible for monoamine metabolism (Heninger, 1996; Jacobsen, 2012). There was also early evidence that compounds that caused depletion of monoamines, like reserpine, which disrupts monoamine vesicle storage, could cause depression, although subsequent studies failed to consistently replicate this finding (Heninger, 1996). Later studies provided evidence that 5-HT and NE were required for sustained therapeutic responses to drug treatments, as selective depletion of either monoamine caused relapse in patients being treated with the corresponding selective reuptake inhibitor (Heninger, 1996).

Evidence based on direct analysis of monoamine levels has also been mixed, with some reports of reduced levels of 5-HT, NE, and/or their metabolites in blood, cerebral spinal fluid, or postmortem brain tissue, although there are also negative reports (Heninger, 1996; Jacobsen, 2012). The data with regard to 5-HT, metabolites, and other functional markers appear to be more consistent when considering severe depression and/or suicide (Jacobsen, 2012). Together these studies indicate that reductions in levels of monoamines are not a generalized trait marker of depression, which is not unexpected given the heterogeneity of depressive illnesses.

The heterogeneity of MDD could have multiple origins, including genetic polymorphisms based on findings from association studies. There is evidence that polymorphisms of the gene for tryptophan hydroxylase, the rate-limiting enzyme for 5-HT synthesis, are associated with depression in a subpopulation of patients (Jacobsen, 2012). Variants of the 5-HT transporter gene, specifically the short, low expressing variant, are associated with anxiety-related traits and increased risk of depression in individuals exposed to early life stress or trauma (Caspi, 2010). This type of gene x environment interaction is thought to play a prominent role in depression as well as other psychiatric illnesses, as the effects of susceptibility genes are expressed when combined with precipitating stressors and/or other comorbid illnesses (see Chapter 37).

Based on this heterogeneity it is not surprising that drugs that act on monoamine systems, including 5-HT selective reuptake inhibitor (SSRI) antidepressants, have limited efficacy with approximately one in three depressed patients responding to the first antidepressant prescribed (Trivedi, 2006). Nevertheless, there is still interest in developing drugs that act on the monoamine systems, with increased emphasis on dual or triple (i.e., 5-HT, NE, and/or dopamine) reuptake inhibitors. While such agents may have fewer side effects than earlier reuptake inhibitors, it is reasonable to question whether such drugs will be more efficacious than currently available antidepressants. The limited efficacy could be due to disease heterogeneity and the restricted role of monoamine depletion in the symptoms of depression, as discussed. In addition, the monoamines are considered to be modulatory neurotransmitter systems (Fig. 32.1), influencing the activity and function of other systems, in contrast to fast-acting glutamate and GABA. This could explain in part the limited efficacy and therapeutic time lag for the actions of antidepressants that work via the monoamine systems. This possibility is supported by recent studies demonstrating that novel antidepressants that act on glutamate neurotransmission (i.e., ketamine) produce rapid antidepressant actions in hard-to-treat depressed patients (Zarate, 2006) (see the following for further discussion of rapid-acting antidepressants and glutamate).

ALTERATIONS OF GLUTAMATE AND GABA IN DEPRESSION

In recent years the focus of depression research has shifted from the monoamine systems to the amino acid neurotransmitters glutamate and GABA. Although the glutamate and GABA systems are often discussed separately, it is useful to consider how they work in concert, as reciprocal interactions are critical for fine control of neuronal circuits and brain function. Notably, tonic firing of GABAergic neurons constrains glutamate transmission and allows for high fidelity point-to-point activation of glutamate activity (Fig. 32.1). The tonic firing of GABA neurons is in turn controlled in part by glutamate receptors on these neurons. The delicate balance of glutamate and GABA transmission is necessary for normal brain function, and disruption of this homeostasis contributes to depression as well as other psychiatric illnesses. Unbalanced signaling can also lead to sustained elevation of glutamate, which can produce excitotoxic neuronal damage and even cell loss.

With this is mind, there is substantial evidence that levels of glutamate and GABA are dysregulated in mood disorders. However, as is often the case with clinical studies of a heterogeneous illness such as depression, there are inconsistencies that could also be related to methodological differences, brain regions examined, medication status, and other variables. With regard to GABA, the prevailing evidence is in favor of a reduction of this neurotransmitter. This includes initial studies of blood plasma and cerebral spinal fluid and later with the development of proton magnetic resonance spectroscopy (MRS) direct evidence for *in vivo* reductions of GABA content in cortical (occipital and frontal) brain regions in depressed patients (Sanacora and Saricicek, 2007). Further studies demonstrated that the GABA deficits measured by MRS are reversed by antidepressant treatments. Postmortem studies also report a loss of GABAergic interneurons in the dorsal lateral PFC (dlPFC) of depressed subjects (Maciag, 2009) and decreased levels of the primary GABA synthesizing enzyme, glutamic acid decarboxylase (Karolewicz, 2010). Imaging studies also demonstrate functional deficits of cortical GABA inhibition (Levinson, 2010).

The evidence for alterations of glutamate transmission is more mixed. Studies of glutamate in blood, CSF, or brain show increases, or no change (reviewed by Yüksel, 2010). Studies using proton MRS have been more consistent. Proton MRS measures levels of Glx, a composite containing mostly glutamate and glutamine (an intermediary metabolite of glutamate) but also some GABA and other metabolites. These studies report decreased levels of Glx in most cortical brain regions of depressed patients, including the anterior cingulate, dlPFC, dorsal medial PFC, ventral medial PFC, amygdala, and hippocampus (Yüksel, 2010). One exception is the occipital cortex, where an increase was reported (Sanacora, 2004). There are also several reports that antidepressant treatments reverse the

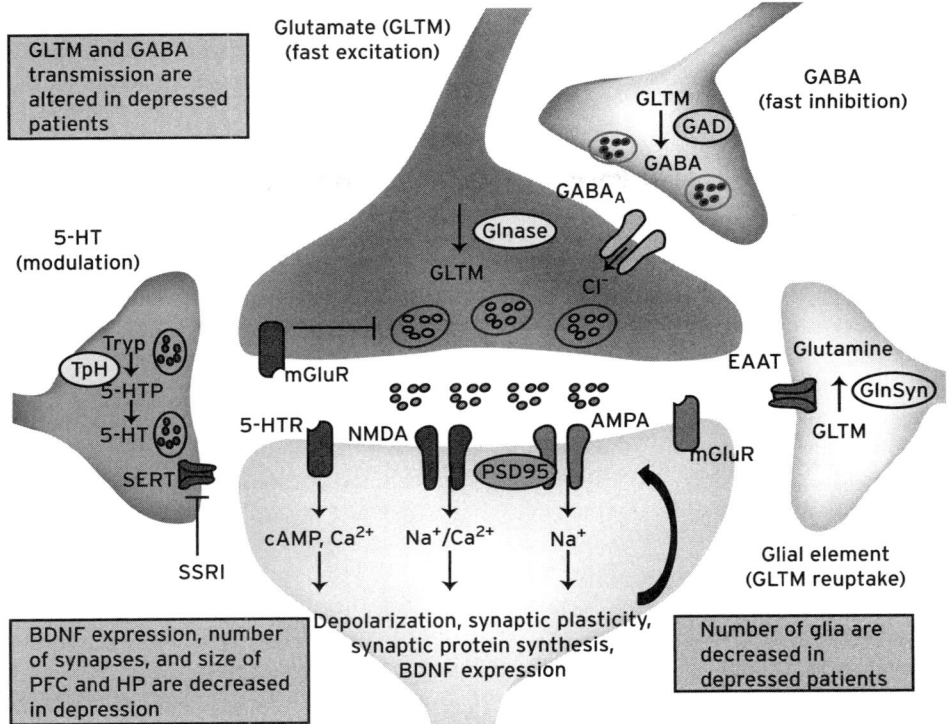

Figure 32.1 Diagram of glutamate transmission and the influence of GABA and 5-HT neurotransmitters, as well as glia. The glutamate, GABA, and 5-HT neurotransmitter systems are coded in dark gray, light shaded gray, and medium gray, respectively; a glial element is also shown on the right. Glutamate transmission is tightly controlled by GABA as well as other synaptic inputs. Glutamine is converted by glutaminase (Glnase) to glutamate, which is then packaged into presynaptic vesicles and released in an activity dependent manner. Glutamate acts on postsynaptic as well as presynaptic receptors, including ionotrophic (i.e., AMPA and NMDA) and metabotropic (e.g., mGluR2/3) subtypes. Activation of AMPA and NMDA receptors, which interact with postsynaptic density proteins (PSD) such as PSD95, leads to influx of Na+ and Ca2+, causing excitatory postsynaptic currents (EPSCs) and eventually depolarization. These pathways also mediate synaptic plasticity, including the insertion of AMPA receptors into the synaptic membrane, which enhances the maturation, stabilization, and function of synapses. Glutamate is cleared from the extracellular space by excitatory amino acid transporters (EAAT) located primarily on glia, where glutamate is converted to glutamine by glutamine synthetase (GlnSyn). Glia cells are also a major source of glutamine for the presynaptic glutamate terminal. GABA and tonic firing of GABAergic neurons provides negative control over glutamate. Glutamate is converted to GABA by glutamic acid decarboxylase (GAD). GABA binds to ionotropic GABA_A receptors, which when activated allow influx of Cl−, resulting in inhibitory postsynaptic currents (IPSCs) and hyperpolarization. 5-HT is a modulatory neurotransmitter that is derived from tryptophan (Tryp), which is converted to 5-hydroxytryptophan (5-HTP) by the rate-limiting enzyme tryptophan hydroxylase (TpH). 5-HT released into the synapse is inactivated by reuptake into the presynaptic terminal by the 5-HT transporter (SERT), which is the target of SSRI antidepressants. Activation of 5-HT receptors (5-HTR) and coupling with G proteins leads to regulation of second messenger systems, including the cAMP cascade and intracellular Ca2+. Alterations in depression include imbalance of glutamate and GABA transmission, decreased expression of BDNF, decreased number of synapses, reduced size of the PFC and hippocampus (HP), and decreased number of glia as indicated.

deficit in levels of Glx. In addition, levels of Glx are increased in patients with bipolar disorder.

Together, the evidence points to a decrease in GABA and glutamate neurotransmission, which could indicate an overall reduction in neuronal function and circuit level control in the brains of MDD patients. This could also be related to the atrophy of neurons and loss of glia in the same cortical and limbic brain regions where neurotransmission is disrupted (see following). The mechanisms that result in decreased neurotransmission, atrophy of neurons, and loss of glia are not known but could be due to an imbalance of glutamate and GABA signaling, resulting in over- or underactivation of neurons. This may occur via loss of the proper balance of activity dependent neurotrophic factor support, and/ or increased glutamate excitotoxicity. The need for proper balance of glutamate and GABA signaling is further highlighted by evidence that the therapeutic action of novel rapid antidepressants is dependent on a transient burst of glutamate transmission. These possibilities are discussed in the following sections.

DISRUPTION OF NEUROPLASTICITY IN DEPRESSION: REVERSAL BY ANTIDEPRESSANT TREATMENT

The loss of glutamate/GABA balance also supports the hypothesis that alterations of neuroplasticity contribute to depression and other stress-related illnesses. Cellular models of neuroplasticity, such as long-term potentiation (LTP) are used to study the mechanisms underlying learning and memory. However, neuroplasticity is a critical process that is involved in many aspects of neuronal adaptation and function. Neuroplasticity refers to the sensing and summation of neurotransmitter signals under a specific set of conditions, resulting in adaptations of synaptic function and architecture, which lead to altered responding upon exposure to the same or related signals. This includes activation of ionotropic glutamate receptors, AMPA (α-amino-3-hydroxy-5-methyl-isoxazole-4-propionic acid) and NMDA (*N*-methyl-D-aspartate), increased intracellular calcium signaling, insertion of glutamate receptors into the synaptic membrane, and stabilization of spine synapses (Fig. 32.1) (the exact mechanisms for synaptic plasticity are reviewed in detail in Chapter 5).

The ability to make the appropriate adaptive response, for example upon exposure to stress or trauma, is critical for proper function of neural circuits that allows for adaptation and resilience to change. Studies in rodent models demonstrate that exposure to chronic stress decreases synaptic plasticity in the PFC and hippocampus (Duman and Aghajanian, 2012). The synaptic plasticity deficits are caused by chronic stress exposure, as a single acute stressor enhances glutamate transmission in the PFC (Yuen, 2012). Conversely, chronic administration of typical antidepressants, such as the highly prescribed SSRIs, increases cellular neuroplasticity determined by studies of hippocampal LTP (Duman and Aghajanian, 2012). Additional evidence is provided by work demonstrating that chronic fluoxetine reinstates ocular dominance plasticity in the adult mouse visual cortex and enhances the extinction of conditioned fear, an active learning process (Karpova, 2011; Maya Vetencourt, 2008). Moreover, SSRI-induced neuroplasticity requires BDNF. These studies are consistent with evidence that glutamate signaling and neurotransmission are altered in depression and in animal models of chronic stress exposure.

STRUCTURAL ABNORMALITIES IN DEPRESSION

In addition to alterations of neurotransmission and plasticity, there is now clear evidence of structural alterations in depression, including changes in the size or volume of cortical and limbic brain regions, as well as ultrastructural changes of the neuronal processes/connections and numbers of neurons and glia. These findings are provided by human brain imaging and postmortem studies as well as animal models of stress and depression.

HUMAN BRAIN IMAGING OF DEPRESSION

There is now consistent evidence from magnetic resonance imaging studies that depression is associated with alterations of the volume or size of several brain regions, notably the PFC and hippocampus (Drevets, 2008; MacQueen, 2011). These brain regions are known to control memory and cognition, which are severely compromised in depressed patients, and are also part of a neural circuit that includes other brain regions that control emotion, anxiety, fear, vegetative, and endocrine responses that are dysregulated in depression (i.e., limbic-cortical-striatal-pallidal-thalamic, with connections to amygdala, hypothalamus, and brainstem structures) (see Chapter 34 on depression circuitry).

Hippocampus, a highly stress-sensitive structure, has been one of the most studied brain regions in MDD patients and in preclinical models of stress. A recent review of imaging studies of over a thousand depressed patients and the same number of controls, demonstrates a consistent reduction in hippocampal size associated with depression (MacQueen, 2011). The smaller volume of hippocampus in depressed patients has been associated with severity and duration of illness and non-response to antidepressant treatment; and conversely there is evidence that treatment response can reverse hippocampal volume deficits. Early life stress and trauma, which are risk factors for depression (see Chapter 44 on early life stress), are also associated with smaller hippocampal volumes. There is evidence that smaller hippocampal volume is observed before the onset of illness in a population of high-risk adolescents.

Prefrontal cortex subregions, including the subgenual PFC, infralimbic, and anterior cingulate cortex, are also altered in depression. Neuroimaging studies demonstrate that decreased volume of these PFC cortical regions occurs at an early stage in depressive illness, and are observed in high-risk young adults, and that the volume deficits progress with length of illness in psychotic depressed patients (Price, 2010). The reductions in subgenual PFC are reported to persist after successful treatment of depressed subjects, but are reversed toward control levels by lithium treatment.

Together these studies demonstrate structural alterations of hippocampus and PFC subregions that are associated with depression. Importantly atrophy of these regions can be attenuated or even reversed with antidepressant treatment. This reversibility is a key feature that distinguishes depression from more permanent structural changes often observed in patients with neurodegenerative disorders. This is also supported by studies in rodent models demonstrating that neuronal atrophy caused by stress is reversible.

Nucleus accumbens and amygdala: In contrast to atrophy of hippocampus and PFC, there is evidence for hypertrophy or increased arbor of neuronal processes in the nucleus accumbens and amygdala in rodent models of depression (Duman and Aghajanian, 2012; Roozendaal, 2009). The nucleus accumbens is part of the mesolimbic dopamine system that controls motivation and reward, and the amygdala regulates emotion and fear. Alterations of these structures in depressed patients have also been identified (Price, 2010). In addition to structural changes, there is evidence for altered metabolic activity and connectivity between the nucleus accumbens, amygdala, PFC, hippocampus, and other cortical and limbic regions implicated in depression. This is consistent with preclinical studies that provide strong evidence for a role of the amygdala and mesolimbic dopamine system in anxiety and mood related behaviors (see Chapter 31).

HUMAN POSTMORTEM STUDIES OF DEPRESSION

The exact cellular changes underlying the volumetric decreases in depression have been difficult to identify and must rely solely on morphometric analysis of neurons in postmortem brain tissue of depressed subjects. These studies have begun to identify changes that are consistent with the brain imaging studies, showing a reduction in the size of neuronal cell bodies, decreased density of neurons, and decreased number of GABAergic interneurons in the dlPFC (Price, 2010; Rajkowska, 2007). The numbers of glia are also decreased in the dlPFC, as well as other cortical structures (Rajkowska, 2007). Postmortem studies of hippocampus report an increased packing density, implying that the neuronal body size is increased in depression. Preclinical studies also demonstrate that stress decreases adult hippocampal neurogenesis (Samuels, 2011). Although decreased neurogenesis has not been observed in postmortem tissue from depressed subjects, there are reports of increased cell birth in subjects treated with antidepressant medications at the time of death (Boldrini, 2012).

The reductions in PFC and hippocampal volume, combined with postmortem evidence for reduced size of neuronal cell bodies suggest that the processes and connections between neurons are also decreased in depression. However, the analysis of synaptic number has been hampered by poor fixation and tissue conditions. The first study to address this question recently reported that the number of synapses, determined by electron microscopy, is decreased in the dlPFC of MDD subjects (Kang, 2012). Supporting evidence for loss of spine synapses is provided by studies reporting decreased levels of synaptic signaling proteins in depressed subjects, including AMPA and NMDA receptor subtypes, presynaptic neurotransmitter vesicle-associated proteins, and postsynaptic structural and functional proteins in the dlPFC, hippocampus, and other forebrain structures (Duman and Aghajanian, 2012). These studies provide strong evidence of disrupted synaptic integrity and function in cortical and limbic brain regions of depressed subjects.

EVIDENCE FOR CELLULAR AND STRUCTURAL ALTERATIONS FROM RODENT STUDIES

The hypothesis that the pathophysiology of depression and stress-related psychiatric illnesses is related to structural alterations has gained significant support from preclinical studies of chronic stress models of depression. There are a number of chronic models that have been developed, including chronic unpredictable stress (CUS), which leads to behavioral anhedonia, a core symptom of depression that is reversed by chronic antidepressant administration, consistent with the therapeutic time lag seen in depressed patients. Chronic social defeat is another well-established model that is characterized by social interaction deficits, as well as anhedonia and vegetative differences, that are also reversed by chronic, but not acute antidepressant treatments (see Chapter 31 on preclinical models). These models contrast with acute helplessness paradigms, such as the forced swim test, in which animals respond rapidly after just a single antidepressant dose, and which are best known for their utility as drug screening paradigms.

Neuronal atrophy: Studies of the hippocampus were the first to demonstrate that chronic immobilization stress causes atrophy of neurons, notably a reduction in the number and length of the apical dendrites of CA3 pyramidal neurons (McEwen, 2012). Subsequent studies of chronic immobilization or CUS also demonstrate atrophy of the apical dendrites of pyramidal neurons in layers II/III and V of medial PFC (Fig. 32.2) (Duman and Aghajanian, 2012; Morrison, 2012). In addition, chronic stress causes a reduction in the number of spine synapses, the primary connection points between neurons, as well as a corresponding decrease in

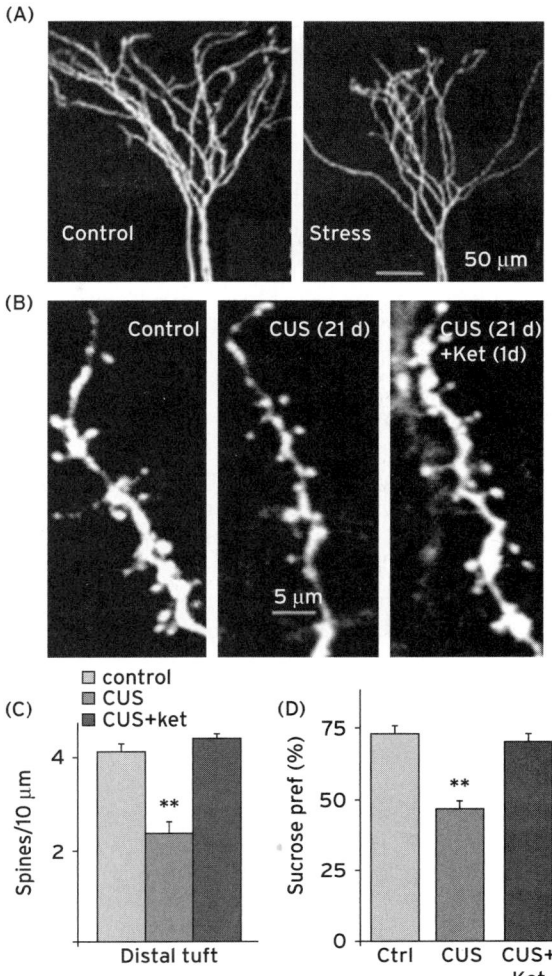

Figure 32.2 *Chronic stress causes atrophy of neurons in the PFC. (A) Shown are representative confocal photomicrographs of layer V pyramidal neurons in the medial PFC labeled with neurobiotin. Chronic immobilization stress (~30 min per day, 7 days) causes a reduction in the number and length of apical dendrites in PFC neurons. (B) CUS (21 days) decreases synaptic connections and produces depressive-like behavior that is rapidly reversed by a single dose of ketamine. Representative confocal images of single dendrites of labeled layer V pyramidal neurons in the medial PFC. CUS decreases the number of dendrites, and a single dose of ketamine rapidly reverses the deficit caused by CUS. (C) Quantitation of the numbers of spines on distal tufts of layer V neurons, further demonstrating the reversal of the CUS spine deficit by ketamine. (D) Influence of CUS ± ketamine on behavior in the sucrose preference test (measured by percent preference for a sucrose solution). The sucrose preference test provides a measure of anhedonia, a core symptom of depression that is rapidly reversed by a single dose of ketamine, compared to long-term administration (three weeks) needed for a typical antidepressant, such as a SSRI.*

neuronal function, demonstrated by a reduction in 5-HT and hypocretin-induced excitatory postsynaptic potentials (EPSPs) (Liu, 2008; Morrison, 2012). These changes are accompanied by altered synaptic glutamate transmission (Popoli, 2011). The atrophy of pyramidal neurons in the PFC is particularly sensitive to stress, with reductions of apical dendrites observed after as little as 30 to 45 minutes of immobilization stress per day for 7 days. Neuronal atrophy caused by stress exposure is reversible, either by removal of stress or with antidepressant treatment, consistent with clinical studies demonstrating that volumetric changes of PFC and hippocampus are reversible with treatment.

As previously discussed, pyramidal neurons of the basolateral amygdala undergo hypertrophy in response to chronic stress exposure (Roozendaal, 2009). This could represent an effect independent of other limbic and cortical structures or could be related to, and influenced by, connections with these regions. Notably, there are reciprocal connections between the PFC and amygdala, with the PFC exerting negative control of amygdala neuronal activity; reduction of the negative feedback from the PFC could account for hypertrophy of amygdala neurons and decreased control of emotion and mood.

Decreased neurogenesis: In addition to neuronal atrophy, stress exposure decreases the birth of new neurons in the adult hippocampus, one of the few neurogenic zones found in the adult brain (the other is the subventricular zone, which gives rise to new neurons in the olfactory bulb) (Samuels, 2011). Neural progenitor cells in the subgranular zone give rise to immature neurons that migrate into the granule cell layer and develop into mature, functional neurons over the course of four to six weeks. Acute or repeated stress exposure decreases the birth of new neurons, and recent studies demonstrate that this stress-induced decrement causes depression-related behaviors in rodents (Snyder, 2011). In contrast, chronic, but not acute administration of all classes of antidepressant treatment increases the birth of new neurons and blocks the effects of stress (Samuels, 2011). Antidepressant treatment is also associated with the birth of new neurons in postmortem hippocampus of MDD subjects (Boldrini, 2012). Moreover, the induction of new neurons in the hippocampus is required for some but not all antidepressant behaviors, linking this cellular process to antidepressant actions. These studies support a role for adult hippocampal neurogenesis in stress, depression, and antidepressant responses.

Glial loss: Decreased number of glia represents one of the most consistently reported postmortem findings in depression, and evidence from rodent stress models is compatible with these findings. This includes studies demonstrating that chronic stress decreases the proliferation of newborn oligodendrocytes in the PFC and astrocytes that express the marker glial fibrillary acidic protein (GFAP) in the PFC and hippocampus (Banasr, 2012). Astrocytes play an important role in the reuptake and termination of glutamate neurotransmitter signaling, as well as metabolism of amino acid neurotransmitters (Fig. 32.1). GFAP+ astrocytes, while capable of proliferation when activated by excitotoxic or mechanical injury, do not typically undergo proliferation under non-activated conditions. Oligodendrocytes are best known for myelination of neurons, but there are also subtypes that have morphological and functional characteristics similar to astrocytes. Oligodendrocyte precursors, labeled with the NG2 proteoglycan, continue to proliferate in the adult brain, and stress decreases the birth of these cells, an effect that could contribute to the decrease observed in depressed subjects. In contrast, chronic antidepressant treatment produces the opposite effect, increasing the number of NG2+ oligodendrocytes (Banasr, 2012).

STRESS-MEDIATED PATHWAYS IN DEPRESSION: THE HYPOTHALAMIC-PITUITARY-ADRENAL AXIS

The mechanisms underlying neuronal atrophy, reduced neurogenesis, and loss of glia are still being characterized, but are related to stress activation of the hypothalamic-pituitary-adrenal (HPA) axis and excess glucocorticoid levels, as well as activation of inflammatory cytokines. These systems then regulate a variety of other pathways that control all aspects of neuronal and glial function and survival, including regulation of growth factors and intracellular signaling cascades. Here we discuss the evidence demonstrating the role of these systems in stress, depression, and treatment response.

ELEVATION OF ADRENAL GLUCOCORTICOIDS IN STRESS AND DEPRESSION

One of the best-studied stress-activated systems is the HPA axis (Holsboer, 2010). Corticotrophin releasing factor (CRF), expressed in neurons in the paraventricular nucleus of the hypothalamus that project to the pituitary and, together with vasopressin, causes release of adrenocorticotrophin hormone (ACTH) into the circulatory system. ACTH then stimulates the biosynthesis and release of glucocorticoids in the adrenal cortex. Clinical studies have provided evidence that HPA activity is elevated in depressed subjects, with reports of increased levels of cortisol, the primary glucocorticoid in humans, and reduced responsiveness to administration of a synthetic glucocorticoid (i.e., dexamethasone suppression test). In fact, a recent extensive review of the literature (354 studies with 18,374 subjects) found that 73% of depressed patients had elevated cortisol levels compared to non-depressed controls (Stetler, 2011).

Glucocorticoids bind to two major types of receptors termed glucocorticoid (GR) and mineralcorticoid (MR), intracellular cytoplasmic receptors that when activated function as transcription factors and regulate expression of a wide range of target genes. MR has a higher affinity for glucocorticoids and mineralcorticoids and serves as the primary signaling receptor under normal, non-stressed physiological conditions, while GR has lower affinity and is only activated by higher, stress-induced levels of glucocorticoids. Both receptors are expressed throughout the brain, but levels of GR are particularly high in the hippocampus, as well as PFC and some other cortical regions. The hippocampus, hypothalamus, and pituitary also respond to glucocorticoids, which provides negative feedback control of HPA-axis release of glucocorticoids. Reductions of this important feedback system, measured in the dexamethasone suppression test, are often reported in depressed subjects, further demonstrating that this key stress response neuroendocrine system is overactivated in MDD (Holsboer, 2010). There is also evidence that levels of CRF are elevated in depressed subjects. In addition to signaling in the HPA axis, CRF and its receptor are expressed in other brain regions, including the amygdala, and have been implicated in the regulation of fear and anxiety, as well as depressive behaviors.

Preclinical studies demonstrate that high levels of glucocorticoids can account for many actions of chronic stress exposure on neurons and glia. Chronic exposure to corticosterone, the active glucocorticoid in rodents, causes atrophy of neurons in the PFC and hippocampus, similar to the effects of chronic stress (McEwen, 2012; Morrison, 2012). Chronic corticosterone exposure, also decreases neurogenesis in the adult hippocampus, and causes reduction of oligodendrocyte proliferation in the PFC (Banasr, 2012; Samuels, 2011). There is also evidence that chronic corticosterone administration decreases the expression of the astrocytic marker, GFAP. Together these findings indicate that elevated glucocorticoid levels could account for the neuronal and glial atrophy caused by chronic stress exposure, and for the atrophy of cortical and limbic brain regions observed in depressed patients.

The findings that stress and glucocorticoids can cause atrophy of neurons and loss of glia are unexpected, as it is difficult to understand the evolutionary advantage of this deleterious effect. However, in nature the stress response is designed to be active only for a transient, brief period of time, during the fight or flight response, and then rapidly return to baseline levels. Acute activation of the stress response systems is required for mobilizing energy and resources to the appropriate organs and tissues to provide a maximum response to danger conditions. However, problems occur when the stress is sustained over long periods of time, as is the case in modern daily human lives filled with stress related to social interactions, work demands, and other environmental conditions, which then results in deleterious effects on brain and many other organ systems.

INFLAMMATORY CYTOKINES AND DEPRESSION

EVIDENCE OF ELEVATED CYTOKINES IN DEPRESSION AND UNDERLYING MECHANISMS

Clinical studies have provided evidence that inflammatory cytokines play a role in the pathophysiology of depression and other mood disorders. Levels of several pro-inflammatory cytokines, including interleukin-1β (IL-1β) and IL-6, as well as tumor necrosis factor-α (TNFα), are increased in the blood of depressed patients compared to control subjects (Miller, 2009). These cytokines cause sickness behavior in rodents, characterized by suppressed locomotor activity, decreased social exploration, decreased food intake, lethargy, and anhedonia, many of which are also observed in depression. Treatment with interferon (IFN), a cytokine that strongly activates the immune system, causes high levels of depressive symptoms (i.e., ~50% of patients) when used as a treatment of certain cancers and viral infections (Raison, 2006). In addition, many illnesses, including diabetes, cancer, and cardiac disease, that have high rates of comorbidity with depression (~20–30%), are characterized by chronic inflammation (see Chapter 37). The inflammatory system can also be activated by psychological stressors, which may account in part for elevation of cytokines in depressed patients (Miller, 2009).

Inflammatory cytokines are released in the peripheral blood system by circulating macrophages, a primary cellular response

element of the innate as well as the adaptive immune system. In addition, inflammatory cytokines are released in the brain from microglial cells, which, like macrophages, are derived from monocytes. Typically, activation of macrophages and microglia occurs via a two-step process: first, via binding of danger substances (e.g., viral, bacterial, etc.) to a toll-like receptor (TLR) that couples to signaling pathways that increase pro-IL-1β gene transcription; and second by substances released during cell damage such as ATP, which activates the inflammasome system resulting in the processing and release of IL-1β. The importance of the latter is highlighted by the ability of IL-1β to act as a primary regulatory of the immune response, as it also leads to increased release of other cytokines such as IL-6 and TNFα.

The mechanisms underlying the release of inflammatory cytokines by psychological stress are less clear, but may involve increased glutamate transmission followed by release of ATP that stimulates microglia in the brain. Another unanswered question is how the peripheral and central inflammatory cytokine systems communicate. Cytokines are large peptides that cannot cross the blood-brain barrier under most conditions, although there may be active uptake, porous regions of the barrier, or conditions that make the barrier leaky and allow cytokines to cross into the brain. It is also notable that inflammatory cytokines are one of the most potent activators of the HPA axis and could contribute to elevated glucocorticoid levels in depression. However, glucocorticoids also suppress the immune system and cytokines, adding another layer of complexity and unanswered questions regarding the interaction and regulation of these related systems in depression.

CONSEQUENCES OF ELEVATED CYTOKINES

Inflammatory cytokines influence a wide range of cellular and neuronal signaling pathways. As is often the case they produce biphasic effects on neuronal systems, characterized by normal physiological responses at low levels but deleterious actions at higher levels caused by stress. For example, both IL-1β and TNFα have been implicated in cellular and behavioral models of learning and memory, but at high doses are known to cause sickness, anxiety, and depressive behaviors in rodent models (Yirmiya, 2011). IL-1β also decreases the birth of new neurons in the adult hippocampus, and blockade of IL-1β signaling with the endogenous antagonist IL-1Ra blocks the antineurogenic, as well as behavioral effects of stress exposure (Koo, 2009).

Inflammatory cytokines such as IL-1β activate the Ikk-nuclear factor-kappaB (NF-κB) signaling pathway, resulting in regulation of many aspects of neuronal function. This includes regulation of gene transcription, such as indoleamine 2,3-dioxygenase (IDO), an enzyme that degrades tryptophan to kynurenine. Earlier studies suggested that this could lead to decreased levels of 5-HT, a product of tryptophan metabolism, but kynurenine is also a precursor of quinolic acid, an NMDA receptor agonist that could cause neurotoxic damage. In addition, Ikk-NFkB signaling in the nucleus accumbens is upregulated by social defeat stress and underlies the morphological alterations caused by stress in this brain region (Christoffel, 2011). Further studies are needed to characterize the mechanisms underlying the behavioral actions of IL-1β, TNFα, and other inflammatory cytokines, as well as the role of these factors in neuronal atrophy and glial loss caused by stress.

INFLAMMATORY CYTOKINE TARGETS FOR ANTIDEPRESSANT THERAPEUTICS

The possibility that inflammatory cytokines can be targeted for the treatment of depression is supported by clinical studies demonstrating that blockade of TNFα, by administration of a neutralizing antibody (i.e., Etanercept), produces an antidepressant response in patients receiving treatment for psoriasis (Miller, 2009) (see Chapter 35). Further studies are needed to replicate this finding and to determine whether blockade of other inflammatory cytokines, such as IL-1β or IL-6 could be useful for the treatment of depression. There is also preclinical evidence that blockade of the ATP-purinergic receptor that activates IL-1β processing and release has antidepressant efficacy in rodent behavioral models. Combined with advanced biomarker testing, these strategies may hold promise for treating depressed patients that present with elevated levels of a specific inflammatory cytokine that could be directly corrected with appropriate antagonist or neutralizing agent.

ROLE OF NEUROTROPHIC FACTOR SUPPORT IN DEPRESSION AND TREATMENT RESPONSE

Activation of the HPA axis and elevation of adrenal glucocorticoids, as well as induction of inflammatory cytokines by stress, results in altered regulation of many neuronal systems that have been implicated in depression. Alterations of neurotrophic factors, particularly BDNF and related signaling pathways have been of particular interest because of the important role that these factors play in the formation and regulation of synapses, as well as the survival and function of neurons. Here we discuss evidence for the role of several key neurotrophic factors in the pathophysiology and treatment of depression. Long-lasting changes in the expression of neurotrophic factors, as well as other signaling molecules, due to epigenetic alterations have also been implicated in depression and treatment response and have been discussed in several excellent reviews (Krishnan, 2008; Sun, 2012).

STRESS DECREASES BDNF EXPRESSION AND SIGNALING: OPPOSING ACTIONS OF ANTIDEPRESSANTS

BDNF is a member of the nerve growth factor family, which also includes neurotrophin 3 and 4. These factors were originally discovered because of the important functions they serve during brain development, guiding the migration and maturation, as well as survival and function of neurons. However, these factors are also expressed in the adult brain, are regulated by neuronal activity, and are involved in synaptic plasticity, and neuronal function and survival (Martinowich, 2007). Initial studies demonstrated that chronic stress exposure decreases the expression of BDNF in the hippocampus and PFC, while chronic antidepressant administration produces the opposite effect and blocks the decreased expression caused by stress (Duman, 2006; Krishnan, 2008). The relevance of these findings is supported by postmortem studies demonstrating that levels of BDNF are decreased in the cerebral cortex of MDD subjects (Duman, 2006). Surprisingly, serum and plasma levels of BDNF are also decreased in depressed patients, and this deficit is reversed with antidepressant treatments (Duman, 2006; Dwivedi, 2010).

The actions of BDNF are mediated by a tyrosine kinase receptor, TrkB, that when stimulated leads to activation of several intracellular pathways including Ras–microtubule-associated protein kinase (MAPK) and phosphatidyl inositol-3 kinase (PI3K)/serine threonine kinase (Akt) (Duman and Voleti, 2012; Martinowich, 2007). These pathways positively influence synaptic maturation and stability via regulation of synaptic protein synthesis and glutamate receptor cycling (Collinridge, 2010; Hoeffer, 2010). Studies of rodent stress models and human postmortem tissue also demonstrate disruption of BDNF-TrkB receptor signaling, including reductions of ERK and Akt pathways in the hippocampus and PFC (Duman and Voleti, 2012; Duric, 2010). Stress and depression also influence BDNF-TrkB signaling by induction of a negative regulator, MAP kinase phosphatase 1, that is sufficient to cause depressive behaviors when expressed in rodent hippocampus (Duric, 2010). Chronic stress also decreases Akt signaling in the mesolimbic dopamine system. Another study has reported that chronic stress inhibits glutamate transmission via ubiquitin/proteasome-mediated degradation of glutamate receptors in the PFC, and that this effect is correlated with cognitive function (Duman and Aghajanian, 2012).

STUDIES OF BDNF MUTANT MICE AND A LOSS OF FUNCTIONAL HUMAN BDNF

GENE POLYMORPHISM

These findings, combined with brain imaging and postmortem studies, have contributed to a neurotrophic hypothesis of depression, which proposes that the neuronal and behavioral deficits caused by stress and depression result from decreased BDNF, and conversely that the actions of antidepressant treatment occur via induction of BDNF. The latter hypothesis is supported by studies demonstrating that the behavioral actions of antidepressants are blocked in BDNF deletion mutant mice, and that BDNF infusion into the hippocampus produces antidepressant responses (Autry, 2012; Duman, 2006).

The hypothesis that loss of BDNF underlies depressive behavior has been more complicated. Studies of mutant mice, including constitutive heterozygous deletion (homozygous mutants are lethal), as well as conditional forebrain deletion mutants have not reported evidence of a depressive phenotype with the exception that female conditional deletion mice show behavioral despair (Autry, 2012; Duman, 2006). However, BDNF deletion mutants are more vulnerable to stress, providing support for a gene x environment interaction, and targeted deletion of BDNF in the hippocampus is sufficient to cause depressive behaviors (Duman and Aghajanian, 2012). In contrast to the PFC and hippocampus, BDNF activity in the mesolimbic dopamine system produces prodepressive effects, demonstrating region-specific actions of this plasticity-related factor (Krishnan and Nestler, 2008). This could also account for the lack of overt behavioral phenotype in constitutive and forebrain deletion mutant mice, in which BDNF deletion in multiple different regions at the same time may have offsetting behavioral consequences.

There is also evidence that BDNF is involved in neuronal deficits caused by stress. In heterozygous deletion mutant mice there is a reduction in number and length of apical dendrites of CA3 pyramidal neurons of the hippocampus, and the effects of chronic stress are occluded, suggesting that BDNF reduction underlies the atrophy of dendrites (Duman and Aghajanian, 2012). There have also been studies of mice with a knockin of a loss of function variant of the BDNF gene, Val66Met, that is found in approximately 30% of humans (Dincheva, 2012). The Met allele decreases the transport of BDNF transcripts to dendrite compartments, where local protein synthesis occurs to support synaptogenesis and neuroplasticity. BDNF Met knockin mice display a reduction of dendrite length and branching, and decreased spine-synapse density, maturity, and function in the hippocampus and/or PFC (Duman and Aghajanian, 2012). Studies in humans demonstrate that carriers of the Met polymorphism have decreased hippocampal volume and reduced executive function and if exposed to early life stress are more vulnerable to depressive symptoms (Duman and Aghajanian, 2012).

OTHER TROPHIC FACTORS IMPLICATED IN STRESS, DEPRESSION AND ANTIDEPRESSANT TREATMENT

There are several other neurotrophic/growth factors that have been implicated in depression, including vascular endothelial growth factor (VEGF), fibroblast growth factor 2 (FGF2), and insulin-like growth factor 1(IGF1). Altered regulation and function of these factors is not surprising given that, like BDNF, they are regulated by neuronal activity, neuroendocrine, and inflammatory factors that are dysregulated by stress and depression. Chronic exposure to stress decreases the expression of VEGF in rodent hippocampus, and levels of FGF2 are decreased in postmortem cerebral cortex of depressed subjects; conversely, antidepressant treatment increases the expression of VEGF and FGF2 in cortical and/or hippocampal brain regions (Duman and Voleti, 2012). In addition, central infusions of VEGF, FGF2, or IGF1 produce antidepressant actions in behavioral models of depression, and blockade of VEGF or FGF2 signaling blocks the response to antidepressant treatments (Duman and Voleti, 2012). These studies demonstrate a complex interaction between these trophic factors and their intracellular signaling pathways, all of which include activation of intracellular tyrosine kinase domains and Ras-MAPK and PI3K-Akt signaling pathways. This overlap may suggest convergence of growth factor receptor signaling on neurons and glia, but it is also possible that different populations of neurons and glia are differentially regulated by these factors. This represents a small number of the growth factors and cytokines that control brain function, and it is likely that there

are other factors and signaling pathways involved in depression and treatment response yet to be discovered.

RAPID-ACTING ANTIDEPRESSANTS INCREASE SYNAPTOGENESIS

Currently available antidepressants that influence monoamine levels require weeks to months to produce a therapeutic response and are only effective in about one-third of patients, and up to two-thirds with multiple trials that can take years. This underscores a major unmet need, particularly for depressed patients at high risk for suicide. In this context, one of the most important findings in the field of depression is the discovery that a single dose of ketamine, an NMDA receptor antagonist, produces rapid antidepressant actions (clinical improvement within two hours) in treatment-resistant depressed patients (Machado-Vieira, 2011). These treatment-resistant patients have failed to respond to two or more typical antidepressants, and the antidepressant response to single-dose ketamine is sustained for 7 to 10 days. Ketamine also produces a rapid antidepressant effect in bipolar depressed patients and decreases suicide ideation. The fast, efficacious actions of ketamine by a completely different mechanism than typical monoamine reuptake inhibitors, NMDA receptor blockade, make this arguably the most exciting advance for depression therapeutics in 50 years. Preclinical studies have demonstrated that ketamine rapidly increases the number and function of synaptic connections, which provides further evidence that synaptogenesis is an important process for the treatment of depression, and that loss of synaptic connections contributes to the pathophysiology of depression (Figs. 32.2 and 32.3).

KETAMINE INCREASES SYNAPTOGENESIS AND mTOR SIGNALING

The profound clinical actions of ketamine have stimulated studies to identify the mechanisms underlying its rapid, efficacious antidepressant actions. These studies have been equally exciting, demonstrating that a single dose of ketamine rapidly increases the formation of new synaptic connections and activates neurotrophic factor translational signaling pathways (Fig. 32.3). A single dose of ketamine increases the number and function of spine synapses in layer V pyramidal neurons of the medial PFC (Li, 2010). Biochemical studies demonstrate that ketamine administration increases levels of synaptic proteins by two hours, indicating that synaptogenesis has started to take place at this early time point, which coincides with the therapeutic response to ketamine. The increase in synaptic number is accompanied by increased number of "mushroom" spines, indicative of mature or stable synapses. At a functional level, there is also an increase in 5-HT and hypocretin-induced excitatory postsynaptic potentials (EPSPs), including increased frequency and amplitude, which are directly correlated with the number and maturation/stability of spine synapses, respectively. Behavioral studies also demonstrate that a single dose of ketamine produces a rapid antidepressant response in the FST, learned helplessness paradigm, and novelty-suppressed feeding

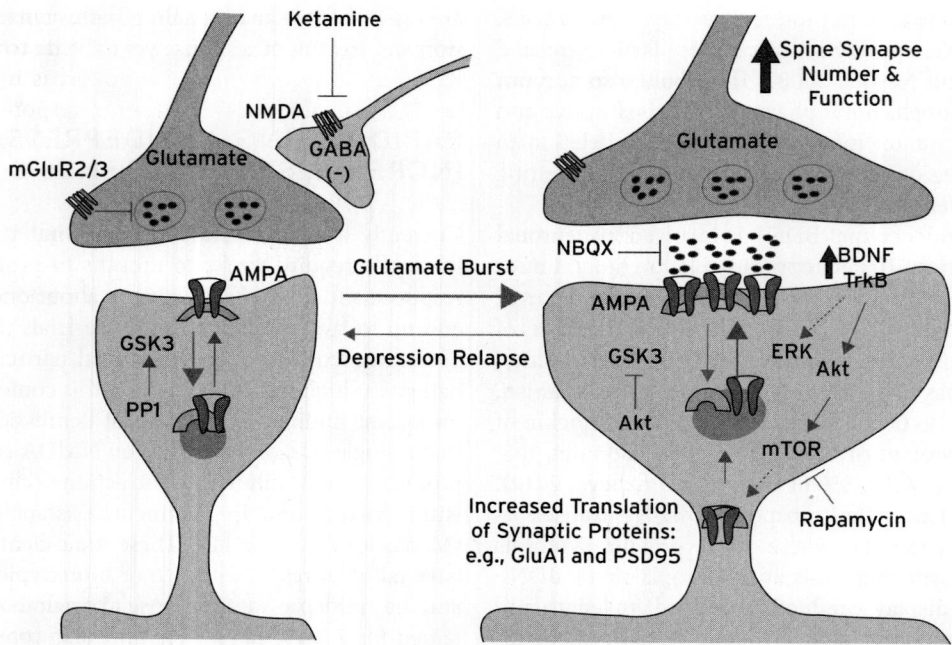

Figure 32.3 *Model for the loss of spine synapses caused by stress and rapid reversal by ketamine. The numbers of synapse connections in the PFC and other structures are maintained by homeostatic mechanisms that contribute to regular mood. This includes cycling of glutamate A1 (GluA1) receptors to and from the synapse. Chronic stress exposure decreases the number of spine synapses, as well as the expression of BDNF, which is thought to contribute to the loss of synapses and neuronal atrophy. GSK3, which is increased in depression, can be activated by protein phosphatase 1 (PP1) and may also contribute to synaptic destabilization, by promoting the internalization of GluA1. Ketamine rapidly increases glutamate transmission and synaptogenesis, resulting in a glutamate burst. The induction of spine synapses requires activation of BDNF/TrkB signaling, and stimulation of the Akt and mTOR pathways, resulting in increased translation of synaptic proteins, including GluA1. The behavioral actions of ketamine are also dependent on inhibition of GSK3, which could occur via stimulation of Akt or by blockade of NMDA receptors and PP1 (not shown). Depressed patients treated with ketamine relapse after 7 to 10 days, possibly due to failure to maintain new synaptic connections, which could be a result of genetic mutations or environmental factors such as sustained or uncontrollable stress.*

test. In addition, a single dose of ketamine rapidly reverses the deficits in synapses and depressive behavior caused by chronic stress exposure (Fig. 32.2), effects that are only observed after chronic administration of a typical antidepressant (Duman and Aghajanian, 2012).

The increase in synaptogenesis is preceded by induction of the mammalian target of rapamycin (mTOR) signaling pathway (Fig. 32.3). This pathway includes a number of up- and downstream elements that allow for summation of hormonal, metabolic, energy, and cell activity signaling to control cellular rates of protein translation. The mTOR system is found throughout the body, and in neurons is located in cell bodies and nerve terminals, where it has been linked to protein synthesis dependent synaptic plasticity (Hoefer and Klann, 2010). A single dose of ketamine rapidly activates the mTOR signaling pathway in preparations of nerve terminals of PFC, including increased levels of the phosphorylated and activated forms of mTOR, p70S6 kinase, and 4-EB-P1 (Li, 2010). This leads to increased translation and levels of synaptic proteins, including glutamate receptor 1 (GluA1), postsynaptic density protein 95 (PSD95), and synapsin 1. Evidence that mTOR signaling is required for the actions of ketamine is provided by studies showing that the synaptogenic and behavioral responses are blocked by preinfusion of the mTOR inhibitor, rapamycin (Li, 2010).

The mechanisms underlying the rapid synaptogenic and mTOR signaling effects of ketamine are still being studied, but there is evidence that these effects require activation of AMPA receptors (Duman and Aghajanian, 2012; Li, 2010). There is also evidence that ketamine causes a rapid and transient "burst" of glutamate transmission in the PFC, possibly resulting from blockade of NMDA receptors on GABAergic interneurons and disinhibition of glutamate transmission (Duman and Aghajanian, 2012). The actions of ketamine are blocked by pretreatment with an AMPA receptor antagonist, and studies in cultured cells demonstrate that AMPA receptor activation results in stimulation of mTOR signaling. The studies in cultured cells also demonstrate that stimulation of mTOR signaling requires the release of BDNF, and studies in BDNF deletion mutant mice or BDNF Val/Met mice demonstrate that BDNF is required for the synaptogenic and behavioral actions of ketamine (Duman and Aghajanian, 2012). The clinical response to ketamine is also significantly reduced in carriers of the Met allele, providing the first evidence that antidepressant responses are influenced by a genetic polymorphism (Laje et al., 2012).

NOVEL KETAMINE-LIKE TARGETS FOR THE TREATMENT OF DEPRESSION

Although ketamine produces rapid and robust antidepressant actions, the psychotomimetic effects and abuse potential of this drug limit its widespread use for the treatment of depression. However, based on the evidence that ketamine acts via the glutamate neurotransmitter system there are several potential targets that could produce ketamine-like actions, without the negative side effects. There is evidence that the NR2B subtype of the NMDA receptor mediates the actions of ketamine, including evidence from preclinical and clinical studies (Duman and Aghajanian, 2012; Li, 2010), and clinical trials are currently underway to further test the efficacy, rapid response, and safety of these agents.

Preclinical studies demonstrating that ketamine causes a transient burst of glutamate suggest that targeting other sites that cause a similar induction of glutamate transmission or directly activate AMPA receptors could produce antidepressant responses. This is supported by studies demonstrating that blockade of Group II metabotropic glutamate receptors (mGluR), which include mGluR2 and 3 (mGluR2/3), that are located presynaptically and regulate the release of glutamate (Fig. 32.1), produce rapid behavioral responses in rodent models that require mTOR signaling (Duman and Aghajanian, 2012; Duman and Voleti, 2012). Studies are currently underway to determine if mGluR2/3 antagonists also produce rapid synaptogenic actions and block or reverse the effects of chronic stress similar to ketamine.

Agents that are direct acting agonists of AMPA receptors cause seizures, but compounds have been developed that are modulators of AMPA receptors and could potentially be used in humans. These agents enhance the opening time or decrease the desensitization of AMPA receptors and thereby serve as positive allosteric modulators (PAMs), also referred to as AMPAkines. There are reports that AMPAkines can produce antidepressant responses in rodent models, and can activate mTOR signaling in cultured neurons (Duman and Aghajanian, 2012). Additional studies are needed to determine if these agents also produce rapid synaptogenic actions and antidepressant responses in CUS models. In addition, it will be important to closely examine the safety and side effect profile of AMPAkines,

as well as other drugs that modulate glutamate transmission, which could also have limitations similar to ketamine.

Another area of research interest is to determine if it is possible to extend the therapeutic response time of a single dose of ketamine. Research studies demonstrate that patients administered ketamine relapse 7 to 10 days after treatment (Machado-Vieira et al., 2011). Work is underway to determine if treatment with another agent after, or even prior to ketamine, could sustain the antidepressant response and thereby negate the need for repeated ketamine administration, which could produce the unwanted side effects. Studies with typical antidepressants, other glutamate compounds, or lithium are currently under investigation.

CONCLUSIONS

Clinical and preclinical studies provide clear evidence of alterations of glutamate and GABA neurotransmission, limbic and cortical brain regions, connectivity, and growth factor and cytokine levels and related signaling pathways. Additional imaging approaches that provide improved static and functional markers of synaptic connections, as well as postmortem studies of ultrastructural changes are needed to further define the abnormal circuitry in depression. There is also evidence for genetic polymorphisms that increase risk for these structural alterations and that are associated with depression, particularly when combined with environmental factors such as lifetime incidence of stress exposure, as well as diet and exercise (Fig. 32.4). Such gene x environment interactions can explain the individual variability and risk for depression. Further studies of single or multiple gene polymorphisms within an individual are needed to better elucidate the basis of depression. Evidence from genetic studies of other psychiatric illnesses, as well as other traits, indicates

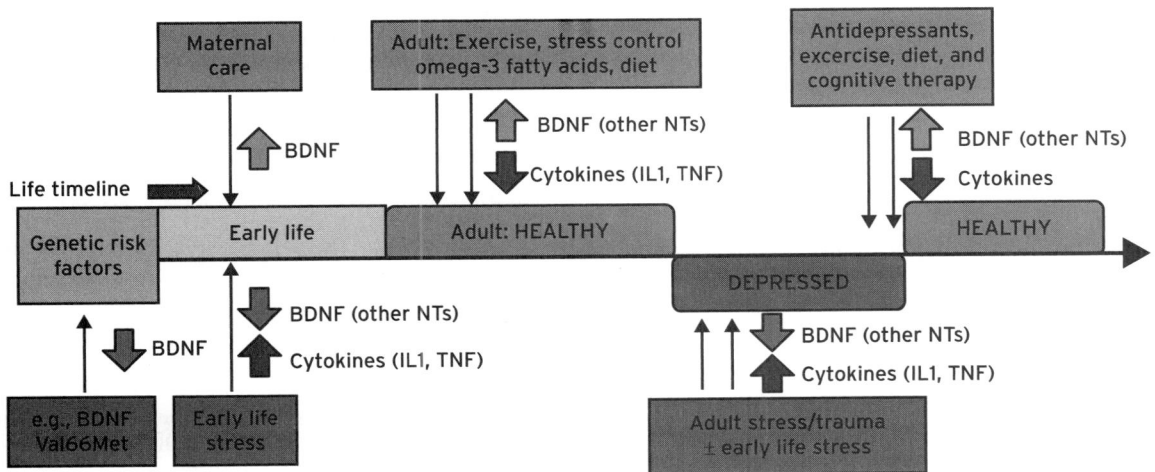

Figure 32.4 Timeline of genetic and environmental factors that regulate neurotrophic factors (NTs) and inflammatory cytokines that influence emotion and mood. Genetic risk factors, such as the BDNF Val/Met polymorphism and stress can exacerbate depressive symptoms, while antidepressants, exercise, and diet may ameliorate depressive symptoms, in part, through regulation of neurotrophic factors and inflammatory cytokines. The up- or downregulation of BDNF and inflammatory cytokines by stress and environmental factors can shift the balance from depressed to healthy, and vice versa. This could explain the heterogeneity of depression, as an individual may have a different combination of genetic risk factors and environmental factors that result in alterations of one or more growth factors and cytokines. Analysis of multiple neurotrophic/growth factors and inflammatory cytokines could provide an individualized signature of depression that would allow targeted, more efficacious treatment strategies (e.g., treatments that increase a particular neurotrophic factor or neutralize/block a specific cytokine).

that there are likely to be hundreds of gene polymorphisms that contribute to depression, accounting for the large degree of heterogeneity of this disorder.

These genetic and environmental factors, however, may have some targets in common, including alterations of the HPA axis, specific neurocircuits, inflammatory cytokines, and neurotrophic factors. While not every case of depression will have the same molecular and cellular signature, evidence is mounting that one or more of these markers (e.g., neurotrophic/growth factors such as BDNF, VEGF, FGF2, and/or IGF1; inflammatory cytokines such as IL-1β, IL6, and/or TNFα) when combined with functional and structural imaging could be used as biomarkers of depressive illness and response to different antidepressant treatments. This could allow for more efficacious, targeted, individualized medicine. For example, blockade or neutralizing a specific inflammatory cytokine that is elevated, or treatments that enhance a specific neurotrophic factor as needed. These approaches, combined with a new generation of ketamine-like agents that are rapid acting, efficacious, and safe, hold promise for a new era for the treatment of depression.

ACKNOWLEDGMENTS

This work is supported by USPHS grants MH45481, by a Veterans Administration National Center Grant for PTSD at the West Haven, Connecticut, VA Medical Center, and the State of Connecticut Department of Mental Health and Addiction Services.

DISCLOSURES

Dr. Duman has served as a consultant and/or provided scientific lectures for Pfizer, Lilly, Johnson & Johnson, Bristol Myers Squibb, Lundbeck, Forest, Taisho, and Roche. Dr. Duman has no conflicts with the material presented in this chapter.

REFERENCES

Autry, A., and Monteggia, L.M. (2012). Brain-derived neurotrophic factor and neuropsychiatric disorders. *Pharmacol. Rev.* 64(2):238–258.

Banasr, M., Dwyer, J.M., et al. (2012). Cell atrophy and loss in depression: reversal by antidepressant treatment. *Curr. Opin. Cell. Biol.* 23(6):730–737.

Boldrini, M., Hen, R., et al. (2012). Hippocampal angiogenesis and progenitor cell proliferation are increased with antidepressant use in major depression. *Biol. Psych.* Epub, ahead of print.

Caspi, A., Hariri, A.R., et al. (2010). Genetic sensitivity to the environment: the case of the serotonin transporter gene and its implications for studying complex diseases and traits. *Am. J. Psychiatry* 167(5):509–527.

Christoffel, D., Golden, S.A., et al. (2011). IκB kinase regulates social defeat stress-induced synaptic and behavioral plasticity. *J. Neurosci.* 31(1):314–321.

Collinridge, G., Peineau, S., et al. (2010). Long-range depression in the CNS. *Nat. Rev. Neurosci.* 11(7):459–473.

Dincheva, I., Glatt, C.E., et al. (2012). Impact of the BDNF Val66Met polymorphism on cognition: implications for behavioral genetics. *Neuroscientist.* Epub, ahead of print.

Drevets, W., Price, J.L., et al. (2008). Brain structural and functional abnormalities in mood disorders: implications for neurocircuitry models of depression. *Brain Struct. Funct.* 213(1–2):93–118.

Duman, R., and Aghajanian, G.K. (2012). Synaptic dysfunction in depression: novel therapeutic targets. *Science* 338(6103):68–72.

Duman, R., and Monteggia, L.M. (2006). A neurotrophic model for stress-related mood disorders. *Biol. Psych.* 59(12):1116–1127.

Duman, R., and Voleti, B. (2012). Signaling pathways underlying the pathophysiology and treatment of depression: novel mechanisms for rapid-acting agents. *Trends. Neurosci.* 35(1):47–56.

Duric, V., Banasr, M., et al. (2010). Negative regulator of MAP kinase is increased in depression and is necessary and sufficient for depressive behavior. *Nat. Med.* 16(11):1328–1332.

Dwivedi, Y. (2010). Brain-derived neurotrophic factor and suicide pathogenesis. *Ann. Med.* 42(2):87–96.

Heninger, G., Delgado, P.L., et al. (1996). The revised monoamine theory of depression: a modulatory role for monoamines, based on new findings from monoamine depletion experiments in humans. *Pharmacopsychiatry* 29(1):2–11.

Hoeffer, C., and Klann, E. (2010). mTOR signaling: at the crossroads of plasticity, memory and disease. *Trends. Neurosci.* 33(2):67–75.

Holsboer, F., and Ising, M. (2010). Stress hormone regulation: biological role and translation into therapy. *Annu. Rev. Psychol.* 61:81–109.

Jacobsen, J., Medvedev, I.O., et al. (2012). The 5-HT deficiency theory of depression: perspectives from a naturalistic 5-HT deficiency model, the tryptophan hydroxylase 2Arg439His knockin mouse. *Philos. Trans. R. Soc. Lond. B Biol. Sci.* 367(1601):2444–2459.

Kang, H., Voleti, B., et al. (2012). Decreased expression of synapse-related genes and loss of synapses in major depressive disorder. *Nat. Med.* 18(9):1413–1417.

Karolewicz, B., Maciag, D., et al. (2010). Reduced level of glutamic acid decarboxylase-67 kDa in the prefrontal cortex in major depression. *Int. J. Neuropsychopharmacol.* 13(4):411–420.

Karpova, N., Pickenhagen, A., et al. (2011). Fear erasure in mice requires synergy between antidepressant drugs and extinction training. *Science* 334(6063):1731–1734.

Kessler, R., Chiu, W.T., et al. (2005). Prevalence, severity, and comorbidity of 12-month DSM-IV disorders in the National Comorbidity Survey Replication. *Arch. Gen. Psych.* 62(6):617–627.

Koo, J., and Duman, R.S. (2009). Evidence for IL-1 receptor blockade as a therapeutic strategy for the treatment of depression. *Curr. Opin. Invest. Drugs* 10(7):664–671.

Krishnan, V., Nestler, E.J. (2008). The molecular neurobiology of depression. *Nature.* 455:894–902.

Levinson, A., Fitzgerald, P.B., et al. (2010). Evidence of cortical inhibitory deficits in major depressive disorder. *Biol. Psych.* 67(5):458–464.

Li, N., Lee, B.Y., et al. (2010). mTOR-dependent synapse formation underlies the rapid antidepressant effects of NMDA antagonists. *Science* 329:959–964.

Liu, R.-J., and Aghajanian, G.K. (2008). Stress blunts serotonin- and hypocretin-evoked EPSCs in prefrontal cortex: role of corticosterone-mediated apical dendritic atrophy. *Proc. Natl. Acad. Sci. USA* 105(1):359–364.

Machado-Vieira, R., Ibrahim, L., et al. (2011). Novel glutamatergic agents for major depressive disorder and bipolar disorder. *Pharmacol. Biochem. Behav.* 100(4):678–687.

Maciag, D., Hughes, J., et al. (2009). Reduced density of calbindin immunoreactive GABAergic neurons in the occipital cortex in major depression: relevance to neuroimaging studies. *Biol. Psych.* 67:465–470.

MacQueen, G., and Frodl, T. (2011). The hippocampus in major depression: evidence for the convergence of the bench and bedside in psychiatric research? *Mol. Psych.* 16(3):252–264.

Martinowich, K., Mannji, H., et al. (2007). New insights into BDNF function in depression and anxiety. *Nat. Neurosci.* 10(9):1089–1093.

Maya Vetencourt, J., Sale, A., et al. (2008). The antidepressant fluoxetine restores plasticity in the adult visual cortex. *Science* 320(5874):385–388.

McEwen, B., Eiland, L., et al. (2012). Stress and anxiety: structural plasticity and epigenetic regulation as a consequence of stress. *Neuropharmacology* 62(1):3–12.

Miller, A., Maletic, V., et al. (2009). Inflammation and its discontents: the role of cytokines in the pathophysiology of major depression. *Biol. Psych.* 65(9):732–741.

Morrison, J., and Baxter, M.G. (2012). The ageing cortical synapse: hallmarks and implications for cognitive decline. *Nat. Rev. Neurosci.* 13(4):240–250.

Popoli, M., Yan, Z., et al. (2011). The stressed synapse: the impact of stress and glucocorticoids on glutamate transmission. *Nat. Rev. Neurosci.* 13(1):22–37.

Price, J., and Drevets, W.C. (2010). Neurocircuitry of mood disorders. *Neuropsychopharmacol.* 35(1):192–116.

Raison, C. L., Capuron, L., et al. (2006). Cytokines sing the blues: inflammation and the pathogenesis of depression [Review]. *Trends Immunol.* 27(1):24–31.

Rajkowska, G., and Miguel-Hidalgo, J.J. (2007). Gliogenesis and glial pathology in depression. *CNS Neurol. Disord. Drug Targets* 6(3):219–233.

Roozendaal, B., McEwen, B.S., et al. (2009). Stress, memory and the amygdala. *Nat. Rev. Neurosci.* 10(6):423–433.

Samuels, B., and Hen, R. (2011). Neurogenesis and affective disorders. *Eur. J. Neurosci.* 33(6):1460–1468.

Sanacora, G., Gueorguieva, R., et al. (2004). Subtype-specific alterations of γ-aminobutyric acid and glutamate in patients with major depression. *Arch. Gen. Psychiatry* 61:705–713.

Sanacora, G., and Saricicek, A. (2007). GABAergic contributions to the pathophysiology of depression and the mechanism of antidepressant action. *CNS Neurol. Disord. Drug Targets* 6:127–140.

Snyder, J., Soumier, A., et al. (2011). Adult hippocampal neurogenesis buffers stress responses and depressive behaviour. *Nature* 476(7361):458–461.

Stetler, C., and Miller, G.E. (2011). Depression and hypothalamic-pituitary-adrenal activation: a quantitative summary of four decades of research. *Psychosom. Med.* 73:114–126.

Sun, H., Kennedy, P.J., et al. (2012). Epigenetics of the depressed brain: role of histone acetylation and methylation. *Neuropsychomacol.* Epub, ahead of print.

Trivedi, M., Rush, A.J., et al. (2006). Evaluation of outcomes with citalopram for depression using measurement-based care in STAR*D: implications for clinical practice. *Am. J. Psych.* 163(1):28–40.

Yirmiya, R., and Goshen, I. (2011). Immune modulation of learning, memory, neural plasticity and neurogenesis. *Br. Behav. Immun.* 25(2):181–213.

Yuen, E., Wei, J., et al. (2012). Repeated stress causes cognitive impairment by suppressing glutamate receptor expression and function in prefrontal cortex. *Neuron* 73(5):962–977.

Yüksel, C., and Öngür, D. (2010). Magnetic resonance spectroscopy studies of glutamate-related abnormalities in mood disorders. *Biol. Psych.* 68(9):785–794.

Zarate, C.J., Singh, J.B., et al. (2006). A randomized trial of an *N*-methyl-D-aspartate antagonist in treatment-resistant major depression. *Arch. Gen. Psych.* 63(8):856–864.

33 | PATHOGENESIS OF DEPRESSION: CLINICAL STUDIES

MAURA A. FUREY, DANIEL C. MATHEWS, AND CARLOS A. ZARATE Jr.

INTRODUCTION

Interest in the biological mechanism of action underlying depression was stimulated largely by serendipitous use of antituberculosis drugs in the 1950s. One of these drugs, imipramine, became the first tricyclic antidepressant medication. Subsequent understanding of this class of drugs led researchers to speculate on the modulatory effects of noradrenergic and serotonergic systems given their ubiquitous presence in the brain. This led to drug discovery efforts including, but not limited to, tricyclic antidepressants (TCAs), monoamine reuptake inhibitors (MAOIs), and serotonin/norepinephrine reuptake inhibitors (SSRIs/SNRIs), representing the primary therapeutic targets in the treatment of depression. While diseases are largely defined by distinct pathophysiologies, depression as a syndrome manifests clinically as a heterogeneous condition, which suggests various or multiple underlying mechanisms of action (Krishnan and Nestler, 2008, 2010).

Since the first antidepressant was introduced, a vast number of agents that regulate serotonin or norepinephrine have been developed, primarily as refinements over previous versions. With the exception of improvements in safety and side effect profiles, no significant progress in the efficacy of one class of antidepressant over another has occurred. Considerable effort has been made in industry, academia, and government to identify alternative drugs targets. Indeed, a number of compounds that produce promising results in preclinical studies failed to translate to an effective antidepressant at the clinical level; examples include NK1 and CRF antagonists (Madaan and Wilson, 2009). There are many reasons for the lack of success in developing novel treatments, most of which are beyond the scope of this chapter. One reason related to the chapter topic is the lack of disease biomarkers that predict clinical efficacy (Leuchter et al., 2010). A biomarker has been defined as "a characteristic that is objectively measured and evaluated as an indicator of normal biological processes, pathogenic processes, or pharmacological responses to a therapeutic intervention" (Frank and Hargreaves, 2003). Recent biomarker development has focused on existing antidepressants, and thus is limited by the inherent limitations of conventional treatments.

A potentially more successful approach would be to study treatments that are radically different from existing antidepressants, such as ketamine and scopolamine, where rapid antidepressant effects are observed in contrast to the slow response time associated with conventional treatments. The rapid clinical response observed with ketamine and scopolamine offers a unique opportunity to evaluate biomarkers quickly with the goal of gaining a better understanding of the pathogenesis of depression and identifying neural signatures of treatment response. Biomarkers can be of great significance as they can prioritize resources and allow for earlier testing in proof-of-concept studies with novel therapeutic agents, especially if a target is well identified. Biomarker studies vary greatly by approach and can target predictors of treatment response based on clinical laboratory markers (e.g., genetic and epigenetic markers, neurotransmitters, hormones, cytokines, neuropeptides, and enzymes), electrophysiological measures (e.g., electroencephalography [EEG] measures, sleep EEG, evoked potentials, magnetic encephalography [MEG], and skin conductance) functional neuroimaging indices (e.g., magnetic resonance imaging [MRI], functional MRI, magnetic resonance spectroscopy [MRS], positron emission tomography [PET], and single photon emission computed tomography [SPECT]), as well as details in clinical history (Wiedemann, 2011).

An improved understanding of the pathogenesis of depression has the potential to contribute to the development of improved therapies. Moreover, insights gained with this strategy would in turn help basic scientists focus on the presumptive molecular and cellular mechanisms that underlie these radically improved treatments. In fact, clinical studies with ketamine have stimulated preclinical research to understand the molecular and cellular underpinnings that might be involved in ketamine's rapid antidepressant effects (Aan Het Rot et al., 2012).

Consequently, this chapter will not review the serotonergic or noradrenergic systems, but instead will selectively summarize recent developments from well-designed clinical trials on other targets, such as the glutamatergic and cholinergic systems. The chapter will also characterize potential biological markers that may predict treatment response to these agents. In this chapter, when available, we review the randomized, placebo-controlled pharmacological trials in MDD and BD that have been conducted exploring these novel targets/systems. We briefly review uncontrolled studies only when the results lead to a randomized controlled clinical trial, and thus the uncontrolled study provides relevant historical context to the testing of the target being explored. We do not review trials with non-pharmacological approaches (e.g., deep brain stimulation and transcranial magnetic stimulation).

THE GLUTAMATERGIC SYSTEM

HISTORY OF THE GLUTAMATERGIC SYSTEM

Understanding the role of glutamatergic neurotransmission has developed gradually over time, particularly when compared to the current levels of interest for research related to the glutamate system and focus on potential applications. High concentrations of glutamate in the brain were first recognized in the 1930s, which led to several trials in the 1940s utilizing dietary glutamate and glutamine for the potential treatment of epilepsy and learning disorders. In the early 1950s, a pivotal animal study demonstrated that an injection of glutamate into the brain of a rat produced convulsions, which led to speculation that glutamate might be a primary excitatory neurotransmitter in the mammalian brain. Subsequent studies demonstrated that glutamate mediated excitatory action via multiple receptors, which were initially classified as N-methyl-D-aspartate (NMDA) and non-NMDA receptors. The latter was subdivided into what are now α-amino-3-hydroxy-5-methyl-4-isoxazolepropionic acid (AMPA) and kainate receptors after learning that agonists and antagonists preferentially interacted with these receptors. By 1977, a study validated NMDA receptors as synaptic receptors, and in the following 20 years key preclinical studies confirmed that NMDA antagonists inhibited long-term potentiation in the hippocampus (important in learning and memory) and mitigated behavioral deficits seen in inescapable stress paradigms comparable to that of clinically effective antidepressants. While much of the early impetus in psychiatry was led by these preclinical studies, recent remarkable clinical observations—particularly the antidepressant effects observed with ketamine—have resulted in increased interest in the identification of potential targets within the complex and dynamic framework of the glutamatergic system (Murrough, 2012; Watkins and Jane, 2006).

GLUTAMATERGIC RECEPTORS AND BASIC PHYSIOLOGY

Glutamate is found in exponentially higher concentrations than monoamines and is considered the most abundant neurotransmitter in the brain. The excitatory effects of glutamate are primarily balanced by another neurotransmitter, γ-aminobutyric acid (GABA), which mediates the greater part of fast inhibitory neurotransmission. This tight regulation of glutamate is of significance as undue glutamate excitotoxicity is implicated in several neuropsychiatric disorders. Most neuronal glutamate is generated either *de novo* via the transamination of α-oxogluturate through the Krebs cycle or by recycling from the glutamate/glutamine cycle. In a simplified model, glutamate acts in three different cell compartments—the presynaptic neuron, postsynaptic neuron, and surrounding glial cells. This model also involves other targets involved in the regulation of synaptic and extrasynaptic glutamate levels. Broadly, glutamate primarily activates diverse ionotropic (NMDA, α-amino-3-hydroxy-5-methyl-4-isoxazolepropionic (AMPA), and kainate (KA) receptors) and eight types of G protein–coupled metabotropic (mGluR) receptors. Other targets include excitatory amino acid transporters (EAATs), which provide glutamate clearance from extracellular space, soluble N-ethylmaleimide-sensitive factor attachment receptor (SNARE) complexes, which are thought to play a role in the structural aspects of synaptic vesicle exocytosis, vesicular glutamate transporters (VGLUTs), which are responsible for the uptake of glutamate into the synaptic vesicle, and cytoplasmic postsynaptic density proteins.

Of note, while glial cells have several functions and far outnumber neurons, they are especially crucial in the clearance and recycling of neurotransmitters, such as glutamate via the glutamate/glutamine cycle. The coupling between glutamatergic neurons and surrounding glial cells is fundamental, as impaired glial cell activity may lead to neuronal toxicity or increased glutamatergic activation. Mounting evidence suggests that frontal cortical areas of subjects with major depression or bipolar disorder have lower numbers of glial cells than non-psychiatric controls. Glial loss in the prefrontal cortex induces depressive-like behaviors similar to chronic stress in preclinical models. Other pathophysiological findings associated with glutamatergic neurotransmission have been drawn from postmortem, gene expression, and neuroimaging studies, such as magnetic resonance spectroscopy (MRS). (For a more complete review of the anatomy of the glutamatergic system and its role in depression and moods disorders, see Machado-Vieira et al., 2012; Machado-Vieira, Manji, 2009.) The complex physiological regulation of glutamate may provide an array of targets for future pharmacologic development and drug discovery.

CLINICAL TRIALS WITH GLUTAMATERGIC AGENTS

Placebo-controlled clinical trials (and select uncontrolled trials) with glutamatergic targets are summarized in Table 33.1.

NMDA ANTAGONISTS—KETAMINE

Of the three major subtypes of ionotropic receptors, NMDA and AMPA receptors have shown compelling evidence of their role in antidepressant action. A significant "proof of concept" translation of NMDA antagonists with MDD patients in clinical trials has been notable particularly with ketamine. Ketamine is a noncompetitive, high affinity NMDA antagonist that was first developed by Parke-Davis in 1963 as a safer anesthetic compared to phencyclidine (PCP). Ketamine is metabolized by the liver into two primary metabolites, norketamine (major metabolite) and dehydronorketamine (DHNK—minor, inactive metabolite) with a half-life of two to two and a half hours. A series of other metabolites of ketamine have been identified recently, some lasting up to three days (Zarate et al., 2012a). Several preclinical studies demonstrated that ketamine produces antidepressant- or anxiolytic-like effects in various behavior models of depression (e.g., forced swim test, tail suspension test, learned helplessness, etc.) (Tokita et al., 2012).

The first reported placebo-controlled, double-blinded, randomized trial ($n = 7$) utilizing a single intravenous (IV) dose of ketamine (0.5 mg/kg infusion over 40 minutes) in patients with MDD demonstrated a significant reduction in depressive symptoms 72 hours postinfusion. Profound but transient cognitive deficits and euphoria also were induced by the ketamine

TABLE 33.1. Controlled trials targeting the glutamatergic system

COMPOUND	SAMPLE	TRIAL DESIGN	RATING SCALE	ADMINISTRATIVE ROUTE	OUTCOME
KETAMINE*					
1. Berman et al. (2000)	MDD (N =6); BPD (N = 1)	Placebo-controlled, double-blind crossover. Single dose of ketamine (0.5 mg/kg)	BDI HDRS-25	Intravenous 0.5 mg/kg	Antidepressant response at 24 hr (25%); 72 hr (50%); significant decrease in HDRS score
2. Zarate et al. (2006)	TRD (N = 18)	Placebo controlled, double-blind, crossover. Single dose of ketamine (0.5 mg/kg)	BDI HDRS-21	Intravenous 0.5 mg/kg	Depressive symptoms improved within 110 minutes; 71% of subjects responded to ketamine; 35% at 7 days
3. DiazGranados et al. (2010)	BPD (N = 18)	Placebo controlled, double-blind, crossover. Single dose of ketamine; (while on therapeutic valproate/lithium dose)	BDI HDRS-17 MADRS	Intravenous 0.5 mg/kg	Depressive symptoms improved within 40 minutes; 71% of the subjects responded to ketamine; 41% response at 24 hr
4. Valentine et al. (2011)	MDD (N = 10)	Placebo lead in (1 week prior to ketamine infusion 0.5 mg/kg). Single blind study.	BDIHDRS-25	Intravenous 0.5 mg/kg	Greatest antidepressant effect of ketamine seen after 2 hours; 40% response at 24hr
5. Zarate et al. (2012)	BPD (N = 15)	Placebo controlled, double-blind, crossover. Single dose of ketamine; (while on therapeutic valproate/lithium dose)	BDI HDRS-17 MADRS	Intravenous 0.5 mg/kg	Depressive symptoms and suicidal ideation improved within 40 minutes; 79% responded to ketamine; 43% response at 24hr
MEMANTINE					
1. Zarate et al. (2006)	MDD (N = 32)	Double-blind, placebo-controlled study; 2 wk placebo lead in; randomized to placebo or memantine; 8 wk study	MADRS	Oral 5–20 mg/d (titrated 5 mg weekly)	No difference in efficacy between placebo and memantine groups
2. Lenze et al. (2011)	Depressed/ apathy symptoms (N = 35)	Placebo-controlled, double-blind, (memantine: 10 mg twice daily), 12 wk study	HDRS	Oral 20 mg/d (Start 10 mg/d; titrated to 20 mg by 2nd week)	No significant improved affective or functional outcome vs. placebo in older adults
3. Anand et al. (2012)	BPD (N = 29)	Placebo-controlled, double-blind, parallel group design; memantine augmentation (5–20 mg/d) to lamotrigine (100 mg+/ day), 8 wk study	HDRS-17	Oral 5–20 mg/d; with 100 mg+ of lamotrigine	Post hoc antidepressant effect with titration of memantine (4 wk); no benefit to memantine augmentation of lamotrigine in BPD depressed patients
RILUZOLE					
1. Mathew et al. (2010)	TRD (N = 26)	Randomized, placebo-controlled, double-blind, continuation trial of riluzole (100–200 mg/day), following single dose ketamine (0.5 mg/kg)	MADRS IDS-C QIDS-SR	Intravenous 0.5 mg/kg ; randomized (to lamotrigine 300 mg pre-infusion;add on riluzole (100–200 mg/d)	65% met response criteria 24 hr post ketamine infusion; 54% met response at 72 hr; no difference in time-to-relapse between add-on riluzole and placebo groups

(Continued)

TABLE 33.1. *(Continued)*

COMPOUND	SAMPLE	TRIAL DESIGN	RATING SCALE	ADMINISTRATIVE ROUTE	OUTCOME
RILUZOLE					
2. Ibrahim *et al.* (2012a)	TRD (N = 42)	Randomized, placebo-controlled, double-blind study, add on Riluzole (100–200 mg/day) after single dose ketamine (0.5 mg/kg)	MADRS BDI HDRS-17	Single dose of ketamine Intravenous 0.5 mg/kg. Add on Riluzole (100–200 mg/day)	Ketamine produced a moderate antidepressant effect through day 28. There was no difference in course of antidepressant effect between ketamine-riluzole and ketamine-placebo groups.
NR2B—SUBUNIT SELECTIVE NMDA ANTAGONISTS					
1. Preskorn *et al.* (2008)	TRD (N = 30)	Open label trial with paroxetine + double-blind single infusion of CP-101,606 or placebo	MADRSHDRS-17 BDI	Paroxetine 40 mg + IV infusion of CP-101,106 (varied dosing)	At day 5 primary outcome measure, 60% met response criteria on MADRS
2. Ibrahim *et al.* (2012b)	TRD (N = 5)	Placebo-controlled, double-blind, crossover pilot (MK-0657); 12 d study	MADRS HDRS-17	MK-0657 (4–8 mg/day); 12 d	Secondary measures (BDI and HDRS) revealed significant antidepressant effects at day 5; no significant antidepressant effects with MADRS (primary outcome measure)
AZD6765 (LOW-TRAPPING, NONSELECTIVE NMDA ANTAGONIST)					
1. Zarate *et al.* (2012)	TRD (N = 22)	Placebo controlled, double-blind, crossover. Single dose of AZD6765 (150 mg)	MADRS	AZD6765, Intravenous 150 mg single dose; 7 d	MADRS scores significant at 80 minutes and remaining up to 110 minutes; 32% overall response with AZD6765. No difference in psychotomimetic effects versus placebo.

* Includes controlled trials only; several other trials (case studies and open-label) have observed antidepressant effects with ketamine infusions.
MDD: Major depressive disorder; BPD: Bipolar disorder- Depressed; TRD: Treatment-resistant depression; BDI: Beck depression inventory; HDRS: Hamilton depression rating scale; MADRS: Montgomery-Asberg depression rating scale; IDSC: Inventory of Depressive Symptomatology Clinical Rating; QIDS-SR: Quick Inventory of Depressive Symptomatology—Self-Report—Response defined as 50% reduction in depression rating scale score.

infusion. A larger double-blind, placebo-controlled, crossover study at the National Institutes of Mental Health (NIMH) replicated these findings by showing that a single ketamine infusion (0.5 mg/kg over 40 minutes) had rapid and relatively sustained antidepressant effects (lasting one to two weeks) in patients with treatment-resistant MDD. Subjects in this study were medication free at least two weeks prior to infusion and on average failed six prior antidepressants. Effect size for the drug difference was large ($d = 1.46$) after 24 hours and moderate to large ($d = 0.68$) after one week. Thirty-five percent of subjects maintained response for at least one week. Adverse effects included perceptual disturbances, confusion, dizziness, euphoria, derealization, and transient elevation in blood pressure with most symptoms peaking at 40 minutes and ceasing 80 minutes postinfusion.

In a similarly designed study, ketamine was added to therapeutic levels of lithium or valproate and also produced rapid antidepressant effects in patients with treatment-resistant bipolar depression. A recent study replicated these latter findings in bipolar depression and also demonstrated that ketamine can rapidly improve suicidal ideation in patients for up to three days following a single intravenous dose ($d = .89$). Similar, albeit uncontrolled, open label and naturalistic studies (e.g., emergency room settings) utilizing ketamine have shown significant and rapid antisuicidal effects in depressed patients. Interestingly, one of these studies had preliminary results showing ketamine to have rapid beneficial effects on suicidal cognition as measured by the Implicit Association Test—a reliable behavioral measure assessing implicit suicidal associations (Price et al., 2009). Taken together, ketamine's use in antisuicidal effects likely will be an area of future interest and research.

Despite ketamine's positive safety profile as a widely used anesthetic agent for children, an important limitation of ketamine's clinical application in larger populations is its acute neuropsychiatric side effects (Green et al., 1998). Equally important are the questions of tolerability and sustained efficacy with repeat ketamine treatments. To this regard, only small, open-label studies have shown ketamine to be fairly well tolerated with repeated/sustained antidepressant effects

(Aan Het Rot et al., 2010; Zanicotti et al., 2012). Frequency of repeat infusions were similar to outpatient ECT scheduling (Monday-Wednesday-Friday) with relapse rates varying significantly after the last dose from 6 days to greater than 45 days (Murrough et al., 2011).

Strategies considered to attenuate ketamine's side effect profile mainly include augmentation with other drugs (pre or post ketamine). In an early study, healthy volunteers were administered haloperidol (5 mg), a typical antipsychotic, two hours prior to a ketamine infusion, but the results were unremarkable (Krystal et al., 1999). More recently, a small ($n = 14$), randomized, double-blind study evaluated the potential of riluzole—an inhibitor of glutamate release (reviewed in Zarate and Manji, 2008)—to prevent postketamine relapse in patients with treatment resistant depression (TRD). The study also assessed whether pretreatment with the anticonvulsant and mood-relapse preventive agent lamotrigine would attenuate the psychotomimetic effects and enhance antidepressant activity of ketamine based on an earlier study showing that lamotrigine attenuated the psychotomimetic side effects in healthy volunteers (Anand et al., 2000). In this study, lamotrigine failed to reduce the transient psychotomimetic side effects associated with ketamine in TRD, or enhance its antidepressant effects. Likewise, riluzole did not differ from placebo in preventing postketamine relapse (Mathew et al., 2010).

A larger, four-week, double-blind, randomized, placebo-controlled study (Ibrahim et al., 2012) also was conducted to evaluate the effect of riluzole use following a single ketamine infusion. Four to six hours after a single infusion of ketamine (0.5 mg/kg), 42 subjects with treatment-resistant MDD were randomized to double-blind treatment with either riluzole (100–200 mg/day; $n = 21$) or placebo ($n = 21$) for four weeks. Although the effect size of improvement with ketamine was initially large and remained moderate throughout the 28-day trial, the difference between the riluzole and placebo treatment groups was not significant for postketamine relapse. These two studies continue to the highlight the complexity of augmentation strategies for both ketamine's tolerability and sustained efficacy.

Despite the attention and interest from ketamine's early trials, the administration of ketamine for use in the clinic remains under study. Larger, controlled trials will be required to evaluate safety with repeated use of ketamine, and continued research will be required to discover successful relapse prevention or strategies to sustain antidepressant effects. Similarly, more studies will be needed to assess whether alternative delivery routes (e.g. intranasal, intramuscular) might improve pharmacokinetics, with continued assessment of optimal dosing regiments, and improved knowledge and understanding of ketamine's underlying mechanism of actions. (All of the previously noted controlled studies, plus those conducted to date in depression, and additional discussion regarding the maintenance of ketamine's antidepressant response, and its effects on suicidal ideation are reviewed in Aan Het Rot et al., 2012; Mathew et al., 2012.)

Putative Molecular Mechanisms Underlying Ketamine's Antidepressant Response

A growing body of preclinical evidence investigating ketamine's rapid antidepressant effects has led to novel findings and an increasing body of knowledge toward the neuroplastic effects of this treatment. In addition to NMDA receptor antagonism, ketamine involves enhanced throughput of AMPA receptors, and some inhibitory effects at muscarinic acetylcholine receptors. Prominent preclinical studies have demonstrated ketamine to rapidly phosphorylate/activate the mammalian target of rapamycin (mTOR) pathway with resulting increased levels of synaptic signaling proteins and synaptic plasticity (e.g., new spine synapse formation) in the prefrontal cortex (PFC) of rodents. Included in this cascade of postsynaptic events, literature discusses mixed results for an increased activation of brain-derived neurotrophic factor (BDNF) with ketamine's antidepressant response. Reduced levels of BDNF have been associated with depression, and BDNF's essential role in cell differentiation, nerve growth, and neuronal survival research makes it a likely area of investigation. Preclinical work by others has also implicated the potential role of glycogen synthase kinase-3 beta (GSK-3β) inhibition in the hippocampus and PFC after ketamine infusions. Patients with MDD are thought to have increased GSK-3β activity, and inhibition of GSK-3β is also thought to play a key role in the therapeutic mechanism of antidepressants and mood stabilizers. Overall, further research will still be required to elucidate the neurobiology underlying ketamine's rapid antidepressant response (Aan Het Rot et al., 2012; Mathew et al., 2012; Murrough, 2012).

Biomarkers of Antidepressant Response to Ketamine

Given the heterogeneity of depression and often "trial and error" approach to current treatments, positive predictors of antidepressant response to ketamine would be of great significance and practical value to both patients and clinicians. Several recent studies are investigating ketamine responders via a multimodal systems level approach, and utilize a range of potential markers from genes to the reversal of the complex behavioral phenotype (i.e., genes, gene expression, synaptic plasticity indices, cellular components, neural circuits, behavioral features of depression) using various experimental methods (neuroimaging, genetics, electrophysiological measures, clinical features, etc.). The goal is to both inform regarding the likelihood of response and provide insights into the mechanisms of action of ketamine. This section will briefly highlight some the more prominent studies.

One neurophysiologic study utilized magnetoencephalography (MEG) to measure rostral anterior cingulate cortex (rACC) activity as drug free patients with MDD were presented with a fearful face paradigm. Previous research has shown that higher pretreatment ACC metabolism predicts antidepressant response in sleep deprivation (also known to induce rapid, but brief antidepressant effects) and several other antidepressant treatments (e.g., SSRIs). In the MEG study, higher pretreatment levels of rACC activity correlated positively with the magnitude of subsequent antidepressant response to a ketamine, while healthy individuals showed reduced activity in this region (Salvadore et al., 2009). Another MEG study incorporating a working memory task demonstrated that patients who showed the least amount of engagement in the pregenual ACC as task difficulty increased showed the largest subsequent response to treatment, within four hours of ketamine administration. Pretreatment functional connectivity between the pregenual ACC and the left amygdala also negatively correlated with the antidepressant following ketamine. These findings concur with functional studies in healthy volunteers, where pgACC regional blood flow increases with emotional tasks, but decreases during cognitive tasks that demand attention. The results suggest that conservation of this pattern may predict better treatment outcome (Salvadore et al., 2010). Both MEG studies overall contribute to the extant literature supporting the role of ACC activity as a promising predictor of response to antidepressant treatment (Pizzagalli, 2011).

Two electrophysiologic studies utilizing sleep measures have also shown interesting findings. One study ($n = 30$, TRD patients) investigated the acute effects of ketamine on depressive symptoms evaluating EEG slow wave activity (SWA), individual slow wave parameters, and plasma BDNF (230 min postinfusion). Earlier research had demonstrated a relationship between SWA and cortical synaptic activity of cortical neurons suggesting its potential role as a surrogate marker of central synaptic plasticity. Decreased production of sleep slow waves is also a core feature observed in depression. Results of the study showed early sleep SWA (during the first non-REM episode) and BDNF levels increased compared to baseline with ketamine responders having changes to BDNF proportional to changes in EEG parameters. Consistent with an earlier finding (Machado-Vieira, Yuan et al., 2009) from the same lab was no difference in BDNF levels from responders and non-responders. The earlier study did note their lack of placebo control and other cautions, such as interpreting peripheral BDNF as a marker of central BDNF. The study overall suggests that sleep SWA parameters and BDNF may serve as future non-invasive measures for testing novel antidepressants and that ketamine increases synaptic strengthening/efficacy (Duncan et al., 2012). Building on the latter study, baseline delta sleep ratio (DSR) was examined to see if it could predict rapid response to a ketamine infusion in individuals with TRD. DSR is the ratio of slow wave activity between the first two non-REM sleep episodes, and this measure has also been shown to be lower in depressed patients than healthy controls. Findings from the study ($n = 30$) showed a significant positive correlation between baseline DSR and reduced MADRS scores from baseline to day 1 (low baseline scores predicted better mood response). These results are notable, as some traditional antidepressants have been found to normalize slow wave sleep and DSR. Sample size was a known limitation of the findings, and larger replications of the study were recommended by the authors. Nevertheless, this preliminary data could lead to DSR being a useful biomarker of response to ketamine in the future (Duncan et al., 2012).

In regard to genetic studies, a recent study ($n = 62$) demonstrated that MDD patients with the Val/Val BDNF allele were more likely to have an increased antidepressant response to ketamine (from baseline HAM-D score to 210/230 min postinfusion) than Met carriers. These results also support previous clinical data, where Val/Val mice exhibited increased antidepressant effect to ketamine (and prefrontal cortex synaptogenesis) on the basis of this single polymorphism. The Val66Met SNP is found in 20–30% of humans and has been linked to psychiatric disorders and impaired trafficking/regulation of BDNF (Laje et al., 2012).

Another innovative approach to study both the pathophysiology of MDD and ketamine response has been proton MRS. This research tool allows for the quantification of amino acid neurotransmitters in the brain, and previous MRS research has shown that GABA and Glx (composite peak formed by glutamate and glutamine) are decreased in the medial and dorsal anterolateral PFC of patients with MDD. Subsequently, 14 drug free patients with MDD who were scanned before receiving a single infusion of ketamine showed an association (230 min postinfusion) between lower Glx/ glutamate ratio (a surrogate marker of glutamine) and a greater improvement in response to ketamine treatment. Pretreatment GABA or glutamate did not correlate with improved depressive symptoms, however pretreatment Glx/glutamate in the dorsomedial/dorsal anterolateral PFC was negatively correlated with improvement in depressive symptoms. As glutamine is primarily localized in glia, the authors hypothesized that the decreased Glx/glutamate ratio may reflect a reduced number of glial cells, further signifying that this "neuropathological construct" (Salvadore et al., 2011) may be associated with antidepressant responsiveness to ketamine.

A potential clinical predictor of response to ketamine is family history of alcohol dependence. It is important to acknowledge that family history could represent a biomarker (i.e., genetic, epigenetic influences) or be the result of environment. A recent study found that patients with MDD who had a family history of alcohol dependence had a better short-term response to ketamine infusion than subjects with no family history of alcohol dependence (Phelps et al., 2009). The positive family history group (FHP) had a significantly higher response rate (67%) at 230 minutes (postinfusion) than the group without alcohol dependence family history (FHN) (18%; $p = .02$). In addition, patients with FHP had fewer dysphoric symptoms postinfusion than those with FHN. Previous clinical studies also found compared to healthy controls, subjects with alcohol dependence experienced fewer perceptual differences and decreased dysphoric mood during ketamine infusion (Krystal et al., 2003). Surprisingly, the healthy controls with a positive family history of alcohol also showed fewer ketamine-induced perceptual alterations (Petrakis et al., 2004). Of note, self-reported history of alcohol use disorders or family history of major depression did not predict response. Possible mechanisms explaining these effects include familial, epigenetic, or genetic variations in the NMDA subunit NR2A, which may have the greatest relevance for human alcohol dependence (Schumann et al., 2008).

Lastly, ketamine infusions in healthy volunteers immediately induced changes similar to those gradually induced by monoaminergic-based antidepressant agents as assessed using quantitative electroencephalography (QEEG). The observed reduction in prefrontal theta cordance (a measure that correlates with cerebral perfusion) may represent a potential marker/predictor for the antidepressant effects of ketamine, a hypothesis that could be tested readily in future studies with depressed populations (Horacek et al., 2010; Hunter et al., 2007).

Overall, increased attention in biomarker research in depression and the field of psychiatry will parallel the trend toward individualized and tailored treatment strategies for patients. The progress toward identifying biomarkers and application of these markers to predict treatment response ultimately will help elucidate the pathogenesis of depression and reduce the all-too-frequent "trial and error" approach for the selection of treatments in depression.

NMDA—SUBUNIT-SELECTIVE NR2B ANTAGONISTS

As noted earlier, non-competitive NMDA receptor antagonists like ketamine and PCP can produce psychotomimetic effects when used acutely. These observations promoted investigation into subunit-selective NMDA receptor agents to potentially mitigate the adverse effects, while promoting a therapeutic effect. Structurally, NMDA receptors are comprised of four tetrameric proteins: 2 NR1 subunits and 2 NR2 subunits. NR2 subunits are further divided by four subtypes: NR2A-D. Prior preclinical and clinical literature demonstrated the NR2B-selective NMDA antagonist. CP-101,606 to be well tolerated without prominent psychotropic side effects in a study evaluating traumatic brain injury (Merchant et al., 1999).

Building on this knowledge, Preskorn and colleagues undertook a "proof of concept" study with a recent randomized, placebo-controlled, double-blind trial, evaluating the antidepressant efficacy of the NR2B subunit-selective NMDA receptor antagonist CP-101,606 in 30 treatment-refractory MDD subjects. The study showed that a single infusion of CP-101,606 administered adjunctively to paroxetine, had greater antidepressant effects as compared with placebo (saline) infusion, with 78% of treated responders maintaining their response (50% reduction in HDRS score) for at least one week after infusion (mean difference, 8.6; 80% confidence interval, −12.3 to −4.5) ($P < 0.10$). The authors did note that the initial dose of 0.75 mg/kg was reduced to 0.5 mg/kg during the study given several initial research subjects experienced moderate to severe dissociative symptoms (Preskorn et al., 2008). All of the initial dissociative reactions resolved within six hours of the discontinuation of the infusion. No clinically significant change in labs was noted, however blood pressure changes similar to ketamine trials were observed (i.e., changes ≥20 mm Hg for diastolic or 30 mm Hg for systolic from baseline). Although the lower dose of CP-101,606 produced a rapid and significant antidepressant response without producing a dissociative reaction, the study highlights the challenges of optimal dosing for similar compounds. More studies will be necessary to replicate these findings and the overall efficacy and safety of compounds selective for the NR2B receptor (Preskorn et al., 2008).

Subsequently, an *oral* formulation of the selective NMDA NR2B receptor antagonist (MK-0657) was administered using a randomized, double-blind, placebo-controlled, crossover pilot study to evaluate the potential antidepressant efficacy and tolerability of this agent in treatment-resistant MDD patients. Following a one-week drug-free period, MDD patients were randomized to receive either MK-0657 monotherapy (4–8 mg/day) or placebo for 12 days. Due to discontinuation of the compound's development by the manufacturer and recruitment challenges, only five patients completed both the MK-0657 and placebo arms of the study. Secondary efficacy scales as assessed by the Hamilton Depression Rating Scale (HAM-D) and Beck Depression Inventory (BDI) demonstrated significant antidepressant effects as early as day 5 in patients receiving MK-0657 compared to placebo; however, no improvement was noted when symptoms were assessed with the primary efficacy measure (MADRS) (Ibrahim et al., 2012). Of note, MK-0657 increased plasma BDNF levels compared to placebo 9 days after treatment was initiated, indicative of a biological effect typically seen with several antidepressants. Although a small study, the role of BDNF may be involved as a potential biomarker of a NR2B antagonist's treatment effect. No dissociative or serious adverse effects were observed. While larger studies will be needed for confirmation, preliminary data suggests that an oral formulation of an NR2B antagonist may have antidepressant properties (Ibrahim et al., 2012).

NMDA (NONSELECTIVE LOW TRAPPING CHANNEL BLOCKER)

More recently, an IV formulation of a low-trapping, non-selective NMDA channel blocker (AZD6765) produced rapid antidepressant effects in a placebo-controlled study in TRD patients. Following a two-week drug-free period, MDD patients received IV infusions of either AZD6765 (150 mg) or saline solution one week apart with a randomized, double-blind, crossover design. Antidepressant effects were seen within 80 minutes with MADRS scores remaining significant for 110 minutes. Results overall demonstrated that 32% of subjects responded to AZD6765, and 15% to placebo at some point in the trial. Furthermore, 18% of patients reached remission on AZD6765 versus 10% on placebo at some point in the study. Interestingly, no difference was observed between the groups with regard to psychotomimetic or dissociative effects (Zarate et al., 2012b). Onset of antidepressant effects were comparable to that of ketamine, but the duration was more short-lived. Subunit selectivity and trapping blockade may explain some AZD6765's observed differences compared to ketamine. Similarly, metabolites of ketamine may contribute to its sustained antidepressant effects (Zarate et al., 2012a). Results from larger placebo-controlled, multicenter trials with AZD6765 are pending (NCT01482221).

OTHER GLUTAMATERGIC MODULATORS: MEMANTINE AND RILUZOLE

Memantine

Memantine, a derivative of amantadine, is already FDA approved for the treatment of moderate to severe Alzheimer's disease and is considered a low-affinity, non-competitive, open-channel NMDA receptor antagonist. Memantine has essentially no psychotomimetic effects at therapeutic doses (5–20 mg/day), a key distinction from ketamine. In addition, memantine has been utilized clinically for over 15 years showing good tolerability in large patient populations. A review of associated preclinical data within depression and anxiety models (e.g., decreased immobility time) is discussed in greater detail by Parsons et al. (1999). Of note, despite amantadine's remarkable antidepressant effects observed in patients with the Borna disease virus, it will not be reviewed in this chapter given a lack of data in any randomized controlled trials and due to its likely involvement with multiple pharmacologic mechanisms (Huber et al., 1999).

Unfortunately, most controlled clinical trials have not demonstrated memantine to have robust antidepressant effects. In an eight-week double blind placebo-controlled trial ($n = 32$), memantine (5–20 mg/day) failed to improve symptoms of depression in patients with MDD (Zarate et al., 2006). More recently, a proof of concept study ($n = 29$) also failed to show any benefit of memantine augmentation (5–20 mg/day) of lamotrigine (stable dose of at least 100 mg/daily for four weeks prior to randomization) for patients with bipolar depression over an eight-week trial (primary outcome time point). However, memantine was observed to have a significant antidepressant effect early on in the treatment (up to four weeks) during its titration (Anand et al., 2012). Lastly, a 12-week, double-blind placebo controlled pilot study ($n = 35$) evaluated memantine (10 mg twice daily) for treatment in late-life depression and apathy after a disabling medical event, but no affective or functional improvement was observed when compared with placebo (Lenze et al., 2011).

With regard to positive outcome trials, a larger study ($n = 80$) alcohol-dependent patients with MDD were randomized to memantine 20 mg/day or escitalopram 20 mg/day. Memantine reduces alcohol cravings in preclinical studies, and alcohol dependence commonly is comorbid with major depression. The study concluded that both treatments significantly reduced depression and anxiety (primary outcome measures) (Muhonen et al., 2008). However, a major limitation of this study was the lack of a placebo control. Alcohol dependence may modulate the antidepressant response that is mediated via NMDA receptors, as long-term alcohol use increases the number (Nagy, 2004) and alters the function of glutamate NMDA receptors (Petrakis et al., 2004). Interestingly, a seven-day, placebo-controlled randomized single-blinded psychopharmacology trial study ($n = 127$) that utilized three different antiglutamatergic strategies (lamotrigine 25 mg 4x/day, memantine 10 mg 3x/day, or topiramate 25 mg 4x/day) for ethanol detoxification demonstrated significant improvements for alcohol withdrawal symptoms and dysphoric mood (Krupitsky et al., 2007).

In an effort to better understand memantine's potential antidepressant role, a recent healthy volunteer model of emotional processing attempted to assess the neuropsychological profile of action associated with memantine (10 mg dose; typical dose in clinical studies is at least 20 mg). Overall, the results suggest that memantine produces an early anxiogenic response in the emotion-potentiated startle similar to that seen in studies considering a single dose of the SSRI citalopram. No other significant difference was observed with emotional or non-emotional information processing. Earlier studies have also shown that SSRI treatments initially increase the emotion-potentiated startle effect with acute administration, but that this effect is reversed after seven daily treatments (Browning et al., 2007; Grillon et al., 2007). Given the study only tested one dose; the authors did note that a future study (to 7 days) may help confirm the current profile of effects and provide more clinical

utility. Nevertheless, the authors also suggest that the limited neuropsychological profile associated with memantine may be consistent with the clinical data previously reported, where memantine is no more effective than placebo (Pringle et al., 2012). As already noted, similar but longer studies would help clarify some of these interpretations.

Riluzole

Riluzole currently is approved by the US Food and Drug Administration for treating amyotrophic lateral sclerosis. This agent crosses the blood-brain barrier and modulates the glutamatergic system by inhibiting glutamate release (via inhibition of voltage-dependent sodium channels) and enhancing both glutamate reuptake and AMPA trafficking and glutamate transporters. Riluzole is thought to have neuroprotective and plasticity enhancing properties given its ability to stimulate neurotrophic factors, such as nerve growth factor (NGF), BDNF, and glial cell line–derived neurotrophic factor (GDNF) in cultured astrocytes. A number of publications also discuss its use in neurodegenerative disorders. Combined with its glutamatergic modulating properties, Riluzole has had increased investigation in off label uses in both psychiatric and neurologic disorders (Zarate and Manji, 2008).

In clinical trials, riluzole monotherapy for depression has been evaluated only in open-label trials. One trial ($n = 19$) with TRD and a one-week medication-free period demonstrated significant improvement in depression during weeks three through six of treatment (50–200 mg/day, mean dose = 168.8 mg/day). Improvements were also seen in scales measuring anxiety. The most common side effects were similar (e.g., headache, gastrointestinal distress, and constipation) to those seen in trials of patients with amyotrophic lateral sclerosis. Similar, positive antidepressant and anxiolytic effects were reported with riluzole (50–200 mg/day) as an augmentation antidepressant agent, but only in smaller open-label trials evaluating effects in bipolar depression, generalized anxiety disorder, and obsessive-compulsive disorder (OCD).

Given some of antidepressant findings of riluzole mentioned, two double-blind, randomized, placebo-controlled studies proceeded to apply riluzole as a potential add-on strategy to maintain ketamine's rapid antidepressant effects (see ketamine section for details). Both studies administered riluzole (100–200 mg/day) orally, and both trials failed to show any difference in time to relapse from placebo after a single ketamine infusion. Nevertheless, both trials did replicate earlier ketamine findings showing it to be well tolerated and having rapid antidepressant effects. Overall, double-blind, placebo-controlled clinical trials will still be necessary to confirm some of the promising findings observed in these open-label studies. For a more systematic review of literature regarding riluzole, see Zarate and Manji (2008).

THE CHOLINERGIC SYSTEM

HISTORY OF THE CHOLINERGIC SYSTEM

The cholinergic system was the first of the neurotransmitters to be identified, and as a result has received a tremendous amount of investigation. Early research characterized the role of the cholinergic system at the neuromuscular junction, in the pathophysiology of Alzheimer's disease, and in cognitive functions including memory and attention. The cholinergic system also is the target of nerve gas, a fact that was accidentally uncovered in Germany in 1936 as researchers were attempting to improve on available insecticides, or organophosphates. These agents target acetylcholinesterase, an enzyme responsible for terminating effects of acetylcholine in the synapse, resulting in continued neural transmission and continued contractions at the neuromuscular junction. After a drop of the potent agent tabun was dropped in the laboratory, the investigator and his assistant began to experience dizziness and severe shortness of breath. These observations led to the development of nerve gas for military purposes during World War II, although it was never used during the war.

The cholinergic neurotransmitter system was implicated in mood disorders in the 1970s, when Janowsky and colleagues demonstrated that the acute administration of the anticholinesterase physostigmine to currently manic bipolar patients results in the rapid development of depressive symptoms (reviewed in Janowsky et al., 1994). Similarly, when physostigmine was administered to currently depressed patients with major depressive disorder, depressive symptoms worsened acutely. Physostigmine produces an increase in available acetylcholine, and thus is non-selective relative to cholinergic receptor type. As a result of this general implication of cholinergic function, interest has been given to both nicotinic and muscarinic cholinergic agents as potential antidepressants. Nonetheless, while the cholinergic system was identified in the early 1970s as a potential target for antidepressant agents, little attention had been given to this system until recently.

CHOLINERGIC RECEPTORS AND BASIC PHYSIOLOGY

The cholinergic neurotransmitter system is supported by two general types of receptors, the nicotinic and the muscarinic receptors (Albuquerque et al., 2009; Pringle et al., 2011). Muscarinic receptors, which are sensitive to muscarine as well as to acetylcholine, are G protein–coupled receptors and thus act through second messenger systems. Five muscarinic subtypes have been described to date, simply called M1 through M5. Muscarinic receptors are located throughout the central nervous system and in the postganglionic neurons of the parasympathetic division of the autonomic nervous system. Nicotinic receptors, which are responsive to nicotine as well as acetylcholine, are ionotropic and thus act by opening or closing ion channels in response to endogenous stimulation by acetylcholine. The nicotinic receptors are made up of five subunits, which surround a central pore. These receptors can be separated broadly based on their location in the nervous system into two subtypes, muscle-type and neuronal-type nicotinic receptor. Muscle-type nicotinic receptors, found at the neuromuscular junction, are either of the embryonic form or the adult form, each with slightly different compositions of the five subunits in the receptors.

The neuronal-type has various combinations of 12 possible receptor subunits.

CLINICAL TRIALS WITH CHOLINERGIC AGENTS

Placebo-controlled clinical trials (and select uncontrolled trials) with cholinergic targets are summarized in Table 33.2.

MUSCARINIC CHOLINERGIC AGENTS

Interest in cholinergic muscarinic agents developed as these receptors explicitly were implicated in aspects of sleep disturbances observed in patients with mood disorders. Specifically, decreased REM latency and increased REM density are observed in this patient population, and these sleep features are mediated through cholinergic muscarinic receptors (reviewed in Janowsky et al., 1994). The pattern of sleep disturbance is consistent with *excessive* muscarinic activity, and thus indicated increased muscarinic cholinergic function in patients with affective disorders.

Biperiden

Early studies looked at the antidepressant properties of a selective M1 antagonist, biperiden (Kasper et al., 1981). In an uncontrolled, open label study evaluating oral biperiden in "severely depressed" patients, the authors report significant improvement in depressive symptoms by the end of study. These findings however did not replicate in a controlled study of biperiden, where no significant benefit was observed over the control condition (Gillin et al., 1995). However, the original study is of interest, as the authors reported that baseline results of a dexamethasome suppression test significantly predicted subsequent clinical response to biperiden.

Scopolamine

More recently, in the context of a dose-finding study designed to evaluate the impact of a muscarinic blocker on cognitive features of mood disorders, unipolar and bipolar patients received intravenous infusions of the cholinergic muscarinic antagonist scopolamine (Furey and Drevets, 2006). Critically, all patients participating in these studies were free of psychoactive medications for a minimum of two weeks, and as patients were not taken off of existing medication, most were free of medications for a longer period of time. Over the course of this three-dose, four-infusion, placebo-controlled pilot study, depressive symptoms notably improved. Despite the small sample size (n = 8), the response was sufficiently large to warrant a clinical trial to properly assess the antidepressant potential of scopolamine.

A clinical trial was conducted (Furey and Drevets, 2006) that included a total of seven infusions, and began with a single-blind placebo lead-in infusion. Patients then were randomized into either a P/S or a S/P series, whereby P = a block of three placebo infusions and S = a block of three scopolamine infusions; these infusions were administered under double-blind conditions. Full clinical assessments always preceded infusions, and one follow-up assessment was obtained three to five days after the last infusion for a total of eight assessments. This crossover design allowed for all patients to receive treatment.

TABLE 33.2. Trials targeting the cholinergic system

COMPOUND	SAMPLE	TRIAL DESIGN	RATING SCALE	ADMINISTRATIVE ROUTE	OUTCOME
SCOPOLAMINE					
1. Furey and Drevets (2006)	MDD (N = 9) BPD (N = 9)	Placebo-controlled, double-blind crossover. A series of 3 drug infusions (4 µg/kg); 4 placebo infusions	MADRS	Intravenous 4 ug/kg	Antidepressant response at first post drug assessment (3–5 days after infusion)
2. Drevets and Furey (2010)	MDD (N = 22)	Placebo-controlled, double-blind crossover. A series of 3 drug infusions (4 µg/kg); 4 placebo infusions	MADRS	Intravenous 4 ug/kg	Antidepressant response at first post drug assessment (3–5 days after infusion)
3. Newhouse et al. (1988)	MDD (N = 9)	Placebo-controlled, double-blind crossover with 3 doses of scopolamine (0.1, 0.25 and 0.5 mg), 1 dose lorazepam (1 mg oral), placebo	BDI; BPRS	Intramuscular (0.1, 0.25 and 0.5 mg)	No antidepressant effect at 120 minutes
4. Gillin et al. (1991)	MDD (N = 9) BPD (N = 1)	Open-label	POMS-Depression Subscale	Intramuscular 0.4 mg for 3 consecutive days	Small but significant antidepressant effect at day 2
BIPERIDEN					
1. Kasper et al. (1981)	MDD (N = 5) BPD (N = 5)	Open-label	HDRS	Oral 6–12 mg/d	Antidepressant effect at study end (30 days) (uncontrolled study)
2. Gillin et al. (1995)	MDD (N = 17) BPD (N = 2)	Placebo-controlled, double-blind, randomized, parallel arm 6-week study	HDRS	Oral 4–12 mg /d	No antidepressant effect vs. placebo
NICOTINE					
1. McClernon et al. (2006)	Non-smokers w/CES-D >10	Placebo-controlled, double-blind, 4-week study	CES-D	Transdermal (3.5 mg/day weeks 1–4; 7 mg/day weeks 2–3)	Reduced depressive symptoms by day 8
2. Salin-Pascual (2002)	MDD (N = 15)	Sleep study with baseline night 1; nicotine patch night 2	HDRS-10	Transdermal 17.5 mg	Ten of 15 patients improved (30% reduction) morning after patch administration
MECAMYLAMINE					
1. George et al. (2008)	MDD (N = 21)	Placebo-controlled, double-blind, 8-week study. Randomized, placebo-controlled, double-blind, 8-week trial	HDRS-17 MADRS	Oral Up to 10 mg/d	Reduction in depressive symptoms vs. placebo by end of study (8 weeks)
2. AstraZeneca (2012)	MDD (N = 145)			Oral 1 or 4 mg TC-5214 or placebo twice dayily; or 60 mg Duloxetine once (active comparator) once daily	
VARENICLINE					
1. Philip et al. (2009)	MDD (N = 12) BPD (N = 5) MDD-NOS (N = 1)	Open-label; 8-week augmentation study (patients currently on stable antidepressant or mood stabilizer regimen)	QIDS-SR	Oral 1 mg- 2x/d	Patients showed significant improvement at study end; significant by week 2. No difference among groups at 8-weeks

MDD: Major depressive disorder; BPD: Bipolar disorder–Depressed; BDI: Beck depression inventory; CES-D—Center for Epidemiological Studies Depression Scale; HDRS: Hamilton depression rating scale; MADRS: Montgomery-Asberg depression rating scale; NOS: Not otherwise specified; QIDS-SR: Quick Inventory of Depressive Symptomatology—Self-Report—Response defined as 50% reduction in depression rating scale score.

A rapid antidepressant response was observed in both the P/S and the S/P patient groups. The P/S group showed little change in MADRS while receiving placebo in the first study block, and subsequently had a significant reduction in MADRS with the first assessment following the first infusion of scopolamine ($F = 94.1$, $p < 0.0001$, Cohen's $d = 3.4$), demonstrating a rapid antidepressant response. Importantly the magnitude of reduction in MADRS increased significantly over the series of three infusions ($p = 0.04$). The S/P group received scopolamine in the first study block, and again showed a significant reduction in MADRS with the first assessment following the first infusion of scopolamine ($F = 34.8$, $p < 0.0001$; Cohen's $d = 2.2$). This group also showed further improvement over the series of three scopolamine infusions suggesting that ($p = 0.002$), together with the P/S group, patients will improve further with additional infusions of scopolamine. In the S/P group, the clinical benefit experienced during the scopolamine infusions in block 1 persisted to the end of the study, demonstrating that the antidepressant effects continue in the absence of additional treatment for at least two weeks. Importantly, the groups differed in study block 1 ($F = 26.7$, $p < 0.0001$; Cohen's $d = 2.7$) demonstrating that drug and placebo separated, and this separation occurred by the first evaluation in study block 1 ($t = 2.5$, $p = 0.02$).

These clinical findings have been replicated (Drevets and Furey, 2010) in an independent sample of patients. The experimental design was unchanged, but the patient sample was limited to patients with major depressive disorder. In this study the overall pattern of rapid antidepressant response was identical, thus providing additional support to these clinical findings. These studies together indicate that the cholinergic muscarinic receptors offer a new neurobiological target for antidepressant treatment that has the potential to produce rapid antidepressant responses.

Patterns of response associated with patient subgroups have been considered in a combined/increased patient sample. In patients studied to date, the magnitude of response is similar for unipolar and bipolar patients, as well as for patients with and without comorbid anxiety disorder. The only patient subgroups that identified differences in response outcome were based on patient gender. While men and women showed significant improvement in symptoms following scopolamine administration, women showed significantly larger responses than men (Furey et al., 2010).

Putative Molecular Mechanism Underlying Scopolamine's Antidepressant Effect

The antidepressant effects observed following scopolamine administration appear to be consistent with the hypothesis that cholinergic hypersensitivity contributes to the pathophysiology of mood disorders. However, the response latency of one to three days together with the persistence of the antidepressant response may suggest that the mechanism of action includes effects beyond the direct influence on muscarinic receptors.

Elevated glutamatergic transmission is associated with the pathophysiology of mood disorders, and like other antidepressant treatments, scopolamine reduces NMDA receptor activity. Muscarinic receptor stimulation enhances NMDA receptor

gene expression (Liu et al., 2004), and thus the increased muscarinic receptor sensitivity seen in mood disorders may lead to increased NMDA receptor activity. In rat brain, the administration of scopolamine has been shown to reduce mRNA concentrations for NMDA receptor types 1A and 2A (Liu et al., 2004), and thus may reduce NMDA receptor activity via this mechanism.

A recently described effect of ketamine on synaptic plasticity (described previously) that is thought to underlie the observed antidepressant effects also has been shown following scopolamine administration (Li et al., 2011-Online). Like ketamine, scopolamine administration in rats activates the mTOR pathway, which leads to increases in synaptic signaling protein expression and increases in the number and function of new spine synapses in prefrontal cortical areas. Rapamycin, which blocks mTOR signaling, disrupts both the scopolamine induced increase in synaptogenesis as well as the antidepressant behavioral response observed in rodent models of depression. The timing and the magnitude of these effects following scopolamine administration are similar to those seen following ketamine administration. The authors hypothesize that increases in mTOR signaling depend on increases in extracellular glutamate levels, and both ketamine and scopolamine have been shown to increase glutamate concentration. This work suggests that the rapid antidepressant effects observed following both scopolamine and ketamine administration may involve influences on synaptic plasticity.

Biomarkers of Antidepressant Response to Scopolamine

Biomarkers of treatment response to scopolamine have been identified using functional neuroimaging. Baseline neuroimaging assessments attained prior to drug administration have been utilized to predict subsequent response to scopolamine. As highlighted earlier, the pursuit and identification of biomarkers of treatment response offers the potential to provide insight into the underlying pathophysiology of mood disorder, and subsequently lead to improved clinical treatment.

The role of the cholinergic system in cognitive functions, and the existing literature on cholinergic modulation during cognitive tasks and functional brain response, renders cognitive studies in patients with cholinergic dysfunction potentially very informative. The role of cholinergic activity in executive functions such as working memory (WM) and attention has been hypothesized to act via stimulus processing mechanisms (reviewed in Furey, 2011). Working memory refers to a process by which information (visual or auditory) is encoded, maintained for a short period of time, and is then used during recall or recognition. The information subsequently is not long available (i.e., no long-term storage). The preclinical literature indicates that increasing cholinergic activity through the direct application of acetylcholine has effects on stimulus processing, and alters signal-to-noise (S/N) mechanisms to enhance the representation of target stimuli. Functional imaging studies in humans also have demonstrated that increased cholinergic function increases response to task-relevant stimuli in visual processing areas, much like an increased S/N at the brain region or brain network level, and results in improved performance on WM and attention tasks. Thus, cholinergic function likely influences cognition by modifying neural representations of task-relevant stimuli.

The role of the cholinergic system specifically in WM processes has been well studied, and the results similarly highlight the impact of cholinergic function specifically on the processing of task-relevant stimuli. The best-characterized cognitive feature in mood disorders is described as a negative processing bias, where negative emotional information is preferentially processed over positive information. The excessive cholinergic activity in mood disorders may underlie this negative processing bias, and potentially could be evident in measures obtained with functional neuroimaging methodologies (reviewed in Furey, 2011).

A WM task was utilized to determine if levels of neural activity to specific stimulus information in visual processing brain areas could predict subsequent treatment response to the cholinergic muscarinic agent, scopolamine (Frankel et al., 2011-Online). A face WM task was used that included two task conditions: one which instructed participants to encode and remember the identity of the face and another which instructed participants to encode and remember the emotional expression in the face. In both conditions, the face to encode was presented, followed by a memory delay period, and then by a test image (Frankel et al., 2011-Online). The task was to indicate if the test image matched the encoded image based on the attended (i.e., identity or emotion) stimulus feature.

Functional magnetic resonance imaging (fMRI) was conducted in patients with MDD and healthy individuals during multiple sessions using the infusion schedule described previously. Blood oxygen-level dependent (BOLD) signal was measured, a surrogate measure of neural activity, as participants performed the two conditions in the WM task. Response magnitude was estimated separately for each task component and for each task condition from the data collected during the baseline session, prior to scopolamine infusions. The BOLD estimates of neural activity were correlated with the magnitude of subsequent treatment response to scopolamine (percent change in MADRS from baseline to study end).

Only the two stimulus processing conditions (i.e., stimulus encoding and test components) when patients were processing emotional expressions in the faces produced significant findings. Importantly, these correlations were observed exclusively in visual processing areas. Specifically, significant negative correlations were observed bilaterally in middle occipital cortex (MOC) between BOLD response and the magnitude of treatment response. While the analyses for the emotion encoding and emotion test components were conducted independently, the areas of significant correlation in MOC were largely overlapping, highlighting the selectivity of these particular brain regions in this effect. Importantly, no correlation emerged when patients were processing the same stimuli but encoding face identity, highlighting the selectivity of this effect to emotion processing.

These findings indicate that in MDD, the baseline, pretreatment levels of neural activity in MOC during the processing of emotional information reflects the potential for a clinical response to scopolamine. These results may suggest that the level of underlying cholinergic dysfunction is expressed in levels of neural response to emotional information, and that this underlying level of cholinergic dysfunction represents a biomarker for subsequent response to a cholinergic muscarinic antagonist agent. Healthy participants on average show higher levels of activity in these same MOC regions than MDD patients. Importantly, those patients who do not respond to scopolamine have BOLD estimates that fall well within the range observed in healthy participants, consistent with the interpretation that those patients who do not respond to scopolamine also do not show processing dysfunction in these areas. Similarly, those who do respond to scopolamine show increased levels of dysfunction in these brain regions at baseline.

BOLD estimates also were obtained from the scanning session that followed the scopolamine infusion, and thus reflects the acute response to muscarinic blockade. To determine the extent to which neural response in visual cortex (with a particular interest in MOC) during the same stimulus processing components of the emotion WM task is susceptible to cholinergic modulation in a manner that predicted treatment outcome, the change in BOLD response was calculated (BOLD drug—BOLD baseline), and this delta BOLD measure was correlated with subsequent treatment response. The change in BOLD response following acute scopolamine administration (thus prior to antidepressant effects) during stimulus processing components of the emotion working memory task also correlated with subsequent treatment response. The brain regions of significance were found to substantially overlap with the MOC regions identified in the analyses described previously (Frankel et al., 2011-Online). These findings may suggest that the visual processing brain regions that show predictive value at baseline also respond to cholinergic modulation in a manner that predicts treatment outcome, an interpretation that would support the conclusion that baseline levels of neural dysfunction in MOC are cholinergically mediated.

NICOTINIC CHOLINERGIC AGENTS
In addition to the early literature implicating cholinergic receptors in general, interest in nicotinic cholinergic receptors as possible targets for antidepressant agents originated based on the observation in 2005 that smoking rates were substantially higher in major depressive disorder (between 40% and 60%) than in the general population (22%) (reviewed in Philip et al., 2010). This observation led to the hypothesis that increased levels of smoking reflected an effort to self-medicate, and that nicotine may have antidepressant effects. Related observations included that smokers with a history of major depression have more difficulty quitting smoking, and patients with depression are at greater risk for developing a major depressive episode during smoking cessation (Philip et al., 2010). Conversely, smokers also have reduced levels of monoamine oxidase (MAO), an enzyme involved in the breakdown of monoamines including serotonin, norepinephrine, and dopamine, which is proposed to result in depressed mood (Philip et al., 2010).

Nicotine
An open label clinical trial using transdermal nicotine in depressed smokers provided some evidence that nicotine may have

potential for producing antidepressant effects (Salin-Pascual, 2002). The authors report that 10 of 15 non-smoking patients with major depressive disorder showed a 30% improvement in depressive symptoms. While the group as a whole did not show a significant response, this change was observed the morning after administration of the nicotine patch, suggesting a potential rapid antidepressant response. Several replications in uncontrolled studies have been reported (reviewed in Salin-Pascual, 2002). A placebo-controlled study also was conducted (McClernon et al., 2006), which showed that depressive symptoms improved by day 8 of nicotine administration, but this study was conducted in a mildly depressed cohort (not reaching criteria for MDD) and thus offers limited utility with regard to implications for patients with depression.

As health concerns prevent the clinical use of nicotine as an antidepressant agent, these clinical findings primarily have led to the evaluation of the antidepressant potential of other agents that target nicotinic receptors. A paradox within this literature does emerge. Some antidepressant medications used clinically for smoking cessation, including bupropion, a norepinephrine and dopamine reuptake inhibitor, and nortriptyline, a tricyclic antidepressant that inhibits reuptake of norepinephrine and serotonin, also have nicotinic antagonistic properties. Thus agents with nicotinic agonist effects and agents with nicotinic antagonist effects reportedly produce antidepressant effects. A potential explanation has been offered (reviewed by Philip et al., 2010), which suggests that nicotine initially activates nicotinic receptors but this activation is rapidly followed by desensitization. Continued binding to the nicotinic receptor potentially leads to ongoing desensitization, which is thought to result in chronic antagonism. Thus, antidepressant effects are thought to result from nicotinic antagonistic action.

Mecamylamine

The potential for the non-selective nicotinic cholinergic receptor antagonist mecamylamine to produce antidepressant effects has been evaluated. In a population of adolescents with Tourette's syndrome and comorbid major depression antidepressant effects were reported, which led to a placebo-controlled clinical trial in patients with MDD (George et al., 2008). MDD patients showing little to no response after receiving a minimum of three months of SSRI treatment were randomized to placebo or mecamylamine (10 mg/d) for an eight-week trial. More patients receiving mecamylamine showed significant improvement (>50% reduction in symptoms) (45%) than those receiving placebo (10%) at end of study, suggesting that MDD patients who are SSRI refractory showed an antidepressant response to mecamylamine.

A double-blind, placebo controlled phase-II study also was conducted with MDD patients who were refractory follow a six-week trial of the SSRI citalopram. Patients were randomized to 5–10 mg/day of mecamylamine or to placebo for a 10-week trial. The group receiving mecamylamine showed more improvement than those receiving placebo (reviewed in Bacher et al., 2009). Nonetheless, a multicenter randomized, double-blind, placebo controlled phase-II study of a non-selective nicotinic receptor antagonist (TC-5214;

S-mecamylamine) failed to show antidepressant efficacy in an eight-week trial (AstraZeneca, 2012), raising questions as to the potential utility of these agents.

Varenicline

In a clinical trial designed to evaluate the effect on smoking cessation, varenicline, a nicotinic agonist, was found to alleviate negative symptoms associated with nicotine withdrawal including depression (reviewed in Philip et al., 2010). This observation lead to an eight-week open label augmentation study in currently depressed patients with MDD or BD who were unresponsive to current treatment. Fourteen of 18 patients completed the study, and showed improvement in depressive symptoms as compared to baseline. Eight patients met criteria for full response, six of whom also met criteria for remission. Interestingly, observed improvement in depressive symptoms correlated with patient smoking cessation (reviewed in Philip et al., 2010).

OTHER POTENTIAL TARGETS AND FUTURE CONSIDERATIONS

While this chapter has focused primarily on the glutamatergic and cholinergic systems given recent promise with rapid acting agents in these respective classes, this should not minimize the research being done in other potential areas including the dysregulation of dopamine neurotransmission (Dunlop and Nemeroff, 2007; Nestler and Carlezon, 2006), the pathophysiology of the hypothalamic-pituitary-adrenal axis (HPA) (Pariante and Lightman, 2008; Wasserman et al., 2010), circadian rhythm regulation (Adrien, 2002; Harvey, 2011), stress hormone regulation (Holsboer and Ising, 2010; Nugent et al., 2011), inflammatory/neuroimmune system (Leonard and Maes, 2012; Miller et al., 2009; Muller et al., 2011), involvement of corticotrophin-releasing factors (Holsboer, 2000; Paez-Pereda et al., 2011), tachykinin/neurokinin (NK-1, NK-2) receptors (Herpfer and Lieb, 2005; Mantyh, 2002), and neurotrophic factors (Autry and Monteggia, 2012; Voleti and Duman, 2012).

Despite advances in the previously mentioned areas, there is still limited success with randomized, placebo-controlled trials with non-monoamine based compounds. For example, corticotropin-releasing factor (CRF, a peptide containing 41 amino acids) and its primary receptor (CRF-1) are well known to regulate behavioral responses to stress. CRF is also distributed throughout the CNS with its interneurons widely localized in the neocortex to areas (prefrontal, cingulate, and insular cortices) well known to be involved in depression and affective disorders. Its relation to impaired regulation of the HPA axis further supports rationale to target this system. While an initial open label trial of NBI-30775/R121919, a non-peptidic tricyclic CRF-1 receptor antagonist with high oral bioavailability and blood-brain barrier penetration, showed initial promising results, clinical development later stopped because of a reversible increase of liver enzymes in healthy controls during an unpublished safety study with high dosages (despite absence of CRF-1 receptor expression in the liver). Phase II controlled clinical trials with CP-316,311 (Pfizer) and BMS-562086 (Bristol-Myers Squibb, pexacerfont) also did not provide therapeutic results over placebo (Paez-Pereda et al., 2011). Results are currently pending regarding SSR-125543A another CRF-1 antagonist with recent completion of a Phase II clinical trial of 580 Russian subjects with MDD (Connolly and Thase, 2012). Despite these lackluster results, published results seem to indicate that CRF-1 receptor antagonism is safe and not intrinsically associated with adverse side effects. Interestingly, it should be noted that none of the mentioned studies included a stratification of patients for HPA abnormalities (Paez-Pereda et al., 2011). Similar to CRF-1 antagonists, NK-1 antagonists have also had disappointing results with a pooled analysis (>2,500 patients) of five, eight-week placebo-controlled clinical trials finding no benefit of the NK-1 antagonist aprepitant over placebo (Connolly and Thase, 2012). Lastly, with regard to inflammation, a recent proof-of-concept study ($n = 60$) demonstrated that tumor necrosis factor (TNF) antagonism does not have generalized efficacy in TRD (Raison et al., 2013). The study incorporated infusions of the TNF antagonist infliximab (5 mg/kg) in a double-blind, placebo-controlled trial and included outpatients that were both medication-free and on a consistent antidepressant regimen. Despite the negative primary findings, an association was observed between high baseline concentrations of the inflammatory biomarker high-sensitivity C-reactive protein (hs-CRP) and subsequent improved response to infliximab. In addition, infliximab-treated patients with a low level of inflammation appeared to do worse than placebo-treated patients. As a result, the study suggests there may be a subgroup of patients with TRD who have increased inflammation and respond to TNF antagonism, but not to placebo. Future development with inflammatory biomarkers may prove promising for personalizing antidepressant treatment. Opium and its derivatives have an extensive history dating several centuries back, both in medicinal and recreational settings. While opioids are utilized largely for the management of pain, endogenous opioid peptides and their receptors have been identified as potential candidates for novel antidepressant treatments given their expression in notable brain areas known to play major roles in affective disorders (e.g., ventral tegmental area, nucleus accumbens [NAc], PFC). Likewise, antidepressants that increase the availability of noradrenaline and serotonin through the inhibition of the reuptake of these monoamines also enhance the opioid pathway (Berrocoso et al., 2009). Of the main receptor subtypes (delta, kappa, mu, and nociceptin), the delta opioid agonists (DOP) are gaining increasing attention, as recent preclinical evidence has provided promising results. DOP agonists have both reduced analgesic properties and less reinforcing/respiratory depression effects than those observed with classic μ receptors (Jutkiewicz, 2006). Currently, two DOP agonist trials (Phase II development) have been completed (AZD-2327 and AZD-7268) for the treatment of MDD with pending efficacy results (Connolly and Thase, 2012). For an excellent and more complete review of novel and emerging drugs/targets for depression, such as sigma receptors, the interested reader should refer to Connolly and Thase (2012).

While barriers to clinical translation for psychiatric drugs are beyond the scope of this chapter, some key issues include the limited predictive value of preclinical models and the ever present challenge of target validation for clinical validity. For example, with CRF-1 antagonism, it is not known if the compounds given in trials are actually blocking CRF-1 receptors in the brain (i.e., target and functional engagement). In this example, we are largely assuming the effects in a preclinical model will extend to functional effects in humans (Potter, 2012). With regard to target validation, a target is often defined as a molecular or cellular structure involved in the pathology of interest that the intervention (e.g., drug) is meant to act on. This is clearly challenging in psychiatry and other CNS areas, as establishing valid targets requires a sound understanding of the underlying pathophysiology. Developing a drug against a specific target can often take several years with escalating costs in the billions of dollars. As a result, "reducing failures early in development is far more important than filling a pipeline with poorly chosen late-stage products likely to fail, and fail expensively" (Smith, 2003). For an optimistic future, collaboration will certainly be required, and an open-source model may provide for more rapid data sharing and better prioritizing of successful targets. Such steps may "de-risk" some of the current barriers for future "bench to bedside" therapeutics. Ideally, continuing advances in other tools such as molecular genetics, systems neuroscience, and translational medicine will lead to innovative tools and biomarkers to ultimately better serve patients suffering with depression and other debilitating disorders. For a more detailed discussion on novel CNS drug development, see Potter (2012).

EXPERIMENTAL MEDICINE

Experimental medicine characterizes a different method designed to understand the pathophysiology underlying mood disorders that merits comment (reviewed in Pringle et al., 2011). This approach proposes a cognitive neuropsychological model to understand antidepressant action, and suggests that pharmacologically mediated changes in emotional processing biases early in treatment contribute to subsequent clinical improvements in mood. Moreover, the delay in treatment response seen following conventional treatment is explained as the time during which the patient learns new associations following social interactions. Much of this work has been conducted in healthy volunteers, demonstrating that conventional antidepressant agents modulate neural responses to emotional information following several days of administration, well before clinical response generally is observed in clinical populations. These findings provide important insights into potential mechanisms of action that require follow-up evaluation in patient groups.

In patient populations, this approach has demonstrated that early in treatment and prior to clinical improvement, antidepressant agents modulate neural responses during emotional processing as measured using fMRI. Similarly, effects on behavioral measures that demonstrate emotional processing biases have been reported at three hours following the first administration of an antidepressant in patients with MDD. As these changes are associated exclusively with drug administration, the question as to whether these early changes predict subsequent clinical response to treatment remains empirical.

CONCLUSION

MDD is a severe, disabling, and potentially life-threatening medical illness that disrupts the lives of millions of individuals worldwide. Despite a considerable number of antidepressant agents developed over the years, significant limitations exist with regard to the utility and efficacy of available drugs. Critically, no specific agent or class of agents has proven to be more efficacious than any other. In addition, a considerable lag in the onset of therapeutic response is observed, often requiring weeks to months for full therapeutic response, thus leaving patients at risk for ongoing impairment and elevated risk of self-harm. Progress in the development of new and better medications that are particularly geared toward accelerating the onset of improvement of depressive symptoms has stalled despite considerable efforts from industry, academia, and government. The translation from targets in preclinical models to clinic populations has not succeeded as of yet in delivering better treatments. One approach for addressing these shortcomings is to focus on new neurophysiological targets, with the goal of identifying rapid acting interventions, and to simultaneously incorporate biomarkers of treatment response to facilitate the understanding of underlying mechanism.

This chapter primarily reviews two drugs that are radically unique and distinct from current antidepressants due to their rapid antidepressant effects; ketamine and scopolamine. Ketamine produces antidepressant effects within hours, while scopolamine produces effects within a few days. Research to date for both drugs is unique in that controlled studies have been conducted and replicated demonstrating rapid antidepressant effects. The inability to replicate clinical experiments recently has been highlighted as a concern in psychiatry. In addition, the evidence showing rapid efficacy of these compounds is augmented with multimodal biomarkers. Using rapid onset antidepressants permits the simultaneous study of multiple biomarkers and thus allows for the examination of biological signatures of rapid improvement using a systems level approach, extending from genes to behavioral phenotype across the cellular, molecular, neurochemical, and circuit domains. This approach permits the careful study of correlations of multiple biomarkers, precisely timed at the onset of antidepressant effects, thus potentially offering an opportunity to obtain greater insight into the molecular and cellular changes that accompany treatment response. In this way, ketamine and scopolamine are experimental tools being used to uncover clues that can then be characterized more precisely to determine what molecular targets are involved in these rapid antidepressant effects. Indeed, this strategy has already led to significant advances in the last several years reinvigorating and solidifying industry, academia, and government partnerships with moving forward toward the development of drugs with a rapid onset of antidepressant action. Specifically with the antidepressant response to ketamine, the systems level approach has led to the identification of genetics correlates associated with SNP on BDNF, molecular correlates identifying the involvement of mTOR, GSK-3 inhibition, and eEF2 as putative targets, the identification of brain areas and brain function associated with clinical improvement, such as increases in slow wave activity during sleep, and cortical excitability gamma power in sensory regions. Although these findings are promising, much more is needed before we gain a comprehensive understanding of biological underpinning of rapid antidepressant effects. These insights will be critical to the development of the next generation of treatments if they are to provide faster, more effective options than existing treatments offer. Similar approaches are being applied to the cholinergic antagonist scopolamine, and we anticipate that data gleaned from this approach will contribute to that of ketamine and other agents with a rapid onset of action to identify the neural and molecular requirements for fast acting treatments.

DISCLOSURES

The authors gratefully acknowledge the support of the Intramural Research Program of the National Institute of Mental Health, National Institutes of Health (IRP-NIMHNIH; Bethesda, MD, USA), and thank the 7SE Research Unit of the NIMH-NIH for their support. Role of funding source: This review was supported by the IRP-NIMH-NIH. The NIMH had no further role in the writing of this chapter, or in the decision to submit the chapter for publication.

The authors gratefully acknowledge the support of the IRP-NIMH-NIH, and the NARSAD Independent Investigator Award and Brain and Behavior Foundation Bipolar Research Award (Dr. Zarate).

Dr. Mathews has no conflict of interest to disclose, financial or otherwise.

Dr. Zarate is listed as a co-inventor on a patent application for the use of ketamine and its metabolites in major depression. Dr. Zarate has assigned his rights in the patent to the US government but will share a percentage of any royalties that may be received by the government.

Dr. Furey is listed as a co-inventor on a patent application for the use of scopolamine and its metabolites in major depression. Dr. Furey has assigned his rights in the patent to the US Government but will share a percentage of any royalties that may be received by the government.

REFERENCES

Aan Het Rot, M., Collins, K.A., et al. (2010). Safety and efficacy of repeated-dose intravenous ketamine for treatment-resistant depression. *Biol. Psychiatry* 67(2):139–145.

Aan Het Rot, M., Zarate, C.A., Jr., et al. (2012). Ketamine for depression: where do we go from here? *Biol. Psychiatry* 15:15.

Adrien, J. (2002). Neurobiological bases for the relation between sleep and depression. *Sleep Med. Rev.* 6(5):341–351.

Albuquerque, E.X., Pereira, E.F., et al. (2009). Mammalian nicotinic acetylcholine receptors: from structure to function. *Physiol. Rev.* 89(1):73–120.

Anand, A., Charney, D.S., et al. (2000). Attenuation of the neuropsychiatric effects of ketamine with lamotrigine: support for hyperglutamatergic effects of N-methyl-D-aspartate receptor antagonists. *Arch. Gen. Psychiatry* 57(3):270–276.

Anand, A., Gunn, A.D., et al. (2012). Early antidepressant effect of memantine during augmentation of lamotrigine inadequate response in bipolar depression: a double-blind, randomized, placebo-controlled trial. *Bipolar Disord.* 14(1):64–70.

AstraZeneca. A study to assess the safety and effect of TC-5214 in patients with major depressive disorder. *ClinicalTrials.gov*. Bethesda (MD): National Library of Medicine (US) 2012. [cited 2013 Jan 03]. Available from: http://www.clinicaltrials.gov/ct2/show/NCT01288079 NLM Identifier: NCT01288079

Autry, A.E., and Monteggia, L.M. (2012). Brain-derived neurotrophic factor and neuropsychiatric disorders. *Pharmacol. Rev.* 64(2):238–258.

Bacher, I., Wu, B., et al. (2009). Mecamylamine—a nicotinic acetylcholine receptor antagonist with potential for the treatment of neuropsychiatric disorders. *Expert. Opin. Pharmacother.* 10(16):2709–2721.

Berman, R.M., Cappiello, A., et al. (2000). Antidepressant effects of ketamine in depressed patients. *Biol. Psychiatry* 47(4):351–354.

Berrocoso, E., Sanchez-Blazquez, P., et al. (2009). Opiates as antidepressants. *Curr Pharm. Des.* 15(14):1612–1622.

Browning, M., Reid, C., et al. (2007). A single dose of citalopram increases fear recognition in healthy subjects. *J. Psychopharmacol.* 21(7):684–690.

Connolly, K.R., and Thase, M.E (2012). Emerging drugs for major depressive disorder. *Exp. Opin. Emerg. Drugs.* 17(1):105–126.

Diazgranados, N., Ibrahim, L., et al. (2010). A randomized add-on trial of an *N*-methyl-D-aspartate antagonist in treatment-resistant bipolar depression. *Arch. Gen. Psychiatry* 67(8):793–802.

Drevets, W.C., and Furey, M.L. (2010). Replication of scopolamine's antidepressant efficacy in major depressive disorder: a randomized, placebo-controlled clinical trial. *Biol. Psychiatry* 67(5):432–438.

Duncan, W.C., Sarasso, S., et al. (2012). Concomitant BDNF and sleep slow wave changes indicate ketamine-induced plasticity in major depressive disorder. *Int. J. Neuropsychopharmacol.* 7:1–11.

Duncan, W.C., Selter, J., et al. (2012). Baseline delta sleep ratio predicts acute ketamine mood response in major depressive disorder. *J. Affect. Disord.* [Epub ahead of print.]

Dunlop, B.W., and Nemeroff, C.B. (2007). The role of dopamine in the pathophysiology of depression. *Arch. Gen. Psychiatry* 64(3):327–337.

Frank, R., and Hargreaves, R. (2003). Clinical biomarkers in drug discovery and development. *Nat. Rev. Drug. Discov.* 2(7):566–580.

Frankel, E.L., Drevets, W.C., et al. (2011-Online). Neural activity in visual processing areas during WM predicts antidepressant response to scopolamine. Paper presented at the Society of Neurosciences.

Furey, M.L. (2011). The prominent role of stimulus processing: cholinergic function and dysfunction in cognition. *Curr. Opin. Neurol.* 24(4):364–370.

Furey, M.L., and Drevets, W.C. (2006). Antidepressant efficacy of the antimuscarinic drug scopolamine: a randomized, placebo-controlled clinical trial. *Arch. Gen. Psychiatry* 63(10):1121–1129.

Furey, M.L., Khanna, A., et al. (2010). Scopolamine produces larger antidepressant and antianxiety effects in women than in men. *Neuropsychopharmacology* 35(12):2479–2488.

George, T.P., Sacco, K.A., et al. (2008). Nicotinic antagonist augmentation of selective serotonin reuptake inhibitor-refractory major depressive disorder: a preliminary study. *J. Clin. Psychopharmacol.* 28(3):340–344.

Gillin, J.C., Lauriello, J., et al. (1995). No antidepressant effect of biperiden compared with placebo in depression: a double-blind 6-week clinical trial. *Psychiatry Res.* 58(2):99–105.

Gillin, J.C., Sutton, L., et al. (1991). The effects of scopolamine on sleep and mood in depressed patients with a history of alcoholism and a normal comparison group. *Biol. Psychiatry* 30(2):157–169.

Green, S.M., Rothrock, S.G., et al. (1998). Intramuscular ketamine for pediatric sedation in the emergency department: safety profile in 1,022 cases. *Ann. Emerg. Med.* 31(6):688–697.

Grillon, C., Levenson, J., et al. (2007). A single dose of the selective serotonin reuptake inhibitor citalopram exacerbates anxiety in humans: a fear-potentiated startle study. *Neuropsychopharmacology* 32(1):225–231.

Harvey, A.G. (2011). Sleep and circadian functioning: critical mechanisms in the mood disorders? *Annu. Rev. Clin. Psychol.* 7:297–319.

Herpfer, I., and Lieb, K. (2005). Substance P receptor antagonists in psychiatry: rationale for development and therapeutic potential. *CNS Drugs* 19(4):275–293.

Holsboer, F. (2000). The corticosteroid receptor hypothesis of depression. *Neuropsychopharmacology* 23(5):477–501.

Holsboer, F., and Ising, M. (2010). Stress hormone regulation: biological role and translation into therapy. *Annu. Rev. Psychol.* 61:81–109, C101–C111.

Horacek, J., Brunovsky, M., et al. (2010). Subanesthetic dose of ketamine decreases prefrontal theta cordance in healthy volunteers: implications for antidepressant effect. *Psychol. Med.* 40(9):1443–1451.

Huber, T.J., Dietrich, D.E., et al. (1999). Possible use of amantadine in depression. *Pharmaco. Psychiatry* 32(2):47–55.

Hunter, A.M., Cook, I.A., et al. (2007). The promise of the quantitative electroencephalogram as a predictor of antidepressant treatment outcomes in major depressive disorder. *Psychiatr. Clin. North. Am.* 30(1):105–124.

Ibrahim, L., Diaz Granados, N., et al. (2012a). Course of improvement in depressive symptoms to a single intravenous infusion of ketamine vs add-on riluzole: results from a 4-week, double-blind, placebo-controlled study. *Neuropsychopharmacology* 37(6):1526–1533.

Ibrahim, L., Diaz Granados, N., et al. (2012b). A randomized, placebo-controlled, crossover pilot trial of the oral selective NR2B antagonist MK-0657 in patients with treatment-resistant major depressive disorder. *J. Clin. Psychopharmacol.* 32(4):551–557.

Janowsky, D.S., Overstreet, D.H., et al. (1994). Is cholinergic sensitivity a genetic marker for the affective disorders? *Am. J. Med. Genet.* 54(4):335–344.

Jutkiewicz, E.M. (2006). The antidepressant-like effects of delta-opioid receptor agonists. *Mol. Interv.* 6(3):162–169.

Krishnan, V., and Nestler, E.J. (2008). The molecular neurobiology of depression. *Nature* 455(7215):894–902.

Krishnan, V., and Nestler, E.J. (2010). Linking molecules to mood: new insight into the biology of depression. *Am. J. Psychiatry* 167(11):1305–1320.

Krupitsky, E.M., Rudenko, A.A., et al. (2007). Antiglutamatergic strategies for ethanol detoxification: comparison with placebo and diazepam. *Alcohol. Clin. Exp. Res.* 31(4):604–611.

Krystal, J.H., D'Souza, D.C., et al. (1999). Interactive effects of subanesthetic ketamine and haloperidol in healthy humans. *Psychopharmacology. (Berl.)* 145(3):193–204.

Krystal, J.H., Petrakis, I.L., et al. (2003). NMDA receptor antagonism and the ethanol intoxication signal: from alcoholism risk to pharmacotherapy. *Ann. NY Acad. Sci.* 1003:176–184.

Laje, G., et al. (2012). Brain-derived neurotrophic factor Val66Met polymorphism and antidepressant efficacy of ketamine in depressed patients. *Biol. Psychiatry* 72:e27–28.

Lenze, E.J., Skidmore, E.R., et al. (2011). Memantine for late-life depression and apathy after a disabling medical event: a 12-week, double-blind placebo-controlled pilot study. *Int. J. Geriatr. Psychiatry* 16(10).

Leonard, B., and Maes, M. (2012). Mechanistic explanations how cell-mediated immune activation, inflammation and oxidative and nitrosative stress pathways and their sequels and concomitants play a role in the pathophysiology of unipolar depression. *Neurosci. Biobehav. Rev.* 36(2):764–785.

Leuchter, A.F., Cook, I.A., et al. (2010). Biomarkers to predict antidepressant response. *Curr. Psychiatry Rep.* 12(6):553–562.

Li, N., Voleti, B., et al. (2011-Online). Rapid antidepressant actions of scopolamine require mTOR signalling and synaptogenesis. Paper presented at the Society for Neurosciences.

Liu, H.F., Zhou, W.H., et al. (2004). [Muscarinic receptors modulate the mRNA expression of NMDA receptors in brainstem and the release of glutamate in periaqueductal grey during morphine withdrawal in rats]. *Sheng Li Xue Bao* 56(1):95–100.

Machado-Vieira, R., Ibrahim, L., et al. (2012). Novel glutamatergic agents for major depressive disorder and bipolar disorder. *Pharmacol. Biochem. Behav.* 100(4):678–687.

Machado-Vieira, R., Manji, H.K., et al. (2009a). The role of the tripartite glutamatergic synapse in the pathophysiology and therapeutics of mood disorders. *Neuroscientist* 15(5):525–539.

Machado-Vieira, R., Yuan, P., et al. (2009b). Brain-derived neurotrophic factor and initial antidepressant response to an *N*-methyl-D-aspartate antagonist. *J. Clin. Psychiatry* 70(12):1662–1666.

Madaan, V., and Wilson, D.R. (2009). Neuropeptides: relevance in treatment of depression and anxiety disorders. *Drug News Perspect.* 22(6):319–324.

Mantyh, P.W. (2002). Neurobiology of substance P and the NK1 receptor. *J. Clin. Psychiatry* 63(Suppl 11):6–10.

Mathew, S.J., Murrough, J.W., et al. (2010). Riluzole for relapse prevention following intravenous ketamine in treatment-resistant depression: a pilot randomized, placebo-controlled continuation trial. *Int. J. Neuropsychopharmacol.* 13(1):71–82.

Mathew, S.J., Shah, A., et al. (2012). Ketamine for treatment-resistant unipolar depression: current evidence. *CNS Drugs* 26(3):189–204.

McClernon, F.J., Hiott, F.B., et al. (2006). Transdermal nicotine attenuates depression symptoms in nonsmokers: a double-blind, placebo-controlled trial. *Psychopharmacology (Berl.)* 189(1):125–133.

Merchant, R.E., Bullock, M.R., et al. (1999). A double-blind, placebo-controlled study of the safety, tolerability and pharmacokinetics of CP-101,606 in patients with a mild or moderate traumatic brain injury. *Ann. NY Acad. Sci.* 890:42–50.

Miller, A.H., Maletic, V., et al. (2009). Inflammation and its discontents: the role of cytokines in the pathophysiology of major depression. *Biol. Psychiatry* 65(9):732–741.

Muhonen, L.H., Lonnqvist, J., et al. (2008). Double-blind, randomized comparison of memantine and escitalopram for the treatment of major depressive disorder comorbid with alcohol dependence. *J. Clin. Psychiatry* 69(3):392–399.

Muller, N., Myint, A.M., et al. (2011). Inflammatory biomarkers and depression. *Neurotox. Res.* 19(2):308–318.

Murrough, J.W. (2012). Ketamine as a novel antidepressant: from synapse to behavior. *Clin. Pharmacol. Ther.* 91(2):303–309.

Murrough, J.W., Perez, A.M., et al. (2011). A case of sustained remission following an acute course of ketamine in treatment-resistant depression. *J. Clin. Psychiatry* 72(3):414–415.

Nagy, J. (2004). Renaissance of NMDA receptor antagonists: do they have a role in the pharmacotherapy for alcoholism? *IDrugs* 7(4):339–350.

Nestler, E.J., and Carlezon, W.A., Jr. (2006). The mesolimbic dopamine reward circuit in depression. *Biol. Psychiatry* 59(12):1151–1159.

Newhouse, P.A., Sunderland, T., et al. (1988). The effects of acute scopolamine in geriatric depression. *Arch. Gen. Psychiatry* 45(10):906–912.

Nugent, N.R., Tyrka, A.R., et al. (2011). Gene-environment interactions: early life stress and risk for depressive and anxiety disorders. *Psychopharmacology (Berl.)* 214(1):175–196.

Paez-Pereda, M., Hausch, F., et al. (2011). Corticotropin releasing factor receptor antagonists for major depressive disorder. *Exp. Opin. Investig. Drugs* 20(4):519–535.

Pariante, C.M., and Lightman, S.L. (2008). The HPA axis in major depression: classical theories and new developments. *Trends. Neurosci.* 31(9):464–468.

Parsons, C.G., Danysz, W., et al. (1999). Memantine is a clinically well tolerated *N*-methyl-D-aspartate (NMDA) receptor antagonist—a review of preclinical data. *Neuropharmacology* 38(6):735–767.

Petrakis, I.L., Limoncelli, D., et al. (2004). Altered NMDA glutamate receptor antagonist response in individuals with a family vulnerability to alcoholism. *Am. J. Psychiatry* 161(10):1776–1782.

Phelps, L.E., Brutsche, N., et al. (2009). Family history of alcohol dependence and initial antidepressant response to an *N*-methyl-D-aspartate antagonist. *Biol. Psychiatry* 65(2):181–184.

Philip, N.S., Carpenter, L.L., et al. (2010). Nicotinic acetylcholine receptors and depression: a review of the preclinical and clinical literature. *Psychopharmacology (Berl.)* 212(1):1–12.

Philip, N.S., Carpenter, L.L., et al. (2009). Varenicline augmentation in depressed smokers: an 8-week, open-label study. *J. Clin. Psychiatry* 70(7):1026–1031.

Pizzagalli, D.A. (2011). Frontocingulate dysfunction in depression: toward biomarkers of treatment response. *Neuropsychopharmacology* 36(1):183–206.

Potter, W.Z. (2012). New era for novel CNS drug development. *Neuropsychopharmacology* 37(1):278–280.

Preskorn, S.H., Baker, B., et al. (2008). An innovative design to establish proof of concept of the antidepressant effects of the NR2B subunit selective *N*-methyl-D-aspartate antagonist, CP-101,606, in patients with treatment-refractory major depressive disorder. *J. Clin. Psychopharmacol.* 28(6):631–637.

Price, R.B., Nock, M.K., et al. (2009). Effects of intravenous ketamine on explicit and implicit measures of suicidality in treatment-resistant depression. *Biol. Psychiatry* 66(5):522–526.

Pringle, A., Browning, M., et al. (2011). A cognitive neuropsychological model of antidepressant drug action. *Prog. Neuropsychopharmacol. Biol. Psychiatry* 35(7):1586–1592.

Pringle, A., Parsons, L., et al. (2012). Using an experimental medicine model to understand the antidepressant potential of the *N*-Methyl-D-aspartic acid (NMDA) receptor antagonist memantine. *J. Psychopharmacol.* 16:16.

Raison, C.L., Rutherford, R.E., et al. (2013) A randomized controlled trial of the tumor necrosis factor antagonist infliximab for treatment-resistant depression: The role of baseline inflammatory biomarkers. *Arch. Gen. Psychiatry* 70(1):31–41.

Salin-Pascual, R.J. (2002). Relationship between mood improvement and sleep changes with acute nicotine administration in non-smoking major depressed patients. *Rev. Invest. Clin.* 54(1):36–40.

Salvadore, G., Cornwell, B.R., et al. (2009). Increased anterior cingulate cortical activity in response to fearful faces: a neurophysiological biomarker that predicts rapid antidepressant response to ketamine. *Biol. Psychiatry* 65(4):289–295.

Salvadore, G., Cornwell, B.R., et al. (2010). Anterior cingulate desynchronization and functional connectivity with the amygdala during a working memory task predict rapid antidepressant response to ketamine. *Neuropsychopharmacology* 35(7):1415–1422.

Salvadore, G., van der Veen, J.W., et al. (2011). An investigation of amino-acid neurotransmitters as potential predictors of clinical improvement to ketamine in depression. *Int. J. Neuropsychopharmacol.* 1:1–10.

Schumann, G., Johann, M., et al. (2008). Systematic analysis of glutamatergic neurotransmission genes in alcohol dependence and adolescent risky drinking behavior. *Arch. Gen. Psychiatry* 65(7):826–838.

Smith, C. (2003). Drug target validation: hitting the target. *Nature* 422(6929):341,343,345 passim.

Tokita, K., Yamaji, T., et al. (2012). Roles of glutamate signaling in preclinical and/or mechanistic models of depression. *Pharmacol. Biochem. Behav.* 100(4):688–704.

Valentine, G.W., Mason, G.F., et al. (2011). The antidepressant effect of ketamine is not associated with changes in occipital amino acid neurotransmitter content as measured by [(1)H]-MRS. *Psychiatry Res.* 191(2):122–127.

Voleti, B., and Duman, R.S. (2012). The roles of neurotrophic factor and Wnt signaling in depression. *Clin. Pharmacol. Ther.* 91(2):333–338.

Wasserman, D., Wasserman, J., et al. (2010). Genetics of HPA-axis, depression and suicidality. *Eur. Psychiatry* 25(5):278–280.

Watkins, J.C., and Jane, D.E. (2006). The glutamate story. *Br. J. Pharmacol.* 147(Suppl 1):S100–S108.

Wiedemann, K. (2011). Biomarkers in development of psychotropic drugs. *Dialogues. Clin. Neurosci.* 13(2):225–234.

Zanicotti, C.G., Perez, D., et al. (2012). Mood and pain responses to repeat dose intramuscular ketamine in a depressed patient with advanced cancer. *J. Palliat. Med.*

Zarate, C.A., Jr., Brutsche, N., et al. (2012a). Relationship of ketamine's plasma metabolites with response, diagnosis, and side effects in major depression. *Biol. Psychiatry* 18:18.

Zarate, C.A., Jr., Mathews, D., et al. (2012b). A randomized trial of a low-trapping nonselective *N*-methyl-D-aspartate channel blocker in major depression. *Biol. Psychiatry.*

Zarate, C.A., and Manji, H.K. (2008). Riluzole in psychiatry: a systematic review of the literature. *Exp. Opin. Drug. Metab. Toxicol.* 4(9):1223–1234.

Zarate, C.A., Jr., Singh, J.B., et al. (2006). A double-blind, placebo-controlled study of memantine in the treatment of major depression. *Am. J. Psychiatry* 163(1):153–155.

34 | NEURAL CIRCUITRY OF DEPRESSION

JOSEPH L. PRICE AND WAYNE C. DREVETS

This review of the neural systems that underlie mood disorders is divided into two main sections dealing with (1) the neuroanatomy of the neural circuits that have been implicated in mood disorders, largely taken from studies of non-human primates, and (2) observations on humans, largely taken from clinical studies. The first section describes circuits linking specific structures that have been implicated in mood disorders, including the ventromedial prefrontal cortex (VMPFC), amygdala and other limbic structures, ventromedial striatum, and medial thalamus. The second section reviews data from *in vivo* neuroimaging and postmortem neuropathological studies of humans with mood disorders in light of the relevant neural circuitry. Finally, observations from the neuroanatomical networks implicated in mood disorders are integrated into neurocircuitry-based models of the pathophysiology of mood disorders aimed at explaining the diverse neurobiological systems that are affected in these conditions and the potential mechanisms underlying neurosurgical and neuromodulation approaches that have proven effective in treatment-refractory depression.

HISTORICAL INTRODUCTION

It has been suggested since the early studies of Broca and Papez that a system of interrelated "limbic" structures, including the hippocampus and amygdala, the anterior and medial thalamus, and the cingulate gyrus, is centrally involved in emotion and emotional expression. Visceral reactions are tightly linked to emotion, often providing the means of emotional expression itself, and it is apparent that these structures are closely connected to visceral control areas in the hypothalamus and brainstem. More recent studies with effective neuroanatomical methods have now defined the circuitry related to emotion in sufficient detail that it is possible to recognize how disorders of this neural mechanism may underlie mood disorders (Price and Drevets, 2010).

The amygdaloid complex of nuclei forms a focal point in the circuitry related to emotion. The connections of the amygdala therefore are a good starting point for understanding emotion-related circuitry. Experiments in rats, cats, and monkeys show that the basal and lateral amygdala have reciprocal connections to orbital and medial prefrontal, insular, and temporal cortical areas, as well as to the mediodorsal thalamic nucleus and the ventromedial striatum (Öngür and Price, 2000). Outputs to hypothalamic and brainstem areas involved directly in visceral control were also found from the central, medial, and other nuclei. These projections include not just the medial and lateral hypothalamus, but also the periaqueductal gray, parabrachial nuclei, and autonomic nuclei in the caudal medulla. The strongest prefrontal cortical projections of the amygdala are with the medial prefrontal cortex (PFC) rostral and ventral to the genu of the corpus callosum, but there are also amygdaloid projections to parts of the orbital cortex, the insula, and the temporal pole and inferior temporal cortex (Fig. 34.1). Other amygdaloid connections are with the entorhinal and perirhinal cortex and hippocampus (subiculum) (Amaral et al., 1992), and the posterior cingulate cortex (Buckwalter et al., 2008).

In the striatum, the amygdaloid projection terminates throughout the ventromedial striatum, including the nucleus accumbens, medial caudate nucleus, and ventral putamen (Öngür and Price, 2000). These striatal areas in turn project to the ventral and rostral pallidum, which itself sends GABAergic axons to the mediodorsal thalamic nucleus (MD). The perigenual PFC also projects to the same ventromedial part of the striatu, and is interconnected to the same region of MD (Öngür and Price, 2000; Price and Drevets, 2010). The connections constitute essentially overlapping cortical-striatal-pallidal-thalamic and amygdalo-striatal-pallidal-thalamic loops (Fig. 34.1). As discussed in the following, these circuits form the core of the neural system implicated in mood disorders.

PREFRONTAL CORTEX (PFC)

In the 1990s, a series of axonal tracing experiments in macaque monkeys more completely defined the cortical and subcortical circuits related to the orbital and medial PFC (OMPFC). Two connectional systems or networks were recognized within the OMPFC, which have been referred to as the "orbital" and "medial prefrontal networks" (Fig. 34.2). The areas within each network are preferentially interconnected with other areas in the same network, and also have common extrinsic connections with other structures (Öngür and Price, 2000) (see following).

Recently, a similar analysis has been made of the organization and connections of the lateral PFC (LPFC). Based on architectonic and connectional analysis, three regions can be recognized in monkeys: a dorsal prefrontal region dorsal to the principal sulcus (DPFC), which is similar to the medial prefrontal network, a ventrolateral region ventral to the principal sulcus (VLPFC), which is related to the orbital prefrontal network, and a caudolateral region just rostral to the arcuate sulcus (CLPFC), which includes the frontal eye fields and is

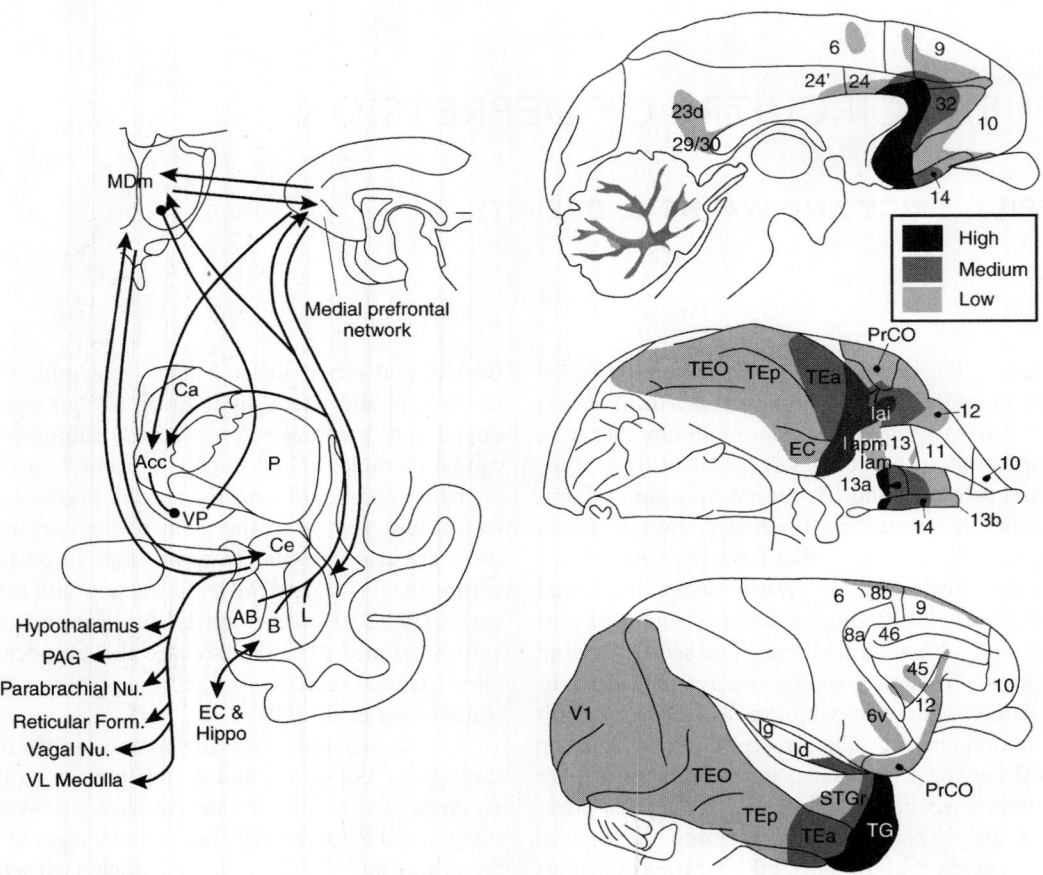

Figure 34.1 *Summary of amygdaloid outputs. Left: Diagram of amygdaloid circuits involving the striatum pallidum medial thalamus and prefrontal cortex and output to the hypothalamus and brainstem. Right: Diagram of areas of the cerebral cortex that receive axonal projections from the amygdala. The dark, medium, and lightly shaded areas represent high, medium, and low density of amygdaloid fibers. (Modified from Amaral et al., 1992, as reproduced by permission from Price and Drevets, 2011.)*

probably part of an attention system (Öngür and Price 2000; Saleem et al., 2008).

ORBITAL PREFRONTAL NETWORK AND VLPFC

The orbital network consists of areas in the central and caudal part of the orbital cortex and the adjacent anterior agranular insular cortex (Fig. 34.2); it does not include the gyrus rectus, nor a small region in the caudolateral orbital cortex. The network is characterized by specific connections with several sensory areas, including primary olfactory and gustatory cortex, visual areas in the inferior temporal cortex (TEa, and the ventral bank of the superior temporal sulcus, or STSv), somatic sensory areas in the dysgranular insula (Id), frontal operculum (Opf), and parietal cortex (area 7b) (Öngür and Price, 2000; Saleem et al., 2008).

Neurophysiological studies have indicated that neurons in the orbital network areas respond to multimodal stimuli (e.g., the sight, flavor, and texture of food stimuli). Notably, these neuronal responses reflect affective as well as sensory qualities of the stimuli. Responses to food stimuli change with satiety (Pritchard et al., 2008; Rolls, 2000), and many neurons code for the presence or expectation of reward (Schultz et al., 1997) or the relative value of stimuli (Padoa-Schioppa and Assad, 2006). Further, lesions of the orbital cortex produce a deficit in the ability to use reward as a guide to behavior (Rudebeck

and Murray, 2008). The orbital network therefore appears to function as a system for assessment of the affective value of multimodal stimuli.

The ventrolateral convexity of the LPFC, is closely related to the orbital network. This "VLPFC system" occupies the cortex ventral to the principal sulcus in monkeys, and includes areas 12l, 12r, 45b, and the ventral part of area 46 (Saleem et al., 2008). These areas are preferentially connected with each other, and to the areas of the orbital network. Further, they have most of the same extrinsic connections as the orbital network, including interconnections with the dysgranular insula, frontal operculum, area 7b, and inferior temporal cortex. The main difference from the medial network is that the VLPFC does not receive direct olfactory or gustatory inputs. These areas of the VLPFC may function to assess value of non-food sensory stimuli.

MEDIAL PREFRONTAL NETWORK AND DPFC

The medial network in the OMPFC is particularly significant for mood disorders. It consists of areas in the vmPFC rostral and ventral to the genu, areas along the medial edge of the orbital cortex, and a small caudolateral orbital region at the rostral end of the insula (Öngür and Price, 2000) (Fig. 34.2). The medial network receives few direct sensory inputs, but it has prominent connections with the amygdala and other limbic

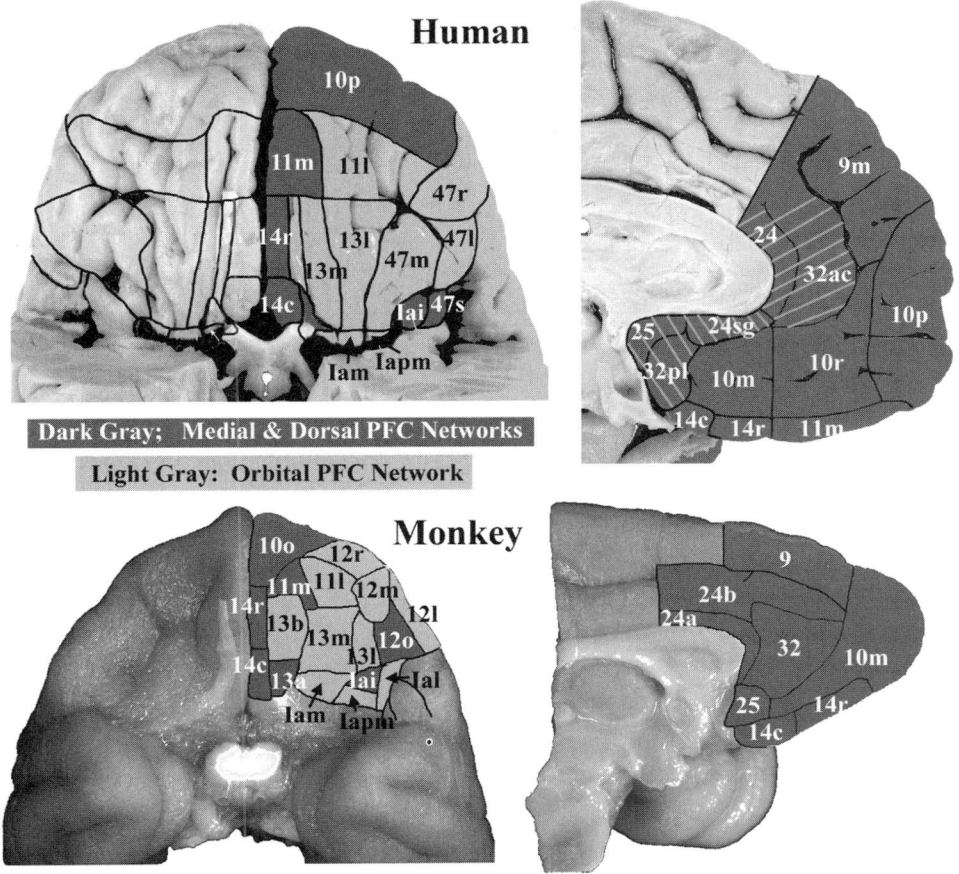

Figure 34.2 *Maps of the orbital and medial surfaces of a human brain (above) and a macaque monkey brain (below), showing architectonic areas as defined in (Öngür et al., 2003) (human) and (Carmichael and Price, 1996) (monkey). The architectonic areas of the OMPFC are grouped into networks or systems based on connectional data (see text). The medial and dorsal prefrontal networks are shaded dark gray, while the orbital network is shaded light gray. Note that the "medial" network includes some areas on the medial orbital surface as well as areas Iai and 47s (the human homologue of monkey 12o), in the lateral orbital cortex. In addition, the regions referred to as the subgenual and pregenual anterior cingulate cortex (sgACC and pgACC) are indicated on the human brain with backwards or forwards slanted stripes.*

structures (Carmichael and Price, 1995a, b), and it is characterized by outputs to visceral control areas in the hypothalamus and periaqueductal gray (PAG). It can be considered a visceromotor system with strong relation to emotion and mood.

The medial network is connected to a very specific set of other cortical regions, particularly the rostral part of the superior temporal gyrus (STGr) and dorsal bank of the superior temporal sulcus (STSd), the anterior and posterior cingulate cortex, and the entorhinal and parahippocampal cortex (reviewed in Price and Drevets, 2010). This corticocortical circuit is distinct from, but complementary to the circuit related to the orbital network.

The medial network is closely related to the areas of the DPFC, on the dorsal medial wall, and the dorsomedial convexity, including area 8b, area 9, the dorsal part of area 46, and the polar part of area 10 (Fig. 34.2). The DPFC is interconnected with itself and with the medial prefrontal network, but less with the VLPFC or CLPFC. It also is connected to the same set of extrinsic cortical areas as the medial network, including the anterior and posterior cingulate cortex, the rostral superior temporal gyrus, and the entorhinal and parahippocampal cortex. Further, there are outputs from areas of the DPFC to the hypothalamus and PAG, so this system can also modulate visceral functions.

The medial network, the DPFC, and the other cortical areas with which they connect, taken together, closely resemble the "default mode network" (DMN), which has been defined by fMRI and functional connectivity MRI (fcMRI) in humans (Raichle et al., 2001) (Fig. 34.3). The DMN is characterized as interconnected areas that are active in a resting state but decrease activity in externally directed tasks. This network has been linked to a variety of self-referential functions such as understanding others' mental state, recollection, and imagination (Buckner et al., 2008).

CAUDOLATERAL PREFRONTAL CORTEX

The caudal part of the LPFC, the caudolateral prefrontal cortex (CLPFC) is largely unrelated to either the medial or orbital networks. It includes the frontal eye fields and adjacent cortex (areas 8av, 8ad, and caudal part of area 46 in the caudal part of the principal sulcus) (reviewed in Price and Drevets, 2010). The extrinsic connections of this system are with the dorsal premotor cortex, the posterior part of the dorsal STS (area TPT), and areas LIP and 7a in the posterior parietal cortex. The CLPFC may be part of the dorsal attention system (Raichle et al., 2001).

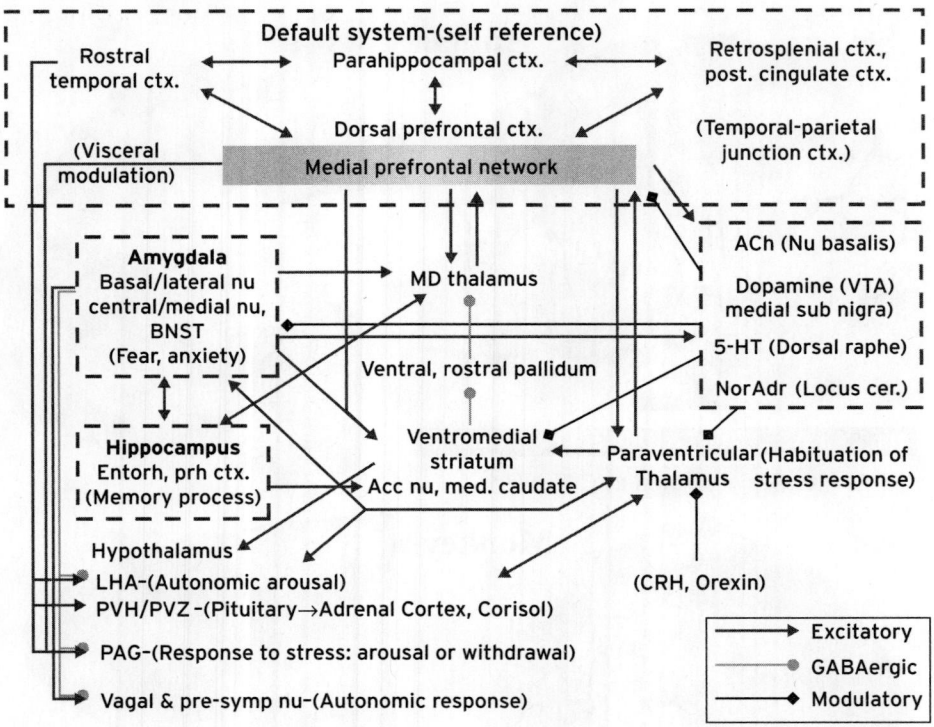

Figure 34.3 Anatomical circuits involving the medial and dorsal prefrontal networks, and the amygdala. Glutamatergic, presumed excitatory, projections are shown with pointed arrows, GABAergic projections are shown with round tipped arrows, and modulatory projections with diamond tipped arrows. In the model proposed herein, dysfunction in the medial prefrontal network and/or in the amygdala results in dysregulation of transmission throughout an extended brain circuit that spans from the cortex to the brainstem, yielding the cognitive, emotional, endocrine, autonomic, and neurochemical manifestations of depression. Intra-amygdaloid connections link the basal and lateral amygdaloid nuclei to the central and medial nuclei of the amygdala and the bed nucleus of the stria terminalis (BNST). Parallel and convergent efferent projections from the amygdala and the medial prefrontal network to the hypothalamus, periaqueductal grey (PAG), nucleus basalis, dorsal raphe, locus coeruleus, and medullary vagal nuclei organize neuroendocrine, autonomic, neurotransmitter, and behavioral responses to stressors and emotional stimuli (Davis and Shi, 1999; LeDoux, 2003). In addition, the medial prefrontal network and amygdala interact with the same cortical-st riatal-pallidal-thalamic loop, through substantial connections both with the accumbens nucleus and medial caudate, and with the mediodorsal and paraventricular thalamic nuclei, which normally function to guide and limit responses to stress. Finally, the medial prefrontal network is a central node in the cortical "default mode network" (DMN) that putatively supports self-referential functions such as mood. Other abbreviations: 5-HT—serotonin; ACh—acetylcholine; Cort.—cortisol; CRH—corticotrophin releasing hormone; Ctx—cortex; NorAdr—norepinephrine; PVN—paraventricular nucleus of the hypothalamus; PVZ—periventricular zone of hypothalamus; STGr—rostral superior temporal gyrus; VTA—ventral tegmental area.

REGIONS WITH EXTENSIVE CONNECTIONS TO MULTIPLE NETWORKS (AREA 45a AND 47s)

Area 45a in the caudal-ventral PFC represents an exception to the dorsal, ventral, and caudal systems of the LPFC. Injections of axonal tracers into this area label connections with areas in all parts of the LPFC. The extrinsic connections resemble those of the dorsal and medial prefrontal systems, but also include the auditory parabelt and belt areas, as well as face areas in the ventral STS. Responses to both faces and species-specific auditory stimuli have been recorded in this region (Romanski, 2007; Tsao et al., 2008). Conceivably this region may represent a multimodal cortex that also is connected to circuits responsible for emotional processing.

AREA 12o/47s

Another area that appears to subserve a similar multimodal processing role with a strong link to emotional processing is area 12o/47s. In monkeys Walker designated the lateral orbitofrontal cortex as area 12, and four subdivisions subsequently

were recognized within this cortex. Brodmann, however, designated approximately the same region in humans as area 47. Because the human area equivalent to the "orbital" part of area 12 (12o) in monkeys is not on the orbital surface but instead lies on the dorsal surface of the lateral orbital gyrus within the horizontal ramus of the lateral sulcus, this region was termed the sulcal part of area 47 (47s). Area 12o/47s shares extensive anatomical connections with several of the regions located on the medial wall (e.g., areas 25, 32pl, 24b, 10m) and in the anterior agranular insula (Iai) that form the medial prefrontal network. Area 12o/47s also projects to visceral control centers in the hypothalamus and periaqueductal gray, and receives auditory or polymodal input from the superior temporal sulcal region similar to the medial prefrontal network (reviewed in Öngür and Price, 2000). Thus area 12o/47s is considered part of the medial prefrontal network that subserves a "visceromotor" or "emotomotor" system that modulates visceral activity in response to affective stimuli. For example, the area corresponding to 47s coactivates within the subgenual ACC during induced sadness (Mayberg et al., 1999). Nevertheless, area

12o/47s also shares extensive connections with the orbital network, providing an interface between sensory integration and emotional expression (Öngür and Price, 2000).

CORTICAL PROJECTIONS TO HYPOTHALAMUS AND BRAINSTEM

Substantial outputs exist from the medial prefrontal network to the hypothalamus, PAG, and other visceral control centers, with the strongest projection from the subgenual cortex (Öngür and Price, 2000; Price and Drevets, 2010). The origin of the projection includes the STGr/STSd and area 9 in the DPFC, which are both connected to the medial network. Electrical stimulation of the medial PFC cause changes in heart rate and respiration, and fMRI studies show that activity in medial PFC correlates with visceral activation related to emotion (reviewed in Price and Drevets, 2010).

Lesions of the VMPFC in humans abolish the automatic visceral response to emotive stimuli (Bechara et al., 2000). Individuals with these lesions also are debilitated in terms of their ability to make appropriate choices, although their cognitive intelligence is intact. To account for such deficits, the "somatic marker hypothesis" proposes that the visceral reaction accompanying emotion serves as a subconscious warning of disadvantageous behaviors (Damasio, 1995). The full basis for this effect is complex, presumably involving the visceral reactions (e.g., sweaty palms, "butterflies" in the gut, etc.), subconscious "as-if" circuits, and circuits such as the cortical-striatal-pallidal-thalamic system. In mood disorders, overactivation of this system (e.g., due to excessive activity in the subgenual cortex) could produce the chronic sense of "unease" that is a common experiential component of depression.

CORTICAL-STRIATAL-THALAMIC CIRCUITS RELATED TO OMPFC

Like other cortical areas, the PFC has specific connections with the striatum and thalamus. These include reciprocal thalamo-cortical connections with the medial part of the mediodorsal thalamic nucleus (MDm). Closely related to these is the cortical-striatal-pallidal-thalamic loop through the ventromedial striatum and connections between the midline thalamic nuclei and the same striatal and cortical areas (Öngür and Price, 2000; Price and Drevets, 2010) (Figs. 34.3, 34.4, and 34.5).

MEDIAL SEGMENT OF MEDIODORSAL THALAMIC NUCLEUS

MDm receives substantial subcortical inputs from many limbic structures, including the amygdala, olfactory cortex, entorhinal cortex, perirhinal cortex, parahippocampal cortex, and subiculum (Öngür and Price, 2000). All of these areas also send direct (non-thalamic) projections to the OMPFC (Öngür and Price, 2000).

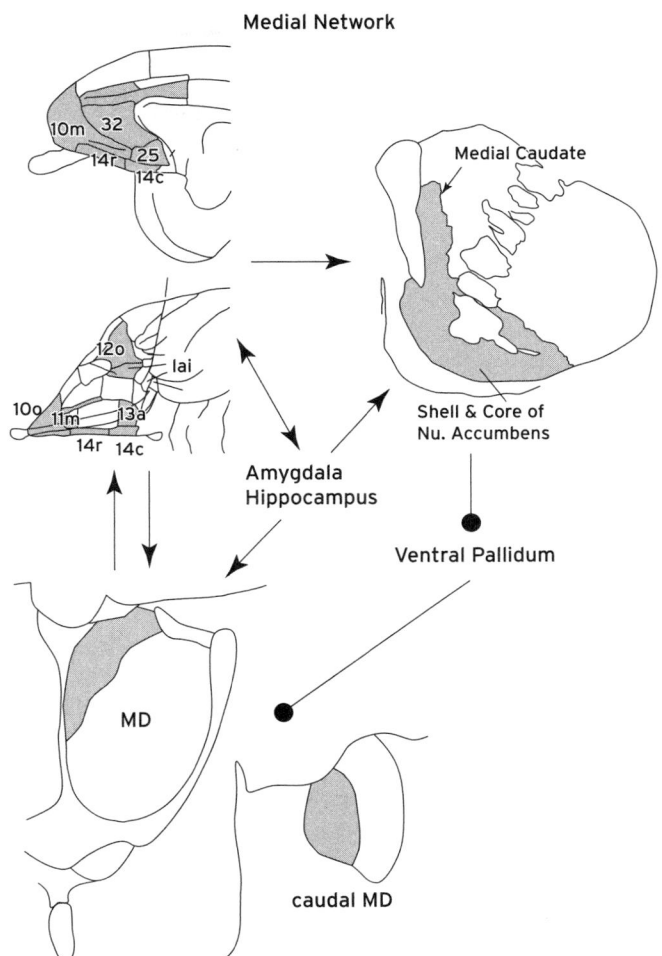

Figure 34.4 *Illustration of the cortical-striatal-pallidal-thalamic loop related to the medial prefrontal network. Note that limbic structures such as the amygdala and hippocampus are also related to several parts of this circuit.*

In addition to these inputs from limbic structures, which are excitatory and probably glutamatergic, MDm also receives GABAergic inputs from the ventral pallidum and rostral globus pallidus (Öngür and Price, 2000) (Figs. 34.3 and 34.4). It can be expected that these convergent but antagonistic inputs would interact to modulate the reciprocal thalamocortical interactions between the OMPFC and MDm. Limbic inputs would promote ongoing patterns of thalamocortical and corticothalamic activity and consistent behavior, while pallidal inputs would interrupt ongoing patterns, allowing a switch between behaviors involving mood, value assessment of objects, and stimulus-reward association. Indeed, lesions of the ventral striatum and pallidum, MD, or the OMPFC have been shown to cause perseverative deficits in stimulus-reward reversal tasks in rats and monkeys, where there is difficulty extinguishing responses to previously rewarded (Ferry et al., 2000). A similar deficit in subjects with mood disorders might be reflected by the difficulty in "letting go" of a negative mood or mind-set long after the resolution of any traumatic events that might have justified it.

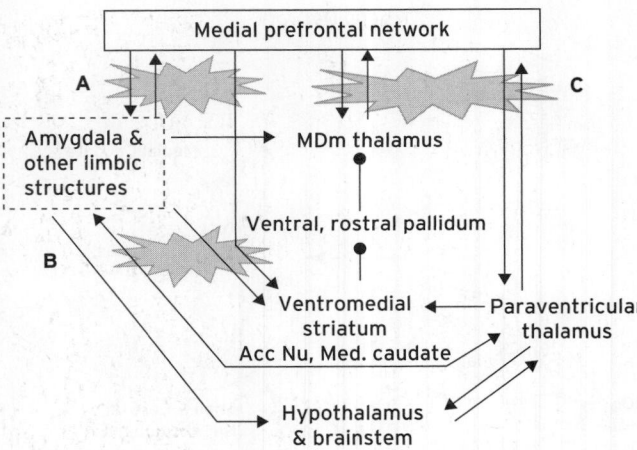

Figure 34.5 *A diagrammatic illustration of the cortical-striatal-pallidal-thalamic loop circuit, involving the medial prefrontal network and the amygdala, together with the ventromedial striatum (nucleus accumbens and medial caudate nuclei), the ventral and rostral globus pallidus, and the medial part of the mediodorsal thalamic nucleus (MDm). The midline paraventricular thalamic nucleus also has prominent connections with the medial network, the ventromedial striatum, and the amygdala, as well as with the hypothalamus and brainstem. The substantial connections from the medial network to the hypothalamus and brainstem are not shown in this figure. The shaded clouds depict areas where the targeted neuromodulation and neurosurgical treatments that have shown benefit in treatment-refractory depression would putatively influence white matter tracts within these circuits. A. Deep brain stimulation of the subgenual anterior cingulate (sgACC; Mayberg et al., 2005) and stereotaxic surgical ablations such as the anterior cingulotomy and prelimbic leukectomy would influence neural afferents and efferents of the sgACC as well as some projections running within the ventral cingulum bundle, thereby modulating or interrupting neurotransmission between the medial prefrontal network and the striatum, the amygdala and other limbic structures, as well as the hypothalamus, PAG, and brainstem stuctures. B. Deep brain stimulation of the ventral capsule/ventral striatum (Malone et al., 2009) and stereotaxic surgical ablations such as the subcaudate tractotomy would influence neural afferents to the ventral striatum emanating from the sgACC and other medial prefrontal network regions (Fig. 34.3) as well as from the amygdala and other limbic structures. C. Deep brain stimulation (Schlaepfer et al., 2008) or surgical lesions (i.e., anterior capsulotomy) administered within the anterior limb of the internal capsule would influence neural projections running between the medial prefrontal network and the mediodorsal thalamic nucleus. (Modified from Price and Drevets, 2012.)*

PREFRONTAL PROJECTIONS TO THE STRIATUM

The OMPFC projects principally to the rostral, ventromedial part of the striatum. The orbital network areas connect to a relatively central region that spans the internal capsule, while the medial network areas project to the nucleus accumbens and the rostromedial caudate nucleus (Öngür and Price, 2000) (Fig. 34.4). The amygdala input to the striatum is essentially coextensive with that of the medial network. These striatal regions, in turn, project to the ventral pallidum, which projects to the portion of MDm that is connected to the medial network areas (Fig. 34.4).

MIDLINE "INTRALAMINAR" NUCLEI OF THALAMUS

In addition to the prefrontal connections with MD, there also are connections with the midline-intralaminar nuclei of the

thalamus, which include the paraventricular thalamic nucleus (PVT), and nuclei that extend ventrally on the midline. These nuclei are reciprocally connected to the medial prefrontal network areas, with little connection to the orbital network, and they have a substantial projection to the same areas of the ventromedial striatum that receives input from the medial network areas (Hsu and Price, 2007) (Fig. 34.4). They also have connections with the amygdala, hypothalamus, and brainstem areas, including the PAG (Fig. 34.3).

Considerable evidence links the PVT to the stress response. In particular, lesions of the PVT facilitate central amygdala neuronal responses to acute psychological stressors and block habituation to repeated restraint stress in rats (Bhatnagar et al., 2002). In humans, habituation to the stress response caused by recurrent hypoglycemia is associated with activity in the midline thalamus (reviewed in Price and Drevets, 2012). It is likely that the role of the PVT is general across many types of stressors.

OVERVIEW OF RECENT OBSERVATIONS IN HUMANS WITH MOOD DISORDERS

Converging evidence from neuroimaging and lesion analysis studies of mood disorders implicates the medial and orbital prefrontal networks along with anatomically related areas of the striatum, thalamus, and temporal lobe previously described in the pathophysiology of depression. Depressed subjects show abnormal hemodynamic responses in both networks during fMRI studies involving reward and emotional processing tasks (reviewed in Murray et al., 2010; Phillips et al., 2008). In addition, however, many of the prefrontal regions that compose the medial network and of the areas of convergence between the medial and orbital networks (i.e., BA 45a, 47s) contain reductions in gray matter and histopathological changes in neuroimaging and/or neuropathological studies of mood disorders. These data support extant neural models of depression positing that dysfunction within the medial network and anatomically related limbic and basal ganglia structures underlies the disturbances in cognition and emotional behavior seen in depression.

NEUROIMAGING ABNORMALITIES IN MOOD DISORDERS

The neuroimaging abnormalities found in mood disorders generally have corroborated hypotheses regarding the neural circuitry of depression that were based initially on observations from the behavioral effects of lesions. Degenerative basal ganglia diseases and lesions of the striatum and orbitofrontal cortex increased the risk for developing major depressive episodes (Folstein et al., 1985; MacFall et al., 2001; Starkstein and Robinson, 1989). Because these neurological disorders affect synaptic transmission through limbic-cortical-striatal-pallidal-thalamic circuits in diverse ways, it was hypothesized that multiple types of dysfunction within these circuits can produce depressive symptoms.

BRAIN STRUCTURAL ABNORMALITIES IN MOOD DISORDERS

Structural abnormalities found in the population of individuals with mood disorders can be distinguished broadly with respect to the age at illness-onset of the sample being considered. Patients with early-onset mood disorders (i.e., first mood episode arising within the initial four to five decades of life) manifest neuromorphometric abnormalities that appear relatively selective for areas within the OMPFC and anatomically related structures within the temporal lobe, striatum, thalamus, and posterior cingulate (reviewed in Price and Drevets, 2010). Cases with affective psychoses also have been differentiated from controls by gray matter loss within the OMPFC (Coryell et al., 2005; MacFall et al., 2001). In contrast, elderly subjects with late-onset depression (i.e., first mood episode arising later than the fifth decade of life) show a higher prevalence of neuroimaging correlates of cerebrovascular disease relative both to age-matched healthy controls and to elderly depressives with an early age at depression-onset (Drevets et al., 2004). MDD and BD cases that have either psychotic features or late-life illness-onset show nonspecific signs of atrophy, such as lateral ventricle enlargement.

Within the OMPFC a relatively consistent abnormality reported in early onset MDD and BD has been a reduction in gray matter in *left* subgenual anterior cingulate cortex (sgACC). This volumetric reduction exists early in illness and in young adults at high familial risk for MDD, yet shows progression in longitudinal studies in samples with psychotic mood disorders (reviewed in Price and Drevets, 2010). Moreover, individuals with more chronic or highly recurrent illness show greater volume loss than those who manifest sustained remission (Fig. 34.6) (Salvadore et al., 2011). The abnormal reduction in

sgACC volume primarily has been identified in mood disordered subjects with evidence for familial aggregation of illness (Hirayasu et al., 1999; Koo et al., 2008; McDonald et al., 2004), suggesting that genetic factors that increase risk for the development of depression also affect neuroplasticity within this region (e.g., Pezawas et al., 2005).

The subgenual cortex areas implicated by volumetric MRI or postmortem neuropathological studies of mood disorders include both the infralimbic cortex (BA 25; e.g. Coryell et al., 2005) and the adjacent sgACC corresponding to BA 24sg (e.g., Drevets et al., 1997; Öngür et al., 1998; Öngür et al., 2003)]. Reductions in gray matter also have been identified consistently in PFC regions that share extensive connectivity with this portion of the medial prefrontal network, such as the BA 47s cortex in BD (Lyoo et al., 2004; Nugent et al., 2006) and BA 45a area of VLPFC in MDD (Bowen et al., 1989), as well as in the caudal orbitofrontal cortex (BA 11), frontal polar/dorsal anterolateral PFC (BA 9,10), hippocampus, parahippocampus and temporopolar cortex in MDD, and in the superior temporal gyrus and amygdala in BD (Coryell et al., 2005; Lyoo et al., 2004; Nugent et al., 2006; Price and Drevets, 2010). Finally, the pituitary and adrenal glands appear enlarged in MDD (Drevets, Gadde et al., 2004; Krishnan et al., 1991), consistent with other evidence that hypothalamic-pituitary-adrenal axis activity is elevated in mood disorders.

Discrepant results exist across studies, conceivably reflecting clinical and etiological heterogeneity extant within the MDD and BD syndromes. For example, in the hippocampus one study reported that reduced volume was limited to depressed women who suffered early-life trauma (Vythilingam et al., 2002), while others reported that hippocampal volume

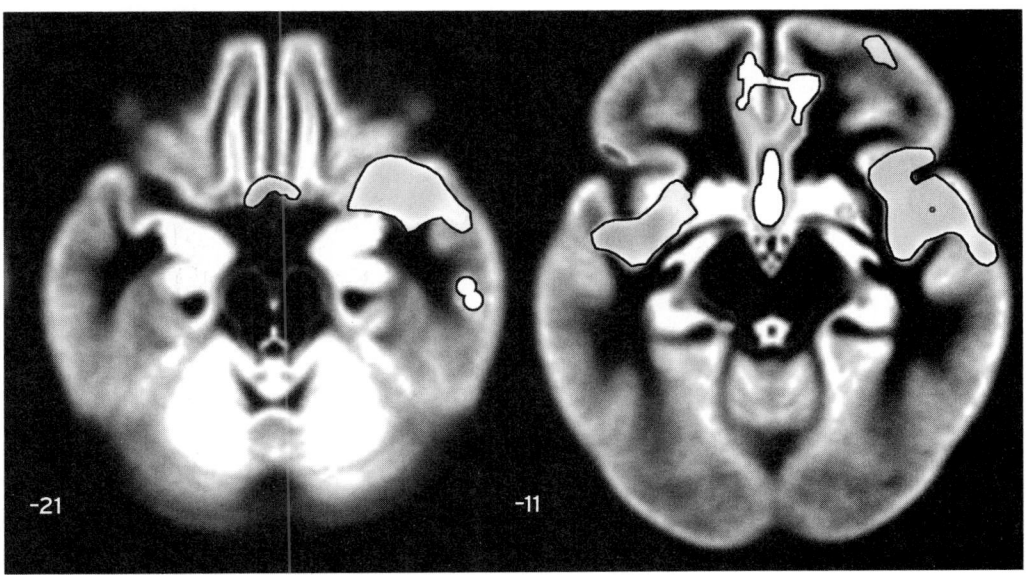

Figure 34.6 Regions where gray matter volume was reduced in unmedicated, currently depressed subjects with major depressive disorder (N = 58) compared to unmedicated, currently remitted MDD subjects (N = 27). The mean time spent in the current major depressive episode for the former group was about four years, and the mean time spent in remission for the latter group was over three years. The depressed group showed reduced gray matter relative to the remitted group in the subgenual and ventromedial prefrontal cortices and the rostral temporal cortex, a pattern that resembles that depicting the density of amygdala projections to the cortex in Fig. 34.1. Results are superimposed on axial slices of the average gray matter map of the 192 subjects participating in this study. The axial slices are located at 21 mm and 11 mm ventral to the bicommissural plane. (Modified from Salvadore et al., 2011.)

correlated inversely with time spent depressed and unmedicated (e.g., Sheline et al., 2003). In addition, the amygdala volume appears abnormally smaller in unmedicated BD subjects, but larger in BD subjects receiving mood stabilizing treatments associated with neurotrophic effects in experimental animals (Savitz et al., 2010).

NEUROPATHOLOGICAL CORRELATIONS WITH NEUROIMAGING ABNORMALITIES

The structural imaging abnormalities found in mood disorders have been associated with histopathological abnormalities in postmortem studies. Such studies report reductions in gray matter volume, thickness, or wet weight in the sgACC, parts of the orbital cortex, and accumbens (reviewed in Price and Drevets, 2010), and greater decrements in volume following fixation (implying a deficit in neuropil) in the hippocampus (Stockmeier et al., 2004) in MDD and/or BD subjects relative to controls. The histopathological correlates of these abnormalities include reductions in glia with no equivalent loss of neurons, reductions in synapses or synaptic proteins, and elevations in neuronal density, in MDD and/or BD samples in the sgACC, and of glial cell counts and density in the pgACC, dorsal anterolateral PFC (BA9), and amygdala (reviewed in Price and Drevets, 2010). The density of non-pyramidal neurons also appears decreased in the ACC and hippocampus in BD (Benes et al., 2001; Todtenkopf et al., 2005) and in the dorsal anterolateral PFC (BA9) in MDD (Rajkowska et al., 2007). Reductions in synapses and synaptic proteins were evident in BD subjects in the hippocampal subiculum/ventral CA1 region, which receives abundant projections from the sgACC (reviewed in Price and Drevets, 2010). Subjects with MDD studied postmortem also manifested dysregulation of synaptic function/structure related genes in the hippocampus and dalPFC, and with a corresponding lower number of synapses in the dorsolateral PFC (Duric et al., 2013; Kang et al., 2012). Notably, Kang et al. (2012) additionally identified a transcriptional repressor, GATA1, that was overexpressed in the dalPFC of MDD subjects, and that when expressed in PFC neurons is sufficient to decrease the expression of synapse-related genes, cause loss of dendritic spines and dendrites, and produce depressive behavior in rat models of depression.

The glial cell type implicated most consistently is the oligodendrocyte (reviewed in Price and Drevets, 2010). The concentrations of oligodendroglial gene products, including myelin basic protein, are decreased in frontal polar cortex (BA 10) and middle temporal gyrus in MDD subjects versus controls, potentially compatible with reductions in white matter volume of the corpus callosum genu and splenium found in MDD and BD. Perineuronal oligodendrocytes also are implicated in mood disorders by electron microscopy and reduced gene expression levels in PFC tissue. Perineuronal oligodendrocytes are immunohistochemically reactive for glutamine synthetase, suggesting they function like astrocytes to take up synaptically released glutamate for conversion to glutamine and cycling back into neurons.

CORRELATIONS WITH RODENT MODELS OF CHRONIC AND REPEATED STRESS

In regions that appear homologous to areas where gray matter reductions are evident in depressed humans (i.e., medial PFC, hippocampus) repeated stress results in dendritic atrophy and dysregulation of synaptic function/structure related gene expression, and these effects can be reversed at least partly by antidepressant drug administration (Banasr and Duman, 2007; Czeh et al., 2006; Duric et al., 2013; McEwen and Magarinos, 2001; Radley et al., 2008; Wellman, 2001). Dendritic atrophy putatively would be observed as a decrease in gray matter volume (Stockmeier et al., 2004). Moreover, both repeated stress and elevated glucocorticoid concentrations impair the proliferation of oligodendrocyte precursors in rodents, leading to reductions in oligodendroglial cell counts (Alonso, 2000; Banasr and Duman, 2007). In rats the stress-induced dendritic atrophy in the medial PFC was associated with impaired modulation of behavioral responses to fear-conditioned stimuli (Izquierdo et al., 2006), suggesting this process can alter emotional behavior.

The similarities between the histopathological changes that accompany stress-induced dendritic atrophy in rats and those found in humans suffering from depression suggest the hypothesis that homologous processes underlie the neuropathological changes in the hippocampal and medial PFC in both conditions (McEwen and Magarinos, 2001). Stress-induced dendritic remodeling depends on interactions between N-methyl-D-aspartate (NMDA) receptor stimulation and glucocorticoid secretion (McEwen and Magarinos, 2001). Notably, the depressive subgroups that show reductions in regional gray matter volume also show evidence of having elevated glutamatergic transmission in the same regions together with increased cortisol secretion (Drevets et al., 2002b). For example, cerebral glucose metabolism largely reflects energetic requirements associated with glutamatergic transmission (Shulman et al., 2004), raising the possibility that excitatory amino acid transmission contributes to the neuropathology of mood disorders (Paul and Skolnick, 2003). Elevated glutamatergic transmission in discrete anatomical circuits may explain the targeted nature of gray matter changes in depression (e.g., selectively affecting *left* sgACC) (Drevets and Price, 2005; McEwen and Magarinos, 2001; Shansky et al., 2009).

INTERRELATIONSHIP BETWEEN FUNCTIONAL AND STRUCTURAL NEUROIMAGING IN DEPRESSION

The co-occurrence of increased glucose metabolism and decreased gray matter within the same regions in mood disorders has been demonstrated most consistently by comparing image data from depressed patients before versus after treatment (e.g., Drevets et al., 2002a) and from remitted patients scanned before versus during depressive relapse (Hasler et al., 2008; Neumeister et al., 2004). In resting metabolic images in contrast, the reduction in gray matter volume in some structures appears sufficiently prominent to produce partial volume effects due to their relatively low spatial resolution of functional brain images. Notably, in some depressed samples the resting metabolism appears *reduced* in the sgACC relative to healthy controls, while in contrast, other studies reported increased metabolic activity in the sgACC in primary or secondary depression, suggesting that these apparent discrepancies may be explained by differing magnitudes of gray matter loss across samples (reviewed in Drevets et al., 2008). Consistent with this hypothesis, in MDD and BD samples who show abnormal reductions of both gray matter volume and metabolism in the sgACC (Drevets et al., 1997), correction of the metabolic data for partial volume (atrophy) effects reveals that metabolism is *increased* in the sgACC in the depressed phase, and decreases to normative levels with antidepressant treatment. This finding is consistent with evidence that the sgACC metabolism decreases during *symptom-remission* induced by a variety of antidepressant treatments (Drevets et al., 1997, 2002a; Holthoff et al., 2004; Mayberg et al., 2000), including electroconvulsive therapy (Nobler et al., 2001) and deep brain stimulation (Mayberg et al., 2005).

EMOTIONAL PROCESSING IN THE MEDIAL PREFRONTAL NETWORK

The sgACC participates generally in the experience and/or regulation of dysphoric emotion. In non-depressed subjects the hemodynamic activity increases in the sgACC during sadness induction, exposure to traumatic reminders, selecting sad or happy targets in an emotional go/no-go study, monitoring of internal states in individuals with attachment–avoidant personality styles, and extinction of fear-conditioned stimuli (reviewed in Price and Drevets 2010). Moreover, enhanced sgACC activity during emotional face processing predicted inflammation-associated mood deterioration in healthy subjects under typhoid vaccine immune challenge (Harrison et al., 2009). Finally remitted MDD subjects show decreased coupling between the hemodynamic responses of the sgACC, rostral superior temporal gyrus, hippocampus, and medial frontal polar cortex during guilt (self-blame) versus indignation (blaming others) (Green et al., 2010) (Fig. 34.7).

The ventral pgACC and vmPFC situated anterior to the sgACC have been implicated in healthy subjects in reward processing, and conversely in depressed subjects, in anhedonia (inability to experience pleasure in or incentive to pursue previously rewarding activities). In healthy humans the BOLD activity in this region correlates positively to ratings of pleasure or subjective pleasantness in response to odors, tastes, water in fluid-deprived subjects, and warm or cool stimuli applied to the hand, and the ventral pgACC shows activity increases in response to dopamine-inducing drugs and during preference judgments (reviewed in Wacker et al., 2009). Conversely in depressed subjects this region showed reduced BOLD activity during reward-learning and higher resting EEG delta current

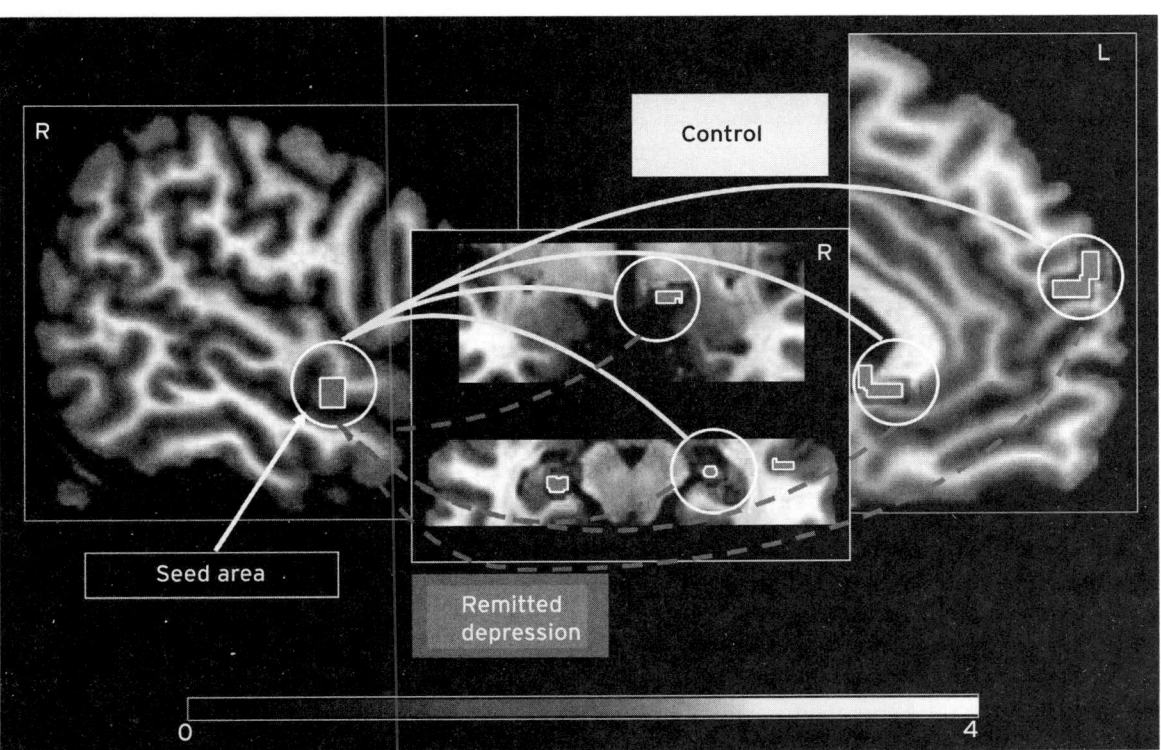

Figure 34.7 *Regions showing decreased coupling with the right superior temporal gyrus during the experience of guilt versus indignation in individuals with remitted MDD compared with healthy controls, including the lateral hypothalamus, hippocampus, medial frontal polar cortex, and subgenual anterior cingulate cortex/septal region. The shaded bar depicts voxel t-values, computed using Statistical Parametric Mapping (SPM) software. (Modified from Green et al., 2010.)*

density (putatively corresponding to decreased resting neural activity) in association with anhedonia ratings (Wacker et al., 2009).

More dorsal regions of the pgACC show physiological responses to diverse types of emotionally valenced or autonomically arousing stimuli. *Higher activity* in the pgACC holds *positive prognostic significance* in MDD, as depressives who improve during antidepressant treatment show abnormally elevated pgACC metabolism, MEG, and EEG activity *prior to treatment* relative to treatment-non-responsive cases or healthy controls (Pizzagalli, 2011).

Moreover, in the supragenual ACC depressed subjects show attenuated BOLD responses versus controls while recalling autobiographical memories (Young et al., 2012), associated with lower subjective arousal ratings experienced during memory recall. Behaviorally, MDD subjects are impaired at generating specific autobiographical memories, particularly when cued by positive words. These deficits were associated with reduced activity in the hippocampus and parahippocampus (Young et al., 2012).

Notably, preclinical evidence indicates that distinct medial prefrontal network structures are involved in opponent processes with respect to emotional behavior (Vidal-Gonzalez et al., 2006). Regions where metabolism correlates positively with depression severity include the sgACC and ventromedial frontal polar cortex; metabolism increases in these regions in remitted MDD cases who experience depressive relapse under catecholamine or serotonin depletion (Hasler et al., 2008; Neumeister et al., 2004) (Fig. 34.8). In contrast, the VLPFC/lateral orbital regions that include BA45a, BA47s and the lateral frontal polar cortex show inverse correlations with depression severity, suggesting they play an adaptive or compensatory role in depression (reviewed in Price and Drevets, 2010).

FUNCTIONAL IMAGING OF LIMBIC STRUCTURES ASSOCIATED WITH THE MEDIAL NETWORK

Subcortical structures that share extensive connections with the medial prefrontal network also show correlations to depressive symptoms. In the accumbens area the elevation of metabolism under catecholamine depletion correlates positively with the corresponding increment in anhedonia ratings (Fig. 34.8). In

Depressive Symptoms (MADRS)

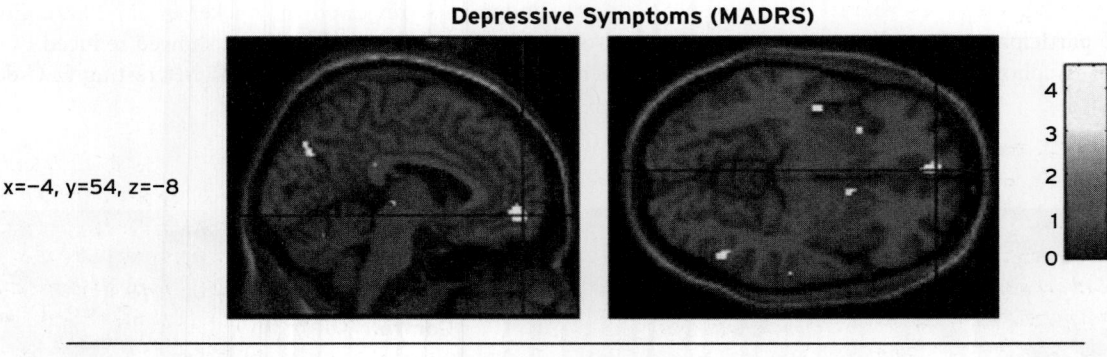

x=−4, y=54, z=−8

Anhedonia (minus-SHAPS)

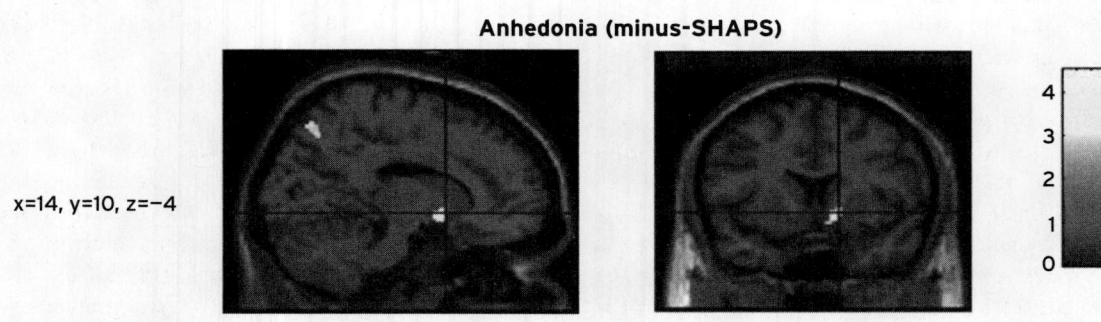

x=14, y=10, z=−4

Figure 34.8 Statistical parametric mapping image sections illustrating catecholamine depletion (CD)–induced metabolic changes and correlations between associated depressive symptoms and regional metabolism displayed on an anatomical MRI brain image in the voxel-wise analyses in a combined group of healthy controls and unmedicated individuals with major depressive disorder in remission (who are prone to develop depressive symptoms under CD produced via alpha-methyl-para-tyrosine administration). Upper Panel: Area where changes in metabolism correlated with CD-induced depressive symptoms (rated using the Montgomery-Asberg Depression Rating Scale) in the ventromedial frontal polar cortex, as shown by voxel t-values corresponding to p < 0.001 in the correlational analysis. Lower Panel: Area where glucose metabolism correlated with CD-induced anhedonia (rated by negative scores from the Snaith-Hamilton Pleasure Scale) in the right accumbens, shown as voxel t-values corresponding to p < 0.005. Coordinates corresponding to the horizontal and vertical axes are listed to the left of each image set, and correspond to the stereotaxic array of Talairach and Tournoux (1988) with the distance denoted in mm from the anterior commissure, with positive x = right of midline, positive y = anterior to the anterior commissure, and positive z = dorsal to a plane containing both the anterior and the posterior commissures. The gray shaded bars indicate voxel t values. (Reproduced by permission from Hasler et al., 2008.)

addition, fMRI studies show that hemodynamic responses of the ventral striatum to rewarding stimuli are decreased in depressives versus controls, and that higher levels of anhedonia are associated with blunted ventral striatal responses to rewarding stimuli in both healthy and depressed subjects (reviewed in Treadway and Zald, 2011). Furthermore, during probabilistic reversal learning, depressed subjects showed impaired reward (but not punishment) reversal accuracy in association with attenuated ventral striatal BOLD response to unexpected reward (Robinson et al, 2012).

In the amygdala glucose metabolic abnormalities appear more selective for depressive subgroups. In the left amygdala, metabolism increased during tryptophan depletion-induced relapse only in MDD subjects homozygous for the long allele of the 5HTT-PRL polymorphism (Neumeister et al., 2006b). In addition, elevated resting amygdala metabolism was reported specifically in depressed subjects classified as BD-depressed, familial pure depressive disease (FPDD), or melancholic subtype (reviewed in Price and Drevets, 2010). These subgroups also shared the manifestation of hypersecreting cortisol under stress, which is noteworthy here because the amygdala plays a major role in driving the stressed component of cortisol release (Drevets et al., 2002). In contrast, task-based hemodynamic responses of the amygdala show a pattern of abnormalities reflecting negative emotional processing biases in depression that appear more generalizable across depressed samples.

FUNCTIONAL NEUROIMAGING CORRELATES OF NEGATIVE EMOTIONAL PROCESSING BIAS IN MDD

Depressed individuals bias stimulus processing toward sad information as evidenced by enhanced recall for negatively versus positively valenced information on memory tests, greater interference from depression-related negative words versus happy or neutral words on emotional stroop tasks, faster responses to sad versus happy words on affective attention shifting tasks and more negative interpretation of ambiguous words or situations (reviewed in Victor et al., 2010). This bias also is evident in neurophysiological indices. Depressed subjects show exaggerated hemodynamic responses of the amygdala to sad words, explicitly or implicitly presented sad faces, and backwardly masked fearful faces, but blunted responses to masked happy faces (Suslow et al., 2010; Victor et al., 2010). A similar pattern of abnormal amygdala responses to masked sad and happy faces is observed in *unmedicated*-remitted subjects with MDD (Neumeister et al., 2006a; Victor et al., 2010) suggesting this abnormality is trait-like. Conversely, antidepressant drug administration shifts emotional processing biases toward the positive direction in both healthy and MDD samples (Geddes et al., 2003; Harmer, 2008; Victor et al., 2010). This shift is in the normative direction, as healthy subjects show a positive attentional bias (Erickson et al., 2005; Sharot et al., 2007; Victor et al., 2010) as well as greater amygdala responses to masked happy versus sad faces (Killgore and Yurgelun-Todd, 2004; Victor et al., 2010).

Taken together these data indicate that both the normative *positive* processing bias in healthy individuals and the pathological *negative* processing bias in MDD occur automatically, below the level of conscious awareness, and are mediated at least partly by rapid, non-conscious processing networks involving the amygdala (Victor et al., 2010). The differential response to masked-sad versus masked-happy faces in the amygdala is associated with concomitant alterations in the hemodynamic responses of the hippocampus, superior temporal gyrus, anterior insula, pgACC, and anterior orbitofrontal cortex (Victor et al., 2010). These regions may participate in setting a context or in altering reinforcement contingencies that conceivably may underlie these biases in MDD.

Similarly, during probabilistic reversal learning depressed MDD subjects showed exaggerated behavioral sensitivity to negative feedback versus controls, in association with blunted BOLD activity in the dorsomedial and ventrolateral PFC during reversal shifting, and absence of the normative deactivation of the amygdala in response to negative feedback (Taylor Tavares et al., 2008). Disrupted top-down control by the PFC over the amygdala thus may result in the abnormal response to negative feedback observed in MDD (Murphy et al., 1999).

IMPLICATIONS FOR NEUROCIRCUITRY-BASED MODELS OF DEPRESSION

Within the larger context of the limbic-cortical-striatal-pallidal-thalamic circuits implicated in the pathophysiology of depression, the basic science literature regarding specific limbic-cortical circuits involving the medial prefrontal network hold clear functional implications to guide translational models. The anatomical projections from the medial prefrontal network to the amygdala, hypothalamus, PAG, locus coeruleus, raphe, and brainstem autonomic nuclei play major roles in organizing the visceral and behavioral responses to stressors and emotional stimuli (Davis and Shi, 1999; LeDoux, 2003) (Fig. 34.4). In rats lesions of the medial PFC enhance behavioral, sympathetic, and endocrine responses to stressors or fear-conditioned stimuli organized by the amygdala (Morgan and LeDoux, 1995; Sullivan and Gratton, 1999). Nevertheless, these relationships appear complex, as stimulation of the amygdala inhibits neuronal activity in the mPFC, and stimulation of infralimbic and prelimbic projections to the amygdala excites intra-amygdaloid GABA-ergic cells that respectively inhibit or excite neuronal activity in the central amygdaloid nucleus (ACe) (Garcia et al., 1999; Likhtik et al., 2005; Perez-Jaranay and Vives, 1991; Vidal-Gonzalez et al., 2006).

For example, the amygdala mediates the *stressed component* of glucocorticoid hormone secretion by disinhibiting CRF release from the hypothalamic paraventricular nucleus (Herman and Cullinan, 1997). Moreover, lesions in the ventral ACC thus increase ACTH and CORT secretion during stress in rats, suggesting that the glucocorticoid response to stress is inhibited by stimulation of glucocorticoid receptors (GR) in this cortex (Diorio et al., 1993). Similarly, in monkeys Jahn et al. (2010) showed that PET measures of the subgenual PFC metabolism consistently predicted individual differences in plasma cortisol concentrations across a range of contexts that varied in stress load. It thus is conceivable that in humans with mood disorders dysfunction within the medial prefrontal network would disinhibit the efferent transmission from the ACe and BNST to the hypothalamus, contributing to elevated stressed cortisol secretion (Price and Drevets, 2010). Compatible with this hypothesis, cortisol hypersecretion in mood disorders has been associated with increased metabolic activity in the amygdala and with reduced gray matter in rostral ACC (Drevets et al., 2002b; Gold et al., 2002; McEwen and Magarinos, 2001; Treadway et al., 2009).

Furthermore, dysfunction of the medial prefrontal network may impair reward learning, potentially contributing to the anhedonia and amotivation manifest in depression. The ACC receives extensive dopaminergic innervation from the VTA and sends projections to the VTA that regulate phasic dopamine (DA) release. In rats, stimulation of these medial PFC areas elicits burst firing patterns in the VTA-DA neurons, while inactivation of the medial PFC converts burst firing patterns to pacemaker-like firing activity (reviewed in Price and Drevets, 2010). The burst firing patterns increase DA release in the accumbens, which is thought to encode information about reward prediction (Schultz et al., 1997). The mesolimbic DA projections from the VTA to the nucleus accumbens shell and the mPFC thus play major roles in learning associations between operant behaviors, or sensory stimuli and reward (Nestler and Carlezon, 2006). If the neuropathological changes in the ACC in mood disorders interfere with the cortical drive on VTA-DA neuronal burst firing activity, they may impair *reward learning*. Compatible with this hypothesis, depressives show attenuated DA release relative to controls in response to unpredicted monetary reward (Martin-Soelch et al., 2008) and fail to develop a response bias toward rewarded stimuli during reinforcement paradigms (reviewed in Treadway and Zald, 2011).

Furthermore, the patterns of physiological activity within the default mode system that involves the medial network are hypothesized to relate to self-absorption or obsessive ruminations (Grimm et al., 2009; Gusnard et al., 2001). In depressed subjects increasing levels of default mode network (DMN) dominance over the putative "task-positive network" (TPN; a group of structures that activate during volitional attention and thought) were associated with higher levels of maladaptive, depressive rumination and lower levels of adaptive, reflective rumination (Hamilton et al., 2011). Crucially, hemodynamic activity increased in the BA47s region in depressed subjects at the onset of increases in TPN activity. It thus was hypothesized that the DMN supports representation of negative, self-referential information in depression, and that activity within the vicinity of BA 47s in conjunction with increased levels of DMN activity may initiate an adaptive engagement of the TPN (Hamilton et al., 2011). Such an adaptive relationship potentially could explain the inverse correlation between depression severity and metabolic activity in BA 47s described previously. Notably, interpersonal psychotherapy, which can reduce depressive symptoms in

MDD, enhanced activity in the vicinity of BA 47s (Brody et al., 2001; Öngür et al., 2003). Cognitive-therapeutic strategies for depression also have been hypothesized to depend on enhancing the function of neural substrates that serve as convergence zones between multiple prefrontal networks, such as BA 47s.

As described earlier, somatic antidepressant treatments also influence activity within the limbic-cortical-striatal-pallidal-thalamic circuitry. Such treatments reduce basal metabolic activity that putatively is pathologically elevated in some limbic and medial prefrontal structures. In addition, however, antidepressant drugs have been shown more specifically to reduce limbic responses to negative or sad stimuli, and in some cases, to additionally enhance such responses to positive stimuli (e.g., Victor et al., 2010). For example, functional imaging studies in depressed humans indicate that metabolism and blood flow decrease in the sgACC/vmPFC in response to chronic treatment with antidepressant drugs, vagus nerve stimulation, or deep brain stimulation of the sgACC or anterior capsule, and activity in the relevant limbic-thalamocortical circuitry also decreases during effective treatment with antidepressant drugs or electroconvulsive therapy (e.g., Mayberg et al., 1999; Mayberg et al., 2005; reviewed in Price and Drevets, 2010). Preliminary reports also indicate that chronic SSRI treatment or deep brain stimulation of the anterior capsule reduces the abnormally elevated metabolism in the accumbens area in MDD or in depression associated with obsessive-compulsive disorder (reviewed in Price and Drevets, 2010). Most notably, the observations that deep brain stimulation (DBS) and neurosurgical lesions placed within the circuits formed by these structures can alleviate treatment refractory depression (TRD) implicate directly the medial prefrontal network and its associated limbic, striatal, and thalamic targets in the mechanisms of antidepressant therapy.

Mayberg et al. (2005) initially demonstrated that DBS applied via electrodes situated in the white matter immediately adjacent to the sgACC produced antidepressant effects in TRD. This site was located in the vicinity of loci where neurosurgically placed lesions had shown efficacy in TRD in association with the prelimbic leukectomy procedure, and also would have involved some white matter tracts interrupted in the anterior cingulotomy procedure (Fig. 34.5). Similarly, Malone et al. (2009) showed that DBS administered within the accumbens area/ventral internal capsule improved depressive symptoms in TRD. This locus targeted by this procedure is in the vicinity of that affected by the subcaudate tractotomy procedure used for TRD. A third site where both DBS and neurosurgical lesions have shown efficacy in TRD is the anterior limb of the internal capsule, an area that had been surgically targeted by the anterior capsulotomy (Schlaepfer et al., 2008). Finally, a fourth site where DBS improved TRD in a single case report is the habenula, an epithalamic structure implicated in the pathophysiology of depression by both preclinical and human neuroimaging studies (Sartorius et al., 2010). Some of the major circuits in which these procedures putatively would modulate or interrupt neurotransmission in mood disorders are depicted in Figure 34.5.

SUMMARY

The results of studies conducted using neuroimaging lesion analysis, and postmortem techniques support models in which the pathophysiology of depression involves dysfunction within an extended network involving the medial prefrontal network and anatomically related limbic, striatal, thalamic, and basal forebrain structures. The abnormalities of structure and function evident within the extended visceromotor network may impair this network's roles in cognitive processes such as reward learning, emotional processing, and autobiographical memory, and may dysregulate visceral, behavioral, and cognitive responses to emotionally salient stimuli and stress, potentially accounting for the disturbances in these domains seen in mood disorders.

DISCLOSURES

Neither author has a potential conflict-of-interest related to this work.

Dr. Price was supported by grant R01 MH070941 from the USPHS/NIMH and Dr. Drevets by funds from the William K. Warren Foundation and by grant R01 MH0XXXX from the NIMH.

REFERENCES

Alonso, G. (2000). Prolonged corticosterone treatment of adult rats inhibits the proliferation of oligodendrocyte progenitors present throughout white and gray matter regions of the brain. *Glia* 31(3):219–231.

Amaral, D.G., Price, J.L., et al. (1992). Anatomical organization of the primate amygdaloid complex. In Aggleton, J.P., ed., The Amygdala: Neurobiological Aspects of Emotion, Memory, and Mental Dysfunction. New York: Wiley-Liss, pp. 1–66.

Banasr, M., and Duman, R.S. (2007). Regulation of neurogenesis and gliogenesis by stress and antidepressant treatment. *CNS Neurol. Disord. Drug Targets* 6(5):311–320.

Bechara, A., Damasio, H., et al. (2000). Emotion, decision making and the orbitofrontal cortex. *Cereb. Cortex* 10(3):295–307.

Benes, F.M., Vincent, S.L., et al. (2001). The density of pyramidal and nonpyramidal neurons in anterior cingulate cortex of schizophrenic and bipolar subjects. *Biol. Psychiatry* 50(6):395–406.

Bhatnagar, S., Huber, R., et al. (2002). Lesions of the posterior paraventricular thalamus block habituation of hypothalamic-pituitary-adrenal responses to repeated restraint. *J. Neuroendocrinol.* 14(5):403–410.

Bowen, D.M., Najlerahim, A., et al. (1989). Circumscribed changes of the cerebral cortex in neuropsychiatric disorders of later life. *Proc. Natl. Acad. Sci. USA* 86(23):9504–9508.

Brody, A.L., Saxena, S., et al. (2001). Regional brain metabolic changes in patients with major depression treated with either paroxetine or interpersonal therapy: preliminary findings. *Arch. Gen. Psychiatry* 58(7):631–640.

Buckner, R.L., Andrews-Hanna, J.R., et al. (2008). The brain's default network: anatomy, function, and relevance to disease. *Ann. NY Acad. Sci.* 1124:1–38.

Buckwalter, J.A., Schumann, C.M., et al. (2008). Evidence for direct projections from the basal nucleus of the amygdala to retrosplenial cortex in the Macaque monkey. *Exp. Brain Res.* 186(1):47–57.

Carmichael, S.T., and Price, J.L. (1995a). Sensory and premotor connections of the orbital and medial prefrontal cortex. *J. Comp. Neurol.* 363:642–664.

Carmichael, S.T., and Price, J.L. (1995b). Limbic connections of the orbital and medial prefrontal cortex in macaque monkeys. *J. Comp. Neurol.* 363:615–641.

Carmichael, S.T., and Price, J.L. (1996). Connectional networks within the orbital and medial prefrontal cortex of macaque monkeys. *J. Comp. Neurol.* 371:179–207.

Coryell, W., Nopoulos, P., et al. (2005). Subgenual prefrontal cortex volumes in major depressive disorder and schizophrenia: diagnostic specificity and prognostic implications. *Am. J. Psychiatry* 162(9):1706–1712.

Czeh, B., Simon, M., et al. (2006). Astroglial plasticity in the hippocampus is affected by chronic psychosocial stress and concomitant fluoxetine treatment. *Neuropsychopharmacology* 31(8):1616–1626.

Damasio, A.R. (1995). Descarte's Error: Emotion, Reason, and the Human Brain. New York, London: Grosset/Putnam, Picador Macmillan.

Davis, M., and Shi, C. (1999). The extended amygdala: are the central nucleus of the amygdala and the bed nucleus of the stria terminalis differentially involved in fear versus anxiety? *Ann. NY Acad. Sci.* 877:281–291.

Diorio, D., Viau, V., et al. (1993). The role of the medial prefrontal cortex (cingulate gyrus) in the regulation of hypothalamic-pituitary-adrenal responses to stress. *J. Neurosci.* 13(9):3839–3847.

Drevets, W.C., Bogers, W., et al. (2002a). Functional anatomical correlates of antidepressant drug treatment assessed using PET measures of regional glucose metabolism. *Eur. Neuropsychopharmacol.* 12(6):527–544.

Drevets, W.C., Price, J.L., et al. (2002b). Glucose metabolism in the amygdala in depression: relationship to diagnostic subtype and plasma cortisol levels. *Pharmacol. Biochem. Behav.* 71(3):431–447.

Drevets, W.C., Gadde, K., et al. (2004). Neuroimaging studies of depression. In: Nestler, E.J., Charney, D.S., Bunney, B.J., eds. The Neurobiological Foundation of Mental Illness, 2nd Edition. New York: Oxford University Press, pp. 461–490.

Drevets, W.C., and Price, J.L. (2005). Neuroimaging and neuropathological studies of mood disorders. In: Wong, M.L., and Licinio, J., eds. Biology of Depression: From Novel Insights to Therapeutic Strategies. Weinheim, Germany: Wiley-VCH Verlag, vol. 1, pp. 427–466.

Drevets, W.C., Price, J.L., et al. (1997). Subgenual prefrontal cortex abnormalities in mood disorders. *Nature* 386(6627):824–827.

Drevets, W.C., Savitz, J., et al. (2008). The subgenual anterior cingulate cortex in mood disorders. *CNS Spectr.* 13(8):663–681.

Duric, V., Banasr, M., et al. (2013). Altered expression of synapse and glutamate related genes in post-mortem hippocampus of depressed subjects. *Int. J. Neuropsychopharmacol.* 16(1):69–82.

Erickson, K., Drevets, W.C., et al. (2005). Mood-congruent bias in affective go/no-go performance of unmedicated patients with major depressive disorder. *Am. J. Psychiatry* 162(11):2171–2173.

Ferry, A.T., Lu, X.C., et al. (2000). Effects of excitotoxic lesions in the ventral striatopallidal-thalamocortical pathway on odor reversal learning: inability to extinguish an incorrect response. *Exp. Brain Res.* 131(3):320–335.

Folstein, M.F., Robinson, R., et al. (1985). Depression and neurological disorders. New treatment opportunities for elderly depressed patients. *J. Affect. Disord. Suppl.* 1:S11–14.

Garcia, R., Vouimba, R.M., et al. (1999). The amygdala modulates prefrontal cortex activity relative to conditioned fear. *Nature* 402(6759):294–296.

Geddes, J.R., Carney, S.M., et al. (2003). Relapse prevention with antidepressant drug treatment in depressive disorders: a systematic review. *Lancet* 361(9358):653–661.

Gold, P.W., Drevets, W.C., et al. (2002). New insights into the role of cortisol and the glucocorticoid receptor in severe depression. *Biol. Psychiatry* 52(5):381–385.

Green, S., Ralph, M.A., et al. (2010). Selective functional integration between anterior temporal and distinct fronto-mesolimbic regions during guilt and indignation. *NeuroImage* 52(4):1720–1726.

Grimm, S., Boesiger, P., et al. (2009). Altered negative BOLD responses in the default-mode network during emotion processing in depressed subjects. *Neuropsychopharmacology* 34(4):932–843.

Gusnard, D.A, Akbudak, E., et al. (2001). Medial prefrontal cortex and self-referential mental activity: relation to a default mode of brain function. *Proc. Natl. Acad. Sci. USA* 98(7):4259–4264.

Hamilton, J.P., Furman, D.J., et al. (2011). Default-mode and task-positive network activity in major depressive disorder: implications for adaptive and maladaptive rumination. *Biol. Psychiatry* 70(4):327–333.

Harmer, C.J. (2008). Serotonin and emotional processing: does it help explain antidepressant drug action? *Neuropharmacology* 55(6):1023–1028.

Harrison, N.A., Brydon, L., et al. (2009). Inflammation causes mood changes through alterations in subgenual cingulate activity and mesolimbic connectivity. *Biol. Psychiatry* 66(5):407–414.

Hasler, G., Fromm, S., et al. (2008). Neural response to catecholamine depletion in unmedicated subjects with major depressive disorder in remission and healthy subjects. *Arch. Gen. Psychiatry* 65(5):521–531.

Herman, J.P., and Cullinan, W.E. (1997). Neurocircuitry of stress: central control of the hypothalamo-pituitary-adrenocortical axis. *Trends. Neurosci.* 20(2):78–84.

Hirayasu, Y., Shenton, M.E., et al. (1999). Subgenual cingulate cortex volume in first-episode psychosis. *Am. J. Psychiatry* 156(7):1091–1093.

Holthoff, V.A., Beuthien-Baumann, B., et al. (2004). Changes in brain metabolism associated with remission in unipolar major depression. *Acta. Psychiatr. Scand.* 110(3:184–194.

Hsu, D.T, and Price, J.L. (2007). Midline and intralaminar thalamic connections with the orbital and medial prefrontal networks in macaque monkeys. *J. Comp. Neurol.* 504(2):89–111.

Izquierdo, A., Wellman, C.L., et al. (2006). Brief uncontrollable stress causes dendritic retraction in infralimbic cortex and resistance to fear extinction in mice. *J. Neurosci.* 26(21):5733–5738.

Jahn, A.L., Fox, A.S., et al. (2010). Subgenual prefrontal cortex activity predicts individual differences in hypothalamic-pituitary-adrenal activity across different contexts. *Biol. Psychiatry* 67(2):175–181.

Kang, H.J., Voleti, B., et al. (2012). Decreased expression of synapse-related genes and loss of synapses in major depressive disorder. *Nat. Med.* 18:1413–1417.

Killgore, W.D., and Yurgelun-Todd, D.A. (2004). Activation of the amygdala and anterior cingulate during nonconscious processing of sad versus happy faces. *NeuroImage* 21(4):1215–1223.

Koo, M.S., Levitt, J.J, et al. (2008). A cross-sectional and longitudinal magnetic resonance imaging study of cingulate gyrus gray matter volume abnormalities in first-episode schizophrenia and first-episode affective psychosis. *Arch. Gen. Psychiatry* 65(7):746–760.

Krishnan, K.R., Doraiswamy, P.M., et al. (1991). Pituitary size in depression. [see comments]. *J. Clin. Endocrin. Met.* 72(2):256–259.

LeDoux, J. (2003). The emotional brain, fear, and the amygdala. *Cell. Mol. Neurobiol.* 23(4–5):727–738.

Likhtik, E., Pelletier, J.G., et al. (2005). Prefrontal control of the amygdala. *J. Neurosci.* 25(32):7429–7437.

Lyoo, I.K., Kim, M.J., et al. (2004). Frontal lobe gray matter density decreases in bipolar I disorder. *Biol. Psychiatry* 55(6):648–651.

MacFall, J.R., Payne, M.E., et al. (2001). Medial orbital frontal lesions in late-onset depression. *Biol. Psychiatry* 49(9):803–806.

Malone, D.A., Jr., Dougherty, D.D, et al. (2009). Deep brain stimulation of the ventral capsule/ventral striatum for treatment-resistant depression. *Biological. Psychiatry* 65(4):267–275.

Martin-Soelch, C., Szczepanik, J., et al. (2008). Lack of dopamine release in response to monetary reward in depressed patients: An 11C-raclopride bolus plus constant infusion PET-study. *Biol. Psychiatry* 63(7 suppl):116S.

Mayberg, H.S., Brannan, S.K., et al. (2000). Regional metabolic effects of fluoxetine in major depression: serial changes and relationship to clinical response. *Biol. Psychiatry* 48(8):830–843.

Mayberg, H.S., Liotti, M., et al. (1999). Reciprocal limbic-cortical function and negative mood: converging PET findings in depression and normal sadness. *Am. J. Psychiatry* 156(5):675–682.

Mayberg, H.S., Lozano, A.M., et al. (2005). Deep brain stimulation for treatment-resistant depression. *Neuron* 45(5):651–660.

McDonald, C., Bullmore, E.T., et al. (2004). Association of genetic risks for schizophrenia and bipolar disorder with specific and generic brain structural endophenotypes. *Arch. Gen. Psychiatry* 61(10):974–984.

McEwen, B.S., and Magarinos, A.M. (2001). Stress and hippocampal plasticity: implications for the pathophysiology of affective disorders. *Hum. Psychopharmacol.* 16(S1):S7–S19.

Morgan, M.A, and LeDoux, J.E. (1995). Differential contribution of dorsal and ventral medial prefrontal cortex to the acquisition and extinction of conditioned fear in rats. *Behav. Neurosci.* 109(4):681–688.

Murphy, F.C., Sahakian, B.J., et al. (1999). Emotional bias and inhibitory control processes in mania and depression. *Psychol. Med.* 29(6):1307–1321.

Murray, E.A., Wise, S.P., et al. (2010). Localization of dysfunction in major depressive disorder: prefrontal cortex and amygdala. *Biol. Psychiatry.* Epub ahead of print.

Nestler, E.J., and Carlezon, W.A., Jr. (2006). The mesolimbic dopamine reward circuit in depression. *Biol. Psychiatry* 59(12):1151–1159.

Neumeister, A., Drevets, W.C., et al. (2006a). Effects of a alpha 2C-adrenoreceptor gene polymorphism on neural responses to facial expressions in depression. *Neuropsychopharmacology* 31(8):1750–1756.

Neumeister, A., Hu, X.Z, et al. (2006b). Differential effects of 5-HTTLPR genotypes on the behavioral and neural responses to tryptophan depletion in patients with major depression and controls. *Arch. Gen. Psychiatry* 63(9):978–986.

Neumeister, A., Nugent, A.C., et al. (2004). Neural and behavioral responses to tryptophan depletion in unmedicated patients with remitted major depressive disorder and controls. *Arch. Gen. Psychiatry* 61(8):765–773.

Nobler, M.S., Oquendo, M.A., et al. (2001). Decreased regional brain metabolism after ect. *Am. J. Psychiatry* 158(2):305–308.

Nugent, A.C., Milham, M.P., et al. (2006). Cortical abnormalities in bipolar disorder investigated with MRI and voxel-based morphometry. *NeuroImage* 30(2):485–497.

Öngür, D., Drevets, W.C., et al. (1998). Glial reduction in the subgenual prefrontal cortex in mood disorders. *Proc. Natl. Acad. Sci. USA* 95(22):13290–13295.

Öngür, D., and Price, J.L. (2000). The organization of networks within the orbital and medial prefrontal cortex of rats, monkeys and humans. *Cereb. Cortex* 10(3):206–219.

Öngür, D., Ferry, A.T., et al. (2003). Architectonic subdivision of the human orbital and medial prefrontal cortex. *J. Comp. Neurol.* 460:425–449.

Padoa-Schioppa, C., and Assad, J.A (2006). Neurons in the orbitofrontal cortex encode economic value. *Nature* 441(7090):223–226.

Paul, I.A., and Skolnick, P. (2003). Glutamate and depression: clinical and preclinical studies. *Ann. NY Acad. Sci.* 1003:250–272.

Perez-Jaranay, J.M., and Vives, F. (1991). Electrophysiological study of the response of medial prefrontal cortex neurons to stimulation of the basolateral nucleus of the amygdala in the rat. *Brain Res.* 564(1):97–101.

Pezawas, L., Meyer-Lindenberg, A., et al. (2005). 5-HTTLPR polymorphism impacts human cingulate-amygdala interactions: a genetic susceptibility mechanism for depression. *Nat. Neurosci.* 8(6):828–834.

Phillips, M.L., Ladouceur, C.D., et al. (2008). A neural model of voluntary and automatic emotion regulation: implications for understanding the pathophysiology and neurodevelopment of bipolar disorder. *Mol. Psychiatry* 13(9):829:833–857.

Pizzagalli, D.A. (2011). Frontocingulate dysfunction in depression: toward biomarkers of treatment response. *Neuropsychopharmacology* 36(1):183–206.

Price, J.L., and Drevets, W.C. (2010). Neurocircuitry of mood disorders. *Neuropsychopharmacology* 35(1):192–216.

Price, J.L., and Drevets, W.C. (2012). Neural circuits underlying the pathophysiology of mood disorders. *Trends Cogn. Neurosci.* 16(1):61–71.

Pritchard, T.C., Nedderman, E.N., et al. (2008). Satiety-responsive neurons in the medial orbitofrontal cortex of the macaque. *Behav. Neurosci.* 122(1):174–182.

Radley, J.J., Rocher, A.B., et al. (2008). Repeated stress alters dendritic spine morphology in the rat medial prefrontal cortex. *J. Comp. Neurol.* 507(1):1141–1150.

Raichle, M.E., MacLeod, A.M., et al. (2001). A default mode of brain function. *Proc. Natl. Acad. Sci. USA* 98(2):676–682.

Rajkowska, G., O'Dwyer, G., et al. (2007). GABAergic neurons immunoreactive for calcium binding proteins are reduced in the prefrontal cortex in major depression. *Neuropsychopharmacology* 32(2):471–482.

Robinson, O.J., Cools, R., et al. (2012). Abnormal reward-related responses in the ventral striatum predict negative affective biases in depression. *Am. J. Psychiatry* 169(2):152–159.

Rolls, E.T. (2000). The orbitofrontal cortex and reward. *Cereb. Cortex* 10(3):284–294.

Romanski, L.M. (2007). Representation and integration of auditory and visual stimuli in the primate ventral lateral prefrontal cortex. *Cereb. Cortex* 17(Suppl 1):i61–69.

Rudebeck, P.H, and Murray, E.A. (2008). Amygdala and orbitofrontal cortex lesions differentially influence choices during object reversal learning. *J. Neurosci.* 28(33):8338–8343.

Saleem, K.S., Kondo, H., et al. (2008). Complementary circuits connecting the orbital and medial prefrontal networks with the temporal, insular, and opercular cortex in the macaque monkey. *J. Comp. Neurol.* 506(4):659–693.

Salvadore, G., Nugent, A.C., et al. (2011). Prefrontal cortical abnormalities in currently depressed versus currently remitted patients with major depressive disorder. *NeuroImage* 54(4):2643–2651.

Sartorius, A., Kiening, K.L., et al. (2010). Remission of major depression under deep brain stimulation of the lateral habenula in a therapy-refractory patient. [Case Reports Letter]. *Biol. Psychiatry* 67(2), e9–e11.

Savitz, J., Nugent, A.C., et al. (2010). Amygdala volume in depressed patients with bipolar disorder assessed using high resolution 3T MRI: the impact of medication. *NeuroImage* 49(4):2966–2976.

Schlaepfer, T.E., Cohen, M.X., et al. (2008). Deep brain stimulation to reward circuitry alleviates anhedonia in refractory major depression. *Neuropsychopharmacology* 33(2):368–377.

Schultz, W., Dayan, P., et al. (1997). A neural substrate of prediction and reward. *Science* 275(5306):1593–1599.

Shansky, R.M., Hamo, C., et al. (2009). Stress-induced dendritic remodeling in the prefrontal cortex is circuit specific. *Cereb. Cortex* 19:2479–2484.

Sharot, T., Riccardi, A.M, et al. (2007). Neural mechanisms mediating optimism bias. *Nature* 450(7166):102–105.

Sheline, Y.I., Gado, M.H., et al. (2003). Untreated depression and hippocampal volume loss. *Am. J. Psychiatry* 160(8):1516–1518.

Shulman, R.G., Rothman, D.L., et al. (2004). Energetic basis of brain activity: implications for neuroimaging. *Trends. Neurosci.* 27(8):489–495.

Starkstein, S.E., and Robinson, R.G. (1989). Affective disorders and cerebral vascular disease. *Br. J. Psychiatry* 154:170–182.

Stockmeier, C.A., Mahajan, G.J., et al. (2004). Cellular changes in the postmortem hippocampus in major depression. *Biol. Psychiatry* 56(9):640–650.

Sullivan, R.M, and Gratton, A. (1999). Lateralized effects of medial prefrontal cortex lesions on neuroendocrine and autonomic stress responses in rats. *J. Neurosci.* 19(7):2834–2840.

Suslow, T., Konrad, C., et al. (2010). Automatic mood-congruent amygdala responses to masked facial expressions in major depression. *Biol. Psychiatry* 67(2):155–160.

Taylor Tavares, J.V., Clark, L., et al. (2008). Neural basis of abnormal response to negative feedback in unmedicated mood disorders. *NeuroImage* 42(3):1118–1126.

Todtenkopf, M.S., Vincent, S.L., et al. (2005). A cross-study meta-analysis and three-dimensional comparison of cell counting in the anterior cingulate cortex of schizophrenic and bipolar brain. *Schizophr. Res.* 73(1):79–89.

Treadway, M.T., Grant, M.M., et al. (2009). Early adverse events, HPA activity and rostral anterior cingulate volume in MDD. *PLoS. One.* 4(3):e4887.

Treadway, M.T., and Zald, D.H. (2011). Reconsidering anhedonia in depression: lessons from translational neuroscience. *Neurosci. Biobehav. Rev.* 35(3):537–555.

Tsao, D.Y., Schweers, N., et al. (2008). Patches of face-selective cortex in the macaque frontal lobe. *Nat. Neurosci.* 11(8):877–879.

Victor, T.A, Furey, M.L., et al. (2010). Relationship of emotional processing to masked faces in the amygdala to mood state and treatment in major depressive disorder. *Arch. Gen. Psychiatry* 67(11):1128–1138.

Vidal-Gonzalez, I., Vidal-Gonzalez, B., et al. (2006). Microstimulation reveals opposing influences of prelimbic and infralimbic cortex on the expression of conditioned fear. *Learn. Mem.* 13(6:728–733.

Vythilingam, M., Heim, C., et al. (2002). Childhood trauma associated with smaller hippocampal volume in women with major depression. *Am. J. Psychiatry* 159(12):2072–2080.

Wacker, J., Dillon, D.G., et al. (2009). The role of the nucleus accumbens and rostral anterior cingulate cortex in anhedonia: integration of resting EEG, fMRI, and volumetric techniques. *NeuroImage* 46(1):327–337.

Wellman, C.L. (2001). Dendritic reorganization in pyramidal neurons in medial prefrontal cortex after chronic corticosterone administration. *J. Neurobiol.* 49(3):245–253.

Young, K.D., Erickson, K., et al. (2012). Functional anatomy of autobiographical memory recall deficits in depression. *Psychol. Med.* 42:345–357.

35 | NEUROBIOLOGY OF DEPRESSION IN LATER LIFE

Anatomy of Melancholia

K. RANGA RAMA KRISHNAN

ABBREVIATIONS

ACC   anterior cingulate cortex
BDNF   brain-derived neurotrophic factor
COMP   catechol-O-methyltransferase
DLPFC   dorsolateral prefrontal cortex
fMRI   functional magnetic resonance imaging
GABA   glycerol and gamma-aminobutyric acid
MRI   magnetic resonance imaging
OFC   orbitofrontal cortex
PFC   prefrontal cortex

INTRODUCTION

"The first of these 'Causes,' which is natural to all, and which no man living can avoid, is old age, which being cold and dry, and of the same quality as melancholy is, must needs cause it." (Burton, 1638).

Depression is common in later life, which was recognized as early as 1638 by Robert Burton (1638). Interestingly he recognized the brain as the possible anatomical location for depression: "but forasmuch as this malady is caused by precedent imagination, with the appetite, to whom spirits obey, and are subject to those principal parts, the brain must needs primarily be misaffected" (Burton, 1638). Large-scale epidemiological work from Kendler et al. (2002, 2006) suggests that multiple pathways can lead to depression in the elderly. These pathways include a strong vascular component (Fig. 35.1). The vascular pathway is one that some have suggested is critical in the development of depression in the elderly.

The study of depression in late life enables an interesting opportunity to dissect the anatomy of melancholia. This is because genetic factors appear to be less important in late-onset depression than in early-onset depression (Krishnan et al., 1988, Maier et al., 1991) and structural vascular or ischemic changes appear to be of greater importance. This is not a new idea. In 1905, Robert Gaupp, a German psychiatrist, described elderly patients with depression secondary to arteriosclerosis, many with persistent apathy and depressed mood (as quoted by Post [1962]). These early findings were based purely on clinical evidence of cerebral vascular lesions, typically strokes. This type of depression was termed arteriosclerotic depression.

More recently, magnetic resonance imaging (MRI) and other imaging techniques have enabled the *in vivo* depiction of subtle and surprisingly widespread structural brain changes in depressed patients. Early studies by our group using MRI suggested that subcortical ischemic changes are more prevalent in patients with late-onset depression, and these changes may play a role in the pathophysiology of this type of depression (Krishnan et al., 1988). This finding has since been replicated in numerous studies (Coffey et al., 1989, 1990; Greenwald et al., 1998; Steffens et al., 1998). This difference has also been demonstrated by Steffens et al. (1999) in community populations with depressive symptoms, thus extending the finding beyond individuals who meet the criteria for major depression. A recent meta-analysis confirmed the consistent increase in vascular disease in elderly depressed patients (Arnone et al., 2012).

We can therefore use these patients as a model to study the neural substrates of unipolar depression due to the occurrence of naturally occurring lesions that relate to depression. The scientific importance of this possibility is obvious: if vascular lesions in the brains of older individuals lead to secondary depressions with clinical characteristics that are similar to primary depressions, then these sites may provide important clues to the brain sites that are involved in depression in general. Lesions disrupt the mood circuit, and this increases the risk of depression by impairing the formation and alternation of stimulus-reward relationships, and by impairing the effect of negative reinforcement and the ability to handle stress.

In this review, we have focused primarily on the brain aspects of depression, but the relationship between vascular disease and depression is complex and most likely bidirectional (see Fig. 35.2). Thus, vascular disease predisposes to depression, but depression may also heighten the risk for vascular disease and worsen the prognosis of vascular disease. A summary of this line of work can be seen in Jiang et al. (2005).

LOCATION OF LESIONS

The first question that arises is: at what locations in the brain do the lesions that relate to depression occur? Figiel et al. (1991) showed that these lesions were more prevalent in patients with late-onset depression than in those with early-onset depression, and they were located in the frontal cortex and basal ganglia regions. Recent data in a large number of patients has identified

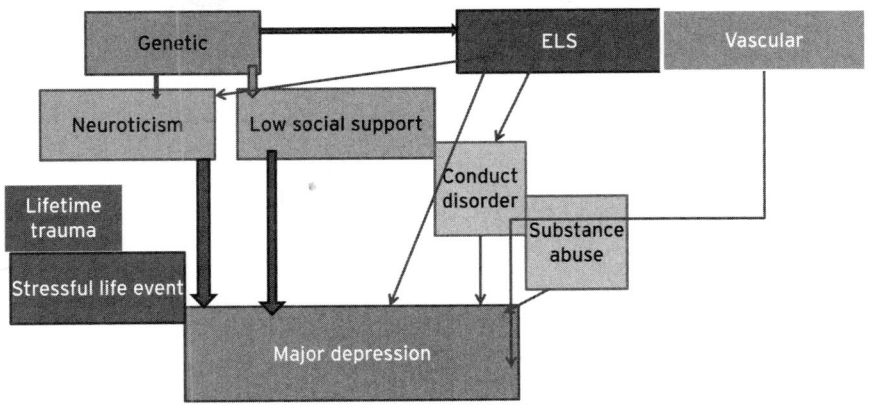

Figure 35.1 Pathways to depression based on large-scale and epidemiological and twin data. Four pathways to depression have been identified: internalizing, externalizing, adversity, and vascular. The basic thrust is that all four pathways to depression lead to structural and functional changes in the neural circuit (described later in text) that lead to risk for depression. Abbreviations: ELS = early life stress. (Simplified and modified from Kendler et al., 2002, 2006.)

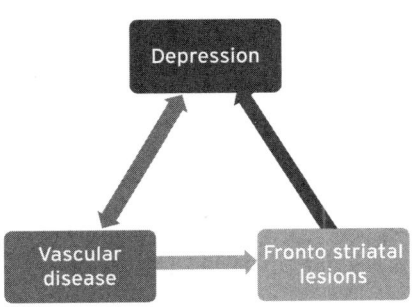

Figure 35.2 Link between vascular disease, lesions, and depression.

the medial orbital prefrontal cortex and the basal ganglia as the regions where the lesions, when present, link to depression (MacFall et al., 2001). This study used statistical parametric mapping to examine the location of lesions in patients and controls to see where the excess lesions were located. Using subtraction mapping, excess lesions were located in the medial orbital frontal cortex and the basal ganglia region.

The next questions that arise are: How do these changes predispose to depression? What neuroanatomical circuits and structural, functional, and biochemical changes are related to the lesions that can lead to depression? Also, what factors lead to the development of these lesions? We will first explore the circuit that affects mood, and then we will explore how these lesions could lead to the development of depression by disrupting the circuit. We will then discuss further the underlying pathophysiology of the lesions.

NEUROANATOMY OF MOOD CIRCUITS

It is not entirely possible to define a mood state in terms of rational, cognitive processes. The mood state, like other emotions, seems to have its own existence in the cognitive state of the individual, often with a momentum that outlasts any triggers it may have had in rational thought (Saper, 1996). Mood is an internal personal state and is, therefore, anthropomorphic. There are inherent difficulties in studying mood in humans through the study of mood in other species. The motoric expression of emotion is recognized in animals and inferences can be drawn about the underlying basis, but these inferences are based on our human experience. Thus, animal models are limited, but they do enable us to evaluate components—especially motoric, that are consistent across species—permitting us to understand relevant biological processes (Saper, 1996).

A mood state is often defined as an emergent property of forebrain connections that supports cognitive processes. These connections, in turn, project to parts of the limbic cortex from which output functions are derived. The limbic cortex, especially the amygdala, is believed to be involved in the evaluation of emotion (LeDoux, 1992). Outputs from the limbic cortex influence cortical processing (cognitive processing), and also regulate sympathetic, parasympathetic, and motoric expressions through mechanisms regulated by the hypothalamus, brainstem, and ventral striatum. These feed-forward mechanisms are important for the development of the momentum that is a common feature of the continued persistence of a mood alteration.

Mayberg (1997) proposed that three brain systems constitute the neurological substrate of depression: (*1*) a dorsal attention-cognitive system composed of the prefrontal cortex (PFC), the anterior cingulate, and the inferior parietal area; (*2*) a ventral vegetative-somatic system composed of the ventral frontal cortex, amygdala, hippocampus, subgenual cingulate, and ventral insula; and (*3*) a rostral cingulate region that integrates the dorsal and ventral systems. Mayberg (1997) proposed that a reciprocal relationship between the dorsal and ventral system regulates mood: sadness and depression decrease activity in the dorsal system and increase activity in the ventral system, and the remission of depression reverses

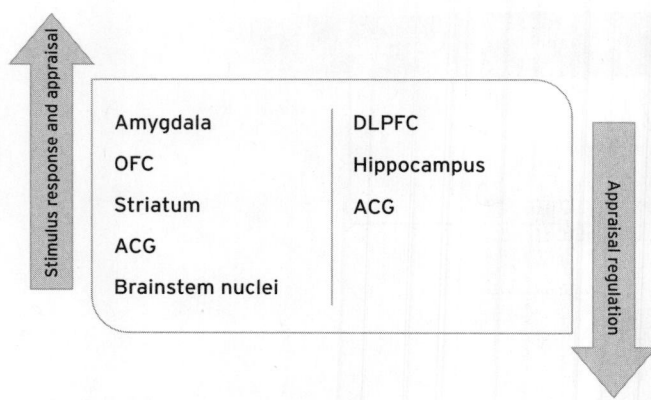

Figure 35.3 Mood circuit. Abbreviations: ACG = anterior cingulate gyrus; DLPFC = dorsolateral prefrontal cortex; OFC = orbitofrontal cortex. (Derived from Philips et al., 2003a.)

these relationships. Studies using functional MRI (fMRI) support this hypothesis (Drevets and Raichle, 1992; Gemar et al., 1996). In these, the amygdala, posteromedial orbitofrontal cortex, and ventral anterior cingulate were activated by the processing of emotional stimuli, but deactivated during attention-demanding cognitive tasks. Conversely, the dorsolateral prefrontal cortex (DLPFC) and dorsal anterior cingulate were activated by cognitive tasks and deactivated during experimentally induced and pathological emotional states. Studies by Drevets and Raichle (1992) and Gemar et al. (1996) are also supportive of such a reciprocal relationship. Phillips et al. (2003a) proposed a more detailed synthesized model (Fig. 35.3).

Three main processes are important for emotion. These are: (1) evaluation and identification emotional significance of the stimulus; (2) production of a specific affective state and its attendant behavior in response to the stimulus; and (3) regulation of the affective state and emotional behavior. The latter may involve inhibiting or modulating the first two processes, ensuring that the emotional experience affective state and generated behaviors are contextually appropriate (Phillips, 2003a).

The ventral system is important for the identification of the emotional significance of a stimulus and the production of an affective state, whereas the dorsal system is important for the regulation of the affective states. A reciprocal functional relationship exists between these two neural systems.

LESIONS DISRUPT BRAIN MOOD CIRCUITS

The basic premise is that structural lesions and functional impairments within the components of the ventral neural system are associated with reduced stimulus-reward relationships and motivation, and are biased toward the perception of negative rather than positive emotions, which leads to apathy, depression, and anhedonia under additional socioenvironmental conditions (Fig. 35.4a). Structural lesions and functional impairments within the dorsal neural system, associated with impairments in executive function, can lead to poor regulation of emotional behavior and perpetuate these phenomena (Fig. 35.4b). Depression can also occur through the disruption of the monoamine system that regulates these two systems.

A recent twin study clearly showed that these lesions can produce atrophy and a decrease in frontal lobe metabolism (DeCarli et al., 1995). This study did not evaluate depression, but it showed that these lesions can produce functional and structural changes (DeCarli et al., 1995; Krishnan et al., 1993)

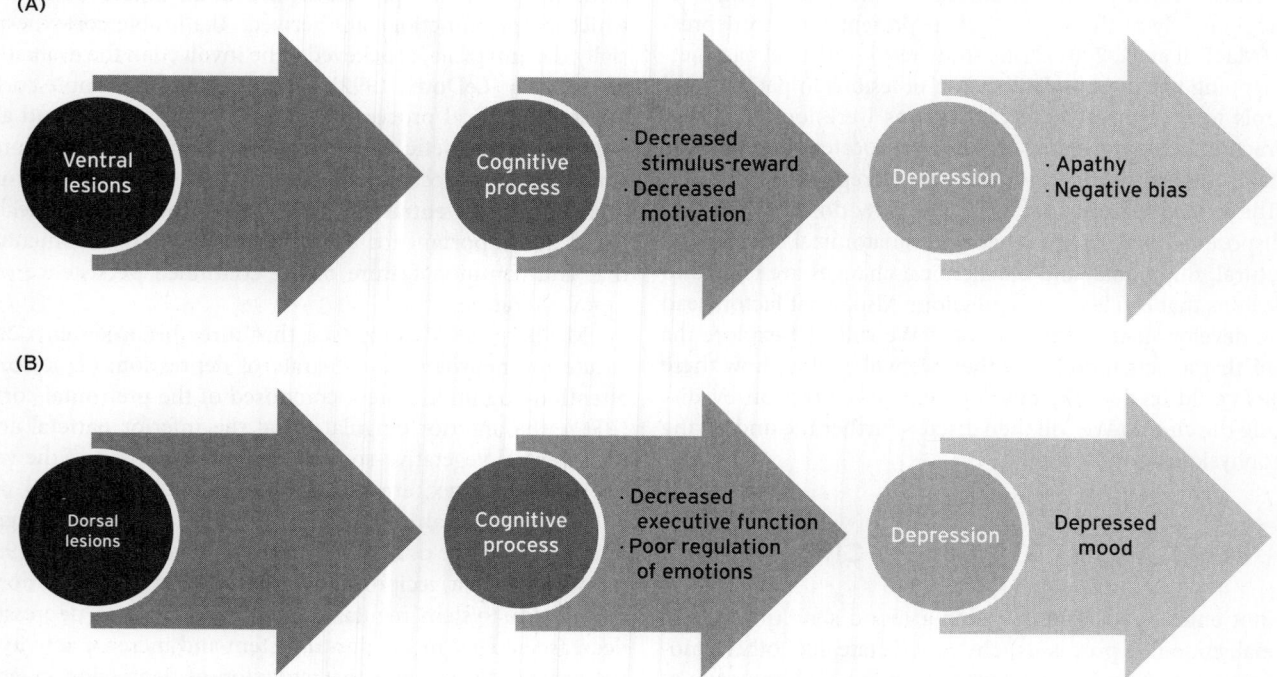

Figure 35.4 Disruption of the mood circuit by lesions in the neural system. (A) Ventral lesions; (B) Dorsal lesions.

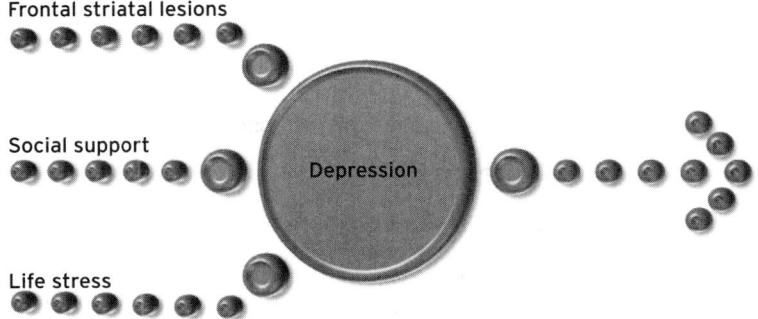

Figure 35.5 *Pathway for depression secondary to vascular disease.*

(Fig. 35.4). Lesions seen in elderly depressed patients are similar to those characterized as of ischemic origin (Taylor et al., 2001). Subcortical vascular disease, silent lacunar infarctions or hyperintense lesions also disrupt prefrontal basal ganglia circuits. These cognitive functions localize to a series of parallel pathways (Tekin and Cummings, 2002) that are tightly segregated, start in the frontal lobe, project to the ventral striatum, pass to the globus pallidus and substantia nigra, and pass through the thalamus back to the frontal lobe. Three of these circuits exhibit behavioral correlates: executive dysfunction (dorsolateral prefrontal circuit), apathy (anterior cingulate circuit), and mood lability and disinhibition (orbitofrontal circuit).

Prefrontal lesions are related to a reduction in caudate volume (Hannestad et al., 2006). In elderly depression, there are both increased lesions of the basal ganglia and an impact of prefrontal lesions on caudate volume (Hannestad et al., 2006; Krishnan et al., 1993). Basal ganglia lesions are related to a reduction in orbitofrontal cortex (OFC) volume. Lesions disrupt white matter tracts and the uncinate appears to be particularly affected in patients with depression, which suggests a disconnection between the amygdala and PFC (Taylor et al., 2008a). These studies suggest that lesions change the circuits that regulate mood. The data generated by these studies clearly supports the notion that when these lesions damage the circuits, it predisposes to depression (Fig. 35.5).

CIRCUIT CHANGES IN ELDERLY DEPRESSION

DORSAL CIRCUIT

DORSOLATERAL PREFRONTAL CORTEX
The dorsolateral part of the PFC forms a neuroanatomical substrate for attention (Puce et al., 1996). This circuit interacts with the cingulate, amygdala, and medial OFC (Carmichael and Price, 1995).

Individuals with DLPFC lesions have deficits on working memory tasks (Bechara et al., 1998), which is consistent with the findings of functional imaging studies regarding DLPFC activation on working memory tasks (Courtney et al., 1997; McCarthy et al., 1994). Reduced superior and middle frontal cortex volumes are reported in geriatric

depression (Ballmaier et al., 2004). Many positron emission tomography studies of depression, mostly conducted in the young, have found DLPFC metabolism to be changed (Drevets et al., 1992; Mayberg et al., 1994). Taylor et al., demonstrated microstructural differences in the white matter of the DLPFC in elderly depressed individuals (Taylor et al., 2004). Initial studies by Rajkowska et al. (1999) also suggest that there is glial pathology in this region in elderly depressed patients. Functional imaging studies in late-life depression demonstrated a reciprocal connectivity between the DLPFC and OFC and persistent deficits in DLPFC functioning in remission (Wang et al., 2008). This supports the concept that even for remitted elderly depressed individuals the DLPFC is not appropriately modulating the response to negative stimuli.

ROSTRAL ANTERIOR CINGULATE CORTEX
The rostral anterior cingulate cortex (ACC) is involved with motor function, cognitive function, and the regulation of arousal and drive states. It has dense projections to the motor cortex and spinal cord, reciprocal connections with the lateral PFC, and extensive afferents from the midline thalamus and brainstem nuclei. The affective division further projects to autonomic brainstem nuclei (Devinsky et al., 1995).

Due to this functional overlap, it has been proposed that the ACC may translate thoughts into action (Ebert and Ebmeier, 1996; Paus et al., 2001). The affective division of the ACC includes the subgenual anterior cingulate (BA 25), BA 33, and the pregenual, dorsal, or rostral anterior cingulate gyrus (rostral regions of BA 24) (Phillips et al., 2003). The caudal supragenual ACC (BA 32) is generally classified as the cognitive division of the ACC, but it may also play a role in mood regulation through its efferents to the amygdala (Philipps et al., 2003). We will discuss the subgenual PFC separately.

Bilateral volume reductions of the ACC have been reported in geriatric depression (Ballmier et al., 2004), and the geriatric depressed population also has been found to have more caudal metabolic deficits (de Asis et al., 2001). Taylor et al. (2004, 2007a) found changes in the fractional anisotropy of the anterior cingulate in geriatric depression. When individuals with geriatric depression perform tasks, there is impairment in ACC response (Wang et al., 2008).

HIPPOCAMPUS

The hippocampus has a complex role in affective regulation and in facilitating or inhibiting defensive behavior and anxiety in response to environmental stimuli (Corcoran et al., 2005; Phillips et al., 2003a; Van Den Hove et al., 2005). Thus, it may have a role in resolving goal conflicts and facilitating exploratory behavior patterns (Phillips et al., 2003a, b).

Some have reported a smaller hippocampal volume in mixed-age groups with depression (Bremner et al., 2000; Frodl et al., 2002; Krishnan et al., 1991; Mervaala et al., 2000; Shah et al., 1998; Sheline et al., 1996), while others have found no difference (Axelson et al., 1993; Hastings et al., 2004; MacQueen et al., 2003; Posener et al., 2003; Vakili et al., 2000). Our group and others have found smaller hippocampal volumes to be associated with recurrent depression (Axelson et al., 1993; Sheline et al., 1999), an earlier age of depression onset (Axelson et al., 1993; Macqueen et al., 2003; Sheline et al., 2003), a longer duration of untreated depression (Sheline et al., 2003), and poorer antidepressant response over one year (Frodl et al., 2004). Similar findings in older depressed populations have been reported, including both positive (Bell-McGinty et al., 2002; Steffens et al., 2000a) and negative studies (Ashtari et al., 1999; Pantel et al., 1997). In the elderly depressed, Steffens et al. (2000a, 2008) found decreased hippocampal volume with depression along with shape of the hippocampus (Qiu et al., 2009; Zhao et al., 2008) and cognitive changes.

VENTRAL CIRCUIT

AMYGDALA

The amygdala is critical for the evaluation of emotions. In animals and humans, bilateral damage to the amygdala results in the organism becoming placid and disinterested in the environment (Aggleton, 1992). In monkeys, bilateral lesions of the amygdala lead to an absence of emotional responses such as fear (LeDoux, 1992). The amygdala has extensive reciprocal projections with the frontal lobe, ventral striatum, thalamus, and cortex, as well as projections with regions that regulate behavioral, autonomic, arousal, and neuroendocrine responses, such as the hypothalamus and brainstem (Cardinal et al., 2002; Morgane et al., 2005). The amygdala is also involved in emotional appraisal and response (Bechara et al., 2003), assigning emotional significance to sensory stimuli (Russchen, 1986) and decision making, and it affects memory consolidation by influencing the hippocampus. The amygdala is necessary for the development of somatic and emotional states from actual environmental stimuli, although such states from secondary inducers such as memories or hypothetical events may be more reliant on the OFC (Bechara et al., 2003).

Neuropathological studies in depressed individuals of mixed ages show reduced glia density and a reduced glia/neuron ratio in the amygdala (Bowley et al., 2002). Structural imaging studies have shown mixed results, with some finding smaller amygdala core nuclei volumes in depressed adults (Sheline et al., 1998) and smaller volumes in adult depressed women (Hastings et al., 2004), whereas others have found no difference in amygdala volumes between depressed and non-depressed adults (Axelson et al., 1993; Frodl et al., 2004). Response to

negative emotional context results in amygdala activation (Hare et al., 2005). Transient sadness results in the activation of the left amygdala (Levesque et al., 2003), which is similar to the increased glucose metabolism in the left amygdala in depression (Drevets et al., 2002). The amygdala interfaces with layers of the OFC in a region that has been shown to have a reduction in pyramidal cell neurons in the elderly (Rajkowska et al., 2005). Imaging studies using the oddball task have also demonstrated that amygdala-OFC-DLPFC circuit activity is altered during depression (Wang et al., 2008).

SUBGENUAL CINGULATE CORTEX

The subgenual ACC has extensive reciprocal connections with several structures, including the OFC, nucleus accumbens, amygdala, and hypothalamus (Carmichael and Price, 1996). These connections likely represent a feedback circuit that regulates the amygdala's response to environmental stimuli, as the ACC can inhibit amygdala function (Rosenkranz et al., 2003).

Smaller left subgenual ACC volumes are seen in depressed individuals (Drevets et al., 1997). Volumetric differences in the left subgenual ACC have also been reported in adult samples with familial affective disorders (Drevets et al., 1997; Hirayasu et al., 1999) and adolescent-onset depression (Botteron et al., 2002). Others have found no differences in the volume of BA 24 or BA 25 in depression (Bremner et al., 2002; Kegeles et al., 2003). Consistent with the positive neuroimaging findings, neuropathological studies demonstrate a reduction in subgenual cingulate volume and a reduction in the number of glia in depressed individuals (Ongur et al., 1998). Sadness results in activation of the subgenual ACC (George et al., 1995; Liotti et al., 2000). Baseline functional imaging studies have found decreased metabolism and cerebral blood flow in the subgenual ACC in depressed individuals (Drevets et al., 2002; Kegeles et al., 2003; London et al., 2004; Mayberg et al., 1994); however, others have found no such difference between depressed and non-depressed individuals (Videbech et al., 2001). It is important to note that if functional imaging data is corrected for the partial volume effect of reduced gray matter volume, the metabolic activity in the subgenual ACC may actually be increased in depressed individuals. Very limited data has been gathered regarding this subject in elderly depressed individuals.

THE ORBITAL PREFRONTAL CORTEX

A variety of studies have implicated the OFC with regard to mood disorders (Bremner et al., 2002). Animal studies have demonstrated that lesions in this region of the PFC produce a behavioral pattern of timidity and reduction in novelty-seeking (Rolls, 1992). The OFC cortex connections have been detailed in a series of elegant studies by Carmichael and Price (1995, 1996). In primates, the orbital cortex has two selected patterns of connectivity that form two networks. One links sensory- and limbic-related areas within the orbital medial PFC. In the second, the orbital cortex is very closely linked to the amygdala. Projections from the medial and dorsal part of the basal nucleus of the amygdala reach areas 1AM, 1APM, 1AU, 13A, and 13M. Other amygdala nuclei also project to the medial orbital frontal cortex. The OFC projects widely upon higher-order multimodal association areas in the frontal, parietal, and temporal lobes (Carmichael and Price, 1995, 1996). The OFC is involved in representing reinforcers and in rapid stimulus-reinforcement learning for both positive and negative reinforcers (Elliott et al., 1997, 1998; Rolls, 2000).

Damage to the OFC impairs the learning and reversal of stimulus-reinforcement associations, and thus impairs the correction of behavioral responses when these are no longer appropriate (Rolls, 1992, 2000). Research with humans and non-human primates with selective damage to the OFC supports the role of these prefrontal territories in reversal learning (changing emotional behavior in response to previously rewarded or punished stimuli) (Anderson et al., 1999; Bechara et al., 1999, 2000). Suppressing negative affect in response to stimuli that previously aroused such emotions can be conceptualized as a form of reversal learning. This suppression of negative affect leads to an inability to correct reward- and punishment-related behaviors, and thus leads to impairments in the ability to modulate emotion. This impaired learning of stimulus-reinforcement associations may explain a key component of severe depression in the elderly, namely apathy. The inability to reverse/extinguish stimulus-reinforcement associations can explain why damage to the OFC impairs the ability to suppress transient sadness (Rolls, 2000). The OFC output pathways to the striatum are believed to be important in the implementation of these functions (Rolls, 1992, 2000).

The intradimensional/extradimensional discrimination task and the Tower of London tasks can be used to assess PFC function (Murphy et al., 1999). These tasks are related to the OFC, and performance on this task has been shown to be deficient in elderly depressed individuals. This task is also impaired during tryptophan depletion (Rogers et al., 1999) and in younger depressed patients (Davidson et al., 2003).

The right OFC exhibits increased activation during attempts to suppress emotional reactions to sad stimuli (Levesque et al., 2003). Using fMRI, depressed individuals have been shown to exhibit less activation in the left lateral OFC in response to negative stimuli (Elliott et al., 2002), as well as differential neural response in the right lateral OFC in response to sad distractors in an emotional go/no-go task (Elliot et al., 2002). Higher choline/creatinine ratios and cytosolic choline/neutral amino acid ratios have been reported in the OFC in depressed adolescents compared to the OFC of healthy adolescents (Steingard et al., 2000).

Hannestad et al. (2006) showed for the first time that the OFC is reduced in size in *elderly* depressed patients and that this change is related to the occurrence of prefrontal lesions. Neuropathological studies in elderly depressed individuals have identified decreases in OFC neuronal size and neuronal and glial densities in depression (Rajkowska et al., 1999). Several neuroimaging studies have reported smaller OFC volumes or smaller OFC gray matter volumes in depressed individuals (Botteron et al., 2002; Lacerda et al., 2004; Lai et al., 2000). Hyperintense lesions within the OFC are also associated with depression in elderly populations (MacFall et al., 2001), and OFC volume is negatively correlated with subcortical gray matter lesion severity (Lee et al., 2003), which supports the theory of orbitofrontal-striatal circuits (Tetkin and Cummings, 2002). OFC volume is related to performance on the Benton

Visual Retention Task and with impaired stimulus-reward relationships, and it is negatively correlated with severity of functional disability (Taylor et al., 2003d). In addition, functional imaging studies have supported the role of OFC in depression (Levesque et al., 2003).

BASAL GANGLIA CIRCUITS

These circuits appear to be of major importance in our understanding of both the motivation and motoric expression of the mood state. The entire cortical mantle projects topographically to the striatum (Alexander and Crutcher, 1990). Thus, in classical reports, the nucleus accumbens and the ventral striatum are considered to be the limbic part of the striatum. The striatal circuits have been well described by Alexander and Crutcher (1990). The ventral striatum projects to the ventral pallidum and then innervates the mediodorsal nucleus of the thalamus, which is reciprocally related to the PFC. The ventral striatum outflow has been conceived as being involved in the regulation of behaviors and thought processes. The striatum is no longer seen as homogeneous, but as consisting of compartments on the basis of connections as well as neurotransmitters. The importance of the basal ganglia is shown by the variety of studies that have implicated it in mood alterations, such as Huntington's disease, Parkinson's disease, Wilson's disease, strokes of the basal ganglia, and so forth (Caine and Shoulson, 1983; Charpier and Deniau, 1997; Folstein et al., 1979; Saint-Cyr et al., 1992; Swerdlow and Koob, 1987). In the elderly, basal ganglia lesions and reduced volume of the caudate are associated with depression. Prefrontal lesions are linked to smaller caudate volume.

SUBCORTICAL ISCHEMIC DISEASE

Subcortical ischemic disease is common in normal elderly patients (Bryan et al., 1999; de Leeuw et al., 2001; Price et al., 1997). The lesions arise in both periventricular and deep white matter and in subcortical gray matter nuclei. The vascular changes are age-related (Awad et al., 1986; Bryan et al., 1997, 1999; Guttmann et al., 1998; Longstreth et al., 1996). Cerebrovascular risk factors, such as hypertension and diabetes, are strongly linked to the development of subcortical ischemic disease (de Leeuw et al., 2002; Fazekas et al., 1988; Liao et al., 1997; Longstreth et al., 1996; Ylikoski et al., 1995). Specific genetic factors also contribute (Schmidt et al., 2000; Viitanen and Kalimo, 2000).

Ischemia negatively affects cognition (Butters et al., 2004) and is associated with disability (Steffens et al., 2002b); either of these factors may also further increase the risk of depression. The lesions are related to medical comorbidity, particularly cerebrovascular risk factors. Greater subcortical lesion severity is associated with hypertension (Dufouil et al., 2001; Fukuda and Kitani, 1995; Liao et al., 1996; Schmidt et al., 1999; Veldink et al., 1998), as well as metabolic factors including hypofolatemia (Iosifescu et al., 2005). The ischemic nature of these lesions has been demonstrated in postmortem studies (Thomas et al., 2002). Interestingly, a recent twin study by Kendler et al. (2009) showed that for older twins, an older age of depression onset in one twin is associated with a higher risk of vascular disease in the other twin, whereas a younger age of

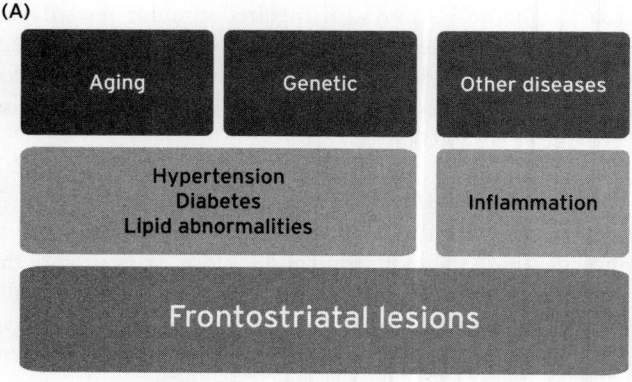

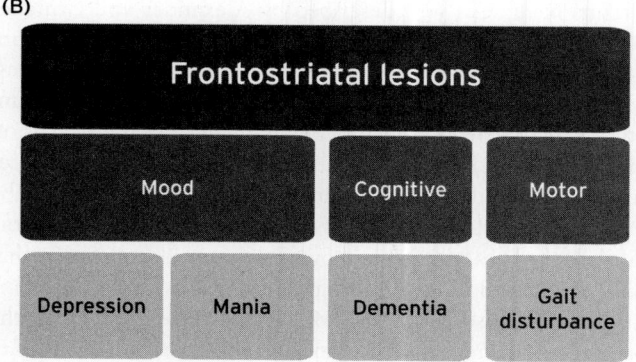

Figure 35.6. *Frontostriatal lesions. (A) Factors leading to frontostriatal lesions; (B) consequences of frontostriatal lesions.*

depression onset in one twin is associated with a higher risk for depression in the other twin (Kendler et al., 2009).

Subcortical vascular disease may have manifold clinical presentations (Kuo and Lipsitz, 2004; Pugh and Lipsitz, 2002) (Fig. 35.6). The clinical presentation for any individual is dependent on lesion location (which determines which neural circuits are affected) and medical illnesses or psychosocial risk factors. Subcortical ischemic disease associated with cognitive impairment is referred to as "vascular cognitive impairment" (O'Brien et al., 2003; Roman and Royall, 1999), and when it is associated with late-life depression, it is referred to as "vascular depression" (Krishnan et al., 1997, 2004; Steffens and Krishnan, 1998; Taylor et al., 2005). Vascular changes can be associated with other psychiatric and medical patterns, including psychosis and visual hallucinations (Breitner et al., 1990; Tonkonogy and Geller, 1999), manic depressive illness (McDonald et al., 1999), gait dysfunction (Whitman, 2001), and urinary incontinence (Sakakibara et al., 1999; Tarvonen-Schroder et al., 1996).

CONSEQUENCES OF SUBCORTICAL ISCHEMIC DEPRESSION

Subcortical ischemic depression is associated with adverse outcomes, including a higher risk for mortality (Baldwin, 2000; Levy et al., 2003) and functional impairment (Krishnan et al., 1997; Sachdev et al., 2005; Steffens et al., 2000a). Subcortical lesions are associated with poor antidepressant outcomes (O'Brien et al., 1998; Papakostas et al., 2005; Simpson et al., 1998) and with the persistence or worsening of depressive

symptoms over time (Steffens et al., 2002b). A poorer depression course is also associated with greater increases in subcortical lesion volume over that time (Taylor et al., 2003c). There may also be a biological gradient, wherein lesions that contribute to depression need to occur in specific regions (Greenwald et al., 1998; MacFall et al., 2001, 2006; Taylor et al., 2003b).

Subcortical ischemic depression also exhibits differences in (*1*) clinical symptoms of depression (Krishnan et al., 2004); (*2*) long-term course of depression, with a higher risk of developing dementia (Baldwin, 2000; Steffens et al., 2000b; Steffens et al., 2004); (*3*) familial pattern of depression (Krishnan et al., 2004); and (*4*) response to antidepressant medications (O'Brien et al., 1998; Papakostas et al., 2005; Simpson et al., 1998).

VASCULAR DEPRESSION AS A DISTINCT SUBTYPE

In the definition of our original proposals for a diagnosis of MRI-defined vascular depression (Krishnan et al., 1997; Steffens and Krishnan, 1998) and refined proposal for subcortical ischemic depression (Krishnan et al., 2004) is the notion that these lesions are causal risk factors for depression. Robins and Guze (1970) proposed formal criteria for establishing the validity of psychiatric diagnoses: (*1*) clinical description; (*2*) laboratory studies (including psychological tests, radiology, and postmortem findings); (*3*) delimitation from other disorders; (*4*) follow-up studies; and (*5*) family studies. However, of the more than 400 entities in the *Diagnostic and Statistical Manual of Mental Disorders*, few meet these criteria, and the concept of discrete disease entities in the psychiatric context may be problematic (Kendell and Gourlay, 1970; Kendell and Jablensky, 2003). One of the hallmarks for symptom- and course-based identification is to demonstrate points of non-overlap between similar syndromes, but the differences between psychiatric diseases are not as distinct as one would like. Any proposal of diagnostic criteria that claims a psychiatric disorder is due to a medical condition should undergo intense scrutiny (Evans, 1978; Hill, 1965).

We have previously proposed other criteria for defining disease (Krishnan, 2005) that may be more applicable to psychiatric disorders. The first criterion is that the condition should be one that leads to a risk for adverse outcomes, specifically mortality or functional impairment. The second criterion is that when an identifiable environmental factor, pathology, or genetic factor can be clearly defined, that factor should be expected to separate the entity from similar entities on at least one of the following domains: (*1*) clinical symptoms; (*2*) course and outcome; (*3*) familial pattern; or (*4*) response to specific treatment.

Subcortical ischemic depression meets these criteria. Given our current understanding of cerebrovascular disease in subcortical ischemic depression, treatment options that address vascular risk factors may prove to be of benefit.

The calcium-channel blocker nimodipine is one potential treatment approach, as studies have shown that it may augment response to antidepressant medications in patients with vascular depression (Taragano et al., 2001, 2005). The cited double-blind studies suggest that nimodipine improves remission rates and improves the odds of sustained response. Testing has not yet been performed to determine whether therapy to prevent the progression of subcortical ischemic disease affects the rates or outcomes of depression, but such a study is needed to examine whether lesions are causal risk factors for depression and to provide a rationale for identifying and treating vascular depression as a separate entity.

GENETICS

As noted multiple times, genetic factors affect many aspects of the development and possibly progression of subcortical ischemic depression (Fig. 35.7). The findings so far are limited to a few candidate genes that we have assessed. They include the gene for serotonin transporter as well as brain-derived neurotrophic factor (BDNF), catechol-O-methyltransferase (COMT) and angiotensin receptor.

SEROTONIN-TRANSPORTER-LINKED PROMOTER REGION

The serotonin-transporter-linked promoter region (5HTTLPR) polymorphism contains either a 44-base pair insertion (long allele or l) or deletion (short allele or s). Compared to the l allele, the s allele is associated with a lower level of 5-HT uptake and transcriptional efficiency of the serotonin transporter. The s allele is associated with reduced gray matter volume in the perigenual cingulate and amygdala (Scherk et al., 2009), resulting in the hypothesis that the 5HTTLPR genotype may affect brain development and be a potential risk for depression and anxiety.

Depressed individuals with the l/l genotype have smaller hippocampal volumes than those without the genotype (Janssen et al., 2004). In older individuals, later depression onset is associated with smaller hippocampal volumes in individuals with the l/l genotype, while an earlier age of depression onset is associated with smaller hippocampal volumes in individuals homozygous for the s allele. Elderly individuals with early-onset depression who are homozygous for the s allele exhibit reduced fractional anisotropy in the left uncinate fasciculus,

the fiber tract that connects the hippocampus and amygdala with the PFC (Taylor et al., 2007b) as well as a lower fractional anisotropy of the frontal gyri white matter. Other structures and links have not been tested, including the amygdalo-thalamic connection, the link between the amygdala and the basal ganglia (putamen), and the indirect pathway through the subthalamic nucleus. Preliminary studies have also shown that 5HTTLPR hetrozygotes have higher rates of subcortical ischemic disease (Steffens et al., 2008). The gene was not related to OFC volume (Taylor et al., 2007b).

BRAIN-DERIVED NEUROTROPHIC FACTOR

In animal models, BDNF appears to protect against cerebral ischemia. In older patients, the BDNF Met66 allele has been found to be associated with greater white matter hyperintensity volumes (Taylor et al., 2007b, 2008c). Depressed individuals have been shown to be more likely to be Met66 allele carriers than are individuals who are not depressed (Taylor et al., 2007b). In addition, although often viewed as a purely environmental construct, the perception of social support may be influenced by genetic factors that in studying the relationship between the BDNF, Val66Met polymorphism and social support measures in older individuals (Taylor et al., 2008c). After controlling for diagnosis and education level, the Met66 allele was associated with lower levels of subjective social support. This supports previous work that genetic factors may influence social support perception (Taylor et al., 2008a; Wang et al., 2012).

ANGIOTENSIN RECEPTOR (AGTR) GENE POLYMORPHISMS

In men, AGTR1 1166A allele homozygotes have shown significantly less change in white matter lesion volume than do 1166C carriers. Men with the AGTR2 3123C allele who report hypertension exhibit less change in white matter lesion volume than do hypertensive men with the 3123A allele, or men without hypertension. No such significant relationships have been found in women. Also, no significant gene-gene or gene-depression interactions have been observed (Taylor et al., 2010). The results are similar to gender differences in the relationship between other renin-angiotensin system polymorphisms and hypertension. It is not known whether these relationships are secondary to the polymorphisms that affect response to antihypertensive medication, or whether antihypertensive medications can slow the progression and lower the risk of morbidity.

METABOLOMIC STUDIES

Metabolomics is the global science of biochemistry. This emerging field enables the detection and quantification of small molecules that are involved in metabolic and signaling pathways. Metabolic signatures for disease and disease treatment could provide valuable biomarkers and insights regarding disease mechanisms. Metabolites that are altered in currently depressed patients compared to controls include several fatty acids, glycerol, and gamma-aminobutyric acid (GABA) (Paige et al.,

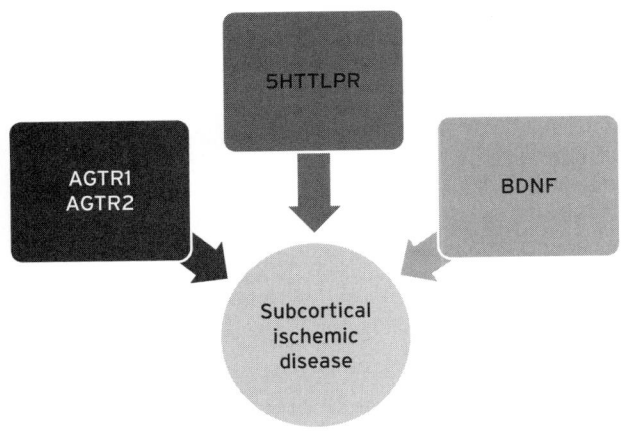

Figure 35.7 Genetic risk factors for subcortical cerebrovascular disease.

2007). Analyses that compared concentrations in remitted and currently depressed patients (Paige et al., 2007) revealed a pattern of metabolite alterations similar to the control versus currently depressed analyses. These observations suggest that the depressed state may be associated with alterations in the metabolism of lipids and neurotransmitters, and that treatment with antidepressants adjusts some of the aberrant pathways in disease so that the patients in remission have a metabolic profile more similar to controls than to the depressed population. These results will need to be examined and validated in larger longitudinal cohorts (Paige et al., 2007).

DEGENERATIVE DISEASE AND LATE-LIFE DEPRESSION

Depression can sometimes be the early stage of a neurodegenerative disorder. This is indeed well known in Huntington's disease. But it can also occur in Alzheimer's and Parkinson's disease.

As in most cases of depression, depressed mood and anhedonia are essential symptoms. Other features that can overlap with the primary disease, such as loss of appetite, sleep disturbance, weight gain, loss of libido, loss of concentration, and fatigue, make diagnosis challenging. However feelings of guilt or worthlessness are not common in these patients. (Aarsland et al., 2009). A robust link between history of depression and increased risk of subsequent development of Parkinson's was identified in a majority of studies (Ishihara and Brayne, 2006). The brain circuits implicated in depression in the context of Parkinson's disease is similar to the mood circuit and lends further credence to the circuit.

Another interreresting aspect of this link is the finding of Lewy body pathology, a known attribute in Parkinson's in patients with late-life depression, thus reinforcing the link and the notion that depression may be a prodrome in Parkinson's (Tsopelas et al., 2011).

A similar story emerges in the context of Alzheimer's disease. Depression is quite common in early Alzheimer's and is also seen as a risk factor for the disease. A common myth was that patients with depression could present with a full dementia syndrome that would be totally reversed with treatment. This is the concept of pseudodementia, considered to be a reversible form of cognitive impairment due to depression. This concept is erroneous. Patients with depression, presenting with severe cognitive impairment, were at a much higher risk of developing dementia (Kral and Emery, 1989). Interestingly there are now reports of increased amyloid pathology (the classic feaure of Alzheimer's) in late-life depressed patients with cognitive impairment thus again reinforcing the link but also highlighting the possibilty that depression can be a prodrome in Alzheimer's (Butters et al., 2008).

SUMMARY

Depressive disorders in the elderly provide a clinical model in which brain lesions are present, and thus they present a clinical patient population which, when coupled with postmortem and transgenic approaches, can increase our understanding of the brain circuits that are involved in mood disorders. It has been proposed that vascular lesions in critical regions of the brain are an important factor in the development of depression in the elderly. The scientific importance of this possibility is obvious: if vascular lesions in the brains of older individuals lead to secondary depressions that have clinical characteristics similar to primary depressions, then these sites may provide important clues to the brain sites involved in depression in general. This has led to a number of crucial findings:

1) OFC and basal ganglia lesions are related to depression;

2) Lesions seen in elderly depressed patients are similar to those characterized as of ischemic origin;

3) Prefrontal lesions are related to a reduction in caudate volume;

4) OFC volume is reduced in depressed patients;

5) Basal ganglia lesions are related to reduction in OFC volume;

6) Lesions disrupt white matter tracts, and the uncinate fasciculus appears to be particularly affected in patients with depression, which suggests fronto-amygdala disconnection;

7) Postmortem cell counts in the OFC among these patients show a reduction in layer-3 pyramidal neurons and layer-5 pyramidal neurons;

8) Postmortem vascular changes, including an increased density of vessels with larger perivascular spaces, are present in the white matter of OFC in elderly patients with depression;

9) BDNF genetic variation is linked to depression and subcortical ischemic disease;

10) A reciprocal interaction between the OFC and DLPFC has been shown using functional imaging;

11) In depressed patients, there is a decreased hemodynamic response in the amygdala, OFC, and striatum in the oddball task during the emotion-distractor condition, and this response is only partially ameliorated following remission;

12) In depressed patients, prefrontal function is impaired in a variety of functional tasks;

13) AGTR1 and AGTR2 genetic variations are linked to the risk of progression of subcortical ischemic disease;

14) Genetic variation in 5HTTLPR is related to lesions and changes in hippocampal volume;

15) Subjective social support, although generally construed as an environmental factor, is also related to change in BDNF genetic variation.

16) Late-life depression can be a prodrome to neurodegenerative disorders such as Alzheimer's and Parkinson's disease.

The net result of these findings is the considerable progress in our understanding of the neural circuits and neuropathology that underlie depression in late life. These findings have an obvious implication in the development of our understanding of other forms of depression.

DISCLOSURE

Dr. Krishnan serves on the Advisory Board of Cenerx, Health Sciences authority and Atentiv. He is Dean Duke NUS, Chairman SCRI and member of the specialist accreditation board Singapore. He is a member of the board for the National Medical Research Council (NMRC) in Singapore. He has stock ownership in Orexigen and indirect holdings in Cenerx. Patents have been licensed to Atentiv.

REFERENCES

Aarsland, D., Marsh, L., et al. (2009). Neuropsychiatric symptoms in Parkinson's disease. *Mov. Disord.* 24:2175–2186.

Aggleton, J.P. (1992). The functional effects of amygdala lesions in humans: a comparison with findings from monkeys. In: Aggleton, J.P., ed., *The Amygdala*. New York: Wiley-Liss, pp. 483–503.

Alexander, G.E., and Crutcher, M.D. (1990). Functional architecture of basal ganglia circuits: Neural substrates of parallel processing. *Trends Neurosci.* 13:266–271.

Anderson, S.W., Bechara, A., et al. (1999). Impairment of social and moral behavior related to early damage in human prefrontal cortex. *Nat. Neurosci.* 2(11):1032–1037.

Arnone, D., McIntosh, A.M., et al. (2012). Magnetic resonance imaging studies in unipolar depression: systematic review and meta-regression analyses. *Eur. Neuropsychopharmacol.* 22(1):1–16.

Ashtari, M., Greenwald, B.S., et al. (1999). Hippocampal/amygdala volumes in geriatric depression. *Psychol. Med.* 29:629–638.

Awad, I.A., Spetzler, R.F., et al. (1986). Incidental subcortical lesions identified on magnetic resonance imaging in the elderly: I. Correlation with age and cerebrovascular risk factors. *Stroke* 17:1084–1089.

Axelson, D.A., Doraiswamy, P.M., et al. (1993). Hypercortisolemia and hippocampal changes in depression. *Psychiatry Res.* 47:163–173.

Baldwin, R.C. (2000). The prognostic significance of abnormalities seen on magnetic resonance imaging in late life depression: clinical outcome, mortality, and progression to dementia at three years. *Int. J. Geriatr. Psychiatry* 15:1097–1104.

Ballmaier, M., Toga, A.W., et al. (2004). Anterior cingulate, gyrus rectus, and orbitofrontal abnormalities in elderly depressed patients: an MRI-based parcellation of the prefrontal cortex. *Am. J. Psychiatry* 161:99–108.

Bechara, A., Damasio, H., et al. (2000). Emotion, decision making and the orbitofrontal cortex. *Cereb. Cortex* 10(3):295–307. Review.

Bechara, A., and Damasio, H. (1999). Different contributions of the human amygdala and ventromedial prefrontal cortex to decision-making. *J. Neurosci.* 19(13):5473–5481.

Bechara, A., Damasio, H., et al. (2003). Role of the amygdala in decision-making. *Ann. NY. Acad. Sci.* 985:356–369.

Bechara, A., Damasio, H., et al. (1998). Dissociation of working memory from decision making within the human prefrontal cortex. *J. Neurosci.* 18:428–437.

Bell-McGinty, S., Butters, M.A., et al. (2002). Brain morphometric abnormalities in geriatric depression: long-term neurobiological effects of illness duration. *Am. J. Psychiatry* 159:1424–1427.

Botteron, K.N., Raichle, M.E., et al. (2002). Volumetric reduction in left subgenual prefrontal cortex in early onset depression. *Biol. Psychiatry* 51:342–344.

Bowley, M.P., Drevets, W.C., et al. (2002). Low glial numbers in the amygdala in major depressive disorder. *Biol. Psychiatry* 52:404–412.

Breitner, J.C., Husain, M.M., et al. (1990). Cerebral white matter disease in late-onset paranoid psychosis. *Biol. Psychiatry* 28:266–274.

Bremner, J.D., Narayan, M., et al. (2000). Hippocampal volume reduction in major depression. *Am. J. Psychiatry* 157:115–117.

Bremner, J.D., Vythilingam, M., et al. (2002). Reduced volume of orbitofrontal cortex in major depression. *Biol. Psychiatry* 51:273–279.

Bryan, R.N., Cai, J., et al. (1999). Prevalence and anatomic characteristics of infarct-like lesions on MR images of middle-aged adults: the atherosclerosis risk in communities study. *AJNR Am. J. Neuroradiol.* 20:1273–1280.

Bryan, R.N., Wells, S.W., et al. (1997). Infarctlike lesion in the brain: prevalence and anatomic characteristics at MR imaging of the elderly–data from the Cardiovascular Health Study. *Radiology* 202:47–54.

Burton, R. (1638). *The Anatomy of Melancholia*. London: Hen, Crisps and Lloyd.

Butters, M.A., Klunk, W.E., et al. (2008). Imaging Alzheimer pathology in late-life depression with PET and Pittsburgh Compound-B. *Alzheimer. Dis. Assoc. Disord.* 22(3):261–268.

Butters, M.A., Whyte, E.M., et al. (2004). The nature and determinants of neuropsychological functioning in late-life depression. *Arch. Gen. Psychiatry* 61:587–595.

Caine, E.D., Shoulson I. (1983). Psychiatric syndrome in Huntington's disease. *Am. J. Psychiatry* 140:728–733.

Cardinal, R.N., Parkinson, J.A., et al. (2002). Emotion and motivation: the role of the amygdala, ventral striatum, and prefrontal cortex. *Neurosci. Biobehav. Rev.* 26:321–352.

Carmichael, S.T., and Price, J.L. (1996). Connectional networks within the orbital and medial prefrontal cortex of macaque monkeys. *J. Comp. Neurol.* 371:179–207.

Carmichael, S.T., and Price, J.L. (1995). Limbic connections of the orbital and medial prefrontal cortex in macaque monkeys. *J. Comp. Neurol.* 363:615–641.

Charpier, S., and Deniau, J.M. (1997). *In vivo* activity-dependent plasticity at cortico-striatal connections: evidence for physiological long-term potentiation. *Proc. Natl. Acad. Sci. USA* 94:7036–7040.

Coffey, C.E., Figiel, G.S., et al. (1989). White matter hyperintensity on MRI clinical and neuroanatomic correlates in the depressed elderly. *J. Neuropsychiat. Clin. Neurosci.* 1:135–144.

Coffey, C.E., Figiel, G.S., et al. (1990). Subcortical hyperintensity on magnetic resonance imaging: A comparison of normal and depressed elderly subjects. *Am. J. Psychiatry* 147:187–189.

Corcoran, K.A., Desmond, T.J., et al. (2005). Hippocampal inactivation disrupts the acquisition and contextual encoding of fear extinction. *J. Neurosci.* 25(39):8978–8987.

Courtney, S.M., Ungerleider, L.G., et al. (1997). Transient and sustained activity in a distributed neural system for human working memory. *Nature* 386:608–611.

Davidson, R.J., Irwin, W., et al. (2003). The neural substrates of affective processing in depressed patients treated with venlafaxine. *Am. J. Psychiatry* 160:64–75.

de Asis, J.M., Stern, E., et al. (2001). Hippocampal and anterior cingulate activation deficits in patients with geriatric depression. *Am. J. Psychiatry* 158:1321–1323.

DeCarli, G., Murphy, D.G.M., et al. (1995). The effect of white matter hyperintensity volume on brain structure, cognitive performance and cerebral metabolism of glucose in 51 healthy adults. *Neurology* 45:2077–2084.

de Leeuw, F.E., de Groot, J.C., et al. (2001). Prevalence of cerebral white matter lesions in elderly people: a population based magnetic resonance imaging study: The Rotterdam Scan Study. *J. Neurol. Neurosurg. Psychiatry* 70:9–14.

de Leeuw, F.E., de Groot, J.C., et al. (2002). Hypertension and cerebral white matter lesions in a prospective cohort study. *Brain* 125:765–772.

Devinsky, O., Morrell, M.J., et al. (1995). Contributions of the anterior cingulate to behaviour. *Brain* 118:279–306.

Drevets, W.C., Bogers, W., et al. (2002). Functional anatomical correlates of antidepressant drug treatment assessed using PET measures of regional glucose metabolism. *Eur. Neuropsychopharmacol.* 12:527–544.

Drevets, W.C., Price, J.L., et al. (1997). Subgenual prefrontal cortex abnormalities in mood disorders. *Nature* 386:824–827.

Drevets, W.C., and Raichle M.E. (1992). Neuroanatomical circuits in depression: implications for treatment mechanisms. *Psychopharmacol. Bull.* 28:261–274.

Drevets, W.C., Videen, T.O., et al. (1992). A functional anatomical study of unipolar depression. *J. Neurosci.* 12:3628–3641.

Dufouil, C., de Kersaint-Gilly, A., et al. (2001). Longitudinal study of blood pressure and white matter hyperintensities. *Neurology* 56:921–926.

Ebert, D., and Ebmeier, K.P. (1996). The role of the cingulate gyrus in depression: from functional anatomy to neurochemistry. *Biol. Psychiatry* 39:1044–1050.

Elliott, R., Rubinsztein, J.S., et al. (2002). The neural basis of mood-congruent processing biases in depression. *Arch. Gen. Psychiatry* 59:597–604.

Elliott, R., Sahakian, B.J., et al. (1997). Abnormal response to negative feedback in unipolar depression: evidence for a diagnosis specific impairment. *J. Neurol. Neurosurg. Psychiatry* 63(1):74–82.

Elliott, R., Sahakian, B.J., et al. (1998). Abnormal neural response to feedback on planning and guessing tasks in patients with unipolar depression. *Psychol. Med.* 28(3):559–571.

Evans, A.S. (1978). Causation and disease: a chronological journey. *Am. J. Epidemiol.* 108:249–258.

Fazekas, F., Niederkor, K., et al. (1988). White matter signal abnormalities in normal individuals: correlation with carotid ultrasonography, cerebral blood flow measurements, and cerebrovascular risk factors. *Stroke* 19:1285–1288.

Figiel, G.S., Krishnan, K.R.R., et al. (1991). Subcortical hyperintensities on brain magnetic resonance imaging: a comparison between late age onset and early onset elderly depressed subjects. *Neurobiol. Aging* 26:245–247.

Folstein, S., Folstein, M.F., et al. (1979). Psychiatric syndromes in Huntington's disease. *Adv. Neurol.* 23:281–289.

Frodl, T., Meisenzahl, E., et al. (2002). Enlargement of the amygdala in patients with a first episode of major depression. *Biol. Psychiatry* 51:708–714.

Frodl, T., Meisenzahl, E.M., et al. (2004). Hippocampal and amygdala changes in patients with major depressive disorder and healthy controls during a 1-year follow-up. *J. Clin. Psychiatry* 65:492–499.

Fukuda, H., and Kitani, M. (1995). Differences between treated and untreated hypertensive subjects in the extent of periventricular hyperintensities observed on brain MRI. *Stroke* 26:1593–1597.

Gemar, M.C., Kapur, S., et al. (1996). Effects of self-generated and sad mood on regional cerebral activity: a PET study in normal subjects. *Depression* 4(2):81–88.

George, M.S., Ketter, T.A., et al. (1995). Brain activity during transient sadness and happiness in healthy women. *Am. J. Psychiatry* 152:341–351.

Greenwald, B.S., Kramer-Ginsberg, E., et al. (1998). Neuroanatomic localization of magnetic resonance imaging signal hyperintensities in geriatric depression. *Stroke* 29:613–617.

Guttmann C.R.G., Jolesz, F.A., et al. (1998). White matter changes with normal aging. *Neurology* 50:972–978.

Hannestad, J., Taylor, W.D., et al. (2006). White matter lesion volumes and caudate volumes in late-life depression. *Int. J. Geriatr. Psychiatry* 21(12):1193–1198.

Hare, T.A., Tottenham, N., et al. (2005). Contributions of amygdala and striatal activity in emotion regulation. *Biol. Psychiatry* 57:624–632.

Hastings, R.S., Parsey, R.V., et al. (2004).Volumetric analysis of the prefrontal cortex, amygdala, and hippocampus in major depression. *Neuropsychopharmacology* 29:952–959.

Hill, A.B. (1965). The environment and disease: association or causation? *Proc. R. Soc. Med.* 58:295–300.

Hirayasu, Y., Shenton, M.E., et al. (1999). Subgenual cingulate cortex volume in first-episdode psychosis. *Am. J. Psychiatry* 156:1091–1093.

Ishihara, L., and Brayne, C. (2006). A systematic review of depression and mental illness preceding Parkinson's disease. *Acta Neurol. Scand.* 113:211–220.

Iosifescu, D.V., Papakostas, G.I., et al. (2005). Brain MRI hyperintensities and one-carbon cycle metabolism in non-geriatric outpatients with major depressive disorder (Part I). *Psychiatry Res.* 140:291–299.

Janssen, J., Pol, H.E.H., et al. (2004). Hippocampal changes and white matter lesions in early-onset depression. *Biol. Psychiatry* 56:825–831.

Jiang, W., Glassman, A., et al. (2005). Depression and ischemic heart disease: what have we learned so far and what must we do in the future? *Am. Heart J.* 150(1):54–78.

Kegeles, L.S., Malone, K.M., et al. (2003). Response of cortical metabolic deficits to serotonergic challenge in familial mood disorders. *Am. J. Psychiatry* 1606:76–82.

Kendell, R.E., and Gourlay, J. (1970). The clinical distinction between psychotic and neurotic depressions. *Br. J. Psychiatry* 117:257–260.

Kendell, R., and Jablensky, A. (2003). Distinguishing between the validity and utility of psychiatric diagnoses. *Am. J. Psychiatry* 160:4–12.

Kendler, K.S., Fiske, A., et al. (2009). Delineation of two genetic pathways to major depression. *Biol. Psychiatry* 65(9):808–811.

Kendler, K.S., Gardner, C.O., et al. (2006).Toward a comprehensive developmental model for major depression in men. *Am. J. Psychiatry* 163(1):115–124.

Kendler, K.S., Gardner, C.O., et al. (2002). Toward a comprehensive developmental model for major depression in women. *Am. J. Psychiatry* 159(7):1133–1145.

Kral V.A., and Emery, O.B. (1989). Long-term follow-up of depressive pseudodementia of the aged. *Can. J. Psychiatry* 34:445–446.

Krishnan, K.R., Doraiswamy, P.M., et al. (1991). Hippocampal abnormalities in depression. *J. Neuropsychiatry Clin. Neurosci.* 3:387–391.

Krishnan, K.R., Hays, J.C., et al. (1997). MRI-defined vascular depression. *Am. J. Psychiatry* 154:497–501.

Krishnan, K.R., McDonald, W.M., et al. (1993). Neuroanatomical substrates of depression in the elderly. *Eur. Arch. Psychiatry Clin. Neurosci.* 243:41–46.

Krishnan, K.R. (2005). Psychiatric disease in the genomic era: rational approach. *Mol. Psychiatry* 10:978–984.

Krishnan, K.R., Taylor, W.D., et al. (2004). Clinical characteristics of magnetic resonance imaging-defined subcortical ischemic depression. *Biol. Psychiatry* 55:390–397.

Krishnan, K.R.R., Goli, V., et al. (1988). Leukoencephalopathy in patients diagnosed as major depressive. *Biol. Psychiatry* 23:519–522.

Kuo, H.K., and Lipsitz, L.A. (2004). Cerebral white matter changes and geriatric syndromes: is there a link? *J. Gerontol. A Biol. Sci. Med. Sci.* 59A:818–826.

Lacerda, A.L., Keshavan, M.S., et al. (2004). Anatomic evaluation of the orbitofrontal cortex in major depressive disorder. *Biol. Psychiatry* 55:353–358.

Lai, T.J., Payne, M.E., et al. (2000). Reduction of orbital frontal cortex volume in geriatric depression. *Biol. Psychiatry* 48(10):971–975.

LeDoux, J.E. (1992). Emotion and the amygdala. In: *The Amygdala*. Aggleton, J.P., ed., New York: Wiley-Liss, pp. 339–352.

Lee, S.H., Payne, M.E., et al. (2003). Subcortical lesion severity and orbitofrontal cortex volume in geriatric depression. *Biol. Psychiatry* 54:529–533.

Levesque, J., Eugene, F., et al. (2003). Neural circuitry underlying voluntary suppression of sadness. *Biol. Psychiatry* 53:502–510.

Levy, R.M., Steffens, D.C., et al. (2003). MRI lesion severity and mortality in geriatric depression. *Am. J. Geriatr. Psychiatry* 11:678–682.

Liao, D., Cooper, L., et al. (1997).The prevalence and severity of white matter lesions, their relationship with age, ethnicity, gender, and cardiovascular disease risk factors: The ARIC Study. *Neuroepidemiology.* 16:149–162.

Liao, D., Cooper, L., et al. (1996). Presence and severity of cerebral white matter lesions and hypertension, its treatment, and its control: the ARIC study. *Stroke* 27:2262–2270.

Liotti, M., Mayberg, H.S., et al. (2000). Differential limbic-cortical correlates of sadness and anxiety in healthy subjects: implications for affective disorders. *Biol. Psychiatry* 48:30–42.

London, E.D., Simon, S.L., et al. (2004). Mood disturbances and regional cerebral metabolic abnormalities in recently abstinent methamphetamine abusers. *Arch. Gen. Psychiatry* 61:73–84.

Longstreth, W.T.J., Manolio, T.A., et al. (1996). Clinical correlates of white matter findings on cranial magnetic resonance imaging of 3301 elderly people: the cardiovascular health study. *Stroke* 27:1274–1282.

MacFall, J.R., Taylor, W.D., et al. (2006). Lobar distribution of lesion volumes in late-life depression: the Biomedical Information Research Network (BIRN). *Neuropsychopharmacology* 31:1500–1507.

MacFall, J.R., Payne, M.E., et al. (2001). Medial orbital frontal lesions in late-onset depression. *Biol. Psychiatry* 49:803–806.

MacQueen, G.M., Campbell, S., et al. (2003). Course of illness, hippocampal function, and hippocampal volume in major depression. *Proc. Natl. Acad. Sci. USA* 100:1387–1392.

Maier, W., Lichtermann, D., et al. (1991). Unipolar depression in the aged: determinants of familial aggregation. *J. Affect. Disord.* 23:53–61.

Mayberg, H.S., Lewis, P.J., et al. (1994). Paralimbic hypoperfusion in unipolar depression. *J. Nucl. Med.* 35:929–934.

Mayberg, H.S. (1997). Limbic-cortical dysregulation: a proposed model of depression. *J. Neuropsychiatry Clin. Neurosci.* 9(3):471–481.

McCarthy, G., Blamire, A.M., et al. (1994). Functional magnetic resonance imaging of human prefrontal cortex activation during a spatial working memory task. *Proc. Natl. Acad. Sci. USA* 91:8690–8694.

McDonald, W.M., Tupler, L.A., et al. (1999). Hyperintense lesions on magnetic resonance images in bipolar disorder. *Biol. Psychiatry* 45:965–971.

Mervaala, E., Fohr, J., et al. (2000). Quantitative MRI of the hippocampus and amygdala in severe depression. *Psychol. Med.* 30:117–125.

Morgane, P.J., Galler, J.R., et al. (2005). A review of systems and networks of the limbic forebrain/limbic midbrain. *Prog. Neurobiol.* 75:143–160.

Murphy, F.C., Sahakian, B.J., et al. (1999). Emotional bias and inhibitory control processes in mania and depression. *Psychol. Med.* 29(6):1307–1321.

O'Brien, J., Ames, D., et al. (1998). Severe deep white matter lesions and outcome in elderly patients with major depressive disorder: follow up study. *BMJ* 317:982–984.

O'Brien, J.T., Erkinjuntti, T., et al. (2003).Vascular cognitive impairment. *Lancet Neurol.* 2:89–98.

Ongur, D., Drevets, W.C., et al. (1998). Glial reduction in the subgenual prefrontal cortex in mood disorders. *Proc. Natl. Acad. Sci. USA* 95:13290–13295.

Paige, L.A., Mitchell, M.W., et al. (2007). A preliminary metabolomic analysis of older adults with and without depression. *Int. J. Geriatr. Psychiatry* 22(5):418–423.

Pantel, J., Schroder, J., et al. (1997). Quantitative magnetic resonance imaging in geriatric depression and primary degenerative dementia. *J. Affect. Disord.* 42:69–83.

Papakostas, G.I., Iosifescu, D.V., et al. (2005). Brain MRI white matter hyper-intensities and one-carbon cycle metabolism in non-geriatric outpatients with major depressive disorder (Part II). *Psychiatry Res.* 140:301–307.

Paus, T. (2001). Primate anterior cingulate cortex: where motor control, drive and cognition interface. *Nat. Rev. Neurosci.* 2:417–424.

Phillips, M.L., Drevets, W.C., et al. (2003a). Neurobiology of emotion perception I: the neural basis of normal emotion perception. *Biol. Psychiatry* 54(5):504–514.

Phillips, M.L., Drevets, W.C., et al. (2003b). Neurobiology of emotion perception II: Implications for major psychiatric disorders. *Biol. Psychiatry* 54(5):515–528.

Posener, J.A., Wang, L., et al. (2003). High-dimensional mapping of the hippocampus in depression. *Am. J. Psychiatry* 160:83–89.

Post, F. (1962). *The Significance of Affective Symptoms in Old Age.* Maudsley Monogr. London: Oxford University Press.

Price, T.R., Manolio, T.A., et al. (1997). Silent brain infarction on magnetic resonance imaging and neurological abnormalities in community-dwelling older adults. The Cardiovascular Health Study. CHS Collaborative Research Group. *Stroke* 28:1158–1164.

Puce, A., Allison, T., et al. (1996). Differential sensitivity of human visual cortex to faces, letterstrings, and textures: a functional magnetic resonance imaging study. *J. Neurosci.* 16(16):5205–5215.

Pugh, K.G., and Lipsitz, L.A. (2002). The microvascular frontal-subcortical syndrome of aging. *Neurobiol. Aging* 23:421–431.

Qiu, A., Taylor, W.D., et al. (2009). APOE related hippocampal shape alteration in geriatric depression. *NeuroImage* 44(3):620–626.

Rajkowska, G., Miguel-Hidalgo, J.J., et al. (2005). Prominent reduction in pyramidal neurons density in the orbitofrontal cortex of elderly depressed patients. *Biol. Psychiatry* 58(4):297–306.

Rajkowska, G., Miguel-Hidalgo, J.J., et al. (1999). Morphometric evidence for neuronal and glial prefrontal cell pathology in major depression. *Biol. Psychiatry* 45(9):1085–1098.

Robins, E., and Guze, S.B. (1970). Establishment of diagnostic validity in psychiatric illness: its application to schizophrenia. *Am. J. Psychiatry* 126:983–987.

Rogers, R.D., Blackshaw, A.J., et al. (1999). Tryptophan depletion impairs stimulus-reward learning while methylphenidate disrupts attentional control in healthy young adults: implications for the mono-aminergic basis of impulsive behaviour. *Psychopharmacol. (Berl.)* 146(4):482–491.

Rolls, E.T. (1992). Neurophysiology and functions of the primate amygdala. In: Aggleton, J.P., ed., *The Amygdala.* New York: Wiley-Liss, pp. 143–165.

Rolls, E.T. (2000). The orbitofrontal cortex and reward. *Cereb. Cortex* 10(3):284–294. Review.

Roman, G.C., and Royall, D.R. (1999). Executive control function: a rational basis for the diagnosis of vascular dementia. *Alzheimer. Dis. Assoc. Disord.* 13:S69–S80.

Rosenkranz, J.A., Moore, H., et al. (2003). The prefrontal cortex regulates lateral amygdala neuronal plasticity and responses to previously conditioned stimuli. *J. Neurosci.* 23:11054–11064.

Russchen, F.T. (1986). Cortical and subcortical afferents of the amygdala complex. *Adv. Exp. Med. Biol.* 203:35–52.

Sachdev, P.S., Wen, W., et al. (2005). White matter hyperintensities are related to physical disability and poor motor function. *J. Neurol. Neurosurg. Psychiatry* 76:362–367.

Saint-Cyr, J.A., Taylor, A.E., et al. (1992). The caudate nucleus: head ganglion of the habit system. In: Vallar, G., Cappa, S.F., Wallesch, C.W., eds., *Neuropsychological Impairments Associate with Sub-cortical Lesions.* Oxford: Oxford University Press, pp. 204–226.

Sakakibara, R., Hattori, T., et al. (1999). Urinary function in elderly people with and without leukoaraiosis: relation to cognitive and gait function. *J. Neurol. Neurosurg. Psychiatry* 67:658–660.

Saper, C.B. (1996). Role of the cerebral cortex and striatum in emotional motor response. *Prog. Brain. Res.* 107:537–550.

Scherk, H., Gruber, O., et al. (2009). 5-HTTLPR genotype influences amygdala volume. *Eur. Arch. Psychiatry Clin. Neurosci.* 259 (4):212–217.

Schmidt, H., Fazekas, F., et al. (2000). Genetic aspects of microangiopathy-related cerebral damage. *J. Neural. Transm. Suppl.* 59:15–21.

Schmidt, R., Fazekas, F., et al. (1999). MRI white matter hyperintensities: three-year follow-up of the Austrian Stroke Prevention Study. *Neurology* 53:132–139.

Shah, P.J., Ebmeier, K.P., et al. (1998).Cortical grey matter reductions associated with treatment-resistant chronic unipolar depression. Controlled magnetic resonance imaging study. *Br. J. Psychiatry* 172:527–532.

Sheline, Y.I., Gado, M.H., et al. (2003). Untreated depression and hippocampal volume loss. *Am. J. Psychiatry* 160:1516–1518.

Sheline, Y.I., Gado, M.H., et al. (1998). Amygdala core nuclei volumes are decreased in recurrent major depression. *Neuroreport* 22:2023–2028.

Sheline, Y.I., Sanghavi, M., et al. (1999). Depression duration but not age predicts hippocampal volume loss in medically healthy women with recurrent major depression. *J. Neurosci.* 19:5034–5043.

Sheline, Y.I., Wang, P.W., et al. (1996). Hippocampal atrophy in recurrent major depression. *Proc. Natl. Acad. Sci. USA* 93:3908–3913.

Simpson, S., Baldwin, R.C., et al. (1998). Is subcortical disease associated with a poor response to antidepressants?: neurological, neuropsychological and neuroradiological findings in late-life depression. *Psychol. Med.* 28:1015–1026.

Steffens, D.C., Bosworth, H.B., et al. (2002a). Subcortical white matter lesions and functional impairment in geriatric depression. *Depress. Anxiety* 15:23–28.

Steffens, D.C., Byrum, C.E., et al. (2000a). Hippocampal volume in geriatric depression. *Biol. Psychiatry* 48:301–309.

Steffens, D.C., Helms, M.J., et al. (1999). Cerebrovascular disease and depression symptoms in the cardiovascular health study. *Stroke* 30:2159–2166.

Steffens, D.C., Krishnan, K.R., et al. (2002b). Cerebrovascular disease and evolution of depressive symptoms in the cardiovascular health study. *Stroke* 33:1636–1644.

Steffens, D.C., and Krishnan, K.R. (1998). Structural neuroimaging and mood disorders: recent findings, implications for classification, and future directions. *Biol. Psychiatry* 43:705–712.

Steffens, D.C., MacFall, J.R., et al. (2000b). Grey-matter lesions and dementia. *Lancet* 356:1686–1687.

Steffens, D.C., Taylor, W.D., et al. (2008). Short/long heterozygotes at 5HTTLPR and white matter lesions in geriatric depression. *Int. J. Geriatr. Psychiatry* 23(3):244–248.

Steffens, D.C., Tupler, L.A., et al. (1998). Magnetic resonance imaging signal hypointensity and iron content of putamen nuclei in elderly depressed patients. *Psychiatry Res.: Neuroimaging* 83:95–103.

Steffens, D.C., Welsh-Bohmer, K.A., et al. (2004). Methodology and preliminary results from the neurocognitive outcomes of depression in the elderly study. *J. Geriatr. Psychiatry Neurol.* 17:202–211.

Steingard, R.J., Yurgelun-Todd, D.A., et al. (2000). Increased orbitofrontal cortex levels of choline in depressed adolescents as detected by *in vivo* proton magnetic resonance spectroscopy. *Biol. Psychiatry* 48:1053–1061.

Swerdlow, N.R., and Koob, G.F. (1987). Dopamine, schizophrenia, mania and depression: toward a unified hypothesis of cortico-striato-pallido-thalamic function. *Behav. Brain Sci.* 10:197–245.

Taragano, F.E., Allegri, R., et al. (2001). A double blind, randomized clinical trial assessing the efficacy and safety of augmenting standard antidepressant therapy with nimodipine in the treatment of "vascular depression." *Int. J. Geriatr. Psychiatry* 16:254–260.

Taragano, F.E., Bagnatti, P., et al. (2005). A double-blind, randomized clinical trial to assess the augmentation with nimodipine of antidepressant therapy in the treatment of "vascular depression." *Int. Psychogeriatr.* 17:487–498.

Tarvonen-Schroder, S., Roytta, M., et al. (1996). Clinical features of leuko-araiosis. *J. Neurol. Neurosurg. Psychiatry* 60:431–436.

Taylor, W.D., Kuchibhatla, M., et al. (2008a). Frontal white matter anisotropy and antidepressant remission in late-life depression. *PLoS One* 3(9):e3267.

Taylor, W.D., MacFall, J.R., et al. (2007a). Structural integrity of the uncinate fasciculus in geriatric depression: Relationship with age of onset. *Neuropsychiatr. Dis. Treat.* 3(5):669–674.

Taylor, W.D., MacFall, J.R., et al. (2004). Late-life depression and microstructural abnormalities in dorsolateral prefrontal cortex white matter. *Am. J. Psychiatry* 161:1293–1296.

Taylor, W.D., MacFall, J.R., et al. (2005).Greater MRI lesion volumes in elderly depressed subjects than in control subjects. *Psychiatry Res.* 139:1–7.

Taylor, W.D., MacFall, J.R., et al. (2003b). Localization of age-associated white matter hyperintensities in late-life depression. *Prog. Neuropsychopharmacol. Biol. Psychiatry* 27:539–544.

Taylor, W.D., Payne, M.E., et al. (2001). Evidence of white matter tract disruption in MRI hyperintensities. *Biol. Psychiatry* 50(3):179–183.

Taylor, W.D., Steffens, D.C., et al. (2010). Angiotensin receptor gene polymorphisms and 2-year change in hyperintense lesion volume in men. *Mol. Psychiatry* 15(8):816–822.

Taylor, W.D., Steffens, D.C., et al. (2003c). White matter hyperintensity progression and late-life depression outcomes. *Arch. Gen. Psychiatry* 60:1090–1096.

Taylor, W.D., Steffens, D.C., et al. (2003d). Smaller orbital frontal cortex volumes associated with functional disability in depressed elders. *Biol. Psychiatry* 53:144–149.

Taylor, W.D., Züchner, S., et al. (2008b). The brain-derived neurotrophic factor VAL66MET polymorphism and cerebral white matter hyperintensities in late-life depression. *Am. J. Geriatr. Psychiatry* 16(4):263–271.

Taylor, W.D., Züchner, S., et al. (2007b). Allelic differences in the brain-derived neurotrophic factor Val66Met polymorphism in late-life depression. *Am. J. Geriatr. Psychiatry* 15(10):850–857.

Taylor, W.D., Züchner, S., et al. (2008c). Social support in older individuals: the role of the BDNF Val66Met polymorphism. *Am. J. Med. Genet. B Neuropsychiatr. Genet.* 147B(7):1205–1201.

Tekin, S., and Cummings, J.L. (2002). Frontal-subcortical neuronal circuits and clinical neuropsychiatry: an update. *J. Psychosom. Res.* 53:647–654.

Thomas, A.J., O'Brien, J.T., et al. (2002). Ischemic basis for deep white matter hyperintensities in major depression. *Arch. Gen. Psychiatry* 59:785–792.

Tonkonogy, J.M., and Geller, J.L. (1999). Late-onset paranoid psychosis as a distinct clinicopathologic entity: magnetic resonance imaging data in elderly patients with paranoid psychosis of late onset and schizophrenia of early onset. *Neuropsychiatry Neuropsychol. Behav. Neurol.* 12:230–235.

Tsopelas,N., Stewart, R., et al. (2011). Neuropathological correlates of late-life depression in older people. *Br. J. Psychiatry* 198:109–114.

Vakili, K., Pillay, S.S., et al. (2000). Hippocampal volume in primary unipolar major depression: a magnetic resonance imaging study. *Biol. Psychiatry* 47:1087–1090.

Van den Hove, D.L., Blanco, C.E., et al. (2005). Prenatal restraint stress and long-term affective consequences. *Dev. Neurosci.* 27(5):313–320.

Veldink, J.H., Scheltens, P., et al. (1998). Progression of cerebral white matter hyperintensities on MRI is related to diastolic blood pressure. *Neurology* 51:319–320.

Videbech, P., Ravnkilde, B., et al. (2001). The Danish PET/depression project: PET findings in patients with major depression. *Psychol. Med.* 31:1147–1158.

Viitanen, M., and Kalimo H. (2000). CADASIL: hereditary arteriopathy leading to multiple brain infarcts and dementia. *Ann. NY Acad. Sci.* 903:273–284.

Wang, L., Krishnan, K.R., et al. (2008). Depressive state- and disease-related alterations in neural responses to affective and executive challenges in geriatric depression. *Am. J. Psychiatry* 165(7):863–871.

Wang, L., Ashley-Koch, A., et al. (2001). Impact of BDNF Val66Met and 5-HTTLPR polymorphism variants on neural substrates related to sadness and executive function. *Genes Brain Behav.* 11(3):352–359.

Whitman, G.T., Tang, Y., et al. (2001). A prospective study of cerebral white matter abnormalities in older people with gait dysfunction. *Neurology* 57:990–994.

Ylikoski, A., Erkinjuntti, T., et al. (1995). White matter hyperintensities on MRI in the neurologically nondiseased elderly: analysis of cohorts of consecutive subjects aged 55 to 85 years living at home. *Stroke* 26:1171–1177.

Zhao, Z., Taylor, W.D., et al. (2008). Hippocampus shape analysis and late-life depression. *PLoS ONE* 3(3):e1837.

36 | GONADAL STEROIDS AND MOOD DISORDERS

DAVID R. RUBINOW, PETER J. SCHMIDT, AND CLAIRE D. CRAFT

Despite lack of recognition until recently of the importance of gonadal steroids in affective regulation, the role of these hormones in mood and behavior can be traced back to the very origins of our understanding of the pathophysiology of mood and behavioral disturbances. Aristotle noted that castration of male birds "when young" not only prevented the development of physical sex characteristics, but also further extinguished sex-specific behaviors such as male singing and sexual interest. In 1849, Berthold observed that the behavioral changes accompanying castration of roosters could be reversed through testicular transplant, leading him to infer that the testes must contain secretions that are responsible for the regulation of behavior. This, and the subsequent work of Charles Brown-Sequard, gave rise to the field of organotherapy, which was based on the premise that the administration of extracts of organs such as the testes and ovaries could treat a variety of mood disorders in humans, ranging from depression to the "anergy of senescence." The use of hormones as psychotropic agents continued after the isolation of estradiol in 1929, when Werner et al. (1934) described the antidepressant efficacy of an estradiol preparation called "theelin" in a study of perimenopausal and early postmenopausal women. This placebo-controlled study established the historical precedent for the use of gonadal steroids for the treatment of depression occurring during periods of reproductive endocrine transition. Throughout much of the 20th century, the possible role of gonadal steroids in affect regulation was inferred from two indirect sources: the twofold greater prevalence of depression in women, and the existence of reproductive endocrine-related mood disorders.

Reproductive endocrine-related mood disorders are affective disturbances that appear in concert with changes in reproductive endocrine activity. They include psychiatric disturbances occurring during menarche, pregnancy or postpartum, the perimenopause, or the menstrual cycle. Also included are disturbances consequent to manipulation of gonadal steroids or reproductive status (e.g., hormone replacement therapy or gonadal suppression). In this chapter, we will review the following: (1) the neurobiology of gonadal steroids; (2) the impact of gonadal steroids on the physiological systems implicated in depression; and (3) the neurobiology of reproductive endocrine-related mood disorders (old models, new models, and therapeutics).

WHAT ARE GONADAL STEROIDS AND WHAT UNDERLIES THEIR BIOLOGICAL EFFECTS?

Gonadal steroids are made in the gonads and adrenals and, like all steroid hormones, are metabolites of cholesterol. They include estradiol (E2), progesterone (P), testosterone (T), as well as precursors (e.g., the androgens DHEA and androstenedione) and metabolites (e.g., the potent androgen, dihydrotestosterone [DHT] and neurosteroid metabolites such as allopregnanolone). As shown in Figure 36.1, T is the immediate precursor of E2. The gonads are under control of the pituitary hormones follicle-stimulating hormone (FSH) and luteinizing hormone (LH), which in turn are under the control of a hypothalamic releasing hormone (GnRH), similar to other neuroendocrine axes. Hormonal changes during the menstrual cycle, the female climacteric (perimenopause), and the menopause are shown in Figure 36.2. In men, blood levels of T and DHT are stable (i.e., not cyclical), albeit with circadian variation and an age-related decrease of plasma levels of 1% per year after age 30. The cellular and molecular effects of gonadal steroids are protean. Many of these effects are mediated by steroid receptors, which, unlike neurotransmitter membrane receptors, are intracytoplasmic proteins that serve as transcription factors. By regulating genomic transcription, gonadal steroids influence the synthesis and metabolism of a wide range of neurotransmitters and neuropeptides.

Both the scope of and variance in the neuroregulatory potential of gonadal steroids are revealed in the details of their signaling effects. First, as the mechanics of transcription became elucidated, it became clear that activated steroid receptors influence transcription not as solitary agents but by forming combinations with other intracellular proteins. These protein–protein interactions are such that an activated receptor might enhance, reduce, initiate, or terminate transcription of a particular gene solely as a function of the specific proteins with which it interacted. The expression or activation state of these proteins—coregulators (coactivators or corepressors)—proved to be tissue specific, thus suggesting the means by which a hormone receptor modulator (e.g., tamoxifen) could act like an (estrogen) agonist in some tissues (e.g., bone) and like an (estrogen) antagonist in others (e.g., breast). In addition to their role in the recruitment of components of the general transcription factor apparatus, many of the coactivator proteins

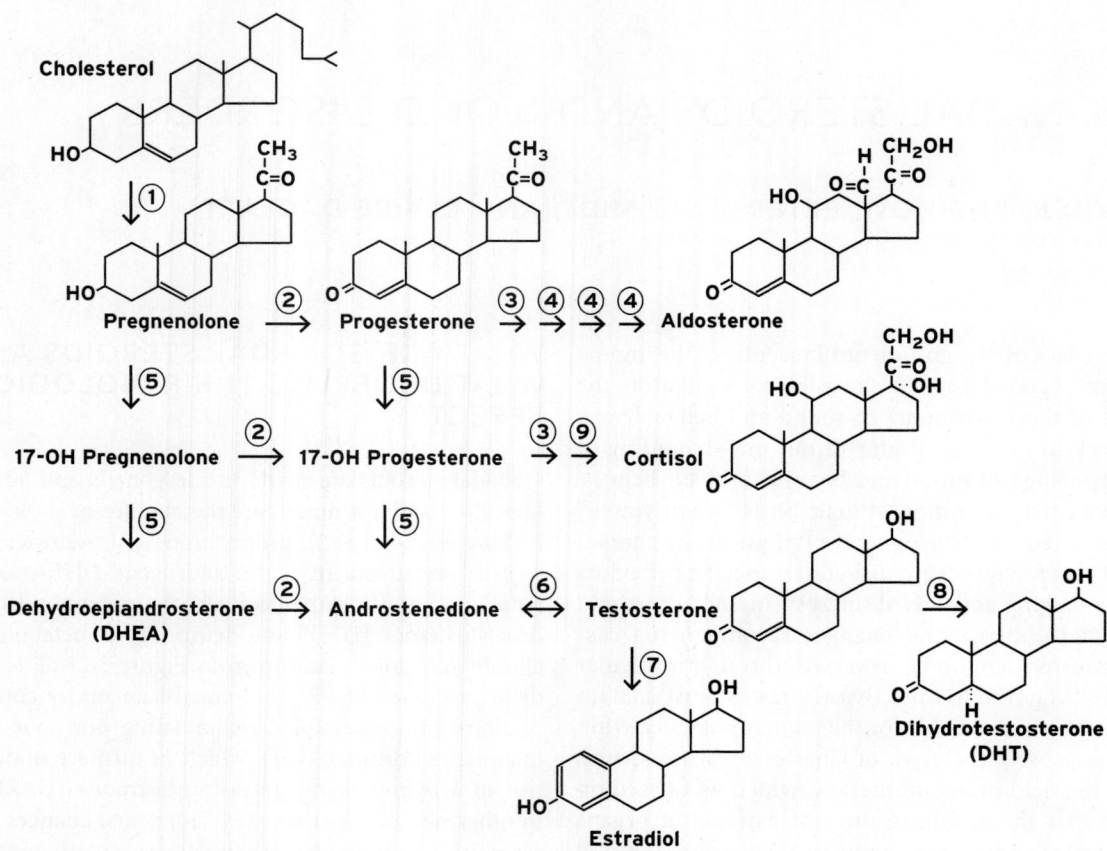

Figure 36.1 *Synthetic pathways for steroid hormones. Circled numbers identify synthetic enzymes: 1 = cytochrome P450 (CYP) 11A (cholesterol desmolase); 2 = 3β-hydroxysteroid dehydrogenase; 3 = CYP21 (21-hydroxylase); 4 = CYP11B2 (11β-hydroxylase, 18-hydroxylase, 18-oxidase); 5 = CYP17 (17α-hydroxylase, 17,20-lyase); 6 = 17β-hydroxysteroid dehydrogenase (or oxidoreductase); 7 = aromatase; 8 = 5α-reductase; 9 = CYP11B1 (11β-hydroxylase).*

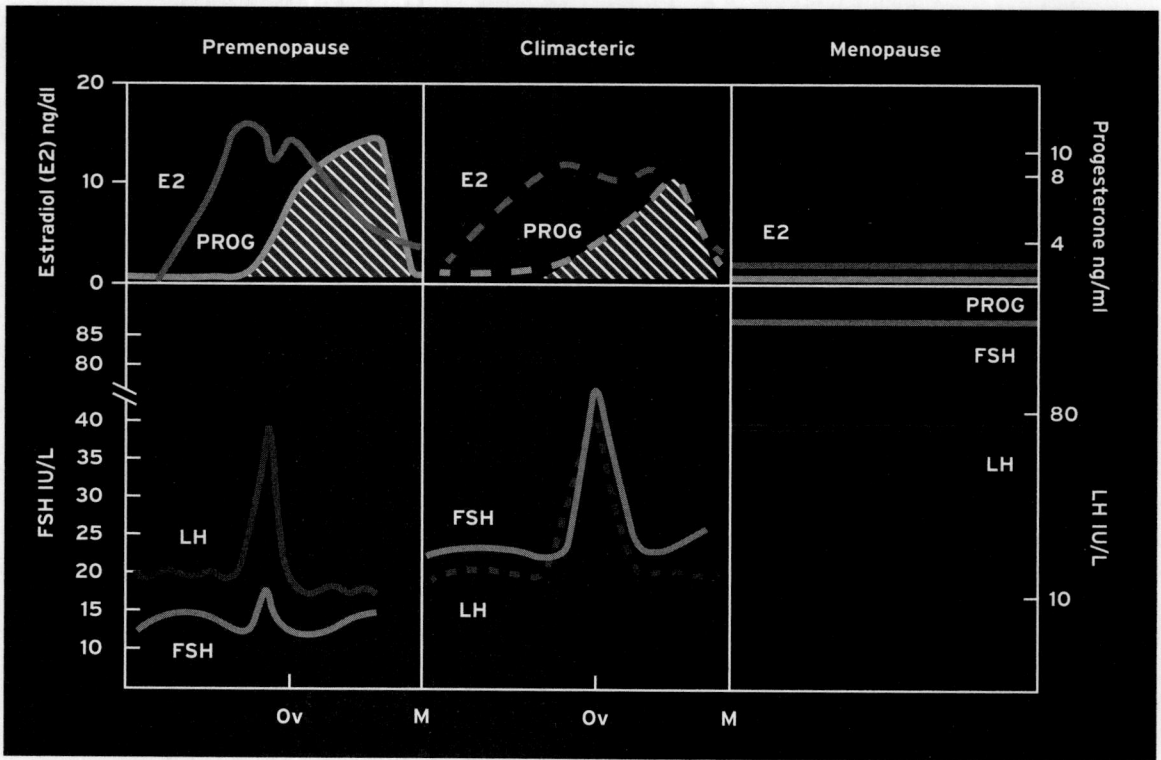

Figure 36.2 *Hormonal changes during the menstrual cycle, the female climacteric (perimenopause), and the menopause.*

have associated enzyme activity (e.g., histone acetylase activity, which facilitates chromatin remodeling and gene transcription). There are 300 or more of these coregulators, and the way in which specific amino acid residues are modified (e.g., phosphorylated) by cell signaling (e.g., hormone binding) determines which other coregulators and transcription factors they recruit, which in turn determines their effect on transcription (McDonnell and Wardell, 2010). Another group of intracellular proteins, the cointegrators, provide a means by which classical hormone receptors can bind to and regulate sites other than hormone response elements (e.g., estrogen receptor [ER] or glucocorticoid receptor [GR] binding cyclic AMP-response element binding [CREB] protein [CBP] and, subsequently, the AP1 binding site), and competition for cointegrator or other transcriptional regulatory proteins appears to be a mechanism by which even ligand-free hormone receptors can influence (e.g., squelch or interfere with) the transcriptional efficacy of other activated hormone receptors. Thus, the intracellular hormone receptor environment as well as the extracellular hormone environment may dictate the response to hormone receptor activation. The binding of a hormone agonist or antagonist in the binding pocket of the receptor alters the conformation of the receptor in such a way as to facilitate or interfere with the binding of coregulatory proteins. Recently, however, additional sites have been identified in the structure of nuclear hormone receptors where other molecules, called nuclear receptor alternate site modifiers (NRAMS), may bind to regulate the actions of hormones.

Second, the hormone receptors were found to exist in different forms. For example, isoforms of the progesterone receptor, PRA and PRB (the latter of which contains a 164 amino acid N-terminal extension), have different distributions and biological actions, and two separate forms of the estrogen receptor, ERα and ERβ, are encoded on different chromosomes (6 and 14, respectively), have different patterns of distribution in the brain, different affinity patterns for certain ligands, and a range of different actions (including those created by ER heterodimers). Further, a variant of ERβ, ERβ2, is expressed in the brain, where it can heterodimerize with the ERα or ERβ receptors and inhibit their transcriptional actions (Thomas and Gustafsson, 2011). The clinical importance of these receptor isoforms is revealed by a variety of studies suggesting that ERβ mediates the antidepressant effects of E2 in animal models as well as exerting proliferative effects in the hippocampus and antiproliferative effects in a variety of peripheral tumor models (e.g., breast, prostate, colon).

Third, a variety of substances (e.g., nerve growth factor, insulin) are capable of activating a steroid receptor even in the absence of ligand. This crosstalk is exemplified by the ability of dopamine to induce lordosis by activating the progesterone receptor.

Fourth, the relatively slow, genomic effects of gonadal steroids have been expanded in two dimensions: time, with a variety of rapid (seconds to minutes) effects observed; and targets, which now include ion channels and a variety of second-messenger systems. Several lines of evidence indicate that the rapid effects of E2 are not likely to be the consequence of nuclear events but rather must be related to events occurring at the cell surface. Both classical and unique ERs

(e.g., ER-X, GPR30) exist in the caveolae or caveolar-like microdomains of membranes where they link to scaffolding proteins (e.g., caveolin-1, flotillin) and multiple signaling molecules, particularly the G proteins, which then activate a wide array of signal transduction systems (reviewed in Zhang et al., 2005). Through alterations in signal transduction or by direct binding, E2 can also regulate ion channel activity (e.g., calcium and potassium channels) and hence, cellular activation (Zhang et al., 2005). The significance of these nongenomic effects is twofold. First, the nongenomic signal may serve to amplify the subsequent genomic effect of the hormone (Vasudevan and Pfaff, 2008). Second, the nongenomic effect on dendritic spines may similarly "prime" the neuron so that closely paired environmental signals are more effectively encoded and "learned" (Srivastava et al., 2011). Finally, the activity of neurotransmitter membrane receptors is acutely modulated by gonadal steroids (e.g., glutamate receptors by E2 and γ-aminobutyric acid [GABA] receptors by the neurosteroid allopregnanolone). Adding to the complexity of the effects described is their tissue- and even cell-specific nature (e.g., E2 increases MAPK in neurons but decreases it in astrocytes).

Fifth, gonadal steroids regulate cell survival. Neuroprotective effects of E2 have been described in neurons grown in serum-free media or those exposed to glutamate, amyloid-β, hydrogen peroxide, ischemia, or glucose deprivation (Dubal and Wise, 2002). Some of these effects appear to lack stereospecificity (i.e., are not classical receptor mediated) and may be attributable to the antioxidant properties of E2, although more recent data support receptor-mediated mechanisms of action. Gonadal steroids may also modulate cell survival through effects on cell survival proteins (e.g., Bcl-2, BAX), MAPK, Akt, or even amyloid precursor protein and Aβ metabolism or through enhancing mitochondrial respiratory efficiency).

Finally, the effects of gonadal steroids do not occur in isolation but, rather, in exquisite interaction with the environment. These environmental influences may include diet and medication, as short-chain fatty acids (including valproic acid) dramatically increase cellular sensitivity to gonadal steroids by amplifying their transcriptional potency through inhibition of histone deacetylase and stimulation of MAPK.

The vicissitudes of gonadal steroids and their receptors, therefore, direct neural architecture and provide the means by which the response of the CNS to incoming stimuli may be altered. The extent to which these effects underlie or contribute to differential pharmacologic efficacy or to behavioral differences observed across individuals is unclear but is of considerable potential relevance for reproductive endocrine-related mood disorders.

HOW DO THE NEUROBIOLOGICAL EFFECTS OF GONADAL STEROIDS OVERLAP THE PATHOPHYSIOLOGY OF DEPRESSION?

The simple answer is that virtually every system implicated in the pathophysiology of depression is regulated by gonadal steroids. For example, as described elsewhere (Rubinow and

Girdler, 2011), E2 "beneficially" modulates the following putative system disturbances in depression:

1. *Neurotransmitter deficiencies*—E2 regulates the synthesis, metabolism, and receptor concentration/trafficking of the classical neurotransmitters implicated in depression (i.e., serotonin, dopamine, and norepinephrine).

2. *Stress*—E2 regulates both basal and stress-induced ACTH and cortisol in animals through effects on GR and corticotropin-releasing hormone (CRH; although P may have more regulatory effects in humans).

3. *Neuroplasticity*—E2 has a significant impact on neuronal plasticity-related processes, acting like antidepressants (and opposite to stress) in stimulating BDNF, a critical growth factor observed to be deficient in depression; increasing activity of the transcription factor cAMP response element-binding protein (CREB) and trkA (neurotrophic tyrosine kinase receptor type 1); and decreasing glycogen synthase kinase (GSK)-3β in rat brain, the same direction of effects as seen with mood stabilizers. Consistent with these effects, as mentioned previously, E2 is neuroprotective in a variety of models, including oxidative damage, glutamate excess, and β-amyloid toxicity.

4. *Cellular energetics*—E2 improves mitochondrial respiratory efficiency and prevents the oxygen free radicals that are believed to adversely affect mitochondrial energetics in depression.

5. *Inflammation*—At multiple levels, E2 prevents or counteracts the proinflammatory processes described as contributing to depression.

6. *Brain systems*—The ability of gonadal steroid hormones to regulate activation in brain regions implicated in depression can be inferred from imaging studies conducted over the menstrual cycle or after gonadal steroid administration.

MENSTRUAL CYCLE EFFECTS

Studies of response to negative visual stimuli have shown significant differences in the response of affective circuitry between menstrual cycle phases and provided clues to the modulatory roles of E2 and P. During the late follicular phase, when E2 levels are at their peak, activity in several limbic, frontal, and hypothalamic regions show a significantly reduced response to negative material compared with the early follicular phase, when E2 levels are low (Goldstein et al., 2005). E2 has been found to modulate affective processing in the dorsolateral prefrontal cortex (dlPFC), where there was significantly increased activation while inhibiting response to positive words during the mid-luteal (high E2) phase of the menstrual cycle.

Menstrual cycle-related differences can also be seen in the orbitofrontal cortex (OFC), which functions in inhibitory control and emotional regulation. In healthy women, OFC responses to negative linguistic stimuli show greater medial activation during the luteal phase than during the follicular phase. Greater medial activation may signify an enhanced emotion-related viscero-motor control circuit activity premenstrually, perhaps indicating a greater need for top-down regulation of a heightened excitability of limbic system premenstrually (Protopopescu et al., 2005).

Negative emotional images produce significantly greater activity in the amygdala and hippocampus during the mid-luteal phase, when P is elevated, than during the early follicular phase, when both E2 and P are at low levels. Similar findings were demonstrated in healthy women in their follicular phase who were administered exogenous P at levels similar to those seen during the mid-luteal phase. These findings suggest that P-mediated effects dominate during the luteal phase, and further suggest that E2 and P may play opposing roles in modulating the brain's arousal circuitry.

The reward circuitry varies in a menstrual cycle-dependent fashion. During reward anticipation, activity in the amygdala and OFC are increased in the follicular phase relative to the luteal phase. At reward delivery, increased follicular phase activity can be observed in the midbrain and striatal areas (Dreher et al., 2007). Additionally, not only does the menstrual cycle regulate cerebral blood flow in brain regions (e.g., amygdala, dlPFC) implicated in depression, but as well it regulates the valence of the stimulus to which brain regions like the OFC react (Protopopescu et al., 2005)

Hormone manipulation studies in humans have shown that normal cognitive-stimulated activation of the dlPFC and cerebral blood flow to that region are suppressed in premenopausal women during pharmacologically induced hypogonadism—an effect that is reversed when gonadal hormones are reintroduced (Berman et al., 1997). E2 also regulates in humans the mesolimbic reward circuitry that is believed disturbed in depression, and it serves to bias toward or against the activation of specific neurocircuitry in animals. For example, it has been demonstrated that stress-induced c-fos expression in various cortical HPA-axis related regions are differentially stress activated in female rats depending on the phase of the estrous cycle. Gonadal steroids may also regulate cognitive-stimulated activity in the subgenual cingulate region (Brodmann area 25; BA25), the region implicated in deep brain stimulation treatment of depression.

The relevance of gonadal steroids in depression is also inferred from the antidepressant effects of E2 in several animal models of depression. Given the well-established role of stress in triggering the onset or exacerbation of depression in humans, preclinical research has focused on behavioral and neuropathological effects of stress to model mechanisms involved in human depression. A number of studies have shown that E2 diminishes "depressive behaviors" in animal models of chronic stress and that the antianxiety and antidepressant effects of E2 are largely mediated through ERβ, an isoform that is abundantly expressed in brain, including the limbic system, the hypothalamus, and the PFC. Additionally, E2 may also influence affective behavior by altering the activity of an extensive array of neuroregulatory proteins. For example, as noted previously, E2 attenuates chronic stress-induced increases in c-fos positive neurons in the paraventricular nucleus of the hypothalamus, similar to the effects seen in rat brain after chronic antidepressant treatment. E2 also attenuates stress-induced sensitization in the limbic system.

The data reviewed in the preceding provide a strong basis for inferring a potential role of gonadal steroids in the etiopathogenesis or treatment of mood disorders, particularly those linked to periods of reproductive endocrine change.

REPRODUCTIVE ENDOCRINE-RELATED MOOD DISORDERS

PREMENSTRUAL DYSPHORIC DISORDER

Premenstrual dysphoric disorder (PMDD) refers to the appearance of mood and behavioral symptoms in the luteal (postovulatory/premenstrual) phase of the menstrual cycle. This disorder is relatively common (about 5% prevalence in women) and is associated with a significant amount of morbidity, estimated at as many as 14.5 million disability-adjusted life years in the United States. Unlike other diagnoses in medicine, PMDD is a time-oriented and not a symptom-oriented diagnosis. The symptoms are relatively nonspecific; rather it is their exclusive appearance during the luteal phase that defines the disorder. As such, the diagnosis cannot be made based on history but instead requires a prospective demonstration that symptoms are confined to the luteal phase, disappearing at or soon after the onset of menses. Although many variations on this theme may potentially exist, use of a more restrictive definition has been necessary to ensure the homogeneity of samples across studies necessary for comparison and generalization of results obtained. Employment of standardized diagnostic guidelines has demonstrated the existence of PMDD and permitted resolution of many (but not all) of the controversies in the literature regarding the neurobiological basis of PMDD.

HORMONE STUDIES OF PMDD

Hormone studies in women with PMDD have employed several different strategies: (1) the measurement of basal hormone levels at selected points in the menstrual cycle; (2) evaluation of dynamic endocrine function employing endocrine challenge paradigms; and (3) the manipulation of menstrual cycle physiology in order to examine the plasticity of the linkage between the menstrual cycle and PMDD symptoms. The most frequently employed strategy has been the comparison of luteal phase basal hormone levels with those from the follicular phase in women with PMDD or with comparable values from a non-PMDD control group.

Comparisons of basal plasma hormone levels (E2, P, T, FSH, and LH) in women with PMDD and controls have revealed no consistent diagnosis-related differences (Rubinow and Schmidt, 2006), suggesting that PMDD is not characterized by abnormal circulating plasma levels of gonadal steroids or gonadotropins or by hypothalamic-pituitary-ovarian axis dysfunction. Several studies do, however, suggest that levels of E2, P, or neurosteroids (e.g., pregnenolone sulfate) may be correlated with symptom severity in women with PMDD.

Studies of a variety of other endocrine factors (e.g., thyroid or HPA axis hormones) in patients with PMDD have been similarly unrevealing. Although isolated significant differences have been reported, neither the diagnostic group-related differences nor their confinement to the luteal phase are consistently observed. Further, for the overwhelming majority of biologic factors for which diagnostic group-related differences have been suggested or demonstrated, the difference is not confined to the luteal phase but rather appears in follicular and luteal phases, thus arguing against their direct role in the expression of a disorder confined to the luteal phase (Rubinow and Schmidt, 2006). Three systems have received special attention for their possible role in PMDD.

SEROTONIN

A variety of observations implicate dysfunction of serotonergic neurons in PMDD. Although investigations utilizing pharmacologic probes to test 5-HT system function in women with PMDD have yielded inconsistent results, treatment studies consistently demonstrate the therapeutic efficacy of serotonin-enhancing agents (e.g., fluoxetine) for many women with PMDD. Additionally, we observed an acute therapeutic response in women with PMDD following oral administration of the 5-HT_{2C} agonist/5HT_{2A} antagonist, m-CPP, as well as a delayed (24 hours) reversal of the efficacy of fluoxetine by the serotonin receptor antagonist metergoline. These data converge to strongly suggest the role of the serotonin system in the pathophysiology of PMDD. As the majority of abnormalities in neuroendocrine response to serotonergic agents in PMDD are observed in both phases of the cycle (and because approximately 40% of women with PMDD do not respond to SSRIs), serotonergic dysfunction cannot be implicated as a direct cause of PMDD. It may, however, convey a vulnerability to mood destabilization in association with changes in gonadal steroids seen during the menstrual cycle.

NEUROSTEROIDS

The 5-α and 5-β reduced metabolites of progesterone (allopregnanolone and pregnanolone, respectively) rapidly and positively modulate the GABA-A receptor in brain and display anxiolytic effects in several animal models. These compounds, shown in Figure 36.3, are intriguing as potentially contributing to PMDD, as their withdrawal (as occurs in the late luteal phase) is associated with anxiety and insensitivity to benzodiazepines. Additionally, cerebral cortical inhibition increases during the luteal phase, a presumed effect of increased allopregnanolone levels and a finding absent in women with PMDD. Further, women with PMDD have blunted allopregnanolone responses to stress and evidence of altered metabolism of P to allopregnanolone (Klatzkin et al., 2006). Nonetheless, studies to date fail to demonstrate any consistent diagnosis-related differences in allopregnanolone or pregnanolone nor any difference in pregnanolone levels in women with PMDD before and after successful treatment with antidepressants.

HPA AXIS

Reports of HPA axis function in PMDD are inconsistent. Compared with controls, blunted HPA axis responses are

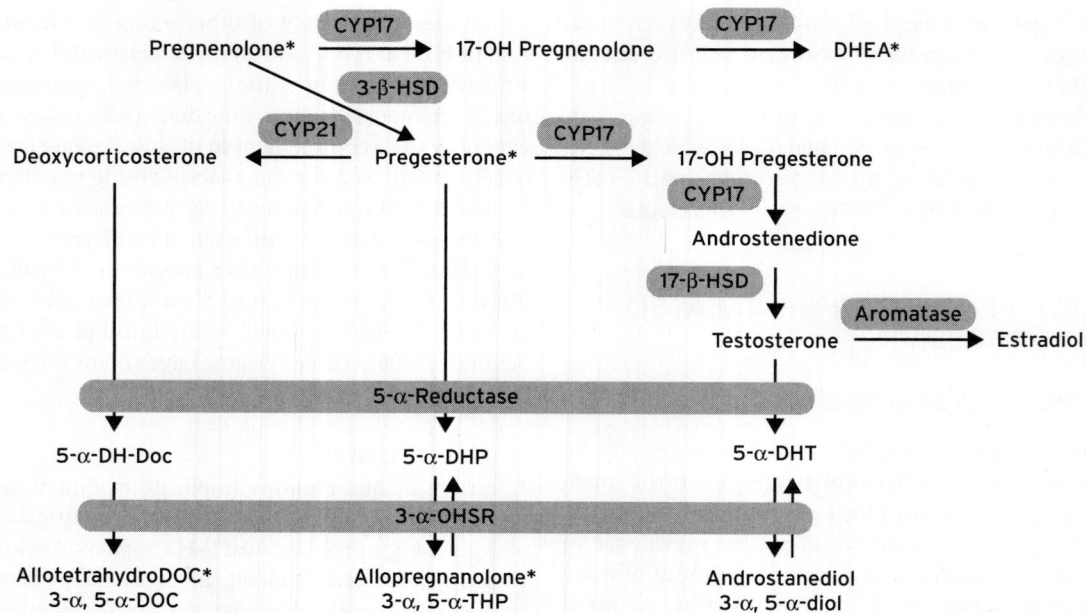

Figure 36.3 *DHEA and progesterone-related neurosteroids. Neurosteroids are marked with *.*

frequently observed, but both enhanced and normal HPA axis function are reported. Most studies employing either an endocrine challenge or serial plasma sampling suggest that the regulation of plasma cortisol and ACTH secretion at the levels of the hypothalamus, pituitary, and adrenal is normal in women with PMDD. Recently, we performed dexamethasone (Dex)/CRH challenge studies during GnRH agonist-induced hypogonadism with and without physiologic levels of E2 and P replacement in women with prospectively confirmed PMDD and in asymptomatic controls. In both women with PMDD and controls, we confirmed the previous findings by Roca and colleagues (2003), who employed an exercise challenge and showed that P but not E2 significantly increased HPA axis responsivity. However, we observed no significant differences between women with PMDD and asymptomatic controls in any measure of HPA axis function. Thus, in contrast to depression, PMDD is characterized by neither abnormal glucocorticoid feedback regulation nor increased central hypothalamic drive. Although stimulation of the HPA axis with psychological stress or with agents that increase serotonergic function has resulted in reported differences between women with PMDD and controls (e.g., blunted HPA response in PMDD), findings again are inconsistent across studies and permit no conclusion of disturbed HPA axis activity in women with PMDD (Lee et al., 2012). Presently, then, there is no clearly demonstrated luteal phase–specific physiologic abnormality in PMDD.

Given the absence of basal or stimulated reproductive endocrine abnormalities or luteal phase–specific biological abnormalities in PMDD, one could reasonably ask whether the luteal phase is required for the expression of PMDD. We answered this question by blinding women with PMDD to menstrual cycle phase with the progesterone antagonist mifepristone (RU-486) combined with either human chorionic gonadotropin (hCG) or placebo. We observed that women with

PMDD experienced their characteristic premenstrual mood state after the mifepristone-induced menses in both groups, despite the presence of an experimentally induced follicular phase in the women receiving mifepristone alone. The mid- to late luteal phase, then, is clearly not required for the appearance of PMDD symptoms. It, nonetheless, remained possible that symptoms could be triggered by hormonal events prior to the mid- to late luteal phase, consistent with reports that the suppression of ovulation results in a remission of PMDD symptoms.

We confirmed the efficacy shown by others of GnRH agonists (e.g., leuprolide acetate [Lupron]) in the treatment of PMDD. Consistent with earlier observations, a therapeutic response was not observed in all patients despite the consistent reduction of gonadal steroid levels to hypogonadal levels. Although the majority of study participants did show a therapeutic response, the mechanism of action remained unclear (e.g., low plasma gonadal steroid levels, consistent gonadal steroid levels, anovulation, suppression of follicular development). This uncertainty was in part addressed by the double-blind, placebo-controlled reintroduction of E2 or P in the study participants in whom Lupron displayed efficacy. The results unequivocally demonstrated the precipitation of a wide range of characteristic symptoms of PMDD during E2 and P addback but not during placebo addback (reviewed in Rubinow and Schmidt, 2006). The combined results from our study and those of earlier studies strongly suggest the role of gonadal steroids in the occurrence of PMDD symptoms despite the absence of evidence for abnormal *levels* of steroid hormones in this disorder. Particularly striking, however, is the observation that controls lacking a history of PMDD and going through the same protocol showed no perturbation of mood during hypogonadism and no mood disturbance during hormonal addback. It would appear, therefore, that women with a history of PMDD are *differentially sensitive* to the mood-perturbing effects of gonadal steroids, as similar steroid manipulations in women without a history of PMDD are without effect.

TRIGGER AND SUSCEPTIBILITY

New neurobiological models: If gonadal steroids trigger PMDD in some women, how do they do so and why not in all women?

Trigger

To determine whether the steroid-induced mood disturbances in women with PMDD are caused by the change in hormone levels or by a permissive effect of elevated hormone levels on expression of an infradian driver, we recently administered Lupron followed by three months of continuous E2 and P replacement. This paradigm demonstrated that it is the change in gonadal steroids that triggers the mood disturbance; that is, reintroduction of gonadal steroids precipitated a self-limited episode with no subsequent dysphoria over the remainder of the three months. These findings suggest that continuous administration of oral contraceptives might, after the first precipitated episode, effectively prevent the recurrence of all other symptoms (due to the stable hormone levels). Possibly consistent with this hypothesis is the recent demonstration of the efficacy of oral contraceptives when administered with a reduced pill-free interval. Several examples exist of the ability of changes in hormones to convey important biological regulatory information. Particularly notable is the demonstration by Shen and colleagues (2005) that withdrawal of allopregnanolone reconfigures hippocampal GABA receptors (changes its subunits) to completely reverse the effects of allopregnanolone on chloride ion conductance, resulting in hippocampal excitability rather than suppression following subsequent exposure to allopregnanolone. The nature of the trigger aside, one must explain why changes in gonadal steroids provoke mood changes only in some women; that is, what is the source of the susceptibility to steroid-induced mood changes?

Susceptibility

There is precedent for inferring that polymorphisms in genes involved in the gonadal steroid signaling pathway or in gonadal steroid-regulated genes may alter the nature or strength of the steroid signal as well as the phenotype. Although some earlier candidate gene studies did not find significant associations with PMDD, we identified a region of the ERα gene (*ESR1*) containing multiple polymorphic alleles that are associated with PMDD (Huo et al., 2007). Further, this association was significant in only those women with the val/val genotype of the COMT Val158Met polymorphism, thus lending support to the idea that the effects of multiple genes may interact in creating a dysphoric behavioral response to normal gonadal steroid levels.

Demonstration of a relationship between genetic variations in *ESR1* and PMDD is very promising for several reasons. First, ERα plays a major role in arousal, the dysfunction of which could underlie somatic, cognitive, and affective symptoms of PMDD. Second, ERα regulates the signaling of neurotransmitter systems implicated in the etiopathogenesis and treatment of PMDD. For example, extensive links exist between E2 and serotonin function, with the latter involved in mood regulation and the selective therapeutic effects of SSRIs in PMDD. At least some of the effects of E2 are mediated through serotonin 1A receptors, which are upregulated through nuclear factor-kappa B (NF-kB) by ERα but not ERβ (Wissink et al., 2001). Third, the ER has clear physiologic relevance in PMDD as the receptor for a hormone that can trigger the onset of symptoms of the disorder. Finally, a speculative model for PMDD can be created based on interactions between E2, ERα, and COMT: The variants in *ESR1* that associate with PMDD do so only in the presence of the COMT val/val polymorphism, which regulates PFC dopamine (as well as participating in the metabolism of E2). E2, which has been shown to provoke symptoms of PMDD, also regulates the activation in brain regions (e.g., PFC, OFC, amygdala, BA25) and brain networks (e.g., reward circuitry) critical to affect as well as the connectivity between the PFC and hippocampus. "Disordered" E2 signaling through ERα, then, could contribute to and combine with reduced PFC dopamine to compromise top-down cortical regulation of affect. Although speculative, this hypothesis receives indirect support from two observations: (*1*) the increased mOFC activation seen normally during the luteal phase is absent in women with PMDD (in association with greater amygdalar response to negative stimuli and less activation of the ventral striatum to positive stimuli); and (*2*) more recently, women with PMDD were found to demonstrate overactivation of the dlPFC on both PET and fMRI compared with control women, with the degree of overactivation significantly correlated with the degree of symptomatic impairment.

SUMMARY

To identify what the study of PMDD may contribute to our understanding of the effects of gonadal steroids on brain and behavior, several observations must be integrated. First, there does not appear to be a disturbance of reproductive endocrine function that underlies PMDD. Second, changes in levels of E2 and P appear to be capable of triggering mood disturbances in a susceptible population; that is, some preexisting vulnerability must explain the capacity of the same biologic stimulus (e.g., gonadal steroids) to elicit a differential behavioral response across groups of people. Third, perturbations of nonreproductive endocrine systems appear capable of precipitating PMDD. Menstrual cycle–related mood disorders may appear in the context of hypothyroidism (with symptoms responsive to thyroid hormone replacement), and provocative and especially treatment studies suggest the relevance of the serotonin system to PMDD. Menstrual cycle–related mood disorders, then, may represent a behavioral state that is triggered by a reproductive endocrine stimulus in those who may be rendered susceptible to behavioral state changes by antecedent experiential events (e.g., history of major depression) or physical or sexual abuse or biological conditions (e.g., hypothyroidism). Treatment can, therefore, be directed to either eliminating the trigger (e.g., ovarian suppression) or correcting the "vulnerability" (e.g., serotonergic antidepressants). Although the means by which alterations in gonadal steroids trigger changes in behavioral state in certain individuals are unclear, it is nonetheless striking that, in contrast to the pathological function of other endocrine systems (e.g., adrenal, thyroid) seen in association with mood disorders, gonadal steroids may precipitate mood disturbances in the context of normal ovarian function. This suggests that further study of the interactions between gonadal steroids and other neuroactive systems may help elucidate general mechanisms underlying affective regulation as well as the physiologic substrate that predisposes certain people to experience reproductive endocrine-related mood disorders.

POSTPARTUM PSYCHIATRIC DISORDERS

Affective syndromes that occur during the postpartum period have traditionally been divided into three categories: (1) postpartum "blues," (2) postpartum depression (PPD), and (3) puerperal psychosis. PPD is associated with more persistent symptoms and a higher rate of morbidity than the "blues" but is less severe (depressions of minor to moderate severity) than postpartum psychotic depressions. The two- to three-month prevalence rates of postpartum depression in studies using conventional diagnostic criteria (e.g., RDC, DSM-III) have been reported to be in the range of 8.2% to 19.2% (Gavin et al., 2005; Wisner et al., 2002). Some studies have reported that the incidence of depression is increased significantly during the first three months after birth as compared with during prepregnancy, pregnancy, or the period after the first postpartum year. Others have disputed this association, arguing that the prevalence of depression during the postpartum period is no greater than that in comparably aged non-puerperal women. In fact, recent epidemiologic studies observed that the last trimester of pregnancy also was associated with an increased prevalence of depression compared with the postpartum. Thus, the peripartum (last trimester and early postpartum) is not associated with an increased prevalence of major or minor depression. Nonetheless, it is not the increased prevalence of depression but the linkage of the onset of depression to a specific phase of reproductive change that distinguishes this condition.

HORMONE STUDIES OF POSTPARTUM DEPRESSION

A number of studies have attempted to determine the relationship between postpartum mood symptoms and gonadal steroid levels by examining basal levels, or changes in levels, during pregnancy and the postpartum period. As reviewed by Bloch and colleagues (2003), most studies of women with PPD showed that plasma E2 and P levels were indistinguishable from controls, although one found higher P in women who went on to develop PPD. In addition to levels of E2 and P, studies have focused on measures that may predict a woman's vulnerability to develop gonadal steroid-induced depression. Examples of such measures include apomorphine-induced growth hormone response and alterations in neurosteroid levels in postpartum psychiatric illness. Wieck and colleagues (1991) demonstrated that an increased growth hormone response to apomorphine on postpartum day four (before the usual onset of illness) was associated with an increased risk of a recurrent episode of depression. The authors speculated that these findings reflected increased sensitivity of central

dopamine receptors, which may be triggered by the sharp fall in circulating E2 concentrations after delivery (i.e., E2 uncouples D2 receptors, with an acute upregulation in D2 receptors possibly resulting in psychiatric disturbance following the sudden postpartum drop in E2 levels). As previously described, neurosteroid metabolites of gonadal steroids are known to have acute, nongenomic modulatory effects at GABA and glutamate receptors. Levels of one such potent P metabolite, allopregnanolone, rise progressively during pregnancy and drop relatively abruptly after parturition (as levels are closely correlated with plasma P levels). Preliminary data (Daly, unpublished data) suggest that women with a history of PPD show a significant correlation between decreasing levels of this anxiolytic neurosteroid and mood symptoms. Pearson-Murphy also has suggested a role for alterations in P metabolites in PPD, with higher levels of 5-α-dihydroprogesterone observed in depressed patients compared with controls during the last trimester of pregnancy (Pearson-Murphy et al., 2001). To summarize the preceding data, no consistent differences in gonadal steroid levels have been demonstrated, either in pregnancy or the postpartum, between women with and those without PPD, suggesting that the condition does not represent a simple gonadal steroid excess or deficiency state.

Higher cortisol levels at the end of pregnancy have been reported in association with more severe blues, and cortisol levels have been shown to correlate with postpartum mood in breastfeeding mothers during the first week postpartum. Most studies, however, have failed to show any association of blues or PPD with plasma or salivary cortisol or with urinary metabolites (reviewed in Bloch et al., 2003).

Abnormalities of CRH-stimulated ACTH (but not cortisol) have been reported in mixed samples of PPD and blues. Magiakou and colleagues (1996) showed that women with the blues or PPD had a more severe and longer-lasting suppression of hypothalamic CRH secretion in the postpartum period than euthymic mothers. Additionally, Bloch et al. (2005) observed greater CRH stimulated cortisol in euthymic women with a history of PPD compared with controls during a hormone add-back state simulating pregnancy. These dynamic abnormalities of the HPA axis suggest that adaptive response to stress may be compromised in women who experience or are susceptible to PPD.

Finally, no clear relationship between thyroid dysfunction and PPD exists, and although thyroid dysfunction may contribute to postpartum mood disorders, other factors would appear to play more defining roles in the development of the condition.

IMAGING STUDIES OF POSTPARTUM DEPRESSION

Differences in the neural processing of affective stimuli have also been reported in women with postpartum depression. When compared with healthy mothers, depressed mothers had significantly diminished dorsomedial prefrontal cortex activity and dorsomedial prefrontal cortical-amygdala connectivity in response to negative emotional faces. Reduced amygdala activity in response to negative emotional faces was associated with greater postpartum depression severity

(Moses-Kolko et al., 2010). This is consistent with a recent report of decreased right amygdala activation in response to threat-related linguistic stimuli in unmedicated women with postpartum depressive symptoms. This pattern is distinct from the cerebral activation associated with unipolar depression.

SUMMARY

Although basal reproductive hormone levels do not distinguish women with PPD from those without the disorder, a role of gonadal steroids in this disorder may nonetheless be inferred from a study that created a scaled-down model of the peripartum in euthymic women with a history of PPD compared with those lacking a history of depression. After suppressing ovarian function with leuprolide acetate, Bloch and colleagues (2000) blindly added back high-dose E2 and P for eight weeks followed by blinded and acute withdrawal of steroid addback. As shown in Figure 36.4, euthymic women with a history of PPD developed depression during high-dose addback, with greater depression demonstrated during the acute withdrawal phase. In contrast, no symptoms of depression were observed in the control group undergoing the same protocol. These findings suggest that, as is the case with PMDD, changes in reproductive steroid signaling can precipitate depression, but only in a susceptible subgroup of women.

It is unclear whether it is prolonged, high dose steroid exposure or steroid withdrawal that is the offending stimulus, perhaps mirroring the clinical observation that the onset of depressive symptoms in some women who develop PPD occurs during pregnancy rather than solely following parturition. Our data would, nonetheless, suggest that alterations in the levels of gonadal steroids are implicated in the development of perinatal depression, either during the period of elevated levels or during withdrawal from such levels. In summary, gonadal steroids appear to play a key role in the development of PPD, but the exact nature of this role has yet to be fully determined. Only a subgroup of women appear to have an underlying biological sensitivity that ultimately manifests as PPD.

PERIMENOPAUSAL DEPRESSION

As with PPD and PMDD, epidemiologic studies observe that only a subgroup of women are at risk for the development of depressive disorders during the menopause transition. Moreover, like PPD, it is unclear whether there is any increased prevalence of depression during the perimenopause compared with other stages of a woman's life. Thus, reproductive aging is not uniformly associated with affective disturbance. Nonetheless, several longitudinal community-based studies have documented an increased risk for depression during the menopause transition compared with the premenopause and the postmenopause, with odds ratios ranging from 1.8 to 2.9 compared with the premenopause (reviewed in Harsh et al., 2009). In particular, two studies (Cohen et al., 2006; Freeman et al., 2006) observed a 2- to 2.5-times greater risk for the first onset of depression during the late menopause transition compared with the premenopause. These data suggest that ovarian aging and the events surrounding the final menstrual period increase vulnerability to depression in some women.

Predictors of vulnerability to perimenopausal depression include longer duration of the menopause transition time, vasomotor symptoms, stressful life events proximate to the menopausal transition, and histories of depression, although none of the characteristics are uniform antecedents to perimenopausal depression. In a small clinic-based longitudinal study, we observed that most depressions appeared during the late stage of the menopause transition, which is characterized by more prolonged hypogonadism than the early perimenopause. Thus the timing suggests an endocrine mechanism related to the perimenopause (E2 withdrawal and/or recent-onset of prolonged hypogonadism) in the pathophysiology of perimenopausal depression. It is possible that fluctuating levels of gonadal steroid hormones interact with individual characteristics (e.g., sensitivity to stress, histories of depression) in some women to increase their vulnerability to develop perimenopausal depression. Individual physiologic or historical characteristics may indeed provide the context in which the response to a biological signal is determined (Rubinow et al., 2002). On the other hand, vulnerability to E2 withdrawal/fluctuations may have a genetic basis, as suggested by the heritability of the puerperal trigger in postpartum disorders (Jones and Craddock, 2007), the heritability of premenstrual symptomatology (Kendler et al., 1992), and the significant association of PMDD with intron 4 SNPs in ERα (Huo et al., 2007).

HORMONE STUDIES OF PERIMENOPAUSAL DEPRESSION

The relevance of changes in pituitary-ovarian function to depression during the perimenopause is suggested by evidence that mood symptoms may change coincidently with FSH levels and that E2 therapy has acute mood-enhancing effects in

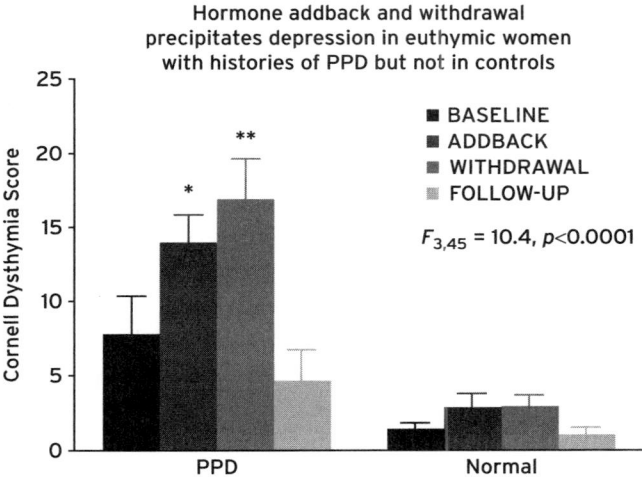

Figure 36.4 Mean Scores on the Cornell Dysthymia Scale before and after estradiol and progesterone replacement in women with a history of postpartum depression (n = 8) and normal controls (n = 8).[a]

[a]Study phases: 8-week baseline, when no medications were administered; 12 weeks of leuprolide-induced ovarian suppression, with addback of estradiol (4–10 mg/day) and progesterone (400–900 mg/day) during the last 8 weeks; 4-week early withdrawal, when estradiol and progesterone were withdrawn but leuprolide continued; and 8-week follow-up, when no medications were administered. * Addback vs. baseline, p < .05. ** Withdrawal vs baseline, p < .01 (Bonferroni corrected t tests)

perimenopausal women with depression (Schmidt et al., 2000; Soares et al., 2001).

Despite a few studies identifying levels of one hormone or another (e.g., estrone, FSH) as different in perimenopausal depressed women compared with controls, subsequent studies have been unable to confirm any diagnosis-related differences in reproductive hormones. A possible exception are the levels of the adrenal androgen dehydroepiandrosterone (DHEA) and its sulfated metabolite, DHEA-S, both of which were observed to be lower in women with perimenopausal depression as well as inversely correlated (DHEA) with symptoms of depression in peri- and postmenopausal women (Rubinow et al., 2002). Limitations of basal hormonal measures notwithstanding, data suggest that depressed perimenopausal women are not distinguished from nondepressed perimenopausal women by being "more" estrogen deficient.

HORMONE THERAPIES FOR PERIMENOPAUSAL DEPRESSION

Multiple reports of increased mood symptoms and depressive disorders during the menopause date back more than 150 years and generated the belief that reversal of these symptoms could be achieved with ovarian hormone replacement. Controversy regarding the antidepressant efficacy of hormone replacement stems almost from its inception and reflects the same methodological inconsistencies that have compromised efforts to determine whether the perimenopause is accompanied by an increase in mood symptoms or depression. Methodological differences of note (other than study design) include menopausal state (perimenopause vs. postmenopause), determination of state (earlier studies used age as a proxy measure), baseline symptomatology (asymptomatic vs. depressive symptoms vs. syndromic depression), and symptom or syndrome measure.

A meta-analytic examination of 26 studies of the effects of HRT on depressed mood revealed a moderate to large effect size of 0.68, showing lower ratings of depressed mood in treated patients compared with controls (Zweifel and O'Brien, 1997). Baseline symptom rating scores were suggestive of syndromal depression in only two of these studies. Twenty-two additional studies have been published since this earlier meta-analysis, nine of which are double-blind and placebo-controlled.

Two general categories of randomized controlled trials have been performed and, as noted in the following, observed findings may differ as a function of the menopausal status of the samples (i.e., postmenopausal vs. perimenopausal):

Non-depressed patients

Among the double-blind, placebo-controlled studies, two had large sample sizes and showed no effect of HRT (conjugated equine estrogen plus medroxyprogesterone acetate) on affective symptoms in postmenopausal women, but subjects in both studies were affectively asymptomatic at baseline or discouraged from participating if menopausal symptoms were present. These studies then provide moderate-strong evidence for a statement of limited clinical value: HRT does not prevent symptoms of depression in an asymptomatic, postmenopausal population. Data from the HERS study suggested that among postmenopausal women, those with menopausal symptoms showed lower depressive symptoms on HRT than those lacking menopausal symptoms.

Depressed patients

Two small randomized, placebo-controlled trials demonstrated the antidepressant efficacy of transdermal E2 in depressed, perimenopausal women. Subjects selected met diagnostic criteria for depression and were followed with standard syndrome rating scales. A study employing similar methodology failed to show antidepressant efficacy of transdermal E2 in a postmenopausal sample. One study did demonstrate antidepressant efficacy of a continuous combined HRT preparation in postmenopausal women selected with diagnostic criteria for the presence of mild-moderate depression. This study was performed by the makers of the HRT preparation and, while methodologically sound, showed a very high drop-out rate (Santen et al., 2010). An additional 14 studies are either observational, open-label, or methodologically compromised, thus providing less compelling evidence regarding the antidepressant efficacy of ERT or HRT. Notwithstanding the small sample sizes in the few well-designed trials in depressed perimenopausal women, there is evidence (low-moderate) for the antidepressant efficacy of E2 in perimenopausal but not postmenopausal women.

SUMMARY

Despite the antidepressant efficacy of E2 and the linkage of perimenopausal depression to a time of E2 withdrawal, we still do not have direct evidence that E2 withdrawal triggers the onset of depression in these women. Preliminary observations from a study of the effects on mood of E2 withdrawal suggest, however, that women with a history of depression during the perimenopause, but not those lacking such a history, experience a recurrence of depressive symptoms when E2 is withdrawn under blinded, placebo-controlled conditions (Schmidt et al., unpublished observation). The ability of fluctuations in hormones during the menopause transition to contribute to the development of depression in vulnerable women is supported by the work of Freeman and colleagues (Freeman et al., 2006). These authors showed that greater variability in E2 concentrations, and not E2 concentrations per se, was associated with both elevated depressive symptomatology as well as diagnosed major depressive disorder during the menopause transition. As with PMDD and PPD, therefore, a reproductive endocrine signal, in this case low or declining E2 levels, can be shown to trigger depression during the perimenopause, but only in a susceptible population.

MIDLIFE DEPRESSION

Midlife also may be associated with the onset of depression in both men and women. Indeed several epidemiologic studies report a recent increase in suicide rates in white men and women during midlife, despite overall stable or declining rates at other stages of life. Depressions that present at midlife can often reflect the onset of medical illness; however, depression at this stage in life also can increase the risk for several midlife-relevant medical illnesses, including heart disease and dementia. Further complicating the picture, the clinical presentation of midlife depression often is focused on symptoms (e.g., low energy, decreased libido, and cognitive decline) that can obscure the underlying depressive illness. The fifth and sixth decades of life are accompanied by several endocrine events related to aging, including changes in growth and metabolism, alterations in HPA axis function, and age-related changes in both gonadal and adrenal androgen secretion. In addition to the precipitous changes in E2 and P in women during the perimenopause, androgen levels—T, DHT, DHEA, and androstenedione—also decrease during midlife in both men and women. However, in contrast to the relatively rapid declines in ovarian E2 and P secretion, androgen secretion declines more gradually in both men and women. Thus declining androgen secretion potentially could lead to a more insidious onset of depressive symptoms. Nonetheless, studies suggest that the age-related decline in androgen secretion occurs in the majority of midlife men and women in the absence of accompanying depression. Thus as with other reproductive endocrine-related depressions, midlife-onset depression could reflect the effects of declining androgen secretion in the context of other individual characteristics that increase a man or woman's risks for depression. However, in midlife depressions the effects of aging on several behaviorally relevant physiologic systems including the HPA axis, insulin-like growth factors, thyroid function, and other metabolic systems must be considered as potential contributors to the onset of depression at this time in life.

ANDROGENS AND MOOD IN MEN

Beginning in the third decade, there is a slow but continuous, age-dependent decline of T levels (1% decrease each year). This decline is more pronounced for free T than for total T, a consequence of the age-associated increase of sex hormone-binding globulin (SHBG) levels. At age 75, mean total T level in the morning is about two-thirds of the mean level at ages 20–30, whereas the mean FT and bioactive T (FT plus albumin bound T) level are only 40% of the mean levels in younger males. The circadian rhythm of plasma T levels, with higher levels in the morning than in the evening, is generally lost in elderly men as well (Kaufman and Vermeulen, 2005).

Plasma androstenedione levels vary between 2 and 8 nmol/liter in adult males aged 20 to 30 years and significantly decline with age. Serum concentrations of DHEA decline more rapidly and more profoundly than those of T—approximately 2% per year (Kaufman and Vermeulen, 2005).

There are three different aspects to the changes in serum testosterone levels in aging men:

1. *Primary testicular changes:* There is a diminished secretory capacity of the Leydig cells in the elderly compared with young men. This decrease in testicular secretory reserve appears to involve a reduction of the number of Leydig cells. Also in rats, all enzymes involved in the synthesis of T are decreased with aging, as is the steroidogenic acute regulatory protein, which is involved in the transport of cholesterol into mitochondria.

2. *Altered neuroendocrine regulation of Leydig cell function:* There is reduced hypothalamic secretion of GnRH, resulting in inadequate stimulation of LH secretion by the pituitary gland.

3. *Increase of plasma SHBG binding capacity:* The decline of the serum levels of FT is accentuated relative to that of total serum T, as a consequence of an age-associated increase of serum SHBG (Kaufman and Vermeulen, 2005).

Findings from cross-sectional and longitudinal studies of testosterone and mood in men have been inconsistent. Studies are fairly equally divided between those that have demonstrated lower T in depressed men than in controls and those that have shown no difference in absolute levels. Inconsistencies in the literature may be due to small sample sizes and different diagnostic assessments of depression in different study samples. However, data are most consistent with the interpretation that if there is any functional effect of MDD on the male HPG-axis, it is likely to be small. Some clinical data suggest that low T, persisting over years, may lead to a chronic, low-grade, depressive illness such as dysthymic disorder rather than to MDD. Nonetheless, caution must be employed in interpreting low T values, in men or women, consequent to the unreliability of assay in the low range.

Early studies on the antidepressant effects of T suggested that a significant number of depressed men responded dramatically to T replacement therapy and relapsed when treatment was discontinued. Standardized psychiatric diagnoses were not used in these studies, however, and baseline hormone levels were not assessed. More recently, a double-blind, randomized trial of T replacement versus placebo in 30 men with MDD and hypogonadism found T replacement indistinguishable from placebo in antidepressant efficacy: 38% responded to T and 41% responded to placebo (Seidman et al., 2001). A study by Pope of 22 hypogonadal men with partial response to SSRIs found that those randomized to T gel had significantly greater improvement in depressive symptoms than subjects randomized to placebo. A subsequent study, also by Pope, of 100 hypogonadal men with partial SSRI response randomized to augmentation with T or placebo gel failed to show a significant difference between groups (Pope, 2010). Most clinical trials of T therapy for depression have included 30 or fewer subjects, too few to reliably detect small antidepressant effects. Overall, systematic trials do not support T as a broadly effective antidepressant. It may be more effective in certain populations, such antidepressant-resistant men or HIV-infected men.

ANDROGENS AND MOOD IN WOMEN

Women experience an approximately 50% drop in T due to loss of ovarian function (the other 50% is adrenal in origin in women). A role for DHEA and DHEA-S in the regulation of mood state has been suggested by both its effects on neural physiology (Baulieu et al., 1998) and its potential synthesis within the central nervous system. Moreover, in clinical trials, DHEA administration has been reported to improve mood in some (Bloch et al., 1999; Wolkowitz et al., 1999), but not all, studies (Wolf et al., 1997). Finally, abnormalities of DHEA secretion have been observed in depressive disorders, with both increased and decreased levels observed relative to non-depressed controls (Heuser et al., 1998). DHEA's potential role in the onset of depression may be particularly relevant at midlife given the declining levels of DHEA production with aging and the accelerated decrease in DHEA levels reported in women, but not men, during midlife (Laughlin and Barrett-Connor, 2000).

CONCLUSIONS

The differential sensitivity to gonadal steroids seen in women with histories of PMDD and PPD (and possibly perimenopausal depression) emphasizes that the response to a biological signal cannot be inferred absent an understanding of the context in which the signal occurs. This context includes current physiological and external environments, prior experience, past history of exposure to the stimulus, and genetic makeup. Data already exist from both animal and human studies in support of the importance of genetic context in determining the response to a reproductive steroid signal. Spearow and colleagues (1999) demonstrated greater than 16-fold differences in sensitivity to E2 (reproductive disruption) across six different mouse strains, with genotype accounting for more of the variation than the hormone dose. Similarly, we observed strain differences in the behavioral impact of E2: antidepressant-like effects in Long Evans but not Wistar rats, and depression-like effects of E2 withdrawal in Wistar but not Long Evans. Finn and colleagues (1997) observed strain/genetic (and task-dependent) differences in behavioral sensitivity to allopregnanolone. Several studies suggest that steroid receptor polymorphisms may alter the steroid signaling pathway (e.g., by increasing transcriptional efficiency) in such a way as to produce or contribute to a different behavioral/phenotypic response to a hormone signal. Indeed, possible genetic susceptibility loci for PMDD and puerperal psychosis have been identified (Huo et al., 2007; Jones and Craddock, 2007). More interesting and compelling, however, are the demonstrations that while both genetic and reproductive steroid effects on behavior exist, their interactions are the most relevant and powerful in determining phenotypic expression. Maguire and Mody (2008) showed that the behavioral effect of a mutation in the delta subunit of the GABA receptor was expressed only in the context of a specific reproductive state—postdelivery—at which time the dams displayed depressive-like behavior and killed their pups. Similarly, the effects of a COMT polymorphism on cognitive performance are entirely dependent on the presence or absence of E2 (Jacobs and D'Esposito, 2011). At the very least, it is time to recognize the importance of context, at the behavioral level no less than at the cellular level, in determining the response to a steroid signal. By understanding the mechanisms underlying the differential sensitivity to gonadal steroids exemplified by women with PMDD, PPD, and perimenopausal depression, we will be in a far better position to answer what is arguably the most important question in behavioral neuroscience: Why do different people respond differently to the same stimulus?

DISCLOSURES

Dr. Rubinow serves on the Editorial Board of *Dialogues in Clinical Neuroscience*, for which he receives compensation. He additionally has served on the Scientific Advisory Board of Azevan Pharmaceuticals, for which he has received stock options. Dr. Rubinow receives no other funding or material support other than his NIMH grant support (three RO1s and a T32 training grant).

Dr. Craft and Dr. Schmidt have no conflicts of interest to disclose.

REFERENCES

Baulieu, E.E., and Robel, P. (1998). Dehydroepiandrosterone (DHEA) and dehydroepiandrosterone sulfate (DHEAS) as neuroactive neurosteroids. *Proc. Natl. Acad. Sci. USA* 95:4089–4091.

Berman, K.F., Schmidt, P.J., et al. (1997). Modulation of cognition-specific cortical activity by gonadal steroids: a positron-emission tomography study in women. *Proc. Natl. Acad. Sci. USA* 94(16):8836–8841.

Bloch, M., Daly, R.C., et al. (2003). Endocrine factors in the etiology of postpartum depression. *Compr. Psychiatry* 44(3):234–246.

Bloch, M., Rubinow, D.R., et al. (2005). Cortisol response to ovine corticotropin-releasing hormone in a model of pregnancy and parturition in euthymic women with and without a history of postpartum depression. *J. Clin. Endocrinol. Metab.* 90:695–699.

Bloch, M., Schmidt, P.J., et al. (1999). Dehydroepiandrosterone treatment of mid-life dysthymia. *Biol. Psychiatry* 45:1533–1541.

Bloch, M., Schmidt, P.J., et al. (2000). Effects of gonadal steroids in women with a history of postpartum depression. *Am. J. Psychiatry* 157:824–930.

Cohen, L.S., Soares, C.N., et al. (2006). Risk for new onset of depression during the menopausal transition: the Harvard study of moods and cycles. *Arch. Gen. Psychiatry* 3:385–390.

Dreher, J.C., Schmidt, P.H., et al. (2007). Menstrual cycle phase modulates reward-related neural function in women. *Proc. Natl. Acad. Sci. USA* 104(7):2465–2470.

Dubal, D.B., and Wise, P.M. (2002). Estrogen and neuroprotection: from clinical observations to molecular mechanisms. *Dialogues Clin. Neurosci.* 4147:149–162.

Finn, D.A., Roberts, A.J., et al. (1997). Genetic differences in behavioral sensitivity to a neuroactive steroid. *J. Pharmacol. Exp. Ther.* 280:820–828.

Freeman, E.W., Sammel, M.D., et al. (2006). Associations of hormones and menopausal status with depressed mood in women with no history of depression. *Arch. Gen. Psychiatry* 63:375–382.

Gavin, N.I., Gaynes, B.N., et al. (2005). Perinatal depression. *Obstet. Gynecol.* 106:1071–1083.

Goldstein, J.M. (2005). Hormonal cycle modulates arousal circuitry in women using fMRI. *J. Neurosci.* 25(40):9309–9316.

Harsh, V., Meltzer-Brody, S., et al. (2009). Reproductive aging, sex steroids, and mood disorders. *Harv. Rev. Psychiatry* 17(2):87–102.

Heuser, I., Deuschle, M., et al. (1998). Increased diurnal plasma concentrations of dehydroepiandrosterone in depressed patients. *J. Clin. Endocrinol. Metab.* 83:3130–3133.

Huo, L., Straub, R.E., et al. (2007). Risk for premenstrual dysphoric disorder is associated with genetic variation in ESR1, the estrogen receptor alpha gene. *Biol. Psychiatry* 62(8):925–933.

Jacobs, E., and D'Esposito, M. (2011). Estrogen shapes dopamine-dependent cognitive processes: implications for women's health. *J. Neurosci.* 31:5286–5293.

Jones, I., and Craddock, N. (2007). Searching for the puerperal trigger: molecular genetic studies of bipolar affective puerperal psychosis. *Psychopharmacol. Bull.* 40:115–128.

Kaufman, J.M., and Vermeulen, A. (2005). The decline of androgen levels in elderly men and its clinical and therapeutic implications. *Endocr. Rev.* 26:833–876.

Kendler, K.S., Silberg, J.L., et al. (1992). Genetic and environmental factors in the aetiology of menstrual, premenstrual and neurotic symptoms: a population-based twin study. *Psychol. Med.* 22(1):85–100.

Klatzkin, R.R., Morrow, A.L., et al. (2006). Histories of depression, allopregnanolone responses to stress, and premenstrual symptoms in women. *Biol. Psychol.* 116(1):2–11.

Laughlin, G.A., and Barrett-Connor, E. (2000). Sexual dimorphism in the influence of advanced aging on adrenal hormone levels: the Rancho Bernardo study. *J. Clin. Endocrinol. Metab.* 85:3561–3568.

Lee, E.E., Nieman, L.K., et al. (2012). ACTH and cortisol response to Dex/CRH testing in women with and without premenstrual dysphoria during GnRH agonist-induced hypogonadism and ovarian steroid replacement. *J. Clin. Endocrinol. Metab.* 97(6):1887–1896.

Magiakou, M.A., Mastorakos, G., et al. (1996). Hypothalamic cortico-releasing hormone suppression during the postpartum period: Implications for the increase in psychiatric manifestations at this time. *J. Clin. Endocrinol. Metab.* 81:1912–1917.

Maguire, J., and Mody, I. (2008). GABA(A)R plasticity during pregnancy: relevance to postpartum depression. *Neuron* 59(2):207–213.

McDonnell, D.P., and Wardell, S.E. (2010). The molecular mechanisms underlying the pharmacological actions of ER modulators: implications for new drug discovery in breast Cancer. *Curr. Opin. Pharmacol.* 10:620–628.

Moses-Kolko, E., Perlman, S., et al. (2010). Abnormally reduced dorsomedial prefrontal cortical activity and effective connectivity with amygdala in response to negative emotional faces in postpartum depression. *Am. J. Psychiatry* 167:1373–1380.

Pearson-Murphy, B.E., Steinberg, S.I., et al. (2001). Neuroactive ring A-reduced metabolites of progesterone in human plasma during pregnancy: elevated levels of 5α-dihydroprogesterone in depressed patients during the latter half of pregnancy. *J. Clin. Endocrinol. Metab.* 86:5981–5987.

Pope, H.G., et al. (2010). Parallel-group placebo-controlled trial of testosterone gel in men with major depressive disorder displaying an incomplete response to standard antidepressant treatment. *J. Clin. Psychopharmacol.* 30(2):126–134.

Protopopescu, X., Pan, H., et al. (2005). Orbitofrontal cortex activity related to emotional processing changes across the menstrual cycle. *Proc. Natl. Acad. Sci. USA* 102(44):16060–16065.

Roca, C.A., Schmidt, P.J., et al. (2003). Differential menstrual cycle regulation of hypothalamic-pituitary-adrenal axis in women with premenstrual syndrome and controls. *J. Clin. Endocrinol. Metab.* 88(7):3057–3063.

Rubinow, D.R., and Girdler, S.S. (2011). Hormones, heart disease, and health: individualized medicine versus throwing the baby out with the bathwater. *Depress. Anxiety* 28:E1–E15.

Rubinow, D.R., and Schmidt, P.J. (2006). Gonadal steroid regulation of mood: the lessons of premenstrual syndrome. *Front. Neuroendocrinol.* 27:210–216.

Rubinow, D.R., Schmidt, P.J., et al. (2002). Gonadal hormones and behavior in women: concentrations versus context. In: Pfaff, D.W., et al., eds., *Hormones, Brain and Behavior* (Vol. 5). New York: Academic Press.

Santen, R.J., Allred, D.C., et al. (2010). Postmenopausal hormone therapy: an Endocrine Society Scientific Statement. *J. Clin. Endocrinol. Metab.* 95(7, Suppl 1):s1–s66.

Schmidt, P.J., Nieman, L., et al. (2000). Estrogen replacement in perimenopause-related depression: a preliminary report. *Am. J. Obstet. Gynecol.* 183:414–420.

Seidman, S.N., Spatz, E., et al. (2001). Testosterone replacement therapy for hypogonadal men with major depressive disorder: a randomized, placebo-controlled clinical trial. *J. Clin. Psychiatry* 62:406–412.

Shen, H., Gong, Q.H., et al. (2005). Short-term steroid treatment increases delta GABA(A) receptor subunit expression in rat CA1 hippocampus: pharmacological and behavioral effects. *Neuropharmacology* 49(5):573–586.

Soares, C.D., Almeida, O.P., et al. (2001). Efficacy of estradiol for the treatment of depressive disorders in perimenopausal women: a double-blind, randomized, placebo-controlled trial. *Arch. Gen. Psychiatry* 58:529–534.

Spearow, J.L., Doemeny, P., et al. (1999). Genetic variation in susceptibility to endocrine disruption by estrogen in mice. *Science* 285(5431):1259–1261.

Srivastava, D.P., Waters, E.M., et al. (2011). Rapid estrogen signaling in the brain: implications for the fine-tuning of neuronal circuitry. *J. Neurosci.* 31:16056–16063.

Thomas, C., and Gustafsson, J.A. (2011). The different roles of ER subtypes in cancer biology and therapy. *Nat. Rev. Cancer* 11:597–608.

Vasudevan, N., and Pfaff, D.W. (2008). Non-genomic actions of estrogens and their interaction with genomic actions in the brain. *Front. Neuroendocrinol.* 29:238–257.

Werner, A.A., Johns, G.A., et al. (1934). Involutional melancholia: probable etiology and treatment. *J. Am. Med. Assoc.* 103(1):13–16.

Wieck, A., Kumar, R., et al. (1991). Increased sensitivity of dopamine receptors and recurrence of affective psychosis after childbirth. *Br. Med. J.* 303:613–616.

Wisner, K.L., Parry, B.L., et al. (2002). Postpartum depression. *N. Engl. J. Med.* 347:194–199.

Wissink, S., van der Burg, B., et al. (2001). Synergistic activation of the serotonin-1A receptor by nuclear factor-kappaB and estrogen. *Mol. Endocrinol.* 15(4):543–552.

Wolf, O.T., Neumann, O., et al. (1997). Effects of a two-week physiological dehydroepiandrosterone substitution on cognitive performance and well-being in healthy elderly women and men. *J. Clin. Endocrinol. Metab.* 82:2363–2367.

Wolkowitz, O.M., Reus, V.I., et al. (1999). Double-blind treatment of major depression with dehydroepiandrosterone. *Am. J. Psychiatry* 156:646–649.

Zhang, L., Sukhareva, M., et al. (2005). Direct binding of estradiol enhances Slack (sequence like a calcium-activated potassium channel) channels' activity. *Neuroscience* 131:275–282.

Zweifel, J., and O'Brien, W. (1997). A meta-analysis of the effect of hormone replacement therapy upon depressed mood. *Psychoneuroendocrinology* 22:189–212.

37 | DEPRESSION AND MEDICAL ILLNESS

TAMI D. BENTON, JOSHUA BLUME, PAUL CRITS-CHRISTOPH, BENOIT DUBÉ, AND DWIGHT L. EVANS

Increasing recognition of the impact of depression on physical health has prompted focused investigation on its diagnosis and treatment. The World Health Organization (WHO) projects that depression will be the leading cause of life lost to disability in 2030, imposing a greater health burden than ischemic heart disease (WHO, 2008). The report also emphasized depression's contribution to morbidity and mortality. Depression is a risk factor for the onset and progression of both physical and social disability (Prince et al., 2007; WHO, 2008). Additionally, individuals with depression and other mental illnesses may develop their health conditions earlier due to behavioral and biological factors related to their mental illnesses, and they may die earlier from comorbid medical illness (Sullivan et al., 2012).

Evidence that adverse health risk behaviors and the presence of depression increases risk for medical disorders, and that the presence of a medical disorder may increase risk for depression has prompted examination of the bidirectional relationship between depression and medical illness (Evans et al., 2005). Further support for these observations has been provided by recent research identifying a potential role for inflammatory responses in the pathophysiology of depression, finding higher levels of pro-inflammatory cytokines, acute phase proteins, chemokines, and cellular adhesion molecules in depression (Blume et al., 2011; Dantzer et al., 2008).

In this chapter, we will review the relevant recent research linking depression and medical illness. We will present an overview of the bidirectional relationship between depression and medical illness. We will review existing research on the possible mechanism for the connection between depression and medical illness, focusing on the connection between depression and several specific medical illnesses (cardiac disease, diabetes, HIV/AIDS, cancer). We then outline basics of the assessment of depression in the context of medical illness. We conclude with a presentation of treatment considerations for depression in specific medically ill populations.

PREVALENCE OF DEPRESSION IN THE MEDICALLY ILL

Depressive disorders are more prevalent among the medically ill when compared to the general population of the United States. The average lifetime prevalence of depression is about 16.6% of the US population and is two times more prevalent in women when compared to men (Kessler et al., 2005). Those with chronic medical illnesses are two to three times more likely to be depressed than age- and gender-matched non-medically ill individuals in community-based primary care settings (Katon, 2011). The prevalence of depression among individuals who are medically ill ranges from 3% to 10% in community and primary care settings and up to 10–14% in inpatient medical settings (Katon, 2003). Prevalence estimates for depressive disorders among those populations with specific medical conditions are even higher, ranging from 20% to 55% (Evans et al., 2005) (Table 37.1).

MECHANISMS OF COMORBIDITY FOR DEPRESSION AND MEDICAL ILLNESS

Recent research examining depression among medically ill populations has sought to link the inflammatory processes underlying specific disorders such as cardiovascular disease, diabetes, and cancer, to those inflammatory processes underlying major depression. Emerging evidence suggests that depressive disorders may be conditions of immune dysregulation, specifically activation of the inflammatory response system (Dowlati et al., 2010; Raison et al., 2009). These theories gain support from the observation that the treatment of patients with cytokines can produce symptoms of depression, antidepressant treatments can reverse those symptoms, and immune system activation is present in some, but not all, individuals with depression. Additionally, cytokine mediated signaling to the brain can influence the production and metabolism of neurotransmitters relevant to mood disorders and its treatments including serotonin, dopamine, and catecholamines (Raison et al., 2009).

A decade of investigation has established the contribution of cytokines to the pathogenesis of depression. Cytokines are proteins and glycoproteins secreted by immune cells that function as signals among and between immune cells. Cytokines are the hormones of the immune system. They can be secreted by immune and nonimmune cells and can affect cells outside of the immune system. They function locally and systemically to modulate and regulate immune functions throughout the body, including those of the central nervous system.

The role of cytokines in the pathogenesis of depression has been confirmed by clinical and experimental observations. Several studies comparing cytokines in people with MDD have found increases in certain cytokines compared to people without MDD (Miller et al., 2009; Raison et al.,

TABLE 37.1. Depression in patients with comorbid medical illness

COMORBID MEDICAL ILLNESS	PREVALENCE RATE (%)
Cardiac disease	17–27
Cerebrovascular disease	14–19
Alzheimer's disease	30–50
Parkinson's disease	4–75
Epilepsy	
Recurrent	20–55
Controlled	3–9
Diabetes	
Self-reported	26
Diagnostic interview	9
Cancer	22–29
HIV/AIDS	5–20
Pain	30–54
Obesity	20–30
General population	10.3

Adapted from Evans et al., 2005, with permission.

2009). Although association does not imply causality, there are many reasons to believe that the abnormalities of inflammation found in depression may contribute to its pathology. Medically ill patients who exhibit immune activation or inflammation secondary to infections, autoimmune diseases, and neoplastic diseases demonstrate higher rates of depression (Nemeroff and Vale, 2005). Cytokines have also been shown to be effective in the treatment of certain cancers, hepatitis C, viral infections, and multiple sclerosis. However, a behavioral syndrome similar to major depression has been observed among these individuals treated with cytokines for the treatment of infectious diseases or cancer. This syndrome referred to as "sickness behavior" is characterized by anhedonia, cognitive dysfunction, anxiety, irritability, psychomotor slowing, anergia, fatigue, anorexia, sleep alterations, and increased sensitivity to pain (Dantzer et al., 2008). Although the exact prevalence is unknown, studies suggest that the incidence of depression associated with cytokine therapy ranges from 0% to 45%, depending on the medical conditions and study designs (Dantzer et al., 2008). Moreover, the behavioral syndrome induced by cytokine treatment has been shown to be responsive to treatment with standard antidepressant medications, suggesting that the behaviors described as the "sickness syndrome" are related to major depression. However, antidepressant treatment has been noted to be more effective on the mood symptoms than on neurovegetative symptoms (Capuron et al., 2002; Constant et al., 2005).

Furthermore, cytokines have been found to influence all of the pathophysiologic domains relevant to depression. Cytokines have been shown to cause alterations in the metabolism of monoamine neurotransmitters relevant to depression, specifically serotonin, dopamine (DA), and norepinephrine (NE); to have stimulatory effects on HPA axis functioning through activation of corticotropin-releasing hormone (CRH) in the amygdala and the hypothalamus; to induce resistance of nervous, endocrine, and immune system tissues to circulating glucocorticoid hormones stimulating the glucocorticoid resistance found in patients with depression; to induce enzymes that metabolize tryptophan the primary precursor of serotonin, and may inhibit pathways involved in thyroid hormone metabolism and to activate NF-kB, a transcription factor that signals the inflammatory cascade in the brain (Dantzer et al., 2008; Irwin and Miller, 2007; Raison et al., 2009).

Despite growing evidence that dysregulation of the immune system may contribute to the pathogenesis of major depression, other studies have found conflicting results or no association between depression and immune parameters or inflammation (Blume et al., 2011; Whooley et al., 2007). One factor that might explain variations between studies is the type of immune system variable or inflammatory marker examined. Pike and Irwin found that, among patients with MDD relative to controls, there was evidence for decreases in NK cell activity (indicating impairment in the immune system) and higher levels of IL-6 (indicating immune activation) (Pike and Irwin, 2006). Furthermore, changes in NK cell activity were not correlated with levels of IL-6, suggesting that depression may have independent effects on these different aspects of the immune system. Alternatively, an emerging literature suggests that while acute inflammation boosts immune defenses, the chronic exposure of immune cells to proinflammatory cytokines may actually result in impaired cellular immunity (Medzhitov, 2008). Thus depression-associated chronic activation of the immune system may lead to immune deficiency resulting in increased vulnerability to cancer and infection (Blume et al., 2011). Miller points out that causality may also operate in the other direction: depression is associated with impaired regulatory T cells, which modulate innate immune responses (Miller, 2010). Thus, depression-associated cellular immune suppression may contribute to chronic inflammation, and the pathogenesis of diseases—such as atherosclerosis and cancer, in which inflammation has been implicated.

Further observations supporting the relationships between chronic inflammation and cellular immune suppression have been demonstrated among two of the most common rheumatologic disorders, rheumatoid arthritis (RA) and systemic lupus erythematosus (SLE). SLE is an autoimmune disorder resulting in tissue and organ damage caused by abnormal immune complexes and T-lymphocytes as well as autoantibodies. RA is characterized by inflammation that primarily affects the synovial tissue of the joints. Both chronic inflammatory disorders have high rates of comorbid depression with prevalence estimates ranging from 13% to 42% in RA (Bruce, 2008) and 10.8% to 39.6% in SLE (Nery et al., 2007), depending on diagnostic methods. Both disorders are characterized by multiorgan systemic involvement affecting the cardiac, vascular, respiratory, and nervous systems. Direct CNS involvement is rare in RA, however neuropsychiatric manifestations are frequent in SLE. The mainstay of treatments for both disorders include anti-inflammatory agents and other immunosuppressant agents.

Chronic inflammation is present in RA and SLE, and both conditions are characterized by a high frequency of infection, possibly related to impaired circulating T-cells leading to immune suppression (Doran et al., 2002; Gladman et al., 2002; Koetz et al., 2000; La Cava, 2008). In addition, impaired T-cell function has been observed in the synovial fluid of individuals with RA, when the T-cells were chronically exposed to TNF alpha (Cope, 2003), and etanercept, an anti TNF-alpha therapy, has been shown to restore T-cell reactivity in patients with RA (Berg et al., 2001; Blume et al., 2011). Dysregulation of immune T-cell tolerance, and decreased numbers and/or functioning of suppressive CD4CD25 T-regulatory cells have been observed in peripheral blood in human models of SLE (La Cava, 2008). Thus, depression associated cellular immune suppression might contribute to inflammation and the pathogenesis of both SLE and RA, as well as atherosclerosis and cancer.

CARDIAC DISEASE

The intimate and clinically relevant connection between depression and cardiovascular disease has been well established. Depression is prevalent across the spectrum of cardiac diseases including coronary artery disease (CAD), unstable angina, acute myocardial infarction, congestive heart failure, and coronary artery bypass graft surgery. Current estimates suggest rates of depression that are significantly higher than in the general population, ranging from 17% to 27% (Rudisch and Nemeroff, 2003). Depressive symptoms increase the risk for the onset of CAD by 1.64-fold. Furthermore, the occurrence of depression within three to four months of a myocardial infarction (MI), predicts a three times greater likelihood of dying in the next year, when compared to individuals without depression following MI (Lett et al., 2004).

Depression appears to be an independent risk factor in cardiac disease, as the connection between depression and cardiac disease does not appear to be due to the association between depression and other known risk factors (e.g., smoking, history of MI). Depression has been found to be a significant predictor of mortality 6 and 18 months following MI, even after adjusting for other risk factors such as left ventricular dysfunction and previous MI (Frasure-Smith et al., 1995).

MECHANISMS OF COMORBIDITY

Several possible mechanisms linking depression to cardiovascular diseases have been proposed. These include inflammation, hypothalamic-pituitary-adrenocortical dysregulation, sympathomedullary hyperactivity, increased platelet activity and aggregation, autonomic dysfunction causing reduced heart rate variability (HRV), and endothelial dysfunction (Celano and Huffman, 2011; Skala et al., 2006).

It is well known that HPA axis dysregulation occurs in depression and that administration of corticosteroids is associated with increases in cardiovascular disease risk factors, including hypercholesterolemia, hypertriglyceridemia, and hypertension. Consistent with this potential mechanism, elevated plasma cortisol has been found to be associated with moderate to severe coronary atherosclerosis in young and middle aged men.

Sympathoadrenal hyperactivity may mediate the relationship between depression and cardiovascular disease through an effect on platelets. Individuals with depression show increased levels of plasma NE in response to cold or orthostatic challenge, which may enhance platelet activity. Some, but not all studies have found platelet hyperactivity in those with MDD. Recent studies of depressed patients with ischemic heart disease show elevated platelet factor 4 and plasma b-thromboglobulin levels (Celano and Huffman, 2011).

Inflammatory responses may partly underlie the relationship between depression and cardiovascular disease. The inflammatory markers IL-6, TNF-a, and C reactive protein (CRP) are associated with cardiovascular and cerebrovascular events, specifically CHD, congestive heart failure, and stroke (Cesari et al., 2003). Increases in circulating levels of IL-6 and CRP are also found in depression (Dowlati et al., 2010). Other studies examining the relationships between depression and inflammation in cardiac disease have found elevations in CRP and serum amyloid A (SAA) in women treated for major depression who are in remission, suggesting a sustained proinflammatory state in women who have clinically recovered and who no longer take antidepressant medications. The authors suggest that the persistence of a "proinflammatory state" might contribute to the increased CAD risk associated with MDD (Kling et al., 2007).

Statins are drugs routinely administered to patients post-MI for their lipid lowering and anti-inflammatory properties. Stafford and Berk investigated the effect of statins on the onset of depression in hospitalized cardiac patients, hypothesizing that the anti-inflammatory effect of statins would serve as prophylaxis against depression. In support of a link among depression, inflammation, and cardiovascular disease, they found that over nine months postdischarge, statins were associated with a 79% reduction in the likelihood of depression (Stafford and Berk, 2011). Recent findings from the Heart and Soul Study suggest that statin use was associated with a 38% decreased odds of developing depression in their sample, further confirming this association (Otte et al., 2012).

Frasure-Smith and colleagues (2007) assessed 702 individuals (602 men) for depression and inflammatory markers (CRP), IL-6, and soluble adhesion molecules at two months postdischarge for an acute coronary syndrome, and then followed them for two years for major adverse cardiac events defined as cardiac death, survived MI or cardiac arrest, and nonelective revascularization. Of this sample, 102 individuals (78 men) experienced at least one major adverse cardiac event. Elevated scores on the Beck Depression Inventory-II (BDI-II) and current major depression were significantly related to major adverse coronary events over two years, and this association was stronger in men than women. The study also found an association between elevated depressive symptoms, CRP, and soluble intercellular adhesion molecules (sICAM-1), but not IL-6, providing some support for the association between depression and inflammation (Frasure-Smith et al., 2007).

Abnormalities of the autonomic nervous system may be another mechanism linking depression and CAD. HRV, a measure of the balance between sympathetic and parasympathetic inputs to the cardiac conduction system, is often reduced in patients with severe CAD or heart failure. Reduced HRV is associated with ventricular arrhythmias and sudden cardiac death (Dekker et al., 2000). Studies that found diminished HRV in depression raised the possibility that HRV might be the link between depression and CAD (Nahshoni et al., 2004; Stein et al., 2000). One study found that HRV partially mediates the relation between depression and increased risk for mortality after acute myocardial infarction (Carney et al., 2005). HRV has also been found to be associated with increased markers of inflammation in patients with heart failure and acute coronary syndromes.

Depression is also associated with endothelial dysfunction, a putative mechanism of atherosclerotic disease. A study of men and women ages 40 to 84 years old concluded that depressed individuals had impaired flow-mediated dilation of the brachial artery—a measure of endothelial function—compared to non-depressed individuals. The use of antidepressant medication was associated with improved endothelial function. Subsequent investigations have corroborated these findings (Cooper et al., 2010; Pizzi et al., 2008, 2009).

Evidence further suggests that depression may worsen the impact of other cardiac factors. In a study examining risks for cardiac mortality following MI, the highest death rates (60%) for patients at 18 months post-MI were found in a subgroup of patients with elevated depressive symptoms and increased numbers of premature ventricular contractions per hour (PVCs) (Frasure-Smith et al., 1995).

Depression can also indirectly increase the risk of CAD. The pessimism and low energy often found in clinical depression can lead individuals to be less adherent to exercise programs, smoking cessation, dietary changes, and pharmacological interventions for CAD (Glazer et al., 2002; Skala et al., 2006; Wang et al., 2002). Failure to adequately address these risk factors may then put the individual with depression at even greater risk for a future cardiac event.

DIABETES MELLITUS

Depression is common among individuals with diabetes. Among the 23.6 million people in the United States diagnosed with diabetes mellitus (DM), 5–15% have type I diabetes (CDC 2008), with type II diabetes (T2DM) being much more prevalent; however, research suggests that rates of depression are elevated in both. People with diabetes are twice as likely to have depression compared with those without diabetes. Prevalence estimates suggest that 10–15% of individuals with DM are currently affected by depression and that 24–29% of individuals with diabetes will be affected by depression during their lifetimes. The presence of depression has been associated with higher symptom burden; poor adherence to medication, diet, and exercise; and higher hemoglobin A1C levels (Markowitz et al., 2011). Depression has also been associated with increased frequency and severity of diabetes complications including retinopathy, nephropathy, neuropathy, macrovascular

complications including coronary vascular diseases, and sexual dysfunction. Furthermore, depression has been associated with an increased risk of all cause mortality in diabetes, among individuals with and without previous cardiovascular disease (Sullivan et al., 2012). Depressive symptoms and heightened distress, absent a major depression diagnosis, have been found to adversely impact diabetes self-care and diabetes control (Markowitz et al., 2011). Depression with diabetes has been associated with increased health care costs (Katon, 2011).

MECHANISMS OF COMORBIDITY

The mechanisms underlying the well-established association between depression and diabetes remain unknown. Studies seeking to understand these associations have focused on the diagnosis and burden of disease management as a risk for the development of depression, suggesting that depression is a consequence of diabetes (Knol et al., 2007) Other studies have suggested that depression is a risk factor for diabetes (Campayo et al., 2010; Golden et al., 2008; Knol et al., 2007).

Studies examining the bidirectional associations between depression and diabetes have provided conflicting results. Longitudinal studies of clinically depressed older adults in the community found depression to be associated with a 65% increased risk for incident diabetes, and that this association was true for untreated depression and persistent and non-severe depression (Campayo et al., 2010). Golden and colleagues examined incident rates for T2DM in men and women with and without depressive symptoms over five years. They found incidence rates for T2DM of 22.0/1,000 person years for those with increased depression symptoms compared with 16.6/1000 person years for those without increased depressive symptoms. Incident rates for elevated depressive symptoms per 1,000 person years were 36.8 for those with normal fasting glucose; 27.9 for those with impaired fasting glucose; 31.2 for untreated T2DM and 61.9 for treated T2DM. They also found a modest association of baseline depressive symptoms with incident T2DM, which were partially attributed to lifestyle. Both untreated T2DM and impaired FG were inversely associated with incident depressive symptoms, but treated T2DM was positively associated with depressive symptoms (Golden et al., 2008).

The Vietnam experience study (Gale et al., 2010) explored the association between fasting glucose, T2DM (diagnosed and undiagnosed), and depression among middle aged men. Subjects with untreated diabetes had nearly double the odds (1.8 95% CI) of developing major depression compared with men with normal FBGs. Men with known diabetes had triple the odds of MDD (3.82 95% CI). Men with undiagnosed and diagnosed T2DM had higher depression scores, suggesting that there is a positive association between T2DM and depression, even for those who are unaware of their disease.

Several, but not all, studies support the hypothesis that increased depression is a consequence of diabetes. Some studies suggest that the psychosocial burden of diabetes may increase risk for depressive symptoms. Other investigators have found that the perceived disability and awareness of having a chronic illness may impose higher levels of psychologic burden for people with diabetes, particularly if they have low levels of social support (Knol et al., 2007). A meta-analysis by Mezuk and colleagues found that people with diabetes have a modest (15%) increased risk for depression compared to those without diabetes, but that depression is associated with a 60% increased risk for T2DM (Mezuk et al., 2008). Another meta-analysis examining depression and diabetes, found a 24% increased risk for incident depression among those diagnosed with diabetes compared to people without diabetes, and that rates of incident diabetes were greater for those with previous depressive episodes (Nouwen et al., 2010). However, investigators discovered that patients with chronic illnesses overall who were frequent users of medical care had similar rates of new depression diagnosis.

Further support for depression as a consequence of diabetes is provided by the Utrecht health project, a longitudinal study of a population of adults in the Netherlands. Knoll and colleagues investigated subjects with impaired fasting glucose and undiagnosed diabetes finding no association with increased depressive symptoms, suggesting that depression results from the diagnosis of diabetes. In this study, those diagnosed with diabetes had a 1.7 times risk for depressive symptoms. After adjusting for the number of chronic diseases, risk for depression was no longer significant (Knol et al., 2007).

Although the biological mechanisms underlying the association between depression and diabetes remain unclear, the evidence strongly suggests a bidirectional relationship.

Depression related physiologic alterations have been associated with increased vulnerability of depressed patients to develop T2DM. Efforts to understand the biological relationships underlying the depression-diabetes link have focused on three potential mechanisms: The hypothalamic pituitary adrenal axis (HPA), counter-regulatory effects of the sympathetic and parasympathetic nervous systems, alterations in glucose transport, and immune activation and inflammation (Musselman et al., 2003).

Psychological stress and depression stimulate activation of the HPA axis and sympathetic nervous systems (SNS), resulting in the release of cortisol and increased catecholamine and cytokine production (Dantzer et al., 2008). The release of these hormones (glucocorticoids, catecholamines, growth hormone, glucagon) stimulating both anabolic and catabolic processes involved in glucose regulation may lead to increased insulin resistance, by counteracting insulin's hypoglycemic effects, thus raising blood glucose levels and increasing the risk for diabetes. Increasing levels of cortisol are associated with redistribution of fat from subcutaneous to increased visceral adipose tissue, which results in central adiposity and dyslipidemia (Champaneri et al., 2010).

Another potential mediator implicated in the relationship between depression and diabetes involves cellular glucose transporters. These transporters facilitate the entry of glucose, a necessary metabolic substrate for all mammalian cells, into cells. Entry of glucose into endothelial cells, astrocytes, and neurons are facilitated by GLUT1 and GLUT3 respectively (Musselman et al., 2003).

Studies using positron emission tomography (PET) and functional magnetic resonance imaging (fMRI), both methods for quantifying neuronal activity in the brain by measuring glucose utilization, have shown decreased glucose utilization in the left lateral prefrontal cortex. PET has also shown a correlation between reduction in LPFC function and depression severity. Further studies are needed to determine whether these alterations in neuronal activity are related to alterations in the glucose transporters. Additionally, since brain glucose consumption does not affect glucose transport, while alterations in plasma glucose does affect glucose transport, further studies will be needed to understand these relationships (Musselman et al., 2003).

Immune activation and cell mediated cytokine production have also been implicated in the relationship between depression and diabetes. Elevations in the proinflammatory cytokines, IL-1, IL-6, and TNF-alpha, have been found in some, but not all, depressed patients (Blume et al., 2011; Dowlati et al., 2010). Proinflammatory cytokine production is also increased in individuals with diabetes (Musselman et al., 2003). Cytokines IL1, IL6, TNF alpha, and IFN gamma, found to induce sickness, exert neural effects that mediate these symptoms.

HIV/AIDS

Meta-analyses of early prevalence studies revealed that those with HIV were nearly twice as likely to have a diagnosis of major depression compared to individuals who were HIV-negative (Ciesla and Roberts, 2001). Prevalence rates of major depression range from about 5% to 20% (Cruess et al., 2003). A number of studies have found that women who were HIV positive may be particularly susceptible to MDD, with rates of current MDD higher in women who are HIV-positive compared to women who were HIV-negative (Evans et al., 2005; Lewis et al., 2010). Large-scale studies of depressive disorders among pediatric patients who are HIV-positive are lacking, but a meta-analysis estimated the prevalence in this population at 25% (Scharko, 2006).

There is considerable evidence that depression impacts the clinical course and treatment of HIV/AIDS. Clinical depression, elevated levels of depressive symptoms, or general psychological stress are associated with poor adherence to antiretroviral treatment, deterioration in psychosocial functioning, more rapid progression of HIV/AIDS, and higher mortality in both men and women before and after the HAART era (Evans et al., 2005; Ickovics et al., 2001; Leserman et al., 2002; Leserman, 2008). One study of over 1,700 women who were HIV-positive followed for 7.5 years found that those with chronic depression had 1.7 times greater odds of dying compared to women without depression (Cook et al., 2004). The impact of depression on mortality remained even after controlling for antiretroviral therapy use, medication adherence, substance abuse, clinical indicators (baseline CD4 count, baseline viral load, baseline HIV symptoms), and demographic factors; the use of mental health services was associated with significantly less AIDS-related mortality.

MECHANISMS OF COMORBIDITY

Although there is now substantial evidence supporting a relationship between depression and HIV disease progression, less is known about the mechanisms underlying this relationship. It is possible that unhealthy lifestyle behaviors may play a mediating role in this relationship between depression and the course of HIV/AIDS, but support for this hypothesis is lacking (Ickovics et al., 2001; Leserman et al., 2002; Leserman, 2003).

Disruption of the HPA axis has been investigated as a possible mediator of the depression-immune relationship. Increased levels of cortisol have been linked to stress and depression in HIV (Gorman et al., 1991), and it is hypothesized that cortisol may adversely influence the immune response and thereby negatively impact HIV disease progression (Evans et al., 2005; Leserman, 2003). In addition, NE has been shown to affect HIV replication (Cole et al., 1998). Another possible mediator is the neuropeptide substance P, which upregulates HIV and is elevated in persons with HIV (Douglas et al., 2001; Ho et al., 1996). The diminished host defense against HIV infection that has been observed in depressed individuals, may result from depression associated alterations in the functioning of killer lymphocytes (NK and cytotoxic T-lymphocytes), thus hastening HIV disease progression (Evans et al., 2002; Ironson et al., 2001; Leserman, 2003). Consistent with this hypothesis, stressful life events, poor social support, and chronic depression have all been associated with more rapid declines in CD4 lymphocyte counts (Burack et al., 1993; Kemeny and Dean, 1995; Kemeny et al., 1995) and progression to AIDS (Ickovics et al., 2001; Leserman et al., 2002; Leserman, 2003, 2008). Recent evidence from ex vivo studies suggest that a SSRI or a substance P antagonist may enhance NK immunity in HIV/AIDS adding further evidence to the potential role for NK cells in the host defense against HIV and the role of depression and antidepressant treatment in HIV disease progression (Evans et al., 2008).

Depression also has an effect on adherence to treatment regimens. Patients with HIV and depressive disorders have greater difficulty in accessing antiretroviral therapy and adhering to treatment once accessed. (Rabkin, 2008).

CANCER

The prevalence of depression is higher among those with cancer than in the general population, and prevalence estimates vary across malignancy types and disease severity. Small sample sizes and non-standardized definitions of depression have also hindered research in this area. The general range of prevalence estimates for MDD among patients with cancer has been reported to be 1.5–50% across studies, with an overall rate of 22–29% (Evans et al., 2005; Raison and Miller, 2003).

The presence of depression in individuals with cancer has been associated with poorer prognosis and increased morbidity and mortality (Evans et al., 2005). A recent meta-analysis of 31 studies found that cancer patients with depressive symptoms had a 25% higher mortality and those with major depression had a 39% greater mortality (Satin et al., 2009). A more recent study by Giese-Davis et al. (2011) suggested that depression is an independent risk factor for survival in cancer and found that a decrease in depressive symptoms was associated with longer survival in a secondary analysis of women with metastatic breast cancer who were treated with supportive-expressive group therapy. An emerging preclinical and clinical literature suggests that immune suppression and immune activation in depression may help explain the effects of depression on cancer survival (Blume et al., 2011).

Recent evidence suggests that proinflammatory cytokines released during tissue damage and destruction resulting from cancer and its treatments may be associated with the onset of depressive symptoms. The inflammatory changes precipitated by these cytokines can have a substantial impact on neurotransmitter function, neuroendocrine function, and behavior, resulting in the "sickness syndrome."

The observation that a significant percentage of patients with cancer treated with the cytokine IFN-a develop a behavioral syndrome with similarities to major depression has been an impetus for the investigations in this area. Cytokine therapies are well known to cause neurobehavioral symptoms including major depression in up to 50% of patients with cancer undergoing cytokine treatment with IFN-a (Capuron et al., 2002; Musselman et al., 2001a) and IL-2 (Capuron et al., 2004). Among patients with cancer, patients with depression and cancer were found to have significantly higher levels of IL-6 compared to patients with cancer and no depression and healthy controls (Musselman et al., 2001b). More recent studies have found associations between specific depressive symptoms and elevated cytokines; for example, some investigators have found elevated IL-6 concentrations in patients with cancer presenting with fatigue and impaired executive functioning (Collado-Hidalgo et al., 2006). Capuron and colleagues (Capuron et al., 2002, 2004) and Musselman et al. (2001a) have described two distinct behavioral syndromes that occur in individuals who become depressed with cytokine therapies. One syndrome is characterized by depressed mood, anxiety, irritability, and memory and attentional disturbances. This syndrome is reported to occur within the first three months of therapy in susceptible individuals (Capuron et al., 2002, 2004; Musselman et al., 2001a). The other syndrome, characterized by the neurovegetative symptoms of fatigue, psychomotor slowing, anorexia, and altered sleep patterns, occurs within the first few weeks of IFN-a therapy and persists at later stages of therapy (Capuron et al., 2002). These two different syndromes are thought to have different responsiveness to antidepressant treatment. The mood and cognitive symptoms were responsive to pretreatment with paroxetine (Capuron et al., 2002) whereas the neurovegetative symptoms were not, suggesting that these systems may have different pathophysiologic pathways.

Although depressive symptoms are very responsive to antidepressant treatment, the neurovegetative symptoms described in the "sickness syndrome" have been less responsive to antidepressant treatments, perhaps requiring a different treatment approach (Capuron et al., 2002; Raison and Miller, 2003).

ASSESSMENT OF DEPRESSION IN MEDICAL ILLNESS

Many psychological and physical factors can make the diagnosis of depression among those with medical illness challenging for the clinician. The classic signs and symptoms such as depressed mood, dysphoric affect, fatigue, pain, psychomotor retardation, anorexia, weight loss, cognitive impairment, and insomnia can represent demoralization or the medical illness itself. Thoughts of death or desire for a hastened death is not a reliable sign for depressive disorders in this population but may represent demoralization. In several studies, demoralization has been associated with lower quality of life and a desire for hastened death (Rackley and Bostwick, 2012). The loss of ability to experience pleasure in many activities may also be the result of physical suffering or disability and not a symptom of depression. Some acute medical conditions, such as hypoactive delirium, or progressive conditions, such as cancers and neurological conditions, have depressive symptoms that may change over time due to the illness or its treatments. Currently, no standardized approach exists for diagnosing depression among individuals who are medically ill. We continue to rely on the mental status examinations and DSM-IV criteria for depression (Evans et al., 2005). Investigators have examined the utility of excluding symptoms that can occur as part of the medical condition and the depressive condition (exclusive approach) versus the more favored inclusive approach that counts all symptoms when making a diagnosis of depression, but the findings have been inconclusive (Newport and Nemeroff, 1998; Raison and Miller, 2003). Fortunately, several well-validated instruments are available to assist the clinician in making the diagnosis of depression in the presence of medical symptoms (Rackley and Bostwick, 2012) (Table 37.2).

TREATMENT OF DEPRESSION IN MEDICAL ILLNESS

Well-controlled trials examining the efficacy of antidepressant treatments among individuals who are medically ill provide strong support for the effective use of antidepressant medications across many medical conditions (Evans et al., 2005). The challenge for the clinician is in choosing a medication that maximizes beneficial side effects while minimizing adverse effects. In the context of medical illness, identifying an effective agent and dosing regimen, whose mechanism of action and side-effect profile will not exacerbate the coexisting medical condition and minimizing polypharmacy can be challenging. The selective serotonin reuptake inhibitors (SSRIs) are widely used for treating depression in medical illness due to their safety and side-effect profiles. They may not only improve depressive symptoms but also result in positive effects on the co-occurring medical illness. For example, fluoxetine has been shown to improve glycemic control in patients with diabetes mellitus (Lustman et al., 2000). Caution in the use of SSRI or serotonin norepinephrine reuptake inhibitors (SNRIs) is warranted under certain circumstances to prevent exacerbation of the medical condition and to prevent the development of potentially serious side effects such as the syndrome of inappropriate antidiuretic hormone secretion (SIADH), platelet dysfunction that can lead to bleeding problems and serotonin syndrome (Turner et al., 2007).

Of greater concern is the potential for drug interactions. Patients with serious medical conditions, particularly the elderly, often receive multiple medications, increasing the risk of drug interactions. The presence of renal or hepatic disease with resulting fluid shifts and weight loss, for example, may affect metabolism and excretion of SSRIs and alter their pharmacokinetics (Beliles and Stoudemire, 1998). Tricyclic antidepressants (TCAs) are effective in the treatment of depression. Despite

TABLE 37.2. Screening tools used for depression in patients who are medically ill

INSTRUMENT	DESCRIPTION	ADVANTAGE/DISADVANTAGE
Center for Epidemiological Studies Depression Scale (CES-D; Radloff, 1977)	20-item self-report instrument of which only four are somatic; recommended cutoff score of 17	Wide use in patients who are medically ill High sensitivity and specificity Lack of consensus on optimal cut scores Positive predictive value low
The Hospital Anxiety and Depression Scale (HADS; Zigmond and Snaith, 1983)	14-item self-report with separate 7-item subscale for depression and anxiety Cutoff scores range from 7 to 21	Brief and highly acceptable to patients Not extensively validated as a screen Lack of consensus about utility of cutoff scores
Beck Depression Inventory-II (BDI-II; Beck et al., 1996)	21-item self-report measure Cutoff scores: 10—mild; 20—moderate; 30—severe	Validated as an accurate self-report measure in patients who are medically ill Less acceptable to patients due to forced-choice format and complex response alternatives Sensitivity and specificity high and positive predictive value high
The Patient Health Questionnaire-9 (PHQ-9; Kroenke and Spitzer., 2002)	9-item self-report depression module of the PHQ Cutoff scores: 5-mild; 10-moderate; 15-moderately severe; 20-severe	Full PHQ well-validated in primary care/medical specialty clinic in United States, Europe, and China Good sensitivity and specificity
Zung Self-Rating Scale for Depression (Zung, 1965)	20-item self report Likert-type scale scores 1–4 with highest possible score of 80 Cutoff scores: >50 for depression	Validated as an accurate self-report measure in patients who are medically ill Good sensitivity and specificity
Hamilton Depression Rating Scale (Hamilton, 1960)	17-item scale; Clinician-administered Cutoff: 10–13 mild; 14–17 moderate; >17 severe	Validated as an accurate measure in patients who are medically ill Good treatment change measure High specificity and sensitivity

evidence of their efficacy in the treatment of depression among patients with medical conditions (Evans et al., 2005), SSRIs and SNRIs have substantially reduced the clinical use of TCAs. SSRIs are more commonly used due to their efficacy, safety, and side-effect profiles. TCAs are strong antagonists of cholinergic, histaminic, and alpha-adrenergic receptors and can affect cardiac conduction, potentially exacerbating medical symptoms.

Like TCAs, monoamine oxidase inhibitors (MAOIs), while effective, are less commonly used due to their abilities to produce hypertensive reactions, drug-drug interactions with common agents such as over-the-counter sympathomimetics and stimulants, and need for tyramine restrictions. A potentially fatal serotonin syndrome, characterized by mental status changes, autonomic instability, and neurotransmitter hyperactivity, may occur when SSRIs or SNRIs are combined with MAOIs, and may be mistaken for disease in the medically ill (Rackley and Bostwick, 2012).

Psychostimulants (methylphenidate and amphetamine-based products) are used to treat depressed patients with medical conditions despite inconsistent data supporting efficacy. These agents have been used due to their ability to rapidly improve mood, motivation, and appetite, and diminish fatigue in patients who are debilitated (Hardy, 2009).

Emerging evidence suggests potential efficacy for other somatic therapies for depression in the medically ill. Neuromodulatory therapies such as electroconvulsive therapy (ECT) and transmagnetic stimulation (TMS) have shown promise for the treatment of depressive symptoms in medical illness. Recent preliminary data suggests IV ketamine, an N-methyl D-aspartate (NMDA) modulator, may rapidly ameliorate treatment-resistant depression in healthy, medically ill, and palliative care patients (Rackley and Bostwick, 2012).

ANTIDEPRESSANT TREATMENTS FOR DEPRESSION IN CARDIAC DISEASE, CANCER, AND HIV

CARDIAC DISEASE

The treatment of depression in the context of cardiac disease has been an area of great interest due to the well-established relationships between CAD, depression, and mortality. Several randomized controlled trials have been suggestive of efficacy and safety of antidepressants in the treatment of depressive disorders in patients with cardiac disease, though efficacy in regard to the progression of the cardiac disease has not been clearly established (Berkman et al., 2003; Glassman et al., 2002, 2009; Honig et al., 2007; Lesperance et al., 2007).

A Cochrane review and meta-analysis found that SSRIs and psychological approaches were effective for the treatment of depression in patients with coronary artery disease (Baumeister et al., 2011). There was no detectible difference in efficacy among various psychological treatments. Hospitalization rates and emergency room visits were reduced in patients treated with SSRIs compared to placebo, however this review was unable to conclude that there was any benefit in mortality, or cardiac events in active treatments compared to placebo. However, another recent meta-analysis did find that treatment with SSRIs is associated with a decrease in the rate of readmission and in the rate of mortality in patients with coronary heart disease (Pizzi et al., 2011).

DIABETES

The known associations of depression and diabetes, and the evidence supporting poor outcomes, have prompted trials examining the efficacy of therapeutic interventions for depression in diabetes. A recent meta-analysis from fourteen RCTs evaluating psychotherapy, pharmacologic interventions, and collaborative care in 1,724 subjects with type 1 and 2 diabetes and depression demonstrated clear effects with moderate effect size for depression treatment. Despite heterogeneity of study settings and treatment outcomes, depression treatments were effective (Markowitz et al., 2011; van der Feltz-Cornelis et al., 2010) for all three interventions in depression and diabetes.

Randomized placebo-controlled trials for fluoxetine, sertraline, paroxetine, and s-citalopram have demonstrated efficacy for the treatment of depression in diabetes (Markowitz et al., 2011). In a fluoxetine trial, significant reductions in depression severity were found for fluoxetine compared to placebo; however, there were no statistically significant differences in HbA1c (Lustman et al., 2000). In another trial with sertraline examining resolution of depression and glycemic control, hazard ratios for the risk of recurrence of depression for the sertraline treated group were significantly lower than for the placebo treated groups, suggesting a greater protection from recurrence of depression. Subjects under 55 years benefited from this prophylactic effect, when compared with a placebo group, but not those over 55 years. There were also improvements in HbA1c levels, however, they did not differ significantly between groups (Markowitz et al., 2011; Williams et al., 2007).

Two studies have examined paroxetine treatment for diabetes. In both studies, investigators studied depressed women who had not achieved optimal control of their type 2 diabetes for changes in depression severity and HbA1c levels, permitting observations of change in glycemic control. One study randomized mildly depressed postmenopausal women to either 10 weeks of a paroxetine or placebo condition. Although no differences were observed between groups with regard to depression scores, there was a statistical trend toward improved HbA1c in the paroxetine treated group when compared with placebo (Paile-Hyvarinen et al., 2007). The second study randomized mildly depressed subjects to six months of treatment with either paroxetine or placebo. HbA1c levels were significantly lower when compared to baseline for the paroxetine treated group when compared to placebo at three months. However, these gains were not maintained at six months. For both studies, depression severity was very low, with small sample sizes limiting power to detect changes in depression severity (Markowitz et al., 2011). There has been one study comparing the efficacy of different SSRIs. In this trial, subjects with T2DM and depression were randomized to either fluoxetine or paroxetine for 12 weeks. Both groups showed significant improvement on depression scores, while the fluoxetine group demonstrated a non-significant decrease in HbA1c levels (Gulseren et al., 2005).

There has been one double blind RCT of a TCA for depression in diabetes. Subjects with T1DM or T2DM and poor glycemic control were randomized to nortriptyline (NT) or placebo for eight weeks. Reductions in depression for the NT group were significantly greater than the placebo group, but not for reductions in HbA1c. NT was discovered to have a direct hyperglycemic effect on further analysis. However, improvements in depression improved glycemic control in both conditions mitigating differences (Markowitz et al., 2011).

An open trial of bupropion for depression with diabetes found that HbA1c levels, BMI, and body fat decreased significantly from baseline. Additionally, reduced BMI and depression severity predicted lower HbA1c levels during maintenance, while only decreased depression severity predicted lower HbA1c. This study, also measured pre- and posttreatment self-care with subjects reporting improvements in self-care during acute and maintenance phases (Markowitz et al., 2011; Williams et al., 2007).

Evidence supporting efficacy of antidepressant medications for depression in diabetes has resulted in increased utilization of SSRIs. However, several studies, but not all, suggest a link between the use of antidepressant medications (SSRIs and TCAs) and the risk for developing T2DM (Andersohn et al., 2009; Pan et al., 2012) while other studies found no association between antidepressant use and DM (Knol et al., 2007). Differing study designs may account for the inconsistencies in these findings.

Recent meta-analysis of treatments for depression in type 1 and type 2 diabetes concluded that psychosocial interventions, particularly cognitive behavioral therapies, are effective in improving depression in patients with diabetes, and in some but not all studies, effective at improving HbA1c levels (Markowitz et al., 2011; van der Feltz-Cornelis et al., 2010).

Collaborative care, an approach utilizing antidepressant and psychosocial interventions using a stepped care algorithm, has been studied in primary care populations. The evidence supports its effectiveness for the treatment of depression in the primary care setting similar to CBT and antidepressant treatments. Additionally, improvements of HbA1c levels and LDL cholesterol levels, were seen with the collaborative care model (Katon et al., 2010; Markowitz et al., 2011; van der Feltz-Cornelis et al., 2010). This approach may be a promising intervention for alleviating depression, and improving self-care and adherence for individuals with diabetes (Katon et al., 2010).

HIV/AIDS

A number of studies have supported the effectiveness of TCAs and SSRIs for treating depression in adults with HIV (Cruess et al., 2003; Rabkin, 2008; Repetto and Petitto, 2008). The TCAs and SSRIs have both shown equal efficacy in head to head studies. In one placebo-controlled study comparing imipramine, paroxetine, and placebo in 75 individuals who were HIV-positive, both agents were equally effective when compared to placebo. However, anticholinergic side effects with imipramine resulted in high dropout rates (48%) for imipramine, compared with 20% for paroxetine and 24% for placebo respectively (Elliott et al., 1998). One small open label study evaluated the efficacy of paroxetine, fluoxetine, and sertraline in HIV seropositive individuals. (Ferrando et al., 1997). Improvements were reported in depression and somatic symptoms related to HIV disease in most patients (83%), but the dropout rates were high (27%). Comparative effectiveness of the three SSRIs could not be evaluated due to the small sample size. One other small uncontrolled study found improvements among clinically depressed HIV seropositive individuals who were treated with paroxetine (Grassi et al., 1997). Preliminary data based on open trials suggests that sustained release bupropion (Theobald et al., 2002) and mirtazapine (Currier et al., 2003) may be effective. Although larger placebo-controlled studies are needed to confirm these findings, existing findings suggest the effectiveness of SSRIs in reducing symptoms of depression in HIV seropositive individuals. A protocol for a Cochrane review has recently been published (Lewis et al., 2010).

TCAs have been found to be ineffective in two studies of HIV-related neuropathy (Saarto and Wiffen, 2010). No data are available on the SNRIs venlafaxine and duloxetine in the treatments of HIV-related neuropathy.

Psychostimulants (methylphenidate and dextroamphetamine) have also been studied in placebo-controlled trials in patients with depression and HIV. There have been two small uncontrolled studies of psychostimulants in the treatment of depression in HIV/AIDS (Fernandez et al., 1995; Wagner et al., 1997), and one small, placebo-controlled study (Wagner and Rabkin, 2000) that showed efficacy. Reductions in depressive symptoms as early as two weeks after initiating treatment have been reported (Wagner et al., 1997). In another study, among patients who were HIV-positive who also had significant levels of fatigue, methylphenidate and pemoline were found to be significantly superior to placebo in decreasing fatigue, and improvement in fatigue was significantly associated with improved quality of life and decreased levels of depression (Breitbart et al., 2001).

Reductions in testosterone levels among individuals with HIV/AIDS can be associated with changes in mood, appetite, and sexual function. In one study enrolling symptomatic patients who were HIV-positive, testosterone treatment was significantly better than placebo at restoring libido and energy, alleviating depressed mood, and increasing muscle mass (Rabkin et al., 2000), and a recent meta-analysis found that testosterone was effective in treating depression in HIV/AIDS (Zarrouf et al., 2009). The adrenal steroid dehydroepiandrosterone (DHEA) has also been evaluated and was effective (Rabkin et al., 2006).

As with other medical and nonmedical populations, the choice of an antidepressant agent in patients with HIV must be guided by the potential for drug-drug interactions and a number of potential interactions have been noted for medications used to treat depression and HIV/AIDS (Watkins et al., 2011).

CANCER

The effectiveness of antidepressants agents, specifically SSRIs and TCAs, for the treatment of depression in individuals with cancer is supported by a number of clinical trials (Evans et al., 2005).

In a small study of major depression among women with breast cancer, comparing the efficacy of an SSRI (paroxetine) to a TCA (desipramine), no differences were found in efficacy compared to placebo (Musselman et al., 2006). In addition to the SSRIs and TCAs, mirtazapine and mianserin have shown promising results in open trials (Costa et al., 1985; Theobald et al., 2002; van Heeringen and Zivkov, 1996). Mirtazapine's potential to cause weight gain might be of benefit for anorexic-cachectic patients with cancer, but should be used cautiously in those already gaining weight from steroids or from chemotherapy (Theobald et al., 2002). SSRIs are generally preferred over TCAs in this population, because of fewer sedative and autonomic side effects. SSRIs and the SNRI venlafaxine have demonstrated positive effects for women without depression who become menopausal after chemotherapy for breast cancer or who have a recurrence of vasomotor symptoms when they discontinue hormone replacement therapy. They have been effective for reducing the number and intensity of hot flashes and night sweats. The potential for drug interactions must be considered in patients with cancer. Recent evidence indicates that antidepressants that inhibit CYP2D6 may adversely affect the metabolism of tamoxifen, and it is recommended that known CYP2D6 inhibitors such as fluoxetine, paroxetine, or buproprion, should be avoided in combination with tamoxifen (Desmarais and Looper, 2009).

As reviewed earlier, another consideration in patients with cancer is depression that can result from certain cancer treatments that activate the immune system. In particular, treatment with IFN-a can cause the onset of new depressive episodes or trigger a recurrence of a previous episode. In a placebo-controlled trial, the use of an antidepressant (paroxetine) at the time of IFN-a treatment was found to reduce the incidence of depressive episodes and reduce the rate of discontinuation of IFN-a treatment (Musselman et al., 2001a). Currently, prophylactic use of antidepressants for patients with cancer is not recommended.

Although studies supporting antidepressant efficacy for psychostimulants (methylphenidate, dextroamphetamine) are lacking, they have been used with patients with cancer to promote a sense of well-being, improve symptoms of depression, increase energy, and improve cognitive function (Rozans et al., 2002). Psychostimulants have also been used to potentiate the analgesic effects of opioids and to counteract their sedative effects (Rozans et al., 2002).

CONCLUSIONS

Depressive disorders are prevalent among those with chronic medical conditions and may increase symptom burden and functional disability, adversely affect self-care and adherence to treatment, and decrease quality of life. Depression is also associated with immune suppression and immune activation. Depression associated cellular immune suppression may be a mechanism whereby depression may adversely effect immune-based diseases such as cancer and AIDS. On the other hand, depression-associated immune activation may be a mechanism whereby depression may have an adverse effect on diseases such as cardiovascular disease and diabetes.

Antidepressant treatments and psychotherapies are effective in the treatment of many of the symptoms of depression in individuals who are medically ill. High rates of depression among the medically ill call for heightened attention to this comorbidity. Depression should be actively identified and targeted for intervention. A number of studies suggest that the treatment of depression in individuals who are medically ill might improve overall medical outcomes or disease progression. Further large-scale studies will be needed to confirm these findings. Future investigation should focus on understanding the immune mechanisms as well as other mechanisms underlying depression and comorbid medical illness. Understanding the mechanisms underlying the associations between depression and medical illness may stimulate the development of novel therapies that provide effective interventions for this complex patient population.

DISCLOSURES

The work of Drs. Benton, Crits-Christoph, Dubé, and Evans, and the training of Dr. Blume, has been funded, in part, by the National Institutes of Health. Dr. Dubé was on the Speaker Bureau of Boehringer Ingelheim in 2009, 2010, and 2011, and has received compensation.

REFERENCES

Andersohn, F., Schade, R., et al. (2009). Long-term use of antidepressants for depressive disorders and the risk of diabetes mellitus. *Am. J. Psychiatry* 166:591–598.

Baumeister, H., Hutter, N., et al. (2011). Psychological and pharmacological interventions for depression in patients with coronary artery disease. *Cochrane Database Syst. Rev.* CD008012.

Beck, A.T., Steer, R.A., et al. (1996). Comparison of Beck depression inventories-IA and -II in Psychiatric Outpatients. *J. Pers. Assess.* 67:588–597.

Beliles, K., and Stoudemire, A. (1998). Psychopharmacologic treatment of depression in the medically ill. *Psychosomatics* 39:S2–S19.

Berg, L., Lampa, J., et al. (2001). Increased peripheral T cell reactivity to microbial antigens and collagen type II in rheumatoid arthritis after treatment with soluble TNFalpha receptors. *Ann. Rheum. Dis.* 60:133–139.

Berkman, L.F., Blumenthal, J., et al. (2003). Effects of treating depression and low perceived social support on clinical events after myocardial infarction: the Enhancing Recovery in Coronary Heart Disease Patients (ENRICHD). Randomized Trial. *JAMA* 289:3106–3116.

Blume, J., Douglas, S.D., et al. (2011). Immune suppression and immune activation in depression. *Brain Behav. Immun.* 25:221–229.

Breitbart, W., Rosenfeld, B., et al. (2001). A randomized, double-blind, placebo-controlled trial of psychostimulants for the treatment of fatigue in ambulatory patients with human immunodeficiency virus disease. *Arch. Intern. Med.* 161:411–420.

Bruce, T.O. (2008). Comorbid depression in rheumatoid arthritis: pathophysiology and clinical implications. *Curr. Psychiatry Rep.* 10:258–264.

Burack, J.H., Barrett, D.C., et al. (1993). Depressive symptoms and CD4 lymphocyte decline among HIV-infected men. *JAMA* 270:2568–2573.

Campayo, A., de Jonge, P., et al. (2010). Depressive disorder and incident diabetes mellitus: the effect of characteristics of depression. *Am. J. Psychiatry* 167:580–588.

Capuron, L., Gumnick, J.F., et al. (2002). Neurobehavioral effects of interferon-alpha in cancer patients: phenomenology and paroxetine responsiveness of symptom dimensions. *Neuropsychopharmacology* 26:643–652.

Capuron, L., Ravaud, A., et al. (2004). Baseline mood and psychosocial characteristics of patients developing depressive symptoms during interleukin-2 and/or interferon-alpha cancer therapy. *Brain Behav. Immun.* 18:205–213.

Carney, R.M., Blumenthal, J.A., et al. (2005). Low heart rate variability and the effect of depression on post-myocardial infarction mortality. *Arch. Intern. Med.* 165:1486–1491.

CDC. (2008). National diabetes fact sheet: general information and national estimates on diabetes in the United States, 2007. U.S. Department of Health and Human Services, Centers for Disease Control and Prevention. Atlanta, GA.

Celano, C.M., and Huffman, J.C. (2011). Depression and cardiac disease: a review. *Cardiol. Rev.* 19:130–142.

Cesari, M., Penninx, B.W., et al. (2003). Inflammatory markers and onset of cardiovascular events: results from the Health ABC study. *Circulation* 108:2317–2322.

Champaneri, S., Wand, G.S., et al. (2010). Biological basis of depression in adults with diabetes. *Curr. Diab. Rep.* 10:396–405.

Ciesla, J.A., and Roberts, J.E. (2001). Meta-analysis of the relationship between HIV infection and risk for depressive disorders. *Am. J. Psychiatry* 158:725–730.

Cole, S.W., Korin, Y.D., et al. (1998). Norepinephrine accelerates HIV replication via protein kinase A-dependent effects on cytokine production. *J. Immunol.* 161:610–616.

Collado-Hidalgo, A., Bower, J.E., et al. (2006). Inflammatory biomarkers for persistent fatigue in breast cancer survivors. *Clin. Cancer Res.* 12:2759–2766.

Constant, E.L., Adam, S., et al. (2005). Effects of sertraline on depressive symptoms and attentional and executive functions in major depression. *Depress. Anxiety* 21:78–89.

Cook, J.A., Grey, D., et al. (2004). Depressive symptoms and AIDS-related mortality among a multisite cohort of HIV-positive women. *Am. J. Public Health* 94:1133–1140.

Cooper, D.C., Milic, M.S., et al. (2010). Adverse impact of mood on flow-mediated dilation. *Psychosom. Med.* 72:122–127.

Cope, A.P. (2003). Exploring the reciprocal relationship between immunity and inflammation in chronic inflammatory arthritis. *Rheumatology (Oxford)* 42:716–731.

Costa, D., Mogos, I., et al. (1985). Efficacy and safety of mianserin in the treatment of depression of women with cancer. *Acta Psychiatr. Scand. Suppl.* 320:85–92.

Cruess, D.G., Evans, D.L., et al. (2003). Prevalence, diagnosis, and pharmacological treatment of mood disorders in HIV disease. *Biol. Psychiatry* 54:307–316.

Currier, M.B., Molina, G., et al. (2003). A prospective trial of sustained-release bupropion for depression in HIV-seropositive and AIDS patients. *Psychosomatics* 44:120–125.

Dantzer, R., O'Connor, J.C., et al. (2008). From inflammation to sickness and depression: when the immune system subjugates the brain. *Nat. Rev. Neurosci.* 9:46–56.

Dekker, J.M., Crow, R.S., et al. (2000). Low heart rate variability in a 2-minute rhythm strip predicts risk of coronary heart disease and mortality from several causes: the ARIC Study. Atherosclerosis Risk In Communities. *Circulation* 102:1239–1244.

Desmarais, J.E., and Looper, K.J. (2009). Interactions between tamoxifen and antidepressants via cytochrome P450 2D6. *J. Clin. Psychiatry* 70:1688–1697.

Doran, M.F., Crowson, C.S., et al. (2002). Frequency of infection in patients with rheumatoid arthritis compared with controls: a population-based study. *Arthritis. Rheum.* 46:2287–2293.

Douglas, S.D., Ho, W.Z., et al. (2001). Elevated substance P levels in HIV-infected men. *AIDS* 15:2043–2045.

Dowlati, Y., Herrmann, N., et al. (2010). A meta-analysis of cytokines in major depression. *Biol. Psychiatry* 67:446–457.

Elliott, A.J., Uldall, K.K., et al. (1998). Randomized, placebo-controlled trial of paroxetine versus imipramine in depressed HIV-positive outpatients. *Am. J. Psychiatry* 155:367–372.

Evans, D.L., Charney, D.S., et al. (2005). Mood disorders in the medically ill: scientific review and recommendations. *Biol. Psychiatry* 58:175–189.

Evans, D.L., Lynch, K.G., et al. (2008). Selective serotonin reuptake inhibitor and substance P antagonist enhancement of natural killer cell innate immunity in human immunodeficiency virus/acquired immunodeficiency syndrome. *Biol. Psychiatry* 63:899–905.

Evans, D.L., Ten Have, T.R., et al. (2002). Association of depression with viral load, CD8 T lymphocytes, and natural killer cells in women with HIV infection. *Am. J. Psychiatry* 159:1752–1759.

Fernandez, F., Levy, J.K., et al. (1995). Effects of methylphenidate in HIV-related depression: a comparative trial with desipramine. *Int. J. Psychiatry Med.* 25:53–67.

Ferrando, S.J., Goldman, J.D., et al. (1997). Selective serotonin reuptake inhibitor treatment of depression in symptomatic HIV infection and AIDS. Improvements in affective and somatic symptoms. *Gen. Hosp. Psychiatry* 19:89–97.

Frasure-Smith, N., Lesperance, F., et al. (1995). Depression and 18 month prognosis after myocardial infarction. *Circulation* 91:999–1005.

Frasure-Smith, N., Lesperance, F., et al. (2007). Depression, C-reactive protein and two-year major adverse cardiac events in men after acute coronary syndromes. *Biol. Psychiatry* 62:302–308.

Gale, C.R., Kivimaki, M., et al. (2010). Fasting glucose, diagnosis of Type 2 diabetes, and depression: the Vietnam experience study. *Biol. Psychiatry* 67:189–192.

Giese-Davis, J., Collie, K., et al. (2011). Decrease in depression symptoms is associated with longer survival in patients with metastatic breast cancer: a secondary analysis. *J. Clin. Oncol.* 29:413–420.

Gladman, D.D., Hussain, F., et al. (2002). The nature and outcome of infection in systemic lupus erythematosus. *Lupus* 11:234–239.

Glassman, A.H., Bigger, J.T., Jr., et al. (2009). Psychiatric characteristics associated with long-term mortality among 361 patients having an acute coronary syndrome and major depression. *Arch. Gen. Psychiatry* 66:1022–1029.

Glassman, A.H., O'Connor, C.M., et al. (2002). Sertraline treatment of major depression in patients with acute MI or unstable angina. *JAMA* 288:701–709.

Glazer, K.M., Emery, C.F., et al. (2002). Psychological predictors of adherence and outcomes among patients in cardiac rehabilitation. *J. Cardiopulm. Rehabil.* 22:40–46.

Golden, S.H., Lazo, M., et al. (2008). Examining a bidirectional association between depressive symptoms and diabetes. *JAMA* 299:2751–2759.

Gorman, J.M., Kertzner, R., et al. (1991). Glucocorticoid level and neuropsychiatric symptoms in homosexual men with HIV infection. *Am. J. Psychiatry* 148:41–45.

Grassi, B., Gambini, O., et al. (1997). Efficacy of paroxetine for the treatment of depression in the context of HIV infection. *Pharmacopsychiatry* 30:70–71.

Gulseren, L., Gulseren, S., et al. (2005). Comparison of fluoxetine and paroxetine in type II diabetes mellitus patients. *Arch. Med. Res.* 36:159–165.

Hamilton, M. (1960). A rating scale for depression. *J. Neurol. Neurosur. PS.* 23:56–62.

Hardy, S.E. (2009). Methylphenidate for the treatment of depressive symptoms, including fatigue and apathy, in medically ill older adults and terminally ill adults. *Am. J. Geriatr. Pharmacother.* 7:34–59.

Ho, W.Z., Cnaan, A., et al. (1996). Substance P modulates human immunodeficiency virus replication in human peripheral blood monocyte-derived macrophages. *AIDS Res. Hum. Retroviruses* 12:195–198.

Honig, A., Kuyper, A.M., et al. (2007). Treatment of post-myocardial infarction depressive disorder: a randomized, placebo-controlled trial with mirtazapine. *Psychosom. Med.* 69:606–613.

Ickovics, J.R., Hamburger, M.E., et al. (2001). Mortality, CD4 cell count decline, and depressive symptoms among HIV-seropositive women: longitudinal analysis from the HIV Epidemiology Research Study. *JAMA* 285:1466–1474.

Ironson, G., Balbin, E., et al. (2001). Relative preservation of natural killer cell cytotoxicity and number in healthy AIDS patients with low CD4 cell counts. *AIDS* 15:2065–2073.

Irwin, M.R., and Miller, A.H. (2007). Depressive disorders and immunity: 20 years of progress and discovery. *Brain Behav. Immun.* 21:374–383.

Katon, W.J. (2003). Clinical and health services relationships between major depression, depressive symptoms, and general medical illness. *Biol. Psychiatry* 54:216–226.

Katon, W.J. (2011). Epidemiology and treatment of depression in patients with chronic medical illness. *Dialogues Clin. Neurosci.* 13:7–23.

Katon, W.J., Lin, E.H., et al. (2010). Collaborative care for patients with depression and chronic illnesses. *N. Engl. J. Med.* 363:2611–2620.

Kemeny, M.E., and Dean, L. (1995). Effects of AIDS-related bereavement on HIV progression among New York City gay men. *AIDS Educ. Prev.* 7:36–47.

Kemeny, M.E., Weiner, H., et al. (1995). Immune system changes after the death of a partner in HIV-positive gay men. *Psychosom. Med.* 57:547–554.

Kessler, R.C., Berglund, P., et al. (2005). Lifetime prevalence and age-of-onset distributions of DSM-IV disorders in the National Comorbidity Survey Replication. *Arch. Gen. Psychiatry* 62:593–602.

Kling, M.A., Alesci, S., et al. (2007). Sustained low-grade pro-inflammatory state in unmedicated, remitted women with major depressive disorder as evidenced by elevated serum levels of the acute phase proteins C-reactive protein and serum amyloid A. *Biol. Psychiatry* 62:309–313.

Knol, M.J., Heerdink, E.R., et al. (2007). Depressive symptoms in subjects with diagnosed and undiagnosed type 2 diabetes. *Psychosom. Med.* 69:300–305.

Koetz, K., Bryl, E., et al. (2000). T cell homeostasis in patients with rheumatoid arthritis. *Proc. Natl. Acad. Sci. USA* 97:9203–9208.

Kroenke, K., and Spitzer, R.L. (2002). The PHQ-9: a new depression diagnostic and severity measure. *Psychiatr. Ann.* 32:509–515.

La Cava, A. (2008). T-regulatory cells in systemic lupus erythematosus. *Lupus* 17:421–425.

Leserman, J. (2003). HIV disease progression: depression, stress, and possible mechanisms. *Biol. Psychiatry* 54:295–306.

Leserman, J. (2008). Role of depression, stress, and trauma in HIV disease progression. *Psychosom. Med.* 70:539–545.

Leserman, J., Petitto, J.M., et al. (2002). Progression to AIDS, a clinical AIDS condition and mortality: psychosocial and physiological predictors. *Psychol. Med.* 32:1059–1073.

Lesperance, F., Frasure-Smith, N., et al. (2007). Effects of citalopram and interpersonal psychotherapy on depression in patients with coronary artery disease: the Canadian Cardiac Randomized Evaluation of Antidepressant and Psychotherapy Efficacy (CREATE). trial. *JAMA* 297:367–379.

Lett, H.S., Blumenthal, J.A., et al. (2004). Depression as a risk factor for coronary artery disease: evidence, mechanisms, and treatment. *Psychosom. Med.* 66:305–315.

Lewis, I.S., Joska, J.A., et al. (2010). Antidepressants for depression in adults with HIV infection (Protocol). *Cochrane Database Syst. Rev.* CD008525.

Lustman, P.J., Freedland, K.E., et al. (2000). Fluoxetine for depression in diabetes: a randomized double-blind placebo-controlled trial. *Diabetes Care* 23:618–623.

Markowitz, S.M., Gonzalez, J.S., et al. (2011). A review of treating depression in diabetes: emerging findings. *Psychosomatics* 52:1–18.

Medzhitov, R. (2008). Origin and physiological roles of inflammation. *Nature.* 454:428–435.

Mezuk, B., Eaton, W.W., et al. (2008). Depression and type 2 diabetes over the lifespan: a meta-analysis. *Diabetes Care* 31:2383–2390.

Miller, A.H. (2010). Depression and immunity: a role for T cells? *Brain Behav. Immun.* 24:1–8.

Miller, A.H., Maletic, V., et al. (2009). Inflammation and its discontents: the role of cytokines in the pathophysiology of major depression. *Biol. Psychiatry* 65:732–741.

Musselman, D.L., Betan, E., et al. (2003). Relationship of depression to diabetes types 1 and 2: epidemiology, biology, and treatment. *Biol. Psychiatry* 54:317–329.

Musselman, D.L., Lawson, D.H., et al. (2001a). Paroxetine for the prevention of depression induced by high-dose interferon alfa. *N. Engl. J. Med.* 344:961–966.

Musselman, D.L., Miller, A.H., et al. (2001b). Higher than normal plasma interleukin-6 concentrations in cancer patients with depression: preliminary findings. *Am. J. Psychiatry* 158:1252–1257.

Musselman, D.L., Somerset, W.I., et al. (2006). A double-blind, multicenter, parallel-group study of paroxetine, desipramine, or placebo in breast cancer patients (stages I, II, III, and IV). with major depression. *J. Clin. Psychiatry* 67:288–296.

Nahshoni, E., Aravot, D., et al. (2004). Heart rate variability in patients with major depression. *Psychosomatics* 45:129–134.

Nemeroff, C.B., and Vale, W.W. (2005). The neurobiology of depression: inroads to treatment and new drug discovery. *J. Clin. Psychiatry* 66(Suppl 7):5–13.

Nery, F.G., Borba, E.F., et al. (2007). Major depressive disorder and disease activity in systemic lupus erythematosus. *Compr. Psychiatry* 48:14–19.

Newport, D.J., and Nemeroff, C.B. (1998). Assessment and treatment of depression in the cancer patient. *J. Psychosom. Res.* 45:215–237.

Nouwen, A., Winkley, K., et al. (2010). Type 2 diabetes mellitus as a risk factor for the onset of depression: a systematic review and meta-analysis. *Diabetologia* 53:2480–2486.

Otte, C., Zhao, S., et al. (2012). Statin use and risk of depression in patients with coronary heart disease: longitudinal data from the heart and soul study. *J. Clin. Psychiatry* 73:610–615.

Pan, A., Sun, Q., et al. (2012). Use of antidepressant medication and risk of type 2 diabetes: results from three cohorts of US adults. *Diabetologia* 55:63–72.

Paile-Hyvarinen, M., Wahlbeck, K., et al. (2007). Quality of life and metabolic status in mildly depressed patients with type 2 diabetes treated with paroxetine: a double-blind randomized placebo controlled 6 month trial. *BMC Fam. Pract.* 8:34–41.

Pike, J.L., and Irwin, M.R. (2006). Dissociation of inflammatory markers and natural killer cell activity in major depressive disorder. *Brain Behav. Immun.* 20:169–174.

Pizzi, C., Mancini, S., et al. (2009). Effects of selective serotonin reuptake inhibitor therapy on endothelial function and inflammatory markers in patients with coronary heart disease. *Clin. Pharmacol. Ther.* 86:527–532.

Pizzi, C., Manzoli, L., et al. (2008). Analysis of potential predictors of depression among coronary heart disease risk factors including heart rate variability, markers of inflammation, and endothelial function. *Eur. Heart J.* 29:1110–1117.

Pizzi, C., Rutjes, A.W., et al. (2011). Meta-analysis of selective serotonin reuptake inhibitors in patients with depression and coronary heart disease. *Am. J. Cardiol.* 107:972–979.

Prince, M., Patel, V., et al. (2007). Global mental health 1—No health without mental health. *Lancet* 370:859–877.

Rabkin, J.G. (2008). HIV and depression: 2008 review and update. *Curr. HIV/AIDS Rep.* 5:163–171.

Rabkin, J.G., McElhiney, M.C., et al. (2006). Placebo-controlled trial of dehydroepiandrosterone (DHEA). for treatment of nonmajor depression in patients with HIV/AIDS. *Am. J. Psychiatry* 163:59–66.

Rabkin, J.G., Wagner, G.J., et al. (2000). A double-blind, placebo-controlled trial of testosterone therapy for HIV-positive men with hypogonadal symptoms. *Arch. Gen. Psychiatry* 57:141–147; discussion 155–156.

Rackley, S., and Bostwick, J.M. (2012). Depression in medically ill patients. *Psychiatr. Clin. North Am.* 35:231–247.

Radloff, L.S. (1977). The CES-D Scale: a self-report depression scale for research in the general population. *Applied Psychological Measurement* 1:385–401.

Raison, C.L., Borisov, A.S., et al. (2009). Activation of central nervous system inflammatory pathways by interferon-alpha: relationship to monoamines and depression. *Biol. Psychiatry* 65:296–303.

Raison, C.L., and Miller, A.H. (2003). Depression in cancer: new developments regarding diagnosis and treatment. *Biol. Psychiatry* 54:283–294.

Repetto, M.J., and Petitto, J.M. (2008). Psychopharmacology in HIV-infected patients. *Psychosom. Med.* 70:585–592.

Rozans, M., Dreisbach, A., et al. (2002). Palliative uses of methylphenidate in patients with cancer: a review. *J. Clin. Oncol.* 20:335–339.

Rudisch, B., and Nemeroff, C.B. (2003). Epidemiology of comorbid coronary artery disease and depression. *Biol. Psychiatry* 54:227–240.

Saarto, T., and Wiffen, P.J. (2010). Antidepressants for neuropathic pain: a Cochrane review. *J. Neurol. Neurosurg. Psychiatry* 81:1372–1373.

Satin, J.R., Linden, W., et al. (2009). Depression as a predictor of disease progression and mortality in cancer patients: a meta-analysis. *Cancer* 115:5349–5361.

Scharko, A.M. (2006). DSM psychiatric disorders in the context of pediatric HIV/AIDS. *AIDS Care* 18:441–445.

Skala, J.A., Freedland, K.E., et al. (2006). Coronary heart disease and depression: a review of recent mechanistic research. *Can. J. Psychiatry* 51:738–745.

Stafford, L., and Berk, M. (2011). The use of statins after a cardiac intervention is associated with reduced risk of subsequent depression: proof of concept for the inflammatory and oxidative hypotheses of depression? *J. Clin. Psychiatry* 72:1229–1235.

Stein, P.K., Carney, R.M., et al. (2000). Severe depression is associated with markedly reduced heart rate variability in patients with stable coronary heart disease. *J. Psychosom. Res.* 48:493–500.

Sullivan, M.D., O'Connor, P., et al. (2012). Depression predicts all-cause mortality: epidemiological evaluation from the ACCORD HRQL substudy. *Diabetes Care* 35:1708–1715.

Theobald, D.E., Kirsh, K.L., et al. (2002). An open-label, crossover trial of mirtazapine (15 and 30 mg) in cancer patients with pain and other distressing symptoms. *J. Pain Symptom Manage.* 23:442–447.

Turner, M.S., May, D.B., et al. (2007). Clinical impact of selective serotonin reuptake inhibitors therapy with bleeding risks. *J. Intern. Med.* 261:205–213.

van der Feltz-Cornelis, C.M., Nuyen, J., et al. (2010). Effect of interventions for major depressive disorder and significant depressive symptoms in patients with diabetes mellitus: a systematic review and meta-analysis. *Gen. Hosp. Psychiatry* 32:380–395.

van Heeringen, K., and Zivkov, M. (1996). Pharmacological treatment of depression in cancer patients. A placebo-controlled study of mianserin. *Br. J. Psychiatry* 169:440–443.

Wagner, G.J., Rabkin, J.G., et al. (1997). Dextroamphetamine as a treatment for depression and low energy in AIDS patients: a pilot study. *J. Psychosom. Res.* 42:407–411.

Wagner, G.J., and Rabkin, R. (2000). Effects of dextroamphetamine on depression and fatigue in men with HIV: a double-blind, placebo-controlled trial. *J. Clin. Psychiatry* 61:436–440.

Wang, P.S., Bohn, R.L., et al. (2002). Noncompliance with antihypertensive medications: the impact of depressive symptoms and psychosocial factors. *J. Gen. Intern. Med.* 17:504–511.

Watkins, C.C., Pieper, A.A., et al. (2011). Safety considerations in drug treatment of depression in HIV-positive patients: an updated review. *Drug. Saf.* 34:623–639.

WHO (2008). The Global Burden of Disease: 2004 Update. World Health Organization. Geneva, Switzerland: WHO Press.

Whooley, M.A., Caska, C.M., et al. (2007). Depression and inflammation in patients with coronary heart disease: findings from the Heart and Soul Study. *Biol. Psychiatry* 62:314–320.

Williams, M.M., Clouse, R.E., et al. (2007). Efficacy of sertraline in prevention of depression recurrence in older versus younger adults with diabetes. *Diabetes Care* 30:801–806.

Zarrouf, F.A., Artz, S., et al. (2009). Testosterone and depression: systematic review and meta-analysis. *J. Psychiatr. Pract.* 15:289–305.

Zigmond, A.S., and Snaith, R.P. (1983). The hospital anxiety and depression scale. *Acta. Psychiatr. Scand.* 67:361–370.

Zung, W.W. (1965). A self-rating depression scale. *Arch. Gen. Psychiat.* 12:63–70.

38 | TREATMENTS FOR DEPRESSION

DAN V. IOSIFESCU, JAMES W. MURROUGH, AND DENNIS S. CHARNEY

INTRODUCTION

Depression encompasses a large number of psychobiological syndromes with the core features of depressed mood and/or loss of interest associated with cognitive and somatic disturbances, which causes significant functional impairment. Clinical depression is distinguished from normal sadness by the severity of associated symptoms and its impact on functional status. Major depressive disorder (MDD) is characterized by one or more episodes of depressed mood, or a loss of interest or pleasure, for a minimum of two weeks, associated with four or more of the following symptoms: appetite disturbance, sleep disturbance, psychomotor agitation or retardation, fatigue or loss of energy, feelings of guilt or worthlessness, poor concentration, suicide attempts, or thoughts of death (American Psychiatric Association, 2000). Frequently, depressed patients present with a chief complaint of chronic pain, fatigue, gastrointestinal problems, anxiety, irritability, or sleep disturbance. The lack of a medical cause for these symptoms should raise the index of suspicion for clinical depression. A full discussion of the diagnosis and symptoms of depression is presented in Chapter 29.

Large epidemiological studies suggest that major depressive disorder is common, with a lifetime prevalence of 16.6%, occurring with approximately twofold higher frequency in women compared to men (Kessler et al., 2005).

Given the high prevalence and morbidity of depression, research efforts for discovery of effective antidepressant treatments span many decades. The first antidepressant agents, iproniazid (Crane, 1956) and imipramine (Kuhn, 1958), were discovered by serendipity, as they had been initially developed for other indications (tuberculosis and psychosis, respectively). Empiric observations about these agents' activity on mood and psychomotor function led to more systematic clinical trials in depressed patients, where they demonstrated clinical efficacy. In further investigations iproniazid was found to inhibit the monoamine oxidase enzyme (involved in the catabolism of serotonin, norepinephrine, and dopamine) while imipramine was shown to inhibit the reuptake of serotonin and norepinephrine (Gershon et al., 1962; Glowinski and Axelrod, 1964). Such insights led directly to the discovery of additional molecules with antidepressant properties—the monoamine oxidase inhibitors (MAOIs) and the tricyclic antidepressants (TCAs)—and to a number of key observations linking the monoamines (serotonin, norepinephrine, and dopamine) to mood, perception, and cognition. This became the basis of the monoamine hypothesis of depression, postulating that basic neurotransmitter imbalances within the brain are the main causes of depression and that medication correcting these imbalances can lead to clinical improvement (Schildkraut, 1965). The support for the monoamine hypothesis came from several observations. The locus coeruleus (the major source of the brain's adrenergic innervations), and the brainstem raphe nuclei (origin of serotonin neurons) have modulatory roles, regulating global functions such as arousal, vigilance, attention, mood, and appetite. Certain drugs, such as reserpine, which deplete the monoamine neurotransmitters, induce a clinical state indistinguishable from depression, thus providing an animal model for the disease. Also, antidepressants such as MAOIs and TCAs increased by different mechanisms the amounts of monoamine neurotransmitters, resulting in clinical relief from depression.

In its most simplistic form, the monoamine hypothesis proved to be an inadequate theory on the biology of depression and the mechanisms of antidepressant drug action. There is a lack of evidence to prove globally diminished levels of noradrenergic or serotonergic neurotransmission characterize depression. Moreover, the effect of most antidepressants in raising the levels of neurotransmitters occurs very fast, in a matter of hours, while the latency for onset of clinical benefit is typically two to four weeks, and for the full clinical effect six to eight weeks. According to more recent understanding of the neurobiological effects of antidepressants, it is possible that changes in monoaminergic neurotransmitters are at the origin of a chain of intracellular second-messenger systems that promote gene regulation and synthesis of neuroprotective factors such as brain-derived neurotrophic factor (BDNF), thereby gradually restoring network function and ultimately mood (Kozisek et al, 2008). By regulating the phosphorylation of the DA- and cAMP-regulated phosphoprotein DARPP-32, antidepressants such as SSRIs also have indirect effects on α-amino-3-hydroxy-5-methyl-4-isoxazolepropionic acid (AMPA) glutamate receptors, which represent a novel therapeutic target in depression (Alt et al., 2006).

However, the monoamine theory had an important role in guiding subsequent efforts for the discovery of novel antidepressants. The understanding that serotonin plays a major role in depression led to focused research for drugs with activity on serotonergic receptors, although antidepressant efficacy has been associated with opposing mechanisms of action (e.g., selective serotonin reuptake inhibitors, SSRIs, versus tianeptine, a selective serotonin reuptake enhancer). SSRIs were the first class of antidepressants specifically researched based on a putative mechanism of action. After the first SSRI, zimelidine, was withdrawn due to side effects, fluvoxamine (first marketed in 1984 in Switzerland) and fluoxetine (marketed in the United States since 1987) became the precursors of a series of other antidepressants with similar monoaminergic mechanisms.

The development of novel antidepressants has been limited by imperfect understanding of the neurobiological mechanisms causing depression and by the biological and clinical heterogeneity of patients with the same diagnosis and by imperfect clinical research methods (e.g., variability in rating scores and limited sensitivity to change in some research instruments, inflation of placebo response rates).

The rational selection of antidepressant treatments requires an understanding of their pharmacological and biological properties (Montgomery, 2007). Partial or inadequate response to antidepressant treatment is common in MDD; only about 30% to 40% of the patients who receive adequate pharmacotherapy will achieve full remission (absence or near absence of symptoms) (Rush et al., 2006). In the Sequenced Treatment Alternatives to Relieve Depression (STAR*D) study only 29% of 2,876 MDD subjects treated with the maximum tolerated dose of citalopram (up to 60 mg) for up to 14 weeks achieved remission (Trivedi et al., 2006). Several clinical variables such as comorbid anxiety disorders (Fava et al., 2008), substance use disorders (Nunes and Levin, 2004), and medical illness (Iosifescu, 2007), have been associated with lower rates of improvement with antidepressant treatments. Non-response to antidepressants is associated with disability and higher medical costs (Simon et al, 2006), and partial response is associated with higher relapse and recurrence rates (Judd et al, 1998). Moreover, it takes 6–12 weeks to fully evaluate the efficacy of an antidepressant treatment. As each new pharmacotherapy is tried, patients are exposed to additional cost, side effect burden, and the potential for loss of function and suicide.

We will focus in this chapter on the pharmacological treatments for major depressive disorder (MDD), while also reviewing somatic treatments, psychotherapies, and natural remedies with proven efficacy in MDD. We will also focus on strategies to use these treatments, alone or in combination, in MDD patients. Finally we will review treatment of depression in special populations such as melancholic, atypical depression, bipolar depression, or psychotic depression.

PHARMACOLOGICAL TREATMENTS (THE ANTIDEPRESSANTS)

Most antidepressants currently available have mechanisms of action involving monoaminergic neurotransmitters. A useful classification is based on their known receptor affinities, despite the fact that significant chemical structural diversity may be present within each class, which in turn may explain significant differences in pharmacokinetics, metabolism, tolerability, or toxicity (see Table 38.1). We will discuss separately major classes of antidepressants (e.g., TCAs, MAOIs, SSRIs, SNRIs), and specific antidepressants not fitting into these classes (e.g., bupropion, mirtazapine). We will then discuss strategies to address treatment non-response, including combinations of antidepressants and other medications used to augment antidepressants (such as lithium, thyroid hormones, atypical antipsychotics).

TRICYCLIC ANTIDEPRESSANTS

Tricyclic antidepressants (TCAs) have been in use for more than 50 years. They are named after their core chemical structure consisting of three rings (two joined benzene rings). The initial TCA, imipramine, with a chemical structure similar to phenothiazines, was discovered in the 1950s and found to be associated with robust clinical improvements in depressed subjects (Kuhn, 1958). The class includes tertiary amine TCAs, which inhibit the reuptake of both norepinephrine and serotonin (members of this class include amitriptyline [Elavil], imipramine [Tofranil], trimipramine [Surmontil], clomipramine [Anafranil], doxepin [Sinequan]), and their demethylated secondary amine derivatives TCAs, with more selective norepinephrine reuptake inhibition (nortriptyline [Pamelor], desipramine [Norpramin], protriptyline [Vivactil], amoxapine [Ascendin]). In addition, maprolitine (Ludiomil) is classified as a tetracyclic.

With the exception of clomipramine, where serotonin reuptake inhibition predominates, all other TCAs inhibit the reuptake of norepinephrine more potently than the reuptake of serotonin (Richelson, 2003). TCAs are also active at multiple other monoamine receptors: to varying degrees TCAs also block histamine H-1 receptors, serotonin 5-HT2 receptors, muscarinic acetylcholine receptors, and α-1 adrenergic receptors (Richelson and Nelson, 1984). This explains their side-effect profile, as described later, and may also explain potential secondary mechanisms of antidepressant effect. Amoxapine is also a dopamine D2 receptor antagonist (which confers both antipsychotic properties and a risk of extrapyramidal side effects (Richelson, 2003).

Although TCAs are generally as effective as the more modern selective serotonin reuptake inhibitors (SSRIs) for depression (Anderson, 2000) and some evidence favors the use of TCAs in severe melancholic depression (Perry, 1996), they are rarely used as first-line treatments due to their inferior side-effect and safety profile in comparison with newer antidepressants. In addition, TCAs have a more established track record than SSRIs in treating a variety of chronic pain conditions, including neuropathies, fibromyalgia, and migraine (Sindrup et al., 2005).

Typical TCA antidepressant doses are 100–300 mg/day (nortriptyline and protriptyline require lower doses). TCA treatment should be initiated with lower doses (e.g., 10 mg/day for imipramine) due to poor tolerability at higher doses. The relationship between serum levels and clinical response varies: while desipramine was reported to have a linear relationship between increasing levels and effectiveness, most other TCAs appear to exhibit an inverse "U" shaped curve, with decreasing efficacy at blood levels above therapeutic range (Perry et al., 1994). Blood levels may be useful in establishing compliance, higher than usual dose requirements (as in chronic smokers), or toxicity due to overdose or drug interactions.

The adverse effect profile of TCAs accounts for the high dropout rate (30–70%) in published studies. Blockade of

TABLE 38.1. Antidepressant blockade of several monoamine transporters and receptors in the human brain. Potency (affinity) data is expressed as the inverse of the equilibrium dissociation constant K_d, multiplied by 10^{-7}. (Data are adapted from Richelson, 2003.)

ANTIDEPRESSANT	SEROTONIN TRANSPORTER INHIBITION	NOREPINEPHRINE TRANSPORTER INHIBITION	SELECTIVITY OF SEROTONIN/ NOREPINEPHRINE UPTAKE BLOCKADE	DOPAMINE TRANSPORTER INHIBITION	ALPHA 1-ADRENORECEPTOR BLOCKADE	DOPAMINE D2 RECEPTOR BLOCKADE	HISTAMINE H1 RECEPTOR BLOCKADE	MUSCARINIC RECEPTOR BLOCKADE	SEROTONIN 5HT-2A RECEPTOR BLOCKADE
Paroxetine	800	2.5	320	0.2	0.029	0.0031	0.0045	0.93	0.0053
Fluoxetine	120	0.41	300	0.028	0.017	0.0083	0.016	0.05	0.48
Sertraline	340	0.24	1400	4	0.27	0.0094	0.0041	0.16	0.01
Fluvoxamine	45	0.077	580	0.011	0.013	0	0.00092	0.0042	0.018
Citalopram	90	0.025	3500	0.0036	0.053	0	0.21	0.045	0.042
Clomipramine	360	2.7	140	0.045	2.6	0.53	3.2	2.7	3.7
Imipramine	70	2.7	27	0.012	1.1	0.05	9.1	1.1	1.2
Amitriptyline	23	2.9	8	0.031	3.7	0.1	91	5.6	3.4
Desipramine	5.7	120	0.05	0.031	0.77	0.0303	0.91	0.5	0.36
Amoxapine	1.7	6.2	0.27	0.023	2	5.6	4	0.1	97
Doxepin	1.5	3.4	0.43	0.0082	4.2	0.042	420	1.2	4
Venlafaxine	11	0.094	120	0.011	0	0	0	0	0
Reboxetine	1.7	14	0.12		0.0084	0.025	0.32	0.015	0.016
Nefazodone	0.5	0.28	2	0.28	3.9	0.11	4.7	0.0091	30
Mirtazipine	0.001	0.021	0.05	0.001	0.02	0.01	700	0.15	6.1
Buproprion	0.011	0.0019	5.8	0.19	0.022	0	0.015	0.0021	0.0011

muscarinic acetylcholine receptors causes dry mouth, blurred vision, constipation, urinary hesitancy, tachycardia, and ejaculatory difficulties. Secondary amine TCAs tend to cause fewer anticholinergic effects than tertiary amine TCAs. TCAs should be avoided in patients with narrow angle glaucoma and prostatic hypertrophy as symptoms related to these conditions may worsen because of anticholinergic effects. Blockade of histamine H-1 receptors may cause sedation, carbohydrate craving, and weight gain. Weight gain with TCAs can be substantial, averaging 1–3 lb per month of treatment. Secondary amine TCAs tend to cause less sedation than tertiary amine TCAs. Alpha-1 adrenergic receptor antagonism may lead to orthostatic hypotension, which can be severe. Nortriptyline is generally thought to be less likely to cause orthostatic hypotension than tertiary amine TCAs. TCAs can block sodium and potassium channels, which can lead to arrhythmogenic and epileptogenic effects, especially in overdose. Cardiac toxicity may occur in susceptible individuals and following TCA overdose. TCAs should be avoided in patients with bifascicular heart block, left bundle branch block, or a prolonged QT interval. TCAs also decrease heart rate variability, which is a risk factor for cardiovascular disease. Baseline and follow-up electrocardiograms should be monitored, especially in older patients or those with cardiac conduction disorders, as well as in pediatric patients.

TCAs have a low threshold for toxicity; overdose of even a one-week supply may be lethal. Due to the lethality after overdose, it may be safer to treat acutely suicidal depressed patients with non-TCA antidepressants or to prescribe limited quantities of TCAs. Cytochrome P450 2D6 inhibitors (such as certain SSRIs) can lead to potentially dangerous increases in TCA blood levels. Manifestations of anticholinergic toxicity may include dilated pupils, blurred vision, dry skin, hyperpyrexia, ileus, urinary retention, confusion, delirium, and seizures. Additionally, arrhythmias, hypotension, and coma may develop. Although TCAs are highly plasma-bound and are not removed by hemodialysis, they are metabolized by hepatic microsomal enzymes. Patients who have overdosed on TCAs may require alkalinization of their serum, pressors, or ventilatory support to maintain survival.

While no longer used as first-line treatment for depression due to their unfavorable side-effect and safety profile, TCAs are effective antidepressants and are commonly used in patients with chronic pain (Sindrup et al., 2005).

MONOAMINE OXIDASE INHIBITORS (MAOIS)

MAOIs act by inhibiting the monoamine oxidase (MAO), an enzyme found on the outer membrane of cellular mitochondria, where it catabolizes intracellular monoamines, including the CNS monoamines: dopamine, norepinephrine, serotonin, and tyramine. In the GI tract and the liver, MAO catabolizes dietary pressor amines, such as dopamine, tyramine, tryptamine, and phenylethylamine. MAO has two forms (MAO-A and MAO-B), with differences in substrate preference, inhibitor specificity, and tissue distribution. MAO-A, which preferentially oxidizes norepinephrine and serotonin, appears in positron emission tomography (PET) studies to be elevated in multiple brain areas in MDD subjects (Meyer et al., 2009), and was considered the therapeutic target of MAOIs in depression.

Older MAOIs such as phenelzine (Nardil), tranylcypromine (Parnate), and isocarboxazid (Marplan), are irreversible inhibitors of both MAO-A and MAO-B. Their chemical structures relate either to the hydrazine class (phenelzine and isocarbaxid) or are related to CNS stimulants (tranylcypromine). Moclobemide is a selective and reversible inhibitor of MAO-A available in Europe. The antiparkinsonian agent, selegiline (Eldepryl), is a more selective MAO-B inhibitor, particularly at low doses (<10 mg/day), but is not effective as an antidepressant at those doses. A newer formulation of transdermal selegiline was shown to minimize the inhibition of MAO-A in the GI tract (30% inhibition) at doses producing maximal MAO-A and MOA-B inhibition in the brain (Wecker et al., 2003). Transdermal selegiline (EmSam) is an effective antidepressant and relatively safer than other orally available MAOIs.

The overall efficacy of MAOIs appears to not differ from that of other antidepressant classes such as SSRIs (Papakostas and Fava, 2006) or TCAs (Thase et al., 1995). In atypical depression (characterized by mood reactivity plus hypersomnia, hyperphagia, extreme fatigue when depressed, and/or rejection sensitivity), MAOIs do appear to be more effective than TCAs (Thase et al., 1995), but it is unclear whether they are more effective than SSRIs.

The older MAOIs are rarely used in clinical practice due to their adverse effects profile (orthostatic hypotension, weight gain, and sexual dysfunction), particularly the need for dietary restrictions (to prevent hypertensive crisis), potentially fatal drug interactions (due to the interaction with sympathomimetic drugs or serotonergic drugs), and toxicity in overdose. Currently the MAOIs are used in individuals with treatment resistant depression, after successive treatment failures with more recent antidepressants.

The most common side effects include postural hypotension, insomnia, agitation, sedation, impotence, delayed ejaculation, or anorgasmia. Others include weight change, dry mouth, constipation, and urinary hesitancy. Peripheral neuropathies have been reported and may be avoided by concomitant therapy with vitamin B6.

When patients on MAOIs ingest dietary amines, rather than being catabolized in the intestines and the liver they are taken up in sympathetic nerve terminals and may cause the release of endogenous catecholamines with resulting adrenergic crises. This is characterized by hypertension, hyperpyrexia, and other adrenergic symptoms such as tachycardia, tremulousness, and cardiac arrhythmias. The amine most commonly associated with these symptoms is tyramine, but others, such as phenylethylalamine and dopamine may be involved. Dietary amines can be avoided by adherence to dietary restrictions and avoiding tyramine-containing foods. The diet must be strictly followed. Patients must be instructed to avoid all matured or aged cheese, fermented or dried meats, such as pepperoni and salami, fava and broad bean pods (not the beans themselves), tap beers, marmite yeast extract, sauerkraut, soy sauce and other soy products, such as tofu and tempe. All meats and cheese must be fresh and must have been stored and refrigerated or frozen properly. Up to two bottles of beer or glasses of wine may be consumed safely; this restriction includes non-alcoholic beers (Walker et al., 1996).

Since endogenous MAO activity does not return to baseline immediately upon MAOI discontinuation, two weeks should transpire before discontinuing the MAOI diet after MAOI discontinuation, or before beginning a contraindicated medication.

Reversible MAOIs such as moclobemide were pursued as a safer alternative to older MAOIs with a lower risk for hypertensive crises, but their antidepressant efficacy was not superior to SSRIs (Papakostas and Fava, 2006). Transdermal selegiline is associated with a lower risk for hypertensive crises although the FDA requires a tyramine-free diet at the higher doses of the patch.

SELECTIVE SEROTONIN REUPTAKE INHIBITORS

Inhibition of the reuptake of serotonin at neuronal synaptic clefts is the immediate mechanism of selective serotonin reuptake inhibitors (SSRIs), which occurs within hours of initiation of SSRI treatment. SSRIs also have effects at other monoamine receptors (such as norepinephrine and dopamine), but their affinity is one to two orders of magnitude higher for the serotonin transporter (Table 38.1) (Richelson, 2003). By blocking serotonin reuptake SSRIs increase the amount of available serotonin in the synaptic cleft, stimulating a large number of serotonin receptors subtypes. However, the immediate effect on serotonin receptors cannot account by itself for antidepressant efficacy; the typical time to clinical improvement in depression for all antidepressant medications, including the SSRIs, is four to eight weeks.

More than 60 double blind placebo-controlled studies support the efficacy of SSRIs in MDD (Papakostas et al., 2006). Available SSRIs include fluoxetine, paroxetine, sertraline, fluvoxamine (in the United States only approved for OCD), citalopram, and escitalopram (the *S*-enantiomer of citalopram). Vilazodone, approved by the FDA in 2011, is a serotonin reuptake inhibitor and a partial agonist of the 5-HT1A receptor. The common dosage regimens of SSRIs are presented in Table 38.2. Although dose-response curves have not been definitively established for the SSRIs, some patients who do not respond at a lower dose may benefit by having their dosage increased. SSRIs are hepatically metabolized and renally excreted; therefore, dose adjustments may be required in patients with reduced liver or renal function.

For reasons of tolerability and their relatively benign side-effect profile (as discussed later), the SSRIs have become the first-line treatment for depressive disorder spectrum illnesses, ranging from dysthymia to major depression. SSRIs are very rarely associated with fatalities even in the presence of large overdoses, unless they are combined with other agents. Several SSRIs may be relatively safe during pregnancy; fluoxetine and sertraline have a larger number of observational studies confirming low rates of fetal malformations or complications, while paroxetine has been associated with an increased risk of congenital heart malformations (Patil et al., 2011). Advantages of SSRIs include a favorable side-effect profile, a broad spectrum of efficacy for comorbid disorders, a low potential for abuse and dependence, safety in overdose, and single daily dosing (with the exception of fluvoxamine).

Disadvantages of SSRIs include side effects and drug–drug interactions by inhibiting the activity of cytochrome P450 isoenzymes. The most common side effects of SSRIs are increased anxiety or "jitteriness" on initial dosing, headaches, agitation, insomnia, nausea (which tends to be worst during early treatment), diarrhea, reduced appetite, weight loss or gain, excessive sweating, headache, insomnia, sedation, dizziness, and sexual dysfunction—including decreased libido, delayed ejaculation, impotence, and anorgasmia. Other side effects include rash, dry mouth, and prolonged bleeding time. SSRIs have been associated with an increased risk of treatment-emergent suicidal ideation in children, adolescents, and young adults (under the age of 25), a side effect shared with other classes of antidepressants.

All currently available SSRIs appear to be equally efficacious for depression. The most significant differences between molecules in this family involve their half-lives and interactions with the cytochrome P 450 isoenzymes. Half-lives vary greatly among the SSRIs. Although an antidepressant's half-life is not relevant to its treatment efficacy or its onset of action, it may be significant in terms of its side effects, its interactions with other agents, and its discontinuation-emergent symptoms. Medications with shorter half-lives may be useful when abrupt discontinuation is desired due to intolerable side effects or to medication interactions, however medications with shorter half-lives are more likely to cause the discontinuation-emergent symptoms (e.g., tachycardia, flu-like symptoms, dizziness, myalgias, anxiety, irritability, worsening of mood, jitteriness, and nausea). An SSRI with a longer half-life is more likely to "self-taper," and may be beneficial for a patient who is apt to miss occasional dosages. Fluoxetine has the longest half-life (two days, while its active metabolite norfluoxetine has a half-life of 7–10 days). Fluoxetine is dosed daily, but due to its long half-life a once-weekly formulation of this drug is also available. Fluvoxamine has the shortest half-life (16 hours) and is the only SSRI requiring twice daily dosing.

Drug interactions: In rare cases, a serotonin syndrome can also occur when SSRIs are combined with monoamine oxidase inhibitors or with relatively serotonergic agents. More commonly, SSRIs may inhibit cytochrome P450 isoenzymes (Manolopoulos et al., 2012). Cytochrome P-450 isoenzymes, including the isoenzymes 1A2, 2C, 2D6, 3A3/4, are a family of heme-thiolate proteins located on microsomal membranes throughout the body. Their mechanism is best known in the liver and bowel wall, where they oxidatively metabolize medications as well as prostaglandins, fatty acids, and steroids. Alteration in function of these isoenzymes may cause clinically significant pharmacokinetic drug-drug interactions, via changes in drug levels. CYP450 2D6 inhibition by several SSRI antidepressants (primarily fluoxetine and paroxetine, but also clinically relevant for sertraline) and by buproprion may lead to increased levels of TCAs, beta-blockers, antiarrhythmics, and several narcotic analgesics (codeine, hydroxycodone, oxycodone, tramadol, dextromethorphan), which are all substrates for this enzyme. Also a potential consequence is inhibition of

TABLE 38.2. Overview of antidepressants used in the United States

PHARMACOLOGIC CLASS	EXAMPLES	DAILY DOSE RANGE (mg)	DOSING SCHEDULE	STARTING DOSE	HALF-LIFE (h)	COMMON ADVERSE EFFECTS	SERIOUS ADVERSE EFFECTS	PREGNANCY CATEGORY
SSRI	Escitalopram (Lexapro)	10–20	q.d.	10	27–32	Class effects: nausea, diarrhea, headache, insomnia, somnolence, sexual dysfunction, weight gain	Class effects: bleeding, seizure, serotonin syndrome, worsening depression or anxiety, suicidal thoughts	C
	Citalopram (Celexa)	20–60	q.d.	10	35			C
	Fluoxetine (Prozac)	10–80	q.d.	10	87			C
	Fluvoxamine (Luvox)*	50–300	q.d.	25	16			C
	Paroxetine (Paxil)	20–50	q.d.	10	21			D
	Sertraline (Zoloft)	50–200	q.d.	25	26			C
	Vilazodone (Viibryd)	20–40	q.d.	10	20			C
SNRI	Venlafaxine (Effexor XR)	75–225	q.d.	37.5	3.6	Class effects: nausea, headache, dry mouth, diarrhea, constipation, dizziness, tremor, sweating, hypertension, blurred vision, sexual dysfunction, tachycardia, hyperlipidemia, urinary hesitancy, orthostatic syncope	Class effects: seizure, serotonin syndrome, suicidal thoughts, bleeding, hyponatremia, glaucoma, hypertension, hepatotoxicity (duloxetine), hyperglycemia	C
	Desvenlafaxine (Pristiq)	50–100	q.d.	50	11			C
	Milnacipran (Savella)*	50–200	b.i.d.	12.5	6–8			C
	Duloxetine (Cymbalta)	60–120	q.d.	60	12			C
TCA	Clomipramine (Anafranil)	25–250	q.d.—b.i.d.	12.5–25	32	Class effects: dry mouth, constipation, urinary retention, somnolence, dizziness, weight gain, sexual dysfunction, orthostasis	Class effects: can be lethal in overdose, cardiac arrhythmia, hematological abnormalities, suicidal thoughts	C
	Doxepine (Sinequan)	75–300	q.d.—b.i.d.	10–25	15			C
	Imipramine (Tofranil)	100–200	q.d.—b.i.d.	10–25	6–18			C
	Maprotiline (Ludiomil)	40–150	q.d.—b.i.d.	10–25	30			B
	Nortriptyline (Pamelor)	15–60	q.d.—b.i.d.	12.5–25	74			D
	Protriptyline (Vivactil)	75–300	q.d.—b.i.d.	5–10	24			C
	Trimipramine (Surmontil)	100–200	q.d.—b.i.d.	10–25	16–40			C
	Desipramine (Norpramin)	75–300	q.d.—b.i.d.	10–25	17			C

(continued)

TABLE 38.2. (*Continued*)

PHARMACOLOGIC CLASS	EXAMPLES	DAILY DOSE RANGE (mg)	DOSING SCHEDULE	STARTING DOSE	HALF-LIFE (h)	COMMON ADVERSE EFFECTS	SERIOUS ADVERSE EFFECTS	PREGNANCY CATEGORY
	Maprotiline (Ludiomil)	40–150	q.d.—b.i.d.	10–25	30			B
	Amoxapine (Asendin)	75–300	q.d.—b.i.d.	10–25	8–30			C
MAOI	Phenelzine (Nardil)	45–90	t.i.d.	15	3	Class effects: dry mouth, constipation, orthostasis, weight gain, sexual dysfunction, somnolence, dizziness, headache	Class effects: can be lethal in overdose, cardiac arrhythmia, hypertensive crisis, myocardial infarction	C
	Tranylcypromine (Parnate)	30–60	b.i.d.	10	3			C
	Isocarboxazid (Marplan)	20–60	bid-qid	10	?			C
	Moclobemide *	300–600	t.i.d.	300	2			C
	Selegiline transdermal (Emsam)	6–12	q.d.	6	1.5			C
Atypical antidepressants	Nefazadone (Serzone)	300–600	b.i.d.	100	3	Somnolence, dizziness, Dry mouth, Nausea, Constipation, Headache, Blurred vision	Hepatotoxicity	C
	Buproprion (Wellbutrin SR, XL)	200–400	b.i.d.	150	12	Agitation, Insomnia, Weight loss, Dry mouth, Headache, Constipation, Tremor	Increased seizure risk	C
	Mirtazapine (Remeron)	30–45	q.d.	15	30	Somnolence, Weight gain, Dizziness, Dry mouth, Constipation, Orthostatic Hypotension		C
	Trazodone (Desyrel)	150–400	q.d.	150	4–9	Sedation, Orthostatic Hypotension, Dizziness, Headache, Dry mouth	Priapism, Arrhythmias	C

* Not FDA approved for the treatment of depression

the conversion of codeine to its active form (morphine) with subsequent reduction of its efficacy. CYP450 3A4 inhibition by fluvoxamine (and the non-SSRI nefazodone) has potential consequences in increased levels of numerous commonly prescribed substrates including carbamazepine, cyclosporine, alprazolam, midazolam, zolpidem, zaleplon, calcium channel blockers, statins, sildenafil, oral contraceptives, and pimozide (arrhythmia risk). CYP450 1A2 inhibition by fluvoxamine may lead to toxicity on clozapine, theophylline, and other 1A2 substrates. CYP450 2C inhibition by fluoxetine, fluvoxamine, or sertraline has a potential for increased levels of anticoagulant (warfarin) and diazepam.

TRAZODONE AND NEFAZODONE

The phenylpiperazine nefazodone and the triazolopyride trazodone are 5-HT$_2$ antagonists. Both inhibit serotonin 5-HT$_{2A}$ receptors; they are also weak inhibitors of serotonin reuptake. Inhibition of postsynaptic 5-HT$_{2A}$ receptors has a synergistic effect with serotonin reuptake inhibition (explaining the antidepressant effects of these molecules as monotherapy and in combination with SSRIs). Trazodone may also act as a serotonin agonist through an active metabolite and it is an antagonist of alpha-1 adrenergic receptors (associated with side effects).

Their antidepressant efficacy appears similar to that of SSRIs in a meta-analysis (Papakostas and Fava, 2007). Usual effective doses for both are 200–600 mg/day. The FDA approved an extended-release version of trazodone in 2010. Both medications have sedative properties and improve sleep continuity (5-HT-2 receptor blockers increase slow-wave sleep). Adrenergic effects of trazodone are associated with orthostatic hypotension. Priapism is a rare side effect of trazodone that requires immediate medical attention. Trazodone may also induce arrhythmias in those with preexisting heart disease. Nefazodone has fewer side effects than trazodone due to lower alpha-1 blockade. It is less likely to cause sexual dysfunction than SSRIs or TCAs, and is less anticholinergic and histaminergic. Common side effects include somnolence, dizziness, dry mouth, nausea, constipation, headache, and amblyopia and blurred vision. Nefazodone has been associated with rare but fatal hepatotoxicity, but remains an effective treatment for depression associated with anxiety.

MIRTAZAPINE (REMERON)

Mirtazapine has a tetracyclic chemical structure (unrelated to the TCAs). It is an antagonist at inhibitory alpha-2 adrenergic auto- and hetero-receptors, leading to increased release of both serotonin and norepinephrine at the synaptic level and increased tonic activation of postsynaptic 5-HT receptors. Mirtazapine also blocks 5HT2 and 5HT3 receptors, it is also a relatively potent histaminergic H-1 receptor antagonist. It does not have significant affinity for cholinergic or postsynaptic adrenergic receptors. Its antidepressant efficacy is comparable with that of SSRIs in a meta-analysis of head-to-head studies (Pakakostas et al., 2008b). Histaminergic receptor antagonism may be related to common side effects including somnolence, weight gain, dizziness, dry mouth, and constipation. Weight gain can be significantly larger compared to other antidepressants. Due to blockade of 5HT2 and 5HT3 receptors, mirtazapine may reduce SSRI-related sexual dysfunction and nausea when administered concomitantly. The drug appears to have no known cardiac toxicity and to be relatively safe in overdose. Mirtazapine is an effective antidepressant, particularly useful in subjects where its effects on increasing sleep and increasing appetite are desirable; it is also preferable due to reduced rate of sexual side effects.

BUPROPION (WELLBUTRIN, WELLBUTRIN SR, XL)

The mechanism of action of bupropion has not been fully elucidated, although it appears to block the reuptake of both dopamine and norepinephrine. Bupropion inhibits the striatal uptake of the selective dopamine transporter (DAT)–binding radioligand (Meyer et al., 2002), but the lack of decrease in cerebrospinal fluid (CSF) levels of homovanilic acid (the primary dopamine metabolite) suggests the activity of bupropion is not primarily related to dopamine reuptake inhibition. Bupropion also has weak affinity for the norepinephrine transporter and increases presynaptic norepinephrine release

(Dong and Blier, 2001). The overall effect appears to be related to an increase in the brain extracellular dopamine and norepinephrine concentrations. Clinically, bupropion has sympathomimetic, stimulant-like effects.

Buproprion appears to be as effective as SSRIs in the treatment of depression (Thase et al., 2005). Its stimulant-like effects suggest it is more effective than SSRIs in treating fatigue associated with depression, while SSRIs appear more effective than bupropion in the treatment of anxious depression. Clinical efficacy was also demonstrated for seasonal affective disorder.

Effective doses range between 200 and 450 mg/day. Common side effects include agitation, insomnia, weight loss, dry mouth, headache, constipation, and tremor. Doses below 450 mg/day are associated with a rate of seizures of 0.4% for its immediate release form and lower for sustained release preparations. However, the risk of seizure markedly increases (2.4%) at doses > 450 mg/day and > 200 mg/dose. Bupropion may be more likely to induce seizures in patients with bulimia nervosa and histories of head trauma. It is generally safe in overdose, though fatalities have been reported. Bupropion is usually safe for patients with cardiac disease, although it may participate in drug interactions. It rarely induces sexual dysfunction and can even be beneficial as an adjunct in SSRI-induced sexual dysfunction. Bupropion is particularly useful for depressed subjects benefiting from its energizing effects (decreasing fatigue, increasing concentration) or from its reduced rate of sexual side effects.

SELECTIVE SEROTONIN NOREPINEPHRINE REUPTAKE INHIBITORS

Selective serotonin norepinephrine reuptake inhibitors (SNRIs) are potent reuptake inhibitors of both serotonin and norepinephrine, neurotransmitters associated with important symptom domains involved in MDD. While this is a simplification, norepinephrine may be related to energy, alertness, attention, and interest, while serotonin to anxiety, obsessions, and compulsions (Nutt, 2008). The SNRI group includes venlafaxine, desvenlafaxine, duloxetine, and milnacipran. Venlafaxine (Effexor, Effexor XR) is a phenylethylamine; it inhibits both serotonin and norepinephrine reuptake at doses above 150 mg, while lower doses only have a clinically significant inhibitory effect on serotonin reuptake. It has very low affinity for histaminergic, cholinergic, and adrenergic receptors. Desvenlafaxine, the major metabolite of venlafaxine, is a more potent reuptake inhibitor of norepinephrine. Duloxetine is a relatively more potent norepinephrine reuptake inhibitor than venlafaxine; it has little affinity for cholinergic or histaminergic receptors. Milnacipran has the highest relative norepinephrine reuptake inhibition in the class. Milnacipran is only approved by the FDA for the treatment of fibromyalgia but is available as an antidepressant in Europe.

Venlafaxine and desvenlafaxine are only 30% protein bound and thus have low likelihood of displacing tightly bound drugs, such as warfarin and phenytoin. Also, both venlafaxine and desvenlafaxine are not potent inhibitors of any cytochrome P450 hepatic enzymes, which results in low risk for pharmacokinetic drug interactions. Desvenlafaxine is also not a substrate for CYP 2D6; therefore it is not subject to drug-drug interactions (its metabolism is not affected by inhibitors or inducers of CYP2D6). Similar to desvenlafaxine, milnacipran undergoes very little hepatic metabolism.

Several meta-analyses have suggested that in aggregate SNRIs are associated with higher rates of remission compared to SSRIs, but the difference appears modest or insignificant from a clinical perspective (Machado and Einarson, 2010). An earlier meta-analysis using the number needed to treat (NNT) statistic suggests nearly 24 patients would need to be treated with SNRIs instead of SSRIs in order to obtain one additional responder (well short of the NNT = 10 suggested as a mark of significant clinical difference between alternate therapies) (Papakostas et al., 2007c). The dual effects of venlafaxine on serotonin and norepinephrine have been used to explain the small increase in remission rates compared to SSRIs (Nemeroff et al., 2008). Duloxetine was shown to be additionally efficacious in the treatment of painful symptoms associated with depression. The dual effect on serotonin and norepinephrine is associated, just as in the case of TCAs, with SNRI efficacy in chronic pain conditions; both duloxetine and milnacipran are effective in the treatment of fibromyalgia.

As a class the SNRIs share many of their side effects. Similar with SSRIs, SNRIs are associated with GI side effects (nausea, diarrhea), insomnia, sedation, sexual dysfunction, headaches, sweating, tremors, dizziness, and weight gain. In contrast to SSRIs, the noradrenergic effects of SNRIs are associated with treatment-emergent hypertension (which is more prominent with venlafaxine and at higher doses), palpitations, and tachycardia. The more potent noradrenergic effects of duloxetine and milnacipran are also associated with dry mouth, constipation, and urinary retention. Abrupt discontinuation of any SNRI may result in withdrawal-related adverse events similar to SSRIs, but the syndrome is most intense with venlafaxine. Hepatotoxicity has been reported with duloxetine and with milnacipran.

As a group of efficacious and relatively well-tolerated antidepressants, SNRIs are frequently used in patients having failed treatment with an SSRI, or even as first-line treatments.

NOREPINEPHRINE REUPTAKE INHIBITORS

Norepinephrine reuptake inhibitors (NRIs) have primary activity by inhibiting the transport (as in the case of reboxetine) or the reuptake of norepinephrine (e.g., atomoxetine). Reboxetine also increases prefrontal cortex dopamine activity. Reboxetine is available as an antidepressant in Europe but not in the United States; its overall antidepressant efficacy appears similar to SSRIs in a meta-analysis (Papakostas et al., 2008a), although in the US phase III trials reboxetine did not separate from placebo. Atomoxetine (Strattera), which is FDA approved for the treatment of attention deficit disorder, has minimal data supporting efficacy in MDD. Both medications share side effects related to noradrenergic effects: dry mouth, nausea, sedation, urinary hesitancy, and tachycardia. At this point the majority of available data appears to favor SSRIs versus NRIs in the treatment of depression.

AGOMELATINE

Agomelatine is an antidepressant with a novel mechanism of action, with melatonin MT1 and MT2 agonist and serotonin 5-HT2C antagonist effects. The 5-HT2C effects appear to be related to increase in prefrontal dopaminergic and noradrenergic activity. Its melatonergic effects appear to be related to improved sleep quality, with no reported daytime drowsiness. It appears to have no affinity for adrenergic, histaminergic, cholinergic, dopaminergic, or other serotonergic receptors. In European studies agomelatine was found to be effective in the treatment of MDD; three out of six placebo-controlled trials have supported the short-term efficacy of agomelatine in MDD. Other studies have shown agomelatine to be as effective as the SSRI paroxetine or the SNRI venlafaxine (Carney and Shelton, 2011). Agomelatine is marketed as an antidepressant in Europe since 2009. Its development in the United States was discontinued in 2011. The phase III US trials provided inconsistent results: in one study the 25 mg dose but not the 50 mg separated from placebo, while in the other study only the 50 mg dose achieved efficacy (Stahl et al., 2010). Agomelatine has a favorable side-effect profile but has been associated with elevated liver transaminases in up to 4% of subjects.

ANTIDEPRESSANT STRATEGIES FOR TREATMENT-RESISTANT DEPRESSION

Given the large variety of available antidepressants and the lack of overwhelming evidence of superior efficacy for any one class, the choice of an initial antidepressant treatment is primarily related to tolerability, safety, and economic factors (cost, insurance formulary). Although many patients with MDD achieve clinical response (defined as 50% improvement of symptoms) to their initial antidepressant treatment, one third to one half of depressed patients fail to respond to antidepressant treatments of adequate dose and duration (Rush et al., 2006a). Treatment-resistant depression (TRD) is generally defined as lack of adequate improvement after two antidepressant treatments used at adequate doses (see Table 38.2) and duration (minimum six weeks). Remission (defined as resolution of symptoms) is an even more important goal; it is associated with improved long-term outcomes and lower relapse rates. The initial evaluation of a subject with TRD should start with a reevaluation of the diagnosis and comorbid illnesses. Bipolar depression would require different pharmacological approaches, as outlined later in this chapter. The presence of comorbid medical (e.g., cardiovascular, diabetes, etc.) and psychiatric illness (e.g., substance abuse, psychosis) has been associated with increased levels of treatment resistance; such comorbidities need to be treated to improve clinical outcomes. Patients who have already failed to respond to two treatments (TRD) experience very low (10–20%) remission rates with their next treatments (defined as near complete resolution of symptoms); for this group of patients there is no single pharmacotherapy showing significant superiority (Rush et al., 2006b, 2009).

Common pharmacological strategies for TRD include antidepressant dose increases/optimization, switches to other antidepressants, combinations of antidepressants, and augmentation of antidepressants with other pharmacological agents. Non-pharmacological strategies include switch or combination treatment with ECT, TMS, or psychotherapy, as discussed later in this chapter. Gradual **dose increases/optimization** to the maximum FDA-recommended doses can be efficacious especially in subjects responding partially to the initial treatment. A **switch to another antidepressant** after the first therapy has been proven ineffective (with discontinuation of the first treatment) has the advantage of maintaining the lower side effect profile associated with monotherapy. The switch can be to another antidepressant in the same class or to a different class. A switch to the same class may be associated with rates of response and remission similar to out of class switches after a single antidepressant failure in the class. In STAR*D Level 2 subjects failing to improve after 12 weeks with the SSRI citalopram had near-identical response rates after switching to the SSRI sertraline compared to switching to the SNRI venlafaxine or to bupropion (Rush et al., 2006b). However, rates of response tend to be lower after failing two antidepressants in the same class, which justifies at that point switching to a different antidepressant class. The disadvantage of switching involves the loss of any benefits of the initial antidepressant treatment; clinical improvement would typically occur only after an adequate duration of treatment with the new antidepressant.

Combination therapy involves the addition of a second antidepressant; the advantages are related to potential pharmacological synergy in mechanisms of action (which may translate in clinical efficacy) and not losing partial benefits associated with the first treatment. The disadvantages relate to an increased side-effect profile (combining side effects of both agents). Commonly used pharmacological combinations are SSRI/SNRI plus bupropion, SNRI/SNRI plus mirtazapine, SSRI plus TCA, and SSRI plus NRI (e.g., reboxetine). While each of these strategies has been associated with adequate rates of success in some studies, a recent study comparing the efficacy of escitalopram monotherapy to the combinations of escitalopram plus bupropion or venlafaxine plus mirtazapine reported no significant differences in the acute (12 weeks) or the longer term (7 months) outcomes (Rush et al., 2011).

Augmentation therapy involves the addition of pharmacological agents (with no proven antidepressant properties as monotherapy) to boost the antidepressant response. Effective augmenting agents include lithium, thyroid hormones, atypical antipsychotics, agents with serotonin 1A activity, and hormonal strategies.

Lithium augmentation was initially proposed after the observation of rapid antidepressant effects after the addition of lithium to TCAs. A meta-analysis of the older studies involving lithium augmentation of TCAs suggested lithium was more efficacious than placebo (Bauer and Dopfmer, 1999), but only 3 studies (with 110 subjects) were determined to involve adequate lithium doses, and lithium effects were assessed after only 2 weeks. More recently, STAR*D level 3 compared lithium or T3 augmentation of antidepressants (sertraline, venlafaxine, or bupropion); numerically lower remission rates were reported for lithium (15.9%) compared to T3 augmentation (24.7%), but the difference was not statistically significant (Nierenberg et al., 2006). Therefore the evidence for the efficacy of lithium as an augmentation is not conclusive. Lithium augmentation of TCAs remains a validated strategy. Adjunctive lithium may be associated with side effects such as tremor, somnolence, sedation, gastrointestinal symptoms (nausea, anorexia, abdominal pain, diarrhea), polyuria, edema, hypothyroidism, weight gain, and cardiac conduction abnormalities.

Atypical antipsychotics are the most extensively researched augmentation strategy in TRD. Given the receptor affinities of atypical antipsychotics, augmentation of SSRIs may increase levels of norepinephrine and/or dopamine in the prefrontal cortex, leading to improved antidepressant response. Randomized controlled studies have been reported with olanzapine, risperidone, quetiapine, and aripiprazole; a meta-analysis of 10 of these studies reported higher response and remission rates among patients who received augmentation with atypical antipsychotics compared to antidepressant monotherapy (Papakostas et al., 2007b). The rate of discontinuation for side effects was 3.5 times higher for patients treated with atypical antipsychotics. Currently three atypical antipsychotics have received FDA approval as augmentation treatments in TRD (aripiprazole, quetiapine XR, and the combination of olanzapine plus fluoxetine). Despite proven efficacy atypical antipsychotic augmentation should be considered in the context of the significant side effect burden of this class of medications, which includes sedation, somnolence, nausea, hyperprolactinemia, dyslipidemia, glucose dysregulation, weight gain, extrapyramidal side effects, neuroleptic malignant syndrome, and tardive dyskinesia.

Selective 5HT1A agonists: initial clinical reports of augmentation of SSRIs with clomipramine or buspirone have led to theories suggesting that increased postsynaptic 5HT1A activity and desensitization of presynaptic 5HT1A autoreceptors play a significant role in the antidepressant mechanisms of multiple monoaminergic antidepressants, particularly SSRIs. Buspirone, a partial agonist at this receptor, appeared as efficacious as bupropion when added to the SSRI citalopram in STAR*D Level 2 (Rush et al., 2009). Pindolol, a beta-adrenergic antagonist and a 5HT1A antagonist, was believed to have augmentation efficacy via effects on presynaptic autoreceptors, but pindolol did not separate from placebo in large randomized studies, possibly due to the low receptor occupancy achieved at the doses tested.

Hormonal strategies as augmentation in TRD:

a) *Thyroid hormones:* Most of the data supporting the efficacy of thyroid hormones as augmentation treatment was derived from studies of TCAs. A meta-analysis of four placebo-controlled studies of triiodothyronine (T3) augmentation of TCAs revealed a non-statistically significant increase in efficacy of T3 versus placebo (Aronson et al., 1996). Limited open data supports the efficacy of T3 augmentation of SSRIs, remission rates with T3 augmentation in STAR*D level 3 were 24.7% and numerically larger than those of lithium (Nierenberg et al., 2006). Side effects include tremors, sweating, nausea, headaches, palpitations, and dry mouth.

b) Estrogens: The role of estrogen receptors has been invoked in the neurobiology of depression, but clinically estrogen augmentation is associated with mixed results. One of two double blind placebo-controlled studies of estrogens in perimenopausal women with TRD reported greater resolution of depressive symptoms with adjunctive estrogens (Ng et al., 2010). Side effects include headache, somnolence, constipation, nausea, and sweating. In a randomized controlled trial the efficacy of adjuvant raloxifene (a selective estrogen receptor modulator) as augmentation in TRD did not differ significantly from placebo.

THE ROLE OF BIOMARKERS IN GUIDING ANTIDEPRESSANT SELECTION AND PREDICTING RESPONSE

Advances in our understanding of genetic, cellular, and brain mechanisms involved in the pathology of mood disorders hold the promise to not only advance our understanding of the pathology of MDD but also to result in specific measures ("biomarkers") to help guide clinical treatment, both generally, by suggesting new molecular and neuroanatomical targets to guide the development of new therapies, and specifically, by guiding clinicians in the selection of existing therapies (i.e., personalized medicine). Over the past few decades, increased capability and availability of genetic, endocrine, neuroimaging, and electrophysiology (EEG) technology has supported efforts to use these as biomarkers of treatment response (e.g., distinguish likely treatment responders from nonresponders with a specific intervention).

The search for such predictors of treatment outcome has cast a very wide net, but while many studies report correlations between specific clinical and/or biological parameters and clinical response to antidepressant treatment, such correlations are not sufficient to define a "predictor of treatment response." An ideal predictor of treatment outcome would be present in many or all patients and would have high (close to 100%) positive and negative predictive values; that is, if the predictor is present, all patients with the predictor would have the outcome of interest, and if the predictor is absent, none would have the outcome (Iosifescu, 2011). To be of clinical utility, the predictor would have to be relatively easy to measure (including cost considerations) and be present either at baseline, before the onset of antidepressant treatment, or early during the treatment (during the first week). Also importantly, research supporting putative predictors would have to report not merely significant statistical associations, but a detailed description of predictor behavior at different cutoff points, such as the area under the receiver-operator characteristic curve, AUROC, a common summary statistic for the goodness of a predictor in a binary classification (see Perlis, 2011, for a discussion of methodological problems in biomarker research).

A large number of studies have explored *genetic markers* as predictors of clinical response to antidepressants in MDD. Many candidate gene studies have been conducted on antidepressant use in MDD, but the results are not yet readily usable in clinical practice, as most of the pharmacogenetic findings for antidepressants have been inconclusive and/or controversial (Narasimhan and Lohoff, 2012). With respect to antidepressant metabolism and drug-drug interaction, the ability to measure CYP450 genes and the known effect of CYP450 enzymes on pharmacokinetics of antidepressants has led to a validated, FDA-approved pharmacogenetic clinical test (AmpliChip CYP450, Roche Diagnostic, Basel, Switzerland). It provides genotypes for the two CYP450 genes CYP2D6 and CYP2C19, allowing clinicians to predict the metabolizer status of a patient, which might influence antidepressant choice and dosing. However, the effect of such metabolic changes on clinical response is inconclusive, and the use of this genotyping test in clinical practice is limited.

Neuroimaging tests have also been studied extensively as potential markers of antidepressant response. Mayberg and colleagues (2000) have reported specific changes in metabolism in subgenual anterior cingulate gyrus in relation to treatment response; such changes were later replicated but found to be present across a variety of antidepressant modalities (and therefore not potentially useful in driving treatment selection). Many other imaging measures proposed have not yet been replicated. Moreover, due to the small size of these studies it is generally difficult to assess the predictive ability of these putative biomarkers (Iosifescu and Lapidus, 2011).

Electrophysiology: Several measures derived from prefrontal analysis of spontaneous electroencephalograms (EEG), evoked potentials, and EEG source localization have been associated with antidepressant response (Iosifescu, 2011). The best developed at this point are spontaneous EEG measures such as the antidepressant treatment response (ATR) index, whose predictive abilities have been replicated in large-scale studies (Iosifescu et al., 2009; Leuchter et al., 2009). EEG-based technologies have considerable advantages as potential clinical predictors. Since EEG is more widely available and cheaper than neuroimaging, it lends itself to studies with larger numbers of subjects (which are required for the validation of any biomarker of treatment response). The translation to clinical practice is also easier with a cheaper, ubiquitous technology (Iosifescu and Lapidus, 2011).

The current development of biomarkers appears to involve large studies where combining a variety of biomarkers (deriving, e.g., from genetics, imaging, or cognition) and clinical characteristics is attempted for improving predictions of a multifactorial process such as treatment response in MDD. Several large-scale clinical trials coupled with biomarker assessments are currently underway, and offer an example of new approaches for biomarker identification and development. One such example is the Emory study "Predictors of Antidepressant Treatment Response," which is assessing genetic and PET imaging predictors of response to antidepressants and behavioral therapy (http://www.ClinicalTrials.gov: NCT00360399).

Another biomarker trial currently underway is the International Study to Predict Optimized Treatment in Depression (iSPOT-D) (http://www.ClinicalTrials.gov: NCT00693849). The study aims to recruit more than 2,000 MDD participants, which will be evaluated clinically, with behavioral tests of cognition and emotion, physiological measures taken during corresponding cognitive and emotional tasks (EEG, event-related potentials, autonomic measures of heart rate, skin, and electromyography), structural and functional imaging (at least 10% of participants), and genotyping. These assessments will be integrated in a standardized assessment battery taken before and eight weeks after randomization to one of three antidepressants (escitalopram, sertraline, or venlafaxine XR).

Another large-scale biomarker study recently started is the Establishing Moderators and Biosignatures of Antidepressant Response for Clinical Care for Depression (EMBARC) study (http://www.ClinicalTrials.gov: NCT01407094), a randomized double blind trial across several US academic centers which will enroll 400 MDD participants, each to be assessed using clinical evaluations, self-report, behavioral tests of cognition, EEG, imaging measures, and genotyping. The study attempts to assess clinical and biological moderators and mediators of treatment response to sertraline versus placebo; non-responders in the first phase will be randomized to sertraline or bupropion.

In summary, there is a high unmet need for objective biomarkers to direct efficient selection of antidepressant treatments, to replace the current "trial and error" process. While no such biomarkers have been currently validated, current large-scale studies offer the promise of analyzing several simultaneously multiple putative biomarkers to detect the most accurate predictors and the relationships between them.

SOMATIC TREATMENTS

Somatic treatments include a large variety of methods of delivering energy directly to the brain (Table 38.3). While electroconvulsive therapy (ECT) is one of the earliest antidepressant treatments, the last decade has seen an important expansion of the somatic treatments used as antidepressant treatments.

ELECTROCONVULSIVE THERAPY

Electroconvulsive therapy (ECT) is a long-standing psychiatric intervention that was introduced as a treatment for schizophrenia in 1938 and became a common treatment for depression in the 1980s. It has been proven effective as an acute treatment option for hard to treat patients, such as those with TRD, psychotic depression, and acute suicidality (Prudic et al., 2004). More than half of patients who receive ECT respond within the first four weeks of treatment (Husain et al., 2004). ECT involves the placement of either one electrode (unilaterally) or two electrodes (bilaterally) on the skull to induce cerebral seizures in anesthetized patients. There has been much debate over the efficacy and safety of different variations of electrode placement and voltage dosage. Evidence has shown that high dosage right unilateral and bilateral ECT seem to be similarly effective, and twice as efficacious as low or moderate dose unilateral ECT; however bilateral electrode placement, most specifically bitemporally, appears to produce increased and more sustained cognitive impairments than unilateral ECT (Kellner et al., 2010). Studies have generally shown response rates of 70–90% in patients across the spectrum of depression severity and with varying treatment history, however, response rates have been lower in patients with severe treatment-resistant depression (Prudic et al., 2004). The majority of patients who do not receive active maintenance treatment will generally relapse in six months to a year following a course of ECT

TABLE 38.3. Somatic treatments for MDD

TREATMENT	FDA APPROVED FOR MDD?	SETTING	INVASIVE	ANESTHESIA REQUIRED?	AREA OF STIMULATION	FORM OF ENERGY
Electroconvulsive therapy (ECT)	Yes (grandfathered)	Inpatient or outpatient procedure	No	Yes	Generalized	Electrical
Repetitive transcranial magnetic stimulation (rTMS)	Yes	Outpatient (office) procedure	No	No	Focal	Magnetic
Vagus nerve stimulation (VNS)	Yes	Surgical implantation followed by outpatient office adjustments	Yes	Yes (for surgery)	Generalized	Electrical
Deep brain stimulation (DBS)	No	Surgical implantation followed by outpatient adjustments	Yes	Yes (for surgery)	Focal	Electrical
Low field magnetic stimulation (LFMS)	No	Outpatient (office) procedure	No	No	Generalized	Magnetic
Magnetic seizure therapy (MST)	No	Inpatient or outpatient procedure	No	Yes	Focal	Magnetic
Transcranial direct current stimulation (tDCS)	No	Office	No	No	Focal	Electrical

(Sackeim et al., 2001). Antidepressant medication therapy reduces the rate of relapse but maintenance ECT is associated with the lowest levels of relapse (approximately 10%; Gagne et al., 2000). ECT is generally considered to be a safe procedure with a low risk of serious medical adverse events, but it is associated in the development of cognitive impairments, specifically memory loss. Cognitive side effects include acute confusion, anterograde amnesia, and retrograde amnesia. While these cognitive side effects are generally considered to be moderate, tolerable, and time-limited, more significant and extensive impairment can result. Continued research is being conducted to examine the possibility of various different dosage and electrode placement combinations having decreased cognitive side effects (Kellner et al., 2010).

A modern variation of ECT is **magnetic seizure therapy** (MST), which involves cortical seizure induction via a magnetic field rather than direct application of electrodes. The goal of MST is to allow a more localized and precise induction of seizures, which may reduce side effects (e.g., cognitive effects) compared to ECT. However small studies so far suggest clinical effects are not different from ECT (Kayser et al., 2011). As in ECT, this technique requires anesthesia and muscle relaxation.

TRANSCRANIAL MAGNETIC STIMULATION

Transcranial magnetic stimulation (TMS) is a brain stimulation technique using electromagnetic induction and a rapidly changing magnetic field to induce weak electric currents, which cause depolarization or hyperpolarization of neurons in specific parts of the brain. The main advantage of TMS is its non-invasiveness and the possibility to stimulate relatively small brain volumes. A variant of TMS, repetitive transcranial magnetic stimulation (rTMS), has been tested as an antidepressant treatment and it is approved in the United States for the treatment of unipolar depression in adults who failed to respond to a single medication trial (O'Reardon et al., 2007). The largest sham-controlled study showed TMS had remission rate superior to sham, but relatively low (14.1% versus 5.1%), with almost 30% of patients achieving remission in the later open-label phase (George et al., 2010). rTMS has moderate effect sizes (0.39) in TRD, similar to those seen with standard pharmacotherapy (Schutter, 2009) and less effective than ECT. In general, rTMS appears to be safe and well tolerated (O'Reardon et al., 2007). Common side effects include headache and scalp pain. Seizures can occur with rTMS, although in less than 0.5% of subjects. More research is needed to determine the optimal stimulation parameters. High frequency (5–20 Hz) stimulation of the left DLPFC has been the technique most studied, while data from low frequency stimulation (1Hz) of right DLPFC are limited.

Other variations of TMS currently researched include techniques with increased brain penetration (*deep TMS*, which can stimulate subcortical brain structures below the 2 cm area accessible with rTMS, or *synchronized TMS*, which allows individualized stimulation at the intrinsic alpha frequency of the subject; for both the efficacy results are still pending).

Low field magnetic stimulation (LFMS) is another investigational method of brain stimulation by an alternating magnetic field. LFMS is based on empirical observations of echo-planar magnetic spectroscopic imaging (EP-MRSI) sequences inducing mood effects, possibly through stimulating effects of weak electromagnetic fields. Pilot studies have shown rapid mood elevating effects in both unipolar and bipolar depressed patients (Rohan et al., 2004). Larger studies, including a multi-site NIMH-sponsored trial (NCT01654796), are ongoing.

SURGICALLY IMPLANTED DEVICES

VAGUS NERVE STIMULATION

Vagus nerve stimulation (VNS) includes a surgical implant that stimulates electrically the ascending branch of left vagus nerve and stimulates the vagal nucleus of the solitary tract, which has widespread projections within the central nervous system, including to the forebrain. In animal models VNS was associated with GABA and noradrenergic effects in the frontal cortex. VNS has been used as an anticonvulsant and was adapted as an antidepressant treatment after positive effects on mood were noticed in patients receiving the treatment for epilepsy. In the pivotal study VNS did not separate from sham in the acute (12-week) period but open continuation for up to 12 months yielded a 27% response rate in highly treatment-resistant patients (George et al., 2005). VNS is FDA approved since 2005 for the treatment of chronic and treatment resistant depression in patients who failed to respond to at least four trials of antidepressants, but the rate of implantations appears low given challenges related to efficacy, surgery, and financial considerations (insurance reimbursement). Side effects for VNS include complications of surgery, neck or jaw pain, hoarseness, or cough.

DEEP BRAIN STIMULATION

Deep brain stimulation (DBS) is an investigational treatment for depression involving direct stimulation of specific subcortical brain areas to affect the brain neurocircuitry of emotional regulation. DBS (which is currently FDA approved for the treatment of essential tremor, Parkinson's, and dystonia) requires surgical implantation of an electrode stimulating the target brain area and connected to an electrical pulse generator. The largest studies investigating DBS in MDD have targeted the subgenual cingulate; a recent report suggests long-term efficacy in a 17 MDD subjects receiving open stimulation (Holtzheimer et al., 2012). Other smaller studies have targeted the ventral anterior internal capsule and the nucleus accumbens; larger controlled studies in several target areas are ongoing.

PSYCHOTHERAPIES

While the space of this chapter does not allow a detailed discussion of psychotherapies, we need to highlight that they represent a first-line treatment for MDD, with cognitive and behavioral therapies (CBT) and interpersonal therapies (IPT) having the most evidence in support of their efficacy in randomized clinical trials (Hollon and Ponniah, 2010). Some data supports the effectiveness of these therapies for prevention of depressive relapse after an initial acute treatment.

COGNITIVE AND BEHAVIORAL THERAPIES

Cognitive and Behavioral Therapies (CBT) includes a family of related treatments involving cognitive and behavioral interventions for MDD. Older meta-analyses have shown a slight advantage for CBT over medications in treating depression; however, methodological limitations in some of these older studies may have favored CBT (Butler et al., 2006). In the large, multisite Treatment of Depression Collaborative Research Program (TDCRP), CBT and medication (imipramine) showed similar efficacy; however, among patients with severe MDD, imipramine was found to be superior to CBT (Elkin et al., 1995). However, in more recent research, CBT and medication were comparable in treating severe depression. CBT and paroxetine were equally effective after 16 weeks of treatment in the treatment of moderate and severe MDD (DeRubeis et al., 2005). Thase and coworkers (2007) reported the results of the second level of the Sequenced Treatment Alternatives to Relieve Depression (STAR*D) study, where MDD subjects received CBT (either alone or as augmentation) after failing an initial trial of citalopram. Patients receiving CBT had similar response and remission rates to patients randomized to medication strategies, but patients receiving drug augmentation had more rapid response than those receiving antidepressant augmentation, while patients receiving CBT monotherapy experienced fewer side effects compared to those assigned to antidepressant monotherapy.

Acute outcomes of CBT and antidepressant medication appear largely comparable, and relapse rates after CBT are comparable to those of individuals maintained on antidepressants after one year and superior to placebo (Hollon et al., 2005). Combining antidepressants and CBT generally yields an advantage over either of the two treatments alone, and may be especially advantageous in more chronic forms of depression (Keller et al., 2000).

INTERPERSONAL THERAPIES

Interpersonal therapy (IPT) is a short-term, manual-based treatment for depression. IPT focuses on interpersonal issues, emphasizing on the way depressive symptoms are related to a person's relationships, including family and peers. The immediate goals of treatment are symptom reduction and improved social adjustment.

Two decades ago a large controlled study suggested that IPT and imipramine were more efficacious than placebo for the more severely depressed individuals, while CBT was not; the entire study sample did not show efficacy differences between treatment modalities (Elkin et al., 1989, 1995). However, in a more recent study CBT was more effective than IPT for the more severely depressed individuals, while the rates of response were comparable between therapies for the entire group and for the subgroups with mild and moderate depression (Luty et al., 2007). IPT was also shown to be more effective than placebo (but less effective than imipramine) in maintaining a group of MDD patients in long-term recovery (Frank et al., 1990). In elderly MDD subjects maintenance with paroxetine was more effective than IPT or placebo for prevention of relapse (Reynolds et al., 2006).

In summary, CBT may be comparable to medication for acute treatment and it provides durable benefits. Combining CBT and pharmacological treatments may be most effective in chronic depression. The efficacy of IPT for acute and maintenance treatment is also supported by several studies (Hollon and Ponniah, 2010).

NATURAL REMEDIES AS ANTIDEPRESSANTS

While the use of natural or "alternative" remedies is popular and increasing in the United States and worldwide, the data supporting their efficacy as antidepressants is limited. The best-studied natural medications for mood disorders are St. John's Wort (hypericum), omega-3 fatty acids, and S-adenosylmethionine (SAMe).

ST. JOHN'S WORT (HYPERICUM)

The extract of the flower of St. John's Wort (*Hypericum perforatum L.*) is widely used for the treatment of depression. Although the extract contains a large number of molecules, the main active components in hypericum are considered to be hypericin and hyperforin. Hypericin does not cross the blood-brain barrier but may have modulatory effects on inflammatory cytokine production (interleukin-6 and interleukin-1β), resulting in a decrease in corticotrophin-releasing hormone. Hyperforin appears to be associated with serotonin reuptake inhibition and norepinephrine and acetylcholine reuptake inhibition (Mischoulon, 2009). Large meta-analyses support the efficacy of St. John's Wort in MDD in comparison with placebo and relatively equivalent efficacy with suboptimal doses of antidepressants, with the most favorable studies all performed in German-speaking countries (Linde et al., 2008). In several large US studies St. John's Wort did not separate from placebo (Freeman et al., 2010). In monotherapy St. John's Wort has a favorable side effect profile; side effects include dry mouth, dizziness, constipation, other gastrointestinal symptoms, confusion, and phototoxicity. St. John's Wort appears to induce cytochrome P450 3A4, resulting in decreased levels of substrates (antiretrovirals, cyclosporines). Other components of hypericum, including flavonoids, are irreversible monoamine oxidase-A inhibitors and cases of serotonine syndrome have been described when St. John's Wort was combined with SSRIs.

OMEGA-3 FATTY ACIDS

Omega-3 fatty acids are polyunsaturated fatty acids with a double bond (C=C), commonly found in marine and nut oils. Their presence in modern diet is decreased due to substitution with omega-6 fatty acids present in vegetable oils. Eicosapentaenoic acid (EPA) and docosahexaenoic acid (DHA) are the two fatty acids with evidence for an antidepressant effect. Proposed mechanisms for the antidepressant effects include their interaction with catecholamine metabolism and inhibition of inflammatory cytokines secretion (prostaglandin E2), leading to decreased corticosteroid release

(Mischoulon, 2009). A recent meta-analysis of 35 randomized controlled trials supports the efficacy of omega-3 fatty acids (in doses ranging from 0.5 to 9.6 g/d) compared to placebo in MDD, but finds the published literature to show significant heterogeneity, likely generated by publication bias (Appleton et al., 2010). There was no clear difference in efficacy between EPA and DHA. The omega-3s appear to be well tolerated and safe. Side effects include gastrointestinal upset, fishy aftertaste, and a small risk of bleeding.

S-ADENOSYLMETHIONINE

S-adenosylmethionine (SAMe) is present in all human cells, including the brain, acting as a methyl donor to membrane phospholipids, myelin, choline, catecholamines, and other molecules important for brain function. It is synthesized from the amino acid l-methionine through the one-carbon cycle; the vitamins folate and B12 are catalysts of this process (folate and B12 deficits have been associated with depression). The mechanism of SAMe's antidepressant effect has been associated with its role as an intermediate for the synthesis of norepinephrine, dopamine, and serotonin (Mischoulon, 2009). A recent systematic review reported that in 7 of 7 controlled trials that parenteral SAMe was more efficacious in MDD than placebo and equal in efficacy to the tricyclic antidepressants (Papakostas, 2009). Four out of 5 controlled trials also support the efficacy of oral SAMe (1600 mg/day). A recent RCT reported SAMe augmentation of SSRIs was more efficacious than placebo (Papakostas et al., 2010). Side effects are uncommon, but occasionally nausea, gastrointestinal upset, and anxiety can occur.

In conclusion, St. John's Wort is supported by evidence of efficacy as monotherapy, but the data is very heterogeneous and the risk of drug interactions should be considered. Limited evidence supports the efficacy of omega-3 fatty acids and SAM-e. Other natural remedies including L-methylfolate and *N*-acetyl cysteine (NAC) are associated with even more limited evidence of efficacy in MDD.

TREATMENT OF DEPRESSION IN SPECIAL POPULATIONS

Depression has a heterogeneous clinical presentation, and several subtypes of depression have been described. While a complete discussion of these subtypes is beyond the scope of this chapter, we will mention the most significant subtypes of depression: psychotic, melancholic, atypical, postpartum, seasonal, and bipolar. The presence of such variations in clinical presentation probably underlies a significant variability in the etiology of depression and does influence treatment decisions, as discussed in the following. Specific treatment strategies for geriatric depression and of depression with comorbid medical illness are addressed in Chapters 35 and 37 of this book.

PSYCHOTIC DEPRESSION

The presence of psychotic symptoms during a major depressive episode is considered a marker of increased severity, even when depressive symptoms are moderate. Psychotic depression is associated with increased rates of recurrence, poor response to antidepressant treatment, and poor outcomes (Rothschild, 2003). Some studies suggest psychotic depression is biologically distinct from non-psychotic MDD, with more significant HPA axis abnormalities (increased cortisol levels, higher rates of non-suppression on the dexamethasone suppression test) and an activation of the dopaminergic system (higher levels of cerebrospinal fluid 5-hydroxyindoleacetic acid and lower serum dopamine-beta-hydroxlyase (which converts dopamine to norepinephrine) (Rothschild, 2003). Recent meta-analyses suggest that while antidepressant or antipsychotic monotherapies are associated with lower rates of response, combined antipsychotic-antidepressant treatment can be more efficacious (Farahani and Correll, 2012). ECT is associated with high rates of treatment response but with relatively rapid loss of response (Prudic et al, 2004) in patients with psychotic depression.

MELANCHOLIC DEPRESSION

Melancholic depression is characterized by severe anhedonia with lack of mood reactivity, severe weight loss or loss of appetite, psychomotor agitation or retardation, early morning awakening, guilt that is excessive, and worse mood in the morning. Biologically, melancholic depression has been associated with enhanced activity of the hypothalamic–pituitary–adrenal (HPA) axis, involving elevated secretion of corticotropin-releasing hormone (CRH), which in turn contributes to sleep abnormalities (Gold and Chrousos, 2002). Clinically, melancholic depression appears associated with higher severity, increased anxiety, and higher rates of suicidality. Cognitive impairments (attention shifting, mental flexibility, decreased memory) are consistently associated with melancholia. Several antidepressants including SSRI and SNRIs appear effective for treating melancholia; ECT is particularly effective in melancholic and severe presentations.

ATYPICAL DEPRESSION

Atypical depression is characterized by persistent mood reactivity, hypersomnia, hyperphagia, leaden paralysis, and rejection sensitivity, although correlation analyses reveal only modest associations between several of the atypical symptoms (Posternak and Zimmerman, 2002). There is a significant degree of overlap with symptoms of bipolar depression. Biologically, several studies suggest reduced activity of the HPA axis and reduced noradrenergic activity in the locus coeruleus. Clinically, atypical depression is associated with a reported preferential response to monoamine oxidase inhibitors compared to TCAs; other studies suggest SSRIs are more efficacious than TCAs in such patients (Stewart et al., 2009). The SSRIs are a preferred first-line therapy in such patients.

POSTPARTUM DEPRESSION

Postpartum depression represents moderate to severe depression experienced by women after giving birth. It occurs in up to 10% of healthy women (but up to 50% in women with previous history of depression) and it is different from the much milder postpartum "blues," a self-limited, non-pathological condition which can occur in 50% to 85% of women in the first 10 days following delivery. The symptoms of postpartum depression appear most often within three months post delivery and are similar to other forms of MDD. Severe forms of postpartum depression are associated with psychosis and represent a psychiatric emergency.

Meta-analyses support the efficacy of psychotherapy (especially IPT and CBT) and of conventional antidepressants (fluoxetine, sertraline, venlafaxine) in the treatment of postpartum depression (Sockol et al., 2011). Postpartum depression has been associated with the significant hormonal fluctuations after delivery, especially the significant decrease in estrogen and progesterone levels. Several studies suggest a role for exogenous estrogen in the treatment of women with postpartum depression (Dennis et al, 2008), but treatment with estrogen has been associated with changes in breast-milk production and with thromboembolic events. Treatment with progesterone is not supported by current evidence.

SEASONAL AFFECTIVE DISORDER

Seasonal affective disorder (SAD, "winter blues") represents a form of recurrent depression with a clear seasonal pattern. Decreased levels of DA transporter in the striatum have been reported in SAD (Neumeister et al., 2001). Bupropion, a dopaminergic antidepressant, appears efficacious as a treatment and for the prevention of seasonal depression episodes (Modell et al., 2005). Studies also support the efficacy of bright light therapy (10,000 lux 30 minutes/day for 8 weeks) and of fluoxetine for the seasonal depression (Lam et al., 2006), while other second-generation antidepressants have only minimal evidence of efficacy (Thaler et al., 2011).

BIPOLAR DEPRESSION

In patients with bipolar disorder, depression is the most frequent clinical problem and the most significant cause of morbidity and dysfunction. Quetiapine (Calabrese et al., 2005) and the olanzapine-fluoxetine combination (OFC) (Tohen et al., 2003) are FDA-approved for the treatment of acute bipolar depression. Lamotrigine is FDA-approved only for prophylaxis of bipolar mood episodes since only one of four controlled studies of lamotrigine for acute bipolar depression has achieved the primary endpoint. Other studies suggest lithium might be an efficacious antidepressant, and that lithium and lamotrigine might be equally efficacious for bipolar depression (Suppes et al., 2008). The usefulness of traditional antidepressants in bipolar patients is more controversial. Most treatment guidelines advocate against using antidepressant monotherapy in bipolar disorder, mainly due to the risk of manic switches and mood cycling. Despite such expert consensus, 50% of bipolar patients receive antidepressant monotherapy as their initial treatment (Baldessarini et al., 2007). While some studies have suggested that antidepressants added to mood stabilizers might have some benefit, in the NIH-funded STEP-BD study ($N = 366$) adding an antidepressant (paroxetine or bupropion) or placebo to a mood stabilizer in bipolar depressed subjects resulted in equally low rates of improvement (23.5% versus 27.3% of subjects achieved recovery on antidepressant versus placebo, respectively) and similar rates of switch to mania (Sachs et al., 2007).

For patients who failed a first-line treatment, lamotrigine appeared to achieve numerically superior efficacy compared to risperidone or inositol, but the differences were not statistically significant due to the low number of patients in the study (Nierenberg et al., 2006b). Only a few small studies support the efficacy of pramipexole (Goldberg et al., 2004), MAOIs (Himmelhoch et al., 1991), or modafinil (Frye et al., 2007) when added to mood stabilizers for the treatment of bipolar depression. Ziprasidone and aripiprazole have failed to demonstrate efficacy in bipolar depression. There is also significant evidence in support of the efficacy of focused psychotherapies (cognitive behavioral therapy, family-focused therapy, and interpersonal and social rhythm therapy) in patients with bipolar disorder (Miklowitz et al., 2007).

NEW AVENUES IN ANTIDEPRESSANT TREATMENT

Given the large disease burden of MDD and the limitations in current treatments, the major goal of current neuropharmacology research is to identify safe and more effective antidepressant treatments. Several such agents currently in development can be broadly classified as monoaminergic, according to their primary mechanism of action. These include triple-reuptake inhibitors (TRIs), which bind to and inhibit all three primary monoamine synaptic reuptake proteins: the serotonin transporter (SERT), the norepinephrine transporter (NET), and the dopamine transporter (DAT). TRIs can be seen as the next logical step in an effort to broaden engagement of the monoamine systems, following the development of serotonin norepinephrine reuptake inhibitors (SNRIs). It remains to be seen, however, if TRIs will confer enhanced efficacy over currently available monoaminergic agents.

Innovative antidepressant drug discovery efforts focus however outside of the monoaminergic by targeting a variety of neural systems and chemical messengers, including the glutamate system, the HPA axis, the galanin and other neuropeptide systems, the melatonin system, inflammatory mediators, and neurogenesis (see Murrough and Charney, 2012, in press, for a recent review of the antidepressant horizon). Recognition of the role of stress-related neuropeptides in preclinical models of depression has prompted investigation into the clinical utility of small-molecule neuropeptide modulators, including corticotropin-releasing hormone (CRH) antagonists and neurokinin (NK) receptor antagonists. However, to date phase II and III RCTs of molecules from both classes of neuropeptide modulators have been disappointing.

The glutamate system in particular may be a fruitful avenue for novel treatment development. In this section we will briefly review the rationale for targeting the glutamate system in mood disorders and highlight the example of the glutamate

N-methyl-D-aspartate (NMDA) receptor (NMDAR) antagonist ketamine as an example of a potentially novel glutamatergic antidepressant (Murrough, 2012). Glutamate is the ubiquitous excitatory neurotransmitter in the brain and is a critical mediator of neuroplasticity and learning and memory. Cortical and limbic brain circuits crucial for cognitive and emotional regulation largely utilize glutamate as the primary neurotransmitter, and maladaptive alterations in synaptic structure and function observed in animal models of stress and depression are seen within glutamatergic pathways (Duman and Voleti, 2012). The extensive plasticity of the glutamate synapse in response to environmental influences suggests a key physiological substrate for the well-known link between environmental stress and depression and the neurotoxic effects of abnormally high levels of glutamate—which may result from stress—is a candidate mechanism for regional reductions in brain volume observed in MDD. These and other data point toward the glutamate system as a principal candidate to target for therapeutic modulation in MDD.

Ketamine is a high-affinity, non-competitive NMDAR antagonist that is currently FDA-approved as an anesthetic agent and is used off-label in the management of chronic pain. The potential antidepressant properties of ketamine were initially highlighted by a series of two small studies (Berman et al., 2000; Zarate et al., 2006), while several controlled and open-label studies conducted subsequently provide support for the rapid antidepressant effects of ketamine (reviewed in Murrough et al., 2012). Acute response rates as high as 70% are observed within 24 hours of a single intravenous infusion, even in patients with TRD. A series of recent basic science studies in animal models highlight alterations of synaptic structure and function as essential aspects of ketamine's antidepressant mechanism of action (Duman and Voleti, 2012). Larger controlled studies of ketamine in depression will be required before a firm conclusion can be drawn regarding the antidepressant efficacy of ketamine. A treatment schedule of repeated administrations of ketamine and relapse prevention strategies following a response to ketamine are currently active areas of investigation.

Non-pharmacological treatments are also an active area of antidepressant research. Those include novel methods utilizing magnetic stimulation (synchronized TMS, deep TMS, LFMS), other forms of non-invasive brain stimulation (e.g., magnetic seizure therapy, transcranial direct current stimulation, near infrared radiation), as well as invasive deep brain stimulation (DBS) with several brain targets. Several of these treatments have shown promise in early studies and are currently undergoing more definitive evaluation.

In conclusion, over the last four decades clinical observations and research have led to the validation of a large number of effective monoaminergic antidepressants, several structured psychotherapies (CBT, IPT), and ECT. However, limitations of current treatments and advances in our understanding of the biology of mood disorders represent the impetus for the major search for new treatments currently underway. A significant number of novel agents, including pharmaceuticals and natural remedies, as well as somatic treatments are currently in development. Potential biomarkers of treatment outcome could also revolutionize current treatment strategies in depression.

DISCLOSURES

Dr. Iosifescu has been for the last three years a consultant to CNS Response, Inc., and Servier. Lifetime he has received research support from Aspect Medical Systems, Forest and Janssen Pharmaceutica, and he has received consulting and speaking honoraria from Cephalon, Eli Lilly, Forest, and Pfizer.

Dr. Murrough has no conflicts of interest to disclose.

Dr. Charney has been named as an inventor on a pending use-patent of ketamine for the treatment of depression. If ketamine were shown to be effective in the treatment of depression and received approval from the Food and Drug Administration for this indication, Dr. Charney and Mount Sinai School of Medicine could benefit financially.

REFERENCES

Alt, A., Nisenbaum, E.S., et al. (2006). A role for AMPA receptors in mood disorders. *Biochem. Pharmacol.* 71(9):1273–1288.

Anderson, I.M. (2000). Selective serotonin reuptake inhibitors versus tricyclic antidepressants: a meta-analysis of efficacy and tolerability. *J. Affect. Disord.* 58(1):19–36.

Appleton, K.M., Rogers, P.J., et al. (2010). Updated systematic review and meta-analysis of the effects of n-3 long-chain polyunsaturated fatty acids on depressed mood. *Am. J. Clin. Nutr.* 91(3):757–770.

American Psychiatric Association. (2000). Diagnostic and Statistical Manual of Mental Disorders DSM-IV-TR. 4th Edition. Washington, DC: Author.

Aronson, R., Offman, H.J., et al. (1996). Triiodothyronine augmentation in the treatment of refractory depression: a meta-analysis. *Arch. Gen. Psychiatry* 53(9):842–848.

Baldessarini, R.J., Leahy, L., et al. (2007). Patterns of psychotropic drug prescription for U.S. patients with diagnoses of bipolar disorders. *Psychiatr. Serv.* 58(1):85–91.

Bauer, M., and Dopfmer S. (1999). Lithium augmentation in treatment-resistant depression: meta-analysis of placebo-controlled studies. *J. Clin. Psychopharmacol.* 19(5):427–434.

Berman, R.M., Cappiello, A., et al. (2000). Antidepressant effects of ketamine in depressed patients. *Biol. Psychiatry* 47:351–354.

Butler, A.C., Chapman, J.E., et al. (2006). The empirical status of cognitive-behavioral therapy: a review of meta-analyses. *Clin. Psychol. Rev.* 26:17–31.

Calabrese, J.R., Keck, P.E., Jr., et al. (2005). A randomized, double-blind, placebo-controlled trial of quetiapine in the treatment of bipolar I or II depression. *Am. J. Psychiatry* 162(7):1351–1360.

Carney, R.M., and Shelton, R.C. (2011). Agomelatine for the treatment of major depressive disorder. *Expert. Opin. Pharmacother.* 12(15):2411–2419.

Crane, G.E. (1956). The psychiatric side-effects of iproniazid. *Am. J. Psychiatry* 112(7):494–501.

Dennis, C.L., Ross, L.E., et al. (2008). Oestrogens and progestins for preventing and treating postpartum depression. *Cochrane Database Syst. Rev.* 4:CD001690.

DeRubeis, R.J., Hollon, S.D., et al. (2005). Cognitive therapy vs. medications in the treatment of moderate to severe depression. *Arch. Gen. Psychiatry* 62:409–416.

Dong, J., and Blier P. et al. (2001). Modification of norepinephrine and serotonin, but not dopamine, neuron firing by sustained bupropion treatment. *Psychopharmacology (Berl.)* 155(1):52–57.

Duman, R.S., and Voleti, B. (2012). Signaling pathways underlying the pathophysiology and treatment of depression: novel mechanisms for rapid-acting agents. *Trends Neurosci.* 35:47–56.

Elkin, I., Gibbons, R.D., et al. (1995). Initial severity and differential treatment outcome in the National Institute of Mental Health Treatment of Depression Collaborative Research Program. *J. Consult. Clin. Psychol.* 63:841–847.

Elkin, I., Shea, M.T., et al. (1989). National Institute of Mental Health Treatment of Depression Collaborative Research Program. General effectiveness of treatments. *Arch. Gen. Psychiatry* 46(11):971–982.

Farahani, A., and Correll, C.U. (2012). Are antipsychotics or antidepressants needed for psychotic depression? A systematic review and meta-analysis of trials comparing antidepressant or antipsychotic monotherapy with combination treatment. *J. Clin. Psychiatry* 73(4):486–496.

Fava, M., Rush, A.J., et al. (2008). Difference in treatment outcome in outpatients with anxious versus nonanxious depression: a STAR*D report. *Am. J. Psychiatry* 165(3):342–351.

Freeman, M.P., Fava, M., et al. (2010). Complementary and alternative medicine in major depressive disorder: the American Psychiatric Association Task Force report. *J. Clin. Psychiatry* 71(6):669–681.

Frank, E., Kupfer, D.J., et al. (1990). Three-year outcomes for maintenance therapies in recurrent depression. *Arch. Gen. Psychiatry* 47(12):1093–1099.

Frye, M.A., Grunze, H., et al. (2007). A placebo-controlled evaluation of adjunctive modafinil in the treatment of bipolar depression. *Am. J. Psychiatry* 164(8):1242–1249.

Gagné, G.G., Jr., Furman, M.J., et al. (2000). Efficacy of continuation ECT and antidepressant drugs compared to long-term antidepressants alone in depressed patients. *Am. J. Psychiatry* 157(12):1960–1965.

George, M.S., Lisanby, S.H., et al. (2010). Daily left prefrontal transcranial magnetic stimulation therapy for major depressive disorder: a sham-controlled randomized trial. *Arch. Gen. Psychiatry* 67(5):507–516.

George, M.S., Rush, A.J., et al. (2005). A one-year comparison of vagus nerve stimulation with treatment as usual for treatment-resistant depression. *Biol. Psychiatry* 58(5):364–373.

Gershon, S., Holmberg, G., et al. (1962). Imipramine hydrochloride: its effects on clinical, autonomic, and psychological functions. *Arch. Gen. Psychiatry* 6:96–101.

Glowinski, J., and Axelrod, J. (1964). Inhibition of uptake of tritiated-noradrenaline in the intact rat brain by imipramine and structurally related compounds. *Nature* 204:1318–1319.

Gold, P.W., and Chrousos, G.P. (2002). Organization of the stress system and its dysregulation in melancholic and atypical depression: high vs low CRH/NE states. *Mol. Psychiatry* 7(3):254–275.

Goldberg, J.F., Burdick, K.E., et al. (2004). Preliminary randomized, double-blind, placebo-controlled trial of pramipexole added to mood stabilizers for treatment-resistant bipolar depression. *Am. J. Psychiatry* 161(3):564–566.

Himmelhoch, J.M., Thase, M.E., et al. (1991). Tranylcypromine versus imipramine in anergic bipolar depression. *Am. J. Psychiatry* 148(7):910–916.

Hollon, S.D., DeRubeis, R.J., et al. (2005). Prevention of relapse following cognitive therapy vs medications in moderate to severe depression. *Arch. Gen. Psychiatry* 62:417–422.

Hollon, S.D., and Ponniah, K. (2010). A review of empirically supported psychological therapies for mood disorders in adults. *Depress. Anxiety* 27(10):891–932.

Holtzheimer, P.E., Kelley, M.E., et al. (2012). Subcallosal cingulate deep brain stimulation for treatment-resistant unipolar and bipolar depression. *Arch. Gen. Psychiatry* 69(2):150–158.

Husain, M.M., Rush, A.J., et al. (2004). Speed of response and remission in major depressive disorder with acute electroconvulsive therapy (ECT): a Consortium for Research in ECT (CORE) report. *J. Clin. Psychiatry* 65(4):485–491.

Iosifescu, D.V. (2007). Treating depression in the medically ill. *Psychiatr. Clin. North Am.* 30(1):77–90.

Iosifescu, D.V. (2011). Electroencephalography-derived biomarkers of antidepressant response. *Harv. Rev. Psychiatry* 19(3):144–154.

Iosifescu, D.V., Greenwald, S., et al. (2009). Frontal EEG predictors of treatment outcome in major depressive disorder. *Eur. Neuropsychopharm.* 19:772–777.

Iosifescu, D.V., and Lapidus, K. (2011). The role of neuroimaging and electrophysiology (EEG) as predictors of treatment response in major depressive disorder. *Clin. Neuropsychiatry* 5(1):47–60.

Judd, L.L., Akiskal, H.S., et al. (1998). A prospective 12-year study of subsyndromal and syndromal depressive symptoms in unipolar major depressive disorders. *Arch. Gen. Psychiatry* 55:694–700.

Kayser, S., Bewernick, B.H., et al. (2011). Antidepressant effects, of magnetic seizure therapy and electroconvulsive therapy, in treatment-resistant depression. *J. Psychiatr. Res.* 45(5):569–576.

Keller, M.B., McCullough, J.P., et al. (2000). A comparison of nefazodone, the cognitive behavioral-analysis system of psychotherapy, and their combination for the treatment of chronic depression. *N. Engl. J. Med.* 342:1462–1470.

Kellner, C.H., Knapp, R., et al. (2010). Bifrontal, bitemporal and right unilateral electrode placement in ECT: randomised trial. *Br. J. Psychiatry* 196(3):226–234.

Kessler, R.C., et al. (2005). Prevalence, severity, and comorbidity of 12-month DSM-IV disorders in the National Comorbidity Survey Replication. *Arch. Gen. Psychiatry* 62(6):617–627.

Kozisek, M.E., Middlemas, D., et al. (2008). Brain-derived neurotrophic factor and its receptor tropomyosin-related kinase B in the mechanism of action of antidepressant therapies. *Pharmacol. Ther.* 117(1):30–51.

Kuhn, R. (1958). The treatment of depressive states with G 22355 (imipramine hydrochloride). *Am. J. Psychiatry* 115(5):459–464.

Lam, R.W., Levitt, A.J., et al. (2006). The Can-STUDY: a randomized controlled trial of the effectiveness of light therapy and fluoxetine in patients with winter seasonal disorder. *Am. J. Psychiatry* 163:805–812.

Leuchter, A.F., Cook, I.A., et al. (2009). Effectiveness of a quantitative electroencephalographic biomarker for predicting differential response or remission with escitalopram and bupropion in major depressive disorder. *Psychiatry Res.* 169:132–138.

Linde, K., Berner, M.M., et al. (2008). St. John's wort for major depression. *Cochrane Database Syst. Rev.* (4):CD000448.

Luty, S.E., Carter, J.D., et al. (2007). Randomised controlled trial of interpersonal psychotherapy and cognitive-behavioural therapy for depression. *Br. J. Psychiatry* 190:496–502.

Machado, M., Einarson TR. (2010). Comparison of SSRIs and SNRIs in major depressive disorder: a meta-analysis of head-to-head randomized clinical trials. *J. Clin. Pharm. Ther.* 35(2):177–188.

Manolopoulos, V.G., Ragia, G., et al. (2012). Pharmacokinetic interactions of selective serotonin reuptake inhibitors with other commonly prescribed drugs in the era of pharmacogenomics. *Drug Metabol. Drug Interact.* 27(1):19–31.

Mayberg, H.S., Brannan, S.K., et al. (2000). Regional metabolic effects of fluoxetine in major depression: serial changes and relationship to clinical response. *Biol. Psychiatry* 48(8):830–843.

Meyer, J.H., Goulding, V.S., et al. (2002). Bupropion occupancy of the dopamine transporter is low during clinical treatment. *Psychopharmacology (Berl.)* 163(1):102–105.

Meyer, J.H., Wilson, A.A., et al. (2009). Brain monoamine oxidase A binding in major depressive disorder: relationship to selective serotonin reuptake inhibitor treatment, recovery, and recurrence. *Arch. Gen. Psychiatry* 66(12):1304–1312.

Miklowitz, D.J., Otto, M.W., et al. (2007). Psychosocial treatments for bipolar depression: a 1-year randomized trial from the Systematic Treatment Enhancement Program. *Arch. Gen. Psychiatry* 64(4):419–426.

Mischoulon, D. (2009). Update and critique of natural remedies as antidepressant treatments. *Obstet. Gynecol. Clin. North Am.* 36(4):789–807.

Modell, J.G., Rosenthal, N.E., et al. (2005). Seasonal affective disorder and its prevention by anticipatory treatment with bupropion XL. *Biol. Psychiatry* 58(8):658–667.

Montgomery, S.A., Baldwin, D.S., et al. (2007). Which antidepressants have demonstrated superior efficacy? A review of the evidence. *Int. Clin. Psychopharmacol.* 22(6):323–329.

Murrough, J.W. (2012). Ketamine as a novel antidepressant: from synapse to behavior. *Clin. Pharmacol. Ther.* 91:303–309.

Murrough, J.W., and Charney D.S. (2012). Is there anything really novel on the antidepressant horizon? *Curr. Psychiat. Rep.* [Epub ahead of print.]

Narasimhan, S., and Lohoff, F.W. (2012). Pharmacogenetics of antidepressant drugs: current clinical practice and future directions. *Pharmacogenomics* 13(4):441–464.

Nemeroff, C.B., Entsuah, R., et al. (2008).Comprehensive analysis of remission (COMPARE) with venlafaxine versus SSRIs. *Biol. Psychiatry* 63(4):424–434.

Neumeister, A., Willeit, M., et al. (2001). Dopamine transporter availability in symptomatic depressed patients with seasonal affective disorder and healthy controls. *Psychol. Med.* 31(8):1467–1473.

Ng, R.C., Hirata, C.K., et al. (2010).Pharmacologic treatment for postpartum depression: a systematic review. *Pharmacotherapy* 30(9):928–941.

Nierenberg, A.A., Fava, M., et al. (2006a). A comparison of lithium and T(3) augmentation following two failed medication treatments for depression: a STAR*D report. *Am. J. Psychiatry* 163(9):1519–1530.

Nierenberg, A.A., Ostacher, M.J., et al. (2006b).Treatment-resistant bipolar depression: a STEP-BD equipoise randomized effectiveness trial of antidepressant augmentation with lamotrigine, inositol, or risperidone. *Am. J. Psychiatry* 163(2):210–216.

Nunes, E.V., and Levin, F.R. (2004). Treatment of depression in patients with alcohol or other drug dependence: a meta-analysis. *JAMA* 291(15):1887–1896.

Nutt, D.J. (2008). Relationship of neurotransmitters to the symptoms of major depressive disorder. *J. Clin. Psychiatry* 69(Suppl E1):4–7.

O'Reardon, J.P., Solvason, H.B., et al. (2007). Efficacy and safety of transcranial magnetic stimulation in the acute treatment of major depression: a multisite randomized controlled trial. *Biol. Psychiatry* 62(11):1208–1216.

Papakostas, G.I. (2009). Evidence for S-adenosyl-L-methionine (SAM-e) for the treatment of major depressive disorder. *J. Clin. Psychiatry* 70(Suppl 5):18–22.

Papakostas, G.I., and Fava M. (2006). A metaanalysis of clinical trials comparing moclobemide with selective serotonin reuptake inhibitors for the treatment of major depressive disorder. *Can. J. Psychiatry* 51(12):783–790.

Papakostas, G.I., and Fava M. (2007a). A meta-analysis of clinical trials comparing the serotonin (5HT)-2 receptor antagonists trazodone and nefazodone with selective serotonin reuptake inhibitors for the treatment of major depressive disorder. *Eur. Psychiatry* 22(7):444–447.

Papakostas, G.I., Homberger, C.H., et al. (2008b). A meta-analysis of clinical trials comparing mirtazapine with selective serotonin reuptake inhibitors for the treatment of major depressive disorder. *J. Psychopharmacol.* 22(8):843–848.

Papakostas, G.I., Mischoulon, D., et al. (2010). S-adenosyl methionine (SAMe) augmentation of serotonin reuptake inhibitors for antidepressant nonresponders with major depressive disorder: a double-blind, randomized clinical trial. *Am. J. Psychiatry* 167(8):942–948.

Papakostas, G.I., Nelson, J.C., et al. (2008a). A meta-analysis of clinical trials comparing reboxetine, a norepinephrine reuptake inhibitor, with selective serotonin reuptake inhibitors for the treatment of major depressive disorder. *Eur. Neuropsychopharmacol.* 18(2):122–127.

Papakostas, G.I., Perlis, R.H., et al. (2006). A meta-analysis of early sustained response rates between antidepressants and placebo for the treatment of major depressive disorder. *J. Clin. Psychopharmacol.* 26(1):56–60.

Papakostas, G.I., Shelton, R.C., et al. (2007b). Augmentation of antidepressants with atypical antipsychotic medications for treatment-resistant major depressive disorder: a meta-analysis. *J. Clin. Psychiatry* 68(6):826–831.

Papakostas, G.I., Thase, M.E., et al. (2007c). Are antidepressant drugs that combine serotonergic and noradrenergic mechanisms of action more effective than the selective serotonin reuptake inhibitors in treating major depressive disorder?: a meta-analysis of studies of newer agents. *Biol. Psychiatry* 62(11):1217–1227.

Patil, A.S., Kuller, J.A., et al. (2011).Antidepressants in pregnancy: a review of commonly prescribed medications. *Obstet. Gynecol. Surv.* 66(12):777–787.

Perlis, R.H. (2011).Translating biomarkers to clinical practice. *Mol Psychiatry* 16:1076–1087.

Perry, P.J. (1996). Pharmacotherapy for major depression with melancholic features: relative efficacy of tricyclic versus selective serotonin reuptake inhibitor antidepressants. *J. Affect. Disord.* 39(1):1–6.

Perry, P.J., Zeilmann, C., et al. (1994).Tricyclic antidepressant concentrations in plasma: an estimate of their sensitivity and specificity as a predictor of response. *J. Clin. Psychopharmacol.* 14(4):230–240.

Posternak, M.A., and Zimmerman, M. (2002). Partial validation of the atypical features subtype of major depressive disorder. *Arch. Gen. Psychiatry* 59:70–76.

Prudic, J., Olfson, M., et al. (2004). Effectiveness of electroconvulsive therapy in community settings. *Biol. Psychiatry* 55(3):301–312.

Reynolds, C.F., 3rd, Dew, M.A., et al. (2006). Maintenance treatment of major depression in old age. *N. Engl. J. Med.* 354:1130–1138.

Richelson, E. (2003). Interactions of antidepressants with neurotransmitter transporters and receptors and their clinical relevance. *J. Clin. Psychiatry* 64 Suppl 13:5–12.

Richelson, E., and Nelson, A. (1984). Antagonism by antidepressants of neurotransmitter receptors of normal human brain *in vitro. J. Pharmacol. Exp. Ther.* 230(1):94–102.

Rohan, M., Parow, A., et al. (2004). Low-field magnetic stimulation in bipolar depression using an MRI-based stimulator. *Am. J. Psychiatry* 161(1):93–98.

Rothschild, A.J. (2003). Challenges in the treatment of depression with psychotic features. *Biol. Psychiatry* 53:680–690.

Rush, A.J., et al. (2006b). Acute and longer-term outcomes in depressed outpatients requiring one or several treatment steps: a STAR*D report. *Am. J. Psychiatry* 163(11):1905–1917.

Rush, A.J., et al. (2009). STAR*D: revising conventional wisdom. *CNS Drugs* 23(8):627–647.

Rush, A.J., Kraemer, H.C., et al. (2006a). Report by the ACNP Task Force on Response and Remission in Major Depressive Disorder. *Neuropsychopharmacology* 31(9):1841–1853.

Rush, A.J., Trivedi, M.H., et al. (2011). Combining medications to enhance depression outcomes (CO-MED): acute and long-term outcomes of a single-blind randomized study. *Am. J. Psychiatry* 168(7):689–701.

Sackeim, H.A., Haskett, R.F., et al. (2001). Continuation pharmacotherapy in the prevention of relapse following electroconvulsive therapy: a randomized controlled trial. *JAMA* 285(10):1299–1307.

Sachs, G.S., Nierenberg, A.A., et al. (2007). Effectiveness of adjunctive antidepressant treatment for bipolar depression. *N. Engl. J. Med.* 356(17):1711–1722.

Schildkraut, J.J. (1965). The catecholamine hypothesis of affective disorders: a review of supporting evidence. *Am. J. Psychiatry* 122(5):509–522.

Schutter, D.J. (2009). Antidepressant efficacy of high-frequency transcranial magnetic stimulation over the left dorsolateral prefrontal cortex in double-blind sham-controlled designs: a meta-analysis. *Psychol. Med.* 39(1):65–75.

Simon, G.E., Khandker, R.K., et al. (2006). Recovery from depression predicts lower health services costs. *J. Clin. Psychiatry* 67(8):1226–1231.

Sindrup, S.H., Otto, M., et al. (2005). Antidepressants in the treatment of neuropathic pain. *Basic. Clin. Pharmacol. Toxicol.* 96(6):399–409.

Sockol, L.E., Epperson, C.N., et al. (2011). A meta-analysis of treatments for perinatal depression. *Clin. Psychol. Rev.* 31(5):839–849.

Stahl, S.M., Fava, M., et al. (2010). Agomelatine in the treatment of major depressive disorder: an 8-week, multicenter, randomized, placebo-controlled trial. *J. Clin. Psychiatry* 71(5):616–626.

Stewart, J.W., McGrath, P.J., et al. (2009). DSM-IV depression with atypical features: is it valid? *NeuroPsychopharmacology* 34(13):2625–2632.

Suppes, T., Marangell, L.B., et al. (2008). A single blind comparison of lithium and lamotrigine for the treatment of bipolar II depression. *J. Affect. Disord.* 111(2–3):334–343.

Thaler, K., Delivuk, M., et al. (2011). Second-generation antidepressants for seasonal affective disorder. *Cochrane Database Syst. Rev.* (12):CD008591.

Thase, M.E., Friedman, E.S., et al. (2007). Cognitive therapy versus medication in augmentation and switch strategies as second-step treatments: a STAR*D report. *Am. J. Psychiatry* 164(5):739–752.

Thase, M.E., Haight, B.R., et al. (2005). Remission rates following antidepressant therapy with bupropion or selective serotonin reuptake inhibitors: a meta-analysis of original data from 7 randomized controlled trials. *J. Clin. Psychiatry* 66(8):974–981.

Thase, M.E., Trivedi, M.H., et al. (1995). MAOIs in the contemporary treatment of depression. *Neuropsychopharmacology* 12(3):185–219.

Tohen, M., Vieta, E., et al. (2003). Efficacy of olanzapine and olanzapine-fluoxetine combination in the treatment of bipolar I depression. *Arch. Gen. Psychiatry* 60(11):1079–1088.

Trivedi, M., Rush, A., et al. (2006). Evaluation of outcomes with citalopram for depression using measurement-based care in STAR*D: implications for clinical practice. *Am. J. Psychiatry* 163(1):28–40.

Walker, S.E., Shulman, K.I., et al. (1996). Tyramine content of previously restricted foods in monoamine oxidase inhibitor diets. *J. Clin. Psychopharmacol.* 16(5):383–388.

Wecker, L., James, S., et al. (2003). Transdermal selegiline: targeted effects on monoamine oxidases in the brain. *Biol. Psychiatry* 54(10):1099–1104.

Zarate, C.A., Jr., Singh, J.B., et al. (2006). A randomized trial of an N-methyl-D-aspartate antagonist in treatment-resistant major depression. *Arch. Gen. Psychiatry* 63:856–864.

SECTION V | ANXIETY DISORDERS

KERRY J. RESSLER

Anxiety disorders affect up to 30% of the population in their lifetime, and a large portion of suicides involve comorbid anxiety. Despite these statistics, anxiety disorders are often underappreciated and understudied. However, beyond the morbidity, mortality, and impairment associated with anxiety is the increasing awareness that these disorders are quite tractable from the perspective of neuroscience. Recent work on the basic neurobiology of fear and fear-related disorders has combined with over 100 years of psychological understanding of conditioned emotional responses and tremendous new tools to dissect the neural circuitry of fear. Together, these approaches have led to very exciting progress into the molecular genetics; cellular and systems neural circuitry; and neural processing, behavioral, and diagnostic implications for the class of mental disorders we call anxiety.

The section begins with an overview of current diagnostic nosology combined with progress in our understanding of etiology, at bio-psycho-social levels, of the shared and different underpinnings of some of these disorders (Chapter 39). This is followed by an update on state-of-the art genetics of anxiety disorders, ranging from heritability studies in large twin samples to recent candidate and hypothesis-neutral-based gene association studies (Chapter 40). Although the genetics of anxiety has somewhat lagged behind other mental disorders, it is widely felt that because of the terrific models to circuitry-level understanding, as genetics catches up, it will be integrated into a scaffold of neural understanding of fear and anxiety, leading to rapid advances.

Progress in the neurobiology of behavior has no greater models of success than work in the area of neurobiology of fear. The central role of amygdala and of other associated brain regions involved in modulating amygdala function are clearly outlined in Chapter 41, which serves as a substrate for many of the subsequent chapters focused on further dissecting the emotion of fear regulation in mammalian systems. Chapter 42 examines the differential roles of the inhibitory GABA receptor population in regulating emotion, fear, and anxiety-like behavior. The inhibitory neuronal population and its accompanying GABA receptors are enormously heterogeneous and complex, and yet the multiple methods of controlling activity, with temporal, spatial, and regional specificity, provide much of the richness of brain function. The most classic anxiolytics such as benzodiazepines, as well as some of the most novel hypnotics and cognitive enhancers, rely on specific targeting of differential GABA subunits. Chapter 43 further dissects regulation of the fear and anxiety modulatory systems by reviewing very recent updates in our understanding of prefrontal cortex control over emotion and anxiety. This chapter, primarily focused on animal models, is complemented by Chapter 45, which updates our understanding of human functional neurocircuitry from the perspective of recent neuroimaging studies of anxiety disorders.

Most anxiety disorders have their antecedent in development. Fascinating new studies in animal models have demonstrated that there are emotional "critical periods" of fear development and inhibition that may be akin to the types of critical periods that the field of neuroscience is familiar with in sensory system development. Chapter 44 outlines some of these new approaches detailing exciting advances in circuit and behavioral systems development.

The final chapters within this section focus on novel and developing treatments for anxiety disorders, including both psychological and cognitive (Chapter 46) and pharmacological approaches (Chapter 47), many of which have been rationally developed based on the preceding understanding of the neurobiology of the circuitry and pharmacology of fear and anxiety-like behaviors. The final two chapters examine the neurobiology and treatment of obsessive-compulsive disorder (Chapter 48) and posttraumatic stress disorder (Chapter 49), two of the most debilitating and refractory anxiety disorders. However, as these chapters illustrate, an enormous amount of progress has been made in recent years related to the neural underpinnings of these disorders, and this advanced understanding is leading to promising new approaches to treatment and prevention. Together, we hope that this entirely new section on anxiety disorders helps the reader appreciate the enormous progress in this area over the last few years. We are very excited that rapid advances in the neurobiology of fear- and anxiety-related behaviors have translated remarkably well to humans. This progress suggests that these disorders may be particularly tractable as affective neuroscience continues to improve, providing a model for other mental illnesses in the translation of basic neuroscience to novel and more powerful treatment and prevention efforts.

SECTION V | ANXIETY DISORDERS

KERRY J. RESSLER

39 | DIAGNOSIS OF ANXIETY DISORDERS

MEGHAN E. KEOUGH, MURRAY B. STEIN, AND PETER P. ROY-BYRNE

THE CURRENT NOSOLOGICAL MODEL

Over the past 60 years, the conceptualization and diagnosis of psychiatric disorders has experienced substantial growth and transformation. Unlike the recent DSMs (*Diagnostic and Statistical Manuals*), the first two editions in 1952 and 1968 did not provide explicit categorical criteria sets and were rooted in the psychodynamic perspective that psychiatric symptoms reflect disguised psychological conflicts rather than disease states (American Psychiatric Association, 1952, 1968). The lack of standardized classification resulted in professionals operating largely based on their own personal beliefs and training, which resulted in substantial variability across individuals and institutions (Mayes and Horowitz, 2005). The publication of the DSM-III (1980) drew from work initiated in 1972 by a group of Washington University researchers (Feighner et al., 1972) and expanded in 1978 as the Research Diagnostic Criteria (RDC) by Spitzer and colleagues (1978). It emphasized an atheoretically derived group of symptom criteria designed to yield reliable diagnoses that, whenever possible, would also predict course of illness, family history, and treatment response (i.e., "predictive validity"). At the time, these investigators also hoped that biological variables might someday be included as diagnostic validators.

While these changes were built upon expanding scientific knowledge, the DSM-III changes also reflected political viewpoints within the mental health field, increased government involvement in mental health research, and pressure from insurance and pharmaceutical companies (Mayes and Horowitz, 2005). Subsequent revisions to the DSM-III and DSM-IV have further attempted to enhance both the reliability and the validity of the diagnostic criteria. One major revision in the DSM-III-R was the removal of the DSM-III hierarchical structure, which among other things, dictated that an individual could not be diagnosed with an anxiety disorder if depressed (American Psychiatric Association, 1980, 1987).

The current nosological model of the modern DSMs, while not without fault, has facilitated significant research growth in the anxiety disorders field over the past three decades, spurring scientific progress in our understanding of pathophysiology and the identification of effective treatments. It has allowed researchers to more reliably conceptualize a population of interest and clinicians to more reliably identify their patients' diagnoses. The DSM is now extensively used around the world by clinicians, researchers, health insurance companies, pharmaceutical companies, funding agencies, and policymakers. This has created a shared language regarding psychiatric illness within and across these different professional stakeholders.

While the modern DSMs have bolstered the conceptualization and treatment of anxiety disorders, the current system continues to fall short of its fundamental goals of establishing a reliable and valid classification of mental disorders. While reliability has been largely achieved with the DSM-III and DSM-IV, a number of issues suggest that the validity of the diagnostic system has yet to be achieved. Among these issues are criticisms that the high rate of comorbidity among the disorders indicates an unwarranted splitting of underlying entities. The polythetic criterion, the requirement that only some criteria be present for diagnostic threshold to be met, has been criticized as resulting in widely disparate symptom presentations for the same diagnosis (i.e., two patients could meet criteria for the same disorder while having few, if any, overlapping symptoms). Others note that many clinically distressed individuals do not meet diagnostic criteria for any of the specific diagnoses, and subsequently, this results in an overreliance on not-otherwise-specified (NOS) diagnoses. Finally, and perhaps most importantly, because the current diagnoses developed apart from genetic and neuroimaging research that seeks to clarify the causes and mechanisms of psychiatric illness, the results of this emerging research do not necessarily align with current diagnostic conceptualizations. The DSM-5, currently in its final stages of development, hopes to address some of these criticisms.

PROPOSED REVISIONS IN DSM-5

BACKGROUND

The American Psychiatric Association is currently in the process of revising the DSM-IV to yield the DSM-5. The revisions are intended to incorporate the wealth of research that the field has generated in the past two decades, to maintain continuity with DSM-IV where possible, and to place the highest priority on clinical utility (American Psychiatric Association 2012a). The process has included preplanning white papers, a series of 13 planning conferences, and appointment of chair, vice-chair, and Work Group members. The DSM-5 development process has made use of systematic literature reviews, several rounds of public feedback, and extensive input from professional and consumer stakeholders. The release and publication of the DSM-5 is projected to coincide with the APA's annual conference in May 2013.

Whereas this chapter is focused on anxiety disorders and the specific changes to these disorders as outlined in what follows, there are a number of general changes that will affect this category. First, the diagnoses previously included in the chapter "Disorders Usually First Diagnosed in Infancy, Childhood, or

Adolescence" are now incorporated into other chapters by noting their developmental continuity with adult disorders. Thus, separation anxiety disorder is now listed first in the anxiety disorders chapter. Second, the current revisions have also placed an emphasis on the additional dimensional assessment of psychiatric disorders. The categorical diagnostic system utilized in the previous DSMs is not being replaced by a dimensional system; however, there is an acknowledgment that measurement-based care that utilizes dimensional measures is feasible and would be of benefit to routine clinical care (Regier et al., 2012). Adding these measures will potentially allow for both a more nuanced conceptualization of patients' psychiatric disorders and a more objective monitoring of patients' progress throughout therapy. Thus, accompanying the proposed revisions of each anxiety disorder is a note of whether a psychometrically sound measure currently exists. In addition, each anxiety disorder includes two newly developed measures that are being tested for these purposes (the first designed to assess the severity of the specific anxiety disorder and the second designed to assess severity across all anxiety disorders).

Revisions to the anxiety disorders chapter were the responsibility of the Anxiety, Obsessive-Compulsive Spectrum, Posttraumatic, and Dissociative Disorders Work Group (referred from this point on in the chapter as the Anxiety Work Group). The Anxiety Work Group commissioned a series of literature reviews that were published in the peer-reviewed journal *Depression and Anxiety*. Proposed recommendations were informed by these reviews as well as secondary data analyses of existing datasets, collection of new data, surveys of experts and input and data provided by advisors and liaisons, DSM-5 Task Force members, other members of the research community, and other stakeholders (Phillips et al., 2010). The overarching approach continues to emphasize a search for associated factors that might "validate" these diagnostic categories, but has expanded beyond symptom measures, course of illness, family history and treatment response, to include, wherever possible, medical and psychiatric illness comorbidities, genetic and environmental risk factors, temperamental and personality antecedents, cognitive and emotional processing response measures, and neurocircuitry.

ANXIETY-RELATED DISORDERS *ON THE MOVE*

OBSESSIVE-COMPULSIVE DISORDER

Obsessive-compulsive disorder (OCD) is characterized by anxiety-provoking obsessions and/or compulsions that are intended to ameliorate anxiety. This disorder is equally common in men and women, yet due to its earlier onset in males, is seen more often in boys than girls. It typically follows a chronic course, and studies indicate a familial risk, with first-degree relatives at higher risk for OCD (American Psychiatric Association 2000).

Much of the discussion regarding OCD and the DSM-5 has surrounded its appropriate placement within the manual. This discussion has considered whether to leave OCD as an anxiety disorder, place it in its own chapter with other disorders from the OC spectrum, or include both anxiety disorders and OCD under the same umbrella category, as is done in the ICD-10,

which places both anxiety disorders and OCD under *neurotic, stress-related, and somatoform disorders* (World Health Organization, 1993). This last option was the favorite of the majority of authors in both the Phillips et al. (2010) and Stein et al. (2010) reviews. However, OCD researchers were mixed regarding their approval (60%) of the removal of OCD from the supraordinate anxiety category (Mataix-Cols et al., 2007), and clinical psychiatrists and "other professionals," largely psychologists, showed a significant difference in opinion (75% agreed versus 40%–45%, respectively). Stein et al. (2010) outlined the research from a series of validators (e.g., neurocircuitry; course of illness; treatment response; and genetic, familial, and environmental risk factors) regarding OCD's appropriate placement. While there are some uniquely distinctive aspects to OCD (involvement of fronto-striatal neurocircuitry and related deficits, a narrower range of effective medications and a clear dose–response pattern to SRI medication response, and a unique association with basal ganglia neurologic disorders), there is still much overlap with anxiety disorders in multiple other domains (e.g., comorbidity, family history). Generally, these results present a mixed picture providing both support for the inclusion of OCD within the anxiety disorders and its removal. Nevertheless, DSM-5 will move OCD to the *Obsessive-Compulsive and Related Disorders* category along with several other disorders including body dysmorphic disorder, hoarding, hair pulling (trichotillomania), and skin picking. These disorders are all characterized by repetitive, anxiety- or dysphoria-inducing thoughts and/or behaviors (designed at reducing the discomfort). While genetic, neural, and biomarker validators that support this new category are few, several other validators link these disorders with OCD or one another, including high comorbidity, similar psychopharmacology and psychotherapy response, and evidence of familial transmission (Phillips et al., 2010).

Proposed changes to the OCD criteria have been made and include moving the two items from the obsessions definition that sought to distinguish obsessions from GAD (generalized anxiety disorder; obsessions are not simply excessive worries regarding life problems) and psychosis (the individual recognized that the obsessional thoughts, impulses, or images are not created by an external force but rather are a product of his or her own mind) and placing them in Criterion D among the other diagnostic hierarchy issues (Leckman et al., 2010). Additionally, the requirement that individuals recognize that their symptoms are excessive was removed, and the poor insight specifier was replaced with specifiers indicting a range of insight (i.e., good or fair insight, poor insight, or absent insight). Finally, suggestions are made for dimensional measures. Previously validated measures include the Yale-Brown Obsessive-Compulsive Scale (Y-BOCS; Goodman et al., 1989), the Florida Obsessive-Compulsive Inventory (FOCI; Storch et al., 2007), and the Brown Assessment of Beliefs Scale (BABS; Eisen et al., 1998). A newly developed five-item questionnaire is also included and currently being tested.

POSTTRAUMATIC STRESS DISORDER

Posttraumatic stress disorder (PTSD) can develop following exposure to a traumatic event and is characterized by reexperiencing the trauma, avoidance of traumatic cues, and increased symptomatic arousal. Evidence suggests that the development of PTSD following trauma is affected by social supports, childhood experiences, personality variables, type of trauma, and preexisting mental disorders (American Psychiatric Association, 2000). Additionally, genetic factors appear to affect the likelihood of developing the disorder (Stein et al., 2002).

Like OCD, much of the DSM-5 focus on PTSD has surrounded its most appropriate placement within the DSM. Stress-related fear circuitry findings from neuroimaging and fear conditioning studies, among other findings, support the retention of PTSD within the anxiety disorders (Friedman et al., 2011a). But PTSD frequently encompasses a broader range of emotions (e.g., numbing, guilt, alienation) than other anxiety disorders and shares a unique precipitating event (all cases are trauma induced). Emphasizing common etiology over symptom similarity, it has been concluded that PTSD should be placed in a newly formed category that includes disorders that are precipitated by a "serious life event" (the *Trauma-and Stressor-Related Disorders*). PTSD's anticipated departure from the anxiety disorders has met strong criticism. Zoellner et al. (2011) note that the "rationale for this shift is unclear, underdeveloped, and unsupported" (p. 853) and delineate four main points that support retaining PTSD as an anxiety disorder: (1) fear is a critical component of PTSD, (2) the treatment of fear and avoidance is central to PTSD as it is with other anxiety disorders, (3) the evidence base does not support a separate category, and (4) reclassification moves the PTSD field away from its well-developed knowledge base.

The diagnostic criteria for PTSD are lengthier than most other diagnoses, and efforts at their improvement have been a frequent focus in previous revisions of the DSM. DSM-5, alas, will do nothing to simplify or shorten the diagnostic criteria. However, several of the proposed revisions to the PTSD criteria within the DSM-5 reflect substantial changes. Criterion A1, defining the nature of the traumatic event, has been retained, but the description of what constitutes an index traumatic event has been articulated in greater detail. Criterion A2, requiring an emotional response of fear, helplessness, or horror in response to the trauma, has been eliminated. One reason for its removal is that some individuals (e.g., military personnel, who in deployment situations are trained *not* to have a response like this) lack this type of emotional response at the time of the event but, nonetheless, can develop PTSD (Friedman et al., 2011b). Because of confirmatory factor analyses that indicate strongest support for a four-factor model (Friedman et al., 2011b), the DSM-5 is proposing splitting the current three-factor model (Criterion B—intrusion, C—avoidance, and D—heightened arousal) into a four-factor model by splitting Criterion C and adding symptoms to the newly formed Criterion D (negative cognitions and mood). There are also a number of other specific changes to the individual criteria. In an effort to enhance cross-cultural applicability of the criteria, the intrusion symptom regarding dreams about the trauma has been revised to include both trauma content or affect about the trauma (Hinton and Lewis-Fernandez, 2011). As the previous C category has been split in two with only two types of avoidance retained, the criteria now require only one to be endorsed. The new category D has two new symptoms, blame and negative emotional state (which, on the face of it, will overlap tremendously with major depressive symptoms), and the previous symptom of a foreshortened future has been expanded to encompass exaggerated negative beliefs and expectations to help expand the applicability to other cultures. Category E also has a new symptom that focuses on reckless and destructive behavior.

Friedman et al. (2011b) also conclude that there is insufficient research to support the acute versus chronic specifier and thus it has been eliminated. However, they conclude that there is support for both a dissociative subtype and a preschool subtype. There is evidence to suggest that individuals whose PTSD is characterized by dissociative symptoms demonstrate distinct prefrontal responses and a decrease in heart rate and skin conductance to trauma cues/memories (Friedman et al., 2011b). Traumatized preschool age children do develop PTSD but at lower rates than other age groups, which likely reflect, at least in part, that the current diagnostic criteria do not accurately capture the disorder among preschoolers. Thus, the revised diagnostic criteria for the preschool subtype is meant to more readily identify PTSD in these young people by being more developmentally sensitive and behaviorally anchored (Scheeringa et al., 2011). For a dimensional measure of PTSD, the Web site suggests the unpublished nine-item National Stressful Events Survey PTSD Short Scale (American Psychiatric Association, 2011).

MIXED ANXIETY/DEPRESSION DISORDER

Mixed anxiety/depression disorder (MADD) is characterized by dysphoric mood that is accompanied by symptoms of both anxiety and depression and is considered to be subordinate to anxiety and mood disorders (not considered if diagnostic criteria for one of these disorders has been met). Empirical work on this disorder and its validators is sparse.

While included as an official diagnosis in the ICD-10, MADD was relegated in DSM-IV to *Criteria Sets and Axes Provided for Further Study* (American Psychiatric Association 2000). Initial versions of the DSM-5 revisions moved MADD to mood disorders. This proposed move was met with intense criticism from a variety of standpoints, including MADD's remarkably poor reliability as well as the paucity of validating data (e.g., First, 2011; Frances, 2012; Wakefield, 2012). On the heels of this criticism, the most recent DSM-5 revisions have moved MADD back to the section reserved for conditions requiring further study (where it had been placed in DSM-IV). This is, admittedly, an unorthodox move on the part of the DSM-5 framers. If the past 20 years was not enough time to study MADD, it seems unlikely that more specific criteria will result in a boon of research. A more judicious approach would have been to delete MADD altogether.

SEPARATION ANXIETY DISORDER

This disorder is expressed as developmentally excessive anxiety in the face of separation from the home or an attachment figure. While it is more common among females, representation among the sexes is equal in clinical samples. The risk of developing separation anxiety disorder is elevated for children of mothers with panic disorder.

Despite clinically significant impairment as children, those with this disorder often do not have a disproportionate rate of anxiety disorders as adults (American Psychiatric Association, 2000).

Because of the redistribution of disorders previously included in the *Disorder Usually First Diagnosed in Infancy, Childhood or Adolescence,* separation anxiety disorder will be included in the *Anxiety Disorders* section of the DSM-5. The literature that the Anxiety Work Group relied upon to make the DSM-5 proposed changes to separation anxiety disorder is not publicly available at this time. But the proposed changes to the diagnosis are available and include removal of the criterion that onset occurs prior to age 18, further differentiating the DSM from the ICD-10 criteria that requires an age of onset prior to 6 (World Health Organization, 1993). The specifier "early-onset" has also been removed.

ANXIETY DISORDERS

AGORAPHOBIA

Agoraphobia (AG) is characterized by a fear of being in situations in which escape may be difficult or in which help may not be readily available. While not *on the move* to a different chapter as are the diagnoses in the previous section, the revisions to the DSM-5 have moved AG from subordinate to panic (i.e., necessarily attributing the avoidance of situations to a fear of panic-related symptoms) to an independent disorder, a status it originally held in the DSM-III. This will be consistent with how agoraphobia is treated by DSM's international counterpart, the ICD (International Classification of Diseases; World Health Organization, 1993).

This decision was made despite remaining questions and controversy, as the authors of the literature review indicate that they reached a consensus in their recommendations but that the consensus was not unanimous (Wittchen et al., 2010). However, the decision was supported by familial genetic data, psychiatric history, patterns of comorbidity, course of illness, treatment response, and reliability (American Psychiatric Association, 2012b). This evidence, reviewed by Wittchen et al. (2010), highlights that AG without panic-like symptoms does occur (in epidemiologic studies) and is associated with significant disability and a persistent course with low rates of spontaneous recovery. Thus, while the majority of AG cases *do* occur in the presence of panic disorder, panic attacks, or panic-like symptoms, that does not uniformly demonstrate that AG is a function of panic.

The proposed criteria for AG are more specific than in DSM-IV to improve differential diagnosis. Criteria A lists five different groups of agoraphobic situations, provides several examples of each group, and requires the endorsement of one situation from two or more groups. Additionally, the new criteria include a six-month duration requirement to avoid unnecessarily pathologizing transient fear. In addition to the two newly developed dimensional measures, The Fear Questionnaire-Agoraphobia Subscale (Marks and Mathews, 1979) is listed as a previously validated dimensional measure, but specific recommendations regarding its use are not included at this time.

PANIC DISORDER

Panic disorder (PD) is characterized by discrete periods of sudden and intense physiological symptoms and fear (i.e., panic attacks [PAs]) that result in persistent concern about additional PAs or a change in behavior (avoidance, emergency department visits, seeking medical diagnostic tests). Age of onset for this disorder varies but is generally between late adolescence and mid-30s. Twin studies suggest a genetic contribution to the disorder, and studies indicated that familial risk is particularly elevated for first-degree relatives of those who developed PD prior to age 20 (American Psychiatric Association, 2000). Early suggestions that PD exhibited a unique pharmacological treatment response are untrue, and notions of unique psychosocial treatment response have been called into question by transdiagnostic cognitive behavioral therapy approaches (e.g., Norton and Philipp, 2008).

As PAs are a crucial piece of PD, the Anxiety Work Group–commissioned review of evidence focused on questions related both to PAs and PD (Craske et al., 2010). It suggested that the symptom "hot flushes" be changed to "heat sensations" to better capture cultural variants in this experience and recommended that culture-specific symptoms be included in the description of PAs but not counted as one of the four required symptoms. The extant evidence did not suggest that a change in the number of symptoms required for a PA is warranted at this time. To reinforce the paroxysmal temporal profile of panic, the wording was changed to indicate that a panic attack reaches "a peak within minutes" and "can occur from a calm state or an anxious state." There was no new evidence exploring validators of panic attack frequency to suggest that the criteria of "recurrent" PAs be modified. Due to the empirical evidence that panic attacks are associated with an increase in symptom severity, comorbidity, suicidality, and treatment resistance of comorbid disorders, a note was added indicating that PAs can serve as a specifier for both anxiety and nonanxiety disorders (e.g., schizophrenia, panic attack specifier). As noted in the previous section, agoraphobia is now a codable disorder, and thus, PD is no longer listed as PD with agoraphobia or PD without agoraphobia.

The DSM-5 Web site identifies the Panic Disorder Severity Scale-Self-Report (Houck et al., 2002) as a dimensional measure that can be utilized to assess PD severity.

SPECIFIC PHOBIA

Specific phobia (SP) is characterized by clinically significant distress or anxiety in response to a specific feared object or situation. While it is more commonly found among women, the sex difference varies by type (e.g., animal and situational). Evidence indicates that familial risk seems to aggregate by type and that blood injection injury–type fears have a particularly strong family link. The symptoms of SP usually first emerge in childhood or midadolescence, and for those that persist into adulthood, remission is infrequent (American Psychiatric Association, 2000). There is some research suggesting neural differences between SP types, but this research remains at a nascent stage (LeBeau et al., 2010).

The diagnostic criteria for SP, which was referred to as simple phobia prior to the DSM-IV, have seen several modifications in preparation for the DSM-5 revisions. The review by LeBeau and colleagues (2010) focused on four main areas: the accuracy and utility of the specific phobia type classification, the validity of test anxiety as a type of SP, the boundary between agoraphobia and SP, and the reliability and utility of the specific phobia criteria. The general conclusion of the review is that the extant literature does support the retention of the specific phobia types as a descriptive option; that little evidence exists either for or against the inclusion of test anxiety as a type of SP; and similarly, that there is insufficient evidence to reclassify agoraphobia as a type of SP. Finally, LeBeau and colleagues (2010) reviewed the SP criteria and made recommendations about rewording and reordering the specific criteria in order to enhance consistency across anxiety disorders and improve clinical utility and ease of use. The criterion that one recognize that his or her fear is excessive or unreasonable has been removed, as it is common for adults to deny that their fear is excessive or unreasonable (LeBeau et al., 2010). Due to research indicating that transient fears and phobias occur among adults (LeBeau et al., 2010), the duration criterion of six months for those under the age of 18 has been extended to all age groups. Currently, the Web site does not recommend any specific dimensional scales for measurement-based care, since most measures assess one specific type of SP; however, two newly developed alternative scales focusing on severity of SP and of anxiety in general are now being tested.

SOCIAL ANXIETY DISORDER

Social anxiety disorder (SAD) is characterized by a marked fear of social and performance situations that often results in avoidance of those situations. Epidemiological data suggest that it is more common among women than men but that the sexes are equally represented in clinical populations. Onset typically occurs by late teens and can be either insidious or abrupt. The course of SAD is typically continuous and lifelong. Increased familial risk among first-degree relatives is particularly strong for the generalized type (American Psychiatric Association, 2000).

Social phobia is currently the official name for this diagnosis, but the term *social anxiety disorder* was added in parentheses following this title in the DSM-IV-TR to reflect that this is a broader diagnosis rather than just a circumscribed phobia (Bogels et al., 2010). Much of the Work Group review focused on the SAD specifiers. The DSM-5 framers have elected to delete the "generalized" specifier for SAD, arguing that there was considerable heterogeneity within this category. Instead, a performance-only specifier was introduced, supported by evidence that there are qualitative differences these individuals demonstrate from others with SAD (later onset, not characterized by childhood factors of shyness or behavioral inhibition, not familial, a stronger physiological response, and more likely to respond to beta blockers). In theory, if an individual with SAD does not meet the performance-only specifier, then he or she would be highly likely to have what had been called *generalized SAD* in DSM-IV. The merits of this change remain to be determined, whereas the disadvantages of disconnecting from two decades of research and over a thousand PubMed references to generalized SAD are obvious.

Selective mutism, listed in DSM-IV as a separate diagnosis in *Disorders Usually First Diagnosed in Infancy, Childhood, or Adolescence*, had tentatively been proposed as a SAD specifier since the majority of those with selective mutism have SAD, there are very high rates of SAD among parents of children with selective mutism, and preliminary treatment evidence suggests that psychological and pharmacological treatments that are effective for SAD are also effective for selective mutism. It was ultimately decided, however, to situate selective mutism as a separate diagnosis within the Anxiety Disorders section, apparently to encourage further attention to factors which may distinguish selective mutism from SAD (e.g., developmental language or speech problems).

Revisions to the SAD criteria also evaluated the comorbidity between SAD and avoidant personality disorder (AVPD), thought by some to be a more severe version of SAD rather than a qualitatively distinct disorder. Alden, Laposa et al. (2002) report that AVPD studies investigating the comorbidity of SAD note an average comorbidity of 42% with SAD, which is considerably lower than one would anticipate if AVPD were synonymous with severe SAD. Genetic studies indicate a link between SAD and AVPD, but this link does not appear to be specific to these two disorders (Bogels et al., 2010). Similarly, psychological and pharmacological treatment studies indicate a similar response style between the two disorders; however, numerous other disorders also respond to these treatments. In addition, there are some indications that AVPD shares links with the schizophrenia spectrum (Bogels et al., 2010). Based in part on these findings, it was concluded that while these two have a high degree of overlap, it is too simplistic to consider AVPD a severe form of SAD (Bogels et al., 2010). Thus, the DSM-5 revisions will not collapse these two disorders.

Additional revisions to the SAD criteria include the expansion of the types of social situations that are avoided to include social interaction, observation, and performance with examples of each provided. To increase the cultural sensitivity of the diagnosis, the feared consequence of offending others has been added to the previously listed fear of negative evaluation. The criteria no longer require the individual to recognize that his or her fear is excessive but does require the fear to be out of proportion to the actual threat posed. This acknowledges that some patients do not see their fear as excessive, but they are clearly not psychotic, and it is sufficient for the clinician to assess the excessiveness of the fear. Finally, the duration criterion of six months has been extended beyond those under the age of 18 to now apply across all age ranges, as it was noted that adults can also experience transient social anxiety, which might result in overdiagnosis.

In addition to the two newly developed dimensional measures, the Web site lists two previously published measures, the Social Phobia Inventory (Connor et al., 2000) and Mini-Social Phobia Inventory (Connor et al., 2001), along with a brief description of each.

GENERALIZED ANXIETY DISORDER

Generalized anxiety disorder (GAD) is characterized by clinically significant worry and anxiety that is disproportionate to the circumstances and persists for at least six months. While adult onset is not uncommon, approximately half of the individuals who present for treatment report childhood or adolescent onset. Course of this disorder is generally chronic but often worsens in times of stress. Twin studies indicate a genetic contribution to the development of GAD (American Psychiatric Association, 2000).

The diagnosis of GAD has been encumbered by poor reliability and substantial comorbidity with mood and anxiety disorders since its first inclusion in DSM-III. Revisions to subsequent versions have attempted to remedy this situation. Likewise, the proposed revisions by Andrews et al. (2010) are meant to further clarify the diagnosis and enhance its reliability. Included in these recommendations was reducing the duration criterion from six to three months as this would substantially increase test–retest reliability and not impact the type of patient included in terms of distress and impairment (Andrews et al., 2010). The criterion that worry is difficult to control has been removed because of a lack of validating support to indicate that it added anything to the criteria (Andrews et al., 2010). Four of the six associated symptoms of worry listed in Criterion C (being easily fatigued, difficulty concentrating or mind going blank, irritability, and sleep disturbance), are nonspecific to GAD and are being proposed for removal, retaining only the two associated symptoms that are specific to the diagnosis (restlessness or feeling keyed up or on edge and muscle tension) to enhance the GAD's discriminant validity, especially from major depressive disorder, which greatly overlaps with these nonspecific symptoms. A list of four behaviors commonly employed by individuals with GAD in an attempt to decrease their worry or ameliorate distressing affect are now proposed for inclusion (e.g., repeatedly seeking reassurance due to worries), one of which needs to be endorsed to meet the diagnostic criteria. When the specific combination of the currently proposed changes was investigated, the prevalence of the disorder increased by 9%. However, these changes did not significantly affect the distress or impairment, indicating that the severity was retained and lending support to these changes (Andrews and Hobbs, 2010). At the time of this writing, it is unclear whether the preceding changes to GAD will be accepted or not. As with the other disorders, a previously published self-report measure of severity, the GAD-7 (Spitzer et al., 2006), is included among the DSM-5 revisions for GAD.

NEED FOR A NEW NOSOLOGICAL FRAMEWORK?

As noted, the central goal of the DSM has been to create a reliable and valid diagnostic system for mental illness that has concurrent and predictive validity. The past several decades have witnessed an increase in the reliability of psychiatric diagnoses and an accumulation of knowledge surrounding associated factors, both clinical and experimental, that might serve as validators. However, much work remains as diagnoses fail to align with recent findings from neuroscience and genetics, the diagnostic boundaries are not consistent with treatment response, and current validators remain relatively limited and lacking specificity.

A recent review nicely outlines the difficulty in identifying consistent validating data to support even the broad distinction of an "anxiety" disorder from other disorders of emotional distress and misery (Craske et al., 2009). Extant evidence does suggest there is some consistency in unique, anxiety-specific findings of distinct self-report measures, elevated sensitivity to threat (based on Pavlovian conditioning paradigms), cognitive bias to threat, and specific anxiety neurocircuitry. However, inconsistency in findings across developmental stages, lack of distinction among the individual anxiety disorders, and some overlap in findings with depressive disorders continue to confound attempts to nail down even the nosological validity of anxiety disorders as a distinct group! The DSM-5 revisions attempt to incorporate new research to bolster the diagnostic system and will likely result in incremental steps toward increased diagnostic validity and reliability, but addressing the evidence base honestly requires that we recognize we are still a long way off from a goal of diagnostic entities that have the kind of pathophysiologic validity of many recognized medical disorders.

The reviews commissioned by the Anxiety Work Group clearly indicate that much empirical work is left to be done. A common theme across these reviews was the call for additional research, and in numerous instances, the authors noted that there was simply insufficient empirical evidence for them to draw conclusions regarding central questions they had been asked to review. Whereas the DSM system is not perfect, it has become indispensable as it helps to bridge researchers and clinicians and is used extensively across settings such as insurance funding, treatment, and legal proceedings (Frances and Widiger, 2012). A system based on clinical description, such as we have, cannot match the validity (and even to some degree, the reliability) of a system based on objective medical tests; however, a mental disorder diagnostic system based on objective tests remains a long-term goal rather than a reality (Bernstein, 2011). The DSM was and is still meant to be a living document that serves as a framework for both research and clinical work that can expand and change based on accumulating knowledge. The mind is very complex, and the lofty goal of carving psychiatric nature at its joints requires more clearly elucidating how it functions and how missteps along its very complicated functioning can result in psychiatric illness.

Kendler has criticized commonly held explanatory models for psychiatric illness and puts forth the need to conceptualize the causes of psychiatric illnesses with "empirically based pluralism" (e.g., Kendler, 2008, 2012). He suggests that psychiatry has had the tendency to inaccurately dichotomize the etiology of disorders because of the influence of Descartes and computer functionalism. Descartes' dualistic approach to psychiatry distinguishes between the mind (thinking) and the brain (physical) as two fundamentally separate entities and, following from this, that disorders are either organic (brain based) or functional (mind based). Similarly, Kendler points out that the advent of the computer era ushered in the functionalist perspective that our functioning runs parallel to that of computers, such that the computer hardware is synonymous with our brain and the software is synonymous with our mind. He suggests that this dichotomous thinking about mind/brain functioning continues to influence our conceptualization of the etiology of psychiatric illness, and beyond it simply being inaccurate, it has impaired our ability to integrate research from multiple domains into our understanding of psychiatric illness. In one of his articles (Kendler, 2012), he makes the case for the inaccuracy of this dualistic perspective by reviewing the biological, psychological, and higher order (social, political, and cultural) etiological effects on major depression, alcohol dependence, and schizophrenia. The presented research indicates that each of the three disorders is affected by factors from each domain and that these factors are not independent but, rather, mediate and moderate each other both within and across domains. Thus, he concludes that understanding the nature of psychiatric illnesses requires an appreciation for the complex interplay between factors from various domains that do not fit into the neat mind/brain divide. He further suggests that a pluralistic view is driven by research and not a priori theory.

On first glance, this view might seem at variance with the notion that psychiatric disorders could be mapped to definitive genetic etiologies tied to neuronal circuit pathophysiologies. However, recent meta-analyses of neuroimaging studies provide tantalizing clues that PTSD, GAD, and MDD share specific neurocircuitry characteristics (hyperactivity of the dorsal anterior cingulate cortex, which is responsible for monitoring and expression of anxiety, and hypoactivity of the ventral anterior cingulate cortex, responsible for extinguishing fear responses) that are distinct from more classic "fear disorders" like panic, social anxiety, and the phobic disorders (Etkin, 2012). Ironically, this does not accord with the proposed DSM-5 changes, as it does not suggest PTSD is unique from all anxiety and mood disorders, nor that GAD is similar to other anxiety disorders.

Related to Kendler's call for an understanding of the complex interplay between factors is NIMH's Research Domain Criteria (RDoC) project (National Institute of Mental Health, 2011). The NIMH has indicated that it will focus its funding priorities on projects that are developed within this framework. It is meant to guide research in a manner that bypasses current diagnostic systems by organizing the focus of research around the following five domains: negative affect (e.g., loss, fear, anxiety), positive affect (e.g., approach motivation, reward learning), cognitive systems (e.g., attention, perception, working memory), systems for social processes (e.g., attachment, imitation), and arousal/regulatory systems. Research into these domains is further structured around specific units of analysis: genes, molecules, cells, circuits, physiology, behavior, self-reports, and paradigms. It is noted that this initial structure is meant to be a starting point that reflects the current state of knowledge and that it will be modified and adjusted as warranted by new research findings (Sanislow et al., 2010). Within this framework, participants would *not* be selected based on current diagnostic categories, but rather, for example, a sample of all patients presenting to an anxiety clinic could be studied to investigate amygdala functioning in response to fearful stimuli (Sanislow et al., 2010). The hope is that by not restricting research to current diagnostic categories research knowledge will develop that is more apt to identify the underlying mechanisms of mental illness. RDoC efforts can be seen as providing a complementary path to that of DSM-5 for the study of mental disorders. It follows that this knowledge would eventually translate into practitioners being able to supplement clinical evaluation with functional or structural imaging, genomic sequencing, or lab-based evaluations of fear conditioning to more effectively determine prognosis and effective treatment (Insel et al., 2010).

As noted (Insel, 2009), the RDoC project is motivated by lofty long-term goals that may prove to dramatically affect the field. However, it also rests on three assumptions: mental illnesses are brain disorders, neural circuit dysfunction can be identified through tools of neuroscience, and genetic and clinical neuroscience research will provide biosignatures that will augment clinical management (Insel et al., 2010). If these assumptions turn out to be valid, then the RDoC project may lead to a revolution in our understanding of anxiety and other forms of mental illness. Until that day, DSM and its latest iteration (DSM-5) will continue to serve as the clinical guidepost for our field.

DISCLOSURES

Dr. Keough has no conflicts of interest to disclose. She currently receives NIMH funding through a National Research Service Award Institutional Training Grant (T32MH082709-01A2).

Dr. Stein is paid as co-editor-in-chief for *UpToDate in Psychiatry*, and as associate editor for the journal *Depression and Anxiety*. His research is funded by NIMH, the VA, and the Department of Defense.

Dr. Roy-Byrne has grant funding from NIDA and NIMH, receives salary for editor-in-chief duties for *Depression and Anxiety*, *UpToDate in Psychiatry*, and Journal Watch Psychiatry, and has received stock options as a consultant and advisor to Valant Medical Solutions, a behavioral health EMR company.

REFERENCES

Alden, L.E., Laposa, J.M., et al. (2002). Avoidant personality disorder: current status and future directions. *J. Pers. Disord.* 16:1–29.

American Psychiatric Association. (1952). Diagnostic and Statistical Manual of Mental Disorders, 1st Edition. Washington, DC: Author.

American Psychiatric Association. (1968). Diagnostic and Statistical Manual of Mental Disorders, 2nd Edition. Washington, DC: Author.

American Psychiatric Association. (1980). Diagnostic and Statistical Manual of Mental Disorders, 3rd Edition. Washington, DC: Author.

American Psychiatric Association. (1987). Diagnostic and Statistical Manual of Mental Disorders, 3rd Edition, Revised. Washington, DC: Author.

American Psychiatric Association. (2000). Diagnostic and Statistical Manual of Mental Disorders, 4th Edition, Text Revision. Washington, DC: Author.

American Psychiatric Association. (2011). Home / proposed revisions / trauma and stressor related disorders // G 03 posttraumatic stress disorder. http://www.dsm5.org/ProposedRevision/Pages/proposedrevision.aspx?rid=165#

American Psychiatric Association. (2012a). Frequently asked questions: why is DSM being revised? http://www.dsm5.org/about/Pages/faq.aspx

American Psychiatric Association. (2012b). Proposed revisions: agoraphobia. http://www.dsm5.org/ProposedRevision/Pages/proposedrevision.aspx?rid=405#

Andrews, G., and Hobbs, M.J. (2010). The effect of the draft DSM-5 criteria for GAD on prevalence and severity. *Aust. N. Z. J. Psychiatry* 44(9):784–790.

Andrews, G., Hobbs, M.J., et al. (2010). Generalized worry disorder: a review of DSM-IV generalized anxiety disorder and options for DSM-V. *Depress. Anxiety* 27(2):134–147.

Bernstein, C.A. (2011). Meta-structure in DSM-5 process. *Psychiatric News* 46(5):7.

Bogels, S.M., Alden, L., et al. (2010). Social anxiety disorder: questions and answers for the DSM-V. *Depress. Anxiety* 27(2):168–189.

Connor, K.M., Davidson, J.R., et al. (2000). Psychometric properties of the Social Phobia Inventory (SPIN): new self-rating scale. *Br. J. Psychiatry* 176:379–386.

Connor, K.M., Kobak, K.A., et al. (2001). Mini-SPIN: a brief screening assessment for generalized social anxiety disorder. *Depress. Anxiety* 14(2):137–140.

Craske, M.G., Kircanski, K., et al. (2010). Panic disorder: a review of DSM-IV panic disorder and proposals for DSM-V. *Depress. Anxiety* 27(2):93–112.

Craske, M.G., Rauch, S.L., et al. (2009). What is an anxiety disorder? *Depress. Anxiety* 26(12):1066–1085.

Eisen, J.L., Phillips, K.A., et al. (1998). The Brown Assessment of Beliefs Scale: reliability and validity. *Am. J. Psychiatry* 155(1):102–108.

Etkin, A. (2012). Neurobiology of anxiety: from neural circuits to novel solutions? *Depress. Anxiety* 29(5):355–358.

Feighner, J.P., Robins, E., et al. (1972). Diagnostic criteria for use in psychiatric research. *Arch. Gen. Psychiatry* 26(1):57–63.

First, M.B. (2011). DSM-5 proposals for mood disorders: a cost-benefit analysis. *Curr. Opin. Psychiatry* 24(1):1–9.

Frances, A. (2012). Newsflash from APA meeting: DSM 5 has flunked its reliability tests. *Psychol. Today*.

Frances, A.J., and Widiger, T. (2012). Psychiatric diagnosis: lessons from the DSM-IV past and cautions for the DSM-5 future. *Annu. Rev. Clin. Psychol.* 8:109–130.

Friedman, M.J., Resick, P.A., et al. (2011a). Classification of trauma and stressor-related disorders in DSM-5. *Depress. Anxiety* 28(9):737–749.

Friedman, M.J., Resick, P.A., et al. (2011b). Considering PTSD for DSM-5. *Depress. Anxiety* 28(9):750–769.

Goodman, W.K., Price, L.H., et al. (1989). The Yale-Brown Obsessive Compulsive Scale: I. development, use, and reliability. *Arch. Gen. Psychiatry* 46(11):1006–1011.

Hinton, D.E., and Lewis-Fernandez, R. (2011). The cross-cultural validity of posttraumatic stress disorder: implications for DSM-5. *Depress. Anxiety* 28(9):783–801.

Houck, P.R., Spiegel, D.A., et al. (2002). Reliability of the self-report version of the panic disorder severity scale. *Depress. Anxiety* 15(4):183–185.

Insel, T., Cuthbert, B., et al. (2010). Research domain criteria (RDoC): toward a new classification framework for research on mental disorders. *Am. J. Psychiatry* 167(7):748–751.

Insel, T.R. (2009). Translating scientific opportunity into public health impact: a strategic plan for research on mental illness. *Arch. Gen. Psychiatry* 66(2):128–133.

Kendler, K.S. (2008). Explanatory models for psychiatric illness. *Am. J. Psychiatry* 165(6):695–702.

Kendler, K.S. (2012). The dappled nature of causes of psychiatric illness: replacing the organic-functional/hardware-software dichotomy with empirically based pluralism. *Mol. Psychiatry* 17(4):377–388.

LeBeau, R.T., Glenn, D., et al. (2010). Specific phobia: a review of DSM-IV specific phobia and preliminary recommendations for DSM-V. *Depress. Anxiety* 27(2):148–167.

Leckman, J.F., Denys, D., et al. (2010). Obsessive-compulsive disorder: a review of the diagnostic criteria and possible subtypes and dimensional specifiers for DSM-V. *Depress. Anxiety* 27(6):507–527.

Marks, I.M., and Mathews, A.M. (1979). Brief standard self-rating for phobic patients. *Behav. Res. Ther.* 17(3):263–267.

Mataix-Cols, D., Pertusa, A., et al. (2007). Issues for DSM-V: how should obsessive-compulsive and related disorders be classified? *Am. J. Psychiatry* 164(9):1313–1314.

Mayes, R., and Horowitz, A.V. (2005). DSM-III and the revolution in the classification of mental illness. *J. Hist. Behav. Sci.* 41(3):249–267.

National Institute of Mental Health. (2011). NIMH Research Domain Criteria (RDoC). URL http://www.nimh.nih.gov/research-funding/rdoc/nimh-research-domain-criteria-rdoc.shtml

Norton, P.J., and Philipp, L.M. (2008). Transdiagnostic approaches to the treatment of anxiety disorders: a quantitative review. *Psychother. Theor. Res. Pract. Train.* 45(2):214–226.

Phillips, K.A., Friedman, M.J., et al. (2010). Special DSM-V issues on anxiety, obsessive-compulsive spectrum, posttraumatic, and dissociative disorders. *Depress. Anxiety* 27(2):91–92.

Phillips, K.A., Stein, D.J., et al. (2010). Should an obsessive-compulsive spectrum grouping of disorders be included in DSM-V? *Depress. Anxiety* 27(6):528–555.

Regier, D.A., Kuhl, E.A., et al. (2012). Research planning for the future of psychiatric diagnosis. *Eur. Psychiatry* 27(7):553–556.

Sanislow, C.A., Pine, D.S., et al. (2010). Developing constructs for psychopathology research: research domain criteria. *J. Abnorm. Psychol.* 119(4):631–639.

Scheeringa, M.S., Zeanah, C.H., et al. (2011). PTSD in children and adolescents: toward an empirically based algorithma. *Depress. Anxiety* 28(9):770–782.

Spitzer, R.L., Endicott, J., et al. (1978). Research diagnostic criteria. *Arch. Gen. Psychiatry* 35:773–782.

Spitzer, R.L., Kroenke, K., et al. (2006). A brief measure for assessing generalized anxiety disorder: the GAD-7. *Arch. Intern. Med.* 166(10):1092–1097.

Stein, D.J., Fineberg, N.A., et al. (2010). Should OCD be classified as an anxiety disorder in DSM-V? *Depress. Anxiety* 27(6):495–506.

Stein, M.B., Jang, K.L., et al. (2002). Genetic and environmental influences on trauma exposure and posttraumatic stress disorder symptoms: a twin study. *Am. J. Psychiatry* 159:1675–1681.

Storch, E.A., Kaufman, D.A., et al. (2007). Florida obsessive-compulsive inventory: development, reliability, and validity. *J. Clin. Psychology* 63(9):851–859.

Wakefield, J.C. (2012). DSM-5: proposed changes to depressive disorders. *Curr. Med. Res. Opin.* 28(3):335–343.

Wittchen, H.U., Gloster, A.T., et al. (2010). Agoraphobia: a review of the diagnostic classificatory position and criteria. *Depress. Anxiety* 27(2):113–133.

World Health Organization. (1993). The ICD-10 Classification of Mental and Behavioural Disorders. Geneva: World Health Organization.

Zoellner, L.A., Rothbaum, B.O., et al. (2011). PTSD not an anxiety disorder? DSM committee proposal turns back the hands of time. *Depress. Anxiety* 28(10):853–856.

40 | GENETICS OF ANXIETY DISORDERS

JAVIER A. PEREZ, TAKESHI OTOWA, ROXANN ROBERSON-NAY,
AND JOHN M. HETTEMA

INTRODUCTION

This chapter provides a broad overview of the state of research in the genetics of the major anxiety disorders (ADs). We will primarily address findings regarding the categorical clinical syndromes as defined in DSM; however, several other human anxiety-related phenotypes (ARPs) are also discussed in relation to these, as indicated by the research data. We conceptually divide the chapter into three main sections: genetic epidemiology (adult and pediatric), human molecular genetics, and animal genetic models. We refer the reader to detailed reviews of the genetics of ADs (Hovatta and Barlow, 2008; Norrholm and Ressler, 2009; Smoller et al., 2009), including a special issue of the *American Journal of Medical Genetics Part C* devoted to this topic (Smoller and Faraone, 2008).

GENETIC EPIDEMIOLOGY OF ADs

In this section, we review the available data on genetic epidemiology of adult ADs. As reviewed in Chapter 12, the "chain of evidence" for genetic investigations begins with family studies, which compare rates of illness in relatives of those who have the condition (case probands) with rates in relatives of healthy controls. Higher rates in the former group of relatives, as parameterized by a relative risk (RR) or odds ratio (OR) greater than 1.0, suggest familial aggregation. The next step relies on either adoption studies (which are not available for ADs) or twin studies to differentiate genetic from within-family environment as sources of aggregation. Twin studies compare resemblance for a condition between members of a twin pair using the fact that identical (monozygotic, MZ) twins share 100% of their genes while nonidentical (dizygotic, DZ) twins share only 50% of their genes on average. One commonly used measure of twin resemblance is the probandwise concordance, that is, the proportion of cotwins of affected index twins who are also affected. If average concordance for MZ pairs is greater than that for DZ pairs, this is evidence for a genetic component to family resemblance. With larger twin samples, one may also estimate the proportion of individual differences due to the effects of genetic factors (heritability). For conditions with substantial heritability, gene finding (linkage or association) studies are undertaken to identify which specific genes contribute to risk.

A 2001 meta-analysis summarized findings across extant family and twin studies for several individual or categories of adult ADs (Hettema et al., 2001). Few family studies have been published since then, as it is now well established that all ADs moderately aggregate in families. More twin studies have been conducted, however, with emphasis on the etiology of comorbidity or developmental risk. While the former meta-analysis is over a decade old, it still provides the most systematic integration of data across primary studies of several of the ADs. We will refer to results of that meta-analysis and augment with data from more recent studies, where available.

FINDINGS FROM FAMILY AND TWIN STUDIES OF ADULT ADs

PANIC DISORDER

As reviewed by Schumacher and colleagues, data from 19 controlled family studies overall support the familial aggregation of panic disorder (PD), with relative risk to first-degree relatives (FDRs) ranging 3–17 (Schumacher et al., 2011). Five of these meeting strict inclusion criteria were analyzed in the meta-analysis, the results of which showed a highly significant association between PD in the proband and PD in FDRs. Summary OR across the five studies was 5.0 (95% CI: 3.0–8.2) and the unadjusted aggregate risk based on 1,356 total FDRs of PD probands was 10.0%, compared with 2.1% in 1,187 control relatives. Additionally, one study suggests higher familial risk associated with early-onset PD in the proband.

The two largest sources of adult twin data for most of the ADs, including PD, are the population-based Virginia Adult Twin Study of Psychiatric and Substance Use Disorders (VATSPSUD), and the Vietnam Era Twin (VET) Registry. The former consists of approximately 9,000 twins from male and female same-sex and opposite-sex pairs born in Virginia, while the latter is of comparable size but contains only U.S. male twins who served during the Vietnam War. The size of these samples permits the use of structural equation modeling to assess the relative contributions of genetics, common family (shared) environment, and individual specific (nonshared) environment to the liability of PD. Both samples reported higher MZ than DZ concordance, suggesting a genetic component to PD, consistent with some prior smaller twin studies. Both VATSPSUD and VET studies estimated heritability of PD to lie between 30% and 40%. The remaining source of individual differences derived from individual specific environment not shared between twins. In addition, the VATSPSUD found no evidence that genetic risk factors for PD significantly differ between men and women.

GENERALIZED ANXIETY DISORDER

Two published family studies of generalized anxiety disorder (GAD) were included in the aforementioned meta-analysis. Both studies, derived from clinical probands, supported the familial aggregation of GAD, and together they show a significant association between GAD in the proband and in their FDRs, with a summary OR of 6.08 (95% CI: 2.5–14.9). Both the VATSPSUD and the VET Registry examined broadened GAD syndromes via twin analyses, with an overall heritability of 31.6% (95% CI: 24–39%) when data from both samples were combined via meta-analysis. Other twin studies report heritability estimates for GAD in this range.

PHOBIAS

Fyer and colleagues performed a series of analyses examining specific phobia (SP), social phobia (SOC), and agoraphobia (AG) and their relationship with each other and PD. They reported higher rates of SP in relatives of SP probands compared with control relatives (31% versus 9%), higher rates of SOC in relatives of SOC probands (16% versus 5%), and higher rates of AG in relatives of AG probands (10% versus 3%). Another family study reported higher rates of AG in relatives of probands with AG compared with control relatives (11.6% versus 4.2%, OR = 3.0). Two studies of SOC found that familial aggregation is primarily due to the generalized subtype. Meta-analysis across family studies found a highly significant association between phobias in the proband and in FDR, with a summary OR of 4.07 (95% CI: 2.7–6.1).

Only two large, adult twin samples have comprehensively examined the genetics of phobias in adults. A series of analyses in the VATSPSUD examining phobic fears and disorders found that twin resemblance was due largely to genetic factors across AG, SOC, and SP, estimating that genetic factors explain from one-third to two-thirds of their individual differences. Similar heritability estimates were recently reported from a study of about 1,400 female twins from the Norwegian Institute of Public Health Twin Panel (NIPHTP) (Czajkowski et al., 2011).

OBSESSIVE-COMPULSIVE DISORDER

As reviewed by Nestadt and colleagues, most of the 15 published family studies of obsessive-compulsive disorder (OCD) support its familial aggregation (Nestadt et al., 2010). Five family studies included in the meta-analysis provided a highly significant association between OCD in the proband and FDRs (summary OR = 4.0, 95% CI: 2.2–7.1), with an unadjusted aggregate risk based on 1,209 total FDRs of OCD probands of 8.2% versus 2.0% in 746 control relatives. Secondary analyses in several of these studies suggest that younger age of onset may further increase familial risk for OCD.

Due to the complex assessment requirements and relatively low prevalence rates of diagnostically defined OCD, many twin studies have only examined broadened phenotypes consisting of OC symptoms or features (reviewed in van Grootheest et al., 2005). A study of OC traits and symptoms assessed by the Leyton Obsessional Inventory in 419 complete pairs from a London-based volunteer twin registry reported heritability estimates of 44% for OC traits and 47% for symptoms, with the remainder of the variance for these measures explained by nonshared environment. Self-report OC symptoms from the Padua Inventory were examined in 527 female twin pairs from the VATSPSUD. Factor analysis identified two major factors accounting for 62% of the variance that appeared to roughly correspond to obsessions and compulsions, with heritabilities of 33% and 26%, respectively.

OCD is a heterogeneous disorder, with several distinct symptom patterns ("dimensions") that can differ widely across patients (Leckman et al., 2001) (see Chapter 48). Preliminary family and twin studies report that these dimensions are individually heritable and might reflect the influence of distinct but correlated underlying genetic factors. This has potentially important implications for molecular genetic studies of OCD (Miguel et al., 2005).

POSTTRAUMATIC STRESS DISORDER

Several recent reviews of the genetics of posttraumatic stress disorder (PTSD) are available in the literature (Afifi et al., 2010; Koenen, 2007). The study of the genetics of PTSD is complicated by the requirement of a specific environmental exposure in its diagnostic criteria. The classification of a subject as not carrying an increased risk for PTSD (i.e., "healthy") is predicated on the condition that they are unaffected only *after* experiencing a significant trauma. Only a handful of published family studies exist, mostly examining general psychopathology in the relatives of PTSD probands to identify correlated familial risk factors. Their overall findings suggest that a family history of either anxiety or depressive disorders or both may increase an individual's risk for developing PTSD after experiencing a significant trauma.

Two twin samples have studied the etiology of risk for PTSD. Self-report symptoms of PTSD from the reexperiencing, avoidance, and hyperarousal clusters were analyzed in 4,042 male twin pairs from the VET Registry (True et al., 1993). The MZ twin correlations were higher than the DZ correlations, and heritabilities in the range of 30–35% were estimated for most of the individual symptoms after controlling for the effects of trauma exposure; nonshared environment explained the remaining variance in liability to PTSD. A second, smaller twin study extended these findings to female subjects and PTSD resulting from civilian traumas (Stein et al., 2002). For pairs in which both twins were exposed to trauma, MZ pairs were more highly correlated than DZ pairs for all of the PTSD symptom clusters, with heritability estimates in a similar range as those from the VET Registry study.

Twin studies have also attempted to estimate the degree to which the effects of genetic and environmental risk factors interact with each other beyond their independent effects on the phenotype (G × E). In other words, does the effect of adverse environmental exposures vary by degree of genetic liability ("genetic control of sensitivity to the environment")? Twin studies have established the importance of G × E effects for ADs (Lau et al., 2007; Silberg et al., 2001a). G × E effects are of particular relevance for PTSD (Afifi et al., 2010; Koenen et al., 2009), since traumatic environmental exposure is a prerequisite for its development. Another layer of complexity comes from twin studies that suggest exposure to many "environmental" experiences is due to behaviors partially driven by their own underlying genetic factors (Kendler and Baker, 2007).

PEDIATRIC ADs

Studies of anxiety in pediatric samples have used varying phenotypic definitions via different types of assessment instruments. These range from broad, often continuous scores for "anxiety" (e.g., Child Behavior Checklist [CBCL]) or anxious temperament, to groups of individual anxiety symptoms (e.g., the Screen for Child Anxiety Related Emotional Disorders [SCARED]), to specific diagnostic syndromes. We will briefly summarize the major findings from these in turn.

Studies of broad anxiety scores in child and adolescent twins report significant but moderate heritability (ranges 20–60%) for the Anxiety Problems scale of the CBCL (Spatola et al., 2010), fears (Rose and Ditto, 1983), state anxiety (Legrand et al., 1999), and anxious/depression scores (Boomsma et al., 2005). Unlike in adult samples, many of these studies also report significant influences of shared family environment.

Few family studies exist using childhood AD probands. A family study of children with ADs, in general, found elevated rates of ADs in their FDRs compared with FDRs of children without an AD (Last et al., 1991), supporting the familial aggregation of pediatric onset ADs. The only specific AD that has been systematically examined for familial aggregation using childhood probands is OCD, with two of the three extant studies reporting higher OR than was typical among studies with adult probands. In concordance with risk estimated from family studies, heritability estimates of OCD in children (45–65%) are generally higher than those from adult studies (reviewed in van Grootheest et al., 2005).

The design of some family studies, rather than attempting to interview all FDRs, limit their assessment to rates of illness in children of affected parents, allowing one to prospectively identify a "high-risk" sample. A meta-analysis of high-risk studies using parental probands with ADs found a significant increase in rates of ADs in general (OR = 3.91) as well as each specific type of AD (OR ranges from 2 to 4) in their offspring (Micco et al., 2009). Rates of OCD are particularly high (OR = 8.7). Interestingly, the rates of major depression (MD) in those offspring are also elevated (OR = 2.67) (see section on comorbidity that follows).

Among specific ADs, separation anxiety disorder (SAD) has received significant research attention, likely owing to its earlier age of onset and frequency. The results for twin studies of SAD have been mixed, with some studies supporting genetic as well as both common and unique environmental events as critical to its expression, while other studies do not observe significant shared environmental factors. An extensive meta-analysis of childhood SAD, which pooled together 18 cohorts with over 30,000 twin subjects, indicated that both genetic (43%) and shared environmental (17%) factors significantly accounted for its familial aggregation (Scaini et al., 2012). Unlike most individual studies, this analysis also possessed adequate power to detect differential heritability estimates between females (52%) and males (26%).

PD has a rather late age of onset compared with some other ADs (median 24 years), although a small subset of adolescents develop PD. Childhood SAD is hypothesized to share etiologic roots with PD, and a recent longitudinal twin study determined that the association between earlier SAD and adult-onset panic was largely explained by common genetic influences between them (Roberson-Nay et al., 2012).

SOC is one of the most prevalent ADs in youth, second only to specific phobias. A study in adolescent female twins reported heritability for SOC of 16% with no significant role for shared environment (Nelson et al., 2000). In a study based on child report using the SCARED, only genetic (53%) and nonshared environmental (47%) influences significantly accounted for variance in self-reported SOC symptoms (Ogliari et al., 2006). An even higher heritability (76%) was reported in a study of 4-year-old twins for the temperamental trait of shyness/behavioral inhibition, a risk factor for SOC (Eley et al., 2003).

DEVELOPMENTAL CHANGES IN GENETIC AND ENVIRONMENTAL RISK FOR ADs

As summarized in Chapters 44 and 71, ADs onset differentially across development, with puberty being a particularly salient time for increase in risk for some new or comorbid conditions. Twin studies conducted in children at different ages or longitudinally can examine the changing effects of genetic and environmental risk factors over time. As reviewed by Franic and colleagues, heritability for anxious/depressive symptoms are highest in early age groups and decrease with age, with correspondingly increasing importance for shared family environment into middle childhood (Franic et al., 2010). However, this trend appears to reverse as children develop through adolescence into adulthood for a range of phenotypes including anxiety symptoms (Bergen et al., 2007). As children age through puberty, family environmental influences decline in significance, consistent with the developmental progression for their sphere of influence from family to peers and beyond.

A longitudinal study of Swedish twins that recorded fear measures at four time points between ages 8 and 20 found that the role of genetic factors salient for fears during middle childhood (ages 8 to 9) subsequently declined over time, with new genetic risk factors coming "online" in early adolescence, late adolescence, and early adulthood (Kendler et al., 2008b). These results suggest that genetic effects for the expression of fear are "developmentally dynamic," from middle childhood through the young adult years. The mechanisms behind changes in genetic influences as a function of age are not well understood, but the findings suggest that certain genes may be differentially activated at different stages of development. While DNA structure is stable across the life span, gene expression and epigenetic processes are dynamic, potentially explaining developmental changes in genetic influences on the manifestation of fear and anxiety.

Longitudinal studies also provide valuable information regarding the genetic basis for developmental unfolding and the fluctuating nature of psychiatric syndromes over time. Some disorders exhibit homotypic continuity, with onsets in childhood and continuing of similar symptom profiles into adulthood (e.g., social phobia); for others, heterotypic continuity (the prediction of a disorder by a different disorder) is observed. In a pediatric twin sample, stable genetic factors explained most of homotypic continuity in childhood anxiety scales in the short age range from seven and nine (Trzaskowski et al., 2011). Looking at genetic risk across fear types (SOC and three types of SP) in the Swedish twin sample cited earlier, there was genetic innovation and attenuation differentially across fear domains. Namely, the major common genetic factor underlying overall fearfulness was stable across development, while new common and fear-specific genetic risk factors emerged over time (Kendler et al., 2008a). In a study of young adults from the NIPHTP, stability of anxiety and depressive symptoms across two time points was mainly attributable to genetic factors, whereas change was primarily related to environmental influences (Nes et al., 2007). As described earlier, a recent longitudinal twin study found heterotypic continuity between childhood SAD and adult-onset panic was best explained by a common genetic vulnerability (Roberson-Nay et al., 2012). In contrast, the genetic factor associated with childhood overanxious disorder (OAD) did not contribute significantly to adult panic. These results indicate that childhood SAD and adult panic share a common genetic diathesis that is not observed for childhood OAD, supporting the hypothesis of a specific genetic heterotypic link among them. However, symptoms of OAD experienced early in life are influenced by the same genes that influence later depressive symptoms (Silberg et al., 2001b), supporting the findings from adult twin studies that OAD/GAD and MD share a common underlying genetic liability (see next section).

SHARED SUSCEPTIBILITY BETWEEN ADs AND OTHER ARPs

Most, but not all, family studies of the ADs reported relative specificity in their familial aggregation; however, this is not the case with twin studies. Studies in the VATSPSUD sample have found genetic and environmental factors are, to a greater or lesser extent, shared across most of the ADs and with other commonly comorbid disorders like MD. The twin studies cited earlier used multivariate modeling to test whether there was a common factor of "phobia proneness" that increased liability across classes of phobic fears and whether it was genetic, environmental, or both in origin. The best fitting models contained both common and disorder-specific genetic and nonshared environmental influences on all of the phobia subtypes examined, with the proportion of genetic variance explained by common genes varying somewhat by disorder and gender. Similar findings were reported in the NIPHTP study cited earlier, although they found evidence for two common genetic factors differentially loading across the phobia subtypes (Czajkowski et al., 2011). Analyses from the VATSPSUD and the Swedish Twin Registry suggest that GAD and MD share the majority of their genetic risk in common but only a modest proportion of environmental risk factors (Kendler et al., 2006).

Several studies from the VATSPSUD tested broader models of comorbidity between the ADs, or between the ADs, MD, and related phenotypes. One such analysis examined the relationships across several ADs: PD, GAD, AG, SOC, and animal and situational SP (Hettema et al., 2005). In the best fitting model, the genetic influences on anxiety susceptibility for both sexes were explained by two additive genetic factors shared across the disorders, with significant disorder-specific genetic risk only for AG. The first factor loaded most strongly on GAD, PD, and AG, while the second loaded primarily on SP. SOC was intermediate, in that it was influenced by both common genetic factors. A similar analysis conducted in NIPHTP identified a single common genetic factor of heritability of 54% that accounted for a large proportion of genetic variance across symptoms of PD, GAD, SP (all types), OCD, and PTSD (Tambs et al., 2009). Only SP and OCD had disorder-specific genetic effects of appreciable magnitude. Analyses from other large twin datasets support the hypothesis of a shared genetic diathesis between the AD phenotypes in adults and children as well as between ADs and MD (reviewed in (Middeldorp et al., 2005)). Similarly, the meta-analysis of high-risk studies cited earlier found no significant differences between risk for anxiety or depression in offspring between parental proband groups with either type of disorder (Micco et al., 2009), suggesting that a nonspecific internalizing diathesis is transmitted to offspring.

Studies have consistently demonstrated associations between high levels of anxiety-related personality traits and increased risk of ADs. Neuroticism and extraversion, two normal traits included in most personality inventories, are generally elevated and lowered, respectively, in subjects with anxiety and depressive disorders; they also likely mediate anxiety-depressive comorbidity (Bienvenu et al., 2001). Twin studies suggest that some of the genetic factors that influence these personality traits overlap those that increase susceptibility for anxiety and depressive disorders. (Bienvenu et al., 2007; Hettema et al., 2006; Kendler et al., 2006).

GENETIC EPIDEMIOLOGY SUMMARY

Overall, genetic epidemiological studies support a moderate level of familial aggregation (OR 4–6) for adult ADs. The source of this familial risk is predominantly genetic in origin, with heritability of about 30–50%. Pediatric ADs are possibly even more highly heritable, with genetic effects dynamically changing throughout development. Twin studies suggest that ADs do not seem to "breed true"; that is, their genetic architecture is not isomorphic with their symptomatic presentations and classifications, sharing risk factors with each other and related phenotypes like depression and anxious personality traits. This helps to explain their patterns of comorbidity as well as their developmental progression.

HUMAN MOLECULAR GENETICS

LINKAGE AND CANDIDATE GENE ASSOCIATION STUDIES

Two main approaches are applied to identify susceptibility genes in human studies: linkage and association studies. Linkage studies are performed in pedigrees with several affected individuals to identify chromosomal loci likely to harbor a gene influencing a biological trait or condition. While effective to identify highly penetrant genes of large effect seen in classic Mendelian disorder, linkage has, with few exceptions, not been very fruitful for most complex phenotypes encountered in medicine, including anxiety. Several linkage studies have been performed for ARPs, with few consistent findings between studies (reviewed in Hovatta and Barlow, 2008; Smoller and Faraone, 2008). Suggestive linkage has been reported for regions on chromosomes 4q, 9q, 13q, 14q, and 22q in PD (reviewed in Maron et al., 2010), 9p in OCD (Nestadt et al., 2010), and 8p for the anxiety-related personality trait of harm avoidance (HA) (Cloninger et al., 1998). A reanalysis of several PD linkage studies supported linkage on chromosomes 4q and 7p (Logue et al., 2012). The most intensively studied ARP using linkage is neuroticism. A recent meta-analysis of all available genome-wide linkage studies of neuroticism using eight independent samples with over 14,000 subjects supported linkage on chromosomes 9, 11, 12, and 14 (Webb et al., 2012). In the same study, similar analysis using a smaller set of samples found suggestive evidence for linkage on chromosomes 1, 5, 15, and 16 for ADs. The results for ADs and neuroticism were moderately but significantly correlated, supporting the results from twin studies suggesting shared genetic susceptibility.

Association studies allow one to test specific genes or markers within genes for their contribution to a phenotype. They may take the form of case-control comparisons in unrelated individuals or family-based transmission tests. To date, most association studies of ADs have focused on candidate genes, which have to be chosen using a priori knowledge, either from their position under a linkage peak or their biologic function as relevant for the pathophysiology of the disease. The most widely studied candidate genes for ADs are genes involved in neurotransmitter systems or related to stress response. In their review, Maron and colleagues summarized more than 350 candidate gene findings for PD, concluding that most of these results remain inconsistent, negative, or not clearly replicated (Maron et al., 2010). Failure to identify susceptibility loci in PD may be due to differences in phenotypic assessment, heterogeneity at the genetic level, and underpowered studies with small sample sizes (issues in association studies of many phenotypes). Several association findings, such as for the genes regulator of G-protein signaling 2 (RGS2), adenosine 2A receptor (ADORA2A), and catechol-O-methyltransferase (COMT), were replicated in other studies, sometimes in other ARPs (Table 40.1). For example, the COMT gene polymorphism (Val158Met) has been implicated in susceptibility to PD by several studies in independent samples. COMT encodes an enzyme metabolizing the monoamine neurotransmitters. The valine (Val) allele shows a significantly higher COMT activity relative to the methionine (Met) allele. A meta-analysis of six case-control studies showed significant association of the COMT 158 Val allele with PD in Caucasian samples and, conversely, a trend toward association of the COMT 158 Met allele with PD in the Asian samples (Domschke et al., 2007). Given the multiple positive findings, COMT seems to be one of the most consistent association findings for ADs.

The other extensively studied gene in genetic studies of ADs, as well as MD, is the serotonin transporter gene (particularly, its promoter length polymorphism, 5HTTLPR), involved in the action of SSRI drugs. The short allele is associated with lower expression of the serotonin transporter gene (SLC6A4)

and, consequently, lower activity of the transporter. Lesch and colleagues initially reported the association of the 5HTTLPR short allele with anxiety-related personality traits (Lesch et al., 1996). Since then, a large number of studies have attempted to replicate the association, but the results have been inconsistent (similar to reports of association between MDD and this polymorphism). Also, meta-analyses of the association studies between the SLC6A4 gene and anxiety-related personality traits are inconclusive: modest overall association with neuroticism as measured by the neuroticism-extraversion-openness personality inventory but no association with HA or neuroticism as measured by the Eysenck Personality Questionnaire (Munafo et al., 2009). Furthermore, a meta-analysis of OCD suggested an association with the long allele in the childhood-onset subgroup and Caucasians (Bloch et al., 2008), whereas a meta-analysis of 10 association studies of PD did not show overall association between 5HTTLPR and PD (Blaya et al., 2007).

Several candidate genes involved in the (hypothalamic-pituitary-adrenal) HPA stress response system have been implicated in PTSD. Binder and colleagues reported significant interactive effects, but no main effects, of polymorphisms in FKBP5, a gene that regulates glucocorticoid receptor sensitivity, and severity of child abuse history in a sample of around 900 primarily African-American adults (Binder et al., 2008). A female-specific association with PTSD and fear discrimination was reported in the same sample for a marker in an estrogen response element of ADCYAP1R1, the gene encoding the receptor for pituitary adenylate cyclase–activating polypeptide (PACAP) (Ressler et al., 2011). Also, PACAP blood levels correlated with PTSD symptoms and startle responses of females in a fear-conditioning paradigm. Other interesting AD–candidate gene associations, some of which were replicated in other studies (Table 40.1), include: (1) overall AD phenotypes with glutamic acid decarboxylase 1 (GAD1) and (2) OCD with both the glutamate transporter (SLC1A1) and brain-derived neurotrophic factor (BDNF) genes.

GENOME-WIDE ASSOCIATION STUDIES

Table 40.2 lists extant Genome-Wide Association Studies (GWAS) of anxiety-related personality traits and ADs. Unlike candidate gene studies, which require a priori knowledge for gene selection, GWAS provides an unbiased survey of common genetic variation across the entire genome (see Chapter 12). The first reported GWAS for an anxiety phenotype was published in 2008 (Shifman et al., 2008) using DNA pooling methods in about 2,000 individuals selected on extremes of neuroticism scores from a cohort of 88,000 people. Among 450,000 SNPs investigated, only one SNP within the phosphodiesterase 4D (PDE4D) gene was replicated in one of three independent samples tested. They concluded that no loci explained more than 1% of variance of the trait and that many loci with small effects account for its heritability. The second neuroticism GWAS was conducted in 1,200 U.S. Caucasian participants, in which the most promising markers were subsequently tested for replication in 1,900 German subjects (van den Oord et al. 2008), demonstrating nearly genome-wide association for

TABLE 40.1. Candidate gene of anxiety disorders and anxiety-related phenotypes showing association in other studies

GENE		LOCATION	PHENOTYPE	FUNCTION
RGS2	Regulator of G-protein signaling 2	1q31.2	PD, PTSD, extraversion	Regulator of G protein signaling
GAD1	Glutamic acid decarboxylase 1	2q31.1	GAD, PD, agoraphobia, social phobia	GABA synthesis
SLC1A1	Glutamate transporter	9p24.2	OCD	Glutamate transmission
BDNF	Brain-derived neurotrophic factor	11p14.1	OCD, harm avoidance	Neurotrophic factor
CCKBR	Cholecystokinin B receptor	11p15.4	PD	Neuropeptide transmission
DRD4	Dopamine receptor D4	11p15.5	OCD, PD, neuroticism	Dopamine neurotransmission
HTR2A	5-hydroxytryptamine receptor 2A	13q14.2	OCD, PD	Serotonin neurotransmission
5HTTLPR	Serotonin transporter	17q11.2	OCD, PTSD, neuroticism	Regulator of serotonin reuptake
COMT	Catechol-O-methyltransferase	22q11.2	PD, anxiety-related personality, phobic anxiety	Catecholamine degradation
ADORA2A	Adenosine A2 receptor	22q11.2	PD	Adenosine regulation

(Adapted from Hovatta and Barlow, 2008.)
PD, panic disorder; OCD, obsessive-compulsive disorder; PTSD, posttraumatic stress disorder; GAD, generalized anxiety disorder

TABLE 40.2. Genome-wide association studies of anxiety disorders and related personality traits

REFERENCE	PHENOTYPE	SAMPLE	GENOTYPING ARRAY(S)	MOST SIGNIFICANT FINDING
Shifman et al. (2008)	Neuroticism (EPQ)	2,054 individuals with extremely high scores on neuroticism	Affymetrix 100 K and 500 K	PDE4D (5q12)
van den Oord et al. (2008)	Neuroticism (EPQ)	1,227 U.S. participants for GWAS; 1,880 German subjects for replication	Affymetrix 500 K	MAMDC1 (15q21)
Otowa et al. (2009, 2010)	Panic disorder	200 cases and 200 controls for GWAS; 558 cases and 566 controls for replication	Affymetrix 500 K	TMEM16B (12p13)
Calboli et al. (2010)	Neuroticism (EPQ)	2,235 individuals from population-based sample	Affymetrix 500 K	NKAIN2 (6q22)
Terracciano et al. (2010)	Neuroticism (NEO-PI)	3,972 individuals from a population within Sardinia	Affymetrix 10 K and 500 K	SNAP25 (20p12)
Erhardt et al. (2011)	Panic disorder	216 cases and 222 controls for GWAS; 693 cases and 693 controls for replication	Illumina 300 K	TMEM132D (12q24)
de Moor et al. (2012)	Neuroticism, extraversion (NEO-PI)	17,375 individuals from 10 samples for discovery (partially overlapped with sample in Terracciano et al., 2010); 3,294 individuals from five samples for replication	Affymetrix 10 K, 250 and 500 K; Illumina 6 K, 317 K, 370 K, 550 K, 610 K, 1 M; Perlegen 600 K	MTR (1q43) for neuroticism; PSAT1 (9q21) for extraversion

EPQ, Eysenck Personality Questionnaire; GWAS, genome-wide association studies; NEO-PI, neuroticism-extraversion-openness personality inventory.

SNPs in *MAMDC1* when combining the two samples. A recent meta-analysis of GWAS for personality traits, combining data from 17,000 subjects, reported genome-wide significant association for traits of openness (near *RASA1* gene on 5q14.3) and conscientiousness (in *KATNAL2* gene on 18q21.1). However, there were no genome-wide significant findings for neuroticism or extraversion (de Moor et al., 2012).

The first AD GWAS was conducted in 200 PD cases and 200 controls in the Japanese population, reporting several potential novel loci for susceptibility to PD (Otowa et al., 2009). However, a follow-up study in a larger sample failed to show any significant association of these genes with PD. The second GWAS of PD, conducted in three German samples, reported two associated SNPs located in *TMEM132D* on 12q24.3 (Erhardt et al., 2011). Risk genotypes for PD were associated with higher *TMEM132D* mRNA expression levels in the frontal cortex. They also demonstrated that *TMEM132D* was associated with anxiety-related behavior using a mouse model of extremes in trait anxiety. Of note, none of these analyses found overlap with previously reported candidate genes, so these results require replication in independent, adequately powered samples.

Several international research collaborations have formed to investigate the genetics of ADs, similar to efforts by the Psychiatric Genetics Consortium for other psychiatric disorders. For example, the Panic International Consortium (PanIC) aims to replicate earlier association findings and to identify new markers using the largest combined sample of PD subjects. The Obsessive-Compulsive Foundation International Genetic Consortium (OCF-ICG) is performing a GWAS of OCD using a sample size of over 3,000 cases and controls. Several groups are also currently conducting large GWAS of PTSD in trauma-exposed subjects. Our group is leading a GWAS meta-analysis, using data from six independent samples from the United States, Europe, and Australia of over 20,000 subjects, to discover novel genes that are responsible for common genetic risk shared across ADs using quantitative anxiety factor scores that, in principle, increase the statistical power to detect genes of small effect.

HUMAN MOLECULAR GENETICS SUMMARY

Linkage studies of ADs have produced inconclusive results, and GWAS have not reached genome-wide significance, to date. This is similar to the experience for a similar psychiatric phenotype, MD (see Chapter 30). This implies that a large number of genes with small effects, rather than a small number of genes of moderate-to-large effects, account for the heritability of these phenotypes. Thus, very large, well-characterized samples and even larger meta-analyses are needed before unambiguous findings will be available. On the other hand, several candidate AD genes have been replicated and confirmed in other ADs, suggesting their pleiotropic effects across these phenotypes. Therefore, we emphasize that very large GWAS using common genetic factors across ADs provide a powerful strategy to identify their susceptibility genes.

ANIMAL MODELS FOR STUDYING THE GENETICS OF ADs

The genetic basis of ADs has been supported by well-established animal models (Jacobson and Cryan, 2010). The human and mouse genome share many common features whereby almost all genes have a respective counterpart. Humans and rodents also share similar autonomic responses and related defensive behaviors to threatening stimuli. Many of these behaviors are modeled and measured in rodents with the use of pharmacologically validated behavioral tasks testing anxiety-like behavior (ALB). Moreover, functional brain mechanisms governing ALB involving regions such as the amygdala and prefrontal cortex (PFC) are phylogenetically well preserved in rodents (see Chapter 41). Thus, while recognizing their obvious limitations, as no animal model can mimic the full spectrum of anxiety in humans, rodents are considered a vital tool for advancing our basic understanding of the genetic and neurobiological basis of AD.

In the last decade, there has been an increase in "translational studies," where human genetic findings are being functionally validated by subsequent work in rodents and vice versa (Sartori et al., 2011). Inbred strains have supported the development of transgenic and knockout (KO) models, while recombinant inbred strains have contributed to the discovery of quantitative trait loci (QTL) associated with ALB. These approaches have been extended with the use of molecular techniques to functionally characterize AD candidate genes. In the following section, we will *(1)* summarize the most current advances in the genetics of AD as supported by research methods in rodent models and *(2)* provide examples on cross-species approaches that have supported and validated genetic research on AD.

GENE IDENTIFICATION THROUGH ANIMAL MODELS OF ANXIETY

To model ARB in rodents, researchers have relied on various paradigms and behavioral tests to assess defensive responses to naturally occurring (e.g., vulnerability to predators) and laboratory-provoked (e.g., tail shock) threats (reviewed in Chapter 41). These can be further be subdivided into conditioned (learned) and unconditioned tests (ethologically based). Unconditioned tests including open field tests (OFTs), elevated plus maze (EPM), and light-dark box (LDB) measure spontaneous or natural responses to innate aversive and threatening stimuli. Conditioning paradigms such as fear conditioning (FC) and fear-potentiated startle (FPS) rely on the learned pairing of a neutral stimulus (i.e., conditioned stimulus; CS) with an aversive stimulus (unconditioned stimulus; US) and subsequent conditioned fear responses (i.e., freezing and startle) are measured during the presence of the CS and absence of the US. Such conditioned responses are hypothesized to model phobias and PTSD.

Inbred mice are a classic tool for investigating the genetic basis of many medical syndromes. Mice from the same strain are almost 100% identical between their respective genomes. Thus, interstrain genetic differences have helped investigate heritable and stable behavioral phenotypes related to anxiety. In Table 40.3, we provide a summary of the various strain differences in ALB measured in different tests. Inbred mice display individual differences in ALB in both conditioned and unconditioned tests. BALB/c, A/J, AKR/J, and S129/SvImJ are known as typically highly anxious strains. Interestingly, the S129/SvImJ strain displays a unique profile for high anxiety in the OFT, LDB, and FC, including an innate inability to extinguish fear. Deficits in fear extinction (FE) of S129/SvImJ are well described (Hefner et al., 2008), in which genetic differences associated with extinction are also correlated with deficiencies in cortico-limbic activation of fear circuitry (see Chapter 41). Thus, it has been hypothesized that genetic

TABLE 40.3. Profile of common inbred mouse strains on anxiety-like behavior

TEST	HIGH ANXIETY	AVERAGE ANXIETY	LOW ANXIETY
Open field	S129/SvlmJ, A/J AKR/J, BALB/c, BALB/CbyJ, DBA/2J		C57BL/6J, FVB/NJ
Elevated zero maze	A/J, AKR/J, BALB/c		
Elevated plus maze	A/J, AKR/J, BALB/c	C57BL/6J, A/J	FVB/NJ
Light-dark box	A/J, BALB/CbyJ, BALB/c, S129/SvlmJ	C57BL/6J, C3H/HeJ	FBV/NJ
Social interaction	A/J, BALB/cByJ, 129S1/SvlmJ	AKR/J, C57BL/6J, C3H/HeJ	FBV/NJ
Conditioned fear and fear extinction (freezing)	S129/SvlmJ, A/J	BALB/CbyJ	C57BL/6J, FVB/NJ

differences accounting for deficits in FE in this strain could account for deficits in the activation of the relevant components of the fear circuit.

The use of inbred strains for investigating genes that may account for polygenic traits of ALB has been extended with the advent of QTL studies. QTL analyses seek to identify an association between a specific phenotype and a marker locus for a set of two or more genes. QTL analysis is commonly carried out by crossing two or more strains followed by subsequent rigorous inbreeding across multiple generations to derive new independent lines. After careful breeding, successive generations of new inbred strains will contain fixed recombination of genes derived from the original gene pool. Profiling of differences in ALB in the recombinant lines such as BXD or AXB/BXA are subsequently used to identify the chromosomal locations related to the phenotype.

QTL strategies of ALB have yielded loci on many mouse chromosomes (1, 4, 5, 7, 8, 9, 10, 11, 13, 14, 18, 19) (reviewed by Flint, 2003). Linkage on chromosome 1, 4, and 15 were consistently found across the three more common ALBs (OFT, EPM, and LDB), where each QTL primarily influenced different phenotypic components: chromosome 1 (exploration), chromosome 4 (activity), and chromosome 15 QTL (avoidance). These three QTLs accounted for almost 21% of the total genetic variance, while genes accounted for 26% of the total phenotypic variance in the analyzed rodent population. Interestingly, the syntenic region on human chromosome 1 coincides with linkage peaks reported for several human ARPs (reviewed in Fullerton, 2006). Further dissection of the chromosome 1 region provided support for three separate murine QTLs (Yalcin et al., 2004), including effects attributable to the *RGS2* gene. *RGS2* has since been reportedly associated with several ADs and ARPs in humans.

It should be noted that QTLs help localize genetic effects to particular chromosomal regions but do not identify specific susceptibility genes; this typically requires further dissection using complementary methods such as gene expression profiling with microarrays. The combination of these approaches, known as expression-QTL (eQTL), is emerging as a promising tool for precise identification of genes underlying many medical phenotypes in rodents. Recent studies have applied these together to mice bred to establish high and low freezing lines presenting differences in FC. After validating gene expression

differences between the selective lines with quantitative polymerase chain reaction (qPCR), a number of genes have been confirmed to be in close proximity to, or within the boundaries of, the behavioral QTLs, including tyrosinase (Tyr) suppressor of Ty 16 homologue (Supt16h), endonucleoside triphosphate diphosphohydrolase4 (Entpd4; aka Lysal1), and diacylglycerol kinase, gamma (Dgkg) (Ponder et al., 2008).

Expression QTL analyses will require further development using recombinant inbred lines. However, inbred strains have been used with high-throughput molecular approaches to determine differences in gene expression associated with ALB. After surveying six inbred mouse strains on the LDB and OFT, Hovatta and colleagues performed gene expression profiling using microarrays to assess global gene expression in several brain regions linked to anxiety (Hovatta et al., 2005). They analyzed gene expression differences across several relevant brain regions between anxious and nonanxious mice across six inbred strains. They identified two novel candidate genes, glyoxalase 1 (Glo1) and glutathione reductase 1 (Gsr), which code for enzymes involved in metabolic pathways regulating oxidative stress. Further validation was demonstrated by viral-mediated gene overexpression and RNA interference (RNAi) knock-down in the target tissues, resulting in increasing or decreasing ALB, respectively.

The study of ALB in rodents has also profited from selective breeding of outbred animals. This strategy enriches for specific traits and enhances their specificity and homogeneity. Subsequent lines obtained after selectively breeding start from the same genetic outbred background, providing an etiologic association between differences in their genome and observed trait differences. Among the most notable selectively bred rodent models of ALB are the high (HAB), normal (NAB), and low (LAB) ALB mouse lines derived from CD-1 outbred mice based on behavioral differences in the EPM. HAB mice also display high anxiety in other unconditioned tests such as LDB and OFT and conditioned tests such as cued and contextual FC. Several candidate genes have been identified in relation to differential ALB between HAB and LAB mice. For example, the C(+40)T SNP in the first exon of the arginine/vasopressin (AVP) peptide precursor gene in LAB mice has been reported to cause an amino acid substitution from alanine to valine at the third position in the signal peptide. This SNP substitution is associated with ALB in an F2 panel of HAB and LAB mice. Sequencing performed within regions 2.5 Kb up- and downstream of the *AVP* gene locus identified several polymorphic loci that differ between the HAB and LAB lines (Bunck et al., 2009). Allele-specific transcription analysis revealed a LAB-specific 75% decrease in transcription rate compared with the HAB-specific allele. AVP expression in the paraventricular nucleus of the hypothalamus was found to correlate with anxiety-like and depression-like behaviors. Moreover, a genotype/phenotype association was shown in an F2 panel, supporting a causal contribution of the *AVP* promoter deletion to ALB.

In the rat, the selectively bred High Responder (bHR) and bred Low Responder (bLR) models are similarly characterized by significant differences in ALB in the OPF, LDB, and EPM. Interestingly, these rats also present significant differences in depression-like behavior, consistent with human studies showing that depression and anxiety share common genetic factors. *Fibroblast Growth Factor-2 (FGF-2)*, a novel gene candidate previously noted to be downregulated in postmortem brains of severely depressed individuals, was shown to regulate, in part, individual differences between bHR and bLR (Perez et al., 2009). The bLRs exhibit significantly low levels of FGF-2 in the hippocampus, but when animals are treated with FGF-2, their ALB resembles that of a bHR. The role of FGF-2 on anxiety has been further supported by a recent report showing that FGF-2 RNAi knockdown in the hippocampus increased ALB. FGF-2 has also been implicated in FE, whereby treatment with FGF-2 has consistently been shown to increase extinction of conditioned fear in both young and adult rats (Graham and Richardson, 2011).

GENE-TARGETING APPROACHES

Genetics of ALB have also been investigated via the development of KO and transgenic mouse models. Similar to human candidate gene studies, many targeted genes were initially selected based on their relevance as pharmacological targets (i.e., monoamine and GABA-ergic genes). More novel gene targets were later developed based on neurobiological findings relevant to ALB. More recently, gene-targeting approaches have served to validate human genetic findings. Thus, throughout the last 15 years, there has been an increase in abundance of KO and transgenic overexpressing mouse models that have demonstrated significantly increasing or decreasing effects on ALB (summarized in Table 40.4). Moreover, the Cre-lox recombination system has enabled conditional and controllable deletions or insertions of genes in specific brain regions, cell types, and at specific time points (for details on the cre-loxP system see Chapter 8: "Transgenic Tools and Animal Models of Mental Illness").

Tissue- and developmentally specific KO methods have been applied in studying serotonin 1A receptor (5HT1A) function in ALB (reviewed by Gordon and Hen, 2004). Serotonin is involved in mood regulation, and drugs acting on the serotonin system are effective in treating anxiety and depressive disorders. Three separate mouse strains with deleted 5-HT1A receptors have consistently exhibited increased anxiety. However, the 5-HT1A receptor is expressed in two separate neuronal populations in the brain: acting as an autoreceptor on serotonin-containing neurons of the raphe nuclei and as a heteroreceptor on neurons in the forebrain. Tissue-specific conditional rescue demonstrated that expression of the 5-HT1A

TABLE 40.4. Effects of gene targeting manipulations in mice showing increased anxiety-like behavior

BIOLOGICAL SYSTEM	TARGET GENE	INCREASED ANXIETY-LIKE BEHAVIOR
Monoamines	5-HT1A (KO)	EPM, OFT, EZM
	5-HT2C (OE)	EPM, OFT
	α2A (KO)	EPM, LDB, FC
	nAChRα4 (KO)	EPM,
	COMT (KO)	LDB, OFT
	D1CT (TG)	LDB, OFT
	D4 (KO)	EPM, LD, OF
	SERT (KO)	EPM, EZM, LDB, OFT, SI
Glutamate	NR2C-2B (RP)	EPM
	GluR1 (KO)	EPM, LDB, SI
	mGluR5 (KO)	EPM, LDB, FE
	mGluR8 (KO)	EPM, OFT
	VGluT1 (HET)	LDB
GABA	GABA-Aγ2 (HET, KO)	EPM, LDB, FC
	GABA-Aγ2L (KO)	EPM
	GABA-B1 (KO)	LDB
	GABA-B2 (KO)	LDB
	GAD65 (KO)	EZM, LDB, OFT, FE
Neuropeptides	BDNFMet (KI)	OFT, EPM
	CB1 (KO)	EPM, LDB, OFT, SI
	CCK (KO)	EPM
	CCK1R (KO)	EPM
	CRH (OE)	EPM, LDB, OFT, SI
	CRH-BP (KO)	EPM, LDB, OFT
	CRH-R2 (KO)	EPM, LDB, OFT
	αER (KO)	OFT, LDB
	GR (OE)	EPM
	Mas (KO)	EPM
	NPSR (KO)	OFT, LDB, EPM
	NPY (KO)	EPM, LD, OFT
	OFQ/N (KO)	EPM, LDB, OFT
	PENK (KO)	EPM, EZM, LDB, OFT, SI, USV
	Ucn (KO)	EPM, OFT
Immune system	IFN-γ (KO)	EPM, OF
	TNF-α (OE)	HB, LD

(continued)

TABLE 40.4. *(Continued)*

BIOLOGICAL SYSTEM	TARGET GENE	INCREASED ANXIETY-LIKE BEHAVIOR
Other	*3xTg-AD* (TG)	LD, OFT
	APP,Sw,Ind (TG)	LDB, OFT
	α-CamKII (OE)	EZM, LDB, OFT, SI
	eNOS (KO)	EPM, OFT
	Fut9 (KO)	EPM, LDB
	Fyn (KO)	EPM, LDB
	PAM (HET)	EZM
	PSA (KO)	EPM, OFT
	Rgs2 (KO)	LDB
	Shn-2 (KO)	OFT
	SF-1 (KO)	EPM, LDB, OFT
	Sim2 (OE)	EZM, OFT, SI
	TAK1/TR4 (KO)	SI, LDB, OFT
	TgNTRK3 (OE)	EPM
	trkbCaMII-CRE (KO)	OFT

(Adapted from Sartori et al., 2011)
Abbreviations: 3xTg-AD: Alzheimer's disease transgenic mice expressing taurine; 5-HT1A: serotonin 1A receptor; 5-HT2C: serotonin 2C receptor; α2A: α2A-adrenergic receptor; α-CamKII: α-calcium/calmodulin-dependent protein kinase II; αER: α-estrogen receptor; APP$_{Sw,Ind}$: Alzheimer's disease transgenic mice expressing human mutant β-amyloid precursor protein; BDNF: Brain-derived neurotrophic factor; CB: cannabinoid receptor; CCK: cholecystokinin; CCK1R: cholecystokinin 1 receptor; CF: conditioned fear; COMT: catechol-O-methyltransferase; CRH: corticotropin-releasing hormone; CRH-BP: CRH binding protein; CRH-R2: CRH 2 receptor; D1CT: expression of a neuropotentiating cholera toxin transgene in dopamine D1 receptor-expressing neurons; D4: dopamine D4 receptor; Dhh: desert hedgehog; eNOS: endothelial nitric oxide synthase; EPM: elevated plus maze; EZM: elevated zero maze; FPS: fear-potentiated startle; Fut9: fucosyltransferase IX; Fyn: Fyn tyrosine kinase; GABA: γ-amino butyric acid; GAD: glutamic acid decarboxylase; GluR1: AMP-A glutamate receptor R1 subunit; GR: glucocorticoid receptor; HB: holeboard test; KI: knockin; KO: knockout; LDB: light-dark box; Mas: Mas proto-oncogene; mGluR: metabotropic glutamate receptor; nAchRα4: α4-nicotinic acetylcholine receptor; NPSR: neuropeptide S receptor; NPY: neuropeptide Y; NR2C-2B: NMDA receptor 2C-2B; OE: overexpression; OFT: open field test; OFQ/N: orphanin FQ, nociceptin; PAM: peptidylglycine α-amidating monooxygenase; PENK: prepro-enkephaline; PSA: puromycin-sensitive aminopeptidase; Rgs2: regulator of G-protein signaling 2; RP: replacement; SERT: serotonin transporter; SF-1: steroidogenic factor-1; Shn-2: Schnurri-2; SI: social interaction; Sim2: single-minded 2 gene; TAK1/TR4: nuclear orphan receptor; TFC: trace fear conditioning; TG: transgenic; TgNTRK3: transgenic mice overexpressing the full-length neurotrophin-3 receptor TrkC; trkB$^{CaMKII-CRE}$: forebrain-specific knockout of the trkB receptor; Ucn: urocortin; USV: stress-induced ultrasonic vocalization; VC: Vogel conflict test; VGlutT1: vesicular glutamate transporter 1.

receptor in the hippocampus and cortex, but not the raphe nuclei, was sufficient to reinstate the anxiety-like phenotype of KO mice. Moreover, using conditional KO techniques, researchers showed that early developmental, but not adulthood, expression of the 5-HT1A receptor is essential for this

behavioral rescue. Together, these results suggest that signaling by serotonin via forebrain 5-HT1A receptor during development is required for normal ALB in adulthood.

The specificity of benzodiazepines (BZDs) on their interaction with the α-subunits of the GABA-A receptor was investigated with the use of genetic knockin methods. The efficacy of BZDs derives from binding and modulating the activity of GABA-A receptors. BZDs bind the α-subunit of the GABA-A receptors, enhancing the efficacy of GABA. There are six isoforms of the α-subunit, two of which are insensitive to BZDs as they lack a conserved histidine residue found in each of the four BZD-sensitive isoforms. By substituting histidine for arginines through targeted mutations on the α1, α2, and α3 subunits, it was demonstrated that α2 was responsible for the anxiolytic effects of diazepam, a BZD, on the LDB and EPM in mice.

We note that transgenic animals have limited utility in characterizing gene function at the molecular level for specific phenotypes like ALB. This is because *(1)* disruption in the expression of a single gene typically has pleiotropic effects on a wide variety of phenotypes, and *(2)* the relationship between any individual gene and a polygenetic phenotype is not isomorphic, by definition. Thus, more integrative cross-species approaches are required to capture the complexity of ALB.

TRANSLATIONAL NEUROGENETICS OF ANXIETY: FROM RODENT TO HUMAN AND BACK

Recent translational studies have attempted to use cross-species approaches to couple neurogenetic findings in humans with rodent models of ALB (Sartori et al., 2011). Besides the efforts of Hovatta and colleagues and the studies on *RGS2* reviewed earlier in this section, other examples exist of research that integrates data across human and rodent studies of anxiety phenotypes to identify novel AD candidate genes. The PD GWAS described in the previous section further validated the genetic association of *TMEM132D* via studies in mice: SNP rs13478518, located in exon 9, was significantly associated with the level of ALB, and upregulation of *TMEM132D* mRNA was observed in the cingulate cortex of HAB mice (Erhardt et al., 2011). A functional polymorphism (Val66Met) of the *BDNF* gene has recently been implicated in fear extinction. Mice expressing the *BDNF* Met allele, which is uncommon in humans, exhibited increased ALB and impaired FE relative to mice expressing the Val allele. Interestingly, similar impairment in FE has also been observed in humans with the Met allele. Using fMRI, impairment in extinction resulting from the Met allele was shown to be accompanied by deficient activity in the ventromedial prefrontal cortex and increased amygdala activation in both human and mice (Soliman et al., 2010). Several other studies have reported genetic effects in human anxiety phenotypes for genes identified from rodent studies (Donner et al., 2008; Hettema et al., 2011; Smoller et al., 2001).

FUTURE DIRECTIONS—EPIGENETICS

Epigenetic mechanisms potentially contribute, at least in part, to some of the observed genetic basis for ADs. As discussed in

Chapter 7, epigenetic modifications involve long-lasting alterations in gene expression that *(1)* are transmissible, *(2)* are affected by environmental factors, and *(3)* do not involve changes to the genome sequence. These are caused by posttranslational alterations including methylation, phosphorylation, and acetylation at specific residues including arginine, histidine, lysine, serine, and threonine. While the mechanisms underlying such effects on anxiety are yet to be determined, the fact that environmental events can alter risk for ADs suggests that epigenetics can play a role. For example, recent rodent studies support the hypothesis that early-life adversity increases risk for the development of psychopathology via negative impact on brain mechanisms underlying emotionality. Altered maternal care of rat pups increases methylation within the promoter region of the glucocorticoid receptor (*GR*) gene (Weaver et al., 2004). GR methylation decreases GR expression during adulthood and is thought to mediate the effects of early-life stress on increased anxiety and HPA axis alterations. Moreover, early life maltreatment leads to methylation of BDNF promoters in the rat, resulting in decreased BDNF expression in the prefrontal cortex into adulthood. Interestingly, early-life adversity in rats leads them to mistreat their own offspring, resulting in significant DNA methylation in the offspring. This underscores the transgenerational impact of such mechanisms on the phenotype and further supports potential non-DNA-mediated inheritance (reviewed in Sartori et al., 2011).

ANIMAL MOLECULAR GENETICS SUMMARY

There exist several well-validated animal models of ALB applicable to the identification of genetic loci underlying AD phenotypes and their biological effects. They provide complementary approaches using selected breeding and manipulations of both genetic and environmental factors not available in humans. The hope is that, like for other complex genetic medical syndromes, bidirectional translational studies between animal models and humans will provide critical insight into the pathophysiological basis of ADs and, ultimately, new targets for intervention.

SUMMARY

The major ADs exhibit moderate familial aggregation and heritability due to genetic risk factors that are common between them as well as those that are disorder specific. Similar findings apply when one expands the phenotypes to include anxiety-related personality traits and some aspects of unipolar depression. Similar to other psychiatric disorders, many candidate gene association studies have been published, with a small set of genes that have been consistently validated for their role in one or more anxiety phenotypes. GWAS of ADs are in their infancy, with only a few published studies so far and more to come in the next few years being conducted by large consortia. Animal studies provide a particularly promising complementary approach to human studies, since animal models for anxiety phenotypes are among the best validated across psychiatry. Several examples already exist of complementary and concurring genetic evidence across species supporting the involvement of particular biological systems in anxiety-related behaviors.

DISCLOSURES

None of the authors have any financial conflicts of interest.

Dr. Perez is supported by NIH grants only: T32MH020030.

Dr. Otowa is supported by a grant from the Japan Society for the Promotion of Science (21-8373).

Dr. Roberson-Nay is supported by NIH grants only: K01MH080953, R01MH098055.

Dr. Hettema is supported by NIH grants only: R01MH087646, R01MH039096, R01MH098055.

REFERENCES

Afifi, T.O., Asmundson, G.J., et al. (2010). The role of genes and environment on trauma exposure and posttraumatic stress disorder symptoms: a review of twin studies. *Clin. Psychol. Rev.* 30:101–112.

Bergen, S.E., Gardner, C.O., et al. (2007). Age-related changes in heritability of behavioral phenotypes over adolescence and young adulthood: a meta-analysis. *Twin. Res. Hum. Genet.* 10:423–433.

Bienvenu, O.J., Brown, C., et al. (2001). Normal personality traits and comorbidity among phobic, panic and major depressive disorders. *Psychiatry Res.* 102:73–85.

Bienvenu, O.J., Hettema, J.M., et al. (2007). Low extraversion and high neuroticism as indices of genetic and environmental risk for social phobia, agoraphobia, and animal phobia. *Am. J. Psychiatry* 164:1714–1721.

Binder, E.B., Bradley, R.G., et al. (2008). Association of FKBP5 polymorphisms and childhood abuse with risk of posttraumatic stress disorder symptoms in adults. *JAMA* 299:1291–1305.

Blaya, C., Salum, G.A., et al. (2007). Lack of association between the Serotonin Transporter Promoter Polymorphism (5-HTTLPR) and Panic Disorder: a systematic review and meta-analysis. *Behav. Brain Funct.* 3:41.

Bloch, M.H., Landeros-Weisenberger, A., et al. (2008). Association of the serotonin transporter polymorphism and obsessive-compulsive disorder: systematic review. *Am. J. Med. Genet. B Neuropsychiatr. Genet.* 147B:850–858.

Boomsma, D.I., van Beijsterveldt, C.E., et al. (2005). Genetic and environmental influences on Anxious/Depression during childhood: a study from the Netherlands Twin Register. *Genes Brain Behav.* 4:466–481.

Bunck, M., Czibere, L., et al. (2009). A hypomorphic vasopressin allele prevents anxiety-related behavior. *PLoS One* 4:e5129.

Cloninger, C.R., Van Eerdewegh, P., et al. (1998). Anxiety proneness linked to epistatic loci in genome scan of human personality traits. *Am. J. Med. Genet.* 81:313–317.

Czajkowski, N., Kendler, K.S., et al. (2011). The structure of genetic and environmental risk factors for phobias in women. *Psychol. Med.* 41:1987–1995.

de Moor, M.H., Costa, P.T., et al. (2012). Meta-analysis of genome-wide association studies for personality. *Mol. Psychiatry* 17:337–349.

Domschke, K., Deckert, J., et al. (2007). Meta-analysis of COMT val158met in panic disorder: ethnic heterogeneity and gender specificity. *Am. J. Med. Genet. B Neuropsychiatr. Genet.* 144B:667–673.

Donner, J., Pirkola, S., et al. (2008). An association analysis of murine anxiety genes in humans implicates novel candidate genes for anxiety disorders. *Biol. Psychiatry* 64:672–680.

Eley, T.C., Bolton, D., et al. (2003). A twin study of anxiety-related behaviours in pre-school children. *J. Child Psychol. Psychiatry* 44:945–960.

Erhardt, A., Czibere, L., et al. (2011). TMEM132D, a new candidate for anxiety phenotypes: evidence from human and mouse studies. *Mol. Psychiatry* 16:647–663.

Flint, J. (2003). Animal models of anxiety and their molecular dissection. *Semin. Cell Dev. Biol.* 14:37–42.

Franic, S., Middeldorp, C.M., et al. (2010). Childhood and adolescent anxiety and depression: beyond heritability. *J. Am. Acad. Child Adolesc. Psychiatry* 49:820–829.

Fullerton, J. (2006). New approaches to the genetic analysis of neuroticism and anxiety. *Behav. Genet.* 36:147–161.

Gordon, J.A., and Hen, R. (2004). Genetic approaches to the study of anxiety. *Annu. Rev. Neurosci.* 27:193–222.

Graham, B.M., and Richardson, R. (2011). Memory of fearful events: the role of fibroblast growth factor-2 in fear acquisition and extinction. *Neuroscience* 189:156–169.

Hefner, K., Whittle, N., et al. (2008). Impaired fear extinction learning and cortico-amygdala circuit abnormalities in a common genetic mouse strain. *J. Neurosci.* 28:8074–8085.

Hettema, J.M., Neale, M.C., et al. (2001). A review and meta-analysis of the genetic epidemiology of anxiety disorders. *Am. J. Psychiatry* 158:1568–1578.

Hettema, J.M., Neale, M.C., et al. (2006). A population-based twin study of the relationship between neuroticism and internalizing disorders. *Am. J. Psychiatry* 163:857–864.

Hettema, J.M., Prescott, C.A., et al. (2005). The structure of genetic and environmental risk factors for anxiety disorders in men and women. *Arch. Gen. Psychiatry* 62:182–189.

Hettema, J.M., Webb, B.T., et al. (2011). Prioritization and association analysis of murine-derived candidate genes in anxiety-spectrum disorders. *Biol. Psychiatry* 70:888–896.

Hovatta, I., and Barlow, C. (2008). Molecular genetics of anxiety in mice and men. *Ann. Med.* 40:92–109.

Hovatta, I., Tennant, R.S., et al. (2005). Glyoxalase 1 and glutathione reductase 1 regulate anxiety in mice. *Nature* 438:662–666.

Jacobson, L.H., and Cryan, J.F. (2010). Genetic approaches to modeling anxiety in animals. *Curr. Top. Behav. Neurosci.* 2:161–201.

Kendler, K.S., and Baker, J.H. (2007). Genetic influences on measures of the environment: a systematic review. *Psychol. Med.* 37:615–626.

Kendler, K.S., Gardner, C.O., et al. (2006). The sources of co-morbidity between major depression and generalized anxiety disorder in a Swedish national twin sample. *Psychol. Med.* 37:453–462.

Kendler, K.S., Gardner, C.O., et al. (2008a). The development of fears from early adolesence to young adulthood: a multivariate study. *Psychol. Med.* 38:1759–1769.

Kendler, K.S., Gardner, C.O., et al. (2008b). A longitudinal twin study of fears from middle childhood to early adulthood: evidence for a developmentally dynamic genome. *Arch. Gen. Psychiatry* 65:421–429.

Koenen, K.C. (2007). Genetics of posttraumatic stress disorder: review and recommendations for future studies. *J. Trauma. Stress* 20:737–750.

Koenen, K.C., Amstadter, A.B., et al. (2009). Gene-environment interaction in posttraumatic stress disorder: an update. *J. Trauma. Stress* 22:416–426.

Last, C.G., Hersen, M., et al. (1991). Anxiety disorders in children and their families. *Arch. Gen. Psychiatry* 48:928–934.

Lau, J.Y., Gregory, A.M., et al. (2007). Assessing gene-environment interactions on anxiety symptom subtypes across childhood and adolescence. *Dev. Psychopathol.* 19:1129–1146.

Leckman, J.F., Zhang, H., et al. (2001). Symptom dimensions in obsessive-compulsive disorder: toward quantitative phenotypes. *Am. J. Med. Genet.* 105:28–30.

Legrand, L.N., McGue, M., et al. (1999). A twin study of state and trait anxiety in childhood and adolescence. *J. Child Psychol. Psychiatry* 40:953–958.

Lesch, K., Bengel, D., et al. (1996). Association of anxiety-related traits with a polymorphism in the serotonin transporter gene regulatory region. *Science* 274:1527–1531.

Logue, M.W., Bauver, S.R., et al. (2012). Multivariate analysis of anxiety disorders yields further evidence of linkage to chromosomes 4q21 and 7p in panic disorder families. *Am. J. Med. Genet. B Neuropsychiatr. Genet.* 159B:274–280.

Maron, E., Hettema, J.M., et al. (2010). Advances in molecular genetics of panic disorder. *Mol. Psychiatry* 15:681–701.

Micco, J.A., Henin, A., et al. (2009). Anxiety and depressive disorders in offspring at high risk for anxiety: a meta-analysis. *J. Anxiety. Disord.* 23:1158–1164.

Middeldorp, C.M., Cath, D.C., et al. (2005). The co-morbidity of anxiety and depression in the perspective of genetic epidemiology: a review of twin and family studies. *Psychol. Med.* 35:611–624.

Miguel, E.C., Leckman, J.F., et al. (2005). Obsessive-compulsive disorder phenotypes: implications for genetic studies. *Mol. Psychiatry* 10:258–275.

Munafo, M.R., Freimer, N.B., et al. (2009). 5-HTTLPR genotype and anxiety-related personality traits: a meta-analysis and new data. *Am. J. Med. Genet. B Neuropsychiatr. Genet.* 150B:271–281.

Nelson, E.C., Grant, J.D., et al. (2000). Social phobia in a population-based female adolescent twin sample: co-morbidity and associated suicide-related symptoms. *Psychol. Med.* 30:797–804.

Nes, R.B., Roysamb, E., et al. (2007). Symptoms of anxiety and depression in young adults: genetic and environmental influences on stability and change. *Twin. Res. Hum. Genet.* 10:450–461.

Nestadt, G., Grados, M., et al. (2010). Genetics of obsessive-compulsive disorder. *Psychiatr. Clin. North Am.* 33:141–158.

Norrholm, S.D., and Ressler, K.J. (2009). Genetics of anxiety and trauma-related disorders. *Neuroscience* 164:272–287.

Ogliari, A., Citterio, A., et al. (2006). Genetic and environmental influences on anxiety dimensions in Italian twins evaluated with the SCARED questionnaire. *J. Anxiety Disord.* 20:760–777.

Otowa, T., Yoshida, E., et al. (2009). Genome-wide association study of panic disorder in the Japanese population. *J. Hum. Genet.* 54:122–126.

Perez, J.A., Clinton, S.M., et al. (2009). A new role for FGF2 as an endogenous inhibitor of anxiety. *J. Neurosci.* 29:6379–6387.

Ponder, C.A., Huded, C.P., et al. (2008). Rapid selection response for contextual fear conditioning in a cross between C57BL/6J and A/J: behavioral, QTL and gene expression analysis. *Behav. Genet.* 38:277–291.

Ressler, K.J., Mercer, K.B., et al. (2011). Post-traumatic stress disorder is associated with PACAP and the PAC1 receptor. *Nature* 470:492–497.

Roberson-Nay, R., Eaves, L.J., et al. (2012). Childhood separation anxiety disorder and adult onset panic attacks share a common genetic diathesis. *Depress. Anxiety* 29:320–327.

Rose, R.J., and Ditto, W.B. (1983). A developmental-genetic analysis of common fears from early adolescence to early adulthood. *Child Dev.* 54:361–368.

Sartori, S.B., Landgraf, R., et al. (2011). The clinical implications of mouse models of enhanced anxiety. *Future Neurol.* 6:531–571.

Scaini, S., Ogliari, A., et al. (2012). Genetic and environmental contributions to separation anxiety: a meta-analytic approach to twin data. *Depress. Anxiety* 29(9):754–761.

Schumacher, J., Kristensen, A.S., et al. (2011). The genetics of panic disorder. *J. Med. Genet.* 48:361–368.

Shifman, S., Bhomra, A., et al. (2008). A whole genome association study of neuroticism using DNA pooling. *Mol. Psychiatry* 13:302–312.

Silberg, J., Rutter, M., et al. (2001a). Genetic moderation of environmental risk for depression and anxiety in adolescent girls. *Br. J. Psychiatry* 179:116–121.

Silberg, J.L., Rutter, M., et al. (2001b). Genetic and environmental influences on the temporal association between earlier anxiety and later depression in girls. *Biol. Psychiatry* 49:1040–1049.

Smoller, J.W., Block, S.R., et al. (2009). Genetics of anxiety disorders: the complex road from DSM to DNA. *Depress. Anxiety* 26:965–975.

Smoller, J.W., and Faraone, S.V. (2008). Genetics of anxiety disorders: complexities and opportunities. *Am. J. Med. Genet. C Semin. Med. Genet.* 148C:85–88.

Smoller, J.W., Rosenbaum, J.F., et al. (2001). Genetic association analysis of behavioral inhibition using candidate loci from mouse models. *Am. J. Med. Genet.* 105:226–235.

Soliman, F., Glatt, C.E., et al. (2010). A genetic variant BDNF polymorphism alters extinction learning in both mouse and human. *Science* 327:863–866.

Spatola, C.A., Rende, R., et al. (2010). Genetic and environmental influences upon the CBCL/6-18 DSM-oriented scales: similarities and differences across three different computational approaches and two age ranges. *Eur. Child Adolesc. Psychiatry* 19:647–658.

Stein, M.B., Jang, K.L., et al. (2002). Genetic and environmental influences on trauma exposure and posttraumatic stress disorder symptoms: a twin study. *Am. J. Psychiatry* 159:1675–1681.

Tambs, K., Czajkowsky, N., et al. (2009). Structure of genetic and environmental risk factors for dimensional representations of DSM-IV anxiety disorders. *Br. J. Psychiatry* 195:301–307.

Terracciano, A., Sanna, S., et al. (2010). Genome-wide association scan for five major dimensions of personality. *Mol. Psychiatry* 15:647–656.

True, W.R., Rice, J., et al. (1993). A twin study of genetic and environmental contributions to liability for posttraumatic stress symptoms. *Arch. Gen. Psychiatry* 50:257–264.

Trzaskowski, M., Zavos, H.M., et al. (2011). Stable genetic influence on anxiety-related behaviours across middle childhood. *J. Abnorm. Child Psychol.* 40(1):85–94.

van den Oord, E.J., Kuo, P.H., et al. (2008). Genomewide association analysis followed by a replication study implicates a novel candidate gene for neuroticism. *Arch. Gen. Psychiatry* 65:1062–1071.

van Grootheest, D.S., Cath, D.C., et al. (2005). Twin studies on obsessive-compulsive disorder: a review. *Twin Res. Hum. Genet.* 8:450–458.

Weaver, I.C., Cervoni, N., et al. (2004). Epigenetic programming by maternal behavior. *Nat. Neurosci.* 7:847–854.

Webb, B.T., Guo, A.Y., et al. (2012). Meta-analyses of genome-wide linkage scans of anxiety-related phenotypes. *Eur. J. Hum. Genet.* 20(10):1078–1084.

Yalcin, B., Willis-Owen, S.A., et al. (2004). Genetic dissection of a behavioral quantitative trait locus shows that Rgs2 modulates anxiety in mice. *Nat. Genet.* 36:1197–1202.

41 | NEUROBIOLOGY OF FEAR AND ANXIETY: CONTRIBUTIONS OF ANIMAL MODELS TO CURRENT UNDERSTANDING

CHRISTOPHER K. CAIN, GREGORY M. SULLIVAN, AND JOSEPH E. LeDOUX

INTRODUCTION

Animal models are *experimental preparations developed in one species for the purpose of studying phenomena occurring in another species* (McKinney 2001). Since human studies are often impractical or unethical, researchers depend on animal models to study the neurobiological mechanisms of fear and anxiety and to evaluate new treatments, especially drugs. There are approximately 100 animal models of fear and anxiety in the literature. We will focus on the models that have contributed most to our current understanding of the neurobiological mechanisms underlying fear and anxiety, and those with the greatest potential to expand our knowledge of pathological anxiety.

Although we will not attempt to summarize the contribution of animal models to the discovery and development of new anxiolytic drugs, it will become apparent that researchers in industry and academia have largely focused on different animal models. We will argue that this strategy, although useful for a time, is now unnecessary and may be impeding progress for both groups. The path forward, in our opinion, is to focus on animal models amenable to studies of the brain circuits and neural processes that mediate threat processing and defensive responding. This may be essential for advancing our understanding of neurobiological processes relevant to anxiety, identifying the causes of pathological anxiety and predicting how drugs may influence these relevant circuits and dysfunctional processes.

LANGUAGE AND CONCEPTUAL FRAMEWORK

A challenge for research on animal models of human psychiatric disorders is developing an appropriate and useful language to relate preclinical and clinical findings. On the one hand, animal models are only useful to the extent that they resemble a human problem, and similar language can improve communication between clinicians and preclinical researchers. On the other hand, these models are limited by differences in the brains of humans and other animals, and imprecision in nomenclature can complicate interpretation and application of preclinical findings. It is particularly important to be clear about which aspects of human anxiety can be studied using animal models. It will also be helpful to define a general conceptual framework for discussing the relationship between fear, anxiety, and animal models of human disorders.

DEFENSIVE RESPONDING, THREAT PROCESSING, AND FEELINGS

Criteria for diagnosing anxiety disorders often use terms that refer to emotional symptoms, such as *afraid, worried, stressed, anxious, distressed,* or *concerned* (DSM-IV-TR 2000). Human anxiety disorders are defined by such emotional symptoms, along with behavioral and physiological symptoms. Because emotional symptoms involve feelings, subjective internal states of consciousness, that are not observable and can only be communicated through language, they are difficult to approach scientifically. Animals with less complex brains are unlikely to experience feelings in the way humans do, and do not possess language to relay feelings. It is therefore extremely important that we resist the temptation to anthropomorphize and view animal models as a tool to reveal mechanisms of feelings; they cannot. Among the perils of such, this can lead to overinterpretation of preclinical results and/or false rejection of animal models that fail to predict human feelings.

A more productive route is to focus on evolutionarily conserved brain systems that detect and respond to threats or actual harm. These systems control the physiological and behavioral defensive responses (DRs) that contribute to anxiety disorder symptoms when dysfunctional. For instance, humans and rats exhibit many of the same behavioral (e.g., freezing, fight, escape), autonomic (e.g., cardiovascular or respiratory), and endocrine (e.g., hormone release) responses when in danger. Core components of the underlying neurocircuitry also show a striking degree of overlap. For example, in both species, the amygdala plays a crucial role in detecting and responding to threats, the hippocampus provides critical contextual information, and the ventromedial prefrontal cortex (vmPFC) can suppress threat responses. The accompanying cellular, hormonal, and molecular processes involved are also remarkably similar. Thus, it is appropriate to model human anxiety-related DRs in other mammals because they are similar, controlled by conserved networks that function unconsciously, and are objectively observable (LeDoux, 2012). Further, human feelings of fear and anxiety depend on DRs. This will be the focus of the chapter. When we have occasion to refer to conscious feelings, these will labeled as fearful feeling, conscious feeling, and so on. In order to make a subtle but important distinction, we will use the term *threat* when referring to responses to cues that predict harm, whereas the broader term *defensive* will refer to responses triggered by threats or actual harm.

TOPOGRAPHY OF DEFENSIVE RESPONDING

Fear and *anxiety* are used in many ways, sometimes interchangeably but sometimes to label distinct reactions to aversive stimulation. *Fear* is usually used to denote a state elicited by clearly defined environmental threats, either innately aversive or learned. This fear state functions to cope with immediate threats and is more intense than anxiety, but also shorter lived. For example, rodents will often freeze when threatened, but freezing subsides quickly when the threat is removed. *Anxiety* often describes threat responding elicited by more diffuse cues. Anxiety states can last longer than fear and function to cope with more distant, or poorly defined, threats. For example, rodents hug the walls in an unfamiliar or brightly lit environment (thigmotaxis), a behavior that likely evolved to thwart detection by predators. Since they often operate on very different time scales, fear responses can be more reflexive, whereas anxiety can include more complex cognitive processes exemplified in humans by anticipation and worry.

Although fear and anxiety often refer to different aspects of threat responding, sometimes mediated by different brain regions, they are not always clearly dissociable in natural situations or laboratory experiments. The distinction is clouded further when one considers drug classifications or diagnostic criteria for human disorders. Therapeutic agents are routinely categorized as *anxiolytic/antianxiety* with no category for *antifear* drugs. Further, although most consider anxiety states to be weaker than fear, many human anxiety disorders are defined by the intensity and form of fear responses. Thus, in addition to anthropomorphic perils, the terms *fear* and *anxiety* fail to clearly define alternate mental states with distinct response profiles. Functional behavior system (FBS) approaches may provide a better framework for considering threat-related defensive responding. Rather than attempt to divide fear and anxiety into separate phenomena, FBS approaches assume that both result from activation of *defense* or *survival circuits* that evolved to protect organisms from harm, especially predators (Blanchard et al., 1989; LeDoux, 2012). For instance, predatory imminence theory (PIT) suggests that DRs are arranged hierarchically along a continuum, and the particular responses elicited depend on the proximity of the threat (Timberlake and Fanselow, 1994). In PIT, threats activate DRs and divert animals from their *preferred activity pattern*. DRs at the low end of the spectrum, like thigmotaxis, are elicited when danger is possible but not imminent. DRs at the high end of the spectrum, like fighting or escape, are elicited by imminent threats, like an attacking predator. DRs function to protect the animal from threats or actual harm, and return the animal to its preferred activity pattern.

FBS approaches are useful because they remove ambiguity in other anxiety/fear distinctions but still capture much of the nuance implicit in other definitions. They nicely explain the progression of defensive responding as threats escalate. Threats that are unlikely, poorly defined, or distant serve to weakly activate survival circuits, resulting in relatively minor deviations from the preferred activity pattern. As threats become more likely, better defined, and closer, survival circuit activation increases, and animals deviate further from their preferred activity pattern. Ultimately, the strongest DR, defensive fighting, is elicited when all earlier responses fail to prevent threat escalation. It should be apparent that weaker DRs can occur over a much greater time frame whereas stronger DRs are often reflexive reactions to immediate threats (Fig. 41.1).

Before proceeding, a brief discussion of triggering stimuli and DR forms is warranted. Some triggering stimuli are innate; however, plasticity in survival circuits allows novel stimuli to gain control of DRs through experience. DRs also reflect an interaction between survival circuit activation and environmental options. For example, animals cannot flee in small laboratory testing chambers with no exits. Lastly, although mammalian DRs are remarkably similar in function and form (Blanchard et al., 1989), the exact behaviors are usually species specific (so-called species-specific defense responses or SSDRs; Timberlake and Fanselow, 1994). This simply means that a mouse will exhibit caution, freeze, flee, or fight differently than a monkey or human. Thus, although survival circuits are highly conserved neural systems for detecting and responding to danger, exact responses are usually unlearned, hard-wired reactions determined by evolution within a particular niche.

ANXIETY MODELS AMENABLE TO NEUROCIRCUIT ANALYSIS

Not all models are amenable to circuit analysis. Animal models can only contribute to our understanding of precise neurobiological mechanisms of defensive responding if a neural circuit mediating specific DRs can be identified and exploited. In line with the FBS approach outlined in the previous section, models amenable to neurocircuit analysis take advantage of discrete, well-defined triggering stimuli and innate, stereotyped DRs. This anchors the behavior to a neural system at the entry to, and exit from, the central nervous system. Models in which the stimulus conditions are diffuse or the responses lack stereotyped expression provide less guidance for studies that seek to identify key structures between the sensory and motor systems that underlie DRs.

Circuits are identified using a number of techniques. For instance, various lesions can demonstrate the necessity of specific brain regions. Disconnection lesions are particularly useful for showing that two different brain regions operate in series within a circuit to mediate a specific behavior. Extracellular recording of single neuronal units in awake, behaving animals is also extremely valuable for identifying information flow in neurocircuits. Other techniques, such as local infusion of drugs, brain stimulation, intracellular recording, or imaging of activity-dependent gene expression and/or energy metabolism, can provide converging evidence for the existence of a defined behavioral neurocircuit. Here it becomes evident why discrete triggering stimuli and

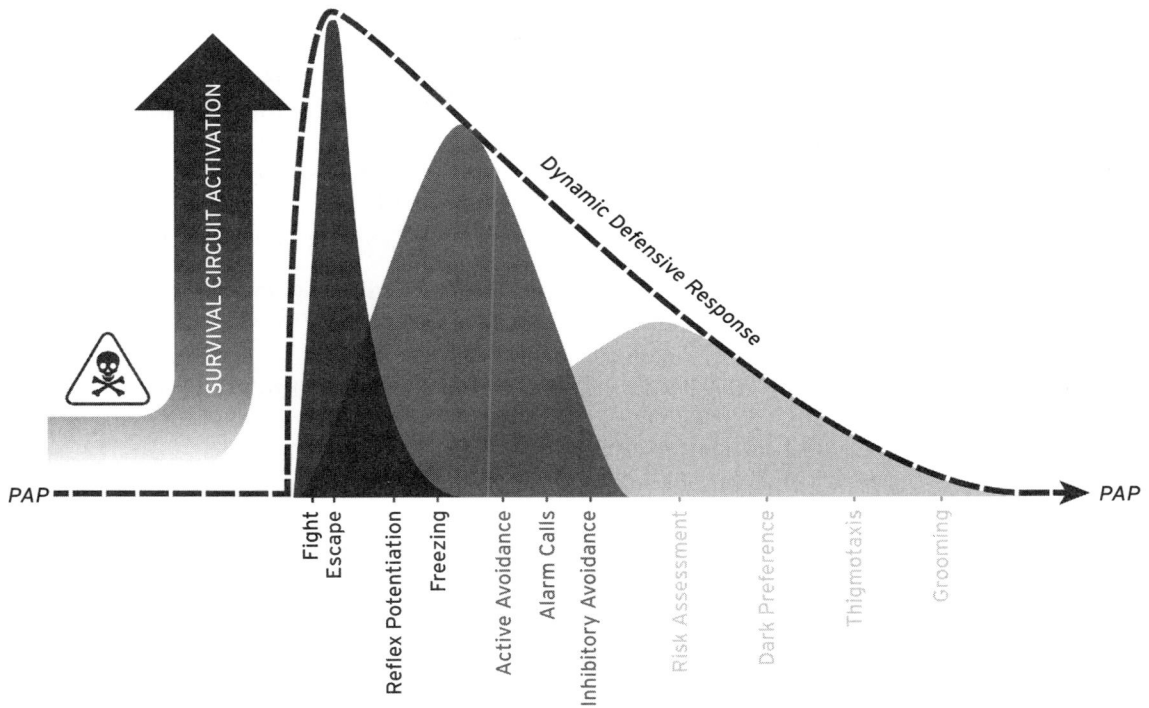

Figure 41.1 *Threats trigger survival circuit activation and initiate defensive responding. Defensive responses function to prevent harm, minimize exposure to threats, and return the organism to its preferred activity pattern (PAP). DRs are organized hierarchically, and more imminent threats lead to greater survival circuit activation; more intense, reflexive DRs; and more total time away from the PAP.*

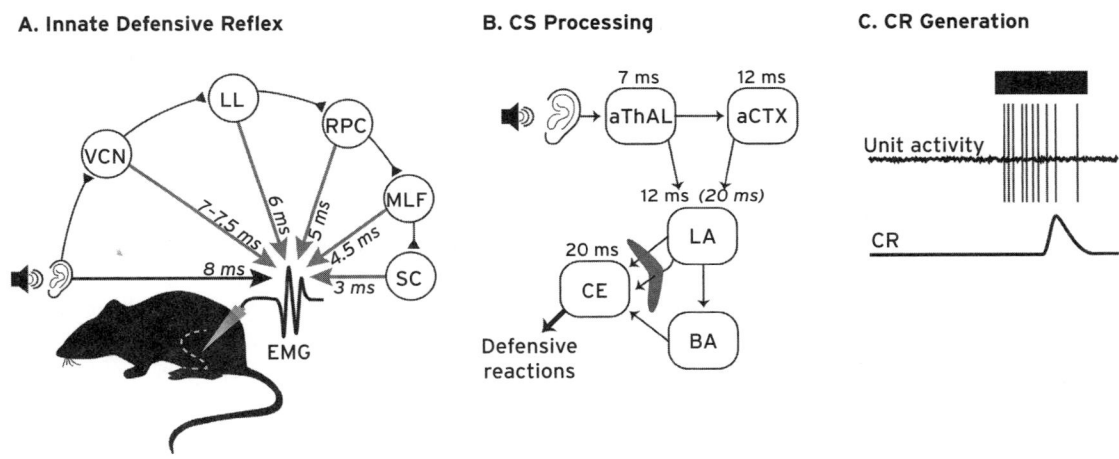

Figure 41.2 *Examples of animal models amenable to neurocircuit analysis. (A) Acoustic startle is an innate, and extremely fast, defensive reflex (8 ms from sound onset to initiation of muscular response). Once lesion studies identified components of the underlying circuit, neural stimulation studies helped establish the order of these nuclei within the circuit, by measuring the latency of startle responding following stimulation (Davis et al., 1982). VCN: ventral cochlear nucleus; LL: lateral lemniscus; RPC: nucleus reticularis pontis caudalis; MLF: medial longitudinal fasciculus; SC: spinal cord. (B) Pavlovian threat processing involves rapid sensory processing and amygdala activation. Recording of CS-evoked neural activity helped identify this core component of the mammalian survival circuit. Again, latency measures helped establish the order of nuclei within the circuit. aThal: auditory thalamus; aCtx: auditory cortex; LA: lateral amgyala; BA: basal amygdala; CE: central amygdala. (C) A very precise neural circuit has been identified for Pavlovian eyeblink conditioning in the cerebellum, and postconditioning, CS-evoked activity in the interpositus nucleus initiates eyeblink CRs (Medina et al., 2002).*

stereotyped responses are so important. By relating the timing of neural responses to the occurrence of stimuli and DRs, one can track information flow through a circuit beginning with stimuli that activate the circuit and ending with neural activity causing precise behavioral responses (Fig. 41.2). Once a circuit is identified, the role of specific brain areas, cells, synapses, molecules, and genes can be elucidated. This strategy, pioneered in studies of invertebrates (e.g., Bailey et al., 2000), has been successfully applied to studies of mammals (Davis et al., 1982; Medina et al., 2002).

NORMAL VERSUS PATHOLOGICAL FEAR AND ANXIETY

Fear and anxiety are normal, adaptive responses to threatening environmental challenges. When threats activate survival circuits, behavior is restricted to responses compatible with SSDRs, and autonomic and endocrine processes divert bodily resources away from nonessential processes (e.g., digestion) and toward systems needed to execute defense (e.g., musculature and brain). Ideally, the degree of activation is proportional to the threat, and an adaptive, or normal, response will subside soon after the threat is gone. This can be illustrated by the contribution of corticosteroids to defensive responding. Aversive stimuli can trigger an endocrine *stress response*. This includes the rapid release of corticosteroids into the peripheral circulation, which has a wide variety of effects on bodily processes, including (*1*) increasing blood glucose and blood pressure, (*2*) enhancing perception and memory, and (*3*) suppressing nonessential immune and reproductive functions. Corticosteroids, through a hypothalamic-pituitary-adrenal (HPA) axis feedback loop, also play a crucial role in limiting the duration of the stress response. The system is rapidly activated to deal with danger and then turned off when the threat is gone. Thus, when functioning properly, threat processing circuits promote survival and maximize time in the preferred activity pattern.

Pathological fear and anxiety can refer to either impaired or facilitated threat responding. For instance, patients with amygdala damage have deficits detecting and responding to threats. Some, like patient S. M., who has no amygdala function due to Urbach-Weithe disease, reportedly also fail to experience fearful feelings (Feinstein et al., 2011). Impaired amygdala function has real-life consequences; S. M. has a history of being victimized and abused, likely a result of her inability to recognize dangerous situations and respond appropriately.

Although rare disorders can produce defensive systems that are pathologically *hyporesponsive*, the vast majority of anxiety disorders involve systems that are *hyperresponsive* (Rosen and Schulkin, 1998). Thus, pathological fear and anxiety usually refer to threat responding that is exaggerated, inappropriate, or prolonged (Fig. 41.3). *Exaggerated* refers to DRs that are stronger than the situation requires. This could mean responding with full-blown stress responses in unfamiliar environments when only vigilance is warranted. Or perhaps responding to an unlikely threat as if it were 100% guaranteed to happen. *Inappropriate* DRs are triggered by stimuli that are not actually dangerous. *Prolonged* refers to DRs, including HPA axis activation, which persist well after the threat is diminished. Together, these factors describe states of fear and anxiety that are more intense, more frequent, and more often present in daily life.

ANIMAL MODELS OF FEAR AND ANXIETY

Since human anxiety disorders are varied and complex, animal models do not typically attempt to mimic full DSM syndromes (McKinney, 2001). Rather, they are adapted to specify and study key components of clinical syndromes. Researchers have approached this problem in many different ways, with varying degrees of success. While much has been learned about threat processing, defensive behavior, and learning in studies of invertebrates and other mammals (Bailey et al., 2000; Kalin, 2004), research on rodents has arguably contributed the most systematic and detailed information and will be the focus here. Ultimately, animal models are judged based on how well they reveal neurobiological mechanisms contributing to human anxiety and how well they predict the efficacy of treatments.

VALIDITY OF ANIMAL MODELS

Validity refers to the degree that a given model is useful for some purpose (McKinney, 2001; Willner, 1991). *Face validity* refers to phenomenological similarities between the model and the human psychiatric condition. Animal models have a high degree of face validity when etiological factors, symptoms, underlying physiology, and treatment effects are similar to the human disorder. *Construct validity* refers to the theoretical rational for linking a process in a model to a process hypothesized to be important in a human disorder. Due to shared aspects of their phylogenetic histories, humans and other animals are often homologous at molecular, cellular, synaptic, and circuitry levels of analysis. Finally, a model is considered to have good *predictive validity* when it can anticipate similar effects in humans. In the realm of drug development,

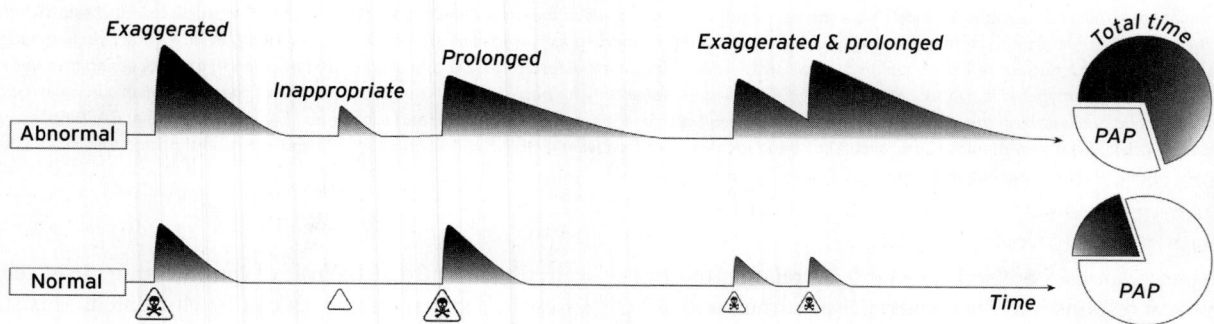

Figure 41.3 *Schematic representation of pathological defensive response profiles. Note that abnormalities reduce the amount of time spent in the preferred activity pattern (PAP).*

predictive validity is the ability to identify and rank drugs for therapeutic efficacy in humans.

Validity arguments are fundamentally epistemological and should not be used as the sole basis for evaluating the usefulness of an animal model. This is summed up nicely here:

> Animal models are tools for our use: They are not developed as part of a beauty contest, with a prize for the most convincing. If a model cannot readily be used, it is of little value, however elegant. Thus, the successful construction of a valid model should not be seen as an end in itself, but as a useful step in the investigation of a scientific problem. As such, validity can be assessed only in relation to the broader objectives of the research program.
>
> WILLNER *(1991)*

This last point is important. Different models may be useful for different purposes, depending on scientific and practical considerations. For instance, a model for rapid screening of drugs may have great predictive validity but little obvious construct validity. However, this could still be useful for developing new treatments, even if it may not be useful for unraveling neurobiological mechanisms of human anxiety. Thus, validity assessments are judgments made with appropriate context and based on available data, not exact measurements.

STATE VERSUS TRAIT ANXIETY

State anxiety is a temporary condition that is elicited by a stimulus or situation. *Trait anxiety* is an enduring condition that occurs across multiple situations or tests but is not necessarily pathological. Usually, tasks that assess trait anxiety are more valuable, as human disorders, and the rodent equivalents, are thought to be fairly stable. Unfortunately, many unconditioned animal models assess state anxiety, as is suggested by the relatively poor reliability in individual performance within or between tasks (Andreatini and Bacellar, 2000).

NORMAL VERSUS ABNORMAL RESPONDING

Most animal models evaluate "normal" fear and anxiety processes, where subjects are grouped and effects are reported as variation around a mean. Preexisting variability, genetic or otherwise, is averaged out. Evaluation of normal behavior is important; however, these studies may not adequately model the processes that cause human anxiety disorders. Anxiety disorders affect only a portion of the population, and for specific disorders like PTSD, only a subset of traumatized individuals develop pathological anxiety (Yehuda, 2007). Thus, animal models that examine abnormal responding, or outliers, may be of particular value. Researchers approach this problem using two basic strategies: (*1*) by performing standard assays but focusing on individuals with abnormal responses that mirror human pathology or (*2*) by introducing manipulations that skew group averages toward an abnormal response profile. Examples of these strategies will be discussed later.

ANIMAL MODELS OF NORMAL FEAR VERSUS ANXIETY

Animal models can be roughly divided into those that have an explicit learning component, and those that do not. Here we will distinguish between *unconditioned* and *conditioned* anxiety models. Note, however, that this terminology is not perfect; some unconditioned assays are referred to as *spontaneous*, *unlearned*, or *innate* anxiety in the literature (Takahashi et al., 2008), and some models involve nonassociative sensitization learning, which is not commonly considered "conditioning." Where relevant, these distinctions will be pointed out.

UNCONDITIONED MODELS

Unconditioned models examine DRs elicited by a novel test situation, not cues associated with prior aversive experience (Blanchard et al., 1989; Takahashi et al., 2008). These assays utilize ethologically relevant behavioral end points that are thought to be sensitive indices of an animal's natural anxiety/fear. Although there are many different unconditioned models of fear and anxiety, in the next section we discuss more commonly used rodent assays.

Innate Aversion to Light or Open Spaces

Rodents are nocturnally active small prey animals, and several popular unconditioned assays capitalize on their natural tendency to avoid brightly lit, open spaces. These assays elicit DRs akin to the *preencounter* behaviors of PIT, which likely evolved to protect animals in uncertain or weakly threatening situations. It has been argued that these weaker DRs reflect a degree of survival circuit activation that, in humans, corresponds to worry or mild anxiety (Craske, 1999; Rau and Fanselow, 2007). Examples are the elevated plus maze (EPM), light/dark, and defensive withdrawal tests. These assays are popular because they are easy to run, are cost-effective, require no learning phase, and reliably predict anxiolytic activity of *some* drugs (e.g., benzodiazepines) in humans. However, the imprecise nature of triggering stimuli (brightness/openness with no clear onset/termination) and resultant DRs (e.g., percentage of time spent in bright/open area, usually over many minutes) make it very difficult to define the underlying neural circuit. Further, these assays are sensitive to subtle variations and often produce inconsistent findings (Hogg 1996). Perhaps most problematic, they often fail to detect activity of nonbenzodiazepine anxiolytics (Kehne and Cain, 2010).

Light-enhanced startle is a related assay, but it has an advantage over those to the preceding because it is amenable to circuit analysis (Davis et al., 1982). In brief, this assay examines how an innate aversion to bright light can potentiate defensive reflexes by influencing neural processing in the well-characterized acoustic startle circuit (see Fig. 41.2). Light-enhanced startle has helped implicate specific brain regions (e.g., bed nucleus of the stria terminalis, or BNST), and molecules (e.g., corticotropin-releasing factor type 1, or CRF1, receptor), in the mediation of anxiety (Walker et al., 2009).

Social Behaviors

The unconditioned social interaction test measures the tendency of one animal to investigate and interact with a novel conspecific when the two are placed in a closed, brightly lit arena (File and Seth, 2003). The separation-induced ultrasonic vocalization model in rat pups is another example. In both tests the eliciting stimulus and resultant response are social in nature. Social anxiety assays have been successfully used to rapidly screen and characterize anxiolytic agents with diverse mechanisms of action, showing some superiority over alternative unconditioned anxiety models. The social interaction test has also been reliable enough to implicate some general brain areas in anxiety, such as the amygdala, hippocampus, and brain stem neuromodulatory centers. However, no precise neural circuit has emerged that would allow for detailed analyses of cellular, synaptic, and molecular mechanisms for these effects. Subtle procedural variations can also cause inconsistent results between laboratories.

Antipredator Models

Given that DRs evolved primarily to protect against predation, stimuli associated with predatory animals are also useful for modeling fear and anxiety (Blanchard et al., 1989; Takahashi et al., 2008). In these assays, predator stimuli are presented to rodents, and DRs ranging from defensive fighting down to weaker responses like risk assessment are measured. Pharmacological studies of antipredator responses have been conducted; however, these assays are primarily used to map the neural circuits underlying innate fear/anxiety, often for comparison with the circuitry mediating conditioned threat responses. Gene expression and lesion studies suggest that unconditioned responses to predator cues depend on slightly different brain regions (e.g., medial amygdala, BNST) from conditioned responses. These assays may be particularly useful for modeling ethologically relevant human phobias (Rosen, 2004).

Summary of Unconditioned Models

Unconditioned fear/anxiety assays are popular for evaluating drugs with anxiolytic potential. However, they may not be ideal models of human psychopathology because most assess state, rather than trait, anxiety, and they can be sensitive to very minor procedural variations (e.g., time of day, lighting conditions). Perhaps more problematic, they are not amenable to circuit analysis and neurobiological studies. The light-enhanced startle and antipredator assays are exceptions. These are unique because response triggers and DRs can be discrete and precisely defined, thus allowing for examination of underlying circuits and neural mechanisms. For instance, light-enhanced startle takes advantage of the known acoustic startle circuit and evaluates how anxiogenic manipulations interact to facilitate defensive reflexes. Antipredator studies have been similarly successful in defining differences between the brain regions mediating learned versus unlearned fear/anxiety. Together unconditioned assays have implicated the extended amygdala, septohippocampal system, PFC, and various brainstem neuromodulator centers (e.g., locus coeruleus or raphe nuclei) in anxiety-like responding (Gray and McNaughton, 2000; Karpova et al., 2011; Knapska et al., 2007), though precise neurobiological mechanisms are still largely unknown.

ASSOCIATIVE CONDITIONING MODELS

Brain systems that detect and respond to threats are not simply innately wired stimulus–response mechanisms; they are also plastic, allowing organisms to learn new predictors of danger. Learning can involve nonassociative and/or associative plasticity. Nonassociative learning occurs when repeated exposure to a single stimulus leads to stronger (sensitization) or weaker (habituation) responding. Both sensitization and habituation have been studied in relation to anxiety, however, usually as modulators of associative responses. We therefore emphasize associative learning processes here.

Associative learning is critical for establishing DRs to novel/innocuous stimuli, and for learning to cope with, or suppress, these responses. Two classes of associative learning with particular relevance to fear and anxiety are *Pavlovian threat conditioning (PTC)* and aversive *instrumental conditioning*. We refer to *conditioned threats* instead of the traditional *conditioned fears* for reasons outlined earlier in the Defensive Responding, Threat Processing, and Feelings section and elsewhere (LeDoux, 2012). PTC is particularly important for many reasons; the conditions for learning are simple, learning is rapid and long-lasting, a basic neurocircuit has been identified, and a great deal is known about the underlying synaptic, cellular, and molecular processes. PTC may also be a prerequisite for other critical forms of anxiety-related learning such as avoidance. Finally, PTC is a powerful tool for investigating how established pathological memories, and/or responses, may be regulated or suppressed through new learning.

Pavlovian Threat Conditioning

Behavioral Aspects of PTC When neutral conditioned stimuli (CSs) are temporally paired with naturally aversive unconditioned stimuli (USs) PTC occurs (Fig. 41.5). Any sensory stimulus can serve as a CS, including social and complex configural cues like contexts, and USs can be any unpleasant or painful stimulus. Auditory CSs and footshock USs are commonly employed in laboratory experiments partly because researchers can precisely control the delivery of these stimuli. Prior to conditioning, subjects respond weakly to the CS. After conditioning, CS-alone presentations elicit a cassette of DRs including freezing, autonomic reactions, neuroendocrine responses, as well as potentiation of somatic reflexes like startle and eyeblink, collectively referred to as conditioned fear/threat responses (CRs; Fig. 41.4). CRs indicate that associative learning took place, provided that similar responses fail to occur when the CS and US are not paired (unpaired) during conditioning. Although CRs can sometimes resemble unconditioned responses to the US (e.g., startle), CRs nearly always take a different form. CRs can be generated with as little as one CS–US pairing and can last a lifetime. PTC also establishes the CS as secondary incentive that can support instrumental avoidance and higher order Pavlovian conditioning (discussed later).

PTC Neurocircuitry The amygdala is a core component of the mammalian threat-processing circuitry and is essential for learning, storing, and expressing PTC memories (Cain and LeDoux, 2008) (Fig. 41.5). It is composed of a dozen or

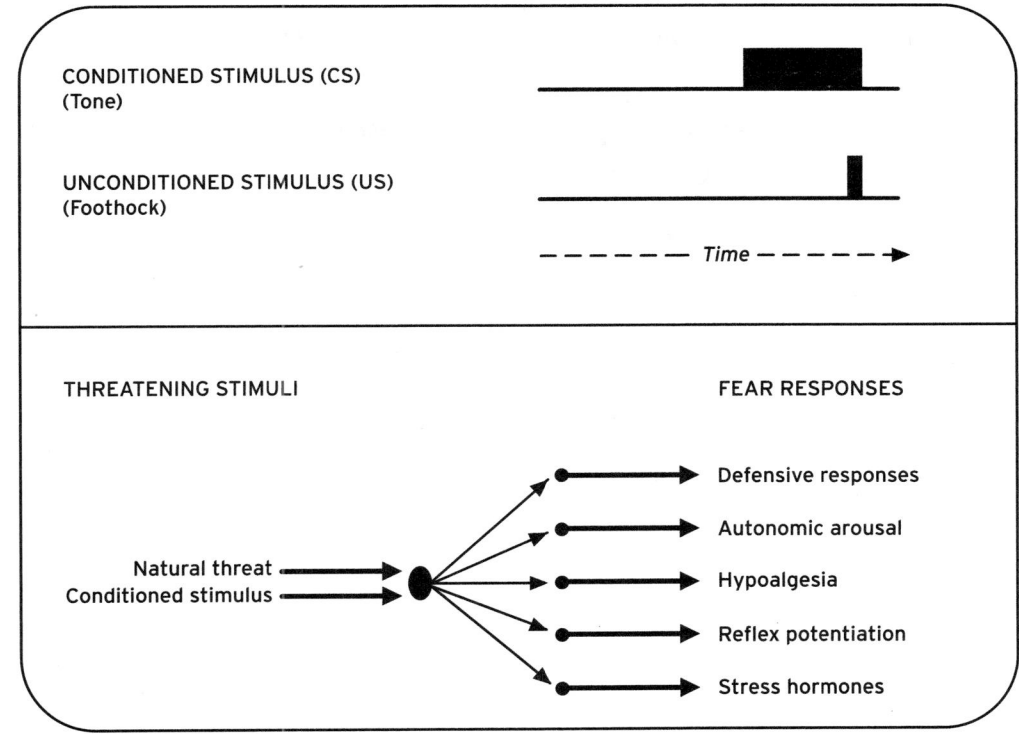

Figure 41.4 *Protocol for inducing Pavlovian threat conditioning and common defensive (fear) responses.*

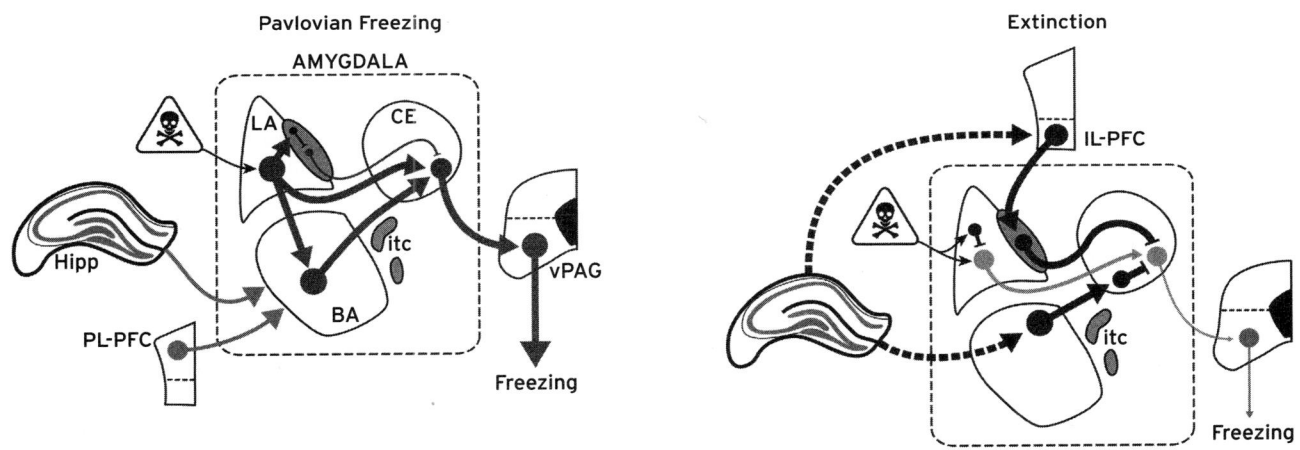

Figure 41.5 *Core neural circuit mediating Pavlovian threat conditioning and extinction. Pavlovian freezing is used as an example for simplicity. (Left) The amygdala plays a critical role in detecting and responding to conditioned threats. Postconditioning, threats activate LA neurons, which in turn activate CE both directly and indirectly (via projections to BA, or to the intercalated cell masses which causes disinhibition of CE). CE outputs project to downstream effector regions (e.g., ventral PAG) that mediate specific DRs (e.g., freezing). Hippocampal inputs to BA provide contextual information, and prelimbic-PFC neurons help sustain conditioned responding over longer intervals. (Right) Extinction learning counteracts threat responding in at least three ways: (1) by strengthening feedforward inhibition in LA, (2) through infralimbic-PFC activation of intercalated cells, and (3) through a subset of BA cells that project to CE interneurons and inhibit CE output. Hippocampus plays a critical role in gating extinction according to context and via connections to il-PFC and BA extinction neurons.*

so bilateral nuclei that reside in the temporal lobes. Of these, three have been the focus of much of the research on PTC: the lateral (LA), central (CE), and basal (BA) nuclei. LA neurons receive converging auditory (CS) and somatosensory (US) information from thalamic and cortical processing regions as early as 12 ms following stimulus onset. LA neurons in turn communicate with CE both directly and indirectly via projections to BA and intercalated cells. Although CE contributes to learning and memory (Gozzi et al., 2010; Haubensak et al., 2010; Wilensky et al., 2006), CE is best known for its role in controlling expression of Pavlovian CRs (Ciocchi et al., 2010; Johansen et al., 2011; Knobloch et al., 2012). BA appears to have a complex role in the expression of CRs that is only beginning to be understood (Amano et al., 2011; Herry et al., 2010). Because the role of LA is best understood, it will be the focus of the discussion here.

LA is essential for learning, consolidation, expression, reconsolidation, extinction, and many other aspects of PTC (Cain and LeDoux, 2008; Johansen et al., 2011). Several recent findings provide especially strong support for the central role of LA in PTC. For instance, using optogenetics we recently demonstrated that artificial PTC memories could be created in rats by pairing standard auditory CSs with depolarization of LA neurons (Johansen et al., 2010). CS presentations after training elicited freezing, even though rats never received any footshocks. Although freezing was weaker than observed after real conditioning with footshock USs, that the rats froze at all was a testament to the importance of LA for PTC learning. Further, lesions of LA conducted 16 months after PTC, nearly the entire adult lifetime of the rat, severely disrupt conditioned freezing (Gale et al., 2004). Finally, using a clever combination of molecular tools, researchers recently demonstrated how a subset of LA neurons (~20%) outcompete their neighbors to store PTC plasticity, and were able to identify and erase PTC memories by ablating only those neurons (Josselyn, 2010). Together these findings firmly implicate LA in the learning, storage, and expression of PTC memories.

Extra-amygdala regions also make important contributions to PTC learning and expression. The hippocampus plays an important role in conditioning to more complex contextual cues, most likely through CS-related projections to BA (Maren and Fanselow, 1995). However, hippocampus plays a time-limited role in expression of contextual CRs; systems-level consolidation processes transfer this memory to more cortical brain regions like the anterior cingulate (Teixeria et al., 2006). Prelimbic PFC also appears to help maintain expression of CRs like freezing even after short-latency neural responses in amygdala adapt during CS presentations (Burgos-Robles et al., 2009).

Synaptic Plasticity in LA Associative pairing of the tone and shock induces synaptic plasticity between CS afferents and LA neurons (for review, see Johansen et al., 2011). PTC also results in synaptic plasticity in structures afferent to the LA (e.g., thalamus, cortex; Quirk et al., 1997; Weinberger, 1995). However, these are unlikely to be essential for threat conditioning at the level of behavior for three reasons: (*1*) inactivation of the LA prevents learning and memory, indicating that these structures alone cannot support PTC, (*2*) plasticity in these afferent structures appears to depend on LA function, and (*3*) conditioning-related plasticity in LA emerges before changes in afferent regions. Together these findings suggest that PTC changes the way a CS is processed in an emotional circuit involving LA, and this plasticity allows the CS to control expression of DRs after the aversive experience (Cain and LeDoux, 2008; Fig. 41.6).

Molecular Mechanisms of PTC in LA With mounting anatomical, physiological, and behavioral evidence implicating the LA in PTC, many researchers have focused their efforts on deciphering the molecular signaling cascades important for learning/memory in this region. The majority of studies employ genetic and pharmacological manipulations coupled with PTC to determine the function of specific molecules. Manipulations carefully timed with respect to training and

testing allow researchers to distinguish between involvement in learning, short-term memory (STM), and long-term memory (LTM) processes. Related studies have also probed the molecular mechanisms of LTP, usually using *in vitro* brain slice preparations while stimulating sensory afferents and recording in the LA. However, we will omit coverage of *in vitro* LTP as this topic has been covered in detail elsewhere and the results are generally in agreement with *in vivo* manipulations. A detailed review of the large body of molecular work related to PTC is beyond the scope of this chapter (for review, see Johansen et al., 2011); however, we will highlight the contributions of a few key molecular players to illustrate how long-lasting plasticity between sensory afferents and LA neurons is achieved.

There appear to be several important molecular stages to PTC-related plasticity in LA. First, receptors and ion channels at the synapse translate presynaptic activity into postsynaptic activation of signaling cascades by elevating intracellular calcium concentrations. NMDA (*N*-methyl-D-aspartate) receptors, L-type calcium channels, and metabotropic glutamate receptors are crucial for this process. αCaMKII (calcium/calmodulin-dependent protein kinase two) is particularly important for short-term memory/plasticity and may covalently modify existing synaptic proteins, like the alpha-amino-3-hydroxy-5-methyl-4-isoxazole propionic acid (AMPA) receptor, to facilitate glutamatergic transmission. PKA (protein kinase A) and MAPK (mitogen-activated protein kinase) are important for long-term memory/plasticity. When activated, they translocate to the nucleus to stimulate CREB (cAMP-responsive element binding protein)-mediated transcription. Long-term changes in synaptic transmission are ultimately achieved by transcription of the appropriate genes, translation of new proteins, and incorporation of these new proteins at the synapse. For instance, the production and synaptic insertion of new AMPA receptors are critical for PTC (Rumpel et al., 2005). Transcription and translation may also help form new synapses between sensory afferents and LA neurons (Ostroff et al., 2010). Together, molecular work in the PTC pathway demonstrates that synaptic receptors/channels, intracellular kinases, and nuclear machinery respond to CS–US pairings in a coordinated fashion to change CS processing in the LA and allow new stimuli to control defensive responding.

Exciting new work illustrates how molecular alterations in amygdala networks can alter threat processing and possibly contribute to human psychopathology. For instance, the discovery of an acid-sensing ion channel in LA that detects CO_2-related changes in pH and elicits DRs has exciting implications for understanding neuropathology in panic disorder, since CO_2-enriched air can precipitate panic attacks (Ziemann et al., 2009). And other studies demonstrate that allelic variants in genes affecting catecholamine catabolism (COMT) and serotonin reuptake (5-HTT) strongly predict hyperresponsiveness of defense-related neurons and behavior, including those responsible for threat conditioning, consistent with the notion of stable trait anxiety (Domschke and Dannlowski, 2010).

Variations of the PTC Procedure The simple PTC procedure described in the preceding is the most common tool for studying fear and anxiety reactions. It is simple because it usually involves discrete, unimodal CSs and USs with few pairings

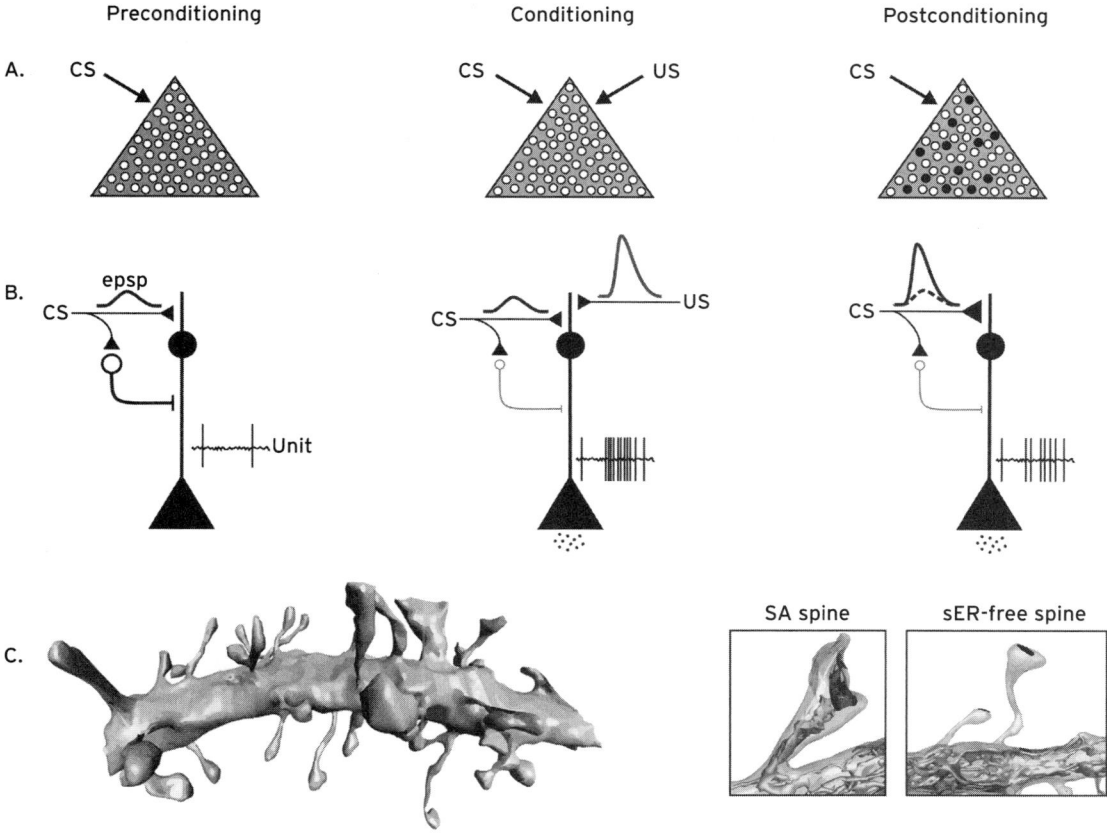

Preconditioning   Conditioning   Postconditioning

A.

B.

C.

SA spine   sER-free spine

Figure 41.6 *The identification of a neurocircuit has greatly facilitated studies of cellular processes important for defensive learning. For instance, approximately 20% of LA neurons outcompete their neighbors during conditioning, via a CREB-dependent mechanism, to learn and store PCT plasticity (A). Prior to conditioning, CS presentations result in weak depolarization of LA neurons and little to no activation of downstream brain areas mediating DRs. However, with CS–US pairings, neurons are strongly depolarized, resulting in initiation of an LTP-like process that strengthens the synapses between CS afferents and LA neurons. Following conditioning, CS presentations strongly depolarize LA neurons, trigger action potentials, and release neurotransmitters to activate downstream brain areas mediating expression of DRs. Recent work suggests the importance neuromodulators like dopamine and norepinephrine to the induction PTC plasticity in LA, both by direct action on excitatory cells and by suppression of feedforward GABAergic inhibition (Ehrlich et al. 2009) (B). Identification of this critical component of the neurocircuit has also allowed for detailed anatomical analyses of LA dendrites (C). For instance, studies using serial electron microscopy to reconstruct segments of LA dendrites after conditioning suggest that larger and more stable spines (SA spines) increase in frequency following conditioning and smaller (smooth ER-free) spines increase postsynaptic density area.*

(<10) given with 100% contingency (all CS and US presentations are paired). There are countless variations on the PTC procedure that could help elucidate specific aspects of fear and anxiety. Here we will mention just a few.

The standard PTC procedure produces robust freezing in rodents, suggesting that CSs can strongly activate survival circuits and produce relatively high-level DRs, similar to those associated with human fear. Recent studies have attempted to model the uncertainty of anxiety more effectively by reducing CS/US contingency, increasing the CS–US delay, or by introducing an interval between the end of the CS and the US. Other variations use complex cues to signal the US, such as contextual stimuli. Much less is known about the neurobiology of these phenomena, but they are promising approaches for unraveling the neural mechanisms of anxiety and structures such as the BNST, hippocampus, and ACC, which have been implicated (Waddell et al., 2006; Walker et al., 2009).

Still another PTC variation assesses how aversive CSs suppress other nondefensive responses such as bar pressing for food. The most common of these assays is called conditioned suppression or the conditioned emotional response (CER) test. These assays are more complicated, require much more training, and have the added layer of food/water deprivation that can muddle interpretation of results. The neural mechanisms of CER and simple PTC are similar, but there are subtle differences. Recently it has been suggested that conditioned suppression is a unique form of Pavlovian-instrument transfer (Balleine and Killcross, 2006) and thus may not be an ideal way to assess PTC directly.

Studies of retrieval-induced learning may also explain the development of some key anxiety disorder symptoms and suggest novel strategies for treatment. As in PTC, cues associated with trauma can reactivate traumatic memories. Such reminders can be severely disruptive, triggering intrusive images and thoughts that accompany a progressive worsening of anxiety symptoms, especially for memory-based disorders like PTSD (Southwick et al., 1999). Preclinical studies indicate that retrieval renders fear memories labile, probably to allow for the incorporation of new information, which is followed by a new consolidation process (reconsolidation). There is ample evidence in the literature that retrieved memories can be reconsolidated in a stronger (fear incubation) or weaker state (Cain et al., 2012). Models that exploit these processes to examine new treatment options will be discussed later.

Summary of Pavlovian Threat Conditioning PTC has arguably enjoyed the most success as an animal model of fear and anxiety. The PTC model has good face, construct, and predictive validity, at least in terms of normal human fear and anxiety. The ability to identify and dissect a basic neural circuit has undoubtedly contributed to this model's success. Procedural variations may even allow for studies of weaker, anxiety-like DRs that were previously thought to require unconditioned anxiety models like the EPM. This system, along with variations in the procedure and/or additional learning phases that depend on PTC, may hold the most potential for modeling key aspects of human pathological anxiety as well.

Instrumental Avoidance Conditioning

Unlike PTC, where subjects learn about relationships between environmental stimuli and react accordingly, instrumental paradigms allow the subjects to *control* exposure to aversive stimuli. There are many variations on the instrumental theme, but here we will focus on two common assay types: passive or inhibitory avoidance (IA) and active avoidance (AA). Avoidance is a hallmark of many human anxiety disorders; however, like fear and anxiety, avoidance mechanisms evolved because they were adaptive and helped protect organisms from threats. But excessive avoidance may interfere with normal functioning and become maladaptive. Here we will discuss normal avoidance and summarize what is known about the underlying neurobiology. Later sections will examine how avoidance can become maladaptive.

Inhibitory Avoidance IA learning involves withholding a response that was previously punished, typically by shock. Although PTC undoubtedly occurs in these situations, the animal has control over exposure to the shock and shock-paired cues; thus, IA is instrumental in nature. There are many obvious parallels between IA and human psychopathology in the realm of anxiety. For example, agoraphobics inhibit actions that expose them to places in which escape would be difficult or embarrassing. Acrophobics inhibit actions that expose them to heights. Some unconditioned assays discussed earlier (e.g., EPM) may also be considered inhibitory avoidance of innately aversive stimuli. Conflict paradigms, like the Vogel test, also fall into this category. In these assays, rats are punished for appetitive actions (e.g., licking a water spout) with US presentations (e.g., shock). Conflict tests are billed as anxiety models, with the "anxiety" response reflected in the ratio between pre- and postpunishment responding (Gray and McNaughton, 2000). IA paradigms are widely used and influential animal models of anxiety and fear. IA tests are commonly used to screen and compare drugs with potential to combat anxiety in humans, primarily because they are very sensitive to benzodiazepine anxiolytics (especially conflict paradigms).

The greatest successes of IA may be its contributions to our understanding of the role neuromodulatory systems play in consolidation of explicit memories and expression of punishment-based memories. Countless drugs have been administered after IA training that either facilitate or impair subsequent memory. Drugs that facilitate IA are seen as cognitive enhancers; those that impair IA may have anxiolytic potential (or be amnestic). The most common finding is that postconditioning amygdala processes modulate the consolidation of explicit memories stored elsewhere in the brain—probably by stimulating neuromodulatory centers (McGaugh, 2004). This is usually demonstrated by infusing drugs directly into the amygdala after IA training and showing LTM effects. Although the neurocircuitry of IA remains somewhat elusive, it is clear that it differs from that of simple Pavlovian PTC; IA depends on extra-amygdala brain regions that are not required for simple PTC (e.g., septohippocampal system), and post-training amygdala manipulations that impair IA have no effect on LTM for PTC (Gray and McNaughton, 2000; Wilensky et al., 2006). As IA may be the most common form of avoidance cited as pathological in human anxiety disorders, more work is clearly needed to precisely define the neural circuits, and synaptic, cellular, and molecular processes mediating this form of instrumental learning.

Active Avoidance For many decades following Pavlov's work, conditional fear and its neural basis were commonly studied with active avoidance protocols (Cain and LeDoux, 2008). In a typical experiment, rats were presented with tone–shock pairings on one side of a two-compartment chamber. Movement to the opposite side (shuttling) terminated the tone and prevented a shock presentation. These avoidance responses (ARs) served as the dependent measure of fear learning, and animals exhibited responses more frequently and with shorter latencies as training progressed.

Avoidance proved to be a difficult paradigm for the analysis and explanation of learning mechanisms. This was partly because AA learning trials were those that successfully avoided the shock, and it was difficult to explain how absence of the US could reinforce the response. Debates still rage about the mechanisms of AA learning; however, one prominent early theory remains, called two-factor, two-process, or sometimes fear theory (Rescorla and Solomon, 1967). In brief, these theories assume that PTC occurs on early training trials, before an AR is acquired. Then, on subsequent trials, fear is aroused by the CS. When an AR is performed, the CS terminates, fear diminishes, and no US is encountered. These theories suggest that fear reduction associated with CS termination somehow reinforces the response. Although still controversial, there are reports that rodents can learn to escape an aversive CS even when no shock is present during training (escape from fear paradigms; e.g., Cain and LeDoux, 2007). These theories are popular with some partly because they provide an entry into the AA neurocircuit through the known Pavlovian threat conditioning circuitry.

Instrumental AA, like PTC and IA, is a normal, adaptive behavior that gives subjects control over threats in dangerous environments. Indeed, AA mechanisms may even contribute to beneficial active coping strategies that prevent unnecessary fear (discussed later). However, like PTC and IA, AA can become maladaptive and contribute to human pathology.

Early studies found that impairing amygdala function disrupts the acquisition and recall of AA, although null effects or even facilitated AA were also reported. More recent investigations, focusing on subregions of the amygdala and other brain structures, paint a clearer picture (Fig. 41.7). Whereas LA and BA are critical for AA learning in several preparations, CE processes appear to constrain or oppose AA learning, possibly because CE mediates competing threat reactions like freezing (Lazaro-Munoz et al., 2010). Interestingly, several labs have shown that the amygdala dependence of AA is transient; when animals are trained beyond asymptotic performance, amygdala lesions no longer impair AA responding (Gabriel et al., 2003). This suggests that with overtraining AA may become habitual and depend on other, extra-amygdala regions. Dorsal striatum and motor cortex have been suggested as sites with possible significance; however, this remains unconfirmed. Recent unpublished findings from our lab also implicate the vmPFC in AA. This makes sense since Pavlovian reactions like freezing must be suppressed to allow for AA learning, and vmPFC is perfectly situated to suppress CE-mediated responses and allow performance of instrumental actions (Amano et al., 2010).

Two bodies of work, one older and one more recent, provide several key insights into how AA learning may be achieved in relation to the PTC circuitry. Michael Gabriel's laboratory implicated amygdala processes in AA very early on, in addition to other brain regions such as the ACC, thalamus, and sensory cortex (Gabriel et al., 2003). Interestingly, measuring training-induced neural activity changes (TIA) during AA training in rabbits, this group showed that LA plasticity precedes plasticity in other regions, and TIA effects in other regions depend on LA plasticity. This emphasizes the importance of LA to AA learning, which is consistent with AA evolving from prior PTC. New studies from multiple laboratories suggest that a distinct population of inhibitory cells in the lateral CE may also play a key role in gating fear (and possibly enabling AA). These interneurons express PKCδ and oxytocin receptors, and function to inhibit the output cells of the medial CE and allow for more active DRs (Ciocchi et al., 2010; Haubensak et al., 2010).

Summary of Instrumental Aversive Conditioning Avoidance has a clear relationship to human anxiety disorders as many are partly defined by excessively avoidant behaviors and thoughts. IA has been widely used to investigate drugs that may have utility in treating human anxiety and has enjoyed reasonable predictive validity. Although IA suffers as a model for studying precise neurobiological mechanisms because it lacks a clearly identified neural circuit, this paradigm has greatly contributed to our understanding of the role that neuromodulators play in consolidation of explicit memories and expression of punishment memories. AA research also has clinical implications, both as a problem (e.g., obsessive-compulsive disorder) and as a potential

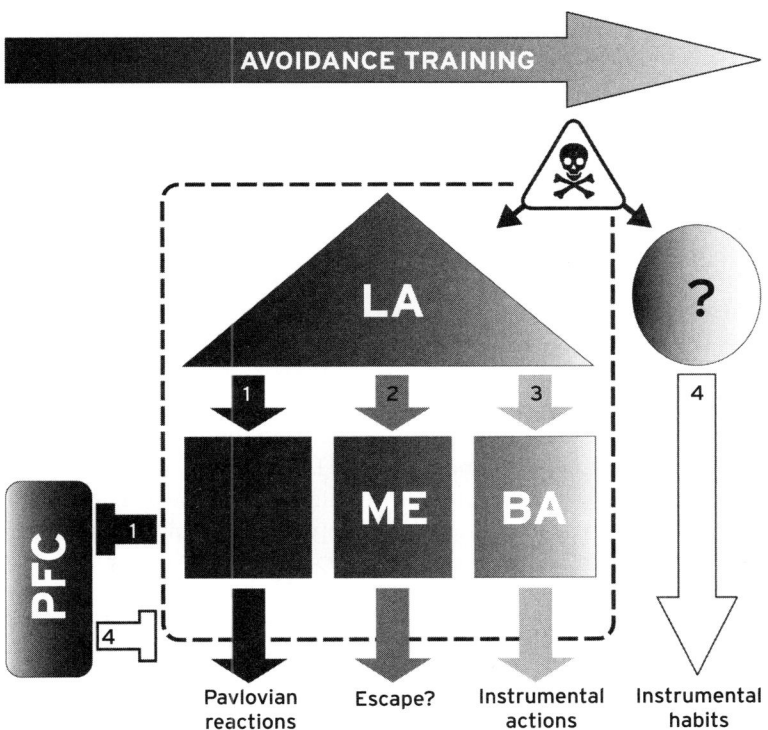

Figure 41.7 *Working model of active avoidance. Early in AA training, failure to avoid leads to PCT trials and Pavlovian reactions mediated by LA and CE (1). CE also suppresses PFC activity. As training progresses, animals may first learn to escape via processes that depend on LA and medial amgydala (ME) (2). Eventually, il-PFC activity suppresses CE outputs and allows for AA learning, which depends on LA and BA processes (3–4). Overtraining of AA responses leads to amygdala-independent, and possibly habitual, AA (4). It is not yet known which brain region(s) mediate overtrained AA behavior; however, striatal and motor systems are likely candidates (Cain and LeDoux., 2008).*

positive coping mechanism (discussed later). However, until recently AA research has stagnated. A resurgence of AA research, conducted using the successful blueprint of PTC, is already providing a much better understanding of the behavior, brain circuits, and neural mechanisms involved. Clearly more research is needed on both forms of avoidance given their role in human pathological anxiety.

Inhibition of Anxiety and Fear

Animal models can also focus on forms of learning that reduce or suppress DRs. The preceding sections described situations where survival circuits are activated and defensive responding is elicited. But as in most systems, what goes up must come down, and the mammalian brain has multiple ways to constrain and/or reverse the activation of defense responses. This is true of both behavioral and physiological responding. Here we will discuss a few key examples.

Negative Feedback in the HPA Axis The hypothalamic-adrenal-pituitary (HPA) axis is a major component of the acute stress response, a highly activated physiological state that prepares the organism by diverting energy and resources from nonessential processes (e.g., digestion) and mobilizing them to prime sensorimotor processes necessary for defensive responding. A properly functioning HPA axis turns itself off once the threat is gone, partly via glucocorticoid-mediated inhibition of hypothalamic and pituitary processes. In some human disorders, dysregulation of the HPA axis is implicated, and stress responding can be prolonged, leading to a number of adverse effects on bodily processes, health, and defensive responding (McEwen, 2004). HPA axis dysregulation can be assessed with tests like the dexamethasone suppression test. These models demonstrate that pathology can result from a failure of inhibition, not just excessive excitation, of DRs (Kehne and Cain, 2010).

Latent Inhibition and Extinction Minor modifications of the basic Pavlovian PTC procedure can profoundly influence the degree of survival circuit activation and the form of defensive responding. PTC occurs because the CS reliably predicts the US, and subsequent CS presentations allow the animal to anticipate unpleasant outcomes. But what if the CS does not always predict the US? In latent inhibition (LI), subjects are first exposed to a series of stimuli with no bad outcome. Then, standard PTC occurs using the same stimuli. DRs to the CS are nearly always weaker than the control condition, where no preexposure to the stimuli occurs. Extinction is a similar procedure but in reverse. Following PTC, subjects are repeatedly exposed to the CS without the anticipated US. This training contradicts the predictive validity of the CS and creates a new inhibitory CS–NoUS association (Bouton et al., 2006). Then, on subsequent trials conditioned responding is greatly diminished, or absent, depending on the amount of training. It is believed that extinction doesn't erase the original CS–US association but, rather, that behavior postextinction is the net result of competition between excitatory and inhibitory CS memories. Thus, one could imagine a scenario where one or both of these processes are impaired, leading to abnormally strong or persistent CRs even if basic PTC processes are normal.

Although some neurobiological studies have been conducted on LI in preclinical models, most of these relate to disorders like schizophrenia, where this learning process is disrupted. However, in the past 15 years there has been an explosion of fear extinction research, and we now know a great deal about its neural mechanisms (Milad and Quirk, 2012) (Fig. 41.5). For instance, vmPFC is essential for rapidly expressing extinction memories. Neural activity in vmPFC increases with extinction training, and electrical or growth factor (BDNF [brain-derived neurotrophic factor]) stimulation of vmPFC can induce extinction. vmPFC projects to inhibitory intercalated cells in the amygdala that can suppress CE-mediated threat reactions. LA and BA also play key roles in extinction learning. Several studies indicate that NMDA receptors, BDNF, calcineurin, MAP kinase, cannabinoid receptors, and GABA (gamma-aminobutyric acid) receptors in these regions participate in fear extinction learning (Myers and Davis, 2007). And BA neurons also appear to select between high- and low-fear states postextinction (Herry et al., 2010). Opioid-mediated input from the periacqueductal gray (PAG) may provide the error signal driving extinction plasticity (McNally et al., 2004). Finally, the hippocampus plays a critical role in the context-dependent expression of fear extinction; extinction is strongest in the place where CS-alone presentations occurred, and the hippocampus provides this critical signal (Bouton et al., 2006). Thus, animal models of extinction are seen by many as critical to understanding human pathological anxiety and barriers to its treatment (Cain et al., 2012; Jovanovic and Ressler, 2010). Indeed, a recent study of fear extinction revealed deficits in fear extinction recall and vmPFC activity when PTSD patients were challenged with an extinguished CS, consistent with preclinical findings (Milad and Quirk, 2012).

Conditioned Inhibition (CI) The CI procedure shares many features with extinction, but unlike extinction, where the CS comes to have ambiguous meaning, CI training produces a stimulus that has purely inhibitory properties. CI training produces a "safety signal" whose presence indicates that no harm will come.

CI learning is complicated and a bit difficult to study, but a few recent publications in rodents suggest that plasticity in the amygdala and striatum play a role. For instance, mice show weakened responses in LA to a conditioned inhibitor, but strengthened responses in the overlying striatum (Rogan et al., 2005). Rats trained similarly show reductions in synapse size in the LA (Ostroff et al., 2010). Thus, like extinction, conditioned inhibitors have the potential to identify safe circumstances and suppress DRs, and dysfunctional CI mechanisms may present as excessive fear/anxiety, even if those processes are operating normally. Impaired CI learning has recently been observed in patients with PTSD (Jovanovic et al., 2012), supporting the notion that dysfunctional inhibitory learning can lead to inappropriate responding (generalization) in anxious people.

ANIMAL MODELS OF PATHOLOGICAL FEAR AND ANXIETY

As discussed, the bulk of animal model research focuses on normal, group-averaged responses in naïve animals. This research is important for gaining a solid understanding of the basic neurobiological processes that operate in human fear and anxiety. However, there is growing appreciation that these models cannot say much about the pathologies causing human disorders, especially if they fail to probe trait anxiety.

Researchers have recognized these problems for years and have taken many different approaches toward improving animal models of human anxiety disorders. Unfortunately, nearly every group uses its own method to coax rats into responding abnormally, which makes comparisons between models extremely difficult. Nevertheless, some important insights have been gained from these efforts, and we will attempt to summarize some major methods for modeling pathological fear and anxiety in animals. The list is not meant to be exhaustive or to suggest that one model is superior to another—it is merely meant to illustrate how researchers have used multimodal or hybrid approaches to examine pathological, rather than normal, defensive responding.

PHYSIOLOGICAL MANIPULATIONS

Physiological models have been used to examine how alterations in survival circuit neurons affect defensive responding. This is usually achieved by delivering chemicals or sensitizing electrical stimulation (i.e., kindling) to induce hyperexcitability in specific brain regions (e.g., amygdala, hypothalamus; Rosen and Schulkin, 1998). For example, models considered relevant to panic disorder (PD) combine treatments with panicogenic drugs with tests of unconditioned or conditioned DRs in rats (Shekhar et al., 2003; Sullivan et al., 2003). In one such model, the respiratory stimulant doxapram is administered prior to threat conditioning. Doxapram induces hyperventilation and panic attacks in most PD patients, by activating carotid body chemoreceptors to produce a (false) visceral signal to the brain of poor air. Doxapram treatment leads to facilitation of PTC, which has been linked to amygdala hyperexcitability and enhanced CRF release in CE. Because the circuitry of PTC is well characterized, it is possible to test the hypothesis that this visceral signal induces panic-like symptoms by altering threat processing in specific amygdala microcircuits.

DEVELOPMENTAL MANIPULATIONS

Developmental models have assessed the effects of early life stress on fearful and anxious behaviors manifested later in life. In rodents, for example, early maternal deprivation permanently alters central CRF systems as well as related behavioral and hormonal responses to stressors throughout life (Sullivan, 2003). Ecologically informed studies of maternal availability have likewise identified similar outcomes in non-human primates. Bonnet macaque monkeys raised in variable foraging demand conditions respond to novel situations with increased anxiety compared with age-matched monkeys raised as low-foraging demand controls. As adults, these monkeys exhibit significant differences in cerebrospinal fluid levels of monoamines, somatostatin, and CRF. These findings agree with evidence from humans that early exposure to severe stress is a risk factor for the development of mood and anxiety disorders (Heim and Nemeroff, 2002). Far less researched, but of equal importance, are indications that mild early-life stressors

can also foster resilience (stress inoculation), perhaps by facilitating vmPFC-mediated inhibition of amygdala and emotional regulation processes (Lyons et al., 2010).

STRESS-ENHANCED FEAR LEARNING IN ADULTS

Behavioral manipulations in adulthood that affect structure and function of survival circuits often involve exposure to acute or chronic stressors that alter defensive responding, especially PTC. These models are sometimes referred to by the abbreviation: stress-enhanced fear learning (SEFL; e.g., Rau and Fanselow, 2007). Stress is achieved in many ways, including restraint, immobilization, cold exposure, electric shock, predator exposure, and underwater submersion. Exposure to these stressors in adulthood increases aggression, alters context-elicited DRs, affects performance on the EPM, and attenuates spatial memory. Restraint stress also facilitates PTC, results in dendritic atrophy in hippocampus and PFC, suppresses neurogenesis in the dentate gyrus, and induces dendritic hypertrophy and sprouting of new synapses in the amygdala (McEwen, 2004). These stress-induced aspects of neural plasticity suggest a putative link between remodeling of defensive circuits and the development of anxiety as modeled in adult rodents. Chronic stress and underwater submersion have also been used in rodent research to mimic the requisite stressful events of traumatic anxiety disorders such as PTSD. Generally speaking, SEFL effects are interpreted as interactions between nonassociative sensitization processes and associative PTC processes. Thus, stressful manipulations may produce hyperexcitability in neural circuits that lower the threshold for defensive responding, and/or enhance PTC learning/consolidation. Such interpretations model key aspects of psychopathology theories in humans, such as Roger Pitman's "overconsolidation" theory of PTSD (for discussion, see Cain et al., 2012).

GENETIC MANIPULATION

Genetic manipulations before assessment of behavioral DRs in rodent models have generally been achieved in two ways. One is selective breeding of rat strains with the goal of enhancing or attenuating particular measures of fear and anxiety. For instance, the Wistar-Kyoto (WKY) rat strain has an extreme AA phenotype that may model aspects of human anxiety disorders. WKY rats show abnormally rapid acquisition in a difficult AA task and also fail to show the normal "warm-up" effect characteristic of other strains (Servatius et al., 2008). The other strategy is creation of transgenic animals that have altered expression of particular genes that code for proteins in brain circuits of interest, and evaluating performance on fear and anxiety assays. An example comes from studies of PTC in the serotonin (5-HT) 1A-receptor knockout mouse. When previously context-conditioned 5-HT1A-null mice are tested in the same context but with novel cues added, they do not exhibit the normal CR decrement seen in wild-type mice (Klemenhagen et al., 2006). This difference in sensitivity to novel stimuli has been likened to a memory bias for threatening cues in an otherwise neutral environment, as may occur in human patients with PD or PTSD. Given the well-described role of hippocampus in providing a representation of context to amygdala, focused investigation of hippocampus–amygdala interactions involving the 5-HT1A receptor is suggested.

Naturally occurring genetic polymorphisms related to anxiety have also been studied, and again, the 5-HT system is implicated. In particular, an insertion/deletion event in the 5-HT transporter linked polymorphic region (5-HTTLPR) is known to produce long (l) and short (s) alleles in humans and rhesus monkeys. *In vitro*, the short allele decreases transcriptional efficiency, which may alter expression of the 5-HT transporter and disrupts control of extracellular concentrations of 5-HT in neural circuits. Humans homozygous for the short allele (s/s) show more anxiety, muscle tension, shyness, and avoidance compared with humans who are homozygous (l/l) or heterozygous (l/s) for the long allele, and greater activation of survival circuits when challenged with threats (Domschke and Dannlowski, 2010).

INDIVIDUAL DIFFERENCES

It has been proposed that consideration be given to individual differences in susceptibility and resilience in animal models of anxiety disorders (Yehuda and LeDoux, 2007). This is particularly important in models for PTSD, as it is well documented that similar exposures to a horrific trauma results in development of PTSD for a relatively small proportion of those exposed. Of note, phenotypic variability in most animal models of fear and anxiety is obscured by the usual practice of reporting the variation around the mean. Recent work shows that "fear reactivity" in conditioned animals is normally distributed in unselected Sprague-Dawley (SD) rats (Yehuda and LeDoux, 2007; Fig. 41.8). When high-fear reactivity rats are extinguished, two additional groups emerge: a fast-extinguishing group and a slow-extinguishing group. The slow-extinguishing group is proposed to have relevance for PTSD, which involves a failure to recover from trauma and is associated with impaired fear extinction recall and reductions in vmPFC activity (Milad and Quirk, 2012).

Related work has recently been conducted with AA in unselected SD rats (Lazaro-Munoz et al., 2010). In many AA studies, a subset of rats show extremely poor AA acquisition and are usually excluded from further analyses. However, these studies demonstrated that poor avoidance was associated with abnormally high expression of competing Pavlovian reactions like freezing. CE lesions that eliminated freezing rescued AA performance without further training. This phenotype may also model a deficit in certain human anxiety disorders, as excessive Pavlovian reactions prevented the poor avoiders from performing a response that could prevent them from harm, even though they had apparently learned that they could avoid harm. Similar to microarray analyses of gene expression in selectively bred rats, these trait-selected rats offer opportunities to correlate gene expression with fearful and anxious phenotypic expression. Thus, models that consider individual phenotypic differences in fearful and anxious responding will likely be among the more effective for modeling anxiety disorders and identifying brain circuits and neuronal processes mediating abnormal anxiety.

MODELS FOCUSED ON TREATMENT AND COPING PROCESSES

Although several of the previous sections allude to implications for treatment of human anxiety disorders, some animal models explicitly attempt to model processes important for learning to suppress, or cope with, fear. The best accepted animal model of treatment learning is extinction. Exciting newer ideas involve disrupting reconsolidation and AA to understand active coping mechanisms for gaining control over threatening circumstances.

Fear Extinction

Extinction processes can be relevant to human treatment in many ways. Generally speaking, extinction training contradicts previously held beliefs or expectations. This creates a new inhibitory memory that competes with a conditioned threat memory for control of behavior. The result is a reduction, or elimination, of conditioned responding. Extinction can be used to reverse expression of both Pavlovian and instrumental CRs, although therapists typically focus on extinction of Pavlovian fear. Consider, for instance, a subject who exhibits pathological avoidance of some fear-eliciting stimulus. The therapist may seek to extinguish fear of this stimulus; however, this can be difficult since avoidance is typically strong, and one cannot extinguish CS

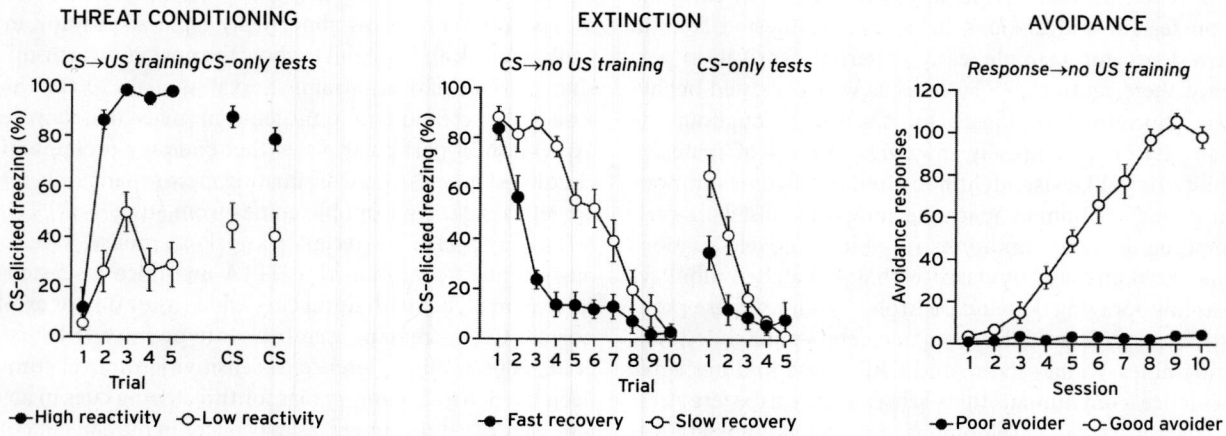

Figure 41.8 *Exploiting natural response variation in key defensive learning tasks may facilitate studies modeling pathological fear/anxiety processes. In each task, the top and bottom 20% are shown.*

fear if the subject avoids the CS altogether. In this case, a therapist may employ response prevention techniques followed by fear extinction. Response prevention means blocking ARs and essentially forcing exposure to the fear-arousing stimulus. Then, exposure, sometimes prolonged exposure (Foa, 2011), is used to extinguish CS fear. If successful, CS fear will diminish along with the motivation to avoid. Extinction is a component of most successful cognitive-behavioral therapies (CBTs) for fear and anxiety disorders, and there is good evidence that extinction-based treatments provide measurable relief to patients with wide-ranging anxiety disorders (Craske, 1999).

Unfortunately, fear extinction has some notable drawbacks. First, some anxiety disorders are accompanied by impairments in fear extinction (Milad and Quirk, 2012). Second, it has been known since Pavlov that extinction memories are "fragile," and more recent preclinical studies reliably show that expression of extinction is transient. The phenomena of renewal, reinstatement, and spontaneous recovery all show how extinction treatments are temporary—CRs return when the context changes, new stressors are experienced, or time passes (Bouton et al., 2006). Thus, it is not surprising that preclinical and clinical researchers have been intensely researching ways to facilitate extinction learning and make it more durable.

Although this topic alone could fill a book, we will highlight several important lines of animal model research that could directly affect the efficacy and permanence of extinction-based therapies. First, many laboratories are investigating how the timing of exposures can enhance extinction. It appears that some degree of temporal massing of CS exposures (sometimes called *flooding*) can enhance initial extinction learning, and once extinction learning begins, sessions spaced out in time facilitate consolidation/LTM (Cain et al., 2003; Li and Westbrook, 2008). Specific variations on this theme have even been reported to produce erasure of PCT memories, presumably by blocking the reconsolidation of reactivated memories with extinction training (Quirk et al., 2010).

Many other studies are evaluating the effects of biological proteins and psychoactive drugs on fear extinction, especially drugs commonly used to treat anxiety (Milad and Quirk, 2012). Several findings are worth highlighting here. First, a number of agents have been found to enhance extinction learning/memory when given before or after CS exposures. These include D-cycloserine, yohimbine, fluoxetine, venlafaxine, valproic acid, cannabidiol, estradiol, corticosterone, and BDNF. Several others have been found to impair fear extinction, most notably benzodiazepines (e.g., valium), blockers of $\alpha 1$ adrenergic (e.g., prazosin) and μ-opioid (e.g., naloxone) receptors (Bernardi and Lattal, 2010; Bouton et al., 2006; McNally et al., 2004). Particularly exciting are findings that extinction therapy can lead to fear memory erasure if combined with appropriate drugs, like SSRIs (Karpova et al., 2011). Such effects suggest that it may be possible to return the defensive circuitry to a developmental state where extinction routinely produces erasure of aversive memories (Quirk et al., 2010). Finally, very recent preclinical studies suggest that deep brain stimulation of specific regions, like vmPFC or ventral striatum, can enhance extinction recall (Rodriguez-Romaguera et al., 2012).

Fear Reconsolidation and Incubation

Interest is gaining in a newer line of preclinical research on the neural mechanisms of reconsolidation and incubation. In brief, memories for conditioned threats become labile when reactivated, perhaps to update the memory trace before it is reconsolidated. This raises the exciting possibility that clinicians can modify or even block the storage of reactivated fear memories. Reconsolidation blockade is typically achieved with drugs that interfere with protein synthesis (Nader et al., 2000); however, these are not suitable for use in humans. Studies are underway to evaluate other ways to blunt reconsolidation. These include drugs that affect protein synthesis and memory such as β-adrenergic receptor blockers (e.g., propranolol; Debiec and LeDoux, 2006), and behavioral interference or extinction procedures (Quirk et al., 2010). In a related phenomenon, fear incubation, recurring activations can enhance reconsolidation processes and produce progressively stronger fear memories—reminiscent of anxiety disorders like PTSD where intrusive memories become progressively more disruptive (Pickens et al., 2009). Although little is known about the neural mechanisms of fear incubation, norepinephrine makes the clearest contribution (Debiec et al., 2011). Reconsolidation can be a double-edged sword when it comes to treatment, however, as cognitive enhancers can cause decreases or increases in threat responding, depending on the amount of CS exposure and the relative recruitment of extinction versus reconsolidation/incubation processes (Lee et al., 2006).

Avoidance, Escape, and Active Coping

A new twist on an old animal model of fear and anxiety suggests that aspects of human active coping can be modeled in laboratory rodents. Although instrumental escape and avoidance are normal and adaptive learning processes, they have a very negative connotation today, partly because they are listed as defining features of many human anxiety disorders. However, escape/avoidance contributions to human pathology reflect the adoption of responses that disrupt life activities, most likely inhibitory avoidance responses that cause one to disengage from the world. Although escape and active avoidance (E-AA) mechanisms can also contribute to pathology, they may represent an ideal way to cope with environmental threats. In E-AA, subjects learn a specific response or action that escapes environmental threats and prevents harm. Thus, E-AA gives subjects control over environmental threats, allowing them to operate in dangerous environments yet stay safe. Lack of control is also a defining feature of many mood and anxiety disorders (DSM-IV 2000). In this sense, adaptive E-AA responses resemble active coping strategies that contribute to resilience and facilitate recovery following trauma (Stewart and Yuen, 2011). Adaptive E-AA responses have some other added benefits, too: they prevent the expression of Pavlovian reactions indicative of human fear and anxiety, and, unlike extinction, this suppression appears to persist, as long as the AA response is available (Cain and LeDoux, 2007; Helmreich et al., 2012; Solomon and Wynne, 1954). AA mechanisms and individual differences were discussed previously, but more research on instrumental E-AA and active coping mechanisms may support another evidence-based treatment method in humans, which may be especially useful for those who respond poorly to other forms of therapy (van der Kolk, 2006).

BEHAVIORAL INHIBITION THEORY OF ANXIETY

In 1982, Jeffrey Gray put forth a theory of anxiety based largely on the notion that classic anxiolytics, like alcohol, barbiturates, and (especially) benzodiazepines, could be useful tools for identifying good animal models of anxiety (Gray and McNaughton, 2000). Since only some DRs were sensitive to these drugs, Gray viewed fear and anxiety as separate response classes, and his definition of anxiety was distinct from that discussed earlier. According to Gray, anxiety reflected a *conflict* between motivations to approach certain stimuli and avoid others. Thus, anxiety was not simply weaker defensive responding to less certain or imminent threats, but a state triggered when one must choose to move toward threats in order to approach other, usually appetitive, goals. For instance, a rat may suppress foraging when presented with a predator odor but still engage in other active behaviors. Gray viewed this *behavioral inhibition (BI)* as distinct from fear-elicited DRs like freezing, which suppress all actions.

BI theory was very influential and affected the development and usage of animal models of anxiety. For instance, benzodiazepines suppressed DRs measured with conflict tests (e.g., Vogel test), IA, and several of the now-popular unconditioned assays (e.g., EPM) but often failed to suppress Pavlovian CRs and AA. Thus, conflict tests, IA, and unconditioned assays were deemed superior animal models of anxiety.

Gray also reasoned that "seat of anxiety" could be identified using brain lesions that produced a behavioral profile similar to the classic anxiolytics. This led to the septohippocampal (SH) theory of BI and anxiety, since lesions of this system impaired punishment effects, IA, and other anxiety-like behaviors in the unconditioned assays. This logic also led Gray to initially reject the notion that the amygdala played a central role in anxiety, since amygdala lesions impaired PCT and AA (unlike the anxiolytic drugs) and sometimes failed to affect the BI assays. In later years, Gray reformulated his theory to include a relatively minor role for the amygdala, mainly because fear-potentiated startle was shown to depend on the amygdala and was also sensitive to anxiolytics from diverse mechanistic classes (Davis, 1990).

Although influential, especially in the realm of drug development, the septohippocampal BI theory has steadily lost ground as new findings accumulate (LeDoux, 2002). First, SH injections of classic anxiolytics often failed to affect BI. Second, the classic anxiolytics all modulated GABAergic neurotransmission, and new anxiolytics were discovered that were effective in treating human anxiety but ineffective in prominent BI models (e.g., β-blockers, $5HT_{1A}$ agonists, SSRIs). Third, an enormous body of research suggested that the core function of the hippocampus related to declarative, spatial/contextual, and working memory, not conflict resolution as proposed by Gray's BI theory. Thus, SH lesion effects could be explained better by theories hypothesizing that this system provided contextual information to the amygdala threat–response system. Fourth, an equally large body of preclinical and clinical work

implicated the amygdala, extended amygdala, and prefrontal cortex in defensive responding and human anxiety. Finally, the septohippocamal physiological mechanism for BI proposed by Gray, theta rhythms, does not appear to play a central role in primate, including human, anxiety. To the contrary, detailed mechanisms of neural processing and plasticity have been discovered in the amygdala, PFC, and hippocampus that can explain the role of neurotransmitter systems, and the action of anxiolytic drugs targeting these systems, in anxiety (see preceding section). These brain regions are now routinely implicated in human anxiety with imaging and neural recordings.

Although BI theory has run into some difficulties, we are not suggesting that the animal models used to support this theory are unrelated to fear and anxiety. Assays that involve punishment, IA, and innately aversive stimuli surely activate survival circuits and DRs relevant to human fear and anxiety. However, recent work strongly suggests that models based on PTC are capable of activating survival circuits to a similar degree, and these models are much better tools for studying the underlying neurobiological mechanisms mediating defensive responding—at both ends of the behavioral spectrum. The notion that approach–avoidance conflicts make a unique contribution to anxiety may still have merit, however, this conflict is probably inherent in all defensive deflections from the preferred activity pattern.

CONCLUSIONS

Current treatments for human pathological anxiety are inadequate; although some individuals respond favorably to psychotherapy and/or pharmacotherapy, both treatment approaches have unacceptably low long-term success rates (Cukor et al., 2010). Meanwhile, the needs of anxiety patients continue to grow, as does the already staggering cost to society (Smith, 2011). Given this unmet need and potential for massive profits, why then are pharmaceutical companies dropping drug development programs for anxiety at an alarming rate? The short answer: it's too risky. When the drug discovery/development process takes 10–20 years, with an average cost of $1.3 billion, these companies are understandably risk averse (Paul et al., 2010). Although there are many contributing factors, the inability of standard animal models to accurately predict efficacy in human anxious populations plays a major role (Smith, 2011).

Generally speaking, preclinical drug discovery leans heavily on pharmacology-based animal models like those used to support BI theory. These benzodiazepine-sensitive assays primarily test conflict behaviors, IA, and unconditioned responses to innately aversive stimuli. Although these assays probe a wide range of anxiety-related behavior, all represent difficult models for studying underlying neural circuits and precise neurobiological mechanisms. Thus, they select for "pharmacologic isomorphism" but often cannot assess the mode of action for new agents, predict enhanced efficacy over current standards, or explain failures in the clinic that could guide future decisions and refine anxiety models (Geyer and Markou, 2002).

In contrast to the recent troubles in drug discovery, studies of the neurobiology of fear and anxiety have had great success over the past few decades (Johansen et al., 2011). This branch of research relies much more heavily on models amenable to neuro-circuit analysis. For instance, Pavlovian threat conditioning uses discrete, controllable stimuli to induce learning, activate survival circuits, and elicit defensive responding. DRs typically studied include reflexive or stereotyped behaviors with clear, measurable onset and termination (Davis, 1990; Medina et al., 2002). These features greatly facilitate circuit analysis by allowing research-ers to relate neural responses to triggering stimuli and behavior. Circuit-based models like PTC have vastly improved our under-standing of the detailed cellular, synaptic, molecular, and genetic contributions to defensive responding and learning.

Although it was once believed that PTC could not elicit the anxiety-like responses that form the basis of many human disorders, recent work suggests otherwise. For instance, condi-tioning with reduced contingency, long duration CSs, complex CSs, or conditioned reinforcers can all produce less imminent/certain threats that elicit anxiety-like responses. Additional train-ing phases can also model inhibitory (e.g., CI or extinction) or instrumental (e.g., AA) learning processes that likely make direct contributions to recovery and coping processes. Perhaps most important, circuit-based models like PTC allow one to hypoth-esize how a new treatment may achieve a positive effect in the context of known neurobiological and psychological processes.

Circuit-based models of anxiety are also consistent with recent efforts to reclassify human mental disorders. There is a growing realization that diagnostic criteria for anxiety dis-orders based on therapist interviews and personal reports of emotional symptoms may not accurately reflect underlying pathology in core anxiety processes. Thus, efforts such as the NIMH Research Domain Criteria Project (RDoC) aim to study basic dimensions of observable behavior and neurobiological measures related to pathological anxiety. The ultimate goal is to provide a knowledge base about core anxiety processes that will inform new diagnoses and treatment approaches. Increasing efforts to apply the preclinical circuit-based approach to new studies in experimental animals and people is likely to facili-tate this process and remove much of the uncertainty associ-ated with subjective emotional measures and models relying too heavily on validation by existing drugs.

DISCLOSURES

Dr. Cain has no conflicts of interest to disclose.

Dr. Sullivan serves as a member of the Scientific Advisory Board of Tonix Pharmaceuticals, Inc. and has served as a con-sultant to Ono Pharma USA, Inc.

Dr. LeDoux has no conflicts of interest to disclose.

REFERENCES

Amano, T., Duvarci, S., et al. (2011). The fear circuit revisited: contribu-tions of the basal amygdala nuclei to conditioned fear. *J. Neurosci.* 31:15481–15489.

Amano, T., Unal, C.T., et al. (2010). Synaptic correlates of fear extinction in the amygdala. *Nat. Neurosci.* 13:489–494.

Andreatini, R., and Bacellar, L.F. (2000). Animal models: trait or state mea-sure? The test-retest reliability of the elevated plus-maze and behavioral despair. *Prog. Neuropsychopharmacol. Biol. Psychiatry* 24:549–560.

Bailey, C.H., Giustetto, M., et al. (2000). Is heterosynaptic modulation essential for stabilizing Hebbian plasticity and memory? *Nat. Rev. Neurosci.* 1:11–20.

Balleine, B.W., and Killcross, S. (2006). Parallel incentive processing: an inte-grated view of amygdala function. *Trends Neurosci.* 29:272–279.

Bernardi, R.E., and Lattal, K.M. (2010). A role for alpha-adrenergic receptors in extinction of conditioned fear and cocaine conditioned place prefer-ence. *Behav. Neurosci.* 124:204–210.

Blanchard, R.J., Blanchard, D.C., et al. (1989). Ethoexperimental approaches to the study of defensive behavior. In: Blanchard, R.J., Brain, P.F., Blanchard, D.C., and Parmigiani, S., eds. Ethoexperimental Approaches to the Study of Behavior. Dordrecht, the Netherlands: Kluwer Academic, pp. 114–136.

Bouton, M.E., Westbrook, R.F., et al. (2006). Contextual and temporal modula-tion of extinction: behavioral and biological mechanisms. *Biol. Psychiatry.* 60:352–360.

Burgos-Robles, A., Vidal-Gonzalez, I., et al. (2009). Sustained conditioned responses in prelimbic prefrontal neurons are correlated with fear expres-sion and extinction failure. *J. Neurosci.* 29:8474–8482.

Cain, C.K., Blouin, A.M., et al. (2003). Temporally massed CS presentations generate more fear extinction than spaced presentations. *J. Exp. Psychol. Anim. Behav. Process.* 29:323–333.

Cain, C.K., and LeDoux, J.E. (2007). Escape from fear: a detailed behavioral analysis of two atypical responses reinforced by CS termination. *J. Exp. Psychol. Anim. Behav. Process.* 33:451–463.

Cain, C.K., and LeDoux, J.E. (2008). Brain mechanisms of Pavlovian and Instrumental Aversive Conditioning. In: Nutt, D.J., Blanchard, R.J., Blanchard, D.C., and Griebel, G., eds. Handbook of Anxiety and Fear. Amsterdam: Elsevier Academic, pp. 103–125.

Cain, C.K., Maynard, G.D., et al. (2012). Targeting memory processes with drugs to prevent or cure PTSD. *Exp. Opin. Investig. Drugs* 21(9):1323–1350.

Ciocchi, S., Herry, C., et al. (2010). Encoding of conditioned fear in central amygdala inhibitory circuits. *Nature* 468:277–282.

Craske, M.G. (1999). Anxiety Disorders: Psychological Approaches to Theory and Treatment. Boulder, CO: Westview Press.

Cukor, J., Olden, M., et al. (2010). Evidence-based treatments for PTSD, new directions, and special challenges. *Ann. NY Acad. Sci.* 1208:82–89.

Davis, M. (1990). Pharmacological and anatomical analysis of fear condition-ing. *NIDA Res. Monogr.* 97:126–162.

Davis, M., Gendelman, D.S., et al. (1982). A primary acoustic startle circuit: lesion and stimulation studies. *J. Neurosci.* 2:791–805.

Debiec, J., Bush, D.E., et al. (2011). Noradrenergic enhancement of reconsoli-dation in the amygdala impairs extinction of conditioned fear in rats: a possible mechanism for the persistence of traumatic memories in PTSD. *Depress. Anxiety* 28:186–193.

Debiec, J., and LeDoux, J.E. (2006). Noradrenergic signaling in the amygdala contributes to the reconsolidation of fear memory: treatment implications for PTSD. *Ann. NY Acad. Sci.* 1071:521–524.

Domschke, K., and Dannlowski, U. (2010). Imaging genetics of anxiety disor-ders. *NeuroImage* 53:822–831.

Ehrlich, I., Humeau, Y., et al. (2009). Amygdala inhibitory circuits and the control of fear memory. *Neuron* 62:757–771.

Feinstein, J.S., Adolphs, R., et al. (2011). The human amygdala and the induc-tion and experience of fear. *Curr. Biol.* 21:34–38.

File, S.E., and Seth, P. (2003). A review of 25 years of the social interaction test. *Eur. J. Pharmacol.* 463:35–53.

Foa, E.B. (2011). Prolonged exposure therapy: past, present, and future. *Depress. Anxiety* 28:1043–1047.

Gabriel, M., Burhans, L., et al. (2003). Consideration of a unified model of amygdalar associative functions. *Ann. NY Acad. Sci.* 985:206–217.

Gale, G.D., Anagnostaras, S.G., et al. (2004). Role of the basolateral amygdala in the storage of fear memories across the adult lifetime of rats. *J. Neurosci.* 24:3810–3815.

Geyer, M.A., and Markou, A. (2002). The role of preclinical models in the development of psychotropic drugs. In: Davis, K.L., Charney, D., Coyle, J.T., and Nemeroff, C., eds. Neuropsychopharmacology: The Fifth Generation of Progress. Philadelphia: Lippincott, Williams, & Wilkins, pp. 445–455.

Gozzi, A., Jain, A., et al. (2010). A neural switch for active and passive fear. *Neuron* 67:656–666.

Gray, J.A., and McNaughton, N. (2000). The Neuropsychology of Anxiety: An Enquiry into the Functions of the Septo-Hippocampal System. New York: Oxford University Press.

Haubensak, W., Kunwar, P.S., et al. (2010). Genetic dissection of an amygdala microcircuit that gates conditioned fear. *Nature* 468:270–276.

Heim, C., and Nemeroff, C.B. (2002). Neurobiology of early life stress: clinical studies. *Semin. Clin. Neuropsychiatry* 7:147–159.

Helmreich, D.L., Tylee, D., et al. (2012). Active behavioral coping alters the behav-ioral but not the endocrine response to stress. *Psychoneuroendocrinology* 37(12):1941–1948.

Herry, C., Ferraguti, F., et al. (2010). Neuronal circuits of fear extinction. *Eur. J. Neurosci.* 31:599–612.

Hogg, S. (1996). A review of the validity and variability of the elevated plus-maze as an animal model of anxiety. *Pharmacol. Biochem. Behav.* 54:21–30.

Johansen, J.P., Cain, C.K., et al. (2011). Molecular mechanisms of fear learning and memory. *Cell* 147:509–524.

Johansen, J.P., Hamanaka, H., et al. (2010). Optical activation of lateral amygdala pyramidal cells instructs associative fear learning. *Proc. Natl. Acad. Sci. USA* 107:12692–12697.

Josselyn, S.A. (2010). Continuing the search for the engram: examining the mechanism of fear memories. *J. Psychiatry Neurosci.* 35:221–228.

Jovanovic, T., Kazama, A., et al. (2012). Impaired safety signal learning may be a biomarker of PTSD. *Neuropharmacology* 62:695–704.

Jovanovic, T., and Ressler, K.J. (2010). How the neurocircuitry and genetics of fear inhibition may inform our understanding of PTSD. *Am. J. Psychiatry* 167:648–662.

Kalin, N.H. (2004). Studying non-human primates: a gateway to understanding anxiety disorders. *Psychopharmacol. Bull.* 38(Suppl. 1):8–13.

Karpova, N.N., Pickenhagen, A., et al. (2011). Fear erasure in mice requires synergy between antidepressant drugs and extinction training. *Science* 334:1731–1734.

Kehne, J.H., and Cain, C.K. (2010). Therapeutic utility of non-peptidic CRF1 receptor antagonists in anxiety, depression, and stress-related disorders: evidence from animal models. *Pharmacol. Ther.* 128:460–487.

Klemenhagen, K.C., Gordon, J.A., et al. (2006). Increased fear response to contextual cues in mice lacking the 5-HT1A receptor. *Neuropsychopharmacology* 31:101–111.

Knapska, E., Radwanska, K., et al. (2007). Functional internal complexity of amygdala: focus on gene activity mapping after behavioral training and drugs of abuse. *Physiol. Rev.* 87:1113–1173.

Knobloch, H.S., Charlet, A., et al. (2012). Evoked axonal oxytocin release in the central amygdala attenuates fear response. *Neuron* 73:553–566.

Lazaro-Munoz, G., LeDoux, J.E., et al. (2010). Sidman instrumental avoidance initially depends on lateral and basal amygdala and is constrained by central amygdala-mediated Pavlovian processes. *Biol. Psychiatry* 67:1120–1127.

LeDoux, J.E. (2002). Synaptic Self: How Our Brains Become Who We Are. New York: Viking.

LeDoux, J.E. (2012). Rethinking the emotional brain. *Neuron* 73:653–676.

Lee, J.L., Milton, A.L., et al. (2006). Reconsolidation and extinction of conditioned fear: inhibition and potentiation. *J. Neurosci.* 26:10051–10056.

Li, S.H., and Westbrook, R.F. (2008). Massed extinction trials produce better short-term but worse long-term loss of context conditioned fear responses than spaced trials. *J. Exp. Psychol. Anim. Behav. Process.* 34:336–351.

Lyons, D.M., Parker, K.J., et al. (2010). Animal models of early life stress: implications for understanding resilience. *Dev. Psychobiol.* 52:402–410.

Maren, S., and Fanselow, M.S. (1995). Synaptic plasticity in the basolateral amygdala induced by hippocampal formation stimulation in vivo. *J. Neurosci.* 15:7548–7564.

McEwen, B.S. (2004). Protection and damage from acute and chronic stress: allostasis and allostatic overload and relevance to the pathophysiology of psychiatric disorders. *Ann. NY Acad. Sci.* 1032:1–7.

McGaugh, J.L. (2004). The amygdala modulates the consolidation of memories of emotionally arousing experiences. *Annu. Rev. Neurosci.* 27:1–28.

McKinney, W.T. (2001). Overview of the past contributions of animal models and their changing place in psychiatry. *Semin. Clin. Neuropsychiatry* 6:68–78.

McNally, G.P., Pigg, M., et al. (2004). Opioid receptors in the midbrain periaqueductal gray regulate extinction of pavlovian fear conditioning. *J. Neurosci.* 24:6912–6919.

Medina, J.F., Christopher Repa, J., et al. (2002). Parallels between cerebellum- and amygdala-dependent conditioning. *Nat. Rev. Neurosci.* 3:122–131.

Milad, M.R., and Quirk, G.J. (2012). Fear extinction as a model for translational neuroscience: ten years of progress. *Annu. Rev. Psychol.* 63:129–151.

Myers, K.M., and Davis, M. (2007). Mechanisms of fear extinction. *Mol. Psychiatry* 12:120–150.

Nader, K., Schafe, G.E., et al. (2000). Fear memories require protein synthesis in the amygdala for reconsolidation after retrieval. *Nature* 406:722–726.

Ostroff, L.E., Cain, C.K., et al. (2010). Fear and safety learning differentially affect synapse size and dendritic translation in the lateral amygdala. *Proc. Natl. Acad. Sci. USA* 107:9418–9423.

Paul, S.M., Mytelka, D.S., et al. (2010). How to improve R&D productivity: the pharmaceutical industry's grand challenge. *Nat. Rev. Drug Discov.* 9:203–214.

Pickens, C.L., Golden, S.A., et al. (2009). Long-lasting incubation of conditioned fear in rats. *Biol. Psychiatry* 65:881–886.

Quirk, G.J., Armony, J.L., et al. (1997). Fear conditioning enhances different temporal components of tone-evoked spike trains in auditory cortex and lateral amygdala. *Neuron* 19:613–624.

Quirk, G.J., Pare, D., et al. (2010). Erasing fear memories with extinction training. *J. Neurosci.* 30:14993–14997.

Rau, V., and Fanselow, M.S. (2007). Neurobiological and neuroethological perspectives on fear and anxiety. In: Kirmayer, L.J., Lemelson, R., and Barad, M., eds. Understanding Trauma: Integrating Biological, Clinical, and Cultural Perspectives. New York: Cambridge University Press, pp. 27–40.

Rescorla, R.A., and Solomon, R.L. (1967). Two process learning theory: relationships between Pavlovian conditioning and instrumental learning. *Psychol. Rev.* 74:151–182.

Rodriguez-Romaguera, J., Do Monte, F.H., et al. (2012). Deep brain stimulation of the ventral striatum enhances extinction of conditioned fear. *Proc. Natl. Acad. Sci. USA* 109:8764–8769.

Rogan, M.T., Leon, K.S., et al. (2005). Distinct neural signatures for safety and danger in the amygdala and striatum of the mouse. *Neuron* 46:309–320.

Rosen, J.B. (2004). The neurobiology of conditioned and unconditioned fear: a neurobehavioral system analysis of the amygdala. *Behav. Cogn. Neurosci. Rev.* 3:23–41.

Rosen, J.B., and Schulkin, J. (1998). From normal fear to pathological anxiety. *Psychol. Rev.* 105:325–350.

Rumpel, S., LeDoux, J., et al. (2005). Postsynaptic receptor trafficking underlying a form of associative learning. *Science* 308:83–88.

Servatius, R.J., Jiao, X., et al. (2008). Rapid avoidance acquisition in Wistar-Kyoto rats. *Behav. Brain Res.* 192:191–197.

Shekhar, A., Sajdyk, T.J., et al. (2003). The amygdala, panic disorder, and cardiovascular responses. *Ann. NY Acad. Sci.* 985:308–325.

Smith, K. (2011). Trillion-dollar brain drain. *Nature* 478:15.

Solomon, R.L., and Wynne, L.C. (1954). Traumatic avoidance learning: the principles of anxiety conservation and partial irreversibility. *Psychol. Rev.* 61:353.

Southwick, S.M., Bremner, J.D., et al. (1999). Role of norepinephrine in the pathophysiology and treatment of posttraumatic stress disorder. *Biol. Psychiatry* 46:1192–1204.

Stewart, D.E., and Yuen, T. (2011). A systematic review of resilience in the physically ill. *Psychosomatics* 52:199–209.

Sullivan, G.M., Apergis, J., et al. (2003). Rodent doxapram model of panic: behavioral effects and c-Fos immunoreactivity in the amygdala. *Biol. Psychiatry* 53:863–870.

Sullivan, R.M. (2003). Developing a sense of safety: the neurobiology of neonatal attachment. *Ann. NY Acad. Sci.* 1008:122–131.

Takahashi, L.K., Chan, M.M., et al. (2008). Predator odor fear conditioning: current perspectives and new directions. *Neurosci. Biobehav. Rev.* 32:1218–1227.

Teixeira, C.M., Pomedli, S.R., et al. (2006). Involvement of the anterior cingulate cortex in the expression of remote spatial memory. *J. Neurosci.* 26:7555–7564.

Timberlake, W., and Fanselow, M.S. (1994). Symposium on behavior systems: learning, neurophysiology, and development. *Psychon. B. Rev.* 1:403–519.

van der Kolk, B.A. (2006). Clinical implications of neuroscience research in PTSD. *Ann. NY Acad. Sci.* 1071:277–293.

Waddell, J., Morris, R.W., et al. (2006). Effects of bed nucleus of the stria terminalis lesions on conditioned anxiety: aversive conditioning with long-duration conditional stimuli and reinstatement of extinguished fear. *Behav. Neurosci.* 120:324–336.

Walker, D.L., Miles, L.A., et al. (2009). Selective participation of the bed nucleus of the stria terminalis and CRF in sustained anxiety-like versus phasic fear-like responses. *Prog. Neuropsychopharmacol. Biol. Psychiatry* 33:1291–1308.

Weinberger, N.M. (1995). Retuning the brain by fear conditioning. In: Gazzaniga, M.S., ed. The Cognitive Neurosciences. Cambridge, MA: MIT Press, pp. 1071–1090.

Wilensky, A.E., Schafe, G.E., et al. (2006). Rethinking the fear circuit: the central nucleus of the amygdala is required for the acquisition, consolidation, and expression of pavlovian fear conditioning. *J. Neurosci.* 26:12387–12396.

Willner, P. (1991). Methods for assessing the validity of animal models of psychopathology. In: Boulton, A., Baker, G., and Martin-Iverson, M., eds. Neuromethods: Animal Models in Psychiatry I. New York: Humana Press, pp. 1–23.

Yehuda, R., and LeDoux, J. (2007). Response variation following trauma: a translational neuroscience approach to understanding PTSD. *Neuron* 56:19–32.

Ziemann, A.E., Allen, J.E., et al. (2009). The amygdala is a chemosensor that detects carbon dioxide and acidosis to elicit fear behavior. *Cell* 139:1012–1021.

42 | DIFFERENTIAL ROLES OF GABA RECEPTORS IN ANXIETY

HANNS MÖHLER

INTRODUCTION

GABA AS SET POINT FOR ANXIETY STATES: GABAERGIC DEFICIT IS CAUSAL FOR ANXIETY

In response to a threat, actual or psychological, evolutionary conserved brain systems orchestrate a physiological and behavioral defensive response. When these brain systems are dysfunctional, feelings of fear and anxiety can reach the pathological level of anxiety disorders. Core features of the underlying neurocircuity include a hyperreactivity of the amygdala as a threat delection system and a hypoactivity of the ventromedial prefrontal cortex as a top-down control for the suppression of a threat response. (Cain, Sullivan, and LeDoux, this volume, Chapter 41). Among the neurotransmitters involved, GABA, the major inhibitory neurotransmitter in the brain, is a critical set point in the fear and anxiety circuits. An acute reduction of GABA transmission causes anxiety. For instance, healthy volunteers experienced panic anxiety when $GABA_A$ receptor function was reduced by the administration of a nonselective benzodiazepine site partial inverse agonist (FG 7142) (Horowski and Dorow, 2002). Pathophysiologically, a defective GABA system is a predisposition to continuing to experience anxiety or fear. Panic anxiety patients show a $GABA_A$ receptor deficit with strongest decrease in cortical areas, in particular in orbitofrontal cortex, insula, and in dorsolateral prefrontal cortex, with the severity of anxiety symptoms correlating with the deficit in $GABA_A$ receptors as shown by [11C] flumazenil PET (Hasler et al., 2008). Furthermore, in combat veterans with PTSD, a dramatic $GABA_A$ receptor deficit (−41%) was apparent in the dorsolateral prefrontal cortex (for review, see Möhler, 2012). Similarly, mutant animals with a targeted constitutive partial reduction of $GABA_A$ receptor, function which mainly affected the hippocampus and cerebral cortex and somewhat the amygdala, displayed a behavior indicative of trait anxiety, reminiscent of generalized anxiety disorder in humans. The animals showed enhanced attention to threat cues, a negative bias to ambiguous cues and a concomitant harm avoidance behavior (Crestani et al., 1999; Earnheart et al., 2007). Conversely, drug-induced enhancement of GABA transmission (benzodiazepines, tiagabine, neurosteroids) exerts anxiolytic activity in the treatment of anxiety disoders (Iosifescu, Murrough, Charney this volume, Chapter 47). The behavioral anxiolytic action of a benzodiazepine such as alprazolam is accompanied by the dampening of the heightened activity of particular anxiety-related brain areas as shown by fMRI in volunteers undergoing an anxiety challenge (cholecytokinin-tetrapeptide i.v.). (Leicht et al., 2013). Thus, anxiety is induced by a reduction of GABA transmission while an enhancement of GABA transmission alleviates anxiety.

BENZODIAZEPINES, A SERVO MECHANISM FOR $GABA_A$ RECEPTOR FUNCTION

Benzodiazepines such as alprazolam are anxiolytics agents with a fast onset of action. They act as positive allosteric modulators of $GABA_A$ receptors. It has long been a mystery how classical benzodiazepines are able to exert anxiolytic activity via a neurotransmitter system as ubiquitous as the GABA system, in particular as these drugs can also act as sedative-hypnotics, muscle relaxants and anticonvulsants. The distinctive pharmacology is largely due to the dose-dependent degree of receptor occupancy in the brain. Generally, anxiolytic activity is achieved at low receptor occupancy (about 20%; Facklam et al., 1992) while sedation and anticonvulsant activity requires higher receptor occupancy levels and correspondingly higher drug doses. The exclusive docking site of these drugs, which was originally termed *benzodiazepine receptor* (Möhler and Okada, 1977), is an allosteric binding site present in all benzodiazepine-sensitive $GABA_A$ receptors (about 80% of all $GABA_A$ receptors), which provides three important features: (*1*) Synapse selectivity: The benzodiazepines do not act unless the GABA-A receptor is activated by GABA drug action and is restricted to operational synapses. (*2*) Ceiling effect: When all $GABA_A$ receptors are fully activated in a synapse, benzodiazepines are unable to increase the peak amplitude of the current response beyond the physiological maximum, a feature that is thought to contribute to the clinical safety of benzodiazepines. (*3*) Bidirectional modulation: Depending on the type of ligand, positive or negative allosteric efficacy in receptor modulation can be achieved. Thus, the pharmacology of ligands of the benzodiazepine site ranges from anxiolytic to anticonvulsant effects for classical benzodiazepine-type ligands (agonists, also termed *positive allosteric modulators*, PAMs) to anxiogenic and convulsant effects of beta-carboline-type ligands (inverse agonists, also termed negative allosteric modulators, NAMs).

Synaptic $GABA_A$ receptors are activated by a brief, nonequilibrium exposure to millimolar GABA (Fig. 42.1). In the presence of a therapeutically active benzodiazepine, the affinity for GABA is increased, which corresponds to a shift of the GABA dose/response curve to the left (i.e., for the same quantum of GABA, more receptors are activated and the amplitude of the GABA response is increased). In keeping with an increase in

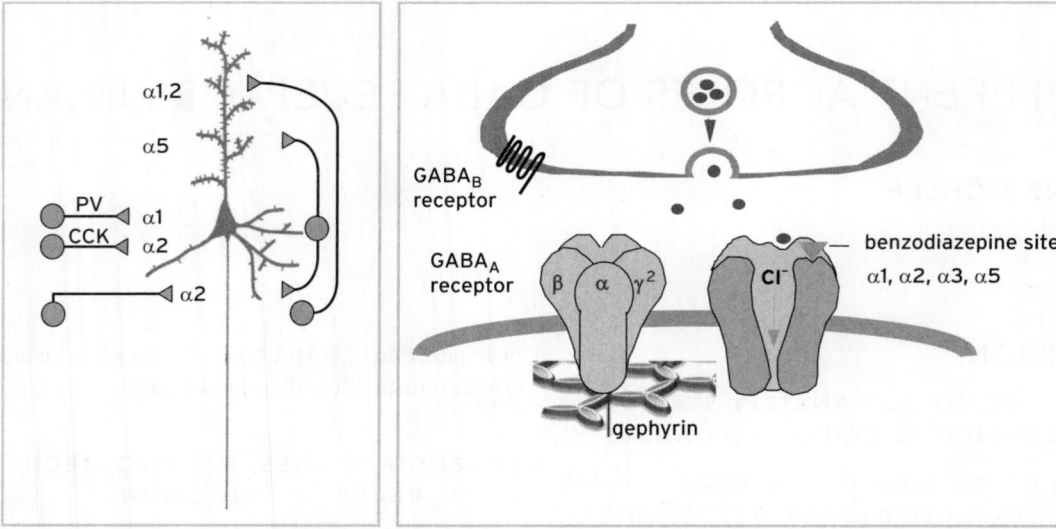

Figure 42.1 *Left: Scheme of the domain-specific innervation of a principal cell by diverse interneurons. Distinct distributions of GABA receptor subtypes are schematically indicated by the type of α-subunit. Right: Scheme of a GABAergic synapse. The heteropentameric GABA$_A$ receptor forms a membrane-spanning chloride ion channel by which GABA (dots) gates fast postsynaptic inhibition. Receptors containing an α$_1$, α$_2$, α$_3$, or α$_5$ subunit in conjunction with a β-subunit (β$_2$, β$_3$) and the γ$_2$ subunit are benzodiazepine sensitive and represent the majority (about 80%) of all GABA$_A$ receptors. Depending on the type of ligand acting at the allosteric modulatory benzodiazepine site, GABA$_A$ receptor function can either be enhanced e.g., by classical benzodiazepines such as diazepam (positive allosteric modulators also termed agonists) or reduced (negative allosteric modulators or inverse agonists, Table 42.2). Besides interacting with the major clustering protein gephyrin, GABA$_A$ receptors undergo regulated trafficking in a dynamic adaption of their cell surface expression (Lüscher et al., 2011). Slow GABAergic inhibition is mediated by G-protein coupled metabotropic GABA$_B$ receptors that cause slow postsynaptic inhibition by opening inwardly rectifying K$^+$ (GiRK) channels (not shown). GABA$_B$ receptors are present presynaptically on some glutamatergic nerve endings (see Fig. 42.3) and, as auto receptors, on some GABAergic interneuron nerve terminal, where they cause inhibition of transmitter release by limiting Ca^{2+} entry.*

affinity, the decay of the spontaneous miniature inhibitory post-synaptic current (mIPSC) is prolonged. However, in various GABA synapses the amplitude of the mIPSCs remained unaltered in the presence of a benzodiazepine agonist, which has been interpreted to indicate that a single quantum of GABA can saturate all GABA$_A$ receptors in the respective synapse and the maximum peak response is not further enhanced by the drug. Nevertheless, even at maximal GABA$_A$ receptor activation, the drug-induced prolongation of individual mIPSCs still remained and resulted in a slightly increased peak amplitude of the compound inhibitory response which is caused by the summation of several mIPSCs. Thus, the action of a benzodiazepine drug appears to be cell- and synapse specific, reflecting local differences in the number of receptors in the cleft or in the GABA concentration released into the cleft. The drug effects will therefore vary with the operational configuration of the GABAergic synapse. Nevertheless, the most pronounced drug effects are expected in synapses operating at suboptimal level, which bodes well for the treatment of pathophysiologies characterized by a reduced GABAergic drive. The action of benzodiazepines on the GABA$_A$ receptor can be compared to the servo mechanism of the brake system in a car. The servo mechanism kicks in only when the brake is activated but does not increase the maximum braking power (for review, see Hajos et al., 2000; Möhler, 2011).

GABA SYSTEMS OPERATE BY DOMAIN-SPECIFIC TARGET INNERVATION

Complex brains have developed highly targeted GABA systems. A wide variety of interneurons dynamically orchestrate the spatiotemporal pattern of network activity. This is largely achieved by the domain-specific innervation of the principal cells to permit an independent regulation of various afferent inputs and the timing of the output (Fig. 42.1). For instance, in the CA1 region of the hippocampus, 21 different classes of GABA interneurons were identified based on their distinct location, morphology, cotransmitter (CCK, SOM), or other marker proteins (parvalbumin [PV], calbindin, calretinin) and activity pattern (Klausberger and Somogyi, 2008). Excitation of PV-positive basket cells can generate neural oscillations over high-frequency ranges, pace them, synchronize participating neurons, and maintain their coherence. Crucial for this property is that basket cells act jointly and have a wide outreach. They are electrically coupled via gap junctions and the axonal arbor of each inhibitory interneuron may contact more than a thousand pyramidal cells. Fast-spiking PV basket cells operate with synapses containing GABA$_A$ receptors, which are geared to high-frequency responses (α$_1$GABA$_A$ receptors). In contrast, the CCK-containing basket cells, which also target the perisomatic compartment, are not fast spiking and operate with structurally different receptors (α$_2$ and α$_3$ GABA$_A$ receptors). Chandelier neurons, which target the axon initial segment of the principal cells in cortex and hippocampus, act as an off-switch by editing the generation and timing of the action potential output and operate with α$_2$GABA$_A$ receptors. Interneurons that preferentially target dendritic sites of pyramidal cells, such as Martinotti cells, influence the synaptic input, by affecting input integration, synaptic plasticity, and the generation of calcium spikes. Sir John Eccles famously wrote, "I always think that inhibition is a sculpturing process. The inhibition, as it were, chisels away at the (…) mass of excitatory action and gives a more specific form to the neuronal performance at every stage of synaptic relay" (Eccles, 1977).

DIVERSITY OF GABA$_A$ RECEPTOR SUBTYPES

The diversity of interneurons is paralleled by a striking diversity of structurally distinct GABA$_A$ receptors. The combinatorial assembly from different subunit classes provides distinct kinetics and pharmacological properties with important consequences for synaptic function and therapeutic drug actions. There is a family of 19 subunits (α_{1-6}, β_{1-3}, γ_{1-3}, δ, ϵ, θ, π, ρ_{1-3}) available for the formation of heteropentameric receptors with a central chloride ion channel pore to be gated by GABA (for review, see Olsen and Sieghart, 2009; Rudolph and Knoflach, 2011). To accommodate the input of diverse interneurons, a principal cell is able to assemble several types of GABA$_A$ receptors and target them to the specific cellular domains and synapses.

The most frequent GABA$_A$ receptor subtype is the $\alpha1$ receptor subtype, assembled from two α_1, two β_2, and one γ_2 subunit (Fig. 42.1). It is highly enriched in synapses and meets the kinetic requirements for high-frequency neurotransmission with a rapid rise and decay time of conductance changes. Correspondingly, fast-spiking PV basket cells drive pyramidal cells via α_1 GABA$_A$ receptors. Other synaptic receptors contain α_2 or α_3 subunits in combination with β_2 or β_3 subunits and the γ_2 subunit. Thus, the predominant receptor subtypes that mediate phasic synaptic inhibition are α_1, α_2, or α_3 GABA$_A$ receptors. Each of these receptors is, however, also found in extrasynaptic plasma membranes, and no receptor subtype has yet been found to have an exclusive synaptic location. This is thought to be largely due to reversible posttranslational modifications that determine the degree of synaptic anchoring of the receptors. However, some GABA$_A$ receptors are excluded from synapses and mediate tonic inhibition by sensing ambient GABA concentrations. They comprise α_5 GABA$_A$ receptors (α_5, β_3, γ_2) and the receptors characterized by a δ subunit, mostly associated with an α_4 or α_6 subunit (Table 42.1) (Mann and Mody, 2010).

Pharmacologically, receptor subtypes are best differentiated by their ability to respond to benzodiazepine drugs. Benzodiazepine-sensitive receptors are those containing an α_1, α_2, α_3, or α_5 subunit in combination with a β_2 or β_3 subunit and a γ_2 subunit with the benzodiazepine binding site being located at the interface between the α and the γ_2 subunit (Fig. 42.1; Table 42.1). Thus, the α_1, α_2, α_3, or α_5 GABA$_A$ receptor subtypes, which represent about 80% of all GABA$_A$ receptors in the brain, mediate the entire repertoire of benzodiazepine actions (anxiolytic action, muscle relaxant, sedative, and anticonvulsant activity). In contrast, GABA$_A$ receptors that contain an α_4 or α_6 subunit are benzodiazepine insensitive, irrespective of the subunits they are associated with (Olsen and Sieghart, 2009; Rudolph and Knoflach, 2011) (Table 42.1).

RESOLVING THE PHARMACOLOGY OF GABA$_A$ RECEPTOR SUBTYPES

Classical benzodiazepines such as diazepam don't differentiate among the four types of benzodiazepine-sensitive GABA$_A$

receptors. It was therefore unknown which part of the spectrum of benzodiazepine actions was mediated by which of the α_1, α_2, α_3, or α_5 receptors *in vivo*. Mouse genetics brought the breakthrough (Rudolph et al., 1999). It was known from recombinant GABA$_A$ receptors that the replacement of a conserved histidine (H) residue in the drug binding pocket by an arginine (R) residue rendered the benzodiazepine-sensitive receptors into benzodiazepine-insensitive receptors. Exploiting this molecular switch, four lines of point-mutated mice were generated, which carried diazepam-insensitive α_1, α_2, α_3, or α_5 subunits, respectively. In these animals, a specific part of the spectrum of benzodiazepine actions was expected to be absent and was therefore attributed to the respective wild-type GABA$_A$ receptor subtype. Importantly, with the exception of the α_5 subunit, the point mutation did not affect the expression or distribution of the receptors nor their response to GABA. It was only when a benzodiazepine drug was administered that the presence of the point mutation manifested itself behaviorally. Thus, GABA$_A$ receptor subtypes became functional markers for the neuronal circuits which mediate selective benzodiazepine actions (Table 42.1) (Möhler, 2011; Rudolph and Knoflach, 2011).

α_1 GABA$_A$ RECEPTORS MEDIATE SEDATION

In mice containing benzodiazepine-insensitive α_1GABA$_A$ receptors (α_1[H101R]), the sedative action of diazepam (measured by locomotor activity) and its anticonvulsant activity (antipentylenetetrazole) was absent, while its anxiolytic effect (measured in the elevated plus maze and the light/dark choice test) and its myorelaxant action (measured by rotarod and horizontal wire test) were fully retained (Rudolph et al., 1999). These results were confirmed in a separate α_1 point mutated mouse line when comparable test conditions were applied (Crestani et al., 2000; McKernan et al., 2000).

Thus, α_1 subunit–containing receptors mediated the sedative but not the anxiolytic action of benzodiazepines. This result provided a rationale for considering the α_1 receptor subtype as a selective target for the development of ligands with sedative-hypnotic activity (Table 42.2). Conversely, GABA$_A$ receptor subtypes other than α_1 were expected to provide a target for developing tranquilizing agents that would lack sedative side effects and largely dependence liability. A new pharmacology was born (see next section).

α_1 GABA$_A$ RECEPTORS LARGELY MEDIATE DEPENDENCE LIABILITY

The dependence liability of classical benzodiazepines is a side effect of medical concern. When wild-type mice were given the choice to consume a drinking solution with or without the benzodiazepine midazolam, a preference for midazolam developed over the course of several days. In mice containing benzodiazepine-insensitive α_1 receptors [(α_1 H101R)], no preference for midazolam developed, pointing to α_1 receptors as the main contributor to dependence liability (Tan et al., 2010). On the cellular level, the preference behavior was attributed to a disinhibition of the reward system represented by dopamine neurons in the ventral tegmental area, activating the reward system. While dopamine neurons

TABLE 42.1. Cellular and subcellular localization of GABA_A receptor subtypes

MAIN SUBUNIT	PROPOSED SUBUNIT REPERTOIRE	BENZODIAZEPINE SITE PHARMACOLOGY	MAJOR SITES OF EXPRESSION	IDENTIFIED NEURONS	SUBCELLULAR LOCALIZATION
α1	α1β2γ2	Major subtype (60% of all GABA_A receptors). Mediates the sedative, amnestic and—to a large extent—the anticonvulsant action and dependence liability of benzodiazepine site agonists.	Cerebral cortex (layers I–VI), hippocampus, amygdala, olfactory bulb, thalamus, basal forebrain, globus pallidus, substantia nigra pars reticulata, inferior colliculus, cerebellum, brainstem	Mitral cells and short-axon cells (olfactory bulb), principal cells and selected interneurons in cerebral cortex and hippocampus, GABAergic neurons in pallidum and substantianigra, thalamic relay neurons, Purkinje cells and granule cells	Synaptic (soma and dendrites) and extrasynaptic in all neurons with high expression
α2	α2β3γ2	Minor subtype (15–20%). Mediates anxiolytic action of benzodiazepine site agonists	Cerebral cortex (layers I–IV), hippocampal formation, amygdala, striatum, olfactory bulb, hypothalamus, superior colliculus, inferior olive, motor nuclei, spinal cord dorsal horn	Principal cells in hippocampal formation and amygdala, spiny stellate striatal neurons, olfactory bulb granule cells, motoneurons, dorsal root ganglion cells and intrinsic dorsal horn neurons	Mainly synaptic; perisomatic location and enriched in axon initial segment of cortical and hippocampal pyramidal cells
α3	α3β2,3γ2	Minor subtype (10–15%). Mediates anxiolytics action of benzodiazepine site agonist although only at high receptor occupancy.	Cerebral cortex (layers V–VI), amygdala, olfactory bulb, thalamic reticular and intralaminar nuclei, superior colliculus, brainstem, spinal cord, locus coeruleus, raphe, medial septum	Tufted cells (olfactory bulb), reticular thalamic neurons, cerebellar Golgi type II cells, serotonergic and catecholaminergic neurons, basal forebrain cholinergic neurons, principal cells in lateral and basolateral amygdala	Mainly synaptic, including some axon initial segments; extrasynaptic in principal cells of the amygdala and in inferior olivary neurons
α4	α4β2,3δ	Less than 5% of all receptors. Insensitive to classical benzodiazepines.	Dentate gyrus, thalamus	Dentate gyrus granule cells	Extrasynaptic
α5	α5β3γ2	Less than 5% of all receptors. Mediates the memory-enhancing effects of benzodiazepine site partial inverse agonists.	Highest in hippocampus, considerably lower in deep cortical layers, amygdala, olfactory bulb, hypothalamus, superior colliculus, superior olivary nucleus, spinal trigeminal nucleus, spinal cord	Pyramidal cells (hippocampus, cerebral cortex), granule cells and periglomerular cells (olfactory bulb), superior olivary neurons, spinal trigeminal neurons	Extrasynaptic in hippocampus, cerebral cortex, and olfactory bulb; synaptic and extrasynaptic in spinal trigeminal nucleus and superior olivary nucleus
α6	α6β2,3γ2; α6β2,3δ	Less than 5% of all receptors. Insensitive to classical benzodiazepines.	Cerebellum, dorsal cochlear nucleus	Granule cells (cerebellum)	Synaptic (cerebellar glomeruli) and extrasynaptic on granule cell dendrites and soma

(Adapted from Fritschy and Brünig, 2003, and Möhler et al., 2002.)

express α3 GABA_A receptors, impinging interneurons themselves express α1 receptors. It is their enhancement by midazolam that apparently provided the overriding input. The ensuing disinhibition of the dopamine neurons is associated with synaptic plasticity processes, which were proposed to underlie drug reinforcement (Tan et al., 2010). The view of α1 receptors being the prime mediator of dependence liability is in line with pharmacological evidence. Ligands that spare α1 receptors but act as partial agonists at α2 and α3 receptors, such as L-838417 or TPA023 (Table 42.2; see following), showed low or no dependence liability in tests of self-administration or place preference in rodents and nonhuman primates (Ator, 2005, 2010; Licata and Rowlett, 2008). Although the partial extent of efficacy of these agents may have contributed to these results, ligands sparing α1 receptors can be expected to have a much reduced dependence liability compared with

TABLE 42.2. Pharmacology of benzodiazepine-sensitive GABA$_A$ receptor subtypes*

DRUG	MAIN ACTIVITY	INTERACTION WITH RECOMBINANT GABA$_A$ RECEPTORS
α$_1$GABA$_A$ RECEPTORS MEDIATE SEDATION		
Zolpidem	Hypnotic	Preferential affinity for α$_1$ subtype[1]
Zaleplone	Hypnotic	Preferential affinity for α$_1$ subtype[1]
Zopiclone	Hypnotic	Preferential affinity for α$_1$ subtype[1]
α$_2$,α$_3$GABA$_A$ RECEPTORS MEDIATE ANXIOLYSIS		
L-838417	Anxiolytic and Antinociceptive	Comparable affinity at α$_1$, α$_2$, α$_3$, α$_5$ subtype[2] Partial agonist at α$_2$, α$_3$, α$_5$ (not α$_1$) subtype
TPA023 (MK0777)	Anxiolytic	Comparable affinity at α$_1$, α$_2$, α$_3$, α$_5$; partial agonist at α$_2$, α$_3$ subtypes; no efficacy at α$_1$, α$_5$ subtypes[3]
NS11394	Anxiolytic and Antinociceptive	Comparable affinity at α$_1$, α$_2$, α$_3$, α$_5$; partial agonist at α$_2$, α$_3$ subtypes; nearly full agonist at α$_5$ subtype[4]
TP003	Anxiolytic	Comparable affinity at α$_1$, α$_2$, α$_3$, α$_5$; full agonist at α$_3$ subtype; acts at high receptor occupancy[5]
α$_5$GABA$_A$ RECEPTORS: PARTIAL INVERSE AGONISTS ENHANCE MEMORY		
L-655 708	Memory enhancer	Partial inverse agonist with preferential affinity for α$_5$ subtype[6]
α$_5$ IA	Memory enhancer	Partial inverse agonist with preferential efficacy at α$_5$ subtype[7]
RO493851	Memory enhancer	Partial inverse agonist with selective affinity and efficacy at α$_5$ receptor subtype[8]

* For further details, see Möhler 2011, 2012.
[1] Dämgen and Lüddens, 1999; [2] McKernan et al., 2000; [3] Atack, 2009; [4] Mirza et al., 2008; [5] Dias et al., 2005; [6] Atack et al., 2006a; [7] Atack 2010; [8] Ballard et al., 2009.

classical benzodiazepines which fail to differentiate between GABA$_A$ receptor subtypes.

α$_2$ GABA$_A$ RECEPTORS MEDIATE ANXIOLYSIS

In mice containing benzodiazepine-insensitive α$_2$ GABA$_A$ receptors (α$_2$H101R), diazepam failed to induce anxiolytics activity (measured in the elevated plus maze test and the light/dark choice test) while its sedative and anticonvulsant activity was fully retained (measured by locomotor activity, rotarod, antipentyleneterazole) (Löw et al., 2000). The lack of anxiolytic activity of diazepam in (α$_2$H101R) mice was confirmed in a conditioned emotional response paradigm (CER) (Morris et al., 2006), in which a conditioning foot shock induces a higher level of stress than in the nonconditioned ethological tests used in the earlier study (Löw et al., 2000).

Thus, the anxiolytic-like action of diazepam is based on the enhancement of α$_2$GABA$_A$ receptor function. Since this receptor population represents only about 15–20% of all GABA$_A$ receptors, it appears to be strategically positioned in anxiety circuits. In cerebral cortex and hippocampus, the α$_2$ GABA$_A$ receptors are largely expressed on pyramidal cells. In the perisomatic domain, these receptors mediate mainly the synaptic inhibitory input arising from CCK-containing basket cells. At the axon initial segment, they mediate the GABAergic input from Chandelier neurons, which exert an output control of the firing pattern of principal cells by being able to suppress action potential propagation (Fig. 42.1).

In the amygdala, α$_2$ GABA$_A$ receptors are prominent throughout. Most conspicuously, the central nucleus (CEA), the output station of the amygdala, contains largely, if not exclusively, α$_2$ GABA$_A$ receptors (Figs. 42.2 and 42.3) (Marowsky et al., 2004). Thus, α$_2$ receptors are in a strategic position to attenuate the output from the CEA to the brain areas, which execute the physiological and hormonal fear and anxiety responses. In addition, α$_2$ GABA$_A$ receptors mediate inhibitory signals in the lateral and basolateral amygdala, areas involved in fear acquisition., The basolateral division also contains α$_1$ receptors. α$_3$ GABA$_A$ receptors are a minor subtype throughout. In humans, the pattern of α$_1$, α$_2$, and α$_3$ receptor subtype expression in the amygdala closely corresponded to that in the mouse (Fig. 42.3). The functional significance of the receptor subtypes for the amygdala microcircuits is described later.

Besides their location in different brain areas, α$_2$ and α$_3$ GABA$_A$ receptors are also found in spinal cord, being located on primary spinal cord afferents and intrinsic spinal neurons. Using the point-mutated mice described earlier, the ability of diazepam to suppress pathological pain was attributed to these receptor subtypes (Knabl et al., 2008). Indeed, using the compound, L-838417, which acts as partial agonist at α$_2$ and α$_3$ receptors (Table 42.2), pain behavior was suppressed in rodent models of inflammatory and neuropathic pain with an efficacy comparable to that of morphine. Furthermore, in contrast to morphine, L-838417, given subchronically, they failed to develop tolerance (Knabl et al., 2008). Thus, new anxiolytic agents acting on α$_{2,3}$ receptor subtypes may, at least partly, have an added antinociceptive potential (Zeilhofer et al., 2009) (Table 42.2).

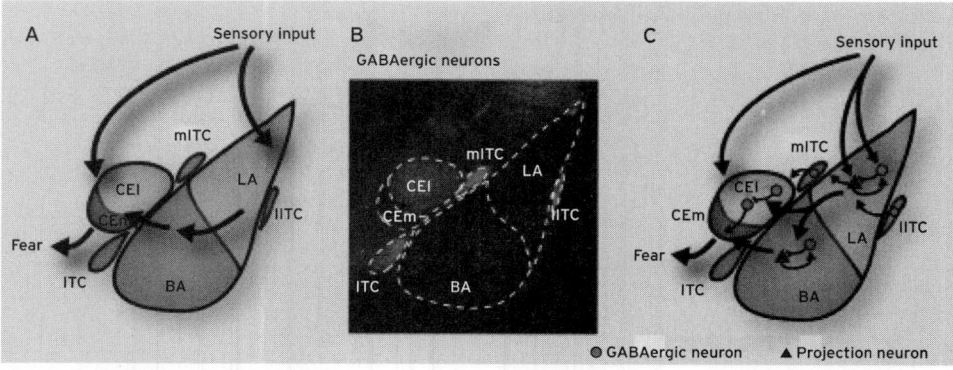

Figure 42.2 *General organization of amygdala circuitry and GABAergic neurons. (A) Scheme of the basic organization and overall flow of information within the amygdaloid complex. LA, lateral amygdala; BA, basal amygdala; CEl, lateral subdivision of the central amygdala; CEm, medial subdivision of the central amygdala (CEA); mITC, medial intercalated cell cluster; lITC, lateral intercalated cell cluster. (B) Coronal brain slice stained for the 67 kD isoform of the GABA synthesizing enzyme glutamic acid decarboxylase (GAD67) illustrating the distribution of GABAergic neurons across the amygdaloid complex. (C) Simplified scheme of the organization and function of inhibitory interneurons in amygdaloid nuclei. In the LA and BA, local interneurons are part of feedforward and feedback circuits and control projection neuron output. The lITCs and mITCs relay feedforward inhibition, which may also participate in controlling CEl output. (Images from Ehrlich et al., 2009 used with permission from Elsevier.)*

α_3 GABA-A RECEPTORS: A BACKUP SYSTEM FOR ANXIOLYSIS

In keeping with the view that the anxiolytic activity of diazepam is mediated via α_2 GABA$_A$ receptors, the anxiolytic response of diazepam remained unaltered when the α_3 receptor was silenced in mice by a point mutation (α_3H126R) (measured in elevated plus maze and light/dark choice test), suggesting that alpha3 receptors do not mediate anxiolytics activity. As expected, the sedative, motor-impairing, and anticonvulsant properties of diazepam were likewise unaltered in this α_3 mutant (Löw et al., 2000). Nevertheless, there is significant

evidence that the α_3 GABA$_A$ receptor subtype contributes to anxiolytic activity. In mice with a benzodiazepine-insensitive α_2 receptor [α_2(H101R) mice], L-838417, a partial agonist acting at the benzodiazepine site of α_2, α_3 and α_5 receptors, showed anxiolytic activity at a somewhat elevated receptor occupancy (tested in elevated plus maze, fear potentiated startle and conditioned emotional response) (McKernan et al., 2000; Morris et al., 2006). These findings pointed to a contribution of receptors other than α_2 receptors to anxiolysis. Indeed, TP003, a full agonist with selective efficacy at α_3 GABA$_A$ receptors displayed anxiolytic activity as measured in an ethological test (elevated

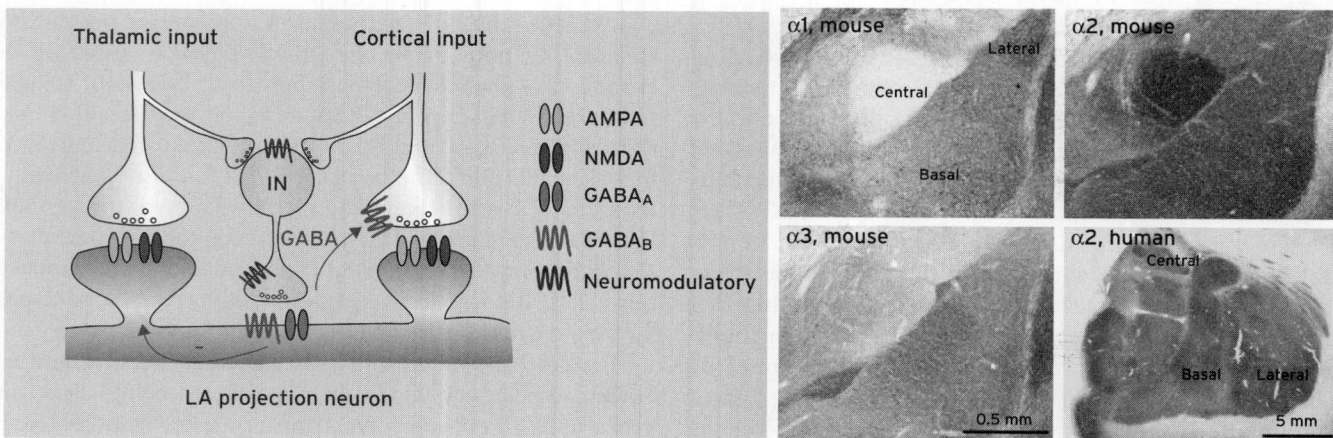

Figure 42.3 *Inhibitory gating of long-term potentiation (LTP) in the lateral amygdala in fear acquisition. Left: Pyramidal projection neurons in the lateral amygdala (LA, gray) receive converging thalamic and cortical sensory afferents. LTP at thalamic and cortical sensory synapses, induced by fear conditioning, is tightly controlled by GABA released from feedforward interneurons (medium gray). At thalamic afferents, this control is predominantly postsynaptic via GABA$_A$ receptors. At cortical afferents, this control is presynaptic via GABA$_B$ receptors. The GABA interneurons are targets of neuromodulators that modify their output activity and thereby gate the induction of LTP by transiently altering the level of pre- and postsynaptic inhibitory drive. By depressing GABA feedforward inhibition, dopamine and noradrenaline enhance LTP, while 5HT reduces LTP (figure from Ehrlich et al., 2009). Right: Immunohistochemical distribution of GABA$_A$ receptor subtypes in the amygdala. In the mouse, the α_2-subunit staining is prominent throughout, in particular in the central nucleus where no α_1 subunit immunoreactivity is detectable. Both subunits produce a diffuse labeling of neuropil in the lateral and basolateral nucleus. The α_3-subunit is detected in the basolateral nucleus and, to a lesser extent, in the lateral and central nuclei (Marowsky et al., 2004, 2012). Similarly, in human amygdala, α_2-subunit staining is prominent throughout and most prevalent in the central and basal nucleus. α_1-subunit staining was prominent only in the lateral nucleus. Minimal staining for α_3-subunits was apparent throughout the amygdala. [Left: Figure from Ehrlich et al., 2009. Right: Data and image of human amygdala courtesy of J. Sung and H. Waldvogel, Centre of Brain Research, University of Auckland, NZ.]*

plus maze in rats) and in a conditioned test paradigm (conditioned emotional response in squirrel monkeys) pointing to α_3 GABA$_A$ receptors as a second target for anxiolysis besides α_2 receptors (Dias et al., 2005).

The two anxiolytic drug targets differ, however, in their systems response sensitivity. Classical benzodiazepines (e.g., diazepam or chlordiazepoxide) show anxiolytic activity, mediated via α_2 receptors, at a low dose when an overall receptor occupancy of 20–25% is reached (Dias et al., 2005; Facklam et al., 1992). In contrast, the level of receptor occupancy required for the minimal effective dose of TP003 (elevated plus maze test) acting at α_3 receptors was 75%, suggesting that three quarters of all α_3 receptors have to be enhanced to reach an anxiolytic response (Dias et al., 2005). The alpha3 receptors are therefore considered to act as a backup system for anxiolytic activity at high receptor occupancy. Presently, most newly developed anxiolytic compounds such as L-838417, TPA023, or NS 11394 interact with both α_2 and α_3 receptors (see next section and Table 42.2). Their primary anxiolytic effect is therefore mediated by α_2 GABA$_A$ receptors while α_3 receptors are recruited in addition when a high receptor occupancy is reached.

α_3 GABA$_A$ receptors are a minor receptor subtype in the brain and are mainly found on catecholaminergic neurons of the brainstem (dopamine, noradrenaline) and basal forebrain cholinergic neurons, which are involved in communicating emotion and vigilance. In the amygdala, α_3 receptors are of minor abundance and, being located extrasynaptically, mediate tonic inhibition of principal cells in the lateral and basolateral domain (Fig. 42.3; Table 42.1) (Marowsky et al., 2012).

α_5 GABA$_A$ RECEPTORS REGULATE HIPPOCAMPUS-DEPENDENT (FEAR) MEMORY

The α_5 GABA$_A$ receptor subtype ($\alpha_5\beta_3\gamma_2$) shows a very restricted expression in the brain with highest density in hippocampus and considerably lower in layer 5 cerebral cortex (Fig. 42.4; Table 42.1). In both regions the receptors are exclusively located extrasynaptically on pyramidal cell dendrites mediating tonic inhibition (Brickley and Mody, 2012). Apparently, the presence of the α_5 subunit seems to override the ability of the γ_2 subunit to promote synaptic localization. Morphologically, being located at the base of the dendritic spines and the adjacent dendritic shaft of hippocampal pyramidal cells, these receptors represent the first inhibitory counterbalance to the incoming excitatory input transmitted through N-methyl-D-aspartate (NMDA) receptors at the dendritic spine synapses (Fig. 42.4).

Synaptic plasticity and learning are often enhanced by a reduction of GABAergic inhibition. Indeed, transgenic mice with a partial knockdown of α_5 receptors showed enhanced performance in the hippocampus-dependent tasks of trace fear conditioning and appetitive conditioning (Crestani et al., 2002; Yee et al., 2004). Mice with a complete deficit of α_5 receptors (α_5 knockout) likewise showed an improved cognitive performance as evident in spatial learning (water maze) concomitant with an enhancement of neural oscillatory synchrony in hippocampal slices (Collinson et al., 2002; Glykys and Mody, 2007). In both α_5 mutant mouse lines, the enhanced behavioral performance was highly selective in that hippocampus-independent learning (delay conditioning, two-way avoidance) remained unaltered compared with wild type. Thus, the α_5 GABA$_A$ receptors in hippocampal pyramidal cells are control elements of the temporal and spatial associative memory. This is the more noteworthy as it is the tonic inhibition that has taken on a critical role in controlling learning and memory performance (Brickley and Mody, 2012). In contrast, the phasic inhibition of hippocampal pyramidal cells is largely mediated via α_2 and α_3 GABA$_A$ receptors. Correspondingly, classical benzodiazepine responses such as sedation or anxiolytic activity are not linked to the α_5 receptor function (for review, see Möhler, 2007). The role of α_5 GABA$_A$ receptors in cognition prompted the development of drugs that selectively target α_5 GABA$_A$ (see later section).

AMYGDALA MICROCIRCUITS FOR ANXIOLYSIS AND THE VOCABULARY OF GABA$_A$ RECEPTOR SUBTYPES

Among the overall circuitry of anxiety and fear, several microcircuits have been identified in which GABA neurons play a key part in the acquisition, storage, and extinction of fear, in particular in the amygdala and cerebral cortex (Fig. 42.2). They provide the first blueprint for the neuronal circuits through

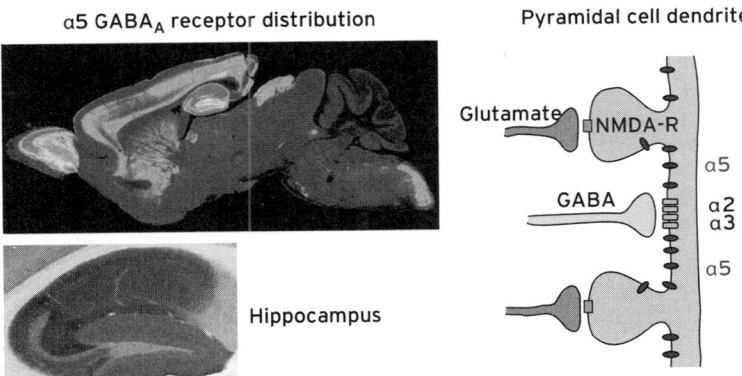

Figure 42.4 Left: Immunohistochemical distribution of the α_5-subunit GABA$_A$ receptor in parasagittal sections of adult mice with the enlargement of the hippocampal formation showing its prominent dendritic localization (Crestani et al., 2002). Right: Schematic distribution of GABA$_A$ receptor subtypes at pyramidal cell dendrites. In balancing the excitatory input, phasic inhibition is mediated via α_2 and α_3 GABA$_A$ receptors, while α_5 GABA$_A$ receptors, located at the base of dendritic spines and the adjacent dendritic shaft, mediate tonic inhibition. (See color insert.)

which α_2 and α_3 GABA$_A$ receptors mediate anxiolytic drug actions.

LATERAL AMYGDALA: LOCAL GABAERGIC CONTROL OF EXPERIENCE-DEPENDENT PLASTICITY

The amygdala is the site for formation and storage of fear memories, frequently investigated in paradigms of fear conditioning, a form of associative learning acquired by temporal coincidence of a neutral conditioned stimulus (CS, e.g., tone) with an unconditioned aversive stimulus (US, foot shock). The lateral amygdala (LA) is responsible for the linking of the conditioned and unconditioned stimulus and thus for the formation of memory of this experience by which the CS gains access to an emotional response circuit. The combination of CS and US requires the formation of long-term potentiation (LTP) of sensory thalamic input onto the neurons in the lateral amygdala (LA), thereby increasing the activity of the LA projection neurons. The LA neurons drive the fear response by projecting to the basolateral (BLA) and central amygdala (CEA) (Fig. 42.2). The LTP process in the LA is under strong GABAergic feedforward control (Fig. 42.3). For instance, infusion of a GABA$_A$ receptor agonist (muscimol) can block fear acquisition. Similarly, intra-amygdala application of a benzodiazepine, restricted largely to the LA and basolateral amygdala (BLA), is sufficient to induce anxiolysis.

Electrophysiologically, monosynaptic IPSCs recorded from pyramidal-shaped principal cells in the lateral and basolateral amygdala (LA/BLA) of the mouse were carried by α_2 subunit–containing GABA$_A$ receptors and to a smaller amount by α_1 subunit–containing receptors (Marowsky et al., 2004), suggesting that the synaptic feedforward inhibition may be largely mediated by α_2GABA$_A$ receptor and provide a major target site for anxiolytic drug action. The α_3GABA$_A$ receptors are expressed throughout LA and BLA, preferentially at extrasynaptic sites mediating tonic inhibition of principal cells (Marowsky et al., 2012). Thus, the LA/BLA is a prominent target for drug-induced anxiolysis based on the enhancement of α_2 and α_3GABA$_A$ receptor function. Thus, by reducing the excitability of LA projection neurons, benzodiazepine-type drugs are able to limit the fear-inducing impact of CS (Fig. 42.3) (for review, see Ehrlich et al., 2009).

The induction of LTP in the lateral amygdala is constrained not only by activation of GABA$_A$ receptors, but also metabotropic GABA$_B$ receptors (Fig. 42.3). The presynaptic GABA$_B$ receptors, which are presumably activated via synaptic GABA spillover, attenuate the release of excitatory neurotransmitter from cortical and thalamic afferents by limiting the entry of Ca^{2+}. In the presence of a GABA$_B$ receptor antagonist, the induction of LTP was facilitated at both cortical and thalamic afferent synapses (Ehrlich et al., 2009). Conversely, anxiolytic activity has been described for GABA$_B$ receptor agonists, although clinical evidence is still lacking.

Presynaptic modulation of GABA neurons by catecholamines in fear acquisition

Under stress and in emotionally charged conditions, dopamine, released from the ventral tegmental area pathway, potentiates amygdala function and enhances aversive conditioning. This is achieved by presynaptic modulation of GABA release in two areas. In the lateral amygdala, dopamine, via presynaptic dopamine D2 receptors, suppresses GABAergic feedforward inhibition and thereby enhances LTP induction by conditioned fear (Fig. 42.3). Various other modulators likewise affect the induction of LTP by targeting the GABA neurons. At the thalamo-LA synapses, besides dopamine, noradrenaline and μ-opioids reduce feedforward GABA inhibition and enhance LTP (Tully et al., 2007). Conversely, other modulators such as 5-hydroxytryptamine (5HT) or gastrin-related peptide enhance GABA inhibition and constrain the induction of LTP (Ehrlich et al., 2009).

A second target for dopamine is the intercalated cell cluster (ITC), a network of paracapsular GABAergic cells that surround the basolateral complex of the amygdala (Fig. 42.2). It provides GABAergic feedforward inhibition into the basolateral and the central amygdala. Dopamine (via D1 receptors) hyperpolarizes these GABA neurons and substantially suppresses their excitability, resulting in disinhibition of the basolateral and central nucleus with an increase in fear responding. Suppression of the paracapsular inhibitory system by dopamine provides a compelling neuronal mechanism for the increased affective behavior observed during stress or other hyperdopaminergic states (Marowsky et al., 2005). The ITC neurons are innervated by cortical fibers and can thus mediate the cortical feed-forward control of the BLA and the CEA (Fig. 42.2). By disinhibiting the BLA and CEA, dopamine promotes amygdala-related behavior and reduces cortical control. Indeed, focal or systemic administration of the D1 receptor antagonist SCH 23390 results in anxiolysis and blocks acquisition and expression of fear.

CENTRAL AMYGDALA: GABA CONTROL OF FEAR EFFECTOR NEURONS

The central nucleus of the amygdala (CEA) is well known as the major output station by which the amygdala determines the expression of fear-related behavior that includes immobility (freezing) and activation of autonomic and neuroendocrine responses (LeDoux, 2000). A microcircuit within the CEA has been identified to be important for both the acquisition as well as the expression of fear (Haubensak et al., 2010). The output neurons, located in the medial subdivision of CEA (CEm) are normally under tight inhibitory control from a population of spontaneously active GABAergic neurons located in the lateral subdivision (CEl) (Fig. 42.2). Diminishing this inhibitory tone through aversive stimuli leads to a disinhibition of the CEm output neurons, which trigger the execution of fear and anxiety responses.

In the CEA, GABAergic inhibition operates largely if not exclusively through α_2GABA$_A$ receptors, the receptor subtype known to mediate benzodiazepine-induced anxiolysis (Löw et al., 2000). Electrophysiologically, diazepam-induced changes in synaptic currents in mouse CEA were found to be exclusively carried by α_2 receptors without a significant contribution form α_1 or α_3 receptors (Marowsky et al., 2004). Immunohistochemically, α_2 receptors, being by far the predominant receptor subtype throughout most of the amygdala

(Fig. 42.3), are almost exclusively expressed in the CEA, with no α_1 receptors being detectable and only a modest amount of α_3 receptors in this nucleus (Marowsky et al., 2004). This pattern of receptor distribution in the mouse was largely confirmed in post-mortem human amygdala. The α_2 receptor is again predominant throughout the amygdala. The CEA and the basal nucleus contain almost exclusively α_2 receptors. The lateral nucleus contains, in addition, α_1 GABA$_A$ receptors. The α_3 receptors are a minor subtype (personal communication, J. Sung and H. Waldvogel, University of Auckland, NZ) (Fig. 42.3). Thus, dampening the output of the CEA via α_2 GABA$_A$ receptors seems to be a major anxiolytic microcircuit, which illustrates the relevance of this particular GABA$_A$ receptor subtype.

Furthermore, both CEl and CEm express high levels of neuropeptides that modulate anxiety and stress-related behavior (Huber et al., 2005). For instance, oxytocin (OT), besides its hormonal functions, exerts strong anxiolytic activity (e.g., in social anxiety), and the CEA has recently been identified as target for its ability to suppress fear. Axonal projections from OT neurons in the hypothalamus reach the CEL. Presumably, by releasing glutamate in addition to OT, a subpopulation of GABA neurons in CEL activates and thereby enhances the inhibition of CEM output neurons (Tovote and Lüthi, 2012). Thus, the anxiolytic activity of OT is based on enhancing the GABAergic inhibition to attenuate the CEA output neurons, an effect mediated by α_2 receptors. There is also an opposing interaction pointing to a convergence of the anxiolytic circuitries of OT and benzodiazepines. A subpopulation of CEl neurons express presynaptic CRF receptors type 1, which respond to the stress hormone CRF (corticotropin releasing factor), suggesting that GABA circuits within the CEA may be a point of convergence of stress and stress-coping (anxiolytic) systems (Ehrlich et al., 2009). In summary, diminishing the activity of CEM output neurons (via α_2 GABA$_A$ receptors) attenuates fear and anxiety responses while increasing CEM output leads to stronger fear responses.

FEAR EXTINCTION: SWITCHING FEAR OFF BY A DISTINCT NEURAL CIRCUIT

Understanding how learned fears are diminished is a valuable contribution to clinical cognitive therapy. Fear extinction is an active learning process eventually leading to the formation of a consolidated extinction memory (Herry et al., 2010). Extinction of conditioned fear is achieved through repeated presentation of the CS in the absence of an aversive unconditioned stimulus rendering the CS as non-aversive. Not only is the amygdala important for the acquisition of fear (see preceding), but also as a site of extinction-associated plasticity. Activating GABAergic neurons in the amygdala is thought to underlie the process of extinction. During extinction, cortical neurons, in conveying the absence of the aversive unconditioned stimulus, are thought to suppress the amygdala output. This is largely achieved by cortical activation of the GABA neurons of the intercalated cell cluster (ITC) which surrounds the amygdala and innervates the basolateral and central nuclei (Fig. 42.2). They act as a switching circuit that can block the fear-induced LTP and guide the change in behavior (Herry et al., 2010). Molecularly, the expression of certain GABA$_A$ receptor subunit genes (α_2 and β_2) was upregulated within hours following extinction training as shown on the mRNA level (Heldt and Ressler, 2007). Since in both the LA and the CEA, α_2 GABA$_A$ receptors play a major role, it might be conceivable that anxiolytics acting on α_2 receptors (sparing sedation via α_1 receptors) may also facilitate fear extinction.

Fear and fear extinction have been recognized in behaving mice to be encoded by distinct populations of basal amygdala neurons termed fear neurons and extinction neurons. After conditioning, fear neurons exhibited increased activity upon CS exposure. In contrast, extinction neurons developed CS responses only during extinction training. Indeed, a decrease in the firing activity of fear neurons and a concomitant increase in activity of extinction neurons preceded the behavioral shift from the fear to the no-fear response upon CS presentation (Herry et al., 2008, 2010). The activation of extinction neurons remained stable for at least one week. However, changing the context resulted in the immediate recovery of the previously conditioned fear response, a process called renewal. The bi-directional switch in behavior between fear extinction and fear renewal is likely to be encoded by discrete neural circuits. They comprise a distributed network with differential connections between the BLA, the mPFC, and hippocampus, the latter being relevant for conveying context information to be associated with the unconditioned stimulus in the amygdala (Ehrlich et al., 2009; see also Cain, Sullivan, and LeDoux, this volume, Chapter 41).

SHIFT FROM PASSIVE FEAR TO ACTIVE COPING

Fear-arousing stimuli elicit a constellation of fear responses through the amygdala, which acts as an interface that triggers freezing, autonomic, and endocrine responses. However, the pathways that initiate this fear behavior can be redirected. Fully fear-conditioned rats were given the option of moving to another place to avoid the conditioned stimulus. The learning of this escape response (i.e., changing the context prevents fear stimulus) engages alternative pathways in the lateral amygdala that circumvent the CEA, as shown by lesion studies. Passive fear responding is replaced by an active coping strategy (Amorapanth et al., 2000; LeDoux and Gorman, 2001). Recently, first insights into the cellular switch between freezing and active coping were made. The inhibition of a particular type of GABA interneuron (type I neuron) in the lateral subdivision of the CEA was shown to be sufficient (via disinhibition of another GABA neuron) to suppress freezing and engage active responses (Gozzi et al., 2010). These findings identify neural circuit that biases fear responses toward active coping strategies. Coping inherently entails a physiologically anxiolytic response by threat avoidance learning.

CORTICAL MICROCIRCUITS FOR ANXIOLYSIS

ANTERIOR CINGULATE CORTEX AND THE RESOLUTION OF CONFLICT

The choice between different options in goal-directed behavior requires a value arbitration. In a conflict situation, upcoming decisions are evaluated as being "good" or "bad" relative to one's expectation. In healthy individuals, the pregenual anterior cingulated cortex (pACC) is involved in cost–benefit evaluations. It communicates the outcome of the evaluation to other brain areas and thereby regulates the emotional response triggered by a conflict situation. The pACC has been implicated in human anxiety disorders and depression (Ressler and Mayberg, 2007).

Generalized anxiety disorder is characterized by continous rumination and worrying. This anxiety behavior relates to risk assessment of a potential threat and crucially involves uncertainty as to the expectancy of the threat. Anxious individuals show a biased evaluation of a situation in that they pay increased attention to threat-related cues and tend to interpret ambiguous stimuli in a threatening manner. These cognitive biases are thought to underlie avoidance behavior (e.g., avoidance of social contact) as a cardinal symptom of anxiety disorders as well as depression. The implication of the pACC was recently tested in a macaque version of an approach–avoidance decision task, which is also used in humans (Amemori and Graybiel, 2012). Visual cues indicated the likelihood of positive outcome (delivery of food) or negative outcome (airpuff) at the end of the trial. The animals varied their decision to approach (reward is worth it) or to avoid (reward is not worth it) depending on the relative sizes of food rewards and airpuffs indicated by the cues at the beginning of the task. By electrical recording, the pACC was found to have an organization of neurons that represented motivationally positive (P) or negative (N) subjective value, respectively. The cost–benefit boundary was set by balanced activity of N-type and P-type neuron populations, flexibly changing depending on the average offers in each task. In one pACC subzone, neurons with negative coding were more numerous, and electrical microstimulation of this subzone, but not elsewhere in the pACC, strongly increased avoidance decisions. Thus, overactivated neurons representing negative motivational values lead to a pessimistic evaluation of future outcome and increased avoidance behavior. In subsequent experiments, a bias toward avoidance persisted even in the absence of the microstimulation. These findings raise the possibility that pACC stimulation could bring about a tonic, persistent state affecting the relative evaluation of cost and benefit.

The uncertainty of a conflict situation frequently induces anxiety. In the approach–avoidance task described earlier, anxiolytic treatment of the animals with diazepam (0.25 mg/kg intramuscularly) fully blocked the negative biasing of the cost–benefit evaluation and the stimulus-induced negative decision making (Amemori and Graybiel, 2012). This result is important as it defines a cellular substrate for the ability of diazepam to reduce negative motivation and reverse a negative biasing of behavior. The diazepam-induced, dampening the stimulus-induced overactivity of N-neurons in the pACC, may possibly be mediated via α_2 GABA$_A$ receptors. In a conflict situation in mice (light/dark test), the anxiolytic action of diazepam was found to be exclusively mediated via α_2 GABA$_A$ receptors (Löw et al., 2000). These results on value arbitration are of major interest not only for anxiety disorders but also for depression, where negative biases in cost–benefit evaluations are part of the pathophysiology. Besides providing a microcircuit for anxiolysis, the results also add support to the GABA hypothesis of major depression where the pACC plays

a critical role (Lüscher et al., 2010; Möhler, 2012; Ressler and Mayberg, 2007).

FEAR LEARNING IN THE AUDITORY CORTEX: A DISINHIBITORY MICROCIRCUIT

Fear memory acquisition (tone/shock association) depends on the amygdala but, depending on the stimulus complexity of the tone, can also engage the auditory cortex. It receives thalamocortical feedforward information and may act as a relay for tone information to down-stream structures such as the amygdala. Fear conditioning causes long-lasting plasticity of CS responses in auditory cortex, which critically involves GABA interneurons (Letzkus et al., 2011). After experiencing the CS, acetylcholine is rapidly released from cholinergic basal forebrain afferents, which activate GABA interneurons in layer 1 (L1) of auditory cortex, which, in turn, inhibit fast-spiking parvalbumin-positive (PV) interneurons in L2/3 of auditory cortex. These PV basket cells in turn provide strong perisomatic inhibition to local pyramidal cells in the L2/3 layer. When stimulation by tone and shock was combined, the activity of pyramidal cells was strikingly enhanced (visualized by Ca-imaging). Disinhibiton of PV interneurons by foot shock probably gates the induction of activity-dependent plasticity in the auditory cortex. The convergence of stimuli and the concomitant auditory cortex disinhibiton are essential for fear learning (Letzkus et al., 2011). The GABA interneurons in L1 are responsive to dopamine and 5HT, indicating that modulatory systems can feed into the cortical microcircuit.

Although an anxiolytic drug was not tested in this paradigm, the disinhibition of the microcircuit in auditory cortex offers a conceptual role for drugs acting on α_2 GABA$_A$ receptors. Being located perisomatically and at the axon initial segment, a drug-induced enhancement of α_2 GABA$_A$ receptors would permit an attenuation of the overactivity of the pyramidal cells without causing sedation via α_1 receptors.

NOVEL DRUGS ACTING ON GABA$_A$ RECEPTOR SUBTYPES

NOVEL ANXIOLYTICS ACTING ON $\alpha_{2,3}$ GABA$_A$ RECEPTOR SUBTYPES

Based on the functional differentiation of GABA$_A$ receptor subtypes *in vivo* by genetic means, the anxiolytic activity of benzodiazepines was attributed to circuits expressing α_2 and α_3 receptors, while sedation was attributed to circuits expressing α_1 receptors (see previous section). These findings gave rise to a new pharmacology based on ligands targeted to the benzodiazepine site of the respective GABA$_A$ receptor subtype. A striking confirmation of the hypothesis that sedation was mediated via α_1 receptors was provided by the sedative hypnotic drugs Zolpidem, Zaleplone, or Zopiclone (Z hypnotics). They invariably show a preferential affinity for α_1 GABA$_A$ receptors (Table 42.2).

Ligands acting at α_2 and/or α_3 GABA$_A$ receptors, sparing α_1 receptors, were expected to act as anxiolytics without inducing sedation. The search for novel nonsedative anxiolytics of this type is ongoing with major challenges for medicinal chemistry. So far, a differentiation of the respective receptor subtypes by affinity (i.e., high affinity for α_2 and/or α_3 receptors versus α_1 receptors) has not yet been achieved. Nevertheless, new ligands have been developed that differentiate between α_1 and α_2 and/or α_3 GABA$_A$ receptors by efficacy although not by ligand affinity (for review, see Möhler, 2011, 2012; Table 42.2). For instance TP003, which displays selective efficacy at α_3 receptors, showed anxiolytic activity, albeit only at high receptor occupancy (Table 42.2) (Dias et al., 2005; see previous section). Major attention was, rather, focused on compounds that act as partial agonists at α_2 and α_3 receptors, sparing α_1 receptors such as L-838417, TPA023, and NS11394. Their anxiolytic activity is mediated primarily via α_2 receptors with α_3 receptors as backup at higher receptor occupancy (see previous section). The best characterized compound is TPA023, for which anxiolytic activity without sedation was firmly demonstrated in a multitude of rodent and monkey models (Atack et al., 2006b; Atack, 2009; Table 42.2). In addition, this compound showed little or no dependence liability, largely by failing to enhance α_1 receptors and possibly also by its partial efficacy (Ator, 2005; Ator et al., 2010; Licata and Rowlett, 2008; see previous section).

Clinical proof of concept

Among the compounds mentioned, TPA023 (MK 0777) reached the stage of clinical development as an anxiolytic drug. In volunteers, TPA023 (0.5 and 1.5 mg) did not affect alertness, postural stability, and memory in contrast to lorazepam (2 mg), which is in line with the absence of overt sedation for TPA023. In patients with generalized anxiety disorder, the anxiolytic activity of TPA023 was validated in proof-of-concept studies (Atack, 2009). TPA023, given over four weeks, was effective with a significantly superior HAM-A scale reduction compared with placebo. TPA023 had a time of onset within the first week of treatment. Unfortunately, due to the formation of cataracts in rodents following long-term treatment, the clinical development of TPA023 was discontinued. Nevertheless, the clinical proof of concept, established for TPA023, is expected to encourage further efforts in developing α_2/α_3 GABA$_A$ receptor modulators as anxiolytic drugs. They are expected to be largely devoid of the side effects of classical benzodiazepines such as sedation and dependence liability.

ANXIOLYTIC ACTION VIA NEUROSTEROIDS

Neuroactive endogenous steroids (neurosteroids) such as the progesterone metabolite allopregnanolone or the corticosterone metabolite $3\alpha,5\alpha$-THDOC, synthesized in both glia and neurons, are able to directly enhance GABA$_A$ receptor function through a neurosteroid binding site present on practically all GABA$_A$ receptors. Neurosteroids, consequently, have anxiolytic, sedative-hypnotic and anticonvulsant properties (Belelli and Lambert, 2005). In patients with panic disorder, neurosteroids were decreased in blood plasma. Stimulating the neurosteroid synthesis was therefore expected to be a novel anti-anxiety treatment strategy. The rate limiting step of neurosteroid synthesis is the transport of cholesterol through the outer mitochondrial membrane, mediated by the translocator protein (18 kD) (TSPO, formerly termed peripheral or mitochondrial benzodiazepine receptor). When a TSPO agonist (XBD173) was administered to human volunteers undergoing an anxiety challenge (cholecystokinin-tetrapeptide i.v.), panic anxiety behavior was suppressed. The anxiolytic effect was indeed mediated by the induction of neurosteroidogenesis since, in rodents, the anxiolytic effect of XBD173 was blocked by finasteride, a 5α-reductase inhibitor of neurosteroid synthesis (Rupprecht et al., 2009). Thus, TSPO as well as the neurosteroid site of GABA$_A$ receptors directly are potential targets for novel types of anxiolytics.

DRUGS ENHANCING MEMORY BY REDUCING $\alpha 5$ GABA$_A$ RECEPTOR FUNCTION

The ability to learn and remember is thought to be encoded at the synaptic level and involves the ability of synapses to undergo long-term changes in synaptic strength. Tonic GABAergic inhibition appears to contribute to this process. Hippocampus-dependent learning and memory was improved when tonic inhibition was reduced based on a partial or full deficit of α_5 GABA$_A$ receptors in transgenic mice (see previous section). This finding pointed to α_5 GABA$_A$ receptors as a potential pharmacological target for the enhancement of cognitive performance (Fig. 42.4). Ligands with only partial efficacy (partial inverse agonists) were considered to be devoid of potential side effects such as proconvulsant activity.

One of the first drugs to be developed was L-655708, a partial inverse agonist with preferential affinity for α_5 GABA$_A$ receptors (Table 42.2). It reduced tonic inhibition, facilitated LTP, induced γ-oscillations in hippocampal CA3, and enhanced performance in the Morris maze without being proconvulsant (Table 42.2). However, its anxiogenic activity, presumably due to its inverse agonistic activity at GABA$_A$ receptors other than α_5 receptors, prevented its use in humans.

Another partial inverse agonist, α_5IA, displayed preferential efficacy (but not affinity) for α_5 GABA$_A$ receptors. It lacked anxiogenic activity and enhanced spatial memory (encoding and recall) in the Morris water maze (Table 42.2) (Atack, 2010). Preclinical renal toxicity prevented further development of this compound.

RO4938581 was the first partial inverse agonist with high selectivity in both affinity and efficacy for α_5GABA$_A$ receptors (Table 42.2) (Ballard et al., 2009). Behaviorally, RO4938581 fully rescued a scopolamine- or diazepam-induced spatial working memory deficit (delayed match to position task or Morris water maze paradigm) in rodents. Furthermore, in monkeys, the performance in an object retrieval task, which is thought to require executive functions, was enhanced by the drug even beyond the physiological level of responding. Thus, such agents hold the promise of novel treatments for various disorders afflicted with learning and memory deficits. They include Down syndrome, Alzheimer's disease, and other neurological and psychiatric disorders.

Indeed, in Ts65Dn mice, a well-characterized murine Down syndrome model, α_5IA improved cognitive performance to the level of euploid controls, as demonstrated in associative and declarative memory tasks. The deficit in spatial learning (Morris water maze) in the Ts65Dn mice was likewise normalized by α_5IA as was the deficit in object recognition (Braudeau et al., 2011). Based on such results, an analogue of RO4938581 was entered into clinical trials with the aim of counteracting the cognitive disabilities of subjects with Down syndrome (http://www.clinicaltrials.gov; drug RG1662; last searched April 7, 2012). Since cognitive deficits are apparent across several disease categories, this type of drug may possibly find multiple indications in psychiatric disorders (Möhler, 2012a).

GABA$_A$ RECEPTOR DRUGS FOR DEPRESSION?

In line with the comorbidity of anxiety disorders and depression, a marked deficit in GABA transmission was not only found in anxiety disorders but also in patients with major depression. It includes a deficit of GABA$_A$ receptors in parahippocampal and in temporal cortex areas, a reduction of GABA neurons in the orbitofrontal cortex, and a reduced level of GABA in occipital brain and cerebrospinal fluid (for review, see Möhler, 2011). In transgenic mice, a partial deficit of GABA$_A$ receptors, which was manifest mainly in hippocampus and cerebral cortex, showed enhanced behavioral inhibitory depression-like responses in tests sensitive to antidepressant drug treatment (novelty-suppressed feeding, forced swim test, tail suppression, sucrose consumption test) concomitant with a deficit in adult hippocampal neurogenesis and a hyperactivity of the HPA (hypothalamic-pituitary-adrenal) axis (Lüscher et al., 2011; Shen at al., 2010). Importantly, the behavioral alterations induced by the partial deficit of GABA$_A$ receptors were reversed by treatment with the antidepressant imipramine, pointing to a close functional link between the GABA- and the monoaminergic system (Lüscher et al., 2011). A partial α_2 GABA$_A$ receptor deficit was recently proposed to contribute to a depression-like phenotype (Vollenweider et al., 2011). Thus, a deficit in the GABA system seems to be a common denominator of both anxiety disorders and depression-like behavior, and the GABA system may therefore offer new therapeutic opportunities for depression. Classical benzodiazepines fail in this respect due to sedation and abuse liability. However, largely lacking these side effects, modulators of α_2, α_3 GABA$_A$ receptors such as TPA023 offer new opportunities to achieve clinically relevant antidepressant activity with the expectation of a rapid onset of action based on alleviating the GABAergic deficits. A major impetus comes from the ability of GABAergic drugs to reverse negative motivation and pessimistic biases by influencing the cost–benefit arbitration in pACC (Amemori and Graybiel, 2012; see previous section), a brain area that is strongly implicated in anxiety disorders and major depression (Ressler and Mayberg, 2007) (for review, see Lüscher et al., 2010, Möhler, 2012b).

DISCLOSURES

Dr. Möhler has no conflicts of interest to disclose.

REFERENCES

Amemori, K.-I., and Graybiel, A.M. (2012). Localized microstimulation of primate pregenual cingulate cortex induces negative decision making. *Nat. Neurosci.* 15:776–784.

Amorapanth, P., LeDoux, J.E., et al. (2000). Different lateral amygdala outputs mediate reactions and actions elicited by a fear-arousing stimulus. *Nat. Neurosci.* 3:74–79.

Atack, J.R. (2009). Subtype-selective GABA$_A$ receptor modulation yields a novel pharmacological profile: the design and development of TPA 023. *Adv. Pharmacol.* 57:137–185.

Atack, J.R. (2010). Preclinical and clinical pharmacology of the GABA$_A$ receptor α5 subtype-selective inverse agonist α5IA. *Pharmacol. Ther.* 125:11–26.

Atack, J.R., Bayley, P.J., et al. (2006a). L-655,708 enhances cognition in rats but is not proconvulsant at a dose selective for alpha5-containing GABA$_A$ receptors. *Neuropharmacol.* 51:1023–1029.

Atack, J.R., Wafford, K., et al. (2006b). TPA023, an agonist selective for α_2- and α_3-containing GABA$_A$ receptors, is a non-sedating anxiolytic in rodents and primates. *J. Pharm. Exp. Ther.* 316:410–422.

Ator, N.A. (2005). Contribution of GABA$_A$ receptor subtype selectivity to abuse liability and dependence potential of pharmacological treatments for anxiety and sleep disorders. *CNS Spectr.* 1:31–39.

Ator, N.A., Atack, J.R., et al. (2010). Reducing abuse liability of GABA$_A$/benzodiazepine ligands via selective partial agonist efficacy at alpha1 and alpha2/3 subtypes. *J. Pharm. Exp. Ther.* 332:4–16.

Ballard, T.M., Knoflach, F., et al. (2009). RO4938581, a novel cognitive enhancer acting at GABA$_A$ alpha5 subunit-containing receptors. *Psychopharmacol. (Berl.)* 202:207–223.

Belelli, D., and Lambert, J. (2005) Neurosteroids: endogenous regulators of the GABA$_A$ receptor. *Nat. Rev. Neurosci.* 6:565–575.

Braudeau, J., Delatour, B., et al. (2011). Specific targeting of the GABA$_A$ receptor α_5 subtype by a selective inverse agonist restores cognitive deficits in Down syndrome mice. *J. Psychopharmacol.* 25:1030–1041.

Brickley, S.G., and Mody, I. (2012). Extrasynaptic GABA$_A$ receptors: their function in the CNS and implications for disease. *Neuron* 73:23–34.

Collinson, N., Kuenzi, F.M., et al. (2002). Enhanced learning and memory and altered GABAergic synaptic transmission in mice lacking the α_5 subunit of the GABA$_A$ receptor. *J. Neurosci.* 22:5572–5580.

Crestani, F., Keist, R., et al. (2002). Trace fear conditioning involves alpha5 GABA-A receptors. *PNAS* 99:8980–8985.

Crestani, F., Lorez, M., et al. (1999). Decreased GABA-A receptor clustering results in enhanced anxiety and a bias for threat cues. *Nat. Neurosci.* 2:823–839.

Crestani, F., Martin, J.R., et al. (2000). Resolving differences in GABA$_A$ receptor mutant mouse studies. *Nat. Neurosci.* 11:1059.

Dämgen, K., and Lüddens, H. (1999). Zaleplon displays a selectivity to recombinant GABA$_A$ receptors different from zolpidem, zopiclone and benzodiazepines. *Neurosci. Res. Commun.* 25:139–148.

Dias, R., Sheppard, W.F., et al. (2005). Evidence for a significant role of alpha3-containing GABA$_A$ receptor in mediating the anxiolytics effects of benzodiazepines. *J. Neurosci.* 25:10682–10688.

Earnheart JC, Schweizer C, et al., (2007) GABAergic control of adult hippocampal neurogenesis in relation to behavior indicative of trait anxiety and depression states. *J. Neurosci.* 27(14):3845–3854.

Eccles, J.C. (1977). The Understanding of the Brain, 2nd Edition. New York: McGraw-Hill.

Ehrlich, I., Humeau, Y., et al. (2009). Amygdala inhibitory circuits and the control of fear memory. *Neuron* 62:757–771.

Facklam, M., Schoch, P., et al. (1992). Relationship between benzodiazepine receptor occupancy and functional effects *in vivo* of four ligands of different intrinsic efficacies. *J. Pharm. Exp. Ther.* 261:1113–1121.

Fritschy, J.M., and Brünig, I. (2003). Formation and plasticity of GABAergic synapses: physiological mechanisms and pathophysiological implications. *Pharmacol.* 98:299–323.

Glykys, J., and Mody, I. (2007). Activation of GABA$_A$ receptors: views from outside the synaptic cleft. *Neuron* 56:763–770.

Gozzi, A., Jain, A., et al. (2010). A neural switch for active and passive fear. *Neuron* 67:656–666.

Hajos, N., Nusser, Z., et al. (2000). Cell type and synapse-specific variability in synaptic GABA$_A$ receptor occupancy. *Eur. J. Neurosci.* 12:810–818.

Hasler, G., Nugent, A.C., et al. (2008). Altered cerebral gamma-aminobutyric acid type A-benzodiazepine receptor binding in panic disorder determined by [11C] flumazenil positron emission. *Arch. Gen. Psychiatry* 65:1166–1175.

Haubensak, W., Kunwar, P.S., et al. (2010). Genetic dissection of an amygdala microcircuit that gates conditioned fear. *Nature* 468:270–276.

Heldt, S.A., and Ressler, K.J. (2007). Training-induced changes in the expression of GABA$_A$-associated genes in the amygdala after the acquisition and extinction of Pavlovian fear. *Eur. J. Neurosci.* 26:3631–3644.

Herry, C., Ciocheci, S., et al. (2008). Switching on and off fear by distinct neuronal circuits. *Nature* 454:600–606.

Herry, C., Ferraguti, F., et al. (2010). Neuronal circuits of fear extinction. *Eur. J. Neurosci.* 31:599–612.

Horowski, R., and Dorow, R. (2002). Anxiogenic, not psychotogenic, properties of the partial inverse benzodiazepine receptor agonist FG 7142 in man. *Psychopharmacology* 162:223–224.

Huber, D., Veinante, P., et al. (2005). Vasopressin and oxytocin excite distinct neuronal populations in the central amygdala. *Science* 308:245–248.

Klausberger, T., and Somogyi, P. (2008). Neuronal diversity and temporal dynamics: the unity of hippocampal circuit operations. *Science* 321:53–57.

Knabl, J., Witschi, R., et al. (2008). Reversal of pathological pain though specific spinal GABA_A receptor subtypes. *Nature* 451:330–334.

LeDoux, J.E. (2000). Emotion circuits in the brain. *Ann. Rev. Neurosci.* 23:155–184.

LeDoux, J.E., and Gorman, J.M. (2001). A call to action: overcoming anxiety through active coping. *Am. J. Psychiatry* 158:1953–1955.

Leicht, G., Mulert, C., et al. (2013). Benzodiazepines counteract rostral anterior cingulated cortex activation induced by cholecystokinin-terapeptide in humans. *Biol. Psychiatry* 73(4):337–344.

Letzkus, J.J., Wolff, S.B.E., et al. (2011). A disinhibitory microcircuit for associative fear learning in auditory cortex. *Nature* 480:331–335.

Licata, S.C., and Rowlett, J.K. (2008). Abuse and dependence liability of benzodiazepine-type drugs: GABA-A receptor modulation and beyond. *Psychopharmacology* 203:539–546.

Löw, K., Crestani, F., et al. (2000). Molecular and neuronal substrate for the selective attenuation of anxiety. *Science* 290:131–134.

Lüscher, B., Fuchs, T., et al. (2011a). GABA_A receptor trafficking-mediated plasticity of inhibitory synapses. *Neuron* 70:385–409.

Lüscher, B., Shen, Q., et al. (2011b). The GABAergic deficit hypothesis of major depressive disorder. *Mol. Psychiatry* 16:383–406.

Mann, E.O., and Mody, I. (2010) Control of hippocampal gamma oscillation frequency by tonic inhibition and excitation of interneurons. *Nat. Neurosci.* 13:205–212.

Marowsky, A., Fritschy, J.M., et al. (2004). Functional mapping of GABA_A receptor subtypes in the amygdala. *Eur. J. Neurosci.* 20:1281–1289.

Marowsky, A., Rudolph, U., et al. (2012). Tonic inhibition in principal cells of the amygdala: a central role for alpha3 subunit-containing GABA_A receptors. *J. Neurosci.* 32:8611–8619.

Marowsky, A., Yomagawa, Y., et al. (2005). A specialized subclass of interneurons mediates dopaminergic facilitation of amygdala function. *Neuron* 48:1025–1037.

McKernan, R.M., Rosahl, T.W., et al. (2000). Sedative but not anxiolytic properties of benzodiazepines are mediated by the GABA_A receptor α1 subtype. *Nat. Neurosci.* 3:587–592.

Mirza, N.R., Larsen, J.S., et al. (2008). NS11394, a unique subtype-selective GABA_A receptor positive allosteric modulator: *in vitro* actions, pharmacokinetic properties and *in vivo* anxiolytics efficacy. *J. Pharmacol. Exp. Ther.* 327:954–968.

Möhler, H. (2007). Molecular regulation of cognitive functions and developmental plasticity: impact of GABA_A receptors. *J. Neurochem.* 102:1–12.

Möhler, H. (2011). The rise of a new GABA pharmacology. *Neuropharmacology.* 60:1042–1049.

Möhler, H. (2012a). Cognitive enhancement by pharmacological and behavioral interventions: the murine Down syndrome model. *Biochem. Pharmacol.* 84:994–999.

Möhler, H. (2012b). The GABA system in anxiety and depression and its therapeutic potential. *Neuropharmacology* 62:42–53.

Möhler, H., Fritschy, J.M., et al. (2002). A new benzodiazepine pharmacology. *JPET* 300:2–8.

Möhler, H., and Okada, T. (1977). Demonstration of benzodiazepine receptors in the central nervous system. *Science* 198:849–851.

Morris, H.V., Dawson, G.R., et al. (2006). Both alpha2 and alpha3 GABA_A receptor subtypes mediate the anxiolytics properties of benzodiazepine-site ligands in the conditioned emotional response paradigm. *Eur. J. Neurosci.* 23:2495–2504.

Olsen, R.W., and Sieghart, W. (2009). GABA_A receptors: subtypes provide diversity of function and pharmacology. *Neuropharmacology* 56:141–148.

Ressler, K.J., and Mayberg, H.S. (2007). Targeting abnormal neural circuits in mood and anxiety disorders: from the laboratory to the clinic. *Nat. Neurosci.* 10:1116–1121

Rudolph, U., Crestani, F., et al. (1999). Benzodiazepine actions mediated by specific γ-aminobutyric acidA receptor subtypes. *Nature* 401:796–800.

Rudolph, U., and Knoflach, F. (2011). Beyond classical benzodiazepines: novel therapeutic potential of GABA_A receptor subtypes. *Nature Rev. Drug Discov.* 10:685–697.

Rupprecht, R., Rammes, G., et al. (2009). Translocator protein (18 kD) as target for anxiolytics without benzodiazepine-like side effects. *Science* 24:490–493.

Shen, Q., Lal, R., et al. (2010). γ-Aminobutyric acid-type A receptor deficits cause hypothalamic-pituitary-adrenal axis hyperactivity and antidepressant drug sensitivity reminiscent of melancholic forms of depression. *Biol. Psychiatry* 68:512–520.

Tan, K.R., Brown, M., et al. (2010). Neural bases for addictive properties of benzodiazepines. *Nature* 463:769–774.

Tovote, P., and Lüthi, A. (2012). Curbing fear by axonal oxytocin release in the amygdala. *Neuron* 73:407–410.

Tully, K., Li, Y., et al. (2007). Norepinephrine enables the induction of associative long-term potentiation at thalamo-amygdala synapses. *Proc. Natl. Acad. Sci. USA* 104:14146–14150.

Vollenweider, I., Smith, K.S., et al. (2011). Antidepressant-like properties of α_2-containing GABA_A receptor. *Behav. Brain Res.* 217:77–80.

Yee, B.K., Hauser, J., et al. (2004). GABA receptors containing the alpha5 subunit mediate the trace effect in aversive and appetitive conditioning and extinction of fear. *Eur. J. Neurosci.* 20:1928–1936.

Zeilhofer, H.U., Möhler, H., et al. (2009). GABAergic analgesia: new insights from mutant mice and subtype-selective agonists. *Trends Pharmacol. Sci.* 30:397–402.

43 | PREFRONTAL CORTEX REGULATION OF EMOTION AND ANXIETY

BRONWYN M. GRAHAM AND MOHAMMED R. MILAD

Emotion regulation encompasses the ability to initiate fight/flight responses to actual threat in the environment. It also encompasses the ability to appropriately inhibit defensive responses when no longer faced with potentially threatening stimuli in order to successfully adapt to and thrive in one's environment—to forage, to seek a mate, and so forth. The adaptive significance of emotion regulation is highlighted by the consequences of instances in which such ability fails. A prime example is anxiety disorders, which affect roughly 30% of the population. People with anxiety disorders exhibit pathological avoidance of perceived threatening situations and cues due to unrealistic beliefs about the probability and cost of negative outcomes associated with such stimuli. Alternatively, they may endure situations with significant distress and typically with the aid of safety behaviors, which serve to maintain irrational beliefs and diminish the person's sense of self-efficacy. At the opposite end of the scale, failures in emotion regulation can also lead to impulsiveness and risky decision making, as is often the case in childhood and adolescent behavioral disorders. Rather than experience too much fear, as observed in anxiety disorders, children with various behavioral disorders exhibit a deficient sense of threat or danger. Despite their differing behavioral profiles, the long-term consequence of both examples of failed emotion regulation is the failure to thrive in one's environment (Fig. 43.1). The normalization of these two extremes of emotion deregulation requires that we first understand how fearful emotions are processed and regulated at a neural level. Once accomplished, advancements can be made toward improving current treatment approaches, as well as developing novel approaches.

The experience and processing of emotion, and its underlying neurobiological substrates, has been a focus of many decades of psychological research. We now have a much more advanced understanding of the mechanisms underlying the perception of fear-relevant stimuli, as well as the induction of species-specific defensive responses in turn. The amygdala is a critical limbic structure underlying these processes in mammals, and several downstream structures have been identified to mediate specific defensive responses (Orsini and Maren, 2012). However, emotion regulation goes beyond mere stimulus–response relationships. Rather than select the best response on the basis of presently available information, emotion regulation (at least in the context of fear and anxiety) involves gauging the extent of potential threat on the basis of present and past experience/knowledge, and integrating such information with short- and long-term motivational goals to decide the most appropriate response. Thus, successful emotion regulation involves the constant updating of threat "schemas" on the basis of learning episodes across time. What are the neurocognitive underpinnings of this ability? Answering this question is not only theoretically important from an evolutionary perspective, but it is also clinically important. If we understand the processes underlying normal/successful emotion regulation, then we can investigate ways to rectify these processes when regulation fails, as described in the previous examples.

As emotion regulation is often considered a "top-down" process involving conscious inhibition over more automatic threat responses, cortical areas like the prefrontal cortex (PFC) have long been suspected to play a crucial role in this ability. With the introduction of neuroimaging to psychiatry research, later reports of deficient PFC activations during presentations of emotional stimuli in various anxiety-disordered cohorts led to hypotheses that the exaggerated fear responses observed in anxiety may be due to failures in PFC inhibition over emotional responses (Etkin and Wager, 2007). However, direct evidence that the PFC was specifically involved in the regulation (not just the processing) of emotions was lacking. More recently, researchers have developed emotional tasks that measure specific aspects of emotion regulation. These tasks have been combined with brain imaging methods in humans, along with lesion, stimulation, and pharmacological manipulations in nonhuman animals, to greater elucidate the contribution of the PFC to emotion regulation. In this chapter we review research on these tasks that explicitly assess the ability to change one's emotional state, either behaviorally through alteration of environmental contingencies, or through cognitive exertion. We discuss how these studies have provided evidence that the PFC plays a regulatory role in the emotions of fear and anxiety, and also how these studies have begun to delineate the exact nature of this role. It is acknowledged that emotion regulation may implicitly occur in many other tasks that simply expose subjects to emotion-eliciting stimuli, and that this research contributed to the push to study PFC contributions to emotion regulation, as noted previously. However, due to the difficulty in interpreting the exact contribution of regulation strategies to the neural activations associated with such tasks, we have largely restricted our discussion to the former tasks. In addition, it is noted that structures other than the PFC have also been implicated in emotion regulation; however, this chapter will focus on the role of the PFC and its interactions with other cortical and subcortical structures involved in emotion processing.

PREFRONTAL CORTEX AND FEAR EXTINCTION

One commonly used method of examining fear and inhibition of fear in the laboratory is Pavlovian conditioning and extinction. In such procedures fear is acquired to an initially neutral conditioned stimulus (CS; e.g., tone or light) through repeated pairings with an aversive unconditioned stimulus (US, e.g., mild electrical shock), until the CS comes to elicit species-specific conditioned fear responses (CRs) on its own. Fear can then be inhibited via extinction training, which involves repeated presentations of the CS without any reinforcement. Subjects typically exhibit long-term retention of extinction memories when again presented the CS at a later

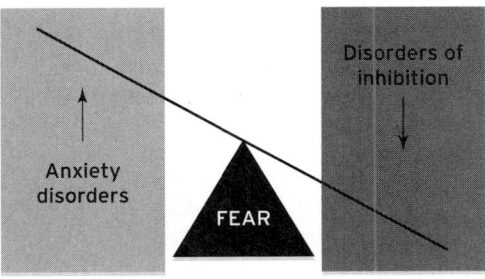

Figure 43.1 *Emotion deregulation can result in too much fear, as is the case in anxiety disorders, or it can result in too little fear, as is the case in disorders of inhibition.*

time (i.e., they exhibit low levels of CRs), although certain manipulations (e.g., change of testing context, exposure to mild stressor, or the mere passage of time) can elicit recovery of fear. Extinction is likely to result from a combination of processes; however, it is widely accepted that extinction largely involves the formation of a new context-dependent memory that coexists and competes with the original fear-conditioning memory (Orsini and Maren, 2012). Thus, when the subject is presented with the (now ambiguous) CS, it must decide the most appropriate course of action on the basis of conflicting past learning episodes (Fig. 43.2). Hence, extinction provides a useful model of emotion regulation, the underlying mechanisms of which can easily be explored across species.

For the past two decades, extinction research has largely centered on the following questions: When the subject is presented with the extinguished CS, what regulates which memory is recalled? How is it determined which response (to fear or not to fear) is elicited (Fig. 43.3)? There are several lines of evidence that support the notion that the ventromedial PFC (vmPFC) is critical to this regulation process, and furthermore, that distinct regions of the vmPFC exert opposing influences on fear expression. Specifically, the prelimbic (PL) division of the vmPFC appears to be necessary for the expression of learned fear. PL inactivation reduces fear responses to conditioned cues and contexts, whereas microstimulation increases conditioned freezing and impairs extinction, and PL neurons exhibit potentiated responses to conditioned cues, the persistence of which is associated with extinction failure (see Milad and Quirk,

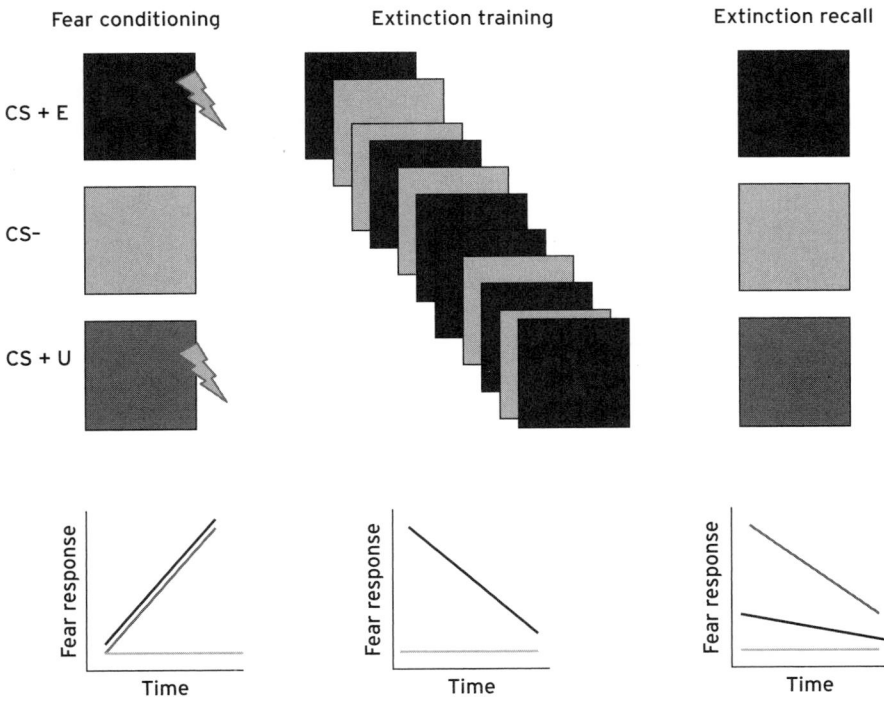

Figure 43.2 *Fear conditioning and extinction protocol. During fear conditioning two stimuli are paired with an aversive outcome (CS+'s), and the third stimuli is unreinforced (CS–). Fear responses generally increase to the CS+'s and remain low to the CS–. During extinction training, one of the CS+'s is extinguished (CS+E) by being repeatedly presented in the absence of the aversive outcome. The other CS+ remains unextinguished (CS+U). Fear responses to the CS+E decrease across training and eventually are comparable to those expressed in the presence of the CS–. During extinction recall, all three CSs are presented. In healthy populations, fear responses are low to the CS+E and the CS–, whereas they are high to the CS+U.*

Rodent

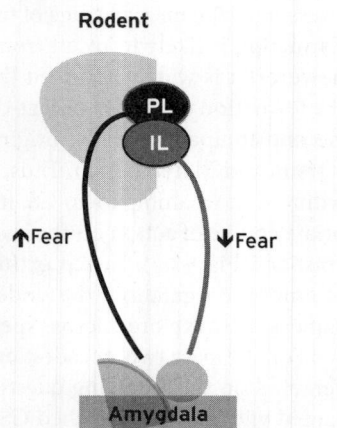

Human

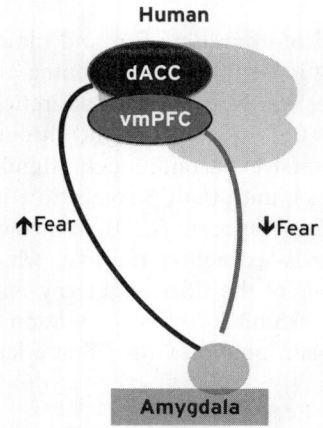

Figure 43.3 Distinct regions of the rodent (prelimbic and infralimbic) and human (ventromedial and dorsal anterior cingulate cortex) PFC increase and decrease expression of conditioned fear, respectively, via interactions with the amygdala.

2012, for review). In contrast, the infralimbic (IL) division of the vmPFC appears to be involved in extinction and/or the expression of extinction memories. Morgan et al. (1993) initially examined the effect of vmPFC lesions (encompassing IL, PL, and some orbital cortices) on acquisition and extinction of conditioned fear. They reported that while vmPFC-lesioned rats exhibited no differences in the acquisition or retention of conditioning, they took a significantly greater number of days to reach the extinction criterion (5 s or less time spent freezing in the presence of the CS). Subsequent studies that have more closely examined the within-session acquisition of extinction reported that vmPFC lesions do not affect the ability to reduce fear within a session but impair the retention of such inhibition the following day (e.g., Lebron et al., 2004; Quirk et al., 2000). Additionally, Quirk et al. (2000) reported that lesions that did not encompass the IL region spared extinction retention, suggesting that the IL region might be necessary to extinction recall. Some studies, however, have reported no effect of vmPFC lesions on fear extinction (e.g., Gewirtz et al., 1997).

The disadvantages of examining the contribution of various structures to a task using lesions are that (a) the role of the structure in the discrete phases of the task is difficult to isolate and (b) there may be some recovery of function or compensation that changes the circuitry involved in the task. To overcome these disadvantages, a second line of studies has used temporary inactivation or inhibition of protein synthesis in the vmPFC at specific points before or after fear extinction. These studies have, by and large, consistently reported impairments in retrieval of extinction memories and, again, have suggested a specific role for the IL in this regard (Orsini and Maren, 2012). While initial studies suggested no effects of vmPFC lesions on the acquisition of extinction learning, a recent study reported that when the IL (but not PL) region of the vmPFC was temporarily inactivated prior to extinction training, rats exhibited a significantly slowed rate of extinction, along with impairments in recall the following day (Sierra-Mercado et al., 2011).

A third line of evidence from rodents has used electrophysiology to measure neural responses to conditioned cues during extinction training and its recall. Milad and Quirk (2002) demonstrated that neural responses to a tone CS increased in the IL region only during the extinction recall, and not the extinction training, phase. Moreover, freezing responses during extinction recall were inversely correlated with IL CS responses, whereas no relation was found for PL CS responses, suggesting a specific role for IL activation in dictating the strength of extinction recall. To provide more direct evidence for this hypothesis, a fourth line of evidence has examined the effects of vmPFC stimulation on extinction. Milad and Quirk (2002) reported that combining CS presentations with IL stimulation reduced freezing during extinction training, and the reduced freezing persisted during extinction recall the following day in the absence of any stimulation, suggesting that IL stimulation enhanced extinction learning or consolidation. Similar results have also been reported in studies that have stimulated thalamic (Herry and Garcia, 2002) or hippocampal (Farinelli et al., 2006) inputs to the vmPFC. In addition, Thompson et al. (2010) demonstrated that IL activation, combined with short exposure to a conditioned context, enhanced the rate of extinction to that context over subsequent days, without inducing extinction in and of itself (i.e., when tested in the context the day after IL activation, all groups exhibited comparable initial levels of freezing). Moreover, the enhanced rate of extinction was also observed when IL activation was combined with exposure to a different aversive context, but not a neutral context. Thompson et al. (2010) suggested that IL activation in the presence of a conditioned context nonspecifically "primes" the extinction circuitry in a way that allows extinction to be acquired more rapidly. In line with this suggestion, Rodriguez-Romaguera et al. (2012) recently demonstrated that deep brain stimulation (DBS) of the ventral striatum in combination with extinction training enhances extinction recall. Interestingly, although DBS without extinction training was ineffective in reducing fear, DBS alone induced plasticity within the IL and PL regions of the vmPFC, as well as regions of the amygdala, leading the authors to suggest that DBS may prime the development of plasticity within the extinction circuitry. It is yet to be determined whether the development of such plasticity within the vmPFC is necessary for the enhancing effects of DBS on extinction.

With the advent of functional magnetic resonance imaging (fMRI) techniques, and spurred on by knowledge advancements from rodent research, the neurocircuitry underlying fear extinction has become a popular target of investigation in humans. Striking cross-species similarity in the networks mediating fear extinction in rodents and humans has been revealed. Humans exhibit increased amygdala and dorsal anterior cingulate (dACC, which appears to be functionally analogous to the PL) activations during fear acquisition and recall (Knight et al., 2004; Phelps et al., 2004), and cortical thickness of the dACC is positively correlated with fear responses during fear conditioning (see Milad and Quirk, 2012, for review). Earlier fMRI studies examining extinction of conditioned fear reported increased orbitofrontal cortex (OFC) activation during extinction training for an aversively conditioned olfactory cue (Gottfried and Dolan, 2004), as well as increased vmPFC activation during recall of an extinguished visual cue (Phelps et al., 2004). Later studies have consistently demonstrated that extinction recall is associated with increased activity in the vmPFC (Milad et al., 2007), and one study reported increased vmPFC activation to an extinguished cue only when it was presented in the extinction context, but not when presented in the original conditioning context (Kalisch et al., 2006). Furthermore, several structural MRI studies have reported a positive correlation between extinction recall and vmPFC thickness (Milad and Quirk, 2012).

Assuming a role for the vmPFC in expression of learned fear and extinction, how exactly does it up- and downregulate fear responses? Anatomically, the vmPFC is well positioned to regulate the activation of limbic structures that are involved in the expression of defensive responses, with the IL sending glutamatergic projections to the amygdala (Quirk et al., 2003), and dorsal regions of the PFC exhibiting positive connectivity with the amygdala (Etkin et al., 2011). One recent study demonstrated a positive functional connectivity between the dorsomedial (dm) PFC and the amygdala during the processing of emotional faces (Robinson et al., 2012). The dmPFC–amygdala coupling strength increased when participants were exposed to fearful faces and told that they may receive a shock, and there was a positive correlation between coupling strength and reaction times in identifying the emotion of the face. Finally, participants with high trait anxiety exhibited greatest dmPFC–amygdala coupling during processing of fearful faces under threat of shock. This suggests that the dorsal regions of the PFC may activate amygdala regions to enhance defensive responses.

With respect to PFC regulation of fear extinction, rodent studies have proved useful in identifying the specific interactions between vmPFC and specific subnuclei of the amygdala due to the ability to record from, stimulate, or lesion anatomically precise areas. Quirk et al. (2003) were the first to demonstrate that mPFC stimulation (on the border between IL and PL) inhibits central amygdala (CeA) neuronal activity in response to insula or basolateral nucleus of the amygdala (BLA) activation. The mPFC is unlikely to inhibit CeA activity via activating inhibitory BLA interneurons, as was originally thought, given that IL projections onto inhibitory interneurons are sparse. Rather, the mPFC may activate the intercalated cells (ITCs) between the BLA and CeA, which send inhibitory projections to the CeA. Indeed, ITC lesions after extinction prevent extinction recall (Likhtik et al., 2008). As these findings from rodent experiments indicate the existence of contrasting contributions of specific amygdala subnuclei in extinction, future fMRI studies will need to make use of high-resolution imaging techniques that can better identify anatomically precise areas to determine the circuits by which vmPFC regulates fear responses during extinction and its recall in humans.

A different line of research that may help inform as to the role of the PFC in fear extinction (and fear regulation more generally) is that which has examined PFC activations during unexpected omissions of the US following presentations of a previously reinforced CS. We reported that whereas an expected shock that eventuates was associated with a decrease in vmPFC activation, an unexpectedly omitted shock was associated with increased dACC activity (Linnman et al., 2011). Another study demonstrated that an unexpectedly omitted shock was associated with ACC and dorsolateral (dl) PFC activations (Dunsmoor and LaBar, 2012). Together with findings from reversal learning paradigms (see next section), these results suggest that the PFC may provide a neural signal for outcome expectancy or further, error detection and signaling. Interestingly, it has been reported that opioid signaling in the periaqueductal gray, which is purported to regulate error detection necessary to extinction paradigms (McNally et al., 2004), mediates mPFC activation during extinction (Parsons et al., 2010), suggesting that the PFC may recruit such information (or be directly involved in processing it) to determine the most appropriate fear response. Furthermore, this research again demonstrates the opposing roles of dorsal from ventral regions of the PFC in emotion regulation.

PREFRONTAL CORTEX AND REVERSAL LEARNING

In addition to the typical Pavlovian conditioning paradigms, investigators have utilized a different experimental approach to examine emotion regulation, namely, reversal learning. This paradigm is useful because it allows for the assessment of how the subject is able to determine the most appropriate response in an ambiguous situation. Reversal learning has been extensively studied in the context of decision making in instrumental (usually rewarding) tasks, in which two different stimuli and/or responses are associated with reward or punishment, respectively, and then halfway through the task the contingencies switch. More recently a variant of this task using fear conditioning has been employed to further explore the processes underlying fear regulation. A typical fear reversal–learning task involves the presentation of two stimuli, one of which is reinforced (CS+, typically paired with shock), while the other is not (CS−). This is termed the "acquisition phase." Halfway through the paradigm, the reinforcement contingencies switch, such that the old CS+ now becomes the CS− (i.e., it is extinguished), whereas the old CS− now becomes the CS+ (i.e., it is now paired with shock). This is termed the "reversal" phase. Fear reversal provides another approach with which to understand flexibility in emotion regulation, and it also allows the examination of two dissociable processes (i.e., fear acquisition and inhibition) in parallel (Fig. 43.4). Schiller et al. (2008) investigated the neural correlates of fear reversal in healthy humans using faces as CSs, and mild electric shock as the US. They reported that during both the acquisition and reversal phases vmPFC activity was slightly and significantly increased during the CS− relative to the CS+ presentations, regardless of whether the stimuli were "new" or "old" CS−'s. However, the increase in vmPFC activity in response to the CS− was significantly greater during the reversal (i.e., extinction) phase than during the acquisition phase. Schiller et al. (2008) suggested that the vmPFC might provide a selective safety signal to indicate which environmental stimuli are safe to ignore. Interestingly, an earlier study using a very similar model of reversal learning reported the exact opposite results, where vmPFC activity increased during presentations of the CS+ compared with the CS−, during both acquisition and reversal phases (Morris and Dolan, 2004). Distinct regions of the right anterior cingulate exhibited segregated patterns of opposing activity: one region that decreased activation when the CS+ became a CS− (i.e., exhibited reversal) and one region (lateral to the previous region) that continued to exhibit increased activation to the CS+ even when it became a CS− (i.e., exhibited nonreversal, or perseveration). Importantly, both studies implicate the vmPFC in switching responses to signal a change in stimulus contingencies; however, the reason for the discrepancy between the studies in terms of the direction of vmPFC activation is unclear.

BEHAVIORAL VERSUS COGNITIVE EMOTION REGULATION

The chapter thus far has focused on tasks that may be considered "behavioral regulation," which involve forming new, or updating existing, representations of CS–US contingencies on the basis of direct experience of the organism. This type of emotion regulation is sometimes conceptualized as "automatic," seeming to occur without input from a declarative (explicit) memory system (Öhman and Mineka, 2001, but see Lovibond and Shanks, 2002). The advantage of such tasks is that they can be easily modeled in the laboratory in both humans and nonhuman animals, and they also reflect the behavioral components of cognitive behavioral therapy (CBT) used to treat a range of disorders with underlying difficulties with emotion regulation. However, emotion regulation in humans can and often does stem from cognitive resources. In such instances, alterations in emotional output can arise without direct experience, merely from altering one's perceptions through reasoning. The next part of this chapter examines cognitive aspects of emotion regulation.

THE PFC AND REAPPRAISAL

Cognitive reappraisal involves the conscious attempt to alter the meaning of an emotionally significant stimulus/event, typically with the goal of downregulating a negative affective

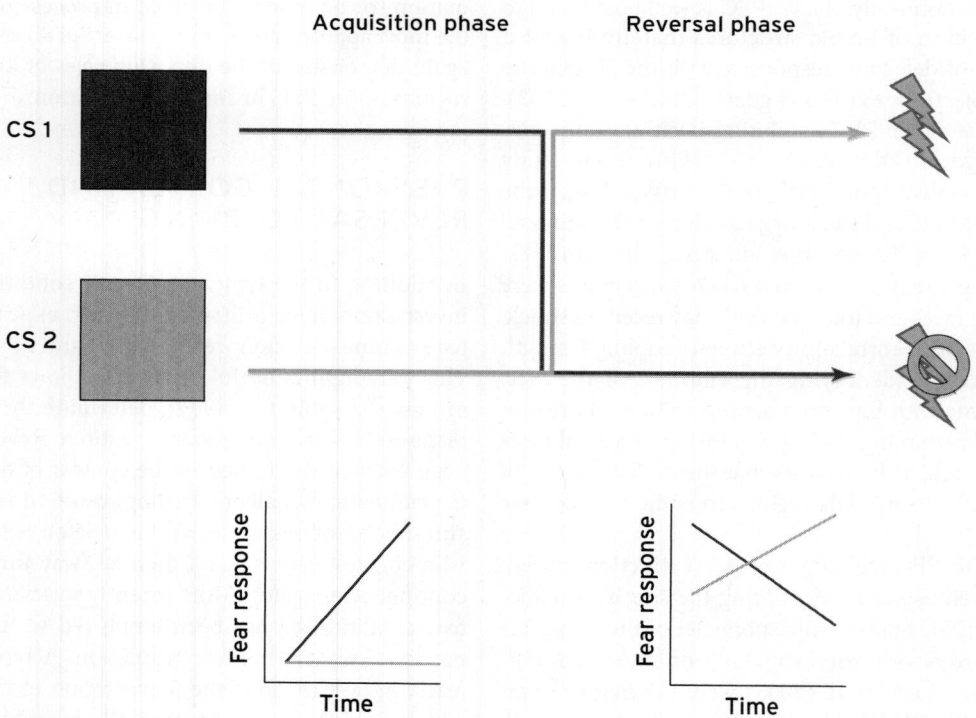

Figure 43.4 Reversal learning protocol. In the acquisition phase, CS1 is paired with an aversive outcome whereas CS2 is unreinforced. Fear responses increase to CS1 and remain low to CS2. In the reversal phase, CS1 is unreinforced (i.e., is extinguished), and CS2 is now paired with an aversive outcome. Fear responses decrease to CS1 and increase to CS2.

response (Gross, 2002). For example, when confronted with an anxiety-provoking stimulus such as a dangerous snake, an individual may attempt to reduce his or her fear by noting that the snake is in an enclosure and therefore very unlikely to escape. Reappraisal is frequently employed in CBT for a range of psychopathologies and often involves the evaluation of all available evidence for one's initial (usually unrealistic) thought, followed by a substitution of the initial thought with one that is more realistic (Smits et al., 2012). Reappraisal capitalizes on humans' unique ability to verbally reason and so is likely to be regulated by higher level cortical structures. It is an indirect means of emotion regulation, in the sense that the emotional response is altered as a consequence of directly modifying attributions of the meaning associated with emotionally relevant stimuli/events. Thus, it fits with the underlying principles of CBT, which holds that emotions are merely reactions to thoughts, by modifying the thought; the emotion is modified in turn.

During the past decade, several studies have started to examine the neurobiological mechanisms underlying cognitive reappraisal. One study examined the use of reappraisal strategies toward classically conditioned cues (images of neutral shapes; Delgado et al., 2008). Following conditioning, participants received nonreinforced presentations of the cues, along with instructions to either attend (pay attention to their natural feelings) or reappraise (imagine something calming in nature, prompted by the color of the cue: e.g., an ocean scene in response to a blue cue). Reappraise trials were associated with reduced skin conductance responses and heightened dlPFC and vmPFC activity relative to attend trials, and a positive correlation was observed between reappraisal success (indexed by reduced skin conductance responses) and dlPFC activation. Interestingly, the vmPFC region activated in this reappraisal task was the same region activated in a previous study that used the same conditioning paradigm but subjected participants to extinction trials rather than reappraisal instructions (Phelps et al., 2004), suggesting the existence of a common neurobiological route for the two different methods of emotion regulation.

Other studies of reappraisal have involved the presentation of innately negative or threatening images with instructions to attend (i.e., pay attention to the image without attempting to control the emotional reaction) or "reappraise"/"decrease" (i.e., think about the image in a more neutral or positive manner). Such studies have revealed that in addition to the vmPFC region that is implicated in fear extinction, reappraisal appears to recruit more lateral regions of the PFC, as also reported by Delgado et al. (2008). For example, a recent meta-analysis concluded that reappraisal use is associated with increased activation of the lateral (including the superior, middle, and inferior frontal gyri, and lateral orbital gyri) and medial (including the superior frontal gyrus and anterior cingulate cortex) prefrontal cortices (Kalisch, 2009; see also Etkin et al., 2011, for review).

Accepting that the PFC is involved in reappraisal, what is the nature of its involvement, and how exactly does it modulate emotional responses? Wager et al. (2008) noted that the PFC may influence emotional responding directly (direct hypothesis), or it may regulate activity of subcortical structures implicated in emotional learning and expression (mediation hypothesis). In support of the mediation hypothesis, several studies have reported that reappraisal success is associated with increased PFC, but decreased amygdala and/or nucleus accumbens, activity (Delgado et al., 2008; Goldin et al., 2008; Phan et al., 2005). Wager et al. (2008) extended these findings in a mediation analysis of the ventrolateral (vl) PFC as a predictor of reappraisal success. They demonstrated that increased amygdala activity was associated with reduced success, whereas increased nucleus accumbens/ventral striatum activity was associated with increased success, and both areas were positively associated with vlPFC activity. Independently, both regions accounted for a part of vlPFC-associated reappraisal success while controlling for the effects attributable to the other. Wager et al.'s (2008) results support the existence of two distinct networks mediated by the vlPFC—one that generates negative affect, and one that downregulates negative affect during reappraisal. The authors therefore concluded that the PFC might be involved in the appraisal process and subsequent recruitment of subcortical regions that up- or downregulate emotional responses, rather than being a constant "dampener" on negative affect as is often assumed.

Other evidence that supports the role of a PFC–amygdala network in reappraisal comes from studies that have exploited individual differences in emotion regulation strategy preference and/or ability. One recent study demonstrated that individuals who were more successful at downregulating emotion exhibited greater inverse functional connectivity between the amygdala and areas of the PFC including the pregenual ACC, OFC, and dm/dlPFC (Lee et al., 2012). Similarly, a different study by Drabant et al. (2009) exposed participants to negative images in the absence of any explicit instructions; thus, participants were free to spontaneously engage in whatever emotion regulation strategy (if any) they chose. The results showed that a greater tendency to use reappraisal in everyday life (as indexed by the Emotion Regulation Questionnaire) was associated with decreased amygdala activation, and increased dl/dmPFC, and lateral OFC activation. These results demonstrate that spontaneous recruitment of reappraisal strategies is associated with similar involvement of neural regions to those involved following instructed recruitment. These results also fit with more recent structural findings demonstrating that high scores on trait measures of cognitive reappraisal positively correlate with dACC, but not ventral ACC, thickness (Giuliani et al., 2011). Emotion regulation is more likely to arise spontaneously rather than in response to explicit cues in everyday life. Thus, these findings provide evidence for the validity of using instructed modes of emotion regulation in the laboratory as a model of such processes as they occur in more natural settings.

From the studies reviewed in this section, it is apparent that while PFC–amygdala (and other subcortical) interactions appear to mediate cognitive reappraisal, lateral and medial, as well as dorsal and ventral, PFC regions have also been implicated in this regard. A focus of more recent research, therefore, has been to disentangle the relative contributions of distinct PFC regions to emotion regulation and their interactions with subcortical structures. It is unlikely that the lateral PFC modulates emotion regulation via direct influence on amygdala activity as robust monosynaptic connections between these two brain regions have not been previously reported (Urry et al., 2006), suggesting an indirect route via additional brain regions. The vmPFC is likely to serve as an intermediate structure given that reciprocal anatomical and functional connections between the lateral PFC and vmPFC have been reported, and the vmPFC has direct anatomical connections with different subnuclei within the amygdala (Kim et al., 2011b; Urry et al., 2006). In view of this, several researchers have suggested that the vmPFC may function as a gateway between phylogenetically newer cortical structures and phylogenetically older subcortical structures to modify emotional responses using higher level cognitive strategies (Delgado et al., 2008). Urry et al. (2006) provided support for this idea by demonstrating that successful reappraisal was associated with greater vmPFC and reduced amygdala activity. Additionally, greater medial frontal gyrus (MFG) activity was associated with greater vmPFC activity when downregulating emotion, and subjects with higher MFG activity showed lower amygdala activity. In a test of mediation, the vmPFC was a significant mediator of the relationship between the MFG and amygdala, whereas the MFG did not mediate the relationship between the vmPFC and amygdala. In other words, the MFG indirectly controlled amygdala activity via the vmPFC, suggestive of the vmPFC's role as a gateway between other cortical areas and the amygdala.

THE PFC AND CONTROLLABILITY

A consistent finding in the clinical anxiety literature is that while many people experience highly traumatic events, only 15–20% of these will ultimately develop an anxiety disorder like PTSD. This highlights the apparent existence of large individual differences with respect to people's response to trauma, or more broadly, people's ability to regulate their emotions following high levels of stress. By examining the differences between people who experience trauma and develop PTSD on the one hand, and people who experience trauma but do not develop any psychopathology on the other, research has identified several factors that may protect against the development of anxiety. Of these, one consistent protective factor relates to perceptions of control. Individuals who hold the belief that they had some amount of control during a traumatic event, or that they have control over their emotional reactions to reminders of the event posttrauma, are far less likely to develop PTSD than are individuals who perceive the traumatic event and/or their reactions to posttrauma reminders to be entirely uncontrollable (Ehlers et al., 2000). In this framework, beliefs of controllability can be viewed as an effective cognitive strategy for emotion regulation.

Although the *perception* of controllability is a cognitive process, much preclinical research has investigated the behavioral and neurophysiological consequences of controllable versus uncontrollable stress in animal models of emotion regulation. In a typical paradigm examining this phenomenon, two groups of subjects are exposed to a series of electrical tail shocks. One group has the ability to terminate the shocks by turning a wheel that is fixed in the chamber. Another group, whose chambers

are yoked to that of the first group, is unable to terminate the shocks, and so receives the same number and duration of shocks as determined by the first group. Despite the fact that both groups receive identical shock experiences and that both procedures induce significant release of stress hormones, the behavioral and neurophysiological characteristics of the two groups differ substantially postshock. Subjects that receive inescapable shock fail to learn how to escape subsequent stressful situations, exhibit potentiated fear during and after fear conditioning, and show large effluxes of serotonin in the dorsal raphe nucleus (DRN; see review by Maier and Watkins, 2010). In contrast, escapable shock does not produce any of these consequences. Moreover, previous experience with escapable shock prevents the behavioral and neurophysiological consequences of later inescapable shock, a phenomenon known as "behavioral immunization" (Maier and Watkins, 2010).

The effects of inescapable shock are dependent on DRN activation, as pharmacological blockade of DRN activity either during inescapable shock or during subsequent behavioral testing prevents escape learning deficits and potentiation of fear conditioning (Maier and Watkins, 2010). Conversely, the effects of escapable shock require the animal to recognize that there is a contingency between its actions and the outcomes, and thus are unlikely to be mediated in the brainstem DRN. Maier and Watkins hypothesized that as the DRN receives almost all its cortical input from the IL and PL, these regions of the vmPFC may regulate the perception of controllable shock. In a series of experiments, they demonstrated that temporary inactivation of the vmPFC during escapable shock increased DRN 5-HT efflux during the procedure, potentiated contextual fear conditioning, and led to deficits in subsequent escape learning (Amat et al., 2005). In other words, inactivation of vmPFC during escapable shock led to all of the consequences of inescapable shock. Importantly, inactivation of the vmPFC did not prevent rats from learning to turn the wheel to terminate the shock. Thus, even though rats did, in fact, learn to escape the shock, they later behaved as if they had received inescapable shock.

In addition to regulating the effects of controllable stress, activation of the vmPFC is also necessary for the immunizing effects of prior experience with control on later consequences of uncontrollability. In a typical behavioral immunization protocol, rats are exposed to escapable shock and then one week later are exposed to inescapable shock, followed by tests for fear conditioning and escape behavior. Amat et al. (2006) demonstrated that inactivation of the vmPFC during escapable shock prevented its immunizing effects on subsequent DRN 5-HT efflux during inescapable shock, potentiated fear conditioning, and escape deficits. In addition, when the vmPFC was inactivated during inescapable shock, this also prevented the immunizing effects of previous exposure to escapable shock.

Perhaps even more convincing, in a later series of experiments, Amat et al. (2008) demonstrated that enhancing vmPFC activity by picrotoxin infusion during inescapable shock prevented the increase in DRN 5-HT efflux, potentiated fear conditioning, and deficits in subsequent escape learning. That is, these rats behaved as if the shock were controllable, despite never being able to actually control the shock during the procedure. In the next experiment, rats were given two sessions of inescapable shock one week apart, followed by behavioral testing. During the first session, half the rats received vmPFC infusion of picrotoxin, thus enhancing vmPFC during the initial inescapable shock session. Remarkably, vmPFC activation during initial inescapable shock abolished the effects of later inescapable shock on 5-HT efflux, fear conditioning, and escape learning. That is, these rats "behaved" as if they had previously been exposed to an escapable stressor. Importantly, vmPFC activation had no effect on wheel-turning behavior during escapable shock.

Together, this experimental series suggests that vmPFC activity is necessary and also sufficient to produce the behavioral and neurophysiological consequences of controllability, and to produce the immunizing effects of prior experience with control. Later, the same group used retrograde tracing to demonstrate that escapable shock, or inescapable shock that was preceded by escapable shock, activates DRN-projecting neurons in the PL of the vmPFC (Baratta et al., 2009). As glutamateric DRN-projecting PL neurons synapse on GABAergic DRN neurons, this suggests that escapable shock may cause vmPFC inhibition over DRN activity, not only during escapable shock, but also during subsequent stressful experiences regardless of their ability to be controlled.

Does the lesser fear exhibited by animals that have previously experienced control indicate that they experience/express less fear, or that they have reduced memory for the fear-conditioning episodes? Fear expression (i.e., the frequency with which a fear behavior is exhibited) is often taken to index the strength of the associative memory. In this sense, the decreased fear conditioning displayed by rats exposed to escapable shock could suggest some blunting of associative memory caused by the vmPFC. However, two findings from Maier and Watkins contradict this interpretation. First, when inescapable shock occurred 24 hours after fear conditioning, these rats still exhibited potentiated freezing at test, even though it is unlikely that the stress procedure could have modulated the memory at such time point (Baratta et al., 2007). Second, inactivation of vmPFC prior to a contextual fear conditioning test in rats that had previously been exposed to escapable shock abolished the blunting effects of escapable shock on fear conditioning (Baratta et al., 2008). These findings suggest that vmPFC activity during controllable/uncontrollable stressful events does not impact the associative strength of subsequent learning episodes; rather, it modulates the expression of fear for any given associative strength. This conclusion fits nicely with research on the role of the vmPFC in fear extinction, which has suggested that the vmPFC may be important in the expression of the fear extinction memory.

The main implication drawn by Maier's group is that the consequences of controllable/uncontrollable shock are not determined by the ability to exert behavioral control over stress per se, but rather by whether vmPFC activity is increased during the time of stress. Subsequent work in humans has demonstrated that individuals who exhibit greater vlPFC activation in anticipation of an uncontrollable painful stimulus report less pain in response to that stimulus and show greater tendencies to engage "acceptance" over "denial" styles of coping,

suggesting that the neural circuitry mediating perceived control has been preserved across species (Salomons et al., 2007). These findings therefore provide strong evidence for the role of the PFC in mediating emotion regulation via enhancing the perception of control. Moreover, the preclinical findings parallel nicely with clinical reports in humans that it is the perception of control over a traumatic event that seems to confer protection from psychopathology rather than the actual ability to exert control (Ehlers et al., 2000).

INTERIM SUMMARY

Though fear extinction, reversal learning, reappraisal, and studies on controllability represent seemingly distinct experimental tools, the involvement of the PFC in these tasks leads to one common behavioral outcome: regulation of inappropriate fear responses. This can be achieved via interactions with the amygdala as in fear extinction, with more lateral and dorsal prefrontal regions during reappraisal, or through the DRN in the case of controllability. The common involvement of the PFC, therefore, leads the organism to make the most advantageous decision to guide its behavior. It can also be argued that there may be some element of reappraisal during fear extinction, and that both reappraisal and fear extinction may confer some element of controllability, and all three involve the altering of perceived or actual contingencies, as modeled by reversal learning. Thus, while investigators often attribute the role of this brain region to a specific task (i.e., PFC and fear extinction), it should be clear to the reader that the PFC is critical for emotion regulation and behavioral choice optimization in a much broader sense (Fig. 43.5).

WHEN REGULATION FAILS

We have so far examined the PFC's involvement in emotion regulation as it occurs in a normally functioning subject. However, there are many instances in which emotion regulation fails. Examining how the PFC functions in circumstances during which emotion regulation fails provides another means of investigating the nature of its involvement in this ability. If the PFC truly is the gateway for successful emotion regulation, then failures in this ability must be associated with aberrant PFC structure and/or function. In the following section, we briefly review rodent and human research that has examined the functioning of the PFC during times of emotion regulation failure, and highlight some of the factors that may influence this process, such as stress and sex hormones. Our review of the clinical studies related to emotion regulation will be very brief as a more thorough examination of this topic will be reported in Chapter 45 by Goodkind, Gyurak, and Etkin.

ANXIETY DISORDERS

Anxiety disorders are characterized by the failure to appropriately regulate fear and anxiety. Neuroimaging tools have

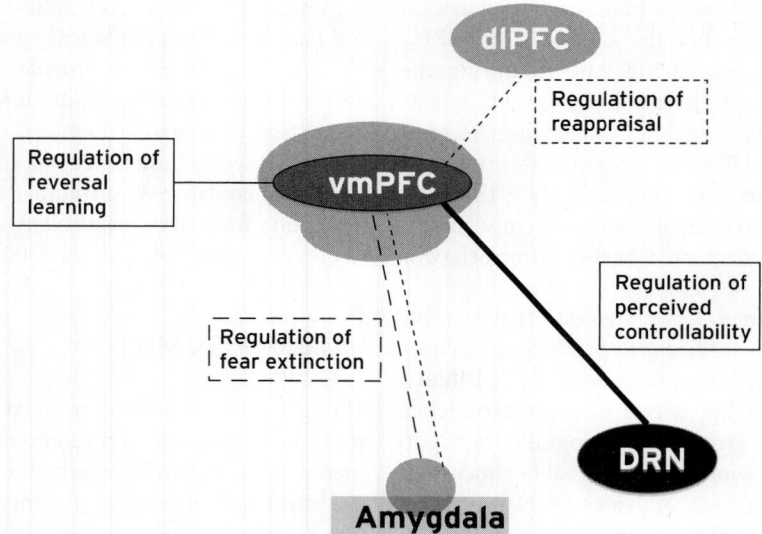

Figure 43.5 *The vmPFC may act as a gateway between phylogenetically newer cortical structures (e.g., dorsal lateral PFC) and phylogenetically older limbic and brainstem structures (e.g., amygdala and dorsal raphe nucleus) to regulate many forms of emotion regulation.*

been used to investigate the underlying pathophysiology of the inappropriate control of fear, in parallel with preclinical investigations that are able to use more invasive means of investigation to gain a more anatomically precise understanding of the mechanisms of emotion regulation. These efforts have led to the identification of a number of brain regions that may contribute to symptoms of anxiety. Not surprisingly, aberrant functioning of regions of the PFC has been identified as a key contributor to the development and maintenance of anxiety. Earlier neuroimaging research examined PFC activations in people with anxiety disorders while viewing fear-relevant and irrelevant images. Such research, known as "symptom provocation studies," has typically reported altered PFC activity in anxious subjects relative to controls; however, the direction of the difference (i.e., increased or decreased activity) has been somewhat inconsistent (Etkin and Wager, 2007). One reason for the variability between studies may be that in the absence of explicit instructions, participants may or may not spontaneously engage in emotion regulation, and if they do, they may differ with respect to the specific emotion regulation strategy engaged, as well as its relative success. We will focus the following discussion on research that has specifically examined neural activations during emotion regulation tasks.

Emotion regulation deficits have been reported in people with anxiety disorders in a range of tasks, including those that tap into behavioral/automatic, as well as cognitive, regulation abilities (Cisler et al., 2010). With respect to the former, conditioning and extinction of fear have been widely examined in clinically anxious populations because the paradigm is thought to reflect the etiology, symptoms, maintenance, and treatment of anxiety disorders to varying degrees. A meta-analysis of earlier studies that focused on fear conditioning and extinction to simple, single cues revealed evidence for moderately enhanced fear responses during both conditioning and extinction in anxious subjects relative to healthy controls (Lissek et al., 2005). Later studies used discriminative conditioning, in

which participants' conditioned responses in the presence of a reinforced cue are compared with those exhibited in the presence of a nonreinforced (safe) cue. Relative to healthy controls, people with PTSD often exhibit heightened fear responses to both types of cues, as well as delayed extinction, suggesting a reduced ability to discriminate between dangerous and safe cues, and another study reported a specific failure in extinction learning in people with panic disorder (see Graham and Milad, 2011, for review). The most recent studies have focused on the ability to retain extinction memories over a longer period (typically 24 hours after extinction training). For example, we have reported that people with PTSD exhibit normal conditioning and extinction learning, but impairments in extinction recall (Milad et al., 2009a).

Similar to extinction, deficits in cognitive reappraisal have also been reported in clinically anxious populations. Such studies typically instruct participants to downregulate their emotional responses to disorder-relevant or innately threatening/negative images. Less success in emotion downregulation, as indexed by self-reports, has been reported in people with PTSD (New et al., 2009) and spider phobia (Hermann et al., 2009).

Might there be common neurobiological underpinnings of anxiety disorder–associated failures in emotion regulation across these tasks? In the case of extinction, there is evidence that heightened activity within the dACC and reduced activity within the vmPFC may be responsible for the enhanced conditioning and reduced extinction observed in PTSD, respectively. For example, using positron emission tomography, Bremner et al. (2005) demonstrated that people with PTSD exhibited heightened behavioral responses during fear acquisition and extinction that were associated with increased resting metabolic activity in the left amygdala and decreased resting metabolic activity in the vmPFC, respectively, compared with healthy controls. We reported that the impaired extinction recall observed in PTSD populations is associated with reduced activity in the vmPFC and hippocampus, but heightened dACC activity to conditioned cues (Milad et al., 2009a) and contexts (Rougemont-Bücking et al., 2011). Replication of these findings in other cohorts/subtypes of anxiety is required to determine whether vmPFC deregulation is characteristic of anxiety as a dimension.

In the case of cognitive reappraisal, the deficits in downregulation among people with PTSD were associated with reductions in lateral PFC activity compared with healthy controls (New et al., 2009). Similarly, participants with spider phobia exhibited decreased rostral ACC and vm/dmPFC activity (but normal vlPFC activity) when attempting to downregulate emotional responses to phobic-relevant fearful images, compared with phobic-irrelevant fearful images (Hermann et al., 2009). Interestingly, no differences in self-report of emotion downregulation via reappraisal were found in people with social anxiety disorder (SAD) compared with healthy controls, but reappraisal was associated with reduced dlPFC and dmPFC activation in SAD participants in response to images of social threat, but not images of physical threat (Goldin et al., 2009).

FACTORS THAT MODULATE EMOTION REGULATION SUCCESS

PERSONALITY

Examining how well variance in emotion regulation ability can be predicted by individual difference factors may potentially lead to the identification of risk factors for disorders associated with emotion regulation failure. To this end, several studies have examined the neural correlates of trait anxiety at rest and during emotion regulation tasks. For example, using diffusion tensor imaging it was shown that high levels of trait anxiety were associated with weaker reciprocal connections between the amygdala and vmPFC (Kim and Whalen, 2009). A later study reported that amygdala resting state activity was positively coupled to vmPFC activity in low-anxious subjects, and negatively coupled to vmPFC activity in high-anxious subjects (Kim et al., 2011c). Together these studies suggest that altered PFC–amygdala functional and structural connectivity may indicate susceptibility to anxiety; however, do these factors covary with emotion regulation success? One recent study examined vmPFC–amygdala activity during cued and contextual fear conditioning tasks in participants with varying levels of trait anxiety (Indovina et al., 2011). High trait anxiety was positively associated with skin conductance responses (i.e., greater arousal) and amygdala response to the conditioned cue, and negatively associated with vmPFC response to both the conditioned cue and context. Moreover, variance in trait anxiety was best accounted for by a model that included amygdala and vmPFC responses (either during the cue or the context). As this task did not include a component of instructed emotion regulation, the authors suggested that low–trait anxious individuals might spontaneously engage the vmPFC–amygdala circuitry involved in emotion downregulation during times of stress. Another study reported that while people high and low in trait anxiety exhibited similar success in reducing negative emotions, reappraisal in high-anxious participants was associated with *greater* engagement of lateral and medial PFC,

suggesting the requirement for greater neural effort to attain the same level of regulation (Campbell-Sills et al., 2011).

STRESS

Stress activates a number of hormones, one of the primary targets of which is the PFC. Numerous studies have demonstrated that chronic stress influences PFC structure and neuronal function in rodents, with chronic stress or corticosterone treatment causing retractions in dendritic length and branch numbers, dendritic spine loss, and reduced neuronal responses to serotonin or dopamine application (see review by Holmes and Wellman, 2009). In light of this, investigations have now turned to the examination of the functional implications of stress effects on the PFC. Several researchers have reported that in rodents chronic stress leads to impairments in fear extinction acquisition (Izquierdo et al., 2006) or extinction recall (Garcia et al., 2008; Knox et al., 2012; Miracle et al., 2006), without altering the acquisition of fear conditioning. The stress-induced impairment in extinction is accompanied by reductions in dendritic branch length in the IL (Izquierdo et al., 2006), reduced mPFC neuronal excitability in response to hippocampal stimulation (Garcia et al., 2008), and a change in the quality of IL–amygdala plasticity (from long-term potentiation to long-term depression; Akirav and Maroun, 2007). Evidence that the chronic stress-induced dendritic remodeling or changes in IL–amygdala pathway plasticity actually causes impairments in extinction, however, is lacking. One recent study reported that IL lesions in rodents prior to chronic stress prevented the impairment in extinction (Farrell et al., 2010), suggesting that IL activity during the stressful experience is necessary for mediating stress effects on subsequent learning episodes. It will be important for future research to investigate whether preventing the impact of stress on PFC morphology and function also prevents extinction impairments, and/or to determine whether a recovery interval following stress (which often reverses the neuronal effects of stress) reduces the impact of stress on extinction. In addition, it will also be useful to extend investigations of stress effects to other modes of emotion regulation, in both rodents and humans.

SEX HORMONES

In addition to stress hormones, sex hormones also appear to modulate emotion regulation. The influence of sex hormones on extinction is receiving increased attention, most likely due to the recognition that women are more vulnerable to anxiety disorders than men (Lebron-Milad et al., 2012). Studies in naturally cycling adult female rodents have revealed that extinction retention is optimal when cycling hormones (e.g., estradiol, progesterone) are high (the proestrus phase of the rat estrous cycle), and extinction retention is significantly impaired when cycling hormones are low (the metestrus phase of the rat estrous cycle) (Chang et al., 2009; Milad et al., 2009b; Zeidan et al., 2011). Similar findings have been reported in healthy, naturally cycling women, where extinction retention is optimal during the midluteal (high estradiol and progesterone) phase of the menstrual cycle, but reduced during the follicular (low-estradiol, progesterone) phase (Milad et al., 2010; Zeidan et al., 2011). A more recent study reported that estradiol levels were negatively correlated with extinction ability and symptom severity in women with PTSD (Glover et al., 2012). We have demonstrated that estrogen's influence on fear extinction appears to be modulated via PFC activation (Zeidan et al., 2011). We reported that the impaired extinction in metestrus female rats is associated with reduced IL, but increased BLA, immediate early gene activity at the time of extinction recall. Moreover, the impaired extinction in follicular women was associated with reduced vmPFC, hippocampal, and amygdala neural responses during extinction recall. A recent fMRI study also found significant differences in vmPFC responding between men and women during extinction recall, supporting the likely influence of sex hormones on the functional responsivity of this brain region during emotion regulation (Lebron-Milad et al., 2012). The impact of sex hormones on the functioning of the PFC during more cognitive forms of regulation, like reappraisal or perceived control over stress, is unknown. However, other research has demonstrated that gender and/or menstrual cycle phase affects recall for emotional films (Ferree et al., 2011), activity of the neural circuitry underlying the stress response (Goldstein et al., 2010), and OFC activity during emotion processing (Protopopescu et al., 2005). Together, these findings suggest that sex hormones may modulate emotion regulation abilities more generally, possibly by altering top-down cortical control over limbic structures.

INFLUENCE OF DEVELOPMENT

Although much is known about the neural and molecular mechanisms underlying fear extinction in adults, much less is known about extinction across development. This is surprising given that anxiety disorders often emerge during adolescence, which is a time of neuronal reorganization within the PFC that is characterized by heightened emotionality and reduced impulse control (Casey et al., 2010). Recent studies have revealed that although adolescent rats exhibit normal acquisition of conditioning and extinction, they exhibit elevated recovery of fear responses the following day (Kim et al., 2011a; McCallum et al., 2010). This deficit can be overcome with extensive extinction training, which has also been observed in adult rats with PFC lesions (Lebron et al., 2004), suggesting that the impaired extinction in adolescent rats may be similarly due to reductions in PFC function during this phase of development. Evidence for the latter idea comes from Kim et al. (2011a), who demonstrated that extinction recall in adolescent rats was associated with reduced phosphorylation of mitogen-activated protein kinase (pMAPK) in the IL compared with adult rats. Moreover, when adolescent rats were overtrained during extinction to prevent impairments in recall, this resulted in increased IL pMAPK at the time of recall.

GENETIC INFLUENCES

In an attempt to determine genetic predispositions to anxiety disorders, several studies have examined the influence of various genetic profiles on tasks of emotion regulation. Conditioning and extinction ability is moderately heritable, accounting for around 35–45% of the variability in conditioning and extinction in a cohort of monozygotic and dizygotic twins (Hettema et al., 2003), which is equivalent to the percentage of variance associated with PTSD that is accounted for by a heritable component. A number of studies have demonstrated that single-nucleotide polymorphisms (SNPs) associated with the serotonin transporter gene (Hartley et al., 2012), the *BDNF* gene (Soliman et al., 2010), and the pituitary adenylate cyclase-activating polypeptide (PACAP; Ressler et al., 2011) are associated with impaired fear extinction and/or discrimination of safety cues. How does genetic variation mediate extinction impairments at a neural level? Preclinical studies that have taken advantage of considerable between- and within-strain differences in extinction abilities have assisted in addressing this question. Hefner et al. (2008) reported that extinction impairments in 129S1 mice were associated with reduced immediate early gene activity in the IL and BLA, and enhanced activity in the CeA, compared with C57BL/6J mice that exhibit normal extinction. Similar findings have been reported for Wistar rats selectively bred for high- and low-anxiety-related behavior (Muigg et al., 2008). High-anxiety rats exhibited impaired extinction learning and recall, and reduced immediate early gene activity in IL and lateral amygdala, and increased activity in the CeA, compared with low-anxiety rats. The neural basis for genetic-associated impairments in rodents may be common in humans, as people with BDNF–SNP associated extinction impairments also exhibit reduced vmPFC, but increased amygdala, activation during extinction (Soliman et al., 2010). Together, these studies suggest that extinction impairments of genetic origin may be due to reduced vmPFC control over subcortical afferents.

FUTURE DIRECTIONS

A focus of future research in the domain of emotion regulation will be to increase the understanding of how the different regions of the PFC interact to mediate emotion regulation and the subcortical structures responsible for emotion processing. Some progress has been made in this area in the study of fear extinction, with different roles for the PL and IL regions becoming increasingly well defined. Similar progress will need to be made in the study of reappraisal. It will be important to address, for example, whether different regions of the PFC are involved in different kinds of reappraisal and/or reappraisal for different types of emotions, and in turn, whether these regions recruit a common mediator, such as the vmPFC, to influence subcortical aspects of emotion processing and expression.

Moving beyond the PFC, it will also be critical for future research on emotion regulation to study the neural circuits involved rather than the activations and contributions of single neural structures in isolation. Such an approach may assist in resolving some inconsistencies in the literature where, for example, some studies have reported decreased activity in the vmPFC in participants with anxiety disorders, whereas others have reported increased activity in the same type of cohort. From the more recent research reviewed here, it is apparent that it may not be the overall activation of distinct neural regions that dictates the emotional output but, rather, the connectivity, or the strength of coupling between two or more regions (in whichever direction), that determines the emotional response. Future research will need to examine structural and functional coupling between proposed circuitries, and how coupling strength changes according to task demands. In addition, it will be useful to examine how the various modulating factors discussed earlier (psychopathology, personality, development, sex, genetics, etc.) affect coupling at a baseline level as well as during various emotion regulation tasks.

DISCLOSURES

Dr. Graham has no conflicts of interests to disclose.

Dr. Milad has received fees from MircoTransponder Inc. in a project not related to the present work. This work was supported by an R01MH081975 (subcontract) and a 1R01MH097880-01 to M. R. M., and an American Australian Association Neurological Fellowship to Dr. Graham.

REFERENCES

Akirav, I., and Maroun, M. (2007). The role of the medial prefrontal cortex-amygdala circuit in stress effects on the extinction of fear. *Neural. Plast.* 2007:30873.

Amat, J., Baratta, M.V., et al. (2005). Medial prefrontal cortex determines how stressor controllability affects behavior and dorsal raphe nucleus. *Nat. Neurosci.* 8:365–371.

Amat, J., Paul, E., et al. (2006). Previous experience with behavioral control over stress blocks the behavioral and dorsal raphe nucleus activating effects of later uncontrollable stress: role of the ventral medial prefrontal cortex. *J. Neurosci.* 26:13264–13272.

Amat, J., Paul, E., et al. (2008). Activation of the ventral medial prefrontal cortex during an uncontrollable stressor reproduces both the immediate and long-term protective effects of behavioral control. *Neuroscience* 154:1178–1186.

Baratta, M.V., Christianson, J.P., et al. (2007). Controllable versus uncontrollable stressors bi- directionally modulate conditioned but not innate fear. *Neuroscience* 146:1495–1503.

Baratta, M.V., Lucero, T.R., et al. (2008). Role of the ventral medial prefrontal cortex in mediating behavioral control-induced reduction of later conditioned fear. *Learn. Mem.* 15:84–87.

Baratta, M.V., Zarza, C.M., et al. (2009). Selective activation of dorsal raphe nucleus-projecting neurons in the ventral medial prefrontal cortex by controllable stress. *Eur. J. Neurosci.* 30:1111–1116.

Bremner, J.D., Vermetten, E., et al. (2005). Positron emission tomographic imaging of neural correlates of a fear acquisition and extinction paradigm in women with childhood sexual-abuse related post-traumatic stress disorder. *Psychol. Med.* 35:791–806.

Campbell-Sills, L., Simmons, A.N., et al. (2011). Functioning of neural systems supporting emotion regulation in anxiety-prone individuals. *NeuroImage* 54:689–696.

Casey, B.J., Duhoux, S., et al. (2010). Adolescence: what do transmission, transition, and translation have to do with it? *Neuron* 67:749–760.

Chang, Y., Yang, C., et al. (2009). Estrogen modulates sexually dimorphic contextual fear extinction in rats through estrogen receptor β. *Hippocampus* 19:1142–1150.

Cisler, J.M., Oltaunji, B.O., et al. (2010). Emotion regulation and the anxiety disorders: an integrative review. *J. Psychopathol. Behav.* 32:68–82.

Delgado, M.R., Nearing, K.I., et al. (2008). Neural circuitry underlying the regulation of conditioned fear and its relation to extinction. *Neuron* 59:829–836.

Drabant, E.M., McRae, K., et al. (2009). Individual differences in typical reappraisal use predict amygdala and prefrontal responses. *Biol. Psychiatry* 65:367–373.

Dunsmoor, J.E., and LaBar, K.S. (2012). Brain activity associated with omission of an aversive event reveals the effects of fear learning and generalization. *Neurobiol. Learn. Mem.* 97:301–312.

Ehlers, A., Maercker, A., et al. (2000). Posttraumatic stress disorder following political imprisonment: the role of mental defeat, alienation, and perceived permanent change. *J. Abnorm. Psychol.* 109:45–55.

Etkin, A., Egner, T., et al. (2011). Emotional processing in anterior cingulate and medial prefrontal cortex. *Trends Cogn. Sci.* 15:85–93.

Etkin, A., and Wager, T.D. (2007). Functional neuroimaging of anxiety: meta-analysis of emotional processing in PTSD, social anxiety disorder, and specific phobia. *Am. J. Psychiatry* 164:1476–1488.

Farinelli, M., Deschaux, O., et al. (2006). Hippocampal train stimulation modulates recall of fear extinction independently of prefrontal cortex synaptic plasticity and lesions. *Learn. Mem.* 13:329–334.

Farrell, M.R., Sayed, J.A., et al. (2010). Lesion of infralimbic cortex occludes stress effects on retrieval of extinction but not fear conditioning. *Neurobiol. Learn. Mem.* 94:240–246.

Ferree, N.K., Kamat, R., et al. (2011). Influences of menstrual cycle position and sex hormone levels on spontaneous intrusive recollections following emotional stimuli. *Conscious. Cogn.* 20:1154–1162.

Garcia, R., Spennato, G., et al. (2008). Hippocampal low-frequency stimulation and chronic mild stress similarly disrupt fear extinction memory in rats. *Neurobiol. Learn. Mem.* 89:560–566.

Gewirtz, J.C., Falls, W.A., et al. (1997). Normal conditioned inhibition and extinction of freezing and fear-potentiated startle following electrolytic lesions of medial prefrontal cortex in rats. *Behav. Neurosci.* 111:712–726.

Giuliani, N.R., Drabant, E.M., et al. (2011). Anterior cingulate cortex volume and emotion regulation: is bigger better? *Biol. Psychology* 86:379–382.

Glover, E.M., Jovanovic, T., et al. (2012). Estrogen levels are associated with extinction deficits in women with posttraumatic stress disorder. *Biol. Psychiatry* 72:19–24.

Goldin, P.R., Manber, T., et al. (2009). Neural bases of social anxiety disorder: emotional reactivity and cognitive regulation during social and physical threat. *Arch. Gen. Psychiatry* 66:170–180.

Goldin, P.R., McRae, K., et al. (2008). The neural bases of emotion regulation: reappraisal and suppression of negative emotion. *Biol. Psychiatry* 63:577–586.

Goldstein, J.M., Jerram, M., et al. (2010). Sex differences in stress response circuitry activation dependent on female hormonal cycle. *J. Neurosci.* 30:431–438.

Gottfried, J.A., and Dolan, R.J. (2004). Human orbitofrontal cortex mediates extinction learning while accessing conditioned representations of value. *Nat. Neurosci.* 7:1145–1153.

Graham, B.M., and Milad, M.R. (2011). The study of fear extinction: implications for anxiety disorders. *Am. J. Psychiatry* 168:1255–1265.

Gross, J.J. (2002). Emotion regulation: affective, cognitive, and social consequences. *Psychophysiology* 39:281–291.

Hartley, C.A., McKenna, M.C., et al. (2012). Serotonin transporter polyadenylation polymorphism modulates the retention of fear extinction memory. *Proc. Natl. Acad. Sci. USA* 109:5493–5498.

Hefner, K., Whittle, N., et al. (2008). Impaired fear extinction learning and corticoamygdala circuit abnormalities in a common genetic mouse strain. *J. Neurosci.* 28:8074–8085.

Hermann, A., Schäfer, A., et al. (2009). Emotion regulation in spider phobia: role of the medial prefrontal cortex. *Soc. Cogn. Affect. Neur.* 4:257–267.

Herry, C., and Garcia, R. (2002). Prefrontal cortex long-term potentiation, but not long-term depression, is associated with the maintenance of extinction of learned fear in mice. *J. Neurosci.* 22:577–583.

Hettema, J.M., Annas, P., et al. (2003). A twin study of the genetics of fear conditioning. *Arch. Gen. Psychiatry* 60:702–708.

Holmes, A., and Wellman, C.L. (2009). Stress-induced prefrontal reorganization and executive dysfunction in rodents. *Neurosci. Biobehav. Rev.* 33:773–783.

Indovina, I., Robbins, T.W., et al. (2011). Fear- conditioning mechanisms associated with trait vulnerability to anxiety in humans. *Neuron* 69:563–571.

Izquierdo, A., Wellman, C.L., et al. (2006). Brief uncontrollable stress causes dendritic retraction in infralimbic cortex and resistance to fear extinction in mice. *J. Neurosci.* 26:5733–5738.

Kalisch, R. (2009). The functional neuroanatomy of reappraisal: time matters. *Neurosci. Biobehav. Rev.* 33:1215–1226.

Kalisch, R., Korenfeld, E., et al. (2006). Context-dependent human extinction memory is mediated by a ventromedial prefrontal and hippocampal network. *J. Neurosci.* 26:9503–9511.

Kim, J.H., Li, S., et al. (2011a). Immunohistochemical analyses of long-term extinction of conditioned fear in adolescent rats. *Cereb. Cortex* 21:530–538.

Kim, M.J., Gee, D.G., et al. (2011b). Anxiety dissociates dorsal and ventral medial prefrontal cortex functional connectivity with the amygdala at rest. *Cereb. Cortex* 21:1667–1673.

Kim, M.J., Loucks, R.A., et al. (2011c). The structural and functional connectivity of the amygdala: from normal emotion to pathological anxiety. *Behav. Brain Res.* 223:403–410.

Kim, M.J., and Whalen, P.J. (2009). The structural integrity of an amygdala–prefrontal pathway predicts trait anxiety. *J. Neurosci.* 29:11614–11618.

Knight, D.C., Smith, C.N., et al. (2004). Amygdala and hippocampal activity during acquisition and extinction of human fear conditioning. *Cogn. Affect. Behav. Neurosci.* 4:317–325.

Knox, D., George, S.A., et al. (2012). Single prolonged stress disrupts retention of extinguished fear in rats. *Learn. Mem.* 19:43–49.

Lebron, K., Milad, M.R., et al. (2004). Delayed recall of fear extinction in rats with lesions of ventral medial prefrontal cortex. *Learn. Mem.* 11:544–548.

Lebron-Milad, K., Abbs, B., et al. (2012). Sex differences in the neurobiology of fear conditioning and extinction: a preliminary fMRI study of shared sex differences with stress-arousal circuitry. *Biol. Mood Anxiety Disord.* 2:7.

Lee, H., Heller, A.S., et al. (2012). Amygdala-prefrontal coupling underlies individual differences in emotion regulation. *NeuroImage* 62:1575–1581.

Likhtik, E., Popa, D., et al. (2008). Amygdala intercalated neurons are required for expression of extinguished fear in rats. *Nature* 454:642–646.

Linnman, C., Rougemount-Bücking, A., et al. (2011). Unconditioned responses and functional fear networks in human classical conditioning. *Behav. Brain Res.* 221:237–245.

Lissek, S., Powers, A.S., et al. (2005). Classical fear conditioning in the anxiety disorders: a meta-analysis. *Behav. Res. Ther.* 43:1391–1424.

Lovibond, P.F., and Shanks, D.R. (2002). The role of awareness in Pavlovian conditioning: empirical evidence and theoretical implications. *J. Exp. Psychol.* 28:3–26.

Maier, S.F., and Watkins, L.R. (2010). Role of the medial prefrontal cortex in coping and resilience. *Brain Res.* 1355:52–60.

McCallum, J., Kim, J.H., et al. (2010). Impaired extinction retention in adolescent rats: effects of D-cycloserine. *Neuropsychopharmacology* 35:2134–2142.

McNally, G.P., Pigg, M., et al. (2004). Opioid receptors in the midbrain periaqueductal gray regulate extinction of Pavlovian fear conditioning. *J. Neurosci.* 24:6912–6919.

Milad, M.R., Igoe, S.A., et al. (2009b). Estrous cycle phase and gonadal hormones influence conditioned fear extinction. *Neuroscience* 164:887–895.

Milad, M.R., Pitman, R.K., et al. (2009a). Neurobiological basis of failure to recall extinction memory in posttraumatic stress disorder. *Biol. Psychiatry* 66:1075–1082.

Milad, M.R., and Quirk, G.J. (2002). Neurons in medial prefrontal cortex signal memory for fear extinction. *Nature* 420:70–74.

Milad, M.R., and Quirk, G.J. (2012). Fear extinction as a model for translational neuroscience: ten years of progress. *Annu. Rev. Psychol.* 63:129–151.

Milad, M.R., Wright, C.I., et al. (2007). Recall of fear extinction in humans activates the ventromedial prefrontal cortex and hippocampus in concert. *Biol. Psychiatry* 62:446–454.

Milad, M.R., Zeidan, M.A., et al. (2010). The influence of gonadal hormones on conditioned fear extinction in healthy humans. *Neuroscience* 168:652–658.

Miracle, A.D., Brace, M.F., et al. (2006). Chronic stress impairs recall of extinction of conditioned fear. *Neurobiol. Learn. Mem.* 85:213–218.

Morgan, M.A., Romanski, L.M., et al. (1993). Extinction of emotional learning: contribution of medial prefrontal cortex. *Neurosci. Lett.* 163:109–113.

Morris, J.S., and Dolan, R.J. (2004). Dissociable amygdala and orbitofrontal responses during reversal fear conditioning. *NeuroImage* 22:372–380.

Muigg, P., Hetzenauer, A., et al. (2008). Impaired extinction of learned fear in rats selectively bred for high anxiety: evidence of altered neuronal processing in prefrontal-amygdala pathways. *Eur. J. Neurosci.* 28:2299–2309.

New, A.S., Fan, J., et al. (2009). A functional magnetic resonance imaging study of deliberate emotion regulation in resilience and posttraumatic stress disorder. *Biol. Psychiatry* 66:656–664.

Öhman, A., and Mineka, S. (2001). Fears, phobias and preparedness: toward an evolved module of fear and fear learning. *Psychol. Rev.* 108:483–522.

Orsini, C.A., and Maren, S. (2012). Neural and cellular mechanisms of fear and extinction memory formation. *Neurosci. Biobehav. Rev.* 36:1773–1802.

Parsons, R.G., Gafford, G.M., et al. (2010). Regulation of extinction-related plasticity by opioid receptors in the ventrolateral periaqueductal gray matter. *Front. Behav. Neurosci.* 4:pii:44.

Phan, K.L., Fitzgerald, D.A., et al. (2005). Neural substrates for voluntary suppression of negative affect: a functional magnetic resonance imaging study. *Biol. Psychiatry* 57:210–219.

Phelps, E.A., Delgado, M.R., et al. (2004). Extinction learning in humans: role of the amygdala and vmPFC. *Neuron* 43:897–905.

Protopopescu, X., Pan, H., et al. (2005). Orbitofrontal cortex activity related to emotional processing changes across the menstrual cycle. *Proc. Natl. Acad. Sci. USA* 102:16060–16065.

Quirk, G.J., Likhtik, E., et al. (2003). Stimulation of medial prefrontal cortex decreases the responsiveness of central amygdala output neurons. *J. Neurosci.* 23:8800–8807.

Quirk, G.J., Russo, G.K., et al. (2000). The role of ventromedial prefrontal cortex in the recovery of extinguished fear. *J. Neurosci.* 20:6225–6231.

Ressler, K.J., Mercer, K.B., et al. (2011). Post-traumatic stress disorder is associated with PACAP and the PAC1 receptor. *Nature* 470:492–497.

Robinson, O.J., Charney, D.R., et al. (2012). The adaptive threat bias in anxiety: amygdala-dorsomedial prefrontal cortex coupling and aversive amplification. *NeuroImage* 60:523–529.

Rodriguez-Romaguera, J., Do Monte, F.H.M., et al. (2012). Deep brain stimulation of the ventral striatum enhances extinction of conditioned fear. *Proc. Natl. Acad. Sci. USA* 109:8764–8769.

Rougemont-Bücking, A., Linnman, C., et al. (2011). Altered processing of contextual information during fear extinction in PTSD: an fMRI study. *CNS Neurosci. Ther.* 17:227–236.

Salomons, T.V., Johnstone, T., et al. (2007). Individual differences in the effects of perceived controllability on pain perception: critical role of the prefrontal cortex. *J. Cogn. Neurosci.* 19:993–1003.

Schiller, D., Levy, I., et al. (2008). From fear to safety and back: reversal of fear in the human brain. *J. Neurosci.* 28:11517–11525.

Sierra-Mercado, D., Padilla-Coreano, N., et al. (2011). Dissociable roles of prelimbic and infralimbic cortices, ventral hippocampus, and basolateral amygdala in the expression and extinction of conditioned fear. *Neuropsychopharmacology* 36:529–538.

Smits, J.A.J., Julian, K., et al. (2012). Threat reappraisal as a mediator of symptom change in cognitive-behavioral treatment of anxiety disorders: a systematic review. *J. Consult. Clin. Psych.* 80:624–635.

Soliman, F., Glatt, C.E., et al. (2010). A genetic variant BDNF polymorphism alters extinction learning in both mouse and human. *Science* 327:863–866.

Thompson, B.M., Baratta, M.V., et al. (2010). Activation of the infralimbic cortex in a fear context enhances extinction learning. *Learn. Mem.* 17:591–599.

Urry, H.L., van Reekum, C.M., et al. (2006). Amygdala and ventromedial prefrontal cortex are inversely coupled during regulation of negative affect and predict the diurnal pattern of cortisol secretion among older adults. *J. Neurosci.* 26:4415–4425.

Wager, T.D., Davidson, M.L., et al. (2008). Prefrontal-subcortical pathways mediating successful emotion regulation. *Neuron* 59:1037–1050.

Zeidan, M.A., Igoe, S.A., et al. (2011). Estradiol modulates medial prefrontal cortex and amygdala activity during fear extinction in women and female rats. *Biol. Psychiatry* 70:920–927.

44 | DEVELOPMENTAL COMPONENTS OF FEAR AND ANXIETY IN ANIMAL MODELS

SIOBHAN S. PATTWELL, ANNE-MARIE MOULY, REGINA M. SULLIVAN, AND FRANCIS S. LEE

INTRODUCTION

Modern advances in psychiatry and neuroscience have uncovered a wealth of knowledge about the underlying neural circuitry implicated in anxiety- and stress-related disorders. As the majority of research has focused on characterizing inappropriate and exaggerated fear responses in the mature adult brain, current clinical treatments have been implemented based on their efficacy in a physiologically mature neural framework. While existing behavioral and psychopharmacological therapies offer significant benefit to adult patients suffering from anxiety disorders, such as posttraumatic stress disorder (PTSD), a comparative lack of knowledge about the development of fear neural circuitry may limit successful treatment outcomes in children and adolescents (Liberman et al., 2006). In addition, early-life environmental and physiological stressors can alter the dynamic nature of this circuitry, highlighting the importance of understanding fear circuitry from early infant development, onward through adolescence, and into adulthood. Importantly, we present data indicating that the developing circuitry underlying fear and anxiety has dynamic developmental periods when fear learning or its expression is prevented. Successful treatment outcomes in children and adolescents will likely need to consider these unique developmental epochs.

NEURAL CIRCUITRY INVOLVED IN FEAR LEARNING AND MEMORY

MODELING FEAR LEARNING IN THE LABORATORY

Behavioral paradigms relying on Pavlovian principles have become standard for studying fear in both humans and nonhuman animals (Pavlov, 1927). Classical conditioning is an attractive model for studying neural mechanisms of fear because learning is rapidly acquired, the memory is long lasting, and stimuli are easily controlled by the experimenter (Sigurdsson et al., 2007). Typically, an inherently threatening and/or unpleasant stimulus, such as an electric shock or aversive noise, serves as an unconditioned stimulus (US), while a previously neutral stimulus, such as a light flicker or tone, serves as the conditioned stimulus (CS). Through pairings of the CS with the US, an association is formed such that the CS becomes predictive of the US. Eventually, after the CS–US association has been learned, presentations of the CS alone are capable of eliciting a fear response that was developed as a result of the US. This conditioned response (CR) is often characterized physiologically by changes in autonomic arousal and behavior, or in the case of the rodent, freezing behavior. Once the CS–US association has been formed, the CR can then be extinguished by giving multiple presentations of the CS alone, in the absence of the US. The initial CS–US pairing is not forgotten during the extinction process, as the fear almost always returns after standard extinction training with renewal, reinstatement, or the passage of time (Bouton et al., 2006). Extinction learning, not to be confused with the process of mere forgetting, is an inhibitory process during which the relationship and expectancy of the CS–US pairing is modified (Sotres-Bayon et al., 2006). By presenting the CS repeatedly, in the absence of any US, one can reevaluate the predictability of the CS, thus learning that a stimulus that was once associated with threat has become safe. Uncovering information behind the mechanisms involved in fear acquisition, and extinction in particular, has wide clinical implications, as the most common and validated treatment for anxiety disorders involves exposure-based therapy, which relies heavily on extinction principles for reevaluating existing contingencies (Rothbaum and Davis, 2003). Strong cross-species preservation of the neural circuitry implicated in fear extinction learning is supported by human and nonhuman animal extinction studies, further bolstering the translational credibility of rodent models for studying fear regulation and extinction.

ACQUISITION AND EXPRESSION OF CONDITIONED FEAR

Decades of probing into the neural circuitry underlying fear learning have yielded data from specified lesion, inactivation, electrophysiological, molecular, and pharmacological studies, confirming the amygdala to be a key structure involved in acquisition of conditioned fear (Milad and Quirk, 2012). During standard auditory cue fear conditioning, both somatosensory and auditory thalamic inputs converge on the lateral nucleus of the amygdala (LA) simultaneously or in close temporal proximity (Collins and Pare, 2000; Sotres-Bayon et al., 2006),

44 DEVELOPMENTAL COMPONENTS OF FEAR AND ANXIETY | 593

such that after repeated pairings, the CS presentations alone are capable of eliciting activity within the LA. See Figure 44.1 for schematic representation of neural circuitry implicated in fear learning and memory.

While the basal (BA) and lateral (LA) nuclei are considered to make up the primary sensory interface involved in fear learning and acquisition, the central (CE) nucleus is the amygdala's interface to fear response systems (Maren, 2001). After integration via the BLA (basolateral amygdala), relevant sensory information responsible for eliciting a behavioral or autonomic response is relayed to the CE through both direct and indirect thalamic and interamygdalar projections (Milad and Quirk, 2012; Sotres-Bayon et al., 2006). After the intraamygdaloid message has been relayed to CE, the CE elicits physiological responses via its divergent projections to downstream efferent structures that target various hypothalamic and brain stem nuclei responsible for engaging autonomic responses such as increased heart rate, blood pressure, respiration, freezing behavior, acoustic startle, and glucocorticoid release (Maren, 2011). Auditory tones or distinct sensory cues are not experienced in isolation, and surrounding contextual and environmental factors have a profound effect on the acquisition of conditioned fear and the resulting fear memory. Projections from the hippocampus, specifically the CA1 region, to the basal nucleus of the amygdala (BA) are implicated in contextual information processing during fear acquisition (Bouton et al., 2006; Phelps and LeDoux, 2005), and lesions to dorsal hippocampus disrupt both acquisition and expression of contextual fear (Kim and Fanselow, 1992; Phillips and LeDoux, 1992). While the CE remains the prime amygdalar site responsible for eliciting autonomic responses and fear behaviors, hippocampus–BA

integration of contextual information can alter downstream CE activity and affect subsequent behaviors. The hippocampus can modulate fear expression by altering contextual fear directly or by influencing amygdala-specific cued fear as animals are capable of using contextual cues to retrieve the meaning of a CS appropriate to a given context (Maren, 2011).

Increased spike firing in amygdala neurons, and long-term potentiation (LTP), or enduring synaptic plasticity, have been shown to occur at synapses in the hippocampus and amygdala during fear conditioning and expression (Milad and Quirk, 2012). Glutamate receptor signaling in the amygdala and hippocampus, through both NMDA and AMPA receptors, has also been shown to be crucial for fear acquisition and expression, further confirming the role of these two structures in fear acquisition and expression. Disruption of various downstream signaling cascades, including protein kinase A (PKA) (Bourtchouladze et al., 1998), mitogen-activated protein kinase (MAPK), and phosphatidylinositol 3 kinase (PI3K) in the amygdala and hippocampus, has also been shown to disrupt learning in both contextual and auditory fear conditioning paradigms (Chen et al., 2005; Schafe et al., 1999).

EXTINCTION OF CONDITIONED FEAR

After CS–US associations have been acquired and consolidated, modifications of the initial fear memory are possible. For example, repeated presentations of the CS (in the absence of any US) may ultimately result in a decreased conditioned fear response and reinterpretation of a formerly threatening cue, transitioning the CS into a nonnoxious stimulus. Through multiple presentations or sessions, this new form of inhibitory

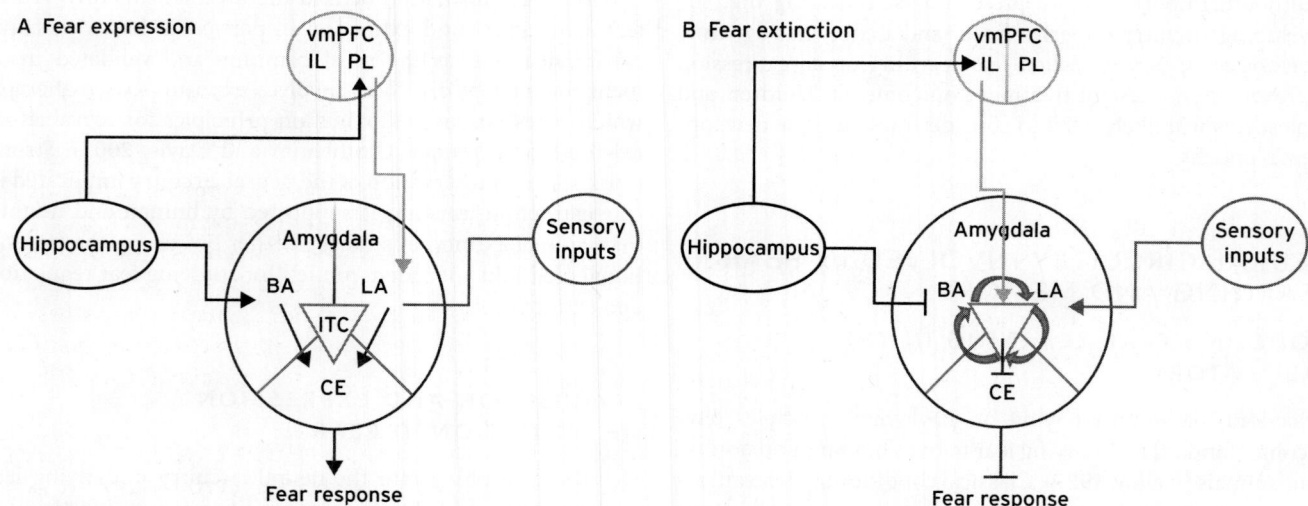

Figure 44.1 Neural circuitry of fear expression and extinction. (A) During acquisition and expression of conditioned fear, projections from PL and thalamic nuclei (mediating converging sensory information) excite LA neurons, while hippocampal projections (mediating contextual inputs) lead to excitation of BA neurons directly or indirectly via connections with PL. LA and BA neurons activate CE output neurons, which project to downstream brain stem and hypothalamic nuclei responsible for mediating physiological responses, resulting in fear expression. (B) During extinction of conditioned fear, hippocampal projections (mediating contextual inputs) lead to divergent excitation of IL neurons and inhibition of BA neurons. IL projections directly activate GABAergic ITC cells within the amygdala. Integration of ITC, BA, and LA inputs during extinction result in a suppression of CE output neurons, resulting in a lack of physiological response and suppression of fear expression. Arrowheads delineate pathway excitation; straight ends delineate pathway inhibition. (BA, basal amygdala; LA, lateral amygdala; CE, central amygdala; vmPFC, ventromedial prefrontal cortex; PL, prelimbic cortex; IL, infralimbic cortex; ITC, intercalated cells). For simplicity, connection arrows are delineated as being unidirectional, although bidirectional projections exist. (Figures adapted from Hormones and Behavior, in press, Pattwell et al.)

learning results in an extinction of the initial conditioned fear memory. While the amygdala itself plays a significant role in extinction learning, lesions to cortical areas have also been shown to interfere with extinction learning, demonstrating that the extinction processes require top-down control and interactions between both cortical and subcortical regions (LeDoux, 2000; Maren and Quirk, 2004).

The prefrontal cortex has been widely accepted to play a role in extinction of conditioned fear, as it is important for adjusting behaviors appropriately when the emotional salience of a given stimulus changes (Sotres-Bayon and Quirk, 2010). The ventromedial prefrontal cortex (vmPFC), in particular, has been shown to be important for making the switch from fear expression to fear inhibition during fear extinction learning and retention of extinction memory (Phelps et al., 2004). Further subdividing this cortical area, distinct subregions within the vmPFC have been differentially implicated in the expression and extinction of conditioned fear in the rodent (Sotres-Bayon and Quirk, 2010). Specifically, the dorsally located prelimbic (PL) cortex is associated with production of conditioned fear responses and expression of conditioned fear behaviors, whereas the more ventrally located infralimbic (IL) cortex is associated with inhibition of conditioned fear responses typically seen during successful extinction learning and upon recall of extinction memory (Myers and Davis, 2007). Importantly, the vmPFC–hippocampus network can modulate extinction learning by picking up on contextual cues present in the surrounding environment (Maren, 2011) and lead to appropriate alterations in plasticity. During repeated presentations of a previously negative CS, in the absence of a US, the vmPFC exerts inhibitory effects on amygdala circuitry, particularly through its excitatory glutamatergic projections to intra-amygdalar inhibitory GABAergic interneurons (Milad and Quirk, 2012; Sotres-Bayon et al., 2006). These inhibitory interneurons, or intercalated cells (ITC cells), receive projections from PL or LA neurons during fear conditioning to relieve inhibition on inhibitory CE neurons, thus resulting in expression of fear and associated autonomic responses. During extinction learning, however, a subset of these ITC cells can be activated by inputs from IL, which together with its modulation by the hippocampus can lead to downstream active inhibition of CE output neurons, thus decreasing fear expression and the associated physiological responses. These complex interactions between the vmPFC, amygdala, and hippocampus during extinction of previously conditioned fear memories are necessary for adjusting behavioral and autonomic responses in rapidly changing environments, and vmPFC–hippocampus–amygdala circuitry is altered in patients with impairments in extinction learning associated with PTSD (Mahan and Ressler, 2011).

DEVELOPMENTAL TRANSITIONS IN FEAR ACROSS THE LIFE SPAN: ECOLOGICAL SIGNIFICANCE

In children and other species, fear responses are developmentally delayed and seemingly emerge when fear expression fits the ecological niche of a particular developmental stage.

The developing fear response continues to be modified and sculpted throughout ontogeny to fit the dynamic needs of the immature organism transitioning to adulthood. This delayed emergence and modification of fear expression has been documented in myriad species, including humans and rodents, for both natural and learned fears. More recently, the neural basis for developmental changes in fear learning has been described in rodents, some of which will be reviewed here. First, we describe the emergence of amygdala-dependent learned fear to the CS odor cue around postnatal (P) day 10, along with its control by corticosterone (CORT) through P15. Second, we describe the emergence of hippocampal–dependent context fear learning around weaning. Together, these results indicate that the emergence of learned fear depends upon the developmental emergence of new brain circuit capabilities. These circuits provide animals with a nervous system and behavioral repertoire adapted to their changing ecological niche from the nest to independence. This approach of defining increased learning ability as the brain matures has been enormously helpful in providing insight into brain function.

More importantly, current developmental research has highlighted the importance of modification of existing fear circuitry to alter the developing animals' behavior to fit the dynamic ecological niche associated with development. We highlight two examples. First, we review literature showing the importance of maternal presence in suppressing fear learning through suppression of amygdala plasticity. Second, we review the surprising recent demonstration of suppressed contextual fear during a brief period during adolescence. These results illustrate the importance of developmental adaptations as animals' move through different ecological niches ranging from a helpless, essentially poikilothermic neonatal pup to the weanling developing skills for independence to the adolescent embarking on an independent life.

DEVELOPMENT OF CUE FEAR: INFANCY TO SEMI-INDEPENDENCE

Research over the past few decades has provided a basic understanding of the ontogeny of fear learning in infant rat pups. It is a history of slowly discovering the importance of assessing learning through pups' ecological niche rather than an immature version of the adult. In the case of infant animals, it is critical to assess fear development within the context of attachment and the infant's dependency on the caregiver for survival.

EARLY-LIFE LIMITATIONS ON FEAR/AVOIDANCE LEARNING: CUE FEAR CONDITIONING

Across species, infant fear learning is characterized by limitations and constraints. For example, during the temporally limited imprinting period in chicks, a moderate electric shock paired with the surrogate caregiver actually enhances following of the surrogate, although this same procedure supports avoidance learning after the imprinting critical period closes. Similarly, pairing of an odor and pain (moderate intensity shock, tail pinch, or rough handling by the caregiver) in rat pup results in a strong learned approach to the odor present during the pain (Camp and Rudy, 1988; Sullivan et al., 2000). This paradoxical preference learning occurs despite a robust pain response in pups. Thus, rat pups have an attenuated-cue fear-learning circuit, but more paradoxically, pups learn to approach odors previously associated with moderate pain. We refer to this early period in pups' life as the Sensitive Period for attachment, which ends at P10, and is illustrated in Figure 44.2. As is discussed in the following, this odor–pain learned approach response seems to have relied not only on a suppressed fear system but also activation of the rat pups' attachment system and learning about the caregiver.

AMYGDALA AND EARLY-LIFE LIMITATIONS ON FEAR/AVOIDANCE LEARNING

Evidence suggests that a lack of amygdala plasticity plays a leading role in pups' attenuated fear learning during the Sensitive Period. Specifically, the amygdala is not recruited during infant learning in controlled classical fear conditioning outside the nest nor within natural learning paradigms with an abusive mother used to deliver the aversive stimuli within the nest (Raineki et al., 2012; Raineki et al., 2010b). As was reviewed previously, in older animals including rodents and humans, the amygdala is a critical brain area for fear learning. At least in very young neonatal pups, lack of amygdala plasticity in early-life learning is due in part to amygdala immaturity, with peak neurogenesis and nuclei subdivision occurring as early as the first week of life, which is quickly followed by peak synaptogenesis at P10-20 (Berdel et al., 1997). Importantly, significant synaptic plasticity, as indicated by amygdala basolateral LTP, emerges at the same age as the emergence of amygdala-dependent fear learning (reviewed in Sullivan and Holman, 2010).

ECOLOGICAL PERSPECTIVE ON EARLY-LIFE LIMITATIONS ON FEAR/AVOIDANCE LEARNING

From an ecological perspective, an attenuated fear–learning system appears to have adaptive value since young rat pups rely on odor learning to support attachment to their mother.

Specifically, in early life, rat pups cannot see or hear and rely on their sense of smell to interact with the mother and attach to her nipples, using the maternal odor. The diet-dependent maternal odor is learned. An evolutionary explanation that we have suggested for this paradoxical learning proposes that it is better for an altricial infant to have a bad caretaker than no caretaker, as an altricial infant rat is dependent upon access to the mother's milk, her warmth, and protection. We further suggest that the fear-learning system is suppressed in early life and that a very broad range of both painful and nurturing stimuli function as a reward to support the learning that is critically important for pup survival (for review, see Sullivan and Holman, 2010).

It should be noted that pups can learn to avoid odors if paired with malaise, such as that produced by a LiCl injection or strong 1.0 mA shock, although unlike the adult, this learning does not depend upon the amygdala (Shionoya et al., 2006; Smotherman, 1982). Together, decades of research indicate that amygdala-dependent fear (cue learning) is not learned by infant rats during the Sensitive Period, although nonamygdala odor avoidance can be learned in perinatal rats provided the aversive stimuli produces malaise (strong shock, LiCl). This failure to engage amygdala plasticity for fear learning is coincident with engagement of the attachment circuitry and paradoxical support of approach/preference learning, despite pups experiencing pain.

DEVELOPMENTAL TRANSITIONS IN CUE FEAR: ROLE OF CORTICOSTERONE

While the developmental emergence of cue fear learning parallels amygdala plasticity and maturation, pharmacological manipulations of pups' CORT proved to be a critical factor in amygdala's functional emergence. Specifically, CORT manipulation uncovered a learning circuit that is malleable by the early environment, which further sculpts the fear learning circuitry to fit pups' ecological niche. As we outline the effects of CORT on pup fear learning, it is important to know that, unlike adults, which mount a robust CORT increase when stressed, infant rats have a Stress Hyporesponsive Period (SHRP) where painful and stressful events typically fail to increase pups'

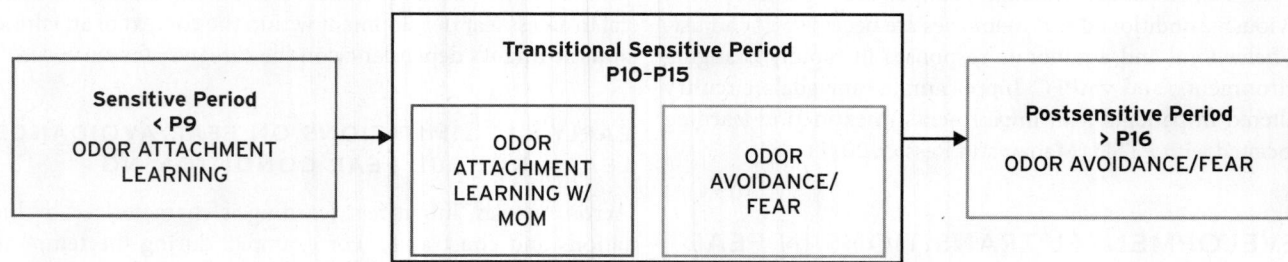

Figure 44.2 *This schematic represents rat pups' developmental transitions associated with odor-0.5mA shock conditioning. Pups have a sensitive period for attachment learning through P9: odor-0.5mA shock conditioning results in a learned odor preference and a new maternal odor used by pups for attachment (illustrated by Dark gray box), regardless of maternal presence. Fear cue learning emerges at P10 but also begins the Transitional Sensitive Period (from P10 to P15) when CORT level can determine whether fear is learned: decreasing CORT either pharmacologically or naturally through maternal presence prevents fear learning and supports attachment learning (Dark gray box), while increasing CORT permits fear learning (Light gray box). Pups P16 and older learn to fear odors previously paired with shock (Light gray box), regardless of maternal presence and represents the Postsensitive Period.*

CORT (Dallman, 2000). Sensory stimulation provided by the mother during nursing and grooming seems to control the pups' SHRP, with prolonged removal of the mother's stimulation (i.e., maternal deprivation procedure) causing increasing CORT, although replacement sensory stimulation returns CORT to normal SHRP levels (VanOers et al., 1998). The SHRP is hypothesized to protect the developing organism from the negative influences of stress hormones, such as reduced brain size that is associated with decreased mitosis, myelination, and granule cell genesis. More recent data outlined here also suggests that the SHRP protects pups from learning to avoid or fear their caregiver during the normal, periodic rough treatment pups receive from mothers as she enters and leaves the nest.

Recently, stress-induced heightened rough maternal care has proven to be an ecologically relevant paradigm that produces a premature elevation in pups' CORT (Gilles et al., 1996). This model relies on insufficient bedding material for the mother's nest building and is a continuous stressor for the mother and pups. The mother repeatedly engages in nest building, which causes her to spend longer time away from her pups, but also to trample on and transport pups more frequently, although pups gain weight normally (Raineki et al., 2012).

CORT modifications and stress have immediate effects on pups' brain and behavior, including determining pups' odor–shock learning: if CORT is elevated, pups learn avoidance/fear, but with low CORT pups learn odor approach/attachment. Specifically, a systemic or intra-amygdala injection of CORT during 0.5mA odor–shock conditioning is sufficient to support amygdala-dependent fear learning in Sensitive Period pups (Moriceau and Sullivan, 2006). Conversely, decreasing CORT, either systemically or when restricted to the amygdala in older pups (P10-16), is capable of reinstating attachment learning and blocking fear. This is in sharp contrast to the modulatory role of CORT in adult fear conditioning, where fear/avoidance learning is simply strengthened or weakened by the level of CORT.

The critical importance of CORT has also been demonstrated in an ecologically significant manner. Specifically, being reared by a mother handling her pups roughly (i.e., insufficient bedding paradigm) can prematurely increase pups' CORT and ends the SHRP early. Specifically, pups reared with this aberrant rearing have early termination of the SHRP but also premature termination of the Sensitive Period and access to amygdala-dependent fear learning (reviewed in Sullivan and Holman, 2010).

Naturalistic suppression of the CORT system is also able to block fear learning in young pups and provides ecological relevance to the important role of CORT. Specifically, attenuation of the shock-induced CORT release has been demonstrated by maternal presence in older animals, a phenomenon known as social buffering. This naturalistic maternal social buffering not only blocks amygdala-dependent fear learning but also reinstates the attachment odor learning of a new maternal odor (Moriceau and Sullivan, 2006). After P15, only fear will be learned during an odor–shock conditioning with maternal presence, and social buffering is no longer sufficient to either block fear or support attachment learning. Furthermore, we have verified the causal

relationship between maternal presence and suppression of a shock-induced CORT release in pups' odor aversion learning by systemic and intra-amygdala CORT infusions, which then permit pups to learn odor aversions even in the presence of the mother (Moriceau and Sullivan, 2006).

DEVELOPMENT OF CONTEXT FEAR LEARNING: WEANING TO PERIADOLESCENCE

Previous work has shown that, in rats, contextual fear learning ontogenetically emerges at weaning age when pups are beginning independent life (Raineki et al., 2010; Rudy, 1993). Other hippocampal-dependent behaviors, such as latent inhibition, spontaneous alternation, and spatial navigation, have been assessed in rat pups and appear to emerge at a slightly younger age (reviewed in Raineki et al., 2010a). It should be noted that contextual fear conditioning is not a unitary phenomenon, nor is the hippocampus the sole supporter of this learning and memory. Indeed, context can be broadly characterized by configural (the environment as a whole or the relationship between environmental elements) and elemental (isolated or specific features or cues in the environment) conditioning, with the latter more dependent upon hippocampus–amygdala interactions. The complexity of context learning and its interaction with the hippocampus and amygdala remains controversial and has received little attention developmentally.

Furthermore, developmental studies have rarely directly assessed the causal relationship between context learning and the hippocampus, which is problematic because contextual fear learning involves structures other than the hippocampus. However, by weaning, the hippocampus seems sufficiently mature for learning-associated plasticity (Benes et al., 1994), and silencing of the hippocampus in postweanling rats abolishes contextual fear learning (Raineki et al., 2010a). The hippocampus is divided into distinct sections and basically a trisynaptic circuit relaying information through the dentate gyrus (DG), CA3, and CA1, with each hippocampal subdivision implicated in different aspects of context fear learning and unique developmental trajectories that continue through adolescence. Importantly, at least a few important neuronal characteristics associated with plasticity do not emerge until the second to third week of life, including LTP and glutamatergic synapses (reviewed in Raineki et al., 2010a). The implications of infant fear memories formed before maturation of the hippocampus and contextual learning has yet to be explored. However, this lack of context constraint on learning likely has implications for fear behaviors that might be appropriate in one place but not another.

ENDURING EFFECTS OF INFANT ODOR–SHOCK AND MATERNAL ODOR LEARNING: CUE AND CONTEXT

Basic and clinical research has long recognized the importance of early-life experience, especially trauma within attachment, in producing particularly pronounced vulnerability to later life psychiatric disorders in humans, as well as rodent and non-human primate animal models (Monk et al., 2003). However, onset of most psychopathologies does not occur until later in life, generally around periadolescence, although possibly expressed as deficits in social behavior early in life (Letcher et al., 2012), which has been modeled in the rodent (Raineki et al., 2012).

The questions of *how* early disruptions to infant attachment effects later behavior remains largely unclear, although nonhuman animal models (maternal separation/deprivation, rearing environment alteration, CORT manipulation, neonatal handling, etc.) have provided a clear link between infant experience, stress, and later life neurobehavioral deficits that appear to target many brain areas, including the amygdala, cerebellum, prefrontal cortex, hippocampus, and stress axis. Since the amygdala and hippocampus are targets of the early life stress, later life fear conditioning is impacted.

The infant odor–shock manipulation described here also appears to target the amygdala. Specifically, experience with paired odor–shock in early life appears to cause not only accelerated maturation of the amygdala and termination of early-life attachment learning sensitive period (Raineki et al., 2012; Raineki et al., 2010b), but also enduring effects related to depressive-like behavior. Importantly, unpaired odor–shock conditioning, which does not produce cue or context learning, producing later life heightened anxiety (reviewed in Sullivan and Holman, 2010), does not alter either early-life attachment learning or later life fear learning (Sevelinges et al., 2011). Thus, the pain of shock is not the critical factor producing many of the enduring effects of infant experience; rather, it is the pairing of the odor–shock and activation of the learning attachment circuitry that is critical for enduring effects. Additional literature, which has modeled early-life adversity using infant shock, suggests that the predictable versus unpredictable manner of early shock influences emotional outcome and learning.

ODOR VALUE: THE IMPORTANCE OF THE INFANT ODOR IS RETAINED INTO LATER LIFE BEHAVIOR—IMPLICATIONS FOR FEAR AND ANXIETY

The attachment odor learned by infants continues to be approached into adulthood, even when it was learned through odor–pain pairings. The odor continues to be used in attachment through reproduction, consistent with other species and imprinting. The infant-learned attachment odors, including those associated with pain, also continue to elicit both enhanced olfactory bulb neural responses and attenuated amygdala activation and conditioned fear into adulthood.

The clinical literature suggests that cues associated with early-life trauma are not always avoided. Indeed, a strong attraction and comfort can sometimes be elicited by the cues associated with early-life maltreatment (Haynes-Seman, 1987). We have begun to explore the value of the odor associated with early-life maltreatment and questioned whether this odor could restore or rescue (bring to control levels) brain and behaviors

in animal models of psychiatric disorders. Specifically, a recent study showed that infant experience with a maltreating mother rat or odor–shock conditioning produced later life depressive-like behaviors, as indicated by performance in the forced swim test and sucrose consumption test (Sevelinges et al., 2011). These depressive-like behaviors were associated with a deficit in paired pulse inhibition in the amygdala, suggesting altered synaptic function. Interestingly, presentation of the shock-associated conditioned maternal odor during both the forced swim test and sucrose test brought performance and amygdala functioning to control levels. We speculated that the odor may have acquired the value of a "paradoxical safety signal," since safety signals reduce conditioned fear responses, normalize forced swim tests (decrease immobility), and normalize amygdala activity. A "safety signal" is typically formed when it predicts the absence of the aversive event in a fear conditioning paradigm and subsequently produces a reduction in fear and/or anxiety and amygdala activity in both humans and rodents (Pollak et al., 2008; Sevelinges et al., 2011). We speculate that, since the mother or her attributes are viewed as a safety signal, and the rat pups' natural maternal odor or learned (odor–shock) maternal odor normalizes their adult depressive-like behavior and amygdala paired pulse inhibition deficit, this odor could be functioning as a safety signal.

BRAIN MATURATION, ANXIETY, AND ADOLESCENCE

The transition between the dependence of childhood to the independence of adulthood is a dynamic developmental period, known as adolescence, associated with emotional, psychological, social, and physical changes, and hormonal fluctuations ultimately leading toward sexual maturity (Schulz et al., 2009; Sisk and Zehr, 2005). The very nature of adolescent development serves to launch an organism toward reproductive success and survival and is associated with increased exploratory behavior and emotional reactivity (Spear, 2000). As such, it is probable that within this adaptive and necessary developmental transition exist neural and behavioral characteristics divergent from those of dependent children and independent adults, which are uniquely specific to the adolescent.

Adolescence, in particular, is a period of increased prevalence of psychopathology (Monk et al., 2003), and it is estimated that over 75% of adults with fear-related disorders met diagnostic criteria as children and adolescents (Kim-Cohen et al., 2003). Prevalence of emotional disorders, and anxiety disorders specifically, is heightened during adolescent years, occurring in as many as 1 in 10 adolescents (Kessler et al., 2005); yet, due to insufficient or inaccurate diagnosis and a dearth of pediatric and adolescent specialized treatments, fewer than one in five anxious children or adolescents are expected to receive treatment for their disorders (Merikangas et al., 2010), leaving a vast number with inadequate or no treatment (Liberman et al., 2006). The inflated frequency of anxiety disorders in pediatric and adolescent populations highlights the importance of recognizing neural mechanisms of fear regulation from a developmental perspective. This increased prevalence for anxiety and affective disorders during adolescence coincides with a period of massive cortical rearrangement that is normatively accompanied by drastic cognitive and behavioral changes (Spear, 2000), and longitudinal studies of brain maturation illustrate a nonlinear process that is not complete until early adulthood (Giedd et al., 1999; Gogtay et al., 2004).

ADOLESCENT FEAR—BEHAVIORAL AND MOLECULAR FINDINGS IN MICE AND HUMANS

As previously outlined in earlier chapter sections, responses in the amygdala and medial prefrontal cortex are inversely related, and decreased functional connectivity between the two regions has been associated with anxiety in adults (Milad and Quirk, 2012). Advances in the developmental neurobiology of emotion regulation have yielded substantial evidence of protracted development of prefrontal regions relative to phylogenetically older regions (Casey et al., 2005). Consistent with developmental changes in structural maturation, immature prefrontal functioning and top-down control of subcortical regions have been observed in adolescents relative to adults during emotional contexts (Hare et al., 2008).

The investigation of learned fear acquisition and extinction across development in humans has previously been limited due to the nature of aversive conditioning paradigms, which often utilize an electric shock as the US. As this US is not as feasible for use with children, various groups have recently employed techniques incorporating loud tones (Craske et al., 2008), aversive airpuffs to the larynx (Grillon et al., 1998), or airpuffs paired with loud screams and aversive faces (Schmitz et al., 2011). Because variations with US delivery and behavioral assessment in humans yield inconsistent results (Glenn et al., 2011), animal models have more recently been relied upon for studying developmental effects of fear learning.

Studies examining the mechanisms of hippocampal-dependent contextual fear and amygdala-dependent cued fear acquisition and extinction in rodent models have traditionally excluded adolescent ages, choosing to focus on earlier developmental ages and adults (Moriceau and Sullivan, 2006; Rudy, 1993). Recently, these previously excluded intermediate ages have been investigated due to the translational relevance of studying fear during adolescent development, when increased prevalence of fear-related disorders typically emerges.

DEVELOPMENT OF CUE FEAR EXTINCTION AND PFC

Building upon studies of structural and functional human brain maturation, a number of translational studies have begun to explore extinction of amygdala-dependent cue fear in rats across development. While cue fear learning emerges during early infancy (Sullivan et al., 2000), adult-like extinction fails to develop until much later. For example, while the mPFC is critical for adult extinction, inactivation of the mPFC

fails to disrupt long-term extinction in preadolescent, P17 rats, suggesting that a system more similar to forgetting may underlie early-life behavioral decrement during an extinction paradigm. Indeed, adult-like mechanisms of extinction appear intact around weaning. Specifically, inactivation of the mPFC fails to disrupt long-term extinction in preadolescent, P17 rats, yet inactivation of mPFC does disrupt this memory in P24 rats (Kim et al., 2009). Extinction training in these young age groups leads to increased levels of pMAPK in both the prelimbic and infralimbic cortices, suggestive of nonspecific, global mPFC activity, as opposed to the inverse pattern of IL/PL activity typically seen with successful adult extinction retention. A similar diffuse activation pattern, with less focal activity, has also been observed in the prefrontal cortex of human children and adolescents during tasks requiring cognitive control (Durston et al., 2006). Developmental studies of innate fear regulation in rodents demonstrate that during innate fear, the mPFC of infant rats is neither active nor responsive while the prelimbic cortex becomes active in preadolescence but does not yet regulate freezing behavior, whereas the PL in adolescents becomes functional, and activity corresponds to an appropriately expressed cued fear response (Chan et al., 2011). These developmentally altered roles in the mPFC are independent of amygdala activity, which suggest that mPFC neural circuitry develops enhanced capacities for fear regulation as an animal matures. In addition, injections of anterograde tracers placed into the BLA of developing rats show that amygdalocortical connectivity is late maturing, with fiber density reaching a plateau circa P45, thus confirming that maturation of this circuit continues into adolescence (Cunningham et al., 2002).

Despite demonstrating equivalent anxiety-like behavior, as assessed by open field, adolescent mice have been shown to exhibit increased acquisition of cued fear compared with preadolescent and adult mice (Hefner and Holmes, 2007). This heightened fear response during adolescence, typically defined in the rodent as the phase surrounding the 10 days prior to sexual maturation at postnatal day P40 (Spear, 2000), has been found to be resistant to extinction (McCallum et al., 2010). Adolescent rats require either twice as many extinction trials or a pharmacological intervention, such as the NMDA-agonist D-cycloserine, to achieve reductions in fear expression comparable to younger or older rats (McCallum et al., 2010). Attenuated fear extinction learning during adolescence is associated with a lack of activity in prefrontal cortex, specifically infralimbic cortex, as assessed by pMAPK immunohistochemistry (Kim et al., 2011) and c-Fos immunohistochemistry (Pattwell et al., 2012) compared with younger and older ages. Electrophysiological recordings at IL and PL synapses across development reveal that a fear conditioning–induced potentiation of PL synapses present in adult mice is absent in adolescent mice. Furthermore, extinction-induced enhancement of IL synaptic plasticity in adult mice is lacking in adolescent mice (Pattwell et al., 2012). Diminished fear extinction, relative to children and adults, has been shown in adolescent humans, with a cued fear-conditioning task involving aversive sounds (Pattwell et al., 2012), and parallels rodent findings as shown in Figure 44.3. Additionally, behavioral tasks using fearful or

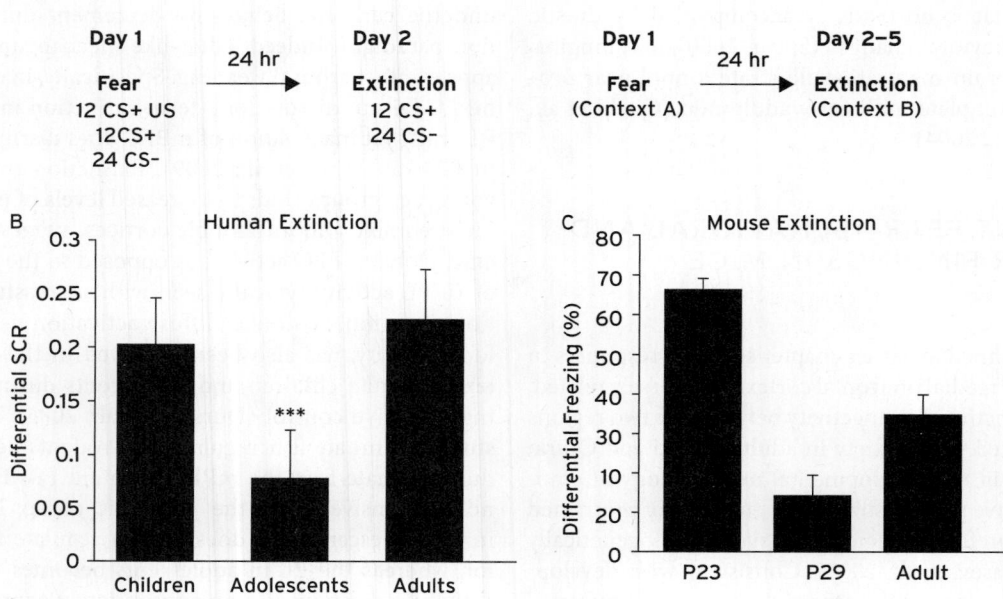

Figure 44.3 *Cued extinction learning and spontaneous recovery across development in mice and humans. (A) Behavioral paradigms for parallel fear conditioning experiments in humans and mice. (B) Analysis of extinction indices ([Averaged first two extinction trials]—[averaged last two extinction trials]) reveals a main effect of age group for humans, such that adolescents display attenuated fear extinction learning compared with children and adults (adolescent 0.05916 ± 0.06904; children 0.25435 ± 0.04839; adults 0. 22510 ± 0.05931). (C) A lack of extinction learning and retention of extinction memory is observed in adolescent mice, as displayed by a significantly decreased differential extinction indices ([Day 1, Tone 1] – [Day 4, Tone 5]) compared with older and younger ages (P23 66.5% ± 2.75; P29 14.72% ± 4.79; P70 35.17% ± 4.89). (Adapted from Figure 1 of Pattwell et al., 2012.)*

screaming faces result in heightened amygdala activity (Hare et al., 2008) and fear learning (Glenn et al., 2011) in adolescent humans, compared with younger children. Taken together, these studies reveal a nonlinear pattern in fear extinction learning and blunted regulation of amygdala-dependent fear responses during fear extinction in adolescents, which may help provide novel insight into the heightened prevalence of anxiety disorders during this period and on treating developing populations with anxiety, as the main form of CBT relies on extinction principles.

The importance of the mPFC in cued extinction learning and extinction retention is widely accepted, and inactivation of the mPFC alone is enough to impair the retrieval of cued extinction memory (Sierra-Mercado et al., 2006). Importantly, and often disregarded, however, is that inactivation of the hippocampus alone before extinction training also leads to impaired retrieval of cued extinction memory the following day, suggesting that mPFC may be an important target of the hippocampus for modulating extinction learning and recalling extinction memory in rodents and humans (Quirk and Mueller, 2008). Furthermore, contextual modulation of amygdala activity requires the hippocampus (Maren, 2011).

It is important to note that in cases where cued extinction retention and the degree of successful extinction are assessed in the same context as where conditioning took place, it may be difficult, even impossible, to claim that poor extinction learning solely results from insufficient vmPFC regulation. Many

of the extinction paradigms in the existing literature fail to account for important hippocampal contributions associated with contextual information. Distinct populations of neurons exist in the BA for triggering the activation of neuronal circuits responsible for integrating sensory and contextual information (Herry et al., 2008). These populations of "fear neurons," and "extinction neurons," as they are called, are differentially connected with the hippocampus and mPFC. Particularly, hippocampal inputs to BA preferentially target the "fear neurons," over the "extinction neurons," suggesting that hippocampal input to these neurons may override the retrieval of cued or contextual extinction memory, a likely contributor to the phenomenon of fear renewal. Fear renewal, or the fear that returns upon experiencing a reminder outside of the extinction context, remains a major obstacle for clinical treatment of anxiety disorder in humans (Mahan and Ressler, 2011) and may be the result of tipping the balance between activation between specific neuronal circuits in the hippocampus and amygdala. This clinical observation lends support for finding better treatment methods, perhaps through further investigation of hippocampally mediated techniques, such as contextual-based extinction.

DEVELOPMENT OF CONTEXTUAL FEAR AND CONTEXTUAL EXTINCTION

From a developmental perspective, the notion of hippocampal involvement in mediating both contextual and cued fear processing is a promising one. While the hippocampal cyto-architecture is well established by 34 weeks *in utero* in the human (Arnold and Trojanowski, 1996), as is noted earlier, development of this structure has been shown to continue through adolescence in both rodents and primates (Benes et al., 1994). Longitudinal scans of children and adolescents, between the ages of 4 and 25 years, reveal that postnatal hippocampal development is not homogenous and that distinct maturational profiles exist for specific subregions (Gogtay et al., 2006). While overall hippocampal volume remains constant throughout these ages, posterior subregions of the hippocampus show volumetric enlargement over time while anterior regions undergo substantial volumetric reductions. The cause of these heterogeneous volume changes remains unknown, but it is hypothesized that they may be due to differences in neuronal proliferation, synaptic production and/or pruning, myelination, or glial alterations and may parallel differences in functional development (Gogtay et al., 2006). Of note, the anterior region of the hippocampus, which exhibits decreases in volume as a function of age, is reciprocally connected to the prefrontal cortex (Cavada et al., 2000), amygdala (Pitkanen et al., 2000), and hypothalamic-pituitary-adrenal axis (Bannerman et al., 2004)—regions implicated in fear and anxiety. This heterogeneous postnatal development of hippocampal subregions, specifically the volumetric decreases observed in the anterior region, correlates with contextual fear data showing that contextual fear expression during preadolescent ages is intact, is temporarily suppressed during adolescence, and then reemerges again during adulthood (Pattwell et al., 2011) (Fig. 44.4), supporting the notion that development is not a linear process in which neural maturation occurs uniformly in one direction or another. Rather, an intricate reciprocal balance

between neural development in one brain region may lead to alterations in another region. Convergent adolescent and adult rodent contextual fear data further highlight the importance of the developing hippocampus in mediating fear responses. The aforementioned literature on human and nonhuman primate hippocampal development suggests a developmentally sensitive fear circuitry model, depicted in Figure 44.5.

A PROPOSED MODEL OF ADOLESCENT NEURAL CIRCUITRY IN FEAR LEARNING AND MEMORY

Crosstalk between CA1 and CA3 regions of the hippocampus is required for contextual fear expression and cued fear extinction in the adult brain. The adult brain integrates specific hippocampally mediated contextual inputs, thalamic sensory inputs, and prefrontal cortical inputs within intra-amygdalar circuits to produce an appropriate behavioral response. As shown in Figure 44.5C and D, the successful retrieval of cued fear memories across preadolescence, adolescence, and adulthood (McCallum et al., 2010; Pattwell et al., 2011, 2012) suggests that sensory inputs to the lateral amygdala (LA) are functional across postnatal development. As adolescent mice are impaired on contextual fear tasks, one possibility is that preadolescent mice rely more heavily on available sensory inputs and are relying solely on elemental cues of odor, texture, and so on, to retrieve the contextual memory rather than its more complex configural elements. The successful retrieval of contextual fear memories during early, preadolescent ages, as previously shown in Pattwell et al. (2011), also suggests that aforementioned age-dependent volumetric decreases in the CA1 region of the hippocampus have yet to occur and a

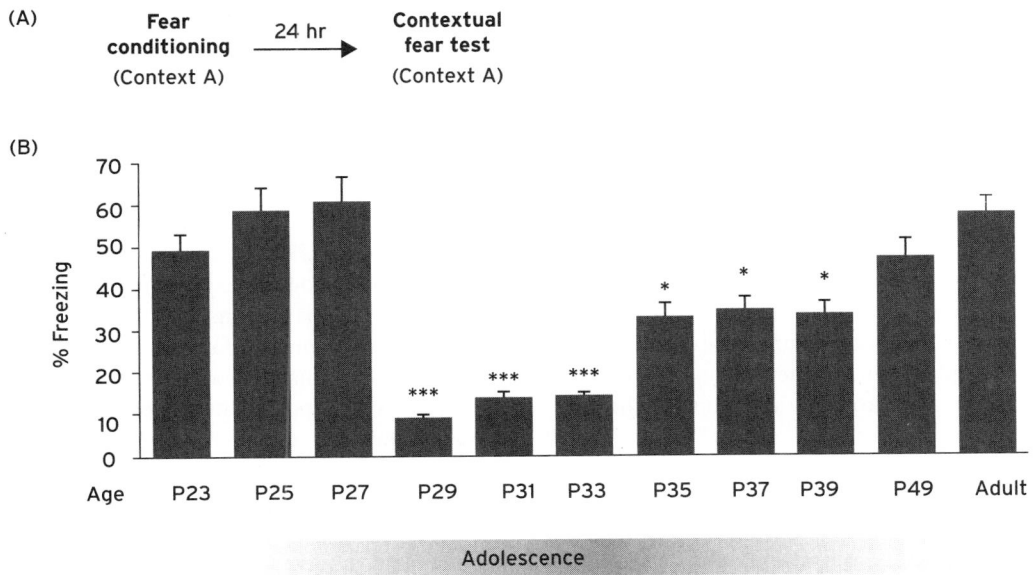

Figure 44.4 Hippocampal-dependent contextual fear memory across adolescent development. (A) Mice of all ages were fear conditioned (fear cond) with three tone–shock pairings. Twenty-four hours later, they were returned to the conditioning context (Context A) and freezing behavior was scored. (B) Adolescent mice (P29–P39) froze significantly less than both younger (P23–P27) and older (P49–P70) mice. All results are presented as a mean ± SEM. determined from analysis of 7–10 mice per group (fear conditioning) and 28 mice per group (novel object placement) (*p < 0.05, ***p < 0.001). (Adapted from Figure 1, Pattwell et al., 2011.)

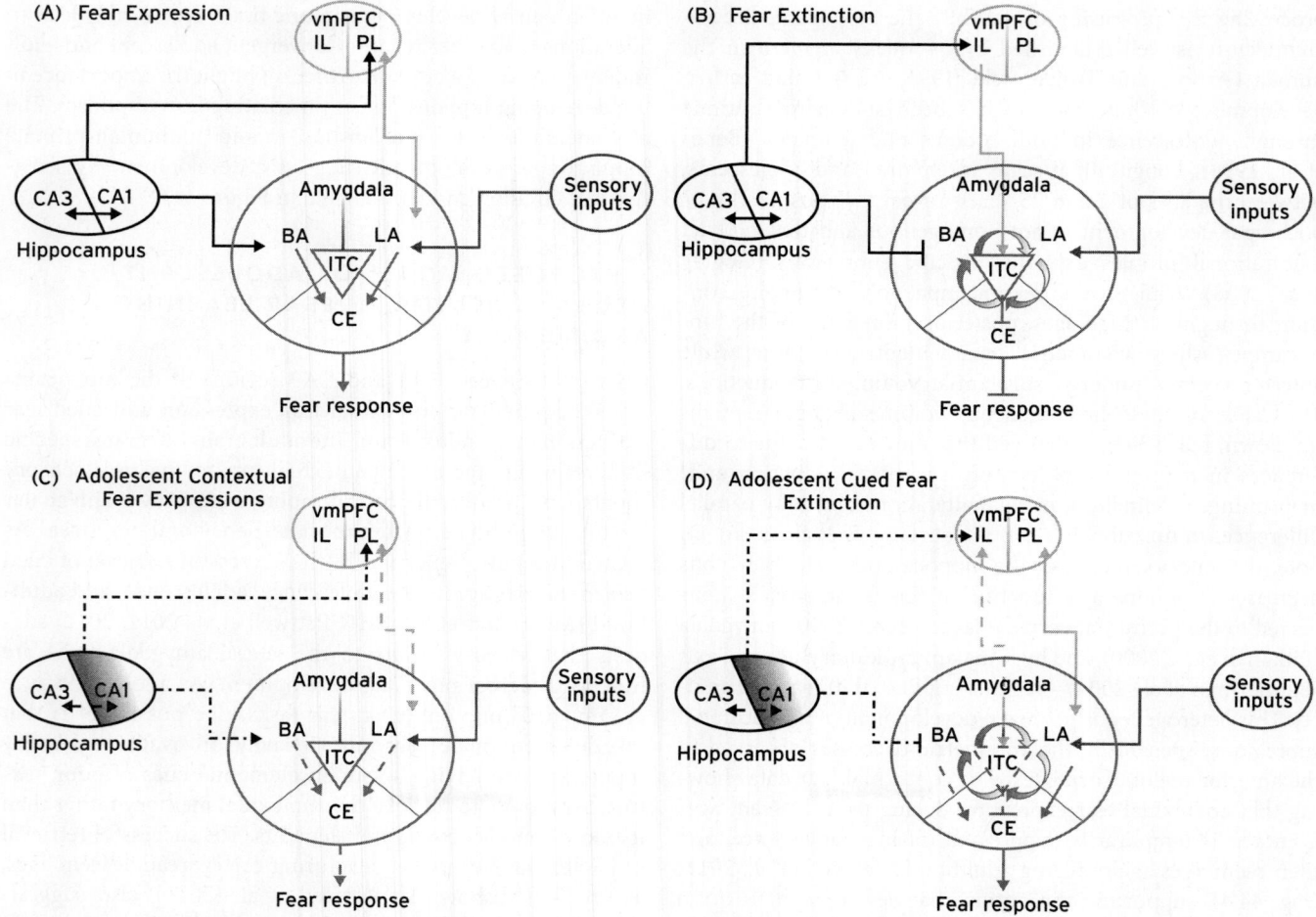

(A) Fear Expression

(B) Fear Extinction

(C) Adolescent Contextual Fear Expressions

(D) Adolescent Cued Fear Extinction

Figure 44.5 *Developmental neural circuitry of fear expression and extinction. Diagrammatic representation of adult neural circuitry implicated in (A) fear expression and (B) fear extinction. (C) A lack of contextual fear expression in adolescent mice can be traced to immature CA1. Without proper CA1–PL and CA1–BA inputs, there is a lack of downstream activation of CE output neurons, resulting in a diminished or suppressed fear response. (Weak signals and low functional connectivity represented by dotted lines.) (D) A lack of CA1 excitatory input to IL combined with a lack of CA1 inhibitory input to BA, typical in cued fear extinction, results in reduced inhibition of CE output neurons, resulting in fear expression and a lack of extinction. Arrowheads delineate pathway excitation; straight ends delineate pathway inhibition (BA, basal amygdala; LA, lateral amygdala; CE, central amygdala; vmPFC, ventromedial prefrontal cortex; PL, prelimbic cortex; IL, infralimbic cortex; ITC, intercalated cells). For simplicity, connection arrows are delineated as being unidirectional, although bidirectional projections exist. (Figures adapted from Hormones and Behavior, in press, Pattwell et al.)*

potential overabundance of active synapses between CA1–PL and CA1–BA allow for successful retrieval and expression of contextual fear. Because rodent data has also shown that bidirectional IL–amygdala synapses are later maturing than PL–amygdala synapses (Chan et al., 2011), it could also be a possibility that the amygdala has not yet received any conflicting IL inputs during preadolescence on contextual fear tests, allowing for PL–amygdala synapse activation. During adolescent development in both rodents and humans, however, vmPFC maturation can be observed (Cunningham et al., 2002; Gogtay et al., 2004), and as IL–amygdala synapses are refined, activity in PL–amygdala circuits must override IL–amygdala inputs, allowing for fear expression. Because CA1–PL connectivity is necessary for this interaction, and because CA1 undergoes volumetric decreases throughout adolescent development (Gogtay et al., 2006), which may be indicative of changes in synaptic pruning or myelination, CA1 inputs to BA and PL are not sufficient for fear expression in adolescent mice

(as represented by the shading out of CA1 and the resulting dotted arrows in Fig. 44.5C and Fig. 44.5D). This hypothesis is also supported by blunted responses in synaptic neurotransmission in BA of P29 mice upon contextual fear tests, as shown via electrophysiological experiments (Pattwell et al., 2011). Importantly, CA1 is responsible for retrieval of fear memories, while CA3 is responsible for fear acquisition and encoding of fear memories. Consistent with behavioral findings, adolescent mice acquire and consolidate contextual fear memories, despite showing impairments in retrieval and expression. Preliminary c-Fos data suggests that CA3 is active during retrieval in adolescent fear-conditioned mice (Pattwell et al., unpublished data), supporting the notion that the fear memory has been encoded and retrieved, allowing for retrieval at later, postadolescent ages when the neural circuitry underlying fear learning and memory has reached stabilized, adult-like structural and functional maturation. Further, it has been shown that inactivation of CA1 can interfere with CA3 communication with extrahippocampal regions (Lee and Kesner, 2004), such as the amygdala. With little or no fear expression and corresponding CA1–PL or CA1–BA inputs, contextual extinction and contextual reconsolidation updates appear to work remarkably well in adolescent mice to persistently attenuate fear memories, possibly due to a lack of CA1 inputs, allowing for intra-amygdalar activation of ITC cells with little or no competing input from CA1 or PL. CA1–vmPFC connectivity has also been shown to be important for retrieval of cued fear extinction, and it is possible that the lack of extinction learning and retention of extinction memory in adolescent mice (McCallum et al., 2010) may result from a similar mechanism, consistent with the developmental role of CA1 maturation in fear learning and integration with IL/PL circuits. Furthermore, due to delayed developmental maturation of cortical GABAergic transmission that extends into adolescence, it is plausible that an imbalance in inhibitory synaptic transmission during adolescence interferes with synaptic plasticity in the mPFC–hippocampus–amygdala network (Kilb, 2011).

CONCLUDING REMARKS

Here we outlined the development of the neural circuitry implicated in fear learning and discussed developmental transitions in fear learning beginning with its emergence and modifications throughout infancy and adolescence. Together, the clinical and basis research suggested that animal models may provide a plausible developmental model of fear neural circuitry that may underlie infant and adolescent fear behaviors. In particular, the development of amygdala-dependent cue fear learning first emerges in midinfancy and followed the emergence of hippocampal contextual fear learning as the infant transitions to independence. Importantly, the fear circuitry of early life needs to be explored within the context of the unique attachment circuitry of early life, where pups must learn an attachment to the caregiver. This highlights the unique importance of social cues from the mother suppressing amygdala-dependent cue learning (Barr et al., 2009; Moriceau and Sullivan, 2006; Sullivan et al., 2000). We also highlighted a unique developmental transition when the contextual fear learning is suppressed during adolescence and reemerges during adulthood (Pattwell et al., 2011). Finally, we review literature on cued fear extinction learning, which appears intact during early ages in both mice and humans, but attenuated during adolescence, and intact again in adulthood (McCallum et al., 2010; Pattwell et al., 2012). Together, these findings suggest a nonlinear pattern in the development of fear learning during infancy and adolescence, which differs from prototypical fear responses associated with both younger and older ages (Casey et al., 2008), and illustrate the importance of assessment of neurobehavioral development within the ecological niche and developmental demands of each developmental period. Infants transition from complete dependence on the caregiver with a gradual transition to independence and learning about the world. The developing organism undergoes multiple transitions during this early-life development with each transition likely requiring some unique features to adapt to the environment. For example, infancy is developmental period of complete dependence on the caregiver, when attachments must be formed for survival and access to food and protections. We suggest that cue fear learning suppression ensures that the infant only learns to approach the caregiver, despite periodic painful interactions with the caregiver. Next, as the animal transitions to the extranest environment, contextual fear learning may become important as the animal learns about spatial characteristics of the environment. However, as the animal approaches adolescence, the suppression of contextual fear learning may provide benefits since increased exploration becomes critical for reproductive success and access to additional resources. Thus, leaving the safety and stability of its environment in search of reproductive success is likely facilitated by a suppression of contextual fear to contribute to the fearlessness required for exploring new environments, typically seen with this age group (Spear, 2000). As specific danger cues are still relevant during this novelty-seeking period, cued fear expression remains intact and resistant to extinction during adolescence. Combined, these behaviors allow the adolescent to remain both exploratory and cautious, thus optimizing chances for survival and success.

As one considers how these transitions in fear learning and expression apply to psychopathology, it is important to understand that aberrant fear behaviors are associated with traumatic situations. Indeed, both infancy and adolescent traumatic experiences have been shown to alter these developmental fear transitions in both basic and clinical studies. The animal literature described here provides insight and clues to potential mechanisms unique to infancy and adolescence, with implications for unique needs for assessment and treatment across development. For example, in infancy, the failure to avoid an abusive caregiver or the failure to show immediate aberrant behavior may not be relied upon as an index of well-being during early life. Another example, in adolescence, notes that the same features of adolescent brain development required for survival may contribute to treatment resistance for disorders such a PTSD or anxiety. If nonlinear development of the neural circuitry implicated in fear learning has evolutionarily primed the adolescent to exhibit attenuated fear extinction, CBT relying on exposure therapy may need to be reconsidered as a treatment option, and new avenues may need to be explored to develop novel treatments for this developmentally distinct period to determine when, during development, specific treatments may be most effective.

DISCLOSURES

Dr. Pattwell has no conflicts of interest to disclose. Funded by NIH HD055177.

Dr. Mouly has no conflicts of interest to disclose. Funded by CNRS & ANR only. Grant Support: PICS Program (CNRS), ANR-07-NEURO-O48, Partner University Fund (PUF).

Dr. Sullivan has no conflicts of interest to disclose. Funded by NIH (DC003906; MH086952; MH091451; DC009910) and Partner University Fund (PUF).

Dr. Lee has no conflicts of interest to disclose. Funded by NIH MH079513 and NS052819.

REFERENCES

Arnold, S.E., and Trojanowski, J.Q. (1996). Human fetal hippocampal development: I. Cytoarchitecture, myeloarchitecture, and neuronal morphologic features. *J. Comp. Neurol.* 367(2):274–292.

Bannerman, D.M., Rawlins, J.N., et al. (2004). Regional dissociations within the hippocampus: memory and anxiety. *Neurosci. Biobehav. Rev.* 28(3):273–283.

Barr, G.A., Moriceau, S., et al. (2009). Transitions in infant learning are modulated by dopamine in the amygdala. *Nat. Neurosci.* 12(11):1367–1369.

Benes, F.M., Turtle, M., et al. (1994). Myelination of a key relay zone in the hippocampal formation occurs in the human brain during childhood, adolescence, and adulthood. *Arch. Gen. Psychiatry* 51(6):477–484.

Berdel, B., Morys, J., et al. (1997). Neuronal changes in the basolateral complex during development of the amygdala of the rat. *Int. J. Dev. Neurosci.* 15(6):755–765.

Bourtchouladze, R., Abel, T., et al. (1998). Different training procedures recruit either one or two critical periods for contextual memory consolidation, each of which requires protein synthesis and PKA. *Learn. Mem.* 5(4–5):365–374.

Bouton, M.E., Westbrook, R.F., et al. (2006). Contextual and temporal modulation of extinction: behavioral and biological mechanisms. *Biol. Psychiatry* 60(4):352–360.

Camp, L.L., and Rudy, J.W. (1988). Changes in the categorization of appetitive and aversive events during postnatal development of the rat. *Dev. Psychobiol.* 21(1):25–42.

Casey, B.J., Getz, S., et al. (2008). The adolescent brain. *Dev. Rev.* 28(1):62–77.

Casey, B.J., Tottenham, N., et al. (2005). Imaging the developing brain: what have we learned about cognitive development? *Trends Cogn. Sci.* 9(3):104–110.

Cavada, C., Company, T., et al. (2000). The anatomical connections of the macaque monkey orbitofrontal cortex: a review. *Cereb. Cortex* 10(3):220–242.

Chan, T., Kyere, K., et al. (2011). The role of the medial prefrontal cortex in innate fear regulation in infants, juveniles, and adolescents. *J. Neurosci.* 31(13):4991–4999.

Chen, X., Garelick, M.G., et al. (2005). PI3 kinase signaling is required for retrieval and extinction of contextual memory. *Nat. Neurosci.* 8(7):925–931.

Collins, D.R., and Pare, D. (2000). Differential fear conditioning induces reciprocal changes in the sensory responses of lateral amygdala neurons to the CS(+) and CS(-). *Learn. Mem.* 7(2):97–103.

Craske, M.G., Waters, A.M., et al. (2008). Is aversive learning a marker of risk for anxiety disorders in children? *Behav. Res. Ther.* 46(8):954–967.

Cunningham, M.G., Bhattacharyya, S., et al. (2002). Amygdalo-cortical sprouting continues into early adulthood: implications for the development of normal and abnormal function during adolescence. *J. Comp. Neurol.* 453(2):116–130.

Dallman, M.F. (2000). Moments in time: the neonatal rat hypothalamo-pituitary-adrenal axis. *Endocrinology* 141(5):1590–1592.

Durston, S., Davidson, M.C., et al. (2006). A shift from diffuse to focal cortical activity with development. *Dev. Sci.* 9(1):1–8.

Giedd, J.N., Blumenthal, J., et al. (1999). Brain development during childhood and adolescence: a longitudinal MRI study. *Nat. Neurosci.* 2(10):861–863.

Gilles, E., Schultz, L., et al. (1996). Abnormal corticosterone regulation in an immature rat model of continuous chronic stress. *Pediatr. Neurol.* 15(2):114–119.

Glenn, C.R., Klein, D.N., et al. (2011). The development of fear learning and generalization in 8–13 year-olds. *Dev. Psychobiol.* 54(7):675–684.

Gogtay, N., Giedd, J.N., et al. (2004). Dynamic mapping of human cortical development during childhood through early adulthood. *Proc. Natl. Acad. Sci. USA* 101(21):8174–8179.

Gogtay, N., Nugent, T.F., III, et al. (2006). Dynamic mapping of normal human hippocampal development. *Hippocampus* 16(8):664–672.

Grillon, C., Dierker, L., et al. (1998). Fear-potentiated startle in adolescent offspring of parents with anxiety disorders. *Biol. Psychiatry* 44(10):990–997.

Hare, T.A., Tottenham, N., et al. (2008). Biological substrates of emotional reactivity and regulation in adolescence during an emotional go-nogo task. *Biol. Psychiatry* 63(10):927–934.

Haynes-Seman, C. (1987). Developmental origins of moral masochism: a failure-to-thrive toddler's interactions with mother. *Child Abuse Negl.* 11(3):319–330.

Hefner, K., and Holmes, A. (2007). Ontogeny of fear-, anxiety- and depression-related behavior across adolescence in C57BL/6J mice. *Behav. Brain Res.* 176(2):210–215.

Herry, C., Ciocchi, S., et al. (2008). Switching on and off fear by distinct neuronal circuits. *Nature* 454(7204):600–606.

Kessler, R.C., Demler, O., et al. (2005). Prevalence and treatment of mental disorders, 1990 to 2003. *N. Engl. J. Med.* 352(24):2515–2523.

Kilb, W. (2011). Development of the GABAergic system from birth to adolescence. *Neuroscientist* 18(6):613–630.

Kim, J.H., Hamlin, A.S., et al. (2009). Fear extinction across development: the involvement of the medial prefrontal cortex as assessed by temporary inactivation and immunohistochemistry. *J. Neurosci.* 29(35):10802–10808.

Kim, J.H., Li, S., et al. (2011). Immunohistochemical analyses of long-term extinction of conditioned fear in adolescent rats. *Cereb. Cortex* 21(3):530–538.

Kim, J.J., and Fanselow, M.S. (1992). Modality-specific retrograde amnesia of fear. *Science* 256(5057):675–677.

Kim-Cohen, J., Caspi, A., et al. (2003). Prior juvenile diagnoses in adults with mental disorder: developmental follow-back of a prospective-longitudinal cohort. *Arch. Gen. Psychiatry* 60(7):709–717.

LeDoux, J.E. (2000). Emotion circuits in the brain. *Annu. Rev. Neurosci.* 23:155–184.

Lee, I., and Kesner, R.P. (2004). Differential contributions of dorsal hippocampal subregions to memory acquisition and retrieval in contextual fear-conditioning. *Hippocampus* 14(3):301–310.

Letcher, P., Sanson, A., et al. (2012). Precursors and correlates of anxiety trajectories from late childhood to late adolescence. *J. Clin. Child Adolesc. Psychol.* 41(4):417–432.

Liberman, L.C., Lipp, O.V., et al. (2006). Evidence for retarded extinction of aversive learning in anxious children. *Behav. Res. Ther.* 44(10):1491–1502.

Mahan, A.L., and Ressler, K.J. (2011). Fear conditioning, synaptic plasticity and the amygdala: implications for posttraumatic stress disorder. *Trends Neurosci.* 35(1):24–35.

Maren, S. (2001). Neurobiology of Pavlovian fear conditioning. *Annu. Rev. Neurosci.* 24:897–931.

Maren, S. (2011). Seeking a spotless mind: extinction, deconsolidation, and erasure of fear memory. *Neuron* 70(5):830–845.

Maren, S., and Quirk, G.J. (2004). Neuronal signalling of fear memory. *Nat. Rev. Neurosci.* 5(11):844–852.

McCallum, J., Kim, J.H., et al. (2010). Impaired extinction retention in adolescent rats: effects of D-cycloserine. *Neuropsychopharmacology* 35(10):2134–2142.

Merikangas, K.R., He, J.P., et al. (2010). Lifetime prevalence of mental disorders in U.S. adolescents: results from the National Comorbidity Survey Replication—Adolescent Supplement (NCS-A). *J. Am. Acad. Child Adolesc. Psychiatry* 49(10):980–989.

Milad, M.R., and Quirk, G.J. (2012). Fear extinction as a model for translational neuroscience: ten years of progress. *Annu. Rev. Psychol.* 63:129–151.

Monk, C.S., McClure, E.B., et al. (2003). Adolescent immaturity in attention-related brain engagement to emotional facial expressions. *NeuroImage* 20(1):420–428.

Moriceau, S., and Sullivan, R.M. (2006). Maternal presence serves as a switch between learning fear and attraction in infancy. *Nat. Neurosci.* 9(8):1004–1006.

Myers, K.M., and Davis, M. (2007). Mechanisms of fear extinction. *Mol. Psychiatry* 12(2):120–150.

Pattwell, S.S., Bath, K.G., et al. (2011). Selective early-acquired fear memories undergo temporary suppression during adolescence. *Proc. Natl. Acad. Sci. USA* 108(3):1182–1187.

Pattwell, S.S., Duhoux, S., et al. (2012). Altered fear learning across development in both mouse and human. *Proc. Natl. Acad. Sci. USA* 109(40):16318–16323.

Pavlov, I.P. (1927). Conditioned Reflexes: An Investigation of the Physiological Activity of the Cerebral Cortex (G. Anrep, Trans.). London: Oxford University Press.

Phelps, E.A., Delgado, M.R., et al. (2004). Extinction learning in humans: role of the amygdala and vmPFC. *Neuron* 43(6):897–905.

Phelps, E.A., and LeDoux, J.E. (2005). Contributions of the amygdala to emotion processing: from animal models to human behavior. *Neuron* 48(2):175–187.

Phillips, R.G., and LeDoux, J.E. (1992). Differential contribution of amygdala and hippocampus to cued and contextual fear conditioning. *Behav. Neurosci.* 106(2):274–285.

Pitkanen, A., Pikkarainen, M., et al. (2000). Reciprocal connections between the amygdala and the hippocampal formation, perirhinal cortex, and postrhinal cortex in rat. A review. *Ann. NY Acad. Sci.* 911:369–391.

Pollak, D.D., Monje, F.J., et al. (2008). An animal model of a behavioral intervention for depression. *Neuron* 60(1):149–161.

Quirk, G.J., and Mueller, D. (2008). Neural mechanisms of extinction learning and retrieval. *Neuropsychopharmacology* 33(1):56–72.

Raineki, C., Cortes, M.R., et al. (2012). Effects of early-life abuse differ across development: infant social behavior deficits are followed by adolescent depressive-like behaviors mediated by the amygdala. *J. Neurosci.* 32(22):7758–7765.

Raineki, C., Holman, P.J., et al. (2010). Functional emergence of the hippocampus in context fear learning in infant rats. *Hippocampus* 20(9):1037–1046.

Raineki, C., Moriceau, S., et al. (2010). Developing a neurobehavioral animal model of infant attachment to an abusive caregiver. *Biol. Psychiatry* 67(12): 1137–1145.

Rothbaum, B.O., and Davis, M. (2003). Applying learning principles to the treatment of post-trauma reactions. *Ann. NY Acad. Sci.* 1008:112–121.

Rudy, J.W. (1993). Contextual conditioning and auditory cue conditioning dissociate during development. *Behav. Neurosci.* 107(5):887–891.

Schafe, G.E., Nadel, N.V., et al. (1999). Memory consolidation for contextual and auditory fear conditioning is dependent on protein synthesis, PKA, and MAP kinase. *Learn. Mem.* 6(2):97–110.

Schmitz, A., Merikangas, K., et al. (2011). Measuring anxious responses to predictable and unpredictable threat in children and adolescents. [Research Support, N.I.H., Intramural]. *J. Exp. Child Psychol.* 110(2):159–170.

Schulz, K.M., Molenda-Figueira, H.A., et al. (2009). Back to the future: the organizational-activational hypothesis adapted to puberty and adolescence. *Horm. Behav.* 55(5):597–604.

Sevelinges, Y., Mouly, A.M., et al. (2011). Adult depression-like behavior, amygdala and olfactory cortex functions are restored by odor previously paired with shock during infant's sensitive period attachment learning. *Dev. Cogn. Neurosci.* 1(1):77–87.

Shionoya, K., Moriceau, S., et al. (2006). Development switch in neural circuitry underlying odor-malaise learning. *Learn. Mem.* 13(6):801–808.

Sierra-Mercado, D., Jr., Corcoran, K.A., et al. (2006). Inactivation of the ventromedial prefrontal cortex reduces expression of conditioned fear and impairs subsequent recall of extinction. *Eur. J. Neurosci.* 24(6):1751–1758.

Sigurdsson, T., Doyere, V., et al. (2007). Long-term potentiation in the amygdala: a cellular mechanism of fear learning and memory. *Neuropharmacology* 52(1):215–227.

Sisk, C.L., and Zehr, J.L. (2005). Pubertal hormones organize the adolescent brain and behavior. *Front. Neuroendocrin.* 26(3–4):163–174.

Smotherman, W.P. (1982). Odor aversion learning by the rat fetus. *Physiol. Behav.* 29(5):769–771.

Sotres-Bayon, F., Cain, C.K., et al. (2006). Brain mechanisms of fear extinction: historical perspectives on the contribution of prefrontal cortex. *Biol. Psychiatry* 60(4):329–336.

Sotres-Bayon, F., and Quirk, G.J. (2010). Prefrontal control of fear: more than just extinction. *Curr. Opin. Neurobiol.* 20(2):231–235.

Spear, L.P. (2000). The adolescent brain and age-related behavioral manifestations. *Neurosci. Biobehav. Rev.* 24(4):417–463.

Sullivan, R.M., and Holman, P.J. (2010). Transitions in sensitive period attachment learning in infancy: the role of corticosterone. *Neurosci. Biobehav. Rev.* 34(6):835–844.

Sullivan, R.M., Landers, M., et al. (2000). Good memories of bad events in infancy. *Nature* 407(6800):38–39.

VanOers, H., Kloet, E.D., et al. (1998). Maternal deprivation effect on the infant's neural stress markers is reversed by tactile stimulation and feeding but not by suppressing corticosterone. *Neuroscience* 18:10171–10179.

45 | FUNCTIONAL NEUROCIRCUITRY AND NEUROIMAGING STUDIES OF ANXIETY DISORDERS

MADELEINE S. GOODKIND, ANETT GYURAK, AND AMIT ETKIN

INTRODUCTION

Fear and anxiety serve adaptive survival functions, signaling to the organism the presence of potential danger in the environment. Fear is the immediate response triggered by a potentially harmful event or object, and anxiety is characterized by prolonged heightened vigilance for looming danger in the environment. The circuitry supporting fear responses is remarkably well preserved phylogenetically across species. Anxiety and fear reactions encompass a wide range of subjective, physiological, behavioral, and cognitive responses that are often experienced subjectively as unpleasant. While the line between functional and pathological fear and anxiety can be vague, once these reactions are present chronically, and to a heightened degree that generalizes to signals beyond those that are objectively dangerous, one sees emergence of clinical anxiety disorders.

Anxiety disorders are among the most common psychiatric disorders, with an estimated one-year prevalence of 18% and a lifetime prevalence of nearly 30% (Kessler et al., 2005). They negatively impact everyday functioning and quality of life (Mendlowicz and Stein, 2000). Anxiety disorders impose a considerable burden on society in terms of both treatment and workplace costs related to absenteeism and lost productivity. Meta-analyses of randomized clinical trials of CBT (cognitive-behavioral therapy) in anxiety yield medium to large effect sizes (e.g., Stewart and Chambless, 2009), however, with a negative correlation between the representativeness of the sample and the effect sizes (Stewart and Chambless, 2009). These data suggest that while in well-controlled situations we are able to provide effective treatment, the effectiveness wanes as situations become more complicated. We are also not yet able to predict who is likely to respond to treatment and why. Thus, given the enormous burden of anxiety disorders to the individual and the community, and the inability of current treatment options to sufficiently alleviate this burden, it is important to bring new tools to bear on understanding the underlying pathophysiology of anxiety disorders to inform and direct treatment. An important route to understanding pathophysiology of anxiety disorders is neuroimaging.

Pathological fear and anxiety responses have traditionally been characterized as resulting from alterations in brain systems that normally control negative emotions, especially fear. Thus, investigating the neural underpinnings of anxiety disorders begins with discussion of fear-related circuitry (see also Graham and Milad in Chapter 43 of this volume for a more in-depth discussion). However, because some anxiety disorders also involve a broader range of emotional disturbances, such as an absence of positive affect or perturbations of other negative emotions (e.g., anger), the constellation of emotional dysfunctions indicates a wider abnormality in emotional systems beyond fear circuitry. Thus, our goal is to present an updated and expanded version of our previously published integrative framework of emotional functioning in anxiety disorders that encompasses disruptions in *emotional reactivity* and highlights deficits in circuits *regulating emotional responses* (Etkin, 2009).

We organize the chapter is as follows: we start by introducing the neural circuitry relevant for fear conditioning and extinction, and emotional reactivity and regulation more broadly, by reviewing relevant neuroimaging studies. We then review neuroimaging studies of social anxiety disorder, specific phobia, generalized anxiety disorder, panic disorder, and posttraumatic stress disorder. We exclude obsessive compulsive disorder from our discussion because it appears to have a distinct neural signature from the other anxiety disorders (Etkin, 2009) and is extensively covered elsewhere in this book (see Ahmari and Simpson, Chapter 48). In each disorder, we highlight areas of disruption or preservation in emotional reactivity and emotion regulation. Although anxiety disorders are highly comorbid with each other (Kessler et al., 2005), they are differentiated by the type of cues that lead to anxious responses, the magnitude of exaggerated fear responses, and whether negative or positive affect are more generally dysregulated. To further diagnostic differentiation, we highlight disorder-specific perturbations within our integrative framework. Similarly, where there are overlaps between disorders, these are also highlighted. With a cross-diagnostic framework in mind, we examine the potential neural markers common to many or all anxiety disorders. This approach is consistent with recent research that finds single disruptions in neural circuitry often cut across many distinct syndromes.

CORE PROCESSES IN ANXIETY DISORDERS: EMOTIONAL REACTIVITY AND REGULATION

CONDITIONED FEAR AS A MODEL OF ANXIETY DISORDERS

Classical conditioning models, extensively studied in experimental animals, have elucidated how emotionally significant events are learned and remembered. In fear conditioning, a neutral stimulus that is paired with an aversive unconditioned stimulus eventually comes to signal the imminent onset of something aversive. Although fear conditioning serves an adaptive and self-preserving function, it is also believed to be implicated in the development of anxiety disorders. Fear extinction is another critical aspect of the conditioning process and refers to diminishing fear response after repeated presentations of the conditioned stimulus alone, without the unconditioned stimulus. This process is thought to reflect fear inhibition rather than unlearning (Phelps et al., 2004). Fear extinction has important implications for understanding both how an adaptive fear response transitions into an anxiety disorder and also for understanding exposure-based psychotherapeutic treatments.

Classical conditioning was first proposed as important for anxiety disorders by Watson and Rayner in their case of "Little Albert" (Watson and Rayner, 1920). In fact, relative to participants without anxiety disorders, people with anxiety disorders show greater conditioned fear responses during both acquisition and extinction phases (Lissek et al., 2005). Moreover, patients with anxiety disorders also show greater subjective and physiological fear reactivity to cues signaling safety (in addition to those that signal an aversive stimulus; Mineka and Oehlberg, 2008), consistent with the hypothesis that these patients are less able to inhibit fear responses when presented with safety signals. As such, a fear conditioning/extinction-based model explains many of the core symptoms of anxiety disorders, such as the hypervigilance for danger and avoidance of cues that provoke anxious cognitions and behaviors. However, many anxiety disorders involve emotional dysfunction beyond simply fear learning. As such, we now consider a broader view of emotion and its regulation.

EMOTIONAL REACTIVITY AND REGULATION

In the previous section, we reviewed fear responsivity. In this section, we expand on this and also include subjective, physiological, and behavioral responses to other negative emotions and to positive emotions. Emotional reactivity refers to the type and magnitude of a response to emotion-eliciting events. Processing emotional information and reacting emotionally involves a large number of cortical and subcortical regions, which have been summarized in recent meta-analyses (Kober et al., 2008; Phan et al., 2002). Emotional reactivity disturbances in anxiety disorders may include excesses of other types of negative emotions (e.g., anger in posttraumatic stress disorder) or diminished positive emotion (e.g., in social anxiety disorder a failure to attend to positive feedback).

Emotion regulation encompasses a wide range of processes. Described by Gyurak and colleagues (2011) as an attempt to influence or modulate the intensity, duration, and type of emotion experienced, regulatory processes include those that happen deliberately and consciously as well as those that occur reflexively and outside of conscious awareness. Examples of the former include changing emotional responses through distraction, reappraisal, distancing, or suppression. In this case, emotion regulation can be antecedent focused, altering emotions before they begin, or response focused, voluntarily modifying the expression of emotions. Antecedent-focused strategies are typically cognitive and include reappraising, detaching from, or distracting oneself from emotional stimuli; response-focused strategies include voluntary suppression of positive or negative emotional reactions. Studies of this type of regulation require participants to deliberately modify how they think about a given situation (e.g., "try to change how you view the situation to feel less negative emotion") or what emotions they express (e.g., "hide your emotional reactions to the situation").

Emotion regulation that occurs automatically (i.e., implicit emotion regulation) is characterized by the lack of a deliberate and conscious emotion regulatory goal, but it results in adaptive changes in behavior and emotional responding. This type of emotion regulation has received less study than explicit regulation. One way implicit emotion regulation has been measured is by using an emotional modification of the traditional Stroop conflict paradigm, in which participants view fear or happy emotional faces with the words "Fear" or "Happy" written across the front. In this task, participants identify the emotion on the face, disregarding the word that is written. Incongruence between the emotion on the face and the written word creates conflict, thereby slowing reaction time to identifying the emotion. This conflict is lessened (and reaction times are quicker) when an incongruent trial is preceded by an incongruent trial, suggesting that a regulatory mechanism is activated in the first incongruent trial and utilized in the second.

CORE STRUCTURES IN EMOTIONAL REACTIVITY AND REGULATION

AMYGDALA

The amygdala is an almond-shaped structure that sits below the temporal lobes and is associated, albeit not exclusively, with the experience of fear and anxiety (see Fig. 45.1). The human amygdala is activated in response to negative emotional stimuli and to unpredictability—cues that lead to feelings and behaviors associated with anxiety in both humans and nonhuman animals (Davis, 2002). Across species, the amygdala signals danger to an organism and provides a basis for avoiding such stimuli in the future. Lesions in the amygdala result in failure to avoid stimuli previously associated with danger (reviewed in Davis, 2002).

The amygdala is activated during the presentation of stimuli indicating fear and, more generally, when organisms are presented with salient, biologically relevant information. Suppression of neuronal activity in the amygdala leads to decreased expression of fear and anxiety across multiple species (Davis, 2002). In human participants, the amygdala is activated when participants view fearful expressions (Phan et al., 2002). Adolphs and colleagues (1995) describe a patient with bilateral calcification of the amygdala who subsequently showed selective deficits in the representation and identification of fearful facial expressions. However, this patient could represent and recognize other basic emotions. Processing of fear-specific stimuli and negative emotional stimuli generally

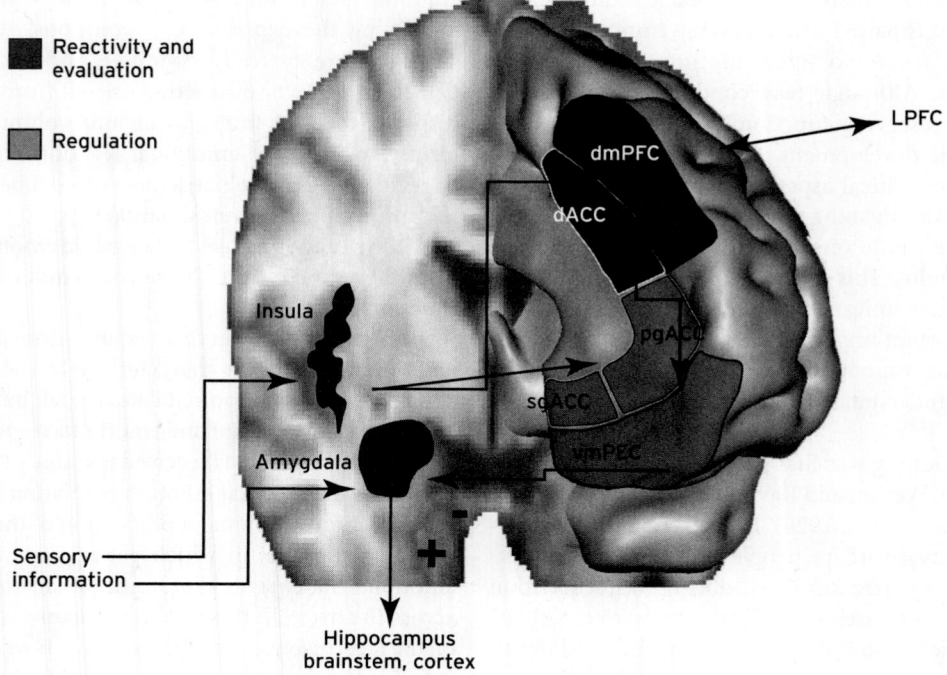

Figure 45.1 *A limbic-medial prefrontal circuit view of emotional processing. Relevant structures are separated into two groups: those involved in emotional reactivity and evaluation and those important for emotion regulation.*

can also occur outside of awareness and this also implicates the amygdala. When healthy participants are shown fearful facial expressions presented too quickly to be perceived, the amygdala is activated (Etkin et al., 2004). Additionally, the degree of amygdala activation correlates positively with self-reported anxiety and individual differences in anxiety (Stein et al., 2007).

The role of the amygdala in monitoring the environment for threatening (e.g., fear cues) and new information (e.g., unpredictable cues) implies a role for this region in hypervigilance, a symptom of many anxiety disorders. Amygdala activity is also associated with the physical reactions that accompany anxiety. In rats, increasing amygdala activity by injecting GABA antagonists leads to increases in blood pressure and heart rate (Sanders and Shekhar, 1991). Electrical stimulation of this region in human participants elicits feelings of fear, anxiety, and apprehension, and direct injection of benzodiazepines into the amygdala has anxiolytic effects (Davis, 2002).

The amygdala is critical in fear conditioning, as demonstrated by fear conditioning studies in experimental animals (Davis, 2002) and in humans (Phelps et al., 2004). The amygdala is activated when participants view stimuli that predict an aversive event, and amygdala lesions in human and experimental animals lead to deficits in conditioned and unconditioned fear (Davis, 2002). For example, lesions in the amygdala result in disrupted Galvanic skin responses during classical fear conditioning tasks (LaBar et al., 1995). In a neuroimaging meta-analysis, we report consistently increased amygdala activation during fear conditioning in healthy subjects (Etkin and Wager, 2007). Additionally, the amygdala is important when changes in conditioned responses occur, such as devaluation of a stimulus when it

is switched to signal aversive rather than appetitive information (Davis, 2002).

The amygdala it not a unitary structure, however, and can be partitioned into multiple subregions, each with specific efferent and afferent projections. Two subregions have been particularly well studied in the context of fear and anxiety, due to their roles in distinct aspects of the fear response. The basolateral amygdala (BLA) is the primary subregion that receives sensory information, coming in from the thalamus and sensory and association cortices, and in turn projects to thalamic and cortical regions, including those that provide input into the BLA (Davis, 2002). Research in rodents has found that the BLA evaluates and encodes the value of a threatening stimulus (Davis, 2002). In rats, the BLA responds differently to odors signaling positive versus negative stimuli and these reactions precede behavioral changes. In humans, the BLA responds to nonconsciously presented fearful emotional expressions (Etkin et al., 2004). Similarly, the lateral ventral amygdala in humans is most responsive to negative stimuli (especially if the stimuli signal impending negative information) (Whalen et al., 2008).

Cortical regions that project to and receive projections from the BLA include those involved in sensory functions and medial prefrontal regions (described in this chapter).

Another critical subregion is the centromedial amygdala (CMA) located dorsal to the BLA in humans, which has primarily subcortical projections, especially those to the brain stem hypothalamus, and periaqueductal gray (PAG) (Pitkanen, 1997). These projections may explain in part the physiological responses associated with fear, as the hypothalamus is important in sympathetic nervous system responding, and the brain stem and PAG with stereotyped species-specific defensive behavior. The CMA elicits these responses to information

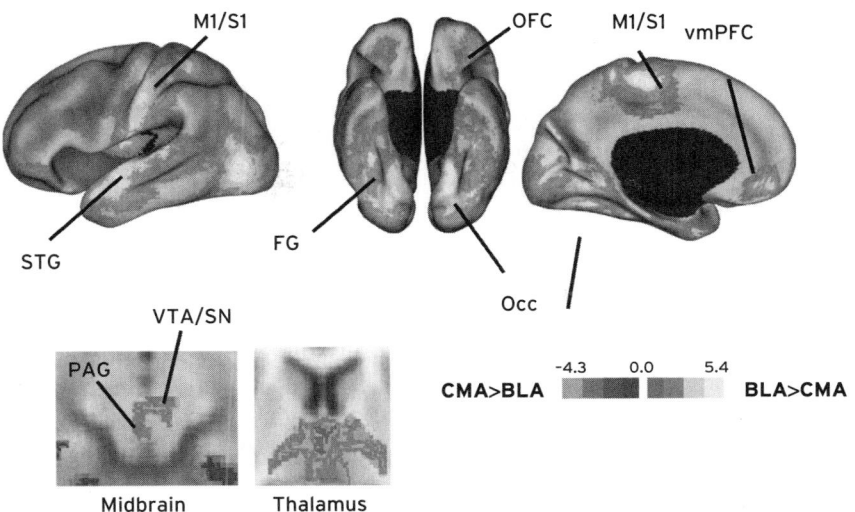

Figure 45.2 *Differential connectivity of the basolateral (BLA) and centromedial (CMA) amygdalar subregions during resting-state fMRI. Findings are from a conjunction of two cohorts of healthy participants. The BLA connectivity was primarily cortical; CMA connectivity was primarily subcortical. Color scales represent t scores for the main effect of region in a voxelwise analysis. Red indicates that BLA connectivity is increased compared with CMA connectivity; blue, CMA connectivity is increased compared with BLA connectivity. FG, fusiform gyrus; M1/S1, primary somatosensory and motor cortices; Occ, occipital cortex; OFC, orbitofrontal cortex; PAG, periaqueductal gray; STG, superior temporal gyrus; vmPFC, ventromedial prefrontal cortex; and VTA/SN, ventral tegmental area/ substantia nigra. (See color insert)*

received from BLA, which represents its primary input. Stimulation of the CMA also results in increased attention, potentially through projections to cholinergic basal forebrain targets, suggesting the importance of this region in arousal in fear and in anxiety disorders. The differentiation between the mostly cortical connections of the BLA and the mostly subcortical connections of the CMA has also been recently demonstrated with human neuroimaging by Etkin and colleagues (2009) (see Fig. 45.2).

INSULA

Another core region in the limbic circuitry is the insula. Like the amygdala, the insula consistently activates in response to negatively valenced emotional stimuli (Phan et al., 2002) and in response to emotionally salient information (Craig, 2009). The positioning of the insula between both limbic and cortical targets makes it an important node in the fear circuit (see Fig. 45.1). The insula is heavily connected with the hypothalamus, PAG, and amygdala; this region receives projections from the amygdala and projects to the anterior cingulate cortex (ACC) (Craig, 2009). Moreover, functional connectivity between the BLA and anterior insula explains 40% of the variance in anxiety levels among control participants (Baur et al., 2012). Interoceptive awareness and monitoring the autonomic nervous system have been consistently linked to this region (Craig, 2009). For example, when attending to their heartbeats, insula activation is greater for individuals with higher levels of anxiety and greater sensitivity to their own bodily responses (Craig, 2009). Internal bodily responses are often perceived by people with anxiety disorders as dangerous, and the encoding of aversive interoceptive cues has been linked to the insula (Craig, 2009).

Individuals with panic disorder show heightened sensitivity to and concern about interoceptive cues, suggesting that the insula may be especially important for understanding this condition, but also of broader relevance to other anxiety disorders.

PERIAQUEDUCTAL GRAY AND HYPOTHALAMUS

These regions are also part of the core limbic circuit and are critical in the regulation of the autonomic nervous system. The PAG is important for active defensive reactions (Davis, 2002). Activation of the PAG correlates with feelings of dread in healthy control participants in the context of impending threat (Mobbs et al., 2007). Stimulating the PAG in experimental animals leads to avoidance, defensive aggression, and cardiovascular reactivity. Stimulation of the PAG in humans leads to cardiovascular reactivity similar to a panic attack. Participants also report experiencing fear and anxiety (along with a desire to stop the stimulation) (Davis, 2002). Moreover, greater activity is seen in the PAG as threats become more proximal (Mobbs et al., 2007). As such, this region is important for rallying the appropriate behavioral response to threat, an important aspect of anxiety and anxiety disorders. The hypothalamus, in particular its ventromedial portion, is heavily connected with the PAG and amygdala and is thought to coordinate and modulate defensive behaviors (Davis, 2002). Panic symptoms or behaviors can be induced by direct stimulation of the ventromedial hypothalamus in humans (Wilent et al., 2010) and experimental animals (Lammers et al., 1998). While the PAG and hypothalamus have not been the focus thus far on studies of clinical anxiety, their roles in the behavioral response to emotional stimuli suggest that they may be quite important.

HIPPOCAMPUS

Early characterization of the limbic system in animals included the hippocampus; however, in humans, this region is most often implicated in memory and has not been heavily studied in anxiety in humans. Human studies of anxiety disorders have also not consistently implicated the hippocampus. However, in a meta-analysis of emotion, Kober and colleagues (2008) found that anterior hippocampal areas contiguous with the amygdala are part of a core limbic group that was consistently activated in emotional tasks. The hippocampus itself, however, is not a unitary structure and can be split into distinct subdivisions. Animal studies have distinguished between dorsal hippocampal regions, important for memory and other cognitive functions, and ventral hippocampal regions, important for anxiety-related behaviors and heavily connected to the amygdala and hypothalamus (Bannerman et al., 2004). In humans, these regions correspond to the posterior hippocampus, which is preferentially connected to the pregenual ACC, posterior cingulate cortex (PCC), and precuneus, and the anterior hippocampus, which is preferentially connected to the amygdala, striatum, dACC, dmPFC, and precentral gyrus (Chen and Etkin, manuscript submitted). Dorsal hippocampal impairments in rodents (i.e., posterior hippocampus in humans) result in deficits in both fear memory and spatial memory (Heldt et al., 2007). Moreover, some molecular perturbations in the dorsal hippocampus can result in normal acquisition of fear memory, but a reduction in the extinction of conditioned fear (Heldt et al., 2007). Rodents with lesions in the ventral hippocampus (i.e., anterior hippocampus in humans) fail to avoid anxiety-provoking situations and show decreased stress responses (via corticosterone response; Kjelstrup et al., 2002). In anxiety disorders, the posterior hippocampus may be important for abnormalities in fear memory and extinction, while the anterior hippocampus may be important in general fear- or anxiety-related behaviors and responses.

PREFRONTAL CORTEX

The prefrontal cortex (PFC) is thought to be critical for the monitoring and regulation of emotion; this includes a very large swath of cortex, which can be meaningfully subdivided into smaller and more clearly differentiated regions. We have previously published a detailed description of prefrontal cortical areas as they relate to negative emotional processing and thus provide a more concise version here (see Etkin et al., 2011 for a review) (see Fig. 45.1).

THE LATERAL PREFRONTAL CORTEX

The dorsolateral (dlPFC) and ventrolateral (vlPFC) prefrontal cortices are commonly associated with emotion regulation (Gyurak et al., 2011). Along with their role in cognitive control and executive functioning, these regions are typically recruited in the context of deliberate, effortful, and conscious regulation of emotion (Gyurak et al., 2011). However, as described earlier, emotion regulation can occur more reflexively and outside of our awareness, and this type of regulation implicates more medial prefrontal regions and is more directly relevant to fear- and anxiety-related regulation (Gyurak et al., 2011).

DORSAL VERSUS VENTRAL MEDIAL FRONTAL CORTEX

Regions of the medial frontal lobes, including the anterior cingulate cortex and medial prefrontal cortex (mPFC) have long been implicated in emotional processes. The original functional distinction between the dorsal and ventral ACC was that of cognitive versus emotional processing. However, consideration of more recent data suggests a more parsimonious distinction between these regions, which places the dorsal ACC (dACC) and dorsomedial prefrontal cortex (dmPFC) as important for the appraisal and expression of negative emotion and the ventral ACC (vACC) and ventromedial prefrontal cortex (vmPFC) as important for emotion regulation. Fear conditioning, and specifically fear acquisition, activates the dACC and dmPFC (Etkin et al., 2011), as does recall of fear memories and generation of fear-instructed fear responses in the absence of having undergone direct fear conditioning. Electrical stimulation of the dACC results in the subjective experience of fear. Moreover, areas of the dACC and dmPFC correlate with sympathetic nervous system activity in general and with interoceptive awareness of heartbeats. Thus, the dACC and dmPFC are critical in the appraisal, experience, and expression of fear. In terms of emotional reactivity more generally, beyond only fear, these regions are involved when participants face ambiguous or emotional conflict. Additionally, these regions are implicated in a number of other emotional situations, including those involving anger, pain, disgust, and rejection. Thus, evaluating emotional stimuli, conflict, and ambiguity involves overlapping neural circuitry as the evaluation and expression of fear. Moreover, these dorsal regions show positive connectivity with the amygdala during emotional tasks, again highlighting the role in emotional reactivity.

Many aspects of regulation draw on the vACC and vmPFC. These regions are important in fear extinction and recalling inhibitory extinction memories a day or more after training. Similarly, the vACC/vmPFC is activated when exposure to a distant threat occurs, suggesting it may be involved in planning adaptive responses, a regulatory function. In contrast to the dACC/dmPFC, the vACC/vmPFC shows a negative correlation with sympathetic activity and with PAG activation. Consistent with the role of these regions in regulating fear, the vACC and vmPFC are also involved in the regulation of other emotions and regulating emotional conflict. Similar to extinction of fear learning, the extinction of appetitive learning activates the vmPFC. Using the emotional conflict task, an incongruent trial that is preceded by an incongruent trial, during which conflict regulation has been increased, activates these ventral regions. Thus, the circuitry involved in the regulation of emotional conflict is comparable to that involved in extinction, likely reflecting a broader role for the vACC/vmPFC in implicit emotion regulation. Of note, the vACC does not regulate conflict arising from nonaffective stimuli, which instead is regulated by lateral PFC regions (Egner et al., 2008). Finally, the vACC/vmPFC shows negative connectivity with the amygdala in a range of tasks. During explicit emotion regulation, the vACC may act as an intermediary between lateral prefrontal regions and the amygdala.

NEUROCIRCUITRY OF ANXIETY IN SPECIFIC DISORDERS

Recent neuroimaging studies have begun to characterize the distinct neural deficits associated with anxiety disorders. For example, in a meta-analysis looking across three anxiety disorders (posttraumatic stress disorder [PTSD], social anxiety disorder [SAD], and specific phobia), we find amygdala and insula hyperreactivity in all three disorders and in control participants during fear conditioning (Etkin and Wager, 2007; see Figs. 45.3 and 45.4). These results point to exaggerated engagement of fear circuitry across anxiety disorders. However, this meta-analysis also points to differences across the three disorders, for example, in regions important for emotion regulation. In the following sections, we review in greater depth the functional neuroimaging literature for similarities and differences across five anxiety disorders (SAD, specific phobia, generalized anxiety disorder, panic disorder, and PTSD). We emphasize those studies that include symptom provocation tasks (e.g., using sounds, images, or scripts to evoke disorder-specific symptoms), fear conditioning, or general emotional reactivity and regulation tasks (e.g., viewing emotional facial expressions).

SOCIAL ANXIETY DISORDER

Social anxiety disorder (SAD), also referred to as generalized social phobia, is a common anxiety disorder in the general community, with a 12-month prevalence of 7% (Kessler et al., 2005). This condition is associated with significant functional impairments and typically has an early onset, with the majority of cases beginning before adulthood. Patients with SAD show negativity biases in terms of the interpretation and recall of social events; the condition is characterized by distorted negative beliefs about oneself and how a person believes he/she will be judged by others (Guyer et al., 2008); as a result, individuals with SAD experience an excessive and unreasonable fear of social interactions in which these individuals anticipate negative evaluation by others. Although some evidence has found that genetics and environment play important roles (Stein et al. 2007), the exact etiology is largely unknown.

Across studies that include symptom provocation tasks or stimuli involving emotional facial expressions, patients with SAD show heightened amygdala activation (Etkin and Wager, 2007). This heightened amygdala reactivity is reported in particular when individuals with SAD view negative or ambiguous (i.e., neutral) emotional expressions (for a review, see Freitas-Ferrari et al., 2010). Among negative emotional expressions, viewing angry and contemptuous emotional faces is associated with increased amygdala activation, including in both the right and left amygdala (Freitas-Ferrari et al., 2010). Results have been mixed regarding whether there are amygdala abnormalities in response to positive emotional stimuli (Phan et al., 2006). Heightened amygdala responses are also seen when individuals with SAD anticipate or perform public speaking tasks (Freitas-Ferrari et al., 2010), read stories depicting social transgressions (Blair et al., 2010), or view phobia-related words (Schmidt et al., 2010). These tasks presumably tap into the core features of the condition, namely, performing publicly and perceiving negative judgment by others.

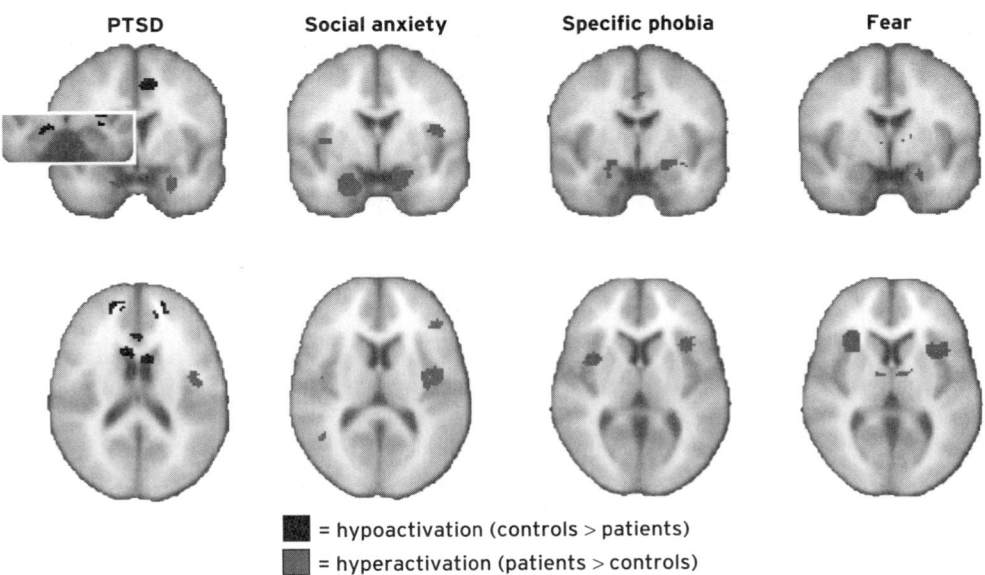

= hypoactivation (controls > patients)

= hyperactivation (patients > controls)

Figure 45.3 *Clusters in which significant hyperactivation or hypoactivation was found in patients with PTSD, social anxiety disorder (SAD), and specific phobia relative to comparison subjects and in healthy subjects undergoing fear conditioning. Notable is common hyperactivation in the amygdala and insula. (Adapted from Etkin and Wager, 2007.)*

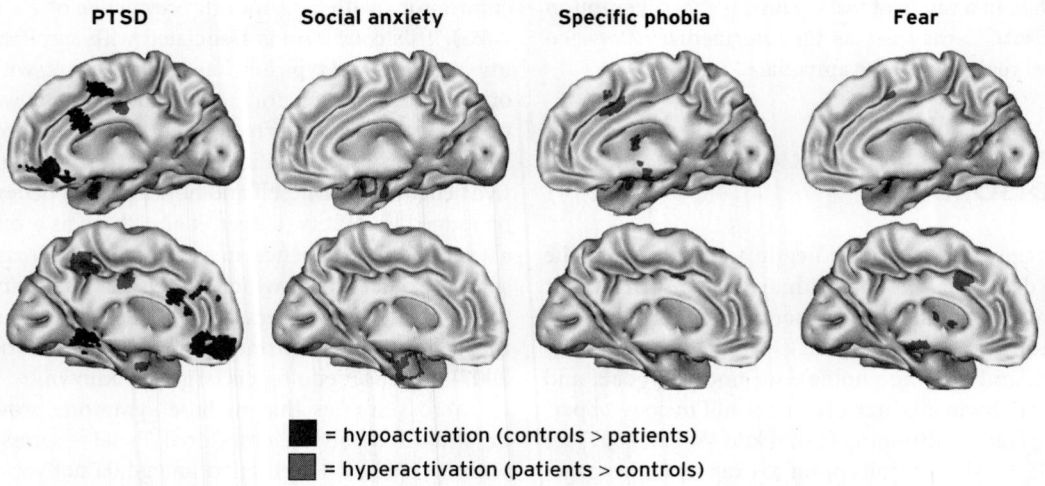

PTSD Social anxiety Specific phobia Fear

■ = hypoactivation (controls > patients)

■ = hyperactivation (patients > controls)

Figure 45.4 *Clusters of significant hyperactivation or hypoactivation in medial prefrontal regions were found in patients with PTSD, social anxiety disorder (SAD), and specific phobia relative to comparison subjects and in healthy subjects undergoing fear. (Adapted from Etkin and Wager, 2007.)*

Similar to many other anxiety disorders, patients with SAD show increased amygdala activity during aversive conditioning, with a peak response occurring later than in control participants (Freitas-Ferrari et al., 2010), suggesting less efficient and dysregulated fear circuitry. The degree of heightened amygdala activation is associated with symptom severity, including the number of DSM-IV symptoms (Battaglia et al., 2012) and the degree of trait anxiety and state social anxiety (Bruhl et al., 2011; Phan et al., 2006). Additionally, greater amygdala reactivity to social, but not physical, threat stimuli is associated with SAD symptom severity (Freitas-Ferrari et al., 2010). Following cognitive-behavioral therapy for SAD, patients show decreased amygdala activity compared with pretreatment levels during a public speaking task (Furmark et al., 2002). The extent of amygdala decrease, along with that in the PAG and left thalamus, correlates with treatment response.

Insula dysfunction is also reported: across studies, patients with SAD show increased insula activation compared with control participants (Etkin and Wager, 2007). For example, increased insula activity has been reported when patients with SAD anticipate public speaking (Freitas-Ferrari et al., 2010), read stories of social transgressions (Blair et al., 2010), view negative emotional expressions (Freitas-Ferrari et al., 2010), and perform working memory tasks (Koric et al., 2011). Additionally, the extent of insula activation correlates with symptoms of SAD (Stein and Stein, 2008) and relates to attending to the meaning of social-phobia-related words (Schmidt et al., 2010). In connectivity analyses, patients with SAD show decreased connectivity between the anterior insula and dACC when viewing fearful emotional expressions (Klumpp et al., 2012), suggesting that exaggerated insula activity may result from insufficient downregulation by cognitive control regions. Previous work highlights the insula's role in interoception (Craig, 2009). Increased insular activation in patients with SAD is thought to reflect a heightened and persistent internal focus on interoceptive cues. For example, patients with SAD often believe that physiological responses to public performance

(such as feeling flushed, sweating, trembling hands) are pronounced and likely to be noticed by others. Treatment often focuses on teaching individuals to objectively evaluate their physiological responses and focus beyond their internal reactions (Huppert et al., 2003).

Frontal lobe differences are also seen in SAD. Specifically, there is evidence for increased vACC activation compared with control participants, particularly when viewing emotional faces (Freitas-Ferrari et al., 2010), and decreases in the vACC following CBT (Furmark et al., 2002). Stein and colleagues (2002) contrast viewing harsh versus accepting emotional faces among individuals with SAD. They report increased activation in the left inferior frontal gyrus and left parahippocampal gyrus in response to negative faces. During a stressful working memory task, patients with SAD and control participants activate lateral frontal regions important for cognitive control; only patients with SAD additionally activate right vlPFC and anterior insular regions (Koric et al., 2011), regions implicated in emotional processing.

However, despite widespread frontal activation during a number of tasks, patients with SAD are less likely to recruit the dlPFC and dACC during cognitive reappraisal tasks (Freitas-Ferrari et al., 2010) and during a measure of top-down attentional control (Blair et al., 2012). Patients with SAD show delayed dlPFC reactivity when faced with autobiographical stories of social anxiety (Freitas-Ferrari et al., 2010). When instructed to cognitively reappraise these autobiographical memories, patients with SAD fail to recruit the dACC and bilateral dlPFC and vlPFC. Greater subjective negative emotion after the reappraisal task (i.e., less successful regulation) is associated with reduced right dlPFC. Moreover, patients with SAD show reduced negative connectivity or even positive connectivity between amygdala and PFC regions (Guyer et al., 2008), suggesting ineffective regulation of the amygdala by prefrontal regions.

Taken together, neuroimaging studies shed light on the heightened and dysregulated emotion seen clinically in patients

TABLE 45.1. Summary of neuroimaging findings in anxiety disorders by brain region. The weight of the arrows reflects the strength of the supporting data. ↔ = evidence for no difference from control participants; ↕ = evidence for both hyperreactivity and hyporeactivity.

BRAIN REGION	ANXIETY DISORDER				
	SAD	Specific phobia	GAD	PD	PTSD
REACTIVITY					
Amygdala	↑	↑	↓↑↔	↑↓	↑↓
Insula	↑	↑		↑	↑
PAG				↑	
Hippocampus				↑	↕
dACC/dmPFC	↓	↑	↕	↑	↑
REGULATION					
dlPFC	↓			↓	
vlPFC	↕		↑	↓	
vACC/vmPFC	↑	↓	↓	↑	↓
Effects seen after treatment	Decreased amygdala and in vACC	Decreased amygdala, insula, dACC; increased vmPFC	Decreased insula	Decreased vACC; increased vlPFC and dlPFC	Decreased amygdala and hippocampus

with SAD and point to increased limbic activation without effective top-down control (see Table 45.1). Patients with SAD show hyperreactivity in the amygdala and insula both to social-anxiety-specific tasks and to emotional faces. It may be the case that for individuals with SAD, emotional facial expressions serve as phobia-specific stimuli due to an increased focus on others' reactions. Dysregulation in frontal lobe regions is also apparent. Patients hyperactivate the vACC and vlPFC when viewing emotional facial expressions and performing cognitive tasks. Thus, they show hyperactivation in regions important for regulation during emotional reactivity and nonemotional tasks. However, during explicit emotion regulation tasks, they fail to recruit lateral prefrontal regions to the extent of control participants. Moreover, these prefrontal regions do not exert sufficient control over limbic areas. Effective cognitive-behavioral treatments exist and seem to normalize many of the emotion circuit problems seen at baseline in patients with SAD.

SPECIFIC PHOBIA

Specific phobia, often called simple phobia, is an anxiety disorder defined by heightened, excessive, consistent, and irrational fear when an individual is faced with or is anticipating a phobia-evoking stimulus. The DSM-IV includes five subtypes of specific phobia: animal (e.g., spiders), natural environment (e.g., heights), blood injection injury (e.g., shots/needles), situational (e.g., flying), and other (e.g., loud sounds). The 12-month prevalence of specific phobia is estimated at 9% (Kessler et al., 2005)

Among neuroimaging studies of specific phobia, both amygdala and insular hyperreactivity are reported (reviewed in Del Casale et al., 2012). While some studies find no differences between patients and control participants in the amygdala (Straube et al., 2006), in a meta-analysis Etkin and Wager (2007) report hyperactivation in the amygdala across studies. Bilateral amygdala hyperactivation is seen when patients with spider phobia consciously view spider stimuli, including when patients view them unconsciously (e.g., using backwardly masked presentations; Lipka et al., 2011) and while simultaneously engaging in a distracting task (Del Casale et al., 2012). Across different subtypes, patients with specific phobia show more rapid time-to-peak activation in the amygdala (Del Casale et al., 2012). Amygdala hyperactivity occurs primarily with phobia-specific stimuli (Del Casale et al., 2012), although there is one report that patients with specific phobia show similar amygdalar reactivity to affective stimuli more broadly (Wendt et al., 2008).

Additional evidence exists for exaggerated emotional reactivity and diminished regulatory ability in specific phobia. Patients with spider phobia show exaggerated insula and dACC activation when faced with spider stimuli, hyperactivation that is not seen after four sessions of cognitive behavioral therapy (Straube et al., 2006). During cognitive reappraisal of emotional stimuli, patients with spider phobia show increased insula and reduced vmPFC/vACC activity (a pattern opposite to that during emotion regulation; Del Casale et al., 2012). This prefrontal disruption is seen only when individuals with spider phobia face spider stimuli and not in response to aversive stimuli generally.

Additionally, insula hyperactivation in response to and in anticipation of phobogenic stimuli is reported (Del Casale et al., 2012). Consistent with these data, after one to four sessions of CBT, patients with specific phobia demonstrate reduced hyperactivity in the amygdala, dACC, and insula compared with baseline (Goossens et al., 2007) and increased vmPFC activation not found in a wait list group over the same time period (Schienle et al., 2007).

As mentioned earlier, the diagnosis of specific phobia encompasses different types of phobias, and specific disruptions across subtypes have not been extensively explored. Two studies address differences in subtypes of specific phobia. In one, patients with the animal subtype show enhanced fear circuitry activation, including the insula and dACC, which is associated with autonomic arousal. In contrast, those with blood injection injury subtype showed activation in the prefrontal and orbitofrontal cortex (Lueken et al., 2011). In another study, patients with blood injection injury phobia have greater activity in the ventral PFC and lower amygdala response compared with patients with animal phobia during symptom provocation (Del Casale et al., 2012). Heightened emotional reactivity may be more common or pronounced in animal phobias compared with others.

Although not fully developed, research in specific phobia reveals increased activation in regions important for emotion generation, such as the amygdala, insula, and the dACC, which is primarily observed only when viewing phobia-specific stimuli. Patients with specific phobia fail to recruit prefrontal regions to effectively regulate phobia-related emotions and to reduce limbic responding to these stimuli (see Table 45.1). As such, abnormalities in processing of phobia-related stimuli resemble those seen in SAD with social evaluation–related stimuli, and in healthy subjects with fear conditioning. Thus, there is common excessive engagement of circuitry involved in fear conditioning and negative emotional processing to disorder-specific stimuli, which fits with a fear conditioning–based conceptualization of these anxiety disorders. Moreover, a small number of sessions of cognitive-behavioral therapy (which can be considered akin to extinction training) leads to decreased activation in limbic regions (e.g., the amygdala and insula) and in the dACC, coupled with increased vmPFC activation, important for emotion and fear regulation. Overall, however, neuroimaging studies indicate less extensive neural disruptions in specific phobia compared with other anxiety disorders, both in terms of the number of brain regions involved and the types of stimuli that elicit hyperreactivity; these disruptions may be more amenable to change with treatment. Although this field is incomplete, there is some evidence that different types of phobias show different neural patterns, with patients with animal phobias showing the most extensive limbic hyperactivation.

GENERALIZED ANXIETY DISORDER

Generalized anxiety disorder (GAD) is an anxiety disorder characterized by frequent worrying that is difficult to control. Over the lifetime, GAD affects nearly 6% of English speakers in the United States (Kessler et al., 2005), has a long duration of symptoms, and negatively impacts relationships, professional functioning, and general well-being (Ballenger et al.,

2001). The clinical presentation of GAD suggests deficits in regulatory abilities, specifically the ability to manage negative affect.

As with other anxiety disorders, amygdala hyperactivation is reported in GAD, though results have been mixed. Nitschke and colleagues (2009) describe exaggerated amygdala responses to the anticipation of both negative and neutral stimuli in individuals with GAD. Additionally, increased response in the amygdala is found in adolescents with GAD, during both conscious and nonconscious viewing of emotional facial expressions (Monk et al., 2008; Shin and Liberzon, 2010). When attending to their own emotional states, children with GAD show greater amygdala responses (McClure et al., 2007). Amygdala activation to nonconsciously processed negative emotional expressions positively correlates with anxiety (Monk et al., 2008), and similarly, greater amygdala activation when viewing emotional faces predicts worse treatment response (McClure et al., 2007; Shin and Liberzon, 2010). Thus, the extent of amygdala hyperactivity may signal both the severity and inflexibility of GAD, again suggesting the presence of primary deficits in emotion regulation. However, this finding may be specific to pediatric GAD as most of these studies include pediatric populations. In contrast, many of the studies in adults report no amygdala activation during symptom provocation tasks (Hoehn-Saric et al., 2004) or comparable or reduced activation in the amygdala to negative stimuli compared with healthy controls (Blair et al., 2012; Shin and Liberzon, 2010) and to patients with other anxiety disorders (Blair et al., 2012).

Patients with GAD also have disrupted amygdala functional connectivity patterns. We examined amygdalar subregion connectivity patterns in patients with GAD and healthy control participants. Within the control group, the CMA subregion of the amygdala had almost exclusively subcortical connectivity during resting state, while the BLA was associated with cortical connectivity (including regions of the occipital lobe, temporal lobe, and prefrontal cortex). Individuals with GAD have decreased differentiability between amygdalar subregions and their targets (Etkin et al., 2009). Thus, amygdalar alterations in GAD may result from abnormal subregional organization, a disruption that may be missed when collapsing across amygdalar subregions. Evidence of other alterations in limbic regions in GAD is limited, with indication that insular activation during symptom provocation declines following medication treatment of GAD and that the degree of decline is associated with symptom improvement (Hoehn-Saric et al., 2004)

Disrupted frontal lobe activation has been reported in GAD in regions important for both the evaluation and regulation of emotional information. In the dACC/dmPFC, evidence is mixed with reports of both increased activation during symptom provocation, emotional, and resting state tasks (Hoehn-Saric et al., 2004; Paulesu et al., 2010) and of decreased activation to emotional faces (Etkin et al., 2010)

Hyperreactivity is also seen in regulatory regions in GAD, such as in the vlPFC when viewing emotional stimuli (Monk et al., 2008; Shin and Liberzon, 2010). During a resting state scan, patients with GAD show greater connectivity between the dlPFC and amygdala (Etkin et al., 2009). Prefrontal activation and prefrontal connectivity to the amygdala has been negatively correlated with symptom severity (Etkin et al., 2009; Shin and Liberzon, 2010), suggesting it may reflect a regulation-related compensation. However, patients with GAD fail to activate the vACC during an implicit regulation task and do not show the expected negative coupling of the vACC with the amygdala during this task (Etkin et al., 2010). Prior to beginning treatment, activity in the vACC to aversive cues and emotional facial expressions positively predicts treatment response (Shin and Liberzon, 2010). Stronger activity in lateral prefrontal regions is consistent with cognitive models of GAD suggesting that worry serves a compensatory function to help individuals avoid or cope with emotional arousal (Behar et al., 2009), in the context of an inability to activate medial regions important for automatic emotion regulation, such as the vACC.

GAD has received less neurobiological study than other anxiety disorders, and areas of preservation and deficit may be clarified with additional research. Thus far, neuroimaging results indicate that adolescents and adults with GAD show both overlapping and distinct neural disruptions. Specifically, limbic functioning in adolescent GAD mirrors that of adults with other anxiety disorders, in particular heightened amygdala activation. In contrast, amygdala reactivity to emotional stimuli is reduced or comparable to control participants among adults with GAD (see Table 45.1). It is unclear exactly when and why this change between adolescence and adult GAD occurs. Decreases in amygdala hyperactivity across development may indicate that individuals with GAD begin to habitually use a cognitive style intended to dampen emotional responses. In terms of the dACC/dmPFC, important for emotional evaluation, there is evidence of both hyperactivation and hypoactivation during emotional tasks in adults with GAD. This dysregulation may indicate attempts to engage cognitive control regions in order to manage excess anxiety. Indeed, worry, the hallmark of GAD, is thought to reflect a cognitive strategy that individuals employ to manage emotions (Behar et al., 2009). In adults, regions implicated in particular in automatic forms of emotion regulation are underactive during GAD, and higher activation in these regulatory regions has been linked to better prognosis. In sum, unlike other anxiety disorders, GAD is not well captured by a fear conditioning model; neuroimaging differences between individuals with GAD and control participants are best accounted for in the context of changes in emotional reactivity and regulation.

PANIC DISORDER

Panic disorder (PD) can be a debilitating condition, with a lifetime prevalence of nearly 5% (Kessler et al., 2005), and nearly 30% of people meeting criteria for having ever had a panic attack. Recurrent, unexpected panic attacks coupled with a concern that they will recur are the hallmarks of the condition, which often runs in tandem with agoraphobia. As with other anxiety disorders that can be described using a traditional fear conditioning model, the fear of the symptom-generating stimuli (in this case, internal physiological sensations) leads to

attempts at avoidance and, consequently, to a generalization of fear. A panic attack is described as intense fear and discomfort, accompanied by multiple physiological symptoms of anxiety, including heart palpitations, sweating, shaking, hot flashes, and shortness of breath. Spontaneous panic attacks are thought to arise from a fear circuitry that is hypersensitive to internal cues or cannot downregulate minor responses. These suggest heightened emotional reactivity and/or inadequate emotion regulation in PD.

Despite the enormous burden both on the individual and the community, neural circuitry research of PD has lagged behind that of other anxiety disorders. Neuroimaging studies find hyperreactivity of the amygdala in response to sensory and visceral stimuli with insufficient top-down regulation by prefrontal regions in PD (reviewed in Shin and Liberzon, 2010). One participant who had a panic attack during imaging showed increased right amygdala (along with right parahippocampal and right putamen) activation (Pfleiderer et al., 2007). In this patient, amygdala activation was associated with increases in heart rate and with insular activation. During PET scanning, patients with PD show increased glucose uptake in the amygdala (Shin and Liberzon, 2010). When presented with panic-specific negative words, patients with PD have heightened amygdala activation (Beutel et al., 2010). However, exaggerated amygdala responses are not found in all studies of PD. Inducing panic attacks pharmacologically does not consistently result in amygdala activation (Shin and Liberzon, 2010). For example, in a study of two patients who had panic attacks during scanning, only one showed amygdala activation while both had significant PFC activity (Dresler et al., 2011). Other studies find no amygdala differences compared with controls (Maddock et al., 2003) or reduced activation in the amygdala when viewing fearful emotional expressions and during anticipatory anxiety (Shin and Liberzon, 2010). These authors suggest that hypoactivity of the amygdala may result from chronic hyperresponsivity, ultimately leading to reduced emotional responses, though this interpretation remains very speculative.

Given the role of the insula in interoception and the role of interoception in panic, it is not surprising that functional imaging studies of PD implicate the insula. Activation increases at the beginning of panic symptoms (Pfleiderer et al., 2007) and is found in both spontaneous and provoked panic attacks (Dresler et al., 2011; Spiegelhalder et al., 2009). The early role of the insula in panic suggests that it may serve as an alarm, communicating information about internal bodily signals. Hippocampal hyperreactivity has been reported during rest (Sakai et al., 2006) and when individuals with PD view negative stimuli (Beutel et al., 2010). The authors suggest that this may reflect patients' preferential attention to and recall of potentially threatening stimuli. The PAG has also been implicated in PD. Electrically stimulating the PAG in patients undergoing neurosurgery results in symptoms similar to that during a panic attack, namely, heart palpitation, hyperventilation, feelings of terror, and a desire to flee (Del-Ben and Graeff, 2009); similar results are found during electrical stimulation of the hypothalamus (Wilent et al., 2010). Antidepressants, which may effectively treat symptoms of PD, are thought to do so via serotonergic inhibition of the PAG. Due to its size and location, the PAG is difficult to image, but likely PAG activation differences have been reported in patients with PD (Shin and Liberzon, 2010). Moreover, Sakai and colleagues (2006) report a correlation between percent change in glucose utilization in midbrain areas "around PAG" during imaging and number of panic attacks over the previous four weeks.

Both neuropsychological and neuroimaging studies find disruptions in PFC functioning in PD. In two cases, damage to the dACC due to surgery or radiation led to panic attacks (Shinoura et al., 2011). Pharmacologically inducing panic leads to activation in the vACC, and middle and superior frontal gyrus (Shin and Liberzon, 2010). Among patients with primary PD, evidence exists for increased frontal lobe activation, in both dorsal and ventral ACC regions and inferior frontal cortex, during directed imagery and when viewing positive images (Shin and Liberzon, 2010). Moreover, these investigators find that responses in the dACC and vACC to happy faces are larger in patients with PD than control participants. Additionally, threat-related material may elicit greater dlPFC activation (Maddock et al., 2003). Successful cognitive-behavioral treatment for PD results in decreased glucose utilization in the left vACC (Sakai et al., 2006). By contrast, others report decreased dACC and vACC activation to fearful faces in untreated PD (Shin and Liberzon, 2010). Additionally, prior to treatment, patients with PD have decreased vlPFC activation to negative stimuli and decreased dlPFC activation to positive stimuli (suggesting widespread lateral prefrontal disruption; Beutel et al., 2010) coupled with high limbic activation; this pattern was normalized after inpatient psychodynamic treatment.

Overall, both *in vivo* symptoms of panic attacks and the condition of PD are associated with hyperreactivity of the insula and often (but not always) the amygdala. Additionally, panic symptoms and PD are associated with exaggerated activation in other regions involved in emotional reactivity that are not consistently implicated in other anxiety disorders, such as the PAG, hippocampus, and hypothalamus (see Table 45.1). The insula and PAG may be more important in PD than other anxiety disorders due to their roles in interoception and sympathetic nervous system activity, two core components of PD. Most of these studies use panic-specific stimuli or correlate activation with panic symptoms, including some that report panic symptoms that occur during scanning. These data suggest exaggerated fear responses in PD coupled with a greater focus on the physiological components of fear. Some evidence also supports hyperactivity in medial prefrontal regions to panic-specific and positive emotional stimuli, but hypoactivation in these areas to fear-specific stimuli. Evidence for lateral prefrontal disruptions is mixed, with some reporting increased activation to threat stimuli, and others reporting decreased activation to positive and negative stimuli (Beutel et al., 2010; Maddock et al., 2003). Given the small number of studies and discrepant findings across studies, further research is needed to explore frontal lobe patterns of hyper- and hypoactivation in PD. As such, it is difficult to draw conclusions about regulatory function in PD, although widespread heightened reactivity suggests deficits in regulatory function.

POSTTRAUMATIC STRESS DISORDER

Posttraumatic stress disorder encompasses a set of symptoms that develop subsequent to exposure to a traumatic event such as threat of death or serious injury to oneself or another person. In the aftermath of a traumatic event, individuals with PTSD develop a constellation of symptoms that fall into three DSM-IV-based categories: reexperiencing (e.g., flashbacks, nightmares), avoidance (attempts to avoid thoughts or situations that are reminders of the trauma), and hyperarousal (e.g., exaggerated startle response and hypervigilance). PTSD is thought to reflect exaggerated and sustained fear conditioning overlaid on a vulnerable state. From a fear conditioning model perspective, PTSD reflects rapid and exaggerated fear learning, coupled with deficient fear extinction and misinterpretation of safe contexts as dangerous. Consequently, those who suffer from PTSD often feel the world is fraught with aversive threat. Symptoms of PTSD are further maintained by a tendency to avoid situations, thoughts, and feelings related to the trauma. There are multiple symptoms of PTSD, however, that do not as readily fit into a fear conditioning framework, and which set it apart from some of the other anxiety disorders. These symptoms include numbing, irritability, anger, and guilt and can be conceptualized as dysregulated negative emotion more broadly.

Extensive research has been published on limbic and prefrontal responses to a range of emotional stimuli in PTSD. We report amygdala hyperactivation in PTSD in our meta-analysis (Etkin and Wager, 2007). Patients with PTSD show amygdalar hyperactivation when viewing emotional expressions (reviewed in Brohawn et al., 2010; Hughes and Shin, 2011), in particular fearful expressions (Hughes and Shin, 2011), including when these stimuli are presented outside of conscious awareness (Hughes and Shin, 2011). The extent of amygdala hyperactivity to emotional facial expressions is also related to symptom severity (Brohawn et al., 2010; Hughes and Shin, 2011). In symptom provocation studies, increased amygdala activity is seen to trauma-related stimuli (e.g., combat-related sounds and combat-related odors [Hughes and Shin, 2011]). Related to core symptomatology in PTSD, patients have heightened amygdala during the construction of negative autobiographical memories (St. Jacques et al., 2011). Consistent with the fear conditioning model of PTSD, amygdala habituation occurs less efficiently in patients with PTSD (Hughes and Shin, 2011), and amygdala activation is stronger during fear extinction in these patients compared with control participants (Milad et al., 2009). Following cognitive-behavioral treatment, patients with PTSD show decreased amygdala activity in response to emotional stimuli, with higher pretreatment amygdala activity relating to less symptom reduction over treatment (Hughes and Shin, 2011).

Despite considerable evidence for amygdala hyperactivation in PTSD, our meta-analysis also suggests that the picture is more complicated (Etkin and Wager, 2007). First, amygdala hyperactivation is found less frequently in PTSD than in SAD or specific phobia. Second, in contrast to SAD and specific phobia, among studies of PTSD, there is evidence for both hyperactivation and hypoactivation in the amygdala. Across studies, a ventral amygdala cluster is hyperreactive and a dorsal cluster is hypoactive. Though precise localization is difficult in the context of a meta-analysis, we speculate that the former relates to the BLA, important for acquiring fear responses and forming emotional memories. The dorsal-posterior cluster may correspond to the CMA, which mediates autonomic and behavioral reactions to threat; hypoactivation in this area may be related to emotional blunting and numbing seen in PTSD. Additionally, these findings and examining amygdala subdivisions individually may help explain the amygdala hypoactivation that has been reported in PD and GAD.

Across studies, insula hyperactivity is seen consistently in PTSD (Etkin and Wager, 2007). Individuals with PTSD show exaggerated insula responses when viewing emotional facial expressions during emotional anticipation and script-driven imagery (Aupperle et al., 2012; Hughes and Shin, 2011) and when retrieving emotional and neutral word pairs (Hughes and Shin, 2011). Greater insula activity during emotional tasks is associated with symptom severity and with reexperiencing occurring during neuroimaging (Hughes and Shin, 2011).

Individuals with PTSD show striking abnormalities in prefrontal cortical functioning, including both hyperactivation and hypoactivation of different regions. Extensive ACC reductions, spanning both dorsal and ventral regions, have been reported in response to symptom provocation and more general emotional tasks (Hughes and Shin, 2011; Lanius et al., 2003). However, consideration of ACC subregions and their functions sheds light on the patterns of hyper- and hypoactivation seen in PTSD. For example, when faced with emotional stimuli, patients with PTSD show increased activation in the dACC and decreased activation in the vACC (Hughes and Shin, 2011). The dACC plays important roles in emotion generation and conflict monitoring, suggesting that hyperactivity here may reflect heightened emotional reactivity in PTSD. Increased dACC activation is reported across tasks in PTSD, such as during trauma-specific words, fear conditioning, and extinction, and at rest (Hughes and Shin, 2011; Rougemont-Bucking et al., 2011). Among survivors of intimate partner violence, dACC activation when viewing male faces is related to hyperarousal symptoms (Hughes and Shin, 2011). Elevated dACC activation may represent a risk factor for PTSD, which is seen in combat veterans with PTSD and their identical, combat-unexposed co-twins without PTSD (Shin et al., 2009).

In contrast, hypoactivation of the vACC in the face of affectively laden stimuli is thought to reflect insufficient regulatory systems in PTSD. Hypoactivation of the vACC and vmPFC is reported in PTSD during traumatic scripts, traumatic imagery, and trauma-related videos (Hughes and Shin, 2011), as well as during negative images generally (Phan et al., 2006). Moreover, this disruption is apparent in adolescent populations with PTSD (Yang et al., 2004). Deficits in emotional processing in PTSD may not be specific to negative emotional stimuli. Patients with PTSD have decreased activity in the vmPFC and nucleus accumbens during reward processing (Sailer et al., 2008). Decreased vmPFC activation has also been found in response to nonemotional stimuli, such as during cognitive tasks (Hughes and Shin, 2011). Activation in the

vmPFC negatively correlates with symptom severity (Hughes and Shin, 2011), and increases in vmPFC activation positively correlate with symptom improvement (Felmingham et al., 2007). Further evidence for inadequate frontal regulation of emotional stimuli comes from functional connectivity studies demonstrating reduced negative coupling between ACC regions and the amygdala (Etkin and Wager, 2007; Sripada et al., 2012).

In healthy control participants, the vmPFC (and an analogous region in experimental animals) has been linked to fear extinction (Phelps et al., 2004). PTSD patients show decreased vACC/vmPFC activation in fear conditioning studies, particularly during fear extinction (Milad et al., 2009) and recall of fear extinction (Milad et al., 2009; Rougemont-Bucking et al., 2011) and in the presence of safety signals (Rougemont-Bucking et al., 2011). Although mostly examined in the context of fear conditioning, vACC deficits likely have more far-reaching implications for emotion dysregulation in PTSD. This region is important for regulating emotional conflict (Etkin et al., 2011), and individuals with PTSD show reduced vACC activation in situations of unexpected emotional conflict (Kim et al., 2008).

Memory difficulties are often reported in PTSD, suggesting a prominent role for the hippocampus. Functional imaging studies of hippocampal activation in PTSD have been mixed. Previous research describes decreased hippocampal activation during script-driven imagery tasks (Hughes and Shin, 2011), memory encoding and retrieval (Hughes and Shin, 2011; Shin et al., 2004), and extinction recall (Milad et al., 2009). Reduction in the integrity of hippocampal function is associated with symptom severity (Hughes and Shin, 2011). However, multiple studies report heightened hippocampal activity in PTSD, including during script-driven imagery and during memory retrieval in emotional contexts (Hughes and Shin, 2011). Hippocampal activation is positively associated with amygdala activation (Brohawn et al., 2010) and symptom severity (Shin et al., 2004), and with decreases in activation following treatment (Felmingham et al., 2007). As previously described, the posterior hippocampus is critical for episodic memory, and the anterior hippocampus is involved in anxiety-related behaviors. Patients with PTSD show decreased connectivity between the posterior hippocampus and regions in the default mode network, such as vACC and PCC, which may relate to the fear memory abnormalities in PTSD, such as intrusive memories and difficulty updating fear memories (Chen and Etkin, manuscript submitted). A similar deficit is seen in activation of these patients in response to a task, which is furthermore related to the traumas being either earlier in life or multiple. By contrast, common decreased connectivity between the anterior hippocampus and dACC is seen in patients with PTSD or GAD. Anterior hippocampal connectivity deficits across these two anxiety disorders may relate to general anxiety responses that are often dysregulated in many anxiety disorders.

Taken together, individuals with PTSD show exaggerated amygdala activation to wide-ranging stimuli, including to consciously and unconsciously presented emotional stimuli, trauma-specific stimuli, autobiographical memories, and fear conditioning. A closer examination suggests that subregions of the amygdala with cortical connections and that are important for the acquisition of fear responses are hyperactive while those with connections to the brainstem and that are important for autonomic responding are hyporeactive. Additional limbic hyperreactivity in PTSD is found in the insula. Given the disruptions in limbic activity when presented with trauma-specific stimuli, fear conditioning, and emotional stimuli more generally, disturbances in emotional reactivity appear more widespread in PTSD than other anxiety disorders. This finding is consistent with the clinical picture of PTSD that includes increased negative affect beyond fear (e.g., guilt, shame, anger, irritability) and reduced positive affect (e.g., emotional numbing or distancing).

In conjunction with limbic hyperactivity, increased responding in the dACC/dmPFC to emotional information reflects heightened reactivity and sensitivity to emotional cues in PTSD. The degree of dACC/dmPFC activation correlates with hyperarousal symptoms and may signal a predisposition to develop PTSD, as indicated by a recent twin study. In contrast, the vACC/vmPFC is consistently hypoactive in PTSD during symptom provocation and fear-conditioning tasks (especially during fear extinction) (see Table 45.1). Decreased responding in the vACC/vmPFC corresponds to inadequate regulation of emotion, such as during fear conditioning and extinction; this alteration in regulatory function tracks with both symptom severity and symptom improvement. Consistent with the clinical picture of PTSD, deficits in emotional circuitry extend beyond those implicated in and in response to fear: patients with PTSD show deficits to wide-ranging negative emotional stimuli and to positive stimuli.

CONCLUSION

The goal of this chapter is to provide a review of relevant neuroimaging findings of anxiety disorders. We introduce a new, expanded framework of our previous model (Etkin, 2009; Etkin, 2010) to catalog neuroimaging findings in the context of emotional reactivity as well as regulation in anxiety disorders. Our updated framework is guided by theory and neuroanatomy simultaneously. As such, we define emotion reactivity deficits as differences seen in behavioral manifestation of emotional responding or neural abnormalities in core limbic structures in response to emotional provocation. Similarly, emotion regulation deficits are defined as behavioral or neural abnormalities in cortical regulatory regions (see Fig. 45.1) in emotion regulation tasks.

Historically, aberrations in fear circuitry have been the guiding framework for research and treatment of anxiety disorders. While this model yields a rich understanding of the neurobiology of anxiety, our new affective science-inspired model shows that it is a minority of anxiety disorders in which disruptions in fear processing account for the entire symptom presentation. In fact, our review suggests that while fear circuit abnormalities are central to many anxiety disorders, there are other emotion reactivity, and very pronounced regulatory, deficits in anxiety pathologies.

Specifically, we found evidence of heightened reactivity in limbic structures in SAD (Etkin and Wager, 2007), but only for socially relevant and not for physical threat-related stimuli. Distinct from other anxiety disorders, SAD is associated with increased activity in the vACC (implicated in automatic emotion regulation) and decreases in lateral PFC regions (associated with deliberate emotion regulation). Neural changes associated with specific phobia are consistent with increased emotion reactivity and decreased regulation, although these deficits appear to be restricted to phobia-specific stimuli. When presented with phobia-specific stimuli, these individuals show increased amygdala, insula, and dACC (all implicated in emotional evaluation and reactivity) with decreased vACC activation (important for automatic emotion regulation). Fewer studies have addressed neural changes associated with GAD. While adolescents with GAD show heightened amygdala activation (similar to other anxiety disorders), adults with GAD often show no changes from control participants or reductions in amygdala activation. This lack of limbic hyperactivation is coupled with dysregulation in frontal regions important for the evaluation (dACC) and regulation (lateral PFC) of emotion. Patients with GAD may be able to engage those regions important for cognitive or deliberate regulation of emotion but fail to activate the vACC important for automatic emotion regulation. PD is characterized by widespread activation in diverse structures implicated in fear responding and in physiological reactivity, such as the amygdala, insula, PAG, and hippocampus, along with decreased activation in prefrontal regions involved in both deliberate and automatic emotion regulation. Finally, increased activity in both limbic and prefrontal regions important for emotional reactivity and evaluation are found in PTSD, along with decreased activation in the vmPFC, an important region in emotion regulation. These patients show heightened reactivity in the amygdala, insula, hippocampus, and dACC and across a wide range of tasks, including symptom provocation, fear conditioning, and emotional stimuli generally (both positive and negative). Within both the amygdala and the hippocampus, deficits in PTSD are more complicated than strictly hypo- or hyperactivation. Within both regions, there are subregions of hyperactivation and of hypoactivation in patients with PTSD.

Thus, it is apparent that there is great deal of variability across anxiety disorders in terms of emotional reactivity. Deficits exist in other affect dimensions than fear, such as social rejection–acceptance in SAD, and anger and numbing in PTSD. In terms of neural deficits, amygdala and insula dysfunctions cut across most anxiety disorders, while other limbic structures showed disorder specificity. We found no evidence of insula deficits in GAD, whereas there were documented cases of hyperactivation in SAD, specific phobia, PD, and PTSD. Abnormalities in the periaqueductal gray and insula appear to be most characteristic of PD due to the role of these structures in interoception.

While emotional hyperreactivity, especially to anxiety-specific stimuli, is a central feature of anxiety disorders, strong reactivity may represent an overactive emotional reactivity system, an underactive regulatory system, or both. As such, in this review we also highlighted those brain regions seen in emotional reactivity generally and those critical for the regulation of emotion. In general, these include core limbic structures in emotional reactivity and connections between these regions and prefrontal cortical areas that play regulatory roles. In this vein, we cataloged pronounced regulatory changes in lateral PFC regions, important for effortful emotion regulation, in SAD, GAD, and PD. Increases in these regions may reflect attempts to compensate for exaggerated emotional reactivity. Strikingly, vACC/vmPFC deficits were seen across nearly all anxiety disorders. The vACC and the vmPFC are richly interconnected with limbic structures, especially the amygdala, and perform implicit emotion regulation. Deficits in activation in these regions may indicate impairments in more automatic, implicit forms of emotion regulatory operations. In summary, our hope is that this review reinforces the utility of an emotional reactivity and regulation framework for understanding and treating anxiety disorders and will inspire future researchers to grow and systematize findings within this model.

DISCLOSURES

Dr. Goodkind has no conflicts of interest to disclose.

Dr. Gyurak has no conflicts of interest to disclose Funding comes from the NIMH.

Dr. Etkin Funding comes from the NIMH, VA, NARSAD and Dana Foundation.

REFERENCES

Adolphs, R., Tranel, D., et al. (1995). Fear and the human amygdala. *J. Neurosci.* 15(9):5879–5891.

Aupperle, R.L., Allard, C.B., et al. (2012). Dorsolateral prefrontal cortex activation during emotional anticipation and neuropsychological performance in posttraumatic stress disorder. *Arch. Gen. Psychiatry* 69(4):360–371.

Ballenger, J.C., Davidson, J.R., et al. (2001). Consensus statement on generalized anxiety disorder from the International Consensus Group on Depression and Anxiety. *J. Clin. Psychiatry* 62(Suppl. 11):53–58.

Bannerman, D.M., Rawlins, J.N.P., et al. (2004). Regional dissociations within the hippocampus: memory and anxiety. *Neurosci. Biobehav. Rev.* 28(3):273–283.

Battaglia, M., Zanoni, A., et al. (2012). Cerebral responses to emotional expressions and the development of social anxiety disorder: a preliminary longitudinal study. *Depress. Anxiety* 29(1):54–61.

Baur, V., Hänggi, J., et al. (2012). Resting-state functional and structural connectivity within an insula-amygdala route specifically index state and trait anxiety. *Biol. Psychiatry.*

Behar, E., DiMarco, I.D., et al. (2009). Current theoretical models of generalized anxiety disorder (GAD): conceptual review and treatment implications. *J. Anxiety Disord.* 23(8):1011–1023.

Beutel, M.E., Stark, R., et al. (2010). Changes of brain activation pre- post short-term psychodynamic inpatient psychotherapy: an fMRI study of panic disorder patients. *Psychiatry Res.* 184(2):96–104.

Blair, K.S., Geraci, M., et al. (2010). Social norm processing in adult social phobia: atypically increased ventromedial frontal cortex responsiveness to unintentional (embarrassing) transgressions. *Am. J. Psychiatry* 167(12):1526–1532.

Blair, K.S., Geraci, M., et al. (2012). Reduced dorsal anterior cingulate cortical activity during emotional regulation and top-down attentional control in generalized social phobia, generalized anxiety disorder, and comorbid generalized social phobia/generalized anxiety disorder. *Biol. Psychiatry.*

Brohawn, K.H., Offringa, R., et al. (2010). The neural correlates of emotional memory in posttraumatic stress disorder. *Biol. Psychiatry* 68(11):1023–1030.

Brühl, A.B., Rufer, M., et al. (2011). Neural correlates of altered general emotion processing in social anxiety disorder. *Brain Res.* 1378:72–83.

Chen, A.C., and Etkin, A. Hippocampal network connectivity and activation differentiates post-traumatic stress disorder from other mood or anxiety disorders. Manuscript submitted for publication.

Craig, A.D.B. (2009). How do you feel: now? The anterior insula and human awareness. *Nat. Rev. Neurosci.* 10(1):59–70.

Davis, M. (2002). Neural circuitry of anxiety and stress disorders. In: Neuropsychopharmacology: 5th Generation of Progress. Philadelphia: Lippincott, Williams, & Wilkins, pp. 931–951.

Del-Ben, C.M., and Graeff, F.G. (2009). Panic disorder: is the PAG involved? *Neural Plast.* 2009.

Del Casale, A., Ferracuti, S., et al. (2012). Functional neuroimaging in specific phobia. *Psychiat. Res.-Neuroim.* 202(3):181–197.

Dresler, T., Hahn, T., et al. (2011). Neural correlates of spontaneous panic attacks. *J. Neural Transm.* 118(2):263–269.

Egner, T., Etkin, A., et al. (2008). Dissociable neural systems resolve conflict from emotional versus nonemotional distracters. *Cereb. Cortex* 18(6):1475–1484.

Etkin, A. (2009). Disrupted amygdalar subregion functional connectivity and evidence of a compensatory network in generalized anxiety disorder. *Arch. Gen. Psychiatry* 66(12):1361.

Etkin, A. (2010). Functional neuroanatomy of anxiety: a neural circuit perspective. *Curr. Top. Behav. Neurosci* 2:251–277.

Etkin, A., and Wager, T.D. (2007). Functional neuroimaging of anxiety: a meta-analysis of emotional processing in PTSD, social anxiety disorder, and specific phobia. *Am. J. Psychiatry* 164(10):1476–1488.

Etkin, A., Egner, T., et al. (2011). Emotional processing in anterior cingulate and medial prefrontal cortex. *Trends Cogn. Sci.* 15(2):85–93.

Etkin, A., Klemenhagen, K.C., et al. (2004). Individual differences in trait anxiety predict the response of the basolateral amygdala to unconsciously processed fearful faces. *Neuron* 44(6):1043–1055.

Etkin, A., Prater, K.E., et al. (2009). Disrupted amygdalar subregion functional connectivity and evidence of a compensatory network in generalized anxiety disorder. *Arch. Gen. Psychiatry* 66(12):1361–1372.

Etkin, A., Prater, K.E., et al. (2010). Failure of anterior cingulate activation and connectivity with the amygdala during implicit regulation of emotional processing in generalized anxiety disorder. *Am. J. Psychiatry* 167(5):545–554.

Felmingham, K., Kemp, A., et al. (2007). Changes in anterior cingulate and amygdala after cognitive behavior therapy of posttraumatic stress disorder. *Psychol. Sci.* 18(2):127–129.

Freitas-Ferrari, M.C., Hallak, J.E.C., et al. (2010). Neuroimaging in social anxiety disorder: a systematic review of the literature. *Prog. Neuropsychopharmacol. Biol. Psychiatry* 34(4):565–580.

Furmark, T., Tillfors, M., et al. (2002). Common changes in cerebral blood flow in patients with social phobia treated with citalopram or cognitive-behavioral therapy. *Arch. Gen. Psychiatry* 59(5):425–433.

Goossens, L., Sunaert, S., et al. (2007). Amygdala hyperfunction in phobic fear normalizes after exposure. *Biol. Psychiatry* 62(10):1119–1125.

Guyer, A.E., Lau, J.Y.F., et al. (2008). Amygdala and ventrolateral prefrontal cortex function during anticipated peer evaluation in pediatric social anxiety. *Arch. Gen. Psychiatry* 65(11):1303–1312.

Gyurak, A., Gross, J.J., et al. (2011). Explicit and implicit emotion regulation: a dual-process framework. *Cognition Emotion* 25(3):400–412.

Heldt, S.A., Stanek, L., et al. (2007). Hippocampus-specific deletion of BDNF in adult mice impairs spatial memory and extinction of aversive memories. *Mol. Psychiatry* 12(7):656–670.

Hoehn-Saric, R., Schlund, M.W., et al. (2004). Effects of citalopram on worry and brain activation in patients with generalized anxiety disorder. *Psychiatry Res.* 131(1):11–21.

Hughes, K.C., and Shin, L.M. (2011). Functional neuroimaging studies of post-traumatic stress disorder. *Exp. Rev. Neurother.* 11(2):275–285.

Huppert, J., Roth, D., et al. (2003). Cognitive-behavioral treatment of social phobia: new advances. *Curr. Psychiatry Rep.* 5(4):289–296.

Kessler, R.C., Chiu, W.T., et al. (2005). Prevalence, severity, and comorbidity of 12-month DSM-IV disorders in the National Comorbidity Survey Replication. *Arch. Gen. Psychiatry* 62(6):617–627.

Kim, M.J., Chey, J., et al. (2008). Diminished rostral anterior cingulate activity in response to threat-related events in posttraumatic stress disorder. *J. Psychiat. Res.* 42(4):268–277.

Kjelstrup, K.G., Tuvnes, F.A., et al. (2002). Reduced fear expression after lesions of the ventral hippocampus. *Proc. Natl. Acad. Sci. USA* 99(16):10825–10830.

Klumpp, H., Angstadt, M., et al. (2012). Insula reactivity and connectivity to anterior cingulate cortex when processing threat in generalized social anxiety disorder. *Biol. Psychol.* 89(1):273–276.

Kober, H., Barrett, L.F., et al. (2008). Functional grouping and cortical-subcortical interactions in emotion: a meta-analysis of neuroimaging studies. *NeuroImage* 42(2):998–1031.

Koric, L., Volle, E., et al. (2011). How cognitive performance-induced stress can influence right VLPFC activation: an fMRI study in healthy subjects and in patients with social phobia. *Hum. Brain Mapp.*

LaBar, K.S., LeDoux, J.E., et al. (1995). Impaired fear conditioning following unilateral temporal lobectomy in humans. *J. Neurosci.* 15(10):6846–6855.

Lammers, J.H., Kruk, M.R., et al. (1988). Hypothalamic substrates for brain stimulation-induced patterns of locomotion and escape jumps in the rat. *Brain Res.* 449(1–2):294–310.

Lanius, R.A., Williamson, P.C., et al. (2003). Recall of emotional states in posttraumatic stress disorder: an fMRI investigation. *Biol. Psychiatry* 53(3):204–210.

Lipka, J., Miltner, W.H.R., et al. (2011). Vigilance for threat interacts with amygdala responses to subliminal threat cues in specific phobia. *Biol. Psychiatry* 70(5):472–478.

Lissek, S., Powers, A.S., et al. (2005). Classical fear conditioning in the anxiety disorders: a meta-analysis. *Behav. Res. Ther.* 43(11):1391–1424.

Lueken, U., Kruschwitz, J.D., et al. (2011). How specific is specific phobia? Different neural response patterns in two subtypes of specific phobia. *NeuroImage* 56(1):363–372.

Maddock, R.J., Buonocore, M.H., et al. (2003). Brain regions showing increased activation by threat-related words in panic disorder. *NeuroReport* 14(3):325–328.

McClure, E.B., Adler, A., et al. (2007). fMRI predictors of treatment outcome in pediatric anxiety disorders. *Psychopharmacology* 191(1):97–105.

Mendlowicz, M.V., and Stein, M.B. (2000). Quality of life in individuals with anxiety disorders. *Am. J. Psychiatry* 157(5):669–682.

Milad, M.R., Pitman, R.K., et al. (2009). Neurobiological basis of failure to recall extinction memory in posttraumatic stress disorder. *Biol. Psychiatry* 66(12):1075–1082.

Mineka, S., and Oehlberg, K. (2008). The relevance of recent developments in classical conditioning to understanding the etiology and maintenance of anxiety disorders. *Acta Psychol.* 127(3):567–580.

Mobbs, D., Petrovic, P., et al. (2007). When fear is near: threat imminence elicits prefrontal-periaqueductal gray shifts in humans. *Science* 317(5841):1079–1083.

Monk, C.S., Telzer, E.H., et al. (2008). Amygdala and ventrolateral prefrontal cortex activation to masked angry faces in children and adolescents with generalized anxiety disorder. *Arch. Gen. Psychiatry* 65(5):568–576.

Nitschke, J.B., Sarinopoulos, I., et al. (2009). Anticipatory activation in the amygdala and anterior cingulate in generalized anxiety disorder and prediction of treatment response. *Am. J. Psychiatry* 166(3):302–310.

Paulesu, E., Sambugaro, E., et al. (2010). Neural correlates of worry in generalized anxiety disorder and in normal controls: a functional MRI study. *Psychol. Med.* 40(1):117–124.

Pfleiderer, B., Zinkirciran, S., et al. (2007). fMRI amygdala activation during a spontaneous panic attack in a patient with panic disorder. *World J. Biol. Psychiatry* 8(4):269–272.

Phan, K.L., Fitzgerald, D.A., et al. (2006). Association between amygdala hyperactivity to harsh faces and severity of social anxiety in generalized social phobia. *Biol. Psychiatry* 59(5):424–429.

Phan, K.L., Wager, T., et al. (2002). Functional neuroanatomy of emotion: a meta-analysis of emotion activation studies in PET and fMRI. *NeuroImage* 16(2):331–348.

Phelps, E.A., Delgado, M.R., et al. (2004). Extinction learning in humans: role of the amygdala and vmPFC. *Neuron* 43(6):897–905.

Pitkänen, A., Savander, V., et al. (1997). Organization of intra-amygdaloid circuitries in the rat: an emerging framework for understanding functions of the amygdala. *Trends Neurosci.* 20(11):517–523.

Rougemont-Bücking, A., Linnman, C., et al. (2011). Altered processing of contextual information during fear extinction in PTSD: an fMRI study. *CNS Neurosci. Ther.* 17(4):227–236.

Sailer, U., Robinson, S., et al. (2008). Altered reward processing in the nucleus accumbens and mesial prefrontal cortex of patients with posttraumatic stress disorder. *Neuropsychologia* 46(11):2836–2844.

Sakai, Y., Kumano, H., et al. (2006). Changes in cerebral glucose utilization in patients with panic disorder treated with cognitive-behavioral therapy. *NeuroImage* 33(1):218–226.

Sanders, S.K., and Shekhar, A. (1991). Blockade of GABAA receptors in the region of the anterior basolateral amygdala of rats elicits increases in heart rate and blood pressure. *Brain Res.* 567(1):101–110.

Schienle, A., Schäfer, A., et al. (2005). Brain activation of spider phobics towards disorder-relevant, generally disgust- and fear-inducing pictures. *Neurosci. Lett.* 388(1):1–6.

Schmidt, S., Mohr, A., et al. (2010). Task-dependent neural correlates of the processing of verbal threat-related stimuli in social phobia. *Biol. Psychol.* 84(2):304–312.

Shin, L.M., Lasko, N.B., et al. (2009). Resting metabolic activity in the cingulate cortex and vulnerability to posttraumatic stress disorder. *Arch. Gen. Psychiatry* 66(10):1099–1107.

Shin, L.M., and Liberzon, I. (2010). The neurocircuitry of fear, stress, and anxiety disorders. *Neuropsychopharmacology* 35(1):169–191.

Shin, L.M., Shin, P.S., et al. (2004). Hippocampal function in posttraumatic stress disorder. *Hippocampus* 14(3):292–300.

Shinoura, N., Yamada, R., et al. (2011). Damage to the right dorsal anterior cingulate cortex induces panic disorder. *J. Affect. Disord.* 133(3):569–572.

Spiegelhalder, K., Hornyak, M., et al. (2009). Cerebral correlates of heart rate variations during a spontaneous panic attack in the fMRI scanner. *Neurocase* 15(6):527–534.

Sripada, R.K., King, A.P., et al. (2012). Altered resting-state amygdala functional connectivity in men with posttraumatic stress disorder. *J. Psychiatry Neurosci.* 37(4):241–249.

St. Jacques, P.L., Botzung, A., et al. (2011). Functional neuroimaging of emotionally intense autobiographical memories in post-traumatic stress disorder. *J. Psychiat. Res.* 45(5):630–637.

Stein, M.B., Simmons, A.N., et al. (2007). Increased amygdala and insula activation during emotion processing in anxiety-prone subjects. *Am. J. Psychiatry* 164(2):318–327.

Stein, M.B., and Stein, D.J. (2008). Social anxiety disorder. *Lancet* 371(9618):1115–1125.

Stewart, R.E., and Chambless, D.L. (2009). Cognitive-behavioral therapy for adult anxiety disorders in clinical practice: a meta-analysis of effectiveness studies. *J. Consult. Clin. Psych.* 77(4):595–606.

Straube, T., Glauer, M., et al. (2006). Effects of cognitive-behavioral therapy on brain activation in specific phobia. *NeuroImage* 29(1):125–135.

Watson, J.B., and Rayner, R. (1920). Conditioned emotional reactions. *J. Exp. Psychol.* 3:1–14.

Wendt, J., Lotze, M., et al. (2008). Brain activation and defensive response mobilization during sustained exposure to phobia-related and other affective pictures in spider phobia. *Psychophysiology* 45(2):205–215.

Whalen, P.J., Johnstone, T., et al. (2008). A functional magnetic resonance imaging predictor of treatment response to venlafaxine in generalized anxiety disorder. *Biol. Psychiatry* 63(9):858–863.

Whalley, M.G., Rugg, M.D., et al. (2009). Incidental retrieval of emotional contexts in post-traumatic stress disorder and depression: an fMRI study. *Brain Cogn.* 69(1):98–107.

Wilent, W.B., Oh, M.Y., et al. (2010). Induction of panic attack by stimulation of the ventromedial hypothalamus. *J. Neurosurg.* 112(6):1295–1298.

Yang, P., Wu, M.-T., et al. (2004). Evidence of early neurobiological alternations in adolescents with posttraumatic stress disorder: a functional MRI study. *Neurosci. Lett.* 370(1):13–18.

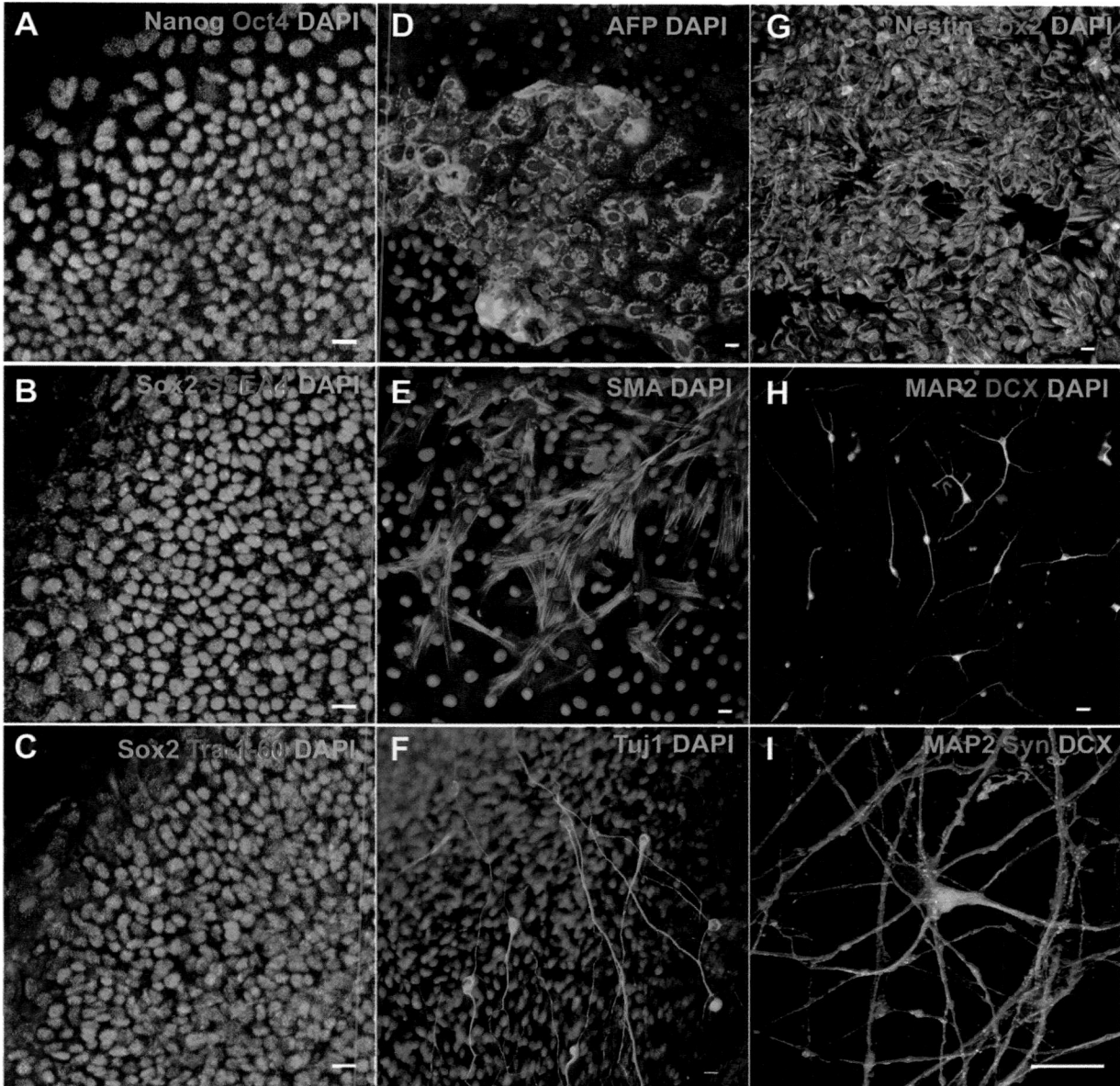

Figure 9.1 Generation of neurons from human iPSCs. (A–C) Confocal images of iPSC colonies expressing pluripotency markers: (A) Nanog (green), Oct4 (red), DAPI (blue); (B) Sox2 (green), SSEA4 (red), DAPI (blue); (C) Sox2 (green), Tra-1–60 (red), DAPI (blue). (D–F) In vitro differentiation into three embryonic germ layers revealed by immunostaining for markers of α-fetoprotein (endoderm) (D), α smooth muscle actin (mesoderm) (E), and Tuj1 (ectoderm) (F). (G–I) Neuronal differentiation: (G) Neural progenitors cells 7 d after neural induction stained for Nestin (green), Sox2 (red), and DAPI (blue); (H) immature neurons 7 d after differentiation, stained for MAP2 (green), DCX (red), and DAPI (blue); (I) 4 week-old neurons stained for MAP2 (green), DCX (blue), and synapsin (red). Scale bar = 20 μm.

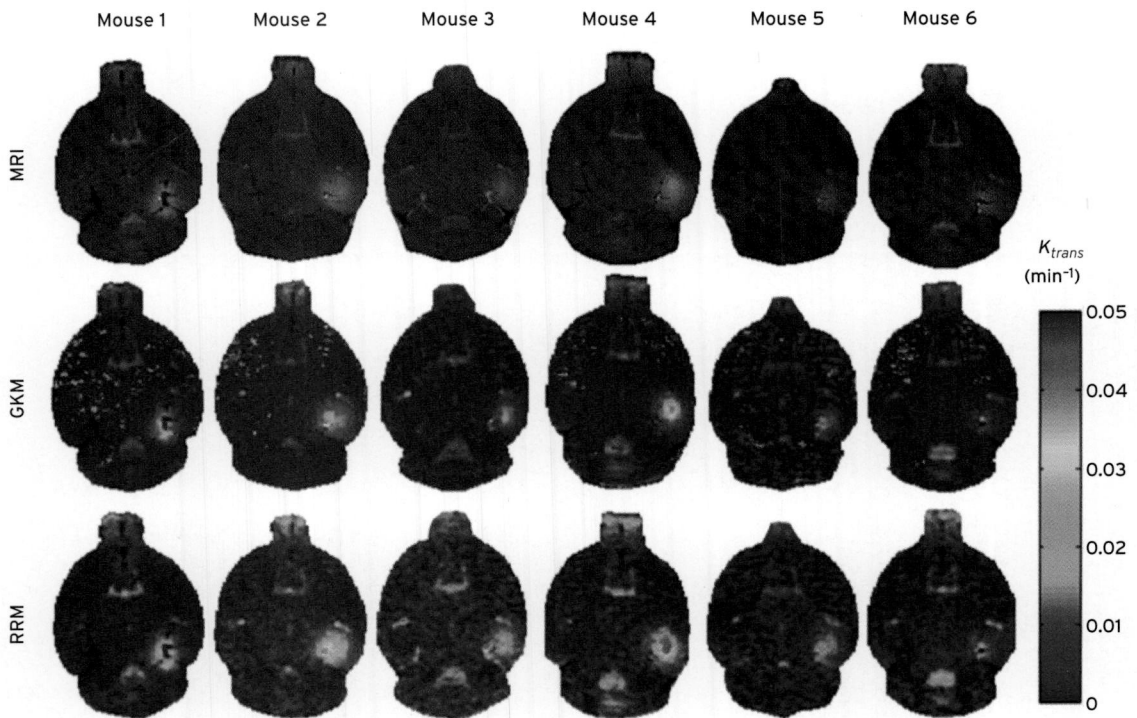

Figure 11.5 *T1 images (first row) and their corresponding permeability maps generated from GKM (second row) and RRM (third row) for all mice. The transverse slice with maximum T1 signal enhancement is selected. The Ktrans values are indicated in the color bar. The maps have been superimposed over the corresponding DCE-MR images. In the case of Mouse 1, the last acquired DCE-MR image is presented instead of a regular T1[61].*

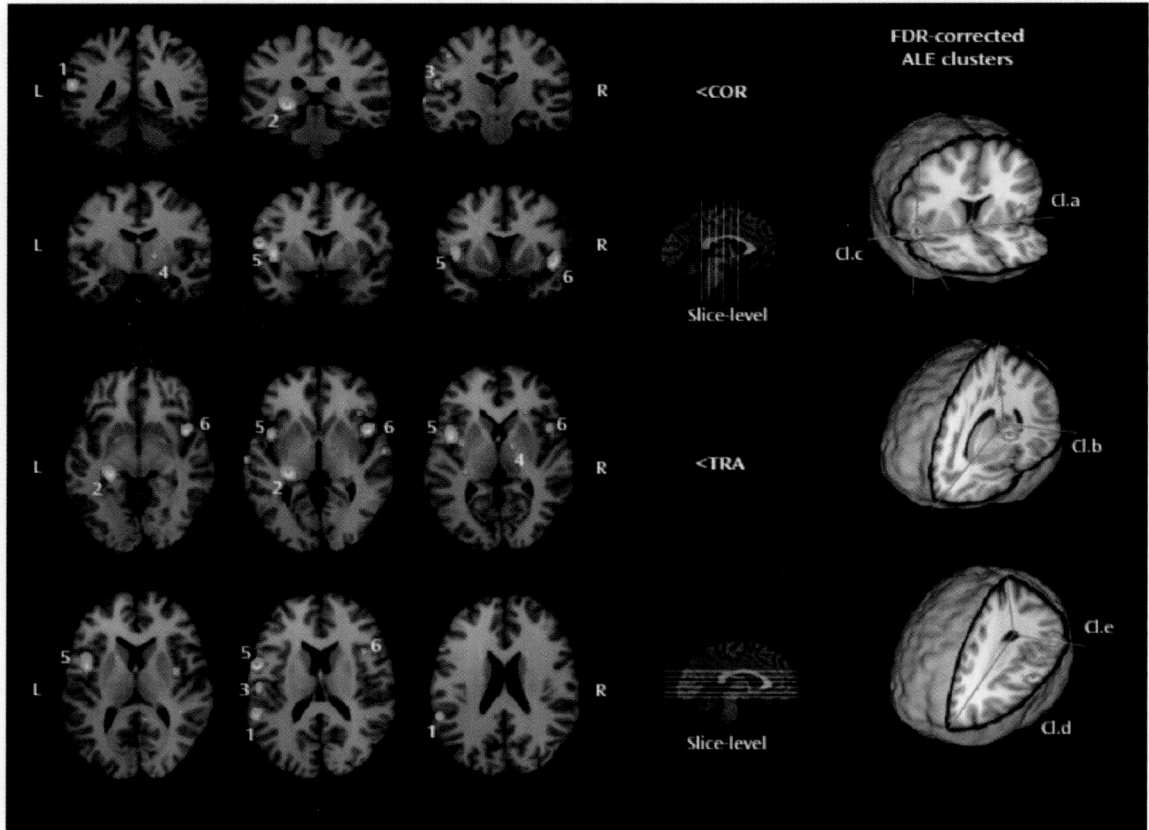

Figure 20.2 *Functional brain activity associated with auditory verbal hallucinations in schizophrenia. The first three columns depict the activation likelihood estimation (ALE) results on coronal (COR) views (upper panel) as well as on transverse (TRA) views (lower panel) of the brain anatomy. The fourth column depicts slice levels shown on sagittal views. The fifth column shows clusters (Cl.a to Cl.e) of consistent activity among patients with schizophrenia spectrum disorders experiencing auditory verbal hallucinations. Reproduced from: Jardri, R., A. Pouchet, et al. (2011). "Cortical activations during auditory verbal hallucinations in schizophrenia: a coordinate-based meta-analysis." The American Journal of Psychiatry 168(1): 73–81; used with permission.*

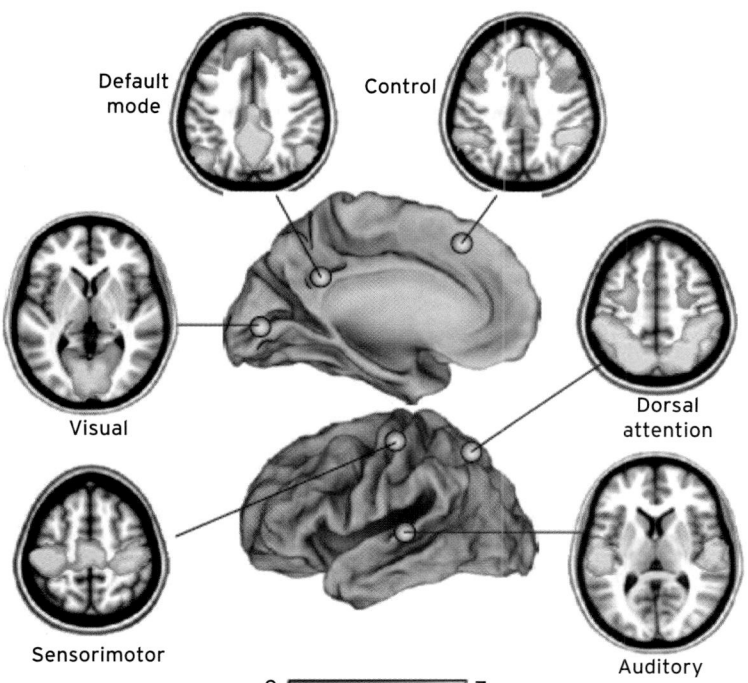

Figure 20.3 Intrinsic neuronal activity of the brain. Correlation of neuronal activity between a seed region (each circle) and the rest of the brain reveals six major networks: visual, sensorimotor, auditory, default mode, dorsal attention, and executive control. The scale numbered 0–7 indicates relative correlation strength. Reproduced from: Zhang, D. and M. E. Raichle (2010). "Disease and the brain's dark energy." Nat.Rev.Neurol. 6(1): 15–28 with permission from Nature Publications Group.

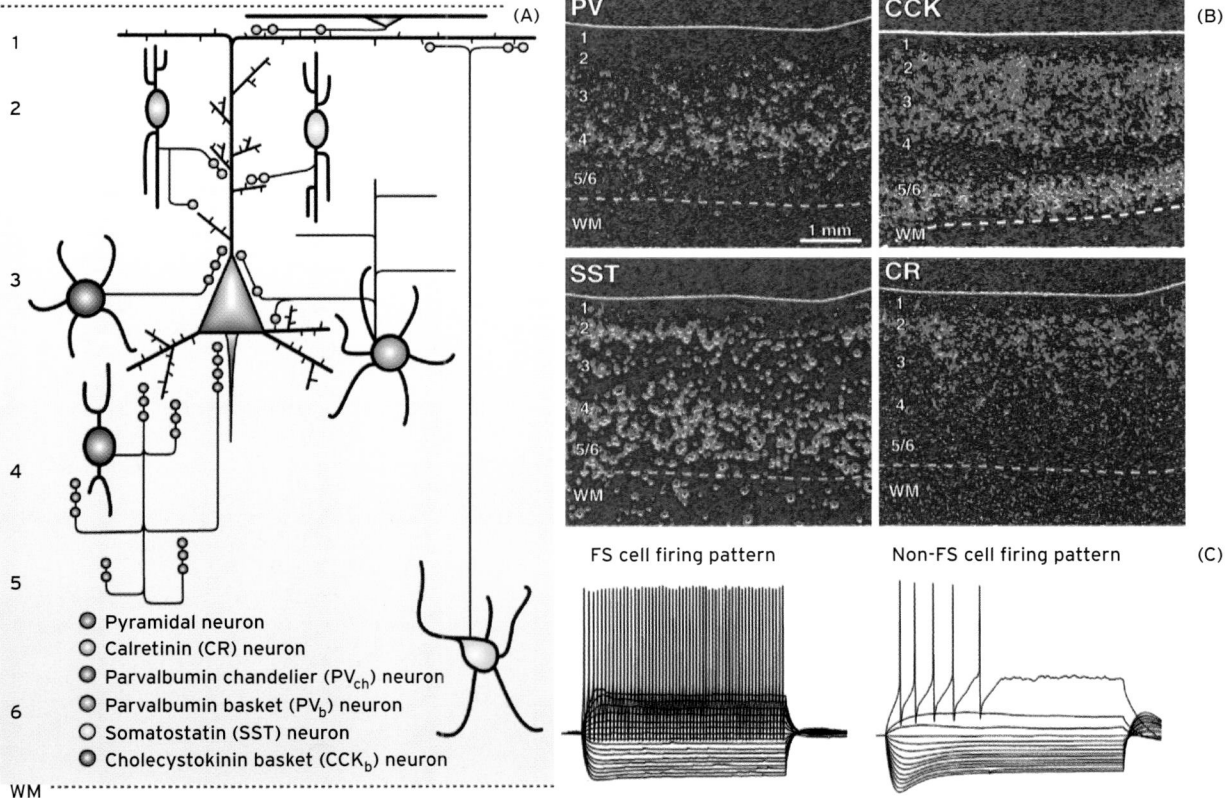

○ Pyramidal neuron
○ Calretinin (CR) neuron
○ Parvalbumin chandelier (PV$_{ch}$) neuron
○ Parvalbumin basket (PV$_b$) neuron
○ Somatostatin (SST) neuron
○ Cholecystokinin basket (CCK$_b$) neuron

Figure 23.1 Diversity of cortical GABA neurons. GABAergic interneurons can be classified based on morphological (A), molecular (B), and electrophysiological (C) properties. Some interneurons express the calcium binding proteins parvalbumin (PV) or calretinin (CR), whereas others contain the neuropeptides somatostatin (SST) or cholecystokinin (CCK). (A) PV and CCK neurons target the perisomatic region of pyramidal cells, while SST and CR neurons target pyramidal neuron dendrites. PV neurons can be divided into chandelier (PV$_{ch}$) and basket (PV$_b$) cells based on their morphology. The axon terminals of PV$_{ch}$ cells exclusively target the pyramidal cell axon initial segment, while the terminals of PV$_b$ cells synapse onto the soma and proximal dendrites. (B) The different interneuron subtypes are distributed distinctively across the layers of the cortex, as evidenced by the different expression patterns of their mRNAs. (C) PV cells exhibit a fast spiking (FS) firing pattern, characterized by a high firing frequency and constant interval between action potentials, while the remaining subclasses are classified as non-FS cells that fire at a lower frequency and exhibit progressively increasing intervals between action potentials. (Image adapted from Gonzalez-Burgos et al. Am J Psychiatry (2007) 164 (1):12; and Hashimoto et al. Mol Psychiatry (2008) 13:147–161.)

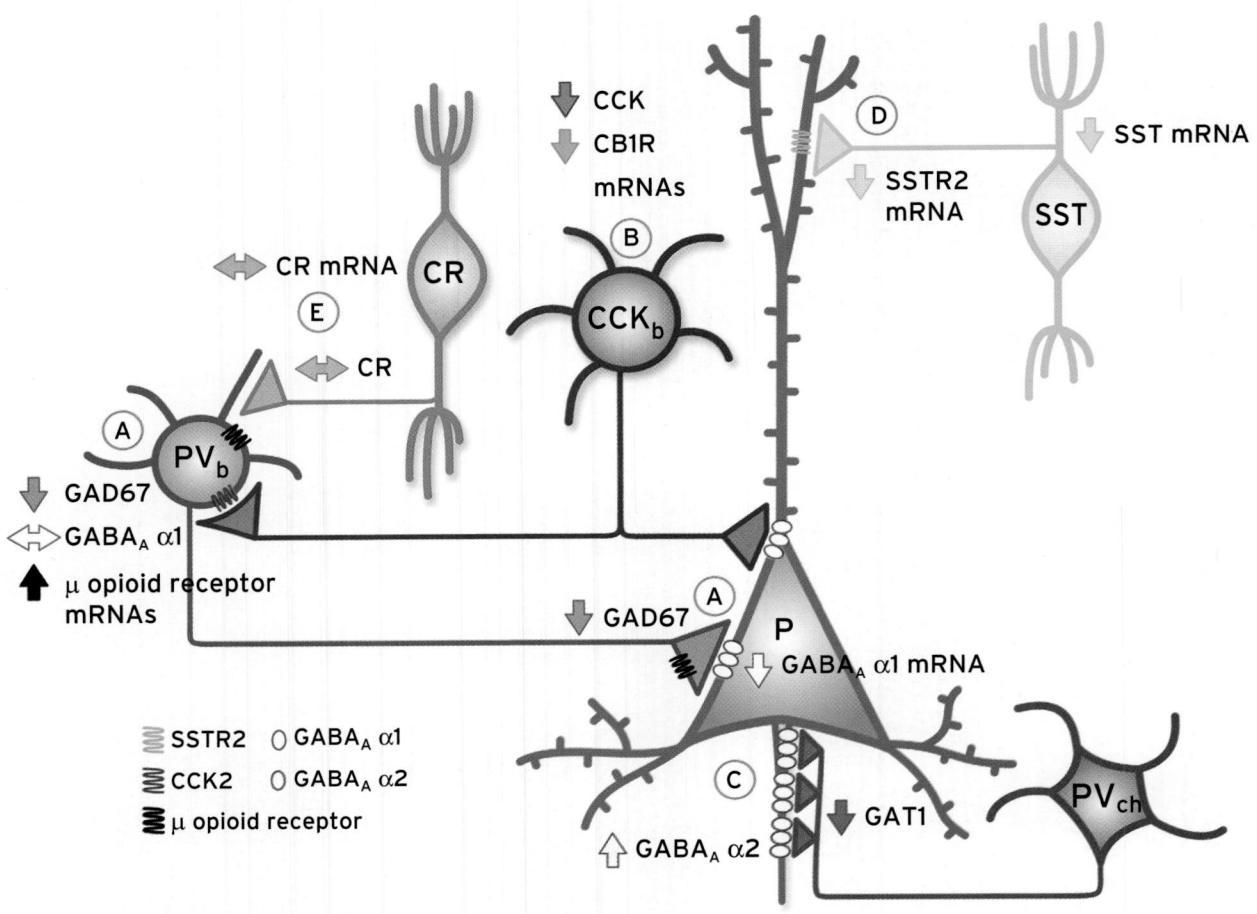

Figure 23.3 Schematic summary of alterations in neuronal circuitry in the PFC of subjects with schizophrenia. (A) The perisomatic inhibition of pyramidal (P) neurons by parvalbumin basket (PV_b) cells is lower due to (1) lower GAD67 mRNA and protein, and therefore less GABA synthesis; (2) higher levels of μ opioid receptor expression in PV_b cells that reduces their activity and suppresses GABA release; (3) reduced expression of cholecystokinin (CCK) mRNA, which stimulates the activity of, and GABA release from, PV_b cells; and (4) less mRNA for, and presumably fewer, postsynaptic GABA_A α1 receptors in pyramidal neurons. (B) The perisomatic inhibition of pyramidal neurons by cholecystokinin-expressing basket (CCK_b) cells is enhanced due to lower levels of CCK and cannabinoid 1 receptor (CB1R) mRNAs that reduce depolarization-induced suppression of inhibition (DSI). Levels of GAD67 in CCK_b cells are unknown, but are thought to be very low, relative to PV cells, in the healthy state. (C) PV-expressing chandelier (PV_ch) cells have decreased GABA membrane transporter 1 (GAT1) protein in their axon terminals and increased postsynaptic GABA_A α2-containing receptors at pyramidal neuron axon initial segments. The levels of GAD67 protein in PV_ch cells in schizophrenia are not known. (D) Somatostatin (SST)-containing cells contain lower mRNA levels of SST, and expression of its receptor, SSTR2, is also lower. Levels of GAD67 in SST cells have not been measured. (E) Calretinin (CR)-containing cells are thought to be unaffected, since levels of CR mRNA and protein are unchanged. GAD67 levels in CR cells are unknown.

		Fusar-Poli2012	Giuliano2012	Combined
Test	Measure			
WAIS-R	Digit Span	-0.39	-0.4	-0.395
	Block design	-0.2	-0.4	-0.3
	Digit Symbol	-0.35	-0.52	-0.435
WMS-R	Logical Memory I	-0.25	-0.49	-0.37
	Visual Repro I (RCFT Imm)	-0.39	NA	-0.39
	Visual Repro II (RCFT Delayed)		-0.16	-0.16
CVLT	Trials 1-5	-0.47	-0.68	-0.575
RAVLT	Sum 1-5	-0.37	-0.47	-0.42
	WCST Total Perseverative Resp	-0.25	-0.36	-0.305
Stroop	Color	NA	-0.25	-0.25
	Color Word	NA	-0.09	-0.09
Finger Tap	RH + LH	-0.09	-0.22	-0.155
Trail Making	A seconds	-0.34	-0.41	-0.375
	B seconds	-0.39	-0.47	-0.43
CPT	Vigilance (total correct)	-0.35	-0.4	-0.375
CFL	FAS Total unique	-0.27	-0.48	-0.375
Animal Naming	Total unique	-0.45	-0.66	-0.555
WRAT-R2	Reading	NA	-0.35	-0.35

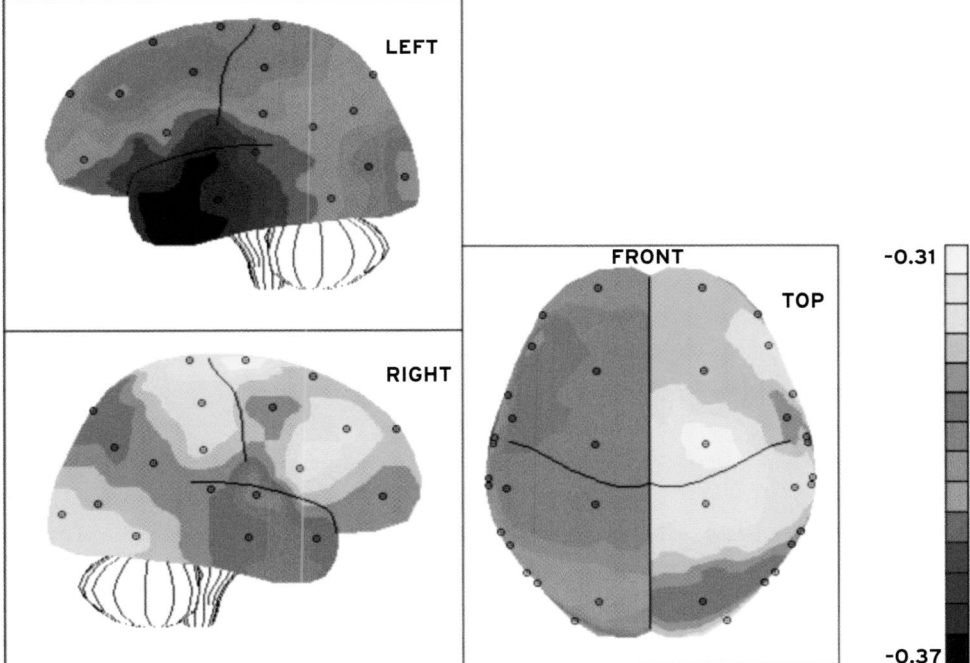

Figure 26.1 *Behavioral Image displays of left hemisphere, right hemisphere, and top view. Values are based on the meta-analyses of tests examined and summarized in the table. The color scale indicates effect sizes of psychosis prone individuals relative to healthy controls.*

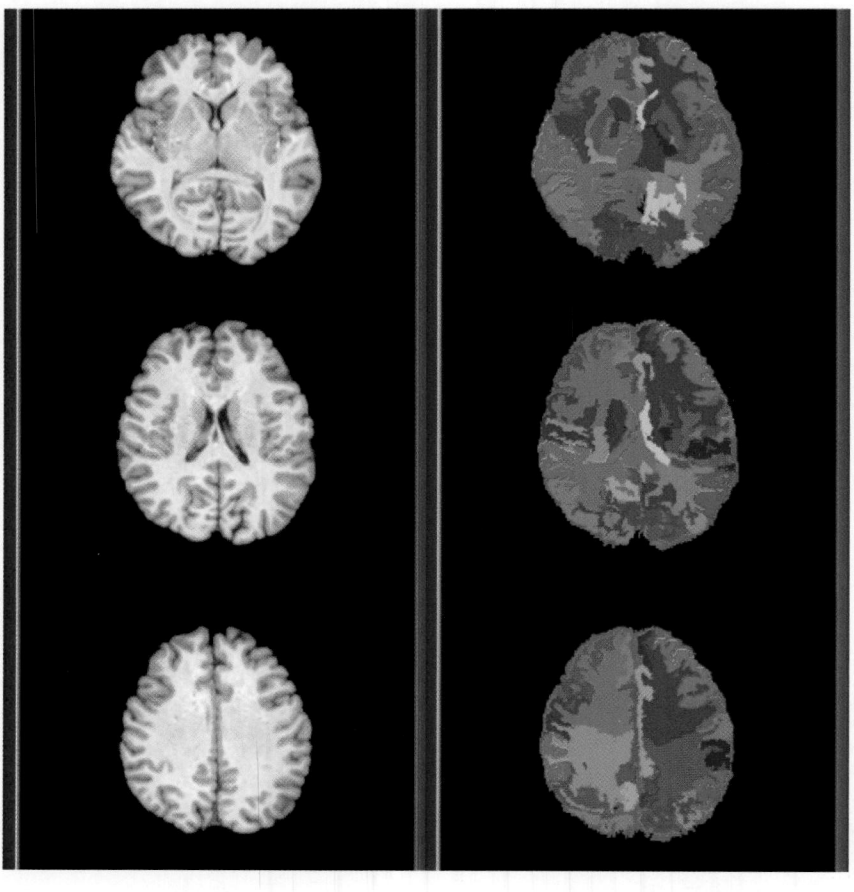

Original Image
(skull removed)

Labelled Image
(each color represents a Region of Interest)

Figure 26.2 MRI template-warping for parcellating regions of interest. A template in which regions are labeled and demarcated is warped into an individual's MRI recording the extent of changes required. As a result, axial slices such as seen on the left are labeled as seen on the right column. Regional volumes can then be calculated for quantitative analysis allowing, for example, comparison between psychosis prone and healthy participants.

FRACTIONAL ANISOTROPY

TRACTOGRAPHY
SUPERIOR LONGITUDINAL FASCICULUS

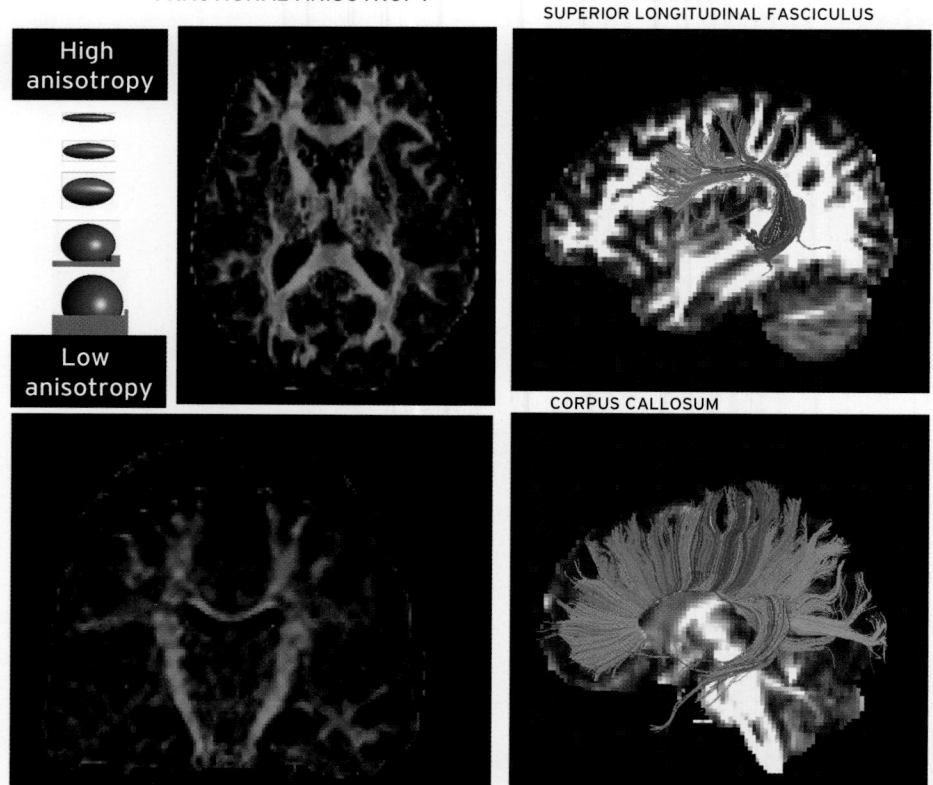

High anisotropy

Low anisotropy

CORPUS CALLOSUM

Figure 26.3 Diffusion tensor imaging (DTI) illustrates fractional anisotropy (left) and tractography (right). Fractional anisotropy reveals white matter architecture while tractography depicts the integrity of fiber tracts.

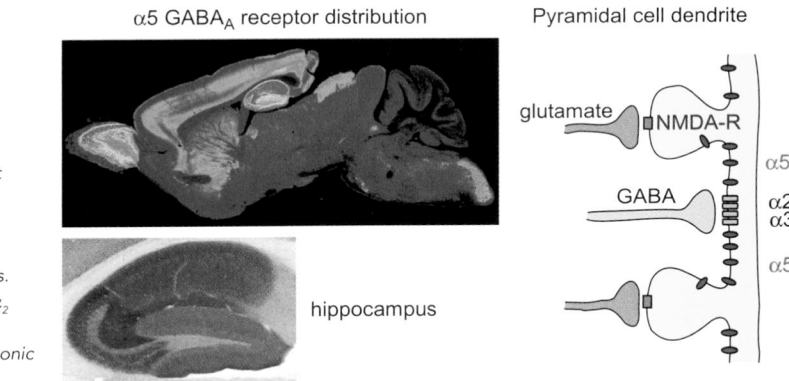

α5 GABA_A receptor distribution

Pyramidal cell dendrite

hippocampus

Figure 42.4 Left: Immunohistochemical distribution of the α_5-subunit GABA_A receptor in parasagittal sections of adult mice with the enlargement of the hippocampal formation showing its prominent dendritic localization (Crestani et al., 2002). Right: Schematic distribution of GABA_A receptor subtypes at pyramidal cell dendrites. In balancing the excitatory input, phasic inhibition is mediated via α_2 and α_3 GABA_A receptors, while α_5 GABA_A receptors, located at the base of dendritic spines and the adjacent dendritic shaft, mediate tonic inhibition.

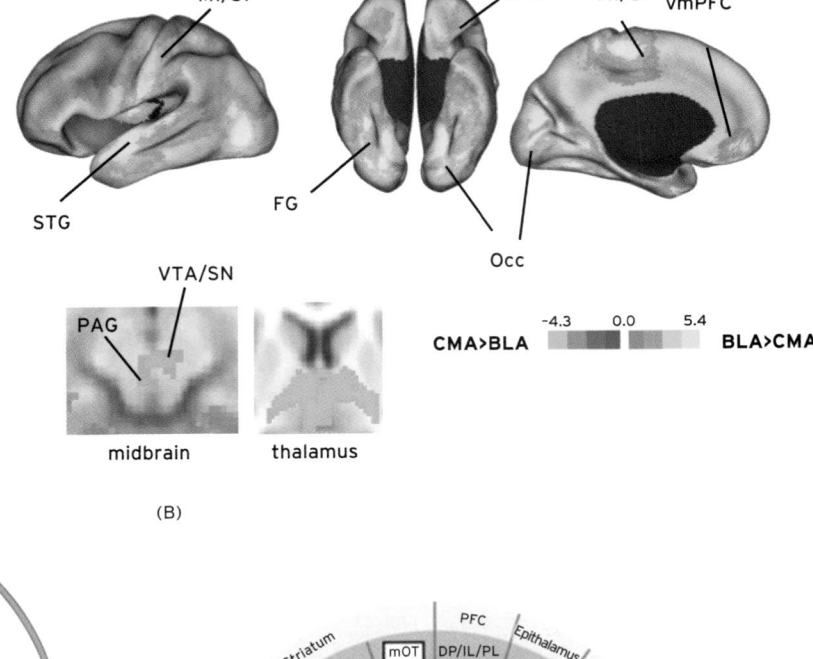

Figure 45.2 Differential connectivity of the basolateral (BLA) and centromedial (CMA) amygdalar subregions during resting-state fMRI. Findings are from a conjunction of two cohorts of healthy participants. The BLA connectivity was primarily cortical; CMA connectivity was primarily subcortical. Color scales represent t scores for the main effect of region in a voxelwise analysis. Red indicates that BLA connectivity is increased compared with CMA connectivity; blue, CMA connectivity is increased compared with BLA connectivity. FG, fusiform gyrus; M1/S1, primary somatosensory and motor cortices; Occ, occipital cortex; OFC, orbitofrontal cortex; PAG, periaqueductal gray; STG, superior temporal gyrus; vmPFC, ventromedial prefrontal cortex; and VTA/SN, ventral tegmental area/substantia nigra.

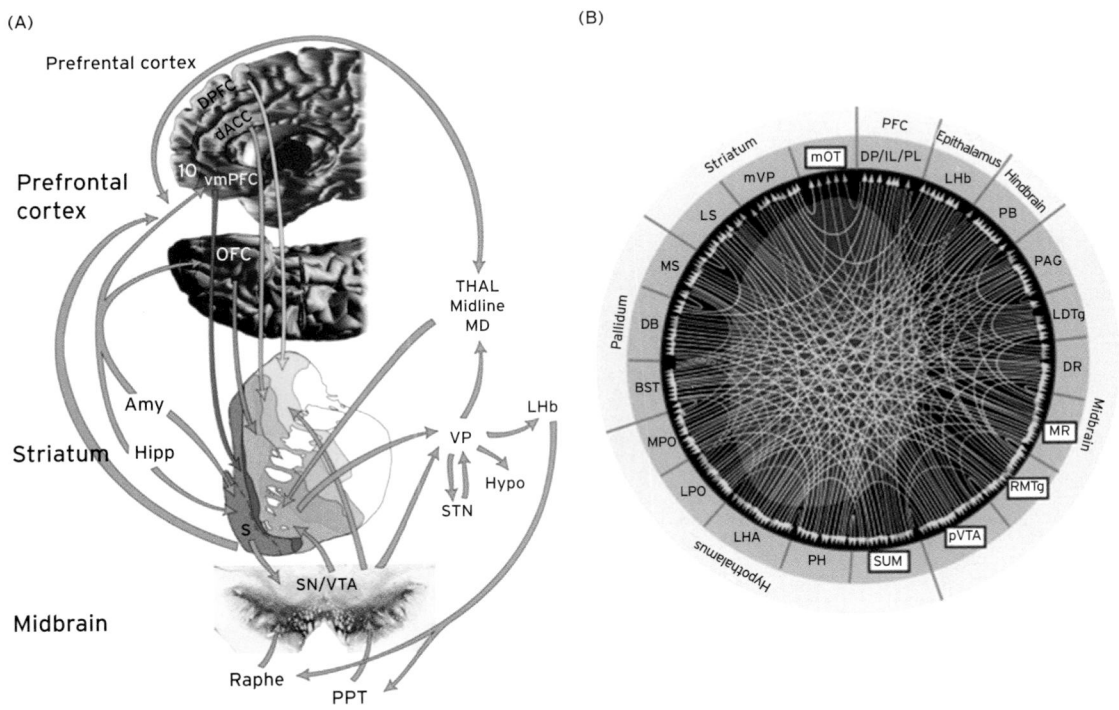

Figure 55.1 The reward circuit and its complexity. (A) Brain regions identified as being key players in the reward circuit, including striatal, midbrain, and prefrontal regions and, more recently, the amygdala, hippocampus, lateral habenula, and brainstem structures. (B) The connectivity between proposed brain reward regions is incredibly complex and has rendered identifying the roles of individual components difficult. Orange lines indicate unidirectional connection and yellow lines reciprocal connections. Purple area represents the medial forebrain bundle, the stimulation of which results in rewarding brain stimulation. (A from Haber S.N., Knutson B. (2010). The reward circuit: linking primate anatomy and human imaging. Neuropsychopharmacology 35:4–26. B from Ikemoto S. (2010). Brain reward circuitry beyond the mesolimbic dopamine system: a neurobiological theory. Neurosci Biobehav Rev 35:129–150.)

A. Healthy Patient

B. MCI Patient with Atrophy

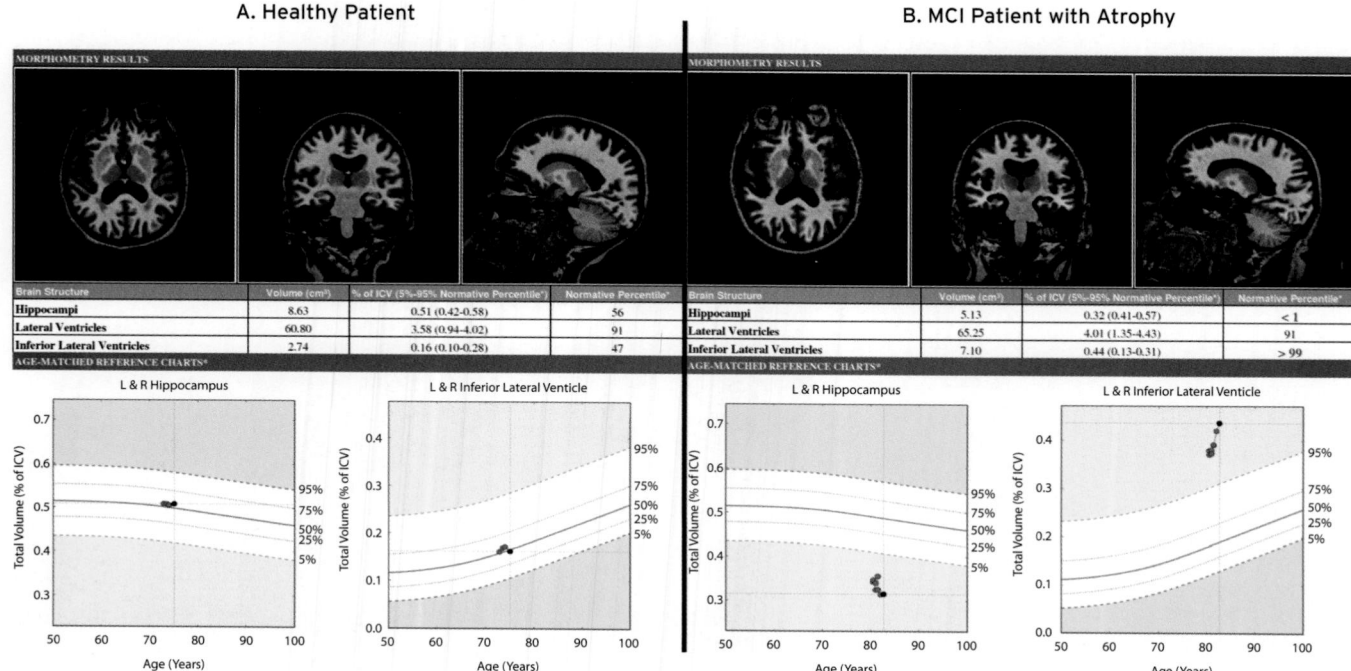

Brain Structure	Volume (cm³)	% of ICV (5%-95% Normative Percentile*)	Normative Percentile*
Hippocampi	8.63	0.51 (0.42-0.58)	56
Lateral Ventricles	60.80	3.58 (0.94-4.02)	91
Inferior Lateral Ventricles	2.74	0.16 (0.10-0.28)	47

Brain Structure	Volume (cm³)	% of ICV (5%-95% Normative Percentile*)	Normative Percentile*
Hippocampi	5.13	0.32 (0.41-0.57)	< 1
Lateral Ventricles	65.25	4.01 (1.35-4.43)	91
Inferior Lateral Ventricles	7.10	0.44 (0.13-0.31)	> 99

Figure 62.1 *Example volumetric reports for two subjects enrolled in a longitudinal quantitative imaging study. (A) A 75-year-old healthy subject who remained stable and was without evidence of hippocampal neurodegeneration or temporal horn enlargement during scanning over two years. (B) An 82-year-old, cognitively impaired subject who progressed from MCI to AD at the third year of follow-up. This patient was a non-carrier of APOE4 genotype who, by CSF testing, had elevated phospho-tau and reduced levels of amyloid beta 42 in cerebrospinal fluid. vMRI shows evidence of hippocampal neurodegeneration and ex vacuo dilatation of the temporal horns during scanning over two years.*

PIB follow-up
from healthy control to MCI/AD

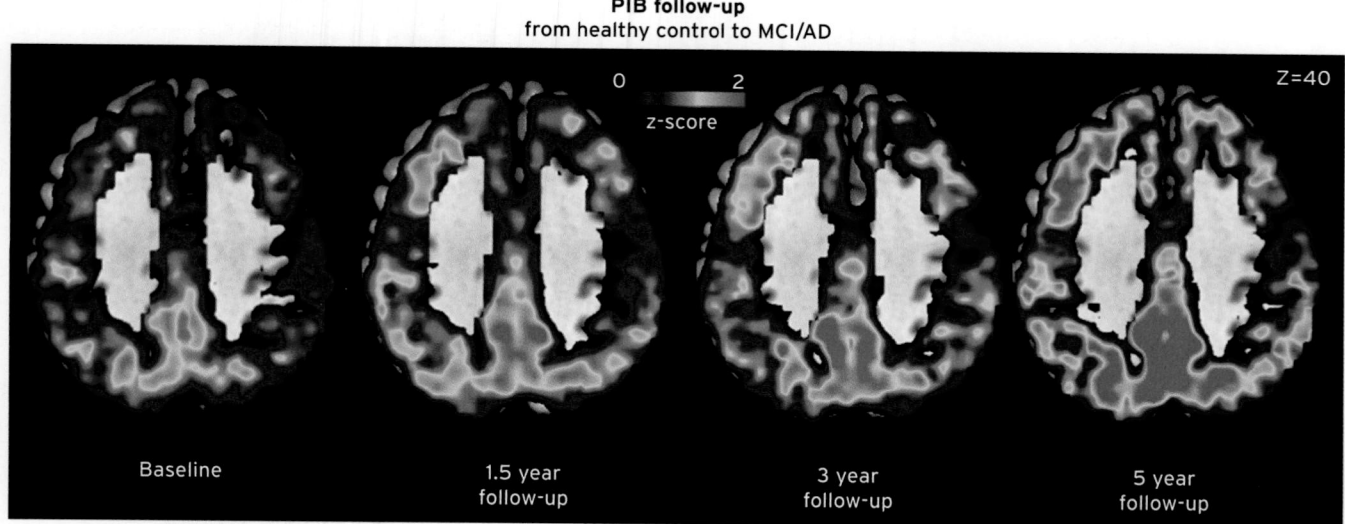

Figure 62.2 *Longitudinal PET amyloid imaging of an individual subject who progressed from healthy to dementia.*

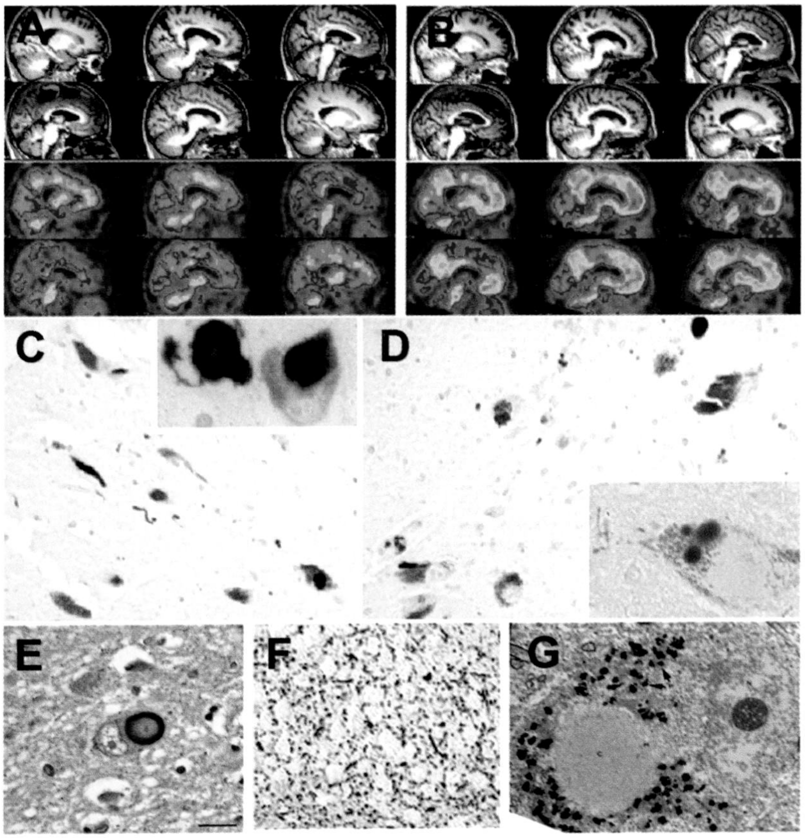

Figure 66.1 Imaging and pathology in lewy body dementia. (A) Sagittal sections of MRI and amyloid imaging in a case of PDD. There is mild cortical atrophy largely sparing the hippocampus. Amyloid imaging reveal minimal to no uptake of the PIB. (B) Sagittal section of MRI and amyloid imaging in a case of mixed LBD and AD. There is slightly more prominent atrophy of the hippocampus with significant uptake of PIB. (C) Photomicrograph of substantia nigra in DLB patient stained with α-synuclein. Note dystrophic neurites. Insert shows higher power magnification of two Lewy bodies in the nigral neurons. (D) Photomicrograph of substantia nigra in PDD patient stained with α-synuclein. Insert shows higher power magnification of a nigral neuron with multiple Lewy bodies. (E) Photomicrograph of Lewy body in the cingulate cortex of a LBD patient stained with α-synuclein. (F) Photomicrograph of dystrophic neurites in the CA 2–3 region of the hippocampus in a LBD patient. (G), Electron micrograph of a Lewy body. Note the dense core (gray) surrounded by a paler halo.

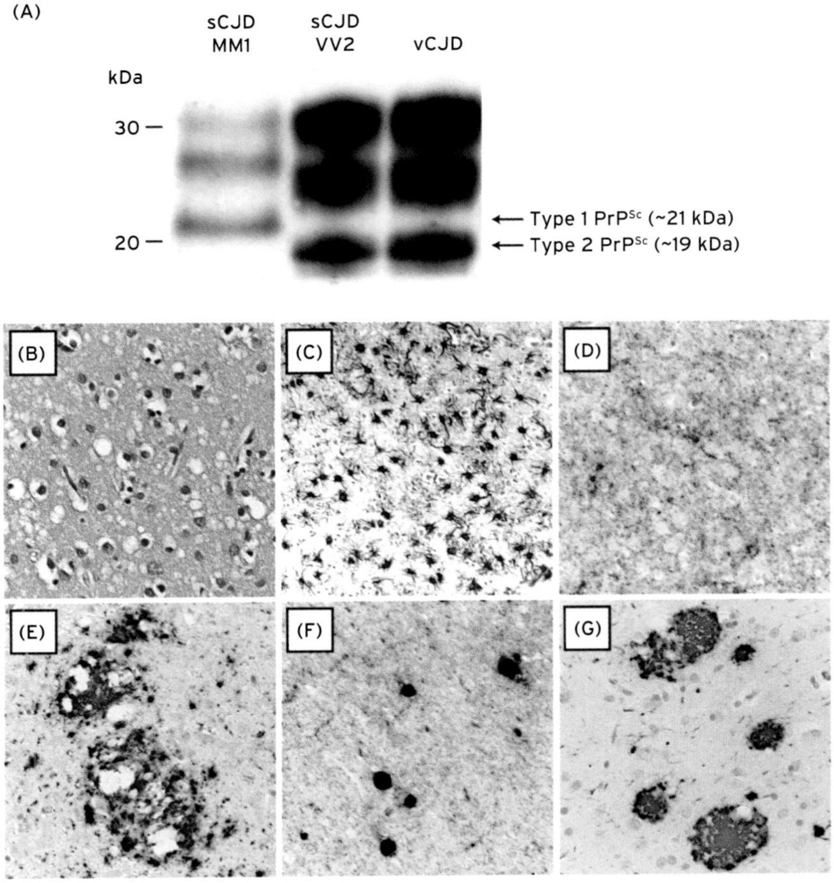

Figure 69.4 Biochemical and neuropathological hallmarks of human prion disease. (A–F) The neuropathological hallmarks of prion disease. Spongiform change (A) and reactive astrocytic gliosis (B) in the parietal cortex of a patient with sporadic CJD (subtype MM1). (C) The synaptic pattern of PrPSc deposition in the frontal cortex of a patient with sporadic CJD exhibiting the MM1 subtype. (D) Perivacuolar PrPSc deposition in the parietal cortex of a patient with MM2 sporadic CJD. (E) Kuru-like PrPSc plaques in the molecular layer of the cerebellum in a patient with MV2 sporadic CJD. (F) PrPSc amyloid plaques in the hippocampus of a GSS patient with the A117V mutation. (G) As revealed by immunoblotting, protease-resistant PrPSc, the biochemical signature of prion disease, is observed in the brains of patients with CJD. In sporadic CJD subtype MM1, type 1 PrPSc is present, whereas type 2 PrPSc is observed in sporadic CJD subtype VV2 and variant CJD.

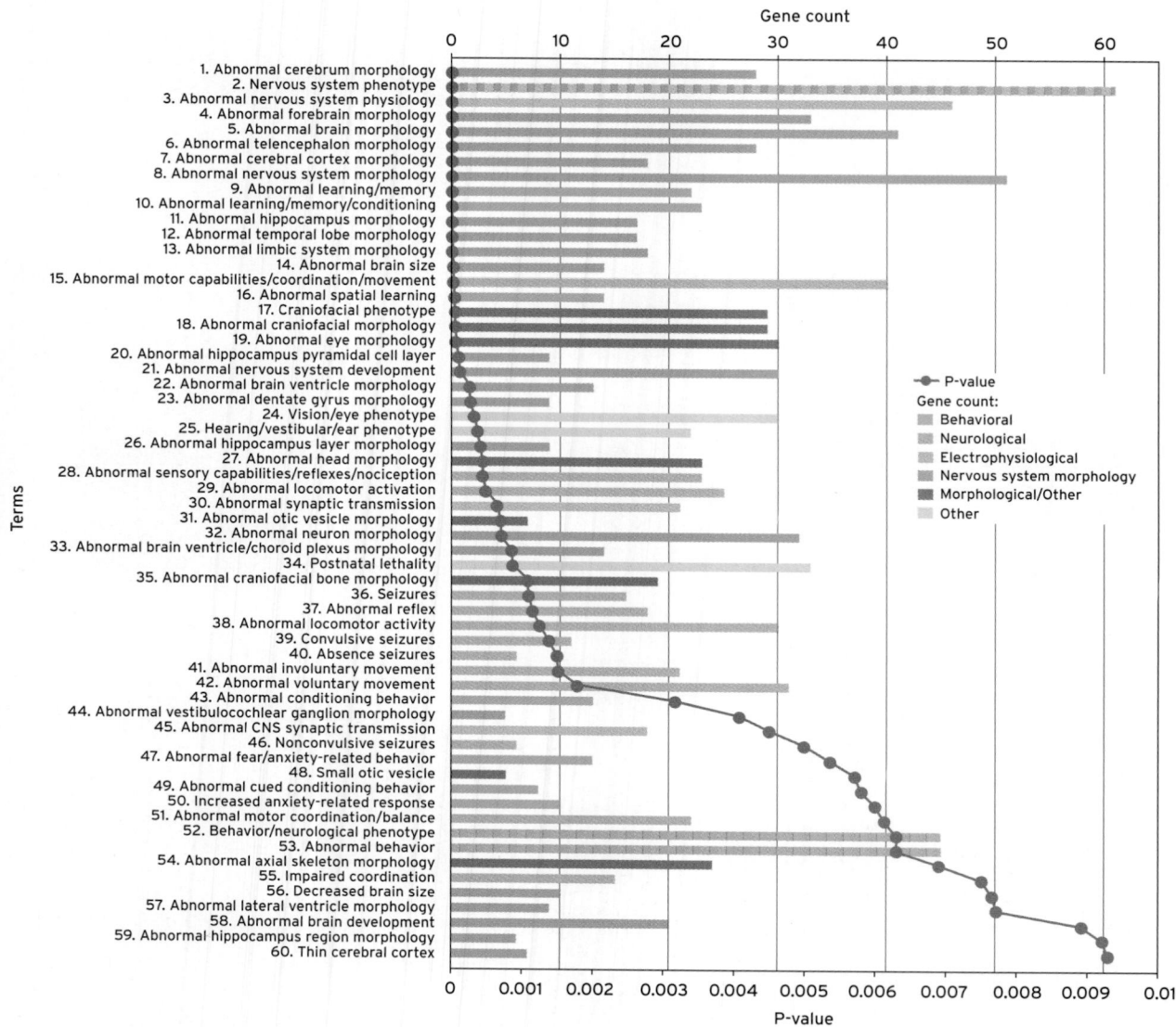

Figure 73.1 *Mouse phenotype categories associated with ASD genes. ASD genes (N = 112) were analyzed for enrichment in mouse phenotypes using ToppGene with a Bonferroni corrected p value cutoff of 0.01. Categories are arranged from most significant and downwards (purple line), and for each category, the number of genes in the ASD112 list for which there were murine models with the associated category are indicated by the length of the horizontal bars (gene count). To highlight differing phenotypic categories, bars are color-coded as indicated in the inset to the figure. Categories relating to nervous system morphology phenotype domains are colored light blue, whereas other morphological categories are colored dark blue, electrophysiological categories are colored pink, neurological categories are colored peach, and higher-order behavioral categories are colored green. Categories corresponding to more than one phenotyping domain are presented as alternating colors, and categories that do not relate to the phenotyping scheme are colored yellow. (Adapted from Buxbaum J.D., Betancur C., Bozdagi O., et al. (2012) Optimizing the phenotyping of rodent ASD models: enrichment analysis of mouse and human neurobiological phenotypes associated with high-risk autism genes identifies morphological, electrophysiological, neurological, and behavioral features. Mol. Autism, 3(1):1.*

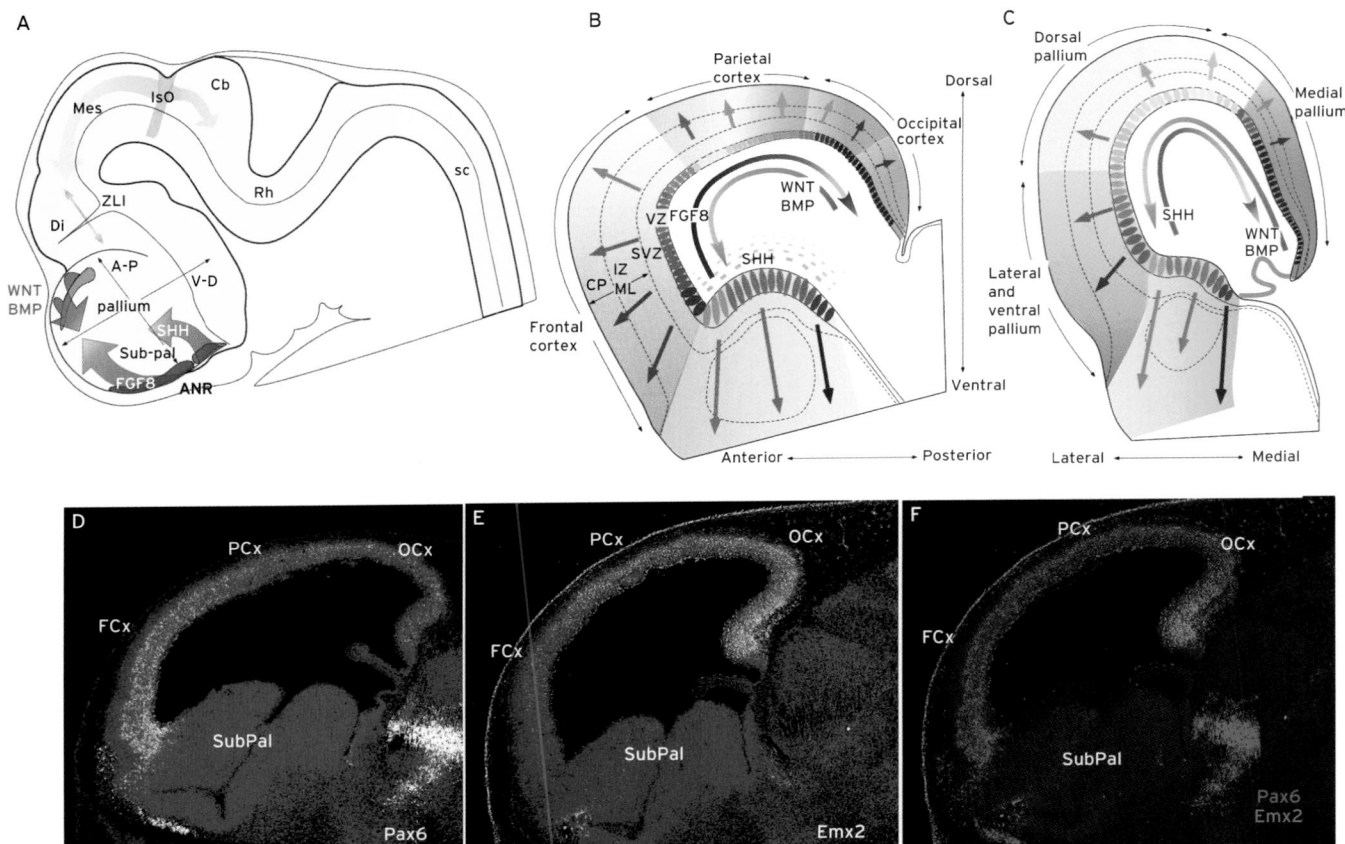

Figure 74.2 *Morphogenetic signals and telencephalic regionalization. (A) Schematic representation of neural tube (lateral view) where the main brain regions have been identified and morphogenetic signals regulating telencephalic regionalization have been represented by colors and arrows. Wnt and Bmp are dorsalizing signals, Fgf8 is a rostralizing signal, and Shh is a ventralizing signal, acting upon dorsal (pallial) telencephalon to specify cortical functional areas in the epithelium. (B,C) Schematic representation of a section in anteroposterior (B) and coronal (C) planes of the dorsal telencephalon (pallium and subpallium) that were color coded in neuroepithelial cells. Colored arrows in the ventricle and the dashed area (B) represent morphogenetic gradients that were translated through the neural wall by radial migration of neural cells into the different cortical regions (radial arrows and color gradient domains). (D–F) Sagittal sections showing the gradient expression pattern of two transcription factors: Pax6 regulated by rostral and ventralizing signals (D), and Emx2 regulated by dorsalizing signals (E). F, A combinatory Photoshop reconstruction of both gradient patterns.*

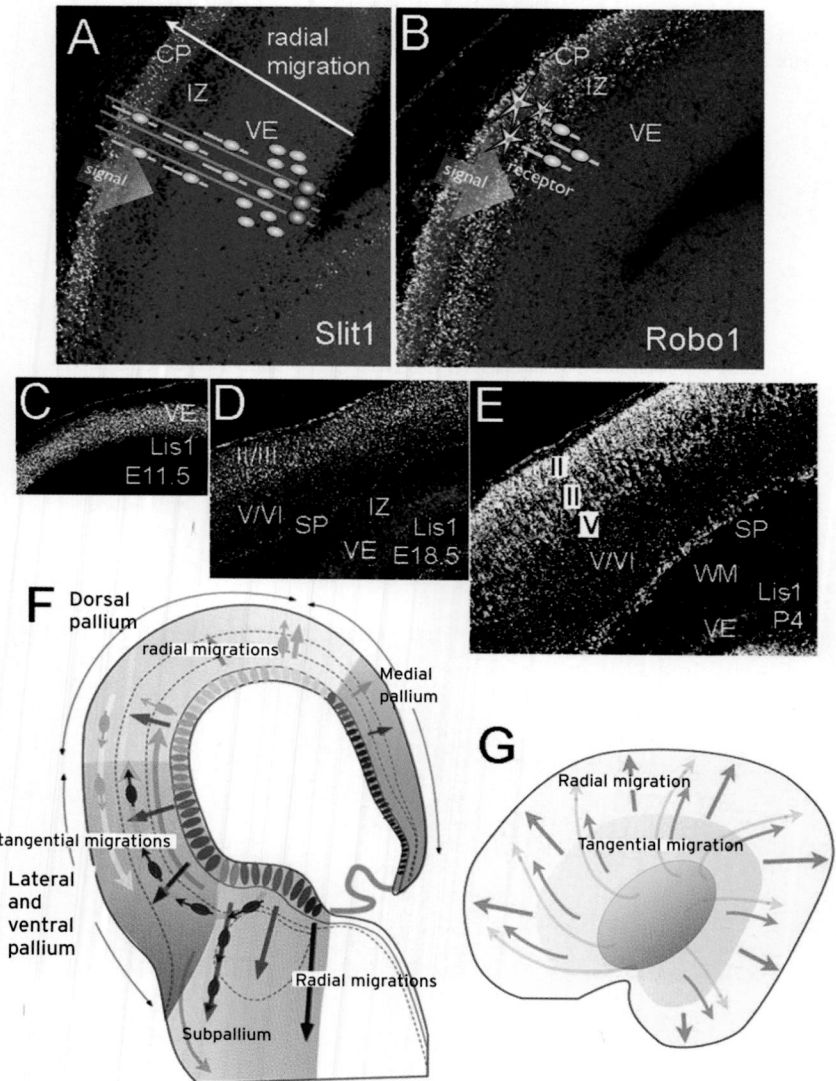

Figure 74.4 *Neuronal migration in the pallium: cortical development. (A,B) Signal: Slit1 expression in E15.5 mouse embryo in the cortical plate. Neural progenitors proliferate in the ventricular epithelium (VE) and subventricular zone (yellow ovoid cells), radial glia cells are schematized in gray with long radial processes crossing the neural wall from ventricular to pail surface. Migrating neurons were distributed in between radial glia processes in the intermediate zone (IZ; yellow ovoid soma with processes) toward the cortical plate (CP). In an equivalent section the receptor of Slit1, Robo1 is expressed in migrating cells of the IZ. (C–E) Expression of Lis1 gene in developing and postnatal mouse cortex. (F) Schematic representation of a coronal section were different lateromedial (ventrodorsal) pallial domains are represented by colored fields. Radial migration is represented by radial arrows and tangential migrations are represented by concentric distributed arrows. Migrating cells were represented by ovoid soma and arrows. (G) Planar representation of the telencephalic vesicle where radial migrations are represented by orange arrows; pallio-pallial tangential migration is represented by grey arrows; subpallio-pallial tangential migration, coming from the subpallium (central orange ovoid).*

Structural and Functional Connectomics

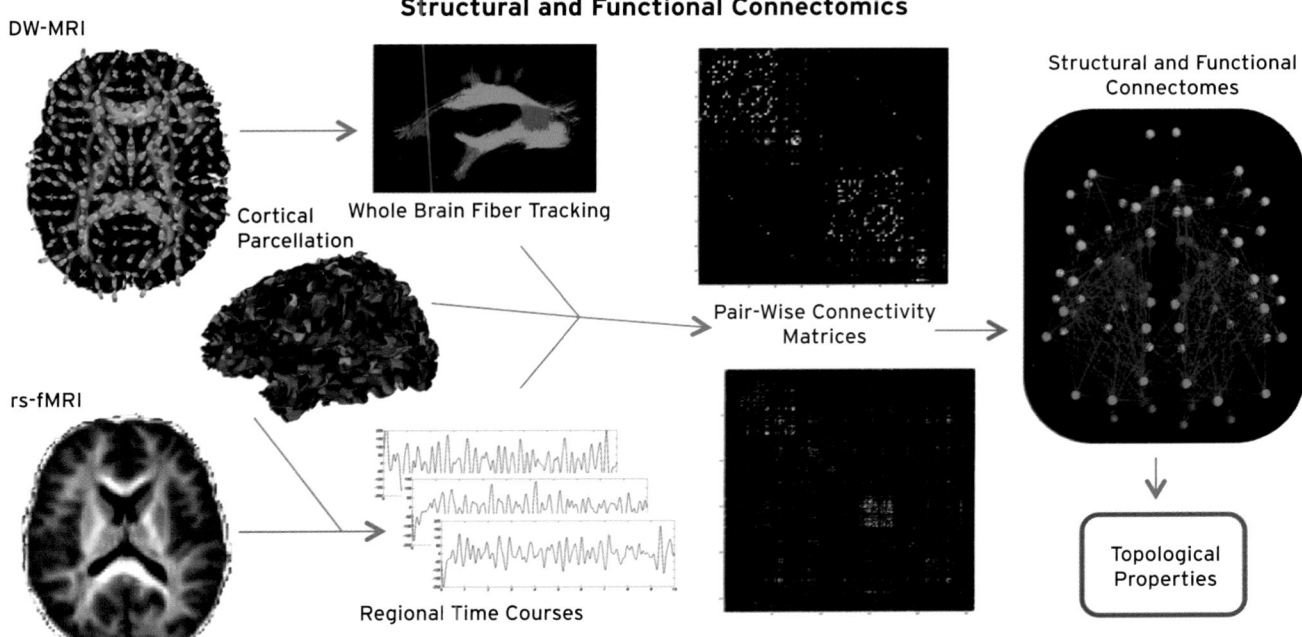

Figure 75.1 *Functional and structural connectomics. The computation of structural and functional connectomes begins with the acquisition of either DW-MRI or rs-fMRI datasets and the parcellation of the cortex into the regions of interest (ROIS). Each modality undergoes specific preprocessing to remove artifacts. For DW-MRI, tractography algorithms are used to identify anatomical pathways connecting the ROIs and information related to these is collected into the pairwise connectivity matrix. Using the rs-fMRI datasets, ROI time courses are extracted and the pairwise connectivity matrix is formed by computing the temporal correlation between each ROI time course. These connectivity matrices can then be combined into a joint structural/functional connectome that can be used in subsequent analysis to represent the brain networks of the subject.*

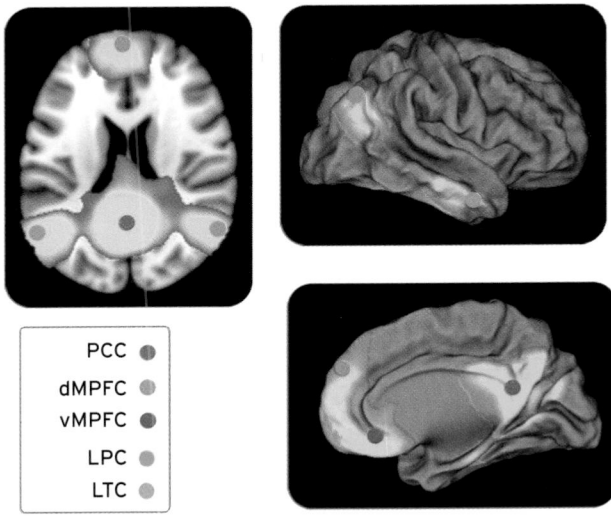

Figure 75.2 *Default mode network. Temporally correlated activity in regions of the default mode network (DMN) has been shown to increase during non–goal-oriented activities and to decrease during goal oriented activities. The areas of the DMN is illustrated via a group averaged (n = 225) temporal correlation map generated by using the posterior cingulate cortex (PCC) as the seed region. The prominent regions of the DMN, the dorsal and ventral medial prefrontal cortexes (dMPFC and vMPFC), the lateral temporal cortex (LTC), and the lateral parietal cortex (LPC) are clearly indicated as being positively correlated with activity in the PCC.*

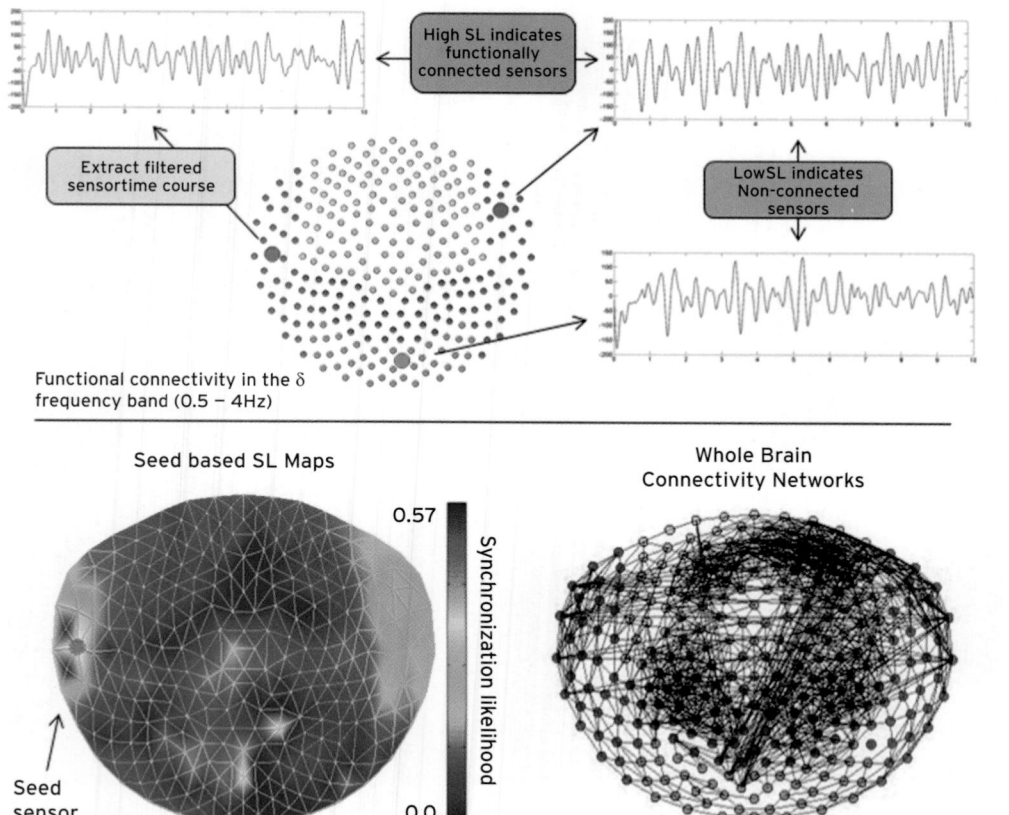

Functional connectivity in the δ
frequency band (0.5 – 4Hz)

Figure 75.3 MEG based functional connectivity. Measuring function connectivity with electrophysiologic modalities like MEG proceeds by extracting time courses of interest from the MEG sensor data. The high temporal resolution of MEG allows users to focus on connectivity within particular frequency bands; for instance, this figure focuses on connectivity in the delta (0.5 to 4 Hz) frequency band. The high resolution also allows for quantifying functional connectivity using complex measures, such as synchronization likelihood (SL). These measures can be computed on time courses from selected regions, shown at the top. Functionally connected sensors, such as those above the right and left motor areas, indicated by purple time courses, have higher SL values, whereas the SL between non-functionally connected regions, such as the occipital lobe and motor areas, have lower SL values. Maps showing connectivity to a particular seed region can also be computed. Similarly, whole brain networks can be determined by examining all of the pair-wise connectivity measures.

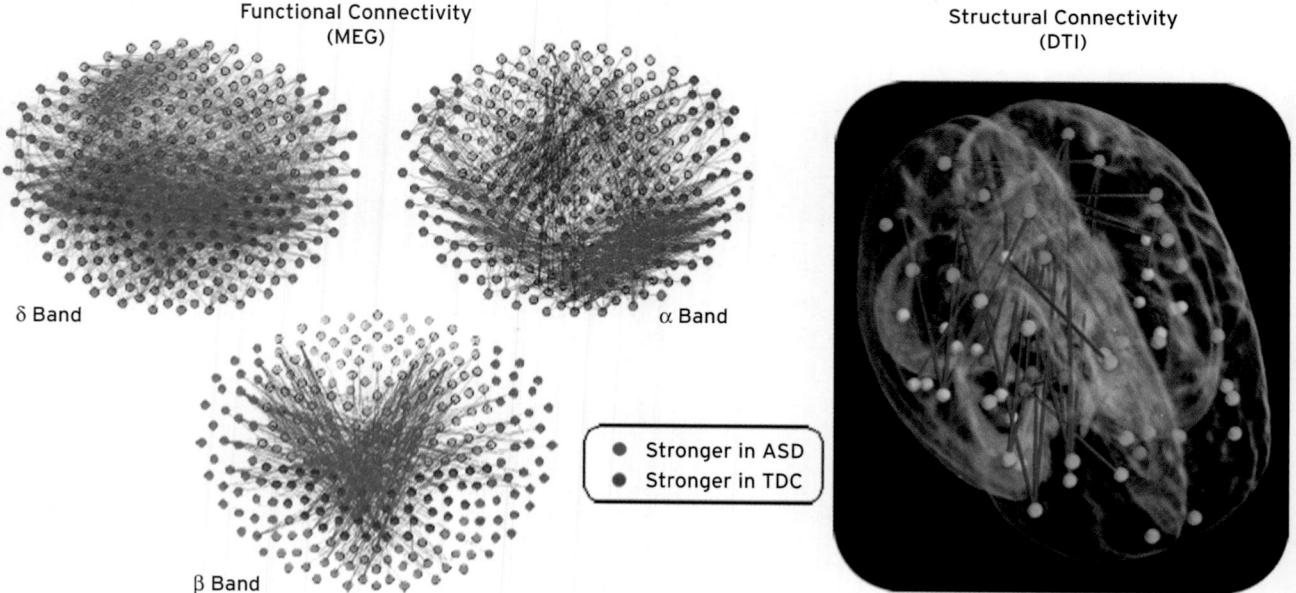

Figure 75.4 Structural and functional connectivity differences between ASD subjects and TDCS. Probabilistic tractography was used to compute DTI-based structural connectivity networks for each subject, which were then subjected to statistical analysis. Synchronization likelihood was used to compute functional connectivity networks in five frequency sub-bands of resting state MEG time courses. Shown are the significant different connections in the δ (0.5 to 4 Hz), α (8 to 13 Hz), and β (13 to 30 Hz). Light gray lines indicate connections that are stronger in the ASD population (predominantly shorter range frontal delta-band connections and posterior alpha-band connections), whereas dark gray lines indicated stronger connections in the TDC population (predominantly longer range and interhemispheric connections).

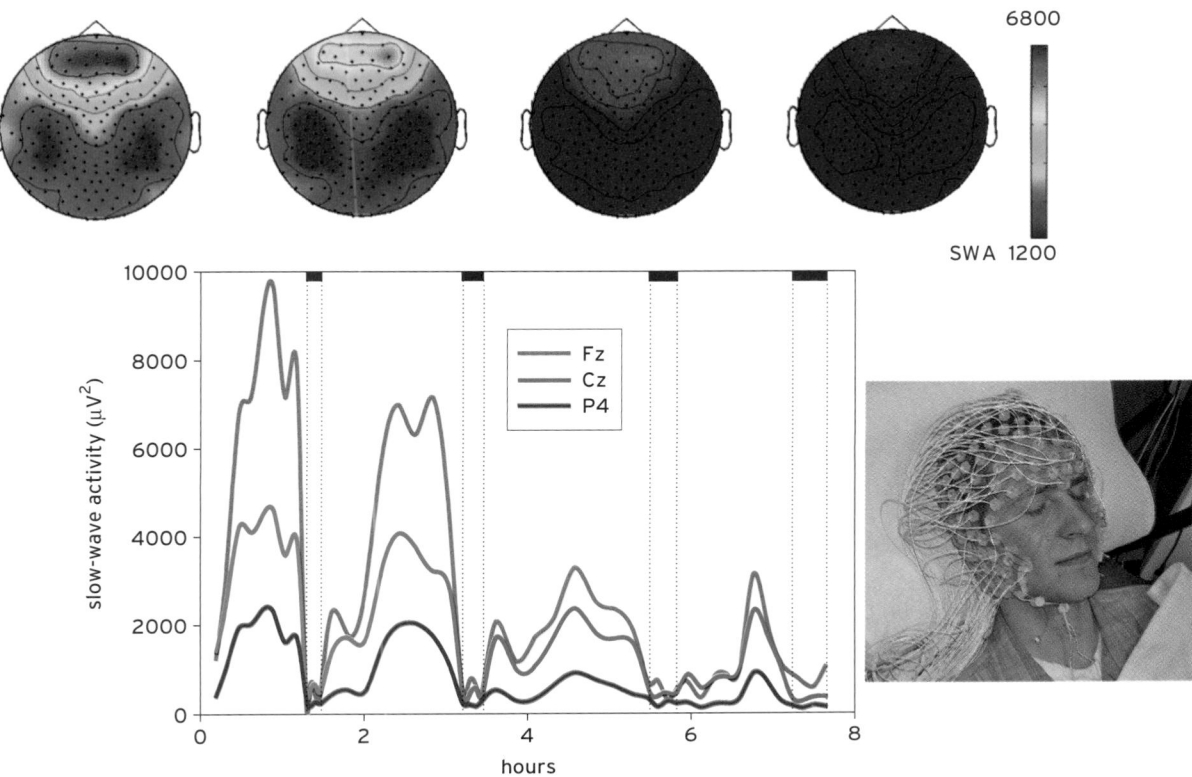

Figure 87.4 Sleep slow waves as a marker of sleep pressure. Bottom panel: During early sleep, at the end of a day of wakefulness, sleep pressure is maximal. This is reflected in frequent and large sleep slow waves, measured here as slow wave activity (power in the 0.5–4 Hz band, in red for a frontal electroencephalogram (EEG) channel, green for a central channel, and blue for an occipital channel). During sleep slow wave activity decreases exponentially, reflecting a reduction of sleep pressure. The transitory drops in slow-wave activity correspond to episodes of rapid-eye-movement (REM) sleep. Top panel: Topographic display of slow wave activity over the scalp for the four sleep cycles. Notice the frontal predominance and the progressive decline in the course of the night.

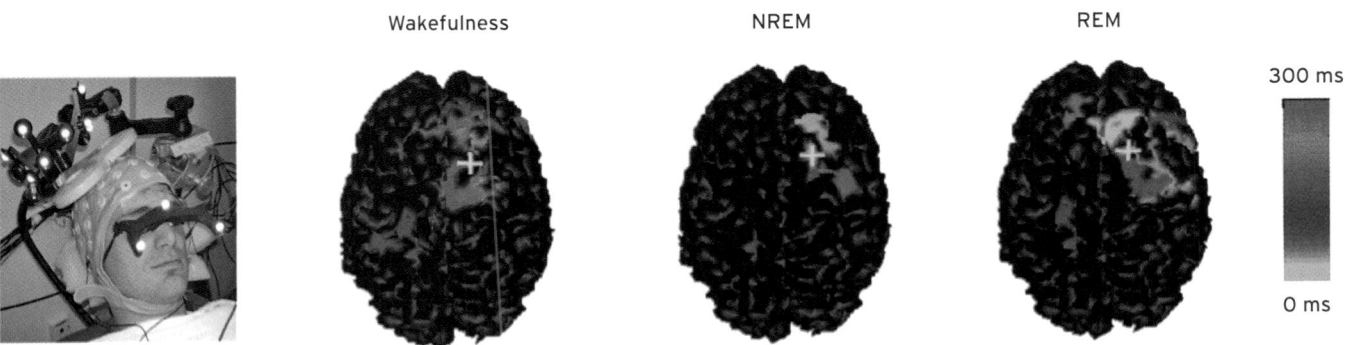

Figure 87.7 Spatiotemporal cortical current maps of transcranial magnetic stimulation (TMS)-induced activity during wakefulness, non-rapid eye movement (NREM), and REM sleep. On the left is the setup for TMS/EEG. From the electroencephalogram (EEG) data, maximum current sources corresponding to periods of significant activations were plotted and color-coded according to their latency of activation (light blue, 0 ms; red, 300 ms). The yellow cross marks the TMS target on the cortical surface. Note the rapidly changing patterns of activation during wakefulness, lasting up to 300 ms and involving several different areas; the brief activation that remains localized to the area of stimulation during NREM sleep; and an intermediate pattern of activation during REM sleep. (From Massimini M., Ferrarelli F., Huber R., et al., 2005. Breakdown of cortical effective connectivity during sleep. Science 309:2228–2232.)

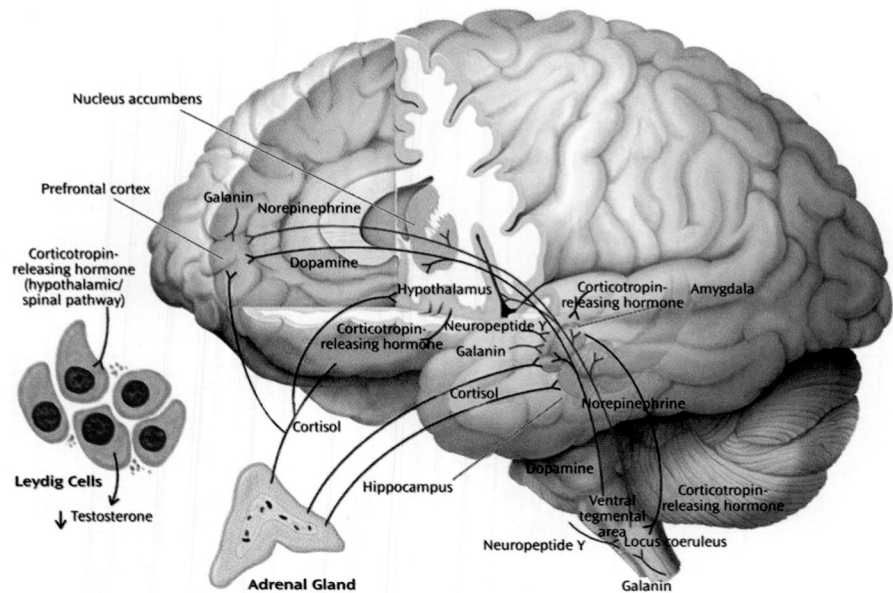

Figure 88.1 Neurochemical response patterns to acute stress. This figure illustrates some of the key brain structures involved in the neurochemical response patterns following acute psychological stress. The functional interactions among the different neurotransmitters, neuropeptides, and hormones are emphasized. The functional status of brain regions such as the amygdala (neuropeptide Y, galanin, corticotropin-releasing hormone [CRH], cortisol, and norepinephrine), hippocampus (cortisol and norepinephrine), locus coeruleus (neuropeptide Y, galanin, and CRH), and prefrontal cortex (dopamine, norepinephrine, galanin, and cortisol) depends upon the balance among multiple inhibitory and excitatory neurochemical inputs. Functional effects may vary depending on the brain region. For example, cortisol increases CRH concentrations in the amygdala and decreases concentrations in the paraventricular nucleus of the hypothalamus. As described in the text, these neurochemical response patterns may relate to resilience and vulnerability to the effects of extreme psychological stress. (Modified and reprinted with permission from Cambridge University Press, 2007.)

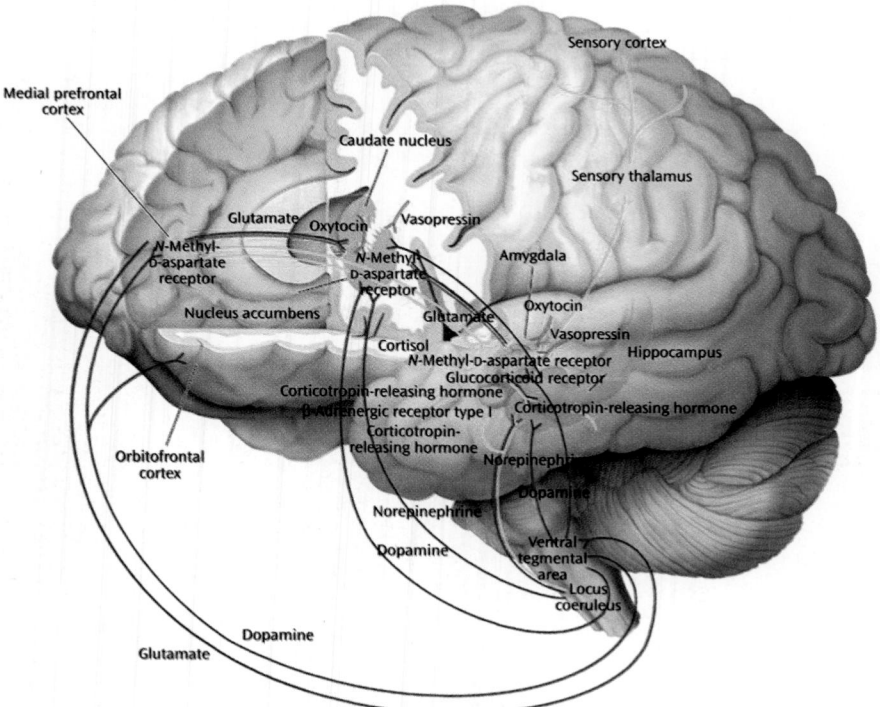

Figure 88.2 Neural circuits associated with reward, fear conditioning, and social behavior. The figure depicts a simplified summary of some of the brain structures and relevant neurochemistry mediating the neural mechanisms of reward (purple paths), fear conditioning and extinction (yellow paths), and social behaviors (blue paths). Only a subset of the many known interconnections among these various regions is shown, and relevant interneurons are not illustrated, yet it can be seen there is considerable overlap in the brain structures associated with these neural mechanisms. This suggests that there may be clinically relevant functional interactions among the circuits. For example, a properly functioning reward circuit may be necessary for the reinforcement of positive social behaviors. An overly responsive fear circuit or impaired extinction process may negatively influence functioning of the reward system. The assessment of these neural mechanisms must be considered in the context of their neurochemical regulation. Alterations in one neurotransmitter, neuropeptide, or hormone system will affect more than one circuit. Several receptors that may be targeted by new anti-anxiety and antidepressant drugs are illustrated. The functional status of these circuits has important influences on stress-related psychopathology and the discovery of novel therapeutics (see text). (Modified and reprinted with permission from Cambridge University Press, 2007.)

46 | NOVEL TREATMENT APPROACHES FOR ANXIETY DISORDERS

ANITA VAN ZWIETEN, GAIL A. ALVARES, AND ADAM J. GUASTELLA

A nxiety is conceptualized as a coherent structure of cognitive and affective components within the defensive motivational system that responds to perceived future threat or danger (Barlow, 2002). This complex system responds to perceived threatening information with cognitive and affective processes, physiological reactions, and behavioral responses, which relate to the well-known defensive behaviors of "freeze, fight, or flight" involved in the fear response (Sullivan et al., 2011). While anxiety is an adaptive response that serves both to alert and prepare the organism for potential threat (Barlow, 2002), pathological anxiety is characterized by its excessive expression across dimensions of duration, frequency, and/or intensity (Barlow, 2002). Anxiety disorders are thereby considered disorders of fear dysregulation (Myers and Davis, 2007).

A remarkable amount of progress has been made in the development of effective and acceptable treatments for anxiety disorders. Although evidence-based psychological and pharmacological treatments exhibit strong clinical efficacy across randomized controlled trials (RCTs), a significant number of individuals do not respond to treatment or relapse after treatment cessation. Such trials may also report overestimated effect sizes due to selection bias, with many complex or comorbid individuals excluded. These, and a number of other issues reviewed subsequently, have led to the surge of interest in recent years toward the need for efficacious and novel approaches in the treatment of anxiety disorders. Key priorities that have been highlighted are the need to identify and target the mechanisms (behavioral, cognitive, neurobiological) that underlie anxiety, as well as to develop comprehensive bio-psycho-social models that take into account factors involved in adherence and treatment response (Etkin, 2012; Taylor et al., 2012). The aim of this chapter, therefore, is to review evidence for recent and promising novel approaches to treat anxiety disorders that extend upon and augment existing best-practice interventions. After a discussion of the current state of evidence-based treatments for anxiety, evidence will be reviewed for several novel pharmacological, cognitive, and technological interventions, with reference to the specific neurobiological mechanisms of anxiety targeted in each. The interventions reviewed in this chapter are summarized in Table 46.2.

CURRENT STATE OF EVIDENCE-BASED TREATMENTS FOR ANXIETY DISORDERS

Existing psychological and pharmacological treatments for anxiety are well established in clinical settings. Although other psychotherapies (such as mindfulness-based therapy) have received some empirical support, cognitive-behavioral therapy (CBT) continues to be the gold standard for psychological treatment of both child and adult anxiety disorders (Butler et al., 2006). CBT aims to redress the maladaptive cognitive, behavioral, and affective patterns related to the focus of an individuals' anxiety. Common components of CBT packages for anxiety include psychoeducation, conscious cognitive restructuring of negatively biased thinking, and behavioral exposure (physical or imaginal) to the focus of anxiety to reduce fear and avoidance (Clark and Beck, 2010). Despite robust empirical support, a number of issues remain. CBT is not universally efficacious, nor is it acceptable to all patients, with considerable rates of non- or partial responders to treatment and treatment nonadherence (Schmidt, 2012). Nonadherence is particularly concerning given that attendance and completion of therapy homework appear to play a role in treatment outcome in treatment with CBT (Taylor et al., 2012). The quality of treatment with CBT also varies depending on the therapist, the therapeutic alliance with the client, and the extent to which the therapist's methods reflect guidelines for evidence-based practice (Collins et al., 2004; Reger and Gahm, 2009).

Pharmacological treatment for anxiety disorders depends upon both the disorder and needs of the individual (see reviews in Bandelow et al., 2012; Ravindran and Stein, 2010). The preferred psychotropic medication across anxiety disorders tends to be selective serotonin reuptake inhibitors or SSRIs (Bandelow et al., 2012), which work to inhibit reuptake at the presynaptic serotonin transporter pump. Overall, their tolerability, efficacy, and safety are good, although drug–drug interactions and side effects during or upon termination of treatment are noted difficulties with SSRI use (Ravindran and Stein, 2010). Serotonin-norepinephrine reuptake inhibitors (SNRIs) are a more recently developed class of medications that work to inhibit the reuptake of serotonin and norepinephrine, with selectivity for the two neurotransmitters varying across dose and drug. They have adequate tolerability and efficacy to be considered alternate first-line treatments to the SSRIs, although again side effects are still a critical limitation (Bandelow et al., 2012). Although both tricyclic antidepressants and mono-amine oxidase inhibitors (MAOIs) have received support in clinical trials with certain anxiety disorders, they are generally considered third- or fourth-line treatment options because of their side effect profiles and tolerability issues (Ravindran and Stein, 2010). Benzodiazepines work to potentiate the action of the inhibitory neurotransmitter γ-aminobutyric acid (GABA) and, although generally effective, carry risks of adverse effects, tolerance, and dependence (Bandelow et al., 2012). Further, they have no recognized antidepressant effects, an important consideration given the high comorbidity between anxiety and mood disorders (Ravindran and Stein, 2010). Other psycho-tropic medications such as anticonvulsants, azapirones, and atypical antipsychotics do not have a sufficient evidence base at this time to justify their use over other anxiolytic agents for anxiety treatment (Ravindran and Stein, 2010). Many patients, however, refuse to undergo pharmacological treatment for their anxiety, and a substantial proportion of those who do consent fail to respond to medication or adhere to their treatment regime (Collins et al., 2004). For many, nonadherence appears to be in part a result of adverse side effects (Taylor et al., 2012).

A recent review of previous meta-analyses found mean dropout rates of 16% and 24% for CBT and serotonergic pharmacotherapy treatment trials, respectively, with mean nonresponse rates of 35% and 30% for the two treatments (Taylor et al., 2012). A common strategy in clinical settings has been to combine psychotherapy and pharmacotherapy, with the assumption that the combination will be more efficacious (Hofmann, 2007; Hofmann et al., 2009). This assumption has either been found to be not empirically supported, or supported only in the case of some disorders and not when one examines longer term outcomes (Hofmann et al., 2009).

There are also issues surrounding access to current treatments for those in need. In particular, CBT is costly to implement and requires regular meetings with a trained clinician, which reduces accessibility for patients from isolated areas, with low socioeconomic status, limited transport, time, or mobility (Collins et al., 2004). These individual psychological and practical barriers seem to contribute to failure to seek treatment and treatment nonadherence (Collins et al., 2004; Taylor et al., 2012). There is also increasing acknowledgment of the difficulty involved in ensuring that empirically supported treatments such as CBT are well disseminated by health care professionals, and the lack of rigorous training in CBT techniques among training and registration programs for psychologists (Collins et al., 2004; Gunter and Whittal, 2010). Epidemiological studies report that up to two-thirds of those experiencing an anxiety disorder in the last 12 months had not used mental health services in that time (Slade et al., 2009). There is, therefore, great potential for improvement in uptake and response rates for both psychotherapy and pharmacotherapy for anxiety. Thus, the development of novel augmentation approaches to existing anxiety treatments has the potential to further enhance the cost effectiveness, accessibility, and efficacy of treatment within the community.

NOVEL PHARMACOLOGICAL APPROACHES

As described previously, substantial research and clinical effort has been placed into the augmentation of psycho-therapy with traditional anxiolytic medications, despite the lack of consistent evidence for substantive additive benefits (Hofmann, 2007). More recently, however, research efforts have been focused on the development of novel pharmacological adjuncts that capitalize on the neurobiological mechanisms involved in overcoming anxiety to augment the learning processes that take place during psychotherapy. Novel compounds that have shown such promise as cognitive enhancers for psychotherapy include yohimbine hydrochloride, gluco-corticoids, and D-cycloserine (DCS; see review in Hofmann et al., 2011).

Much of our current understanding of psychological anxiety treatments, and exposure therapy in particular, is based on associative Pavlovian fear conditioning and extinction models (Sullivan et al., 2011). In brief, fear conditioning involves a harmless stimulus (*conditioned stimulus*, CS) being repeatedly paired with an innately aversive stimulus (*unconditioned stimulus*, US) that naturally elicits a fear response (*unconditioned response*, UCR). This can include the initiation of reflexes (e.g., startle and eyeblink responses), release of stress hormones, defensive behaviors, and autonomic arousal (Sullivan et al., 2011). After repeated pairings, the CS comes to elicit the same innate fear response as the US, known as the *conditioned response* (CR). This conditioned response in animal models is used as an experimental analogue of the human fear response (Barlow, 2002). In order to eliminate this learned fear response, the CS is presented repeatedly without the aversive US (Myers and Davis, 2002). This process is known as extinction and is a major component of successful anxiety reduction (Barlow, 2002).

It is likely that there are multiple neural mechanisms involved in fear extinction (Myers and Davis, 2002; see reviews in Myers and Davis, 2007). Fear conditioning involves the formation of an excitatory association between the mental representations of the CS and US (Myers and Davis, 2007). Extinction appears to involve more than a mere forgetting or even "unlearning" of this maladaptive association; rather, it additionally includes the formation of a new competing association that inhibits the excitatory association representing the learned fear response (Myers and Davis, 2002). Evidence in support of this view shows that the fear response can return after the US is unexpectedly presented again (termed *reinstatement*), when contexts change (renewal) or may spontaneously reappear after a length of time (Myers and Davis, 2007). Hence, while successful extinction alleviates fear in one context, this may only be temporary and may not generalize to other contexts.

There appear to be a number of structures involved in fear conditioning and extinction. In particular, a substantial body of evidence in animals and humans points to the amygdala (especially the basolateral complex or BLA), as well as prefrontal cortical structures including the medial prefrontal cortex (mPFC), orbital cortex, and insula in humans and the prelimbic and infralimbic cortices in rats (see reviews in

Bishop, 2007; Myers and Davis, 2002, 2007; Sullivan et al., 2011). The amygdala plays a central role in threat processing and is generally acknowledged to be critical to the acquisition and expression of conditioned fear, serving not only as the site where sensory CS and US information converges but also that from which efferent projections initiate the various (autonomic, endocrine, and behavioral) aspects of the conditioned fear response (Bishop, 2007; Sullivan et al., 2011). Animal studies implicate plasticity within the BLA in the formation of memory traces for fear conditioning and fear extinction (Charney, 2003; Myers and Davis, 2007), through the process of long-term potentiation. Neuroimaging studies have consistently demonstrated amygdala activation during fear conditioning (Etkin and Wager, 2007; Rauch et al., 2003). There is evidence to suggest that prefrontal cortical structures may modulate amygdala activity, such that the amygdala is involved in rapid fear conditioning and responses to salient stimuli while prefrontal cortical structures control more complex cognitive processing of fear stimuli, prediction of outcomes, and moderation of behavioral responses according to instrumental contingencies (Charney, 2003). N-methyl-D-aspartate (NMDA) receptors, which are activated by the neurotransmitter glutamate, play a key role in memory and learning (Hofmann et al., 2006). Extinction acquisition, and thus the overcoming of the fear response, involves activation of NMDA receptors in the amygdala, while plasticity within the mPFC contributes to extinction consolidation and inhibition of the fear response (Bishop, 2007; Sullivan et al., 2011). That is, the mPFC is crucial for short- and long-term memory of extinction learning. Although the role of the hippocampus in fear responses and fear- and extinction-related memory, particularly in relation to contextual fear conditioning and expression of extinction learning (Sullivan et al., 2011), has been well demonstrated in animals, its role in human fear has not yet been extensively investigated (Etkin, 2012).

GLUCOCORTICOIDS

Glucocorticoids (cortisol in humans and corticosterone in most animals) are a class of steroid hormones that are the major component of adaptive stress responses. Stressful situations produce a range of automatic, behavioral, and endocrine responses, including activation of the hypothalamic–pituitary–adrenal (HPA) axis. The end product of HPA axis activation is increased endogenous glucocorticoid levels that act to increase blood glucose levels, break down protein and fat, and increase inflammatory responses. Later, they also inhibit further HPA axis activity (Tsigos and Chrousos, 2002). Importantly, glucocorticoids play a critical role in learning and memory processes, particularly for emotional stimuli, through their actions at glucocorticoid receptors found in high density in the hippocampus, amygdala, and frontal lobes (Myers and Davis, 2007).

While endogenous levels of glucocorticoids increase in response to stress in both animal and human models, acutely administered glucocorticoid agonists selectively enhance and impair memory processes. In rats, glucocorticoid administration dose-dependently enhances memory consolidation of new information when given prior to or immediately after

extinction training, and impairs memory retrieval for stored aversive information (de Quervain et al., 2009). In humans, exogenous administration of cortisol facilitates extinction processes and impairs retrieval of stored fear memories. The effects of cortisol on memory are most strongly observed for emotionally arousing stimuli. Glucocorticoid administration has been shown to enhance memory consolidation and impair recall of words across a number of contexts, with strongest effects observed in the context of emotional arousal (as reviewed in Wolf, 2008).

Results of placebo-controlled clinical studies to date suggest that glucocorticoid administration may enhance the extinction of clinical fear. In one study, acute administration of cortisone to social anxiety patients prior to a psychosocial stressor reduced self-reported fear across the task (Soravia et al., 2006). For those participants given placebo, individuals with higher endogenous cortisol exhibited less subjective fear, which suggests that higher levels of cortisol may buffer fear in stressful situations. In the same article, the authors also reported that acute hydrocortisone progressively reduced fear induced by pictures of spiders among individuals with arachnophobia. Further, this effect was maintained two days after the last administration, implying a long-term memory consolidation effect. In patients with chronic posttraumatic stress disorder (PTSD), daily low-dose cortisol reduced intensity of reexperiencing symptoms, physiological distress, and frequency of nightmares (Aerni et al., 2004). Lastly, acute cortisol administered in conjunction with exposure-based therapy resulted in significantly fewer fear symptoms at both posttreatment and one-month follow-up in acrophobia patients (de Quervain et al., 2011). Cumulative evidence from preclinical and clinical studies therefore provides promising initial support for the suggestion that both acute and repeated doses of cortisol may reduce anxiety symptoms. Further, more recent evidence suggests that cortisol may enhance consolidation of newly learned associations after successful exposure therapy, implying that an augmentative approach involving combination with exposure-based therapy may provide the strongest clinical effects.

YOHIMBINE HYDROCHLORIDE

Yohimbine, an African plant derivative, is a dietary supplement often used to treat sexual dysfunction and to metabolize fat. A selective competitive α2 adrenergic autoreceptor antagonist, yohimbine acts on the noradrenergic system to modulate the formation and maintenance of emotional and fear memories (Myers and Davis, 2007). In particular, yohimbine increases norepinephrine levels in the hippocampus, amygdala, and prefrontal cortex, areas known to mediate fear extinction (reviewed in Holmes and Quirk, 2010).

Initial preclinical findings indicated that mice treated with yohimbine prior to extinction retained cued and contextual extinction memories, even when tested drug-free the next day (Cain et al., 2004). Paradoxically, yohimbine seems to increase arousal and anxiety in both animals and humans. This finding sparked interest into the ways in which the compound could be used as an adjunct for behavioral exposure-based therapies, especially in relation to treatment-resistant anxiety disorders. That is, Cain et al. (2004) argued that yohimbine may be able to enhance the acute effects of exposure-based treatments where other treatments have failed. However, studies have shown that rats administered yohimbine significantly reduce freezing behavior after extinction but fail to eliminate this fear memory, as return of freezing is evident when tested out of the original context (Morris and Bouton, 2007). This suggests that gains may be context specific and return of fear may occur upon leaving the therapeutic context.

In terms of clinical utility in humans, a study in participants with claustrophobia demonstrated that although acutely administered yohimbine did not initially improve the efficacy of *in vivo* exposure sessions, at a one-week follow-up yohimbine participants exhibited significantly reduced fear (Powers et al., 2009). This is consistent with animal findings suggestive of stronger effects of yohimbine on memory consolidation after extinction than on initial extinction learning. In a recent study, individuals with a fear of flying were given yohimbine or placebo prior to five virtual reality exposure sessions (Meyerbroeker et al., 2012). Results indicated that while noradrenaline activity was increased by yohimbine as expected, no additional effect of the active drug was found on measures of anxiety or treatment outcome. However, an important caveat is that no follow-up assessment was conducted. Given the findings from the previous study by Powers et al., time of assessment seems to be a critical factor in determining the success of facilitatory effects of yohimbine on exposure therapy. Thus, preliminary evidence suggests that although yohimbine may enhance the outcomes of exposure-based therapies for anxiety disorders, this seems to be only evident after a period of consolidation or in specific contexts, which may limit potential clinical applications.

D-CYCLOSERINE (DCS)

DCS is a partial agonist of the glycine binding site in the NMDA receptor complex, which acts to cofacilitate glutamatergic activation of the receptor (Hofmann et al., 2006). In contrast with the drugs combined with psychotherapy in previous augmentation studies, DCS does not appear to have a direct anxiolytic or anxiogenic effect. Rather, acute doses of DCS appear to augment learning during extinction and thus facilitate exposure therapy (Norberg et al., 2008). It appears that DCS has two facilitatory effects on neuroplasticity in extinction training: first, it facilitates NMDA-dependent potentiation of GABA neurons within the BLA to enhance the learning that normally takes place during extinction, and second, it facilitates NMDA-dependent depotentiation of glutamate neurons in the amygdala (Krystal, 2012). It has been suggested that this second "depression-like" action may reduce the risk of reinstatement of the fear response as well as enhance extinction (Krystal, 2012).

EMPIRICAL EVIDENCE
DCS administered systemically or into the amygdala prior to conditioned fear extinction facilitates memory consolidation in

rats, with antagonists to the NMDA glycine binding site blocking these effects (as reviewed in Davis et al., 2006; Hofmann, 2007). Rodent studies indicate that DCS is most effective when given immediately before or after extinction training, which suggests that it works to moderate memory consolidation (Myers and Davis, 2007; Norberg et al., 2008). Research also suggests that DCS may not only enhance fear extinction for target CSs, but also reduce fear responses to other stimuli that have been previously paired with the aversive US but are not specifically targeted in extinction training (Richardson et al., 2004). That is, DCS may promote generalized fear extinction. One way in which these results have been interpreted is that DCS works to devalue the mental representation of the feared US (Ledgerwood et al., 2005). It suggests that DCS may work not only to speed up fear extinction (see Norberg et al., 2008) but also to enhance the strength of the effect. DCS may also reduce the risk of relapse after exposure-based therapy, as it has been shown to reduce reinstatement of fear responses following extinction training in rodents (Hofmann, 2007; Richardson et al., 2004). In conjunction with observed effects of DCS on protein expression and synaptic activity in the amygdala from rodent studies, it has been suggested that this indicates DCS promotes erasure of the fear memory (Myers and Davis, 2007).

Based on the parallels between extinction training and exposure therapy, it was hypothesized that DCS could be utilized as a novel adjunctive treatment to enhance learning in exposure-based psychotherapy (Davis et al., 2006; Myers and Davis, 2007). A number of RCTs to date investigating the use of DCS as an adjunct to exposure therapy in clinical anxiety populations have demonstrated promising initial findings (reviewed in Guastella and Alvares, 2012). Of note, the use of DCS has been examined in social anxiety disorder, specific phobias, PTSD, panic disorder, and obsessive-compulsive disorder (OCD). A recent meta-analysis by Norberg et al. (2008) found a moderate to large effect size favoring use of DCS over placebo when added to extinction or exposure therapy across both animal and clinical human studies. Examining the studies separately, the effect for animal studies was larger, more significant, and more robust. The clinical human studies exhibited a moderate yet significant effect size.

The most consistent positive results for DCS-facilitated exposure therapy have been observed in RCTs for social anxiety disorder and specific phobia, which are reviewed in Hofmann et al. (2006) and Guastella and Alvares (2012). The first adjunctive DCS study with exposure-based treatment, conducted by Ressler and colleagues (2004), demonstrated that DCS facilitated reductions in subjective fear after virtual reality treatment for fear of heights. This immediate effect generalized to improved outcomes at one-week and three-month follow-up assessments, with greater numbers of self-exposures to real-world heights among those receiving DCS, indicative of greater clinical efficacy outside of a therapeutic context. Two RCTs for social anxiety disorder have demonstrated similar results. In the first, Hofmann and colleagues demonstrated that DCS administered prior to four exposure sessions significantly reduced self-reported social anxiety symptoms compared with placebo, with the greatest difference observed at a one-month follow-up assessment. We replicated these findings in what is currently the largest study of DCS in combination with exposure therapy to treat an anxiety disorder. Fifty-six social anxiety patients received either DCS or placebo prior to four exposure-based therapy sessions. DCS-administered patients reported fewer social fear and avoidance symptoms, fewer dysfunctional cognitions, and greater overall improved functioning in everyday life posttreatment. Moderate effect sizes were found on most measures, and near-significant effects suggested that fewer DCS-treated patients may have dropped of treatment in comparison with placebo. Further, treatment effects emerged early, with differences between drug groups emerging at the third exposure session. These studies demonstrated a positive relationship between DCS enhancement of therapy outcomes and the amount of learning achieved between exposure therapy sessions. Notably, indirect evidence suggests that the greater the amount of learning achieved within exposure therapy sessions, the greater the effectiveness of DCS in combination with exposure therapy (Guastella and Alvares, 2012).

Despite the success from social anxiety and specific phobia clinical trials, more mixed results have been reported for OCD and panic disorder, with several studies reporting beneficial effects of DCS only in more symptomatic patients or at midtreatment, but not posttreatment or follow-up (Guastella and Alvares, 2012). Two studies administered DCS adjunctively to an exposure-based protocol for OCD, finding that while some moderate gains emerged midtreatment, these disappeared by the end of the 10 sessions (Kushner et al., 2007; Wilhelm et al., 2008). This suggests that DCS may be useful in speeding up or enhancing the effectiveness of the initial phase of exposure-based treatment (Guastella and Alvares, 2012), and is in agreement with mixed findings from panic disorder clinical trials. It further indicates that DCS may be sensitive to the number of administrations. Indeed, multiple DCS administrations prior to extinction training appears to reduce its potential efficacy (Parnas et al., 2005), implying a potential tolerance of NMDA-R sites associated with chronic administration. Such a tolerability effect may, in part, explain some of the inconclusive findings from OCD clinical trials. It may also be that, for some patients, ceiling effects emerge in terms of treatment efficacy. For example, in a recent study examining the combination of DCS with exposure-based therapy in PTSD patients (de Kleine et al., 2012), no significant effect of DCS was found on symptom reduction across the total sample. However, subgroup analyses suggested beneficial effects of DCS for regular, as opposed to early, completers of exposure-based therapy. As suggested by the authors, this may imply that only more severe patients are likely to benefit from DCS augmentation, while others recover relatively quickly from exposure-based therapy alone.

DIRECTIONS FOR FUTURE RESEARCH

Although RCTs of DCS in anxiety disorders have shown promising findings, conclusions about the outcomes of DCS-facilitated exposure therapy from these studies are limited by a number of factors such as study design heterogeneity, dosage, timing of administration, and number of adjunctive therapy sessions (Guastella and Alvares, 2012). These factors have been summarized in Table 46.1.

Given that the drug absorbs relatively slowly and takes approximately two to four hours to reach peak plasma levels, it has been suggested that null effects in some studies could reflect administration too soon before therapy to facilitate learning (Krystal, 2012). Studies are therefore needed that directly compare the effectiveness of DCS administered at different times relative to exposure, and administration before versus after therapy. Rodent studies indicate significant effects of DCS even when administered a relatively long time after extinction training. One advantage of administration after therapy is that DCS could be given only in sessions where within-session extinction has actually occurred, and thus where there is learning to consolidate, in order to minimize the risk of tolerance effects following chronic administration (Norberg et al., 2008). Administration only after successful exposure therapy sessions may therefore further enhance potential efficacy and treatment acceptability in the clinic.

An additional factor is that of dose; systematic dose–response studies with DCS are needed to determine the optimal dose for each administration. Most previous human studies have used 50 mg, and few have directly compared the effects of administering doses of varying levels (Guastella and Alvares, 2012; Norberg et al., 2008). It has also been suggested that prior exposure to antidepressants may limit DCS efficacy

TABLE 46.1. Administration and dosage factors that may influence the effects of DCS administration on learning in exposure therapy

FACTOR	RELATIONSHIP WITH EFFECTS OF DCS
Time of administration relative to therapy	Has been used successfully with administration both before and after exposure therapy. Greater time interval between administration and therapy appears to reduce efficacy, although window yet to be clearly defined (Myers and Davis, 2007; Norberg et al., 2008).
Chronic versus isolated administration	Evidence indicates that repeated chronic administration reduces or eliminates beneficial effects of DCS on extinction learning (Hofmann, 2007). Optimal number of doses and interval between doses yet to be established.
Dose	Unclear, yet to be systematically investigated (Guastella and Alvares, 2012; Hofmann, 2007; Norberg et al., 2008).
Previous use of other medications	Rodent studies suggest that previous use of antidepressants may reduce efficacy of DCS (Hoffmann, 2007; Norberg et al., 2008).

on NMDA receptor functioning. For example, rodents previously administered with the antidepressant imipramine exhibit reduced DCS facilitation of extinction training (Norberg et al., 2008). Further research is needed to investigate whether this also occurs with other drugs commonly coadministered in clinical practice, such as benzodiazepines or SSRIs, and to investigate whether these effects are short- or long-term in nature (Hofmann, 2007).

Further, it appears that DCS is best used in isolated doses; both preclinical rodent and clinical human studies indicate that any beneficial effects become less pronounced or disappear across repeated or chronic administration (Davis et al., 2006; Hofmann, 2007). This may reflect tolerance effects or a modification of the structure and function of the NMDA receptor complex through repeated activation (Davis et al., 2006; Richardson et al., 2004). Although available evidence indicates that acute administration is most effective and efficacy declines with repeated administration, the optimal number of doses and interval between repeated administration of DCS still needs to be defined (Hofmann, 2007).

NOVELTY AND CLINICAL POTENTIAL

Bearing in mind a number of factors that may limit initial conclusions about its efficacy in clinical practice, the findings of these RCTs provide the strongest evidence to suggest that DCS enhances exposure-based therapy for disorders that respond strongly to CBT, such as specific phobias and social anxiety. Novel augmentative approaches to anxiety treatment have a number of clinical benefits over traditional approaches. Speeding treatment response allows for efficient treatment delivery, benefitting both the patient and therapist. Augmentation of exposure therapy with DCS may also enhance the therapeutic response in treatment no-responders, especially for those who demonstrate insufficient learning of the required safety associations for successful fear extinction (Norberg et al., 2008). This may result in more cost-effective outcomes and decrease attrition rates across services. An additional perspective comes from stepped care models, in which treatments that are less intensive in terms of cost or therapist time are used as first-line treatments and more intensive treatments are reserved for either nonresponders to first-line treatment or patients initially identified as potential nonresponders (Bower and Gilbody, 2005). Such a model offers the potential to tailor treatment level to patient characteristics and severity in order to reduce costs and enhance efficacy. Considered within this framework, DCS could be utilized as a second-line treatment for individuals who do not initially respond to exposure-based protocols. The real potential for DCS is that, for a limited cost, it may substantially improve a simple evidence-based treatment, thus making an already relatively effective intervention more accessible and efficient.

NOVEL COGNITIVE APPROACHES

Cognitive models of anxiety emphasize that biased or irrational cognitive processes (thoughts, attitudes, beliefs, and information processes) and consequent maladaptive emotions and behaviors are crucial etiological and maintenance factors in anxiety (Clark and Beck, 2010). Many contemporary learning theories go beyond purely behavioral accounts to acknowledge additional cognitive factors in anxiety, such as social and observational learning, CS–US contingencies and expectancies, and perceived control and predictability (Barlow, 2002). However, cognitive models differ in that cognitive processes are seen as a cause rather than merely a consequence of pathological anxiety (Clark and Beck, 2010). As reviewed by Clark and Beck (2010), the strength of cognitive models is bolstered by neurobiological evidence concerning the extensive connections between the amygdala and the hippocampal and higher order cortical structures (prefrontal, anterior cingulate, and orbital cortical regions) involved in conscious cognitive processes as well as the role of these structures in moderating fear responses and contextual fear conditioning.

Cognitive processes have formed a key target in the treatment of anxiety for quite some time, particularly in the form of cognitive-behavioral therapy, which, as mentioned earlier, is currently the "gold standard" in terms of psychological treatments for anxiety. As reviewed by Porto et al. (2009), neuroimaging studies suggest that treatment with CBT is associated with changes in the activity of neural areas identified as playing a critical role in the fear response (including the insula, anterior cingulate cortex, prefrontal cortex, amygdala, and hippocampal regions).

More recently, the cognitive anxiety literature has focused on the potential role of biases in information processes (including attention, interpretation, memory, imagery, and appraisal) in the etiology and maintenance of anxiety (see recent reviews in Beard, 2011; Macleod and Mathews, 2012). Attentional and interpretive biases toward threatening information among clinically anxious individuals are well supported by empirical evidence. A substantial body of evidence (see Bar-Haim et al., 2007; Ouimet, Gawronski, and Dozois, 2009) indicates that, relative to healthy controls, clinically anxious populations tend to preferentially attend to threatening (as opposed to nonthreatening) stimuli (i.e., display an *attentional bias*), and to interpret ambiguous information as threatening rather than positive (i.e., display an *interpretive bias*). For instance, a socially anxious individual might be more likely to attend to others' negative facial expressions and also more likely to interpret ambiguous body language in a negative manner (e.g., as a sign of distaste for themselves rather than unrelated situational factors; see Beard, 2011). Based on the hypothesis that these biases may play a role in the etiology and/or maintenance of the anxiety disorders, they have been proposed as a potential target mechanism for novel anxiety treatment approaches (Beard, 2011). As the majority of research thus far has focused on the modification of attentional and interpretive biases, these will form the focus of the present section.

According to biased competition models, attention is mediated by both automatic deployment through a "bottom-up," amygdala-based threat evaluation system that directs attention toward salient stimuli, and a more flexible "top-down," prefrontal cortical attentional control signal that is evoked when there are conflicting demands placed on attention (see reviews in Bishop, 2007; Browning et al., 2010a). These signals direct processing resources in the sensory and association cortices toward the preferred stimulus. It has been argued that the biased competition model used to account for attentional processes can also be applied to the interpretation of ambiguous stimuli, such that competition between alternate interpretations is resolved through the interaction of an amygdala-based threat evaluation system and a top-down prefrontal control system (Bishop, 2007). It appears that both automatic and controlled cognitive processes are involved in attention and interpretation (Bar-Haim et al., 2007; Mathews, 2012; Ouimet et al., 2009).

In a meta-analytic study, Bar-Haim et al. (2007) found that attentional bias toward threat is robust across anxiety disorders for both consciously perceived stimuli and stimuli presented outside of awareness. Attention consists of three primary stages: orientation and engagement, disengagement, and avoidance (Ouimet et al., 2009), with biases toward threat observed among clinically anxious individuals at all three stages. That is, during earlier stages of processing anxious individuals are likely to preferentially allocate attention to threat (facilitated attention). Once engaged they are also likely to experience trouble disengaging from threatening stimuli to focus on other stimuli (difficulty disengaging). Finally, at later, more strategic stages of processing they may be seen to divert attention away from threatening stimuli (attentional avoidance), which is hypothesized to maintain anxiety by preventing elaborative processing that reduces the threatening value of the stimulus (Bar-Haim et al., 2007).

As Bishop (2007) notes, the literature concerning the neurocircuitry of attentional and interpretive processes in anxiety is less developed than that of fear conditioning and extinction learning. However neurobiological evidence from animal models and neuroimaging studies in humans implicate perturbations in both the amygdala-based and prefrontal fear systems when explaining biased information processing (see reviews in Bishop, 2007; Hofmann et al., 2012). More specifically, pathological anxiety is hypothesized to involve both hyperactivation of the amygdala-based threat evaluation system and insufficient downregulation of the fear response by prefrontal control mechanisms. This neurobiological perturbation results in heightened activation of threat-related representations and failure to activate nonthreatening representations, and has been used to account for both interpretive and attentional biases in the literature (Bishop, 2007; Cisler and Koster, 2010). Cisler and Koster (2010) have proposed that hyperactivity of the amygdala-based system is likely to account for automatic vigilance and facilitated attention to threat, while failure of the higher order prefrontal system to downregulate amygdala activity and direct attention to task-relevant stimuli may explain difficulty disengaging from threat. The attentional avoidance component of attentional biases also appears to reflect activity in the prefrontal region, through its role in strategic emotion regulation. Similarly, in their cognitive-neurobiological information-processing model, Hofmann et al. (2012) also emphasize the role of

subcortical networks in hypervigilance and facilitated attention to threat and prefrontal cortical structures in higher order regulation of anxiety responses.

COGNITIVE BIAS MODIFICATION—CBM

Recognition of the association between information processing biases and pathological anxiety led to the development of cognitive bias modification treatments for anxiety disorders. These treatments aim to modify these biases to subsequently alleviate anxiety symptoms.

ATTENTION BIAS MODIFICATION (CBM-A)

Attention bias modification focuses specifically on retraining attentional biases toward threat (see Bar-Haim, 2010, for an overview). Typically, this is done using a "dot-probe task" (depicted in Fig. 46.1), where participants are asked to discriminate between two variants of a probe (e.g., "." and "..") and respond by pressing the corresponding one of two keyboard keys. These probes are presented behind two stimuli (e.g., words or pictures), one threatening and one neutral. In the original task, developed to assess attentional biases, the target probe is presented behind the threatening stimulus 50% of the time. A threat bias is indicated when participants are faster to identify probes presented behind a threatening stimulus relative to those presented behind a neutral stimulus.

An extension of the dot-probe task manipulates or retrains this attentional bias toward threat. In the modified paradigm, the target probe is presented consistently behind either the threatening (attend-threat training) or neutral (avoid-threat

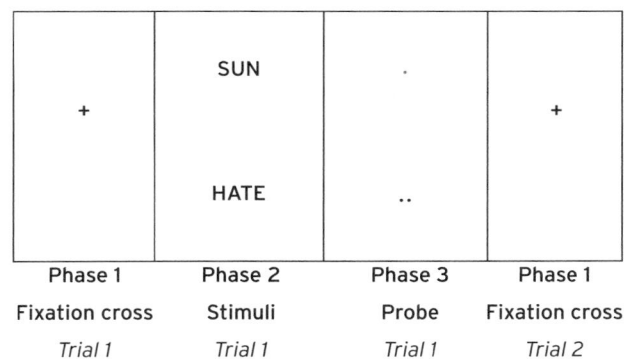

Phase 1	Phase 2	Phase 3	Phase 1
Fixation cross	Stimuli	Probe	Fixation cross
Trial 1	*Trial 1*	*Trial 1*	*Trial 2*

Figure 46.1 *A typical protocol for attentional bias assessment or training using the dot-probe paradigm. A typical dot-probe attention bias task, where the target probe is the single dot (denoted in gray). The participant is instructed to fixate on the cross, then press the keyboard key that corresponds to the location of the target probe, and finally refixate on the cross for the start of the next trial. Between the presentation of the cross and the probe, two emotionally valenced stimuli are presented in the locations where the probes will appear. In attentional bias assessment (or control training with no contingency), the target probe appears behind the threatening and neutral stimuli with equal probability (i.e., 50% of the time for each). In avoid-threat attentional bias training, the target probe is always presented behind the nonthreatening stimulus. In attend-threat training, the target probe is always presented behind the threatening stimulus.*

training) stimulus. Since attending to the relevant stimulus results in the correct identification of the target probe, repeated trials should implicitly train the individual to preferentially allocate attention either toward or away from threat, depending on the training contingency.

INTERPRETIVE BIAS MODIFICATION (CBM-I)

Interpretive biases can be assessed in two broad ways (as reviewed in Mathews and MacLeod, 2005). Online measures assess interpretations at the time of encountering ambiguous information, usually by assessing latency to read targets that either confirm or disconfirm possible threatening interpretations of ambiguous primes. Targets that confirm the participant's interpretation of the ambiguous prime are read or identified more quickly than those than disconfirm their interpretation. Offline measures assess interpretations either before or after encountering ambiguous information, usually through self-report. Studies using offline measures have consistently shown a negative interpretive bias in clinically anxious populations, while those using online measures have found mixed results but generally support either the presence of a negative interpretive bias or the absence of the emotionally positive bias often present in nonanxious controls (Mathews and MacLeod, 2005).

A common means of CBM-I involves the presentation of a series of ambiguous homographs or situations, followed by a word fragment target that must be completed after reading the stimulus (Beard, 2011). The emotional valence of the ambiguous stimulus can only be interpreted by using the subsequent target. The individual can be compelled to interpret these ambiguous stimuli in either a negative or positive manner through the consistent presentation of word fragment targets that relate to either the negative or positive interpretation. Thus, over repeated trials, the participant develops a positive or negative interpretive bias.

EMPIRICAL EVIDENCE

Many CBM studies have been conducted under a diathesis-stress model of anxiety, which suggests that CBM may reduce what is known as stress reactivity or vulnerability (i.e., the level of anxiety in response to a stressor) but not necessarily anxiety symptoms per se. Hence, the beneficial effects of CBM on anxiety should only be apparent once patients are exposed to a stressor (Hallion and Ruscio, 2011). Empirical studies have therefore investigated the impact of CBM on anxiety symptoms either immediately posttraining or in reaction to a stressor (laboratory-induced or naturalistic). A number of recent reviews have been conducted to consolidate findings from previous CBM-A studies (Bar-Haim, 2010; Hakamata et al., 2010) and CBM studies more generally (Beard, 2011; Macleod and Mathews, 2012).

CBM-A

The majority of CBM-A studies conducted thus far have employed a modified dot-probe paradigm (Macleod and Mathews, 2012). Studies in nonclinical populations compare avoid-threat training to either an attend-threat or a no-training placebo control (no training contingency) condition. While these studies have consistently demonstrated that it is possible to induce an attentional bias toward or away from threat, the impact of CBM-A on anxiety scores posttraining and in response to a stressor have been mixed (Beard, 2011). More specifically, there is stronger evidence in support of reduced stress reactivity (i.e., anxiety in response to a stressor) following avoid-threat training than there is for reductions in posttraining state and trait anxiety. In clinical populations, CBM-A studies have thus far been conducted in generalized anxiety disorder (GAD) and social anxiety disorder (SAD) patients, typically allocated to either avoid-threat or a no-training placebo control. As reviewed in Bar-Haim (2010) and Macleod and Mathews (2012), these studies have consistently demonstrated that CBM-A can be used to retrain attentional biases away from threat toward neutral information. Furthermore, significant reductions in both anxiety symptoms and stress reactivity have been found for those participants allocated to avoid-threat training. These outcomes have been found following both single- and multisession attention training, and shown to persist over time to follow-up assessment up to 4 months later (Macleod and Mathews, 2012). Hakamata et al. (2010) recently conducted a meta-analysis of 12 CBM-A studies employing the dot-probe paradigm (among nonclinical populations, GAD, and SAD patients), including only studies where the control group was a no-training placebo rather than attend-threat training. This analysis demonstrated a large and significant effect size of avoid-threat training on attention bias. It also found a medium and significant effect on anxiety symptoms (relative to control training placebo). It is important to note, however, that the effect on anxiety symptoms included both posttraining measures of anxiety symptoms and measures of anxiety symptoms following exposure to a stressor (i.e., stress reactivity). Effect sizes for the impact of CBM-A on anxiety symptoms did not differ significantly between patients and nonclinical samples. Interestingly, the effect of CBM-A on magnitude of attention bias change (but not on magnitude of anxiety symptom change) was significantly moderated by the number of sessions involved. For attention bias change, a greater number of sessions was associated with a greater amount of change. However, these findings are tentative given the small number of studies concerned.

CBM-I

As reviewed in Beard (2011) and Macleod and Mathews (2012), single- and multiple-session versions of CBM-I have been used in nonclinical populations to successfully induce positive and negative interpretive biases. In these studies, interpret-positive and interpret-negative training have been compared with each other or to a no-training placebo control. Although a few studies have reported null findings, others have found significant reductions in outcome measures (state and trait anxiety and/or stress reactivity) for those allocated to the interpret-positive condition. Studies in GAD patients and populations with high trait or state anxiety (including worry, social anxiety, spider fear, and trait anxiety) have compared the impact of single- or multiple-session interpret-positive training versus a no-training placebo control on stress reactivity and anxiety symptoms. In both clinical and nonclinical populations, interpretive bias modification from single-session training has been shown to persist over time up to 24 hours later, the longest time period investigated thus far (Macleod and Mathews, 2012). In terms of clinical outcomes, several studies have found that interpret-positive training induces a positive interpretive bias and reduces state and trait anxiety, anxiety symptoms, and/or stress reactivity. However, results have been mixed depending on the specific anxiety disorder and outcome measure concerned. First, CBM-I has not yet been shown to significantly reduce spider fear (Macleod and Mathews, 2012). Further, its effect on posttraining anxiety versus stress reactivity is still unclear. Some studies have shown significant reductions in state and trait anxiety from CBM-I but no effect on specific anxiety symptoms (e.g., social anxiety scales) or stress reactivity, while others have found the opposite (Beard, 2011).

Hallion and Ruscio (2011) recently conducted a meta-analysis to examine the effect of CBM (both CBM-I and CBM-A) on cognitive biases and anxiety symptoms posttraining and poststressor across both anxiety and depression. Their review included both clinical and nonclinical populations and, unlike Hakamata et al., did not exclude CBM-A studies using an alternative to the dot-probe paradigm or those comparing avoid-threat training to attend-threat training rather than a no-training placebo. Across anxiety and depression, this comprehensive review found a significantly larger effect of CBM on interpretive biases (medium effect size) than on attention biases (small effect size). After correcting for publication bias, the effect of CBM on anxiety and depression symptoms was significant following exposure to a stressor (with a small effect size), but not immediately posttraining. This echoes the mixed findings of narrative reviews outlined previously in relation to the effect of CBM on posttraining anxiety versus stress reactivity, although again it is important to bear in mind the inclusion of studies concerning both anxious and depressive symptoms. When anxiety studies were examined separately, there was a small but significant effect of CBM on symptoms both posttraining and after exposure to a stressor.

HYPOTHESIZED MECHANISM OF ACTION

A key assumption of CBM and associated models of anxiety is that information processing biases are a causal factor in the etiology and maintenance of anxiety disorders rather than merely a consequence of anxiety (Hallion and Ruscio, 2011). That is, CBM assumes that information processing biases precipitate negative thoughts and subsequent maladaptive behavioral and emotional patterns. This assumption about the causal role of information processing biases in anxiety disorders requires further empirical validation. Prospective studies have provided preliminary support, demonstrating that information processing biases are capable of predicting the presence and severity of anxiety disorders, as well as stress reactivity (as reviewed in Beard, 2011; Mathews and MacLeod, 2005). These associations

could, however, be a product of a third stable personality variable that predicts both cognitive biases and anxiety outcome measures (Mathews and MacLeod, 2005). Further support comes from the results of intervention studies outlined earlier, which have shown that CBM can be used both to modify cognitive biases (toward and away from threat) and accordingly increase or reduce anxiety levels. Further, in their CBM-A review Hakamata et al. (2010) reported a strong correlation between the degree of attention bias change and the degree of change in anxiety scores that approached significance. Again, however, it is possible that change in anxiety symptoms is not mediated by change in cognitive biases but by some other associated factor. In their meta-analysis of CBM for anxiety and depression, Hallion and Ruscio (2011) found that change in cognitive biases did not significantly moderate the effect of CBM on symptoms, although the effect did approach significance. They note that this finding should be interpreted cautiously given the diverse array of trials included in their analysis, and indeed a substantial number of individual trials have demonstrated that change in cognitive biases mediated change in anxiety symptoms (Beard, 2011). Together, existing evidence provides partial support for a causal role of biased information processing in anxiety and a meditational role of cognitive bias change in clinical outcomes of CBM interventions.

Preliminary research has been conducted to explore the neurobiological mechanisms underlying change following CBM-A. It has been suggested that CBM-A may serve to modify attentional control processes, as opposed to the more "bottom-up" threat evaluation processes (Bar-Haim, 2010; Beard, 2011). As reviewed in Beard (2011), Derryberry and Reed (2002) have shown that anxious individuals with strong attentional control do not show an attentional bias, which suggests that attentional control moderates the relationship between attention bias and anxiety. Further, neurobiological evidence suggests that CBM-A may serve to modify attention through effects on prefrontal attentional control processes (Browning et al., 2010a). A first CBM-A neuroimaging study (Browning et al., 2010b) among healthy individuals found significant differences in the activity of prefrontal cortical, but not amygdala-based, structures between those who had completed attend- versus avoid-threat training in a subsequent task. Further, Koster et al. (2010) found that avoid-threat CBM-A influenced late but not early stages of threat processing, hypothesizing that the procedure influences later stage attentional avoidance rather than earlier hypervigilance and facilitated attention processes.

Little is known at present about the specific mechanism of action by which CBM-I modifies interpretive processes. Some research has been conducted to explore whether artifacts are responsible for the changes in interpretive bias that occur. Evidence suggests that they do not simply reflect a response bias or demand effects induced by repeated trials, they are not fully accounted for by semantic priming effects alone, nor are they entirely dependent on changes in mood and state anxiety that may occur as a result of exposure to emotionally salient stimuli during training (Beard, 2011; Macleod and Mathews, 2012). It appears that active generation of interpretations rather than mere passive processing is necessary for CBM-I to have a significant impact on anxiety levels (Beard, 2011). Mathews (2012) has suggested that this highlights a potential mechanism of action for CBM-I, specifically the acquisition of a particular processing style for emotionally salient information. That is, through interpretive training the individual may learn a new style of seeking and selecting specific types of emotional meanings, which is then unintentionally elicited and implemented when encountering subsequent ambiguous events in real life.

NOVELTY AND CLINICAL POTENTIAL

The critical finding from CBM-A trials has been evidence that these procedures produce treatment effect sizes comparable to traditional psychological and pharmacological interventions for anxiety, while requiring relatively minimal time and clinician input (MacLeod et al., 2009). In the future, computerized bias modification therapy could be made accessible on a range of technological platforms such as personal computers and mobile phones, and even over the Internet, for patients who are unable or unwilling to attend in-person therapy sessions. In this way, it offers the potential to address many practical barriers to participation in therapy. Furthermore, its convenience, accessibility, and low operating costs may be particularly beneficial in terms of facilitating ongoing practice and engagement in treatment and so potentially reducing the risk of attrition and relapse and promoting maintenance of treatment gains (Bar-Haim, 2010). The outcomes from CBM trials imply that it may also be useful as an adjunct to CBT, with the potential to be used as a preparatory step to exposure-based CBT in more severe patients, to reduce anxiety to a point where they can participate in behavioral experiments (MacLeod et al., 2009). CBM-A may also be a useful adjunctive treatment to psychotropic medications for anxiety (Browning et al., 2010a), or integrated into stepped-care models as a preliminary step for patients who are seen to require less intensive intervention. However, as cautioned by Macleod and Mathews (2012), there is not yet sufficient evidence to suggest that CBM can be used as a stand-alone treatment for anxiety disorders. Further, a first study of Internet-delivered CBM-A (Carlbring et al., 2012) published this year found it had no significant effect on social anxiety symptoms and general anxiety levels among individuals with social anxiety disorder. Thus, further investigation into the impact of delivery mode on treatment outcome for CBM is needed before implementation of Internet-based CBM treatment programs.

DIRECTIONS FOR FUTURE RESEARCH

Many potential avenues for improving both efficacy and utility of CBM remain. Further exploration into the role of other information processing biases aside from interpretation and attention (such as memory, imagery, and appraisal) in anxiety, and the development of relevant bias modification therapies, should be undertaken (Macleod and Mathews, 2012). It may well be that the type of CBM offered to patients could be customized to their particular information processing

biases (MacLeod et al., 2009). It has also been proposed that the impact of CBM could be boosted by using training packages targeted at modifying multiple cognitive biases (Hallion and Ruscio, 2011). Although a recent pilot study (Beard et al., 2011) found that a combined interpretive and attentional CBM training package significantly improved anxiety symptoms and speech performance among SAD patients, it remains to be seen whether this combination approach results in significantly greater symptom reduction than programs targeting one type of cognitive bias.

Future studies should also focus on using cognitive theory and knowledge of the cognitive mechanisms underpinning anxiety to enhance the efficacy of CBM. At present, technology is being used to enhance CBM through the development of programs delivered through the Internet or smartphones, meaning that patients can be exposed to treatment over extended periods of time and across multiple settings (Macleod and Mathews, 2012). The possibility of using novel pharmacological compounds, such as DCS, to enhance the potency of bias modification interventions is also being investigated (Behar et al., 2010). Another possible means of enhancing efficacy involves the modification of specific components of CBM. This could include the tailoring of stimuli to the specific informational domains related to each anxiety disorder (such as faces or other socially relevant stimuli in CBM-A for social anxiety; see Hakamata et al., 2010; MacLeod et al., 2009), based on findings that patients' information processing biases are most evident when assessed on stimuli related to their particular disorder.

Finally, in CBM, participants are generally not explicitly informed of the training contingency but instead implicitly learn it through the completion of repeated trials. Hence, although some CBT packages also include attentional training or interpretive restructuring exercises, a crucial distinction between CBM and these CBT exercises is that CBM aims to implicitly retrain information processing biases rather than to consciously challenge and modify thoughts and behaviors (Beard, 2011). An area for further investigation is the impact of adding explicit instructions to CBM training, which may either facilitate or impair learning of the training contingency (Bar-Haim, 2010; MacLeod et al., 2009). As outlined in Macleod and Mathews (2012), only two CBM-A studies to date have compared explicit and implicit instruction conditions, reporting contradictory findings such that explicit instruction either enhanced or eliminated the therapeutic effects of CBM-A on anxiety.

Therefore, the grounding of CBM in cognitive theory means that it has immense potential to be developed and enhanced as a treatment for anxiety. The strength of this approach will be further bolstered by integration with neuroimaging techniques and circuitry models of both cognitive processes and the etiology and maintenance of anxiety disorders. As the neurocircuitry of these cognitive processes (attention and interpretation) and the ways in which they are altered among individuals suffering from pathological levels of anxiety are better understood, CBM interventions can be developed that specifically aim to rectify these perturbations (such as enhancing prefrontal control of attention).

NOVEL DELIVERY APPROACHES— INTERNET THERAPY

One of the key barriers to treatment response outlined in the introduction to this chapter is the failure to successfully engage some individuals. The use of technology (particularly the Internet or computers) to deliver psychotherapy is a practical means of addressing this issue. Internet- and computer-based psychotherapy (ICT) programs involve the delivery of structured psychotherapy modules through a computer located at a clinic (computer-based), or remotely via the Internet on the patient's personal computer or smartphone (Internet-based). The anonymity and potential accessibility of ICT may overcome common practical barriers to seeking and participating in therapy such as unwillingness, fear of stigma, lack of time, mobility or transport, or isolated geographical location (Andrews et al., 2010; Schmidt, 2012). In this way, approaches such as ICT are a means of engaging patients in the therapeutic learning required to successfully modify fear circuitry and overcome their anxiety. ICT programs also offer the potential to provide a consistent standard of treatment (Reger and Gahm, 2009) that is independent of the success of a therapeutic alliance or the expertise of an individual therapist and may therefore maximize the potential for positive outcomes. Furthermore, ICT can be flexibly integrated into a patients' lifestyle and offers the potential for constant review of the treatment program in order to consolidate the learning taking place during treatment (Spek et al., 2007), which may also enhance efficacy and reduce risk of relapse. From a practical perspective, Internet-based treatments also offer the potential to reduce the economic burden placed on the health care system (Spek et al., 2007).

Clinician involvement in ICT ranges from entirely self-directed programs, with or without reminders and technical help from a therapist or nonclinical technician (*minimal assistance*), to clinician-directed programs with feedback and/ or advice as patients progress through the program (Andrews et al., 2010; Spek et al., 2007). Minimal assistance does not involve clinical feedback or the establishment of a therapeutic relationship but mere facilitation of the patient's independent progress through the program (Spek et al., 2007). Contact from a therapist or technician may be in person or via phone, post, or e-mail. The majority of ICT programs that have been tested thus far have been based on a cognitive-behavioral therapeutic framework (Andersson et al., 2007). Accumulating evidence from RCTs of cognitive-behavioral ICT programs for anxiety disorders is promising. Spek et al. (2007) conducted a meta-analysis of seven treatment trials comparing Internet-based CBT with nontreatment control groups (waiting list, self-monitoring, or information control) for adults with panic disorder and social anxiety disorder, finding a large reduction in anxiety symptoms. There is also evidence from several studies that gains from ICT are maintained over time to follow-up assessment (Andrews et al., 2010). More recently, Reger and Gahm (2009) separately examined the effect sizes for ICT compared with wait list, placebo, and therapist-delivered treatment-as-usual (TAU) conditions. In their analyses ICT programs were significantly more effective than both

placebo (ES = 0.88) and wait list control (ES = 0.77) conditions, and there was no significant difference between ICT and therapist-delivered TAU. However, as reviewed in (Reger and Gahm, 2009), the conclusions of these studies are limited by both their heterogeneity and key methodological limitations such as small sample sizes, high dropout rates, and failure to use wait list control conditions.

ICT may prove especially useful as an initial treatment step in stepped-care models or as an adjunct to in-person CBT or pharmacological treatments. One key priority in future ICT research should be to establish the relationship between extent of clinician assistance and treatment outcome, with a view to balancing the potential cost savings associated with more self-directed programs with issues of risk management, motivation, and compliance according to the needs of the individual. The nature of this relationship is yet to be established. Andersson et al. (2007) found a strong and significant correlation between clinician contact and treatment outcome for ICT programs, and Spek et al. (2007) suggested programs with assistance had lower heterogeneity and greater effect sizes than those without. Meanwhile, Reger and Gahm (2009) found no significant effect of clinician assistance on the outcome of ICT programs, although this was based on a categorical comparison of programs with and without clinician assistance. Future studies should include a continuous measure of level of clinician assistance as a matter of course to address this issue.

Moreover, the ICT interventions that have been developed to date have largely been an extension of existing models of psychotherapy (CBT in particular), simply delivered in a new modality. While this has value in terms of determining whether traditional CBT can be successfully administered over the Internet or in other formats, it does not focus more broadly on what treatment strategies can be delivered via technology to produce the best clinical outcomes. Future interventions should capitalize on the practical advantages of self-delivered ICT, while targeting different cognitive and neurobiological mechanisms underlying anxiety disorders, rather than merely trying to replicate what takes place in the therapy room.

COST EFFECTIVENESS AND ACCEPTABILITY OF NOVEL INTERVENTIONS

Following on from further empirical and theoretical validation, effectiveness trials will now need to be undertaken with these novel treatment approaches in order to investigate their potential translation into clinical practice. Compared with patients enrolled in many RCTs, patient populations are less homogenous and exhibit significant comorbidity with other psychiatric disorders, which may play a role in treatment nonresponse. Outside the laboratory, it may also be difficult to regulate specific aspects of treatment regimes, such as timing of administration and the nature of exposure therapy, in the case of DCS (Guastella and Alvares, 2012). Similarly, cost effectiveness and acceptability to key stakeholders are important factors to consider when evaluating new treatment approaches and are reviewed in the next section.

DCS

As larger scale RCTs of DCS are only now beginning to emerge, there is limited evidence surrounding its acceptability and cost effectiveness. If, as empirical results suggest, DCS can be used to enhance clinical efficacy and/or the speed and efficiency of treatment, it may improve patient satisfaction and treatment outcomes and reduce attrition to enhance both the cost effectiveness and acceptability of exposure-based therapy (Norberg et al., 2008). No studies have examined the cost effectiveness of DCS-augmented CBT or compared it with nonaugmented CBT. In relation to acceptability, it appears that DCS is well tolerated with minimal side effects (Hofmann et al., 2006). Furthermore, one study (Kushner et al., 2007) that compared attrition rates for exposure therapy with and without DCS found that dropout rates were six times greater among those who did not receive DCS, hypothesized to be attributable to greater symptom reduction among the DCS group.

CBM

Although the cost effectiveness of CBM has not yet been studied specifically, it has the potential to be an effective treatment for anxiety that requires minimal therapist input and time and has relatively low operating costs. In a recent review of CBM (Beard, 2011), the authors note that the relatively low attrition rates in previous studies (0–8%) may not be an indication of the acceptability of CBM in the "real world" due to the incentive of participant reimbursement. In their own pilot study assessing multisession CBM (combined CBM-A and CBM-I) in real treatment settings without remuneration, Beard et al. (2011) reported a substantially greater attrition rate (33%), although those patients who completed the program reported high levels of satisfaction on a standardized questionnaire. Qualitative results of CBM studies indicate that treatment credibility is an issue (see review in Beard, 2011); as CBM involves implicit retraining using repeated practice on a cognitive task, it may be viewed by some patients as monotonous, obscure, or pointless. These concerns are particularly relevant to CBM-A, which appears to have lower perceived face validity than CBM-I (Beard et al., 2011). Unfortunately, negative attitudes are likely to influence not only the likelihood of uptake but also the success of treatment, given that perceived treatment credibility and treatment preferences are known to play a key role in adherence (Taylor et al., 2012) and treatment outcome (Collins et al., 2004).

One important final consideration relates to the generalizability, longevity, and real-world applicability of laboratory treatment effects for CBM. Consideration of context-specific learning effects has led to the development of home-based training programs to promote transfer of learning to naturalistic environments (Macleod and Mathews, 2012). However, more work needs to be done to assess the generalizability of treatment gains across a variety of stimuli, particularly given that many studies have assessed bias change using the same cognitive task on which participants were trained (MacLeod et al., 2009). Those studies that have included independent measures of cognitive biases to assess generalizability have reported mixed results (Beard, 2011). Future studies should also focus on incorporating longer term assessment of cognitive biases, and the development of bias modification programs designed to maximize the duration of bias change (e.g., using spaced learning and booster sessions) (Macleod and Mathews, 2012).

ICT

Although at face value ICT would seem to reduce costs by minimizing the amount of therapist time required, the use of minimal therapies such as ICT may in fact result in cost shifting to other sectors and encourage patients to seek supplementary interventions (Bower and Gilbody, 2005). Interestingly, the sole cost effectiveness analysis that has been conducted thus far suggested that ICT is competitively cost effective (McCrone et al., 2004). Of particular concern in terms of acceptability of ICT is the issue that should ICT programs be implemented as a preliminary stage to in-person therapy in a stepped-care approach, patients may view ICT as an inferior and less "personal" treatment option (Andersson et al., 2007). Results thus far have been mixed, with concerningly low uptake rates and substantial variation in attrition rates across the various ICT trials that have been conducted. Overall, self-reported patient satisfaction tends to be relatively high among those who have used the treatment (see review in Waller and Gilbody, 2009). However, individuals who have chosen to participate in ICT trials may be more computer literate or amenable to computer-delivered treatments than the general population, and thus satisfaction from such self-selecting samples should be considered with caution. Clearly, treatment acceptability among broader samples should be a focus of future research.

CONCLUSION

As summarized in Table 46.2, the novel treatment approaches explored here differ greatly in terms of their nature and the specific mechanisms of anxiety they target. However, they share a common goal of harnessing knowledge of the cognitive, behavioral, and neurobiological mechanisms underlying anxiety to enhance treatment outcomes.

Future research should continue to assess and further improve the clinical efficacy, cost effectiveness, and acceptability of these interventions. In particular, their efficacy across different anxiety disorders needs to be established to inform evidence-based treatment guidelines. As outlined in Table 46.3, most evidence for the efficacy of these interventions is either still forthcoming or has exhibited mixed results.

Aside from further refining and extending these existing novel approaches, future research should continue within this translational framework to capitalize on our growing understanding of the anxiety disorders and extend our reach with further novel augmentative approaches. A particular emphasis should be placed on understanding the effects of interventions on underlying fear neurocircuitry, the ways in which this circuitry may be different among individuals with anxiety disorders, and which aspects may be modified to produce therapeutic outcomes. Furthermore, there is now a growing and substantial

TABLE 46.2. Proposed therapeutic mechanism of action and neural target site for each of the novel pharmacological, cognitive, and technological interventions reviewed in this chapter

INTERVENTION	(POTENTIAL) THERAPEUTIC EFFECT	PROPOSED TARGET SITE/ NEURAL MECHANISM OF ACTION
Cortisol	Impairs retrieval of fear memories, enhances consolidation of fear extinction training/exposure therapy (Wolf, 2008)	Acts on glucocorticoid receptors; impaired retrieval relates to medial temporal lobe activity (Wolf, 2008); fear extinction mediated by the basolateral amygdala (Myers and Davis, 2007)
Yohimbine	Enhances learning in fear extinction training/exposure therapy (Holmes and Quirk, 2010)	α2-adrenoreceptor antagonist in the hippocampus, amygdala, and prefrontal cortex; increases extracellular norepinephrine (Holmes and Quirk, 2010)
DCS	Enhances learning in fear extinction training/exposure therapy (Davis et al., 2006)	Cofacilitates glutamatergic activation of NMDA receptors in the amygdala at glycine binding site (Davis et al., 2006)
CBM-A	Reduces threat-related attention bias (Bar-Haim, 2010)	Not yet well established; may modify prefrontal activity (Beard, 2011)
CBM-I	Reduces threat-related interpretive bias (Mathews, 2012)	Not yet established
ICT	Depends on therapeutic framework. For CBT-based interventions, aims to modify distorted cognitions and maladaptive behavior patterns.	Not yet established

TABLE 46.3. State of current evidence for the effectiveness of each novel intervention in the reduction of anxiety symptoms across the various anxiety disorders

	GAD	SAD	SPECIFIC PHOBIA	PTSD	OCD	PANIC DISORDER
Cortisol	—	✓	✓	✓	—	—
Yohimbine	—	—	?	—	—	—
DCS	—	✓	✓	?	?	?
CBM-A	✓	✓	—	—	—	—
CBM-I	✓	—	—	—	—	—
ICT	✓	✓	✓	?	?	✓

✓ indicates that trials to date have supported effectiveness of this intervention; ? indicates insufficient or mixed evidence from trials to date; — indicates that this intervention has not been studied in relation to this disorder.

body of evidence concerning the role of genetic and environmental factors in the etiology and maintenance of anxiety (as reviewed in Hamilton and Fyer, 2009). As research in this area expands, a better understanding of the interactions between genetic and environmental risk factors in the neuroplastic changes that underpin pathological anxiety will facilitate the delivery of preventative and early-stage interventions targeted toward at-risk groups. Such early-stage interventions are a critical step in improving the outcomes of anxiety treatment. For both existing and future treatment approaches, these interindividual genetic and neurobiological differences are likely to be a key predictor of treatment response, providing a potential means to target efficacious interventions to the right individuals.

DISCLOSURES

The chapter authors have no conflicts of interest to declare.

REFERENCES

Aerni, A., Traber, R., et al. (2004). Low-dose cortisol for symptoms of post-traumatic stress disorder. *Am. J. Psychiatry* 161(8):1488–1490.

Andersson, G., Carlbring, P., et al. (2007). Internet-delivered treatments with or without therapist input: does the therapist factor have implications for efficacy and cost? [Report]. *Exp. Rev. Pharmacoecon. Outcomes Res.* 7(3):291–297.

Andrews, G., Cuijpers, P., et al. (2010). Computer therapy for the anxiety and depressive disorders is effective, acceptable and practical health care: a meta-analysis. *PLoS ONE* 5(10):e13196.

Bandelow, B., Sher, L., et al. (2012). Guidelines for the pharmacological treatment of anxiety disorders, obsessive–compulsive disorder and post-traumatic stress disorder in primary care. *Int. J. Psychiatry Clin. Pract.* 16(2):77–84.

Bar-Haim, Y. (2010). Research review: attention bias modification (ABM): a novel treatment for anxiety disorders. *J. Child Psychol. Psychiatry* 51(8):859–870.

Bar-Haim, Y., Lamy, D., et al. (2007). Threat-related attentional bias in anxious and nonanxious individuals: a meta-analytic study. *Psychol. Bull.* 133(1):1–24.

Barlow, D. (2002). *Anxiety and Its Disorders: The Nature and Treatment of Anxiety and Panic.* New York: Guildford Press.

Beard, C. (2011). Cognitive bias modification for anxiety: current evidence and future directions. *Exp. Rev. Neurother.* 11(2):299–311.

Beard, C., Weisberg, R.B., et al. (2011). Combined cognitive bias modification treatment for social anxiety disorder: a pilot trial. *Depress. Anxiety* 28(11):981–988.

Behar, E., McHugh, R.K., et al. (2010). d-Cycloserine for the augmentation of an attentional training intervention for trait anxiety. *J. Anxiety Disord.* 24(4):440–445.

Bishop, S.J. (2007). Neurocognitive mechanisms of anxiety: an integrative account. *Trends Cogn. Sci.* 11(7):307–316.

Bower, P., and Gilbody, S. (2005). Stepped care in psychological therapies: access, effectiveness and efficiency. *Br. J. Psychiatry* 186(1):11–17.

Browning, M., Holmes, E., Harmer, C. (2010a). The modification of attentional bias to emotional information: a review of the techniques, mechanisms, and relevance to emotional disorders. *Cogn. Affect. Behav. Neurosci.* 10(1):8–20.

Browning, M., Holmes, E.A., Murphy, S.E., (2010b). Lateral prefrontal cortex mediates the cognitive modification of attentional bias. *Biol. Psychiatry* 67(10):919–925.

Butler, A., Chapman, J., et al. (2006). The empirical status of cognitive-behavioral therapy: a review of meta-analyses. *Clin. Psychol. Rev.* 26(1):17–31.

Cain, C.K., Blouin, A.M., et al. (2004). Adrenergic transmission facilitates extinction of conditional fear in mice. *Learn. Mem.* 11(2):179–187.

Carlbring, P., Apelstrand, M., et al. (2012). Internet-delivered attention bias modification training in individuals with social anxiety disorder: a double blind randomized controlled trial. *BMC Psychiatry* 12:66–80.

Charney, D.S. (2003). Neuroanatomical circuits modulating fear and anxiety behaviors. *Acta Psychiatr. Scand.* 108:38–50.

Cisler, J.M., and Koster, E.H. (2010). Mechanisms of attentional biases towards threat in anxiety disorders: an integrative review. *Clin. Psychol. Rev.* 30(2):203–216.

Clark, D.A., and Beck, A. (2010). *Cognitive Therapy of Anxiety Disorders: Science and Practice.* New York: Guildford Press.

Collins, K.A., Westra, H.A., et al. (2004). Gaps in accessing treatment for anxiety and depression: challenges for the delivery of care. *Clin. Psychol. Rev.* 24(5):583–616.

Davis, M., Ressler, K., et al. (2006). Effects of D-cycloserine on extinction: translation from preclinical to clinical work. *Biol. Psychiatry* 60(4):369–375.

de Kleine, R., Hendriks, G.-J., et al. (2012). A randomized placebo-controlled trial of d-cycloserine to enhance exposure therapy for posttraumatic stress disorder. *Biol. Psychiatry* 71(11):962–968.

de Quervain, D.J.F., Aerni, A., et al. (2009). Glucocorticoids and the regulation of memory in health and disease. *Front. Neuroendocrinol.* 30(3):358–370.

de Quervain, D.J.F., Bentz, D., et al. (2011). Glucocorticoids enhance extinction-based psychotherapy. *Proc. Natl. Acad. Sci.* 108(16):6621.

Derryberry D, Reed MA. (2002). Anxiety-related attentional biases and their regulation by attentional control. *Journal of Abnormal Psychology,* 111(2):225–36.

Etkin, A. (2012). Neurobiology of anxiety: from neural circuits to novel solutions? *Depress. Anxiety* 29(5):355–358.

Etkin, A., and Wager, T. (2007). Functional neuroimaging of anxiety: a meta-analysis of emotional processing in PTSD, social anxiety disorder, and specific phobia. *Am. J. Psychiatry* 164(10):1476–1488.

Guastella, A., and Alvares, G. (2012). D-Cycloserine. In: Hofmann, S., ed. *Psychobiologial Approaches for Anxiety Disorders: Treatment Combination Strategies.* West Sussex, UK: Wiley-Blackwell, pp. 75–90.

Gunter, R.W., and Whittal, M.L. (2010). Dissemination of cognitive-behavioral treatments for anxiety disorders: overcoming barriers and improving patient access. *Clin. Psychol. Rev.* 30(2):194–202.

Hakamata, Y., Lissek, S., et al. (2010). Attention bias modification treatment: a meta-analysis toward the establishment of novel treatment for anxiety. *Biol. Psychiatry* 68(11):982–990.

Hallion, L.S., & Ruscio, A.M. (2011). A meta-analysis of the effect of cognitive bias modification on anxiety and depression. *Psychol. Bull.* 137(6):940–958.

Hamilton, S., and Fyer, A.J. (2009). The molecular genetics of anxiety disorders. In: Charney, D.S., and Nestler, E.J., eds. *Neurobiology of Mental Illness, 3rd Edition.* New York: Oxford University Press, pp. 585–602.

Hofmann, S.G. (2007). Enhancing exposure-based therapy from a translational research perspective. *Behav. Res. Ther.* 45:1987–2001.

Hofmann, S.G., Ellard, K.K., et al. (2012). Neurobiological correlates of cognitions in fear and anxiety: a cognitive-neurobiological information-processing model. *Cognition Emotion* 26(2):282–299.

Hofmann, S.G., Pollack, M.H., et al. (2006). Augmentation treatment of psychotherapy for anxiety disorders with D-cycloserine. *CNS Drug Reviews* 12(3–4):208–217.

Hofmann, S.G., Sawyer, A.T., et al. (2009). Is it beneficial to add pharmacotherapy to cognitive-behavioral therapy when treating anxiety disorders? A meta-analytic review. *Int. J. Cogn. Ther.* 2(2):160–175.

Hofmann, S.G., Smits, J.A.J., et al. (2011). Cognitive enhancers for anxiety disorders. *Pharmacol. Biochem. Behav.* 99(2):275–284.

Holmes, A., and Quirk, G. J. (2010). Pharmacological facilitation of fear extinction and the search for adjunct treatments for anxiety disorders: the case of yohimbine. *Trends Pharmacol. Sci.* 31(1):2–7.

Koster, E.H., Baert, S., et al. (2010). Attentional retraining procedures: manipulating early or late components of attentional bias? *Emotion* 10(2):230–236.

Krystal, J.H. (2012). Enhancing prolonged exposure therapy for posttraumatic stress disorder with D-cycloserine: further support for treatments that promote experience-dependent neuroplasticity. *Biol. Psychiatry* 71(11):932–934.

Kushner, M.G., Kimb, S.W., et al. (2007). D-Cycloserine augmented exposure therapy for obsessive-compulsive disorder. *Biol. Psychiatry* 62(8):835–838.

Ledgerwood, L., Richardson, R., et al. (2005). D-Cycloserine facilitates extinction of learned fear: effects on reacquisition and generalized extinction. *Biol. Psychiatry* 57(8):841–847.

MacLeod, C., Koster, E.H., et al. (2009). Whither cognitive bias modification research? Commentary on the special section articles. *J. Abnorm. Psychol.* 118(1):89–99.

Macleod, C., and Mathews, A. (2012). Cognitive bias modification approaches to anxiety. *Annu. Rev. Clin. Psychol.* 8:189–217.

Mathews, A. (2012). Effects of modifying the interpretation of emotional ambiguity. *J. Cogn. Psychology* 24(1):92–105.

Mathews, A., and MacLeod, C. (2005). Cognitive vulnerability to emotional disorders. *Annu. Rev. Clin. Psychol.* 167(1):167–195.

McCrone, P., Knapp, M., et al. (2004). Cost-effectiveness of computerised cognitive behavioural therapy for anxiety and depression in primary care: randomised controlled trial. *Br. J. Psychiatry* 185(55):55–62.

Meyerbroeker, K., Powers, M.B., et al. (2012). Does yohimbine hydrochloride facilitate fear extinction in virtual reality treatment of fear of flying? A randomized placebo-controlled trial. *Psychother. Psychosom.* 81(1):29–37.

Morris, R.W., and Bouton, M.E. (2007). The effect of yohimbine on the extinction of conditioned fear: a role for context. *Behav. Neurosci.* 121(3):501.

Myers, K.M., and Davis, M. (2002). Behavioral and neural analysis of extinction. *Neuron* 36(4):567–584.

Myers, K.M., and Davis, M. (2007). Mechanisms of fear extinction. *Mol. Psychiatry* 12:120–150.

Norberg, M.M., Krystal, J.H., et al. (2008). A meta-analysis of D-cycloserine and the facilitation of fear extinction and exposure therapy. *Biol. Psychiatry* 63(12):1118–1126.

Ouimet, A.J., Gawronski, B., et al. (2009). Cognitive vulnerability to anxiety: a review and an integrative model. *Clin. Psychol. Rev.* 29(6):459–470.

Parnas, A.S., Weber, M., et al. (2005). Effects of multiple exposures to D-cycloserine on extinction of conditioned fear in rats. *Neurobiol. Learn. Mem.* 83(3):224–231.

Porto, P.R., Oliveira, L., et al. (2009). Does cognitive behavioral therapy change the brain? A systematic review of neuroimaging in anxiety disorders. *J. Neuropsychiatry Clin. Neurosci.* 21(2):114–125.

Powers, M.B., Smits, J.A.J., et al. (2009). Facilitation of fear extinction in phobic participants with a novel cognitive enhancer: a randomized placebo controlled trial of yohimbine augmentation. *J. Anxiety Disord.* 23(3):350–356.

Rauch, S.L., Shin, L.M., et al. (2003). Neuroimaging studies of amygdala function in anxiety disorders. *Ann. NY Acad. Sci.* 985(1):389–410.

Ravindran, L., and Stein, M. (2010). The pharmacologic treatment of anxiety disorders: a review of progress. *J. Clin. Psychiatry* 71(7):839–854.

Reger, M.A., and Gahm, G.A. (2009). A meta-analysis of the effects of internet- and computer-based cognitive-behavioral treatments for anxiety. *J. Clin. Psychology* 65(1):53–75.

Ressler, K.J., Rothbaum, B.O., et al. (2004). Cognitive enhancers as adjuncts to psychotherapy: use of D-cycloserine in phobic individuals to facilitate extinction of fear. *Arch. Gen. Psychiatry* 61(11):1136–1144.

Richardson, R., Ledgerwood, L., et al. (2004). Facilitation of fear extinction by D-cycloserine: theoretical and clinical implications. *Learn. Mem.* 11(5):510–516.

Schmidt, N. B. (2012). Innovations in the treatment of anxiety psychopathology: introduction to a special series. *Behav. Ther.* 43(3):465–467.

Slade, T., Johnston, A., et al. (2009). 2007 National Survey of Mental Health and Wellbeing: methods and key findings. *Aust. N. Z. J. Psychiatry* 43(7):594–605.

Soravia, L.M., Heinrichs, M., et al. (2006). Glucocorticoids reduce phobic fear in humans. *Proc. Natl. Acad. Sci.* 103(14):5585–5590.

Spek, V., Cuijpers, P., et al. (2007). Internet-based cognitive behaviour therapy for symptoms of depression and anxiety: a meta-analysis. *Psychol. Med.* 37:319–328.

Sullivan, G., Debiec, J., et al. (2011). The neurobiology of fear and anxiety: contributions of animal models to current understanding. In: Charney, D.S., and Nestler, E.J., eds. *Neurobiology of Mental Illness, 3rd Edition*. New York: Oxford University Press, pp. 603–626.

Taylor, S., Abramowitz, J., et al. (2012). Non-adherence and non-response in the treatment of anxiety disorders. *J. Anxiety Disord.* 26(5):583–589.

Tsigos, C., and Chrousos, G.P. (2002). Hypothalamic-pituitary-adrenal axis, neuroendocrine factors and stress. *J. Psychosom. Res.* 53(4):865–871.

Waller, R., and Gilbody, S. (2009). Barriers to the uptake of computerized cognitive behavioural therapy: a systematic review of the quantitative and qualitative evidence. *Psychol. Med.* 39:705–712.

Wilhelm, S., Buhlmann, U., et al. (2008). Augmentation of behavior therapy with D-cycloserine for obsessive-compulsive disorder. *Am. J. Psychiatry* 165:335–341.

Wolf, O.T. (2008). The influence of stress hormones on emotional memory: relevance for psychopathology. *Acta Psychol.* 127(3):513–531.

47 | PHARMACOTHERAPY OF ANXIETY DISORDERS

JAMES W. MURROUGH, DAN V. IOSIFESCU, AND
DENNIS S. CHARNEY

INTRODUCTION

Anxiety disorders are among the most prevalent mental disorders in the United States and are associated with a high degree of morbidity and public health costs (Kessler et al., 2005a). Approximately one in four adults will suffer from an anxiety disorder at some point in their lives. Anxiety disorders often have an age of onset in young adulthood or before and are frequently comorbid with general medical disorders and other psychiatric disorders. General risk factors for the development of an anxiety disorder include a temperamental trait described as behavioral inhibition—increased physiological reactivity and anxious behaviors observed in some children in response to unfamiliar surroundings—female gender, family history, and exposure to certain types of environmental stress in childhood or adulthood. Chapter 40 of this volume provides a thorough discussion of the genetics of anxiety disorders.

There are seven primary anxiety disorders defined in the Diagnostic and Statistical Manual of Mental Disorder—Fourth Edition, Text Revision (DSM-IV-TR): panic disorder, specific phobia, social phobia, obsessive-compulsive disorder (OCD), posttraumatic stress disorder (PTSD), acute stress disorder, and generalized anxiety disorder (GAD) (American Psychiatric Association, Task Force on DSM-IV, 2000). The current chapter will focus on the pharmacotherapeutic treatment of panic disorder, PTSD, GAD, and social phobia. The treatment of OCD is discussed by Dr. H. Blair Simpson in Chapter 48 and will not be reviewed here. Acute stress disorder is characterized by symptoms similar to those of PTSD that occur immediately following a traumatic event and will not be discussed separately from PTSD. Finally, specific phobia will not be discussed since there is a minimal role for pharmacotherapy for this disorder.

Other anxiety disorders defined in the DSM-IV-TR are considered to be secondary to either the direct physiological result of another medical condition (anxiety disorder due to a general medical condition: e.g., hyperthyroidism) or the direct physiological consequence of a substance (substance-induced anxiety disorder: e.g., withdrawal from alcohol or a sedative/hypnotic medication). These important secondary causes of anxiety disorders will not be discussed in depth; however, it is critical that these disorders be considered in the diagnostic assessment of the patient who presents with anxiety. The residual category termed "anxiety disorder not otherwise specified"

is included in the DSM to enable patients who present with prominent anxiety symptoms and functional impairment but who do not meet the criteria for a specific anxiety disorder to be diagnosed. Chapter 39 of this volume provides a complete discussion of the diagnosis of anxiety disorders.

A general approach to the evaluation and treatment of anxiety disorders is presented in Table 47.1. A complete diagnostic assessment—including medical and psychiatric history, vital signs, physical exam, and laboratory or other tests if indicated—should precede initiation of a treatment intervention. As mentioned earlier, particularly important to consider in the differential diagnosis of a patient who presents with anxiety symptoms are general medical disorders and substance use disorders. Other important principles relevant to the diagnosis and treatment of anxiety disorders include the establishment of a therapeutic alliance, provision of psychoeducation and counseling, and ongoing assessment of treatment adherence (Table 47.1). For most patients, first-line treatment will consist of an evidence-based trial of a medication, a psychotherapeutic modality (e.g., cognitive-behavioral therapy ([CBT]), or a combination of the two. If the treatment is effective, it should generally be continued for at least 6–12 months in the case of pharmacotherapy while some prescribed forms of CBT are considerably shorter. If the initial treatment modality is either partially effective or ineffective, then the treating clinician must determine the next best treatment step for the particular patient. Pharmacotherapeutic next-step options typically consist of augmentation—the addition of another agent to increase the effectiveness of the primary agent, or combination—the addition of a second antianxiety agent, or switching agents (Table 47.1).

An overview of U.S. Food and Drug Administration (FDA)-approved pharmacotherapeutic agents available to the clinician for the treatment of anxiety disorders is presented in Table 47.2. As will be reviewed in detail in the following text for specific anxiety disorders, serotonin-selective reuptake inhibitors (SSRIs) and serotonin-norepinephrine reuptake inhibitors (SNRIs) are usually considered first-line medication treatment. Older monoaminergic agents—including the tricyclic antidepressants (TCAs) and monoamine oxidase inhibitors (MAOIs)—are often efficacious but are usually reserved for second-line treatment due to safety and tolerability issues. The benzodiazepines (BZDs) play an important role in the treatment of some anxiety disorders; however, these agents, too, are usually reserved for second-line or adjunctive use due

TABLE 47.1. Approach to the treatment of anxiety disorders

1. Diagnostic Assessment

   Complete medical and psychiatric history.

   Assess for general medical or substance-related causes of anxiety symptoms.

   Obtain laboratory (e.g., TSH) or other diagnostic tests if indicated by history.

   Establish working diagnosis of a primary anxiety disorder after ruling out secondary causes.

   Establish presence or absence of comorbid psychiatric, medical, or substance use disorders.

2. Develop therapeutic alliance with patient to facilitate adherence to treatment.

3. Provide initial and ongoing psychoeducation to facilitate adherence to treatment.

4. Initiate first-line pharmacotherapeutic or psychotherapeutic treatment.

5. If initial treatment is effective, continue treatment for a minimum of 6 to 12 months, depending on clinical situation.

6. If initial treatment is ineffective:

   Assess adherence to treatment, provide psychoeducation, address potential barriers to treatment adherence, optimize therapeutic alliance.

   Reassess primary diagnosis and presence of comorbid psychiatric, medical, or substance use disorders.

   Consider switch to alternative first-line treatment option or augment current treatment with another evidence-based treatment option.

7. If first-line treatment options are ineffective:

   Identify potential specific psychosocial stressors that may respond to nonmedical intervention.

   Recommend evidence-based psychotherapy if not already tried.

   Consider second-line treatment options based on clinical circumstances and patient preference.

   Pursue ongoing diagnostic reevaluation and adherence monitoring

to tolerability and abuse liability issues. Benzodiazepines act by binding to a specific site on the gamma-aminobutyric acid (GABA)-A receptor and increasing the inhibitory effect associated with GABA binding. Other pharmacological agents, including anticonvulsants and atypical antipsychotics, have been investigated in different anxiety disorders, and the evidence to date generally does not support their use as first-line treatments; however, they may represent appropriate options in refractory patients.

While there has been an increasing recognition of the public health burden of anxiety disorders, historically there has been relatively little research focus on the development of new treatments. Most of the treatments for anxiety disorders are based on medications developed for the treatment of major depressive disorder (MDD). New research focusing on targets outside of the monoamine system—e.g., amino acid, neurohormonal, and neuropeptide systems—may yield novel and much needed treatment interventions for these common disorders.

PANIC DISORDER

OVERVIEW

Panic disorder (PD) is characterized by recurrent, unexpected panic attacks with attendant adverse behavioral effects between attacks (American Psychiatric Association, Task Force on DSM-IV, 2000). Panic attacks are periods of intense fear that peak within 10 minutes but can continue on for much longer. The intense fear is typically accompanied by physical symptoms such as heart palpitations, sweating, shortness of breath, chest pain or tightness, nausea, and dizziness. Sensations of choking or smothering and/or derealization during a panic attack are also common. By definition, the panic attacks are not due to the direct physiological effects of a substance or a general medical condition—both of which are important for the clinician to consider in the differential diagnosis of panic disorder. Ongoing worry about the implications of the panic attacks and/or anxiety about experiencing another unprovoked attack characterizes the disorder, and a duration of at least one month of persistent concern is required for the diagnosis. Individuals diagnosed with panic disorder may or may not also have agoraphobia—anxiety about and avoidance of situations where escape may be difficult.

Panic disorder affects between 1% and 3% of the U.S. population and is associated with significant morbidity and public health costs (Kessler et al., 2005b). Increased health care utilization is common in patients with panic disorder, and the presence of the illness places individuals at elevated risk for suicide (Perna et al., 2011). Overall there is good evidence for the efficacy of both pharmacotherapeutic and psychotherapeutic treatments for panic disorder, although there is still significant room for improvement to current treatment options. While evidence supports both approaches as first-line treatment, this chapter will focus on pharmacotherapeutic approaches.

FIRST-LINE PHARMACOTHERAPY

There is good evidence for the efficacy of SSRIs, SNRIs, TCAs, and BZDs in the treatment of panic disorder (American Psychiatric Association, 2009; McHugh et al., 2009). The 2009 American Psychiatric Association practice guideline on the treatment of panic disorder found that there was insufficient evidence to recommend one of these therapeutic options over the others (American Psychiatric Association, 2009). Given their relative tolerability, safety, and efficacy, a trial of an SSRI or SNRI for the patient with panic disorder is a pragmatic first treatment step. As always, factors specific to a particular case will guide treatment selection, including patient preference and the presence of comorbid medical or psychiatric conditions.

TABLE 47.2. Overview of pharmacotherapy for anxiety disorders

PHARMACOLOGIC CLASS	EXAMPLES	MOLECULAR TARGET(S)	FDA-APPROVED INDICATIONS	DOSE RANGE	HALF-LIFE	COMMON ADVERSE EFFECTS	SERIOUS ADVERSE EFFECTS	PREGNANCY CATEGORY
SSRI	Escitalopram	SERT	GAD	10–20 mg daily	27–32 hours	Nausea, diarrhea, headache, insomnia, somnolence, sexual dysfunction (class effects)	Bleeding, seizure, serotonin syndrome, worsening depression or anxiety, suicidal thoughts (class effects)	C
	Fluoxetine	SERT	OCD, PD	20–60 mg daily	4–6 days	Class effects	Class effects	C
	Fluvoxamine	SERT	OCD, SP	100–300 mg daily	16 hours	Class effects	Class effects	C
	Paroxetine	SERT	GAD, OCD, PD, PTSD, SP	20–50 mg daily	33 hours	Class effects	Class effects	D
	Sertraline	SERT	OCD, PD, PTSD, SP	50–200 mg daily	26 hours	Class effects	Class effects	C
SNRI	Duloxetine	SERT, NET	GAD	60–120 mg daily	12 hours	SSRI class effects, hypertension	SSRI class effects, hypertensive crisis, hepatitis	C
	Venlafaxine	SERT, NET	GAD, PD, SP	75–225 mg daily	5 hours	SSRI class effects, hypertension	SSRI class effects, hypertensive crisis, hepatitis	C
BZD	Alprazolam	GABA-AR	Anxiety (nonspecific), PD	1–4 mg daily	11–16 hours	Somnolence, cognitive problems, appetite change, fatigue (class effects)	Stevens-Johnson syndrome, hepatic dysfunction, withdrawal seizure (class effects)	D
	Chlordiazepoxide	GABA-AR	Anxiety (nonspecific)	15–40 mg daily	24–48 hours	Class effects	Class effects, hepatitis, agranulocytosis	?
	Clonazepam	GABA-AR	PD	1–4 mg daily	30–40 hours	Class effects	Class effects	D
	Diazepam	GABA-AR	Anxiety (nonspecific)	2–10 mg daily	15–20 hours	Class effects	Class effects, neutropenia	D
	Lorazepam	GABA-AR	Anxiety (nonspecific)	1–6 mg daily	12–14 hours	Class effects	Class effects	D
	Oxazepam	GABA-AR	Anxiety (nonspecific)	30–120 mg daily	6–11 hours	Class effects	Class effects	?

(continued)

TABLE 47.2. (*Continued*)

PHARMACOLOGIC CLASS	EXAMPLES	MOLECULAR TARGET(S)	FDA-APPROVED INDICATIONS	DOSE RANGE	HALF-LIFE	COMMON ADVERSE EFFECTS	SERIOUS ADVERSE EFFECTS	PREGNANCY CATEGORY
TCA	Clomipramine	SERT, NET, mACh, alpha1, H1	OCD, PD	25–250 mg daily	32 hours	Dry mouth, constipation, urinary retention, somnolence, dizziness, weight gain, sexual dysfunction, orthostasis (class effects)	Can be lethal in overdose, cardiac arrhythmia, hematological abnormalities, suicidal thoughts (class effects)	C
	Doxepine	SERT, NET, mAChR, A1R, H1R	Anxiety (nonspecific)	75–300 mg daily	15 hours	TCA class effects	TCA class effects	C
	Imipramine	SERT, NET, mAChR, A1R, H1R	PD	100–200 mg daily	6–18 hours	TCA class effects	TCA class effects	C
MAOI	Phenelzine	MAO	PD	45–90 mg daily	12 hours	Dry mouth, constipation, orthostasis, weight gain, sexual dysfunction, somnolence, dizziness, headache (class effects)	Can be lethal in overdose, cardiac arrhythmia, hypertensive crisis, myocardial infarction	?
Antihistamine	Hydroxyzine	H1R	Anxiety (nonspecific)	200–400 mg daily	20 hours	Sedation, dry mouth, dizziness, headache	Hypotension, cardiac arrhythmia, respiratory depression	C
Other	Buspirone	5-HT1AR	Anxiety (nonspecific)	20–60 mg daily	2–3 hours	Nausea, dizziness, headache	Myocardial infarction (rare), stroke (rare)	B

A1R, alpha-adrenergic type 1 receptor; BZD, benzodiazepines; GABA, gamma-aminobutyric acid; GABA-AR, GABA type A receptor; H1R, histamine type 1 receptor; MAO, monoamine oxidase; MAOI, MAO inhibitor; mAChR, muscarinic acetylcholine receptor; NET, norepinephrine transporter; OCD, obsessive-compulsive disorder; PD, panic disorder; SERT, serotonin transporter; SP, social phobia; SNRI, serotonin norepinephrine reuptake inhibitor; SSRI, selective serotonin reuptake inhibitor; TCA, tricyclic antidepressant; 5-HT, 5-hydroxy-tryptamine; 5HT1AR, 5-HT type 1A receptor.

The SSRIs fluoxetine, paroxetine, and sertraline are FDA approved for the treatment of panic disorder, as is the SNRI venlafaxine. Three meta-analytic reviews of SSRIs in panic disorder support the efficacy of these interventions (Bakker et al., 2002; Mitte, 2005; Otto et al., 2001). In one example, an analysis of 12 placebo-controlled trials found a mean effect size for acute treatment outcome for SSRIs relative to placebo of 0.55 (Otto et al., 2001). A study including 664 patients with panic disorder randomized to venlafaxine extended-release (ER) 75 mg or 150 mg daily, paroxetine 40 mg daily, or placebo for up to 12 weeks found response rates of 77–80% for the venlafaxine and paroxetine groups compared with 56% for the placebo group (Pollack et al., 2007). Studies comparing different agents in the SSRI class to each other or to venlafaxine have generally not found support for the efficacy of one agent over another (see Freire et al., 2011 for review).

SSRIs and SNRIs are generally safe and well tolerated in this and other anxiety disorder populations. The most commonly reported side effects include sleep changes, nausea, headache, sleep problems, and sexual dysfunction (see Table 47.2). Importantly, patients with panic disorder may be particularly sensitive to transient increases in anxiety that are sometimes observed at the initiation of treatment or upon a dosage increase with an SSRI or SNRI agent. Psychoeducation represents an important component of the treatment in this regard. Adjunctive treatment with BZD at the outset of treatment with an SSRI or SNRI to mitigate this increase in anxiety may also be indicated, as discussed in more detail next.

SECOND-LINE/OTHER APPROACHES

The BZDs alprazolam and clonazepam are FDA approved for the treatment of panic disorder. BZDs are potent anxiolytic medications that can result in substantial symptom relief for patients with panic and other anxiety disorders when used appropriately (American Psychiatric Association, 2009; Ballenger et al., 1988). BZDs have the advantage of a more rapid onset of action compared with SSRIs or other monoaminergic agents, although data supporting their longer term efficacy is more limited. Alprazolam has a short half-life and a rapid onset of action, particularly desirable when rapid relief from a developing panic attack is the treatment goal. Clonazepam has a longer half-life and is more suited to standing dosing as opposed to as-needed (e.g., "prn") use. See Table 47.1 for a description of commonly prescribed BZD medications. Principal disadvantages associated with the use of BZDs in panic or other anxiety disorders include their well-known abuse liability and the predictable development of tolerance, the need for dose escalation, and prominent withdrawal effects. Somnolence and cognitive problems are additional adverse effects characteristic of this drug class.

As mentioned in the preceding section, patients may experience a temporary increase in anxiety following initiation of treatment with an SSRI or SNRI agent. Another limitation commonly observed with monoaminergic treatments is a delay in onset of therapeutic effect of several weeks. BZDs can, therefore, have an important therapeutic role as adjunctive treatment to a first-line agent. Goddard et al.

showed that coadministration of low-dose clonazepam with sertraline in the treatment of panic disorder resulted in a significantly greater proportion of responders in the sertraline/clonazepam compared with the sertraline/placebo group at the end of one week (41% compared with 4%) (Goddard et al., 2001). Notably, the groups did not differ in response rate by the end of the study. These data support the common clinical practice of initiating a BZD agent concurrently with an SSRI or SNRI at the outset of the treatment and then tapering the BZD after three to four weeks and continuing the first-line agent.

The TCAs clomipramine and imipramine are FDA approved for the treatment of panic disorder, and several early studies have established the efficacy of these agents in reducing the frequency and intensity of panic attacks (Bakker et al., 2002; Perna et al., 2011). The TCAs are considered second-line agents for the treatment of panic disorder—as well as other anxiety disorders—primarily due to their side effect burden. For example, a meta-analysis including 2,367 patients compared SSRIs with TCAs and found that the proportion of patients free of panic attacks did not differ while the number of dropouts was significantly lower in the group of patients treated with SSRIs compared with TCAs (18% vs. 31%, respectively) (Bakker et al., 2002). Commonly observed adverse effects for this drug class are attributable to blockade of the muscarinic acetylcholine receptor (e.g., dry mouth, constipation, urinary retention) or the alpha-adrenergic or histamine receptors (e.g., somnolence, orthostasis, weight gain). Serious adverse reactions such as cardiac arrhythmia can occur and TCAs can be fatal in overdose. Despite the potential for side effects, a trial of a TCA is warranted in patients who fail to demonstrate an adequate response to first-line therapy.

The MAOI phenelzine is approved for the treatment of panic disorder and represents an important third- or fourth-line agent for refractory patients. MAOIs irreversibly inhibit the enzyme monoamine oxidase and result in a net increase in monoamine availability in the synapse. The use of MAOIs is restricted by the need to maintain a low-tyramine diet and the risk of (potentially fatal) hypertensive crisis and drug–drug interactions. Moclobemide—a reversible MAOI (RIMA [reversible inhibitors of monoamine oxidase A]) not currently available in the United States—has some efficacy data in panic disorder and does not have the same strict dietary restrictions and safety liability as the irreversible MAOIs.

There is currently no controlled evidence supporting the use of anticonvulsant medications in panic disorder. RCTs examining the efficacy of the anticonvulsants gabapentin and tiagabine in panic disorder have been conducted, and these studies did not find support for the use of these agents.

There is a paucity of evidence available to the clinician to help determine the next treatment step in the management of panic disorder in the event that first-line pharmacotherapy fails. Given the evidence supporting the efficacy of specific psychotherapeutic interventions for panic disorder, this option should be considered at the top of the treatment algorithm. If a partial response is gained with an SSRI or SNRI, upward dose titration and/or augmentation with psychotherapy or a BZD may represent a pragmatic therapeutic step. If no response is achieved with a first-line agent after appropriate treatment duration (at least four to six weeks) and dose escalation, then a switch to a second first-line agent is an appropriate step. TCAs, MAOIs, or other agents (e.g., anticonvulsants) may be reserved for more refractory cases.

POSTTRAUMATIC STRESS DISORDER

OVERVIEW

Posttraumatic stress disorder is a disabling condition that develops in a subset of individuals exposed to extreme psychological stress. The disorder is characterized by intrusive reexperiencing of traumatic memories along with symptoms of increased arousal and avoidance of stimuli associated with the trauma (American Psychiatric Association, Task Force on DSM-IV, 2000). By definition, the symptoms must be present for more than one month and be associated with significant distress and functional impairment. PTSD is increasingly being recognized as a major public health problem, and the alarming rates of PTSD and associated sequelae—including suicide attempts and completed suicide—observed in U.S. soldiers returning from combat portend the urgent need to identify effective treatments.

The estimated lifetime prevalence of PTSD in the United States is 7.8% according to the National Comorbidity Survey, with women being approximately twice as likely to suffer from PTSD compared with men (10.4% vs. 5.0%, respectively) (Kessler et al., 1995). The estimated lifetime prevalence of trauma exposure is 60.7% for men and 51.2% for women. Therefore, while trauma exposure is very common, development of PTSD is relatively less so. It is estimated that 79% of women and 88% of men with PTSD have also been diagnosed with at least one other psychiatric disorder—most frequently MDD, other anxiety disorders, and substance use disorders (Pratchett et al., 2011).

FIRST-LINE PHARMACOTHERAPY

Two SSRIs—sertraline and paroxetine—are approved by the FDA for the treatment of PTSD, and SSRIs are generally recommended by practice guidelines as first-line pharmacotherapy for the disorder (American Psychiatric Association, 2004). In an early positive, 12-week RCT (randomized controlled trial) comparing sertraline with placebo, the response rate was 53% for drug compared with 32% for placebo (Brady et al., 2000) and similar data are available for paroxetine (Marshall et al., 2001). Sertraline was found to be more effective than placebo at preventing relapse in a 28-week relapse prevention study (Davidson et al., 2001). In contrast, a more recent acute-phase RCT comparing sertraline to placebo conducted in a Veterans Affairs (VA) setting was negative (Friedman et al., 2007). Some data are also available in support of the SNRI venlafaxine in the treatment of PTSD. Importantly, a report from the Institute of Medicine (IOM) found that the existent evidence was inadequate to support the efficacy of SSRIs or other pharmacotherapy in PTSD (Institute of Medicine, 2008). A *Cochrane Review* of pharmacotherapy for PTSD including

35 RCTs and 4,597 participants did support the use of SSRIs as first-line medication treatment; however, it also acknowledged that there exist significant gaps in the evidence base (Stein et al., 2006). Responder status from 13 trials included in the *Cochrane Review* demonstrated overall superiority of medication compared with placebo: relative risk 1.49 (95% CI: 1.28, 1.73).

The data just reviewed paints a sobering picture of the current state of pharmacotherapy for PTSD, and new, more effective treatments are clearly needed for this disability disorder. Although not the focus of the current review, it is important to note that specific psychotherapeutic interventions—most notably, exposure therapy—have relatively strong evidence for efficacy in PTSD and may be considered a first-line treatment for PTSD. For example, in contrast to its conclusions regarding pharmacotherapy, the IOM report described earlier found sufficient evidence to conclude that exposure therapy is effective for PTSD (Institute of Medicine, 2008).

SECOND-LINE/OTHER APPROACHES

As noted preceding, exposure therapy or related CBT approaches should be considered for patients with PTSD early in the treatment algorithm, particularly if a patient does not respond adequately to a trial of an SSRI. Regarding second-line pharmacotherapeutic options, some evidence exists supporting the use of MAOIs, TCAs, BZDs, atypical antipsychotics, or anticonvulsants in the treatment of PTSD (see Baker et al., 2009 for review). The TCA amitriptyline has weak evidence for efficacy while desipramine was not found to be effective. One trial comparing the MAOI phenelzine with the TCA, imipramine, or placebo found support for both drugs, although another study investigating phenelzine in PTSD was negative.

BZDs can be used to target specific anxiety symptoms, hyperarousal, or insomnia associated with PTSD. Well-controlled data supporting the overall efficacy of BZD in the treatment of PTSD, however, is lacking, and tolerance and abuse potential issues limit the role of these medications. Studies investigating the use of BZDs immediately following trauma were not favorable. A small amount of research investigating alpha-adrenergic antagonists—prazosin, in particular—provides some support for their use in treating nightmares and sleep disturbance associated with PTSD (Raskind et al., 2003).

Atypical antipsychotic medication is frequently used as an adjunctive treatment in PTSD when first-line agents fail to yield a complete response. Risperidone has been the focus of the majority of research in PTSD with several smaller studies suggesting a beneficial effect of the addition of risperidone to an SSRI or SNRI. A recent, large, six-month RCT of adjunctive risperidone in PTSD conducted in a VA setting, however, did not find a significant advantage of risperidone over placebo (Krystal et al., 2011). In the same study, risperidone was associated with significantly greater adverse events compared with placebo, including weight gain, fatigue, and somnolence. The data reviewed in the preceding, along with consideration of potentially serious longer term adverse effects associated with atypical antipsychotic agents, including tardive dyskinesias and metabolic syndrome, must be weighed against potentially therapeutic gains when considering risperidone or other antipsychotic agents as a treatment option for refractory PTSD.

Several studies investigating the use of anticonvulsants in PTSD have been conducted with generally discouraging results. Topiramate, tiagabine, and valproate have failed to demonstrate clear efficacy in PTSD in controlled study designs. Several case series and open studies of anticonvulsants have yielded favorable results, suggesting that these agents may help in select cases.

In summary, the evidence base for effective treatments in PTSD is unfortunately limited, and new treatments for this disabling condition are urgently needed. SSRIs and exposure therapy have the best efficacy evidence, but a significant proportion of patients will remain symptomatic with currently available treatments. The evidence supporting the use of TCAs, MAOIs, BZDs, anticonvulsants, atypical antipsychotics, or other agents is quite limited.

GENERALIZED ANXIETY DISORDER

OVERVIEW

Generalized anxiety disorder (GAD) is characterized by excessive anxiety and worry occurring more days than not for at least six months (American Psychiatric Association, Task Force on DSM-IV, 2000). By definition, the worry is difficult to control, is out of proportion to real or perceived external factors, and is associated with three or more of the following six symptoms: restlessness, fatigue, difficulty concentrating, irritability, muscle tension, or sleep disturbance. To meet criteria for the disorder, the symptoms must cause clinically significant distress or impairment in social, occupational, or other important areas of functioning, and the disturbance must not be due to the direct physiological effects of a general medical condition or substance.

GAD is a common disorder, with a lifetime prevalence of 5–6% in the general population, and is more common in women than in men (approximately 2:1). Notably, GAD is one of the most common psychiatric disorders in primary care settings and is associated with increased utilization of health services. The disorder has a high rate of comorbidity with mood and other anxiety disorders, as well as with substance use and general medical conditions. It is estimated that nearly 50% of patients with GAD also meet criteria for MDD. The high rate of comorbidity between GAD and MDD and symptomatic overlap have led to the idea that these syndromes may be different manifestations of the same disorder, although there continues to be debate regarding this issue.

FIRST-LINE PHARMACOTHERAPY

More than a dozen RCTs of drugs in the SSRI class support the use of SSRIs as first-line pharmacotherapy for GAD (Baldwin et al., 2011; Kapczinski et al., 2003). Escitalopram and paroxetine have an FDA indication for the treatment of GAD and good controlled data also exist for sertraline. Response rates for SSRIs of between 60% and 75% are generally reported in RCTs, compared with response rates of between 40% and 60%

for placebo (Baldwin et al., 2011). In a study by Rickels et al. where outpatients with GAD ($N = 566$) were randomized to eight weeks of paroxetine at 20 or 40 mg/day or placebo, response rates were 62%, 68%, and 46% for patients receiving 20 mg, 40 mg, or placebo, respectively (Rickels et al., 2003). Data also support the longer term efficacy of SSRIs in sustaining treatment effects over a period of six months (Stocchi et al., 2003).

In addition to that of SSRIs, good controlled data also support the use of SNRIs as a first-line treatment option in GAD. The SNRIs venlafaxine ER and duloxetine both carry FDA indications for the treatment of GAD and observed response rates and drug–placebo differences in RCTs generally similar to what is observed in trials of SSRIs (Baldwin et al., 2011). In one study, patients with GAD ($n = 377$) were randomized to venlafaxine ER 75, 150, or 225 mg/day or placebo for eight weeks, and resulting analysis indicated that patients had significant reductions in illness severity under venlafaxine ER compared with placebo conditions (Rickels et al., 2000). A second RCT including 251 patients with GAD assessed longer term efficacy of venlafaxine ER over six months and found response rates of 69% or higher in the active drug group compared with 42–46% in the placebo group (Gelenberg et al., 2000). Duloxetine has demonstrated efficacy comparable to venlafaxine for GAD (Hartford et al., 2007), although longer term maintenance studies of duloxetine in GAD have not been conducted to date.

As reviewed in previous sections, SSRI and SNRI medications have favorable tolerability profiles. Alerting patients to the common, usually transient, adverse effects of these medication classes—including nausea, headache, changes in sleep, and nervousness—is an important component of psychoeducation and will facilitate treatment adherence. Transient nervousness, jitteriness, or worsening of anxiety at the onset of treatment with an SSRI or SNRI may be a particular concern for this patient population. In addition to psychoeducation, short-term treatment with low-dose BZD at the outset of treatment, as described next, may be a fruitful pharmacotherapeutic strategy.

Considering the safety, efficacy, and tolerability of SSRIs and SNRIs, these drugs represent first-line treatment for GAD.

SECOND-LINE/OTHER APPROACHES

There is limited data available to guide clinicians regarding next best steps for treatment in patients with GAD who manifest an inadequate response to first-line therapy. There is fair evidence for BZDs, the azapirone buspirone, TCAs, and the anticonvulsant agent pregabalin in the treatment of GAD. Weak evidence also exists for other anticonvulsants (e.g., valproic acid), antihistamines (e.g., hydroxyzine), and atypical antipsychotics (e.g., quetiapine). CBT is an important therapeutic consideration for patients with GAD, especially if they have not responded to a prior first-line medication trial.

The rapid and robust anxiolytic effects of BZDs make this class of drugs an important component of the treatment armamentarium for GAD. A key early RCT comparing diazepam with trazodone and imipramine found that diazepam was associated with the most improvement in anxiety during the first two weeks of treatment (Rickels et al., 1993). In contrast, during weeks three through eight, imipramine was superior to diazepam in the proportion of patients achieving moderate or marked symptom improvement (73% vs. 66%). Given the limitation of BZD therapy discussed in the preceding sections, including sedation, cognitive disturbance, and abuse or dependence liability, these agents should be used judiciously in the treatment of GAD. Specific circumstances that may be particularly suited to the use of BZDs include short-term use as an adjunct to antidepressant medication or in patients who are refractory to first-line treatments after consideration of the risk:benefit ratio for the individual patient. Patients with a history of substance use disorder may be particularly vulnerable to the abuse or dependence liability of BZDs, and additional caution should be used in this patient population.

The azapirone buspirone is a unique partial agonist at the 5-HT$_{1A}$ receptor and is FDA approved for the treatment of GAD. Buspirone and other azapirones have demonstrated superiority to placebo in the treatment of GAD in a number of large RCTs (Chessick et al., 2006). Despite reasonable controlled evidence for its efficacy, buspirone is not generally considered a first-line treatment for GAD, in part due to its relatively slow onset of action, tolerability issues at higher doses, and some data suggesting inferiority to antidepressant or BZD treatment options (Davidson et al., 1999).

As referenced earlier, there is some data for the effectiveness of TCAs, imipramine in particular, in the treatment of GAD (Rickels et al., 1993). Potential advantages of TCAs over BZDs include their ability to treat symptoms of both anxiety and depression and the absence of potential for abuse and physiological dependence. As a class, TCAs are generally reserved for patients who have failed other treatment strategies, owing to safety and tolerability issues related to this class of medications. As discussed in previous sections, pharmacological blockade of muscarinic, histamine, and alpha-adrenergic receptors limit their use. The utility of TCAs is also limited by their cardiotoxic potential and lethality in overdose.

Pregabalin, a voltage-dependent calcium channel modulator approved for the adjunctive treatment of seizure disorder, has fair efficacy data for the treatment of GAD from several RCTs (Montgomery et al., 2006; Rickels et al., 2005). In one study, patients were randomized to four weeks of treatment with pregabalin, 300 mg, 450 mg, or 600 mg per day, alprazolam, 1.5 mg per day, or placebo, and results indicated that both pregabalin and alprazolam produced significant reductions in anxiety compared with placebo (Rickels et al., 2005). A second study randomized patients with GAD ($n = 421$) to six weeks of double-blind treatment with pregabalin 400 mg or 600 mg per day, venlafaxine 75 mg per day, or placebo and found both pregabalin and venlafaxine to be more effective than placebo in decreasing anxiety symptoms (Montgomery et al., 2006).

A recent effect size analysis of treatments for GAD—including SSRIs, SNRIs, BZDs, buspirone, hydroxyzine, and pregabalin—yielded an overall effect size of 0.39 for all drugs versus placebo (Hidalgo et al., 2007). Drug-specific effect sizes, listed from largest to smallest effect, were as follows: pregabalin: 0.50, hydroxyzine: 0.45, SNRI: 0.42, BZD: 0.38, SSRI: 0.36, buspirone: 0.17. While this analysis provides some interesting insights and suggests that overall our current treatments for GAD vary from modestly to poorly effective, methodological limitations inherent in effect size analysis limit specific conclusions that can be drawn.

In summary, first-line pharmacotherapy for GAD—including SSRIs and SNRIs—provides substantial symptomatic relief in many but not all patients with GAD. Second-line treatment options include BZDs, buspirone, TCAs, pregabalin, and hydroxyzine, among other agents. Future research is required to establish the optimal treatment approach for patients who do not respond to a first-line treatment trial.

SOCIAL PHOBIA

OVERVIEW

Social phobia—also known as social anxiety disorder—is a common and potentially disabling anxiety disorder with a lifetime estimated prevalence of approximately 12% (Kessler et al., 2005b). The disorder is characterized by marked anxiety in reaction to social or performance situations, often leading to avoidance behavior (American Psychiatric Association, Task Force on DSM-IV, 2000). By definition, exposure to the feared social situation nearly always provokes anxiety, and the resulting avoidance, anxious anticipation, or distress interferes significantly with the person's social or occupational functioning. Comorbidity is common, and social phobia often precedes the onset of other disorders, in particular MDD and substance use disorders. (Stein and Stein, 2008). The disorder often begins in childhood or early adolescence and has been associated with the heritable temperament trait behavior inhibition.

FIRST-LINE PHARMACOTHERAPY

More than two dozen RCTs of SSRIs or SNRIs support the use of these medications as first-line pharmacotherapy in social phobia (de Menezes et al., 2011; Stein et al., 2004; Stein and Stein, 2008). Fluvoxamine, paroxetine, sertraline, and venlafaxine have FDA approval for the treatment of social phobia. In the case of paroxetine trials, reported response rates for active drug vary from 55% to 72% compared with response rates for placebo between 8% and 50% (Stein and Stein, 2008a). Reported response rates are similar for other SSRIs and venlafaxine. A *Cochrane Review* including 36 RCTs and 4,268 patients with social phobia demonstrated short-term superiority of medication over placebo with a relative risk of nonresponse of 0.63 (95% CI: 0.55, 0.72) (Stein et al., 2004). For SSRIs in particular, the relative risk of nonresponse was 0.67 (95% CI: 0.59, 0.76). A recent quantitative meta-analysis including 27 RCTs aimed to compare efficacy between members of the SSRI, SNRI, and atypical antidepressant classes and found paroxetine, sertraline, fluvoxamine, escitalopram, and venlafaxine to be consistently more effective than placebo (de Menezes et al., 2011). The superiority of drug over placebo was less convincing for other agents, including citalopram, mirtazapine, and nefazodone.

Fewer data exist concerning the effectiveness of longer-term treatment in social phobia. The *Cochrane Review* just described included three maintenance studies and five relapse prevention studies and found some support for longer term treatment (relative risk of nonresponse was 0.58 [95% CI: 0.39, 0.85] and 0.33 [95% CI: 0.22, 0.49], respectively). Considering the safety, efficacy, and tolerability of SSRIs, these drugs—along with the SNRI venlafaxine—represent first-line treatment for social phobia.

SECOND-LINE/OTHER APPROACHES

A series of early studies established the efficacy of the MAOI phenelzine in the treatment of social phobia (Blanco et al., 2002). For example, an RCT including 85 patients with social phobia found a 64% response rate in the phenelzine group compared with 23% in the placebo group (Liebowitz et al., 1992). Despite safety and tolerability issues related to irreversible MAOIs, a trial of phenelzine or other MAOI should be considered in cases where patients fail to achieve response to first-line treatment. The RIMA moclobemide has some efficacy evidence from RCTs in social phobia conducted in Europe. To date there have been no RCTs published of TCAs in social phobia.

There is limited data to support the use of BZDs in the treatment of social phobia. An early 10-week RCT found support for clonazepam (mean dose 2.4 mg/day) with a 78% response rate in the active arm compared with a 20% response rate in the placebo arm while evidence for the efficacy of alprazolam or other BZDs was less favorable (Blanco et al., 2002). Given the predictable disadvantages of chronic BZD therapy, this class of medication should be used judiciously and reserved for treatment-refractory cases.

Several studies have investigated the role of anticonvulsants in social phobia and have yielded generally negative results. RCTs of levetiracetam, gabapentin, and pregabilin have failed to demonstrate superiority of these agents over placebo. A small amount of evidence exists for the atypical antipsychotic quetiapine in social phobia.

As with other anxiety disorders, CBT has been shown to be effective for patients with social phobia and should be considered as part of the treatment plan, particularly if first-line pharmacotherapy has been ineffective. An interesting and potentially important line of research focuses on using glutamate-based pharmacotherapy to enhance the effectiveness of CBT. An initial RCT conducted in 27 patients with social phobia investigated the efficacy of combining the glutamatergic *N*-methyl-D-aspartate (NMDA) receptor agonist D-cycloserine with exposure therapy and found that patients receiving D-cycloserine in addition to exposure therapy reported significantly less social anxiety compared with patients receiving exposure therapy plus placebo (Hofmann et al., 2006). While these results are preliminary and await replication, the strategy of leveraging pharmacotherapy to enhance learning-based treatments represents a novel and potentially powerful treatment approach to anxiety disorders in the future.

CONCLUSIONS AND FUTURE DIRECTIONS

Substantial progress has been made over the past several decades in the treatment of anxiety disorders. Large RCTs support the efficacy of SSRIs and in some cases SNRIs in the treatment of many of the anxiety disorders, including panic disorder, GAD, and social phobia. Second-, third-, or fourth-line agents for the different anxiety disorders include TCAs, MAOIs, BZDs, buspirone, anticonvulsants, or atypical antipsychotics wherein the evidence base is less than optimal. Despite their superiority compared with placebo, the effect sizes for first-line agents in most anxiety disorders are only modest, and a substantial number of patients suffering from anxiety disorders do not gain full relief from their symptoms with currently available treatments. In the case of PTSD, the situation is particularly concerning, and there is current uncertainty regarding the effectiveness of any medication in the treatment of this potentially disabling disorder. Taken together, improved treatments for anxiety disorders represent a critical unmet public health need.

Significant progress in neuroscience is illuminating potential new avenues of treatment discovery and novel targets from rational drug development. The rapidly developing neuroscience related to fear and anxiety is described in several chapters in the current volume, including Chapters 41, 42, 43, 44, 45, 48 and 49. Compounds with novel mechanisms of action currently in development for anxiety disorders include corticotropic releasing factor antagonists, neurokinin receptor antagonists, a variety of glutamate modulators, and glucocorticoid modulators. The endocannabinoid system has recently emerged as an interesting target in PTSD and other anxiety disorders. Continued progress in basic and translational neuroscience is expected to meet the need for new, more effective treatments for patients suffering from these disorders.

DISCLOSURES

Dr. Iosifescu has consulted for CNS Response, Inc. and has received grant/research support through Mount Sinai School of Medicine from Brainsway, Euthymics Bioscience Inc., Neosync, and Shire.

Dr. Murrough is supported by a Career Development Award from the National Institute of Mental Health (K23MH094707) and by the Brain and Behavior Research Foundation (NARSAD Young Investigator Award) and the American Foundation for Suicide Prevention.

Dr. Charney has been named as an inventor on a pending use-patent of ketamine for the treatment of depression. If ketamine were shown to be effective in the treatment of depression and received approval from the Food and Drug Administration for this indication, Dr. Charney and Mount Sinai School of Medicine could benefit financially.

REFERENCES

American Psychiatric Association. (2004). Practice Guideline for the Treatment of Patients with Acute Stress Disorder and Posttraumatic Stress Disorder. Washington, DC: Author.

American Psychiatric Association. (2009). Practice Guideline for the Treatment of Patients with Panic Disorder, 2nd Edition. Washington, DC: Author.

American Psychiatric Association. Task Force on DSM-IV. (2000). Diagnostic and Statistical Manual of Mental Disorders: DSM-IV-TR, 4th Edition, Text Revision. Washington, DC; New York: Author.

Baker, D.G., Nievergelt, C.M., et al. (2009). Post-traumatic stress disorder: emerging concepts of pharmacotherapy. *Exp. Opin. Emerg. Drugs* 14(2):251–272.

Bakker, A., van Balkom, A.J., et al. (2002). SSRIs vs. TCAs in the treatment of panic disorder: a meta-analysis. *Acta Psychiatr. Scand.* 106(3):163–167.

Baldwin, D.S., Waldman, S., et al. (2011). Evidence-based pharmacological treatment of generalized anxiety disorder. *Int. J. Neuropsychopharmacol.* 14(5):697–710.

Ballenger, J.C., Burrows, G.D., et al. (1988). Alprazolam in panic disorder and agoraphobia: results from a multicenter trial: I. Efficacy in short-term treatment. *Arch. Gen. Psychiatry* 45(5):413–422.

Blanco, C., Antia, S.X., et al. (2002). Pharmacotherapy of social anxiety disorder. *Biol. Psychiatry* 51(1):109–120.

Brady, K., Pearlstein, T., et al. (2000). Efficacy and safety of sertraline treatment of posttraumatic stress disorder: a randomized controlled trial. *JAMA* 283(14):1837–1844.

Chessick, C.A., Allen, M.H., et al. (2006). Azapirones for generalized anxiety disorder. *Cochrane Database Syst. Rev. (Online)* (3)(3):CD006115.

Davidson, J., Pearlstein, T., et al. (2001). Efficacy of sertraline in preventing relapse of posttraumatic stress disorder: results of a 28-week double-blind, placebo-controlled study. *Am. J. Psychiatry* 158(12):1974–1981.

Davidson, J.R., DuPont, R.L., et al. (1999). Efficacy, safety, and tolerability of venlafaxine extended release and buspirone in outpatients with generalized anxiety disorder. *J. Clin. Psychiatry* 60(8):528–535.

de Menezes, G.B., Coutinho, E.S., et al. (2011). Second-generation antidepressants in social anxiety disorder: meta-analysis of controlled clinical trials. *Psychopharmacol.* 215(1):1–11.

Freire, R.C., Hallak, J.E., et al. (2011). New treatment options for panic disorder: clinical trials from 2000 to 2010. *Exp. Opin. Pharmacother.* 12(9):1419–1428.

Friedman, M.J., Marmar, C.R., et al. (2007). Randomized, double-blind comparison of sertraline and placebo for posttraumatic stress disorder in a department of veterans affairs setting. *J. Clin. Psychiatry* 68(5):711–720.

Gelenberg, A.J., Lydiard, R.B., et al. (2000). Efficacy of venlafaxine extended-release capsules in nondepressed outpatients with generalized anxiety disorder: a 6-month randomized controlled trial. *JAMA* 283(23):3082–3088.

Goddard, A.W., Brouette, T., et al. (2001). Early coadministration of clonazepam with sertraline for panic disorder. *Arch. Gen. Psychiatry* 58(7):681–686.

Hartford, J., Kornstein, S., et al. (2007). Duloxetine as an SNRI treatment for generalized anxiety disorder: results from a placebo and active-controlled trial. *Int. Clin. Psychopharmacol.* 22(3):167–174.

Hidalgo, R.B., Tupler, L.A., et al. (2007). An effect-size analysis of pharmacologic treatments for generalized anxiety disorder. *J. Psychopharmacol.* 21(8):864–872.

Hofmann, S.G., Meuret, A.E., et al. (2006). Augmentation of exposure therapy with D-cycloserine for social anxiety disorder. *Arch. Gen. Psychiatry* 63(3):298–304.

Institute of Medicine. (2008). Treatment of Posttraumatic Stress Disorder: An Assessment of the Evidence. Washington, DC: National Academies Press.

Kapczinski, F., Lima, M.S., et al. (2003). Antidepressants for generalized anxiety disorder. *Cochrane Database Syst. Rev. (Online)* (2)(2):CD003592.

Kessler, R.C., Berglund, P., et al. (2005). Lifetime prevalence and age-of-onset distributions of DSM-IV disorders in the national comorbidity survey replication. *Arch. Gen. Psychiatry* 62(6):593–602.

Kessler, R.C., Chiu, W.T., et al. (2005). Prevalence, severity, and comorbidity of 12-month DSM-IV disorders in the national comorbidity survey replication. *Arch. Gen. Psychiatry* 62(6):617–627.

Kessler, R.C., Sonnega, A., et al. (1995). Posttraumatic stress disorder in the national comorbidity survey. *Arch. Gen. Psychiatry* 52(12):1048–1060.

Krystal, J.H., Rosenheck, R.A., et al. (2011). Adjunctive risperidone treatment for antidepressant-resistant symptoms of chronic military service-related PTSD: a randomized trial. *JAMA* 306(5):493–502.

Liebowitz, M.R., Schneier, F., et al. (1992). Phenelzine vs atenolol in social phobia: a placebo-controlled comparison. *Arch. Gen. Psychiatry* 49(4):290–300.

Marshall, R.D., Beebe, K.L., et al. (2001). Efficacy and safety of paroxetine treatment for chronic PTSD: a fixed-dose, placebo-controlled study. *Am. J. Psychiatry* 158(12):1982–1988.

McHugh, R.K., Smits, J.A., et al. (2009). Empirically supported treatments for panic disorder. *Psychiatric Clin. North Am.* 32(3):593–610.

Mitte, K. (2005). A meta-analysis of the efficacy of psycho- and pharmacotherapy in panic disorder with and without agoraphobia. *J. Affect. Disord.* 88(1):27–45.

Montgomery, S.A., Tobias, K., et al. (2006). Efficacy and safety of pregabalin in the treatment of generalized anxiety disorder: a 6-week, multicenter, randomized, double-blind, placebo-controlled comparison of pregabalin and venlafaxine. *J. Clin. Psychiatry* 67(5):771–782.

Otto, M.W., Tuby, K.S., et al. (2001). An effect-size analysis of the relative efficacy and tolerability of serotonin selective reuptake inhibitors for panic disorder. *Am. J. Psychiatry* 158(12):1989–1992.

Perna, G., Guerriero, G., et al. (2011). Emerging drugs for panic disorder. *Exp. Opin. Emerg. Dr.* 16(4):631–645.

Pollack, M., Mangano, R., et al. (2007). A randomized controlled trial of venlafaxine ER and paroxetine in the treatment of outpatients with panic disorder. *Psychopharmacol.* 194(2):233–242.

Pratchett, L.C., Daly, K., et al. (2011). New approaches to combining pharmacotherapy and psychotherapy for posttraumatic stress disorder. *Exp. Opin. Pharmacother.* 12(15):2339–2354.

Raskind, M.A., Peskind, E.R., et al. (2003). Reduction of nightmares and other PTSD symptoms in combat veterans by prazosin: a placebo-controlled study. *Am. J. Psychiatry* 160(2):371–373.

Rickels, K., Downing, R., et al. (1993). Antidepressants for the treatment of generalized anxiety disorder: a placebo-controlled comparison of imipramine, trazodone, and diazepam. *Arch. Gen. Psychiatry* 50(11):884–895.

Rickels, K., Pollack, M.H., et al. (2005). Pregabalin for treatment of generalized anxiety disorder: a 4-week, multicenter, double-blind, placebo-controlled trial of pregabalin and alprazolam. *Arch. Gen. Psychiatry* 62(9):1022–1030.

Rickels, K., Pollack, M.H., et al. (2000). Efficacy of extended-release venlafaxine in nondepressed outpatients with generalized anxiety disorder. *Am. J. Psychiatry* 157(6):968–974.

Rickels, K., Zaninelli, R., et al. (2003). Paroxetine treatment of generalized anxiety disorder: a double-blind, placebo-controlled study. *Am. J. Psychiatry* 160(4):749–756.

Stein, D.J., Ipser, J.C., et al. (2004). Pharmacotherapy for social phobia. *Cochrane Database Syst. Rev. (Online)* (4)(4):CD001206.

Stein, D.J., Ipser, J.C., et al. (2006). Pharmacotherapy for post traumatic stress disorder (PTSD). *Cochrane Database Syst. Rev. (Online)* (1)(1):CD002795.

Stein, M.B., and Stein, D.J. (2008). Social anxiety disorder. *Lancet* 371(9618):1115–1125.

Stocchi, F., Nordera, G., et al. (2003). Efficacy and tolerability of paroxetine for the long-term treatment of generalized anxiety disorder. *J. Clin. Psychiatry* 64(3):250–258.

SUSANNE E. AHMARI AND H. BLAIR SIMPSON

INTRODUCTION

OCD IS A DISABLING ILLNESS

Obsessive-compulsive disorder (OCD) is characterized by recurrent intrusive thoughts, images, or impulses (obsessions) that cause anxiety or distress, and repetitive mental or behavioral acts (compulsions). The obsessions and compulsions are time consuming (e.g., more than an hour a day), are distressing, and interfere with functioning. Compulsions are typically performed in response to an obsession (e.g., fears of contamination leading to washing rituals), with the aim of reducing the distress triggered by obsessions or to prevent a feared event (e.g., becoming ill). However, these compulsions are either not connected in a realistic way or are clearly excessive (e.g., showering many hours each day). Of note, compulsions are not performed with a primary purpose of deriving pleasure, although some individuals experience the relief from anxiety that accompanies the compulsive behavior as pleasurable.

With a lifetime prevalence of up to 2–3% (i.e., two to three times more common than schizophrenia), the World Health Organization has identified OCD as one of the world's 10 leading causes of illness-related disability. This is largely due to the fact that OCD typically starts in childhood or adolescence, persists throughout a person's life, and produces substantial impairment in functioning due to the severe and chronic nature of the illness (Koran, 2000). In addition, OCD has a significant financial impact, with the most recent report indicating that treatment and management of OCD costs several billions of dollars a year in the United States alone.

KEY CLINICAL FEATURES OF OCD

Onset of OCD usually occurs in adolescence or early adulthood; however, a subgroup of OCD patients, a majority of them male, have symptom onset in childhood. Some childhood-onset OCD may have a different clinical course and a different underlying neurobiology than adult-onset OCD.

Though all OCD patients have obsessions and/or compulsions, specific content of the obsessions and compulsions differs between individuals. However, certain themes are common, including forbidden or taboo thoughts (e.g., aggressive, sexual, and religious obsessions and related compulsions), cleaning (fears of contamination and related cleaning rituals), harm (fears of harm to oneself or others and checking compulsions), symmetry (symmetry obsessions and repeating, ordering, and counting compulsions), and hoarding (obsessive collecting and maintaining of worthless objects). These different themes,

also known as symptom dimensions, are similar across different cultures, are relatively consistent over time in adults with OCD, and may be associated with different neural substrates (Leckman et al., 2010). Importantly, individuals often have symptoms in more than one dimension, suggesting that the dimensions do not represent discrete subtypes.

Patients may also differ significantly in their level of insight into the irrationality of their obsessions and compulsions. Level of insight can be classified as good/fair (the patient recognizes that the beliefs are definitely or probably not true, e.g., that compulsions are not effective at warding off feared consequences), poor (the patient thinks the beliefs are probably true), or absent (the patient is completely convinced the beliefs are true, thus bordering on a delusional belief in the reality of the obsessions). Notably, level of insight can fluctuate over the course of illness (Leckman et al., 2010).

OCD has significant comorbidity with other psychiatric illnesses, particularly major depressive disorder (MDD: 61% current; 85% lifetime), other anxiety disorders (range: 24.5–69.6%), and Tourette's disorder (range: 7–59%). Notably, there is evidence that OCD patients with comorbid tic disorder may be a biologically distinct entity, with earlier age of onset, greater prevalence in males, different neurochemical and neurobiological features, and distinct treatment response. In addition, OCD is very prevalent in individuals with anorexia/bulimia (37%) and schizophrenia (8–32%) (Leckman et al., 2010).

ETIOLOGY OF OCD

Though our understanding of the etiology underlying OCD is quite limited, it is an area of very active investigation. Current evidence implicates both genetic and environmental factors in development of OCD, though the importance of particular factors is still unclear. It is crucial to identify specific pathogenic insults and/or protective factors; we may then be able to intervene early in development to prevent onset of this severe and chronic illness.

GENETIC FACTORS

Twin and family studies suggest that there is genetic susceptibility to OCD. In addition, this genetic vulnerability may be greater in pediatric onset OCD, since there is greater heritability in this population (genetic influences in the range of 45–65% in pediatric OCD vs. 27–47% in adult-onset OCD [Pauls, 2008]). These findings have been followed up by candidate gene studies (over 60 studies from 1998 to 2008); many of these candidate gene studies focused on genetic loci associated with serotonin, dopamine, and glutamate, based on their hypothesized roles in the etiology of OCD. In addition, genome-wide linkage and association studies have recently been performed. In the next section, we will review selected findings from candidate gene studies and genome-wide association studies that may have implications for the pathophysiology underlying OCD.

Glutamate

SLC1A1 To date, the only consistently replicated genetic finding in OCD is an association with the neuronal glutamate transporter *SLC1A1* (protein known as EAAT3 or EAAC1) (see Wu et al., 2012 for review). Findings cluster in the 3′ gene region, with most evidence for association with the rs301430C allele. In cell models and brain tissue, this allele is associated with increased *SLC1A1* expression, suggesting that overexpression contributes to OCD susceptibility. Coding variants in *SLC1A1* are very rare (3/1400 subjects screened) and do not clearly segregate with OCD. Thus, noncoding polymorphisms most likely account for the association of *SLC1A1* with OCD.

GRIN2B Other genetic association studies have less consistently implicated *GRIN2B*, a gene that encodes the NR2B subunit of the NMDA glutamate receptor (see Wu et al., 2012, for review). The NR2B subunit is an important contributor to synaptic plasticity, since incorporation of the subunit renders NMDA receptors more permeable to calcium. In 2004, Arnold et al. found that both a GRIN2B polymorphism and one additional haplotype were associated with OCD. Further support for a GRIN2B role in OCD comes from magnetic resonance spectroscopy studies in OCD patients that have demonstrated an association between GRIN2B polymorphisms and glutamatergic concentrations in the anterior cingulate cortex. Overall, the association of NR2B with OCD is consistent with the theory that glutamatergic dysfunction underlies OCD pathophysiology. However, NR2B deficits throughout the brain would be expected to lead to significant abnormalities in global functioning, since NMDA receptors are essential for basic neurobiological functions necessary for learning and memory, including long-term potentiation. It is therefore more likely that NR2B functional abnormalities in specific brain regions account for the genetic association with OCD.

Grik2 Another glutamatergic gene that has been implicated in OCD is the ionotropic glutamate receptor gene, *Grik2* (see Wu et al., 2012, for review). In an initial association study, a secondary analysis indicated that a Grik2 polymorphism was undertransmitted in OCD patients. A follow-up candidate gene study found that a particular haplotype at this same locus was significantly associated with OCD. Further investigation is required to determine if this association is robust and biologically significant.

Serotonin

Serotonin-1b Receptor (5-HT1B) Several lines of evidence suggest that abnormalities in 5-HT1B receptor function (known as the 5-HT1D receptor in the human literature) play a role in

OCD (reviewed in Hemmings and Stein 2006). Pharmacological challenge studies found that acute activation of 5-HT1B receptors with the specific agonist sumatriptan can cause a transient worsening of OCD symptoms. In contrast, case reports suggest that chronic administration of 5-HT1B agonists can lead to a reduction in OCD symptoms possibly through receptor desensitization. Finally, some studies show a genetic association between a variant of the *5-HT1B* receptor gene and OCD. While a role of *5-HT1B* gene variants in susceptibility to OCD is not consistently supported, there is tentative support for the idea that such variants could be related to OCD severity. It is not clear whether the inconsistencies in the literature are due to small sample size, methodological problems inherent in challenge paradigms, dose of challenge agents, or differences between OCD patient samples. Nevertheless, in aggregate, the data point to 5-HT1B abnormalities in some OCD patients.

Serotonin-2A Receptor (5-HT2A) A positive association has been inconsistently reported between the A allele of the 5-HT2A receptor and OCD. However, though preliminary PET studies supported a link between 5-HT2A receptors and OCD, a more recent study did not find differences in 5-HT2A binding between OCD patients and controls (Simpson et al., 2011). There is still the possibility that 5-HT2A receptor polymorphisms may be linked to OCD symptomatology or treatment response, but the evidence is weaker than for other polymorphisms.

Serotonin Transporter There have been many studies examining the potential association between the serotonin transporter polymorphism (5-HTTLPR) and OCD. Though some family-based association studies have reported an association between the 5-HTTLPR long allele and OCD, these findings have been inconsistently replicated—in fact, a 2007 meta-analysis found an association between the 5-HTTLPR short allele and OCD susceptibility. A more recent meta-analysis (Bloch et al., 2008) demonstrated an association between the long allele and OCD in specific subgroups, including childhood onset OCD; however, this was only found in the stratified meta-analysis and did not retain significance in the overall meta-analysis. The significance of 5-HTTLPR in OCD etiology remains unclear.

ENVIRONMENTAL FACTORS

Many studies have suggested a role for environmental factors in the etiology of both childhood- and adult onset OCD, but it has been difficult to establish direct links. In this section, we review environmental theories with the strongest evidence.

Infectious

Acute onset of OCD symptoms in children has been observed; this syndrome has been associated with environmental factors, including various infectious agents and a postinfectious autoimmune syndrome. There has been some support for a specific association between infection with group A β-hemolytic streptococcus and onset of an autoimmune disorder that triggers OCD; this is commonly known as PANDAS (Pediatric Autoimmune Neuropsychiatric Disorder Associated with

Streptococcal Infections). However, this association remains controversial, as other infectious agents may also trigger an acute neurospsychiatric syndrome. This is a topic of active research (Singer et al., 2012).

Hormonal

There have been multiple reports of premenstrual and post-partum exacerbation of OCD, suggesting that hormonal fluctuations may play a role in either the onset or the exacerbation of OCD symptoms. A majority of these studies were limited by the fact that they were retrospective analyses and did not directly assess hormone levels (McGuinness et al., 2011). However, they complement findings from the neurocognitive literature demonstrating that prepulse inhibition deficits, which are observed in OCD patients, are most pronounced during phases of elevated progesterone (i.e., late pregnancy and premenstrual).

Psychological Trauma

Though rare, there have been reports of acute OCD onset in adults following exposure to traumatic events. Until recently, these studies had consisted of case reports and case series in chronic OCD patients whose trauma had occurred a significant amount of time before initiation of the study, leading to uncertainty about the timing of symptom onset, and possible conflation of OCD and PTSD symptoms. A recent study addressed this problem by assessing five veterans with new onset OCD shortly after combat and found a suggestive link between the

traumatic events and the initiation of OCD symptoms (Fostick et al., 2012). Interestingly, these OCD symptoms continued to evolve independently of the initial environmental trigger, such that rituals were no longer related to thoughts associated with the trauma.

NEUROBIOLOGY OF OCD

Although the etiology of OCD is unknown, many studies have investigated the brain mechanisms underlying OCD symptoms. Development of modern neuroimaging technology has led to a dramatic increase in our understanding of the neurobiology of OCD over the past 20 years. In the next section, we will discuss findings from studies that have used this technology to examine neuroanatomy, circuit function, and neurochemistry in OCD. Together, these findings have converged to implicate cortico-striato-thalamo-cortical circuits in the pathophysiology of OCD.

OVERVIEW OF CORTICO-STRIATO-THALAMO-CORTICAL (CSTC) CIRCUITS

Cortico-striato-thalamo-cortical circuits (Fig. 48.1) have been implicated in many higher order cognitive functions, including allocation of attention, executive functioning (e.g., inhibition of impulsive behavior), and modulation of motor activity. Anatomical studies in both humans and nonhuman primates

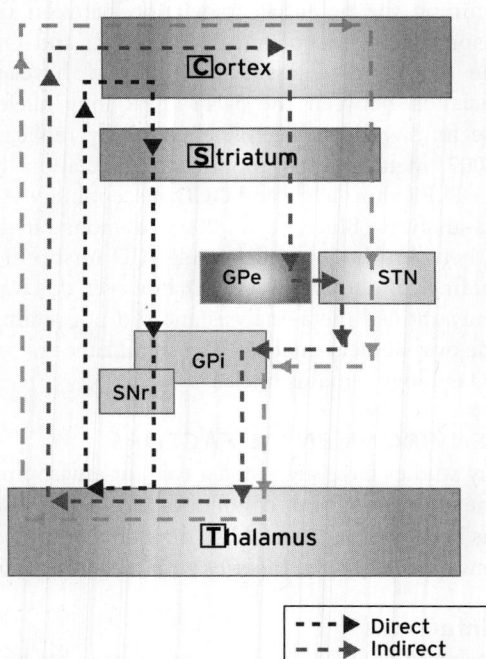
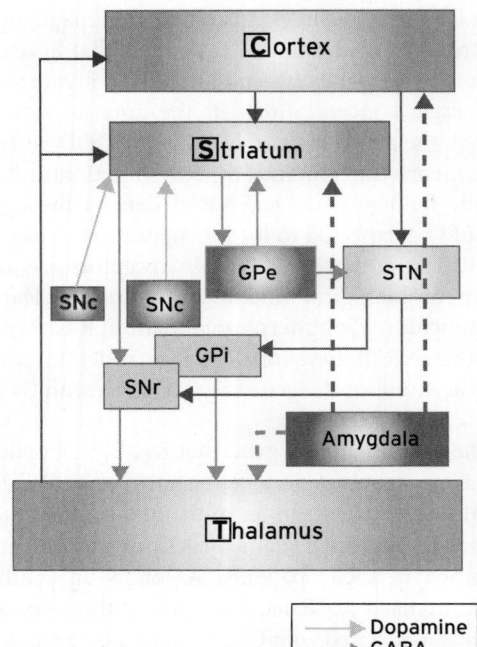

Figure 48.1 Cortico-striatal-thalamo-cortical (CSTC) loops. Circuit diagrams of CSTC loops. (left) It is hypothesized that multiple parallel CSTC circuits connecting the cortex and basal ganglia subserve different neural functions. Three examples of parallel loops are the direct pathway, hyperdirect pathway, and indirect pathway. SNr substantia nigra, pars reticulata; GPe globus pallidus externa; GPi globus pallidus interna, STN subthalamic nucleus. (right) Glutamate and GABA serve as the main neurotransmitter systems underlying communication within CSTC loops. However, other brain regions/neurotransmitter systems play significant modulatory roles (dashed lines), including ventral tegmental area (VTA) (dopamine), substantia nigra pars compacta (SNc) (dopamine), and amygdala (glutamate and GABA).

have demonstrated that CSTC circuits are composed of multiple parallel and interconnected loops that connect frontocortical and subcortical brain areas (Parent and Hazrati, 1995). These loops are comprised of (1) glutamatergic corticostriatal projections synapsing onto striatal medium spiny neurons, (2) GABAergic medium spiny neurons projecting to the output structures of the basal ganglia (globus pallidus pars internalis [GPi] and substantia nigra pars reticulata [SNr]), (3) GABAergic output neurons from GPi and SNr projecting to thalamus, and (4) glutamatergic neurons from thalamus connecting back to cortical areas. Within the striatum, medium spiny neurons can connect to GPi/SNr through either the direct (striatonigral) or indirect (striatopallidal) pathways. In a simplified framework, these anatomically distinct pathways are thought to oppose each other, resulting in inhibition of thalamus through activation of the indirect pathway, or disinhibition by activation of the direct pathway.

It is thought that different sets of CSTC loops may be responsible for dictating particular motor and cognitive functions, and it has been suggested that this selectivity is determined by the particular frontocortical area included in the loop (Pennartz et al., 2009). Functional imaging studies support this hypothesis, indicating that different cognitive functions are subserved by distinct CSTC circuits, and that disruption of these circuits occurs in multiple psychiatric disorders. Multiple models have been proposed suggesting that the interplay between frontocortical areas and basal ganglia determines which behaviors are performed, and which are screened out as being "undesirable." In particular, it is hypothesized that changing the balance of activity between direct and indirect pathways can either promote or inhibit the selection of appropriate behavior sequences. Dysfunction in screening out "undesirable" behavior sequences would potentially lead to symptomatology. An accumulation of evidence specifically implicates CSTC dysfunction in OCD pathophysiology.

NEUROANATOMY

Anatomical findings suggest that abnormalities in the orbitofrontal cortex (OFC), anterior cingulate cortex (ACC), and striatum contribute to pathogenesis of OCD, as reviewed in Pittenger et al. (2011). The largest structural MRI study to date reported reduced gray matter in the OFC and increased gray matter in the ventral striatum, a structure intimately connected with the OFC. A recent meta-analysis including 14 structural studies of both pediatric and adult patients with OCD reported reduced volumes of the left ACC and bilateral OFC, and increased thalamic volumes bilaterally, but no differences in basal ganglia volumes relative to control samples. Thus, structural abnormalities in a CSTC circuit involving the OFC, ACC, and striatum have been repeatedly demonstrated in OCD, although exact findings have varied across studies. This is supported by neurosurgical studies that demonstrate symptom reduction after surgical interventions disrupting connections between frontocortical and subcortical areas. In addition, successful deep brain stimulation (DBS) for treatment-refractory OCD typically targets connections between prefrontal cortex and striatum, and is often accompanied by reduced OFC activity as measured by PET.

FUNCTIONAL NEUROIMAGING (RESTING STATE, SYMPTOM PROVOCATION, AND PRE-/POSTTREATMENT STUDIES)

Functional PET and fMRI neuroimaging studies in OCD have implicated the OFC, ACC, caudate nucleus (specifically the head), and thalamus in OCD, brain regions linked by well-described neuroanatomical connections as described in the previous section (reviewed in Pittenger et al., 2011). In resting studies, OCD subjects have hyperactivity in OFC, and, to a lesser extent, caudate, ACC, and thalamus. When their symptoms are provoked, OCD subjects have increased activity relative to baseline in the OFC, caudate, ACC, and, to a lesser extent, thalamus. In studies that examined OCD patients before and after treatment, most found that successful SRI or cognitive behavioral therapy treatment was associated with reduced activity in the OFC or caudate, and to a lesser extent the ACC.

COGNITIVE ACTIVATION STUDIES

In recent years, there has been a shift toward performing imaging studies in OCD patients using cognitive activation paradigms; studies of executive functions have been particularly emphasized. Many neurocognitive tasks have been used (for a comprehensive list, see Maia et al., 2008). Some of the evidence for differences between OCD patients and controls comes from three studies that found that OCD subjects aberrantly recruited the hippocampus during an implicit sequence-learning task, while healthy participants recruited the striatum; behavioral performance was the same across groups. These findings suggest that OCD patients have dysfunction in the striatal portions of CSTC circuits known to mediate normal implicit sequence learning. However, the link between this deficit in implicit sequence learning and OCD pathogenesis and/or symptomatology remains unclear, since hippocampal activation was not correlated with the severity of global OCD symptoms or specific symptom dimensions. In addition, several studies have demonstrated hyperactivity of the dorsal anterior cingulate cortex (dACC) in OCD patients during performance of tasks that probe brain activity during error monitoring and/ or conflict resolution, suggesting that this region might function differently in OCD (Milad and Rauch, 2012). Other studies have used go/no-go tasks to assess inhibitory control processes in OCD, with some finding greater OFC activation compared with controls (Elliott et al., 2010) and others reporting less activation compared with controls in inferior frontal regions (Roth et al., 2007). Greater frontostriatal activation has recently been demonstrated in unmedicated OCD compared with control participants during the engagement of control and conflict resolution on the Simon task (Marsh et al., 2009). The findings from these studies are inconsistent, likely due to differences in the tasks used and neural processes that they measure, in addition to differences in the patient samples.

NEUROCHEMISTRY

Based on the specific efficacy of SRIs for the treatment for OCD (see "Treatment of OCD" section for further details), it has been hypothesized for over 20 years that serotonergic dysfunction plays a central role in the pathophysiology of OCD (Insel et al., 1985). As a result, many neurochemical studies in OCD have focused on the serotonergic system (reviewed in Goddard et al., 2008; Koo et al., 2010). Studies of peripheral markers of serotonin (5-HT) function (e.g., receptor binding in the blood) or of concentrations of 5-HT metabolites in cerebral spinal fluid have produced inconsistent results. Furthermore, it is not clear that these markers accurately reflect brain 5-HT function. Pharmacological challenge studies in OCD have used a variety of challenge agents (e.g., mCPP, MK-212, fenfluramine, metergoline, ipsapirone, buspirone, tryptophan, and sumatriptan/ zolmitriptan). Findings suggest that there is altered 5-HT function in OCD. However, these challenge studies have been unable to pinpoint the exact 5-HT abnormality, and many findings have not been consistently replicated.

Finally, neuroimaging studies have examined the distribution of serotonin transporters (5-HTT) and 5-HT2A receptors in the brains of OCD patients. With regard to 5-HTT binding, three SPECT studies found three disparate results (increased, decreased, and no differences in midbrain 5-HTT binding). Using PET, we found no differences in 5-HTT binding between OCD patients and controls in striatal, limbic, or midbrain regions, which are the brain areas that could be reliably assessed with the PET ligand used (Simpson et al., 2003). In addition, we found that there are no differences in 5-HT2A binding between OCD patients and controls (Simpson et al., 2011).

Abnormalities in regulation of dopamine signaling have also been implicated in OCD (see Koo et al., 2010 for review). Specifically, it has been hypothesized that dopaminergic abnormalities exist in some OCD patients based on findings that antipsychotic medications augment SRI response in up to 50% of OCD patients. However, SPECT studies investigating the dopaminergic system have led to inconsistent or unreplicated findings in small samples.

A current leading model also proposes that OCD symptoms result either directly or indirectly from increased glutamatergic signaling in corticostriatal pathways (reviewed in Pittenger et al., 2011). Both clinical and preclinical evidence supports this "hyperglutamatergic" hypothesis of OCD symptomatology. Rosenberg et al. (2000) initially found that glutamatergic compounds measured by magnetic resonance spectroscopy (MRS) were increased in the caudate nucleus of SRI-naïve children with OCD. This led to speculation that OCD patients have abnormalities in glutamatergic-serotonergic neurotransmission and to the initial development of hyperglutamatergic models of OCD. Additional MRS studies in OCD patients have demonstrated increased GLX (a combination of glutamate and glutamine) concentrations in the OFC and caudate; levels correlate with symptom severity and are decreased after effective treatment with paroxetine. In addition, as described in the preceding, genetic studies have found associations between the glutamate transporter SLC1A1 and OCD. An association was also found between a polymorphism in the NMDA receptor (NR2B) and decreased ACC glutamate in pediatric OCD. Finally, case studies and open label trials demonstrate efficacy of glutamatergic agents in reducing OCD symptoms—namely,

NMDA antagonists including memantine and riluzole (though unexpectedly there is also evidence for symptom relief following treatment with an NMDA agonist, glycine).

In summary, it is likely that abnormalities in multiple different neurotransmitter systems are related to the generation and resolution of OCD symptoms. There is good evidence that abnormalities in serotonin, dopamine, and glutamate signaling are associated with OCD. However, the following issues remain unclear: (1) the precise circuit localization of neurochemical abnormalities, (2) their role in either the generation or resolution of OCD symptoms, and (3) when they have their effects during development.

WORKING MODEL OF OCD PATHOPHYSIOLOGY

Based on the findings previously reviewed, several brain models of OCD have been proposed (reviewed in Saxena et al., 2001; Ting and Feng, 2011). While the models differ in specific details, they share the idea that obsessions and compulsions result from a malfunctioning neural circuit that includes the orbitofrontal (and sometimes the cingulate) cortex, caudate nucleus, and thalamus. The models differ in how this circuit malfunctions and/or is affected by SRIs. Some models try to account for different potential subtypes of OCD. For example, Baxter et al. (2001) proposed that tic-related and non-tic-related OCD have different patterns of striatal pathophysiology. More recently, because different OCD symptom dimensions (e.g., symmetry and ordering vs. washing and cleaning) have been associated with different patterns of neural activity in OFC, ACC, and caudate on PET scans, some have proposed that different symptom dimensions have different underlying neural substrates.

A leading model proposes that different populations of striatal medium spiny neuron projections differentially regulate the direct and indirect basal ganglia pathways, ultimately leading to alterations in motor behavior and stereotypies. Given the known functions of the direct pathway (including the striatum, globus pallidus interna, and substantia nigra) and indirect pathway (including the striatum, globus pallidus externa, and subthalamic nucleus) in modulating thalamic input to the cortex and in generating motor patterns, this has led to the hypothesis that OCD is due to excess activity in the direct versus indirect orbitofrontal-subcortical pathways. This increased direct pathway activity leads to decreased inhibition of the thalamus, and decreased filtering of intrusive thoughts and images to the cortex. Ritualistic compulsions are then triggered.

Another model that could be consistent with direct versus indirect pathway imbalance proposes that OCD symptoms result from increased glutamatergic signaling in corticostriatal pathways (see Pittenger et al., 2011). There is both clinical and preclinical evidence supporting this "hyperglutamatergic" hypothesis of OCD symptomatology, as discussed in detail in the preceding. The accumulation of evidence that increased cortical glutamatergic activity is linked to OCD symptoms has led to the suggestion that increased glutamatergic activity in specific cortical areas (OFC and ACC) may lead to generation of intrusive thoughts and images in the cortex that override other sensorimotor input; this, in turn, could trigger ritualistic compulsions driven by the striatum through persistent activation of the direct pathway.

Though models of OCD have typically focused on abnormalities in CSTC circuitry, there has recently been a call for investigation of the role of other brain regions in OCD pathophysiology (Milad and Rauch, 2012). Specifically, CSTC models do not generally provide an explanation for the increased anxiety observed in OCD. However, exaggerated responses in the amygdala, a structure classically associated with anxiety and fear, have typically been observed after the presentation of OCD-specific stimuli. In addition, although the dACC has been classically associated with conflict monitoring (and therefore linked to obsessions in OCD), there is also recent evidence that it plays a role in the expression of fear responses. Hyperactivation of the dACC could therefore lead to increased anxiety and fear responses observed in OCD patients. It may therefore be necessary to integrate other brain structures, such as the amygdala or the dACC, to provide a satisfying explanatory model of OCD.

CHALLENGES IN STUDYING OCD CIRCUITRY

The field of OCD research has faced significant difficulties with study replication. This has been particularly evident in studies of neurophysiologic task performance. One of the most reliable abnormalities in OCD is prepulse inhibition (PPI) deficits, which have now been found in three studies from independent groups (although another group failed to find the deficit). However, this level of consistency has not been demonstrated with other neurophysiologic tasks. For example, there are significant discrepancies in the field on tests of executive function, motor speed, visual memory, and response inhibition using tasks such as Spatial Working Memory, Stockings of Cambridge, and Stop-Signal Reaction Time (Simpson et al., 2006). Many different factors may contribute to the difficulties with replication. For example, a recent study found that up to 25% of OCD patients reported significant OCD-related anxieties and motivational difficulties during neurophysiologic task performance. The self-reported symptoms and decreased motivation were significantly associated with objective performance deficits on the tasks (Moritz et al., 2012). Thus, cognitive deficits may not necessarily reflect a uniform neurobiological abnormality (as would be expected in an endophenotype) but, instead, may be state dependent. It is therefore possible that a single patient may have vastly different performance depending on his or her level of acute symptomatology at the time of testing. Though this could be related to disease-specific deficits, it could also be due to a more general difficulty with allocation of attentional resources during symptom flares.

Another possible complicating factor is heterogeneity of clinical phenotype that may reflect heterogeneity in the underlying neural substrate (Mataix-Cols et al., 2005). For example, OCD patients differ in the content of their symptoms (also known as symptom dimensions—e.g., washers versus checkers), their comorbidity (e.g., tic versus non-tic-related OCD), and the course of illness (e.g., early versus late onset). Attempts to identify homogeneous subgroups in OCD based on a single clinical feature have had limited success. To address this issue, a dimensional model of OCD has been proposed. In this model, OCD is composed of several different and potentially overlapping symptom dimensions, each with its own associated clinical features and with possible differences in neurobiology. This model has been supported by some imaging studies, indicating that different patterns of brain activity are associated with different symptom dimensions. Thus, different OCD subtypes could have different core neurobiologic deficits leading to differences in imaging findings and neurophysiologic task performance.

PRECLINICAL STUDIES OF OCD

There have been numerous attempts to establish rodent models of OCD, since valid animal models will assist in the dissection of the molecular and cellular pathophysiology of the illness (see Wang et al., 2009 for review). Though it is now generally accepted that no one animal model will be able to recreate all aspects of a complex neuropsychiatric disorder such as OCD, it is possible to create powerful models that mimic particular aspects of a disorder (e.g., symptoms, medication responses, imaging findings, genetic abnormalities). However, it is important for these models to be carefully assessed to determine their relevance to the human disorder.

One method for judging clinical relevance is to determine the extent of face, predictive, and construct validity of a particular animal model. Face validity refers to the phenomenologic similarity between the phenotype measured in the mouse and human symptomatology. It is generally considered to be the least rigorous method for validating an animal model, since the assessment is relatively subjective, and identical phenotypes can be produced by different underlying biological processes. Predictive validity is the ability of a model to make accurate predictions about the human phenomenon of interest. Though typically understood as the ability of a model to replicate effects of medications, it also refers to its ability to make accurate predictions about the impact of environmental variables on the disorder being studied. Construct validity refers to how well an animal model mimics pathophysiologic constructs that are thought to underlie the disorder in question. These constructs can include things such as genetic abnormalities or circuit dysfunction. Though construct validity is inherently limited in OCD due to our nascent understanding of the disorder, rodent models based on construct validity are valuable tools for testing and generating new hypotheses about underlying pathology. In the next section, we will provide a brief overview of established OCD animal models and discuss the validity associated with each.

MODELING SYMPTOMS

Many OCD animal models have emphasized face validity based on stereotypy and compulsivity. These include marble burying, barbering (repetitive hair biting and pulling), acral paw-lick (repetitive paw-licking in dogs), zoo-related stereotypies (e.g., pacing around cages), and pharmacologically induced compulsive checking. In addition, behavioral paradigms have been established in rodents that generate (1) perseverative lever pressing in the absence of reward, and (2) persistent revisiting of unrewarded arms in a T-maze (i.e., impaired reversal learning). Furthermore, pharmacologic studies in wild-type rats have demonstrated that striatal injections of an NMDA-antagonist led to increased perseveration on a T-maze delayed alternation task. Finally, a recently developed model capitalizes on the fact that injection of 5-HT1B agonists in mice leads to both PPI deficits (also observed in OCD patients) and perseverative behavior; unlike other models discussed here, this model exhibits strong predictive validity for the chronic time course and high SRI dose necessary for human OCD treatment response. Finally, the deer mouse, an ethological model of OCD, also has strong face validity. At baseline, deer mice demonstrate repetitive running, jumping, and flipping behaviors. *In vivo* microdialysis in corticostriatal projections was performed to investigate the molecular correlates of these repetitive behaviors. These studies found that increased glutamate directly preceded stereotypic behaviors in these mice, supporting the idea that glutamatergic abnormalities may lead to OCD symptomatology.

MODELING GENETIC ABNORMALITIES

Transgenic technology has enabled the generation of animal models of OCD based on alteration of specific genes (see Ting and Feng, 2011 for comprehensive review). This increasingly advanced technology allows investigators to upregulate or downregulate genes of interest in specific regions of the brain that have been implicated in OCD. Thus, the function of candidate genes identified in human studies can be directly tested in mice. This allows for dissection of molecular and cellular mechanisms that may underlie OCD pathophysiology.

As discussed earlier, the identification of candidate genes in OCD has been difficult, since the field has been hampered by a lack of replication in genetic studies. However, there is increasing interest in the role of glutamate system genes in OCD pathophysiology. This is due in large part to the fact that the only consistently replicated genetic finding in OCD is an association with the neuronal glutamate transporter *SLC1A1* (see Wu et al., 2012 for review). Based on findings that *SLC1A1* overexpression contributes to OCD susceptibility, we are in the process of making a transgenic mouse that yields tissue-specific *SLC1A1* overexpression. This will allow us to directly address the molecular, cellular, and behavioral impact of changes in expression of this OCD candidate gene.

OCD animal models have also been unexpectedly generated following disruption of genes not previously implicated in OCD. For example, knockout of the developmentally expressed *Hoxb8lox* gene leads to perseverative grooming, while disruption of the serotonin 2C receptor leads to perseverative chewing. However, the link between disruption of these genes and the human OCD phenotype remains unclear. There is somewhat stronger evidence that two other knockout mouse models may have relevance to OCD. In a recent elegant study, Welch et al. (2007) used a transgenic approach to knock out SAPAP3, a corticostriatal postsynaptic density protein. Knockouts had excessive grooming leading to facial lesions, similar to some OCD subgroups (contamination fears/washing rituals). In addition, these mice demonstrated abnormal glutamatergic signaling at corticostriatal synapses (increased NMDA-dependent fEPSPs (excitatory post-synaptic potentials) and decreased AMPA-dependent fEPSPs) that correlated with the OCD-related behaviors. Overgrooming and the electrophysiologic changes

were eliminated after either lentiviral-mediated SAPAP3 rescue in corticostriatal synapses or acute treatment with low-dose fluoxetine. In another study, Shmelkov et al. (2010) performed targeted inactivation of the *Slitrk5* gene, a postsynaptic density transmembrane protein that is one of a family of genes implicated in Tourette's and obsessive-compulsive spectrum disorders. Slitrk5 knockout mice demonstrate several OCD-relevant behaviors that are reversed by chronic treatment with the serotonin-reuptake inhibitor fluoxetine, including increased anxiety and perseverative grooming behaviors; this lends predictive validity to the model. Notably, knockout of Slitrk5 also led to selective overactivation of orbitofrontal cortex; this parallels findings in human OCD patients.

For both SAPAP3 and Slitrk5 knockouts, the challenge of linking these findings back to the human disorder remains. For example, the SAPAP3 knockout phenotype may be more consistent with pathological skin picking than OCD: a recent human genetics study found no association of SAPAP3 SNPs with OCD in a clinical sample but did find associations with grooming disorders such as pathologic skin picking, nail biting, and/ or trichotillomania. Preliminary evidence from Slitrk5 genetic studies is promising, indicating the presence of rare Slitrk5 genetic variants in OCD patients; however, these findings still need to be validated (F. Lee, personal communication). Regardless, both of these studies clearly demonstrated a link between molecular changes at corticostriatal synapses and repetitive pathological behaviors. These studies therefore yield new insights into possible molecular and cellular mechanisms underlying OCD.

MODELING CIRCUIT ABNORMALITIES

New technology development now facilitates the generation of OCD animal models based on manipulation of specific neural circuits. These technologies allow direct translation of human neuroimaging findings into mice. This approach was first elegantly demonstrated through the generation of D1CT-7 transgenic mice. In this transgenic line, the active subunit of cholera toxin was placed under the regulation of the D1 receptor promoter (D1CT-7 transgenic mice). Thus, the stimulatory subunit of cholera toxin was expressed in a subset of D1-positive neurons, leading to constitutive hyperactivation of these neurons. This mouse model therefore had strong overactivation in prefrontal-cortex and striatal neurons, similar to observations from OCD imaging studies. These mice demonstrated baseline perseverative climbing, leaping, and biting behaviors that were exacerbated by increased NMDA-dependent glutamatergic transmission, yielding a model with strong construct validity.

Other new technologies can also be used to mimic circuit abnormalities seen in human imaging studies (reviewed in Rogan and Roth, 2011). For example, there have been recent significant advances in precise modulation of activity of neural circuits using light-activated microbial ion channel proteins. The development of this optogenetic technology has focused on channelrhodopsin-2, an excitatory sodium channel gated by 470 nm blue light; and halorhodopsin, an inhibitory chloride pump gated by 580 nm yellow light. By specifically expressing and stimulating these light-activated proteins, distinct neural populations can be rapidly activated or inhibited without affecting neighboring cells. We are currently using this technology to directly translate imaging findings from OCD patients into rodents. In addition, technology has been recently developed that allows for cell type–specific expression of mutant G-protein coupled receptors (GPCRs) that can be activated by administration of inert small molecules. These mutant GPCRs are known as DREADDs (Designer Receptors Rxclusively Activated by Designer Drugs). Whereas optogenetic technology allows for rapid and specific activation and inhibition, DREADD technology yields more sustained but specific activation and inhibition that may better mirror pathophysiologic processes.

FUTURE DIRECTIONS

The examples discussed in the preceding demonstrate the power of using animal model systems to explore the molecular and cellular pathology underlying OCD. In addition, by capitalizing on new technologies, we may be able to develop more refined disease models through precise control of neural activity. However, these examples also highlight the importance of critically evaluating mouse models to determine if they are truly relevant to the disorder of interest—in this case, OCD. Ongoing studies in our group are identifying translatable probes of neural circuits that are reliably abnormal in OCD patients. Using these neural circuit probes, we can better determine clinical relevance of our animal models. These types of studies will help ensure that dissection of molecular and

cellular abnormalities in animal models will ultimately yield information relevant for the development of new treatments.

TREATMENT OF OCD

Although the etiology and pathophysiology of OCD are still under study, evidence-based treatments for OCD have been developed in the absence of unclear mechanisms of action. These treatments can lead to remission of symptoms in up to 50% of patients. First-line treatments recommended by the American Psychiatric Association (American Psychiatric Association, 2007) include pharmacotherapy with serotonin reuptake inhibitors (SRIs), and cognitive-behavioral therapy (CBT) consisting of exposure and response prevention (Fig. 48.2). These two treatments are described next along with other strategies that are used when these first-line treatments do not suffice.

PHARMACOTHERAPY FOR OCD

SEROTONIN REUPTAKE INHIBITORS

OVERVIEW

The only medications proven effective as monotherapy for OCD in multisite randomized controlled trials are serotonin reuptake inhibitors (SRIs). SRIs include clomipramine, a tricyclic antidepressant, and the selective serotonin reuptake

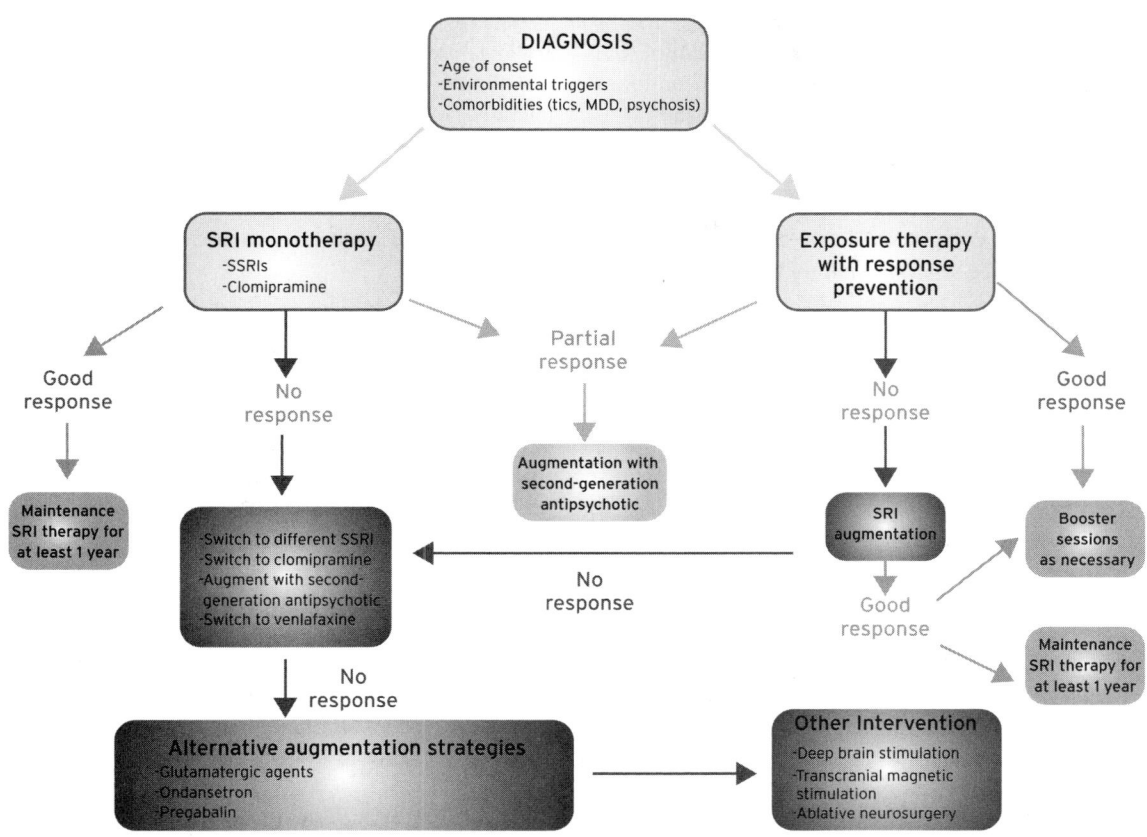

Figure 48.2 OCD treatment guidelines. OCD treatment guidelines are based on APA recommendations. After diagnosis, flowchart outlines treatment algorithims for individual and combined pharmacotherapy and exposure therapy. Alternative interventions for treatment-refractory OCD are also indicated.

inhibitors (i.e., fluoxetine, fluvoxamine, sertraline, paroxetine, citalopram, and escitalopram). All but citalopram and escitalopram are currently approved by the Food and Drug Administration for the treatment of OCD. Though the mechanism of action of SRIs in OCD is unknown, it was initially thought that their efficacy was linked to the direct modulation of serotonin levels. However, more recent hypotheses propose that SRIs modulate CSTC circuit function through action on serotoninergic heteroreceptors, which in turn control levels of glutamate, GABA, and dopamine.

In general, serotonin reuptake inhibitors lead to improvement in 40–60% of people with OCD, and OCD patients who receive an adequate trial will achieve on average a 20–40% reduction in their OCD symptoms (reviewed in Simpson, 2010). Thus, serotonin reuptake inhibitors typically lead to amelioration rather than elimination of symptoms. Various issues arise when treating OCD with serotonin reuptake inhibitors that are discussed in the following sections: which one to try first, what dose to use, the time to response, how to manage potential side effects, and the recommended duration of treatment.

COMPARATIVE EFFICACY

Serotonin reuptake inhibitors are not thought to differ from each other in efficacy for OCD, with the possible exception of clomipramine. Clomipramine, a tricyclic antidepressant, is both a serotonin reuptake inhibitor and a norepinephrine reuptake inhibitor. In meta-analyses, clomipramine has greater effects than the other serotonin reuptake inhibitors. However, the clomipramine studies were done earlier in time than the studies using the selective serotonin reuptake inhibitors and thus likely included more treatment-naïve samples. In head-to-head comparisons, clomipramine has not been found to be superior to fluoxetine, fluvoxamine, or paroxetine.

Practice guidelines (American Psychiatric Association, 2007) recommend that patients first be started on a selective serotonin reuptake inhibitor because they have a better side effect profile than clomipramine (as described in the next section). If there is no response, they should be switched to another selective serotonin reuptake inhibitor and, if satisfactory symptom reduction is not achieved, eventually tried on clomipramine. To determine which selective serotonin reuptake inhibitor to try first, the clinician should consider prior treatment response, safety and acceptability of particular side effects for the individual patient (see the next section), and the potential for drug–drug interactions.

DOSE

Clinical trials of fluoxetine, paroxetine, and citalopram that randomized patients to different doses of the same medication (i.e., fixed-dose studies) found that higher doses produced a higher response rate and/or greater degree of improvement than lower doses; one fixed-dose study of sertraline did not find significant differences between the effects of 50 and 200 mg/day. Based on these data, the American Psychiatric Association's Practice Guidelines (2007) recommend the following usual target doses for adults with OCD: fluoxetine, 40–60 mg/day; fluvoxamine, 200 mg/day; paroxetine, 40–60 mg/day; sertraline, 200 mg/day; citalopram, 40–60 mg/day (note: the FDA no longer recommends citalopram above 40 mg/day because of dose-dependent QT prolongation); escitalopram, 20 mg/day; clomipramine, 100–250 mg/day (see Table 48.1). These therapeutic doses of SRIs for OCD tend to be higher than the doses used for treatment of other anxiety disorders and depression. It is advised that patients start at a low dose for tolerability (e.g., fluoxetine 10 or 20 mg/day) and that the dose be increased every week or every other week (as tolerated) to doses at least as high as listed in the preceding (with

TABLE 48.1. Dosage guidelines for OCD pharmacotherapy in adult patients. Starting dose, FDA-approved dose, and usual maximum dose for OCD are based on the American Psychiatric Association's Practice Guidelines (2007). If patients do not respond to the usual maximum dose, OCD specialists will often try higher doses.

DRUG CLASS	MEDICATION	STARTING DOSE (in mg)	FDA-APPROVED DOSE (in mg)	USUAL MAXIMUM DOSE (in mg) FOR OCD PATIENTS	MAXIMUM DOSE (in mg) USED IN CLINICAL PRACTICE (NORMALLY INITIATED BY SPECIALISTS)
Selective serotonin reuptake inhibitors (SSRIs)	Fluoxetine	40	60	80	120
	Paroxetine	20	40	60	100
	Sertraline	50	200	300	400
	Citalopram***	20	20–40	60–80***	120
	Escitalopram	10	30	40	60
	Fluvoxamine	50	100–200	300	450
Tricyclic antidepressants	Clomipramine	25	250	250	<500 ng/mL by blood levels

***Note that the FDA no longer recommends citalopram above 40 mg/day because of dose-dependent QT prolongation and Torsades de Pointes. Patients with pre-existing congestive cardiac failure, brady-arrhythmias or predisposition to hypokalemia or hypomagnesemia are at increased risk of developing these cardiac abnormalities, and should therefore be monitored closely, ideally in conjunction with a cardiologist. Recommended medication dosage for treatment of OCD in adults (18–65).

the exception now of citalopram) before deciding that a patient is resistant to any particular serotonin reuptake inhibitor.

When patients do not respond to the doses outlined, doses even higher have been tried in clinical practice (e.g., fluoxetine, 120 mg/day; paroxetine, 100 mg/day). For example, Ninan et al. (2006) randomized patients who had not responded to 16 weeks of sertraline (titrated from 50 mg/day to 200 mg/day) to continued sertraline (200 mg/day) or to increased sertraline (250–400 mg/day). Although the high-dose group had significantly more improvement than the lower dose group, the difference in additional improvement was clinically modest, and both groups were still left with clinically significant symptoms. Thus, increasing selective serotonin reuptake inhibitors to higher than recommended doses may be effective for certain OCD patients, but this strategy is not useful for all.

TIME TO RESPONSE

Many of the randomized controlled trials of serotonin reuptake inhibitors for OCD did not show a significant difference between placebo and active medication before six weeks. Thus, an adequate trial has been defined as the maximum dose tolerated for a minimum of six weeks (American Psychiatric Association, 2007). This usually amounts to an 8–12 week trial overall given usual titration schedules. Preclinical studies have found that therapeutic response to serotonin reuptake inhibitors corresponds to the time course of desensitization of inhibitory serotonin receptors. It has thus been suggested that delayed receptor desensitization in the OFC accounts for the delay in treatment response seen in OCD patients (Moritz et al., 2012). It is important to explain this delayed response to treatment to patients so that they don't prematurely stop their serotonin reuptake inhibitor.

SIDE EFFECTS

Selective serotonin reuptake inhibitors are generally well tolerated. Potential side effects include gastrointestinal problems (e.g., nausea or diarrhea), agitation, sleep disturbances (e.g., insomnia, vivid dreams), increased tendency to sweat, and sexual side effects (e.g., decrease in libido, trouble ejaculating, delayed orgasm). In addition, weight gain or fatigue can occur (reviewed in Simpson, 2010). There are also clinical reports of specific side effects with certain agents that are presumed due to their unique pharmacological characteristics (e.g., more sedation and constipation due to the mild anticholinergic effects of paroxetine, more anorexia and activation due to the 5HT2C antagonism of fluoxetine). Thus, it is possible for a patient to tolerate one serotonin reuptake inhibitor, but not another.

As mentioned, the FDA has recently issued a safety warning for citalopram because of data that it causes dose-dependent QT interval prolongation, which can cause Torsades de Pointes, ventricular tachycardia, and sudden death. Thus, citalopram is no longer recommended for use in patients with congenital long QT syndrome, bradycardia, hypokalemia, hypomagnesismia, recent acute myocardial infarction, or uncompensated heart failure. Citalopram is also not recommended for use in patients who are taking other drugs that prolong the QT interval. QT interval prolongation was not observed with escitalopram (the S-isomer of citalopram).

The other serotonin reuptake inhibitor with known effects on the heart is clomipramine. In addition to being a serotonin and norepinephrine reuptake inhibitor, clomipramine blocks muscarinic cholinergic receptors, H1 histamine receptors, alpha1 adrenergic receptors, and sodium channels in the heart and brain. Thus, in addition to the side effects described for selective serotonin reuptake inhibitors, clomipramine can cause anticholinergic effects (e.g., dry mouth, constipation, delayed urination), antihistamine effects (e.g, sedation, weight gain), antiadrenergic effects (e.g., orthostatic hypotension), and cardiac conduction abnormalities or seizures.

DURATION OF TREATMENT

Clinical trials that treat with medications for a certain period of time and then randomly assign responders to either continue on that medication or be switched to pill placebo (i.e., double-blind drug discontinuation studies) help determine the risk of relapse if medication is stopped. Several double-blind discontinuation studies in adults with OCD (reviewed in Fineberg et al., 2012; Simpson, 2010) examined different serotonin reuptake inhibitors, used different designs (e.g., length of follow-up, procedure for placebo substitution) and had different relapse definitions. The studies came to different conclusions about the risk of relapse if medication is stopped. For example, relapse rates (or discontinuation due to insufficient clinical response) after double-blind switch to placebo ranged from a high of 89% within 7 weeks for clomipramine, to a low of 24% within 28 weeks for sertraline. Given the limited number of studies and the methodological differences, the risk of relapse remains unclear. Practice guidelines (American Psychiatric Association, 2007) recommend that an OCD patient who has improved during an adequate trial of a serotonin reuptake inhibitor should stay on that medication for one to two years and that if the medication is discontinued, it should be slowly tapered (e.g., 10–25% every one to two months).

If stopped abruptly, serotonin reuptake inhibitors can lead to a drug discontinuation syndrome. This can include flulike symptoms (e.g., dizziness, nausea/vomiting, headache, and lethargy) as well as agitation, insomnia, myoclonic jerks, and paresthesias (Tamam and Ozpoyraz, 2002; Zajecka et al., 1997). Drugs with a shorter half-life (e.g., paroxetine) are more likely to cause this than those with a longer half-life and an active metabolite (e.g., fluoxetine).

ROLE OF VENLAFAXINE AND DULOXETINE IN THE TREATMENT OF OCD

Like clomipramine, venlafaxine and duloxetine are both serotonin and norepinephrine reuptake inhibitors. Because they inhibit serotonin reuptake, both are presumed effective for the treatment of OCD. Other than two case reports, the only published study of duloxetine in OCD to date is a case series of four patients with OCD who had either a partial or no response to an SRI; after being switched to duloxetine up to 120 mg/day, three responded to duloxetine (Dell'osso et al., 2008). Larger controlled studies are needed to confirm this preliminary observation.

Venlafaxine has been studied more extensively, but the findings from different studies are conflicting (reviewed in Simpson, 2010). The only randomized controlled trial of venlafaxine in OCD found no significant difference between venlafaxine and placebo. However, the sample was small ($n = 30$), the maximum dose was 225 mg/day, and the trial was only eight weeks long. Other randomized controlled trials have compared venlafaxine (or venlafaxine XR) with either paroxetine or clomipramine. These trials were limited by the lack of a placebo group, but each was 12 weeks in length and used higher doses of venlafaxine (e.g., 225–300 mg/day). In both studies, venlafaxine was as efficacious as the serotonin reuptake inhibitor with which it was compared. Finally, in a crossover study of nonresponders, when paroxetine nonresponders were switched to venlafaxine, only 3 of 16 (19%) responded, whereas when venlafaxine nonresponders were switched to paroxetine, 15 of 27 (56%) responded. These findings suggest that paroxetine is more efficacious than venlafaxine in patients with limited response to the other medication.

In sum, venlafaxine is often tried in clinical practice in OCD patients who have not responded to several selective serotonin reuptake inhibitors and cannot tolerate clomipramine. However, the evidence supporting the use of venlafaxine in OCD is not as strong as the evidence for the serotonin reuptake inhibitors, and there is little data supporting the use of duloxetine. Neither is approved by the Food and Drug Administration for the treatment of OCD.

LIMITATIONS OF SEROTONIN REUPTAKE INHIBITORS IN THE TREATMENT OF OCD

Although they are the only medications proven effective as monotherapy for OCD, serotonin reuptake inhibitors have important limitations: only up to 65% of people will respond to an adequate trial, the typical response is a 20–40% reduction in symptoms, and patients can relapse if the medication is discontinued. Because many OCD patients will have a clinically meaningful but modest reduction in symptoms and others will have no response (e.g., <25% reduction in symptoms), clinicians who treat OCD patients will commonly be faced with both problems.

One strategy is to switch to another SRI (e.g., if there is no response to the first) and to eventually switch to clomipramine. The American Psychiatric Association's Practice Guidelines suggest that up to 50% of patients might respond to a second SRI trial but that the rate of response diminishes as the number of failed trials increases (American Psychiatric Association, 2007). Switching to venlafaxine or duloxetine is another option; however, the data for both agents is limited (as reviewed earlier). Mirtazapine, shown in a small double-blind discontinuation study to reduce OCD symptoms, is another possibility (Koran et al., 2005). However, the efficacy of switching either to another SRI or to another agent as monotherapy has not been well studied, and there are limited data to support this strategy.

Another strategy with more data to support it is to include additional treatments in ongoing SRI treatment to augment SRI response. SRI augmentation strategies are discussed in the following.

SRI AUGMENTATION STRATEGIES

Randomized controlled trials support the addition of antipsychotics or the addition of CBT consisting of exposure and response prevention. Many other augmenting agents have also been tried, as reviewed next (see Simpson, 2010 for review).

ANTIPSYCHOTIC AUGMENTATION

Haloperidol, risperidone, quetiapine, olazapine, and aripiprazole have all been shown in randomized controlled trials to augment the effects of serontonin reuptake inhibitors. There are also negative findings from studies of these agents, although this may be due to methodological issues (reviewed in Fineberg et al., 2012). A systematic review of antipsychotic augmentation (Bloch et al., 2006), which combined nine double-blind, randomized controlled clinical trials involving 278 subjects, concluded that about one-third of OCD patients will be helped by antipsychotic augmentation. The strongest evidence supports the use of haloperidol or risperidone. Some data suggest that the patients most likely to respond to antipsychotic augmentation may be those with a minimal response to an SRI and/or those with comorbid tic disorders.

Given the delayed onset of action of serotonin reuptake inhibitors in OCD, it is recommended that antipsychotic augmentation only be implemented after an OCD patient has failed to respond to a maximal dose of a serotonin reuptake inhibitor for at least 12 weeks (American Psychiatric Association, 2007). Low antipsychotic doses appear effective (e.g., <3 mg for risperidone or the equivalent), and the time to response is about two to four weeks. Given that only some OCD patients will respond to antipsychotic augmentation, the antipsychotic should be terminated after one month of intervention in those who do not clearly benefit. This minimizes the known risks of antipsychotic exposure, which can include metabolic syndrome, tardive dyskinesia, and neuroleptic malignant syndrome.

Questions remain about the use of antipsychotics in OCD, including whether some agents are more effective than others, their long-term efficacy, and the risk of relapse upon discontinuation. One small retrospective study suggested that 13 of 15 patients had a resurgence of OCD symptoms when their antipsychotic was discontinued.

CBT AUGMENTATION

Two randomized controlled trials have demonstrated the benefit of adding CBT consisting of exposure and response prevention to OCD patients with clinically significant symptoms despite an adequate SRI trial. The specific components of this treatment are described in detail in the following. In the first study, Tenneij et al., 2005) compared the effects of continuing medication (paroxetine or venlafaxine) versus adding exposure and response prevention in patients who had mild OCD symptoms. Adding exposure and response prevention (eighteen 45-minute sessions over 6 months) was superior to medication alone, but the effects were modest. In the second study, Simpson et al. (2008) recruited patients on an adequate dose for at least 12 weeks of any serotonin reuptake inhibitor who still had clinically significant OCD symptoms. Patients were randomized to exposure and response prevention or to stress management therapy as a control therapy; both treatments included seventeen 90-minute sessions delivered over eight weeks. Patients who received exposure and response therapy had a significantly greater decrease in symptoms, and significantly more achieved minimal symptoms at the end of treatment (33% versus 4%). These effects were maintained in many at six-month follow-up.

Together, these findings support the use of exposure and response prevention in augmenting the effects of serotonin reuptake inhibitors in OCD. The addition of exposure and response prevention is clearly safer than the addition of antipsychotics, given the known risks of the latter (Marder et al., 2004). On the other hand, exposure and response prevention is not widely available, it is more time consuming, and some patients refuse it because it requires exposures to feared stimuli.

OTHER AGENTS

Many other medications have been tested as adjunctive agents to serotonin reuptake inhibitors in OCD (reviewed in Fineberg et al., 2012; Simpson, 2010). Although promising in case reports or open trials, several did not show clear efficacy in small placebo-controlled trials, including lithium, buspirone, clonazepam, L-triiodothyronine, pindolol, and desipramine (American Psychiatric Association, 2007). The initially promising effects of other augmentation agents await confirmation in large randomized controlled trials (as reviewed in Fineberg, 2012; Simpson, 2010), including clomipramine, morphine sulfate, pregabalin (Oulis et al., 2011), celecoxib (Sayyah et al., 2011), dextroamphetamine, and ondansetron. Medications that modulate the glutamatergic system or that might enhance learning from cognitive-behavioral therapy have been a recent area of study, as described in what follows.

NOVEL MEDICATIONS FOR OCD THAT TARGET BRAIN MECHANISMS

Because of the limitations of serotonin reuptake inhibitors, new medications continue to be tried in OCD. Because of data from human genetic studies, human imaging studies, and animal models of OCD that glutamatergic abnormalities in corticostriatal circuits might underlie OCD symptoms (as reviewed previously in this chapter), medications that modulate the glutamate system have been a recent focus of study. Various agents, each thought to modulate glutamate in different ways, have shown some promise in case reports, open-label studies, or small controlled trials either as monotherapy or as an adjunct to SRIs (reviewed in Pittenger et al., 2011). These include N-acetylcysteine (an animoacid derivative that reduces synaptic glutamate; Lafleur et al., 2006), memantine (a noncompetitive NMDA receptor antagonist), topiramate, riluzole (an antiglutamatergic agent that reduces glutamatergic neurotransmission in several ways), and minocycline. A case report demonstrated rapid resolution of obsessions in a treatment-resistant patient after IV ketamine infusion (Rodriguez et al., 2011). Though this initial finding must be explored in a larger controlled study, the possibility of a rapidly acting treatment for OCD is exciting.

Historically, medications have been used to target OCD symptoms directly. However, a novel approach is to use medication to enhance learning from psychotherapy. One of the best examples is the use of D-cycloserine (a partial agonist at the N-methyl-D-aspartate receptor), which is known to facilitate fear extinction in animal models. D-cycloserine is being paired with CBT that is focused on exposure techniques like exposure and response prevention, with the goal of enhancing extinction learning. This is described in more detail in the next section.

PSYCHOTHERAPY FOR OCD

COGNITIVE-BEHAVIORAL THERAPY

OVERVIEW

In addition to SRI pharmacotherapy, CBT is the other recommended first-line treatment for adults with OCD and the only first-line treatment recommended for pediatric OCD (see Rodriguez and Simpson, 2010, for review). Historically, CBT has evolved from two traditions: (*1*) CBT that relies primarily on behavioral techniques such as exposure and response prevention, known as exposure therapy, or ERP or EX/RP; and (*2*) CBT that relies primarily on cognitive techniques, such as identifying, challenging, and modifying faulty beliefs. Of these two, ERP-based CBT has the strongest evidence in OCD. However, it is important to note that ERP routinely includes some informal CT techniques (e.g., a discussion of fear-related thoughts and beliefs) and that CBT typically includes behavioral experiments, which are similar to exposure techniques. Thus, there is an overlap between these two forms of CBT. In clinical practice, cognitive and behavioral techniques are often combined.

EXPOSURE AND RESPONSE PREVENTION

CBT consisting of exposure and response prevention (called EX/RP or ERP in the literature and ERP in this chapter) involves *in vivo* (i.e., actual) exposures to feared situations, imaginal exposure to feared consequences, and ritual prevention, in which patients refrain from compulsive rituals (see Rodriguez and Simpson, 2010). For example, a patient with contamination obsessions and washing rituals is coached to confront feared contaminants (e.g., by touching objects in public restrooms), to imagine touching feared contaminants, and to refrain from washing rituals. For ERP to work, the therapist tailors the exposure exercises to the varied obsessive fears of patients with OCD (e.g., fear of contamination, fear of harm befalling themselves or others, fear of perverse sexual or religious thoughts, fear of not doing something just right). There are two main theories about the mechanisms underlying effective ERP. From a behavioral perspective, it is thought that repeated prolonged exposures to triggering situations while preventing conditioned rituals leads to extinction of conditioned fear responses (i.e., compulsions) through habituation. Over time, this leads to decreases in anxiety even in the face of obsessional thoughts. From a cognitive perspective, it is thought that ERP helps OCD patients eradicate dysfunctional beliefs (such as overestimation of threat in a particular situation), by providing information that leads to correction of faulty associations.

ERP therapy has been shown to be superior when compared with other treatments and control conditions in randomized controlled trials (as reviewed by Rodriguez and Simpson, 2010; Simpson, 2010) including pill placebo, anxiety management therapy, self-guided relaxation therapy, therapist-guided progressive muscle relaxation, and wait list control. ERP is also effective at augmenting response to SRI medications, as described previously. Up to 70% of patients who enter ERP treatment will respond to it, and up to 50% will achieve minimal symptoms after acute treatment. Importantly, not only does ERP lead to acute improvement in OCD symptoms, but many patients can also maintain their gains over time.

Several factors appear to affect ERP outcome (as reviewed by Rodriguez and Simpson, 2010), including the number and intensity of sessions, patient adherence with ERP procedures, comorbidities (e.g., severe depression, comorbid posttraumatic stress disorder), and degree of insight. Further study is required to determine if addressing these factors prior to or during ERP treatment leads to better outcomes. Data suggest that providing relapse prevention techniques helps patients to maintain the gains of ERP therapy. In addition, how patients adhere to acute treatment is a robust predictor of long-term outcome (Simpson et al., 2012).

In sum, after acute treatment with ERP (either with or without concomitant SRIs), up to half of patients will achieve minimal symptoms and many can maintain their gains after acute treatment ends. This is quite remarkable given the typically chronic and impairing nature of OCD.

COGNITIVE THERAPY FOR OCD

Cognitive therapy (CT), another form of cognitive-behavioral therapy, has also been used in OCD. In CT, patients and therapist work together to identify distorted patterns of thinking that lead to emotional reactions and then challenge and alter their ways of thinking in order to change their emotional response. Clinical trials have compared CT with ERP. However, separating these treatments can be procedurally difficult because many ERP protocols include informal cognitive techniques (e.g., relapse prevention, cognitive restructuring during exposures), and standard CT includes behavioral experiments that can resemble exposures. Clinical trials that have tried to separate these treatments suggest that CT that includes behavioral interventions is similar in efficacy to ERP when it is not optimally delivered (e.g., 45-minute weekly sessions, self-guided exposure) (reviewed in Rodriguez and Simpson, 2010). An open trial suggested that CT in the absence of behavioral experiments can help some OCD patients. However, given the limited data for CT alone, ERP remains the recommended first-line psychotherapy for OCD (APA Practice Guidelines).

LIMITATIONS OF CBT IN THE TREATMENT OF OCD

Even though CBT consisting of exposure and response prevention is a very effective treatment for OCD, it also has important limitations. The therapy requires a substantial time commitment on the part of the patient and is labor intensive. It requires full adherence with treatment procedures to achieve full effects. To complete treatment, patients have to be willing to tolerate high levels of anxiety during the exposure procedures. In addition, certain types of OCD patients (e.g., those with prominent hoarding symptoms or with mental, unobservable compulsions that the therapist can't directly observe) may have a poorer response to standard ERP procedures. Finally, one of the biggest hurdles is that ERP is not widely available, and many patients therefore do not have access to it.

Because ERP is challenging for many patients, approaches such as motivational interviewing and modification of treatment-interfering cognitive beliefs are used to improve treatment adherence (Simpson et al., 2012). Another approach for maximizing ERP efficacy stems from animal research: using medications to enhance what patients learn during exposures. As previously mentioned, one of the best examples is the use of D-cycloserine (a partial agonist at the N-methyl-D-aspartate receptor), which is known to facilitate fear extinction in animal models. There are three published studies of the effects of D-cycloserine augmentation of ERP in OCD; these are reviewed in Simpson, 2010. In two, D-cycloserine reduced the time to response. A reanalysis of the data from one study confirmed that D-cycloserine does not change overall effectiveness of ERP but speeds up the time to response.

The problem of access to ERP is also being addressed. For example, Web-based platforms have recently been developed that deliver ERP over the Internet; minimal therapist support is provided by e-mail or phone. Andersson et al. (2012) found that this Web-based ERP therapy was significantly better than an attention control condition delivered by the Internet and led to clinically meaningful improvement in OCD symptoms.

In sum, CBT consisting of exposure and response prevention is a first-line treatment for OCD, and research is underway to make it not only more accessible but also more efficacious for different types of patients with OCD.

SURGICAL AND OTHER TREATMENTS FOR OCD

OVERVIEW

A subset of OCD patients do not respond to the pharmacologic and psychotherapy treatment strategies described in the previous sections. To be designated as treatment refractory according to current clinical trial guidelines, patients must have failed at least three adequate trials of SRIs for at least three months at the maximum tolerated dose; at least one augmentation trial with clomipramine, a neuroleptic, or clonazepam; and at least one ERP trial performed in combination with pharmacotherapy. These treatment-refractory patients are then potential candidates for neurosurgical intervention. Up to 10% of patients fit into this category. Most modern neurosurgical techniques take advantage of the fact that OCD symptoms are associated with abnormal neuronal activity in CSTC circuits. These techniques share the same general approach—i.e., attempting to decrease symptoms via disruption of CSTC circuits at circuit nodes. However, the exact targets for surgical interventions vary from study to study, since target selection and side effect minimization are active areas of investigation. In this section, we will review currently available procedures, including ablation/radiosurgery, deep brain stimulation, electroconvulsive therapy (ECT), and transcranial magnetic stimulation (TMS). Some of these procedures have not only been used to treat OCD, but are also increasingly being used to study brain mechanisms underlying OCD (e.g., see Sheth et al., 2012).

SURGERY

MRI-guided stereotactic neurosurgical lesions in the anterior limb of the internal capsule, the anterior cingulate, and/or the subcaudate region appear to be beneficial in the treatment of highly refractory OCD. These lesions can be generated either using traditional MRI-guided stereotactic neurosurgery, or radiosurgery (i.e., gamma knife), which does not require a craniotomy. The fact that symptom relief can be generated through intervention at multiple points in the CSTC circuit provides further evidence that hyperactive CSTC circuits may lead to OCD symptomatology.

DEEP BRAIN STIMULATION

Deep brain stimulation (DBS) is being investigated as an experimental surgical therapy in treatment-resistant OCD (reviewed in Greenberg et al., 2010). DBS requires craniotomy to implant stimulating electrodes in specific brain targets and is therefore an invasive procedure. However, because it is nonablative, it permits flexible and largely reversible modulation of brain function. Conceptually, it may therefore permit normalization of abnormal activity patterns seen in OCD patients by "resynchronizing" circuit activity. Though DBS shows promise, optimal brain targets continue to be refined to avoid side effects, and the underlying mechanism of action remains unknown. Of note, all current targets are consistent with the theory that CSTC pathology underlies OCD symptoms. Though DBS is sometimes performed in the anterior limb of the internal capsule, target regions in the ventral capsule/ventral striatum (VC/VS) are currently the primary location under investigation for treatment-refractory OCD. A recent meta-analysis examining the combined long-term results of DBS in 26 OCD patients demonstrated clinically significant symptom reductions and functional improvement in approximately two-thirds of the patients. At last follow-up, 73% of patients had at least a 25% Y-BOCS improvement. Based on these results, the FDA has approved the use of DBS in OCD patients as a humanitarian device exemption. However, general utility of DBS based on long-term efficacy in large, controlled clinical trials remains to be determined.

OTHER

TRANSCRANIAL MAGNETIC STIMULATION (TMS)

TMS is a neurophysiologic technique that permits noninvasive stimulation of cortical structures. Magnetic stimulation frequencies and strengths can be altered to generate either stimulatory or inhibitory effects on neural transmission. There have been several treatment targets that have been investigated in OCD. To date, the main area of investigation has been the prefrontal cortex (PFC). Initial data from Greenberg et al. (1997) suggested that a single session of stimulation of the right PFC led to a decrease in compulsive urges that lasted for eight hours. However, a recent meta-analysis of the three studies of TMS in prefrontal regions in OCD did not demonstrate overall efficacy (see Slotema et al., 2010). These conclusions may be limited due to differences in the studies, including geometry of the TMS coil and frequency of stimulation. Though TMS is therefore not currently recommended as a standard treatment for OCD, it is still being investigated as an experimental treatment. For example, based on evidence for hyperactivity in the supplemental motor area (SMA) in OCD, an open label study was performed to investigate the use of low-frequency SMA TMS in OCD patients. In the follow-up randomized sham-controlled trial, response rate (i.e., >25% reduction in Y-BOCS scores) in treatment-refractory OCD patients was 67% compared with sham responses of 22% (see Mantovani et al., 2010). Ongoing studies continue to investigate SMA as a potential TMS treatment target.

ELECTROCONVULSIVE THERAPY (ECT)

Because there has been limited investigation into the efficacy of ECT in OCD, it is not currently recommended as a treatment by the APA practice guidelines unless there is a comorbid condition (e.g., severe major depression) for which ECT is effective.

CONCLUSIONS

In summary, OCD is a severe, chronic, and disabling illness that is highly prevalent. Though we still have a limited understanding of the etiology and pathophysiology of OCD, these are very active areas of research. Accumulated evidence from both clinical and preclinical studies suggests that there is dysregulation of activity in CSTC circuits, particularly in connections between prefrontal cortical regions and striatum. This evidence lends both experimental and theoretical support to the idea that multiple neurotransmitter systems and neuromodulators play a role in OCD pathophysiology, including GABA, dopamine, and glutamate (which has the strongest support from genetic studies). It is also necessary to investigate whether other circuits more specifically related to anxiety and fear extinction (e.g., cortico-amygdala connections) are dysfunctional in OCD. Though it is still unclear whether/how circuit abnormalities lead to symptomatology, new technologies such as optogenetics are allowing us to directly investigate these questions in animal models.

The only medications proven to be effective for monotherapy in OCD are the serotonin reuptake inhibitors. Although helpful for many patients, some patients do not respond, and many achieve only a partial response and are left with clinically meaningful residual symptoms. Proven augmentation strategies include the addition of antipsychotics and/or CBT consisting of exposure and response prevention; exposure and response prevention is also a highly effective monotherapy for patients who are able to complete it. For patients who do not respond to serotonin reuptake inhibitors, cognitive-behavioral therapy, or the combination of an SRI and either CBT or an antipsychotic medication, alternative strategies can be tried; however, evidence supporting these alternatives is limited. Ongoing studies are investigating novel treatment strategies that target underlying brain mechanisms, and determining how currently accepted treatments should be sequenced for maximum efficacy.

DISCLOSURES

Dr. Ahmari has no conflicts of interest to disclose. She is funded by NIMH, the Irving Institute for Clinical and Translational Research, and the Louis V. Gerstner, Jr., Foundation. NIMH: K08MH087718-01A1; Irving Institute Pilot Award; Gerstner Scholar Grant.

In the past three years, Dr. Simpson has received medication at no cost from Janssen Pharmaceuticals for an NIMH-funded study, consulting fees from Pfizer Inc. for advice regarding the medication Lyrica, and research funds from Neuropharm Ltd. and from Transcept Pharmaceuticals to conduct clinical trials of novel medications for OCD. In addition, she receives grant support from the NIMH.

REFERENCES

American Psychiatric Association. (2007). Practice guideline for the treatment of patients with obsessive-compulsive disorder. *Am. J. Psychiatry* 164:1–56.

Andersson, E., Enander, J., et al. (2012). Internet-based cognitive behaviour therapy for obsessive-compulsive disorder: a randomized controlled trial. *Psychol. Med.* 42:2193–2203.

Baxter, L.R., Clark, L.C., et al. (2001). Cortical-subcortical systems in the mediation of obsessive-compulsive disorder. In: Lichter, D.G., and Cummings, J.L., eds. Frontal-Subcortical Circuits in Psychiatric and Neurological Disorders. New York: Guilford Press, pp. 207–230.

Bloch, M.H., Landeros-Weisenberger, A., et al. (2006). A systematic review: antipsychotic augmentation with treatment refractory obsessive-compulsive disorder. *Mol. Psychiatry* 11(7):622–632.

Bloch, M.H., Landeros-Weisenberger, A., et al. (2008). Meta-analysis of the symptom structure of obsessive-compulsive disorder. *Am. J. Psychiatry* 165(12):1532–1542.

Dell'osso, B., Mundo, E., et al. (2008). Switching from serotonin reuptake inhibitors to duloxetine in patients with resistant obsessive compulsive disorder: a case series. *J. Psychopharmacol.* 22(2):210–213.

Elliott, R., Agnew, Z., et al. (2010). Hedonic and informational functions of the human orbitofrontal cortex. *Cereb. Cortex* 20(1):198–204.

Fineberg, N.A., Brown, A., et al. (2012). Evidence-based pharmacotherapy of obsessive-compulsive disorder. *Int. J. Neuropsychopharmacol.* 15:1173–1191.

Fostick, L., Nacasch, N., et al. (2012). Acute obsessive compulsive disorder (OCD) in veterans with posttraumatic stress disorder (PTSD). *World J. Biol. Psychiatry* 13(4):312–315.

Goddard, A.W., Shekhar, A., et al. (2008). Serotoninergic mechanisms in the treatment of obsessive-compulsive disorder. *Drug Discov. Today* 13(7–8):325–332.

Greenberg, B.D., George, M.S., et al. (1997). Effect of prefrontal repetitive transcranial magnetic stimulation in obsessive-compulsive disorder: a preliminary study. *Am. J. Psychiatry* 154:867–869.

Greenberg, B.D., Rauch, S.L., et al. (2010). Invasive circuitry-based neurotherapeutics: stereotactic ablation and deep brain stimulation for OCD. *Neuropsychopharmacology* 35(1):317–336.

Hemmings, S.M., and Stein, D.J. (2006). The current status of association studies in obsessive-compulsive disorder. *Psychiatr. Clin. North Am.* 29(2):411–444.

Insel, T.R., Mueller, E.A., et al. (1985). Obsessive-compulsive disorder and serotonin: is there a connection? *Biol. Psychiatry* 20(11):1174–1188.

Koo, M.S., Kim, E.J., et al. (2010). Role of dopamine in the pathophysiology and treatment of obsessive-compulsive disorder. *Expert Rev. Neurother.* 10(2):275–290.

Koran, L.M. (2000). Quality of life in obsessive-compulsive disorder. *Psychiatr. Clin. North Am.* 23(3):509–517.

Koran, L.M., Gamel, N.N., et al. (2005). Mirtazapine for obsessive-compulsive disorder: an open trial followed by double-blind discontinuation. *J. Clin. Psychiatry* 66(4):515–520.

Lafleur, D.L., Pittenger, C., et al. (2006). N-acetylcysteine augmentation in serotonin reuptake inhibitor refractory obsessive-compulsive disorder. *Psychopharmacology* 184(2):254–256.

Leckman, J.F., Denys, D., et al. (2010). Obsessive-compulsive disorder: a review of the diagnostic criteria and possible subtypes and dimensional specifiers for DSM-V. *Depress. Anxiety* 27(6):507–527.

Maia, T.V., Cooney, R.E., et al. (2008). The neural bases of obsessive-compulsive disorder in children and adults. *Dev. Psychopathol.* 20(4):1251–1283.

Mantovani, A., Simpson, H.B., et al. (2010). Randomized sham-controlled trial of repetitive transcranial magnetic stimulation in treatment-resistant obsessive-compulsive disorder. *Int. J. Neuropsychopharmacol.* 13(2):217–227.

Marder, S.R., Essock, S.M., et al. (2004). Physical health monitoring of patients with schizophrenia. *Am. J. Psychiatry* 161(8):1334–1349.

Marsh, R., Maia, T.V., et al. (2009). Functional disturbances within frontostriatal circuits across multiple childhood psychopathologies. *Am. J. Psychiatry* 166(6):664–674.

Mataix-Cols, D., Rosario-Campos, M.C., et al. (2005). A multidimensional model of obsessive-compulsive disorder. *Am. J. Psychiatry* 162(2):228–238.

McGuinness, M., Blissett, J., et al. (2011). OCD in the perinatal period: is postpartum OCD (ppOCD) a distinct subtype? A review of the literature. *Behav. Cogn. Psychother.* 39(3):285–310.

Milad, M.R., and Rauch, S.L. (2012). Obsessive-compulsive disorder: beyond segregated cortico-striatal pathways. *Trends Cogn. Sci.* 16(1):43–51.

Moritz, S., Hottenrott, B., et al. (2012). Effects of obsessive-compulsive symptoms on neuropsychological test performance: complicating an already complicated story. *Clin. Neuropsychol.* 26(1):31–44.

Ninan, P.T., Koran, L.M., et al. (2006). High-dose sertraline strategy for nonresponders to acute treatment for obsessive-compulsive disorder: a multicenter double-blind trial. *J. Clin. Psychiatry* 67(1):15–22.

Oulis, P., Mourikis, I., et al. (2011). Pregabalin augmentation in treatment-resistant obsessive-compulsive disorder. *Int. Clin. Psychopharmacol.* 26(4):221–224.

Parent, A., and Hazrati, L.N. (1995). Functional anatomy of the basal ganglia: I. the cortico-basal ganglia-thalamo-cortical loop. *Brain Res. Brain Res. Rev.* 20(1):91–127.

Pauls, D.L. (2008). The genetics of obsessive compulsive disorder: a review of the evidence. *Am. J. Med. Genet. C Semin. Med. Genet.* 148C(2):133–139.

Pennartz, C.M., Berke, J.D., et al. (2009). Corticostriatal interactions during learning, memory processing, and decision making. *J. Neurosci.* 29(41):12831–12838.

Pittenger, C., Bloch, M.H., et al. (2011). Glutamate abnormalities in obsessive compulsive disorder: neurobiology, pathophysiology, and treatment. *Pharmacol. Ther.* 132(3):314–332.

Rodriguez, C.I., Kegeles, L.S., et al. (2011). Rapid resolution of obsessions after an infusion of intravenous ketamine in a patient with treatment-resistant obsessive-compulsive disorder. *J. Clin. Psychiatry* 72(4):567–569.

Rodriguez, C.I., and Simpson, H.B. (2010). Evidence-based treatment for patients with OCD: questions and controversies. In: Simpson, H.B., Neria, Y., Lewis-Fernandez, R., and Schneier, F., eds. Anxiety Disorders: Theory, Research, and Clinical Perspectives. Cambridge, UK: Cambridge University Press, pp. 249–260.

Rogan, S.C., and Roth, B.L. (2011). Remote control of neuronal signaling. *Pharmacol. Rev.* 63(2):291–315.

Rosenberg, D.R., MacMaster, F.P., et al. (2000). Decrease in caudate glutamatergic concentrations in pediatric obsessive-compulsive disorder patients taking paroxetine. *J. Am. Acad. Child Adolesc. Psychiatry* 39(9):1096–1103.

Roth, R.M., Saykin, A.J., et al. (2007). Event-related functional magnetic resonance imaging of response inhibition in obsessive-compulsive disorder. *Biol. Psychiatry* 62(8):901–909.

Saxena, S., Bota, R.G., et al. (2001). Brain-behavior relationships in obsessive-compulsive disorder. *Semin. Clin. Neuropsychiatry* 6(2):82–101.

Sayyah, M., Boostani, H., et al. (2011). A preliminary randomized double-blind clinical trial on the efficacy of celecoxib as an adjunct in the treatment of obsessive-compulsive disorder. *Psychiatry Res.* 189(3):403–406.

Sheth, S.A., Mian, M.K., et al. (2012). Human dorsal anterior cingulate cortex neurons mediate ongoing behavioural adaptation. *Nature* 9:218–221.

Shmelkov, S.V., Hormigo, A., et al. (2010). Slitrk5 deficiency impairs cortico-striatal circuitry and leads to obsessive-compulsive-like behaviors in mice. *Nat. Med.* 16:598–602.

Simpson, H.B., Marcus, S.M., et al. (2012). Patient adherence to cognitive behavioral therapy predicts long-term outcome in obsessive-compulsive disorder. *J. Clin. Psych.* 73:1265–1266.

Simpson, H.B. (2010). Pharmacological treatment of obsessive-compulsive disorder. *Curr. Top. Behav. Neurosci.* 2:527–543.

Simpson, H.B., Foa, E.B., et al. (2008). A randomized, controlled trial of cognitive-behavioral therapy for augmenting pharmacotherapy in obsessive-compulsive disorder. *Am. J. Psychiatry* 165:621–630.

Simpson, H.B., Lombardo, I., et al. (2003). Serotonin transporters in obsessive-compulsive disorder: a positron emission tomography study with [(11)C]McN 5652. *Biol. Psychiatry* 54(12):1414–1421.

Simpson, H.B., Rosen, W., et al. (2006). Are there reliable neuropsychological deficits in obsessive-compulsive disorder? *J. Psychiatr. Res.* 40(3):247–257.

Simpson, H.B., Slifstein, M., et al. (2011). Serotonin 2A receptors in obsessive-compulsive disorder: a positron emission tomography study with [11C]MDL 100907. *Biol. Psychiatry* 70(9):897–904.

Singer, H.S., Gilbert, D.L., et al. (2012). Moving from PANDAS to CANS. *J. Pediatr.* 160(5):725–731.

Slotema, C.W., Blom, J.D., et al. (2010). Should we expand the toolbox of psychiatric treatment methods to include Repetitive Transcranial Magnetic Stimulation (rTMS)? A meta-analysis of the efficacy of rTMS in psychiatric disorders. *J. Clin. Psychiatry* 71(7):873–884.

Tamam, L., and Ozpoyraz, N. (2002). Comorbidity of anxiety disorder among patients with Bipolar I Disorder in remission. *Psychopathology* 35(4):203–209.

Tenneij, N.H., van Megen, H.J., et al. (2005). Behavior therapy augments response of patients with obsessive-compulsive disorder responding to drug treatment. *J. Clin. Psychiatry* 66(9):1169–1175.

Ting, J.T., and Feng, G. (2011). Neurobiology of obsessive-compulsive disorder: insights into neural circuitry dysfunction through mouse genetics. *Curr. Opin. Neurobiol.* 21(6):842–848.

Wang, L., Simpson, H.B., et al. (2009). Assessing the validity of current mouse genetic models of obsessive-compulsive disorder. *Behav. Pharmacol.* 20(2):119–133.

Welch, J.M., Lu, J., et al. (2007). Cortico-striatal synaptic defects and OCD-like behaviours in Sapap3 mutant mice. *Nature* 448:894–900.

Wu, K., Hanna, G.L., et al. (2012). The role of glutamate signaling in the pathogenesis and treatment of obsessive-compulsive disorder. *Pharmacol. Biochem. Behav.* 100(4):726–735.

Zajecka, J., Tracy, K.A., et al. (1997). Discontinuation symptoms after treatment with serotonin reuptake inhibitors: a literature review. *J. Clin. Psychiatry* 58(7):291–297.

49 | NEUROBIOLOGY AND TREATMENT OF PTSD

KAREN E. MURRAY, ORION P. KEIFER JR., KERRY J. RESSLER,
SETH DAVIN NORRHOLM, AND TANJA JOVANOVIC

INTRODUCTION

Experiencing an extremely traumatic event, such as combat or violent assault, can lead to posttraumatic stress disorder (PTSD). PTSD is the fourth most common psychiatric diagnosis (Breslau et al., 1998) and is defined by three primary symptom clusters (Fig. 49.1) following an event that elicited fear, helplessness, or horror (Criterion A) (APA, 2000). The first cluster of symptoms (Criterion B) includes reexperiencing of the traumatic event through intrusive thoughts, nightmares, flashbacks, and related phenomena that are often produced by reminders of the traumatic event. The second cluster (Criterion C) is characterized by avoidance symptoms including loss of interest in social situations and emotional detachment. The third cluster (Criterion D) includes psychophysiological reactivity in response to trauma-related stimuli including exaggerated startle, hypervigilance, elevated perspiration, and shortness of breath. Finally, PTSD is defined by the mentioned symptoms lasting for more than 30 days after the trauma exposure, given that the initial response to trauma may resolve itself within one month's time. This chapter will explore vulnerability and resilience factors for developing PTSD, describing several theoretical frameworks for the disorder, as well as examining the animal model systems, differential pathways, and brain regions identified as involved in the disorder, and finally the available treatments for patients with PTSD.

MORBIDITY AND EPIDEMIOLOGY OF PTSD

Current estimates report that 37–92% of all people will be exposed to a severe traumatic event during their lifetime (Breslau et al., 1998). Given the high rates of trauma exposure, the prevalence of PTSD is relatively low, affecting approximately only 10% of the general population, with women being twice as likely to develop PTSD as men (Kessler et al., 1995). The rates of lifetime PTSD are closer to 40% in highly exposed trauma populations, such as low-income urban populations (Breslau et al., 1998). Recent studies have demonstrated a steep dose–response curve between trauma frequency and PTSD symptom severity such that the more traumatic events a person experiences, the greater the intensity of PTSD symptoms (Binder et al., 2008).

PTSD is a heterogeneous disorder, and some patients may present higher symptom severity in one domain compared

with another, and other patients may only exhibit lower intensity levels along the spectrum of PTSD symptoms. Recent papers highlighted the importance of treating patients who exhibit some but not all of the requisite PTSD symptoms across clusters for a full PTSD diagnosis (subsyndromal PTSD), suggesting that a "one-size-fits-all" treatment approach is often inadequate (Norrholm and Jovanovic, 2010). Furthermore, the neurobiological underpinnings of the different symptoms may not overlap (Hopper et al., 2007), suggesting that different "subtypes" of PTSD may have different treatment targets. Finally, PTSD is frequently comorbid with other disorders, such as depression, substance abuse, and other anxiety disorders (Kessler et al., 1995). Taken together, these issues result in a complex phenotype of PTSD, one that is difficult to model in animal research and does not easily lend itself to treatment outcome studies. However, several laboratory paradigms have shown promise in testing different elements of the PTSD syndrome—from aspects of risk and resilience, fear consolidation and expression, memory discrimination versus generalization, and differential symptom clusters. Although these cannot encompass the full complexity of the disorder, they provide useful tools to evaluate its different aspects. Next we outline theoretical frameworks for PTSD and describe several animal model systems and laboratory paradigms derived from these theoretical bases.

THEORETICAL FRAMEWORK FOR TRANSLATIONAL STUDIES OF PTSD

Several theorists have proposed that fear-conditioning processes are involved in the etiology and maintenance of PTSD. This model suggests that through Pavlovian conditioning, neutral cues (conditioned stimuli, CSs) present at the time of the trauma (the unconditioned stimulus, US) acquire the ability to elicit a conditioned fear reaction that can be triggered when the person subsequently encounters these or similar cues in his or her environment. Consistent with this hypothesis, emotional and physiological reactivity to stimuli resembling the original traumatic event (even years after the event's occurrence) is a prominent characteristic of PTSD and has been reliably replicated in the laboratory (Orr et al., 2002). Additionally, overgeneralization of trauma-related stimuli or situations, that is, an impaired ability to discriminate between danger and safety cues, can lead to hypervigilance and exaggerated startle

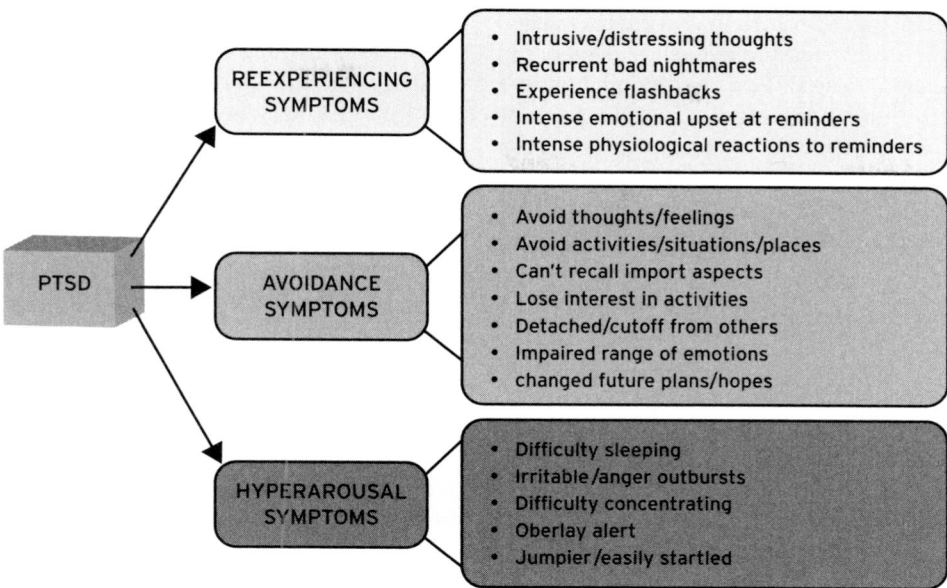

Figure 49.1 Symptom clusters in posttraumatic stress disorder (PTSD). The syndrome of PTSD includes the following clusters of symptoms following the experiencing of a traumatic event that elicits fear, helplessness, or horror (DSM-IV Criterion A). The clusters include reexperiencing symptoms (Criterion B), avoidance symptoms (Criterion C), and hyperarousal symptoms (Criterion D).

responses that are part of the hyperarousal symptom cluster (Mahan and Ressler, 2012), depicted in Figure 49.2.

Conceptualizing PTSD within the framework of fear conditioning affords the use laboratory paradigms, such as fear inhibition and fear extinction, to better understand altered fear processing and to develop better treatments for this dysregulation. As noted earlier, most trauma victims show fear-related reactions immediately after the traumatic event, but these effects diminish over time in most traumatized individuals. The reduction in fear-related behavior over time is similar to extinction and may indicate that the development of chronic PTSD represents a failure of such fear extinction (Norrholm et al., 2011). Such an inability to extinguish conditioned fear may be due to a complex gene × environment interaction

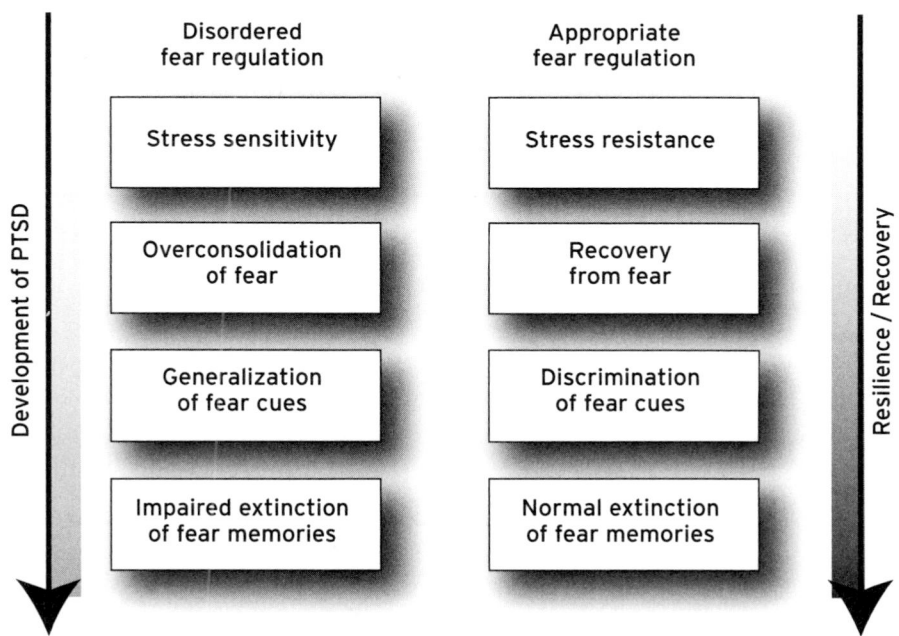

Figure 49.2 Disordered fear regulation in posttraumatic stress disorder (PTSD). Individuals with PTSD typically show increased sensitization to stress, overgeneralization of fear to irrelevant stimuli, and impaired extinction of fear memories. Individuals who demonstrate resilience to PTSD, and/or who recover from traumatic/stressful experiences, are able to better discriminate between fearful and nonfearful stimuli. Further, those with disordered fear regulation may also have impairment of extinction of fearful memories, further contributing to the lack of recovery as seen in PTSD. (Adapted from Mahan and Ressler, 2012.)

between one's individual predisposition(s) and environmental factors such as early life stress and the frequency, degree, and intensity of the traumatic event(s). Fear conditioning offers a unique framework for translational studies because it can be modeled in animal experiments. Given the richness of the animal literature, the neural underpinnings of fear conditioning are well understood, and PTSD research can capitalize on these findings (Jovanovic and Ressler, 2010).

ANIMAL MODEL SYSTEMS OF PTSD

Studies of PTSD in humans have several logistical and ethical limitations, such as the lack of control over the extent and level of trauma exposure, or the inability to match individuals based on past trauma history. Animal models provide the opportunity for increased experimental flexibility and control of trauma exposure in order to examine causal relationships in PTSD. While model systems of mental illness are discussed in other chapters, here we briefly describe animal models of relevance to PTSD.

FEAR CONDITIONING MODEL

As described in the preceding, PTSD patients have dysregulated fear responses including overgeneralization of the conditioned response, fear extinction deficits, and impaired safety signal learning (Mahan and Ressler, 2012). Fear conditioning and extinction are a widely used paradigm used in

many species, including humans (Mahan and Ressler, 2012). The deficits in fear extinction observed in several studies of PTSD patients are particularly important for animal models of PTSD treatment. As shown in Figure 49.3, fear extinction is a laboratory analogue of exposure therapy (Rothbaum and Davis, 2003). Manipulating rodent models using behavioral, pharmacological, lesion, or genetic techniques is useful in elucidating molecules and brain structures that are necessary for normal extinction. For example, brain-derived neurotrophic factor (BDNF) is one of the molecules that has been identified as having a role in fear conditioning and has been studied in rodent models (Andero et al., 2011). Therefore, compounds thought to act on BDNF can be administered during fear conditioning or extinction sessions to rodent models to assess their potential for PTSD treatment. Please see Chapter 41 in this volume for further details on understanding fear in animal model systems.

REPEATED CHRONIC STRESS MODEL

While the fear conditioning model can be used to examine extinction deficits in PTSD, other animal models can mimic the trauma exposure in order to examine the etiology of the human illness. Many PTSD patients experience repeated exposure to unpredictable traumatic events, particularly in combat-related PTSD. Therefore, a rodent model using chronic variable stress (CVS) provides a unique tool (McGuire et al., 2010). McGuire and colleagues described the CVS paradigm followed by a recovery period (CVS-R). The CVS model is characterized by

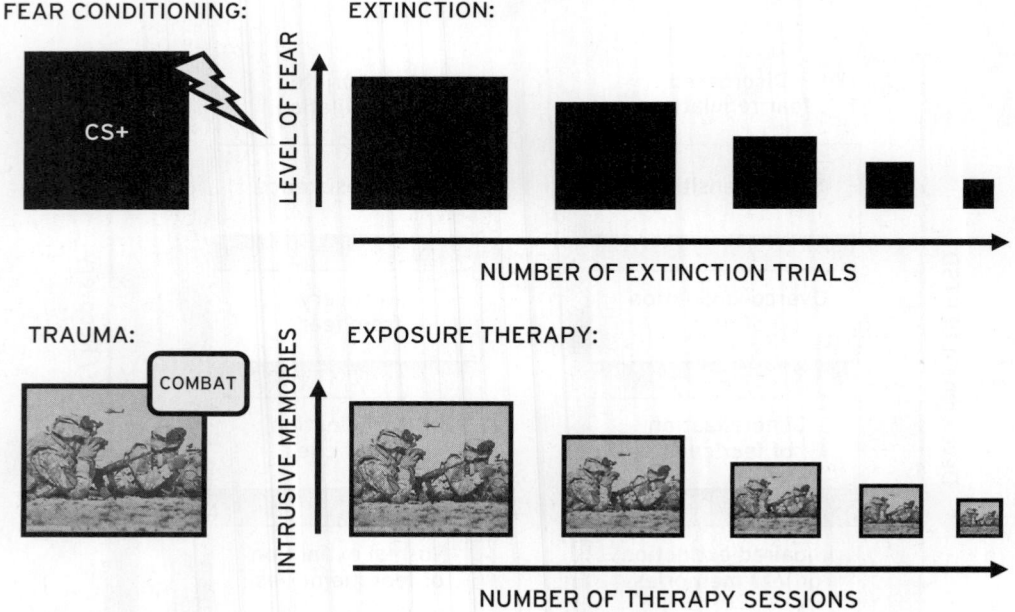

Figure 49.3 Parallels between fear conditioning and extinction in preclinical studies and trauma and exposure therapy in the treatment of PTSD. (Top) Fear conditioning, through the combination of a previously neutral conditioned stimulus (CS) combined with an aversive unconditioned stimulus (e.g., foot shock), leads to high levels of fear expression. However, with repeated reexposure to the CS in the absence of the aversive stimulus, a process known as extinction, the CS no longer elicits substantial levels of fear. (Bottom) Fear conditioning models of PTSD suggest that the cues that are associated with the aversive trauma experience, for example, the sights, sounds, and smells related to trauma exposure, come to elicit fearful intrusive memories, even if they are only somewhat related to the initial trauma (such as with fear generalization). Repeated exposure to these memories and trauma cues over time, through psychotherapy, leads to extinction and symptom reduction.

a week of various stressors, such as cold swim, warm swim, or hypoxia followed by an assessment of the rat's fear-conditioned responses, weight changes, or molecular changes in the tissue.

SINGLE PROLONGED STRESS MODEL

Although some PTSD patients experience chronic or repeated trauma exposure, such as prisoners of war, within-theater refugees, and military personnel, other PTSD patients experience a single trauma, such as people who develop PTSD after a natural disaster or terrorist attack. For the latter situation, the CVS model may not properly mimic the human experience. The single prolonged stress (SPS) model, developed by Liberzon and colleagues in the late 1990s (Liberzon et al., 1997) exposes the rodent to a single stressor followed by a period of rest before assessing the rodent's responses. SPS has been accepted as a valid model because it elicits neuroendocrine changes similar to those observed in PTSD patients (reviewed in Yamamoto et al., 2009). SPS consists of a quick succession of restraint, swim, and loss of consciousness stressors, followed by a week of rest period prior to further testing. This delay period is thought to function as the duration criterion for PTSD inasmuch as it allows for the separation of adaptive versus pathological responses to trauma (Yamamoto et al., 2009).

DIFFERENTIAL PATHWAYS TO PTSD

The discrepancy in prevalence rates of trauma exposure and PTSD suggests resiliency in the majority of individuals, indicating the presence of "risk factors" that increase vulnerability in those who develop PTSD in the aftermath of trauma (Fig. 49.4). These factors can be environmental, such as early life stress during development (Heim and Nemeroff, 2001), as well as genetic, as shown by several recent gene-by-environment interaction studies (Binder et al., 2008). It should be noted that there are also "resilience factors" that reduce the likelihood of PTSD, even after severe trauma exposure; these include environmental factors, such as social support (Charney, 2004) and genetic factors (Binder et al., 2008).

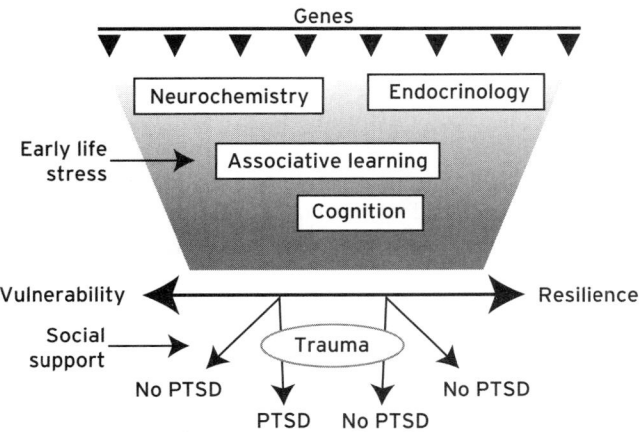

Figure 49.4 *Interaction of genetics, biology, and environment in regulating vulnerability versus resilience following trauma.*

DEVELOPMENTAL TRAUMA—CHILD ABUSE AND MALTREATMENT

The impact of early adverse events on mental health has been established for more than a decade: early-life stress (ELS) is a predictor of adult depression, while ELS and adult trauma are both predictors of PTSD (Nemeroff et al., 2006). A rodent model of ELS in which neonates were repeatedly separated from their mothers found long-term effects on the hypothalamic-pituitary-adrenal (HPA) axis (Plotsky and Meaney, 1993). Similarly, women who were abused in childhood show increased HPA reactivity to a psychosocial stressor (Heim and Nemeroff, 2001). The hormones of the HPA axis, including corticotrophin-releasing hormone (CRH), can have anxiogenic effects and are some of the most replicated neuroendocrine alterations found in PTSD.

Childhood abuse and maltreatment can have especially pervasive negative psychiatric outcomes. Chen and colleagues (2010) reviewed the prevalence of lifetime diagnosis of psychiatric disorders and sexual abuse and reported a significant association of childhood sexual abuse with later PTSD even after controlling for factors such as socioeconomic status, relationship to the abuser, and number of abuse episodes. Maltreatment before the age of 12, including physical abuse and neglect, produces significant increases in adulthood diagnosis of PTSD (Gilbert et al., 2009). With rates of child abuse ranging from 4–35% in high-income countries such as the United States and the United Kingdom, the persistent effects manifested in PTSD and other psychiatric illnesses create a long-lasting public health burden (Gilbert et al., 2009). Further, as discussed later in this chapter, childhood abuse interacts with genetic vulnerabilities to increase the severity of PTSD symptoms.

GENETIC VULNERABILITY

Although twin data support the importance of genetic inheritance in vulnerability to PTSD (Koenen et al., 2003), there are few studies that have found main effects of candidate gene(s) related to PTSD. This dearth of studies arises from the complexity of the phenotype, the difficulty of defining groups with comparable traumatic exposure, and the high comorbidity with other psychiatric disorders (Nemeroff et al., 2006). However, the fact that a majority of individuals experience a trauma in their lifetime but only a subset develop PTSD is suggestive of a strong genetic component. Identifying these genetic risk factors for PTSD may provide future avenues to personalize treatment in vulnerable individuals with recent exposure to trauma. Next we describe a number of candidate genes, identified to date, with the most robust effects on PTSD.

FKBP5

FKBP5 is a cochaperone protein that interacts with hsp90 and regulates glucocorticoid receptor (GR) sensitivity. Binder and colleagues (2008) identified several single-nucleotide polymorphisms (SNPs) within the *FKBP5* gene (rs9296158, rs3800373, rs1360780, rs9470080) that were linked to adult PTSD symptoms in patients with a history of child abuse. In the largest candidate gene study of PTSD at that time, this group has shown a gene × environment (G × E) effect of the polymorphisms in

FKBP5 with a history of childhood maltreatment to predict level of adult PTSD symptoms in a traumatized civilian sample (Binder et al., 2008). There have been several replications of this finding since its initial description. Notably, no main effects were found for the *FKBP5* genotype directly associating with PTSD symptoms, nor was there an effect of the gene interacting with adult trauma levels. These data suggest that the interaction of trauma, perhaps during a developmental critical period, with the HPA-stress related genes increases vulnerability for PTSD.

CRHR1

The corticotropin-releasing hormone receptor (CRHR1) is also a part of the GR system and involved in HPA axis regulation. A polymorphism in the *CRHR1* gene has been linked to PTSD associated with child abuse (Amstadter et al., 2011). CRHR1 polymorphisms have also been recognized as a risk factor for depressive symptoms in adults with a history of child abuse (Bradley et al., 2008). CRHR1 polymorphisms as a risk factor for both PTSD and depression symptoms suggest that the *CRHR1* gene plays a role in a PTSD depression phenotype.

5HTTLPR

The serotonin transporter gene's promoter region has a polymorphism that results in short and long alleles. In one of the greatest breakthroughs in psychiatry in the last decade that illustrates gene–environment interactions, Caspi and colleagues (2003) reported that 5HTTLRP is associated with symptoms of depression but only in stressed individuals. This early G × E discovery fueled investigations of the same polymorphism with PTSD. Kilpatrick and colleagues (2007) identified a G × E interaction predictive of PTSD in an analysis of individuals exposed to 2004 hurricanes in South Florida. As part of this same hurricane study, it was also reported that the short allele of the 5-HTTLPR polymorphism was associated with decreased risk of PTSD in low-risk environments but increased risk of PTSD in high-risk environments (Amstadter et al., 2009), suggesting that social environment modifies the effect of 5-HTTLPR genotype on PTSD risk. Several groups have now identified that individuals who are homozygous for the short allele are more likely to develop PTSD (Mercer et al., 2012) and are less likely to respond to PTSD treatment (Bryant et al., 2010). This gene also remains of interest because the serotonin transporter is the site of action for a class of compounds used to treat PTSD patients' symptoms, as discussed later in this chapter.

COMT

A functional polymorphism of the gene coding for catechol-*O*-methyltransferase (COMT), an enzyme that catalyzes the breakdown of norepinephrine and dopamine, in which valine (Val) has been substituted by methionine (Met) at codon 158, is associated with lower enzyme activity. *COMT* is primarily expressed in the prefrontal cortex and hippocampus (Matsumoto et al., 2003) and represents the principal synaptic dopamine-clearing mechanism in these brain regions. Recent work has implicated the *COMT* Val[158]Met polymorphism in the development of PTSD following repeated traumatic exposure (Kolassa et al., 2010).

PACAP

Pituitary adenylate cyclase–activating polypeptide (PACAP) coordinates normal physiological stress reactions. PACAP and corticotrophin-releasing hormone work together in limbic brain areas to modulate anxiety-like behavior (Hammack et al., 2010). We have recently shown that blood levels of PACAP and a SNP within its PAC1 receptor (PAC1R) may be critical mediators of response to psychological trauma. The *PAC1R* gene has an SNP (rs2267735) in its putative estrogen response element that is predictive of PTSD (Ressler et al., 2011). Specifically this SNP appears to be a risk factor in females but not males. This sex effect is particularly interesting because females are more likely to develop PTSD (Kessler et al., 1995). So while the *PACAP receptor* is not the only gene identified to have a PTSD risk SNP, it may be an important factor in the development of the disorder in females.

NEUROBIOLOGY OF PTSD FROM HUMAN NEUROIMAGING STUDIES

The last two decades of neuroimaging work have pointed to a functional neurocircuitry of PTSD that highly overlaps with the neuroanatomical substrates of fear described in animal studies. The primary neuroimaging techniques used in humans have been magnetic resonance imaging (MRI) and positron emission tomography (PET). A number of areas have been implicated in PTSD; however, the sections that follow highlight the most replicated findings, focusing on the hippocampus, amygdala, medial prefrontal cortex, and insula. Although the early studies of brain structure and function were limited with regard to spatial resolution, recent advances in imaging methodology have allowed for more fine-grained analyses of subcomponents of these areas.

HIPPOCAMPUS

The hippocampus plays an integral role in memory formation and context conditioning (see Fig. 49.5). In one of the earliest neuroimaging studies in PTSD, Bremner and colleagues, taking advantage of both the clear anatomical boundaries of the hippocampus in MRI and the known deficits in memory associated with PTSD (reviewed in Bremner et al., 2008), compared hippocampal volume between the Vietnam combat veterans with PTSD and healthy controls. There was a significant reduction of 8% in the right hippocampus, a rather surprising finding in a functional psychiatric disease as opposed to an organic disease (e.g., neurodegenerative disease like Alzheimer's disease). To ensure the effect was not specific to combat-related PTSD, it was also shown that the effects were replicated in PTSD patients with a history of childhood sexual and physical abuse, who demonstrated a 12% reduction in the volume of the left hippocampus (Bremner et al., 2008). However, around the same time De Bellis and colleagues (1999) examined maltreated children with PTSD using MRI and found a reduction in overall cerebral volume in PTSD compared with matched controls, but they did not find hippocampal volume differences after correcting for overall brain volume. Nevertheless, to date

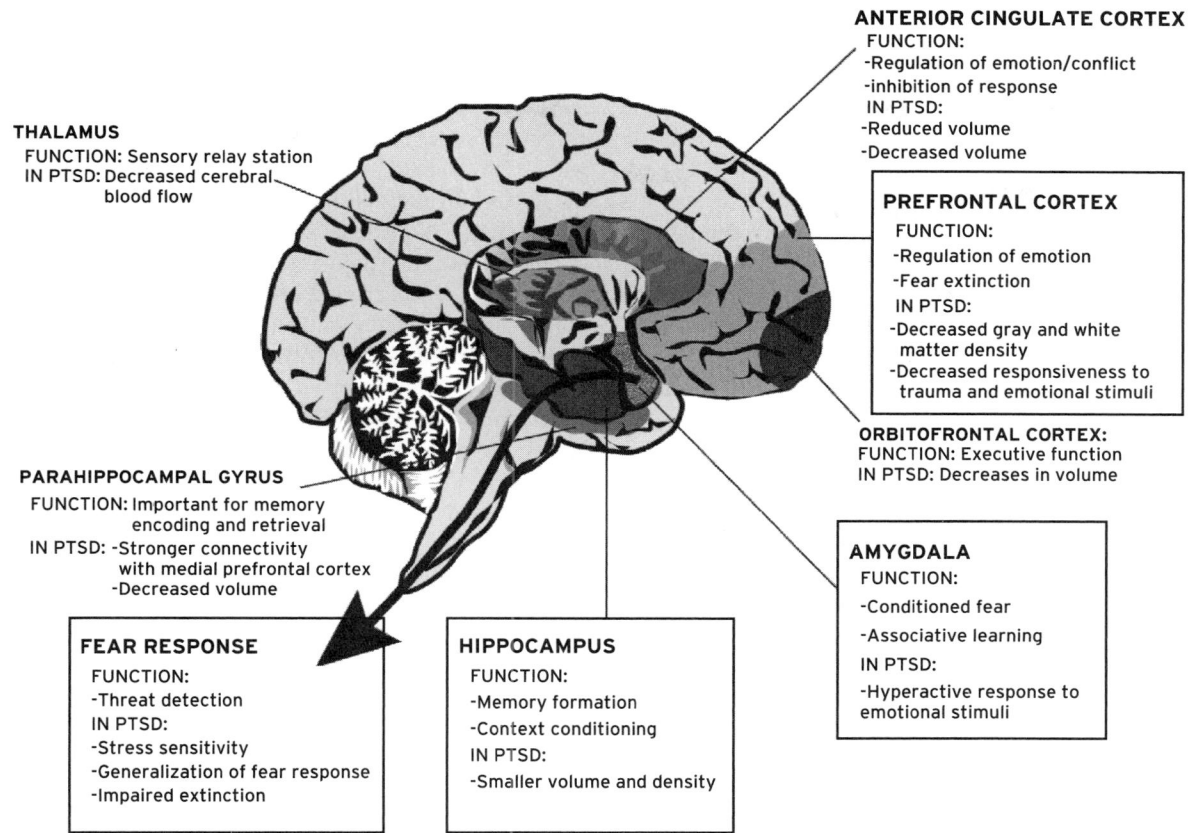

THALAMUS
FUNCTION: Sensory relay station
IN PTSD: Decreased cerebral blood flow

ANTERIOR CINGULATE CORTEX
FUNCTION:
-Regulation of emotion/conflict
-inhibition of response
IN PTSD:
-Reduced volume
-Decreased volume

PREFRONTAL CORTEX
FUNCTION:
-Regulation of emotion
-Fear extinction
IN PTSD:
-Decreased gray and white matter density
-Decreased responsiveness to trauma and emotional stimuli

ORBITOFRONTAL CORTEX:
FUNCTION: Executive function
IN PTSD: Decreases in volume

PARAHIPPOCAMPAL GYRUS
FUNCTION: Important for memory encoding and retrieval
IN PTSD: -Stronger connectivity with medial prefrontal cortex
-Decreased volume

AMYGDALA
FUNCTION:
-Conditioned fear
-Associative learning
IN PTSD:
-Hyperactive response to emotional stimuli

FEAR RESPONSE
FUNCTION:
-Threat detection
IN PTSD:
-Stress sensitivity
-Generalization of fear response
-Impaired extinction

HIPPOCAMPUS
FUNCTION:
-Memory formation
-Context conditioning
IN PTSD:
-Smaller volume and density

Figure 49.5 *Structure and function of brain regions differentially involved in PTSD. Brain regions with the most up-to-date evidence to support their role in PTSD are highlighted, along with their presumptive roles, supported by preclinical and clinical studies in fear regulation. (Adapted from Mahan and Ressler, 2012.)*

reduced hippocampal volume has been one of the most widely replicated findings in adult PTSD patients relative to trauma controls and healthy controls (Woon et al., 2010). Recent studies using higher resolution imaging techniques have indicated that reductions in specific subregions of the hippocampus, such as the cornu ammonis 3 (CA3) and dentate gyrus, are associated with PTSD (Wang et al., 2010). A question of particular interest, and source of some controversy, has been delineating whether a smaller hippocampus is a predisposing factor for developing PTSD, or induced by the stress of trauma exposure and PTSD. The strongest evidence for the former is a twin study by Pitman and colleagues showing reduced hippocampal volume in PTSD patients as well as their monozygotic twins who were unexposed to trauma (Gilbertson et al., 2002). Evidence for the latter, beyond the work in children, comes from a longitudinal study that found decreased gray matter density in the hippocampus using voxel-based morphometry in response to stressful life events (Papagni et al., 2011).

PTSD is also associated with alterations in hippocampal function. The first study to show deficits in hippocampal blood flow/activation in PTSD patients was conducted by Bremner and colleagues (2008), using personalized trauma scripts during PET imaging in women with childhood sexual abuse. Interestingly, and in partial contradiction (with notable differences in experimental and imaging setups) to Bremner's work, Shin and colleagues (2006) observed an increase in left hippocampal activity using an fMRI emotional stroop paradigm with combat-related words in PTSD patients compared with controls. However, again using PET, Bremner and colleagues (2008) showed that healthy controls had increased blood flow to the left hippocampus compared with PTSD patients during a declarative working memory task. A recent review of functional neuroimaging in PTSD concluded that the relationship between PTSD symptoms and hippocampal activation may be dependent on the type of task employed (Hughes and Shin, 2011).

AMYGDALA

Based on the extensive work in animal models, the amygdala is known to play a central role in regulating fear responses to threatening and emotional stimuli (Davis, 1992). This area in the limbic system is also activated in humans in response to emotional cues (Phan et al., 2002). Unlike studies of the hippocampus, studies investigating amygdala volume in PTSD patients have no evidence of volume differences in the amygdala; however, the results show significant lateralization asymmetry (Woon and Hedges, 2009). In a final note on amygdala volume, at least one study showed bilateral volume reduction in PTSD patients who were part of the Tokyo subway attacks when compared with those survivors who did not develop PTSD (Rogers et al., 2009).

The strongest evidence for the role of the amygdala in PTSD comes from functional neuroimaging studies. As early as 1996, Rauch and colleagues (1996) used PET imaging to show that the right amygdala was more active in PTSD patients during a traumatic script-driven imagery condition compared with a neutral condition. Studies using fMRI have also found hyperactivation in the amygdala in PTSD patients compared with controls using emotionally salient stimuli such as fearful faces (Phan et al., 2002; Shin et al., 2006). Focusing on temporal dynamics, Protopopescu and colleagues (2005) analyzed early and late epochs of fMRI blood oxygen level–dependent (BOLD) responses, suggesting that the time course of the amygdala response is also altered in PTSD. Specifically, the study found greater initial amygdala reactivity to trauma-related words in PTSD patients compared with other words. Furthermore, PTSD patients did not show normal sensitization and habituation patterns of amygdala responses over repeated presentations of stimuli throughout the MRI session. Similar results were found by Shin and colleagues (2006) with regard to happy, fearful, and neutral faces.

The final line of evidence for the amygdala's involvement in PTSD comes from surgical case reports. For example, Adami and colleagues (2006) reported a case of a left amygdala-hippocampectomy in an epileptic patient with a history of childhood sexual abuse, but no PTSD. Two weeks after surgery, the patient manifested PTSD symptoms, suggesting a potential importance of the structural integrity of these regions for resilience to trauma. Similarly, Smith and colleagues (2008) reported on a patient who developed PTSD after a motor vehicle accident that occurred two years after having the left amygdala removed. Taken together, these studies strongly suggest that the amygdala is one of the crucial neuroanatomical areas involved in PTSD, and that patients exhibit exaggerated amygdala activity in response to emotional cues and trauma reminders.

MEDIAL PREFRONTAL CORTEX

The prefrontal cortex (PFC) has long been thought to play a role in behavioral inhibition. More than a decade ago, animal studies reported that lesions of the medial PFC (mPFC) prior to original fear conditioning retard extinction to a tone (Morgan et al., 1993). The prefrontal cortex can be subdivided into medial and orbitofrontal PFC. The anterior cingulate cortex (ACC), also referred to frequently as Brodmann areas 24 and 32, is part of the PFC and has both rostral and dorsal components. Brain development studies of healthy children and adolescents have indicated robust changes in gray and white matter in the prefrontal cortex, with gray matter decreasing and white matter increasing in volume from ages 9–18 (Giedd and Rapoport, 2010). A volumetric study that stratified PTSD and control subjects by sex demonstrated significant sex-by-group effects, with smaller cerebral volumes and corpus callosum in PTSD males (De Bellis and Keshavan, 2003). Using both volumetric and voxel-based morphometry (VBM) methods, Carrion and colleagues (2008) showed an increase in PFC volume and gray matter density in adolescents with PTSD. A number of studies to date have found reduction in gray matter volume and density in the ACC related to PTSD (Sekiguchi et al., 2012).

While the orbitofrontal cortex has more recently gained a lot of attention with regard to PTSD, some of the earliest evidence of its functional involvement was shown in the study by Rauch and colleagues (1996). Using PET during traumatic script-driven imagery, this study showed that combat veterans with PTSD demonstrate increased activation in the OFC and the ACC. Shin and colleagues (2006) found reduced medial PFC activity in PTSD patients compared with controls using different paradigms and trauma populations during PET imaging.

Several neuroimaging studies have used different paradigms that specifically activate the PFC; the simplest and most commonly used tasks involve response inhibition. Such tasks have been used in subjects with PTSD using fMRI measures (Carrion et al., 2008). This task reliably indicates decreased activation in PTSD subjects compared with controls in the rostral ACC, located at the genu of the corpus callosum. A recent meta-analysis of imaging studies during emotion processing in PTSD, social anxiety, and specific phobia indicated that the rostral ACC is less active in PTSD patients relative to controls, an effect not found in other anxiety disorders (Etkin and Wager, 2007). Studies that have examined functional connectivity between the PFC and the amygdala have demonstrated impaired inhibition of the amygdala in PTSD (Lanius et al., 2004). Finally, larger rostral ACC volume was found to predict positive outcomes to cognitive-behavior therapy for PTSD (Bryant et al., 2008).

INSULA

Located at the junction of the frontal and temporal lobes the insular cortex (Brodmann area 13) is another prominent cortical area associated with PTSD. This structure is involved in interoceptive stimuli and has been linked to processing of painful or noxious sensations (Critchley et al., 2004). Structural changes in the insula have been largely understudied but highly consistent in demonstrating decreased volume and gray matter density in PTSD patients compared with controls (Chen et al., 2006).

The early PET studies using script-driven imagery showed increased activation in the right insular cortex in PTSD patients when listening to traumatic scripts compared with neutral scripts (Rauch et al., 1996). Recent functional studies using various paradigms with emotional stimuli have found mixed results: some have found increased insula activation in PTSD compared with controls (Hopper et al., 2007), while others have found the inverse relationship (Bremner et al., 2008). Some of the discrepancies may be due to the type of stimuli used; in particular, studies that have used sensation-related cues have found increased insula activation in PTSD. For example, in a study of the role in olfaction in PTSD, Vermetten et al. (2007) showed that the smell of diesel fumes and hydrogen sulfide significantly increased insula activation in the PTSD patients compared with controls. Similarly, a recent study of neural correlates of painful stimulation found that women with PTSD resulting from domestic violence had increased insula activation (Strigo et al., 2010). Increased insula activation seems to be somewhat specific to PTSD; an fMRI study of script-driven imagery found that PTSD patients without comorbid depression showed this increase, which patients with both disorders did not (Lanius et al., 2007).

TREATMENT OF PTSD

PTSD is a heterogeneous and highly disabling mental disorder that requires the tailoring of treatment strategies according to the needs of each patient. Future treatment strategies for PTSD may be governed by a shift toward personalized medicine based on an individual's environmental risk factors, genotypes, or gene expression patterns. As outlined earlier, the identification of potential genetic variants that increase susceptibility for developing psychiatric illness would be a particularly important tool for advancing treatment options for PTSD and related anxiety disorders. Current treatment regimens typically involve the combination of psychotherapy and pharmacotherapy (Friedman, 2006). Figure 49.6 shows a flowchart of treatment strategies for PTSD.

PSYCHOTHERAPEUTIC APPROACHES

The first-line, nonpharmacological treatment approach for PTSD has traditionally been psychological treatments including psychoeducation, individual psychotherapy, and group psychotherapy (Friedman, 2006). Psychoeducation, which is not intended to be a stand-alone intervention, is designed to provide a patient with information regarding the nature and course of PTSD to a traumatized individual presenting with PTSD-related symptoms (Friedman, 2006). Individual psychotherapy is aimed at specific PTSD symptom clusters and includes cognitive behavioral therapy (CBT) techniques such as prolonged exposure (PE) (Rothbaum et al., 2000) and cognitive processing therapy (CPT). Of these, only exposure-based psychotherapy has met criteria for evidence-based treatment by the Institute of Medicine in 2008.

COGNITIVE BEHAVIOR THERAPY

The primary purpose of CBT is to deconstruct the PTSD-related aberrant thinking patterns that underlie avoidance. Effective PE techniques include imaginal and *in vivo* exposure to stimuli that are related to the traumatic event and a patient's memories of this event (Rothbaum et al., 2000). Imaginal exposure therapy requires the patient to narrate his or her traumatic experience during weekly sessions that continue for 8–10 weeks. An important step in imaginal exposure is for the patient to face contexts directly related to his or her traumatic experience during *in vivo* contact.

EXPOSURE THERAPY

Prolonged exposure therapy, which is based on the learning principles of fear extinction, requires repeated exposure to cues associated with the traumatic event within a safe, therapeutic context (Rothbaum et al., 2000). This repeated exposure might

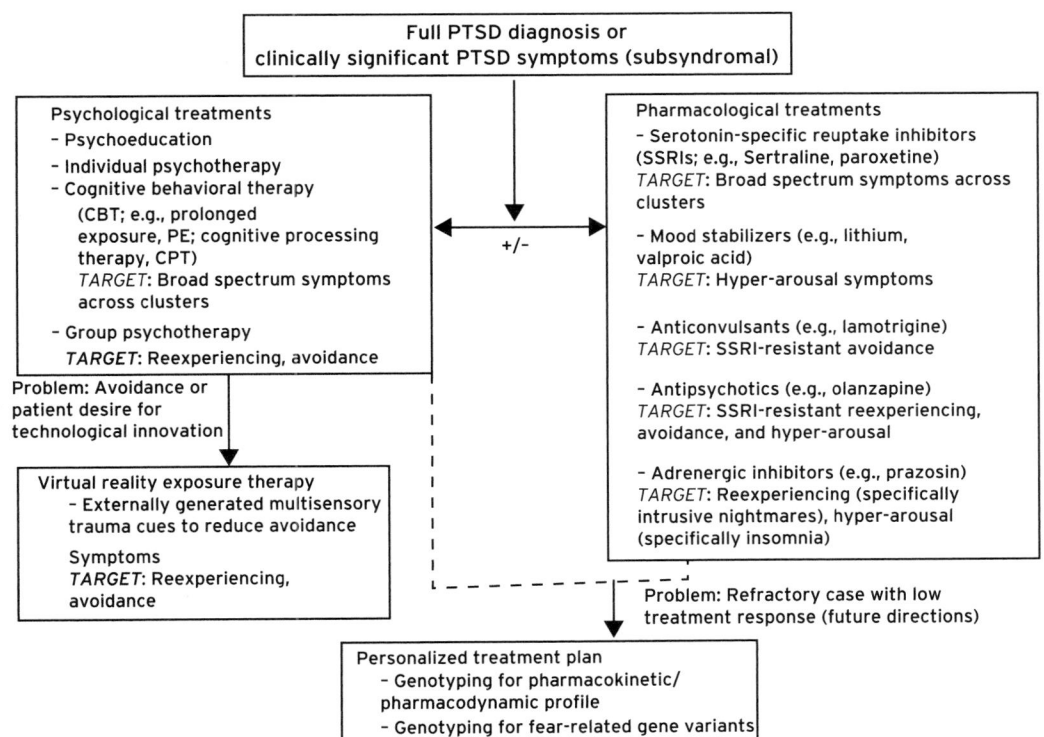

Figure 49.6 Treatment options for posttraumatic stress disorder (PTSD). Current PTSD treatment options include both psychological treatments (including CBT, exposure therapy, virtual reality exposure therapy, and other forms of individual and group talk therapy) and pharmacological (primarily SSRIs, mood stabilizers, and adrenergic blockers). (Adapted from Norrholm and Jovanovic, 2010.)

take the form of recorded self-narrations of the traumatic event coupled with cognitive measures to reduce the fear responses (anxiety symptoms) associated with the reminders. Exposure therapy is thought to rely on the same learning-based neural processes that underlie extinction learning as outlined previously (Fig. 49.3). Recent work has focused on the use of virtual reality exposure (VRE) therapy to treat combat-related PTSD (Gerardi et al., 2008). With this type of treatment, veterans are exposed to a virtual combat scenario (e.g., Iraq, Afghanistan) that includes cues such as explosions, insurgents, improvised explosive devices (IEDs), darkness, smoke, and low-flying aircraft. This type of therapy provides direct exposure to the feared stimuli, but without the negative outcomes experienced in combat. The novel approach of VRE represents an innovative alternative to traditional prolonged exposure methodologies.

PHARMACOLOGICAL APPROACHES

Many of the pharmacological studies that have informed drug treatments for PTSD have significant limitations including small sample size and reduced power, a lack of double-blinding and randomization, and inconsistent dosing regimens (Choi et al., 2010). In fact, a recent Institute of Medicine of the National Academies report concluded that there was insufficient evidence to support efficacy of pharmacological treatment for PTSD. In spite of these limitations, several classes of drugs have been used in the treatment of symptoms of this disorder. Multiple drug classes, including antipsychotics, anticonvulsants, adrenergic-inhibitors, opioids, and benzodiazepines, were rated according to the empirical support behind their therapeutic value for treating PTSD (Choi et al., 2010).

The first-line approach for pharmacological interventions for PTSD is antidepressants such as selective serotonin reuptake inhibitors (SSRIs; e.g., sertraline) and serotonin-norepinephrine reuptake inhibitors (SNRIs; e.g., venlafaxine) (Ravindran and Stein, 2010). Prescription drug treatments for PTSD target specific symptoms as required by clinical need. For example, antidepressants aid in elevating general mood and anxiety (and treating comorbid depression) whereas anticonvulsants, antipsychotics, anxiolytics, and adrenergic inhibitors may be used to treat specific symptoms such as irritability, intrusive thoughts, and insomnia (Ravindran and Stein, 2010).

Novel pharmacological approaches that enhance fear extinction are currently being evaluated for treatment efficacy in PTSD. The use of D-cycloserine (DCS), a partial N-methyl-D-aspartate (NMDA) receptor agonist, as a potential treatment for PTSD arose as a result of numerous preclinical studies implicating NMDA glutamate receptor activity in learning and memory processes. DCS has recently been investigated in combination with VRE therapy for the fear of heights (Ressler et al., 2004) along with a number of other fear-related disorders. After treatment, those patients that received DCS in combination with VRE showed greater improvement compared with those who received placebo and VRE. DCS is currently being investigated as adjunct to exposure therapy in panic disorder, social anxiety disorder, OCD, and PTSD. Additionally, other methods of augmenting NMDA receptor activity in conjunction with extinction are now being explored.

Several pharmacological agents are being tested as early-intervention agents in the immediate aftermath of trauma for their potential in preventing PTSD. For example, glucocorticoids such as hydrocortisone were found to reduce PTSD symptoms and traumatic memories when administered in the emergency room (de Quervain and Margraf, 2008). Although this intervention is showing promise, the sample sizes are still too small. Another similarly acting drug, propranolol, which is involved in memory consolidation (Pitman et al., 2002), is being explored for its potential in treating PTSD symptoms, but large-size, controlled studies of this compound are still lacking, so no conclusions can be made. Other approaches hope to target reconsolidation, a period of potential vulnerability of fear memories to disruption, in the "erasure" of specific fear memories after a trauma. Overall, it is hoped that a further understanding of the molecular mechanisms of fear processing and extinction, as outlined in Figure 49.2, will lead to a number of more powerful ways to combine pharmacotherapy with the specific learning processes underlying recovery from fear and resilience.

NEUROBIOLOGICAL TARGETS FOR TREATMENT

There is an emerging body of literature assessing treatment-related structural and functional changes in the neural underpinnings of mental disorders. An early study using SPECT imaging pre- and posttreatment with SSRIs found significant changes in ACC and hippocampus after 12 weeks of treatment (Carey et al., 2004), and a more recent study found similar SSRI treatment effects in the orbitofrontal cortex using PET imaging during script-driven imagery (Fani et al., 2011). SSRIs have also shown efficacy in increasing hippocampus volume in PTSD patients (Vermetten et al., 2003). In a recent study of Iraq and Afghanistan combat soldiers with PTSD who underwent exposure therapy, increased neural activation in the ACC in response to treatment was associated with greater clinical improvement, even in the absence of large changes in PTSD symptoms (Roy et al., 2010). Interestingly, repeated high-frequency transcranial magnetic stimulation over the dorsolateral prefrontal cortex ameliorated PTSD core symptoms beyond sham stimulation or slow frequency stimulation (Cohen et al., 2004). In summary, these studies suggest neuroplasticity in the hippocampus, amygdala, and PFC with the potential for treatment-related modifications in activity (e.g., successfully attenuating amygdala-driven fear responses). Such findings offer great promise for improving available treatments for PTSD.

CONCLUSION

As this chapter details, PTSD is a common psychiatric disorder that has given rise to numerous clinical and animal model studies to understand both the disorder itself and how to treat it. As a disorder that is in part explained by disruption of normal fear regulation, it provides a particularly interesting and exciting intersection of the molecular neurobiology of fear processing that is being rapidly understood in animal models. The convergence of data from such preclinical studies with human neuroimaging, neurophysiology, and genetic studies in humans is being combined with fear-modification therapies such as exposure therapy in human patients. Future work will build on the knowledge of animal fear studies, including greater understanding of consolidation, reconsolidation, and extinction processes, as well as genetic analyses and human neuroimaging studies to better treat and prevent PTSD in at-risk individuals.

DISCLOSURES

Ms. Murray, Mr. Keifer, Dr. Norrholm and Dr. Jovanovic declare no conflict of interest to disclose.

Dr. Ressler is a founding member of Extinction Pharmaceuticals/ Therapade Technologies to develop d-cycloserine, a generically available compound, for use to augment the effectiveness of psychotherapy. He has received no equity or income from this relationship within at least the last 3 years.

This work was supported by NIMH, NIH, Howard Hughes Medical Institute, and the Burroughs Wellcome Fund.

REFERENCES

Adami, P., König, P., et al. (2006). Post-traumatic stress disorder and amygdala-hippocampectomy. *Acta Psychiatr. Scand.* 113:360–363.

American Psychological Association. (2000). DSM-IV-TR: Diagnostic and Statistical Manual of Mental Disorders. Washington, DC: Author.

Amstadter, A.B., Nugent, N.R., et al. (2009). Genetics of PTSD: fear conditioning as a model for future research. *Psychiatric Annals* 39(6):358–367.

Amstadter, A.B., Nugent, N.R., et al. (2011). Corticotrophin-releasing hormone type 1 receptor gene (CRHR1) variants predict posttraumatic stress disorder onset and course in pediatric injury patients. *Dis. Markers* 30(2–3):89–99.

Andero, R., Heldt, S.A., et al. (2011). Effect of 7,8-dihydroxyflavone, a small-molecule TrkB agonist, on emotional learning. *Am. J. Psychiatry* 168:163–172.

Binder, E.B., Bradley, R.G., et al. (2008). Association of FKBP5 polymorphisms and childhood abuse with risk of posttraumatic stress disorder symptoms in adults. *JAMA* 299:1291–1305.

Bradley, R.G., Binder, E.B., et al. (2008). Influence of child abuse on adult depression: moderation by the corticotropin-releasing hormone receptor gene. *Arch. Gen. Psychiatry* 65:190–200.

Bremner, J.D., Elzinga, B., et al. (2008). Structural and functional plasticity of the human brain in posttraumatic stress disorder. *Prog. Brain Res.* 167:171–186.

Breslau, N., Kessler, R.C., et al. (1998). Trauma and posttraumatic stress disorder in the community: the 1996 Detroit Area Survey of Trauma. *Arch. Gen. Psychiatry* 55:626–632.

Bryant, R.A., Felmingham, K., et al. (2008). Rostral anterior cingulate volume predicts treatment response to cognitive-behavioural therapy for posttraumatic stress disorder. *J. Psychiatry Neurosci.* 33:142–146.

Bryant, R.A., Felmingham, K.L., et al. (2010). Preliminary evidence of the short allele of the serotonin transporter gene predicting poor response to cognitive behavior therapy in posttraumatic stress disorder. *Biol. Psychiatry* 67:1217–1219.

Carey, P., Warwick, J., et al. (2004). Single photon emission computed tomography (SPECT) of anxiety disorders before and after treatment with citalopram. *BMC Psychiatry* 4:30.

Carrion, V.G., Garrett, A., et al. (2008). Posttraumatic stress symptoms and brain function during a response-inhibition task: an fMRI study in youth. *Depress. Anxiety* 25:514–526.

Caspi, A., Sugden, K., et al. (2003). Influence of life stress on depression: moderation by a polymorphism in the 5-HTT gene. *Science* 301:386–389.

Charney, D.S. (2004). Psychobiological mechanisms of resilience and vulnerability: implications for successful adaptation to extreme stress. *Am. J. Psychiatry* 161:195–216.

Chen, L.P., Murad, M.H., et al. (2010). Sexual abuse and lifetime diagnosis of psychiatric disorders: systematic review and meta-analysis. *Mayo Clin. Proc.* 85:618–629.

Chen, S., Xia, W., et al. (2006). Gray matter density reduction in the insula in fire survivors with posttraumatic stress disorder: a voxel-based morphometric study. *Psychiatry Res.* 146:65–72.

Choi, D.C., Rothbaum, B.O., et al. (2010). Pharmacological enhancement of behavioral therapy: focus on posttraumatic stress disorder. *Curr. Top. Behav. Neurosci.* 2:279–299.

Cohen, H., Kaplan, Z., et al. (2004). Repetitive transcranial magnetic stimulation of the right dorsolateral prefrontal cortex in posttraumatic stress disorder: a double-blind, placebo-controlled study. *Am. J. Psychiatry* 161:515–524.

Critchley, H.D., Wiens, S., et al. (2004). Neural systems supporting interoceptive awareness. *Nat. Neurosci.* 7:189–195.

Davis, M. (1992). The role of the amygdala in fear and anxiety. *Ann. Rev. Neurosci.* 15:353–375.

De Bellis, M.D., and Keshavan, M.S. (2003). Sex differences in brain maturation in maltreatment-related pediatric posttraumatic stress disorder. *Neurosci. Biobehav. Rev.* 27:103–117.

De Bellis, M.D., Keshavan, M.S., et al. (1999). A.E. Bennett Research Award: developmental traumatology: Part II. Brain development. *Biol. Psychiatry* 45:1271–1284.

de Quervain, D.J.F., and Margraf, J. (2008). Glucocorticoids for the treatment of post-traumatic stress disorder and phobias: A novel therapeutic approach. *Eur. J. Pharmacol.* 583:365–371.

Etkin, A., and Wager, T. (2007). Functional neuroimaging of anxiety: a meta-analysis of emotional processing in PTSD, social anxiety disorder, and specific phobia. *Am. J. Psychiatry* 164:1476–1488.

Fani, N., Ashraf, A., et al. (2011). Increased neural response to trauma scripts in posttraumatic stress disorder following paroxetine treatment: a pilot study. *Neurosci. Lett.* 491:196–201.

Friedman, M. (2006). Post-traumatic and Acute Stress Disorders: The Latest Assessment and Treatment Strategies. Kansas City, MO: Dean Psych Press.

Gerardi, M., Rothbaum, B.O., et al. (2008). Virtual reality exposure therapy using a virtual Iraq: case report. *J. Trauma. Stress* 21:209–213.

Giedd, J.N., and Rapoport, J.L. (2010). Structural MRI of pediatric brain development: what have we learned and where are we going? *Neuron* 67:728–734.

Gilbert, R., Widom, C.S., et al. (2009). Burden and consequences of child maltreatment in high-income countries. *Lancet* 373:68–81.

Gilbertson, M.W., Shenton, M.E., et al. (2002). Smaller hippocampal volume predicts pathologic vulnerability to psychological trauma. *Nat. Neurosci.* 5:1242–1247.

Hammack, S., Roman, C., et al. (2010). Roles for pituitary adenylate cyclase-activating peptide (PACAP) expression and signaling in the bed nucleus of the stria terminalis (BNST) in mediating the behavioral consequences of chronic stress. *J. Mol. Neurosci.* 42:327–340.

Heim, C., and Nemeroff, C.B. (2001). The role of childhood trauma in the neurobiology of mood and anxiety disorders: preclinical and clinical studies. *Biol. Psychiatry* 49:1023–1039.

Hopper, J.W., Frewen, P.A., et al. (2007). Neural correlates of reexperiencing, avoidance, and dissociation in PTSD: symptom dimensions and emotion dysregulation in responses to script-driven trauma imagery. *J. Trauma. Stress* 20:713–725.

Hughes, K.C., and Shin, L.M. (2011). Functional neuroimaging studies of post-traumatic stress disorder. *Exp. Rev. Neurother.* 11:275–285.

Jovanovic, T., and Ressler, K.J. (2010). How the neurocircuitry and genetics of fear inhibition may inform our understanding of PTSD. *Am. J. Psychiatry* 167:648–662.

Kessler, R.C., Sonnega, A., et al. (1995). Posttraumatic stress disorder in the national comorbidity survey. *Arch. Gen. Psychiatry* 52:1048–1060.

Kilpatrick, D.G., Koenen, K.C., et al. (2007). The serotonin transporter genotype and social support and moderation of posttraumatic stress disorder and depression in hurricane-exposed adults. *Am. J. Psychiatry* 164:1693–1699.

Koenen, K.C., Lyons, M.J., et al. (2003). A high risk twin study of combat-related PTSD comorbidity. *Twin Res.* 6:218–226.

Kolassa, I.-T., Kolassa, S., et al. (2010). The risk of posttraumatic stress disorder after trauma depends on traumatic load and the catechol-O-methyltransferase Val158Met polymorphism. *Biol. Psychiatry* 67:304–308.

Lanius, R.A., Frewen, P.A., et al. (2007). Neural correlates of trauma script-imagery in posttraumatic stress disorder with and without comorbid major depression: a functional MRI investigation. *Psychiatry Res.* 155:45–56.

Lanius, R.A., Williamson, P.C., et al. (2004). The nature of traumatic memories: a 4-T fMRI functional connectivity analysis. *Am. J. Psychiatry* 161:36–44.

Liberzon, I., Krstov, M., et al. (1997). Stress-restress: effects on ACTH and fast feedback. *Psychoneuroendocrinology* 22:443–453.

Mahan, A.L., and Ressler, K.J. (2012). Fear conditioning, synaptic plasticity and the amygdala: implications for posttraumatic stress disorder. *Trends Neurosci.* 35:24–35.

Matsumoto, M., Weickert, C.S., et al. (2003). Catechol *O*-methyltransferase mRNA expression in human and rat brain: evidence for a role in cortical neuronal function. *Neuroscience* 116:127–137.

McGuire, J., Herman, J.P., et al. (2010). Enhanced fear recall and emotional arousal in rats recovering from chronic variable stress. *Phys. Behav.* 101:474–482.

Mercer, K.B., Orcutt, H.K., et al. (2012). Acute and posttraumatic stress symptoms in a prospective gene x environment study of a university campus shooting. *Arch. Gen. Psychiatry* 69(1):89–97.

Morgan, M.A., Romanski, L.M., et al. (1993). Extinction of emotional learning: contribution of medial prefrontal cortex. *Neurosci. Lett.* 163:109–113.

Nemeroff, C.B., Bremner, J.D., et al. (2006). Posttraumatic stress disorder: a state-of-the-science review. *J. Psychiat. Res.* 40:1–21.

Norrholm, S.D., and Jovanovic, T. (2010). Tailoring therapeutic strategies for treating posttraumatic stress disorder symptom clusters. *Neuropsychiatr. Dis. Treat.* 6:517–532.

Norrholm, S.D., Jovanovic, T., et al. (2011). Fear extinction in traumatized civilians with posttraumatic stress disorder: relation to symptom severity. *Biol. Psychiatry* 69:556–563.

Orr, S.P., Metzger, L.J., et al. (2002). Psychophysiology of post-traumatic stress disorder. *Psychiat. Clin. N. Am.* 25:271–293.

Papagni, S.A., Benetti, S., et al. (2011). Effects of stressful life events on human brain structure: a longitudinal voxel-based morphometry study. *Stress* 14:227–232.

Phan, K.L., Wager, T., et al. (2002). Functional neuroanatomy of emotion: a meta-analysis of emotion activation studies in PET and fMRI. *NeuroImage* 16:331–348.

Pitman, R.K., Sanders, K.M., et al. (2002). Pilot study of secondary prevention of posttraumatic stress disorder with propranolol [see comment]. *Biol. Psychiatry* 51:189–192.

Plotsky, P.M., and Meaney, M.J. (1993). Early, postnatal experience alters hypothalamic corticotropin-releasing factor (CRF) mRNA, median eminence CRF content and stress-induced release in adult rats. *Mol. Brain Res.* 18:195–200.

Protopopescu, X., Pan, H., et al. (2005). Differential time courses and specificity of amygdala activity in posttraumatic stress disorder subjects and normal control subjects. *Biol. Psychiatry* 57:464–473.

Rauch, S.L., Van der Kolk, B.A., et al. (1996). A symptom provocation study of posttraumatic stress disorder using positron emission tomography and script-driven imagery. *Arch. Gen. Psychiatry* 53:380–387.

Ravindran, L.N., and Stein, M.B. (2010). Pharmacotherapy of post-traumatic stress disorder. *Curr. Top. Behav. Neurosci.* 2:505–525.

Ressler, K.J., Mercer, K.B., et al. (2011). Post-traumatic stress disorder is associated with PACAP and the PAC1 receptor. *Nature* 470:492–497.

Ressler, K.J., Rothbaum, B.O., et al. (2004). Cognitive enhancers as adjuncts to psychotherapy: use of D-cycloserine in phobic individuals to facilitate extinction of fear. *Arch. Gen. Psychiatry* 61:1136–1144.

Rogers, M.A., Yamasue, H., et al. (2009). Smaller amygdala volume and reduced anterior cingulate gray matter density associated with history of post-traumatic stress disorder. *Psychiat. Res.-Neuroim.* 174:210–216.

Rothbaum, B.O., and Davis, M. (2003). Applying learning principles to the treatment of post-trauma reactions. *Ann. NY Acad. Sci.* 1008:112–121.

Rothbaum, B.O., Meadows, E.A., et al. (2000). Cognitive-behavioral therapy. In: Foa, E.B., et al., eds. Effective Treatments for Posttraumatic Stress Disorder: Practice Guidelines from the International Society for Traumatic Stress Studies. New York: Guilford Press, pp. 60–83.

Roy, M.J., Francis, J., et al. (2010). Improvement in cerebral function with treatment of posttraumatic stress disorder. *Ann. NY Acad. Sci.* 1208:142–149.

Sekiguchi, A., Sugiura, M., et al. (2012). Brain structural changes as vulnerability factors and acquired signs of post-earthquake stress. *Mol. Psychiatry.* [Epub ahead of print.]

Shin, L.M., Rauch, S.L., et al. (2006). Amygdala, medial prefrontal cortex, and hippocampal function in PTSD. *Ann. NY Acad. Sci.* 1071:67–79.

Smith, S.D., Abou-Khalil, B., et al. (2008). Posttraumatic stress disorder in a patient with no left amygdala. *J. Abnorm. Psychol.* 117:479–484.

Strigo, I.A., Simmons, A.N., et al. (2010). Neural correlates of altered pain response in women with posttraumatic stress disorder from intimate partner violence. *Biol. Psychiatry* 68:442–450.

Vermetten, E., Schmahl, C., et al. (2007). Positron tomographic emission study of olfactory induced emotional recall in veterans with and without combat-related posttraumatic stress disorder. *Psychopharmacol. Bull.* 40:8–30.

Vermetten, E., Vythilingam, M., et al. (2003). Long-term treatment with paroxetine increases verbal declarative memory and hippocampal volume in posttraumatic stress disorder. *Biol. Psychiatry* 54:693–702.

Wang, Z., Neylan, T.C., et al. (2010). Magnetic resonance imaging of hippocampal subfields in posttraumatic stress disorder. *Arch. Gen. Psychiatry* 67:296–303.

Woon, F.L., and Hedges, D.W. (2009). Amygdala volume in adults with posttraumatic stress disorder: a meta-analysis. *J. Neuropsychiatry Clin. Neurosci.* 21:5–12.

Woon, F.L., Sood, S., et al. (2010). Hippocampal volume deficits associated with exposure to psychological trauma and posttraumatic stress disorder in adults: a meta-analysis. *Prog. Neuropsychopharmacol. Biol. Psychiatry* 34:1181–1188.

Yamamoto, S., Morinobu, S., et al. (2009). Single prolonged stress: toward an animal model of posttraumatic stress disorder. *Depress. Anxiety* 26:1110–1117.

SECTION VI | SUBSTANCE USE DISORDERS

ANTONELLO BONCI AND NORA D. VOLKOW

More than 80 million Americans have experienced use of nicotine and other drugs of abuse at a level that can create potentially harmful effects. This is why substance abuse and addiction represent a massive burden to society. The negative effects on health result from both the direct pharmacological effects of abused drugs and from the ways in which they are self-administered. A perfect example is the use of non-sterile needles, which has been linked to the increased incidence of transmission of HIV as well as of hepatitis B and C. Additional disorders that all too commonly result from drug use range from lung cancer and cirrhosis to the exacerbation of psychiatric disorders. Moreover substance use disorders (SUD) produce significant and long-term modifications in brain function and behavior that can create havoc in the individuals' life and in social systems including the enormous costs from lost educational opportunities, lost productivity, and associated accidents and the legal repercusions from their use. As a result of direct pharmacological effects and illegal drug trafficking, drugs are also a major cause of violence and crime. The nine chapters included in this section provide a comprehensive overview of the state of the art and the most recent discoveries in the many fields of investigations related to SUD, ranging from basic science to the most recent clinical discoveries.

The first chapter of this section (Chapter 50) provides a comprehensive review of the current animal models used to study drug reward and addiction. During the past decade, the field of behavioral neuroscience has produced more and more sophisticated non-human addiction models, which have greatly expanded our understanding of the complex cadre of symptoms that affect substance abusers. These models are particularly important because it is imperative for neuroscientists to understand the complex interactions between neuronal activity and behavioral aspects of addiction such as craving, drug self-administration, and relapse to drug seeking, which are influenced by environmental exposures (i.e., stressors) and genetics. Likewise, our understanding of the cellular and molecular mechanisms that underlie addictive behaviors has made tremendous progress since the last edition of this book, and will be discussed in Chapter 51. For example, it is well accepted now that drugs of abuse produce many forms of long-term memories at the cellular level, and that these cellular memories play a variety of roles in reorganizing the circuits of the brain and in solidifying pathological, addictive behaviors. Chapter 52 will discuss the recent expansion of knowledge on human genetic studies to better understand some of the fundamental questions that shape the very nature of SUD. This new knowledge includes the role of genetics in drug experimentation and addiction, the

mechanisms by which genetics mediate these effects through their modulation of brain development and function, and how this in turn influences response to the environment (i.e., drugs and stress) in ways that enhance susceptibility or support resilience toward SUD. Chapter 53 focuses on the importance of studying SUD during development, including characterizing the features that render the adolescent brain particularly susceptible to substance abuse.

Chapters 54, 55, and 56 provide a comprehensive review of the technological advances in brain imaging (PET, SPECT, fMRI, and spectroscopic imaging studies) and how these have been used to study the effects of drugs in the human brain. Technology has been used to understand the toxic effects of various drug classes, the mechanisms underlying the rewarding effects of drugs, and the neuroadaptations associated with repeated drug exposure that underlie the addictive process. More recently, studies have started to investigate how genes that increase vulnerability to SUD affect the anatomy, connectivity, and function of the human brain and what functional characteristics of the human brain in turn are associated with enhanced vulnerability (i.e., decreased prefrontal function and decreased striatal D2 receptors).

The many fields of neuroscience focused on SUD described above not only inform us on how the various brain regions are affected by drug exposure and natural rewards, but they have also generated novel therapeutic targets to inhibit drug reward to mitigate symptoms of addiction and prevent relapse. These targets and therapies are discussed in Chapter 57, wherein the authors review the complex issue of bringing novel and promising therapeutic targets from the bench to the bedside. Finally, in Chapter 58, Denise Kandel and coauthors will review recent data on the epidemiology of substance use disorders from both comparative and developmental perspectives, including a discussion of adolescence as a particularly vulnerable period for developing SUD.

The challenges facing investigators parallel those faced by researchers in the addiction field over the last 20 years to a degree, but maintain certain distinctions. A remaining challenge is the integration of discovery from the preclinical to the clinical, and then its translation into interventions that can be used to prevent, treat, and revert the adverse effects of drugs to the human brain. Success in animal models will require that these models more comprehensively emulate the complexity of social systems that influence drug taking and the transition to addiction in humans. Such models should also take into account the complex interactions among environment, genes, development, and the pharmacology of the abused drug, as well as the relevance of studies on different species to human neurobiology. In clinical neuroscience, a new challenge is the standardization of protocols for image acquisition and phenotypic characterization of patients with SUD and their normative that will allow for the integration of imaging and genetic/epigenetic data sets from independent laboratories. Despite these challenges, the opportunities for discovery are greater than they have ever been. The enhanced access to larger databases, more powerful technologies, and a greater understanding of the molecular, cellular, and functional connectivity of the brain allow us to address neurobiological questions that we would have not been able to do 10 years ago. In parallel, an enhanced awareness of the importance of translating neuroscientific findings into the clinic is likely to accelerate the use of that knowledge for more effective interventions for the prevention and treatment of SUD.

50 | ANIMAL MODELS OF ADDICTION

RAFAEL MALDONADO, J. DAVID JENTSCH, BRIGITTE L. KIEFFER, AND
CHRISTOPHER J. EVANS

rug addiction, or substance use disorder (SUD), is a chronic brain disease characterized by the compulsive use of drugs, loss of control over drug-taking in spite of their adverse consequences, and relapse even after long periods of drug abstinence (Koob and Volkow, 2010; O'Brien et al., 1998). Substance use disorder is considered the result of a series of transitions from voluntary use in search of a hedonic effect, to loss of control over this behavior, and ultimately to compulsive behavior (Everitt et al., 2008). Important in the context of mental illness is the high comorbidity of depressive illness and anxiety with SUD and that drugs of abuse taken acutely often alleviate symptoms of these afflictions, yet during abstinence the symptoms of depression and anxiety are exacerbated. Indeed, SUD is comorbid with many psychiatric diseases (clinically referred to as dual diagnosis), including schizophrenia, where incidence of both cigarette and cannabinoid smoking is exceptionally high (Santucci, 2012). In current research of SUD, animal models recapitulate the phenotypes contributing to abuse susceptibility through initial drug taking, habitual drug taking, abstinence, and finally relapse (Fig. 50.1). These models have begun to unravel the molecular, cellular, and behavioral adaptations regulating addictive behaviors in research, which has greatly enriched our understanding of the neurocircuitry mediating learning, motivation, mood, and stress (Koob and Volkow, 2010; Russo et al., 2010). This chapter systematically explores animal models that contribute insights to the addiction cycle as outlined in Figure 50.1. We first cover models assessing reward-related and reinforcement behaviors. We follow this with descriptions of models for abstinence and relapse, and new genetic models that increasingly are facilitating addiction research. Finally, we discuss animal model contributions to susceptibility for initiating additive behaviors.

Maladaptive patterns of reward-seeking and -taking involving natural rewards have been reported to share similarities with those observed in drug addicts. Animal models have revealed that natural rewards activate the mesocorticolimbic system, which mediates the hedonic and motivational aspects of different rewarding stimuli in a manner very similar to drugs of abuse. Repeated activation of this reward pathway leads to neuroadaptive changes that are involved in the progressive behavioral changes caused by natural rewards and drugs. Similar structural plasticity changes in the mesocorticolimbic system have recently been reported after repeated exposure to natural rewards, such as highly caloric food (Johnson and Kenny, 2010), palatable food (Guegan et al., 2012), or sex (Pitchers et al., 2010), all of which can drive the development of compulsive behavior. The similarities and differences among the behavioral disorders promoted by drugs and natural rewards represent a complex and fascinating topic that has been investigated in animal models. Although this area is out of the scope of this chapter, it has been reviewed elsewhere (Olsen, 2011).

MODELS OF REWARD AND REINFORCEMENT

Animal models of reward and reinforcement are the fundamental tools for substance abuse research. Drug consumption is promoted and maintained by the rewarding and reinforcing properties of the drug. These rewarding effects play a crucial role in the initiation of the addictive processes (Koob and Le Moal, 2008). However, it is important to note that although drug consumption is a requirement for the development of addiction, drug intake does not necessarily induce an addicted state. In fact, addiction is defined as a chronic relapsing mental disease and is difficult to comprehensively mimic with the animal models currently available. Most of the animal models described in this chapter have been designed for evaluating particular properties of drugs leading to the development of this disease (reward/reinforcing properties) or some specific manifestations of the disease (tolerance, withdrawal, or relapse).

Animal models for reward and reinforcement use either investigator administration of drug (non-contingent), or self-administration of drug (contingent) in which drug taking is under the control of the animal (Fig. 50.2). Contingent or non-contingent administration paradigms can elicit different behavioral responses that can be reflected at the level of neuronal adaptations. The analysis of drug-induced changes in dendritic spine density and dendritic branching that controls inter-neuronal communication is one example in which differential adaptations in multiple brain regions depend on whether the drug is given contingently or non-contingently (Robinson and Kolb, 2004). Human addictions are most effectively recapitulated in contingent models. However, the value of non-contingent models should not be discounted because they can provide information on adaptations that occur only because of the presence of the drug as well as insight into a subset of reward-related behaviors using uncomplicated drug administration procedures.

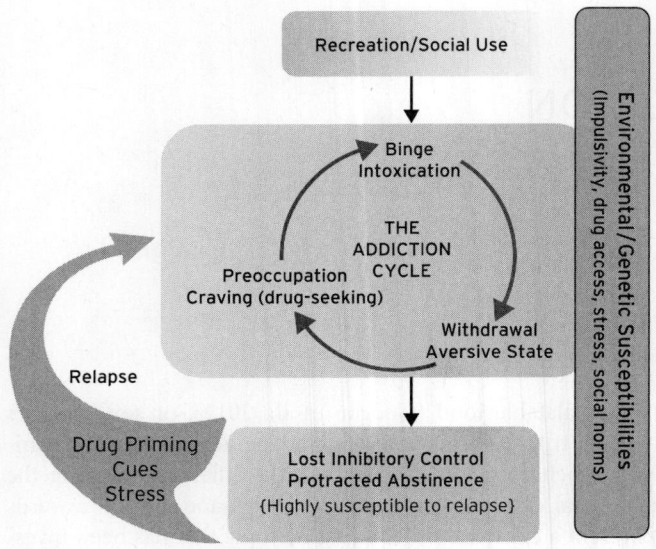

Figure 50.1 *Addiction cycle. In addicted individuals, recreational drug use switches to compulsive drug intake. The addiction cycle typically includes intoxication/withdrawal/craving episodes (Koob and Volkow, 2010). Exiting the cycle requires maintenance of abstinence. Drug abstinence is characterized by a negative affect that strongly contributes to relapse and is often triggered by drug cues, the drug itself, or stress. All aspects of the cycle are subject to modification by genetic–environment interactions.*

All animal models measuring reinforcement and reward require learning. Some acute models of drug administration engage only goal-directed learning, whereas others engage habit learning after extensive repetition of drug administration paradigms. Animal studies in recent years have identified different brain circuitry mediating goal-directed and habit learning with circuitry between the medial prefrontal cortex and dorsomedial striatum mediating goal-directed learning and the sensory-motor cortex to the dorsolateral striatum mediating habit learning (Balleine and O'Doherty, 2010). Reinforcement assays require instrumental actions to obtain the reward, and a learning curve is necessary to develop the instrumental association between an action (e.g., lever push, nose poke, or eye movement) and its contingent effect. Reinforcement can be demonstrated by an increase in responding to a rewarding stimulus (positive reinforcement) or responding to avoid or delay an aversive stimulus (negative reinforcement), and animals will clearly work for both. Models of drug self-administration may not readily distinguish between these two motivational states given that the cycle of addiction includes a dysphoric phase as a consequence of absence of the drug (see Fig. 50.1). Furthermore, certain intrinsic aspects of the models may be aversive (e.g., the anxiety of a novel environment or surgery for catheterization) and the drug may relieve these aversive components as a result of anxiolytic, analgesic, or dissociative properties. Modeling the relief of an aversive stimulus has important implications for certain aspects of human behavior in which amelioration of pain, depression, or anxiety favor drug use. However, the circuitry recruited for euphoric reward will undoubtedly differ from the circuitry recruited to obfuscate an aversive stimulus (Koob and Volkow, 2010).

SELF-ADMINISTRATION

Self-administration methods are considered the most reliable and predictive animal models to directly evaluate the

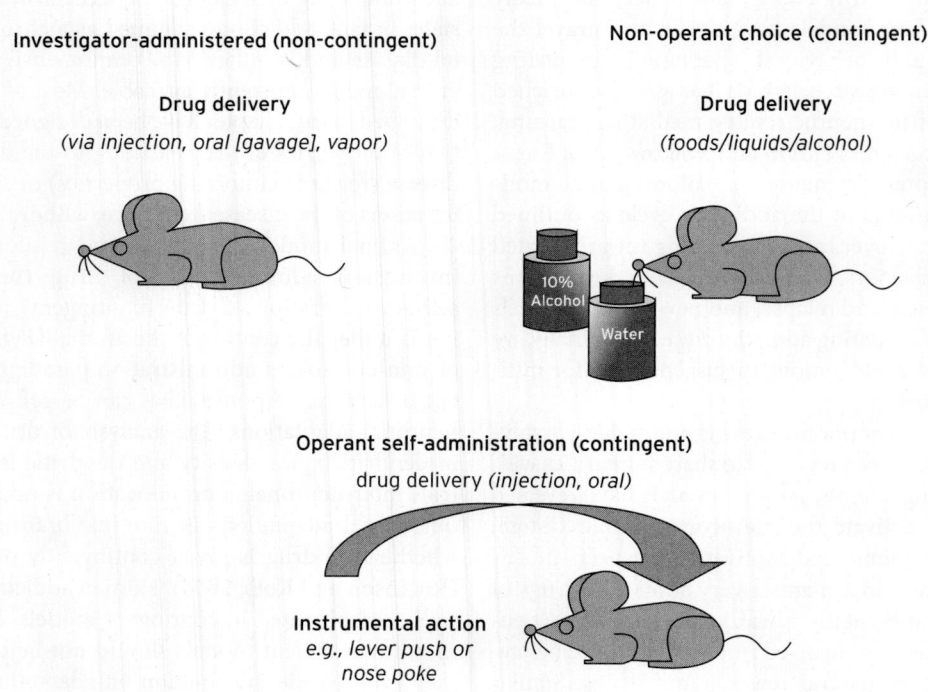

Figure 50.2 *Drug administration.*

reinforcing properties of a drug. These procedures mimic drug-taking behavior in humans and are widely used by many researchers. The neurobiological mechanisms involved in drug self-administration in animals are assumed to be similar to those underlying drug intake in humans (Maldonado et al., 2011). Operant and non-operant procedures can be used in these self-administration models. Non-operant paradigms involve the consumption of a freely available drug, are centered on the amount of drug consumed, and are restricted in rodents to oral self-administration. These non-operant methods are widely used to study alcohol-rewarding effects, and they have also been used less frequently with other drugs of abuse, such as nicotine, cocaine, amphetamine, and morphine (Sanchis-Segura and Spanagel, 2006). Oral ethanol non-operant self-administration procedures present high reliability and predictive value as models of human alcohol consumption. Indeed, rodents drink alcohol when using the oral route, whereas they hardly consume this drug through other routes of self-administration (Sanchis-Segura and Spanagel, ·2006; Spanagel and Zieglgansberger, 1997). In contrast, rodents show only modest motivation to self-administer other drugs by the oral route, including opioids or psychostimulants (Meisch, 2001), and very specific and sometimes biased procedures are required to induce their oral consumption. Therefore, the behavioral responses evaluated in those particular situations do not necessarily reflect the rewarding properties of these drugs. In the most currently used oral alcohol self-administration procedures, rodents have simultaneous access to two bottles, one containing an aqueous alcohol solution and another containing water (Spanagel and Zieglgansberger, 1997). The consumption of alcohol in these paradigms is greatly influenced by the genetic background and animal species used. The alcohol concentration represents another critical factor that can even bias the outcome because low concentrations may have a mild-sweet taste, whereas overly high concentrations have an aversive flavor (Sanchis-Segura and Spanagel, 2006). Other critical factors in these paradigms are the temporal accessibility to alcohol (Vengeliene et al., 2012), and the kind and number of available bottles and/or other reinforcers (Tordoff and Bachmanov, 2003). In general, alcohol consumption increases when rodents are given restricted access to the drug (e.g., every other day) or a higher number of alternative alcohol solutions are presented.

Operant paradigms require that the animal performs an instrumental response to self-administer the drug. In these models, the animal learns to maintain a behavioral response, typically by pressing a lever or nose poking in a hole, to obtain a positive reinforcer (drug delivery) that is delivered contingently after completion of the schedule requirement (Maldonado et al., 2011). The operant chamber levers and nose poking holes also transmit operant response. The response in the active manipulandum is linked to the delivery of the drug, whereas the response in the inactive manipulandum results in the delivery of the drug vehicle or lacks any programmed consequence. These operant procedures are considered by most researchers to be reliable models of

drug consumption in humans with a high predictive value. The route of administration most commonly used in these operant procedures is intravenous delivery of all the prototypical drugs with the exception of alcohol, which usually requires the delivery of an oral solution. However, these operant procedures are not specifically associated with any route of administration, and multiple additional routes have been successfully used, such as intracranial, intraventricular, or intragastric delivery.

Different single and complex schedule requirements to obtain the reinforcer can be programmed in these operant paradigms. The schedules most frequently used are the fixed ratio and progressive ratio schedule of reinforcement programs. Under a fixed ratio schedule, the drug is delivered each time a preselected number of responses are completed in the active manipulandum. Under the progressive ratio schedule, the response requirement to deliver the drug escalates according to an arithmetic progression. The common index of performance evaluated in this last schedule is the highest number of responses that the animal accomplishes to obtain a single infusion of drug (the break point), which provides information about its motivation for the drug. The analysis of this instrumental response provides valuable data about different behavioral aspects of drug consumption. After acquisition of the operant task, the behavioral response can be extinguished by exposing the animals to an additional training in which the reward is no longer available. The operant behavior to seek the drug can be then reinstated by using different stimuli.

Rodents typically maintain an operant behavior to self-administer all the prototypical drugs of abuse, including opioids, psychostimulants, synthetic drugs, nicotine, and cannabinoids (Maldonado et al., 2011). In the case of cannabinoids, rodents self-administer synthetic cannabinoids but not Δ9-tetrahydrocannabinol, the main psychoactive component in *Cannabis sativa*, which is only self-administered by monkeys (Tanda et al., 2000). In rodents, these operant self-administration models were first validated in rats, and then adapted to mice. Reliable operant models of acquisition and relapse of morphine, cocaine, ecstasy, alcohol, nicotine, and synthetic cannabinoids self-administration are also now available in mice (Martin-Garcia et al., 2009; Mendizabal et al., 2006; Soria et al., 2008). Application of these new models to the different lines of genetically modified mice will yield more insights in the future.

CONDITIONED PLACE PREFERENCE

In these paradigms, the subjective effects of a drug are repeatedly paired to a previously neutral stimulus. Through this repeated conditioning process, the neutral stimulus acquires the ability to act as a conditioned stimulus, and the animal will prefer or avoid this conditioned stimulus depending on the rewarding or aversive effects produced by the drug (Fig. 50.3). The most commonly used paradigms apply a spatial environmental stimulus as the conditioned stimulus and the animal will show a conditioned place preference or aversion for the

A

B

C

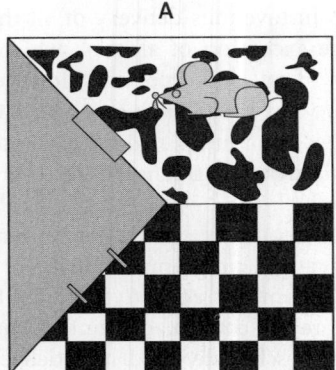
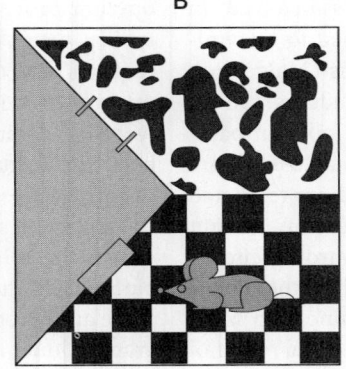
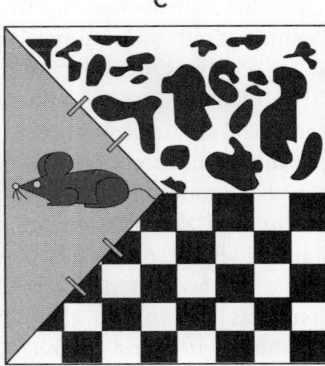

Figure 50.3 (A) *Drug administered non-contingently (repeated three to five times on alternate days) and the animal confined to one compartment ("cow pattern" in this example but the side would be a randomized group). (B) Drug vehicle given to the animal confined to the other compartment ("checked pattern") on alternate days from drug. (C) Animal put in the neutral chamber (gray triangle) with access to both the drug- and vehicle-paired compartments.*

environment associated with the effects of the drug or its withdrawal. Although a conditioned approach/avoidance toward specific stimuli can also occur in humans as a result of drug consumption (Bardo and Bevins 2000), the place conditioning paradigms are not primarily intended to model any particular feature of human behavior. These paradigms mainly represent an indirect assessment of the rewarding or aversive effects of a drug or its withdrawal, by measuring the response of the animal toward the conditioned stimulus. Drugs of abuse display a differential ability to produce conditioned place preference. Opioids and psychostimulants easily produce robust place preference over a wide range of experimental conditions, whereas other drugs, such as ethanol, cannabinoids, or nicotine, produce more inconsistent results. The caveats of the place preference assay are many, with issues of memory function, circadian rhythm, and that the animals non-contingently receive the drug in a novel environment, which has consequences for eliciting stress. Despite this, conditioned place preference has been an informative and widely utilized behavioral model for understanding parameters that disrupt or enhance the rewarding effects of abused drugs.

INTRACRANIAL SELF-STIMULATION

Intracranial electric self-stimulation (ICSS) procedures were essential in the discovery of the brain reward circuits. These paradigms are now widely used to study the effects of acute and chronic drugs of abuse administration and withdrawal in the activity of the reward circuits (Sanchis-Segura and Spanagel, 2006). In this paradigm, animals are trained to maintain an operant behavior so as to obtain an electric pulse through an electrode that has been previously implanted in a reward-related brain site, most frequently the lateral hypothalamic area. The threshold of the minimal current needed to promote intracranial electric self-stimulation is estimated. A drug that stimulates the reward circuit will decrease this threshold, which is related to its rewarding properties, whereas a drug having aversive effects will enhance the minimal current required to maintain the self-stimulation (Markou and Koob, 1993). The ICSS threshold

increases after prolonged drug administration and during withdrawal. This is interpreted as a desensitized reward system and parallels other behavioral and imaging evidence that SUD can, over time, attenuate the basal functioning of the dopaminergic reward circuitry (Kenny, 2007).

MODELS OF WITHDRAWAL AND RELAPSE

Withdrawal from drugs of abuse can be an important aspect of SUD because withdrawal can promote a state at both the behavioral and cellular level that supports negative reinforcement. Drug withdrawal has multiple phenotypes, including physical symptoms, craving, and the modulation of affect (Koob and Volkow, 2010). Symptoms of acute and protracted withdrawal are sensitizers for relapse and can serve as major drivers for the addiction cycle (see Fig. 50.1). Although the acute physical withdrawal behaviors caused by individual drugs appear very different, the prolonged withdrawal phenotype (negative affect, craving behavior, and vulnerability to stress) begin to emerge as common phenotypes. This is reflected by merging transcript profiles in the extended amygdala, one of the brain regions involved in emotional responses following protracted abstinence of several drugs of abuse (Le Merrer et al., 2012).

PHYSICAL WITHDRAWAL

Depressant drugs such as opioids, alcohol, or benzodiazepines have dramatic acute withdrawal symptoms. In the case of alcohol and benzodiazepines these result in seizures, which can be lethal. In acute withdrawal from opioids, there are a classical set of physical symptoms that can be readily measured in rodents and include jumping, wet dog shakes, weight loss, paw tremors, diarrhea, and piloerection. In the most frequently used model of opioid withdrawal, the symptoms are triggered by administration of an opioid receptor antagonist such as naloxone. Similar antagonist-precipitated withdrawal assays have been used for measures of nicotine and cannabinoid physical withdrawal, although the symptoms are considerably less robust than opioid withdrawal (Trigo et al., 2010). Cocaine and other psychostimulants do not elicit physical withdrawal symptoms that can be easily measured in animal models or human subjects. This demonstrates that physical withdrawal is not a predicate for addiction.

WITHDRAWAL AND AFFECTIVE STATE/CRAVING

Although many studies have focused on the physical aspects of withdrawal, the affective state and drug craving (the desire to attain the drug state) are aspects that deserve focus, given their role in triggering relapse and modeling the primary mental affliction of SUD. In the case of opioid withdrawal, antagonist precipitation cannot be used to assess changes in affect because antagonists such as naloxone and naltrexone are highly aversive in rodents that have never been exposed to an opioid drug. This aversion in drug-naïve mice has been shown to be caused by a constitutive hedonic tone as a result of proenkephalin-derived opioid peptides activating mu-opioid receptors (Skoubis et al., 2005). Affective state and craving is best modeled in animals simply withdrawn from the drug. Recent studies have assessed animals during both acute and protracted withdrawal. Significantly, although physical signs of withdrawal diminish rapidly and within a few days after opioid withdrawal, some phenotypes strengthen, including social interaction deficits and depressive phenotypes (Goeldner et al., 2011). The strengthening of such behaviors after protracted abstinence is associated with deficits in serotonin and can be reversed with the serotonin membrane transporter blocker fluoxetine. Incubation after acute withdrawal also enhances drug-seeking induced by drug-related stimuli (Weiss, 2010).

RELAPSE

Relapse susceptibility is an extremely persistent and robust phenotype in both humans and animals (Wikler and Pescor, 1970) and can get progressively stronger in response to some triggers during abstinence (Weiss, 2010). Relapse models in animals first require the animal to learn a drug self-administration task, although a place-preference paradigm could also be used. The animal receives extinction training so as to erode the established associations, followed by test sessions in which behavior spontaneously recovers or is reinstated by a drug-related cue, the drug, or stress (Sinha et al., 2011). The use of extinction training is not an optimum method to reduce drug-seeking behavior because it does not accurately recapitulate the human experience and, in fact, changes the underlying neuroadaptations mediating drug-seeking and -taking. However, without extinction, extinguishing drug-seeking may not be practically feasible given the strength and longevity of reward-related behaviors. In humans, relapse happens when the motivation to abstain is overwhelmed by the motivation to take the drug. This stands in contrast to animal models in which the motivation to take the drug overwhelms extinction-related learning. New research should focus on the development of models that emphasize conflict between the motivational states that excite and inhibit drug-taking and the role for cognitive control circuitry in these circumstances.

MODELS OF DRUG ADDICTION

As discussed, the animal models available for evaluating drug reward and reinforcement, as well as withdrawal, have been very useful in clarifying the neurobiological basis of drug taking and specific features of the addictive process. However, addiction is a chronic relapsing disorder characterized by compulsive drug use maintained despite adverse consequences for the user (O'Brien et al., 1998). Behavioral models that resemble the main diagnostic criteria for addiction have only recently been studied using animal models. Two independent research groups have validated behavioral models of compulsive drug-seeking in rodents, resembling addictive behavior in humans (Belin et al., 2008; Deroche-Gamonet et al., 2004; Vanderschuren and Everitt, 2004). These models evaluate the persistence of drug-seeking and -taking in the face of punishment, resistance to extinction, and exaggerated motivation to obtain the drug. In one animal model, the motivation for the drug determined by the break point (the maximal amount of work that the animal performs before cessation of responding) was abnormally high under these conditions. Indeed, a break point greater than 500 operant actions to obtain a single cocaine injection in "addict rats" was reported in these models (Deroche-Gamonet et al., 2004). Although there is significant promise in this area of work, it remains relatively underutilized and studied.

GENETIC ANIMAL MODELS FOR ADDICTION RESEARCH

Multiple studies in humans (family twin and adoption studies) point to a major genetic component in the etiologies of SUD (Ho et al., 2010). Rodent models have been developed to identify genes and pathways related to this disease. Three major approaches are well exampled in alcohol research (Crabbe, 2008). The first approach has used inbred lines with different SUD propensity. A second approach has used genetic selection for phenotypes related to SUD. A third approach has been the targeted modification of the genome, a strategy that has probably been the most informative in identification of relevant primary targets and reward-dependent mechanisms. What is becoming clear from genetic association analysis in both human and animal subjects is that SUD is an exceptionally complex disorder with multiple genetic contributions that modify susceptibility to different drugs and different aspects of the disorder in selective environments (Ho et al., 2010). This complexity of genetic contribution and interaction with environment makes human analysis an ominous task requiring large cohorts for valid analysis. However, recently the identification of one locus in a cluster of nicotinic receptors, the *CHRNA5-A3-B4* cluster on chromosome 15, has been repeatedly associated with both lung cancer and smoking (Bierut, 2010). Ongoing research is elucidating how this locus modulates disease susceptibility in animal models with genetically down- or up-regulated levels of the nicotinic receptor subunits in this area of the genome (Fowler et al., 2011; Gallego et al., 2012).

During the past decade there has been an explosion of genetically modified mouse models to determine the effects of specific genes on SUD. The endogenous opioid system provides an outstanding example of progress that can be achieved with targeted modification of genome (Le Merrer et al., 2009). The genetic ablation of the mu-opioid receptor (mu knockout mice) eliminates the place preference, self-administration, and analgesic effects of drugs such as morphine and fentanyl. Intriguingly the mu knockouts additionally exhibit diminished or abolished reward-associated behaviors for nicotine, alcohol, and cannabinoids, which do not directly activate opioid receptors. These data are suggestive of the recruitment of the endogenous opioid system for the rewarding experience by several non-opioid drugs. Indeed proenkephalin knockout mice, which lack one of the three precursors of endogenous opioid peptides, exhibit the same reduced-reward phenotype as mu-opioid receptor knockout mice.

Genetically modified mice have also contributed to our understanding of the dark side of addiction. Kappa-opioid receptor knockout mice as well as mice null for the gene encoding kappa-opioid receptor ligands (prodynorphin), both exhibit a phenotype of reduced stress (Bruchas et al., 2010). Mice null for the endogenous kappa-opioid system do not show stress-induced relapse for cocaine and relieve the aversive component of tetrahydrocannabinol in place preference assays (Maldonado et al., 2011). Kappa antagonists are now a major focus for drug development for the treatment of relapse and other stress-related disorders. The era of developing new animal models by genetic modification has not ended and the new era of conditional knockout and knockin models are revealing cell types, circuits, and brain regions involved in selective aspects of SUD. Furthermore, as genetic analysis begins to reveal new genes of interest, such as in the case of the alpha 5 nicotinic receptor for smoking, animal models provide the tools to understand the genetic influence mechanistically and perhaps enlighten therapeutic approaches.

ANIMAL MODELS OF ADDICTION SUSCEPTIBILITY

A variety of biological and environmental factors have been hypothesized to prospectively (causally) influence SUD. These hypothesized relationships can often be studied in a controlled, experimental manner in animal models because of the capacity to selectively manipulate all factors but the one under study and prospectively examine the characteristics of the phenotypic relationship. These procedures overcome the confounds associated with covariation of phenotypes (Lynch et al., 2002) in human subjects as well as the limitations of purely retrospective analyses.

SEX

In many ways, the potential for animal models of vulnerability to drug abuse is best demonstrated by studies of sex effects on drug reinforcement. In most Western societies, the use of licit and illicit substances with addiction liability is more common in males than females (Lynch et al., 2002). On the other hand, it has been suggested that among those persons who sample the drug, the development of a compulsive, clinically significant form of drug-seeking and -taking occurs more readily in females (Lynch et al., 2002). Because of the absence of social factors that likely inhibit drug sampling in human females, rodent models are useful in interrogating the influence of purely biological dimensions of sex on the phases of drug use, abuse, and dependence that follow initial sampling. Significantly, female rats have been shown, in multiple laboratories and using multiple preparations, to more readily acquire drug self-administration, self-administer larger amounts of drug, to reinstate drug self-administration, and develop inflexible patterns of drug intake (Lynch et al., 2002; Perry and Carroll, 2008). Subsequent studies have revealed the partial contributions of estrogenic hormones to these differences (Lynch et al., 2002), but it remains unknown how genetic aspects of sex contribute to gender differences. These results demonstrate the potential for animal models to reveal important biological predetermining factors, particularly when those factors are sometimes overridden by environmental or psychosocial factors.

BIOBEHAVIORAL PHENOTYPES

Substance use disorders cosegregate with a number of biobehavioral preclinical or clinical phenotypes. One such relationship is the apparent comorbidity between SUD and several mental disorders, including attention deficit/hyperactivity disorder (ADHD) (Groman et al., 2009). Children diagnosed with ADHD are at greater risk for the development of a SUD during their lifetime, particularly if they are not successfully medicated. There are many theories regarding the causal basis of this comorbidity. On one hand, some argue that substance use in the teenage and adult years represents a form of "self-medication" in which patients consume nicotine and/or stimulants because of their ability to remediate inattentive and/or hyperactive symptoms. A different view, however, is that individuals with ADHD are susceptible for substance misuse because they exhibit novelty seeking, behavioral impulsivity, and/or differential reward sensitivity, which independently predispose them for dyscontrolled reward-seeking behaviors (Groman et al., 2009). These and other phenotypes that segregate with SUD may represent predisposing factors that are worthy of causal and biological dissection in animal models.

NOVELTY-SEEKING

Novelty-seeking traits in humans—defined as the propensity to be attracted to environments associated with novelty, sensation, and/or risk—are associated with SUD, and novelty reactivity in rats has been conceptually linked with novelty-seeking in humans (Dellu et al., 1996). One of the earliest demonstrations that traits related to novelty reactivity predict individual differences in response to illicit substances of abuse was that, in outbred rats, the magnitude of the locomotor response evoked by a novel environment positively predicted subsequent acquisition of an instrumental response reinforced by drugs (Piazza et al., 1989). This relationship is present in both male and female subjects, and is under genetic control in that it can be enriched by breeding for the phenotype. So-called "high responders" (in the novel environment) are therefore more susceptible to the reinforcing effects of stimulants and opiates under some circumstances.

On the other hand, psychomotor reactivity to novelty may only be one dimension of novelty-seeking in humans because the trait is primarily defined as the propensity to seek out and participate in novel and exciting circumstances. With that in mind, it is interesting that individual differences in novelty preference or novelty reinforcement in rats has also been linked to drug self-administration phenotypes in a manner that extends beyond the explanatory value of simple novelty reactivity (Belin et al., 2011), suggesting that the overall relationship is quite complex.

IMPULSIVITY

Novelty-seeking has been conceptually linked to another dimension of temperament often referred to as impulsivity—a tendency to act or react with limited forethought and/or a tendency of one's behavior to be driven by immediate, rather than delayed, outcomes associated with behavior (Evenden, 1999). High impulsivity is itself a phenotype that segregates with SUD and that likely explains the dysregulated pattern of drug intake in some individuals with drug abuse and dependence (Jentsch and Taylor, 1999). Because of evidence that exposure to drugs of abuse is sufficient to elicit impulsive patterns of responding (Izquierdo and Jentsch, 2012; Jentsch and Taylor, 1999), it was unclear that impulsivity in SUD was a preexisting vulnerability factor.

Recent studies in rodents, however, have dramatically clarified this view. Rapid response impulsivity (acting without forethought) and impulsive choice (diminished sensitivity to delayed, as opposed to immediate, outcomes) both predict high liability for drug self-administration (Dalley et al., 2007; Izquierdo and Jentsch, 2012; Perry and Carroll, 2008), although different aspects of impulsivity have been revealed to dissociably relate to distinct aspects of self-administration (e.g., initial acquisition versus motivation to consume the drug versus escalation versus extinction versus reinstatement). Impulsivity traits in animal models are under genetic control and are linked to reduced dopamine D2-like receptor availability/function in brain (Dalley et al., 2007; Laughlin et al., 2011). Although all the details of this relationship remain to be exposed, it is clear that a multidimensional model that incorporates both the phenotypic complexity of impulsivity and drug reinforcement is required. In this sense, the results of the animal models not only generally clarify the causal nature of the relationship between impulsivity and drug abuse phenotypes, but can also generate new hypotheses about the behavioral and molecular architecture of this relationship that can be subsequently tested in humans.

REWARD SENSITIVITY

It has been suggested that individual differences in the positive subjective response to reward is an independent predictor of liability for SUD and that so-called reward sensitivity can be phenotypically indexed by specific behavioral paradigms, such as the sweet flavor preference (Carroll et al., 2008). In other words, high preference for sweet flavors indicates high reward sensitivity, and the hypothesis is that reward sensitivity in turn translates into individual differences in sensitivity to drug reward and/or reinforcement. In a comprehensive series of studies, Carroll and colleagues have provided empirical support for this hypothesis in rat models. Saccharin preference (a phenotype that indicates sweet, but not calorie, preference) is a genetically influenced trait, in the sense that it can be enriched by breeding for the phenotype. Rats bred for high saccharin preference more readily self-administer cocaine and opioids, compared with rats bred for low saccharin preference, with a greater effect in females than males (Perry and Carroll, 2008).

SUMMARY

The concept that animal models can disambiguate the causal nature of the relationship between putative biological and behavioral susceptibility factors and SUD is not new, but recent years have seen a dramatic increase in the sophisticated use of these systems to do so. For those relationships now exposed (e.g., among novelty-seeking, impulsivity, reward sensitivity, and drug self-administration), it is now possible to begin taking apart the genetic, molecular, and circuit mechanisms that mediate the relationship. Presumably, these biological factors are useful for a variety of reasons, including their ability to serve as biomarkers of risk and as targets for prevention of SUD.

DISCLOSURES

Dr. Maldonado receives financial support and/or research contracts from Laboratorios Esteve SA, Ferrer SA, Pharmaleads, and a grant from Marató TV3. He currently holds a patent under exploitation by Panlab SA.

Dr. Jentsch and Dr. Evans have no conflicts of interest to disclose. They are both funded by the NIDA and NINDS.

Dr. Kieffer has no conflicts of interests to disclose. She is funded by academic institutions (CNRS, INSERM and Université de Strasbourg and the National Institutes of Health (National Institute of Drug Addiction, grant #05010 and National Institute on Alcohol Abuse and Alcoholism, grant #16658).

REFERENCES

Balleine, B.W., and O'Doherty, J.P. (2010). Human and rodent homologies in action control: corticostriatal determinants of goal-directed and habitual action. *Neuropsychopharmacology* 35(1):48–69.

Bardo, M.T., and Bevins, R.A. (2000). Conditioned place preference: what does it add to our preclinical understanding of drug reward? *Psychopharmacology* 153(1):31–43.

Belin, D., Berson, N., et al. (2011). High-novelty-preference rats are predisposed to compulsive cocaine self-administration. *Neuropsychopharmacology* 36(3):569–579.

Belin, D., Mar, A.C., et al. (2008). High impulsivity predicts the switch to compulsive cocaine-taking. *Science* 320(5881):1352–1355.

Bierut, L.J. (2010). Convergence of genetic findings for nicotine dependence and smoking related diseases with chromosome 15q24-25. *Trends Pharmacol. Sci.* 31(1):46–51.

Bruchas, M.R., Land, B.B., et al. (2010). The dynorphin/kappa opioid system as a modulator of stress-induced and pro-addictive behaviors. *Brain Res.* 1314:44–55.

Carroll, M.E., Morgan, A.D., et al. (2008). Selective breeding for differential saccharin intake as an animal model of drug abuse. *Behav. Pharmacol.* 19(5–6):435–460.

Crabbe, J.C. (2008). Review: neurogenetic studies of alcohol addiction. *Philos. Trans. R. Soc. Lond. B Biol. Sci.* 363(1507):3201–3211.

Dalley, J.W., Fryer, T.D., et al. (2007). Nucleus accumbens D2/3 receptors predict trait impulsivity and cocaine reinforcement. *Science* 315(5816): 1267–1270.

Dellu, F., Piazza, P.V., et al. (1996). Novelty-seeking in rats: biobehavioral characteristics and possible relationship with the sensation-seeking trait in man. *Neuropsychobiology* 34(3):136–145.

Deroche-Gamonet, V., Belin, D., et al. (2004). Evidence for addiction-like behavior in the rat. *Science* 305(5686):1014–1017.

Evenden, J.L. (1999). Varieties of impulsivity. *Psychopharmacology* 146(4):348–361.

Everitt, B.J., Belin, D., et al. (2008). Review. Neural mechanisms underlying the vulnerability to develop compulsive drug-seeking habits and addiction. *Philos. Trans. R. Soc. Lond. B Biol. Sci.* 363(1507):3125–3135.

Fowler, C.D., Lu, Q., et al. (2011). Habenular alpha5 nicotinic receptor subunit signalling controls nicotine intake. *Nature* 471(7340):597–601.

Gallego, X., Molas, S., et al. (2012). Overexpression of the CHRNA5/A3/B4 genomic cluster in mice increases the sensitivity to nicotine and modifies its reinforcing effects. *Amino Acids* 43(2):897–909.

Goeldner, C., Lutz, P.E., et al. (2011). Impaired emotional-like behavior and serotonergic function during protracted abstinence from chronic morphine. *Biol. Psychiatry* 69(3):236–244.

Groman, S.M., James, A.S., et al. (2009). Poor response inhibition: at the nexus between substance abuse and attention deficit/hyperactivity disorder. *Neurosci. Biobehav. Rev.* 33(5):690–698.

Guegan, T., Cutando, L., et al. (2012). Operant behavior to obtain palatable food modifies neuronal plasticity in the brain reward circuit. *Eur. Neuropsychopharmacol.*

Ho, M.K., Goldman, D., et al. (2010). Breaking barriers in the genomics and pharmacogenetics of drug addiction. *Clin. Pharmacol. Ther.* 88(6):779–791.

Izquierdo, A., and Jentsch, J.D. (2012). Reversal learning as a measure of impulsive and compulsive behavior in addictions. *Psychopharmacology* 219(2):607–620.

Jentsch, J.D., and Taylor, J.R. (1999). Impulsivity resulting from frontostriatal dysfunction in drug abuse: implications for the control of behavior by reward-related stimuli. *Psychopharmacology* 146(4):373–390.

Johnson, P.M., and Kenny, P.J. (2010). Dopamine D2 receptors in addiction-like reward dysfunction and compulsive eating in obese rats. *Nat. Neurosci.* 13(5):635–641.

Kenny, P.J. (2007). Brain reward systems and compulsive drug use. *Trends Pharmacol. Sci.* 28(3):135–141.

Koob, G.F., and Le Moal, M. (2008). Review. Neurobiological mechanisms for opponent motivational processes in addiction. *Philos. Trans. R. Soc. Lond. B Biol. Sci.* 363(1507):3113–3123.

Koob, G.F., and Volkow, N.D. (2010). Neurocircuitry of addiction. *Neuropsychopharmacology* 35(1):217–238.

Laughlin, R.E., Grant, T.L., et al. (2011). Genetic dissection of behavioral flexibility: reversal learning in mice. *Biol. Psychiatry* 69(11):1109–1116.

Le Merrer, J., Becker, J.A., et al. (2009). Reward processing by the opioid system in the brain. *Physiol. Rev.* 89(4):1379–1412.

Le Merrer, J., Befort, K., et al. (2012). Protracted abstinence from distinct drugs of abuse shows regulation of a common gene network. *Addict. Biol.* 17(1):1–12.

Lynch, W.J., Roth, M.E., et al. (2002). Biological basis of sex differences in drug abuse: preclinical and clinical studies. *Psychopharmacol. (Berl.).* 164(2):121–137.

Markou, A., and Koob, G.F. (1993). Intracranial self-stimulation thresholds as a measure of reward. In: Sahgal, A., ed. *Behavioral Neuroscience: A Practical Approach.* New York: Oxford University Press, pp. 93–115.

Martin-Garcia, E., Barbano, M.F., et al. (2009). New operant model of nicotine-seeking behaviour in mice. *Int. J. Neuropsychopharmacol.* 12(3):343–356.

Meisch, R.A. (2001). Oral drug self-administration: an overview of laboratory animal studies. *Alcohol* 24(2):117–128.

Mendizabal, V., Zimmer, A., et al. (2006). Involvement of kappa/dynorphin system in WIN 55,212-2 self-administration in mice. *Neuropsychopharmacology* 31(9):1957–1966.

O'Brien, C.P., Childress, A.R., et al. (1998). Conditioning factors in drug abuse: can they explain compulsion? *J. Psychopharmacol.* 12(1):15–22.

Olsen, C.M. (2011). Natural rewards, neuroplasticity, and non-drug addictions. *Neuropharmacology* 61(7):1109–1122.

Perry, J.L., and Carroll, M.E. (2008). The role of impulsive behavior in drug abuse. *Psychopharmacology* 200(1):1–26.

Piazza, P.V., Deminiere, J.M., et al. (1989). Factors that predict individual vulnerability to amphetamine self-administration. *Science* 245(4925):1511–1513.

Pitchers, K.K., Balfour, M.E., et al. (2010). Neuroplasticity in the mesolimbic system induced by natural reward and subsequent reward abstinence. *Biol. Psychiatry* 67(9):872–879.

Robinson, T.E., and Kolb, B. (2004). Structural plasticity associated with exposure to drugs of abuse. *Neuropharmacology* 47(Suppl 1):33–46.

Russo, S.J., Dietz, D.M., et al. (2010). The addicted synapse: mechanisms of synaptic and structural plasticity in nucleus accumbens. *Trends Neurosci.* 33(6):267–276.

Sanchis-Segura, C., and Spanagel, R. (2006). Behavioural assessment of drug reinforcement and addictive features in rodents: an overview. *Addict. Biol.* 11(1):2–38.

Santucci, K. (2012). Psychiatric disease and drug abuse. *Curr. Opin. Pediatr.* 24(2):233–237.

Sinha, R., Shaham, Y., et al. (2011). Translational and reverse translational research on the role of stress in drug craving and relapse. *Psychopharmacology* 218(1):69–82.

Skoubis, P.D., Lam, H.A., et al. (2005). Endogenous enkephalins, not endorphins, modulate basal hedonic state in mice. *Eur. J. Neurosci.* 21(5):1379–1384.

Soria, G., Barbano, M.F., et al. (2008). A reliable method to study cue-, priming-, and stress-induced reinstatement of cocaine self-administration in mice. *Psychopharmacology* 199(4):593–603.

Spanagel, R., and Zieglgansberger, W. (1997). Anti-craving compounds for ethanol: new pharmacological tools to study addictive processes. *Trends Pharmacol. Sci.* 18(2):54–59.

Tanda, G., Munzar, P., et al. (2000). Self-administration behavior is maintained by the psychoactive ingredient of marijuana in squirrel monkeys. *Nat. Neurosci.* 3(11):1073–1074.

Tordoff, M.G., and Bachmanov, A.A. (2003). Influence of the number of alcohol and water bottles on murine alcohol intake. *Alcohol Clin. Exp. Res.* 27(4):600–606.

Trigo, J.M., Martin, E.-Garcia, et al. (2010). The endogenous opioid system: a common substrate in drug addiction. *Drug Alcohol Depen.* 108(3):183–194.

Vanderschuren, L.J., and Everitt, B.J. (2004). Drug seeking becomes compulsive after prolonged cocaine self-administration. *Science* 305(5686):1017–1019.

Vengeliene, V., Noori, H.R., et al. (2013). The use of a novel drinkometer system for assessing pharmacological treatment effects on ethanol consumption in rats. *Alcohol Clin. Exp. Res.* 37(Suppl 1):E322–E328.

Weiss, F. (2010). Advances in animal models of relapse for addiction research. In: Kuhn, C.M., and Koob, G.F., eds. *Advances in the Neuroscience of Addiction.* Boca Raton, FL: CRC Press.

Wikler, A., and Pescor, F.T. (1970). Persistence of "relapse-tendencies" of rats previously made physically dependent on morphine. *Psychopharmacologia* 16(5):375–384.

51 | CELLULAR AND MOLECULAR MECHANISMS OF ADDICTION

KATHRYN J. REISSNER AND PETER W. KALIVAS

The social, economic, and public health impact of addiction to drugs of abuse is well addressed throughout this volume. Indeed, the public health cost of addiction to substances both legal and illicit places tremendous burden on the individual and society. The estimated monetary cost of addiction within the United States reaches $500 billion per year (Abuse, 2011; Koob et al., 2009; Uhl and Grow, 2004). Of the 2.4 million deaths in the United States in 2000, more than 450,000 were attributed to smoking, 67,000 to alcohol-related deaths, and nearly 10,000 to illicit drug use (Keeney, 2008). In 2009, illicit drug-related deaths had increased to nearly 37,000 per annum (Kochanek et al., 2011). These statistics underscore the importance of understanding and treating addiction disorders. Thus, a majority priority of addiction research is to investigate the nature of drug-dependent pathology at the behavioral, neuroanatomical, and cellular levels, as they contribute to the biological mechanisms responsible for the transition from social use through stages of abuse and compulsive drug seeking.

Addiction to drugs of abuse is characterized not only by increased motivation to obtain the drug, but also by decreased motivation to obtain natural reward and loss of control over behavior. The enduring changes that occur in regions of reward neurocircuitry and mediate the drug seeking characteristic of an addiction disorder occur over time and repeated exposures. Drug use typically escalates in a series of steps beginning with social use and transitions to regulated relapse, which is followed by compulsive relapse (Kalivas and O'Brien, 2008) (Fig. 51.1). In this chapter we will discuss the cellular and molecular changes and engagement of neural circuits that occur loosely on a timescale correlated with stages of use and drug seeking, and consider how these changes may mediate the uncontrollable drive to use that characterizes an addiction disorder. It is however important to note that these are not clear delineations. For example, although we present pronounced dopamine (DA) signaling as a hallmark feature associated with reinforcing effects of social drug use, dopaminergic mechanisms persist throughout all stages of addition disorder.

NEUROCIRCUITRY OF ADDICTION

STAGE I: REWARD NEUROCIRCUITRY AND SOCIAL USE

An overview of the neurocircuitry of addiction is essential for any discussion of the cellular and molecular mechanisms, because identifying relevant brain loci of change is imperative. The elucidation of the neurocircuitry of addiction has underscored the growing appreciation that addiction involves a pathology of reward learning (Hyman et al., 2006; LaLumiere and Kalivas, 2007). Reward learning can be defined as the adaptive associations between the environment and rewarding stimuli (e.g. food, sex, social interaction), and in a broader context includes the modulation of reward learning by motivational drive and decision making. Reward learning is a critical component of survival and evolutionary success, governing the necessary associations of reinforcement with context and behavior.

Early understanding of the neurocircuitry of reward learning was provided by the seminal work of Olds and Milner, who described the rewarding effects of electrical self-stimulation, with most pronounced effects in regions of the brain including the septum and tegmentum (Olds and Milner, 1954). Subsequent studies by Olds and others identified a number of other reward centers, most particularly along the medial forebrain bundle, which extends from the ventral tegmental area (VTA) through the lateral hypothalamus to the nucleus accumbens (Wise, 1998) (Fig. 51.2).

Shortly thereafter in 1957, Arvid Carlsson determined that dopamine (DA) functions as a neurotransmitter in the brain, as opposed to simply as a precursor for norepinephrine (Carlsson et al., 1957). This finding allowed for the inclusion of DA among the signaling candidates responsible for the activation of reward circuitry. A number of subsequent studies performed in the 1970s and 1980s determined that anatomical or pharmacological inhibition of DA signaling was found to impair a myriad of reward-related behaviors including feeding, electrical stimulation, sexual contact, and ultimately, pursuit of drugs of abuse (for review, see Wise, 1998, 2004). These studies established the framework within which to investigate dopaminergic mechanisms of reinforcement and hypotheses of addiction neurobiology.

By the late 1980s it had become clear that the reward pathway was multisynaptic, that DA antagonists blocked the rewarding effects of brain stimulation, and that the majority of drugs of abuse caused release of DA within the mesolimbic projections, particularly into the nucleus accumbens (NAc) (Di Chiara and Imperato, 1988; Wise and Rompre, 1989). Thus, the rewarding effects of drugs of abuse have been attributed to an increase in DA signaling within the mesolimbic reward centers of the brain, particularly the NAc and prefrontal cortex

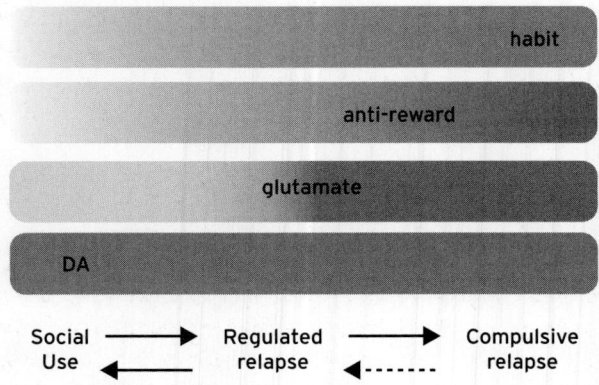

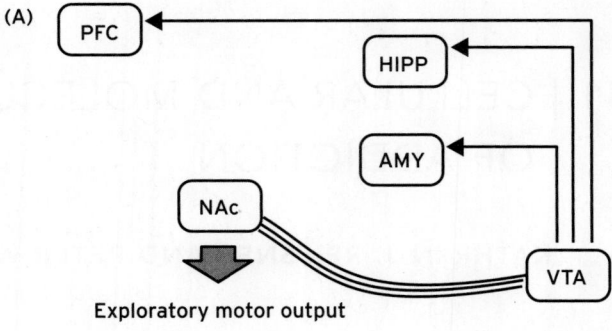

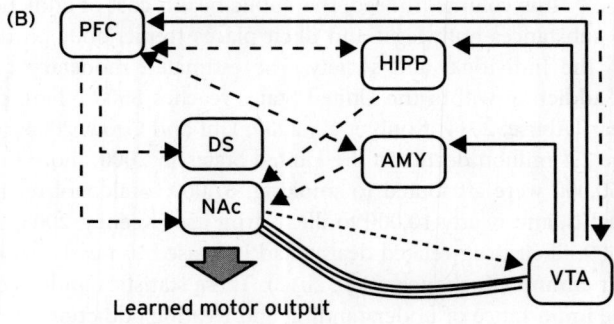

Figure 51.1 *Behavior stages in the development of an addiction disorder overlaid with corresponding categories of cellular changes. Extension of darker shading indicates the engaged or continued requirement for each mechanism in stages of addiction development. Changes in DA signaling are observed after an acute exposure to many drugs of abuse, and continue to be observed following multiple exposures (solid dark gray). Over time and repeated exposures/withdrawal, changes in glutamatergic signaling and plasticity are also observed, and contribute to the development of regulated drug seeking. As drug abuse continues, the brain "anti-reward" system is activated, and ultimately dorsal striatal habit circuitry, in the later stages of compulsive relapse. (Adapted from Kalivas P.W., O'Brien C. 2008. Drug addiction as a pathology of staged neuroplasticity. Neuropsychopharmacology, 33: 166–180.)*

Figure 51.2 *Reward and addiction neurocircuitry. Established circuit connections in the neuropathology of drug abuse are shown. Solid lines indicate DA transmission, dashed lines indicate glutamatergic transmission, dotted line represents GABA; arrows indicate directionality of neurotransmission. (A) Ascending reward neurocircuitry engaged by both natural rewards and isolated exposure to drugs of abuse. Triplet lines indicate median forebrain bundle. (B) Additional nuclei and structures are engaged following repeated drug exposure and mediate regulated relapse and increasingly compulsive drug seeking behavior. Enduring adaptations emerge within these structures, which underlie the pathophysiology of addiction. AMY, amygdala; DS, dorsal striatum; HIPP, hippocampus; NAC, nucleus accumbens; PFC, prefrontal cortex; VP, ventral pallidum; VTA, ventral tegmental area. For clarity, not included are nuclei included in the section on additional structures. For further discussion of the neurocircuitry of addiction, see Feltenstein and See, 2008; Koob and Volkow, 2010; McGinty et al., 2011.*

(PFC). Drug-dependent DA release in the NAc and PFC, as well as the amygdala and hippocampus, is now known to be a critical mediator of the rewarding effects of drugs of abuse, a necessary early step in the development of addiction disorders, the mechanisms of which will be discussed in depth in the following section.

STAGE 2: REGULATED RELAPSE

Because activation of the mesocorticolimbic DA system mediates responsiveness to the effects of drugs of abuse as well as natural rewards, the development of changes within the structures receiving DA following chronic drug exposure can mediate elements of drug craving and seeking, which are associated with the appearance of regulated relapse (Feltenstein and See, 2008). In particular, the NAc is a structure receiving input from not only the VTA, but also from the PFC, amygdala, and hippocampus, and is a critical mediator of reward seeking (Feltenstein and See, 2008; Mogenson et al., 1980) (see Fig. 51.2). The NAc is comprised of core and shell subcompartments, from which GABAergic projections are sent to the ventral pallidum, which in turn project back to the NAc and VTA, as well as to the subthalamic nucleus and the dorsomedial nucleus of the thalamus.

The NAc core and shell differ with respect to histological markers, and afferent and efferent connectivity (Ambroggi et al., 2011). Moreover, the cellular consequences of drug exposure differ in the NAc subcompartments, and consequently these subregions may mediate different elements of the addiction process (Peters et al., 2008). In the absence of drug exposure, the NAc core is associated with instrumental behaviors and is functionally connected with motor output systems,

whereas the shell plays a role in emotional modulation and appetitive motivations (Kelley, 2004; Sesack and Grace, 2010).

The prefrontal cortex is another major recipient of DA from the VTA, and inactivation of the PFC impairs drug self-administration and relapse related behaviors (McLaughlin and See, 2003). Regions within the PFC implicated in the neuropathology of addiction include the prelimbic cortex (PL), orbitofrontal cortex (OFC), and anterior cingulate cortex. Relapse-related behaviors of animals trained to self-administer drugs of abuse, followed by drug-abstinent extinction training, is particularly dependent on the activation of the synapse between the PL and NAc core (Kalivas et al., 2005; McLaughlin and See, 2003). Importantly, the PFC as well as the NAc send projections back to the VTA to regulate continued firing of DA neurons under adaptive learning conditions.

The amygdala is another major mesolimbic DA recipient and is composed of nuclei including the basolateral amygdala (BLA), central nucleus, medial nucleus, and cortical nucleus

(Freese and Amaral, 2009). With respect to drug cue-dependent relapse in preclinical animal models, synaptic connections between the BLA and NAc core, as well as the PL and NAc core, appear to be particularly important (Feltenstein and See, 2008). In addition, the extended amygdala is a composite of structures including the central nucleus of the amygdala, the bed nucleus of the stria terminalis, and the NAc shell, which are largely associated with stress-induced relapse to drug seeking (Kalivas and McFarland, 2003).

STAGE III: COMPULSIVE DRUG SEEKING

The compulsive drug-seeking characteristic of addiction is further associated with brain stress systems including the extended amygdala (comprised of the central nucleus of the amygdala, bed nucleus of the stria terminalis, and the NAc shell), and the hypothalamic–pituitary–adrenal (HPA) axis (composed of the paraventricular nucleus of the *h*ypothalamus, the anterior lobs of the *p*ituitary gland, and the *a*drenal gland). The extended amygdala and the HPA axis secrete neuropeptides and stress hormones, most notably corticotropin-releasing hormone (CRF), orexin, dynorphin, and vasopressin (Koob, 2008). The action of these molecules affects the physiology of structures affiliated with anti-reward systems and become activated during and following cessation of drug use (Koob and Le Moal, 2005). In particular CRF is released into the VTA in response to stress (Koob, 2008; Sarnyai et al., 2001). Release of CRF onto VTA dopaminergic neurons exerts a number of cellular effects including increased excitability and enhanced NMDA receptor mediated synaptic currents (Borgland et al., 2010). Preclinical models of stress reveal release of CRF into the VTA and consequent increased release of DA. These effects, as well as stress-induced reinstatement of drug seeking, are blocked by administration of a CRF receptor antagonist in the VTA (Borgland et al., 2010; Wang et al., 2005).

ADDITIONAL BRAIN CIRCUITS

Brain regions beyond those described earlier whose activation and/or inactivation may contribute to addiction-related behaviors include the habenula, insula, and septum. The habenula is located medial and posterior to the thalamus and projects to the VTA and substantia nigra pars compacta (SNc), and receives inputs from structures including the lateral hypothalamus, septum and dorsal striatum (Hikosaka, 2010). Stimulation of neurons within the lateral habenula inhibits activation of DA neurons in the SNc and VTA (Fowler et al., 2011). Accordingly, lateral habenula neurons fire in the absence of an expected reward to inhibit VTA DA release (McGinty et al., 2011). Thus, the lateral habenula has been proposed to serve as a control center for negative reward prediction. However, rats will seek electrical stimulation of the lateral habenula, and lesions of the lateral habenula decrease self-stimulation of the lateral hypothalamus and VTA (McGinty et al., 2011).

The insula, also known as the insular cortex, is a region of the cerebral cortex outside the PFC, located between the frontal and temporal lobes, that is associated with interoception and decision making (Naqvi and Bechara, 2009). Interoception refers to a perception of state of being, often considered as a measure of well-being, and is influenced by external environmental stimuli as well as internal awareness of emotions, stress, and energy level. The insula receives input from a number of structures implicated in addiction pathology including the anterior cingulate cortex, ventromedial PFC, amygdala, and ventral striatum. Activation of the insula is associated with craving for nicotine, cocaine, alcohol, and heroin; moreover, inactivation of the insula in preclinical animal models impairs measures of relapse to nicotine and methamphetamine (Naqvi and Bechara, 2010).

Lastly, the septum was one of the earliest structures identified by Olds and Milner in their original self-stimulation study (Olds and Milner, 1954); however, comparatively little work in animal models of reward learning and drug abuse has been performed since then. The lateral septum projects to the lateral hypothalamic orexin field, and inhibition of the lateral septum blocks conditioned place preference to cocaine (Aston-Jones et al., 2010; Sartor and Aston-Jones, 2012).

Comparatively little is currently known about cellular events induced in these structures by exposure to drugs of abuse, even though they have been clearly implicated in the neurocircuitry of addiction and illustrate the complexity of neuroanatomical substrates of reward-related behaviors and pathologies. The preponderance of data in the cellular biology of addiction show changes in the NAc and VTA, which are in some cases both necessary and sufficient to drive drug seeking, even following extended abstinence. These studies provide important insight into molecular mechanisms of addiction and craving, and will be the primary focus of the remainder of this chapter. Nonetheless, it is important to acknowledge that drug-dependent changes in the structures previously described almost certainly contribute to the complex cellular dynamics that comprise an addiction disorder.

RECEPTOR-MEDIATED SIGNALING

STAGE I: SOCIAL USE

As mentioned previously, exposure to most drugs of abuse results in pharmacological release of DA from the VTA onto neurons within the PFC, NA, amygdala, and hippocampus. However, although acute hyperdopaminergia is a common mechanism of the rewarding effects of most drugs of abuse, it occurs via distinct mechanisms (Nestler, 2005; Woolverton and Johnson, 1992). For example, psychostimulants cocaine and (meth)amphetamine lead to a surge of DA by inhibiting and reversing the activity of the dopamine transporter (Torres et al., 2003). Opiates stimulate opiate receptors (mu, kappa, delta), which reduce GABAergic inhibition on DA-releasing neurons of the VTA, whereas nicotine causes DA release through signaling downstream of nicotinic acetylcholine receptors on VTA neurons (Cami and Farre, 2003; Mansvelder and McGehee, 2002; Woolverton and Johnson, 1992). The primary psychoactive ingredient in marijuana, Δ9 tetrahydrocannabinol (THC), binds to endogenous CB_1 cannabinoid receptors, which are coexpressed on GABAergic neurons that innervate the VTA (Robbe et al., 2001). Thus, akin to opiate-mediated inhibition of GABAergic input to the VTA, marijuana also leads to decreased inhibition onto dopaminergic neurons. It is important to note that the pleasurable, reinforcing effects of drugs including opiates and THC are not exclusive to the effects of DA, and that not all drugs of abuse have profound effects on DA (e.g., non-DAergic mechanisms contribute to the effects of alcohol and benzodiazepines) (Wise, 2004). However, the initiation of cellular mechanisms that contribute to a generalized substance abuse disorder are believed to be mediated by repeated excessive hyperdopaminergia.

SIGNALING INDUCED BY DA RECEPTOR ACTIVATION

Increased DA signaling following drug use or natural rewards is observed in structures which receive afferent input from the VTA; of particular relevance are the PFC, NAc, amygdala, and hippocampus (Koob and Volkow, 2010). Importantly, although this response subsides with repeated exposures to natural rewards, increased DA signaling is pharmacologically stimulated with each exposure to drug (Cami and Farre, 2003; LaLumiere and Kalivas, 2007). This critical difference may underlie the initiation of pathology by drugs of abuse as opposed to natural rewards.

Dopamine receptors are members of the D1 (D1 and D5) or D2 (D2S, D2L, D3, and D4) G-protein coupled receptor families, and are positively and negatively coupled to adenylyl cyclase, respectively. With respect to the cellular effects of drugs of abuse, one of the most widely studied DA receptor effector molecules is *Dopamine and cAMP-Regulated Phosphoprotein of 32 kDa* (DARPP-32) (Svenningsson et al., 2005) (Fig. 51.3). DARPP-32 is highly expressed in medium spiny neurons of the striatum, including the NAc. Activation of DARPP-32 by PKA phosphorylation leads to inhibition of the phosphatase PP1, which controls the phosphorylation state of a number of signal transduction molecules. DARPP-32 is also a substrate for cyclin-dependent kinase 5 (Cdk5/p35), which in turn inhibits the ability of PKA to phosphorylate DARPP-32. Both acute and chronic exposure to cocaine, amphetamine, opiates, nicotine, and alcohol modulate the phosphorylation of DARPP-32, and DARPP-32 knockout mice demonstrate altered behavioral responses, including locomotor sensitization and place preference, to cocaine, amphetamine, and alcohol, as well as self-administration of ethanol (Fienberg and Greengard, 2000; Fienberg et al., 1998; Risinger et al., 2001). One of the cellular roles of DARPP-32 activation is modulation of gene transcription by control of transcription factors. Indeed, activation CREB (cAMP response element binding protein), c-Fos, and ΔFosB, three transcription factors all heavily implicated in the cellular mechanism of addiction, are decreased in DARPP-32 knockout mice in response to DA (Svenningsson et al., 2000, 2005; Yan et al., 1999). These important pathways will be discussed more extensively in the section on transcriptional mechanisms of addiction.

STAGES II & III: RELAPSE

Over time and repeated exposures, social use may progress to regulated relapse (Kalivas and O'Brien, 2008). Continued use is associated with the engagement of receptors and signaling

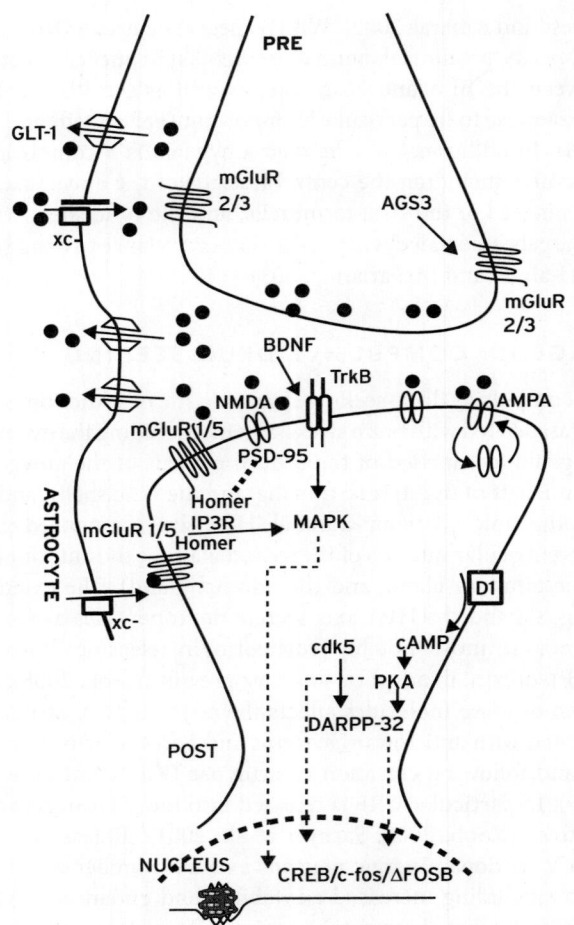

Figure 51.3 *Receptor-mediated signaling pathways affected by acute and chronic exposure to drugs of abuse. Representative pathways shown in a schematic medium spiny neuron (MSN) of the NAc, surrounded by astrocytes expressing glutamate transporter GLT-1 and glutamate antiporter system xc-. Arrows indicate directionality of glutamate transport or molecular signaling. Shown on the presynaptic face, activator of G-protein signaling 3 (AGS3) proteins are upregulated following multiple drugs of abuse. AGS3 proteins are inhibitory to Gi coupled receptors, such as GluR2/3 receptors, and thus increased expression promotes synaptic glutamate release probability in the PFC-NAc synapse. On the postsynaptic side, activation of D1 receptors leads to stimulation of adenylyl cyclase and enhanced cAMP production, leading to increased PKA activity. D2 receptors are inhibitory to ac activation and are expressed in MSN populations independent of D1-expressing neurons in the NAc. Both PKA and cdk5 activity are regulated by chronic cocaine, and both phosphorylate numerous substrates, including DARPP-32. DARPP-32 exerts downstream effects on transcription, as evidenced by decreased activation of CREB, FosB, and ΔFosB in DARPP-32 mice (Svenningsson et al., 2005). Both scaffolding and signaling molecules linked to iGluR and mGluR receptors are also influenced by chronic drug use. In particular, expression of Homer proteins is regulated by cocaine use. Homer proteins bind to the C-terminal tail of postsynaptic group I mGluR proteins and share an indirect interaction with NMDA receptor binding protein PSD-95. Not shown are additional scaffolding proteins of the postsynaptic density which form glutamate receptor complexes, including AMPA receptors. Membrane trafficking of AMPA receptors is also affected by chronic drug use, indicated by cyclic arrows. The coordinated activity of many signaling proteins including MAPK, PKA, and DARPP-32 influence activity of transcriptional regulators in the nucleus via activation of transcription factors including CREB, c-fos/ΔFosB, NFkB. Chromatin remodeling is also strongly affected by chronic cocaine exposure, via modifications to both DNA and histones, allowing for increased (or decreased) promoter availability for transcription factor binding. Depiction of histone octamer wrapped in DNA is schematized at bottom. For additional discussion of these and other pathways, see Dietz et al., 2009; Kalivas, 2009; McGinty et al., 2010; Robison and Nestler, 2011; Thomas et al., 2008.*

pathways beyond DA, most notably glutamate and neuropeptides, which may mediate the next behavioral stage of addiction, regulated relapse. Repeated drug use results in repeated release of DA from the VTA into structures described earlier, most notably the PFC, NAc, and amygdala (see Fig. 51.2). In parallel, for the addiction-vulnerable individual, repeated social use leads to regulated relapse associated with seeking out of the drug. Repeated exposures also lead to a variety of changes in glutamatergic signaling pathways, associated with a disruption of glutamate homeostasis (Baker et al., 2003).

GLUTAMATE HOMEOSTASIS HYPOTHESIS OF ADDICTION

Glutamate homeostasis refers to the regulation of extracellular glutamate in the synaptic and perisynaptic environment by both glia and neurons. Extracellular glutamate levels regulate synaptic activity and plasticity, and thus disruptions of glutamate homeostasis can have considerable effect on synaptic strength and function (Danbolt, 2001; Haydon, 2001; Kalivas, 2009). Basal levels of glutamate, which are predominantly extrasynaptic in origin, are reduced in the NA core of rats following long-term cocaine self-administration but not heroin or alcohol administration (Baker et al., 2003; LaLumiere and Kalivas, 2008; McFarland et al., 2003; Melendez et al., 2005). This reduction in extrasynaptic glutamate, in turn, provides less tonic inhibition of the mGluR2/3 receptors that are located on the presynaptic glutamatergic terminals (Moran et al., 2005). Less tonic inhibition in turn results in increased synaptic transmission in response to a drug-related stimulus, and contributes to the potentiated glutamate release observed in the NAc following a cocaine prime in withdrawn animals trained to self-administer cocaine. The cocaine prime- or stress-induced increase in glutamate is prevented by inactivation of the dorsal medial prefrontal cortex (mPFC) (McFarland et al., 2003, 2004) indicating an important regulatory role for the dorsal mPFC following long-term cocaine self-administration. A similar glutamate overflow occurs during reinstated heroin-seeking that also depends on mPFC activation (LaLumiere and Kalivas, 2008).

The regulation of extrasynaptic glutamate is predominantly dependent on the coordinated activity of the cystine-glutamate exchanger (system xc-) and high affinity glutamate transporters (Baker et al., 2002; McBean, 2002; Reissner and Kalivas, 2010) (see Fig. 51.3). Release of glutamate is accomplished by system xc-, in which one molecule of glutamate is released in exchange for the uptake of one extracellular cystine molecule. The exchanger exists as a heterodimer of a light catalytic subunit xCT and heavy subunit 4F2. Expression of the catalytic subunit xCT is decreased following cocaine self-administration in animals, resulting in decreased basal extracellular glutamate in the NAc of cocaine-withdrawn rats (Baker et al., 2002; Knackstedt et al., 2010a). Glutamate uptake from the extracellular space is primarily accomplished by the high affinity glutamate transporters. Expression of the astroglial glutamate transporters, EAAT2/GLT-1 and EAAT1/GLAST are also decreased following cocaine, heroin, and nicotine self-administration, thus compromising the ability of NAc synapses to accommodate the potentiated glutamate release observed during relapse to cocaine seeking in rats (Knackstedt et al., 2010a; Reissner et al., 2011).

Expression of xCT and GLT1 can be restored by treatment with N-acetylcystine and ceftriaxone, which also inhibits relapse in the reinstatement/self-administration animal model (Baker et al., 2003; Zhou and Kalivas, 2008; Knackstedt et al., 2010a).

RELAPSE IS MEDIATED BY GLUTAMATE RECEPTOR ACTIVITY

Considerable evidence supports a role for striatal glutamate receptors in the reinforcement of long-lasting drug-seeking behaviors (Uys and Reissner, 2011). Specifically, three main lines of evidence implicate ionotropic glutamate receptor involvement in addictive behaviors in a rat self-administration model of addition. First, a drug prime following self-administration of either cocaine or heroin followed by extinction results in potentiated glutamate release in the NAc (Baker et al., 2003; LaLumiere and Kalivas, 2008). Second, glutamatergic PFC-NAc synapses exist in a baseline potentiated state following self-administration and withdrawal (Kourrich et al., 2007; Moussawi et al., 2009). Third, inhibition of α-amino-3-hydroxyl-5-methyl-4-isoxazole-propionate (AMPA)-type glutamate receptors in the NAc inhibits self-administration and reinstatement to cocaine and heroin, whereas activation of these receptors potentiates drug seeking (Backstrom and Hyytia, 2007; Cornish and Kalivas, 2000; Di Ciano and Everitt, 2001; LaLumiere and Kalivas, 2008; Ping et al., 2008; Suto et al., 2009). These findings collectively suggest a glutamate receptor-dependent mechanism in the neuroplasticity of addiction and underscore the involvement of glutamatergic mechanisms of relapse.

IONOTROPIC GLUTAMATE RECEPTORS

Ionotropic glutamate receptors are of the AMPA, N-methyl-D-aspartic acid (NMDA), and kainite receptor types (Dingledine et al., 1999). AMPA receptors exist as homo- or heterotetramers, most often composed of set sets of two subunits (GluR1, GluR2 GluR3, GluR4). Increases in synaptic strength are largely associated with increased surface expression of AMPA receptors, particularly GluR1, whereas conversely, decreases in synaptic strength are caused by internalization or decreased surface expression (Kauer and Malenka, 2007). In addition, receptor subunit composition can affect the biophysics of glutamate-mediated currents; for example, all AMPA receptors not containing GluR2 subunits are permeable to calcium; however, GluR2-containing AMPA receptors are calcium impermeable.

A number of studies using preclinical animal models have revealed complex AMPA receptor dynamics in different stages of self-administration, extinction/abstinence, and relapse (for review, see Wolf and Ferrario, 2010). In one seminal study, although no change in AMPA receptor expression was observed one day after the end of self-administration, an increase in surface and total GluR1 receptors was found 45 days after the last cocaine self-administration session (Conrad et al., 2008). Moreover, a functional increase in GluR2-lacking receptors was found in the NAc following self-cocaine administration at this time point, indicating a role for GluR2-lacking receptors in the incubation of cocaine craving (Grimm et al., 2001; Lu et al., 2004).

Changes in GluR1 and GluR2 trafficking are also observed after an acute drug challenge following chronic abuse and withdrawal. For example, thirty minutes after a cocaine challenge, increased surface expression of GluR1 is observed in the NAc shell (Anderson et al., 2008). Moreover, increased GluR2 phosphorylation (consistent with internalization) was also observed 30 minutes after a cocaine prime (Famous et al., 2008), collectively suggesting a mechanism in which, in a self-administration model of addition, a cocaine challenge leads to an increase in surface GluR1 in exchange for surface GluR2 (Wolf and Ferrario, 2010). Numerous studies have also found effects on expression of NMDA receptor subunits following exposure to cocaine, and effects of NMDA receptor agonists and antagonists on drug-seeking behaviors (Huang et al., 2009; Ma et al., 2009; Schmidt and Pierce, 2010). The dynamics of both NMDA and AMPA receptors that occur within the reward circuitry following prolonged drug use, withdrawal, and relapse indicate a complex and critical contribution to cellular mechanisms of addiction.

METABOTROPIC GLUTAMATE RECEPTORS

In addition to ionotropic glutamate receptors, metabotropic glutamate receptors also contribute to mechanisms of neuroplasticity associated with addiction to drugs of abuse. Group I mGluRs include mGluR1 and mGluR5 receptors, which are excitatory Gq-coupled receptors and are localized predominately postsynaptically (Shigemoto et al., 1997). In contrast, group II receptors (mGluR2 and mGluR3) are Gi/Go-coupled, and are predominantly presynaptic (Shigemoto et al., 1997; Tamaru et al., 2001; Testa et al., 1998). Presynaptic group II mGluRs are inhibitory to synaptic transmission (Anwyl, 1999; Cartmell and Schoepp, 2000) as are group III receptors (mGluR4-8).

Reflecting the differential expression and effects on cellular activity, group I and group II mGluR receptors exert opposing effects on the drug-dependent cellular physiology and drug-seeking behaviors. Inhibition of group I mGluRs, particularly mGluR5, has been thoroughly described as inhibitory to drug seeking (Backstrom et al., 2004; Besheer et al., 2008; Carroll, 2008; Gass et al., 2009; Kumaresan et al., 2009; Liechti and Markou, 2008; Paterson and Markou, 2005; Platt et al., 2008). And in support of this, mGluR5 knockout mice demonstrate no cocaine-induced changes in locomotor activity, and do not self-administer cocaine (Chiamulera et al., 2001).

Alternatively, mGluR2/3 activation is inhibitory to drug-seeking behaviors associated with several drugs of abuse including heroin, cocaine, nicotine, and alcohol (Bossert et al., 2005, 2006; Liechti et al., 2007; Moussawi and Kalivas, 2010; Peters and Kalivas, 2006; Xie and Steketee, 2009; Zhao et al., 2006). Genetic deletion of mGluR2 receptors results in increased behavioral sensitization and conditioned place preference following exposure to cocaine (Morishima et al., 2005). Moreover, a reduction of group II mGluR receptor function has been observed following exposure to multiple drugs of abuse, including cocaine and nicotine (Liechti et al., 2007; Xi et al., 2002; Xie and Steketee, 2008).

Akin to the cellular signaling pathways initiated by D1 and D2 receptor stimulation, glutamate receptor engagement following repeated use leads to changes in signaling pathways downstream of glutamate receptors, both ionotropic and metabotropic (see Fig. 51.3). After extended drug use and withdrawal, it is in some cases not entirely clear whether relevant signaling cascades are dependent on activation of DA or glutamate receptors, or both, or whether specific cascades may be particularly relevant for some or all of the behavioral stages discussed. Nonetheless, the following pathways are central to the behavioral pathology of relapse in the drug-dependent animal and provide critical insight into the cell biology of drug abuse.

For example, Homer 1a is an immediate early gene that is rapidly upregulated in response to an acute exposure to cocaine (Brakeman et al., 1997). In neurons, Homer proteins are found in the glutamatergic postsynaptic density where they serve both scaffolding and signaling roles, binding directly to a number of proteins including group I metabotropic glutamate receptors, inositol trisphosphate receptors (IP3R), Shank, and dynamin III (Lu et al., 2007; Tu et al., 1998; Tu et al., 1999) (see Fig. 51.3).

Although the immediate early splice variant of Homer is upregulated following exposure to cocaine, the constitutively-expressed form of Homer, Homer 1, demonstrates more complex regulation. Homer 1 is decreased following experimenter-administered cocaine, but upregulated in the NAc after extinction, but not abstinence, following cocaine self-administration (Knackstedt et al., 2010b; Szumlinski et al., 2006a, 2006b). Genetic deletion of Homer proteins leads to reduced extrasynaptic glutamate, similarly as does chronic cocaine exposure (see preceding), and increased sensitivity to the physiological effects of cocaine in the Homer1 KO mice is rescued by viral-mediated overexpression of Homer proteins (Szumlinski et al., 2004).

G protein-coupled signaling pathways are also highly affected by exposure to drugs of abuse. Activator of G-protein signaling 3 (AGS3) is a member of the AGS family of proteins, which function to facilitate G-protein coupled receptor (GPCR) activation of heterotrimeric G-proteins (Lanier, 2004). AGS3 is upregulated following chronic exposure to cocaine, opiates, and alcohol, and is required for reinstatement in the self-administration model of addiction (Bowers et al., 2004, 2008; Fan et al., 2009; Yao et al., 2005).

Brain derived neurotrophic factor (BDNF) mediated signaling represents another seminal pathway influenced by drugs of abuse, particularly cocaine (McGinty et al., 2010). Although cocaine-mediated BDNF expression in the NAc promotes drug seeking (Graham et al., 2007), an infusion of BDNF in the PFC following self-administration is sufficient to suppress reinstatement behavior several weeks later (Whitfield et al., 2011). BDNF receptor binding leads to conversion of several signaling pathways that influence gene expression, particularly via changes in CREB-mediated transcription, via mitogen activated protein kinase (MAPK) (Robison and Nestler, 2011; Russo et al., 2009). Contributions of transcriptional regulation by CREB are discussed in more detail subsequently, in the section on transcriptional mechanisms.

CELLULAR PHYSIOLOGY

STAGE I: SYNAPTIC PLASTICITY IN THE VENTRAL TEGMENTAL AREA

Changes in synaptic strength are believed to represent a cellular mechanism for behavioral plasticity, particularly memory formation (Mayford et al., 2012). Accordingly, changes in synaptic strength within the VTA are observed after natural rewards (Chen et al., 2008; Stuber et al., 2008) as well as drugs of abuse (Ungless et al., 2001). The most widely used measure for increased synaptic strength is long-term potentiation (LTP), which typically reflects an increased presentation of AMPA currents relative to NMDA currents in the glutamatergic EPSC. A single noncontingent exposure to many drugs of abuse results in LTP in the VTA lasting for 5–10 days, an effect that is not seen with fluoxetine or carbamazepine (Saal et al., 2003; Ungless et al., 2001). This LTP is mediated by the biphasic insertion of homomeric GluR1 AMPA receptors, followed by insertion of GlluR2/3-containing AMPA receptors (Stuber et al., 2010). More enduring increases in synaptic strength in the VTA have been observed following extended self-administration of cocaine, for at least three months after cessation of drug use (Chen et al., 2008).

STAGE II: PLASTICITY WITHIN THE NUCLEUS ACCUMBENS

In contrast to the VTA, changes in synaptic strength are not observed in the NAc following a single cocaine exposure (Chen et al., 2010; Thomas et al., 2001). However, potentiated synapses are observed in the NAc core *in vivo* after self-administration and extinction training (Moussawi et al., 2009) and are depressed in the NAc shell 24 hours following a cocaine challenge after noncontingent administration and abstinence (Thomas et al., 2001). Importantly, despite changes in baseline synaptic strength following drug history, synapses are resistant to protocols that normally induce synaptic plasticity (Martin et al., 2006; Moussawi et al., 2009).

Although the results obtained from these studies are complex, they also illustrate two fundamentally important points about the nature of drug abuse and synaptic plasticity. First, chronic self-administration of drugs of abuse leads to enduring changes in synaptic strength throughout the mesocorticolimbic system, and second, drug-exposed synapses are resistant to adaptive changes in synaptic strength.

Interestingly, evidence suggests that the plasticity in the VTA observed after acute cocaine is mechanistically linked to the plasticity observed in the NAc following chronic exposure (Mameli et al., 2009). By manipulating mGluR1 function in the VTA, Mameli et al. (2009) were able to extend the duration of LTP in the VTA following a single injection of cocaine and consequently observe synaptic depression in the NAc that would otherwise not be observed following a single cocaine exposure.

Importantly, changes in synaptic strength have also been observed in other structures receiving synaptic input from the VTA, notably the amygdala and PFC (Luscher and Malenka, 2011; Stuber et al., 2010). In addition, while the majority of studies on synaptic strength within the mesolimbic system have been performed following exposure to cocaine, increases in synaptic strength have been reported in the NAc core following a heroin challenge after chronic self-administration and extinction (Shen et al., 2011) and cannabinoids elicit LTD in the NAc and hippocampus (Han et al., 2012; Robbe et al., 2002). Moreover, a considerable body of evidence indicates that alcohol results in changes in synaptic strength in a number of structures including the PFC, NAc, and hippocampus (Abernathy et al., 2010; Kroener et al., 2012; Mishra et al., 2012). These findings underscore the importance of circuitry in the cellular biology of addiction, and the cumulative effect of chronic hyperdopaminergia on glutamatergic plasticity. A current challenge of the field, then, is to determine whether restoration of synaptic plasticity may provide a cellular target for behavioral and pharmacotherapeutic intervention for addiction (Chen et al., 2010).

CHANGES IN STRUCTURAL PLASTICITY

Beyond changes in functional synaptic strength, morphological synaptic changes are also observed in response to multiple drugs of abuse, including opiates, nicotine, alcohol, and psychostimulants (Robinson and Kolb, 2004; Russo et al., 2010). Intriguingly however, psychostimulants and opiates, which exert markedly different physiological effects, also exert generally opposing baseline effects on cell body size and spine size and density; whereas psychostimulant use leads to increases in the number and size of dendritic spines, opiate exposure leads to decreases (Russo et al., 2010). However, a drug challenge following withdrawal from both drugs leads to a transient increase in spine head size (Shen et al., 2009, 2011).

Several studies have reported an increase in overall spine size and/or density in the NAc following exposure to cocaine (Dumitriu et al., 2012; Ferrario et al., 2005; Lee et al., 2006; Norrholm et al., 2003; Pulipparacharuvil et al., 2008; Shen et al., 2009). Moreover, following an acute cocaine challenge, dynamic changes in the morphology of dendritic spines are observed in animals with a chronic cocaine (but not saline) history (Shen et al., 2009). These changes are associated with changes in the expression of cytoskeletal proteins within the postsynaptic density, and indicate that a cocaine history results in a priming of synapses leading to enhanced responsiveness following later exposure to drug (Dietz et al., 2012; Shen et al., 2009; Toda et al., 2006). Moreover, the nature of spine changes in the NAc varies between neurons which express D1 versus D2 DA receptors (Lee et al., 2006). After extended exposure to cocaine, although dendritic spine density was increased in both populations, enduring changes were only observed in D1-positive neurons. Interestingly, animals receiving an acute cocaine exposure following chronic saline did not demonstrate these effects, indicating that changes in spine morphology likely do not mediate acute effects associated with social drug use, but develop over time and with repeated use.

STAGE III: LOSS OF COGNITIVE CONTROL

In the progression of an addiction disorder, following a period of regulated relapse and escalating drug use, the individual becomes preoccupied with pursuit of drug (Kalivas and O'Brien, 2008; Koob and Volkow, 2010). This stage of addiction is associated with a continued compulsive drive to obtain and use drugs, despite often clear and adverse consequences. It is likely that many of the cellular changes previously outlined are responsible not only for the craving responsible for regulated relapse (Stage II) but contribute to the transition to behaviors associated with a true addiction to drugs of abuse. There are however, further changes that are in particular attributed to uncontrolled pursuit of drug use.

For example, one of the hallmark features of an addiction disorder is loss of cognitive or executive control. This is reflected in brain scans from human addicts following abuse of a myriad of drugs, in which a decreased baseline in metabolic activity is observed in subregions of the PFC including the OFC, cingulate gyrus, and dorsolateral prefrontal cortex (Volkow et al., 2004, 2007a). Because these regions of the PFC are important for cognitive and executive control, decreased metabolic function may indicate impaired cognitive control in the addicted individual (Spiga et al., 2008; Volkow et al., 2004). Interestingly, in a number of structures showing impaired activity at baseline, activity is increased during presentation of a drug-associated cue (Volkow et al., 2005). The cue-induced increased activity in the OFC has been correlated with craving caused by drug paraphernalia or memories or drug use (Childress et al., 1999; Grant et al., 1996; Martin-Soelch et al., 2001; Wang et al., 1999). Thus, although hypoactivity in regions of the PFC may well contribute to diminished cognitive capability in the addicted user, these same regions may be overactive in the uncontrolled drive to use.

To understand the cellular mechanisms of addiction, it is important thus to consider what mechanism(s) may underlie these changes in metabolic activity. Although this remains largely unclear, the decrease in baseline activity correlates with a decrease of dopamine D2 receptor availability in the striatum (Volkow et al., 1993, 2002, 2007a, 2007b). Receptor availability assessed by PET imaging provides an indication of radiolabeled ligand-receptor interaction and can be affected by density of receptors, or by increased endogenous neurotransmitter levels (Nader and Czoty, 2005). The decrease in D2 receptor availability persists for up to four months in drug abstinent addicts, by which time all subjects had relapsed (Volkow et al., 1990). The decrease in D2 receptor availability correlated with decreased basal activation state of the OFC and reports of dysphoria (Volkow et al., 1993), suggesting that D2 availability may contribute to activation state and/or affect of the addicted individual. This point is particularly relevant, given the frequent reports by abstinent addicts that drug seeking is fueled by the desire to escape negative affect (Koob, 2009). Interestingly, a decrease in D2/3 receptor availability is also observed in rhesus macaque monkey and rats following extended cocaine self-administration (Dalley et al., 2009; Dalley et al., 2011; Nader et al., 2006).

Besides a decrease in cognitive control, compulsive drug seeking is also associated with powerful activation of habit circuitry (Everitt and Robbins, 2005; Gerdeman et al., 2003). This concept was briefly introduced within the neurocircuitry of addiction section. Decreased activation of prefrontal regions responsible for goal directed behavior is exchanged for increased dominance of established drug-seeking habits. Whereas adaptations earlier in the addiction process occur in regions of the ventral striatum, particularly NAc, over time engagement of the habit circuitry including the dorsal striatum is observed (Belin and Everitt, 2008). At the cellular level, ascending cortical loops exist between the ventral and dorsal striatum that may be responsible for this transition (Belin and Everitt, 2008; Haber et al., 2000; Ikemoto, 2007; Voorn et al., 2004). Indeed, changes in dendritic spine morphology in the dorsal striatum have been observed months after methamphetamine cessation (Cuzon Carlson et al., 2011; Jedynak et al., 2007).

In conclusion to considering the cellular physiology of addiction, it is worthwhile to make note of developing technologies that will enable interrogation of more sophistication hypotheses. For example, techniques in optogenetics have been developed to investigate cellular mechanisms of reinforcement and addiction. Optogenetics utilizes the technology of light-activated channels to control cellular activity, and is discussed in detail in the Emerging Technologies section of this edition. Transgenic or viral-mediated expression of channelrhodopin or halorhodopsin related proteins, respectively, allow for activation or silencing of cells with a high degree of spatial and temporal control (Fenno et al., 2011; LaLumiere, 2011). Use of optogenetics has recently begun to shed light on the cellular neuroscience of neurological diseases including mental illness, in particular anxiety and addiction (Bernstein and Boyden, 2011; Cao et al., 2011). For example, Lobo et al. (2010) expressed channelrhodopsin-2 selectively in D1- or D2-expressing neurons in the NAc, to control activation selectively in D1+ or D2+ neurons. Activation of D1+ neurons coincident with cocaine led to an increase in cocaine-conditioned place preference (CPP), whereas activation of D2+ neurons led to a reduction in time spent in the cocaine-paired chamber relative to controls, thus illustrating antagonizing roles for D1+ and D2+ neurons in the responsiveness to the rewarding effects of cocaine. In addition, optogenetic stimulation within the VTA has revealed a central role for DA firing patterns in the induction of CPP, as well as for control of reward consummatory behavior by specific populations of VTA GABA neurons respectively (Tsai et al., 2009; van Zessen et al., 2012). Finally, optical inhibition of the projection from the mPFC to the NAc core prevents cocaine reinstatement (Stefanik et al., 2013).

TRANSCRIPTIONAL MECHANISMS OF ADDICTION

TRANSCRIPTIONAL REGULATORS: ΔFosB AND CREB

Acute exposure to drugs of abuse, particularly cocaine, is known to activate expression of immediate early genes including FosB and Homer 1a (Brakeman et al., 1997; Young et al., 1991). However, these effects are transient and do not appear to exert enduring cellular effects that mediate lasting drug craving. In contrast, transcription factors ΔFosB and CREB are activated by multiple drug exposures and have been implicated in the chronic effects of repeated drug use (Robison and Nestler, 2011). CREB (cAMP response element binding proteins) is responsible for transcription of hundreds to thousands of genes, many of which have been implicated in addiction to drugs of abuse (Barco and Marie, 2011). Activation of CREB is observed in response to alcohol, cocaine, methamphetamine, and nicotine, whereas biphasic effects on CREB activation have been reported in response to opiate exposure and withdrawal. Functional studies have indicated complex roles for CREB in the drug-associated behaviors following exposure to multiple classes of drugs, as well as in related behaviors including depression, anxiety, and stress response (Briand and Blendy, 2010; Carlezon et al., 2005). Thus, the engagement of CREB is likely not restricted to the pharmacological effects of drugs, but also to the contribution of environment and affect to drug seeking behaviors as well.

Similar to CREB, the transcription factor ΔFosB has been heavily implicated in the enduring adaptations induced by numerous drugs of abuse (Carlezon et al., 2005; McClung et al., 2004). An enduring increase in expression of ΔFosB is observed following chronic exposure to cocaine, morphine, amphetamine, nicotine, ethanol, as well as various types of stress and natural rewards. Although most Fos family proteins are short-lived immediate early genes, the ΔFosB variant exhibits unique protein stability, and thus increased expression can accumulate and endure for a period of weeks following chronic drug administration (McClung et al., 2004). Importantly, ΔFosB can act as a transcriptional activator or repressor, and exerts influence over the expression of a wide variety of genes following a chronic (versus acute) regimen of cocaine administration (McClung and Nestler, 2003).

EPIGENETIC MECHANISMS OF ADDICTION

Beyond control of transcriptional expression through the activity of transcription factors, epigenetic mechanisms provide genetic control of addiction related behaviors. From Greek for over, outer, or above (epi), epigenetics refers to a change in gene function that is not caused by changes in DNA sequence (Haig, 2004; Maze and Nestler, 2011). Examples of epigenetic changes include DNA methylation and histone modifications that regulate chromatin structure and consequently influence gene expression. Accumulating studies from the early 2000s indicate considerable epigenetic involvement in controlling experience dependent plasticity and behavior (Borrelli et al., 2008; Day and Sweatt, 2011). Because many epigenetic changes can be long lasting, through the lifespan of the animal and in many cases directly or indirectly inherited by offspring, these changes have been proposed to reflect a cellular marker for the changes in gene expression which persist long after cessation of drug use (Tsankova et al., 2007).

Chromatin regulation by post-translational modification of histones includes phosphorylation, acetylation, and methylation (Maze and Nestler, 2011). Acute and chronic exposure to cocaine leads to histone modifications associated with regulation of gene expression. In particular, acetylation of histones H3 and H4 leads to increased transcription, because

the posttranslational modification masks a charge-dependent interaction between histones and DNA, allowing opening of the chromatin (Maze and Nestler, 2011). Histone acetylation is reversed by histone deacetylases (HDACs). Pharmacological inhibition or genetic suppression of HDACs potentiates the locomotor effects of cocaine as well as time spent in a drug-associated context; conversely, viral overexpression of HDAC4 or HDAC5 (Class II HDACs) has the opposite effect, indicating behavioral effects for global histone acetylation modification (Kumar et al., 2005; Renthal et al., 2007). In contrast, manipulation of a class III HDAC has the opposite behavioral effect (Renthal et al., 2009). Further, HDAC inhibition given post drug exposure facilitates extinction of CPP and reduces CPP reinstatement, indicating that histone modification may influence learning of drug associations, as well as the rewarding effects (Malvaez et al., 2010). Importantly, genes whose expression is regulated following chronic exposure to cocaine, including BDNF and cdk5, demonstrated histone H3 acetylation following chronic cocaine use, which remains elevated one week following withdrawal (Kumar et al., 2005). Changes in the physical association of ΔFosB and CREB with promoters of genes in which histone acetylation was present was observed for a number of genes (Renthal et al., 2009), thereby supporting the importance of these transcription factors in the regulation of cocaine-dependent targets, as discussed earlier.

Opposite to the activity of HDACs, histone acetyltransferases (HATs) are responsible for adding acetyl groups to proteins, including H3. CREB binding protein (CBP) is an example of such a HAT. Deletion of CBP in the NAc leads to decreased histone acetylation and locomotor responses to cocaine as well as inhibition of CPP (Malvaez et al., 2011). Notably, this effect of inhibition of CBP HAT activity on CPP is opposite to that observed following HDAC inhibition, previously described.

Studies investigating the inhibition of HDAC activity in a self-administration paradigm have yielded complex results (Maze and Nestler, 2011). Although results from CPP studies suggest that HDAC inhibition should increase cocaine self-administration, multiple studies have yielded conflicting results indicating both increased and decreased responsiveness to cocaine (Romieu et al., 2008; Romieu et al., 2011; Sun et al., 2008; Wang et al., 2005). These conflicting results underscore the importance of which experimental paradigm is used; for example in this case variables included use of different HDAC inhibitors, method of inhibitor administration, and time of inhibition relative to training and drug administration.

In contrast to histone acetylation, histone methyltransferase activity is decreased following chronic cocaine exposure (Maze et al., 2010). Moreover, genetic diminution of histone methyltransferase G9a in the NAc increased response to social defeat stress and cocaine CPP, whereas overexpression of G9a protected against cocaine-dependent social avoidance and led to decreased preference for cocaine CPP (Covington et al., 2011; Maze et al., 2010).

Last, beyond epigenetic histone modifications, direct DNA methylation can also affect gene expression. Three weeks following cocaine exposure or social defeat stress, an increase in DNA methylating enzyme Dnmt3 was observed in the NAc

(LaPlant et al., 2010). Interestingly, overexpression of Dnmt3 appears to be inhibitory to cocaine CPP and increases depressive behavioral symptoms in mice, suggesting that DNA methylation of Dnmt3 targets represents an adaptive mechanism against the cellular consequences of stress or cocaine. This and related hypotheses will continue to be tested and provide important insight into the long-term cellular mechanisms of addiction.

It remains to be seen to what degree epigenetic mechanisms are engaged following exposure to drugs in addition to cocaine. However, the escalation of studies in this area underscores the importance of genetic mechanisms of addiction, and will continue to provide important insight into mechanisms of reward learning, as well as the long-lasting changes responsible for relapse to drug seeking.

CONCLUSIONS

Chronic exposure to drugs of abuse leads to enduring changes at the levels of behavior, neural circuitry, synaptic strength, dendritic size, cellular signaling, and gene expression. Presumably, these levels of analysis share a functional relationship; thus, an understanding of cellular and molecular mechanisms of addiction can provide insight into circuit and behavioral changes. As such, identification of the cellular mechanisms responsible for controlled, social drug use, as well the ability of drugs to usurp adaptive reward learning in exchange for maladaptive drug seeking, remains essential as we move toward development of effective behavioral and pharmacotherapeutic treatments for addiction.

DISCLOSURES

Dr. Reissner and Dr. Kalivas have no conflicts of interest to disclose. They are funded by NIDA. Current grant support: P50 DA015369 (PWK), R01 DA012513 (PWK), R01 DA003906 (PWK), and K99 DA031790 (KJR).

REFERENCES

Abernathy, K., Chandler, L.J., et al. (2010). Alcohol and the prefrontal cortex. *Int. Rev. Neurobiol.* 91:289–320.

Abuse NIDA. (2011). Drug Facts: Understanding Drug Abuse and Addiction. http://www.drugabuse.gov/publications/drugfacts/understanding-drug-abuse-addiction

Ambroggi, F., Ghazizadeh, A., et al. (2011). Roles of nucleus accumbens core and shell in incentive-cue responding and behavioral inhibition. *J. Neurosci.* 31:6820–6830.

Anderson, S.M., Famous, K.R., et al. (2008). CaMKII: a biochemical bridge linking accumbens dopamine and glutamate systems in cocaine seeking. *Nat. Neurosci.* 11:344–353.

Anwyl, R. (1999). Metabotropic glutamate receptors: electrophysiological properties and role in plasticity. *Brain Res. Brain Res. Rev.* 29:83–120.

Aston-Jones, G., Smith, R.J., et al. (2010). Lateral hypothalamic orexin/hypocretin neurons: a role in reward-seeking and addiction. *Brain Res.* 1314:74–90.

Backstrom, P., Bachteler, D., et al. (2004). mGluR5 antagonist MPEP reduces ethanol-seeking and relapse behavior. *Neuropsychopharmacology* 29:921–928.

Backstrom, P., and Hyytia, P. (2007). Involvement of AMPA/kainate, NMDA, and mGlu5 receptors in the nucleus accumbens core in cue-induced reinstatement of cocaine seeking in rats. *Psychopharmacology (Berl.)* 192:571–580.

Baker, D.A., McFarland, K., et al. (2003). Neuroadaptations in cystine-glutamate exchange underlie cocaine relapse. *Nat. Neurosci.* 6:743–749.

Baker, D.A., Xi, Z.X., et al. (2002). The origin and neuronal function of *in vivo* nonsynaptic glutamate. *J. Neurosci.* 22:9134–9141.

Barco, A., and Marie, H. (2011). Genetic approaches to investigate the role of CREB in neuronal plasticity and memory. *Mol. Neurobiol.* 44:330–349.

Belin, D., and Everitt, B.J. (2008). Cocaine seeking habits depend upon dopamine-dependent serial connectivity linking the ventral with the dorsal striatum. *Neuron* 57:432–441.

Bernstein, J.G., and Boyden, E.S. (2011). Optogenetic tools for analyzing the neural circuits of behavior. *Trends. Cogn. Sci.* 15:592–600.

Besheer, J., Faccidomo, S., et al. (2008). Regulation of motivation to self-administer ethanol by mGluR5 in alcohol-preferring (P) rats. *Alcohol Clin. Exp. Res.* 32:209–221.

Borgland, S.L., Ungless, M.A., et al. (2010). Convergent actions of orexin/hypocretin and CRF on dopamine neurons: emerging players in addiction. *Brain Res.* 1314:139–144.

Borrelli, E., Nestler, E.J., et al. (2008). Decoding the epigenetic language of neuronal plasticity. *Neuron* 60:961–974.

Bossert, J.M., Busch, R.F., et al. (2005). The novel mGluR2/3 agonist LY379268 attenuates cue-induced reinstatement of heroin seeking. *Neuroreport* 16:1013–1016.

Bossert, J.M., Gray, S.M., et al. (2006). Activation of group II metabotropic glutamate receptors in the nucleus accumbens shell attenuates context-induced relapse to heroin seeking. *Neuropsychopharmacology* 31:2197–2209.

Bowers, M.S., Hopf, F.W., et al. (2008). Nucleus accumbens AGS3 expression drives ethanol seeking through G betagamma. *Proc. Natl. Acad. Sci. USA* 105:12533–12538.

Bowers, M.S., McFarland, K., et al. (2004). Activator of G protein signaling 3: a gatekeeper of cocaine sensitization and drug seeking. *Neuron* 42:269–281.

Brakeman, P.R., Lanahan, A.A., et al. (1997). Homer: a protein that selectively binds metabotropic glutamate receptors. *Nature* 386:284–288.

Briand, L.A., and Blendy, J.A. (2010). Molecular and genetic substrates linking stress and addiction. *Brain Res.* 1314:219–234.

Cami, J., and Farre, M. (2003). Drug addiction. *N. Engl. J. Med.* 349:975–986.

Cao, Z.F., Burdakov, D., et al. (2011). Optogenetics: potentials for addiction research. *Addict. Biol.* 16:519–531.

Carlezon, W.A., Jr., Duman, R.S., et al. (2005). The many faces of CREB. *Trends Neurosci.* 28:436–445.

Carlsson, A., Lindqvist, M., et al. (1957). 3,4-Dihydroxyphenylalanine and 5-hydroxytryptophan as reserpine antagonists. *Nature* 180:1200.

Carroll, F.I. (2008). Antagonists at metabotropic glutamate receptor subtype 5: structure activity relationships and therapeutic potential for addiction. *Ann. NY Acad. Sci.* 1141:221–232.

Cartmell, J., and Schoepp, D.D. (2000). Regulation of neurotransmitter release by metabotropic glutamate receptors. *J. Neurochem.* 75:889–907.

Chen, B.T., Bowers, M.S., et al. (2008). Cocaine but not natural reward self-administration nor passive cocaine infusion produces persistent LTP in the VTA. *Neuron* 59:288–297.

Chen, B.T., Hopf, F.W., et al. (2010). Synaptic plasticity in the mesolimbic system: therapeutic implications for substance abuse. *Ann. NY Acad. Sci.* 1187:129–139.

Chiamulera, C., Epping-Jordan, M.P., et al. (2001). Reinforcing and locomotor stimulant effects of cocaine are absent in mGluR5 null mutant mice. *Nat. Neurosci.* 4:873–874.

Childress, A.R., Mozley, P.D., et al. (1999). Limbic activation during cue-induced cocaine craving. *Am. J. Psychiatry* 156:11–18.

Conrad, K.L., Tseng, K.Y., et al. (2008). Formation of accumbens GluR2-lacking AMPA receptors mediates incubation of cocaine craving. *Nature* 454:118–121.

Cornish, J.L., and Kalivas, P.W. (2000). Glutamate transmission in the nucleus accumbens mediates relapse in cocaine addiction. *J. Neurosci.* 20:RC89.

Covington, H.E., 3rd, Maze, I., et al. (2011). A role for repressive histone methylation in cocaine-induced vulnerability to stress. *Neuron* 71:656–670.

Cuzon Carlson, V.C., Seabold, G.K., et al. (2011). Synaptic and morphological neuroadaptations in the putamen associated with long-term, relapsing alcohol drinking in primates. *Neuropsychopharmacology* 36:2513–2528.

Dalley, J.W., Everitt, B.J., et al. (2011). Impulsivity, compulsivity, and top-down cognitive control. *Neuron* 69:680–694.

Dalley, J.W., Fryer, T.D., et al. (2009). Modelling human drug abuse and addiction with dedicated small animal positron emission tomography. *Neuropharmacology* 56(Suppl 1):9–17.

Danbolt, N.C. (2001). Glutamate uptake. *Prog. Neurobiol.* 65:1–105.

Day, J.J., and Sweatt, J.D. (2011). Epigenetic mechanisms in cognition. *Neuron* 70:813–829.

Di Chiara, G., and Imperato, A. (1988). Drugs abused by humans preferentially increase synaptic dopamine concentrations in the mesolimbic system of freely moving rats. *Proc. Natl. Acad. Sci. USA* 85:5274–5278.

Di Ciano, P., and Everitt, B.J. (2001). Dissociable effects of antagonism of NMDA and AMPA/KA receptors in the nucleus accumbens core and shell on cocaine-seeking behavior. *Neuropsychopharmacology* 25:341–360.

Dietz, D.M., Dietz, K.C., et al. (2009). Molecular mechanisms of psychostimulant-induced structural plasticity. *Pharmacopsychiatry* 42 (Suppl)1:S69–S78.

Dietz, D.M., Sun, H., et al. (2012). Rac1 is essential in cocaine-induced structural plasticity of nucleus accumbens neurons. *Nat. Neurosci.* 15:891–896.

Dingledine, R., Borges, K., et al. (1999). The glutamate receptor ion channels. *Pharmacol. Rev.* 51:7–61.

Dumitriu, D., Laplant, Q., et al. (2012). Subregional, dendritic compartment, and spine subtype specificity in cocaine regulation of dendritic spines in the nucleus accumbens. *J. Neurosci.* 32:6957–6966.

Everitt, B.J., and Robbins, T.W. (2005). Neural systems of reinforcement for drug addiction: from actions to habits to compulsion. *Nat. Neurosci.* 8:1481–1489.

Famous, K.R., Kumaresan, V., et al. (2008). Phosphorylation-dependent trafficking of GluR2-containing AMPA receptors in the nucleus accumbens plays a critical role in the reinstatement of cocaine seeking. *J. Neurosci.* 28:11061–11070.

Fan, P., Jiang, Z., et al. (2009). Up-regulation of AGS3 during morphine withdrawal promotes cAMP superactivation via adenylyl cyclase 5 and 7 in rat nucleus accumbens/striatal neurons. *Mol. Pharmacol.* 76:526–533.

Feltenstein, M.W., and See, R.E. (2008). The neurocircuitry of addiction: an overview. *Br. J. Pharmacol.* 154:261–274.

Fenno, L., Yizhar, O., et al. (2011). The development and application of optogenetics. *Annu. Rev. Neurosci.* 34:389–412.

Ferrario, C.R., Gorny, G., et al. (2005). Neural and behavioral plasticity associated with the transition from controlled to escalated cocaine use. *Biol. Psychiatry* 58:751–759.

Fienberg, A.A., and Greengard, P. (2000). The DARPP-32 knockout mouse. *Brain Res. Brain Res. Rev.* 31:313–319.

Fienberg, A.A., Hiroi, N., et al. (1998). DARPP-32: regulator of the efficacy of dopaminergic neurotransmission. *Science* 281:838–842.

Fowler, C.D., Lu, Q., et al. (2011). Habenular alpha5 nicotinic receptor subunit signalling controls nicotine intake. *Nature* 471:597–601.

Freese, J.L., and Amaral, D.G. (2009). Neuroanatomy of the primate amygdala. In: Whalen, P.J., and Phelps, E.A., eds. The Human Amygdala. New York: Guilford Press, pp. 3–42.

Gass, J.T., Osborne, M.P., et al. (2009). mGluR5 antagonism attenuates methamphetamine reinforcement and prevents reinstatement of methamphetamine-seeking behavior in rats. *Neuropsychopharmacology* 34:820–833.

Gerdeman, G.L., Partridge, J.G., et al. (2003). It could be habit forming: drugs of abuse and striatal synaptic plasticity. *Trends Neurosci.* 26:184–192.

Graham, D.L., Edwards, S., et al. (2007). Dynamic BDNF activity in nucleus accumbens with cocaine use increases self-administration and relapse. *Nat. Neurosci.* 10:1029–1037.

Grant, S., London, E.D., et al. (1996). Activation of memory circuits during cue-elicited cocaine craving. *Proc. Natl. Acad. Sci. USA* 93:12040–12045.

Grimm, J.W., Hope, B.T., et al. (2001). Neuroadaptation. Incubation of cocaine craving after withdrawal. *Nature* 412:141–142.

Haber, S.N., Fudge, J.L., et al. (2000). Striatonigrostriatal pathways in primates form an ascending spiral from the shell to the dorsolateral striatum. *J. Neurosci.* 20:2369–2382.

Haig, D. (2004). The (dual) origin of epigenetics. *Cold Spring Harb. Symp. Quant. Biol.* 69:67–70.

Han, J., Kesner, P., et al. (2012). Acute cannabinoids impair working memory through astroglial CB1 receptor modulation of hippocampal LTD. *Cell* 148:1039–1050.

Haydon, P.G. (2001). GLIA: listening and talking to the synapse. *Nat. Rev. Neurosci.* 2:185–193.

Hikosaka, O. (2010). The habenula: from stress evasion to value-based decision-making. *Nat. Rev. Neurosci.* 11:503–513.

Huang, Y.H., Lin, Y., et al. (2009). *In vivo* cocaine experience generates silent synapses. *Neuron* 63:40–47.

Hyman, S.E., Malenka, R.C., et al. (2006). Neural mechanisms of addiction: the role of reward-related learning and memory. *Annu. Rev. Neurosci.* 29:565–598.

Ikemoto, S. (2007). Dopamine reward circuitry: two projection systems from the ventral midbrain to the nucleus accumbens-olfactory tubercle complex. *Brain Res. Rev.* 56:27–78.

Jedynak, J.P., Uslaner, J.M., et al. (2007). Methamphetamine-induced structural plasticity in the dorsal striatum. *Eur. J. Neurosci.* 25:847–853.

Kalivas, P.W. (2009). The glutamate homeostasis hypothesis of addiction. *Nat. Rev. Neurosci.* 10:561–572.

Kalivas, P.W., and McFarland, K. (2003). Brain circuitry and the reinstatement of cocaine-seeking behavior. *Psychopharmacology (Berl.)* 168:44–56.

Kalivas, P.W., and O'Brien, C. (2008). Drug addiction as a pathology of staged neuroplasticity. *Neuropsychopharmacology* 33:166–180.

Kalivas, P.W., Volkow, N., et al. (2005). Unmanageable motivation in addiction: a pathology of prefrontal-accumbens glutamate transmission. *Neuron* 45:647–650.

Kauer, J.A., and Malenka, R.C. (2007). Synaptic plasticity and addiction. *Nat. Rev. Neurosci.* 8:844–858.

Keeney, R.L. (2008). Personal decisions are the leading cause of death. *Oper. Res.* 56:1335–1347.

Kelley, A.E. (2004). Ventral striatal control of appetitive motivation: role in ingestive behavior and reward-related learning. *Neurosci. Biobehav. Rev.* 27:765–776.

Knackstedt, L.A., Melendez, R.I., et al. (2010a). Ceftriaxone restores glutamate homeostasis and prevents relapse to cocaine seeking. *Biol. Psychiatry* 67:81–84.

Knackstedt, L.A., Moussawi, K., et al. (2010b). Extinction training after cocaine self-administration induces glutamatergic plasticity to inhibit cocaine seeking. *J. Neurosci.* 30:7984–7992.

Kochanek, K.D., Xu, J., et al. (2011). Deaths: preliminary data for 2009. *Nat. Vital Stat. Rep.* 59:1–51.

Koob, G.F. (2008). A role for brain stress systems in addiction. *Neuron* 59:11–34.

Koob, G.F., Kenneth Lloyd, G., et al. (2009). Development of pharmacotherapies for drug addiction: a Rosetta stone approach. *Nat. Rev. Drug Discov.* 8:500–515.

Koob, G.F., and Le Moal, M. (2005). Plasticity of reward neurocircuitry and the "dark side" of drug addiction. *Nat Neurosci* 8:1442–1444.

Koob, G.F. (2009). Neurobiological substrates for the dark side of compulsivity in addiction. *Neuropharmacology* 56 (Suppl 1):18–31.

Koob, G.F., and Volkow, N.D. (2010). Neurocircuitry of addiction. *Neuropsychopharmacology* 35:217–238.

Kourrich, S., Rothwell, P.E., et al. (2007). Cocaine experience controls bidirectional synaptic plasticity in the nucleus accumbens. *J. Neurosci.* 27:7921–7928.

Kroener, S., Mulholland, P.J., et al. (2012). Chronic alcohol exposure alters behavioral and synaptic plasticity of the rodent prefrontal cortex. *PLoS One* 7:e37541.

Kumar, A., Choi, K.H., et al. (2005). Chromatin remodeling is a key mechanism underlying cocaine-induced plasticity in striatum. *Neuron* 48:303–314.

Kumaresan, V., Yuan, M., et al. (2009). Metabotropic glutamate receptor 5 (mGluR5) antagonists attenuate cocaine priming- and cue-induced reinstatement of cocaine seeking. *Behav. Brain Res.* 202:238–244.

LaLumiere, R.T. (2011). A new technique for controlling the brain: optogenetics and its potential for use in research and the clinic. *Brain Stimul.* 4:1–6.

LaLumiere, R.T., and Kalivas, P.W. (2008). Glutamate release in the nucleus accumbens core is necessary for heroin seeking. *J. Neurosci.* 28:3170–3177.

LaLumiere, R.T., and Kalivas, P.W. (2007). Reward and drugs of abuse. In: Kesner, R.P., and Martinez, J.L., eds. Neurobiology of Learning and Memory. San Diego, CA: Academic Press, pp. 459–482.

Lanier, S.M. (2004). AGS proteins, GPR motifs and the signals processed by heterotrimeric G proteins. *Biol. Cell* 96:369–372.

LaPlant, Q., Vialou, V., et al. (2010). Dnmt3a regulates emotional behavior and spine plasticity in the nucleus accumbens. *Nat. Neurosci.* 13:1137–1143.

Lee, K.W., Kim, Y., et al. (2006). Cocaine-induced dendritic spine formation in D1 and D2 dopamine receptor-containing medium spiny neurons in nucleus accumbens. *Proc. Natl. Acad. Sci. USA* 103:3399–3404.

Liechti, M.E., Lhuillier, L., et al. (2007). Metabotropic glutamate 2/3 receptors in the ventral tegmental area and the nucleus accumbens shell are involved in behaviors relating to nicotine dependence. *J. Neurosci.* 27:9077–9085.

Liechti, M.E., and Markou, A. (2008). Role of the glutamatergic system in nicotine dependence : implications for the discovery and development of new pharmacological smoking cessation therapies. *CNS Drugs* 22:705–724.

Lobo, M.K., Covington, H.E., 3rd, et al. (2010). Cell type-specific loss of BDNF signaling mimics optogenetic control of cocaine reward. *Science* 330:385–390.

Lu, J., Helton, T.D., et al. (2007). Postsynaptic positioning of endocytic zones and AMPA receptor cycling by physical coupling of dynamin-3 to Homer. *Neuron* 55:874–889.

Lu, L., Grimm, J.W., et al. (2004). Incubation of cocaine craving after withdrawal: a review of preclinical data. *Neuropharmacology* 47 (Suppl 1):214–226.

Luscher, C., and Malenka, R.C. (2011). Drug-evoked synaptic plasticity in addiction: from molecular changes to circuit remodeling. *Neuron* 69:650–663.

Ma, Y.Y., Cepeda, C., et al. (2009). The role of striatal NMDA receptors in drug addiction. *Int. Rev. Neurobiol.* 89:131–146.

Malvaez, M., Mhillaj, E., et al. (2011). CBP in the nucleus accumbens regulates cocaine-induced histone acetylation and is critical for cocaine-associated behaviors. *J. Neurosci.* 31:16941–16948.

Malvaez, M., Sanchis-Segura, C., et al. (2010). Modulation of chromatin modification facilitates extinction of cocaine-induced conditioned place preference. *Biol. Psychiatry* 67:36–43.

Mameli, M., Halbout, B., et al. (2009). Cocaine-evoked synaptic plasticity: persistence in the VTA triggers adaptations in the NAc. *Nat. Neurosci.* 12:1036–1041.

Mansvelder, H.D., and McGehee, D.S. (2002). Cellular and synaptic mechanisms of nicotine addiction. *J. Neurobiol.* 53:606–617.

Martin, M., Chen, B.T., et al. (2006). Cocaine self-administration selectively abolishes LTD in the core of the nucleus accumbens. *Nat. Neurosci.* 9:868–869.

Martin-Soelch, C., Leenders, K.L., et al. (2001). Reward mechanisms in the brain and their role in dependence: evidence from neurophysiological and neuroimaging studies. *Brain Res. Brain Res. Rev.* 36:139–149.

Mayford, M., Siegelbaum, S.A., et al. (2012). Synapses and memory storage. *Cold Spring Harb. Perspect. Biol.* 4:1–18.

Maze, I., and Nestler, E.J. (2011). The epigenetic landscape of addiction. *Ann. NY Acad. Sci.* 1216:99–113.

Maze, I., Covington, H.E., 3rd, et al. (2010). Essential role of the histone methyltransferase G9a in cocaine-induced plasticity. *Science* 327:213–216.

McBean, G.J. (2002). Cerebral cystine uptake: a tale of two transporters. *Trends Pharmacol. Sci.* 23:299–302.

McClung, C.A., and Nestler, E.J. (2003). Regulation of gene expression and cocaine reward by CREB and DeltaFosB. *Nat. Neurosci.* 6:1208–1215.

McClung, C.A., Ulery, P.G., et al. (2004). DeltaFosB: a molecular switch for long-term adaptation in the brain. *Brain Res. Mol. Brain Res.* 132:146–154.

McFarland, K., Davidge, S.B., et al. (2004). Limbic and motor circuitry underlying footshock-induced reinstatement of cocaine-seeking behavior. *J. Neurosci.* 24:1551–1560.

McFarland, K., Lapish, C.C., et al. (2003). Prefrontal glutamate release into the core of the nucleus accumbens mediates cocaine-induced reinstatement of drug-seeking behavior. *J. Neurosci.* 23:3531–3537.

McGinty, J.F., Whitfield, T.W., Jr., et al. (2010). Brain-derived neurotrophic factor and cocaine addiction. *Brain Res.* 1314:183–193.

McGinty, V.B., Hayden, B.Y., et al. (2011). Emerging, reemerging, and forgotten brain areas of the reward circuit: notes from the 2010 Motivational Neural Networks conference. *Behav. Brain Res.* 225:348–357.

McLaughlin, J., and See, R.E. (2003). Selective inactivation of the dorsomedial prefrontal cortex and the basolateral amygdala attenuates conditioned-cued reinstatement of extinguished cocaine-seeking behavior in rats. *Psychopharmacology (Berl.)* 168:57–65.

Melendez, R.I., Hicks, M.P., et al. (2005). Ethanol exposure decreases glutamate uptake in the nucleus accumbens. *Alcohol Clin. Exp. Res.* 29:326–333.

Mishra, D., Zhang, X., et al. (2012). Ethanol disrupts the mechanisms of induction of long-term potentiation in the mouse nucleus accumbens. *Alcohol Clin. Exp. Res.* 36:2117–2125.

Mogenson, G.J., Jones, D.L., et al. (1980). From motivation to action: functional interface between the limbic system and the motor system. *Prog. Neurobiol.* 14:69–97.

Moran, M.M., McFarland, K., et al. (2005). Cystine/glutamate exchange regulates metabotropic glutamate receptor presynaptic inhibition of excitatory transmission and vulnerability to cocaine seeking. *J. Neurosci.* 25:6389–6393.

Morishima, Y., Miyakawa, T., et al. (2005). Enhanced cocaine responsiveness and impaired motor coordination in metabotropic glutamate receptor subtype 2 knockout mice. *Proc. Natl. Acad. Sci. USA* 102:4170–4175.

Moussawi, K., and Kalivas, P.W. (2010). Group II metabotropic glutamate receptors (mGlu2/3) in drug addiction. *Eur. J. Pharmacol.* 639:115–122.

Moussawi, K., Pacchioni, A., et al. (2009). N-acetylcysteine reverses cocaine-induced metaplasticity. *Nat. Neurosci.* 12:182–189.

Nader, M.A., and Czoty, P.W. (2005). PET imaging of dopamine D2 receptors in monkey models of cocaine abuse: genetic predisposition versus environmental modulation. *Am. J. Psychiatry* 162:1473–1482.

Nader, M.A., Morgan, D., et al. (2006). PET imaging of dopamine D2 receptors during chronic cocaine self-administration in monkeys. *Nat. Neurosci.* 9:1050–1056.

Naqvi, N.H., and Bechara, A. (2009). The hidden island of addiction: the insula. *Trends Neurosci.* 32:56–67.

Naqvi, N.H., and Bechara, A. (2010). The insula and drug addiction: an interoceptive view of pleasure, urges, and decision-making. *Brain Struct. Funct.* 214:435–450.

Nestler, E.J. (2005). Is there a common molecular pathway for addiction? *Nat. Neurosci.* 8:1445–1449.

Norrholm, S.D., Bibb, J.A., et al. (2003). Cocaine-induced proliferation of dendritic spines in nucleus accumbens is dependent on the activity of cyclin-dependent kinase-5. *Neuroscience* 116:19–22.

Olds, J., and Milner, P. (1954). Positive reinforcement produced by electrical stimulation of septal area and other regions of rat brain. *J. Comp. Physiol. Psychol.* 47:419–427.

Paterson, N.E., and Markou, A. (2005). The metabotropic glutamate receptor 5 antagonist MPEP decreased break points for nicotine, cocaine and food in rats. *Psychopharmacology (Berl.)* 179:255–261.

Peters, J., and Kalivas, P.W. (2006). The group II metabotropic glutamate receptor agonist, LY379268, inhibits both cocaine- and food-seeking behavior in rats. *Psychopharmacology (Berl.)* 186:143–149.

Peters, J., LaLumiere, R.T., et al. (2008). Infralimbic prefrontal cortex is responsible for inhibiting cocaine seeking in extinguished rats. *J. Neurosci.* 28:6046–6053.

Ping, A., Xi, J., et al. (2008). Contributions of nucleus accumbens core and shell GluR1 containing AMPA receptors in AMPA- and cocaine-primed reinstatement of cocaine-seeking behavior. *Brain Res.* 1215:173–182.

Platt, D.M., Rowlett, J.K., et al. (2008). Attenuation of cocaine self-administration in squirrel monkeys following repeated administration of the mGluR5 antagonist MPEP: comparison with dizocilpine. *Psychopharmacology (Berl.)* 200:167–176.

Pulipparacharuvil, S., Renthal, W., et al. (2008). Cocaine regulates MEF2 to control synaptic and behavioral plasticity. *Neuron* 59:621–633.

Reissner, K.J., and Kalivas, P.W. (2010). Using glutamate homeostasis as a target for treating addictive disorders. *Behav. Pharmacol.* 21:514–522.

Reissner, K.J., Uys, J.D., et al. (2011). AKAP signaling in reinstated cocaine seeking revealed by iTRAQ proteomic analysis. *J. Neurosci.* 31:5648–5658.

Renthal, W., Kumar, A., et al. (2009). Genome-wide analysis of chromatin regulation by cocaine reveals a role for sirtuins. *Neuron* 62:335–348.

Renthal, W., Maze, I., et al. (2007). Histone deacetylase 5 epigenetically controls behavioral adaptations to chronic emotional stimuli. *Neuron* 56:517–529.

Risinger, F.O., Freeman, P.A., et al. (2001). Motivational effects of ethanol in DARPP-32 knock-out mice. *J. Neurosci.* 21:340–348.

Robbe, D., Alonso, G., et al. (2001). Localization and mechanisms of action of cannabinoid receptors at the glutamatergic synapses of the mouse nucleus accumbens. *J. Neurosci.* 21:109–116.

Robbe, D., Bockaert, J., et al. (2002). Metabotropic glutamate receptor 2/3-dependent long-term depression in the nucleus accumbens is blocked in morphine withdrawn mice. *Eur. J. Neurosci.* 16:2231–2235.

Robinson, T.E., and Kolb, B. (2004). Structural plasticity associated with exposure to drugs of abuse. *Neuropharmacology* 47 (Suppl 1):33–46.

Robison, A.J., and Nestler, E.J. (2011). Transcriptional and epigenetic mechanisms of addiction. *Nat. Rev. Neurosci.* 12:623–637.

Romieu, P., Deschatrettes, E., et al. (2011). The inhibition of histone deacetylases reduces the reinstatement of cocaine-seeking behavior in rats. *Curr. Neuropharmacol.* 9:21–25.

Romieu, P., Host, L., et al. (2008). Histone deacetylase inhibitors decrease cocaine but not sucrose self-administration in rats. *J. Neurosci.* 28:9342–9348.

Russo, S.J., Dietz, D.M., et al. (2010). The addicted synapse: mechanisms of synaptic and structural plasticity in nucleus accumbens. *Trends Neurosci.* 33:267–276.

Russo, S.J., Mazei-Robison, M.S., et al. (2009). Neurotrophic factors and structural plasticity in addiction. *Neuropharmacology* 56 (Suppl 1):73–82.

Saal, D., Dong, Y., et al. (2003). Drugs of abuse and stress trigger a common synaptic adaptation in dopamine neurons. *Neuron* 37:577–582.

Sarnyai, Z., Shaham, Y., et al. (2001). The role of corticotropin-releasing factor in drug addiction. *Pharmacol. Rev.* 53:209–243.

Sartor, G.C., and Aston-Jones, G.S. (2012). A septal-hypothalamic pathway drives orexin neurons, which is necessary for conditioned cocaine preference. *J. Neurosci.* 32:4623–4631.

Schmidt, H.D., and Pierce, R.C. (2010). Cocaine-induced neuroadaptations in glutamate transmission: potential therapeutic targets for craving and addiction. *Ann. NY Acad. Sci.* 1187:35–75.

Sesack, S.R., and Grace, A.A. (2010). Cortico-Basal Ganglia reward network: microcircuitry. *Neuropsychopharmacology* 35:27–47.

Shen, H., Moussawi, K., et al. (2011). Heroin relapse requires long-term potentiation-like plasticity mediated by NMDA2b-containing receptors. *Proc. Natl. Acad. Sci. USA* 108:19407–19412.

Shen, H.W., Toda, S., et al. (2009). Altered dendritic spine plasticity in cocaine-withdrawn rats. *J. Neurosci.* 29:2876–2884.

Shigemoto, R., Kinoshita, A., et al. (1997). Differential presynaptic localization of metabotropic glutamate receptor subtypes in the rat hippocampus. *J. Neurosci.* 17:7503–7522.

Spiga, S., Lintas, A., et al. (2008). Addiction and cognitive functions. *Ann. NY Acad. Sci.* 1139:299–306.

Stefanik, M.T., Moussawi, K., et al. (2013). Optogenetic inhibition of cocaine seeking in rats. *Addict. Biol.* 18:50–53.

Stuber, G.D., Hopf, F.W., et al. (2010). Neuroplastic alterations in the limbic system following cocaine or alcohol exposure. *Curr. Top. Behav. Neurosci.* 3:3–27.

Stuber, G.D., Klanker, M., et al. (2008). Reward-predictive cues enhance excitatory synaptic strength onto midbrain dopamine neurons. *Science* 321:1690–1692.

Sun, J., Wang, L., et al. (2008). The effects of sodium butyrate, an inhibitor of histone deacetylase, on the cocaine- and sucrose-maintained self-administration in rats. *Neurosci. Lett.* 441:72–76.

Suto, N., Ecke, L.E., et al. (2009). Control of within-binge cocaine-seeking by dopamine and glutamate in the core of nucleus accumbens. *Psychopharmacology (Berl.)* 205:431–439.

Svenningsson, P., Fienberg, A.A., et al. (2000). Dopamine D(1) receptor-induced gene transcription is modulated by DARPP-32. *J. Neurochem.* 75:248–257.

Svenningsson, P., Nairn, A.C., et al. (2005). DARPP-32 mediates the actions of multiple drugs of abuse. *AAPS J.* 7:E353–E360.

Szumlinski, K.K., Abernathy, K.E., et al. (2006a). Homer isoforms differentially regulate cocaine-induced neuroplasticity. *Neuropsychopharmacology* 31:768–777.

Szumlinski, K.K., Dehoff, M.H., et al. (2004). Homer proteins regulate sensitivity to cocaine. *Neuron* 43:401–413.

Szumlinski, K.K., Kalivas, P.W., et al. (2006b). Homer proteins: implications for neuropsychiatric disorders. *Curr. Opin. Neurobiol.* 16:251–257.

Tamaru, Y., Nomura, S., et al. (2001). Distribution of metabotropic glutamate receptor mGluR3 in the mouse CNS: differential location relative to pre- and postsynaptic sites. *Neuroscience* 106:481–503.

Testa, C.M., Friberg, I.K., et al. (1998). Immunohistochemical localization of metabotropic glutamate receptors mGluR1a and mGluR2/3 in the rat basal ganglia. *J. Comp. Neurol.* 390:5–19.

Thomas, M.J., Beurrier, C., et al. (2001). Long-term depression in the nucleus accumbens: a neural correlate of behavioral sensitization to cocaine. *Nat. Neurosci.* 4:1217–1223.

Thomas, M.J., Kalivas, P.W., et al. (2008). Neuroplasticity in the mesolimbic dopamine system and cocaine addiction. *Br. J. Pharmacol.* 154:327–342.

Toda, S., Shen, H.W., et al. (2006). Cocaine increases actin cycling: effects in the reinstatement model of drug seeking. *J. Neurosci.* 26:1579–1587.

Torres, G.E., Gainetdinov, R.R., et al. (2003). Plasma membrane monoamine transporters: structure, regulation and function. *Nat. Rev. Neurosci.* 4:13–25.

Tsai, H.C., Zhang, F., et al. (2009). Phasic firing in dopaminergic neurons is sufficient for behavioral conditioning. *Science* 324:1080–1084.

Tsankova, N., Renthal, W., et al. (2007). Epigenetic regulation in psychiatric disorders. *Nat. Rev. Neurosci.* 8:355–367.

Tu, J.C., Xiao, B., et al. (1999). Coupling of mGluR/Homer and PSD-95 complexes by the Shank family of postsynaptic density proteins. *Neuron* 23:583–592.

Tu, J.C., Xiao, B., et al. (1998). Homer binds a novel proline-rich motif and links group 1 metabotropic glutamate receptors with IP3 receptors. *Neuron* 21:717–726.

Uhl, G.R., and Grow, R.W. (2004). The burden of complex genetics in brain disorders. *Arch. Gen. Psychiatry* 61:223–229.

Ungless, M.A., Whistler, J.L., et al. (2001). Single cocaine exposure *in vivo* induces long-term potentiation in dopamine neurons. *Nature* 411:583–587.

Uys, J.D., and Reissner, K.J. (2011). Glutamatergic neuroplasticity in cocaine addiction. *Prog. Mol. Biol. Transl. Sci.* 98:367–400.

van Zessen, R., Phillips, J.L., et al. (2012). Activation of VTA GABA neurons disrupts reward consumption. *Neuron* 73:1184–1194.

Volkow, N.D., Fowler, J.S., et al. (1990). Effects of chronic cocaine abuse on postsynaptic dopamine receptors. *Am. J. Psychiatry* 147:719–724.

Volkow, N.D., Fowler, J.S., et al. (1993). Decreased dopamine D2 receptor availability is associated with reduced frontal metabolism in cocaine abusers. *Synapse* 14:169–177.

Volkow, N.D., Fowler, J.S., et al. (2002). Role of dopamine, the frontal cortex and memory circuits in drug addiction: insight from imaging studies. *Neurobiol. Learn. Mem.* 78:610–624.

Volkow, N.D., Fowler, J.S., et al. (2004). Dopamine in drug abuse and addiction: results from imaging studies and treatment implications. *Mol. Psychiatry* 9:557–569.

Volkow, N.D., Fowler, J.S., et al. (2007a). Dopamine in drug abuse and addiction: results of imaging studies and treatment implications. *Arch. Neurol.* 64:1575–1579.

Volkow, N.D., Wang, G.J., et al. (2005). Activation of orbital and medial prefrontal cortex by methylphenidate in cocaine-addicted subjects but not in controls: relevance to addiction. *J. Neurosci.* 25:3932–3939.

Volkow, N.D., Wang, G.J., et al. (2007b). Profound decreases in dopamine release in striatum in detoxified alcoholics: possible orbitofrontal involvement. *J. Neurosci.* 27:12700–12706.

Voorn, P., Vanderschuren, L.J., et al. (2004). Putting a spin on the dorsal-ventral divide of the striatum. *Trends Neurosci.* 27:468–474.

Wang, B., Shaham, Y., et al. (2005). Cocaine experience establishes control of midbrain glutamate and dopamine by corticotropin-releasing factor: a role in stress-induced relapse to drug seeking. *J. Neurosci.* 25:5389–5396.

Wang, G.J., Volkow, N.D., et al. (1999). Regional brain metabolic activation during craving elicited by recall of previous drug experiences. *Life Sci.* 64:775–784.

Whitfield, T.W., Jr., Shi, X., et al. (2011). The suppressive effect of an intra-prefrontal cortical infusion of BDNF on cocaine-seeking is Trk receptor and extracellular signal-regulated protein kinase mitogen-activated protein kinase dependent. *J. Neurosci.* 31:834–842.

Wise, R.A., and Rompre, P.P. (1989). Brain dopamine and reward. *Annu. Rev. Psychol.* 40:191–225.

Wise, R.A. (1998). Drug-activation of brain reward pathways. *Drug Alcohol. Depend.* 51:13–22.

Wise, R.A. (2004). Dopamine, learning and motivation. *Nat. Rev. Neurosci.* 5:483–494.

Wolf, M.E., and Ferrario, C.R. (2010). AMPA receptor plasticity in the nucleus accumbens after repeated exposure to cocaine. *Neurosci. Biobehav. Rev.* 35:185–211.

Woolverton, W.L., and Johnson, K.M. (1992). Neurobiology of cocaine abuse. *Trends Pharmacol. Sci.* 13:193–200.

Xi, Z.X., Ramamoorthy, S., et al. (2002). Modulation of group II metabotropic glutamate receptor signaling by chronic cocaine. *J. Pharmacol. Exp. Ther.* 303:608–615.

Xie, X., and Steketee, J.D. (2009). Effects of repeated exposure to cocaine on group II metabotropic glutamate receptor function in the rat medial prefrontal cortex: behavioral and neurochemical studies. *Psychopharmacology (Berl.)* 203:501–510.

Xie, X., and Steketee, J.D. (2008). Repeated exposure to cocaine alters the modulation of mesocorticolimbic glutamate transmission by medial prefrontal cortex Group II metabotropic glutamate receptors. *J. Neurochem.* 107:186–196.

Yan, Z., Feng, J., et al. (1999). D(2) dopamine receptors induce mitogen-activated protein kinase and cAMP response element-binding protein phosphorylation in neurons. *Proc. Natl. Acad. Sci. USA* 96:11607–11612.

Yao, L., McFarland, K., et al. (2005). Activator of G protein signaling 3 regulates opiate activation of protein kinase A signaling and relapse of heroin-seeking behavior. *Proc. Natl. Acad. Sci. USA* 102:8746–8751.

Young, S.T., Porrino, L.J., et al. (1991). Cocaine induces striatal c-fos-immunoreactive proteins via dopaminergic D1 receptors. *Proc. Natl. Acad. Sci. USA* 88:1291–1295.

Zhao, Y., Dayas, C.V., et al. (2006). Activation of group II metabotropic glutamate receptors attenuates both stress and cue-induced ethanol-seeking and modulates c-fos expression in the hippocampus and amygdala. *J. Neurosci.* 26:9967–9974.

Zhou, W., and Kalivas, P.W. (2008). N-acetylcysteine reduces extinction responding and induces enduring reductions in cue- and heroin-induced drug-seeking. *Biol. Psychiatry* 63:338–340.

52 | THE GENETIC BASIS OF ADDICTIVE DISORDERS

DAVID GOLDMAN

Addictions share mechanisms subject to both genetic and environmental influences. Conversely, environmental, genetic, and psychophysiological vulnerability factors and individual choice play important, but differing roles, in addicted individuals, including ones addicted to the same agent. The inheritance of addictions ranges from moderate (40%) to high (70%), representing consequences of alleles (sequence variants) shared by descent. At all phases of the multistep process of addiction, gene × environment interactions, including correlations between gene and environment, shape vulnerability. However, neither exposure nor consequent dependence necessarily leads to addiction. Many individuals use addictive agents without becoming addicted. Physical dependence (tolerance) often occurs to drugs administered in the course of medical care, followed by withdrawal and no consequent addiction.

Genetic susceptibility and resilience to addiction are attributable to alleles that are both substance-specific (e.g., variants that alter metabolism) and non-specific. Alleles that moderate reward, stress resiliency and executive cognitive control are among the factors that are non-specific to any particular agent. Cross-inheritance and shared etiology also partly explain the tendency of addictions to co-occur with other psychiatric diseases. From verified examples, alleles that alter propensity and resilience to addiction are diverse in molecular mechanisms, as well as in their abundances and effect sizes. Some are common, but most are probably rarer, and the strongest effects are probably produced by rarer alleles.

The genetic evolutionary context of addiction is poorly understood. However, there is as yet no evidence that vulnerability and protective alleles were directly selected by addiction itself, except in artificially selected model organisms wherein it must be admitted that the effects of selection are often surprisingly rapid. However, certain alleles that alter propensity to addiction appear to have been maintained at high frequency by balanced selection. These include alcohol metabolic enzyme variants in *ADH1B* and *ALDH2*, as well as alleles that alter cognition and emotion. Many common alleles that increase liability probably have counterbalancing positive values, if not in modern times then in the past. Certain genes influencing propensity to addiction can be accurately described as genes "for" behavior, although their effects on vulnerability to addictions may be secondary.

Three pathways to identify genes that alter propensity to addictions are candidate gene approaches, candidate gene approaches targeted to relevant psychophysiology and genome-wide approaches. The latter two paradigmatic methods

have been partially successful and are to some extent convergent, as genome-wide approaches are applied to psychophysiology and mechanisms of genes identified by GWA (genome-wide association) are defined. The combination of genetic tools with neuroscience techniques such as brain imaging enables exploration of mechanisms by which alleles alter risk. Functional alleles that partially account for interindividual differences in stress resiliency, and thereby addiction, are found at *SLC6A4*, *COMT*, *NPY*, and *MAOA*, all having been linked to activity of brain regions mediating stress response and emotion. Linkage analysis, including GWA, has enabled the hypothesis-free search for common variants moderating vulnerability. Via GWA, Asp398Asn, a common missense variant of *CHRNA5*, was discovered to influence risk of smoking and lung cancer consequent to smoking. Confirmation of this discovery validated the potential of GWA in addictions. However, at an early stage when GWA has been applied to relatively small numbers of samples, crudely phenotyped samples, and samples of heterogeneous origins, more than 95% of the genetic variance (heritability) in propensity remains unexplained, and replicated gene findings are primarily from candidate gene analyses.

The predictive value of any particular allele or genotype is low. The primary reasons for mismatch between heritability and strength of effect of individual alleles are twofold. Variation in several psychophysiologic processes including drug metabolism, sensation, reward, anxiety and resilience, and executive cognition contribute to vulnerability, and each is itself a manifestation of the action of many genes in contexts of exposure. Second, addictions are currently defined as end-stage diagnoses, and the effects of genetic variants are diluted or confounded when queried against an amalgam of phenotypes with different etiologies. Recent advances in genomics including massively parallel sequencing at low cost have opened the possibility for systematic searches for rare variants that may have stronger effects. For example, stop codons moderating addiction through the mechanism of impulsivity, also a risk factor in other psychiatric diseases, have been discovered within both *MAOA* and *HTR2B*.

The predictive value of genotypes for treatment response will determine their value for development of personalized medicine, one goal of gene identification being individualization of prevention and treatment of addictions. Genotypes may have different predictive value for treatment response than for diagnosis, and the use of genetic predictors will require controlled studies with predefined treatment outcomes. However, and in advance of these prospective clinical trials, genotypes have been identified that appear useful for predicting treatment response for alcoholism and nicotine addiction. For example, an *OPRM1* variant is associated with treatment response to naltrexone in alcoholism, and altered brain reward responses.

Addictions, including substance use disorders (SUDs), follow exposure to a wide variety of agents, and addictions are a worldwide phenomenon sparing no culture. Exposure to a diverse array of agents may lead to an *addicted state* through partially overlapping neurobiological pathways. However, although most or all people are exposed to addictive agents at multiple points in their lives only a minority become addicted. Even tolerance and dependence are not equivalent to addiction. For example, most patients receiving opioid drugs do not become addicted, although temporary tolerance and dependence are elicited. In both vulnerable and resilient (less vulnerable) individuals, repetitive exposures induce long-lasting neuroadaptive changes that alter behavior. In some individuals, tolerance, craving, withdrawal, and motivational shifts lead to persistent and uncontrolled patterns of use that constitute addiction. Addiction accesses different vulnerability mechanisms. Initially, motivation to drug seeking is driven by impulsivity and positive reward. Later, compulsivity and negative affect may more strongly motivate use. As defined in DSM IV, and probably in the next DSM, addictions are "end-stage" diagnoses based on behavior that began to emerge years earlier from preexisting vulnerability and exposure. The trajectory of addiction culminates in long-lasting and potentially irreversible neuroadaptive changes and constellations of behaviors and social impairments. Both the probability of initial use and progression are influenced by the nature of the addictive agent including its mode of administration, distribution, metabolism, and psychoactive properties, by intrinsic factors such as sex, age, age at first use, preexisting addictive disorder or other mental illness, and by extrinsic factors including parenting and childhood adversity, peer influences, social support and drug availability. Genes act within a matrix of factors.

Progress has been made to define clinical categories of addicted individuals who may also be more likely to share mechanisms of vulnerability, and both developmental trajectory and personality features have been incorporated into these schema. Genetic liability to addiction varies both quantitatively and qualitatively across the lifespan. Quantitatively, peer influences and family environment are most important for initial exposure and early patterns of use, and genetic factors and psychopathology are more important in the transition to problematic use. During adolescence the heritability of addiction rises, peaking in young adulthood and declining again in older age (Kendler et al., 2008). Qualitatively, childhood conduct disorder and antisocial behavior are associated with early abuse and dependence. These behaviors were incorporated into the Type I/Type II typology for alcoholism together with early age of onset and personality factors reflecting variation in brain function (Cloninger, 1987). The role of conduct disorder and antisociality on the one hand and anxiety on the other have long been recognized and some addiction-associated behaviors have been broadly described as internalizing (associated with behavioral inhibition), and others as externalizing (associated with disinhibition). However, regardless of whether they are antisocial and impulsive, addicted individuals, for example

alcoholics, tend to be anxious (Ducci et al., 2007). Overall, their greater anxiety may be caused by drug-induced allostatic change. Therefore it is important that adoptive studies and twin studies have pointed to the genetic transmission of vulnerability via both the externalizing and internalizing domains of behavior.

INHERITANCE OF ADDICTIONS

Family, adoption, and twin studies convergently establish the existence of genetic variation that determines genetic liability to addictions. Weighted mean heritabilities for addictions computed from large, epidemiologically ascertained cohorts of twins point to moderate to high heritabilities (0.39–0.72) (Goldman et al., 2005). These heritability values are within-population estimates and have not been deflated by including pairs of related individuals who would specifically capture variation in vulnerability that occurs across countries or across time, for example when an addictive agent becomes more readily available and vulnerability shifts as it might for example when use of an addictive agent is legalized. Both "no pathological drug use" and "initiation of use" are heritable, indicating that genetic variation also influences initiation (Kendler et al., 1999). Paradoxically, easing access to addicted agents may increase heritability by decreasing the environmental variance.

MODE OF INHERITANCE

Heritability directly implicates genes in causation; however, any particular heritable trait may be intractable to genetic analysis because of complexity of causation. In contrast, less heritable traits that are more narrowly defined or closer to the action of a gene may be more successfully parsed at the level of specific genetic loci that contribute to them. Therefore, two somewhat interrelated themes of this chapter are the mode of inheritance of addictions and the deconstruction (or redefinition) of addictions using neuroscience phenotypes on which genes may act more directly.

Genetic complexity arises from incomplete penetrance of alleles, phenocopies, variable expressivity, pleiotropy, gene–environment interactions, genetic heterogeneity, polygenicity, and epistasis. An epistatic model in which combinations of genetic variants determine addiction would seem consistent with the complex molecular architecture of the brain. However it is also possible that the molecular complexity of behavior could lead to a high degree of heterogeneity of genetic causation, with additive effects of the vulnerability variants. Epistatic interaction between alleles will tend to produce high MZ:DZ (monozygotic/dizygotic) twin concordance ratios, with identical twins resembling each other on the basis of common sharing of a constellation of variants but dizygotic twins being discordant because of the likelihood that some essential element of the constellation is not transmitted to the co-twin, disrupting the genotypic combination. For example if several dominantly acting alleles at different loci are required, the odds of this genotype being shared in a monozygotic co-twin would be 100% but the odds of sharing in a dizygotic co-twin (or full sibling) would be $(1/2)^n$, where n is the number of alleles. Incompatible with the epistatic model, the risk of addiction in dizygotic twins and first-degree relatives of addicted probands (index cases) has been found to fall off proportionally to degree of relationship, rather than exponentially. For example, MZ:DZ concordance ratios are approximately 2:1 for various addictive disorders (Goldman et al., 2005). Also there is enhanced risk in individuals with first-degree relatives who are addicted, regardless of whether they have been adopted away in infancy. Two factors complicating this interpretation of MZ/DZ ratios are assortative mating, which can increase the likelihood of multilocus allelic combinations in first degree relatives, and multiple allelic combinations that might lead to the same phenotype. However, under the epistatic model there is as yet no good explanation for the linear correspondence between risk and degree of relationship to an affected proband.

A critical test of the epistatic model is the additivity of alleles with proven relationship to addiction. However, as yet few addiction genes have been identified. Perhaps by chance, but perhaps because additively acting loci are in some way more easily discovered, gene × gene interactions in addictions are thus far consistent with the genetic heterogeneity and gene-gene additivity models. Two missense variants in ADH1B (Arg48) and ALDH2 (Lys487) diminish risk of alcoholism via alcohol-induced flushing. Surprisingly, these alleles act additively (Thomasson et al., 1991) despite the fact that they affect consecutive steps in alcohol metabolism. Functional loci within HTR3B and the serotonin transporter (SLC6A4) together alter serotonin function but appear to act additively on risk for alcoholism comorbid with other SUDs (Enoch et al., 2011). Two variants associated with nicotine addiction, one in the CHRNA5-CHRNA3-CHRNB4 nicotinic acetylcholine receptor subunit cluster found by GWA and the other in the TTC12-ANKK1-DRD2 cluster, which includes DRD2, a dopamine receptor important in nicotine reward apparently, also appear to act additively (Ducci et al., 2011). The discovery of epistatic interactions in addiction may await the detection of novel loci as well as measurement of new addiction-related phenotypes on which allele effects may be epistatic; however, the quantitative genetic (transmission) and molecular genetic (gene action) data available thus far do not support reconception of addiction to take into account epistasis.

CHANGES IN GENE EFFECTS ACROSS THE LIFESPAN

The risk, heritability, and specific factors that determine vulnerability to addiction vary across the lifespan and during development. Heritabilities of alcoholism, cannabis addiction, and nicotine addiction are low in early adolescence but gradually increase, peaking in young adulthood and declining with older age (Kendlet et al., 2008). Reciprocally, family environment is most important in childhood and declines as adolescents increasingly shape their social environment. For addictions, and perhaps paradoxically, genotype becomes relatively more important as people are able to make their own choices and shape their environments in line with intrinsic predisposition.

Another explanation for the greater importance of inheritance in older children is that some genetic factors are important only after repetitive exposure to addictive agents. An intriguing possibility is that some alleles only alter responses of the adult or adolescent brain. CHRNA5-CHRNA3-CHRNB4 genotypes have been reported to exert a stronger effect on smoking behavior in adulthood than in adolescence and to moderate the risk of a severe nicotine addiction in people who have already initiated use. In contrast, the TTC12-ANKK1-DRD2 and MAOA genes appear to influence personality characteristics, such as novelty seeking and impulsivity, that promote initiation of use (Ducci et al., 2012).

SHARED AND UNSHARED INHERITANCE

Addictive disorders tend to co-occur (Kessler et al., 1997). However, the observation of comorbidity is insufficient to demonstrate causality. For example, comorbidity could be caused by common environmental factors, or the first addiction could increase the risk of the second. Comorbidity sometimes can arise because of the pleitropic action of a single allele—one variant/multiple manifestations. The question of shared and agent-specific pathways to addiction will ultimately be answered at the level of individual genetic loci, some that alter risk for addiction to a specific agent and others that alter a mechanism, or mechanisms, common to multiple addictive agents. Substance-specific genes include metabolic enzymes for alcohol (ALDH2, ADH1B) and nicotine (CYP) as well as genes encoding gatekeeper molecules such as drug receptors (e.g. nicotinic receptors). Other genes influence mechanisms intrinsic to the action of multiple addictive agents or modulate an individual's likelihood of exposure or ability to quit.

Diverse aspects of addiction neurobiology that have been discovered to be modulated by functional genetic variation include anxiety, resilience, impulsivity, and reward. The genes implicated include rare stop codons and other functional variation in monoamine oxidase A (MAOA) and the serotonin HTR2B receptor, a serotonin transporter (SLC6A4) VNTR (HTTLPR) and a catechol-O-methyl transferase (COMT) missense variant Val158Met. These loci are also implicated in the shared genetic liability between addictions and other psychiatric diseases, and connect the inheritance of addictions to variation in specific aspects of brain function. Nevertheless, few genes influencing addiction vulnerability have been discovered, and therefore most knowledge of the relative importance of shared and unshared factors in inheritance is from quantitative studies of inheritance. Fortunately, these quantitative studies have been highly informative for the overall importance of shared and unshared genetic vulnerability factors.

Adoption, family, and twin studies distinguish between correlation and causation by measuring cross-transmission (Goldman and Bergen, 1998). Several large, methodologically sound twin studies have detected substantial cross-transmission of risk of addictions. For example, the risks of alcoholism and smoking are cross-transmitted. There is apparently more than one shared factor. In the Virginia twin sample two shared factors were found, one being identified as an illicit agent factor relevant to cannabis and cocaine dependence and the second being a licit agent factor mainly explaining vulnerability to alcohol, caffeine, and nicotine (Kendler et al., 2007).

Addictions are also cross-transmitted with other mental illnesses with which they are frequently comorbid. Addictions are cross-transmitted with externalizing disorders, including conduct disorder (CD), antisocial personality disorder, borderline personality disorder, and attention deficit hyperactivity disorder (ADHD) (Kendler et al., 2003; Krueger et al., 2002). Preexisting CD and ADHD are risk factors for addiction. Anxiety and depression may be preexisting or consequent (Kendler et al., 2003). Some longitudinal studies have also found that anxiety disorders and anxiety-related personality traits predict alcohol problems in adolescents and young adults. The connection between addictions and internalizing disorders is interwoven with the role of genes in resilience, stress exposure being a powerful determinant of both addictions and internalizing disorders, as discussed next.

GENE × ENVIRONMENT INTERACTION IN ADDICTION

Two ways gene–environment independence is frequently violated are gene by environment interaction and gene by environment correlation.

GENE × ENVIRONMENT CORRELATION

Genotypes modulate the likelihood of exposures leading to correlation (r) of gene and environment, and creating a "genetics of the environment." Note that gene × environment correlation is caused by a unidirectional interaction, environment not modulating genotype, although it may lead to widespread epigenetic change modulating gene expression. An example of gene × environment correlation is the ability of *CHRNA5* Asn398 to increase risk of lung cancer (Thorgeirsson et al., 2008) via its influence on heavy smoking, thereby leading to increased exposure of the lung to carcinogens. However, and as a possible example of pleiotropy, nicotine could also directly modulate cancer risk at the cellular level.

GENE × ENVIRONMENT INTERACTION

The effect of an environmental exposure can be modified by genotype (Caspi and Moffitt, 2006). Again, gene × environment interaction is caused by a unidirectional interaction, environment not modulating genotype, although it may lead to widespread epigenetic change modulating gene expression. Childhood adversity is an important risk factor for addiction and comorbid diseases, including antisocial personality disorder (ASPD), CD, borderline personality disorder, and anxiety disorders. As discovered by Rutter and others, not all people exposed to severe early trauma develop psychopathology, indicating differences in resiliency. Loci modifying stress resiliency are likely to be numerous and are at this point largely unknown. Several that have been identified are monoamine oxidase A (*MAOA*) (Ducci et al., 2008), the serotonin transporter (*SLC6A4*) (Caspi et al., 2003; Hariri et al., 2002), *COMT*

(Zubieta et al., 2003), neuropeptide Y (*NPY*, an anxiolytic neuropeptide) (Zhou et al., 2008), and *FKBP5* (an accessory protein for the glucocorticoid receptor) (Binder et al., 2008). These are functional loci, and most have been demonstrated to alter the relevant molecular and neuroscience-based intermediate phenotypes for stress response and emotion, as will next be discussed.

INTERMEDIATE PHENOTYPES IN ADDICTION

One strategy to discover gene effects for complex diseases that are amalgams of distinctly different pathologies is to split the lumped disease phenotypes or deconstruct them into etiologic components.

If it were readily feasible to parse addictions into subtypes based on clinical features, this would undoubtedly have already been done, because of the burden to society that addictions pose, and commendable efforts have been made in this area. However only a few clinical subtypes (e.g., Cloninger Type I/ Type II) have been identified; these subtypes are themselves amalgams. Additional measures are needed. These include measures that do not reflect causal processes but are indicators of severity or response; for example, neuroimaging and neuropsychological indicators can track long-term damage consequent to exposure and that may impede recovery. These can be termed biomarkers. Other measures are intermediate phenotypes that access mediating mechanisms of genetic and environmental influences on the brain. For addictions these would include measures of emotional response and stress resiliency, reward, executive cognitive control and impulsivity, and metabolism and pharmacodynamic response. Furthermore, heritable, disease-associated, intermediate phenotypes are termed endophenotypes (Gottesman and Gould, 2003). Whether a particular biomarker, intermediate phenotype, or endophenotype is useful clinically or in genetic studies depends on multiple factors, including measurement properties, frequency, sensitivity, specificity, independence from other measures, and whether the measurement can be practically obtained from living patients or populations and families seen in the clinic or that might be enrolled in genetic studies.

Alcohol-induced flushing is an intermediate phenotype that is practically useful both clinically and for genetic studies. It is a protective alcohol-related endophenotype influenced by specific alleles mediating variation in ethanol metabolism, as will be discussed. Flushing is a clinically accessible, pharmacokinetic endophenotype that can be more thoroughly characterized and explained via psychophysiological measures, assays of alcohol metabolism, and genotyping of the variants that alter alcohol metabolism. Low pharmacodynamic response to alcohol is a genetically influenced intermediate phenotype that predicts enhanced risk (Heath et al., 1999). Level of response is mainly a result of intrinsic pharmacodynamic variation in neuronal response to alcohol rather than variation in metabolism (Schuckit et al., 1998). Some functional variants have been associated with low response to alcohol, including variants in the serotonin transporter gene (*SLC6A4*) and the gene encoding the α6 subunit of the gamma-aminobutyric acid receptor A (*GABRA6*) (Hu et al., 2005). However, the genetic origins of variation in alcohol response are largely, or even entirely, unknown.

Many other intermediate phenotypes relevant to addictions are known, and several have been shown to be more strongly influenced by gene action than addiction itself. Focusing on brain-related measures, electrophysiologic, neuropsychologic, neuroendocrinologic, and neuroimaging measures have been tied to addictions. Electrophysiologic measures including both baseline EEG and evoked responses are both addiction-associated and heritable, baseline EEG power in different spectral bands being highly heritable (van Beijsterveldt and van Baal, 2002). Neuroimaging accesses the structure and activity of circuits underlying emotion, reward, and craving. Studies incorporating neuroimaging have indirectly linked genes to processes and neuronal networks relevant in addiction. Interindividual differences in emotional response are predicted by amygdala activation after exposure to emotional imagery and stressful stimuli, and thus the study of fMRI-detected metabolic activation of amygdala and functionally related regions such as hippocampus has captured effects of genes that influence emotion (Bevilacqua and Goldman, 2011). As will be discussed, *SLC6A4* and *MAOA* are among the genes influencing emotion and more strongly amygdala activation. Activations of frontal cortex by executive cognitive tasks are modulated by genetic variants of both *COMT* and *MAOA*, thus providing an important clue, again by indirect means, to impairments in impulse control that are important in predisposition to addiction. Recently it was discovered that a functional polymorphism of the mu-opioid receptor gene (*OPRM1 Asn398Asp*) modulates activation of the ventral striatum by reward, and this same polymorphism has directionally consistent effects on naltrexone response in alcoholics treated with this medication (Anton et al., 2008; Oslin et al., 2003) and controversial effects on risk of addictions. Depending on the properties of intermediate phenotypes including proximity to gene action, measurement error, and specificity, they offer an important starting point for unraveling the genetics of addiction, and arguably most of the successes in gene identification are directly tied to intermediate phenotypes and functional alleles that alter them in ways that are directionally consistent with physiology.

GENE IDENTIFICATION FOR ADDICTION

In candidate gene studies, genes influencing relevant physiology are rationally selected based on pathways, mechanisms and molecules of addiction or the pharmacokinetics and pharmacodynamics of the drug. A functional locus may be identified and specifically studied, representing a candidate locus, or allele. In genome-wide studies, the genome is interrogated in hypothesis-free fashion via an expanding array of methods including GWA, linkage in families, and genome and exome sequencing. For addictions, genes have primarily been identified via the candidate gene approach. However, GWA and deep sequencing has yielded several "hits," including a functional locus altering nicotine addiction vulnerability. Both methods

are increasingly convergent as detailed information is developed on the locations of functional elements, for example in the ENCODE project, which aims to identify the functional elements genome-wide.

ALCOHOL METABOLIZING GENES: *ADH1B* AND *ALDH2*

Polymorphisms of alcohol dehydrogenase IB (ADH1B) and aldehyde dehydrogenase 2 (ALDH2) influence alcohol consumption and risk of alcohol use disorders as well as damage secondary to alcohol exposure. In adults these enzymes catalyze consecutive steps in ethanol metabolism although other enzymes including catalase and cytochrome P450 also play significant roles. Acetaldehyde, the product of ADH, is toxic and potently releases histamine thereby triggering flushing, an aversive reaction that can include headache, nausea, and palpitations. If aldehyde dehydrogenase is blocked by medications including metronidazole and disulfiram (a drug that is actually used to help alcoholics maintain abstinence), flushing follows the ingestion of small quantities of alcohol. Acetaldehyde is a mutagen, leading to increased risk of upper GI cancer in moderate drinkers who carry the dominantly acting *ALDH2* Lys487 allele, as some 500 million people do (Brooks et al., 2009).

At *ADH1B*, the His48 allele increases catalytic efficiency of the enzyme. In East Asian populations both *ADH1B* His48 and *ALDH2* Lys487 are highly abundant, and His48 is present in many individuals of Jewish ancestry. A protective effect of His48 on alcohol dependence has been demonstrated in European and African populations as well as East Asians, in whom this relationship was originally observed (Bierut et al., 2012), and both the *ADH1B* and *ALDH2* flushing alleles are associated with enhanced risk of upper GI cancers.

The *ADH1B* and *ALDH2* His48 and Lys487 alleles are ancient in the human lineage. They occur on characteristic and highly diverged haplotypes at these genes, are found at high frequency in particular populations, and are unlikely to have been selected to high frequency to protect against alcoholism. It has been hypothesized that they have been selected to high frequencies in East Asians because of their ability to alter susceptibility to protozoal infections, including infections of the gut such as amebiasis (Goldman and Enoch, 1990). This hypothesis is unproven; however, metronidazole is used to treat protozoal infections and potently inhibits aldehyde dehydrogenase.

GENES MODERATING MONOAMINE NEUROTRANSMITTERS

Monoamine neurotransmitters modulate emotionality, cognition, and reward. Therefore, it would be predicted that genes that contain functional loci that can alter function of monoamine neurotransmitters should alter liability to addiction. Congruently, catechol-*O*-methyltransferase (COMT) and the serotonin transporter (SLC6A4), and MAOA (as already mentioned) have been implicated in vulnerability to addiction and other psychiatric diseases that share these etiologic mechanisms.

COMT plays an important role in the regulation of dopamine in the prefrontal cortex and metabolizes dopamine, norepinephrine, and other catechols in various brain regions. The Val158Met polymorphism alters COMT activity via an effect on enzyme stability, the Met158 allele being three- to fourfold less active (Lachman et al., 1996). Because of the higher activity of the Val158 allele, it is predicted that it leads to lower frontal dopamine levels, and it has been associated with dopamine-modulated cognitive differences including inefficient frontal lobe function as seen by neuroimaging (Egan et al., 2001). Amphetamine improved executive cognitive function in val/val homozygotes, but not met/met homozygotes indicating that baseline dopamine levels of val/val homozygotes may be suboptimal for frontal cortical function (Mattay et al., 2003). Reciprocally, and leading to *COMT* being called a Warrior versus Worrier gene (Goldman, 2012), the Met158, allele has been associated with decreased stress resilience and increased emotionality, including anxiety in women (Enoch et al., 2003). Met 158 was associated with increased pain–stress induced brain activations as well a slower pain threshold and stronger affective response to pain (Zubieta et al., 2003). The evidence for association of *COMT* to addiction is mixed, including negative studies, studies implicating Val158, and others implicating Met158 (Tammimaki and Mannisto, 2010). These divergent results may be reconciled if the Val158Met polymorphism, which does affect behavior, has countervailing effects on different mechanisms of vulnerability to addiction. The Val158 allele was in excess among methamphetamine, nicotine, and polysubstance addicts (Vandenbergh et al., 1997). On the other hand, the Met158 allele was more common in late-onset alcoholics in Finland (Tiihonen et al., 1999).

Via reuptake, the serotonin transporter (SLC6A4) regulates synaptic serotonin. Reflecting the diverse effects of this neurotransmitter on mood, appetite, and impulse control, serotonin-specific reuptake inhibitors are widely prescribed for a variety of different mental illnesses. HTTLPR, a polymorphism located in the promoter region of this gene and involving variable numbers of an imperfect repeat located in tandem (a VNTR), probably remains the most studied locus in psychiatric genetics. Three relatively common HTTLPR alleles are functional, altering transcriptional efficiency (Hu et al., 2006) and expression of the transporter expression in the brain (Heinz et al., 2000). Reduction of function HTTLPR genotypes has been associated with anxiety, depression, and alcoholism, but inconsistently in the case of each disease. Overall, the predictive effect of HTTLPR on any clinically measured behavior is modest. However, the effects appear stronger in the context of stress exposure moderating impact of stressful life events on depression and suicidal behavior. Carriers of low-transcribing HTTLPR genotypes exhibited more depression and suicidality following stressful life events (Csapi et al., 2003).

Although contradictory meta-analyses have not clarified the GxE relationship of HTTLPR to behavior, neuroscience evidence has supported a role for *HTTLPR* regulation of emotion and response to stress, and provided clues to mechanism. Low activity HTTLPR genotypes predict stronger metabolic responses of brain regions intrinsically involved in processing of emotional stimuli and predict smaller volumes of some of these structures and diminished connectivity with regions that modulate their activity. The low-activity "s" allele predicts increased amygdala reactivity to emotional stimuli under the passive viewing condition (Hariri et al., 2002) and also predicts reduced amygdala volume and reduced functional coupling between the amygdala and ventromedial prefrontal cortex (Heinz et al., 2005). The effects of reduction of function serotonin transporter alleles on emotion have been validated in two animal models. An orthologous polymorphism designated rs-5HTTLPR is found in the Rhesus macaque (*Macaca mulatta*). In macaques, early life stress exposure together with rs-HTTLPR again leads to enhanced stress response and emotionality later in life. Carriers of the low-expression genotype that were separated from their mothers at an early age were more stress reactive and drank more alcohol later in life (Barr et al., 2004), a difference that appears to be in part mediated by the hypothalamic–pituitary–adrenal axis.

GENOMIC APPROACHES IN ADDICTIONS

GENOME-WIDE ASSOCIATION

Genome-wide association is a genomic approach to the analysis of genetically influenced traits that queries all genes and unknown functional genetic elements in a hypothesis-free way for their potential effects. The importance of hypothesis-free, global approaches is emphasized by discoveries by the ENCODE consortium and others that there are many previously unrecognized functional elements in the genome, and many of these have poorly understood regulatory functions. Furthermore, GWA, when performed with appropriate attention to confounds such as ethnic stratification and other systematic errors that can upward bias statistical results, and with confirmation and validation, for example by identification of the functional locus, is a direct route to making causal inferences about the roles of genes in behavior. In other words, the implication of the genetic linkage is more than correlational: a locus, or one nearby the linked locus, modulates the behavior. The genome-wide significance threshold is usually approximately 10^{-8} corresponding to a single locus *p* value of 0.05. Within this statistical framework, GWA will detect the effects of common alleles (MAF >5%) of at least moderate effect (e.g., odds ratio >1.2), requiring thousands of cases and controls for such small effect sizes. As later discussed, less common alleles have been linked to addictions by resequencing and by linkage studies in families and founder populations in whom particular rare alleles are common. A salient advantage of GWA is that data can be combined across studies using a common pool of SNPs that are either directly genotyped or imputable.

Addictions GWA has yielded a confirmed functional locus for nicotine addiction, located in the *CHRNA5-CHRNA3-CHRNB4* gene-cluster on chromosome 15 (Bierut et al., 2007; Thorgeirsson et al., 2008). These genes encode subunits of the nicotinic acetylcholine receptor (nAChR), which is a ligand-gated ion channel activated by nicotine. A functional locus influencing nicotine addiction was identified in this region. *CHRNA5* Asp398Asn alters nicotine dependence/heavy smoking, pleasurable response to smoking, smoking quantity, and smoking persistence (Bierut et al., 2007; Thorgeirsson et al., 2008), as well as secondary susceptibilities to lung cancer and

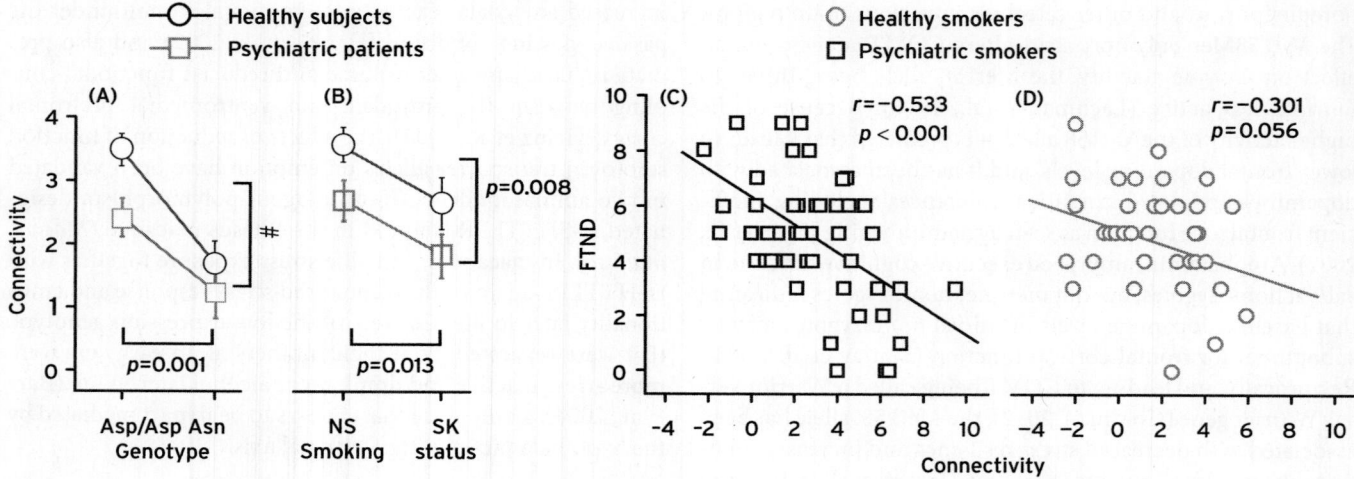

Figure 52.1 *The CHRNA5 Asn398 allele, identified as a risk factor in nicotine addiction by GWA, predicts weakness of a dorsal anterior cingulate/ventral striatal circuit whose weakness predicts nicotine craving. Right panel: Strength of the circuit, as measured by resting state functional connectivity (rsFC) predicts nicotine craving. Middle panel: the CHRNA5 Asn398 allele predicts smoking status. Left panel: The Asn398 allele predicts weaker connectivity of the circuit. (From Hong et al. (2010). A genetically modulated, intrinsic cingulate circuit supports human nicotine addiction. Proc Natl Acad Sci U S A. 107(30):13509–13514.)*

vascular disease (Amos et al., 2008) and smoking cessation (Munafo et al., 2011). The locus has a modest effect on addiction itself. Each copy of Asn398 accounts for ~0.5% of the variance in cigarettes smoked/day but more strongly predicts the strength of connectivity between anterior cingulate and ventral striatum (Hong et al., 2010) a circuit that in turn modulates nicotine craving, as shown in Figure 52.1.

Furthermore, (α4β2)$_2$α5 receptors that differed only in containing the *CHRNA5* Asn398 allelic form had altered response to agonist. Other studies have shown that Asp398 lowers calcium permeability and increases short-term desensitization, but does not alter receptor sensitivity to activation (Kuryatov et al., 2011). Whether the Asp398Asn polymorphism alters nicotine response or connectivity of reward circuits, or both, remains an open question.

For alcohol consumption, a meta-analysis of GWA in 12 European populations, totaling 26,316 individuals, identified the autism susceptibility 2 gene (*AUTS2*). The SNP implicated may moderate AUTS2 expression in prefrontal cortex, and expression of *AUTS2* (Schumann et al., 2011). Several genome-wide significant loci were identified for resting EEG traits that are addiction-associated (Hodgkinson et al., 2010), illustrating the power of combining GWAS with intermediate phenotypes.

RARE AND UNCOMMON VARIANTS

The common disease/common variant paradigm has been disturbed by the failure of GWA to account for a substantial portion of inherited variation of complex disease, and by discovery of extensive rare and uncommon genetic variation in humans. These rarer variants of stronger effect may account for a large portion of genetic vulnerability to common diseases. Advances in DNA sequencing technologies facilitate the detection of rare variants; however, the full impact of this approach depends on study of effects of these variants in founder populations and families where they are common, statistical combination of

multiple rare allele with the same probable functional impact, and further development and use of other convergent information such as evidence of effect on molecular function or effects of homologous variants in model organisms including the mouse.

Rare variants relevant to addiction are known within the serotonin receptor 2B gene (*HTR2B*) (Bevilacqua et al., 2011), *MAOA* (Brunner et al., 1993), and *CYP*, the *CYP2A6* variants even predicting fMRI responses to smoking cues (Tang et al., 2012). Both *HTR2B* and *MAOA* influence impulsivity, findings involving these genes having close parallels in animal models, and the *CYP* alleles have pharmacogenetic effects on response to nicotine that are also lawfully expected due to alteration of nicotine metabolism.

MAOA, located on the X chromosome, encodes monoamine oxidase A, which metabolizes monoamine neurotransmitters including norepinephrine, dopamine, and serotonin. The main effect of a common allele leading to lower MAOA expression is enhanced impulsivity, an important mediating trait in addictions. A stop codon found in eight males in one Dutch family led to impulsivity, carrier females being unaffected (Brunner et al., 1993) A common *MAOA* variable-number tandem repeat polymorphism can lead to lower MAOA enzyme activity and has been a model for understanding the role of context in gene effects on complex behaviors in which impulsivity plays an important role. Gene × environment interaction was observed in a longitudinally studied cohort of boys, with the lower expression allele and childhood adversity together predicting vulnerability to conduct disorder (Caspi et al., 2002) as confirmed by others. In women, who unlike males can be heterozygous for the low activity *MAOA* allele, results are mixed, and may depend on severity of adversity. A parallel GxE effect on ASPD was observed in a sample of Native American women with a combined effect of childhood sexual abuse and low activity MAOA genotype on risk of both alcoholism and ASPD (Ducci et al., 2008), and an allele dosage effect in the presence of childhood sexual abuse. Complicating the relationship of MAOA to impulsivity and aggression are other releasers of these behaviors. Testosterone independently predicts aggression, but males with high expression *MAOA* genotypes did not show the effect, which was limited to males with the low expression *MAOA* genotype that is apparently permissive for this behavior (Sjoberg et al., 2008). Similarly, *MAOA* genotype can interact with alcohol consumption, another disinhibitor of behavior (Tikkanen et al., 2009), and as will next be described, alcohol consumption also leads to impulsive aggression in carriers of a stop codon in *HTR2B* (Bevilacqua et al., 2010).

HTR2B is a serotonin receptor that, in part because of genetic studies implicating it in behavior, has been discovered to be widely expressed in the brain wherein it is found on approximately 40% of dopamine neurons in VTA, where it regulates dopamine release (L. Maroteaux, submitted). A stop codon disabling *HTR2B* (Q20*) is common in Finland, but rare or absent in other populations surveyed worldwide. The stop codon is linked to severe impulsive aggression, ASPD, and alcoholism, with an effect on impulsive aggression that is strongly modulated, or dependent, on inebriation. This *HTR2B* stop codon was discovered by sequencing impulsive and aggressive offenders who underwent psychiatric evaluation because of the extreme nature of their crimes. The stop codon is several times as common in these individuals as in Finnish controls, and is cotransmitted with impulsive behavior, including alcoholism, in families. Carriers of the stop codon who committed violent crimes did so while inebriated with alcohol, and were cognitively normal. In the Finnish population, most carriers are unaffected, indicating the *20 is a factor in impulsive behavior and addiction but not sufficient itself. *Htr2b* −/− mice exhibit higher novelty seeking and impulsivity, and enhanced responses to activating drugs including a D1 dopamine receptor agonist and cocaine.

Variants, many of which are rare, of *CYP2A6* (cytochrome P450, Family 2, subfamily A, polypeptide 6) alter risk of nicotine addiction via metabolism, the enzyme accounting for 70% of initial nicotine metabolism.

CONCLUSIONS

Vulnerability to addictive agents is widespread because addictive agents activate natural reward systems and abuse is kindled by variations in executive cognitive control and emotional response that are widespread in populations. Addictive agents of a variety of types are readily accessible, and in fact access is increasing, with legalization of gambling and marijuana, development of designer drugs and new ways to administer drugs, and the nearly universal availability of the internet and electronic devices to which people can become addicted. For these reasons, it seems paradoxical that addictions are moderately to highly heritable. However, there are many sources of resilience against addiction. These include social norms, positive family and peer influences, the diversity of rewarding activities available to most people, and conscious decisions to reduce harm and limit exposures. Because there are many routes to addictions, protective and predisposing genetic variants have diverse

actions. Furthermore, no single genetic variant is likely to be highly predictive for an addiction, and indeed no highly predictive locus emerged from GWA studies that provide a global view of the relative contribution of individual loci.

Our state of knowledge of the complex causal landscape of genetic effects on addictions is limited and insufficient for diagnostic prediction. However, the status quo is subject to change. Although it would be unwise to predict a timeline, it is likely that addictions will be redefined via a combination of neuroscience-based measures, improved understanding of the behavioral interface with the environment, and by cataloging the genetic variations that influence risk and understanding their mechanisms.

Addiction is a categorical end-diagnosis, assuming a cutoff between normal and abnormal, although many non-addicted individuals have the same predisposing factors and even subthreshold addictive behaviors. Other complex diagnostic amalgams, syndromes, and chief complaints have been successfully refined and redefined at the etiological level. For example, deafness was deconstructed and reconstructed into a series of better defined diseases through a combination of clinical, neuroanatomic, psychophysiologic, cellular, and genetic approaches. We recognize that the same functional consequence—namely hearing loss—has many distinct causes ranging from exposure to chemicals and loud noises to adverse panoply of genetic variants, with profound implications for prevention and intervention. As compared to the ear, the brain is a more complex organ. However, the brain's structures, functions, and outputs, both behavioral and molecular, are increasingly amenable to measurement, and as discussed earlier, the genetic study of these measures, many which represent intermediate phenotypes for addiction, offers a different and potentially better path to the identification of genes that alter vulnerability, as illustrated (Fig. 52.2). However, and as also indicated in the figure, because addictions are clinically defined, the genes that exert large effects on intermediate phenotypes such as executive cognition, stress resilience, and reward may not be strong clinical predictors of addictions as presently defined. In similar fashion, none of the deafness genes explains a large portion of deafness as a whole.

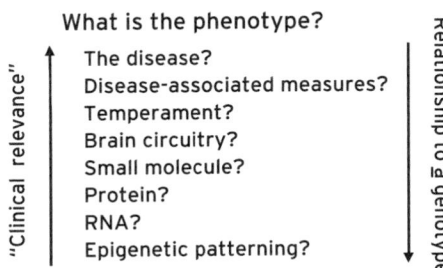

Figure 52.2 As presently defined, addictions are heritable but remote to the action of particular genes. This is because of intervening effects of environmental context and different mechanisms of vulnerability. These mechanisms, including differences in brain emotional response, reward, executive cognitive function, and drug metabolism have become partially accessible in the form of molecular and psychophysiologic intermediate phenotypes.

What might be the impact of gene identification in addiction? The *CFTR* gene does not strongly predict pneumonia, or fever, because it is found in only a fraction of patients presenting with these problems. However, *CFTR* is the defining factor in cystic fibrosis, a disease that with fuller understanding also involves pancreatic insufficiency, infertility, and non-genetic factors that critically shape clinical course. Although a gene therapy for cystic fibrosis has not emerged, careful attention to non-genetic factors in cystic fibrosis patients has revolutionized the care, and clinical course, of this distinct genetically defined subgroup. The same general approach may also be effective in addictions—the genetically-based diagnosis serving to identify a population to which intensive intervention has to be targeted. For addictions, there are now some positive indications that identification of specific genetic influences is a step towards individualization of treatment. For example, a common functional missense variant of the mu-opioid receptor (OPRM1 Asn40Asp) is associated with altered reward function (Ramchandani et al., 2011) and alcoholic carriers of the Asp40 allele showed greater clinical improvement when treated with the opioid antagonist naltrexone (Anton et al., 2008; Oslin et al., 2003). Similarly, CHRNA5 Asn398Asp (Munafo et al., 2011) and other genes have been reported to influence response to smoking cessation treatment.

In conclusion, addictions are multistage, chronic, and relapsing diseases with heritabilities that range from 0.39 (hallucinogens) to 0.72 (cocaine). Genes influence each stage of the disease. Because addictions are in parts volitional, inborn, and determined by experience, they pose unique medical and moral challenges. The genetic basis of addictions is largely unknown; however the inheritance of addictions and knowledge of a few specific genes altering vulnerability have established that these are illnesses that can be understood via neuroscience-based chains of causality. Neither heritability of addictions nor the existence of addiction genes establishes that addictions are diseases, because many benign traits are also heritable, but inheritance and gene discoveries point to chains of causality that lead some people and not others to addiction. Many putative addiction genes have been discovered by association studies although few appear are well-validated. Encouragingly, among the small group of genes whose effects appear validated (e.g., *OPRM1, ADH1B, ALDH2, MAOA, SLC6A4, NPY, COMT, CHRNA5* and *CYP2A6*) are several that have potential clinical utility, for example to understand alcohol-related flushing and upper GI cancer risk (*ADH1B* and *ALDH2*), variation in nicotine metabolism (*CYP26*), and naltrexone treatment response (*OPRM1*). These genes act through a variety of mechanisms: by altering drug metabolism, by altering affinity of receptors for addictive drugs (*CHRNA5*, which may also alter circuitry of reward), and by altering stress response, emotion, and behavioral control, as do genes such as *MAOA, NPY, HTR2B, COMT,* and *HTTLPR*. The genes that influence addiction repeat and enhance broader themes in the neuroscience of addiction.

DISCLOSURES

Dr. Goldman has no conflicts of interest to disclose.

REFERENCES

Amos, C.I., Wu, X., et al. (2008). Genome-wide association scan of tag SNPs identifies a susceptibility locus for lung cancer at 15q25.1. *Nat. Genet.* 40(5):616–622.

Anton, R.F., Oroszi, G., et al. (2008). An evaluation of mu-opioid receptor (OPRM1) as a predictor of naltrexone response in the treatment of alcohol dependence: results from the Combined Pharmacotherapies and Behavioral Interventions for Alcohol Dependence (COMBINE) study. *Arch. Gen. Psychiatry* 65(2):135–144.

Barr, C.S., Newman, T.K., et al. (2004). Interaction between serotonin transporter gene variation and rearing condition in alcohol preference and consumption in female primates. *Arch. Gen. Psychiatry* 61(11):1146–1152.

Bevilacqua, L., and Goldman, D. (2011). Genetics of emotion. *Trends Cogn. Sci.* 15:401–408.

Bevilacqua, L., Doly, S., et al. (2011). A population-specific HTR2B stop codon predisposes to severe impulsivity. *Nature* 468(7327):1061–1066.

Bierut, L.J., Goate, A.M., et al. (2012). ADH1B is associated with alcohol dependence and alcohol consumption in populations of European and African ancestry. *Mol. Psychiatry* 4:445–450.

Bierut, L.J., Madden, P.A., et al. (2007). Novel genes identified in a high-density genome wide association study for nicotine dependence. *Hum. Mol. Genet.* 16(1):24–35.

Binder, E.B., Bradley, R.G., et al. (2008). Association of FKBP5 polymorphisms and childhood abuse with risk of posttraumatic stress disorder symptoms in adults. *JAMA* 299(11):1291–1305.

Brooks, P.J., Goldman, D., et al. (2009). Alleles of alcohol and acetaldehyde metabolism genes modulate susceptibility to oesophageal cancer from alcohol consumption. *Hum. Genomics* 3(2):103–105.

Brunner, H.G., Nelen, M., et al. (1993). Abnormal behavior associated with a point mutation in the structural gene for monoamine oxidase A. *Science* 262(5133):578–580.

Caspi, A., and Moffitt, T.E. (2006). Gene–environment interactions in psychiatry: joining forces with neuroscience. *Nat. Rev. Neurosci.* 7(7):583–590.

Caspi, A., McClay, J., et al. (2002). Role of genotype in the cycle of violence in maltreated children. *Science* 297(5582):851–854.

Caspi, A., Sugden, K., et al. (2003). Influence of life stress on depression: moderation by a polymorphism in the 5-HTT gene. *Science* 301(5631):386–389.

Cloninger, C.R. (1987). Neurogenetic adaptive mechanisms in alcoholism. *Science* 236(4800):410–416.

Ducci, F., Enoch, M.A., et al. (2007). Increased anxiety and other similarities in temperament of alcoholics with and without antisocial personality disorder across three diverse populations. *Alcohol* 41(1):3–12.

Ducci, F., Enoch, M.A., et al. (2008). Interaction between a functional MAOA locus and childhood sexual abuse predicts alcoholism and antisocial personality disorder in adult women. *Mol. Psychiatry* 13(3):334–347.

Ducci, F., Kaakinen, M., et al. (2011). TTC12-ANKK1-DRD2 and CHRNA5-CHRNA3-CHRNB4 influence different pathways leading to smoking behavior from adolescence to mid-adulthood. *Biol. Psychiatry* 69:650–660.

Egan, M.F., Goldberg, T.E., et al. (2001). Effect of COMT Val108/158 Met genotype on frontal lobe function and risk for schizophrenia. *Proc. Natl. Acad. Sci. USA* 98(12):6917–6922.

Enoch, M.A., Gorodetsky, E., et al. (2011). Functional genetic variants that increase synaptic serotonin and 5-HT3 receptor sensitivity predict alcohol and drug dependence. *Mol. Psychiatry* 16(11):1139–1146.

Enoch, M.A., Xu, K., et al. (2003). Genetic origins of anxiety in women: a role for a functional catechol-O-methyltransferase polymorphism. *Psychiatr. Genet.* 13(1):33–41.

Goldman, D., and Bergen, A. (1998). General and specific inheritance of substance abuse and alcoholism. *Arch. Gen. Psychiatry* 55(11):964–965.

Goldman, D., and Enoch, M.A. (1990). Genetic epidemiology of ethanol metabolic enzymes: a role for selection. *World. Rev. Nutr. Diet.* 63:143–160.

Goldman, D., Oroszi, G., et al. (2005). The genetics of addictions: uncovering the genes. *Nat. Rev. Genet.* 6(7):521–532.

Goldman, D. (2012). Our Genes, Our Choices. Boston: Elsevier.

Gottesman, I.I., and Gould, T.D. (2003). The endophenotype concept in psychiatry: etymology and strategic intentions. *Am. J. Psychiatry* 160(4):636–645.

Hariri, A.R., Mattay, V.S., et al. (2002). Serotonin transporter genetic variation and the response of the human amygdala. *Science* 297(5580):400–403.

Heath, A.C., Madden, P.A., et al. (1999). Genetic differences in alcohol sensitivity and the inheritance of alcoholism risk. *Psychol. Med.* 29(5):1069–1081.

Heinz, A., Braus, D.F., et al. (2005). Amygdala-prefrontal coupling depends on a genetic variation of the serotonin transporter. *Nat. Neurosci.* 8(1):20–21.

Heinz, A., Jones, D.W., et al. (2000). A relationship between serotonin transporter genotype and *in vivo* protein expression and alcohol neurotoxicity. *Biol. Psychiatry* 47(7):643–649.

Hodgkinson, C.A., Enoch, M.A., et al. (2010). Genome-wide association identifies candidate genes that influence the human electroencephalogram. *Proc. Natl. Acad. Sci. USA* 107(19):8695–8700.

Hong, L.E., Hodgkinson, C.A., et al. (2010). A genetically modulated, intrinsic cingulate circuit supports human nicotine addiction. *Proc. Natl. Acad. Sci. USA* 107(30):13509–13514.

Hu, X., Oroszi, G., et al. (2005). An expanded evaluation of the relationship of four alleles to the level of response to alcohol and the alcoholism risk. *Alcohol Clin. Exp. Res.* 29(1):8–16.

Hu, X.Z., Lipsky, R.H., et al. (2006). Serotonin transporter promoter gain-of-function genotypes are linked to obsessive-compulsive disorder. *Am. J. Hum. Genet.* 78(5):815–826.

Kendler, K.S., Karkowski, L.M., et al. (1999). Genetic and environmental risk factors in the aetiology of illicit drug initiation and subsequent misuse in women. *Br. J. Psychiatry* 175:351–356.

Kendler, K.S., Myers, J., et al. (2007). Specificity of genetic and environmental risk factors for symptoms of cannabis, cocaine, alcohol, caffeine, and nicotine dependence. *Arch. Gen. Psychiatry* 64(11):1313–1320.

Kendler, K.S., Prescott, C.A., et al. (2003). The structure of genetic and environmental risk factors for common psychiatric and substance use disorders in men and women. *Arch. Gen. Psychiatry* 60(9):929–937.

Kendler, K.S., Schmitt, E., et al. (2008). Genetic and environmental influences on alcohol, caffeine, cannabis, and nicotine use from early adolescence to middle adulthood. *Arch. Gen. Psychiatry* 65(6):674–682.

Kessler, R.C., Crum, R.M., et al. (1997). Lifetime co-occurrence of DSM-III-R alcohol abuse and dependence with other psychiatric disorders in the National Comorbidity Survey. *Arch. Gen. Psychiatry* 54(4):313–321.

Krueger, R.F., Hicks, B.M., et al. (2002). Etiologic connections among substance dependence, antisocial behavior, and personality: modeling the externalizing spectrum. *J. Abnorm. Psychol.* 111(3):411–424.

Kuryatov, A., Berrettini, W., et al. (2011). Acetylcholine receptor (AChR) alpha5 subunit variant associated with risk for nicotine dependence and lung cancer reduces (alpha4beta2)alpha5 AChR function. *Mol. Pharmacol.* 79(1):119–125.

Lachman, H.M., Papolos, D.F., et al. (1996). Human catechol-O-methyltransferase pharmacogenetics: description of a functional polymorphism and its potential application to neuropsychiatric disorders. *Pharmacogenetics* 6(3):243–250.

Mattay, V.S., Goldberg, T.E., et al. (2003). Catechol O-methyltransferase val158-met genotype and individual variation in the brain response to amphetamine. *Proc. Natl. Acad. Sci. USA* 100(10):6186–6191.

Munafo, M.R., Johnstone, E.C. (2011). CHRNA3 rs1051730 genotype and short-term smoking cessation. *Nicotine Tob. Res.* 13: 982–988.

Oslin, D.W., Berrettini, W., et al. (2003). A functional polymorphism of the mu-opioid receptor gene is associated with naltrexone response in alcohol-dependent patients. *Neuropsychopharmacology* 28(8):1546–1552.

Ramchandani, V.A., Umhau, J., et al. (2011). A genetic determinant of the striatal dopamine response to alcohol in men. *Mol. Psychiatry* 16(8):809–817.

Schuckit, M.A. (1998). Biological, psychological and environmental predictors of the alcoholism risk: a longitudinal study. *J. Stud. Alcohol.* 59(5):485–494.

Schumann, G., Coin, L.J., et al. (2011). Genome-wide association and genetic functional studies identify autism susceptibility candidate 2 gene (AUTS2) in the regulation of alcohol consumption. *Proc. Natl. Acad. Sci. USA* 108(17):7119–7124.

Sjoberg, R.L., Ducci, F., et al. (2008). A non-additive interaction of a functional MAO-A VNTR and testosterone predicts antisocial behavior. *Neuropsychopharmacology* 33(2):425–430.

Tammimaki, A.E., and Mannisto, P.T. (2010). Are genetic variants of COMT associated with addiction? *Pharmacogenet. Genomics.* 20(12):717–741.

Tang, D.W., Hello, B., et al. (2012). Genetic variation in CYP2A6 predicts neural reactivity to smoking cues as measured using fMRI. Neuroimage. 60(4):2136–2143.

Thomasson, H.R., Edenberg, H.J., et al. (1991). Alcohol and aldehyde dehydrogenase genotypes and alcoholism in Chinese men. *Am. J. Hum. Genet.* 48(4):677–681.

Thorgeirsson, T.E., Geller, F., et al. (2008). A variant associated with nicotine dependence, lung cancer and peripheral arterial disease. *Nature* 452(7187):638–642.

Tiihonen, J., Hallikainen, T., et al. (1999). Association between the functional variant of the catechol-O-methyltransferase (COMT) gene and type 1 alcoholism. *Mol. Psychiatry* 4(3):286–289.

Tikkanen, R., Sjoberg, R.L., et al. (2009). Effects of MAOA-genotype, alcohol consumption, and aging on violent behavior. *Alcohol Clin. Exp. Res.* 33(3):428–434.

van Beijsterveldt, C.E., and van Baal, G.C. (2002). Twin and family studies of the human electroencephalogram: a review and a meta-analysis. *Biol Psychol.* 61(1–2):111–138.

Vandenbergh, D.J., Rodriguez, L.A., et al. (1997). High-activity catechol-O-methyltransferase allele is more prevalent in polysubstance abusers. *Am. J. Med. Genet.* 74(4):439–442.

Zhou, Z., Zhu, G., et al. (2008). Genetic variation in human NPY expression affects stress response and emotion. *Nature* 452(7190):997–1001.

Zubieta, J.K., Heitzeg, M.M., et al. (2003). COMT val158met genotype affects mu-opioid neurotransmitter responses to a pain stressor. *Science* 299(5610):1240–1243.

53 | BRAIN DEVELOPMENT AND THE RISK FOR SUBSTANCE ABUSE

KRISTINA CAUDLE AND B.J. CASEY

An estimated 22.4 million Americans have used illicit drugs in the last month, representing nearly 9% of the population (NSDUH, 2011), and individuals between the ages of 16 to 25 years show the highest rates of illicit substance use. The sharp rise in substance use during adolescence underscores the importance of understanding risk for addiction. Changes in the brain during this developmental period and variation in these changes across individuals may predict who is at risk for substance abuse, enabling the prevention of later dependence. This chapter provides an overview of how the brain circuitry involved in addiction changes across development, and how this may identify who may be most at risk and when they may be most vulnerable.

Addiction is the persistent use of a substance or engagement in a behavior to alter mood despite the adverse consequences of that substance or behavior. Traditionally, addiction research has focused on alcohol, tobacco, and drug use, especially illicit drug use, but recently compulsive behaviors including gambling, gaming, and overeating that are similar in many ways to alcohol and drug dependency have begun to be examined (Gold et al., 2009; Kourosh et al., 2010; Lee, 2012; Reynaud et al., 2010; Weinstein, 2010; Weinstein and Lejoyeux, 2010). At the core of each of these behaviors is an experience of craving and a loss of control that leads to persistence of the behavior, and ultimately addiction.

A theory for why individuals engage in addiction-prone behaviors is for their pleasurable or positive mood-altering effects. According to this hedonic hypothesis, drugs serve as rewards that elicit approach behavior and induce pleasure, increasing the frequency and intensity of consumption. In addiction, it is thought that the behavior becomes pathologically persistent in an attempt to maintain these rewarding effects (Volkow et al., 2011), as well as to avoid the negative outcomes associated with withdrawal symptoms (Robinson and Berridge, 2003). This chapter examines how brain circuitry underlying impulse control and sensitivity to rewards change across development and vary among individuals.

ADDICTION CIRCUITRY

A prominent neurobiological model of addiction is that addictive substances and behaviors act upon the brain's "reward" circuitry, either directly or indirectly, by flooding the brain with the neurotransmitter dopamine (Volkow et al., 2011). Although several neurotransmitter systems have been implicated in addiction (Fleckenstein et al., 2007; Howell and Kimmel, 2008), increased levels of dopamine are thought to mediate the reinforcing effects (Volkow et al., 2012). Dopamine is released in response to rewards like food, sex, and drugs. Over time, dopamine activity shifts from the rewards themselves to the cues that predict those rewards (Hollerman and Schultz, 1998; Mirenowicz and Schultz, 1994). When a reward is greater than expected, the firing of dopaminergic neurons increases (Schultz et al., 1997), increasing motivation towards the reward via a learning mechanism referred to as prediction error. Prediction error is the difference between an expected reward value and the actual value of that reward (Arias-Carrion and Poppel, 2007). In addiction, cues that come to be associated with the substance of abuse lead to increases in dopamine, rather than the substance itself (Volkow et al., 2011). Unlike healthy individuals, addicts show a blunting of dopamine increases to stimulants, presumably due to their history of prior use and increases in striatal dopamine in response to drug-specific cues. The discrepancy between the expectation of the drug effects and the blunted response in addicts is thought to maintain drug taking in an attempt to achieve the expected reward (Volkow et al., 2011).

The most important brain-reward circuit involved in addiction is comprised of the dopamine-containing neurons in the ventral tegmental area of the midbrain and their target areas in the limbic forebrain, in particular, the ventral striatum and prefrontal cortex (Haber, 2003; Nestler, 2004; Volkow et al., 2011). The majority of studies have focused on the ventral striatum and its role in reinforcing effects in addiction (Breiter et al., 1997; Ito et al., 2002, 2004). This region is an important part of the reward circuit responsible for assigning value to current rewards and learning to predict future events. These value signals are broadcast to prefrontal control regions to help guide future behavior (Knutson et al., 2001; O'Doherty et al., 2002). An imbalance in the communication between regions involved in reinforcement learning and those that underlie cognitive control has been suggested to contribute to addiction. Accordingly, drugs of abuse are thought to "hijack" the systems associated with the rewarding properties of drugs of abuse and lead to less regulation of behavior by prefrontal control regions (Bechara, 2005).

BRAIN DEVELOPMENT

The portrayal of addiction, as an imbalance between brain regions involved in cognitive control and those that are involved in reward processes, parallels aspects of typical behavioral and brain development. Specifically, adolescent brain development has been characterized by a tension between early-emerging bottom-up striatal regions that express exaggerated reactivity to motivational stimuli and later-maturing top-down cortical control regions (Casey et al., 2008; Ernst et al., 2006, 2009; Geier and Luna, 2009; Steinberg, 2008). This bottom-up system that has been associated with reward-seeking and risk-taking behavior gradually loses its competitive edge with the progressive emergence of top-down regulation during development. With age and experience, the connectivity between these regions is strengthened and provides a mechanism for top-down modulation of the subcortically driven reward behavior. Empirical support for this model comes from the differential neurochemical, structural, and functional development in cortical and subcortical regions.

Significant dopaminergic changes occur across development. There is a peak in D1 and D2 receptor density in the striatum during early adolescence (Benes et al., 2000; Brenhouse et al., 2008; Galvan et al., 2005), whereas this peak does not emerge until later in prefrontal cortex (Cunningham et al., 2008; Tseng and O'Donnell, 2007). This differential timeline in the peak of D1 and D2 receptor density in the striatum and cortex may result in an imbalance between these systems.

REGIONAL DIFFERENCES IN BRAIN DEVELOPMENT

Findings from both human and nonhuman primate studies provide evidence for different time courses in regional postnatal brain development. These changes are illustrated in Figure 53.1. Following cell proliferation, differentiation, and migration there is a rapid overproduction of synapses relative to its adult state (Rakic, 1974). Although this process of synaptogenesis appears to occur concurrently across diverse regions of the non-human primate cerebral cortex (Rakic et al., 1986), the plateau and subsequent decrease in synapses varies by brain regions. The plateau and pruning phases of association cortical regions (e.g. prefrontal cortex) are relatively protracted compared with others (e.g., sensorimotor and subcortical regions; Bourgeois et al., 1994; Huttenlocher and Dabholkar, 1997). Positron emission tomography studies of glucose metabolism show similar patterns of development, with local metabolic rates paralleling the time course of overproduction and subsequent pruning of synapses (Chugani et al., 1987). Human studies using magnetic resonance imaging show a significant decrease in cortical gray matter by approximately 12 years in prefrontal and association cortices that is preceded by earlier maturing development in sensorimotor and subcortical regions (Giedd et al., 1999; Gotgay et al., 2004; Sowell et al., 1999; Sowell et al., 2002). Together these studies support different time courses in the development of brain regions implicated in higher cognitive function relative to those involved in sensorimotor and primitive emotive functions.

Whereas gray matter changes appear to peak during childhood and adolescences, cerebral white matter shows a gradual increase well into adulthood, especially in prefrontal white matter tracts (Klingberg et al., 1999). The protracted development of prefrontal and association cortices, along with white matter fiber tract development in this circuitry, contributes to children's developing capacity for cognitive control (Klingberg et al., 1999; Liston et al., 2006). Variability in the myelination and regularity of prefrontal white matter fibers also contribute

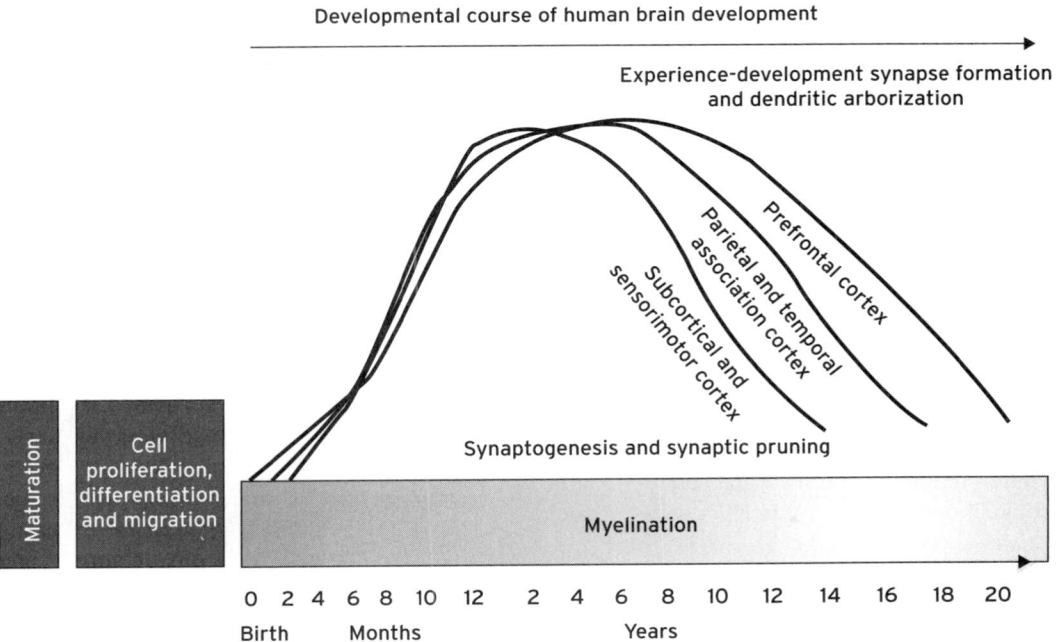

Figure 53.1 Regional brain development. Cell proliferation, differentiation, and migration is followed by rapid formation of synapses that subsequently plateau and decline to adult levels at different time points in development and increases in myelination well into adulthood. (Adapted from Casey et al., 2005. Imaging the developing brain: what have we learned about cognitive development? Trends Cogn. Sci., 9(3): 104–110.)

to individual differences in cognitive control and have been linked to disorders of cognitive control like attention deficit hyperactivity disorder (ADHD).

To more directly examine functional neural circuits underlying the development of cognitive control and reward sensitivity across development, a means of assessing, *in vivo*, the developmental physiological course of behavior is needed. Functional magnetic resonance imaging (fMRI) provides this ability (Logothetis et al., 2001). Understanding how brain function changes during adolescence, relative to both childhood and adulthood, and how these changes vary across individuals is essential in predicting risk for later substance abuse and dependence. This chapter reviews recent human imaging work supporting the emerging view of adolescence as characterized by a tension between early-emerging bottom-up subcortical brain regions that express exaggerated reactivity to reward related cues and later-maturing top-down cognitive control regions involved in self-control.

Human functional imaging studies show dramatic changes in corticostriatal circuitry across development. Children recruit distinct but often larger, more diffuse brain regions when performing cognitive control tasks than do adults. The pattern of activity within brain regions central to cognitive control performance, such as prefrontal cortex, becomes more focal or fine-tuned based on cross-sectional (Brown et al., 2004) and longitudinal studies (Durston et al., 2004). This pattern of activity is suggestive of development within, and refinement of, projections to and from, the prefrontal cortex with maturation. Recent developmental functional connectivity data (Kelly et al., 2009) is consistent with this observation of diffuse correlations among frontal brain regions in children, whereas adults exhibit more focal connections with distal regions. This development of the prefrontal cortex is associated with age-related improvement in cognitive control (Asato et al., 2010; Astle and Scerif, 2009; Casey et al., 2007; Durston et al., 2006; Forbes and Dahl, 2010; Liston et al., 2006; Luna et al., 2001; Luna et al., 2010; Romeo, 2003).

While the prefrontal cortex shows protracted development, well into adulthood, striatal regions sensitive to novelty and reward appear to develop earlier (Bunge et al., 2002; Liston et al., 2006). One of the first studies to examine reward-related circuitry from early childhood to adulthood (Galvan et al., 2006) used a task previously developed to examine the role of reward magnitude on dopamine firing in nonhuman primates (Cromwell and Schultz, 2003). They found that the ventral striatum was sensitive to varying magnitudes of monetary reward, exhibiting monotonic increases with increasing reward amounts. This response was exaggerated during adolescence, relative to both childhood and adulthood. Moreover, a positive association between ventral striatal activity to large rewards and the likelihood of engaging in risky behavior such as substance use was shown (Galvan et al., 2007). These findings are consistent with the adult imaging literature showing an association between ventral striatal activity and risky choices (Kuhnen and Knutson, 2005; Matthews et al., 2004).

Several groups have shown heightened activation of the ventral striatum in anticipation and/or receipt of rewards in adolescents compared to adults (Ernst et al., 2005; Galvan et al., 2006; Geier et al., 2010; Van Leijenhorst et al., 2010). This heightened striatal activity and increased reward seeking during adolescence has been associated with heightened dopaminergic prediction error responsivity (Cohen et al., 2010). It should be noted that others report hyporesponsiveness during adolescence in the ventral striatum (e.g., Bjork et al., 2004). Regardless, both hyper- and hyporesponsiveness to rewards and drug-related cues have been implicated in substance use disorders. Heightened responses to drugs potentially increase use, whereas dampened responses to drug-related cues appear to maintain use.

Ventral striatal activity does not appear to be associated with impulse control (Galvan et al., 2007). Instead, impulsivity is negatively correlated with age. Studies of clinical populations characterized by impulsivity problems such as ADHD support these findings. Specifically, individuals with ADHD have reduced activity in prefrontal regions compared to controls when performing impulse control tasks (Casey et al., 2007; Epstein et al., 2007; Vaidya et al., 1998) but do not show heightened responses to incentives in the striatum to rewards (Scheres et al., 2007). Treatment with stimulants that increase the availability of dopamine by blocking the dopamine transporter leads to increases in frontostriatal activity and enhanced impulse control. Together these findings provide support for a dissociation between reward sensitivity and impulsivity both neurally and developmentally, with the former showing a curvilinear developmental pattern and the latter a linear pattern of development.

Only recently have studies begun to examine how rewarding cues can differentially influence impulse control across development. Somerville and colleagues imaged children, adolescents, and adults while they performed an impulse control task with appetitive social cues (happy faces) and neutral cues. The ability to inhibit a response to a rare neutral cue showed steady improvement with age. However, on trials for which the individual had to resist approaching appetitive social cues, adolescents failed to show the expected age-dependent improvement (Fig. 53.2A). Relative to neutral cues, adolescents made more commission errors to these appetitive social cues than did adults or children. This performance decrement during adolescence was paralleled by heightened activity in the ventral striatum (Fig. 53.2B and C). Conversely, activation in the inferior frontal gyrus was associated with overall performance and showed a linear pattern of change with age.

As drug use among teens typically occurs with peers, a number of studies have begun to examine how differential development of cognitive control and motivational systems impact susceptibility to peer influences. These studies find that adolescents relative to adults make riskier decisions when a peer is present as opposed to when alone (Gardner and Steinberg, 2005). This performance is paralleled by heightened activity in the ventral striatum for adolescents relative to adults (Chein et al., 2011). These findings suggest that peers have reinforcing effects on behavior that are represented at the level of the ventral striatum. Moreover, the differential development of reward and cognitive control processes during adolescence suggests that this period of development may be prone to addictive behaviors.

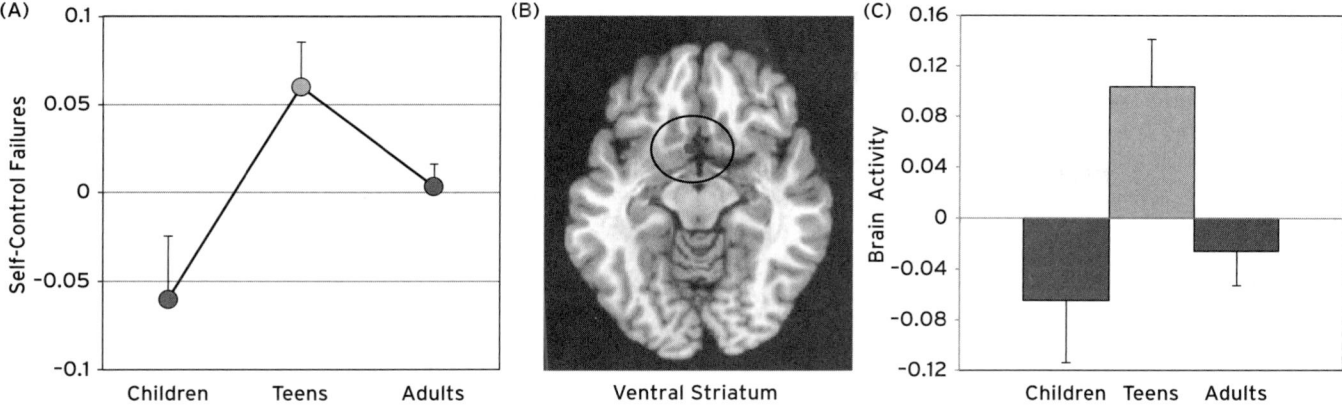

Figure 53.2 *Developmental differences in self control. (A) Adolescents have more self control failures (commission errors) when inhibiting responses to appetitive cues than do adults or children. (B) Localization of ventral striatal activity when inhibiting responses to appetitive cues. (C) Adolescents show greater ventral striatal activity when inhibiting responses to appetitive cues. (Adapted from Somerville et al., 2011.)*

RISK FACTORS FOR ADDICTION

ADOLESCENCE

Adolescence clearly marks a period of increased experimentation with drugs and alcohol (Hardin and Ernst, 2009) with alcohol being the most abused of illegal substances by teens (Johnston et al., 2009; Windle et al., 2008; Witt, 2010). Early use of these substances, such as alcohol, is a reliable predictor of later dependence and abuse (Grant and Dawson, 1997). Alcohol and substances of abuse, including cocaine and cannabinoids, have been shown to have reinforcing properties. These substances influence mesolimbic dopamine transmission with acute activations of neurons in frontolimbic circuitry rich in dopamine, including the ventral striatum (French et al., 1997; Maldonado and Rodriguez de Fonseca, 2002; Volkow et al., 2002).

The use of these substances may exacerbate enhanced ventral striatum responses resulting in strengthening of reinforcement properties to certain drugs (Hardin and Ernst, 2009). As such, drugs of abuse may "hijack" systems associated with drug incentives like the ventral striatum, and lead to down-regulation of top-down prefrontal control regions (Robinson and Berridge, 1993, 2003, 2008).

Few studies have examined functional brain activity in response to drug or alcohol related stimuli (i.e., pictures of alcohol) in adolescents (Nagel et al., 2005), although this is a growing area of research (Brown and Tapert, 2004). Studies of high-risk populations (e.g., familial load of alcohol dependence) suggest impairments in prefrontal functioning are apparent prior to drug use exposure (e.g., McQueeny et al., 2009; Medina et al., 2008) and predict later substance use (Pulido et al., 2010; Tapert et al., 2003). Poorer top down prefrontal control prior to drug exposure may set up a long-term course of alcohol and drug abuse well beyond adolescence (Monti et al., 2005; Pulido et al., 2010).

A heightened sensitivity to rewarding effects of drugs and alcohol and diminished sensitivity to negative effects has been postulated as a reason for why adolescence may be a specific developmental window of increased risk for addiction. The majority of empirical work on developmental use of drugs and alcohol has been performed in animals, given ethical constraints on performing such studies in humans. These studies have shown that adolescent rodents, unlike adults, are less sensitive to the negative effects of alcohol like motor impairment, sedation, acute withdrawal, and "hangover effects" of ethanol (Doremus et al., 2003; Pautassi et al., 2008; Spear and Varlinskaya, 2005). These findings are important because they suggest that many of the effects that serve as cues to limit intake in adults are not present in adolescents (Windle et al., 2008). In an early behavioral study of the effects of alcohol in 8- to 15-year-old boys of low and high familial risk (Behar et al., 1983), the most significant finding was little, if any, behavioral change or impairment on tests of intoxication—even after given doses that had been intoxicating in an adult population. In parallel, adolescents seem more sensitive to positive influences of alcohol, such as social facilitation, which may further encourage alcohol and substance use (Varlinskaya and Spear, 2002). Most substance and alcohol use occurs in social situations in adolescents (Steinberg, 2008), potentially pushing them towards greater alcohol and drug use when their peers value this behavior.

INDIVIDUAL TRAITS

One potential risk factor for substance use and abuse is vulnerability in resisting temptation or self-control. Low self-control have been linked to increased sensitivity to stimulant drugs in both humans (Nigg et al., 2006; Tarter et al., 2003) and rats (Yates et al., 2012). Lapses in this ability have been suggested to be at the very core of suboptimal choices (Eigsti et al., 2006; Mischel et al., 1989) including those related to substance use and abuse (Bechara and Van Der Linden, 2005). This ability can be measured in childhood simply by assessing how well the child can resist an immediate reward (e.g., a cookie) in favor of a larger reward later (e.g., two cookies). Although individuals vary in this ability to control one's impulses or delay gratification, even as adults, developmental studies suggest there are temporal windows in which an individual may be particularly susceptible to temptations.

The ability to wait for reward has been demonstrated to buffer against the development of a variety of dispositional physical and mental health vulnerabilities in middle age, including higher body mass index and illicit substance use, even when controlling for childhood social environment and child health (Kubzansky et al., 2009; Mischel and Ayduk, 2004; Mischel et al., 1988; Rodriguez et al., 1989). The relative lifetime stability in the capacity to resist temptation or control impulses was recently shown in a 40-year longitudinal study. Specifically, individuals who, as a group, had more difficulty delaying gratification at four years of age continued to show reduced self-control abilities 40 years later. These individuals exhibited more difficulty as adults in suppressing responses to positive social cues during a go/no-go impulse control task (Casey et al., 2011) (Fig. 53.3A). A subset of these high- and low-delaying individuals was imaged during performance of the go/no-go task. Whereas the prefrontal cortex differentiated between no-go and go trials to a greater extent in high delayers, the ventral striatum showed an exaggerated response in low delayers that paralleled their behavioral performance (Fig. 53.3B–C). These findings suggest that sensitivity to rewarding cues can influence an individual's ability to suppress thoughts and actions and that control systems may be "hijacked" by reward systems, rendering control systems unable to appropriately modulate behavior. Similar analogies of imbalances between these neural systems in the literature suggest that addiction (Bechara, 2005) and adolescence (Chein et al., 2011; Galvan et al., 2006; Somerville et al., 2011) may be contexts during which cognitive control may be particularly vulnerable to salient reward-related cues.

Because addictive substances and behaviors alter mood, the role of positive and negative affect have been examined as risk factors for addiction (Cheetham et al., 2010; Robinson and Berridge, 2003). Individuals who are high in positive affect are more likely to engage in risky behavior, such as drug use, whereas individuals low in positive affect may initially use substances because of a lack of responsiveness to natural positive rewards (Cyders and Smith, 2008). Individuals who are more reactive to negative cues and tend to engage in risky behaviors when distressed are also at high risk for substance abuse, especially during adolescence (Cyders and Smith, 2008). Individual differences in impulse control and reactivity to affective or emotional states appear to impact different core features of substance use disorders (Dawe and Loxton, 2004). High reactivity and approach behavior predicts the propensity to initiate drug use, whereas high impulsivity predicts the development of persistent and compulsive addiction-like behavior in the face of aversive outcomes (Belin et al., 2008).

PRIOR EXPOSURE

Differential sensitivities to positive and negative properties of substances of abuse have been postulated to underlie risk for addiction. A contributing factor to these sensitivities is the role of prior exposure on the brain and behavior. We focus on two developmental windows of exposure. First, we review the risk of later substance abuse caused by exposure to stimulants (cocaine) during fetal development. Second, we review the effects of stimulant medications during postnatal periods of childhood and adolescence on risk for substance abuse.

EFFECTS OF PRENATAL EXPOSURE ON LATER SUBSTANCE ABUSE

The fetal brain may be especially vulnerable to substances introduced through maternal consumption. Prenatal substance exposure to stimulants has a wide range of possible effects on the developing brain, depending on the dosage and timing in fetal development. Specifically, animal studies show that prenatal exposure to cocaine leads to lasting anatomical alterations in dopamine-rich prefrontal cortical regions (Stanwood et al., 2001a, 2001b). These effects appear to be specific to embryonic days 16–25 in the rabbit when the onset of D1 dopamine receptor expression occurs and there is a peak in corticogenesis (Stanwood et al., 2001a). These changes result in a reduction rather than an increase in reinforcing properties of stimulants and in an increased tolerance for substances of

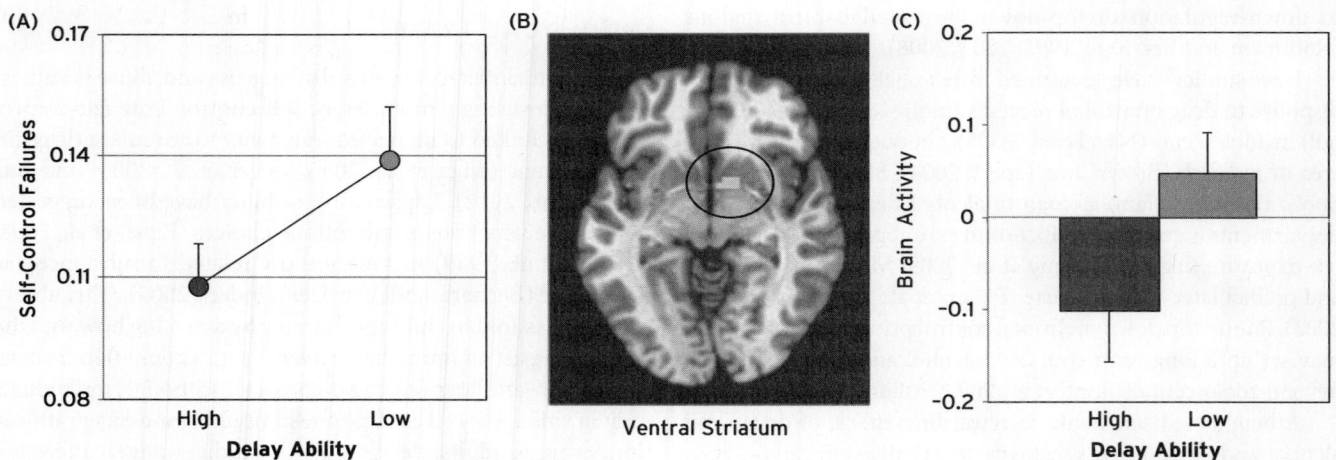

Figure 53.3 Individual differences in self control. (A) Individuals who had difficulty delaying gratification (low delay ability) as 4 year olds have more self control failures when inhibiting responses to appetitive cues 40 years later. (B) Localization of ventral striatal activity when inhibiting responses to appetitive cues. (C) Adults with low delay ability show greater ventral striatal activity when inhibiting responses to appetitive cues than do adults with high delay ability. (Adapted from Casey et al., 2011.)

abuse such as cocaine as adults (Slamberova et al., 2011). These findings suggest one potential pathway to addiction, given that both drug tolerance and hyporeactivity to substances of abuse have been linked to substance use dependence.

The human literature on prenatal exposure to substances of abuse is less clear. Cognitive and behavioral deficits have been associated with prenatal exposure to cocaine that may put these individuals at risk for later substance abuse. For example, children with prenatal cocaine exposure have problems of inattention and impulsivity (Kable et al., 2008; Li et al., 2009) that are in and of themselves risk factors for substance use. Together the human and animal research suggest that prenatal exposure to stimulants like cocaine alter reward circuitry and function, thus impacting both reactivity to substances and impulse control, both of which increase the risk for later substance abuse.

EFFECTS OF STIMULANT MEDICATION ON LATER SUBSTANCE ABUSE

Given the high comorbidity of addiction with other mental disorders, a clinical concern has been whether treating individuals with medications such as stimulants may enhance their propensity toward substances of abuse, especially in the case of treating developing populations. Some of the most common drugs prescribed in childhood and adolescence are stimulants for ADHD such as methylphenidate. The clinical concerns in using this standard treatment revolve around three major considerations. First, methylphenidate has pharmacological effects similar to drugs of abuse like cocaine, in increasing the availability of dopamine in the ventral striatum (Volkow and Swanson, 2008). Second, this treatment often begins in early adolescence—a period of increased risk for substance use disorders (Casey and Jones, 2010). Third, independent of stimulant treatment, ADHD is a risk factor for substance use dependence (Wilens et al., 2011), which may be attributable to poor impulse control and/or a drive to self-medicate with dopamine-augmenting stimulants. These concerns underscore the need to understand the long-term effects of stimulant medication on the developing brain and on risk for later substance abuse.

The human literature on studies of children with ADHD who were treated with stimulant medications has found no clear evidence for an increase in later substance use disorders. Rather the findings have been mixed, with some studies suggesting sensitization to such substances later (Hartsough and Lambert, 1987; Lambert and Hartsough, 1998; Lambert et al., 2006) and others suggesting protective or no effects of stimulant treatment on later substance use or dependence (Barkley et al., 2003; Biederman et al., 2008; Faraone and Wilens, 2003; Faraone et al., 1997; Katusic et al., 2005; Mannuzza et al., 2003; Mannuzza et al., 2008; Paternite et al., 1999; Wilens et al., 2003). Two recent studies of nonhuman primates, both of which mimic therapeutic methylphenidate administration in human periadolescence, showed no effect in either physical development or proclivity for cocaine self-administration (Gill et al., 2012; Soto et al., 2012). However, recent evidence in humans suggests that age of stimulant treatment onset may be an important factor influencing later substance abuse in treated ADHD patients. Specifically, the earlier the treatment,

the more of a protective effect against later substance abuse, whereas later treatment has little if any effect (Mannuzza et al., 2008).

Animal studies have tried to clarify the mixed clinical findings of methylphenidate treatment effects on later substance abuse. These studies suggest that the potential effects of stimulant exposure on future substance use might be dependent on the timing, dose, and administration of stimulants. For example, administering low doses of methylphenidate that more closely mirror typical plasma levels in therapeutic uses in humans increases cocaine (Brandon et al., 2001) and methamphetamine self-administration (Schindler et al., 2011) whereas high doses do not. Rats administered either intermittent or continuous methylphenidate during adolescence showed a differential effect, wherein intermittent administration increased cocaine sensitivity, and continuous administration decreased cocaine sensitivity (Griggs et al., 2010). Finally, administering stimulants during adolescence to spontaneously hypertensive rats, a proposed animal model of ADHD, results in the rats reaching cocaine self-administration faster than non-spontaneously hypertensive rats and in an increase in cocaine uptake in the prefrontal cortex (Harvey et al., 2011). Thus, a number of variables may moderate how stimulant treatment, such as that seen in methylphenidate treatment of ADHD, may influence later substance abuse and dependence. These variables include the age and duration of methylphenidate treatment, the dosage and type of stimulant treatment (continuous vs. intermittent), and even the presence or absence of ADHD phenotype. Not all children or adolescents who are treated with methylphenidate meet ADHD diagnostic criterion, and clinical status may impact how therapeutic stimulant administration may interact with the dopaminergic system.

CONCLUSIONS

Addiction affects millions each year, with adolescence being a particularly vulnerable period of risk. This chapter has provided an overview of recent human imaging and animal studies of adolescent brain development to help further elucidate who may be most at risk for developing a substance abuse problem and when they may be most vulnerable. Figure 53.4 illustrates how individual, environmental, and developmental factors may enhance the reinforcing effects of drugs in the ventral striatum and decrease self-regulatory capacity of the prefrontal cortex, potentially leading to greater risk for substance abuse and dependence.

Exposure to drugs of abuse is a fundamentally risky proposition. Initial use can represent a gamble with a long-term, highly disruptive, substance use disorder, with immensely high personal and societal costs. Understanding who is most at risk to develop a substance use disorder within a population is valuable, as it may allow earlier interventions and better outcomes. Psychological traits, such as impulsivity and self-control, influence how likely one is to become a substance user or dependent. These traits are closely tied to neural signatures in dopamine rich reward circuitry, especially in the ventral striatum and prefrontal cortex.

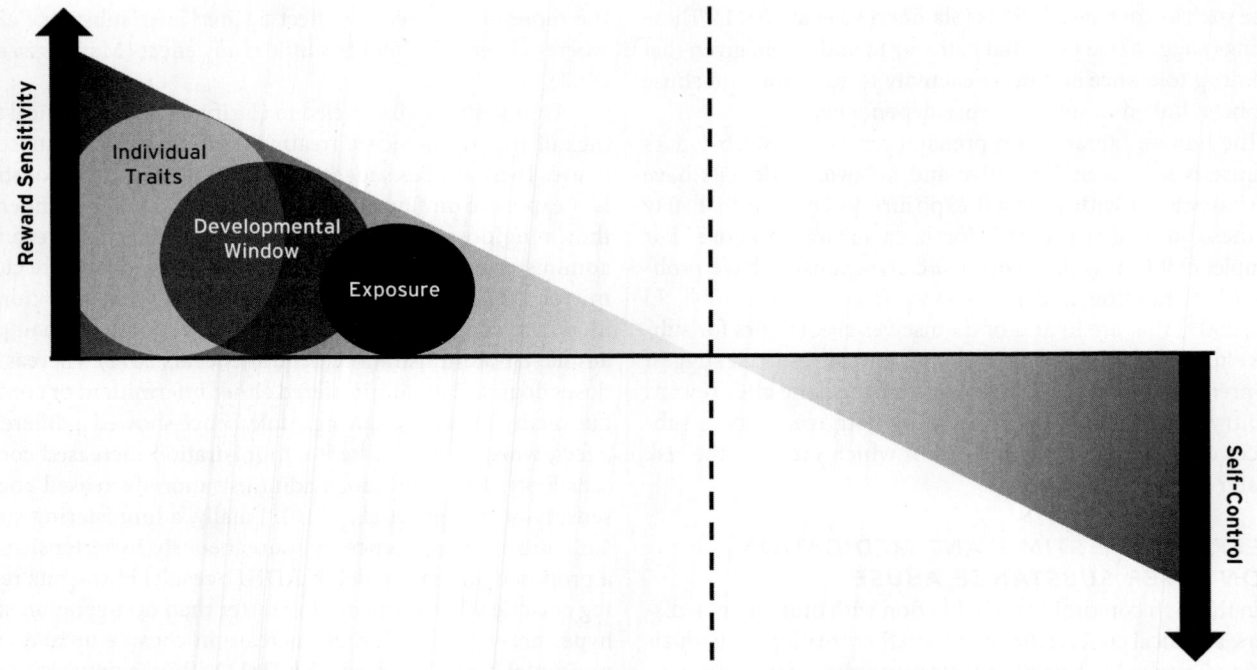

Figure 53.4 *Risk factors for addiction. Individual traits, developmental windows, and drug exposure can combine to increase the appetitive response associated with the reinforcing effects of drugs to decrease self-regulatory capacity, potentially leading to greater risk for substance abuse and dependence.*

Windows of development enhance vulnerability to substance exposure. These include periods of development when there are significant changes in dopamine receptor expression (fetal development) and peak density (adolescence). Adolescents as a group are also more likely to try drugs for the first time, and may be uniquely susceptible to developing substance dependencies because of an imbalance between structural and functional development of subcortical regions (involved in motivation and reinforcement learning) relative to prefrontal cortical regions (involved in impulse control).

The effects of drug exposure on neurotransmitter systems involved in motivation, reward, and learning are complex, changing both between individuals and across the lifespan. These factors, including brain structure, personal exposure history, and personality traits such as impulse control and reward sensitivity, involved in the response to stimulant exposure combine to form a multifactored risk profile for substance abuse. The better these risk factors are understood, the more effectively substance use disorders can be managed, treated, and ultimately prevented.

DISCLOSURES

The chapter authors have no conflicts of interest to disclose. Dr. Casey is funded by NIH and the MacArthur Foundation only. Grant Support: NIH (R01 HD069178, RC2 DA029475, P50-MH079513) and the MacArthur Foundation.

Dr. Caudle is funded by the MacArthur Foundation only. Grant Support: MacArthur Foundation.

REFERENCES

Arias-Carrion, O., and Poppel, E. (2007). Dopamine, learning, and reward-seeking behavior. *Acta Neurobiol. Exp.* 67(4):481–488.

Asato, M.R., Terwilliger, R., et al. (2010). White matter development in adolescence: a DTI study. *Cereb. Cortex* 20(9):2122–2131.

Astle, D.E., and Scerif, G. (2009). Using developmental cognitive neuroscience to study behavioral and attentional control. *Dev. Psychobiol.* 51(2):107–118.

Barkley, R.A., Fischer, M., et al. (2003). Does the treatment of attention-deficit/hyperactivity disorder with stimulants contribute to drug use/abuse? A 13-year prospective study. *Pediatrics* 111(1):97–109.

Bechara, A. (2005). Decision making, impulse control and loss of willpower to resist drugs: a neurocognitive perspective. *Nat. Neurosci.* 8(11):1458–1463.

Bechara, A., and Van Der Linden, M. (2005). Decision-making and impulse control after frontal lobe injuries. *Curr. Opin. Neurol.* 18(6):734–739.

Behar, D., Berg, C.J., et al. (1983). Behavioral and physiological effects of ethanol in high-risk and control children: a pilot study. *Alcohol Clin. Exp. Res.* 7(4):404–410.

Belin, D., Mar, A.C., et al. (2008). High impulsivity predicts the switch to compulsive cocaine-taking. *Science* 320(5881):1352–1355.

Benes, F.M., Taylor, J.B., et al. (2000). Convergence and plasticity of monoaminergic systems in the medial prefrontal cortex during the postnatal period: implications for the development of psychopathology. *Cereb. Cortex* 10(10):1014–1027.

Biederman, J., Monuteaux, M.C., et al. (2008). Stimulant therapy and risk for subsequent substance use disorders in male adults with ADHD: a naturalistic controlled 10-year follow-up study. *Am. J. Psychiatry* 165(5):597–603.

Bjork, J.M., Knutson, B., et al. (2004). Incentive-elicited brain activation in adolescents: similarities and differences from young adults. *J. Neurosci.* 24(8):1793–1802.

Bourgeois, J.P., Goldman-Rakic, P.S., et al. (1994). Synaptogenesis in the prefrontal cortex of rhesus monkeys. *Cereb. Cortex* 4(1):78–96.

Brandon, C.L., Marinelli, M., et al. (2001). Enhanced reactivity and vulnerability to cocaine following methylphenidate treatment in adolescent rats. *Neuropsychopharmacology* 25(5):651–661.

Breiter, H.C., Gollub, R.L., et al. (1997). Acute effects of cocaine on human brain activity and emotion. *Neuron* 19(3):591–611.

Brenhouse, H.C., Sonntag, K.C., et al. (2008). Transient D1 dopamine receptor expression on prefrontal cortex projection neurons: relationship to enhanced motivational salience of drug cues in adolescence. *J. Neurosci.* 28(10):2375–2382.

Brown, S.A., and Tapert, S.F. (2004). Adolescence and the trajectory of alcohol use: basic to clinical studies. *Ann. NY Acad. Sci.* 1021:234–244.

Brown, T.T., Lugar, H.M., et al. (2004). Developmental Changes in Human Cerebral Functional Organization for Word Generation. *Cereb. Cortex* 15(3):275–290.

Bunge, S.A., Dudukovic, N.M., et al. (2002). Immature frontal lobe contributions to cognitive control in children: evidence from fMRI. *Neuron* 33(2):301–311.

Casey, B.J., Epstein, J.N., et al. (2007). Frontostriatal connectivity and its role in cognitive control in parent-child dyads with ADHD. *Am. J. Psychiatry* 164(11):1729–1736.

Casey, B.J., Getz, S., et al. (2008). The adolescent brain. *Dev. Rev.* 28(1):62–77.

Casey, B.J., and Jones, R.M. (2010). Neurobiology of the adolescent brain and behavior: implications for substance use disorders. *J. Am. Acad. Child Adolesc. Psychiatry* 49(12):1189–1201; quiz 1285.

Casey, B.J., Somerville, L.H., et al. (2011). Behavioral and neural correlates of delay of gratification 40 years later. *Proc. Natl. Acad. Sci. USA* 108(36):14998–15003.

Casey, B.J., Tottenham, N., et al. (2005). Imaging the developing brain: what have we learned about cognitive development? *Trends Cogn. Sci.* 9(3):104–110.

Cheetham, A., Allen, N.B., et al. (2010). The role of affective dysregulation in drug addiction. *Clin. Psychol. Rev.* 30(6):621–634.

Chein, J., Albert, D., et al. (2011). Peers increase adolescent risk taking by enhancing activity in the brain's reward circuitry. *Developmental Sci.* 14(2):F1–10.

Chugani, H.T., Phelps, M.E., et al. (1987). Positron emission tomography study of human brain functional development. *Ann. Neurol.* 22(4):487–497.

Cohen, J.R., Asarnow, R.F., et al. (2010). A unique adolescent response to reward prediction errors. *Nat. Neurosci.* 13(6):669–671.

Cromwell, H.C., and Schultz, W. (2003). Effects of expectations for different reward magnitudes on neuronal activity in primate striatum. *J. Neurophysiol.* 89(5):2823–2838.

Cunningham, M.G., Bhattacharyya, S., et al. (2008). Increasing interaction of amygdalar afferents with GABAergic interneurons between birth and adulthood. *Cereb. Cortex* 18(7):1529–1535.

Cyders, M.A., and Smith, G.T. (2008). Emotion-based dispositions to rash action: positive and negative urgency. *Psychol. Bull.* 134(6):807–828.

Dawe, S., and Loxton, N.J. (2004). The role of impulsivity in the development of substance use and eating disorders. *Neurosci. Biobehav. Rev.* 28(3):343–351.

Doremus, T.L., Brunell, S.C., et al. (2003). Anxiogenic effects during withdrawal from acute ethanol in adolescent and adult rats. *Pharmacol. Biochem. Behav.* 75(2):411–418.

Durston, S., Davidson, M.C., et al. (2006). A shift from diffuse to focal cortical activity with development. *Developmental Sci.* 9(1):1–8.

Durston, S., Hulshoff Pol, H.E., et al. (2004). Magnetic resonance imaging of boys with attention-deficit/hyperactivity disorder and their unaffected siblings. *J. Am. Acad. Child Adolesc. Psychiatry* 43(3):332–340.

Eigsti, I.M., Zayas, V., et al. (2006). Predicting cognitive control from preschool to late adolescence and young adulthood. *Psychol. Sci.* 17(6):478–484.

Epstein, J.N., Casey, B.J., et al. (2007). ADHD- and medication-related brain activation effects in concordantly affected parent-child dyads with ADHD. *J. Child Psychol. Psychiatry* 48(9):899–913.

Ernst, M., Nelson, E.E., et al. (2005). Amygdala and nucleus accumbens in responses to receipt and omission of gains in adults and adolescents. *NeuroImage* 25(4):1279–1291.

Ernst, M., Pine, D.S., et al. (2006). Triadic model of the neurobiology of motivated behavior in adolescence. *Psychol. Med.* 36(3):299–312.

Ernst, M., Romeo, R.D., et al. (2009). Neurobiology of the development of motivated behaviors in adolescence: a window into a neural systems model. *Pharmacol. Biochem. Behav.* 93(3):199–211.

Faraone, S.V., Biederman, J., et al. (1997). Is comorbidity with ADHD a marker for juvenile-onset mania? *J. Am. Acad. Child Adolesc. Psychiatry* 36(8):1046–1055.

Faraone, S.V., and Wilens, T. (2003). Does stimulant treatment lead to substance use disorders? *J. Clin. Psychiatry* 64 (Suppl 11):9–13.

Fleckenstein, A.E., Volz, T.J., et al. (2007). New insights into the mechanism of action of amphetamines. *Annu. Rev. Pharmacol. Toxicol.* 47:681–698.

Forbes, E.E., and Dahl, R.E. (2010). Pubertal development and behavior: hormonal activation of social and motivational tendencies. *Brain Cogn.* 72(1):66–72.

French, E.D., Dillon, K., et al. (1997). Cannabinoids excite dopamine neurons in the ventral tegmentum and substantia nigra. *NeuroReport* 8(3):649–652.

Galvan, A., Hare, T.A., et al. (2005). The role of ventral frontostriatal circuitry in reward-based learning in humans. *J. Neurosci.* 25(38):8650–8656.

Galvan, A., Hare, T.A., et al. (2006). Earlier development of the accumbens relative to orbitofrontal cortex might underlie risk-taking behavior in adolescents. *J. Neurosci.* 26(25):6885–6892.

Galvan, A., Hare, T., et al. (2007). Risk-taking and the adolescent brain: who is at risk? *Developmental Sci.* 10(2):F8–F14.

Gardner, M., and Steinberg, L. (2005). Peer influence on risk taking, risk preference, and risky decision making in adolescence and adulthood: an experimental study. *Dev. Psychol.* 41(4):625–635.

Geier, C., and Luna, B. (2009). The maturation of incentive processing and cognitive control. *Pharmacol. Biochem. Behav.* 93(3):212–221.

Geier, C.F., Terwilliger, R., et al. (2010). Immaturities in reward processing and its influence on inhibitory control in adolescence. *Cereb. Cortex* 20(7):1613–1629.

Giedd, J.N., Blumenthal, J., et al. (1999). Brain development during childhood and adolescence: a longitudinal MRI study. *Nat. Neurosci.* 2(10):861–863.

Gill, K.E., Pierre, P.J., et al. (2012). Chronic treatment with extended release methylphenidate does not alter dopamine systems or increase vulnerability for cocaine self-administration: a study in nonhuman primates. *Neuropsychopharmacology* 37(12):2555–2565.

Gold, M.S., Graham, N.A., et al. (2009). Food addiction? *J. Addict. Med.* 3(1):42–45.

Gotgay, N., Giedd, J., et al. (2004). Dynamic mapping of human cortical development during childhood through early adulthood. *Proc. Natl. Acad. Sci. USA* 21(101):8174–8179.

Grant, B.F., and Dawson, D.A. (1997). Age at onset of alcohol use and its association with DSM-IV alcohol abuse and dependence: results from the National Longitudinal Alcohol Epidemiologic Survey. *J. Subst. Abuse* 9:103–110.

Griggs, R., Weir, C., et al. (2010). Intermittent methylphenidate during adolescent development produces locomotor hyperactivity and an enhanced response to cocaine compared to continuous treatment in rats. *Pharmacol. Biochem. Behav.* 96(2):166–174.

Haber, S.N. (2003). The primate basal ganglia: parallel and integrative networks. *J. Chem. Neuroanat.* 26(4):317–330.

Hardin, M.G., and Ernst, M. (2009). Functional brain imaging of development-related risk and vulnerability for substance use in adolescents. *J. Addict. Med.* 3(2):47–54.

Hartsough, C.S., and Lambert, N.M. (1987). Pattern and progression of drug use among hyperactives and controls: a prospective short-term longitudinal study. *J. Child Psychol. Psychiatry* 28(4):543–553.

Harvey, R.C., Sen, S., et al. (2011). Methylphenidate treatment in adolescent rats with an attention deficit/hyperactivity disorder phenotype: cocaine addiction vulnerability and dopamine transporter function. *Neuropsychopharmacology* 36(4):837–847.

Hollerman, J.R., and Schultz, W. (1998). Dopamine neurons report an error in the temporal prediction of reward during learning. *Nat. Neurosci.* 1(4):304–309.

Howell, L.L., and Kimmel, H.L. (2008). Monoamine transporters and psychostimulant addiction. *Biochem. Pharmacol.* 75(1):196–217.

Huttenlocher, P.R., and Dabholkar, A.S. (1997). Regional differences in synaptogenesis in human cerebral cortex. *J. Comp. Neurol.* 387(2):167–178.

Ito, R., Dalley, J.W., et al. (2002). Dopamine release in the dorsal striatum during cocaine-seeking behavior under the control of a drug-associated cue. *J. Neurosci.* 22(14):6247–6253.

Ito, R., Robbins, T.W., et al. (2004). Differential control over cocaine-seeking behavior by nucleus accumbens core and shell. *Nat. Neurosci.* 7(4):389–397.

Johnston, L., O'Malley, P., et al. (2009). Monitoring the Future National Results on Adolescent Drug Usage: Overview of Key Findings 2008. Bethesda, MD: National Institute on Drug Abuse.

Kable, J.A., Coles, C.D., et al. (2008). Physiological responses to social and cognitive challenges in 8-year olds with a history of prenatal cocaine exposure. *Dev. Psychobiol.* 50(3):251–265.

Katusic, S.K., Barbaresi, W.J., et al. (2005). Psychostimulant treatment and risk for substance abuse among young adults with a history of attention-deficit/hyperactivity disorder: a population-based, birth cohort study. *J. Child Adolesc. Psychopharmacol.* 15(5):764–776.

Kelly, A.M., Di Martino, A., et al. (2009). Development of anterior cingulate functional connectivity from late childhood to early adulthood. *Cereb. Cortex* 19(3):640–657.

Klingberg, T., Vaidya, C.J., et al. (1999). Myelination and organization of the frontal white matter in children: a diffusion tensor MRI study. *NeuroReport* 10(13):2817–2821.

Knutson, B., Fong, G.W., et al. (2001). Dissociation of reward anticipation and outcome with event-related fMRI. *NeuroReport* 12(17):3683–3687.

Kourosh, A.S., Harrington, C.R., et al. (2010). Tanning as a behavioral addiction. *Am. J. Drug Alcohol Ab.* 36(5):284–290.

Kubzansky, L.D., Martin, L.T., et al. (2009). Early manifestations of personality and adult health: a life course perspective. [Multicenter Study]. *Health Psychol.* 28(3):364–372.

Kuhnen, C.M., and Knutson, B. (2005). The neural basis of financial risk taking. *Neuron* 47(5):763–770.

Lambert, N.M., and Hartsough, C.S. (1998). Prospective study of tobacco smoking and substance dependencies among samples of ADHD and non-ADHD participants. *J. Learn Disabil.* 31(6):533–544.

Lambert, N.M., McLeod, M., et al. (2006). Subjective responses to initial experience with cocaine: an exploration of the incentive-sensitization theory of drug abuse. *Addiction* 101(5):713–725.

Lee, B. (2012). Addiction: a runaway phenomenon of our time? *JABTR* 1(1).

Li, Z., Coles, C.D., et al. (2009). Prenatal cocaine exposure alters emotional arousal regulation and its effects on working memory. *Neurotoxicol. Teratol.* 31(6):342–348.

Liston, C., Watts, R., et al. (2006). Frontostriatal microstructure modulates efficient recruitment of cognitive control. *Cereb. Cortex* 16(4):553–560.

Logothetis, N.K., Pauls, J., et al. (2001). Neurophysiological investigation of the basis of the fMRI signal. *Nature* 412(6843):150–157.

Luna, B., Padmanabhan, A., et al. (2010). What has fMRI told us about the development of cognitive control through adolescence? *Brain Cogn.* 72(1):101–113.

Luna, B., Thulborn, K.R., et al. (2001). Maturation of widely distributed brain function subserves cognitive development. *NeuroImage* 13(5):786–793.

Maldonado, R., and Rodriguez de Fonseca, F. (2002). Cannabinoid addiction: behavioral models and neural correlates. *J. Neurosci.* 22(9):3326–3331.

Mannuzza, S., Klein, R.G., et al. (2003). Does stimulant treatment place children at risk for adult substance abuse? A controlled, prospective follow-up study. *J. Child Adol. Psychop.* 13(3):273–282.

Mannuzza, S., Klein, R.G., et al. (2008). Age of methylphenidate treatment initiation in children with ADHD and later substance abuse: prospective follow-up into adulthood. *Am. J. Psychiatry* 165(5):604–609.

Matthews, S.C., Simmons, A.N., et al. (2004). Selective activation of the nucleus accumbens during risk-taking decision making. *NeuroReport* 15(13):2123–2127.

McQueeny, T., Schweinsburg, B.C., et al. (2009). Altered white matter integrity in adolescent binge drinkers. *Alcohol Clin. Exp. Res.* 33(7):1278–1285.

Medina, K.L., McQueeny, T., et al. (2008). Prefrontal cortex volumes in adolescents with alcohol use disorders: unique gender effects. *Alcohol Clin. Exp. Res.* 32(3):386–394.

Mirenowicz, J., and Schultz, W. (1994). Importance of unpredictability for reward responses in primate dopamine neurons. *J. Neurophysiol.* 72(2):1024–1027.

Mischel, W., and Ayduk, O. (2004). Willpower in a cognitive-affective processing system: the dynamics of delay of gratificaton. In: Baumeister, R., and Vohs, K., eds. Handbook of Self-Regulation: Research, Theory, and Applications. New York: Guildford, pp. 99–129.

Mischel, W., Shoda, Y., et al. (1988). The nature of adolescent competencies predicted by preschool delay of gratification. *J. Pers. Soc. Psychol.* 54(4):687–696.

Mischel, W., Shoda, Y., et al. (1989). Delay of gratification in children. *Science* 244(4907):933–938.

Monti, P.M., Miranda, R., Jr., et al. (2005). Adolescence: booze, brains, and behavior. *Alcohol Clin. Exp. Res.* 29(2):207–220.

Nagel, B.J., Schweinsburg, A.D., et al. (2005). Reduced hippocampal volume among adolescents with alcohol use disorders without psychiatric comorbidity. *Psychiatry Res.* 139(3):181–190.

Nestler, E.J. (2004). Historical review: Molecular and cellular mechanisms of opiate and cocaine addiction. *Trends Pharmacol. Sci.* 25(4):210–218.

Nigg, J.T., Wong, M.M., et al. (2006). Poor response inhibition as a predictor of problem drinking and illicit drug use in adolescents at risk for alcoholism and other substance use disorders. *J. Am. Acad. Child Adolesc. Psychiatry* 45(4):468–475.

NSDUH. (2011). Results from the 2010 National Survey on Drug Use and Health: Summary of National Findings. NSDUH Series H-41 (pp. 11–4658). Rockville, MD: US Department of Health and Human Services.

O'Doherty, J.P., Deichmann, R., et al. (2002). Neural responses during anticipation of a primary taste reward. *Neuron* 33(5):815–826.

Paternite, C.E., Loney, J., et al. (1999). Childhood inattention-overactivity, aggression, and stimulant medication history as predictors of young adult outcomes. *J. Child Adol. Psychopharmacol.* 9(3):169–184.

Pautassi, R.M., Myers, M., et al. (2008). Adolescent but not adult rats exhibit ethanol-mediated appetitive second-order conditioning. *Alcohol Clin. Exp. Res.* 32(11):2016–2027.

Pulido, C., Brown, S.A., et al. (2010). Alcohol cue reactivity task development. *Addict. Behav.* 35(2):84–90.

Rakic, P. (1974). Neurons in rhesus monkey visual cortex: systematic relation between time of origin and eventual disposition. *Science* 183(123):425–427.

Rakic, P., Bourgeois, J.P., et al. (1986). Concurrent overproduction of synapses in diverse regions of the primate cerebral cortex. *Science* 232(4747):232–235.

Reynaud, M., Karila, L., et al. (2010). Is love passion an addictive disorder? *Am. J. Drug Alcohol Ab.* 36(5):261–267.

Robinson, T.E., and Berridge, K.C. (2003). Addiction. *Annu. Rev. Psychol.* 54:25–53.

Robinson, T.E., and Berridge, K.C. (2008). Review. The incentive sensitization theory of addiction: some current issues. *Philos. Trans. R. Soc. Lond. B Biol. Sci.* 363(1507):3137–3146.

Robinson, T.E., and Berridge, K.C. (1993). The neural basis of drug craving: an incentive-sensitization theory of addiction. *Brain Res. Brain Res. Rev.* 18(3):247–291.

Rodriguez, M.L., Mischel, W., et al. (1989). Cognitive person variables in the delay of gratification of older children at risk. *J. Pers. Soc. Psychol.* 57(2):358–367.

Romeo, R.D. (2003). Puberty: a period of both organizational and activational effects of steroid hormones on neurobehavioural development. [Review]. *J. Neuroendocrinol.* 15(12):1185–1192.

Scheres, A., Milham, M.P., et al. (2007). Ventral striatal hyporesponsiveness during reward anticipation in attention-deficit/hyperactivity disorder. *Biol. Psychiatry* 61(5):720–724.

Schindler, C.W., Gilman, J.P., et al. (2011). Comparison of the effects of methamphetamine, bupropion, and methylphenidate on the self-administration of methamphetamine by rhesus monkeys. *Exp. Clin. Psychopharm.* 19(1):1–10.

Schultz, W., Dayan, P., et al. (1997). A neural substrate of prediction and reward. *Science* 275(5306):1593–1599.

Slamberova, R., Schutova, B., et al. (2011). Does prenatal methamphetamine exposure affect the drug-seeking behavior of adult male rats? *Behav. Brain Res.* 224(1):80–86.

Somerville, L.H., Hare, T., et al. (2011). Frontostriatal maturation predicts cognitive control failure to appetitive cues in adolescents. *J. Cogn. Neurosci.* 23(9):2123–2134.

Soto, P.L., Wilcox, K.M., et al. (2012). Long-term exposure to oral methylphenidate or dl-amphetamine mixture in peri-adolescent rhesus monkeys: effects on physiology, behavior, and dopamine system development. *Neuropsychopharmacology* 37(12):2566–2579.

Sowell, E.R., Thompson, P.M., et al. (1999). Localizing age-related changes in brain structure between childhood and adolescence using statistical parametric mapping. *NeuroImage* 9(6 Pt 1):587–597.

Sowell, E.R., Trauner, D.A., et al. (2002). Development of cortical and subcortical brain structures in childhood and adolescence: a structural MRI study. *Dev. Med. Child Neurol.* 44(1):4–16.

Spear, L.P., and Varlinskaya, E.I. (2005). Adolescence: alcohol sensitivity, tolerance, and intake. *Recent Dev. Alcohol.* 17:143–159.

Stanwood, G.D., Washington, R.A., and Levitt, P. (2001a). Identification of a sensitive period of prenatal cocaine exposure that alters the development of the anterior cingulate cortex. *Cereb. Cortex* 11(5):430–440.

Stanwood, G.D., Washington, R.A., Shumsky, J.S., et al. (2001b). Prenatal cocaine exposure produces consistent developmental alterations in dopamine-rich regions of the cerebral cortex. *Neuroscience* 106(1):5–14.

Steinberg, L. (2008). A social neuroscience perspective on adolescent risk-taking. *Dev. Rev.* 28(1):78–106.

Tapert, S.F., Cheung, E.H., et al. (2003). Neural response to alcohol stimuli in adolescents with alcohol use disorder. *Arch. Gen. Psychiatry* 60(7):727–735.

Tarter, R.E., Kirisci, L., et al. (2003). Neurobehavioral disinhibition in childhood predicts early age at onset of substance use disorder. *Am. J. Psychiatry* 160(6):1078–1085.

Tseng, K.Y., and O'Donnell, P. (2007). Dopamine modulation of prefrontal cortical interneurons changes during adolescence. *Cereb. Cortex* 17(5):1235–1240.

Vaidya, C.J., Austin, G., et al. (1998). Selective effects of methylphenidate in attention deficit hyperactivity disorder: a functional magnetic resonance study. *Proc. Natl. Acad. Sci. USA* 95(24):14494–14499.

Van Leijenhorst, L., Gunther Moor, B., et al. (2010). Adolescent risky decision-making: neurocognitive development of reward and control regions. *NeuroImage* 51(1):345–355.

Varlinskaya, E.I., and Spear, L.P. (2002). Acute effects of ethanol on social behavior of adolescent and adult rats: role of familiarity of the test situation. *Alcohol Clin. Exp. Res.* 26(10):1502–1511.

Volkow, N.D., Fowler, J.S., et al. (2002). Role of dopamine, the frontal cortex and memory circuits in drug addiction: insight from imaging studies. *Neurobiol. Learn. Mem.* 78(3):610–624.

Volkow, N.D., and Swanson, J.M. (2008). Does childhood treatment of ADHD with stimulant medication affect substance abuse in adulthood? *Am. J. Psychiatry* 165(5):553–555.

Volkow, N.D., Wang, G.J., et al. (2012). Food and drug reward: overlapping circuits in human obesity and addiction. *Curr. Top. Behav. Neurosci.* 11:1–24.

Volkow, N.D., Wang, G.J., et al. (2011). Addiction: beyond dopamine reward circuitry. *Proc. Natl. Acad. Sci. USA* 108(37):15037–15042.

Weinstein, A., and Lejoyeux, M. (2010). Internet addiction or excessive internet use. *Am. J. Drug Alcohol Ab.* 36(5):277–283.

Weinstein, A.M. (2010). Computer and video game addiction—a comparison between game users and non-game users. *Am. J. Drug Alcohol Ab.* 36(5):268–276.

Wilens, T.E., Faraone, S.V., et al. (2003). Does stimulant therapy of attention-deficit/hyperactivity disorder beget later substance abuse? A meta-analytic review of the literature. *Pediatrics* 111(1):179–185.

Wilens, T.E., Martelon, M., et al. (2011). Does ADHD predict substance-use disorders? A 10-year follow-up study of young adults with ADHD. *J. Am. Acad. Child Adolesc. Psychiatry* 50(6):543–553.

Windle, M., Spear, L.P., et al. (2008). Transitions into underage and problem drinking: developmental processes and mechanisms between 10 and 15 years of age. *Pediatrics* 121(Suppl 4):S273–289.

Witt, E.D. (2010). Research on alcohol and adolescent brain development: opportunities and future directions. *Alcohol* 44(1):119–124.

Yates, J.R., Marusich, J.A., et al. (2012). High impulsivity in rats predicts amphetamine conditioned place preference. *Pharmacol. Biochem. Behav.* 100(3):370–376.

CHELSEA L. ROBERTSON, STEVEN M. BERMAN, AND EDYTHE D. LONDON

MOLECULAR IMAGING METHODS AND THEIR APPLICATION IN STUDIES OF ADDICTION

Positron emission tomography (PET) and single photon emission computed tomography (SPECT) are nuclear medicine techniques that allow minimally invasive *in vivo* measurements of biochemical processes and pharmacokinetics. Molecules of interest can be radiolabeled and administered at tracer doses, allowing measurements without perturbing the systems under study. Both techniques can be used to assess functional activity, indexed by global and regional cerebral blood flow and/or metabolism, and how they change with various conditions or treatments. In addition, viability or function in neurotransmitter systems can be evaluated through imaging radiotracer binding to specific neurotransmitter receptors, transporters, and enzymes to assess neurotransmitter turnover. Although PET generally produces images with higher resolution and provides greater flexibility in radiotracer synthesis, SPECT has the advantage of using radiotracers with a longer half-life, reducing the need for onsite radiosynthesis (Cumming et al., 2012).

Molecular imaging of brain function started with the introduction of 2-deoxy-1-[C-14]glucose ([C-14]-2DG) to quantify local cerebral glucose metabolism, relying on the role of glucose as the major substrate for oxidative brain metabolism (Sokoloff et al., 1977). Autoradiographic studies of cerebral glucose metabolism in rodents were extended to human assesments with the development of 2-deoxy-2-[F-18]-fluoro-D-glucose ([F-18]FDG) (Som et al., 1980) to be combined with PET (Phelps et al., 1979; Reivich et al., 1979). Soon thereafter, cerebral blood flow could be measured in humans with PET, using [O-15]-labeled water (Mintun et al., 1984), reflecting the vascular response to energy demand produced by neural activity. Given the two-minute half-life of [O-15], repeated measurements were possible within minutes, offering greater time resolution than the [F-18]-FDG method, which measures glucose metabolism over the first 10–15 minutes after administration of the radiotracer. Cerebral perfusion measurements also were possible with SPECT, using radiolabeled N-isopropyl[I-123]-p-iodoamphetamine (IMP) (Kuhl et al., 1982); later [Tc-99m]-D,L-hexamethylpropyleneamine oxime (HMPAO) (Nickel et al., 1989) became the most commonly used tracer for SPECT measurements of cerebral blood flow (Mathew and Wilson 1991). Studies using markers of blood flow and glucose metabolism can provide quantitative maps of global and regional cerebral blood flow or metabolic rates for glucose, respectively.

Since 1986, when [C-11]N-methylspiperone was introduced as a PET radiotracer for human studies of D2/D3 dopamine receptors (Wong et al., 1986), many other radiotracers have become available for the visualization and quantification of neurotransmitter systems (Table 54.1). Over the last few decades, molecular neuroimaging has extended the knowledge about addiction that had been derived from invasive studies in rodents (Wise and Bozarth, 1987). The human studies using PET and SPECT, which are described later, have provided information about vulnerability to addiction, and brain abnormalities at various stages of the addiction cycle (Fig. 54.1). These findings have contributed to the current view of addiction and potential therapeutic interventions.

VULNERABILITY TO ADDICTIVE DISORDERS

Much attention has focused on why some people become addicts while others do not. This interest was fueled by observations of the fate of Vietnam War veterans who returned home after using heroin and becoming opioid-dependent during their tours of duty. It was estimated that 35–38% of US soldiers used heroin during the Vietnam War (Robins, 1993). Twenty percent of those using heroin reported physical dependence in Vietnam, but only 5% of those remained addicted in the first year after returning home. Because socioeconomic variables or effectiveness of treatment strategy did not explain the differences in outcome (Robins, 1993), the importance of biological factors was apparent. Three decades later, research has included studies of genetic polymorphisms associated with substance dependence, with positive evidence for roles of opioid (Nelson et al., 2012), nicotinic acetylcholine (Hartz et al., 2012), and dopamine receptors (Noble, 2003).

Molecular imaging has also provided insight regarding vulnerability to addiction, with a primary focus on the dopamine system. An important observation in this regard was the demonstration that lower levels of striatal dopamine D2/D3 receptor binding than in healthy controls subjects accompanies addictions and is often correlated with severity of the disorder (Martinez and Narendran, 2010; Volkow et al., 2004). Lower than control dopamine D2/D3 receptor availability was found in striata of research subjects dependent on various drugs, including alcohol, cocaine, and opioids. A recent PET study confirmed a previous report that light-smoking men also exhibit lower striatal D2/D3 receptor availability than non-smoking men, but there were no difference between

RADIOTRACER TARGET	RADIOTRACER COMMON NAME	RADIOTRACER CHEMICAL NAME
D2/D3 dopamine receptor	[C-11]N-methylsprioperidol	[C-11]-8-[4-(4-fluorophenyl)-4-oxo-butyl]-1-phenyl-1,3,8-triazaspiro[4.5]-decan-4-one
	[C-11]raclopride	3,5-dichloro-N-[[(2S)-1-ethylpyrrolidin-2-yl]methyl]-2-hydroxy-6-([C-11]methoxy)benzamide
	[F-18]fallypride	(S)-5-(3-[F-18]-fluoropropyl)-2,3-dmethoxy-N-[[(2S)-(2-propenyl)-2-pyrrolidinyl]methyl]benzamide
	[C-11]FLB457	[C-11](S)-N-((1-ethyl-2-pyrrolidinyl)methyl)-5-bromo-2,3-dimethoxybenzamide
	[F-18]fluoroclebopride ([F-18]FCP)	4-amino-5-chloro-N-[1-(4-[F-18]-fluoranylbenzyl)-4-piperidyl]-2-methoxy-benzamide
	[I-123]epidipride	(S)-N-[(l-methyl-2-pyrrolidinyl)methyl 5-[I-123]iodo-2,3-dimethyl benzamide
	[I-123]iodobenzamide ([I-123]IBZM)	(S)-(−)-2-hydroxy-3-[I-123]-iodo-6-methoxy-N[(1-ethyl-2-pyrrolidinyl)methyl]-benzamide
Dopamine transporter (DAT)	[C-11]methylphenidate	[C-11]-methyl phenyl(piperidin-2-yl)acetate
	[C-11]cocaine	[C-11]-methyl (1R,2R,3S,5S)-3-(benzoyloxy)-8-methyl-8-azabicyclo[3.2.1]octane-2-carboxylate
	[C-11]WIN35428 ([C-11]CFT)	2-beta-carbomethoxy-3-beta-(4-fluorophenyl)-[N-[C-11]-methyl]tropane
	[I-123]PE2I	N-(3-[I-123]-iodoprop-2E-enyl)-2β-carboxymethoxy-3β-(4-methylphenyl)nortropane
	[I-123]β-CIT	Beta-carbomethoxy-3-beta-4-[I-123]-iodophenyltropane
Vesicular monoamine transporter (VMAT)	[C-11]dihydrotetrabenazine ([C-11]DTBZ)	[C-11]2-hydroxy-3-isobutyl-9,10-dimethoxy-1,3,4,6,7-hexahydro-11βH-benzo[a]-quinolizine
Dopamine synthesis capacity	[F-18]FDOPA	6-[F-18]fluoro-L-dihydroxyphenylalanine
D1/D5 dopamine receptor	[C-11]NNC112	[C-11]-chloro-5-(7-benzofuranyl)-7-hydroxy-3-methyl-2,3,4,5-tetra-hydro-lH-3 benzazepine
	[C-11]SCH23390	[C-11]-7-chloro-3-methyl-1-phenyl-1,2,4,5-tetrahydro-3-benzazepin-8-ol
D3 dopamine receptor	[C-11]PHNO	[C-11]-4-propyl-3,4,4a,5,6,10-beta-hexahydro-2H-naphtho[1,2-beta][1,4] oxazin-9-ol
Serotonin transporter (SERT)	[C-11]McN5652	[C-11]-6β-(4-methylthiophenyl)-1,2,3,5,6α,10β-hexahydropyrrolo[2,1-α] isoquinoline
	[C-11]DASB	[C-11]-N,N-dimethyl-2-(2-amino-4-cyanophenylthio)benzylamine
	[C-11]ADAM	[C-11]-2-[2-(dimethylaminomethylphenylthio)]-5-iodophenylamine
	[I-123]β-CIT	2-beta-carbomethoxy-3-beta-(4-[I-123]-iodophenyl)-tropane
Serotonin 1A receptor	[C-11]WAY100635	[C-11]N-[2-[4-(2-methoxyphenyl)-1-piperazinyl]-ethyl]-N-2-pyridinylcyclohexanecarboxamide
	[F-18]MPPF	4-[F-18]-N-[2-[4-(2-methoxyphenyl)piperazin-1-yl]ethyl]-N-pyridin-2-ylbenzamide
Serotonin 2A receptor	[F-18]altanserin	3-[2-[4-(4-[F-18]fluorobenzoyl)piperidin-1-yl]ethyl]-2-sulfanylidene-1H-quinazolin-4-one
Mu-opiate receptor	[C-11]carfentanil	[C-11]-4-((1-oxopropyl)-phenylamino)-1-(2-phenylethyl)- 4-piperidinecarboxylic acid methyl
	[F-18]cyclofoxy	6-desoxy-6-beta-[F-18]-fluoronaltrexone

(continued)

TABLE 54.1. (*Continued*)

RADIOTRACER TARGET	RADIOTRACER COMMON NAME	RADIOTRACER CHEMICAL NAME
Kappa-opiate receptor	[C-11]-GR103545	[C-11]-4-methoxycarbonyl-2-[(1-pyrrolidinylmethyl]-1-[(3,4-dichlorophenyl)-acetyl]-piperidine
Nicotinic acetylcholine receptor (nAChR)	[F-18]-2F-A85380 ([F-18]2FA)	2-[F-18]fluoro-3-(2(S)azetidinylmethoxy)pyridine
	[F-18]-6F-A85380 ([F-18]6FA)	6-[F-18]fluoro-3-(2(S)-azetidinylmethoxy)pyridine
	[I-123]-5-iodo-A-85380	5-[I-123]-3-(2(S)-azetidinylmethoxy)pyridine
MAO(A)	[C-11]-clorgyline	[C-11]*N*-[3-(2,4-dichlorophenoxy)propyl]-*N*-methyl-prop-2-yn-1-amine
MAO(B)	[C-11]-deprenyl-d2	[C-11](*R*)-*N*-methyl-*N*-(1-phenylpropan-2-yl)prop-1-yn-3-amine
Type 1 cannabinoid receptor (CB1)	[C-11]-OMAR ([C-11]JHU75528)	1-(2, 4-dichlorophenyl)-4-cyano-5-(4-[C-11]-methoxyphenyl)-*N*-(piperidin-1-yl)-1H-pyrazole-3-carboxamide
	[F-18]-FMPEP-d2	(3*R*,5*R*)-5-(3-[F-18]fluoromethoxy-D2)phenyl)-3-((*R*)-1-phenyl-ethylamino)-1-(4-trifluoromethyl-phenyl)-pyrrolidin-2-one
GABA(A) receptor	[C-11]-flumazenil	[C-11]-ethyl 8-fluoro-5-methyl-6-oxo-5,6-dihydro-4H-benzo[f]imidazo[1,5-a][1,4]-diazepine-3-carboxylate
	[I-123]-iomazenil	Ethyl 7-[I-123]-iodo-5-methyl-6-oxo-5,6-dihydro-4H-imidazo[1,5-alpha][1,4]-benzodiazepine-3-carboxylate
Cerebral perfusion	[I-123]-iodoamphetamine ([I-123]IMP)	*N*-isopropyl[I-123]-*p*-iodoamphetamine
	[Tc-99m]-HMPAO	[Tc-99m]-D,L-hexamethylpropyleneamine oxime
	[O-15]-Water	
Glucose metabolism	[F-18]-fluorodeoxyglucose ([F-18]FDG)	2-deoxy-2-[F-18]fluoro-D-glucose

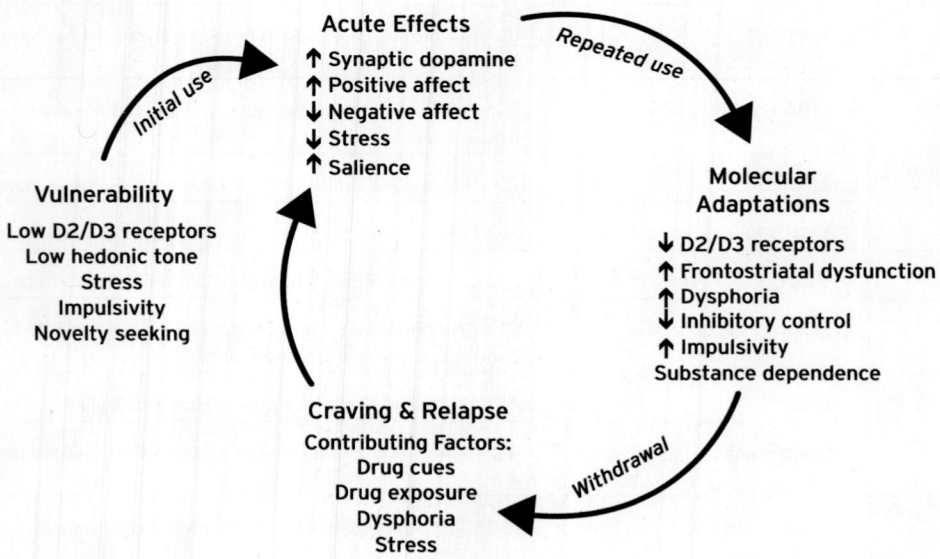

Figure 54.1 Factors that confer vulnerability to addiction increase reward and decrease punishment associated with early use of addictive substances. Acute drug effects increase the salience of drug-related cues and promote chronic use. Chronic use causes additional adaptations in risk-related biobehavioral systems, favoring continued drug abuse.

smoking and non-smoking women (Brown et al., 2012). In pathologically obese subjects, striatal D2/D3 receptor availability was also below control levels, and inversely related to body mass index (Wang et al., 2004). The extent to which these differences in D2/D3 receptor availability pre-date addiction was not clear, but as indicated in the following, several lines of evidence support a role for dopaminergic dysfunction as a vulnerability factor for substance abuse.

Early PET findings of dopamine D2/D3 receptor deficits in addictive disorders led to the hypothesis that a defect in striatal dopaminergic reward circuits promoted a Reward Deficiency Syndrome characterized by anhedonia and a dysfunctional impulsive-addictive-compulsive trajectory of behaviors (Blum et al., 1995). The premise was that those who suffer from a Reward Deficiency Syndrome engage in behaviors that augment dopaminergic activity, in some cases substituting one reward for another to satisfy a dopaminergic deficit. Such reward substitution is exemplified by unusually high caloric intake by methamphetamine addicts during their first month of drug abstinence, their caloric intake during the initial week being negatively correlated with striatal D2/D3 dopamine receptor availability (Zorick et al., 2012) (see Fig. 54.2).

Molecular imaging studies also have investigated effects of stress, gender, family history of addictive disorders, specific gene variants, and personality traits proposed as intermediate phenotypes associated with vulnerability to substance abuse. Novelty-seeking (Sweitzer et al., 2012), impulsivity (Verdejo-Garcia et al., 2008) and exposure to stress (Cumming et al., 2011; Dalley et al., 2011; Sinha 2008) have been linked to substance abuse in both humans and animal models; and most relevant investigations support the view that dopaminergic hypofunction, as assessed by amphetamine-induced dopamine release or striatal D2/D3 receptor availability, confers vulnerability for addictive disorders. For example, both impulsivity and lifetime stress were associated with blunted amphetamine-induced dopamine release (Oswald et al., 2005). Although high stress blunted dopamine release at all levels of impulsivity, high impulsivity was associated with rating intravenous amphetamine as being more pleasant, while high stress was associated with ratings of less pleasant responses.

PET findings in humans have supported a link between novelty-seeking and an exaggerated response to amphetamine. Novelty-seeking was inversely related to the availability of D2/D3 dopamine receptors in the midbrain, measured with [F-18]fallypride, as well as a heightened subjective response to amphetamine administration and striatal dopamine release, suggesting an important role of dopamine D2/D3 autoreceptors in the midbrain (Buckholtz et al., 2010; Zald et al., 2008). Novelty-seeking and impulsivity also have been associated with sensitization of amphetamine-induced striatal dopamine release, measured using [C-11]raclopride and PET (Boileau et al., 2006). More recently, a SPECT study found a positive correlation of novelty-seeking with striatal D2/D3 receptor availability (Huang et al., 2010). Extrastriatal dopamine D2/D3 receptors have also been associated with at-risk personality traits. A study using [C-11]FLB457 and PET found that

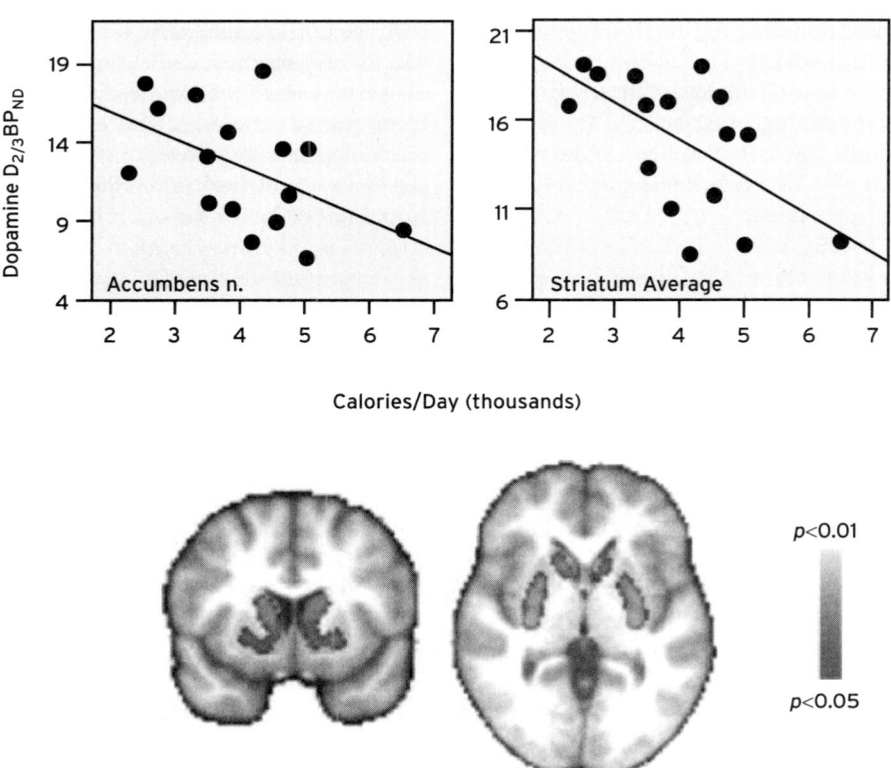

Figure 54.2 Top: Correlations of striatal dopamine D2/D3 receptor availability (BP_ND) with daily caloric intake (kcalories/day) in abstinent methamphetamine-dependent participants, N = 16. Bottom: Voxelwise regression of D2/D3 BP_ND on kcalories/day. Statistical maps are shown with results thresholded at Threshold-Free Cluster Enhancement (TFCE)-corrected p < 0.05, and displayed in radiological orientation. Vertical gradient bar indicates p-values.

novelty-seeking was negatively correlated with D2/D3 receptor availability in the insular cortex (Kaasinen et al., 2004).

Rats that were bred for high levels of impulsivity self-administered greater amounts of intravenous cocaine and nicotine than rats with low levels of impulsivity. PET revealed lower levels of ventral striatal D2/D3 receptor availability in high-impulsive rats, and the dopaminergic receptor deficit was correlated with the degree of impulsivity (Dalley et al., 2011). These findings are concordant with a human study in which self-reported impulsivity was negatively correlated with striatal D2/D3 receptor availability in healthy control subjects as well as methamphetamine-dependent subjects, with a more robust effect in the addict sample (Lee et al., 2009).

PET studies have provided evidence that high levels of striatal D2/D3 dopamine receptors may protect against drug abuse. For example, when methylphenidate, a stimulant with a mechanism of action similar to that of cocaine, was administered to healthy control subjects, an inverse relationship was found between D2/D3 receptor availability and subjective drug experience. Individuals with high D2/D3 receptor availability reported more unpleasant effects, suggesting a lower risk of drug self-administration (Volkow et al., 2002). This idea was supported by work using animal models (Cumming et al., 2011; Gould et al., 2012), showing that striatal D2/D3 receptor availability, quantified in drug-naïve rhesus monkeys with PET and [F-18] FCP, was negatively correlated with cocaine self-administration. Furthermore, adenoviral-mediated increased expression of striatal D2 receptors decreased alcohol self-administration in rats (Thanos et al., 2001).

The identification of high striatal D2/D3 dopamine receptor availability as a protective factor was further supported by observations that despite association of alcoholism with low striatal D2/D3 receptors, non-alcoholics with a strong family history of alcoholism have higher striatal D2/D3 receptors than non-alcoholics from low-risk families (Volkow et al., 2006a), suggesting that this neurochemical phenotype may protect against alcohol dependence. This view is consistent with results from a PET study with [F-18]FDG examining the hedonic effects of drinking ethanol versus placebo beverages in non-alcoholic men with and without a genetic allele conferring reduced D2/D3 receptor availability (London et al., 2009). Ethanol decreased anxiety and fatigue in men with the allele, but increased these measures in men without it. Reduction of anxiety and fatigue in men carrying the allele was associated with greater glucose metabolism in the orbitofrontal cortex and less activity in subcortical structures implicated in anxiety, fatigue and craving. Hedonic changes in men without the allele were unrelated to metabolic activity.

Animal studies of dominance hierarchies have provided insight into other factors, particularly environmental stressors, that contribute to drug abuse vulnerability. Social dominance and subordinance in animals are considered forms of environmental enrichment and stress, respectively (reviewed in Cumming et al., 2011; Gould et al., 2012). Dominant social status was associated with higher [C-11]raclopride binding than subordinate social status in animals. After a stressful encounter with a stranger, [F-18]FDG and PET revealed a greater increase in mesocorticolimbic glucose metabolism in dominant than in subordinate monkeys. After the encounter, dominant monkeys chose fewer cocaine injections and more food rewards than subordinate monkeys (Gould et al., 2012). The development of social dominance in group cages increased dopamine D2/D3 receptor availability by approximately 20%, with no change in the subordinates. Dominant male monkeys subsequently self-administered less cocaine than subordinates, suggesting protection against the reinforcing properties of cocaine. In contrast, dominant female monkeys chose more cocaine injections than female subordinate monkeys (Gould et al., 2012).

These results link impulsivity and novelty-seeking in non-addicted subjects to both pleasant subjective effects and striatal dopamine release elicited by addictive drugs. Sensitivity to drug-induced reward may increase vulnerability for initiation and early abuse of addictive substances. Ethical considerations limit the extent to which vulnerability may be manipulated in humans, but animal findings, in combination with demonstrations of drug-induced response as a function of genotype and inferences from genetic association studies, suggest that preexisting levels of dopaminergic signaling combine with personality traits and environmental conditions or stress to influence risk for substance abuse disorders.

ACUTE EFFECTS OF ADDICTIVE DRUGS: REWARD AND REINFORCEMENT

Although drugs of abuse from different chemical classes differ in some of their effects on mood and feeling state, they all produce positive subjective effects that reinforce drug-taking, and thereby promote addiction. These effects involve multiple neural systems, but a large body of evidence, primarily derived from animal studies, supported the idea that drug-related reinforcement requires dopaminergic neurotransmission (Di Chiara and Imperato, 1988; Everitt and Robbins, 2005; Koob, 1992). Molecular brain imaging has demonstrated that an increase in intrasynaptic dopamine within the striatum is also important in human drug abuse.

Fluctuations in synaptic dopamine and other neurotransmitters can be measured using PET and SPECT, based on the principle that endogenous neurotransmitters compete with radiotracers for receptor binding (Laruelle, 2000; Martinez and Narendran, 2010). With respect to dopamine dynamics, [C-11]raclopride and [F-18]fallypride have been used with PET and [I-123]IBZM was used with SPECT to measure extracellular dopamine dynamics as a function of physiological and/or pharmacological state (Laruelle, 2000; Riccardi et al., 2006). Molecular imaging has been combined with microdialysis in nonhuman primates to show that changes in radiotracer binding mostly reflect changes in extracellular dopamine levels (Laruelle et al., 1997b), but that the sensitivity of PET is lower than that of microdialysis, a 1% decrease in [C-11]raclopride binding potential corresponding to a 44% change measured with microdialysis (Breier et al., 1997). With an intravenous amphetamine challenge, [C-11]raclopride and PET revealed up to a 40% decrease in receptor binding potential indexed by the ratio B_{max}/K_d (Laruelle et al., 1997a, 1997b) despite evidence that intravenous amphetamine (1.5 mg/kg) increases extracellular dopamine concentrations more than 100-fold (Laruelle et al., 1997b). Notably, many factors contribute to insensitivity and problems in collecting reproducible and accurate measurements of intrasynaptic dopamine concentrations using radiotracers. These include D2/D3 receptor affinity state (Laruelle 2000), receptor internalization (Skinbjerg et al., 2010), receptor polymerization (Logan et al., 2001), and timing of dopamine release and radiotracer equilibration. Also important are methodological details, such as the time window for data collection and the kinetic modeling approach.

Despite these caveats, molecular imaging has shown that all classes of abused drugs increase intrasynaptic dopamine concentrations in the ventral striatum of human subjects. These findings were obtained with PET using amphetamine (Drevets et al., 2001), cocaine (Schlaepfer et al., 1997), cigarette smoking (Brody et al., 2004), alcohol (Boileau et al., 2003), and opiates (Spreckelmeyer et al., 2011). PET studies with [C-11] raclopride have provided mixed findings regarding ventral striatal dopamine release by Δ9-tetrahydrocannibinol (THC) (Bossong et al., 2009; Stokes et al., 2009). Such molecular imaging studies allow for the linking of acute biochemical effects of drugs with simultaneous changes in mood and feeling state. In this way, it has been used to directly relate change in intrasynaptic dopamine with feelings of drug-liking and euphoria after exposure to intravenous amphetamine (Drevets et al., 2001), intravenous methylphenidate (Volkow et al., 2001c), and cigarette smoking (Barrett et al., 2004).

The effects of various drugs and treatments on striatal dopamine dynamics are under genetic control. Examples of such effects have been derived from studies of cigarette smoking. In one study, dopamine release from smoking a cigarette, inferred from decreases in the binding of [C-11]raclopride, was influenced by polymorphisms in genes that influence dopamine function and metabolism (Brody et al., 2006b). In another study, using similar methodology, striatal dopamine release after cigarette smoking was modulated by the mu opioid receptor A118G polymorphism, carriers of the G allele showed a stronger response to cigarette smoking than those homozygous for the more common A allele (Domino et al., 2012).

Similar methology has been used to detect increased release of endogenous opioids from PET studies showing reductions in the binding of [C-11]carfentanil after administration of various drugs of abuse. This has been observed after the administration of oral amphetamine (Colasanti et al., 2012), oral alcohol (Mitchell et al., 2012), and smoked cigarettes (Scott et al., 2007), highlighting the importance of opiate signaling in the effects of these drugs. In this regard, direct interactions between opioid and dopaminergic neurotransmission in rats have shown that nicotine-induced dopamine release in the nucleus accumbens depends on activation of mu-opioid receptors in the ventral tegmental area (Tanda and Di Chiara, 1998).

Pharmacokinetic profile and route of administration can have substantial effects on subjective experience and dopamine dynamics. For example, a PET study of dopamine transporter occupancy, measured using [C-11]cocaine, found that at the time of peak plasma levels after unlabeled cocaine administration,

DAT occupancy was comparable after intravenous, smoked and intranasal administration, but that self-ratings of "high" were greater after smoking than after administration by the other routes (Volkow et al., 2000). This suggested that the speed of drug delivery to the brain influences the subjective response to cocaine. These results are corroborated by the relationship between the rate of uptake of cocaine analogs into the brain and their reinforcing properties in a self-administration paradigm in non-human primates, such that the drugs with faster brain uptake produced greater levels of responding relative to the drugs with slower brain uptake (cited in Howell and Murnane, 2011). Collectively, these studies show how the route of administration and pharmacokinetic properties of drugs are key elements mediating the subjective, reinforcing, and behavioral effects of abused drugs, and thus their addictive potential.

In addition to measuring drug-induced changes in specific neurotransmission, PET and SPECT can measure changes in cerebral blood flow and glucose metabolism. Quantitative global measures as well as values normalized to global or other (e.g., activity in the slice) values have been used. As measures of glucose metabolism and perfusion are positively linked (Roy and Sherrington, 1890), they provide indices of neural activity that require oxidative metabolism. Glucose is the primary metabolic substrate in the adult brain, and perfusion follows metabolic activity to deliver glucose and oxygen. Similar to fMRI, these methods do not resolve the contributions of different neurotransmitter systems to the signal, nor do they separate the effects in afferents from those in intrinsic neurons or dendrites of receptive neurons.

Some of the earliest assessments of acute changes in cerebral function involved [F-18]FDG PET studies of changes in cerebral glucose metabolism produced by euphorigenic doses of morphine (30 mg, intramuscularly) and cocaine (40 mg, intravenously), administered to research participants reporting recent use of heroin or cocaine (London et al., 1990a, 1990b). Self-reports of positive subjective effects of morphine coincided with a 10% decrease in global cerebral glucose metabolism, not unexpected given the sedative effects of opiates. Decreases in telencephalic regions were significant, and the decrement was greater in the frontal than occipital cortex, consistent with the distribution of mu-opioid receptors observed with [C-11]carfentanil in humans (Frost et al., 1990); however, the reductions in glucose metabolism were not correlated with subjective responses.

Cocaine also produced a global decrease in glucose metabolism (London et al., 1990b), which initially seemed incompatible with the behavioral stimulant effects. However, global decreases in glucose utilization and/or cerebral blood flow after administration of most drugs of abuse, including ethanol (de Wit et al., 1990; Volkow et al., 1988b), opiates (London et al., 1990a), benzodiazepines (de Wit et al., 1991), and nicotine (Domino et al., 2000b; Stapleton et al., 2003; Zubieta et al., 2001), were subsequently revealed by PET. SPECT studies with [Tc-99m]HMPAO showed an acute effect of cocaine to reduce global perfusion (Wallace et al., 1996), which was related to ratings of subjective experience (Pearlson et al., 1993). The mechanism by which abused drugs reduce global glucose metabolism and blood flow is unknown.

These effects observed in humans were inconsistent with observations from earlier animal studies, potentially reflecting species differences or poor matching of doses or drug histories. Cocaine reduced cerebral glucose metabolism in human subjects with substantial drug experience, but produced dose-related increases in glucose metabolism in dopaminergic brain regions and the cerebellar vermis of naïve rats studied using the autoradiographic [C-14]2DG method (London et al., 1986; Porrino et al., 1988). Acute cocaine administration to cynomolgus monkeys decreased glucose utilization in a discrete set of cortical and subcortical limbic structures (Lyons et al., 1996), resembling decrements found in humans (London et al., 1990b). Subsequent PET studies of rhesus monkeys trained to self-administer cocaine employed the [F-18]FDG method (cited in Howell and Murnane, 2011). Absolute quantification was not reported, but normalized voxelwise analyses revealed that the initial dose of cocaine produced relative increases in glucose metabolism in the prefrontal cortex. With increasing cocaine exposure, relative effects extended throughout frontal cortex and striatum, demonstrating the importance of prior drug history and identifying brain regions that are progressively affected by increasing drug exposure. Normalized blood flow maps in nonhuman primates after cocaine administration also showed relative increases in the dorsolateral prefrontal cortex (cited in Howell and Murnane, 2011), indicating selective activation of regions with dopaminergic enervation, and suggesting that dopaminergic transmission may underlie cocaine-induced increases in neuronal activity.

Similar to observation with cocaine, nicotine administration shows marked species differences in its effect on local cerebral glucose metabolism. In rats, dose-related increases in nicotine-induced local cerebral glucose metabolism (London et al., 1988) were observed in a pattern that generally followed the distribution of high-affinity nAChRs reported by earlier studies using autoradiographic ligand binding sites with [H-3]nicotine (London et al., 1985) thus linking the nicotine binding sites to nicotine-induced changes in neuronal function. Noninvasive imaging of nAChRs in the human brain *in vivo* is important for elucidating the role of these receptors in response to nicotine administration. Development of specific radioligands targeting nAChRs (β2-containing) for use with SPECT (Fujita et al., 2003) and PET (Kimes et al., 2003) in humans were used to show high levels of binding in the thalamus, cerebellum, putamen, pons, and cerebral cortices, indicating that species differences in nAChR distribution may underlie the differential response to nicotine.

Intravenous or intranasal (spray) nicotine administration in human subjects, like other stimulants, decreased global glucose metabolism (Domino et al., 2000b; Stapleton et al., 2003) and perfusion (Zubieta et al., 2001). Normalized data have revealed relative increases in glucose metabolism (Domino et al., 2000b) and blood flow (Domino et al., 2000a; Zubieta et al., 2001) in thalamus and other regions with high nACHR binding (Fujita et al., 2003; Kimes et al., 2003), suggesting that regional nicotine-induced changes in glucose metabolism are mediated by nAChRs. Increases in normalized regional cerebral blood flow, measured with [O-15]water and PET, in the left frontal cortex, anterior cingulate (Rose et al., 2003) dorsolateral prefrontal cortex, orbitofrontal cortex, and striatum after nicotine administration (Domino et al., 2000a) further support the role of nAChRs in nicotine-induced neuronal activation. One to two puffs of a cigarette result in over 50% occupancy of brain nAChRs in smokers studied using PET and [F-18]2FA (Brody et al., 2006a), and this occupancy lasts for over three hours. In combination with data showing that secondhand smoke produces 20% occupancy of nAChRs (Brody et al., 2011), these findings demonstrate that low doses of nicotine occupy a substantial proportion of brain nAChRs, and thereby can influence brain function.

In summary, molecular imaging studies of acute administration of abused drugs have confirmed the importance of striatal dopamine release in the rewarding properties of these drugs. Molecular imaging studies of the time course of drug effects have shown the importance of rapid actions with respect to striatal dopamine and drug-induced euphoria. In the case of cigarette smoking, PET has been used to reveal a mismatch between duration of nAChR receptor occupancy and smoking behavior, presenting questions regarding the molecular basis for the frequency of smoking among nicotine-dependent smokers. In addition, studies on the effects of secondhand smoke have shown how PET may be useful in guiding policy decisions regarding smoking.

MOLECULAR ADAPTATIONS TO CHRONIC DRUG EXPOSURE

Over the course of the past two decades, the focus of human drug abuse research have moved from the acute effects of drugs of abuse to persistent neurochemical alterations that promote the maintenance of addiction. Mounting evidence indicates that drug abuse produces adaptations within neural circuits that process reward, react to stress, and mediate executive functions (Broft and Martinez, 2012; Koob and Volkow, 2010). Drug-induced increases in synaptic dopamine cannot fully explain the changes observed during the shift from drug use to addiction in vulnerable individuals (Volkow et al., 2011), or the sequential neuroadaptations that follow repeated drug exposure (Everitt and Robbins, 2005). These transitions involve dopaminergic, serotonergic, nicotinic cholinergic, and endogenous opioid systems (Table 54.2).

A consistent finding relates to lower levels of striatal D2/D3 dopamine receptors in research participants who had abused drugs compared to controls (Broft and Martinez, 2012). Chronic users of cocaine (Volkow et al., 1990), methamphetamine (Lee et al., 2009), alcohol (Volkow et al., 1996), opiates (Wang et al., 1997), or nicotine (Brown et al., 2012; Fehr et al., 2008) all display deficits in striatal D2/D3 dopamine receptor availability. Similar observations have been made in behavioral addictive disorders, such as pathological obesity (Wang et al., 2004). This commonality across several addictive disorders raises questions regarding the extent to which low D2/D3 receptor availability predates drug abuse, or is an effect of chronic drug exposure.

Whereas ethical restrictions limit direct evaluation of this question in humans, molecular imaging studies of nonhuman

TABLE 54.2. Findings from molecular imaging studies of human substance abuse: adaptations and/or preexisting differences

RADIOTRACER TARGET	NICOTINE		COCAINE		ALCOHOL		METHAMPHETAMINE		OPIATES
Striatal dopamine D2/D3 receptors	↓	Fehr et al. (2008); Brown et al. (2012)#	↓	Volkow et al. (1993); Martinez et al. (2004)	↓	Volkow et al. (1996); Heinz et al. (2005b)	↓	Volkow et al. (2001b); Lee et al. (2009)	↓	Wang et al. (1997); Zjistra et al. (2008)
Striatal dopamine transporter (DAT)	⊘	Staley et al. (2001)	↑	Malison et al. (1998)	↓	Repo et al. (1999)	⊘	Volkow et al. (2001a)	↓	Shi et al. (2008)
	↓	Leroy et al. (2011)			⊘	Volkow et al. (1996)			⊘	Cosgrove et al. (2010)
Striatal dopamine synthesis	↑	Salokangas et al. (2000)^	↓	Baxter et al. (1988); Wu et al. (1997)	⊘	Heinz et al. (2005b)				
Presynaptic dopaminergic element			↓	Volkow et al. (1997)	↓	Martinez et al. (2005)	↓	Wang et al. (2011)	↓	Martinez et al. (2012)
Striatal vesicular monoamine			↓	Narendran et al. (2012)	↓	Gilman et al. (1998)	↓	Johanson et al. (2006)		
Transporter 2 (VMAT2)							↑	Boileau et al. (2008)		
Serotonin transporter (SERT)	↑	Staley et al. (2001)#	↑	Jacobsen et al. (2000)	↓	Heinz et al. (1998)	↓	Sekine et al. (2006)	⊘	Cosgrove et al. (2010)
					⊘	Martinez et al. (2009b)				
Subcortical mu opiate receptor	↓	Scott et al. (2007)^	↑	Zubieta et al. (1996)^	↑	Heinz et al. (2005a)				
Cortical mu opiate receptor			↑	Gorelick et al. (2005)	↓	Bencherif et al. (2004)^			↑	Zubieta et al. (2000)^

↓: substance abusing participants < control
↑: substance abusing participants > control
⊘: substance abusing participants not different from control
^: study conducted in males only
#: results observed in males only

primates have provided useful information. Vervet monkeys exposed to a methamphetamine dosing regimen designed to mimic human consumption of the drug showed significant decreases in striatal D2/D3 receptor availability using [F-18] fallypride and PET after two weeks of methamphetamine exposure. These deficits persisted for at least seven weeks after cessation of treatment (Groman et al., 2012), indicating deleterious effects that are long-lasting. In another study, baseline striatal D2/D3 receptor availability, measured using [F-18]FCP, in rhesus monkeys was inversely related to rates of subsequent cocaine self-administration, but irrespective of baseline levels, chronic exposure to cocaine significantly reduced D2/D3 receptor availability (cited in Howell and Murnane, 2011). Taken together, these findings indicate that the apparent D2/D3 receptor deficiencies in human research participants who abuse addictive drugs reflect both a vulnerability to drug abuse and a consequence of chronic drug use.

Although abnormalities in D2/D3 dopamine receptor binding in addiction are well documented, findings regarding the dopamine transporter (DAT) have been less consistent. One report showed low levels of DAT binding using [C-11] WIN35428 in methamphetamine-dependent individuals (McCann et al., 1998). In another study, DAT binding recovered with at least one year of abstinence (Volkow et al., 2001a). A direct relationship between the recovery of DAT and duration of abstinence (Sekine et al., 2001) suggested that reductions in striatal DAT associated with methamphetamine dependence may reflect short-term, drug-induced neuroadaptations.

SPECT studies of recently detoxified alcoholics using [I-123]PE2I found lower striatal DAT binding compared to control subjects (Repo et al., 1999). In a study using [I-123]β-CIT, DAT binding availability returned to control levels after four weeks if participants abstained from drinking (Laine et al., 1999). In contrast, a small PET study using [C-11] D-threo-methylphenidate ($N = 5$) showed no differences in striatal DAT binding between alcohol-dependent and healthy subjects (Volkow et al., 1996). That study reported a lower D2/D3 receptor to DAT binding ratio in the alcohol-dependent group, suggesting that chronic alcohol abuse may disrupt the balance between pre- and postsynaptic dopaminergic function. Changes in DAT levels in alcoholism may be transient adaptations that typically recover with abstinence.

Striatal DAT has also been studied with respect to nicotine dependence and heroin abuse. A SPECT study using [I-123]β-CIT revealed no differences in DAT availability between smokers and nonsmokers (Staley et al., 2001). However, a PET study examining DAT using [C-11]PE2I binding in cannabis and tobacco smokers showed significantly less striatal DAT binding availability in participants who smoked both substances compared to subjects who smoked neither. Furthermore, tobacco-only smokers showed a trend towards lower striatal DAT binding than the control group (Leroy et al., 2011). SPECT studies using [I-123]β-CIT showed no differences in striatal DAT binding between heroin addicts and controls (Cosgrove et al., 2010), but higher binding in cocaine-dependent subjects than controls (Malison et al., 1998). A later PET study using [C-11] CFT found lower striatal DAT availability in opiate-dependent subjects than in control subjects, even after an abstinence period of six months (Shi et al., 2008).

Sample sizes and differences in tracers and techniques must be considered when interpreting DAT findings, but variation in the abstinence period may be particularly important. As DAT is subject to regulation by drugs that alter synaptic dopamine concentrations (Vander Borght et al., 1995), the length of abstinence from dopamine-modulating drugs may substantially influence measures of DAT. This issue has encouraged the use of other markers of dopaminergic terminal integrity, such as the vesicular monoamine transporter (VMAT2), which are less sensitive than DAT to pharmacological alterations (Narendran et al., 2012; Vander Borght et al., 1995). VMAT2 is present in all monoaminergic neurons and has been assessed in substance-dependent groups.

Lower striatal VMAT2 was seen postmortem in former methamphetamine abusers (Wilson et al., 1996), and PET studies using [C-11]dihydrotetrabenazine to assess striatal VMAT2 *in vivo* showed lower levels in participants with severe alcohol-dependence (Gilman et al., 1998), cocaine-dependence (Narendran et al., 2012) and methamphetamine-dependence even after three months of abstinence (Johanson et al., 2006). In another study, however, the same tracer showed that recently abstinent methamphetamine-dependent individuals had greater VMAT2 binding availability than controls (Boileau et al., 2008). As drugs such as alpha-methylparatyrosine and d-amphetamine, which affect endogenous vesicular dopamine, modulate striatal VMAT2 binding in rats (Tong et al., 2008), a paradoxical increase in VMAT2 in early abstinence from methamphetamine (Boileau et al., 2008) may result from transient methamphetamine-induced alterations in vesicular dopamine concentration (Tong et al., 2008). Indeed, consideration of time since last drug use revealed VMAT2 increases relative to control subjects only in those who had most recently used methamphetamine (<12 days) (Boileau et al., 2008). Collectively, these findings suggest that increased VMAT2 may be a transient response to drug exposure and the reduction in VMAT2 binding observed after longer abstinence may indicate lasting damage to neuronal terminals as a consequence of drug use.

Quantification of endogenous vesicular dopamine pools can be inferred from molecular imaging studies of drug-induced dopamine release and depletion. Levels of endogenous dopamine in the brain can be reduced by alpha-methyl-*para*-tyrosine (AMPT), which inhibits tyrosine hydroxylase, the rate-limiting enzyme in the dopamine biosynthesis pathway (Brogden et al., 1981). PET and SPECT studies have estimated endogenous dopamine levels inferred from changes in D2/D3 receptor availability before and after AMPT treatment (Laruelle et al., 1997a). Using PET and [C-11]raclopride, the AMPT paradigm was used to examine endogenous dopamine levels in cocaine-dependent and healthy participants (Martinez et al., 2009a). Cocaine-dependent subjects had lower levels of endogenous dopamine, reflected in a 6% increase in D2/D3 receptor availability in the cocaine-dependent group as compared to an 11% increase in the control group. Therefore, group differences in D2/D3 receptor binding reported using [C-11]raclopride in cocaine-dependent participants (Martinez et al., 2004; Volkow et al., 1993) may have been underestimated because of interference by endogenous dopamine (more so in control than in cocaine-dependent subjects).

PET studies also have suggested that cocaine dependence is associated with diminished activity of the presynaptic element of dopaminergic neurons. A PET and [C-11]raclopride study of the effect of methylphenidate, which blocks reuptake of released dopamine, showed smaller changes in D2/D3 receptor availability in cocaine-dependent than in healthy subjects (Volkow et al., 1997). Similar findings were obtained in studies of heroin- (Martinez et al., 2012), methamphetamine dependence (Wang et al., 2011) and alcohol dependence (Martinez et al., 2005). In light of the findings from studies with AMPT, a smaller response to a methylphenidate challenge in substance-dependent groups may reflect low endogenous dopamine (Martinez et al., 2009a) in addition to reduced presynaptic activity. This view is consistent with lower rates of striatal dopamine synthesis, as measured by [F-18]DOPA uptake, in recently abstinent cocaine-dependent (Baxter et al., 1988; Wu et al., 1997) and alcohol-dependent subjects (Salokangas et al., 2000) relative to controls.

Alterations to the dopaminergic signaling system in substance dependence also occur via neurotransmitter metabolism. Monoamine oxidase A (MAOA) and monoamine oxidase B (MAOB), are both involved in dopamine degradation (Riederer et al., 1987). In cigarette smokers, levels of each are reduced between 30 and 40% (Fowler et al., 1996a, 1996b), as measured with PET using [C-11]clorgyline (MAOA) and [C-11]deprenyl-D2 (MAOB). Inhibition of MAOA and B by cigarette smoking results in enhanced dopaminergic activity and may represent an additional mechanism by which nicotine provides reinforcement. MAO inhibition by smoking is temporary because normalization of enzymatic activity occured after approximately four weeks of abstinence (Rose et al., 2001). Because MAOA also regulates central serotonergic activity, impaired MAOA activity in smokers may contribute to antidepressant effects of cigarette smoking, and depressive symptoms during nicotine withdrawal. Because MAOA breaks down monoamines linked to mood, and persons with major depression are more likely both to smoke and to have difficulty stopping (Covey et al., 1998), MAOA inhibition should be considered as a link between smoking and depression (Fowler et al., 1996b).

Although dopaminergic markers generally show deficits across addictive disorders, findings regarding other neurotransmitter systems are more variable. Alcohol abuse has been studied with molecular probes for the GABA and serotonin systems. Alcohol-dependent subjects had lower $GABA_A$ receptor binding than controls, as shown using [I-123]iomazenil and SPECT (Abi-Dargham et al., 1998; Lingford-Hughes et al., 1998) and [C-11]flumazenil and PET (Gilman et al., 1996). Alcohol-dependent subjects showed less serotonin transporter availability using [I-123]βCIT and SPECT (Heinz et al., 1998). In a seperate PET study, alcohol-dependent subjects showed no differences relative to control subjects in serotonin transporter availability, using the tracer [C-11]DASB or 5-HT1A receptor availability using [C-11]WAY100635 (Martinez et al., 2009b).

Deficits in serotonin transporter (SERT) availability, assessed with PET and [C-11]McN5652, were seen in subcortical brain regions of methamphetamine- (Sekine et al., 2006) and alcohol-dependent subjects (Heinz et al., 1998). In rhesus monkeys, SERT binding was studied with PET and [C-11]DASB after chronic self-administration of cocaine (cited in Howell and Murnane, 2011). SERT availability differed as a function of cocaine self-administration where monkeys with a history of cocaine exposure showed higher levels of striatal SERT than drug-naive monkeys. This result resembled findings in cocaine-dependent humans (Jacobsen et al., 2000), indicating that chronic cocaine exposure may increase striatal SERT binding.

Few human molecular imaging studies have examined endogenous opioid systems in addiction, and most of the relevant information has come from studies of mu-opiate receptors. Using PET and [C-11]carfentanil, it was shown that one- to four-day abstinent cocaine-dependent subjects had higher mu-receptor binding than controls in the cingulate, frontal cortex, caudate, and thalamus, persisting up to 12 weeks of abstinence (Gorelick et al., 2005; Zubieta et al., 1996). PET studies using [C-11]carfentanil have shown greater mu-receptor binding availability in the ventral striatum of alcohol-dependent subjects (Heinz et al., 2005a), with deficits also observed in cortical mu-receptor availability (Bencherif et al., 2004). Heroin-dependent subjects had higher mu-receptor availability in the anterior cingulate and inferior frontal cortex relative to control subjects (Zubieta et al., 2000). Endogenous opiate-receptor signaling represents an important facet of substance dependence because many studies show relationships between mu-receptor levels and drug craving (Gorelick et al., 2005; Zubieta et al., 1996) and substance abuse treatment outcomes (Ghitza et al., 2010). An increasing body of literature supports a role of dynorphin and kappa-opioid receptors in addiction (Shippenberg et al., 2001), but further investigations of abuse-related plastic changes within the endogenous opiate signaling system are needed to draw conclusions that can improve addiction treatment strategies. Development and application of specific radiotracers, such as [C-11]GR103545 to image kappa-opiate receptors (Schoultz et al., 2010), may yield valuable new information.

Motivated by the high prevalence of cigarette smoking worldwide, much attention has been paid to adaptations of nicotinic acetylcholine receptors (nAChRs) in the brains of cigarette smokers (Sharma and Brody, 2009). These receptors modulate the release of transmitter from presynaptic terminals on several types of neurons (Wonnacott, 1997). Nicotine-induced stimulation of nAChRs on dopaminergic neurons increases extracellular dopamine levels in the nucleus accumbens (Nisell et al., 1994). Alterations in nAChRs observed using molecular imaging techniques have been important in development of nicotine-cessation therapies. Chronic nicotine administration upregulates nAChRs in rodents (Koylu et al., 1997), as has been shown in human postmortem studies (Benwell et al., 1988) and *in vivo* with the tracer 2-[F-18]fluoro-A-85380 (Mukhin et al., 2008). [I-123]5-iodo-A-85380 was used with SPECT to show that β2* nAChR availability was elevated in the striatum and cerebral cortex of one-week abstinent smokers, relative to nonsmokers, and was correlated with the days since last cigarette (Staley et al., 2006). A SPECT study using the same tracer, showed that β2* nAChR availability returned to baseline after 21 days of abstinence (Mamede et al., 2007). These findings indicate that when smokers quit smoking, upregulation of the receptors normally activated by nicotine persists for several weeks. Greater β2* nAChR availability during this period may impact the ability of smokers to maintain abstinence.

SPECT imaging, using [I-123]5-iodo-A-85380, showed higher β2* nAChR binding in the striatum and cerebellum of male smokers, compared to nonsmokers, but no detectable difference between female smokers and nonsmokers (Cosgrove et al., 2012). This study corroborated the observation that nAChRs were upregulated in male but not female rats (Koylu et al., 1997). Notably, men and women show differences in the smoking-induced upregulation of nAChRs, which may be useful in treating nicotine dependence. The lack of nAChR upregulation suggests that females may respond better to medications that do not target nAChRs than to nicotine replacement or varenicline (Cosgrove et al., 2012).

Molecular adaptations to substance abuse have also been evaluated using PET and SPECT measurements of blood flow and glucose metabolism. An early PET study of blood flow measured with [O-15]water showed large focal deficits in the prefrontal cortex of cocaine-dependent relative to control subjects (Volkow et al., 1988a). A SPECT study using [Tc-99m]HMPAO found focal decreases in perfusion of the frontal cortex and basal ganglia (Holman et al., 1991). Glucose metabolism, measured with [F-18]FDG and PET, showed deficits in frontal cortical regions, relative to control subjects, with no recovery after three–four months of cocaine abstinence (Volkow et al., 1992). Similar deficits in global and relative glucose metabolism were noted in three-week abstinent alcohol-dependent men (Volkow et al., 1994). Although relative metabolism in the basal ganglia recovered somewhat during abstinence, it was still abnormal after detoxification. A repeat study in women showed no differences from controls in cerebral glucose metabolism associated with alcohol dependence (Wang et al., 1998). The women, however, had markedly lower rates of alcohol use than the men in the previous study (Volkow et al., 1994), which may contribute to the apparent sex difference.

Regional cerebral glucose metabolism in fourteen-day abstinent intravenous cocaine users with histories of poly-substance abuse was lower than in control subjects. The poly-substance abusers showed lower absolute metabolic rates for glucose in lateral occipital gyrus and higher normalized metabolic rates in temporal and frontal cortices, including orbitofrontal cortex (Stapleton et al., 1995). Cocaine-dependent subjects had higher rates of orbitofrontal cortex glucose metabolism than controls after one week of abstinence, but metabolism normalized after four weeks (Volkow et al., 1991). Compared to control subjects, methamphetamine-dependent participants (4–7 days abstinent) had lower glucose metabolism in the anterior cingulate and insular corticies, and higher glucose metabolism in the lateral orbitofrontal cortex, middle and posterior cingulate, amygdala, ventral striatum, and cerebellum (London et al., 2004). In both cocaine-dependent and methamphetamine-dependent subjects, orbitofrontal glucose metabolism was negatively correlated with striatal D2/D3 receptor availability (Volkow et al., 1993, 2001b), suggesting a mechanistic link between orbitofrontal function and striatal dopaminergic transmission in stimulant dependence. These findings support a model in which dysfunction of frontal circuits that inhibit the striatal dopaminergic reward system, combined with deficient striatal dopaminergic transmission, may promote behaviors that perpetuate the cycle of addictive disorders (Volkow and Fowler, 2000).

PET and SPECT studies of molecular adaptations in substance use disorders have extended preclinical findings to humans. Most studies have focused on the dopamine system. Dopaminergic deficits are consistently reported in substance dependence, suggesting that they contribute to initiation and/or maintenance of the addictive process. Imaging of serotonin, nicotinic, and opiate receptor signaling have not yet yielded as consistent a picture.

PERSISTENT STATES: FACTORS CONTRIBUTING TO RELAPSE

Drug addiction is associated with intense craving or desire to consume the relevant drug, and reduced motivation to seek other forms of reinforcement (Parvaz et al., 2011). Even after prolonged periods of abstinence, craving triggered by reminders of substance abuse, such as relevant people, places, or things, can overcome attempts to maintain sobriety. Studies in animals have revealed an important role of striatal dopamine in the conditioned responses that model craving (Everitt and Robbins, 2005), and molecular neuroimaging has been used to extend this work to delineate the circuits and neurotransmitter systems that mediate drug craving in humans.

SPONTANEOUS CRAVING DURING ABSTINENCE

The period of early abstinence has been a focus of study because most treatment for addiction begins at this time (Huber et al., 1997). PET with [F-18]FDG showed elevated glucose metabolism in the basal ganglia and orbitofrontal cortex during the first week of abstinence from chronic cocaine, and orbitofrontal

cortical metabolism was correlated with self-rated cocaine craving (Volkow et al., 1991). Newly abstinent cocaine abusers had higher mu-opioid receptor binding than control subjects in the dorsal striatum, thalamus, anterior cingulate, and fronto-temporal cortices, as assessed with PET and [C-11]carfentanil (Zubieta et al., 1996). Craving was correlated with binding of the radiotracer in amygdala, anterior cingulate, and frontotemporal cortices. In a later study, craving on the first day of cocaine abstinence was correlated with mu-opioid receptor binding in the anterior cingulate, prefrontal, temporal, and parietal cortices (Gorelick et al., 2005). Correlations were significant between craving and mu-opioid receptor binding in the left frontal and right temporal/parietal cortex for up to six days. These findings contrasted with a report that mu-opioid receptor binding in the right dorsolateral prefrontal cortex, right anterior frontal cortex, and right parietal cortex in alcohol dependent subjects was lower than control values, and that the deficit was associated with alcohol craving (Bencherif et al., 2004). The literature points to involvement of frontostriatal regions as well as more extended corticolimbic circuitry in spontaneous craving for cocaine as well as upregulation of the mu-opioid system.

Other studies have focused on striatal dopamine D2/D3 receptors. In abstinent alcoholics, alcohol craving was inversely related to striatal D2/D3 receptor availability, measured using [F-18]fallypride, and to dopamine synthesis capacity in the putamen, as indexed by [F-18]FDOPA uptake (Heinz et al., 2005b). In contrast, an [F-18]fallypride PET study of 24-hour abstinent, heavy cigarette smokers found no relationship of cigarette craving to D2/D3 receptor availability, but when the participants were tested without forced abstinence from smoking, craving was positively correlated with D2/D3 receptor availability in the ventral striatum, but negatively with D2/D3 receptor availability in the anterior cingulate and inferior temporal cortices (cited in Parvaz et al., 2011), suggesting that cigarette craving may be maintained by region-specific shifts in D2/D3 receptor availabilities.

CUE-ELICITED CRAVING

The first imaging study of cue-elicited drug craving used [F-18] FDG and PET, and showed increased glucose metabolism in a network of corticolimbic regions implicated in memory when abstinent cocaine-abusing participants viewed videotapes of drug-related objects, compared to a session in which they viewed a neutral videotape (Grant et al., 1996). The cue-related increase in craving was correlated with a metabolic increase in dorsolateral prefrontal cortex, amygdala, and cerebellum. Expansion of this work (Bonson et al., 2002) showed that cocaine cues elicited a higher degree of craving than previously reported and resulted in activation of lateral amygdala, lateral orbitofrontal cortex, dorsolateral prefrontal cortex, and cerebellum. Activation in these regions and the insular cortex was correlated with self-reported craving, suggesting that activity within a network that integrates emotional and cognitive aspects of memory links environmental cues with cocaine craving. Similar methodology was used in a study of cue-induced craving for cigarettes (Brody et al., 2002). In the active-cue video condition, smokers had greater increases in relative glucose metabolism than nonsmokers in the perigenual anterior cingulate cortex. Craving was correlated with glucose metabolism in the orbitofrontal, dorsolateral, anterior insular, and right sensorimotor cortices, suggesting potential therapeutic targets for treatments designed to reduce cigarette craving.

Studies of cue-induced craving have also used [O-15]water and PET to measure cerebral blood flow. In the first of these studies, cocaine abusers exhibited greater activation, indexed by blood flow in the amygdala and anterior cingulate cortex, but lower blood flow in the caudate nucleus and globus pallidus when they viewed a cocaine-related video than when viewing a neutral video (Childress et al., 1999). In another study, script-guided imagery of autobiographical memories was used to generate cocaine craving and was compared to a control condition of neutral memory recall during PET data acquisition (Kilts et al., 2001). Compared with the neutral condition, drug craving activated the bilateral (right greater than left) amygdala, left insula and anterior cingulate gyrus, and right subcallosal gyrus and nucleus accumbens. A subsequent study of cue-induced craving in opiate-dependent subjects who listened to autobiographical scripts of an episode of craving and a neutral episode while undergoing a PET scan with the tracer [O-15]water revealed cue-induced activation in the left medial prefrontal and left anterior cingulate cortices, and activation of the orbitofrontal cortex was correlated with craving ratings (Daglish et al., 2001). When similar methods were used to study heroin addicts, the "urge-to-use" heroin after viewing heroin-related as compared with neutral videotapes was correlated with blood flow increases in portions of the inferior frontal/orbitofrontal cortices, precuneus, and insula (cited in Parvaz et al., 2011). These findings show the involvement of a corticolimbic network, including brain regions important for decision-making, in generating or experiencing craving in response to relevant environmental cues.

Dopaminergic modulation of cue-elicited craving was revealed in a study using [C-11]raclopride and PET to measure change in intrasynaptic dopamine concentrations, inferred from changes in [C-11]raclopride binding, in cocaine-dependent subjects viewing cocaine-related videotapes. Subjects who reported craving for cocaine had larger cue-induced decreases in dopamine D2/D3 receptor availability than those who did not report craving. Furthermore, the magnitude of change in intrasynaptic dopamine concentrations in the putamen was positively correlated with the intensity of cocaine craving (Wong et al., 2006). Comparable results were found in a similar study (Volkow et al., 2006b) wherein cue-induced decreases in [C-11]raclopride binding in the dorsal striatum were largest in the most severely addicted participants. Similar heroin-related videotapes elicited greater dopamine release in the right putamen of opiate-dependent subjects, relative to controls, with dopamine release being correlated with chronic craving and anhedonia, in a SPECT study of D2/D3 receptor availability (Zijlstra et al., 2008). Evidence of cue-elicited dopamine release in the dorsal striatum, a region implicated in habit learning, suggests that dopaminergic transmission in this region is a fundamental component of how craving maintains addiction.

DRUG-ELICITED CRAVING

An early SPECT study used [Tc-99m]HMPAO to examine blood flow in alcoholics after craving was elicited by a low non-pharmacological dose of alcohol (cited in Hommer, 1999). An increase in blood flow in the right caudate was correlated with the increase in craving for alcohol. Similarly, in a study of hospitalized patients who had chronically abused cocaine, methylphenidate increased glucose metabolism measured with [F-18]FDG and PET in frontal cortex, thalamus, and cerebellum, with the increases in right orbitofrontal cortex and caudate metabolism positively correlated with increased craving (cited in Hommer, 1999). These correlations add to substantial literature on the link between orbitofrontal cortex and striatal function in evaluating and responding to potential rewards.

In a novel PET study on the effects of secondhand smoke, the tracer [F-18]2FA was used to label the β2 subtype of nicotinic acetylcholine receptors (nAChRs) (Brody et al., 2011). After one hour of moderate exposure to second-hand smoke, smokers reported increased craving, and the specific binding volume of distribution of the radiotracer was reduced by ~19%, corresponding to occupancy of β2 nAChRs by nicotine. The thalamic nAChR occupancy in smokers by secondhand smoke was correlated with the alleviation of craving by subsequent smoking. This link between the amount of nicotine delivered and the response to subsequent smoking suggested that secondhand smoke primes a smoker to receive greater negative reinforcement from smoking.

Finally, a PET study using [C-11]raclopride showed that reducing serotonin transmission via acute tryptophan depletion increased cocaine-elicited craving and cocaine-induced striatal dopamine release in non-dependent intranasal cocaine users (Cox et al., 2011). Neither craving nor striatal dopamine release were altered by tryptophan depletion prior to placebo administration. These observations suggested that low serotonergic transmission may increase craving and dopaminergic responses to cocaine, indicating a possible mechanism by which individuals with low serotonergic transmission may be at elevated risk for substance use disorders.

Generally, the findings presented here suggest that craving, whether it is spontaneous, cue-induced, or drug-induced, involves corticostriatal and more generally corticolimbic circuitry. These data suggest that the orbitofrontal cortex is involved in the induction of craving in several substance-dependence disorders. As the orbitofrontal cortex and other regions of the prefrontal cortex are involved in salience attribution, inhibitory control, emotion regulation, and decision-making (London et al., 2000), dysregulation in the frontal cortex may enhance the motivational value of the drug of abuse and may lead to loss of control over drug intake (Goldstein and Volkow, 2002). Notably, deficits in D2/D3 receptor availability in stimulant-dependent subjects are related to low rates of glucose metabolism in the orbitofrontal cortex (Volkow et al., 1993, 2001b), suggesting a mechanistic link between striatal dopaminergic dysfunction and frontal metabolism.

A study highlighting the importance of frontostriatal dysfunction and inhibition studied cocaine-dependent subjects that were instructed to inhibit craving actively while viewing a cocaine-related video (cited in Parvaz et al., 2011). Successful inhibition of craving was associated with decreased glucose metabolism in the right nucleus accumbens and increased metabolism in right inferior frontal cortex, suggesting that strengthening frontostriatal regulation could be a useful goal and biomarker of therapeutic interventions.

CONCLUSIONS

Animal models of substance dependence have helped to elucidate the neurobiological mechanisms involved in the reinforcing effects of addictive drugs in human subjects and have provided a foundation for studying the biological basis of drug addiction. However, there remains a degree of uncertainty regarding the extent to which these observations coincide with relevant addiction-related processes in humans. Molecular imaging approaches can be instrumental in providing direct evidence of the analogous biological processes and behaviors in humans.

The progress of the molecular imaging field in addiction is principally driven by the development of novel radiotracers to image integral components of neurochemistry, with the goal of developing targeted interventions for substance abuse disorders. Within the dopaminergic system, agonist-based tracers targeting D2/D3 dopamine receptors designed to distinguish between high- and low-affinity receptor configurations will be instrumental in elucidating dopamine receptor dynamics as a mechanism of functional state of the receptor. New tracers targeting the glutamate, cannabinoid, and kappa-opioid systems in humans will allow for the expansion of concepts surrounding the integral role for these neurotransmitters in addiction that were constructed using evidence from animal models.

Finally, molecular imaging tools enable the examination of biological processes as a function of genotype, which is essential for understanding the processes by which genes affect the vulnerability or resilience of an individual to addiction. Furthermore, effectiveness of future treatment interventions designed to strengthen and restore brain areas affected by chronic drug use can be assessed using molecular imaging to track progressive changes in the relevant brain systems during the course of treatment and recovery.

DISCLOSURES

Dr. Robertson, Dr. Berman, and Dr. London have no conflicts to disclose. Their work is funded by NIDA and the Friends Research Institute only.

REFERENCES

Abi-Dargham, A., Krystal, J.H., et al. (1998). Alterations of benzodiazepine receptors in type II alcoholic subjects measured with SPECT and [123I] iomazenil. *Am. J. Psychiatry* 155:1550–1555.

Barrett, S.P., Boileau, I., et al. (2004). The hedonic response to cigarette smoking is proportional to dopamine release in the human striatum as measured by positron emission tomography and [11 C]raclopride. *Synapse* 54:65–71.

Baxter, L.R., Jr., Schwartz, J.M., et al. (1988). Localization of neurochemical effects of cocaine and other stimulants in the human brain. *J. Clin. Psychiatry* 49(Suppl):23–26.

Bencherif, B., Wand, G.S., et al. (2004). Mu-opioid receptor binding measured by [11C]carfentanil positron emission tomography is related to craving and mood in alcohol dependence. *Biol. Psychiatry* 55:255–262.

Benwell, M.E., Balfour, D.J., et al. (1988). Evidence that tobacco smoking increases the density of (-)-[3H]nicotine binding sites in human brain. *J. Neurochem.* 50:1243–1247.

Blum, K., Sheridan, P.J., et al. (1995). Dopamine D2 receptor gene variants: association and linkage studies in impulsive-addictive-compulsive behaviour. *Pharmacogenetics* 5:121–141.

Boileau, I., Assaad, J.M., et al. (2003). Alcohol promotes dopamine release in the human nucleus accumbens. *Synapse* 49:226–231.

Boileau, I., Dagher, A., et al. (2006). Modeling sensitization to stimulants in humans: an [11C]raclopride/positron emission tomography study in healthy men. *Arch. Gen. Psychiatry* 63:1386–1395.

Boileau, I., Rusjan, P., et al. (2008). Increased vesicular monoamine transporter binding during early abstinence in human methamphetamine users: Is VMAT2 a stable dopamine neuron biomarker? *J. Neurosci.* 28:9850–9856.

Bonson, K.R., Grant, S.J., et al. (2002). Neural systems and cue-induced cocaine craving. *Neuropsychopharmacology* 26:376–386.

Bossong, M.G., van Berckel, B.N., et al. (2009). Delta 9-tetrahydrocannabinol induces dopamine release in the human striatum. *Neuropsychopharmacology* 34:759–766.

Breier, A., Su, T.P., et al. (1997). Schizophrenia is associated with elevated amphetamine-induced synaptic dopamine concentrations: evidence from a novel positron emission tomography method. *Proc. Natl. Acad. Sci. USA* 94:2569–2574.

Brody, A.L., Mandelkern, M.A., et al. (2002). Brain metabolic changes during cigarette craving. *Arch. Gen. Psychiatry* 59:1162–1172.

Brody, A.L., Mandelkern, M.A., et al. (2006a). Cigarette smoking saturates brain alpha 4 beta 2 nicotinic acetylcholine receptors. *Arch. Gen. Psychiatry* 63:907–915.

Brody, A.L., Mandelkern, M.A., et al. (2006b). Gene variants of brain dopamine pathways and smoking-induced dopamine release in the ventral caudate/nucleus accumbens. *Arch. Gen. Psychiatry* 63:808–816.

Brody, A.L., Mandelkern, M.A., et al. (2011). Effect of secondhand smoke on occupancy of nicotinic acetylcholine receptors in brain. *Arch. Gen. Psychiatry* 68:953–960.

Brody, A.L., Olmstead, R.E., et al. (2004). Smoking-induced ventral striatum dopamine release. *Am. J. Psychiatry* 161:1211–1218.

Broft, A., and Martinez, D. (2012). Neurochemical imaging of addictive disorders. In: Gründer, G., ed. Neuromethods: Molecular Imaging in the Clinical Neurosciences, vol. 71. New York: Humana Press, pp. 249–271.

Brogden, R.N., Heel, R.C., et al. (1981). α-methyl-*p*-tyrosine: a review of its pharmacology and clinical use. *Drugs* 21:81–89.

Brown, A.K., Mandelkern, M.A., et al. (2012). Sex differences in striatal dopamine D2/D3 receptor availability in smokers and non-smokers. *Int. J. Neuropsychopharmacol.* 15(7):989–994.

Buckholtz, J.W., Treadway, M.T., et al. (2010). Dopaminergic network differences in human impulsivity. *Science* 329:532.

Childress, A.R., Mozley, P.D., et al. (1999). Limbic activation during cue-induced cocaine craving. *Am. J. Psychiatry* 156:11–18.

Colasanti, A., Searle, G.E., et al. (2012). Endogenous opioid release in the human brain reward system induced by acute amphetamine administration. *Biol. Psychiatry* 72:371–377.

Cosgrove, K.P., Esterlis, I., et al. (2012). Sex differences in availability of β2*-nicotinic acetylcholine receptors in recently abstinent tobacco smokers. *Arch. Gen. Psychiatry* 69:418–427.

Cosgrove, K.P., Tellez-Jacques, K., et al. (2010). Dopamine and serotonin transporter availability in chronic heroin users: a [(1)(2)(3)I]beta-CIT SPECT imaging study. *Psychiatry Res.* 184:192–195.

Covey, L.S., Glassman, A.H., et al. (1998). Cigarette smoking and major depression. *J. Addict. Dis.* 17:35–46.

Cox, S.M., Benkelfat, C., et al. (2011). Effects of lowered serotonin transmission on cocaine-induced striatal dopamine response: PET [(1)(1)C]raclopride study in humans. *Br. J. Psychiatry* 199:391–397.

Cumming, P., and Böning, G. (2012). Overview of positron emission tomography (PET) and single photon emission computed tomography (SPECT) methodologies. In: *Advances in Neurobiology*, Vol. 4. New York: Springer, pp. 255–270.

Cumming, P., Caprioli, D., et al. (2011). What have positron emission tomography and "Zippy" told us about the neuropharmacology of drug addiction? *Br. J. Pharmacol* 163:1586–1604.

Daglish, M.R., Weinstein, A., et al. (2001). Changes in regional cerebral blood flow elicited by craving memories in abstinent opiate-dependent subjects. *Am. J. Psychiatry* 158:1680–1686.

Dalley, J.W., Everitt, B.J., et al. (2011). Impulsivity, compulsivity, and top-down cognitive control. *Neuron* 69:680–694.

de Wit, H., Metz, J., et al. (1991). Effects of ethanol, diazepam and amphetamines on cerebral metabolic rate: PET studies using FDG. *NIDA Res. Monogr.* 105:61–67.

de Wit, H., Metz, J., et al. (1989). The effects of 0.8 g/kg ethanol on cerebral metabolism and mood in normal volunteers. *NIDA Res. Monogr.* 95:450.

Di Chiara, G., and Imperato, A. (1988). Drugs abused by humans preferentially increase synaptic dopamine concentrations in the mesolimbic system of freely moving rats. *Proc. Natl. Acad. Sci. USA* 85:5274–5278.

Domino, E.F., Evans, C.L., et al. (2012). Tobacco smoking produces greater striatal dopamine release in G-allele carriers with mu opioid receptor A118G polymorphism. *Prog. Neuropsychopharmacol. Biol. Psychiatry* 38:236–240.

Domino, E.F., Minoshima, S., et al. (2000a). Nicotine effects on regional cerebral blood flow in awake, resting tobacco smokers. *Synapse* 38:313–321.

Domino, E.F., Minoshima, S., et al. (2000b). Effects of nicotine on regional cerebral glucose metabolism in awake resting tobacco smokers. *Neuroscience* 101:277–282.

Drevets, W.C., Gautier, C., et al. (2001). Amphetamine-induced dopamine release in human ventral striatum correlates with euphoria. *Biol. Psychiatry* 49:81–96.

Everitt, B.J., and Robbins, T.W. (2005). Neural systems of reinforcement for drug addiction: from actions to habits to compulsion. *Nat. Neurosci.* 8:1481–1489.

Fehr, C., Yakushev, I., et al. (2008). Association of low striatal dopamine d2 receptor availability with nicotine dependence similar to that seen with other drugs of abuse. *Am. J. Psychiatry* 165:507–514.

Fowler, J.S., Volkow, N.D., et al. (1996a). Inhibition of monoamine oxidase B in the brains of smokers. *Nature* 379:733–736.

Fowler, J.S., Volkow, N.D., et al. (1996b). Brain monoamine oxidase A inhibition in cigarette smokers. *Proc. Nal. Acad. Sci.* 93:14065.

Frost, J.J., Mayberg, H.S., et al. (1990). Comparison of [11 C]diprenorphine and [11 C]carfentanil binding to opiate receptors in humans by positron emission tomography. *J. Cereb. Blood Flow Metab.* 10:484–492.

Fujita, M., Ichise, M., et al. (2003). Quantification of nicotinic acetylcholine receptors in human brain using [125 I]5-I-A-85380 SPET. *Eur. J. Nucl. Med. Mol. Imaging* 30:1620–1629.

Ghitza, U.E., Preston, K.L., et al. (2010). Brain mu-opioid receptor binding predicts treatment outcome in cocaine-abusing outpatients. *Biol. Psychiatry* 68:697–703.

Gilman, S., Koeppe, R.A., et al. (1996). Positron emission tomographic studies of cerebral benzodiazepine-receptor binding in chronic alcoholics. *Ann. Neurol.* 40:163–171.

Gilman, S., Koeppe, R.A., et al. (1998). Decreased striatal monoaminergic terminals in severe chronic alcoholism demonstrated with (+)[11C]dihydrotetrabenazine and positron emission tomography. *Ann. Neurol.* 44:326–333.

Goldstein, R.Z., and Volkow, N.D. (2002). Drug addiction and its underlying neurobiological basis: neuroimaging evidence for the involvement of the frontal cortex. *Am. J. Psychiatry* 159:1642–1652.

Gorelick, D.A., Kim, Y.K., et al. (2005). Imaging brain mu-opioid receptors in abstinent cocaine users: time course and relation to cocaine craving. *Biol. Psychiatry* 57:1573–1582.

Gould, R.W., Porrino, L.J., et al. (2012). Nonhuman primate models of addiction and PET imaging: dopamine system dysregulation. *Curr. Top. Behav. Neurosci.* 11:25–44.

Grant, S., London, E.D., et al. (1996). Activation of memory circuits during cue-elicited cocaine craving. *Proc. Natl. Acad. Sci. USA* 93:12040–12045.

Groman, S.M., Lee, B., et al. (2012). Dysregulation of d2-mediated dopamine transmission in monkeys after chronic escalating methamphetamine exposure. *J. Neurosci.* 32:5843–5852.

Hartz, S.M., Short, S.E., et al. (2012). Increased genetic vulnerability to smoking at CHRNA5 in early-onset smokers. *Arch. Gen. Psychiatry* 69:854–860.

Heinz, A., Ragan, P., et al. (1998). Reduced central serotonin transporters in alcoholism. *Am. J. Psychiatry* 155:1544–1549.

Heinz, A., Reimold, M., et al. (2005a). Correlation of stable elevations in striatal mu-opioid receptor availability in detoxified alcoholic patients with alcohol craving: a positron emission tomography study using carbon 11-labeled carfentanil. *Arch. Gen. Psychiatry* 62:57–64.

Heinz, A., Siessmeier, T., et al. (2005b). Correlation of alcohol craving with striatal dopamine synthesis capacity and D2/3 receptor availability: a combined [18F]DOPA and [18F]DMFP PET study in detoxified alcoholic patients. *Am. J. Psychiatry* 162:1515–1520.

Holman, B.L., Carvalho, P.A., et al. (1991). Brain perfusion is abnormal in cocaine-dependent polydrug users: a study using technetium-99m-HM-PAO and ASPECT. *J. Nucl. Med.* 32:1206–1210.

Hommer, D.W. (1999). Functional imaging of craving. *Alcohol Res. Health* 23:187–196.

Howell, L.L., and Murnane, K.S. (2011) Nonhuman primate positron emission tomography neuroimaging in drug abuse research. *J. Pharmacol. Exp. Ther.* 337:324–334.

Huang, H.Y., Lee, I.H., et al. (2010). Association of novelty seeking scores and striatal dopamine D(2)/D(3) receptor availability of healthy volunteers: single photon emission computed tomography with (1)(2)(3)i-iodobenzamide. *J. Formos. Med. Assoc.* 109:736–739.

Huber, A., Ling, W., et al. (1997). Integrating treatments for methamphetamine abuse: a psychosocial perspective. *J. Addict. Dis.* 16:41–50.

Jacobsen, L.K., Staley, J.K., et al. (2000). Elevated central serotonin transporter binding availability in acutely abstinent cocaine-dependent patients. *Am. J. Psychiatry* 157:1134–1140.

Johanson, C.E., Frey, K.A., et al. (2006). Cognitive function and nigrostriatal markers in abstinent methamphetamine abusers. *Psychopharmacology (Berl.)* 185:327–338.

Kaasinen, V., Aalto, S., et al. (2004). Insular dopamine D2 receptors and novelty seeking personality in Parkinson's disease. *Mov. Disord.* 19:1348–1351.

Kilts, C.D., Schweitzer, J.B., et al. (2001). Neural activity related to drug craving in cocaine addiction. *Arch. Gen. Psychiatry* 58:334–341.

Kimes, A.S., Horti, A.G., et al. (2003). 2-[18 F]f-a-85380: PET imaging of brain nicotinic acetylcholine receptors and whole body distribution in humans. *FASEB J.* 17:1331–1333.

Koob, G.F. (1992) Drugs of abuse: anatomy, pharmacology and function of reward pathways. *Trends Pharmacol. Sci.* 13:177–184.

Koob, G.F., and Volkow, N.D. (2010). Neurocircuitry of addiction. *Neuropsychopharmacology* 35:217–238.

Koylu, E., Demirgoren, S., et al. (1997). Sex difference in up-regulation of nicotinic acetylcholine receptors in rat brain. *Life Sci.* 61:PL 185–190.

Kuhl, D.E., Barrio, J.R., et al. (1982). Quantifying local cerebral blood flow by *N*-isopropyl-*para*-[123I]iodoamphetamine (IMP) tomography. *J. Nucl. Med.* 23:196–203.

Laine, T.P., Ahonen, A., et al. (1999). Dopamine transporters increase in human brain after alcohol withdrawal. *Mol. Psychiatry* 4:189–191, 04–05.

Laruelle, M., D'Souza, C.D., et al. (1997a). Imaging D2 receptor occupancy by endogenous dopamine in humans. *Neuropsychopharmacology* 17:162–174.

Laruelle, M., Iyer, R.N., et al. (1997b). Microdialysis and SPECT measurements of amphetamine-induced dopamine release in nonhuman primates. *Synapse* 25:1–14.

Laruelle, M. (2000). Imaging synaptic neurotransmission with *in vivo* binding competition techniques: a critical review. *J. Cereb. Blood Flow Metab.* 20:423–451.

Lee, B., London, E.D., et al. (2009). Striatal dopamine d2/d3 receptor availability is reduced in methamphetamine dependence and is linked to impulsivity. *J. Neurosci.* 29:14734–14740.

Leroy, C., Karila, L., et al. (2011). Striatal and extrastriatal dopamine transporter in cannabis and tobacco addiction: a high-resolution PET study. *Addict. Biol.* 17:981–990.

Lingford-Hughes, A.R., Acton, P.D., et al. (1998). Reduced levels of GABA-benzodiazepine receptor in alcohol dependency in the absence of grey matter atrophy. *Br. J. Psychiatry* 173:116–122.

Logan, J., Fowler, J.S., et al. (2001). A consideration of the dopamine D2 receptor monomer-dimer equilibrium and the anomalous binding properties of the dopamine D2 receptor ligand, N-methyl spiperone. *J. Neural. Transm.* 108:279–286.

London, E.D., Berman, S.M., et al. (2009). Effect of the TaqIA polymorphism on ethanol response in the brain. *Psychiatry Res.* 174:163–170.

London, E.D., Broussolle, E.P., et al. (1990a). Morphine-induced metabolic changes in human brain. Studies with positron emission tomography and [fluorine 18]fluorodeoxyglucose. *Arch. Gen. Psychiatry* 47:73–81.

London, E.D., Cascella, N.G., et al. (1990b). Cocaine-induced reduction of glucose utilization in human brain. A study using positron emission tomography and [fluorine 18]-fluorodeoxyglucose. *Arch. Gen. Psychiatry* 47:567–574.

London, E.D., Connolly, R.J., et al. (1988). Effects of nicotine on local cerebral glucose utilization in the rat. *J. Neurosci.* 8:3920–3928.

London, E.D., Ernst, M., et al. (2000). Orbitofrontal cortex and human drug abuse: functional imaging. *Cereb. Cortex* 10:334–342.

London, E.D., Simon, S.L., et al. (2004). Mood disturbances and regional cerebral metabolic abnormalities in recently abstinent methamphetamine abusers. *Arch. Gen. Psychiatry* 61:73–84.

London, E.D., Waller, S.B., et al. (1985). Autoradiographic localization of [3H] nicotine binding sites in the rat brain. *Neurosci. Lett.* 53:179–184.

London, E.D., Wilkerson, G., et al. (1986). Effects of L-cocaine on local cerebral glucose utilization in the rat. *Neurosci. Lett.* 68:73–78.

Lyons, D., Friedman, D.P., et al. (1996). Cocaine alters cerebral metabolism within the ventral striatum and limbic cortex of monkeys. *J. Neurosci.* 16:1230–1238.

Malison, R.T., Best, S.E., et al. (1998). Elevated striatal dopamine transporters during acute cocaine abstinence as measured by [123I] beta-CIT SPECT. *Am. J. Psychiatry* 155:832–834.

Mamede, M., Ishizu, K., et al. (2007). Temporal change in human nicotinic acetylcholine receptor after smoking cessation: 5IA SPECT study. *J. Nucl. Med.* 48:1829–1835.

Martinez, D., Broft, A., et al. (2004). Cocaine dependence and D2 receptor availability in the functional subdivisions of the striatum: relationship with cocaine-seeking behavior. *Neuropsychopharmacology* 29:1190–1202.

Martinez, D., Gil, R., et al. (2005). Alcohol dependence is associated with blunted dopamine transmission in the ventral striatum. *Biol. Psychiatry* 58:779–786.

Martinez, D., Greene, K., et al. (2009a). Lower level of endogenous dopamine in patients with cocaine dependence: findings from PET imaging of D(2)/D(3) receptors following acute dopamine depletion. *Am. J. Psychiatry* 166:1170–1177.

Martinez, D., Slifstein, M., et al. (2009b). Positron emission tomography imaging of the serotonin transporter and 5-HT(1A) receptor in alcohol dependence. *Biol. Psychiatry* 65:175–180.

Martinez, D., and Narendran, R. (2010). Imaging neurotransmitter release by drugs of abuse. *Curr. Top. Behav. Neurosci.* 3:219–245.

Martinez, D., Saccone, P.A., et al. (2012). Deficits in dopamine D(2) receptors and presynaptic dopamine in heroin dependence: commonalities and differences with other types of addiction. *Biol. Psychiatry* 71:192–198.

Mathew, R.J., and Wilson, W.H. (1991). Substance abuse and cerebral blood flow. *Am. J. Psychiatry* 148:292–305.

McCann, U.D., Wong, D.F., et al. (1998). Reduced striatal dopamine transporter density in abstinent methamphetamine and methcathinone users: evidence from positron emission tomography studies with [11C] WIN-35,428. *J. Neurosci.* 18:8417–8422.

Mintun, M.A., Raichle, M.E., et al. (1984). Brain oxygen utilization measured with O-15 radiotracers and positron emission tomography. *J. Nucl. Med.* 25:177–187.

Mitchell, J.M., O'Neil, J.P., et al. (2012). Alcohol consumption induces endogenous opioid release in the human orbitofrontal cortex and nucleus accumbens. *Sci. Transl. Med.* 4:116ra6.

Mukhin, A.G., Kimes, A.S., et al. (2008). Greater nicotinic acetylcholine receptor density in smokers than in nonsmokers: a PET study with 2-18F-FA-85380. *J. Nucl. Med.* 49:1628–1635.

Narendran, R., Lopresti, B.J., et al. (2012). *In vivo* evidence for low striatal vesicular monoamine transporter 2 (VMAT2) availability in cocaine abusers. *Am. J. Psychiatry* 169:55–63.

Nelson, E.C., Lynskey, M.T., et al. (2012). Association of OPRD1 polymorphisms with heroin dependence in a large case-control series. *Addict. Biol.* [EPub ahead of print, April 13 2012]. http://onlinelibrary.wiley.com.

Nickel, O., Nagele-Wohrle, B., et al. (1989). RCBF-quantification with 99mTc-HMPAO-SPECT: theory and first results. *Eur. J. Nucl. Med.* 15:1–8.

Nisell, M., Nomikos, G.G., et al. (1994). Systemic nicotine-induced dopamine release in the rat nucleus accumbens is regulated by nicotinic receptors in the ventral tegmental area. *Synapse* 16:36–44.

Noble, E.P. (2003). D2 dopamine receptor gene in psychiatric and neurologic disorders and its phenotypes. *Am. J. Med. Genet. B Neuropsychiatr. Genet.* 116B:103–125.

Oswald, L.M., Wong, D.F., et al. (2005). Relationships among ventral striatal dopamine release, cortisol secretion, and subjective responses to amphetamine. *Neuropsychopharmacology* 30:821–832.

Parvaz, M.A., Alia-Klein, N., et al. (2011). Neuroimaging for drug addiction and related behaviors. *Rev. Neurosci.* 22:609–624.

Pearlson, G.D., Jeffery, P.J., et al. (1993). Correlation of acute cocaine-induced changes in local cerebral blood flow with subjective effects. *Am. J. Psychiatry* 150:495–497.

Phelps, M.E., Huang, S.C., et al. (1979). Tomographic measurement of local cerebral glucose metabolic rate in humans with (F-18)2-fluoro-2-deoxy-D-glucose: validation of method. *Ann. Neurol.* 6:371–388.

Porrino, L.J., Domer, F.R., et al. (1988). Selective alterations in cerebral metabolism within the mesocorticolimbic dopaminergic system produced by acute cocaine administration in rats. *Neuropsychopharmacology* 1:109–118.

Reivich, M., Kuhl, D., et al. (1979). The [18 F]fluorodeoxyglucose method for the measurement of local cerebral glucose utilization in man. *Circ. Res.* 44:127–137.

Repo, E., Kuikka, J.T., et al. (1999). Dopamine transporter and D2-receptor density in late-onset alcoholism. *Psychopharmacology (Berl.)* 147:314–318.

Riccardi, P., Li, R., et al. (2006). Amphetamine-induced displacement of [18F] fallypride in striatum and extrastriatal regions in humans. *Neuropsychopharmacology* 31:1016–1026.

Riederer, P., Konradi, C., et al. (1987). Localization of MAO-A and MAO-B in human brain: a step in understanding the therapeutic action of L-deprenyl. *Adv. Neurol.* 45:111–118.

Robins, L.N. (1993). The sixth Thomas James Okey Memorial Lecture. Vietnam veterans' rapid recovery from heroin addiction: a fluke or normal expectation? *Addiction* 88:1041–1054.

Rose, J.E., Behm, F.M., et al. (2001). Platelet monoamine oxidase, smoking cessation, and tobacco withdrawal symptoms. *Nicotine Tob. Res.* 3:383–390.

Rose, J.E., Behm, F.M., et al. (2003). PET studies of the influences of nicotine on neural systems in cigarette smokers. *Am. J. Psychiatry* 160:323–333.

Roy, C.S., and Sherrington, C.S. (1890). On the regulation of the blood supply of the brain. *J. Physiol.* 11:85–108.

Salokangas, R.K., Vilkman, H., et al. (2000). High levels of dopamine activity in the basal ganglia of cigarette smokers. *Am. J. Psychiatry* 157:632–634.

Schlaepfer, T.E., Pearlson, G.D., et al. (1997). PET study of competition between intravenous cocaine and [11C]raclopride at dopamine receptors in human subjects. *Am. J. Psychiatry* 154:1209–1213.

Schoultz, B.W., Hjornevik, T., et al. (2010). Evaluation of the kappa-opioid receptor-selective tracer [(11)C]GR103545 in awake rhesus macaques. *Eur. J. Nucl. Med. Mol. Imaging* 37:1174–1180.

Scott, D.J., Domino, E.F., et al. (2007). Smoking modulation of mu-opioid and dopamine D2 receptor-mediated neurotransmission in humans. *Neuropsychopharmacology* 32:450–457.

Sekine, Y., Iyo, M., et al. (2001). Methamphetamine-related psychiatric symptoms and reduced brain dopamine transporters studied with PET. *Am. J. Psychiatry* 158:1206–1214.

Sekine, Y., Ouchi, Y., et al. (2006). Brain serotonin transporter density and aggression in abstinent methamphetamine abusers. *Arch. Gen. Psychiatry* 63:90–100.

Sharma, A., and Brody, A.L. (2009). *In vivo* brain imaging of human exposure to nicotine and tobacco. *Handb. Exp. Pharmacol.* 192:145–171.

Shi, J., Zhao, L.Y., et al. (2008). PET imaging of dopamine transporter and drug craving during methadone maintenance treatment and after prolonged abstinence in heroin users. *Eur. J. Pharmacol.* 579:160–166.

Shippenberg, T.S., Chefer, V.I., et al. (2001). Modulation of the behavioral and neurochemical effects of psychostimulants by kappa-opioid receptor systems. *Ann. NY Acad. Sci.* 937:50–73.

Sinha, R. (2008). Chronic stress, drug use, and vulnerability to addiction. *Ann. NY Acad. Sci.* 1141:105–130.

Skinbjerg, M., Liow, J.S., et al. (2010). D2 dopamine receptor internalization prolongs the decrease of radioligand binding after amphetamine: a PET study in a receptor internalization-deficient mouse model. *NeuroImage* 50:1402–1407.

Sokoloff, L., Reivich, M., et al. (1977). The [14C]deoxyglucose method for the measurement of local cerebral glucose utilization: theory, procedure, and normal values in the conscious and anesthetized albino rat. *J. Neurochem.* 28:897–916.

Som, P., Atkins, H.L., et al. (1980). A fluorinated glucose analog, 2-fluoro-2-deoxy-D-glucose (F-18): nontoxic tracer for rapid tumor detection. *J. Nucl. Med.* 21:670–675.

Spreckelmeyer, K.N., Paulzen, M., et al. (2011). Opiate-induced dopamine release is modulated by severity of alcohol dependence: an [(18)F]fallypride positron emission tomography study. *Biol. Psychiatry* 70:770–776.

Staley, J.K., Krishnan-Sarin, S., et al. (2001). Sex differences in [123I]beta-CIT SPECT measures of dopamine and serotonin transporter availability in healthy smokers and nonsmokers. *Synapse* 41:275–284.

Staley, J.K., Krishnan-Sarin, S., et al. (2006). Human tobacco smokers in early abstinence have higher levels of beta2* nicotinic acetylcholine receptors than nonsmokers. *J. Neurosci.* 26:8707–8714.

Stapleton, J.M., Gilson, S.F., et al. (2003). Intravenous nicotine reduces cerebral glucose metabolism: a preliminary study. *Neuropsychopharmacology* 28:765–772.

Stapleton, J.M., Morgan, M.J., et al. (1995). Cerebral glucose utilization in polysubstance abuse. *Neuropsychopharmacology* 13:21–31.

Stokes, P.R., Mehta, M.A., et al. (2009). Can recreational doses of THC produce significant dopamine release in the human striatum? *NeuroImage* 48:186–190.

Sweitzer, M.M., Donny, E.C., et al. (2012). Imaging genetics and the neurobiological basis of individual differences in vulnerability to addiction. *Drug Alcohol Depend.* 123(Suppl 1):S59–S71.

Tanda, G., and Di Chiara, G. (1998). A dopamine-mu1 opioid link in the rat ventral tegmentum shared by palatable food (Fonzies) and non-psychostimulant drugs of abuse. *Eur. J. Neurosci.* 10:1179–1187.

Thanos, P.K., Volkow, N.D., et al. (2001). Overexpression of dopamine D2 receptors reduces alcohol self-administration. *J. Neurochem.* 78:1094–1103.

Tong, J., Wilson, A.A., et al. (2008). Dopamine modulating drugs influence striatal (+)-[11C]DTBZ binding in rats: VMAT2 binding is sensitive to changes in vesicular dopamine concentration. *Synapse* 62:873–876.

Vander Borght, T., Kilbourn, M., et al. (1995). The vesicular monoamine transporter is not regulated by dopaminergic drug treatments. *Eur. J. Pharmacol.* 294:577–583.

Verdejo-Garcia, A., Lawrence, A.J., et al. (2008). Impulsivity as a vulnerability marker for substance-use disorders: review of findings from high-risk research, problem gamblers and genetic association studies. *Neurosci. Biobehav. Rev.* 32:777–810.

Volkow, N.D., Chang, L., et al. (2001a). Loss of dopamine transporters in methamphetamine abusers recovers with protracted abstinence. *J. Neurosci.* 21:9414–9418.

Volkow, N.D., Chang, L., et al. (2001b). Low level of brain dopamine D2 receptors in methamphetamine abusers: association with metabolism in orbitofrontal cortex. *Am. J. Psychiatry* 158:2015–2021.

Volkow, N.D., and Fowler, J.S. (2000). Addiction, a disease of compulsion and drive: involvement of the orbitofrontal cortex. *Cereb. Cortex* 10:318–325.

Volkow, N.D., Fowler, J.S., et al. (1990). Effects of chronic cocaine abuse on postsynaptic dopamine receptors. *Am. J. Psychiatry* 147:719–724.

Volkow, N.D., Fowler, J.S., et al. (1991). Changes in brain glucose metabolism in cocaine dependence and withdrawal. *Am. J. Psychiatry* 148:621–626.

Volkow, N.D., Fowler, J.S., et al. (1993). Decreased dopamine D2 receptor availability is associated with reduced frontal metabolism in cocaine abusers. *Synapse* 14:169–177.

Volkow, N.D., Fowler, J.S., et al. (2004). Dopamine in drug abuse and addiction: results from imaging studies and treatment implications. *Mol. Psychiatry* 9:557–569.

Volkow, N.D., Hitzemann, R., et al. (1992). Long-term frontal brain metabolic changes in cocaine abusers. *Synapse* 11:184–190.

Volkow, N.D., Mullani, N., et al. (1988a). Cerebral blood flow in chronic cocaine users: a study with positron emission tomography. *Br. J. Psychiatry* 152:641–648.

Volkow, N.D., Mullani, N., et al. (1988b). Effects of acute alcohol intoxication on cerebral blood flow measured with PET. *Psychiatry Res.* 24:201–209.

Volkow, N.D., Wang, G.J., et al. (1994). Recovery of brain glucose metabolism in detoxified alcoholics. *Am. J. Psychiatry* 151:178–183.

Volkow, N.D., Wang, G.J., et al. (1996). Decreases in dopamine receptors but not in dopamine transporters in alcoholics. *Alcohol Clin. Exp. Res.* 20:1594–1598.

Volkow, N.D., Wang, G.J., et al. (1997). Decreased striatal dopaminergic responsiveness in detoxified cocaine-dependent subjects. *Nature* 386:830–833.

Volkow, N.D., Wang, G.J., et al. (2000). Effects of route of administration on cocaine induced dopamine transporter blockade in the human brain. *Life Sci.* 67:1507–1515.

Volkow, N.D., Wang, G., et al. (2001c). Therapeutic doses of oral methylphenidate significantly increase extracellular dopamine in the human brain. *J. Neurosci.* 21:RC121.

Volkow, N.D., Wang, G.J., et al. (2002). Brain DA D2 receptors predict reinforcing effects of stimulants in humans: replication study. *Synapse* 46:79–82.

Volkow, N.D., Wang, G.J., et al. (2006a). High levels of dopamine D2 receptors in unaffected members of alcoholic families: possible protective factors. *Arch. Gen. Psychiatry* 63:999–1008.

Volkow, N.D., Wang, G.J., et al. (2006b). Cocaine cues and dopamine in dorsal striatum: mechanism of craving in cocaine addiction. *J. Neurosci.* 26:6583–6588.

Volkow, N.D., Wang, G.J., et al. (2011). Addiction: beyond dopamine reward circuitry. *Proc. Natl. Acad. Sci. USA* 108:15037–15042.

Wallace, E.A., Wisniewski, G., et al. (1996). Acute cocaine effects on absolute cerebral blood flow. *Psychopharmacology (Berl.)* 128:17–20.

Wang, G.J., Smith, L., et al. (2011). Decreased dopamine activity predicts relapse in methamphetamine abusers. *Mol. Psychiatry* 17:918–925.

Wang, G.J., Volkow, N.D., et al. (1997). Dopamine D2 receptor availability in opiate-dependent subjects before and after naloxone-precipitated withdrawal. *Neuropsychopharmacology* 16:174–182.

Wang, G.J., Volkow, N.D., et al. (1998). Regional cerebral metabolism in female alcoholics of moderate severity does not differ from that of controls. *Alcohol Clin. Exp. Res.* 22:1850–1854.

Wang, G.J., Volkow, N.D., et al. (2004). Similarity between obesity and drug addiction as assessed by neurofunctional imaging: a concept review. *J. Addict. Dis.* 23:39–53.

Wilson, J.M., Kalasinsky, K.S., et al. (1996). Striatal dopamine nerve terminal markers in human, chronic methamphetamine users. *Nat. Med.* 2:699–703.

Wise, R.A., and Bozarth, M.A. (1987). A psychomotor stimulant theory of addiction. *Psychol. Rev.* 94:469–492.

Wong, D.F., Gjedde, A., et al. (1986). Quantification of neuroreceptors in the living human brain. I. Irreversible binding of ligands. *J. Cereb. Blood Flow Metab.* 6:137–146.

Wong, D.F., Kuwabara, H., et al. (2006). Increased occupancy of dopamine receptors in human striatum during cue-elicited cocaine craving. *Neuropsychopharmacology* 31:2716–2727.

Wonnacott, S. (1997). Presynaptic nicotinic ACh receptors. *Trends Neurosci.* 20:92–98.

Wu, J.C., Bell, K., et al. (1997). Decreasing striatal 6-FDOPA uptake with increasing duration of cocaine withdrawal. *Neuropsychopharmacology* 17:402–409.

Zald, D.H., Cowan, R.L., et al. (2008). Midbrain dopamine receptor availability is inversely associated with novelty-seeking traits in humans. *J. Neurosci.* 28:14372–14378.

Zijlstra, F., Booij, J., et al. (2008). Striatal dopamine D2 receptor binding and dopamine release during cue-elicited craving in recently abstinent opiate-dependent males. *Eur. Neuropsychopharmacol.* 18:262–270.

Zorick, T., Lee, B., et al. (2012). Low striatal dopamine receptor availability linked to caloric intake during abstinence from chronic methamphetamine abuse. *Mol. Psychiatry* 17:569–571.

Zubieta, J., Greenwald, M.K., et al. (2000). Buprenorphine-induced changes in mu-opioid receptor availability in male heroin-dependent volunteers: a preliminary study. *Neuropsychopharmacology* 23:326–334.

Zubieta, J., Lombardi, U., et al. (2001). Regional cerebral blood flow effects of nicotine in overnight abstinent smokers. *Biol. Psychiatry* 49:906–913.

Zubieta, J.K., Gorelick, D.A., et al. (1996). Increased mu opioid receptor binding detected by PET in cocaine-dependent men is associated with cocaine craving. *Nat. Med.* 2:1225–1229.

55 | BRAIN, REWARD, AND DRUG ADDICTION

VANI PARIYADATH, MARTIN P. PAULUS, AND ELLIOT A. STEIN

Substance abuse and dependence have an enormous impact on society. For example, according to the Substance Abuse and Mental Health Services Administration (SAMHSA; http://www.samhsa.gov/), in the United States, the lifetime prevalence of substance abuse or dependence in adults is over 15%. Estimates of the overall costs of drug and alcohol abuse in the United States exceed $600 billion annually (National Institute on Drug Abuse, 2011). In 2006, an estimated 20.4 million Americans aged 12 or older used illicit drugs over the past month, which represents 8.3% of the population aged 12 years or older (SAMHSA). According to another SAMHSA report, 14.8 million individuals reported using marijuana in the past month, with an additional 9.6 million persons who used illicit drugs other than marijuana.

Addiction occurs rarely as an isolated disease entity. Instead, there is significant comorbidity between substance dependence with most mood disorders and anxiety disorders (Reske and Paulus, 2008). Interestingly, only a minority of individuals with substance use disorders seek treatment (Reske and Paulus, 2008). Psychiatric comorbidity has a profound influence on course and outcome. Individuals with substance use disorders and posttraumatic stress disorder, relative to those with substance use disorders only, are more impaired, have greater psychosocial problems, and show a more severe course (Reske and Paulus, 2008). Similarly, comorbid antisocial personality disorder results in earlier onset of substance use disorders, greater multisubstance use, poorer outcomes, more severe course, and other psychosocial dysfunctions (Reske and Paulus, 2008). The complex neural basis of addiction is complicated by three major factors. First, addiction is a highly dynamic disorder that undergoes frequent transition from intense use to sobriety. Second, psychiatric comorbidity has profound influences on the course and neurobiology of drug addiction. Finally, and of particular relevance here, both reward-related processes as well as negative reinforcement processes are thought to contribute to the various stages of drug addiction.

Reward is a complex construct that entails a feeling and an action. Components of reward include the hedonic aspects, that is, the degree to which a stimulus is associated with pleasure, and the incentive motivational aspects, that is, the degree to which a stimulus induces an action towards obtaining it (Berridge and Robinson, 2003). Typically, the feeling is described as pleasurable or positive and the actions comprise behavior aimed to approach the stimulus that is associated with reward. However, importantly, both feeling and action are highly dependent on the homeostatic state of the individual (Craig, 2002). Few other topics in neuroscience have received as much attention in the last 60 years as the brain's reward system, and yet much of its function remains poorly understood. With more sophisticated technology and tools for studying brain reward circuitry, an increasingly complex yet still ambiguous picture has emerged. A more thorough understanding of this intricate system may yield a better appreciation of the challenges facing addiction research and treatment outcome improvement. We thus begin with a brief introduction of the reward system before reviewing the current literature on addiction neuroimaging.

REPRESENTATION OF REWARD IN THE BRAIN

Since the seminal study from Olds and Milner (1954) establishing that rats would move to a specific place in an open field to obtain electrical stimulation of certain brain areas, it has been established that there exists a neural system, which were originally conceptualized as centers, whose activation appears to signal positive rewarding effects. In the intervening decades, pharmacological, electrophysiological, and neuroimaging studies have helped delineate an extensive reward circuit that spans striatal, midbrain and prefrontal regions (Fig. 55.1A).

Research on the reward circuit has revolved around midbrain dopaminergic neurons, along with the structures they enervate (Haber and Knutson, 2010). This includes the mesolimbic pathway or the dopaminergic nerve bundle that originates mostly in the ventral tegmental area in the midbrain and projects to multiple limbic structures, the mesocortical pathway that projects to frontal cortical regions, and the nigrostriatal pathway that extends primarily between the substantia nigra and the dorsal striatum. Although we have a limited understanding of their specific roles, other subcortical regions have now been identified as being central to reward processing including the lateral habenula and the amygdala (Haber and Knutson, 2010). When probing the reward circuit in humans on a systems level, functional magnetic resonance imaging (fMRI) studies have highlighted the orbitofrontal cortex, amygdala, nucleus accumbens, ventral tegmental area, and hypothalamus as responding to abused drugs and other positive reinforcing stimuli (Haber and Knutson, 2010). Extracting the specific roles of these nodes within the reward circuit is made complicated by the extensive forward and backward projections between them (Ikemoto, 2010; Fig. 55.1B), as

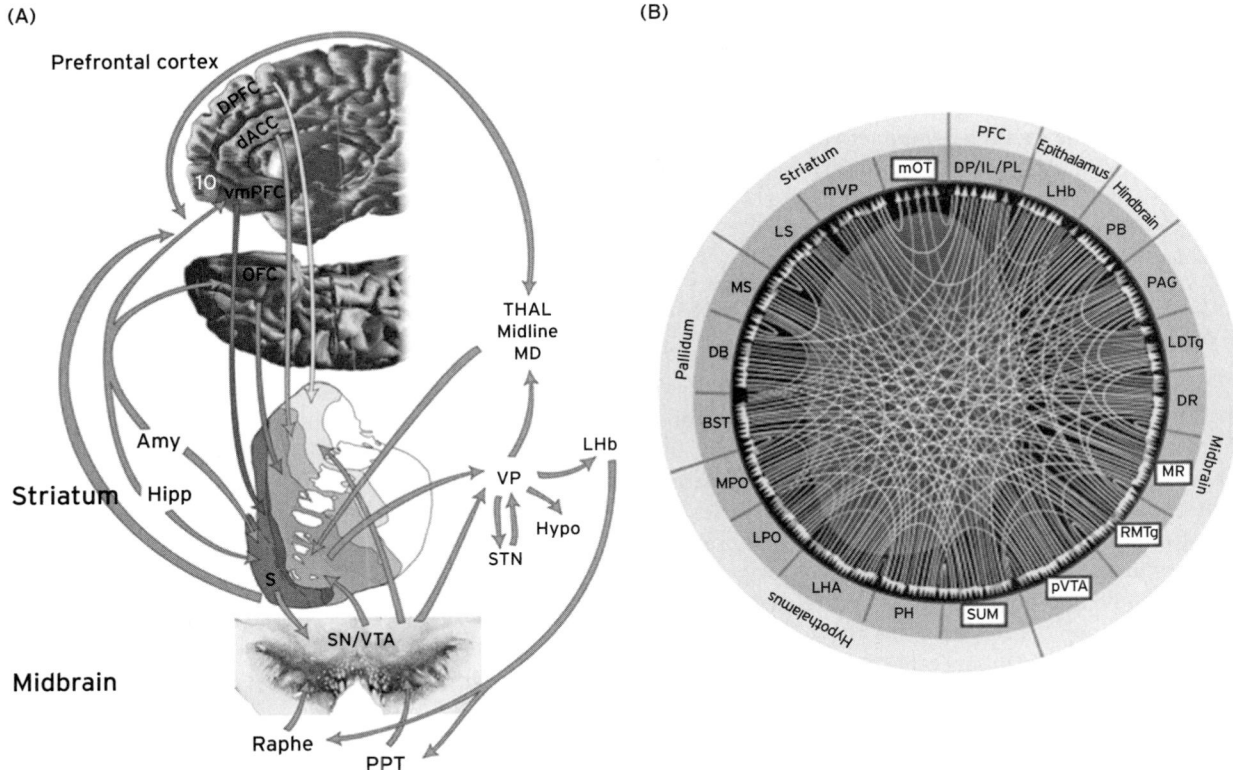

Figure 55.1 *The reward circuit and its complexity. (A) Brain regions identified as being key players in the reward circuit, including striatal, midbrain, and prefrontal regions and, more recently, the amygdala, hippocampus, lateral habenula, and brainstem structures. (B)The connectivity between proposed brain reward regions is incredibly complex and has rendered identifying the roles of individual components difficult. Orange lines indicate unidirectional connection and yellow lines reciprocal connections. Purple area represents the medial forebrain bundle, the stimulation of which results in rewarding brain stimulation. (A from Haber S.N., Knutson B. (2010). The reward circuit: linking primate anatomy and human imaging. Neuropsychopharmacology 35:4–26. B from Ikemoto S. (2010). Brain reward circuitry beyond the mesolimbic dopamine system: a neurobiological theory. Neurosci Biobehav Rev 35:129–150.) (See color insert.)*

well as the complexity introduced by the interaction of different neurotransmitter systems and their associated receptor machinery.

NEUROTRANSMITTER SYSTEMS INVOLVED IN REWARD PROCESSING

THE DOPAMINE HYPOTHESIS OF REWARD

Arguably, the most influential model for dopamine function has stemmed from the anhedonia hypothesis, which suggested that dopamine signals the pleasure experienced from food and other natural and artificial rewards (Wise, 2008). However, dopamine receptor antagonists do not diminish the appetitive value of rewards, as would be expected from the anhedonia model, but instead affects the animal's ability to act upon these value computations (Berridge, 2007). In the last 30 years, the anhedonia hypothesis has faced severe opposition and undergone revisions, but there is no denying the impact it has had on successive theories of motivation and dopamine function (Wise, 2008).

A second school of thought posits that dopaminergic neurons in the ventral tegmental area (VTA) reflect a reward prediction error: These neurons fire phasically in response to an unexpected reward, and, after learning has taken place, in response to the omission of an expected reward, but not to an expected reward itself. Curiously, after multiple presentations of a paired cue and reward, these neurons shift their time of firing from the onset of the reward to that of the cue predicting the reward (Schultz et al., 1997). Reinforcement learning models have emphasized the difference between the encoding of the reward itself and the reward prediction error, and have provided the field with quantitative tools for understanding dopaminergic function. For example, temporal difference learning models have contributed a precise basis for the temporal evolution of the dopamine signal as learning of cue-reward associations takes place (Niv et al., 2005).

An alternative viewpoint holds that there are two components to the response to reward: one is "liking," which corresponds to the pleasure experienced from a reward, and the other is "wanting" or incentive salience that relates to the attractiveness of the reward (Berridge, 2007). To assay the former, researchers have focused on facial palatability responses to appetitive (e.g., sweet tasting) and aversive (e.g., bitter tasting) stimuli (Steiner et al., 2001). Humans and a wide range of animals display a distinct, reproducible facial response to both types of stimuli, for example, gaping in response to bitter tasting stimuli and tongue protrusions in response to sweet tasting ones. Importantly, these liking responses are not influenced by dopamine modulations (Berridge, 2007). Instead, dopamine seems to play a role in the wanting of rewarding stimuli, such that elevated dopamine levels in the synapse (e.g., in hyperdopaminergic mutant mice) bring about increased wanting of the reward, measured by the willingness to work for it (Berridge, 2007). In this sense, the wanting component of the reward signal corresponds to the reward prediction error, whereas the liking component resembles the hedonic aspect of reward described in early models of dopamine function.

MOVING BEYOND THE DOPAMINE HYPOTHESIS OF REWARD AND PREDICTION ERROR

Although much effort has been spent on elucidating the precise function of dopamine, many important questions about reward processing remain unanswered. While the role of this neurotransmitter, especially within the basal ganglia, carries important implications for the effects of drugs of abuse, it is clearly far from a simple mediator of reward in the brain, as was once presumed. Perhaps only by deemphasizing the role of dopamine can further progress on reward-related disorders like addiction be made. To this end, this chapter offers a brief exploration of the research linking other major neurotransmitters to reward learning.

The neurotransmitter system best positioned to enhance addiction research is probably glutamate, an excitatory neurotransmitter localized within over half of all synapses in the brain. Within the reward circuit, glutamate-dopamine interactions appear to play an important role in synaptic plasticity in the striatum (Wang et al., 2012), and in frontostriatal communication (Taber and Fibiger, 1995). Some view such interactions as a promising new avenue of research, especially in the context of such psychiatric disorders as drug addiction (Wang et al., 2012).

There is also emerging evidence to suggest that dopamine and serotonin work in opposition to each other (Cools et al., 2011). Although earlier models proposed a symmetric relationship for dopamine and serotonin centered around reward and punishment learning, a more nuanced framework has emerged wherein the two neurotransmitters control the interaction between reward/punishment and behavioral activation/inhibition (Cools et al., 2011). Dopamine is thought to behave in complex ways pre- and post-synaptically to effect changes in synaptic function through two main groups of receptors, categorized as D1-like (D1 and D5) and D2-like (D2, D3, and D4) receptor families (De Mei et al., 2009). Serotonin's function may seem labyrinthine in comparison because it employs at least 14 different receptor subtypes (Hoyer et al., 2002).

Finally, recent research suggests that GABAergic neurons play an important role in reward processing as well, and, as with other neurotransmitters, this role is mediated through its interactions with dopaminergic neurons (Parker et al., 2011). Recently, GABAergic neurons have been shown to encode expected reward, such that they remain persistently active between the presentation of the cue and the reward (Cohen et al., 2012). Taken together, it seems apparent that a better understanding of neurotransmitter interactions within the reward circuit is needed in the field.

OUTSIDE THE BASAL GANGLIA

A drive-by observer of reward-related research may be forgiven for mistaking the basal ganglia for being the beginning and end of reward processing since a vast majority of research has focused on this body, especially in terms of dopaminergic function. Even so, there is currently no unified theory for basal ganglia function, and the story only grows murkier as the series of parallel circuits that form corticobasal ganglia-thalamocortical loops are taken into account (Alexander et al., 1986). As research has ventured beyond the basal ganglia, new and unexpected players have emerged, and given their prominent roles in non–reward-related functions, it has been suggested that reward be understood within a larger framework of animal behavior (Hikosaka et al., 2008). Because a detailed understanding of the basal ganglia has thus far not significantly improved understanding of drug addiction to the extent one might have predicted, it seems particularly pertinent to extend the roles of other subcortical and cortical nodes within the reward circuit.

AMYGDALA AND REWARD PROCESSING

By the middle of the twentieth century, it was evident that the amygdala plays a central role in emotional processing, but ensuing research resulted in some confusion as important differences in the distinct subareas of the amygdala had not yet been fully appreciated (LeDoux, 2007). Currently, there is much debate on whether the amygdala is really a single structural or functional unit, but studies on Kluver-Bucy syndrome and fear conditioning have suggested a general role for emotional processing, with an emphasis on fear. The lateral nucleus, in particular, has long been emphasized in fear learning, but, along with the basal and central amygdala, is now also considered important for reward learning and motivation more generally (LeDoux, 2007).

Within the context of this review, it is important to note that the amygdala seems to represent reward- and punishment-related predictions (Roesch et al., 2010), and is likely involved in associative learning in general (Murray, 2007). Whereas dopaminergic activity in the VTA closely resembles a neural prediction error (Schultz et al., 1997), amygdalar neurons behave as though they signal a different entity—associability, or the amount of attention devoted to cues (Li et al., 2011). Per the Pearce-Hall model of associative learning, the associability of a cue is determined by the positive or negative surprise accompanying previous presentations of that cue (Pearce and Hall, 1980), and likely modulates the rate at which learning from prediction errors takes place. Electrophysiological studies in animals (Roesch et al., 2010) and an fMRI study in humans (Li et al., 2011) have revealed similar computations taking place within the amygdala. Although much work is required to elucidate the precise role of the amygdala in reward learning and how it is made possible, it is evident that these learning-related computations have important implications for reward processing "upstream" in the prefrontal cortex (Hampton et al., 2007).

THE CONTRIBUTIONS OF THE LATERAL HABENULA TO REWARD PROCESSING

Although there is strong evidence for dopamine's role in positive surprise, there is much less support for its role in disappointment, which can be considered another important brain signal for reward-related processing. Thus, midbrain dopaminergic neurons code for positive prediction errors, but show relatively weak response to negative prediction errors (Schultz et al., 1997), suggesting that the latter is maintained elsewhere. From primate studies, we now know that habenular neurons show a transient dip in firing rate in response to cues predictive of rewards (Matsumoto and Hikosaka, 2007). Further, the lateral habenula has been shown to drive dopaminergic activity in the midbrain (Ji and Shepard, 2007) via GABAergic neurons in the rostromedial mesopontine tegmental nucleus (Jhou et al., 2009). Critically, the lateral habenula responds to the absence of a reward (Matsumoto and Hikosaka, 2007), or the presence of a punishment (Matsumoto and Hikosaka, 2007), suggesting an opponent role for the habenula vis-à-vis midbrain dopaminergic function.

THE ROLE OF THE MEDIAL PREFRONTAL CORTEX—EXPECTATION AND VIOLATION OF EXPECTATIONS

The medial prefrontal cortex (mPFC) frequently plays a prominent role in models for various cognitive processes, and reward learning models are no exception The anterior cingulate cortex (ACC) in particular appears to encode anticipated, experienced, and fictive reward conditions (Hayden et al., 2009; Matsumoto et al., 2003), much like the dopaminergic neurons that project to it (Williams and Goldman-Rakic, 1993). However, although dopaminergic signaling follows a narrow dynamic range—positive prediction errors are represented as increases in firing rate, but negative prediction errors are encoded as a slight decrease in firing (Schultz et al., 1997)—the ACC may employ distinct neuronal populations for encoding positive and negative prediction errors whereby each type of prediction error is encoded as an increase in firing rate (Matsumoto et al., 2007). The ACC has also been suggested to set the learning rate in reinforcement learning-type models by mediating the degree to which stimulus-response outcomes will influence future behavior (Rushworth and Behrens, 2008). Human fMRI data suggest that the ACC may be involved in determining when to predict outcome based on experience over an extended history, and when to make predictions from recent events (i.e., the ACC assesses volatility in the environment) (Behrens et al., 2007). The ACC has also enjoyed prominence for its putative role in error detection and conflict monitoring (Kerns et al., 2004), both of which would influence reward learning in a broader fashion.

In general, the mPFC has proven difficult to deconstruct because it appears to participate in different roles depending on experimental context and methodology, but one attempt at presenting a unifying model for the mPFC's function posits that the mPFC is essentially an action-outcome predictor (Alexander and Brown, 2011). Neurons here signal predictions for the outcome of an action, and its expected timing, through its firing rate, which is then inhibited by the outcome itself. The strongest signal here is thus observed when the expected outcome does not take place at the expected time; in other words, the ACC might be signaling negative surprise (Alexander and Brown, 2011). This model succeeds at reconciling several seemingly conflicting pieces of data on the mPFC, and places certain aspects of reward learning within the larger context of surprise and predictability.

THE ORBITOFRONTAL CORTEX AND VALUE ESTIMATION

There is near-consensus that the orbitofrontal cortex (OFC) is involved in the representation of decision-value. Data in support of such a role for the OFC in decision-making comes from rat, monkey, and human studies, all of which indicate OFC activation that correlates with behavioral measures of goal values (Wallis, 2007). One school of thought holds that the OFC explicitly signals goal-value (Montague and Berns, 2002), which it computes through its interconnections with the basolateral amygdala and the striatum (Rushworth et al., 2007).

To further appreciate the role of the OFC in reward processing, we need first differentiate between two types of decision-making systems—the rigid model-free system that maintains cached values representing a summary of its decision-value, and the flexible model-based system that computes these decision-values as and when needed from a model of the environment built from experience (Daw et al., 2005). Although dopaminergic activity together with dorsal striatal dopaminergic projections are thought to facilitate model-free learning (Daw et al., 2005), some evidence indicates that the OFC is critical for model-based representation (Schoenbaum et al., 2011). In this view, the OFC is not signaling value per se, but states relevant to reward that may be used to derive value (Schoenbaum et al., 2011). Reminiscent of the previous section on the ACC, the OFC in this framework is involved in processing not just reward, but all events that pertain to the reward, and it does so in a predictive manner (Schoenbaum et al., 2011).

Based on the preceding discussion, the reward system can be seen as a complex piece of computational machinery, with several vulnerable regions wherein the system could become dysregulated. Drug addiction is one such example of how disruptions in reward mechanisms can lead to disastrous consequences.

ADDICTION AND THE REWARD SYSTEM

One reason the mesolimbic dopamine system has attracted so much attention in addiction research is that all drugs of abuse—psychostimulants, opiates, alcohol, nicotine, and cannabinoids—appear to act on this system (Pierce and Kumaresan, 2006). For example, several commonly used drugs of abuse have been shown to enhance synaptic strength at excitatory synapses on midbrain dopaminergic neurons

(Saal et al., 2003). Behavioral investigations in animal models following pharmacological manipulations have revealed that the reinforcing effects of drugs of abuse are mediated at least in part by increased dopamine transmission in the nucleus accumbens (Pierce and Kumaresan, 2006). Although it remains to be determined whether these effects are sufficient to cause drug addiction, altered dopaminergic function may be critical at certain stages of the addiction process.

THE INITIATION . . .

Just as with natural rewards, acute administration of drugs of abuse have been show to activate critical neural elements of the reward circuit (Breiter et al., 1997), and produce subjective feelings of pleasure and well-being. Novelty-seeking, a trait that is one of the best available predictors of drug use, has been shown to be inversely associated with D2-like receptor availability in the midbrain (Zald et al., 2008). Also, PET Imaging studies have revealed a link between D2-like receptor availability and the intensity of the subjective high from and the "liking" (Volkow et al., 2002) of methylphenidate administration. Specifically, lower D2 receptor levels lead to higher drug liking scores, and thus likely facilitate repeated use of the drug.

. . . AND TRANSITION TO COMPULSIVE USE

Along with the putative link between dopamine function and reward liking, there is evidence to suggest a role for extracellular dopamine levels following drug administration and drug wanting (Berridge, 2007). One model of addiction suggests that drug-induced increase in dopamine transmission results in a prediction error signal that cannot be compensated, which in turn leads to an ever-increasing value estimate for the drug with repeated drug administration (Redish, 2004). Everitt and Robbins have suggested that the transition from voluntary drug use to compulsive use is mediated by a shift in control from the prefrontal cortex to the striatum over drug-seeking behavior, with concomitant shifts from ventral to more dorsal striatal control circuits (Everitt and Robbins, 2005).

Concurrent with neural changes in the basal ganglia, impaired prefrontal function may underlie the transition to compulsive drug use. For example, the impaired response inhibition and salience attribution model posits that addiction is a syndrome characterized by attributing increased salience to drugs and drug-related cues, at the expense of other reinforcers, and decreased impulse control (Goldstein and Volkow, 2011). In this model, impaired prefrontal cortex functioning plays a crucial role in some of the cognitive and emotional deficits observed in the disease. Some researchers have focused on the OFC in particular, emphasizing drug (cocaine specifically) induced changes here that result in increased non-flexible or "model-free" drug-seeking behaviors (Lucantonio et al., 2012).

INDIVIDUAL DIFFERENCES IN THE REWARD SYSTEM AND THE RISK FOR ADDICTION

While all drugs of abuse influence the mesolimbic dopaminergic system, and have reinforcing effects, only about 20%

of individuals who experiment with drugs go on to become addicted to them (Odgers et al., 2008). In recent years, addiction models have evolved to accommodate individual differences in susceptibility to drug addiction. For animal models, this has translated into a shift from focusing on passive drug effects, or simply the willingness to self-administer drugs, to satisfying "addiction-life criteria" (Deroche-Gamonet et al., 2004). Through such modified paradigms, it is now appreciated that increased vulnerability to drug addiction may arise, for example, from decreased D2-like receptor function in the striatum (Dalley et al., 2007) or midbrain (Buckholtz et al., 2010) dopaminergic neurons resulting in deficits in impulse control. Relatedly, increased risk for drug addiction could arise from individual differences in the attribution of incentive salience to drug-related cues (Flagel et al., 2010). A recent study suggests that impaired glutamate receptor-mediated plasticity in the prefrontal cortex may also confer risk to future drug addiction (Kasanetz et al., 2012). As mentioned previously, there are differences in the sensitivity to the reinforcing effects of drugs of abuse (Volkow et al., 2002). Because these studies were performed on non-dependent individuals, it is possible that genetically determined receptor levels predispose some individuals to be more sensitive to initial acute drug effects, supporting a gene x environment risk for addiction. These neural differences could play into susceptibility at the initiation phase of drug addiction, but not necessarily toward the transition to compulsive use.

NEGATIVE REINFORCEMENT AND DRUG ADDICTION

In addition to the neural mechanisms underlying positive reinforcement and how they might relate to drug addiction, drug-seeking behavior is also a function of negative reinforcement (Wise, 1988) as best conceptualized by antireward system mechanisms (Koob and Le Moal, 2008). Taking an aspirin for headaches or leaving home early for work to avoid traffic are daily examples of negative reinforcement. Negative reinforcement is at work when an individual is in or anticipates a negatively valued state and acts to terminate this state. The degree to which negative reinforcement controls behavior is determined by the change of frequency of different types of behavior as a function of the negative state. Reinforcers act via brain-related processes in several different ways: (1) activating neural substrates of approach or escape responses, (2) producing rewarding or aversive internal states, and (3) modulating information that has been stored in memory. As reviewed by Baker and colleagues (Baker et al., 2004), addicted individuals are thought to take drugs to escape or avoid aversive states such as withdrawal or stress. Baker has argued that the addicted individual learns to detect the interoceptive cues of the negative feelings that occur whenever drug levels begin to fall in the body, and acts to avoid the negative affect caused by these falling levels. Both interruptions of drug use or the presence of stressors generate a strong negative affective state, which enters consciousness and fosters renewed drug use. Therefore, negative affect is proposed to have the greatest motivational impact on drug use among addicted users, is closely linked to withdrawal symptoms, and fosters learning by means of negative reinforcement. Baker further argues that signs of incipient withdrawal-induced negative affect are detected interoceptively, which subsequently serve as discriminative stimuli for instrumental behaviors. In addition, external stimuli that become associated with such discriminative interoceptive stimuli may function as conditioned stimuli. Therefore, both aversive internal states and conditioned (external) stimuli are important antecedents to non-adaptive behaviors (e.g. compulsive drug use).

EXAMPLES OF NEGATIVE REINFORCEMENT IN DRUG ADDICTION

Several studies provide compelling behavioral evidence for negative reinforcement mechanisms in addictive disorders, for example, in methamphetamine use (Simons et al., 2008) and alcohol consumption (Johnson et al., 2008). Direct evidence for different susceptibility to negative reinforcement has been mixed. Some have reported that increased anxiety sensitivity, a measure of the increased anticipation of aversive events, is a significant predictor of substance abuse (Wagner, 2001). There have been some experimental attempts to examine the effect of drug use on reinforcement and learning behavior. For example, chronic smokers made choices on a learning task that were not guided by error signals derived from counterfactuals (i.e., possible but not actual outcomes) despite ongoing and robust neural activation to these fictive errors (Chiu et al., 2008). Others have found that negative affect in smokers increases selective attention to drug cues and urge to smoke (Bradley et al., 2007). Finally, individuals with ventromedial frontal damage show selectively disrupted ability to learn from negative feedback (Wheeler and Fellows, 2008). However, much needs to be done to specifically link negative reinforcement processes to specific brain regions in drug-addicted individuals.

MODELS OF NEGATIVE REINFORCEMENT AND ADDICTION

Several negative reinforcement models have been proposed for drug addiction. As reviewed by Eissenberg (2004), withdrawal-based negative reinforcement models emphasize that avoidance or suppression of drug withdrawal by drug self-administration increases the likelihood of future drug self-administration. In comparison, classical conditioning models propose that stimuli that predict drug administration are important for the regulation of the internal milieu. Therefore, negative reinforcement may be particularly important for the avoidance of potential withdrawal rather than escape from existing withdrawal. One may even go as far as stating that the degree of drug dependence is related to the strength of the conditioned response (i.e., a stronger conditioned response is evidence for a greater dependence). Similar to Baker (Baker et al., 2004), Eissenberg emphasizes that in addition to exteroceptive cues, interoceptive stimuli (e.g., drug onset cues) may be particularly important in dependence development because these interoceptive cues predict the drug effect

perhaps more reliably than any external drug-associated cues. Self-medication models of drug dependence highlight the role that a drug of abuse might play in helping the user to escape or avoid emotional distress or negative affect that predates the initial drug use episode (Eissenberg, 2004). Importantly, negative affect is thought to not be a consequence of repeated drug use but instead is hypothesized to predate the initial drug use episode. Finally, opponent-process models of drug dependence propose that internal reward processes are set awry by drug use and that drug-induced increases in reward threshold yield compulsive drug self-administration (Solomon, 1980). These models have in common that a proposed interoceptive state is driven out of balance (or stability) and leads to non-adaptive restorative behaviors that are driven by the intent to reduce a negatively valenced state.

DRUG ADDICTION—A DYNAMIC ILLNESS

A central characteristic of addictive behaviors is their chronically relapsing nature (Miller, 1996). Relapse is a complex process and includes multiple dimensions such as the process prior to reuse of the drug, the event of using the drug, the level to which the use returns, and the consequences associated with use. Several models that stress cognitive behavioral, person–situation interactional, cognitive appraisal, and outcome expectation factors have been put forth to explain the process of relapse (Connors et al., 1996). These models differ in the extent to which the focus is on the person (decreased self-efficacy), the situation (exposure to high-risk environments), and/or their interaction (insufficient mobilization of coping skills) (Connors et al., 1996). On the other hand, psychobiological models of relapse have been based on opponent process and acquired motivation theories, craving or loss of control, urges or craving, withdrawal, and kindling processes (Reske and Paulus, 2008). These models focus on the fact that brain reward systems become sensitized to drugs and drug-associated stimuli (Robinson and Berridge, 2000) resulting in increased drug-wanting, which increase the susceptibility to relapse. Some investigators have suggested that relapse is best understood as having multiple and interactive determinants that vary in their temporal proximity from and their relative influence on relapse. Therefore, an adequate assessment and prediction model must be sufficiently comprehensive to include theoretically relevant variables from each of the multiple domains and different levels of potential predictors (Connors et al., 1996). Others have pointed out that relapse is not a binary but a continuous outcome across multiple dimensions (Miller, 1996), which include the threshold, duration, prior sobriety level, number of substances involved, and consequences. Moreover, relapse encompasses a multidimensional response pattern with (1) the occurrence of negative life events; (2) cognitive appraisal variables including self-efficacy, expectancies, and motivation for change; (3) subject coping resources; (4) craving (Bechara and Van der Linden, 2005) experiences; and (5) affective/mood status (Miller, 1996).

Some investigators have suggested that aberrant learning processes within subcortical circuitry underlie aspects of observations that: (*1*) drug-seeking behavior becomes compulsive and habitual and (*2*) propensity for relapse to drug-seeking can be manifest even after long periods of sobriety (Everitt et al., 2001). Others have suggested that substance use disorders are consequences of imbalances between overactive "impulsive" amygdala systems, which signal pain or pleasure of immediate prospect, and weakened "reflective" prefrontal cortex system for signaling pain or pleasure of future prospect (Bechara, 2005). In particular, drugs and/or conditioned stimuli associated with the availability of drugs are thought to overwhelm the goal-driven cognitive resources important for exercising the willpower to resist drugs. Finally, some have argued that substance dependence is characterized by an overvaluing of drug reinforcers associated with an undervaluing of alternative reinforcers in combination with deficits in inhibitory control (Goldstein and Volkow, 2011). Based on animal experiments, Koob and LeMoal have conceptualized substance dependence or addiction as a cycle of increasing dysregulation of brain reward systems, which leads to compulsive drug use and a loss of control over drug taking. Both, sensitization and counter-adaptation processes contribute to this hedonic homeostatic dysregulation. The neurobiological mechanisms involved include the mesolimbic dopamine system, opioid peptidergic systems, and brain and hormonal stress systems (Koob and Le Moal, 2008). Based on these views, it is clear that brain processes that are candidates for monitoring clinical states involve learning, drug and conditioned cue-related processing, homeostatic regulation, inhibition, and decision making.

NEGATIVE REINFORCEMENT AND THE DYNAMIC STATE OF ADDICTION

Koob and colleagues (for a recent review, see Koob and Le Moal, 2008) have pointed out that negative reinforcement may be one of the key processes that leads to the transition from impulsive to compulsive drug use, which results in an addiction cycle that is comprised of three stages: (*1*) preoccupation and anticipation (of drug taking), (*2*) binge and/or intoxication (of the drug), and (*3*) withdrawal or negative affect (as a consequence of lack of drug). They propose a cycle of increasing dysregulation of brain reward/anti-reward mechanisms and suggest that whereas the positive reinforcement system is driven mainly by dopaminergic mechanisms, negative reinforcement systems may rely on the stress response, which is closely linked to the cortisol and corticotropin releasing hormone system. Finally, an allostatic state (i.e., an unstable set point) emerges because of the loss of function in the reward systems and recruitment of the brain stress or anti-reward systems. The opponent process model and its adaptation to drug addiction is not unlike the proposal by Baker and colleagues (Baker et al., 2004) of two types of urge networks: a positive-affect network, which is activated associatively and nonassociatively by appetitive stimuli; and a negative-affect network, which is activated associatively and nonassociatively by non-appetitive stimuli or consequences (e.g., punishment, signals of punishment, frustrating lack of reward), and by withdrawal and signals of withdrawal. Sinha and colleagues have reported that stress is closely linked to craving, drug-taking behavior, and relapse

(Sinha et al., 2011). These authors have conceptualized stress as internal and external events or stimuli that exert demands or load on the organism and demand mounting of adaptive resources in response to stressors. Brain regions such as the amygdala, hippocampus, insula, and orbitofrontal, medial prefrontal, and cingulate cortices are involved in the perception and appraisal of emotional and stressful stimuli (Sinha et al., 2011). The interplay among reward and anti-reward, appetitive, and aversive systems, with many of the characteristics of the interoceptive system, supports the idea that drug addiction is a dynamically dysregulated homeostatic disease.

WHAT CAN NEUROIMAGING TELL US ABOUT RISK, PREVENTION, AND TREATMENT OF ADDICTION?

In the following we describe some recent and ongoing efforts to apply what we have learned about addiction to improving treatment outcome and in preventing future substance dependence in current users.

A NEURAL MEASURE OF ADDICTION SEVERITY

Not all addicts are created equal; overall about 40–60% of addicted individuals undergoing treatment relapse within a year following discharge from treatment (McLellan, 2002); in the case of nicotine addiction, the recidivism rate can reach 95% (Cigarette smoking among adults—United States, 2000). One of the best predictors of response to treatment for cigarette smokers is the Fagerström Test for Nicotine Dependence (FTND). Functional magnetic resonance imaging is well-positioned to provide a neural predictor of treatment outcome because it provides a quick, non-invasive measure of anatomical integrity and neural function at a system level in humans. For example, functional connectivity strength (as measured through temporal correlations in the blood oxygen level-dependent (BOLD) fMRI signal between brain regions in the absence of task performance) of a dorsal ACC-ventral striatum circuit correlates with FTND scores in smokers and is not modified in the presence of a nicotine patch, used routinely (but generally unsuccessfully) in smoking cessation programs (Fig. 55.2*A*; Hong et al., 2009). Critically, this feature is related to a single nucleotide polymorphism in the cholinergic gene encoding the α5 subunit—CHRNA5 (Hong et al., 2010), and underscores the need to better understand the role of regions that express α5-rich nicotinic receptors (e.g., the habenula) in nicotine addiction (De Biasi and Dani, 2011). In general, the identification of such neural correlates of severity of addiction may allow investigation of the neurobiological changes that are required for recovery from addiction, and to tailor treatment interventions accordingly.

TREATMENT-CENTERED APPROACHES

Recovery from addiction is typically assessed through duration of complete abstinence from drug use (e.g. clean urine tests), and many forms of addiction-treatment are labeled

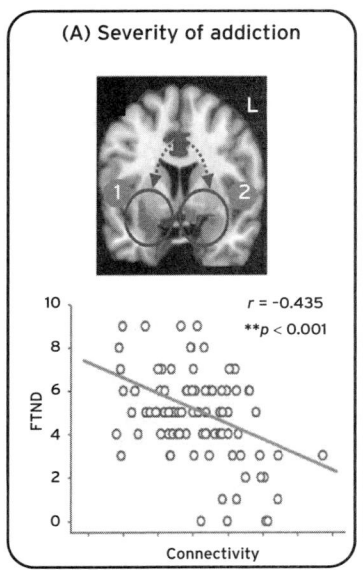

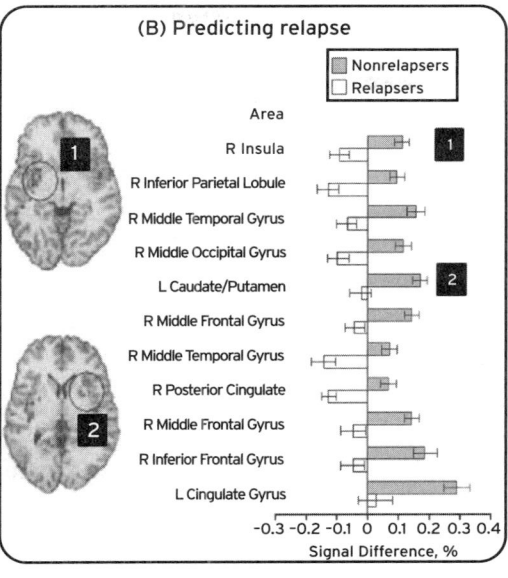

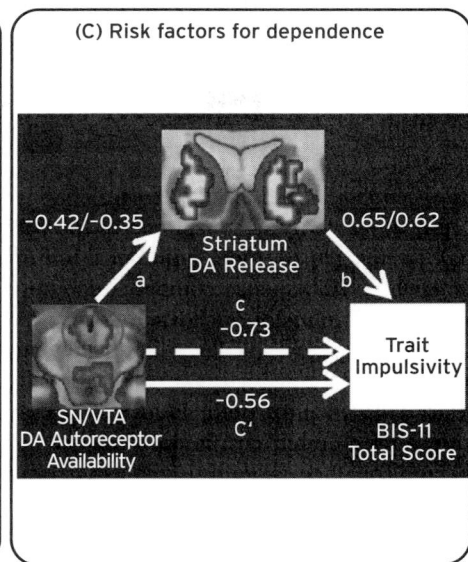

Figure 55.2 *Examples of how neuroimaging may aid addiction research. (A) Uncovering the neural mechanisms determining the severity of addiction—resting state functional connectivity in dorsal ACC-striatal circuits (upper panel) is inversely correlated with severity of nicotine addiction as assayed through the Fagerstrom Test for Nicotine Dependence or FTND. (B) Identifying neural biomarkers for predicting relapse in substance-dependent individuals—fMRI activation patterns in regions including the insula (1) and striatum (2) during a binary forced choice task predicts relapse in methamphetamine-dependent individuals. (C) Identifying neural risk factors for future substance dependence—midbrain D2 receptor availability, measured through PET, is linked to trait impulsivity, likely via increased stimulated dopamine release in the striatum. (A from Hong et al., 2010. B from Paulus et al., 2005. C from Buckholtz et al., 2010.)*

as unsuccessful based on relapse rates within 6–12 months following discharge (McLellan, 2002). But some have questioned this approach and suggested moving toward a model similar to other chronic diseases, such as diabetes, that report similar relapse rates following treatment cessation. In this framework, the success of an intervention would rest on the frequency and severity of addiction-related symptoms and the patient's ability to resume a functional life under an extended treatment plan and not complete abstinence (McLellan, 2002). To extend the chronic disease analogy, recovery from addiction might then better be assayed through intermittent or continuous monitoring of biomarkers—by measuring the addiction equivalent of blood sugar levels. Currently, no reliable neural markers of recovery from addiction exist, but non-invasive neuroimaging methods and behavioral tests could be designed to serve this purpose. As a step in this direction, fMRI activation in the insula, posterior cingulate, and temporal cortex during a simple two-choice prediction task has been shown to predict relapse in methamphetamine-dependent individuals (Fig. 55.2B; Paulus et al., 2005). More recently, an fMRI based cue-reactivity signal has been proposed as a potential signature of relapse vulnerability (Janes et al., 2010).

Similarly, some treatments for addiction might be deemed unsuccessful if only a subset of patients benefit from them; this outcome too needs further consideration, as multiple treatment approaches matched to individual endophenotypes (i.e., personalized medicine) may lead to overall better outcomes. If so, the need appears to be better assessment tools of individual differences that merit differential treatment intervention, and to carry out prescription accordingly. The FTND, for example, predicts which patients stand to benefit from faster delivery

nicotine replacement medications (Stapleton and Sutherland, 2011), and pretreatment rate of nicotine metabolism, as measured by a nicotine metabolite ratio, can predict the efficacy of nicotine replacement therapy (Lerman et al., 2006). Again, a more detailed understanding of the neural underpinnings to these pretreatment differences—through neuroimaging, genetics, and behavioral metrics—may allow for customized and possibly more efficacious treatment plans. For example, fMRI activation in the insula, posterior cingulate, and temporal cortex during a simple two-choice prediction task has been shown to predict relapse in methamphetamine-dependent individuals. For example, reaction time performance in a simple social stressor task can predict how nicotine or varenicline (Chantix) modulates amygdalar reactivity, and both brain and behavioral responses identify different subgroups of smokers and differentiate them from non-smokers (Sutherland et al., 2013). A similar approach might benefit our understanding of another promising addiction-treatment—the GABA receptor agonist, Baclofen (Franklin et al., 2009).

Aside from providing tools for monitoring efficacy of treatment, fMRI could potentially offer a line of treatment itself. Real-time fMRI, which involves providing patients with immediate feedback of their BOLD activity, has shown potential in the treatment of pain. This technique could potentially be harnessed for alleviating symptoms (e.g., craving), or to ameliorate addiction-related cognitive deficits (e.g., impulse control), and could be used in conjunction with behavioral therapy to enhance treatment efficacy. However the available data using real time feedback is still extremely preliminary. Nevertheless, efforts to apply real-time fMRI to treatment of addiction have commenced (Childress et al., 2010), and this technique remains a promising new tool in the field.

IDENTIFYING RISK FOR FUTURE SUBSTANCE DEPENDENCE

As alluded to previously, the risk for substance dependence is not equal in all individuals—about one in five individuals who experiment with drugs go on to become dependent (Odgers et al., 2008). Major inroads would be made to understand addiction through better understanding of the variability in the transition from drug use to dependence. For one, it may help in the development of individualized, customized treatment of addiction. Second, a better understanding of addiction vulnerability may assist in guiding early treatment interventions. Third, identifying individuals who are at increased risk for future substance abuse would be a first step towards improved preventative measures. Finally, how certain life experiences could serve as protective factors against future substance dependence in the face of increased susceptibility could be approached.

At present, the most promising avenue for research on vulnerability to addiction is trait impulsivity, which is generally considered a core component of substance use disorders. In rats, deficits in impulse control have been shown to predict the transition from repeated use to stimulant dependence (Belin et al., 2008). Human and animal studies have pointed to a link between impulse control and D2-like receptor function in the ventral striatum and midbrain (Belin et al., 2008; Buckholtz et al., 2010; Fig. 55.2C), and low D2/D3 receptor function may drive a predisposition to stimulant dependence (Belin et al., 2008). More recently, a study employed diffusion tensor imaging in siblings of substance-dependent individuals, who presumably carry some genetic risk for addiction, found differences in white matter tract integrity in frontal areas that correlated with behavioral impulsivity measures (Ersche et al., 2012). Genetic and neuroimaging approaches to understanding other addiction-related traits such as novelty seeking (Zald et al., 2008) are progressing, and suggest a promising new direction for addiction research.

RESHAPING ADDICTION RESEARCH

Much has been uncovered regarding the neural mechanisms underlying the learning and representation of reward in the brain, but the precise roles of various components of the reward circuit remain poorly understood. Addiction research, in particular, may benefit from shifting the spotlight from dopamine-centered processing to less traditional members of the circuitry underlying positive and negative reinforcement, such as the insula, habenula, and orbitofrontal cortex. Also, a more comprehensive understanding of the interactions between these nodes is needed, especially in the context of addiction. Neuroimaging offers a valuable tool in this regard by allowing functional connectivity between multiple regions simultaneously, even in the absence of cognitive tasks. This functionality may prove especially useful for uncovering the complex interactions between reward and anti-reward systems. Finally, a recurring recent theme in addiction research is the appreciation of individual differences, especially in terms of vulnerability to addiction, reactivity to acute drug administration, and response to treatments. A continued appreciation of these individual differences may go a long way toward achieving breakthroughs in the field.

DISCLOSURES

Drs. Stein and Pariyadath have no conflicts of interest to disclose. They are funded entirely by the NIDA-IRP.

Dr. Paulus has no conflicts of interest to disclose. Grant Support: This work was supported by grants from the Veterans Administration and the National Institute on Drug Abuse (R01-DA016663, P20-DA027834, R01-DA027797, and R01-DA018307 to Martin Paulus).

REFERENCES

Alexander, G.E., DeLong, M.R., et al. (1986). Parallel organization of functionally segregated circuits linking basal ganglia and cortex. *Annu. Rev. Neurosci.* 9:357–381.

Alexander, W.H., and Brown, J.W. (2011). Medial prefrontal cortex as an action-outcome predictor. *Nat. Neurosci.* 14:1338–1344.

Baker, T.B., Piper, M.E., et al. (2004). Addiction motivation reformulated: an affective processing model of negative reinforcement. *Psychol. Rev.* 111:33–51.

Bechara, A. (2005). Decision making, impulse control and loss of willpower to resist drugs: a neurocognitive perspective. *Nat. Neurosci.* 8:1458–1463.

Bechara, A., and Van der Linden, M. (2005). Decision-making and impulse control after frontal lobe injuries. *Curr. Opin. Neurol.* 18:734–739.

Behrens, T.E., Woolrich, M.W., et al. (2007). Learning the value of information in an uncertain world. *Nat. Neurosci.* 10:1214–1221.

Belin, D., Mar, A., et al. (2008). High impulsivity predicts the switch to compulsive cocaine-taking. *Science* 320:1352–1355.

Berridge, K.C. (2007). The debate over dopamine's role in reward: the case for incentive salience. *Psychopharmacology (Berl.)* 191:391–431.

Berridge, K.C., and Robinson, T.E. (2003). Parsing reward. *Trends Neurosci.* 26:507–513.

Bradley, B.P., Garner, M., et al. (2007). Influence of negative affect on selective attention to smoking-related cues and urge to smoke in cigarette smokers. *Behav. Pharmacol.* 18:255–263.

Breiter, H.C., Gollub, R.L., et al. (1997). Acute effects of cocaine on human brain activity and emotion. *Neuron* 19:591–611.

Buckholtz, J., Treadway, M., et al. (2010). Dopaminergic network differences in human impulsivity. *Science* 329:532.

Childress, A.R., Magland, J.F., et al. (2010). Rapid Control of a Screen Cursor by Thought: A Whole-Brain Classifier for Real-Time fMRI Feedback Training of Cognitive Control. San Diego, CA: Society for Neuroscience.

Chiu, P.H., Lohrenz, T.M., et al. (2008). Smokers' brains compute, but ignore, a fictive error signal in a sequential investment task. *Nat. Neurosci.* 11:514–520.

Cohen, J.Y., Haesler, S., et al. (2012). Neuron-type-specific signals for reward and punishment in the ventral tegmental area. *Nature* 482:85–88.

Connors, G.J., Maisto, S.A., et al. (1996). Conceptualizations of relapse: a summary of psychological and psychobiological models. *Addiction* 91(Suppl):S5–13.

Cools, R., Nakamura, K., et al. (2011). Serotonin and dopamine: unifying affective, activational, and decision functions. *Neuropsychopharmacology* 36:98–113.

Craig, A.D. (2002). How do you feel? Interoception: the sense of the physiological condition of the body. *Nat. Rev. Neurosci.* 3:655–666.

Daw, N.D., Niv, Y., et al. (2005). Uncertainty-based competition between prefrontal and dorsolateral striatal systems for behavioral control. *Nat. Neurosci.* 8:1704–1711.

De Biasi, M., and Dani, J.A. (2011). Reward, addiction, withdrawal to nicotine. *Annu. Rev. Neurosci.* 34:105–130.

De Mei, C., Ramos, M., et al. (2009). Getting specialized: presynaptic and postsynaptic dopamine D2 receptors. *Curr. Opin. Pharmacol.* 9:53–58.

Deroche-Gamonet, V., Belin, D., et al. (2004). Evidence for addiction-like behavior in the rat. *Science* 305:1014–1017.

Eissenberg, T. (2004). Measuring the emergence of tobacco dependence: the contribution of negative reinforcement models. *Addiction* 99(Suppl 1):5–29.

Ersche, K.D., Jones, P.S., et al. (2012). Abnormal brain structure implicated in stimulant drug addiction. *Science* 335:601–604.

Everitt, B.J., Dickinson, A., et al. (2001). The neuropsychological basis of addictive behaviour. *Brain Res. Brain Res. Rev.* 36:129–138.

Everitt, B.J., and Robbins, T.W. (2005). Neural systems of reinforcement for drug addiction: from actions to habits to compulsion. *Nat. Neurosci.* 8:1481–1489.

Flagel, S.B., Robinson, T.E., et al. (2010). An animal model of genetic vulnerability to behavioral disinhibition and responsiveness to reward-related cues: implications for addiction. *Neuropsychopharmacology* 35:388–400.

Franklin, T.R., Harper, D., et al. (2009). The GABA B agonist baclofen reduces cigarette consumption in a preliminary double-blind placebo-controlled smoking reduction study. *Drug Alcohol Depend.* 103:30–36.

Goldstein, R.Z., and Volkow, N.D. (2011). Dysfunction of the prefrontal cortex in addiction: neuroimaging findings and clinical implications. *Nat. Rev. Neurosci.* 12:652–669.

Haber, S.N., and Knutson, B. (2010). The reward circuit: linking primate anatomy and human imaging. *Neuropsychopharmacology* 35:4–26.

Hampton, A.N., Adolphs, R., et al. (2007). Contributions of the amygdala to reward expectancy and choice signals in human prefrontal cortex. *Neuron* 55:545–555.

Hayden, B.Y., Pearson, J.M., et al. (2009). Fictive reward signals in the anterior cingulate cortex. *Science* 324:948–950.

Hong, L.E., Gu, H., et al. (2009). Association of nicotine addiction and nicotine's actions with separate cingulate cortex functional circuits. *Arch. Gen. Psychiatry* 66:431–441.

Hong, L.E., Hodgkinson, C.A., et al. (2010). A genetically modulated, intrinsic cingulate circuit supports human nicotine addiction. *Proc. Natl. Acad. Sci. USA* 107:13509–13514.

Hoyer, D., Hannon, J.P., et al. (2002). Molecular, pharmacological and functional diversity of 5-HT receptors. *Pharmacol. Biochem. Behav.* 71:533–554.

Ikemoto, S. (2010). Brain reward circuitry beyond the mesolimbic dopamine system: a neurobiological theory. *Neurosci. Biobehav. Rev.* 35:129–150.

Janes, A.C., Pizzagalli, D.A., et al. (2010). Brain reactivity to smoking cues prior to smoking cessation predicts ability to maintain tobacco abstinence. *Biol. Psychiatry* 67:722–729.

Jhou, T.C., Geisler, S., et al. (2009). The mesopontine rostromedial tegmental nucleus: a structure targeted by the lateral habenula that projects to the ventral tegmental area of Tsai and substantia nigra compacta. *J. Comp. Neurol.* 513:566–596.

Ji, H., and Shepard, P.D. (2007). Lateral habenula stimulation inhibits rat midbrain dopamine neurons through a GABA(A) receptor-mediated mechanism. *J. Neurosci.* 27:6923–6930.

Johnson, K.A., Zvolensky, M.J., et al. (2008). Linkages between cigarette smoking outcome expectancies and negative emotional vulnerability. *Addict. Behav.* 33:1416–1424.

Kasanetz, F., Lafourcade, M., et al. (2012). Prefrontal synaptic markers of cocaine addiction-like behavior in rats. *Mol. Psychiatry.* [Epub ahead of print.]

Kerns, J.G., Cohen, J.D., et al. (2004). Anterior cingulate conflict monitoring and adjustments in control. *Science* 303:1023–1026.

Koob, G.F., and Le Moal, M. (2008). Review. Neurobiological mechanisms for opponent motivational processes in addiction. *Philos. Trans. R. Soc. Lond. B Biol. Sci.* 363:3113–3123.

LeDoux, J. (2007). The amygdala. *Curr. Biol.* 17:R868–874.

Lerman, C., Tyndale, R., et al. (2006). Nicotine metabolite ratio predicts efficacy of transdermal nicotine for smoking cessation. *Clin. Pharmacol. Ther.* 79:600–608.

Li, J., Schiller, D., et al. (2011). Differential roles of human striatum and amygdala in associative learning. *Nat. Neurosci.* 14:1250–1252.

Lucantonio, F., Stalnaker, T.A., et al. (2012). The impact of orbitofrontal dysfunction on cocaine addiction. *Nat. Neurosci.* 15:358–366.

Matsumoto, M., and Hikosaka, O. (2007). Lateral habenula as a source of negative reward signals in dopamine neurons. *Nature* 447:1111–1115.

Matsumoto, M., Matsumoto, K., et al. (2007). Medial prefrontal cell activity signaling prediction errors of action values. *Nat. Neurosci.* 10:647–656.

Matsumoto, K., Suzuki, W., et al. (2003). Neuronal correlates of goal-based motor selection in the prefrontal cortex. *Science* 301:229–232.

McLellan, A.T. (2002). Have we evaluated addiction treatment correctly? Implications from a chronic care perspective. *Addiction* 97:249–252.

Miller, W.R. (1996). What is a relapse? Fifty ways to leave the wagon. *Addiction* 91(Suppl):S15–S27.

Montague, P.R., and Berns, G.S. (2002). Neural economics and the biological substrates of valuation. *Neuron* 36:265–284.

Murray, E.A. (2007). The amygdala, reward and emotion. *Trends Cogn. Sci.* 11:489–497.

National Institute on Drug Abuse. (2011). Drug Facts: Understanding Drug Abuse and Addiction. http://www.drugabuse.gov/publications/drugfacts/understanding-drug-abuse-addiction

Niv, Y., Duff, M.O., et al. (2005). Dopamine, uncertainty and TD learning. *Behav. Brain Funct.* 1:6.

Odgers, C., Caspi, A., et al. (2008). Is it important to prevent early exposure to drugs and alcohol among adolescents? *Psychol. Sci.* 19:1037–1044.

Olds, J., and Milner, P. (1954). Positive reinforcement produced by electrical stimulation of septal area and other regions of rat brain. *J. Comp. Physiol. Psychol.* 47:419–427.

Parker, J.G., Wanat, M.J., et al. (2011). Attenuating GABA(A) receptor signaling in dopamine neurons selectively enhances reward learning and alters risk preference in mice. *J. Neurosci.* 31:17103–17112.

Paulus, M.P., Tapert, S.F., et al. (2005). Neural activation patterns of methamphetamine-dependent subjects during decision making predict relapse. *Arch. Gen. Psychiatry* 62:761–768.

Pearce, J.M., and Hall, G. (1980). A model for Pavlovian learning: variations in the effectiveness of conditioned but not of unconditioned stimuli. *Psychol. Rev.* 87:532–552.

Pierce, R.C., and Kumaresan, V. (2006). The mesolimbic dopamine system: the final common pathway for the reinforcing effect of drugs of abuse? *Neurosci. Biobehav. Rev.* 30:215–238.

Redish, A. (2004). Addiction as a computational process gone awry. *Science* 306:1944–1947.

Reske, M., and Paulus, M.P. (2008). Predicting treatment outcome in stimulant dependence. *Ann. NY Acad. Sci.* 1141:270–283.

Robinson, T.E., and Berridge, K.C. (2000). The psychology and neurobiology of addiction: an incentive-sensitization view. *Addiction* 95 (Suppl 2):S91–117.

Roesch, M.R., Calu, D.J., et al. (2010). Neural correlates of variations in event processing during learning in basolateral amygdala. *J. Neurosci.* 30:2464–2471.

Rushworth, M.F., and Behrens, T.E. (2008). Choice, uncertainty and value in prefrontal and cingulate cortex. *Nat. Neurosci.* 11:389–397.

Rushworth, M.F., Behrens, T.E., et al. (2007). Contrasting roles for cingulate and orbitofrontal cortex in decisions and social behaviour. *Trends Cogn. Sci.* 11:168–176.

Saal, D., Dong, Y., et al. (2003). Drugs of abuse and stress trigger a common synaptic adaptation in dopamine neurons. *Neuron* 37:577–582.

Schoenbaum, G., Takahashi, Y., et al. (2011). Does the orbitofrontal cortex signal value? *Ann. NY Acad. Sci.* 1239:87–99.

Schultz, W., Dayan, P., et al. (1997). A neural substrate of prediction and reward. *Science* 275:1593–1599.

Simons, J.S., Dvorak, R.D., et al. (2008). Methamphetamine use in a rural college population: associations with marijuana use, sensitivity to punishment, and sensitivity to reward. *Psychol. Addict. Behav.* 22:444–449.

Sinha, R., Shaham, Y., et al. (2011). Translational and reverse translational research on the role of stress in drug craving and relapse. *Psychopharmacology (Berl.)* 218:69–82.

Solomon, R.L. (1980). The opponent-process theory of acquired motivation: the costs of pleasure and the benefits of pain. *Am. Psychol.* 35:691–712.

Stapleton, J.A., and Sutherland, G. (2011). Treating heavy smokers in primary care with the nicotine nasal spray: randomized placebo-controlled trial. *Addiction* 106:824–832.

Steiner, J.E., Glaser, D., et al. (2001). Comparative expression of hedonic impact: affective reactions to taste by human infants and other primates. *Neurosci. Biobehav. Rev.* 25:53–74.

Sutherland, M.T., Carroll, A.J., et al. (2013). Down-regulation of amygdala and insula functional circuits by varenicline and nicotine in abstinent cigarette smokers. *Biol. Psychiatry* S0006-3223(13)00137-6.

Taber, M.T., and Fibiger, H.C. (1995). Electrical stimulation of the prefrontal cortex increases dopamine release in the nucleus accumbens of the rat: modulation by metabotropic glutamate receptors. *J. Neurosci.* 15:3896–3904.

Volkow, N.D., Wang, G.J., et al. (2002). Brain DA D2 receptors predict reinforcing effects of stimulants in humans: replication study. *Synapse* 46:79–82.

Wagner, M.K. (2001). Behavioral characteristics related to substance abuse and risk-taking, sensation-seeking, anxiety sensitivity, and self-reinforcement. *Addict. Behav.* 26:115–120.

Wallis, J.D. (2007). Orbitofrontal cortex and its contribution to decision-making. *Annu. Rev. Neurosci.* 30:31–56.

Wang, M., Wong, A.H., et al. (2012). Interactions between NMDA and dopamine receptors: a potential therapeutic target. *Brain Res.* 1476:154–163.

Wheeler, E.Z., and Fellows, L.K. (2008). The human ventromedial frontal lobe is critical for learning from negative feedback. *Brain* 131:1323–1331.

Williams, S.M., and Goldman-Rakic, P.S. (1993). Characterization of the dopaminergic innervation of the primate frontal cortex using a dopamine-specific antibody. *Cereb. Cortex* 3:199–222.

Wise, R.A. (1988). The neurobiology of craving: implications for the understanding and treatment of addiction. *J. Abnorm. Psychol.* 97:118–132.

Wise, R.A. (2008). Dopamine and reward: the anhedonia hypothesis 30 years on. *Neurotox. Res.* 14:169–183.

Zald, D.H., Cowan, R.L., et al. (2008). Midbrain dopamine receptor availability is inversely associated with novelty-seeking traits in humans. *J. Neurosci.* 28:14372–14378.

56 | MAGNETIC RESONANCE SPECTROSCOPY STUDIES IN SUBSTANCE ABUSERS

LINDA CHANG, CHRISTINE C. CLOAK, AND JOHN L. HOLT

Magnetic resonance spectroscopy (MRS) is a quantitative technique that has been used in chemistry laboratories to identify chemical structures since the 1950s. More recently, MRS has become a useful imaging modality that can be applied both *in vivo* noninvasively and ex vivo in tissue extracts. Therefore, MRS is particularly useful as a clinical translational tool for evaluations and longitudinal monitoring of brain abnormalities associated with various brain disorders, including addiction to drugs. When performed *in vivo*, MRS can be performed in a select voxel (or volume of interest), which is typically referred to as localized or single voxel MRS, or across a grid of voxels in a slice to form an image of the metabolite of interest as in MRS imaging (MRSI) (Fig. 56.1). More advanced techniques also allow multiple slices of metabolite maps to be obtained with MRSI, so that a larger portion of the brain can be assessed.

Although the overwhelming majority of MRS studies in brain disorders focus on the proton (^{1}H) resonances associated with various brain metabolites and chemicals, resonances from other atomic nuclei also can be measured with MRS. Molecules with other nuclei include many that are relevant to neurobiology and neuropharmacology (e.g., lithium [^{7}Li], carbon [^{13}C], fluorine [^{19}F], sodium [^{23}Na], and phosphorus [^{31}P]). Owing to the requirement of specialized MRS equipment (e.g., specific coils), costs, and limited expertise, however, only few studies have employed the other nuclei, specifically ^{31}P MRS or ^{13}C MRS, to study brain abnormalities associated with drug abuse. We will discuss these MRS studies and how they can provide additional insights into the neuropathophysiology associated with major categories of drugs abused. At the end of the chapter, we will also compare and contrast how the brain may be affected by these different types of drugs, and some technical issues to be considered in the use of MRS to assess brain changes and to monitor treatment effects.

BRAIN METABOLITES MEASURED WITH MAGNETIC RESONANCE SPECTROSCOPY

Proton MRS can measure several major brain metabolites (see Fig. 56.1). The concentrations of these metabolites represent neuronal or glial cellular density or health, and hence are useful for assessing possible brain alterations associated with drug exposure or abuse. The metabolites observable with MRS are different from those measured in most other neurochemical assays. Specifically, ^{1}H-MRS detects proton resonances from metabolites that are found in large (millimolar) quantities, whereas most of the neurochemicals measured in basic science research laboratories are in much smaller quantities (e.g., less than micromolar concentrations). Typical brain metabolites observed include N-acetylaspartate (NAA) at 2.02 ppm, glutamate (Glu) at 2.1–2.5 ppm with overlapping resonances from glutamine (Gln) and gamma amino butyric acid (GABA), total creatine (tCR) at 3.03 and 3.94 ppm, choline-containing compounds (Cho) at 3.2 ppm, myoinositol (MI) at 3.56 ppm, and less often lactate (Lac) at 1.35 ppm.

NAA is a putative neuronal marker, because it is found primarily in mature neurons and is reduced in conditions of neuronal damage or loss (Birken and Oldendorf, 1989). NAA is localized primarily in the neuronal cytosol and is the second most abundant amino acid in the brain. Although NAA is not known to have specific neurophysiological properties, it serves as an acetyl donor, an initiator of protein synthesis or a carbon transfer source across the mitochondrial membrane (Tsai and Coyle, 1995). Therefore, lower NAA has been reported in brain disorders that are associated with neuronal injury or mitochondrial dysfunction. Lower than normal brain NAA levels were reported in hypoxia, cerebral infarction, head trauma, dementias, chronic HIV infection, neurodegenerative disorders, and some individuals with substance abuse (Schuff et al., 2006) as described in the following.

Glu is an amino acid involved in the tricarboxylic acid cycle and is the major excitatory neurotransmitter in the CNS. Since the majority of the neurons in the brain are glutamatergic, Glu levels typically correlate well with NAA levels on MRS. Excess amounts of Glu in the extracellular spaces have been associated with neurotoxicity and cell death (McDonald and Johnston, 1990; Plaitakis and Shashidharan, 2000). However, Glu levels measured on MRS typically represent the neuronal cytosolic Glu pool, which is much larger than the extracellular pool. The proton resonances from Glu overlaps with those of glutamine and GABA, forming an overlapping range of resonances often reported as Glx; therefore, specialized MRS techniques are often required to measure Glu. These techniques include two-dimensional MRS or echo time (TE)-averaged point resolved spectroscopy (PRESS). The proton resonances from Glu are readily observed with shorter echo times (<50 ms) on MRS, which is more easily performed with localized MRS, rather than MRSI.

GABA, which is derived from Glu, is the predominant inhibitory neurotransmitter in the CNS and is often altered

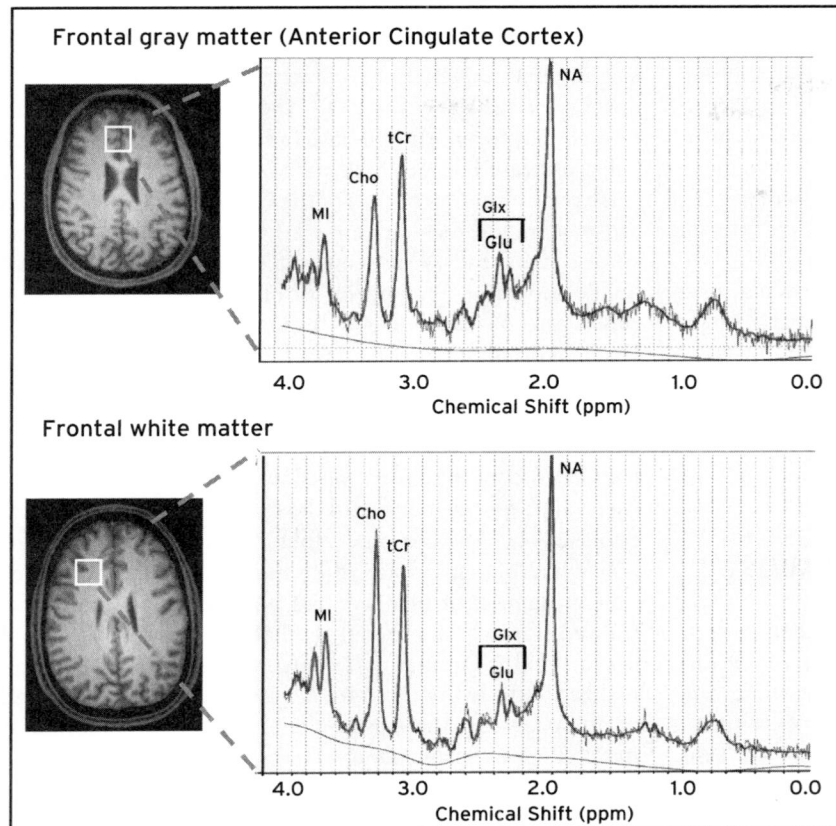

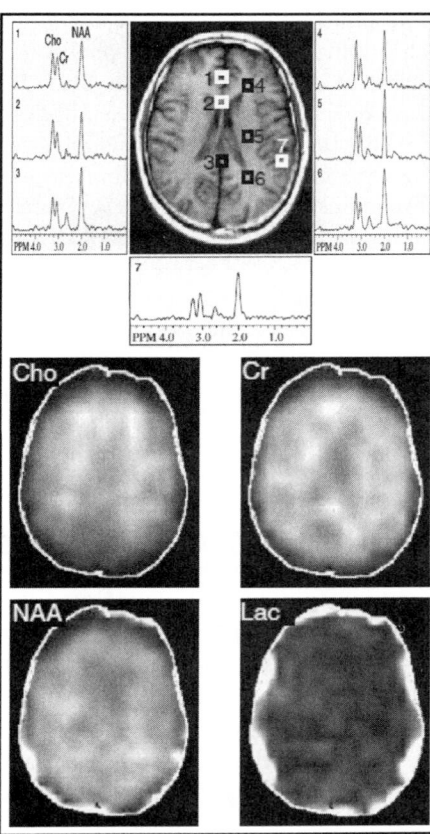

Figure 56.1 Left: Localized MR spectroscopy from a 40-year-old healthy man, showing voxel locations in the frontal gray matter (top) and frontal white matter (bottom) and the corresponding MR spectra with the major brain metabolite levels from these brain regions. Note higher N-acetyl compounds (NA) levels in the frontal gray matter, but higher choline (Cho) levels in the frontal white matter. Right: 2D MRSI data showing regional variability of metabolite concentrations in the different spectra (top) and spectroscopic images of choline-containing compounds (Cho); creatine (Cr); NA, which includes N-acetylaspartate (NAA); and lactate (Lac) across the brain slice (bottom). (Right panel is modified from Barker P.B., Lin D.D. (2006). In vivo proton MR spectroscopy of the human brain. Prog Nucl Mag Res Sp 49:99–128; permission to use obtained from Dr. Peter Barker and from Elsevier.)

in psychiatric or neurological disorders (Chang et al., 2003). Specialized editing techniques (e.g., J-resolved spectroscopy or MEGA-PRESS) are also needed to subtract out the much larger overlapping resonances from the total creatine resonances (at 3.0 ppm) or from Glx (~1.9 ppm) in order to detect the very small GABA resonances. Therefore, very few studies have been performed to evaluate GABA levels in substance-dependent individuals.

The Cho peak on MRS comprises the water-soluble choline-containing compounds, mainly free choline, phosphocholine, and glycerophosphocholine. These compounds are found in the pathways of synthesis and breakdown of choline-containing phospholipids; therefore, Cho is often increased in conditions associated with increased cell membrane turnover and breakdown, such as neoplasms, demyelinating conditions (e.g., multiple sclerosis), cerebral infarction, and even in neuroinflammatory or neuroinfectious conditions (e.g., infections with HIV or JCV). Cho is also found to be three times higher in glia than in neurons (Brand et al., 1993). Therefore, in conditions that glial activation are prominent, such as in psychostimulant users, Cho may be elevated as well.

MI is an organic osmolyte and a putative glial marker (Ross et al., 1992). *In vitro* studies showed that MI is present in high levels in glia, particularly astrocytes, but lower levels are found in neuronal cells (Brand et al., 1993). Therefore, gliosis, with reactive glial proliferation including microglia, during brain degeneration or neuroinflammation, might lead to increased MI concentrations, often along with increased Cho and tCR. MI also is involved in plasma membrane metabolism and is enzymatically converted to inositol triphosphate (IP_3), an important intracellular second messenger (Worley et al., 1987). A defect or interference of this pathway also might result in a change in the MI concentration. Elevated MI levels have been noted in brain injury, infections, and degeneration (Mader et al., 2008). However, the proton resonances from MI are not visible on MRS studies performed with long echo-times (>100 ms). Therefore, short-echo time MRS studies are preferable in most instances and are more easily performed with localized MRS than with MRSI.

The proton resonance for tCR (at 3.0 ppm) includes free creatine and phosphocreatine, which likely reflects high-energy phosphate metabolism because phosphocreatine is involved in adenosine triphosphate (ATP) synthesis (Miller, 1991). tCR is often used as a reference metabolite in MRS studies because it was once thought to be relatively constant even in disease states; however, changes in tCR levels have been reported in multiple brain disorders as well as in substance abusers, as noted in the following.

Phosphocreatine (PCr) can also be measured with ^{31}P MRS, which additionally can assess phosphomonoesters (PME), inorganic phosphate, phosphodiesters (PDE), and three resonances associated with ATP (i.e., gamma-ATP, alpha-ATP, and beta-ATP). These phosphorous metabolites provide insights to the integrity of cellular energy stores, as well as cellular membrane composition and turnover. Several studies used ^{31}P MRS to evaluate these energetic metabolites in individuals during methadone-maintenance (see discussion following). Last, ^{13}C MRS can be used to study the metabolism of particular neurochemicals because the precursors of these chemicals can be enriched with ^{13}C, and the levels of the metabolic products can be measured. One example is ^{13}C-glutamate, which has been used to assess the neuronal health in individuals dependent on stimulants.

MAGNETIC RESONANCE SPECTROSCOPY STUDIES IN PSYCHOSTIMULANT ABUSE

Psychostimulants typically refer to several drugs that are commonly abused; these include but are not limited to cocaine, amphetamines (i.e., amphetamine, methamphetamine, and MDMA), and methylphenidate. MRS studies of stimulant users demonstrated abnormalities in brain metabolites associated with neurons, glia, and cellular metabolism. Findings often vary by the amount used, time since last use, and age of exposure to the stimulant drug.

MRS STUDIES IN COCAINE USERS

Several MRS studies of adult cocaine users have reported cerebral metabolite alterations (Table 56.1). Specifically, lower levels of the neuronal marker NAA were found in the anterior cingulate cortex (ACC) (Chang et al., 1999b) and thalamus (Li et al., 1999). Because the majority of neurons are glutamatergic, it is not surprising that Glu/tCR was also lower in the ACC of cocaine users, especially in those with a longer duration of cocaine use (Yang et al., 2009). In the same frontal region (ACC), cocaine users showed higher glial response with elevated MI, which also correlated with the duration of cocaine use (Chang et al., 1997). However, elevated tCR levels were found in both parietal (Chang et al., 1997; O'Neill et al., 2001b) and frontal white matter (Chang et al., 1997), as well as the ACC of cocaine users, especially in men (Chang et al., 1999b). The etiology of the elevated tCR is unclear, but similarly elevated tCR was also observed in children with prenatal cocaine exposure (Smith et al., 2001a). Although glial cells contain higher levels of tCR than neurons, the elevated tCR did not always coincide with the same brain regions that showed higher glial marker MI. Elevated tCR in the frontal lobe has been correlated with the frequency of cocaine use (Chang et al., 1997). In children with prenatal cocaine exposure, the higher frontal white matter tCR suggest aberrant cellular metabolism; however, these children had normal NAA, which indicated normal neuronal function and density (Smith et al., 2001a).

Although metabolites measured with MRS typically reflect cellular changes, one study found that acute cocaine administration induced increases in basal ganglia Cho and NAA, showing a transient effect at lower doses, but greater and more sustained increases in these metabolites at higher doses (Christensen et al., 2000). The investigators of this study posited that cocaine might have induced osmotic stress, which led to increased intracellular water and hence increased transverse relaxation times (T2*) of the Cho and NAA, via cocaine's action as an indirect dopamine D1 receptor agonist. However, since cocaine causes vasoconstriction, probably via its effects on the dopamine receptors on the blood vessels, the tissue concentrations of these metabolites may be increased within the voxel accordingly.

Studies that evaluated individuals who abused both cocaine and alcohol found even greater neurotoxic effects than those who abused cocaine only. For instance, prefrontal cortex GABA concentrations were lower than normal in cocaine users, and were even lower in those who also used alcohol (Ke et al., 2004). Another study found that cocaine using alcoholics had higher frontal white matter choline, indicative of cellular damage or turnover, but non-alcoholic cocaine users showed normal Cho levels. Furthermore, lower NAA in the dorsolateral prefrontal cortex of cocaine users partially normalized with abstinence from alcohol (Meyerhoff et al., 1999), again suggesting that some of the metabolite abnormalities may reflect transient neuronal dysfunction rather than neuronal loss. Because alcohol abuse is very common among cocaine-dependent subjects, and cocaine is not known to be neurotoxic from preclinical studies, findings from these studies suggest that the metabolite abnormalities observed in prior MRS studies may primarily be caused by alcohol abuse or the synergistic effects of alcohol and cocaine (e.g., the neurotoxic effects of cocaethylene).

Few MRS studies evaluated the effects of pharmacological treatment for cocaine dependence. One small study found that the GABA levels in the prefrontal cortex of cocaine users increased after pramipexole treatment, but the GABA levels were not related to treatment success (Streeter et al., 2005). A preliminary study also found that cocaine users showed normalized glutamate levels after N-acetylcysteine treatment (Schmaal et al., 2012).

MRS STUDIES IN METHAMPHETAMINE-DEPENDENT INDIVIDUALS

MRS studies of methamphetamine (METH) users (Table 56.2) consistently reported metabolite alterations that suggest neuronal or cell membrane injury, but the findings vary depending on the age of the subjects, amount METH used, and duration of abstinence. Abstinent METH-dependent individuals showed lower NAA in the basal ganglia regions (Chang et al., 2005; Ernst et al., 2000), and those with the greatest cumulative METH usage had the lowest NAA in their frontal white matter (Ernst et al., 2000; Sung et al., 2007). Glial activation with elevated MI was also found in the frontal lobe regions (Chang et al., 2005; Ernst et al., 2000; Sung et al., 2007). Some of these metabolite alterations might normalize with longer duration of abstinence, since subjects with longer duration of abstinence had higher NAA (Sung et al., 2007). The one small

TABLE 56.1. MRS studies in cocaine users

REFERENCE	SUBJECTS (DURATION ABSTINENCE)	METHODS	BRAIN REGIONS	FINDINGS
Chang et al., *Biol. Psychiatry* 1997	26 cocaine (0–2 years) 26 controls	1.5 T STEAM concentrations and ratios	ACC, frontal WM	Cocaine users had higher frontal WM tCR and MI. tCR correlated positively with frequency of use; MI correlated positively with duration of use.
Chang et al., *Am. J. Psychiatry* 1999	64 cocaine (>5 months) 58 controls	1.5 T PRESS concentrations and ratios	ACC, frontal WM	Cocaine users had lower NAA and MI in the ACC, as well as higher frontal WM MI. In the frontal WM of cocaine users, only males showed elevated tCR, whereas females showed elevated MI.
Li et al., *Biol. Psychiatry* 1999	21 cocaine (active users) 13 control	1.5 T PRESS concentrations and ratios	BG, thalamus	Cocaine users had lower NAA, NAA/tCR, and Cho/tCR in thalamus.
Meyerhoff et al., *Addict. Biol.* 1999	7 cocaine (16 weeks) 15 cocaine + alcohol users 11 controls	1.5 T 2 slice MRSI integrals and ratios	29 spectra (subcortical and periventricular)	Both cocaine user groups showed lower NAA and NAA/tCR in DLPFC, and lower NAA/tCR and NAA/Cho in central WM. WM Cho/tCR was associated with longer duration of cocaine + alcohol use. Partial NAA recovery with abstinence from alcohol.
Christensen et al., *Biol. Psychiatry* 2000	30 recreational cocaine users given acute cocaine dose	1.5 T PRESS peak area	Basal ganglia	Both 0.2 and 0.4 mg/kg cocaine did not alter tCR or water peak areas. 0.2 mg/kg cocaine induced small, reversible increases in Cho and NAA. 0.4 mg/kg cocaine induced larger, sustained increases in Cho and NAA. No changes following placebo.
O 'Neill et al., *Addict Biol.* 2001	8 cocaine 12 alcohol 17 cocaine + alcohol (5–39 weeks) 13 controls	1.5 T 2 slice MRSI concentrations	11 cortical regions of interest	Alcohol groups had lower gray-matter NAA than non-alcohol groups throughout the brain. Cocaine users had higher posterior parietal WM tCR than non-cocaine users.
Smith et al., *Pediatrics* 2001	14 prenatal cocaine 12 unexposed (3–16 years old)	1.5 T PRESS concentrations	Frontal WM, BG	Cocaine exposed children had higher FWM tCR and normal NAA.
Ke et al., *Psychiatry Res.* 2004	12 cocaine 23 cocaine + alcohol users (active users) 20 controls	1.5T 2D J-resolved normalized to est. tCR	Prefrontal cortex	Cocaine users had lower than normal GABA concentrations. Cocaine alcohol users had even lower GABA levels.
Streeter et al., *Psychopharmacology* 2005	28 cocaine [9 pramipexole 9 venlafaxine 10 placebo]	1.5T 2D J-resolved normalized to est. tCR	Prefrontal cortex	Compared to placebo treatment, pramipexole treated subjects showed increased GABA levels, and venlafaxine subjects showed only a trend for increased GABA levels. GABA levels were not related to treatment success (+/−urine).
Yang et al., *Psychiatry Res.* 2009	14 cocaine (active users) 14 controls	3 T TE-averaged PRESS ratios	ACC	Cocaine users showed lower than normal Glu/tCR that correlated with years of cocaine use. In both groups, Glu/tCR also correlated with NAA/tCR, which decreased with age.
Schmaal et al., *Neuropsycho-pharmacology* 2012	8 cocaine (<6 months; in treatment) 14 controls	3 T PRESS concentrations	Left dorsal ACC	Baseline, cocaine users had higher Glu than controls. After 1 dose (2400 mg) NAC, Glu reduced in the cocaine group but unchanged in controls. Higher baseline Glu was associated with higher Barratt Impulsiveness Scale scores; both were predictive of greater NAC-induced Glu reduction.

Notes: ACC, anterior cingulate cortex; BG, basal ganglia; GM, gray matter; NAC, *N*-acetylcysteine; WM, white matter

TABLE 56.2. MRS studies in methamphetamine users

REFERENCE	SUBJECTS (AVERAGE DURATION ABSTINENCE)	MRS METHODS	BRAIN REGIONS STUDIED	FINDINGS
Ernst et al., *Neurology* 2000	26 METH (>2 weeks) 24 controls	1.5 T PRESS concentrations and ratios	ACC, frontal WM, BG	METH users had lower BG and FWM NAA than controls. Frontal WM NAA correlated inversely with lifetime METH used. METH users also had lower BG tCR, and higher ACC Cho and MI.
Smith et al., *Neurology* 2001	12 prenatal METH 14 controls (3–16 years old)	1.5 PRESS concentrations and ratios	Frontal WM, BG	METH-exposed had higher tCR than unexposed children in striatum but normal NAA and behavior.
Sekine et al., *Neuropsycho-pharmacology* 2002	13 METH (1.5 year) 11 controls	1.5 T PRESS ratios	Left and right BG	METH users had lower tCR/Cho than controls in both BG. tCR/Cho correlated with the duration of METH use and with positive BPRS symptoms.
Chang et al., *Am. J. Psychiatry* 2005	24 METH+HIV 44 HIV 36 METH (>1 week) 39 controls	1.5 T PRESS concentrations	ACC, frontal WM, BG	METH users had lower FWM and BG NAA, but higher ACC choline and MI. HIV(+) subjects had lower ACC NAA and tCR but higher FWM MI than HIV(–) subjects. HIV+METH showed additive deleterious effects on NAA in all three regions, on tCR in the BG, and on MI in the FWM.
Nordahl et al., *Arch. Gen. Psychiatry* 2005	8 METH (>1 year) 16 METH (<6 month) 13 controls	1.5T PRESS ratios	ACC, PVC	METH users had low ACC NAA/tCR. ACC Cho/NAA values were high in the METH users with <6 months abstinence but not in those with >1 year abstinence. tCR did not differ between groups.
Salo et al., *Biol. Psychiatry* 2007	36 METH (>3 weeks) 16 controls	1.5 T PRESS ratios	ACC, PVC	METH users performed worse on the Stroop Interference task. ACC NAA/tCR was lower and Cho/NAA was higher in the METH users than controls. ACC NAA/tCR correlated with Stroop performance in the METH group only.
Sung et al., *Drug Alcohol Depend* 2007	9 METH (<6 months) 21 METH (>6 months) 20 controls	3 T PRESS concentrations	ACC, frontal WM	METH users had higher FWM MI than controls, and those with >100 gram lifetime dose had lower FWM NAA than those who used less. FWM NAA correlated inversely with the cumulative METH dose. ACC NAA in METH users correlated negatively with the cumulative METH dose and positively with the duration of abstinence.
Taylor et al., *J. Neurovirol* 2007	40 METH+HIV 66 HIV 48 METH 51 controls	1.5 T PRESS concentrations	ACC frontal WM, BG	HIV subjects had lower ACC and FWM NAA, and those with lower CD4 counts and higher plasma HIV viral loads had lower ACC and BG NAA. Plasma viral load correlated with FWM NAA and ACC and FWM MI in HIV+METH. Duration of METH use was associated with higher ACC Cho and higher BG MI.
Ernst and Chang, *J. Neuroimm. Pharmacol.* 2008	25 METH (<1 month) 12 METH (after 5 months) 28 controls	1.5 T PRESS concentrations and ratios	ACC, frontal WM, BG	METH users <1 month of abstinence had lower ACC Glx. Abstinence duration positively correlated with ACC and FWM Glx. After five months, changes in ACC Glx tended to increase with longer duration of abstinence. Subjects with craving symptoms had lower ACC Glx than those without craving.
Chang et al., *NeuroImage* 2009	49 Prenatal METH 49 controls (3–4 years old)	3 T PRESS concentrations	ACC, frontal WM, BG, thalamus	METH-exposed children had higher FWM tCR, NAA, and GLX, but lower thalamic MI, than unexposed. METH girls but not boys had higher FWM NA. METH children had poorer VMI scores. which correlated with thalamic MI.

(continued)

TABLE 56.2. (Continued)

REFERENCE	SUBJECTS (AVERAGE DURATION ABSTINENCE)	MRS METHODS	BRAIN REGIONS STUDIED	FINDINGS
Yoon et al., *Neuropsycho-pharmacology* 2010	16 METH treated with CDP-choline 15 METH with placebo	3 T PRESS concentrations	ACC	Over four-weeks of CDP-choline treatment for METH dependence, the rate of change in ACC NAA and Cho levels was greater with CDP-choline treatment than with placebo. Changes in ACC NAA but not Cho levels were positively associated with the number of negative urine results in CDP-choline-treated patients.
Sailasuta et al., *J. Cereb. Blood Flow Metab.* 2010	5 METH (>7 days) 5 controls	1.5 T ^{13}C MRS ratios	ACC	Steady-state bicarbonate concentrations showed no group difference. Glial ^{13}C-bicarbonate production rate (~glial TCA cycle) was reduced to 36% of normal in METH users.
Salo et al., *Drug Alcohol Depend* 2011	30 METH (<6 months) 17 (1–5 years) 24 controls	1.5 T PRESS ratios	ACC, PVC	Short-term abstinent METH users had higher ACC-Cho/NAA than controls, and lower ACC-NAA/tCR ithan both controls and long-term abstinent METH users. No differences between controls and the long-term abstinent group
Salo et al. *Neuropsychologia* 2011	51 METH (25 months) 22 controls	1.5 T PRESS ratios	ACC, PVC	Meth subjects had lower ACC NAA/tCR, inverse correlations between PVC and ACC NAA/tCR and spatial interference on the Spatial Stroop Attention task.
Cloak et al., *Drug Alcohol Depend* 2011	54 adolescent METH (days to years) 53 controls	3 T PRESS concentrations	ACC, frontal WM, BG, thalamus	METH males and female controls showed age-dependent increases in FWM tCR. Only male controls showed age-dependent increase in ACC choline, which was associated with faster performance on the Stroop Interference task. Male METH users had slowest performance on the Stroop Interference task and did not show age-appropriate levels of ACC choline.

Notes: ACC, anterior cingulate cortex; BG, basal ganglia; GM, gray matter; PVC, primary visual cortex; WM, white matter

study that used ^{13}C MRS to evaluate the incorporation of ^{13}C in the tricarboxylic acid cycle found lower glial ^{13}C-bicarbonate production in METH users, but the sample size is too small to yield conclusive interpretations (Sailasuta et al., 2010).

Methamphetamine use is prevalent among HIV-infected individuals. MRS studies that evaluated the combined effects of METH and HIV consistently found additive effects of lower NAA levels in the frontal white matter (WM) and basal ganglia, as well as elevated myoinositol (Chang et al., 2005; Taylor et al., 2007). These findings demonstrate that METH use may exacerbate the neurotoxic effects of HIV, especially in the striatum.

A few studies evaluated METH subjects longitudinally to assess for possible treatment effects on brain metabolite abnormalities. Cell membrane turnover with elevated Cho/NAA in recently abstinent METH subjects may normalize with longer duration of abstinence (>one year) (Nordahl et al., 2005). In addition, Glx, which is the sum of Glu, Gln, and GABA, was lower in those during early abstinence but may normalize or become elevated with more than five months of abstinence (Ernst and Chang, 2008). In addition, METH users treated with cytidine-5'-diphosphate choline, but not those given placebo, for one month showed increased NAA and choline levels, and greater increased NAA levels were associated with more negative urine results (Yoon et al., 2010). These findings suggest that alteration in the neuronal marker NAA may be reversible and that MRS may be useful for monitoring treatment effects.

These metabolite alterations might be related to behavioral consequences in METH users. For example, low basal ganglia tCR/Cho levels were associated with more psychiatric symptoms, even in abstinent METH users (Sekine et al., 2002). Lower ratios of NAA/tCR in the ACC also correlated with poorer executive function (Salo et al., 2007). In addition, abstinent METH subjects with the lowest ACC Glx had the greatest craving symptoms (Ernst and Chang, 2008). Because craving is an important symptom for relapse, Glx levels may be a useful marker for predicting relapse.

Unlike the consistent findings of possible neurotoxicity of chronic long-term METH abuse, acute dextroamphetamine administration to humans showed no metabolite changes in the ACC (McGrath et al., 2008), but increased glial metabolite ratio MI/tCR and PME/bATP in the temporal lobe (Silverstone et al., 2002). These changes may reflect a glial response to the drug, which may be transient or reversible.

Although many chronic METH users first used METH during their teenage years, only one MRS study evaluated brain metabolite levels in adolescent METH users. In contrast to the lower NAA found in the adults, these younger subjects showed normal NAA levels, which may be because of their lower cumulative lifetime doses. However, these young METH users showed less steep age-dependent increases in their frontal lobe metabolites (frontal white matter tCR in the females and ACC choline in the males), and the young male METH users also showed poorer executive function (Cloak et al., 2011). In contrast, children with prenatal METH exposure showed elevated tCR in the basal ganglia (Smith et al., 2001b) and the frontal white matter (Chang et al., 2009), which is similar to children with prenatal cocaine exposure (Smith et al., 2001a). The girls with prenatal METH exposure additionally showed elevated frontal white matter NAA. These children also showed lower glial metabolite MI in the thalamus that correlated with poorer visual motor integration performance (Chang et al., 2009). Taken together, the neurotoxic effects of METH on the developing brain varied based on age of exposure and sex.

ECSTASY (3,4-METHYLENEDIOXY-N-METHYLAMPHETAMINE)

Findings from MRS studies of ecstasy users are somewhat conflicting (Table 56.3). Early MRS studies reported higher glial marker MI in the parietal white matter of ecstasy users that correlated with estimated lifetime usage of the drug (Chang et al., 1999a), as well as lower frontal gray matter NAA/tCR and NAA/Cho, both also correlated negatively with the estimated lifetime use (Reneman et al., 2002). Because lower ratios of NAA/tCR and NAA/Cho may reflect normal NAA and higher tCR and Cho, these findings may suggest glial activation or response in the brains of ecstasy users. Such glial response may or may not represent toxic effects to the neurons. However, another study found that lower NAA/tCR was associated with impaired memory in ecstasy users (Reneman et al., 2001), which suggested that the drug might have "neurotoxic" effects with cognitive consequences. However, more recent prospective studies, with larger sample size and similar comparison subjects who used multiple substances but not ecstasy, failed to find metabolite abnormalities on MRS in those who used ecstasy, despite alterations in other imaging measures (de Win et al., 2007, 2008a, 2008b). Even small studies that focused on metabolite levels in the hippocampus found little (Daumann et al., 2004) or no (Obergriesser et al., 2001) differences between the ecstasy users and comparison subjects. Two studies of polydrug users who used ecstasy also found no differences between the ecstasy users and comparison subjects (Cowan et al., 2007), but noted an association between lower frontal cortex NAA/tCR and more lifetime marijuana use in this population (Cowan et al., 2009). Taken together, the brain metabolite levels are relatively normal in ecstasy users, except for possible increased glial metabolites in some individuals. Given the extremely common co-abuse of other psychostimulants and marijuana in ecstasy users, these glial responses also might have resulted from other drugs abused. Because preclinical studies of MDMA showed that the drug primarily affects the serotonergic nerve terminals, MRS does not appear to be the most sensitive imaging method for detecting the neurotoxic effects of ecstasy.

MRS STUDIES OF INHALANT (TOLUENE, ORGANIC SOLVENTS) ABUSE OR EXPOSURE

Few studies have addressed the neurotoxic effects of inhalant or solvent abuse using MRS. This is partly due to the transient usage pattern of inhalants or solvents by youths. Toluene and organic solvents are readily accessible to adolescents because they are common ingredients in household cleaning solutions, paint thinner, or glue. These inhalant or solvent abusers tend to progress to abusing other illicit drugs as adults. A few MRS studies evaluated individuals who abused inhalants, while others assessed individuals who had environmental (i.e., work place) exposure to chemicals that have abuse potential. Similar to other drugs of abuse, MRS studies showed metabolite abnormalities in inhalant users that reflect both neuronal and glial abnormalities. In addition, oxygen deprivation during the inhalation process also may exacerbate the neurotoxicity. A study of workers exposed to organic solvents on a daily basis found higher Cho/tCR in the parietal white matter, thalamus, and basal ganglia, and their duration of exposure correlated with metabolite abnormalities in the basal ganglia (Alkan et al., 2004). A case study of a woman who had abused toluene showed lower NAA/tCR in the centrum semiovale (Noda et al., 1996). This finding was validated in a larger study of individuals who abused toluene (paint-thinner), and showed lower NAA/tCR in the parietal and cerebellar white matter, as well as higher than normal MI/tCR in the same brain regions, especially in those with longer duration of abuse (Aydin et al., 2003). A similar study of toluene abusers found elevated Cho/tCR and Cho/NAA in the basal ganglia, and those with higher Cho/tCR ratios in the left basal ganglia had more psychiatric symptoms (Takebayashi et al., 2004). Therefore, findings from these few MRS studies clearly demonstrated the neurotoxic effects of toluene abuse, with evidence for glial activation and possible neuronal injury in the white matter and the striatum.

MRS STUDIES OF OPIATE USERS

Multiple MR studies of opiate-dependent individuals found brain abnormalities, including altered brain activation, structural neuroimaging abnormalities, and neuropsychological deficits. In particular, these brain abnormalities were typically found in the prefrontal brain regions of opiate-dependent individuals (Licata and Renshaw, 2010). However, only a few MRS studies evaluated opiate-dependent subjects (Table 56.4).

TABLE 56.3. MRS studies in ecstasy (MDMA) users

REFERENCE	SUBJECTS (DURATION ABSTINENCE)	MRS METHODS	BRAIN REGIONS STUDIED	FINDINGS
Chang et al., *J. Magn. Reson Imaging* 1999	22 MDMA (>2 weeks) 37 controls	1.5 T PRESS concentrations and ratios	Occipital GM, parietal WM ACC	MDMA users had higher than normal MI in parietal WM, which correlated with cumulative lifetime dose.
Reneman et al., *Biol. Psychiatry* 2001	8 MDMA (>1 week) 7 controls	1.5 T PRESS ratios	Prefrontal cortex, occipital GM, parietal WM	MDMA users had poorer word recall than controls and their prefrontal NAA/tCR correlated with delayed recall (on RAVLT).
Obergriesser et al., *Eur. Arch. Psychiatry Clin. Neurosci.* 2001	5 MDMA (variable) 5 controls	1.5 T MRSI PRESS concentrations and ratios	Slice centered around hippocampus	No group differences.
Reneman et al., *AJNR Am. J. Neuroradiol.* 2002	15 MDMA (>1 week) 12 controls	1.5 T PRESS ratios	ACC, occipital GM, parietal WM	MDMA users had lower NAA/tCr and NAA/Cho in ACC, which negatively correlated with lifetime use.
Daumann et al., *Neurosci. Lett.* 2004	13 MDMA (>1 week) 13 controls	1.5 T PRESS ratios	ACC, occipital GM, hippocampus	MDMA users showed only a trend for lower NAA/tCR in left hippocampus.
Cowan et al., *Psychiatry Res.* 2007	9 MDMA + polydrug (>3 weeks) 7 polydrug	4 T PRESS ratios	occipital GM	No group differences. MDMA user group used more other drugs.
de Win et al., *Neuropsychopharmacology* 2007	28 MDMA (before and after 8 weeks)	1.5 T PRESS concentrations and ratios	Frontal GM, occipital GM, frontoparietal WM	No group differences in brain metabolites, but lower regional blood volume in dorsolateral frontal cortex of MDMA subjects.
de Win et al., *Brain* 2008	59 novel MDMA users (19 weeks) 56 controls	1.5 T PRESS concentrations and ratios	Frontal GM, occipital GM, frontoparietal WM	No group differences in brain metabolites; lower rCBF in striatum and lower FA in several brain regions of MDMA users.
de Win et al., *Br. J. Psychiatry* 2008	33 MDMA + polydrug (8 weeks) 38 polydrug	1.5 T PRESS, ratios	Frontal GM, occipital GM, frontoparietal WM	No group difference in MRS metabolites or ADC. Ecstasy users showed abnormalities in thalamus on other studies (lower [123I]b-CIT binding, lower fractional anisotropy, and higher cerebral blood volume).

Notes: ACC: anterior cingulate cortex, GM: gray matter, WM: white matter

Patients enrolled in opioid maintenance therapy (OMT) with either methadone or buprenorphine have been studied with both ^{13}P MRS and ^{1}H MRS. ^{13}P MRS studies showed that methadone maintenance patients had elevated percentage of phosphomonoester in the white matter after seven days of treatment (Christensen et al., 1996; Kaufman et al., 1999), peaking between 15 and 28 days on treatment (Silveri et al., 2004), and normalized compared with controls following an average of 137 weeks of treatment (Kaufman et al., 1999). Reduced percentage of phosphocreatine was observed after seven days on treatment (Kaufman et al., 1999; Silveri et al., 2004), with continued decreases as a function of treatment duration up to 28 days (Silveri et al., 2004), and remained lower than controls after 137 weeks of treatment (Kaufman et al., 1999). Additionally, percentage of nucleotide triphosphates (β-NTP) and percentage of total nucleotide phosphates were lower than normal in the brains of cocaine and heroin-dependent individuals (Christensen et al., 1996). These findings indicated that cerebral energy metabolism is significantly altered during opiate withdrawal and methadone maintenance.

Studies using ^{1}H MRS further showed evidence of neuronal injury, with lower frontal gray matter (GM) NAA (Haselhorst et al., 2002) and lower dorsal ACC NAA and Glx (Yucel et al., 2007). Possible cell membrane turnover was also implicated with higher Cho in frontal WM of OMT subjects (Hermann et al., 2012a). Such cell membrane turnover may result from neurotransmitter release or adaptation associated with neuroplasticity. ACC Glu concentration also correlated with the number of previous withdrawals, whereas Glx decreased with age in controls but increased with age in opiate-dependent subjects (Hermann et al., 2012a). Investigators from this study suggested that these findings may be related to a hyperglutamatergic state associated with more frequent withdrawals, which might result in kindling of withdrawal symptoms after repeated withdrawal episodes.

TABLE 56.4. Brain metabolite abnormalities associated with opiate use or dependence

REFERENCE	SUBJECTS (DURATION ABSTINENCE)	MRS METHODS	BRAIN REGIONS STUDIED	FINDINGS
Christensen et al., *Magn. Reson. Med.* 1996	9 polysubstance (2–7 days) 11 controls	1.5 T ^{31}P MRS-ISIS % metabolite	Frontooccipital GM slice, frontal WM slice	Polysubstance abusers. showed higher %PME, but lower %β-NTP and %NP in GM.
Kaufman et al., *Psychiatr. Res. Neuroimag.* 1999	15 MMT (7 at 39 weeks; 8 at 137 weeks) 16 controls	1.5 T ^{31}P MRS-ISIS % metabolite	Frontooccipital GM slice	MMT subjects showed higher %PME and %PDE, but lower %PCr. Short-term MMT had higher %PME and %PDE, but lower %PCr. Long-term MMT had lower %PCr despite continued drug use.
Haselhorst et al., *Neurology* 2002	12 opiate-dependent (10 IV methadone 2 heroin) 12 controls	1.5 T ^{1}H MRS PRESS concentration	Frontal GM, frontal WM	Opiate-dependent subjects had lower NAA in GM but not in WM.
Silveri et al., *Psychiatr. Res. Neuroimag.* 2004	43 MMT (0–7, 8–14, or 15–28 days) 15 controls	1.5 T ^{31}P MRS-ISIS % metabolite	Axial slice (including frontal-occipital and BG)	MMT subjects had lower %PCr and higher %PDE. %PCr decreased and %PME increased with treatment duration.
Yucel et al. *Mol. Psychiatr.* 2007	24 opiate-dependent (24 hours) 24 controls	3 T ^{1}H MRS-PRESS concentration	Dorsal ACC	Opiate-dependent patients (10 on methadone, 14 on buprenorphine) had lower Glx and NAA in dorsal ACC.
Hermann et al., *Addict. Biol.* 2012	17 opiate-dependent 20 controls	3 T PRESS concentration	ACC, frontal WM	OD patients (11 on methadone, 6 on buprenorphine) had ACC Glu concentration that correlated with number of previous withdrawals. Glx decreased with age in controls, but increased with age in OD subject.

METABOLITE ABNORMALITIES IN BRAIN REGIONS WITH OPIOID-INDUCED LEUKOENCEPHALOPATHY

REFERENCE	SUBJECTS (DURATION ABSTINENCE)	MRS METHODS	BRAIN REGIONS STUDIED	FINDINGS
Kriegstein et al., *Neurology* 1999	3 heroin inhalation 1 control	1.5 T PRESS ratios	Cortical and cerebellar	Low NAA/tCR and Cho/tCR in GM in abnormal WM of 2 of 3 subjects. High cerebellar Lac/tCR in 1 patient
Vella et al., *Neuropediatrics* 2003	1 heroin-inhalation once only (8 days and 6 months) 5 controls	1.5 T PRESS concentration	Centrum semiovale supraventricular WM, occipital GM	Day 8: Lower than normal NAA, Cho, Glu, and higher Lac in centrum semiovale and superventricular WM, and tCR, MI in SV WM. At 6 months: Lower NAA and higher Gln in centrum semiovale.
Bartlett et al., *Brit. J. Radiol.* 2005	2 heroin-inhalation 1 cocaine-inhalation	1.5 T not specified ratios	Occipital WM	Abnormal WM in heroin users showed higher Lac/tCR, MI/tCR, and lower NAA/tCR. The cocaine patient had higher Lac/tCR, Cho/Cr and lipids.
Offiah & Hall, *Clin. Radiol.* 2008	5 of 6 heroin-inhalation No control	1.5 T PRESS visual reading	In abnormal WM	All 5 patients showed relative reduced NAA, Cho, and presence of Lactate doublet (TE 144 ms) in abnormal WM.
Salgado et al., *Am. J. Neuroradiol.* 2010	1 methadone overdose (27 days)	1.5 T ratios	Frontal WM	Markedly lower relative level of NAA, elevated relative level of Cho, and presence of lactic acid in abnormal WM.

Notes: ACC: anterior cingulate cortex, GM: gray matter, WM: white matter

In addition to the MRS studies in opiate-dependent individuals without gross structural brain abnormalities, several case reports or small series have used MRS to evaluate heroin-induced spongiform leukoencephalopathy, which is a rare condition resulting from inhalation of heroin vapors (aka "chasing the dragon"). These patients typically showed lactate and lower brain metabolite in the abnormal white matter regions. Specifically, lower levels of NAA (Kriegstein et al., 1999; Offiah and Hall, 2008; Vella et al., 2003), NAA/tCR (Bartlett and Mikulis, 2005); tCR (Vella et al., 2003); Cho, Glu, and MI (Vella et al., 2003); as well as higher Lac (Offiah and Hall, 2008; Kriegstein et al., 1999; Vella et al., 2003), or Lac/tCR (Bartlett and Mikulis, 2005) were found in brain regions showing leukoencephalopathy. A longitudinal case study of a

16-year-old boy who inhaled heroin only once showed bilateral leukoencephalopathy with reduced levels of brain metabolites and presence of lactate eight days later, and the reduced NAA and elevated Gln persisted at six months (Vella et al., 2003). Similarly, methadone-induced leukoencephalopathy showed relatively lower NAA, elevated Cho and presence of Lac (Salgado et al., 2010), whereas a case of cocaine-induced leukoencephalopathy showed only elevated Lac/tCR, Cho/tCR and lipids (Bartlett and Mikulis, 2005).

Taken together, findings from these ^{13}P MRS and ^{1}H MRS studies suggest opiate abuse may lead to increased cell membrane turnover (elevated percentage of PDE and percentage of PME, and Cho), possibly related to neuronal damage (lower NAA) and alterations in cerebral metabolism (lower percentage of PCr and presence of lactate). However, interpretations of these findings are confounded by several factors. First, with the exception of patients with drug-induced leukoencephalopathy, most patients were enrolled in OMT. Variability in scan days from dosing of methadone may affect cerebral metabolism and/or phospholipids, especially in early treatment prior to methadone tolerance. Additionally, many subjects had active polydrug abuse or dependence (cocaine, amphetamine, barbiturates, alcohol, etc.), which may additionally alter MRS detectable metabolites. Finally, the lifestyles of these patients may make accurate histories difficult to obtain (Yucel et al., 2007). More studies are needed to determine whether MRS may be useful for monitoring the efficacy of treatments in these individuals.

BRAIN METABOLITES ABNORMALITIES IN ALCOHOL USE DISORDERS

The neuropathological consequences of alcohol use disorders (AUD) include neuronal loss in the dorsolateral frontal cortex, cerebellum, and hypothalamus (Harding et al., 1997; Korbo, 1999; Kril and Halliday, 1999), glial abnormalities in the hippocampi, and dorsolateral prefrontal cortex, (Harper, 2009; Miguel-Hidalgo et al., 2002), as well as reductions in density of both neuronal and glial cells in the orbitofrontal cortex (Miguel-Hidalgo et al., 2006) (Table 56.5). Based on these neuropathological findings, most ^{1}H MRS studies were evaluated for neuronal loss (NAA), cellular (Cho), glial (MI), and metabolic (tCR) alterations in the frontal lobes, cerebellum, and subcortical regions. Almost all ^{1}H MRS studies of recently detoxified alcohol-dependent (RDA) individuals within two weeks of detoxification found consistent evidence of neuronal loss or injury, with lower NAA levels, lower NAA/tCR or NAA/Cho in the frontal lobe GM (Fein et al., 1994; O'Neill et al., 2001a), frontal WM (Bartsch et al., 2007; Durazzo et al., 2004; Durazzo et al., 2008; Ende et al., 2005; Gazdzinski et al., 2008a; Jagannathan et al., 1996; Schweinsburg et al., 2001), cerebellum (Bendszus et al., 2001; Jagannathan et al., 1996; Parks et al., 2002; Seitz et al., 1999), anterior cingulate cortex (Mon et al., 2012), parietal lobe (O'Neill et al., 2001a), and thalamus (Jagannathan et al., 1996). Only one study of individuals during early (three to five days) abstinence reported normal levels of frontal WM NAA (Parks et al., 2002). Another major metabolite abnormality in RDA subjects is lower Cho levels and lower Cho/Cr or Cho/NAA, which were found in the cerebellum (Bartsch et al., 2007; Ende

et al., 2005; Seitz et al., 1999), frontal WM (Ende et al., 2005), anterior cingulate cortex (Lee et al., 2007; Mon et al., 2012), and the occipital region (Modi et al., 2011). The lower Cho or Cho/tCR ratios suggest alterations in myelin or cell membrane, or decreased cellular synthesis. Additionally, elevated MI concentrations, suggestive of glial activation, have been reported in the thalamus and ACC (Schweinsburg et al, 2000), as well as in the frontal and parietal WM (Schweinsburg et al., 2001).

MRS also may be useful for predicting relapse because the odds of relapse to alcohol use within 6–12 months were greater in those with lower NAA in the temporal GM and frontal WM and lower Cho in the frontal GM (Durazzo et al., 2008). A more recent study further confirmed that relapsers had significantly lower NAA than non-relapsers in many brain regions, including the dorsolateral prefrontal cortex (DLPFC), ACC, insula, cerebellar vermis, and the corona radiata; therefore, the authors speculated that connectivity of components of the rewards system may be impaired in those at risk for relapse (Durazzo et al., 2010). A small study that evaluated patients with bipolar disorder with and without alcoholism found only higher Glx levels in the DLPFC in the bipolar subjects, whereas those with alcoholism actually had normal brain metabolites despite their worse outcome and treatment refractoriness for their bipolar symptoms (Nery et al., 2010).

Recent studies have investigated the role of Glu and its metabolite Gln in AUD. Glu has been implicated in both AUD neuropathology and in the development of alcohol dependence. Young (<40 years old) RDA subjects abstinent for two weeks, without gross brain atrophy on MRI (GM, WM, and CSF volumes), showed significantly lower than normal ACC tCR, Cho, and Glu/tCR (Lee et al., 2007). Some of these metabolite abnormalities might be transient because older subjects (>40 years) with longer histories of AUD showed lower than normal NAA, Glu, and tCR in the ACC at baseline, mild elevation of Glu during early abstinence, and normalization of these metabolite abnormalities four weeks later (Mon et al., 2012). Furthermore, despite lower than normal Glu and Gln in RDA subjects, those who had been abstinent for at least one year also showed normal brain metabolite levels. Finally, in a placebo-controlled study of acamprosate, decreased Glu/tCR ratios were found only in the RDA subjects who were on acamprosate after four weeks, but not in the placebo treated RDA subjects. Because acamprosate is a medication approved for the treatment of alcohol dependence that reduces craving and relapse, the decreased Glu/tCR ratio after treatment may be a potential surrogate marker for future studies. Unfortunately, craving and relapse measures were not evaluated in relation to the changes in Glu/tCR in the subjects studied, and no correlations with CSF glutamate or other clinical measures were performed. Nevertheless, the various studies that evaluated brain GLX or glutamate demonstrated that MRS may be useful to evaluate the altered brain glutamatergic system in alcoholics, which may represent the effects of alcohol consumption or a predisposing susceptibility to AUD.

Several studies suggested that much of the neuropathological damage associated with AUD is reversible. With sustained abstinence, recovery has been observed in WM volume (Monnig et al., 2012), GM volume (Sullivan and Pfefferbaum,

TABLE 56.5. Brain changes associated with AUD: selected MRS studies

REFERENCE	SUBJECTS (DURATION ABSTINENCE)	MRS METHODS	BRAIN REGIONS STUDIED	FINDINGS
Seitz et al., *Alcohol Clin. Exp. Res.* 1999	11 RDA (3–6 days) 10 controls	1.5 T STEAM ratios	Cerebellar vermis	Compared with controls subjects, RDA subjects had lower NAA/tCR at TE = 135 msec and lower Cho/tCR at TE = 5 msec.
Behar et al., *Am. J. Psychiatry* 1999	5 RDA (34 days) 5 hepatic encephalopathy 10 controls	2.1 T homonuclear editing short-TE	Occipital GM	GABA is lower in RDA and HE subjects than in controls.
Schweinsberg et al., *Alcohol Clin. Exp. Res.* 2001	37 RDA (average 28 days) 15 controls	1.5 T PRESS concentration	Frontal WM Parietal WM	RDA subjects have lower FWM NAA and higher MI in FWM and PWM.
Bendszus et al., *Am. J. Neuroradiol.* 2001	17 RDA (1–3 days and 36–39 days) 12 controls	1.5 T PRESS ratios	Midline frontal lobe Cerebellum	Low NAA/tCR in frontal lobes and cerebellum at day 1–3, but significant increases after 1 month.
O'Neill et al., *Alcohol Clin. Exp. Res.* 2001	12 recovering alcoholics (128 weeks) 8 active heavy drinkers	1.5 T MRSI concentration	Frontal, Parietal, Remainder	Recovering alcoholics had fewer WM lesions and more GM volumes, but no difference in brain metabolites, compared with heavy drinkers.
Parks et al., *Alcohol Clin. Exp. Res.* 2002	31 RDA (3–5 days, 3 weeks and 3 months) 12 controls	1.5 T PROBE-P concentration	Vermis Frontal WM	No group differences in WM at 3–5 days, but RDA had lower NAA and Cho in cerebellum. 11 RDA subjects who remained abstinent at 3 months had increases in cerebellar NAA.
Ende et al., *Biol. Psychiatry* 2005	33 RDA (3 weeks, 3 months, 6 months) 30 controls	1.5 T spin echo multislice	DLPFC GM, WM, Vermis	RDA had lower Cho in frontal lobe and cerebellum, and low NAA in frontal WM. Cho increased at 3 months; no differences between 3 months and 6 months.
Ende et al., *NeuroImage* 2006	24 very light use 18 moderate use	1.5 T PRESS	Frontal WM, ACC, Cerebellum	Frontal WM and ACC Cho correlate with alcohol consumption.
Bartsch et al., *Brain* 2007	15 RDA (5 days and 6 weeks) 10 controls	1.5 T PRESS concentration	Frontomesial, Cerebellum	RDA had low frontal NAA and low cerebellar Cho. Increases in both at 6 weeks.
Durazzo et al., *Alcohol Alcoholism* 2008	26 RDA abstainers (1 month) 44 RDA resumers	1.5 T MRSI concentration	Frontal WM, BG, Cerebellar vermis	Lower NAA in temporal GM and frontal WM and lower Cho in frontal GM predicted relapse within 6–12 months.
Gazdzinski et al., *Alcohol* 2008a	35 RDA (1 week) 32 HD 38 controls	1.5 T MRSI concentration	Major lobes, Subcortical nuclei, Midbrain, Vermis	RDA had lower NAA, Cho, and MI than non-treated heavy drinkers.
Durazzo et al., *J. Stud. Alcohol Drugs* 2010	51 RDA (1 week) 33 resumers 26 controls	1.5 T MRSI concentration	DLPFC, Insula, ACC, Vermis, Superior corona radiata	RDA with lower NAA and tCR were more prone to relapse within 6–12 months.
Nery et al., *J. Psychiatr. Res.* 2010	22 ALC with BD 26 BD 54 controls	1.5 T PRESS concentration	DLPFC	ALC subjects with BD had normal Glu levels, whereas non-ALC BD subjects had higher Glx levels than other groups.
Umhau et al., *Arch. Gen. Psychiatry* 2010	33 RDA (4 days and 25 days after treatment) 15 RAD+Acamprosate 18 RDA on placebo	3 T TE-Avg PRESS ratios	ACC	RDA treated with acamprosate showed decreased Glu/tCR in the ACC but not RDA treated with placebo.
Yeo, et al. *Biol. Psychiatry* 2011	146 RDA (≤21 days)	1.5 T PRESS concentration	ACC	Number and length of copy number variation deletions correlated with lower ACC NAA, tCR, MI, and Glx.

(continued)

TABLE 56.5. *(Continued)*

REFERENCE	SUBJECTS (DURATION ABSTINENCE)	MRS METHODS	BRAIN REGIONS STUDIED	FINDINGS
Hermann et al., *Biol. Psychiatry* 2011	47 RDA (1 and 14 days) 57 controls	3T PRESS concentration	ACC	Both RDA and animals had higher Glu and Glu/Gln during acute withdrawal in prefrontal GM. Elevated Glu and Glu/Gln normalized after a few weeks.
Modi et al., *Eur. J. Radiol.* 2011	9 RDA (1 week) 13 controls	1.5 T PRESS ratios	Occipital lobe	RDA had higher Cho/tCR in occipital lobe.
Thoma et al., *Neuropsychopharacology* 2011	6 RDA (1 year) 7 current AUD 17 controls	3T PRESS concentration	ACC	Lower Glu and higher Gln were found in both RDA and current AUD subjects than in controls. However, the two AUD groups did not differ on any of the brain metabolites.
Mon et al., *Drug Alcohol Depend* 2012	20 RDA (9 days) 36 RDA (34 days) 16 light drinkers	4T STEAM and MEGA PRESS concentration	ACC, POC, and DLPFC cortices	At baseline, compared with LD subjects, RDA subjects had lower tCR, Cho, and NAA in the ACC, but normal Glu and MI. After 5 weeks of abstinence no differences were noted between RDA and LD subjects. 11 RDA scanned at both time points had increased ratios of Glu, NAA, and Cho to water in the ACC, and of Glu to water in the POC.

Notes: ACC, anterior cingulate cortex; BG, basal ganglia; DLPFC, dorsolateral prefrontal cortex; GM, gray matter; POC, Parietooccipital cortex; WM, white matter; RDA, recently detoxified alcoholic

2005) and cognitive function (see following). When compared with control subjects after 35 to 39 days (Bendszus et al., 2001; Mon et al., 2012), or three months of abstinence (Ende et al., 2005), RDA subjects showed relatively normal levels of frontal (ACC) NAA, Glu, and Cho (Mon et al., 2012), NAA/tCR (Bendszus et al., 2001), frontal GM and WM Cho (Ende et al., 2005), cerebellar Cho/NAA (Martin et al., 1995), NAA/tCR and Cho/tCR (Bendszus et al., 2001), and Cho levels (Ende et al., 2005). In longitudinal follow-up studies of RDA subjects who were scanned after three days, three weeks, and three months of abstinence, frontal WM metabolites were normal at three days, whereas the cerebellar NAA and volume were lower at baseline but continued to increase toward normalization at three months, suggesting that the cerebellum is particularly sensitive, and may recover slower from the alcohol induced brain injury (Parks et al., 2002).

BRAIN METABOLITE ABNORMALITIES IN AUD ARE RELATED TO COGNITIVE PERFORMANCE

Alcohol may induce cognitive impairments, particularly in the learning and memory domains, which may be associated with alterations in brain metabolites measured with ^{1}H MRS. For example, deficits in delayed recall on the Hopkins Verbal Learning Test were negatively correlated with occipital GABA plus homocarnosine in RDAs (Behar et al., 1999), and improvements in verbal learning assessed on day 2 and day 38 of abstinence were correlated with increases in frontal NAA/tCR (Bendszus et al., 2001). Furthermore, levels of the glial marker MI in either the ACC or the parietal cortex of RDA subjects negatively correlated with verbal learning, delayed visual memory, visuomotor scanning speed, and visuospatial memory, after 2 days of abstinence, and with auditory-verbal learning after 35 days of abstinence (Mon et al., 2012). Additionally, poorer short-term memory function was associated with lower Glu/tCR in the ACC of young RDA who had no evidence of GM or WM atrophy (Lee et al., 2007). Furthermore, poorer visuospatial learning was associated with higher DLPFC Glx after 2 days of abstinence, but with higher Cho on day 35 of abstinence, whereas poorer working memory was associated with higher glial marker MI also on day 35 (Mon et al., 2012). However, the degree of improvement on these cognitive measures from day 2 to day 35 did not correlate with changes in metabolite concentrations (Mon et al., 2012). Moreover, the neuronal marker NAA also may predict cognitive performance. In one study, cerebellar NAA/tCR in RDA subjects correlated with their performance on the Concentration Load test both after 2 days and after 38 days of abstinence (Bendszus et al., 2001). In heavy drinkers, the lower than normal frontal WM NAA also correlated with poorer executive and working memory functioning (Meyerhoff et al., 2004).

BRAIN METABOLITE ABNORMALITIES IN TREATMENT-NAIVE AUD

Most studies were performed on RDA subjects, who may not be representative of the majority (85%) of people with AUD who do not seek treatment (Gazdzinski et al., 2008a). RDA subjects typically have more severe medical and psychiatric comorbidities (Meyerhoff et al., 2013), and may have up to 50% greater lifetime alcohol consumption (Fein and Landman, 2005). Lifetime consumption of alcohol is an important consideration, because even light to moderate drinkers without AUD showed reductions in frontal Cho levels that correlated with alcohol consumption within 90 days of their MRS (Ende et al., 2006). The few studies that compared current heavy drinkers (HD) to RDA and healthy controls reported conflicting results. Surprisingly, RDA participants typically showed lower brain metabolite levels than HD subjects. For example, although NAA, Cho, tCR, or MI were typically lower in HD subjects than in controls (Gazdzinski et al., 2008a), including HD subjects with a negative family history of AUD, the brain metabolite abnormalities in these HD subjects were less severe than those observed in RDA individuals (Meyerhoff et al., 2004). In contrast, although both current drinkers and AUD subjects who had been abstinent for one year showed lower brain Glu and higher Gln than controls, both AUD subject groups showed no differences in NAA, tCR, Cho, MI, Gln, or Glx in their ACC (Thoma et al., 2011). Similarly, despite group differences in regional brain volumes and the amount of white matter lesions, recovering alcoholics (median abstinence 128 weeks) and active heavy drinkers showed no differences in their brain metabolites in any brain regions studied (O'Neill et al., 2001a). Therefore, MRS may not be sensitive for differentiating the brain health of HD and RDAs. However, the lack of differences between RDA, HD, and control subjects in these two studies might have resulted from normalization of the brain metabolites in the RDAs following abstinence.

ALCOHOL USE WITH TOBACCO SMOKING

Cigarette smoking is the most common comorbidity among drug users, including those with AUD. Up to 80% of alcohol-dependent individuals regularly smoke (Romberger and Grant, 2004) and 50–90% are dependent on nicotine (Daeppen et al., 2000). Only a few MRS studies specifically evaluated brain metabolite abnormalities in tobacco smokers. One study of current tobacco smokers showed lower hippocampal NAA, and their ACC Cho correlated with lifetime nicotine exposure (Gallinat et al., 2007). Another study of tobacco smokers who "slipped" or relapsed from smoking cessation (with nicotine replacement therapy) showed lower baseline Glu/tCR, GABA/tCR, and Cho/tCR than those who were able to remain abstinent from the treatment (Mashhoon et al., 2011). Therefore, these metabolite ratios may be useful for predicting treatment outcomes (Table 56.6).

Smoking appeared to have additive effects with alcohol use in that RDA subjects who smoked had the lowest metabolite concentrations. RDA subjects with greater alcohol consumption also smoked more and had worse neuropsychological performance (Durazzo et al., 2004). Furthermore, after one month of abstinence, compared with RDA subjects who smoked (sRDA), non-smoking RDA (nsRDA) subjects showed greater increases (normalization) in medial temporal lobe Cho and NAA (Gazdzinski et al., 2008b), frontal WM NAA and Cho, and thalamic Cho (Durazzo et al., 2006).

Additionally, diffusion tensor imaging indicated lower than normal fractional anisotropy in brain regions of RDA subjects who showed lower NAA concentrations (Durazzo et al., 2006), as well as in the frontal WM, superior corona radiata, and adjacent WM in sRDA, but not nsRDA subjects (Wang et al., 2009). Therefore, comorbid tobacco smoking with alcohol use may lead to greater brain metabolite abnormalities, which may be related to the direct neurotoxic effects from these comorbid conditions, or indirect effects from hypoxia associated with smoking. Prior studies of individuals with AUD often did not account for concurrent tobacco smoking. Because NAA and Cho may normalize in alcohol users who became abstinent, but not in AUD with concurrent tobacco smoking, some of the metabolite abnormalities found in subjects with AUD may be caused by comorbid tobacco smoking.

MRS STUDIES IN MARIJUANA SMOKERS

Marijuana or cannabis smoking is also very common among drug users and is often used for medicinal purposes. Medicinal marijuana use is now legal in more than half of the United States. Few studies have used MRS to measure brain metabolites in chronic marijuana users (see Table 56.6). Because marijuana use is common among HIV-infected individuals, one study evaluated the independent and combined effects of chronic marijuana use in subjects with or without HIV-infection. Regardless of HIV-infection status, abstinent marijuana users showed lower levels of basal ganglia NAA, Cho, and glutamate, but elevated thalamic tCR (Chang et al., 2006). Similarly, young men who smoked marijuana daily showed mild memory and attention impairments and lower levels of NAA/tCR in the dorsolateral prefrontal cortex, and the NAA/tCR levels in their lentiform nuclei positively correlated with hair cannabidiol levels (indicative of amount of marijuana smoked recently) (Hermann et al., 2007). A small 2D MRS study of marijuana-dependent young men reported lower than normal global MI/tCR levels (from one large voxel that included basal ganglia, thalamus, hippocampus, and surrounding regions) (Silveri et al., 2011). Furthermore, young regular marijuana users showed lower levels of glutamate, NAA, tCR, and MI in the ACC; however, some of these marijuana users were also heavy alcohol users and/or were medicated for depression (Prescot et al., 2011). Last, a study of polydrug users who used ecstasy and marijuana found only an association between lower frontal cortex NAA/tCR and more lifetime marijuana use but not with other drug use (Cowan et al., 2009). Taken together, the few studies that evaluated brain metabolite changes in chronic marijuana users found decreased neuronal and/or glial metabolites in the basal ganglia and in the frontal lobe. Longitudinal studies are needed to evaluate the relationship between marijuana use and brain metabolite abnormalities, and whether these alterations are reversible or may normalize with longer duration of abstinence. Because marijuana is often used by adolescents, when their brains are still undergoing development, future evaluations should assess the

TABLE 56.6. MRS studies in tobacco (TOB) or marijuana (MJ) smokers or exposure

REFERENCE	SUBJECTS (DURATION ABSTINENCE)	METHODS	BRAIN REGIONS	FINDINGS
Epperson et al., *Biol. Psychiatry* 2005	16 TOB (48 hours) 20 controls	2.1 T J-edit GABA concentration est. from tCR	Occipital GM	Short-term TOB abstinence did not affect GABA. Female TOB had reduced GABA during the follicular phase but no cyclicity in GABA levels across the menstrual cycle. Male TOB users had normal GABA levels.
Gallinat et al., *J. Clin. Psycho-pharmacol.* 2007	13 TOB (current) 13 controls	3 T PRESS concentration	ACC, HIPC	TOB smokers had lower NAA in the hippocampus, whereas their ACC Cho correlated positively with pack years smoked.
Durazzo et al., *Alcohol Clin. Exp. Res.* 2004	14 TOB+alcohol (1 wk) 7 TOB10 alcohol (1 wk) 19 controls	1.5 T MRSI 3 slices concentration	3 cortical, 4 WM, 5 other regions	Alcohol effect: lower frontal NAA and lower frontal, parietal, and thalamic Cho. TOB+alcohol had lower FWM and midbrain Cho than alcohol. TOB effect: lower midbrain NAA and choline and CBV. Correlations with cognitive measures varied by group.
Durazzo et al., *Alcohol Clin. Exp. Res.* 2006	14 TOB+alcohol (1 month) 9 TOB11 alcohol (1 month) 20 controls	1.5 T 3 slice (subcortical and cortical) MRSI concentration	3 cortical, 4 WM, 5 other regions	After 1 month of abstinence from alcohol, PWM Cho increased in the alcohol group and PWM NAA decreased in the TOB+alcohol group. Metabolite/cognition correlations varied between alcohol and TOB+alcohol.
Mason et al., *Biol. Psychiatry* 2006	7 TOB+alcohol (1–13 days) 5 TOB5 alcohol (2–7 days) 3 controls	2.1 T J-edit GABA concentration est. from tCR	Occipital GM	At 1-week sobriety, GABA was higher in alcohol users relative to others but normalized after 1 month. Glx was higher in smokers.
Gazdzinski et al., *Psychiatry Res.* 2008	13 TOB+alcohol 11 alcohol (both at 6 and 32 days) 14 controls	1.5 T 1 slice MRSI concentration	Slice centered around HIPC	Hippocampal NAA Cho and MI increased to near normal levels after 1-month alcohol abstinence for alcohol group but not TOB+alcohol group. Cho changes positively correlated with memory changes.
Wang et al., *NMR Biomed.* 2009	26 TOB+alcohol (1 month) 22 alcohol (1 month) 26 controls (light drinkers)	1.5 T MRSI–3 slices concentration	7 WM regions	TOB+alcohol had lower NAA in frontal WM with abnormal fractional anisotropy (FA) on DTI. Alcohol users had normal NAA. No NAA group differences were detected in FWM with normal FA on DTI.
Mashhoon et al., *Prog. Neuropsycho-pharmacol. Biol. Psychiatry* 2011	9 TOB on NRT (5 relapse, 4 6-wks abstinent)	4 T 2D_J PRESS Ratios	Dorsal ACC, occipital GM	Subjects who relapsed had lower baseline dACC Glu/tCR, GABA/tCR, and Cho/tCR compared with abstinent subjects.
Chang et al., *J. Neuroimm. Pharmacol.* 2012	26 prenatal TOB24 controls age 3–4 years	3 T PRESS concentration	ACC, Frontal WM, BG, thalamus	Prenatal TOB exposed children had higher ACC Glx. Those with highest Glx had poorest vocabulary and visual motor integration.
MRS IN MARIJUANA SMOKERS				
Chang et al., *J. Neuroimm. Pharmacol.* 2006	24 MJ (0–2 yrs) 21 HIV21 HIV+MJ (0–2 years) 30 controls	4 T PRESS concentration	ACC, Frontal WM, BG thalamus	MJ users had lower NAA, Cho, and Glu in BG but elevated tCR in thalamus. MJ users, but not HIV+MJ, also had lower Glu in FWM.
Hermann et al., *Biol. Psychiatry* 2007	12 active MJ users 10 controls	1.5 T MRSI 3 slices ratio	HIPC, frontal WM, BG, thalamus, DLPFC, ACC	MJ users had lower NAA/tCR in DLPFC; NAA/tCR in BG correlated with hair cannabidiol. MJ users had poor cognitive performance.
Cowan et al., *Pharmacol. Biochem, Behav.* 2009	17 polydrug (>4 days)	3 T PRESS ratio	Occipital GM, temporal WM, LFC	NAA/tCR in LFC correlated inversely with lifetime marijuana use only, but not with other drugs used (MDMA, alcohol, or cocaine).

(continued)

TABLE 56.6. (*Continued*)

REFERENCE	SUBJECTS (DURATION ABSTINENCE)	METHODS	BRAIN REGIONS	FINDINGS
Silveri et al., *Psychiatry Res.* 2011	15 active MJ users 10 controls	4T 2D:MRSICSI-PRESS ratio	1 slice: temporal, parietal, occipital lobes, thalamus, BG	Correlations between global MI/tCR, impulsivity and mood symptoms varied between groups. Correlations with frequency of use, age of first use, impulsivity, and mood, differed between MJ and controls.
Prescot et al., *NeuroImage* 2011	17 active MJ users 17 controls	3 T PRESS concentration	ACC	MJ users had lower Glu, NAA, tCR and MI but no differences in GM/WM/CSF content.

Notes: ACC, anterior cingulate cortex; BG, basal ganglia; DLPFC, dorsolateral prefrontal cortex; GM, gray matter; HIPC, hippocampus; NRT, nicotine replacement therapy; TOB, tobacco; WM, white matter

impact of marijuana usage on brain metabolites or cognitive changes during brain development.

SUMMARY MRS FINDINGS IN VARIOUS DRUGS OF ABUSE AND DRUG DEPENDENCE

MRS can detect neurochemical alterations that reflect neuronal loss, dysfunction, or glial activation associated with various drugs of abuse. Specifically, neuronal markers such as NAA and Glu or Glx are shown to be lower than normal in many brain regions of the drug users discussed in the preceding, except for those who used ecstasy. Decreased NAA often correlated with the cumulative exposure of the drug, cognitive performance, severity of psychiatric symptoms, and may even predict the likelihood of relapse (e.g., in alcoholics). However, NAA levels also may normalize with longer duration of abstinence from alcohol or methamphetamine use, which indicates that some of the neuronal injury may be reversible. The magnitude of the lower NAA levels are typically in the range of 5–7%, which are less than those found in neurodegenerative disorders, such as frontotemporal dementia (>25%) and Alzheimer's disease (>10%), or in neuroinflammatory conditions such as multiple sclerosis (up to >30%, especially in secondary progressive disease) and chronic HIV infection (5–20%). However, such decreased NAA may differ across brain regions and may vary greatly depending on the stage of the disease (Table 56.7).

Similarly, the glial marker MI is often elevated in the white matter of drug users which may reflect glial activation or neuroinflammation associated with drug abuse. Specifically, elevated MI has been reported in the white matter of psychostimulant (cocaine, methamphetamine, and ecstasy) users, inhalant users, opiate-dependent individuals, and alcoholics. The magnitude of the elevated MI in drug users (10–15%) are only slightly less than those observed in neuroinflammatory responses associated with other chronic brain disorders. For example, MI is often elevated in patients with chronic HIV infection (up by 10–20%) or neurodegenerative disorders such as Alzheimer's disease (also 10–20%, depending on the brain region), but may be higher in those with more acute neuroinflammation such as progressive multiple sclerosis (10–35%). Limited data on cocaine or marijuana users reported lower MI in the ACC, but these subjects might have had other confounding variables (e.g., depression).

Because tCR and choline compounds are in both neurons and glia, their levels are more variable depending on the brain regions assessed, usage patterns, or duration of abstinence. tCR was consistently found to be elevated in the white matter of adult cocaine users and in children with prenatal exposure to either cocaine or methamphetamine, although most of these individuals also had tobacco exposure. In contrast, adult methamphetamine users showed lower tCR levels in both the basal ganglia and white matter, and alcoholics also showed lower tCR in the DLPFC and WM, especially during early abstinence and in those who relapsed. Since tCR reflects energetic metabolites, its level may reflect the energy states of the brains of drug users during various states of recovery.

Glutamate or Glx levels, which reflect primarily Glu, tended to be lower during early abstinence (e.g., in methamphetamine users and RDA), but may normalize with longer duration of abstinence, with pharmacotherapy (e.g., RDA treated with acamprosate), and may also correlate with number of withdrawals (e.g., in opiate users). Glx is also elevated in the frontal lobes of tobacco smokers, individuals with AUD, and in those with prenatal stimulant exposure. However, quantitative measurements of Glx and Glu are often less reliable than other metabolites, and are not possible with studies performed using longer echo times. Therefore, better techniques are needed for future analyses (see the following). The few studies that evaluated GABA also found reduced levels in cocaine and alcohol dependent individuals, and the lower levels may predict relapse (e.g., tobacco smoking). This plethora of studies demonstrate that MRS provides valuable *in vivo* neuropathological assessment of the brains of drug addicted individuals, which may be useful both for initial assessments but may also be used as a surrogate marker to predict treatment outcome or relapse to drug use.

TECHNICAL CONSIDERATIONS AND FUTURE DIRECTIONS

MRS complements other neuroimaging techniques well because it can often be acquired with structural imaging, which is required for voxel placements for MRS studies. This approach was used in a study of alcohol users (Wang et al., 2009); the investigators used diffusion tensor imaging to assess axonal integrity, which demonstrated abnormal fractional anisotropy,

TABLE 56.7. Brain metabolite abnormalities (in selected brain regions) associated with drugs of abuse or exposure

BRAIN METABOLITES	COCAINE	AMPHETAMINE/ METHAMPHETAMINE	ECSTASY (MDMA)	INHALANTS/ SOLVENTS	OPIATES	MARIJUANA	ALCOHOL	TOBACCO
NAA or NAA/tCR	⇓ (ACC, thalamus, DLPFC, WM); ⇑ (BG—acute)	⇓ (BG, FWM, ACC) correlated with usage or behavior; ⇑ prenatal exp (FWM)	Normal	⇓ (PWM, cerebellum)	⇓ (GM, dorsal ACC); ⇓⇓⇓ in leukoencephalopathy	⇓ (DLPFC, ACC, BG)	⇓ (most brain regions), in relapsers; may normalize with abstinence	⇓ (hippocampi, midbrain)
tCR or %PCr	⇑ (FWM) in both adults and prenatal exposed; sex-differences ⇑ (PWM)	⇓ (BG, FWM); ⇑ prenatal exposure (BG, FWM)			⇓ (GM) decreased with MMT	⇓ (ACC); ⇑ (THL)	⇓ (DLPFC, WM, Vermis) in relapsers; may normalize with abstinence	
Choline or Cho/ tCR Cho/NAA	⇓ (TH); ⇑ (BG-acute)	⇓ (ACC, BG); ⇑ (ACC)		⇓ (thalamus, BG, PWM); correlated with psychiatric symptoms	⇓ in leukoencephalopathy	⇓ (BG)	⇓ (FGM, ACC, cerebellum); normalized with abstinence ⇑ (OGM)	⇓ ACC in relapsers; ⇑ (FWM, vermis, midbrain); correlated with pack years
Myoinositol or MI/ tCR	⇑ (FWM) correlated with duration; sex-differences ⇓ (ACC)	⇑ (ACC, FWM); ⇑ after dextro-amphetamine ⇓ prenatal (thalamus)	⇑ (PWM) correlation with lifetime dose	⇑ (PWM, cerebellum)	⇑ (OWM)	⇓ (ACC)	⇑ (thalamus, ACC, FWM, PWM)	
Glx or Glx/tCR		⇓ or ⇑ (ACC and FWM) vary with duration of abstinence ⇑ prenatal exp (FWM)			⇓ (dorsal ACC)		⇑ (DLPFC)	⇑ ACC (prenatal) ⇑ (OGM)
Glutamate (Glu) or Glu/tCR	⇓ or ⇑ (ACC) ⇓ correlated with duration				Correlated with times withdrawal	⇓ (ACC, BG)	⇑ or ⇓ (ACC) ⇓ (ACC) after acamprosate	⇓ ACC in those who relapse
GABA or GABA/ tCR	⇓ (PFC)						⇓ (Occipital)	⇓ ACC in relapsers
Lac or Lac/tCR					Only in leukoencephalopathy			
%PDE or %PME					⇑ (GM) with MMT			
%B-NTP or %NP					⇓ (GM) with MMT			

Notes: ACC, anterior cingulate cortex; BG, basal ganglia; CBV, cerebellar vermis; DLPFC, dorsolateral prefrontal cortex; GM, gray matter; POC, Parieto-occipital cortex; RDA, recently detoxified alcoholic; WM, white matter and selected brain regions for MRS evaluation from previously collected MRSI. Therefore, MRSI has the advantage that once the data are collected, selected brain regions can be queried retrospectively. However, because of the magnetic field inhomogeneity from different tissues across the brain, localized MRS often allows better assessments of brain metabolite concentrations in selected brain regions, especially at short-echo time acquisitions (<100 ms). This is important because some of the metabolite resonances are visible only at shorter echo time MRS (e.g., myoinositol, glutamate, lactate, lipids).

Aside from technical issues related to the MRS acquisition, many clinical variables may influence the metabolite measurements. For example, the duration of abstinence from the drug use, the cumulative amount of drug exposure, age of the drug exposure, and comorbid drug use (e.g., tobacco or marijuana smoking) all may affect the brain metabolite levels. Therefore, study designs and interpretations of the metabolite levels from MRS need to include these variables. Furthermore, normal variations in brain metabolites can be caused by sex differences (e.g., men have higher choline than women in the frontal WM) and age-dependent changes (e.g., tCR increase and Glu decrease with age), which need to be controlled when evaluating brain metabolite abnormalities in drug users.

Future studies with advanced MRS techniques may further assess other neurochemicals that may be affected with drug dependence. For example, glutathione levels can be measured to assess the oxidative capacity of brain tissue using MEGA-PRESS or 2-D MRS techniques. Similarly, glutamate levels are difficult to delineate and may be better assessed using these same techniques. Given the abundance of glutamatergic neurons and the important role of glutamate in addiction, more MRS studies to evaluate this neurochemical are needed. More studies are also needed to determine whether MRS may be a useful surrogate marker for predicting treatment outcomes. MRS may be used along with other neuroimaging techniques as endophenotypes to evaluate genetic variations or deletions on how the brain may be impacted by drugs of abuse (e.g., rare copy number deletions in AUD [Yeo et al., 2011]) and to predict the likelihood of relapse, which may guide treatment approaches. Because MRS can be performed noninvasively in both humans and in animals, it can be a powerful research tool for clinical-translational studies, especially those that require longitudinal assessments (e.g., MRS were performed in both humans and rodents during alcohol withdrawal and abstinence [Hermann et al., 2012b]).

DISCLOSURES

Dr. Chang has no conflicts of interest to disclose. Dr. Chang is funded by the National Institutes of Health (K24-DA016170, R24-DA027318, R01-DA035659, U54-NS056883).

Dr. Cloak has no conflicts of interest to disclose. Dr Cloak is funded by the National Institutes of Health (K01-DA021203), and the Hawaii CommunityFoundation (Geist Foundation: 12ADVC-51341).

Dr. Holt has no conflicts of interest to disclose.

REFERENCES

Alkan, A., Kutlu, R., et al. (2004). Occupational prolonged organic solvent exposure in shoemakers: brain MR spectroscopy findings. *Magn. Reson. Imaging* 22:707–713.

Aydin, K., Sencer, S., et al. (2003). Single-voxel proton MR spectroscopy in toluene abuse. *Magn. Reson. Imaging* 21:777–785.

Bartlett, E., and Mikulis, D.J. (2005). Chasing "chasing the dragon" with MRI: leukoencephalopathy in drug abuse. *Br. J. Radiol.* 78:997–1004.

Bartsch, A.J., Homola, G., et al. (2007). Manifestations of early brain recovery associated with abstinence from alcoholism. *Brain* 130:36–47.

Behar, K.L., Rothman, D.L., et al. (1999). Preliminary evidence of low cortical GABA levels in localized 1H-MR spectra of alcohol-dependent and hepatic encephalopathy patients. *Am. J. Psychiatry* 156:952–954.

Bendszus, M., Weijers, H.G., et al. (2001). Sequential MR imaging and proton MR spectroscopy in patients who underwent recent detoxification for chronic alcoholism: correlation with clinical and neuropsychological data. *Am. J. Neuroradiol.* 22:1926–1932.

Birken, D.L., and Oldendorf, W.H. (1989). N-acetyl-L-aspartic acid: a literature review of a compound prominent in 1H-NMR spectroscopic studies of brain. *Neurosci. Biobehav. Rev.* 13:23–31.

Brand, A., Richter-Landsberg, C., et al. (1993). Multinuclear NMR studies on the energy metabolism of glial and neuronal cells. *Dev. Neurosci.* 15:289–298.

Chang, L., Cloak, C.C., et al. (2003). Magnetic resonance spectroscopy studies of GABA in neuropsychiatric disorders. *J. Clin. Psychiatry* 64 (Suppl 3):7–14.

Chang, L., Cloak, C., et al. (2009). Altered neurometabolites and motor integration in children exposed to methamphetamine *in utero*. *Neuroimage* 48:391–397.

Chang, L., Cloak, C., et al. (2006). Combined and independent effects of chronic marijuana use and HIV on brain metabolites. *J. Neuroimmune Pharmacol.* 1:65–76.

Chang, L., Ernst, T., et al. (1999a). Cerebral (1)H MRS alterations in recreational 3, 4-methylenedioxymethamphetamine (MDMA, "ecstasy") users. *J. Magn. Reson. Imaging* 10:521–526.

Chang, L., Ernst, T., et al. (2005). Additive effects of HIV and chronic methamphetamine use on brain metabolite abnormalities. *Am. J. Psychiatry* 162:361–369.

Chang, L., Ernst, T., et al. (1999b). Gender effects on persistent cerebral metabolite changes in the frontal lobes of abstinent cocaine users. *Am. J. Psychiatry* 156:716–722.

Chang, L., Mehringer, C.M., et al. (1997). Neurochemical alterations in asymptomatic abstinent cocaine users: a proton magnetic resonance spectroscopy study. *Biol. Psychiatry* 42:1105–1114.

Christensen, J.D., Kaufman, M.J., et al. (2000). Proton magnetic resonance spectroscopy of human basal ganglia: response to cocaine administration. *Biol. Psychiatry* 48:685–692.

Christensen, J.D., Kaufman, M.J., et al. (1996). Abnormal cerebral metabolism in polydrug abusers during early withdrawal: a 31P MR spectroscopy study. *Magn. Reson. Med.* 35:658–663.

Cloak, C.C., Alicata, D., et al. (2011). Age and sex effects levels of choline compounds in the anterior cingulate cortex of adolescent methamphetamine users. *Drug Alcohol Depend.* 119:207–215.

Cowan, R.L., Bolo, N.R., et al. (2007). Occipital cortical proton MRS at 4 Tesla in human moderate MDMA polydrug users. *Psychiatry Res.* 155:179–188.

Cowan, R.L., Joers, J.M., et al. (2009). N-acetylaspartate (NAA) correlates inversely with cannabis use in a frontal language processing region of neocortex in MDMA (Ecstasy) polydrug users: a 3 T magnetic resonance spectroscopy study. *Pharmacol. Biochem. Behav.* 92:105–110.

Daeppen, J.B., Smith, T.L., et al. (2000). Clinical correlates of cigarette smoking and nicotine dependence in alcohol-dependent men and women: the Collaborative Study Group on the Genetics of Alcoholism. *Alcohol Alcohol.* 35:171–175.

Daumann, J., Fischermann, T., et al. (2004). Proton magnetic resonance spectroscopy in ecstasy (MDMA) users. *Neurosci. Lett.* 362:113–116.

de Win, M.M., Jager, G., et al. (2008a). Sustained effects of ecstasy on the human brain: a prospective neuroimaging study in novel users. *Brain* 131:2936–2945.

de Win, M.M., Jager, G., et al. (2008b). Neurotoxic effects of ecstasy on the thalamus. *Br. J. Psychiatry* 193:289–296.

de Win, M.M., Reneman, L., et al. (2007). A prospective cohort study on sustained effects of low-dose ecstasy use on the brain in new ecstasy users. *Neuropsychopharmacology* 32:458–470.

Durazzo, T.C., Gazdzinski, S., et al. (2004). Cigarette smoking exacerbates chronic alcohol-induced brain damage: a preliminary metabolite imaging study. *Alcohol Clin. Exp. Res.* 28:1849–1860.

Durazzo, T.C., Gazdzinski, S., et al. (2006). Brain metabolite concentrations and neurocognition during short-term recovery from alcohol dependence: preliminary evidence of the effects of concurrent chronic cigarette smoking. *Alcohol Clin. Exp. Res.* 30:539–551.

Durazzo, T.C., Gazdzinski, S., et al. (2008). Combined neuroimaging, neurocognitive and psychiatric factors to predict alcohol consumption following treatment for alcohol dependence. *Alcohol Alcohol.* 43:683–691.

Durazzo, T.C., Pathak, V., et al. (2010). Metabolite levels in the brain reward pathway discriminate those who remain abstinent from those who resume hazardous alcohol consumption after treatment for alcohol dependence. *J. Stud. Alcohol Drugs* 71:278–289.

Ende, G., Walter, S., et al. (2006). Alcohol consumption significantly influences the MR signal of frontal choline-containing compounds. *NeuroImage* 32:740–746.

Ende, G., Welzel, H., et al. (2005). Monitoring the effects of chronic alcohol consumption and abstinence on brain metabolism: a longitudinal proton magnetic resonance spectroscopy study. *Biol. Psychiatry* 58:974–980.

Epperson, C.N., O'Malley, S., et al. (2005). Sex, GABA, and Nicotine: The impact of smoking on cortical GABA levels across the menstrual cycle as measured with proton magnetic resonance spectroscopy. *Biol. Psychiatry.* 57:44–48.

Ernst, T., Chang, L., et al. (2000). Evidence for long-term neurotoxicity associated with methamphetamine abuse: A 1H MRS study. *Neurology* 54:1344–1349.

Ernst T, Chang L. (2008). Adaptation of brain glutamate plus glutamine during abstinence from chronic methamphetamine use. *J. Neuroimmune Pharmacol.* 3(3):165–172.

Fein, G., and Landman, B. (2005). Treated and treatment-naive alcoholics come from different populations. *Alcohol* 36:19–26.

Fein, G., Meyerhoff, D.J., et al. (1994). 1H magnetic resonance spectroscopic imaging separates neuronal from glial changes in alcohol-related brain atrophy. In: Lancaster, F.E., ed. Alcohol and Glial Cells. Bethesda, MD: National Institutes of Health, National Institute on Alcohol Abuse and Alcoholism, pp. 227–241.

Gallinat, J., Lang, U.E., et al. (2007). Abnormal hippocampal neurochemistry in smokers: evidence from proton magnetic resonance spectroscopy at 3 T. *J. Clin. Psychopharmacol.* 27:80–84.

Gazdzinski, S., Durazzo, T.C., et al. (2008a). Are treated alcoholics representative of the entire population with alcohol use disorders? A magnetic resonance study of brain injury. *Alcohol* 42:67–76.

Gazdzinski, S., Durazzo, T.C., et al. (2008b). Chronic cigarette smoking modulates injury and short-term recovery of the medial temporal lobe in alcoholics. *Psychiatry Res.* 162:133–145.

Harding, A.J., Wong, A., et al. (1997). Chronic alcohol consumption does not cause hippocampal neuron loss in humans. *Hippocampus* 7:78–87.

Harper, C. (2009). The neuropathology of alcohol-related brain damage. *Alcohol Alcohol.* 44:136–140.

Haselhorst, R., Dursteler-MacFarland, K.M., et al. (2002). Frontocortical N-acetylaspartate reduction associated with long-term i.v. heroin use. *Neurology* 58:305–307.

Hermann, D., Frischknecht, U., et al. (2012a). MR spectroscopy in opiate maintenance therapy: association of glutamate with the number of previous withdrawals in the anterior cingulate cortex. *Addict. Biol.* 17:659–667.

Hermann, D., Sartorius, A., et al. (2007). Dorsolateral prefrontal cortex N-acetylaspartate/total creatine (NAA/tCR) loss in male recreational cannabis users. *Biol. Psychiatry* 61:1281–1289.

Hermann, D., Weber-Fahr, W., et al. (2012b). Translational magnetic resonance spectroscopy reveals excessive central glutamate levels during alcohol withdrawal in humans and rats. *Biol. Psychiatry* 71:1015–1021.

Jagannathan, N.R., Desai, N.G., et al. (1996). Brain metabolite changes in alcoholism: an *in vivo* proton magnetic resonance spectroscopy (MRS) study. *Magn. Reson. Imaging* 14:553–557.

Kaufman, M.J., Pollack, M.H., et al. (1999). Cerebral phosphorus metabolite abnormalities in opiate-dependent polydrug abusers in methadone maintenance. *Psychiatry Res.* 90:143–152.

Ke, Y., Streeter, C.C., et al. (2004). Frontal lobe GABA levels in cocaine dependence: a two-dimensional, J-resolved magnetic resonance spectroscopy study. *Psychiatry Res.* 130:283–293.

Korbo, L. (1999). Glial cell loss in the hippocampus of alcoholics. *Alcohol Clin. Exp. Res.* 23:164–168.

Kriegstein, A.R., Shungu, D.C., et al. (1999). Leukoencephalopathy and raised brain lactate from heroin vapor inhalation ("chasing the dragon"). *Neurology* 53:1765–1773.

Kril, J.J., and Halliday, G.M. (1999). Brain shrinkage in alcoholics: a decade on and what have we learned? *Prog. Neurobiol.* 58:381–387.

Lee, E., Jang, D.P., et al. (2007). Alteration of brain metabolites in young alcoholics without structural changes. *Neuroreport* 18:1511–1514.

Li, S.J., Wang, Y., et al. (1999). Neurochemical adaptation to cocaine abuse: reduction of N-acetyl aspartate in thalamus of human cocaine abusers. *Biol. Psychiatry* 45:1481–1487.

Licata, S.C., and Renshaw, P.F. (2010). Neurochemistry of drug action: insights from proton magnetic resonance spectroscopic imaging and their relevance to addiction. *Ann. NY Acad. Sci.* 1187:148–171.

Mader, I., Rauer, S., et al. (2008). (1)H MR spectroscopy of inflammation, infection and ischemia of the brain. *Eur. J. Radiol.* 67:250–257.

Martin, P.R., Gibbs, S.J., et al. (1995). Brain proton magnetic resonance spectroscopy studies in recently abstinent alcoholics. *Alcohol Clin. Exp. Res.* 19:1078–1082.

Mashhoon, Y., Janes, A.C., et al. (2011). Anterior cingulate proton spectroscopy glutamate levels differ as a function of smoking cessation outcome. *Prog. Neuropsychopharmacol. Biol. Psychiatry* 35:1709–1713.

Mason, G.F., Petrakis, I.L., et al. (2006). Cortical Gamma-Aminobutyric acid levels and the recovery from ethanol dependence: Preliminary evidence of modification by cigarette smoking. *Biol. Psychiatry.* 59:85–93.

McDonald, J.W., and Johnston, M.V. (1990). Physiological and pathophysiological roles of excitatory amino acids during central nervous system development. *Brain Res. Brain Res. Rev.* 15:41–70.

McGrath, B.M., McKay, R., et al. (2008). Acute dextro-amphetamine administration does not alter brain myo-inositol levels in humans and animals: MRS investigations at 3 and 18.8 T. *Neurosci. Res.* 61:351–359.

Meyerhoff, D.J., Bloomer, C., et al. (1999). Cortical metabolite alterations in abstinent cocaine and cocaine/alcohol-dependent subjects: proton magnetic resonance spectroscopic imaging. *Addict. Biol.* 4:405–419.

Meyerhoff, D.J., Blumenfeld, R., et al. (2004). Effects of heavy drinking, binge drinking, and family history of alcoholism on regional brain metabolites. *Alcohol Clin. Exp. Res.* 28:650–661.

Meyerhoff, D.J., Durazzo, T.C., et al. (2013). Chronic alcohol consumption, abstinence and relapse: brain proton magnetic resonance spectroscopy studies in animals and humans. *Curr. Top. Behav. Neurosci.* 13:511–540.

Miguel-Hidalgo, J.J., Overholser, J.C., et al. (2006). Reduced glial and neuronal packing density in the orbitofrontal cortex in alcohol dependence and its relationship with suicide and duration of alcohol dependence. *Alcohol Clin. Exp. Res.* 30:1845–1855.

Miguel-Hidalgo, J.J., Wei, J., et al. (2002). Glia pathology in the prefrontal cortex in alcohol dependence with and without depressive symptoms. *Biol. Psychiatry* 52:1121–1133.

Miller, B.L. (1991). A review of chemical issues in 1H NMR spectroscopy: N-acetyl-L-aspartate, creatine and choline. *NMR Biomed.* 4:47–52.

Modi, S., Bhattacharya, M., et al. (2011). Brain metabolite changes in alcoholism: localized proton magnetic resonance spectroscopy study of the occipital lobe. *Eur. J. Radiol.* 79:96–100.

Mon, A., Durazzo, T.C., et al. (2012). Glutamate, GABA, and other cortical metabolite concentrations during early abstinence from alcohol and their associations with neurocognitive changes. *Drug Alcohol Depend.* 125:27–36.

Monnig, M.A., Tonigan, J.S., et al. (2012). White matter volume in alcohol use disorders: a meta-analysis. *Addict. Biol.* 10.1111/j.1369-1600.2012.00441.x. [Epub ahead of print.]

Nery, F.G., Stanley, J.A., et al. (2010). Bipolar disorder comorbid with alcoholism: a 1H magnetic resonance spectroscopy study. *J. Psychiatr. Res.* 44:278–285.

Noda, S., Yamanouchi, N., et al. (1996). Proton MR spectroscopy in solvent abusers. *Ann. NY Acad. Sci.* 801:441–444.

Nordahl, T.E., Salo, R., et al. (2005). Methamphetamine users in sustained abstinence: a proton magnetic resonance spectroscopy study. *Arch. Gen. Psychiatry* 62:444–452.

O'Neill, J., Cardenas, V.A., et al. (2001a). Effects of abstinence on the brain: quantitative magnetic resonance imaging and magnetic resonance spectroscopic imaging in chronic alcohol abuse. *Alcohol Clin. Exp. Res.* 25:1673–1682.

O'Neill, J., Cardenas, V.A., et al. (2001b). Separate and interactive effects of cocaine and alcohol dependence on brain structures and metabolites: quantitative MRI and proton MR spectroscopic imaging. *Addict. Biol.* 6:347–361.

Obergriesser, T., Ende, G., et al. (2001). Hippocampal 1H-MRSI in ecstasy users. *Eur. Arch. Psychiatry Clin. Neurosci.* 251:114–116.

Offiah, C., and Hall, E. (2008). Heroin-induced leukoencephalopathy: characterization using MRI, diffusion-weighted imaging, and MR spectroscopy. *Clin. Radiol.* 63:146–152.

Parks, M.H., Dawant, B.M., et al. (2002). Longitudinal brain metabolic characterization of chronic alcoholics with proton magnetic resonance spectroscopy. *Alcohol Clin. Exp. Res.* 26:1368–1380.

Plaitakis, A., and Shashidharan, P. (2000). Glutamate transport and metabolism in dopaminergic neurons of substantia nigra: implications for the pathogenesis of Parkinson's disease. *J. Neurol.* 247(Suppl 2):II25–II35.

Prescot, A.P., Locatelli, A.E., et al. (2011). Neurochemical alterations in adolescent chronic marijuana smokers: a proton MRS study. *Neuroimage* 57:69–75.

Reneman, L., Majoie, C.B., et al. (2002). Reduced N-acetylaspartate levels in the frontal cortex of 3,4-methylenedioxymethamphetamine (Ecstasy) users: preliminary results. *Am. J. Neuroradiol.* 23:231–237.

Reneman, L., Majoie, C.B., et al. (2001). Prefrontal N-acetylaspartate is strongly associated with memory performance in (abstinent) ecstasy users: preliminary report. *Biol. Psychiatry* 50:550–554.

Romberger, D.J., and Grant, K. (2004). Alcohol consumption and smoking status: the role of smoking cessation. *Biomed. Pharmacother.* 58:77–83.

Ross, B., Kreis, R., et al. (1992). Clinical tools for the 90s: magnetic resonance spectroscopy and metabolite imaging. *Eur. J. Radiol.* 14:128–140.

Sailasuta, N., Abulseoud, O., et al. (2010). Glial dysfunction in abstinent methamphetamine abusers. *J. Cereb. Blood Flow Metab.* 30:950–960.

Salgado, R.A., Jorens, P.G., et al. (2010). Methadone-induced toxic leukoencephalopathy: MR imaging and MR proton spectroscopy findings. *Am. J. Neuroradiol.* 31:565–566.

Salo, R., Nordahl, T.E., et al. (2007). Attentional control and brain metabolite levels in methamphetamine abusers. *Biol. Psychiatry* 61:1272–1280.

Salo, R., Buonocore, M.H., et al. (2011). Extended findings of brain metabolite normalization in MA-dependent subjects across sustained abstinence: a proton MRS study. *Drug Alcohol Depend.* 113:133–138.

Salo, R., Nordahl, T.E., et al. (2011). Spatial inhibition and the visual cortex: a magnetic resonance spectroscopy imaging study. *Neuropsychologia.* 49:830–838.

Schmaal, L., Veltman, D.J., et al. (2012). N-acetylcysteine normalizes glutamate levels in cocaine-dependent patients: a randomized crossover magnetic resonance spectroscopy study. *Neuropsychopharmacology* 37:2143–2152.

Schuff, N., Meyerhoff, D.J., et al. (2006). N-acetylaspartate as a marker of neuronal injury in neurodegenerative disease. *Adv. Exp. Med. Biol.* 576:241–262; discussion 361–363.

Schweinsburg, B.C., Taylor, M.J., et al. (2001). Chemical pathology in brain white matter of recently detoxified alcoholics: a 1H magnetic resonance spectroscopy investigation of alcohol-associated frontal lobe injury. *Alcohol Clin. Exp. Res.* 25:924–934.

Schweinsburg, B.C., Taylor, M.J., et al. (2000). Elevated myo-inositol in gray matter of recently detoxified but not long-term abstinent alcoholics: a preliminary MR spectroscopy study. *Alcohol Clin. Exp. Res.* 24:699–705.

Seitz, D., Widmann, U., et al. (1999). Localized proton magnetic resonance spectroscopy of the cerebellum in detoxifying alcoholics. *Alcohol Clin. Exp. Res.* 23:158–163.

Sekine, Y., Minabe, Y., et al. (2002). Metabolite alterations in basal ganglia associated with methamphetamine-related psychiatric symptoms. A proton MRS study. *Neuropsychopharmacology* 27:453–461.

Silveri, M.M., Jensen, J.E., et al. (2011). Preliminary evidence for white matter metabolite differences in marijuana-dependent young men using 2D J-resolved magnetic resonance spectroscopic imaging at 4 Tesla. *Psychiatry Res.* 191:201–211.

Silveri, M.M., Pollack, M.H., et al. (2004). Cerebral phosphorus metabolite and transverse relaxation time abnormalities in heroin-dependent subjects at onset of methadone maintenance treatment. *Psychiatry Res.* 131:217–226.

Silverstone, P.H., O'Donnell, T., et al. (2002). Dextro-amphetamine increases phosphoinositol cycle activity in volunteers: an MRS study. *Hum. Psychopharmacol.* 17:425–429.

Smith, L.M., Chang, L., et al. (2001a). Brain proton magnetic resonance spectroscopy and imaging in children exposed to cocaine in utero. *Pediatrics* 107:227–231.

Smith, L.M., Chang, L., et al. (2001b). Brain proton magnetic resonance spectroscopy in children exposed to methamphetamine in utero. *Neurology* 57:255–260.

Streeter, C.C., Hennen, J., et al. (2005). Prefrontal GABA levels in cocaine-dependent subjects increase with pramipexole and venlafaxine treatment. *Psychopharmacology (Berl.)* 182:516–526.

Sullivan, E.V., and Pfefferbaum, A. (2005). Neurocircuitry in alcoholism: a substrate of disruption and repair. *Psychopharmacology (Berl.)* 180:583–594.

Sung, Y.H., Cho, S.C., et al. (2007). Relationship between N-acetyl-aspartate in gray and white matter of abstinent methamphetamine abusers and their history of drug abuse: a proton magnetic resonance spectroscopy study. *Drug Alcohol Depend.* 88:28–35.

Takebayashi, K., Sekine, Y., et al. (2004). Metabolite alterations in basal ganglia associated with psychiatric symptoms of abstinent toluene users: a proton MRS study. *Neuropsychopharmacology* 29:1019–1026.

Taylor, M.J., Schweinsburg, B.C., et al. (2007). Effects of human immunodeficiency virus and methamphetamine on cerebral metabolites measured with magnetic resonance spectroscopy. *J. Neurovirol.* 13:150–159.

Thoma, R., Mullins, P., et al. (2011). Perturbation of the glutamate-glutamine system in alcohol dependence and remission. *Neuropsychopharmacology* 36:1359–1365.

Tsai, G., and Coyle, J.T. (1995). N-acetylaspartate in neuropsychiatric disorders. *Prog. Neurobiol.* 46:531–540.

Umhau, J.C., Momenan, R., et al. (2010) Effect of acamprosate on magnetic resonance spectroscopy measures of central glutamate in detoxified alcohol-dependent individuals. *Arch. Gen. Psychiatry* 67(10):1069–77.

Vella, S., Kreis, R., et al. (2003). Acute leukoencephalopathy after inhalation of a single dose of heroin. *Neuropediatrics* 34:100–104.

Wang, J.J., Durazzo, T.C., et al. (2009). MRSI and DTI: a multimodal approach for improved detection of white matter abnormalities in alcohol and nicotine dependence. *NMR Biomed.* 22:516–522.

Worley, P.F., Baraban, J.M., et al. (1987). Inositol trisphosphate receptor localization in brain: variable stoichiometry with protein kinase C. *Nature* 325:159–161.

Yang, S., Salmeron, B.J., et al. (2009). Lower glutamate levels in rostral anterior cingulate of chronic cocaine users: A (1)H-MRS study using TE-averaged PRESS at 3 T with an optimized quantification strategy. *Psychiatry Res.* 174:171–176.

Yeo, R.A., Gangestad, S.W., et al. (2011). Rare copy number deletions predict individual variation in human brain metabolite concentrations in individuals with alcohol use disorders. *Biol. Psychiatry* 70:537–544.

Yoon, S.J., Lyoo, I.K., et al. (2010). Neurochemical alterations in methamphetamine-dependent patients treated with cytidine-5′-diphosphate choline: a longitudinal proton magnetic resonance spectroscopy study. *Neuropsychopharmacology* 35:1165–1173.

Yucel, M., Lubman, D.I., et al. (2007). A combined spectroscopic and functional MRI investigation of the dorsal anterior cingulate region in opiate addiction. *Mol. Psychiatry* 12:611, 691–702.

57 | PHARMACOTHERAPY OF SUBSTANCE USE DISORDERS

JANE B. ACRI AND PHIL SKOLNICK

OVERVIEW

There has been a dramatic retreat from research and development of medications to treat psychiatric disorders over the past four to five years (Brady and Insel, 2012; Jarvis, 2012; Paul et al., 2010). Moreover, the development of pharmacotherapies to treat substance use disorders (SUDs) has traditionally lagged well behind efforts to develop novel medicines to treat other psychiatric disorders, including schizophrenia, depression, and anxiety. Thus, despite remarkable progress in our understanding of the neurobiological bases of drug abuse (Koob and Volkow, 2010), there are no approved pharmacotherapies to treat either stimulant (e.g., cocaine, methamphetamine) or cannabis abuse. Moreover, approved pharmacotherapies to treat other SUDs (e.g., opiates, tobacco) are far from ideal. For example, no more than 20% of smokers are able to sustain long term (12 month) abstinence, despite the availability of multiple options to treat tobacco dependence (nicotine replacement therapies, bupropion, and varenicline). Although heroin abuse remains a significant public health issue, abuse of prescription opioids is far more pervasive, with approximately 2% of the US population (age 12 and older) reporting nonmedical use of prescription opiates during the past month (2010 National Survey On Drug Use and Health; http://oas.samhsa.gov/nsduhLatest.htm). Here too, progress in developing medications to treat opiate addiction has been incremental, with reformulations of long approved medications (e.g., depot naltrexone, and implantable buprenorphine) aimed at enhancing adherence the most significant therapeutic advances in this area. This lack of progress is attributable, in large part, to a lack of interest (and investment) by the pharmaceutical industry. There are multiple factors that contribute to this indifference, ranging from a perceived small market size (translating to a lack of return on investment) to the perception of a high regulatory bar for approval, as detailed in the following.

ECONOMIC CONSIDERATIONS

The development of a new chemical entity, from the laboratory through FDA approval, generally requires more than 15 years and a capital outlay estimated between $1 and 2 billion (Paul et al., 2010). More recently, it has been argued that these values grossly underestimate the true costs of bringing a drug to market, which may range from $4 to 11 billion (http://www.forbes.com/sites/matthewherper/2012/02/10/the-truly-staggering-cost-of-inventing-new-drugs/). Given the cost and risks associated with drug development, a perceived small market size is one of the reasons most often given for the limited interest in developing medications to treat SUDs. However, with several available treatment options including methadone, Subutex®, and Vivitrol®, annual sales well in excess of $1 billion for Suboxone® (a combination of sublingual naloxone and buprenorphine that discourages abuse) belie the notion that the treatment of SUDs is not an attractive market. Perhaps even more compelling is an estimate of the market size for a first in class medication to treat cocaine use disorders. Based on a 2009 survey by SAMSHA, 1.6 million Americans used cocaine in the past month. If this population, rather than the much larger (>5 million) cohort who reported using cocaine in the past year is considered as the target treatment group, and 20% of this cohort seek treatment, the potential market is 320,000 patients. Assuming treatment duration of six months to achieve abstinence at a cost of $700/month, annual sales for this medication would be in excess of $1.2 billion. Although both the cost and duration of treatment are clearly assumptions, the current cost of Vivitrol® (approximately $1,200/month) can be viewed as a valid comparator. Thus, many third-party payors will reimburse because of the favorable health and economic outcomes compared with other types of maintenance therapy (Baser et al., 2011).

Most drug candidates for the treatment of SUDs are repurposed compounds that have either been approved, are currently in development, or have failed in another indication. Because of the contraction of research and development in psychiatry, there may be a bumper crop of "parked" molecules available with the potential to treat SUDs on the near-term horizon. These compounds were in various stages of development that were either halted for strategic reasons, and cannot be out-licensed or otherwise monetized. Although repurposing is clearly a less costly strategy than a *de novo* development campaign, approval would nonetheless require multiple, double-blind, placebo-controlled efficacy trials. Although off label prescribing of drugs is an option, FDA approval (amounting to a change in current labeling) is important both for reimbursement by third payors and establishing treatment guidelines. In the absence of patent protection, the effectiveness of a repurposing strategy is questionable, absent some form of de jure economic incentives such as a period of market exclusivity.

DIFFICULTIES IN EXECUTING A CLINICAL CAMPAIGN

Pharmacotherapy trials in SUDs pose unique challenges that can dampen sponsor enthusiasm. Thus, treatment centers specializing in SUDs are often either not equipped or trained to conduct a trial based on good clinical practice guidelines that are essential for FDA approval. Patients with SUDs, particularly intravenous drug users, often have comorbid conditions, including HIV and hepatitis C. If these individuals are enrolled in a trial, concomitant medications administered to these patients such as cocktails of antiretroviral therapies (Perelson et al., 1997) pose formidable drug interaction challenges. In addition, interpretation of negative data in SUD trials may be confounded by low rates of medication adherence. When monitored by measurement of drug levels in urine, the compliance rate has been reported at less than 40% in a trial examining the effects of vigabatrin in cocaine use disorder (http://ir.catalystpharma.com press release 9.30.2009). In contrast, compliance assessed by self- report/pill count was ~85%. This trial failed to replicate an earlier study (Brodie et al., 2009) demonstrating that vigabatrin produced a significant increase (28% vs. 7.5% in placebo) in the percentage of abstinent individuals at end of study. However, the Brodie et al. (2009) study required three weekly in-clinic doses of vigabatrin, whereas the study with a negative outcome was an outpatient trial. In a study assessing the efficacy of modafinil in treating methamphetamine use disorder, Anderson et al. (2012) recently reported very low agreement (intraclass correlation coefficient, 0.21) between compliance assessed by pill count/self-report (93% rate of compliance) and weekly measurement of modafinil in urine. Approximately 10% of the subjects never had detectable levels of modafinil in urine during the entire 12 week trial. Thus, it is perhaps not surprising there were no significant differences between the modafinil and placebo groups on either primary or secondary outcomes. Noncompliance is an important and often overlooked issue in both the conduct of clinical trials (Czobor and Skolnick, 2011) and real world practice (Cutler and Everett, 2010), but may be viewed as particularly cogent in the absence of approved medications to treat cocaine, methamphetamine and cannabis use disorders.

REGULATORY HURDLES

In contrast to other psychiatric disorders, medication trials in SUDs can assess efficacy with a biomarker measuring the abused substance in a biological matrix such as urine. A clean (drug-free) urine (generally sampled two–three times/week during an in clinic visit) is generally taken as prima facie evidence that a medication is effective in reducing or eliminating drug use. Many contemporary medications trials look at group means (i.e., the percentage of patients with drug free urine) over the course of a study (Heinzerling et al., 2010; Jayaram-Lindstrom et al., 2008; Shearer et al., 2009).

Although positive signals have been reported from this type of analysis (e.g., naltrexone reducing the percentage of patients with cocaine-positive urines during the course of a 12-week trial; see Fig. 57.1), the FDA currently views an analysis based on success/failure, rather than reduction in group means, as an acceptable outcome measure (Winchell et al., 2012). The success must be clinically meaningful, preferably defined by a period of abstinence that lasts through the end of treatment (reviewed in Donovan et al., 2012; McCann and Li, 2011). Blunting of subjective ratings related drug effects such as liking and wanting as well as reductions in craving scale scores (e.g., Jayaram-Lindstrom et al., 2008) would not likely be viewed as a primary outcome measure unless associated with a salutary outcome for the patient (Donovan et al., 2012).

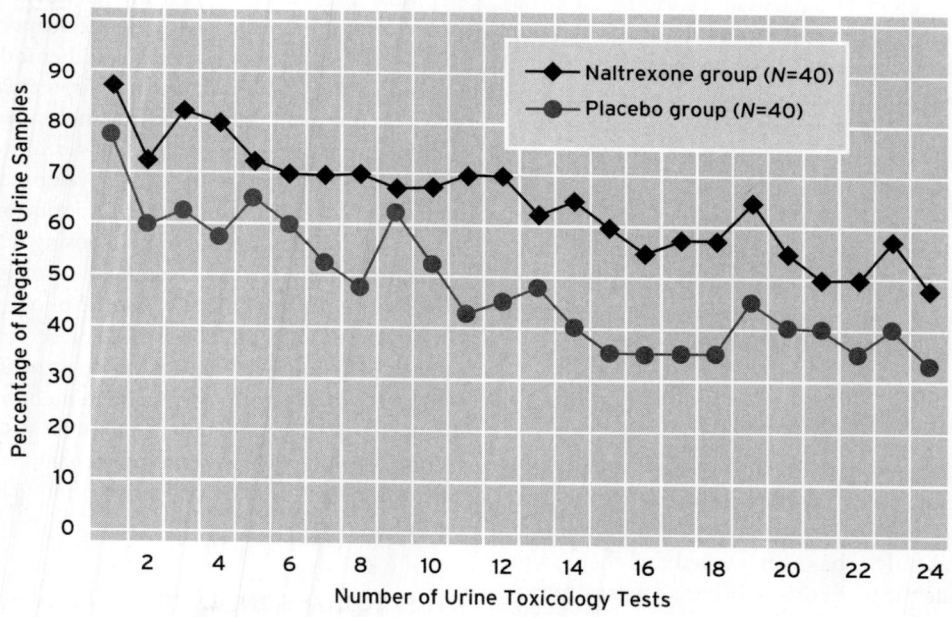

Figure 57.1 *Percentage of negative urine samples in the naltrexone (N =40) and placebo (N =40) groups during a 12-week trial for the treatment of amphetamine dependence (Intent to treat analysis). The FDA does not accept analyses based on reduction in group means but currently views an analysis based on success/failure, defined as a period of abstinence at the end of the trial as a clinically meaningful endpoint (Winchell et al., 2012). (Data and Image from Jayaram-Lindstrom N, Hammarberg A, Beck O, and Franck J. 2008 with permission from the American Psychiatric Association.)*

Abstinence may be viewed as analogous to remission in other psychiatric disorders. When viewed in this context, abstinence may be considered a very high, perhaps unattainable or unrealistic endpoint for a medication, even if combined with psychotherapy (Donovan et al., 2012). Certainly, drugs have been approved for the treatment of other psychiatric disorders (e.g., schizophrenia) if there is a statistically significant improvement in a subset of symptoms (e.g., positive symptoms) absent complete remission. However, a compelling counterargument can be made that this analogy is flawed, because no amount of an illegal substance can be linked to a beneficial health outcome. Indeed, for this reason, sustained abstinence is the primary outcome measure in contemporary smoking cessation trials (Hatsukami et al., 2011). Although many experts have proposed reduced use as an acceptable outcome in clinical trials (Donovan et al., 2012), reduced use per se (e.g., a 50% reduction in the frequency or amount of cocaine used) may not provide clear expectations for the prescriber or patient. Further, it may not be realistic to expect reimbursement by third party payors for a medication that results in reduced use, absent evidence that reduced use will produce a tangible, measurable benefit for the patient (and thereby reduce health costs for the insurer). Certainly, drugs such as varenicline that have been approved for smoking cessation produce a significantly higher rate of long-term abstinence compared with placebo (Fagerstrom et al., 2012). There are also notable examples of producing short-term abstinence to cocaine (vigabatrin; Brodie et al., 2009) and methamphetamine (bupropion; McCann and Li, 2011) compared with placebo in double-blind, placebo-controlled trials, but these studies require replication.

OTHER ISSUES

There are other issues that have prevented the pharmaceutical industry from viewing SUDs (other than smoking cessation medications) as an attractive market. Often mentioned are the negative aspects of linking a company's name and reputation with the use of illegal substances. A fragmented advocacy, sending mixed, and often contradictory and polarizing messages (" … why substitute one addiction for another") about treatment of SUDs also can intimidate potential investors. Nonetheless, the commercial success of a medication like Suboxone®, which entered an arguably crowded space (including methadone, buprenorphine, and naloxone), may serve as an impetus for investment, especially in SUDs for which there are no approved medications.

ANIMAL MODELS

There is no single animal model that can either adequately capture all aspects and stages of SUDs (e.g., reward, conditioning, craving, acquisition, maintenance, withdrawal) or that is necessarily predictive of clinical efficacy. Thus, targets and compounds are viewed as high value if they are active in several models, and when studies in genetically engineered animals (e.g., when the gene encoding the target is silenced) are consistent with results from these models. Several commonly used animal models are briefly discussed in the following text. There are variations of each procedure, and there is an ongoing debate regarding the aspects of drug abuse that each model captures, as well as their appropriateness and predictive validity to evaluate potential medications (Koob et al., 2004). Treatments for SUDs are only considered effective if they alter drug-taking behavior in humans, rather than addressing the theoretical constructs of addiction, compulsion, or dependence. Therefore, compounds that selectively alter the behavior of drug taking in animals might be effective in altering drug taking in humans, whether or not the model has captured all aspects of addiction.

The etiology of human drug abuse cannot be adequately modeled in animals beyond one significant and overriding factor, exposure to the drug of abuse. When animals are exposed to a drug of abuse, they undergo behavioral changes that are consistent with those that occur in humans: drug seeking and drug taking. In self-administration models, animals exposed to drugs of abuse will develop consistent patterns of behavior that result in self-administration depending on the drug, dose, duration of action, route of administration, operant training schedule, length of the session, and a number of additional environmental factors (see Mello and Negus, 1996 for review) (Fig. 57.2). It is the intrinsic reinforcing effects of the drug that maintain self-administration behavior, based on the observations that animals do not self-administer psychoactive drugs not producing pleasurable effects in humans (e.g., haloperidol, imipramine, or topiramate) (Balster, 1991; Brady et al., 1984; Griffiths and Balster, 1979). The self-administration model has been used to demonstrate the efficacy of FDA-approved medications for smoking (Le Foll et al., 2011; Levin et al., 2012; O'Connor et al., 2010), alcohol (Jimenez-Gomez et al., 2011), and opioids (Harrigan and Downs, 1981; Negus, 2006; Winger et al., 1992), but must be used with appropriate controls for non-specific effects. The examples of effective medications that reduce self-administration in animals suggest that use of the method has predictive validity, but the literature is rife with studies that either did not incorporate appropriate controls for sedating or other non-specific effects; or that did not address the dose of drug being self-administered in the test.

The conditioned place preference model utilizes Pavlovian conditioning processes in which environmental stimuli are coupled to administration of a drug of abuse resulting in a "preference" for the specific environment in which the drug was experienced. In this procedure, animals are placed in one distinctive chamber following an injection of drug, and in another distinctive chamber following administration of saline. After several pairings of drug and saline with their respective chambers, animals given free choice to roam between the two chambers will spend proportionally more time in the drug-paired chamber. This is generally interpreted as indicative of the intrinsic rewarding effect of the drug of abuse in which the chamber itself becomes a conditioned stimulus and a conditioned reward (see Schechter and Calcagnetti, 1998; Tzschentke, 2007, for reviews).

Animal models of relapse have been developed in part because cocaine use has been described as a chronic, relapsing

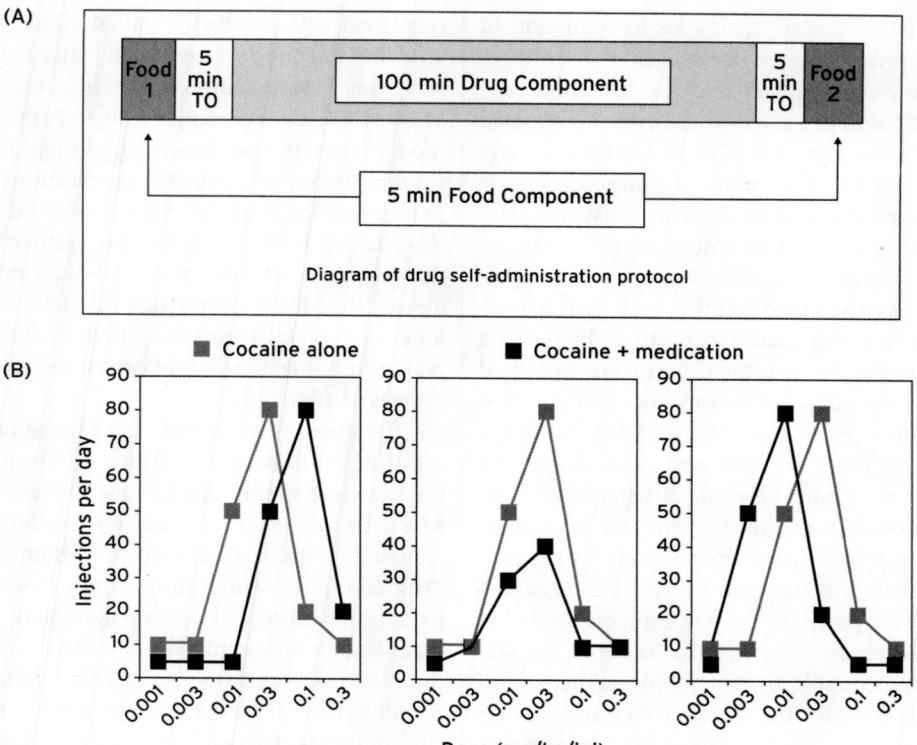

(A)

| Food 1 | 5 min TO | 100 min Drug Component | 5 min TO | Food 2 |

5 min Food Component

Diagram of drug self-administration protocol

(B)

■ Cocaine alone   ■ Cocaine + medication

Dose (mg/kg/inj)

Injections per day

Figure 57.2 (A) A self-administration protocol in which animals that are trained to self-administer cocaine also have the opportunity to lever press for food pellets after test medication administration but before exposure to cocaine (Food 1), and then again after exposure to cocaine (Food 2). This paradigm allows comparisons between changes in rates of lever pressing for food and cocaine in response to the same dose of test drug and in the same session. This is an important control for compounds that might reduce lever pressing for cocaine because of generalized CNS depression or motor impairment. (B) Illustration of the importance of assessing a test compound against the entire inverted-U shaped dose–effect curve of cocaine, in order to understand the nature of decreases in responding for the "peak" dose of cocaine, which can occur as a result of rightward, downward, or leftward shifts in the cocaine dose–effect curve. An assessment of a test compound against one dose of cocaine may yield misleading results. (Adapted from Mello N.K., and Negus S.S., 1996. Preclinical evaluation of pharmacotherapies for treatment of cocaine and opioid abuse using drug self-administration procedures. Neuropsychopharmacology 14 (6): 375–424.)

disorder based on epidemiological and experimental evidence that users can maintain abstinence for short periods of time, but typically report a resumption of use despite good intentions to remain abstinent. In clinical studies, the "triggers" for relapse have been described by self-report, and increasingly, by imaging studies aimed at addressing craving in humans. Although the contingencies involved in animal reinstatement studies and human relapse are not parallel, it is compelling that the same types of stimuli produce reinstatement in animals and reports of craving in humans. These so-called triggers consist of a priming effect of the drug (Gawin and Kleber, 1986, O'Brien et al., 1998), exposure to psychological stress (Fox et al., 2011; Sinha, 2001), and environmental stimuli or cues (Childress et al., 1993).

Relapse models (see Fig. 57.3) use variations of several behavioral paradigms. Most commonly, operant self-administration techniques are used, although there is an increasing use of the conditioned place preference paradigm for this purpose (Itzhak and Martin, 2002; Mueller and Stewart, 2000; Mueller et al., 2002). Most of the operant models involve training animals to self-administer a drug of abuse, followed by extinction or forced abstinence and subsequent reinstatement testing. That is, after a period of training in which responding reaches stable levels, animals undergo a period of either forced abstinence

where there is no opportunity to self-administer, or extinction, during which time lever pressing is not followed by drug availability, until responding reaches very low levels. Finally, animals are tested following exposure to one of the relapse triggers, and responding is said to be reinstated if lever-pressing ensues (see Bossert et al., 2005 and Epstein et al., 2006 for reviews).

A model called the "incubation of craving" examines the number of lever presses following different periods of forced abstinence, and has produced responses that increase over time in response to cues, but not to drug primes (Lu et al., 2004). This model can also be used to examine effects of compounds for possible clinical utility in blocking resumption of drug taking after a period of drug unavailability.

TARGETS FOR SUBSTANCE USE DISORDERS

Based on preclinical studies in established animal models of self-administration (Mello and Negus, 1996) and relapse (Epstein et al., 2006), multiple targets for intervention have been identified (Koob et al., 2009; Vocci et al., 2005). These targets range from "classical" biogenic amine receptors (e.g., Bubar and Cunningham, 2008; Heidbreder and Newman, 2010) that

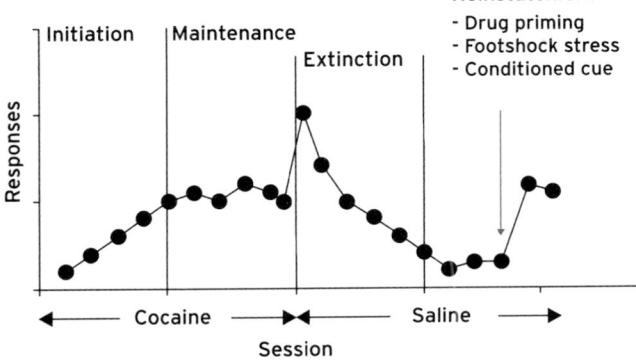

Figure 57.3 *Schematic diagram of operant reinstatement model illustrating the phases of training and the point at which testing occurs. During the initiation phase, animals are trained to self-administer cocaine and then subsequently maintained at stable levels of responding for a specified period of time. Then cocaine is replaced by saline in the infusion pump and animals undergo experimental "extinction," during which time the cocaine is absent and responding gradually falls to low level for a specified period of time. On the test day, animals are exposed to one of the three reinstatement triggers, which could be (1) a priming dose of cocaine, (2) an intermittent footshock stressor, or (3) a cue that was previously paired with cocaine infusions such as a light or tone. Any of these stimuli can reinstate responding at least to maintenance levels and usually higher. Doses of a test compound can be administered prior to the reinstatement trigger to determine if a compound can block reinstatement. Control studies of the effects of the test compound under extinction conditions for food responding are assessed in a different group of animals in order to control for non-specific effects on lever pressing behavior as a result of motor impairment or CNS depression.*

have long been linked to other psychiatric disorders to DNA modification (epigenetic) strategies (Adachi and Monteggia, 2009; Renthal et al., 2009; Robison and Nestler, 2011) and biological approaches (Skolnick and Volkow, 2011) aimed at limiting the entrance of abused substance (e.g., nicotine, cocaine) into the central nervous system (Fahim, 2011; Shen and Kosten, 2011). Although converging lines of evidence indicate that many of these targets may be valid, a significant subset may not be "druggable." From a drug development perspective, this means that it is not possible (within the known chemical space) to synthesize a compound with sufficient specificity, druglike (e.g., favorable solubility, absorption, metabolism, and distribution profile) and safety characteristics. From a biological perspective, a target may be so widely distributed and play such a fundamental role in cell homeostasis, that chronic target engagement (as would be required in toxicology and carcinogenicity studies) would result in unacceptable safety margins for an indication in SUDs.

Given the large number of potential targets and indications, molecules active in several models of SUDs (e.g., self-administration, cue- and prime-induced relapse) and against multiple substances of abuse (e.g., cocaine, nicotine) are of the highest potential value. There are several targets with molecules that fulfill these criteria, but among this subset, few have drug candidates that are sufficiently advanced (or approved) to enable a clinical test of the hypothesis. Several of the most promising targets that fulfill these criteria are described later.

TYPE 5 METABOTROPIC GLUTAMATE RECEPTORS

Type 5 metabotropic glutamate receptor antagonists and negative allosteric modulators (mGluR5) bind to a subclass of Group 1 metabotropic glutamate receptors and these compounds modulate glutamatergic neurotransmission in brain regions that converging lines of evidence have linked to CNS disorders (see Conn, 2003; Schoepp, 2001 for reviews). Over the past decade, accumulating evidence has begun to elucidate the role of glutamate, and specifically, mGluR5 receptors in SUDs (see Olive, 2009, that for review). Several compounds representative of this class that have been tested in animal models have produced effects suggestive of efficacy for SUDs.

Data implicating mGluR5 receptors in drug abuse-related behaviors date back to 2001, when it was first reported that mice lacking the mGluR5 receptor exhibited an impaired locomotor stimulant response to cocaine, and further, failed to acquire cocaine self-administration (Chiamulera et al., 2001). During the past decade, several compounds that have been widely used as research tools for this mechanism have been tested in animal models relevant to SUDs for alcohol, nicotine, cocaine, and methamphetamine.

MPEP (2-methyl-6-[phenylethynyl]-pyridine) and MTEP (3-[2-methyl-1,3-thiazol-4-yl]ethynyl]-pyridine), two compounds originally developed by Merck, have been valuable as research tools because they are relatively selective for mGluR5. Both are negative allosteric modulators, but MTEP is more potent and selective than MPEP (Lea and Faden, 2006). These compounds have been used extensively to both characterize the function of the mGluR5 receptor, and study its role in models of drug abuse. A few examples are described next.

There are multiple studies using MPEP and MTEP in models of cocaine self-administration, reinstatement, and conditioned place preference. Tessari et al. (2004) and Kenny et al. (2003) have reported that MPEP reduces operant cocaine self-administration in rodents while having no effect on responding for food. Responding for food is generally used as a control for impairment in lever pressing produced by CNS depression. In relapse models in which animals no longer produce an operant response after extinction training, reinstatement by a cocaine priming injection can be reduced in monkeys (Lee et al., 2005; Platt et al., 2008) and reinstatement by a cocaine cue can be reduced in rats (Backstrom and Hyytia, 2006) by MPEP and MTEP. Finally, in models of cocaine-conditioned place preference in which animals seek an environment previously paired with cocaine, MPEP administered during conditioning dose dependently reduced the acquisition of the preference (McGeehan and Olive, 2003), as well as its reinstatement.

Schroeder et al. (2005) have shown that MPEP dose dependently reduced operant ethanol drinking in rats without affecting inactive lever presses. Similarly, Cowen et al. (2005) reported that MTEP reduced operant self-administration of ethanol by both Fawn-Hooded rats and an inbred strain of alcohol-preferring (iP) rats. In a model of relapse in rats, Backstrom et al. (2004) reported that MPEP dose-dependently reduced responding stimulated by cues previously associated alcohol and therefore reduced reinstatement of ethanol self-administration.

The data using nicotine as the drug of abuse are similarly compelling. Paterson et al. (2003), Tessari et al. (2004), and Palmatier et al. (2008) have all reported that MPEP reduced nicotine self-administration in rats, and similarly, Tessari et al. (2004) and Bespalov et al. (2005) have reported that MPEP decreases responding for nicotine prime and nicotine cue in reinstatement models.

Taken together, these and other studies suggest that mGluR5 negative allosteric modulators should be evaluated in SUDs. There are several compounds of this class that have been advanced to clinical studies for various indications according to publicly available information including pharmaceutical research services (http://www.Thomson-pharma.com), pharmaceutical company websites, and http://www.clinicaltrials.gov. Fenobam is a compound developed in the 1970s that had been evaluated first as an anxiolytic, and more recently, as a treatment for Fragile X type mental retardation (Berry-Kravis et al., 2009), recently designated an orphan disease. Other compounds that have either reached Phase I or Phase II for Fragile X include Mavoglurant (Novartis), STX106 (Seaside Therapeutics), and RO-4917523 (Roche). Dipraglurant (Addex) has completed a Phase IIa safety and exploratory efficacy trial for levodopa-induced dyskinesia in Parkinson's disease, and RG07090 (Roche/Chugai Pharmaceuticals) may be in clinical trials for treatment-resistant depression. It is likely that one or more of these compounds will become available for proof-of-concept trials in substance abuse disorders.

Fenobam, for example, has been tested both in animal models of anxiety, and in small, Phase II trials for anxiety. In animal models, fenobam was shown to reverse stress-induced hypothermia at doses of 20 and 30 mg/kg in mice, and it was reported to have anxiolytic effects in the Vogel test at a dose of 30 mg/kg in rats (Porter et al., 2005). It also was shown to increase punished responding in the Geller-Seifter test with an MED of 10 mg/kg (Porter et al., 2005). In a human trial conducted at St. Mary's Hospital in Montreal, nine patients were randomized to fenobam, nine to diazepam, and eleven to placebo. The study lasted five weeks, during which time fenobam was compared to both placebo and diazepam. Over the five weeks of the study, fenobam and diazepam were not significantly different, and both were superior to placebo. Dosing of fenobam began at 100 mg, and subjects were individually titrated. Most adverse events occurred at doses of 200 and 300 mg/day of fenobam (Pecknold et al., 1982) but for the most part, fenobam was well-tolerated. Fenobam was additionally reported to be effective in patients with severe anxiety (Pecknold, 1980).

National Institute on Drug Abuse (NIDA) contract studies have suggested that fenobam sulfate blocks cocaine-priming induced reinstatement at a dose of 60 mg/kg, although the effect was not behaviorally selective. Other NIDA laboratories have shown the same dose reduces cocaine self-administration and cocaine seeking in response to cues in an incubation of craving model (Xi and Gardner, in preparation). These doses are somewhat higher than those that produced anxiolytic effects in animal studies (Porter et al., 2005), suggesting that doses in humans that resulted in anxiolysis may be slightly below an effective dose for substance use disorders.

5HT2 RECEPTORS

Serotonergic neurotransmission is mediated through a family of receptors that include both G-protein coupled receptors and ligand-gated ion channels. Serotonin has been implicated in many CNS functions including mood, appetite, sleep, and cognition. Moreover, serotonin is an important modulator of dopaminergic function, with serotonergic projections to most of the major dopaminergic pathways including the nigrostriatal, mesolimbic, and mesocortical. Both 5HT2A and 5HT2C receptors modulate the release of dopamine via glutamatergic and GABAergic mechanisms that have not been fully elucidated (see Alex and Pehek, 2007, for review).

These receptors have also been implicated in modulating the behavioral effects of cocaine and nicotine (Grottick et al., 2001, Levin et al., 2011), and specifically, compounds that either stimulate 5HT2C receptors or block 5HT2A receptors have been shown to attenuate the effects of drugs of abuse in relevant animal models (see Bubar and Cunningham, 2008, for review).

Serotonin 2A and 2C receptors are widely expressed throughout the brain, and can be pre- or postsynaptic, although they appear to be largely postsynaptic. Both have distinct expression patterns on dopaminergic, glutamatergic, and GABAergic neurons, and appear to modulate the function of dopaminergic pathways originating in the VTA through multiple mechanisms (see Bubar and Cunningham, 2008, for review). Compounds acting at these receptors have also been shown to modulate psychostimulant-induced dopamine efflux and the resulting changes in behavior. Engagement of these receptors elicits opposite effects on cocaine-evoked dopamine release, with 5HT2A antagonists reducing, and 5HT2C antagonists enhancing release, respectively (Broderick et al., 2004; De Deurwaerdere et al, 2004; Leggio et al., 2009). Such opposing actions have been demonstrated in behavioral studies using measures of cocaine-induced locomotor stimulation; drug discrimination, self-administration, and reinstatement (see Bubar and Cunningham, 2008, for review).

The research tools that have been most widely used to delineate the function of these receptors include M100907 (volinanserin) and ketanserin, 5HT2A antagonists, and WAY 163909 and Ro 60-0175, 5HT2C agonists. Volinanserin was in clinical development as an antipsychotic in the 1990s, and again more recently as a sleep aid. It has been used extensively by the research community as M100907.

Although Fletcher et al. (2002) originally reported that the selective 5HT2A antagonist M100907 did not decrease rates of responding for cocaine or nicotine in rats, a selective reduction of cocaine self-administration across the dose-effect curve of cocaine by M100907 has been observed in primates (unpublished NIDA contract studies). The non-selective 5HT2A antagonist, ketanserin, has been reported to decrease nicotine self-administration in rats (Levin et al., 2008). The effects of 5HT2A antagonists in reinstatement models have also been reported. Pockros et al. (2011) reported that microinfusion of M100907 into the ventromedial prefrontal cortex attenuated cocaine cue induced reinstatement, and Nic Dhonnchadha et al. (2009) reported reductions in cue induced reinstatement after systemic treatment with M100907. Fletcher et al. (2012)

recently reported that M100907 reduced both nicotine prime and cue induced reinstatement in rats. NIDA contract studies are also consistent with reported decreases in cue reinstatement, with no effect on cocaine primed reinstatement following treatment with M100907. Controls for impairment of lever pressing demonstrated that the blockade of cocaine cue reinstatement was not the result of motor impairment.

5HT2C receptor activation can recapitulate many of the behavioral effects of 5HT2A receptor blockade. The 5HT2C receptor agonist, WAY 163909, dose dependently reduced cocaine self-administration in rats, and also blocked cocaine cue-induced reinstatement at doses lower than those that suppress locomotor behavior, suggesting that these effects are not attributable to a generalized suppression of behavior (Cunningham et al., 2011). Another 5HT2C agonist, Ro60-0175, has been reported to reduce nicotine self-administration (Grottick et al., 2001) as well as both cue and primed-reinstatement in rats (Fletcher et al., 2012). It also reduced cocaine self-administration and prime-induced reinstatement in squirrel monkeys (Manvich et al., 2012). In NIDA contract studies, Ro60-0175 was shown to reduce cocaine-prime induced reinstatement, and lorcaserin, a selective 5HT2C agonist developed as a treatment for obesity (Hurren and Berlie, 2011) reduced both methamphetamine prime- and cue-reinstatement. Lorcaserin also has been reported to reduce nicotine self-administration in rats, after both acute and repeated administration, without altering responding for food (Levin et al., 2011). Similarly, Higgins et al. (2012) reported that lorcaserin decreased nicotine self- administration and reinstatement at similar doses to those that affected palatable food, a model related to the obesity indication.

Taken together, these findings indicate that 5HT2A antagonists and 5HT2C agonists may be useful for treating SUDs. Several of these compounds that have advanced to human studies, including 5HT2A antagonists volinanserin and eplivanserin for sleep disorders (Sanofi-Aventis), APD 125 for sleep disorders (Arena Pharmaceuticals), and pimavanserin for psychosis associated with Parkinson's disease (Acadia Pharmaceuticals). Two 5HT2C agonists that have advanced to humans, are vabicaserin for psychosis (Wyeth/Pfizer) and lorcaserin (Belviq), which was recently approved for the treatment of obesity (Arena Pharmaceuticals). Compounds either approved, or in late-phase clinical studies could potentially become available for testing in SUDs (e.g., lorcaserin, pimavanserin). The development of several of these compounds (e.g., vabicaserin, volinanserin) has been halted, making treatment of SUDs an attractive rescue indication, for a potential licensee, given the market size.

Volinanserin was originally developed as an antipsychotic, and was found to block amphetamine stimulated locomotor activity (commonly used as a screen for antipsychotic efficacy) at doses that did not effect locomotor activity alone (see Schmidt et al., 1995 for review). The proposed clinical dose for antipsychotic activity, based on 90% occupancy of 5HT2A receptors, was 20 mg daily, which resulted in plasma concentrations of 18 ng/ml (Talvik-Lotfi et al., 2000). Volinanserin was subsequently dropped from development after it failed to demonstrate an antipsychotic effect compared to haloperidol

(de Paulis 2001). Subsequently, it was developed a second time for sleep maintenance. No data are publically available regarding efficacy for this indication, but receptor occupancy studies suggest dosing was in the range of 20 mg (Grunder et al., 1997; Teegarden et al., 2008). Doses effective in animal studies of cocaine reinstatement were well below 0.1 mg/kg (Nic Dhonnchadha et al., 2009), suggesting that efficacy for substance use disorders may occur at doses lower than those that have been tested in the clinic.

Lorcaserin was effective in reducing weight at doses of 10–20 mgs daily, and was generally well-tolerated in two clinical trials (Hurren and Berlie, 2011). In the first trial, completers who achieved greater than 5% body weight reductions were taking daily doses of 10 (12.8%), 15 (19.5%), and 20 mg/day (31.2%) (Smith et al., 2009). In the second trial, which was larger and multisite, at the end of one year, 47.5% of patients in the lorcaserin group (20 mg/day) and 20.3% in the placebo group lost 5% or more of body weight (Smith et al., 2010). Effects in animal models of food intake and obesity were obtained at doses ranging from 9 to 36 mg/kg (Smith et al., 2008); whereas in animal models of SUDs it was effective at doses up to 1.0 mg/kg. These differences in potency may be the result of differences in route of administration (oral vs. subcutaneous dosing). Nonetheless, these data suggest that lorcaserin would be effective in SUDs at or below doses that were effective for weight loss.

BIOLOGICALS

Substance abuse disorder is the only area in psychiatry currently amenable to the use of biologicals as therapy. Because two proof of principle studies in humans (reviewed in Hatsukami et al., 2011; Shen and Kosten, 2011) have yielded promising results, these studies will be overviewed here. The principle underlying biological approaches to treat SUDs is pharmacokinetic: preventing or slowing the entry of abused substance into the central nervous system. There are three principal strategies for developing biologicals as pharmacotherapies: (1) vaccines that result in the production of antibodies directed toward a specific drug of abuse, (2) monoclonal antibodies directed toward a specific drug of abuse, and (3) genetically engineered enzymes that catalyze the degradation of a specific drug of abuse.

VACCINES

Vaccines directed against nicotine, cocaine, and heroin are in various stages of development (see reviews by Fahim et al., 2011; Koob et al., 2011; Shen and Kosten, 2011). Perhaps the major obstacle to developing vaccines directed against drugs of abuse is that these low molecular weight molecules are not inherently antigenic (i.e., they are not recognized by the immune system). In order to render a small molecule antigenic, the strategy most often employed is chemical modification of the abused substance so that it is capable of covalently bonding to a protein that is now recognized as "foreign" by the immune system. As exemplified by the nicotine vaccine NicVax®, the parent molecule is first chemically converted to 3′aminomethynicotine, and it is this molecule that covalently bonds (in the presence of succinaldehyde) to both the amino acid side chains and terminal amino groups of a recombinant protein (Exoprotein A) from Pseudomonas aeruginosa (Fahim et al., 2011). An amino acid deletion to this recombinant carrier protein renders it nontoxic, but highly antigenic (Fahim et al., 2011). One proof of concept study with this nicotine vaccine (NicVax®) yielded a positive efficacy signal in a subset of smokers with the highest levels of antinicotine antibodies (Hatsukami et al., 2011). In this cohort (subjects with the highest tertile of antibodies), a significantly higher level of sustained end of trial (eight weeks) abstinence was reported compared with placebo (24.6% vs. 12%, $p = 0.024$). However, this vaccine failed to achieve its primary endpoint in two Phase III trials (http://www.nabi.com). No additional details have been publicly disclosed by the sponsor. Other companies have engineered nicotine vaccines with the potential to yield higher antibody titers, and at least one of these is currently in clinical development (http://www.select-abio.com). There has been one reported clinical study examining the efficacy of a cocaine vaccine. This vaccine is a cocaine derivative that was linked to an inactivated form of cholera toxin B (Shen and Kosten, 2011). In a 24-week double-blind, placebo-controlled trial, Martell et al. (2009) reported significantly more cocaine-free urine samples during weeks 9–16 in methadone-maintained patients with the highest tertile of anticocaine antibody levels compared with either subjects with lower antibody levels or placebo (45% vs. 35%, respectively). A second efficacy trial with this vaccine is currently in progress. At least one alternative approach, coupling a cocaine analog to a disrupted adenovirus, has yielded very high antibody levels and anticocaine effects (blocking reinforcing and psychostimulant actions) in animals (Hicks et al., 2011; Koob et al., 2011; Skolnick and Volkow, 2011; Wee et al., 2012). This vaccine has the potential for translation to the clinic, whereas other vaccines (e.g., for heroin) are in preclinical development (Stowe et al., 2011).

Despite attempts to make highly antigenic and effective vaccines, based on the clinical data obtained to date, additional innovation is required. Thus, five injections were required for both the successful proof of concept study with NicVax (Hatsukami et al., 2011) as well as the Martell et al. (2009) study using a cocaine vaccine. Compared with other commercial vaccines, a product requiring five vaccinations administered over a period spanning several months is far from ideal. It has been noted (Shen and Kosten, 2011) that although the cocaine vaccine used in the Martell et al. (2009) study produced robust antibody responses to cholera toxin B in every patient, far lower levels of anticocaine antibodies were produced in a significant proportion of subjects. Clearly, strategies aimed at producing higher levels of drug-directed antibodies in response to a vaccine, including newer, more powerful adjuvating agents (both the Nabi and Celtic vaccines used an alum adjuvant), will be required to make a commercially viable product.

MONOCLONAL ANTIBODIES

Although the vaccines described here all require multiple immunizations to produce therapeutic levels of antibodies (Hatsukami et al., 2011; Koob et al., 2011; Martell et al., 2009), this passive immunization strategy is effective upon administration. The most advanced monoclonal antibody is directed against methamphetamine (Owens et al., 2011), with first-in-human studies in progress. Perhaps the major drawback of passive immunization strategies is the need to readminister the monoclonal antibody because of a limited biological half-life. However, it is now feasible (http://www.xencor.com) to genetically engineer mABs with significantly longer biological half-lives, which could ultimately lower the treatment costs of this approach.

ENGINEERED ENZYMES

Cocaine is hydrolyzed in plasma by butyrylcholinesterase. Point mutation studies have demonstrated it is possible to increase the rate of catalysis in an engineered butyrylcholinesterase by more than 1,000-fold compared with the wild type enzyme. This enzyme is capable of reducing the pharmacological actions of cocaine in animals (e.g., administration blocks cocaine lethality as well as cocaine primed reinstatement of drug-seeking behavior) (Brimijoin, 2011; Gao et al., 2005 review). Teva Pharmaceutical is pursuing the development of an engineered esterase (presentation by Dr. M. Bassan at CPDD, June 2012). Like mABs, proteolysis of an engineered butyrylcholinesterase limits its biological half-life, requiring frequent (perhaps weekly or bimonthly) injections. However, gene transfer of an engineered butyrylcholinesterase using an adenoviral vector can produce high levels of this enzyme (that was sustained in rats for several months). This strategy was recently reported (Anker et al., 2012) to block reinstatement to cocaine for up to six months.

There are both advantages and disadvantages to treating SUDs using biological approaches. Among the most compelling reasons to develop these as therapeutics is the potential for a long-lived protective effect, requiring a patient to make one good decision to receive a biological therapy, compared with one (or multiple) daily decisions to remain compliant with traditional pharmacotherapies. The specificity of an effective biologic such a heroin vaccine could dramatically reduce its use, but would neither preclude a patient from receiving maintenance therapy nor prevent the abuse of a structurally unrelated opiate, such as oxycodone. The ability of a patient to circumvent a specific therapy by taking drugs other than the one targeted by the biologic (e.g., an effective cocaine vaccine would not preclude abuse of heroin) is a limitation of these biological approaches. However, this is also a limitation of current medications, exemplified by the use of cocaine while on methadone maintenance therapy (Martell et al., 2009).

Active immunization therapies currently in clinical trials can take weeks or months before antibody titers reach pharmacologically relevant levels (Hatsukami et al., 2011; Martell et al., 2009). This therapeutic lag, along with the requirement for multiple immunizations and high patient expectations of a cure, could negatively impact the commercial success of such a product. Nonetheless, biological approaches represent appealing alternatives that have the potential to change the practice of addiction medicine.

CONCLUSIONS

The contraction of research and development in psychiatry has produced a bumper crop of parked compounds that cannot be either out-licensed or otherwise monetized. This contraction, in combination with a new appreciation of the market potential in treating SUDs, may facilitate the repurposing of compounds developed for other indications. There may be unprecedented opportunities in both the short- and midterm horizons for translating some of the targets identified by preclinical research as promising for the treatment of SUDS. In addition, biological approaches are now viewed as a viable alternative to small molecules. In the case of vaccines, improvements in antibody specificity and titer through the use of more immunogenic recombinant proteins and better adjuvants will be required for commercially viable products. Similarly, genetically engineered monoclonal antibodies and catalytic enzymes with improved biological half-lives also have the potential to transform future addiction treatment and, based on development costs, may be more attractive than small molecules.

Clearly, the pharmaceutical and biotechnology sectors must be more engaged in order to address the need for SUD treatments. Both the funding and expertise required for drug development are simply beyond the scope of academia and the public sector. Despite progress in understanding the neurobiology and genetics of substance abuse, the investment required to bring a molecule to market remains feasible only for the private sector, barring a paradigm shift toward public-private partnerships, government-sponsored cooperative agreements, or other models in which the financial risks are shared or blunted.

DISCLOSURES

Dr. Acri and Dr. Skolnick have no conflicts of interest to disclose. The authors are full time employees of the National Institute on Drug Abuse, National Institutes of Health.

REFERENCES

Adachi, M., and Monteggia, L.M. (2009). Synergistic interactions between histone deacetylase inhibitors and drugs of abuse. *Neuropsychopharmacology* 34(13):2619–2620.

Alex, K.D., and Pehek, E.A. (2007). Pharmacologic mechanisms of serotonergic regulation of dopamine neurotransmission. *Pharmacol. Ther.* 113(2):296–320.

Anderson, A.L., Li, S.H., et al. (2012). Modafinil for the treatment of methamphetamine dependence. *Drug Alcohol Depend.* 120(1–3):135–141.

Anker, J.J., Brimijoin, S., et al. (2012). Cocaine hydrolase encoded in viral vector blocks the reinstatement of cocaine seeking in rats for 6 months. *Biol. Psychiatry* 71(8):700–705.

Backstrom, P., Bachteler, D., et al. (2004). mGluR5 antagonist MPEP reduces ethanol-seeking and relapse behavior. *Neuropsychopharmacology* 29(5): 921–928.

Backstrom, P., and Hyytia, P. (2006). Ionotropic and metabotropic glutamate receptor antagonism attenuates cue-induced cocaine seeking. *Neuropsychopharmacology* 31(4):778–786.

Balster, R.L. (1991). Drug abuse potential evaluation in animals. *Br. J. Addict.* 86(12):1549–1558.

Baser, O., Chalk, M., et al. (2011). Cost and utilization outcomes of opioid-dependence treatments. *Am. J. Manag. Care* 17(Suppl 8):S235–S248.

Berry-Kravis, E., Hessl, D., et al. (2009). A pilot open label, single dose trial of fenobam in adults with fragile X syndrome. *J. Med. Genet.* 46(4):266–271.

Bespalov, A.Y., Dravolina, O.A., et al. (2005). Metabotropic glutamate receptor (mGluR5) antagonist MPEP attenuated cue- and schedule-induced reinstatement of nicotine self-administration behavior in rats. *Neuropharmacology* 49(Suppl 1):167–178.

Bossert, J.M., Ghitza, U.E., et al. (2005). Neurobiology of relapse to heroin and cocaine seeking: an update and clinical implications. *Eur. J. Pharmacol.* 526(1–3):36–50.

Brady, J.V., Griffiths, R.R., et al. (1984). Abuse liability and behavioral toxicity assessment: progress report from the behavioral biology laboratories of the Johns Hopkins University School of Medicine. *NIDA Res. Monogr.* 49:92–108.

Brady, L.S., and Insel, T.R. (2012). Translating discoveries into medicine: psychiatric drug development in 2011. *Neuropsychopharmacology* 37(1):281–283.

Brimijoin, S. (2011). Interception of cocaine by enzyme or antibody delivered with viral gene transfer: a novel strategy for preventing relapse in recovering drug users. *CNS Neurol. Disord. Drug Targets* 10(8):880–891.

Broderick, P.A., Olabisi, O.A., et al. (2004). Cocaine acts on accumbens monoamines and locomotor behavior via a 5-HT2A/2C receptor mechanism as shown by ketanserin: 24-h follow-up studies. *Prog. Neuropsychopharmacol. Biol. Psychiatry* 28(3):547–557.

Brodie, J.D., Case, B.G., et al. (2009). Randomized, double-blind, placebo-controlled trial of vigabatrin for the treatment of cocaine dependence in Mexican parolees. *Am. J. Psychiatry* 166:1269–1277.

Bubar, M.J., and Cunningham, K.A. (2008). Prospects for serotonin 5-HT2R pharmacotherapy in psychostimulant abuse. *Prog. Brain Res.* 172:319–346.

Chiamulera, C., Epping-Jordan, M.P., et al. (2001). Reinforcing and locomotor stimulant effects of cocaine are absent in mGluR5 null mutant mice. *Nat. Neurosci.* 4(9):873–874.

Childress, A.R., Hole, A.V., et al. (1993). Cue reactivity and cue reactivity interventions in drug dependence. *NIDA Res. Monogr.* 137:73–95.

Conn, P.J. (2003). Physiological roles and therapeutic potential of metabotropic glutamate receptors. *Ann. NY Acad. Sci.* 1003:12–21.

Cowen, M.S., Djouma, E., et al. (2005). The metabotropic glutamate 5 receptor antagonist 3-[(2-methyl-1,3-thiazol-4-yl)ethynyl]-pyridine reduces ethanol self-administration in multiple strains of alcohol-preferring rats and regulates olfactory glutamatergic systems. *J. Pharmacol. Exp. Ther.* 315 (2):590–600.

Cunningham, K.A., Fox, R.G., et al. (2011). Selective serotonin 5-HT(2C) receptor activation suppresses the reinforcing efficacy of cocaine and sucrose but differentially affects the incentive-salience value of cocaine- vs. sucrose-associated cues. *Neuropharmacology* 61(3):513–523.

Cutler, D.M., and Everett, W. (2010). Thinking outside the pillbox: medication adherence as a priority for health care reform. *N. Engl. J. Med.* 362(17):1553–1555.

Czobor, P., and Skolnick, P. (2011). The secrets of a successful clinical trial: compliance, compliance, and compliance. *Mol. Interv.* 11(2):107–110.

DeDeurwaerdere, P., Navailles, S., et al. (2004). Constitutive activity of the serotonin2C receptor inhibits in vivo dopamine release in the rat striatum and nucleus accumbens. *J. Neurosci.* 24(13):3235–3241.

dePaulis, T. (2001). M-100907 (Aventis). *Curr. Opin. Investig. Drugs* 2(1):123–132.

Donovan, D.M., Bigelow, G.E., et al. (2012). Primary outcome indices in illicit drug dependence treatment research: systematic approach to selection and measurement of drug use end-points in clinical trials. *Addiction* 107(4):694–708.

Epstein, D.H., Preston, K.L., et al. (2006). Toward a model of drug relapse: an assessment of the validity of the reinstatement procedure. *Psychopharmacology (Berl.)* 189(1):1–16.

Fagerstrom, K., Russ, C., et al. (2012). The Fagerstrom test for nicotine dependence as a predictor of smoking abstinence: a pooled analysis of varenicline clinical trial data. *Nicotine Tob. Res.* 14(12):1467–1473.

Fahim, R., Kessler, P., et al. (2011). Nicotine vaccines. *CNS Neurol. Disord. Drug Targets* 10:905–915.

Fletcher, P.J., Grottick, A.J., et al. (2002). Differential effects of the 5-HT(2A) receptor antagonist M100907 and the 5-HT(2C) receptor antagonist SB242084 on cocaine-induced locomotor activity, cocaine self-administration and cocaine-induced reinstatement of responding. *Neuropsychopharmacology* 27(4):576–586.

Fletcher, P.J., Rizos, Z., et al. (2012). Effects of the 5-HT(2C) receptor agonist Ro60-0175 and the 5-HT(2A) receptor antagonist M100907 on nicotine self-administration and reinstatement. *Neuropharmacology* 62(7):2288–2298.

Fox, H.C., Bergquist, K.L., et al. (2011). Selective cocaine-related difficulties in emotional intelligence: relationship to stress and impulse control. *Am. J. Addict.* 20(2):151–160.

Gao, Y., Atanasova, E., et al. (2005). Gene transfer of cocaine hydrolase suppresses cardiovascular responses to cocaine in rats. *Mol. Pharmacol.* 67(1):204–211.

Gawin, F.H., and Kleber, H.D. (1986). Abstinence symptomatology and psychiatric diagnosis in cocaine abusers. Clinical observations. *Arch. Gen. Psychiatry* 43(2):107–113.

Griffiths, R.R., and Balster, R.L. (1979). Opioids: similarity between evaluations of subjective effects and animal self-administration results. *Clin. Pharmacol. Ther.* 25(5 Pt 1):611–617.

Grottick, A.J., Corrigall, W.A., et al. (2001). Activation of 5-HT(2C) receptors reduces the locomotor and rewarding effects of nicotine. *Psychopharmacology (Berl.)* 157(3):292–298.

Grunder, G., Yokoi, F., et al. (1997). Time course of 5-HT2A receptor occupancy in the human brain after a single oral dose of the putative antipsychotic drug MDL 100,907 measured by positron emission tomography. *Neuropsychopharmacology* 17(3):175–185.

Harrigan, S.E., and Downs, D.A. (1981). Pharmacological evaluation of narcotic antagonist delivery systems in rhesus monkeys. *NIDA Res. Monogr.* 28:77–92.

Hatsukami, D.K., Jorenby, D.E., et al. (2011). Immunogenicity and smoking-cessation outcomes for a novel nicotine immunotherapeutic. *Clin. Pharmacol. Ther.* 89(3):392–399.

Heidbreder, C.A., and Newman, A.H. (2010). Current perspectives on selective dopamine D(3) receptor antagonists as pharmacotherapeutics for addictions and related disorders. *Ann. NY Acad. Sci.* 1187: 4–34.

Heinzerling, K.G., Swanson, A.N., et al. (2010). Randomized, double-blind, placebo-controlled trial of modafinil for the treatment of methamphetamine dependence. *Drug Alcohol Depend.* 109 (1–3):20–29.

Hicks, M.J., De, B.P., et al. (2011). Cocaine analog coupled to disrupted adenovirus: a vaccine strategy to evoke high-titer immunity against addictive drugs. *Mol. Ther.* 19(3):612–619.

Higgins, G.A., Silenieks, L.B., et al. (2012). The 5-HT(2C) Receptor agonist lorcaserin reduces nicotine self-administration, discrimination, and reinstatement: relationship to feeding behavior and impulse control. *Neuropsychopharmacology* 37(5):1177–1191.

Hurren, K.M., and Berlie, H.D. (2011). Lorcaserin: an investigational serotonin 2C agonist for weight loss. *Am. J. Health Syst. Pharm.* 68(21):2029–2037.

Itzhak, Y., and Martin, J.L. (2002). Cocaine-induced conditioned place preference in mice: induction, extinction and reinstatement by related psychostimulants. *Neuropsychopharmacology* 26(1):130–134.

Jarvis, L.M. (2012). Tough times for neuroscience R & D. *Chem. Eng. News* 90(12):22–25.

Jayaram-Lindstrom, N., Hammarberg, A., et al. (2008). Naltrexone for the treatment of amphetamine dependence: a randomized, placebo-controlled trial. *Am. J. Psychiatry* 165(11):1442–1448.

Jimenez-Gomez, C., Winger, G., et al. (2011). Naltrexone decreases D-amphetamine and ethanol self-administration in rhesus monkeys. *Behav. Pharmaco.* 22(1):87–90.

Kenny, P.J., Paterson, N.E., et al. (2003). Metabotropic glutamate 5 receptor antagonist MPEP decreased nicotine and cocaine self-administration but not nicotine and cocaine-induced facilitation of brain reward function in rats. *Ann. NY Acad. Sci.* 1003:415–418.

Koob, G.F., and Volkow, N.D. (2010). Neurocircuitry of addiction. *Neuropsychopharmacology* 35(1):217–238.

Koob, G.F., Ahmed, S.H., et al. (2004). Neurobiological mechanisms in the transition from drug use to drug dependence. *Neurosci. Biobehav. Rev.* 27(8):739–749.

Koob, G., Hicks, M.J., et al. (2011). Anti-cocaine vaccine based on coupling a cocaine analog to a disrupted adenovirus. *CNS Neurol. Disord. Drug Targets* 10(8):899–904.

Koob, G.F., Kenneth Lloyd, G., et al. (2009). Development of pharmacotherapies for drug addiction: a Rosetta Stone approach. *Nat. Rev. Drug Discov.* 8(6):500–515.

Lea, P.M., and Faden, A.I. (2006). Metabotropic glutamate receptor subtype 5 antagonists MPEP and MTEP. *CNS Drug Rev.* 12(2):149–166.

Lee, B., Platt, D.M., et al. (2005). Attenuation of behavioral effects of cocaine by the Metabotropic Glutamate Receptor 5 Antagonist 2-Methyl-6-(phenylethynyl)-pyridine in squirrel monkeys: comparison with dizocilpine. *J. Pharmacol. Exp. Ther.* 312(3):1232–1240.

LeFoll, B., Chakraborty-Chatterjee, M., et al. (2012). Varenicline decreases nicotine self-administration and cue-induced reinstatement of nicotine-seeking behaviour in rats when a long pretreatment time is used. *Int. J. Neuropsychopharmacol.* 15(9):1265–1274.

Leggio, G.M., Cathala, A., et al. (2009). Serotonin2C receptors in the medial prefrontal cortex facilitate cocaine-induced dopamine release in the rat nucleus accumbens. *Neuropharmacology* 56(2):507–513.

Levin, E.D., Johnson, J.E., et al. (2011). Lorcaserin, a 5-HT2C agonist, decreases nicotine self-administration in female rats. *J. Pharmacol. Exp. Ther.* 338(3):890–896.

Levin, E.D., Slade, S., et al. (2008). Ketanserin, a 5-HT2 receptor antagonist, decreases nicotine self-administration in rats. *Eur. J. Pharmacol.* 600(1–3):93–97.

Levin, M.E., Weaver, M.T., et al. (2012). Varenicline dose dependently enhances responding for nonpharmacological reinforcers and attenuates the reinforcement-enhancing effects of nicotine. *Nicotine Tob. Res.* 14(3):299–305.

Lu, L., Grimm, J.W., et al. (2004). Incubation of cocaine craving after withdrawal: a revew of preclinical data. *Neuropharmacology* 47(Suppl 1):214–226.

Manvich, D.F., Kimmel, H.L., et al. (2012). Effects of serotonin 5-ht2c receptor agonists on the behavioral and neurochemical effects of cocaine in squirrel monkeys. *J. Pharmacol. Exp. Ther.* 341(2):424–434.

Martell, B.A., Orson, F.M., et al. (2009). Cocaine vaccine for the treatment of cocaine dependence in methadone-maintained patients: a randomized, double-blind, placebo-controlled efficacy trial. *Arch. Gen. Psychiatry* 66(10):1116–1123.

McCann, D.J., and Li, S.H. (2012). A novel, nonbinary evaluation of success and failure reveals bupropion efficacy versus methamphetamine dependence: reanalysis of a multisite trial. *CNS Neurosci. Ther.* 18(5):414–418.

McGeehan, A.J., and Olive, M.F. (2003). The mGluR5 antagonist MPEP reduces the conditioned rewarding effects of cocaine but not other drugs of abuse. *Synapse* 47(3):240–242.

Mello, N.K., and Negus, S.S. (1996). Preclinical evaluation of pharmacotherapies for treatment of cocaine and opioid abuse using drug self-administration procedures. *Neuropsychopharmacology* 14(6):375–424.

Mueller, D., and Stewart, J. (2000). Cocaine-induced conditioned place preference: reinstatement by priming injections of cocaine after extinction. *Behav. Brain Res.* 115(1):39–47.

Mueller, D., Perdikaris, D., et al. (2002). Persistence and drug-induced reinstatement of a morphine-induced conditioned place preference. *Behav. Brain Res.* 136(2):389–397.

Negus, S.S. (2006). Choice between heroin and food in nondependent and heroin-dependent rhesus monkeys: effects of naloxone, buprenorphine, and methadone. *J. Pharmacol. Exp. Ther.* 317(2):711–723.

Nic Dhonnchadha, B.A., Fox, R.G., et al. (2009). Blockade of the serotonin 5-HT2A receptor suppresses cue-evoked reinstatement of cocaine-seeking behavior in a rat self-administration model. *Behav. Neurosci.* 123(2):382–396.

O'Brien, C.P., Childress, A.R., et al. (1998). Conditioning factors in drug abuse: can they explain compulsion? *J. Psychopharmacol.* 12(1):15–22.

O'Connor, E.C., Parker, D., et al. (2010). The alpha4beta2 nicotinic acetylcholine-receptor partial agonist varenicline inhibits both nicotine self-administration following repeated dosing and reinstatement of nicotine seeking in rats. *Psychopharmacology (Berl.)* 208(3):365–376.

Olive, M.F. (2009). Metabotropic glutamate receptor ligands as potential therapeutics for addiction. *Curr. Drug Abuse Rev.* 2(1):83–98.

Owens, S.M., Atchley, W.T., et al. (2011). Monoclonal antibodies as pharmacokinetic antagonists for the treatment of (+)-methamphetamine addiction. *CNS Neurol. Disord. Drug Targets* 10:892–898.

Palmatier, M.I., Liu, X., et al. (2008). Metabotropic glutamate 5 receptor (mGluR5) antagonists decrease nicotine seeking, but do not affect the reinforcement enhancing effects of nicotine. *Neuropsychopharmacology* 33(9):2139–2147.

Paterson, N.E., Semenova, S., et al. (2003). The mGluR5 antagonist MPEP decreased nicotine self-administration in rats and mice. *Psychopharmacology (Berl.)* 167(3):257–264.

Paul, S.M., Mytelka, D.S., et al. (2010). How to improve R&D productivity: the pharmaceutical industry's grand challenge. *Nat. Rev. Drug Discov.* 9(3):203–214.

Pecknold, J.C., McClure, D.J., et al. (1980). Fenobam in anxious outpatients. *Curr. Ther. Res.* 27:119–123.

Pecknold, J.C., McClure, D.J., et al. (1982). Treatment of anxiety using fenobam (a nonbenzodiazepine) in a double-blind standard (diazepam) placebo-controlled study. *J. Clin. Psychopharmacol.* 2(2):129–133.

Perelson, A.S., Essunger, P., et al. (1997). Decay characteristics of HIV-1-infected compartments during combination therapy. *Nature* 387(6629):188–191.

Platt, D.M., Rowlett, J.K., et al. (2008). Attenuation of cocaine self-administration in squirrel monkeys following repeated administration of the mGluR5 antagonist MPEP: comparison with dizocilpine. *Psychopharmacology (Berl.)* 200(2):167–176.

Pockros, L.A., Pentkowski, N.S., et al. (2011). Blockade of 5-HT2A receptors in the medial prefrontal cortex attenuates reinstatement of cue-elicited cocaine-seeking behavior in rats. *Psychopharmacology (Berl.)* 213(2–3):307–320.

Porter, R.H., Jaeschke, G., et al. (2005). Fenobam: a clinically validated nonbenzodiazepine anxiolytic is a potent, selective, and noncompetitive mGlu5 receptor antagonist with inverse agonist activity. *J. Pharmacol. Exp. Ther.* 315(2):711–721.

Renthal, W., Kumar, A., et al. (2009). Genome-wide analysis of chromatin regulation by cocaine reveals a role for sirtuins. *Neuron* 62(3):335–348.

Robison, A.J., and Nestler, E.J. (2011). Transcriptional and epigenetic mechanisms of addiction. *Nat. Rev. Neurosci.* 12(11):623–637.

Schechter, M.D., and Calcagnetti, D.J. (1998). Continued trends in the conditioned place preference literature from 1992 to 1996, inclusive, with a cross-indexed bibliography. *Neurosci. Biobehav. Rev.* 22(6):827–846.

Schmidt, C.J., Sorensen, S.M., et al. (1995). The role of 5-HT2A receptors in antipsychotic activity. *Life Sci.* 56(25):2209–2222.

Schoepp, D.D. (2001). Unveiling the functions of presynaptic metabotropic glutamate receptors in the central nervous system. *J. Pharmacol. Exp. Ther.* 299(1):12–20.

Schroeder, J.P., Overstreet, D.H., et al. (2005). The mGluR5 antagonist MPEP decreases operant ethanol self-administration during maintenance and after repeated alcohol deprivations in alcohol-preferring (P) rats. *Psychopharmacology (Berl.)* 179(1):262–270.

Shearer, J., Darke, S., et al. (2009). Modafinil for methamphetamine dependence. *Addiction* 104:224–233.

Shen, X., and Kosten, T.R. (2011). Immunotherapy for drug abuse. *CNS Neurol. Disord. Drug Targets* 10:876–879.

Sinha, R. (2001). How does stress increase risk of drug abuse and relapse? *Psychopharmacology (Berl.)* 158(4):343–359.

Skolnick, P., and Volkow, N.D. (2011). Magic bullets and arrows: biologic approaches to treat substance use disorders. *CNS Neurol. Disord. Drug Targets* 10(8):864.

Smith, B.M., Smith, J.M., et al. (2008). Discovery and structure-activity relationship of (1R)-8-chloro-2,3,4,5-tetrahydro-1-methyl-1H-3-benzazepine (Lorcaserin), a selective serotonin 5-HT2C receptor agonist for the treatment of obesity. *J. Med. Chem.* 51(2):305–313.

Smith, S.R., Prosser, W.A., et al. (2009). Lorcaserin (APD356), a selective 5-HT(2C) agonist, reduces body weight in obese men and women. *Obesity (Silver Spring)* 17(3):494–503.

Smith, S.R., Weissman, N.J., et al. (2010). Multicenter, placebo-controlled trial of lorcaserin for weight management. *N. Engl. J. Med.* 363(3):245–256.

Stowe, G.N., Schlosburg, J.E., et al. (2011). Developing a vaccine against multiple psychoactive targets: a case study of heroin. *CNS Neurol. Disord. Drug Targets* 10:865–875.

Talvik-Lotfi, M., Nyberg, S., et al. (2000). High 5HT2A receptor occupancy in M100907-treated schizophrenic patients. *Psychopharmacology (Berl.)* 148(4):400–403.

Teegarden, B.R., Al, S.H., et al. (2008). 5-HT(2A) inverse-agonists for the treatment of insomnia. *Curr. Top. Med. Chem.* 8(11):969–976.

Tessari, M., Pilla, M., et al. (2004). Antagonism at metabotropic glutamate 5 receptors inhibits nicotine- and cocaine-taking behaviours and prevents nicotine-triggered relapse to nicotine-seeking. *Eur. J. Pharmacol.* 499(1–2):121–133.

Tzschentke, T.M. (2007). Measuring reward with the conditioned place preference (CPP) paradigm: update of the last decade. *Addict Biol.* 12(3–4):227–462.

Vocci, F.J., Acri, J., et al. (2005). Medication development for addictive disorders: the state of the science. *Am. J. Psychiatry* 162(8):1432–1440.

Wee, S., Hicks, M.J., et al. (2012). Novel cocaine vaccine linked to a disrupted adenovirus gene transfer vector blocks cocaine psychostimulant and reinforcing effects. *Neuropsychopharmacology* 37(5):1083–1091.

Winchell, C., Rappaport, B.A., et al. (2012). Reanalysis of methamphetamine dependence treatment trial. *CNS Neurosci. Ther.* 18(5):367–368.

Winger, G., Skjoldager, P., et al. (1992). Effects of buprenorphine and other opioid agonists and antagonists on alfentanil- and cocaine-reinforced responding in rhesus monkeys. *J. Pharmacol. Exp. Ther.* 261(1):311–317.

58 | EPIDEMIOLOGY OF SUBSTANCE USE DISORDERS

DENISE B. KANDEL, MEI-CHEN HU, AND PAMELA C. GRIESLER

The epidemiology of drug use in the general population includes two distinct streams of research. The more common stream measures consumption patterns by asking individuals whether they have ever used specific classes of drugs, and, if so, how frequently they have done so. The second stream, and one implemented more rarely, measures the extent of problematic drug use by asking individuals about behaviors and symptoms that meet criteria for a substance use disorder.

Currently, the most extensive data on substance use disorders in the US population are provided by four national surveys implemented since 2001. The ongoing National Survey on Drug Use and Health (NSDUH-Substance Abuse and Mental Health Services Administration [SAMHSA], 2011) surveys respondents 12 years of age and older annually. This survey also provides excellent data on patterns of use. The National Epidemiologic Survey on Alcohol and Related Conditions (NESARC) (Compton et al., 2005; Conway et al., 2006; Grant et al., 2004a, 2004b), carried out in 2001–2002, and the National Comorbidity Survey Replication (NCS-R) (Kessler et al., 2005a, 2005b), carried out in 2001–2003, surveyed adults 18 years and older. The National Comorbidity Survey for Adolescents (NCS-A) (Kessler et al., 2012a, 2012b), carried out in 2001–2004, surveyed youths 13–18 years old. These surveys have different strengths and weaknesses and generate somewhat different estimates of rates of substance use and substance use disorders and their comorbidity with other psychiatric disorders in the population.

In this chapter, we present data on the epidemiology and phenomenology of substance use disorders from comparative and developmental perspectives. We discuss six issues:

- The definition and measurement of substance use disorders and characteristics of existing epidemiological studies

- The prevalence of substance use and substance use disorders for legal drugs (cigarettes, alcohol), illegal drugs (marijuana, cocaine), and non-medical use of prescribed psychoactive drugs in different studies among adults and adolescents

- The prevalence of substance use disorders by age, gender, and race/ethnicity

- The comorbidity of substance use disorders with other psychiatric disorders

- Developmental stages of involvement in drugs

- Adolescence as a critical exposure period

The data presented in the chapter are based on publications from these studies and secondary analyses of the data sets that we implemented to illustrate points for which the documentation was not available in published reports.

DEFINITION AND MEASUREMENT OF SUBSTANCE USE DISORDERS

The currently available data on rates of disorders are based on the diagnostic criteria for substance use disorders specified by the fourth edition of the *Diagnostic and Statistical Manual of Mental Disorders* (DSM-IV and DSM-IV-TR; American Psychiatric Association, 1994, 2000). The DSM-IV covers two maladaptive patterns of substance use: abuse, and dependence (addiction); abuse is less severe than dependence and is diagnosed only if criteria for dependence are not met. The criteria for dependence have evolved over the past 30 years with a shift of emphasis from the necessary physiological criteria of tolerance and withdrawal to behavioral criteria for compulsive use. Tolerance and withdrawal form two of the seven potential criteria (Koob et al., 2008: p. 354). Three criteria need to be experienced within a 12-month period in order for the diagnosis of a substance dependence disorder to be made. The seven criteria are: (1) tolerance; (2) withdrawal; (3) impaired control, the substance taken in larger amounts or over a longer period than intended; (4) unsuccessful quit attempts; (5) time spent obtaining, using the substance, or recovering from its effects; (6) neglect of important social, occupational, or recreational activities; (7) continued use despite persistent or recurrent physical or psychological problems caused or exacerbated by the substance. These criteria closely resemble those outlined by the *International Statistical Classification of Diseases and Related Health Problems* (ICD-10; World Health Organization, 1992). In both systems, the specific withdrawal symptoms vary across drugs (Koob et al., 2008: p. 354). Withdrawal from cannabis (marijuana) is not included as a criterion although a cannabis withdrawal "syndrome is now well established (Budney et al., 2003)." (Koob et al., 2008: p. 355) As noted by Hughes (2006), generic criteria are based in part on shared genotype across different drugs, common underlying neurobiological processes, as well as by common behavioral correlates, such as antisocial syndromes (Compton et al., 2005; Koob et al., 2008: p. 354; Nelson et al., 1999).

Abuse is a distinct diagnostic category that excludes individuals who meet criteria for dependence. Abuse requires recurrent substance use during a twelve-month period resulting

TABLE 58.1. Lifetime and last 12-month prevalence of nonmedical substance use among persons aged 18 and older in NSDUH 2010, NESARC 2001–2002 and NCS-R, and persons aged 12–17 in NSDUH 2010 and 13–17 in NCS-A

SUBSTANCE USE	(1) LIFETIME RATES OF USE AMONG PERSONS 18+			(2) LAST 12-MONTH RATES OF USE AMONG PERSONS 18+			(3) LIFETIME RATES OF USE AMONG PERSONS 12/13–17		(4) LAST 12-MONTH RATES OF USE AMONG PERSONS 12/13–17	
	NSDUH % (95% CI)	NESARC % (95% CI)	NCS-R % (95% CI)	NSDUH % (95% CI)	NESARC % (95% CI)	NCS-R % (95% CI)	NSDUH % (95% CI)	NCS-A % (95% CI)	NSDUH % (95% CI)	NCS-A % (95% CI)
Alcohol	87.7 (87.0–88.4)	82.7 (81.5–83.9)	91.7 (89.7–93.3)	70.4 (69.5–71.3)	65.4 (64.3–66.6)	62.3[a] (59.4–65.1)	35.4 (34.5–36.3)	58.5 (55.7–61.3)	28.5 (27.6–29.5)	22.0[a] (20.2–24.1)
Tobacco (Nicotine)[b]	73.4 (72.6–74.1)	46.9 (45.4–48.4)	73.6 (71.0–76.0)	34.5 (33.8–35.3)	27.7 (26.6–28.8)	31.3 (29.7–32.9)	25.3 (24.4–26.3)	33.8 (31.7–36.1)	18.2 (17.4–19.1)	12.9 (11.4–14.5)
Cigarettes	68.9 (68.1–69.7)	—	—	28.5 (27.7–29.4)	—	—	20.6 (19.7–21.5)	—	14.2 (13.5–15.0)	—
Cigarettes (100+ ever)	44.3 (43.4–45.3)	43.7 (42.3–45.0)	—	24.9 (24.2–25.6)	24.3 (23.4–25.2)	—	4.6 (4.2–5.1)	—	4.5 (4.1–4.9)	—
Any Illicit Drug	49.5 (48.5–50.4)	22.8 (21.8–23.8)	44.2 (42.0–46.4)	15.0 (14.5–15.6)	6.2 (5.8–6.6)	11.0 (10.0–12.1)	25.8 (24.8–26.8)	23.2 (20.5–26.2)	19.6 (18.7–20.4)	16.2 (14.3–18.4)
Marijuana	44.5 (43.6–45.4)	20.6 (19.6–21.6)	42.4 (40.3–44.4)	11.3 (10.9–11.8)	4.1 (3.8–4.4)	9.5 (8.6–10.4)	17.2 (16.3–18.1)	22.1 (19.4–25.0)	14.1 (13.3–15.0)	14.1 (12.3–16.0)
Cocaine	16.3 (15.8–16.9)	6.1 (5.7–6.6)	16.2 (15.0–17.6)	1.9 (1.7–2.1)	0.6 (0.5–0.7)	1.6 (1.2–2.2)	1.5 (1.3–1.8)	2.0 (1.5–2.7)	1.0 (0.8–1.2)	1.0 (0.7–1.4)
Heroin	1.7 (1.5–2.0)	0.3 (0.3–0.4)	—	0.3 (0.2–0.3)	0.0 (0.0–0.1)	—	0.2 (0.1–0.3)	—	0.1 (0.1–0.2)	—
Inhalants	8.8 (8.4–9.2)	1.7 (1.6–1.9)	—	0.5 (0.4–0.6)	0.1 (0.1–0.2)	—	8.2 (7.7–8.9)	—	3.6 (3.2–4.0)	—
Hallucinogens	16.1 (15.5–16.6)	5.8 (5.4–6.3)	—	1.7 (1.5–1.8)	0.6 (0.5–0.7)	—	4.1 (3.7–4.5)	—	3.1 (2.7–3.4)	—
Analgesics	14.2 (13.7–14.8)	4.7 (4.4–5.2)	—	4.8 (4.5–5.0)	1.8 (1.6–2.0)	—	9.1 (8.5–9.8)	—	6.2 (5.7–6.8)	—
Tranquilizers	9.3 (8.9–9.7)	3.4 (3.2–3.7)	—	2.2 (2.0–2.4)	0.9 (0.8–1.1)	—	3.0 (2.7–3.3)	—	1.9 (1.7–2.2)	—
Stimulants	8.4 (7.9–8.9)	4.7 (4.2–5.1)	—	1.0 (0.9–1.2)	0.5 (0.4–0.6)	—	2.0 (1.8–2.4)	—	1.3 (1.1–1.5)	—
Sedatives	3.3 (3.0–3.6)	4.1 (3.8–4.4)	—	0.3 (0.3–0.4)	1.2 (1.1–1.4)	—	0.7 (0.6–0.9)	—	0.4 (0.3–0.6)	—
Total N	(39,259)	(43,093)	(5,692)	(39,259)	(43,093)	(5,692)	(18,614)	(9,525)	(18,614)	(9,525)

Notes: Secondary analysis of data sets.
[a] Asked of those who ever consumed at least 12 drinks in a year.
[b] Based on having ever smoked at least 100 cigarettes, or 50+ cigars, or 50+ times pipes, or used snuff or chewing tobacco 20+ times lifetime in NESARC. Last 12-month question asked of those who ever smoked tobacco daily for a two-month period in NCS-R and NCS-A.

in at least one of four harmful consequences: failure to fulfill major role obligations at work, school, or home; hazardous use, such as driving an automobile or operating a machine when impaired by substance use; legal problems, for example, arrests for substance-related disorderly conduct; and continued use despite social or interpersonal problems caused by the substance.

The criteria for tobacco (nicotine) dependence are the same as for alcohol and illicit drugs. Abuse does not apply to tobacco.

These definitions differ substantively from those in the fifth edition (DSM-5) of the American Psychiatric Association, which will become the standard as of 2013. In the DSM-5, the distinction between abuse and dependence will be eliminated and, for all substances including tobacco, the criteria for drug disorder will be 2 out of 11 criteria (Hasin, 2012a, 2012b; O'Brien, 2011; Schuckit, 2012). This decision was based on secondary analysis of several large-scale epidemiological data sets. Craving was considered, in addition to the seven traditional DSM-IV criteria. The methods used to determine the relationship between abuse and dependence included factor analysis to establish unidimensionality, item response theory to assess the relationship of abuse to dependence criteria, criterion/item characteristic curves to examine the severity and discrimination of each criterion relative to each other, and total information curves to allow comparisons of two or more sets of criteria (Hasin, 2012a; Hasin et al., 2012; Saha et al., 2012). The evidence suggested that abuse and dependence formed one disorder. Craving was added as a diagnostic criterion but legal difficulties was eliminated (O'Brien, 2011), leaving a total of 11 criteria. Based on analyses of existing data sets, this definition is expected to generate rates of substance use disorders similar to those derived from combining rates of DSM-IV dependence and abuse. However, the rates will in all likelihood be higher than the rates of DSM-IV dependence discussed in this chapter, which do not include abuse.

LIMITATIONS OF MEASUREMENT: DIFFERENCES ACROSS SURVEYS

There are important differences among the surveys regarding the measurement of drug use, drug abuse, and drug dependence. Methodological features affect comparability across studies, the rates they each report, and lead to substantial variations in prevalences.

Discrepancies in estimates of prevalence and the correlates of substance use and substance use disorders between the NSDUH and NESARC were discussed in detail by Grucza et al. (2007). A discussion of NSDUH methodology compared with other surveys is also provided by Hedden et al. (2012). Two limitations of the assessments regarding alcohol and illicit drugs implemented by the National Comorbidity Studies, both the replication among adults (NCS-R) and the adolescent survey (NCS-A), have also previously been highlighted (Cottler, 2007; Grant et al., 2007). In the NCS, abuse symptoms were used as a screen so that respondents were not asked the dependence questions unless they had endorsed at least one abuse symptom. Because in the DSM-IV abuse symptoms are not required for the dependence diagnosis, this strategy results in an underestimate of dependence in the population. As illustrated by NESARC, a substantial number of individuals meet criteria for dependence although they are negative for abuse, 33.7% for those dependent on alcohol and 22.4% for those dependent on an illicit drug (Hasin and Grant, 2004; Hasin et al., 2005). The underestimate is especially pronounced among women and minorities. Second, in the NCS the assessment of abuse and dependence on marijuana and other illicit drugs was made for different illicit drugs as a group rather than for each drug separately, thereby creating a generic diagnosis of drug abuse or drug dependence, rather than one that was drug specific, as specified by the DSM-IV (Cottler, 2007). Asking about symptoms for drugs as a group may have led to underestimates of reports compared with asking about each drug separately. The principal investigators of the NCS-R and NCS-A studies acknowledged the validity of the first criticism but not the second (Kessler and Merikangas, 2007).

A third limitation of the NCS, not previously noted, pertains to the assessment of nicotine dependence. Among smokers, assessment was restricted to those who had smoked daily for a two-month period. This reduced the number of smokers eligible to report symptoms of dependence. Craving, a symptom that is not part of the DSM-IV definition, was included first in a list of eight criteria of nicotine dependence; tolerance and withdrawal were listed second and third. The logic and skip patterns of the interview schedule resulted in the inclusion of two different groups among those defined as nicotine dependent: (1) tobacco users who endorsed the first three criteria, but who were not asked the remaining five criteria, and (2) tobacco users who had endorsed up to two criteria among the first three and were asked all remaining five criteria. Finally, the definition of nicotine dependence applied to adolescents (NCS-A) did not apply the DSM-IV requirement that three symptoms be experienced within a 12-month time frame.

There are additional differences in the assessment of drug use and the eligibility of respondents for answering abuse and dependence questions across surveys. In NESARC, respondents were asked which illicit drugs they had used from a list of ten drug classes. Non-medical use of medically prescribed drugs was listed first; the last class included "any other medicines or drugs (not otherwise defined)." More detailed questions about drug-specific patterns of use were then asked for each drug reported to have been used. Symptoms of dependence were ascertained first without reference to any drugs. Respondents were then asked which "medicines or drugs did this happen with?" during the last 12 months, and before the last 12 months. The NSDUH asked only about symptoms experienced in the last 12 months but not lifetime. In NESARC, being a smoker was defined as having ever smoked at least 100 cigarettes. The nicotine dependence questions were ascertained in this restrictive group of smokers, whereas the NSDUH asked these questions of anyone who had ever smoked, even if only a puff. As noted earlier, in the NCS the last 12-month smoking and nicotine dependence questions were restricted to individuals who had smoked daily for at least two months. The alcohol abuse and dependence questions were restricted to those who had ever drunk 12 drinks in a year.

TABLE 58.2. Lifetime and last 12-month prevalence of substance abuse and dependence among persons aged 18 and older in NSDUH 2010 (N = 39,259), NESARC 2001–2002 (N = 43,093), and NCS-R (N = 5,692)

SUBSTANCE ABUSE/ DEPENDENCE	(1) LIFETIME RATES		(2) LAST 12-MONTH RATES			(3) LIFETIME RATES AMONG LIFETIME USERS		(4) LAST 12-MONTH RATES AMONG 12-MONTH USERS			(5) LAST 12-MONTH RATES AMONG LIFETIME ABUSE/ DEPENDENT	
	NESARC[a] % (95% CI)	NCS-R[b] % (95% CI)	NSDUH[c] % (95% CI)	NESARC[d] % (95% CI)	NCS-R[e] % (95% CI)	NESARC % (95% CI)	NCS-R % (95% CI)	NSDUH % (95% CI)	NESARC % (95% CI)	NCS-R % (95% CI)	NESARC % (95% CI)	NCS-R % (95% CI)
Alcohol Abuse[f]	17.8 (16.8–18.9)	7.8[g] (7.1–8.6)	3.9 (3.6–4.2)	4.7 (4.3–5.0)	1.6[g] (1.4–2.0)	21.5 (20.5–22.6)	8.5 (7.7–9.3)	5.5 (5.2–6.0)	7.1 (6.6–7.7)	2.6 (2.2–3.1)	24.0 (22.8–25.3)	21.0 (18.0–24.3)
Alcohol Dependence[f]	12.5 (11.8–13.2)	5.4 (4.8–6.1)	3.4 (3.2–3.7)	3.8 (3.5–4.1)	1.3 (1.0–1.8)	15.1 (14.3–15.9)	5.9 (5.3–6.6)	4.9 (4.5–5.3)	5.8 (5.4–6.3)	2.2 (1.6–2.9)	30.5 (28.6–32.4)	24.8 (19.1–31.5)
Drug (Illicit) Abuse	7.7 (7.3–8.2)	4.9[h] (4.3–5.6)	0.7 (0.6–0.9)	1.4 (1.2–1.5)	0.8[h] (0.6–1.1)	33.9 (32.7–35.3)	11.1 (9.7–12.7)	5.0 (4.2–5.8)	22.2 (20.2–24.2)	7.4 (5.5–10.0)	15.7 (14.1–17.4)	16.5 (13.1–20.7)
Drug (Illicit) Dependence	2.6 (2.4–2.9)	3.0 (2.6–3.6)	1.8 (1.6–2.0)	0.6 (0.5–0.7)	0.4 (0.3–0.7)	11.3 (10.5–12.3)	6.9 (6.0–8.0)	12.1 (10.9–13.4)	10.1 (8.7–11.7)	3.8 (2.4–5.8)	24.2 (21.1–27.6)	13.6 (8.9–20.2)
Any Substance Use Disorder, not including Nicotine Dependence	32.3 (30.8–33.9)	14.6 (13.6–15.8)	8.9 (8.5–9.4)	9.4 (8.7–9.9)	3.6 (3.0–4.4)	38.9 (37.3–40.4)	15.9 (14.8–17.1)	12.4 (11.8–13.1)	14.2 (13.5–14.9)	5.8 (4.8–6.9)	28.9 (27.9–30.0)	24.8 (21.5–28.6)
Nicotine Dependence[i,j]												
Tobacco	17.7 (16.8–18.7)	8.2 (7.5–9.1)	—	12.8 (12.0–13.6)	4.0 (3.5–4.6)	37.8 (36.6–39.0)	11.2 (10.1–12.4)	—	46.1 (44.7–47.6)	12.9 (11.3–14.7)	72.0 (70.5–73.5)	49.0 (43.9–54.0)
Cigarettes	—	—	9.8 (9.4–10.3)	—	—	—	—	34.5 (33.2–35.8)	—	—	—	—
Cigarettes (100+ ever)	17.1 (16.2–18.1)	—	9.8 (9.3–10.2)	12.3 (11.6–13.1)	—	39.2 (37.9–40.5)	—	39.2 (37.7–40.7)	49.7 (48.2–51.3)	—	72.0 (70.5–73.5)	—
Any Substance Use Disorder, including Nicotine Dependence	38.4 (36.7–40.1)	19.5 (18.1–21.0)	16.7 (16.1–17.4)	18.8 (17.9–19.8)	7.2 (6.2–8.0)	44.7 (43.1–43.6)	20.8 (19.4–22.3)	21.9 (21.1–22.8)	26.2 (25.1–27.1)	10.1 (8.9–11.4)	49.0 (47.9–50.2)	36.1 (33.0–39.3)

Notes: Italicized figures from published articles. Non-italicized from secondary analysis of data sets.
[a] Compton et al. (2005); [b] Kessler et al. (2005b); [c] SAMHSA (2011); [d] Grant et al. (2004b); [e] Kessler et al. (2005a).
[f] Asked of those who consumed at least 12 drinks in a year in NCS-R.
[g] Published figures = 13.2%, 3.1%. We assume that these include alcohol dependence.
[h] Published figures = 7.9%, 1.4%. We assume that these include illicit drug dependence.
[i] DSM-IV in NCS-R and NESARC; last 30 days NDSS in NSDUH.
[j] Based on having ever smoked at least 100 cigarettes, or 50+ cigars, or 50+ times pipes, or used snuff or chewing tobacco 20+ times lifetime in NESARC. Asked of those who ever smoked tobacco daily for a two-month period in NCS-R.

There are also differences in mode of survey administration that impact on the resulting rates of self-reported drug behavior. Of the surveys, NSDUH is the only anonymous one. In addition, the assessment of lifetime symptoms based on retrospective reports may lead to undercounts compared with repeated prospective assessments (Moffitt et al., 2010).

Thus, existing surveys have different strengths and weaknesses. NESARC has the most systematic assessment of substance use disorders and psychiatric disorders. The repeated annual NSDUH surveys provide the best data on patterns of use of legal and illegal drugs in the population. They also include detailed DSM-IV assessments of abuse and dependence on alcohol, specific illicit drugs, and the non-medical use of medically prescribed drugs for the last 12 months but not lifetime. Nicotine dependence is measured by the NDSS (Shiffman et al., 2004) rather than the DSM-IV. Anonymity in the NSDUH may have led to higher rates of self-reported drug use than in NESARC, whereas differences in instrumentation may have led to higher rates of last 12-month substance use disorder among the self-acknowledged drug users in NESARC than NSDUH. The NSDUH surveys respondents as of age 12, making possible comparisons between adolescents and adults. The nature of the NCS-R and NCS-A assessments greatly limit the quality of the data collected on substance use disorders, although they allow comparisons between adults and adolescents, because the same methodology (although flawed) was implemented in both surveys.

We implemented extensive secondary analyses of the four data sets in order to increase comparability across studies. For reasons of confidentiality, the public use NSDUH data included 84.5% of the original sample, so that in certain instances the figures in this chapter differ very slightly from published ones. To increase comparability of NCS with the other surveys, we reran NCS data on abuse excluding cases that met criteria for dependence. We also applied the DSM-IV requirement of experiencing three criteria within a 12-month period for nicotine dependence in NCS-A. We included nicotine dependence in summary measures of drug disorder for all the surveys. Finally, we excluded respondents 18 years old from the NCS-A sample to obtain a sample 13–17 years old and increase comparability with the sample of adolescents 12–17 years old in NSDUH.

Taking into account the issues discussed earlier, the data presented by any one study must be interpreted with caution. Comparisons across studies are subject to many limitations.

PREVALENCE OF SUBSTANCE USE AND DISORDERS

PREVALENCE OF SUBSTANCE USE AND DISORDERS AMONG ADULTS

The lifetime and last 12-month prevalence of use of specific substances in the NSDUH, NESARC, and NCS-R for persons aged 18 and over are presented in the first two panels of Table 58.1.

The rates of use for alcohol are very similar across the three studies, whereas those for tobacco and illicit drugs (as a group) are similar in the NSDUH and NCS-R, but much lower in NESARC (see Table 58.1, Panels 1 and 2). The discrepancy

for tobacco is explained by the fact that, in NESARC, smoking at least 100 cigarettes lifetime was required to be defined as a smoker. Yet, 36% of smokers in the NSDUH never smoked 100 cigarettes. When restricted to those who smoked at least 100 cigarettes, the rate in NSDUH is identical to NESARC. It is not clear why the overall rates of lifetime or last year illicit drug use in NESARC are half those of the other two surveys. Lack of anonymity may be one explanation. The discrepancies are especially large for cocaine, with 16.3% and 16.2% in NSDUH and NCS-R, respectively, reporting lifetime use compared with only 6.1% in NESARC (see Table 58.1, Panel 1) (see Grucza et al., 2007). Despite these differences in absolute rates across studies, the relative rankings for overall prevalence of use are the same. Alcohol is the substance that is used most widely, followed by tobacco and illicit drugs. Half the adults 18 and over in the United States have used an illicit drug, including non-medical use of a prescribed drug, representing 113 million individuals in 2010. Of these drugs, marijuana is the most prevalent, followed by cocaine; almost three times as many individuals have ever used marijuana as have used cocaine (Table 58.1, Panel 1). The higher rates in NSDUH and NCS-R than NESARC increase the base of individuals eligible for being asked the questions relevant to drug abuse and dependence and the absolute number identified as meeting criteria for abuse or dependence.

Lifetime and last 12-month rates of abuse or dependence in the total adult population, lifetime rates among lifetime users of each drug, last 12-month rates among last 12-month users, and last 12-month rates among lifetime abusers or dependents are presented in Table 58.2. None of the published reports from the studies include nicotine dependence in any substance use disorder. This is a serious omission inasmuch as tobacco is one of the two most addictive substances that are used, second to heroin. Table 58.2 presents rates of abuse and dependence separately for alcohol, illicit drugs as a group, nicotine, any substance use disorder as reported in the literature (Row 5), and rates including nicotine dependence that we calculated from secondary analysis of the public use data (Row 9). The conditional rates among users specify the risk of abusing or becoming dependent on a drug among those who consumed the drug in their lifetime or the last 12 months. The conditional rates of last 12-month abuse or dependence among those who met lifetime criteria index chronicity of abuse or dependence.

Except for illicit drug dependence, the rates of lifetime and last 12-month abuse and dependence for all drug classes in the total adult population and among last 12-month users were consistently the lowest in NCS-R (Table 58.2, Panels 1, 2 and 4).

In NESARC, close to 40% of the population 18 years old and over ever met criteria for a substance disorder (abuse and/or dependence), including nicotine dependence; 17.7% met criteria for nicotine dependence, 12.5% for alcohol dependence, 2.6% for illicit drug dependence (Table 58.2, Panel 1). The 12-month rates were 80% to 28% lower than lifetime rates. Slightly less than 20% of the population met criteria for a substance use disorder within the last year in NESARC, a rate very similar to the NSDUH (Table 58.2, Panel 2). The proportion meeting criteria for abuse or substance dependence on a given drug among individuals who used the drug varied greatly across drug classes. Across all surveys, conditional upon lifetime use, nicotine emerged as the most addictive of the substances, with 37.8% of tobacco users in NESARC meeting criteria for lifetime dependence (Table 58.2, Panel 3). This compares with 28.2% among heroin users (Compton et al., 2005). Among last year users, however, heroin emerged as the most addictive substance in NSDUH, followed by tobacco, sedatives, cocaine, and analgesics. The ranking in NESARC, wherein heroin could not be ranked because of the small number of users, was tobacco, cocaine, and stimulants (data not presented). The conditional last 12-months rates among last 12-month users were the highest in NESARC for any substance use disorder with or without nicotine (Table 58.2, Panel 4), although there were differences among specific illicit substances. The rates were higher in NESARC than NSDUH for cocaine and stimulants, lower for analgesics and sedatives, and the same for alcohol, marijuana, inhalants, hallucinogens, and tranquilizers (data not presented). The proportion of individuals with an alcohol-related disorder among those who consumed alcohol in the last year was among the lowest of any of the substances. However, because so many individuals consume alcohol, this percentage translates into a large number of affected individuals. Detailed comparison across drug classes could not be made in the NCS-R.

Substance use disorders are chronic disorders. As illustrated by NESARC, close to half of those who met lifetime abuse or dependence criteria on any substance still experienced these symptoms within the last year (Table 58.2, Panel 5). These rates could not be calculated for NSDUH, which only measured last 12-months abuse and dependence. While rates of chronicity of dependence are consistently lower in NCS-R than NESARC, the patterns across drug classes are identical. Nicotine is by far the most chronic of the addictions, with 72.0% of tobacco users in NESARC meeting criteria for last 12-month dependence among those who ever met lifetime criteria. Chronicity is slightly higher for dependence on alcohol (30.5%) than illicit drugs (24.2%) (Table 58.2, Panel 5). Chronicity of dependence is also relatively high among those who consume prescribed drugs non-medically, especially analgesics (data not presented).

PREVALENCE OF SUBSTANCE USE AND DISORDERS AMONG ADOLESCENTS

The behavior of adults 18 years old and over could be compared with that of adolescents 12–17 years old in NSDUH and 13–17 years old in NCS-A. Except for inhalants, the prevalence of lifetime use of various substances is lower among adolescents than adults, with wide differences across substances (Table 58.1, Panels 3 and 4). Although the absolute rates differ between NCS-A and NSDUH, the patterns are strikingly similar in both surveys. As illustrated by NSDUH, the lifetime adolescent rates for alcohol and any tobacco use are about 40% and those for any illicit drug about 50% of those observed among adults, and only 10% for use of 100 cigarettes or more. There are great variations across specific illicit drugs in the ratio of adolescent to adult prevalence rates. Inhalants is the only drug class for which the rates are the same. With respect

to last 12-month use, the age patterns reverse for illicit drugs, where adolescents have higher rates than adults, 19.6% versus 15.0% in NSDUH and 16.2% versus 11.0% in NCS.

The overall rates of any substance use disorders among lifetime users are the same among adolescents and adults, although there are differences across substances. Lifetime dependence on illicit drugs among lifetime users is higher among adolescents, whereas tobacco dependence is lower than among adults (NCS, Tables 58.2 and 58.3, Panel 3). The last 12-month rates among 12-month users are consistently higher among adolescents than adults in both surveys, except for tobacco dependence in NSDUH (Tables 58.2 and 58.3, Panel 4). The differences are greater in NCS-A than NSDUH, where three times as many adolescents (31.0%) as adults (10.1%) meet criteria for any substance use disorder among those who used those drugs within the last 12 months (NCS, Tables 58.2 and 58.3, Panel 4). Persistence is also much higher among adolescents than adults (Tables 58.2 and 58.3, Panel 5), reflecting the fact that duration since onset of drug use is much shorter for adolescents than adults.

COMORBIDITY OF USE AND DISORDERS ACROSS SUBSTANCES

Consideration of each drug class by itself underestimates the extent of drug use in the population because many individuals use more than one class of drugs. Thus, in 2010, only 8.2% of the population aged 18 and over had not experimented with any substance; 44.2% had experimented with all three major classes: alcohol, tobacco, and illicit drugs (based on NSDUH 2010).

Similarly, substance use disorders on multiple drugs tend to cooccur. In NESARC, 40.3% of individuals 18 and over who met criteria for abuse or dependence on one drug class also met criteria for abuse or dependence for at least another drug; 11.7% met criteria for two other substances. The highest comorbidity was between dependence on an illicit drug and dependence on alcohol (70%) or nicotine (69%) (secondary analysis of NESARC). Yet, only a minority of addicted individuals have been treated for their addiction (Compton et al., 2007).

PREVALENCE OF SUBSTANCE USE AND DISORDERS BY AGE, GENDER, RACE/ ETHNICITY

There are important differences in the prevalence of use and substance use disorders in different subgroups in the population, but the patterns are not necessarily consistent across surveys. Age differences were examined in all four surveys, but only in NSDUH and NESARC for gender and race/ ethnicity.

AGE

Differences between adolescents and adults were discussed earlier. Adulthood itself can be differentiated into periods. Four age

TABLE 58.3. Lifetime and last 12-month prevalence of substance abuse and dependence among persons aged 12–17 in NSDUH 2010 (N = 18,614) and aged 13–17 in NCS-A (N = 9,525)

SUBSTANCE ABUSE/ DEPENDENCE	(1) LIFETIME RATES NCS-A % (95% CI)	(2) LAST 12-MONTH RATES NSDUH % (95% CI)	NCS-A % (95% CI)	(3) LIFETIME RATES AMONG LIFETIME USERS NCS-A % (95% CI)	(4) LAST 12-MONTH RATES AMONG 12-MONTH USERS NSDUH % (95% CI)	NCS-A % (95% CI)	(5) LAST 12-MONTH RATES AMONG LIFETIME ABUSE/ DEPENDENT NCS-A % (95% CI)
Alcohol Abuse[a]	4.4 (3.9–5.0)	2.9 (2.6–3.3)	3.2 (2.8–3.7)	7.6 (6.7–8.6)	10.3 (9.1–11.5)	14.4 (12.8–16.2)	72.5 (66.7–77.6)
Alcohol Dependence[a]	1.3 (1.0–1.6)	1.7 (1.4–2.0)	1.0 (0.7–1.3)	2.1 (1.8–2.6)	5.8 (5.0–6.8)	4.3 (3.3–5.8)	76.2 (59.5–87.5)
Drug (Illicit) Abuse	6.8 (5.8–8.0)	2.2 (1.9–2.5)	4.5 (3.7–5.4)	29.3 (27.1–31.7)	11.1 (9.7–12.7)	26.1 (23.1–29.4)	65.3 (56.9–72.8)
Drug (Illicit) Dependence	1.7 (1.3–2.2)	2.5 (2.3–2.8)	1.1 (0.8–1.6)	7.2 (5.9–8.8)	13.0 (11.8–14.3)	6.7 (5.0–9.0)	67.3 (52.6–79.3)
Any Substance Use Disorder, not including Nicotine Dependence	10.6 (9.3–12.0)	7.3 (6.8–8.0)	7.8 (6.9–8.9)	17.7 (15.9–19.6)	21.8 (20.3–23.4)	28.3 (25.9–30.7)	74.0 (68.5–78.9)
Nicotine Dependence[b,c]	2.6 (2.0–3.3)	—	2.0 (1.6–2.7)	7.5 (6.1–9.3)	—	15.9 (12.7–19.6)	79.8 (70.3–86.8)
Cigarettes	—	1.8 (1.5–2.0)	—	—	12.4 (10.7–14.3)	—	—
Cigarettes (100+ ever)	—	1.6 (1.4–1.8)	—	—	35.8 (31.6–40.3)	—	—
Any Substance Use Disorder, including Nicotine Dependence	11.3 (9.9–12.8)	8.0 (7.4–8.7)	8.7 (7.7–9.9)	18.9 (16.9–21.0)	22.5 (20.9–24.1)	31.0 (28.6–33.6)	77.3 (72.0–81.9)

Notes: Based on secondary analysis of data sets.
[a] Asked of those who ever consumed at least 12 drinks in a year in NCS-A.
[b] DSM-IV in NCS-A; last 30 days NDSS in NSDUH.
[c] Asked of those who ever smoked tobacco daily for a two-month period in NCS-A.

groups (ages 12/13–17 to ages 50+) could be differentiated in NSDUH and NCS and three age groups (ages 18–25 to 50+) in NESARC. Rates of last 12-month use by age in the population are presented in Figure 58.1A–C, and rates of last 12-month dependence among last 12-month users are presented in Figure 58.1D–F. Age-related trends are presented for tobacco users in NCS, and for all cigarette users in NSDUH as well as for those who smoked at least 100 cigarettes, the NESARC definition of being a smoker, to maximize comparability between the two surveys.

Age-related patterns are very similar across the surveys, although the absolute rates of use or dependence may differ. The prevalence of substance use varies greatly by age. With the exception of tobacco (cigarettes), age-related differences are stronger for use in the population than for dependence among those who used a particular substance.

Rates of use of all substances increase sharply throughout adolescence, and decline also sharply from ages 18–25 for illicit drugs (see Fig. 58.1A–C). Use of cigarettes declines more slowly; the decline for those who smoked at least 100 cigarettes occurs at older ages. In NSDUH and NESARC, the prevalence of drinking alcohol remains at fairly stable levels from ages 18 to 49, when rates start to decline. In NCS-R, rates decline as of ages 26–34.

Among last 12-month users, age-related patterns for dependence differ from those for use itself (see Fig. 58.1D–F). For all cigarette users (NSDUH), conditional rates of nicotine dependence rise sharply from adolescence to the mid-thirties and then more slowly thereafter (see Fig. 58.1D). Rates of nicotine dependence (for those who smoked 100 cigarettes or more or used tobacco daily) change little with age in NSDUH and NCS but decline as of age 35–49 in NESARC (see Fig. 58.1D–F). The rates of alcohol dependence decline gradually as of ages 18–25, except for a sharp drop from ages 18–25 to 26–34 in NESARC. In the three surveys, the conditional rates of dependence on illicit drugs decline slowly over time as of age 18–25 (see Fig. 58.1D–F).

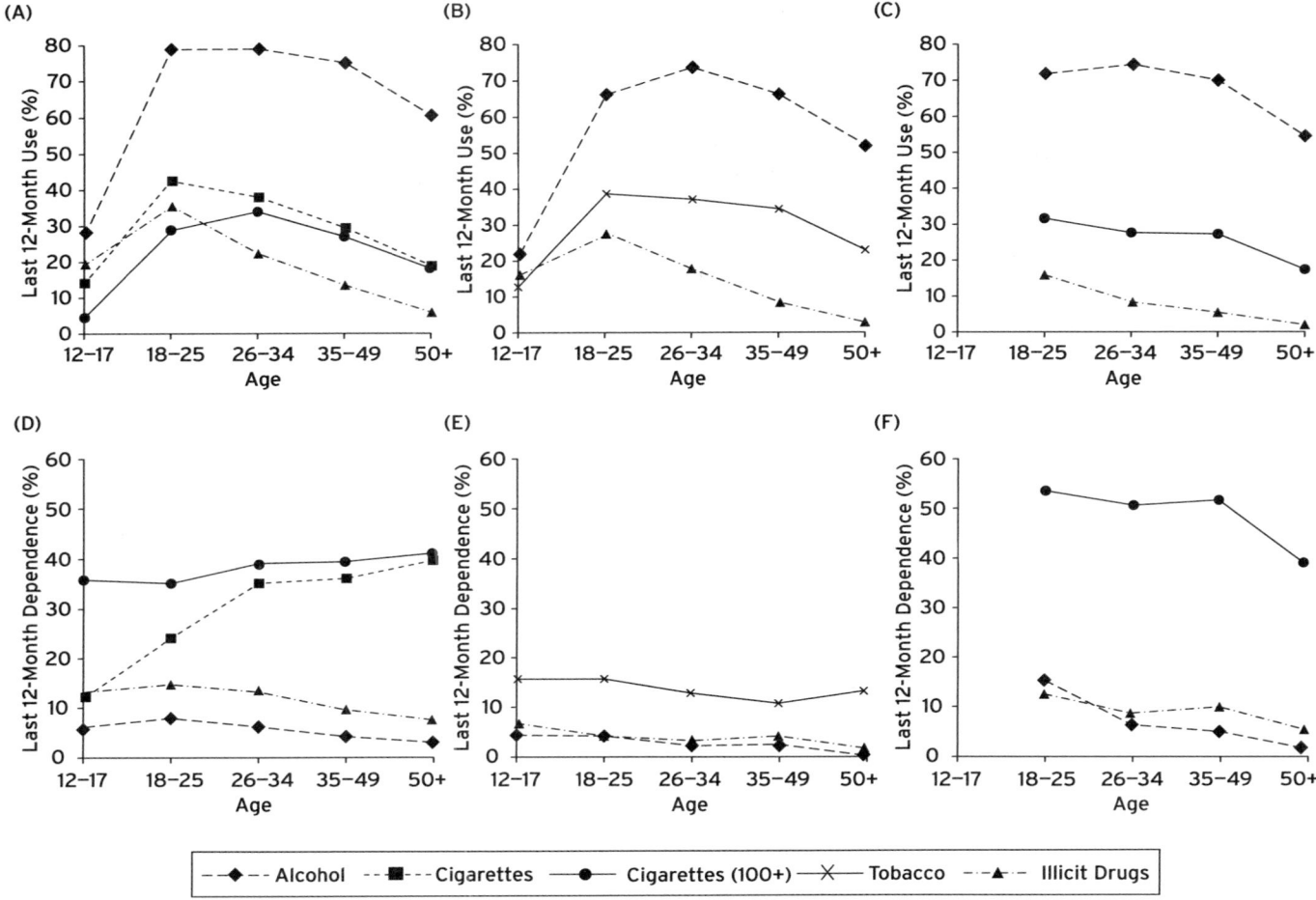

Figure 58.1 Prevalence of last 12-month use by age of alcohol and illicit drugs in (A) NSDUH, (B) NCS-R, NCS-A, (C) NESARC; of any cigarettes (NSDUH); of any cigarettes 100+ lifetime (NSDUH, NESARC); or of tobacco (NCS-R, NCS-A); and prevalence of last 12-month dependence by age among last 12-month users in (D) NSDUH, (E) NCS-R, NCS-A, (F) NESARC.

GENDER

Gender patterns for substance use and substance use disorders are similar in NSDUH and NESARC (Table 58.4). For all substances, including nonmedical use of psychotherapeutics, males have consistently higher rates of use than females, with the rates higher by 10–20% for alcohol, and 50–60% higher for tobacco and all illicit drugs combined. Gender differences are especially pronounced for marijuana and cocaine.

Among drug users, the rates of abuse and dependence on alcohol and illicit drugs are also consistently higher for males than females, except for nicotine, for which the rates of dependence are the same for males and females in NSDUH but significantly higher for females than males in NESARC (see Table 58.4). Combining all substances, the conditional rates of overall substance use disorders, including nicotine, are 39% higher in NSDUH and 28% higher in NESARC among males than females.

RACE/ETHNICITY

Racial/ethnic differences in patterns of substance use and disorders in the population are similar in NESARC and NSDUH (Table 58.5). In both surveys, Asians have the lowest rates of use and disorder for every drug class, except for tobacco dependence and illicit drug abuse in NESARC. In NESARC, whites have the highest rates of any group for alcohol abuse and nicotine dependence; African-Americans and Hispanics have the highest rates of illicit drug dependence. In the NSDUH, ethnic patterns are less consistent. Whites have much higher rates of nicotine dependence among last 12-month smokers than any other racial/ethnic group. African-Americans tend to have higher rates of dependence on illicit drugs than any other group. The most striking differences are the higher rates of alcohol use and nicotine dependence among whites than any other group, and the higher rate of dependence on illicit drugs among African-Americans (see Table 58.5).

COMORBIDITY OF SUBSTANCE USE DISORDERS WITH PSYCHIATRIC DISORDERS

"There is extensive comorbidity between addiction and mental illness, as documented by NESARC. Among individuals

TABLE 58.4. Last 12-month prevalence of nonmedical substance use and last 12-month DSM-IV abuse and dependence among last 12-month users aged 18 and older by gender in NSDUH 2010 and NESARC 2001–2002

LAST 12-MONTH	NSDUH MALES %	NSDUH FEMALES %	NESARC MALES %	NESARC FEMALES %
SUBSTANCE USE				
Alcohol	74.2	66.9***	71.8	59.6***
Tobacco (Nicotine)[a]	42.8	26.7***	33.9	22.0***
Cigarettes	31.9	25.3***	—	—
Cigarettes (100+ ever)	27.7	22.2***	27.2	21.6***
Any Illicit Drug	18.5	11.8***	7.8	4.8***
Marijuana	14.6	8.2***	5.6	2.6***
Cocaine	2.7	1.2***	0.8	0.3***
Any Substance	81.5	72.7***	78.6	65.5***
Total N	(18,339)	(20,920)	(18,518)	(24,575)
DSM-IV ABUSE/DEPENDENCE AMONG LAST 12-MONTH USERS OF EACH SUBSTANCE				
Alcohol Abuse	7.8	3.2***	9.7	4.3***
Alcohol Dependence	5.9	3.9***	7.5	3.9***
Nicotine Dependence[a, b]				
Tobacco	—	—	41.8	52.3***
Cigarettes	33.9	35.1	—	—
Cigarettes (100+ ever)	38.7	39.8	47.1	52.8***
Drug (Illicit) Abuse	5.9	3.7***	25.2	17.7***
Drug (Illicit) Dependence	12.6	11.3	11.2	8.4*
Any Substance Use Disorder, including Nicotine Dependence	25.5	18.3***	29.3	22.9***

Notes: Secondary analysis of data sets. *p < .05, **< .01, ***< .001, differences between males and females.
[a] Based on having ever smoked at least 100 cigarettes, or 50+ cigars, or 50+ times pipes, or used snuff or chewing tobacco 20+ times lifetime in NESARC.
[b] DSM-IV in NESARC; last 30 days NDSS in NSDUH.

with a diagnosis of abuse or dependence on illicit drugs, 40.9% met criteria for mood disorder, 29.9% for anxiety disorder (Conway et al., 2006), 18.3% for antisocial personality disorder, and 57.5% for any psychiatric disorder (unpublished analysis). The rates were at least 50% higher among those who met criteria specifically for illicit drug dependence (i.e., 61.7% for mood, 47.2% for anxiety, 32.9% for antisocial personality, and 78.2% for any psychiatric disorder) (Koob et al., 2008: p. 362) (Table 58.6). The rates among those dependent on alcohol or nicotine were similar and lower than those for the seven classes of illicit drugs that were considered. For alcohol dependence, the rates were 40.0% for mood, 32.3% for anxiety, 14.3% for antisocial personality, and 55.9% for any disorder. Comorbidity rates among those dependent on nicotine were similar to those dependent on alcohol, namely 36.6%, 30.8%, 11.2%, and 52.2%, respectively. The associations between psychiatric disorders and substance dependence are highly statistically significant for all substances and all classes of psychiatric disorders. The associations are somewhat higher with mood than anxiety disorders, and much higher—by a factor of two or three—with antisocial personality than mood or anxiety disorders" (Koob et al., 2008: p. 362) with odds ratios ranging from 15 to 23 for illicit drugs (Table 58.6). Among the mood disorders, mania has the highest association with dependence for every illicit drug, as does panic with agoraphobia among anxiety disorders (Conway et al., 2006, see Tables 4 and 5).

For all three broad classes of psychiatric disorders, the lower the overall prevalence of dependence on a specific substance in the population, the greater its comorbidity with psychiatric disorders (Compton et al., 2005; Conway et al., 2006).

"A particularly strong comorbidity, observed in clinical samples but not in the general population, because of the small numbers of affected individuals, is that of schizophrenia with smoking and nicotine dependence. Rates of smoking are three to four times higher among schizophrenics than in the general population and higher than among individuals diagnosed with other psychiatric disorders (Kumari and Postma, 2005; Volkow, 2009; Wing et al., 2012). Smoking may represent self-medication for the cognitive and negative symptoms prominent in schizophrenia, given the interaction of nicotine with dopaminergic and glutamatergic transmitter systems (de Leon and Diaz, 2005; Kumari and Postma, 2005).

As suggested by Compton et al. (2005), the strong association with antisocial personality disorder across various substances may reflect an underlying comorbidity factor rather than substance specific links. This has important implications regarding the potential commonality of selected mechanisms and genetic factors underlying substance use disorders and psychiatric disorders, especially antisocial personality disorder." (Koob et al., 2008: p. 362)

To the extent that gender differences appear, comorbidity of psychiatric disorders with substance use disorders is consistently higher among females than males. Comorbidity is higher for any mood disorder with alcohol and nicotine dependence, and for antisocial personality with alcohol, nicotine,

TABLE 58.5. Last 12-month prevalence of substance use and last 12-month DSM-IV abuse and dependence among last 12-month users aged 18 and older by race/ethnicity in NSDUH 2010 and NESARC 2001–2002

LAST 12-MONTH	NSDUH				NESARC			
	WHITE %	AA %	HISPANIC %	ASIAN %	WHITE %	AA %	HISPANIC %	ASIAN %
SUBSTANCE USE								
Alcohol	74.5[a]	62.1[b]	63.5[b]	54.6[c]	69.3[a]	53.0[b]	59.9[c]	47.5[d]
Tobacco (Nicotine)[e]	36.2[a]	34.2[a]	30.8[b]	18.8[c]	29.9[a]	24.7[b]	19.9[c]	13.9[d]
Cigarettes	29.3[a]	28.5[a]	27.9[a]	15.7[b]	—	—	—	—
Cigarettes (100+ ever)	26.6[a]	24.3[a]	20.2[b]	12.2[c]	25.9[a]	22.1[b]	18.7[c]	18.2[c]
Any Illicit Drug	15.0[a]	16.6[a]	14.7[a]	8.9[b]	6.4[a]	6.1[a]	5.2[b]	4.1[c]
Marijuana	11.4[a]	14.0[b]	10.1[a]	5.3[c]	4.2[a]	4.6[b]	3.3[c]	2.0[d]
Cocaine	1.9[ab]	1.6[ac]	2.5[b]	1.0[c]	0.5[a]	0.6[b]	0.7[b]	0.2[c]
Any Substance	81.1[a]	69.6[b]	69.5[b]	58.9[c]	75.8[a]	60.3[b]	64.6[c]	50.5[d]
Total N	(25,211)	(4,735)	(5,982)	(1,471)	(25,133)	(8,130)	(8,308)	(1,124)
DSM-IV ABUSE/DEPENDENCE AMONG LAST 12-MONTH USERS OF EACH SUBSTANCE								
Alcohol Abuse	5.6[a]	4.2[b]	6.8[a]	3.3[b]	7.3[a]	6.2[b]	6.6[b]	4.0[c]
Alcohol Dependence	4.6[a]	5.9[b]	5.8[b]	2.8[c]	5.6[a]	6.5[b]	6.6[b]	4.1[c]
Nicotine Dependence[e, f]								
Tobacco	—	—	—	—	48.3[a]	41.8[b]	31.6[c]	36.5[d]
Cigarettes	39.7[a]	27.2[b]	16.9[c]	19.1[c]	—	—	—	—
Cigarettes (100+ ever)	43.6[a]	31.1[b]	22.4[c]	24.4[bc]	52.5[a]	44.6[b]	32.8[c]	45.5[ab]
Drug (Illicit) Abuse	4.0[a]	6.1[b]	8.6[c]	6.5[abc]	22.0[ab]	25.9[c]	20.3[a]	23.4[b]
Drug (Illicit) Dependence	11.2[a]	17.5[b]	12.2[a]	8.2[a]	9.1[a]	12.6[b]	13.1[b]	5.1[c]
Any Substance Use Disorder, including Nicotine Dependence	22.9[a]	21.1[ab]	19.4[b]	10.9[c]	27.2[a]	26.2[b]	20.4[c]	15.0[d]

Notes: Secondary analysis of data sets.
AA = African-American.
[abcd] Racial/ethnic groups with different superscripts in the same row from the same data set were significantly different at $p < .05$.
[e] Based on having ever smoked at least 100 cigarettes, or 50+ cigars, or 50+ times pipes, or used snuff or chewing tobacco 20+ times lifetime in NESARC.
[f] DSM-IV in NESARC; last 30 days NDSS in NSDUH.

and any illicit drug dependence (Compton et al., 2005; Grant et al., 2004a; Unpublished analysis of NESARC; data not presented). There are several gender differences in the association of specific anxiety and mood disorders with specific illicit drug disorders (see Conway et al., 2006). "Although rates of psychiatric disorders vary substantially across racial/ethnic groups, the association between alcohol dependence and illicit drug dependence with mood and anxiety disorders is similar among whites, African-Americans, Hispanics, and Asians (Smith et al., 2006)." (Koob et al., 2008: p. 362) Hispanics have the highest rate of mood disorder comorbid with nicotine dependence, while African-Americans have the lowest, and Asians the highest, rates of antisocial personality disorder comorbid with nicotine and illicit drug dependence (unpublished analysis of NESARC).

DEVELOPMENT OF PSYCHIATRIC COMORBIDITY WITH DRUG DEPENDENCE

"These cross-sectional associations do not inform on developmental processes underlying comorbidity, whether mental illness follows and causes drug dependence or whether drug dependence follows and causes mental illness. For some cases, mental illness and addiction may cooccur independently (Grant et al., 2004b); for others, there might be a sequential relationship. The direction of causality between psychiatric disorders and dependence is ambiguous because both pathways of influence have been documented. For instance, among adolescents and young adults, when drug use and psychiatric disorders have their onset, depression, social anxiety, and

TABLE 58.6. Lifetime comorbidity of dependence (percentages and unadjusted odds ratios) on alcohol, nicotine, and illicit drugs with three classes of psychiatric disorders among persons aged 18 and older in NESARC 2001–2002 (N = 43,093)

SUBSTANCE DEPENDENCE	ANY MOOD[a]		ANY ANXIETY[a]		ANTISOCIAL PERSONALITY[b]		ANY PSYCHIATRIC DISORDER	
	%	OR	%	OR	%	OR	%	OR
Alcohol dependence	40.0	3.3	32.3	2.7	14.3	7.8	55.9	3.6
Nicotine dependence	36.6	3.1	30.8	2.7	11.2	6.2	52.2	3.3
Drug (illicit) dependence[c]	61.7	7.1	47.2	4.9	32.9	16.7	78.2	9.1
Marijuana	60.5	6.5	48.5	5.0	38.0	18.7	79.8	6.5
Cocaine	62.5	7.1	45.0	4.3	34.2	15.1	78.3	8.8
Opioids	72.9	11.2	60.9	8.2	39.5	18.0	86.0	14.8
Hallucinogens	73.6	11.6	55.5	6.5	40.2	18.3	89.9	21.2
Tranquilizers	72.1	10.7	59.9	7.8	45.8	23.0	86.8	15.8
Stimulants	64.3	7.5	50.3	5.3	37.8	17.1	82.0	11.0
Sedatives	68.4	9.0	58.4	7.4	43.3	20.9	85.1	13.7

Notes: Italicized figures from published articles.
[a] Conway et al., 2006, Tables 4 & 5.
[b] Compton et al., 2005, Table 3.
[c] Also includes heroin, inhalants, and other drugs.

disruptive disorders predict the onset of smoking and nicotine dependence (Breslau et al., 2004; Karp et al., 2006; Kessler, 2004), but prior smoking and nicotine dependence also predict depression, disruptive disorders, panic attacks and disorder, and agoraphobia (Boden et al., 2010; Breslau et al., 2004; Isensee et al., 2003; Klungsøyr et al., 2006)." (Koob et al., 2008: p. 362) Analysis that we conducted in a longitudinal sample of adolescent smokers (mean age 16.7) indicated that DSM-IV psychiatric disorders preceded and, for the most part, predicted the onset of nicotine dependence, while nicotine dependence rarely predicted psychiatric disorder (Griesler et al., 2008, 2011). Anxiety, mood, and disruptive disorders had their onset at least 2.5 years before nicotine dependence. Psychiatric disorders started, on average, between ages 10.6 and 11.7, tobacco use at age 13, the first symptom of nicotine dependence at age 14.3, and full nicotine dependence at age 14.7. Panic disorder, attention-deficit hyperactivity disorder, and oppositional defiant disorder predicted the onset of nicotine dependence; nicotine dependence predicted the onset of oppositional defiant disorder. Depression and nicotine dependence did not predict each other. In adults, psychiatric disorders predicted persistent course of alcohol, nicotine, and illicit drug dependence but substance use disorders did not predict persistence of mood or anxiety disorders (Hasin and Kilcoyne, 2012).

The mechanisms underlying the comorbidity between substance use disorders and psychiatric disorders are not properly understood. Both classes of disorder may be caused by shared genetic or environmental factors. "It is likely that different neurobiological factors are involved in comorbidity depending on its development. When mental illness is followed by dependence on some types of drugs, comorbidity might reflect self-medication. However, when drug dependence is followed by mental illness, chronic drug exposure itself may lead to changes in the brain that would increase the risk for mental illness, particularly in persons with genetic vulnerability. For example, the high prevalence of smoking after individuals become depressed could reflect the antidepressant effects of nicotine and of monoamine oxidase A (MAOA) and B (MAOB) inhibition by cigarette smoking (Fowler et al., 2003)." (Koob et al., 2008: p. 362)

DEVELOPMENTAL STAGES OF INVOLVEMENT IN DRUGS

"Not only are there regular patterns of cooccurrence of use and dependence across drugs, but there are regular sequences of progression from the use of one drug class to another. The existence of a developmental sequence of involvement in drugs is one of the best replicated findings in the epidemiology of drug use (Kandel, 2002). In the United States and other Western societies, a regular sequence of progression has consistently been found. The use of cigarettes or alcohol precedes the use of marijuana and, in turn, the use of marijuana precedes the use of other illicit drugs (Fig. 58.2). Very few individuals among those who have tried cocaine have not previously used marijuana (2%), cigarettes (3.6%), or alcohol (2.2%) (based on NSDUH 2010). The majority (66.8%) of individuals have used alcohol or cigarettes prior to marijuana use or at the same age. Such behavioral regularities have given rise to the gateway hypothesis" (Koob et al., 2008: p. 360) to emphasize that certain drugs serve as gateways for the use of other substances. The drugs used earlier increase the risk of using other drugs. Even now, when rates of marijuana use among

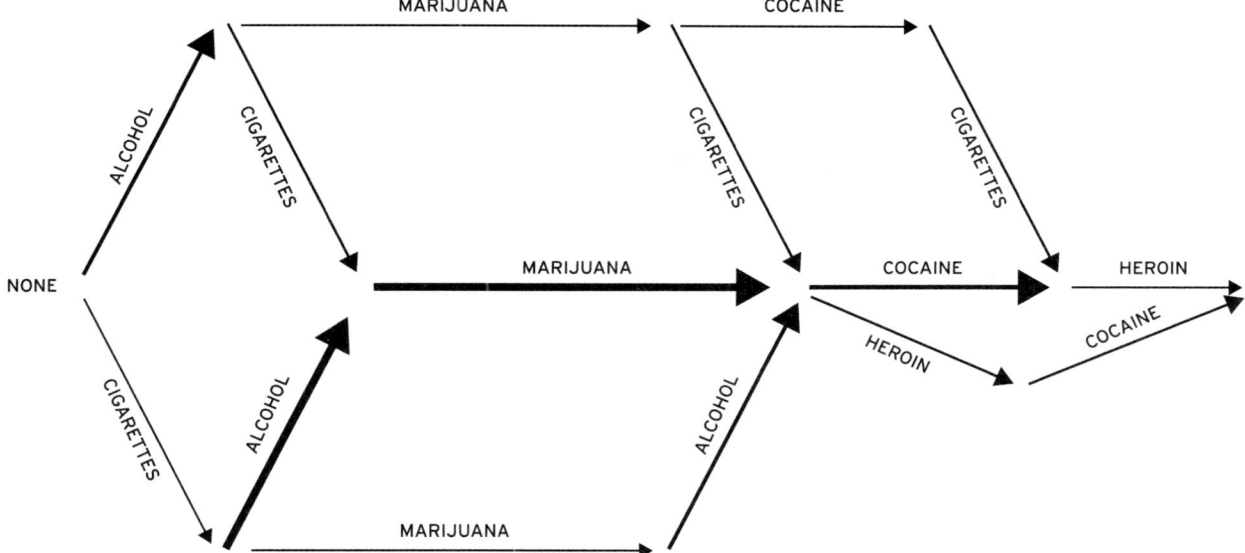

Figure 58.2 Pathways of drug involvement.

young people have greatly increased and even surpass slightly those of cigarette use, the majority of those who have experimented with marijuana or cocaine had first experimented with cigarettes or alcohol. Thus, among high school seniors in the 2010 *Monitoring the Future* (MTF) Survey, 42.2% ever smoked cigarettes, 71.0% ever drank alcohol, 43.8% ever used marijuana or hashish, and 5.5% ever used cocaine (Johnston et al., 2010). Yet, 54.8% had started smoking cigarettes or using alcohol prior to using marijuana and 33.7% had started using these drugs in the same grade; only 8.6% of marijuana users had started to use marijuana before smoking or drinking alcohol; 2.9% had only used marijuana. Parallel percentages for cocaine are 73.3% who smoked or drank alcohol prior to starting using cocaine; 19.9% started in the same grade, and 6.8% used cocaine prior to cigarettes or alcohol (unpublished analysis of MTF).

However, since publication of the original observation in 1975 (Kandel, 1975; Kandel and Faust, 1975), "surprisingly little progress has been made in addressing fundamental questions that derive from the finding that the use of one class of drug is followed by the use of another class. We still do not know (1) whether the use of a class of drugs used first, such as tobacco, is a cause of the use of the second class, such as cocaine, or whether the sequence is determined exclusively by availability of the drug or other social factors; and (2) what biological mechanisms underlie this progression in drug use. Although epidemiological studies have established the sequence between substances and specified their association, epidemiological studies cannot establish a causal progression nor can they identify the underlying cellular and molecular mechanisms that could contribute to the gateway sequence of drug use." (Koob et al., 2008: p. 360)

To obtain biological insights into the transition from nicotine to cocaine in the development of drug abuse and address how gateway drugs exert their effects, Kandel and colleagues at Columbia University have bridged the epidemiology of drug

abuse and molecular biology by developing a mouse model of this epidemiological sequence so as to explore the behavioral, physiological, and molecular genetic mechanisms underlying the gateway sequence. Animal models can provide a rigorous test of drug use progression in which drug-taking behavior can be observed in relation to well-defined prior experiences with specific drugs, independently of any social or legal constraints regulating and defining drug use. In mice, one can readily control the order in which drugs are taken so that the order is the only determinant of outcome. Alternate specifications of the sequential order of drug presentation can help resolve the possibility that the ordered use between any two drugs is only determined by social factors related to availability of different substances.

Most drugs of abuse exert their addictive effects through effects on the striatum (Thomas et al., 2001). The nucleus accumbens (NAc) in the ventral striatum is critical for reward and addiction and is a site of convergence and integration of rewarding input from dopaminergic neurons in the ventral tegmental area (VTA) and glutamatergic input from the amygdala and the prefrontal cortex. The core of the NAc is made up primarily of GABAergic inhibitory spiny neurons. The NAc sends inhibitory feedback to the dopaminergic cells of the VTA. Reduction of excitatory input to the NAc is thought to decrease inhibitory output from the NAc to the VTA and thereby contribute, through disinhibition, to the increased reward and enhanced locomotion activation observed after cocaine administration (Kauer and Malenka, 2007).

We examined in mice how sequential administration of nicotine and cocaine alters locomotor sensitization and conditioned place preference, two addiction-related behaviors that are modulated by drugs of abuse, and three physiological and molecular markers in the nucleus accumbens of the striatum: synaptic plasticity; transcription of FosB, an immediate response gene implicated in addiction to many drugs of abuse and in the response to other rewarding stimuli; and histone acetylation in chromatin (Levine et al., 2011).

Pretreatment of mice with nicotine for seven days increased the response to cocaine. Locomotor sensitization was increased by 98%, conditioned place preference by 78%, and cocaine-induced reduction in long-term potentiation (LTP) by 24%. Responses to cocaine were altered only when nicotine was administered first, and nicotine and cocaine were then administered concurrently. Reversing the order of drug administration was ineffective. Cocaine had no effect on nicotine-induced behaviors and synaptic plasticity. We found that nicotine by itself induced only a small increase in FosB expression in the striatum. However, nicotine also inhibited histone deacetylase (HDAC) activity, leading to a more widespread acetylation of histones at a larger number of genome locations in the striatum than did cocaine alone, thereby creating an environment that was primed for the induction of a number of genes. This ability of nicotine to hyperacetylate chromatin widely by inhibiting HDACs was not shared by cocaine, which caused a more local and transient acetylation. When a second drug of abuse, in this case cocaine, was given to animals after nicotine exposure, the higher histone acetylation levels led to greater activation of FosB and, likely, other genes.

Further, we found that a histone deacetylase inhibitor simulated the actions of nicotine by priming the response to cocaine and enhancing FosB gene expression and LTP depression in the nucleus accumbens. Conversely, in a genetic mouse model characterized by reduced histone acetylation, the effects of cocaine on LTP were diminished. We achieved a similar effect by infusing a low dose of theophylline, an activator of histone deacetylase, into the nucleus accumbens.

Cocaine must be administered to the animals while they are actively exposed to nicotine. These results from mice prompted an analysis of epidemiological data, which indicated that most cocaine users initiate cocaine use after the onset of smoking and while actively still smoking, and that initiating cocaine use after smoking increases the risk of becoming dependent on cocaine, consistent with our data from mice.

HDAC activators may be of potential clinical utility in the treatment of addiction because they could decrease FosB expression in response to cocaine. Modifying HDAC activators so that they target the striatum specifically would be particularly desirable because systemic treatments with HDAC activators or histone acetyltransferase inhibitors are likely to have cognitive and other deleterious effects.

DEVELOPMENTAL FACTORS: ADOLESCENCE AS A CRITICAL EXPOSURE PERIOD

"Normal developmental processes may result in higher risk for drug use at certain stages of the life cycle than others and experimentation with drugs at a particular stage of the life cycle may have lifelong consequences for subsequent extensiveness and chronicity of use. Epidemiological data on patterns of drug use in human populations as well as animal studies support the notion of critical developmental periods for drug behavior (Purves et al., 2001). Experimentation most often starts in adolescence, as does addiction (Wagner and Anthony, 2002), a period when the brain is still undergoing significant developmental changes (Dahl and Spear, 2004)." (Koob et al., 2008: p. 363) The rates of drug use increase dramatically during adolescence. Rates of use of different substances double from early to late adolescence, as illustrated by *Monitoring the Future*, a national study of drug use among high school students. In 2011, lifetime rates of use in the 8th, 10th, and 12th grades for alcohol were 33.1%, 56.0%, and 70.0%, respectively; for cigarettes, 18.4%, 30.4%, and 40.0%; and for any illicit substances, 20.1%, 37.7%, and 49.9% (Johnston et al., 2011).

"Although the effects of drugs of abuse during this stage of development have not been adequately investigated, initial exposure in adolescence is associated with more chronic and intensive use, and greater risk of developing a substance use disorder (e.g., nicotine dependence, alcoholism, or dependence on illicit drugs) when cigarette smoking, drinking, or the use of illicit drugs starts early during adolescence compared with initiation at older ages (Hingson et al., 2006; Kandel, 2003; Kandel and Chen, 2000; Volkow, 2006)." (Koob et al., 2008: p. 363) In NESARC, 47% of those who reported having started drinking before age 14 became dependent on alcohol compared with 9% of those who started drinking at age 21 or older (Hingson et al., 2006). In NSDUH, 12.8% of those who had first started using marijuana before age 15 met criteria for last year dependence on an illicit drug within the last year compared with 2.6% of those who first started using marijuana at age 18 or older (SAMHSA, 2011: p. 72). As we described in the preceding, the rates of drug abuse or dependence among drug users are higher among adolescents than adults. "Normal adolescent-specific behaviors (such as risk-taking, novelty-seeking, response to peer pressure) increase the propensity of experimenting with legal and illegal drugs (Spear, 2000), which might reflect incomplete development of brain regions (e.g., myelination of frontal lobe regions) involved in the processes of executive control and motivation (Sowell et al., 2003).

The importance of adolescence as a critical developmental risk period for drug involvement and substance dependence is supported by work on rodents, which documents the greater vulnerability of adolescent than adult animals to various drugs. For example, in rats, exposure to nicotine during adolescence is associated with greater nicotine self-administration than first exposure in adulthood, a difference that persists when the adolescent rats reach adulthood (Levin et al., 2003). Adolescent rats appear to be more sensitive than adults to the rewarding actions of nicotine (Belluzzi et al., 2004)." (Koob et al., 2008: p. 363) Similarly, nicotine pretreatment leads to enhanced cocaine self-administration and locomotor activity in response to cocaine in adolescent but not adult rats (McQuown et al., 2007, 2009). Drug exposure during adolescence might result in different neuroadaptations from those during adulthood. In rodents, exposure to nicotine during the period corresponding to adolescence, but not adulthood, leads to alterations in cholinergic systems in the cerebral cortex, midbrain, and hippocampus

(Abreu-Villaca et al., 2003), including changes in nicotine receptors and enhancement of the reinforcing responses to nicotine (Adriani et al., 2003). "In addition, enhanced expression of plasticity-related genes following injection of nicotine in adolescent compared with adult rats has been observed throughout the brain, especially the forebrain (Schochet et al., 2005). Similar vulnerabilities in adolescence compared with adulthood have been reported for alcohol (Rezvani and Levin, 2004; Ristuccia and Spear, 2005)" (Koob et al., 2008: p. 363), amphetamines (McPherson and Lawrence, 2006), and morphine (White and Holtzman, 2005). Future research should allow clarification of whether neurobiological changes are the reason adolescents appear to become addicted to nicotine with lower nicotine exposure than adults (Kandel and Chen, 2000). Similarly, future research will allow us to determine if the increased neuroadaptations to alcohol during adolescence compared with adulthood (Slawecki and Roth, 2004) explains the greater vulnerability to alcoholism in individuals who start using alcohol early in life (Grant et al., 2001).

CONCLUSIONS

Data currently available to assess the extent of substance use disorders in the United States have many shortcomings and make comparison and replication across studies difficult. To overcome some of the limitations, we implemented secondary analyses of data from four surveys: NSDUH, NESARC, NCS-R, and NCS-A. The use of legal and illegal drugs in the United States is pervasive. In 2010, more than 90% of the adult population had ever used at least one substance and 45% of adolescents had done so (NSDUH). In 2001–2002, close to 40% of adult lifetime substance users met criteria for any lifetime substance use disorder, whether abuse or dependence on alcohol, nicotine, or an illicit drug. The highest lifetime rates of dependence were observed for nicotine dependence (17.7%), followed by alcohol (12.5%) and illicit drugs (2.6%) (NESARC). Adolescence appears to be a period of high risk for substance use disorders among those who have experimented with legal and illegal substances. Although the lifetime and last 12-month prevalence of use is lower among adolescents than adults, except for last 12-month use of illicit drugs, the rates of lifetime disorders among lifetime users are similar among adolescents and adults (NCS). The rates are even higher for last 12-month disorders among last 12-month adolescent users than adult users both in NCS and NSDUH, with the exception of dependence on nicotine among all cigarette users in NSDUH. Ages 18–25 represent the period of highest drug use prevalence for most substances. Whereas use of cigarettes and illicit drugs peaks in early adulthood at ages 18–25, the use of alcohol stabilizes through the late forties, when it starts its decline. The rates of dependence among users tend to remain flat for cigarette smokers and, as of age 18–25, to decline but slowly for users of other substances throughout adulthood.

Nicotine represents the most serious public health problem of the drugs that are used because not only does it affect almost a fifth of the population but it is also the most chronic of the addictions, with more than 70% of adults who ever experienced symptoms of nicotine dependence reporting such symptoms within the last year. Furthermore, individuals who experiment with tobacco are more likely subsequently to experiment with illicit drugs, such as marijuana and cocaine. Recent work carried out using mice models identified molecular effects of nicotine on the brain that could explain its chronicity and its effects on other substances. Nicotine primes the response to cocaine by inhibiting histone deacetylase activity, causing global histone acetylation in the striatum, thereby inducing transcriptional activation of the *FosB* gene implicated in addiction. Understanding the pathways involved in this process may lead to the development of drugs that would impact in the addictive process.

Substance abuse and dependence are highly comorbid with other psychiatric disorders, especially among those who meet criteria for dependence on an illicit drug. In that group, close to 80% also meet criteria for a mood, anxiety, or antisocial personality disorder. The comorbidity between substance use disorders and psychiatric disorders is especially strong for antisocial personality disorder. Common biological and environment factors may underlie the observed associations between these two classes of disorder. Although much work remains to be done to understand the direction of causality between psychiatric and substance use disorders, it would appear that psychiatric disorders are more likely a cause of substance use disorders than substance use disorders are a cause of psychiatric disorders. Research on adolescents suggests that psychiatric disorders are more likely to precede and lead to substance use disorders than the reverse. Similarly, among adults, psychiatric disorders, in particular mood and anxiety disorders, predict persistence of substance use disorders but not the reverse.

Early onset of drug use during adolescence leads to more extensive and chronic use than later onset postadolescence, highlighting the importance of implementing prevention and educational efforts in that developmental period.

The use of animal models, imaging, and longitudinal epidemiological studies, in which individuals can be followed at relatively closely spaced intervals and for a long period of time, would help resolve some of the questions that are raised by the abuse of drugs in the population.

DISCLOSURES

No conflicts of interest to disclose for any of the authors. Support was provided by grant K05-DA0081 from the National Institute on Drug Abuse to Denise Kandel.

ACKNOWLEDGMENTS

Sections of this chapter were previously published in Koob, G.F., Volkow, N.D., et al. (2008). Pathophysiology of addiction. In Tasman, A., Kay, J., Lieberman, J.A., First, M.B., and Maj, M., eds., *Psychiatry*, 3rd ed., vol. 1. West Sussex, England: Wiley, pp. 354–378.

REFERENCES

Abreu-Villaca, Y., Seidler, F.J., et al. (2003). Short-term adolescent nicotine exposure has immediate and persistent effects on cholinergic systems: critical periods, patterns of exposure, dose thresholds. *Neuropsychopharmacology* 28(11):1935–1949.

Adriani, W., Spijker, S., et al. (2003). Evidence for enhanced neurobehavioral vulnerability to nicotine during periadolescence in rats. *J. Neurosci.* 23(11):4712–4716.

American Psychiatric Association. (1994). Diagnostic and Statistical Manual of Mental Disorders, 4th Edition. Washington, DC: Author.

American Psychiatric Association. (2000). Diagnostic and Statistical Manual of Mental Disorders, Text Revision, 4th Edition. Washington, DC: Author.

Belluzzi, J.D., Lee, A.G., et al. (2004). Age-dependent effects of nicotine on locomotor activity and conditioned place preference in rats. *Psychopharmacology* 174(3):389–395.

Boden, J.M., Fergusson, D.M., et al. (2010). Cigarette smoking and depression: tests of causal linkages using a longitudinal birth cohort. *Br. J. Psychiatry* 196(6):440–446.

Breslau, N., Novak, S.P., et al. (2004). Psychiatric disorders and stages of smoking. *Biol. Psychiatry* 55(1):69–76.

Budney, A.J., Moore, B.A., et al. (2003). The time course and significance of cannabis withdrawal. *J. Abnorm. Psychol.* 112(3):393–402.

Compton, W.M., Conway, K.P., et al. (2005). Prevalence, correlates, and comorbidity of DSM-IV antisocial personality syndromes and alcohol and specific drug use disorders in the United States: results from the National Epidemiologic Survey on Alcohol and Related Conditions. *J. Clin. Psychiatry* 66(6):677–685.

Compton, W.M., Thomas, Y.F., et al. (2007). Prevalence, correlates, disability, and comorbidity of DSM-IV drug abuse and dependence in the United States: results from the National Epidemiologic Survey on Alcohol and Related Conditions. *Arch. Gen. Psychiatry* 64(5):566–576.

Conway, K.P., Compton, W., et al. (2006). Lifetime comorbidity of DSM-IV mood and anxiety disorders and specific drug use disorders: results from the National Epidemiologic Survey on Alcohol and Related Conditions. *J. Clin. Psychiatry* 67(2):247–257.

Cottler, L.B. (2007). Drug use disorders in the National Comorbidity Survey: have we come a long way? *Arch. Gen. Psychiatry* 64(3):380–381.

Dahl, R.E., and Spear, L.P. (2004). Adolescent Brain Development: Vulnerability and Opportunities. New York: New York Academy of Sciences.

de Leon, J., and Diaz, F.J. (2005). A meta-analysis of worldwide studies demonstrates an association between schizophrenia and tobacco smoking behaviors. *Schizophr. Res.* 76(2–3):135–157.

Fowler, J.S., Logan, J., et al. (2003). Monoamine oxidase and cigarette smoking. *Neurotoxicology* 24(1):75–82.

Grant, B.F., Compton, W.M., et al. (2007). Errors in assessing DSM-IV substance use disorders. *Arch. Gen. Psychiatry* 64(3):379–380.

Grant, B.F., Hasin, D.S., et al. (2004a). Nicotine dependence and psychiatric disorders in the United States: results from the National Epidemiologic Survey on Alcohol and Related Conditions. *Arch. Gen. Psychiatry* 61(11):1107–1115.

Grant, B.F., Stinson, F.S., et al. (2004b). Prevalence and co-occurrence of substance use disorders and independent mood and anxiety disorders: results from the National Epidemiologic Survey on Alcohol and Related Conditions. *Arch. Gen. Psychiatry* 61(8):807–816.

Grant, B.F., Stinson, F.S., et al. (2001). Age at onset of alcohol use and DSM-IV alcohol abuse and dependence: a 12-year follow-up. *J. Subst. Abuse* 13(4):493–504.

Griesler, P.C., Hu, M.C., et al. (2008). Comorbidity of psychiatric disorders and nicotine dependence among adolescents: findings from a prospective, longitudinal study. *J. Am. Acad. Child Adolesc. Psychiatry* 47(11):1340–1350.

Griesler, P.C., Hu, M.C., et al. (2011). Comorbid psychiatric disorders and nicotine dependence in adolescence. *Addiction* 106(5):1010–1020.

Grucza, R.A., Abbacchi, A.M., et al. (2007). Discrepancies in estimates of prevalence and correlates of substance use and disorders between two national surveys. *Addiction* 102(4):623–629.

Hasin, D.S. (2012a, April 17). DSM-V Substance Use Disorders. Paper presented at the Drugs and Society Seminar, Columbia University, New York.

Hasin, D.S. (2012b). Combining abuse and dependence in DSM-5. *J. Stud. Alcohol Drugs* 73(4):702–704.

Hasin, D.S., Fenton, M.C., et al. (2012). Analyses related to the development of DSM-5 criteria for substance use related disorders: 2. proposed DSM-5 criteria for alcohol, cannabis, cocaine and heroin disorders in 663 substance abuse patients. *Drug Alcohol Depen.* 122(1–2):28–37.

Hasin, D.S., and Grant, B.F. (2004). The co-occurrence of DSM-IV alcohol abuse in DSM-IV alcohol dependence: results of the National Epidemiologic Survey on Alcohol and Related Conditions on heterogeneity that differ by population subgroup. *Arch. Gen. Psychiatry* 61(9):891–896.

Hasin, D.S., Hatzenbueler, M., et al. (2005). Co-occurring DSM-IV drug abuse in DSM-IV drug dependence: results from the National Epidemiologic Survey on Alcohol and Related Conditions. *Drug Alcohol Depen.* 80(1):117–123.

Hasin, D.S., and Kilcoyne, B. (2012). Comorbidity of psychiatric and substance use disorders in the United States: current issues and findings from the NESARC. *Curr. Opin. Psychiatry* 25(3):165–171.

Hedden, S., Gfroerer, J., et al. (2012). The NSDUH Data Review: Comparison of NSDUH Mental Health Data and Methods with Other Data Sources. Rockville, MD: U.S. Department of Health and Human Services, Substance Abuse and Mental Health Services Administration, Center for Behavioral Health Statistics and Quality.

Hingson, R.W., Heeren, T., et al. (2006). Age at drinking onset and alcohol dependence: age at onset, duration, and severity. *Arch. Pediat. Adol. Med.* 160(7):739–746.

Hughes, J.R. (2006). Should criteria for drug dependence differ across drugs? *Addiction* 101(Suppl 1):134–141.

Isensee, B., Wittchen, H.U., et al. (2003). Smoking increases the risk of panic: findings from a prospective community study. *Arch. Gen. Psychiatry* 60(7):692–700.

Johnston, L.D., O'Malley, P.M., et al. (2010, December 14). National press release: Marijuana use is rising; ecstasy use is beginning to rise; and alcohol use is declining among U.S. teens. Ann Arbor: University of Michigan News Service.

Johnston, L.D., O'Malley, P.M., et al. (2011, December 14). National press release: Marijuana use continues to rise among U.S. teens, while alcohol use hits historic lows. Ann Arbor: University of Michigan News Service.

Kandel, D.B. (1975). Stages in adolescent involvement in drug use. *Science* 190(4217):912–914.

Kandel, D.B. (2002). Stages and Pathways of Drug Involvement: Examining the Gateway Hypothesis. Cambridge, UK: Cambridge University Press.

Kandel, D.B. (2003). The Natural History of Smoking and Nicotine Dependence. Paper presented at the Proceedings of the Royal Society of Canada 2002 Symposium on Addictions: Impact on Canada, Ottawa, Ontario, Canada.

Kandel, D.B., and Chen, K. (2000). Extent of smoking and nicotine dependence in the United States: 1991–1993. *Nicotine Tob. Res.* 2(3):263–274.

Kandel, D.B., and Faust, R. (1975). Sequence and stages in patterns of adolescent drug use. *Arch. Gen. Psychiatry* 32(7):923–932.

Karp, I., O'Loughlin, J., et al. (2006). Risk factors for tobacco dependence in adolescent smokers. *Tob. Control* 15(3):199–204.

Kauer, J.A., and Malenka, R.C. (2007). Synaptic plasticity and addiction. *Nat. Rev. Neurosci.* 8(11):844–858.

Kessler, R.C. (2004). The epidemiology of dual diagnosis. *Biol. Psychiatry* 56(10):730–737.

Kessler, R.C., Avenevoli, S., et al. (2012a). Prevalence, persistence, and sociodemographic correlates of DSM-IV disorders in the National Comorbidity Survey Replication Adolescent Supplement. *Arch. Gen. Psychiatry* 69(4):372–380.

Kessler, R.C., Avenevoli, S., et al. (2012b). Lifetime co-morbidity of DSM-IV disorders in the U.S. National Comorbidity Survey Replication Adolescent Supplement (NCS-A). *Psychol. Med.* 42(9):1–14.

Kessler, R.C., Berglund, P., et al. (2005a). Lifetime prevalence and age-of-onset distributions of DSM-IV disorders in the National Comorbidity Survey Replication. *Arch. Gen. Psychiatry* 62(6):593–602.

Kessler, R.C., Chiu, W.T., et al. (2005b). Prevalence, severity, and comorbidity of 12-month DSM-IV disorders in the National Comorbidity Survey Replication. *Arch. Gen. Psychiatry* 62(6):617–627.

Kessler, R.C., and Merikangas, K.R. (2007). Drug use disorders in the National Comorbidity Survey: have we come a long way? In reply. *Arch. Gen. Psychiatry* 64(3):381–382.

Klungsøyr, O., Nygard, J.F., et al. (2006). Cigarette smoking and incidence of first depressive episode: an 11-year, population-based follow-up study. *Am. J. Epidemiol.* 163(5):421–432.

Koob, G.F., Volkow, N.D., et al. (2008). Pathophysiology of addiction. In: Tasman, A., Kay, J., Lieberman, J.A., First, M.B., and Maj, M., eds. Psychiatry, 3rd Edition, Volume 1. West Sussex, UK: Wiley, pp. 354–378.

Kumari, V., and Postma, P. (2005). Nicotine use in schizophrenia: the self-medication hypotheses. *Neurosci. Biobehav. Rev.* 29(6):1021–1034.

Levin, E.D., Rezvani, A.H., et al. (2003). Adolescent-onset nicotine self-administration modeled in female rats. *Psychopharmacology* 169(2):141–149.

Levine, A., Huang, Y., et al. (2011). Molecular mechanism for a gateway drug: epigenetic changes initiated by nicotine prime gene expression by cocaine. *Sci. Transl. Med.* 3(107):107ra109.

McPherson, C.S., and Lawrence, A.J. (2006). Exposure to amphetamine in rats during periadolescence establishes behavioural and extrastriatal neural sensitization in adulthood. *Int. J. Neuropsychopharmacol.* 9(4):377–392.

McQuown, S.C., Belluzzi, J.D., et al. (2007). Low dose nicotine treatment during early adolescence increases subsequent cocaine reward. *Neurotoxicol. Teratol.* 29(1):66–73.

McQuown, S.C., Dao, J.M., et al. (2009). Age-dependent effects of low-dose nicotine treatment on cocaine-induced behavioral plasticity in rats. *Psychopharmacology* 207(1):143–152.

Moffitt, T.E., Caspi, A., et al. (2010). How common are common mental disorders? Evidence that lifetime prevalence rates are doubled by prospective versus retrospective ascertainment. *Psychol. Med.* 40(6):899–909.

Nelson, C.B., Rehm, J., et al. (1999). Factor structures for DSM-IV substance disorder criteria endorsed by alcohol, cannabis, cocaine and opiate users: results from the WHO reliability and validity study. *Addiction* 94(6):843–855.

O'Brien, C. (2011). Addiction and dependence in DSM-V. *Addiction* 106(5):866–867.

Purves, D., Augustine, G.J., et al. (2001). Neuroscience, 2nd Edition. Sunderland, MA: Sinauer.

Rezvani, A.H., and Levin, E.D. (2004). Adolescent and adult rats respond differently to nicotine and alcohol: motor activity and body temperature. *Int. J. Dev. Neurosci.* 22(5–6):349–354.

Ristuccia, R.C., and Spear, L.P. (2005). Sensitivity and tolerance to autonomic effects of ethanol in adolescent and adult rats during repeated vapor inhalation sessions. *Alcohol Clin. Exp. Res.* 29(10):1809–1820.

Saha, T.D., Compton, W.M., et al. (2012). Analyses related to the development of DSM-5 criteria for substance use related disorders: 1. toward amphetamine, cocaine and prescription drug use disorder continua using Item Response Theory. *Drug Alcohol Depen.* 122(1–2):38–46.

Schochet, T.L., Kelley, A.E., et al. (2005). Differential expression of arc mRNA and other plasticity-related genes induced by nicotine in adolescent rat forebrain. *Neuroscience* 135(1):285–297.

Schuckit, M.A. (2012). Editor's corner: editorial in reply to the comments of Griffith Edwards. *J. Stud. Alcohol Drugs* 73(4):521–522.

Shiffman, S., Waters, A., et al. (2004). The nicotine dependence syndrome scale: a multidimensional measure of nicotine dependence. *Nicotine Tob. Res.* 6(2):327–348.

Slawecki, C.J., and Roth, J. (2004). Comparison of the onset of hypoactivity and anxiety-like behavior during alcohol withdrawal in adolescent and adult rats. *Alcohol Clin. Exp. Res.* 28(4):598–607.

Smith, S.M., Stinson, F.S., et al. (2006). Race/ethnic differences in the prevalence and co-occurrence of substance use disorders and independent mood and anxiety disorders: results from the National Epidemiologic Survey on Alcohol and Related Conditions. *Psychol. Med.* 36(7):987–998.

Sowell, E.R., Peterson, B.S., et al. (2003). Mapping cortical change across the human life span. *Nat. Neurosci.* 6(3):309–315.

Spear, L.P. (2000). The adolescent brain and age-related behavioral manifestations. *Neurosci. Biobehav. Rev.* 24(4):417–463.

Substance Abuse and Mental Health Services Administration [SAMHSA]. (2011). Results from the 2010 National Survey on Drug Use and Health: Summary of National Findings (NSDUH Series H-41, HHS Publication No. [SMA] 11-4658). Rockville, MD: Author.

Thomas, M.J., Beurrier, C., et al. (2001). Long-term depression in the nucleus accumbens: a neural correlate of behavioral sensitization to cocaine. *Nat. Neurosci.* 4(12):1217–1223.

Volkow, N.D. (2006). Altered pathways: drug abuse and age of onset. *Add. Prof.* 4(3):26, 29.

Volkow, N.D. (2009). Substance use disorders in schizophrenia: clinical implications of comorbidity. *Schizophr. Bull.* 35(3):469–472.

Wagner, F.A., and Anthony, J.C. (2002). From first drug use to drug dependence: developmental periods of risk for dependence upon marijuana, cocaine, and alcohol. *Neuropsychopharmacology* 26(4):479–488.

White, D.A., and Holtzman, S.G. (2005). Periadolescent morphine exposure alters subsequent behavioral sensitivity to morphine in adult rats. *Eur. J. Pharmacol.* 528(1–3):119–123.

Wing, V.C., Wass, C.E., et al. (2012). A review of neurobiological vulnerability factors and treatment implications for comorbid tobacco dependence in schizophrenia. *Ann. NY Acad. Sci.* 1248:89–106.

World Health Organization. (1992). International Statistical Classification of Diseases and Related Health Problems, 10th revision. Geneva: Author.

SECTION VII | DEMENTIA

DAVID M. HOLTZMAN

Although Alzheimer's disease (AD) was first described clinically and pathologically more than 100 years ago, it has only been over the last 30 years that clinicians and scientists have been able to unravel many of the scientific underpinnings of AD as well as several of the other causes of dementia. Because AD causes or contributes to dementia in about 30 million people worldwide and because of better overall medical care, we are facing a looming crisis. It is predicted that unless an effective therapy is developed, the prevalence of AD will triple over the next 30 to 40 years. An underlying principle that has emerged is that most neurodegenerative diseases, including AD, Parkinson disease, frontotemporal dementias, and prion diseases, appear to be disorders of protein aggregation in which normally soluble proteins become insoluble and accumulate in the brain, leading to neurotoxicity. Important clinical, genetic, and diagnostic advances, as well as a better understanding of pathophysiology, have led the field to the point where we are now poised to make important contributions to modify the course of different dementing diseases. There is even the possibility of delaying or preventing dementia.

Chapters 59 to 69 deal with various aspects of AD, which cause or contribute to approximately 70% to 75% of cases of dementia. In Chapter 59, Hassenstab, Burns, and Morris provide an update on the clinical and neuropsychological features of AD. They emphasize the importance of obtaining a history from a knowledgeable informant in determining whether an individual has developed cognitive impairment and if so, provide clinical and psychological methods to accurately quantify current cognitive and functional status. Utilizing purely clinical techniques, diagnosis of dementia caused by AD can be made quite accurately though imaging (see Chapter 62 by Brewer, Sepulcre, and Johnson) and fluid biomarker techniques (see Chapter 63 by Fagan) are proving to be very useful adjuncts. Structural and functional neuroimaging techniques are demonstrating the time course of changes in brain structure and function in relation to the clinical onset and progression of disease. Both measures appear to begin to become abnormal a few years before the onset of detectable cognitive change. Amyloid imaging as well as CSF measures of Aβ42 appear to detect the onset of amyloid deposition in the brain as long as 10 to 15 years before cognitive decline and an increase in CSF tau, which occurs a few years before cognitive decline, marks the onset of neurodegeneration. These imaging and fluid biomarker techniques strongly add to both diagnostic and prognostic accuracy and will likely be very valuable in assisting in the enrollment of participants in both treatment and secondary prevention trials that are just beginning.

In Chapter 60, Tanzi describes how the discovery of different genes that cause dominantly inherited AD has revolutionized our understanding of AD by pointing us to which pathways are key in disease causation. These studies clearly point to the role of Aβ in instigating disease in that mutations in *PS1*, *PS2*, and *APP* almost all cause an increase in production in either all Aβ species or more commonly an increase in production of Aβ42. Further, *APOE*, the most important genetic risk factor for AD, also influences Aβ metabolism, not by increasing synthesis but by influencing its aggregation and clearance. Additional new genetic risk factors have been uncovered and how they impact disease is still being sorted out. In Chapter 61, Morgan describes how researchers have taken advantage of the knowledge of the genes that cause or contribute to AD by creating many different genetic mouse models in which various pathological and behavioral phenotypes that mimic aspects of AD can be seen. This has been a colorful and productive area of research and is beginning to reap benefits, as disease modifying therapies are now being tested in humans based on promising data coming from these different models.

Although currently no therapies have been proved to delay the onset or slow the cognitive decline in AD, in Chapter 64 Sano and Neugroschl describe the current pharmacological therapies that have been shown to improve the symptoms of AD, including cholinesterase inhibitors and memantine, as well as results from a host of other studies. In Chapter 65, Grill and Cummings describe the very exciting work that is emerging on potential disease-modifying therapies for AD. Many different small molecules and biological therapies such as antibodies that target Aβ have shown promising preclinical data in animals. These treatments are in both early as well as later trials in AD. Additional targets such as tau and inflammation are also beginning to be tested now and in the near future.

A variety of other diseases contribute to or lead to dementia in addition to AD. The most common neurodegenerative diseases in individuals greater than age 65 outside of AD are dementia with Lewy bodies and dementia in Parkinson disease, described by Karantzoulis and Galvin in Chapter 66. These disorders feature the accumulation of synuclein in the brain. Many cases also feature Aβ accumulation. Another very common contributor to dementia either alone or more frequently in combination with AD is vascular dementia, described in Chapter 68 by Chui. Although not a frequent cause of dementia in the elderly, frontotemporal dementia (FTD) is a common cause of dementia in individuals less than 60 years of age. In Chapter 67, Naasan and Miller beautifully describe the varied clinical and neuroimaging features of FTD, which present with either behavioral or language abnormalities. Importantly, the genetics and pathology of FTD clearly show it to be more than one disease, in which different genes and proteins can contribute. Improvements in diagnostic and biomarkers methods in this area should allow for promising treatment development as pathophysiological mechanisms emerge. Finally, although not a common cause of dementia, Chapter 70 by Watts and Geschwind describes diseases caused by prions. These diseases can cause rapidly progressive dementia in both humans and animals. Some of the major insights into a variety of neurodegenerative diseases have emerged from studies of prion disease, which can be both genetic and infectious.

It is clear that a major public health crisis is in the process of emerging because of the fact that lifespan is increasing and with that, dementing disorders, especially AD, are becoming more and more common. We have seen a clinical and scientific revolution in this area over the last 30 years in that the genetic and pathophysiological basis for these disorders is now much better understood. This is leading to the emergence of better diagnostic methods as well as promising disease-modifying therapies. It seems likely that over the next decades there will be a real chance that effective therapies for AD and other neurodegenerative diseases will become a reality. That day cannot come too soon.

59 | CLINICAL AND NEUROPSYCHOLOGICAL FEATURES OF ALZHEIMER'S DISEASE

JASON HASSENSTAB, JEFFREY BURNS, AND JOHN C. MORRIS

Alois Alzheimer reported in a meeting of German psychiatrists in 1906 his conclusion that a pathologic brain process, marked by microscopic lesions now recognized as amyloid plaques and neurofibrillary tangles, was responsible for the dementia and psychosis experienced for years by a woman before she died at age 55. His report generated little enthusiasm or interest from the audience and for many years thereafter what became known as Alzheimer's disease (AD) was considered to be an unusual presenile dementing disorder and garnered little attention. Studies in the 1960s, however, by Bernard Tomlinson, Gary Blessed, and Martin Roth in Great Britain (Tomlinson et al., 1968, 1970) showed conclusively that the neuropathology of the presenile disorder was identical to that of the far more numerous older cases of "senile dementia," thus establishing that AD is the same clinicopathologic disorder regardless of its age at onset. Based on this knowledge, Robert Katzman in 1976 correctly presaged the rapidly increasing prevalence and malignancy of AD (Katzman, 1976).

Alzheimer's disease is by far the most common cause of dementia and is present in 77% of demented individuals (Barker et al., 2002). It is strongly age-associated and thus typically is a disorder of older adulthood: 7% of persons affected by AD are age 65 to 74, 53% are 75 to 84, and 40% are 85 and older (Hebert et al., 2003). The prevalence of AD doubles every five years after the age of 65, affecting as many as 47% of people 85 years and older (Evans, 1987). Increased life expectancy in the United States and other developed countries has fueled an unprecedented growth in the elderly population that, in the absence of truly effective therapies, ensures continued dramatic increases in the prevalence of AD. In the United States alone, costs of caring for individuals with AD are estimated to be over $200 billion annually (Alzheimer's Association, 2012). Although these figures very likely are underestimates given that AD is considerably underrecognized in clinical practice (Lavery et al., 2007) and on death certificates (Wachterman et al., 2008), the number of cases of AD, currently estimated to be 5.3 million in the United States, are expected to nearly triple over the next 50 years (Hebert, 2001).

This chapter reviews the clinical and neuropsychological characteristics and course of dementia caused by AD with a focus on its earliest symptomatic stages, because the typical person affected by AD is not profoundly demented (48% of individuals affected by AD are mildly demented, 31% are moderately demented, and only 21% are severely demented [Hebert et al., 2003]). The chapter is written from the viewpoint of the clinician. It addresses the variability in current sets of clinical diagnostic criteria for AD and provides the rationale for the use of biological markers (biomarkers) to aid in moving the diagnostic process from a syndromic to a quantitative basis. Full discussions of biomarkers are found elsewhere in this section (imaging, Chapter 62; fluid, Chapter 63). Similarly, other illnesses that are considered in the differential diagnosis of AD dementia are addressed (dementia with Lewy bodies, Chapter 66; frontotemporal dementia, Chapter 67; vascular dementia, Chapter 68; prion disease, Chapter 69) and therapeutic approaches for AD dementia are the focus of Chapters 64 and 65. Genetic factors for AD are fully discussed in Chapter 60.

PATHOPHYSIOLOGY OF ALZHEIMER'S DISEASE

Alzheimer's disease is defined histopathologically by the presence of the hallmark lesions of plaques and neurofibrillary tangles (NFTs). Plaques are composed of extracellular beta-amyloid (Aβ) peptide deposited in the cerebral cortex as amorphous aggregates (diffuse plaques) and those with degenerating dendrites that contain hyperphosphorylated tau aggregates (neuritic plaques). NFTs are intracellular fibrillar aggregates of the hyperphosphorylated form of the microtubule-associated protein tau. NFTs are not specific for AD, suggesting that they may represent a secondary response to neuronal injury, at least in some instances. On the other hand, there is a strong association of Aβ plaques with AD. Down Syndrome and autosomal dominantly inherited AD, caused by deterministic mutations (or duplications) in the *amyloid precursor protein (APP)*, *presenilin 1 (PSEN1)*, and *presenilin 2 (PSEN2)* genes are rare but highly penetrant genetic causes of AD and are linked mechanistically by the overproduction of Aβ or an alteration in the ratio of the Aβ42 isoform to Aβ40. Hence, Aβ dysregulation (e.g., overproduction, reduced clearance, altered processing) is hypothesized as a critical "upstream" factor in the pathogenesis of AD (Hardy and Selkoe, 2002). When AD dementia is present, however, NFTs correlate more strongly with cognitive dysfunction than do plaques, perhaps because NFTs are more associated with synaptic and neuronal injury. The full-blown AD process involves many other pathologic factors, including neuroinflammation, microglial activation, oxidative stress, and cell cycle abnormalities, that may contribute to disease progression. Although the precise cause(s) of AD remain unknown (Small and Duff, 2008), recent evidence of a gene mutation that results in inhibition of the proteolytic processing of APP into amyloidogenic peptides is associated with reduced incidence of cognitive decline and AD dementia in older adults, providing additional support for the amyloid hypothesis of AD (Jonsson et al., 2012).

Several sets of criteria for the neuropathological diagnosis of AD, based on the recognition of plaques and NFTs, have been developed but emphasize slightly different facets, such as whether diffuse and neuritic plaques or only neuritic plaques are considered (Nelson et al., 2012). A consensus panel now has recommended standard guidelines for the neuropathological assessment of AD and for its clinicopathologic correlations (Hyman et al., 2012). These new guidelines recognize a preclinical stage of AD, wherein Aβ deposits appear to accumulate over many years as plaques in the cerebral cortex in the absence of symptoms (Price and Morris, 1999). This preclinical stage is hypothesized as a clinically silent pathologic cascade resulting in increasing synaptic and neuronal loss that eventually produces the symptomatic stage (Jack et al., 2010; Perrin et al., 2009). This hypothesis also suggests that attempts to treat individuals with symptomatic AD may require a combination of drugs that target the multiple pathophysiologic mechanisms involved in the cascade. Because (presumably) irreversible neuronal loss already is substantial in medial temporal lobe structures by the time AD symptoms first appear (Price et al., 2001), detection of preclinical AD (before the brain is badly damaged) is desirable to enable possible "secondary prevention" strategies where therapeutic interventions aim to delay or possibly even prevent the appearance of symptomatic AD.

THE ALZHEIMER'S DISEASE CONTINUUM

Work groups convened by the National Institute on Aging (NIA) and the Alzheimer's Association (AA) to revise clinical diagnostic criteria for symptomatic AD proposed a continuum that begins with the preclinical AD stage and then gradually manifests with subtle symptoms of mild cognitive impairment that then progresses to fully developed AD dementia. Compelling support for the AD continuum comes from a study of dominantly inherited AD. Representing less than 1% of all AD, individuals from families with autosomal dominant AD (ADAD) are at 50% risk of inheriting a causative mutation for AD (i.e., in the PSEN1, PSEN2, or APP genes) from their affected biological parent. Virtually all mutation carriers (MCs) will develop symptomatic AD, generally at the same age as their affected parent (the mean age of symptom onset in ADAD families is ~46 years), whereas their sibling non-carriers have no more risk for AD than the general population. The Dominantly Inherited Alzheimer Network (DIAN) has demonstrated that abnormal levels of Aβ42 (the most pathogenic isoform of Aβ) measured in the cerebrospinal fluid (CSF) begin in asymptomatic MCs about 20–25 years prior to estimated age at onset (AAO) for symptomatic AD (Bateman et al., 2012). Cerebral

deposits of fibrillar Aβ are detected with molecular imaging about 15 years prior to estimated AAO, as are abnormalities in CSF levels of tau protein (and of its phosphorylated species); volumetric brain loss also is detected by magnetic resonance imaging (MRI) about 15 years prior to estimated AAO. Brain hypometabolism and deficits in episodic memory performance occur about 10 years before estimated AAO, and global cognitive impairment begins about 5 years before estimated AAO (Bateman et al., 2012). These findings are consistent with a continuous pathologic cascade in preclinical AD that ultimately manifests as symptomatic AD and suggest that abnormalities in Aβ metabolism begin more than two decades before symptomatic onset of AD. This provides a potential "window" for prevention therapies in asymptomatic individuals who are destined to develop symptomatic AD and further offers the opportunity to directly test the amyloid hypothesis with clinical trials of anti-Aβ monotherapies in asymptomatic MCs with preclinical AD. The extent to which these observations in DIAN extrapolate to the far more common "sporadic" form of late onset AD is unknown. Because abnormal biomarkers were present in DIAN only in MCs destined to develop symptomatic AD, however, it is likely that the same biomarker abnormalities in cognitively normal older adults also will predict symptomatic AD if the individuals continue to live.

CLINICAL DIAGNOSTIC CRITERIA FOR ALZHEIMER'S DISEASE

In 1984 uniform clinical diagnostic criteria were introduced by a Work Group convened by the National Institute on Neurological and Communicative Disorders and Stroke and the Alzheimer's Disease and Related Disorders Association (NINCDS-ADRDA) (McKhann et al., 1984). These criteria provided the basis for the accurate recognition of the clinical disorder. The application of these clinical criteria firmly established AD as the dominant cause of dementia. The NINCDS-ADRDA criteria for the diagnosis of probable AD have been the underpinnings of AD clinical trials and research for over 25 years. To incorporate new knowledge resulting from this research, NIA-AA work groups recently updated these criteria. The new criteria recognize AD as a neuropathological entity that progresses from an asymptomatic stage (preclinical AD; Sperling et al., 2011) to a prodromal symptomatic stage (mild cognitive impairment; Albert et al., 2011) to the fully expressed AD dementia syndrome (McKhann et al., 2011). By definition, preclinical AD presently is detected solely by biomarkers, antecedent to symptomatic stages of AD. Only the clinical diagnosis of symptomatic AD, encompassing MCI and AD dementia, is addressed here.

MILD COGNITIVE IMPAIRMENT

The term mild cognitive impairment (MCI) was introduced to characterize the boundary of aging and dementia (Flicker et al., 1991). The earliest symptoms of AD are insidious and almost all patients with AD progress through a stage of subtle cognitive impairment that may not interfere importantly with daily functioning. Clinical criteria for MCI were intended to characterize this prodromal stage, prior to the diagnosis of overt dementia (Petersen et al., 1995). Because MCI was not defined as a clinicopathologic entity, however, it can represent the earliest symptomatic stage of many underlying pathologies (not all of which necessarily progress to dementia) and thus MCI is heterogeneous in nature with highly variable outcomes.

The revised criteria for MCI move toward providing an etiologic diagnosis for this condition when it is considered to be a symptomatic predementia phase of AD (Albert et al., 2011). These criteria nominally appear consistent with consensus criteria for MCI published in 2004 (Winblad et al., 2004) and require: (1) a change in cognition, self-reported or noted by an observer; (2) objective impairment in one or more cognitive domains; (3) independence in functional activities; and (4) absence of dementia (because functional independence is preserved). Unfortunately, the revised criteria for MCI broaden the definition of "independence in functional activities" to include "mild problems performing complex tasks...such as paying bills, preparing a meal, or shopping" and allow reliance on aids and assistance to accomplish these tasks to qualify

as "independent." Because the differentiation of MCI from dementia rests solely on the criterion of functional independence (McKhann et al., 2011), this blurring of what represents "independence" leaves the diagnostic distinction entirely to the individual judgment of the clinician, resulting in nonstandard and arbitrary classifications (Morris, 2012). The "problematic" threshold for distinguishing the "essentially preserved" functional activities in MCI from the subtle functional deficits that accompany the milder stages of AD dementia (Petersen, 2004), combined with the heterogeneity of MCI, have left the field struggling to characterize this condition. In response, some investigators have recommended that the term "MCI" be replaced by etiological diagnoses, particularly when AD is believed to be the underlying causative disorder as determined by an appropriate clinical phenotype and/or by biomarker evidence (Dubois et al., 2010; Morris, 2012) (Table 59.1).

ALZHEIMER'S DISEASE DEMENTIA

Revised criteria for probable AD dementia include the presence of dementia and no evidence for other dementing conditions

TABLE 59.1. Current versions of lexicons and diagnostic criteria for Alzheimer's disease

---

1. Diagnostic and Statistical Manual of Mental Disorders, 4th Edition, Text Revision (DSM-IV-TR[1]; 2000)
   Criteria for AD: the development of memory impairment and deficits in executive function, language, praxis, and/or perception that represent a decline from previous functioning, impair social or occupational activities, have a gradual onset and progression, and are not attributable to another disease

---

2. International Working Group for New Research Criteria for the Diagnosis of AD (Dubois et al., 2010)
   Alzheimer's disease: use of this term is restricted to the clinical disorder, encompassing the full symptomatic spectrum from predementia to dementia. The diagnosis is established by the presence of episodic memory loss and imaging or cerebrospinal fluid (CSF) biomarker evidence of AD. The term "AD" can be subdivided into "prodromal AD" (predementia stage of AD) when instrumental activities of daily living (IADLs) are preserved and "AD dementia" when the cognitive loss interferes with IADLs
   AD pathology: the neurobiologic changes responsible for AD, regardless of whether the clinical disorder is present
   Mild Cognitive Impairment (MCI): cognitive impairment that is too mild to interfere with IADLs but for which no attributable disease can be discerned

---

3. National Institute on Aging-Alzheimer's Association Workgroups on Diagnostic Guidelines for AD (Albert et al., 2011; McKhann et al., 2011; Sperling et al., 2011)
   Dementia: encompass the spectrum of dementia, from the mildest to most severe stages, and defined as cognitive deficits that represent a decline from previous levels of function and interfere with IADLs
   AD dementia: meets criteria for dementia, and cognitive decline is marked by insidious onset with progressive worsening and other illnesses that can explain or contribute to the cognitive loss are absent. Biomarker evidence for AD may enhance confidence in the clinical diagnosis, but such evidence is not presently ready to be incorporated into the routine diagnostic process
   MCI due to AD: concern about cognitive change (either self-reported or from an informant or observer), impaired performance in one or more cognitive domains, and independence in IADLs (distinguishing this condition from dementia). However, "independence" is expansively operationalized to include problems in performing IADLs and to include dependence on aids or assistance to function in daily life. AD biomarkers may be used to increase certainty that AD pathology is the cause of MCI, although currently there remain limitations in how biomarker evidence is interpreted.
   Preclinical AD: AD is defined as the underlying neuropathologic disorder and represents a continuum of pathophysiologic changes that eventually result in cognitive decline. Biomarkers of AD pathology provide hypothetical staging categories for preclinical AD (i.e., when cognitive symptoms and decline are undetectable by current clinical methods but AD lesions are present in the brain)

---

4. Washington University (Morris, 2012)
   Alzheimer's disease: the neurodegenerative brain disorder, regardless of clinical status, that results in a continuous process of synaptic and neuronal deterioration
   - AD is characterized by two major stages:
     – Preclinical (asymptomatic)
     – Symptomatic
   - Symptomatic AD is defined by intra-individual cognitive decline that interferes (from subtle to severe) with daily function. It can be subclassified on severity of symptoms:
     – Incipient (prodromal; MCI)
     – Dementia

---

[1]DSM-5 is scheduled for publication in 2013.

(neurologic disorders or medical comorbidities) or medications that can substantively impair cognition (Table 59.1). When there is an atypical course or an etiologically mixed presentation, possible AD dementia is diagnosed. These criteria recognize advances in AD biomarkers and, when deemed appropriate by the clinician, encourage their use to enhance confidence that the etiology of the dementia syndrome is AD. Biomarkers reflect either the molecular pathology of AD or the presumed downstream effects of the underlying pathology (Table 59.2). The primary use of AD biomarkers currently remains in investigational studies but increasingly will become optional diagnostic tools. Indeed, the Food and Drug Administration in April 2012 approved the use of the ^{18}F amyloid imaging tracer, florbetapir, for the indication of "brain imaging of amyloid plaques in patients…being evaluated for AD and other causes of cognitive decline" ("FDA Approves Amyvid®," 2012). Nonetheless, much work is needed before the clinical utility of AD biomarkers for diagnostic considerations can be fully realized. A biomarker should detect a fundamental feature of AD neuropathology and should be validated using histopathologically confirmed AD cases. A biomarker should be precise in that it should detect AD early in its course and distinguish it from other dementias. Both the sensitivity and specificity of an AD biomarker should be at least 80%, with a positive predictive value approaching 90%. Biomarkers represent continuous biological processes, yet the cutpoints to define a "positive" or "negative" test impose an artificial dichotomous outcome on this continuum and will occasionally produce ambiguous or indeterminate results. There is a great need to standardize both the CSF and imaging biomarkers across laboratories. Practicing physicians have varying degrees of access to AD biomarkers, and reimbursement procedures have yet to be established. An ideal biomarker should be reliable, non-invasive, simple to perform, and inexpensive. The ultimate "test" will be to determine the utility of AD biomarkers in the clinic (Schoonenboom et al., 2012). Although the

revised criteria for AD dementia do not recommend the use of biomarkers for routine diagnostic purposes, other proposed criteria now require biomarker evidence for the diagnosis of AD (Dubois et al., 2010).

DIAGNOSTIC APPROACH TO ALZHEIMER'S DISEASE DEMENTIA

Because biomarkers have not yet been established for clinical practice, clinical methods currently provide the key information needed to diagnose AD dementia and create a differential diagnosis: history taking, mental status testing, and neurological examination. The diagnosis of AD dementia at present rests on the documentation of (1) intraindividual cognitive decline that (2) interferes with daily function.

HISTORY TAKING

Serial cognitive testing provides objective evidence of progressive cognitive decline but such data rarely are available in the acute patient care setting. Fortunately, the observations of a knowledgeable informant also are sensitive and reliable for detecting meaningful intraindividual cognitive decline that characterizes dementia (Carr et al., 2000). Whenever possible, therefore, a person who knows the patient well should be interviewed to assess whether the individual's current levels of cognitive function represent a decline from previously attained levels. In this way, the patient serves as his or her own control and mitigates the fact that specific cognitive strengths and weaknesses and activities of daily life vary widely among individuals. Factors that can influence cognitive test performance, such as literacy and educational attainment, native language, and cultural background, also are minimized. Even in the early stages of AD dementia, most patients lack insight into their cognitive problems. Patient self-report thus is less reliable that the report of an informant (Carr et al., 2000).

The Clinical Dementia Rating (CDR) is an informant-based clinical assessment and dementia staging instrument that is widely used in research settings to determine the presence of absence of dementia and, when present, its severity (Morris, 1993). Semistructured interviews are conducted by an experienced clinician independently with the informant and the patient to assess the patient's abilities in each of six domains: memory, orientation, judgment and problem solving, function in community affairs, home and hobbies, and personal care. Incorporated into the interviews are portions of the Dementia Scale (informant) and Information-Memory-Orientation test (patient) (Blessed et al., 1968), and also included are an aphasia battery, medical and psychiatric histories, and medication inventory. Using all information, the clinician rates each of the six CDR domains along five levels of impairment from none to maximal (rated as 0, 0.5, 1, 2, and 3). Combining the domain scores in accordance with a scoring algorithm produces a global CDR score, where 0 indicates cognitive normality and 0.5, 1, 2, and 3 indicate very mild, mild, moderate, and severe dementia.

The CDR is the primary global staging instrument for the Uniform Data Set (UDS; Morris et al., 2006; Weintraub

TABLE 59.2. Biomarkers for AD

BIOMARKERS FOR THE MOLECULAR PATHOLOGY OF AD

Cerebrospinal fluid
    Reduced levels of amyloid β-42 (Aβ$_{42}$)
    Elevated levels of total tau or phosphorylated tau (p-tau)

Positron emission tomography (PET)
    Retention in cerebral cortex of amyloid tracers such as [^{11}C] Pittsburgh
    Compound B (PIB) or [^{18}F] Florbetapir (Amyvid®)

BIOMARKERS FOR THE CONSEQUENCES OF AD PATHOLOGY
PET   Hypometabolism in temporoparietal cortex as demonstrated by decreased [^{18}F] fluorodeoxyglucose (FDG) uptake

Structural magnetic resonance imaging (MRI)
    Volume loss in:
        Hippocampus
        Medial, basal, lateral temporal lobe
        Medial parietal lobe
        Whole brain

et al., 2009), which, since 2005 has been the standard clinical and cognitive instrument for the evaluation of all cognitively normal control participants and individuals with MCI and AD dementia at the federally funded Alzheimer's Disease Centers (ADCs). Also included in the UDS are additional informant-based scales that capture other aspects of dementia, including neuropsychiatric features (Neuropsychiatric Inventory; Cummings et al., 1994), and functional abilities (Functional Assessment Questionnaire; Pfeffer et al., 1982). Mood and depression are assessed in the patient with the Geriatric Depression Scale (Yesavage et al., 1983). Few practitioners, however, have the training and expertise, much less the time, to administer the UDS or derive the CDR. A derivative of the informant portion of the semistructured interview used to score the CDR is the Ascertain Dementia 8 (AD8; Galvin et al., 2005), a brief eight-item questionnaire that can be used in practice settings as a dementia screening tool.

The AD8 can be completed in two to three minutes and can be administered in person or by telephone; it also can be self-administered by the informant. The eight questions (Table 59.3) ask whether there has been a change due to cognitive decline in the ability of the patient to perform daily tasks. Scores of 2 or more on the AD8 provide good discrimination between cognitive normality and even early-stage AD dementia with a positive predictive value of 87% (Galvin et al., 2005). Poor performance on the AD8 corresponds to biomarker evidence of AD dementia (Galvin et al., 2010). However, the AD8 is a screening, not a diagnostic, instrument and should be used to identify persons who would benefit from an evaluation for possible dementia.

NEUROPSYCHOLOGICAL TESTING

MENTAL STATUS TESTS

Standard cognitive testing can be very useful at the bedside. The ideal information for detecting dementia comes not from a comparison of an individual's cognitive performance with others (i.e., comparison of individual performance with normative values derived from age- and education-matched controls), but from whether an individual has declined from his/her past abilities. Such information is best captured at an initial evaluation by a careful history. Bedside cognitive testing is often accomplished using mental status tests, such as the Mini Mental State Examination (MMSE; Folstein et al., 1975). The MMSE is widely used and has modest sensitivity but fair specificity for detecting dementia (Galvin et al., 2005). The accuracy of the MMSE depends on the age, cultural background, and educational level of the individual. A standard cutpoint score of 23 or less as indicative of dementia has poor accuracy in individuals with education levels at the low and high end of the spectrum (Galvin et al., 2005). In addition, individuals who receive a clinical diagnosis of MCI often score in the normal range for elderly adults (Ismail et al., 2010). The Montréal Cognitive Assessment (MoCA; Nasreddine et al., 2005) is another popular bedside mental status examination that was designed to be more sensitive to frontal and subcortical pathology and to detect cognitive changes in individuals who score in the normal range on the MMSE. Like the MMSE, the MoCA has been validated in several languages and cultures. Some reports show the MoCA to be superior to the MMSE in sensitivity and specificity for detecting MCI and AD (Freitas et al., 2011).

NEUROPSYCHOLOGICAL EVALUATION

Although mental status tests can be useful to screen for the presence of global cognitive difficulties, they are not designed to detect the subtle cognitive changes seen in early symptomatic AD and can be strongly affected by the demographic characteristics of the patient. Mental status tests also cannot provide a comprehensive assessment of specific domains of cognitive functioning, which can be critical for differential diagnosis, tracking change over time, and for treatment planning. A full neuropsychological evaluation is useful when there is a question of more subtle cognitive impairment, or when a more thorough assessment of cognitive strengths and weaknesses is necessary. Neuropsychological evaluations are also indicated when attempting to establish the cognitive fitness or competency of an individual with dementia to perform activities of daily living, including working and driving, and their capacity to make medical, legal, and financial decisions (Moberg and Kniele, 2006). In moderate to severe AD (CDR 2–3), neuropsychological assessment becomes less useful, because patients with advanced AD have pronounced global cognitive deficits that preclude testing. A typical neuropsychology referral involves history taking with the patient and often an informant, and several hours of testing using standardized measures of cognitive functioning. The neuropsychologist then compares the cognitive profile of the individual to normative data (see section on normative data in neuropsychological assessment for more information) and generates a report describing the cognitive profile and the most likely contributing factors, and may include recommendations for treatment. Tests administered usually include an estimate of premorbid functioning and assessments of fluid and crystallized intelligence, attention, working memory, processing speed, visuospatial skills, language, executive functioning, and several aspects of

TABLE 59.3. The AD8: dementia screening interview to differentiate aging and dementia

Is there repetition of questions, stories, or statements?

Are appointments forgotten?

Is there poor judgment (e.g., buys inappropriate items, poor driving decisions)?

Is there difficulty with financial affairs (e.g., paying bills, balancing checkbook)?

Is there difficulty in learning or operating appliances (e.g., television remote control, microwave oven)?

Is the correct month or year forgotten?

Is there decreased interest in hobbies and usual activities?

Is there overall a problem with thinking and/or memory?

Note: Report only a change ccaused by memory and thinking difficulties. (Source: Galvin et al., 2005.)

memory. Mood and personality assessments may also be completed. Neuropsychologists are typically Ph.D. level clinical psychologists who, in addition to training in psychopathology and psychotherapy, have completed specialized internship and fellowship training in neuropsychological assessment. As such, they are well suited for assessment of mood and personality and can play a valuable role in differential diagnosis.

NEUROLOGICAL EXAMINATION

The neurological examination is a standard part of the assessment of a patient with dementia to detect neurological deficits and signs that may suggest possible causes of dementia. In typical AD dementia, the neurological examination is nonfocal and generally unremarkable, particularly in the mild-moderate stages. In more advanced AD dementia, the apparent inability to cooperate may result in gegenhalten (oppositional resistance) when limb muscles are passively stretched. Cortical release signs (suck and grasp reflexes) may be elicited in late-stage AD dementia, and not infrequently there are mild extrapyramidal signs (usually bradykinesia and gait and tone abnormalities) and occasionally myoclonus. The risk of seizures is increased in advanced AD dementia (Romanelli et al., 1990) but seizures are uncommon in the mild-moderate stages (Irizarry et al., 2012).

Aphasia (language dysfunction), apraxia (disordered purposeful movement, distinct from paresis), and agnosia (disordered perception) may develop in later stages of AD dementia. For individuals with milder stages of dementia, deficits in these areas usually are limited to word-finding difficulty for names of people and objects (dysnomia) and perhaps constructional apraxia (i.e., visuospatial impairment as manifested by poor clock drawing performance). Occasionally, AD dementia presents as an asymmetric ("focal") cortical syndrome. Unexplained language dysfunction with relative sparing of memory may indicate the presence of a variant of frontotemporal lobar degeneration, such as nonfluent progressive aphasia or semantic dementia, but atypical AD also can cause progressive aphasia. AD also can present as posterior cortical dysfunction (Renner et al., 2004). The dysfunction can include partial or full examples of the disconnection syndrome, alexia without agraphia (generally involving pathology in the left occipital lobe and splenium of the corpus callosum) and Gerstmann syndrome (dyscalculia, agraphia, right-left disorientation, and finger agnosia), implicating pathology in the left parietal lobe. In one series of 100 "focal" cortical syndrome cases that were examined postmortem, 34 of 100 were attributed to histopathological AD and close to one-half (12 of 26) of the cases with progressive aphasia had neuropathologic AD (Alladi et al., 2007). Visual agnosias include Balint syndrome, where there is failure to properly synthesize all components in the visual field (simultanagnosia) owing to bilateral occipitoparietal pathology that occasionally can be AD (Graff-Radford et al., 1993).

LABORATORY EVALUATION

Depression, B12 deficiency, polypharmacy, and hypothyroidism are not infrequent disorders in older adults and have been associated with cognitive impairment. Screening for these treatable disorders is recommended in the evaluation of possible contributors to dementia (Knopman et al., 2001). Treatment of these disorders is unlikely to completely reverse cognitive deficits. Nevertheless, the high frequency of these co-morbidities and the potential for at least partial amelioration of cognitive symptoms justifies screening.

RADIOLOGICAL EVALUATION

STRUCTURAL IMAGING

Structural neuroimaging, either MRI or non-contrast computed tomography, is recommended to evaluate potential causes of dementia (Knopman et al., 2001). Up to 5% of patients with dementia have imaging evidence for brain neoplasms, subdural hematomas, communicating hydrocephalus, or other structural lesions that may contribute to the cognitive symptoms. Although not specific for AD, neuroanatomic changes consistently have been linked with AD brain pathology and MRI volumetrics are increasingly being used as a "downstream" biomarker for AD dementia that indirectly detects cell loss and AD neuropathological burden (Du et al., 2003; Jack et al., 2002). Cerebral atrophy also is associated with normal aging (Fotenos et al., 2005). Programs have been developed to indicate whether the degree of quantitative volumetric loss (either regional, such as for the hippocampus, or whole brain) falls in the range of "normal" or "pathologic" atrophy.

PHENOMENOLOGY OF ALZHEIMER'S DISEASE DEMENTIA

COURSE

Alzheimer's disease is a uniformly fatal disorder. The duration of AD dementia, from initial appearance of symptoms until death, averages 7 to 10 years, although shorter and longer periods of survival are not uncommon. Staging of dementia generally describes three levels of severity: very mild/mild (corresponding to CDR 0.5 and CDR 1), moderate (CDR 2), and advanced (CDR 3). Although an inevitably progressive disorder, the rate of progression of AD dementia is stage-dependent such that the less the dementia severity, the slower the rate of progression. For example, the median time to progression to a higher CDR score was 3.07 years for CDR 0.5 individuals with AD dementia versus 2.41 years for CDR 1 individuals (Williams et al., 2012). Older age and the presence of the ε4 allele of *apolipoprotein E* (*APOE*) are associated with more rapid progression (Cosentino et al., 2008; Williams et al., 2012).

FEATURES OF VERY MILD/MILD ALZHEIMER'S DISEASE DEMENTIA

The evaluation seldom is sought by the patient, who typically is unaware that there is a "problem," but most often by family or friends. The clinical hallmark of AD dementia is impairment in the learning and retention of new knowledge, such that details of events and conversations are not recalled and questions and statements often are repeated. Performance for autobiographical memory, where the individual's ability to correctly recall events (independently related by the family) in which s/he had recently participated is assessed, is at least as informative for memory function as brief memory tests (Dreyfus et al., 2010). Patients may have difficulty in remembering appointments or to take their medications and often demonstrate misplacement of items without independent retrieval. Temporal and geographical disorientation may result in forgetting the date or day of the week and difficulty in navigating unfamiliar areas. Executive dysfunction is manifested by less facility in organizing information and in impaired decision-making. There is less ability to perform cognitively demanding behaviors, such as operating a motor vehicle or managing the household finances (Table 59.4). Although language skills generally are preserved, difficulties with word retrieval are common and may result in slow, hesitant speech. Personality generally is maintained, although family and friends may note that the affected individual is "quieter" or withdrawn, especially in social settings. Many activities in the community (shopping; attending religious services) and at home (cooking; laundry) still may be performed, if less well than previously, without assistance from others and self-care tasks (dressing, grooming, bathing, toileting) generally are completed independently. Hence, to the casual observer the affected person looks and acts normally, and it is only those who know the person well who are aware of the decline from previously attained levels of cognition and function.

TABLE 59.4. Alzheimer's disease dementia clinical phenotype: mild stage

Gradual onset and progression
Informant report
Frequent repetition, misplaced items, difficulty recalling names
Functional impairment
Driving (failure to maintain lane; minor accidents; poor navigation)
Operation of appliances (e.g., remote controlled devices)
Household finances; cooking; shopping
Affected individual
Impaired insight
Impaired recall of recent events
Poor judgment
Keys
Decline from prior levels
Consistency of problems
Interference with daily function
Probe for intraindividual cognitive decline
Ask if a "problem" represents a change from prior abilities
Obtain concrete examples of how cognitive problems interfere with everyday function
Use judgment
Discordance of informant report vs. individual performance
Alzheimer dementia phenotype can be present in high-functioning persons who still perform well on tests
Individual's self-report of whether or not there are cognitive problems often is unreliable

FEATURES OF MODERATE ALZHEIMER'S DISEASE DEMENTIA

Progressive decline in cognitive and functional abilities now necessitates supervision for almost all aspects of the individual's daily life, and the dementia is obvious even to people who do not know the patient well. New information quickly is forgotten, and recall of even highly learned information may be impaired. Attention also is impaired and the patient is more distractible, with the consequence that attempted tasks are not completed. Disorientation for even familiar settings may result in the individual failing to recognize a home they have visited many times. Elopement is a serious risk as the patient cannot find the way home nor communicate appropriately to others where they live or with whom. Judgment and problem solving abilities are notably impaired, such that it is unsafe for the individual to be home alone because of safety and security concerns (e.g., leaving the doors unlocked; inviting strangers into the house; failing to turn off the stove burners; acquiesce to solicitations for money). The affected individual also must be accompanied in all activities outside of the home. Although the individual may engage in some basic tasks, including cooking, cleaning, and self-care, these generally require supervision. Although patients may continue to dress themselves, supervision may be needed to ensure that the patient does not repeatedly wear the same soiled clothes or put them on improperly; prompting often is needed to have them bathe. Medications must be administered to the patient. The increased dependence of the patient often results in considerable burden for the primary caregiver, who most often is the spouse or adult child of the patient, and negatively affects the caregiver's health. Additional care often is sought from unpaid (family and friends) and paid caregivers. Institutionalization also may be considered, particularly when there is frequent incontinence, wandering, or behavioral abnormalities.

ADVANCED ALZHEIMER'S DISEASE DEMENTIA

Patients in the advanced stages of AD dementia lack comprehension, may no longer remember loved ones, and fail to recognize their home or other familiar surroundings. They lose the ability to perform even simple activities of daily living. Night and day are confused. Eventually patients become near-mute and nonambulatory and require total care for dressing, hygiene, eating, and toilet functions as sphincter control is lost. The patient ultimately succumbs to medical complications such as inanition, aspiration, pneumonia, and sepsis arising from urinary tract infections or decubitus ulcers.

NEUROPSYCHIATRIC FEATURES

Neuropsychiatric and behavioral symptoms are common in AD dementia and contribute to the clinical profile of the disease. Neuropsychiatric problems do not occur in all persons with AD dementia, but generally emerge during the moderate stage of dementia. Neuropsychiatric symptoms can be subclassified as mood disturbances, psychosis (delusions and hallucinations), and personality changes and are observed in a majority of patients with dementia (Sink et al., 2005). Neuroimaging and pathological studies have demonstrated that neuropsychiatric and behavioral symptoms reflect associations with regional pathology as indicated by discrete areas of atrophy, hypometabolism or decreased blood flow (Bruen et al., 2008). For instance, patients with apathy are more likely to have disproportionate dysfunction in the medial frontal and anterior cingulate regions, whereas agitation is higher in those with increased NFT burden in the left orbitofrontal cortex.

The relationship of AD and depression is complicated, but 30% or more of individuals with AD dementia will have at least some depressive features, although the percent meeting criteria for major affective disorder is much lower (Olin et al., 2002). Depressive symptoms in individuals with AD may be a manifestation of pathology in the locus ceruleus and the substantia nigra and thus may be an early symptom of AD pathology (Bruen et al., 2008). Importantly, effectively treating depression can have an impact on the severity of cognitive-related disability, and a low threshold for treatment of depressive symptoms in patients with cognitive impairment is important as some associated cognitive impairments may be improved (McNeil, 1999).

Agitation and aggression are particularly difficult to manage. Agitation represents disruptive psychomotor activity. Hallucinations and delusions occur in about 30% of cases at some point during the course of the illness (Lyketsos et al., 2002). Visual hallucinations are a key feature of dementia with Lewy bodies but are less common in AD and, when present, generally occur in the later stages. Delusions of spousal infidelity and theft are common. Misidentification syndromes such as the Capgras syndrome or reduplicative paramnesia can also occur. Capgras syndrome is the belief that a family member or friend has been replaced by an identical appearing impostor. Reduplicative paramnesia is the delusion that a place (such as one's house) has been duplicated in and exists in two or more places. For instance, the patient may believe their house is somewhere else and that the house they are in is identical to their own. Treating these distressing neuropsychiatric symptoms should first seek to identify the possible physical, social, and environmental precipitants and to remove or reverse them. When non-pharmacologic interventions fail, atypical antipsychotics may provide some relief from agitation or psychosis but randomized clinical trials generally fail to demonstrate benefit (Sink et al., 2005). Metaanalyses indicate that the use of antipsychotics in elderly patients with dementia is associated with increased mortality, primarily related to cardiovascular events.

BIOMARKERS FOR ALZHEIMER'S DISEASE

An autopsy study of 919 individuals with a clinical diagnosis of AD dementia at federally-funded ADCs found that the clinical diagnosis was relatively inaccurate, with mismatches between the clinical and neuropathologic diagnoses in 16.7% of cases (Beach et al., 2012). Although it is possible that the ADCs were referred more complicated cases than are encountered in routine practice, the expertise of these tertiary care centers might

be expected to compensate and yield more accurate diagnoses. Hence, diagnostic misclassification is not inconsiderable for cases of presumed AD dementia. The advent of biomarkers of the molecular pathology of AD is anticipated to improve clinical diagnostic accuracy. Biomarkers also may provide more precise and sensitive measures of disease progression and may allow shorter trials with smaller sample sizes by using biomarkers as surrogate end points. For example, in early symptomatic AD, individuals who were most likely to cognitively decline rapidly were identified by CSF markers for AD (Snider et al., 2009), potentially helping to reduce the number of participants needed to demonstrate a drug effect in trials of MCI and early-stage AD individuals.

Despite promising results, biomarkers must be shown to be at least as accurate as clinical diagnosis alone before their role in the routine assessment in patients with cognitive impairment can be determined. It is likely that a panel of biomarkers rather than a single test will have the most utility for the diagnosis of AD and, in cognitively normal persons, for predicting who will progress to symptomatic AD (de Leon et al., 2001). A major remaining problem for the field is the lack of standardization of the analytic techniques to determine CSF biomarkers. Even the time of collection of CSF is important as CSF $A\beta42$ levels have diurnal fluctuations (Batemen et al., 2007). Different assay platforms also introduce variability. Harmonization of laboratory measurements are needed to minimize current intercenter variations in CSF assays (Mattsson et al., 2011).

Although there remains some uncertainty as to precisely how biomarkers will ultimately be incorporated into the standard evaluation of cognitive impairment, a variety of biomarker measures are currently available for the practicing physician and may provide clinically relevant information in specific circumstances. Measures of amyloid and tau in CSF are commercially available. Although the PET radioligand [11]C Pittsburgh Compound B (PIB; Klunk et al., 2004) has dominated amyloid imaging research because it enters the human brain rapidly and has very high selectivity and nanomolar affinity for $A\beta$ plaques, it has a half-life of only 20 minutes. Its use is thus limited to medical centers with on-site cyclotrons and ^{11}C radiochemistry expertise. Tracers labeled with ^{18}F have a longer half-life (close to two hours) and allow for wider distribution from commercial producers.

Amyloid imaging with ^{18}F florbetapir now is commercially available for detecting the presence of cerebral amyloid deposits in individuals with cognitive decline and additional ^{18}F amyloid tracers are in development. Structural neuroimaging techniques are becoming readily available for volumetric quantification. The use of biomarkers to aid the clinical evaluation of individuals with cognitive impairment is likely to accelerate in coming years. Early recognition of disease will be increasingly important if disease modifying therapies are developed, in particular because those therapies are likely to have greatest efficacy early in the course of disease before major neurodegeneration has occurred.

Alzheimer's disease is associated with a number of modifiable risk factors. Cardiovascular risk factors such as diabetes, hypertension, and hypercholesterolemia are associated with a higher risk of developing AD, whereas lifestyle factors such as physical activity, diet (low fat consumption, moderate alcohol consumption, Mediterranean diet), and cognitive engagement are associated with a lower risk of developing AD. These observations suggest that interventions designed to modify these factors may influence AD risk. The observational nature of the data and methodological limitations of the studies, however, limit the scientific quality of the data and make them insufficient for drawing firm conclusions on the association of any modifiable risk factor with cognitive decline or AD. Further studies are necessary, including long-term population-based studies and randomized controlled trials to further investigate these strategies. Intriguing but nonsignificant data from a population-cohort study suggests that age-adjusted dementia incidence may be declining (Schrijvers et al., 2012). This observation would be consistent with a concept that risk of dementia may be modifiable by trends in social (increased years of education) and medical (better treatment of cardiovascular disease) factors; it also is inconsistent with dementia as an inevitable consequence of aging (Larson and Langa, 2012).

NEUROPSYCHOLOGICAL FEATURES OF ALZHEIMER'S DISEASE

The limbic structures, including the hippocampus and entorhinal cortex, are among the brain regions involved in the earliest stage of symptomatic AD, with increasing involvement of frontal, temporal, and parietal cortices as the disease progresses (e.g., Bondi et al., 2008; Braak and Braak, 1991). In line with this, numerous studies have shown that episodic memory tasks typically are the first to evidence change in symptomatic AD and the structures underlying episodic memory function (medial temporal lobe, precuneus, and other limbic areas) are the first to show changes in volume, connectivity, and task-related brain activity (Bondi et al., 2008; Buckner et al., 2009). These changes also are excellent predictors of disease state (Putcha et al., 2011; Yassa et al., 2011). The AD dementia syndrome is thus characterized by prominent episodic memory deficits with rapid forgetting of material, executive dysfunction, and additional deficits in certain aspects of language, visuospatial abilities, and attention.

Subtle declines in episodic memory in older adults may precede the recognition of symptomatic AD (see Bondi et al., 2008 for review). The traditional view that the first cognitive change is represented by episodic memory deficits may not always be the case. As Storandt (2008) notes, a circularity bias exits when group designations such as MCI are based on neuropsychological status. For example, if a diagnosis of MCI is contingent on episodic memory deficits, it is not surprising that affected individuals most often exhibit significant differences in episodic memory. Longitudinal cognitive and clinical assessments over several years in individuals who subsequently had AD confirmed that deficits occur in non-episodic memory domains in over one-third of cases (Storandt, 2008; Storandt et al., 2006). Personality changes, difficulties with executive or visuospatial functions, slowing of psychomotor speed, or combinations of these appeared to mark initial cognitive decline in some persons (Johnson et al., 2009; Storandt, 2008). Information about intraindividual changes that is gathered from collateral sources also detected subtle cognitive decline that was so minimal it did not meet the cutoffs used to classify MCI. Similarly, others have reported that persons without dementia but with notable personality changes were much more likely to develop dementia two years later (see Storandt, 2008, for review).

Difficulties with attention and executive functioning commonly occur in patients at early stages of AD, and continue to worsen with the progression of the disease. It may be the case that early episodic memory deficits are a result of multiple factors, including difficulty with attention and executive functioning mechanisms. Attention and executive functioning represent somewhat overlapping constructs with many aspects, but the processes of inhibitory control and maintenance of task sets appear to play a critical role in early AD (Buckner, 2004; Storandt, 2008). Neuropsychological tasks that emphasize these processes are very sensitive indicators of the early stage of symptomatic AD. For example, the Stroop test (Stroop, 1935) and the Trail Making test (Reitan, 1992) are good examples of measures that assess these processes. The incongruent condition of the Stroop test requires the patient to inhibit a more salient overlearned response (reading a word) in favor of a less salient response (naming the contrasting ink color). Patients with symptomatic AD, even at early stages, will perform much more slowly and make more errors on this task compared with the baseline conditions where they are asked to simply read words or name color blotches (Amieva et al., 2004). Similarly, individuals with symptomatic AD will have considerable difficulty on the Trail Making B test, which requires them to switch between one overlearned task to another overlearned task to connect a series of numbers and letters (Albert, 2008).

NORMATIVE DATA IN NEUROPSYCHOLOGICAL ASSESSMENT

Clinical assessment of an individual can be understood as having two distinct forms. An idiographic approach considers the individual as a unique agent with characteristics that set him or her apart from other individuals and refers to theories that are applicable to that specific case. In contrast, the nomothetic approach describes general laws of functioning that apply to all individuals and groups of individuals (Persons and Tompkins, 1997). Neuropsychological assessment emphasizes the nomothetic approach, in that a patient's score on a cognitive test is compared to the average performance of a larger group of demographically similar individuals who are typically free from disease. This larger group is referred to as a normative data set and may include individuals with a wide range of demographics (e.g., ages, educational achievement) and linguistic and ethnic backgrounds. In addition to healthy normative data sets, a patient's score can be compared to disease- (e.g., MCI or dementia) or cohort- (e.g., inpatients, on/off medications, age-groups) specific normative data sets. Normative data often are provided by the authors or publishers of a particular test or by other investigators attempting to validate an instrument in a particular clinical population. Attending carefully to the selection of normative data sets for clinical application is critical for interpretation of raw test scores. Normative data can be quite heterogeneous in terms of the size and demographics of the sample, and the time at which the data were collected may introduce cohort effects. Normative data sets are not consistent in accounting for potential moderator variables such as education, gender, or cultural and linguistic backgrounds (Manly, 2008). Also, generalizability may be compromised by geographic limitations, because the samples may be representative of a certain region or collection of disparate regions in the United States or elsewhere (Kalechstein et al., 1998). Differences between these normative samples can significantly alter interpretation of test results. Kalechstein, van Gorp, and Rapport (1998) applied different sets of normative data to scores on commonly used cognitive tests for a group of individuals of various ages and education levels. Interpretation of performance was drastically affected depending on which set of normative data were used for comparison. In the most extreme cases, a score from a single test could span as many as four clinical classifications (e.g., Average, Low Average, Borderline, and Impaired). In other words, the percentile rank for a score on a single test could range from greater than the 25th percentile (Average) to less than the 2nd percentile (Impaired), depending on which normative data set was used for comparison.

Several studies have noted that many individuals continue to perform well on cognitive tests despite having substantial neuropathological abnormalities that ultimately lead to symptomatic AD (Knopman et al., 2003; Price et al., 2009; Schmitt et al., 2000). These individuals tend to be more educated, have larger brain volumes, and may be more socially engaged (James et al., 2011; Roe et al., 2011; Scarmeas and Stern, 2003). This phenomenon has been described as a reserve capacity that may prolong the prodromal period of AD (Roe et al., 2011). However, others have noted that an overreliance on insensitive cognitive tests and the relatively few studies that track intraindividual change may fail to detect subtle cognitive decline in these individuals. Although serial neuropsychological evaluation is ideal for assessment of intraindividual change, this may be impractical for a number of reasons. Thus, most referrals for neuropsychological assessment provide a cross-sectional view of cognitive functioning. Without a careful history taking, which should include the patient and a reliable informant, it is possible that an apparently normal-looking cognitive profile may actually represent a significant decline from a former level of cognitive functioning (Fig. 59.1). This is often the case for high-functioning individuals.

Storandt and Morris (2010) describe an ascertainment bias, which highlights methodological issues related to determining the clinical diagnosis of dementia. They point out that many studies of so-called "cognitive reserve" have used insensitive mental status examinations as the only outcome measures. They also note that individuals who already have early cognitive impairment are included in normative samples, thereby lowering the group mean and reducing the sensitivity to detect impairment (Fig. 59.2). In a carefully assessed sample that was followed through autopsy confirmation of AD, application of commonly used standard deviation cutoffs of −1.0 or −1.5 on episodic memory tests detected only 23% and 44%, respectively, of patients who later developed AD. When this same sample was compared with a robust control group composed of individuals who never progressed to CDR greater than 0, sensitivity and specificity increased greatly but still was inaccurate in over 30% of cases (Storandt and Morris, 2010). These findings underscore the need for development of robust normative data, and also emphasize that an approach that uses standard deviation cutoff scores for classification may not be ideal, even with very robust normative data.

One potential solution is the development of a single comprehensive set of normative data that would include a large, demographically and geographically diverse sample with complete biomarker and neuroimaging data. Cerebrospinal fluid analytes and neuroimaging markers (including structural and functional MRI, amyloid imaging, and white matter imaging) could be used to identify individuals most likely to develop AD and classify them appropriately in the normative data set. An individual's cognitive profile could then be compared with the normative group that is free of detectable AD neuropathology

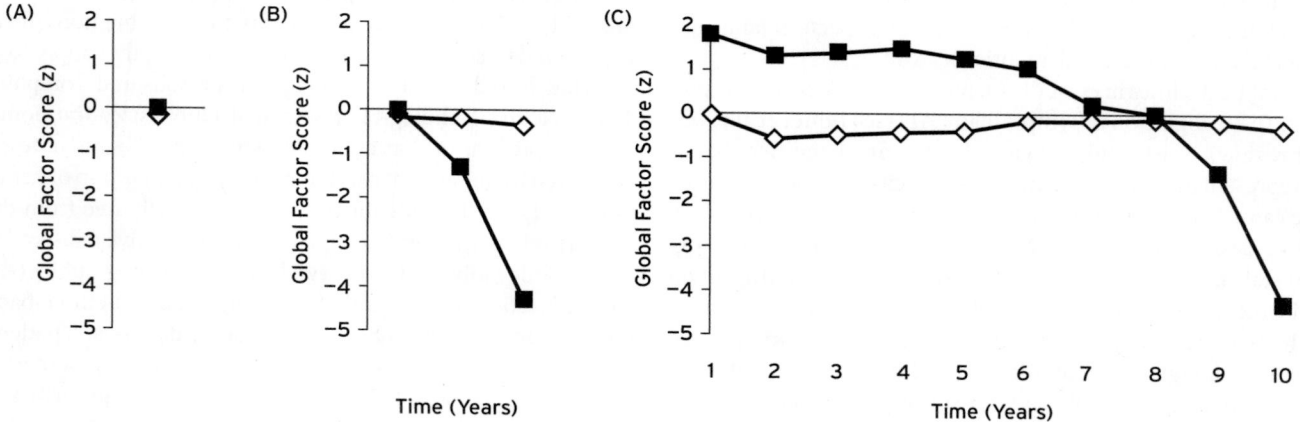

Figure 59.1 *Global factor Z-score cognitive trajectories for two individuals seen over 10 annual follow-up visits. (A) At follow-up visit 8, both individuals score very close to the mean of the reference sample, indicating "normal" cognitive performance. (B) In subsequent assessments, one individual (filled black squares) declined at visit 9 to approximately 1.5 standard deviations below the mean performance of the reference sample and at visit 10 to over four standard deviations below the mean of the reference sample. (C), Cognitive performance at assessments prior to visit 8 for the same individual (filled black squares) reveal that decline had begun well before visit 8. Based on visit-specific neuropsychological performance alone, this individual might be considered as "cognitively normal" (visit 8) or "mild cognitive impairment" (visit 9), but neither of these considerations can be supported once intraindividual decline is taken into account. (Courtesy of Storandt, M.)*

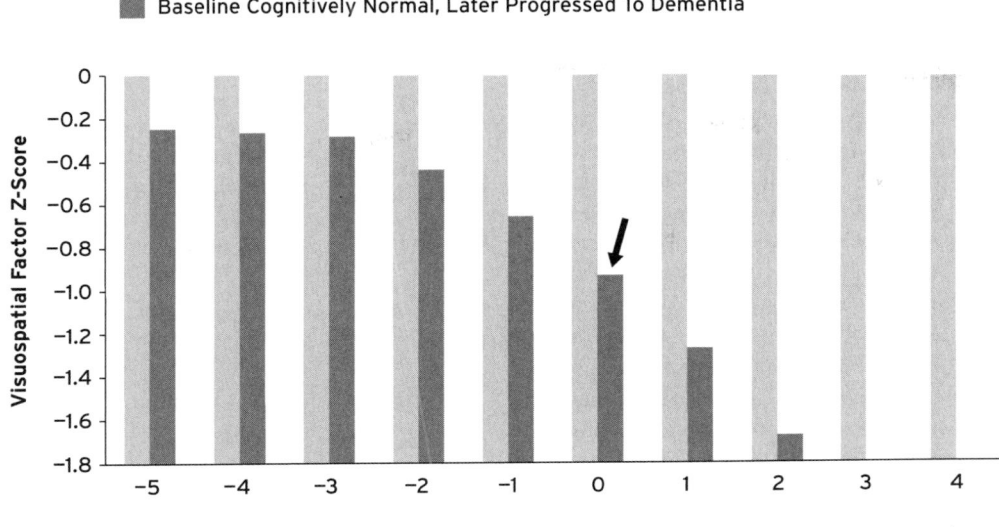

Figure 59.2 *Longitudinal change in visuospatial domain factor scores in older adults who were cognitively normal at entry. The stable cognitively normal group never progressed to a CDR > 0. The autopsy-confirmed group began to decline 3 years prior to receiving a clinical diagnosis of dementia at year 0 (black arrow). Please note that the x-axis (time in years) is only applicable to the Stable group. Including asymptomatic persons with preclinical AD artificially lowers normative values. As a result, means and cutpoints used to detect impairment are too low. (Johnson et al., 2009.)*

and could also be compared with a group with AD neuropathology but who show no clinical symptoms. However, this would be a costly and likely impractical endeavor making a set of "local norms" an appealing option (Kalechstein et al., 1998). Local norms would have the advantage of being ideally similar to the group to which each individual would be compared.

NEUROPSYCHOLOGICAL ASSESSMENT OF ALZHEIMER'S DISEASE IN DIVERSE POPULATIONS

The tremendous growth of ethnic minorities in the United States and Western Europe places increasing emphasis on the need for cognitive measures and normative data that are appropriate to adequately assess individuals of different ethnic, cultural, and linguistic backgrounds. Neuropsychology is in a position to benefit from advances in psychometric methods that move beyond the scrutinizing of between-group test score discrepancies, yet the vast majority of traditional neuropsychological measures commonly in use have not been properly validated for use in minority populations (Manly, 2008; Pedraza and Mungas, 2008). Thus, making diagnostic decisions using neuropsychological tests can be problematic when used on individuals who are not white, have at least two years of college education, are native English speakers, and from at least the midlevels of socioeconomic status (see Manly, 2008 for review). There have been large-scale efforts to develop normative data sets (see Pedraza and Mungas, 2008 for review), but there is still insufficient normative data for the two largest ethnic minorities groups in the United States, blacks and Hispanics. As such, classification accuracy rates for ethnic minorities using traditional normative data sets, especially for difficult diagnoses like prodromal AD, are unacceptable. Pedraza and Mungas (2008)

found that using traditional cutoff values of −1.0 standard deviations below the mean for a primarily white sample resulted in classification of 24% to 56% of cognitively normal blacks as cognitively impaired. Results were dramatically improved when using ethnically-specific normative data from Mayo's Older African American Normative Studies (MOAANS; Lucas et al., 2005). Even when the most likely moderator variables such as age, gender, education, and ethnic backgrounds are taken into account either statistically as covariates or through use of specific normative data sets, other factors can significantly influence cognitive test performance. In a seminal manuscript, Manly and colleagues (Manly et al., 2002) found that using reading level as a proxy for quality of educational attainment largely attenuated differences in neuropsychological test performance between older blacks and whites. These findings appear to extend to blacks with AD. Chin and colleagues (Chin et al., 2012) found that controlling for quality of education using a reading level score, even after including reported years of education as a covariate, attenuated observed differences between blacks and white Non-Hispanics with AD on every neuropsychological test included in the analyses, as well as performance on mental status examinations. Interestingly, the attenuating effect remained after consideration of differences in functional impairment and disease duration, suggesting that use of reading level as a proxy for quality of education is a powerful predictor of neuropsychological performance even in patients with substantial clinical symptoms of AD.

Normative data sets that include mixed ethnicities may provide more accurate performance estimates for ethnic minorities than norms based exclusively on whites. However, grouping people of diverse ethnic backgrounds together may diminish the impact of cultural variables that are unique to particular ethnicities (Lucas et al., 2005). Persons of different ethnic backgrounds may approach the testing situation with different experiences and attitudes that can significantly affect performance. Participants may not be accustomed to the emphasis on speeded performance or have limited familiarity with the wording used in test instructions or test questions (Lucas et al., 2005). Thus, there have been several large-scale attempts to create racially and ethnicity-specific normative data sets in efforts to circumvent these issues; however, this approach has not been without some controversy. Pedraza and Mungas (2008) summarize several arguments against race- or ethnicity-specific normative data sets. Some argue that use of separate norms may ignore underlying factors that contribute to between group differences, such as educational quality. Others argue that use of separate norms reinforces the assumption that race is a biological rather than a socially constructed distinction; another position is that use of separate norms promotes a fundamental misunderstanding about why the discrepancies exist.

DISCLOSURES

Dr. Jason Hassenstab reports that neither he nor his family owns stock or has equity interest (outside of mutual funds or other externally directed accounts) in any pharmaceutical or biotechnology company. Research support from the Charles F. and Joanne Knight Alzheimer's Disease Research Center and the National Institutes of Health (K23DK094982).

Dr. Jeffrey Burns reports research support from the National Institutes of Health (R01AG034614, R01AG03367, P30AG035982, U10NS077356, UL1TR000001). Dr. Burns also receives research support for clinical trials from Jannsen, Wyeth, Danone, Pfizer, Baxter, Avid Radiopharmaceuticals, and Merck. Dr. Burns serves as a consultant for PRA International, has served as an expert witness for legal cases involving decision-making capacity, and has received royalties from publishing Early Diagnosis and Treatment of Mild Cognitive Impairment (Wiley Press, 2008) and Dementia: An Atlas of Investigation and Diagnosis (Clinical Publishing, Oxford, England, 2007).

Dr. John C. Morris reports that neither he nor his family owns stock or has equity interest (outside of mutual funds or other externally directed accounts) in any pharmaceutical or biotechnology company. Dr. Morris has participated or is currently participating in clinical trials of antidementia drugs sponsored by the following companies: Janssen Immunotherapy, and Pfizer. Dr. Morris has served as a consultant for the following companies: Eisai, Esteve, Janssen Alzheimer Immunotherapy Program, Glaxo-Smith-Kline, Novartis, and Pfizer; and receives research support from Eli Lilly/Avid Radiopharmaceuticals.

REFERENCES

Albert, M. (2008). Neuropsychology of Alzheimer's disease. *Handb. Clin. Neurol.* 88:511–525.

Albert, M.S., DeKosky, S.T., et al. (2011). The diagnosis of mild cognitive impairment due to Alzheimer's disease: recommendations from the National Institute on Aging-Alzheimer's Association workgroups on diagnostic guidelines for Alzheimer's disease. *Alzheimers Dement.* 7:270–279.

Alladi, S., Xuereb, J., et al. (2007). Focal cortical presentations of Alzheimer's disease. *Brain* 130:2636–2645.

Alzheimer's Association. (2012). Alzheimer's disease facts and figures. *Alzheimers Dement.* 8:131–168.

Amieva, H., Phillips, L.H.. (2004). Inhibitory functioning in Alzheimer's disease. *Brain* 127:949–964.

Barker, W.W., Luis, C.A., et al. (2002). Relative frequencies of Alzheimer disease, Lewy body, vascular and frontotemporal dementia, and hippocampal sclerosis in the State of Florida Brain Bank. *Alzheimer Dis. Assoc. Disord.* 16:203–212.

Bateman, R.J., Xiong, C., et al. (2012). Clinical and biomarker changes in dominantly inherited Alzheimer's disease. *N. Engl. J. Med.* 367:795–804.

Bateman R.J., Wen G., et al. (2007). Fluctuations of CSF amyloid-beta levels: implications for a diagnostic and therapeutic biomarker. *Neurol.* 68:666–669.

Beach, T.G., Monsell, S.E., et al. (2012). Accuracy of the clinical diagnosis of Alzheimer disease at National Institute on Aging Alzheimer Disease Centers, 2005–2010. *J. Neuropathol. Exp. Neurol.* 71:266–273.

Blessed, G., Tomlinson, B.E., et al. (1968). The association between quantitative measures of dementia and of senile change in the cerebral grey matter of elderly subjects. *Br. J. Psychiatry* 114:797–811.

Bondi, M.W., Jak, A.J., et al. (2008). Neuropsychological contributions to the early identification of Alzheimer's disease. *Neuropsychol. Rev.* 18:73–90.

Braak, H., and Braak, E. (1991). Neuropathological stageing of Alzheimer-related changes. *Acta Neuropathol.* 82:239–259.

Bruen, P.D., McGeown, W.J., et al. (2008). Neuroanatomical correlates of neuropsychiatric symptoms in Alzheimer's disease. *Brain* 131:2455–2463.

Buckner, R.L. (2004). Memory and executive function in aging and AD: multiple factors that cause decline and reserve factors that compensate. *Neuron* 44:195–208.

Buckner, R.L., Sepulcre, J., et al. (2009). Cortical hubs revealed by intrinsic functional connectivity: mapping, assessment of stability, and relation to Alzheimer's disease. *J. Neurosci.* 29:1860–1873.

Carr, D.B., Gray, S., et al. (2000). The value of informant versus individual's complaints of memory impairment in early dementia. *Neurology* 55:1724–1727.

Chin, A.L., Negash, S., et al. (2012). Quality, and not just quantity, of education accounts for differences in psychometric performance between African Americans and white non-Hispanics with Alzheimer's disease. *J. Int. Neuropsychol. Soc.* 18:277–285.

Cosentino, S., Scarmeas, N., et al. (2008). APOE epsilon 4 allele predicts faster cognitive decline in mild Alzheimer disease. *Neurology* 70:1842–1849.

Cummings, J.L., Mega, M., et al. (1994). The Neuropsychiatric Inventory: comprehensive assessment of psychopathology in dementia. *Neurology* 44:2308–2314.

de Leon, M.J., Convit, A., et al. (2001). Prediction of cognitive decline in normal elderly subjects with 2-[(18)F]fluoro-2-deoxy-D-glucose/positron-emission tomography (FDG/PET). *Proc. Natl. Acad. Sci. USA* 98:10966–10971.

Dreyfus, D.M., Roe, C.M., et al. (2010). Autobiographical memory task in assessing dementia. *Arch. Neurol.* 67:862–866.

Du, A.T., Schuff, N., et al. (2003). Atrophy rates of entorhinal cortex in AD and normal aging. *Neurology* 60:481–486.

Dubois, B., Feldman, H.H., et al. (2010). Revising the definition of Alzheimer's disease: a new lexicon. *Lancet Neurol.* 9:1118–1127.

Evans, J.G. (1987). The onset of dementia. *Ann. Acad. Med. Singap.* 16:271–276.

FDA Approves Amyvid. (2012). PRNewswire 2012: 1–4. http://www.prnewswire.com/news-releases/fda-approves-amyvid-florbetapir-f-18-injection-for-use-in-patients-being-evaluated-for-alzheimers-disease-and-other-causes-of-cognitive-decline-146497155.html

Flicker, C., Ferris, S.H., et al. (1991). Mild cognitive impairment in the elderly: predictors of dementia. *Neurology* 41:1006–1009.

Folstein, M.F., Folstein, S.E., et al. (1975). "Mini-mental state." A practical method for grading the cognitive state of patients for the clinician. *J. Psychiatr. Res.* 12:189–198.

Fotenos, A.F., Snyder, A.Z., et al. (2005). Normative estimates of cross-sectional and longitudinal brain volume decline in aging and AD. *Neurology* 64:1032–1039.

Freitas, S., Simões, M.R., et al. (2011). Montreal Cognitive Assessment: validation study for mild cognitive impairment and Alzheimer disease. *Alzheimer Dis. Assoc. Disord.* [Epub ahead of print].

Galvin, J.E., Fagan, A.M., et al. (2010). Relationship of dementia screening tests with biomarkers of Alzheimer's disease. *Brain* 133:3290–3300.

Galvin, J.E., Roe, C.M., et al. (2005). The AD8: a brief informant interview to detect dementia. *Neurology* 65:559–564.

Graff-Radford, N.R., Bolling, J.P., et al. (1993). Simultanagnosia as the initial sign of degenerative dementia. *Mayo Clin. Proc.* 68:955–964.

Hardy, J., and Selkoe, D.J. (2002). The amyloid hypothesis of Alzheimer's disease: progress and problems on the road to therapeutics. *Science* 297:353–356.

Hebert, L.E. (2001). Is the risk of developing Alzheimer's disease greater for women than for men? *Am. J. Epidemiology* 153:132–136.

Hebert, L.E., Scherr, P.A., et al. (2003). Alzheimer disease in the US population: prevalence estimates using the 2000 census. *Arch. Neurol.* 60:1119–1122.

Hyman, B.T., Phelps, C.H., et al. (2012). National Institute on Aging-Alzheimer's Association guidelines for the neuropathologic assessment of Alzheimer's disease. *Alzheimers Dement.* 8:1–13.

Irizarry, M.C., Jin, S., et al. (2012). Incidence of new-onset seizures in mild to moderate Alzheimer disease. *Arch. Neurol.* 69:368–372.

Ismail, Z., Rajji, T.K., et al. (2010). Brief cognitive screening instruments: an update. *Int. J. Geriatr. Psychiatry* 25:111–120.

Jack, C.R., Dickson, D.W., et al. (2002). Antemortem MRI findings correlate with hippocampal neuropathology in typical aging and dementia. *Neurology* 58:750–757.

Jack, C.R., Jr., Knopman, D.S., et al. (2010). Hypothetical model of dynamic biomarkers of the Alzheimer's pathological cascade. *Lancet Neurol.* 9:119–128.

James, B.D., Wilson, R.S., et al. (2011). Late-life social activity and cognitive decline in old age. *J. Int. Neuropsychol. Soc.* 17:998–1005.

Johnson, D.K., Storandt, M., et al. (2009). Longitudinal study of the transition from healthy aging to Alzheimer disease. *Arch. Neurol.* 66:1254–1259.

Jonsson, T., Atwal, J.K., et al. (2012). A mutation in APP protects against Alzheimer's disease and age-related cognitive decline. *Nature* 488:96–99.

Kalechstein, A.D., van Gorp, W.G., et al. (1998). Variability in clinical classification of raw test scores across normative data sets. *Clin. Neuropsychol.* 12:339–347.

Katzman, R. (1976). The prevalence and malignancy of Alzheimer disease: a major killer. *Alzheimers Dement.* 4:378–380.

Klunk, W.E., Engler, H., et al. (2004). Imaging brain amyloid in Alzheimer's disease with Pittsburgh Compound-B. *Ann. Neurol.* 55:306–319.

Knopman, D.S., DeKosky, S.T., et al. (2001). Practice parameter: diagnosis of dementia (an evidence-based review). Report of the Quality Standards Subcommittee of the American Academy of Neurology. *Neurology* 56:1143–1153.

Knopman, D.S., Parisi, J.E., et al. (2003). Neuropathology of cognitively normal elderly. *J. Neuropathol. Exp. Neurol.* 62:1087–1095.

Larson, E.B., and Langa, K.M. (2012). Aging and incidence of dementia: a critical question. *Neurology* 78:1452–1453.

Lavery, L.L., Lu, S.-Y., et al. (2007). Cognitive assessment of older primary care patients with and without memory complaints. *J. Gen. Intern. Med.* 22:949–954.

Lucas, J.A., Ivnik, R.J., et al. (2005). Mayo's Older African Americans Normative Studies: normative data for commonly used clinical neuropsychological measures. *Clin. Neuropsychol.* 19:162–183.

Lyketsos, C.G., Lopez, O., et al. (2002). Prevalence of neuropsychiatric symptoms in dementia and mild cognitive impairment: results from the cardiovascular health study. *JAMA* 288:1475–1483.

Manly, J.J. (2008). Critical issues in cultural neuropsychology: profit from diversity. *Neuropsychol. Rev.* 18:179–183.

Manly, J.J., Jacobs, D.M., et al. (2002). Reading level attenuates differences in neuropsychological test performance between African American and White elders. *J. Int. Neuropsychol. Soc.* 8:341–348.

Mattsson, N., Andreasson, U., et al. (2011). The Alzheimer's Association external quality control program for cerebrospinal fluid biomarkers. *Alzheimers Dement.* 7:386–395.e6.

McKhann, G., Drachman, D., et al. (1984). Clinical diagnosis of Alzheimer's disease: report of the NINCDS-ADRDA Work Group under the auspices of Department of Health and Human Services Task Force on Alzheimer's Disease. *Neurology* 34:939–944.

McKhann, G.M., Knopman, D.S., et al. (2011). The diagnosis of dementia due to Alzheimer's disease: recommendations from the National Institute on Aging-Alzheimer's Association workgroups on diagnostic guidelines for Alzheimer's disease. *Alzheimers Dement.* 7:263–269.

McNeil, J.K. (1999). Neuropsychological characteristics of the dementia syndrome of depression: onset, resolution, and three-year follow-up. *Clin. Neuropsychol.* 13:136–146.

Moberg, P.J., and Kniele, K. (2006). Evaluation of competency: ethical considerations for neuropsychologists. *Appl. Neuropsychol.* 13:101–114.

Morris, J.C. (2006). Alzheimer's disease and mild cognitive impairment. In: Morris, J.C., Galvin, J.E., and Holtzman, D.M., eds. *Handbook of Dementing Illnesses*, 2nd Edition. New York: Taylor & Francis, pp. 191–208.

Morris, J.C. (2012). Revised criteria for mild cognitive impairment may compromise the diagnosis of Alzheimer disease dementia. *Arch. Neurol.* 69:700–708.

Morris, J.C. (1993). The Clinical Dementia Rating (CDR): current version and scoring rules. *Neurology* 43:2412–2414.

Morris, J.C., Weintraub, S., et al. (2006). The Uniform Data Set (UDS): clinical and cognitive variables and descriptive data from Alzheimer Disease Centers. *Alzheimer Dis. Assoc. Disord.* 20:210–216.

Nasreddine, Z.S., Phillips, N.A., et al. (2005). The Montreal Cognitive Assessment, MoCA: a brief screening tool for mild cognitive impairment. *J. Am. Geriatr. Soc.* 53:695–699.

Nelson, P.T., Alafuzoff, I., et al. (2012). Correlation of Alzheimer disease neuropathologic changes with cognitive status: a review of the literature. *J. Neuropathol. Exp. Neurol.* 71:362–381.

Olin, J.T., Katz, I.R., et al. (2002). Provisional diagnostic criteria for depression of Alzheimer disease: rationale and background. *Am. J. Geriatr. Psychiatry* 10:129–141.

Pedraza, O., and Mungas, D. (2008). Measurement in cross-cultural neuropsychology. *Neuropsychol. Rev.* 18:184–193.

Perrin, R.J., Fagan, A.M., et al. (2009). Multimodal techniques for diagnosis and prognosis of Alzheimer's disease. *Nature* 461:916–922.

Persons, J.B., and Tompkins, M.A. (1997). Cognitive-behavioral case formulation. In: Eells, T.D., ed. *Handbook of Psychotherapy Case Formulation*. New York: Guilford Press, pp. 314–339.

Petersen, R.C. (2004). Mild cognitive impairment as a diagnostic entity. *J. Intern. Med.* 256:183–194.

Petersen, R.C., Smith, G.E., et al. (1995). Apolipoprotein E status as a predictor of the development of Alzheimer's disease in memory-impaired individuals. *JAMA* 273:1274–1278.

Pfeffer, R.I., Kurosaki, T.T., et al. (1982). Measurement of functional activities in older adults in the community. *J. Gerontol.* 37:323–329.

Price, J.L., Ko, A.I., et al. (2001). Neuron number in the entorhinal cortex and CA1 in preclinical Alzheimer disease. *Arch. Neurol.* 58:1395–1402.

Price, J.L., McKeel, D.W., et al. (2009). Neuropathology of nondemented aging: presumptive evidence for preclinical Alzheimer disease. *Neurobiol. Aging* 30:1026–1036.

Price, J.L., and Morris, J.C. (1999). Tangles and plaques in nondemented aging and "preclinical" Alzheimer's disease. *Ann. Neurol.* 45:358–368.

Putcha, D., Brickhouse, M., et al. (2011). Hippocampal hyperactivation associated with cortical thinning in Alzheimer's disease signature regions in non-demented elderly adults. *J. Neurosci.* 31:17680–17688.

Reitan, R.M. (1992). *Trail Making Test: Manual for Administration and Scoring [Adults].* Tucson, AZ: Reitan Neuropsychology Laboratory.

Renner, J.A., Burns, J.M., et al. (2004). Progressive posterior cortical dysfunction: a clinicopathologic series. *Neurology* 63:1175–1180.

Roe, C.M., Fagan, A.M., et al. (2011). Cerebrospinal fluid biomarkers, education, brain volume, and future cognition. *Arch. Neurol.* 68:1145.

Romanelli, M.F., Morris, J.C., et al. (1990). Advanced Alzheimer's disease is a risk factor for late-onset seizures. *Arch. Neurol.* 47:847–850.

Scarmeas, N., and Stern, Y. (2003). Cognitive reserve and lifestyle. *J. Clin. Exp. Neuropsychol.* 25:625–633.

Schmitt, F.A., Davis, D.G., et al. (2000). "Preclinical" AD revisited: neuropathology of cognitively normal older adults. *Neurology* 55:370–376.

Schoonenboom, N.S.M., Reesink, F.E., et al. (2012). Cerebrospinal fluid markers for differential dementia diagnosis in a large memory clinic cohort. *Neurology* 78:47–54.

Schrijvers, E.M.C., Verhaaren, B.F.J., et al. (2012). Is dementia incidence declining?: Trends in dementia incidence since 1990 in the Rotterdam Study. *Neurology* 78:1456–1463.

Sink, K.M., Holden, K.F., et al. (2005). Pharmacological treatment of neuropsychiatric symptoms of dementia: a review of the evidence. *JAMA* 293:596–608.

Small, S.A., and Duff, K. (2008). Linking Abeta and tau in late-onset alzheimer's disease: a dual pathway hypothesis. *Neuron* 60:534–542.

Snider, B.J., Fagan, A.M., et al. (2009). Cerebrospinal fluid biomarkers and rate of cognitive decline in very mild dementia of the Alzheimer type. *Arch. Neurol.* 66:638–645.

Sperling, R.A., Aisen, P.S., et al. (2011). Toward defining the preclinical stages of Alzheimer's disease: recommendations from the National Institute on Aging-Alzheimer's Association workgroups on diagnostic guidelines for Alzheimer's disease. *Alzheimers Dement.* 7:280–292.

Storandt, M. (2008). Cognitive deficits in the early stages of Alzheimer's disease. *Curr. Dir. Psychol. Sci.* 17:198–202.

Storandt, M., Grant, E.A., et al. (2006). Longitudinal course and neuropathologic outcomes in original vs revised MCI and in pre-MCI. *Neurology* 67:467–473.

Storandt, M., and Morris, J.C. (2010). Ascertainment bias in the clinical diagnosis of Alzheimer disease. *Arch. Neurol.* 67:1364–1369.

Stroop, J.R. (1935). Studies of interference in serial verbal reactions. *J. Exp. Psychol.* 18:643–662.

Tomlinson, B.E., Blessed, G., et al. (1970). Observations on the brains of demented old people. *J. Neurol. Sci.* 11:205–242.

Tomlinson, B.E., Blessed, G., et al. (1968). Observations on the brains of non-demented old people. *J. Neurol. Sci.* 7:331–356.

Wachterman, M., Kiely, D.K., et al. Reporting dementia on the death certificates of nursing home residents dying with end-stage dementia. *JAMA* 300:2608–2610.

Weintraub, S., Salmon, D., et al. (2009). The Alzheimer's Disease Centers' Uniform Data Set (UDS): the neuropsychologic test battery. *Alzheimer Dis. Assoc. Disord.* 23:91–101.

Williams, M., Storandt, M., et al. (2012). Progression of Alzheimer disease as measured by Clinical Dementia Rating sum of Boxes scores. *Alzheimers Dement.*

Winblad, B., Palmer, K., et al. (2004). Mild cognitive impairment: beyond controversies, towards a consensus: report of the International Working Group on Mild Cognitive Impairment. *J. Intern. Med.* 256:240–246.

Yassa, M.A., Mattfeld, A.T., et al. (2011). Age-related memory deficits linked to circuit-specific disruptions in the hippocampus. *Proc. Natl. Acad. Sci.* 108:8873–8878.

Yesavage, J.A., Brink, T., et al. (1983). Development and validation of a geriatric depression screening scale: a preliminary report. *J. Psychiatr. Res.* 17:37–49.

60 | THE GENETICS OF ALZHEIMER'S DISEASE

RUDOLPH E. TANZI

Over the past three decades, considerable progress has been made in the identification of genetic risk factors for Alzheimer's disease (AD). However, the challenges have been immense. First, although one of the key features of AD is familial aggregation and family history is the second greatest risk factor for AD, the genetics of AD are complex and heterogeneous (reviewed in Bertram et al., 2009; Bertram et al., 2010; Tanzi and Bertram, 2005). Second, a definitive diagnosis of AD requires a postmortem neuropathological examination of the brain. The quality of any genetic study depends on the validity and reliability of the phenotypes used. In considering "affection status" as a phenotype, it needs to be emphasized that any AD cohort consisting of living patients may be "contaminated" with non-AD cases of dementia (e.g., frontotemporal lobar dementia). A third challenge is that AD strikes late in life, usually after the age of 70 years. Thus, in family-based genetic studies, parental DNA is rarely if ever available. Moreover, family history, as related by family members may not be accurate. Despite these challenges, genetic discoveries in AD have provided the first and most vital clues regarding the causes of AD. For decades after Alois Alzheimer described the disease in the autopsied brain of a demented female patient in her 50s, our understanding of the etiology and pathogenesis was limited to what could be garnered from the pathological aftermath of the disease. The advent of the first AD genes in the 1980s and 1990s provided us with the first solid clues regarding the etiology and pathogenic events of AD along with strategies for treating and preventing this devastating disease.

EARLY-ONSET FAMILIAL ALZHEIMER'S DISEASE

Based on twin and family studies, approximately 80% of AD includes the inheritance of specific genetic factors as part of its etiology (Gatz et al., 2006). The existence of relatively large multigenerational early-onset familial Alzheimer's disease (EO-FAD) families helped to make the EO-FAD genes the "low hanging fruit" in AD gene discovery. Roughly 5% of AD is EO-FAD, which can be caused by well over 200 rare, fully penetrant mutations in three different genes. In 1987, we and others isolated the gene encoding the amyloid β (A4) protein precursor (APP), (Goldgaber et al., 1987; Kang et al., 1987; Tanzi et al., 1987a; Tanzi et al., 1988a), and physically and genetically mapped it to chromosome 21 (Tanzi et al., 1987a). The cloning of APP was made possible by the publication of the amino acid sequence of the amyloid β-protein by Glenner and

Wong (1984) and Masters et al (1985). In their paper, Glenner and Wong predicted that the gene responsible for making the "β-protein," as they called it, would be on chromosome 21 and carry mutations causing AD. More importantly, Glenner first proposed that AD is a cerebral form of amyloidosis, in which the accumulation of cerebral amyloid β-protein drives all subsequent pathology. Glenner's β-protein hypothesis was subsequently reinterpreted and reported eight years later as the "amyloid cascade hypothesis" of AD (Hardy and Higgins, 1992), and was further refined in later years (Hardy and Selkoe, 2002; Tanzi and Bertram, 2005).

When we and others used the Aβ amino acid sequence (Glenner's β-protein and Masters' A4) to clone the APP gene (Goldgaber et al., 1987; Kang et al., 1987, Tanzi et al., 1987a, Tanzi et al., 1988), the first AD candidate gene had been identified. Concurrent with the isolation of the APP gene, we also reported in that same issue of *Science*, evidence for genetic linkage of EO-FAD to genetic markers on chromosome 21 in the vicinity of APP (St George-Hyslop et al., 1987). From 1982 to 1987, Paul Watkins and I had been working in the laboratory of James Gusella at MGH to isolate the first single nucleotide polymorphisms (SNP) on chromosome 21, called restriction fragment length polymorphisms (RFLPs). These were used to build a complete genetic map of this chromosome (Tanzi et al., 1988b). At that same time, we had been collecting some of the largest, multi-generational EO-FAD families and started testing them for genetic linkage to chromosome 21 in 1983.

After testing the first two EO-FAD families (of Canadian and Italian descent), no genetic linkage of AD was observed for the SNPs on our genetic linkage map of chromosome 21. Later, two more EO-FAD families (of German and Russian descent) were added to the study, and Peter St George-Hyslop and Jonathan Haines had taken over the project as I turned my own efforts to cloning the first AD candidate gene, APP. At the same time that we and others had reported the identification and characterization of the APP gene, St George-Hyslop and Haines claimed to find linkage to chromosome 21 in the vicinity of the APP gene near marker D21S1 (St George-Hyslop et al., 1987). Disappointingly, soon after, we showed that the same four large EO-FAD families apparently linked to markers on chromosome 21 near APP exhibited absolutely no genetic linkage to APP (Tanzi et al., 1987b). Van Broeckhoven et al. also reported lack of linkage of EO-FAD to APP in other EO-FAD families (Van Broeckhoven et al., 1987). Importantly, in both of papers, APP was ruled from linkage in the specific EO-FAD families tested, however, we did not rule out APP as a candidate gene for other cases of AD. Later the four EO-FAD families reported to be linked to chromosome 21 were shown to actually be linked to an EO-FAD locus on chromosome 14q24 and were ultimately demonstrated to carry mutations in the presenilin 1 (*PSEN1*) gene (Sherrington et al., 1995).

So, although the original genetic linkage of EO-FAD to chromosome 21 (St George-Hyslop et al., 1987) was spurious, ironically, it prompted other groups, including that of John Hardy, to test other EO-FAD families for genetic linkage of EO-FAD to our DNA markers (RFLPs) on chromosome 21. And some of those families exhibited genuine linkage to our chromosome 21 map RFLP markers that we had shared with John Hardy. In 1991, the first EO-FAD mutation was found in *APP* by re-sequencing those independent chromosome 21-linked EO-FAD families (Goate et al., 1991). However, this was not the first disease mutation reported in *APP*. Prior to the Goate et al. (1991) paper, Frangione et al. had already reported the first pathogenic mutation in APP (Levy et al., 1990). Levy et al. (1990) sequenced exons 16 and 17 of *APP*, which encode the Aβ domain, and uncovered the first pathogenic mutation in APP, which was responsible for Dutch hereditary cerebral hemorrhage with amyloidosis, sometimes referred to as a vascular form of AD. Goate et al. (1991) took a similar approach on their chromosome 21-linked families by resequencing the same two *APP* exons, to find the first EO-FAD mutation (London mutation; V717I) in *APP*.

Less than a year after the elucidation of the first *APP* mutations, it became clear that mutations in *APP* accounted for a very tiny proportion of EO-FAD (Tanzi et al., 1992). In 1995, several EO-FAD mutations were found in *PSEN1* (Sherrington et al., 1995) on chromosome 14. Shortly afterward, we reported a homolog of *PSEN1* called presenilin (*PSEN2*) (Levy-Lahad et al., 1995) on chromosome 1 and showed that it contained the N141I mutation in Volga-German EO-FAD families. This was subsequently confirmed by Rogaev et al. (1995). To date, 30 mutations (plus duplications) have been reported for *APP*, 185 for *PSEN1*, and 14 for *PSEN2* (Alzheimer's Disease & Frontotemporal Dementia Mutation Database; http://www.molgen.ua.ac.be/ADMutations). Generally, the EO-FAD mutations in *APP*, *PSEN1*, and *PSEN2* and duplication of *APP* are fully penetrant for causing AD (Table 60.1). However, we recently reported the first case of non-penetrant *APP* duplication (Hooli et al., 2012).

The vast majority of the more than 200 EO-FAD mutations in *APP*, *PSEN1*, and *PSEN2* lead to increase in the ratio of Aβ42:Aβ40 (Scheuner et al., 1996; Tanzi and Bertram, 2005). The increase in relative levels of Aβ42 then promotes the aggregation of the peptide into β-amyloid (Jarrett et al., 1993). Three years after the discovery of the presenilins in 1995, they were shown to act as aspartyl proteases that carry out γ-secretase cleavage of APP in it transmembrane domain to produce Aβ (reviewed in Tanzi and Bertram, 2005). Based on these collective findings, we have been collaborating with Steve Wagner (UCSD) to develop a class of highly promising AD drugs known as γ-secretase modulators, which are aimed at reversing this ratio. (Kounnas et al, 2010).

GENETICS OF LATE-ONSET ALZHEIMER'S DISEASE

The most common form of the disease is defined by onset after 65 years and is referred to as LOAD. Unlike EO-FAD, which is characterized by classic Mendelian inheritance most often in an autosomal dominant manner, LOAD exhibits a genetically complex pattern of inheritance. Risk for most cases of LOAD involve the influence of both genetic and life exposure factors. The most highly confirmed risk factor for LOAD is the ε4 variant of the apolipoprotein E gene (*APOE*) (Strittmatter et al, 1993) on chromosome 19. The three major variants of *APOE* are based on combinations of amino acids 112 and 158 (ε2: Cys_{112}/Cys_{158}; ε3: Cys_{112}/Arg_{158}; ε4: Arg_{112}/Arg_{158}). A single copy of the ε4-allele increases AD risk by about four-fold, whereas two copies increase risk by greater than 10-fold. In contrast, the ε2-allele of *APOE* is protective (Corder et al., 1994). Functionally, APOE is believed to play a role in the clearance of Aβ from the brain (reviewed in Kim et al., 2009).

For a decade or more after the report of association of LOAD with *APOE*, hundreds of genes were tested for association with AD leading to endless series of replications and refutations. Lars Bertram, colleagues, and I started an online database called AlzGene.org (http://www.alzgene.org) (Bertram and Tanzi, 2008; Bertram et al., 2007) to summarize and display these findings in a systematic and objective manner. In addition, AlzGene.org presents metaanalysis results for AD candidate genes that have been tested in at least four independent case-control samples. The strongest association with LOAD on AlzGene is obtained with *APOE*. Roses et al. (2010) recently proposed that additional genes near *APOE* might also influence risk for AD. One of these is a poly-T variant in the gene for the translocase of outer mitochondrial membrane 40 homolog (*TOMM40*), which is in strong linkage disequilibrium with *APOE*, mapping only ~2,000 basepairs away. The "long"

TABLE 60.1. Early-onset familial Alzheimer's disease genes

GENE	PROTEIN	CHROMOSOME	MUTATIONS	CONSEQUENCE
APP	Amyloid β (A4) Protein Precursor	21q21	30 (duplication)	Elevated $Aβ_{42}/A_{40}$ ratio Increased Aβ production Enhanced Aβ aggregation
PSEN1	Presenilin 1	14q24	185	Elevated $Aβ_{42}/Aβ_{40}$ ratio
PSEN2	Presenilin 2	1q31	14	Elevated $Aβ_{42}/Aβ_{40}$ ratio

poly-T repeats were reported to be associated with earlier onset of AD. This creates a conundrum because it is highly unlikely that both *APOE* and *TOMM40*, sitting right next door to each other, both contribute to AD risk. Given the choice of whether the real AD gene there is *APOE* or *TOMM40*, functional studies strongly support *APOE* as the actual AD gene in this region based on its ability to affect cerebral Aβ clearance (reviewed in Kim et al., 2009). Moreover, in our own family-based studies of AD, the statistical signal strength of the association of *APOE* with AD is 15 orders of magnitude higher than that observed for any of other genes in the *APOE* region, including *TOMM40* (unpublished data).

Although most studies searching for novel AD genes after the report of the association with *APOE* employed candidate gene searches, more genome-wide association studies (GWAS) have become more common. In GWAS, up to one million SNPs (along with single copy probes to detect copy number variants) are tested for genetic association with disease risk and phenotypes including age-of-onset, biomarkers, imaging results, and neuropathological endpoints. The first genome-wide significant GWAS finding of a gene associated with LOAD was with the gene encoding GRB2-associated binding protein 2 (*GAB2*; Reiman et al., 2007). However, the association was only deemed "genome-wide significant" following post hoc stratification by APOE. The association was followed by a series of replications and refutations. Functionally, *GAB2* has been proposed to affect both tau phosphorylation (Reiman et al., 2007) and Aβ production (Nizzari et al., 2007).

A year after the *GAB2*, we reported the first genes to exhibit genome-wide significant association with AD without stratification on *APOE*. To achieve this, we employed family-based GWAS (Bertram et al, 2008) and reported three AD genes candidates containing SNPs that exhibited genome-wide significance for association AD. These included *ATXN1* (ataxin 1), *CD33* (siglec 3), and an uncharacterized locus on chromosome 14 (GWA_14q31.2). *ATXN1* can carry an expanded poly-glutamine repeat that causes spinocerebellar ataxia type 1. *ATXN1* also affects Aβ levels by regulating levels of β-secretase, the rate-limiting enzyme for Aβ production (Zhang et al., 2010). *CD33* is a sialic acid-binding, immunoglobulin-like lectin that regulates the innate immune system (Crocker et al., 2007), including inflammation. We recently showed that Aβ has the microbiological properties of an antimicrobial peptide, used in the brain's innate immune system (Soscia et al., 2010). Thus, control of the brain's innate immune system by molecules like CD33, might also regulate Aβ levels via clearance by microglial cells.

In 2009, two of the largest case-control GWAS carried out to date (Harold et al., 2009; Lambert et al., 2009) led to three novel AD genes: *CLU* (clusterin; apolipoprotein J), *CR1* (complement component [3b/4b] receptor 1), and *PICALM* (phosphatidylinositol binding clathrin assembly protein). However, the effect sizes of the AD-associated SNPs in these genes are tiny (i.e. increasing or decreasing risk by ~1.15-fold). In contrast, APOE-ε4 increases risk for AD by ~4-fold and 15-fold, for one or two alleles, respectively. Functionally, *CLU* is likely involved in importing Aβ from plasma back into the brain (DeMattos et al., 2004; Nuutinen et al., 2009). In contrast, APOE exports the peptide out of the brain into the plasma. *PICALM*

is involved in clathrin-mediated endocytosis (Tebar et al., 1999; Treusch et al., 2011), and *CR1*, like *CD33*, plays a role in the innate immune system (Khera and Das, 2009). In 2010, another case-control GWAS (Seshadri et al., 2010) reported association with the gene for bridging integrator 1 (*BIN1*), which had actually been reported to be associated with AD in an earlier study (Lambert et al., 2009). The AD-associated SNP in *BIN1* also has a very small effect size on AD risk with an allelic odds ratio of ~1.15. *BIN1* is expressed in the CNS and like PICALM, plays a role in receptor-mediated endocytosis (Pant et al., 2009).

In 2011, two more case-control GWAS reported four more AD candidate genes including *CD2AP*, *MS4A6A/MS4A4E*, *EPHA1*, and *ABCA7* (Hollingworth et al., 2011; Naj et al., 2011). These studies also identified a second AD-associated SNP in *CD33* providing strong support for our previously reported genome-wide significant association of *CD33* with AD three years earlier (Bertram et al., 2008). Thus, in addition to the four original AD genes, *APP*, *PSEN1*, *PSEN2*, and *APOE*, 11 more AD genes (*CD33*, *GWA_14q31.2*, *ATXN1*, *CLU*, *PICALM*, *CR1*, *BIN1*, *ABCA7*, *MS4A6E/MS4A4E*, *CD2AP*, and *EPHA1*) harbor SNPs that exhibit genome-wide significance for association with LOAD (Table 60.2).

The predicted and known functions of the AD genes fall into four basic categories: Aβ metabolism, lipid metabolism, innate immunity, and cellular signaling. With the identification of the original 4 and 11 novel confirmed AD genes, we hope to answer some key remaining questions regarding the etiology and pathogenesis of AD. First, which genes besides APP, PSEN1 and PSEN2 affect the production of Aβ? Based on our own data these would minimally include *ATXN1* (Zhang et al., 2010). Second, which genes besides APOE affect the clearance of Aβ in the brain? These would likely include *CLU* and according to our own unpublished preliminary data, *CD33*, based on its ability to activate microglial degradation of Aβ. Other AD candidate genes that activate microglia to clear Aβ may also be involved (e.g. CR1).

The excessive accumulation of Aβ in the brain is believed to trigger tauopathy and tangles, followed by neurodegeneration and inflammation. The ability of excess accumulation of

TABLE 60.2. Late-onset Alzheimer's disease genes

GWAS	DESIGN	GENES EXHIBITING GENOME-WIDE SIGNIFICANT ASSOCIATION WITH LOAD
Reiman, 2007	Case-control	APOE, GAB2
Bertram, 2008	Family-based	APOE, ATXN1, CD33, GWA_14q31
Lambert, 2009	Case-control	APOE, CLU, CR1
Harold, 2009	Case-control	APOE, CLU, PICALM
Seshadri, 2010	Case-control	APOE, BIN1
Naj, 2011	Case-control	MS4A6A/MS4A4E, EPHA1, CD33, CD2AP
Hollingworth, 2011	Case-control	ABCA7, MS4A6A/MS4A4E, EPHA1, CD33, CD2AP

cerebral Aβ to trigger tauopathy likely involves aberrant signaling and could therefore involve *PICALM, BIN1, CD2AP* (Treusch et al., 2011). Neurodegeneration accompanied by tauopathy and excess Aβ accumulation must also induce inflammatory pathways to complete the course of neuronal cell death and synapse loss initially triggered by excessive Aβ accumulation in the brain. It is likely that AD genes involved in the innate immune system (e.g. *CD33, CLU, MS4A6E/MS4A4E,* and *EPHA1*) play a role here. Thus, so far, the known AD genes and newly confirmed AD gene candidates from GWAS fit fairly nearly into an overall pathogenic pathway in which excessive accumulation of Aβ leads to tauopathy and neurodegeneration followed by inflammation ultimately resulting in catastrophic loss of neurons and synapses leading to dementia (Tanzi and Bertram, 2005).

ADAM10: FIRST LOAD GENE WITH RARE PATHOGENIC MISSENSE MUTATIONS

Late-onset AD has been associated with common genetic variants, which, with the exception of *APOE*, exert small effects on risk. However, our laboratory recently reported two rare, highly penetrant mutations for LOAD (Kim et al., 2008), located in the *ADAM10* gene. *ADAM10* encodes the major α-secretase in the brain, which cleaves within the Aβ domain of APP to preclude β-amyloid formation We reported two rare (7 of 1000 LOAD families) LOAD mutations in *ADAM10*: Q170H and R181G. Both are located in the prodomain region and lead to AD at roughly 70 years old. Both mutations severely impair *ADAM10*'s ability to cleave at the α-secretase site of APP *in vitro* (Kim et al., 2008) and these effects have now been confirmed *in vivo* (unpublished observations). To date, these are the first and only highly penetrant, rare mutations reported for LOAD. These findings underscore the critical need for whole genome or whole exome sequencing to identify other rare functional DNA variants causing LOAD, perhaps with high penetrance as we have observed for the novel LOAD mutations in *ADAM10*.

CONCLUSIONS

Over the past three decades, the identification and characterization of the AD genes have elucidated the etiology and pathogenesis of AD. Studies of these genes have also provided valuable clues regarding treatment and prevention of AD (reviewed in Bertram and Tanzi, 2010; Tanzi and Bertram, 2005). Following the initial discovery of the first four established AD genes, *APP, PSEN1, PSEN2,* and *APOE*, AD GWAS aimed at identifying additional AD genes (reviewed in Bertram et al., 2009, 2010) have introduced a new era of AD genetics. However, the new LOAD genes coming out of GWAS carry SNPs that generally have only small effect sizes. It is almost certain that in most, if not all cases, these SNPs are not the functional variants affecting risk for AD. Fortunately, the development of powerful sequencing technologies such as whole genome sequencing should allow us to identify the actual functional variants in the

novel AD genes emerging from GWAS, as well as in the original AD genes. The eventual elucidation of the actual functional variants in these genes (as we have found in *ADAM10*) will allow for more meaningful biological and translational studies as well as novel animal models for AD. In this way, genetic studies of AD will continue to inform and guide new treatment strategies for preventing and treating this terrible disease.

DISCLOSURES

Dr. Tanzi serves as a consultant to Prana Biotechnology. Eisai, Genomind, Probio Drug, Abide, and EcoEos. He also has a financial interest in Prana Biotechnology, Neurogenetic Pharmaceuticals, Evolutionary Genomics, Neuroptix, Abide, and Genomind.

REFERENCES

Bertram, L., and Tanzi, R.E. (2005). The genetic epidemiology of neurodegenerative disease. *J. Clin. Invest.* 115(6):1449–1457.

Bertram, L., and Tanzi, R.E. (2008). Thirty years of Alzheimer's disease genetics: systematic meta-analyses herald a new era. *Nat. Rev. Neurosci.* 9:768–778.

Bertram, L., and Tanzi, R.E. (2009). Genome-wide association studies in Alzheimer's disease. *Hum. Mol. Genet.* 18(R2):R137–R145.

Bertram, L., Lange, C., et al. (2008). Genome-wide association analysis reveals putative Alzheimer's disease susceptibility loci in addition to APOE. *Am. J. Hum. Genet.* 83(5):623–632.

Bertram, L., Lill, C.M., et al. (2010). The genetics of Alzheimer disease: back to the future. *Neuron* 68(2):270–281.

Bertram, L., McQueen, M.B., et al. (2007). Systematic meta-analyses of Alzheimer disease genetic association studies: the AlzGene database. *Nat. Genet.* 39(1):17–23.

Corder, E.H., Saunders, A.M., et al. (1994). Protective effect of apolipoprotein E type 2 allele for late onset Alzheimer disease. *Nat. Genet.* 7:180–184.

Crocker, P.R., Paulson, J.C., et al. (2007). Siglecs and their roles in the immune system. *Nat. Rev. Immunol.* 7(4):255–266.

DeMattos, R.B., Cirrito, J.R., et al. (2004). ApoE and clusterin cooperatively suppress Abeta levels and deposition: evidence that ApoE regulates extracellular Abeta metabolism *in vivo. Neuron* 41:193–202.

Gatz, M., Reynolds, C.A., et al. (2006). Role of genes and environments for explaining Alzheimer disease. *Arch. Gen. Psychiat.* 63:168–174.

Glenner, G.G., and Wong, C.W. (1984). Alzheimer's disease and Down's syndrome: sharing of a unique cerebrovascular amyloid fibril protein. *Biochem Biophys. Res. Comm.* 122:1131–1135.

Goate, A., Chartier-Harlin, M.C., et al. (1991). Segregation of a missense mutation in the amyloid precursor protein gene with familial Alzheimer's disease. *Nature* 349(6311):704–706.

Goldgaber, D., Lerman, M.I., et al. (1987). Characterization and chromosomal localization of a cDNA encoding brain amyloid of Alzheimer's disease. *Science* 235:877–880.

Hardy, J.A., and Higgins, G.A. (1992). Alzheimer's disease: the amyloid cascade hypothesis. *Science* 256:184–185.

Hardy, J., and Selkoe, D.J. (2002). The amyloid hypothesis of Alzheimer's disease: progress and problems on the road to therapeutics. *Science* 297:353–356.

Harold, D., Abraham, R., et al. (2009). Genome-wide association study identifies variants at CLU and PICALM associated with Alzheimer's disease. *Nat. Genet.* 41(10):1088–1093.

Hollingworth, P., Harold, D., et al. (2011). Common variants at ABCA7, MS4A6A/MS4A4E, EPHA1, CD33 and CD2AP are associated with Alzheimer's disease. *Nat. Genet.* 43(5):429–435.

Hooli, B.V., Mohapatra, G., et al. (2012). Role of common and rare APP DNA sequence variants in Alzheimer disease. *Neurology* 78(16):1250–1257.

Jarrett, J.T., Berger, E.P., et al. (1993). The carboxy terminus of the beta amyloid protein is critical for the seeding of amyloid formation: implications for the pathogenesis of Alzheimer's disease. *Biochemistry* 32:4693–4697.

Kang, J., Lemaire, H.G., et al. (1987). The precursor of Alzheimer's disease amyloid A4 protein resembles a cell-surface receptor. *Nature* 325:733–736.

Khera, R., and Das, N. (2009). Complement Receptor 1: disease associations and therapeutic implications. *Mol. Immunol.* 46(5):761–772.

Kim, J., Castellano, J.M., et al. (2009). Overexpression of low-density lipoprotein receptor in the brain markedly inhibits amyloid deposition and increases extracellular A beta clearance. *Neuron* 64(5):632–644.

Kim, M., Suh, J., et al. (2009). Potential late-onset Alzheimer's disease-associated mutations in the ADAM10 gene attenuate α-secretase activity. *Hum Mol Genet.* 18(20):3987–3996.

Kounnas, M.Z., Danks, A.M., et al. (2010). Modulation of γ-secretase reduces β-amyloid deposition in a transgenic mouse model of Alzheimer's disease. *Neuron* 67(5):769–780.

Lambert, J., Heath, S., et al. (2009). Genome-wide association study identifies variants at CLU and CR1 associated with Alzheimer's disease. *Nat. Genet.* 41(10):1094–1099.

Levy, E., Carman, M.D., et al. (1990). Mutation of the Alzheimer's disease amyloid gene in hereditary cerebral hemorrhage, Dutch type. *Science* 248:1124–1126.

Levy-Lahad, E., Wasco, W., et al. (1995). Candidate gene for the chromosome 1 familial Alzheimer's disease locus. *Science* 269(5226):973–977.

Masters, C.L., Simms, G., et al. (1985). Amyloid plaque core protein in Alzheimer disease and Down syndrome. *Proc. Natl. Acad. Sci. USA* 82:4245–4249.

Naj, A.C., Jun, G., et al. (2011). Common variants at MS4A4/MS4A6E, CD2AP, CD33 and EPHA1 are associated with late-onset Alzheimer's disease. *Nat. Genet.* 43(5):436–441.

Nizzari, M., Venezia, V., et al. (2007). Amyloid precursor protein and Presenilin1 interact with the adaptor GRB2 and modulate ERK 1,2 signaling. *J. Biol. Chem.* 282(18):13833–13844.

Nuutinen, T., Suuronen, T., et al. (2009). Clusterin: a forgotten player in Alzheimer's disease. *Brain. Res. Rev.* 61(2):89–104.

Pant, S., Sharma, M., et al. (2009). AMPH-1/Amphiphysin/Bin1 functions with RME-1/Ehd1 in endocytic recycling. *Nat. Cell Biol.* 11(12):1399–1410.

Reiman, E.M., Webster, J.A., et al. (2007). GAB2 alleles modify Alzheimer's risk in APOE epsilon4 carriers. *Neuron* 54(5):713–720.

Rogaev, E.I., Sherrington, R., et al. (1995). Familial Alzheimer's disease in kindreds with missense mutations in a gene on chromosome 1 related to the Alzheimer's disease type 3 gene. *Nature* 376(6543):775–778.

Roses, A.D., Lutz, M.W., et al. (2010). A TOMM40 variable-length polymorphism predicts the age of late-onset Alzheimer's disease. *Pharmacogenomics J.* 10:375–384.

Scheuner, D., Eckman, C., et al. (1996). Secreted amyloid beta-protein similar to that in the senile plaques of Alzheimer's disease is increased *in vivo* by the presenilin 1 and 2 and APP mutations linked to familial Alzheimer's disease. *Nat. Med.* 2:864–870.

Seshadri, S., Fitzpatrick, A.L., et al. (2010). Genome-wide analysis of genetic loci associated with Alzheimer disease. *JAMA* 303(18):1832–1840.

Sherrington, R., Rogaev, E.I., et al. (1995). Cloning of a gene bearing missense mutations in early-onset familial Alzheimer's disease. *Nature* 375(6534):754–760.

Soscia, S.J., Kirby, J.E., et al. (2010). The Alzheimer's disease-associated amyloid beta-protein is an antimicrobial peptide. *PLoS ONE* 5(3):e9505.

St George-Hyslop, P.H., Tanzi, R.E., et al. (1987). The genetic defect causing familial Alzheimer's disease maps on Chromosome 21. *Science* 235:885–890.

Strittmatter, W.J., Saunders, A.M., et al. (1993). Apolipoprotein E: high-avidity binding to beta-amyloid and increased frequency of type 4 allele in late-onset familial Alzheimer disease. *Proc. Natl. Acad. Sci. USA* 90(5):1977–1981.

Tanzi, R.E., Gusella, J.F., et al. (1987a). Amyloid beta protein gene: cDNA, mRNA distribution, and genetic linkage near the Alzheimer locus. *Science* 235(4791):880–884.

Tanzi, R.E., St George-Hyslop, P.H., et al. (1987b). The genetic defect in familial Alzheimer's disease is not tightly linked to the amyloid beta protein gene. *Nature* 329:156–157.

Tanzi, R.E., Haines, J.L., et al. (1988a). Genetic linkage map of human chromosome 21. *Genomics* 3:129–136.

Tanzi, R.E., McClatchey, A.I., et al. (1988b). Protease inhibitor domain encoded by an amyloid protein precursor mRNA associated with Alzheimer's disease. *Nature* 331:528–530.

Tanzi, R.E., Vaula, G., et al. (1992). Assessment of β-amyloid protein precursor gene mutations in a large set of familial and sporadic Alzheimer disease cases. *Am. J. Hum. Genet.* 51:273–282.

Tanzi, R.E., and Bertram, L. (2005). Twenty years of the Alzheimer's disease amyloid hypothesis: a genetic perspective. *Cell* 120(4):545–555.

Tebar, F., Bohlander, S.K., et al. (1999). Clathrin assembly lymphoid myeloid leukemia (CALM) protein: localization in endocytic-coated pits, interactions with clathrin, and the impact of overexpression on clathrin-mediated traffic. *Mol. Biol. Cell* 10(8):2687–2702.

Treusch, S., Hamamichi, S., et al. (2011). Functional links between Aβ toxicity, endocytic trafficking, and Alzheimer's disease risk factors in yeast. *Science* 334(6060):1241–1245.

Van Broeckhoven, C., Genthe, A.M., et al. (1987). Failure of familial Alzheimer's disease to segregate with the A4-amyloid gene in several European families. *Nature* 329:153–155.

Zhang, C., Browne, A., et al. (2010). Loss of function of ATXN1 increases amyloid beta-protein levels by potentiating beta-secretase processing of beta-amyloid precursor protein. *J. Biol. Chem.* 285(12):8515–8526.

61 | EXPERIMENTAL ANIMAL MODELS OF ALZHEIMER'S DISEASE

DAVE MORGAN

This meta-review will summarize the history and current state of the science in the use of animals to glean insights into the causes and to assist in identifying meaningful treatments for Alzheimer's disease (AD). As such it will refer readers to more detailed reviews on specific topics as needed and not to the original works to any great extent. Moreover this review will focus on experimental models of Alzheimer's disease that are based on the pathology of that disease and not merely the symptoms (e.g., memory loss).

PURPOSE OF ANIMAL MODELS

For virtually every known human malady there have been attempts to understand the disease better using systems that can be manipulated either more conveniently, more precisely, or more ethically than similar manipulations in human subjects. There are two primary goals of the animal models. The first is to provide a platform in which to study the basic mechanisms underlying the disease. This more detailed understanding can occur at molecular, cellular, tissue, organs, or systems level within the organism. Rarely do the models mimic all aspects of the human disorder. This is particularly true for AD. However, because of our capacity to manipulate the animal models, we can test hypotheses regarding the causes and processes generating the disorder.

A second rationale for animal models is to use them to identify treatments, often pharmacological, to consider for evaluation in the human disease. Importantly, these two roles do not require the same types of models. For example drugs designed to have symptomatic benefit may be tested quite readily in models that have the same physiological changes as the disorder in question, irrespective of how those changes developed. Streptozocin induced diabetes is one example. This toxin is not a pathogenic mechanism normally causing the disease in man, yet can create a model to evaluate certain types of drugs intended to benefit diabetics.

In the field of Parkinson disease the use of animal models reflecting the pathology of the disease has been a mainstay of investigations since the 1960s. The 6-hydroxydopamine lesion model mimics the dopaminergic deficit that is found in Parkinson disease. This has facilitated the development of the number of dopamine enhancing medications and surgical interventions (cells, electrical stimulation, lesions) that have proven beneficial in the treatment of Parkinson disease. In the 1980s the MPTP model was developed as a possible explanation of the pathogenic mechanisms involved in Parkinson disease. This model also has permitted the development of medications of benefit in treating Parkinson. However more recently the identification that synuclein is a key component in the pathophysiology of Parkinson disease has led to the conclusion that the MPTP model probably only is mechanistically valid for the few individuals inadvertently exposed to this toxin. Instead it is now the case that a number of new models based on the rare genetic causes of parkinsonism are providing a valuable adjunct to the symptomatic models. The hope is these new models may be recapitulating some of the pathogenic mechanisms of the sporadic disease.

ANIMAL MODELS OF ALZHEIMER'S DEMENTIA BASED ON THE CHOLINERGIC HYPOTHESIS

In the middle 1970s two groups of British neurochemists led by David Bowen and Peter Davies independently identified a decrease in markers of the cholinergic system in Alzheimer's disease (AD) postmortem tissue. Importantly, the brain regions that were most affected by AD were the regions of the neocortex and the perirhinal area including the hippocampus (Mesulam, 2004). Other regions of the brain such as the striatum and the thalamus were relatively unaffected in AD patients compared to age-matched controls. This was the first indication that the cholinergic system played a role in the symptoms of Alzheimer's disease analogous, in some ways, to the role of the dopaminergic system in Parkinson disease. These neurochemical observations were followed shortly by anatomical measurements within the forebrain nuclei known to contain the cholinergic neurons. These include the nucleus basalis magnocellularis, the medial septum, and the diagonal band of Broca. These cholinergic nuclei are the regions known to project to the neocortex and the perirhinal regions including the hippocampus.

There is a large and extensive literature relating the acetylcholine system in the central nervous system to learning and memory function. In the 1970s David Drachman and his collaborators demonstrated that cholinergic antagonists such as scopolamine were capable of decreasing learning and memory performance in rats (Hasselmo, 2006). One important control used by this group was to test methylscopalamine and demonstrate that there were no learning and memory performance deficits caused by this drug. Methylscopolamine fails to cross the blood-brain barrier. Thus it has all of the autonomic nervous system effects that scopolamine has, yet lacks central cholinergic blockade. These groups also reported that the effects of scopolamine could be reversed by coadministration of cholinergic agonists such as carbachol or cholinesterase inhibitors. More recent work has shown that selective muscarinic antagonists, selective nicotinic antagonists, and drugs that block choline uptake into the nerve terminal also can impair learning and memory function in animals. Another important feature of anticholinergic drugs is that the memory deficits observed are qualitatively similar to those that are observed with AD. That is, the drugs tend to disrupt the acquisition of new information while sparing the recollection of previously learned information. This is similar to early-stage Alzheimer patients who show impairment of short term or working forms of memory yet have intact recollection of events that occurred many years prior to the onset of their memory deficits. Moreover, there is a correlation between the degree of cholinergic marker reduction and cognitive dysfunction in Alzheimer patients at autopsy (Mesulam, 2004).

Consistent with the psychopharmacology studies, lesions of the cholinergic neurons in the basal forebrain generally lead to impairments of learning and memory functions. Cholinergic neuron lesions have been achieved by electrocoagulation, excitotoxin injections, fimbria-fornix transections, and more selective cholinergic lesions using 192-IgG saponin (Casamenti et al., 1998; Yamada and Nabeshima, 2000). This latter agent is a conjugate of an immunoglobulin and a toxin. The antibody binds the p75 nerve growth factor receptor that exists largely on cholinergic neurons. The saponin is internalized and released to cause the death of the cholinergic neurons in the basal forebrain. These lesions cause memory deficits that can be reversed by cholinomimetic drugs or treatments that promote cholinergic neuron survival such as nerve growth factor (Yamada and Nabeshima, 2000). Somewhat surprisingly, the more selective the lesion is for the cholinergic neurons within these basal forebrain nuclei the less impact this has on learning and memory function in the rats or other animals in which these lesions are performed. Instead it appears that the major impact of these cholinergic selective lesions is on attentional processes rather than learning and memory per se (Blokland, 1995). It should be noted that sufficient attention is essential for the acquisition of new information and this may underlie a large component of the deficits observed both in the animal models as well as in Alzheimer patients when testing learning and memory performance.

The evidence provided by the pharmacology experiments combined with the results observed in the lesion studies led to the *cholinergic hypothesis* of the memory dysfunction in AD. In the early 1980s this was proposed most clearly by Ray Bartus, arguing that the cholinergic model of geriatric memory dysfunction would provide a convenient system in which to identify drugs that could later be used to treat Alzheimer's disease.

Based largely on the evidence detailed in the preceding, the first cholinesterase inhibitor was tested in human Alzheimer patients by Summers. This initial drug, Tacrine, showed a modest cognitive benefit but was approved as the first available agent to treat AD. However, liver toxicity in a substantial number of patients has led to it being replaced by newer agents. The second-generation cholinesterase inhibitors, donepezil, rivastigmine, and galantamine have become the primary approach to treating Alzheimer's disease. Although these drugs have frustratingly modest impact on disease symptoms, unlike the dopaminergic drugs in Parkinson, they do provide some benefit and have been argued to delay institutionalization by up to two years. There also remain opportunities to improve the use of these medications using a personalized medicine approach to identify those individuals who will respond to each cholinesterase inhibitor optimally. This is based on the observation that although only one-third of patients respond to the first cholinesterase inhibitor they are administered, approximately one-half of those non-responders will respond to one of the other cholinesterase inhibitors that are available (Auriacombe et al., 2002).

AMYLOID INJECTION MODELS

Early studies on cultured primary neurons found that incubation with Aβ could kill these cultured cells at μM concentrations. This rapidly led to attempts in the early 1990s to generate a model of Aβ neurotoxicity *in vivo* by injecting Aβ into the brain. The first attempts had very mixed results (Harkany et al., 1999; Yamada and Nabeshima, 2000). Several groups reported some apparent toxicity and occasional neuron loss, whereas others reported only minimal effects. Some of these early studies examined the effects of Aβ25–35 peptide or Aβ1–40. This was largely because of the early challenges in synthesizing the 1–42 peptide, and the greater costs of the longer synthetic peptides. Aβ25–35 was a low cost means of rapidly generating amyloid fibrils, although it is not found *in vivo* at meaningful concentrations. Nonetheless, parsing the studies on the basis of the Aβ sequence does not resolve the diverse outcomes. One suggestion was that effects of Aβ25–35 were only transient, compared with Aβ1–42 (Harkany et al., 1999). Another general observation was that infusions of Aβ using osmotic pumps generally caused larger effects that endured longer than acute bolus injections (Harkany et al., 1999). Our own work in this area identified that the heparan sulfate proteoglycan, perlecan, promoted the formation of Aβ-congophilic deposits when infused into the hippocampus of young rats. This was associated with dramatic activation of astrocytes and microglia. However, after several years of experience in evaluating this preparation, we finally concluded that these deposits did not cause significant neurotoxicity (Holcomb et al., 2000). Parallel, but unpublished work concluded the same for combinations of Aβ with apolipoprotein E or alpha-1 antichymotrypsin. Instead, these infusions resulted in large congophilic aggregates (several hundred μm), which would then gradually be cleared by microglia leaving a vacuole at the site of the infusion.

In studies that did report an impact of intracranial Aβ, the most common observations were memory deficits in mice or rats. The groups led by Giancarlo Pepeu and Tibor Harkany found that the most sensitive neurons to the toxicity of infused Aβ were the cholinergic neurons (Chambon et al., 2011). Reasonably consistent declines in rat cholinergic markers in cerebral cortex and hippocampus were found following either direct injections into cholinergic nuclei or infusions into the ventricles. Some studies also found that ventricular infusions of Aβ peptides *in vivo* would lead to defective long-term potentiation in ex vivo slices from these mice (Yamada and Nabeshima, 2000). Finally, the age of the organism appears to be a meaningful consideration. Bruce Yankner's group found that of aged rats, aged rhesus, and young rhesus, only the aged rhesus monkeys demonstrated neuronal loss after injections of fibrillar (but not soluble) Aβ into the cortex (Geula et al., 1998).

The introduction of the transgenic mouse models in the mid-1990s, coupled with frustrations in identifying a consistent means of producing toxicity with Aβ application, led many to abandon these direct injection approaches. Although the precise reasons for the inconsistency between and often within a research team are not resolved, Pat May and others commented on the lot to lot inconsistency for most synthetic Aβ preparations (Yamada and Nabeshima, 2000). Moreover, we are now increasingly aware that there are different aggregations states of Aβ, with the intermediate sized aggregates, oligomers, likely being more toxic to neurons than the monomers or the fibrils. As indicated in Table 61.1, there are some distinct advantages of the direct administration approach. Given the advances in peptide synthesis, and availability of recombinant peptides, some of the lot to lot variability plaguing early studies may be avoided. Moreover, we now have reasonably well characterized means of producing stable aggregated forms of Aβ intermediates that may produce more reliable impacts on neuronal activity. Certainly, for drug targets designed to interfere with events downstream of Aβ action, the intracranial injections may be more useful screening systems than transgenic mice.

TRANSGENIC MOUSE MODELS OF AMYLOIDOGENESIS

AMYLOID PRECURSOR PROTEIN TRANSGENIC MICE

Probably the most studied models relevant to Alzheimer's disease are those which overproduce the Aβ peptide. These mice derive from oocyte injection of a construct containing multiple copies of the human amyloid precursor protein (APP) gene (often as concatemers). Overexpression of human APP leads to overproduction of Aβ via the processing of the APP protein. The excess Aβ leads to a variety of changes, some of which are consistent with observations in AD. These models have proven very useful in (1) understanding the mechanisms leading to the production and clearance of the Aβ peptide *in vivo* and (2) screening agents suggested as potential amyloid lowering therapeutics.

George Glenner's publication of the amino acid sequence of vascular amyloid led within a year to the identification by four independent groups that the sequence was contained within the APP gene. This launched a number of campaigns to produce transgenic mice overexpressing this protein in hopes of creating a mouse model of AD. The seminal observation by John Hardy and Alison Goate that mutations in APP could lead to familial Alzheimer's disease provided further impetus to this effort, and suggested modifications that could increase the likelihood of success.

However, obtaining a successful mouse model proved exceedingly challenging. Some early approaches employed constructs directly expressing the Aβ sequence. One of these was first described in a paper in *Science*. These mice had low levels of transgene expression, but as they aged developed some punctate staining seen with anti-Aβ antisera, which were interpreted as amyloid deposits. However, neuropathologists noted these did not resemble amyloid plaques in AD, but instead appeared to be artifacts typically observed in the C57BL6 mice (used as background strain) as they aged (Greenberg et al., 1996). Additional scrutiny revealed the control mice for the published study were considerably younger than the transgenic mice. Subsequent work revealed that the non-transgenic mice of this background also developed these histological artifacts. This paper was later retracted.

Another approach was to express the C terminal 100 amino acids of the APP sequence. This essentially provided a peptide that has the N terminus produced by the beta secretase cleavage. Subsequent processing by gamma secretase would result in release of the Aβ peptide. A paper was published in *Nature* that presented micrographs that recapitulated all of the histological changes found in AD: amyloid plaques and neurofibrillary tangles. However, shortly after publication, neuropathologists noticed that the micrographs shown were not from mouse brain, but appeared to be AD brain tissue. Subsequent evaluation of

TABLE 61.1. Advantages and disadvantages of direct Aβ administration models

ADVANTAGES	DISADVANTAGES
• Can examine multiple species • Studies can be conducted rapidly with minimal colony maintenance expense • Have known time when toxicity initiates. Can measure time course to determine if there is spontaneous recovery or permanent damage • Can use different variants of Aβ • Can measure the physical state of the administered material (monomer, oligomer, fibril) • Can control dose • Can evaluate the effects of host age	• Doses used are likely in excess of those found *in vivo* • Requires surgical intervention/anesthesia • Injected material can be cleared quickly • Aβ will form a concentration gradient from the site of administration (nonuniform dose) • Aβ largely extrasynaptic as opposed to synaptically released *in vivo* • Problems with consistency of lots/preparations of Aβ

the sections by Don Price revealed they were indeed human in origin, and the paper was retracted (Greenberg et al., 1996). This series of events led one of the coauthors, Gerry Higgins, a coauthor of the original amyloid cascade hypothesis manuscript with John Hardy, to stop working in the Alzheimer field. As a personal anecdote, the author of this chapter recalls a casual conversation with Dr Higgins about this mouse shortly after publication. His enthusiasm for its use as a model and willingness to share it suggests he was unaware that the data published in *Nature* were not genuinely from the transgenic mice he had collected.

Another early mouse used full length APP with a neuron-specific enolase promoter. These mice, developed at the biotechnology firm Scios-Nova, expressed some Aβ, but the histology did not resemble the amyloid deposits found in the AD brain. The author of this chapter recalls having to be "educated" regarding what a plaque was on tissue sections we had stained with anti-Aβ antisera in tissue from these mice. It was a faint cloud of staining which might easily be taken as artifact. Nonetheless, these mice did exhibit memory deficits, a point of relevance to be discussed later. There are a number of other transgenic mice that were reported in the early 1990s that were attempts to model the amyloid pathology of AD, but none of these produced the plaque pathology found in the postmortem AD tissue. These are summarized nicely in Greenberg et al. (1996). There were probably thousands more oocytes injected and progeny born without phenotypes that were never reported in publications.

The first mouse to demonstrate amyloid deposition that resembled that found in AD was reported by Games et al. (1995). These mice used a minigene construct to produce multiply spliced forms of APP and the platelet derived growth factor promoter (which, in spite of its name, drives high expression in neurons). The APP sequence included the Indiana mutation near the gamma secretase site, which increased the production of Aβ ending at residue 42 relative to residue 40. These mice produced APP at almost ten-fold excess over endogenous levels. These mice also developed both diffuse and compact fibrillar amyloid deposits as they aged. Furthermore, there was a characteristic activation of microglial cells near the compacted deposits and activation of astrocytes surrounding the deposits. They also induced dystrophic neurite formation near the compacted plaques, all of which were similar to the pathology found in AD. This so called "PDAPP" mouse has been used extensively by Athena/Elan, Lilly, and their collaborators for evaluating potential treatments for AD. An interesting back story on this mouse, to this author's understanding, is that it was originally generated at a small biotech in Worcester, Massachusetts called Exemplar by Sam Wadsworth and colleagues. Shortly after the production of the line, the company's deteriorating finances led to attempts to license the mouse, but they did not yet have any histopathology demonstrating their success. Given the history of APP transgenics up to that time, a number of companies offered the opportunity refused to license or purchase the mouse until Athena neuroscience (now Elan) obtained the line. Another important component of this episode is that before the paper was published in *Nature*, histological sections were sent to Don Price, a neuropathologist who played a role in debunking the two earlier transgenic mouse claims that were retracted. His verification that these amyloid deposits were authentic was crucial to the acceptance of the conclusions.

Shortly after the publication of the Games et al., 1995 paper, additional transgenic models came to light that had remarkably similar forms of amyloid pathology. The mouse described by Karen Hsiao (now Karen Hsiao Ashe) and her group expressed APP with a Swedish mutation under the control of the prion promoter (Hsiao et al., 1996). The Swedish mutation increases beta secretase cleavage, increasing both C terminal length variants of Aβ. This mouse also deposited both diffuse and compacted amyloid, but most importantly, also demonstrated impaired learning and memory. Dr. Ashe has been exceedingly generous in making these mice available for academic research, and through licensing via the Mayo clinic, for pharmaceutical company research, even as she has weathered legal challenges. At this time they are probably the most frequently investigated model of amyloid deposition (Elder et al., 2010).

A report on a third mouse was published in 1997 (Sturchler-Pierrat et al., 1997) that used an APP construct with a Swedish mutation driven by the Thy-1 promoter. This mouse has been largely used extensively by Novartis and their collaborators. A fourth mouse model from David Borchelt used a construct very similar to that used by Karen Ashe (Borchelt et al., 1996). Although it is certainly the case that one can find differences among these different models, they all share some striking features. First, they all have both diffuse and compact fibrillar amyloid (although the ratios vary, discussed later). They all have a strong microglial reaction within the plaque core for the compacted deposits (but not the diffuse). They all have astrocytic activation in the periphery of the compacted deposits. They all have dystrophic neurites that stain for many of the same markers as dystrophic neurites in AD (including phospho-tau, although they do not have paired helical filaments of tau). Also somewhat surprising is they all, at least initially, deposit amyloid in those regions most associated with pathology in AD; the hippocampus and the neocortex. Again, the relative distributions may be different, but they do not show compacted deposits in cerebellum or brainstem until the animals age considerably. Interestingly, another mouse with the Thy-1 promoter that expresses only Aβ with a truncation at amino acid 3 (glutamine; p3E Aβ; TBA2 mouse) initially produces pathology in the cerebellum, rather than forebrain (Crews et al., 2010). This would imply that it is not the promoter, but the processing of APP that directs the initial forebrain pathology in these models.

Some other useful mice soon followed. The TgCRND8 mouse from Peter St George-Hyslop's group is a very aggressive model. This mouse carries the Swedish and Indiana mutations driven by the prion promoter. These mice develop plaques by 3 months of age and have a 50% lethality by 12 months (Balducci and Forloni, 2011; Kobayashi and Chen, 2005). A pair of mice generated by Lennart Mucke's group, called J9 and J20, also have some useful properties. These two lines share the same construct, a combined Swedish and Indiana mutant driven by the PDGF promoter. These two lines vary considerably in expression and one can be used to study the phenotypes associated with low expression (and delayed onset of deposition) and the other to study the phenotype of an aggressively depositing mouse model. Although a number of reviewers believe that the promoter is important in the differences among different lines, there are many other factors influencing expression. These include insertion site and copy number. In our own work with the Tg2576 line, we encountered a sudden appearance of mice in studies that had little amyloid deposition relative to the other mice in the same experimental group. This was outside the range of variability over the prior five years. Fortunately, we had information on transgene copy number collected at genotyping and necropsy and were able to determine that all these mice with reduced phenotype had reduced copy number. Through our genealogy records for the colony, we were able to trace this back to a single male mouse who was, unfortunately, exceptionally fertile. We then walked forward and culled all mice derived from this sire to minimize the influence of this low copy number on the variance in the colony phenotype.

In some lines, the first deposits are stained by Thioflavin S or Congo red, have dystrophic neurites and activated glial in their vicinity. Later these mice develop the less intensely stained diffuse deposits. These lines include the PDAPP and Tg2576 lines (Bloom et al., 2005; Gordon et al., 2002). Conversely, there are some lines such as the J20, that develop the diffuse deposits first, then later establish the compacted plaques (Kobayashi and Chen, 2005). The diffuse deposits stain with anti-Aβ antisera but not Thioflavin S and Congo red. They also lack the reactive glial cells. In some lines (Tg2576), there are some brain regions that only develop diffuse deposits (striatum). Additionally, many of the mice also develop cerebral amyloid angiopathy. These deposits are along the arterioles and arteries penetrating the parenchyma of the neocortex from the meninges. These deposits follow the ring-like contours of smooth muscle around the arterioles and can be stained by Congo red and Thioflavin S (Duyckaerts et al., 2008).

The C terminus of Aβ ends predominantly at amino acid 40 and, to a lesser extent, 42. The longer form of Aβ has a greater propensity to form aggregates *in vitro* (Greenberg et al., 1996). When antisera specific for Aβ40 or Aβ42 are used to stain brain sections from transgenic lines, the diffuse deposits are labeled exclusively by Aβ42 and not Aβ40. The compacted deposits are stained by both Aβ40 and Aβ42 specific antibodies, whereas the cerebral amyloid angiopathy stains almost exclusively with the Aβ40 antisera. This pattern is very similar to that in Alzheimer cases at autopsy (Duyckaerts et al., 2008).

Different mutations affect the ratio of Aβ42/40. Most mutations in the C terminus of Aβ (London, Indiana) bias the gamma secretase cleavage towards the long form of the Aβ peptide. As such they alter the ratio without altering the total amount of Aβ produced. The N terminal Swedish double mutation increases beta secretase cleavage relative to alpha secretase. This leads to increases in both Aβ40 and Aβ42, with no change in the ratio in newborn mice. This can modify the subsequent extent of Aβ deposition into the various compartments of the brain. For example, the PDAPP mouse, which only carries the Indiana mutation, at maturity, has a large amount of diffuse deposits, but relatively few compacted deposits (Bloom et al., 2005). Further

there is very little amyloid angiopathy in this mouse. The Tg2576 mouse, which only expresses the Swedish mutation, has a large compacted plaque load relative to diffuse, and develops amyloid angiopathy. The APP23 mouse, which carries the Swedish mutation also has a very large number of compacted plaques and severe amyloid angiopathy, often with spontaneous cerebrovascular hemorrhage (Hock and Lamb, 2001).

One mutation of APP in the mid-domain region, known as the Dutch mutation, causes hereditary cerebral amyloidosis with hemorrhage characterized by severe cerebral amyloid angiopathy. This mutation does not alter amyloid processing, but appears to have a higher rate of fibril formation and possibly reduced clearance rates relative to wild type Aβ. Mice generated by Mathias Jucker's group carrying this mutation driven by the Thy1 promoter develop primarily amyloid angiopathy, presumably owing to the preserved ratio of Aβ42/40, replicating the human disease (Balducci and Forloni, 2011). However, when crossed with a mouse containing a mutation in presenilin 1 (PS1), which increased the amount of Aβ42, these mice now deposited amyloid in compacted and diffuse deposits; therefore, one can argue it is the 40/42 ratio, not the Dutch mutation leading to the excess vascular pathology in these mice (relative to parenchymal) (McGowan et al., 2006).

In order to address the question of the relative importance of Aβ40 versus Aβ42 in amyloid deposition, Mike Hutton and Todd Golde's group developed two mouse lines using the BRI fusion proteins which only overproduced 40 or 42. The BRI construct is cleaved after synthesis to release the Aβ molecule, so one caveat is this peptide is not generated through normal APP processing. The mice overproducing Aβ42 developed deposits in all three loci; compacted, diffuse and vascular. The mice overproducing Aβ40 developed no deposits. This argues that all forms of deposition still require Aβ42 to seed the formation of fibrils found in compacted and vascular amyloid. Interestingly, when the BRI-40 and BRI-42 mice are crossed, the expression of Aβ40 in the crossed mice reduces the overall amount of pathology seen in the BRI-42 mouse line, arguing that Aβ40 can inhibit fibril formation to some extent (Elder et al., 2010).

The great majority of mouse lines modeling amyloidogenesis have found it necessary to have considerable APP overexpression (greater than fivefold over endogenous). This has been achieved by insertion of multiple copies of the transgenes (concatamers) and use of heterologous promoters to drive high levels of expression. However, these promoters do not mimic the spatial and temporal pattern of expression of endogenous APP. Two models have been developed to avoid the heterologous promoter issue. One is the production of a yeast artificial chromosome mouse containing the entire 300 kb human APP gene. The wild type version of this mouse produced human APP but failed to result in deposition. However, introduction of the Swedish mutation produced the R1–40 mouse line, which does develop many of the same deposits as the cDNA or minigene based transgenics. These mice have the advantage of proper APP cellular, regional and developmental regulation of expression and RNA splicing, permitting the same mRNA variants as found in the human brain (Hock and Lamb, 2001). These mice also develop memory deficits as they age.

Another approach at generating amyloid depositing mice has used gene targeting technology to knock-in the human Aβ sequence with a Swedish mutation into the mouse APP gene. Alone, this APP knock-in model does not result in amyloid deposits, but when crossed with a mouse containing a knocked-in PS1 mutation, these mice develop robust plaque pathology (Hock and Lamb, 2001). These mice were developed at Cephalon, and have not been widely disseminated. However, the absence of APP over expression and the appropriate regulation of the modified gene provide important information and reduce the caveats associated with transgenic models in exploring the regulation of APP and PS1 expression by AD-like pathology (Crews et al., 2010).

AMYLOID PRECURSOR PROTEIN TRANSGENIC LINES CROSSED WITH OTHER LINES

In October of 1996, Karen Ashe published her paper in *Science* regarding the Tg2576 APP transgenic mouse line (Hsiao et al., 1996) and Karen Duff and John Hardy published their paper on a PS1 transgenic mouse line that overproduced mouse Aβ42, yet failed to develop amyloid deposits (Duff et al., 1996). Although most PS1 mutant mice have minimal phenotype (Kobayashi and Chen, 2005), there are reports of increased sensitivity to neurotoxic insults (Elder et al., 2010). Within a month of these two publications, Dr. Ashe had shared her mouse with Hardy and Duff at the University of South Florida (USF) and a cross between these mice was initiated. Before the first progeny were mature, Dr. Hardy was recruited to the Mayo Clinic in Jacksonville with Dr. Duff, yet the mice remained at USF. Our research team at USF then characterized these crossed APP+PS1 mice, and identified a considerable synergy of the combined mouse (termed by us as APP+PS1) with respect to amyloid deposition, with first deposits moved to three to four months of age from nine to eleven months in the APP only mice (Holcomb et al., 1998). A parallel observation was made by David Borchelt's group at Hopkins (Borchelt et al., 1997) with largely the same outcomes. These crosses demonstrated that the mutation in APP and the mutations in PS1 appeared to both be active through the processing of APP with the final common outcome the generation of more Aβ42. Interestingly, these crossed mice have been designated with a variety of arithmetic operators (APP-PS1; APP/PS1; APPxPS1; PSAPP) We remained convinced because the two transgenes are added together, not subtracted, divided or multiplied, that APP+PS1 is the appropriate designation, but recognize this convention is unlikely to hold sway. These doubly transgenic lines have also become widely disseminated through the Mayo Clinic and USF. The Borchelt group generously provided their mice to the Jackson Laboratories where they can be purchased commercially. The Tg2576 mouse is also now commercially available through Taconic. Of further interest is the fact that the widely used Swedish mutation was sequenced in Tampa in laboratories rented by USF. In a recent court decision, ownership of the Swedish mutation patent was transferred from the Alzheimer's Institute of America with Michael Mullan as sole inventor, to USF and the University of London, with John Hardy named as coinventor (this ruling is under appeal). Thus USF, although a minor player overall, has had significant impact in the area of mouse models for amyloid deposition.

Another informative cross was to breed the APP mice onto a BACE1 (beta secretase) null condition. By deleting the BACE1 gene, Aβ was not produced. Thus one could discern those aspects of the APP mouse phenotype which were due to Aβ deposition from those due to APP overexpression, or the presence of the mutation. The APPxBACE1$^{-/-}$ mice fail to develop amyloid deposits, as expected, and also fail to develop memory impairments. There are some effects of the BACE1 null condition, such as impaired myelination during development, but the general absence of phenotype implies that BACE1 inhibition could be relatively free of adverse events (PS1 null mice are embryonic lethal; Kobayashi and Chen, 2005). Conversely, crossing APP mice with a line overexpressing BACE1 leads to accelerated amyloid deposition (Kobayashi and Chen, 2005). Crossing an APP mouse line with mice overexpressing ADAM-10, an enzyme capable of alpha-secretase cleavage, leads to reduced amyloid pathology and diminished phenotype, presumably due to increased competition with endogenous BACE1 for APP substrate (Duyckaerts et al., 2008).

BEHAVIORAL CHANGES IN AMYLOID PRECURSOR PROTEIN TRANSGENIC MICE

The Tg2576 mouse was the first line to develop memory deficits associated with amyloid deposits similar to those in Alzheimer patients (Hsiao et al., 1996). The PDAPP mouse, develops an early atrophy of the hippocampus and corpus callosum prior to any amyloid deposits (Bloom et al., 2005), which made observation of amyloid-associated behavioral changes challenging, although ultimately these could be discerned on top of the developmental atrophy using a working memory approach (Chen et al., 2000). In our own research, the Tg2576 or APP+PS1 lines have been shown in multiple studies to have decreased performance on spatial navigation tasks that was correlated with the amount of amyloid deposition (mostly Congophilic plaques in cortex and or hippocampus; Gordon et al., 2001). Hence, this impairment of learning, often found in early stage Alzheimer cases, is an important component of the amyloid depositing mouse phenotype.

MORRIS WATER MAZE

The most common method of evaluating memory in APP mice has been the Morris water maze. This task involves use of a pool in which a hidden platform is submerged that mice are expected to find in order to escape the need to swim. The task takes place in a room with salient extramaze cues (probably the most critical one being the investigator) and the mouse is expected to use these extramaze cues to determine the location of the hidden platform. The task is performed with multiple trials per day (four consecutive trials are common) over multiple days (10 is common). At the end or on intermediate days, the mice are administered a "probe" trial, in which the platform is removed and the specificity with which the mouse attempts to find the platform in its prior location is measured. Typically, mice will decrease the time required to find the hidden platform with increased training (decreased latency) until reaching some minimum time (typically 10–15 seconds). One potential concern with the latency measure is that it can be confounded by swim speed of the mouse. To rule this out, distance traveled can also be measured with computerized equipment. A common measure of retention on the probe trial is percent of time spent swimming in the pool quadrant previously containing the probe. However, there are many other measures developed with computerized tracking equipment (e.g. platform crossings, learning index) that can be used to assess performance on the probe trial. One factor rarely mentioned is that the probe trial is really an extinction trial (no reward is administered). Some animals, not finding the platform where it previously was located, might logically decide to search elsewhere, yet this would be scored as failure to learn. Another problem with this task is that the mice are expected to apply a spatial hypothesis to solving the problem (which the vast majority do). However, some mice might instead learn to swim in a circle a certain distance from the edge of the pool and stumble upon the platform by chance. Although this works equally well for the mouse, it again is judged as failure to learn. Intriguingly, mice with hippocampal lesions, or blind mice, do reduce latency over trials on this task. However, they do poorly on the probe trials because they are not applying a spatial hypothesis to solving the problem.

OBJECT RECOGNITION

Another oft used task is the object recognition task. Advantages of this task are that it requires little specialized equipment (the Morris maze often uses computerized equipment to measure learning) and can be performed in a much shorter time than the Morris water maze task. This task involves placing the mouse into a new environment in which there are one or two objects within the environment. During the exploration of this novel environment the mouse will encounter and presumably learn about these objects. Sometime later (usually the same day, but sometimes 24 hours later) the mouse is reintroduced to the same novel environment but this time with one object being from the previous encounter and another object for which the mouse lacks prior exposure. The assumption is that the mouse wishes to seek novelty and will spend more time exploring the novel object than time spent exploring the previously encountered object. The ratio of time attending to novel versus old object is called the recognition index. Periods of exposure run from 60 to 300 seconds for these sessions in the novel environment. One problem with this approach is the assumption that the APP mouse seeks novelty to the same extent as non-APP mice. However, there are indications that APP mice develop neophobia (Duyckaerts et al., 2008). If the mice are scared of the novel object, they may not show increased attention toward it and be deemed memory deficient. However, the difference is really one of motivation. This confound can be easily addressed by an independent measure of neophobia. One such measure is to water deprive mice for 12 hours and administer two water bottles, one with standard water and the other with water sweetened with 0.1% saccharin. Noting the relative consumption from the two bottles over 60 minutes is an independent measure of neophobia (which in the form of bait shyness is a great asset to a mouse in the wild). If mice lack neophobia, yet demonstrate no preference for the new object, then one can more safely infer a true memory deficiency. A final comment from our experience: the amount of time mice spend attending to objects in total is relatively small (less than 20% of the time in the environment). Our work found that the difference between six seconds and eight seconds was often all that separated the APP and non-transgenic littermates in this task. As "attending to the object" is a very subjective measure, it is essential that the rater be blind to the identity of the mice being evaluated (preferably via videotape with multiple raters). Variants of this task include use of spatial location as the difference between the first and second exposures to the new environment (one object moves and the other remains in place) or use of other mice as the objects (social recognition). This latter task has a great deal of ethological validity, and mice do spend more time attending to other mice than they do to inanimate objects.

FEAR CONDITIONING

Another task often used to determine memory loss in APP mice is fear conditioning. This task has the advantage of being relatively rapid to perform (three five-minute sessions), but does require expensive equipment. In this task mice are introduced to a novel environment with a grid floor that can be electrified. After two minutes they are administered first a tone followed by a foot shock, Often this is repeated a second time within the same session. The environment has sensors that can detect if the mouse is "freezing" (not moving, a typical response to threat in a mouse). Usually the next day mice are once again introduced to the novel environment in which they were shocked the day before. Once again freezing is measured and mice that learned the task well are expected to freeze for the majority of the five-minute session, or at least during the first few minutes. This is called contextual fear conditioning. Typically the day after testing for context mice are placed in a completely different environment and administered the tone. Again, freezing is measured in response to this cue, referred to as cued conditioning. Lesion studies in rats have demonstrated that the contextual conditioning is a hippocampal-dependent task, whereas the cued conditioning is dependent on the amygdala. Often the APP mice are shown to be deficient in the contextual component of this task, leading investigators to conclude there is a memory deficit. However, the majority of APP mouse lines show excessive activity in open field tasks and increased numbers of arm choices in Y-maze alternation testing. They skitter. Thus one would like to have some independent measure of the capacity for freezing to be convinced that the deficit is truly failure to recognize the context in the fear conditioning recall test. One means of achieving this is to see no difference in response to the cued conditioning trial between the APP mice and non-transgenic littermates. However, rarely is this critical control presented in publications, and on some occasions

APP mice are deficient in this response as well as the response to the context. Drugs which increase or decrease the propensity towards immobility will have impact on the readout for this task without requiring an impact on the learning process. Rarely are these potential confounds considered.

RADIAL ARM WATER MAZE

When our group began working in earnest with APP and APP+PS1 mice in the late 1990s, we were fortunate to have in the Psychology department at USF David Diamond. Diamond had developed a variant of the Morris maze using rats, which overcame some of the caveats regarding the task. Essentially he superimposed the radial arm maze, used often in dry form for learning in rats, onto the water maze pool. This provided swim alleys within the pool which mice could enter. The hidden platform was placed near the end of one of these arms and the number of incorrect arm entries (errors) could be used to evaluate the degree to which mice have learned the platform location. An advantage over the traditional Morris maze is that mice are forced to use a spatial strategy to solve the problem so long as the starting location for each trial is varied (swimming in a circle does not solve the problem). The number of errors (incorrect arm entries) is relatively independent of swim speed; moreover, the task has a broad dynamic range. In the Morris maze probe trial, a well learned mouse may swim 60% in the target quadrant versus 25% for the clueless mouse. In the radial arm water maze, chance performance is four–five errors, whereas a well-learned mouse performs at less than one error (on average). Intermediate performance (two to three errors) can be resolved statistically with reasonable sample sizes ($N = 10$), and rate of learning (trials to criterion) can also be assessed. When we first used this task with APP mice, we developed a working memory version of the task, with four massed trials followed 30 minutes later by a fifth "probe" trial (although the platform remained in the pool). The idea was to measure registration of learning in the first four with failure of recall on the fifth trial. We have yet to see this occur (memory impaired mice never learn on the first four trials). This was a working memory task because each day the platform location was moved. Mice had to find the new location on trial 1, and recall that during the succeeding trials that day.

One drawback of this working memory approach was the need for 10–14 consecutive days of training to obtain criterion learning (less than one error on trials four and five). The labor involved in 70 trials per mouse was extensive. Towards reducing this burden, we have developed a two-day variant of the procedure that is a reference memory version of task (the original Morris maze is a reference memory task). A detailed methods paper has been published describing the testing procedures (Alamed et al., 2006). In this version of the task mice are run in cohorts of four mice (counterbalanced amongst treatment and genotype groups). Mice are given 15 trials on day one and another 15 on day two. However, mice are rested in between each trial as other cohort mates perform, and a second cohort is interspersed every five trials to decrease fatigue and permit consolidation. These changes to a spaced practice format have permitted us to identify criterion learning (less

than one error) by midway through the second day of training (about 22 trials) in non-transgenic mice. If additional challenge is needed to resolve subtle memory differences, mice can be administered reversal training on a third day (new platform location). Finally, mice are given a series of trials in an open pool with a visible platform, just to confirm that mice are capable of performing the task.

This task also has confounds. One confound is mice that fail to swim, or do so slowly. A mouse that swims in circles in the center of the pool, fails to make errors. But, this does not mean it has learned. To overcome this confound, we "charge" mice one error for every 15 seconds (out of 60 total seconds) they fail to make an arm entry. This admittedly contrived correction would give a non-performing mouse four errors (dead mice do not perform perfectly). Mice that consistently fail to swim (25% of trials) are culled from further analysis. Hence, this approach is an alternative to the other widely used tasks mentioned previously. It measures spatial navigation, imposes a use of a spatial strategy, can permit independent verification of performance capability, requires minimal equipment (small pool, flowerpot platforms, and aluminum or plexiglass inserts to form alleys). It is intermediate in the number of trials and short in the number of consecutive days required to commit to testing. Still, it is a single measure of behavioral performance and should be included in the context of a behavioral test battery with sensory and motor function tasks. There are a number of other behavioral tasks that can be used in assessing memory in APP mice (conditioned food aversion; passive avoidance, Barnes maze, among others), but none of them is a perfect test of memory independent of performance or motivational confounds. Given the range of such tasks, it is remarkable how consistently APP mice perform poorly on these tasks (Kobayashi and Chen, 2005).

One of the surprising findings in the APP mice is that the memory deficits do not appear to be directly caused by the amyloid deposits visible histologically. There are several building lines of evidence that suggest the cognitive deficits in these mice are due to some variant of Aβ that is present, likely in soluble form, before the first deposits have developed. One is that for many of the lines, impaired memory can be found at ages prior to observable deposits (Kobayashi and Chen, 2005), including an early mouse line from Scios-Nova, that never developed traditional amyloid deposits (Greenberg et al., 1996).

A second observation, pioneered by Karen Ashe's group, is that although individual mouse memory performance correlates with amyloid deposits within an age group, the memory loss does not grow increasingly worse as the mice age. This is consistent with there being a variable rate of Aβ production in each mouse that affects multiple pools of Aβ. Thus mice overproducing oligomeric Aβ would also be expected to deposit more amyloid, but the oligomer level could remain stable with age, resulting in a constant level of memory disturbance. One 56 kDa oligomer of Aβ (predicted to be a 12 mer) shows a strong correlation with Morris maze performance over a range of ages (Elder et al., 2010). In addition, injection of extracts enriched for this 12 mer cause memory impairments in rats.

A third observation is treatments that rescue memory function without any further reductions in amyloid deposition.

Antibodies against the Aβ peptide can be administered for short durations and rescue memory without impacting the number of amyloid deposits (in young and middle aged mice; our work in 20-month-old and greater mice has not found this to be true). Presumably, these soluble forms of Aβ will be the first ones accessible to the antibodies, permitting a rapid reversal of the memory impairment caused by these variants (Kobayashi and Chen, 2005). Treatment with BDNF similarly can lead to reversal of memory deficits, with no impact on the amyloid loads (Gotz et al., 2011). All of this has led to a hypothesis that Aβ when produced in excess overloads synapses, impairing their function (Jaworski et al., 2010). Thus, modest reduction in soluble Aβ steady-state levels could have profound impact on memory performance by relieving this overload.

There are a number of physiological changes observed in APP mouse brain. In general, long-term potentiation (LTP) is reduced and/or basal synaptic transmission is impaired, but this is not true for all models studied thus far (Balducci and Forloni, 2011). Interestingly, extracts of APP mouse brains containing dimeric forms of Aβ can induce LTP loss in non-transgenic mice. Most mice have minimal brain atrophy. In PDAPP mice there is some atrophy very early in development, but this does not progress as the mice age and develop memory problems (Bloom et al., 2005). The vast majority of mice have minimal neuron loss. However a few lines are reported to have considerable loss in hippocampus, or select cortical regions, but not the widespread atrophy and loss of brain volume found in AD (Elder et al., 2010). Synapse loss in selected brain regions is common in APP mice. The Tg2576 mouse has minimal loss of synaptic markers, but others show losses of synaptophysin, MAP2, and synaptic spines (Duyckaerts et al., 2008). In a number of models, this can be detected before the first deposits of Aβ appear. Often this is in association with a transient increase in intracellular Aβ, although some still question if this is instead APP (Balducci and Forloni, 2011). Given the data that the memory loss in these mice precedes deposition, it would seem plausible to propose that some soluble form of Aβ impacts synaptic function leading to impaired learning and memory. However, this inhibition appears reversible and can be overcome by a variety of treatments, without requiring concomitant reductions in the total amount of amyloid deposited in the brain.

TAU DEPOSITING MICE

Although more appropriately considered models of frontotemporal dementia or other tauopathies than Alzheimer's disease, the co-occurrence of both amyloid and tau pathology in Alzheimer victims makes brief consideration of these models appropriate here. Like APP mice, early models of tau overexpression failed to reproduce a number of the histological features of tauopathies, especially neurofibrillary tangles (NFTs). However, Mike Hutton's observation that mutations in tau were responsible for some cases of frontotemporal dementia led to development of transgenic lines expressing mutated forms of tau. These produced the first models of tauopathy with development of a full spectrum of abnormal tau aggregates and neurodegeneration (Gotz et al., 2011). Surprisingly,

a large number of these mice caused neuropathology in the spinal cord and brain stem, with minimal involvement of the forebrain (Elder et al., 2010).

A major step in sequencing the pathology of Alzheimer's disease came from studies increasing amyloid deposition in tau transgenic lines either by direct injection or crosses with APP mice. This led to increases in forebrain tau pathology in association with amyloid deposits (Gotz et al., 2011; McGowan et al., 2006). Mathias Jucker's group showed that extracts from APP mouse brains could perform similarly (Gotz et al., 2011). Studies with anti-Aβ antibodies in the 3x Tg mouse of Frank LaFerla (APP, PS1, and tau mutations) observed that reductions of Aβ were paralleled by reduction in early stage tau pathology (but not later-stage tau pathlogy), inferring that in this mouse the tau pathology was being driven by Aβ. Moreover, Mucke' group has shown that breeding the APP mouse onto a tau null background leads to intact learning and memory, in spite of a full spectrum of amyloid pathology (Elder et al., 2010). This would suggest that even the APP phenotype is mediated through effects on tau.

One mouse that has aggressive tauopathy is the Tg4510, developed by Jada Lewis and Karen Ashe. This mouse drives mutant tau expression with a regulatable promoter. The transcription factor for the regulator is driven by the CaM kinase 2 promoter, thus producing tau overexpression largely in forebrain neurons (where CaM kinase 2 is expressed) and delaying production until after birth. These mice develop abnormal tau pathology within neurons by three months, memory loss and neuron loss by six months, and continued brain atrophy to nine months (Santacruz et al., 2005). Interestingly, turning off the overexpression of tau with doxycycline at five months can reverse the memory loss and atrophy, but does not arrest the further development of NFTs, implying these are not responsible for these aspects of the phenotype. There have been oligomeric forms of tau identified that may be related to this memory loss (Gotz et al., 2011). Our own work with this mouse has reproduced the severe atrophy that develops such that stereotaxic coordinates need to be adjusted for the age of the mouse. Upon removal the brain is obviously smaller, and ultimately the mice become moribund and cannot be tested behaviorally, even though they can continue to survive for several months.

COMPARISONS OF TRANSGENIC MOUSE MODELS TO ALZHEIMER'S DISEASE

Few argue that the mutant APP overexpression mouse models fully mirror the pathology found in Alzheimer's disease. At least superficially, there is no abnormal tau pathology (without adding tau mutations), there is no neuron loss, nor is there brain atrophy (Table 61.2). There is synapse loss, but this is modest compared to AD and is apparently reversible. There is no substantial loss of forebrain cholinergic neurons that seems characteristic of AD. Still, the physiological appearance of amyloid deposits, the distribution of different Aβ length variants into vascular, diffuse, and compacted deposits appears qualitatively similar. The activation of microglia, centered within the plaques, and the activated astrocytes surrounding the plaques

TABLE 61.2. Advantages and disadvantages of transgenic models of amyloidogenesis

ADVANTAGES	DISADVANTAGES
• Resembles AD histopathologically • Utilizes the normal APP processing machinery to synthesize, release, and degrade Aβ • Progressive development of the phenotype with age • Observe deficits in learning and memory which resemble those in early AD • Models are reasonably consistent across individual mice	• Requires use of mutations; may not be relevant to sporadic AD • Requires overexpression of APP. May overload cellular compartments • Cognitive deficits precede amyloid deposition in mice. In AD, amyloid deposits precede cognitive changes • Incomplete pathology; no neuron loss, no NFT, no atrophy • No deficits in the cholinergic neurotransmitter system

are very similar to Alzheimer cases. Moreover, the first appearance is in the hippocampus and cortical structures, as opposed to brainstem, spinal cord, and cerebellum as found for tau transgenic mice.

However, there are differences even in those structures that appear similar. Roher has pointed out that the plaques in APP mice are "soft." They are soluble in strong detergents, unlike those from Alzheimer postmortem cases. This results in only small amounts of racemized, isomerized, and cross-linked Aβ within the APP mouse plaques. Some of these changes require the simple passage of time (not dependent upon biological age) and mice are not sufficiently long lived. Furthermore, Roher claims the transgenic mice have minimal quantities of oligomeric forms of Aβ (Kokjohn and Roher, 2009).

Perhaps the most concerning issue regards the mismatches between timing of pathology and memory dysfunction. Data clearly show that that humans develop considerable amyloid deposition years before the first detectable symptoms of the disease become manifest. However, the data in mice argue that the memory deficits appear before the deposits. Moreover, at least in the APP mice, these memory deficits do not progress like human AD to involve all neuronal functions. Our experience with Tg2576 mice is that there is modest attrition in the transgenic offspring until 15 months of age (about 25%). However after that time they lead a normal lifespan. We have studies demonstrating antibody reversal of memory loss as late as 28 months of age in this line (Wilcock et al., 2004b). At this point, we have not found treatments reversing memory loss in AD cases, ever.

In the opinion of this author, these mice are rightfully studied as models of amyloidogenesis (first denoted by Price). If one's scientific question regards amyloid deposition, perhaps even the relative deposition into specific compartments, the models would seem to be adequate. They have predicted well the outcomes of immunotherapy studies, with increased vascular amyloid and microhemorrhage associated with clearance of parenchymal deposits (Boche and Nicoll, 2008; Wilcock et al., 2004a). Importantly, this would not have been observed had we evaluated middle-aged mice instead of aged mice (Li et al., 2012). However, it is likely that the severe cognitive dysfunction in AD results from more degeneration than found in the APP mice. The relentless progressive decline from short-term memory to profound dementia, is considerably more dramatic than anything found in APP mice (even those with added tau transgenes). Some have argued the APP mice to be possibly models of the earliest stages of mild cognitive impairment, or

perhaps models of accelerated aging in mice (Ashe and Zahs, 2010).

The tau mice may be better as models of later stages of the disease. There is profound neuron loss and brain atrophy in these models. It is likely the later features in AD result from consequences of tauopathy rather than amyloid. Thus, the tau models may be better for predicting the outcomes of therapeutic trials directed at reducing the rate of atrophy, or protecting neurons and synapses, than the APP mice.

The emerging view is that mouse models can duplicate certain aspects of Alzheimer's disease. The processing of APP is likely very similar in mouse and man. Drugs intended to attack this target are likely to find the APP models good predictors of hitting that target. However, they are not models of Alzheimer's disease. As such it is folly to predict, in the absence of human data, that amyloid reductions will benefit patients or that drugs benefitting APP mice will benefit patients. That is a question being addressed by the multitude of trials with antiamyloid agents. It is likely that one or more of these will successfully lower amyloid and we can ascertain at what disease stage, if any, this approach can be used to slow disease course. Other models represent other components of the AD pathogenesis. The tau models are emerging as the next line of investigation, and development of therapeutics to attack this pathology are in the early phases. Undoubtedly, the mouse models of tauopathy will have benefit in this regard, but will need to be interpreted with the same caveats as for amyloid depositing animals.

Time will tell.

DISCLOSURE

Dr. Morgan is supported by the following grants; NIH AG-18478, AG-04418, AG-15490, NS-76308; Alzheimer's Association 10-174448.

REFERENCES

Alamed, J., Wilcock, D.M., et al. (2006). Two-day radial-arm water maze learning and memory task; robust resolution of amyloid-related memory deficits in transgenic mice. *Nat. Protoc.* 1:1671–1679.

Ashe, K.H., and Zahs, K.R. (2010). Probing the biology of Alzheimer's disease in mice. *Neuron* 66:631–645.

Auriacombe, S., Pere, J.J., et al. (2002). Efficacy and safety of rivastigmine in patients with Alzheimer's disease who failed to benefit from treatment with donepezil. *Curr. Med. Res. Opin.* 18:129–138.

Balducci, C., and Forloni, G. (2011). APP transgenic mice: their use and limitations. *Neuromolecular. Med.* 13:117–137.

Blokland, A. (1995). Acetylcholine: a neurotransmitter for learning and memory? *Brain Res. Rev.* 21:285–300.

Bloom, F.E., Reilly, J.F., et al. (2005). Mouse models of human neurodegenerative disorders: requirements for medication development. *Arch. Neurol.* 62:185–187.

Boche, D., and Nicoll, J.A. (2008). The role of the immune system in clearance of Abeta from the brain. *Brain Pathol.* 18:267–278.

Borchelt, D.R., Ratovitski, T., et al. (1997). Accelerated amyloid deposition in the brains of transgenic mice coexpressing mutant presenilin 1 and amyloid precursor protein. *Neuron* 19:939–945.

Borchelt, D.R., Thinakaran, G., et al. (1996). Familial Alzheimer's disease-linked presenilin 1 variants elevate Abeta1–42/1–40 ratio *in vitro* and *in vivo*. *Neuron* 17:1005–1013.

Casamenti, F., Prosperi, C., et al. (1998). Morphological, biochemical and behavioural changes induced by neurotoxic and inflammatory insults to the nucleus basalis. *Int. J. Dev. Neurosci.* 16:705–714.

Chambon, C., Wegener, N., et al. (2011). Behavioural and cellular effects of exogenous amyloid-beta peptides in rodents. *Behav. Brain Res.* 225:623–641.

Chen, G., Chen, K.S., et al. (2000). A learning deficit related to age and beta-amyloid plaques in a mouse model of Alzheimer's disease. *Nature* 408:975–979.

Crews, L., Rockenstein, E., et al. (2010). APP transgenic modeling of Alzheimer's disease: mechanisms of neurodegeneration and aberrant neurogenesis. *Brain Struct. Funct.* 214:111–126.

Duff, K., Eckman, C., et al. (1996). Increased amyloid-beta42(43) in brains of mice expressing mutant presenilin 1. *Nature* 383:710–713.

Duyckaerts, C., Potier, M.C., et al. (2008). Alzheimer disease models and human neuropathology: similarities and differences. *Acta Neuropathol.* 115:5–38.

Elder, G.A., Gama Sosa, M.A., et al. (2010). Transgenic mouse models of Alzheimer's disease. *Mt. Sinai J. Med.* 77:69–81.

Games, D., Adams, D., et al. (1995). Alzheimer-type neuropathology in transgenic mice overexpressing V717F beta-amyloid precursor protein. *Nature* 373:523–527.

Geula, C., Wu, C., et al. (1998). Aging renders the brain vulnerable to amyloid B-protein neurotoxicity. *Nat. Med.* 4:827–831.

Gordon, M.N., Holcomb, L.A., et al. (2002). Time course of the development of Alzheimer-like pathology in the doubly transgenic PS1+APP mouse. *Exp. Neurol.* 173:183–195.

Gordon, M.N., King, D.L., et al. (2001). Correlation between cognitive deficits and Abeta deposits in transgenic APP+PS1 mice. *Neurobiol. Aging* 22:377–385.

Gotz, J., Eckert, A., et al. (2011). Modes of Abeta toxicity in Alzheimer's disease. *Cell. Mol. Life Sci.* 68:3359–3375.

Greenberg, B.D., Savage, M.J., et al. (1996). APP transgenesis: approaches toward the development of animal models for Alzheimer disease neuropathology. *Neurobiol. Aging* 17:153–171.

Harkany, T., Hortobagyi, T., et al. (1999). Neuroprotective approaches in experimental models of beta-amyloid neurotoxicity: relevance to Alzheimer's disease. *Prog. Neuropsychopharmacol. Biol. Psychiatry* 23:963–1008.

Hasselmo, M.E. (2006). The role of acetylcholine in learning and memory. *Curr. Opin. Neurobiol.* 16:710–715.

Hock, B.J., Jr., and Lamb, B.T. (2001). Transgenic mouse models of Alzheimer's disease. *Trends Genet.* 17:S7–12.

Holcomb, L., Gordon, M.N., et al. (1998). Accelerated Alzheimer-type phenotype in transgenic mice carrying both mutant amyloid precursor protein and presenilin 1 transgenes. *Nat. Med.* 4:97–100.

Holcomb, L.A., Gordon, M.N., et al. (2000). A beta and perlecan in rat brain. Glial activation, gradual clearance and limited neurotoxicity. *Mech. Ageing Dev.* 112:135–142.

Hsiao, K., Chapman, P., et al. (1996). Correlative memory deficits, Abeta elevation, and amyloid plaques in transgenic mice. *Science* 274:99–102.

Jaworski, T., Dewachter, I., et al. (2010). Alzheimer's disease: old problem, new views from transgenic and viral models. *Biochim. Biophys. Acta* 1802:808–818.

Kobayashi, D.T., and Chen, K.S. (2005). Behavioral phenotypes of amyloid-based genetically modified mouse models of Alzheimer's disease. *Genes Brain Behav.* 4:173–196.

Kokjohn, T.A., and Roher, A.E. (2009). Amyloid precursor protein transgenic mouse models and Alzheimer's disease: understanding the paradigms, limitations, and contributions. *Alzheimers Dement.* 5:340–347.

Li, Q., Lebson, L., et al. (2012). Chronological age impacts immunotherapy and monocyte uptake independent of amyloid load. *J. Neuroimmune Pharmacol.* 7:202–214.

McGowan, E., Eriksen, J., et al. (2006). A decade of modeling Alzheimer's disease in transgenic mice. *Trends Genet.* 22:281–289.

Mesulam, M. (2004) The cholinergic lesion of Alzheimer's disease: pivotal factor or side show? *Learn. Mem.* 11:43–49.

Morgan, D., Diamond, D.M., et al. (2000). A beta peptide vaccination prevents memory loss in an animal model of Alzheimer's disease. *Nature* 408:982–985.

Price, D.L., Wong, P.C., et al. (2000). The value of transgenic models for the study of neurodegenerative diseases. *Ann. NY Acad. Sci.* 920:179–191.

Santacruz, K., Lewis, J., et al. (2005). Tau suppression in a neurodegenerative mouse model improves memory function. *Science* 309:476–481.

Sturchler-Pierrat, C., Abramowski, D., et al. (1997). Two amyloid precursor protein transgenic mouse models with Alzheimer disease-like pathology. *Proc. Natl. Acad. Sci. USA* 94:13287–13292.

Wilcock, D.M., Rojiani, A., et al. (2004a). Passive immunotherapy against Abeta in aged APP-transgenic mice reverses cognitive deficits and depletes parenchymal amyloid deposits in spite of increased vascular amyloid and microhemorrhage. *J. Neuroinflamm.* 1:24.

Wilcock, D.M., Rojiani, A., et al. (2004b). Passive amyloid immunotherapy clears amyloid and transiently activates microglia in a transgenic mouse model of amyloid deposition. *J. Neurosci.* 24:6144–6151.

Yamada, K., and Nabeshima, T. (2000). Animal models of Alzheimer's disease and evaluation of anti-dementia drugs. *Pharmacol. Ther.* 88:93–113.

62 | STRUCTURAL, FUNCTIONAL, AND MOLECULAR NEUROIMAGING BIOMARKERS FOR ALZHEIMER'S DISEASE

JAMES B. BREWER, JORGE SEPULCRE, AND KEITH A. JOHNSON

Alzheimer disease (AD) is currently a major public health challenge and one that poses an even greater threat for the future as the population ages. The role of neuroimaging in AD diagnosis and in the general assessment of cognitive impairment in the elderly has greatly evolved over the past two decades. In the past, structural neuroimaging was used merely to support the physical exam in the exclusion of focal lesions that could contribute to a patient's cognitive impairment. In most cases, any such discrete lesion sufficient to impair cognition would also be detectable through a careful examination, so the majority of clinical neuroimaging interpretations were negative and unhelpful. In fact, the added benefit of neuroimaging used in this manner was, and continues to be, controversial, as evidenced by variation in professional society guidelines regarding the use of neuroimaging in this setting (Knopman et al., 2001; Rabins et al., 2007). However, the development of magnetic resonance imaging (MRI) and positron emission tomography (PET) biomarkers that directly assess the degree of regional neurodegeneration or dysfunction and, more recently, neuroimaging biomarkers that assess pathological hallmarks of AD have brought transformative change to the field and shifted interest to earlier pathophysiological events. While much effort remains focused on the study of AD dementia and mild cognitive impairment (MCI), now preclinical stages have become a major focus. The move toward expanding the scope of inquiry into preclinical stages and younger age groups is motivated in part by the recognition that the presymptomatic phase of the illness is of 10–20 years duration and in part by the related need to enable earlier disease modifying intervention. The evolving view of AD pathophysiology has recently been fueled by rapid developments in amyloid-beta (Aβ) imaging and fluid biomarkers; however, simultaneous advances have been realized in other types of AD biomarkers. Neuroimaging biomarkers are now routinely incorporated into AD clinical trials and are increasingly used in clinical practice. This chapter will broadly describe the development and use of these biomarkers as they relate to AD.

ESTIMATES OF NEURODEGENERATION IN ALZHEIMER'S DISEASE

QUANTITATIVE MAGNETIC RESONANCE IMAGING BIOMARKERS

VOLUMETRIC MAGNETIC RESONANCE IMAGING

The slowly progressive neurodegeneration of AD is reflected in brain structural changes that can be appreciated at the macroscopic level. Medial temporal regions, such as the entorhinal cortex and hippocampus, are typically affected earliest, consistent with the hallmark memory problems that usually accompany disease onset. Macroscopic structural change broadly mirrors the pathological spread of the disease, with atrophy subsequently apparent in lateral temporal as well as medial and lateral parietal association cortex followed by frontal regions and, finally, primary sensorimotor cortices (McDonald et al., 2009). Though the changes are slow, over time the accumulation of atrophy is readily apparent to visual inspection (Fox et al., 1996; Scheltens et al., 1992).

Thus, in the absence of a suitable biofluid marker of neural damage and the unacceptable invasiveness of brain biopsy, a great deal of research has focused on the promise of neuroimaging and direct visualization of brain structure to assess the likelihood of neurodegeneration in individual patients. Typically, such approaches have leveraged the improvements in image quality afforded by MRI, though the quantitative nature of computed tomography (CT), including high spatial fidelity, and recent advances in achievable image spatial resolution, tissue contrast, and overall quality might suggest future promise for CT in quantitative assessment of neurodegeneration. The discussion that follows regarding structural neuroimaging will nonetheless focus on approaches using MRI.

Direct assessment of putative brain atrophy can make use of semiquantitative approaches to rate severity of volume loss or employ tools for quantification of brain structure volumes, volumetric MRI (vMRI), to provide measurements that could be tracked over time or compared to a normative database (for review, see Jack, 2011). In clinical practice, volumetrics may inform the clinical assessment by either supporting or calling into question the impression, previously based solely on clinical history and examination, that neurodegenerative disease is present and possibly causing the complaint (Fig. 62.1).

It is not surprising that the hippocampus has been targeted as the structure most likely to provide a reliable volumetric biomarker of neurodegeneration in AD. Damage to hippocampal tissue is severe early in the disease and, owing to its somewhat cylindrical structure, hippocampal borders are relatively easy to delineate for volume measurement. However, it should be noted that hippocampal atrophy is not specific to AD, nor is all AD associated with severe hippocampal atrophy (for review of focal variants of AD, see Kramer and Miller, 2000). Some degree of hippocampal volume loss is expected even in healthy aging, and the structure's volume is further correlated with overall intracranial volume. Thus, the effects of age and intracranial volume, and possibly gender and race, must be accounted for. An individual's prior history of brain trauma, alcoholism, drug abuse, and vascular risk factors such as hypertension and smoking, would also likely influence the measure, so it is unlikely that a distinct "cutoff" in hippocampal volume could be identified that will reliably predict AD risk across patients.

Instead, hippocampal volume is more likely to be useful as a measure that helps assess the likelihood that neurodegeneration is present rather than a diagnostic for AD. As such, the measure should be seen by treating physicians as one additional data point to assist in their clinical impression. Most clinicians are familiar with tests that shape, rather than define, a clinical impression, and such tests are valuable nonetheless. An example might be the measurement of hemoglobin in the setting of a patient complaint of fatigue. A normal hemoglobin directs attention to etiologies other than anemia, and a finding of low hemoglobin supports, but does not assure, that anemia is causing the fatigue. The assessment and management depend heavily on the clinical setting and ancillary factors associated with the measurement. In practical terms, this means that the relevance of a vMRI finding to a particular case will be determined by the treating physician, rather than by the radiologist. However, the radiologist can provide additional qualitative information from the images that lend further value to the quantitative information.

Despite intense focus on translation of hippocampal volumetry to the clinical realm for AD assessment, ancillary measures of atrophy may be critical to improve interpretability of hippocampal volume. Several research groups have examined the value of combining regional volumetric measures across cortical and subcortical structures to more completely describe the spatial pattern of changes associated with AD (Davatzikos et al., 2008; Dickerson et al., 2009; McEvoy et al., 2009; Vemuri et al., 2011). A pattern with broad consistency across techniques emerges, where atrophy is prominent in medial and lateral temporal and parietal regions, moderate in frontal regions, and minimal in primary sensorimotor regions. The combination of regions, naturally, improves classifier sensitivity and specificity beyond that achieved through the use of a single region. However, the ability to translate such advanced approaches to the clinical environment has

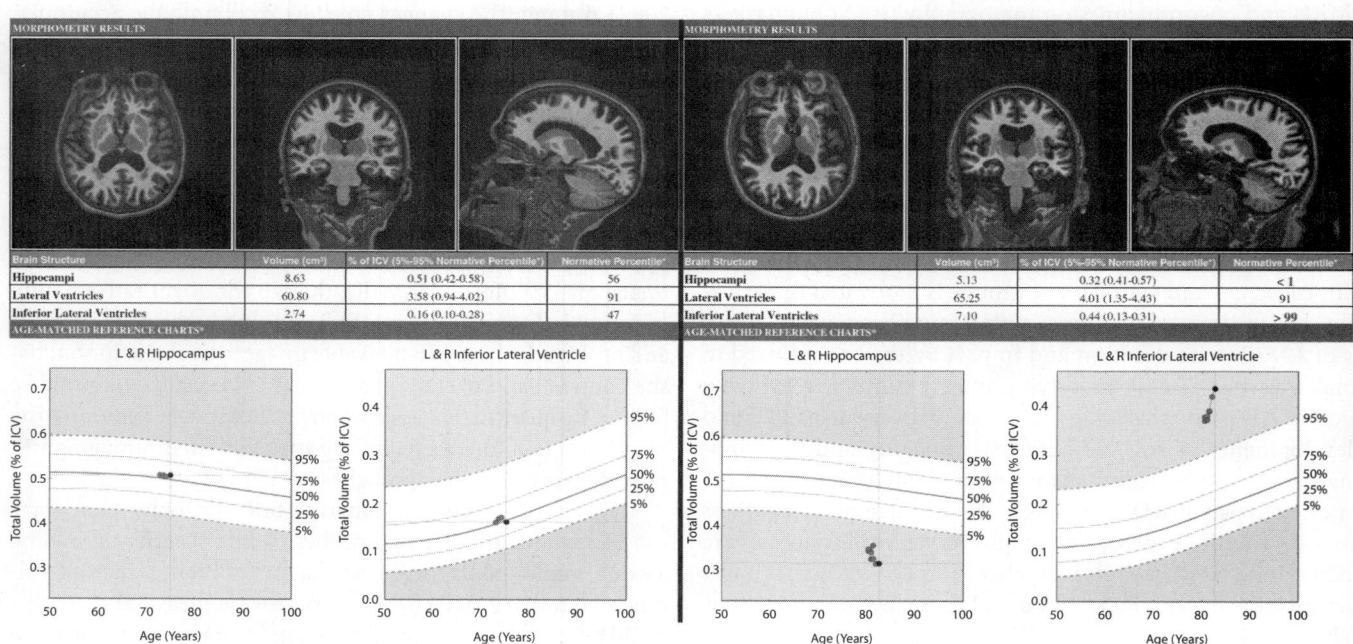

Figure 62.1 Example volumetric reports for two subjects enrolled in a longitudinal quantitative imaging study. (A) A 75-year-old healthy subject who remained stable and was without evidence of hippocampal neurodegeneration or temporal horn enlargement during scanning over two years. (B) An 82-year-old, cognitively impaired subject who progressed from MCI to AD at the third year of follow-up. This patient was a non-carrier of APOE4 genotype who, by CSF testing, had elevated phospho-tau and reduced levels of amyloid beta 42 in cerebrospinal fluid. vMRI shows evidence of hippocampal neurodegeneration and ex vacuo dilatation of the temporal horns during scanning over two years. (See color insert.)

not yet been demonstrated and may not be practical. In particular, those that rely on support vector machines to obtain data-derived regions with highest classifier performance might be overly reliant on features of the data set used to train the classifier, and so performance may not necessarily generalize to the wider population seen in clinical practice. Further, given anatomical variation in cortical folding, derivation of regional cortical volume or thickness is more challenging and computationally expensive than derivation of volumes for most subcortical structures, such as the hippocampus and ventricular subregions.

Indeed, some contextual information about a hippocampal volume measurement can be provided by additionally assessing temporal horn volume. Hippocampal and wider medial temporal lobe (MTL) degeneration is often associated with *ex vacuo* expansion of the temporal horn of the lateral ventricle. Therefore, temporal horn volumetry with comparison to normative values can provide complementary evidence of concurrent *ex vacuo* dilatation of this ventricular structure. Such a finding could support that the individual's hippocampus was previously larger and had undergone degeneration, as opposed to having been congenitally small. Further, measurement of the entire ventricular system and its relationship to norms can assist interpretation of the temporal horn volume. The combination of measures would inform assessment of likelihood that the temporal horn enlargement is more specifically due to regional *ex vacuo* changes (if, along with low hippocampal volume, only the temporal horn is abnormally large), rather than due to general ventricular system expansion (if both temporal horn and the entire ventricular system are abnormally large). Evidence of MTL-focused atrophy might provide an early sign of neurodegenerative disease, including AD, which typically affects these structures first. Table 62.1 provides examples of possible clinical interpretations when hippocampal, temporal horn, and overall lateral ventricle volumes are examined in combination.

Finally, it should be noted that, even when a typical pattern is noted or when markedly out of the normal range, a single measurement in time cannot definitively point to a neurodegenerative etiology, since many of the aforementioned traumatic or congenital factors are associated with low volumes of structures not seen to progressively deteriorate. Therefore, the most powerful evidence for ongoing neurodegeneration might be demonstration of accelerated progressive deterioration in structure volumes through longitudinal imaging. Thus, beyond comparing a patient's brain to a normative database, a patient's brain volumes would be quantitatively compared to those measured for that individual at a prior time. Differences in scanner hardware and software adds significant variability to measures of very subtle volume change across time, and, even at a single site, equipment changes are frequent in clinical practice, so this remains a significant challenge to obtaining accurate measurement of change across time. To be most relevant to clinical practice, meaningful information would need to be obtained across a relatively brief period of follow-up, preferably around one year. This would require highly robust methods, including correction for subtle scanner-specific distortions that could assess anatomical changes with high enough precision to reliably distinguish across individual subjects miniscule differences in rate of atrophy (e.g., hippocampal volume loss ranges from 1–5% across healthy elderly, MCI, and AD). Such precision is a significant challenge, particularly if the equipment changes between scans. Nevertheless, equipment manufacturers are becoming more aware of the potential value of quantitative neuroimaging, which lends hope that procedures could be standardized to improve accuracy of measurements despite equipment and software variability.

Though several caveats remain to be considered, working groups gathered through efforts of the Alzheimer's Association and the National Institute on Aging recently published guidelines for revised diagnostic criteria for AD and MCI that incorporate vMRI and other biomarkers (Albert et al., 2011; McKhann et al., 2011). Tools for vMRI have already been established in large radiological practices to assess the degree to which an individual's brain structure volumes fit within the normative range adjusted for age, sex, and intracranial volume. Relatively recent Food and Drug Administration approval of an automated vMRI tool has permitted further research of its applicability in unselected clinical cohorts encountered through everyday practice as well as in the highly selected cohorts studied in AD clinical trials.

DIFFUSION-WEIGHTED IMAGING

Magnetic resonance physics allows flexible approaches to examine water molecule behavior within tissue. Structural neuroimaging may focus on achieving high anatomical detail through examining magnetic contrast related to tissue content, itself, or it may focus on measuring more general effects on contrast due to surrounding tissue structure or magnetic properties. In diffusion-weighted imaging, the effect that surrounding tissue structure has on water movement is paramount. MRI contrast can be achieved by examining the degree of water movement within the region; water movement is restricted by surrounding anatomy, and the more restricted, the greater the signal. In directional diffusion weighted imaging, such as diffusion tensor imaging or diffusion spectrum imaging, both the magnitude and direction of water movement is collected, informing whether water movement is more hindered in one direction versus another.

As white matter tracts in the brain are one of the major anatomical features that might direct water to diffuse in one direction (parallel the white matter) relative to another (perpendicular to the white matter), directional diffusion weighted imaging has become a favored research tool with which to examine white matter integrity in neurodegenerative diseases such as AD (for review, see Oishi et al., 2011). Indeed prior cognitive research has described AD as a disease of "disconnection" between disparate cortical brain areas, so the ability to examine fiber tract disruption is a compelling reason to examine the effects of AD on white matter tracts as evidenced by changes in diffusion-weighted signal.

However, it remains to be seen whether degeneration of fiber tracts is best measured through changes in directionality, as opposed to magnitude, of diffusion. When comparing impaired patients to healthy controls, studies have found regional group differences in fractional anisotropy, a measure

TABLE 62.1. Influence of temporal horn and lateral ventricle measures on the interpretation of volumetric MRI (vMRI) findings

EXAMPLE SEGMENTED MRI	EXAMPLE VMRI FINDINGS	HIPPOCAMPUS	TEMPORAL HORN	LATERAL VENTRICLE	INTERPRETATION
	Brain Structure — Volume (cm³) — % of ICV (5%-95% Normative Percentile) — Normative Percentile Hippocampi 8.64 / 0.54 (0.45-0.60) / 55; Lateral Ventricles 33.32 / 2.07 (0.98-3.65) / 55; Inferior Lateral Ventricles 2.57 / 0.16 (0.11-0.28) / 45. AGE-MATCHED REFERENCE CHARTS (L & R Hippocampus; L & R Inferior Lateral Ventricle)	Normal (not atrophied)	Normal (not enlarged)	Normal (bot enlarged)	Normal scan: does not support neurodegeneration
	Hippocampi 7.33 / 0.43 (0.46-0.61) / <1; Lateral Ventricles 38.70 / 2.17 (0.82-3.11) / 76; Inferior Lateral Ventricles 2.26 / 0.13 (0.09-0.26) / 36. AGE-MATCHED REFERENCE CHARTS (L & R Hippocampus; L & R Inferior Lateral Ventricle)	Low volume	Normal	Normal	Low hippocampal volume without ex vacuo dilatation: possibly congenitally small hippocampi. Follow to establish presence and trajectory of volume change.
	Hippocampi 5.05 / 0.37 (0.43-0.58) / <1; Lateral Ventricles 38.76 / 2.87 (0.97-3.44) / 83; Inferior Lateral Ventricles 4.50 / 0.33 (0.11-0.27) / >99. AGE-MATCHED REFERENCE CHARTS (L & R Hippocampus; L & R Inferior Lateral Ventricle)	Low volume	High volume	Normal	Low hippocampal volume and suggestive of local ex vacuo dilatation: supports MTL-focused neurodegenerative etiology

	Low volume	High volume	High volume	
AGE-MATCHED REFERENCE CHARTS	Low volume	High volume	High volume	Low hippocampal volume and suggestive of global ex vacuo dilatation: supports neurodegenerative etiology, but may or may not be MTL-focused

Brain Structure	Volume (cm³)	% of ICV (5%-95% Normative Percentile)	Normative Percentile
Hippocampi	7.34	0.42 (0.46-0.61)	< 1
Lateral Ventricles	63.95	3.62 (0.55-2.99)	> 99
Inferior Lateral Ventricles	6.17	0.35 (0.09-0.25)	> 99

	Normal	High volume	High volume	
AGE-MATCHED REFERENCE CHARTS	Normal	High volume	High volume	Normal hippocampal volume with enlarged ventricular system: does not support hippocampal neurodegeneration. Possible expansion of overall ventricular system without MTL-focused ex vacuo changes.

Brain Structure	Volume (cm³)	% of ICV (5%-95% Normative Percentile)	Normative Percentile
Hippocampi	7.81	0.53 (0.44-0.60)	52
Lateral Ventricles	60.13	4.07 (1.15-3.90)	> 99
Inferior Lateral Ventricles	5.18	0.35 (0.12-0.29)	> 99

of directional diffusion, yet some studies have found even more robust differences in mean diffusivity, a directionless measure of diffusion magnitude. Neurodegeneration in AD seems more likely to cause loss of fibers within defined tracts rather than a shift in direction of those tracts. Thus directional measures, though useful for identifying tract location, might be less powerful for detecting tract degeneration than simpler measures of diffusion magnitude. Further, the directional diffusion signal can be influenced by a number of subtle factors, so export of this tool to the clinical realm will face a number of challenges, not least of which will be the development of normative ranges for determining whether a patient's scan is normal or abnormal when placed in context with the general healthy population. Nevertheless, the approach shows promise as a technique that shows a complementary anatomy not seen in conventional structural imaging.

FUNCTIONAL MAGNETIC RESONANCE IMAGING

Though other approaches exist, most functional MRI is based on the Blood Oxygen Level-Dependent (BOLD) effect, which allows MRI sensitivity to variations in relative levels of oxyhemoglobin and deoxyhemoglobin that vary in association with regional brain activity (for review, see Brown, Perthen, Liu, & Buxton, 2007). Given the probability that changes in neural function precede frank neurodegeneration and changes in structure, functional MRI (fMRI) has been studied extensively as a potential biomarker to identify the earliest brain changes associated with AD. Broadly, methods applied to fMRI can be divided into two categories: task-dependent fMRI and task-free, or "resting-state," fMRI (rsfMRI).

In task-dependent fMRI, subjects in the scanner might be asked to perform a defined "activation" task that alternates with or occurs separately from a "control" task while BOLD signal is recorded. The control task differs from the activation task in a way that is designed to isolate and identify the brain activity linked to a targeted cognitive function, which is a cognitive function used during the activation task, but not during the control task. This "cognitive subtraction" technique suffers from a number of factors that limit interpretation, particularly when applied to a diseased population. For example, an observed signal difference between AD and controls might be related to uncontrolled variation in task difficulty or attentional resources that must be dedicated to performing the task, despite matched performance across groups. This adds to more general concerns about factors of subject motion and brain atrophy that must be accounted for in all neuroimaging biomarkers of AD. Such factors might be particularly problematic for fMRI biomarkers, because the effect of confounders can be amplified by the analysis approach (Seibert and Brewer, 2011).

In rsfMRI, subjects are instructed to simply lie still in the scanner, perhaps with guidance to keep their eyes open throughout the session, but functional data are nonetheless collected without regard to any specific mental activity. Instead, it is the interregional correlation in BOLD signal fluctuations that provides the marker of interest. The pattern of interregional correlation is remarkably consistent, in that signal from a particular brain region tends to be tightly linked with signal from other regions that show relatively stable correlations across subjects and scanning sessions. These stable interregional correlations have been termed "functional connectivity" and the phrase "functional network" is often used to refer to regions linked by their covariance in BOLD signal. Several distinct functional networks have been described, including the attentional/salience network of bilateral frontal regions and anterior cingulate gyrus, the sensorimotor network of bilateral primary motor and sensory cortex, and the default mode network of medial and lateral parietal, medial and lateral temporal, and medial frontal cortex.

The latter default network is the most studied and, owing to its remarkable overlap with the spatial distribution of amyloid deposition and atrophy in AD (Buckner et al., 2009; Greicius et al., 2004; Raichle et al., 2001; Sepulcre et al., 2010), has garnered the most interest for its potential as an early biomarker of the disease. A consistent finding is that interregional correlations in the default network are reduced in AD. However, concerns remain about the general effects of atrophy and motion on the ability to identify functional correlations themselves. A more compelling finding is the identification of default network reductions in amyloid positive individuals who are asymptomatic, who would not be expected to exhibit large differences in atrophy or motion from those who are amyloid negative (Sperling et al., 2009). Default network correlations have been noted even to be reduced in individuals gene positive for autosomal dominant AD before symptoms have begun (Sperling et al., 2012). Such findings suggest the tremendous potential for fMRI as an early biomarker of AD, though its translation to use in the clinical setting will require a great deal more research.

MAGNETIC RESONANCE SPECTROSCOPY

Magnetic resonance spectroscopy (MRS) has long showed promise for detection of regional chemical changes associated with neurodegeneration, inflammation, or gliosis, and so it has been a technique of interest for detecting such changes in AD. It provides information about relative concentrations of key chemicals, such as N-acetylaspartate, creatinine, and myoinositol, and there is strong evidence that the regional concentration of these chemicals varies with the neurodegeneration seen in AD (for review, see Tran et al., 2009). While specialized research laboratories have consistently demonstrated robust discrimination between clinical groups, suggesting potential value in assessment of individual cases, improved standardization of approach is needed before MRS can be widely applied in multisite clinical trials or generally in the clinical setting.

POSITRON EMISSION TOMOGRAPHY

FLUORODEOXYGLUCOSE IMAGING

CLINICAL USE OF FLUORODEOXYGLUCOSE PET

Fluorodeoxyglucose (FDG) PET is a marker of brain metabolism with limited but established utility in differentiating AD from other brain pathologies that manifest as cognitive impairment. Under normal circumstances, the physiological level of glucose use reflected by FDG PET is due primarily to regional synaptic activity, and FDG uptake in nonhuman primates has been correlated with levels of synaptophysin in histological studies (Rocher et al., 2003). Since glucose consumption is by far the major contributor to the brain's energy budget, FDG uptake reflects the full range of brain energy requirements, including protein and lipid synthesis, as well as maintenance of electrochemical gradients used in neural activity (Raichle et al., 2001). Alterations in synaptic activity detectable with FDG reflect chronic synaptic dysfunction (or loss) as well as perturbed functional status observed within shorter time intervals, such as during specific cognitive or motor task performance.

Fluorodeoxyglucose metabolism is assessed regionally with PET so that anatomic patterns of relative hypometabolism may be both visually evident and expressed quantitatively; quantification may involve arterial blood sampling or may alternatively use internal tissue reference standards. No single pathognomonic FDG PET finding specifies the presence of the clinical syndrome of AD dementia or the presence of AD pathology. However, the anatomic pattern of relative FDG hypometabolism in AD is characteristic and is considered to be an endophenotype of AD, that is, a consistently affected hypometabolic group of brain structures that has been strongly associated with both the clinical syndrome of AD dementia and the postmortem finding of definite AD (Jagust et al., 2007). The AD endophenotype of FDG hypometabolism comprises the posterior midline cortices of the parietal (precuneus) and posterior cingulate, the inferior parietal lobule, posterolateral portions of the temporal lobe, hippocampus, and medial temporal cortices (Foster et al., 1983; Minoshima et al., 1997). This pattern is present in AD, is linearly related to dementia severity, and is associated with subsequent clinical decline and conversion to AD (Chetelat et al., 2003; Jagust et al., 2007). It is seen less severely or consistently in MCI, and to some extent, in Aβ positive normal elderly (Caselli et al., 2008; Cohen et al., 2009; Langbaum et al., 2009). Because the AD-like pattern of FDG hypometabolism is associated both with the clinical features of established AD dementia, and with AD pathology at postmortem (Jagust et al., 2007), it may be used to differentiate AD from frontotemporal lobar degeneration (FTLD) and to some extent from dementia with Lewy bodies (DLB). Specifically, it is typical to find frontotemporal hypometabolism in FTLD, and occipital—in addition to the AD-like temporoparietal—hypometabolism, in DLB. Other applications have been proposed for FDG PET, particularly to detect individuals who are likely to develop AD dementia in the future (Chetelat et al., 2003); however, this has not yet been successfully implemented in clinical practice.

UNDERSTANDING THE ALZHEIMER'S DISEASE BRAIN WITH FLUORODEOXYGLUCOSE

In recent years neuroimaging techniques such as FDG PET and fMRI that are capable of revealing different aspects of the brain function have provided key insights about functional organization and its spatial distribution in AD. For instance, the metabolic-anatomic endophenotype of AD described earlier is sometimes asymmetric and predominantly temporoparietal in the early stages, but later progresses to involve prefrontal and heteromodal areas largely overlapping with the aforementioned default mode network.

As AD progresses from presymptomatic to established AD dementia, regional glucose metabolism gradually worsens (Bateman et al., 2012; Jack, 2011) and the spatial pattern of progression may be conditioned by anatomic interconnectivity, in parallel with the progression of pathological processes (Arnold et al., 1991; Pearson and Powell, 1989). AD neurodegeneration involves specific functional networks of the human brain (Greicius et al., 2004; Seeley et al., 2009), and this feature has led to a new reformulation of the old hebbian principal: "not only neurons that fire together wire together, but also neurons that wire together die together" (Sepulcre et al., 2012). It may be possible to track FDG metabolic changes along specific anatomic pathways that relate to underlying pathologic progression, and also to relate these findings to evidence of regional atrophy (Villain et al., 2010).

Some investigators have reported that FDG hypometabolism is detectable along the AD trajectory prior to the appearance of cognitive symptoms and signs of neurodegeneration in individuals at increased risk for AD (Jack et al., 2010; Jagust et al., 2006). Thus, the AD-like pattern of hypometabolism or hypoperfusion predicts cognitive decline in subjects that eventually convert to AD (Jagust et al., 2006) and in carriers of autosomal dominant AD mutations (Bateman et al., 2012; Johnson et al., 2012). It is also associated with the progression of the clinical dementia rating scale sum-of-boxes in both AD and MCI subjects (Chen et al., 2010). Importantly, several studies have found that glucose alterations are not merely caused by concurrent atrophy, and therefore regional FDG reduction is an independent piece of information in AD (Johnson et al., 2012). Moreover, FDG metabolism continues to decline even in advanced stages of the disease when other pathological factors reach a plateau (Engler et al., 2006; Jack et al., 2010). It is likely that these declines reflect the combined effects of several potentially overlapping processes; these include specific genetic effects, mitochondrial dysfunction, oxidative stress, excitotoxicity, synaptic and neuronal failure triggered by Aβ, neurofibrillary tangle accumulation, and/or other factors, together with other downstream degenerative processes. It is likely that FDG PET is sensitive to several components of the neurodegenerative process, and thus separate biomarker representation may be required to track specific processes.

Finally, several studies have shown that FDG hypometabolism matches, to some extent, the brain distribution of amyloid deposits, particularly in the default mode network (Cohen et al., 2009; Engler et al., 2006; Klunk et al., 2004). However, this relationship is not settled and other groups have not found meaningful or strong associations particularly at later stages of the disease (Furst et al., 2012; Rabinovici et al., 2010). In general, glucose hypometabolism in frontal regions is less evident than in temporoparietal cortex, whereas amyloid uptake is usually somewhat greater in frontal regions (Klunk et al., 2004).

Therefore, the association of amyloid deposition with reductions of glucose utilization remains unclear. Many important challenges remain unsolved in AD research and one of them is the integration of structural, functional, and molecular neuroimaging findings.

SUMMARY AND LIMITATIONS OF FLUORODEOXYGLUCOSE PET

FDG PET is a widely available technology that may help diagnostic accuracy in neurodegenerative illnesses, particularly when earlier stages of cognitive impairment are possibly due to AD pathology or to FTLD. However, further work is needed to determine the diagnostic value of FDG when assessing preclinical stages of AD. Like other imaging biomarkers, FDG does not indicate clear spatial patterns that distinguish between normal aging and MCI or AD (Caselli et al., 2008; Chetelat et al., 2003; Langbaum et al., 2009). As with these other modalities, the observed heterogeneity in FDG patterns of metabolism may be the result of individual differences, particularly in cognitive reserve, or comorbid conditions of aging such as vascular disease, as well as to idiosyncratic factors. Neural dysfunction likely precedes neurodegenerative changes, and so FDG PET holds great promise for monitoring cognitive transition from preclinical to established AD (Furst et al., 2012; Jack et al., 2010), Nevertheless, the sensitivity of FDG PET relative to that of vMRI remains to be established despite the existence of head-to-head comparisons performed in the same patients (Karow et al., 2010). Sensitivity of a biomarker depends not only on acquisition modality, but also on analysis techniques, which continue to evolve. Therefore, it is still unknown which variable will best be associated with cognitive symptoms for continued translation into clinical use in the earliest stages of disease. Although the availability of FDG PET has increased dramatically over the past decade and the standardization of methods has improved substantially, costs of PET technology remain high, and cost effectiveness in dementia diagnosis has been difficult to demonstrate.

AMYLOID IMAGING

CLINICAL USE OF AMYLOID IMAGING

Amyloid-β (Aβ) dysmetabolism and subsequent deposition is a defining neuropathological feature of AD (Braak and Braak, 1991; Selkoe, 2006), and the ability to detect brain Aβ deposits during life has revolutionized clinical research in AD (Klunk et al., 2004). The *in vivo* visualization of brain Aβ deposition with amyloid PET is virtually equivalent to demonstration of the pathology at autopsy, as has been repeatedly demonstrated (Bacskai et al., 2003; Ikonomovic et al., 2008; Klunk et al., 2004; Sojkova et al., 2011) for rare exceptions, see Klunk, 2011). Amyloid PET detects fibrillar amyloid because PET tracers bind to the beta-sheet protein structure that forms when Aβ polymerizes (Ikonomovic et al., 2008). Amyloid PET can thus detect the Aβ that is a major component of the damage occurring in patients with cognitive impairment caused by AD and is always seen in AD dementia patients at autopsy. A negative amyloid PET scan generally indicates very few or no amyloid deposits and greatly reduces the likelihood that any cognitive

impairment is caused by AD. A positive scan indicates that moderately to severely elevated numbers of β-amyloid deposits are present. A fundamental concept of amyloid PET is that the images indicate presence of Aβ deposits, but do not reliably distinguish between normal, MCI, and AD dementia, and thus do not relate directly to these traditional clinical diagnostic categories (Johnson et al., 2012). In other words, it is critically important to note that a positive amyloid PET scan does not by itself establish any clinical diagnosis, including that of AD dementia. The test may be positive in normal older individuals as well as in other clinical entities such as DLB.

The highly stereotyped anatomic pattern of amyloid PET ligand binding to areas of high connectivity forms the basis for the amyloid PET endophenotype of AD (Arnold et al., 1991; Braak and Braak, 1991; Buckner et al., 2009). Thus, areas that are highly interconnected, such as precuneus, posterior cingulate, inferior parietal and lateral temporal cortices (i.e., portions of the DMN), are typically affected, but the earliest and most heavily involved is often the middle frontal cortex, which is part of the cognitive control network. The time course of amyloid deposition typically involves these vulnerable regions; however, there is substantial variability in regional deposition at early stages, and at later stages, additional brain regions including primary cortices are also affected.

Most published reports to date involve the C-11-labeled agent *N*-methyl 11C-2-(4-methylaminophenyl)-6-hydroxyb enzothiazole, also known as Pittsburgh Compound-B (PIB; half-life 20 minutes) (Klunk et al., 2004). Other compounds made with the more convenient F-18 radio-label (half-life 110 minutes) are increasingly available for research and even clinical use (Johnson et al., 2012).

The reported correspondence of amyloid positivity with traditional clinical diagnoses is as follows: more than 90% of clinically diagnosed AD patients and approximately 60% of MCI patients are classified as amyloid positive with PET (Johnson et al., 2012). Similar proportions have been reported using CSF biomarkers of Aβ (Fagan et al., 2007).

Longitudinal studies are just now emerging, but when MCI subjects have been followed over one to three years after PET, approximately one-half of those who were amyloid positive at baseline converted to AD dementia and approximately 10% of the amyloid negative subjects converted to AD dementia. These studies are ongoing, and continued clinical and histopathological follow-up will be required because it is possible that the clinical diagnoses would not be confirmed at autopsy.

A substantial fraction of apparently healthy, elderly cognitively normal subjects have Aβ deposits detected by PET (10% to 50%) (Jack et al., 2010; Johnson et al., 2012), and such individuals are termed preclinical AD based on the hypothesis that the progressive accumulation of amyloid places them at higher risk for developing clinical syndrome of AD dementia (Jack et al., 2010). The magnitude and timing of such risk remains the subject of active investigation; however, several AD prevention clinical trials are proceeding on the basis of AD risk defined in this way. The analysis of early changes and preclinical stages of AD is critical to understand the transition to symptomatic forms of the disease. Recent data have shown a continuum of accumulation of *in vivo* amyloid protein from

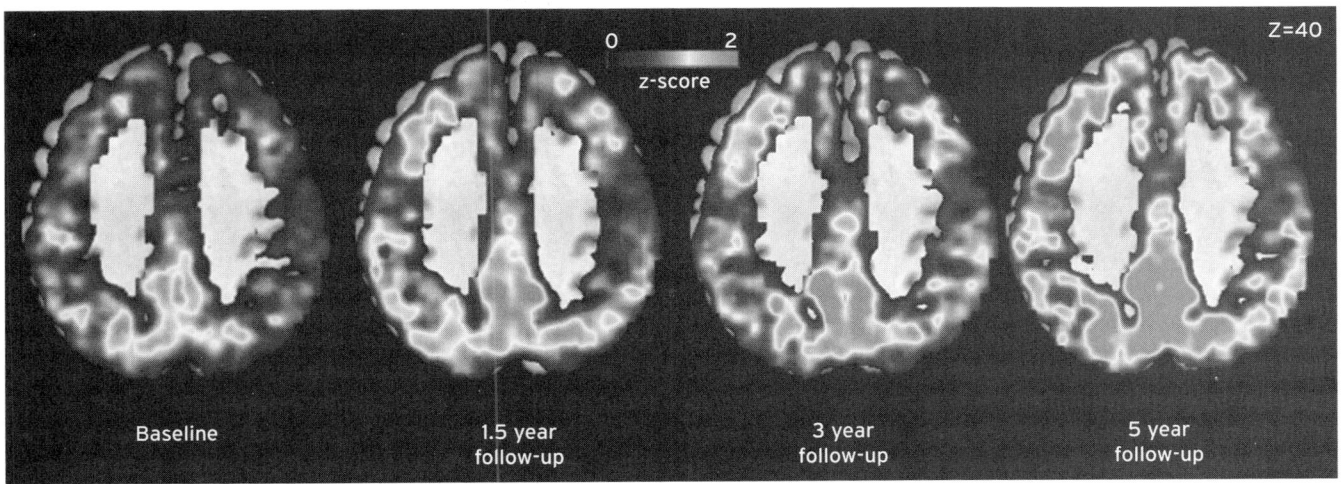

Figure 62.2 Longitudinal PET amyloid imaging of an individual subject who progressed from healthy to dementia. (See color insert.)

early stages (i.e., elderly cognitively normal controls) to symptomatic phases of the disease (Jack et al., 2010; Villain et al., 2012; Villemagne et al., 2011) (see Fig. 62.2).

Amyloid PET may have substantial clinical utility in differential diagnosis of established dementia, particularly in younger individuals in whom the prognosis and clinical management would differ depending on the underlying pathology. For example, the underlying pathology of FTLD does not involve Aβ, and amyloid PET is reported to be negative in clinical FTLD that has been confirmed at autopsy (Rabinovici et al., 2011). Other entities in the differential diagnosis of dementia that could potentially be informed by amyloid PET include late life depression or other psychiatric disorder with cognitive impairment, prion disease (Villemagne et al., 2009) and semantic dementia with tauopathy (Drzezga et al., 2008). The situation for parkinsonian dementing syndromes is somewhat more complex, because amyloid deposition is a common but not universal feature of DLB, and may or may not be seen in Parkinson's disease with dementia (Gomperts et al., 2008). Similarly, posterior cortical atrophy (Migliaccio et al., 2009), progressive aphasia (Rabinovici et al., 2008) and corticobasal syndrome (Rabinovici et al., 2011) present substantial clinical and histopathological heterogeneity and may not at present be distinguishable with amyloid PET.

SUMMARY AND LIMITATIONS OF AMYLOID IMAGING

Amyloid PET is an emerging technology and the FDA approved an amyloid radiotracer, Florbetapir F18, in April of 2012. At the time of this writing (mid-2012), amyloid PET has not been widely deployed in clinical practice. Whatever clinical value that could be expected is entirely dependent upon the availability of good quality images and accurate interpretation. Although clinical FDG PET scanning is generally available for nonbrain indications, experience with brain imaging is quite variable and depends on local circumstances.

Since essentially no one is free of risk for developing amyloid deposition, the clinical utility of amyloid PET could theoretically extend to nearly any circumstance in which the underlying basis of suspected neurodegenerative disease could be Aβ. However, the high cost of PET and its uncertain impact on clinical management have limited enthusiasm for widespread adoption of (both FDG and) amyloid PET when expert dementia specialist evaluation is available. While utility at this time remains to be precisely defined, the availability of disease modifying AD therapy will almost certainly change the level of demand. At present, appropriate use criteria are still being discussed and refined, but would optimally integrate amyloid PET technology into the existing framework of dementia evaluation, so that amyloid status can be placed in the appropriate context of medical, neurological, neuropsychological, and neuroimaging data.

ADNI AND STANDARDIZATION OF NEUROIMAGING BIOMARKERS

The successful incorporation of neuroimaging biomarkers into multi-site clinical trials has relied upon unprecedented levels of collaboration across the major equipment manufacturers to identify approaches that would yield consistency sufficient to provide meaningful enrichment and outcome measures. Much of the groundwork for these efforts was provided through the Alzheimer's Disease Neuroimaging Initiative (ADNI). The ADNI included an intensive preparatory phase to develop and assess image preprocessing steps that would enhance longitudinal stability of the measures. Variability across imaging sites, manufacturers, and equipment upgrades remains a source of noise in multi-site imaging studies, but the preparatory phase of ADNI and its cross-institutional collaborative efforts were critical to establishing the potential for the incorporation of neuroimaging biomarkers in large-scale clinical trials, which is already nearly universal. As of April 2012, 298 papers were published or in press using the ADNI study open access data, and the image repository had dispensed more than one million image downloads (http://www.adni-info.org/scientists/Pdfs/09_Green_Data_and_Publications.pdf). Since the initial ADNI study, a number of spinoff and continuation studies

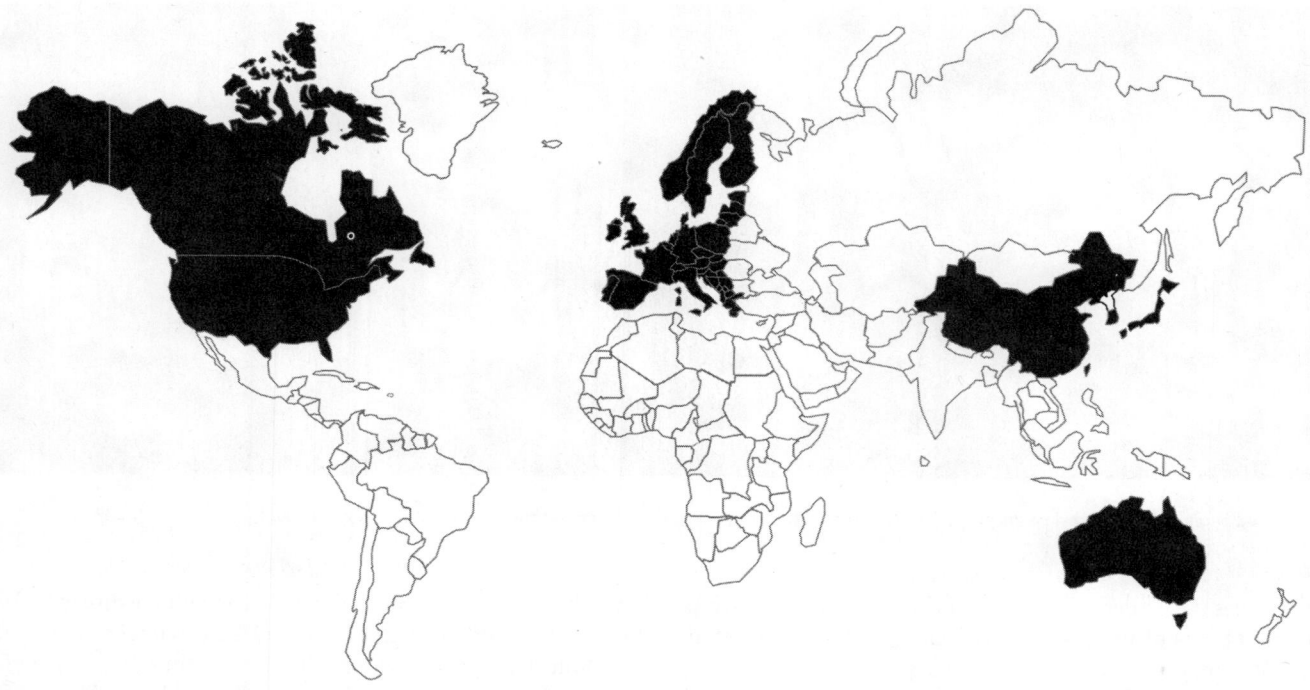

Figure 62.3 Map representation of worldwide studies examining biomarkers of AD. Multisite imaging and biofluid biomarker studies are planned or underway in Europe, China, Taiwan, South Korea, Japan, and Australia. These studies were influenced by the pivotal ADNI study in North America. (Source: World map template from http://presentationmagazine.com.)

have begun within and beyond the field of AD. As further testament to the success and influence of the study, a number of international efforts have begun that have been modeled on the methods of ADNI (Fig. 62.3).

ADDED VALUE OF BIOMARKERS IN COMBINATION

A significant advance attributable to ADNI and its readily available dataset is the more complete description of the regional structural and metabolic changes associated with AD, a finding that has been consistent across a number of analysis approaches. Results from ADNI have suggested that structural, metabolic, and amyloid biomarkers may be used in a complementary manner, given a putative temporal progression of biomarker positivity across the development of the disease (Jack et al., 2010). Such hypothesized progression of disease markers in typical, late onset, AD remains, as yet, unsupported through directed experimentation and therefore highly controversial, but several studies that have examined a combination of biomarkers for predicting progression of symptoms toward dementia have found them to provide additive information that may be related to differential sensitivity and dynamic changes that vary with disease stage. Specifically, it appears that amyloid deposition is detectable 10–20 years before the onset of symptoms, whereas tau positivity within the CSF and vMRI changes are relatively concurrent with cognitive changes detectable with specialized neuropsychological testing (see, e.g., Heister et al., 2011; Bateman et al., 2012). Thus, while amyloid positivity suggests that a patient is at higher risk for development of AD, atrophy or hypometabolism suggests that

the patient has entered the neurodegenerative stage of disease and is at risk for imminent clinical decline (Fig. 62.4).

The apparent complementary and differential disease-stage sensitivity of amyloid testing and vMRI or FDG PET provides additional leverage for clinical trial design, such that amyloid testing can be incorporated at screening to enrich the trial with subjects that have objective evidence of the targeted disease (or even the targeted protein), and baseline vMRI or FDG PET can provide complementary information about disease stage. Further, the imaging studies provide information that is relatively independent from and orthogonal to the cognitive complaint that led to subject selection, whereas cognitive measures provide information that overlaps with complaint and so could yield positive results even for etiologies that are not neurodegenerative. Consistent with this, studies using ADNI data have shown remarkable power advantages for enrichment based on baseline atrophy that could not have been achieved using any of the available cognitive measures from ADNI (McEvoy et al., 2010). As such, quantitative PET and MRI neuroimaging show promise for enriching clinical trials of prodromal AD with individuals likely to progress to AD and to decline in the period of study (Jack et al., 2008; Kovacevic et al., 2009; McEvoy et al., 2009).

In addition to potential usages in clinical trial enrichment, vMRI and amyloid biomarkers appear to provide complementary secondary outcome measures when acquired across time. Neuroimaging of brain structure through vMRI provides a measure that does not vary based on day-to-day fluctuations in the cognitive abilities of subjects that are caused by wakefulness, medication effects, motivation, and the like, and it has been shown to be less variable across time than cognitive

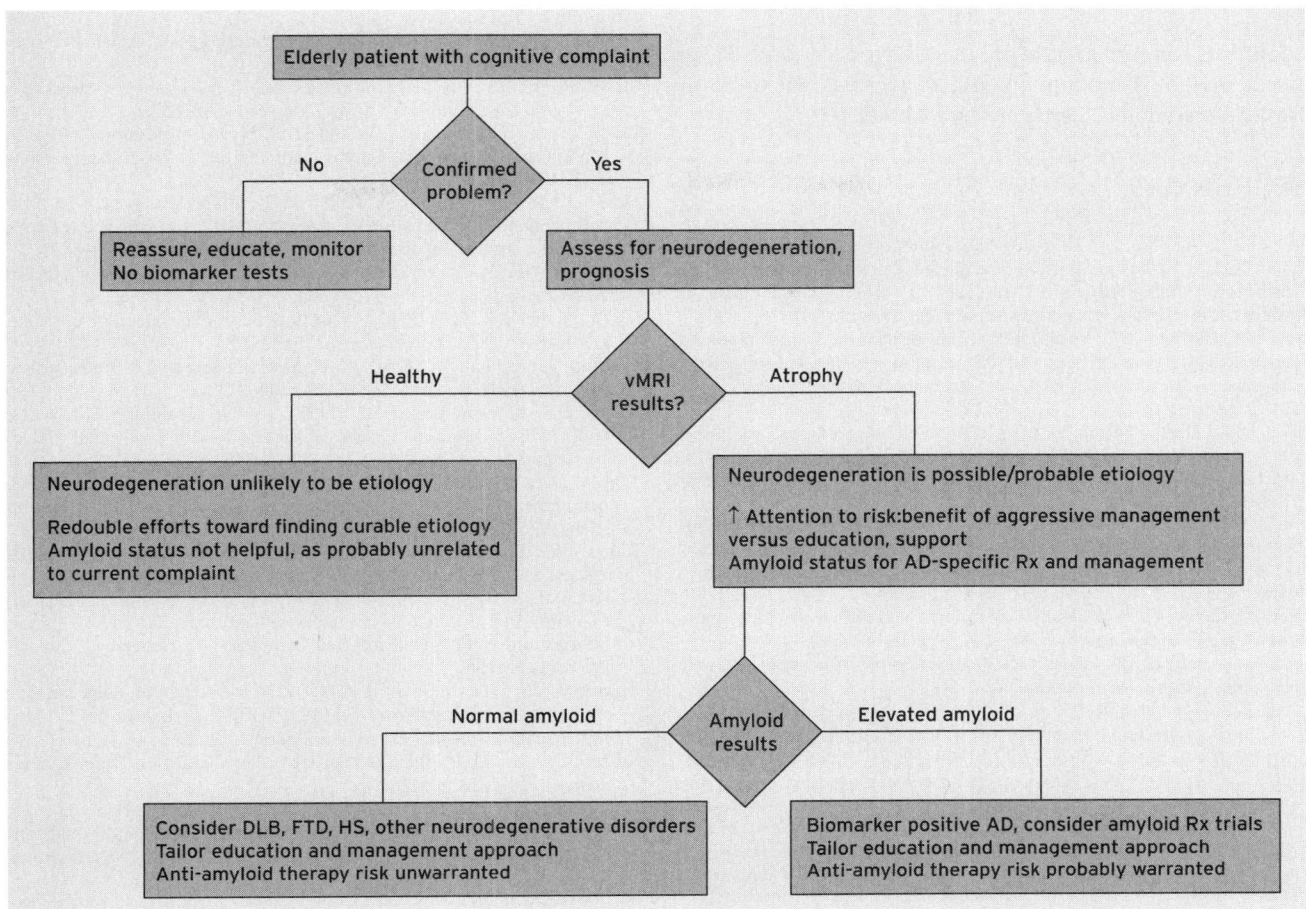

Figure 62.4 *Example decision tree presenting one approach to incorporating vMRI and amyloid biomarkers in clinical practice. HS, Hippocampal sclerosis. (McEvoy, L.K., & Brewer, J.B. (2012). Biomarkers for the clinical evaluation of the cognitively impaired elderly: amyloid is not enough. Imag Med, 4(3), 14.)*

measures (Weiner et al., 2012). Amyloid measures, though less sensitive to disease progression, may support putative effects of the therapy on disease pathology. The combination of regional amyloid measures with regional measures of brain atrophy may be especially powerful, because changes in amyloid burden can be colocalized with structural neuroimaging to examine interactions between amyloid and atrophy as well as a study drug's effects on each. Neuroimaging biomarkers might therefore support claims that a medication's effect on cognition is likely due to halted neurodegeneration or reduction of pathological burden rather than due to a brief symptomatic benefit.

CONCLUSIONS

Neuroimaging in the assessment of the elderly with cognitive impairment has changed from its previously limited role, in ruling out discrete lesions, to an integral role, in quantitatively assessing the cardinal components of neurodegeneration, neural dysfunction, and pathological burden observable in AD. Both MRI and PET benefit from wide flexibility in application, given the various anatomical, functional, and pathological features that might be assessed with each. The path toward clinical application was guided primarily by large scale, multisite

pharmaceutical trials, in which a more direct assessment of the effects of therapies was sought. Such efforts demonstrated the feasibility of obtaining these measures across sites in clinical practice, though a great deal of work remains to determine how best to integrate the information into clinical assessment, and how each can be used to inform predictive prognosis and guide management in individual patients (Brewer, 2009). Though publicly accessible databases of clinical trial enrollees have assisted in these efforts, the recent availability of highly standardized acquisition techniques and FDA-approved quantitative imaging approaches will allow such research to proceed in the unselected populations encountered in clinical practice.

DISCLOSURES

Dr. Brewer is supported by NINDS K02 NS067427, NIA U01 AG10483, NIA P50 AG005131, NIA R01 AG034062. He is an investigator for and receives research funds from Janssen Alzheimer Immunotherapy. He also has received research funds from General Electric Medical Foundation; holds stock options in Cortechs Labs., Inc; and has served on advisory boards for Elan, Avanir, Bristol-Myers-Squibb, and Lilly Biomarker Business Unit.

Dr. Sepulcre has no conflicts of interest to disclose.

Dr. Johnson has served as a site investigator for Avid, Pfizer, Janssen, Bristol-Myers-Squibb, and as a consultant to Bayer, Bristol-Myers-Squibb, Genzyme, and Siemens.

REFERENCES

Albert, M.S., DeKosky, S.T., et al. (2011). The diagnosis of mild cognitive impairment due to Alzheimer's disease: recommendations from the National Institute on Aging-Alzheimer's Association workgroups on diagnostic guidelines for Alzheimer's disease. *Alzheimers Dement.* 7(3):270–279.

Arnold, S.E., Hyman, B.T., et al. (1991). The topographical and neuroanatomical distribution of neurofibrillary tangles and neuritic plaques in the cerebral cortex of patients with Alzheimer's disease. *Cereb. Cortex* 1(1):103–116.

Bacskai, B.J., Hickey, G.A., et al. (2003). Four-dimensional multiphoton imaging of brain entry, amyloid binding, and clearance of an amyloid-beta ligand in transgenic mice. *Proc. Natl. Acad. Sci. USA* 100(21):12462–12467.

Bateman, R.J., Xiong, C., et al. (2012). Clinical and biomarker changes in dominantly inherited Alzheimer's disease. *N. Engl. J. Med.* 367(9):795–804.

Braak, H., and Braak, E. (1991). Neuropathological stageing of Alzheimer-related changes. *Acta Neuropathol.* 82(4):239–259.

Brewer, J.B. (2009). Fully-automated volumetric MRI with normative ranges: translation to clinical practice. *Behav. Neurol.* 21(1):21–28.

Brown, G.G., Perthen, J.E., et al. (2007). A primer on functional magnetic resonance imaging. *Neuropsychol. Rev.* 17(2):107–125.

Buckner, R.L., Sepulcre, J., et al. (2009). Cortical hubs revealed by intrinsic functional connectivity: mapping, assessment of stability, and relation to Alzheimer's disease. *J. Neurosci.* 29(6):1860–1873.

Caselli, R.J., Chen, K., et al. (2008). Correlating cerebral hypometabolism with future memory decline in subsequent converters to amnestic pre-mild cognitive impairment. *Arch. Neurol.* 65(9):1231–1236.

Chen, K., Langbaum, J.B., et al. (2010). Twelve-month metabolic declines in probable Alzheimer's disease and amnestic mild cognitive impairment assessed using an empirically pre-defined statistical region-of-interest: findings from the Alzheimer's Disease Neuroimaging Initiative. *Neuroimage* 51(2):654–664.

Chetelat, G., Desgranges, B., et al. (2003). Mild cognitive impairment: Can FDG-PET predict who is to rapidly convert to Alzheimer's disease? *Neurology* 60(8):1374–1377.

Cohen, A.D., Price, J.C., et al. (2009). Basal cerebral metabolism may modulate the cognitive effects of Abeta in mild cognitive impairment: an example of brain reserve. *J. Neurosci.* 29(47):14770–14778.

Davatzikos, C., Fan, Y., et al. (2008). Detection of prodromal Alzheimer's disease via pattern classification of magnetic resonance imaging. *Neurobiol. Aging* 29(4):514–523.

Dickerson, B.C., Bakkour, A., et al. (2009). The cortical signature of Alzheimer's disease: regionally specific cortical thinning relates to symptom severity in very mild to mild AD dementia and is detectable in asymptomatic amyloid-positive individuals. *Cereb. Cortex* 19(3):497–510.

Drzezga, A., Grimmer, T., et al. (2008). Imaging of amyloid plaques and cerebral glucose metabolism in semantic dementia and Alzheimer's disease. *Neuroimage* 39(2):619–633.

Engler, H., Forsberg, A., et al. (2006). Two-year follow-up of amyloid deposition in patients with Alzheimer's disease. *Brain* 129(Pt 11):2856–2866.

Fagan, A.M., Roe, C.M., et al. (2007). Cerebrospinal fluid tau/beta-amyloid(42) ratio as a prediction of cognitive decline in nondemented older adults. *Arch. Neurol.* 64(3):343–349.

Foster, N.L., Chase, T.N., et al. (1983). Alzheimer's disease: focal cortical changes shown by positron emission tomography. *Neurology* 33(8):961–965.

Fox, N.C., Freeborough, P.A., et al. (1996). Visualisation and quantification of rates of atrophy in Alzheimer's disease. *Lancet* 348(9020):94–97.

Furst, A.J., Rabinovici, G.D., et al. (2012). Cognition, glucose metabolism and amyloid burden in Alzheimer's disease. *Neurobiol. Aging* 33(2):215–225.

Gomperts, S.N., Rentz, D.M., et al. (2008). Imaging amyloid deposition in Lewy body diseases. *Neurology* 71(12):903–910.

Greicius, M.D., Srivastava, G., et al. (2004). Default-mode network activity distinguishes Alzheimer's disease from healthy aging: evidence from functional MRI. *Proc. Natl. Acad. Sci. USA* 101(13):4637–4642.

Heister, D., Brewer, J.B., et al. (2011). Predicting MCI outcome with clinically available MRI and CSF biomarkers. *Neurology* 77(17):1619–1628.

Ikonomovic, M.D., Klunk, W.E., et al. (2008). Post-mortem correlates of *in vivo* PiB-PET amyloid imaging in a typical case of Alzheimer's disease. *Brain* 131(Pt 6):1630–1645.

Jack, C.R., Jr. (2011). Alliance for aging research AD biomarkers work group: structural MRI. *Neurobiol. Aging* 32(Suppl 1):S48–S57.

Jack, C.R., Jr., Knopman, D.S., et al. (2010). Hypothetical model of dynamic biomarkers of the Alzheimer's pathological cascade. *Lancet Neurol.* 9(1):119–128.

Jack, C.R., Jr., Lowe, V.J., et al. (2008). 11C PiB and structural MRI provide complementary information in imaging of Alzheimer's disease and amnestic mild cognitive impairment. *Brain* 131(Pt 3):665–680.

Jagust, W., Gitcho, A., et al. (2006). Brain imaging evidence of preclinical Alzheimer's disease in normal aging. *Ann. Neurol.* 59(4):673–681.

Jagust, W., Reed, B., et al. (2007). What does fluorodeoxyglucose PET imaging add to a clinical diagnosis of dementia? *Neurology* 69(9):871–877.

Johnson, K.A., Fox, N.C., et al. (2012). Brain imaging in Alzheimer disease. *Cold Spring Harb. Perspect. Med.* 2(4):a006213.

Karow, D.S., McEvoy, L.K., et al. (2010). Relative capability of MR imaging and FDG PET to depict changes associated with prodromal and early Alzheimer disease. *Radiology* 256(3):932–942.

Klunk, W.E. (2011). Amyloid imaging as a biomarker for cerebral beta-amyloidosis and risk prediction for Alzheimer dementia. *Neurobiol. Aging* 32(Suppl 1):S20–S36.

Klunk, W.E., Engler, H., et al. (2004). Imaging brain amyloid in Alzheimer's disease with Pittsburgh Compound-B. *Ann. Neurol.* 55(3):306–319.

Knopman, D.S., DeKosky, S.T., et al. (2001). Practice parameter: diagnosis of dementia (an evidence-based review). Report of the Quality Standards Subcommittee of the American Academy of Neurology. *Neurology* 56(9):1143–1153.

Kovacevic, S., Rafii, M.S., et al. (2009). High-throughput, fully automated volumetry for prediction of MMSE and CDR decline in mild cognitive impairment. *Alzheimer Dis. Assoc. Disord.* 23(2):139–145.

Kramer, J.H., and Miller, B.L. (2000). Alzheimer's disease and its focal variants. *Semin. Neurol.* 20(4):447–454.

Langbaum, J.B., Chen, K., et al. (2009). Categorical and correlational analyses of baseline fluorodeoxyglucose positron emission tomography images from the Alzheimer's Disease Neuroimaging Initiative (ADNI). *Neuroimage* 45(4):1107–1116.

McDonald, C.R., McEvoy, L.K., et al. (2009). Regional rates of neocortical atrophy from normal aging to early Alzheimer disease. *Neurology* 73(6):457–465.

McEvoy, L.K., and Brewer, J.B. (2012). Biomarkers for the clinical evaluation of the cognitively impaired elderly: amyloid is not enough. *Imag. Med.* 4(3):14.

McEvoy, L.K., Edland, S.D., et al. (2010). Neuroimaging enrichment strategy for secondary prevention trials in Alzheimer disease. *Alzheimer Dis. Assoc. Disord.* 24(3):269–277.

McEvoy, L.K., Fennema-Notestine, C., et al. (2009). Alzheimer disease: quantitative structural neuroimaging for detection and prediction of clinical and structural changes in mild cognitive impairment. *Radiology* 251(1):195–205.

McKhann, G.M., Knopman, D.S., et al. (2011). The diagnosis of dementia due to Alzheimer's disease: recommendations from the National Institute on Aging-Alzheimer's Association workgroups on diagnostic guidelines for Alzheimer's disease. *Alzheimers Dement.* 7(3):263–269.

Migliaccio, R., Agosta, F., et al. (2009). Clinical syndromes associated with posterior atrophy: early age at onset AD spectrum. *Neurology* 73(19):1571–1578.

Minoshima, S., Giordani, B., et al. (1997). Metabolic reduction in the posterior cingulate cortex in very early Alzheimer's disease. *Ann. Neurol.* 42(1):85–94.

Oishi, K., Mielke, M.M., et al. (2011). DTI analyses and clinical applications in Alzheimer's disease. *J. Alzheimers Dis.* 26(Suppl 3):287–296.

Pearson, R.C., and Powell, T.P. (1989). The neuroanatomy of Alzheimer's disease. *Rev. Neurosci.* 2(2):101–122.

Rabinovici, G.D., Furst, A.J., et al. (2010). Increased metabolic vulnerability in early-onset Alzheimer's disease is not related to amyloid burden. *Brain* 133(Pt 2):512–528.

Rabinovici, G.D., Jagust, W.J., et al. (2008). Abeta amyloid and glucose metabolism in three variants of primary progressive aphasia. *Ann. Neurol.* 64(4):388–401.

Rabinovici, G.D., Rosen, H.J., et al. (2011). Amyloid vs FDG-PET in the differential diagnosis of AD and FTLD. *Neurology* 77(23):2034–2042.

Rabins, P.V., Blacker, D., et al. (2007). American Psychiatric Association practice guideline for the treatment of patients with Alzheimer's disease and other dementias, second edition. *Am. J. Psychiatry* 164(12 Suppl):5–56.

Raichle, M.E., MacLeod, A.M., et al. (2001). A default mode of brain function. *Proc. Natl. Acad. Sci. USA* 98(2):676–682.

Rocher, A.B., Chapon, F., et al. (2003). Resting-state brain glucose utilization as measured by PET is directly related to regional synaptophysin levels: a study in baboons. *Neuroimage* 20(3):1894–1898.

Scheltens, P., Leys, D., et al. (1992). Atrophy of medial temporal lobes on MRI in "probable" Alzheimer's disease and normal ageing: diagnostic value and neuropsychological correlates. *J. Neurol. Neurosurg. Psychiatry* 55(10):967–972.

Seeley, W.W., Crawford, R.K., et al. (2009). Neurodegenerative diseases target large-scale human brain networks. *Neuron* 62(1):42–52.

Seibert, T.M., and Brewer, J.B. (2011). Default network correlations analyzed on native surfaces. *J. Neurosci. Methods* 198(2):301–311.

Selkoe, D.J. (2006). The ups and downs of Abeta. *Nat. Med.* 12(7):758–759; discussion 759.

Sepulcre, J., Liu, H., et al. (2010). The organization of local and distant functional connectivity in the human brain. *PLoS Comput. Biol.* 6(6):e1000808.

Sepulcre, J., Sabuncu, M.R., et al. (2012). Network assemblies in the functional brain. *Curr. Opin. Neurol.* 25(4):384–391.

Sojkova, J., Driscoll, I., et al. (2011). *In vivo* fibrillar beta-amyloid detected using [11C]PiB positron emission tomography and neuropathologic assessment in older adults. *Arch. Neurol.* 68(2):232–240.

Sperling, R.A. (2012). Presentation of Resting fMRI results from DIAN. Alzheimer's Association International Conference, Vancouver, BC.

Sperling, R.A., Laviolette, P.S., et al. (2009). Amyloid deposition is associated with impaired default network function in older persons without dementia. *Neuron* 63(2):178–188.

Tran, T., Ross, B., et al. (2009). Magnetic resonance spectroscopy in neurological diagnosis. *Neurol. Clin.* 27(1):21–60, xiii.

Vemuri, P., Simon, G., et al. (2011). Antemortem differential diagnosis of dementia pathology using structural MRI: Differential-STAND. *NeuroImage* 55(2):522–531.

Villain, N., Chetelat, G., et al. (2012). Regional dynamics of amyloid-beta deposition in healthy elderly, mild cognitive impairment and Alzheimer's disease: a voxelwise PiB-PET longitudinal study. *Brain* 135(Pt7):2126–2139.

Villain, N., Fouquet, M., et al. (2010). Sequential relationships between grey matter and white matter atrophy and brain metabolic abnormalities in early Alzheimer's disease. *Brain* 133(11):3301–3314.

Villemagne, V.L., McLean, C.A., et al. (2009). 11C-PiB PET studies in typical sporadic Creutzfeldt-Jakob disease. *J. Neurol. Neurosurg. Psychiatry* 80(9):998–1001.

Villemagne, V.L., Pike, K.E., et al. (2011). Longitudinal assessment of Abeta and cognition in aging and Alzheimer disease. *Ann. Neurol.* 69(1):181–192.

Weiner, M.W., Veitch, D.P., et al. (2012). The Alzheimer's Disease Neuroimaging Initiative: a review of papers published since its inception. *Alzheimers Dement.* 8(Suppl 1):S1–S68.

63 | FLUID BIOMARKERS FOR ALZHEIMER'S DISEASE

ANNE M. FAGAN

Alzheimer disease (AD), the most common cause of dementia in the elderly, is a progressive and fatal neurodegenerative disorder that currently affects ~10.6 million people in the United States and Europe, with projected estimates reaching epidemic proportions (15.4 million) by the year 2030 (http://www.alz.org/national/documents/Facts_Figures_2011.pdf). Alzheimer's disease leads to a loss of memory, cognitive function, and ultimately independence, causing a heavy personal toll on patients and their families and a tremendous financial burden on health care systems globally. Indeed, the cost for care of AD patients in 2011 in the United States alone was over $183 billion, with projected annual costs increasing to $1 trillion by the year 2050 unless effective disease-modifying treatments are developed (Brookmeyer et al., 2011).

At present, a definitive diagnosis of AD can only be obtained at autopsy, requiring postmortem identification of the presence of two hallmark brain lesions: extracellular deposits of the β-amyloid peptide (amyloid plaques) and intraneuronal accumulations of hyperphosphorylated tau protein (neurofibrillary tangles). A clinical diagnosis of AD during life is based on guidelines established in 1984 by the National Institute of Neurological Disorders and Stroke—Alzheimer's Disease and Related Disorders Association (NINCDS-ADRDA) (McKhann et al., 1984). Unfortunately, the accuracy of current clinical AD diagnostic methods to predict pathologic diagnoses, though promising in some specialized dementia centers and clinics, is generally quite low; a recent study involving research participants ($N > 900$) evaluated in more than 30 Alzheimer's Disease Centers in the United States reports sensitivities ranging from 70.9% to 87.3% and specificities from 44.3% to 70.8% (depending on the specific histopathological diagnostic criteria employed) (Beach et al., 2012). This variable and inadequate performance is particularly troubling given the high level of expertise of the clinicians in such specialized AD centers. Diagnostic accuracies in secondary or primary care settings are likely even lower. Therefore, there is an urgent need for objective tests that can increase diagnostic accuracy in the shorter term, to aid in the design and evaluation of treatment efficacy of clinical trials, and in the longer term, for individual patient care.

Another imperative is early disease diagnosis. To date clinical trials of AD therapeutics have been unsuccessful in reversing, halting, or even slowing cognitive decline (see Chapters 65 and 66 in this book). A widely held belief is that some of this failure is because of the exclusive enrollment of individuals who already exhibit mild or moderate dementia, stages of AD that are accompanied by robust neuronal cell death.

At even earlier stages of the disease (very mild dementia and mild cognitive impairment due to AD), neuron loss in certain vulnerable brain regions is already severe (Price et al., 2001). Thus, it is critical to diagnose individuals at very early disease stages—and enroll them in clinical trials—in order to identify and apply therapies that have the best chance of preserving *normal* cognitive function.

ALZHEIMER'S DISEASE IS A CHRONIC DISEASE

The past several years have brought about an appreciation of the chronic, evolving nature of AD pathogenesis in large part because of advances in the AD biomarker field. The clinical construct of mild cognitive impairment (MCI) (Petersen et al., 1999), defined by impairments in cognitive abilities (compared with age-matched normative values) but that are below the threshold considered to be "dementia," has been hypothesized to represent a transition between healthy aging and AD dementia for those with AD pathology. Furthermore, clinicopathologic correlation studies support the notion of a long asymptomatic (preclinical) stage of the disease, with brain pathology estimated to begin years, even decades, prior to significant neuronal cell death and the appearance of *any* behavioral signs or symptoms, including MCI (Price et al., 2009). This appreciation has fueled a paradigm shift in therapeutic goals from disease "cure" (considered to be virtually impossible in the "end-stage" dementia stage associated with significant neuron loss), to halting, delaying, or even preventing cognitive decline due to AD pathology in the very early, even preclinical/presymptomatic, stages of the disease.

FLUID BIOMARKERS OF ALZHEIMER'S DISEASE

Given the current limitations of clinical diagnostic accuracy during the preclinical and early clinical stages of the disease, fluid (and imaging) biomarkers of AD pathologies are currently being sought. A biomarker is defined as a characteristic that is objectively measured and evaluated as an indicator of normal biological processes, pathogenic processes, or pharmacological responses to a therapeutic intervention (Biomarkers Definitions Working Group, 2001). As such, a biomarker can be used to guide clinical diagnosis (diagnostic), estimate disease risk or prognosis (prognostic), evaluate disease stage, and monitor progression and/or response to therapy (theragnostic) (Blennow et al., 2010). Because cerebrospinal fluid (CSF) is in direct contact with the extracellular space of the brain, biochemical changes in the brain are reflected in the CSF. Therefore, CSF is considered an optimal source for AD biomarkers. Indeed, analysis of CSF has yielded the most promising biomarker candidates and has also provided important insights into the temporal ordering of neuropathological changes during the normal course of the disease. Although CSF collection via lumbar puncture is considered by some an invasive procedure, its risks are similar to those of standard venipuncture when performed by a trained clinician. Furthermore, when using atraumatic (Sprotte) spinal needles, the incidence of postlumbar puncture headache is low (<2%) in older individuals, including those with mild to moderate AD (Peskind et al., 2009).

CEREBROSPINAL FLUID MARKERS OF CORE ALZHEIMER'S DISEASE PATHOLOGIES

Ideally, a core biomarker should reflect the underlying pathology of a disease. One of the challenges in AD (and most neurodegenerative diseases) is that biomarker validation requires comparison of fluid collection during life with neuropathological findings at autopsy (the current gold standard for diagnosis), and the time lag between CSF collection and autopsy makes such comparisons difficult. Because the 42 amino acid form of the Aβ peptide (Aβ42) and the tau protein are the primary components of amyloid plaques and neurofibrillary tangles, respectively, the levels of these proteins in CSF have been assessed as potential biomarkers of these core pathologic features. Normally Aβ is produced by neurons and subsequently cleared from brain interstitial fluid into the CSF and blood via passive and active transport processes. In AD, this normally soluble Aβ peptide aggregates to form insoluble, higher-order structures with β-pleated sheet confirmation, termed β-amyloid. The mechanism(s) by which this aggregation occurs in AD continues to be the focus of much research and likely involves alterations in the production and/or clearance of the peptide. In AD, levels of CSF Aβ42 have been shown to negatively correlate with amyloid plaque load at autopsy (Strozyk et al., 2003; Tapiola et al., 2009) as well as more recently in the living brain as determined by amyloid imaging using positron emission tomography (PET) with amyloid-binding compounds (Klunk, 2011; Villemagne & Rowe, 2012). The most widely accepted explanation for the reduced CSF level of Aβ42 in AD is that the aggregation of Aβ into plaques (and thus retention in the brain parenchyma) results in less Aβ being available to diffuse into the CSF.

Tau is a microtubule-associated protein expressed predominantly by neurons in the brain, where it functions to stabilize microtubules (among other less known functions). In AD, for unknown reasons, tau becomes hyperphosphorylated, thus impairing its ability to bind microtubules. As a result, tau forms structures called paired helical filaments, which aggregate to form intracellular neurofibrillary tangles. However, although the presence of tangles is required for the neuropathologic diagnosis of AD, they are also observed in other neurodegenerative conditions (i.e., tauopathies) such as frontotemporal lobar degeneration (FTLD). Tangles also increase in normal aging, albeit to a much lesser extent. Levels of CSF tau increase in AD (Blennow et al., 2010; Olsson et al., 2011; Sunderland et al., 2003), supporting the notion of it being a marker of tangles. However, levels also increase markedly (but transiently) in acute disorders such as stroke and brain trauma, with the magnitude of the increase positively correlating with the size of the damage (Hesse et al., 2001; Neselius et al., 2012; Stern et al., 2011). Levels are also highly elevated in Creutzfeldt-Jakob disease (CJD), a neurodegenerative disease involving rapid neuronal degeneration (VanHarten et al., 2011). These observations suggest that CSF tau is a more general marker of neuronal cell death. In contrast, levels of hyperphosphorylated tau species (p-tau) increase in AD but not in CJD (VanHarten et al., 2011) or in response to traumatic injury, thus supporting the idea of p-tau being a more specific marker of tangles in AD. Consistent with this notion, elevated CSF p-tau levels positively correlate with tangle pathology at autopsy (Buerger et al., 2006).

DIAGNOSTIC PERFORMANCE IN ALZHEIMER'S DISEASE DEMENTIA

Because the current criteria for the clinical diagnosis of AD requires the presence of dementia (McKhann, et al., 1984), the majority of biomarker studies have evaluated the performance of analytes in differentiating individuals with dementia believed to be due to AD from individuals with no dementia. In such analyses, elevated CSF levels of tau and p-tau (~300%) and reduced levels of Aβ42 (~50%) perform quite well, typically with sensitivities and specificities above 80% (Blennow et al., 2010). Combined analyses of these biomarkers (e.g., high levels of tau(s) in the presence of low Aβ42) perform better than any single biomarker on its own (Galasko et al., 1998; Maddalena et al., 2003). Importantly, CSF levels of these markers are normal in several other disorders that are often accompanied by cognitive impairment such as depression and Parkinson's disease (Blennow, 2004). CSF p-tau, in particular, can aid in the differentiation of AD from other dementias, such as frontotemporal dementia (FTD) and Lewy body dementia (LBD) (Hampel et al., 2004). However, the overall diagnostic performance of these CSF biomarkers to discriminate AD dementia from dementia caused by other pathologies is not optimal, likely reflecting the relative abundance of mixed pathologies in people presenting with dementia (Halliday et al., 2011), as well as inaccuracies in differential clinical diagnosis, especially at early disease stages.

DIAGNOSTIC PERFORMANCE IN PRODROMAL ALZHEIMER'S DISEASE

Development of disease-modifying drugs for AD likely requires testing in patient populations at very early disease stages. This critical interest in early diagnosis coupled with the appreciation of the long time period (estimated to be 10–20 years), during which AD pathology develops prior to clinical or cognitive symptoms of dementia, has fueled efforts to identify biomarkers of AD pathology prior to the onset of dementia. As a group, cohorts of individuals clinically diagnosed with MCI (defined by impairments in cognitive abilities compared with age-matched normative values but at levels that are below the threshold considered to be "dementia") typically display mean AD biomarker profiles of CSF Aβ42, tau and p-tau intermediate to those of cohorts with AD dementia and non-demented controls (Blennow et al., 2010; Weiner et al., 2012). However, there is significant overlap between individuals in the MCI and the other diagnostic groups, with approximately two-thirds displaying profiles consistent with AD pathology and one-third appearing in the normal range (Shaw et al., 2009). Such heterogeneity likely reflects differences in the underlying etiology of the cognitive impairments. Indeed, longitudinal studies in several international cohorts have shown that the combination of low CSF Aβ42 and high CSF tau and p-tau is highly predictive of which MCI cases will progress to AD dementia (Buchhave et al., 2012; Mattsson et al., 2009; Shaw et al., 2009; Visser et al., 2009), as well as their rate of cognitive decline (Snider et al., 2009). Such studies have prompted a proposal for the use of these CSF biomarkers to define (probabilistically) the underlying etiology of MCI cases in research as well as clinical settings (Albert et al., 2011) (see the following).

DIAGNOSTIC/PROGNOSTIC PERFORMANCE IN ASYMPTOMATIC (PRECLINICAL) ALZHEIMER'S DISEASE

The ultimate goal in AD therapy, to *prevent* cognitive decline (prior to irrevocable neuronal cell loss), provides a unique challenge because, by definition, clinical measures will be unable to identify individuals in this presymptomatic phase. Therefore, the use of validated disease biomarkers will be required for such patient identification. Clinicopathologic studies have shown that roughly one-third of cognitively normal elderly individuals who come to autopsy meet the histopathologic criteria for AD (Price et al., 2009). Data from more recent biomarker studies in large cohorts of cognitively normal individuals confirm this finding; a similar proportion of cognitively normal elders exhibit low levels of CSF Aβ42, and low levels correlate with the presence of cortical amyloid as detected by PET amyloid imaging (Fagan et al., 2009). A subset of cognitively normal elders also displays high levels of CSF tau and/or p-tau in the setting of reduced levels of Aβ42. Importantly, the combination of these pathologic markers (e.g., as estimated by the ratio of CSF tau(s)/Aβ42) has been shown to be highly predictive of future cognitive decline (to MCI as well as to AD dementia) within three to five years in these cognitively normal individuals (Fagan et al., 2007; Li et al., 2007). Recent data from members of families with known AD-causing mutations indicate that robust alterations in CSF Aβ42 and tau(s) can be observed in asymptomatic mutation carriers ~15 to potentially 25 years prior to their predicted age of symptom onset (defined as the age at which their parent developed symptoms) (Bateman et al., 2012). Because mutation carriers will go on to develop AD dementia with a virtual 100% certainty, these data strongly support the feasibility of using CSF markers as predictors of future dementia. The precise timing of such changes in the presymptomatic stage of the more common "sporadic" form of the disease is currently a topic of much investigation and will be important to consider if an AD diagnosis is ever to be made in the absence of cognitive symptoms (Sperling et al., 2011).

THE NEED FOR NOVEL BIOMARKERS

Despite the association between the levels of these established CSF analytes and underlying AD pathology, measures of biomarker accuracy for clinical diagnosis vary widely among studies. Such variability underscores the need for the development of additional biomarkers that will, either on their own or in combination with more established core markers, increase diagnostic accuracy. Novel biomarkers are also needed that will identify additional processes involved in AD pathogenesis, such as markers of neuroinflammation and early neuronal stress and dysfunction prior to overt cell death. Given that other neurodegenerative conditions (e.g., FTLD, LBD, vascular dementia [VaD], progressive supranuclear palsy, hippocampal sclerosis) can present with AD-like clinical symptoms, and individuals with AD frequently have comorbid pathologies, additional markers are needed that can aid in differential diagnosis and identify cases with mixed pathologies. Markers will also be required to define the pathophysiological stages of AD (in parallel with clinical stages; preclinical, MCI due to AD, AD dementia) and identify those individuals at increased risk of rapid cognitive decline.

The pathophysiology of AD is complex. In addition to the hallmark lesions of β-amyloid plaques and neurofibrillary tangles, AD pathology includes gliosis/neuroinflammation, oxidative damage, synaptic dysfunction/loss, and eventually neuronal cell death (Fig. 63.1; Table 63.1). Because the sophistication and power of proteomics technology has evolved tremendously over the last decade, proteins comprise the vast majority of novel candidate markers of such processes. Individually, many candidates show utility for differentiating cohorts of AD dementia cohorts and "controls," and many of these also show potential to improve upon the diagnostic accuracy of Aβ42, tau, and p-tau (Fagan and Perrin, 2012). A shorter list of candidates shows potential to track disease progression, and even some have been reported to predict rate of cognitive decline. Although a detailed discussion of all the individual candidates is beyond the scope of this chapter, general categorical mentioning is warranted.

Several promising CSF biomarkers are related to the processing of the amyloid precursor protein (APP) and the metabolism and amyloidogenesis of Aβ itself; these include soluble fragments of APP, APP cleaving and transport enzymes, truncated and oligomeric Aβ species, and several Aβ-binding proteins. As potential markers of tangles, levels of tau species that are phosphorylated at different amino acid residues (e.g., serine 231 vs. 181) are also being explored, especially for differential diagnosis. Potential CSF markers of synapse loss and/or neurodegeneration include several members of the granin family of dense core vesicle proteins, synaptic adhesion molecules and neuron-specific proteins. One neuron-specific marker that warrants discussion because of its great promise is visinin-like protein 1 (VILIP-1), which is a neuron-specific calcium sensor protein. Like tau, the level of VILIP-1 in the CSF is elevated in AD (Lee et al., 2008; Tarawneh et al., 2011) and, when combined with CSF Aβ42, is a strong predictor of future cognitive decline in very mild AD dementia/MCI and cognitively normal controls (Tarawneh et al., 2011; Tarawneh et al., 2012), potentially performing even better than the tau/Aβ42 ratio. Perhaps not unexpectedly, levels of CSF VILIP-1

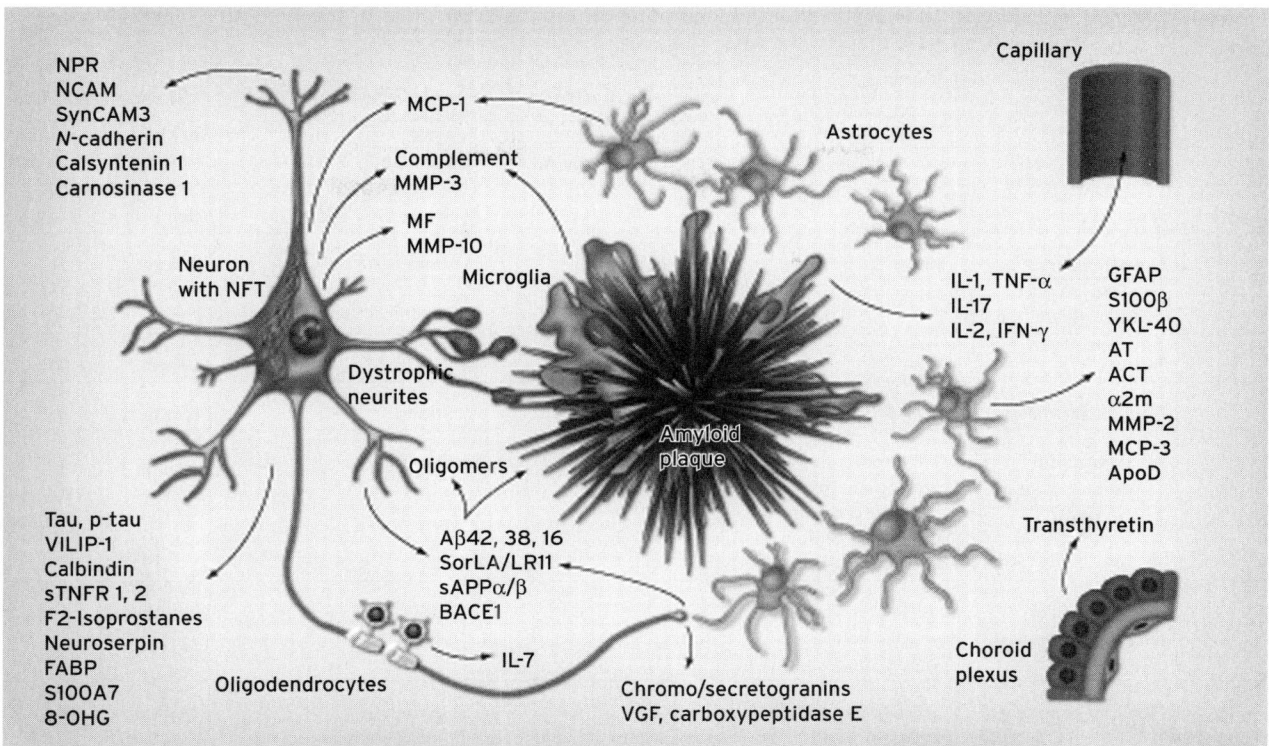

Figure 63.1 *Schematic histological representation of origins of upcoming and established CSF biomarkers. Synaptic adhesion molecules, other neuronal proteins, and dense core vesicle proteins generally decline in AD, perhaps reflecting synapse loss (upper left, bottom center, respectively). Other neuronal proteins (bottom left), including tau and p-tau, and oxidation products increase in AD and may reflect neuronal injury. Also produced by neurons, Aβ42 (center, left) preferentially oligomerizes and partitions into plaques, but other proteins associated with the processing of the amyloid precursor protein (APP), including shorter Aβ species, soluble fragments of APP, and secreted processing enzymes such as β-APP cleaving enzyme (BACE I), do not. Different subsets of neuroinflammatory molecules are secreted by each of the parenchymal cells represented here; neurons selectively produce macrophage migration inhibiting factor (MIF) and matrix metalloproteinase-10 (MMP-10) (upper center), but share responsibility with microglial cells for MMP-3 and factors of complement. Microglial cells themselves produce most of the other cytokines and chemokines (upper right), though many of these can also cross the blood brain barrier from the periphery. Among the neuroinflammatory mediators of greater significance as potential biomarkers, oligodendroglial cells produce IL-7 (lower left), and astrocytes produce MMP-2 and YKL-40 (center right). Astrocytes are also responsible for shedding some intrinsic proteins (glial fibrillary acidic protein [GFAP] and S100β) and for secreting many other miscellaneous proteins implicated in AD pathogenesis. Transthyretin (lower right), one of the most abundant proteins in the CSF, is produced principally by the choroid plexus. Not pictured are many other candidate biomarker molecules for which the cell(s) of origin are unknown (e.g., miRNAs), not specific (e.g., cystatin C), or too prolific (e.g., astrocyte products), prohibiting the inclusion of all their relevant secreted products. (Reprinted with permission from Fagan, A., and Perrin, R. (2012). Upcoming candidate cerebrospinal fuid biomarkers of Alzheimer's disease. Biomarkers Med, 6, 455–476.)*

are positively correlated with tau, and both are increased in response to stroke and acute traumatic brain injury (Laterza et al., 2006). Whether VILIP-1 provides diagnostic or prognostic value beyond that of tau in AD remains to be determined.

A broad array of neuroinflammatory molecules with known or hypothesized neurotoxic and/or neuroprotective roles have also been identified as potential AD CSF biomarkers; these include complement proteins, proteases and their inhibitors, cytokines and their receptors, chemokines, and markers of astrogliosis. Although neuroinflammation and gliosis are not specific to AD, markers of such inflammatory processes may be useful as part of a biomarker panel. Several apolipoproteins in CSF have shown AD-associated changes, some of which may be involved in Aβ metabolism and/or fibrillogenesis. Again, although not specific for AD, markers of pathological oxidative processes such as modified lipid species (e.g., F2-isoprostanes) and nucleic acids (e.g., 8-OHG), may have a role in early stage diagnosis, prognosis, and biomarker outcomes in clinical trials. "Metabolome" screens and surveys

of micro RNAs in CSF are also being investigated but are still in the method development phase.

PLASMA BIOMARKERS

There is widespread interest in identifying blood-based biomarkers of AD since blood is more easily obtained than CSF in routine clinical settings. Unfortunately, efforts to discover reliable AD biomarkers in blood have yielded little success, but it is unclear whether this failure reflects the true biology of the disease or limitations of current analytical methods. The most obvious candidate, and hence the one most extensively examined, is plasma Aβ (see Table 63.1). Unfortunately, findings from the many published studies are contradictory (Mayeux and Schupf, 2011). Some groups report slightly higher plasma levels of either Aβ42 or Aβ40 in AD, although with broad overlap between AD and control groups, whereas most studies find no change. Some studies report that a high level of plasma Aβ42, or a high Aβ42/Aβ40 ratio, is an indicator

TABLE 63.1. Summary of fluid biomarker candidates and their potential uses as determined by the strength of empirical research support

	PATHOGENIC PROCESS	BIOMARKER	DIAGNOSTIC UTILITY		PROGNOSTIC UTILITY		THERAGNOSTIC UTILITY	
			RESEARCH SUPPORT	DIRECTION IN AD	RESEARCH SUPPORT	DIRECTION IN AD	RESEARCH SUPPORT	DIRECTION IN AD
CSF: core	Amyloid plaques	Aβ42	Strong	↓	Some	↓	Some	↓↑*
	Neurofibrillary tangles/ neurodegeneration	Tau	Strong	↑	Weak	↑	Some	↓
	Tangles	P-tau	Strong	↑	Weak	↑	Some	↓
	Plaques and Tangles	Tau/Aβ42	Strong	↑	Strong	↑	Not tested	n.a.
CSF: non-core	Aβ metabolism	APP fragments, APP cleaving enzymes/ transport proteins, Aβ-binding proteins, other Aβ species	Some	↓↑	Some	↑	Strong	↓↑*
	Synapse loss or neurodegeneration	Dense core vesicle, synaptic adhesion, neuron-specific proteins	Some strong	↓↑	Some strong	↑	Not tested	n.a.
	Neuroinflammation	Complement proteins, proteases and inhibitors, cytokines and receptors, chemokines, astrocyte proteins	Some/ exploratory	↓↑	Some	↑	Not tested	n.a.
	Oxidative stress	Oxidized lipids and nucleic acids	Some	↑	Some	↑	Some	↓
	Cellular metabolism	Metabolome	Some/ exploratory	↓↑	Not tested	n.a.	Not tested	n.a.
	Gene expression and/or RNA stability	Micro-RNAs (miRNAs)	Some/ exploratory	↓↑	Not tested	n.a.	Not tested	n.a.
Plasma/ serum	Aβ metabolism	Aβ40	Some	↓↑	Some	↑	Some strong	↓
		Aβ42	Some	↑	Some	↓↑	Some strong	↓
		Aβ42/Aβ40	Some	↑	Some	↑	Some	↓
	Various (panels)	Growth factors, signaling and inflammatory markers	Some/ exploratory	↓↑	Some/ exploratory	↓↑	Not tested	n.a.
	Autoimmunity	Autoantibodies	Strong/ exploratory	↓↑	Not tested	n.a.	Not tested	n.a.

* Direction is therapeutic agent-specific

of increased risk for future AD; however, other studies have reported the opposite. These discouraging results may be due to the fact that the majority of plasma Aβ is derived from peripheral tissues (especially platelets), and does not reflect brain Aβ turnover or metabolism. Observations of a lack of correlation between plasma Aβ species and brain amyloid load as determined by *in vivo* amyloid imaging (Fagan et al., 2009) are consistent with this notion. It is conceivable, however, that the binding of Aβ to various proteins in plasma may result in epitope masking and other analytical interference, thus impairing the ability of current assays to accurately measure Aβ levels in blood-derived samples. Alternate analytical methodologies are being explored.

Other studies have utilized hypothesis-driven approaches (such as screening with predetermined protein arrays) or exploratory proteome-based methods in plasma and serum from AD and control groups, as has been performed in CSF (see Table 63.1). Multivariate analyses of several defined panels have identified groups of proteins (notably growth factors and proteins involved in signaling or inflammation) that discriminate clinical groups (AD vs. controls) (Doecke et al., 2012; Hu et al., 2012; Nagele et al., 2011; O'Bryant et al., 2011; Ray et al., 2007) Unfortunately, some results have not been replicated, whereas others require additional validation in independent cohorts. Furthermore, the reported accuracies are inferior to those observed for the core AD CSF markers (Aβ42, tau, p-tau). Another more recent approach uses libraries of known peptides or, in a novel assay, synthetic, unnatural "peptoids," to screen serum samples from AD and control individuals for potential disease-related autoantibodies (Reddy et al., 2011). The reported diagnostic accuracies are impressive, rivaling those of the core CSF markers, although the results need to be replicated

in larger and better characterized cohorts before definitive conclusions can be drawn. Such studies are in progress.

POTENTIAL USE OF FLUID BIOMARKERS OF ALZHEIMER'S DISEASE

The field of AD biomarker research has made tremendous progress over the past decade, not only leading to more accurate disease diagnosis and prognosis in research participants, but also providing a window into the trajectories of neuropathologic changes over the normal course of the disease, especially during the long asymptomatic (presymptomatic, preclinical) phase. Results from many cross-sectional studies support a model in which dynamic reductions in CSF Aβ42 (indicative of the presence of amyloid plaques) occur early in the pathologic

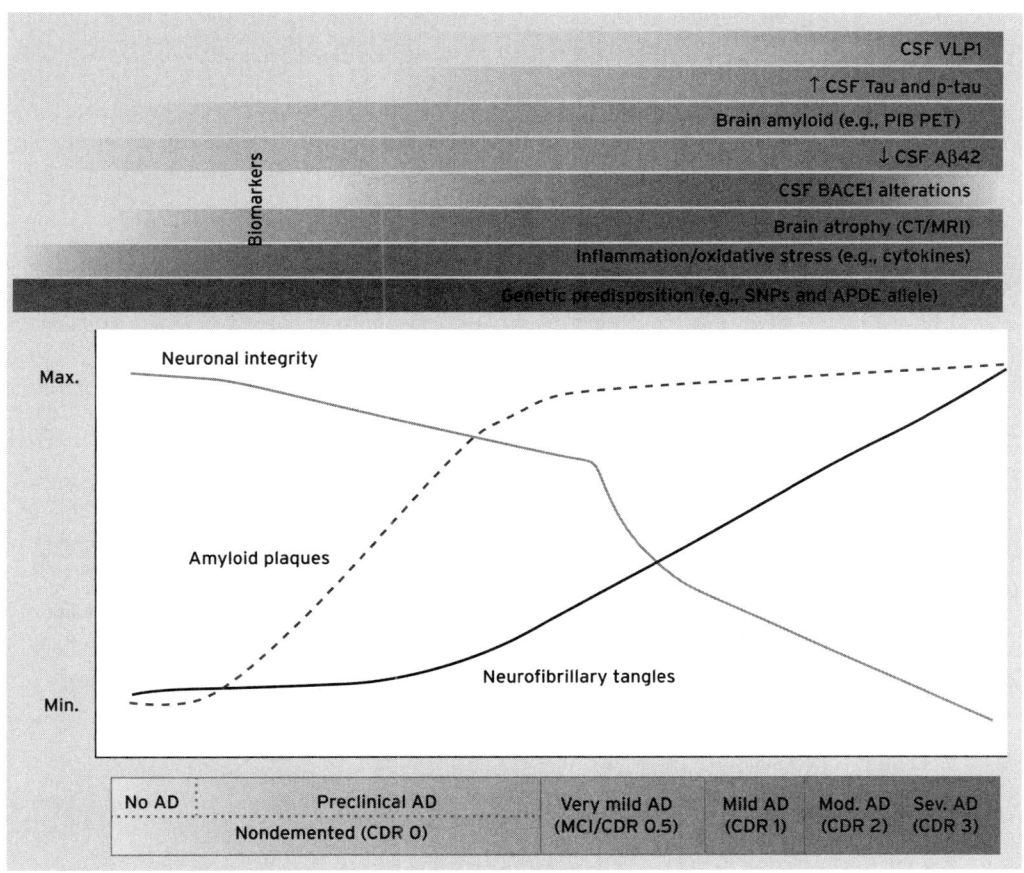

Figure 63.2 Hypothesized trajectory of AD pathologic changes as evidenced by CSF and imaging biomarkers. The clinical stages of AD, described as very mild dementia or mild cognitive impairment (MCI), mild, moderate, and severe, correspond to the Clinical Dementia Rating (CDR) scores of 0.5, 1, 2, and 3, respectively. These symptomatic stages are associated with abundant amyloid plaques (dashed line), the gradual accumulation of neurofibrillary tangles (dark gray line), and synaptic and neuronal loss in certain brain regions (light gray line). During the "preclinical" stage of AD (estimated to range from ~10–20 years), the Aβ42 peptide aggregates to form amyloid plaques in asymptomatic individuals (CDR 0) and is hypothesized to damage neuronal processes and synapses. Dementia onset is associated with significant neuronal cell death in vulnerable brain regions. These pathologic changes can be measured by biochemical examination of cerebrospinal fluid (CSF), and/or a variety of radiological imaging modalities (e.g., computed tomography [CT], magnetic resonance imaging [MRI], and amyloid imaging [PIB PET]). The most promising CSF biomarkers to date have been Aβ42 and tau species, which show diagnostic and prognostic utility. VILIP-1 as a potential marker of neuronal death and BACE 1 as an indicator of Aβ production warrant further study, as do panels of inflammatory markers and markers of oxidative stress. Genetic variations (e.g., single nucleotide polymorphisms [SNPs]) may also be considered biomarkers that allow the earliest possible estimation of risk. (Reprinted with permission from Fagan, A., and Holtzman, D. (2010). Cerebrospinal fluid biomarkers of Alzheimer's disease. Biomarkers Med, 4, 51–63.)

cascade (during the asymptomatic/preclinical phase) and do not change substantially during the subsequent symptomatic phase, whereas an elevation in CSF tau is a biomarker of downstream neurodegenerative pathologies that are dynamic later in the course of the disease, as people approach and move through the symptomatic phase (Jack et al., 2010; Perrin et al., 2009) (Fig. 63.2). Consistent with this model, cognitive decline is more closely related to biomarkers of neuronal injury than amyloid load. Investigation of longitudinal change in biomarkers within individuals over time, especially during middle-age, will be required to test this model and is currently underway.

Although measurements of CSF levels of Aβ42, tau, and p-tau in clinic patients can already be obtained by physicians, these measures are not part of the current clinical criteria for the diagnosis of AD dementia; however, this may soon change. The current clinical diagnostic criteria for AD were developed more than 25 years ago by the National Institute of Neurological and Communicative Disorders and Stroke and the Alzheimer's Disease and Related Disorders (NINCDS-ADRDA) Work Group (McKhann et al., 1984). The criteria depend largely on the exclusion of causes other than AD for dementia. These criteria state that a diagnosis of AD cannot be made until the patient has dementia, which is defined as "cognitive symptoms severe enough to interfere with social or occupational activities." The DSM-IV criteria, which are used for routine diagnosis, also require that a patient demonstrate dementia before a diagnosis of AD is possible (American Psychiatric Association, 2000). Given that dementia is the end-stage of the disease and disease-modifying therapies will likely have the most benefit if administered earlier in the disease process, new criteria for different stages of AD have recently been proposed by three National Institute on Aging and the Alzheimer Association Workgroups (Albert et al., 2011; McKhann et al., 2011; Sperling et al., 2011). Similar revisions have been proposed by others (Dubois et al., 2010). These criteria have been developed, in principle, to permit a diagnosis of AD in earlier disease stages, and involve assessment of cognition as well as biomarkers, including MRI, PET, and CSF markers, in order to increase the confidence of AD being the underlying etiology of a clinical impairment. More detailed guidelines are currently being discussed to establish if and how the use of biomarkers can be implemented in clinical practice, not only in the presence of dementia (Fig. 63.3) but at earlier disease stages, such as MCI (Fig. 63.4), or even before the development of any dementia symptoms (Fig. 63.5).

In the shorter (and present) term, biomarkers are being used in AD secondary prevention trials of potential disease-modifying therapies. Levels of CSF Aβ42, tau, and/or p-tau are being used to: (1) enrich the number of patients who actually have underlying AD pathology (diagnostic), (2) stratify patients according to the presence and/or the amount of underlying pathology (prognostic), and (3) assess therapeutic target engagement and monitor the effects of treatment on downstream pathogenic events (theragnostic). Not only will this approach result in an overall reduction in required patient numbers, trial duration, and cost, but it is also expected to provide information particularly suitable for making go/no-go decisions whether to move candidate therapies forward into large and expensive Phase II and III trials.

CHALLENGES AND FUTURE DIRECTIONS

The AD biomarker field is faced with several challenges it must overcome in order to move promising analytes into clinical practice. From a methodological perspective, biomarker

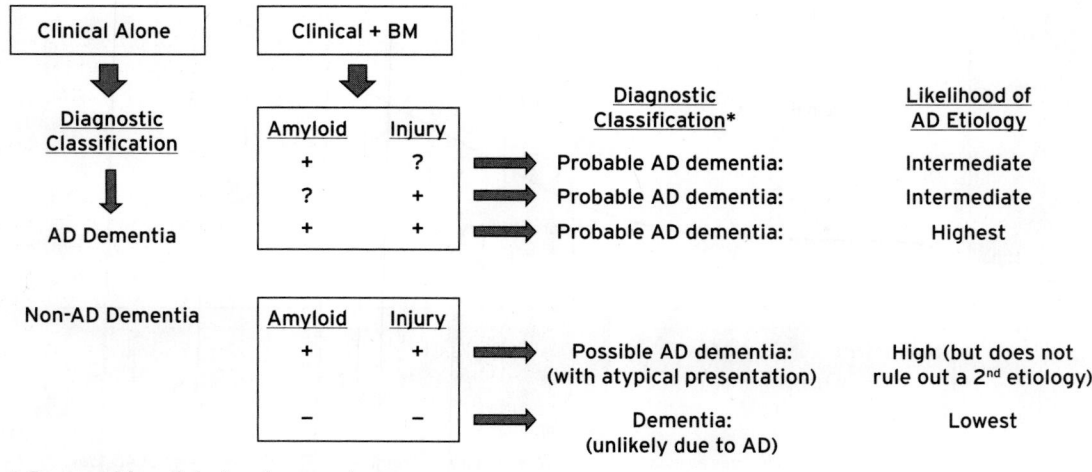

Figure 63.3 Proposed diagnostic classifications of AD dementia according to clinical criteria alone compared with clinical criteria plus AD pathology-related biomarkers. The addition of biomarker (BM) information to clinical evaluation permits an assessment of probability (likelihood) that dementia symptoms are caused by underlying AD pathobiological processes. Positive amyloid markers include low levels of CSF Aβ42 and/or positive amyloid PET. Positive neuronal injury markers include high levels of CSF tau, glucose hypometabolism via FDG-PET, and/or atrophy via structural MRI. Still evolving are standards for determining biomarker positivity, evaluations of potential rankings of the various fluid and imaging markers for identifying underlying disease processes, and decision making in cases of indeterminant or conflicting fluid and imaging markers within a biomarker category. These criteria are proposed for clinical and research use. (From McKhann, G., Knopman, D., Chertkow, H., Hyman, B., Jack, C., Kawas, C., et al. (2011). The diagnosis of dementia due to Alzheimer's disease: Recommendations from the National Institute on Aging and the Alzheimer's Association Workgroup. Alzheimers Dement, 7, 263–269.)

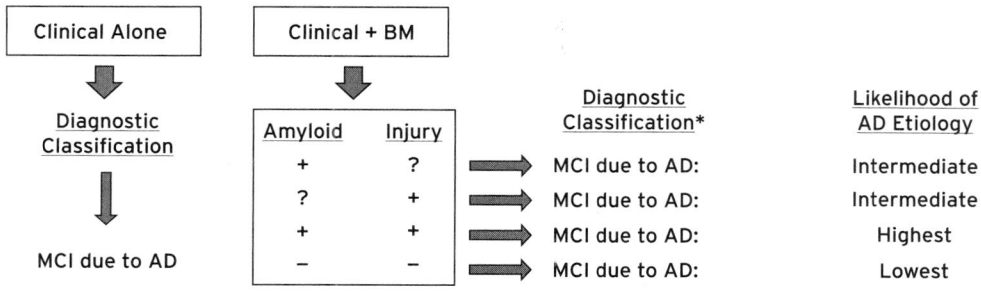

Figure 63.4 *Proposed diagnostic classifications of Mild Cognitive Impairment (MCI) according to clinical criteria alone compared with clinical criteria plus AD pathology-related biomarkers. The addition of biomarker (BM) information to clinical evaluation permits an assessment of probability (likelihood) that MCI is caused by underlying AD pathobiological processes. Positive amyloid markers include low levels of CSF Aβ42 and/or positive amyloid PET. Positive neuronal injury markers include high levels of CSF tau, glucose hypometabolism via FDG-PET, and/or atrophy via structural MRI. Still evolving are standards for determining biomarker positivity, evaluations of potential rankings of the various fluid and imaging markers for identifying underlying disease processes, and decision making in cases of indeterminant or conflicting fluid and imaging markers within a biomarker category. These criteria are proposed for clinical and research use. (From Albert, M., DeKosky, S., Dickson, D., Dubois, B., Feldman, H., Fox, N., et al. (2011). The diagnosis of mild cognitive impairment due to Alzheimer's disease: Recommendations from the National Institute on Aging-Alzheimer's Association workgroups on diagnostic guidelines for Alzheimer's disease. Alzheimers Dement, 7, 270–279.)*

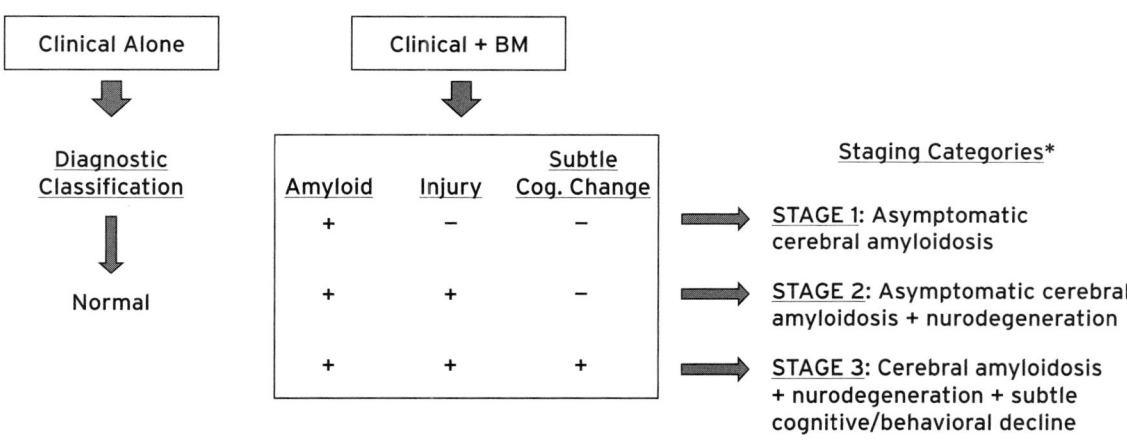

Figure 63.5 *Proposed staging of preclinical AD according to clinical criteria alone compared with clinical criteria plus AD pathology-related biomarkers. Use of biomarker (BM) information in asymptomatic individuals permits an assessment of the presence of AD pathobiological processes. Positive amyloid markers include low levels of CSF Aβ42 and/or positive amyloid PET. Positive neuronal injury markers include high levels of CSF tau, glucose hypometabolism via FDG-PET, and/or atrophy via structural MRI. Subtle cognitive change awaits definition but may include declines in episodic memory and/or non-memory cognitive domains. Still evolving are standards for determining biomarker positivity, evaluations of potential rankings of the various fluid and imaging markers for identifying underlying disease processes, and decision making in cases of indeterminant or conflicting fluid and imaging markers within a biomarker category. It is important to note that these criteria are proposed for research use only. (From Sperling, R., Aisen, P., Beckett, L., Bennett, D., Craft, S., Fagan, A., et al. (2011). Toward defining the preclinical stages of Alzheimer's disease: Recommendations from the National Institute on Aging and the Alzheimer Association Workgroup. Alzheimer's Dement, 7, 280–292.)*

candidates must be validated in large, well-characterized research cohorts, with care taken to evaluate the potential impact of important AD-related covariates such as age, gender, and *APOE* genotype (the strongest genetic risk factor for AD). For the most part, this has been accomplished for the core CSF markers Aβ42, tau, and p-tau. However, protocol and assay standardization for these analytes must still be achieved in order to maximize biomarker sensitivity and reliability. For example, because potential diurnal variations in CSF Aβ levels have been reported (Bateman et al., 2007), sample collection and processing procedures must be standardized. In addition, significant between-assay and within-assay performance inconsistencies must be overcome (Mattsson et al., 2011), and worldwide standardization efforts toward this goal are currently underway. Such assays need to eventually be transformed into platforms with high-throughput capabilities. Given the long preclinical stage of AD, biomarker validation should define sensitivity and specificity (and associated positive and negative predictive values) for underlying AD pathology, not merely clinical diagnosis that is often inaccurate. To date, very few studies have been able to correlate biomarkers in antemortem samples with results of histologic postmortem examination, and the time interval between the two evaluations can be large. Thus, cross-sectional studies employing only clinical measures must be large to compensate for the loose correlation between functional and pathological decline. Methods to image neurofibrillary tangles and inflammatory responses *in vivo* are currently being developed and will be very informative for providing pathologic validation for CSF markers (Fodero-Tavoletti et al., 2011). Evaluation of biomarker utility for differential diagnosis in cohorts with known underlying non-AD pathologies (FTLD, LBD, VaD, etc.) is also needed. Characterizing the change in biomarker profiles within individuals with disease progression, both in terms of underlying pathology as well as the severity of clinical symptoms, will be important for disease staging purposes, and large, longitudinal AD biomarker studies are currently underway in the United States and abroad. It is likely that changes in analyte levels within individuals over time may be more useful as biomarkers than baseline measures alone.

It is predicted that combinations of biomarkers will prove most useful for disease diagnosis (presence vs absence of AD pathology) and prognosis (predicting cognitive decline), within modalities or between modalities (e.g., fluids and imaging) (Perrin et al., 2009). Ongoing studies that collect multiple types of biomarker data will be critical for that assessment. The combination of CSF Aβ42 and tau (total and/or phosphorylated tau species) will likely remain the essential biomarker panel to aid in AD diagnosis and prognosis because they represent core features of AD pathology. However, markers of more general neurodegenerative processes (e.g., neuroinflammation, synaptic loss/dysfunction) may eventually complement CSF Aβ42 and tau(s) for AD diagnosis, prognosis, and staging. Novel markers of other neurodegenerative pathologies (e.g., Lewy bodies, TDP-43-inclusions, α-synuclein inclusions, etc.) are still needed to aid in differential diagnosis as well as for diagnosing mixed dementias. Specific markers for non-AD dementias have received somewhat less research attention owing to limited CSF collections, but several efforts focused on LBD and FTD are underway and will facilitate such biomarker discovery. It remains to be determined whether any viable plasma biomarkers will emerge in the near future, but many research groups are actively engaged in the search, given the clinical appeal of diagnostic blood tests.

CONCLUSIONS

The AD field is experiencing an exciting evolution, both in its appreciation of the dynamic nature of the disease and the development of therapeutic strategies aimed at truly modifying the underlying disease pathogenic processes (as opposed to simply ameliorating dementia symptoms), and biomarkers have been at the forefront of these paradigm shifts. The core CSF analytes, Aβ42, tau, and p-tau, have not only withstood the test of time in identifying individuals with AD dementia, but they have also been shown to strongly predict the development of future cognitive decline in individuals at very early, predementia stages. Importantly, the AD biomarker signature of low CSF Aβ42 and high tau/p-tau can be detected in individuals while they are still cognitively normal, thus providing a potential window for therapeutic interventions aimed at *preventing* cognitive decline, not just delaying or halting it once impairments are already clinically apparent. The field is also actively researching novel biomarker candidates (in CSF and plasma/serum) that will aid in discriminating AD from non-AD neurodegenerative diseases (differential diagnosis) and those that will identify additional processes involved in AD pathogenesis (e.g., markers of neuroinflammation and early neuronal stress and dysfunction prior to overt cell death). Multiplexed panels of biomarkers will likely be informative for pathophysiological disease staging (in parallel with clinical stages; preclinical, MCI due to AD, AD dementia) and identifying individuals at increased risk of rapid cognitive decline. A better understanding of the temporal trajectories of disease pathogenic processes will inform the design of clinical trials and the evaluation of efficacy of proposed disease-modifying therapies. Eventually the hope is to bring validated biomarkers to the clinic in order to increase diagnostic accuracy in symptomatic individuals and prognostic accuracy in individuals at early disease stages and perhaps even prior to any cognitive symptoms. Realization of this goal requires worldwide standardization of biomarker protocols, consensus among researchers and clinicians regarding the clinical utility of assessing biomarkers in patient care settings, and eventually the endorsement and adoption of such procedures and practices into global health care systems. Given the large and expanding aging population, we cannot afford to wait.

DISCLOSURES

Dr. Fagan is supported by grants from the National Institute of Aging of the National Institutes of Health (P01 AG03991, P01 AG026276, and U01 AG032438), the Hope Center for Neurological Disorders, the Alzheimer's Association, and the DIAN Pharma Consortium. She is a member of the Alzheimer's Disease CSF Biomarker Development Advisory Board for Roche and the U.S. Alzheimer's Disease Advisory Board for Lilly USA. No conflicts of interest exist.

REFERENCES

Albert, M., DeKosky, S., et al. (2011). The diagnosis of mild cognitive impairment due to Alzheimer's disease: recommendations from the National Institute on Aging-Alzheimer's Association workgroups on diagnostic guidelines for Alzheimer's disease. *Alzheimers Dement.* 7:270–279.

American Psychiatric Association. (2000). Diagnostic and Statistical Manual of Mental Disorders, Text Revision, 4th Edition. Washington, DC: Author.

Bateman, R., Wen, G., et al. (2007). Fluctuations of CSF amyloid-beta levels: implications for a diagnostic and therapeutic biomarker. *Neurology* 68:666–669.

Bateman, R., Xiong, C., et al. (2012). Clinical, cognitive, and biomarker changes in the Dominantly Inherited Alzheimer Network. *NEJM* 367:795–804.

Beach, T., Monsell, S., et al. (2012). Accuracy of the clinical diagnosis of Alzheimer disease at National Institute on Aging Alzheimer Disease Centers, 2005–2010. *J. Neuropathol. Exp. Neurol.* 71:266–273.

Biomarkers Definitions Working Group. (2001). Biomarkers and surrogate endpoints: preferred definitions and conceptual framework. *Clin. Pharmacol. Ther.* 69:89–95.

Blennow, K. (2004). Cerebrospinal fluid protein biomarkers for Alzheimer's disease. *NeuroRx* 1:213–225.

Blennow, K., Hampel, H., et al. (2010). Cerebrospinal fluid and plasma biomarkers for Alzheimer's disease. *Nature Rev. Neurol.* 6:131–144.

Brookmeyer, R., Evans, D., et al. (2011). National estimates of the prevalence of Alzheimer's disease in the United States. *Alzheimers Dement.* 1:61–73.

Buchhave, P., Minthon, L., et al. (2012). Cerebrospinal fluid levels of β-amyloid 1–42, but not of tau, are fully changed already 5 to 10 years before the onset of Alzheimer Dementia. *Arch. Gen. Psychiatry* 69:98–106.

Buerger, K., Ewers, M., et al. (2006). CSF phosphorylated tau protein correlates with neocortical neurofibrillary pathology in Alzheimer's disease. *Brain* 129:3035–3041.

Doecke, J., Laws, S., et al. (2012). Blood-based protein biomarkers for diagnosis of Alzheimer disease. *Arch. Neurol.* 69:1318–1325.

Dubois, B., Feldman, H., et al. (2010). Revising the definition of Alzheimer's disease: a new lexicon. *Lancet Neurol.* 9:1118–1127.

Fagan, A., and Holtzman, D. (2010). Cerebrospinal fluid biomarkers of Alzheimer's disease. *Biomarkers Med.* 4:51–63.

Fagan, A., Mintun, M., et al. (2009). Cerebrospinal fluid tau and ptau$_{181}$ increase with cortical amyloid deposition in cognitively normal individuals: implications for future clinical trials of Alzheimer's disease. *EMBO Mol. Med.* 1:371–380.

Fagan, A., and Perrin, R. (2012). Upcoming candidate cerebrospinal fluid biomarkers of Alzheimer's disease. *Biomarkers Med.* 6:455–476.

Fagan, A., Roe, C., et al. (2007). Cerebrospinal fluid tau/Aβ42 ratio as a prediction of cognitive decline in nondemented older adults. *Arch. Neurol.* 64:343–349.

Fodero-Tavoletti, M., Okamura, N., et al. (2011). 18F-THK523: a novel *in vivo* tau imaging ligand for Alzheimer's disease. *Brain* 134:1089–1100.

Galasko, D., Chang, L., et al. (1998). High cerebrospinal fluid tau and low amyloid β42 levels in the clinical diagnosis of Alzheimer's disease and relation to apolipoprotein E genotype. *Arch. Neurol.* 55:937–945.

Halliday, G., Holton, J., et al. (2011). Neuropathology underlying clinical variability in patients with synucleinopathies. *Acta Neuropathol.* 122:187–204.

Hampel, H., Buerger, K., et al. (2004). Measurement of phosphorylated tau epitopes in the differential diagnosis of Alzheimer disease: a comparative cerebrospinal fluid study. *Arch. Gen. Psychiatry* 1:95–102.

Hesse, C., Rosengren, L., et al. (2001). Transient increase in total tau but not phospho-tau in human cerebrospinal fluid after acute stroke. *Neurosci. Lett.* 297:187–190.

Hu, W., Holtzman, D., et al. (2012). Plasma multianalyte profiling in mild cognitive impairment and Alzheimer disease. *Neurol.* 79:897–905.

Jack, C., Knopman, D., et al. (2010). Hypothetical model of dynamic biomarkers of the Alzheimer's pathological cascade. *Lancet Neurol.* 9:119–128.

Klunk, W. (2011). Amyloid imaging as a biomarker for cerebral β-amyloidosis and risk prediction for Alzheimer dementia. *Neurobiol. Aging* 32 (Suppl 1):S20–36.

Laterza, O., Modur, V., et al. (2006). Identification of novel brain biomarkers. *Clin. Chem.* 52:1713–1721.

Lee, J., Blennow, K., et al. (2008). The brain injury biomarker VLP-1 is increased in the cerebrospinal fluid of Alzheimer disease patients. *Clin. Chem.* 54:1617–1623.

Li, G., Sokal, I., et al. (2007). CSF tau/Aβ42 ratio for increased risk of mild cognitive impairment: a follow-up study. *Neurology* 69:631–639.

Maddalena, A., Papassotiropoulos, A., et al. (2003). Biochemical diagnosis of Alzheimer disease by measuring the cerebrospinal fluid ratio of phosphorylated tau protein to beta-amyloid peptide42. *Arch. Neurol.* 60:1202–1206.

Mattsson, N., Andreasson, U., et al. (2011). The Alzheimer's Association external quality control program for cerebrospinal fluid biomarkers. *Alzheimers Dement.* 7:386–395.

Mattsson, N., Zetterberg, H., et al. (2009). CSF biomarkers and incipient Alzheimer disease in patients with mild cognitive impairment. *JAMA* 302:385–393.

Mayeux, R., and Schupf, N. (2011). Blood-based biomarkers for Alzheimer's disease: plasma Aβ40 and Aβ42, and genetic variants. *Neurobiol. Aging* 32(Suppl 1):S10–19.

McKhann, G., Drachman, D., et al. (1984). Clinical diagnosis of Alzheimer's disease: report of the NINCDS-ADRDA Work Group under the auspices of Department of Health and Human Services Task Force on Alzheimer's Disease. *Neurology* 34:939–944.

McKhann, G., Knopman, D., et al. (2011). The diagnosis of dementia due to Alzheimer's disease: recommendations from the National Institute on Aging and the Alzheimer's Association Workgroup. *Alzheimers Dement.* 7:263–269.

Nagele, E., Han, M., et al. (2011). Diagnosis of Alzheimer's disease based on disease-specific autoantibody profiles in human sera. *PLoS One* 6(8):e23112.

Neselius, S., Brisby, H., et al. (2012). CSF-biomarkers in Olympic boxing: diagnosis and effects of repetitive head trauma. *PLoS One* 7(4):e33606. Epub 2012 Apr 4.

O'Bryant, S., Xiao, G., et al. (2011). A blood-based screening tool for Alzheimer's disease that spans serum and plasma: findings from TARC and ADNI. *PLoS One* 6(12):e28092. Epub 2011 Dec 7.

Olsson, B., Zetterberg, H., et al. (2011). Biomarker-based dissection of neurodegenerative diseases. *Prog. Neurobiol.* 95:520–534.

Perrin, R., Fagan, A., et al. (2009). Multi-modal techniques for diagnosis and prognosis of Alzheimer's disease. *Nature* 461:916–922.

Peskind, E., Nordberg, A., et al. (2009). Safety of lumbar puncture procedures in patients with Alzheimer's disease. *Curr. Alzheimer Res.* 6:290–292.

Petersen, R., Smith, G., et al. (1999). Mild cognitive impairment: clinical characterization and outcome. *Arch. Neurol.* 56:303–308.

Price, J., Ko, A., et al. (2001). Neuron number in the entorhinal cortex and CA1 in preclinical Alzheimer's disease. *Arch. Neurol.* 58:1395–1402.

Price, J., McKeel, D., et al. (2009). Neuropathology of nondemented aging: presumptive evidence for preclinical Alzheimer disease. *Neurobiol. Aging* 30:1026–1036.

Ray, S., Britschgi, M., et al. (2007). Classification and prediction of clinical Alzheimer's diagnosis based on plasma signaling proteins. *Nat. Med.* 13:1359–1362.

Reddy, M., Wilson, R., et al. (2011). Identification of candidate IgG biomarkers for Alzheimer's disease via combinatorial library screening. *Cell* 144:132–142.

Shaw, L., Vanderstichele, H., et al. (2009). Cerebrospinal fluid biomarker signature in Alzheimer's disease neuroimaging initiative subjects. *Ann. Neurol.* 65:403–413.

Snider, B., Fagan, A., et al. (2009). Cerebrospinal fluid biomarkers and rate of cognitive decline in very mild dementia of the Alzheimer type. *Arch. Neurol.* 66:638–645.

Sperling, R., Aisen, P., et al. (2011). Toward defining the preclinical stages of Alzheimer's disease: recommendations from the National Institute on Aging and the Alzheimer Association Workgroup. *Alzheimer's Dement.* 7:280–292.

Stern, R., Riley, D., et al. (2011). Long-term consequences of repetitive brain trauma: chronic traumatic encephalopathy. *PM&R* 3(10 Suppl 2):S460–467.

Strozyk, D., Blennow, K., et al. (2003). CSF Abeta 42 levels correlate with amyloid-neuropathology in a population-based autopsy study. *Neurology* 60:652–656.

Sunderland, T., Linker, G., et al. (2003). Decreased β-amyloid1-42 and increased tau levels in cerebrospinal fluid of patients with Alzheimer's disease. *JAMA* 289:2094–2103.

Tapiola, T., Alafuzoff, I., et al. (2009). Cerebrospinal fluid b-amyloid 42 and tau proteins as biomarkers of Alzheimer-type pathologic changes in the brain. *Arch. Neurol.* 66:382–389.

Tarawneh, R., D'Angelo, G., et al. (2011). Visinin-like protein 1: a novel prognostic biomarker in Alzheimer's disease. *Ann. Neurol.* 70:274–285.

Tarawneh, R., Lee, J., et al. (2012). CSF VILIP-1 predicts rates of cognitive decline in early Alzheimer disease. *Neurology* 10:709–719.

VanHarten, A., Kester, M., et al. (2011). Tau and p-tau as CSF biomarkers in dementia: a meta-analysis. *Clin. Chem. Lab. Med.* 49:353–366.

Villemagne, V., and Rowe, C. (2012). Long night's journey into the day: amyloid-β imaging in Alzheimer's disease. *J. Alzheimers Dis.* 33(Suppl 1):S349–S359.

Visser, P., Verhey, F., et al. (2009). Prevalence and prognostic value of CSF markers of Alzheimer's disease pathology in patients with subjective cognitive impairment or mild cognitive impairment in the DESCRIPA study: a prospective cohort study. *Lancet Neurol.* 8:619–627.

Weiner, M., Veitch, D., et al. (2012). The Alzheimer's Disease Neuroimaging Initiative: a review of papers published since its inception. *Alzheimers Dement.* 8(Suppl 1):S1–68.

64 | CURRENT THERAPIES FOR ALZHEIMER'S DISEASE

MARY SANO AND JUDITH NEUGROSCHL

The awareness of cognitive loss and dementia has grown dramatically in the past 20 years. The most common etiology of dementia is Alzheimer's disease (AD), a neurodegenerative condition characterized by progressive cognitive and functional deterioration. Alzheimer's disease has an estimated prevalence of approximately 5.2 million in the United States (Alzheimers Association, 2012), with an estimated 36 million people worldwide currently suffering with dementias (Prince et al., 2011). The CDC has estimated that the US population older than age 65 will more than double from 2010 to 2050, with the population older than 85 more than tripling (Administration on Aging, 2010). Age is the greatest risk factor for Alzheimer's disease and other dementias, thus the number of individuals with dementia will continue to rapidly rise unless significant advances are made. In January 2011, the National Alzheimer's Project Act was signed into law in the United States, establishing a national project to facilitate and coordinate research efforts on Alzheimer treatment and prevention and to improve diagnosis and coordination of care, particularly in minority populations.

Although five medications representing two classes of drugs were approved by the US FDA for the treatment of Alzheimer's disease since 1994, there have been no approved agents since 2003. However, several randomized trials have provided additional information about the efficacy of these FDA-approved medications in subgroups of patients with AD. The development of these agents preceded the most current approaches to diagnosis including imaging confirmation of cerebral amyloid, which might yield a somewhat different patient population in trials. This specificity of diagnosis may or may not change the efficacy of the current agents. Currently there are approximately 330 trials registered in the US and recruiting subjects for the treatment of AD and there are over a thousand that have been registered and completed.

This chapter will review the pharmacology underlying the currently approved treatments, and the data supporting efficacy. Several approaches have also been well studied in rigorously conducted clinical trials, which have increased our knowledge about what primarily does not work. These include hormones, agents that modify cardiovascular and metabolic risk as well as a number of vitamins and nutritional approaches. We also review this evidence.

FDA-APPROVED TREATMENTS FOR ALZHEIMER'S DISEASE

CHOLINESTERASE INHIBITORS

Acetylcholine has long been known to effect memory. Reductions in the activities of acetylcholinesterase and choline acetyltransferase, enzymes involved in the synthesis and degradation of acetylcholine, were found in brain tissues from Alzheimer's disease patients (Davies and Maloney, 1976). According to the cholinergic hypothesis of Alzheimer's disease, the destruction of cholinergic neurons in the basal forebrain and the resulting deficit in central cholinergic transmission contribute substantially to the cognitive deficits and behavioral symptoms observed in patients suffering from AD (Bartus et al., 1982).

After its release into the synaptic cleft the acetylcholine is degraded rapidly by the hydrolytic activity of cholinesterases, the most prominent being acetyl-cholinesterase, although butyryl-cholinesterase can also hydrolyze acetylcholine in the human brain (Mesulam et al., 2002). Inhibition of cholinesterases leads to an increase of acetylcholine concentration in the synaptic cleft and is thought to enhance cholinergic transmission and ameliorate cholinergic deficit. In 1983 the first acetyl-cholinesterase inhibitor (AChEI) was approved (tacrine [Cognex]). It was not well tolerated, with four times per day dosing, reversible hepatocellular injury in up to 50% of patients (Watkins et al., 1994), and significant procholinergic side effects of nausea, vomiting, and diarrhea. The three other AChEIs donepezil, rivastigmine, and galantamine, were released between 1996 and 2001 and have very similar efficacy. They have slightly different mechanisms of action. For example, rivastigmine also inhibits butyrylcholinesterase, and galantamine is an allosteric modulator of the nicotinic receptor. In general, these medications tend to effect a 3–18 month improvement in cognitive functioning, followed by deterioration along a parallel path. Rivastigmine has received an additional indication for dementia caused by Parkinson's disease (Olin et al., 2010). Systematic reviews of all available randomized, double-blind, multicenter and placebo-controlled studies by the Cochrane Collaboration showed moderate benefits of cholinesterase inhibitors on cognitive, behavioral, and functional symptoms (e.g., Birks, 2006), and they are considered standard of care for patients with Alzheimer's disease by the American Academy of Neurology (Doody, 2005).

Originally, AChEIs were approved for the treatment of patients with mild-to-moderate disease. However, since 2007 the indications have been expanded to severe dementia. There have been numerous studies supporting the efficacy of donepezil (Cummings et al., 2010), rivastigmine (Farlow et al., 2011), galantamine (Burns et al., 2009), with significant cognitive effects for all medications in severe AD. Continuing treatment into moderate and severe AD also has been shown to improve cognition and function over placebo, in a one year trial of patients with moderate to severe AD who were randomized to either continue or stop donepezil and add either placebo or active memantine. Combined treatment did not suggest an additional benefit (Howard et al., 2012). A similar positive finding was seen in trials of galantamine withdrawal (Gaudig et al., 2011). Of note, a trial examining the use of donepezil for agitation in AD did not show a significant placebo medication difference, although interestingly about 20% in both groups had a greater than 30% reduction in agitation scores (Howard et al., 2007).

Some of the cholinesterase inhibitors have been tried in higher doses (Farlow et al., 2010; Grossberg et al., 2011), with donepezil receiving FDA approval for a 23-mg formulation of Aricept in moderate to severe AD. Although there were data showing mild benefit in cognition there was no statistically significant difference in global functioning, a requirement for FDA approval, and significantly more procholinergic side effects such as nausea and vomiting, suggesting that the risk benefit ratio does not support the use of this higher dose. Other studies have suggested that the side effects are most pronounced in the first few weeks of treatment (Tariot et al., 2012), but given the lack of improvement in global functioning there is debate as to the true benefit of this dose.

Another significant question is the utility and efficacy of AChEIs in mild cognitive impairment (MCI). To date, trials of cholinesterase inhibitors in MCI have not shown a significant effect on progression to AD (Petersen et al., 2005; Winblad et al., 2008), but some studies have suggested that they may delay the conversion (Petersen et al., 2005) or possibly have a differential effect on subgroups based on genetics or gender (Ferris et al., 2009).

Recently, a placebo-controlled trial of a Chinese herb, Huperzine A, which is a cholinesterase inhibitor, was conducted in 210 individuals with mild-to-moderate AD. Huperzine A did not meet the primary efficacy endpoints of cognition, functional, or global change (Rafii et al., 2011).

There are numerous areas for further study concerning the cholinesterase inhibitors that will be facilitated by greater understanding of biomarkers in this disease as well as the newly available amyloid imaging. One is whether early or even presymptomatic treatment affects the course of disease, amyloid deposition, and/or later functional changes. As the prodromal stages of AD are better defined, this will open up many avenues of inquiry concerning the AChEIs as well as various other treatment strategies.

MEMANTINE

Glutamate is the main excitatory neurotransmitter in the central nervous system and a physiological level of glutamate-receptor activity is essential for normal brain function. Glutamate excitotoxicity, mediated through excessive activation of N-methyl-D-aspartate (NMDA) receptors is believed to play a role in the neuronal cell death observed in Alzheimer's disease and other neurodegenerative diseases by causing increases in intracellular calcium which then triggers downstream events that cause cell death (Hynd et al., 2004). Thus, NMDA-receptor antagonists may have a therapeutic potential for neuronal protection from glutamate-mediated neurotoxicity.

Memantine is a low-to-moderate affinity, voltage-dependent, noncompetitive NMDA receptor antagonist with rapid gating kinetics (Danysz et al., 2000). Its fast on/off kinetics and low-to-moderate affinity are key to memantine's action because it ameliorates the effects of excessive glutamate while preserving the physiologic activation of NMDA-receptors required for learning and memory. Like other NMDA-receptor antagonists, memantine at high concentrations can inhibit mechanisms of synaptic plasticity that are believed to underlie learning and memory, but studies have shown that at lower, clinically relevant concentrations memantine actually promotes synaptic plasticity and preserves or enhances memory in animal models of Alzheimer's disease (Johnson and Kotermanski, 2006).

Memantine was approved in the United States for treatment of moderate to severe AD in 2003, and the FDA rejected a request to extend its approval to mild AD in 2005. Systematic reviews of all available randomized, double-blind, multicenter and placebo-controlled studies by the Cochrane Collaboration showed that memantine treatment resulted in significant benefits in cognitive, functional, and behavioral assessments in the treatment group compared with placebo in patients with moderate to severe Alzheimer's disease (McShane et al., 2006). It is usually well tolerated; adverse effects included confusion, insomnia, and headache that occurred in a small percentage of the study participants (Tariot et al., 2004).

Memantine does not affect the inhibition of acetylcholinesterase by cholinesterase inhibitors. It is well tolerated with cholinesterase inhibitors, (Choi et al., 2011; Tariot et al., 2004). In some studies, memantine was shown to enhance AChEI therapy (Atri et al., 2008; Tariot et al., 2004), whereas others have not seen an effect (Choi et al., 2011; Howard et al., 2012).

The question of whether memantine affects the rate of decline in mild AD is being addressed in a current trial (http://clinicaltrials.gov ID: NCT00235716). This study examines the effect of vitamin E 2,000 IU, versus vitamin E plus memantine, versus memantine, versus placebo in a group of approximately 600 individuals with mild-to-moderate AD over the course of up to four years to see if the rate of decline is modified. Data collection began in August 2007, and was expected to be completed in the fall of 2012.

OTHER TREATMENT STRATEGIES

Based on epidemiologic studies and basic science research, a number of FDA-approved drugs, as well as vitamins, supplements, medical foods, and herbal medications have been considered in the treatment of AD.

ANTIINFLAMMATORY DRUGS

A number of lines of evidence supported the hypothesis that neuronal damage caused by increased immune system activity is a mechanism of AD pathogenesis. Increased concentrations of cytokines, acute phase reactants, and complement protein have been found on autopsy in the brains of Alzheimer patients compared with aged matched controls (e.g., Bauer et al., 1992; Fillit et al., 1991). Senile plaques are often surrounded by activated astrocytes and microglia cells and can also induce activation of the complement cascade (McGeer and McGeer, 2001). Epidemiologic studies looking at the risk for AD have suggested that use of nonsteroidal antiinflammatory or corticosteroids lessened the risk of developing Alzheimer's disease (e.g., Hayden et al., 2007; McGeer and McGeer, 2007).

Cyclooxygenase (COX) enzymes mediate the conversion of arachidonic acid to prostaglandins, which are crucial components of the proinflammatory process. The main target of nonsteroidal antiinflammatory drugs (NSAIDs) is COX enzymes. The inducible COX isoform, COX2, is upregulated in the brains of patients with AD (Yasojima et al., 1999), suggesting that NSAIDs might be beneficial in AD by reducing neurotoxic inflammation. A subset of NSAIDs have been found to lower Aβ levels independently of COX enzyme activity, apparently by directly modulating γ-secretase activity, which enzymatically cleaves Aβ from its larger precursor protein (Weggen et al., 2001). Flurizan (tarenflurbil) was shown to be effective in modulating γ-secretase activity and ultimately in selective Aβ42 lowering in animal models. In a phase II study the agent had no effect on a group of cognitive outcomes in mild-to-moderate AD, but a post hoc analysis showed some benefit at the highest dose for those with the mildest disease (Wilcock et al., 2008). This finding led to an 18-month phase III trial, which was also negative (Green et al., 2009). This is particularly interesting in light of the fate of semagacestat (LY450139), a gamma secretase inhibitor, which was shown to worsen patient outcomes more than placebo in two phase III trials (NCT00762411 and NCT00594568) (Lilly, 2010).

There have been a number of clinical trials that have examined a variety of antiinflammatory agents ranging from NSAIDS to prednisone, which have unfortunately shown no benefit as a treatment for AD (discussed in Aisen, 2008). Primary and secondary prevention trials with NSAIDS have also been negative (e.g., Lyketsos et al., 2007; Thal et al., 2005). In addition, the dropouts from many of these trials have been high, owing to significant side effects of NSAID use such as renal insufficiency and gastrointestinal intolerance or, more seriously, gastrointestinal bleeding. A trial of 2,538 elderly patients without AD called the Alzheimer's Disease Anti-inflammatory Prevention Trial, has led to a number of publications suggesting a possible deleterious cognitive effect with both naproxen and celecoxib (Lyketsos et al., 2007). Although the trial was halted early, observation was continued for two subsequent years, and models have been reported to explain the findings based on disease stage and rapidity of decline. All of these analyses are post hoc and many characterize subjects in idiosyncratic ways, leaving doubt to their value (Breitner et al., 2011; Leoutsakos et al., 2012).

ANTIOXIDANTS

Oxidative stress and free radicals have been implicated in cell damage and aging in general, and in neurodegenerative diseases in particular, including MCI and AD (Lovell and Markesbery, 2007). Vitamin C and E have been found to protect from oxidative DNA damage (Huang et al., 2000) and vitamin E protects nerve cells from amyloid-β peptide toxicity (Behl et al., 1992).

Several population-based prospective observational studies that have used questionnaires to monitor the intake of vitamins C and E on the risk of developing dementia revealed mixed results (Boothby and Doering, 2005). A placebo-controlled, clinical trial of vitamin E and selegiline in patients with moderately advanced Alzheimer's disease was conducted by the Alzheimer's Disease Cooperative Study (Sano et al., 1997). Subjects in the vitamin E group were treated with 2,000 IU of vitamin E. The results indicated that vitamin E may slow functional deterioration. A more recent study looking at markers of oxidation in the CSF of patients with AD treated with vitamins E and C, and alphalipoic acid (ALA); or coenzyme Q3; or placebo (Galasko et al., 2012) showed no effect on CSF Abeta or tau and although the vitamin E/C/ALA group had lower CSF oxidative markers, they also showed worse mini mental scores over the four months. Other clinical trials with vitamin E were conducted in patients with MCI (2002; Petersen et al., 2005) that failed to demonstrate a significant difference in the rate of progression to Alzheimer's disease between the vitamin E and placebo group.

Unfortunately there are safety concerns with the use of vitamin E. A clinical trial of long-term vitamin E supplementation studying the effects on cardiovascular events and cancer showed no effect on cancer or major cardiovascular events but an increase in the risk of heart failure (Lonn et al., 2005). A metaanalysis of randomized controlled trials examined the potential dose-response relationship between vitamin E supplementation and total mortality showed dose-dependent and significantly increased all-cause mortality with the use of vitamin E (Miller et al., 2005). Recent recommendations are therefore not to advocate the use of vitamin E in individuals at risk or affected by Alzheimer's disease (Ames and Ritchie, 2007).

Interest remains in clarifying the risk/protective effects of vitamin E and two important ongoing studies will be informative. There is a current trial mentioned previously (http://clinicaltrials.gov ID: NCT00235716) looking at the effect of either vitamin E 2,000 IU versus memantine vs. a combination or placebo, in approximately 600 individuals for up to four years, to see if the rate of decline is affected. Another trial is an "add-on" (called PREADVISE [http://clinicaltrials.gov ID: NCT00040378]) to a trial evaluating the use of vitamin E and/or selenium, to prevent prostate cancer (the SELECT trial with 35,533 participants). This trial was halted in 2008 because there was a nonsignificant increased risk of prostate cancer in the vitamin E group, and a nonsignificant increased risk of type 2 diabetes in the selenium only group (Lippman et al., 2009). The PREADVISE study continues to follow more than 5,000 individuals who had been taking vitamin E 400 IU alone or in combination with 200 mcg of selenium, or placebo, and will evaluate their effect on developing risk.

B VITAMINS/LOWERING HOMOCYSTEINE

Elevated plasma homocysteine levels are a risk factor for cardiovascular disease and stroke (e.g., Bostom et al., 1999; Stampfer et al., 1992) and may be related to an increased risk of Alzheimer's disease (Seshadri et al., 2002). Deficiencies of folic acid and vitamin B12 and B6 intake increase homocysteine plasma levels. Folic acid and vitamin B12 are needed for the conversion of homocysteine to methionine, and vitamin B6 is needed for the conversion of homocysteine to cysteine. High dietary intake of folic acid and vitamin B12 and B6 decreased homocysteine levels in adults (2005). Theories about how homocysteine might act as a risk factor for AD range from potentiating Abeta production (Zhang et al., 2009) or toxicity to vascular-related effects.

A recent longitudinal cohort study reported higher folate intake decreased the risk of incident Alzheimer's disease independent of levels of vitamin B6 and B12 (Luchsinger et al., 2007). However, metaanalyses of clinical trials addressing the influence of folic acid, vitamin B6, and vitamin B12 intake failed to show any beneficial effect on cognitive function (e.g., Malouf and Grimley Evans, 2008). Furthermore, two clinical trials on folic acid and vitamins B6 and B12 failed to show any reduction of the risk of major cardiovascular events and stroke (Bonaa et al., 2006; Lonn et al., 2006). To see if lowering homocysteine in patients with AD would change the course of the illness, an 18-month prospective trial in 400 mild-to-moderate AD patients was done. The intervention (folate and vitamins B6 and B12) was quite successful at lowering homocysteine, but it did not slow cognitive decline, with no difference between the active and placebo groups on the rate of change of a cognitive measure (ADAS-cog) (Aisen et al., 2008). This was confirmed in a recent two-year trial looking at both vascular dementia and AD (Kwok et al., 2011).

Prevention trials have also been generally negative. One study of supplementation over a three-year period in nondemented older individuals selected on the basis of relatively high homocysteine levels indicated a favorable influence on cognitive function (Durga et al., 2007), whereas a two-year study in older individuals not selected on the basis of homocysteine levels did not (McMahon et al., 2006). Another trial of two years of vitamin supplementation in hypertensive men confirmed that lowering homocysteine did not significantly alter the risk of cognitive decline, either in the whole sample, or when individuals with baseline high homocysteine were analyzed separately. Of the 299 patients assessed at baseline, 73 were followed a mean of 7.7 years for long-term follow-up, and again no significant differences were seen, although a trend toward less cognitive impairment was seen in the treatment arm (Ford et al., 2010).

Overall there is no convincing evidence that supplementation of B vitamins significantly changes either risk of AD or subsequent decline in AD, although it remains possible that lowering homocysteine in individuals with high levels at baseline might decrease risk.

OMEGA-3 FATTY ACIDS

Several epidemiologic studies showed a protective effect of increased fish consumption and omega-3 fatty acid intake for the development of Alzheimer's disease (Barberger-Gateau et al., 2002; Morris et al., 2003). Docosahexaenoic acid (DHA) is an omega-3 polyunsaturated fatty acid found in some marine algae as well as fish. These fatty acids are a component of synaptic plasma membranes. Animal research suggests a number of roles in the brain including neuroprotection, affecting the rate of signal transduction, and regulating gene expression.

A Cochrane metaanalysis of all available biological, epidemiological, and observational data suggested a protective effect of omega-3 fatty acids (Lim et al., 2006), but the author concluded that until there was significant randomized prospective data, no conclusions could be drawn. Since then clinical trials have been published examining both AD treatment, as well as dementia prevention.

One placebo-controlled treatment trial demonstrated that in 204 patients treated over a year, no effect was seen in patients with mild-to-moderate stage disease, but in a subset with very mild AD (MMSE >27), omega-3 fatty acids slowed cognitive decline, as evaluated by MMSE (Freund-Levi et al., 2006). An 18-month trial followed 402 patients with mild-to-moderate AD who had low dietary intake of DHA at baseline who were given either DHA or placebo. The two outcome measures, a cognitive outcome (ADAS-Cog) and a global one (Clinical Dementia Rating Scale Sum of Boxes), as well as other behavioral outcome measures, did not differ between the placebo and active group, and in a subset of 102 patients who underwent volumetric MRI there was no difference in the rate of brain atrophy (Quinn et al., 2010).

Other trials have looked at DHA for primary and secondary prevention. A trial looking at high- and low-dose DHA and eicosapentaenoic acid (EPA) in 302 cognitively healthy older adults (MMSE >21), showed no cognitive benefit over the 26 weeks of the trial (van de Rest et al., 2008). A six-month trial of DHA versus placebo in 485 elderly patients with a memory complaint using a visuospatial episodic memory test as the primary outcome measure demonstrated significantly fewer errors in the treatment group, as compared with their baseline scores (Yurko-Mauro et al., 2010). However, a large trial of 1,748 individuals aged 45–80 at risk for cognitive decline because of a history of myocardial infarction, unstable angina, or ischemic stroke, did not show any significant effects on cognitive function after four years of treatment with either B vitamins (folate, B6, and B12); omega-three fatty acids (EPA and DHA); B vitamins and omega-3 fatty acids; or placebo (Andreeva et al., 2011).

Overall, the majority of data suggests that omega-3 fatty acids do not significantly alter the course of AD. The possibility remains that it may have an effect in individuals with only memory complaints. Given the short duration (six months) of that one positive trial, it is impossible to say anything about secondary prevention, although clearly in cardiovascular at-risk groups there was no benefit over four years.

GINKGO

Extracts of the leaves of the maidenhair tree, ginkgo biloba, have long been used in China, but also in several European countries as a traditional medicine for various disorders of health. A one-year randomized placebo-controlled treatment trial of 309 AD patients demonstrated a modest improvement on some measures (Le Bars et al., 1997), although two later six-month trials of 214 (van Dongen et al., 2000) and 513 (Schneider et al., 2005) patients, showed no benefit. Two recent metaanalyses of ginkgo for the treatment of AD suggested that overall there was a modest treatment effect, but again the trials were very heterogeneous concerning duration and patients included in the trials, as well as outcomes (Janssen et al., 2010; Weinmann et al., 2010). A Cochrane review in 2009 called the research on ginkgo is at best "inconsistent and unconvincing" (Birks and Grimley Evans, 2009).

In terms of prevention, the best trial to date was a placebo-controlled trial of gingko. Evaluations were done at six-month intervals for incident dementia. In this trial, 3,069 elderly individuals, approximately 16% of whom met criteria for MCI at the start of the trial, were followed for a median of six years. The rates of all-cause dementia, AD, as well as conversion to dementia from MCI were not statistically different in the two groups. In addition, there was no improvement on any secondary outcome, such as overall morbidity (DeKosky et al., 2008), nor did it have any effect on cognitive decline in any cognitive domain (Snitz et al., 2009).

The overall results are at best inconsistent (Schneider, 2008) and the British Association for Psychopharmacology concluded that ginkgo cannot be recommended for the prevention or treatment of AD (O'Brien and Burns, 2011).

CURCUMIN

Because curcumin has antiinflammatory and antioxidant properties, it has engendered interest in the AD community. In animal models it was found to decrease brain amyloid plaques (e.g., Frautschy et al., 2001)). A population-based cohort study found better cognition in elderly Asian subjects with high curcumin consumption (Ng et al., 2006). A small clinical trial in Hong Kong did not show any significant cognitive results (Baum et al., 2008). A trial has been completed in the United States and results were negative, but the preparation of curcumin was poorly absorbed with little to no curcumin found in the bloodstream of participants (Ringman et al., 2008). Additional trials with other formulations are planned, such as a trial (http://clinicaltrials.gov ID: NCT01383161) that began recruitment in March 2012, looking at the effect of curcumin in 50–90 year olds with a cognitive complaint but no dementia over the course of 18 months.

RESVERATROL

Several observational studies have demonstrated that moderate consumption of wine is associated with a lower incidence of Alzheimer's disease. Wine is enriched in antioxidant compounds, with potential neuroprotective activities. Resveratrol, a polyphenol that occurs in abundance in grapes and red wine, is used by the plant to defend itself against fungal and other attacks. In the early 1990s the presence of resveratrol was detected in red wine wherein it is suspected to afford antioxidant and neuroprotective properties (Miller and Rice-Evans, 1995) and therefore to contribute to the beneficial effects of red wine consumption on neurodegeneration (Savaskan et al., 2003). In animal studies, resveratrol has a variety of antiaging effects, including extending the lifespan in *C. elegans* (Wood et al., 2004). In mice, it seemed to improve a variety of aging outcomes (bone health, cholesterol, coordination), but did not increase longevity (Pearson et al., 2008).

Resveratrol promotes intracellular degradation of Abeta via a mechanism that involves the proteasome (Marambaud et al., 2005), and it protected rats from Abeta-induced neurotoxicity (Huang et al., 2011). Resveratrol does not influence the Abeta-producing enzymes and therefore does not inhibit Abeta generation. In a transgenic Alzheimer model of Abeta amyloidosis, resveratrol significantly reduced amyloid plaque formation (Karuppagounder et al., 2009). A small clinical trial of low dose resveratrol in patients with Alzheimer's disease has shown encouraging results (Blass and Gibson, 2006), and another low-dose trial was recently completed (http://clinicaltrials.gov ID: NCT00678431). A large multicenter clinical trial of high dose resveratrol (ID: NCT01504854) began recruiting in May 2012.

MEDICAL FOODS

Medical foods for Alzheimer's disease have been marketed over the past decade. A medical food is defined as a specially formulated and processed product (as opposed to a naturally occurring food) required for the dietary management of the patient under medical supervision, which cannot be achieved by normal diet. This category of products does not undergo premarket review or approval by the FDA. Also individual medical food products do not have to be registered with FDA. However, ingredients used in medical foods must be approved or exempted food additives, and ingredients are "Generally Recognized as Safe" (GRAS). Axona (previously known as Ketasyn) is an example of a Medical Food marketed for AD. The product proposes to provide an alternative energy source for the production of glucose in the brain through a proprietary formulation of caprylic triglycerides that increases plasma concentrations of ketone bodies. A clinical trial in mild-to-moderate AD demonstrated improvement in a cognitive test, though not in other outcomes (Henderson et al., 2009).

Another medical food, Souvenaid, which is not currently available in the United States, has been used in clinical trials for AD. The development of this product is based on the notion that coadministration of rate-limiting precursors for membrane phosphatide synthesis, such as the nucleotide uridine, omega-3 polyunsaturated fatty acids, and choline, can restore synapses, increase hippocampal dendritic spines, and surrogate markers of new synapses. In a "proof of concept," placebo-controlled study of 212 drug naive subjects with AD, Souvenaid improved scores on a delayed memory score but not on other cognitive and functional measures (Scheltens et al., 2010). In a preliminary report of the The Souvenir II, a 24-week international study of 259 individuals with AD, Souvenaid significantly improved the memory domain of a neuropsychological test battery. No significant intervention effect was observed on other cognitive or functional outcomes (Scheltens et al., 2011). The S-Connect study, a 24-week randomized, controlled, double-blind study conducted in the United States in 527 subjects with AD who were on standard drug therapy reported no differences in any cognitive or functional outcome (Shah et al., 2011). Since it is likely that most individuals with AD will receive treatment with conventional medication, there is no indication that supplementation with medical foods has an additive benefit on clinical outcomes. Additionally, there are no trials of treatment in those who have failed other medications.

It is noteworthy that nether the mechanisms of intervention nor the efficacy of medical foods are well established, and are not supported. Despite this, the use of nutritional and dietary supplements in the United States is extensive. It is estimated that 65% of adults are self-described supplement users, according to a 2009 survey conducted by Ipsos-Public Affairs for the Council for Responsible Nutrition (Hlasney, 2009). Thus, patients and families are likely to be exploring these treatment options.

GONADAL HORMONAL TREATMENT OF DEMENTIA

Interest in a beneficial role on cognition and prevention of dementia for gonadal hormone, specifically estrogen and testosterone, has a long history with little to recommend these agents. As treatments for dementia there is little positive data to support a role for estrogen. A comprehensive metaanalysis of trials assessing forms of estrogen in the treatment of AD identified seven studies with over 350 women (Hogervorst et al., 2009). The cumulative summary of these results indicates worsening on clinical global measures, verbal memory, and finger tapping. Since that review several other trials have been described. A randomized trial using transdermal estrogen for up to three months in a small study of postmenopausal women with AD (N = 43) described improvements in visual and semantic memory (Wharton et al., 2011). Also a 12-month trial with low-dose estradial with norethisterone in women

with AD (N = 65) yielded non-signficant treatment differences on cognitive outcomes, although a benefical treatment effect on mood was noted in those who did not possess the ApoE ε4 allele (Valen-Sendstad et al., 2010). In a small study of women with mild-to-moderate (N = 27) cognitive impairment, otherwise unspecified, Yamada et al. (2010) found improved cognition and function with six months of treatment with dehydroepiandrosterone, which increased plasma testosterone (Yamada et al., 2010).

In a randomized, double-blind, placebo-controlled design, women with surgically induced menopause (N = 50; mean [SD] age, 54.0 [2.9] years) received estradiol valerate in combination with testosterone undecanoate or placebo. The women were assessed with a self-report questionnaire regarding memory and neuropsychological tests for verbal and spatial episodic memory and incidental learning at baseline, at the time of crossover, and after completion of treatment. Results indicate testosterone had a negative effect on immediate but not delayed recall. Overall no treatment benefit was noted (Moller et al., 2010). Taken together, there is little consistent evidence that there is a benefit to estrogen or testosterone treatment in women with AD.

Several studies have examined testosterone in males with AD, though the trials have been small and brief. In one small study (N = 16) using testosterone in the form of hydroalcoholic gel (75 mg) applied topically for 25 weeks, there were no differences in cognition or behavior but a benefit was seen in the patient's quality of life as reported by a caregiver. (Lu et al., 2006). In another small (N = 32) study of men with AD or MCI treated with intramuscular injections of 100 mg T enanthate for six weeks, improvements compared to placebo were seen in spatial memory and constructional tests (Cherrier et al., 2005).

A third small study (N = 10) of hypogonadal males (total testosterone <240 ng/dl or 7 nmol/l) with AD examined the effect of treatment with intramuscular testosterone, 200 mg every two weeks for up to a year compared with placebo. Benefits on global cognitive measures were seen on the ADAS cog and the Mini-Mental State Exam. Prostate-specific antigen levels were also elevated (Tan and Pu, 2003).

Although the focus of this chapter is treatments for dementia and Alzheimer's disease, there have been several studies to assess the value of estrogen and testosterone in non-demented males to protect against cognitive decline or to enhance cognitive function. Several reviews are recommended (Wharton et al., 2011; Yamada et al., 2010); most report little evidence of a benefit in cognition or dementia prevention.

MODIFICATION OF CARDIOVASCULAR RISK FACTORS AS A TREATMENT OF DEMENTIA

Traditionally, AD has been thought to be a primary neurodegenerative disorder and not of vascular origin. However, many discussions of AD incidence and prevalence have included references to the vascular contributions to the symptoms of dementia (e.g., Barnes and Yaffe, 2011; Schrijvers et al., 2012).

Cardiovascular risk factors are highly prevalent in the elderly population and rarely exist in isolation. Diabetes mellitus, hypertension, hyperlipidemia, and coronary artery disease often coexist, and this constellation of cardiovascular risk factors has been found to increase the risk for cognitive decline, vascular dementia, and AD (Luchsinger and Mayeux, 2004). The risk of AD has been found to increase with the number of vascular risk factors present in an individual (Luchsinger et al., 2005). However, many randomized clinical trials have been conducted to capture this benefit but to date few have succeeded in demonstrating that treatments for hypertension, hyperlipidemia, or diabetes can modify cognitive decline, incident dementia, or the trajectory of AD. These approaches are summarized as follows.

CHOLESTEROL LOWERING

A 2009 Cochrane review of two randomized trials of cholesterol lowering agents in adults with cardiovascular risks, with primary outcomes for reducing cardiovascular events, described the absence of benefit on cognition and dementia prevention (McGuinness, Craig et al., 2009). In the most recent trial with pravastatin (PROPSER), there was no effect on cognition or incident dementia despite robust assessment (Trompet et al., 2010), despite the fact that cognitive tests showed a significant decline over time, confirming sensitivity to cognitive deterioration with age. The review concludes that despite biological feasibility, there is good evidence from RCTs that statins given in late life to individuals at risk of vascular disease have no effect in preventing AD or dementia.

Another series of studies examined the effect of statins on improving the cognitive deterioration of individuals with AD who did not have cardiovascular risk factors. A study using atorvastatin, which does not have CNS penetration (Feldman et al., 2010) as well as a study with simvastatin, which does (Sano et al., 2011), had similarly negative results. Both showed no benefit on any cognitive, functional, or clinical outcome, despite evidence of significant lipid lowering, although both studies demonstrated acceptable safety. The efficacy of statins for preventing cardiovascular events prevents the ethical conduct of studies to assess the effects of these agents on cognition among individuals with AD who do have cardiovascular risks. Although these agents have efficacy for reducing events that are associated with cognitive impairment, there is no evidence of direct clinical or cognitive benefit in AD.

ANTIHYPERTENSIVES

Hypertension is a well-known risk factor for cardiovascular disease and stroke, and thus for vascular dementia. Vascular contribution to AD has been proposed and neuropathological studies suggest that these are independent and additive (Launer et al., 2008). However, the treatment of hypertension is not so clearly associated with a reduction in risk of dementia or a benefit in cognition. Treatment trials usually use a combination of agents from several classes to achieve maximum control of hypertension, including diuretics, ACE inhibitors, angiotensin receptor blockers, and calcium channel blockers.

In a comprehensive review of antihypertensive treatment trials, four were identified that assessed incident dementia as an outcome (McGuinness, Todd et al., 2009). This metaanalysis found no treatment-related differences in incident dementia, despite a trend in that direction in three of the four trials. Three of the four also assessed cognitive change as an outcome, with only one trial, Hypertension in the Very Elderly Trial (HYVET-COG), showing a trend in the positive direction (Peters et al., 2008). A recent report, modeling the effect over longer intervals indicated persistence of the small benefit with treatment (Peters et al., 2010).

In a recent metaanalysis of more than 60,000 cases, vascular dementia was considered separately from all other dementias and the results detected a benefit of antihypertensive treatment on vascular dementia but not on other dementias (Chang-Quan et al., 2011). It is important to note that in these large-scale trials the dementia diagnosis is a clinical one and seldom includes technologies that assess the underlying pathology of amyloid, tau, or synaptic loss and dysfunction. Thus these trials might have yielded different results in subsets of individuals with specific AD pathology.

While the direct benefit of medications to lower cardiovascular risk on cognitive outcomes does not support its use to prevent or treat AD, evidence-based medicine indicates these agents should be used to treat cardiovascular disease. Yet there is evidence that patients with AD and related disorders are undertreated with these agents (Rattinger et al., 2012).

TREATMENTS FOR DIABETES MELLITUS

The association between cognitive impairment and dementia and diabetes has been supported by many epidemiological studies. In type II diabetes, cognitive impairment mainly affects learning and memory, mental speed, and flexibility (Allen et al., 2004). The association between diabetes mellitus and AD is particularly strong among carriers of the apolipoprotein ε4 (ApoE4) allele (Peila et al., 2002). Treatments for diabetes, including insulin, have been studied in large and small randomized clinical trials with mixed results. Two categories of studies are of note: one includes the treatment of individuals with diabetes with antidiabetic agents and assesses the impact on cognition and dementia. Sato et al. described a six-month, randomized trial in patients with AD and type II diabetes mellitus treated with 15–30 mg pioglitazone daily ($N = 21$) or not ($N = 21$) (Sato et al., 2011). While cognitive improvement over baseline was reported in the treated group but not the placebo group, no drug placebo comparison was conducted. A secondary analysis, comparing diabetic and non-diabetic patients with The ACCORD-MIND study examined the cognitive effect of intensive versus standard glucose lowering of individuals with type II diabetes, aged 49–79. No benefit on memory, attention, or executive function was observed (Launer et al., 2011). The authors indicate that intensive antidiabetic therapy is not recommended to reduce the adverse effects of diabetes on the brain.

The other category of studies assesses individuals with AD to determine if typical antidiabetic drugs can improve symptoms or modify disease course. Two phase 3 studies evaluated the safety and efficacy of the peroxisome proliferator-activated receptor gamma agonist, rosiglitazone, in nondiabetic patients with AD. More than 2,000 subjects were enrolled, with one cohort receiving concomitant AD medications and the other not. There was no effect on cognition or other clinical measures and no interaction with ApoEε4 (Harrington et al., 2011). Studies with Piaglitazone, though smaller and fewer, show comparable results (Geldmacher et al., 2011). Small single site studies have indicated that insulin, administered by infusion or intranasally, may have some cogntive benefits. One study found a benefit with infused insulin in individuals with mild cognitive impairment who were ApoE ε4 carriers (Watson et al., 2009). Another larger study (N = 100) of individuals with MCI found better scores on memory with a low dose (20/mg) of intranasal insulin but poorer performance at a higher dose (Craft et al., 2012). This result will be explored in a larger trial in AD which was recently funded.

CONCLUSIONS

Although there are few currently FDA-approved treatments for AD, the data on the cholinesterase inhibitors consistently show robust although modest effect on cognitive improvement across disease severity. Some data suggest that higher doses provide greater effect, though this is limited by side effects. Memantine has shown less robust effects and primarily in moderate to severely impaired populations, but not in more mild individuals. A large current trial is again looking at effects in milder disease stages.

Despite the very significant need, no novel treatments have been approved over the past nine years. Although future research is likely aiming at prevention strategies, the challenge of treating symptomatic AD will continue to persist, given increased longevity. Novel approaches that target hallmark pathology may or may not have an effect at the fully symptomatic stage. New approaches may include addressing synaptic dysfunction and cell death, which should be relevant at a wide range of disease severity.

Future development of therapeutics for AD will undoubtedly include treatments for symptomatic individuals who are considered to have prodromal AD, and later trials will probably turn to those with no symptoms but who have imaging biomarkers that may prove to be associated with AD development later in life.

Although risk reduction of competing conditions has been proposed as an effective approach for the treatment and prevention of AD (Barnes and Yaffe, 2011), population-based studies suggest that these risks may already be well managed (Schrijvers et al., 2012), mitigating (Langa et al., 2008) the expectation of further benefit. Thus only new therapeutics hold a hope for true improvement.

DISCLOSURES

Dr. Sano reports that she has been a paid advisor/consultant to Eli Lilly, Esai, Medivation, Medpace, Nutricia, Sanofi-Aventis, and Takeda. Dr. Sano reports she has been an unpaid advisor to Merck.

Dr. Neugroschl has no conflicts of interest to disclose.

REFERENCES

Administration on Aging, Department of Health and Human Services. (2010). Projected Future Growth of Older Population. http://www.aoa.gov/aoaroot/aging_statistics/future_growth/future_growth.aspx.

Aisen, P.S. (2008). The inflammatory hypothesis of Alzheimer disease: dead or alive? *Alzheimer Dis. Assoc. Disord.* 22(1):4–5.

Aisen, P.S., Schneider, L.S., et al. (2008). High-dose B vitamin supplementation and cognitive decline in Alzheimer disease: a randomized controlled trial. *JAMA* 300(15):1774–1783.

Allen, K.V., Frier, B.M., et al. (2004). The relationship between type 2 diabetes and cognitive dysfunction: longitudinal studies and their methodological limitations. *Eur. J. Pharmacol.* 490(1–3):169–175.

Alzheimers Association. (2012). 2012 Alzheimer's disease facts and figures. *Alzheimers Dement.* 8(2):131–168.

Ames, D., and Ritchie, C. (2007). Antioxidants and Alzheimer's disease: time to stop feeding vitamin E to dementia patients? *Int. Psychogeriatr.* 19(1):1–8.

Andreeva, V.A., Kesse-Guyot, E., et al. (2011). Cognitive function after supplementation with B vitamins and long-chain omega-3 fatty acids: ancillary findings from the SU.FOL.OM3 randomized trial. *Am. J. Clin. Nutr.* 94(1):278–286.

Atri, A., Shaughnessy, L.W., et al. (2008). Long-term course and effectiveness of combination therapy in Alzheimer disease. *Alzheimer Dis. Assoc. Disord.* 22(3):209–221.

Barberger-Gateau, P., Letenneur, L., et al. (2002). Fish, meat, and risk of dementia: cohort study. *BMJ* 325(7370):932–933.

Barnes, D.E., and Yaffe, K. (2011). The projected effect of risk factor reduction on Alzheimer's disease prevalence. *Lancet Neurol.* 10(9):819–828.

Bartus, R.T., Dean, R.L., 3rd, et al. (1982). The cholinergic hypothesis of geriatric memory dysfunction. *Science* 217(4558):408–414.

Bauer, J., Ganter, U., et al. (1992). The participation of interleukin-6 in the pathogenesis of Alzheimer's disease. *Res. Immunol.* 143(6):650–657.

Baum, L., Lam, C.W., et al. (2008). Six-month randomized, placebo-controlled, double-blind, pilot clinical trial of curcumin in patients with Alzheimer disease. *J. Clin. Psychopharmacol.* 28(1):110–113.

Behl, C., Davis, J., et al. (1992). Vitamin E protects nerve cells from amyloid beta protein toxicity. *Biochem. Biophys. Res. Commun.* 186(2):944–950.

Birks, J. (2006). Cholinesterase inhibitors for Alzheimer's disease. *Cochrane Database Syst. Rev.* (1):CD005593.

Birks, J., and Grimley Evans, J. (2009). Ginkgo biloba for cognitive impairment and dementia. *Cochrane Database Syst. Rev.* (1):CD003120.

Blass, J.P., and Gibson, G.E. (2006). Correlations of disability and biologic alterations in Alzheimer brain and test of significance by a therapeutic trial in humans. *J. Alzheimers Dis.* 9(2):207–218.

Bonaa, K.H., Njolstad, I., et al. (2006). Homocysteine lowering and cardiovascular events after acute myocardial infarction. *N. Engl. J. Med.* 354(15):1578–1588.

Boothby, L.A., and Doering, P.L. (2005). Vitamin C and vitamin E for Alzheimer's disease. *Ann. Pharmacother.* 39(12):2073–2080.

Bostom, A.G., Rosenberg, I.H., et al. (1999). Nonfasting plasma total homocysteine levels and stroke incidence in elderly persons: the Framingham Study. *Ann. Intern. Med.* 131(5):352–355.

Breitner, J.C., Baker, L.D., et al. (2011). Extended results of the Alzheimer's disease anti-inflammatory prevention trial. *Alzheimers Dement.* 7(4):402–411.

Burns, A., Bernabei, R., et al. (2009). Safety and efficacy of galantamine (Reminyl) in severe Alzheimer's disease (the SERAD study): a randomised, placebo-controlled, double-blind trial. *Lancet Neurol.* 8(1):39–47.

Chang-Quan, H., Hui, W., et al. (2011). The association of antihypertensive medication use with risk of cognitive decline and dementia: a meta-analysis of longitudinal studies. *Int. J. Clin. Pract.* 65(12):1295–1305.

Cherrier, M.M., Matsumoto, A.M., et al. (2005). Testosterone improves spatial memory in men with Alzheimer disease and mild cognitive impairment. *Neurology* 64(12):2063–2068.

Choi, S.H., Park, K.W., et al. (2011). Tolerability and efficacy of memantine add-on therapy to rivastigmine transdermal patches in mild to moderate Alzheimer's disease: a multicenter, randomized, open-label, parallel-group study. *Curr. Med. Res. Opin.* 27(7):1375–1383.

Collaboration, H.L.T. (2005). Dose-dependent effects of folic acid on blood concentrations of homocysteine: a meta-analysis of the randomized trials. *Am. J. Clin. Nutr.* 82(4):806–812.

Craft, S., Baker, L.D., et al. (2012). Intranasal insulin therapy for Alzheimer disease and amnestic mild cognitive impairment: a pilot clinical trial. *Arch. Neurol.* 69(1):29–38.

Cummings, J., Jones, R., et al. (2010). Effect of donepezil on cognition in severe Alzheimer's disease: a pooled data analysis. *J. Alzheimers Dis.* 21(3):843–851.

Danysz, W., Parsons, C.G., et al. (2000). Neuroprotective and symptomatological action of memantine relevant for Alzheimer's disease: a unified glutamatergic hypothesis on the mechanism of action. *Neurotox. Res.* 2(2–3):85–97.

Davies, P., and Maloney, A.J. (1976). Selective loss of central cholinergic neurons in Alzheimer's disease. *Lancet* 2(8000):1403.

DeKosky, S.T., Williamson, J.D., et al. (2008). Ginkgo biloba for prevention of dementia: a randomized controlled trial. *JAMA* 300(19):2253–2262.

Doody, R.S. (2005). Refining treatment guidelines in Alzheimer's disease. *Geriatrics* (Suppl):14–20.

Durga, J., van Boxtel, M.P., et al. (2007). Effect of 3-year folic acid supplementation on cognitive function in older adults in the FACIT trial: a randomised, double blind, controlled trial. *Lancet* 369(9557):208–216.

Farlow, M.R., Grossberg, G.T., et al. (2011). Rivastigmine transdermal patch and capsule in Alzheimer's disease: influence of disease stage on response to therapy. *Int. J. Geriatr. Psychiatry* 26(12):1236–1243.

Farlow, M.R., Salloway, S., et al. (2010). Effectiveness and tolerability of high-dose (23 mg/d) versus standard-dose (10 mg/d) donepezil in moderate to severe Alzheimer's disease: a 24-week, randomized, double-blind study. *Clin. Ther.* 32(7):1234–1251.

Feldman, H.H., Doody, R.S., et al. (2010). Randomized controlled trial of atorvastatin in mild to moderate Alzheimer disease: LEADe. *Neurology* 74(12):956–964.

Ferris, S., Lane, R., et al. (2009). Effects of gender on response to treatment with rivastigmine in mild cognitive impairment: a post hoc statistical modeling approach. *Gend. Med.* 6(2):345–355.

Fillit, H., Ding, W.H., et al. (1991). Elevated circulating tumor necrosis factor levels in Alzheimer's disease. *Neurosci. Lett.* 129(2):318–320.

Ford, A.H., Flicker, L., et al. (2010). Vitamins B(12), B(6), and folic acid for cognition in older men. *Neurology* 75(17):1540–1547.

Frautschy, S.A., Hu, W., et al. (2001). Phenolic anti-inflammatory antioxidant reversal of Abeta-induced cognitive deficits and neuropathology. *Neurobiol. Aging* 22(6):993–1005.

Freund-Levi, Y., Eriksdotter-Jonhagen, M., et al. (2006). Omega-3 fatty acid treatment in 174 patients with mild to moderate Alzheimer disease: OmegAD study: a randomized double-blind trial. *Arch. Neurol.* 63(10):1402–1408.

Galasko, D.R., Peskind, E., et al. (2012). Antioxidants for Alzheimer disease: a randomized clinical trial with cerebrospinal fluid biomarker measures. *Arch. Neurol.* 69(7):836–841.

Gaudig, M., Richarz, U., et al. (2011). Effects of galantamine in Alzheimer's disease: double-blind withdrawal studies evaluating sustained versus interrupted treatment. *Curr. Alzheimer Res.* 8(7):771–780.

Geldmacher, D.S., Fritsch, T., et al. (2011). A randomized pilot clinical trial of the safety of pioglitazone in treatment of patients with Alzheimer disease. *Arch. Neurol.* 68(1):45–50.

Green, R.C., Schneider, L.S., et al. (2009). Effect of tarenflurbil on cognitive decline and activities of daily living in patients with mild Alzheimer disease: a randomized controlled trial. *JAMA* 302(23):2557–2564.

Grossberg, G.T., Olin, J.T., et al. (2011). Dose effects associated with rivastigmine transdermal patch in patients with mild-to-moderate Alzheimer's disease. *Int. J. Clin. Pract.* 65(4):465–471.

Harrington, C., Sawchak, S., et al. (2011). Rosiglitazone does not improve cognition or global function when used as adjunctive therapy to AChE inhibitors in mild-to-moderate Alzheimer's disease: two phase 3 studies. *Curr. Alzheimer Res.* 8(5):592–606.

Hayden, K.M., Zandi, P.P., et al. (2007). Does NSAID use modify cognitive trajectories in the elderly? The Cache County study. *Neurology* 69(3):275–282.

Heart Protection Study Collaborative Group. (2002). MRC/BHF Heart Protection Study of antioxidant vitamin supplementation in 20,536 high-risk individuals: a randomised placebo-controlled trial. *Lancet* 360(9326):23–33.

Henderson, S.T., Vogel, J.L., et al. (2009). Study of the ketogenic agent AC-1202 in mild to moderate Alzheimer's disease: a randomized, double-blind, placebo-controlled, multicenter trial. *Nutr. Metab.* 6:31.

Hlasney, E. (2009). Consumer Confidence in Dietary Supplements Rises in 2009. http://www.crnusa.org/CRNPR2009CRNConsumerSurvey_Usage Confidence. html.

Hogervorst, E., Yaffe, K., et al. (2009). Hormone replacement therapy to maintain cognitive function in women with dementia. *Cochrane Database Syst. Rev.* (1):CD003799.

Howard, R.J., Juszczak, E., et al. (2007). Donepezil for the treatment of agitation in Alzheimer's disease. *N. Engl. J. Med.* 357(14):1382–1392.

Howard, R., McShane, R., et al. (2012). Donepezil and memantine for moderate-to-severe Alzheimer's disease. *N. Engl. J. Med.* 366(10):893–903.

Huang, H.Y., Helzlsouer, K.J., et al. (2000). The effects of vitamin C and vitamin E on oxidative DNA damage: results from a randomized controlled trial. *Cancer Epidemiol. Biomarkers Prev.* 9(7):647–652.

Huang, T.C., Lu, K.T., et al. (2011). Resveratrol protects rats from Abeta-induced neurotoxicity by the reduction of iNOS expression and lipid peroxidation. *PLoS One* 6(12):e29102.

Hynd, M.R., Scott, H.L., et al. (2004). Glutamate-mediated excitotoxicity and neurodegeneration in Alzheimer's disease. *Neurochem. Int.* 45(5):583–595.

Janssen, I.M., Sturtz, S., et al. (2010). Ginkgo biloba in Alzheimer's disease: a systematic review. *Wien. Med. Wochenschr.* 160(21–22):539–546.

Johnson, J.W., and Kotermanski, S.E. (2006). Mechanism of action of memantine. *Curr. Opin. Pharmacol.* 6(1):61–67.

Karuppagounder, S.S., Pinto, J.T., et al. (2009). Dietary supplementation with resveratrol reduces plaque pathology in a transgenic model of Alzheimer's disease. *Neurochem. Int.* 54(2):111–118.

Kwok, T., Lee, J., et al. (2011). A randomized placebo controlled trial of homocysteine lowering to reduce cognitive decline in older demented people. *Clin. Nutr.* 30(3):297–302.

Langa, K.M., Larson, E.B., et al. (2008). Trends in the prevalence and mortality of cognitive impairment in the United States: is there evidence of a compression of cognitive morbidity? *Alzheimers Dement.* 4(2):134–144.

Launer, L.J., Miller, M.E., et al. (2011). Effects of intensive glucose lowering on brain structure and function in people with type 2 diabetes (ACCORD MIND): a randomised open-label substudy. *Lancet Neurol.* 10(11):969–977.

Launer, L.J., Petrovitch, H., et al. (2008). AD brain pathology: vascular origins? Results from the HAAS autopsy study. *Neurobiol. Aging* 29(10):1587–1590.

Le Bars, P.L., Katz, M.M., et al. (1997). A placebo-controlled, double-blind, randomized trial of an extract of Ginkgo biloba for dementia. North American EGb Study Group. *JAMA* 278(16):1327–1332.

Leoutsakos, J.M., Muthen, B.O., et al. (2012). Effects of non-steroidal anti-inflammatory drug treatments on cognitive decline vary by phase of pre-clinical Alzheimer disease: findings from the randomized controlled Alzheimer's Disease Anti-inflammatory Prevention Trial. *Int. J. Geriatr. Psychiatry* 27(4):364–374.

Lilly. (2010, August 17). Lilly halts development of semagacestat for Alzheimer's disease based on preliminary results of Phase III clinical trials. http://newsroom.lilly.com/releasedetail.cfm?ReleaseID=499794.

Lim, W.S., Gammack, J.K., et al. (2006). Omega 3 fatty acid for the prevention of dementia. *Cochrane Database Syst. Rev.* (1):CD005379.

Lippman, S.M., Klein, E.A., et al. (2009). Effect of selenium and vitamin E on risk of prostate cancer and other cancers: the Selenium and Vitamin E Cancer Prevention Trial (SELECT). *JAMA* 301(1):39–51.

Lonn, E., Bosch, J., et al. (2005). Effects of long-term vitamin E supplementation on cardiovascular events and cancer: a randomized controlled trial. *JAMA* 293(11):1338–1347.

Lonn, E., Yusuf, S., et al. (2006). Homocysteine lowering with folic acid and B vitamins in vascular disease. *N. Engl. J. Med.* 354(15): 1567–1577.

Lovell, M.A. and Markesbery, W.R. (2007). Oxidative damage in mild cognitive impairment and early Alzheimer's disease. *J. Neurosci. Res.* 85(14):3036–3040.

Lu, P.H., Masterman, D.A., et al. (2006). Effects of testosterone on cognition and mood in male patients with mild Alzheimer disease and healthy elderly men. *Arch. Neurol.* 63(2):177–185.

Luchsinger, J.A., and Mayeux, R. (2004). Cardiovascular risk factors and Alzheimer's disease. *Curr. Atheroscler. Rep.* 6(4):261–266.

Luchsinger, J.A., Reitz, C., et al. (2005). Aggregation of vascular risk factors and risk of incident Alzheimer disease. *Neurology* 65(4):545–551.

Luchsinger, J.A., Tang, M.X., et al. (2007). Relation of higher folate intake to lower risk of Alzheimer disease in the elderly. *Arch. Neurol.* 64(1):86–92.

Lyketsos, C.G., Breitner, J.C., et al. (2007). Naproxen and celecoxib do not prevent AD in early results from a randomized controlled trial. *Neurology* 68(21):1800–1808.

Malouf, R., and Grimley Evans, J. (2008). Folic acid with or without vitamin B12 for the prevention and treatment of healthy elderly and demented people. *Cochrane Database Syst. Rev.* (4):CD004514.

Marambaud, P., Zhao, H., et al. (2005). Resveratrol promotes clearance of Alzheimer's disease amyloid-beta peptides. *J. Biol. Chem.* 280(45):37377–37382.

McGeer, P.L., and McGeer, E.G. (2001). Inflammation, autotoxicity and Alzheimer disease. *Neurobiol. Aging* 22(6):799–809.

McGeer, P.L., and McGeer, E.G. (2007). NSAIDs and Alzheimer disease: epidemiological, animal model and clinical studies. *Neurobiol. Aging* 28(5):639–647.

McGuinness, B., Craig, D., et al. (2009). Statins for the prevention of dementia. *Cochrane Database Syst. Rev.* (2):CD003160.

McGuinness, B., Todd, S., et al. (2009). Blood pressure lowering in patients without prior cerebrovascular disease for prevention of cognitive impairment and dementia. *Cochrane Database Syst. Rev.* (4):CD004034.

McMahon, J.A., Green, T.J., et al. (2006). A controlled trial of homocysteine lowering and cognitive performance. *N. Engl. J. Med.* 354(26):2764–2772.

McShane, R., Areosa Sastre, A., et al. (2006). Memantine for dementia. *Cochrane Database Syst. Rev.* (2):CD003154.

Mesulam, M., Guillozet, A., et al. (2002). Widely spread butyrylcholinesterase can hydrolyze acetylcholine in the normal and Alzheimer brain. *Neurobiol. Dis.* 9(1):88–93.

Miller, E.R., 3rd, Pastor-Barriuso, R., et al. (2005). Meta-analysis: high-dosage vitamin E supplementation may increase all-cause mortality. *Ann. Intern. Med.* 142(1):37–46.

Miller, N.J., and Rice-Evans, C.A. (1995). Antioxidant activity of resveratrol in red wine. *Clin. Chem.* 41(12 Pt 1):1789.

Moller, M.C., Bartfai, A.B., et al. (2010). Effects of testosterone and estrogen replacement on memory function. *Menopause* 17(5):983–989.

Morris, M.C., Evans, D.A., et al. (2003). Consumption of fish and n-3 fatty acids and risk of incident Alzheimer disease. *Arch. Neurol.* 60(7):940–946.

Ng, T.P., Chiam, P.C., et al. (2006). Curry consumption and cognitive function in the elderly. *Am. J. Epidemiol.* 164(9):898–906.

O'Brien, J.T., and Burns, A. (2011). Clinical practice with anti-dementia drugs: a revised (second) consensus statement from the British Association for Psychopharmacology. *J. Psychopharmacol.* 25(8):997–1019.

Olin, J.T., Aarsland, D., et al. (2010). Rivastigmine in the treatment of dementia associated with Parkinson's disease: effects on activities of daily living. *Dement. Geriatr. Cogn. Disord.* 29(6):510–515.

Pearson, K.J., Baur, J.A., et al. (2008). Resveratrol delays age-related deterioration and mimics transcriptional aspects of dietary restriction without extending life span. *Cell Metab.* 8(2):157–168.

Peila, R., Rodriguez, B.L., et al. (2002). Type 2 diabetes, APOE gene, and the risk for dementia and related pathologies: the Honolulu-Asia Aging Study. *Diabetes* 51(4):1256–1262.

Peters, R., Beckett, N., et al. (2008). Incident dementia and blood pressure lowering in the Hypertension in the Very Elderly Trial cognitive function assessment (HYVET-COG): a double-blind, placebo controlled trial. *Lancet Neurol.* 7(8):683–689.

Peters, R., Beckett, N., et al. (2010). Modelling cognitive decline in the Hypertension in the Very Elderly Trial [HYVET] and proposed risk tables for population use. *PLoS One* 5(7):e11775.

Petersen, R.C., Thomas, R.G., et al. (2005). Vitamin E and donepezil for the treatment of mild cognitive impairment. *N. Engl. J. Med.* 352(23):2379–2388.

Prince, M., Bryce, R., et al. (2011). World Alzheimer Report 2011: The Benefits of Early Diagnosis and Intervention. London: Alzheimer's Disease International.

Quinn, J.F., Raman, R., et al. (2010). Docosahexaenoic acid supplementation and cognitive decline in Alzheimer disease: a randomized trial. *JAMA* 304(17):1903–1911.

Rafii, M.S., Walsh, S., et al. (2011). A phase II trial of huperzine A in mild to moderate Alzheimer disease. *Neurology* 76(16):1389–1394.

Rattinger, G.B., Dutcher, S.K., et al. (2012). The effect of dementia on medication use and adherence among medicare beneficiaries with chronic heart failure. *Am. J. Geriat. Pharmacother.* 10(1):69–80.

Ringman, J.M., Frautschy, S.A., et al. (2012). Oral curcumin for Alzheimer's disease: tolerability and efficacy in a 24-week randomized, double blind, placebo-controlled study. *Alzheimers Res. Ther.* 4(5):43. [Epub ahead of print]

Sano, M., Bell, K.L., et al. (2011). A randomized, double-blind, placebo-controlled trial of simvastatin to treat Alzheimer disease. *Neurology* 77(6):556–563.

Sano, M., Ernesto, C., et al. (1997). A controlled trial of selegiline, alpha-tocopherol, or both as treatment for Alzheimer's disease: the Alzheimer's Disease Cooperative Study. *N. Engl. J. Med.* 336(17):1216–1222.

Sato, T., Hanyu, H., et al. (2011). Efficacy of PPAR-gamma agonist pioglitazone in mild Alzheimer disease. *Neurobiol. Aging* 32(9):1626–1633.

Savaskan, E., Olivieri, G., et al. (2003). Red wine ingredient resveratrol protects from beta-amyloid neurotoxicity. *Gerontology* 49(6):380–383.

Scheltens, P., Twisk, J.W., et al. (2011). Souvenaid® Improves Memory in Drug-Naïve Patients with Mild Alzheimer's Disease: Results from a Randomized, Controlled, Double-Blind Study (Souvenir II). San Diego, CA: CtAD.

Scheltens, P., Kamphuis, P.J., et al. (2010). Efficacy of a medical food in mild Alzheimer's disease: a randomized, controlled trial. *Alzheimers Dement.* 6(1):1–10 e11.

Schneider, L.S. (2008). Ginkgo biloba extract and preventing Alzheimer disease. *JAMA* 300(19):2306–2308.

Schneider, L.S., DeKosky, S.T., et al. (2005). A randomized, double-blind, placebo-controlled trial of two doses of Ginkgo biloba extract in dementia of the Alzheimer's type. *Curr. Alzheimer Res.* 2(5):541–551.

Schrijvers, E.M., Verhaaren, B.F., et al. (2012). Is dementia incidence declining?: Trends in dementia incidence since 1990 in the Rotterdam Study. *Neurology* 78(19):1456–1463.

Seshadri, S., Beiser, A., et al. (2002). Plasma homocysteine as a risk factor for dementia and Alzheimer's disease. *N. Engl. J. Med.* 346(7):476–483.

Shah, R., Kamphuis, P.J., et al. (2011). Souvenaid® as an Add-On Intervention in Patients with Mild to Moderate Alzheimer's Disease Using Alzheimer's Disease Medication: Results from a Randomized, Controlled, Double-Blind Study (S-Connect). San Diego: CtAD.

Snitz, B.E., O'Meara, E.S., et al. (2009). Ginkgo biloba for preventing cognitive decline in older adults: a randomized trial. *JAMA* 302(24):2663–2670.

Stampfer, M.J., Malinow, M.R., et al. (1992). A prospective study of plasma homocyst(e)ine and risk of myocardial infarction in US physicians. *JAMA* 268(7):877–881.

Tan, R.S., and Pu, S.J. (2003). A pilot study on the effects of testosterone in hypogonadal aging male patients with Alzheimer's disease. *Aging Male* 6(1):13–17.

Tariot, P.N., Farlow, M.R., et al. (2004). Memantine treatment in patients with moderate to severe Alzheimer disease already receiving donepezil: a randomized controlled trial. *JAMA* 291(3):317–324.

Tariot, P., Salloway, S., et al. (2012). Long-term safety and tolerability of donepezil 23 mg in patients with moderate to severe Alzheimer's disease. *BMC Res. Notes* 5(1):283.

Thal, L.J., Ferris, S.H., et al. (2005). A randomized, double-blind, study of rofecoxib in patients with mild cognitive impairment. *Neuropsychopharmacol.* 30(6):1204–1215.

Trompet, S., van Vliet, P., et al. (2010). Pravastatin and cognitive function in the elderly: results of the PROSPER study. *J. Neurol.* 257(1):85–90.

Valen-Sendstad, A., Engedal, K., et al. (2010). Effects of hormone therapy on depressive symptoms and cognitive functions in women with Alzheimer disease: a 12 month randomized, double-blind, placebo-controlled study of low-dose estradiol and norethisterone. *Am. J. Geriatr. Psychiatry* 18(1):11–20.

van de Rest, O., Geleijnse, J.M., et al. (2008). Effect of fish oil on cognitive performance in older subjects: a randomized, controlled trial. *Neurology* 71(6):430–438.

van Dongen, M.C., van Rossum, E., et al. (2000). The efficacy of ginkgo for elderly people with dementia and age-associated memory impairment: new results of a randomized clinical trial. *J. Am. Geriatr. Soc.* 48(10):1183–1194.

Watkins, P.B., Zimmerman, H.J., et al. (1994). Hepatotoxic effects of tacrine administration in patients with Alzheimer's disease. *JAMA* 271(13):992–998.

Watson, G.S., Baker, L.D., et al. (2009). Effects of insulin and octreotide on memory and growth hormone in Alzheimer's disease. *J. Alzheimers Dis.* 18(3):595–602.

Weggen, S., Eriksen, J.L., et al. (2001). A subset of NSAIDs lower amyloidogenic Abeta42 independently of cyclooxygenase activity. *Nature* 414(6860):212–216.

Weinmann, S., Roll, S., et al. (2010). Effects of Ginkgo biloba in dementia: systematic review and meta-analysis. *BMC Geriatr.* 10:14.

Wharton, W., Baker, L.D., et al. (2011). Short-term hormone therapy with transdermal estradiol improves cognition for postmenopausal women with Alzheimer's disease: results of a randomized controlled trial. *J. Alzheimers Dis.* 26(3):495–505.

Wilcock, G.K., Black, S.E., et al. (2008). Efficacy and safety of tarenflurbil in mild to moderate Alzheimer's disease: a randomised phase II trial. *Lancet Neurol.* 7(6):483–493.

Winblad, B., Gauthier, S., et al. (2008). Safety and efficacy of galantamine in subjects with mild cognitive impairment. *Neurology* 70(22):2024–2035.

Wood, J.G., Rogina, B., et al. (2004). Sirtuin activators mimic caloric restriction and delay ageing in metazoans. *Nature* 430(7000):686–689.

Yamada, S., Akishita, M., et al. (2010). Effects of dehydroepiandrosterone supplementation on cognitive function and activities of daily living in older women with mild to moderate cognitive impairment. *Geriatr. Gerontol. Int.* 10(4):280–287.

Yasojima, K., Schwab, C., et al. (1999). Distribution of cyclooxygenase-1 and cyclooxygenase-2 mRNAs and proteins in human brain and peripheral organs. *Brain Res.* 830(2):226–236.

Yurko-Mauro, K., McCarthy, D., et al. (2010). Beneficial effects of docosahexaenoic acid on cognition in age-related cognitive decline. *Alzheimers Dement.* 6(6):456–464.

Zhang, C.E., Wei, W., et al. (2009). Hyperhomocysteinemia increases beta-amyloid by enhancing expression of gamma-secretase and phosphorylation of amyloid precursor protein in rat brain. *Am. J. Pathol.* 174(4):1481–1491.

65 | DISEASE-MODIFYING THERAPIES FOR ALZHEIMER'S DISEASE

JOSHUA D. GRILL AND JEFFREY CUMMINGS

Alzheimers disease (AD) is an age-related progressive neurodegenerative disorder. It is the most common cause of dementia, underlying 60–70% of all cases of late-onset cognitive decline. In the United States alone, more than 5 million persons are afflicted with AD and the prevalence is increasing. Whereas modern medicine has seen significant decline in deaths resulting from human immunodeficiency virus/acquired immunodeficiency syndrome, stroke, heart disease, and prostate and breast cancer, AD-related death has sharply risen. Alzheimer's disease is the sixth leading cause of death in the United States. The association of AD with age is marked; disease risk doubles for every five years of life beginning after age 60. With the recent explosion of the baby boomer generation into retirement age and the expected increases of the world's elderly population, an epidemic of AD is upon us. More than 30 million patients have dementia worldwide and the global prevalence of AD will double every 20 years (Ferri et al., 2005). The progressive course of AD eventually results in complete dependence and a high burden of care. The cost of this care is substantial, estimated at $180 billion annually in the United States, with worldwide expectations of unsustainable increases in cost. Thus, finding interventions that can reduce the burden associated with AD represents one of the most important scientific challenges in medical research.

The previous chapters in this section have described the substantial increases in understanding AD over the last several decades. The clinical phenomenology of AD is now well characterized and understood to include the slow and unrelenting progression of dementia, as well as a decade-long period of silent and then prodromal disease that eventually leads to clinical dementia. These predementia phases are characterized by accumulation of pathological substrates in the brain and initial neurodegeneration and may represent the ideal time of treatment.

Significant discoveries related to the genetic, molecular, and cellular underpinnings of AD have also been described in the preceding text. These discoveries have led to the identification of a wide array of therapeutic targets. Despite this, few drugs have achieved regulatory approval. Moreover, none of the approved drugs impact the underlying course of AD, instead providing mild improvement related to AD symptoms.

This chapter describes the state of the science of the pursuit of therapies that are capable of slowing the course of disease and, if started early enough, can impact the impending epidemic of AD. Specifically, the chapter:

- Defines disease modification and discuss its demonstration in the setting of AD clinical trials

- Presents the current state of trial design and outcome choices for studies of new potential disease-modifying agents

- Identifies the challenges to disease-modifying trials and how they may differ depending upon the clinical population enrolled

- Reviews findings from AD trials and how they contribute to the current understanding of potential disease modification and trial conduct

- Describes the current understanding of AD pathology and classes of drug candidates for disease-modification

- Presents the identified targets and candidate agents for potential disease-modifying therapies for AD

DEFINING DISEASE MODIFICATION

Many current clinical trials for AD address the pathophysiology of the disorder using pharmacologic targets affecting Aβ, tau-protein related mechanisms, mitochondrial function, neuroprotection, apoptosis, or neuroregenerative strategies (Salloway et al., 2008). These "disease-modifying" interventions aim to prevent, delay the onset, or slow the progression of the disease process. Neuroregenerative strategies or interventions that rescue dysfunctional but not moribund neurons could theoretically produce an improvement in function. These mechanism-based strategies are generally contrasted with symptomatic interventions that aim to compensate for deteriorating neural systems function but do not slow or ameliorate the underlying disease process. Neurotransmitter-related interventions, for example, are viewed as compensatory and not disease-modifying interventions.

No specific consensus definition of disease modification has evolved. Katz (2008) suggested that a strong definition of disease-modification is "a therapy that affects the underlying pathology and structure of the disease." Cummings (2006) suggested that a disease-modifying agent is a pharmacological treatment that intervenes in the neurobiological processes that lead been suggested that define synchronization in a more general context (Quian Quiroga et al., 2002). The majority of these methods make use of time-delay embedding to compute feature vectors, for example, a vector consisting of the next n time points of a signal, at each time point. These vectors are used to describe the short time dynamics of the underlying system that is being measured. Information regarding the synchronization of two signals can be extracted by examining how these feature vectors repeat within each, and how the repeatability patterns of each signal are correlated. One of the more widely utilized measures of generalized synchronization is synchronization likelihood (SL) (Montez et al., 2006). The SL technique assumes that two signals are synchronized if the repetition pattern of one signal coincides with the repetition pattern of the second signal. Suppose that the number of pattern repetitions in each of the two signals is n_{ref} and the number of time instants that is shared between the two patterns of repetitions is n_{k1k2} then SL is defined as n_{k1k2}/n_{ref}, which is a measure of coupling between the two signals. Figure 75.3 shows SL connectivity maps between different regions of the brain.

LIMITATIONS

As with the fMRI- and structural-based measures of connectivity, the use of electrophysiology in determining the likelihood of connections is not without limitations. In most cases, the connectivity methods described in the preceding have been used on time courses acquired directly from the MEG or EEG sensors. These sensors measure fluctuations in the magnetic fields or electrical potentials at the surface of the head. The activity of multiple brain regions contribute to the measured surface field, hindering the direct brain-level interpretation of sensor-level connectivity (Schoffelen and Gross, 2009), because the recordings of two sensors may be driven by a single brain region leading to a false detection of connectivity.

A number of source localization methods exist (Salmelin and Baillet, 2009) that determine time courses for specific regions of the brain, opening up the possibility of performing connectivity analysis within the source space, avoiding the interpretation issues that pervade the analysis of sensor-level connectivity. Methods include multiple regional source current dipole modeling, spatial filtering with beamformers, and L1- and L2-minimum norm estimation. Care, however, must be taken when choosing a source localization methodology, as many methods make assumptions about the statistical relationship between the time series of the computed sources and may have a significant effect on the measured connectivity.

APPLICATIONS IN NEURODEVELOPMENTAL DISORDERS

The study and quantification of brain connectivity offers researchers unique insight into the structure, organization, and fidelity of the neuronal circuits that facilitate our cognitive functions and complex behavior. Recently, there has been a change in the perspective concerning the biological underpinnings of many neuropsychiatric disorders. Increasingly, the models of these disorders, specifically developmental disorders, are moving away from focusing on the localized dysfunction of specific anatomical regions. Instead, these models stress the interconnectedness of the functional units of the brain, hypothesizing that the etiology of many disorders arises from abnormal network patterns of communication and connectivity.

As connectivity based analysis methods have advanced to the point where neuronal connectivity can routinely be investigated *in vivo*, its successful use in illuminating the underlying processes of several neurological and neurodegenerative diseases has become more pronounced. Although this field is in its infancy, it is evident that it holds considerable promise, motivating its increased adoption within clinical research programs. Here we highlight some of the insights these approaches have garnered into normal development, as well as, into developmental disorders such as autism spectrum disorders, schizophrenia, attention deficit/hyperactivity disorder, obsessive compulsive disorder, and Tourette syndrome.

TYPICAL DEVELOPMENT

The investigation of normal brain development is a very active area of research. The overarching goal is that by better characterizing and understanding normal neuronal development, we are better able to identify deviations, such as delays or periods of accelerated growth, from normal developmental progression that are associated with particular disorders (Shaw et al., 2010). Furthermore, an increased understanding of the interactions between genetic and environmental factors and development trajectories, better enables researchers to identify the underlying biological factors that drive deviations from this process and thus may illuminate underlying endophenotypes of specific disorders.

Although longitudinal studies focused on structural connectivity are still rare, there have been a number of cross-sectional studies to investigate WM development. DTI lifespan studies have shown that FA values in WM increase during adolescence and early adulthood, peaking roughly around 33 years of age (Hasan et al., 2007). This parabolic increase is followed by an equally gradual decrease. Not all fiber pathways develop with identical FA trajectories; pathways connecting the frontal and temporal lobe develop latest (Lebel et al., 2012), whereas those thought to involve more critical processing, such as, the corpus callosum (CC), the inferior longitudinal fasciculus (ILF), and the fornix develop earlier.

Structural connectome models have also been utilized to study differences in the organizational and topological properties of the neural networks with age. Gong et al. (2009) focused on changes across the entire adult lifespan (19 to 84 years), finding decreases in cortical regional efficiency, particularly in the parietal and occipital neocortex, with increases in the frontal and temporal regions. Global efficiencies did not show significant changes. Hagmann et al. (2010) focused on childhood and adolescent development (2 to 18 years), finding increases in global efficiency, node strength, and decreases in clustering electrophysiological time courses (Sakkalis, 2011), and so will not be recapitulated here. Additional methodologies have been developed that take better advantage of the temporal resolution available, which we introduce briefly in the following.

PARTIAL DIRECTED COHERENCE

Like Granger causality, partial directed coherence (PDC) is an effective connectivity technique that seeks to measure directed (causal) relationships between the time series of two regions. It accomplishes this by using a multivariate vector autoregression (MVAR) model. As opposed to GC, based on VAR models, which only examine the relationship between two autoregressive models, the utilization of an MVAR model estimates a full linear model, including interactions between all of the time courses. For instance, let the set of all the regional time courses be represented as $x(t) = [x_1(t),\ldots,x_n(t)]^T$, where $x_1(t)$ is the time course for region 1 and so on. The MVAR model is

$$x(t) = \sum_{i=1}^{p} A_i x(t-i) + \varepsilon(t),$$

where A_i is the matrix of mixing coefficients, including the interaction terms, and $\varepsilon(t)$ is a multivariate Gaussian noise. In contrast with GC, a time domain approach, PDC is defined in the frequency domain. It requires the computation of the Fourier transform of the set coefficient matrices (A_is), resulting in a coupling matrix defined across the frequency domain ($A(f)$). The PDC between any two channels is then computed from this Fourier transform (Sameshima and Baccala, 1999) as

$$\frac{\overline{A}_{ij}(f)}{\left(\overline{A}_{i:}^{H}(f)\overline{A}_{j:}(f)\right)^{\frac{1}{2}}}$$

where $\overline{A}(f) = I - A(f)$ and H represents conjugate transpose matrix operation.

MAGNITUDE SQUARED COHERENCE

Magnitude squared coherence (MSC) is the second most widely used method for examining functional connectivity from either MEG or EEG signals, after linear cross correlation. The MSC between two time courses $x(t)$ and $y(t)$ is defined as

$$MSC_{xy}(f) = \frac{\left|S_{xy}(f)\right|^2}{S_{xx}(f)S_{yy}(f)},$$

where $S_{xy}(f)$ is the cross spectral density function, the Fourier transform of the cross correlation between $x(t)$ and $y(t)$, and $S_{yy}(f)$ and $S_{xx}(f)$ are the respective autospectral density functions. Magnitude squared coherence provides a means to quantify the similarity between the time courses at each frequency. Typically, Welch's method is used to compute the cross and auto spectral density functions. This consists of dividing $x(t)$

and $y(t)$ into a number of segments by appropriate windowing techniques and then using the discrete FT in each segment. The frequency response is then averaged, across all the segments, to generate the MSC(f). During this process, care must be taken to ensure the stationarity of both time series during each segment.

PHASE SYNCHRONIZATION: THE PHASE LOCKING VALUE

In addition to the linear methods like cross-correlation, ICA and MSC that have been discussed, a group of non-linear methods have developed out of the field of nonlinear dynamics and chaos theory (Stam, 2005). Of this group, the phase locking value (PLV) has emerged as a prominent choice to measure the phase synchrony between two signals. Phase synchrony is defined when the difference between the instantaneous phase, $\phi(t)$, of the two signals, x and y, being compared, remains constant, $|\phi_x(t) - \phi_y(t)| = const$. The instantaneous phase of each signal can be estimated using either the Hilbert transform or via wavelet convolution (Ghuman et al., 2011). Once the instantaneous phases have been estimated, the PLV can be computed as

$$PLV = \left|\frac{1}{N}\sum_{k=0}^{N-1} e^{i\left(\phi_x(k\Delta t) - \phi_y(k\Delta t)\right)}\right|$$

where N is the length of the signal, Δt is the sampling period, and $|.|$ represents the magnitude of a complex number. The PLV generates a normalized number, between 0 and 1, which is sensitive to the stability of the phase relationship between the two signals.

CROSS MUTUAL INFORMATION

Cross mutual information is able to capture both linear and non-linear relationships between time series by measuring their interdependence using concepts derived from information theory. The mutual information of two observations (X, Y) is defined as

$$I(X,Y) = \sum_{y}\sum_{x} p(x,y)\log\left(\frac{p(x,y)}{p_x(x)p_y(y)}\right)$$

where $p(x,y)$ is the joint probability distribution of X and Y, and $p_x(x)$ and $p_y(y)$ are marginal probability distributions. This computation is typically difficult because of the need to correctly estimate these probability distributions (Tsiaras et al., 2011).

GENERALIZED SYNCHRONIZATION

In addition to measuring the synchrony between time signals with respect to their phases, a number of approaches have relegates fMRI to the investigation of relatively slowly changing signals, hindering its ability to quantify higher-frequency synchronizations. Furthermore, regional differences in the time course and shape of hemodynamic response function of the brain's vascular system (Ances et al., 2008), in principle, additionally confound measures of connectivity derived from such signals.

MEASURING CONNECTIVITY WITH ELECTROPHYSIOLOGY

Unlike the preceding fMRI-based neuroimaging methods, which are sensitive to secondary measures of neural activity such as the hemodynamic response, the magnetic and electrical signals measured by MEG and EEG are directly generated by neural activity. There are two clear benefits to using MEG/EEG for measuring functional and effective connectivity. First, the direct sensitivity to neuronal activity decreases the dependence on metabolic activity and vascular response, which can confound fMRI measurements. Second, and more important,

the high temporal resolution of these methods, typically less than 1 ms, allows much better characterization of the temporal dynamics of neuronal systems. As the methodologies for determining functional and effective connectivity are largely based on determining statistical relationships between the time courses of different brain regions, the increased temporal resolution offered by these electrophysiological methods makes them excellent choices to the investigation of neuronal connectivity (Fig. 75.3). Furthermore, the collection of data with high temporal resolution allows separate characterization of activity in different spectral bands (e.g., delta 0.5 to 4 Hz, alpha 8 to 13 Hz), as well as assessment of such phenomena as cross-frequency coupling (or phase-amplitude coupling), wherein activity in one frequency band may be modulated by activity in another.

Electrophysiology has been used to investigate brain connectivity since the 1960s. During this time the methods that have been utilized to investigate it have grown in complexity to take better advantage of the available high temporal resolution. In addition to their use in fMRI, all the mentioned functional connectivity analysis methodologies are applicable to

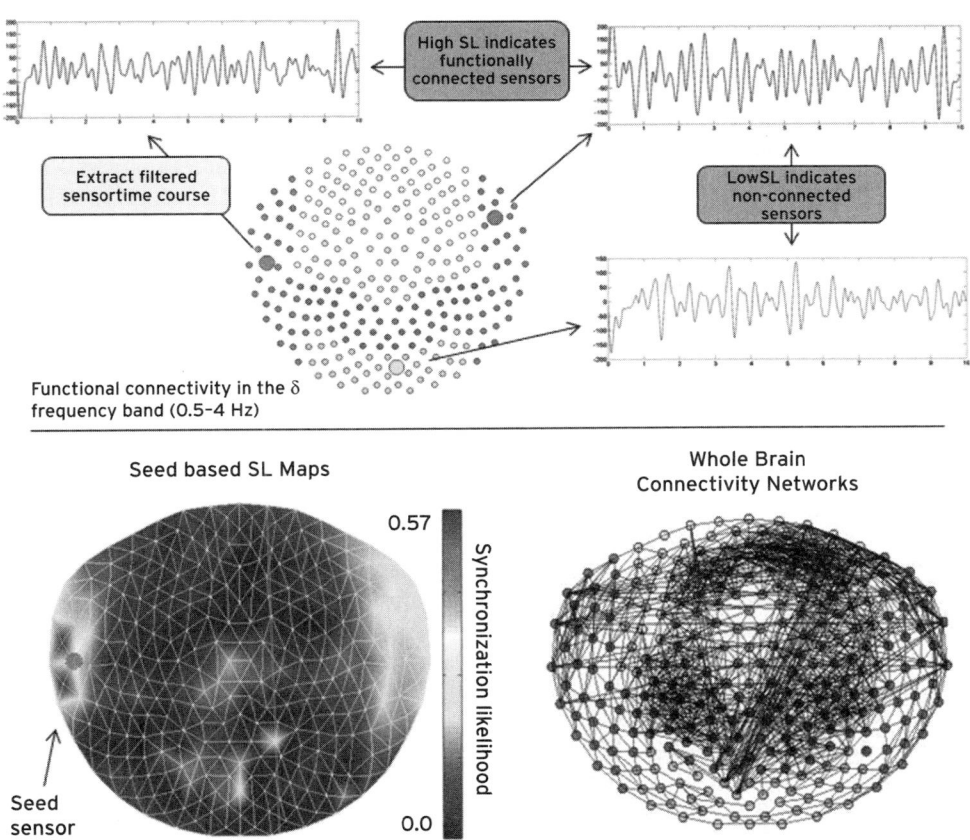

Figure 75.3 *MEG based functional connectivity. Measuring function connectivity with electrophysiologic modalities like MEG proceeds by extracting time courses of interest from the MEG sensor data. The high temporal resolution of MEG allows users to focus on connectivity within particular frequency bands; for instance, this figure focuses on connectivity in the delta (0.5 to 4 Hz) frequency band. The high resolution also allows for quantifying functional connectivity using complex measures, such as synchronization likelihood (SL). These measures can be computed on time courses from selected regions, shown at the top. Functionally connected sensors, such as those above the right and left motor areas, indicated by purple time courses, have higher SL values, whereas the SL between non-functionally connected regions, such as the occipital lobe and motor areas, have lower SL values. Maps showing connectivity to a particular seed region can also be computed. Similarly, whole brain networks can be determined by examining all of the pair-wise connectivity measures. (See color insert).*

determining the statistically optimal set of parameter values that best fit the observed data. When the model being fit includes interactions among different anatomical regions, the values of these parameters can tell us the degree to which these areas are interacting. It is important to recognize that the central goal of DCM is not necessarily to examine the effect elicited by an experimental condition, but serve as a means of comparing the possibility of alternative biologically meaningful models. Thus one of its principal applications is the investigation of models in which many regions interact to elicit a particular response.

Although there is considerable flexibility in the types of models that can be used, there are a number of traits that are common across many DCMs. First, DCMs are, by definition, dynamic; part of the modeling centers around describing, either linearly or nonlinearly, the temporal dynamics of the underlying neuronal responses. Second, DCMs describe how the dynamics in one region interacts with that of another region and is modulated by experimental stimuli or spontaneous activity. The final central piece of any DCM model is a biologically realistic forward model relating the unobserved neuronal response to the observed fMRI response. In fMRI-based studies, these models typically attempt to describe the local hemodynamic response to the underlying activity via a realistic vascular model that incorporates properties such as vascular expansion, arterial volume, and blood flow. One of the principal strengths of DCMs is the ability to compare different models based on their suitability to account for various datasets, leading to improvements in hemodynamic models, as well as models of brain connectivity.

GRANGER CAUSALITY

As opposed to techniques such as DCM, which require the testing/validation of full models, data-driven techniques do not make any assumptions about the underlying model or require a priori information concerning the spatiotemporal interactions of the various regions. Granger causality mapping is a data-driven approach that uses vector autoregressive (VAR) models of fMRI time courses extracted from two brain regions to quantify the ability of one time series to predict the other. Granger causality is built explicitly around the ideas of temporal precedence, if including past time points from region x's time series improves the prediction of the current value of a different region y's time series, then x can be thought of as causing y. In fMRI this process can be used to compute Granger causality maps (GCMs) that indicate the causal sources or targets of a preselected seed region (Roebroeck et al., 2005).

Granger causality makes use of VAR modeling to model each time series,

$$x(t) = \sum_{i=1}^{p} A_i x(t-i) + \varepsilon(t),$$

where A_i is the set of mixing coefficients at time lag i and $\varepsilon(t)$ is white noise. The core of the VAR model is that the current value of the time series $x(t)$ is modeled as a linear combination of the most recent p values. For two such time series, the Granger causality can be computed in terms of their respective VAR models. It should be noted that although the predominant use of Granger causality has centered on the VAR models, it is possible to formulate it in a more general nonlinear modeling framework (Stephan and Roebroeck, 2012).

LIMITATIONS

All of the fMRI-based connectivity methodologies discussed here have utilized the BOLD signal time series to examine the dependence or synchrony between anatomically disparate regions, each arriving at some measure of connectivity. In the case of fMRI-based functional connectivity, in which statistical relationships between time courses are used to determine the degree of connectivity, it is important to consider the existence of nuisance signals that may obfuscate the underlying neuronal signal and lead to spurious findings.

Because of the low temporal sampling rate of fMRI (around 0.5 Hz), many of the relatively higher-frequency components of cardiac and respiratory oscillations are aliased into the low-frequency rs-fMRI data set (<0.1 Hz), leading to spurious connectivity findings, because these signals affect the global signal. Although these are certainly of concern, because they are global signals, their effect can be adequately mitigated by regressing each voxel's time course with the mean global time course or from the mean time course of central WM regions in which no neuronal activity is occurring.

The primary nuisance signal revolves around the possible confounds that arise from subject motion. As can be imagined, even small amounts of motion, on the order of a few millimeters, can cause pronounced changes in the signal values of many voxels. Furthermore, because these signal changes are caused by gross subject motion, they are coincident in time and can lead to increases in temporal correlation. Recently, the effect of motion has been experimentally demonstrated to have significant impact of rs-fMRI–based connectivity measures (Satterthwaite et al., 2012; Van Dijk et al., 2012). This issue is particularly acute, as compliance in neuropsychiatric patient populations is generally more difficult, resulting in higher degrees of motion in patient populations than in control populations, introducing possible systematic biases into the connectivity analysis. Thus if there are group differences (patients vs. controls or younger vs. older subjects) in motion, there may appear to be group differences in functional connectivity. Whether these are authentic functional connectivity differences or entirely spurious consequences of the motion differences requires more thorough analysis (Van Dijk et al., 2012).

A final issue that is important to consider is that the BOLD signal is a direct measure of the hemodynamic response, which is coupled to the underlying neuronal activity via metabolism. Because the hemodynamic response is slow, compared with the underlying neuronal activity, it typically obfuscates the high temporal dynamics of the underlying neuronal signal. Thus fMRI is limited not only by scanner sampling rate, but also ultimately by the physiological origin of the signals. This

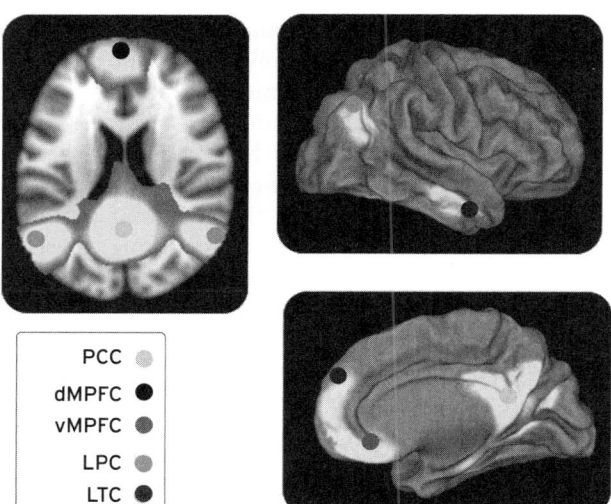

Figure 75.2 Default mode network. Temporally correlated activity in regions of the default mode network (DMN) has been shown to increase during non–goal-oriented activities and to decrease during goal oriented activities. The areas of the DMN is illustrated via a group averaged (n = 225) temporal correlation map generated by using the posterior cingulate cortex (PCC) as the seed region. The prominent regions of the DMN, the dorsal and ventral medial prefrontal cortexes (dMPFC and vMPFC), the lateral temporal cortex (LTC), and the lateral parietal cortex (LPC) are clearly indicated as being positively correlated with activity in the PCC. (See color insert).

posterior cingulate cortex. Figure 75.2 illustrates the DMN computed from 225 healthy subjects; rs-fMRI datasets from each subject were first spatially aligned. A seed region was placed in the posterior cingulate cortex and used to generate correlation maps to the other voxels of the brain. The average correlation map is shown in Figure 75.2, clearly identifying the main regions participating in the DMN. Connectivity between these regions has been robustly demonstrated in subjects not performing specific tasks (Fox and Raichle, 2007), and deactivated during the performance of goal-orientated tasks. Although the biological function of the DMN remains unresolved, its relationship to a number of neurodevelopmental disorders has become a major topic of research.

FUNCTIONAL CONNECTOMICS

A number of more holistic approaches have been put forth, seeking to examine the simultaneous interaction of many regions. Similar to the generation of structural connectomes, functional connectomes have been extracted from rs-fMRI (Yeo et al., 2011). As with the structural connectome, the functional connectome depends on a predefined set of regions (see Fig. 75.1). Time courses are extracted from each region and a correlation matrix is constructed, called the functional connectome. Clustering algorithms can be applied to identify highly interconnected subnetworks, or hierarchical topological maps of a subject's functional connectivity. Alternatively, topological properties, such as small worldedness, can be computed from these matrices (as in the diffusion-based structural connectivity matrices) and used to summarize the overall

functional connectivity patterns of the subject (Rubinov and Sporns, 2010). Table 75.1 shows some of the local and global properties that can be computed from these network matrices and used for subsequent statistical analysis of functional connectivity, analogous to structural connectivity.

INDEPENDENT COMPONENT ANALYSIS

An additional technique used for analyzing rs-fMRI data is the utilization of independent component analysis (ICA) to automatically discover highly interconnected networks of brain activity (Calhoun et al., 2008). As opposed to relying on a priori seed regions, ICA makes use of sophisticated algorithms to simultaneously analyze the entire rs-fMRI dataset (the time series of every voxel), and to decompose it into statistically independent components. This process yields spatial maps for each component, in addition to the time series for that component, allowing both the spatial extent and the temporal properties of each component to be characterized and analyzed. The temporal properties of fMRI noise and signal arising from neuro-anatomical systems are typically quite different, allowing ICA to isolate the two. Although this trait is extremely useful, it is typically up to the user to identify which component is noise and which correspond to actual networks, introducing the possibility for user bias. Relatedly, the results of ICA are often dependent on the number of components that are used in the decomposition. These issues combined with the vagaries introduced by the complexity of the decomposition process, can make biological interpretation of spatial maps and time series returned by ICA difficult. As a tool for hypothesis generation (for subsequent more focused exploration), this methodology, nonetheless, has considerable utility and promise.

Other approaches have been proposed to extract the dominant components and networks for resting state connectivity matrices. One popular approach is to attempt to increase the biological interpretation of the resulting components by imposing certain traits that are expected from physiologically based networks. For instance, by ensuring a decomposition that promotes positive connection values (Ghanbari et al., 2012), methods can be developed that extract subnetworks with direct connectivity interpretability. Similarly, decomposition algorithms can be developed that seek to identify components that maximally distinguish between patient and control populations (Batmanghelich et al., 2012), possibly shedding light on the neurologic underpinnings of disease.

DYNAMIC CAUSAL MODELING

Dynamic causal models (DCMs) are generative models of brain responses (Friston et al., 2003). They are used to describe the relationship between the unobserved neuronal states and the measured fMRI time courses. These models are governed by parameters that are constrained by a prior distribution that reflects empirical knowledge about the range of possible parameter values. Fitting a model to a given dataset involves

This scale discrepancy leads to many voxels containing tissue of diverse microstructure, encompassing complex fiber organization and geometry. Current estimates suggest that as many as two-thirds of the WM voxels (Behrens et al., 2007) show evidence of multiple, differently oriented fiber populations. Thus the models that are used to represent this organization must be able to accurately capture all of this complexity. The DT is able to accurately measure a single diffusion direction, making it well equipped to handle many of the major fiber pathways in the brain. However, in regions where multiple fibers intersect, more complex models are needed to reflect these geometries. Although a number of such models have been put forward, including high angular resolution diffusion imaging (HARDI) and diffusion spectrum imaging (DSI), there is no consensus on the optimal acquisition protocol and the analytic modeling.

Related to the issues arising from low spatial resolution and modeling is the need to improve our understanding of the biological basis for many of the diffusion scalars that are routinely used as measures of connectivity (Jones, 2010). For instance decreases in the FA of voxels containing only a single well-organized fiber population may have different root causes than observed FA decreases in voxels containing multiple fiber populations, each with different orientation.

Finally, as the field of structural connectomics matures, and studies move beyond examining topological properties of brain networks to investigating these networks on a connection by connection basis, the biological basis of these connection strengths and the topological measures computed from the networks will need to be investigated. There will also need to be a search for consensus in determining the optimal combination of tractography (Bastiani et al., 2012) methods, region parcellations (Zalesky et al., 2010), and connectivity measures (Bassett et al., 2011) to be used to create and analyze the network.

FUNCTIONAL MAGNETIC RESONANCE IMAGING–BASED CONNECTIVITY

Functional magnetic resonance imaging (fMRI) is a magnetic resonance imaging technique that is used to measure brain activity by detecting changes in the flow and oxygenation of blood. The blood-oxygen-level-dependent (BOLD) signal contrast provided by fMRI allows researchers to investigate the hemodynamic response to local increases in oxygen metabolism caused by neuronal activity. Images of these hemodynamic responses are acquired, typically every one to three seconds generating a time series for fMRI data. The high spatial resolution of fMRI (typically, 2 to 3 mm) makes it extremely well suited for investigating the roles and functions of brain regions, offering valuable insights into the functional segregation of the brain. With the broadening of research interests beyond basic functional localization, novel fMRI analysis methodologies have been developed that strive to characterize and quantify the degree of functional integration and communication that occurs between brain regions.

There are two experimental paradigms that are often used in fMRI investigations of neural connectivity. The most widely used fMRI-based connectivity methodology, resting state fMRI (rs-fMRI), centers on quantifying the degree of temporal synchrony between distant brain regions, during rest (Biswali, 1995), typically over the course of two to five minutes. Low-frequency (<0.1 Hz) BOLD signals of distant gray matter regions have been shown to have strong correlations through a wide variety of resting states, including eyes closed, or eyes open with simple fixation. The initial rs-fMRI studies (Biswal et al., 1995) demonstrated high correlation of the low-frequency BOLD signals between the left and right primary motor network areas, illustrating not only that these signals were able to capture the spontaneous activity that occurs during rest, but that regions known to functionally interact have similar temporal signatures at rest. Subsequent studies have successfully replicated this finding in the motor cortex, but also demonstrated high temporal correlations between regions of other known functional networks, such as the primary visual network, auditory network, and higher-order cognitive networks (Rosazza and Minati, 2011).

Alternatively, a number of studies focus on quantifying the neural connectivity between distant brain regions while the subject is actively performing a specified task. By manipulating the task being performed, experimenters can exert a degree of control over which cognitive processes and neural networks are being activated during a specific experiment. Although many connectivity analysis methods are applicable to either experimental paradigm, often particular analysis methods have been adopted based on the type of fMRI data used. For instance, the majority of studies using the *functional connectivity* measures, temporal correlation, independent component analysis, and so on, have focused on measuring intrinsic connectivity that occurs during rest. The *effective connectivity* measures, like dynamic casual modeling (DCM) and Granger causality (GC), which attempt to capture directional or causal nature of the interactions between different regions, have typically made greater use of the task-driven paradigm.

TEMPORAL CORRELATION

Several techniques have been described seeking to identify the spatial patterns of functional connectivity based on the BOLD signal. The most straightforward of these involves extracting the time series from a seed region of interest (ROI) and determining the temporal cross-correlation between this signal and those extracted from other brain voxels. This process generates maps of voxels that are functionally connected with the seed region. Although the dependence of an a priori definition of the seed region hinders the simultaneous investigation of multiple systems or the exploration the interaction of many regions, it does facilitate the simple extraction of networks with known function or those affected by certain pathologies.

One of the brain networks most studies using ROI-based temporal correlations focus on is the default mode network (DMN). The DMN is a network of brain regions including the medial prefrontal cortex, medial temporal lobe, and the

TABLE 75.1. Topological properties of connectivity networks

GLOBAL FEATURES	LOCAL FEATURES (DEFINED ON NODE *l*)
Density $D = \dfrac{\sum_{i \in N, j \in N, j \neq i} a_{ij}}{N(N-1)}$	Degree $k_i = \sum_{j \in N} a_{ij}$
Characteristic path length $$C = \frac{1}{n} \sum_{i \in N} \frac{\sum_{j \in N, j \neq i} d_{ij}^{w}}{n-1}$$	Local efficiency $$\eta_i = \frac{1}{2} \sum_{i \in N} \frac{\sum_{j,h \in N, j \neq i} \left(w_{ij} w_{ij} \left[d_{jh}^{w}(N_i)^{-1} \right] \right)^{\frac{1}{3}}}{k_i (k_i - 1)}$$
Global efficiency $$E = \frac{1}{n} \sum_{i \in N} \frac{\sum_{j \in N, j \neq i} \left(d_{ij}^{w} \right)^{-1}}{n-1}$$	Vulnerability $V_i = \dfrac{E - E^i}{E}$ E_i is the global efficiency without node i
Modularity $$Mod = \sum_{u \in M} \left[e_{uv} - \left(\sum_{u \in M} e_{uv} \right)^2 \right]$$ M is the number of modules, e_{uv} is the links proportion connecting nodes in modules u to module v	Betweenness centrality $$B_i = \frac{1}{(n-1)(n-2)} \sum_{h,j \in N, h \neq j, j \neq i, h \neq i} \frac{\rho_{hj}(i)}{\rho_{hj}}$$ $\rho_{hj}^{(i)}$ is number of shortest paths between h and j passing through i
Transitivity $T = \dfrac{\sum_{i \in N} 2t_i}{\sum_{i \in N} k_i (k_i - 1)}$	Strength $k_i^{w} = \sum_{j \in N} w_{ij}$
Assortativity $A = \dfrac{l^{-1} \sum_{i,j \in L} k_i k_j - \left[l^{-1} \sum_{i,j \in L} 0.5(k_i + k_j) \right]^2}{l^{-1} \sum_{i,j \in L} 0.5(k_i^2 + k_j^2) - \left[l^{-1} \sum_{i,j \in L} 0.5(k_i + k_j) \right]^2}$	**LEGEND** N is set of all nodes, n is number of nodes, d_{ij} is shortest path between i and j, a_{ij} is the connection status between i and j, w is weight of link, t_i is the number of triangles around i, L is set of all links, and l is number of links.

The *density* of the network is the ratio of the number of found connections to the total possible number of connections and is a general measure of how overtly connected the network is. The *characteristic path length* is the average number of connections required to connect any pair of regions. Finally, the *global efficiency* is related to how well the nodes are able to communicate. Similarly, there are three measures that capture the modularity of the network: *modularity*, *transitivity*, and *assortativity*. Topological measures can also be used to examine local (regional) features as well. These include local versions of *efficiency* and *degree*, as well as measures that focus on the resilience (*betweenness centrality*) and fault tolerance (*vulnerability*) of the entire network to disruptions of a particular region.

VOXEL- AND TRACT-BASED CONNECTIVITY

A second approach to the investigation of *structural connectivity* has focused on identifying population differences in DW-MRI derived scalar measures (most typically FA) used for representing local white matter tissue fidelity. (Note: It is not appropriate to generally consider this "integrity," as there are normal developmental changes in microstructural organization that should not be interpreted as changes in "integrity" with its associated semantic interpretation.) Localizing these differences enables the identification of altered white matter tissue structure and the ability to infer differences in the connectivity of the pathways passing through those regions. There are a number of spatial scales in which this approach has been successfully used. Population differences have been investigated at both the voxel and regional level, by aligning the images of each subject to a common spatial coordinate frame or anatomical atlas and then performing group-wise statistical analysis at each voxel or on average scalar measures extracted from each atlas defined region. Similar approaches have been undertaken, using fiber tractography to define specific anatomically relevant pathways, such as the acoustic radiations, which are then used to define regions for statistical analysis, as discussed, or alternatively, statistical differences in scalar indices can be investigated along the length of the pathway (Goodlett et al., 2009).

LIMITATIONS

DW-MRI allows researchers to infer the organizational structure of neuronal WM that is largely governed by the underlying organization of axonal fibers. Although it is sensitive to these small structures, the spatial resolution of DW-MRI images is generally on the order of 2 mm. Thus the signals that are measured, as well the models that are used to represent the local structures, are all ensemble averages of the many fiber bundles contained in each voxel.

NETWORK MODELS: THE STRUCTURAL CONNECTOME

The structural connectome (Hagmann et al., 2007; Sporns et al., 2005), is a network model of the brain consisting of a set of interconnected brain regions that are chosen a priori. For each pair of regions, the degree of structural connectivity between them is computed using tractography algorithms (Bastiani et al., 2012). These tractography algorithms are used to extract complete fiber pathways from the directional information, for instance, the eigenvectors of the DT model, obtained from the DW-MRI model at each voxel. The simplest of these algorithms works by starting at a seed location and moving in the direction indicated by the DW-MRI model. This deterministic process is repeated until the pathway leaves the white matter or until other stopping criteria are met, such as visiting a subthreshold FA location or generating a pathway with a large turning angle. More complex tractography methods also exist. Some use probabilistic methods to determine the next step taken in each pathway, whereas others seek to determine the most efficient path between any of the regions.

By seeding these algorithms at locations in the white matter determined by parcellation algorithms, the set of fibers that traverse the brain can be modeled. The end points of each computed fiber can then be used to examine the structural connections between the cortical and subcortical regions. A number of measures have been proposed to quantify the degree of structural connectivity. The most straightforward simply counts the fibers connecting two regions, essentially treating each computed fiber as a surrogate for an axonal bundle. Other approaches compute path integrals of scalar indices, such as FA, along each fiber connecting two regions yielding measures representing the fidelity of the structural connection between them. This information, coalesced in the *structural connectome*, allows the investigation of the global patterns of structural connections (Hagmann et al., 2007; Sporns, 2011). Figure 75.1 pictorially depicts the steps of parcellation, tractography, and network matrix generation, in creating a structural connectome. The structural connectome also provides an initial network representation of brain connectivity that is amenable to additional mathematical and graph theoretical analysis.

In addition to the statistical analysis of each individual connectivity strength (Zalesky et al., 2010a), a task made difficult by the large number of possible pairwise connections, these networks have been investigated using topological properties (Rubinov and Sporns, 2010), such as small worldedness and characteristic path length. Topological measures can be used to summarize the local and global properties of the connectome and provide a key to the understanding of the organization of the structural connectivity in individuals or how this organization can be affected by development or pathology. Table 75.1 lists some of the local and global properties that have been computed from these connectivity matrices that represent the network.

The most common of these topological properties are the global measures, which provide a single number to quantify the overall connectivity of a subject. There are three global measures used to capture the efficiency of the connectome.

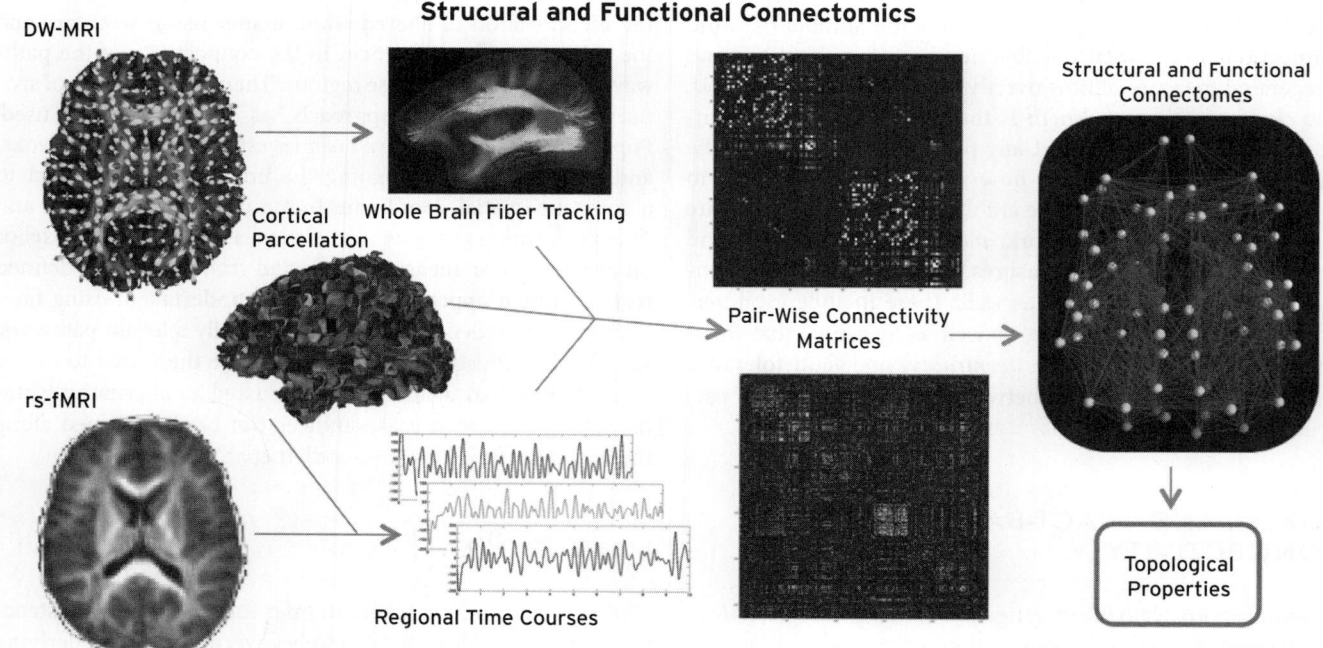

Figure 75.1 Functional and structural connectomics. The computation of structural and functional connectomes begins with the acquisition of either DW-MRI or rs-fMRI datasets and the parcellation of the cortex into the regions of interest (ROIS). Each modality undergoes specific preprocessing to remove artifacts. For DW-MRI, tractography algorithms are used to identify anatomical pathways connecting the ROIs and information related to these is collected into the pairwise connectivity matrix. Using the rs-fMRI datasets, ROI time courses are extracted and the pairwise connectivity matrix is formed by computing the temporal correlation between each ROI time course. These connectivity matrices can then be combined into a joint structural/functional connectome that can be used in subsequent analysis to represent the brain networks of the subject. (See color insert).

the vast interconnectedness of the brain and attempting to measure the structural and functional connectivity between distinct regions, the utilization of these methodologies enable the realization of a more holistic picture of brain function as it relates to normal and pathological development. This effort is the logical extension of the research focused on investigating functional segregation of the brain and essentially seeks to understand the means of information transfer between these functional units, as well as how this information transfer can be modulated by development and/or pathology.

The direct signaling between distant brain regions is achieved via the afferent and efferent axonal fibers that project between them. Action potentials traveling down these axons synapse on the dendrites of neurons in the destination regions. Although the exact investigation of this anatomical connectivity, at the axonal/synaptic scale, is difficult because of the dynamic nature of synaptic connections and the small spatial scales involved, the investigation of *structural connectivity* at the scale of axonal fiber bundles is possible via a careful modeling of the neuronal white matter. Alternatively, methods have been developed that focus on using spatiotemporal patterns of functional activity to investigate connectivity in the brain. Two types of methods have been proposed that take this second approach. The first, quantifies the *functional connectivity* between two regions based on the statistical relationship (Friston et al., 1993) of their respective functional activity time courses. Alternatively, the second method, *effective connectivity*, attempts to move beyond identifying regions that show similar patterns of activity. It seeks to quantify the causal influence that one neural assembly has over another (Friston et al., 1994) allowing for various hypotheses of neural communication to be tested.

A number of neuroimaging modalities have been used to non-invasively investigate brain connectivity and function. Both *functional* and *effective connectivity* rely on temporal measurements of neuronal activity, which are available from a number of modalities. Of these functional modalities, we focus on those that have been widely adopted, namely, fMRI and the methods of electrophysiology, MEG and EEG. These three methods are inherently non-invasive, requiring no additional contrast agents, and interestingly offer the most extreme tradeoffs between spatial and temporal resolution. The excellent spatial resolution provided by fMRI (2 to 3 mm) allows for the detailed investigation of interregional connectivity, but suffers from its low temporal resolution (typically one to three seconds). Alternatively, EEG and MEG possess excellent temporal resolution (<1 ms), which facilitates an in-depth investigation of neuronal dynamics, but with limited spatial resolution (roughly mm-cm). In contrast, only diffusion weighted MRI (DW-MRI) is able to provide *in vivo* information relating to structural connectivity. This section provides an overview of the methods and imaging modalities that enable the investigation of brain connectivity.

STRUCTURAL CONNECTIVITY

DW-MRI has emerged as the most prominent *in vivo* imaging methodology used to investigate neuronal white matter (WM) organization and fidelity. The contrast provided by DW-MRI is sensitive to the diffusion of water molecules as they traverse through their microenvironment. Cell membranes and other obstacles impede this motion, reducing the measured signal along directions perpendicular to these boundaries. By acquiring a set of DW-MRI images, each sensitive to the diffusion in different directions, insight can be gained relating to the local diffusion process and, in turn, into the local microstructure that gives rise to it. For instance, in highly ordered tissues such as those consisting of bundles of coaligned axons, the diffusion process is less restricted along the axonal pathway than perpendicular to it, resulting in anisotropic (directed) diffusion, whereas in less ordered tissues, in which the diffusion barriers are more randomly oriented, there is no dominant orientation of the diffusion process, resulting in an isotropic or spherical diffusion process.

At present, the most prominent form of DW-MRI, diffusion tensor imaging (DTI), consists of modeling the local diffusion process with a Gaussian distribution fully characterized by a 3×3 symmetric matrix, the diffusion tensor (DT). An eigensystem analysis can be used to diagonalize the DT, identifying the principal diffusion directions (the eigenvectors), as well as the diffusivity in those directions (the eigenvalues, λs). This yields information concerning both the shape and orientation of the diffusion process. Additionally, many scalars have been introduced to quantify the amount of anisotropic diffusion that is present in each voxel. For instance, linear anisotropy (CL), planar anisotropy (CP), and spherical anisotropy (CS), have been proposed (Westin et al., 2002) to measure different types of anisotropy in each voxel. However, the most widely accepted measure remains the fractional anisotropy (FA) (Basser and Pierpaoli, 1996). Fractional anisotropy is defined at each imaging voxel, in terms of the eigenvalues of the local DT as

$$FA = \sqrt{\frac{3}{2} \frac{(\lambda_1 - \bar{\lambda})^2 + (\lambda_2 - \bar{\lambda})^2 + (\lambda_3 - \bar{\lambda})^2}{\lambda_1^2 + \lambda_2^2 + \lambda_3^2}}$$

where $\bar{\lambda}$ is the mean of the eigenvalues.

Fractional anisotropy is a measure of the local severity of the diffusion anisotropy and is often used as a surrogate measure for tissue fidelity/integrity, owing to its relationship with axon myelination (Madler et al., 2008) within WM regions.

The DT model is not the only DW-MRI model currently being used to capture aspects of WM tissue structure and organization. More complex approaches have also been proposed (Tuch, 2004) that have similar goals of capturing the directionality and shape of the diffusion process and thus of the underlying anatomical microstructure. These methods typically require the acquisition of additional data, with prolonged acquisition times, and therefore have only recently been explored within clinical research.

There are two analysis pathways that utilize DW-MRI to investigate structural brain connectivity. The first uses network models to represent the structural interconnectedness of the brain, while the second infers deficiencies in connectivity from group based statistical analysis of diffusion measures such as fractional anisotropy.

75 | FUNCTIONAL CONNECTIVITY: APPLICATION TO DEVELOPMENTAL DISORDERS

LUKE BLOY, RAGINI VERMA, AND TIMOTHY P.L. ROBERTS

MOTIVATION FOR FUNCTIONAL CONNECTIVITY

The human brain consists of approximately 100 billion neurons, organized into a vastly complex network of interconnections. This network, consisting of both local neural circuits and long distance fiber pathways, is thought to provide the anatomical substrate allowing for the distributed interactions between brain regions (Hagmann et al., 2007; Sporns, 2011). Although neural anatomy has been extensively studied using cerebral dissection, relatively little is known about this complex set of connections, which mediate brain function and give rise to the richness of human behavior and experience. Chemical tracing, in which markers are locally injected into the cortex and their subsequent distribution is observed, has facilitated the probing of this network, yielding connectivity information in many animal models (Markov et al., 2011). However, the invasiveness of this technique necessarily precludes its use in human subjects, particularly within a clinical setting.

Noninvasive imaging (Kwong et al., 1992) and electrophysiological techniques have been developed to probe specific aspects of brain function and dysfunction, providing exquisite spatial maps of functional centers (typically using task-performance functional magnetic resonance imaging [fMRI]) and temporal characteristics, such as evoked response components and their amplitude modulation and latency shifts (typically using electroencephalography [EEG], or its magnetic counterpart, magnetoencephalography [MEG]). However, these descriptions are inadequate in fully accommodating the complex dynamic interplay, in space, time, and frequency band, that represents our present understanding of brain functional activity, in terms of structurally and functionally connected networks of neuronal ensembles. The evolution of non-invasive imaging techniques, in order to provide such descriptions, can be seen to have advanced from single-modality methods of identifying functional localization, specialization, and segregation, through real-time measures of activity itself (in terms of neuronal current amplitude and oscillatory power), through multimodality integration of structural, spatial, functional, and spectro-temporal approaches.

Thus, when considering the brain as a dynamic system, it is perhaps more appropriate to progress from brain "maps" toward brain "movies," allowing the time domain to represent the spatially distinct, but interacting, activity fluctuations. But what underlies the communication and connectivity between these spatially separate centers, or nodes, of activity? To address this question, the concepts of "connectomes" have been introduced, first to describe the node-to-node structural connectivity (for pairwise nodes distributed throughout the brain), and more recently to describe the relationship between activity at such pairs of nodes (Sporns, 2011). Experimentally, this approach to establishing the nature and complexity of functional connectivity draws primarily on resting state scans, either using functional MRI (rs-fMRI) or EEG/MEG, with a variety of measures of connectivity being constructed (perhaps, the simplest is a simple correlation of two regions' time courses), ultimately feeding mathematical models of connectivity (often drawing upon graph theoretical constructs) and quantification.

Although there are many compelling rationales for taking this approach to *describe* the functional relationships within the healthy brain, as well as in disease/neuropsychiatric disorders, it is worth considering how functional connectivity might be mediated at the cellular and molecular level. The inhibitory activity of the neurotransmitter γ-aminobutyric acid (GABA) released by inhibitory interneurons, upon the excitatory pyramidal cells (driven primarily by the excitatory neurotransmitter glutamate) might well be a source of modulation of local circuit activity, with measureable short- and long-range sequelae. Thus by observing (at a macroscopic level) the nature of functional connectivity, we might be able to infer (at a microscopic level) regional imbalance in excitation/inhibition, with the prospect of gaining molecular insights into the neurobiological basis of disease, and with the longer-term goal of identifying targets (at a molecular as well as substrate level) for novel interventions. Although this remains a hypothesis, both speculative and incomplete, this argument provides an additional motivation for a comprehensive and detailed, spatio-spectro-temporal characterization of human brain functional connectivity.

MEASURING NEURONAL CONNECTIVITY

The last two decades have seen the development of a number of analysis techniques seeking to move beyond the localization and identification of brain regions that are utilized during specific neurological processes. These new approaches focus on elucidating the degree of interconnectedness between disparate brain regions involved in these processes. By acknowledging von Bohlen Und Halbach, O. (2010). Dendritic spine abnormalities in mental retardation. *Cell Tissue Res.* 342:317–323.

Webber, C., Hehir-Kwa, J.Y., et al. (2009). Forging links between human mental retardation-associated CNVs and mouse gene knockout models. *PLoS Genet* 5:e1000531.

Weitz Doerfer, R., Dierssen, M., et al. (2001). Fetal life in Down syndrome starts with normal neuronal density but impaired dendritic spines and synaptosomal structure. *J. Neural. Trans.* 61:59–70.

West, A.E., and Greenberg, M.E. (2011). Neuronal activity-regulated gene transcription in synapse development and cognitive function. *Cold Spring Harb. Perspect. Biol.* 3:6.

Wright, G.J., and Washbourne, P. (2011). Neurexins, neuroligins and LRRTMs: synaptic adhesion getting fishy. *J. Neurochem.* 117:765–778.

Yin, D.M., Chen, Y.J., et al. (2012). Synaptic dysfunction in schizophrenia. *Adv. Exp. Med. Biol.* 970:493–516.

Yuste, R. (2011). Dendritic spines and distributed circuits. *Neuron* 71:772–781.

Zhang, Z., Jiao, Y.Y., et al. (2011). Developmental maturation of excitation and inhibition balance in principal neurons across four layers of somatosensory cortex. *Neuroscience* 174:10–25.

Zoghbi, H.Y. (2003). Postnatal neurodevelopmental disorders: meeting at the synapse? *Science* 302:826–830.

Frotscher, M. (2010). Role for Reelin in stabilizing cortical architecture. *Trends Neurosci.* 33:407–414.

Fukuchi-Shimogori, T., and Grove, E.A. (2001). Neocortex patterning by the secreted signaling molecule FGF8. *Science* 294:1071–1074.

Gatto, C.L., and Broadie, K. (2010). Genetic controls balancing excitatory and inhibitory synaptogenesis in neurodevelopmental disorder models. *Front. Syn. Neurosci.* 2:4.

Giedd, J.N., Blumenthal, J., et al. (1999). Brain development during childhood and adolescence: a longitudinal MRI study. *Nat. Neurosci.* 2:861–863.

Giedd, J.N., and Rapoport, J.L. (2010). Structural MRI of pediatric brain development: what have we learned and where are we going? *Neuron* 67:728–734.

Glantz, L.A., and Lewis, D.A. (2000). Decreased dendritic spine density on prefrontal cortical pyramidal neurons in schizophrenia. *Arch. Gen. Psychiatry* 57:65–73.

Goellner, B., and Aberle, H. (2012). The synaptic cytoskeleton in development and disease. *Dev. Neurobiol.* 72:111–125.

Graff, J., and Mansuy, I.M. (2008). Epigenetic codes in cognition and behaviour. *Behav. Brain Res.* 192:70–87.

Grilli, M., Ferrari Toninelli, G., et al. (2003). Alzheimer's disease linking neurodegeneration with neurodevelopment. *Funct. Neurol.* 18:145–148.

Grove, E.A., and Fukuchi-Shimogori, T. (2003). Generating the cerebral cortical area map. *Annu. Rev. Neurosci.* 26:355–380.

Guerrini, R., and Marini, C. (2006). Genetic malformations of cortical development. *Exp. Brain. Res.* 173:322–333.

Hamasaki, T., Leingartner, A., et al. (2004). EMX2 regulates sizes and positioning of the primary sensory and motor areas in neocortex by direct specification of cortical progenitors. *Neuron* 43:359–372.

Harrison, P.J., and Weinberger, D.R. (2005). Schizophrenia genes, gene expression, and neuropathology: on the matter of their convergence. *Mol. Psychiatry* 10:40–68; image 45.

Hippenmeyer, S., Youn, Y.H., et al. (2010). Genetic mosaic dissection of Lis1 and Ndel1 in neuronal migration. *Neuron* 68:695–709.

Hoeffer, C.A., Dey, A., et al. (2007). The Down syndrome critical region protein RCAN1 regulates long-term potentiation and memory via inhibition of phosphatase signaling. *J. Neurosci.* 27:13161–13172.

Hoftman, G.D., and Lewis, D.A. (2011). Postnatal developmental trajectories of neural circuits in the primate prefrontal cortex: identifying sensitive periods for vulnerability to schizophrenia. *Schizophr. Bull.* 37:493–503.

Insel, T.R. (2010). Rethinking schizophrenia. *Nature* 468:187–193.

Kendler, K.S., Kuhn, J.W., et al. (2005). The interaction of stressful life events and a serotonin transporter polymorphism in the prediction of episodes of major depression: a replication. *Arch. Gen. Psychiatry* 62:529–535.

Kessler, R.C., Amminger, G.P., et al. (2007). Age of onset of mental disorders: a review of recent literature. *Curr. Opin. Psychiatry* 20:359–364.

Knickmeyer, R.C., Gouttard, S., et al. (2008). A structural MRI study of human brain development from birth to 2 years. *J. Neurosci.* 28:12176–12182.

Kohl, M.M., and Paulsen, O. (2010). The roles of GABAB receptors in cortical network activity. *Adv. Pharmacol.* 58:205–229.

Krueger, R.F., and South, S.C. (2009). Externalizing disorders: cluster 5 of the proposed meta-structure for DSM-V and ICD-11. *Psychol. Med.* 39:2061–2070.

Lewis, D.A., Curley, A.A., et al. (2012). Cortical parvalbumin interneurons and cognitive dysfunction in schizophrenia. *Trends Neurosci.* 35:57–67.

Linhoff, M.W., Lauren, J., et al. (2009). An unbiased expression screen for synaptogenic proteins identifies the LRRTM protein family as synaptic organizers. *Neuron* 61:734–749.

Lockett, G.A., Wilkes, F., et al. (2010). Brain plasticity, memory and neurological disorders: an epigenetic perspective. *Neuroreport* 21:909–913.

Lott, I.T., and Dierssen, M. (2010). Cognitive deficits and associated neurological complications in individuals with Down's syndrome. *Lancet Neurol.* 9:623–633.

Maffei, A., and Turrigiano, G. (2008). The age of plasticity: developmental regulation of synaptic plasticity in neocortical microcircuits. *Prog. Brain Res.* 169:211–223.

Malhotra, D., and Sebat, J. (2012). CNVs: harbingers of a rare variant revolution in psychiatric genetics. *Cell* 148:1223–1241.

Marin, O. (2012). Interneuron dysfunction in psychiatric disorders. *Nat. Rev. Neurosci.* 13:107–120.

Marino, J., Schummers, J., et al. (2005). Invariant computations in local cortical networks with balanced excitation and inhibition. *Nat. Neurosci.* 8:194–201.

Martinez de Lagran, M., Benavides-Piccione, R., et al. (2012). Dyrk1a influences neuronal morphogenesis through regulation of cytoskeletal dynamics in mammalian cortical neurons. *Cereb. Cortex* 22(12):2867–2877.

McEwen, B.S., Eiland, L., et al. (2012). Stress and anxiety: structural plasticity and epigenetic regulation as a consequence of stress. *Neuropharmacology* 62:3–12.

McGrath, J.J., Feron, F.P., et al. (2003). The neurodevelopmental hypothesis of schizophrenia: a review of recent developments. *Ann. Med.* 35:86–93.

Michel, G.F. (2012). Using knowledge of development to promote recovery of function after brain damage. *Dev. Psychobiol.* 54:350–356.

Miyashita-Lin, E.M., Hevner, R., et al. (1999). Early neocortical regionalization in the absence of thalamic innervation. *Science* 285:906–909.

Molnar, Z., and Clowry, G. (2012). Cerebral cortical development in rodents and primates. *Prog. Brain Res.* 195:45–70.

Murphy, B.K., and Miller, K.D. (2009). Balanced amplification: a new mechanism of selective amplification of neural activity patterns. *Neuron* 61:635–648.

Nicol-Benoit, F., Le-Goff, P., et al. (2012). Epigenetic memories: structural marks or active circuits? *CMLS* 69:2189–2203.

Niere, F., Wilkerson, J.R., et al. (2012). Evidence for a fragile X mental retardation protein-mediated translational switch in metabotropic glutamate receptor-triggered Arc translation and long-term depression. *J. Neurosci.* 32:5924–5936.

Penzes, P., and Rafalovich, I. (2012). Regulation of the actin cytoskeleton in dendritic spines. *Adv. Exp. Med. Biol.* 970:81–95.

Pombero, A., Bueno, C., et al. (2011). Pallial origin of basal forebrain cholinergic neurons in the nucleus basalis of Meynert and horizontal limb of the diagonal band nucleus. *Development* 138:4315–4326.

Pouille, F., Marin-Burgin, A., et al. (2009). Input normalization by global feedforward inhibition expands cortical dynamic range. *Nat. Neurosci.* 12:1577–1585.

Puelles, L., and Rubenstein, J.L. (2003). Forebrain gene expression domains and the evolving prosomeric model. *Trends Neurosci.* 26:469–476.

Purpura, D.P. (1974). Dendritic spine "dysgenesis" and mental retardation. *Science* 186:1126–1128.

Rash, B.G., Lim, H.D., et al. (2011). FGF signaling expands embryonic cortical surface area by regulating Notch-dependent neurogenesis. *J. Neurosci.* 31:15604–15617.

Rice, D.P. (2005). Craniofacial anomalies: from development to molecular pathogenesis. *Curr. Mol. Med.* 5:699–722.

Rodger, J., Salvatore, L., et al. (2012). Should I stay or should I go? Ephs and ephrins in neuronal migration. *Neurosignals* 20:190–201.

Rubenstein, J.L., and Merzenich, M.M. (2003). Model of autism: increased ratio of excitation/inhibition in key neural systems. *Genes Brain Behav.* 2:255–267.

Shankle, W.R., Rafii, M.S., et al. (1999). Approximate doubling of numbers of neurons in postnatal human cerebral cortex and in 35 specific cytoarchitectural areas from birth to 72 months. *Pediatr. Dev. Pathol.* 2:244–259.

Siddiqui, T.J., and Craig, A.M. (2011). Synaptic organizing complexes. *Curr. Opin. Neurobiol.* 21:132–143.

Storm, E.E., Garel, S., et al. (2006). Dose-dependent functions of Fgf8 in regulating telencephalic patterning centers. *Development* 133:1831–1844.

Tabares-Seisdedos, R., Escamez, T., et al. (2006). Variations in genes regulating neuronal migration predict reduced prefrontal cognition in schizophrenia and bipolar subjects from mediterranean Spain: a preliminary study. *Neuroscience* 139:1289–1300.

Takahashi, N., Sakurai, T., et al. (2011). Linking oligodendrocyte and myelin dysfunction to neurocircuitry abnormalities in schizophrenia. *Prog. Neurobiol.* 93:13–24.

Tau, G.Z., and Peterson, B.S. (2010). Normal development of brain circuits. *Neuropsychopharmacol.* 35:147–168.

Terauchi, A., Johnson-Venkatesh, E.M., et al. (2010). Distinct FGFs promote differentiation of excitatory and inhibitory synapses. *Nature* 465:783–787.

Urbanska, M., Swiech, L., et al. (2012). Developmental plasticity of the dendritic compartment: focus on the cytoskeleton. *Adv. Exp. Med. Biol.* 970:265–284.

Urdinguio, R.G., Sanchez-Mut, J.V., et al. (2009). Epigenetic mechanisms in neurological diseases: genes, syndromes, and therapies. *Lancet Neurol.* 8:1056–1072.

Valnegri, P., Sala, C., et al. (2012). Synaptic dysfunction and intellectual disability. *Adv. Exp. Med. Biol.* 970:433–449.

van Bokhoven, H. (2011). Genetic and epigenetic networks in intellectual disabilities. *Annu. Rev. Genet.* 45:81–104.

van Spronsen, M., and Hoogenraad, C.C. (2010). Synapse pathology in psychiatric and neurologic disease. *Curr. Neurol. Neurosci. Rept.* 10:207–214.

Vogels, T.P., and Abbott, L.F. (2007). Gating deficits in model networks: a path to schizophrenia? *Pharmacopsychiatry* 40(Suppl 1):S73–77.

BOX 74.1 NEURODEVELOPMENTAL DISORDERS REVISITED

The translation of discoveries in basic neuroscience to clinical problems has been frustrating owing in part to the reliance on categorical, symptom-based diagnostic systems, such as the Diagnostic and Statistical Manual of Mental Disorders (DSM; http://www.dsm5.org/) and the International Classification of Diseases (ICD). These systems have been very useful for increasing the reliability of clinical diagnoses, but could complicate the search for genetic, behavioral, and neural elements that define etiology and pathogenetic mechanisms. An alternative conceptualization and classification has been proposed in the Research Domain Criteria initiative (RDoC; http://www.nimh.nih.gov/research-funding/rdoc/index.shtml). The Research Domain Criteria initiative is aimed at establishing new ways of classifying psychopathology based on dimensions of observable behavior and neurobiological measures.

Since 2007, the diagnostic and categorization criteria in psychiatry have been extensively revised based on comprehensive review of scientific advancements, targeted research analyses, and clinical expertise. The release of the final, approved DSM-5 is expected in May 2013. In DSM-5 the category of Neurodevelopmental Disorders contains diagnoses that were listed in DSM-IV under the chapters of Disorders Usually First Diagnosed in Infancy, Childhood, or Adolescence, and Anxiety Disorders. Among the recent revisions is the proposal to now include two superordinate categories of Language Disorder and Speech Disorder and one category for Social Communication Disorder. Speech Disorder now includes specifiers for the specific type of speech difficulty. Learning Disorder has been changed to Specific Learning Disorder, and the previous types of Learning Disorders (Dyslexia, Dyscalculia, and Disorder of Written Expression) are no longer being recommended. The type of Learning Disorder will instead be specified as noted in the diagnosis. Finally, a category of ADHD Not Elsewhere Classified has been added (see Table 74.I). The RDoC scheme, in contrast, is represented as a two-dimensional matrix with rows representing the "dimensions of observable behavior and neurobiological measures," such as "cognition" that includes attention, perception, working memory, declarative memory, language behavior, and cognitive (effortful) control, and columns representing various "units" (levels) of analysis, including genes, molecules, cells, circuits, behaviors, or paradigms (see Table I in Sarah et al., 2012).

DISCLOSURES

Dr. Dierssen's laboratory is supported by the Spanish Ministry of Science and Innovation SAF2010-16427, FIS PS09102673-(CureFXS), and PI11/00744, Jerôme Lejeune Foundation, Fundación Areces and Alicia Koplowitz, FRAXA Foundation and Generalitat de Catalunya SGR1313 and CIBERER, an initiative of the Instituto de Salud Carlos III (ISCIII). The funders had no role in preparation of the manuscript.

Dr. Martínez. The funders had no role in preparation of the manuscript.

REFERENCES

Altafaj, X., Ortiz-Abalia, J., et al. (2008). Increased NR2A expression and prolonged decay of NMDA-induced calcium transient in cerebellum of TgDyrk1A mice, a mouse model of Down syndrome. *Neurobiol. Dis.* 32:377–384.

Arango, C., Moreno, C., et al. (2008). Longitudinal brain changes in early-onset psychosis. *Schizophr. Bull.* 34:341–353.

Aronica, E., Becker, A.J., et al. (2012). Malformations of cortical development. *Brain Pathol.* 22:380–401.

Attwood, B.K., Patel, S., et al. (2012). Ephs and ephrins: emerging therapeutic targets in neuropathology. *Int. J. Biochem. Cell. Biol.* 44:578–581.

Barkovich, A.J., Kuzniecky, R.I., et al. (2005). A developmental and genetic classification for malformations of cortical development. *Neurology* 65(12):1873–1887.

Bayes, A., van de Lagemaat, L.N., et al. (2011). Characterization of the proteome, diseases and evolution of the human postsynaptic density. *Nat. Neurosci.* 14:19–21.

Best, T.K., Cramer, N.P., et al. (2012). Dysfunctional hippocampal inhibition in the Ts65Dn mouse model of Down syndrome. *Exp. Neurol.* 233:749–757.

Betancur, C., Sakurai, T., et al. (2009). The emerging role of synaptic cell-adhesion pathways in the pathogenesis of autism spectrum disorders. *Trends Neurosci.* 32:402–412.

Bhardwaj, R.D., Curtis, M.A., et al. (2006). Neocortical neurogenesis in humans is restricted to development. *Proc. Natl. Acad. Sci. USA* 103:12564–12568.

Birke, G., and Draguhn, A. (2010). No simple brake: the complex functions of inhibitory synapses. *Pharmacopsychiatry* 43(Suppl 1):S21–31.

Bosch, M., and Hayashi, Y. (2012). Structural plasticity of dendritic spines. *Curr. Opin. Neurobiol.* 22:383–388.

Bottos, A., Rissone, A., et al. (2011). Neurexins and neuroligins: synapses look out of the nervous system. *Cell. Mol. Life. Sci.* 68:2655–2666.

Buxbaum, J.D. (2009). Multiple rare variants in the etiology of autism spectrum disorders. *Dia. Clin. Neurosci.* 11:35–43.

Bystron, I., Blakemore, C., et al. (2008). Development of the human cerebral cortex: Boulder Committee revisited. *Nat. Rev. Neurosci.* 9:110–122.

Cardoso, C., Leventer, R.J., et al. (2003). Refinement of a 400-kb critical region allows genotypic differentiation between isolated lissencephaly, Miller-Dieker syndrome, and other phenotypes secondary to deletions of 17p13.3. *Am. J. Hum. Genet.* 72:918–930.

Carvalho, T.P., and Buonomano, D.V. (2009). Differential effects of excitatory and inhibitory plasticity on synaptically driven neuronal input-output functions. *Neuron* 61:774–785.

Chelly, J., Khelfaoui, M., et al. (2006). Genetics and pathophysiology of mental retardation. *Eur. J. Hum. Genet.* 14:701–713.

Chi, C.L., Martinez, S., et al. (2003). The isthmic organizer signal FGF8 is required for cell survival in the prospective midbrain and cerebellum. *Development* 130:2633–2644.

Coghlan, S., Horder, J., et al. (2012). GABA system dysfunction in autism and related disorders: from synapse to symptoms. *Neurosci. Biobehav. Rev.* 36:2044–2055.

Colasante, G., Collombat, P., et al. (2008). Arx is a direct target of Dlx2 and thereby contributes to the tangential migration of GABAergic interneurons. *J. Neurosci.* 28:10674–10686.

Courchesne, E., Pierce, K., et al. (2007). Mapping early brain development in autism. *Neuron* 56:399–413.

Cruikshank, S.J., Lewis, T.J., et al. (2007). Synaptic basis for intense thalamocortical activation of feedforward inhibitory cells in neocortex. *Nat. Neurosci.* 10:462–468.

D'Arcangelo, G. (2006). Reelin mouse mutants as models of cortical development disorders. *Epilepsy Behav.* 8:81–90.

Day, J.J., and Sweatt, J.D. (2011). Epigenetic modifications in neurons are essential for formation and storage of behavioral memory. *Neuropsychopharmacol.* 36:357–358.

Dierssen M. (2012). Down syndrome: the brain in trisomic mode. *Nat. Rev. Neurosci* 13(12):844–858.

Dierssen, M., Herault, Y., et al. (2009). Aneuploidy: from a physiological mechanism of variance to Down syndrome. *Physiol. Rev.* 89:887–920.

Dierssen, M., and Ramakers, G.J. (2006). Dendritic pathology in mental retardation: from molecular genetics to neurobiology. *Genes Brain Behav.* 5 (Suppl 2):48–60.

Dong, W.K., and Greenough, W.T. (2004). Plasticity of nonneuronal brain tissue: roles in developmental disorders. *Ment. Retard. Dev. Disabil. Res. Rev.* 10:85–90.

Feinberg, I. (1990). Cortical pruning and the development of schizophrenia. *Schizophr. Bull.* 16:567–570.

Feinberg, I. (1982). Schizophrenia: caused by a fault in programmed synaptic elimination during adolescence? *J. Psychiatr. Res.* 17:319–334.

disruption of the balance between excitation and inhibition produced by interneuron reduction has been suggested to lead to gating defects that are related to cognitive impairment (Vogels and Abbott, 2007).

Little is known how the E/I ratio is dynamically adjusted through the postnatal critical periods, when the strength of excitatory and inhibitory synapses is rapidly changing. Some authors have suggested that the tightly regulated E/I ratios in adults' cortex is a result of drastic changes in relative weight of inhibitory but not excitatory synapses during critical period, and the local inhibitory structural changes are the underpinning of altered E/I ratio across postnatal development (Zhang et al., 2011). Mutation of genes that normally sculpt and maintain the excitatory/inhibitory balance results in severe dysfunction, causing neurodevelopmental disorders including autism, schizophrenia, and ID (van Spronsen and Hoogenraad, 2010; Yin et al., 2012). For example, altered GAD67 expression is found in postmortem brain tissue from individuals affected of several neurodevelopmental disorders and those with childhood-onset schizophrenia, suggesting interneuron anomalies. Postmortem studies revealed that neurons in autistic patients present reduced level of glutamic acid decarboxylase (GAD), the rate-limiting enzyme in GABA synthesis. GABAA receptors are also reduced at mRNA and protein levels, showing altered α1–5 and β1 subunits in the parietal cortex (Brodmann area [BA]), α1 in the frontal cortex (BA 9), and α1 and β3 in the cerebellum of autistic patients postmortem tissue (Coghlan et al., 2012). Genetic studies of subjects with ASD show abnormalities among gene loci containing synaptic imbalance candidates, including the GABA β3 receptor subunit and genes encoding the neurorexin, neuroligin, and Shank proteins (Kohl and Paulsen, 2010). Such mutations may result in defective synaptic connections and/or functional synaptogenesis, leading to the selective loss of either excitatory or inhibitory synapses, without compensatory changes, or genetic conditions that actively favor the formation or maintenance of one class of synapse relative to the other.

In fact, the E/I imbalance may also affect the shape of the dendritic spines, because the plastic changes in the neuronal cytoskeleton are triggered in mature neurons in response to excitatory neurotransmission (for review see Bosch and Hayashi, 2012). Glutamate is one of the excitatory neurotransmitters that can induce long-term potentiation (LTP) mainly driving the strengthening of the connection between a presynaptic and postsynaptic neuron for a long period. The binding of glutamate to the N-methyl-D-aspartic (NMDA) receptor increases Ca^{2+} levels and triggers short-lasting activation of proteins, such as CamKII, that can phosphorylate the α-amino-3-hydroxy-5-methyl-4-isoxazolepropionic acid (AMPA) receptor to modulate insertion of more AMPA receptors at the postsynaptic membrane. The gain or loss of AMPA receptors at the postsynaptic membrane is related to the strength of the synapse and also the morphology of the spines. Long-term depression (LTD) is the opposite process, being the weakening of the synapse, reflected by a reduced number of ion receptors at the postsynaptic membrane. Glutamatergic synapses also undergo dynamic changes during postnatal brain maturation.

These activity-dependent rearrangements of the actin network mediate structural changes of dendritic spines and can be mediated by certain proteins. For example, activity-regulated cytoskeleton-associated protein (Arc) (also termed Arg3.1) is an immediate-early gene (IEG) induced in response to sensory experience, learning, LTP, spatial exploration, and novelty, and might be a good candidate for the excessive AMPA receptor internalization. It has been suggested that Arc is an mRNA target of FMRP and that the protein levels of Arc are increased in the absence of FMRP. Arc synthesis is required for mGluR-LTD induction by increasing the AMPA receptor internalization rate. Therefore, Arc may play a major role in the excessive AMPA receptor internalization and altered protrusion morphology in FXS (Niere et al., 2012). Genetic factors involved in these processes might function in synaptic plasticity, learning, enrichment, exercise, and neurogenesis. Also, the DSCR1 gene overexpressed in fetal and adult DS brains inhibits calcineurin, which is involved in synaptic plasticity and has a role in the transition from short- to long-term memory through perturbation in long-term potentiation and long-term depression (Hoeffer et al., 2007). Other interesting examples are drebrin, an actin-binding protein thought to regulate assembly and disassembly of actin filaments, thereby changing the shape of spines, the levels of which are reduced in the early second trimester in the brains of patients with Down syndrome (Weitzdoerfer et al., 2001) and Dyrk1A (Altafaj et al., 2008; Martinez de Lagran et al., 2012), and are associated with altered synaptic plasticity and learning and memory deficits. Changes in levels of expression of these genes may lead to changes in the timing and synaptic interaction between neurons during development, which can lead to suboptimal functioning of neural circuitry and signaling at that time and in later life.

CONCLUSIONS

Brain development is a non-linear dynamic process in which small initial differences may yield large later effects. The basic layout of the brain is established by genetic programs and intrinsic activity and is actively refined by the environment as well as gene–environment interaction. This takes place in an age-sensitive manner with underlying mechanisms including developmental changes in gene expression, epigenetic modifications, synaptic arborization, pruning, and behavioral maturation. A hypothesis that is gaining predominance proposes that a spectrum of diseases such as schizophrenia, autism, and intellectual disabilities may have common deficits that explain their overlapping phenotypes and genetics. In this context, the idea is gaining support that the disruption of general developmental processes, alteration of the establishment of neural circuits in the developing brain and neural plasticity, or the imbalance of excitation and inhibition in specific neural circuits might be responsible for some of the clinical features of these disorders. Recent studies in animal models demonstrate that the molecular basis of such disorders is linked to common defects in development leading to schizophrenia, autism, or intellectual disabilities (Box 74.1).

Different mental retardation–associated genes have been identified that encode modulators of the Rho GTPases. Disturbances in these genes can lead to mental retardation and—on the morphological level—to alterations in dendritic spines (von Bohlen Und Halbach, 2010). A good example is Down syndrome (for a comprehensive review see Dierssen et al., 2009). Postmortem studies show that patients with Down syndrome start their lives with an apparently normal neuronal architecture that progressively degenerates, showing reduced dendrites and degenerative changes in older age. Significantly, abnormalities of synaptic density and length, fewer contact zones, a reduction of dendritic spines, and shorter basilar dendrites are observed in Down syndrome brains. Several candidate genes within the Down syndrome critical region are involved in synaptic plasticity with particular impact on dendritic function and spine motility and plasticity. Among those, DSCR1, DYRK1A, or ITSN1 may be candidates to explain the dendritic spine functional and structural alterations. Interestingly, Intersectin controls local formation and branching of actin filaments and Dyrk1A phosphorylates actin-binding proteins, and may also have a role in shaping the interaction of the spine membrane with the actin cytoskeleton (see Dierssen et al., 2009, 2012).

EXCITATORY/INHIBITORY IMBALANCE

In the mammalian cortex roughly 80% of neurons are excitatory (pyramidal cells) and 20% are inhibitory interneurons (Rubenstein and Merzenich, 2003). Pyramidal cells specialize in transmitting information between different cortical areas and from cortical areas to other regions of the brain, whereas interneurons primarily contribute to local neural assemblies, where they provide inhibitory input and shape synchronized oscillations. Complex brain circuitries comprise hierarchical networks of these excitatory and inhibitory neurons (for a review see Birke and Draguhn, 2010). Establishing and maintaining the appropriate ratio of excitatory versus inhibitory synapses is a critical factor that enables circuit threshold definition and balances output responsiveness. In fact, excitation and inhibition are balanced globally in cortical networks but their ratio may vary dramatically with brain region, development, or aging, and ratios do not necessarily reflect the excitation-inhibition synaptic balance per individual neuron. Balance between feedback or feedforward inhibition and recurrent excitation can give rise to balanced network amplification (Carvalho and Buonomano, 2009; Murphy and Miller, 2009) or stability (Marino et al., 2005). In sensory cortices, such a balance serves to increase temporal precision and reduce the randomness of cortical operation (Cruikshank et al., 2007; Pouille et al., 2009).

Excitatory and inhibitory synapses show divergent features. Excitatory synapses target on mature mushroom-shaped spines containing a prominent postsynaptic density (PSD) after preferential contacting with an exploratory filopodium. In contrast, inhibitory GABAergic synapses are present on dendritic shafts, nerve cell somata, and axon initial segments, lacking postsynaptic thickening, and arise from axon–dendrite contacts with no apparent protrusive activity. At the ultrastructural level, excitatory contacts are asymmetric with an electron-dense postsynaptic density opposing a presynaptic active zone, whereas inhibitory contacts appear relatively symmetrical, with presynaptic vesicles clustered opposite a synaptic cleft without a robust postsynaptic density. During developmental stages neural circuit development is regulated by the balance of excitatory and inhibitory neurotransmission (Zhang et al., 2011), so that disruption of this balance leads to aberrant states, which cause severe dysfunction when chronically unresolved (Marin, 2012).

An increased ratio of excitation/inhibition (E/I) is observed in sensory, mnemonic, social, and emotional systems of autistic patients where it is thought to contribute to the prevalence of poor signal-to-noise ratios, resulting in hyperexcitable, non-tunable cortical circuits (Gatto and Broadie, 2010). These results suggest a shift in the excitation–inhibition ratio favoring an elevated preponderance of glutamatergic connections with inhibitory insufficiency. Excitation-dominant synaptic imbalance may underlie the pathophysiology of other intellectual disabilities. Fragile X syndrome exhibits significant GABAergic deficits leading to hyperexcitability as well as synaptic imbalance neurophysiology (Coghlan et al., 2012). The opposite is observed in Down syndrome (Dierssen et al., 2009; Dierssen, 2012). Various Down syndrome mouse models exhibit a reduced ratio of hippocampal excitation–inhibition, leading to overinhibition with an increased number of inhibitory synapses as well as a reduced density of excitatory synapses. Moreover, large morphological changes are seen in the granular cell dentate gyrus to the CA3 pathway in Ts65Dn mice along with a reduction in synapse density, and reduction of mushroom spines with multivesicular bodies in the middle molecular layer of dentate gyrus. As a consequence, the Ts65Dn dentate gyrus shows enhanced GABAergic synaptic transmission, owing to increased presynaptic release of GABA and increased postsynaptic GABAB receptor–Kir3.2 signaling (Best et al., 2012).

Abnormal GABAergic neurotransmission in the prefrontal cortex of individuals with schizophrenia has also been suggested to cause the cognitive disturbances (Lewis et al., 2012). Indeed, deficits in cortical inhibition have been reported both *in vivo* and in analyses of postmortem brain tissue from patients with schizophrenia, and cognitive functions such as working memory, which is clearly altered in schizophrenic patients, seems to depend on normal interneuron performance. It was originally suggested that the GABAergic deficits that are observed in schizophrenia might be caused by a deficit in the number of interneurons in the prefrontal and cingulate cortices that was speculated to reduce GABAergic inputs to pyramidal cells. The subsequent finding that such patients had increased GABAA receptor binding activity in pyramidal cells was thought to be consistent with this idea, but other studies failed to find similar interneuron reductions in all individuals with schizophrenia. It is now accepted that GABAergic deficits preferentially occur at the level of specific synapses. Interneurons mediate the precise gating of information through specific signaling pathways by controlling—both spatially and temporally—the amounts of excitatory and inhibitory inputs that individual neurons receive. Thus, the

Recent studies have identified leucine-rich repeat transmembrane neuronal proteins LRRTMs to be trans-synaptic partners for neurexins (Linhoff et al., 2009). LRRTM1 and LRRTM2 are glutamatergic postsynaptic proteins and bind α and β neurexins and compete with neuroligin-1 for an overlapping face of β-neurexin (–S4). Given their broadly overlapping expression patterns, neuroligin-1, LRRTM1, and LRRTM2 are likely to coexist at many glutamatergic postsynaptic sites (Wright and Washbourne, 2011). Other proteins have also been well documented for their role in experience-dependent plasticity such as ephrins and EphRs or the Wnt family and could thus be good candidates for neurodevelopmental disorders (Attwood et al., 2012). Other synaptogenic proteins have not been systematically studied but associations were also found for LRRTM1 and GluRδ1 with schizophrenia and SynCAM1, SHANK3, and CNTNAP2 with autism.

SPINE PATHOLOGY

A close look onto the surfaces of the dendritic processes of neurons allows the observation of small protrusions called dendritic spines, small protrusions (<2 Am) that contain postsynaptic densities (PSD), which are major sites of excitatory synapse. Typically, adult dendritic spines are composed of a bulbous head with a thin neck. In younger neurons, dendritic shafts are covered by thin, long protrusions called dendritic filopodia, which are thought to be precursors of spines. Filopodia typically lack "heads," whereas mature spines have a distinct head and neck, giving rise to different morphologies named mushroom-like, stubby, thin, and branched. At the cellular level, the primary function of dendritic spines is to compartmentalize local synaptic signaling pathways and restrict the diffusion of postsynaptic molecules, insulating signaling molecules to a specific PSD. Dendritic spines and filopodia show rapid actin-based motility in the time scale of seconds (Yuste, 2011). This confers highly dynamic properties to the spines, which morphology can change very rapidly upon different types of stimulation by remodeling the architecture of their actin cytoskeleton (Penzes and Rafalovich, 2012).

During brain development, the initial dendritic arborization and outgrowth of dendritic spines precede synapse formation, and the number and morphology of the spines change dramatically as synaptic contacts mature. This happens as a response to environmental inputs, activity, and experience that strengthen the immature synaptic connections. On the contrary, inactive synapses become weaker and are eventually eliminated (use it or lose it). Thus, elimination of spines and change of their morphology also seem to be essential to establish neuronal circuits in early life.

Abnormal protrusion morphology in different brain areas seems to be a hallmark of many syndromic or non-syndromic mental disorders (van Spronsen and Hoogenraad, 2010; von Bohlen Und Halbach, 2010). The first link between neurodevelopmental disorders (e.g., ID) and aberrant spines was reported by Purpura (1974) and showed a significant increase of abnormally long, thin spines on dendrites of cortical neurons in children with ID. Later, many ID syndromes have been reported presenting alterations in spine morphology

and synapse number and have been linked to mutations in synaptic proteins involved directly or indirectly in the stabilization of the spine structure, including different signaling pathways, epigenetic regulators, and local mRNA translation at the synapse (Dierssen and Ramakers, 2006). For example, as stated, mutations in synaptic scaffolding protein SHANK3 and adhesion molecules neuroligin-3 and -4 have been linked to autism spectrum disorder but further evidence also suggests that other neurodevelopmental disorders involve defects in the regulation of actin cytoskeleton (Dierssen and Ramakers, 2006; Goellner and Aberle, 2012; von Bohlen Und Halbach, 2010). For example, the schizophrenia risk factor DISC1 regulates dendritic spine morphology via Rac1 and mutations in the cofilin kinase PAK3 (p21-activated kinase) gene lead to X-linked mental retardation. Moreover, decreased levels of PAK3 relate to synaptic dysfunction in Alzheimer's disease and possibly FXS, and PAK3 inhibition in mice causes cofilin pathology and memory impairment, consistent with a potential causal role of PAK defects in cognitive deficits in Alzheimer's disease. The inability to preserve the spine structure causes profound alterations in neural circuit formation and can thus alter information processing, learning, and memory, and produce behavioral impairment (Lott and Dierssen, 2010). However, whether this phenotype is a cause or derives from the mental disturbance and whether we can use this feature as a translational end point to investigate the therapeutic effects of pharmacological interventions are still open questions.

Besides altered spinogenesis, altered spine pruning can also account for mis-wired circuit formation. In 1982, Feinberg (Feinberg, 1982, 1990) proposed that schizophrenia is a disease of aberrant synaptic pruning, based on findings of progressive postnatal "synaptic pruning" and aberrant synaptic elimination in early adolescence. This hypothesis was further expanded by the proposal that hyperpruning of collateral axons in the prefrontal cortex and defective pruning of certain brain structures leads to the aberrant connectivity of schizophrenia. This was further demonstrated by Golgi-impregnation studies revealing a region- and disease-specific decrease in dendritic spine density in dorsolateral prefrontal cortex layer III pyramidal cells in subjects with schizophrenia (Glantz and Lewis, 2000). Aberrant synaptic conductance and/or efficacy in schizophrenics are also observed in the subcortical gray matter, where striatal spines were reduced in size by approximately 30%. Another good example of pruning alterations is Fragile X syndrome (FXS). In a FXS mouse model, the *Fmr1* knockout mice, the persistent increase in spine density in dentate gyrus in the absence of a defined pruning period argues for a role of FMRP in processes controlling developmental pruning. However, the disruption of the regulation of forming, stabilizing, or removing dendritic spines is a common phenotype in many neurodevelopmental disorders. Changes in the cytoskeletal structure are important for the protrusion morphology and play a role in many forms of ID that have been related to LIMK1, oligophrenin-1, PAK3, and ARHGEF6. Small GTPases, such as Rho, Rac, and Cdc42, are proteins known for their effects on the actin cytoskeleton and microtubule organization.

epigenome have been demonstrated to be critical factors in a number of cognitive and behavioral disorders (Lockett et al., 2010). The epigenetic mechanisms that contribute to these deficits include the deregulation of essential components of the epigenetic machinery, alterations in the expression of genes important for cognition and behavior by epigenetic mechanisms, instability at trinucleotide repeats, and the breakdown of major epigenetic processes such as imprinting and X-chromosome inactivation. Some illustrative examples include Rett syndrome (caused by mutations in the methylated DNA binding protein MecP2), Rubinstein-Taybi syndrome (caused by mutations in the histone acetyltransferase CBP), and Coffin-Lowry syndrome (caused by mutations in histone phosphorylase; see Urdinguio et al., 2009 for a review).

NEURAL PLASTICITY AS A COMMON MECHANISM IN NEURODEVELOPMENTAL DISORDERS

Neural plasticity can be defined as the ability of a neuron or network to functionally or structurally alter in response to changes in input or activity. During the postnatal period, but also in infancy and adolescence, neural plasticity is one important mechanism in circuit development and refinement. Often, an outcome of neuronal plasticity is a structural plasticity manifested as a change of neuronal morphology (Urbanska et al., 2012). The number and branching pattern of dendrites are strictly correlated with the function of a particular neuron and the geometry of the connections it receives. The development of proper dendritic tree morphology depends on the interplay between genetic programming and extracellular signals. Spinogenesis is also an important target for structural plasticity. Spines are tiny actin-rich dendritic protrusions that harbor excitatory synapses. If plasticity mechanisms operate abnormally—either through long-lasting epigenetic modifications or disruption of functional mechanisms—neuronal networks improperly develop in response to activity-dependent experience. In psychiatric disorders and ID syndromes, plasticity malfunction leads to aberrant morphology and/or number of excitatory dendritic spines, a sign that is considered pathognomonic of ID, suggesting important changes in structural plasticity. Of course, the birth, death, and cellular characteristics of neurons, as well as the formation and reformation of their axons, dendrites, and synapses are also possible contributing factors.

In fact, most neurodevelopmental disorders can be considered synaptic plasticity disorders, in which different genomic causes result in abnormal synaptic development. Accumulation of this abnormal synaptic development, over time, leads to a characteristic and consistent behavioral and/or cognitive phenotype (Zoghbi, 2003).

SYNAPTOGENIC PROTEINS IN MENTAL ILLNESS

As described, neurons are connected by synapses in complex networks that regulate specific physiological and behavioral outcomes in adulthood. For this reason, circuit development is considered a fundamental unit for regulating specific physiological and behavioral outcomes in adulthood. Synapses are the basic units of neural connectivity and communication in the brain in which synaptic transmission relies on the coordinated function of highly specialized structures on both sides of the cleft, involving membranous organelles, cytoskeleton, and vast protein networks. Postsynaptic neurotransmitter receptors, with associated scaffolding and signaling molecules, should be precisely aligned on the dendrite opposite chemically matched presynaptic vesicles with regulated release and recycling machinery in the axon. If we consider that a typical neuron may contain 1,000 to 10,000 synapses, and each synapse contains more than 1,000 protein components (Bayes et al., 2011) and that the complex neuronal networks derived from this connectivity will regulate behavioral outcomes in a dynamic manner, it becomes clear that synaptogenesis is a highly sensitive process.

Multiprotein complexes in the synapse are organized into molecular networks that detect and respond to patterns of neural activity. These synaptic organizing proteins mediate plasticity and dynamic synaptic changes during postnatal brain maturation and contribute to synaptic specificity, pairing specific presynaptic and postsynaptic cells, and controlling where and when synapses are formed (Siddiqui and Craig, 2011) and destroyed. Many synaptogenic genes are at high risk for predisposing to neurodevelopmental disorders (Valnegri et al., 2012; van Bokhoven, 2011). Synaptic gene alterations include copy number variants, protein-truncating frame shifts, and function-altering missense variants, some de novo, contributing to the disease through pre- and/or postsynaptic alterations. Although in the last two decades a number of synaptic genes have been discovered whose mutations cause ID and a number of neuropsychiatric disorders, we are still far from identifying the impact of these mutations on brain development and neuronal function. One prominent example is the so-called synaptic organizing proteins, which include synaptic adhesion complexes and secreted factors (Betancur et al., 2009). The synaptogenic adhesion complexes are composed of transmembrane presynaptic and postsynaptic partners that bind in trans across the cleft, as in presynaptic neurexin (NRXN) and postsynaptic neuroligin, for example (Bottos et al., 2011). Such cleft-spanning synaptic organizing complexes often have bidirectional activity, inducing presynaptic and postsynaptic differentiation, and mediating cell adhesion and alignment of the pre- and postsynaptic specializations. Since the initial linkage of mutations in neuroligins 3 and 4 to autism, evidence has rapidly accumulated for the contribution of neuroligin and neurexin variants to disorders such as schizophrenia and ID. NRXN bind multiple structurally diverse partners across the cleft. Neuroligin-1 is the major glutamatergic neuroligin and binds only β-neurexins. Neuroligin-2 functions specifically at GABAergic synapses and appears to bind all neurexins. Of particular interest is the replicated finding of SHANKS deficits, which directly implicates glutamatergic synapse dysfunction in both autism and Asperger syndrome (Buxbaum, 2009). This finding is supported by the replicated findings with NRXN1 and NLGNS/4, which can also play a role in excitatory synapse formation, maintenance, and plasticity. NRXN1 deletions have been associated with autistic spectrum disorders, and confer risk for schizophrenia, suggesting an etiological overlap between both disorders.

2006). Although it was estimated that most of the genes remain to be discovered, a table of known monogenic causes of mental retardation shows that neuronal migration and synaptic function–related genes predominated over other functions. Therefore, we can speculate about the importance of neuronal connectivity (synaptogenesis) with or without evident migratory alterations during human development as a substrate of mental retardation and/or predisposition to develop a mental disease. Copy number variants in developmental genes controlling principal neurodevelopmental processes, such are brain regionalization, neural cell migration/differentiation, and synaptogenesis have been postulated underlying the neurobiological roots of mental disorder predisposition (Insel, 2010; Malhotra and Sebat, 2012).

POSTNATAL NEURAL DEVELOPMENT

As discussed, the major developmental processes in the human telencephalon following closure of the neural tube are neuronal proliferation, astrocytic proliferation, neuronal migration, neurite (i.e., axonal and dendritic) growth, neuronal apoptosis, axon myelination, synaptogenesis, and neurite pruning. All of these processes begin during gestation, but the development of the brain circuitry requires the coordination of a complex set of postnatal neurodevelopmental events, such as neurite proliferation, axonal myelination, neurite pruning, and synaptogenesis, which exert their major effects during postgestational development (Giedd and Rapoport, 2010). Thus, the early postnatal period is crucial for brain development. The newborn brain at two to four weeks of age is approximately 36% the size of an adult brain and grows to about 80% of adult size by two years of age (Knickmeyer et al., 2008). Possibly, this dramatic brain growth is not primarily caused by postnatal cortical neurogenesis and neuronal migration (Bhardwaj et al., 2006; Shankle et al., 1999), but by the expansion of glia and myelination. At two to four weeks of age, the primary cortical areas, including motor, somatosensory, visual, and auditory cortices are well defined, but instead, association cortices at this age can be less clearly identified. Thus, the development of gray matter connections, especially in sensorimotor and visual cortices and the onset of myelination, drives the striking development of the brain during the perinatal and early postnatal period.

ENVIRONMENTAL INFLUENCES ON BRAIN DEVELOPMENT

During development, neural networks are shaped by experience-dependent processes that selectively strengthen and prune connections, creating and restructuring synaptic maps, or even changing dendritic architecture locally. The final neuronal circuits, primary mediators of the brain's diverse functional capacities, and their connectivity, rely on experience-dependent sculpting (Maffei and Turrigiano, 2008; Tau and Peterson, 2010). This environmental sensitivity is especially important during the so-called critical periods; sensitive temporal windows of elevated plasticity allowing the structural consolidation of neuronal circuits and their connectivity. It was long believed that the potential for organization or reorganization existed only during these critical periods in early development, so that over time neural connections become more stable, forming widely distributed, interconnected networks involving balanced excitation and inhibition and structural stabilizers such as myelin. However, the successful treatments for adults with stroke or amblyopia suggest that the potential for circuit reorganization persists well into adulthood; thus, the final neuronal circuits are neither present at birth nor are they invariant through life (Michel, 2012). Besides, it has been proposed that each functional modality (from basic visual processing to language and social skills) has a different postnatal "critical" period.

Thus, the early postnatal and infancy periods are times of opportunity, but also of great vulnerability for the developing brain. Early disruption of proper sensory or social experiences results in mis-wired circuits that will respond suboptimally to normal experiences in the future. These deviations of the typical trajectories of maturation of neural circuits can also be caused by genetic alterations intrinsically impairing the response of the system to the environment, or to the combined effects of adverse experience on genetically abnormal brain maturation, leading to pathogenesis through both genetic and epigenetic mechanisms.

In this scenario, epigenetic mechanisms reveal as a critical determinant in disease predisposition and outcome. The term epigenetics has referred to heritable traits that are not mediated by changes in DNA sequence, and more broadly to any change in gene function not associated with sequence variation and promoted by the environment to influence or "program" gene expression or patterns that may or may not be heritable (Nicol-Benoit et al., 2012). Although often restricted to chromatin modifications specifying the sets of genes to be expressed or repressed, epigenetic mechanisms also include other gene expression controllers, such as noncoding RNAs, including microRNAs. Increasing evidence shows epigenetic processes are widespread in the brain and undergo dynamic regulation in both the developing and postmitotic neurons. Epigenetic gene control is in fact an intrinsic mechanism for normal tissue development. The epigenetic marking of chromatin provides a ubiquitous means for cells to shape and maintain their identity, and to react to environmental stimuli via specific remodeling. In mature, differentiated neurons in the central nervous system, epigenetic codes are critical for basic cellular processes such as synaptic plasticity, and play critical roles in encoding experience and environmental stimuli into stable, behaviorally meaningful changes in gene expression (Day and Sweatt, 2011; Graff and Mansuy, 2008).

In humans, because maturation processes in the brain continue well into adolescence, the influence of the epigenetic programming on disease risk and pathogenesis is critical. For example, early life environmental threats, such as stress (McEwen et al., 2012), influence the long-term outcome of neurodevelopmental disorders. Mutations in epigenetic components are associated with multisystem disease syndromes in human beings, all of which involve the nervous system; thus, the alteration of the epigenetic machinery may be a common process in many neurological diseases. In fact, anomalies in the

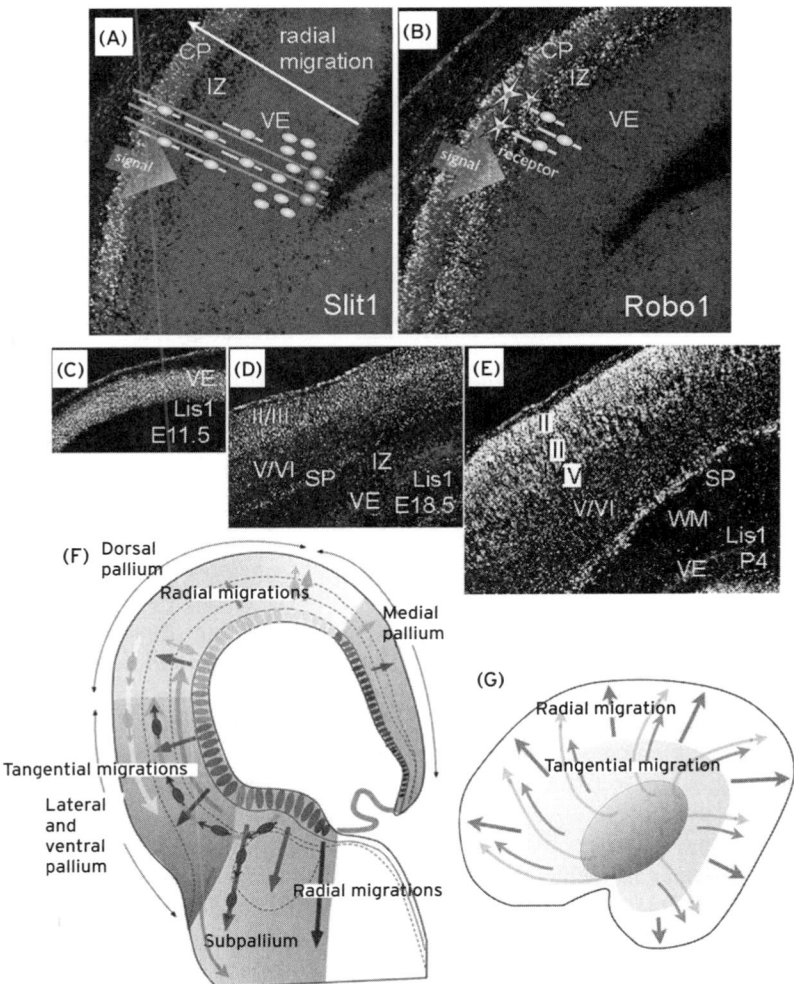

Figure 74.4 *Neuronal migration in the pallium: cortical development. (A,B) Signal: Slit1 expression in E15.5 mouse embryo in the cortical plate. Neural progenitors proliferate in the ventricular epithelium (VE) and subventricular zone (yellow ovoid cells), radial glia cells are schematized in gray with long radial processes crossing the neural wall from ventricular to pail surface. Migrating neurons were distributed in between radial glia processes in the intermediate zone (IZ; yellow ovoid soma with processes) toward the cortical plate (CP). In an equivalent section the receptor of Slit1, Robo1 is expressed in migrating cells of the IZ. (C–E) Expression of Lis1 gene in developing and postnatal mouse cortex. (F) Schematic representation of a coronal section were different lateromedial (ventrodorsal) pallial domains are represented by colored fields. Radial migration is represented by radial arrows and tangential migrations are represented by concentric distributed arrows. Migrating cells were represented by ovoid soma and arrows. (G) Planar representation of the telencephalic vesicle where radial migrations are represented by orange arrows; pallio-pallial tangential migration is represented by grey arrows; subpallio-pallial tangential migration, coming from the subpallium (central orange ovoid). (See color insert).*

of *RELN* (OMIM 600514) results in a type of lissencephaly with severe cortical and cerebellar malformation (Norman-Roberts type lissencephaly; revised by D'Arcangelo, 2006). Genetic and biochemical studies using mouse mutants suggest that the Lis1 protein may participate in the Reelin signaling pathway, controlling cortical development by its interaction with the dynein system and, therefore, neuronal motility.

A recent classification proposed for developmental cortical malformations in humans by Barkovich and co-workers have listed the human genetic mutations identified as malformations owing to abnormal neuronal migration (Barkovich et al., 2005). Most of the genes identified in human's cortical malformations also have been proved as functionally relevant to neuronal migration in mice; suggesting that in these situations the mouse models are of great value for analyzing the physiopathological mechanisms of these human diseases (Webber

et al., 2009). Indeed, it is of special relevance that alterations in the Reelin-dependent genetic cascade activate complex molecular interactions regulating cell migration and microtubule transport. Mutation in some of the molecules involved in this interactive cascade produced important alterations in cell migration and, subsequently, in cortical structure, characterized phenotypically by different degrees of cortical dysplasia, such as the double-cortex syndrome within lissencephaly spectrum (Cardoso et al., 2003), whereas mutations in some other molecules (e.g., DSC1) or moderate genetic alteration of lissencephaly critical region genes produce functional alterations without important structural malformation that may manifest as schizophrenic or bipolar disease symptoms. A recent metaanalysis showed that more than 290 genes have been involved in mental retardation associated with syndromes and metabolic or neurological disorders (Chelly et al., for instructively guiding the process of synapse development. These effects of neuronal activity are transduced in part through regulation of a set of activity-dependent transcription factors that coordinate a program of gene expression required for the formation and maturation of synapses (West and Greenberg, 2011). A number of human neurodevelopmental disorders have been linked to anomalies in the expression of these activity-regulated genes, such as Fragile X syndrome, Angelman syndrome, and ASD, in which it seems that excitatory and inhibitory synaptic equilibrium in the cortical regions is distorted. Indeed, the transcription of these activity-dependent genes regulates the fine-tuning of the adequate distribution of ion channels in specific neuronal populations. This is the case of *GYRK2* (*KCNJ6*), a gene regulating GABAergic (inhibitory synaptic function) in the substantia nigra, thalamus, and hippocampus. It has been related to familial Parkinson disease and Down syndrome functional alterations (Fig. 74.3*H–J*).

A mechanistic model can be proposed to understand brain regionalization in which morphogenetic signals from different organizer regions interact in regulative networks to establish initial territories of specified progenitor cells, establishing the molecular domains in which specific functional areas will develop (see Fig. 74.2). Then, the same or different signals, acting at different temporospatial scales, may stabilize the final molecular codes in these regions and regulate the production of specific cell types. Then, young neural cell follows specific migratory patterns of radial and/or tangential movements to generate the cellular diversity of neural structures. This cellular diversity is required for the establishment of neuronal connectivity networks and intercellular trophic support (e.g., neuron–glia interactions). Eventually, ambient influences, acting through posttranscriptional mechanisms, can modify the structural and functional properties of such neural systems, both in positive (adaptive) or negative (toxic) directions (see following sections).

NEURAL MIGRATION IN THE CORTEX AND SYNAPTOGENESIS DURING EMBRYONIC STAGES

The neurons and glial progenitors generated from the ventricular and subventricular layers of the pallium migrated to populate specific radial strata in the mantle layer (Fig. 74.4*F,G*). This migration is known as radial migration because it follows the radial axis in the brain wall, and migrating young neurons are guided to the pial (external) surface by radial glia fibers (Fig. 74.4*A*). In the pallium the first migration from the ventricular progenitors form a cellular layer known as the cortical plate (50 to 54 gestation days in humans), which represents the primordium of the cortex (embryonic days 12.5 to 15.5 in mouse development). Then at three months of gestation in human embryos the cells of layers IV, V, and VI are generated and migrate into the cortical plate (Fig. 74.4*D*), which correspond to E15.5 to 18.5 in mouse development. Structural maturation beyond this time is complex and varies in the different regions of the pallium, following a general lateromedial gradient; that is, starting from the lateral pallium (allocortex)

at 70 to 80 days and progressing dorsally. Although the superficial neurons (layers II and III) are still generating, the neurons in the cortical plate become grouped into the six layers, corresponding to those of the adult cortex between six and seven gestational months (Fig. 74.4*E*; perinatal development in the mouse cortex). Intercalated with or after radial migration, other directions also can be followed by migratory neural cells, which do not follow radial glia axis and are known as tangential migration (Fig. 74.4*F,G*; revised in Molnar and Clowry, 2012).

We previously described that cellular migrations are essential processes necessary to develop cellular diversity in brain areas and require precisely coordinated movements in time and space. Cell–cell and cell–substrate interactions underlie the guidance mechanisms of these migrations during brain development, by signal–receptor interaction coded by ephrins and their receptors (revised in Rodger et al., 2012), SLIT proteins, ROBO receptors (see Fig. 74.4*A,B*), neuregulin1, and ErB4 receptors, as well as FGF8 and FGF receptors (FgfR; Pombero et al., 2011). Finally, positioning of cells in the specific layers of growing cortical areas is dependent on the Reelin (RELN) signaling cascade generated from Cajal-Retzuis cells, which are produced very early in development in layer I (revised in Frotscher, 2010). Actually, the RELN signal is received in migrating cells by apolipoprotein E (Apo-ER2) or very low-density lipoprotein (VLDLR) receptors and transduced by tyrosine phosphorylation of the Disabled-1 (DAB1) protein. Disruption of the *RELN* gene in humans results in severe brain abnormalities, including lissencephaly and cerebellar hypoplasia, and patients show ataxia, ID, and seizures. It is interesting to note that important tangential migration of neurons coming from the subpallial ganglionic eminences generate early cortical GABAergic interneurons, starting to invade the pallium at six weeks of gestation and generating deep layer interneurons (predominant from six to 15 gestation weeks), whereas during the second half of gestation, the cortical subventricular and subgranular zones (progenitor proliferating layers especially prominent in primates and humans) originate locally the most numerous superficial interneurons, which are completed by interneurons in layer I that originate in the cortical surface by the subpial granular layer (revised in Bystron et al., 2008).

Developmental defects in neuronal positioning and synaptic connectivity are commonly found in neurological and psychiatric diseases, and they are believed to underlie many cognitive and affective disorders (Barkovich et al., 2005; Harrison and Weinberger, 2005; Tabares-Seisdedos et al., 2006). Several mouse mutants are currently available that model at least some aspects of human developmental brain disorders that might be related to similar structural alterations. With the identification of the genes mutated in these animals and the study of the cellular basis of their phenotypes, we have taken significant strides toward an understanding of the mechanisms controlling proper brain development and the consequences of their dysfunction. In particular, mouse mutants deficient in the *Reelin* and *Lis1* expressions have provided valuable insights into the mechanisms of cortical development. Absence of *Reelin* expression in the spontaneous mutant mouse reeler leads to extensive defects in neuronal position and dendrite development. In humans, loss

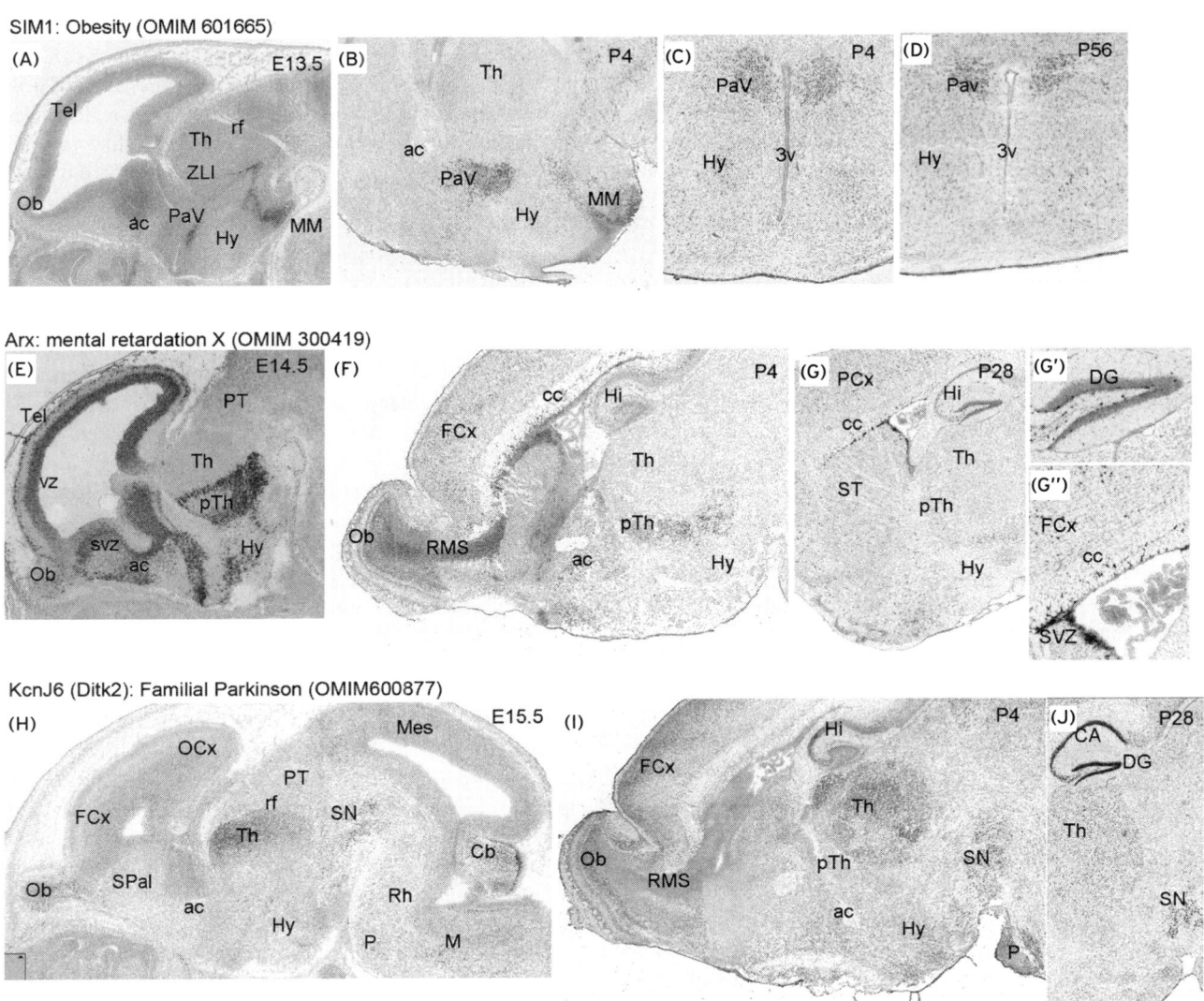

Figure 74.3 *Gene expression patterns in mouse brain (from developing mouse brain in the Allen Brain Atlas website: http://www.brain-map.org/.)*
(A–D) Hypothalamic expression of Sim1 gene at embryonic (E13.3; A, sagittal section) and postnatal P4 (B, sagittal sections; C: coronal section) and P56 (coronal section) in the paraventricular nucleus (PaV). (E–G) Expression pattern of Arx gene at embryonic (E14.5), and postnatal stages (P28) in sagittal sections. G' and G''
are high-power pictures of (G) where Arx transcripts accumulated in subgranular cells of the dentate gyrus (DG) in the hippocampus, subependymal region (SVZ), and cortical cells above corpus callosum (cc). (H–J) Expression pattern of KcnJ6 gene in the developing (H) and postnatal (I,J) thalamus (Th), hippocampus (Hi, CA, and DG) and substantia nigra (SN). ac, anterior commissure; cc, corpus callosum; DG, dentate gyrus; FCx, frontal cortex; Hy, hypothalamus; Mes, mesencephalon; MM, mammillare nuclei; OB, olfactory bulb; OCx, occipital cortex; P, pons; PaV, paraventricular nucleus; PT, pretectum; pTh, prethalamus; rf, retroflexus tract; RMS, rostral migratory stream; SN, substantia nigra; SPal, subpallium; SVZ, subventricular zone; ST, atriatum; Th, thalamus; vz, ventricular zone; ZLI, zona limitans; 3V, third ventricle.

for neocortical areal specification, in which neocortical progenitor cells become patterned by extracellular signals into molecular domains that in turn generate area-specific neurons. The protomap is thought to be underpinned by spatial differences in progenitor cell identity that is reflected by regional specific genes at the transcriptional level (Fukuchi-Shimogori and Grove, 2001; Grove and Fukuchi-Shimogori, 2003). Furthermore, cross-regulation among the rostral (FGF-signal dependent), dorsal (BMP- and WNT-signal dependent), and ventral (SHH-signal dependent) secondary inductive centers plays an essential role in patterning the early telencephalon. Modulation of this cross-regulation has the potential to regulate the relative size of structures whose morphogenesis is controlled by a given patterning center (Hamasaki et al., 2004). For instance, a reduction in FGF8 signaling reduces the ratio of the frontal motor versus sensory regions of the neocortex. Therefore, controlling the relative strength and range of a given patterning signal may provide a fundamental mechanism to modify the relative sizes of brain subdivisions during evolution and in disease states. Nevertheless, very little is known about the underlying processes that generate local reduction or lack of progenitors in specific cortical regions, as is the case of schizencephaly, in which mutations of *EMX2, SIX3,* and *SHH* have been reported (Aronica et al., 2012).

Once the developmental processes have operated, both spontaneous and sensory-driven neural activity are essential regulate the establishment of the common complex structural pattern of the developing brain in vertebrates. Distinct neural and glial identities are acquired by neuroepithelial cells according to their relative positions in the neural tube wall, through a progressive restriction of their histogenetic potential, under the influence of local environmental signals. Evidence for controlling morphogenetic processes at specific locations of the developing neural crest and neural tube has suggested the concept of morphogenetic organizers. Such centers regulate by their own signaling the choices of identity and regional polarity of neural precursors in neighboring neuroepithelial regions and may even function as target-derived presynaptic organizers to specify the type of synaptic terminals (Terauchi et al., 2010).

Three regions in the neural plate and tube have been identified as putative secondary organizers (Fig. 74.2A). Two of these organizers control prosencephalic regionalization: the anterior neural ridge (ANR) at the anterior end of the neural plate, and the zona limitans intrathalamicae (ZLI) in the middle of the diencephalon. In addition, the isthmic organizer (IsO) at the mid-hindbrain boundary controls mesencephalic and rostral rhombencephalic (including cerebellar) regionalization. To focus the present chapter on mental function related structures, we describe only the mechanisms of anterior prosencephalic regionalization and concentrate on the function of the anterior neural ridge (ANR).

ANTERIOR NEURAL RIDGE

The most anterior secondary organizer, the ANR, is a morphologically indistinct median sector at the junction between the neural plate and non-neural ectoderm. The ANR controls prosencephalic regionalization and proliferation and it was demonstrated that some genes expressed in this region control others that are necessary for telencephalic and hypothalamic specification (Fig. 74.2A). In particular, the *Fgf8* gene is expressed very early in ANR cells, and has been shown to be crucial for specification of the anterior areas of the forebrain and telencephalon. *Fgf8* hypomorphic mutations in both mouse and zebrafish result in a small telencephalon and midline anomalies. Prosencephalic regionalization by FGF8 signal operates at least in part through inhibition of *Otx2* and *Emx2* expression, in cooperation with BMP4, WNT, and SHH signaling molecules. Modifications in this interactive molecular network originate important anomalies in brain and skull development. For instance, decreasing FGF activity caused by mutations in FGF receptors (FGFR1 and FGFR2) produces severe brain alterations and different forms of craniosynostosis (including Apert syndrome; OMIM 101200) (revised in Chi et al., 2003; Rice, 2005; Storm et al., 2006). Less severe alterations in this FGF signaling have been described in hypogonadotropic hypogonadism (OMIM 146110), Jackson–Weiss syndrome (OMIM 123150), Kallmann syndrome 2 (OMIM 147950), Pfeiffer syndrome (OMIM 101600), and Trigonocephaly 1 (OMIM 190440). These syndromic forms of FGF signaling anomalies show limb and cephalic patterning alterations (because of FGF expression in ectodermal apical ridge of the limb bud and branchial arches), together different degrees of sensorial—hearing and smelling—deficits (because of the requirement of

FGF signaling in cephalic placode development). Moreover, different degrees of developmental retardation and ID (with or without telencephalic structural phenotype) are also present that can be attributed to anomalies in cortical regionalization derived from expansion deficits of the cortical surface (Rash et al., 2011). Morphogenetic influences derived from secondary organizers regulate progenitor proliferation in the developing cortex. For instance, ID can be associated with anomalies in the regulation of centrosomic distribution and mitotic spindle orientation of neuroepithelial precursors, disrupting spatial and temporal rates of neuronal progenitor proliferation and differentiation, and causing a reduction of normal cortical surface and cerebral volume. Alterations of these processes course with primary microcephaly—MCPH1 gene (MIM 251200)—or secondary microcephaly associated to neural migration alterations: LIS1 (OMIM 601545) and NDEL1 (OMIM 607538) (Guerrini and Marini, 2006; Hippenmeyer et al., 2010).

Another gene coding morphogenetic information is sonic hedgehog (SHH), which is expressed in the subpallium slightly later than Fgf8 expression in the ANR. Abundant data suggest that SHH signaling is both necessary and sufficient for the specification of the ventral pattern throughout the nervous system. After abundant experimental demonstrations in animal models, it is widely accepted that normal patterning in the telencephalon depends on the "ventral" repression of GLI3 function by SHH and, and conversely on the "dorsal" repression of SHH signaling by GLI3. Different types of *GLI3* mutations in humans produce craniofacial and brain anomalies together with other patterning anomalies. The SHH signal in the subpallium has also been shown to be involved in the regulatory activity of NKX2.1, a homeodomain gene required for the development of the telencephalic subpallium as well as the hypothalamus, the latter being ventral part of the forebrain (see Fig. 74.1). The *DLX2* gene codes for a transcription factor expressed in the subpallium, prethalamus, and thalamus, and regulates the expression of *ARX* (Colasante et al., 2008) in prosencephalic progenitors (Fig. 74.3E–G). It is an essential gene in the proliferation and migration of neural progenitors. Mutations of *ARX* frequently have been involved in X-linked ID (OMMIM 300419) and epilepsy. The hypothalamus is the main brain center regulating homeostasis by controlling autonomous nervous and hormonal systems, where molecular patterns define neurons with specific functional properties; for instance, SIM1 is a transcription factor expressed in the hypothalamus, in the paraventricular hypothalamic nucleus (Fig. 74.3A–D). SIM1 haploinsufficiency is associated with hyperphagia and obesity. In addition, in close relation to this ventral signal coded by *SHH*, a longitudinal column of epithelial progenitors is specified along the whole neural tube to produce oligodendroglial progenitors, revealed by the expression of PLP/dm20, PDGFalpha, and OLIG1/2. Although very little is known about the underlying physiopathological mechanisms, extensive knowledge has been accumulated about myelin developmental anomalies in relation to mental disorders and ID (Dong and Greenough, 2004; Takahashi et al., 2011).

All these recent findings on the molecular regionalization of the neuroepithelium support the protomap model is a frequent malformation commonly associated with multiple human syndromes of genetic origin, including Joubert syndrome, DiGeorge syndrome, Waardenburg syndrome, and orofaciodigital syndrome, some of which have psychiatric manifestations, as well as toxic agents associated with another tube defect, folate sensitivity.

NEURAL TUBE REGIONALIZATION

The discovery that putative regulatory genes (mainly coding for transcription factors) are expressed in regionally restricted patterns in the developing forebrain has provided new tools for defining histogenetic domains and their boundaries at higher resolution (see Fig. 74.1; Puelles and Rubenstein, 2003). This molecular regionalization has unveiled the morphological significance of numerous gene expression patterns in the neural tube, suggesting the existence of molecular subdivisions of the main AP and DV zones, representing histogenetically specified domains of neural precursors. Genetic alterations associated with brain regionalization anomalies frequently occur with important structural alterations in brain morphogenesis that

finally appear as congenital malformations such as holoprosencephaly (OMIM 236100; caused by combinations of mutations in genes as *SIX3*; Fig. 74.1), *ZIC2*, and *GLI2*, which are transcription factors coding for positional information in the prosencephalon at early stages of neural tube development. But smaller genetic alterations underlying copy number variants could produce subtle variations in regionalization that modify regional morphogenesis and synaptogenesis of the affected region, which may represent a predisposition to develop intellectual disabilities and/or psychiatric disorders (revised in Malhotra and Sebat, 2012).

The longitudinal study of this molecular/structural causal association in the neural tube of experimental models has shown how the expression of particular genes is directly related to neural morphogenetic and cytogenetic development. For instance *Gbx2* expression in mouse embryos is associated with the generation of thalamic neurons, which develop into the thalamocortical projection (Fig. 74.2) (Miyashita-Lin et al., 1999), whereas *Lhx8* and *Tbr1* expression are associated with the development of basal forebrain cholinergic neurons (Pombero et al., 2011). Thus, elaborated cellular interactions

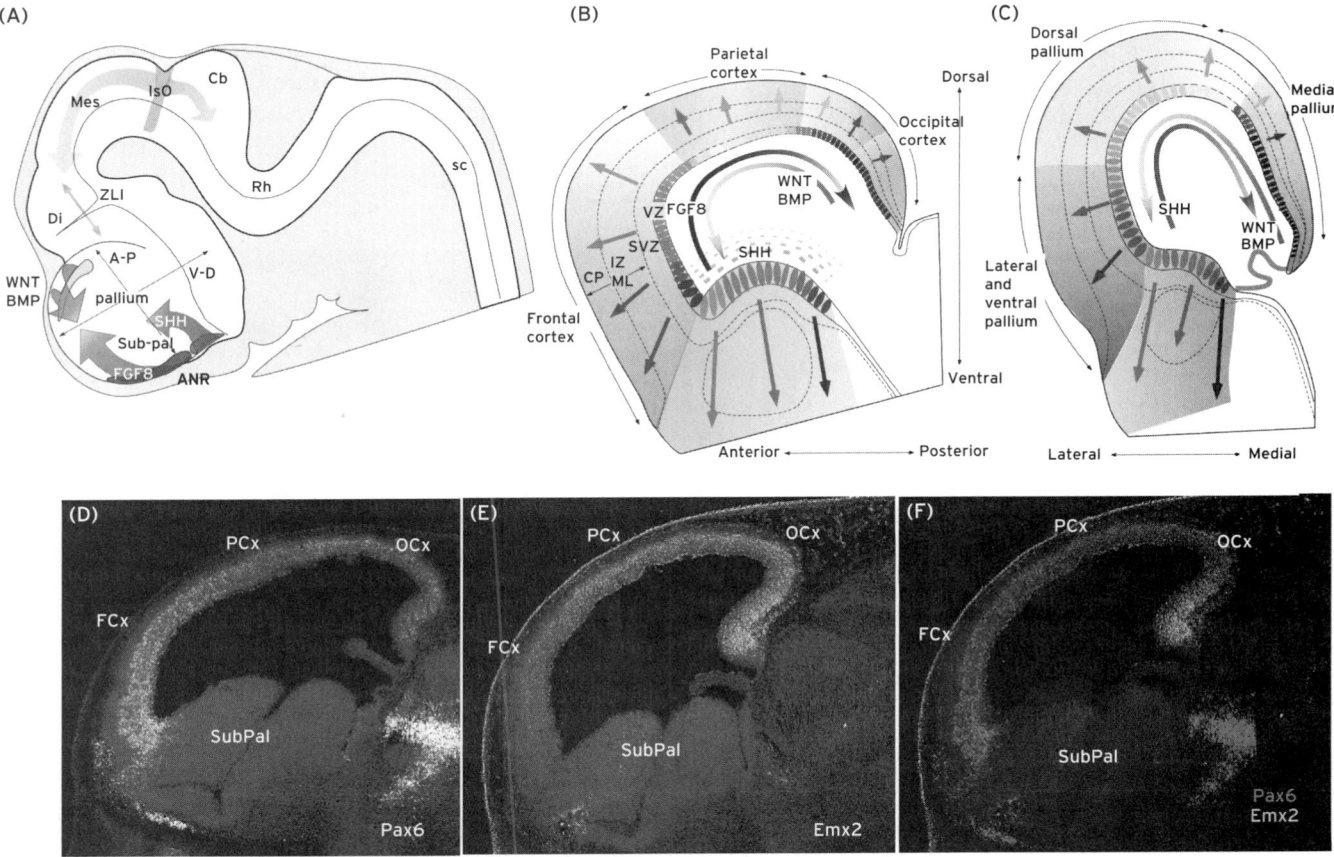

Figure 74.2 *Morphogenetic signals and telencephalic regionalization. (A) Schematic representation of neural tube (lateral view) where the main brain regions have been identified and morphogenetic signals regulating telencephalic regionalization have been represented by colors and arrows. Wnt and Bmp are dorsalizing signals, Fgf8 is a rostralizing signal, and Shh is a ventralizing signal, acting upon dorsal (pallial) telencephalon to specify cortical functional areas in the epithelium. (B,C) Schematic representation of a section in anteroposterior (B) and coronal (C) planes of the dorsal telencephalon (pallium and subpallium) that were color coded in neuroepithelial cells. Colored arrows in the ventricle and the dashed area (B) represent morphogenetic gradients that were translated through the neural wall by radial migration of neural cells into the different cortical regions (radial arrows and color gradient domains). (D–F) Sagittal sections showing the gradient expression pattern of two transcription factors: Pax6 regulated by rostral and ventralizing signals (D), and Emx2 regulated by dorsalizing signals (E). F, A combinatory Photoshop reconstruction of both gradient patterns. (See color insert).*

TABLE 74.1. Disorders that are currently proposed for the diagnostic category of Neurodevelopmental Disorders in DSM-5

A 00–01 Intellectual Developmental Disorders
A 00 Intellectual Developmental Disorder
A 01 Intellectual or Global Developmental Delay Not Elsewhere Classified
A 02–04 Communication Disorders
A 02 Language Disorder
A 03 Speech Disorder
A 04 Social Communication Disorder
A 05 Autism Spectrum Disorder
A 05 Autism Spectrum Disorder
A 06–07 Attention Deficit/Hyperactivity Disorder
A 06 Attention Deficit/Hyperactivity Disorder
A 07 Attention Deficit/Hyperactivity Disorder Not Elsewhere Classified
A 08 Specific Learning Disorder
A 08 Specific Learning Disorder

the time the posterior end of the neural tube closes, secondary bulges—the optic vesicles—have extended laterally from each side of the developing forebrain. Then the prosencephalon becomes subdivided into the anterior secondary prosencephalon (telencephalon and hypothalamus) and the more caudal diencephalon.

Anomalies of neurulation normally generate severe malformations in the embryos and are classified as dysraphias. Several genetic anomalies have been detected underlying these malformations, including mutations in *VANGL1* and *VANGL2* (OMIM 610132 and 600533, respectively) as well as *SCRIB* (OMIM 607733) and *SHH* (OMIM 600725). When the process of fusion of neural folds does not occur at any level of the neural grove craniorachischisis results. When the closure skipped areas localize at different levels, anencephaly, exencephaly, or meningomyelocele (from rostral to caudal) results.

After the posterior neuropore closes (28 days of gestation), the second phase of caudal neural tube formation begins. This process requires the formation of the caudal cell mass. Neural progenitors differentiate around vesicles in contact with caudal neural tube, and then these vesicles coalesce and fuse with the central canal (30 to 50 days of gestation); and finally there is a regressive process in the tail (50 to 100 days of gestation). Abnormal development of the caudal neural tube formation generates defects of closure and malformation in the lumbo-sacrococcygeal levels of the spinal cord: myelocystocele, diastematomyelia, and myelomeningocele. Myelomeningocele

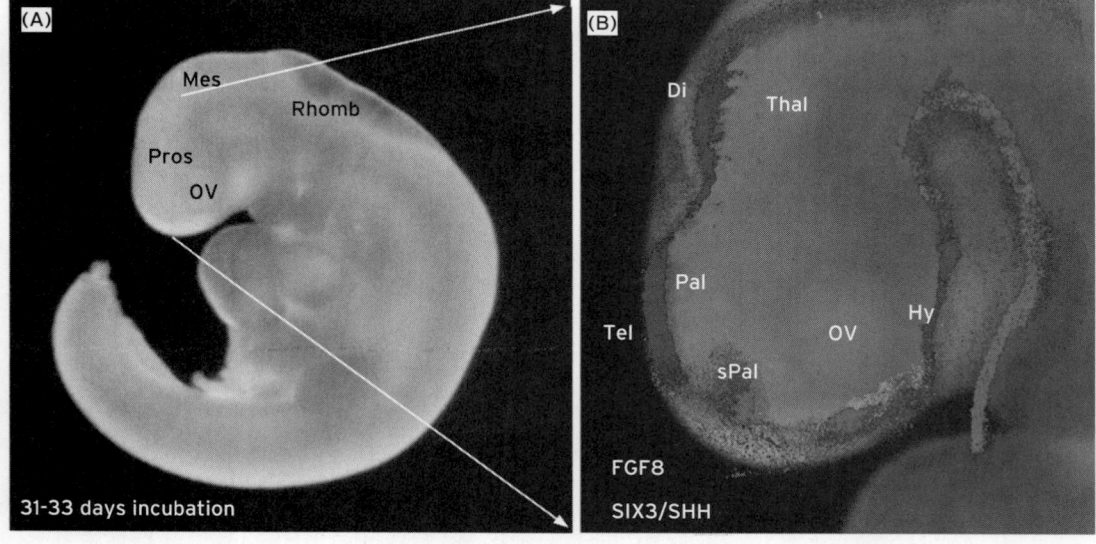

Figure 74.1 Human embryo at postneurulation stage. (A) Lateral view of a human embryo of 31–32 days of incubation. The main brain regions were detected: Prosencephalon (Pros), mesencephalon (Mes), rhombencephalon (Rhomb) and optic vesicle (OV). (B) Magnification of the anterior brain area where different gene expression patterns have been represented by different gray shades. The expression patterns were translated from mouse embryos sections at equivalent stage of neural tube development (E11.5). Di, diencephalon; Hy, hypothalamus; OV, optic vesicle; Pal, pallium; sPal, subpallium; Tel, telencephalon; Thal, thalamus. (Data from Developing Mouse Brain in the Allen Brain Atlas website: http://www.brain-map.org/.)

74 | NEUROPATHOLOGY AND SYNAPTIC ALTERATIONS IN NEURODEVELOPMENTAL DISORDERS

MARA DIERSSEN AND SALVADOR MARTÍNEZ

The term neurodevelopmental disorder has been classically restricted to intellectual disability (ID) (Table 74.1). However, epidemiological studies increasingly demonstrate that most psychiatric disorders begin during childhood or adolescence (Kessler et al., 2007). Moreover, even though the notion of critical periods is still accepted, our concept of development in temporal terms has dramatically changed in the last years, and neurodevelopment now is considered to encompass the period from fetal life into adolescent brain maturation and synaptic pruning. This change in our conceptualization of neurodevelopment has led to an increased interest in understanding the role of neurodevelopmental processes, not only in ID, but also in mental illnesses such as schizophrenia and autism spectrum disorders (Kendler et al., 2005; McGrath et al., 2003). Mental disorders that become symptomatic in childhood or adolescence are affected by early environmental conditions that may interact with genetic risk factors. This increases the potential to identify genes leading to deviations from normal development, at prodromal stages in which intervention might be particularly useful.

Significantly, neurodevelopmental disorders have been found to share a number of similarities in terms of common genetic risks, co-occurrence of neurodevelopmental symptom domains, cognitive processing deficits, early onset, and chronic course. Schizophrenia, autism, and intellectual disabilities, for example, are spectrums of diseases with broad sets of causes that have overlapping phenotypes and genetics, which is suggestive of common deficits. Other disorders of childhood and adolescence, such as attention deficit/hyperactivity disorder (ADHD), eating disorders, or the separation anxiety disorders (Krueger and South, 2009), may not overlap in terms of risks and manifestations.

Structural brain development in healthy children follows complex, regionally heterochronous trajectories (Giedd et al., 1999). In gray matter development, whether measured by cortical volume or thickness, there is a phase of early increase, followed by a late childhood/adolescent phase of adjustment, before the cortex settles into adult dimensions. White matter has a more sustained pattern of expansion, persisting through adolescence. Given the complexities of these trajectories and their exquisite genetic control, it is not surprising that small disturbances can result in disturbances in cognition, affect, and behavior. For example, a disorder may be characterized by a delay in the pattern of typical development, or may be associated with differences in the temporal occurrence of the neural changes. Another possibility is a more profound deviance in the basic shape of the typical developmental trajectory. Obviously, these anomalies are not mutually exclusive. (A trajectory could incorporate elements of delay but also be altered in speed.) Anomalies in developmental trajectories are linked with ADHD or schizophrenia (Arango et al., 2008; Hoftman and Lewis, 2011), but also autism (Courchesne et al., 2007) and neurodegenerative disorders (Grilli et al., 2003).

This chapter gives a general view of the fetal and postnatal development that can be disrupted in an age-sensitive manner. It also discusses some of the common cellular and molecular targets that may explain similarities and differences in the phenotypes and comorbidity.

THE PRENATAL DEVELOPMENT OF THE REGIONAL DIVERSITY OF THE BRAIN

NEURAL TUBE FORMATION

The structural and functional complexity of the brain derives from precise orchestration of molecular and cellular mechanisms regulating the main developmental processes of neural progenitors: proliferation, differentiation, and synaptogenesis, in a temporospatial pattern defined into the matrix of embryonic development and perinatal life. The vertebrate central nervous system originates from the embryonic dorsal ectoderm. Differentiation of the neural plate epithelium from the ectoderm constitutes the first phase of complex processes called gastrulation and neurulation, which culminates in the formation of the neural tube.

Neurulation is a fundamental event of embryogenesis that culminates in the formation of the neural tube, which is the precursor of the brain and spinal cord. The bending of the neural plate involves the elevation of the neural folds establishing a trough-like space called the neural groove (20 days of gestation), which becomes the lumen of the primitive neural tube after closure of the neural groove (between 22 and 28 days of gestation). With the closure of anterior and posterior neuropores, the first phase of neural tube formation is completed, and internal cavities of the neural tube are no longer in connection with amniotic fluid. In addition, the neural folds generate the specialized cells of the neural crest. Then the most anterior portion of the neural tube balloons into three primary vesicles: the forebrain (prosencephalon), midbrain (mesencephalon), and hindbrain (rhombencephalon; Fig. 74.1). By

Li, H.H., Roy, M., et al. (2009). Induced chromosome deletions cause hypersociability and other features of Williams-Beuren syndrome in mice. *EMBO Mol. Med.* 1(1):50–65.

Martynyuk, A.E., van Spronsen, F.J., et al. (2010). Animal models of brain dysfunction in phenylketonuria. *Mol. Genet. Metab.* 99 (Suppl 1):S100–S105.

Muehlmann, A.M., and Lewis, M.H. (2012). Abnormal repetitive behaviours: shared phenomenology and pathophysiology. *J. Intellect. Disabil. Res.* 56(5):427–440.

Parker, S.E., Mai, C.T., et al. (2010). Updated national birth prevalence estimates for selected birth defects in the United States, 2004–2006. *Birth Defects Res. A Clin. Mol. Teratol.* 88:1008–1016.

Patterson, P.H. (2012). Maternal infection and autism. *Brain Behav. Immun.* 26(3):393.

Paylor, R., Glaser, B., et al. (2006). Tbx1 haploinsufficiency is linked to behavioral disorders in mice and humans: implications for 22q11 deletion syndrome. *Proc. Natl. Acad. Sci.* 103:7729–7734.

Qin, M., Entezam, A., et al. (2011). A mouse model of the fragile X premutation: effects on behavior, dendrite morphology, and regional rates of cerebral protein synthesis. *Neurobiol. Dis.* 42(1):85–98.

Robertson, H.R., and Feng, G. (2011). Annual research review: transgenic mouse models of childhood-onset psychiatric disorders. *J. Child Psychol. Psychiatry* 52(4):442–475.

Rooms, L., and Kooy, R.F. (2011). Advances in understanding fragile X syndrome and related disorders. *Curr. Opin. Pediatr.* 23(6):601–606. Review.

Ropers, H.H. (2008). Genetics of intellectual disability. *Curr. Opin. Genet. Dev.* 18(3):241–250.

Roubertoux, P.L., and Carlier, M. (2010). Mouse models of cognitive disabilities in trisomy 21 (Down syndrome). *Am. J. Med. Genet. C Semin. Med. Genet.* 154C(4):400–416. Review.

Rueda, N., Flórez, J., et al. (2012). Mouse models of Down syndrome as a tool to unravel the causes of mental disabilities. *Neural Plast.* 2012:584071.

Russell, V.A. (2011). Overview of animal models of attention deficit hyperactivity disorder (ADHD). *Curr. Protoc. Neurosci.* 9:35.

Russell, V.A. (2007). Reprint of "Neurobiology of animal models of attention-deficit hyperactivity disorder." *J. Neurosci. Meth.* 166(2):I–XIV.

Sakurai, T., Dorr, N.P., et al. (2010). Haploinsufficiency of Gtf2i, a gene deleted in Williams Syndrome, leads to increases in social interactions. *Autism Res.* 4(1):28–39.

Schmeisser, M.J., Ey, E., et al. (2012). Autistic-like behaviours and hyperactivity in mice lacking ProSAP1/Shank2. *Nature* 486(7402):256–260.

Scorza, C.A., and Cavalheiro, E.A. (2011). Animal models of intellectual disability: towards a translational approach. *Clinics (Sao Paulo)* 66(Suppl 1):55–63. Review.

Sontag, T.A., Tucha, O., et al. (2010). Animal models of attention deficit/hyperactivity disorder (ADHD): a critical review. *Atten. Defic. Hyperact. Disord.* 2(1):1–20.

Spencer, C.M., Alekseyenko, O., et al. (2011). Modifying behavioral phenotypes in Fmr1KO mice: genetic background differences reveal autistic-like responses. *Autism Res.* 4(1):40–56.

State, M.W. (2010). The genetics of child psychiatric disorders: focus on autism and Tourette syndrome. *Neuron* 68(2):254–269.

Vacano, G.N., Duval, N., et al. (2012). The use of mouse models for understanding the biology of down syndrome and aging. *Curr. Gerontol. Geriatr. Res.* 2012:717315.

van der Kooij, M.A., and Glennon, J.C. (2007). Animal models concerning the role of dopamine in attention-deficit hyperactivity disorder. *Neurosci. Biobehav. Rev.* 31(4):597–618.

Wang, L., Simpson, H.B., et al. (2009). Assessing the validity of current mouse genetic models of obsessive-compulsive disorder. *Behav. Pharmacol.* 20(2):119–133.

Willemsen, R., Levenga, J., et al. (2011). CGG repeat in the FMR1 gene: size matters. *Clin. Genet.* 80(3):214–225.

Zang, J.B., Nosyreva, E.D., et al. (2009). A mouse model of the human Fragile X syndrome I304N mutation. *PLoS Genet* 5:e1000758.

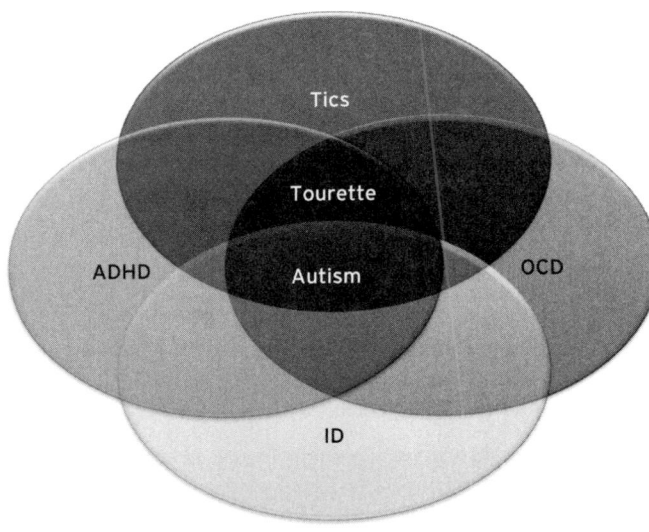

Figure 73.2 Example of how behaviors from multiple psychiatric disorders may overlap and form complex relationships. ADHD, attention deficit/hyperactivity disorder; ID, intellectual disability; OCD, obsessive-compulsive disorder.

by a combination of modes of inheritance (i.e., owing to different causes or ASD subtypes that remain to be defined), epigenetic effects, or a combination of genetic and environmental factors. Thus far, approximately 20% of ASD has been linked to genetic causes (Betancur, 2011). As the immense heterogeneity of ASD symptoms, severity, onset, and genetic etiology unfolds, animal models, as described in the preceding may offer a means for unraveling the underlying pathophysiology of ASD and developing functional or novel therapeutics.

Interestingly, many of the observed symptoms are shared across multiple psychiatric disorders. For example some form of anxiety can occur with many of the mentioned disorders. An example of how characteristics may overlap between disorders is illustrated in Fig. 73.2. This overlap may suggest that either shared pathways underlie multiple disorders or there are various pathways underlying a given behavior that can be disrupted in multiple ways.

As these animal models improve, they will continue to provide insight into candidate genes for disorders and the neurological pathways underlying the observed phenotypes, as well as help to identify therapeutic targets for future development. Evidence for the reversibility of phenotypes in several animal models at birth or even in adults provides hope that despite the occurrence of these disorders during a critical developmental time period, systems underlying these conditions may be highly plastic, thereby allowing multiple opportunities for therapeutic intervention.

ACKNOWLEDGMENTS

This work was supported by the Baylor IDDRC, the Baylor Fragile X Center, and Autism Speaks. AMT, SV, and SMH all contributed equally to this chapter.

DISCLOSURES

Dr. Paylor has no conflicts of interest to disclose. He is funded by NIH, Autism Speaks, CHDI, and Seaside Therapeutics.

Dr. Thomas has no conflicts of interest to disclose (no independent funding sources).

Dr. Veeraragavan has no conflicts of interest to disclose (no independent funding sources).

Dr. Hamilton has no conflicts of interest to disclose (no independent funding sources).

REFERENCES

Arime, Y., Kubo, Y., et al. (2011). Animal models of attention-deficit/hyperactivity disorder. *Biol. Pharm. Bull.* 34(9):1373–1376.

Baker, K.B., Wray, S.P., et al. (2010). Male and female Fmr1 knockout mice on C57 albino background exhibit spatial learning and memory impairments. *Genes Brain Behav.* 9:562–574.

Bakker, C.E., Verheij, C., et al. (1994). Fmr1 knockout mice: a model to study fragile X mental retardation. *Cell* 78:23–33.

Bessa, C., Lopes, F., et al. (2012). Molecular genetics of intellectual disability. In: Tan, U., ed. Latest Findings in Intellectual and Developmental Disabilities Research. Intech. http://www.intechopen.com/books/mostdownloaded/latest-findings-in-intellectual-and-developmental-disabilities-research.

Betancur, C. (2011). Etiological heterogeneity in autism spectrum disorders: more than 100 genetic and genomic disorders and still counting. *Brain Res.* 1380:42–77.

Betancur, C., Sakurai, T., et al. (2009). The emerging role of synaptic cell-adhesion pathways in the pathogenesis of autism spectrum disorders. *Trends Neurosci.* 32(7):402–412.

Bhogal, B., and Jongens, T.A. (2010). Fragile X syndrome and model organisms: identifying potential routes of therapeutic intervention. *Dis. Model. Mech.* 3(11–12):693–700. Review.

Buxbaum, J.D., Betancur, C., et al. (2012). Optimizing the phenotyping of rodent ASD models: enrichment analysis of mouse and human neurobiological phenotypes associated with high-risk autism genes identifies morphological, electrophysiological, neurological, and behavioral features. *Mol. Autism* 3(1):1.

Chao, H.T., Chen, H., et al. (2010). Dysfunction in GABA signalling mediates autism-like stereotypies and Rett syndrome phenotypes. *Nature* 468(7321):263–269.

Chiurazzi, P., Schwartz, C.E., et al. (2008). XLMR genes: update 2007. *Eur. J. Hum. Genet.* 16(4):422–434.

Das, I., and Reeves, R.H. (2011). The use of mouse models to understand and improve cognitive deficits in Down syndrome. *Dis. Model. Mech.* 4(5):596–606.

De Rubeis, S., Fernández, E., et al. (2012). Molecular and cellular aspects of mental retardation in the Fragile X syndrome: from gene mutation/s to spine dysmorphogenesis. *Adv. Exp. Med. Biol.* 970:517–551. Review.

Dölen, G., Carpenter, R.L., et al. (2010). Mechanism-based approaches to treating fragile X. *Pharmacol. Ther.* 127(1):78–93.

Felling, R.J., and Singer, H.S. (2011). Neurobiology of Tourette syndrome: current status and need for further investigation. *J. Neurosci.* 31(35):12387–12395.

Guris, D.L., Fantes, J., et al. (2001). Mice lacking the homologue of the human 22q11.2 gene CRKL phenocopy neurocristopathies of DiGeorge syndrome. *Nature Genet.* 27:293–298.

Hagerman, R., Lauterborn, J., et al. (2012). Fragile X syndrome and targeted treatment trials. *Results Probl. Cell. Differ.* 54:297–335. Review.

Haydar, T.F., and Reeves, R.H. (2012). Trisomy 21 and early brain development. *Trends Neurosci.* 35(2):81–91.

Khwaja, O.S., and Sahin, M. (2011). Translational research: Rett syndrome and tuberous sclerosis complex. *Curr. Opin. Pediatr.* 23(6):633–6339.

Krueger, D.D., Osterweil, E.K., et al. (2011). Cognitive dysfunction and prefrontal synaptic abnormalities in a mouse model of fragile X syndrome. *Proc. Natl. Acad. Sci. USA* 108:2587–2592.

Kwon, C.H., Luikart, B.W., et al. (2006). Pten regulates neuronal arborization and social interaction in mice. *Neuron* 50(3):377–388.

Lana-Elola, E., Watson-Scales, S.D., et al. (2011). Down syndrome: searching for the genetic culprits. *Dis. Model. Mech.* 4(5):586–595.

no specific genes have been confirmed as risk factors (State, 2010). Despite the lack of known susceptibility genes for TS, the generation of several animal models has been useful in elucidating potential mechanisms underlying TS.

Animal models with face validity exhibit behaviors analogous to the motor tics observed in human patients, including motor stereotypies, sequential super-stereotypy, circling, repetitive grooming, and self-injurious behaviors. Alternatively, other models have been constructed based on the known pathophysiology of TS (Felling and Singer, 2011). Abnormalities within the dopaminergic system have been identified in individuals with TS (Muehlmann and Lewis, 2012). Even though levels of dopamine or its primary metabolites appear normal, other dopaminergic system abnormalities have been found, including increased dopamine transporters in the caudate and putamen, elevated putamen dopamine release, increased D_2 receptor sensitivity, and decreased caudate volumes that seem to correlate with symptom severity. Therefore, animal models have been created based on the hypothesis that abnormal regulation of synaptic dopamine and signaling within basal ganglia circuits may play a role in the pathogenesis of TS.

PSYCHOSTIMULANT MODEL

Psychostimulants that exhibit dopaminergic-enhancing properties also may result in people experiencing tics. Therefore, these drugs are used in rodent models to investigate behavioral phenomena such as motor stereotypies as well as the brain structures believed to underlie these behaviors, including basal ganglia circuitry.

DOPAMINE TRANSPORTER KNOCKDOWN MOUSE

A mouse model containing a knockdown mutation of the dopamine transporter gene (DAT-KD mouse) effectively expresses 10% normal DAT levels and results in a 170% rise in extracellular dopamine within the striatum. DAT-KD mice exhibit hyperactivity, perseverative walking patterns, and stereotypic grooming sequences that are resistant to interruption. On the contrary, this model fails to demonstrate tic-like motor stereotypies and therefore models more closely perseverative-type behaviors.

D1 RECEPTOR CHOLERA TOXIN TRANSGENIC MODEL

D1CT-7 transgenic mice express an intracellular form of cholera toxin that is under the control of the D_1 promoter in a subset of neurons containing D_1 receptors that are active in sensorimotor, orbitofrontal, corticostriatal, and limbic circuits. These mice display compulsive behaviors, including repetitive climbing, digging, leaping, and grooming. Furthermore, they exhibit TS-relevant phenotypes such as juvenile-onset tics that are effectively reduced following administration of clonidine, a treatment used to suppress tics in humans. Although these behaviors demonstrate face validity for the model, mutants

also express an increased susceptibility to seizures, a phenotype uncommon for those with TS (Felling and Singer, 2011; Wang et al., 2009).

MONKEY FOCAL STRIATAL DISINHIBITION

One hypothesis asserts that tics are produced by abnormal focal disinhibition of striatal neurons. Disinhibition of the putamen in monkeys using $GABA_A$ antagonists results in motor tics, thereby supporting the involvement of the striatum in tic production.

AUTOIMMUNE MODELS

Another hypothesis proposes that TS may in part result from dysfunction of the immune system. Some studies have injected sera or IgG from TS patients into rodent striatum, but this approach has been met with conflicting results. Some report elevations in stereotypic-like behaviors, whereas others report no effects. Another model is based on findings that some children with TS experience a worsening of their symptoms following streptococcal infections or those with no prior history suddenly present with symptoms following similar infections. Immunization of mice with Group A β-hemolytic streptococcal (GABHS) can induce motor-related disturbances that correlate with IgG deposits in deep cerebellar nuclei. This model, however, is geared to elucidate the mechanisms by which GABHS may alter neuronal function, and is therefore not specifically targeted toward understanding TS.

OTHER MODELS

Other psychiatric disorders of childhood onset may include schizophrenia, obsessive/compulsive disorder, anxiety, and mood disorder. The reader is encouraged to visit other units in this book covering these conditions.

CONCLUSIONS

Despite the complexity of psychiatric disorders, much has been learned from the animal models currently available. Even though it is unlikely that a "perfect" model will ever be created embodying every aspect of a disorder, as more information is gathered regarding underlying pathologies, current models can be improved upon, bringing us closer to understanding these disorders. In fact the first genetic rat models for autism and other neurodevelopmental disorders were generated in 2011. Although their validity as models have yet to be established, these lines hold the promise of providing additional novel insights that complement the basic research already being carried out in mouse lines.

The multitude of models available to researchers for a given disorder illustrates not only the complexity in creating a model for a complex psychiatric disorder, but also the seeming difficulty in creating a single model supports the contention that many of these disorders are likely multifactorial. For instance, ASD prevalence rates are likely caused rats with high blood pressure, which produced a rat model that not only develops hypertension over time, but also exhibits each of the three core ADHD symptoms: hyperactivity, impulsivity, and poor sustained attention. The SHR also has been found to exhibit dysfunctions within the dopaminergic system, consistent with findings that individuals with ADHD demonstrate dopamine-related abnormalities. More specifically, SHR exhibits impaired dopamine release and reduced expression of the dopamine transporter (DAT) gene. Furthermore, SHR demonstrate enhanced norepinephrine release, thereby implicating the noradrenergic system. It is important to mention that hypertension in untreated ADHD patients has not been reported. Therefore an attempt was to separate the hypertensive phenotype from the more ADHD-related phenotypes with the creation of a WKHA rat. However, even though WKHA rats are hyperactive and hypersensitive to stress, they lack predictive validity because methylphenidate (a clinically used psychostimulant) causes a further increase rather than a decrease in locomotion.

Mice lacking functional neurokinin-1 (NK1) receptors through knockout strategies for the tachykinin-1 receptor gene display hyperactivity that is ameliorated by both D-amphetamine (a clinically used psychostimulant) and methylphenidate. Inattentive and impulsive phenotypes have also been described, supporting the face validity for this model. These mice also exhibit dysfunction in the regulation of dopaminergic, noradrenergic, and serotonergic transmission.

DAT knockout (DAT-KO) mice reportedly exhibit hyperactivity, impulsiveness, and increased inattention. Both D-amphetamine and methylphenidate alleviate hyperactivity. Although extracellular dopamine is elevated, dopamine release appears to be decreased. Some have questioned the relevance as a model for ADHD since DAT-knockdown mice (expressing 10% normal levels of DAT) display stereotypies in addition to hyperactivity and impulsivity, which is not consistent with ADHD but instead is suggestive as a model for Tourette syndrome.

Children with high levels of thyroid-stimulating hormone (TSH) and resistance to thyroid hormone exhibit symptoms of ADHD. Mice expressing a mutated human thyroid receptor demonstrate all three ADHD-related phenotypes. Methylphenidate can reduce the hyperactivity, and abnormalities in dopamine turnover have been found in this model.

The coloboma mutant mouse contains mutations in the genes for the synaptosomal-associated protein-25 (SNAP-25) and phospholipase C β-1 (PLC β-1), both of which are important for synaptic function. Polymorphisms of SNAP-25, a protein that assists in the fusion of synaptic vesicles to the plasma membrane during neurotransmitter release, have been found to be associated with ADHD. Coloboma mice display hyperactivity and impulsivity, consistent with ADHD. Even though δ-amphetamine reduced ADHD-related symptoms in coloboma mice, methylphenidate was unable to do the same, thereby questioning the predictive validity for this model.

Other genetically based models include the Naples high excitability (NHE) rat, poor performers in the five-choice serial reaction time (5-CSRT) task, and mutant mice for Grin1, a gene encoding a subunit of the NMDA receptor. Grin1-mutant mice are hyperactive, NHE rats exhibit hyperactivity and inattentiveness, whereas animals selected for deficiencies in sustained attention as poor performers during the 5-CSRT task display inattentiveness and impulsivity, but no hyperactivity. Interestingly, dysfunction in dopamine function is associated with poor performers in the 5-CSRT task. Further studies are required to determine the relevance of these models to ADHD.

CHEMICAL MODELS OF ATTENTION DEFICIT/HYPERACTIVITY DISORDER

Neonatal exposure to 6-hydroxydopamine (6-OHDA) in rats has been used as a model for ADHD. They display hyperactivity and impaired spatial learning, which improves with methylphenidate or D-amphetamine treatment; however, they exhibit no impulsiveness. Decreases in dopamine and DAT have been reported as well as increases in serotonin and serotonin transporter binding. Hyperactivity can be ameliorated with inhibitors of norepinephrine and serotonin transporters, supporting a role for these systems in the observed hyperactivity phenotype.

Prenatal or early postnatal exposure to a variety of chemical compounds has been proposed to increase the risk for developing ADHD, including exposure to nicotine, ethanol, and polychlorinated biphenyls. Prenatal or early postnatal exposure to nicotine or ethanol induces hyperactivity in rodents. Associated dopaminergic changes also have been identified: ethanol exposure leads to decreases in dopamine and DAT expression and nicotine exposure can decrease levels of dihydroxyphenylacetic acid (DOPAC) and alter dopamine turnover.

ENVIRONMENTAL MODELS OF ATTENTION DEFICIT/HYPERACTIVITY DISORDER

There are some indications that hypoxia during birth may increase the risk of ADHD. Hypoxia induced in neonatal rats leads to hyperactivity. Furthermore, D_1 receptor levels are reportedly increased in this model, along with alterations in dopamine, serotonin, and norepinephrine levels; however, DAT expression appears to be unaltered. Further studies are required to confirm its validity as a model for ADHD.

The diversity of animal models proposed illustrates the diversity in potential causes for ADHD. Although it remains to be clarified how relevant each of these models is to the human manifestation of ADHD, these models have helped to begin elucidating the mechanisms underlying behavioral phenomena relevant to ADHD. These animal studies have highlighted the potential importance of not only the dopaminergic system, but also that of the noradrenergic and serotonergic systems. Behavioral phenotypes giving rise to ADHD may likely culminate as a result of complex interactions between multiple monoaminergic neurotransmitter systems.

TOURETTE SYNDROME

Tourette syndrome (TS) is a condition characterized by uncontrollable audible and/or motor tics. Even though studies have suggested that genetics plays a critical role in the cause of TS, of the availability of tools to manipulate their expression, including receptor antagonists and molecular inhibitors. Some of the molecular targets include metabotropic glutamate receptor (mGluR 5) antagonists, GABA agonists, NMDA receptor antagonists, muscarinic receptor antagonists, and PAK inhibitors, to name a few. A number of these molecules are currently being tested in preclinical and clinical trials, suggesting the validity of these model systems in therapeutic applications (Dolen et al., 2010; Hagerman et al., 2012; Rooms and Kooy, 2011).

X-LINKED LISSENCEPHALY

Another example of an X-linked ID is lissencephaly that occurs because of mutations in *Dcx*, which encodes doublecortin, a microtubule associated protein playing an important role in growth of neuronal processes. Although the *Dcx* knockout mice show normal neocortical lamination and neocortical neurogenesis, they show abnormalities in hippocampal lamination. The *Dcx* mutants also exhibit impairments in contextual and cued fear conditioning (Bessa et al., 2012).

Both FXS and X-linked lissencephaly represent syndromic models of ID in which the cognitive impairments are associated with clinical and biological features. The non-syndromic models represent the second category, in which cognitive impairment is the only manifestation of the disease. The non-syndromic models are valuable tools in identifying genes and pathways involved in cognitive processes. One of the genes involved in non-syndromic ID is *Gdi1*, which encodes a rabGDP-dissociation inhibitor and has been shown to be important for neuronal maturation. Although the *Gdi1* knockout mice show normal behavior outcomes in most assays, they exhibit impairments in short-term memory and abnormal social behavior (Bessa et al., 2012). The *Gdi1* mouse model acts as an important tool in understanding the mechanism underlying cognitive processes.

INBORN ERRORS OF METABOLISM

Metabolic disorders are caused by mutations in genes encoding enzymes, resulting in reduced enzyme activity, leading to toxic buildup of metabolites in the system. Intellectual disability is commonly seen in metabolic disorders along with other behavioral problems, including ataxia, seizures, and motor problems. The most common metabolic disorder associated with ID is phenylketonuria (PKU), with an incidence of 1:10,000 in the general population.

MOUSE MODELS OF PHENYLKETONURIA

Phenylketonuria is a metabolic disorder caused by mutations in phenylalanine hydroxylase gene (PAH) that is essential for metabolism of phenylalanine (Phe) in the system, which converts phenylalanine to tyrosine. Phenylketonuria results in the toxic accumulation of phenylalanine in the body. Phenylketonuria presents with a number of clinical features, including intellectual disability, abnormal gait, eczema, epilepsy, abnormalities in executive function, learning and memory defects, and autism. One of the best-known treatments for PKU is dietary restriction of phenylalanine. Initially, mouse and rat models of PKU were created by artificially increasing Phe concentration by Phe supplements or enzyme inhibitors. But a true genetic model of PKU was created by ENU mutagenesis of the BTBR mice. The BTBR-Pah^{enu2} mice carries a point mutation in the PAH gene and has best construct validity. Some of the phenotypes in the Pah^{enu2} mice includes light pigmentation, increased Phe concentration in the blood, and reduced levels of Tyr, all of which are seen in human patients. The mouse model also recapitulates some of the human behavioral phenotypes, including short-term memory defects, and impairments in procedural memory and motor defects. Thus, Pah^{enu2} mice provide a very valuable tool to improve our understanding of the genetics and neurobiology of PKU in humans (Martynyuk et al., 2010).

ENVIRONMENTAL MODELS OF INTELLECTUAL DISABILITY

A number of environmental factors cause ID, including prenatal exposure of the fetus to toxic substances, radiation, infection, and malnutrition, suggesting the heterogeneity of this disorder. Treatment of pregnant rats with methyazoxymethanol (MAM) represents a good animal model of environmental cause of ID. Offsprings of MAM-treated rats showed a number of cognitive defects and hyperactivity. Animal models of lead exposure have also been shown to cause cognitive impairments. Also animal models of congenital toxoplasmosis, congenital rubella syndrome, and fetal alcohol syndrome are being tested as models of ID (Scorza and Cavalheiro, 2011).

ATTENTION DEFICIT/HYPERACTIVITY DISORDER

Attention deficit hyperactivity disorder (ADHD) is a highly heritable and heterogeneous disorder that is characterized by three behavioral phenotypes: hyperactivity, impulsiveness, and impaired sustained attention. It likely results from complex gene–gene and/or gene–environment interactions, although an exact etiology for ADHD remains highly elusive. A number of animal models have been proposed, each falling within one of three general categories of insult to the biological system: genetic, chemical, and environment. Cumulatively, findings from these multiple models will hopefully provide insight to the pathophysiology for this heterogeneous disorder. This section is aimed at highlighting some of the models used for ADHD-related research. More in-depth coverage of these and other models is discussed in several reviews (Arime et al., 2011; Russell, 2007; Russell, 2011; Sontag et al., 2010; van der Kooij and Glennon, 2007).

GENETIC MODELS OF ATTENTION DEFICIT/ HYPERACTIVITY DISORDER

Probably one of the most well-studied and characterized models is the spontaneously hypertensive rat (SHR). This model was created through the selective inbreeding of Wistar-Kyoto knockout mice have shown a number of DGS phenotypes, including in cranial and cardiac anomalies (Guris et al., 2001). Another example is the *Df1* knockout mouse, which exhibits learning and memory and sensorimotor gating abnormalities (Paylor et al., 2006). These mouse models have enabled us to better understand the mechanism underlying DGS.

FRAGILE X SYNDROME

Fragile X syndrome (FXS) is the most common form of X-linked intellectual disability and accounts for about 10% to 20% of all inherited IDs (Chiurazzi et al., 2008). Fragile X syndrome presents with a wide spectrum of physical abnormalities, including prominent protruding ears, elongated face, macroorchidism, and behavioral abnormalities, including hyperactivity, obsessive-compulsive behavior, aggression, self-injurious behavior, alterations in sensorimotor gating, cognitive impairments, and abnormal social behavior. Several magnetic resonance imaging (MRI) studies have reported neuroanatomical abnormalities and generalized seizures in patients with FXS (Hagerman et al., 2012).

MOUSE MODELS OF FRAGILE X SYNDROME

FMR1*KO MOUSE MODEL*

To understand the function of FMRP and the disease mechanism in FXS, a *Fmr1* knockout (*Fmr1*KO) mouse model was created in 1994 by the Dutch-Belgium Fragile X consortium (Bakker et al., 1994), and this model has been widely used in studying FXS. The *Fmr1*KO mice (both males and females) are viable and fertile and did not show any gross morphological abnormalities. Microscopic examination of the brain in the *Fmr1*KO revealed dendritic spine abnormalities in different brain regions, which recapitulates the spine abnormalities observed in patients with FXS (Rubeis et al., 2012). Electrophysiological studies revealed enhanced long-term depression (LTD) mediated by the metabotropic glutamate receptor 5 (mGluR5) and the M1 muscarinic acetylcholine receptor (mAChR) in the *Fmr1*KO mice (Dolen et al., 2010). One of the most consistent phenotypes seen in *Fmr1*KO mice is macroorchidism, which recapitulates the macroorchidism phenotype seen in patients with FXS. Behavioral abnormalities in *Fmr1*KO mice include increased locomotor activity and impairment, acoustic startle response, and sensorimotor gating deficits. Mutant mice exhibited a decreased startle response and an enhanced PPI response to sound stimulus when measured using whole body flinch protocol. However, this phenotype is opposite of what has been reported in patients with FXS, who exhibit enhanced startle response and decreased PPI when measured using an eye-blink conditioning protocol. They also show abnormal social behavior, alterations in social and non-social anxiety, and mild learning and memory impairments (Baker et al., 2010; Krueger et al., 2011; Spencer et al., 2011).

POINT MUTATION MODEL

The second mouse model, the *Fmr1*I304N mice, carries a single missense mutation (I304N), resulting in a substitution of isoleucine (Ile) to asparagine (Asn) in the *Fmr1* gene, has been reported in a severely affected FXS patient with a normal repeat length and an unmethylated CPG island who presented with an IQ below 20 and severe macroorchidism. Behavioral analysis in the *Fmr1*I304N mutant mice photocopied the null mutation, including increased activity, decreased acoustic startle response, and increased susceptibility to AGS (Zang et al., 2009). Thus, the I304N point mutation model provides a valuable model to understand FXS behaviors and to test and validate treatments for FXS.

YAC TRANSGENIC MICE

An FMR1 YAC transgenic mouse model containing a 450 kb region of the human Xq27.3 region with the entire *FMR1* gene was created to investigate the function of FMRP and to assess the therapeutic potential of introducing FMRP in the *Fmr1*KO mice. Introducing FMRP in the KO mice rescued a number of phenotypes including macroorchidism, activity and anxiety measures, prepulse inhibition, social behavior, and audiogenic seizures. However, transgenic expression of FMRP overcorrected some of the behaviors, including activity and anxiety in the WT animals expressing the YAC transgene (Willemsen et al., 2011). There are a number of mouse models that carry CGG repeat expansion similar to the human disorders, including the CGG repeat knockin (KI) mouse model, with a portion of the mouse *Fmr1* gene along with the repeat tract replaced with a human *FMR1* permutation with (CGG) 98 repeats. The KI mice showed increased activity and less anxiety in the open field assay, impaired learning and memory in the passive avoidance assay, and defects in social interaction (Qin et al., 2011). The neurohistological and behavioral phenotypes observed suggests that the KI mice provide a useful tool to study the mechanism of instability and pathogenesis of FXTAS.

OTHER MODELS

Apart from mouse models of FXS, a drosophila model exists that recapitulates some of the salient features seen in FXS. Anatomically the null mutants are normal; however, they do exhibit enlarged testes as seen in humans and mouse models with a loss of FMRP. Behaviorally, loss of dFMR1 expression can lead to flight/motor defects, erratic activity with bouts of hyperactivity, abnormal circadian cycle, and courtship behavior defects. Orthologues of all three *FMR1*-related genes have been identified in zebrafish, and thus morpholino antisense oligonucleotide repression of *fmr1* mRNA translation in zebrafish embryos was utilized to study FXS and were phenotypically normal, making it not a suitable model to study FXS (Bhogal and Jongens, 2010).

THERAPEUTIC IMPLICATIONS

Over the last decade the *Fmr1* KO mouse model has been used in the identification of molecular pathways thought to play a role in the pathogenesis of FXS. As a result, specific molecules have been identified as potential therapeutic targets, not only because of their probable involvement in FXS, but also because

MOUSE MODELS OF DOWN SYNDROME

A number of different mouse models of TRS21 have been created based on syntenies between human chromosome 21 (HSA21) and mouse chromosomes 10 (Mmu10), 16 (MMu16), and 17 (Mmu17). Overall, the DS mouse models fall under two broad categories: (1) chromosomal trisomy that includes mice trisomic for chromosomal regions syntenic to HSA21 and (2) transgenic mice overexpressing select dosage-sensitive genes present on HSA21 (Vacano et al., 2012).

CHROMOSOMAL TRISOMY

The first mouse model of DS termed Ts16 was created by spontaneous robertsonian translocation resulting in animals trisomic for Mmu16. But these embryos died *in utero*, making it unsuitable for studying various aspects of DS. However, biochemical studies conducted on cell lines derived from Ts16 have been used to study some of the biological processes, including apoptosis (Vacano et al., 2012). Another major disadvantage with this mouse model is that Mmu16 is syntenic with some regions on HSA3, 8, and 16; hence, these animals are trisomic for a number of genes not present on HSA21, suggesting that this might not be the ideal model of DS. The second model of TRS21 is the Ts65Dn mouse model, a partial trisomy of Mmu16 encompassing a portion of HSA21. These mice are trisomic for about 96 genes syntenic to HSA21 and also trisomic for about 60 centromeric genes on Mmu17. These mice exhibit a number of features seen in patients with DS including craniofacial abnormalities such as hypoplasia of the proximal facies, brachycephaly, altered skull and mandibles, hydrocephaly, tremors and seizures, and degeneration of basal cholinergic forebrain, which has been shown to contribute to dementia seen in patients with DS. They also exhibit congenital heart defects, myeloproliferative disorders, decreased bone density, and show altered incidence of certain cancers (Rueda et al., 2012; Vacano et al., 2012). Some of the behavioral abnormalities include hyperactivity and learning and memory defects (Das and Reeves, 2011). This model seems to exhibit good face validity in spite of not exhibiting perfect construct validity. The Ts65Dn mouse model has been used to investigate therapeutic potential of a number of drug targets, including memantine, which has been shown to improve learning and memory in mutant mice (Rueda et al., 2012).

Another example of a partial trisomic model is the Ts1Cje mouse model, which is a partial trisomy of Mmu16 for a region that contains about 74 genes syntenic to HSA21. These mutants show enlarged brain ventricles and decreased neurogenesis. Learning and memory defects in these mutants are less severe compared with the Ts65Dn mutants. The Ts1Rhr mouse model is trisomic for the DS critical region encompassing about 33 genes and has been created by chromosome engineering. These animals exhibited a number of behavioral and neurophysiological phenotypes that are characteristic of DS but some of the phenotypes were found to be less severe compared with Ts65Dn mouse model (Roubertoux and Carlier, 2010). To model the trisomy of HSA21 syntenic to Mmu17, the Ts1Yah mouse model was created, which is trisomic for 12 genes in the Mmnu17

region. These animals exhibit learning and memory defects in the Y arm maze and novel object recognition, but show improved performance in the Morris water maze, suggesting the variation and complexity of DS phenotypes (Rueda et al., 2012). Also, mouse models that are trisomic for the complete HSA21 syntenic regions on Mmu16 (Dp (16)1Yep/+), Mmu17 (Dp (17)1Yep/+), and Mmu10 (Dp (10)1Yep/+) were created. However, the mouse model that exhibits perfect construct validity is the Dp(10)1Yep/+; Dp(16)1Yep/+; Dp(17)1Yep/+ mouse model, which is trisomic for the entire HSA21 syntenic region on Mmu10, 16, and 17. The mutants exhibit several DS phenotypes, suggesting that this model has good face validity as well (Vacano et al., 2012). The Tc1 or the human transchromosomal mouse model has the entire human HSA21 stably introduced into the mouse genome. The Tc1 model has been shown to exhibit several phenotypes observed in individuals with DS.

OVER-EXPRESSION OF DOSAGE-SENSITIVE GENES

The second category of mouse model comprises dosage-sensitive genes that have been implicated in causing DS phenotypes (Lana-Elola et al., 2011). A few examples of dosage sensitive genes on HSA21 implicated in various DS phenotypes are as follows: (1) Learning and memory: amyloid precursor protein (APP), dual-specificity tyrosine-(Y)-phosphorylation regulated kinase 1A (DYRK1A), synaptojanin 1 (SYNJ1); (2) motor coordination: DYRK1A, APP; (3) cardiac defects: collagen VI alpha-1 (COL6A1), Down syndrome cell adhesion molecule (DSCAM); (4) increased incidence of cancer: v-ets erythroblastosis virus E26 oncogene homolog 2 (ETS2); (5) craniofacial abnormalities: ETS2. Transgenic over-expression and knockout models of these genes have provided a valuable tool in understanding the development of DS phenotypes. However, it is important to consider the genetic background of the mouse models because the phenotypes show variability across different strains of mice.

Overall, the chromosomal trisomic models have provided a valuable tool to recapitulate human DS phenotypes and led to the identification of a number of dosage-sensitive genes that play important roles in contributing to DS. These models have also enabled us to develop novel therapeutic strategies for treatment of DS phenotypes.

DIGEORGE SYNDROME

DiGeorge syndrome (DGS) results from a deletion of chromosome 22q11.2 that is characterized by neonatal hypocalcaemia, susceptibility to infection, hypoplasia of parathyroid glands, cardiac malformation, short stature, mild to moderate learning difficulties, cleft lip, deafness, low set ears, and slant eyes. A variety of psychiatric problems have also been reported, including schizophrenia and depression (Bessa et al., 2012). *Tbx1* knockout mice displayed a wide range of developmental anomalies recapitulating some of the DGS phenotypes in humans, including hypoplasia of the thymus and parathyroid glands, cardiac outflow tract abnormalities, abnormal facial structures, and cleft palate. Another gene implicated is the CRKL and *Crkl* genes Reelin, an extracellular matrix protein, Dishevelled-1, involved in the WNT signaling pathway, Engrailed-2, a neurodevelopmentally important transcription factor, and contactin associated protein-like 2, a neurexin family cell adhesion molecule.

ENVIRONMENTAL MODELS FOR AUTISM SPECTRUM DISORDER

Maternal infection during the first trimester is increasingly becoming recognized as a risk factor for ASD. Rodent models of maternal infection have been generated through respiratory infection via influenza virus or administration of maternal immune activating (MIA) substances such as polyinosine:cytosine (poly(I:C)) and lipopolysaccharide (LPS) (Patterson, 2012). Offspring from these models exhibit ASD-related phenotypes such as impaired social and communication behaviors and increased stereotyped behaviors in addition to non–core symptom behaviors. Cellular deficits present in MIA models include histopathological changes, altered dopaminergic neurochemistry, Purkinje cell disruption, and synaptic communication between hippocampus and prefrontal cortex, and in LPS models include altered hippocampal cell density and dendritic arbors, as well as a variety of synaptic input, response, and plasticity impairments (Patterson, 2012).

Valproic acid (VPA) intake during pregnancy increases ASD susceptibility in offspring, thus administration of VPA to pregnant rodents, most commonly rats, serves as another prominent environmental model for ASD. In rat models numerous behavioral abnormalities are observed in offspring, including ASD-like behaviors such as reduced social interaction, increased repetitive behaviors, and altered sensitivity to sensory stimuli, in addition to relevant physiological changes in microcircuit connectivity, immune abnormalities, and synaptic alterations in the lateral amygdaloid nucleus (Patterson, 2012).

AUTISM SPECTRUM DISORDER MOUSE MODELS IN SUMMARY

There are numerous additional mouse models relevant to ASD that already exist and are still being engineered because of the tremendous genetic variability underlying the disorder. Although not every model, or even all of the aspects of a few models, can be thoroughly captured in this discussion, an expert review of mouse and human phenotypes in ASD provides some broad insights into what we have learned from mouse models of ASD. Buxbaum and colleagues performed an unbiased assessment to identify what phenotypes were enriched in mouse models of 112 ASD causal genes (see Fig. 73.1). Interestingly, they found that social domain deficits (as assayed) were minimally observed, suggesting that broad neurological examinations in mice are important for best understanding the gene functions. Additionally, electrophysiological alterations were present, absent, and directionally divergent across models, suggesting that a hypothesis of a simple imbalance in excitation and inhibition is too broad based on currently compiled data. Certainly, the study of the etiology

of ASD is still in its infancy and as the number of proposed susceptibilities grows along with their animal model counterparts, research studies and the comparisons and conclusions drawn across them will benefit greatly from some level of standardization across genetic backgrounds and assays.

As approximately 80% of ASD cases claim no discernible cause, face validity–based models may still provide novel targets to assess for in human ASD, but cumulatively should be considered with caution as insults unrelated to human ASD may phenocopy ASD-related phenotypes in mice. Ultimately, as additional genes or environmental insults are implicated in ASD, construct validity–based models will continue to allow for increased understanding of specific gene and neural circuitry contributions to physiology and behavior.

INTELLECTUAL DISABILITY

Intellectual disability (ID), previously known as mental retardation, is one of the most common central nervous system impairments, affecting 1% to 3% of the general population. Intellectual disability is characterized by failure to develop normal intellectual functioning, limitations in adaptive behavior including communication and social skills, and most important, the cognitive impairments occur before 18 years of age. The diagnosis of ID is based on cognition, language and social skills, and modeling the cognitive phenotypes in an animal, understanding the manifestation of the phenotypes and interpretation of the behavioral outcomes become very challenging (Ropers, 2008). The causes of ID are heterogeneous, and both genetic and environmental factors have been shown to play important roles. Therefore, based on the causal agents the animal models of ID can be classified into two broad categories: (1) genetic models and (2) environmental models.

The genetic causes of ID include chromosomal abnormalities (e.g., Down syndrome), microdeletions (e.g., Williams–Beuren, DiGeorge, Prader–Willi, Angelman), and coding abnormalities in single genes (e.g., Fragile X syndrome) (Bessa et al., 2012). This section highlights some of the most important animal models of ID.

DOWN SYNDROME

Down syndrome (DS), caused by human trisomy 21, is the most common genetic cause of intellectual disability, affecting 1 in 750 newborns (Parker et al., 2010). Patients with DS present a wide range of clinical features, including craniofacial abnormalities, cardiac defects, hypotonia, gastrointestinal defects, increased incidence of childhood leukemia, and dementia at later stages of life. One of the hallmarks of DS is intellectual disability, which affects 100% of the individuals with IQs ranging from 30 to 70. Some of the cognitive deficits include impairment in long-term memory, spatial memory, and problems in acquiring new skills. The current hypothesis for the pathogenesis of DS is that the phenotypes are caused by extra copies of dosage-sensitive genes present on chromosome 21 (Haydar and Reeves, 2012; Rueda et al., 2012).

seizures, and electroencephalogram abnormalities. TSC1, TSC2, and Pten KO mouse models were successfully improved on a number of measures including seizure, cognition, neuronal hypertrophy, and hippocampal synaptic plasticity by targeting this pathway with pharmacological agents such as rapamycin (Betancur et al., 2009).

SYNDROMIC DISORDER MODELS

Fragile X syndrome is one of the most significant known genetic causes of ASD because approximately 30% of persons with FXS also satisfy the requirements for an ASD diagnosis. Numerous animal models of FXS exist with various behavioral phenotypes (described previously), but few of these reproducibly recapitulate ASD-relevant traits. For instance, the *Fmr1* gene was knocked out on six different mouse genetic backgrounds (hybrid strains) and only knockout (KO) mice on a C57/B6 x DBA/2J background showed consistent ASD-relevant traits of decreased social interactions, altered ultrasonic communication, and stereotypic/repetitive behaviors (Spencer et al., 2011). Thus, all animal models for FXS may not necessarily translate as ideal models for studying ASD. It is possible that, as most ASD-linked genetic insults exhibit incomplete penetrance because of human genetic variability, the same may hold true for animal models.

RETT SYNDROME

Loss-of-function mutations in the gene encoding methyl-CpG-binding protein 2 (MECP2) cause Rett syndrome (RTT), a neurological disorder defined by a period of apparently normal development followed by the manifestation of various behavioral and physiological symptoms including hand stereotypies, loss of verbal skills, motor impairments, poor sociability, and respiratory problems. *Mecp2* mutations can also lead to other neurodevelopmental disorders including cognitive disorders, childhood-onset schizophrenia, and a subset of persons with Rett syndrome also meet the diagnostic criteria for ASD. Thus consequences of loss of MECP2 from animal models yield potential insights into a variety of neurodevelopmental disorders. Numerous mouse models of RTT, including tissue and time-specific models, have demonstrated the molecular and phenotypic consequences of loss of Mecp2. These phenotypes include abnormal gait, limb stereotypies (reminiscent of hand-clasping observed in humans with RTT), seizures, cardiorespiratory irregularities, altered social interactions, anxiety, learning and memory deficits, growth failure, and early death (Khwaja and Sahin, 2011). Autism-like phenotypes, including repetitive behaviors, were specifically observed in a mouse model in which *Mecp2* expression was uniquely disrupted in only GABAergic neurons (Chao et al., 2010). Additionally, mice with a full loss of *Mecp2* and mice expressing a truncated version of *Mecp2* exhibit fewer numbers of synaptic connections, synaptic plasticity deficits, and spine morphology defects (Robertson and Feng, 2011). It is encouraging that separate postnatal applications, reactivation of *Mecp2* gene expression, systemic treatment with an active peptide fragment of insulin-like growth factor 1, and treatment with ampakine CX546 (although more

limited), have been demonstrated to rescue abnormal phenotypes in *Mecp2*-deficient mouse models (Betancur et al., 2009; Khwaja and Sahin, 2011).

15q11-13 DUPLICATION/DELETION SYNDROME

Perturbations of chromosomal region 15q11-13 have been implicated in several neurodevelopmental disorders depending on the genes and allele (maternal or paternal) affected, including Angelman syndrome, Prader-Willi syndrome, and ASD. This region includes genes such as the imprinted ubiquitin ligase *Ube3A* and $GABA_A$ receptor subunit genes. Mice modeling the loss of these genes individually exhibit a wide variety of behavioral deficits. For instance, data from several labs indicate that *Gabrb3* KO mice have impaired social interaction and nesting, repetitive circling behaviors, impaired learning and memory, increased tactile sensitivity, hyperactivity, and increased seizure susceptibility (Robertson and Feng, 2011). A paternal 15q11-13 duplication mouse model of ASD, duplicating a 6.3-Mb analogous murine chromosomal region, replicates the full spectrum of ASD core symptoms resulting in altered communication (ultrasonic vocalization measures elevated pups and decreased in adults), reduced social interest, and a deficit in behavioral flexibility (poor reversal learning in the Morris water maze and Barnes test).

WILLIAMS–BEUREN SYNDROME

Williams–Beuren syndrome (WBS) is a genetic deletion disorder characterized by prominent physical and cognitive attributes including hypersociability. Although children with WBS pursue social interactions, they often have difficulty maintaining friendships. Williams–Beuren syndrome mouse models, generated through deletion of chromosome 7q11.23 regions defining the disorder, exhibit phenotypes that remarkably parallel the human phenotypes, including physical deficits, craniofacial dysmorphism, body and brain growth retardation, and disrupted motor coordination, as well as social/cognitive impairments, hypersociability in social approach, direct social interaction and social choice, and mild intellectual disability (Li and Roy, 2009). A second study that disrupted only a single gene in the mouse WBS locus, *Gtf2i*, also observed increased social interactions and a lack of habituation to a social partner (Sakurai et al., 2010). When considered together, findings of hypersociability in WBS mouse models combined with decreased social behaviors observed in models of ASD causal genes correlatively suggest mouse models of human social disorders may indeed be informative at the mechanistic level and may provide a unique opportunity for comparisons attempting to identify molecular substrates underlying the directionally divergent behaviors.

Many single-gene candidate and rare syndromic models exist exhibiting various combinations of ASD-related behavior and/or pathology (see Betancur, 2011 for extensive review of genes and syndromes implicated in ASD). Several additional genetic mouse models of ASD that show promising phenotypes include mice with induced expression deficits of the

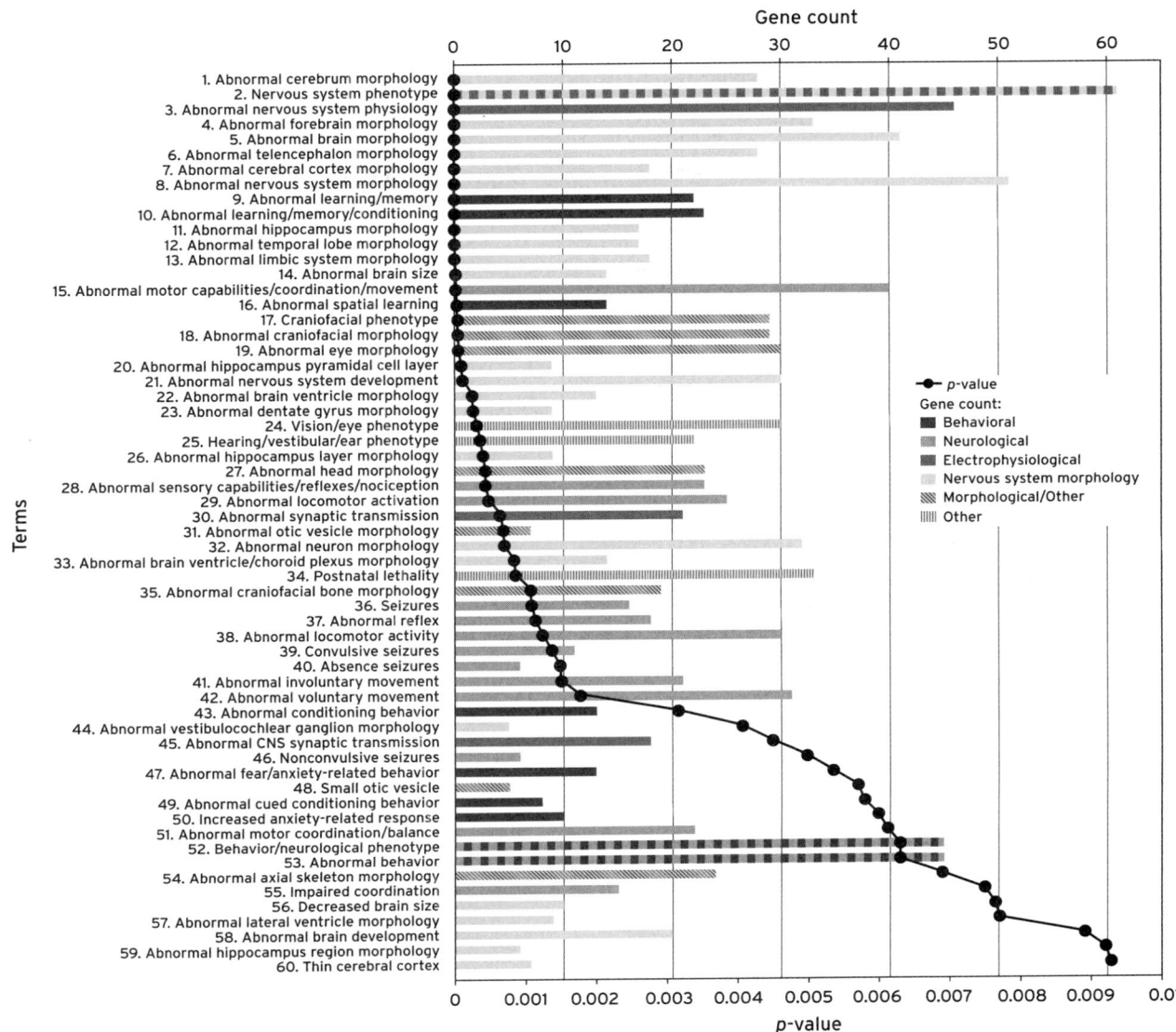

Figure 73.1 Mouse phenotype categories associated with ASD genes. ASD genes (N = 112) were analyzed for enrichment in mouse phenotypes using ToppGene with a Bonferroni corrected p value cutoff of 0.01. Categories are arranged from most significant and downwards (purple line), and for each category, the number of genes in the ASD112 list for which there were murine models with the associated category are indicated by the length of the horizontal bars (gene count). To highlight differing phenotypic categories, bars are color-coded as indicated in the inset to the figure. Categories relating to nervous system morphology phenotype domains are colored light blue, whereas other morphological categories are colored dark blue, electrophysiological categories are colored pink, neurological categories are colored peach, and higher-order behavioral categories are colored green. Categories corresponding to more than one phenotyping domain are presented as alternating colors, and categories that do not relate to the phenotyping scheme are colored yellow. (Adapted from Buxbaum J.D., Betancur C., Bozdagi O., et al. (2012) Optimizing the phenotyping of rodent ASD models: enrichment analysis of mouse and human neurobiological phenotypes associated with high-risk autism genes identifies morphological, electrophysiological, neurological, and behavioral features. Mol. Autism, 3(1):1. (See color insert).

models may provide useful insights into this neurodevelopmental disorder.

TUBEROUS SCLEROSIS COMPLEX

Approximately 1% of children with ASD have tuberous sclerosis complex (TSC). Although full knockout of the *Tsc1* gene in mice leads to limited viability, heterozygous loss of *Tsc1* or *Tsc2* in mice results in TSC-like behaviors, including several related to ASD, specifically impaired learning and memory, social behaviors, and pup vocalizations, as well as disrupted

synaptic plasticity (Khwaja and Sahin, 2011). However, despite the relevant behavioral abnormalities, the hallmark anatomic abnormalities of TSC are not present in these mouse models. Through *in vitro* as well as mouse model–based studies, the mammalian target of rapamycin (mTOR) pathway has been strongly implicated in both TSC and PTEN-related disorders. *PTEN* mutations have been identified in individuals with ASD (Betancur, 2011). In the *Pten* condition null mouse model of ASD, reciprocal social interaction deficits and impaired PPI have been reported (Kwon et al., 2006). This model also exhibits brain abnormalities similar to those observed in humans with PTEN disruptions such as macrocephaly, spontaneous

TABLE 73.1. *(Continued)*

BEHAVIOR TEST	DESCRIPTION
OTHER	
Delayed Reinforcement	Measures the ability to wait for a preferred reinforcer (ex. water) over the immediately available less-preferred reinforce (ex. quinine). The time for the preferred reinforcer increases with each trial.
Reaction-Time Task	Measures the number of nose poke entries to receive a reward during a cued time period
Home Cage Activity	Measures the amount of total, horizontal, and vertical activity in a home cage environment to test for habituation
Latent Inhibition	Measures the impaired performance during an active avoidance task when test training includes exposure to the cued stimulus but without any reinforcement contingencies
Open Field Activity	Measures the amount of total, horizontal, and vertical activity in a novel environment; other activities including stereotypic or repetitive patterns of movement can also be assessed
Pre-pulse Inhibition/ Sensory Motor Gating	Measures the inhibition of a reflexive acoustic startle response to be inhibited when weaker stimuli are presented before the startle stimulus
Acoustic Startle	Measures the startle response to a loud auditory stimulus
Hot Plate	Measures the latency to respond to a heated plate as an index of thermal sensitivity
Von Frey Hairs	Measures a withdrawal response from mechanical stimulation to determine a tactile detection threshold
Running Wheels	Measures the amount and duration of activity in a 24-hour period. Manipulation of light and dark cycles can allow for measuring circadian rhythm based on activity patterns over several months

(Adapted from Robertson H.R., Feng G. (2011) Annual research review: transgenic mouse models of childhood-onset psychiatric disorders. *J. Child Psychol. Psychiatry*, 52(4):442–475.)

and utilized for characterizing ASD models, particularly assays in the social, repetitive, and other domains listed in Fig. 73.1. Based on assessment of ASD phenotypes in both humans and mice with disruptions in ASD genes, defined groups of changes have been identified leading researchers to stress that five levels of analysis should be considered when investigating or reviewing mouse ASD models: (*1*) molecular assays, (*2*) nervous system morphology, (*3*) electrophysiological assays, (*4*) neurological assays, and (*5*) higher-order behavioral assays (Buxbaum et al., 2012).

Current mouse models for ASD can be divided into three general groups of (*1*) genetic models–based on genes believed to contribute to ASD, (*2*) environmental models–based on environmental or pharmacological insults that have been linked to ASD, and (*3*) behavioral models–based on engineered or naturally occurring animal models whose behaviors appear to parallel core features present in human ASD. Although the study of behavioral models will undoubtedly lead to a better understanding of biological mechanisms underlying specific phenotypes, this discussion focuses on construct validity-based models.

CANDIDATE-GENE–BASED MODELS FOR AUTISM SPECTRUM DISORDERS

A number of synaptic genes have been implicated in ASD (Betancur, 2011). For instance, some of the earliest gene candidate models for ASD, based on identification of single gene disruptions in humans, include models in which the postsynaptic neuroligin (NLGN) and presynaptic neurexin (NRXN) families of cell adhesion proteins have been disrupted, including NLGN1, NLGN3, NLGN4X, and NRXN1 (Betancur

et al., 2009). The most well-studied NLGN model is a NLGN3 knockin mouse replicating a human point mutation. Variable behaviors were identified by different groups. Autism spectrum disorder–like phenotypes of impaired social interactions and altered synaptic transmission (enhanced inhibitory transmission) were observed by one group, whereas a second group failed to observe any social deficits, but did observe decreased pup USVs (Betancur et al., 2009; Robertson and Feng, 2011). Neither group observed deficits in repetitive behaviors. NLGN3 and NLGN4 KO mice showed impairments in domains of social and communication behaviors, but not repetitive behaviors, whereas NLGN1 and NRXN1 KO mice showed elevated repetitive grooming behavior. They also, respectively, showed synaptic alterations of impaired hippocampal LTP and hippocampal excitatory transmission (Robertson and Feng, 2011).

The shank family of proteins, particularly SHANK3, which operate in the postsynaptic density as intracellular binding partners of NLGNs, have also been implicated in ASD, as well as schizophrenia. Although SHANK3 KO mice have shown mild autism-like phenotypes, SHANK2 KO mice exhibited ionotropic glutamate receptor up-regulation, fewer dendritic spines, decreased basal synaptic transmission, and altered excitatory currents. Behaviorally they exhibited ASD-like abnormalities in social behaviors, vocalization, and increased repetitive behaviors. Of clinical relevance, the authors identified that social and vocalization changes were caused by alterations in synaptic glutamate receptor expression, suggesting that ASD therapies might benefit from a better understanding of underlying synaptopathic phenotypes (Schmeisser et al., 2012). Additionally, the gene *Shank3* is included in the deletion region identified in 22q13.3 deletion syndrome (Phelan-McDermid syndrome) and is thought to be major causative factor; thus, SHANK KO

TABLE 73.1. Common behavior tests used to characterize rodent models of childhood onset psychiatric disorders

BEHAVIOR TEST	DESCRIPTION
ANXIETY/FEAR	
Active/Passive Avoidance	Measures the avoidance of an area where a foot shock was given. Passive avoidance required the mouse to not enter the area where the foot shock was presented. Active avoidance requires the mouse to exit the area where the foot shock was presented upon a cue
Contextual Fear Conditioning	Measures the amount of freezing when placed in an environment where a previous negative stimulus (foot shock) was given
Elevated Plus Maze	Measures time spent in the open arm versus protected arm of a cross-shaped arena
Elevated Zero Maze	Measures time spent in the open area versus protected area of a circular arena
Light Dark Emergence	Measures latency to emerge from the dark chamber to the light chamber. Also measure total time spent in light and dark chambers, and activity levels in these chambers
Open Field	Measures time spent in the center of the open field arena versus the perimeter or corners of the arena
Reward/Aversion	Measures the latency to obtain a reward in the presence of an aversive stimulus (ex. predator urine, brightly lit novel arena)
REPETITIVE/STEREOTYPICAL BEHAVIORS	
Marble Burying	Measures the number of marbles buried as a result of compulsive digging or shifting in bedding
Non-nutritive Chewing	Measures amount of chewing of non-nutritive clay or substances
Repetitive Grooming	Measures number of grooming sessions and total time spent grooming in a 24-hour period. Also measures time spent grooming relative to other adaptive behaviors (eating, sleeping)
DEPRESSION	
Learned Helplessness	Measures latency to escape a foot shock after repetitive training with foot shock in an inescapable chamber
Porsolt Forced Swim	Measures the time spent in vigorous swimming relative to the time spent floating in a tall cylinder filled with water
Tail Suspension	Measures the time spent struggling relative to the time spent immobile when suspended by the tail
LEARNING AND MEMORY	
Barnes Maze	Measures the ability to learn the location of an escape hole in a circular maze with 18 evenly spaced holes using spatial environmental cues
Morris Water Maze	Measures the ability to learn the location of a hidden platform using extra-maze spatial environmental cues
Radial Arm	Measures the number of entries into one of eight arms that are baited with food or water using spatial environmental cues; may tap into cognitive preservation
T-Maze/Y-Maze	Measures the correct initial entry into an alternating arm of the maze bated with food or water using spatial environmental cues; may tap into cognitive preservation
SOCIAL PARADIGMS	
Nest Building	Evaluates size and organization of nest building; may also assess procedural cognitive function
Pairing in Novel Environment	Measures amount of social approach of two mice paired in a novel environment
Resident Intruder	Measures amount of social approach when an intruder mouse is introduced into the home cage of the test mouse following social isolation
Social Approach-Partitioned	Measures amount of time spent near the partition dividing the test mouse from either a stranger or known mouse
Social Approach-Three Chamber	Measures amount of time spent in an empty chamber versus a chamber containing a stranger mouse. Second trial measures the time spent in the chamber with a known mouse versus a stranger mouse versus an empty chamber
Social Recognition	Measures the amount of social interaction between the test mouse and a second mouse on the first and subsequent exposures
Ultrasonic Vocalization-Adults	Measures the number and duration of ultrasonic vocalizations of male mice exposed to female mice in estrous OR male mice during a resident intruder test
Ultrasonic Vocalization- Neonates	Measures the number and duration of ultrasonic vocalizations of pups during brief isolation from the dam and/or littermates

(continued)

73 | ANIMAL MODELS IN PSYCHIATRIC DISORDERS OF CHILDHOOD ONSET

RICHARD PAYLOR, ALEXIA M. THOMAS, SURABI VEERARAGAVAN, AND SHANNON M. HAMILTON

Research conducted to elucidate the mechanisms underlying psychiatric disorders occurs with greater flexibility of manipulation using animal models. This is particularly true with childhood disorders, in which human samples available to researchers are not only limited, but there are also ethical considerations regarding the ability of children to provide informed consent. Cellular and *in vitro* assays and computer-based models offer alternative strategies to elucidate mechanisms underlying cellular processes. However, it must be considered that many neurological disorders are characterized by complex alterations in behavior that are likely the culmination of multiple pathways and networks spanning the brain. Therefore, it is important to bear in mind that studies of these behavioral components may be best modeled at the whole organismal level.

How are animal models designed or chosen to represent complex human psychiatric disorders? For those disorders in which the etiology is known, models can be more easily constructed; for example, by genetic perturbation or chemical/environmental insult based on the known etiology. Unfortunately, for many disorders little is known regarding the underlying pathology, and other methods must be used to choose suitable models for study. In these cases a model is often chosen based on its ability to mimic the human condition phenotypically. For psychiatric disorders this relies heavily on characterization of rodent behavior. At present there are many tools available to investigate rodent behaviors that span multiple behavioral domains, as indicated in Table 73.1. However, it must be kept in mind that behaviors in rodent models are likely not completely analogous to human behavior.

Regardless of how a model is created, each one must meet certain criteria to be considered relevant for the study of a particular disorder. Currently, the accepted standard in ascertaining the appropriateness of a model is how well it conforms to three criteria: face validity, construct validity, and predictive validity.

A model with face validity is one in which the characteristics observed in that model parallel those made in humans with the disorder. These characteristics may be at the molecular, cellular, or behavioral level. Construct validity requires that a model recapitulate known etiological factors of the disease (e.g., genetic or environmental). Genetic studies, including gene association and linkage studies, have implicated genes for particular disorders that can then be targeted for investigation

using transgenic animal models. Predictive validity refers to the expectation that one will be able to make predictions about the human condition based on the animal model. For example, pharmacological treatments effectively implemented in human patients would be expected to demonstrate similar effectiveness in a proposed animal model. In order to increase confidence in evaluating the potential effectiveness of novel therapies in human patients, it is important to have already established predictive validity in the model.

Although models that fit all three validity criteria are favored over those that meet only one or two, critical insights into behavioral pathways may still be made for those models not meeting full validation status. This is important considering that many psychiatric conditions have no known cause.

This chapter highlights the major animal models currently employed in the research of childhood-onset psychiatric disorders.

AUTISM SPECTRUM DISORDERS

MODELING AUTISM SPECTRUM DISORDERS IN ANIMALS

Modeling autism spectrum disorders (ASDs) in animals is challenging on several counts. (*1*) Autism spectrum disorder is defined by human behaviors. These include a number of diagnostic criteria, particularly in the domains of social interaction and social communication behavior, which are uniquely human. Additionally, behavioral traits exhibited across the ASD spectrum are highly variable both in terms of the presence (number and type) of traits individuals exhibit and the magnitude of each trait's expression. (*2*) The majority of instances of ASD remain idiopathic. Known genetic causes of ASD are highly complex with no single insult likely contributing to more than approximately 2% of all ASD cases and most contributing to less than 0.005%. Even for instances in which a genetic insult can be identified, the underlying pathology remains undiscovered. Thus, there are currently no biomarkers available for validating any animal model of ASD.

Despite these difficulties, significant progress has been made in identifying behaviors and pathologies relevant to ASD that are assayable in animals, particularly in rodent models. Because the majority of these models are rodent, that is this section's focus. Many behavioral assays have been proposed

CONCLUSIONS

In examination of the epigenetic mechanisms that may contribute to neurodevelopmental disease risk, the necessity for and value in studies using valid animal models in which variables such as environmental conditions, temporal specificity, and offspring sex can be evaluated. The transmission of epigenetic marks to future generations through reprogramming of the germ cells adds to the complexity in establishing causal links between disease presentation and fetal antecedents in clinical and epidemiological studies. In looking at offspring phenotypic changes, it is clear that although some phenotypes terminate with the first generation, others will be transmitted across multiple generations (Dunn et al., 2011). The degree to which there is true transgenerational "epigenetic" involvement in a given end point is determined by the ability for that mark to be erased and re-established outside of a re-exposure or continuation of the insult. Further, the sex-specificity of transgenerational epigenetic programming requires examination at both the level of transmission of an effect as well as the inheritance of it. In other words, can both mom and dad pass on the trait? And do both male and female offspring inherit it? Maternal exposure to aversive environments such as maternal stress, infection, or obesity results in a variety of phenotypes that have different transmission characteristics as they pass through the generations. Information about maternal experience, in the form of changes in hormonal milieu, can be transmitted via the placenta to the fetal compartment producing a direct action on the developing embryo (Dunn et al., 2011) (see Fig. 72.1).

In addition to ascertaining the transmission and generational passage of epigenetic marks, understanding the cell type specificity and involvement is also helpful in determining in what tissue an effect might occur as windows of developmental vulnerability to environmental challenges may be tissue specific (Fig. 72.2). Somatic tissues may be acutely programmed, leading to changes in health outcomes in the first generation. However, if prenatal insults do not directly affect the germline, the phenotype will terminate with this generation. Phenotypes that persist through the second generation but not a third may relate to the programming of the primordial germ cells during the initial maternal insult, and acquired transient epigenetic marks only capable of passing through a single generation. Thus, transmission of an epigenetic trait does not demonstrate a fully integrated, transgenerational

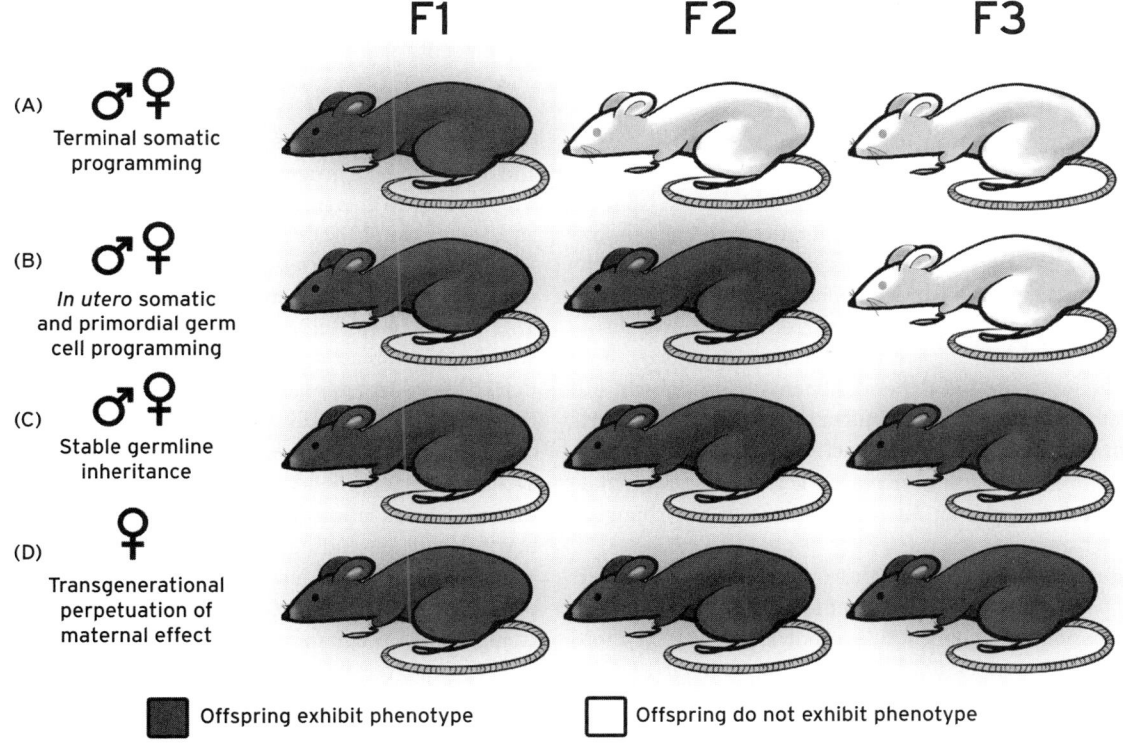

Figure 72.2 Modes of transgenerational epigenetic transmission. Several mechanisms for transgenerational epigenetic transmission are possible, as exemplified here in dark gray. Dark gray mice represent a changed phenotype, whereas white mice represent the "normal" end point, indicating that the phenotype has not been transmitted to that generation. The sex symbols at left indicate the maternal or paternal lineage capable of transmitting phenotypes in the indicated manner. (A) In utero somatic programming may acutely affect tissue and brain development in the fetus, initiating a developmental trajectory that results in an adult phenotype that is not transmitted into the next generation. (B) In addition to in utero somatic programming, changes in the maternal environment can acutely program primordial germ cells, resulting in transmission of the phenotype into the second generation. In this scenario, germ cells must be directly exposed to a maternal insult. (C) In utero exposure is sufficient to stably alter the germline of offspring, resulting in many generations of transmission without the need for re-exposure to the original maternal insult. (D) Transgenerational phenotypes may occur through a maternal effect wherein programming during gestation or through exposure to altered maternal behavior results in an adult phenotype in female offspring. The presence of this phenotype during pregnancy in the mother can in turn acutely program the next generation, perpetuating the transgenerational trait.

folate, an important methyl donor shown to regulate levels of methylation of non-imprinted genes during pregnancy, thus shifting more broadly the epigenetic landscape (Bale, 2011).

Evidence from animal models of maternal stress supports an important regulatory role of the placenta in mediating effects between the maternal and fetal compartments. In early prenatal stress studies, a sex-specific effect of stress on placental epigenetic machinery was shown in which maternal stress increased expression of DNMT1 and the methyl binding protein, MeCP2, in males (Bale, 2011). Previous studies in mice have reported that regulation of placental methylation patterns is predictive of similar embryonic changes critical in neurodevelopment. Recent studies examining early life stress found similar changes for MeCP2 expression and methylation in the brains of first- and second-generation stressed mice (Bale, 2011). Further, maternal stress in mice has reported significant increases in the expression of genes important in growth and development including PPARα, IGFBP-1, GLUT4, and HIF3α in male but not female placentas (Bale et al., 2010). Mechanistically, the link between maternal stress and changes in placental gene expression may involve direct or indirect actions of stress hormones. As an example, stress-induced glucocorticoids increase expression of PPARα, and PPARα in turn drives expression of IGFBP-1, suggesting one mechanism whereby maternal stress could directly affect placental gene expression patterns directly relevant to embryo development. In addition, reductions in growth factors have been linked to affective and neurodevelopmental disorders, and IGFBP-1 is known to down-regulate genes involved in embryonic growth. Thus, as one example these studies suggest that an elevation in placental IGFBP-1 with a consequent decrease in available growth factors during critical developmental periods could impart a sex-specific effect on male fetal programming. Alterations in oxygen and nutrient availability have also been associated with inflammation, and there is an established association between placental inflammatory events and an increased risk for affective disorders, schizophrenia, and autism (Bale et al., 2010). How these placental outcomes are sex dependent remains unknown, but may be related to a protective or buffering mechanism of genes on the X chromosome. Because X inactivation occurs to a much lesser extent in the placenta, increased gene dosage in female placentas could underlie an altered response to the changing maternal environment.

The ability for maternal stress hormones (cortisol or corticosterone) to gain access to and affect fetal brain development is highly dependent on placental levels of 11β-hydroxysteroid dehydrogenase-2 (11β-HSD2), the placental barrier enzyme that converts glucocorticoids to their inactive metabolite. At the interface of the maternal:fetal circulation is the syncytiotrophoblastic cells that express high levels of 11β-HSD2, and function to exclude the majority of maternal active glucocorticoids before they reach the fetal compartment. Typically, in early-mid gestation, fetal blood has greater than 10-fold lower cortisol levels than maternal blood (O'Donnell et al., 2009). Environmental perturbations that would serve to decrease 11β-HSD2 expression could then expose the fetus to higher levels of active glucocorticoids. Such evidence has been reported in animal models in which pharmacological blockade of 11β-HSD2 was administered during pregnancy and resulted in significant increases in glucocorticoid receptors in the amygdala of the offspring as adults (Holmes et al., 2006). Genetic disruption of placental/fetal 11β-HSD2 to reduce its expression was also found to produce offspring with higher levels of anxiety-like behaviors. Perturbations in maternal diet are also known to affect placental 11β-HSD2 where a low protein diet during pregnancy significantly decreased its activity, supporting again a link between nutritionally deficiencies and stress axis changes (O'Donnell et al., 2009).

Fetal antecedents such as high fat diet or obesity and maternal stress have also been associated with increases in placental inflammation (O'Donnell et al., 2009; Frias et al., 2011). Cytokine production in the placenta can increase markers of immune activation in the developing fetus or disrupt overall placental function, producing long-term programming changes in the offspring. In macaques, maternal high-fat diet increased placental inflammatory cytokines and expression of Toll-like receptor-4 (Frias et al., 2011). Similarly, high-fat diets in rodents during pregnancy have also shown significant increases in placental inflammatory cytokines, supporting a change in appropriate placental function in response to an unhealthy environment. Timing of these effects is also important in predicting outcomes. For instance, maternal immune activation during early gestation can result in a failure for implantation to occur, whereas mid-gestation inflammation in the placenta has been linked to schizophrenia and ASD-like phenotypes (Hsiao and Patterson, 2012).

Critical epigenetic processes occur within the placenta as part of the regulation for normal development and function, and disruptions in programmatic changes in the chromatin have been linked to increased disease risk for the offspring (Hsiao and Patterson, 2012). Chromatin remodeling complexes and DNA methyltransferases (DNMTs) are necessary for epigenetic reprogramming that occurs in pre-implantation development. This highly regulated process produces competent embryos and the trophoblastic cells of the placenta. The same epigenetic marks found in fetal tissue including DNA methylation, miRNAs, and histone modifications have also been reported in placental tissue. Studies have established unique roles for DNMT isoforms during pre-implantation in the placenta to maintain uniform methylation imprints in all embryonic and extraembryonic cells, including the placenta (Ackerman et al., 2012). Recent studies have identified miRNAs that are specific to the placenta, where their expression pattern appears to dynamically change across pregnancy in humans and rodents. As these miRNAs are also released from the placenta and are detectable in the maternal serum encased in microvesicles, there is potential to classify them as biomarkers of placental function. The necessity of miRNA expression in placental development has been established, in which mice deficient in the Argonaut-2 gene, a protein component of the RNA-induced silencing complex (RISC), show abnormal placenta function resulting in embryonic lethality (Ackerman et al., 2012). The placental miRNA environment also appears to be susceptible to perturbations resulting from such insults as hypoxia, immune activation, and dietary challenges, supporting a likely role for miRNAs in programmatic changes that are poised to alter fetal development.

responsive to the hormonal status of the animal (McCarthy et al., 2009). One mechanism by which estrogen is thought to modulate methylation is through its effects on DNMT gene expression and activity levels. These effects are brain region specific, providing yet another level of control for sex differences to progress and ultimately affect systems outcomes such as stress responsivity. Estradiol can also directly alter histone modifications, including actions on histone deacetylases (HDACs) (McCarthy et al., 2009). A single postnatal administration of an HDAC inhibitor in males during the critical window disrupted programming of the sexually dimorphic BNST, a brain region important in stress neurocircuitry. In addition, the broad epigenetic programming effect of estrogen has been shown for dramatic shifts in the miRNA environment in the developing brain. In the early postnatal mouse brain, males and females have significant differences in expression patterns of the 250 most abundant miRNAs. These sex differences were dependent on the conversion of testosterone to estradiol in males, as a single administration of an aromatase inhibitor on postnatal day 1 completely shifted the normal male pattern to that of females (Morgan and Bale, 2011). These studies provide substantial evidence for epigenetic mechanisms for steroid hormones to impact neurodevelopment, producing dramatic and important sex differences. However, these mechanisms are also vulnerable to perturbations in the environment, shifting "normal" developmental patterns and trajectories. As described, maternal stress and infection have both been associated with dysmasculinizing phenotypes, suggesting that a disruption at some level in male sexual differentiation or gonadal development occurs that alters testosterone production during the organizational period.

INTRICACIES OF THE PLACENTAL CONTRIBUTION TO FETAL PROGRAMMING

The developing placenta is an intriguing candidate tissue for mechanistic examination of epigenetic programming, as it is a rapidly developing and sex-specific endocrine tissue that continues to respond to the dynamic maternal milieu throughout pregnancy. The placenta serves as the critical messenger between the maternal and embryonic compartments, and therefore is poised to be influenced by perturbations occurring in pregnancy by a number of mechanisms, including alterations in: (1) nutrient and oxygen transport, (2) inflammatory responses, and (3) epigenetic programming (Bale et al., 2010) (Fig. 72.1). Tight control of placental and embryonic epigenetic machinery is critical during gestation when a wave of genome demethylation before *de novo* re-methylation by DNA methyltransferases, establishment of imprints, and sex determination occurs, identifying novel targets as highly vulnerable to maternal disturbances that could result in embryonic reprogramming. For instance, inflammatory cytokines can directly affect levels and activity of DNA methyltransferases (DNMT), as well as regulate placental receptors and transporters for

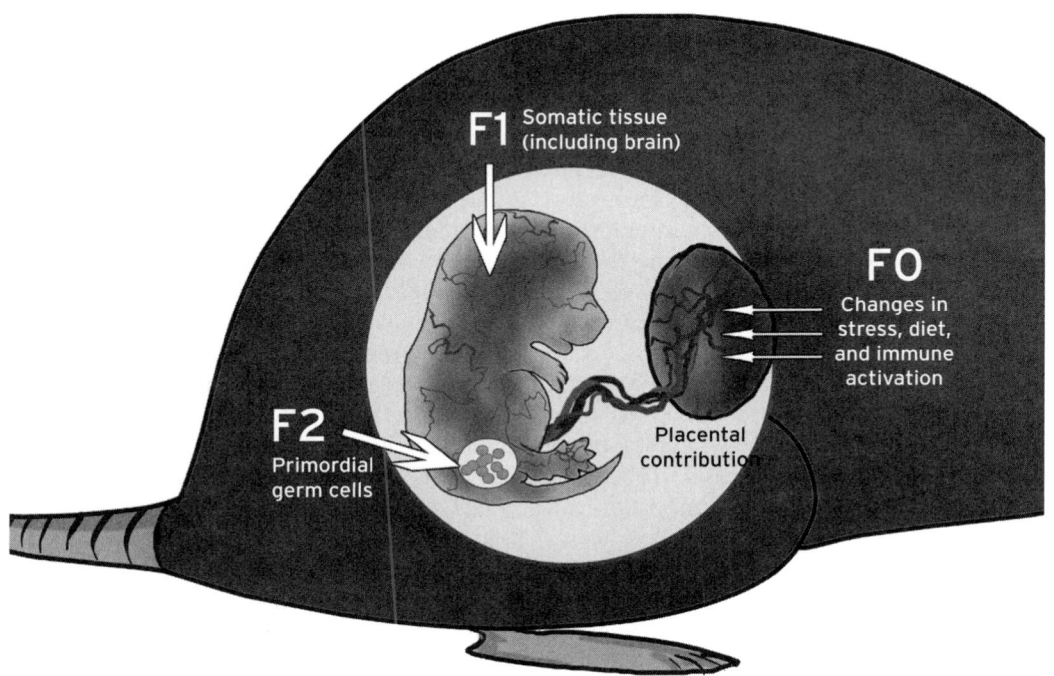

Figure 72.1 *Intersection of prenatal insult and developmental timing to program tissue targets and affect subsequent generations. Information regarding maternal stress, infection, or diet perturbations, in the form of changes in hormonal milieu, is transmitted from the maternal compartment to the fetal compartment via the placenta. The dynamic process and trajectory of fetal development provides a temporal specificity for responses to fetal antecedents. Acute programming of somatic tissues can lead to changes in long-term health outcomes in the first generation. In addition, the primordial germ cells, which contribute genetic and epigenetic information to the second generation, are also present and can undergo reprogramming during embryonic development. Thus, a truly "transgenerational epigenetic" mark must be present into a third generation. In addition, embryo sex plays an important role in determining how an insult may become part of the epigenome and passed on to future generations.*

Newschaffer et al., 2007). However, when further separated for cognitive impairment, this bias was even further increased for ASD without mental retardation to 5.5:1, suggesting that distinct underlying mechanisms or predisposing factors may be involved. As exposure to maternal stress before 32 weeks' gestation has been suggested as a potential contributing factor to ASD (Beversdorf et al., 2005), understanding the role sex plays in the specificity of response to stress during development may provide unique insight as to disease etiology. A recent report detected a significant effect of maternal depression during pregnancy on offspring postnatal anxiety development, particularly in males (Gerardin et al., 2010). These studies support both a sex- and temporal-specificity in the association between maternal stress and offspring disease. Although there are many factors that likely contribute to sex differences in disease predisposition, sex-specific responses to fetal antecedents occurring during sensitive windows of development may promote long-term programming effects that underlie such disease biases. Along these lines, structural brain volume analyses using functional magnetic resonance imaging (fMRI) in male and female patients with schizophrenia have confirmed a disruption of the normal sexual dimorphism of the brain, including the dimorphic ratio of orbitofrontal cortex to amygdala where male schizophrenic patients showed a phenotypically more female pattern in these brain regions (Bale et al., 2010).

The brain develops in the face of combined and opposing forces of resiliency and vulnerability. The central factors important in resilience, ongoing neurogenesis, migration, myelination, differentiation, and synaptogenesis are the same processes subject to derailment, which can promote lasting consequences. The complex interplay of genetics, early experience, and later environment underlies the weak but consistent heritability of numerous neurodevelopmental disorders. The developing brain is organized by developmental hormone exposure, with males experiencing elevated testosterone levels during normal testes development. Aromatization of this testosterone to estradiol in the brain drives masculinization, an active process affecting cell differentiation and connectivity in the brain. Estrogenic involvement in cell death and cell birth in the developing nervous system is a critical component in programming the sexually dimorphic brain (McCarthy et al., 2009). The variety of mechanisms evoked by estradiol during development provides numerous avenues for disruption of the active process of masculinization. Programming of important regulatory brain regions, such as the neuroendocrine hypothalamus, via steroid hormone effects on cell migration patterns during early development may also contribute to sex differences in disease susceptibility (Bale et al., 2010).

In rodent models, studies have taken advantage of the ability to manipulate the early postnatal critical window to examine the organizational effects on long-term stress responsivity, resulting in an established sex difference in stress responsivity in adult mammals. Similar to outcomes reported with prenatal stress exposure, hippocampal GR expression was altered in female offspring masculinized at birth by a single injection of testosterone, supporting the importance of the male testosterone surge in normal wiring of these pathways (Bale, 2011). In addition, the early postnatal period is a sensitive window

during which hormonal exposure produces organizational effects on maturation of the serotonin system, potentially leading to long-term changes in adult stress sensitivity. In addition to the early critical period of programming, the rise in testosterone beginning in puberty exerts modulatory actions on neurotransmitter systems critical in regulation of stress physiology and coping. Such systems affected included serotonergic and γ-aminobutyric acid (GABA)-ergic (Bitran et al., 1993). Therefore, the coordinated impact of masculinization at both time periods may interact with components of sex chromosomes to orchestrate a complete "normal" male phenotype. Neuropsychiatric disease predisposition may then involve a mismatch between brain organizational programming and activational hormones.

Similar to models of maternal stress, there is also evidence to support that offspring programming responses to maternal immune activation are also sex dependent. For example, male offspring of pregnant rats challenged with LPS late in gestation showed significant deficits in PPI, whereas females were unaffected by this insult (Howerton and Bale, 2012). Similarly, male but not female mice exposed during late gestation to the viral mimic Poly I:C displayed behavioral and cognitive inflexibility, key negative symptoms in schizophrenia. These sex-dependent programming effects were associated with significant reductions in glutamate content in the prefrontal cortex in the males exposed to the prenatal immune activation (Meyer et al., 2011).

Little is currently understood regarding how offspring sex may influence the epigenetic response to a changing maternal environment. It is likely that sex-specific responses to fetal antecedents during sensitive windows of development contribute to these differences. Studies in animal models of prenatal stress have begun providing interesting clues as to the timing and mechanisms involved in how perturbations in the maternal milieu may have sex specificity in their effects on the developing brain (Bale et al., 2010). The disruption of sex-dependent processes is a common theme in the prenatal stress literature. Sex differences in neurodevelopment are the result of both genetic sex and circulating gonadal hormones. One of the first papers modeling prenatal stress in rats found that chronic restraint during the final week of gestation disrupted male sex behavior (Ward, 1972). Late gestational restraint stress has also been shown to disrupt the organizational perinatal testosterone surge, reduce adult testis size, shorten anogenital distance, and block the differentiation of sexually dimorphic brain nuclei in males (Bale, 2011). Similarly, male mice exposed to maternal stress during early gestation have reduced testis size and testosterone levels and a shortened anogenital distance as adults, supporting a disruption in their normal masculinization. Such outcomes demonstrate potential sex-specific mechanisms for changes in the programming of the sexually dimorphic brain despite a shared intrauterine environment.

There are many epigenetic mechanisms by which estrogen promotes and drives sex differences in the developing brain. During the critical window of brain sexually dimorphic brain programming, estradiol can broadly act to alter DNA methylation patterns, including that of its own estrogen receptor alpha (ERα), effectively shaping the landscape to be more or less including increased expression and reduced DNA methylation of the promoter regions of key dopaminergic genes in the ventral tegmental area, prefrontal cortex, and nucleus accumbens (Vucetic et al., 2010). Mechanistically, one of the ways in which protein deficiency may produce changes in the offspring brain is via an intersection with immune activation. For instance, in a rat model of maternal low protein, increased levels of the proinflammatory cytokines TNFα and IL-6 were found in the placenta, again suggesting that common pathways may be involved in programming offspring disease risk.

It is also clear that pregnancy undernutrition is a stressor, and likely elevates maternal stress responsivity. In rats, maternal 50% food restriction during late pregnancy increased maternal plasma corticosterone levels and fetal adrenal weights. Offspring subsequently showed changes in hippocampal GRs and HPA axis sensitivity similar to that reported in maternal stress models (Lesage et al., 2001). Similar results were found in a guinea pig model of maternal nutrient restriction of 48 hours of food deprivation in which both maternal and fetal cortisol levels were elevated during late gestation, and GRs were reduced in the offspring hypothalamus and hippocampus as adults (Lingas et al., 1999).

MATERNAL HIGH-FAT DIET AND OBESITY MODELS

Because the organization of neural circuits controlling energy balance takes shape during perinatal life, considerable attention has focused on the developing hypothalamus, the source of neuroendocrine control, including that of stress regulation. Interestingly, the adipocyte hormone leptin, which is dramatically increased in the obese state, plays a vital role in directing development of hypothalamic projections in and around the arcuate nucleus. Moreover, secretion of leptin both within the fetus and from the placenta during development changes in response to the nutritional environment. Leptin signaling is thus poised to influence the developing brain regarding maternal over- or undernutrition via distinct actions on two functionally divergent neuronal populations, the anorexigenic pro-opiomelanocortin (POMC) and orexigenic neuropeptide Y (NPY) neurons (Bale et al., 2010). Target projections of these neurons include the paraventricular nucleus and the lateral hypothalamus, hypothalamic regions that exert widespread regulatory control over homeostatic functions throughout life. Such studies have perhaps identified specific modes of neurodevelopmental programming whereby the wiring of the hypothalamus is determined through endocrine signals. In addition, mice fed a high-fat diet throughout pregnancy produce offspring with altered DNA methylation patterns in dopaminergic and opioid genes and behaviors, suggesting that an obese maternal environment programs offspring with reward pathway dysregulation that may ultimately influence mood and affect (Li et al., 2010).

As mentioned, there is convincing evidence for a likely intersection between maternal dietary challenges and immune activation. In both rodents and nonhuman primates, studies have demonstrated increased inflammatory processes in important brain regions in offspring born to mothers on a high-fat or obesogenic diets. Rat offspring from a dam fed a high-saturated fat diet during pregnancy showed significant levels of activated microglia in their hippocampus at birth that remained high throughout life, consistent with an increased basal neuroinflammatory tone (Bilbo and Tsang, 2010). These offspring also displayed increased anxiety-like behaviors and reduced performance ability in a spatial learning and memory task, supporting a likely contribution of local immune factors such as proinflammatory cytokines in disrupting normal brain function and stress processing. Further, in the nonhuman primate, offspring from macaque mothers fed a high fat diet for four years before pregnancy showed substantial increases in proinflammatory cytokines and activated microglia in their hypothalamus during the third trimester (Grayson et al., 2010). Female offspring in these studies also demonstrated high levels of social anxiety and fear of novelty as infants (Sullivan et al., 2010). Results from these studies support a potential link between maternal nutritional intake throughout pregnancy and increased neuroinflammation in the developing brain and long-term changes in behaviors relevant to neurodevelopmental disease.

Epigenetic mechanisms, which exert lasting effects on gene expression and can be heritable, are a particularly intriguing target when examining links between the perinatal nutritional environment and offspring metabolic phenotype. For example, foods high in choline cause marked changes in DNA methylation, which, in turn, alter long-term gene expression. Studies have demonstrated that choline deficiency during pregnancy produced alterations in histone methylation and subsequent changes in gene expression in mice (Bale et al., 2010). Pregnant dams fed choline-deficient diets during late gestation produced offspring with diminished progenitor cell proliferation and increased fetal hippocampus apoptosis, altered hippocampal angiogenesis, insensitivity to long-term potentiation as adults and decreased visual-spatial and auditory memory. These changes in fetal brain development were associated with epigenetic alterations in DNA and histone methylation in the fetal hippocampus. Similarly, studies using changes in mouse coat color as a marker of dietary and nutrient influence on epigenetic regulation of the *agouti* locus demonstrated how relatively minor changes in DNA methylation can produce a profound phenotypic impact (Waterland, 2003). Such studies support the ultimate mechanistic impact for minor dietary and nutritional fluctuations during key points in development.

FETAL SEX AS A FACTOR IN EPIGENETIC PROGRAMMING

Epidemiological studies linking fetal antecedents with long-term disease risk have established gender as an important determinant in disease severity and onset. As an example, pregnant mothers exposed during their second trimester to the stress of the 1940 invasion of The Netherlands had male, but not female, offspring with an increased risk of schizophrenia (van Os and Selten, 1998). Further, many neurodevelopmental disorders have a strong sex bias, including ASD with an overall sex ratio of 4.3:1 for boys-to-girls (as reviewed in very limited nesting and bedding material as a stressor in the postpartum environment, epigenetic changes were identified within the adult offspring hippocampus where the ability of a transcriptional repressor to bind to the silencing region of the stress gene, CRF, was found, thus altering the ability of these offspring to appropriately respond to and cope during stress experience as adults (Korosi et al., 2010).

Animal models have also examined transgenerational outcomes demonstrating germ cell programming from stress exposure in both the prenatal and postnatal environments. Prenatally, studies in mice have shown that males exposed to stress *in utero* and presenting with increased stress sensitivity themselves as adults, can pass on this phenotype to their male offspring (Morgan and Bale, 2011). In examination of the brain miRNA environment, it was found that there were significant differences in the expression of a number of these noncoding RNAs in these second-generation males, supporting an epigenetic target of maternal stress that was present into the second generation not requiring subsequent re-exposure to the insult. Similarly, in a mouse early postnatal stress model, offspring continued to present with a depressive-like phenotype through three generations, with comparable changes detected in DNA methylation in the germline of these mice (Franklin et al., 2010). These studies showing interactions of the environment with the genome at the level of placing long-lasting epigenetic marks in the chromatin that remain through cell divisions and across generations, support the susceptibility of the germline to external influences that could increase the disease susceptibility in subsequent generations.

MATERNAL INFECTION AND IMMUNE ACTIVATION

Numerous animal models of maternal infection show similar relationships with that reported in epidemiological studies in which maternal immune activation during pregnancy produced offspring endophenotypes associated with neurodevelopmental disorders, including ASD and schizophrenia (Meyer et al., 2011). Such studies have utilized several models, including maternal influenza viral infection, injection of the pathogen mimics Poly I:C and lipopolysaccharide (LPS), and the proinflammatory cytokine IL-6 (Howerton and Bale, 2012). The most consistent phenotype produced in these models is a deficit in offspring pre-pulse inhibition (PPI) in response to an acoustic startle, a change that is reversed by the administration of the antipsychotic drugs haloperidol or clozapine. Sensorimotor gating deficiencies, phenotypes measured by PPI, are commonly associated with schizophrenia, and have also been demonstrated in numerous other psychiatric or affective disorders such as obsessive compulsive disorder, Tourette syndrome, and posttraumatic stress disorder, and thus are highly relevant endophenotypes in which potential epigenetic mechanisms can be explored. Again, highlighting the importance of gestational timing for the impact of fetal insults in producing long-term outcomes, a single administration of the proinflammatory cytokine, IL-6, at mid-gestation in mice was sufficient to produce significant deficits in both PPI and latent inhibition. Maternal immune activation in rodents using a low dose of LPS during mid-gestation also produced offspring with deficits in PPI, and these offspring also exhibited enlarged ventricles, a hallmark of schizophrenia (Hsiao and Patterson, 2012).

The mechanism and potential epigenetic involvement in maternal immune activation programming of the offspring developing brain is not clear. Certainly, maternal cytokines have direct access to the placenta, the intermediary tissue that serves to protect the developing fetus, and have also been detected in the amniotic fluid following maternal immune challenge (Howerton and Bale, 2012). Therefore, there are likely direct as well as indirect downstream targets of these maternally produced cytokines that are involved in programming changes in the fetal brain. Of note, uteroplacental inflammation is sufficient to produce an increase in expression of apoptotic markers, including caspase-3 and -4 in Purkinje cells of the fetal ovine cerebellum, similar to the Purkinje cell loss reported in ASD and schizophrenia brains (Hsiao and Patterson, 2012). These results suggest that a contributing mechanism for maternal infection to alter brain development involves immune effectors at the level of the placenta. Interestingly, studies in mice and rats have clearly demonstrated that pregnant dams treated with viral "mimics" have reported features of schizophrenia in their offspring, supporting that a replicating virus is not required to transmit these programming outcomes, and that the array of pathogens that may promote inflammatory processes is great.

MATERNAL DIET: LOW PROTEIN AND HIGH FAT

Molecular and phenotypic evidence for programming effects of altered maternal nutrition including protein restriction, high fat diet, and methyl donor supplementation on brain development has been collected from extensive studies in animal models. In general, consequences of maternal dietary manipulations on first generation offspring reflect those observed in humans, although the extent of phenotypes, mechanisms, and sex-specific outcomes vary depending on the diet, timing of exposure, and model organism examined (Bale et al., 2010).

INTRAUTERINE GROWTH RESTRICTION AND LOW PROTEIN MODELS

Rodent models have demonstrated an important link between the maternal nutritional availability and offspring brain development, especially for models of maternal low protein that typically induce an intrauterine growth restriction (IUGR) phenotype (Dunn et al., 2011). In mice, a protein deficient diet throughout pregnancy and lactation produced profound changes in offspring reward-related behaviors as adults in which IUGR mice showed a reduced preference for a palatable sucrose solution and hyperactivity in response to an acute cocaine injection, such reduced reward sensitivity or anhedonia is an endophenotype of affective disorders, including depression and anxiety. These behavioral changes were associated with programming differences in reward circuitry stress responsivity (behavioral or physiological), cognitive performance, spatial learning, and social behaviors. Many of these outcomes have been pharmacologically validated, with human pharmaceuticals having known efficacies in mental health disorders. These studies provide a wealth of opportunities to manipulate the animals' environment while controlling all other variables so as to identify important mechanisms involved in epigenetic programming and brain development.

In examining the prenatal or intrauterine environment, animal studies have examined factors such as maternal stress exposure, infection, and dietary changes (high fat, or low protein) and their impact on offspring outcomes during specific developmental windows and as adults. Postnatal environments have also been studied for promoting changes in maternal care that are associated with long-term effects on offspring brain and behavior. Transgenerational effects have been examined in these models to determine potential epigenetic programming that involves the germ cells, potentially altering future generations' disease susceptibility. An additional benefit provided by animal models is the ability to examine the temporal specificity for effects of fetal antecedents. Because fetal organ and tissue development occurs over the course of gestation, it follows that the impact of a given insult would depend on the stage at which it occurred. Thus, by more closely examining these specific periods of development, greater insight has been obtained as to points of increased vulnerability, as well as the potential for improved interventions and biomarker identification in predicting neurodevelopmental disorder risk. Animal models hold the greatest promise to accomplish this for their ability to control and study necessary variables such as genetic background and life experience, while manipulating the environment during specific windows of development.

PROGRAMMING EFFECTS OF EARLY STRESS EXPOSURE

PRENATAL STRESS

Stress pathway dysregulation is the most pervasive symptom in neuropsychiatric disease, and both clinical and basic research has identified factors important in the developmental programming and maturation of this system, as well as the sensitive periods during which perturbations may be disruptive. Animal models examining maternal stress have provided mechanistic insight into the long-term programming of important endophenotypes. As in humans, outcomes from maternal stress studies in animals have varied depending upon the stressors utilized, the outcomes examined, and timing of the stress event during pregnancy (Bale, 2011). Overall, in mice, rats, guinea pigs, and nonhuman primates, prenatal stress increases the sensitivity of the offspring HPA stress axis, anxiety-like and depressive-like behaviors, and cognitive deficits; all endophenotypes associated with neuropsychiatric disease.

Although prenatal stress has been broadly associated with offspring disease, the developing nervous system is unlikely to show uniform vulnerability to perturbations over the course of gestation. To compare maternal stress experience across early, mid, or late pregnancy on programming of offspring stress

regulation, a chronic stress model in mice determined that early gestation (days 1 to 7 of the 20- to 21-day gestation in mice) resulted in male offspring with an increased stress-sensitive phenotype as adults (Mueller and Bale, 2008). These males had elevated amygdalar CRF, and reduced hippocampal glucocorticoid receptors (GR). Epigenetic analyses determined that DNA methylation changes of these genes correlated with their expression. Interestingly, similar outcomes have been reported following gestational glucocorticoid exposure on offspring GR expression and promoter methylation, suggesting potential common mechanisms and points of vulnerability that may relate to direct or indirect actions of glucocorticoids during brain development (Bale, 2011).

A prenatal stress model in the guinea pig has similarly explored the timing specificity of prenatal stress using short periods of daily flashing light as a maternal stress beginning on embryonic day E50 or E60 of the 70-day guinea pig gestation. Although stress beginning at E50 resulted in increased anxiety-like behaviors, elevated basal corticosterone levels, and lower hippocampal GR in adults, stress beginning at E60 failed to produce these outcomes (Kapoor et al., 2008). Overall, these results support epidemiological findings as to the importance of temporal specificity for maternal stress programming of offspring.

POSTNATAL STRESS

Rodent models examining the early postnatal window of brain development have produced a great deal of evidence for the effects of both enhanced and fragmented maternal care producing long-term effects on the developing brain. Meaney et al. have contributed a wealth of information to the field as to the epigenetic programming that occurs in early life related to the quality of maternal care (Hackman et al., 2010; Meaney, 2001). This group characterized a rat model in which dams had either high or low levels of early postnatal maternal care—defined as high or low licking and grooming. In this model, the postnatal interactions of the dam with her litter determined the behaviors of the offspring as adults, in which high licking and grooming offspring showed reduced levels of anxiety-like behaviors and diminished HPA stress axis activity. The epigenetics involved in these outcomes, at least in part, appeared related to the DNA methylation status of the GR in the hippocampus of these offspring. High licking and grooming mothers produced enhanced tactile stimulation of their pups, resulting in increased expression of specific transcription factors during brain development that ultimately dictate expression levels of GR. This is one example, then, of a gene that is epigenetically programmed during early development lasting into adulthood and having a potential impact on shaping offspring stress responsivity.

In contrast to models of stress resilience, chronic postnatal stress can promote cognitive *decline* via functional and structural programming of specific brain regions, including the hippocampus. These studies suggest that the magnitude of stress exposure may determine its long-lasting effects, such that modest postnatal stress may promote resilience, whereas severe or chronic stress may set in motion mechanisms that contribute to stress-related neurodevelopmental disease (Bale et al., 2010). For instance, in a model in which dams are provided

Although maternal infection, stress, and undernutrition differentially affect the developing fetus, there are likely shared underlying mechanisms contributing to an increased vulnerability to MDD, including effects on the developing stress neurocircuitry (Bale et al., 2010).

As the brain continues to mature and develop well into adolescence, appreciation of the influences of the postnatal environment on programming of disease risk is necessary. Studies of the long-term consequences of adverse early childhood experience have unequivocally revealed that adults exposed to child abuse and/or neglect are at a greater risk for the lifetime development of affective disorders. In clinical studies, there is clear evidence for long-term neurobiological, neuroendocrine, and immune alterations following exposure to early life adverse events during critical periods in brain development (Bale, 2011). In addition, plasma stress hormone levels in response to relatively mild stressors are markedly increased in patients who have experienced early life trauma, including sexual or physical abuse.

In humans and non-human primates, hypersecretion of the stress hormone corticotropin-releasing factor (CRF), as detected in the cerebrospinal fluid (CSF), has been found years after the initial period of stress exposure during early life. Similar results were found in clinical studies in which women with a history of child abuse and/or neglect exhibit hyperactivity of the hypothalamic–pituitary–adrenal (HPA) axis in the Trier Social Stress test and increased CSF CRF concentrations. In addition, these patients exhibited decreased CSF concentrations of oxytocin, a peptide shown to be important in social biology and bonding, increased proinflammatory cytokines such as IL-6, and reduced hippocampal volume as measured

by structural magnetic resonance imaging (Bale et al., 2010; Heim et al., 2009, 2010). Further supporting a gene x environment interaction for development of affective disorders is the growing evidence of a genetic predisposition that underlies a stress-sensitive phenotype, thereby increasing the likelihood for stress experience throughout life, and elevating the risk for disease presentation (Kendler, 1998).

What is clear from examination of the epidemiological literature is that although a relatively small number of fetal antecedents (e.g., stress, infection, dietary challenges) have been linked with the neuropsychiatric disorders discussed in the preceding, what distinguishes the outcomes is likely the timing of the exposure/insult combined with the genetic background and fetal sex of the individual. How these factors independently or combined can act to influence neurodevelopmental programming is best examined using animal models.

THE ANIMAL MODELS

The incredible complexity of neuropsychiatric diseases makes the generation of relevant and beneficial animal models difficult; but without these models, mechanistic studies are nearly impossible. Evaluation and diagnosis of a mental health disorder requires a clinical conversation with a patient so as to assess specific criteria. Obviously, this is not possible in an animal. Therefore, rather than producing models of diseases in their entirety, an alternate approach has been to focus on important aspects, or endophenotypes, of the disease that can be more clearly measured in animals (Table 72.1). Examples include

TABLE 72.1. Summary of animal models being examined in relation to early life exposure and long-term outcomes of endophenotypes relevant to neuropsychiatric disease

ANIMAL MODEL	HUMAN DISEASE	ENDOPHENOTYPE EXAMINED	CITATION
Maternal infection	Schizophrenia, OCD, PTSD, Tourette	Sensory motor deficits (PPI)	Bilbo (2010), Hsiao and Patterson (2012)
Maternal immune activation	Schizophrenia	Enlarged ventricles	Hsiao and Patterson (2012)
Uteroplacental inflammation	Schizophrenia, ASD	Purkinje cell loss	Hsiao and Patterson (2012), Howerton and Bale (2012)
Postnatal neglect	Anxiety	Anxiety-like behaviors, hippocampal GR, hypothalamic CRF	Meaney (2001), Korosi (2010), Hackman (2010)
Postnatal stress	Depression	Stress reactivity and coping, depression-like behaviors	Franklin (2010), Bale (2010)
Prenatal stress	Schizophrenia, ASD	Male specific stress sensitivity, cognitive deficits	Kapoor (2008), Mueller (2008), Morgan (2011)
IUGR; low protein	Depression	Anhedonia	Vucetic (2010)
Caloric restriction	Affective disorders	Stress reactivity and coping, hippocampal GR expression	Bale (2010), Lesage (2001), Lingas (1999)
Maternal obesity	ASD, Anxiety	Anxiety-like behaviors, social anxiety, raphe TPH2 expression	Sullivan (2010), Vucetic (2010), Li (2010)

antibody to *Toxoplasma gondii* in maternal serum taken during pregnancy was also associated with a twofold increased risk of schizophrenia (Brown, 2012; Mortensen et al., 2007). Maternal genital reproductive infections around the time of conception have also been reported to have a fivefold increase in schizophrenia risk. Clinical studies examining neural end points have found an association of prenatal infection with deficits in executive function and morphological changes in schizophrenia patients (Brown, 2012). More specifically, neuroimaging findings indicated that prenatal infection was related to enlargement of the cavum septum pellucidum and diminished intracranial volume in these cases (Brown et al., 2009a).

Similar to the contributions made by maternal stress or infection to offspring development and programming, maternal diet directly regulates fetal growth, epigenetic programming, and disease risk. Epidemiological studies have repeatedly found an increased risk of schizophrenia in offspring from mothers exposed to severe caloric restriction or famine. In addition to the volume of epidemiological reports demonstrating intergenerational consequences of maternal starvation, obesity, and metabolic syndrome during pregnancy, the first data pointing to molecular mechanisms are now beginning to emerge. Periods of famine affecting human populations for well-defined durations afford the potential to track effects of undernutrition during pregnancy on offspring outcome. Findings stemming from the Dutch Hunger Winter of 1944–1945 reveal consequences ranging from glucose intolerance, increased coronary heart disease, altered stress responsiveness, and schizophrenia for the adult offspring of pregnancies occurring during a period of reduced caloric availability and increased psychological stress (Brown and Susser, 2008; Ravelli et al., 1976). These outcomes have been associated with changes detected in circulating growth factors and alterations in DNA methylation patterns of several genes, including the imprinted gene, insulin-like growth factor-2 (IGF-2) (Bale et al., 2010). These findings were detected 60 years following the famine exposure, supporting the long-lasting programming effects of the epigenetic marks. Interestingly, data from the Dutch Hunger Winter and the nineteenth century Swedish famine revealed that severe caloric restriction during pregnancy has transgenerational consequences in which even the second generation of offspring had increased neonatal adiposity, and overall lower quality health as adults when their mothers were exposed to famine (Brown and Susser, 2008), suggesting that epigenetic marks in germ cells must have occurred during the initial insult exposure.

Although most epidemiological studies have focused on offspring outcomes following periods of famine or malnutrition during pregnancy, our changing landscape is shifting the focus to effects of maternal overnutrition. Certainly, transgenerational epigenetics may be contributing to the rapid amplification of obesity rates and human height observed in recent generations (Bale et al., 2010). In addition, predisposing subsequent generations to these traits through epigenetic inheritance may compound the rate at which phenotypes progress. Maternal obesity has also been associated with a two- to threefold increased risk for schizophrenia in the offspring from two separate birth cohorts (Khandaker et al., 2012).

AUTISM SPECTRUM DISORDERS

Many factors have been examined as potential fetal antecedents related to an increased risk for autism spectrum disorders (ASD), including stress and infectious and immune disturbances (Brown, 2012). Although genome-wide association studies (GWAS) and other genetic analyses studies have identified candidate ASD susceptibility genes, more recent work in identical and fraternal twin pairs with autism showed that genetics accounted for less of the disease risk than did the shared environment (Angelidou et al., 2012). Such analyses support the critical importance for consideration of the interaction between genetic susceptibility and potential environmental insults that may produce epigenetic changes in neurodevelopment. Studies using the Danish Medical Birth Register found an association between viral infection resulting in hospitalization in the first trimester of pregnancy and a threefold increase in ASD risk. In a prospective study by the Early Markers for Autism, in which the presence of 17 cytokines was assayed in maternal serum and related to offspring ASD diagnosis, the authors found that specific cytokines, including IL-4, IL-5, and IFNγ, were increased at mid-gestation in mothers of children diagnosed with ASD. Prospective studies have also reported associations between amniotic fluid levels of specific cytokines such as TNFα, IL-4, and IL-5 with an increased risk for ASD (as reviewed in Brown, 2012).

Maternal stress has also been associated with an increased risk for ASD, including stress exposure at 21 to 32 weeks of gestation, and postnatal stressors such as the death of a relative in the first six months of life (Angelidou et al., 2012). However, in a metaanalysis by Gardner et al. on combined studies published since 2007, only four factors appear to consistently increase the risk for ASD: advanced maternal age, advanced paternal age, being first born, and having a mother born outside North America, Europe, or Australia (Gardener et al., 2009). A recent follow-up metaanalysis study from this group has added interactions of factors including umbilical cord complications, fetal distress, birth trauma, and a low five-minute Apgar score with increased risk for ASD (Gardener et al., 2011). What is clear is that more information and controlled prospective studies are still needed for confirming links between maternal stress or infection with ASD risk (Guinchat et al., 2012).

AFFECTIVE DISORDERS

There is growing evidence supporting an association between fetal risk factors and affective disorder predisposition, likely involving early epigenetic shifts in developmental trajectories. Birth cohort studies have identified prenatal conditions, including maternal immune and stress responses, as significant risk factors for major depressive disorder (MDD) (Bale et al., 2010). For instance, second trimester maternal exposure to type A$_2$/Singapore influenza significantly increased the risk for unipolar and bipolar disorders in a cohort of Finnish and British adults. In addition, maternal exposure to famine during the second and third trimesters elevated offspring lifetime risk for MDD, supporting an important link between maternal nutrition and offspring neurodevelopment that may also relate to maternal stress resulting from insufficient food sources.

72 | EPIGENETICS IN EARLY LIFE PROGRAMMING

TRACY L. BALE

Fetal antecedents such as maternal stress, infection, or dietary challenges have long been associated with an increased disease risk, capable of affecting multiple generations. The mechanisms through which such determinants contribute to disease development likely involve complex and dynamic relationships between the maternal environment, the endocrine placenta, and the epigenetic programming of the developing embryo itself. Although an appreciation for the importance of the epigenome in offspring disease predisposition has evolved, the incredible variability in critical factors such as gestational timing of insults, sex of the fetus, and maternal genetics make clear interpretations difficult. However, animal models have proved highly informative in providing the best knowledge yet as to just how dynamically responsive the epigenome is, and in determining important mechanisms that shape and reprogram the developing brain. This chapter discusses the epidemiological and clinical evidence and supportive animal models related to environmental influences on neurodevelopmental and neuropsychiatric disease risk.

Historically, the term epigenetics has referred to heritable traits that are not mediated by changes in DNA sequence. More recently, epigenetics has been used more broadly to refer to any change in gene function not associated with sequence variation (Jiang et al., 2008) and has been embraced by the neuroscience community as a means by which we can integrate a role for the environment to influence or "program" gene expression or patterns that may or may not be heritable (Borrelli et al., 2008; Sweatt, 2009). Epigenetic mechanisms typically involve biochemical modifications of the DNA or histones such as methylation or acetylation, as well as noncoding RNAs, including microRNAs. Increasing evidence notes that numerous types of chromatin modifications, referred to as chromatin remodeling, are widespread in the brain and undergo dynamic regulation in both the developing and adult nervous system (Tsankova et al., 2007).

FETAL ANTECEDENTS AND PROGRAMMING IN NEURODEVELOPMENTAL DISORDERS: CLINICAL AND EPIDEMIOLOGICAL STUDIES

Although evidence points to a strong genetic component in risk factors for neurodevelopmental diseases, in which the concordance rate for schizophrenia in monozygotic twins is between 50% and 60%, and 40% to 90% of the variance in autism risk is attributed to genetic heritability, new studies have focused on the potential contributions of epigenetic factors (Brown, 2012). The interactions between the rapidly changing intrauterine environment and the genetic background of the developing fetus produce epigenetic programming changes at the level of transcription, ultimately shaping developmental trajectories. Birth cohort studies examining specific maternal exposures to stress, infection, and dietary challenges have provided the clearest evidence to date for the critical role such fetal antecedents play in disease risk, and the temporal specificity for exposure windows of susceptibility. These large registries allow prospective studies to be conducted, which greatly aids in the accuracy of exposure reporting and confirmation, and the collection of biological materials to be analyzed as potential biomarkers for genetic/epigenetic factors associated with susceptibility. In the following, evidence from clinical and epidemiological studies is described related to specific neurodevelopmental diseases and our current knowledge of fetal antecedents that increase risk for these disorders.

SCHIZOPHRENIA

Prenatal and early life events such as maternal stress and infection have been associated with an increased risk of schizophrenia (Brown, 2012). Studies from large birth cohorts in which clinical, neurocognitive, and neuroimaging measures have been obtained revealed strong associations between *in utero* exposure to stress, infections, hypoxia, starvation, and an increased risk for schizophrenia (Bale, 2011; Susser et al., 2008), including disturbances of executive function, working memory, verbal memory, and structural brain abnormalities among offspring with schizophrenia (Brown et al., 2009b). In support of a temporal specificity to the effects of fetal antecedents on long-term outcomes in neurodevelopmental disorders, a recent epidemiological study reported a significant association between maternal stress experienced during the first trimester of pregnancy with an increased risk of schizophrenia in males (Khashan et al., 2008). Prospective birth cohort studies have suggested that such stress exposures may act by altering brain developmental trajectories involving epigenetic modifications, the evidence for which in humans, however, is currently lacking.

Maternal infection and immune disturbances during pregnancy have a strong association with offspring schizophrenia risk. Influenza exposure during early or mid-gestation produced a three-fold increased risk for schizophrenia compared with controls (Brown, 2012). The presence of elevated IgG

State, M.W. (2011). The genetics of Tourette disorder. *Curr. Opin. Genet. Dev.* 21(3):302–309.

Stefansson, H., Rujescu, D., et al. (2008). Large recurrent microdeletions associated with schizophrenia. *Nature* 455(7210):232–236.

Sultana, R., Yu, C.E., et al. (2002). Identification of a novel gene on chromosome 7q11.2 interrupted by a translocation breakpoint in a pair of autistic twins. *Genomics* 80(2):129–134.

Szafranski, P., Schaaf, C.P., et al. (2010). Structures and molecular mechanisms for common 15q13.3 microduplications involving CHRNA7: benign or pathological? *Hum. Mutat.* 31(7):840–850.

Szatmari, P., Paterson, A.D., et al. (2007). Mapping autism risk loci using genetic linkage and chromosomal rearrangements. *Nat. Genet.* 39(3):319–328.

Ullmann, R., Turner, G., et al. (2007). Array CGH identifies reciprocal 16p13.1 duplications and deletions that predispose to autism and/or mental retardation. *Hum. Mutat.* 28(7):674–682.

van Bon, B.W., Balciuniene, J., et al. (2011). The phenotype of recurrent 10q22q23 deletions and duplications. *Eur. J. Hum. Genet.* 19(4):400–408.

van Bon, B.W., Mefford, H.C., et al. (2009). Further delineation of the 15q13 microdeletion and duplication syndromes: a clinical spectrum varying from non-pathogenic to a severe outcome. *J. Med. Genet.* 46(8):511–523.

Vissers, L.E., de Ligt, J., et al. (2010). A *de novo* paradigm for mental retardation. *Nat. Genet.* 42(12):1109–1112.

von der Lippe, C., Rustad, C., et al. (2011). 15q11.2 microdeletion: seven new patients with delayed development and/or behavioural problems. *Eur. J. Med. Genet.* 54(3):357–360.

Vu, T.H., Coccaro, E.F., et al. (2011). Genomic architecture of aggression: rare copy number variants in intermittent explosive disorder. *Am. J. Med. Genet. B Neuropsychiatr. Genet.* 156B(7):808–816.

Walsh, T., McClellan, J.M., et al. (2008). Rare structural variants disrupt multiple genes in neurodevelopmental pathways in schizophrenia. *Science* 320(5875):539–543.

Walters, R.G., Jacquemont, S., et al. (2010). A new highly penetrant form of obesity due to deletions on chromosome 16p11.2. *Nature* 463(7281):671–675.

Weiss, L.A., Shen, Y., et al. (2008). Association between microdeletion and microduplication at 16p11.2 and autism. *N. Engl. J. Med.* 358(7):667–675.

Willatt, L., Cox, J., et al. (2005). 3q29 microdeletion syndrome: clinical and molecular characterization of a new syndrome. *Am. J. Hum. Genet.* 77(1):154–160.

Williams, N.M., Zaharieva, I., et al. (2010). Rare chromosomal deletions and duplications in attention-deficit hyperactivity disorder: a genome-wide analysis. *Lancet* 376(9750):1401–1408.

Xu, B., Roos, J.L., et al. (2008). Strong association of *de novo* copy number mutations with sporadic schizophrenia. *Nat. Genet.* 40(7):880–885.

Yan, W., Jacobsen, L.K., et al. (1998). Chromosome 22q11.2 interstitial deletions among childhood-onset schizophrenics and "multidimensionally impaired." [Case Reports]. *Am. J. Med. Genet.* 81(1):41–43.

Zhang, D., Cheng, L., et al. (2009). Singleton deletions throughout the genome increase risk of bipolar disorder. *Mol. Psychiatry* 14(4):376–380.

Iossifov, I., Ronemus, M., et al. (2012). *De novo* gene disruptions in children on the autistic spectrum. *Neuron* 74(2):285–299.

Itsara, A., Cooper, G.M., et al. (2009). Population analysis of large copy number variants and hotspots of human genetic disease. *Am. J. Hum. Genet.* 84(2):148–161.

Jacquemont, S., Reymond, A., et al. (2011). Mirror extreme BMI phenotypes associated with gene dosage at the chromosome 16p11.2 locus. *Nature* 478(7367):97–102.

Karayiorgou, M., Morris, M.A., et al. (1995). Schizophrenia susceptibility associated with interstitial deletions of chromosome 22q11. *Proc. Natl. Acad. Sci. USA* 92(17):7612–7616.

Kiholm Lund, A.B., Hove, H.D., et al. (2008). A 15q24 microduplication, reciprocal to the recently described 15q24 microdeletion, in a boy sharing clinical features with 15q24 microdeletion syndrome patients. *Eur. J. Med. Genet.* 51(6):520–526.

Kim, H.G., Kishikawa, S., et al. (2008). Disruption of neurexin 1 associated with autism spectrum disorder. *Am. J. Hum. Genet.* 82(1):199–207.

Klopocki, E., Graul-Neumann, L.M., et al. (2008). A further case of the recurrent 15q24 microdeletion syndrome, detected by array CGH. *Eur. J. Pediatr.* 167(8):903–908.

Knight, S.J., Regan, R., et al. (1999). Subtle chromosomal rearrangements in children with unexplained mental retardation. *Lancet* 354(9191):1676–1681.

Koolen, D.A., and de Vries, B.B.A. (1993). KANSL1-related intellectual disability syndrome. In: Pagon, R.A., Bird, T.D., Dolan, C.R., Stephens, K., and Adam, M.P., eds. GeneReviews™ [Internet]. Seattle: University of Washington. 2010 Jan 26 [updated 2013 Jan 10].

Koolen, D.A., Sharp, A.J., et al. (2008). Clinical and molecular delineation of the 17q21.31 microdeletion syndrome. *J. Med. Genet.* 45(11):710–720.

Koolen, D.A., Vissers, L.E., et al. (2006). A new chromosome 17q21.31 microdeletion syndrome associated with a common inversion polymorphism. *Nat. Genet.* 38(9):999–1001.

Kumar, R.A., KaraMohamed, S., et al. (2008). Recurrent 16p11.2 microdeletions in autism. *Hum. Mol. Genet.* 17(4):628–638.

Leonard, H., and Wen, X. (2002). The epidemiology of mental retardation: challenges and opportunities in the new millennium. *Ment. Retard Dev. Disabil. Res. Rev.* 8(3):117–134.

Lisi, E.C., Hamosh, A., et al. (2008). 3q29 interstitial microduplication: a new syndrome in a three-generation family. *Am. J. Med. Genet. A* 146A(5):601–609.

Locke, D.P., Sharp, A.J., et al. (2006). Linkage disequilibrium and heritability of copy-number polymorphisms within duplicated regions of the human genome. *Am. J. Hum. Genet.* 79(2):275–290.

Loirat, C., Bellanne-Chantelot, C., et al. (2010). Autism in three patients with cystic or hyperechogenic kidneys and chromosome 17q12 deletion. *Nephrol. Dial. Transplant* 25(10):3430–3433.

Lynch, M. (2010). Rate, molecular spectrum, and consequences of human mutation. *Proc. Natl. Acad. Sci. USA* 107(3):961–968.

Malhotra, D., McCarthy, S., et al. (2011). High frequencies of *de novo* CNVs in bipolar disorder and schizophrenia. *Neuron* 72(6):951–963.

Marshall, C.R., Noor, A., et al. (2008). Structural variation of chromosomes in autism spectrum disorder. *Am. J. Hum. Genet.* 82(2):477–488.

McCarthy, S.E., Makarov, V., et al. (2009). Microduplications of 16p11.2 are associated with schizophrenia. *Nat. Genet.* 41(11):1223–1227.

Mefford, H.C., Cooper, G.M., et al. (2009). A method for rapid, targeted CNV genotyping identifies rare variants associated with neurocognitive disease. *Genome Res.* 19(9):1579–1585.

Mefford, H.C. (2009). Genotype to phenotype-discovery and characterization of novel genomic disorders in a "genotype-first" era. *Genet Med.* 11(12):836–842.

Mefford, H.C., Rosenfeld, J.A., et al. (2011). Further clinical and molecular delineation of the 15q24 microdeletion syndrome. *J. Med. Genet.* 49(2):110–118.

Mefford, H.C., Rosenfeld, J.A., et al. (2012). Further clinical and molecular delineation of the 15q24 microdeletion syndrome. *J. Med. Genet.* 49(2):110–118.

Mefford, H.C., Sharp, A.J., et al. (2008). Recurrent rearrangements of chromosome 1q21.1 and variable pediatric phenotypes. *N. Engl. J. Med.* 359(16):1685–1699.

Mefford, H., Shur, N., et al. (1993). 15q24 Microdeletion Syndrome. In: Pagon, R.A., Bird, T.D., Dolan, C.R., Stephens, K., and Adam, M.P., eds. GeneReviews™ [Internet]. Seattle: University of Washington. 2012 Feb 23.

Mefford, H.C., Yendle, S.C., et al. (2011). Rare copy number variants are an important cause of epileptic encephalopathies. *Ann. Neurol.* 70(6):974–985.

Miller, D.T., Adam, M.P., et al. (2010). Consensus statement: chromosomal microarray is a first-tier clinical diagnostic test for individuals with developmental disabilities or congenital anomalies. *Am. J. Hum. Genet.* 86(5):749–764.

Miller, D.T., Shen, Y., et al. (2008). Microdeletion/duplication at 15q13.2q13.3 among individuals with features of autism and other neuropsychiatirc disorders. *J. Med. Genet.* 46(4):242–248.

Moreno-De-Luca, D., Mulle, J.G., et al. (2010). Deletion 17q12 is a recurrent copy number variant that confers high risk of autism and schizophrenia. *Am. J. Hum. Genet.* 87(5):618–630.

Murthy, S.K., Nygren, A.O., et al. (2007). Detection of a novel familial deletion of four genes between BP1 and BP2 of the Prader-Willi/Angelman syndrome critical region by oligo-array CGH in a child with neurological disorder and speech impairment. *Cytogenet. Genome Res.* 116(1–2):135–140.

Nagamani, S.C., Erez, A., et al. (2010). Clinical spectrum associated with recurrent genomic rearrangements in chromosome 17q12. *Eur. J. Hum. Genet.* 18(3):278–284.

Najmabadi, H., Hu, H., et al. (2011). Deep sequencing reveals 50 novel genes for recessive cognitive disorders. *Nature* 478(7367):57–63.

Neale, B.M., Kou, Y., et al. (2012). Patterns and rates of exonic *de novo* mutations in autism spectrum disorders. *Nature* 485(7397):242–245.

Ng, S.B., Bigham, A.W., et al. (2010). Exome sequencing identifies MLL2 mutations as a cause of Kabuki syndrome. *Nat. Genet.* 42(9):790–793.

Noor, A., Whibley, A., et al. (2010). Disruption at the PTCHD1 Locus on Xp22.11 in autism spectrum disorder and intellectual disability. *Sci. Transl. Med.* 2(49):49ra68.

O'Roak, B.J., Deriziotis, P., et al. (2011). Exome sequencing in sporadic autism spectrum disorders identifies severe *de novo* mutations. *Nat. Genet.* 43(6):585–589.

O'Roak, B.J., Vives, L., et al. (2012). Sporadic autism exomes reveal a highly interconnected protein network of *de novo* mutations. *Nature* 485(7397):246–250.

Pagnamenta, A.T., Wing, K., et al. (2009). A 15q13.3 microdeletion segregating with autism. *Eur. J. Hum. Genet.* 17(5):687–692.

Pinto, D., Pagnamenta, A.T., et al. (2010). Functional impact of global rare copy number variation in autism spectrum disorders. *Nature* 466(7304):368–372.

Ramalingam, A., Zhou, X.G., et al. (2011). 16p13.11 duplication is a risk factor for a wide spectrum of neuropsychiatric disorders. *J. Hum. Genet.* 56(7):541–544.

Ramocki, M.B., Bartnik, M., et al. (2010). Recurrent distal 7q11.23 deletion including HIP1 and YWHAG identified in patients with intellectual disabilities, epilepsy, and neurobehavioral problems. *Am. J. Hum. Genet.* 87(6):857–865.

Ravnan, J.B., Tepperberg, J.H., et al. (2006). Subtelomere FISH analysis of 11 688 cases: an evaluation of the frequency and pattern of subtelomere rearrangements in individuals with developmental disabilities. *J. Med. Genet.* 43(6):478–489.

Redon, R., Ishikawa, S., et al. (2006). Global variation in copy number in the human genome. *Nature* 444(7118):444–454.

Ropers, H.H. (2010). Genetics of early onset cognitive impairment. *Annu. Rev. Genomics Hum. Genet.* 11:161–187.

Rosenfeld, J.A., Coppinger, J., et al. (2009). Speech delays and behavioural problems are the predominant features in individuals with developmental delays and 16p11.2 microdeletions and microduplications. *J. Neurodevelop. Disord.* 2:26–38.

Sanders, S.J., Ercan-Sencicek, A.G., et al. (2011). Multiple recurrent De Novo CNVs, including duplications of the 7q11.23 Williams Syndrome Region, are strongly associated with autism. *Neuron* 70(5):863–885.

Sanders, S.J., Murtha, M.T., et al. (2012). *De novo* mutations revealed by whole-exome sequencing are strongly associated with autism. *Nature* 485(7397):237–241.

Sebat, J., Lakshmi, B., et al. (2007). Strong association of *de novo* copy number mutations with autism. *Science* 316(5823):445–449.

Sebat, J., Lakshmi, B., et al. (2004). Large-scale copy number polymorphism in the human genome. *Science* 305(5683):525–528.

Sharp, A.J., Hansen, S., et al. (2006). Discovery of previously unidentified genomic disorders from the duplication architecture of the human genome. *Nat. Genet.* 38(9):1038–1042.

Sharp, A.J., Mefford, H.C., et al. (2008). A recurrent 15q13.3 microdeletion syndrome associated with mental retardation and seizures. *Nat. Genet.* 40(3):322–328.

Sharp, A.J., Selzer, R.R., et al. (2007). Characterization of a recurrent 15q24 microdeletion syndrome. *Hum. Mol. Genet.* 16(5):567–572.

Shaw-Smith, C., Pittman, A.M., et al. (2006). Microdeletion encompassing MAPT at chromosome 17q21.3 is associated with developmental delay and learning disability. *Nat. Genet.* 38(9):1032–1037.

Shinawi, M., Liu, P., et al. (2010). Recurrent reciprocal 16p11.2 rearrangements associated with global developmental delay, behavioural problems, dysmorphism, epilepsy, and abnormal head size. *J. Med. Genet.* 47(5):332–341.

the variants that have a large effect on risk are rare variants, and each is found in only a very small percentage of affected individuals. The most frequent risk variants in each disorder are found in only approximately 1% of patients. Finally, one of the most intriguing themes to emerge is that some large-effect genetic risk factors are shared among multiple disorders.

The vast genetic heterogeneity for each of these disorders will complicate clinical diagnostics, and thoughtful consideration must be given to how to approach risk assessment and diagnostics in the clinic. However, the rapid pace of discovery in childhood psychiatric disorders, a group of conditions that has been largely intractable so far, lends hope for the future. Many risk genes and regions have been discovered, and a goal of future research should be to investigate the common pathways that appear to be important for normal brain development and function.

DISCLOSURE

Dr. Mefford serves on the SFARI Gene Advisory Board. She receives grant support from National Institutes of Health and the Burroughs Wellcome Fund.

REFERENCES

Addington, A.M., Gauthier, J., et al. (2011). A novel frameshift mutation in UPF3B identified in brothers affected with childhood onset schizophrenia and autism spectrum disorders. [Case Reports Letter]. *Mol. Psychiatry* 16(3):238–239.

Addington, A.M., and Rapoport, J.L. (2009). The genetics of childhood-onset schizophrenia: when madness strikes the prepubescent. [Review]. *Curr. Psychiatry Repts.* 11(2):156–161.

American Psychiatric Association. (2000). Diagnostic Criteria from DSM-IV-TR. Washington, DC: American Psychiatric Association.

Andrieux, J., Dubourg, C., et al. (2009). Genotype-phenotype correlation in four 15q24 deleted patients identified by array-CGH. *Am. J. Med. Genet. A* 149A(12):2813–2819.

Bachmann-Gagescu, R., Mefford, H.C., et al. (2010). Recurrent 200-kb deletions of 16p11.2 that include the SH2B1 gene are associated with developmental delay and obesity. *Genet. Med.* 12(10):641–647.

Balciuniene, J., Feng, N., et al. (2007). Recurrent 10q22-q23 deletions: a genomic disorder on 10q associated with cognitive and behavioral abnormalities. *Am. J. Hum. Genet.* 80(5):938–947.

Ballif, B.C., Sulpizio, S.G., et al. (2007). The clinical utility of enhanced subtelomeric coverage in array CGH. *Am. J. Med. Genet. A* 143A(16):1850–1857.

Ballif, B.C., Theisen, A., et al. (2008). Expanding the clinical phenotype of the 3q29 microdeletion syndrome and characterization of the reciprocal microduplication. *Mol. Cytogenet.* 1(1):8.

Barak, T., Kwan, K.Y., et al. (2011). Recessive LAMC3 mutations cause malformations of occipital cortical development. *Nat. Genet.* 43(6):590–594.

Battaglia, A., Novelli, A., et al. (2009). Further characterization of the new microdeletion syndrome of 16p11.2-p12.2. *Am. J. Med. Genet. A* 149A(6):1200–1204.

Bedoyan, J.K., Kumar, R.A., et al. (2010). Duplication 16p11.2 in a child with infantile seizure disorder. *Am. J. Med. Genet. A* 152A(6):1567–1574.

Ben-Shachar, S., Lanpher, B., et al. (2009). Microdeletion 15q13.3: a locus with incomplete penetrance for autism, mental retardation, and psychiatric disorders. *J. Med. Genet.* 46(6):382–388.

Ben-Shachar, S., Ou, Z., et al. (2008). 22q11.2 distal deletion: a recurrent genomic disorder distinct from DiGeorge syndrome and velocardiofacial syndrome. *Am. J. Hum. Genet.* 82(1):214–221.

Bijlsma, E.K., Gijsbers, A.C., et al. (2009). Extending the phenotype of recurrent rearrangements of 16p11.2: deletions in mentally retarded patients without autism and in normal individuals. *Eur. J. Med. Genet.* 52(2–3):77–87.

Brunetti-Pierri, N., Berg, J.S., et al. (2008). Recurrent reciprocal 1q21.1 deletions and duplications associated with microcephaly or macrocephaly and developmental and behavioral abnormalities. *Nat. Genet.* 40(12):1466–1471.

Burnside, R.D., Pasion, R., et al. (2011). Microdeletion/microduplication of proximal 15q11.2 between BP1 and BP2: a susceptibility region for neurological dysfunction including developmental and language delay. *Hum. Genet.* 130(4):517–528.

Caliskan, M., Chong, J.X., et al. (2011). Exome sequencing reveals a novel mutation for autosomal recessive non-syndromic mental retardation in the TECR gene on chromosome 19p13. *Hum. Mol. Genet.* 20(7):1285–1289.

Chahrour, M.H., Yu, T.W., et al. (2012). Whole-exome sequencing and homozygosity analysis implicate depolarization-regulated neuronal genes in autism. *PLoS Genetics* 8(4):e1002635.

Chakrabarti, S., and Fombonne, E. (2005). Pervasive developmental disorders in preschool children: confirmation of high prevalence. *Am. J. Psychiatry* 162(6):1133–1141.

Chakrabarti, S., and Fombonne, E. (2001). Pervasive developmental disorders in preschool children. *JAMA* 285(24):3093–3099.

Ching, M.S., Shen, Y., et al. (2010). Deletions of NRXN1 (neurexin-1) predispose to a wide spectrum of developmental disorders. *Am. J. Med. Genet. B* 153B(4):937–947.

Christiansen, J., Dyck, J.D., et al. (2004). Chromosome 1q21.1 contiguous gene deletion is associated with congenital heart disease. *Circ. Res.* 94(11):1429–1435.

Claes, L., Ceulemans, B., et al. (2003). *De novo* SCN1A mutations are a major cause of severe myoclonic epilepsy of infancy. *Hum. Mutat.* 21(6):615–621.

Cook, E.H., Jr., Lindgren, V., et al. (1997). Autism or atypical autism in maternally but not paternally derived proximal 15q duplication. *Am. J. Hum. Genet.* 60(4):928–934.

Descartes, M., Franklin, J., et al. (2008). Distal 22q11.2 microduplication encompassing the BCR gene. *Am. J. Med. Genet. A* 146A(23):3075–3081.

El-Hattab, A.W., Smolarek, T.A., et al. (2009). Redefined genomic architecture in 15q24 directed by patient deletion/duplication breakpoint mapping. *Hum. Genet.* 126(4):589–602.

Elia, J., Gai, X., et al. (2010). Rare structural variants found in attention-deficit hyperactivity disorder are preferentially associated with neurodevelopmental genes. . *Mol. Psychiatry* 15(6):637–646.

Elia, J., Glessner, J.T., et al. (2012). Genome-wide copy number variation study associates metabotropic glutamate receptor gene networks with attention deficit hyperactivity disorder. *Nat. Genet.* 44(1):78–84.

Endele, S., Rosenberger, G., et al. (2010). Mutations in GRIN2A and GRIN2B encoding regulatory subunits of NMDA receptors cause variable neurodevelopmental phenotypes. *Nat. Genet.* 42(11):1021–1026.

Gauthier, J., Champagne, N., et al. (2010). *De novo* mutations in the gene encoding the synaptic scaffolding protein SHANK3 in patients ascertained for schizophrenia. *Proc. Natl. Acad. Sci. USA* 107(17):7863–7868.

Gilissen, C., Arts, H.H., et al. (2010). Exome sequencing identifies WDR35 variants involved in Sensenbrenner syndrome. *Am. J. Hum. Genet.* 87(3):418–423.

Girirajan, S., Rosenfeld, J.A., et al. (2010). A recurrent 16p12.1 microdeletion supports a two-hit model for severe developmental delay. *Nat. Genet.* 42(3):203–209.

Glessner, J.T., Wang, K., et al. (2009). Autism genome-wide copy number variation reveals ubiquitin and neuronal genes. *Nature* 459(7246):569–573.

Grozeva, D., Kirov, G., et al. (2010). Rare copy number variants: a point of rarity in genetic risk for bipolar disorder and schizophrenia. *Arch. Gen. Psychiatry* 67(4):318–327.

Hamdan, F.F., Daoud, H., et al. (2010). *De novo* mutations in FOXP1 in cases with intellectual disability, autism, and language impairment. *Am. J. Hum. Genet.* 87(5):671–678.

Hannes, F.D., Sharp, A.J., et al. (2009). Recurrent reciprocal deletions and duplications of 16p13.11: the deletion is a risk factor for MR/MCA while the duplication may be a rare benign variant. *J. Med. Genet.* 46(4):223–232.

Harvard, C., Strong, E., et al. (2011). Understanding the impact of 1q21.1 copy number variant. *Orphanet J. Rare Dis.* 6:54.

Hempel, M., Rivera Brugues, N., et al. (2009). Microdeletion syndrome 16p11.2-p12.2: clinical and molecular characterization. *Am. J. Med. Genet. A* 149A(10):2106–2112.

Hinney, A., Scherag, A., et al. (2011). Genome-wide association study in German patients with attention deficit/hyperactivity disorder. *Am. J. Med. Genet. B Neuropsychiatr. Genet.* 156B(8):888–897.

Hogart, A., Wu, D., et al. (2010). The comorbidity of autism with the genomic disorders of chromosome 15q11.2-q13. *Neurobiol. Dis.* 38(2):181–191.

Hoischen, A., van Bon, B.W., et al. (2010). *De novo* mutations of SETBP1 cause Schinzel–Giedion syndrome. *Nat. Genet.* 42(6):483–485.

Iafrate, A.J., Feuk, L., et al. (2004). Detection of large-scale variation in the human genome. *Nat. Genet.* 36(9):949–951.

International Schizophrenia Consortium. (2008). Rare chromosomal deletions and duplications increase risk of schizophrenia. *Nature* 455(7210):237–241.

though several candidate genes remain promising. The *SLITRK1* gene is located near the breakpoint of a *de novo* inversion in a patient with Tourette syndrome and is involved in neurite outgrowth. Subsequent sequencing studies revealed three affected individuals with rare mutations, although follow-up studies have yielded varying results. The *CNTNAP2* gene was disrupted in three affected individuals from one family. This gene is an attractive candidate because it has been implicated in ASD and ID as well. Finally, in one family, two affected boys carry a maternally inherited *NLGN4X* deletion. *NLGN4X* is also involved in ASD and ID (State, 2011).

OTHER CHILDHOOD-ONSET PSYCHIATRIC DISORDERS

There has been one study of 90 individuals with intermittent explosive disorder (IED), which is characterized by episodes of aggression in which the individual acts impulsively, with a response that is grossly out of proportion with the associated stressors. Two patients were each found to have a rare CNV, suggesting that rare CNVs may play a role in the etiology of IED. One of the CNVs was a deletion of 1q21, which has also been seen in patients with ID, ASD, and schizophrenia (Vu et al., 2011). Bipolar disorder is a severe mood disorder characterized by alternating episodes of mania and depression. In some cases, age of onset is before age 18. There have been several studies to identify rare CNVs in patients with bipolar disorder (Grozeva et al., 2010; Malhotra et al., 2011; Zhang et al., 2009). One study included 107 patients with childhood onset. Six of 107 childhood onset patients had one or more *de novo* CNVs, and the rate of *de novo* CNVs was significantly higher in early onset compared with adult onset disease (Malhotra et al., 2011).

SHARED GENETIC SUSCEPTIBILITY

The discovery of rare genetic variants has been made possible by technological advances that allow efficient, genome-wide investigations in large numbers of patients and controls. These technologies have changed the direction of disease gene discovery, facilitating unbiased, hypothesis-free studies, compared with targeted and candidate gene studies of the past. One important outcome has been the simultaneous discovery of the same risk variant in different patient cohorts.

There are several examples of rare recurrent CNVs that appear to confer risk of several different psychiatric conditions (Mefford, 2009) (Table 71.7). Deletions and duplications of 16p11.2 were first described in patients with ASD and remain an important risk factor for this condition. However, it is now clear that the deletion is enriched in patients with developmental delay and ID. The duplication is important for schizophrenia and perhaps epilepsy. Deletions of 15q13.3 were first recognized in patients with ID, most of whom also had seizures. Additional studies of patients with epilepsy showed the deletion is enriched (and more frequent) in this patient population. Furthermore, it is also a risk factor for schizophrenia

TABLE 71.7. Copy number variations associated with risk for multiple conditions

CNV REGION	DISEASES ASSOCIATED WITH DELETION	DISORDERS ASSOCIATED WITH DUPLICATION
1q21.1	ID, SCZ, EP, ASD, IED	ID, ASD, CHD
3q29	ID, SCZ	ID
15q11.2	ID, SCZ, EP	—
15q13.3	ID, ASD, SCZ, EP	ID
16p11.2	ID, ASD	ID, ASD, SCZ
16p13.11	ID, ASD, SCZ	ADHD
17q12	ID, ASD, SCZ	EP
22q11	ID, SCZ	ID

ADHD, attention deficit/hyperactivity disorder; ASD, autism spectrum disorder; EP, epilepsy; ID, intellectual disability; IED, intermittent explosive disorder; SCZ, schizophrenia.

and autism. Another example comes from 1q21.1 deletions and duplication. Both are found in patients with ID or ASD, and deletions are enriched in patients with schizophrenia. Together, these results highlight the fact that the genetic architecture of each of these disorders is not distinct. Rather, there are probably many genes and pathways that, when disrupted, increase the risk of abnormal brain functioning. Whether the outcome is ASD, ID, schizophrenia, or a combination likely depends on genetic background and perhaps other epigenetic or environmental factors. Non-recurrent CNVs have also revealed genes and genomic regions that confer risk for various disorders. Deletions involving *NRXN1*, for example, have been reported in ASD and schizophrenia. Although deletions are occasionally seen in controls, the frequency is greater in cohorts of affected individuals. Similar conclusions about shared genetic risk can be drawn from rare SNVs. There are several genes that cause ID syndromes that can also cause ASD. For example, *FMR1* mutations, which are one of the most common causes of ID, are also found in boys with autism. The recent discovery of *de novo* mutations in *SCN1A*, *SCN2A*, and *GRIN2B* in ASD highlight a shared genetic susceptibility to ASD and epilepsy, as mutations in *SCN1A*, *SCN2A*, and *GRIN2A*, a close relative of *GRIN2B*, most often cause epilepsy syndromes that are also associated with ID.

CONCLUSIONS

Recent advances in genomic technologies have revolutionized the field of rare variant discovery. Numerous large investigations using these technologies have led to rapid advances in our understanding of genetic risk for various psychiatric conditions, and common themes have emerged. Each disorder that has been studied exhibits significant genetic heterogeneity. Therefore, despite the large number of patients that have been studied, only a small proportion of the genetic risk factors have been identified, and additional work is required. Most of microdeletions, the 22q11 deletion is associated with a wide range of cognitive abilities and other associated findings. It is one of the most common genetic factors associated with schizophrenia of adult onset as well as COS (Karayiorgou et al., 1995). All of these early studies were targeted and investigated the 22q11 region but not the rest of the genome.

The first genome-wide CNV studies in schizophrenia took place in 2008 and firmly established the role of both recurrent and non-recurrent CNVs in the genetic etiology of schizophrenia (International Schizophrenia Consortium, 2008; Stefansson et al., 2008; Walsh et al., 2008). Specifically, *de novo* mutations are more common in patients with sporadic schizophrenia. Furthermore, several recurrent CNVs are found at an increased frequency in patients with schizophrenia when compared with population controls, and all are associated with other neuropsychiatric conditions (see the following). Although the majority of studies have been performed in adults, at least two studies have looked specifically at COS. One study of 83 cases of COS found an excess of large (>150 kb) CNVs in affected children (Walsh et al., 2008). A deletion disrupting *NRXN1* was present in a pair of monozygotic twin children concordant for schizophrenia; similar deletions have been reported in adult-onset schizophrenia. Two children harbored recurrent duplications of 16p11.2. Another study of 96 patients with COS confirmed the importance of 22q11 deletions in this patient group and also identified a *NRXN1* deletion and two 16p11.2 duplications among other CNVs (Addington and Rapoport, 2009). Comparison of CNVs found in adult-onset disease compared with COS suggests that there are some shared risk factors, including 22q11 deletions, 16p11.2 duplications, and *NRXN1* deletions. Whether there are additional factors that influence age-of-onset or genetic variants that are specific to the childhood-onset form will require additional studies.

RARE SINGLE NUCLEOTIDE VARIATIONS IN CHILDHOOD ONSET SCHIZOPHRENIA

As for other psychiatric conditions, candidate genes have been studied individually in an attempt to identify rare variants associated with schizophrenia. In a study of several hundred candidate genes in 28 probands with COS, a maternally transmitted frameshift mutation in the X-linked gene *UPF3B* was identified in two brothers with COS, ASD, and ADHD (Addington et al., 2011). Mutations in the same gene are associated with ID. In a targeted analysis of the *SHANK3* gene, 2/185 affected individuals had a *de novo* mutation. In one family, three affected brothers shared the same mutations, likely as a result of germline mosaicism (Gauthier et al., 2010). As discussed, mutations in *SHANK3* are also important for autism risk.

Exome sequencing in sporadic cases of adult-onset schizophrenia suggests a role for *de novo* mutations (Xu et al., 2008). Notably, the 40 *de novo* mutations that were found in 27 patients were all in different genes, again supporting the notion that there is extensive genetic heterogeneity. Exome sequencing studies have not yet been published for COS, but it would not be surprising to find a similar role for severe *de novo* mutations as suggested by the finding of a *de novo* mutation in SHANK3 in a patient with COS (Gauthier et al., 2010).

ATTENTION DEFICIT/HYPERACTIVITY DISORDER

Attention deficit hyperactivity disorder (ADHD) affects up to 5% of children and is characterized by motor hyperactivity, inattention, and impulsivity. The heritability of ADHD is approximately 0.8 (Hinney et al., 2011). Although GWAS have yielded inconsistent results, CNV studies have identified several genomic regions and pathways that may be important in the genetic etiology of ADHD. No exome sequencing studies have been performed in ADHD yet.

As for other childhood neuropsychiatric disorders, CNV studies in ADHD reveal an enrichment of rare CNVs in affected children. One study identified rare recurrent CNVs involving glutamate receptors in approximately 10% of cases across multiple cohorts (Elia et al., 2012). In another study, there was a clear excess of large, rare CNVs in children with ADHD compared to healthy controls (Williams et al., 2010). Duplications of 16p13.11—also seen in ID, schizophrenia, and ASD—were specifically enriched in this cohort (Table 71.6).

TOURETTE SYNDROME

Rare genetic variants have also been found in Tourette syndrome, a childhood-onset disorder characterized by multiple motor tics and one or more phonic tics. Historically, chromosome abnormalities in isolated patients or families have been used to identify potential genomic regions that are important for Tourette syndrome. To date, there has been a single genome-wide study of CNVs in 11 patients with Tourette syndrome. In that study, there was no enrichment of CNVs in cases versus controls, but several CNVs that have been implicated in other neuropsychiatric disorders were found in patients with Tourette syndrome, including a 1q21 deletion and two deletions involving *NRXN1*, lending further support for shared genetic susceptibility among multiple neuropsychiatric conditions. Single nucleotide variation studies in candidate genes have been relatively unrevealing,

TABLE 71.6. Copy number variation studies in attention deficit/hyperactivity disorder

STUDY	N	FINDINGS
Elia et al. (2012)	1013 ADHD 4,105 healthy children	Metabotropic glutamate receptor gene networks enriched (GRM family)
Williams et al. (2010)	366 ADHD 1,047 controls	Increased rate of large, rare CNVs in ADHD; excess of 16p13.11 dups
Elia et al. (2010)	335 ADHD 2,026 controls	Rare inherited CNVs enriched for genes also associated with ASD, schizophrenia, Tourette syndrome, including *A2BP1*, *AUTS2*, *CNTNAP2*, *IMMP2L*, *GRM5*

SINGLE NUCLEOTIDE VARIATIONS IN AUTISM SPECTRUM DISORDERS

Although there is ample evidence for a genetic contribution to ASD, identification of true "autism genes" has been slow. Certainly there are many genetic syndromes in which a significant proportion of affected individuals have features of ASD (see Table 71.3). Some of the most important players are *MECP2* (Rett syndrome), *FMR1* (Fragile X syndrome), *SHANK3* (Phelan-McDermid syndrome/22q13.3 deletion syndrome), *PTEN* (*PTEN* macrocephaly syndrome), and *TSC2* (tuberous sclerosis) among others. Clearly this supports the notion that a subset of genes and pathways are important for ASD risk.

Identifying genes that play a clear role in idiopathic or non-syndromic ASD have been more elusive, and the discovery of genetic variants that confer risk for ASD has been approached from multiple directions. Large chromosomal rearrangements in individual patients can provide clues to genomic regions that are important for risk and are often reported as case studies in the literature. For example, the *AUTS2* gene was described as a possible autism gene after it was found to be disrupted by an inversion breakpoint in monozygotic twins concordant for autism (Sultana et al., 2002). *SHANK3* emerged as an ASD risk gene by comparing overlapping deletions in patients with 22q13 deletions. More comprehensive analyses have been carried out since the introduction of genome-wide array technologies, and the role of rare CNVs is discussed in the following. Some candidate genes have been studied individually using standard sequencing techniques to look for rare variants in modest patient cohorts. Finally, MPS has recently been employed for genome-wide discovery of rare, *de novo* SNVs that may be causative in some patients.

Recently, exome sequencing has been employed to investigate the role of rare *de novo* variants in ASD (Table 71.5) (Chahrour et al., 2012; Iossifov et al., 2012; Neale et al., 2012; O'Roak et al., 2011, 2012; Sanders et al., 2012). All support a role for rare, protein-altering *de novo* mutations in the genetic etiology of ASD. However, they also highlight the significant genetic heterogeneity that underlies ASD risk. In one of the first studies, exome sequencing was performed in 20 trios (O'Roak et al., 2011), and compelling *de novo* mutations in four of the 20 children were identified within genes that are known to be involved in brain development: *FOXP1* (Hamdan et al., 2010), *GRIN2B* (Endele et al., 2010), *SCN1A* (Claes et al., 2003), and *LAMC3* (Barak et al., 2011). Three large studies used exome sequencing in a total of 622 children with ASD (209 trios (O'Roak et al., 2012), 175 trios (Neale et al., 2012), 238 families (Sanders et al., 2012). There were eighteen genes in which two or more patients had a *de novo* non-synonymous change across the studies. Mutations in three of the genes were nonsense, splice, or frameshift. Another study performed exome sequencing in 343 simplex families and found 59 genes with *de novo*, likely gene-disrupting mutations (Iossifov et al., 2012) but none with a mutation in more than one patient. Based on their results, they estimate that there are 350 to 400 ASD susceptibility genes. Finally, one study has used exome sequencing to investigate a recessive model for autism in 16 families and identified several potential candidate genes (Chahrour et al., 2012).

CHILDHOOD ONSET SCHIZOPHRENIA

Childhood onset schizophrenia (COS) is a rare and severe form of schizophrenia with onset of symptoms before age 18. Because of similarities with other neuropsychiatric disorders and the progressive and evolving symptoms, COS can be difficult to diagnose early. Although there have been several studies aimed at identifying rare variants in adult-onset schizophrenia, fewer have been targeted specifically to COS. We briefly discuss the support for rare variants in schizophrenia generally, with a focus on studies that address COS.

RARE COPY NUMBER VARIATIONS IN CHILDHOOD ONSET SCHIZOPHRENIA

Early studies in COS highlighted the role of 22q11 deletions in affected individuals (Yan et al., 1998). Like many

TABLE 71.5. Exome studies in autism spectrum disorder

STUDY	N	FINDINGS	KEY GENES IMPLICATED
O'Roak et al. (2011)	20 trios sporadic ASD	21 *de novo* mutations (11 protein altering)	*FOXP1, GRIN2B, SCN1A, LAMC3*
O'Roak et al. (2012)	209 trios 1703 cases for validation of 6 genes	126 *de novo* disruptive mutations; 49 map to B-catenin/chromatin remodeling network	*CHD8, NTNG1, GRIN2B, LAMC3, SCN1A*
Neale et al. (2012)	175 trios 935 cases for validation in 3 genes	46.3% carry *de novo* disruptive variant	*CHD8, KATNAL2*
Sanders et al. (2012)	238 families, 200 including a discordant sibling, total of 928 individuals	279 *de novo* coding mutations	2 samples with *de novo* nonsense mutation in *SCN2A*
Iossifov et al. (2012)	343 simplex families	Increase in *de novo* gene-disrupting mutations in affected vs unaffected	
Chahrour et al. (2012)	16 probands	Recessive inheritance model	*UBE3B, CLTCL1, MCKAP5L, ZNF18*

be validated in additional samples, but the study provides a framework for evaluation of recessive forms of ID.

AUTISM SPECTRUM DISORDERS

Autism spectrum disorders (ASD), estimated to affect as many as 1/150 to 1/100 children (Chakrabarti and Fombonne, 2001, 2005), share common features of impaired social relationships, impaired language and communication, and repetitive behaviors or a narrow range of interests. Children with ASD often have comorbid conditions, including ID (approximately 70%) and epilepsy (approximately 25%), and most require lifelong social and educational support. Evidence for a strong genetic component comes from family and twin studies. In addition, many genetic syndromes caused by single gene mutations or chromosomal rearrangements are associated with ASD (Table 71.3). Therefore, extensive studies have been performed to identify the genes and genomic regions that have a large effect on genetic risk for ASD. We focus on the most recent findings from genome-wide approaches.

COPY NUMBER VARIATIONS IN AUTISM SPECTRUM DISORDER

Rare CNVs clearly play a role in the genetic etiology of ASD. One of the first CNVs to be associated with ASD was duplication of 15q11-q13, the same region associated with Prader-Willi and Angelman syndromes when deleted. Duplication of this region, which contains maternally and paternally imprinted genes, is associated with ASD when maternally inherited or derived, but not when paternally inherited (Cook et al., 1997) and is responsible for 1–3% of ASD (Hogart et al., 2010). More recently, genome-wide array technologies have been used extensively for CNV discovery in ASD. Since 2007 numerous studies have each identified multiple rare, often *de novo* variants in affected individuals that are either not present or present at a much lower frequency in unaffected individuals (Table 71.4). Together, these studies indicate that there is a strong association between *de novo* CNVs and ASD, especially in the case of simplex families where only one child is affected.

A number of recurrent CNVs are associated with an increased risk for ASD. One of the first regions to be strongly associated with ASD was 16p11.2 (Kumar et al., 2008; Marshall et al., 2008; Weiss et al., 2008). The 16p11.2 region is approximately 550 kb and contains 25 annotated genes, although which gene or combination of genes contribute to the ASD phenotype is not yet known. Deletion or duplication of 16p11.2 can be found in up to 0.5% to 1% of children with ASD, but it is now clear that the same CNVs are also significant risk factors for ID (Bijlsma et al., 2009; Mefford et al., 2009; Shinawi et al., 2010), schizophrenia (McCarthy et al., 2009), epilepsy (Bedoyan et al., 2010; Mefford et al., 2011), and obesity (Jacquemont et al., 2011; Walters et al., 2010). Recurrent deletions of the 15q24 region cause a syndrome characterized by moderate to severe delays, including significant speech delays; many patients are also described as having ASD characteristics as well (Andrieux et al., 2009; El-Hattab et al., 2009; Klopocki et al., 2008; Mefford et al., 1993; Mefford et al., 2011; Sharp et al., 2007). As for ID, there are recurrent CNVs that seem to confer risk for ASD as well as other disorders, including 15q13.3 deletions (Ben-Shachar et al., 2009; Miller et al. 2008; Pagnamenta et al., 2009), 16p13.11 deletions and duplications (Ramalingam et al., 2011; Ullmann et al., 2007), and 17q12 deletions (Loirat et al., 2010; Moreno-De-Luca et al., 2010; Nagamani et al., 2010) (see the following).

Non-recurrent CNVs can be important for identifying specific genes that might be important for ASD risk. Multiple CNVs within the *NRXN1* gene have been reported in affected individuals (Ching et al., 2010; Glessner et al., 2009; Kim et al., 2008; Szatmari et al., 2007). Although deletions within the gene are also seen in some control studies, the frequency of *NRXN1* deletions is greater in cases compared to controls. This suggests that such deletions confer risk but are not completely penetrant. Deletions involving the *PTCHD1* gene highlight this gene's potential role in ASD (Noor et al., 2010; Pinto et al., 2010) as well.

TABLE 71.3. Examples of genetic syndromes in which autism spectrum disorder is a prominent feature

SYNDROME	CAUSATIVE GENE	INHERITANCE
Fragile X syndrome	FMR1	XLR
Tuberous sclerosis	TSC2	AD
PTEN macrocephaly	PTEN	AD
Sotos syndrome	NSD1	AD
Rett syndrome	MECP2	XLD
Timothy syndrome	CACNA1C	AD

TABLE 71.4. Key copy number variation studies in autism spectrum disorder

STUDY	CASES/CONTROLS	FINDINGS
Sebat et al. (2007)	118 sporadic ASD 77 familial ASD 196 controls	*De novo* CNVs significantly associated with sporadic ASD
Szatmari et al. (2007)	1181 multiplex families	Linkage + CNVs Neurexins implicated
Weiss et al. (2008)	751 multiplex ASD families 18,834 controls	16p11.2 deletion and duplication significantly associated with ASD
Marshall et al. (2008)	427 ASD cases 500 controls	*De novo* CNVs important for ASD
Pinto et al. (2010)	996 ASD 1287 controls	Higher genic CNV burden in cases
Sanders et al. (2011)	1124 ASD families	Large, *de novo* CNVs, including duplications at 7q11.23, confer significant risk

et al., 2007). All 15q24 deletions described to date are *de novo*, and common features include variable developmental delay and ID that is usually moderate to severe; severe speech delays or absent speech; dysmorphic features, including a high anterior hairline, prominent forehead, and downslanting palpebral fissures; joint laxity; and hypotonia. Many patients also have some features of autism spectrum disorders. The 15q24 deletions have variable breakpoints and range in size, but most include a region of 1.1-Mb that is thought to be the critical region for the phenotype.

In addition to the syndromic microdeletions described in the preceding, several recurrent microdeletions and duplications have been associated with ID but also with a wider range of phenotypic features and severity. Examples include 1q21.1 deletions and duplications (Brunetti-Pierri et al., 2008; Christiansen et al., 2004; Mefford et al., 2008), 16p11.2 deletions and duplications (Battaglia et al., 2009; Bijlsma et al., 2009; Hempel et al., 2009; Rosenfeld et al., 2009; Shinawi et al., 2010), 15q13.3 deletions (Ben-Shachar et al., 2009; Sharp et al., 2008; van Bon et al., 2009), 15q11.2 deletions (Mefford et al., 2009; Murthy et al., 2007; von der Lippe et al., 2011) and 16p13.11 deletions and duplications (Hannes et al., 2009; Mefford et al., 2009; Ullmann et al., 2007). Each of these CNVs is associated with a significant risk for ID, but is also associated with risk for at least one other psychiatric condition including schizophrenia, autism, ADHD, and/or epilepsy (see the following).

Numerous non-recurrent deletions and duplications have also been described in cohorts of patients with ID. Because they are non-recurrent—often unique—it can be difficult to accumulate a series of patients so as to identify common features. Pathogenicity is generally determined because of the inheritance (*de novo*), size (large), or gene content (many or at least one known disease gene) of a given CNV (Miller et al., 2010). In some cases, overlapping deletions are frequent enough to describe common features. Such is the case for overlapping deletions involving 1p36, 9q34, distal 22q11, 22q13 and others.

SINGLE NUCLEOTIDE VARIATIONS IN INTELLECTUAL DISABILITY

There are numerous single-gene causes of ID and syndromes associated with ID, many of which are discussed elsewhere in this volume. Early discoveries of genes responsible for ID relied on family-based genetic linkage studies and DNA sequencing. Because X-linked forms of ID can be transmitted through unaffected females in families, allowing pedigree analysis, a large effort has focused on identifying genes on the X chromosome, and mutations in more than 90 X-linked genes are now known to cause ID, accounting for about 10% of cases (Ropers, 2010). Autosomal genes have been more difficult to identify, because there are few familial forms of ID. Indeed, it is thought that the majority of moderate to severe ID is caused by *de novo* mutations, which cannot be detected by linkage mapping. However, new sequencing technologies are facilitating gene discovery in this previously intractable form of inheritance.

Exome sequencing has been used to identify the genes responsible for many disorders since 2009, including Kabuki syndrome (Ng et al., 2010), Schinzel–Giedion syndrome (Hoischen et al., 2010), Sensenbrenner syndrome (Gilissen et al., 2010), and others. One approach that has been quite successful is exome sequencing in "trios" of one affected child and two unaffected parents. The goal of trio analysis is to identify the small number of *de novo* sequence changes that are present in the affected child but not in either parent. The trio approach is efficient because, on average, it is predicted that each exome will have less than one *de novo* mutation that changes an amino-acid (Lynch, 2010). At least one study has applied exome sequencing in trios to identify causes of nonsyndromic ID (Table 71.2) (Vissers et al., 2010). In 10 affected individuals without a family history of ID, they identified nine true *de novo* variants (in nine different genes) in six individuals. Two patients each had a *de novo* mutation in a known ID gene. In four other cases, patients had a *de novo* variant in a plausible candidate gene. It must be noted that additional studies are required to confirm that the candidate genes truly play a role in ID. However, the results indicate that trio analysis is an efficient method to detect *de novo* mutations and novel candidate genes. These results also highlight the genetic heterogeneity in ID, as no two patients had *de novo* mutations in the same gene.

Exome sequencing has also been used to investigate causes of autosomal recessive ID (see Table 71.2). In one study, investigators sequenced the exomes of two parents with multiple affected children to look for heterozygous deleterious mutations within a 2-Mb linkage region (Caliskan et al., 2011). They identified a mutation in the gene *TECR* that was homozygous in all affected children. In another study, investigators set out to tackle autosomal recessive ID in 136 consanguineous families (Najmabadi et al., 2011). Using linkage data for their families that narrowed the genomic regions of interest, they captured the subset of exons within linkage regions for each family rather than sequencing the entire exome. They found mutations in 23 known ID genes in 26 families, providing a definitive diagnosis. In the remaining families, they identified 50 novel candidate genes, each with a homozygous mutation in a single family. Clearly, these candidate genes need to

TABLE 71.2. Exome sequencing studies in intellectual disability

DISORDER	GENE	INHERITANCE PATTERN	REFERENCE
Kabuki syndrome	*MLL2*	*De novo*, AD	Ng et al. (2010)
Schinzel-Giedion	*SETBP1*	*De novo*, AD	Hoischen et al. (2010)
Nonsyndromic sporadic ID	Multiple	*De novo*, AD	Vissers et al. (2010)
Recessive ID	*TECR*	AR, consanguineous	Caliskan et al. (2011)
Recessive ID	Multiple	AR, consanguineous	Najmabadi et al. (2011)

AD, autosomal dominant; AR, autosomal recessive.

Replication—Adolescent Supplement (NCS-A). *J. Am. Acad. Child Adolesc. Psychiatry* 49(10):980–989.

Neale, B.M., Kou, Y., et al. (2012). Patterns and rates of exonic *de novo* mutations in autism spectrum disorders. *Nature* 485(7397):242–245.

Nichols, P.L. (1984). Familial mental retardation. *Behav. Genet.* 14(3):161–170.

Nolan, E.E., Gadow, K.D., et al. (2001). Teacher reports of DSM-IV ADHD, ODD, and CD symptoms in schoolchildren. *J. Am. Acad. Child Adolesc. Psychiatry* 40(2):241–249.

O'Roak, B.J., Vives, L., et al. (2012). Sporadic autism exomes reveal a highly interconnected protein network of *de novo* mutations. *Nature* 485(7397):246–250.

Ozonoff, S., Young, G.S., et al. (2011). Recurrence risk for autism spectrum disorders: a Baby Siblings Research Consortium study. *Pediatrics* 128(3):e488–495.

Pappert, E.J., Goetz, C.G., et al. (2003). Objective assessments of longitudinal outcome in Gilles de la Tourette's syndrome. *Neurology* 61(7):936–940.

Pedersen, A., Pettygrove, S., et al. (2012). Prevalence of autism spectrum disorders in Hispanic and non-Hispanic white children. *Pediatrics* 129(3):e629–635.

Piven, J., Harper, J., et al. (1996). Course of behavioral change in autism: a retrospective study of high-IQ adolescents and adults. *J. Am. Acad. Child Adolesc. Psychiatry* 35(4):523–529.

Piven, J., Palmer, P., et al. (1997). Broader autism phenotype: evidence from a family history study of multiple-incidence autism families. *Am. J. Psychiatry* 154(2):185–190.

Plomin, R., DeFries, J., et al. (2008). Behavioral Genetics, 5th Edition. New York: Worth.

Ripke, S., Sanders, A.R., et al. (2011). Genome-wide association study identifies five new schizophrenia loci. *Nat. Genet.* 43(10):969–976.

Risch, N., and Merikangas, K. (1996). The future of genetic studies of complex human diseases. *Science* 273(5281):1516–1517.

Robinson, E.B., Koenen, K.C., et al. (2011a). Evidence that autistic traits show the same etiology in the general population and at the quantitative extremes (5%, 2.5%, and 1%). *Arch. Gen. Psychiatry* 68(11):1113–1121.

Robinson, E.B., Munir, K., et al. (2011b). Stability of autistic traits in the general population: further evidence for a continuum of impairment. *J. Am. Acad. Child Adolesc. Psychiatry* 50(4):376–384.

Rohde, L.A., Biederman, J., et al. (1999). ADHD in a school sample of Brazilian adolescents: a study of prevalence, comorbid conditions, and impairments. *J. Am. Acad. Child Adolesc. Psychiatry* 38(6):716–722.

Ronald, A., Happe, F., et al. (2006). Genetic heterogeneity between the three components of the autism spectrum: a twin study. *J. Am. Acad. Child Adolesc. Psychiatry* 45(6):691–699.

Ronald, A., and Hoekstra, R.A. (2011). Autism spectrum disorders and autistic traits: a decade of new twin studies. *Am. J. Med. Genet. B Neuropsychiatr. Genet.* 156B(3):255–274.

Ronald, A., Simonoff, E., et al. (2008). Evidence for overlapping genetic influences on autistic and ADHD behaviours in a community twin sample. *J. Child Psychol. Psychiatry* 49(5):535–542.

Rosenberg, R.E., Daniels, A.M., et al. (2009). Trends in autism spectrum disorder diagnoses: 1994–2007. *J. Autism Dev. Disord.* 39(8):1099–1111.

Russell, G., Steer, C., et al. (2010). Social and demographic factors that influence the diagnosis of autistic spectrum disorders. *Soc. Psychiatry Psychiatr. Epidemiol.* 46(12):1283–1293.

Rutter, M.L. (2011). Progress in understanding autism: 2007–2010. *J. Autism Dev. Disord.* 41(4):395–404.

Sachidanandam, R., Weissman, D., et al. (2001). A map of human genome sequence variation containing 1.42 million single nucleotide polymorphisms. *Nature* 409(6822):928–933.

Sanders, S.J., Ercan-Sencicek, A.G., et al. (2011). Multiple recurrent de novo CNVs, including duplications of the 7q11.23 Williams syndrome region, are strongly associated with autism. *Neuron* 70(5):863–885.

Sanders, S.J., Murtha, M.T., et al. (2012). *De novo* mutations revealed by whole-exome sequencing are strongly associated with autism. *Nature* 485(7397):237–241.

Scott, F.J., Baron-Cohen, S., et al. (2002). The CAST (Childhood Asperger Syndrome Test): preliminary development of a UK screen for mainstream primary-school-age children. *Autism* 6(1):9–31.

Sebat, J., Levy, D.L., et al. (2009). Rare structural variants in schizophrenia: one disorder, multiple mutations; one mutation, multiple disorders. *Trends Genet.* 25(12):528–535.

Shattuck, P.T., Roux, A.M., et al. (2012). Services for adults with an autism spectrum disorder. *Can. J. Psychiatry* 57(5):284–291.

Shattuck, P.T., Seltzer, M.M., et al. (2007). Change in autism symptoms and maladaptive behaviors in adolescents and adults with an autism spectrum disorder. *J. Autism Dev. Disord.* 37(9):1735–1747.

Simonoff, E., Pickles, A., et al. (2008). Psychiatric disorders in children with autism spectrum disorders: prevalence, comorbidity, and associated factors in a population-derived sample. *J. Am. Acad. Child Adolesc. Psychiatry* 47(8):921–929.

Singer, H.S. (2005). Tourette's syndrome: from behaviour to biology. *Lancet Neurol.* 4(3):149–159.

Skuse, D.H. (2007). Rethinking the nature of genetic vulnerability to autistic spectrum disorders. *Trends Genet.* 23(8):387–395.

Skuse, D.H. (2009). Is autism really a coherent syndrome in boys, or girls? *Br. J. Psychol.* 100(Pt 1):33–37.

Skuse, D.H., Mandy, W.P., et al. (2005). Measuring autistic traits: heritability, reliability and validity of the Social and Communication Disorders Checklist. *Br. J. Psychiatry* 187:568–572.

St Pourcain, B., Mandy, W.P., et al. (2011). Links between co-occurring social-communication and hyperactive-inattentive trait trajectories. *J. Am. Acad. Child Adolesc. Psychiatry* 50(9):892–902.

Starr, E., Szatmari, P., et al. (2003). Stability and change among high-functioning children with pervasive developmental disorders: a 2-year outcome study. *J. Autism Dev. Disord.* 33(1):15–22.

Still, G.F. (1902). Some abnormal psychical conditions in children: the Goulstonian lectures. *Lancet* (1):1008–1012.

Sukhodolsky, D.G., Scahill, L., et al. (2003). Disruptive behavior in children with Tourette's syndrome: association with ADHD comorbidity, tic severity, and functional impairment. *J. Am. Acad. Child Adolesc. Psychiatry* 42(1):98–105.

Svensson, A.C., Lichtenstein, P., et al. (2007). Fertility of first-degree relatives of patients with schizophrenia: a three generation perspective. *Schizophr. Res.* 91(1–3):238–245.

Szatmari, P., Bryson, S., et al. (2009). Similar developmental trajectories in autism and Asperger syndrome: from early childhood to adolescence. *J. Child Psychol. Psychiatry* 50(12):1459–1467.

Szatmari, P., Bryson, S.E., et al. (2000). Two-year outcome of preschool children with autism or Asperger's syndrome. *Am. J. Psychiatry* 157(12):1980–1987.

Szatmari, P. (2011). Is autism, at least in part, a disorder of fetal programming? *Arch. Gen. Psychiatry* 68(11):1091–1092.

Talkowski, M.E., Rosenfeld, J.A., et al. (2012). Sequencing chromosomal abnormalities reveals neurodevelopmental loci that confer risk across diagnostic boundaries. *Cell* 149(3):525–537.

Tarpey, P.S., Smith, R., et al. (2009). A systematic, large-scale resequencing screen of X-chromosome coding exons in mental retardation. *Nat. Genet.* 41(5):535–543.

Uher, R. (2009). The role of genetic variation in the causation of mental illness: an evolution-informed framework. *Mol. Psychiatry* 14(12):1072–1082.

Volkmar, F., Cook, E., Jr., et al. (1999). Summary of the practice parameters for the assessment and treatment of children, adolescents, and adults with autism and other pervasive developmental disorders. American Academy of Child and Adolescent Psychiatry. *J. Am. Acad. Child Adolesc. Psychiatry* 38(12):1611–1616.

Vorstman, J.A., Staal, W.G. et al. (2006). Identification of novel autism candidate regions through analysis of reported cytogenetic abnormalities associated with autism. *Mol. Psychiatry* 11(1):1, 18–28.

Weiss, L.A., Shen, Y., et al. (2008). Association between microdeletion and microduplication at 16p11.2 and autism. *N. Engl. J. Med.* 358(7):667–675.

Weschler, D., Golombok, J., et al. (1992). Manual for the Weschler Intelligence Scale for Children, 3rd Edition. Sidkup, UK: Psychological Corporation.

Williams, E., Thomas, K., et al. (2008). Prevalence and characteristics of autistic spectrum disorders in the ALSPAC cohort. *Dev. Med. Child Neurol.* 50(9):672–677.

Williams, N.M., Franke, B., et al. (2012). Genome-wide analysis of copy number variants in attention deficit hyperactivity disorder: the role of rare variants and duplications at 15q13.3. *Am. J. Psychiatry* 169(2):195–204.

Williams, N.M., Zaharieva, I., et al. (2010). Rare chromosomal deletions and duplications in attention-deficit hyperactivity disorder: a genome-wide analysis. *Lancet* 376(9750):1401–1408.

Wolraich, M.L., Hannah, J.N., et al. (1998). Examination of DSM-IV criteria for attention deficit/hyperactivity disorder in a county-wide sample. *J. Dev. Behav. Pediatr.* 19(3):162–168.

71 | RARE VARIANTS OF SUBSTANTIAL EFFECT IN PSYCHIATRIC DISORDERS OF CHILDHOOD ONSET

HEATHER C. MEFFORD

Psychiatric disorders in children carry a significant financial and social burden for affected children and their families. Examples include autism, intellectual disability, attention deficit/hyperactivity disorder (ADHD), childhood-onset schizophrenia, and bipolar disorder. For parents, these diagnoses also carry a psychological burden as questions about etiology and recurrence risk arise. The evidence for genetic contribution to these disorders is extensive and stems from family and twin studies. In fact, early genetic studies focused on linkage analysis in rare, large families with multiple affected family members. However, for all of these disorders, such large families are rare; rather, the inheritance pattern for most psychiatric disorders is complex and does not follow a simple mendelian inheritance pattern.

Two hypotheses have been put forth concerning the genetics of such disorders. One suggests that multiple common genetic variants each contribute a small increased risk for disease. Genome-wide association studies (GWAS) are designed to identify common single nucleotide variants that are more frequent in affected versus unaffected individuals and have been carried out for many psychiatric disorders. Results of GWAS are varied, but in most cases, a single nucleotide change that is found to be associated with disease confers only a slight increased risk for disease. The rare variant hypothesis, on the other hand, puts forth that some rare genetic variants have a large effect on disease risk. Each variant may be individually quite rare—even absent from control populations—but the collection of rare variants together explain a large portion of genetic risk. This chapter focuses on the identification of rare variants that have a large effect on genetic risk for childhood psychiatric disorders.

GENETIC VARIANTS AND THE TECHNOLOGIES THAT DETECT THEM

Over the past five to ten years, advances in technology have enabled genome-wide discovery of both common and rare genetic variation. Here we consider two general classes of variation: single nucleotide variants (SNVs) and copy number variants (CNVs; Fig. 71.1). Single nucleotide variants are DNA changes involving a single base pair (e.g., an A to G change) that can be found be in noncoding or coding regions of the genome. Single nucleotide variants that vary from the reference genome in 5% or more of the population are termed single nucleotide polymorphisms (SNPs) and occur at an average frequency of one per kilobase throughout the genome.

Copy number variants are defined as deletions or duplications of a stretch of DNA when compared with the reference human genome and may range in size from a kilobase (kb) to several megabases (Mb) or even an entire chromosome (trisomies and monosomies). Copy number variants can involve multiple, one or no genes. As with SNVs, some CNVs are polymorphisms. Multiple studies of large control cohorts have shown that some regions of the genome are tolerant of copy number changes, and that every individual carries many copy number changes that are, for the most part, benign (Iafrate et al., 2004; Itsara et al., 2009; Locke et al., 2006; Redon et al., 2006; Sebat et al., 2004). Copy number variants come in two basic flavors: recurrent and non-recurrent (Fig. 71.1). Recurrent CNVs are those that arise by non-allelic homologous recombination (NAHR) during meiosis. The breakpoints of recurrent CNVs lie in large duplicated blocks of sequence flanking the CNV event, so the breakpoints of recurrent CNVs in unrelated individuals will be essentially identical. In contrast, non-recurrent CNVs have breakpoints that generally lie within unique sequence and do not occur because of predisposing genomic architecture. There are several different mechanisms by which non-recurrent CNVs can arise including non-homologous end joining (NHEJ) and fork stalling and template switching (FoSTeS). Although two unrelated individuals may have overlapping non-recurrent CNVs, they are unlikely to have the same breakpoints. Significantly, comparison of overlapping non-recurrent CNVs in individuals with similar phenotypes can lead to narrowing of the critical region for a given phenotype (see Fig. 71.1).

Three technologies developed over the past several years have transformed our ability to efficiently detect genetic variation across the entire genome: array comparative genomic hybridization (CGH), SNP genotyping arrays, and massively parallel sequencing. Array CGH technology was developed to detect copy number changes throughout the genome. Although initial studies were performed in population controls to determine the "CNV landscape" in normal individuals, the technology was rapidly applied to large cohorts of individuals with ID, autism, and other disorders to detect disease-causing CNVs. Single nucleotide polymorphism genotyping arrays were developed to genotype up to several million common SNPs simultaneously and have been used extensively for GWAS. It was also recognized that SNP microarray data could be used to detect CNVs, facilitating CNV discovery in cohorts that had already been genotyped for GWAS. Both array CGH and SNP

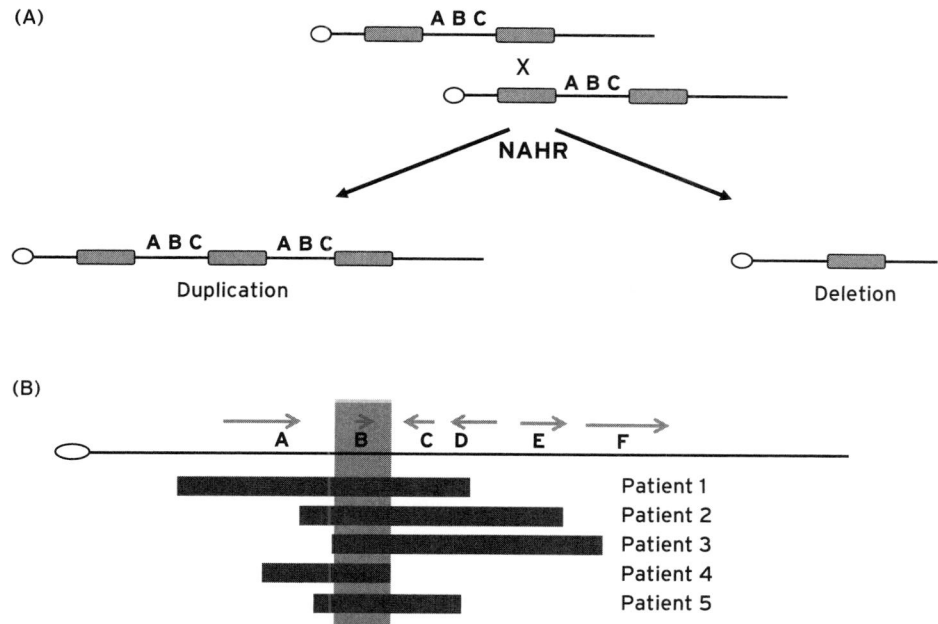

Figure 71.1 *Schematic representation of recurrent (A) and non-recurrent (B) copy number changes. (A) Recurrent CNVs usually arise by non-allelic homologous recombination (NAHR) during meiosis. Light Gray blocks represent large duplicated blocks of sequence where mis-alignment can occur. Recombination, represented by the "X," causes duplication or deletion of the sequence between the duplicated blocks. "A B C" represent genes within the region that are deleted or duplicated as a result. (B) Non-recurrent CNVs are represented by dark gray horizontal bars, each with different proximal and distal breakpoints. Comparison of overlapping, non-recurrent CNVs in individuals with similar phenotypes can lead to narrowing of the critical region for a given phenotype, represented by the gray shading over gene "B."*

microarrays have been used extensively to investigate the role of CNVs in disease and are also used in clinical laboratory settings for diagnostic testing.

Although common SNPs can be genotyped with SNP microarrays, rare SNVs cannot, although recurrent rare SNV are now being incorporated into microarrays. The technology that has enabled efficient detection of rare SNVs is massively parallel or "next-generation" sequencing. Massively parallel sequencing (MPS) involves highly parallelized sequencing of millions of short DNA fragments from the genome. Indeed, an entire genome can be sequenced using MPS in a matter of weeks. A more efficient approach, and one that has now been employed extensively for disease gene discovery, is to sequence only the approximately 1% of the genome that is protein-coding, termed the exome. There are two main reasons for sequencing the exome as opposed to the whole genome when looking for disease-associated variants. First, the majority of known variants that cause mendelian disorders occur in coding sequence, whereas a minority is found in non-coding regions of the genome. Second, variants within coding exons are readily interpretable. That is, it is fairly straightforward to determine whether a given nucleotide change will result in a change in the protein. Interpretation of variants in noncoding regions is much more difficult.

All of these technologies have been used to investigate the role of genetic and genomic variation in various neuropsychiatric illnesses, and three consistent themes have emerged. First, each disorder exhibits significant genetic heterogeneity. That is, the number of genes and genomic loci that confer disease risk is extensive, and unrelated patients are more likely to

have unique, rather than shared, genetic risk factors. A second and related theme is that the genetic factors involved in disease risks of large effect are rare, rather than common, variants. This is true for both SNVs and CNVs, with *de novo* variants playing an important role. Finally, large-scale studies across diverse disorders have revealed shared genetic susceptibility factors for disorders once thought to be distinct. In some respects, this shared genetic susceptibility is not surprising. Indeed, there is considerable comorbidity as children with ID often have autistic features; children with schizophrenia may exhibit ASD features before onset of psychosis; children with ASD may have ID or seizures, and so forth. With the technologies described earlier, genome-wide studies of rare variants in each of these disorders are illuminating specific genomic regions and genes that confer shared genetic susceptibility. This will shed light on common pathways for normal brain development and function, providing insight into potential therapies. This chapter discusses recent advances in the discovery of rare genetic variants that confer risk for childhood-onset psychiatric disorders including intellectual disability, autism, childhood-onset schizophrenia, attention deficit hyperactivity disorder, and Tourette syndrome.

INTELLECTUAL DISABILITY

Intellectual disability (ID) affects 1% to 2% of individuals and is characterized by significant limitations in both intellectual functioning and adaptive behavior that begins before the age of 18 years (American Psychiatric Association., 2000; Leonard and Wen, 2002). Although a diagnosis of ID is usually made in late childhood or early adulthood when IQ testing reveals an IQ of less than 70, most individuals with ID are identified early in childhood with concerns about developmental delays that may include any or all of motor, cognitive, and speech delays. A thorough discussion of ID syndromes is presented elsewhere (see Chapter 76). Here, we will discuss more recent discoveries made possible by array CGH, SNP microarrays and exome sequencing.

COPY NUMBER VARIATIONS IN INTELLECTUAL DISABILITY

It has long been known that chromosomal copy number changes can cause ID. One of the earliest examples, and still one of the most important causes of ID, is the presence of an extra copy of chromosome 21 resulting in Down syndrome. Intellectual disability syndromes caused by recurrent deletions were recognized as cytogenetic techniques improved and fluorescent in situ hybridization (FISH) techniques became available. Examples of well-known ID syndromes cause by recurrent microdeletions include Prader-Willi syndrome (paternal deletion of 15q11-q13), Angelman syndrome (maternal deletion of 15q11-q13), Smith-Magenis syndrome (deletion of 17p11.2), and velocardiofacial syndrome (deletion of 22q11.2). Fluorescent in situ hybridization studies of subtelomeric regions near the ends of chromosomes highlighted the importance of unbalanced subtelomeric rearrangements, which cause 2.5% to 5% of ID (Ballif et al., 2007; Knight et al., 1999; Ravnan et al., 2006). These early studies were targeted to specific regions of the genome. In most cases, a suspected diagnosis could be confirmed or ruled out with a FISH study for a specific deletion. Subtelomeric studies targeted multiple regions at once, but still assayed only a small portion of the genome.

In approximately 2004, the introduction of array CGH and SNP arrays for CNV detection facilitated unbiased, genome-wide discovery of CNVs in patients with ID, paving the way for an unprecedented rate of discovery of novel ID syndromes associated with both recurrent and non-recurrent CNVs. Since 2006, more than 20 novel recurrent deletion and duplication syndromes have been described in patients with ID (Table 71.1), along with many more non-recurrent deletions and duplications. Two examples of recently described recurrent deletions that are highly penetrant and associated with syndromic features are microdeletions of 17q21.31 and 15q24. Heterozygous deletions of 17q21.31 are always *de novo* and are associated with moderate to severe ID, hypotonia, facial dysmorphic features, occasional cardiac and renal abnormalities, seizures, and a generally happy disposition (Koolen et al., 2006; Koolen and de Vries, 1993; Sharp et al., 2006; Shaw-Smith et al., 2006). The deletion is 500 to 650 kb in size, is not detectable by routine karyotyping, and has never been seen in healthy controls. The prevalence is estimated to be approximately 1/16,000 (Koolen et al., 2008). Deletions of 15q24 are much rarer, but patients with 15q24 microdeletions also appear to be syndromic (Andrieux et al., 2009; El-Hattab et al., 2009; Klopocki et al., 2008; Mefford et al., 1993; Mefford et al., 2011; Sharp

TABLE 71.1. Novel recurrent deletion and duplication syndromes in intellectual disability*

GENOMIC LOCATION	COORDINATES (HG19) FOR CRITICAL REGION	REPRESENTATIVE REFERENCES
1q21.1 del	Chr1: 146.5–147.5	Brunetti-Pierri et al. (2008), Mefford et al. (2008), Harvard et al. (2011)
1q21.1 dup	Chr1: 146.5–147.5	Brunetti-Pierri et al. (2008), Mefford et al. (2008), Harvard et al. (2011)
3q29 del	Chr3: 195.8–197.4	Willatt et al. (2005), Ballif et al. (2008)
3q29 dup	Chr3: 195.8–197.4	Ballif et al. (2008), Lisi et al. (2008)
7q11.23 distal del	Chr7: 75.1–76.1	Ramocki et al. (2010)
10q22q23 del	Chr10: 81.5–89.0	Balciuniene et al., (2007), van Bon et al. (2011)
15q11.2 del	Chr15: 22.8–23.1	Burnside et al. (2011), von der Lippe et al. (2011)
15q13.3 del	Chr15: 31.3–32.5	Sharp et al. (2008), van Bon et al. (2009)
15q13.3 dup	Chr15: 31.9–32.5	Szafranski et al. (2010)
15q24 del	Chr15: 74.4–75.5	Sharp et al. (2007), Mefford et al. (2012)
15q24 dup	Chr15: 74.4–75.5	Kiholm Lund et al. (2008)
16p11.2 (prox) del	Chr16: 29.6–30.2	Bijlsma et al. (2009), Shinawi et al. (2010)
16p11.2 (prox) dup	Chr16: 29.6–30.2	Shinawi et al. (2010)
16p11.2 (distal) del	Chr16: 28.8–29.1	Bachmann-Gagescu et al. (2010)
16p12 del	Chr16: 21.9–22.5	Girirajan et al. (2010)
16p13.11 del	Chr16: 15.0–16.3	Ullmann et al. (2007), Hannes et al. (2009), Mefford et al. (2009)
16p13.11 dup	Chr16: 15.0–16.3	Ullmann et al. (2007), Mefford et al. (2009)
17q12 del	Chr17: 34.8–36.3	Moreno-De-Luca et al. (2010), Nagamani et al. (2010)
17q21.3 del	Chr17: 43.7–44.3	Koolen et al. (2008)
22q11.2 distal del	Chr22: 21.8–23.7	Ben-Shachar et al. (2008)
22q11.2 distal dup	Chr22: 21.8–23.7	Descartes et al. (2008)

*Newly described syndromes since 2006.
del, deletion; dup, duplication.

Charman, T., Pickles, A., et al. (2011b). IQ in children with autism spectrum disorders: data from the Special Needs and Autism Project (SNAP). *Psychol. Med.* 41(3):619–627.

Charman, T. (2011c). Commentary: glass half full or half empty? Testing social communication interventions for young children with autism: reflections on Landa, Holman, O'Neill, and Stuart. *J. Child Psychol. Psychiatry* 52(1):22–23.

Coffey, B.J., and Park, K.S. (1997). Behavioral and emotional aspects of Tourette syndrome. *Neurol. Clin.* 15(2):277–289.

Collins, F.S., Guyer, M.S., et al. (1997). Variations on a theme: cataloging human DNA sequence variation. *Science* 278(5343):1580–1581.

Constantino, J.N., Davis, S.A., et al. (2003). Validation of a brief quantitative measure of autistic traits: comparison of the social responsiveness scale with the autism diagnostic interview-revised. *J. Autism Dev. Disord.* 33(4):427–433.

Constantino, J.N., Lajonchere, C., et al. (2006). Autistic social impairment in the siblings of children with pervasive developmental disorders. *Am. J. Psychiatry* 163(2):294–296.

Constantino, J.N., and Todd, R.D. (2003). Autistic traits in the general population: a twin study. *Arch. Gen. Psychiatry* 60(5):524–530.

Constantino, J.N., Zhang, Y., et al. (2010). Sibling recurrence and the genetic epidemiology of autism. *Am. J. Psychiatry* 167(11):1349–1356.

Croen, L.A., Grether, J.K., et al. (2011). Antidepressant use during pregnancy and childhood autism spectrum disorders. *Arch. Gen. Psychiatry* 68(11):1104–1112.

Dawson, G., Rogers, S., et al. (2010). Randomized, controlled trial of an intervention for toddlers with autism: the Early Start Denver Model. *Pediatrics* 125(1):e17–23.

Deary, I.J., Yang, J., et al. (2012). Genetic contributions to stability and change in intelligence from childhood to old age. *Nature* 482(7384):212–215.

Eaves, L.C., and Ho, H.H. (1996). Brief report: stability and change in cognitive and behavioral characteristics of autism through childhood. *J. Autism. Dev. Disord.* 26(5):557–569.

Einfeld, S.L., Ellis, L.A., et al. (2011). Comorbidity of intellectual disability and mental disorder in children and adolescents: a systematic review. *J. Intellect. Dev. Disabil.* 36(2):137–143.

Elsabbagh, M., Divan, G., et al. (2012). Global prevalence of autism and other pervasive developmental disorders. *Autism Res.* 5(3):160–179.

Faraone, S.V., Biederman, J., et al. (2006). The age-dependent decline of attention deficit hyperactivity disorder: a meta-analysis of follow-up studies. *Psychol. Med.* 36(2):159–165.

Faraone, S.V., Perlis, R.H., et al. (2005). Molecular genetics of attention-deficit/hyperactivity disorder. *Biol. Psychiatry* 57(11):1313–1323.

Faraone, S.V., Sergeant, J., et al. (2003). The worldwide prevalence of ADHD: is it an American condition? *World Psychiatry* 2(2):104–113.

Feinstein, A.R. (1970). The pre-therapeutic classification of comorbidity in chronic disease. *J. Chron. Dis.* (23):455–468.

Folstein, S.E., and Piven, J. (1991). Etiology of autism: genetic influences. *Pediatrics* 87(5 Pt 2):767–773.

Fombonne, E. (2003). Epidemiological surveys of autism and other pervasive developmental disorders: an update. *J. Autism Dev. Disord.* 33(4):365–382.

Fountain, C., Winter, A.S., et al. (2012). Six developmental trajectories characterize children with autism. *Pediatrics* 129(5):e1112–1120.

Ganz, M.L. (2007). The lifetime distribution of the incremental societal costs of autism. *Arch. Pediatr. Adolesc. Med.* 161(4):343–349.

Gillberg, C., and Billstedt, E. (2000). Autism and Asperger syndrome: coexistence with other clinical disorders. *Acta Psychiatr. Scand.* 102(5):321–330.

Gilles de la Tourette, G., Goetz, C.G., et al. (1982). Etude sur une affection nerveuse caracterisee par de l'incoordination motrice accompagnee d'echolalie et de coprolalie. *Adv. Neurol.* 35:1–16.

Gimpel, G.A., and Kuhn, B.R. (2000). Maternal report of attention deficit hyperactivity disorder symptoms in preschool children. *Child Care Health Dev.* 26(3):163–176; discussion 176–169.

Girirajan, S., Brkanac, Z., et al. (2011). Relative burden of large CNVs on a range of neurodevelopmental phenotypes. *PLoS Genet.* 7(11):e1002334.

Goodman, R., Ford, T., et al. (2000). Using the Strengths and Difficulties Questionnaire (SDQ) to screen for child psychiatric disorders in a community sample. *Br. J. Psychiatry* 177:534–539.

Grados, M.A., and Mathews, C.A. (2009). Clinical phenomenology and phenotype variability in Tourette syndrome. *J. Psychosom. Res.* 67(6):491–496.

Graetz, B.W., Sawyer, M.G., et al. (2001). Validity of DSM-IV ADHD subtypes in a nationally representative sample of Australian children and adolescents. *J. Am. Acad. Child Adolesc. Psychiatry* 40(12):1410–1417.

Hallmayer, J., Cleveland, S., et al. (2011). Genetic heritability and shared environmental factors among twin pairs with autism. *Arch. Gen. Psychiatry* 68(11):1095–1102.

Hansson, S.L., Svanstrom Rojvall, A., et al. (2005). Psychiatric telephone interview with parents for screening of childhood autism: tics, attention-deficit hyperactivity disorder and other comorbidities (A-TAC): preliminary reliability and validity. *Br. J. Psychiatry* 187:262–267.

Haworth, C.M., Wright, M.J., et al. (2010). The heritability of general cognitive ability increases linearly from childhood to young adulthood. *Mol. Psychiatry* 15(11):1112–1120.

Hudziak, J.J., Heath, A.C., et al. (1998). Latent class and factor analysis of DSM-IV ADHD: a twin study of female adolescents. *J. Am. Acad. Child Adolesc. Psychiatry* 37(8):848–857.

International HapMap Consortium. (2005). A haplotype map of the human genome. *Nature* 437(7063):1299–1320.

Irving, C., Basu, A., et al. (2008). Twenty-year trends in prevalence and survival of Down syndrome. *Eur. J. Hum. Genet.* 16(11):1336–1340.

Kimura, M., and Ota, T. (1973). The age of a neutral mutant persisting in a finite population. *Genetics* 75(1):199–212.

King, M., and Bearman, P. (2009). Diagnostic change and the increased prevalence of autism. *Int. J. Epidemiol.* 38(5):1224–1234.

Knapp, M., Romeo, R., et al. (2009). Economic cost of autism in the UK. *Autism* 13(3):317–336.

Kuntsi, J., Rijsdijk, F., et al. (2005). Genetic influences on the stability of attention-deficit/hyperactivity disorder symptoms from early to middle childhood. *Biol. Psychiatry* 57(6):647–654.

Kurlan, R., McDermott, M.P., et al. (2001). Prevalence of tics in schoolchildren and association with placement in special education. *Neurology* 57(8):1383–1388.

Lander, E.S., and Schork, N.J. (1994). Genetic dissection of complex traits. *Science* 265(5181):2037–2048.

Larsson, H., Anckarsater, H., et al. (2011a). Childhood attention-deficit hyperactivity disorder as an extreme of a continuous trait: a quantitative genetic study of 8,500 twin pairs. *J. Child Psychol. Psychiatry* 53(1):73–80.

Larsson, H., Anckarsater, H., et al. (2012). Childhood attention-deficit hyperactivity disorder as an extreme of a continuous trait: a quantitative genetic study of 8,500 twin pairs. *J. Child Psychol. Psychiatry* 53(1):73–80.

Larsson, H., Dilshad, R., et al. (2011b). Developmental trajectories of DSM-IV symptoms of attention-deficit/hyperactivity disorder: genetic effects, family risk and associated psychopathology. *J. Child Psychol. Psychiatry* 52(9):954–963.

Leibson, C.L., Katusic, S.K., et al. (2001). Use and costs of medical care for children and adolescents with and without attention-deficit/hyperactivity disorder. *JAMA* 285(1):60–66.

Lejeune, J., Turpin, R., et al. (1959). [Mongolism; a chromosomal disease (trisomy)]. *Bull. Acad. Natl. Med.* 143(11–12):256–265.

Leonard, H., and Wen, X. (2002). The epidemiology of mental retardation: challenges and opportunities in the new millennium. *Ment. Retard Dev. Disabil. Res. Rev.* 8(3):117–134.

Lewontin, R. (1972). The apportionment of human diversity. In: Dobzhansky, T., Hecht, M.K., and Steere, W.C., eds. Evolutionary Biology, 6th Edition. New York: Appleton-Century-Crofts, pp. 381–398.

Lichtenstein, P., Carlstrom, E., et al. (2010). The genetics of autism spectrum disorders and related neuropsychiatric disorders in childhood. *Am. J. Psychiatry* 167(11):1357–1363.

Lord, C., Risi, S., et al. (2006). Autism from 2 to 9 years of age. *Arch. Gen. Psychiatry* 63(6):694–701.

Lord, C., and Schopler, E. (1985). Differences in sex ratios in autism as a function of measured intelligence. *J. Autism Dev. Disord.* 15(2):185–193.

Lossie, A.C., and Driscoll, D.J. (1999). Transmission of Angelman syndrome by an affected mother. *Genet. Med.* 1(6):262–266.

Lundstrom, S., Chang, Z., et al. (2012). Autism spectrum disorders and autisticlike traits: similar etiology in the extreme end and the normal variation. *Arch. Gen. Psychiatry* 69(1):46–52.

Maj, M. (2005). "Psychiatric comorbidity": an artefact of current diagnostic systems? *Br. J. Psychiatry* 186:182–184.

Malhotra, D., and Sebat, J. (2012). CNVs: harbingers of a rare variant revolution in psychiatric genetics. *Cell* 148(6):1223–1241.

Mathews, C.A., and Grados, M.A. (2011). Familiality of Tourette syndrome, obsessive-compulsive disorder, and attention-deficit/hyperactivity disorder: heritability analysis in a large sib-pair sample. *J. Am. Acad. Child Adolesc. Psychiatry* 50(1):46–54.

McCarthy, S.E., Makarov, V., et al. (2009). Microduplications of 16p11.2 are associated with schizophrenia. *Nat. Genet.* 41(11):1223–1227.

McGovern, C.W., and Sigman, M. (2005). Continuity and change from early childhood to adolescence in autism. *J. Child Psychol. Psychiatry* 46(4):401–408.

Mefford, H.C., Batshaw, M.L., et al. (2012). Genomics, intellectual disability, and autism. *N. Engl. J. Med.* 366(8):733–743.

Merikangas, K.R., He, J.P., et al. (2010). Lifetime prevalence of mental disorders in U.S. adolescents: results from the National Comorbidity Survey case of severe ID, it appears to play a reduced role in idiopathic ASDs and has not been documented to contribute substantially to ADHD or TD. The high heritability of the latter three, particularly ASD and ADHD, suggests some substantial role for inherited and somewhat more common variation. If we contrast the published efforts to date in ASD, ADHD, and TD with those in schizophrenia (as well as particularly polygenic and complex non-psychiatric diseases and phenotypes such as type 2 diabetes, coronary artery disease, and adult stature), a consistent pattern emerges. In all of these cases with similar high heritabilities, early GWAS studies of one to a few thousand cases failed to reject the null hypothesis that any common variants were associated to disease risk. Much larger collaborative studies that followed, however, were able to define many distinct and replicated associated loci. In each case, these studies provided novel insight into the biology of the diseases in question. This is of course not proof that such insights will be forthcoming in childhood neuropsychiatric disorders, but the productivity of schizophrenia GWAS after early "failure" suggests that further investment may be warranted in tandem with the focus on rare variation.

CONCLUSIONS

Research approaches that integrate the levels of evidence introduced in the preceding sections are likely to improve the efficacy of genetic inquiries into child neuropsychiatric conditions. Behaviorally defined disorders are characterized by enormous genetic complexity, and inferences drawn from epidemiological and family data, as well as classic genetic theory, can be used in concert to begin parsing that variation. The ASD literature presented here provides an example of such a collaborative logical trajectory. Autism spectrum disorders as currently defined exist across a broad range of severities, including phenotypes that both do and do not confer substantial reproductive disadvantage. Although the etiological structure of the disorders is unlikely to fall cleanly along these phenotypic lines, family and twin data are consistent with such a pattern in that they suggest that ASDs exist in both familial and non-familial forms (and likely in the space in between). These patterns can be used to justify a tandem approach of genetic investigation, focusing on both common and rare variants, consistent with the relationship between genetic architecture and reproductive disadvantage, as it has been observed more broadly within genomic inquiry.

Large sample, multidisciplinary collaborations designed to uncover the biology underlying neuropsychiatric disorders in children are already in progress. Following lessons from the progress emerging from larger, adult psychiatric consortia, it is very likely that continued efforts along these lines will be necessary to elucidate the complete genetic architecture of each disorder, as well as to progress to a full understanding of the relationship between etiologically linked phenotypes.

DISCLOSURES

Dr. Daly's research into childhood psychiatric disorders is currently funded through grants from the NIMH and NHGRI and a philanthropic gift from the Gerstner Foundation. In the past year Dr. Daly has consulted with Pfizer, Inc. and Eisai Pharmaceuticals. Grant Support: R01 NS 059727 NIH; 1R01 DK083756-1 NIH/NIEHS; 2P30DK043351-21 NIH/NIDDK; R01AI091649-01AI NIH/NIAID; 1R01MH09443201 NIH/NIMH; 5R01DK064869-09 NIH/NIDDK; 1R01MH089208-01 NIH/NIMH; 1R01MH094469 NIH/NIMH; P40 RR12305 NIH/NCBI; U01HG006569 NIH/NHGRI; I5-A523 Starr Cancer Consortium.

Dr. Neale has no conflicts of interest to disclose. He is funded by the NIMH, the Gerstner Foundation, and the Stanley Center for Psychiatric Research. Grant support: 5R01MH080403-03S1 NIH/NIMH; 1R01MH09443201 NIH/NIMH; 1R01MH089208-01 NIH/NIMH; 1R01MH094469 NIH/NIMH.

Dr. Robinson has no conflicts of interest to disclose. She is funded by Massachusetts General Hospital.

REFERENCES

Anderson, D.K., Lord, C., et al. (2007). Patterns of growth in verbal abilities among children with autism spectrum disorder. *J. Consult. Clin. Psychol.* 75(4):594–604.

APA. (2000). Diagnostic and Statistic Manual of Mental Disorders, 4th Edition. Washington, DC: American Psychological Association.

Baird, G., Simonoff, E., et al. (2006). Prevalence of disorders of the autism spectrum in a population cohort of children in South Thames: the Special Needs and Autism Project (SNAP). *Lancet* 368(9531):210–215.

Barbaresi, W.J., and Olsen, R.D. (1998). An ADHD educational intervention for elementary schoolteachers: a pilot study. *J. Dev. Behav. Pediatr.* 19(2):94–100.

Barkley, R.A., Fischer, M., et al. (2004). Young adult follow-up of hyperactive children: antisocial activities and drug use. *J. Child Psychol. Psychiatry* 45(2):195–211.

Baron-Cohen, S., Scott, F.J., et al. (2009). Prevalence of autism-spectrum conditions: UK school-based population study. *Br. J. Psychiatry* 194(6):500–509.

Baumgaertel, A., Wolraich, M.L., et al. (1995). Comparison of diagnostic criteria for attention deficit disorders in a German elementary school sample. *J. Am. Acad. Child Adolesc. Psychiatry* 34(5):629–638.

Betancur, C. (2011). Etiological heterogeneity in autism spectrum disorders: more than 100 genetic and genomic disorders and still counting. *Brain Res.* 1380:42–77.

Biederman, J., Faraone, S., et al. (1996). Predictors of persistence and remission of ADHD into adolescence: results from a four-year prospective follow-up study. *J. Am. Acad. Child Adolesc. Psychiatry* 35(3):343–351.

Biederman, J., Mick, E., et al. (2000). Age-dependent decline of symptoms of attention deficit hyperactivity disorder: impact of remission definition and symptom type. *Am. J. Psychiatry* 157(5):816–818.

Biederman, J., Petty, C.R., et al. (2010). Adult psychiatric outcomes of girls with attention deficit hyperactivity disorder: 11-year follow-up in a longitudinal case-control study. *Am. J. Psychiatry* 167(4):409–417.

Brugha, T.S., McManus, S., et al. (2011). Epidemiology of autism spectrum disorders in adults in the community in England. *Arch. Gen. Psychiatry* 68(5):459–465.

Cavanna, A.E., David, K., et al. (2012). Predictors during childhood of future health-related quality of life in adults with Gilles de la Tourette syndrome. *Eur. J. Paediatr. Neurol.* 16(6):605–612.

Cavanna, A.E., Servo, S., et al. (2009). The behavioral spectrum of Gilles de la Tourette syndrome. *J. Neuropsychiatry Clin. Neurosci.* 21(1):13–23.

Centers for Disease Control and Prevention. (2012). Prevalence of autism spectrum disorders: Autism and Developmental Disabilities Monitoring Network, 14 sites, United States, 2008. *MMWR Surveill. Summ.* 61(3):1–19.

Chakrabarti, S., and Fombonne, E. (2005). Pervasive developmental disorders in preschool children: confirmation of high prevalence. *Am. J. Psychiatry* 162(6):1133–1141.

Charman, T. (2011a). The highs and lows of counting autism. *Am. J. Psychiatry* 168(9):873–875.

also occasionally seen bearing the mutations. Accordingly, although risk conferred is quite high (approximate odds ratios of 10 to 20), the penetrances for any specific outcome are generally less than 50%. In these two properties, the risk variants discovered in large case-control studies (generally focusing on large, idiopathic population samples of cases) seem distinct from those relevant to the rare mendelian genomic syndromes. Such syndromes usually are caused by high penetrance events and have an extremely specific set of comorbidities and features that make them clinically recognizable often in advance of conclusive genetic testing.

Related to this, a considerable number of specific, single-gene genetic syndromes have been described that feature unusually high rates of ID or ASD (Betancur, 2011). Although some of these are rare and apparently fully penetrant entities such as Rett syndrome, a severe form of autism most often caused by mutations in one copy of MECP2 or CDKL5 on one X chromosome in girls (these mutations are usually lethal prenatally in boys), most have far less than complete penetrance. Noteworthy examples among these in the case of ASDs include Fragile X and tuberous sclerosis complex (TSC) (Folstein and Piven, 1991), specific and long-identified Mendelian syndromes with high rates of ASD. Similar to the CNVs described in the preceding, however, fewer than 50% of cases manifest ASDs. Although many such rare genetic syndromes are now identified, taken in total they likely explain only a small percentage of idiopathic ASDs.

Figure 70.1 shows the relationship between effect size and frequency for CNVs associated to ASD and the first common variants identified in schizophrenia at genome-wide significance. The CNVs clearly confer much greater risk, but are only present in a small fraction of cases. The common variants are selected from schizophrenia, to illustrate the effect sizes of common variants typical of psychiatric phenotypes. As sample sizes continue to increase for GWAS for these traits, further clues are likely to be revealed in the biological basis of these diseases.

The massively parallel genome sequencing technologies that have become available since 2010 have it possible to sequence the roughly 1% of the human genome that encodes proteins (the exome). Autism spectrum disorders are among the first disorders for which this approach has been utilized in substantial numbers of cases and indeed, by sequencing parents and children, recent studies have documented excesses of *de novo* loss-of-function mutations in cases when compared with either control individuals (Sanders et al., 2012) or mutational expectations (Neale et al., 2012; O'Roak et al., 2012). Although these early studies suggest that only a minority (<20%) of cases harbor relevant spontaneously arising mutations, they do have the ability to pinpoint specific genes relevant to ASD risk. Overall, however, these studies reinforce estimates from the CNV work that hundreds of genes likely contribute to ASD risk. Although large-scale studies have not yet been performed in the other childhood psychiatric disorders, earlier studies of X-linked mental retardation (Tarpey et al., 2009) similarly concluded that relevant mutations are likely distributed across many genes, resulting in a situation that will inevitably require considerable sample sizes on which to provide clarity.

As noted, GWAS has far and away been the most productive avenue toward insight into the genetics of unquestionably polygenic common diseases. Common variation, as assessed by GWAS, has yet to provide compelling findings in the case of any of the childhood neuropsychiatric disorders. Although the role of rare and spontaneous mutations may well dominate in the

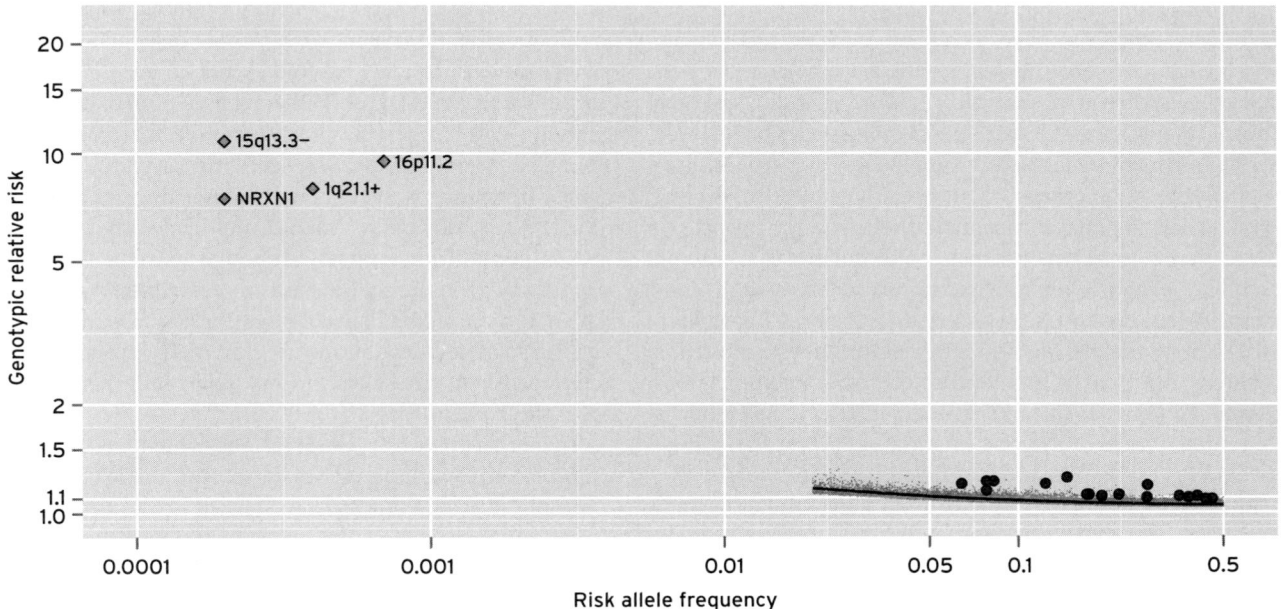

Figure 70.1 The risk allele frequency is plotted against the genotypic relative risk for the copy number variations identified in autism spectrum disorder along with single nucleotide polymorphisms associated at genome-wide significance for schizophrenia. The specific copy number variations identified are 15q33.3 deletion, deletions at NRXN1, 1q21.1 duplications, and both deletions and duplications at 16p11.2 (Malhotra and Sebat, 2012). These events confer strong risk to ASD in contrast to the identified genome-wide significant loci from schizophrenia (Ripke et al., 2011). (Thanks to P.F. Sullivan for concept and underlying data.)

genetic associations have been defined since the first GWAS studies were initiated in 2005–2006 and, in the vast majority of cases, the associations were novel and therefore harbored unique insights into the pathogenesis of disease. It is noteworthy that most of these discoveries emerged in diseases and phenotypes only when very large sample sizes were assessed, often after initial smaller studies had not revealed any replicable, significant associations. Thus, a collective picture that has emerged from GWAS studies is one of extreme polygenicity for the complex disorders studied in which individual contributing alleles are of extremely modest effect and provide little predictive information about individual risk. Collectively, however, they can reveal novel insights into the pathways and processes of disease.

Negative reproductive selection is likely to be acting on severe forms of autism and intellectual disability (Uher, 2009). Although formal studies estimating the specific degree of reproductive disadvantage associated with these conditions have not been conducted, it is widely accepted that individuals with these phenotypes produce offspring far less often than the population average. Bolstered by classical examples of the role of major sporadic chromosomal anomalies in similar phenotypes such as Down syndrome, this observation has led to a substantial and sensible focus on the role of spontaneously arising (so-called de novo) DNA variants in ASD and ID. At the same time, large GWAS studies have also been undertaken, and draw considerable hope from the example of schizophrenia. Schizophrenia has a similar prevalence and estimated selective disadvantage (approximately 50% reduced fecundity) (Svensson et al., 2007). Genome-wide association studies of schizophrenia have proved, at large sample sizes, to be able to demonstrate specific compelling associations and to establish a significant global role for common as well as rare variation. It is not incongruous that common variation can be associated to a common and reproductively deleterious phenotype. In the case of extremely polygenic phenotypes, an obligate relationship between allele frequency and reproductive advantage is precluded by each of: the modest contributions of individual loci; unknown interactions that may exist among genes or between genes and environmental factors; and the other (perhaps positive) phenotypic outcomes that may be influenced by some of the risk variation. Take for example the predominant role of common variation in type I diabetes, and the mix of common, rare, and de novo variation in Hirschsprung disease—both conditions that had extreme selection against them owing to high lethality before modern medical interventions developed in the last century. The genetic architecture of these conditions does not stand in stark violation of fundamental principles but is likely representative of the mix of variation types that will be uncovered in childhood neuropsychiatric disease.

The insights attained to date from the early studies of both common and rare DNA variation are outlined in the next section and more thoroughly delineated in subsequent sections of the book. Of note, the accepted negative selection attributable to ID and ASD does not carry over into ADHD and TD, where no perceived reproductive disadvantage resides. As noted, however, strong etiological overlaps likely exist between each of these disorders. We fully expect that overlap to manifest

itself in considerable shared genetic risk factors of both a common and rare variety.

EMPIRICAL INSIGHTS INTO THE GENETIC ARCHITECTURE OF CHILDHOOD PSYCHIATRIC DISORDERS

The most compelling evidence compiled to date with respect to neuropsychiatric disorders of childhood onset surrounds the role of large and predominantly spontaneously arising chromosomal abnormalities and copy number variants. Down syndrome (trisomy 21) is the most common and widely recognized karyotypic abnormality associated with ID but, in recent years, many such findings have emerged as substantial components of both ASD and ID more broadly. Many additional syndromes (e.g., Prader–Willi/Angelman, Williams syndrome, DiGeorge/velocardiofacial syndrome) result from specific recurrent copy number variants. Genome-wide, gross chromosomal abnormalities (Sanders et al., 2011; Vorstman et al., 2006) and even balanced translocations (Talkowski et al., 2012) have been documented as strongly enriched in both ID and ASD. However, as most such events are rare and seen only in individual cases, certainty is generally lacking that individual events are causative. In addition, because these events are most often large and delete, duplicate, or disrupt many genes, biological insights have been slow to emerge in many cases.

Recent surveys (Girirajan et al., 2011) have clearly demonstrated that the burden of CNVs in ID is considerably greater than in ASDs. In particular, large CNVs (>1 Mb) are observed in four to five times as many instances of ID-related phenotypes than in ASDs, although the distinction between syndromic and non-syndromic forms of ID is not always made, and there could be more CNVs associated with syndromic ID (or ASDs). Overall, rare CNVs (seen in roughly 2% of the general population) are observed in 10% of ASD cases and 16% of IDs. A more modest, roughly twofold excess of rare CNVs has also been observed in ADHD (Williams et al., 2010, 2012). Thus, emerging data suggest a convincing role for rare, primarily spontaneous, CNVs but to significantly varying degrees. The highest frequency is in ID, then to lesser degrees respectively in ASD + ID, ASD alone, ADHD, and likely other less deleterious childhood phenotypes. Although it is still early in the use of many genomic analysis techniques (e.g., GWAS, genome sequencing), it seems plausible that these observations represent the relative contribution of extremely rare and de novo variation versus more common, older inherited variation across these phenotypes.

Two other important observations, which are also likely to extend to other variation types, have been made convincingly as sample sizes and studies have grown across many distinct clinical end points. First, the majority of CNVs that have been associated with ASDs have independently been demonstrated to confer risk to other, apparently unrelated phenotypes such as schizophrenia or epilepsy (Sebat et al., 2009). This suggests pointedly that most of these mutations confer risk to a very broad set of phenotypes, rather than a clinically specific one. Second, for most of these CNVs, healthy adult controls are subclinical behavioral impairment. In other words, pleiotropy may extend to levels of affectation. It is believed that both common and rare genetic variants influence liability toward autism and ADHD, so these possibilities cannot be disentangled in the context of phenotypic family data.

PHENOTYPIC AND ETIOLOGIC RELATIONSHIPS AMONG CHILDHOOD PSYCHIATRIC DISORDERS

Neuropsychiatric disorders of childhood appear together far more often than predicted by chance. Among the phenotypes discussed in this chapter, most individuals with ASDs meet criteria for additional developmental or behavioral disorders such as ADHD, anxiety disorders, or intellectual disabilities (Gillberg and Billstedt, 2000; Lichtenstein et al., 2010; Simonoff et al., 2008; Volkmar et al., 1999). Intellectual disabilities themselves are similarly associated with an increased risk for a wide range of mental health conditions (Einfeld et al., 2011), and Tourette syndrome often co-occurs with ADHD and OCD (Mathews and Grados, 2011).

Twin and molecular genetic studies suggest that shared genetic risk factors are contributing substantially to the disorders' co-occurrence. Using the twin method, Lichtenstein et al. (2010) estimated that ASDs share approximately three-fourths of their genetic variance with ADHD, one-half of their genetic variance with intellectual disabilities, and one-third of their genetic variance with tic disorder. The authors further noted that the genetic influences on ADHD are highly correlated with those on tic disorder, a finding that has since been replicated in family studies (Mathews and Grados, 2011). Molecular genetic analyses have similarly indicated that the etiological influences on child neuropsychiatric disorders are unlikely to exclusively predict the phenotypes circumscribed by the DSM. For example, virtually every genetic variant that has been associated with ASDs is also associated with intellectual disabilities (Betancur, 2011); several of the notable rare variants are also risk factors for other major psychiatric disorders (McCarthy et al., 2009; Weiss et al., 2008).

Genetic relationships between the disorders raise questions about research approach. More often than not, investigations into ASDs, ADHD, and Tourette are conducted independently. This model is consistent with the classical approach to comorbidity, a term originally designed to indicate distinct, co-occurring medical problems (Feinstein, 1970). The etiological overlap described in the preceding section, however, suggests that conceptualizing multiple psychiatric disorders as comorbid could be "artificially splitting a complex clinical condition into several pieces" (Maj, 2005).

Large multidisorder research initiatives, such as the Psychiatric Genomics Consortium (PGC), are able to investigate etiological factors that may be shared across neuropsychiatric conditions. With the identification of genetic risk factors, broadly phenotyped samples provide the opportunity to potentially shed insight into the disorders' underlying biological and behavioral processes.

REPRODUCTIVE DISADVANTAGE AND GENETIC ARCHITECTURE

Reproductive disadvantage provides a major influence on the genetic architecture of disorders that are, on average, associated with reduced fecundity. In the simplest case, autosomal-recessive diseases that are lethal in childhood are defined by allelic spectra consisting of rare mutations. This occurs because of the consistently lower than chance probability of the alleles being passed on in each generation. Generally, such genetic variants are seen at less than 0.1% in population frequency, but they can be significantly more frequent in instances in which an advantage is conferred to heterozygote carriers (e.g., Hb mutations that confer resistance to malaria in heterozygotes but sickle cell disease in homozygotes). These alleles may also have been previously favorably selected in alternate environmental conditions or appeared recently in bottlenecked or isolated populations (e.g., Finns, Ashkenazi Jews, Quebecois from Saguenay-Lac St. Jean), where they received a chance boost to high frequency and are still early in the many hundreds of generations selection takes to inexorably push them down. As a consequence, gene mapping efforts in diseases associated with reproductive disadvantage are designed with a focus on rare and spontaneously arising variation.

By contrast, and consistent with classical theory (Kimura and Ota, 1973), humans have limited genetic variation. Considering two copies of the human genome, the heterozygosity rate for single nucleotide polymorphisms (SNPs) is approximately one in 1,000 bases (Sachidanandam et al., 2001) and roughly 90% of those heterozygous sites in each individual are common DNA variants. The variants are typically seen in multiple, diverse populations and show evidence of having existed for thousands of generations (Lewontin, 1972; International Hapmap Consortium, 2005). High frequency of an allele does not by any means rule it out as a contributing factor in diseases with reproductive disadvantage. However, it does indicate that the allele itself is not under strong selective disadvantage and limits the individual impact it could have in a reproductively deleterious phenotype. It is also important to note that mildly deleterious alleles can persist at intermediate allele frequencies, particularly under the conditions described that moderate the relationship between selection and frequency.

With these observations in mind, human genetics has been drawn to the common disease-common variant hypothesis, which suggests a role for common DNA polymorphisms (>1% in population frequency) in the genetic architecture of common and complex human diseases (Collins et al., 1997; Lander and Schork, 1994; Risch and Merikangas, 1996). This hypothesis produced the subsequent proposal that genome-wide association studies (GWAS) of common human diseases might yield, for the first time, specific genetic insights into complex human disease. Genome-wide association studies are powered by massively parallel array–based genotyping technologies that permit the evaluation of hundreds of thousands of common DNA variants simultaneously. Alongside the construction of maps of common variation and linkage disequilibrium patterns across the genome, GWAS has delivered myriad insights into common diseases. As of the end of 2011, more than 1,500 exist as extreme positions of phenotypic continua (Larsson et al., 2011a; Lundstrom et al., 2012; Robinson et al., 2011a). This section reviews some of that evidence, concentrating on studies that link the genetic influences on major behavioral impairment to typical variation in traits of those disorders (e.g., autistic behavior, traits of hyperactivity/inattentiveness).

Because intelligence is measured on a continuum, much like height or weight, it is natural to think of intellectual disability as an extreme position on that distribution. The point below which an individual meets criteria for ID, however, is in many ways arbitrary, a problem common to categorical cutoffs superimposed on continuous distributions. Although an IQ of 70 is typically employed as the clinical threshold (APA, 2000), there is no clear biological or phenotypic break point that indicates where the boundary of "meaningfully" disordered cognition should lie. In other words, identifying the position on the IQ distribution below which a person has ID is no simpler than identifying the position on the height distribution above which a person is tall.

Only recently have researchers begun to consider the degree to which major psychiatric disorders may similarly exist as extreme positions on behavioral distributions. Diseases like autism and ADHD have traditionally been thought of as categorical clinical entities that one either has or does not have. However, traits typical of many behavioral disorders occur commonly at subthreshold levels in the general population as well as "deficits" characterizing many of these clinical phenotypes (Constantino and Todd, 2003; Goodman et al., 2000; Ronald et al., 2008; Skuse et al., 2005).

Autistic traits provide a useful example as they have been studied extensively over the last decade. Autistic trait measures are designed to capture the extent to which an individual manifests characteristics of the clinical ASD phenotype. These measures aim to assess the extent of social impairment, communication impairment, and restricted and repetitive behaviors and interests that a person displays (Constantino et al., 2003; Scott et al., 2002). When autistic trait scores are estimated in large samples of people in the general population, the distribution is typically skewed. The bulk of the population displays few if any autism-like behaviors, with a declining distribution to individuals that endorse a high number of traits, at or above the level that is on average associated with clinical ASD (Robinson et al., 2011a, 2011b). Using these trait measures, however, does not reveal a distinction between the clinical and subclinical levels of autism-like behavior. This pattern mimics the IQ distribution leading to intellectual disability (Constantino and Todd, 2003; Ronald et al., 2006).

Traits of ADHD can be measured in a similar way (Hansson et al., 2005) using a variety of instruments. The Conner's Rating Scale, for example, aims to assess the presence and severity of symptoms recognized in the clinical phenotype. The Swan Rating Scale, in contrast, attempts to characterize individuals on a more normal scale of activity level, impulsivity, and attention. Consequently, the distribution of the Conner's ADHD scale tends to be J-shaped, whereas the Swan is considerably more normally distributed. For each of these measures,

children with an ADHD diagnosis lie within the most affected tail (Larsson et al., 2011a).

The study of general population traits will only be informative with respect to disease processes if there is an etiological link between the extreme or categorical phenotype (e.g., ASDs) and the behavioral continuum (e.g., autistic traits in the general population). In the case of both ASDs and ADHD, evidence is building that such a link exists. Empirically, there is a high degree of consistency between clinically significant and subclinical levels of impairment. Much like the ASD diagnosis, autistic trait scores in the general population are highly stable over time (Robinson et al., 2011b; St Pourcain et al., 2011). Longitudinal studies of traits of ADHD suggest similar coherence with the clinical diagnosis (Biederman et al., 1996, 2000; Faraone et al., 2006).

On the whole, traits of ADHD are moderately stable across development (Kuntsi et al., 2005; Larsson et al., 2011b).

Many studies suggest a shared etiology between Robinson the clinical phenotypes of ASDs and ADHD and their respective behavioral continua. If autism and ADHD are extreme positions on quantitative distributions, two primary conditions should hold. The estimated heritability of traits of each disorder should be approximately equivalent to the estimated heritability of the clinical phenotype, and a clinical diagnosis should predict increased trait scores in family members of the proband. With respect to overall heritability, there is a substantial body of literature suggesting that this is the case. Like ASDs, autistic traits are moderately to highly heritable (Ronald and Hoekstra, 2011). Similarly, like ADHD, traits of hyperactivity and inattentiveness are consistently highly heritable (Larsson et al., 2011a). Autism spectrum disorders and ADHD also show the predicted pattern of increased trait burden in family members. In the case of ASDs, it has been noted for more than a decade that the family members of people with autism, on average, display more autistic traits than the family members of people without autism (Constantino et al., 2006, 2010; Piven et al., 1997). Twin studies can be used to examine the extent to which that pattern might be secondary to genetic influences that are shared between levels of affectation. Two large, general population twin studies recently reported evidence of strong genetic overlap between severely impairing autistic behavior and subclinical autistic traits (Lundstrom et al., 2012; Robinson et al., 2011a). In a similar analysis, Larsson et al. (2012) evidenced a genetic link between clinically diagnosed ADHD and traits typical of the disorder as they are distributed continuously.

These patterns can be interpreted in a number of ways and, in so doing, it is important to bear in mind the established etiological heterogeneity of neuropsychiatric conditions (Betancur, 2011). On the one hand, etiological overlap between the clinical (extreme) phenotype and the continuum could be interpreted as evidence that relevant *common* genetic variants act across the behavioral distribution, influencing both normal trait variation in the general population and the probability with which an individual will meet criteria for clinical disorder. On the other, these results are also consistent with the model in which *rare* (and potentially unique), familial genetic variants that increase risk for autism and ADHD can also predict had yet to become common (Brugha et al., 2011). Studies such as these do not, however, preclude the possibility of a "true" increase in prevalence, and the degree to which current data may reflect such a trend is unknown.

The estimated prevalence of certain types of intellectual disability, discussed in the preceding, may also change with diagnostic climate. Although ID to ASD diagnostic substitution does not account for the majority of the increase in ASD prevalence, it has clearly made a substantial contribution. Using data from the California Department of Developmental Services, King and Bearman (2009) estimated that one-fourth of the observed increase in ASD prevalence in California between 1992 and 2005 was a direct consequence of diagnostic exchange between ID and ASD (King and Bearman, 2009). These changes are likely to have implications for the etiological structure and pathophysiological heterogeneity of ASDs.

The male to female ratio among individuals with an ASD diagnosis is approximately 4:1. The overall ratio, however, obscures a substantial sex by IQ interaction in the population distribution of the disorder. Among individuals with ASDs who have very low IQ, the male to female ratio is closer to 2:1. In cases with above average IQ, the ratio is much higher, likely 6:1 or above (Fombonne, 2003; Skuse, 2009). This trend has held constant across the period of prevalence increase (Lord and Schopler, 1985). Because much of the recent diagnostic expansion has occurred within the high functioning range (Rutter), several population-based studies have begun to report overall male:female ratios that are higher than 4:1 (Brugha et al., 2011; Williams et al., 2008). Although some of the sex by IQ interaction likely reflects greater ascertainment probabilities in boys (Russell et al., 2010), above average cognitive abilities do appear to confer greater ASD protection to women (at least as the diagnostic category is currently defined). Although the data are strong that some etiological overlap exists between ASDs and ID, ascertainment considerations do preclude a conclusive interpretation of population data. In fact, it has been proposed that the observed correlation between ID and ASD could be in part explained by the fact the presence of both in an individual dramatically increases the chance of the individual being ascertained owing to severe impairment (Skuse, 2007). This thesis is not inconsistent with the high rate of identification of IQ-normative ASD in adults who were not ascertained as children in the Brugha study (Brugha et al., 2011).

Autism spectrum disorders have long been considered among the most heritable of neuropsychiatric conditions. Through the period of diagnostic expansion, most twin studies of ASDs have suggested that the disease category is at least 60% heritable (Ronald and Hoekstra, 2011). However, the largest of those studies, both conducted recently, have noted a trend that reinforces the possibility of both genetic and environmental influence on autistic behavior (Hallmayer et al., 2011; Rosenberg et al., 2009). Rosenberg et al. (2009) and Hallmayer et al. (2011) reported that the dizygotic (DZ) twin of an individual with ASD has approximately a 30% chance of being diagnosed with autism him- or herself. This figure suggests that ASD recurrence in DZ twins may be higher than that estimated for regular siblings (Constantino et al., 2010; Ozonoff et al., 2011). This is notable because DZ twins are no more genetically similar than regular siblings. Some of the estimated difference may be caused by higher ascertainment probabilities among twins (e.g., because twins are the same age, they are more likely to be assessed by the same clinician at the same time). There is also a possibility that the registries employed for these studies are not representative of the population as a whole, and families with multiple affected twins were more likely to participate than families with only one affected child. However, elevated DZ twin risk may also suggest that ASDs, in part, reflect environmental exposures during fetal development (Szatmari, 2011). The nature of such possible exposures, and the manner in which they interact with genetic vulnerability, are important areas of future research (Croen et al., 2011).

ATTENTION DEFICIT/HYPERACTIVITY DISORDER

The estimated prevalence of ADHD varies substantially based on age at assessment, informant (clinician, parent, teacher, self, or some combination), country, and diagnostic criteria. Using DSM-IV criteria, the estimated prevalence ranges from 5.8% in Brazil (Rohde et al., 1999) to 7.5% in Australia (Graetz et al., 2001) and 17% in Germany (Baumgaertel et al., 1995). In Sweden, using the Autism-Tics, ADHD, and Other Comorbidities inventory, prevalence was estimated at 1.8% with a 2.5-fold enrichment in boys compared with girls (Lichtenstein et al., 2010). In the United States, prevalence estimates range between 9.5% and 16% (Hudziak et al., 1998; Gimpel and Kuhn, 2000; Nolan et al., 2001), but can be lower when functional impairment is taken into consideration (Wolraich et al., 1998).

The estimated heritability of ADHD is consistently high. Faraone and colleagues conducted a metaanalysis of diagnostic and dimensional assessments of ADHD determining a mean estimate of 76% for heritability across 20 different twin studies conducted in the United States, the European Union, and Australia with point estimates ranging from approximately 60% to more than 95% (Faraone et al., 2005).

TOURETTE DISORDER

The prevalence of Tourette disorder is estimated between 0.1% and 1% with the expanded phenotype of tic disorder estimated to be between 3% and 12% (Kurlan et al., 2001; Lichtenstein et al., 2010; Singer, 2005). In a large population cohort of twins from Sweden, tic disorder is estimated to be significantly heritable, with a point estimate of 56% (95%; CI, 37–68%) (Lichtenstein et al., 2010). Some estimates for Tourette disorder alone are lower (32%) (Mathews and Grados, 2011).

CHILDHOOD PSYCHIATRIC DISORDERS AS THE EXTREMES OF NORMAL TRAIT VARIATION

A growing body of population-based studies suggests that, like mild intellectual disabilities, ASDs and ADHD may et al., 2000). However, even though some children with ASDs experience growth in specific skills (Fountain et al., 2012), the great majority continue to manifest the core symptoms of the disorder throughout their lives (McGovern and Sigman, 2005; Piven et al., 1996; Szatmari et al., 2009). The population of adults with an ASD diagnosis is growing rapidly, and further study is needed to understand their range of functioning and need for services (Shattuck et al., 2012).

ATTENTION DEFICIT/HYPERACTIVITY DISORDER

Longitudinal studies of ADHD have suggested that approximately 40% of patients continue to meet full criteria for ADHD in early adulthood and approximately 60% manifest residual symptoms (Faraone et al., 2006). Although the disorder as a whole is moderately stable over time, there is evidence for varying stability among ADHD's phenotypic domains. Multiple studies have noted greater persistence of inattentive as compared with hyperactive/impulsive symptomology (Biederman et al., 2000; Larsson et al., 2011b). However, few studies have assessed persistence beyond the age of 25. Children diagnosed with ADHD have significantly higher rates of arrest for both misdemeanor and felony charges than children without an ADHD diagnosis, although the samples in which this has been investigated are predominantly male (Barkley et al., 2004). In a longitudinal study of girls diagnosed with ADHD, higher rates of all major classes of psychopathology were found (Biederman et al., 2010).

TOURETTE DISORDER

Typically, vocal and motor tic symptoms peak during early puberty and tend to diminish in adulthood. Even though symptoms ease in adulthood, an estimated 90% of patients with Tourette continue to experience tics (Pappert et al., 2003). Tic severity in childhood has been shown to be inversely correlated with health-related quality of life (Cavanna et al., 2012).

HERITABILITY AND PREVALENCE OF CHILDHOOD PSYCHIATRIC DISORDERS

INTELLECTUAL DISABILITY

Unlike the other developmental phenotypes discussed in this chapter, intellectual disability is currently defined by a quantitative measure. Intelligence is assessed on a continuum in the general population, and IQ scores are standardized such that they are normally distributed around an empirically derived population average. The DSM-IV defines intellectual disability as an IQ score more than two standard deviations below the mean—accordingly corresponding with the lowest scoring 2.5% of individuals, an inherent marker of prevalence (APA, 2000).

Although the population rate of ID is stable under the DSM-IV definition, there can be fluctuation in the commonality of specific ID-associated syndromic conditions. For example, Down syndrome remains the most significant single, identified cause of major cognitive impairment (Mefford et al., 2012),

but its prevalence varies by time period and geographic region. Like many spontaneous genetic events, the incidence of chromosomal disorders like DS varies significantly with parental age and likely with other sociodemographic and environmental factors (Irving et al., 2008).

It is difficult to estimate the heritability of ID given its limited prevalence and etiologic heterogeneity. IQ itself is moderately to highly heritable (Haworth et al., 2010), and evidence suggests that at least mild ID represents the low end of typical variation (Plomin et al., 2008). However, the etiologic structure of ID is likely to vary across levels of severity (Nichols, 1984). The empirical basis for this model is drawn from family studies showing that the siblings of children with mild cognitive disabilities had, on the whole, below-average IQs themselves. The siblings of children with severe ID, by contrast, were on average IQ-normative. This pattern suggests that the genetic sources of rare and severe cognitive impairments are more likely to be sporadic, and the genetic sources of more common and mild cognitive impairments more likely to be familial.

On the whole, severe ID is considered to be significantly less heritable than most common neuropsychiatric conditions (or indeed nearly all medical and anthropometric traits in general) (Plomin et al., 2008). Although some inherited genetic causes have been identified (Lossie and Driscoll, 1999), there are a variety of clear environmental risk factors that can induce major cognitive impairment (e.g., trauma, infection, poisoning, or malnutrition before, during, or after birth, early childhood diseases). Furthermore, many of the documented genetic influences are large-scale spontaneous chromosomal anomalies, which themselves can be environmentally induced (Mefford et al., 2012). Such a heterogeneous etiology necessitates that inherited factors explain a smaller proportion of variance for ID than many other common medical phenotypes.

AUTISM SPECTRUM DISORDERS

The estimated prevalence of ASDs has increased dramatically over four decades in the United States and the United Kingdom, and is currently approximated at around 1% in both countries (Baird et al., 2006; Baron-Cohen et al., 2009; CDC, 2012; Elsabbagh et al., 2012). The increase in measured prevalence is at least in large part secondary to definitional expansion and greater diagnostic awareness. Neither Asperger syndrome nor pervasive developmental disorder not otherwise specified (PDD-NOS) were included in the DSM description of autism until the text's fourth edition (1994), and recent studies suggest that the probability of ASD ascertainment continues to grow within certain US populations (Pedersen et al., 2012; "Prevalence of autism spectrum disorders—Autism and Developmental Disabilities Monitoring Network, 14 sites, United States, 2008"). A recent UK study highlighted the probable importance of changes to the definition and study of ASDs in prevalence estimation. Using modern clinical criteria and research methods, Brugha et al. (2011) found that the prevalence of ASDs among UK adults was also approximately 1%. Because ASDs are typically lifelong phenotypes, this suggests that these adults would have met *current* clinical criteria as children but were not diagnosed because ascertainment

40% to 60% of children with ASDs have concomitant intellectual disabilities, and it is estimated that an even larger fraction require lifelong external supports (Chakrabarti and Fombonne, 2005; Charman et al., 2011b; Centers for Disease Control and Prevention, 2012). For each patient, the lifetime societal costs associated with an ASD diagnosis are estimated to be $3.2 to $5 million in the United States and £0.8 to £1.2 in the United Kingdom (Ganz, 2007; Knapp et al., 2009).

These costs become staggering in aggregate, especially given the growing frequency of ASD diagnoses. The prevalence of ASDs and their apparent rise in incidence has been a point of enormous contention in recent years and is discussed in the following section. Current estimates place the prevalence of ASDs at approximately 1% today in both the United States and the United Kingdom (Baron-Cohen et al., 2009; CDC, 2012).

ATTENTION DEFICIT/HYPERACTIVITY DISORDER

Excess levels of activity along with difficulties in attention and impulse control have been characterized in children for more than a century (Still, 1902). Three subtypes of ADHD are recognized in the DSM-IV: (1) hyperactive/impulsive, (2) inattentive, and (3) combined type, reflecting endorsed criteria in both categories. Examples of ADHD symptoms include interrupting, always being on the go, fidgeting and difficulty sitting still (which reflect the hyperactive/impulsive dimension), as well as difficulty completing tasks, an inability to maintain focus on an activity, and flipping focus (which reflects the inattention dimension). In developing the DSM-5, the psychiatric community is moving to abandon the distinction between the three subtypes in favor of a single construct. This is motivated in large part by the strong phenotypic correlation between the two dimensions, both among patients and the population at large (Larsson et al., 2011b).

Attention deficit/hyperactivity disorder is one of the most common psychiatric disorders of childhood, affecting an estimated 4% to 12% of children worldwide. Approximately 40% of cases are estimated to persist into adulthood, but method of assessment substantially impacts estimated adult prevalence. Self-report measures tend to be least reliable and yield the most restrictive estimates (Faraone et al., 2003). Attention deficit/hyperactivity disorder predicts a range of behaviors and outcomes in both childhood and adulthood that carry a societal cost. Children and adults with ADHD are more likely to be disruptive in school environments, have lower educational attainment, and higher rates of substance use, sexually transmitted diseases, criminality, incarceration, and incurred health care costs. In 2006, worldwide costs of ADHD were estimated to be between $77.5 and $115.9 billion annually because of the costs of treatment and more significantly lost productivity and indirect social costs (Barbaresi and Olsen, 1998; Leibson et al., 2001).

TOURETTE DISORDER

Tourette disorder (TD) and the related phenotype of tic disorder are characterized by uncontrolled movements, speech, or actions. Tourette was originally proposed in 1885 by Georges Gilles de la Tourette as a phenotype that included multiple motor tics and at least one vocal tic (Gilles de la Tourette et al., 1982). Motor tics span from simple movements such as eye blinking to complex movements including jumping or body contortions. Vocal tics similarly vary from simple tics of throat clearing or sniffing to more complex tics, including syllables, words, coprolalia (undesired vocalization of profanities), echolalia (uncontrolled repetition of what other people say), and palilalia (repetition of one's own words) (Singer, 2005). In the DSM-IV, a Tourette diagnosis requires both motor and vocal tics persisting for a year or longer. When only vocal or motor tics are present, the patient is considered to have tic disorder, with presentation for less than a year considered transient and longer than a year considered chronic (APA, 2000). Onset of these phenotypes is primarily in childhood and is typically most severe during development.

Tourette Disorder and tic disorder are somewhat unusual as psychiatric phenotypes in that neither deficit nor difficulty resulting from the behaviors is necessary to define the disorder. Nevertheless, patients with these disorders experience increased average levels of anxiety and depression (Coffey and Park, 1997; Sukhodolsky et al., 2003). In addition to greater stress, patients with TD have higher rates of ADHD, obsessive compulsive disorder (OCD), and other neuropsychiatric phenotypes (Cavanna et al., 2009; Grados and Mathews, 2009). These comorbidities are well documented but poorly understood. (A discussion of the genetics of anxiety disorders including OCD is found in Chapter 41.)

TRAJECTORIES INTO ADULTHOOD FOR THOSE DIAGNOSED WITH CHILDHOOD PSYCHIATRIC DISORDERS

INTELLECTUAL DISABILITY

Although individuals with developmental disabilities can benefit from early intervention strategies (Charman, 2011c; Dawson et al., 2010), measured intelligence is, on the whole, stable following early childhood (Plomin et al., 2008). Recent evidence suggests that the common genetic influences on intelligence are highly consistent across the lifespan (Deary et al., 2012). The rare, sporadic genetic events associated with major cognitive impairment—e.g., Down syndrome and Fragile X syndrome—similarly influence cognition across the life course (Plomin et al., 2008). However, because of the great heterogeneity within the ID diagnostic category, there is also likely to be substantial variation in developmental trajectories both within and between etiologically distinct sets of cases.

AUTISM SPECTRUM DISORDERS

Studies in clinical populations have suggested that there is substantial heterogeneity in the developmental trajectory of ASDs (Eaves and Ho, 1996; Fountain et al., 2012; Lord et al., 2006; Starr et al., 2003). Improvements are common; for example, gains are often made in the domain of verbal fluency (Anderson et al., 2007; Shattuck et al., 2007; Szatmari

70 | EPIDEMIOLOGY OF NEUROPSYCHIATRIC AND DEVELOPMENTAL DISORDERS OF CHILDHOOD

ELISE B. ROBINSON, BENJAMIN M. NEALE, AND MARK J. DALY

Psychiatric and developmental disorders of childhood onset have been studied for much of the twentieth century. There is an emerging recognition, however, that neuropsychiatric conditions affecting children are rising in estimated prevalence and place an enormous burden on parents, educators, and the health care system (Charman, 2011a; King and Bearman, 2009). Although this rise in prevalence likely contains elements of diagnostic changes, greater awareness of these disorders, and true changes in incidence, there is little doubt that psychiatric and developmental disorders among children are a major concern to society today. A recent survey of more than 10,000 US adolescents concluded that there is nearly a 50% lifetime childhood prevalence of one or more DSM-IV mood, anxiety, or behavioral disorders (excluding eating and substance abuse disorders) and that more than 20% of children meet the definition of severe impairment (Merikangas et al., 2010).

It has become increasingly common for traditionally "adult" psychiatric disorders, such as bipolar disorder or major depression, to be diagnosed in children. However, the focus of this chapter is classical childhood neuropsychiatric conditions whose diagnosis requires the presence of symptoms before age 18 within the DSM-IV-TR framework (APA, 2000). We consider four major diagnostic categories falling within these specifications and highlight the major diagnosis within each—specifically, intellectual disability (ID; formerly referred to as mental retardation and referred to as learning disability in Europe), pervasive developmental disorders (autism spectrum disorders [ASDs]), hyperactive and inattentive behavior (attention deficit/hyperactivity disorder [ADHD]), and tic disorders (Tourette disorder [TD]). Within this first subsection, we address the epidemiology, heritability, and implied genetic architecture within each diagnostic category. We draw synergies and overlaps where appropriate and articulate the connection between traditional diagnostic categories and common behavioral and cognitive traits.

Some of these connections bear relevance to the fifth edition of the DSM, currently under development. In the DSM-IV, the central approach for disease classification is one of categorical symptoms without an empirical basis for diagnostic thresholds. In construction of the DSM-5, the recognition of a continuum underpinning some psychiatric illnesses is growing, exemplified by the planned adoption of autism spectrum disorder in place of a discrete diagnosis within the Pervasive Developmental Disorders category. This shift recognizes a robust literature on more quantitative approaches to neuropsychiatric phenotypes and may influence estimates of disease prevalence. We discuss several implications of assessing psychiatric traits with a dimensional approach in the following, particularly as they relate to genetic architecture.

DEFINITION AND IMPACT OF CHILDHOOD PSYCHIATRIC AND DEVELOPMENTAL DISORDERS

INTELLECTUAL DISABILITY

Intellectual disability and the formal diagnosis of mental retardation in the DSM-IV are characterized by intellectual functioning that is substantially below average and significant limitations in adaptive behavior with onset before the age of 18 (APA, 2000). Approximately 2% of people worldwide meet criteria for IDs. Most individuals with a diagnosis require some level of assisted services throughout adulthood, although there is considerable inter-individual variability in the degree of impairment.

Intellectual functioning is most often assessed via IQ tests (e.g., the Wechsler Intelligence Scales for Children) (Weschler et al., 1992). Intellectual disability is traditionally defined as a score below 70 (at or below two standard deviations below the mean). Although some people with IDs are not diagnosed until mid- or late-childhood, most are identified early in life subsequent to parental concerns about developmental delays (Leonard and Wen, 2002). The genetic sources of certain syndromic cases of ID have long been recognized (Lejeune et al., 1959), but in most cases the cause of cognitive impairment is unknown. Intellectual disability in general is accepted to have numerous genetic and non-genetic causes, representing the end result of a defect in any number of many possible elements of central nervous system (CNS) development.

AUTISM SPECTRUM DISORDERS

Autism spectrum disorders (ASDs) are a system of neurodevelopmental conditions with onset before age three, characterized by impairments in social interaction and communication, along with significantly restricted interests and repetitive behaviors (APA, 2000). Although ASDs vary widely in phenotypic expression, they are universally impairing and present an enormous burden to affected individuals and their families. Approximately discoveries in childhood-onset psychiatric disorders, many models are emerging with construct validity, which in turn provide manifest evidence for specific neuropathobiological substrates for such disorders.

Neuropathobiology in mental illness can be considered on both the micro and macro scale. Recurrent findings in the more severe neurodevelopmental disorders are pathological changes in synaptic structure and function that lead to disruption of plasticity and synchronicity (see Chapter 74). Dierssen and Martínez put these findings in a developmental perspective and examine additional neuronal mechanisms underlying neurodevelopmental disorders. These sorts of perturbations are reflected in changes in functional connectivity in many child psychiatric disorders (see Chapter 75). With enhanced neuroimaging modalities, coupled with advanced biostatistical algorithms, we now have the ability to interrogate and understand systems level processes in the brain. With magnetic resonance spectroscopy, molecular alterations can be mapped to other imaging changes in an entirely non-invasive manner, allowing for an examination of the neurotransmitter/synaptic (micro) and systems levels (macro) alterations at the same time.

Intellectual disability syndromes (see Chapter 76) and ASD (see Chapter 77) can arise from genetic variation as well as from prenatal and perinatal insults. Hundreds of genes and loci are implicated with these two disorders, and there is strong evidence for overlapping risk genes and loci, implying shared origins of ID and ASD. Understanding how multiple genes come together in canonical and newly identified molecular networks is an exciting and challenging field of endeavor summarized in both Chapters 76 and 77. Such pathway analysis holds the promise of identifying "driver" genes that control the state of a neural network and, as such, these genes have potential to be optimal therapeutic targets.

Attention deficit/hyperactivity disorder (see Chapter 78), as well as tic disorders (see Chapter 79), represents disorders not associated with strong reproductive disadvantage and hence are likely to have differing risk architecture from disorders such as intellectual disability or ASD. However, more is known about specific neurobiological systems, with important roles for the attentional circuitry in ADHD and cortico-striato-thalamo-cortical circuitry in TD. Rare genetic variation has been associated with ADHD and TD, and has implicated specific neurotransmitter systems, including some unexpected ones, such as histamine in TD.

We end with a look forward. The emerging molecular insights into psychiatric disorders of childhood onset has led to important cell and animal models, which in turn have driven new neurobiological understandings of these disorders and identified potential novel therapeutic avenues. These potential treatments, previously unpredicted by the state of our knowledge but implicated from these translational approaches, are being evaluated in several clinical trials, summarized briefly in Chapter 80.

SECTION VIII | PSYCHIATRIC DISORDERS OF CHILDHOOD ONSET

JOSEPH D. BUXBAUM

There have been remarkable breakthroughs in our conceptualization of mental illness in the past few years, particularly in the areas of etiology and pathobiology. Nowhere is this more apparent than in neuropsychiatric disorders of childhood onset. The genomic architecture of these disorders includes rare genetic variation of major effect, allowing for the creation of cell and animal models with strong construct validity. In turn, results from these experimental model systems have provided the scientific basis for clinical trials using neurobiologically driven novel therapeutics. Given the current strengths of our research tools, genes are more tractable to discovery, but genes do not tell the entire story and the role of non-genic factors remains to be better elucidated. Important markers of environment, most broadly defined, are the epigenetic changes that regulate gene expression. Elegant and creative studies in this domain are leading to a better understanding of the interactions among environment, genes, and the epigenome and how the environment can sculpt the expression of genes in a manner with long-lasting and even trans-generational impact. Co-incident with these discoveries of molecular etiology, the advent of enhanced imaging and other techniques have not only increased our understanding of the neural processes underlying diverse mental disorders but are leading to important biomarkers for determining clinical subgroups, as well as monitoring clinical course and response to treatment, providing a window on the neural basis of successful and unsuccessful interventions, whether behavioral or pharmacological.

This section charts these advances, focusing on select disorders falling within the DSM-5 Neurodevelopmental Disorders group. We do not, however, wish to imply that there is necessarily an unambiguous distinction between the neuropsychiatric disorders of childhood onset discussed here and other disorders discussed elsewhere in this book. Many psychiatric disorders can onset either in childhood and adulthood (e.g., anxiety and mood disorders) or are likely to be neurodevelopmental in origin (e.g., anxiety, psychosis). Truly, as William Wordsworth said, "The Child is father to the man," and processes that occur in early development and childhood and adolescence lay a foundation for mental health and mental illness in later life.

The chapters in this section can be arranged into two groups, reflecting either broad findings in neurodevelopmental disorders when viewed from a given perspective, or specific neurodevelopmental psychiatric conditions.

Chapter 70 presents the state of the art regarding the epidemiology of childhood onset psychiatric disorders, summarizing current knowledge related to epidemiology, heritability, and implied genetic architecture within each diagnostic category. One important theme discussed in this chapter is how reproductive disadvantage influences the genetic architecture of neurodevelopmental disorders associated with reduced fecundity, and hence a role for rare and spontaneously arising variation in such disorders. Such variation can be associated with intermediate or major effects, and occur on all genomic scales, from aneuploidy, through copy number variation (CNV), to single nucleotide variation (SNV), as discussed in by Mefford (see Chapter 71). The role of CNV in both human variation and mental illness was little known until just a few years ago and we have already reached a point at which CNV screening is a standard component in the clinical evaluation of individuals with unexplained intellectual disability (ID) and/or autism spectrum disorder (ASD). With the widespread availability of massively parallel sequencing (MPS; also termed next- or second-generation sequencing), the role of SNV in neurodevelopmental disorders will become clearer in the next few years, as will screening for such variation. Examples of CNV and SNV in specific disorders are found in the chapters on ID, ASD, Tourette syndrome, and tic disorders (TD), and attention deficit/hyperactivity disorder (ADHD).

Epigenetics, although difficult to study in disorders of the brain, likely has a great or greater impact on dynamic neural processes, when compared to genetic variation. In Chapter 72 Bale notes epigenetics encompasses change in gene function not associated with sequence variation and represents a means by which we can integrate a role for the environment to influence or "program" gene expression. Animal model systems demonstrate that epigenetics is a mechanism by which well-known associations of maternal stress, infection, or dietary challenges can increase risk for psychiatric illness at later times and be transmitted to subsequent generations, and we are learning about other important neuropsychiatric phenotypes modulated by epigenetics.

Animal models (see Chapter 73) provide opportunities for hypothesis testing and for evaluating novel therapeutics. In addition, these models have a special place in disorders of the brain for generating hypotheses because neuronal tissue from human subjects is not typically accessible before death, except in rare cases of neurosurgery (not typically associated with psychiatric illness). Given the growing genetic and molecular

Tschampa, H.J., Neumann, M., et al. (2001). Patients with Alzheimer's disease and dementia with Lewy bodies mistaken for Creutzfeldt–Jakob disease. *J. Neurol. Neurosurg. Psychiatry* 71(1):33–39.

Vitali, P., Maccagnano, E., et al. (2011). Diffusion-weighted MRI hyperintensity patterns differentiate CJD from other rapid dementias. *Neurology* 76(20):1711–1719.

Vitali, P., Migliaccio, R., et al. (2008). Neuroimaging in dementia. *Semin. Neurol.* 28(4):467–483.

Wall, C.A., Rummans, T.A., et al. (2005). Psychiatric manifestations of Creutzfeldt–Jakob disease: a 25-year analysis. *J. Neuropsychiatry Clin. Neurosci.* 17(4):489–495.

Watts, J.C., Balachandran, A., et al. (2006). The expanding universe of prion diseases. *PLoS Pathog.* 2(3):e26.

Watts, J.C., Giles, K., et al. (2012). Spontaneous generation of rapidly transmissible prions in transgenic mice expressing wild-type bank vole prion protein. *Proc. Natl. Acad. Sci. USA* 109(9): 3498–3503.

Watts, J.C., and Westaway, D. (2007). The prion protein family: diversity, rivalry, and dysfunction. *Biochim. Biophys. Acta* 1772(6):654–672.

Webb, T.E., Poulter, M., et al. (2008). Phenotypic heterogeneity and genetic modification of P102L inherited prion disease in an international series. *Brain* 131(Pt 10):2632–2646.

WHO. (1998, 9–11 February). Global Surveillance, Diagnosis and Therapy of Human Transmissible Spongiform Encephalopathies: Report of a WHO Consultation. Paper presented at the World Health Organization: Emerging and Other Communicable Diseases, Surveillance and Control, Geneva.

Will, R., Alpers, M., et al. (2004). Infectious and sporadic prion diseases. In: Prusiner, S., ed. Prion Biology and Diseases, 2nd Edition. Cold Spring Harbor, NY: Cold Spring Harbor Laboratory Press, pp. 629–671.

Will, R.G. (2003). Acquired prion disease: iatrogenic CJD, variant CJD, kuru. *Br. Med. Bull.* 66, 255–265.

Will, R.G., Alperovitch, A., et al. (1998). Descriptive epidemiology of Creutzfeldt–Jakob disease in six European countries, 1993–1995. EU Collaborative Study Group for CJD. *Ann. Neurol.* 43(6):763–767.

Will, R.G., Ironside, J.W., et al. (1996). A new variant of Creutzfeldt-Jakob disease in the UK. *Lancet* 347(9006):921–925.

Will, R. (2004). Variant Creutzfeldt-Jakob disease. *Folia Neuropathol.* 42 (Suppl A):77–83.

Young, G.S., Geschwind, M.D., et al. (2005). Diffusion-weighted and fluid-attenuated inversion recovery imaging in Creutzfeldt–Jakob disease: high sensitivity and specificity for diagnosis. *Am. J. Neuroradiol.* 26(6):1551–1562.

Zerr, I., Kallenberg, K., et al. (2009). Updated clinical diagnostic criteria for sporadic Creutzfeldt–Jakob disease. *Brain* 132(Pt 10):2659–2668.

Zou, W.Q., Puoti, G., et al. (2010). Variably protease-sensitive prionopathy: a new sporadic disease of the prion protein. *Ann. Neurol.* 68(2):162–172.

Appleby, B.S., Appleby, K.K., et al. (2009). Characteristics of established and proposed sporadic Creutzfeldt–Jakob disease variants. *Arch. Neurol.* 66(2):208–215.

Atarashi, R., Satoh, K., et al. (2011). Ultrasensitive human prion detection in cerebrospinal fluid by real-time quaking-induced conversion. *Nat. Med.* 17(2):175–178.

Barash, J.A. (2009). Clinical features of sporadic fatal insomnia. *Rev. Neurol. Dis.* 6(3):E87–93.

Brown, K., and Mastrianni, J.A. (2010). The prion diseases. *J. Geriatr. Psychiatry Neurol.* 23(4):277–298.

Brown, P., Brandel, J.P., et al. (2006). Iatrogenic Creutzfeldt–Jakob disease: the waning of an era. *Neurology* 67(3):389–393.

Brown, P., Cathala, F., et al. (1986). Creutzfeldt–Jakob disease: clinical analysis of a consecutive series of 230 neuropathologically verified cases. *Ann. Neurol.* 20(5):597–602.

Brown, P., Gibbs, C.J., Jr., et al. (1994). Human spongiform encephalopathy: the National Institutes of Health series of 300 cases of experimentally transmitted disease. *Ann. Neurol.* 35(5):513–529.

Brown, P., Preece, M., et al. (2000). Iatrogenic Creutzfeldt–Jakob disease at the millennium. *Neurology* 55(8):1075–1081.

Budka, H., Aguzzi, A., et al. (1995). Neuropathological diagnostic criteria for Creutzfeldt–Jakob disease (CJD) and other human spongiform encephalopathies (prion diseases). *Brain Pathology* 5(4):459–466.

Bueler, H., Aguzzi, A., et al. (1993). Mice devoid of PrP are resistant to scrapie. *Cell* 73(7):1339–1347.

Buganza, M., Ferrari, S., et al. (2009). The oldest old Creutzfeldt–Jakob disease case. *J. Neurol. Neurosurg. Psychiatry* 80(10):1140–1142.

Bugiani, O., Giaccone, G., et al. (2000). Neuropathology of Gerstmann–Straussler–Scheinker disease. *Microsc. Res. Tech.* 50(1):10–15.

Chapman, T., McKeel, D.W., Jr., et al. (2000). Misleading results with the 14-3-3 assay for the diagnosis of Creutzfeldt-Jakob disease. *Neurology* 55(9):1396–1397.

Chohan, G., Llewelyn, C., et al. (2010). Variant Creutzfeldt–Jakob disease in a transfusion recipient: coincidence or cause? *Transfusion* 50(5):1003–1006.

Colby, D.W., and Prusiner, S.B. (2011). Prions. *Cold Spring Harb. Perspect. Biol.* 3(1):a006833.

Collins, S.J., Sanchez-Juan, P., et al. (2006). Determinants of diagnostic investigation sensitivities across the clinical spectrum of sporadic Creutzfeldt–Jakob disease. *Brain* 129(Pt 9):2278–2287.

Corato, M., Cereda, C., et al. (2006). Young-onset CJD: age and disease phenotype in variant and sporadic forms. *Funct. Neurol.* 21(4):211–215.

Cummings, J.L. (1997). The neuropsychiatric inventory: assessing psychopathology in dementia patients. *Neurology* 48(5 Suppl 6):S10–16.

Forner, S., Wong, K., et al. (2011). Cross-sectional neuropsychiatric inventory (NPI) analysis comparing sporadic Jakob-Creutzfeldt (sCJD) disease to other neurodegenerative diseases. [Abstract]. *Neurology* 76(9):A622.

Gambetti, P., Parchi, P., et al. (1995). Fatal familial insomnia and familial Creutzfeldt–Jakob disease: clinical, pathological and molecular features. *Brain Pathol.* 5(1):43–51.

Geschwind, M.D. (2009). Clinical trials for prion disease: difficult challenges, but hope for the future. *Lancet Neurol.* 8(4):304–306.

Geschwind, M.D., Haman, A., et al. (2007). Rapidly progressive dementia. *Neurol. Clin.* 25(3):783–807.

Geschwind, M.D., Josephs, K.A., et al. (2007). A 54-year-old man with slowness of movement and confusion. *Neurology* 69(19):1881–1887.

Geschwind, M.D., Kuryan, C., et al. (2010). Brain MRI in sporadic Jakob–Creutzfeldt disease is often misread. *Neurology* 74(Suppl 2):A213.

Geschwind, M.D., Martindale, J., et al. (2003). Challenging the clinical utility of the 14-3-3 protein for the diagnosis of sporadic Creutzfeldt–Jakob disease. *Arch. Neurol.* 60(6):813–816.

Gibbs, C.J., Jr. (1992). Spongiform encephalopathies—slow, latent, and temperate virus infections—in retrospect. In: Prusiner, S.B., Collinge, J., Powell, J., and Anderton, B., eds. Prion Diseases of Humans and Animals. London: Ellis Horwood, pp. 53–62.

Giovagnoli, A.R., Di Fede, G., et al. (2008). Atypical frontotemporal dementia as a new clinical phenotype of Gerstmann–Straussler–Scheinker disease with the PrP-P102L mutation: description of a previously unreported Italian family. *Neurol. Sci.* 29(6):405–410.

Goldfarb, L.G., Petersen, R.B., et al. (1992). Fatal familial insomnia and familial Creutzfeldt–Jakob disease: disease phenotype determined by a DNA polymorphism. *Science* 258(5083):806–808.

Hall, D.A., Leehey, M.A., et al. (2005). PRNP H187R mutation associated with neuropsychiatric disorders in childhood and dementia. *Neurology* 64(7):1304–1306.

Hamlin, C., Puoti, G., et al. (2012). A comparison of tau and 14-3-3 protein in the diagnosis of Creutzfeldt–Jakob disease. *Neurology* 79(6):547–552.

Heath, C.A., Cooper, S.A., et al. (2010). Validation of diagnostic criteria for variant Creutzfeldt–Jakob disease. *Ann. Neurol.* 67(6):761–770.

Hohler, A.D., and Flynn, F.G. (2006). Onset of Creutzfeldt–Jakob disease mimicking an acute cerebrovascular event. *Neurology* 67(3):538–539.

Holman, R.C., Belay, E.D., et al. (2010). Human prion diseases in the United States. *PLoS One* 5(1):e8521.

Hsich, G., Kenney, K., et al. (1996). The 14-3-3 brain protein in cerebrospinal fluid as a marker for transmissible spongiform encephalopathies. *N. Engl. J. Med.* 335(13):924–930.

Johnson, D.Y., Dunkelberger, D.L., et al. (2012). Sporadic Jakob–Creutzfeldt disease presenting as primary progressive aphasia. *Arch. Neurol.* 1–4.

Katscher, F. (1998). It's Jakob's disease, not Creutzfeldt's. *Nature* 393(6680):11.

Kong, Q., Surewicz, W.K., et al. (2004). Inherited prion diseases. In: Prusiner, S.B., ed. Prion Biology and Diseases, 2nd Edition. Cold Spring Harbor, NY: Cold Spring Harbor Laboratory Press, pp. 673–775.

Kovacs, G.G., Horvath, S., et al. (2009). Genetic Creutzfeldt–Jakob disease mimicking variant Creutzfeldt–Jakob disease. *J. Neurol. Neurosurg. Psychiatry* 80(12):1410–1411.

Kovacs, G.G., Puopolo, M., et al. (2005). Genetic prion disease: the EUROCJD experience. *Hum. Genet.* 118(2):166–174.

Kretzschmar, H.A., Ironside, J.W., et al. (1996). Diagnostic criteria for sporadic Creutzfeldt–Jakob disease. *Arch. Neurol.* 53(9):913–920.

Kropp, S., Schulz-Schaeffer, W.J., et al. (1999). The Heidenhain variant of Creutzfeldt–Jakob disease. *Arch. Neurol.* 56(1):55–61.

Ladogana, A., Puopolo, M., et al. (2005). Mortality from Creutzfeldt–Jakob disease and related disorders in Europe, Australia, and Canada. *Neurology* 64(9):1586–1591.

Laplanche, J.L., Hachimi, K.H., et al. (1999). Prominent psychiatric features and early onset in an inherited prion disease with a new insertional mutation in the prion protein gene. *Brain* 122(Pt 12):2375–2386.

Mead, S. (2006). Prion disease genetics. *Eur. J. Hum. Genet.* 14(3):273–281.

Mead, S., Webb, T.E., et al. (2007). Inherited prion disease with 5-OPRI: phenotype modification by repeat length and codon 129. *Neurology* 69(8):730–738.

Murray, K., Ritchie, D.L., et al. (2008). Sporadic Creutzfeldt–Jakob disease in two adolescents. *J. Neurol. Neurosurg. Psychiatry* 79(1):14–18.

Parchi, P., Giese, A., et al. (1999). Classification of sporadic Creutzfeldt–Jakob disease based on molecular and phenotypic analysis of 300 subjects. *Ann. Neurol.* 46(2):224–233.

Peretz, D., Supattapone, S., et al. (2006). Inactivation of prions by acidic sodium dodecyl sulfate. *J. Virol.* 80(1):322–331.

Polymenidou, M., Stoeck, K., et al. (2005). Coexistence of multiple PrPSc types in individuals with Creutzfeldt-Jakob disease. *Lancet Neurol.* 4(12):805–814.

Prusiner, S.B. (2012). Cell biology: a unifying role for prions in neurodegenerative diseases. *Science* 336(6088):1511–1513.

Prusiner, S.B. (1998). Prions. *Proc. Natl. Acad. Sci. USA* 95(23): 13363–13383.

Rabinovici, G.D., Wang, P.N., et al. (2006). First symptom in sporadic Creutzfeldt–Jakob disease. *Neurology* 66(2):286–287.

Sanchez-Juan, P., Green, A., et al. (2006). CSF tests in the differential diagnosis of Creutzfeldt–Jakob disease. *Neurology* 67(4):637–643.

Satoh, J., Kurohara, K., et al. (1999). The 14-3-3 protein detectable in the cerebrospinal fluid of patients with prion-unrelated neurological diseases is expressed constitutively in neurons and glial cells in culture. *Eur. Neurol.* 41(4):216–225.

Scott, M.R., Will, R., et al. (1999). Compelling transgenetic evidence for transmission of bovine spongiform encephalopathy prions to humans. *Proc. Natl. Acad. Sci. USA* 96(26):15137–15142.

Seipelt, M., Zerr, I., et al. (1999). Hashimoto's encephalitis as a differential diagnosis of Creutzfeldt–Jakob disease. *J. Neurol. Neurosurg. Psychiatry* 66(2):172–176.

Shiga, Y., Miyazawa, K., et al. (2004). Diffusion-weighted MRI abnormalities as an early diagnostic marker for Creutzfeldt–Jakob disease. *Neurology* 63:443–449.

Steinhoff, B.J., Zerr, I., et al. (2004). Diagnostic value of periodic complexes in Creutzfeldt-Jakob disease. *Ann. Neurol.* 56(5):702–708.

Tateishi, J., Kitamoto, T., et al. (1996). Experimental transmission of Creutzfeldt–Jakob disease and related diseases to rodents. *Neurology* 46(2):532–537.

Telling, G.C., Parchi, P., et al. (1996). Evidence for the conformation of the pathologic isoform of the prion protein enciphering and propagating prion diversity. *Science* 274(5295):2079–2082.

Telling, G.C., Scott, M., et al. (1995). Prion propagation in mice expressing human and chimeric PrP transgenes implicates the interaction of cellular PrP with another protein. *Cell* 83(1):79–90.

PRION STRAINS AND STRAIN TYPING OF HUMAN PRION DISEASES

One of the greatest challenges to the protein-only hypothesis is derived from the existence of distinct "strains" of prions. Prion strains are defined as distinct prion isolates that exhibit differences in incubation period, neuropathological lesion profile in the brain, pattern of PrP^{Sc} deposition, and/or biochemical properties of PrP^{Sc} when propagated in a given species. In viruses or bacteria, different strains arise from mutations in their nucleic acid genomes, which confer novel properties to the infectious agent. Prion strains, however, can occur in the absence of any genetic material and without any changes to the amino acid sequence of PrP. Instead, it is thought that prion strains arise from distinct conformations of PrP^{Sc} (Telling et al., 1996). Thus, subtle changes to the "shape" of the PrP^{Sc} molecule can engender vastly different biochemical and neuropathological properties.

For human prion diseases, the most common way of differentiating different prion strains is by examining the biochemical properties of PrP^{Sc}. The biochemical hallmark of CJD is the presence of protease-resistant prion protein in the brain. Whereas PrP^{C} in healthy brain tissue is completely degraded by treatment with a protease such as proteinase K (PK), PrP^{Sc} is usually partially resistant to PK digestion, leaving behind the portion of PrP corresponding to the aggregated core of the protein. Protease-resistant PrP is most commonly detected in brain homogenate from CJD patients by immunoblotting using an antibody to detect PK-resistant PrP species. Following PK digestion, three PrP bands are typically visible, which correspond to di-, mono-, and un-glycosylated forms of PrP^{Sc}. Different prion strains can be ascertained by the relative ratios of the three PrP^{Sc} glycoforms as well as by the size of the unglycosylated PrP^{Sc} fragment. Using the most common nomenclature, there are two common sizes of PrP^{Sc} fragments, an approximately 21-kDa band referred to as type 1 PrP^{Sc} and an approximately 19-kDa band referred to as type 2 PrP^{Sc} (see Fig. 69.4G) (Parchi et al., 1999). For example, vCJD and FFI are classified as exhibiting type 2 PrP^{Sc}, whereas type 1, type 2, or both types of PrP^{Sc} can exist in sporadic CJD.

For sporadic CJD, prion strain types are classified according to the codon 129 genotype and the PrP^{Sc} type. There are at least six possible combinations (MM1, MM2, MV1, MV2, VV1, and VV2), where the two letters denote which polymorphic variant of PrP is present on the two copies of chromosome 20 (methionine [M] or valine [V]) and the number indicates whether type 1 or 2 PrP^{Sc} is present (Parchi et al., 1999). Of these six possibilities, at least five constitute distinct strains of sCJD (MM1, MM2, MV2, VV1, and VV2) (see Table 69.1). The MM1 and VV2 subtypes are the most common, whereas VV1 is by far the rarest. In general, sporadic CJD occurs more often in individuals who are homozygous for the codon 129 polymorphism (i.e., MM or VV). This is likely because the conformational conversion of PrP^{C} into PrP^{Sc} occurs more efficiently when identical PrP molecules are present. To complicate matters, although it was initially thought that patients with sCJD only had either type 1 or 2 PrP^{Sc} present in the brain, it is now known that some patients have both type 1 and 2 PrP^{Sc} (Polymenidou et al., 2005). How these MM1/2, VV1/2, and MV1/2 patients present is still not clear.

Protease-resistant PrP^{Sc} molecules that resemble those observed in sCJD are present in some but not all GSS cases. More common in GSS are smaller PK-resistant fragments of PrP that are approximately 14 and 7 kDa in size. These likely correspond to the protease-resistant core of the PrP amyloid plaques observed in GSS patients. A recently described sporadic prion disease in humans, termed variably protease sensitive prionopathy (VPSPr), is also characterized by atypical smaller protease-resistant PrP fragments, and might represent a sporadic version of GSS (Zou et al., 2010).

TREATMENT OF PRION DISEASES

Current management of prion diseases is largely symptomatic. Although many drugs have been effective at stopping or eliminating prion disease in cell culture and even in animal models when given before or near the time of prion inoculation, no drugs have been curative to date when given at a clinically meaningful time point after inoculation (to model sCJD). Drugs that are effective only before the disease has progressed, might however be helpful in presymptomatic gPrD or persons at high risk for acquired/variant CJD because of known exposure. A treatment trial in Germany with flupirtine showed some mild cognitive improvement in sCJD, but no effect on survival. Although quinacrine showed some promise *in vitro*, it failed to improve survival in an observational study of human prion disease in the United Kingdom and our own sCJD treatment trial in the United States (Geschwind, 2009). A treatment trial with doxycycline in Italy and France was completed in 2012 and showed no benefit. There is great effort to identify new treatments by high throughput drug screening, and other approaches, such as siRNA therapy to knock down the PrP^{C} substrate for PrP^{Sc}, are being actively studied in laboratories around the world (Brown and Mastrianni, 2010). Perhaps even more hopeful and exciting are recent data suggesting that other more common neurodegenerative diseases, such as Alzheimer's disease, Parkinson disease, and frontotemporal dementia/ALS, might spread within the brain via a prion-like mechanism. Thus, drugs that work for one condition, might be helpful in other neurodegenerative diseases as well (Prusiner, 2012).

DISCLOSURES

Dr. Watts receives grant support from the NIH NINDS and NIA.

Dr. Geschwind receives grant support from the NIH NIA. Dr. Geschwind has served as a consultant for MedaCorp and Gerson Lehrman Group and has served on the advisory board for Lundbeck.

REFERENCES

Alner, K., Hyare, H., et al. (2011). Distinct neuropsychological profiles correspond to distribution of cortical thinning in inherited prion disease caused by insertional mutation. *J. Neurol. Neurosurg. Psychiatry* 83(1):109–114.

NEUROPATHOLOGY OF FATAL FAMILIAL INSOMNIA

The most striking aspect of FFI is that the neuropathology is largely confined to the thalamus. In the anterior ventral and mediodorsal nuclei of the thalamus there is widespread neuronal loss and associated reactive astrocytic gliosis. Neuronal loss and gliosis are also observed in the inferior olives. Spongiform change is comparatively mild in FFI, but sometimes can be found in the cerebral cortex of patients with long disease duration. Compared with sCJD, the amount of PrP^{Sc} deposition in the brain is minimal (Gambetti et al., 1995). One form of sCJD, MM2-thalamic, has a similar pathological appearance to FFI, with some clinical overlap. Some have called this form sporadic fatal insomnia (sFI) (Barash, 2009).

NEUROPATHOLOGY OF KURU

Because the predominant clinical characteristic of Kuru is ataxia, it is not surprising that the most severely affected brain region in this disease is the cerebellum, in which large numbers of PrP-containing amyloid plaques can be found in the granule cell layer. These are associated with loss of granule cells, loss of Purkinje cells, and an intense activation of Bergmann radial glial cells. Milder neuropathological changes, including spongiform degeneration, are also observed in other regions of the brain.

PRION REPLICATION AND THE SPECIES BARRIER

Prions replicate using a process called template-directed misfolding. When a PrP^{Sc} molecule encounters a PrP^{C} molecule, it causes PrP^{C} to refold into an identical copy of PrP^{Sc} (Colby and Prusiner, 2011). These newly formed PrP^{Sc} molecules then serve as additional templates for converting more PrP^{C} molecules, allowing the infectious PrP^{Sc} form to propagate. This conformational conversion is thought to occur on the surface of the cell or within an endocytic compartment. The spontaneous (non-templated) conversion of PrP^{C} into PrP^{Sc} is an exceedingly rare event, likely owing to a large energy barrier between the two conformational isoforms of PrP.

Binding of PrP^{Sc} to PrP^{C} can be highly specific. For instance, hamster PrP^{Sc} is very ineffective at converting mouse PrP^{C} into mouse PrP^{Sc} and vice versa. When prions from one species are inoculated into an unrelated species, very inefficient disease transmission is observed, which is characterized by a low disease transmission rate and prolonged incubation periods. This is what is referred to as the species barrier for prion replication (Prusiner, 1998). The species barrier is encoded primarily by the amino acid sequence of PrP in a given species. For example, whereas normal mice are generally resistant to CJD prions, transgenic mice expressing human PrP in their brains are highly susceptible to CJD and other human prion strains (Telling et al., 1995).

The species barrier has important consequences for human health. Whereas there is no evidence that scrapie or CWD can be transmitted to humans (e.g., through the consumption of prion-contaminated meat from sheep or deer), consumption of BSE-contaminated meat has led to about 226 prion disease cases of variant CJD (vCJD), mostly in the United Kingdom and France (http://www.cjd.ed.ac.uk/data.html), as discussed earlier. Thus, BSE is one strain of prion that can more readily cross the species barrier. Indeed, BSE prions are also known to infect cats.

PRION TRANSMISSION AND DETECTION

The gold standard for demonstrating prion infectivity in a biological sample is to perform an animal bioassay. In a laboratory setting, the most efficient method for transmitting prion disease is to intracerebrally inject brain material from a sick animal into a young recipient animal (Watts et al., 2006). After a long incubation period (typically four to six months for various strains of mouse-adapted prions), the inoculated animals will exhibit clinical signs typical of prion disease and eventually progress to death within a few weeks. In mice, prion disease also can be transmitted via the oral and intraperitoneal routes of exposure, although the incubation times are longer than for intracerebral injections. Scrapie and CWD are known to be horizontally transmissible in nature (i.e., the disease can be transmitted from animal to animal under non-experimental conditions). Although the precise mechanism of inter-animal transmission remains to be established, prions are known to exist in the saliva and feces of CWD-infected deer. In contrast, there is little evidence to suggest that CJD is horizontally transmissible under normal conditions. Little or no prion infectivity has been found in biologically accessible fluids in CJD patients, including blood and urine. One notable exception is vCJD, in which secondary transmission of the disease through blood transfusion appears to have occurred (Brown and Mastrianni, 2010).

Although animal bioassays provide a definitive test for prions, they are time consuming and expensive. Consequently, numerous *in vitro* tests have been developed for detecting the presence of misfolded prion protein. Using a PrP-specific antibody, PrP^{Sc} deposits can be detected in formalin-fixed brain sections by immunohistochemistry, providing that a denaturing treatment has been performed to remove PrP^{C} and enhance the immunoreactivity of PrP^{Sc}. Similarly, protease-resistant PrP can be detected in brain homogenate by Western blotting using an anti-PrP antibody. More recently, two techniques have been developed that permit prions to be amplified in a test tube. Protein misfolding cyclic amplification (PMCA) and real-time quaking-induced conversion (RT-QuIC) can both be used to amplify and detect minute quantities of prions present in a sample, analogous to the polymerase chain reaction (PCR) technique that is used to detect trace amounts of specific DNA sequences (Atarashi et al., 2011).

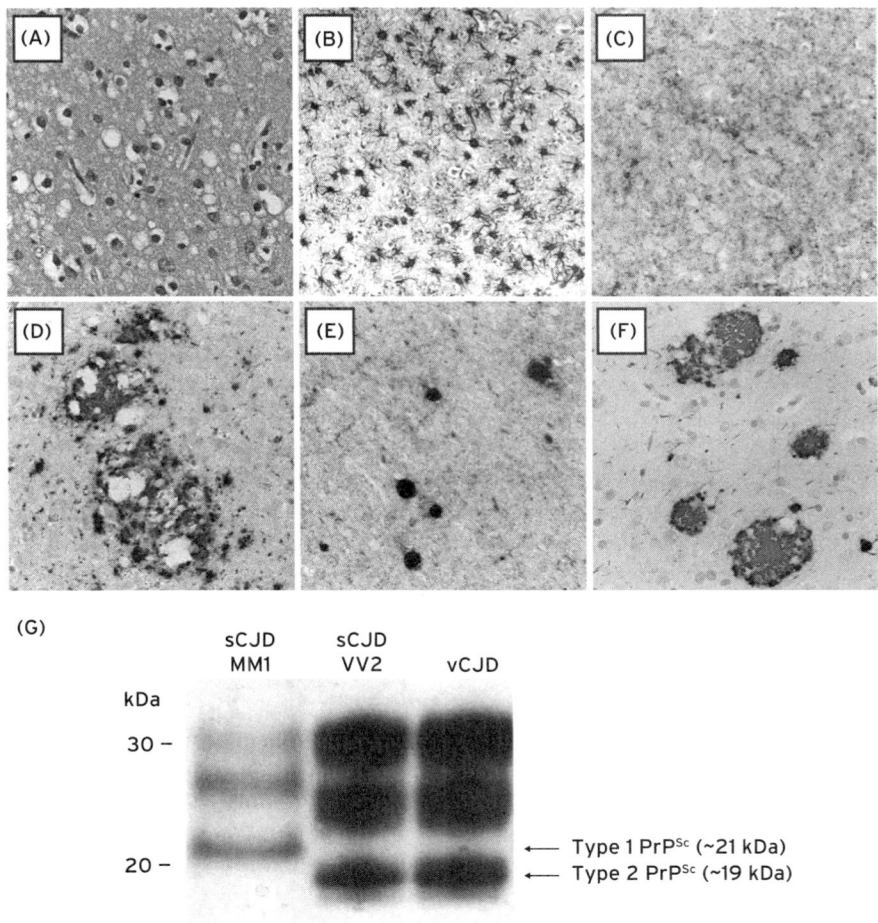

Figure 69.4 *Biochemical and neuropathological hallmarks of human prion disease. (A–F) The neuropathological hallmarks of prion disease. Spongiform change (A) and reactive astrocytic gliosis (B) in the parietal cortex of a patient with sporadic CJD (subtype MM1). (C) The synaptic pattern of PrPSc deposition in the frontal cortex of a patient with sporadic CJD exhibiting the MM1 subtype. (D) Perivacuolar PrPSc deposition in the parietal cortex of a patient with MM2 sporadic CJD. (E) Kuru-like PrPSc plaques in the molecular layer of the cerebellum in a patient with MV2 sporadic CJD. (F) PrPSc amyloid plaques in the hippocampus of a GSS patient with the A117V mutation. (G) As revealed by immunoblotting, protease-resistant PrPSc, the biochemical signature of prion disease, is observed in the brains of patients with CJD. In sporadic CJD subtype MM1, type 1 PrPSc is present, whereas type 2 PrPSc is observed in sporadic CJD subtype VV2 and variant CJD. (See color insert.)*

as well as perivacuolar PrP^{Sc} deposition in brain regions containing spongiform change. Spongiform change, PrP^{Sc} deposition, and reactive astrocytic gliosis tend to co-localize in the brain, arguing that PrP^{Sc} deposition is responsible for the neuronal damage. The location and intensity of the neuropathological changes vary between the different molecular subtypes of sporadic CJD. For instance, the "synaptic" pattern of PrP^{Sc} deposition is most common in the MM1 subtype of CJD, whereas focal plaque-like PrP^{Sc} deposits are typically found in the VV2 subtype. Likewise, Kuru-like PrP^{Sc} plaques are most commonly found in the MV2 subtype, but perivacuolar PrP^{Sc} deposits are found in the MM2 subtype. The neuropathology of most fCJD cases generally resembles that of sCJD. The most prominent feature of vCJD is the presence of large numbers of PrP-containing amyloid plaques in the brain, including so-called "florid plaques," in which PrP^{Sc} deposits are surrounded by vacuolation, giving a flower-like appearance (Brown and Mastrianni, 2010). Intense vacuolation is also observed in patients with vCJD, allowing them to be further differentiated from GSS pathologically.

NEUROPATHOLOGY OF GERSTMANN–STRÄUSSLER–SCHEINKER SYNDROME

The defining neuropathological feature of GSS is the presence of PrP-containing amyloid plaques in the brain. The morphology and location of the plaques vary according to the specific GSS-causing mutation in *PRNP*. Although there is widespread neuronal loss in the brains of patients with GSS, there is minimal spongiform degeneration and reactive astrocytic gliosis is mostly associated with the amyloid plaques. Interestingly, neurofibrillary tangles (NFTs) composed of hyperphosphorylated tau protein are also found in some patients with GSS, such as those linked to the mutations F198S or Y145Stop. Neurofibrillary tangles are one of the two pathological hallmarks of Alzheimer's disease. The amyloid plaques in GSS contain aggregated PrP; however, not Aβ as occurs in Alzheimer's disease. Some GSS cases, such as those caused by the Y145Stop mutation, also exhibit prominent deposition of PrP amyloid along the walls of cerebral blood vessels, leading to a condition known as cerebral amyloid angiopathy (Bugiani et al., 2000).

spongiform encephalopathy (BSE or mad cow disease) or, in a few cases, blood transfusion from asymptomatic patients who were unknowing carriers of vCJD (Brown and Mastrianni, 2010). Cattle are thought to have contracted BSE from being fed scrapie-infected sheep products used as feed (Scott et al., 1999). Compared with sCJD, patients with vCJD are generally younger, with a median age of around 27 (range 12 to 74 years) and most patients have been less than 50 years old. The mean disease duration is longer, about 14.5 months, versus about seven months for sCJD. Relevant to this text, early psychiatric symptoms are quite prominent and more characteristic in vCJD than even sCJD (Wall et al., 2005; Rabinovici et al., 2006). Diagnostic criteria for vCJD are shown in Table 69.4 (Heath et al., 2010). Significantly, profound psychiatric features typically are an early and prominent feature of the disease, often occurring several months before obvious neurological symptoms. Painful paresthesias, usually persistent through the disease course, often occur in vCJD, although such pain rarely is seen in other prion diseases. The EEG does not show the classic periodic sharp wave complexes, except in rare cases at the end of the disease. Cerebrospinal biomarkers, such as 14-3-3, NSE, and t-tau, appear to be even less sensitive in vCJD than in sCJD (Sanchez-Juan et al., 2006). The best diagnostic marker currently is the brain MRI, which usually shows the "pulvinar sign," in which the pulvinar (posterior thalamus) is brighter than the anterior putamen on T2-weighted or DWI MRI (see Fig. 69.2A,B). This MRI pattern is very rare in the other prion diseases (Vitali et al., 2008). More specific tests are under development, including detecting vCJD prions in the blood and/or CSF.

The younger age of onset, MRI findings, prominent early psychiatric features, persistent painful sensory symptoms, and possible chorea help differentiate vCJD from sCJD. As with sCJD, definitive diagnosis of vCJD is based on neuropathological evidence of PrP^Sc in brain biopsy or autopsy. Unlike most other human prion diseases, in which prions are found primarily in the central nervous system, in vCJD prions are found in high numbers in the lymphoreticular system, including the appendix, tonsils, and other lymphoid tissue. Variant CJD is still exceedingly rare, with only about 226 cases identified worldwide through late 2012 (http://www.eurocjd.ed.ac.uk). Curiously, all but approximately two cases of vCJD have been MM at codon 129; two have been MV, suggesting that methionine homozygosity confers increased risk for vCJD (Brown and Mastrianni, 2010). It appears that the initial epidemic of vCJD has leveled off, with only a few new cases per year recently. There is, however, concern that an increase in cases will occur in the future either through blood transmission or longer latency, such as in MV or VV individuals (Brown and Mastrianni, 2010).

NEUROPATHOLOGY OF HUMAN PRION DISEASES

There are four neuropathological hallmarks of prion disease: spongiform (vacuolar) degeneration, neuron death, reactive astrocytic gliosis, and deposition of misfolded prion protein in the brain (Budka et al., 1995). The signature pathology in these diseases is the presence of extensive vacuolation of the brain parenchyma (spongiform change), giving it a Swiss cheese–like appearance (see Fig. 69.4A). Although reactive astrocytic gliosis is a general marker for CNS damage, it is notable in that it is present to a much greater extent in prion diseases than in other neurodegenerative disorders such as Alzheimer's disease and Parkinson disease (see Fig. 69.4B). Although PrP^Sc deposition is present in almost all cases of prion disease, the type and pattern of deposition can vary greatly among individual classes of human prion diseases (see Fig. 69.4C–F). For instance, cerebral amyloid plaques composed of aggregated PrP^Sc are found in patients with GSS and vCJD, whereas PrP^Sc deposition is more granular or "punctate" in nature in patients with CJD.

NEUROPATHOLOGY OF CJD

More than 95% of patients with sporadic CJD exhibit spongiform degeneration in the cerebral cortex. This is associated with an intense reactive astrocytic gliosis. In contrast to Kuru and GSS, only 5% to 10% of patients with sporadic CJD exhibit mature PrP-containing amyloid plaques. Non-amyloid PrP^Sc deposition, however, is much more common, with frequent evidence for "synaptic" or punctate deposition in the cortex

TABLE 69.4. Diagnostic criteria for variant CJD

DEFINITE	I	
1A and neuropathological confirmation of vCJD[a]		A Progressive neuropsychiatric disorder
		B Duration of illness >6 months
		C Routine investigations do not suggest an alternative diagnosis
PROBABLE		D No history of potential iatrogenic exposure
I and 4/5 of II and IIIA and IIIB		E No evidence of a familial form of prion disease
Or		
I and IV A[b]	II	
		A Early psychiatric symptoms[c]
POSSIBLE		B Persistent painful sensory symptoms[d]
I and 4/5 of II and III A		C Ataxia
		D Myoclonus or chorea or dystonia
		E Dementia
	III	
		A EEG does not show the typical appearance of sporadic CJD[e] in the early stages of illness
		B Bilateral pulvinar high signal on MRI scan
	IV	
		A Positive tonsil biopsy[b]

[a] Spongiform change and extensive PrP deposition with florid plaques throughout the cerebrum and cerebellum
[b] Tonsil biopsy is NOT recommended routinely, nor in cases with EEG appearances typical of sCJD, but may be useful in suspect cases in which the clinical features are compatible with vCJD and MRI does not show bilateral I pulvinar high signal
[c] Depression, anxiety, apathy, withdrawal, delusions
[d] This includes both frank pain and or dysesthesia
[e] The typical appearance of the EEG in sporadic CJD consists of generalized triphasic periodic complexes at approximately one per second. These may occasionally be seen In the late stages of vCJD
(Borrowed with permission from Heath et al. Ann. Neurol, 67(6): 761–770.)

testing typically shows frontal-executive impairment in almost all cases and many patients have visuospatial, naming, and memory difficulty (Alner et al., 2011).

Another gPrD of particular interest to this chapter is caused by the *PRNP* mutation H187R, of which only a few families have been reported. The first reported family presented with early-onset dementia and other motor features classic for CJD. Another family had childhood or adolescent onset of neuropsychiatric features in more than one-half of patients. Some of the common neuropsychiatric disorders include suicide attempts, pedophilia, pyromania, and kleptomania. Rarely there was developmental delay or mental retardation. Dementia often began in the early thirties, and progressed slowly over a decade or longer. Early cognitive features include frontal-executive dysfunction (including disinhibition) and poor insight. Later aphasia (often fluent), ideomotor apraxia, visuospatial dysfunction, extrapyramidal symptoms, as well as chorea and stereotypies occurred (Hall et al., 2005). This mutation sometimes presents with a more variable pathology that is not necessarily consistent with GSS (Brown and Mastrianni, 2010).

FATAL FAMILIAL INSOMNIA

Fatal familial insomnia (FFI) is one of the rarest gPrDs and is caused by a single *PRNP* point mutation, D178N, with codon 129 having methionine (129M) on the same chromosome (*cis*) (see Fig. 69.3). Patients with D178N but *cis* valine at codon 129 (129V) usually present with fCJD, clinically more similar to sCJD than to FFI. Fatal familial insomnia usually presents at a mean age of the late forties (48 to 49; range, 20 to 72) with progressive, severe insomnia occurring for several months before the onset of other features, such as dysautonomia (e.g., tachycardia, hyperhidrosis, hyperpyrexia), with motor and cognitive problems variably appearing later in the illness. Average survival is about 18 months (range, 7 to 33 months), slightly longer than most patients with sCJD (Brown and Mastrianni, 2010; Kong et al., 2004).

In our practice, after appropriate genetic counseling for autosomal-dominant neurological disease (http://www.hdfoundation.org/html/hdsatest.php), we test every patient suspected to have prion disease for gPrD by analyzing for a *PRNP* mutation. This genetic testing is usually done by blood test, or if done postmortem, by extraction of DNA from fresh-frozen tissue. Because many gPrDs appear similar to sCJD and can have obscured family histories, this testing is important after the appropriate genetic counseling.

DIAGNOSTIC TESTS IN GENETIC PRION DISEASES

In general, EEG, CSF, and MRI are less sensitive in gPrDs than in sCJD. In fCJD, depending on the mutation, the EEG often shows PSWCs (in later stages). The CSF biomarkers (14-3-3, NSE, t-tau) in fCJD often are elevated, but with typically lower sensitivity than in sCJD (Sanchez-Juan et al., 2006). Magnetic resonance images, again depending on the mutation, show

overlapping findings with sCJD. Some mutations, however, have particular patterns. E200K typically shows symmetrical, prominent striatal hyperintensity, with less prominent cortical ribboning (Vitali et al., 2008). The V180I mutation often shows cortical ribboning with minimal or absent deep nuclei hyperintensities. (The EEG typically lacks PSWCs.) In GSS, the EEG usually only shows slow waves and not PSWCs. Cerebrospinal fluid typically does not show elevated biomarkers (Sanchez-Juan et al., 2006), probably because GSS is not a very rapidly progressive dementia, like sCJD, and these biomarkers are probably more markers of rapid neuronal injury (Geschwind et al., 2003). Magnetic resonance imaging usually does not show the deep nuclei hyperintensities and cortical ribboning seen in sCJD and many patients with fCJD. There are GSS mutations, however, in which some patients have some of these CJD-like MRI findings, although for unclear reasons other patients with the same mutation might not have these MRI abnormalities (Vitali et al., 2011). In FFI, EEG usually just shows slowing, but not PSWCs. Brain MRI, including diffusion-weighted imaging, is usually normal, but FDG-PET imaging reveals thalamic and cingulate hypometabolism, often even before disease onset. Cerebrospinal fluid biomarkers in general have very low sensitivity in FFI.

ACQUIRED CJD

Acquired prion diseases occur because prion diseases typically are transmissible and infectious. Acquired forms include Kuru (now essentially extinct, occurring in the Fore tribe in Papua, New Guinea because of endocannibalism), iatrogenic CJD (iCJD), and the highly publicized variant CJD (vCJD), occurring primarily in the United Kingdom and France, caused by consumption of bovine spongiform encephalopathy (BSE or mad cow disease) contaminated beef and about five cases by blood transfusion (Brown and Mastrianni, 2010).

As prions are proteins, typical sterilization methods that kill viruses and bacteria do not denature proteins (Prusiner, 1998). Inactivation requires other methods or longer times at higher pressure and temperatures than typically used for standard sterilization (Peretz et al., 2006). Inadequate decontamination has led to approximately 400 cases of iatrogenic CJD (iCJD) from the use of cadaveric-derived human pituitary hormones (mostly human growth hormone), dura mater for grafts, cornea for transplants, as well as the re-use of "sterilized" EEG depth electrodes implanted directly into the brain and other neurosurgical equipment, and now blood transfusion from vCJD (Brown and Mastrianni, 2010; Brown et al., 2000; Will, 2003). Most of the pituitary-derived (human grown hormone [hGH]) cases occurred in France, the United Kingdom, and the United States. Methods have since been instituted to prevent prion transmission through such hormones (Brown et al., 2000). Fortunately, the number of iCJD cases is declining (Brown et al., 2006).

The most notorious form of CJD is variant CJD (vCJD), which was first identified in 1995 (Will et al., 1996). In most cases it is caused by inadvertent ingestion of bovine

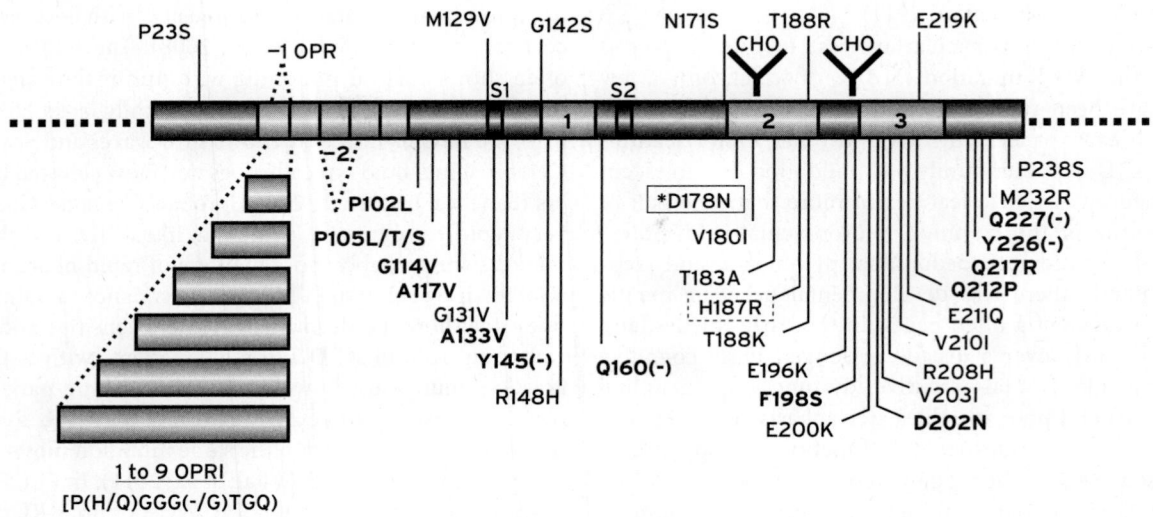

DISEASE-ASSOCIATED
MUTATIONS

Figure 69.3 *General organization of human prion protein (PRP) and related mutations and polymorphisms. The 762 base pair (bp) open-reading frame of PRNP encodes the 253 amino acid protease-sensitive, cellular isoform (PrP^C). Nuclear magnetic resonance (NMR) studies predict 3 a-helices (H1, H2, and H3), and 2 b strands (S1 and S2). Asn-linked glycosylation sites (CHO) occur at residues 181 and 197. The octapeptide repeat segment extends between residues 51 and 91. Pathogenic mutations and polymorphisms of the PRNP gene are represented below and above the schematic, respectively. A single octapeptide repeat deletion and a small number of single bp changes are considered non-pathogenic polymorphisms, some of which act as phenotypic modifiers, most notably, residue 129. Octapeptide repeat insertions (OPRI) of 1 to 9, excluding 3, are pathogenic, as are *30 bp changes. Letters preceding the numbers indicate the normal amino acid residue for the position and letters following the numbers designate the new residue caused by the mutation. Bold mutations are associated with Gerstmann–Sträussler–Scheinker syndrome (GSS); the remainder cause Creutzfeldt–Jakob disease (CJD).* D178N is associated with either CJD or familial fatal insomnia (FFI), depending on the allelic codon 129 sequence (Met = FFI; Val = CJD). H187R displays variable pathology in the limited cases reported. Amino acid letter designations are as follows: A, alanine; D, aspartate; E, glutamate; F, phenylalanine; H, histidine; I, isoleucine; K, lysine; L, leucine; P, proline; Q, glutamine; R, arginine; S, serine; T, threonine; V, valine; Y, tyrosine; (–), stop signal. (Borrowed from Brown and Mastrianni 2011 J. Ger. Psych. Neuro with permission from Sage Publications The prion diseases. J. Geriatr. Psychiatry Neurol, 23(4), 277–298.)*

FAMILIAL CJD

More than 15 mutations cause familial CJD (fCJD). Most are point (missense) mutations, but some are insertion mutations and a deletion (Kong et al., 2004; Mead, 2006). Most fCJD patients present similarly to sCJD with overlapping clinical MRI and EEG findings. The most common fCJD mutation worldwide is E200K (Mead, 2006), found most commonly among Libyan Jews and Czechs (Kovacs et al., 2009). Many other *PRNP* mutations are presented in Figure 69.3.

GERSTMANN–STRÄUSSLER–SCHEINKER

Gerstmann–Sträussler–Scheinker (GSS) syndrome is caused by at least 10 *PRNP* mutations, including several missense mutations, a stop mutation, and insertion mutations (OPRI) (see Fig. 69.3). Generally OPRI mutations with five or more additional octapeptide repeats (repeats of 24 base pairs) present with a GSS phenotype with a long duration of several years, whereas OPRI mutations with four or fewer repeats present phenotypically as CJD, with lower penetrance as well. There are many exceptions, however (Kong et al., 2004; Mead, 2006). The age of onset for GSS mutations is often under the age of 65, typically in one's fifties or younger. As noted, GSS often starts with a slowly progressive ataxic and/or parkinsonian disorder.

Cognitive impairment often comes later, although some mutations present with early dementia and/or behavioral abnormalities. There is, however, considerable phenotypic variability within and between mutations and families (Giovagnoli et al., 2008; Kong et al., 2004; Webb et al., 2008). Because of the slow course (up to several years), persons with GSS can be mistaken to have other neurodegenerative or even neuropsychiatric conditions such as multiple system atrophy, spinocerebellar ataxias, idiopathic Parkinson disease, AD, or Huntington disease (Alner et al., 2011; Laplanche et al., 1999; Mead, 2006).

Of the 8 OPRI mutations causing GSS, an atypical form of GSS caused by an 8-octapeptide repeat insertion mutation (OPRI-8) results in prominent early neuropsychiatric features, often in the patient's late twenties, with a long disease course of several years. Patients are often hospitalized early in psychiatric institutions. Psychiatric features often include mania or mania-like features (Laplanche et al., 1999). Patients with 6-OPRI mutations often have a premorbid or early-onset psychological/personality disorder characterized by irritability, short temper, aggression, antisocial behavior, and aggression. Arrests and other involvement with police are common. These symptoms often predate onset of obvious neurological symptoms, which typically occurs in one's thirties with quite variable survival of less than one year to more than a decade. Cognitive

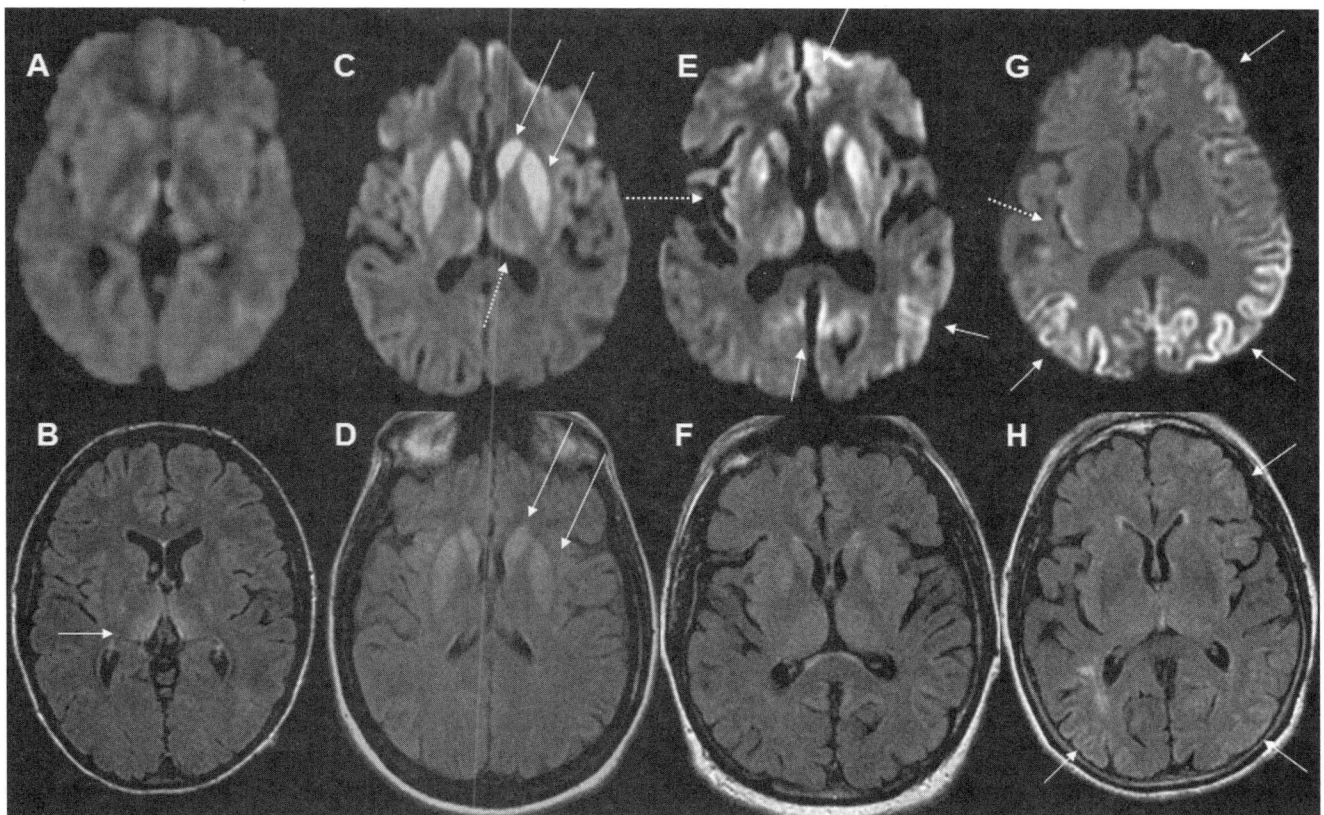

Figure 69.2 *MRI findings in CJD. (A,B) A patient with probable variant CJD and three common MRI patterns in sporadic CJD: (C,D) predominantly subcortical, (E,F) both cortical and subcortical, and (G,H) predominantly cortical. Note that in sporadic CJD the abnormalities are always (C,E,G) more evident on DWI than (D,F,H) on FLAIR images. (A,B) An MRI of a 21-year-old woman with probable variant CJD showing bilateral thalamic hyperintensity in the mesial pars (mainly dorsomedian nucleus) and posterior pars (pulvinar) of the thalamus, the so-called double hockey stick sign. Also note the pulvinar sign, with the posterior thalamus (pulvinar) being more hyperintense than the anterior putamen. The three sporadic CJD cases are pathology proved. (C,D) An MRI of a 52-year-old woman showing strong hyperintensity in bilateral striatum (solid arrows, both caudate and putamen) and slight hyperintensity in mesial and posterior thalamus (dotted arrow). (E,F) An MRI of a 68-year-old man showing hyperintensity in bilateral striatum (note anteroposterior gradient in the putamen, which is commonly seen in CJD), thalamus, right insula (dotted arrow), anterior and posterior cingulate gyrus (arrow, L > R), and left temporal-parietal-occipital junction (arrow). (G,H) An MRI of a 76-year-old woman showing a diffuse hyperintense signal mainly in the bilateral parietal and occipital cortex, right posterior insula (dashed arrow) and left inferior frontal cortex (arrow), but no significant subcortical abnormalities. CJD, Creutzfeldt–Jakob disease; DWI, diffusion-weighted imaging; FLAIR, fluid-attenuated inversion recovery; MRI, magnetic resonance imaging. (Borrowed from Vitali et al. Neuroimaging in dementia. Semin. Neurol. Sep 2008;28(4):467–483 with permission from Thieme Publishing Group.)*

history of prion disease; often this is because relatives were misdiagnosed with other neuropsychiatric or other conditions, such as alcoholic dementia. In some cultures, it is common for families to hide their medical history. In some mutations such as E200K in Slovakia, however, there is a negative family history because of reduced mutation penetrance (Kovacs et al., 2005).

As noted, historically, there have been three major classifications of gPrDs, largely based on clinical and pathological characteristics: fCJD, GSS, and FFI. These classifications are not absolute because some mutations have features that blend fCJD and GSS. More important, these classifications predate identification of the *PRNP* gene and thus genetic classification (Mead, 2006). Patients with gPrD typically have a younger age of onset (typically approximately in their forties to sixties), a slower progressive course, and a longer life span (typically a few years) than sCJD patients, but this varies greatly among mutations. Depending on the *PRNP* mutation and other genetic and epigenetic factors, some

gPrDs present virtually identically (clinically and pathologically) to sCJD, with rapid onset of clinical symptoms and short survival of weeks to months (Kong et al., 2004; Mead, 2006). In general, fCJD presents like classic sCJD with rapidly progressive dementia, with ataxia, other motor problems and myoclonus. GSS usually has a slower progression over a few years, often with early ataxia and other cerebellar features, sometimes early behavioral features, and dementia later in the course. The course of FFI usually presents with intractable insomnia, dysautonomia, hallucinations, and motor signs.

Some less common *PRNP* mutations, such as V180I, result in an older age of onset, in one's seventies or eighties. gPrDs often have variable presentations and disease courses within the same mutation, and sometimes, even within the same family. As noted, the codon 129 polymorphism within *PRNP* as well as other polymorphisms (see Fig. 69.3) often effect the presentation of gPrDs (Brown and Mastrianni, 2010; Kong et al., 2004; Mead, 2006; Mead et al., 2007).

TABLE 69.3. (Continued)

MAJOR AND MINOR BEHAVIORAL FEATURES	sCJD	
MAJOR SUBCATEGORY	% OF ALL sCJD CASES (N = 84)	PERCENT OF sCJD WITH THE MAJOR BEHAVIOR
Only tactile	1	3
Only auditory	4	10
Any two	6	16
All three types	2	6
Disturbing	15	42

*Unlike Table 69.2, frequencies in this table are for any subjects with these symptoms (not just symptoms occurring at least weekly, as in Table 69.2).

fluid samples, this study did not allow for legitimate comparison between biomarkers. Nevertheless, they found the sensitivity and specificity of the 14-3-3 to be 85% and 84%, t-tau (cutoff greater than 1,300 pg/ml) 86% and 88%, NSE 73% and 95%, and S100β 82% and 76%, respectively (Sanchez-Juan et al., 2006). The same methodological problems were also present in a more recent 2010 survey of the UK surveillance

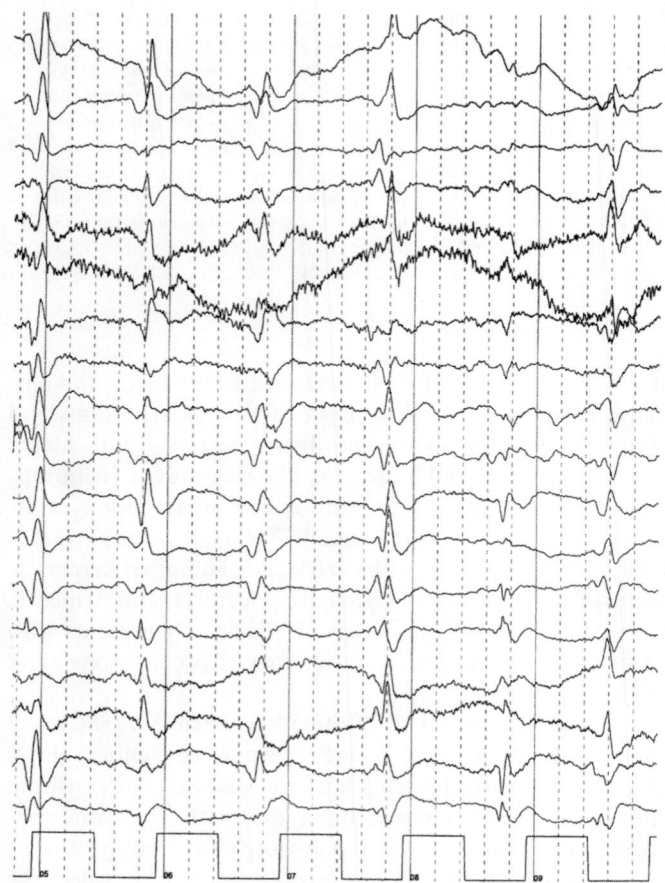

Figure 69.1 *Diagnostic EEG in CJD. Electroencephalogram showing 1-Hz periodic sharp wave complexes (PSWCs) consistent with CJD.*

center data; however, they did a separate analysis of cases in which both 14-3-3 and t-tau protein were tested in the same samples. The sensitivity and specificity for 14-3-3 and t-tau tested in the same samples were 85% and 74% for 14-3-3 and 81% and 85% for t-Tau (Chohan et al., 2010).

MAGNETIC RESONANCE IMAGING IN SCJD

Diffusion weighted imaging (DWI) MRI has higher sensitivity for sCJD than either electroencephalogram or 14-3-3 protein (Shiga et al., 2004; Vitali et al., 2008; Young et al., 2005; Zerr et al., 2009). Magnetic resonance imaging typically shows cortical gyral hyperintensities (cortical ribboning) on fluid attenuated inversion recovery (FLAIR) and especially DWI sequences (Vitali et al., 2011). These same sequences, as well as standard T2 sequences, also often reveal hyperintensities in the deep nuclei (the caudate, putamen, and less often the thalamus). Diffusion weighted imaging has a higher sensitivity than FLAIR for sCJD (Vitali et al., 2011). Figure 69.2C–H shows some typical MRI patterns in sCJD.

When CJD is suspected, a brain MRI with diffusion (DWI and attenuated diffusion coefficient map [ADC map]) and FLAIR sequences should be obtained (Vitali et al., 2008). Even at major medical centers, many radiologists are not familiar with the MRI findings indicative of CJD, and a majority of sCJD MRIs are misread (Geschwind et al., 2010). Diagnostic MRI criteria for sCJD have been proposed. Some allow the use of FLAIR or DWI and do not include abnormalities in the frontal lobes (Zerr et al., 2009), whereas others require diffusion abnormalities and do not exclude frontal lobe involvement (Vitali et al., 2008).

DIAGNOSTIC TESTS ON THE HORIZON FOR CJD

Although not yet in clinical practice, newer *in vitro* assays such as the protein misfolding cyclic amplification (PMCA) assay and modifications of this assay are on the horizon (see Prion Transmission and Detection). In these assays, a very small amount of fluid (e.g., blood or CSF) or brain tissue suspected to contain prions is mixed with PrP^C (recombinant or from normal brain) and subjected to alternating series of incubations and either shaking or sonication. PrP^Sc is amplified and more easily detected by transforming the PrP^C substrate into PrP^Sc (see Prion Transmission and Detection) (Atarashi et al., 2011; Brown and Mastrianni, 2010).

GENETIC PRION DISEASES

Genetic prion diseases (gPrDs) were discussed previously (Prion Diseases: Basic Concepts) More than 40 mutations, including point mutations, stop codons, insertions, and deletions, have been identified to cause gPrD (Fig. 69.3). Testing and diagnosis can be achieved through DNA testing of blood while a patient is alive or through autopsy tissue. Despite the typically high penetrance (100% for most mutations), more than 60% of patients with gPrD do not have a positive family

TABLE 69.2. Frequency of UCSF sCJD cohort patients exhibiting behaviors from the neuropsychiatric inventory (NPI) at least once a week

BEHAVIOR FROM THE NPI OBSERVED ≥ ONCE/WEEK	PERCENT OF sCJD SUBJECTS (N = 84)
Eating behavior	68
Apathy	63
Anxiety	55
Sleep disturbance	53
Aberrant motor	49
Agitation	44
Depression	43
Delusions	34
Irritability	32
Hallucinations	23
Euphoria	18
Disinhibition	17

TABLE 69.3. Analysis of frequency of any occurrence of five common behaviors in sCJD*

MAJOR AND MINOR BEHAVIORAL FEATURES	sCJD	
MAJOR SUBCATEGORY	% OF ALL sCJD CASES (N = 84)	PERCENT OF sCJD WITH THE MAJOR BEHAVIOR
Change in eating habits	71% (N = 60)	
Loss of appetite	25	35
Increase in appetite	20	28
Weight loss	39	55
Weight gain	18	25
Change eating behavior	16	22
Change food preferences	35	48
Sleep disturbances	55% (N = 46)	
Less sleep	48	87
Increased sleep	4	7
Unspecified	4	7
Aberrant motor	50% (N = 42)	
Pacing	23	45
Rummaging	20	40
Repeatedly taking on/off clothes	13	26
Handling buttons or picking	27	55
Fidgeting	31	62
Delusions	45% (N = 38)	
In danger	20	45
Others stealing from them	19	42
Cheating spouse	5	11
Unwelcome visitors in home	13	29
Family will abandon them	6	13
Their house not their home	6	13
TV/magazine figures present in their home	11	24
Hallucinations	37% (N = 31)	
Any visual	31	84
Any auditory	8	23
Any tactile	7	19
Only visual	23	61

(continued)

conditions (Satoh et al., 1999). When initially published in 1996, the 14-3-3 was reported to have 100% sensitivity and 96% specificity, but this study was limited by small sample size and poor controls (Hsich et al., 1996). Subsequent larger European studies have found this protein to have a sensitivity and specificity of about 85%, but control patients might not have been sufficiently characterized in some of these studies (Collins et al., 2006; Sanchez-Juan et al., 2006). A more recent analysis in the United Kingdom showed cerebrospinal fluid 14-3-3 sensitivity of 86% and specificity of 74% in a pathologically confirmed cohort (Chohan et al., 2010). Recent data in a large US cohort from the US National Prion Disease Pathology Surveillance Center (NPDPSC) showed the 14-3-3 Western blot only had a receiver operating characteristic area under the curve (ROC AUC) value of 0.68 (Hamlin et al., 2012), which is rather poor (a test with perfect sensitivity and specificity would be 1.0). Many feel that the 14-3-3 protein is merely a marker of rapid neuronal injury and has little specificity for sCJD. It is important to realize that cerebrospinal fluid 14-3-3 protein is elevated in many non-prion neurological conditions resulting in neuronal injury including multiple sclerosis, encephalitis, Alzheimer's disease, and stroke (Geschwind et al., 2003).

Total-tau (t-tau), neuron specific enolase (NSE), and the astrocytic protein S100β are also used as cerebrospinal fluid biomarkers for sCJD diagnosis. The sensitivity and specificity of these biomarkers for sCJD varies greatly among studies. One large multicenter European study retrospectively examined the sensitivity and specificity of four biomarkers: 14-3-3, t-tau, NSE, and S100β. Because not all patients underwent all four tests, nor were the tests performed in the same cerebrospinal

Cognitive problems are often among the first symptoms in sCJD, and typically include mild confusion, memory loss, and difficulty concentrating, organizing, or planning (Appleby et al., 2009; Rabinovici et al., 2006). Motor manifestations of CJD include extrapyramidal symptoms (bradykinesia, dystonia, tremor), cerebellar symptoms (gait or limb ataxia), and in many patients myoclonus (sudden jerking movements of the limbs or trunk) (Brown et al., 1986). Whereas the cognitive and certainly motor symptoms are obvious, behavioral/psychiatric features are common (Brown et al., 1986) and often early but are more subtle, and might not be what bring patients to medical attention (Rabinovici et al., 2006). These are discussed further in the section Neuropsychiatric Features of sCJD. Prodromal signs often include constitutional symptoms (i.e., fatigue, malaise, headache, dry cough, lightheadedness, vertigo), which occur in at least one-third of patients (Brown et al., 1986). Visual symptoms, such as blurred or double vision, cortical blindness, or other perceptual problems, occur as the first symptom in about 5% (Rabinovici et al., 2006), as early symptoms in about 15% (Brown et al., 1986), and in almost one-third of patients throughout the disease course (Brown et al., 1986). These symptoms likely are caused by problems with processing of visual information in the brain rather than retinal or cranial nerve abnormalities. Higher cortical signs, such as aphasia, neglect, or apraxia (inability to perform learned movements), owing to cortical dysfunction are present early in 15% and through the disease course in almost one-half of patients (P. Brown et al., 1986). Sensory symptoms, such as numbness, tingling, and/or pain are less well-recognized symptoms, and are probably under-reported given the magnitude of the other symptoms in sCJD. They occur about 10% of sCJD patients but often are very early symptoms (Brown et al., 1986; Rabinovici et al., 2006; Will et al., 2004). Painful dysesthesias, a more common feature (included in clinical diagnostic criteria for vCJD) might also occur in some patients with sCJD (Rabinovici et al., 2006).

Various clinical subtypes of sCJD also have been described, including a visual-onset form (Heidenhain variant; Kropp et al., 1999), an ataxic-onset form (Brownell-Oppenheimer; Brown et al., 2010), and recently an "affective variant" (Appleby et al., 2009). In the Heidenhain form typically the first symptom(s) are visual disturbances, such as blurred vision, visual field restriction, illusions, visual hallucinations, and even cortical blindness. Patients with the Heidenhain variant tend to have typical EEG findings, often have MM1 molecular classification, and shorter disease duration than other sCJD forms (Appleby et al., 2009; Kropp et al., 1999). In the Brownell-Oppenheimer variant of sCJD, patients have isolated ataxia at onset. These patients tend to not have classic EEG findings of PSWCs and the brain MRI often shows T2/FLAIR and DWI hyperintensity in the caudate and putamen (see Diagnostic Tests for sCJD) (Appleby et al., 2009). Behavioral/affective features of sCJD are discussed in Neuropsychiatric Features of sCJD.

NEUROPSYCHIATRIC FEATURES OF sCJD

Although sCJD generally is thought of as a cognitive and motor disorder, psychiatric symptoms often are prominent and are under-recognized as early, if not the very first symptoms. Early behavioral and psychiatric symptoms in sCJD might include irritability, agitation, depression, apathy, aberrant motor behavior, aggression, anxiety, and unspecified personality changes (Rabinovici et al., 2006). Table 69.2 shows the frequency of a various neuropsychiatric behaviors from the Neuropsychiatric Inventory (NPI) (Cummings, 1997) occurring at least once per week in our UCSF cohort of 84 probable and definite patients with sCJD (M. D. Geschwind et al., 2007; Forner et al., 2011). Eating behaviors were the most common, occurring in about two-thirds of patients, and were usually eating less/losing weight (Tables 69.2 and 69.3). Apathy, anxiety, and sleep disturbances (typically insomnia) were the next most frequent neuropsychiatric behaviors, followed by aberrant motor behavior (repetitive behaviors, such as taking on/ off clothes), agitation, and depression. When hallucinations occurred, they were usually visual. Table 69.3 shows details of five major NPI behaviors (change in eating habits, sleep disturbances, aberrant motor behavior, delusions, and hallucinations) occurring at any frequency (not just at least weekly, as in Table 69.2) in a UCSF sCJD cohort. More than half of sCJD patients had sleep problems, usually insomnia. Half of the patients had aberrant motor behaviors. Although only about 25% of subjects had hallucinations occurring at least once per week (see Table 69.2), 37% had hallucinations of any frequency (see Table 69.3). Auditory and tactile hallucinations occurred in less than 10% of patients. Some patients had multiple modalities of hallucinations. Delusions were even more common than hallucinations, and were often paranoid (Forner et al., 2011).

DIAGNOSTIC TESTS FOR sCJD

ELECTROENCEPHALOGRAM IN sCJD

The diagnostic electroencephalogram finding in sCJD consists of sharp or triphasic waves (periodic sharp wave complexes or PSWCs) occurring every 0.5 to 2 seconds (Fig. 69.1) (Brown and Mastrianni, 2010). This electroencephalogram is found in only two-thirds of sCJD patients and often is present only late in the disease course. Other neurological conditions, however, such as Alzheimer's disease, dementia with Lewy bodies (DLB), toxic-metabolic and anoxic encephalopathies, progressive multifocal leukoencephalopathy, and Hashimoto encephalopathy, also can have PSWCs on electroencephalogram (Seipelt et al., 1999; Tschampa et al., 2001). In most sCJD patients, the electroencephalogram typically first shows focal or diffuse slowing (Steinhoff et al., 2004).

CEREBROSPINAL FLUID TESTS IN sCJD

The clinical utility of cerebrospinal fluid biomarkers is somewhat controversial, in part because of varying degrees of sensitivity and specificity around the world. The 14-3-3 protein was one of the first CSF proteins touted as a diagnostic marker for CJD, but many feel it has limited sensitivity and specificity (Chapman et al., 2000; Geschwind et al., 2003) because it is found elevated in many non-prion neurological

From 1999 to 2002, mortality from CJD in Europe, Canada, and Australia was estimated to be 1.67/million for all prion cases and 1.39 for sCJD (Ladogana et al., 2005). In the United States, with about 300 million people, there are about 300 cases per year, but this number varies considerably from year to year (Holman et al., 2010). Because sCJD tends to fluctuate within a relatively narrow age range, and most persons in developed countries will live to the age at which CJD usually occurs (see sCJD: Clinical Features) a person's lifetime risk of dying from sCJD is estimated to be about 1 in 10,000s, much higher than the incidence (across all age groups) of 1 to 1.5 per million.

CLINICAL FEATURES

One of the difficulties in the diagnosis of prion diseases is that they may present with many varied neurological and psychiatric symptoms, and each patient presents differently, likely depending on where in that patient's brain the prions begin to accumulate. Most patients with sCJD and fCJD present with cognitive impairment (eventually dementia), movement disorders (e.g., myoclonus), and coordination problems (e.g., ataxia) (Brown and Mastrianni, 2010) and/or psychiatric symptoms (Brown et al., 1986). Visual symptoms are also common. Unfortunately, psychiatric features have been given a lower profile in much of the neurological literature and diagnostic criteria. The following section discusses the major clinical and laboratory aspects of various prion diseases.

sCJD: CLINICAL FEATURES

Sporadic CJD typically is characterized by rapidly progressive dementia, with a median survival of seven to eight months. (More than 90% of patients die within the first year of disease.) The typical age of onset, however, is generally quite narrow; the unimodal peak mean age of onset is around 68 years (Brown et al., 1986). Most persons with CJD are more than 65 years old (Holman et al., 2010). Occurrence of sCJD at less than the forties or later than the mid-seventies is uncommon (Corato et al., 2006; Will, 2004), but the range of onset of sCJD is quite wide, from teenagers (Murray et al., 2008)—the youngest to our knowledge is a 12-year-old diagnosed recently in Spain (M. Geschwind, personal communication)—to a 98-year-old in Italy (Buganza et al., 2009).

Diagnostic criteria for sCJD are often divided by increasing likelihood of diagnosis into possible, probable, and definite categories. The most commonly used criteria are World Health Organization revised criteria (WHO, 1998). For possible sCJD, they require dementia plus any two of the four combinations of symptoms:

1. Myoclonus

2. Pyramidal/extrapyramidal features

3. Visual/cerebellar features

4. Akinetic mutism (not moving, not speaking)

To meet probable criteria, patients must meet possible and also have positive laboratory evidence of either a characteristic electroencephalogram (EEG) (showing about one hertz periodic sharp wave complexes [PSWCs]) or a positive/elevated CSF 14-3-3 protein (see Diagnostic Tests for sCJD) (WHO, 1998). The pyramidal symptoms are motor findings on exam, such as hyperreflexia, focal weakness, or an extensor response. Extrapyramidal symptoms typically include rigidity, slowed movement (bradykinesia), tremor, or dystonia and are caused by problems in the basal ganglia or its connections. Akinetic mutism is the end stage of the disease when patients are mute and without purposeful movement (WHO, 1998). Definite sCJD diagnosis requires neuropathological evidence of CJD (Kretzschmar et al., 1996; WHO, 1998). One problem with WHO-based clinical diagnostic criteria for possible and probable sCJD is that they were designed for epidemiological purposes to identify cases by record review that had not had definitive pathological diagnosis. These criteria were not designed to diagnosis patients early or when first presenting to a physician's office. Thus, in our experience, many patients will not meet Revised WHO criteria until later in the disease course.

The addition of brain MRI to probable sCJD criteria was proposed in 2007 (Geschwind, Haman et al., 2007; Geschwind, Josephs et al., 2007), and in 2009, Modified European probable sCJD criteria allowed inclusion of brain MRI as a supportive ancillary test. Note that there are errors in the listed symptoms in these European criteria as initially published; dementia was supposed to be required for all cases and is not in the choice of four possible symptoms, and myoclonus was inadvertently left out (Zerr et al., 2009) (see Magnetic Resonance Imaging in sCJD).

The clinical presentation of sCJD is highly variable. Most commonly the first symptoms are cognitive or cerebellar (Brown et al., 1986; Rabinovici et al., 2006). Onset is typically subacute, but rarely is acute or strokelike (Hohler and Flynn, 2006). As noted by epidemiological diagnostic criteria, motor features such as ataxia and other cerebellar dysfunction and extrapyramidal and pyramidal symptoms are quite common. These are often the first symptoms that bring patients to medical attention. Symptoms of sCJD vary widely, but typically include cognitive changes (dementia), behavioral and personality changes, difficulties with movement and coordination, visual symptoms, and constitutional symptoms (Brown et al., 1986, 1994; Rabinovici et al., 2006). Although most patients with sCJD progress rapidly over weeks to months from the first obvious symptoms to death, a large minority survive for a year or longer, sometimes surviving for two to three years (Johnson et al., 2012; Parchi et al., 1999). The presentation and duration of sCJD are in part affected by the molecular classification of patients based on their polymorphism at codon 129 in PRNP (see Prion Diseases: Basic Concepts) and the prion typing based on Western blot of brain tissue (see Prion Strains and Strain Typing of Human Prion Diseases) (Parchi et al., 1999). The ultimate, final stage of sCJD is usually an akinetic-mute state (no purposeful movement and not speaking) (WHO, 1998). Most patients with prion disease, as with other neurodegenerative dementias, eventually die from aspiration pneumonia.

TABLE 69.1. Human prion diseases

CLASS	DISEASE	*PRNP* MUTATION	AVERAGE AGE OF ONSET (YR)	AVERAGE DISEASE DURATION	PROTEASE-RESISTANT PRP	PRPSc NEUROPATHOLOGY
Sporadic	sCJD MM1/MV1	None	65	4 mo	Type 1	Predominantly non-amyloid "synaptic" PrPSc deposition
	sCJD MM2	None	64	16 mo	Type 2	Perivacuolar PrPSc deposits
	sCJD MM2-thalamic (sporadic fatal insomnia)	None	52	16 mo	Type 2	Mild PrPSc deposition in the thalamus
	sCJD MV2	None	60	17 mo	Type 2	Kuru-like plaques
	sCJD VV2	None	61	6 mo	Type 2	Focal plaque-like PrPSc deposits
	sCJD VV1	None	44	21 mo	Type 1	Mild "synaptic" PrPSc deposition
	VPSPr	None	67	30 mo	Variable presence of smaller PrPSc fragments	Granular and "synaptic" PrPSc deposits
Genetic	gCJD	Many (i.e., E200K, D178N-V129, V210I)	39–59 (mutation dependent)	6–14 mo (mutation dependent)	Type 1 or Type 2	Similar to typical sporadic CJD
	GSS	Many (i.e., P102L, A117V, F198S, Y145Stop)	Mutation dependent	5–6 yr	Smaller PrPSc fragments (~7–14 kDa)	PrPSc amyloid plaques, PrPSc amyloid angiopathy with certain mutations
	FFI	D178N-M129	49	11 mo	Type 2	Mild PrPSc deposition in the thalamus
Acquired	Iatrogenic CJD	None	N/A	4 mo	Type 1 or Type 2	Dependent on source of contamination and route of infection
	vCJD	None	28	13 mo	Type 2	Florid PrPSc plaques
	Kuru	None	N/A	12 mo	Type 1 or Type 2	Kuru plaques

truncations (Mead, 2006). Because the mutations are not clustered within a specific region of the PrP amino acid sequence, ascertaining the causal link between mutation and disease has been difficult. Although it is unlikely that all mutations act by the same mechanism, it is generally thought that mutant PrP^C is more likely to misfold and spontaneously adopt the PrP^{Sc} conformation than non-mutant PrP^C, greatly enhancing the probability of prion disease initiation. The clinical phenotype of the disease (i.e., CJD vs. GSS vs. FFI) is dependent on the mutation present in PrP and whether M129 or V129 is also present on the mutant protein. For instance, the D178N mutation in *PRNP* causes FFI if present in conjunction with the M129 polymorphism or fCJD if present in conjunction with the V129 polymorphism (Goldfarb et al., 1992).

The third forms of human prion diseases, which account for less than approximately 1% of all cases, are the acquired or infectious forms. Acquired forms of the disease occur when small amounts of PrP^{Sc} are introduced into the body by either dietary or iatrogenic (introduced by medical treatment) routes.

This PrP^{Sc} "seed" then prompts the conversion of PrP^C in the host, which initiates the process of prion disease. Currently, the most well-known human prion disease of this form is variant CJD (vCJD), acquired largely through the consumption of BSE (Brown and Mastrianni, 2010). Other examples include iatrogenic CJD caused by the implantation of prion-contaminated dura mater grafts, treatment with contaminated human pituitary hormones, such as growth hormone, and the use of improperly sterilized (i.e., treated in a way to kill viruses and bacteria, but not sufficient to denature prions) neurosurgical instruments (Brown et al., 2000; Brown et al., 2006; Will et al., 2004).

EPIDEMIOLOGY

The incidence of human prion diseases is about 1 to 1.5 per million per year in most developed countries, with some variability between countries and from year to year (Will et al., 1998).

position 129 of the protein, giving rise to the M129 or V129 PrP allotypes. The codon 129 polymorphism is a critical determinant of susceptibility to a variety of prion diseases (Parchi et al., 1999). Under normal conditions, PrP is expressed at high levels in the brain and at lower levels in peripheral tissues but does not cause disease. This form of the protein is referred to as PrP^C (cellular PrP) and is a precursor of disease-associated forms of PrP. PrP^C is typically found in cholesterol-rich microdomains of the cell membrane referred to as lipid rafts. The N-terminal domain of PrP contains a series of octapeptide repeats that allow PrP^C to bind copper ions. Expansion of the octarepeat domain in PrP causes certain forms of genetic prion disease, called octapeptide repeat insertion (OPRI) mutations, classified clinically either as fCJD or GSS depending on the number of repeats present and their clinical–pathological features (see Genetic Prion Diseases). Although the function of PrP^C in the brain under normal conditions remains contentious, it appears to play roles in neuroprotection, olfactory behavior, and/or the maintenance of peripheral nerve myelination (Watts and Westaway, 2007).

During prion disease, PrP^C undergoes a conformational (structural) transition into a pathologically misfolded isoform referred to as PrP^{Sc} (PrP Scrapie) (Colby and Prusiner, 2011). PrP^{Sc} is the infectious, neurotoxic, and disease-causing form of the prion protein and has vastly different biochemical and structural properties than PrP^C. The atomic structure of PrP^C has been solved using nuclear magnetic resonance (NMR) spectroscopy, revealing that PrP^C is a predominantly α-helical protein with an intrinsically disordered N-terminal domain (Colby and Prusiner, 2011). In contrast, although the high-resolution structure of PrP^{Sc} has not yet been obtained, PrP^{Sc} is enriched in β-sheet content and is generally more insoluble, more prone to aggregate into higher-order structures such as amyloid fibrils, and more resistant to protease digestion than PrP^C. The fact that PrP can fold into at least two completely different conformations (PrP^C and PrP^{Sc}) was a highly novel assertion; it was previously believed that only a single tertiary structure was possible for a given amino acid sequence.

Several lines of evidence argue strongly that the protein-only hypothesis is the most reasonable explanation for the properties of prion disease. First, PrP is absolutely required for prion disease because mice that lack the prion protein are resistant to prions (Bueler et al., 1993). Second, transgenic mice over-expressing certain mutant or wild-type PrP molecules develop neuropathological changes reminiscent of prion disease and propagate infectious prions in their brains (Watts et al., 2012). The "final" proof of the protein-only hypothesis has recently been achieved via the generation of "synthetic prions" from recombinant prion protein produced in bacteria, proving that no nucleic acids are required for the creation of prion infectivity (Colby and Prusiner, 2011).

NOMENCLATURE OF JAKOB–CREUTZFELDT DISEASE

The naming of CJD is a bit confusing, and somewhat controversial, so it helps to briefly review some of the history. In 1921 and

1923 Alfons Jakob published four papers describing five unusual cases of rapidly progressive dementia. He stated that his cases were nearly identical to a single case report of a young woman published in 1920 by his professor Hans Creutzfeldt. This disease was referred to for many decades as Jakob's or Jakob-Creutzfeldt disease until Clarence J. Gibbs, a prominent researcher in the field, started using the term Creutzfeldt–Jakob disease because the acronym was closer to his own initials, CJ (Gibbs, 1992). The patients whom Jakob described, however, were quite different from Creutzfeldt's case, which did not have what we now call prion disease, and only two of Jakob's five cases actually had prion disease (Katscher, 1998). Thus, the name of for prion disease probably should be Jakob's disease, or possibly Jakob–Creutzfeldt disease. We use the term Jakob–Creutzfeldt disease and the acronym therefore probably should be JCD, but in our experience we have noted that many clinicians mistakenly think the JC virus (the source of progressive multifocal leukoencephalopathy; PML) is the cause of or associated with prion disease and even test for the JC virus working up a suspected prion case. Therefore, unfortunately we continue to use the term CJD for Jakob's disease. This chapter uses the term CJD.

FORMS OF HUMAN PRION DISEASE: MODES OF ACQUISITION

Human prion diseases are unique in that they can manifest through three completely distinct modes of acquisition (Table 69.1). The most common forms of human prion diseases, which accounts for approximately 85% to 90% of all cases, are the sporadic disorders, including sporadic CJD (sCJD). In sporadic cases, there is no evidence of a genetic cause (including no mutations in *PRNP*) and no evidence of any environmental and/or iatrogenic risk factors suggesting that the disease arose spontaneously. Although the exact molecular details underlying the cause of sporadic CJD remain unclear, it is thought to arise from the spontaneous misfolding of PrP^C into PrP^{Sc}.

This conversion likely happens on rare occasions in the healthy brain because the cellular quality control machinery is capable of degrading the newly formed PrP^{Sc} molecules and thus prevents the initiation of prion disease. As the brain ages, however, quality control mechanisms might begin to malfunction, increasing the probability that larger quantities of PrP^{Sc} form spontaneously. In rare cases, once a critical amount of PrP^{Sc} has been reached, the cellular degradation machinery is no longer able to keep up with prion replication, and the pathogenic cascade of prion disease commences. This explains why sporadic CJD occurs most frequently in older individuals and why the disease is very rare.

The second forms of human prion diseases, accounting for approximately 10% to 15% of all cases, are the genetic forms such as fCJD, GSS, and FFI. In these genetic prion diseases (gPrDs), a mutation in the *PRNP* gene results in the production of a mutant PrP molecule. These mutations are inherited in an autosomal-dominant fashion. Only a single copy of the mutant gene is necessary for prion disease to occur. Many different types of mutations in *PRNP* cause genetic prion disease, including point mutations, insertions, deletions, and

69 | CLINICAL FEATURES AND PATHOGENESIS OF PRION DISEASE

JOEL C. WATTS AND MICHAEL D. GESCHWIND

A BRIEF HISTORY OF PRION DISEASES

The first recognized prion disease in humans was Jakob–Creutzfeldt disease (CJD), a rapidly progressive neurodegenerative disorder of the central nervous system (CNS) in which patient death often occurs within a few months of the appearance of clinical symptoms. At the time of its first description in the early twentieth century by Alfons Jakob, who referred to a case originally described by Hans Creutzfeldt (see Nomenclature of Jakob–Creutzfeldt Disease), the cause of CJD remained completely unknown, and little research was conducted on CJD because of its rarity. The first clue toward the nature of CJD came when it was recognized that brains from patients who had died of CJD resembled the brains of patients with Kuru, a neurodegenerative disorder that affected the Fore tribe of Papua New Guinea (Prusiner, 1998). The neuropathology of both CJD and Kuru resembled that of scrapie, a neurodegenerative disease of sheep known to be transmissible between animals. This led to idea that CJD and Kuru might also be transmissible in a laboratory setting, and indeed it was demonstrated that brain extracts from CJD or Kuru patients could transmit disease to non-human primates after long incubation periods. This class of diseases is now often referred to as transmissible spongiform encephalopathies (TSEs) because of their infectious nature and unique neuropathological features. Other TSEs include bovine spongiform encephalopathy (BSE), also known as mad cow disease, in cattle, and chronic wasting disease (CWD), a TSE of deer, elk, and moose that occurs in free ranging animals. Although rare, TSEs are invariably fatal disorders. No treatment or vaccine exists for this class of diseases (Prusiner, 1998).

The nature of the infectious agent responsible for TSEs remained a scientific curiosity for many years. The vast majority of infectious human diseases are caused by exposure to parasites, bacteria, or viruses. All of these agents require an informational molecule such as DNA or RNA, which is essential for their persistence and spread. Because of the atypical nature of TSEs in that a prolonged period exists between exposure to the disease and the onset of clinical symptoms, it was assumed that a "slow" or "unconventional" virus was the cause of these disorders, and thus for many years they were considered to be caused by "slow viruses." Mounting evidence, however, argued that procedures known to inactivate viruses, such as formalin treatment, nuclease treatment, or ultraviolet irradiation, had little effect on the TSE agent, whereas procedures known to destroy proteins decreased the infectivity of the agent. Furthermore, no immune response was observed in patients with CJD, as would be expected if a foreign viral genome was present in the body. The critical breakthrough came in 1982 when Stanley Prusiner successfully purified the TSE agent from infected hamster brains and found that preparations that were highly enriched for infectivity contained a single protein but no nucleic acid. He coined the term prion to denote a *proteinaceous infectious* particle that replicates in the absence of a nucleic acid (Prusiner, 1998). This protein-only hypothesis was met with great skepticism because all previously known infectious agents, including bacteria and viruses, required a nucleic genome for replication. The concept of prions is now, however, widely accepted, and the protein-only hypothesis has been proved beyond a reasonable doubt. For his discovery of prions, Stanley Prusiner was awarded the 1997 Nobel Prize in Physiology or Medicine (Prusiner, 1998).

This chapter uses the general term prion disease instead of TSEs. This is for several reasons: (1) The term spongiform is not quite accurate neuropathologically because the pathological feature is actually vacuolation (see Neuropathology of Human Prion Diseases); (2) a few prion diseases have little or no vacuolation (Brown and Mastrianni, 2010); and (3) some prion diseases are either very difficult to transmit or have not been reliably shown to transmit (Tateishi et al., 1996).

PRION DISEASES: BASIC CONCEPTS

The protein-only hypothesis posits that infectious prions are composed of a single protein: the prion protein (PrP). The PrP is encoded by the *PRNP* gene, which is found on chromosome 20 in humans. Mutations in *PRNP* cause genetic prion diseases, often classified as familial CJD (fCJD), Gerstmann-Sträussler-Scheinker syndrome (GSS), or fatal familial insomnia (FFI). *PRNP* directs the synthesis of an approximately 250–amino acid protein that is posttranslationally modified by the removal of N- and C-terminal signal sequences and the addition of one or two asparagine-linked sugars. Following synthesis in the endoplasmic reticulum, PrP is transported to the cell surface, where it is tethered to the cell membrane of neurons by a glycosylphosphatidylinositol (GPI) anchor. In humans, there are two major polymorphic variants of PrP, with either methionine or valine residues encoded at

[Research Support, Non-U.S. Gov't]. *J. Neurol. Neurosurg. Psychiatry* 80(4):366–370.

Mayda, A.V., and DeCarli, C. (2009). Vascular cognitive impairment: prodrome to VaD? In: Wahlund, L.-O., Erkinjuntti, T., and Gauthier, S., eds. Vascular Cognitive Impairment in Clinical Practice. Cambridge, UK: Cambridge University Press, pp. 11–31.

McGuinness, B., Todd, S., et al. (2009). Blood pressure lowering in patients without prior cerebrovascular disease for prevention of cognitive impairment and dementia. [Meta-Analysis Review]. *Cochrane Database Syst. Rev.* (4):CD004034.

McKhann, G.M., Knopman, D.S., et al. (2011). The diagnosis of dementia due to Alzheimer's disease: recommendations from the National Institute on Aging-Alzheimer's Association workgroups on diagnostic guidelines for Alzheimer's disease. *Alzheimers Dement.* 7(3):263–269.

Mehagnoul-Schipper, D.J., Colier, W.N., et al. (2001). Reproducibility of orthostatic changes in cerebral oxygenation in healthy subjects aged 70 years or older. [Research Support, Non-U.S. Gov't]. *Clin. Physiol.* 21(1):77–84.

Moody, D.M., Santamore, W.P., et al. (1991). Does tortuosity in cerebral arterioles impair down-autoregulation in hypertensives and elderly normotensives? A hypothesis and computer model. [In Vitro]. *Clin. Neurosurg.* 37:372–387.

Ovbiagele, B. (2010). Optimizing vascular risk reduction in the stroke patient with atherothrombotic disease. [Review]. *Med. Princ. Pract.* 19(1):1–12.

Palumbo, V., Boulanger, J.M., et al. (2007). Leukoaraiosis and intracerebral hemorrhage after thrombolysis in acute stroke. *Neurology* 68(13): 1020–1024.

Peters, R., Beckett, N., et al. (2008). Incident dementia and blood pressure lowering in the Hypertension in the Very Elderly Trial cognitive function assessment (HYVET-COG): a double-blind, placebo controlled trial. *Lancet Neurol.* 7(8):683–689.

Peters, N., Opherk, C., et al. (2005). The pattern of cognitive performance in CADASIL: a monogenic condition leading to subcortical ischemic vascular dementia. *Am. J. Psychiatry* 162(11):2078–2085.

Poggesi, A., Pantoni, L., et al. (2011). 2001–2011: A decade of the LADIS (Leukoaraiosis And DISability) study: what have we learned about white matter changes and small-vessel disease? *Cerebrovasc. Dis.* 32(6):577–588.

Pohjasvaara, T., Mantyla, R., et al. (1999). Clinical and radiological determinants of prestroke cognitive decline in a stroke cohort. *J. Neurol. Neurosurg. Psychiatry* 67(6):742–748.

Prabhakaran, S., Wright, C.B., et al. (2008). Prevalence and determinants of subclinical brain infarction: the Northern Manhattan Study. *Neurology* 70(6):425–430.

Qiu, C., Xu, W., et al. (2010). Vascular risk profiles for dementia and Alzheimer's disease in very old people: a population-based longitudinal study. [Research Support, Non-U.S. Gov't]. *J. Alzheimers Dis.* 20(1):293–300.

Randomised trial of a perindopril-based blood-pressure-lowering regimen among 6,105 individuals with previous stroke or transient ischaemic attack. (2001). [Clinical Trial Multicenter Study Randomized Controlled Trial Research Support, Non-U.S. Gov't]. *Lancet* 358(9287):1033–1041.

Ravaglia, G., Forti, P., et al. (2005). Incidence and etiology of dementia in a large elderly Italian population. [Research Support, Non-U.S. Gov't]. *Neurology* 64(9):1525–1530.

Reed, B.R., Mungas, D.M., et al. (2004). Clinical and neuropsychological features in autopsy-defined vascular dementia. *Clin. Neuropsychol.* 18(1):63–74.

Reitz, C., Tang, M.X., et al. (2010). A summary risk score for the prediction of Alzheimer disease in elderly persons. [Research Support, N.I.H., Extramural Research Support, Non-U.S. Gov't]. *Arch. Neurols.* 67(7):835–841.

Roman, G.C., Erkinjuntti, T., et al. (2002). Subcortical ischaemic vascular dementia. *Lancet Neurol.* 1(7):426–436.

Roman, G.C., Tatemichi, T.K., et al. (1993). Vascular dementia: diagnostic criteria for research studies. Report of the NINDS-AIREN International Workshop. *Neurology* 43(2):250–260.

Ronnemaa, E., Zethelius, B., et al. (2011). Vascular risk factors and dementia: 40-year follow-up of a population-based cohort. *Dement. Geriatr. Cogn. Disord.* 31(6):460–466.

Sacco, R.L. (2007). The 2006 William Feinberg lecture: shifting the paradigm from stroke to global vascular risk estimation. [Lectures Research Support, N.I.H., Extramural]. *Stroke* 38(6):1980–1987.

Sanossian, N., and Ovbiagele, B. (2009). Prevention and management of stroke in very elderly patients. [Research Support, Non-U.S. Gov't Review]. *Lancet Neurol.* 8(11):1031–1041.

Schmidt, R., Fazekas, F., et al. (1999). MRI white matter hyperintensities: three-year follow-up of the Austrian Stroke Prevention Study. *Neurology* 53(1):132–139.

Schmidt, R., Ropele, S., et al. (2010). Diffusion-weighted imaging and cognition in the leukoariosis and disability in the elderly study. [Comparative Study Multicenter Study Research Support, Non-U.S. Gov't]. *Stroke* 41(5):e402–e408.

Schneider, J.A., Aggarwal, N.T., et al. (2009). The neuropathology of older persons with and without dementia from community versus clinic cohorts. *J. Alzheimers Dis.* 18(3):691–701.

Schneider, J.A., Arvanitakis, Z., et al. (2007). Mixed brain pathologies account for most dementia cases in community-dwelling older persons. *Neurology* 69(24):2197–2204.

Schneider, J.A., Wilson, R.S., et al. (2004). Cerebral infarctions and the likelihood of dementia from Alzheimer disease pathology. *Neurology* 62(7):1148–1155.

Sheline, Y.I., Pieper, C.F., et al. (2010). Support for the vascular depression hypothesis in late-life depression: results of a 2-site, prospective, antidepressant treatment trial. [Comparative Study Controlled Clinical Trial Multicenter Study Research Support, N.I.H., Extramural]. *Arch. Gen. Psychiatry* 67(3):277–285.

Silbert, L.C., Dodge, H.H., et al. (2012). Trajectory of white matter hyperintensity burden preceding mild cognitive impairment. *Neurology* 79(8):741–747.

Silbert, L.C., Howieson, D.B., et al. (2009). Cognitive impairment risk: white matter hyperintensity progression matters. *Neurology* 73(2):120–125.

Skoog, I., Lithell, H., et al. (2005). Effect of baseline cognitive function and antihypertensive treatment on cognitive and cardiovascular outcomes: Study on COgnition and Prognosis in the Elderly (SCOPE). [Comparative Study Multicenter Study Randomized Controlled Trial Research Support, Non-U.S. Gov't]. *Am. J. Hypertens.* 18(8):1052–1059.

Smith, E.E., and Greenberg, S.M. (2009). Beta-amyloid, blood vessels, and brain function. *Stroke* 40(7):2601–2606.

Spence, J.D. (2010). Secondary stroke prevention. [Review]. *Nat. Rev. Neurol.* 6(9):477–486.

Srikanth, V.K., Quinn, S.J., et al. (2006). Long-term cognitive transitions, rates of cognitive change, and predictors of incident dementia in a population-based first-ever stroke cohort. [Comparative Study Research Support, Non-U.S. Gov't]. *Stroke* 37(10):2479–2483.

Troncoso, J.C., Zonderman, A.B., et al. (2008). Effect of infarcts on dementia in the Baltimore longitudinal study of aging. [Comparative Study Research Support, N.I.H., Extramural Research Support, N.I.H., Intramural Research Support, Non-U.S. Gov't]. *Ann. Neurol.* 64(2):168–176.

Vermeer, S.E., Den Heijer, T., et al. (2003a). Incidence and risk factors of silent brain infarcts in the population-based Rotterdam Scan Study. *Stroke* 34(2):392–396.

Vermeer, S.E., Prins, N.D., et al. (2003b). Silent brain infarcts and the risk of dementia and cognitive decline. *N. Engl. J. Med.* 348(13):1215–1222.

White, L., Petrovitch, H., et al. (2002). Cerebrovascular pathology and dementia in autopsied Honolulu-Asia Aging Study participants. *Ann. NY Acad. Sci.* 977:9–23.

et al., 2012; Horiuchi et al., 2010). In contrast, angiotensin converting enzyme inhibitors decrease activation of both AT1 and AT2 receptors. In a recent pilot study, candesartan was associated with greater improvement in tests sensitive to executive dysfunction than hydrochlorothiazide or lisinopril (Hajjar et al., 2012). Protection of endothelial and neuronal cells may represent promising new strategies to ameliorate VCI.

DISCLOSURE

Dr. Chui has no conflicts of interest to disclose. She is funded by NIA only. Grant Support: NIH (P01-AG12435; P50 AG05142).

REFERENCES

Acciarresi, M., De Rango, P., et al. (2011). Secondary stroke prevention in women. [Research Support, Non-U.S. Gov't Review]. *Womens Health* 7(3):391–397.

Alexopoulos, G.S., Meyers, B.S., et al. (1997). "Vascular depression" hypothesis. [Research Support, U.S. Gov't, P.H.S. Review]. *Arch. Gen. Psychiatry.* 54(10):915–922.

Allan, L.M., Rowan, E.N., et al. (2011). Long term incidence of dementia, predictors of mortality and pathological diagnosis in older stroke survivors. [Research Support, Non-U.S. Gov't]. *Brain* 134(Pt 12):3716–3727.

Armario, P., and de la Sierra, A. (2009). Antihypertensive treatment and stroke prevention: are angiotensin receptor blockers superior to other antihypertensive agents? [Research Support, Non-U.S. Gov't Review]. *Ther. Adv. Cardiovasc. Dis.* 3(3):197–204.

Beach, T.G., Wilson, J.R., et al. (2007). Circle of Willis atherosclerosis: association with Alzheimer's disease, neuritic plaques and neurofibrillary tangles. [Research Support, N.I.H., Extramural Research Support, Non-U.S. Gov't]. *Acta Neuropathol.* 113(1):13–21.

Bennett, D.A., Wilson, R.S., et al. (1990). Clinical diagnosis of Binswanger's disease. *J. Neurol. Neurosurg. Psychiatry* 53(11):961–965.

Cervera, A., Amaro, S., et al. (2012). Oral anticoagulant-associated intracerebral hemorrhage. [Review]. *J. Neurol.* 259(2):212–224.

Chobanian, A.V., Bakris, G.L., et al. (2003). Seventh report of the Joint National Committee on Prevention, Detection, Evaluation, and Treatment of High Blood Pressure. [GuidelinePractice Guideline Research Support, U.S. Gov't, P.H.S.]. *Hypertension* 42(6):1206–1252.

Chui, H.C., Victoroff, J.I., et al. (1992). Criteria for the diagnosis of ischemic vascular dementia proposed by the State of California Alzheimer's Disease Diagnostic and Treatment Centers. *Neurology* 42(3 Pt 1):473–480.

Chui, H.C., Zarow, C., et al. (2006). Cognitive impact of subcortical vascular and Alzheimer's disease pathology. *Ann. Neurol.* 60(6):677–687.

Chui, H.C., Zheng, L., et al. (2012). Vascular risk factors and Alzheimer's disease: are these risk factors for plaques and tangles or for concomitant vascular pathology that increases the likelihood of dementia? An evidence-based review. *Alzheimers Res. Ther.* 4(1):1.

Cordoliani-Mackowiak, M.A., Henon, H., et al. (2003). Poststroke dementia: influence of hippocampal atrophy. *Arch. Neurol.* 60(4):585–590.

Das, R.R., Seshadri, S., et al. (2008). Prevalence and correlates of silent cerebral infarcts in the Framingham offspring study. *Stroke* 39(11):2929–2935.

Debette, S., Beiser, A., et al. (2010). Association of MRI markers of vascular brain injury with incident stroke, mild cognitive impairment, dementia, and mortality: the Framingham Offspring Study. *Stroke* 41(4):600–606.

Decarli, C., Massaro, J., et al. (2005). Measures of brain morphology and infarction in the Framingham heart study: establishing what is normal. *Neurobiol. Aging* 26(4):491–510.

Dichgans, M., Mayer, M., et al. (1998). The phenotypic spectrum of CADASIL: clinical findings in 102 cases. *Ann. Neurol.* 44(5):731–739.

Diener, H.C., Sacco, R.L., et al. (2008). Effects of aspirin plus extended-release dipyridamole versus clopidogrel and telmisartan on disability and cognitive function after recurrent stroke in patients with ischaemic stroke in the Prevention Regimen for Effectively Avoiding Second Strokes (PRoFESS) trial: a double-blind, active and placebo-controlled study. *Lancet Neurol.* 7(10):875–884.

Duering, M., Righart, R., et al. (2012). Incident subcortical infarcts induce focal thinning in connected cortical regions. *Neurology* 79(20):2025–2028.

Erkinjuntti, T., Inzitari, D., et al. (2000). Research criteria for subcortical vascular dementia in clinical trials. *J. Neural. Transm. Suppl.* 59:23–30.

Fratiglioni, L., Launer, L.J., et al. (2000). Incidence of dementia and major subtypes in Europe: a collaborative study of population-based cohorts. Neurologic Diseases in the Elderly Research Group. [Multicenter Study]. *Neurology* 54(11 Suppl 5):S10–S15.

Gold, G., Bouras, C., et al. (2002). Clinicopathological validation study of four sets of clinical criteria for vascular dementia. [Research Support, U.S. Gov't, P.H.S.]. *Am. J. Psychiatry* 159(1):82–87.

Goldstein, L.B., Bushnell, C.D., et al. (2011). Guidelines for the primary prevention of stroke: a guideline for healthcare professionals from the American Heart Association/American Stroke Association. [Practice Guideline]. *Stroke* 42(2):517–584.

Gorelick, P.B., Scuteri, A., et al. (2011). Vascular contributions to cognitive impairment and dementia: a statement for healthcare professionals from the American Heart Association/American Stroke Association. *Stroke* 42(9):2672–2713.

Hachinski, V., Iadecola, C., et al. (2006). National Institute of Neurological Disorders and Stroke-Canadian Stroke Network vascular cognitive impairment harmonization standards. *Stroke* 37(9):2220–2241.

Hachinski, V.C., Iliff, L.D., et al. (1975). Cerebral blood flow in dementia. *Arch. Neurol.* 32(9):632–637.

Hajjar, I., Hart, M., et al. (2012). Effect of antihypertensive therapy on cognitive function in early executive cognitive impairment: a double-blind randomized clinical trial. [Comparative Study Letter Randomized Controlled Trial Research Support, N.I.H., Extramural Research Support, Non-U.S. Gov't]. *Arch. Intern. Med.* 172(5):442–444.

Honig, L.S., Kukull, W., et al. (2005). Atherosclerosis and AD: analysis of data from the US National Alzheimer's Coordinating Center. [Research Support, N.I.H., Extramural Research Support, Non-U.S. Gov't Research Support, U.S. Gov't, P.H.S.]. *Neurology* 64(3):494–500.

Horiuchi, M., Mogi, M., et al. (2010). The angiotensin II type 2 receptor in the brain. [Review]. *JRAAS* 11(1):1–6.

Jeerakathil, T., Wolf, P.A., et al. (2004). Stroke risk profile predicts white matter hyperintensity volume: the Framingham Study. *Stroke* 35(8):1857–1861.

Jouvent, E., Viswanathan, A., et al. (2007). Brain atrophy is related to lacunar lesions and tissue microstructural changes in CADASIL. *Stroke* 38(6):1786–1790.

Kales, H.C., Maixner, D.F., et al. (2005). Cerebrovascular disease and late-life depression. [Research Support, U.S. Gov't, Non-P.H.S. Review]. *Am. J. Geriat. Psychiat.* 13(2):88–98.

Kavirajan, H., and Schneider, L.S. (2007). Efficacy and adverse effects of cholinesterase inhibitors and memantine in vascular dementia: a meta-analysis of randomised controlled trials. *Lancet Neurol.* 6(9):782–792.

Knopman, D.S., Rocca, W.A., et al. (2002). Incidence of vascular dementia in Rochester, Minn, 1985–1989. [Research Support, U.S. Gov't, P.H.S.]. *Arch. Neurol.* 59(10):1605–1610.

Kokmen, E., Whisnant, J.P., et al. (1996). Dementia after ischemic stroke: a population-based study in Rochester, Minnesota (1960–1984). *Neurology* 46(1):154–159.

Launer, L.J., Hughes, T.M., et al. (2011). Microinfarcts, brain atrophy, and cognitive function: the Honolulu Asia Aging Study Autopsy Study. [Research Support, N.I.H., Extramural Research Support, N.I.H., Intramural]. *Ann. Neurol.* 70(5):774–780.

Lee, M., Saver, J.L., et al. (2012). Does achieving an intensive versus usual blood pressure level prevent stroke? [Comparative Study Meta-Analysis]. *Ann. Neurol.* 71(1):133–140.

Leys, D., Henon, H., et al. (2005). Poststroke dementia. [Research Support, Non-U.S. Gov't Review]. *Lancet Neurol.* 4(11):752–759.

Longstreth, W.T., Jr., Arnold, A.M., et al. (2005). Incidence, manifestations, and predictors of worsening white matter on serial cranial magnetic resonance imaging in the elderly: the Cardiovascular Health Study. *Stroke* 36(1):56–61.

Longstreth, W.T., Jr., Dulberg, C., et al. (2002). Incidence, manifestations, and predictors of brain infarcts defined by serial cranial magnetic resonance imaging in the elderly: the Cardiovascular Health Study. *Stroke* 33(10):2376–2382.

Lopez, O.L., Kuller, L.H., et al. (2005). Classification of vascular dementia in the Cardiovascular Health Study Cognition Study. [Research Support, N.I.H., Extramural Research Support, U.S. Gov't, P.H.S.]. *Neurology* 64(9):1539–1547.

Lopez, O.L., Kuller, L.H., et al. (2003). Evaluation of dementia in the cardiovascular health cognition study. [Research Support, U.S. Gov't, P.H.S.]. *Neuroepidemiology* 22(1):1–12.

Massaro, J.M., D'Agostino, R.B., Sr., et al. (2004). Managing and analysing data from a large-scale study on Framingham offspring relating brain structure to cognitive function. [Comparative Study Research Support, U.S. Gov't, P.H.S.]. *Stat. Med.* 23(2):351–367.

Matsui, Y., Tanizaki, Y., et al. (2009). Incidence and survival of dementia in a general population of Japanese elderly: the Hisayama study.

in MMSE were noted in the active versus placebo arms (i.e., PROGRESS and PRoFESS) (Diener et al., 2008; "Randomised trial…," 2001). This lack of evidence may reflect limitations in clinical trial design, because studies have been relatively short in duration (two–four years), have employed insensitive cognitive outcome measures (i.e., Mini-Mental State Examination), and have been stopped early because of effective but preemptive reduction of other vascular endpoints.

The Joint National Commission-7 (Chobanian et al., 2003) recommended more intensive blood pressure (BP) targets for patients with diabetes or kidney disease. The opposite may be true for individuals with extensive leukoaraiosis, in whom more liberal BP targets may be appropriate. Patients who have severe small-artery disease and compromised autoregulatory reserve may be at increased risk for ischemia, if blood pressure is abruptly lowered by postural changes (orthostatic hypotension) (Mehagnoul-Schipper et al., 2001) or overly aggressive

antihypertensive treatment. In a metaanalysis of 11 clinical trials, achieving an SBP less than 130 mmHg compared with 130 to 139 mmHg appears to provide additional stroke protection only among people with risk factors but no established cardiovascular disease (Lee et al., 2012). Higher risk of hemorrhage has been reported with administration of tPA (Palumbo et al., 2007) or anticoagulant drugs (Cervera et al., 2012) in patients with leukoaraiosis. Additional research using dynamic measures of vasoreactivity, cerebral perfusion, and integrity of the blood–brain barrier, may help set BP parameters for special subgroups of patients with significant white matter disease.

It is possible that beyond their effects on lowering blood pressure, angiotensin receptor blockers may be have selective benefits for VCI. Angiotensin receptor blockers selectively block angiotensin receptor type 1 (AT1) and increase relative activation of AT2 receptors, which may protect endothelial cells and neurons (Fig. 68.6) (Armario and de la Sierra, 2009; Hajjar

Figure 1. Forest plot of comparison: 1 Incidence of dementia, outcome: 1.1 Number of cases of dementia

Study or Subgroup	Active Treatment Events	Total	Placebo Events	Total	Weight	Odds Ratio M-H, Fixed, 95% CI	Odds Ratio M-H, Fixed, 95% CI
HYVET 2008	126	1687	137	1649	51.6%	0.89 [0.69, 1.15]	
SCOPE 2003	62	2477	57	2460	22.4%	1.08 [0.75, 1.56]	
SHEP 1991	37	2365	44	2371	17.4%	0.84 [0.54, 1.31]	
Syst Eur 1997	11	1238	21	1180	8.6%	0.49 [0.24, 1.03]	
Total (95% CI)		7767		7660	100.0%	0.89 [0.74, 1.07]	
Total events	236		259				

Heterogeneity: Chi^2 = 3.63, df = 3 (p = 0.30); I^2 = 17%
Test for overall effect: Z = 1.25 (p = 0.21)

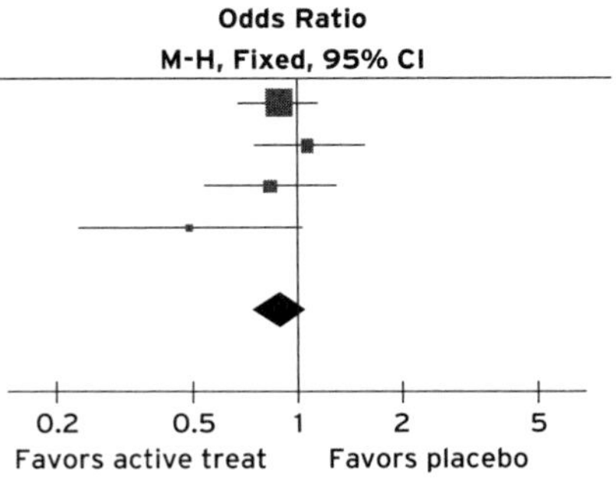

0.2 0.5 1 2 5
Favors active treat   Favors placebo

Figure 3. Forest plot of comparison: 2 Cognitive change from baseline, outcome: 2.1 Change in MMSE

Study or Subgroup	Active Treatment Mean	SD	Total	Placebo Mean	SD	Total	Weight	Mean Difference IV, Fixed, 95% CI	Mean Difference IV, Fixed, 95% CI
HYVET 2008	0.7	4	1687	-1.1	3.9	1649	18.9%	1.80 [1.53, 2.07]	
SCOPE 2003	-0.49	4.07	2477	-0.64	4.07	2409	26.1%	0.15 [-0.08, 0.38]	
Syst Eur 1997	0.08	1.76	1238	0.01	2.15	1180	55.1%	0.07 [-0.09, 0.23]	
Total (95% CI)			5402			5238	100.0%	0.42 [0.30, 0.53]	

Heterogeneity: Chi^2 = 126.25, df = 2 (p < 0.00001); I^2 = 98%
Test for overall effect: Z = 7.03 (p < 0.00001)

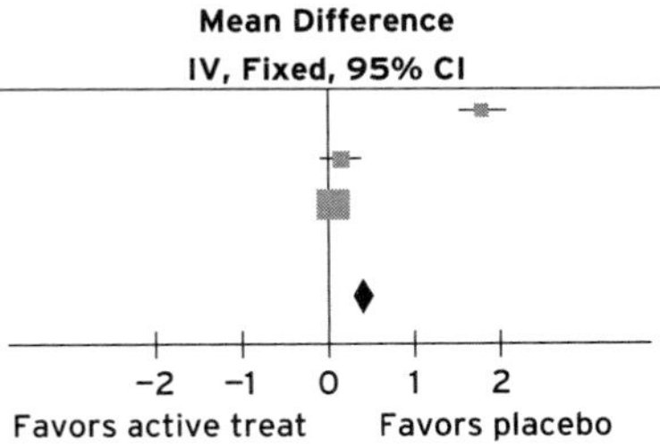

-2 -1 0 1 2
Favors active treat   Favors placebo

Figure 4. Forest plot of comparison: 3 Blood pressure level, outcome: 3.1 Change in systolic blood pressure level (mmHg)

Study or Subgroup	Active Treatment Mean	SD	Total	Placebo Mean	SD	Total	Weight	Mean Difference IV, Fixed, 95% CI	Mean Difference IV, Fixed, 95% CI
HYVET 2008	-29.6	15.3	1687	-14.6	18.5	1649	23.5%	-15.00 [-16.15, -13.85]	
SCOPE 2003	-21.7	22.38	2468	-18.5	22.38	2455	20.0%	-3.20 [-4.45, -1.95]	
SHEP 1991	-26.4	17.9	1966	-14.5	20.3	1890	21.4%	-11.90 [-13.11, -10.69]	
Syst Eur 1997	-23	16	2398	-13	17	2297	35.0%	-10.00 [-10.95, -9.05]	
Total (95% CI)			8519			8291	100.0%	-10.22 [-10.78, -9.66]	

Heterogeneity: Chi^2 = 194.69, df = 3 (p < 0.00001); I^2 = 98%
Test for overall effect: Z = 35.80 (p < 0.00001)

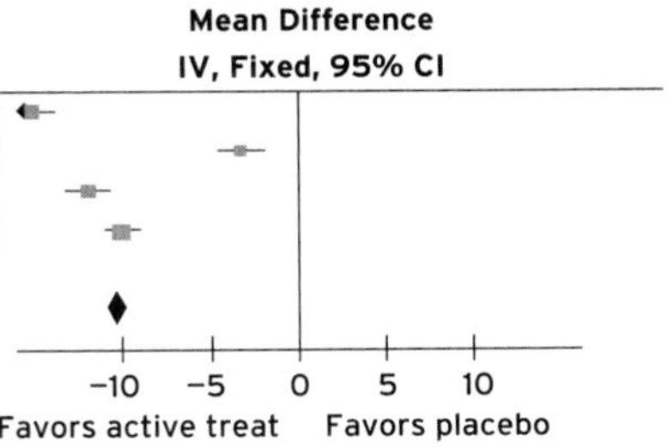

-10 -5 0 5 10
Favors active treat   Favors placebo

Figure 68.7 Forest plot of comparison. (Reproduced with permission from McGuinness, B., Todd, S., Passmore, P., and Bullock, R. (2009). Blood pressure lowering in patients without prior cerebrovascular disease for prevention of cognitive impairment and dementia [Meta-Analysis Review]. Cochrane Database Syst Rev, (4), CD004034 Courtesy of Ihab Hajjar.)

TABLE 68.6. Primary and secondary prevention trials that included a cognition outcome measure

	ANTI-HYPERTENSIVE MEDICATION	FOLLOW-UP	OUTCOME	MAIN RESULTS FOR DEMENTIA	p VALUE
PRIMARY PREVENTION					
SHEP (1991) N = 4736	Diuretic (chlorthalidone) and/ or beta-blocker (atenolol) or reserpine	4.5	– –	16% reduction in dementia	n.s.
Syst-Eur (1998) N = 2418	Ca-channel blocker (dihydropyridine) with or without enalapril maleate and/ or diuretic (hydrochlorothiazide)	2.0	MMSE	50% (0 to 76%) reduction in dementia	0.05
SCOPE (2003) N = 4937	ARB (candesartan cilexetil) and/ or diuretics	3.7	MMSE	7% increased risk in active arm (but only 3.2/1.6 mmHg reduction in BP in treatment vs. control arm)	>0.20
HYVET (2008) N = 3336	Diuretic (indapamide) with or without ACEI (perindopril)	2.2	MMSE	14% (−9 to 23%) reduction in dementia. (Trial stopped early because of significant reduction in stroke and mortality)	0.2
SECONDARY PREVENTION					
PROGRESS (2003) N = 6104	ACEI (perindopril) with or without diuretic (indapamide)	4.0	MMSE	12% (−8 to 28%) reduction in dementia	0.2
PRoFESS (2008) N = 20332	ARB (telmisartan)	2.4	MMSE	No reduction of the risk of dementia	0.48

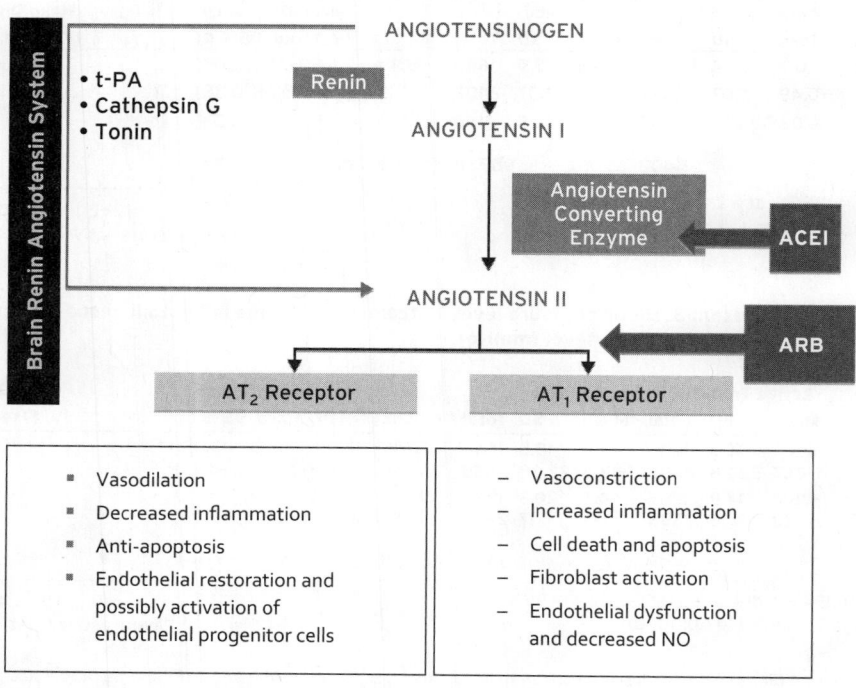

Figure 68.6 ARB selectively blocks AT1 receptor. (Reproduced with permission from The Cochrane Collaboration.)

TABLE 68.5. Randomized clinical trials of antihypertensive drugs for prevention of stroke in the elderly

	N	MEAN AGE (SD, RANGE OR AGE CUT-OFF)	POPULATION STUDIED	INTERVENTION	FOLLOW-UP	RRR (95% CL) FOR STROKE	EFFECT IN ELDERLY	COMMENTS
PROGRESS	6105	64 (10, 26–91)	History of stroke or transient ischemic attack	Perindopril-based with indapamide add-on vs placebo-based	4 years	28% (17 to 38) for perindopril	Not reported	There was a 43% RRR in stroke for perindopril plus indapamide, which drove the positive result
LIFE	9193	67 (7, 55–80)	Essential hypertension and left ventricular hypertrophy	Losartan-based vs atenolol-based	4.8 years	2 5% (11 to 37) for losartan	Stroke reduction only seen in those aged ≥65 years	Equal reduction of blood pressure with losartan and atenolol
ACCESS	342	68 (9, 50–85)	Acute ischemic stroke	Candesartan vs placebo	12 months	32% (NS)	Not reported	Equal reduction of blood pressure in both groups but a 53% RRR for mortality and vascular events favoring candesartan
HOPE	9297	66 (7, >55)	Vascular disease or diabetes mellitus and one vascular risk factor	Ramipril vs placebo	4.5 years	32% (16 to 44) for ramipril	Elderly (>75years) had a 31% RRR of stroke[34]	Only modest reduction in blood pressure (3.8/2.8 mmHg)
ALLHAT	33357	67 (8, >55)	Hypertension and one other coronary risk factor	Chlorthalidone vs. amlodipine vs. lisinopril	4.9 years	7% (-7 to 18); NS	Not reported	Most required multi-drug regimen
SHEP	4736	71 (not reported, ≥60)	Isolated systolic hypertension and age ≥60 years	Chlorthalidone vs placebo with atenolol add-on	4.5 years	36% (18 to 52) for chlorthalidone and atenolol	Stroke incidence was lower in the 13–7% aged ≥80 years	Active treatment was associated with fewer myocardial infarctions and a trend towards lower mortality
Syst-Eur	4695	70 (6.7, ≥60)	Isolated systolic hypertension and age >60 years	Nitrendipine with enalapril and hydrochlorothiazide add-on vs matching placebos	2 years	44% (14 to 63) for active treatment	33% risk reduction in stroke for those aged ≥80 years	Active treatment was associated with 50% reduction in dementia
MOSES	1405	68 (10, <85)	Hypertension and history of stroke	Eprosartan vs nitrendipine	2.5 years	25% (3 to 42) for eprosartan	Not reported	Equal reductions in blood pressure between the groups
PRoFESS	20332	66 (9, ≥55)	History of stroke or transient ischemic attack	Telmisartan vs placebo	2.5 years	None	Not reported	Largest secondary stroke prevention trial
HYVET	3845	84 (3, 80–100)	Systolic blood pressure >160 mmHg	Indapamide with perindopril add-on vs. placebo	1.8 years	30% (-1 to 51) for active treatment	All participants aged ≥80 years	Blood pressure with treatment 15.0/6.1 mmHg lower
SCOPE	4964	76 (not reported, 70–89)	Age 70–89 years and systolic blood pressure 160–179 mmHg or diastolic blood pressure 90–99 mmHg	Candesartan vs. placebo	3.8 years	28% (1 to 47) for candesartan	All participants aged 70–89 years	No difference in blood pressure reported among groups

ACCESS, Acute Candesartan Cilexetil Therapy in Stroke Survivors; ALLHAT, Antihypertensive and Lipid-Lowering Treatment to Prevent Heart Attack Trial; HOPE, Heart Outcomes Prevention Evaluation study. HYVET, HYpertension in the Very Elderly Trial; LIFE, Losartan Intervention For Endpoint reduction in hypertension study; MOSES, Morbidity and Mortality After Stroke, Eprosartan Compared With Nitrendipine for Secondary Prevention; NS, non-significant; PRoFESS, Prevention Regimen for Effectively Avoiding Second Strokes; PROGRESS = Perindopril Protection Against Recurrent Stroke Study. RRR = relative risk reduction; SCOPE, Study on Cognition and Prognosis in the Elderly; SHEP, Systolic Hypertension in the Elderly Program. Syst-Eur, Systolic Hypertension in Europe study.

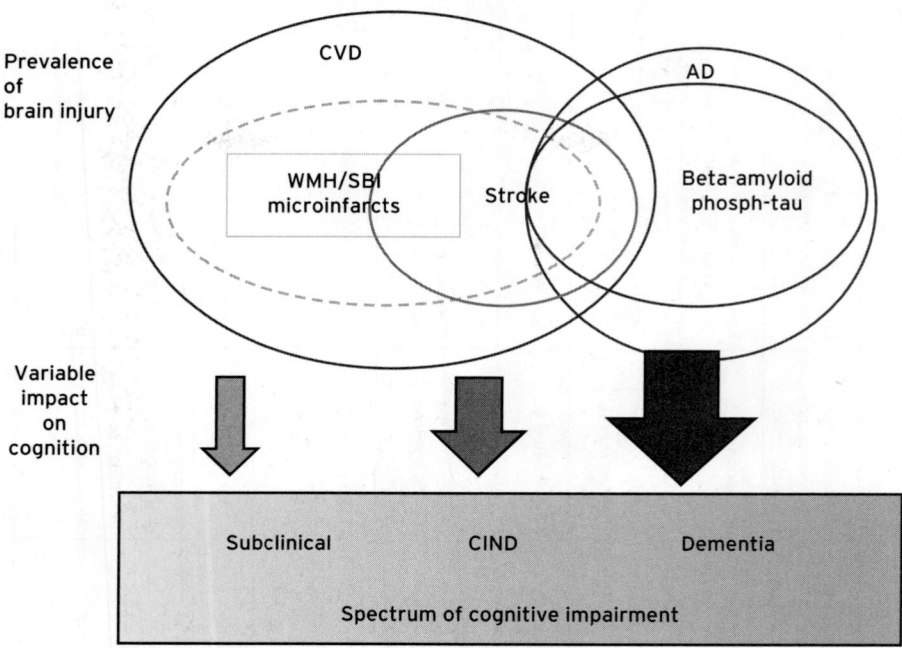

Differential burden of CVD & AD on cognitive function

Figure 68.5 *Differential burden of CVD and AD on cognitive function.*

through clinical trials shows significant reductions in risk of stroke, although the benefits are not as large as among younger subjects (Table 68.5) (Sanossian and Ovbiagele, 2009).

Based on our understanding of the pathogenesis of VCI, it stands to reason that risk reduction for stroke will generalize to risk reduction for VCI. In fact, whereas the benefits of antihypertensive treatment in reducing the risk of stroke are compelling, evidence-based data vis-à-vis reduction of VCI is relatively modest. Only small reductions in VCI were observed in a metaanalysis of four double-blind placebo-controlled primary prevention trials of antihypertensive medication (i.e., SHEP, Syst-Eur, HYVET, and SCOPE) (Table 68.6; Fig. 68.7) (McGuinness et al., 2009). In two anti-hypertensive trials for the secondary prevention of stroke, only modest differences

TABLE 68.4. Importance of secondary stroke interventions

INTERVENTION	REDUCTION IN RISK OF RECURRENT STROKE (%)	TIME FRAME FOR RISK REDUCTION	PROPORTION OF PATIENTS WHO WOULD BENEFIT (%)
Smoking cessation	≈50	6 months to several years	25
Mediterranean diet	60	4 years	100
Blood pressure control	40–50	3 years	60
Exercise	25–30	2 years	80
Antiplatelet agents	25–30	2 years	85
Lipid-lowering drugs	20–30	4 years	75
Pioglitazone for diabetes	47	3 years	20
Vitamins (B^)	25–35	2–4 years	30
Carotid endarterectomy for severe symptomatic carotid stenosis	67	2 years	10
Anticoagulants for atrial fibrillation	50	1 year	15

Interventions are ranked in approximate order of importance (most important first), as determined by the combination of the magnitude of effect of the intervention and the proportion pf patients presenting with transient ischemic attack or ischemic stroke who stand to benefit from each measure. (Spence, J. D. (2010). Secondary stroke prevention. [Review]. *Nat. Rev. Neurol.*, 6(9), 477–486.)

TABLE 68.3. Correlations between CVD and AD: longitudinal aging cohort with autopsy

FIRST AUTHOR/ STUDY	ORIGINAL SAMPLE	AUTOPSY SAMPLE	AD PATHOLOGY	CEREBRAL INFARCTS
Peila, 2002 Honolulu Asia Aging Study 1991	Community-based Japanese-American males N = 3734	216 autopsies/ 521 deaths (42.5%)	**Negative:** *Type 2 diabetes* was not associated with cortical neuritic plaques (RR 0.8, 95% CI [0.5,1.4] or tangles (RR 1.0 [0.6–2.4])	**Positive:** *Type 2 diabetes* was associated with higher risk of large infarcts (RR 1.8, 95% CI [1.1, 3.0]).
Arvanitakis, 2006 Religious Orders Study	Older Catholic nuns, priests, or brothers N = 1060	233 autopsies (94%)	**Negative:** *Diabetes* was not related to global AD pathology score, or to specific measures of neuritic plaques, diffuse plaques or tangles, or to amyloid burden or tangle density.	**Positive:** *Diabetes* (present in 15% subjects) was associated with an increased odds of infarction (OR = 2.47, 95% CI [1.16, 5.24]).
Wang, 2009 Adults Changes in Thought	Health Maintenance Organization N = 2581	250/1167 deaths (21.4%)	**Negative:** *Hypertension* in mid-life was not associated with plaques and tangles	**Positive:** Among persons < 80, each 10 mmHg increase in SBP was associated with 1.15 [1.0–1.33] increased risk of ≥2 microinfarcts.
Ahtilouoto, 2010 Vaanta 85%+ Study	Community-based, elderly longitudinal study N = 553	N = 291 (48% of total cohort) (Age = 92+ years)	**Negative:** History of *diabetes mellitus* was less likely to have beta-amyloid (OR = 0.48 [0.23–0.98]) and tangles (OR 0.72 [0.39, 1.33])	**Positive:** History of *diabetes mellitus* was more likely to have cerebral infarcts (OR [95% CI] 1.88 [1.06, 3.34])
Dolan, 2010 Baltimore Longitudinal Study on Aging	**Longitudinal cohort study with autopsy** N of incident dementia cohort = 1236 (Kawas, 2000[8])	N = 200 (16% of incident cohort) (87.6 ±7.1 years)	**Negative:** <u>No</u> relationship between the degree of *atherosclerosis* in intracranial, aorta, or heart and the degree of Alzheimer-type brain pathology	**Positive:** Intracranial *atherosclerosis* significantly increased the odds of infarcts (OR = 1.8 [1.2, 2.7]) and for dementia, independent of cerebral infarction
Richardson, 2012 Cognitive Function and Ageing Study (CFAS)	Community-based Longitudinal cohort study with autopsy N = 18,231	N = 456 Age range 66–103 years	**Negative:** Medicated *hypertension* was associated with less severe neocortical tangles (OR = 0.5, 95% CI = 0.3–0.8) and cerebral amyloid angiopathy (OR = 0.5, 95% CI = 0.3–0.8).	**Positive:** Medicated *hypertension* was associated with increased microinfarcts (OR = 2.1, 95% CI = 1.3–3.7). Heart attack was associated with increased microinfarcts (OR = 2.1, 95% CI = 1.2–3.9).

(Chui, H.C., Zheng, L., Reed, B.R., et al. (2012). Vascular risk factors and Alzheimer's disease: are these risk factors for plaques and tangles or for concomitant vascular pathology that increases the likelihood of dementia? An evidence-based review. *Alzheimers Res. Ther.* 4(1):1.)

the symptomatic treatment of VCI. Clinical trials of cognitive-enhancing medications approved for the treatment of AD (e.g., acetylcholinesterase inhibitors and memantine) have also shown beneficial effects in subjects with VCI (Kavirajan and Schneider, 2007). But it was unclear whether these beneficial effects result from the concomitant presence of AD pathology or specific effects on VCI. Vascular brain injury is commonly associated with depression (Alexopoulos et al., 1997; Kales et al., 2005). Treatment with antidepressant medications (e.g., selective serotonin uptake inhibitors) is warranted, although responses in patients with VBI may be less gratifying (Sheline et al., 2010).

Overwhelming evidence indicates that early identification and reduction of VRF is effective for the primary or secondary prevention of stroke. Interventions include antihypertensives, statins, glycemic control, antiplatelet medications, revascularization procedures, and lifestyle modification (smoking cessation, exercise, and diet education). Recommendations for primary prevention (American Heart Association/American Stroke Association Guidelines [Goldstein et al., 2011]) and secondary prevention of ischemic stroke (Table 68.4) (Acciarresi et al., 2011; Ovbiagele, 2010; Spence, 2010) have been recently reviewed. Among the very elderly, targeted reduction of vascular risk factors (e.g., hypertension and hyperlipidemia)

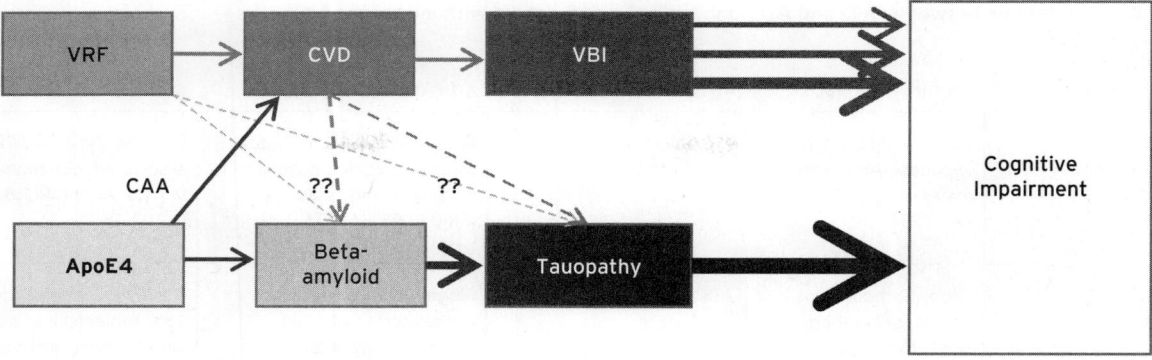

Figure 68.4 *Impact of vascular risk factors and Alzheimer's disease on cognition.*

risk factors for plaques and tangles, or are they promoting subclinical VBI that make symptoms of dementia appear earlier? (Fig. 68.4).

Positive associations between intracranial atherosclerosis and severity of plaques and tangles have been reported from several Alzheimer's disease brain banks (Beach et al., 2007; Honig et al., 2005). However, in a recent evidence-based review (Chui et al., 2012), no representative, prospective autopsy studies have shown significant positive associations between diabetes mellitus, hypertension, or intracranial atherosclerosis and AD pathology (i.e., plaques or tangles) (Table 68.3). The authors concluded that at the present time, there is no compelling evidence to show that vascular risk factors increase AD pathology. The alternate, but also unproven possibility remains that arteriosclerosis promotes *subclinical* VBI, thereby increasing the likelihood of dementia and in some cases making symptoms present earlier.

It is difficult to determine to what extent cognitive impairment may be caused by stroke versus concomitant AD. Estimates of the proportion of patients with poststroke dementia who also have underlying AD vary widely between 19% and 61%. (Leys et al., 2005) About 15% to 30% of persons with poststroke dementia have a history of dementia before stroke (Pohjasvaara et al., 1999; Cordoliani-Mackowiak et al., 2003) and approximately one-third have significant medial temporal atrophy. In the Lille study, the incidence of dementia three years after stroke was significantly greater in those patients with versus without medial temporal atrophy (81% vs. 58%) (Cordoliani-Mackowiak et al., 2003). Taken together, these finding suggest that-approximately one-third of cases AD may contribute to dementia in patients poststroke.

COGNITIVE IMPACT OF VBI AND AD: ADDITIVE OR SYNERGISTIC?

Converging evidence suggests an additive effect of VBI and AD on cognitive function. In the Cognitive Function in Aging Study some degree of neocortical neurofibrillary pathology was found in 61% of demented ($N = 100$) and 34% of non-demented individuals ($N = 109$). Vascular lesions were equally common in both groups, although the proportion with multiple vascular lesions was higher in the demented group (46% vs. 33%). In the Religious Order study ($N = 153$),

each unit of AD pathology increased the odds of dementia by 4.40-fold and the presence of one or more infarctions independently increased the odds of dementia by 2.80-fold. There was no interaction between AD pathology and infarctions to further increase the likelihood of dementia ($p = 0.39$) (Schneider et al., 2004). In the Baltimore Longitudinal Study of Aging Autopsy Program (BLSA) ($N = 179$), a logistic regression model indicated that AD pathology alone accounted for 50% of the dementia, and hemispheral infarcts alone or in conjunction with AD pathology accounted for 35% (Troncoso et al., 2008). In a longitudinal study of SIVD, severity of AD pathology and presence of hippocampal sclerosis were the strongest predictors of dementia, whereas subcortical VBI exerted a significantly weaker effect (Chui et al., 2006). In the Honolulu Asia Aging Study, microinfarcts and neurofibrillary tangles were the strongest predictors of cognitive status, with microinfarcts having a greater impact in persons without dementia and tangles exerting the stronger influence in dementia (Launer et al., 2011).

Taken together, these findings suggest a model in which the attributable risk of cognitive impairment is the sum of various pathological lesions (including aging, and vascular and neurodegenerative changes) weighted by their differential impact on cognition minus cognitive reserve:

$$CI = age + (A*AD + B*VBI + C*Other\ pathology\ldots)$$
$$- (A1*Edu + A2*Other\ reserve)$$

Alzheimer's disease pathology has a relatively large and consistent impact A on cognition, whereas VBI has a highly variable impact B on cognition, depending on location, size, and number. Strategic infarcts by definition are associated with high impact on cognition. Of interest, microinfarcts (which may be numerous and widespread) also appear to contribute relatively greater deleterious effects (Fig. 68.5).

WHAT IS THE BEST WAY TO PREVENT OR TREAT VASCULAR COGNITIVE IMPAIRMENT?

At the present time, there are no medications specifically approved by the Food and Drug Administration for

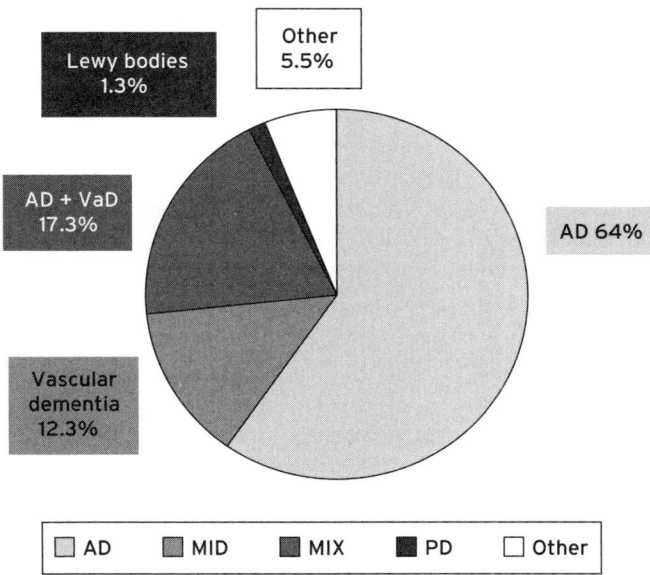

Figure 68.2 Causes of senile dementia.

after age 85, the rates were 7, 1, and 4 (Fig. 68.3). Thus, the incidences of AD, mixed dementia, and other types of dementia (but not VD) rose with increasing age, particularly after the age of 85 years (Matsui, et al., 2009). Similar incidence rates of AD and VaD (2/100 person years and 1/100 person years at age 85) were reported in Conselice, Italy, based on clinical diagnostic classifications (i.e., did not include mixed cases) (Ravaglia et al., 2005). Lower rates for VaD were reported in Rochester, MN (0.3 per 100 person years at age 85 years), as well as in earlier European metaanalysis without neuroimaging studies (Fratiglioni et al., 2000), which also did not include mixed cases.

In a poststroke dementia study (Allan et al., 2011), the incidence of delayed dementia was calculated to be 6.32 cases per 100 person years. The most robust predictors of dementia

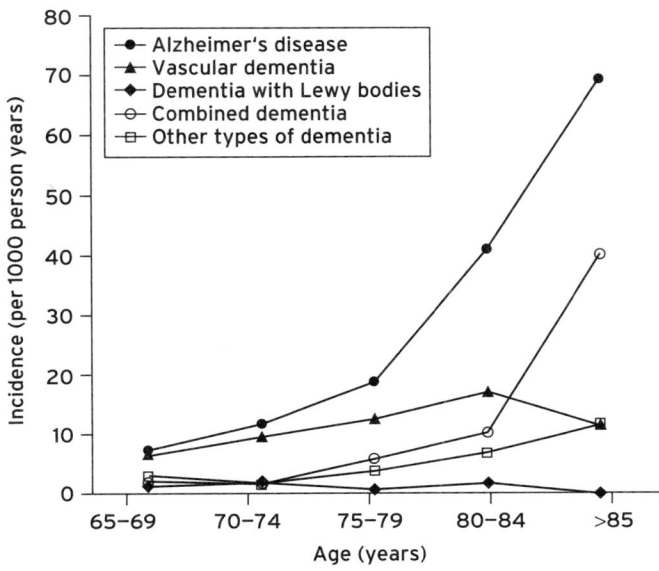

Figure 68.3 Incidence of dementia subtypes. (Reproduced with permission from BMJ Publishing Group Ltd.)

included low baseline Cambridge Cognitive Examination executive function and memory scores, Geriatric Depression Scale score and three or more cardiovascular risk factors. Autopsy findings suggested that 75% or more of the demented stroke survivors met criteria for VaD. But demented subjects tended to exhibit marginally greater neurofibrillary pathology, including tauopathy and Lewy bodies and microinfarcts, than nondemented stroke survivors, again underscoring the relevance and contributions of mixed pathologies.

WHAT IS THE RELATIONSHIP BETWEEN CVD AND AD?

MIXED VASCULAR BRAIN INJURY/ AD PATHOLOGIES

Mixed vascular and neurodegenerative pathologies are commonly found in community-based autopsy studies. In the Honolulu Asia Aging Study of Japanese-American men, 25% of dementia cases had mixed pathologies, compared with 57% with primarily AD, and 53% with primarily microinfarcts (White et al., 2002). In the Religious Orders Study (Schneider et al., 2007) and community-based elderly autopsies series (Schneider et al., 2009), mixed pathologies was more common than AD or infarcts alone. Among the first 209 autopsy cases from the Cognitive Function in Aging Study (CFAS), both cerebrovascular (78%) and Alzheimer type (70%) pathologies were common.

The frequent concurrence of VBI and AD in the same person, especially with advancing age, prompts several questions. Does the concurrence of two distinct pathologies (VBI and AD) represent the chance occurrence of two common age-associated pathologies? How do CVD and AD influence or interact with each other, in terms of pathogenesis, presentation, diagnosis, prognosis, and treatment. Do vascular risk factors increase the risk of AD? Can treatment of vascular risk factors prevent AD?

In the following discussions of CVD and AD we refer to arteriosclerosis, the most prevalent form of CVD, and to VRF for stroke associated with arteriosclerosis (e.g., hypertension, diabetes mellitus, hyperlipidemia, smoking). We do not include cerebral amyloid angiopathy, a common vasculopathy, which shares with parenchymal AD pathology a strong association with the apolipoprotein E ε4 allele (Smith and Greenberg, 2009).

PATHOGENESIS OF VBI AND AD: CROSSING OR PARALLEL PATHWAYS?

Recently, the concept that risk factors for arteriosclerosis are also risk factors for Alzheimer's disease has gained traction. This hypothesis has been driven largely by some (Qiu et al., 2010; Reitz et al., 2010), but not all (Ronnemaa et al., 2011), epidemiologic studies wherein recognized risk factors for arteriosclerosis (e.g., diabetes mellitus, hypertension, hyperlipidemia, and aggregated vascular risk factors) are associated with increased risk of incident clinically-diagnosed Alzheimer's disease. These data suggest two possibilities: Are vascular risk factors also based on features of the clinical history and examination (e.g., abrupt onset, stepwise progression, emotional incontinence, focal neurologic signs and symptoms) associated with clinical stroke.

The threshold for detecting VBI was lowered dramatically with the arrival of MRI in the 1980s. Numerous second generation criteria for VaD appeared, incorporating results of neuroimaging: DSM, ICD, ADDTC, and NINDS-AIREN criteria. These criteria share several elements in common, but differ in operational definition: (1) requirement for cognitive impairment, (2) evidence of vascular brain injury, and (3) operational criteria linking VBI to cognitive impairment.

A diagnosis of probable VaD by NINDS-AIREN criteria requires a temporal association between the onset of stroke and cognitive decline (Roman et al., 1993). Evidence of two infarcts outside of the cerebellum suffices for a diagnosis of probable IVD by ADDTC criteria (Chui et al., 1992; Lopez et al., 2005) The number of subjects classified as VCI may differ two- to fourfold depending upon diagnostic criteria, (Knopman et al., 2002; Lopez et al., 2003, 2005) with NINDS-AIREN criteria being most conservative and ADDTC criteria most liberal. ICD-10 and DSM-5 feature minor variations on these past themes.

Clinical criteria have also been proposed for subtypes of VCI, including subcortical vascular dementia (SVD) (Erkinjuntti et al., 2000) and Binswanger syndrome (Bennett et al., 1990). Recently, criteria have been proposed for the clinical diagnosis of vascular cognitive impairment not meeting criteria for dementia (Vascular CIND) (Gorelick et al., 2011).

In evidence-based medicine, accuracy of clinical criteria is measured against a reference standard. Accuracy of clinical criteria for AD is assessed against a neuropathological gold standard (e.g., CERAD criteria, NIA-Reagan criteria). In the case of VCI, there is still no agreed upon gold standard for the diagnosis. Bearing these limitations in mind, comparisons between clinical criteria versus neuropathological criteria for VaD (e.g., evidence of VBI in three lobes of the cerebral hemisphere) show limited sensitivity, but high specificity. Positive likelihood ratios range from 3 to 5 (Gold et al., 2002), wherein modest changes in pre- to posttest probability may be seen.

NEUROPATHOLOGICAL EVALUATION

Although neuropathology excels in the characterization of CVD and VBI, there is lack of consensus about how to apportion cognitive impairment to evidence of VBI, AD, or other pathologies found on neuropathological evaluation. Thus, as mentioned in the preceding, there are no consensus criteria for the neuropathological diagnosis of VCI (Hachinski et al., 2006). On the other hand, guidelines to harmonize the neuropathological evaluation for VBI have been published (Hachinski et al., 2006), hopefully laying the foundation for future diagnostic paradigms.

Neuropathological examination provides valuable information regarding the presence and severity of CVD, VBI, neurodegenerative and mixed pathologies. Neuropathologic evaluation elucidates the type and severity of CVD (e.g., atherosclerosis, arteriolosclerosis, amyloid angiopathy), and the severity, location, and size of VBI, including microinfarcts (too small to be seen by current 1.5 or 3 tesla MRI). Neuropathological examination greatly enhances our ability to identify cases with relatively pure versus mixed vascular and neurodegenerative pathologies by disclosing the presence and severity of amyloid plaques, tau-associated neurofibrillary degeneration, alpha-synuclein associated Lewy bodies, and TDP-43 intracytoplasmic inclusions. Better methods are needed to quantify the severity of diffuse white matter lesions, multiple microinfarcts, which are hallmarks of VBI, as well as synaptic loss, which may be a common underlying denominator of cognitive decline.

DYNAMIC AND FUNCTIONAL NEUROIMAGING: FUTURE ADVANCES IN DIAGNOSIS?

The advent of new structural and dynamic MRI sequences (e.g., diffusion tensor, fMRI, perfusion) promises additional advances for the detection and characterization of VCI. Diffusion tensor imaging/tractography provides a measure of white matter integrity. Resting fMRI provides a noninvasive measure of functional brain connectivity. Arterial spin labeling allows noninvasive and readily available measure of cerebral perfusion (compared with contrast arteriography or $H_2(^{15}O)$ PET. This may advance characterization of vasoreactivity in response to physiologic stressors (e.g., hypercapnea, orthostasis). With these additional advances in neuroimaging, we anticipate new approaches to the prevention and diagnosis of vascular cognitive impairment that include measures of vascular endothelial cell function and earlier recognition of the brain at risk.

WHAT IS THE INCIDENCE OF VCI AND MIXED VBI/AD?

Vascular brain injury is the second most common cause of dementia, after Alzheimer neurodegeneration. In the Cardiovascular Health Study 69% of cases with incident dementia were classified as Alzheimer's disease (AD), 11% as vascular dementia (VaD), 16% as both, and 4% as other types of dementia (Fig. 68.2) (Lopez et al., 2003). There is considerable variability in the incidence rates of vascular dementia (VaD) reported in the literature, depending upon methodological differences (e.g., diagnostic criteria, neuroimaging, neuropathology), threshold for cognitive impairment, as well as demography (e.g., age, ethnicity, education, and gender). Although neuroimaging increases the detection of VBI (McKhann et al., 2011), the cost may become prohibitive for large-scale epidemiology studies. Neuropathology improves the diagnosis of AD, VaD, and especially mixed pathology. Few studies have set the threshold for diagnosis of VCI at the level of mild cognitive impairment.

The Hisayama study (Matsui et al., 2009) stands out as a rare population-based study in Japan with a high autopsy rate (80%), where diagnostic classifications were informed by clinical, neuroimaging, and neuropathologic findings. Between ages 80 to 85 years, the annual incidence of AD, VD, and mixed AD/VD were approximately 4, 2, and 1 per 100 person years, respectively;

TABLE 68.2. Main findings from the LADIS study concerning the role of neuroimaging features in clinical aspects

CLINICAL CORRELATES	MRI LESIONS (PARAMETER)	RESULTS
Functional status	Baseline severe WMC	– Association with worse functional status – Independent predictor of disability
Cognition	Baseline severe WMC	– Association with worse score on MMSE and ADAS – Association with worse cognitive performances on global tests of cognition, executive functions, speed and motor control, attention, naming and visuoconstructional praxis – Independent predictor of dementia and cognitive impairment
	Progression of WMC	– Association with decrease in executive function score
	Number of lacunar infarcts	– Association with worse score on MMSE and ADAS
	Location of lacunar infarcts	– Thalamus location associated with worse cognitive performances (MMSE and compound scores for speed and motor control, and executive functions)
	Number of new lacunes	– Association with deterioration in executive functions, speed and motor control
	SIVD[1]	– Independent predictor of decline in cognitive performances and of dementia
	MTA severity	– Association with mild cognitive deficits (MMSE <26); additional effect with severe WMC – Predictor of Alzheimer's disease
	Corpus callosum atrophy	– Association with worse cognitive performances – Regional association with cognitive performances: anterior with deficits of attention and executive functions, isthmus sub region with semantic verbal fluency – Independent predictor of dementia and motor impairment
	Changes in mean diffusivity of normal appearing white matter	– Association with cognitive dysfunction
Mood	Baseline WMC severity	– Association with depressive symptoms – Independent predictor of depressive mood and depressive episodes
	WMC location	– Deep WMC associated with depressive symptoms – Frontal and temporal regions associated with depressive symptoms
	Location of lacunar infarcts	– Association of basal ganglia lesions with depressive symptoms
Motor performances	Baseline severe WMC	– Association with worse motor performances – Association with falls and balance disturbances
	WMC location	– Periventricular and deep frontal WMC associated with falls – Deep frontal WMC associated with balance disturbances
Urinary problems	Baseline severe WMC	– Association with urinary urgency

SIVD, Small-vessel ischemic disease.
[1] Defined as severe WMC (Fazekas scale grade 3) plus at least one lacuna or moderate WMC (Fazekas scale grade 2) plus > 5 lacunes

SVD caused by a relatively rare autosomal dominant mutation in Notch 3 gene (Dichgans et al., 1998), neuropsychological testing shows impairments in tests sensitive to speed and executive function (verbal fluency, digit symbol substitution, trails B) (Peters et al., 2005). In CADASIL, cognitive decline correlated with increased mean diffusivity, progressive atrophy, and infarct volume, rather than WMH or microbleeds (Jouvent et al., 2007). Among neuropathologically-defined cases followed prospectively with psychometrically-matched measures of executive and memory function, SIVD cases showed relatively similar levels of impairment in memory and executive function (only 9% showed predominant executive dysfunction) (Reed et al., 2004). In contrast, 67% of AD cases and 64% of mixed cases presented with a profile of predominant memory impairment. This autopsy study suggests that although executive dysfunction is common, predominant dysexecutive profile (i.e., greater than memory impairment) may not be a sensitive diagnostic marker for sporadic SVD.

HOW ACCURATE IS THE DIAGNOSIS OF VASCULAR COGNITIVE IMPAIRMENT?

CLINICAL CRITERIA

Diagnostic criteria for VCI have evolved as new imaging modalities have come on line. In 1975, the likelihood that dementia was caused by multiple infarctions (vs. primary neuronal degeneration), was operationalized using the Hachinski Ischemic Score (Hachinski et al., 1975). Points were assigned

TABLE 68.1. (Continued)

PATHOGENETIC MECHANISM	HISTORY	NEUROPSYCHOLOGICAL PROFILE	STRUCTURAL MRI	MRI EXAMPLE
Microvascular stenosis or hypoperfusion	May be slowly progressive (e.g., Binswanger syndrome) Gait apraxia Urinary urgency	Slowed processing speed Executive dysfunction	Periventricular and deep white matter hyperintensities	
Microvascular hemorrhage	May be clinically silent	Subtle changes on neuropsychological testing depending upon location within functional network	Location in subcortical gray matter suggests arteriolosclerosis Hemosiderin related microbleeds Location at gray white junction suggests CAA	

type of vasculopathy, coexisting neurodegenerative processes, and cognitive reserve.

SILENT BRAIN ISCHEMIA

Structural MRI reveals evidence of asymptomatic VBI, including silent brain infarcts (SBI), white matter hyperintensities (WMH), and microbleeds. The designation *subcortical ischemic vascular disease* (SIVD) describes cases of WMH and SBI located in subcortical gray and white matter. Gradient echo MR sequences may give evidence of small microbleeds, another often asymptomatic manifestation of VBI.

The prevalence of SBI on MRI in community-based samples varies between 5.8% and 17.7% with an average of 11%, depending on age, ethnicity, presence of comorbidities, and imaging techniques (Das et al., 2008). In the Framingham study, prevalence of SBI between the fifth and seventh decades of life is approximately 10%, but increases rapidly in the eighth decade to 17% and in the ninth decade to nearly 30%. Silent brain infarcts are most often located in the basal ganglia (52%), followed by other subcortical (35%) and cortical areas (11%) (Das et al., 2008). Risk factors for SBI are generally the same as those for clinical stroke (Das et al., 2008; Prabhakaran et al., 2008)

White matter hyperintensities are even more common and are generally present in most individuals older than 30 years of age (Decarli et al., 2005), increasing steadily in extent with advancing age. Also, WMH share risk factors with stroke (Jeerakathil et al., 2004). Age-specific definitions of extensive WMH can be created (Massaro et al., 2004) and prove useful in defining risk for VCI in a community cohort (Debette et al., 2010).

Numerous studies have examined the cross-sectional relationship between MRI evidence of VBI and cognitive ability. A recent review (Mayda and DeCarli, 2009) of a large number of epidemiological studies summarizes cognitive and behavioral effects of both SCI and WMH on cognition. The presence of SBI more than doubles the risk of dementia and risk of stroke (Vermeer, Den Heijer et al., 2003a; Vermeer, Prins et al., 2003b). WMH are associated with decline in the modified Mini-Mental State Exam and the digit symbol substitution test (Longstreth et al., 2002, 2005), incident MCI, dementia, and death (Mayda and DeCarli, 2009).

Recent data suggests that progression of WMH is an even better predictor of persistent cognitive impairment than baseline white matter lesion burden (Schmidt et al., 1999; Silbert et al., 2009). In the Leukoaraiosis and DISability (LADIS) study the, severity of white matter lesions (WML) was associated with diminished executive function, depression, decreased balance and more falls, and urinary incontinence over 10 years of follow-up (Table 68.2) (Poggesi et al., 2011). Longitudinal quantitative MR studies in a relatively healthy elderly cohort showed that acceleration of WMH burden preceded the onset of mild cognitive impairment by a decade (Silbert et al., 2012).

SUBCORTICAL VASCULAR DEMENTIA

At a certain threshold, subcortical ischemic vascular disease becomes clinically symptomatic. The cognitive profile associated with subcortical vascular dementia (SVD) is said to be characterized by greater impairment in executive compared to memory domains, as well as apathy and depression (Roman et al., 2002). Indeed in CADASIL, a relatively pure form of

TABLE 68.1. VCI phenotype depends on pathogenetic mechanism and location of VBI

PATHOGENETIC MECHANISM	HISTORY	NEUROPSYCHOLOGICAL PROFILE	STRUCTURAL MRI	MRI EXAMPLE
Macrovascular occlusion	Sudden onset	Depends on location within functional networks Strategic locations include left angular gyrus, inferomesial temporal, mesial frontal, anterior and dorsomedial thalamus, anterior limb of internal capsule, left capsular genu, and caudate nuclei.	Wedge-shaped territorial infarcts	
Macrovascular stenosis or hypoperfusion	Sudden onset	Transcortical aphasias	Border-zone infarcts in major end arterial zones	
Macrovascular hemorrhage	Sudden onset Signs of increased intracranial pressure	Depends on location within functional networks	Location in basal ganglia, thalamus, brainstem and cerebellum suggests arteriolosclerosis Lobar location suggests CAA, malformations.	
Microvascular occlusion	May be clinically silent	Subtle changes on neuropsychological testing depending upon location within functional networks	Lacunar infarcts Incomplete infarcts Silent brain infarct (microinfarcts escape MRI detection at 1.5 or 3T MRI)	

(continued)

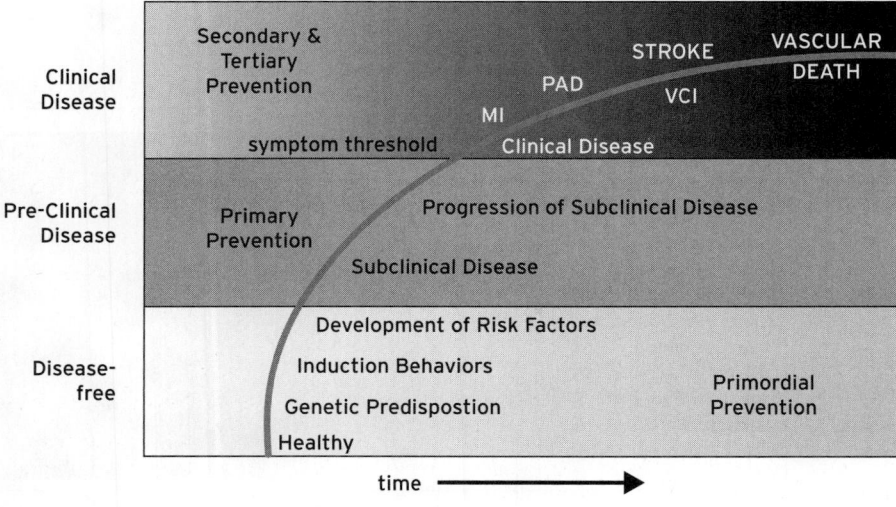

Figure 68.1 Global vascular risk. (Reproduced with Permission from the American Heart Association.)

differences in cerebral blood flow, assuming normal blood content of oxygen and glucose, and (3) the duration of hypoperfusion. Energy requirements are higher for neurons than glia. Blood flow declines as the length of the vessel increases and the radius of the vessel decreases. (Moody et al., 1991) Local cerebral blood flow is lowest in the periventricular and deep white matter—regions perfused by long, narrow, end-arterioles with no collaterals (Moody et al., 1991)

Two regional patterns of infarction are recognized. When a single artery is narrowed or occluded, the maximal extent of ischemic injury occurs in the *center* of the corresponding arterial territory. When perfusion pressure drops across several arteries, maximum injury takes place at the *border zones* between overlapping arteries and at the *end zones* of terminal arteries. This scenario may occur when: (1) systemic blood pressure drops below autoregulatory reserve, (2) intracranial pressure exceeds mean arterial pressure, or (3) there is severe stenosis of multiple arteries (e.g., hypertensive arteriolosclerosis or amyloid angiopathy). In cases of severe stenotic small artery disease, the periventricular and deep white matter border zones (despite lower oxygen requirements by oligodendroglia and axons) are at risk for chronic ischemia and incomplete infarction.

HETEROGENEITY OF CLINICAL PHENOTYPE

The phenotype of VCI and VaD is highly variable (Table 68.1). In the preimaging era, multiinfarct dementia was described as an abrupt onset and stepwise decline in cognitive function, with focal and patchy deficits in higher cortical function (e.g., aphasia, neglect, visual-spatial, executive). *Strategic infarct dementia* referred to cases where a single infarct in certain locations (e.g., anterior or dorsomedial nucleus of the thalamus; head of the caudate, genu of the internal capsule) resulted in impairment in multiple cognitive domains. *Binswanger's syndrome* represents a triad of slowly progressive dementia, early gait disturbance, and urinary incontinence caused by severe arteriolosclerosis of deep penetrating arteries, leading to demyelination of the periventricular and deep cerebral white matter.

The location of VBI is undoubtedly a major determinant of its impact on cognition and behavior. Subcortical lacunes and white matter changes disrupt frontal-subcortical loops and are associated with impairment in executive function. Left middle cerebral artery infarcts impact language faculties, whereas right middle cerebral artery infarcts cause neglect and deterioration of visual-spatial ability. Widespread small vessel disease (e.g., white matter encephalopathy) compromises the attentional matrix and processing speed (Schmidt et al., 2010). Newer imaging techniques such as fMRI and diffusion-weighted tractography promise more precise mapping of VBI onto relevant cognitive and behavior al networks (Duering et al., 2012), and future advances in understanding of the relationship between VBI and VCI.

POSTSTROKE DEMENTIA

Approximately 25–30% of persons meet criteria for dementia three months after hospitalization for first stroke. In addition, the risk of developing dementia in the subsequent one to two years following a stroke is double the general population. In a community-based study of stroke, the prevalence of dementia was 30% immediately after stroke. The incidence of new onset dementia increased from 7% after one year to 48% after 25 years (Kokmen et al., 1996). Long-term mortality is two to six times higher in patients with poststroke dementia, after adjustment of demographic factors, associated cardiac diseases, stroke severity, and stroke recurrence (for review, see Leys et al., 2005). Risk of dementia was higher with increased age, fewer years of education, diabetes mellitus, atrial fibrillation, and recurrent stroke (Srikanth et al., 2006). Among neuroimaging findings, silent cerebral infarcts, white matter changes, and global and medial temporal lobe atrophy are associated with increased risk of poststroke dementia (Leys et al., 2005). Left hemisphere, anterior and posterior cerebral artery distribution, multiple infarcts, and strategic infarcts have been associated with greater risk of dementia (Allan et al., 2011). Thus, differential risk for cognitive impairment is not straightforward, but appears to be related to number, location, underlying

68 | PATHOGENESIS, DIAGNOSIS, AND TREATMENT OF VASCULAR AND MIXED DEMENTIAS

HELENA CHANG CHUI

Cerebrovascular disease (CVD) is the second most common contributor to cognitive impairment in late life. Its impact on cognition and behavior is highly variable, depending on the location and extent of vascular brain injury (VBI) in relation to relevant functional networks. A diagnostic approach based on symptomatic profile (e.g., sudden onset, stepwise progression, executive dysfunction, apathy, depression) applies to a typical subset of patients. Alternative approaches based on structural imaging (e.g., MRI) have improved sensitivity for detecting presymptomatic VBI, thereby allowing earlier identification and treatment of vascular risk factors.

Vascular cognitive impairment (VCI) is currently the umbrella term encompassing both mild cognitive impairment and more severe dementia due to vascular brain injury and cerebrovascular disease. It subsumes other appellations including multiinfarct dementia, Binswanger's syndrome, poststroke dementia, vascular dementia (VD, VaD), ischemic vascular dementia (IVD), subcortical vascular dementia (SVD, SIVD), and vascular cognitive impairment not meeting criteria for dementia (Vascular CIND).

With advancing age, concurrent CVD and neurodegenerative pathologies (e.g., amyloid plaques, neurofibrillary tangles, synucleinopathy) become increasingly likely. Alzheimer pathology is associated with progressive loss of cognitive function, whereas the effect of VBI is variable. Sensitive and specific biomarkers for the major pathologies in late life are needed to identify each type of pathology. There is a widely held presumption that reduction of vascular risk will diminish vascular contributions to cognitive impairment.

Vascular cognitive impairment represents one manifestation in the larger realm of global vascular risk, including stroke, myocardial infarction, and peripheral artery disease (Fig. 68.1) (Sacco, 2007)). Ideally, reduction of global vascular risk should commence before the appearance of symptomatic clinical disease. In the case of VCI, neuroimaging offers a means of identifying the brain at risk. As imaging modalities become even more versatile and dynamic, they may offer new approaches to diagnosis as well as surrogate outcome measures for the prevention and treatment of VCI.

This chapter addresses five empirical questions of clinical relevance to VCI: (*1*) What is the pathogenesis of vascular cognitive impairment? (*2*) How accurate is the diagnosis of VCI? (*3*) What is the incidence and prevalence of vascular cognitive impairment? (*4*) What is the relationship between VBI and AD? (*5*) What is the best way to prevent or treat VCI?

The reader is also referred to a recent consensus statement for health care professionals on vascular cognitive impairment published by the American Heart Association/American Stroke Association (Gorelick et al., 2011) and the recommendations for Harmonization of Vascular Cognitive Impairment by the National Institute for Neurological Disease and Stroke and the Canadian Stroke Network (Hachinski et al., 2006).

WHAT IS THE PATHOGENESIS OF VASCULAR COGNITIVE IMPAIRMENT?

Vascular cognitive impairment embodies the construct that vascular risk factors (VRF) lead to cerebrovascular disease (CVD), which leads to parenchymal brain injury (VBI) that leads to cognitive impairment (VCI). There are a plethora of VRFs, CVDs, and mechanisms leading to VBI. There is also tremendous variability in the level of impact VBI imposes on cognition.

$$VRF \rightarrow CVD \rightarrow VBI \rightarrow ?VCI$$

The most prevalent types of CVD are atherosclerosis, arteriolosclerosis, and cerebral amyloid angiopathy (CAA). Other less common forms include vasculitis, fibromuscular dysplasia, malformations, and the like. CADASIL (cerebral autosomal dominant arteriopathy subcortical infarcts and leukoencephalopathy) is a relatively rare but pure example of small vessel disease. The cerebrovascular tree may be compromised secondarily by heart disease (e.g., cardiac embolism or heart failure).

Substrate transport and barrier protection are two main functions of the cerebrovascular system. Inadequate delivery of oxygen and glucose to support the basic metabolic needs of brain cells (neurons, astrocytes, oligodendroglia) results in VBI. Narrowing or occlusion of blood vessels leads to ischemic infarction; leakage or rupture of blood vessels to hemorrhage. Clinical investigations focus predominantly on acute and focal stroke syndromes. Less is known about chronic, repeated, or widespread compromise of the cerebral vascular tree or to bidirectional molecular transport across the blood-brain-barrier at the microvascular level.

Ischemia refers to conditions in which tissue perfusion and supply of vital substrate (i.e., oxygen and glucose) are inadequate to support cell metabolism. The balance between supply and demand is influenced by: (*1*) differences in oxygen and glucose requirements of individual brain cells, (*2*) regional

Mesulam, M.M. (1982). Slowly progressive aphasia without generalized dementia. *Ann. Neurol.* 11(6):592–598.

Mesulam, M.M. (2001). Primary progressive aphasia. *Ann. Neurol.* 49(4):425–432.

Miller, B.L., Cummings, J.L., et al. (1991). Frontal lobe degeneration: clinical, neuropsychological, and SPECT characteristics. *Neurology* 41(9):1374–1382.

Mioshi, E., Kipps, C.M., et al. (2009). Activities of daily living in behavioral variant frontotemporal dementia: differences in caregiver and performance-based assessments. *Alzheimer Dis. Assoc. Disord.* 23(1):70–76.

Neary, D., Snowden, J.S., et al. (1998). Frontotemporal lobar degeneration: a consensus on clinical diagnostic criteria. *Neurology* 51(6):1546–1554.

Neary, D., Snowden, J.S., et al. (2000). Cognitive change in motor neurone disease/amyotrophic lateral sclerosis (MND/ALS). *J. Neurol. Sci.* 180(1–2):15–20.

Neary, D., Snowden, J.S., et al. (1990). Frontal lobe dementia and motor neuron disease. *J. Neurol. Neurosur. Psychiatry* 53(1):23–32.

Neumann, M., Rademakers, R., et al. (2009). A new subtype of frontotemporal lobar degeneration with FUS pathology. *Brain* 132(Pt 11):2922–2931.

Neumann, M., Sampathu, D.M., et al. (2006). Ubiquitinated TDP-43 in frontotemporal lobar degeneration and amyotrophic lateral sclerosis. *Science* 314(5796):130–133.

Pa, J., Possin, K.L., et al. (2010). Gray matter correlates of set-shifting among neurodegenerative disease, mild cognitive impairment, and healthy older adults. *JINS* 16(4):640–650.

Papageorgiou, S.G., Kontaxis, T., et al. (2009). Frequency and causes of early-onset dementia in a tertiary referral center in athens. *Alzheimer Dis. Assoc. Disord.* 23(4):347–351.

Perry, R.J., and Miller, B.L. (2001). Behavior and treatment in frontotemporal dementia. *Neurology* 56(11 Suppl 4):S46–51.

Peters, F., Perani, D., et al. (2006). Orbitofrontal dysfunction related to both apathy and disinhibition in frontotemporal dementia. *Dement. Geriatr. Cogn. Disord.* 21(5–6):373–379.

Pick, A. (1892). Uber die beziehungen der senilen hirnatropie zur aphasie [Pertaining to senile brain-atrophy and aphasia]. *Prag. Med. Wchnschr.* 17:165–167.

Piguet, O., Petersen, A., et al. (2011). Eating and hypothalamus changes in behavioral-variant frontotemporal dementia. *Ann. Neurol.* 69(2):312–319.

Poljansky, S., Ibach, B., et al. (2011). A visual [18F]FDG-PET rating scale for the differential diagnosis of frontotemporal lobar degeneration. *Eur. Arch. Psychiatry Clin. Neurosci.* 261(6):433–446.

Pollock, B.G., Mulsant, B.H., et al. (2002). Comparison of citalopram, perphenazine, and placebo for the acute treatment of psychosis and behavioral disturbances in hospitalized, demented patients. *Am. J. Psychiatry* 159(3):460–465.

Possin, K.L., Brambati, S.M., et al. (2009). Rule violation errors are associated with right lateral prefrontal cortex atrophy in neurodegenerative disease. *JINS* 15(3):354–364.

Rabinovici, G.D., Jagust, W.J., et al. (2008). Abeta amyloid and glucose metabolism in three variants of primary progressive aphasia. *Ann. Neurol.* 64(4):388–401.

Rademakers, R., Baker, M., et al. (2007). Phenotypic variability associated with progranulin haploinsufficiency in patients with the common 1477C→T (Arg493X) mutation: an international initiative. *Lancet Neurol.* 6(10):857–868.

Rankin, K.P., Gorno-Tempini, M.L., et al. (2006). Structural anatomy of empathy in neurodegenerative disease. *Brain* 129(Pt 11):2945–2956.

Rankin, K.P., Mayo, M.C., et al. (2011). Behavioral variant frontotemporal dementia with corticobasal degeneration pathology: phenotypic comparison to bvFTD with pick's disease. *J. Mol. Neurosci.* 45(3):594–608.

Rascovsky, K., Hodges, J.R., et al. (2011). Sensitivity of revised diagnostic criteria for the behavioural variant of frontotemporal dementia. *Brain* 134(Pt 9):2456–2477.

Ratnavalli, E., Brayne, C., et al. (2002). The prevalence of frontotemporal dementia. *Neurology* 58(11):1615–1621.

Rebeiz, J.J., Kolodny, E.H., et al. (1967). Corticodentatonigral degeneration with neuronal achromasia: a progressive disorder of late adult life. *T. Am. Neurol. Assoc.* 92:23–26.

Renton, A.E., Majounie, E., et al. (2011). A hexanucleotide repeat expansion in C9ORF72 is the cause of chromosome 9p21-linked ALS-FTD. *Neuron* 72(2):257–268.

Rizzu, P., Van Swieten, J.C., et al. (1999). High prevalence of mutations in the microtubule-associated protein tau in a population study of frontotemporal dementia in the Netherlands. *Am. J. Hum. Genet.* 64(2):414–421.

Roberson, E.D., Hesse, J.H., et al. (2005). Frontotemporal dementia progresses to death faster than Alzheimer disease. *Neurology* 65(5):719–725.

Rohrer, J.D., Guerreiro, R., et al. (2009). The heritability and genetics of frontotemporal lobar degeneration. *Neurology* 73(18):1451–1456.

Rosen, H.J., Allison, S.C., et al. (2005). Neuroanatomical correlates of behavioural disorders in dementia. *Brain* 128(Pt 11):2612–2625.

Rosen, H.J., Allison, S.C., et al. (2006). Behavioral features in semantic dementia vs other forms of progressive aphasias. *Neurology* 67(10):1752–1756.

Rosen, H.J., Wilson, M.R., et al. (2006). Neuroanatomical correlates of impaired recognition of emotion in dementia. *Neuropsychologia* 44(3):365–373.

Rosso, S.M., Donker Kaat, L., et al. (2003). Frontotemporal dementia in the Netherlands: patient characteristics and prevalence estimates from a population-based study. *Brain* 126(Pt 9):2016–2022.

Sampathu, D.M., Neumann, M., et al. (2006). Pathological heterogeneity of frontotemporal lobar degeneration with ubiquitin-positive inclusions delineated by ubiquitin immunohistochemistry and novel monoclonal antibodies. *Am. J. Pathol.* 169(4):1343–1352.

Seelaar, H., Kamphorst, W., et al. (2008). Distinct genetic forms of frontotemporal dementia. *Neurology* 71(16):1220–1226.

Seeley, W.W., Bauer, A.M., et al. (2005). The natural history of temporal variant frontotemporal dementia. *Neurology* 64(8):1384–1390.

Seeley, W.W., Crawford, R.K., et al. (2009). Neurodegenerative diseases target large-scale human brain networks. *Neuron* 62(1):42–52.

Seeley, W.W., Zhou, J., et al. (2012). Frontotemporal dementia: what can the behavioral variant teach us about human brain organization? *Neuroscientist* 18(4):373–385.

Sha, S.J., Takada, L.T., et al. (2012). Frontotemporal dementia due to C9ORF72 mutations: clinical and imaging features. *Neurology* 79(10):1002–1011.

Snowden, J.S., Bathgate, D., et al. (2001). Distinct behavioural profiles in frontotemporal dementia and semantic dementia. *J. Neurol. Neurosur. Psychiatry* 70(3):323–332.

Stevens, M., van Duijn, C.M., et al. (1998). Familial aggregation in frontotemporal dementia. *Neurology* 50(6):1541–1545.

Suarez, J., Tartaglia, M.C., et al. (2009). Characterizing radiology reports in patients with frontotemporal dementia. *Neurology* 73(13):1073–1074.

Tapia, L., Milnerwood, A., et al. (2011). Progranulin deficiency decreases gross neural connectivity but enhances transmission at individual synapses. *J. Neurosci.* 31(31):11126–11132.

Urwin, H., Josephs, K.A., et al. (2010). FUS pathology defines the majority of tau- and TDP-43-negative frontotemporal lobar degeneration. *Acta Neuropathol.* 120(1):33–41.

van Swieten, J.C., and Heutink, P. (2008). Mutations in progranulin (GRN) within the spectrum of clinical and pathological phenotypes of frontotemporal dementia. *Lancet Neurol.* 7(10):965–974.

Whitwell, J.L., Josephs, K.A., et al. (2011). Altered functional connectivity in asymptomatic MAPT subjects: a comparison to bvFTD. *Neurology* 77(9):866–874.

Whitwell, J.L., Weigand, S.D., et al. (2012). Neuroimaging signatures of frontotemporal dementia genetics: C9ORF72, tau, progranulin and sporadics. *Brain* 135(Pt 3):794–806.

Womack, K.B., Diaz-Arrastia, R., et al. (2011). Temporoparietal hypometabolism in frontotemporal lobar degeneration and associated imaging diagnostic errors. *Arch. Neurol.* 68(3):329–337.

Woolley, J.D., Gorno-Tempini, M.L., et al. (2007). Binge eating is associated with right orbitofrontal-insular-striatal atrophy in frontotemporal dementia. *Neurology* 69(14):1424–1433.

Woolley, J.D., Khan, B.K., et al. (2011). The diagnostic challenge of psychiatric symptoms in neurodegenerative disease: rates of and risk factors for prior psychiatric diagnosis in patients with early neurodegenerative disease. *J. Clin. Psychiatry* 72(2):126–133.

Yener, G.G., Leuchter, A.F., et al. (1996). Quantitative EEG in frontotemporal dementia. *Clin. EEG* 27(2):61–68.

Zamboni, G., Huey, E.D., et al. (2008). Apathy and disinhibition in frontotemporal dementia: insights into their neural correlates. *Neurology* 71(10):736–742.

Zhou, J., Greicius, M.D., et al. (2010). Divergent network connectivity changes in behavioural variant frontotemporal dementia and alzheimer's disease. *Brain* 133(Pt 5):1352–1367.

Chow, T.W., Miller, B.L., et al. (1999). Inheritance of frontotemporal dementia. *Arch. Neurol.* 56(7):817–822.

Davies, R.R., Kipps, C.M., et al. (2006). Progression in frontotemporal dementia: identifying a benign behavioral variant by magnetic resonance imaging. *Arch. Neurol.* 63(11):1627–1631.

Deakin, J.B., Rahman, S., et al. (2004). Paroxetine does not improve symptoms and impairs cognition in frontotemporal dementia: a double-blind randomized controlled trial. *Psychopharmacol.* 172(4):400–408.

DeJesus-Hernandez, M., Mackenzie, I.R., et al. (2011). Expanded GGGGCC hexanucleotide repeat in noncoding region of C9ORF72 causes chromosome 9p-linked FTD and ALS. *Neuron* 72(2):245–256.

Eslinger, P.J., Moore, P., et al. (2012). Apathy in frontotemporal dementia: behavioral and neuroimaging correlates. *Behav. Neurol.* 25(2):127–136.

Foster, N.L., Heidebrink, J.L., et al. (2007). FDG-PET improves accuracy in distinguishing frontotemporal dementia and Alzheimer's disease. *Brain* 130(Pt 10):2616–2635.

Galton, C.J., Patterson, K., et al. (2000). Atypical and typical presentations of Alzheimer's disease: a clinical, neuropsychological, neuroimaging and pathological study of 13 cases. *Brain* 123(Pt 3):484–498.

Garcin, B., Lillo, P., et al. (2009). Determinants of survival in behavioral variant frontotemporal dementia. *Neurology* 73(20):1656–1661.

Gibb, W.R., Luthert, P.J., et al. (1990). Clinical and pathological features of corticobasal degeneration. *Adv. Neurol.* 53:51–54.

Gibb, W.R., Luthert, P.J., et al. (1989). Corticobasal degeneration. *Brain* 112(Pt 5):1171–1192.

Gislason, T.B., Sjogren, M., et al. (2003). The prevalence of frontal variant frontotemporal dementia and the frontal lobe syndrome in a population based sample of 85 year olds. *J. Neurol. Neurosur. Psychiatry* 74(7):867–871.

Gorno-Tempini, M.L., Dronkers, N.F., et al. (2004). Cognition and anatomy in three variants of primary progressive aphasia. *Ann. Neurol.* 55(3):335–346.

Gorno-Tempini, M.L., Hillis, A.E., et al. (2011). Classification of primary progressive aphasia and its variants. *Neurology* 76(11):1006–1014.

Greicius, M.D., Geschwind, M.D., et al. (2002). Presenile dementia syndromes: an update on taxonomy and diagnosis. *J. Neurol. Neurosur. Psychiatry* 72(6):691–700.

Greicius, M.D., Krasnow, B., et al. (2003). Functional connectivity in the resting brain: a network analysis of the default mode hypothesis. *Proc. Natl. Acad. Sci. USA* 100(1):253–258.

Hassan, A., Parisi, J.E., et al. (2011). Autopsy-proven progressive supranuclear palsy presenting as behavioral variant frontotemporal dementia. *Neurocase* 18(6):478–488.

Hauw, J.J., Daniel, S.E., et al. (1994). Preliminary NINDS neuropathologic criteria for Steele-Richardson-Olszewski syndrome (progressive supranuclear palsy). *Neurology* 44(11):2015–2019.

Herrmann, N., Black, S.E., et al. (2011). Serotonergic function and treatment of behavioral and psychological symptoms of frontotemporal dementia. *Am. J. Geriatr. Psychiatry* 20(9):789–797.

Hodges, J.R., Davies, R.R., et al. (2004). Clinicopathological correlates in frontotemporal dementia. *Ann. Neurol.* 56(3):399–406.

Hodges, J.R., and Patterson, K. (1996). Nonfluent progressive aphasia and semantic dementia: a comparative neuropsychological study. *JINS* 2(6):511–524.

Hodges, J.R., Patterson, K., et al. (1992). Semantic dementia: progressive fluent aphasia with temporal lobe atrophy. *Brain* 115(Pt 6):1783–1806.

Hornberger, M., Geng, J., et al. (2011). Convergent grey and white matter evidence of orbitofrontal cortex changes related to disinhibition in behavioural variant frontotemporal dementia. *Brain* 134(Pt 9):2502–2512.

Hornberger, M., Piguet, O., et al. (2008). Executive function in progressive and nonprogressive behavioral variant frontotemporal dementia. *Neurology* 71(19):1481–1488.

Hou, C.E., Yaffe, K., et al. (2006). Frequency of dementia etiologies in four ethnic groups. *Dement. Geriatr. Cogn. Disord.* 22(1):42–47.

Houlden, H., Baker, M., et al. (2001). Corticobasal degeneration and progressive supranuclear palsy share a common tau haplotype. *Neurology* 56(12):1702–1706.

Hu, W.T., Chen-Plotkin, A., et al. (2010). Novel CSF biomarkers for frontotemporal lobar degenerations. *Neurology* 75(23):2079–2086.

Huey, E.D., Goveia, E.N., et al. (2009). Executive dysfunction in frontotemporal dementia and corticobasal syndrome. *Neurology* 72(5):453–459.

Huey, E.D., Putnam, K.T., et al. (2006). A systematic review of neurotransmitter deficits and treatments in frontotemporal dementia. *Neurology* 66(1):17–22.

Hutton, M., Lendon, C.L., et al. (1998). Association of missense and 5'-splice-site mutations in tau with the inherited dementia FTDP-17. *Nature* 393(6686):702–705.

Ikeda, M., Ishikawa, T., et al. (2004). Epidemiology of frontotemporal lobar degeneration. *Dement. Geriatr. Cogn. Disord.* 17(4):265–268.

Johnson, J.K., Diehl, J., et al. (2005). Frontotemporal lobar degeneration: demographic characteristics of 353 patients. *Arch. Neurol.* 62(6):925–930.

Josephs, K.A., Whitwell, J.L., et al. (2008). Progressive aphasia secondary to Alzheimer disease vs FTLD pathology. *Neurology* 70(1):25–34.

Josephs, K.A., Whitwell, J.L., et al. (2011). Gray matter correlates of behavioral severity in progressive supranuclear palsy. *Mov. Disord.* 26(3):493–498.

Kerchner, G.A., Tartaglia, M.C., et al. (2011). Abhorring the vacuum: use of Alzheimer's disease medications in frontotemporal dementia. *Exp. Rev. Neurother.* 11(5):709–717.

Kertesz, A., Martinez-Lage, P., et al. (2000). The corticobasal degeneration syndrome overlaps progressive aphasia and frontotemporal dementia. *Neurology* 55(9):1368–1375.

Kertesz, A., McMonagle, P., et al. (2005). The evolution and pathology of frontotemporal dementia. *Brain* 128(Pt 9):1996–2005.

Khan, B.K., Woolley, J.D., et al. (2012b). Schizophrenia or neurodegenerative disease prodrome? Outcome of a first psychotic episode in a 35-year-old woman. *Psychosomatics* 53(3):280–284.

Khan, B.K., Yokoyama, J.S., et al. (2012a). Atypical, slowly progressive behavioural variant frontotemporal dementia associated with C9ORF72 hexanucleotide expansion. *J. Neurol. Neurosur. Psychiatry* 83(4):358–364.

Kipps, C.M., Hodges, J.R., et al. (2009). Combined magnetic resonance imaging and positron emission tomography brain imaging in behavioural variant frontotemporal degeneration: refining the clinical phenotype. *Brain* 132(Pt 9):2566–2578.

Kipps, C.M., Nestor, P.J., et al. (2007). Behavioural variant frontotemporal dementia: not all it seems? *Neurocase* 13(4):237–247.

Knopman, D.S., Petersen, R.C., et al. (2004). The incidence of frontotemporal lobar degeneration in Rochester, Minnesota, 1990 through 1994. *Neurology* 62(3):506–508.

Komori, T. (1999). Tau-positive glial inclusions in progressive supranuclear palsy, corticobasal degeneration and pick's disease. *Brain Pathol.* 9(4):663–679.

Kompoliti, K., Goetz, C.G., et al. (1998). Clinical presentation and pharmacological therapy in corticobasal degeneration. *Arch. Neurol.* 55(7):957–961.

Kramer, J.H., Jurik, J., et al. (2003). Distinctive neuropsychological patterns in frontotemporal dementia, semantic dementia, and Alzheimer disease. *Cogn. Behav. Neurol.* 16(4):211–218.

Le Ber, I., Guedj, E., et al. (2006). Demographic, neurological and behavioural characteristics and brain perfusion SPECT in frontal variant of frontotemporal dementia. *Brain* 129(Pt 11):3051–3065.

Lebert, F., Stekke, W., et al. (2004). Frontotemporal dementia: a randomised, controlled trial with trazodone. *Dement. Geriatr. Cogn. Disord.* 17(4):355–359.

Lee, S.E., Rabinovici, G.D., et al. (2011). Clinicopathological correlations in corticobasal degeneration. *Ann. Neurol.* 70(2):327–340.

Lindau, M., Jelic, V., et al. (2003). Quantitative EEG abnormalities and cognitive dysfunctions in frontotemporal dementia and Alzheimer's disease. *Dement. Geriatr. Cogn. Disord.* 15(2):106–114.

Lomen-Hoerth, C., Anderson, T., et al. (2002). The overlap of amyotrophic lateral sclerosis and frontotemporal dementia. *Neurology* 59(7):1077–1079.

Lund and Manchester Groups. (1994). Clinical and neuropathological criteria for frontotemporal dementia. *J. Neurol. Neurosur. Psychiatry* 57(4):416–418.

Mackenzie, I.R., Baborie, A., et al. (2006). Heterogeneity of ubiquitin pathology in frontotemporal lobar degeneration: classification and relation to clinical phenotype. *Acta Neuropathol.* 112(5):539–549.

Mackenzie, I.R., Neumann, M., et al. (2011). A harmonized classification system for FTLD-TDP pathology. *Acta Neuropathol.* 122(1):111–113.

Majounie, E., Renton, A.E., et al. (2012). Frequency of the C9orf72 hexanucleotide repeat expansion in patients with amyotrophic lateral sclerosis and frontotemporal dementia: a cross-sectional study. *Lancet Neurol.* 11(4):323–330.

Massey, L.A., Micallef, C., et al. (2012). Conventional magnetic resonance imaging in confirmed progressive supranuclear palsy and multiple system atrophy. *Mov. Disord.* 27(14):1754–1762.

Mercy, L., Hodges, J.R., et al. (2008). Incidence of early-onset dementias in Cambridgeshire, United Kingdom. *Neurology* 71(19):1496–1499.

Merrilees, J. (2007). A model for management of behavioral symptoms in frontotemporal lobar degeneration. *Alzheimer Dis. Assoc. Disord.* 21(4):S64–S69.

Merrilees, J., Dowling, G.A., et al. (2012). Characterization of apathy in persons wth frontotemporal dementia and the impact on family caregivers. *Alzheimer Dis. Assoc. Disord.* [Epub ahead of print]

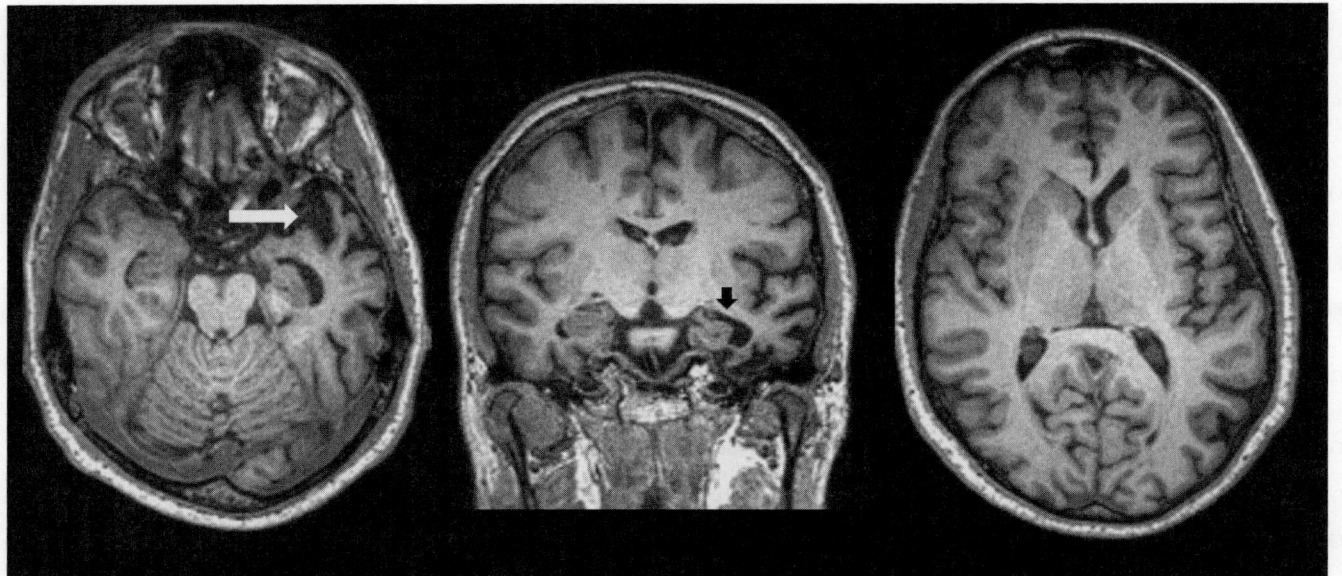

Figure 67.2 Ms. Y's MRI reveals left anterior temporal lobe volume loss in axial (right) and coronal (middle) planes on T1 sequences (arrows). There is relative preservation of other brain structures (left).

She had no memory, executive function, visuospatial, motor, or behavioral complaints. She continued to be independent in her activities of daily living. Her family history was unremarkable.

On exam, Ms. Y was appropriately groomed. Her speech output was increased, fluent, and grammatically intact, with word-finding difficulties and frequent questioning of the meaning of words. She had difficulties naming objects around the room. She spelled "cough" as "coff," "knot" as "naught" or "note," "choir" as "cwier," and she could not spell "yacht." She named only four out of 15 items on a naming test and could point to the correct picture describing a word in five out of 16 cases. Her visuospatial and executive functions skills were intact. She has mild difficulties on verbal learning tasks likely confounded by her inability to understand the meaning of the words. She performed well on visual memory tasks. Her neurological examination was otherwise unremarkable.

Her MRI is shown in Figure 67.2 and reveals left anterior temporal lobe parenchymal volume loss with relative preservations of other brain structures. There is only a slight volume loss in the right anterior temporal lobe.

This case illustrates the typical presentation of svPPA. The history and exam are usually focally localizing to the anterior temporal lobe through a predominant deficit of loss of word and object knowledge. Behavioral disturbances arise when more right anterior temporal lobe structures become involved. The underlying pathology is almost always that of TDP-43. Notice that in most cases the family history is unremarkable as this is the least genetic related disorder of all FTDs.

DISCLOSURES

Dr. Naasan has no conflicts of interest to disclose.

Dr. Miller receives grant support from the NIH/NIA and has nothing to disclose related to this chapter. Dr. Miller serves as a consultant for TauRx, Allon Therapeutics and Siemens Medical Solutions. He has also received a research grant from Novartis. He is on the board of directors for the John Douglas French Foundation for Alzheimer's Research and for The Larry L. Hillblom Foundation.

REFERENCES

Alladi, S., Xuereb, J., et al. (2007). Focal cortical presentations of Alzheimer's disease. *Brain* 130(Pt 10):2636–2645.

Bian, H., Van Swieten, J.C., et al. (2008). CSF biomarkers in frontotemporal lobar degeneration with known pathology. *Neurology* 70(19 Pt 2):1827–1835.

Boeve, B.F., Lang, A.E., et al. (2003). Corticobasal degeneration and its relationship to progressive supranuclear palsy and frontotemporal dementia. *Ann. Neurol.* 54(Suppl 5):S15–19.

Boxer, A.L., Garbutt, S., et al. (2012). Saccade abnormalities in autopsy-confirmed frontotemporal lobar degeneration and Alzheimer disease. *Arch. Neurol.* 69(4):509–517.

Brun, A. (1987). Frontal lobe degeneration of non-Alzheimer type: I. neuropathology. *Arch. Gerontol. Geriat.* 6(3):193–208.

Brunnstrom, H., Gustafson, et al. (2009). Prevalence of dementia subtypes: A 30-year retrospective survey of neuropathological reports. *Arch. Gerontol. Geriat.* 49(1):146–149.

Buckner, R.L., Snyder, A.Z., et al. (2005). Molecular, structural, and functional characterization of Alzheimer's disease: Evidence for a relationship between default activity, amyloid, and memory. *J. Neurosci.* 25(34):7709–7717.

Cairns, N.J., Bigio, E.H., et al. (2007). Neuropathologic diagnostic and nosologic criteria for frontotemporal lobar degeneration: consensus of the consortium for frontotemporal lobar degeneration. *Acta Neuropathol.* 114(1):5–22.

Caselli, R.J., Windebank, A.J., et al. (1993). Rapidly progressive aphasic dementia and motor neuron disease. *Ann. Neurol.* 33(2):200–207.

Caso, F., Cursi, M., et al. (2012). Quantitative EEG and LORETA: valuable tools in discerning FTD from AD? *Neurobiol. Aging* 33(10):2343–2356.

Caso, F., Gesierich, B., et al. (2012). Nonfluent/agrammatic PPA with in-vivo cortical amyloidosis and pick's disease pathology. *Behav. Neurol.* 26(1–2):95–106.

Chemali, Z., Schamber, S., et al. (2012). Diagnosing early onset dementia and then what? A frustrating system of aftercare resources. *Int. J. Gen. Med.* 5:81–86.

Chemali, Z., Withall, A., et al. (2010). The plight of caring for young patients with frontotemporal dementia. *Am. J. Alzheimers Dis. Other Demen.* 25(2):109–115.

told her that he will be waiting for her in the car to go visit his daughter. He has become more self-centered and cares less about others' needs.

His daughter also describes ritualistic behavior. For example, he enjoys saluting the sun and the moon. When he walks through a room, he high-fives the walls, the tables, and the chairs that are on his way, sometimes kissing the back of the chairs. His attention to grooming has diminished and he now wears the same clothes over and over again until they are worn down. He uses the bathroom frequently during the day without necessarily urinating. Moreover, he compulsively sticks his tongue out. He often repeats catch phrases as well as tunes that he sings or whistles constantly regardless of the social setting. He is described as impulsive. In addition, he has been having paranoid delusions for the past three years. He checks that all the doors are locked and there are no people hiding under the beds.

Regarding his eating behavior, at the onset of the disease he had a decreased appetite and lost some weight. He had decreased interest in the gourmet food he usually enjoyed. He started craving sweets and could eat candy all day. In addition, he was drinking more and smoking cigars.

In terms of memory complaints, Mr. X often asked the same question repeatedly. He forgot plans and errands. In terms of executive functions, he had difficulties with planning and organization, multi-tasking, concentration, judgment, and problem-solving. His fiancée in fact does all the finances and sorts his mail. His language and visuospatial domains were spared.

Mr. X does not report any memory, cognitive, or behavioral complaints when asked.

He has no pertinent family history except for alcoholism in his father and a non-specific behavioral syndrome in his paternal uncle with onset at 40 years old. His grandfather was diagnosed with Alzheimer's disease.

On physical examination, Mr. X was wearing a green sweater, worn-out jeans, and tennis shoes. His behavior was childish and he giggled throughout the exam. He asked to leave the room multiple times to use the bathroom. He stuck out his tongue multiple times at the examiner. His neurological examination was essentially normal except for a mild increase in tone of his left arm. On his neuropsychology testing, he had difficulties with tasks of verbal and visual memory, as well as a decreased performance on design fluency with relative sparing of other domains.

His MRI revealed bilateral orbitofrontal, bilateral insular, bilateral caudate, bilateral anterior temporal, and bilateral hippocampal volume loss, with generally worse parenchymal loss on the right than on the left (Fig. 67.1).

This case illustrates the typical presentation of a patient with bvFTD. Mr. X fulfills five out of the six criteria for the clinical diagnosis of bvFTD (see Table 67.2) with the exception of executive deficits on neuropsychology testing, possibly because of sparing of the dorsolateral structures. This case also demonstrates that patients with classical bvFTD can also have memory impairments and that the presence of short-term memory loss should not preclude the diagnosis.

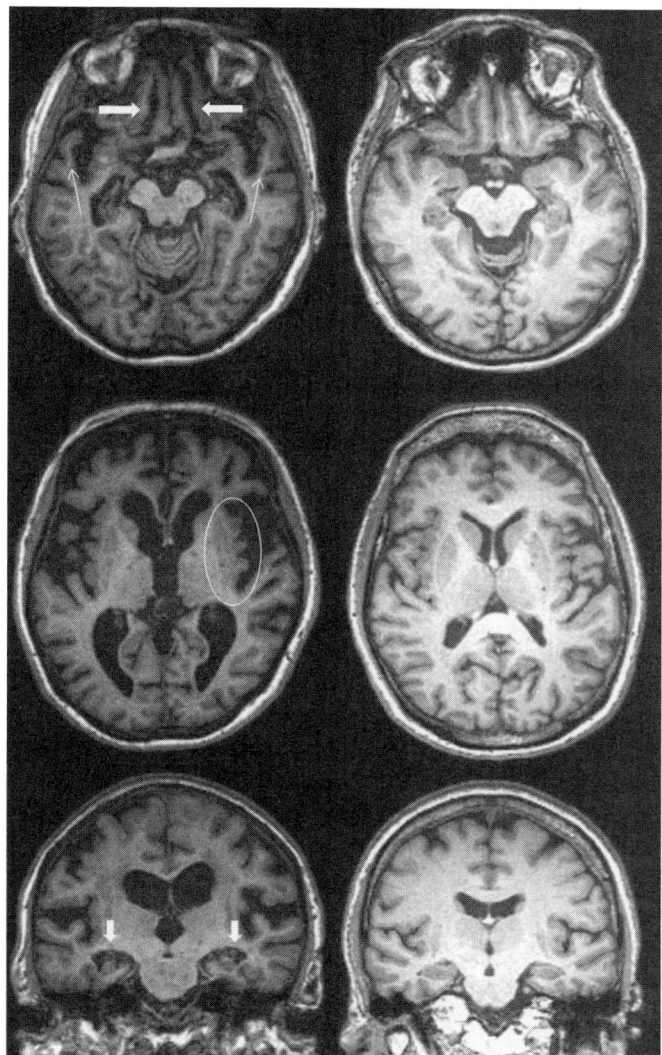

Figure 67.1 Mr. X magnetic resonance image (MRI) (left) as compared with a normal control (right) shows bilateral orbitofrontal (thick arrows) and anterior temporal (thin arrows) parenchymal volume loss (top images), bilateral insular volume loss (oval, middle images), and bilateral hippocampal volume loss (arrows, bottom images). In this figure, all sequences are T1-weighted and the right side of the MRI images corresponds to the right hemisphere.

CASE 2

Ms. Y is a 50-year-old right-handed woman who presented to the clinic with a chief complaint of "forgetting words and names," which started five years ago. This was first noticeable when she was reading stories to her two-year-old boy and she could not come up with the names of animals depicted in the story books, such as "rabbit" or "squirrel." She initially was able to describe the words she could not come up with, but became worse over time. For example, she would say "the word that starts with H and that pushes things against the wall as opposed to screwing." She also had difficulties recalling names of famous actors and names of cities. Moreover, she often asked about the meaning of words but had no difficulties comprehending and participating in general conversations.

(continued)

21%) compared with patients with sporadic bvFTD (approximately 10%) (Sha et al., 2012). Measurements of gray matter atrophy by voxel-based morphometry analysis of MRI images of 76 subjects with bvFTD revealed differences in brain parenchymal volume loss across subjects with different genetic mutations: symmetric atrophy in dorsolateral, medial orbitofrontal, anterior temporal, parietal, occipital, and cerebellar regions was associated with mutations in the C9orf72, whereas anteromedial temporal atrophy was associated with mutations in the MAPT gene and temporoparietal atrophy with mutations in the progranulin gene (Whitwell et al., 2012).

TREATMENT

The treatment for FTD is complex and calls for a multidisciplinary approach. Perhaps the first approach for treatment focuses on the education of patients and their caregivers (Merrilees, 2007). The understanding that abnormal behavior stems from a brain dysfunction can be difficult to grasp and caregivers may become quickly tired and frustrated. It is crucial for caregivers to develop strategies to help effectively interact with patients suffering from FTD and to keep them safe from the faulty judgment that inherently accompanies their disease (Perry and Miller, 2001). Social support services including support groups, home health aides, and a day care center can provide a healthy environment in which patients with FTD, especially in more advanced stages, can continue to have a good quality of life, especially in the absence of more structured institutions and nursing homes to care for a young population with a dementing illness (Chemali et al., 2010; Chemali et al., 2012).

The pharmacological treatment of FTD can be divided into symptomatic or disease-modifying therapy. Disease-modifying treatments would ideally target the underlying molecule associated with the respective pathology. For that reason, specific clinicopathological correlations are important to differentiate among diseases that would respond to a specific disease-modifying agent. For example, if a drug were to target TDP-43 pathology, it would be crucial to differentiate between cases of bvFTD that have TDP-43 as their underlying pathology as opposed to tau. Such treatments are currently not available. The results of a large multicenter clinical trial of PSP (a tauopathy) with davunetide, a microtubule stabilizing small peptide, were reported in December of 2012. The study failed to detect an effect on primary outcome measures. Similarly, a trial for patients with progranulin mutations is contemplated for 2013.

Because FTD is associated with many aberrant behaviors that might be troublesome to patients, their caregivers, and their surroundings, symptomatic therapy, although not curative, is important for a healthy patient–caregiver dynamic. It also provides control to patients that might be considered disruptive to others, especially in assisted living and nursing home settings. Both selective serotonin-reuptake inhibitors (SSRIs) and antipsychotic medications have been used in the symptomatic treatment of FTD. Indeed, autopsy and imaging studies seem to suggest that there is a serotonergic deficit in patients with FTD, possibly related to the neural projections from the raphe nuclei to the frontal cortex (Huey et al., 2006). There are also PET and SPECT studies that implicate deficiencies in the dopaminergic systems, especially in the striatum, in FTD (Huey et al., 2006).

From the SSRIs, paroxetine (Paxil©) was the most studied in FTD. It was shown to improve behavior symptoms such as disinhibition and compulsions at a dose of 20 mg per day (Kerchner et al., 2011); however, because of its anticholinergic effect, paroxetine may worsen cognitive symptoms (Deakin et al., 2004). On the other hand, citalopram (Celexa©) has very little anticholinergic effect and had been successfully used in the treatment of behavioral symptoms in AD patients (Pollock et al., 2002). It was also shown to decrease behavioral symptoms in patients with FTD at a dose of 30 mg daily (Herrmann et al., 2011). Trazodone at a dose of 150 to 300 mg daily also helps control agitation and eating disorders in patients with FTD (Lebert et al., 2004). Antipsychotic medications such as olanzapine and risperidone have been used in the treatment of agitation and disinhibition in FTD. However, there is little evidence-based support for their use and the high risk of extrapyramidal symptoms argues against their use (Kerchner et al., 2011).

CASE 1

Mr. X is a 73-year-old right-handed man who presented to the clinic with his daughter and his fiancée. He was at baseline an accomplished man, holding a PhD in sociology and working in an academic setting until retirement. His ex-wife was a biology professor and had been deceased for more than 15 years. He met his current fiancée eight years ago after flirtatiously following her into a restaurant. His daughter describes him previously as a sophisticated man. She feels that at baseline her father was gregarious and outgoing, while being respectful.

Four years ago, Mr. X started making rude remarks to friends and strangers who attended his weekly movie night. In fact, he ended a friendship with a long-term woman after insulting her and calling her derogatory names in front of other guests. His social decorum declined since and his daughter describes him now as having "no filter," telling people rude remarks to their faces. During the renewal of his driving license one year ago, he quarreled with his examiner and failed the test. He has also been walking up to strangers, starting conversations and touching them inappropriately; for example, hugging them. Furthermore, he is losing interest in activities he usually enjoyed doing such as fishing. He does not enjoy movies anymore but watches TV shows. His symptoms have all been slowly progressive over time.

Mr. X has lost the ability to be empathic and attentive to other people's needs and emotions. Once, his fiancée was having a bout of diverticulitis with severe vomiting and he simply

(continued)

associated with mutations in the valosin-containing protein gene. Because different pathologies and genetic factors might invoke different treatment options in the future, it is important to recognize the diversity of these pathologies and the clinical clues that allow a differentiation between them.

FUS

A small number of patients with FTD have a pathology that stains positive with ubiquitin antibodies but lack a TDP-43 (or tau) pathology. These were found to have fused in sarcoma (FUS) protein (Neumann et al., 2009), which was later found to be the underlying pathology in 5% to 10% of patients presenting with bvFTD (Seelaar et al., 2008; Urwin et al., 2010). Patients with the FTLD-FUS pathology present with a severe behavioral syndrome at a younger age, with a mean of 41 years old, accompanied by a high prevalence of psychotic symptoms and very little motor symptoms until much later in the disease (Urwin et al., 2010).

GENETICS

The genetics of FTD was a focus of interest in the past decade. Although roughly 40% of the cases have a family history, around 10% have an autosomal dominant pattern of genetic heritability (Rohrer et al., 2009). The bvFTD group has the largest proportion of familial cases while svPPA has the least.

MAPT

The microtubule-associated protein tau gene (*MAPT*), located on chromosome 17, was identified in 1998 as a culprit for a subset of familial Pick disease then termed FTD and parkinsonism (Hutton et al., 1998). The gene was found to carry a mutation in 17.8% of patients with clinically determined FTD and 43% of those with a positive family history in the Netherlands (Rizzu et al., 1999). In other series, it was found in 32% of patients with FTD and a positive family history, whereas only rare in the absence of family history (Rosso et al., 2003). In more recent case series mutations in *MAPT* was found in roughly 3% to 14% of patients with FTD (Rohrer et al., 2009; Seelaar et al., 2008). In our series it accounts for approximately 17% of all our familial forms of FTD.

These patients tend to have symmetrical frontal and anterior temporal atrophy; therefore, bvFTD is the most common clinical presentation (Rohrer et al., 2009). The typical age at the time of presentation is around 50 years, although patients have been seen with much earlier and later years of onset. Gene carriers were found to exhibit alteration of the functional connectivity in the default mode network (DMN) similar to that seen in patients with bvFTD who are also carriers of the mutation. This finding, in the absence of clinical symptoms or evidence of atrophy on structural imaging, suggests that a change in functional connectivity may be an early sign of the disease (Whitwell et al., 2011).

GRN

Mutations in the progranulin gene (*PGRN*), also located on chromosome 17, vary in frequency and are found in 1% to 16% of patients with FTD (Rohrer et al., 2009). They account for approximately 8% of all of our familial forms of FTD. The mean age of onset in patients with a GRN mutation is usually higher than that of patients with an MAPT mutation averaging around 62 years of age (Seelaar et al., 2008). Most of the GRN mutations cause nonsense-mediated decay of granulin so that no protein is produced by one chromosome. This is called haploinsufficiency, and patients with the mutation produce approximately 50% of the normal levels of progranulin (Rademakers et al., 2007).

Patients with GRN mutations tend to have an asymmetrical neurodegenerative condition that begins in the frontal or temporal region and spreads out along one hemisphere. Many are diagnosed with bvFTD or nfvPPA, whereas others are suspected of having CBS or Alzheimer's disease because of the spread into posterior brain regions. Additionally, the parkinsonian features found in some individuals lead them to be diagnosed with Parkinson disease.

Studies in knockout rat hippocampal cultures show that low progranulin levels reduce neural connectivity by decreasing the number of synapses and length of axons (Tapia et al., 2011). Interestingly, the number of neuronal vesicles per synapse was increased, similarly to observations in brains of patients with FTD and harboring the GRN mutation. The whole progranulin molecule seems to work as a neuronal growth factor that works at the neuronal level via the sortilin receptor, whereas it is broken down into smaller granulins molecules that activate inflammation. Histone deacetylase inhibitors increase the production of progranulin from the normal chromosome offering hope for a therapy for FTD related to this mutation.

C9ORF72

In the past two decades, several families with FTD-MND were reported, the genetic culprit being an autosomal dominant mutation that linked to a locus on chromosome 9. In 2011, a noncoding GGGGCC hexanucleotide expansion in the gene called C9orf72 was described and found to be strongly associated with the disease (DeJesus-Hernandez et al., 2011; Renton et al., 2011). It became the most common genetic mutation in familial FTD (11.7% of cases) and familial ALS (23.5% of cases). The expansion was found in 7% of Caucasians with sporadic ALS and 39.3% of Caucasians with familial ALS. In FTD, the expansion is found in 6% of individuals of European ancestry in the sporadic form and 24.8% in the familial form. It accounts for approximately two-thirds of our familial cases of FTD. Data for non-Caucasian ethnic groups is scarce but it has been reported in Asians. The mutation was found to have very strong penetrance with the typical age of onset in the sixth decade (Majounie et al., 2012).

Clinically, patients with the C9 mutation often present similarly to patients with sporadic bvFTD. In our series we found a higher prevalence of delusions in C9 carriers (approximately pathology-confirmed study, FDG-PET was found to be reliable among different raters and aid in the differentiation between FTD and AD pathology (Womack et al., 2011). In FTD, it shows hypometabolism of frontal, anterior cingulate, and anterior temporal regions, whereas hypometabolism of temporoparietal and posterior cingulate regions was observed in AD (Foster et al., 2007; Poljansky et al., 2011). With the advent of biomarkers such as Pittsburgh Compound-B PET for the detection of amyloidosis in the brain, it is imperative to recognize that co-pathologies can occur and the pathologic diagnosis of Alzheimer's disease should not be conclusive in patients with a positive PiB-PET and an otherwise clinical presentation of FTD (Caso, Gesierich et al., 2012).

ELECTROENCEPHALOGRAM

Electroencephalograms (EEG) may help distinguish FTD from AD, especially when using quantitative analysis and other computational methods (Caso et al., 2012; Lindau et al., 2003; Yener et al., 1996). Yet, EEG is not used in the routine diagnosis of FTD.

CEREBROSPINAL FLUID MARKERS

Measurement of tau and amyloid-β42 in the cerebrospinal fluid (CSF) of patients with neurodegenerative diseases is helpful in differentiating FTD from AD. In AD, amyloid-β42 levels are low with tau levels being elevated. In FTD, the ratio of tau/amyloid-β42 is significantly lower than in AD because of preserved amyloid-β42 levels. Using a cutoff of 1.06, the tau/amyloid-β42 ratio has a 79% sensitivity and a 97% specificity in discriminating between the two neurodegenerative conditions (Bian et al., 2008); however, this finding has not been validated in neuropathology-confirmed series. Measurements of other biomarkers in CSF continue to be investigated, especially for the differentiation of different pathological subtypes of FTD such as FTD-TDP43 and FTD-tau (see the following) (Hu et al., 2010).

HISTOPATHOLOGY

The major pathological hallmark of FTLD is atrophy of the frontal and anterior temporal lobes with microvacuolation and astrogliosis observed in affected areas on hematoxylin and eosin staining. In early pathological studies, cases that lacked the Pick disease pathology were roughly 80% and formed a group of unknown pathological etiologies that did not have typical Alzheimer's disease pathology. This group was initially termed frontal lobe degeneration of non-Alzheimer type.

Over the past two decades, neuropathologists have deciphered many distinct histopathologies that can underlie a pathological diagnosis of what is now referred to as frontotemporal lobar degeneration. These can be broadly classified according to the predominant abnormal protein deposition found on immunohistochemistry, and more specifically categorized according to the pattern of protein deposition. The two major proteins with which FTLD is associated are tau

(FTLD-tau) and TAR DNA-binding protein 43 (TDP-43; FTLD-TDP).

TAU

3-R TAU

The term Pick disease now refers to an FTLD pathology with observable Pick bodies that consist of intraneuronal argyrophilic inclusions. Pick bodies are mainly composed of abnormal three-repeat tau protein aggregates and stain strongly with antibodies against the tau protein on immunohistochemistry. In pathological series, Pick disease is found in roughly 15% to 20% of patients with FTD (Brun, 1987; Rosso et al., 2003).

4-R TAU

Corticobasal degeneration was initially described as a Pick-like pathology of corticodentatonigral degeneration with neuronal achromasia (Rebeiz et al., 1967). Later, its specific histopathology was described as ballooned neurons, neuronal loss, astrocytosis, and tau-positive neuronal and glial inclusions with the presence of coiled bodies and axonal and dendritic threads consisting of four-repeat tau protein isoforms (Gibb et al., 1989a; Gibb et al., 1990; Komori, 1999; Houlden et al., 2001), associated with an H1/H1 haplotype (Houlden et al., 2001). Progressive supranuclear palsy is another pathology related to four-repeat tau protein depositions and is summarized in the preceding.

TDP-43

One of the major non–tau-related pathologies of FTLD was initially termed FTLD-U for the presence of ubiquitin. In the past decade, pathological studies uncovered the implication of a protein called TAR DNA-binding protein 43 (TDP-43) as one of the major pathologies in FTLD-U (for ubiquitin) and FTD-MND (Neumann et al., 2006).

Three distinct histological patterns of FTLD with TDP-43 pathology were recognized based on the morphology and anatomical distribution of neuronal inclusions (Mackenzie et al., 2006; Sampathu et al., 2006). A unified classification was proposed in 2011 and another category was added based on emerging studies (Mackenzie et al., 2011). Each of the four subtypes was found to correlate well with different clinical and genetic forms of FTD. FTLD-TDP 43 type A consists of many neuro-cytoplasmic inclusions (NCI) and short dystrophic neuritis (DN) predominantly in layer 2 of the cortex, and correlates mostly with the clinical syndrome of bvFTD and PNFA, especially in *GRN* mutation cases. FTLD-TDP 43 type B consists mostly of moderate NCI and only few DN found in all layers of the cortex, and correlates mostly with bvFTD and FTD-MND, especially linked to *C9orf72* mutation cases. FTLD-TDP 43 type C consists mostly of numerous long DN and only few NCI predominantly in layer 2 of the cortex, and correlates best with svPPA. Finally, FTLD-TDP 43 type D consists of many lentiform neuronal intranuclear inclusions and many short DN in all layers of the cortex, and correlates best with the familial syndrome of inclusion body myopathy with Paget disease of bone and frontotemporal dementia, which is svPPA quickly spreads to) in the manifestation of these symptoms. When the predominant presentation is behavioral, then the syndrome is that of right-sided predominant svPPA. In a longitudinal study of patients with either the right or left predominant svPPA, it was found that the disease spread to the contralateral temporal lobe within three years so that patients with initial language problems develop the behavioral disturbances later on and vice versa (Seeley et al., 2005). Both progressed to a more frontal type of behavioral disturbance within seven years.

Brain atrophy in svPPA localizes to the anterior temporal lobes bilaterally and can involve both lateral and medial aspects of the temporal lobe, including the inferior, middle, and superior temporal gyrus (Gorno-Tempini et al., 2004). The clinical presentation of svPPA strongly indicates an underlying pathology of TDP-43 type C.

LOGOPENIC VARIANT OF PRIMARY PROGRESSIVE APHASIA

Patients with the logopenic variant of PPA (lvPPA) have a deficit in phonological memory, often erroneously termed echoic memory. Phonological memory allows a person to hold short-term information by "repeating" and "hearing" it in his or her mind, such as when given a phone number to dial. Patients with lvPPA have a slow and syntactically simple speech with many word-finding difficulties. They have difficulties repeating and comprehending long sentences, regardless of their syntactic difficulties. Patients with lvPPA can have difficulty with calculation and with memory tasks (Gorno-Tempini et al., 2004). Brain atrophy localizes to the angular gyrus and posterior aspects of the middle temporal gyrus (Gorno-Tempini et al., 2004). The underlying pathology of lvPPA appears to be that of plaques and tangles similar to that seen in classical Alzheimer's disease (Alladi et al., 2007; Josephs et al., 2008). Also, neuroimaging using Pittsburgh compound-B PET demonstrated that these patients have an amyloid deposition pattern similar to that seen in classical Alzheimer's disease (Rabinovici et al., 2008). In fact, lvPPA is now considered another "atypical" presentation of the more classically memory-predominant presentation of Alzheimer's disease.

CORTICOBASAL SYNDROME

Corticobasal syndrome (CBS) is clinically characterized by asymmetrical basal ganglia symptoms manifesting as parkinsonism, rigidity, akinesia, tremor; and cortical symptoms manifesting as apraxia, myoclonus, cortical sensory loss, and alien limb (Gibb, Luthert, & Marsden, 1989b; Kompoliti et al., 1998; Boeve et al., 2003). The clinical syndrome and the pathological diagnosis of corticobasal degeneration (CBD, discussed in the following) were used interchangeably for decades. Yet, CBS and CBD are two distinct entities. Corticobasal degeneration, a neuropathologically defined entity, a four-repeat tauopathy with distinctive cortical and subcortical tau aggregates has variable clinical presentations; and, CBS, a clinical syndrome, is associated with a wide spectrum of underlying pathologies (AD, CBD, PSP, or TDP-43) (Lee et al., 2011). The clinical presentation of patients with CBD pathology is variable but includes nfvPPA, bvFTD, and an executive motor disorder with prominent difficulties with gait. Patients who initially present with clinical bvFTD and are found to have CBD pathology on autopsy tend to be more apathetic than have florid disinhibition, are more anxious, and have a more dorsal and milder pattern of frontal atrophy when compared with patients with bvFTD who end up having a pathology of Pick disease (Rankin et al., 2011).

PROGRESSIVE SUPRANUCLEAR PALSY

Progressive supranuclear palsy is a neurodegenerative disorder that is pathologically defined by the presence of neurofibrillary tangles and neuropil threads in brainstem, basal ganglia, and cerebellar nuclei associated with abnormal four repeat tau protein deposition (Hauw et al., 1994). The most common clinical presentation is that of Richardson syndrome and includes postural instability, gait imbalance, multiple falls, and supranuclear gaze palsy that primarily affects vertical saccades. However, around 5% of patients may present with a behavioral syndrome similar to that of bvFTD without any sign of parkinsonism, falls, or eye movement abnormality until much later in the disease (Hassan et al., 2011; Josephs et al., 2011). These signs should be examined carefully in patients presenting with bvFTD because they may point to the diagnosis of PSP. Vertical saccade abnormalities in particular have been found to have a high predictability of PSP pathology (Boxer et al., 2012). Magnetic resonance imaging might reveal only mild frontotemporal atrophy with or without the classical decrease in midbrain size.

IMAGING AND OTHER DIAGNOSTIC METHODS

MAGNETIC RESONANCE IMAGING

Magnetic resonance imaging (MRI) is pivotal in reaching a more objective and neuroanatomically guided diagnosis in FTD. Patients with bvFTD usually have bilateral frontal and temporal atrophy with the earliest changes apparent in frontoinsular structures and other regions of the salient network (Seeley et al., 2009, 2012; Suarez et al., 2009). Nearly all patients referred with bvFTD show prominent frontally predominant atrophy, a finding that is often ignored in reports from radiologists (Suarez et al., 2009). Non-fluent variant primary progressive aphasia shows atrophy in the left perisylvian region, whereas svPPA shows parenchymal volume loss in left (or right) anterior temporal lobe (Gorno-Tempini et al., 2004). Patients with CBS show asymmetrical peri-rolandic dorsal atrophy, whereas those with PSP may show midbrain atrophy and a "hummingbird" sign on sagittal T1 resulting from atrophy of the midbrain tegmentum with a relative preservation of the pons (Massey et al., 2012).

POSITRON EMISSION TOMOGRAPHY

Fluorodeoxyglucose positron emission tomography (FDG-PET) may help in confirming a diagnosis of FTD. In a atrophy seen in patients with the progressive type (Davies et al., 2006; Kipps et al., 2007). Further functional imaging with fluorodeoxyglucose-positron emission tomography (FDG-PET) displays no hypometabolism in frontal brain regions (Kipps et al., 2009). Patients with the phenocopy often have a much longer survival and seldom get institutionalized, as opposed to their progressive counterparts who usually advance to death or institutionalization within three to four years (Davies et al., 2006; Garcin et al., 2009). Few of these cases that have come to autopsy have been reported in the literature as lacking the pathological changes typically seen in FTLD (Kertesz et al., 2005), however, there is not yet a large number of autopsies to definitively classify these patients as lacking a clear neurodegenerative process.

Recently the discovery of the C9ORF72 gene as implicated in the pathogenesis of FTD led to some re-examination of patients previously labeled as phenocopy. It was found that two out of four patients with the bvFTD phenocopy diagnosis harbored the mutation, raising concerns that there might in fact be an underlying neurodegenerative process in at least a subset of these slowly progressive patients (Khan, Yokoyama et al., 2012b).

PRIMARY PROGRESSIVE APHASIA

Primary progressive aphasia should be diagnosed when a patient experiences a progressive decline in language in which other cognitive domains and behavior are relatively spared for two years (Mesulam, 1982). The hallmark of the PPAs is a predominant deficit in conversational skills and language with an initial relative sparing of other cognitive and behavioral domains such as memory, executive functions, and visuospatial skills (Mesulam, 1982, 2001). Care must be taken when assessing other cognitive domains in a patient who has a primary language deficit because language greatly influences virtually all other cognitive functions. As an example, a person who does not understand the meaning of words may have difficulty memorizing them on verbal learning tasks.

Initial studies found that a primary language deficit can be the presenting clinical syndrome of many underlying brain pathologies, including FTLD, corticobasal degeneration, progressive supranuclear palsy, Creutzfeldt–Jakob disease, and Alzheimer's disease (Galton et al., 2000; Kertesz et al., 2000; Neary et al., 1998). In the past decade, a clearer understanding of primary language disorders divided their clinical presentation into three primary subtypes, each with a different clinical presentation and a distinct focal neuroanatomical correlate (Gorno-Tempini et al., 2004). Each subtype also provides clues for the prediction of the underlying pathological neurodegenerative process. The classification criteria for PPA set forth by an international group of PPA investigators are summarized in Table 67.2 (Gorno-Tempini et al., 2011).

NON-FLUENT VARIANT OF PRIMARY PROGRESSIVE APHASIA

Non-fluent variant of primary progressive aphasia (nfvPPA) is characterized by difficulties in speech production including agrammatism, an effortful, slow speech and/or apraxia of speech, defined as presence of speech initiation difficulties, sound distortion or substitution, and deletion or transposition of syllables (Gorno-Tempini et al., 2004; Hodges and Patterson, 1996; Neary et al., 1998). This can be apparent in spontaneous speech or when patients are given a polysyllabic word to say multiple times in a row. Phonemic paraphasias such as faulty syllable sequencing (amadant for adamant) or improper usage of phoneme (bumble for mumble) can occur. Patients are usually aware of their deficits and may try to correct their pronunciation errors, which often leads to frustration.

In addition to these deficits in language production, difficulty in understanding complex sentences with difficult grammatical syntax may indicate agrammatism in comprehension. Single-word comprehension is typically preserved and patients with nvfPPA perform within normal limits on word comprehension tasks (Gorno-Tempini et al., 2004). Patients with nfvPPA are the most likely to have motor findings on their neurological examination consisting of rigidity, and slowing and reduced dexterity, usually observable in the right arm (Gorno-Tempini et al., 2004). Brain atrophy is mostly localized to the left perisylvian region, and more specifically to the pars opercularis and pars triangularis (Gorno-Tempini et al., 2004). The clinical presentation of nfvPPA usually points to an underlying pathology of CBD or TDP-43 type A (see the following).

SEMANTIC VARIANT OF PRIMARY PROGRESSIVE APHASIA

The semantic variant of primary progressive aphasia (svPPA) (see Case 2 later in chapter) was initially described in its left predominant form, which presents with a loss of knowledge of words and objects in the setting of a relatively preserved speech production (fluent speech) and grammar both in production and comprehension (Gorno-Tempini et al., 2004; Hodges et al., 1992). Surface dyslexia can occur and is defined as the inability to recognize (and correctly read) irregular words, sounding them out instead. For example, a patient with surface dyslexia might read choir as chore. Similarly, spelling errors resulting from the inability to recognize words also occurs: in a word such as orchestra, the "ch" is pronounced and yacht is spelled like "yat.'" Patients with svPPA perform poorly on confrontation naming and word recognition tasks. In fact, their speech often contains non-specific words such as thing or animal to circumvent words that they have lost the meaning of (Gorno-Tempini et al., 2004). Conversational speech is usually comprehended, although patients may ask about the meaning of a specific word in conversation. Patients with svPPA usually exhibit no motor findings on their neurological examination (Gorno-Tempini et al., 2004).

Patients with svPPA often develop more behavioral changes in the course of their disease than do those with other subtypes of PPA (Rosen et al., 2006). Prominent features of these behavioral manifestations include loss of empathy, irritability, mental rigidity, and compulsive behavior, as well as disruption of sleep, appetite, and libido, likely speaking for the role of the anterior temporal lobe and the orbital frontal cortex (where they mostly progressed to mixed within four years of disease duration (Le Ber et al., 2006).

Patients with bvFTD can make rude remarks or gestures without regard for other people's feelings. They are often described as becoming self-centered and losing the ability to understand the feelings of others. Families often describe insensitivity to someone else's illness or injury. Patients become emotionally distant and detached. This often creates a toxic dynamic for couples. Also, because the majority of the patients present at a younger age, children who may be in their early teenage years, or even younger, may complain that their father or mother had become less affectionate and less involved in their schooling and upbringing. Neuroanatomical correlates of empathy include the right anterior temporal and medial frontal regions in a large-scale correlation study by voxel-based morphometry analysis of magnetic resonance imaging (MRI) data (Rankin et al., 2006). Also, by similar methods, an impaired recognition of emotions, and specifically negative emotions such as sadness, correlated with right lateral inferior temporal and right middle temporal gyri (Rosen et al., 2006).

Patients with bvFTD can become obsessed with specific thoughts and display compulsory behavior, which may be either simple or complex. For example, there may be repetitive picking, chewing, lip smacking, or pacing; there may also be constant locking and unlocking, as well as rituals that can be bizarre in nature. Compulsions can also manifest as hoarding. Mental rigidity occurs and patients may become less flexible to changes in plans or routines. Examples include exercising at a specific hour every day, eating specific types of food at specific times of the day, and taking the same route when walking their dogs.

Informants often describe hyperorality and inability to refrain from eating, even after satiety is achieved. A change in diet and more specifically a craving for sweets is often reported, as well as eating non-food items. The excessive, compulsive eating can result in weight gain. Hyperorality can also manifest in excessive drinking of alcohol, smoking, or chewing gum. Hyperorality despite reported satiety was found to correlate with right orbitofrontal, insular, and striatal regions, supporting the hypothesis that this circuitry is involved in higher gustatory integration and internal satiety signaling (Woolley et al., 2007). In another study, overeating correlated with loss of tissue in the posterior hypothalamus (Piguet et al., 2011).

Neuropsychological testing in patients with bvFTD primarily reveals deficits in executive functions (Kramer et al., 2003), with a relative sparing of verbal and visual memory and performance that is error prone and perseverative. It is important to recognize that episodic memory can be impaired in bvFTD (Hodges et al., 2004), even in early stages, and especially in some genetic forms of the disease that involve the progranulin gene (van Swieten and Heutink, 2008). Rule violation errors on neuropsychological testing correlated with tissue loss in the right lateral prefrontal cortex (Possin et al., 2009). In contrast, executive function tasks seem to be more diffuse and invoke attention, and visuospatial and language networks. Specific tasks of the executive function testing can localize to a specific region of the brain. Verbal fluency, in which patients are asked to generate the maximum number of words they can think of that start with a specific letter in one minute, correlated with

tissue loss in the left perisylvian cortex, while card-sorting tasks with the left dorsolateral prefrontal cortex (Huey et al., 2009). Set shifting tasks such as trails-making correlated with tissue loss in prefrontal and posterior parietal regions (Pa et al., 2010). Patients with bvFTD usually have relatively spared performances on verbal and visual memory tasks as well as visuospatial tasks.

With new emerging neuroimaging techniques, it is proposed that neurodegenerative diseases may involve various regions of the brain that operate together and are collectively referred to as brain networks. For example, the default mode network, including the posterior cingulate, medial temporal, lateral temporoparietal, and dorsal medial prefrontal regions, is thought to be involved in Alzheimer's disease (Greicius et al., 2003; Buckner et al., 2005). Seeley and colleagues have shown prominent deficits in functional connectivity in other networks such as the salience using task free functional MRI and this promising technique is likely to become standard in the assessment of patients with bvFTD (Seeley et al., 2009; Seeley et al., 2012; Zhou et al., 2010).

FRONTOTEMPORAL DEMENTIA AND MOTOR NEURON DISEASE

The co-association of FTD and ALS is now accepted at a clinical, neuropathological, and genetic level (Caselli et al., 1993; Lomen-Hoerth et al., 2002; Neary et al., 1990; Neary et al., 2000). Patients with frontotemporal dementia and motor neuron disease (FTD-MND) have the typical features of bvFTD that are either preceded or shortly followed by typical features of ALS. Perhaps one of the features that should make the clinician suspicious of MND with bvFTD is the lack of weight gain that classically comes with hyperorality, but instead, there is loss of weight resulting from muscle atrophy and diminished desire to swallow. Also, patients with FTD-MND have the highest frequency of concomitant psychotic symptoms, including delusions and hallucinations, which are less common in more classical forms of bvFTD. Familial FTD-MND was found to correlate with a genetic mutation on chromosome 9 and, in recent years, the culprit gene, C9ORF72, was discovered (see next section).

BEHAVIORAL VARIANT OF FRONTOTEMPORAL DEMENTIA "PHENOCOPY"

After the publication of diagnostic criteria for bvFTD, a group of patients was identified that fulfilled the criteria without necessarily progressing to a clinically defined dementia state, frequently plateauing at mild stages of the disease (Davies et al., 2006). These patients are referred to as bvFTD "phenocopies" because they display the "phenotype" of the disease, presumably without evidence of an underlying neurodegenerative process. These patients also score better on measures of activities of daily living as compared to patients with bvFTD (Mioshi et al., 2009). On neuropsychology testing, executive functions that are usually impaired in bvFTD may be spared in patients with the phenocopy (Hornberger et al., 2008). Magnetic resonance imaging is usually normal and does not reveal the typical pattern of frontal lobe

TABLE 67.2. Diagnostic consensus criteria for FTD and PPA

TABLE 67.2. (*Continued*)

BEHAVIORAL VARIANT OF FRONTOTEMPORAL DEMENTIA (BVFTD)

I. Possible bvFTD (three out of the six following symptoms [a–f] should be present to meet criteria)
  A. Early behavioral disinhibition
  B. Early apathy or inertia
  C. Early loss of sympathy or empathy
  D. Early perseverative, steryotyped, or compulsive/ritualistic behavior
  E. Hyperorality and dietary changes
  F. Neuropsychological profile: executive/generation deficits with relative sparing of memory and visuospatial functions
II. Probable bvFTD (all of the following [a–c] must be present)
  A. Meets criteria for possible bvFTD
  B. Exhibits significant functional decline
  C. Imaging results consistent with bvFTD
III. Exclusion Criteria
  A. Pattern of deficits is better accounted for by other non-degenerative nervous system or medical disorders
  B. Behavioral disturbance is better accounted for by a psychiatric diagnosis
  C. Biomarkers strongly indicative of Alzheimer's disease or other neurodegenerative process

PRIMARY PROGRESSIVE APHASIA (PPA)

I. Inclusion Criteria (All of a-c must be present)
  A. Most prominent clinical feature is difficulty with language
  B. Deficits are the principal cause of impaired daily living activities
  C. Aphasia should be the most prominent deficit at symptom onset and for the initial phases of the disease
II. Exclusion Criteria
  A. Pattern of deficits is better accounted for by other non-degenerative nervous system or medical disorders
  B. Cognitive disturbance is better accounted for by a psychiatric diagnosis
  C. Prominent initial episodic memory, visual memory, and visuo-perceptual impairments
  D. Prominent initial behavioral disturbances
III. Diagnostic Criteria for Non-fluent/Agrammatic Variant PPA (PNFA for progressive non-fluent aphasia)
  A. Clinical diagnosis of NFAV-PPA
    1. Agrammatism in language production
    2. Effortful, halting speech with apraxia of speech
    3. Impaired comprehension of syntactically complex sentences
    4. Spared single-word comprehension
    5. Spared object knowledge
  B. Imaging-supported NFAV-PPA
    1. Clinical diagnosis of NFAV-PPA
    2. Imaging showing one or more of:
      a. Predominant left posterior fronto-insular atrophy on MRI
      b. Predominant left posterior fronto-insular hypoperfusion or hypometabolism on SPECT of PET
IV. Diagnostic Criteria for Semantic Variant PPA (svPPA)
  A. Clinical diagnosis of SV-PPA
    1. Poor confrontation naming
    2. Impaired single-word comprehension
    3. Poor object knowledge
    4. Surface dyslexia and/or dysgraphia
    5. Spared repetition
    6. Spared motor speech (no distortions) and grammar
  B. Imaging-supported SV-PPA
    1. Clinical diagnosis of SV-PPA
    2. Imaging showing one or more of:
      a. Predominant anterior temporal lobe atrophy on MRI
      b. Predominant anterior temporal hypoperfusion or hypometabolism on SPECT or PET

(continued)

V. Diagnostic Criteria for Logopenic Variant PPA (LPA for logopenic progressive aphasia)
  A. Clinical diagnosis of LV-PPA
    1. Impaired single-word retrieval in spontaneous speech
    2. Impaired repetition of sentences and phrases
    3. Speech (phonological) errors in spontaneous speech and naming
    4. Spared single-word comprehension and object knowledge
    5. Spared motor speech (no distortions)
    6. Absence of frank agrammatism
  B. Imaging supported diagnosis of LV-PPA
    1. Clinical diagnosis of LV-PPA
    2. Imaging must show one of:
      a. Predominant left posterior perisylvian or parietal atrophy on MRI
      b. Predominant left posterior perisylvian or parietal hypoperfusion or hypometabolism on SPECT or PET

BEHAVIORAL VARIANT OF FRONTOTEMPORAL DEMENTIA

Patients with the behavioral variant of frontotemporal dementia (see Case 1 later in chapter) often present initially to the psychiatry clinic with what appears to be a mania or depression, or to a marriage counselor because of marital problems. The first presenting symptom is often one of disinhibition and social inappropriateness (Miller et al., 1991). As an example, patients might become overly friendly, approaching strangers and starting conversations that are too personal or explicit. Excessive trust of strangers coupled with a difficulty in making sound judgments, can particularly make these individuals vulnerable to exploitation, both sexually and financially. In fact, many spouses may report that their loved ones were the subjects of an online or telephone prank involving investing suspicious amounts of money in unfounded organizations. Symptoms of disinhibition correlate mainly with a pattern of atrophy in the orbitofrontal cortex but can also involve the subgenual cingulate, medial prefrontal, and anterior temporal cortex, as well as the white matter tracts connecting those regions, as measured by voxel-based morphometry and diffusion tensor imaging analysis (Hornberger et al., 2011; Peters et al., 2006; Rosen et al., 2005).

Apathy, social withdrawal, and decreased motivation are often reported (Rosen et al., 2005). Informants may report a decrease in interest for previous hobbies and a general attitude of indifference. In an objective assessment of daytime activity using a wristwatch that measures motion, patients with bvFTD spent 25% of their day immobile compared with their caregivers, who spent 11% of their day immobile (Merrilees et al., 2012). Apathy was found to correlate with reduced gray matter density in the right dorsolateral prefrontal cortex, right ventromedial superior frontal gyrus, right anterior cingulate, right lateral orbitofrontal cortex, right caudate, right temporoparietal junction, and right posterior inferior and middle temporal gyri (Eslinger et al., 2012; Rosen et al., 2005; Zamboni et al., 2008). A subclassification of bvFTD presentations, separating between predominantly disinhibited and predominantly apathetic, was suggested in the past (Snowden et al., 2001); however, it was shown that most cases are often mixed, and if not,

TABLE 67.1. Clinical subtypes of frontotemporal dementia

	BVFTD	PNFA	SVPPA	LPA	CBS	PSP
Classical clinical presentation	Behavioral changes including disinhibition, lack of empathy, apathy, obsessions and ritualistic behavior, overeating, and executive problems	Non-fluent speech with agrammatism and apraxia of speech; usually with sparing of repetition, object, and word knowledge	Word finding difficulties with loss of individual word meaning and object knowledge; usually with fluent speech and spared grammar	Difficulty with spontaneous word retrieval and phonological memory loop with impaired repetition and intact grammar and semantic knowledge	Asymmetric parkinsonism, tremor, and rigidity with possible alien hand, dystonia, and apraxia	Postural imbalance, eye movement abnormalities, and parkinsonism
Patterns of atrophy on MRI	Bilateral frontal and/or temporal	Left frontoinsular and opercular	Left (and/or right) anterior temporal lobe	Left angular gyrus	Unilateral peri-rolandic dorsal	Midbrain atrophy
Associated pathology	Tau: 3R (Pick disease), 4R (CBD or PSP); TDP-43: Type A (in GRN mutations), B (in C9 mutations), C or D	Tau: 3R (Pick disease), 4R (CBD or PSP) TDP-43: Type A	TDP-43: Type C	AD pathology (plaques and tangles)	Tau: 4R (CBD most common, PSP) AD pathology TDP-43	Tau: 4R (PSP)

AD, Alzheimer's disease; bvFTD, behavioral variant frontotemporal dementia; CBD, corticobasal degeneration; CBS, corticobasal syndrome; FTD, frontotemporal dementia; LPA, logopenic progressive aphasia; PNFA progressive non-fluent aphasia; PSP, progressive supranuclear palsy; svPPA, semantic variant of primary progressive aphasia; TDP, TAR DNA binding protein.

Lund-Manchester criteria was calculated at 3% (Gislason et al., 2003).

Frontotemporal dementia seems to peak in the sixth and seventh decades. The incidence of FTD was reported to be 2.2, 3.3, and 8.9 per 100,000 person-years in the age groups of 40 to 49, 50 to 59, and 60 to 69, respectively, as compared with 0.0, 3.3, and 88.9 for AD (Knopman et al., 2004). In the United Kingdom, the incidence of FTD in the age group of 45 to 64 was found to be 3.5 per 100,000 person-years as compared with 4.2 for AD (Mercy et al., 2008). The age of onset in FTD can vary according to the specific subtype of the disease. It is generally between 50 and 60 years of age and might be dependent on the underlying pathology and on genetic factors (Johnson et al., 2005; Rosso et al., 2003; Seelaar et al., 2008). Although patients with the bvFTD appear to have the earliest onset, patients with svPPA have an earlier onset than those with PNFA (Johnson et al., 2005).

In a study of the California State Alzheimer's Disease Centers the frequency of FTD as a clinical diagnosis was different across ethnic differences: 4.2% in Asians and Pacific Islander and 4.7% in Caucasians, but was significantly less in Blacks (1.5%) and Latinos (2.4%) (Hou et al., 2006). Sadly most of this data was collected during the 1980s and 1990s when FTD was severely neglected and underdiagnosed in the United States, accounting for the low prevalence in this study.

The evidence for gender differences in FTD is conflicting. Although some studies report no significant differences (Hou et al., 2006; Ikeda et al., 2004; Mercy et al., 2008; Papageorgiou et al., 2009), others suggest that there is a male predominance in the behavioral and semantic subtypes and a female predominance in the non-fluent aphasia group (Ratnavalli et al., 2002; Johnson et al., 2005). Frontotemporal dementia is strongly familial, and patients with FTD were reported to have a family history of dementia in 10% to 38% of the cases (Chow et al., 1999; Stevens et al., 1998). Psychiatric illnesses in these families, including major depression and schizoaffective disorders, were reported in 33% of patients with FTD (Chow et al., 1999).

Although the typical survival of patients with Alzheimer's disease from the time of diagnosis to death is reported to be seven to 13 years from symptom onset (Garcin et al., 2009; Roberson et al., 2005), the survival of patients with FTD is shorter, ranging from 3.4 years for patients with bvFTD to closer to six years for those with semantic variant primary progressive aphasia (Roberson et al., 2005).

CLINICAL PRESENTATIONS AND DIAGNOSTIC CRITERIA

BEHAVIORAL VARIANT OF FRONTOTEMPORAL DEMENTIA

Behavioral variant of frontotemporal dementia (bvFTD) is the most common subtype of FTD (Johnson et al., 2005). An international consortium revised and published new criteria for the diagnosis of bvFTD in 2011 and compared their sensitivity with the previous criteria set forth by Neary in 1998 in 137 pathology confirmed cases of FTLD (Rascovsky et al., 2011). The new criteria were superior to the previous ones in picking up possible and probable bvFTD when it corresponded to a pathological diagnosis of FTLD. These criteria are summarized in Table 67.2.

Often bvFTD patients have little insight into their problems and interviewing an informant is essential in diagnosing bvFTD. In fact, in early stages, the diagnosis can be completely missed if patients are interviewed without an informant, and they can have an intact cognitive performance on routine neuropsychology testing (Miller et al., 1991).

67 | CLINICAL FEATURES AND PATHOGENESIS OF FRONTOTEMPORAL DEMENTIA

GEORGES NAASAN AND BRUCE MILLER

First described by Pick in 1892 as frontal lobe dementia, frontotemporal dementia (FTD) was neglected
for almost a century before re-emerging as a clinically
important neurodegenerative disease. It is the second most
common dementia in patients under the age of 65 and the
third, after Alzheimer's disease (AD) and dementia with
Lewy bodies (DLB), in the elderly population. In neuropathological studies, frontotemporal lobar degeneration
(FTLD) was found to be the third leading neuropathological
diagnosis of neurodegenerative diseases with a prevalence of
4% after AD (42%) and vascular disease (VD; 23.7% isolated
and 21.6% in combination with AD) (Brunnstrom et al.,
2009).

Frontotemporal dementia (FTD) is used to describe a
group of clinical syndromes that are caused by frontal and/or
temporal lobe dysfunction with a relative preservation of the
posterior brain structures that are typically involved in AD and
DLB. The clinical presentation of FTD is insidious and slowly
progressive. The predominant symptom can be behavioral
changes (orbitofrontal, medial frontal, and/or anterior temporal lobe), executive function impairment (dorsolateral frontal),
and/or language impairment (perisylvian, frontoinsular, or
anterior temporal lobe) giving rise to various clinical subtypes
that are summarized in Table 67.1.

The term frontotemporal lobar degeneration (FTLD)
refers to the pathological syndrome associated with predominant frontal and/or temporal lobe atrophy (Cairns et al., 2007).
Most FTLD cases show neuronal aggregates of tau, TDP-43, or
FUS. Some FTD subtypes overlap with other neurological syndromes, including amyotrophic lateral sclerosis (ALS) in frontotemporal dementia with motor neuron disease (FTD-MND)
(Caselli et al., 1993; Lomen-Hoerth et al., 2002; Neary et al.,
1990; Neary et al., 2000) and parkinsonism in corticobasal
syndrome (CBS) and progressive supranuclear palsy (PSP).
Novel genetic mutations in familial and sporadic cases of FTD
have been identified in the past decade and their implications
continue to be a major subject of research.

Frontotemporal dementia represents a disorder of behavior
that is caused by neurodegeneration, and this concept can be
difficult for physicians to understand. Often, FTD is ascribed
to conditions of the "psyche," without making an attempt to
understand them as caused by degeneration in specific brain
structures. In addition, patients with FTD may present fairly
young, sometimes in their young adulthood, which is the

typical age at presentation for many psychiatric disorders such
as schizophrenia and bipolar disease.

Many examples of FTD being misdiagnosed as a psychiatric disorder are reported in the literature and expose the medical and social burdens of a misdiagnosis on patients and their
caregivers (Khan et al., 2012). Approximately 30% of patients
with a neurodegenerative disease are initially erroneously
diagnosed as having a psychiatric illness, especially when the
predominant presentation is behavioral issues (Woolley et al.,
2011).

EPIDEMIOLOGY AND DEMOGRAPHICS

The prevalence and incidence of FTD is variably reported
and has been difficult to ascertain, partly because of the
heterogeneity of the clinical syndromes and the pathological diagnoses that the terms FTD and FTLD encompass. It is
likely that all of the previous studies have underestimated the
true prevalence of FTD for a variety of reasons. First, many
patients with FTD never get diagnosed and end up in mental institutions or prisons. Additionally, the co-association
of FTD with memory difficulty, parkinsonian movement
disorders, and amyotrophic lateral sclerosis means that even
when a neurodegenerative disorder is recognized, many FTD
patients are classified as having another neurodegenerative
condition.

Studies conducted by European investigators suggested that
the prevalence of a clinical frontal-lobe predominant dementia
was between 12% and 16% at autopsy (Brun, 1987; Greicius
et al., 2002). The release of the Lund-Manchester criteria for
the diagnosis of FTD in 1994 (The Lund and Manchester
Groups, 1994), followed later by the publication of the Neary
criteria in 1998, helped to establish a clinical framework from
which researchers could attempt to determine the epidemiology of the disease (Neary et al., 1998). By applying those clinical criteria, the prevalence of FTD in the United Kingdom was
found to be similar to that of AD in the age group of 45 to 65
and was estimated at 15 per 100,000 (Ratnavalli et al., 2002). In
the Netherlands, the prevalence of FTD was found to be lower
and peaked between the ages of 60 to 69 at 9.4 per 100,000. It
was roughly four in 100,000 for the age groups 50 to 59 and 70
to 79 (Rosso et al., 2003). For individuals age 85 and greater,
the prevalence of the frontal variant of FTD according to the

Walker, Z., Jaros, E., et al. (2007). Dementia with Lewy bodies: a comparison of clinical diagnosis, FP-CIT single photon emission computed tomography imaging and autopsy. *J. Neurol. Neurosurg. Psychiatry* 78:1176–1181.

Weiner, M.F., Hynan, L.S., et al. (2003). Can Alzheimer's disease and dementias with Lewy bodies be distinguished clinically? *J. Geriatr. Psychiatry Neurol.* 16:245–250.

Weisman, D., and McKeith, I. (2007). Dementia with Lewy bodies. *Semin. Neurol.* 27:42–47.

Whitwell, J.L., Weigand, S.D., et al. (2007). Focal atrophy in dementia with Lewy bodies on MRI: a distinct pattern from Alzheimer's disease. *Brain* 130:708–719.

Woods, S.P., and Troster, A.I. (2003). Prodromal frontal/executive dysfunction predicts incident dementia in Parkinson's disease. *J. Int. Neuropsychol. Soc.* 9:17–24.

Yong, S.W., Yoon, J.K., et al. (2007). A comparison of cerebral glucose metabolism in Parkinson's disease, Parkinson's disease dementia and dementia with Lewy bodies. *Eur. J. Neurol.* 14:1357–1362.

Yoshita, M., Taki, J., et al. (2001). A clinical role for [(123)I]MIBG myocardial scintigraphy in the distinction between dementia of the Alzheimer's-type and dementia with Lewy bodies. *J. Neurol. Neurosurg. Psychiatry* 71:583–588.

Zaccai, J., McCracken, C., et al. (2005). A systematic review of prevalence and incidence studies of dementia with Lewy bodies. *Age Ageing* 34:561–566.

Klatka, L.A., Louis, E.D., et al. (1996). Psychiatric features in diffuse Lewy body disease: a clinicopathologic study using Alzheimer's disease and Parkinson's disease comparison groups. *Neurology* 47:1148–1152.

Koeppe, R.A., Gilman, S., et al. (2008). Differentiating Alzheimer's disease from dementia with Lewy bodies and Parkinson's disease with (+)-[11C] dihydrotetrabenazine positron emission tomography. *Alzheimers Dement.* 4:S67–S76.

Kruger, R., Kuhn, W., et al. (1998). Ala30Pro mutation in the gene encoding alpha-synuclein in Parkinson's disease. *Nat. Genet.* 18:106–108.

Lambon Ralph, M.A., Powell, J., et al. (2001). Semantic memory is impaired in both dementia with Lewy bodies and dementia of Alzheimer's type: a comparative neuropsychological study and literature review. *J. Neurol. Neurosurg. Psychiatry* 70:149–156.

Leplow, B., Dierks, C., et al. (1997). Remote memory in Parkinson's disease and senile dementia. *Neuropsychologia* 35:547–557.

Lim, S.M., Katsifis, A., et al. (2009). The 18F-FDG PET cingulate island sign and comparison to 123I-beta-CIT SPECT for diagnosis of dementia with Lewy bodies. *J. Nucl. Med.* 50:1638–1645.

Lockhart, A., Lamb, J.R., et al. (2007). PIB is a non-specific imaging marker of amyloid-beta (Abeta) peptide-related cerebral amyloidosis. *Brain* 130:2607–2615.

Matsui, H., Udaka, F., et al. (2005). N-isopropyl-*p*-123I iodoamphetamine single photon emission computed tomography study of Parkinson's disease with dementia. *Intern. Med.* 44:1046–1050.

McKeith, I., Del Ser, T., et al. (2000). Efficacy of rivastigmine in dementia with Lewy bodies: a randomised, double-blind, placebo-controlled international study. *Lancet* 356:2031–2036.

McKeith, I., Fairbairn, A., et al. (1992). Neuroleptic sensitivity in patients with senile dementia of Lewy body type. *BMJ* 305:673–678.

McKeith, I., Mintzer, J., et al. (2004). Dementia with Lewy bodies. *Lancet Neurol.* 3:19–28.

McKeith, I., O'Brien, J., et al. (2007). Sensitivity and specificity of dopamine transporter imaging with 123I-FP-CIT SPECT in dementia with Lewy bodies: a phase III, multicentre study. *Lancet Neurol.* 6:305–313.

McKeith, I.G. (2000a). Clinical Lewy body syndromes. *Ann. NY Acad. Sci.* 920:1–8.

McKeith, I.G. (2000b). Spectrum of Parkinson's disease, Parkinson's dementia, and Lewy body dementia. *Neurol. Clin.* 18:865–902.

McKeith, I.G., Dickson, D.W., et al. (2005). Diagnosis and management of dementia with Lewy bodies: third report of the DLB Consortium. *Neurology* 65:1863–1872.

McKeith, I.G., Grace, J.B., et al. (2000). Rivastigmine in the treatment of dementia with Lewy bodies: preliminary findings from an open trial. *Int. J. Geriatr. Psychiatry* 15:387–392.

Molloy, S., McKeith, I.G., et al. (2005). The role of levodopa in the management of dementia with Lewy bodies. *J. Neurol. Neurosurg. Psychiatry* 76:1200–1203.

Monsch, A.U., Bondi, M.W., et al. (1992). Comparisons of verbal fluency tasks in the detection of dementia of the Alzheimer type. *Arch. Neurol.* 49:1253–1258.

Namba, H., Fukushi, K., et al. (2002). Positron emission tomography: quantitative measurement of brain acetylcholinesterase activity using radiolabeled substrates. *Methods* 27:242–250.

Nishioka, K., Wider, C., et al. (2010). Association of alpha-, beta-, and gamma-synuclein with diffuse lewy body disease. *Arch. Neurol.* 67:970–975.

Noe, E., Marder, K., et al. (2004). Comparison of dementia with Lewy bodies to Alzheimer's disease and Parkinson's disease with dementia. *Mov. Disord.* 19:60–67.

O'Brien, J.T., Colloby, S., et al. (2004). Dopamine transporter loss visualized with FP-CIT SPECT in the differential diagnosis of dementia with Lewy bodies. *Arch. Neurol.* 61:919–925.

O'Brien, J.T., Colloby, S.J., et al. (2007). Alpha4beta2 nicotinic receptor status in Alzheimer's disease using 123I-5IA-85380 single-photon-emission computed tomography. *J. Neurol. Neurosurg. Psychiatry* 78:356–362.

O'Brien, J.T., Colloby, S.J., et al. (2008). Nicotinic alpha4beta2 receptor binding in dementia with Lewy bodies using 123I-5IA-85380 SPECT demonstrates a link between occipital changes and visual hallucinations. *Neuroimage* 40:1056–1063.

O'Brien, J.T., Paling, S., et al. (2001). Progressive brain atrophy on serial MRI in dementia with Lewy bodies, AD, and vascular dementia. *Neurology* 56:1386–1388.

Ohtake, H., Limprasert, P., et al. (2004). Beta-synuclein gene alterations in dementia with Lewy bodies. *Neurology* 63:805–811.

Oide, T., Tokuda, T., et al. (2003). Usefulness of [123I]metaiodobenzylguanidine ([123I]MIBG) myocardial scintigraphy in differentiating between Alzheimer's disease and dementia with Lewy bodies. *Intern. Med.* 42:686–690.

Okereke, C.S., Kirby, L., et al. (2004). Concurrent administration of donepezil HCl and levodopa/carbidopa in patients with Parkinson's disease: assessment of pharmacokinetic changes and safety following multiple oral doses. *Br. J. Clin. Pharmacol.* 58(Suppl 1):41–49.

Olson, E.J., Boeve, B.F., et al. (2000). Rapid eye movement sleep behaviour disorder: demographic, clinical and laboratory findings in 93 cases. *Brain* 123(Pt 2):331–339.

Parkkinen, L., Pirttila, T., et al. (2008). Applicability of current staging/categorization of alpha-synuclein pathology and their clinical relevance. *Acta Neuropathol.* 115:399–407.

Polymeropoulos, M.H., Lavedan, C., et al. (1997). Mutation in the alpha-synuclein gene identified in families with Parkinson's disease. *Science* 276:2045–2047.

Rabinovici, G.D., Furst, A.J., et al. (2007). 11C-PIB PET imaging in Alzheimer disease and frontotemporal lobar degeneration. *Neurology* 68:1205–1212.

Ricci, M., Guidoni, S.V., et al. (2009). Clinical findings, functional abilities and caregiver distress in the early stage of dementia with Lewy bodies (DLB) and Alzheimer's disease (AD). *Arch. Gerontol. Geriatr.* 49:e101–e104.

Ridha, B.H., Josephs, K.A., et al. (2005). Delusions and hallucinations in dementia with Lewy bodies: worsening with memantine. *Neurology* 65:481–482.

Rowe, C.C., Ackerman, U., et al. (2008). Imaging of amyloid beta in Alzheimer's disease with 18F-BAY94-9172, a novel PET tracer: proof of mechanism. *Lancet Neurol.* 7:129–135.

Sabbagh, M.N., Hake, A.M., et al. (2005). The use of memantine in dementia with Lewy bodies. *J. Alzheimers Dis.* 7:285–289.

Samuel, W., Caligiuri, M., et al. (2000). Better cognitive and psychopathologic response to donepezil in patients prospectively diagnosed as dementia with Lewy bodies: a preliminary study. *Int. J. Geriatr. Psychiatry* 15:794–802.

Sanchez-Ramos, J.R., Ortoll, R., et al. (1996). Visual hallucinations associated with Parkinson disease. *Arch. Neurol.* 53:1265–1268.

Shimada, H., Hirano, S., et al. (2009). Mapping of brain acetylcholinesterase alterations in Lewy body disease by PET. *Neurology* 73:273–278.

Shimizu, S., Hanyu, H., et al. (2005). Differentiation of dementia with Lewy bodies from Alzheimer's disease using brain SPECT. *Dement. Geriatr. Cogn. Disord.* 20:25–30.

Simard, M., van Reekum, R., et al. (2000). A review of the cognitive and behavioral symptoms in dementia with Lewy bodies. *J. Neuropsychiatry Clin. Neurosci.* 12:425–450.

Simard, M., van Reekum, R., et al. (2003). Visuospatial impairment in dementia with Lewy bodies and Alzheimer's disease: a process analysis approach. *Int. J. Geriatr. Psychiatry* 18:387–391.

Sinforiani, E., Zangaglia, R., et al. (2006). REM sleep behavior disorder, hallucinations, and cognitive impairment in Parkinson's disease. *Mov. Disord.* 21:462–466.

Spiegel, J. (2010). Diagnostic and pathophysiological impact of myocardial MIBG scintigraphy in Parkinson's disease. *Parkinsons Dis.* 2010:295346.

Spiegel, J., Mollers, M.O., et al. (2005). FP-CIT and MIBG scintigraphy in early Parkinson's disease. *Mov. Disord.* 20:552–561.

Suzuki, M., Kurita, A., et al. (2006). Impaired myocardial 123I-metaiodobenzylguanidine uptake in Lewy body disease: comparison between dementia with Lewy bodies and Parkinson's disease. *J. Neurol. Sci.* 240:15–19.

Tateno, M., Kobayashi, S., et al. (2008). Comparison of the usefulness of brain perfusion SPECT and MIBG myocardial scintigraphy for the diagnosis of dementia with Lewy bodies. *Dement. Geriatr. Cogn. Disord.* 26:453–457.

Tiraboschi, P., Salmon, D.P., et al. (2006). What best differentiates Lewy body from Alzheimer's disease in early-stage dementia? *Brain* 129:729–735.

Touchon, J., Bergman, H., et al. (2006). Response to rivastigmine or donepezil in Alzheimer's patients with symptoms suggestive of concomitant Lewy body pathology. *Curr. Med. Res. Opin.* 22:49–59.

Trinh, N.H., Hoblyn, J., et al. (2003). Efficacy of cholinesterase inhibitors in the treatment of neuropsychiatric symptoms and functional impairment in Alzheimer disease: a meta-analysis. *JAMA* 289:210–216.

Wada-Isoe, K., Kitayama, M., et al. (2007). Diagnostic markers for diagnosing dementia with Lewy bodies: CSF and MIBG cardiac scintigraphy study. *J. Neurol. Sci.* 260:33–37.

Walker, M.P., Ayre, G.A., et al. (2000). Quantification and characterization of fluctuating cognition in dementia with Lewy bodies and Alzheimer's disease. *Dement. Geriatr. Cogn. Disord.* 11:327–335.

Walker, Z., Costa, D.C., et al. (2002). Differentiation of dementia with Lewy bodies from Alzheimer's disease using a dopaminergic presynaptic ligand. *J. Neurol. Neurosurg. Psychiatry* 73:134–140.

Walker, Z., Grace, J., et al. (1999). Olanzapine in dementia with Lewy bodies: a clinical study. *Int. J. Geriatr. Psychiatry* 14:459–466.

REFERENCES

Aarsland, D., and Kurz, M.W. (2010). The epidemiology of dementia associated with Parkinson's disease. *Brain Pathol.* 20:633–639.

Aarsland, D., Litvan, I., et al. (2003). Performance on the dementia rating scale in Parkinson's disease with dementia and dementia with Lewy bodies: comparison with progressive supranuclear palsy and Alzheimer's disease. *J. Neurol. Neurosurg. Psychiatry* 74:1215–1220.

Aarsland, D., Perry, R., et al. (2005). Neuroleptic sensitivity in Parkinson's disease and parkinsonian dementias. *J. Clin. Psychiatry* 66:633–637.

Ala, T.A., Hughes, L.F., et al. (2002). The Mini-Mental State exam may help in the differentiation of dementia with Lewy bodies and Alzheimer's disease. *Int. J. Geriatr. Psychiatry* 17:503–509.

Allan, L.M., Ballard, C.G., et al. (2007). Autonomic dysfunction in dementia. *J. Neurol. Neurosurg. Psychiatry* 78:671–677.

Almeida, O.P., Burton, E.J., et al. (2003). MRI study of caudate nucleus volume in Parkinson's disease with and without dementia with Lewy bodies and Alzheimer's disease. *Dement. Geriatr. Cogn. Disord.* 16:57–63.

Ballard, C.G., Aarsland, D., et al. (2002). Fluctuations in attention: PD dementia vs DLB with parkinsonism. *Neurology* 59:1714–1720.

Ballard, C., Holmes, C., et al. (1999). Psychiatric morbidity in dementia with Lewy bodies: a prospective clinical and neuropathological comparative study with Alzheimer's disease. *Am. J. Psychiatry* 156:1039–1045.

Ballard, C., Ziabreva, I., et al. (2006). Differences in neuropathologic characteristics across the Lewy body dementia spectrum. *Neurology* 67:1931–1934.

Barber, R., McKeith, I.G., et al. (2001). A comparison of medial and lateral temporal lobe atrophy in dementia with Lewy bodies and Alzheimer's disease: magnetic resonance imaging volumetric study. *Dement. Geriatr. Cogn. Disord.* 12:198–205.

Beyer, M.K., Larsen, J.P., et al. (2007). Gray matter atrophy in Parkinson disease with dementia and dementia with Lewy bodies. *Neurology* 69:747–754.

Boeve, B.F., Silber, M.H., et al. (2004). REM sleep behavior disorder in Parkinson's disease and dementia with Lewy bodies. *J. Geriatr. Psychiatry Neurol.* 17:146–157.

Boeve, B.F., Silber, M.H., et al. (2007). Pathophysiology of REM sleep behaviour disorder and relevance to neurodegenerative disease. *Brain* 130:2770–2788.

Bohnen, N.I., Kaufer, D.I., et al. (2003). Cortical cholinergic function is more severely affected in parkinsonian dementia than in Alzheimer disease: an *in vivo* positron emission tomographic study. *Arch. Neurol.* 60:1745–1748.

Braak, H., Del Tredici, K., et al. (2003). Staging of brain pathology related to sporadic Parkinson's disease. *Neurobiol. Aging* 24:197–211.

Bradshaw, J., Saling, M., et al. (2004). Fluctuating cognition in dementia with Lewy bodies and Alzheimer's disease is qualitatively distinct. *J. Neurol. Neurosurg. Psychiatry* 75:382–387.

Bronnick, K., Ehrt, U., et al. (2006). Attentional deficits affect activities of daily living in dementia-associated with Parkinson's disease. *J. Neurol. Neurosurg. Psychiatry* 77:1136–1142.

Buchman, V.L., Adu, J., et al. (1998). Persyn, a member of the synuclein family, influences neurofilament network integrity. *Nat. Neurosci.* 1:101–103.

Burton, E.J., Karas, G., et al. (2002). Patterns of cerebral atrophy in dementia with Lewy bodies using voxel-based morphometry. *Neuroimage* 17:618–630.

Burton, E.J., McKeith, I.G., et al. (2004). Cerebral atrophy in Parkinson's disease with and without dementia: a comparison with Alzheimer's disease, dementia with Lewy bodies and controls. *Brain* 127:791–800.

Calderon, J., Perry, R.J., et al. (2001). Perception, attention, and working memory are disproportionately impaired in dementia with Lewy bodies compared with Alzheimer's disease. *J. Neurol. Neurosurg. Psychiatry* 70:157–164.

Collerton, D., Burn, D., et al. (2003). Systematic review and meta-analysis show that dementia with Lewy bodies is a visual-perceptual and attentional-executive dementia. *Dement. Geriatr. Cogn. Disord.* 16:229–237.

Colloby, S.J., Firbank, M.J., et al. (2008). A comparison of 99mTc-exametazime and 123I-FP-CIT SPECT imaging in the differential diagnosis of Alzheimer's disease and dementia with Lewy bodies. *Int. Psychogeriatr.* 20:1124–1140.

Colloby, S.J., Firbank, M.J., et al. (2011). Alterations in nicotinic alpha4beta2 receptor binding in vascular dementia using (1)(2)(3)I-5IA-85380 SPECT: comparison with regional cerebral blood flow. *Neurobiol. Aging* 32:293–301.

Colloby, S.J., Pakrasi, S., et al. (2006). *In vivo* SPECT imaging of muscarinic acetylcholine receptors using (R,R) 123I-QNB in dementia with Lewy bodies and Parkinson's disease dementia. *Neuroimage* 33:423–429.

Cormack, F., Aarsland, D., et al. (2004). Pentagon drawing and neuropsychological performance in Dementia with Lewy Bodies, Alzheimer's disease, Parkinson's disease and Parkinson's disease with dementia. *Int. J. Geriatr. Psychiatry* 19:371–377.

Cousins, D.A., Burton, E.J., et al. (2003). Atrophy of the putamen in dementia with Lewy bodies but not Alzheimer's disease: an MRI study. *Neurology* 61:1191–1195.

Cummings, J.L., Darkins, A., et al. (1988). Alzheimer's disease and Parkinson's disease: comparison of speech and language alterations. *Neurology* 38:680–684.

Donnemiller, E., Heilmann, J., et al. (1997). Brain perfusion scintigraphy with 99mTc-HMPAO or 99mTc-ECD and 123I-beta-CIT single-photon emission tomography in dementia of the Alzheimer-type and diffuse Lewy body disease. *Eur. J. Nucl. Med.* 24:320–325.

Duda, J.E., Giasson, B.I., et al. (2002). Novel antibodies to synuclein show abundant striatal pathology in Lewy body diseases. *Ann. Neurol.* 52:205–210.

Edison, P., Rowe, C.C., et al. (2008). Amyloid load in Parkinson's disease dementia and Lewy body dementia measured with [11C]PIB positron emission tomography. *J. Neurol. Neurosurg. Psychiatry* 79:1331–1338.

Emre, M. (2003). Dementia associated with Parkinson's disease. *Lancet Neurol.* 2:229–237.

Emre, M., Aarsland, D., et al. (2007). Clinical diagnostic criteria for dementia associated with Parkinson's disease. *Mov. Disord.* 22:1689–1707; quiz 1837.

Ferman, T.J., Smith, G.E., et al. (2006). Neuropsychological differentiation of dementia with Lewy bodies from normal aging and Alzheimer's disease. *Clin. Neuropsychol.* 20:623–636.

Friedman, J.H., and Fernandez, H.H. (2002). Atypical antipsychotics in Parkinson-sensitive populations. *J. Geriatr. Psychiatry Neurol.* 15:156–170.

Galvin, J.E., Malcom, H., et al. (2007). Personality traits distinguishing dementia with Lewy bodies from Alzheimer disease. *Neurology* 68:1895–1901.

Galvin, J.E., Pollack, J., et al. (2006). Clinical phenotype of Parkinson disease dementia. *Neurology* 67:1605–1611.

Gilbert, P.E., Barr, P.J., et al. (2004). Differences in olfactory and visual memory in patients with pathologically confirmed Alzheimer's disease and the Lewy body variant of Alzheimer's disease. *J. Int. Neuropsychol. Soc.* 10:835–842.

Gomperts, S.N., Rentz, D.M., et al. (2008). Imaging amyloid deposition in Lewy body diseases. *Neurology* 71:903–910.

Hansen, L., Salmon, D., et al. (1990). The Lewy body variant of Alzheimer's disease: a clinical and pathologic entity. *Neurology* 40:1–8.

Hanyu, H., Shimizu, S., et al. (2006). Comparative value of brain perfusion SPECT and [(123)I]MIBG myocardial scintigraphy in distinguishing between dementia with Lewy bodies and Alzheimer's disease. *Eur. J. Nucl. Med. Mol. Imaging* 33:248–253.

Harding, A.J., Broe, G.A., et al. (2002). Visual hallucinations in Lewy body disease relate to Lewy bodies in the temporal lobe. *Brain* 125:391–403.

Higuchi, M., Tashiro, M., et al. (2000). Glucose hypometabolism and neuropathological correlates in brains of dementia with Lewy bodies. *Exp. Neurol.* 162:247–256.

Hu, X.S., Okamura, N., et al. (2000). 18F-fluorodopa PET study of striatal dopamine uptake in the diagnosis of dementia with Lewy bodies. *Neurology* 55:1575–1577.

Huber, S.J., Shuttleworth, E.C., et al. (1986). Dementia in Parkinson's disease. *Arch. Neurol.* 43:987–990.

Hurtig, H.I., Trojanowski, J.Q., et al. (2000). Alpha-synuclein cortical Lewy bodies correlate with dementia in Parkinson's disease. *Neurology* 54:1916–1921.

Ikonomovic, M.D., Klunk, W.E., et al. (2008). Post-mortem correlates of *in vivo* PiB-PET amyloid imaging in a typical case of Alzheimer's disease. *Brain* 131:1630–1645.

Ishii, K., Imamura, T., et al. (1998). Regional cerebral glucose metabolism in dementia with Lewy bodies and Alzheimer's disease. *Neurology* 51:125–130.

Iwai, A., Masliah, E., et al. (1995). The precursor protein of non-A beta component of Alzheimer's disease amyloid is a presynaptic protein of the central nervous system. *Neuron* 14:467–475.

Jellinger, K.A. (2008). Re: In dementia with Lewy bodies, Braak stage determines phenotype, not Lewy body distribution. *Neurology* 70:407–408.

Johnson, D.K., and Galvin, J.E. (2011). Longitudinal changes in cognition in Parkinson's disease with and without dementia. *Dement. Geriatr. Cogn. Disord.* 31:98–108.

Johnson, D.K., Morris, J.C., et al. (2005). Verbal and visuospatial deficits in dementia with Lewy bodies. *Neurology* 65:1232–1238.

Katz, I.R., Jeste, D.V., et al. (1999). Comparison of risperidone and placebo for psychosis and behavioral disturbances associated with dementia: a randomized, double-blind trial. Risperidone Study Group. *J. Clin. Psychiatry* 60:107–115.

Kehagia, A.A., Barker, R.A., et al. (2010). Neuropsychological and clinical heterogeneity of cognitive impairment and dementia in patients with Parkinson's disease. *Lancet Neurol.* 9:1200–1213.

olanzapine have been shown to control psychosis and agitation in AD in randomized trials. Although low doses of risperidone (0.5 mg) and olanzapine (2.5 mg) are usually well tolerated and do not usually result in motor deterioration (Katz et al., 1999), motor deterioration may still be seen in advanced LBD (Walker et al., 1999).

Quetiapine and clozapine are preferred treatment options when pharmacological intervention is warranted. Randomized, placebo-controlled studies showing significant improvement of psychosis without worsening of motor symptoms has only been shown with clozapine (Friedman and Fernandez, 2002). However, given the potentially fatal adverse event of agranulocytosis and need for blood monitoring, it is not a first-line treatment. Apiprazole has not been studied in LBD but it has been shown to be effective in PD and AD and may be considered in LBD if needed. Quetiapine has become a popular treatment of psychosis in LBD given the low incidence of motor deterioration and its ability to control visual hallucinations at low doses. Efficacy and tolerability have been documented in both PD and DLB (Friedman and Fernandez, 2002). It is worth noting that hallucinations that are non-threatening to the patient and do not disturb function may not require pharmacological intervention. Rapid eye movement sleep behavior disorder generally responds to low doses of clonazepam before sleep.

ACETYLCHOLINESTERASE INHIBITORS FOR BEHAVIORAL SYMPTOMS

A metaanalysis of six large trials in AD showed a small but significant benefit for AChEIs in treating neuropsychiatric symptoms (Trinh et al., 2003). There also appears to be a differential effect of AChEIs on different psychiatric symptoms, with psychosis, agitation, wandering, and anxiety being the most consistently responsive. In a large multicenter trial, rivastigmine resulted in a 30% improvement from baseline in psychiatric symptoms (McKeith et al., 2000). In a case-control study of rivastigmine, treatment was associated with a reduction in NPI scores, hallucinations, and sleep disorders compared with AD. There were lower rates of apathy, anxiety, delusions, and hallucinations in the treatment group compared with controls. It is not clear whether this effect on behavior is owing to drug effect or more severe behavioral pathology in LBD.

AUTONOMIC DYSFUNCTION

Management of orthostatic hypotension includes relatively simple measures such as leg elevation, elastic stockings, increasing salt and fluid intake, and if not medically contraindicated, avoiding medications that can exacerbate orthostasis. Medications such as midodrine or fludrocortisone can be used in the event that such simple measures fail. Midodrine is a vasoconstrictor and side effects include urine retention and supine hypertension. Fludrocortisone has mineralocorticoid activity and causes fluid retention.

Medications with anticholinergic activity, including oxybutynin, tolterodine tartrate, bethanechol chloride, and propantheline can be used to treat urinary urgency, frequency, and urge incontinence. Because they can potentially exacerbate cognitive problems, these medications should be used cautiously. Because LBD is more common in men, the risk of producing urinary retention in the setting of prostatic hypertrophy should be considered.

Constipation can usually be treated by exercise and dietary modifications. Laxatives, stool softeners, and mechanical disimpaction may be needed. The prokinetic effect of cholinergic stimulation by AChEIs might improve these symptoms in some patients.

CONCLUSIONS

Lewy body disorders are a common cause of dementia in elderly people, characterized by varying degrees of cognitive, behavioral, affective, movement, and autonomic dysfunction in older adults. The LBD syndromes are associated with the accumulation of Lewy bodies in subcortical, limbic, and neocortical regions and are characterized clinically by progressive dementia, parkinsonism, cognitive fluctuations, and visual hallucinations. Whether or not PDD and DLB reflect the same underlying disorder whose differences in symptom presentation are merely the end product of the underlying brain region(s) affected earlier or later in the disease course is the subject of much controversy. For now, current diagnostic criteria for PDD and DLB advise that clinical distinctions be maintained ("one year rule") even though they are pathologically similar. From a neuropsychological perspective, PDD and DLB are more readily distinguished from AD than from each other. It is hoped that the identification of a prodrome of PDD may improve our understanding of the earliest cognitive changes associated with LBD. This information can then be used in conjunction with biomarkers to diagnose these disorders earlier, as well as aid in the prediction and monitoring of treatment response and development of more selective therapeutic agents. Public awareness campaigns that specifically address LBD are also hoped for, as these may aid in generating interest and understanding of this group of dementias, and maybe even stimulate efforts to develop appropriate supportive programs and services for patients and their family caregivers.

DISCLOSURES

Dr. Karantzoulis has no conflicts of interest to disclose. She serves as co-investigator for one NIH grant (R01 AG040211-A1) and one Michael J. Fox Foundation for Parkinson Research award. She does not receive financial compensation or salary support from any pharmaceutical company.

Dr. Galvin is funded by grants from the NIH, Michael J Fox Foundation, Alzheimer Association, New York State Department of Health, and Morris and Alma Schapiro Fund. Dr. Galvin serves as a consultant for Pfizer, Eisai, Baxter, Accera, Novartis, and Forest. He does mold stock or any equity in any pharmaceutical company.

of patients with LBD experience significant perceptions of burden that is heightened by behavioral and emotional problems present early on in LBD (depression, irritability, hallucinations, delusions, sleep disturbances, nightmares, and unusual sleep movements), impaired ADLs, sense of isolation, and challenges with the diagnostic experience. Significantly, the level of subjective burden among this group of caregivers was noted to be higher than what is typically endorsed among caregivers of AD or mixed diagnostic groups. These data suggest that future interventions targeting each of these challenges are needed for caregivers of patients with LBD.

THERAPEUTIC APPROACHES

There are no approved therapies specifically for LBD; however, there is ample evidence in the literature regarding the use of medications approved for other disorders for the treatment of the various symptoms of LBD.

COGNITIVE SYMPTOMS

Acetylcholinesterase inhibitors (AChEIs) may be especially useful in the treatment of LBD. These medications, including donepezil (Aricept), rivastigmine (Exelon), and galantamine (Razadyne ER or Reminyl) block the breakdown of acetylcholine within the synapse, thereby prolonging its effect on postsynaptic receptors. AChEIs are generally well tolerated at their standard dosing. Primary side effects are gastrointestinal (e.g., nausea, vomiting, diarrhea, anorexia, weight loss); other side effects can include insomnia, vivid dreams, leg cramps, and urinary frequency.

It has been suggested that treatment with AChEIs may be more effective in DLB than AD because of early and prominent central nervous system cholinergic dysfunction in this group (Touchon et al., 2006). In one study, patients with DLB showed greater treatment improvement in cognition relative to AD patients, although the difference between the two groups was not significant (Samuel et al., 2000). Only a few clinical trials for the use of AChEIs in LBD have been conducted and most guidelines are based on case reports and extension of therapeutic trials in AD. Three independent clinical studies of AChEI treatment using donepezil, galantamine, and rivastigmine in patients with LBD suggest that AChEIs improve cognitive and neuropsychiatric measures, with no significant increase in EPS with AChEI use. Rivastigmine was the first AChEIs to be given European and American marketing approval for patients with mild to moderate PDD. Currently, there is no compelling evidence that any one AChEI is better than the other.

The NMDA antagonist memantine, another treatment modality approved for use in AD, has not yet been tested in large, randomized, controlled studies in PDD. Results have been variable in a few case reports or case series in patient with DLB, with both worsening (Ridha et al., 2005) and improvement (Sabbagh et al., 2005) noted. Good tolerability and possible benefits have been reported in a small case series of patients with PDD.

MOTOR SYMPTOMS

There are no controlled clinical trials that have yet evaluated the treatment of motor features in DLB. There are reports of small series of patients with DLB whose motor impairments were successfully treated with L-dopa (Molloy et al., 2005). Levodopa is more effective in treating motor impairments in idiopathic PD than DLB. Dopamine agonists are associated with more side effects, especially drug-induced psychosis, even at low doses. Given this risk and because the motor impairments may be mild, the recommendation is to treat the movement disorder only if the motor symptoms interfere with function. Antiparkinsonism medicines should be initiated at the lowest possible dose and increased with caution. There have been reports of increased adverse events with the combined use of L-dopa and cholinesterase inhibitors in PD (Okereke et al., 2004).

Other PD medications such as amantadine, catechol-O-methyltransferase inhibitors, monoamine oxidase inhibitors, and anticholinergics tend to exacerbate cognitive impairment and should ideally be avoided. Furthermore, the cognitive impairment in DLB makes them poor candidates for DBS. Cholinesterase inhibitors can potentially worsen parkinsonism. In a study of rivastigmine in PD, approximately 10% of patients treated with rivastigmine had worsening of tremor (I. McKeith et al., 2000). However, their overall motor function was not significantly different between the treatment and placebo groups (I. McKeith et al., 2000).

BEHAVIORAL SYMPTOMS

As discussed, behavioral symptoms frequently accompany LBD. Clinical experience suggests that nonpharmacological treatment approaches should be considered first, including evaluating for physical ailments that may be provoking behavioral disturbances (e.g., fecal impaction, pain, or decubitus ulcers). Avoidance or reduction of doses of other medications that can potentially cause agitation should also be attempted. Both anxiety and depression are common occurrences in LBD. Generally speaking, when medications are needed to modify behaviors, they should be used for the shortest duration possible. Benzodiazepines are better avoided given their risk of sedation and paradoxical agitation.

There have been no randomized, controlled studies of antidepressants in patients with PDD. In one systematic review, amitriptyline was found to be the only compound with evidence of efficacy in PD depression; however, tricyclic antidepressants such as amitriptyline should be avoided in patients with PDD because of their anticholinergic effects.

ANTIPSYCHOTICS

Visual hallucinations have been considered predictors of a good response to AChEIs (I. McKeith et al., 2004). Classical neuroleptics (e.g., haloperidol) are best avoided in DLB because they may worsen motor function and even potentially result in life-threatening neuroleptic sensitivity. Experience with atypical antipsychotics in LBD has been mixed. Risperidone and decreases in the frontal and temporal lobes of PDD and DLB, and relative increases in the uptake of both ligands in the occipital lobe, with the nicotinic ligand uptake being higher in DLB subjects with recent hallucinations (O'Brien et al., 2008). However, these changes are likely not specific to DLB because an increase in nicotinic binding in the occipital lobe has also been observed in vascular dementia (Colloby et al., 2011) and decreases have been noted in the frontal and temporal lobes in AD (O'Brien et al., 2007). The data are not yet compelling enough to suggest that PET and SPECT imaging looking at cholinergic activity could be used diagnostically in LBD.

METAIODOBENZYLGUANIDINE MYOCARDIAL SCINTIGRAPHY

[^{123}I] Metaiodobenzylguanidine myocardial scintigraphy is a noninvasive technique that was developed to evaluate the local myocardial sympathetic nerve damage, primarily in heart disease, and has only recently been used in LBD. The rationale for its use is that impairment of the peripheral sympathetic nervous system can occur even in the earliest clinical stage of PD (Spiegel et al., 2005). In addition, cardiovascular autonomic dysfunction is common in DLB (Allan et al., 2007). The early disturbance in the sympathetic nervous system can be detected by reduced MIBG uptake on myocardial scintigraphy independent of the duration of the disease.

A number of studies have demonstrated reduced MIBG uptake (heart to mediastinum ratio) in DLB relative to patients with AD and normal controls, with impressive accuracy for discriminating DLB from AD. Most studies performed measurement of both early (15- to 30-minute) and late (three- to four-hour) MIBG uptake, with the late image ratio typically resulting in better diagnostic accuracy. Several studies have found no correlation of MIBG scintigraphy with disease severity or duration of DLB or AD (Oide et al., 2003; Suzuki et al., 2006; Yoshita et al., 2001). Studies comparing MIBG scintigraphy and occipital hypoperfusion on SPECT have reported MIBG scintigraphy to be more sensitive in detecting DLB (Hanyu et al., 2006; Tateno et al., 2008). Also, MIBG scintigraphy has been reported to be more sensitive than cerebrospinal fluid (CSF) p-tau in terms of differentiating between DLB and AD (Wada-Isoe et al., 2007). No comparison with FP-CIT imaging has so far been carried out. However, one potential advantage of MIBG over FP-CIT is that myocardial MIBG can distinguish PD and DLB from atypical parkinsonian syndromes such as multiple system atrophy, corticobasal degeneration, and progressive supranuclear palsy (Spiegel, 2010), because in PD and DLB, the myocardial sympathetic damage is predominantly postganglionic, whereas in other parkinsonian syndromes, the preganglionic structures are mainly affected, resulting in normal MIBG uptake.

POSITRON EMISSION TOMOGRAPHY AMYLOID IMAGING

Over the past five years or so, amyloid imaging has emerged as important neuroimaging tool in studies of brain aging and dementia. Pittsburgh compound B (PIB) is currently the most widely studied amyloid imaging agent. *In vitro*, PIB has been shown to bind specifically to extracellular and vascular fibrillar Aβ deposits in postmortem AD brains (Ikonomovic et al., 2008; Lockhart et al., 2007). At PET tracer concentrations, PIB does not significantly bind to other protein aggregates such as neurofibrillary tangles or Lewy bodies, and hence may be useful for diagnostically discriminating between AD and non–Aβ dementias (Rabinovici et al., 2007; Rowe et al., 2008).

As discussed, LBD is characterized at autopsy by the presence of subcortical and cortical LBs with a substantial burden of amyloid pathology also possible (Ballard et al., 2006). A limited number of PET studies have examined the amyloid burden in DLB and PDD *in vivo* (Edison et al., 2008; Gomperts et al., 2008). Edison et al. (2008) showed that in DLB, mean brain PIB uptake was significantly higher than that in controls, whereas uptake in PDD was comparable to controls and PD patients without dementia (Fig. 66.1). None of the patients with PD showed any evidence of increased cortical amyloid deposition. Gomperts et al. (2008) revealed that cortical amyloid burden as measured by PIB was higher in DLB than in PDD, but similar to that in AD. It may be that global cortical amyloid burden is high in DLB but lower and less frequent in PDD. Pittsburgh compound B imaging may prove to be useful to distinguish AD from PDD, but not AD from DLB.

CAREGIVER ISSUES

Lewy body dementia not only affects the individual diagnosed with the illness, but also has a profound impact on his or her caregivers, families, and friends. Those close to the patient have to learn to assist with the behavioral and emotional symptoms that accompany LBD, which are more pronounced and manifest earlier than in AD, as well as with the motor impairment, falls, and overall higher levels of disability than with other types of dementia (Ricci et al., 2009). Lewy body dementia caregivers also have to struggle through the often years-long challenge of obtaining an accurate diagnosis and adequate medical care for their relative.

The Lewy Body Dementia Association recently conducted an Internet survey of caregiver burden in LBD. Respondents were 611 people who stated that they were actively involved in the care of their relative with LBD. Results of this survey showed that in contrast to AD, many more LBD caregivers are women and are more often the spouse of the affected person. This difference likely reflects that fact that LBD is slightly more common in men than women, whereas AD is more common in women. Caregivers also reported many barriers in obtaining a diagnosis for their loved ones, with most having seen multiple physicians over more than a year before their relative was diagnosed with LBD and with more than three-fourths of persons with LBD given a different diagnosis at first.

Using these data from the Lewy Body Dementia Association, Leggett et al. (2011) were able to examine levels of stress and burden among caregivers of patients with LBD. Subjective burden was assessed with a 12-item short version of the Zarit Burden Interview. The results showed that caregivers

(Burton et al., 2002, 2004); this contrasts with the reported occipital hypometabolism/hypoperfusion noted with PET/SPECT studies, respectively. Longitudinal rates of whole-brain atrophy in PDD and DLB are probably intermediate between healthy aging and AD (O'Brien et al., 2001; Whitwell et al., 2007).

A robust MR finding in DLB and PDD is that of relative preservation of the medial temporal lobe when compared with AD (Barber et al., 2001; Burton et al., 2002; Whitwell et al., 2007); this holds promise as a diagnostic marker in differentiating AD from DLB (see Fig. 66.1).

Subcortical changes in terms of striatal atrophy have also been described in DLB. Putamen atrophy has been reported in DLB relative to AD (Cousins et al., 2003), but no significant differences were detected in caudate nucleus (Almeida et al., 2003; Cousins et al., 2003).

FUNCTIONAL IMAGING

OCCIPITAL HYPOPERFUSION AND HYPOMETABOLISM

Single-photon emission computed tomography (SPECT) studies in PD (Matsui et al., 2005) and DLB (Donnemiller et al., 1997) indicate reduced occipital perfusion relative to other cortical areas. It has been suggested that reduced flow in the medial occipital lobe, including the cuneus and the lingual gyrus, can discriminate LBD from AD, with a sensitivity and specificity of 85% (Shimizu et al., 2005). The possibility that parietal lobe perfusion is more severely reduced rather than occipital lobe hypoperfusion in DLB has also been raised (Ishii et al., 1998), which may be caused by the dopaminergic and/or cholinergic impairment in this region.

The use of PET scanning with markers such as [18F] fluorodeoxyglucose ([18F] FDG) shows metabolic reductions have been observed in the visual association cortex in DLB not evident in AD (Higuchi et al., 2000). A multicenter study examining ([18F] FDG PET measures in the differential diagnosis of dementia, including AD, frontotemporal dementia (FTD), and DLB reported hypometabolism in the parieto-temporal and posterior cingulate cortices in AD, more prominent hypoperfusion in the occipital lobe in DLB, and more prominent hypometabolism in the frontal/temporal cortices in FTD. These cortical abnormalities discriminated DLB from AD with a sensitivity of 71% and a specificity of 95%. In another study, occipital hypometabolism and relative preservation of the posterior cingulate gyrus distinguished DLB from patients with AD with a sensitivity of 77% and a specificity of 80% (Lim et al., 2009). Greater metabolic decrease in the anterior cingulate has also been shown in DLB than PDD (Yong et al., 2007).

STRIATAL DOPAMINE LOSS

Nigrostriatal degeneration, with profound reductions in the striatal dopamine transporter, has consistently been found in patients with DLB at autopsy. Nigrostriatal integrity is assessed *in vivo* with specific ligands, such as 123I-FP-CIT in SPECT imaging, which binds to dopamine transporter and [11C] dihydrotetrabenazine in PET imaging, which binds to the vesicular monamine transporter T2 series.

Reduced striatal dopamine transporter uptake in DLB but not in AD has been shown in SPECT studies, which may aid in differential diagnosis (O'Brien et al., 2004; Walker et al., 2002). A large multicenter study examining 123I-FP-CIT SPECT in DLB reported a sensitivity of 78% for detecting probable DLB and a specificity of 90% for excluding non-LBD, primarily AD (McKeith et al., 2007). In another study, 123I-FP-CIT imaging was in line with postmortem diagnoses in 19 of 20 cases, and was more precise than clinical diagnosis (Walker et al., 2007). However, 123I-FP-CIT is limited in that it does not discriminate DLB from other atypical parkinsonian syndromes. Nevertheless, head-to-head analyses comparing 123I-FP-CIT imaging to other imaging modalities including ([18F] FDG-PET have shown superior diagnostic accuracy with 123I-FP-CIT imaging (Colloby et al., 2008; Lim et al., 2009).

Positron emission tomography studies have also been used to evaluate nigrostriatal dopaminergic degeneration in DLB. Reduction of striatal dopamine uptake was observed in patients with DLB using [18F] fluorodopa, with a sensitivity of 86% and a specificity of 100%, although this study was limited by a small sample size (Hu et al., 2000). These findings were confirmed in a later study using [11C] dihydrotetrabenazine, which also showed significantly reduced uptake in caudate nucleus and anterior and posterior putamen in DLB and PD compared with patients with AD and normal controls (Koeppe et al., 2008).

The latest revision of the International Consensus Criteria for DLB indicates that low dopamine transporter uptake in basal ganglia demonstrated by SPECT or PET imaging is a feature that in addition to a single core feature can support a diagnosis of probable DLB (I.G. McKeith et al., 2005). The National Institute for Health and Clinical Experience also recommends that 123I-FP-CIT SPECT imaging may be particularly helpful when the diagnosis of DLB is unclear. Likewise, the European Federation of Neurological Societies (EFNS) guidelines also recommend the use of dopaminergic SPECT to differentiate between DLB and AD (Hort et al., 2010), the only imaging category to reach level A category of evidence.

CHOLINERGIC MARKERS

Brain cholinergic function can be estimated *in vivo* by measuring acetylcholinesterase (ACh) activity by PET using radiolabeled ACh analogues (Namba et al., 2002). Acetylcholinesterase is an enzyme that degrades ACh into the inactive metabolites choline and acetate. Several studies have demonstrated that cortical ACh activity is more severely and extensively reduced in the cerebral cortex, especially in the medial occipital cortex in DLB and PDD in comparison with AD, in which deficits were more prominent in the temporal cortex (Bohnen et al., 2003; Shimada et al., 2009).

Nicotinic and muscarinic receptors are subclasses of ACh receptors, implicated in memory and cognitive processes. Imaging of muscarinic receptors (Colloby et al., 2006) and nicotinic receptors (O'Brien et al., 2008) with SPECT has revealed

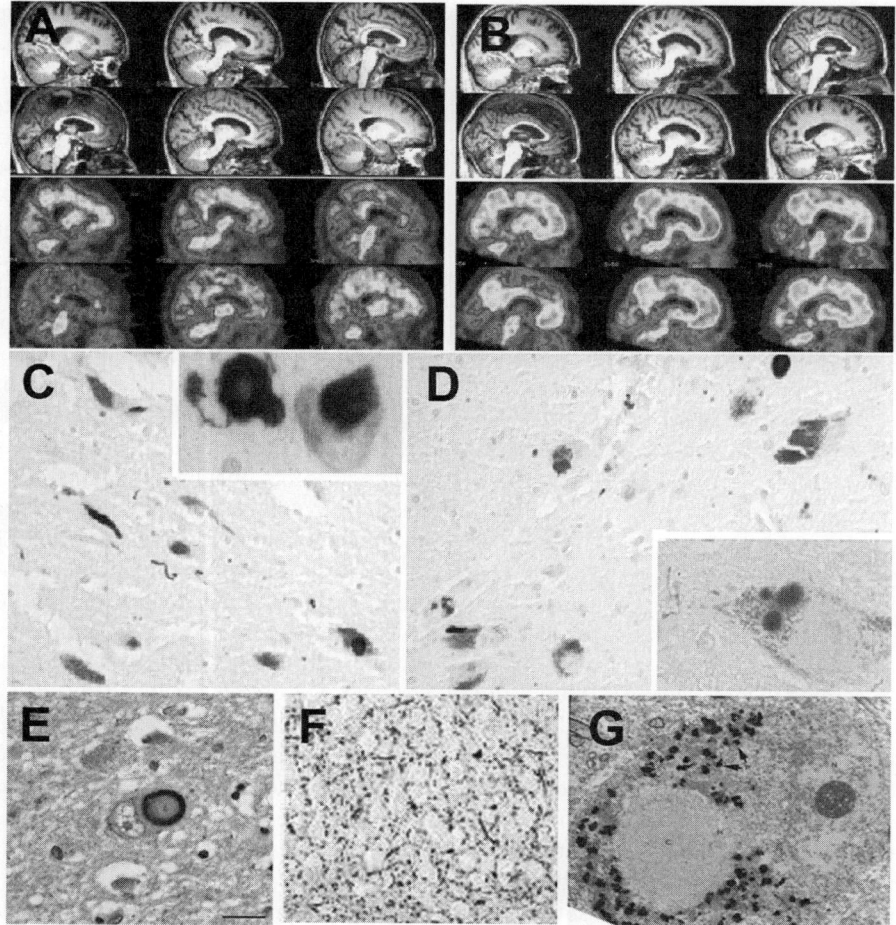

Figure 66.1 Imaging and pathology in lewy body dementia. (A) Sagittal sections of MRI and amyloid imaging in a case of PDD. There is mild cortical atrophy largely sparing the hippocampus. Amyloid imaging reveal minimal to no uptake of the PIB. (B) Sagittal section of MRI and amyloid imaging in a case of mixed LBD and AD. There is slightly more prominent atrophy of the hippocampus with significant uptake of PIB. (C) Photomicrograph of substantia nigra in DLB patient stained with α-synuclein. Note dystrophic neurites. Insert shows higher power magnification of two Lewy bodies in the nigral neurons. (D) Photomicrograph of substantia nigra in PDD patient stained with α-synuclein. Insert shows higher power magnification of a nigral neuron with multiple Lewy bodies. (E) Photomicrograph of Lewy body in the cingulate cortex of a LBD patient stained with α-synuclein. (F) Photomicrograph of dystrophic neurites in the CA 2–3 region of the hippocampus in a LBD patient. (G), Electron micrograph of a Lewy body. Note the dense core (gray) surrounded by a paler halo. (See color insert.)

in patients with both sporadic and familial DLB. From a susceptibility marker on chromosome 4q21-23 that segregated with the PD phenotype in Italian and Greek kindreds, A53T (Polymeropoulos et al., 1997) and A30P (Kruger et al., 1998) were the first two missense mutations in α-synuclein associated with familial Parkinson disease.

α-synuclein is a member of a larger family of synuclein proteins, which also includes β- and γ-synuclein. Like α-synuclein, β-synuclein has recently been implicated in PD and DLB pathogenesis, but its precise role in disease is still emerging. β-synuclein is highly localized to presynaptic sites in neocortex, hippocampus, and thalamus (Iwai et al., 1995) and it may act as a biological negative regulator of α-synuclein. Two novel β-synuclein point mutations, P123H and V70M, were found in highly conserved regions of the β-synuclein gene in respective familial (P123H) and sporadic (V70M) DLB index cases (Ohtake et al., 2004), where abundant LB pathology and α-synuclein aggregation was present without β-synuclein aggregation.

Unlike the other synuclein family members, γ-synuclein or persyn is largely expressed in the cell bodies and axons of primary sensory neurons, sympathetic neurons, and motor neurons as well as in brain (Buchman et al., 1998). γ-synuclein is the most recent synuclein member to be linked to LBD neuropathology and the least well understood. Single-nucleotide polymorphisms in all three synucleins have been associated with sporadic DLB, most prominently γ-synuclein (Nishioka et al., 2010).

STRUCTURAL MAGNETIC RESONANCE IMAGING

A diffuse pattern of global gray matter atrophy including temporal, parietal, middle, and inferior frontal gyri and occipital lobe has been reported in DLB, similar to AD (Beyer et al., 2007; Burton et al., 2004). Most volumetric studies have not found a significant occipital structural change in DLB

SLEEP DISORDERS

Many patients with LBD have parasomnias. Most common is REM sleep behavioral disorder (RBD), which tends to begin concurrently or after the onset of parkinsonism or dementia (Boeve et al., 2007). Rapid eye movement sleep behavioral disorder is marked by lack of normal muscle atonia that prevents movements (other than eye movements) during REM sleep in the presence of excessive activity while dreaming; this can result in vocalizations and sometimes wildly violent behavior. Rapid eye movement sleep behavioral disorder may be idiopathic or may be associated with LBD and other synucleinopathies. Patients may be unaware of the disorder and the history is therefore often dependent on the patient's bed partner. Rapid eye movement sleep behavioral disorder is more commonly found in men in their fifties and may precede the clinical signs associated with LBD by many years. Parkinson disease patients with RBD show impairments of some logical abilities as compared with subjects without RBD (Sinforiani et al., 2006). There are, however, no longitudinal studies confirming RBD as a risk factor for PDD. On the other hand, excessive daytime sleepiness has been reported to be a risk factor for PDD (Olson et al., 2000).

NEUROLOEPTIC SENSITIVITY

Patients with DLB are notorious for their neuroleptic sensitivity. Reactions are observed in 30% to 50% of patients with DLB and are characterized by sudden onset of impaired sensitivity, acute confusion, psychotic episodes, and exacerbation of parkinsonism symptoms such as rigidity and immobility (I. McKeith et al., 1992). In some cases, these reactions can lead to death within several days. One survey (Aarsland et al., 2005) revealed a 58% frequency of neuroleptic sensitivity to olanzapine, with lower rates with clozapine (11%) and thioridazine (6%). These data support the notion of unacceptable safety profiles for some neuroleptics in LBD. Patients with DLB also tend to be activated by sedatives and awakened by sleep medications (Rogan and Lippa, 2002). Severe neuroleptic sensitivity has been reported in up to 40% of patients with PDD exposed to neuroleptic drugs (Aarsland et al., 2005).

NEUROPATHOLOGY

The main identifying pathological features of LBD are cortical and subcortical LBs and Lewy neurites (LNs). Lewy bodies are spherical intracytoplasmic protein deposits around the nucleus and throughout the dendrite of subcortical and cortical neurons. They consist of filamentous protein granules composed of α-synuclein and ubiquitin, and are surrounded by a halo of neurofilaments. Cortical LB sites include the cingulate gyrus, entorhinal cortex, insular cortex, frontal cortex, and amygdala (Fig. 66.1).

The different forms of LBD can have variations as to the extent and spread of α-synuclein pathology and variable amount of AD pathology (see Fig. 66.1). For both PDD and DLB, staging/classification systems based on semiquantitative assessment of the distribution and progression pattern of α-synuclein pathology are used that are considered to be linked to clinical symptoms.

In PD, a six-stage system is suggested to indicate a predictable sequence of lesions with ascending progression from medullary and olfactory nuclei to the cortex (Braak et al., 2003) (see Table 66.3). Braak stages 1 and 2, with LB pathology involving medulla oblongata and pontine tegmentum, are considered asymptomatic or presymptomatic and may explain the early nonmotor symptoms (autonomic and olfactory). Braak stages 3 and 4, involving extension of LB pathology to midbrain and basal prosencephalon and mesocortex, has been correlated to clinical symptomatic stages. The terminal Braak stages 5 and 6, characterized by widespread neocortical LB degeneration, are correlated with significant cognitive decline associated with severe parkinsonism (Hurtig et al., 2000).

Dementia with Lewy bodies, according to consensus pathological guidelines, by semiquantitative scoring of α-synuclein pathology (LB density and distribution) in specific brain regions, is distinguished into three phenotypes: brainstem, limbic, and diffuse cortical. Concomitant AD-type pathology is also considered. Generally speaking, the more neocortical LBs and the lower the Braak stage, the more likely the patient will meet the criteria for DLB, whereas higher Braak stages and non-neocortical LBs are associated with a lower likelihood of obtaining DLB diagnosis. In one review of 88 autopsy-confirmed cases, identification of clinical DLB was inversely proportional to Braak staging of neurofibrillary pathology. It should be noted that clinician sensitivity was still poor regardless of classification scheme (Weisman and McKeith, 2007). Neuronal loss in the substantia nigra is greater in PDD than in DLB, whereas beta-amyloid patterns are more consistent in DLB. α-synuclein pathology is also greater in the striatum in DLB than PDD (Duda et al., 2002).

In PDD, Galvin et al. (2006) identified three neuropathological profiles when comparing autopsy reports of 103 cases followed longitudinally. Roughly one-third of PDD was found to be caused by neocortical LBs without evidence of AD pathology. Another one-third had abundant senile plaques and neurofibrillary tangles meeting criteria for both PD and AD. The final group had only brainstem pathology comprising LBs. These data are in line with the staging paradigm proposed by Braak and colleagues, suggesting that PD pathology begins in the lower brainstem and spreads in a caudal-rostral fashion (Braak et al., 2003). Importantly, recent studies have revealed exceptions to the general order of progression suggested by Braak and colleagues (e.g., Jellinger, 2008; Parkkinen et al., 2008).

GENETICS

In the past decade, tremendous advances have been made in understanding the genetic factors influencing the pathogenesis of LBD. Compelling evidence for a genetic basis for both PD and DLB followed the discovery of mutations in the α-synuclein gene (PARK1/4) in patients with autosomal dominant familial PD, and subsequently, mutations were identified

Delusions also occur in 56% of patients with DLB at first presentation and 65% at some point in their illness. Delusions tend to be more common in DLB than in PDD or AD. Paranoid, Capgras (believing individuals are replaced by identical imposters), and "phantom boarder" (unseen individuals residing in one's home) are among the most common delusions. Misidentification syndromes appear to be particularly prevalent in DLB, occurring in up to 40% of patients, compared with 10% in AD (Ballard et al., 1999). It is not yet clear whether misidentification delusions are also characteristic of PDD.

Depression is common in both PDD and DLB and there is equivocal evidence as to whether base rates of depressed mood and major depression differ between these disorders and AD (Ferman et al., 2006). A history of depression has been reported in 58% of persons with PDD, 50% of patients with DLB, and in 14% of AD cases coming to autopsy (Klatka et al., 1996). Risk factors for depression include early onset PD, presence of hallucinations or delusions, and an akinetic rigid presentation (vs a tremor predominant variant). The incidence of depression appears to be unrelated to the presence or absence of dementia or the severity of motor impairment (I. G. McKeith, 2000a). Anxiety and apathy co-occur, with depression in 40% and 15% of patients with PD, respectively. Apathy is also common in DLB, particularly with more severe dementia.

PERSONALITY CHANGES

Personality changes in DLB tend to occur with auditory and visual hallucinations and include diminished emotional responsiveness, resignation of hobbies, increased apathy, and purposeless hyperactivity (Galvin et al., 2007). Using principal components analysis, Galvin and his colleagues were able to identify three general personality traits in DLB. The first were irritable traits (accounting for almost 33% of the variance) and included increased rigidity, egocentricity, loss of concern, coarsening of affect, and impaired emotional control. The second were a passive group of traits (this explained just more than 12% of the variance) and included diminished emotional responsiveness, relinquished hobbies, growing apathy, and purposeless activity. The third reflected disinhibition (this explained an additional 10.4% of the variance) and included inappropriate hilarity and sexual misdemeanor. Using this three-factor structure, patients with DLB were more likely to manifest personality traits associated with passive personality traits than patients with AD. Using receiver operating characteristic curves, these authors also showed that the passive personality traits discriminated between AD and DLB, whereas both the irritable set of traits and those reflecting disinhibition were uncommon in both groups.

COGNITIVE FLUCTUATIONS

Fluctuations in cognition are one of the hallmarks of DLB, seen in 15% to 80% of patients with DLB (Ballard et al., 2002).

Cognitive fluctuations are also common in PDD and may be as frequent as in DLB (Ballard et al., 2002). These often involve waxing and waning of cognition, attention, concentration, functional abilities, or arousal in the absence of any clear precipitant. They are often described as episodes of behavioral confusion, inattention, hypersomnolence, and incoherent speech alternating with episodes of lucidity and capable task performance. Patients may be described as staring into space or being dazed and the episodes can last minutes to days, varying from alertness to stupor. An extreme form of fluctuations may occur when patients are found mute and unresponsive for a few minutes.

Given the large variability in the description and quantifications of fluctuations in patients with LBD, a number of scales have been developed, including the Clinical Assessment of Fluctuation and the One Day Fluctuation Assessment Scale, and the Mayo Fluctuations Questionnaires (Ferman et al., 2006). The Mayo scale describes four features of fluctuations that can reliably distinguish DLB from AD or normal aging. Three or four features of this composite occurred in 63% of patients who had DLB compared with 12% of those who had AD and 0.5% of normally functioning elderly people. The presence of three or four of these features yielded a positive predictive value of 83% for the clinical diagnosis of DLB against an alternate diagnosis of AD.

AUTONOMIC DYSFUNCTION

Autonomic dysfunction is a common clinical sign in LBD. Autonomic features tend to occur later in the disease course of DLB, although there have been some cases with early and prominent involvement. Symptomatic orthostasis is probably the most serious manifestation of autonomic dysfunction, observed in approximately 15% of patients with DLB. Other features include decreased sweating, excessive salivation (sialorrhea), seborrhea, heat intolerance, urinary dysfunction, constipation or diarrhea, and erectile dysfunction or impotence. In fact, constipation may precede any cognitive or motor symptoms by more than a decade. Patients with DLB also have a higher frequency of carotid hypersensitivity than elderly patients or those with AD. There is also evidence of cardiac denervation by MIBG scintigraphic scanning, a finding not seen in AD.

Autonomic dysfunction tends to occur in the late stages of PD and is related to disease severity and duration. Approximately one-third of patients have clinical features of autonomic dysfunction, although estimation of the prevalence of autonomic dysfunction is compounded by factors such as the use of antiparkinsonian medications. Most common in PD are decreased gastrointestinal ability and bladder dysfunction. Also common is constipation and there is a risk of more serious complications including intestinal pseudoobstruction and toxic megacolon. Other common features include bladder dysfunction with urgency, frequency and incontinence, and sexual dysfunction (decreased libido and erectile dysfunction). Symptomatic orthostasis is more common in association with cognitive impairment in PDD.

consolidation and storage, with significant improvement noted with cuing in LBD relative to AD (Burn, 2006). The more severe amnestic deficits in AD relative to LBD likely reflects the greater burden of neurofibrillary tangles in the entorhinal cortex and surrounding medial temporal lobe regions in AD.

Some studies have suggested better recall on verbal memory tests (including the California Verbal Learning Test; Simard et al., 2000; Logical Memory subtest of the Wechsler Memory Scale-Revised; Calderon et al., 2001; memory subtest on the Dementia Rating Scale; Aarsland et al., 2003) among patients with DLB than those with AD, but this has not been consistently reported, possibly because of the difficulty in isolating pure forms of DLB from LBD cases caused by concurrent AD pathology. Dementia with Lewy bodies tends to co-occur with AD in 80% of cases, with only 20% having pure DLB. Patients with pure Lewy body pathology have better verbal memory skills than those with pure AD or mixed DLB/AD (Johnson et al., 2005). Patients with pure AD and mixed DLB/AD show equivalent degrees of impairment on verbal memory testing. In contrast, combined AD and Lewy body pathology appears to have an additive effect on visual memory skills.

Remote memory may also be affected by PDD (Huber et al., 1986; Leplow et al., 1997). Contrary to patients with AD who typically show a temporal gradient in their memories (with greater impairment noted for recent than remote information), the memory loss in PDD tends to be equally severe across past decades. Recognition of famous faces (a measure of remote memory) may be comparably impaired in DLB and AD (Gilbert et al., 2004).

LANGUAGE

Patients with DLB generally show milder naming deficits than patients with AD on measures of confrontation naming and there are group differences in terms of error profiles (Williams et al., 2007). The naming deficits may become progressively more severe with disease progression in DLB. Patients with AD are more likely to make more semantic errors on confrontation naming testing than patients with DLB, whereas those with DLB make significantly more visuoperceptual errors than patients with AD. The disproportionate visuospatial dysfunction described in DLB may contribute to reduced ability to perceive objects accurately, leading secondarily to errors in naming. Measures of generative fluency have also proved to be useful in differentiating AD from DLB. Patients with DLB are equally impaired in category and letter fluency, whereas patients with AD perform significantly better with letters than categories (Lambon et al., 2001). This may be related to underlying mechanisms: whereas patients with AD have degraded semantic networks or retrieval difficulties affecting semantic networks, attentional and executive impairments likely contribute to the difficulties with word search and retrieval in DLB subjects.

The language impairments in PDD also tend to be mild, with aphasia being a rare occurrence. Verbal fluency impairments are reliably observed in PDD and the deficits tend to be greater in PDD than AD (Cahn-Weiner et al., 2002). Mild deficits on measures of semantic fluency have also been reported (Monsch et al., 1992). Additional features of language impairment in PDD include decreased content of spontaneous speech, impaired naming, shorter phrase length, and dysarthria (Cummings et al., 1988).

BEHAVIORAL AND NEUROPSYCHIATRIC FEATURES

Neuropsychiatric features such as hallucinations and delusions are common in LBD, elicited primarily via informant ratings and less on formal diagnostic criteria. Perhaps most widely used of the informant ratings in LBD is the Neuropsychiatric Inventory (NPI; Cummings et al., 1988). Approximately 61% of PD patients exhibit neuropsychiatric disturbances. The most common features are depression (38%), hallucinations (27%), delusions (6%), anxiety (40%), sleep disturbances (60–90%), and sexual misdemeanor (5% to 10%). Galvin et al. (2006) found that visual hallucinations were the strongest single predictor of developing dementia in patients with PD and increased the risk of developing dementia 20-fold.

The phenomenology of visual hallucinations is similar in PDD and DLB. Visual hallucinations tend to be well formed, detailed, most commonly involving anonymous people (often described by the patient and dysmorphic or small), although they may also involve family members, animals, body parts, and machines. Hallucinations can occur in other modalities, including auditory, tactile, and olfactory. Auditory hallucinations are less common and generally not present in the absence of visual hallucinations. Hallucinations may be frightening and it is difficult to convince the patient that they are not real. This may pose safety problems, as the patient will feel that he or she will be attacked or have his or her home invaded.

Patients with DLB are more likely to show psychiatric symptoms and have more functional impairment at the time of initial evaluation than patients with AD. Visual hallucinations are typically present early in the course of the disease and do not diminish in later periods. In an analysis of autopsy-confirmed cases, hallucinations and delusions were more frequent with LB pathology (75%) than AD (21%) at the time of the initial clinical evaluation (Weiner et al., 2003). This was also true for those cases with mixed DLB and AD (53%) pathology relative to AD alone. The occurrence of visual hallucinations in the first four years after dementia onset has a positive and negative predictive value for DLB of 81% and 79%, respectively (Ferman et al., 2006).

There is a strong association between visual hallucinations and cholinergic depletion in the temporal cortex and the basal forebrain (Harding et al., 2002). Visual hallucinations may predict a good response to cholinesterase inhibitors (I. McKeith et al., 2004). The hallucinations of DLB do not seem to correlate with the dose of levodopa (L-dopa) or the occurrence of motor fluctuations seen with dopaminergic therapy (Sanchez-Ramos et al., 1996); however, hallucinations may be elicited or worsened with dopaminergic medications. Other suggested mechanisms for visual hallucinations include dysregulation of rapid eye movement (REM) sleep with the intrusion of dreams into wakefulness (Boeve et al., 2004).

TABLE 66.3. Cognitive profiles comparing Lewy body dementia to Alzheimer's disease

	ALZHEIMER'S DISEASE	LEWY BODY DEMENTIA
Episodic memory		
Free recall	+++	++
Recognition	+++	—
Prompting	x	√
Intrusions	+++	+++
Semantic memory (naming)	++	+
Procedural memory	—	+
Working memory	++	+++
Insight	+++	+
Attention	++	+++
Executive functions	++ typical Alzheimer's disease +++ frontal variant	+++
Visuospatial skills	++ typical Alzheimer's disease +++ posterior variant	+++

+ mild impairment; ++ moderate impairment; +++ early and severe impairment; + mild impairment;
— no significant impairment; x not helpful; √ helpful.

whether letters or shapes are used, Patients with LBD perform more poorly than AD patients. Additionally, the demonstration of greater attentional impairment and variability in reaction times in DLB relative to AD may be the function of the executive and visuospatial demands of the tasks (Bradshaw et al., 2004). Attentional deficits are important determinants of the inability to perform instrumental and physical activities of daily living, even after controlling for age, sex, motor function, and other cognitive profiles (Bronnick et al., 2006).

Early frontal/executive dysfunction may be predictive of incident PDD (Woods and Troster, 2003) and is considered a core feature of PDD (Emre et al., 2007). Executive functions comprise a number of cognitive skills (planning, abstraction, conceptualization, mental flexibility, insight, judgment, self-monitoring, and regulation) and are central to adaptive, goal-directed behavior. The executive dysfunction seen in patients with LBD includes impaired judgment, organization, and planning (Kehagia et al., 2010). These patients are also more susceptible to distraction and have difficulty engaging in a task and shifting from one task to another. They tend to perform more poorly on Stroop, card sorting, and phonemic verbal fluency tasks than comparably demented patients with AD (Calderon et al., 2001). In general, executive impairments tend to be worse in LBD than AD (Collerton et al., 2003; Simard et al., 2000).

The neurochemical basis of executive dysfunction is likely to be multifactorial in nature and associated with dopaminergic,

cholinergic, and noradrenergic deficits; although further study is required, increasing evidence from imaging and autopsy studies highlights the importance of cortical cholinergic loss (Emre, 2003).

VISUOSPATIAL/CONSTRUCTION

Visuospatial deficits are common in LBD and represent a very early and sensitive marker of PDD, especially when LB pathology and AD are mixed (Johnson and Galvin, 2011). Visuospatial changes are varied and can manifest across measures of facial recognition, spatial memory spatial planning, object-form perception, visual attention, visual orientation, and constructional praxis. Several studies have shown greater impairments in LBD than AD on visuospatial and constructional tasks (Collerton et al., 2003; Noe et al., 2004; Simard et al., 2003). Even brief-screening tests, such as pentagon copying from the Mini Mental State Examination (MMSE; Folstein et al., 2001) have been reported to be greater in LBD than AD (Ala et al., 2002; Cormack et al., 2004).

On complex figure copy tests, performance of patients with DLB is known to be affected partially by disrupted visual spatial perception and partially because of reduced frontally mediated skills such as organization, planning, and working memory. Furthermore, impairments on constructional tasks likely reflect more than just the motor demands of the tasks and the motor impairments of LBD, as these patients also show greater impairments than patients with AD on visual perceptual tasks without significant motor demands (Calderon et al., 2001) and even after controlling for the motor slowing characteristic in PDD (Johnson and Galvin, 2011). Subjects with DLB performed more poorly than patients with AD not only in size and form discrimination and visual counting, but also in recognizing overlapping figures. Studies have linked visual perceptual deficits in DLB to visual hallucinations (Mori et al., 2000); that is, those patients with visual hallucinations performed significantly worse on the overlapping figures test and performed worse in size and form discrimination than those subjects with DLB without visual hallucinations. Mosimann et al. (2004) also found that among patients with DLB and PDD, those with visual hallucinations performed significantly worse than those without hallucinations on tasks of angle, object-form, and space-motion discrimination. Because visual hallucinations are among the strongest predictors of DLB and PDD (Galvin 2006; Tiraboschi et al., 2006), the neuropsychological assessment of visual perceptual and constructional functions is important in suspected DLB and PDD and their differentiation from AD.

MEMORY

Generally speaking, patients with LBD perform better on episodic memory tasks than patients with AD. Memory may be spared early on in LBD and manifest as the disease progresses. Memory deficits are the presenting problem in 67% of patients with PDD, which is fewer than the number of patients with DLB (94%) and AD (100%) (Noe et al., 2004). The nature of the memory deficit in LBD differs from that noted in AD as it tends to be one of retrieval rather than encoding and/or functioning. The cognitive profile is one of mixed subcortical and cortical cognitive impairments that are often indistinguishable from PDD. Although the rate of dementia progression was once considered to be more rapid in DLB relative to AD, this has not been a consistent finding in the literature.

There is no one sign or symptom that definitively distinguishes PDD from DLB. Current clinical criteria for DLB distinguish PDD only by the temporal requirement that the dementia manifests more than 12 months after the onset of motor signs; if dementia precedes or is concurrent with parkinsonism, then DLB is diagnosed. In one study of 100 participants (10 nondemented controls, 40 patients with PD, 15 with DLB, and 35 with AD) enrolled in a longitudinal study of memory and aging, Galvin et al. (2006) found that postural instability is more common in PDD than DLB, whereas sexual disinhibition, alexia, and naming problems were more common in DLB relative to PDD. Galvin et al. also found that the presence of these features, whether at first evaluation or at any point in the course of PD, was highly predictive of PDD and the development of LBs at autopsy.

The core features of DLB include fluctuating cognition, recurrent well-formed visual hallucinations, and spontaneous parkinsonism. Extrapyramidal signs, including bradykinesia, facial masking, and rigidity are the most frequent signs of parkinsonism and can vary in severity. Resting tremor is not common. Parkinsonism is usually bilateral. There tends to be more axial rigidity and facial masking in DLB than in idiopathic PD.

Additional clinical features suggestive of DLB were also identified in the revised criteria. These include rapid eye movement sleep behavior disorder (RBD), severe neuroleptic sensitivity, and low dopamine transporter uptake in the basal ganglia demonstrated by single photon emission computed tomography (SPECT) or positron emission tomography (PET) imaging. Often present but not specific features of DLB include repeated falls and syncope, transient and unexplained loss of consciousness, autonomic dysfunction, hallucinations in other modalities, systematized delusions, depression, relative preservation of medial temporal lobe structures on structural neuroimaging, reduced occipital activity on functional neuroimaging, prominent slow wave activity on electroencephalogram (EEG), and low uptake iodine-123 metaiodobenzylguanidine (MIBG) myocardial scintigraphy.

According to the revised DLB consortium criteria, two core features (or one core feature and one suggestive feature) are sufficient for a diagnosis of probable DLB; one core feature or one or more suggestive feature is suggestive for a diagnosis of possible DLB (I. G. McKeith et al., 2005). As with AD, definitive diagnosis of DLB rests on brain autopsy following death. Although these features may support the clinical diagnosis of DLB, they lack diagnostic specificity and can be seen in other neurodegenerative disorders. These criteria permit 83% sensitivity and 95% specificity for the presence of neocortical LBs (I. G. McKeith, 2000b). These criteria are also more predictive of cases with pure or diffuse LB pathology than those with concomitant AD pathology, and fail to reliably differentiate between pure DLB (which is rare) and the more common mixed forms of DLB and AD. There are currently no definitive radiological or biological markers available to support a diagnosis of DLB.

EPIDEMIOLOGY OF LEWY BODY DEMENTIA

The precise number of people with LBD remains unclear. The point prevalence of dementia in PD is close to 30% and the incidence rate is increased at four to six times relative to controls. The cumulative percentage is very high, with at least 75% of PD patients who survive more than 10 years likely to develop dementia (Aarsland and Kurz, 2010). The mean time from disease onset of PD to dementia is approximately 10 years. However, there are considerable variations, and some patients develop dementia early in the disease course. Old age, more severe motor symptoms (in particular, gait and postural disturbances), mild cognitive impairment at baseline, and visual hallucinations are reliably identified as risk factors for early dementia.

Prevalence estimates of DLB range from 0% to 5% in the general population and from 0% to 30.5% of all dementia cases (Zaccai et al., 2005). Very few studies have looked at the incidence rates in DLB. Miech et al. (2002) found the incidence of DLB to be about 0.1% in the general population, and 3% for all new dementia cases.

NEUROPSYCHOLOGICAL FEATURES OF LEWY BODY DEMENTIA

Neuropsychological evaluation has provided clinicians and researchers with profiles of cognitive strengths and weaknesses that help to define LBD, as well as distinguish LBD from AD. It is important to keep in mind that neuropsychological tests often tap a number of different domains and the reasons that patients may perform poorly on any given test for any number of reasons. Unfortunately, the underlying cognitive processes of widely used neuropsychological measures have yet to be elucidated more precisely. Generally speaking, cognitive symptoms in LBD include a combination of cortical and subcortical impairment; this is contrasted with a classic cortical profile of impairment predominant in AD. See Table 66.3 for a summary of the neuropsychological deficits differentiating LBD from AD.

ATTENTION AND EXECUTIVE FUNCTION

Lewy body dementia is typified by impairments in attention and executive functions. Marked attentional disturbance in DLB may serve as the basis of fluctuating cognition that is characteristic of DLB (Walker et al., 2000). A range of experimental, screening, and clinical neuropsychological measures have been used to compare attention in LBD relative to AD. Few studies have shown group differences on digit span tasks (Hansen et al., 1990). Rather, more consistent group differences emerge on more complex attentional tasks, such as those requiring mental control, visual search and set shifting, and visual selective attention. On cancellation tasks, regardless of

TABLE 66.1. Clinical diagnostic criteria for Parkinson disease dementia

Core features (required for both probable or possible PDD)	Diagnosis of PD according to UK Brain Bank (Queen Square) criteria Dementia with insidious onset and slow progression in the context of of PD diagnosis, defined by: • Impairment of more than one domain of cognition • Impairment represents a decline from premorbid functioning • Impairment in day-to-day functioning not caused by motor or autonomic dysfunction
Associated features (typical cognitive profile in at least two of the four domains + at least one behavioral symptom = probable PDD; atypical cognitive profile in one or more domains = possible PDD, and behavioral disturbance may or may not be present)	*Cognition* Impaired attention, may fluctuate within/across days Impaired executive functions (e.g., planning, conceptualization, initiation, rule finding, set maintenance or shifting, mental speed) Impaired visuospatial functions (e.g., visual-spatial orientation, perception, or construction) Impaired memory (typically with benefit from cuing, better recognition than recall) Preserved language (some difficulties with word-finding and complex sentence comprehension may be present) *Behavior* Apathy Changes in mood and personality (including depression and anxiety) Delusions, typically of paranoid type Hallucinations, mainly visual, complex, and well formed Excessive daytime sleepiness/somnolence
Features making the diagnosis of PDD uncertain (none of these features can be present when diagnosing probable PDD; one or two features can be present when diagnosing possible PDD)	Another abnormality capable of impairing cognition, but judged not to be the cause of the dementia (e.g., vascular disease on neuroimaging) Time interval between onset of motor and cognitive symptoms is unknown
Supportive features (commonly present but lacking diagnostic specificity)	Cognitive and behavioral abnormality occurs solely in the context of other conditions, such as confusional state owing to systemic disease or intoxication, or major depressive disorder Features consistent with probable vascular dementia per NINDS-AIREN criteria

PD, Parkinson disease; PDD, Parkinson disease dementia.
From Emre, M., Aarsland, D., Brown, R. (2007). Clinical diagnostic criteria for dementia associated with Parkinson's disease. *Mov Disord, 22*, 1689–1707; quiz 1837.

TABLE 66.2. Revised clinical diagnostic criteria for dementia with Lewy bodies

Central feature	Progressive cognitive decline that interferes with social and occupational function
Core features (any two core features = probable DLB; any one = possible DLB)	Fluctuating cognition Recurrent visual hallucinations Spontaneous features of parkinsonism
Suggestive features (one or more + a core feature = probable DLB; one or more with no core feature = possible DLB)	REM sleep behavior disorder Severe neuroleptic sensitivity Decreased tracer uptake in striatum on SPECT dopamine transporter imaging or on MIBG myocardial scintigraphy
Supportive features (commonly present but lacking diagnostic specificity)	Repeated falls and syncope Transient, unexplained loss of consciousness Severe autonomic dysfunction Hallucinations in other modalities Systematized delusions Depression Relative preservation of mesial temporal lobe structures on CT/MRI Reduced occipital activity on SPECT/PET imaging Prominent slow waves on EEG with temporal lobe transient sharp waves

CT, computed tomography; DLB, dementia with lewy bodies; EEG, electroencephalograph; MIBG, metaiodobenzylguanidine; MRI, magnetic resonance imaging; REM, rapid eye movement; SPECT; single photon emission computed tomography.
McKeith, I. G., Dickson, D. W., Lowe, J., Emre, M., O'Brien, J. T., Feldman, H., Cummings, J., Duda, J. E., Lippa, C., Perry, E. K., Aarsland, D., Arai, H., Ballard, C. G., Boeve, B., Burn, D. J., Costa, D., Del Ser, T., Dubois, B., Galasko, D., Gauthier, S., Goetz, C. G., Gomez-Tortosa, E., Halliday, G., Hansen, L. A., Hardy, J., Iwatsubo, T., Kalaria, R. N., Kaufer, D., Kenny, R. A., Korczyn, A., Kosaka, K., Lee, V. M., Lees, A., Litvan, I., Londos, E., Lopez, O. L., Minoshima, S., Mizuno, Y., Molina, J. A., Mukaetova-Ladinska, E. B., Pasquier, F., Perry, R. H., Schulz, J. B., Trojanowski, J. Q., & Yamada, M. (2005). Diagnosis and management of dementia with Lewy bodies: third report of the DLB Consortium. *Neurology, 65*, 1863–1872.

66 | LEWY BODY DEMENTIAS

STELLA KARANTZOULIS AND JAMES E. GALVIN

Lewy body dementia (LBD) is an umbrella term for two related diagnoses, Parkinson disease dementia (PDD), and dementia with Lewy bodies (DLB). Lewy body dementia is now recognized as the second most common cause of dementia after Alzheimer's disease (AD). The Lewy Body Dementia Association estimates that there are between 1 and 2 million Americans with LBD. Lewy body dementia symptoms can closely resemble the more widely recognized dementia syndrome of AD but can be distinguished with identification of the visuospatial, executive, and attentional components of dementia (rather than the marked episodic memory impairment that characterizes AD), together with evidence of parkinsonism, visual hallucinations, and rapid eye movement sleep behavioral disorder (RBD). Cognitive fluctuations, although quite specific for LBD, can be difficult to elicit even at specialized centers given the lack of standardized questionnaires validated in large populations. Additional suggestive features incorporated in the consensus criteria for LBD that may facilitate diagnosis include depression, hallucinations in other modalities, syncope and frequent falls, transient and unexplained loss of consciousness, severe autonomic dysfunction, alterations in personality and behavior, relative preservation of medial temporal lobe structures on structural neuroimaging, reduced occipital activity on functional neuroimaging, and low uptake myocardial scintigraphy. Management of LBD currently rests on both pharmacological (cholinesterase inhibitors, N-methyl-D-aspartate antagonists, antiparkinsonism agents; atypical antipsychotics used with caution) and nonpharmacological (therapeutic environment, psychological and social support, physical activity, behavioral management strategies, caregivers' education and support) therapy options for its many cognitive, neuropsychiatric, motor, autonomic, and sleep disturbances.

WHAT IS LEWY BODY DEMENTIA?

Over the past two decades, research has suggested that Lewy bodies (LBs) found in up to 40% of autopsied brains (Galvin et al., 2006) play a significant role in the spectrum of diseases that have come to be known as the Lewy body dementias (LBD). Lewy body dementias include Parkinson disease dementia and dementia with Lewy bodies. This chapter uses the term Lewy body dementia to describe the syndrome of LB disorders, and the terms Parkinson disease dementia and dementia with Lewy bodies when citing specific experimental and clinical data.

Parkinson disease (PD), one of the most common movement disorders of the elderly, affects one in 100 individuals greater than 60 years of age and 4% to 5% of older adults greater than 85 years of age (roughly 1.5 million Americans). Parkinson disease is characterized by the cardinal motor features of rigidity, bradykinesia, and tremor at rest. Historically, cognitive problems were not considered to be important features of PD. In his famous text, James Parkinson (1755–1824) stated, "by the absence of any injury to the senses and to the intellect that the morbid state does not extend to the encephalon." It is now well recognized that cognitive impairment and dementia in the setting of PD are common and are two of the most debilitating symptoms associated with the disease. There is strong evidence that dementia not only has significant clinical consequences for PD patients in terms of increased disability, risk for psychosis, reduced quality of life, and increased mortality, but also results in a greater stress and burden of caring for patients with PDD and higher disease-related costs resulting from increasing chances of nursing home admission (Emre, 2003).

According to clinical diagnostic criteria (Table 66.1), PDD is a dementia syndrome that develops in the context of established PD (Emre et al., 2007). Like AD, PDD has an insidious onset with slow progression, and is defined as having impairment in more than one cognitive domain, representing a decline from prior levels. The deficits must be severe enough to affect daily social or occupational functioning or personal care and the deficits must be independent of the impairment resulting from motor or autonomic symptoms (Emre et al., 2007).

A wide variety of cognitive impairments have been reported in PDD, even early in the course of the disease. To date, the relationship between onset of initial deficits and subsequent decline to dementia has not been clearly established. Preliminary evidence suggests that an intermediate stage (PD-MCI) with predominant visuospatial and executive impairments may exist for one to three years (Johnson and Galvin, 2011). The neuropathology of PDD is controversial and it remains unknown whether or not dementia in PD occurs alone or only in the presence of other dementing disorders such as DLB and AD.

Dementia with Lewy bodies is now considered to be the second most common cause of dementia in elderly people. An international consortium on DLB resulted in revised criteria for the clinical and pathological diagnosis of DLB incorporating new information about the core clinical features and improved methods for their assessment (I. G. McKeith et al., 2005) (Table 66.2). Dementia with Lewy bodies, like all dementias, is characterized by a progressive reduction in cognitive

Jack, C.R., Jr., Slomkowski, M., et al (2003). MRI as a biomarker of disease progression in a therapeutic trial of milameline for AD. *Neurology* 60(2):253–260.

Jelic, V., Kivipelto, M., et al. (2006). Clinical trials in mild cognitive impairment: lessons for the future. *J. Neurol. Neurosurg. Psychiatry* 77:429–438.

Katz, R. (2004). Biomarkers and surrogate markers: an FDA perspective. *NeuroRx* 1:189–195.

Katz, R. (2008). Food and Drug Administration regulation. *CNS Spectr.* 13:10.

Kawas, C.H., Clark, C.M., et al. (1999). Clinical trials in Alzheimer disease: debate on the use of placebo controls. *Alzheimer Dis. Assoc. Disord.* 13(3):124–129.

Keller, C., Kadir, A., et al. (2011). Long-term effects of galantamine treatment on brain functional activities as measured by PET in Alzheimer's disease patients. *J. Alzheimers Dis.* 24(1):109–123.

Kins, S., Crameri A., et al. (2001). Reduced protein phosphatase 2A activity induces hyperphosphorylation and altered compartmentalization of tau in transgenic mice. *J. Biol. Chem.* 276(41):38193–38200.

Lannfelt, L., Blennow, K., et al. (2008). Safety, efficacy, and biomarker findings of PBT2 in targeting Abeta as a modifying therapy for Alzheimer's disease: a phase IIa, double-blind, randomised, placebo-controlled trial. *Lancet Neurol.* 7(9):779–786.

Liu, L., Drouet, V., et al. (2012). Trans-synaptic spread of tau pathology *in vivo*. *PLoS One* 7(2):e31302.

Mega, M.S., Dinov, I.D., et al. (2005). Metabolic patterns associated with the clinical response to galantamine therapy: a fludeoxyglucose f 18 positron emission tomographic study. *Arch. Neurol.* 62(5):721–728.

Meilandt, W.J., Cisse, M., et al. (2009). Neprilysin overexpression inhibits plaque formation but fails to reduce pathogenic Abeta oligomers and associated cognitive deficits in human amyloid precursor protein transgenic mice. *J. Neurosci.* 29(7):1977–1986.

Mohs, R.C., Doody, R.S., et al. (2001). A 1-year placebo-controlled preservation of function survival study of donepezil in AD patients. *Neurology* 57:481–488. Erratum in: *Neurology* 57:1942.

Morris, J.C., Roe, C.M., et al. (2009). Pittsburgh compound b imaging and prediction of progression from cognitive normality to symptomatic Alzheimer disease. *Arch. Neurol.* 66:1469–1475.

Nagahara, A.H., Merrill, D.A., et al. (2009). Neuroprotective effects of brain-derived neurotrophic factor in rodent and primate models of Alzheimer's disease. *Nat. Med.* 15(3):331–337.

Necula, M., Breydo L., et al. (2007). Methylene blue inhibits amyloid Abeta oligomerization by promoting fibrillization. *Biochemistry* 46(30):8850–8860.

Nitsch, R.M., Deng, M., et al. (2000). The selective muscarinic M1 agonist AF102B decreases levels of total Abeta in cerebrospinal fluid of patients with Alzheimer's disease. *Ann. Neurol.* 48(6):913–918.

Orgogozo, J.M., Gilman, S., et al. (2003). Subacute meningoencephalitis in a subset of patients with AD after Abeta42 immunization. *Neurology* 61(1):46–54.

Ostrowitzki, S., Deptula, D., et al. (2012). Mechanism of amyloid removal in patients with Alzheimer disease treated with gantenerumab. *Arch. Neurol.* 69(2):198–207.

Rascol, O., Fitzer-Attas, C.J., et al. (2011). A double-blind, delayed-start trial of rasagiline in Parkinson's disease (the ADAGIO study): prespecified and post-hoc analyses of the need for additional therapies, changes in UPDRS scores, and non-motor outcomes. *Lancet Neurol.* 10:415–423.

Reiman, E.M., Langbaum, J.B., et al. (2010). Alzheimer's prevention initiative: a proposal to evaluate presymptomatic treatments as quickly as possible. *Biomarkers Med.* 4(1):3–14.

Relkin, N.R., Szabo, P., et al. (2008). 18-month study of intravenous immunoglobulin for treatment of mild Alzheimer disease. *Neurobiol. Aging* 30(11):1728–1736.

Ridha, B.H., Anderson, V.M., et al. (2008). Volumetric MRI and cognitive measures in Alzheimer disease: comparison of markers of progression. *J. Neurol.* 255(4):567–574.

Rinne, J.O., Brooks, D.J., et al. (2010). 11C-PiB PET assessment of change in fibrillar amyloid-beta load in patients with Alzheimer's disease treated with bapineuzumab: a phase 2, double-blind, placebo-controlled, ascending-dose study. *Lancet Neurol.* 9(4):363–372.

Roberson, E.D., Scearce-Levie, K., et al. (2007). Reducing endogenous tau ameliorates amyloid beta-induced deficits in an Alzheimer's disease mouse model. *Science* 316(5825):750–754.

Sabbagh, M.N., Richardson, S., et al. (2008). Disease-modifying approaches to Alzheimer's disease: challenges and opportunities—lessons from donepezil therapy. *Alzheimers Dement.* 4:S109–118.

Sadowski, M.J., Pankiewicz, J., et al. (2006). Blocking the apolipoprotein E/amyloid-beta interaction as a potential therapeutic approach for Alzheimer's disease. *Proc. Natl. Acad. Sci. USA* 103(49):18787–18792.

Saito, T., Iwata, N., et al. (2005). Somatostatin regulates brain amyloid beta peptide Abeta42 through modulation of proteolytic degradation. *Nat. Med.* 11(4):434–439.

Salloway, S., Mintzer, J., et al. (2008). Disease-modifying therapies in Alzheimer's disease. *Alzheimers Dement.* 4(2):65–79.

Salloway, S., Sperling, R., et al. (2009). A phase 2 multiple ascending dose trial of bapineuzumab in mild to moderate Alzheimer disease. *Neurology* 73(24):2061–2070.

Sano, M., Grossman, H., et al. (2008). Preventing Alzheimer's disease: separating fact from fiction. *CNS Drugs* 22(11):887–902.

Schneider, A., and Mandelkow, E. (2008). Tau-based treatment strategies in neurodegenerative diseases. *Neurotherapeutics* 5(3):443–457.

Schneider, L.S., Olin, J.T., et al. (1997). Eligibility of Alzheimer's disease clinic patients for clinical trials. *J. Am. Geriatr. Soc.* 45(8):923–928.

Serrano-Pozo, A., William, C.M., et al. (2010). Beneficial effect of human anti-amyloid-beta active immunization on neurite morphology and tau pathology. *Brain* 133(Pt 5):1312–1327.

Sperling, R., Salloway, S., et al. (2012). Amyloid-related imaging abnormalities in patients with Alzheimer's disease treated with bapineuzumab: a retrospective analysis. *Lancet Neurol.* 11(3):241–249.

Sperling, R.A., Aisen, P.S., et al (2011). Toward defining the preclinical stages of Alzheimer's disease: recommendations from the National Institute on Aging-Alzheimer's Association workgroups on diagnostic guidelines for Alzheimer's disease. *Alzheimers Dement.* 7:280–292.

Tariot, P.N., Cummings, J., et al. (2009). The ADCS Valproate Neuroprotection Trial: primary efficacy and safety results. *Alzheimers Dement.* 5(4):P84–P85.

Vellas, B., Aisen, P.S., et al. (2011). Prevention trials in Alzheimer's disease: an EU-US task force report. *Prog. Neurobiol.* 95(4):594–600.

Wagner, J.A., Williams, S.A., et al. (2007). Biomarkers and surrogate end points for fit-for-purpose development and regulatory evaluation of new drugs. *Clin. Pharmacol. Ther.* 81(1):104–107.

Weinreb, O., Amit, T., et al. (2011). A novel anti-Alzheimer's disease drug, ladostigil neuroprotective, multimodal brain-selective monoamine oxidase and cholinesterase inhibitor. *Int. Rev. Neurobiol.* 100:191–215.

Wild, K., Howieson, D., et al. (2008). Status of computerized cognitive testing in aging: a systematic review. *Alzheimers Dement.* 4(6):428–437.

Wischik, C., and Staff, R. (2009). Challenges in the conduct of disease-modifying trials in AD: practical experience from a phase 2 trial of Tau-aggregation inhibitor therapy. *J. Nutr. Health Aging* 13(4):367–369.

Yu, Y.J., Zhang, Y., et al. (2011). Boosting brain uptake of a therapeutic antibody by reducing its affinity for a transcytosis target. *Sci. Transl. Med.* 3(84):84ra44.

GlaxoSmithKline, Janssen, Lilly, Lundbeck, MedAvante, Medivation, Medtronics, Merck, Neurokos, Neurotrax, Novartis, Otsuka, Pfizer, Prana, QR Pharma, Sonexa, Takeda, and UBC. He owns stock in ADAMAS, Prana, Sonexa, MedAvante, Neurotrax, and Neurokos. He has been a speaker for Eisai, Forest, Janssen, Novartis, Pfizer, Lundbeck. Dr. Cummings has provided expert witness consultation regarding olanzapine and ropinirole.

REFERENCES

Aisen, P.S., Andrieu, S., et al. (2011). Report of the task force on designing clinical trials in early (predementia) AD. *Neurology* 76:280–286.

Albert, M.S., DeKosky, S.T., et al. (2011). The diagnosis of mild cognitive impairment due to Alzheimer's disease: recommendations from the National Institute on Aging-Alzheimer's Association workgroups on diagnostic guidelines for Alzheimer's disease. *Alzheimers Dement.* 7:270–279.

Arendash, G.W., Mori T., et al. (2009). Caffeine reverses cognitive impairment and decreases brain amyloid-beta levels in aged Alzheimer's disease mice. *J. Alzheimers Dis.* 17(3):661–680.

Bales, K.R., Verina T., et al. (1997). Lack of apolipoprotein E dramatically reduces amyloid beta-peptide deposition. *Nat. Genet.* 17(3):263–264.

Bateman, R.J., Aisen P.S., et al. (2011). Autosomal-dominant Alzheimer's disease: a review and proposal for the prevention of Alzheimer's disease. *Alzheimers Res. Ther.* 2(6):35.

Bateman, R.J., Munsell, L.Y., et al. (2006). Human amyloid-beta synthesis and clearance rates as measured in cerebrospinal fluid *in vivo*. *Nat. Med.* 12(7):856–861.

Bateman, R.J., Siemers, E.R., et al. (2009). A gamma-secretase inhibitor decreases amyloid-beta production in the central nervous system. *Ann. Neurol.* 66(1):48–54.

Blennow, K., Zetterberg, H., et al. (2012). Effect of immunotherapy with bapineuzumab on cerebrospinal fluid biomarker levels in patients with mild to moderate Alzheimer disease. *Arch. Neurol.* 69(8):1002–1010.

Blurton-Jones, M., Kitazawa M., et al. (2009). Neural stem cells improve cognition via BDNF in a transgenic model of Alzheimer disease. *Proc. Natl. Acad. Sci. USA* 106(32):13594–13599.

Bodick, N., Forette, F., et al. (1997). Protocols to demonstrate slowing of Alzheimer disease progression. Position paper from the International Working Group on harmonization of dementia drug guidelines. The disease progression sub-group. *Alzheimer Dis. Assoc. Disord.* 3:50–53.

Braak, H., and Del Tredici, K. (2011). Alzheimer's pathogenesis: is there neuron-to-neuron propagation? *Acta Neuropathol.* 121(5):589–595.

Burton, E.J., Mukaetova-Ladinska, E.B., et al. (2012). Quantitative neurodegenerative pathology does not explain the degree of hippocampal atrophy on MRI in degenerative dementia. *Int. J. Geriatr. Psychiatry* 27(12):1267–1274.

Cabrol, C., Huzarska M.A., et al. (2009). Small-molecule activators of insulin-degrading enzyme discovered through high-throughput compound screening. *PLoS One* 4(4):e5274.

Cheng, I.H., Scearce-Levie K., et al. (2007). Accelerating amyloid-beta fibrillization reduces oligomer levels and functional deficits in Alzheimer disease mouse models. *J. Biol. Chem.* 282(33):23818–23828.

Clark, C.M., Xie, S., et al. (2003). Cerebrospinal fluid tau and beta-amyloid: how well do these biomarkers reflect autopsy-confirmed dementia diagnoses? *Arch. Neurol.* 60(12):1696–1702.

Committee for Medicinal Products for Human Use. (2008). Guideline on medicinal products for the treatment of Alzheimer's disease and other dementias. *European Medicines Agency.*

Congdon, E.E., Wu, J.W., et al. (2012). Methylthioninium chloride (methylene blue) induces autophagy and attenuates tauopathy *in vitro* and *in vivo*. *Autophagy* 8(4):609–622.

Craft, S., Baker L.D., et al. (2012). Intranasal insulin therapy for Alzheimer disease and amnestic mild cognitive impairment: a pilot clinical trial. *Arch. Neurol.* 69(1):29–38.

Cramer, P.E., Cirrito, J.R., et al. (2012). ApoE-directed therapeutics rapidly clear beta-amyloid and reverse deficits in AD mouse models. *Science* 335(6075):1503–1506.

Cummings, J.L. (2011a). Alzheimer's disease clinical trials: changing the paradigm. *Curr. Psychiatry Rep.* 13(6):437–442.

Cummings, J.L. (2011b). Biomarkers in Alzheimer's disease drug development. *Alzheimers Dement.* 7(3):e13–44.

Cummings, J.L. (2006). Challenges to demonstrating disease-modifying effects in Alzheimer's disease clinical trials. *Alzheimers Dement.* 2:263–271.

Cummings, J.L. (2009). Defining and labeling disease-modifying treatments for Alzheimer's disease. *Alzheimers Dement.* 5:406–418.

Cummings, J.L. (2008). Optimizing phase II of drug development for disease-modifying compounds. *Alzheimers Dement.* 4(Suppl 1):S15–20.

Cummings, J.L. (2010). What can be inferred from the interruption of the semagacestat trial for treatment of Alzheimer's disease? *Biol. Psychiatry* 68(10):876–878.

Cummings, J., Reynders R., et al. (2011). Globalization of Alzheimer's disease clinical trials. *Alzheimers Res. Ther.* 3(4):24.

Desikan, R.S., McEvoy L.K., et al. (2012). Amyloid-beta-associated clinical decline occurs only in the presence of elevated P-tau. *Arch. Neurol.* 69(6):709–713.

Divinski, I., Mittelman, L., et al. (2004). A femtomolar acting octapeptide interacts with tubulin and protects astrocytes against zinc intoxication. *J. Biol. Chem.* 279(27):28531–28538.

Dubois, B., Feldman, H.H., et al. (2010). Revising the definition of alzheimer's disease: a new lexicon. *Lancet Neurol.* 9:1118–1127.

Edland, S.D., Emond J.A., et al. (2010). NIA-funded Alzheimer centers are more efficient than commercial clinical recruitment sites for conducting secondary prevention trials of dementia. *Alzheimer Dis. Assoc. Disord.* 24(2):159–164.

Elias-Sonnenschein, L.S., Viechtbauer, W., et al. (2011). Predictive value of APOE-ε4 allele for progression from MCI to AD-type dementia: a meta-analysis. *J. Neurol. Neurosurg. Psychiatry* 82(10):1149–1156.

Engler, H., Forsberg, A., et al. (2006). Two-year follow-up of amyloid deposition in patients with Alzheimer's disease. *Brain* 129 (Pt 11):2856–2866.

Eriksdotter Jonhagen, M., Nordberg A., et al. (1998). Intracerebroventricular infusion of nerve growth factor in three patients with Alzheimer's disease. *Dement. Geriatr. Cogn. Disord.* 9(5):246–257.

Fan, J., Donkin J., et al. (2009). Greasing the wheels of Abeta clearance in Alzheimer's disease: The role of lipids and apolipoprotein E. *Biofactors* 35(3):239–248.

Ferri, C.P., Prince, M., et al. (2005). Global prevalence of dementia: A delphi consensus study. *Lancet* 366:2112–2117.

Fleisher, A.S., Truran, D., et al. (2011). Chronic divalproex sodium use and brain atrophy in Alzheimer disease. *Neurology* 77(13):1263–1271.

Fox, N.C., Black, R.S., et al. (2005). Effects of Abeta Immunization (AN1792) on MRI measures of cerebral volume in Alzheimer disease. *Neurology* 64(9):1563–1572.

Gozes, I., Morimoto, B.H., et al. (2005). NAP: research and development of a peptide derived from activity-dependent neuroprotective protein (ADNP). *CNS Drug Rev.* 11(4):353–368.

Grill, J.D., and Cummings, J.L. (2010). Current therapeutic targets for the treatment of Alzheimer's disease. *Exp. Rev. Neurother.* 10(5):711–728.

Grill, J.D., and Karlawish, J. (2010). Addressing the challenges to successful recruitment and retention in Alzheimer's disease clinical trials. *Alzheimers Res. Ther.* 2(6):34.

Grill, J.D., Di, L., et al. (2012a). Estimating sample sizes for predementia Alzheimer's trials based on the Alzheimer's Disease Neuroimaging Initiative. *Neurobiol. Aging* 34(1):62–72.

Grill, J.D., Karlawish, J., et al. (2012b). Risk disclosure and preclinical Alzheimer's disease clinical trial enrollment. *Alzheimers Dement.*

Grill, J.D., Monsell, S., et al. (2012c). Are patients whose study partners are spouses more likely to be eligible for Alzheimer's disease clinical trials? *Dement. Geriatr. Cogn. Disord.* 33:334–340.

Grill, J.D., Raman, R., et al. (2012d). Effect of study partner on the conduct of Alzheimer disease clinical trials. *Neurology.* [Epub ahead of print].

Hampel, H., Ewers, M., et al. (2009). Lithium trial in Alzheimer's disease: a randomized, single-blind, placebo-controlled, multicenter 10-week study. *J. Clin. Psychiatry* 70(6):922–931.

He, G., Luo, W., et al. (2010). Gamma-secretase activating protein is a therapeutic target for Alzheimer's disease. *Nature* 467(7311):95–98.

Heister, D., Brewer, J.B., et al. (2011). Predicting MCI outcome with clinically available MRI and CSF biomarkers. *Neurology* 77(17):1619–1628.

Holmes, C., Boche, D., et al. (2008). Long-term effects of Abeta42 immunisation in Alzheimer's disease: follow-up of a randomised, placebo-controlled phase I trial. *Lancet* 372(9634):216–223.

Iqbal, K., Alonso Adel, C., et al. (2002). Significance and mechanism of Alzheimer neurofibrillary degeneration and therapeutic targets to inhibit this lesion. *J. Mol. Neurosci.* 19(1–2):95–99.

Jack, C.R., Jr., Knopman, D.S., et al. (2010). Hypothetical model of dynamic biomarkers of the Alzheimer's pathological cascade. *Lancet Neurol.* 9:119–128.

peptide and the active component of the glial-derived activity dependent neuroprotective protein (ADNP). NAP stabilizes microtubules and can reduce tau phosphorylation (Divinski et al., 2004). NAP reduced AD pathology in mouse models and has reached clinical investigation in an intranasal form (Gozes et al., 2005).

NEUROPROTECTION

Neuroprotection is defined here as including therapeutic strategies that aim to increase neuronal and synaptic survival in the face of AD pathology. Many neuroprotective strategies are independent of the actual mechanisms of cell and synapse loss. Epidemiological findings suggest AD-preventing properties for the NSAIDs and the cholesterol-lowering drugs (Sano et al., 2008). If these agents indeed prevent AD, the mechanisms by which they do so are unknown. As discussed, NSAIDs may alter proteolytic processing of APP, but AD pathology also includes a significant inflammatory component. Similarly, cholesterol may be involved in Aβ processing and statin therapy may impact AD pathology. Despite this and the epidemiologic results, prospective randomized trials in mild-to-moderate AD have failed to confirm disease-slowing properties for the NSAIDs diclofenac, misoprostol, rofecoxib, or naproxen; or for the HMG-CoA reductase inhibitors atorvastatin and simvastatin. Additionally, rofecoxib was no better than placebo at delaying conversion to dementia in MCI, and primary prevention trials of naproxen and celecoxib were halted for safety reasons (Sano et al., 2008).

Other therapies target the mechanisms by which cells die. Given that age is the strongest risk factor for AD, cellular aging is one logical correlate for study and the production of reactive oxygen species (ROS) in particular may be critical both in normal aging and AD. ROS may penetrate cellular mitochondria, and Aβ-dependent and independent mitochondrial dysfunction has been implicated in AD. The mitochondrial membrane stabilizer, latrepirdine (Dimebon, dimebolin) showed early promise in a small phase II trial, but two larger phase III studies failed to confirm latrepirdine's efficacy (Cummings, 2010). Other antioxidant compounds remove ROS and demonstrated preclinical efficacy in AD models, but trial results are generally mixed. One study suggested a delay in the time to severe AD (as measured with the CDR) in patients treated with vitamin E, but other trials have suggested no benefit (Sano et al., 2008). Sirtuins are another family of compounds believed to have antioxidant and potential Aβ-lowering properties. A large phase II trial of resveratrol, the sirtuin found in red wine and the skin of red grapes, is currently underway.

Both neuronal survival and apoptotic cell death are critical to proper CNS development and this process is largely dependent upon neurotrophic factor regulation. Because of their potent survival effects in development, neurotrophic factors are logical treatment candidates in neurodegenerative disease. Trophic factor therapies face a variety of challenges, most specifically size that limits penetration of the CNS and intolerability related to potent off-target effects (Eriksdotter Jonhagen et al., 1998). To address both of these challenges, neurosurgical delivery of gene transfer technology can be applied. An ongoing clinical development program uses neurosurgery to deliver adeno-associated virus (AAV)-delivered nerve growth factor DNA to the trk-A receptor-expressing cholinergic neurons of nucleus basalis of Meynert. These cells provide cholinergic supply to the neocortex and hippocampus and are known to degenerate early in the disease. Their enhanced survival may increase cholinergic tone and slow disease progression. Similarly, in a primate model, gene transfer to the entorhinal cortex with brain-derived neurotrophic factor (BDNF) DNA enhances memory performance (Nagahara et al., 2009).

Cell-based therapies for AD present unique challenges. The synapse and cell loss in AD is widespread, making replacement unlikely. Recent animal studies suggest that replacement may not be necessary, however, to achieve therapeutic efficacy. In triple transgenic mice, stem cell therapy resulted in increased hippocampal synaptic density, possibly as a result of increased BDNF signaling (Blurton-Jones et al., 2009).

CONCLUSIONS

Alzheimers disease is one of the most important areas of medical research. Without improvements in treatment options and earlier intervention AD will bankrupt world health care systems. No treatment can slow the course of AD, but a wide range of targets for potential disease-modifying therapies have been identified and many candidate drugs are in development. Clinical trials will be essential to finding disease-modifying drugs, but face a variety of challenges. As trials move earlier in disease, the reliance on standards set in dementia trials may hinder success. Improved outcome measures, surrogate biomarkers, and better means of enrolling samples are critically needed. Despite these challenges, optimism exists for the numerous compounds that have entered or will soon begin clinical study. The field is on the cusp of disease-modifying therapies, which may act as catalysts for continued improvement in therapeutics, implementation of trials to delay cognitive impairment, and amelioration of the human and financial toll associated with AD.

DISCLOSURES

Dr. Grill has received grant/research support from the National Institute on Aging (AG016570), the Alzheimer's Association (NIRG-12-242511), the John Douglas French Foundation, the Sidell-Kagan Foundation, and as a site investigator for clinical trials sponsored by Elan, Genentech Janssen Alzheimer Immunotherapy, Bristol-Myers Squibb, Medivation, Pfizer, and the Alzheimer's Disease Cooperative Study (ADCS). He has served as a paid consultant to Avanir Pharmaceuticals and Phloronol Inc.

Dr. Cummings owns the copyright of the Neuropsychiatric Inventory. He has provided consultation to Abbott, Acadia, ADAMAS, Anavex, Astellas, Avanir, Avid, Baxter, Bayer, Bristol-Myers Squibb, Eisai, Elan, EnVivo, Forest, GE, Genentech, the rates of occurrence of ARIA and its subtypes, as well as how often ARIA results in symptoms. It is likely that these rates will differ among candidate therapies and some antibodies are being developed specifically with the goal of improving the profile. Preliminary data suggest that ARIA may be most likely in areas of substantial Aβ removal.

While most antibodies in development for AD are monoclonal and specifically target a particular fragment of the Aβ peptide, polyclonal antibodies may also remove Aβ and provide clinical efficacy. Plaques in the brains of untreated AD patients are decorated with IgG antibodies, which elicit a microglial response, and an inverse relationship exists between IgG level and plaque burden in AD patients. Therapeutic use of naturally produced autoantibodies in the form of intravenous immunoglobulin (IVIg) as treatment for AD is a current area of clinical investigation. Treatment with IVIg increased plasma and decreased CSF levels of Aβ in a study of eight AD patients (Relkin et al., 2008). There is a large multisite clinical trial of IVIg in the United States and a second trial is planned.

One hypothetical mechanism by which immunotherapies reduce Aβ is through transport across the blood–brain barrier (BBB). Apolipoproteins do not cross the BBB, but play a role in Aβ transport and may regulate passage of Aβ between the CNS and the periphery. Beside age, APOE genetic status is the most well established risk factor for AD. The extent to which the different isoforms of ApoE bind Aβ is debated (Fan et al., 2009). ApoE ε4 likely decreases passage of Aβ from brain to blood. Mouse models that overproduce and deposit Aβ, when combined with transgenic animals that lack ApoE, have reduced Aβ deposition (Bales et al., 1997). Synthesized compounds that prevent ApoE binding to Aβ reduce plaque deposition and memory impairment in animal models of AD (Sadowski, Pankiewicz et al. 2006). Alternatively, in another mouse model, the FDA-approved cutaneous T-cell lymphoma drug, bexarotene, demonstrated rapid plaque clearance and behavioral improvement. Bexarotene targets ApoE and liver X receptors and is being considered for clinical development for AD (Cramer et al., 2012).

One proposed mechanism by which ApoE regulates brain Aβ is by facilitating passage across the BBB via the low-density lipoprotein receptor-related protein (LRP). Antibodies against the LRP reduce Aβ efflux from the brain, and peripheral administration of soluble LRP as a mechanism to pull Aβ out of the brain has been proposed as a potential therapy. Alternatively, because Aβ travels bidirectionally, it may be useful to prevent its entry to the CNS from peripheral sources. The receptor for advanced glycation end-products (RAGE) is a multiligand receptor that binds Aβ with high affinity. Preventing ligands from binding RAGE lowers brain levels of Aβ. RAGE-inhibiting compounds are in development, though the first major phase II trial of a RAGE inhibitor failed to demonstrate efficacy and may have resulted in cognitive worsening, relative to placebo.

TAU

The second pathognomonic hallmark of AD is the neurofibrillary tangle (NFT). NFTs can be used to stage AD severity, based on a stereotypical progression that begins in the entorhinal cortex and parahippocampal gyrus and progresses to include neocortical regions. Pathological studies have found the correlation between NFT pathology and disease progression to be stronger than that for neuritic plaque burden.

Neurofibrillary tangles are intracellular, composed of condensed hyperphosphorylated paired helical filaments of the microtubule-associated protein tau (MAPtau or tau). Although phosphorylation of tau is critical to its normal function, hyperphosphorylated tau (phospho-tau) aggregates into paired helical filaments rather than binding to microtubules. The resulting instability disrupts axonal transport and may result in neuronal injury and cell death, though neurons may live a decade or longer with neurofibrillary tangles (Braak and Del Tredici, 2011).

Abnormally high levels of phosphorylated or total tau in the CSF are indicators of neurodegenerative disease or injury. Clinical examinations suggest that abnormalities in Aβ do not predict cognitive decline unless p-tau levels are also abnormal (Desikan et al., 2012). In basic science models, tau is essential to AD and reducing tau can alleviate Aβ-dependent cognitive impairment (Roberson et al., 2007). Given that tau is a constitutive part of the cytoplasm of neurons, removal of cytoplasmic tau is not a realistic target. Staging of tau pathology in postmortem AD brains and a mouse model in which abnormal tau expression is limited to the entorhinal cortex but still develops pathology throughout the limbic structures (Liu et al., 2012) suggest that tau is transsynaptically transported, perhaps underlying the anatomic spread of AD pathology. Investigational therapies aim to stabilize tau or to prevent its hyperphosphorylation, aggregation, or spread between cells.

Several classes of agents, including anthraquinones, polyphenols, aminothienopyridazines, and phenothiazines, may prevent tau aggregation. Wischik and colleagues have begun clinical development of the phenothiazine methylene blue as a treatment for AD (Wischik and Staff, 2009) The initial clinical trial of this agent failed to meet its prespecified endpoints but long-term observations and biomarker studies suggested possible benefit. Clinical development in AD continues. Methylene blue may reduce tau levels through autophagy (Congdon et al., 2012) and preventing tau fibril formation.

Reducing hyperphosphorylation might slow AD. Small molecule inhibitors of glycogen synthase kinase 3 beta (GSK-3β) and the cyclin-dependent kinase-5 (cdk5), both of which phosphorylate tau at multiple sites, are logical candidates to prevent NFT development (Schneider and Mandelkow, 2008). Lithium and valproate inhibit GSK-3β, but large controlled studies have failed to confirm initial promising results from small open label studies (Hampel et al., 2009; Tariot et al., 2009). Caffeine also inhibits GSK-3β (Arendash et al., 2009).

Drugs that dephosphorylate tau may offer an alternative approach. Protein phosphatase 2A (PP2A) is decreased in AD and inhibition can cause tau hyperphosphorylation, tangle-like pathology, and behavioral impairment in animal models (Kins et al., 2001). Multiple PP2As exist and candidates capable of increasing PP2A activity, potentially through targeting upstream regulators, are logical (Iqbal et al., 2002), though no such candidates have reached clinical testing. NAP is an 8 amino acid the non-amyloidogenic pathway by enhancing the activity of α-secretase. Few compounds have been identified that successfully activate α-secretase. Laboratory studies have suggested such activating effects for muscarinic ACh receptor agonists. M_1 and M_3 receptor agonism may regulate APP processing. In one small uncontrolled trial of 19 AD patients, mean decline in CSF Aβ was observed after treatment with an M_1 agonist (Nitsch et al., 2000).

AMYLOID BETA DEGRADATION

Endogenous Aβ degradation occurs through activity of neprilysin (also known as neutral endopeptidase), insulin-degrading enzyme (IDE), endothelin-converting enzyme, angiotensin-converting enzyme, metalloproteinase 9, and as many as 15 other recently identified proteinases. Neprilysin and IDE are thought to be the primary regulators of Aβ degradation and are reduced in AD. Studies in transgenic mouse models suggest that degrading enzyme activity is dose-dependently related to AD pathology and may be a suitable target for new treatments, but that targeting multiple degrading enzymes may be needed to ensure that treatment effect is not washed out by compensatory pathways. For example, APP transgenic mice that overexpress the neprilysin transgene demonstrate increased Aβ degradation but not behavioral improvement (Meilandt et al., 2009). Mice engineered to overexpress neprilysin and IDE, alternatively, have reduced Aβ levels, reduced astrogliosis, microgliosis, and dystrophic neurites, and improved spatial memory.

Targeting molecular regulators of Aβ degrading enzyme levels *in vivo* may be more readily accomplished. Saito and colleagues identified somatostatin receptors as a potential regulator of neprilysin activity (Saito et al., 2005), and Cabrol and colleagues recently completed a high-throughput screen in which they identified multiple small molecule activators of IDE (Cabrol et al., 2009).

ANTIAGGREGATION AND IMMUNOTHERAPIES

In the CNS, Aβ is prone to aggregation. Dimers, trimers, and other high-molecular-weight combinations of Aβ may provide a compelling treatment target, since transgenic animals with reduced plaque burden but high oligomer levels do not demonstrate behavioral improvement (Cheng et al., 2007). Small molecules may specifically inhibit oligomerization (Necula et al., 2007), fibrillization, or both, and it remains unclear which (if any) is optimal for slowing the course of AD.

The only antiaggregation agent tested in a large phase III trial—tramiprosate—failed to demonstrate efficacy, but a variety of other agents that aim specifically to prevent the oligomerization of Aβ are in development. Cyclohexanehexol (also known as AZD-103 and ELND-005) prevents oligomerization *in vitro*, improved behavioral performance in a mouse model of AD, and was tolerated in a human phase I trial. A metal protein attenuating compound, PBT2, is believed to prevent Aβ oligomerization by chelating copper and zinc, which have been proposed as critical to this process. The compound demonstrated initial efficacy in AD, lowering CSF levels of

Aβ and mitigating cognitive deterioration, relative to placebo (Lannfelt et al., 2008).

Aβ plaques may be deleterious to synaptic function and can be removed from the brain. Several types of immunotherapies have demonstrated an ability to reduce fibrillar amyloid burden, as measured by amyloid PET, and AD immunotherapies represent the most active area of disease-modifying trials.

Active vaccination with a synthetic full-length Aβ peptide (AN1792) in 300 mild AD patients initially suggested a clinical benefit in participants who received therapy and generated antibodies against Aβ but was halted because of a 6% incidence of T-cell mediated meningoencephalitis. Although analysis of the primary outcomes at the time of trial interruption demonstrated no drug–placebo difference, long-term follow up of survivors suggested a benefit in activities of daily living among antibody responders. Long-term follow-up to autopsy of the first subjects to die demonstrated that there was no impact on the rate of progression to severe dementia, but that responders demonstrated substantial and sometimes complete removal of plaque burden. Pathological examination has also suggested an impact on hyperphosphorylated tau and dystrophic neurites in the hippocampus of antibody responders (Serrano-Pozo et al., 2010). These findings have challenged the validity of Aβ plaques as a target in AD. Aβ vaccinations modified to remove T-cell activity, consisting primarily of peptide fragments, are in clinical development.

The initial active vaccination studies sparked initiation of robust passive immunotherapy development programs. Treatment with antibody therapy should avoid the T-cell mediated response that was believed to underlie meningoencephalitis in the AN1792 studies. Furthermore, since only a portion of patients administered the vaccine responded by generating antibodies, passive immunotherapy is hypothesized to increase the proportion of patients who respond to therapy. Several not mutually exclusive hypotheses for the mechanism of action of anti-Aβ antibodies have been proposed and studied in animal models. In such studies, passive immunization has been demonstrated to result in enhanced breakdown of Aβ through activation of microglia and some antibodies appear to serve as a "peripheral sink" binding Aβ in the blood and creating a flow of Aβ out of the brain.

Multiple antibodies in development for AD have demonstrated ability to reduce fibrillar Aβ burden, as measured by amyloid PET (Ostrowitzki et al., 2012), and one has been shown to alter tau levels in the CSF (Blennow et al., 2012). Ongoing studies will determine if these biological drug effects are associated with reduced cognitive decline. In the first phase III studies, the monoclonal antibody bapineuzumab was reported to not meet its primary outcome measures in mild-to-moderate AD. It will be important to know whether the antibody was efficacious in reducing amyloid plaques in this trial. Although no safety issues related to meningoencephalitis have been observed with passive immunotherapies to date, antibody treatments do result in symptomatic and asymptomatic amyloid-related imaging abnormalities (ARIA), which have been categorized as consisting of vasogenic edema and effusion changes (ARIA-E) or the deposition of hemosiderin indicating microhemorrhages (ARIA-H) (Sperling et al., 2012). Ongoing trials will determine pathologies first identified by Alzheimer himself, the amyloid beta (Aβ) protein that accumulates in neuritic plaques within the cortical parenchyma, and tau, the microtubule-associated protein intrinsic to every neuron that becomes hyperphosphorylated and condensed in neurofibrillary tangles. Most small molecules target specific molecular components of the cascade of events that lead to the formation of these brain pathologies (candidates are described further in the following).

Alternatively, treatments may target the cellular processes associated with disease, be they downstream or independent of plaques and tangles. Such targets include the known inflammation associated with AD; cellular metabolism and production of reactive oxygen species that may accompany AD and normal aging; mitochondrial functioning or misfunctioning as part of neurodegenerative disease; apoptosis and apoptosis-associated genes and cell cycling molecules; and genes or proteins that may result in neuroprotection. Despite a plethora of possible molecular targets, these therapies can largely be distilled to a single goal: preventing neuron and synapse loss in the AD brain. Once such synapse loss has occurred, which is likely to have begun by the time of prodromal AD or before, regenerative strategies may be necessary if a return to baseline function is to be achieved. Replenishing tissue through stem cell treatment, cell transplants, or treatment with neurotrophic factors that increase endogenous neurogenesis may offer such promise, though successful neuroregeneration remains a distant goal.

Most agents have more than one mechanism of action. Off-target action may be responsible for side effects of some agents. Off-target effects may also lead to repurposing agents for non-AD indications.

DISEASE-MODIFYING TREATMENTS— CLASSES AND AGENTS

Aβ PRODUCTION

Neuritic plaques are pathognomonic to AD, and the Aβ protein that accumulates in the plaques is a primary target for disease-modifying AD drug development. Central to the amyloid hypothesis is the abnormal proteolytic processing of the amyloid precursor protein (APP). Initial cleavage of APP occurs by either α- or β-site enzymes. In either case, the produced C-terminal fragment is subsequently modified by gamma secretase within the transmembrane region. If the α-secretase product is cleaved by gamma secretase, the resulting protein fragment (p3) is believed to be non-toxic. In contrast, the product of sequential beta-site cleavage enzyme (BACE) and gamma secretase cleavages are a variety of Aβ peptide species ranging in size from ~37–43 amino acids in length. Aβ40 is the most abundant species and Aβ42 is less abundant but very important from the disease standpoint. Aβ42 is especially prone to aggregation and concentrated in the core of neuritic plaques. Recent evidence suggests that high molecular weight species of Aβ aggregated together (e.g., consisting of 2 to 20 Aβ molecules), collectively referred to as oligomers, may represent the most synapto- or neurotoxic forms of Aβ.

Several candidate drugs targeting Aβ are now in clinical development. Many of these drugs directly target APP or molecules involved in its proteolytic processing. Posiphen is a positive enantiomer of phenserine, the acetylcholinesterase inhibitor. Though it has no cholinergic activity, Posiphen reduces expression of APP and subsequently lowers Aβ in culture and animal models. Clinical studies of Posiphen are ongoing.

Small molecules that inhibit or modulate the enzymes critical to the amyloidogenic pathway may reduce levels of Aβ and therefore slow disease course. Because it represents the most upstream cleavage step, BACE (also known as β-secretase and memapsin-2) may represent an ideal target to halt production of all pathologic posttranslational APP products. The activity of BACE on APP, however, requires multisite binding and successful inhibition may require large molecules (>500Da) that cross the blood–brain barrier with difficulty. Small lipophilic agents able to access the CNS have been developed and clinical trial results are pending. Alternatively, basic science studies have linked BACE-neutralizing antibodies to transferrin receptor antibodies as a novel mechanism of transporting larger molecules including antibodies into the CNS (Yu et al., 2011).

Gamma secretase inhibitors have been more approachable for small molecule drug development; candidates have reached clinical testing. Gamma secretase is a four-part complex, consisting of the membrane proteins presenilin-1 or -2, nicastrin, Aph-1, and Pen-2. Presenilin serves as the catalytic subunit and is critical to APP proteolysis, but also to function of other transmembrane proteins including the Notch signaling receptor. As a result, presenilin knockouts are lethal and potent nonselective gamma secretase (and Notch) inhibitors lack tolerability sufficient for clinical use. Semagacestat, the non-selective gamma secretase inhibitor in development by Eli Lilly Pharmaceuticals had phase III studies halted because of unacceptable levels of skin cancer and other adverse events, including worsening cognition. Other gamma secretase-targeting drugs remain under clinical study. For these drugs to be successful, activity must sufficiently lower Aβ to have clinical impact (though to what extent is unknown) without causing significant off-target side effects. Alternatively, recent basic studies have identified other targets related to gamma secretase that include a protein critical to this secretase activity (He et al., 2010).

An alternate mechanism by which Aβ production may be lowered without directly preventing APP cleavage by gamma secretase is the modulation of gamma secretase activity, such that the postcleavage product is an alternate-length peptide fragment. The obvious benefit of drugs with such mechanisms of action is that they may have therapeutic effect without altering Notch activity. Several compounds with gamma secretase modulating activity have been identified, including some nonsteroidal anti-inflammatory drugs (NSAIDS). R-flurbiprofen is a non-NSAID gamma secretase modulator that was demonstrated as being no different from placebo on any outcome measure in a large phase III mild-to-moderate clinical trial. Penetration of the CNS by the agent may have been insufficient. Several other gamma secretase-modulating compounds have been identified and may soon enter clinical development.

Another mechanism to reduce Aβ levels in the CNS would be to enhance alternate processing of APP through not be advanced, at least in patients with mild-to-moderate AD exposed at this dose (Cummings, 2010). More experience with gamma secretase inhibitors is needed before concluding whether these side effects are inevitably associated with gamma secretase inhibition or unique to semagacestat.

It is important to understand a compound as well as possible before advancing it to phase III pivotal trials. Phase III trials are large, long, and expensive. Agents not likely to succeed in phase III should not be advanced. Phase II trials large enough to show a drug–placebo difference are as large as phase III trials. Drug development programs often combine phases II and III (Cummings, 2008) in a II/III design, anticipating using the data for registration purposes. Alternatives to this approach include greater use of adaptive trial designs in phase II to adjust for duration, doses, and side effects, and greater use of biomarkers in phase II to insure patient selection, target engagement, and disease modification. Biomarkers may show disease modification in shorter times or with smaller populations than required for demonstration of clinical evidence of disease modification (Jack et al., 2003). Positive biomarker effects will de-risk a phase III program but do not guarantee its success since the predictive validity of biomarkers is currently unknown.

DISEASE-MODIFYING TREATMENTS OVERVIEW AND CLASSIFICATION

Many types of treatments are in development as disease-modifying therapies for AD and have advanced to the point of clinical testing (Table 65.3) (Grill and Cummings, 2010). They have various targets, potential mechanisms of action, and modes of administration. As is the case for any therapy targeting the CNS, candidate treatments must be able to penetrate the blood–brain barrier if on-target activity is to be achieved. Therefore, many drug candidates for AD are small molecules and are being developed as oral medications. The unique biology of AD, however, presents additional challenges, and many promising agents in clinical trials utilize alternate modes of administration. These include small peptides, such as davunetide (AL-108), a potentially neuroprotective agent that is administered intranasally. Similarly, a recent study of intranasal insulin administration suggested possible symptomatic efficacy in early AD (Craft et al., 2012). An active vaccination, AN-1792, was tested in phase I and phase II trials and served as a catalyst to development of a variety of immunotherapies, including some that are currently in development as intramuscular injections. Several candidate passive immunotherapies are in development and administered through intravenous infusion or subcutaneous injection. Finally, some treatments such as gene transfer and cell-based therapies are administered directly to the brain.

The broad range of modes of administration of these AD candidate therapies are paralleled by a variety of targets and mechanisms of action. Many small molecules aim to alter protein processing of one of the abnormally folded and accumulated proteins in the brains of AD patients. These include the two abnormally processed proteins responsible for the hallmark

TABLE 65.3. Classes and examples of emerging therapies for the treatment of Alzheimer's disease

CLASS	MECHANISM	EFFECT OR AGENT
Anti-amyloid therapies	Decrease APP expression	Posiphen
	Increase Aβ metabolism	Neprilysin/IDE stimulators
	BACE inhibition	MK-8931; LY-2811376
	Gamma secretase inhibition	BMS708163
	Gamma secretase modulation	EVP-0962
	Alpha-secretase enhancement	M1 agonists
	Aggregation inhibitors	AZD-103/ELND-005; PBT2
	Monoclonal antibodies	Bapineuzumab; solanezumab; gantenerumab; crenezumab
	Polyclonal antibodies	IVIg
	Active vaccination	CAD-106; ACC-001
	BBB transport inhibitors (to brain)	RAGE inhibitors
	BBB transport facilitators (to blood)	LRP enhancement
	ApoE expression increase	Bexarotene
Anti-tau therapies	Aggregation inhibitors	Methylene blue
	Kinase inhibitors	GSK-3β inhibitors
	Phosphatases	Protein phosphatase 2A (PP2A) enhancers
	Microtubule stabilization	AL-108
Neuroprotective agents	Anti-inflammatory agents	NSAIDs
	Antioxidants	Resveratrol; curcumin; vitamin E
	PPAR gamma agonists	Pioglitazone; rosiglitazone
	Trophic factors	NGF and BDNF-like molecules
Regenerative approaches	Stem cell therapies	Cell replacement; generation of support cells

APP, amyloid precursor protein; BBB, blood–brain barrier; BDNF, brain derived neurotrophic factor; LRP, lipoprotein receptor-related protein; NGF, nerve growth factor; NSAIDs, nonsteroidal antiinflammatory drugs investigators, and the general public. The wide consensus is in favor of the use of surrogate consent for the majority of AD trial scenarios and most current trials will enroll patients if there is a spouse, family member, or another person identified in an advanced directive that can provide informed consent on behalf of the patient. This varies only slightly from trial-to-trial; for example, the ongoing ADCS-conducted trial of nerve growth factor (NGF) gene transfer delivery to the basal forebrain will enroll only patients with capacity to provide informed consent. Greater variability exists on a state-by-state basis regarding who can provide informed consent in the patient's stead and trialists are referred to their local regulatory bodies to determine a decision tree for this issue. Informed consent practices vary among nations and must be carefully monitored in global trials.

With the successful development of the cholinesterase inhibitors, a brief debate over the ethics of placebo controlled AD trials occurred (Kawas et al., 1999). This debate subsided, in large part because of the recognition that the available medications were only symptomatic. Thus, withholding these medications for the sake of a trial is not seen to have long-term ramifications on patient health. Moreover, trials examining agents anticipated to possibly have disease-modifying properties will generally enroll patients on symptomatic AD drugs, provided that they are maintained on stable doses. It is unclear how this landscape may change in the scenario of approval of the first disease-modifying AD drugs. Further, as trials have become more global in their conduct, AD drug development may bring the ethical challenge of developing a drug where it may not be made readily available, if proven effective.

Despite the management of ethical matters in dementia trials, the initiation of prodromal and preclinical AD trials brings new challenges. As discussed, the testing of agents in predementia populations will be critical to disease understanding, testing the amyloid hypothesis, and effectively treating and defraying the cost of AD. Ethical challenges must not derail predementia AD trials. However, a variety of ethical issues remain understudied in the setting of predementia trials. For example, these trials will enroll MCI or asymptomatic patients at highest risk for AD. The language that should be used to describe the criteria for entry (preclinical AD, at risk for AD, and the like) is uncertain; few prospective studies of long-term outcomes related to biomarker positivity are available to guide study conduct, including informed consent; and how enrolled participants (or those deemed ineligible) will interpret risk information is unknown. The strongest guidance for delivering risk information has been provided by the Risk Evaluation and Education for AD study, which randomized cognitively normal participants with a family history of AD to learn their *APOE* genotype or not. In this study, learning *APOE* genotype did not cause depression or anxiety, but those who were informed they were ε4 carriers were more likely than those who learned they were non-carriers to begin taking vitamins and supplements. Grill, Raman et al. (2012b) have recently shown in a qualitative study that persons in a hypothetical situation of learning they are at increased risk for AD will approach the decision of whether to participate in AD prevention trials differently—more frequently citing a desire to lower their personal AD risk

and less frequently citing logistical barriers to participation. The ethical issues surrounding predementia trials are in need of future research to more adequately address each of these issues.

LESSONS LEARNED FROM TRIALS

There have been no successful phase III trials for any disease-modifying compound of any neurodegenerative disorder. All trials conducted to date have failed to show a compelling, consistent, and repeatable drug–placebo difference. In some cases, trial conduct is impugned and the efficacy of the drug in the clinical trial was inadequately tested. In others, appropriately conducted clinical trials failed to show a drug–placebo difference or there was an emergence of unacceptable side effects (Cummings, 2010). It is important to distinguish between failed trials and failed drugs because failed trials cannot provide evidence for or against a specific pathway or specific intervention. Hallmark features of failed trials include a failure of decline in the placebo group, failure to demonstrate a drug–placebo difference with the active comparator (typically donepezil), and excessive variability in measures (Table 65.2).

A well-conducted trial that fails to show a drug–placebo difference is valuable in demonstrating that the agent is not effective in this particular population, at this specific dose, used for this specific period of time. Trials answer very limited questions. Trials are focused experiments that can answer only limited questions and do not provide evidence of a possible effect in a different population, dose, or exposure duration.

A well-conducted trial that demonstrates excessive and unacceptable side effects also provides valuable information on whether to advance a molecule. The increased cognitive and functional decline and increased emergence of skin cancer associated with semagacestat—the gamma-secretase inhibitor—exemplifies a well-conducted trial in which adverse events were demonstrated suggesting that the agent should

TABLE 65.2. Approach to trials that fail to show a drug–placebo difference

Failed trials
No placebo decline or placebo improvement
No drug–placebo difference in an active comparator arm (e.g., donepezil)
High measurement variability or site-to-site inconsistency
Failed drugs
Lack of efficacy
• Did not cross the blood–brain barrier
• Dose too low
• Lack of effect on target
Unacceptable side effects

RETENTION

Retention of enrolled participants is as important as their initial recruitment. Ethical guidelines outline the voluntary nature of research participation and ensure participant rights to withdraw consent and cease participation at any time. Therefore, participant retention begins with the recruitment process; investigators should enroll only participants likely to complete the trial. Like slow enrollment, high dropout can render a trial underpowered to examine the primary scientific question. Alternatively, skewed dropout can lead to scientific error. For example, were a symptomatic drug to lead to increased dropout throughout the trial (and the trial analyzed using the last observation carried forward analysis), the results could be misinterpreted as representing a disease-modifying effect.

Alzheimer's disease dementia trials reported in the literature have demonstrated an approximately 75% retention rate (Grill and Karlawish, 2010). Mild cognitive impairment trials have had a lower mean rate of retention, with dropout ranging from 40% to 50%, rendering these trials far more challenging to interpret (Jelic et al., 2006). MCI trials of cholinesterase inhibitors have been hypothesized to suffer high dropout as a result of drug side effects, since dropout is higher in the group randomized to drug. Trial retention in early (preclinical) disease will be critical, as these trials are likely to require long durations. Though existing primary AD prevention trials have had good retention rates, most have employed benign interventions and infrequent visits (e.g., annual) and may not provide optimal guidance for preclinical AD studies. Preclinical trials studies are likely to employ riskier interventions that require more frequent assessment of safety.

Retrospective analyses have examined factors that predict trial dropout. In the ADCS MCI trial of donepezil and vitamin E, Edland and colleagues found that minority participants were more likely to drop out than non-Hispanic white participants and non-married participants were more likely to drop out than married participants (Edland et al., 2010). In a recent examination of six ADCS dementia trials, Grill, Raman et al. (2012d) observed dropout rates of 25% for patients with spouse partners, 32% for those with adult child partners, and 34% for those with other study partners. Edland and colleagues also observed a significantly higher rate of drop out at commercial trial sites, relative to academic sites. We recently observed a similar (though not statistically significant) difference between academic and non-academic sites in the rate of trial completers in a phase II mild-to-moderate dementia trial.

REPRESENTATIVE SAMPLES

Another major challenge in AD disease-modifying trials is increasing the representativeness of trial samples. Alzheimer's disease trials enroll predominantly highly educated non-Hispanic White participants who are joined in their participation by spouse caregivers. Faison and colleagues examined minority participation in a sample of trials conducted over a ten-year period and observed less than 10% participation in ADCS trials and less than 3% participation in industry-sponsored trials. It is critical to increase the diversity of AD trial samples, especially because African Americans and Hispanics may be at increased risk for AD. Lower education has also been suggested as a risk factor for AD, though trial samples generally are of high education levels. Similarly, 67% of participants enrolled in a sample of ADCS trials did so with a spouse study partner (Grill, Raman et al., 2012d), despite the observation that in the U.S. most AD patients receive care from non-spouse family members.

GLOBALIZATION

Given the frequent struggles of AD trials to meet enrollment goals, there is an increasing need to conduct trials outside of the United States, where abundant samples of (especially treatment naïve) AD patients may exist. The majority of AD trials now include international (non-US) sites (Cummings et al., 2011). The conduct of clinical trials in a wide variety of global regions is associated with a variety of challenges. Life expectancy and access to health care vary substantially across global regions. Such variance is likely to manifest in differences in survival especially in the setting of longer trials, may affect the probability of adverse events, and may impact the representativeness of trial results. Mean levels of education also are considerably different among global regions that conduct AD trials. In addition to potential implications related to education-associated differences in AD progression, educational differences have substantial impact on the psychometric properties of cognitive outcome measures. Other challenges to interpreting global AD trials include potential differences in genetics among populations under study, including drug metabolism and AD risk genes; differences in attitudes toward AD diagnosis or biomarker procedures; and cultural differences in caregiving (and subsequent implications to trial outcome measures that rely on an informant). Finally, the availability of qualified investigators and nation-specific differences in trial regulations may hinder successful disease-modifying trials conducted globally.

TRIAL ETHICS

A number of ethical issues are raised in AD trials. Whether a patient suffering cognitive impairment is capable of providing truly informed consent and how to assess which patients are and which are not capable remains a challenging issue. Having capacity is not an all-or-none phenomenon. At one time, a patient may have capacity to make one decision (what they would like to eat for dinner) but lack the capacity to make another decision (whether to enroll in a high-risk trial). A variety of capacity scales exist and trials and the institutions in which they are conducted often standardize the metrics for assessing the patients' understanding of the trial.

For trials that may directly benefit the patients or advance the science of the field, proxies may provide surrogate consent for AD patients that lack it. The use of surrogate consent has substantial research support. Many studies have examined the attitudes toward surrogate consent of patients regarding their future selves, caregivers and families regarding patients, expert

TABLE 65.1. Potential roles of biomarkers in clinical trials (examples of biomarker applications)

Patient selection
Amyloid imaging
Hippocampal atrophy
CSF with low Aβ42 or elevated tau/phospho-tau
APOEε4 allele
Target engagement
Stable isotope labeled kinetics (SILK)
Serum Aβ40 or Aβ42
Amyloid imaging
Efficacy
Whole brain atrophy or ventricular enlargement
FDG PET
CSF tau/phosphor-tau
Amyloid imaging
Cytokines
Isoprostanes
Side-effect monitoring
MRI for effusions and microhemorrhages
Liver function tests and other safety measures

An important use of biomarkers is to support disease modification with proposed disease-modifying intervention. Reduced atrophy on MRI, reduced hypometabolism on FDG PET, and reduced CSF tau or phospho-tau compared with placebo groups in a placebo-controlled clinical trial would be evidence of disease modification. Isoprostane and cytokine measures might also reflect disease-modifying activity of therapeutic candidates. Neuronal injury biomarkers promise to be better measures of disease modification than amyloid biomarkers because amyloid measures such as CSF Aβ and amyloid imaging have had limited relationships to cognitive decline and dementia (Engler et al., 2006).

Biomarkers have an important role in detecting adverse events associated with antidementia therapies. Encephalitis associated with AN1792 was evident on MRI scans (Orgogozo et al., 2003) and MRI is used to follow amyloid related imaging abnormalities (ARIA), hemorrhagic type (ARIA-H) and ARIA effusion (ARIA-E), associated with immunotherapy and possibly with other amyloid related interventions (Salloway et al., 2009; Sperling et al., 2012).

A biomarker tightly linked to the mechanism of action of a drug might be approved in combination with the agent as a "theranostic" combination. For example, if an AD population with a specific genotype was identified as responding to a specific intervention, the test for the genotype might be approved together with use of the intervention conditional on the presence of the associated biological abnormality.

CHALLENGES TO DISEASE-MODIFYING TRIALS

Disease-modifying trials for AD face many unique barriers to success. Throughout, this chapter has addressed the many challenges to disease-modifying trial design. This section outlines some of the specific challenges to successful disease-modifying trial conduct.

RECRUITMENT

Essentially all clinical trials struggle to meet their recruitment goals. For most trials, the actual exceeds the planned time to complete study enrollment. In other cases, slow enrollment of sufficient numbers of suitable trial candidates can require study amendment (to add sites or altered inclusion/exclusion criteria), render a trial underpowered, or stop a trial entirely. Some barriers to trial enrollment are ubiquitous. These include low trial awareness, low rates of primary care (and even specialty) referrals to trials, and patient skepticism of research.

Alzheimer's disease trial enrollment has many specific barriers (Grill and Karlawish, 2010). AD is a disease of the elderly and older patients are less likely to qualify for trials. The average American over the age of 60 takes 6–12 prescription medications and, especially in early phase trials, such medications may be prohibited by protocols. Elderly patients also suffer a variety of comorbidities that may prevent trial participation. These include cancers, diabetes (especially if uncontrolled), hypertension (especially if uncontrolled), and other problems that impact cognition, mobility, or independence. In fact, based on data from the State of California's Alzheimer's Disease Diagnostic and Treatment Centers, Schneider and colleagues estimated that less than 10% of AD patients are eligible for AD trials (Schneider et al., 1997). Using data from the National Alzheimer's Coordinating Center, Grill and colleagues found that approximately 25% of participants in that large natural history study met generalized disease-modifying trial criteria for eligibility (Grill, Monsell et al., 2012c). Of eligible patients, only a portion will be aware of and interested in trials.

Less is known about the barriers to participation in disease-modifying trials in earlier (predemence) disease. In MCI/prodromal trials, a major barrier to enrollment is that few patients have received a diagnosis. Community screens inevitably identify a large number of patients with cognitive impairment, but after identification, there are no guarantees that these patients will be eligible or interested in trial participation. For example, those identified as MCI in community screens would need to undergo testing for AD biomarkers because entry criteria for prodromal AD trials and patient attitudes toward these biomarker testing procedures may be a barrier to participation (Grill et al., 2012b). Little is known about the barriers to disease-modifying trials in asymptomatic at-risk/preclinical populations.

et al., 2011). The CDR-sob may represent a logical choice as a single outcome. The CDR includes memory, cognition, and function; it lacks behavioral measures included in other global assessments. In very mild AD, the CDR is internally valid, sensitive to change over time, and requires fewer trial participants than do cognitive outcome measures. In trials of the earliest AD patients, however, which will enroll asymptomatic at risk or preclinical populations, the CDR-sob may not achieve the necessary sensitivity. Ongoing discussions and research aim to identify and develop unique metrics to quantify the earliest cognitive impairments in AD. For example, the planned API prevention trial in autosomal dominant mutation carriers, the proposed ADCS A4 trial in asymptomatic preclinical participants, and the pioglitazone trial are likely to use newly developed composite measures of cognition.

SECONDARY OUTCOMES IN DISEASE-MODIFYING TRIALS

Alzheimer's disease trials include a large variety of secondary outcome measures. The neuropsychiatric inventory is the most commonly included metric of behavioral symptoms. Behavioral symptoms occur in 75% of AD patients and few safe treatment options adequately manage these symptoms. Importantly, even in the prodromal stages of AD, behavioral symptoms are common and behavior tends both to worsen in severity and change in type over the course of AD. Both earlier and later stage trials therefore generally include the neuropsychiatric inventory.

Global and functional measures such as the CDR, MMSE, and ADCS-ADL, if not used as coprimary outcomes in a given trial, are often included as secondary outcomes. Scales that will support the registration and use of a drug if it is approved also are commonly incorporated into disease-modifying trials. These include scales of quality of life (QoL). In particular, the QoL-AD has been developed for use in AD studies and is now commonly incorporated. Three variants of the QoL-AD exist: the patient's assessment of patient QoL, the caregiver assessment of patient QoL, and the caregiver assessment of caregiver QoL. A variety of other scales measure the burden of care: these include the Dependence Scale.

Increasingly, sponsors may need to anticipate data required by payers to inform decisions regarding adopting drugs, placing them on formularies, and reimbursing their costs. The Resource Utilization in Dementia scale examines caregiver time spent supervising and assisting the patient with ADLs. This and other pharmacoeconomic tools are needed to provide insight into the clinical meaningfulness of treatment effects.

COMPUTERIZED OUTCOMES

Computerized cognitive assessment batteries may bring additional sensitivity and convenience to outcomes assessment in disease-modifying trials. Sufficient data now exist to support use of computerized measures in elderly populations, including the development of age normative data. These batteries are associated with reduced variance and may afford smaller sample sizes, especially in early phase trials. Although computerized testing affords standardized administration and response/reaction time measurements, the correlations between computerized tests and activities of daily living are less established (Wild et al., 2008). A major strength (and rationale for development) of computerized batteries is to increase sensitivity to very mild changes in cognition. In theory, batteries could use adaptive testing and item response theory to examine cognitive ability more efficiently, though none of the currently available systems uses such technology. Computerized cognitive testing systems include the NeuroTrax Mindstreams system, the Cambridge Neuropsychological Test Automated Battery, and the CogState.

PATIENT-REPORTED OUTCOMES

The FDA has recently provided guidance recommending the use of patient-reported outcomes (PRO) as supportive for the demonstration of drug efficacy. As is implied by their names, PROs require no interpretation from a clinician. The PRO in cognitive impairment (PROCOG) has been developed for possible use in disease-modifying trials. The PROCOG has been validated in MCI and AD and was designed to assess cognition, as well as behavior, function, and quality of life.

BIOMARKERS FOR CLINICAL TRIALS

Neuroimaging and fluid biomarkers are discussed in Chapters 62 and 63, respectively. The characteristics of biomarkers will not be reviewed here. Biomarkers can have multiple roles in clinical trials (Table 65.1). State or trait markers might be used for clinical trial enrollment. APOE ε4 is a trait marker of increased risk for AD. Patients with MCI who are ε4 carriers are more likely to progress to AD than those who are not ε4 carriers. APOE ε4 carrier status could be used to enrich a population of MCI patients likely to progress to AD (Elias-Sonnenschein et al., 2011). State biomarkers can be used for enrollment also. Asymptomatic individuals who have positive amyloid imaging for example, might be considered at risk for progression to symptomatic AD (Dubois et al., 2010; Sperling et al., 2011). Similarly, low CSF Aβ42 or low Aβ42 and high tau or phospho-tau could also be used as biological measures that would enrich an asymptomatic or MCI population likely to progress to AD dementia (Heister et al., 2011). Biomarkers could also be used to further enrich a population in ways that would match the proposed mechanism of action of an intervention. For example, patients with high serum isoprostane levels might be appropriate candidates for antioxidant interventions, or patients with high cytokine levels might be appropriate candidates for anti-inflammatory interventions (Cummings, 2011a).

Biomarkers can be used to demonstrate target engagement and proof of mechanism. Stable isotope labeled kinetics (SILK) (Bateman et al., 2006) can be used to show inhibition of amyloid production by secretase inhibitors (Bateman et al., 2009). SILK is valuable for demonstrating target engagement of agents that affect Aβ reduction or clearance. The long-term relationship and clinical outcomes related to these relatively brief physiologic measures has not yet been established.

Mohs and colleagues demonstrated in a one-year trial of moderate AD patients that donepezil delayed the time to functional decline, relative to placebo, as measured by the functional assessment and change scale. This trial, especially in combination with the results of the donepezil MCI trial, display the possibility for symptomatic benefit to imitate disease modification. Longer studies, at least 18-months, and combined clinical and biological support are necessary to support a claim of disease modification in AD.

SLOPE CHANGE

The progressive nature of AD presents an opportunity to examine drug effect on disease course. In contrast to endpoint comparisons, slope analyses examine drug effect throughout the course of study, in effect using the entire course of the trial as an outcome. Drug ability to slow the *rate* of cognitive decline over time serves as the primary outcome. The phase III trial of tarenflurbil included a prespecified slope analysis as a secondary outcome, with the aim of supporting a claim of disease modification, though the drug failed to demonstrate efficacy. Statistical slope analyses are complicated and challenging, due in large part to the nonlinear progression of disease and the influence of outliers (see the following). Placebo response and potential symptomatic effects, especially at trial initiation, can further complicate these analyses. Nevertheless, slope analyses may be sufficient for a disease-modifying label for the European Medicines Agency; the US Food and Drug Administration (FDA) has not, as yet, agreed that successful demonstration of altered disease slope of decline is sufficient for this claim.

CLINICAL OUTCOME MEASURES FOR DISEASE-MODIFYING TRIALS

The registration trials of the available symptomatic AD treatments provided a roadmap to drug approval that has subsequently been embraced by regulatory agencies, investigators, and sponsors. This has been particularly relevant in the choice of clinical outcome measures. To receive marketing approval from the FDA, a new AD drug must demonstrate efficacy on coprimary outcomes, including one cognitive measure and one functional or global measure. The *standard* approach to trial designs and outcome choices may soon require amending, however. It remains unclear if this approach is optimal in disease-modifying trials that aim at new targets, test medications with unique mechanisms of action, that depend more on biomarkers, and that ultimately incorporate more challenging (and beneficial) objectives, including early symptomatic and presymptomatic intervention.

COGNITIVE OUTCOME MEASURES

Successful registration trials in mild-to-moderate populations have utilized the ADAS-cog. The ADAS-cog is a 70-point instrument that examines memory, orientation, comprehension of language and commands, naming, word finding, and ideational and constructional praxis. The ADAS-cog lacks linearity when used as a longitudinal or cross-sectional measure

of disease severity. In early or late dementia, the annual change in the ADAS-cog is minimal, relative to that observed in mild-to-moderate dementia. This issue is particularly critical in trials that move earlier in disease with the goal of intervention at a stage of minimal neuropathological burden. An 80-point version of the ADAS-cog that includes a delayed recall task (ADAS12) is available and multiple lines of evidence suggest increased sensitivity for the ADAS12 in MCI and prodromal AD populations, relative to the standard ADAS-cog. A 13-item version of the ADAS-cog includes executive measures.

Few trials in mild-to-moderate AD have implemented other cognitive outcomes. The neuropsychological test battery (NTB) was developed as alternative to the ADAS-cog, attempting to account for some of its weaknesses (the standard version of the ADAS-cog largely fails to examine attention, working memory, and executive function). Preliminary analyses of psychometric properties and longitudinal change in early AD suggested that the NTB may be more sensitive than the ADAS-cog to cognitive change in early AD. Administrative demands of the NTB are high. In moderate-to-severe dementia, only the severe impairment battery has been used in trials to successfully demonstrate cognitive efficacy.

GLOBAL AND FUNCTIONAL OUTCOMES

The most common choice of second coprimary outcome measure for AD trials has been the ADCS-activities of daily living (ADCS-ADL) scale. Similar scales include the Disability Assessment for Dementia and Functional Assessment Questionnaire. The overriding principle behind each of these informant-based scales is impairment to basic and instrumental ADLs and a sensitivity to detect further impairment, slowing of that decline, or improvement with treatment.

Alternatively, some AD dementia trials have incorporated the CDR as a global outcome. This scale includes assessment of memory and function and may offer greater sensitivity in milder populations, including MCI and prodromal AD. The CDR can be examined as an outcome measure in two capacities. A global staging score can be calculated using a scoring algorithm that weights memory (relative to the other components: orientation, judgment and problem solving, community affairs, home and hobbies, and self-care). Alternatively, the six components or "boxes" can be treated equally and summed (sum of the boxes score, CDR-sob).

Another commonly used global scale is the Clinician Interview Based Impression of Change plus caregiver input (CIBIC+). This tool compares the outcomes at prespecified intervals to baseline global severity. The interview assesses cognition, function, and behavior. The CIBIC+ has generally been used in shorter trials (3 and 6 months) and the CDR-sob in longer-duration trials (12 and 18 months).

OUTCOME CHOICES IN FUTURE DISEASE-MODIFYING TRIALS

With the evolution of AD research and the realization of the need for trials earlier in the disease, use of single outcome measures to demonstrate drug efficacy has been proposed (Aisen even in dementia trials, may facilitate improved sample homogeneity. Even the application of biological criteria, however, is not a guarantee of sample homogeneity. For example, amyloid PET may label some Lewy body dementia patients (and may fail to label some AD patients). Furthermore, a large portion (20–40%) of AD patients suffer vascular comorbidity and a smaller portion (<5%) may suffer comorbid neurodegenerative disease. Only through combined clinical and biological criteria (including MRI exclusion of those with vascular pathology likely to contribute to cognitive impairment) can enrollment of an appropriate and homogeneous sample be achieved. Evolving biomarkers may allow further narrowing of populations to better match biological subtype and mechanism of action of the test compound.

CLINICAL OUTCOMES IN DISEASE-MODIFYING TRIALS

Dependent upon the trial design and the population enrolled, a large number of clinical outcome scenarios may be used to examine if a drug or other treatment is capable of altering the natural history of AD. As yet, there is no clear preferred outcome choice for disease-modifying AD trials. Broadly categorized, these trials either directly examine efficacy or test the ability of a drug to delay a milestone. For each choice, primary comparison is versus placebo. An active comparison is sometimes included as a means of assessing trial quality. A trial with donepezil that did not demonstrate a donepezil-placebo difference would be regarded skeptically.

DRUG–PLACEBO DIFFERENCE AT TRIAL END

The most straightforward outcome metric for assessing drug efficacy is to compare the group randomized to drug to the group randomized to placebo at trial end. This parallel design assumes successful randomization (otherwise the groups might not be equivalent at baseline, complicating analyses and interpretation). In most trials to date, mean group changes from baseline were compared, rather than cross-sectional comparisons at trial completion. The parallel group design has been used in most mild-to-moderate or moderate-to-severe AD dementia trials, including those that resulted in the regulatory approval of the cholinesterase inhibitors and memantine.

DELAY IN ONSET OF MILD COGNITIVE IMPAIRMENT

When enrolling asymptomatic patients, a delay-to-milestone approach can be used, incorporating the mean time to a diagnosis of MCI as the outcome or using a survival-type design. Both primary prevention trials (enrolling community based samples with no clinical or biological sign of disease) and secondary prevention trials (enrolling "asymptomatic at risk" or "preclinical AD") could use the MCI construct as an outcome. If the mean time to MCI diagnosis is delayed or a significantly lower proportion of subjects randomly assigned to the active medication fulfills MCI criteria at a predetermined time point, the claim of

delay of disability would be supported. As with all predementia disease-modifying trials, there is currently little guidance on the choice of trial length. A resulting potential challenge is that insufficient numbers of subjects may develop cognitive impairment to provide adequate statistical power to examine a drug effect. Adaptive designs with variable lengths determined by prespecified outcomes are one solution to this problem. To support a claim of disease modification, the delay in MCI should be supported by delay in progression of biomarkers.

DELAY IN ONSET OF DEMENTIA

Trials enrolling MCI populations can examine a treatment's ability to delay dementia onset. Several trials have employed this design, including trials of rofecoxib, rivastigmine, and donepezil and vitamin E (Jelic et al., 2006). These trials employed fulfillment of NINCDS-ADRDA criteria for possible or probable AD or fulfillment of NINCDS-ADRDA and DSM-IV-TR criteria for AD as primary outcomes. In most cases, assessment of progression to dementia was performed every three months. In the trial of donepezil and vitamin E, there was a suggestion after one year that fewer participants assigned to donepezil had progressed to dementia than in the placebo group (secondary outcome). By three years (the time point of the primary outcome assessment), however, there was no difference in the proportion of participants who had progressed to dementia between the groups. A primary outcome at one-year (or a one-year trial) might have concluded drug efficacy or inappropriately concluded a disease-modifying effect. No other MCI trial has observed even a trend toward disease modification. In the trials of rofecoxib and rivastigmine, fewer than expected participants progressed to dementia (in both the treatment and the placebo groups). The rofecoxib trial was halted prior to completion because of this low conversion rate and high drop out. The rivastigmine trial was subsequently extended to permit examination of the primary outcome. Symptomatic benefit will delay onset of dementia and by themselves the delay to dementia designs do not establish disease modification. These challenges encountered in the cholinesterase inhibitor dementia progression trials demonstrate the importance of trial planning and adequate data support for trial design decisions.

DELAY IN OTHER MILESTONES

Besides delay to diagnostic outcomes (onset of dementia or onset of MCI), AD trials have examined other milestones and the ability of a drug to delay the onset of those milestones. Two very large trials in MCI examined progression to a global CDR score greater than or equal to 1 (mild dementia, see the following) as a primary outcome. The rofecoxib MCI trial discussed earlier incorporated this endpoint as a secondary outcome. Other trials enrolling dementia populations, such as that examining vitamin E and selegiline, have incorporated a time to global CDR score 3 (severe dementia), loss of activities of daily living (ADLs), institutionalization, or death. An ADCS study of valproic acid enrolled moderate AD patients with no history of agitation or psychosis and investigated the drug's ability to reduce (relative to placebo) the time to emergence of such symptoms.

TRIALS ENROLLING ASYMPTOMATIC PATIENTS AT GREATEST BIOLOGICAL RISK

Disease-modifying trials can identify and enroll cognitively normal older persons who demonstrate AD biomarkers. At autopsy, approximately 20–40% of cognitively normal elderly (age 65 or older) meet criteria for neuropathological diagnosis of AD. Amyloid PET imaging reveals a similar proportion of *amyloid positive* older living individuals who, at the time of scanning, have no cognitive impairment. A growing literature supports the inclusion of such patients in disease-modifying trials, because they are at substantially increased risk to develop cognitive impairment and symptomatic AD. For example, in one study of 159 nondemented participants with follow-up periods ranging from one to five years, amyloid PET positivity at baseline was associated with a hazard ratio of 4.85 [95% CI: 1.2–19.0] for progression to AD dementia (Morris et al., 2009).

The first trial enrolling biomarker positive cognitively normal older participants is being planned. The *anti-amyloid in asymptomatic AD (A4)* trial will enroll amyloid PET positive volunteers age 70 or older and randomize to placebo or amyloid immunotherapy. These patients have been described as asymptomatic at risk (Dubois et al., 2010) or preclinical AD (Sperling et al., 2011). The length of the asymptomatic phase of AD is unknown, and one challenge for the A4 trial is to determine an optimal study length. Too short of a trial would not permit examination of prevention or delay of onset of cognitive impairment as an outcome. Alternatively, amyloid biomarker positive patients experience greater and more rapid change in other biomarkers, such as brain volume and metabolic rate, but such outcome measures are unlikely to satisfy FDA requirements for approval (see previous). Validation of biomarkers in demented populations may lead to a regulatory pathway for demonstration of disease modification in asymptomatic patients (Aisen et al., 2011). Another potential pitfall of preclinical AD trials is that they will require very large numbers of subjects and are likely to encounter high rates of screen failures for biomarker criteria for entry (Grill, Di et al., 2012a).

TRIALS ENROLLING SYMPTOMATIC PATIENTS

Most disease-modifying trials are conducted in impaired patients. DuBois and colleagues describe the earliest symptomatic phase of disease as "prodromal AD." Prodromal AD patients demonstrate episodic memory impairment (adjusted for education) and AD biomarkers. Recent trials have applied these criteria for entry. Prodromal AD trials have used Aβ biomarkers (low CSF Aβ42, high ratio of CSF tau/CSF Aβ42, or amyloid PET).

The development of criteria for prodromal AD was in part the result of challenges previously met by trials enrolling patients with mild cognitive impairment (MCI). MCI is based only on clinical criteria for impairment of memory or other cognitive domains (generally 1 to 1.5 standard deviations below age- and education-adjusted norms). MCI trials that examined the rate of conversion to AD dementia as a primary outcome measure frequently met lower than expected rates of conversion, necessitating trial extension in some cases. No trial succeeded in demonstrating a therapeutic effect in MCI patients. MCI is a heterogeneous disorder with several underlying pathologies and diverse clinical outcomes. Many observational studies have shown that MCI patients demonstrating AD biomarkers are at greatest risk for progression to AD dementia and proposed research criteria have incorporated biomarker support to the diagnosis of MCI caused by AD (Albert et al., 2011). The use of prodromal AD criteria obviates the need for the MCI construct.

The majority of AD trials have enrolled patient populations meeting criteria for dementia and mild-to-moderate AD. As discussed, the most commonly applied diagnostic criteria are those developed by the NINCDS-ADRDA. Criteria for mild-to-moderate severity are frequently defined using the Mini-Mental State Examination (MMSE), typically set at MMSE 14–26. Most AD patients will meet these criteria at the time of dementia diagnosis or shortly thereafter and for approximately the next three to five years. By the time of AD dementia diagnosis, most but not all AD patients will be readily identifiable on multiple AD biomarkers. Recent work suggests that some biomarkers such as amyloid PET may reach a plateau (peak level of abnormality) by the time of AD dementia diagnosis (Jack et al., 2010). Such findings suggest that this phase of AD biology may already be too advanced for targeted treatments to be successful. Alternatively, biomarkers such as hippocampal volume, cortical thickness, and FDG PET metabolism appear to decline linearly through the dementia phase of AD. Therapeutic strategies able to arrest this decline may therefore still be able to modify the natural history of disease, rescuing brain tissue or function. Since no trial for disease-modifying agents has succeeded in any AD populations, it is premature to conclude which population are most treatment responsive.

AD trials have been conducted in more impaired patients, including moderately demented (e.g., global CDR = 2) or severely demented patients (e.g., defined as minimum MMSE of 5–7 and maximum MMSE defined as 14–17). The capacity of severely demented patients to sign informed consent or complete cognitive outcome assessments is diminished. For many families, these trials represent a last attempt to find alternative therapy, often out of desperation. Successful disease modification that fails to provide clinical improvement in severely demented patients, however, presents a serious ethical dilemma; the likely outcome is prolongation of a significantly compromised state.

CHALLENGES RELATED TO TRIAL SAMPLES

Trial inclusion and exclusion criteria are designed to ensure a homogeneous sample and facilitate interpretation of trial results. Trials that enroll heterogeneous samples face significant challenges. Mild-to-moderate AD dementia trial populations are often wide-ranging in age, requiring various stratifications as part of randomization strategies (e.g., age, genotype, site, MMSE). These trials may also have enrolled heterogenous populations in terms of disease biology. Most AD dementia trials have applied clinical criteria without biomarker requirements related to disease diagnosis. It is likely that a portion of trial participants do not suffer from AD, but instead some other underlying pathology, potentially affecting trial internal validity. The application of biomarker criteria,

(Ridha et al., 2008). The correlation of a biomarker with a clinical outcome is necessary but not sufficient evidence to establish that the biomarker and clinical outcomes reflect a common mechanism. Most drugs have multiple effects, some known and some unknown. Biomarker and clinical effects could be mediated by different pathways or could even have opposite effects. Establishing the relationship between a biomarker and a clinical outcome will take experience across multiple clinical trials and multiple therapeutic mechanisms (Katz, 2004).

To incorporate a biomarker in a clinical trial and be included in the package insert labeling of a therapeutic agent, the biomarker must go through a qualification process with review by the FDA. Decisions about how the biomarker is best included in the trial and how biomarker data will be managed in data analysis plan (Cummings, 2011b; Wagner et al., 2007) must be prespecified.

The use of biomarkers as an outcome for treatment in prevention trials including patients who are without symptoms is under consideration (Aisen et al., 2011; Vellas et al., 2011). A surrogate marker would have predictive value for a drug–placebo difference on a clinical outcome. No biomarker has risen to surrogate status. Although biomarkers have been shown to correlate with clinical measures, none have been shown to predict clinical outcomes. An incremental evolutionary approach is most likely to succeed in developing surrogate measures over time. Showing that a biomarker change predicts a clinical outcome in a mildly affected patient population would be a step towards incorporating the biomarker in a trial of asymptomatic individuals. The biomarker might eventually replace the clinical outcome and serve as a surrogate. This is a multiyear, multitrial process.

Clinical trial outcomes used in conjunction with biomarkers in trials of disease-modifying agents might include a drug–placebo difference at trial conclusion, delay in milestones, increasing drug–placebo difference or time, and change in slope of decline (discussed in more detail in the following).

POPULATIONS CONSIDERED FOR DISEASE-MODIFYING TRIALS

AD is traditionally described as a disease with a progressive clinical course over 8–12 years, ultimately resulting in complete dependence and then death. Fulfillment of the National Institute on Neurological and Communicative Disorders and Stroke-Alzheimer's Disease and Related Dementias Association (NINCDS-ADRDA) criteria for probable AD has been used as an inclusion criterion in most trials. The NINCDS-ADRDA criteria are purely clinical and incorporate the concept of dementia. A patient must demonstrate memory impairment and impairment to another domain of cognition, and these cognitive impairments must affect the patient's ability to perform activities of daily living and not be better accounted for by another possible cause. The cognitive impairment must be progressive and present for at least six months.

The course of AD, however, spans 20 years and includes a period of biological onset that precedes dementia. Recent improvements to AD criteria incorporate biomarkers, increase diagnostic accuracy, and facilitate earlier diagnosis—including before criteria for dementia are met. Differing nomenclatures and clinical and biological criteria for the phases of AD have been proposed. Disease-modifying trials can use these criteria as an initial means for defining the population to be studied and can enroll any sample of patients with AD, be they asymptomatic, mildly symptomatic, or demented. The group of patients to be included is decided based on trial goals.

TRIALS ENROLLING ASYMPTOMATIC PATIENTS AT GREATEST GENETIC RISK

Alzheimer's disease can be predicted with certainty from conception in a fraction of cases. Autosomal dominant AD results from gene mutations to the *amyloid precursor protein (APP)*, *presenilin-1*, and *presenilin-2* genes. Within families that carry these mutations, there is a 50% heritability, 100% penetrance, and substantial consistency in the age of symptom onset. This creates an opportunity for trial designs that initiate therapy at an approximate time frame preceding clinical onset to examine drug potential to delay that onset. Two major international programs are currently underway with the objective of better characterizing this familial form of AD and conducting prevention trials (Bateman et al., 2011; Reiman et al., 2010). The Dominantly Inherited Alzheimer's Network includes seven US sites, one UK site, and three Australian sites. The AD Prevention Initiative (API) is a collaboration between US and Colombian investigators that follows the largest known kindred of familial AD, a cohort of *presenilin-1* mutation carriers in Antioquia, Colombia. Asymptomatic offspring will be enrolled (non-randomly assigning non-carriers to placebo). Crenezumab, a monoclonal antibody targeting Aβ, is the candidate agent to be studied in this cohort.

A second component of the API proposes trials in those at greatest genetic risk for the sporadic form of AD: carriers of the ε4 allele of the *apolipoprotein E (APOE)* gene. *Apolipoprotein E* was the first identified and remains the strongest known genetic risk factor for sporadic AD. Three alleles have been identified: ε2, ε3, and ε4. The ε3 allele is most common among the general population. Hetero- and homozygotic carriers of ε4 are at significantly increased risk for sporadic AD. Current studies estimate up to a 12-fold increased risk associated with ε4 homozygosity (see http://www.alzgene.org/). Furthermore some ε4 carriers, by middle age, demonstrate AD-like abnormalities on functional MRI, FDG PET, and amyloid PET. Therefore, enrollment of ε4 carriers is an enrichment strategy.

Takeda and Zinfandel pharmaceuticals are conducting a prevention trial in which patients are selected on the basis of risk associated with *APOE* and *TOMM40* carrier status for specific age strata. Those at highest risk are assigned to pioglitazone or placebo and those at low risk are assigned to placebo.

For each genetic risk strategy, it is unknown what proportion of asymptomatic patients will meet biomarker criteria for trial entry (see the following) and at what time points. The overlap between genetics and biology is substantial, but imperfect. Combined biomarker and genetic inclusion criteria are feasible.

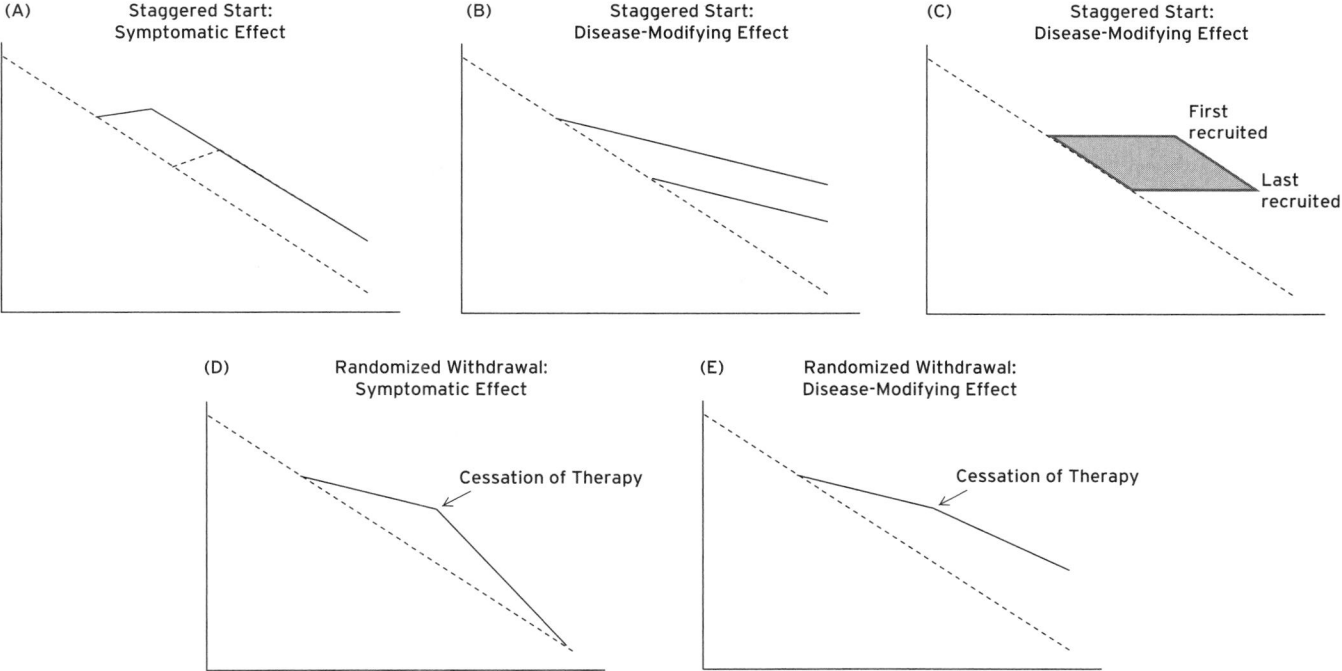

Figure 65.1 (A) Staggered start design with symptomatic effect shown. (B) Staggered start design with disease-modifying effect shown. (C) Natural history staggered start with observations collected over the course of the recruitment period. (D) Randomized withdrawal design with symptomatic effect shown. (E) Randomized withdrawal design with disease-modifying effect shown.

has occurred (Fig. 65.1D), whereas a withdrawal group that continues to remain above the expected level has experienced disease modification (Fig. 65.1E). The randomized withdrawal design is subject to the same uncertainties as the randomized start design. The duration of treatment and the duration of observation off treatment are both uncertain.

These designs have rarely been implemented in neurodegenerative disorders due to their complexities and uncertainties. When used in a Parkinson's disease trial, the results did not lead to a clear-cut conclusion, interpretation (Rascol et al., 2011), and/or new labeling.

Delay of disability is consistent with disease modification but can be achieved with symptomatic therapy (Mohs et al., 2001). Delay of milestones is not conclusive evidence of disease modification.

Use of biomarkers in conjunction with clinical outcomes is an alternative for establishing that an agent has changed the underlying biology of the disorder. Most biomarkers are inferential in that they represent imaging findings, electrophysiological observations, or peripheral indicators of a central process. The central process itself is undocumented. Although MRI correlates with nerve cell loss, nerve cell loss does not account for all the variance of MRI atrophy (Burton et al., 2012). This suggests that other as yet unidentified factors account for some aspects of MRI atrophy. Atrophy is also common across neurodegenerative disorders, is not specific to AD, does not identify a mechanism of action of an intervention, and does not indicate a specific change in pathology. Similarly, FDG PET is a measure of metabolism, a non-specific indicator of synaptic activity. A beneficial effect of an intervention on FDG PET compared with placebo would indicate improved

neuronal and synaptic function in the treatment group, but would not establish the mechanism for such improvement. Symptomatic agents may improve FDG PET activity in AD (Keller et al., 2011; Mega et al., 2005). Amyloid PET provides specific information on deposited fibrillar amyloid in the cortex, and its removal can be demonstrated by amyloid imaging in clinical trials (Rinne et al., 2010; Ostrowitzki et al., 2012). However, fibrillar amyloid may be a nontoxic species of Aβ and removal of fibrillar amyloid does not necessarily predict cognitive benefit (Holmes et al., 2008). Fibrillar Aβ is a proxy for the amyloidogenic process and possibly the presence of neurotoxic oligomers. It is not necessarily a direct measure of a neurotoxic species or the effect on neuronal and synaptic function. Serum and CSF measures such as Aβ40 and Aβ42 or CSF tau and phospho-tau are measures of cellular products and processes that have migrated from the interstitial space of the brain across the blood-brain or brain–CSF barrier and into the serum or CSF. Measures of these elements provide indirect reflections of the processes leading to cell death and dysfunction (Clark et al., 2003) but are not direct brain measures. Biomarkers are indirect and inferential measures of the basic processes leading to cell death and dementia.

To be supportive of a disease-modifying effect, the response of a biomarker (drug–placebo difference) should be correlated with the clinical outcomes. Biomarkers chosen as key outcomes should correlate with the primary clinical outcomes. For example, hippocampal atrophy may be a good choice to support a diagnosis of AD, but whole brain atrophy or ventricular enlargement may correlate better with trial outcomes such as Alzheimer's Disease Assessment Scale-Cognitive Subscale (ADAS-Cog) and Clinical Dementia Rating (CDR) to cell death and produces a corresponding clinical response. This definition is essentially identical to that of the European Medicines Agency (EMA) (Committee for Medicinal Products for Human Use, 2008) that states that "for regulatory purposes a disease-modifying effect will be considered when the pharmacologic treatment delays the underlying pathological or pathophysiological disease processes and when this is accompanied by an improvement of clinical signs and symptoms of the dementing condition." The EMA goes on to suggest a two-step approach in which the first step depends on delaying the course of the progression of the disease based on clinical signs and symptoms and leading to the limited claim of delay of disability. If these results are supported by a convincing package of biological and/or neuroimaging data (e.g., slowing, delay in the progression of brain atrophy) a full claim of disease modification can be considered.

The distinction between disease-modifying and symptomatic compounds cannot be drawn sharply. Some agents have dual action—such as ladostigil with cholinesterase inhibition plus monoamine oxidase inhibition (Weinreb et al., 2011)—and agents such as cholinesterase inhibitors that are viewed as largely symptomatic may have modest disease-modifying effects (Sabbagh et al., 2008).

Disease modification from a clinical trialist or regulatory point of view may differ from that of a practicing physician or patient and caregiver. Patients and caregivers would likely see a therapy that slows clinical progression but does not produce improvement of symptoms as less than successful.

The terminology of disease modification is typically not used in regulatory language appearing in the package insert for a medication. Interferon beta-1a, for example, has clinical and biomarker support as a disease-modifying intervention for multiple sclerosis. Its label reads, "to slow the accumulation of physical disability and decrease the frequency of exacerbations." Similarly, etanercept has clinical and biomarker evidence of disease modification for rheumatoid arthritis. Its label notes its utility for "inhibiting the progression of structural damage and improving physical function" (Cummings, 2009). Regulatory terminology for AD interventions with clinical and biomarker evidence of disease modification will likely have similar trial-specific labeling regarding reduction in loss of cognition and function with supporting evidence from a specified biomarker.

The FDA tends to avoid mechanism-related terminology. The language for the indication for the use of a cholinesterase inhibitor is "for the treatment of mild-to-moderate Alzheimer's disease" and does not stipulate that this is symptomatic or disease-modifying therapy (Katz, 2008).

The development of therapies targeting the pathophysiology and biology of AD has led many companies to adopt trial outcomes that will support labeling related to disease modification. Two strategies have been discussed in this context. The randomized withdrawal design and the randomized start design can theoretically demonstrate delay of progression in the absence of a biomarker. However, the statistical and ethical issues involved in these designs (Bodick et al., 1997; Rascol et al., 2011) have led to rare use of this approach. These are discussed in more detail in the following.

For practical purposes of constructing clinical trials and demonstrating disease-modifying properties of an intervention, a combination of a clinical trial demonstrating a drug–placebo difference in clinical outcomes and accompanied by a related drug–placebo difference in key biomarker outcomes is typically used. The terminology for the indication will likely reflect the clinical trial outcomes, such as reduction in loss of cognition and activities of daily living and corresponding improvement in a biomarker indicative of the biology of the disease such as atrophy on magnetic resonance imaging (MRI), amyloid burden on amyloid imaging, brain-metabolism on fluorodeoxyglucose positron emission tomography (FDG PET), or spinal fluid measures such as cerebrospinal fluid (CSF) Aβ42, tau, or phospho-tau. There remains substantial uncertainty about exactly how a regulatory agency such as the FDA will view data from biomarkers included in clinical trials of disease-modifying compounds (Katz, 2004). Paradoxical effects have confounded clinical trial interpretation; the observation that patients in the AN 1792 trial (active vaccination comprised of Aβ42) with a more robust antibody response had greater atrophy was unanticipated (Fox et al., 2005). Similarly in a trial of divalproex designed to show disease modification with a kinase inhibitor, there was greater MRI atrophy in the treatment than the placebo group (Fleisher et al., 2011). These observations complicate the planning for optimal use of biomarkers in trials.

DEMONSTRATING DISEASE MODIFICATION IN CLINICAL TRIALS

CLINICAL TRIAL DESIGNS

Two clinical trial designs have been suggested as adequate to indicate disease modification: These are the staggered start design and the randomized withdrawal design (Bodick et al., 1997). In the staggered start design, individuals are randomized to drug or placebo at study onset (Fig. 65.1A). After a defined interval, individuals in the placebo arm are switched to active treatment. If the switched group "catches up" with the original treatment group, then no disease modification has been demonstrated and a symptomatic benefit is concluded. On the other hand, if the delayed treatment group fails to "catch up" with the original treatment group, this suggests that the disease has been modified in the group first randomized to therapy (Fig. 65.1B). There are several uncertainties with this design. It is unclear how long of a therapeutic exposure might be required to establish therapeutic benefit, and likewise it is unclear how long of an observation period would be required to determine if the delayed start group has "caught up" with the original therapy group.

A novel interpretation of the delayed start design is the observation that in any recruitment period some patients begin early after the trial is initiated and some may begin as long as twelve months later (e.g., in a twelve-month recruitment period). Patients recruited later in the trial can be compared with patients recruited earlier in the trial. This allows a statistical "staggered start" analysis (Fig. 65.1C) (Hendrix S., personal communication).

The randomized withdrawal design is based on the fact that a group withdrawn from therapy will decline to the level of function expected of a placebo group if no disease modification coefficient. This suggests that the overall effect of development on structural network properties is increased network integration and decreased segregation.

This theme of decreased local connectivity, combined with an increase in long-range connectivity as we mature from childhood through adolescence, is also borne out from the rs-fMRI literature. Studies focusing on the DMN in children have shown that although the anatomical regions participating in the DMN are the same as in adults, there are differences in the degree of connectivity between them, specifically lower connectivity between the mPFC and the PCC was seen in children (Supekar et al., 2010). Similar findings have emerged from studies focused on more global connectivity patterns. In a metaanalysis of rs-fMRI (Power et al., 2010), studies focused on connectivity within specific age groups illustrate the general trend of decreasing local (short-range) connectivity and increasing global (long-range) connectivity with age (Fair et al., 2009). Development has also been investigated using electrophysiology, for instance, EEG-based connectivity as measured with synchronization likelihood showed a similar developmental trajectory as those measured using WM volume (Smit et al., 2012), whereas topological properties were indicative of a decrease in randomness with development.

SCHIZOPHRENIA

One of the dominant hypotheses concerning the etiology of schizophrenia centers on disruptions of neuronal connectivity (Bullmore et al., 1997), making the study of brain connectivity of particular interest. As with normal development, the focus of many structural connectivity studies has been on identifying differences in regional measures of WM fidelity, typically FA, between schizophrenic and control populations. The most consistent of these findings indicate abnormal tissue structure in the cingulate, the CC and frontal WM, whereas the superior longitudinal fasciculus (SLF), the inferior fronto-occipital fasciculus (IFOF), and the uncinate fasciculus have also been implicated. Topological analysis of whole brain structural connectivity networks of schizophrenic patients as compared with controls has also been performed, demonstrating decreases in global network efficiency with decreases in regional efficiency found in frontal regions and limbic regions (Wang et al., 2012; Zalesky et al., 2011).

fMRI-based connectivity methodologies have also been extensively used in the study of schizophrenia. Evidence for dysconnectivity in schizophrenia has been found involving various brain regions (Honey et al., 2005; Zhou et al., 2007). Network-based differences have also been observed, for instance those involving the prefrontal/temporal regions and the DMN (Whitfield-Gabrieli et al., 2009). Additionally, a number of whole brain functional connectome studies have demonstrated altered topological properties in the networks of schizophrenics. In general these studies have found that the complex brain networks in schizophrenia are less hierarchical, have decreased small-world indices, and are less efficiently wired (Lynall et al., 2010).

Connectivity analysis, using MEG- and EEG-based measures, has also been performed. Mutual information computed between EEG time courses, acquired during rest, showed significant increases both within and between hemispheres. Magnetoencephalography-based mutual information demonstrated a relationship between connectivity in the β band and performance in a working memory task (Bassett et al., 2009). Finally, there is a growing body of evidence of altered γ oscillations in schizophrenia (Gandal et al., 2012). For instance, a sensor-based EEG study using phase locking and coherence during a gestalt perception task (Spencer et al., 2003) demonstrated deficits in γ synchrony as well as abnormal coherence patterns.

AUTISM SPECTRUM DISORDERS

The autism spectrum disorders (ASDs) are developmental disorders characterized by impaired social interaction, impaired communication abilities, and repetitive behaviors. Increasingly, they are being viewed as disorders of functional networks (Welsh et al., 2005). There is a growing body of neuroimaging research supporting the hypothesis that ASD could be a disorder of impaired or altered connectivity (Courchesne and Pierce, 2005), specifically, a decrease in the long-range connectivity between the frontal lobe and the rest of the brain and an increase short-range intrafrontal lobe connectivity.

DW-MRI studies of ASD have shown alterations in local WM organization. Although there has been some variability in reported findings, the predominant pattern is one of compromised WM of the frontal and temporal lobes (Ameis et al., 2011; Sundaram et al., 2008). Tract and region-based analysis has implicated the ILF, IFOF, and SLF (Nagae et al., 2012), in addition to differences in the CC and, to a lesser extent, the cortical spinal tract. These findings clearly suggest altered structural connectivity between the frontal and temporal lobes.

Rs-fMRI studies have also generated evidence of altered connectivity in ASD. Studies focusing on the DMN have shown the regions of the DMN to be less strongly connected (Weng et al., 2010) in subjects with ASD compared with controls. Decreases in the connectivity of social and emotional processing networks have also been observed using rs-fMRI (Ebisch, et al., 2011). Decreased functional connectivity in ASD between frontal and posterior regions has been found as well during a variety of tasks (Just et al., 2012).

Finally, studies using electrophysiology to measure connectivity in ASD have also been undertaken. Electroencephalograph-based studies of sensor level MSC (Murias et al., 2007b) have indicated both increased and decreased connectivity in a number of frequency bands. Decreases in delta band functional connectivity, measured using synchronization likelihood between frontal and occipital EEG sensors has also been demonstrated (Barttfeld et al., 2011). Magnetoencephalography-based connectivity in ASD has been investigated using mutual information, PDC and MSC, with the goal of extracting useful biomarkers (Tsiaras et al., 2011) potentially able to aid in

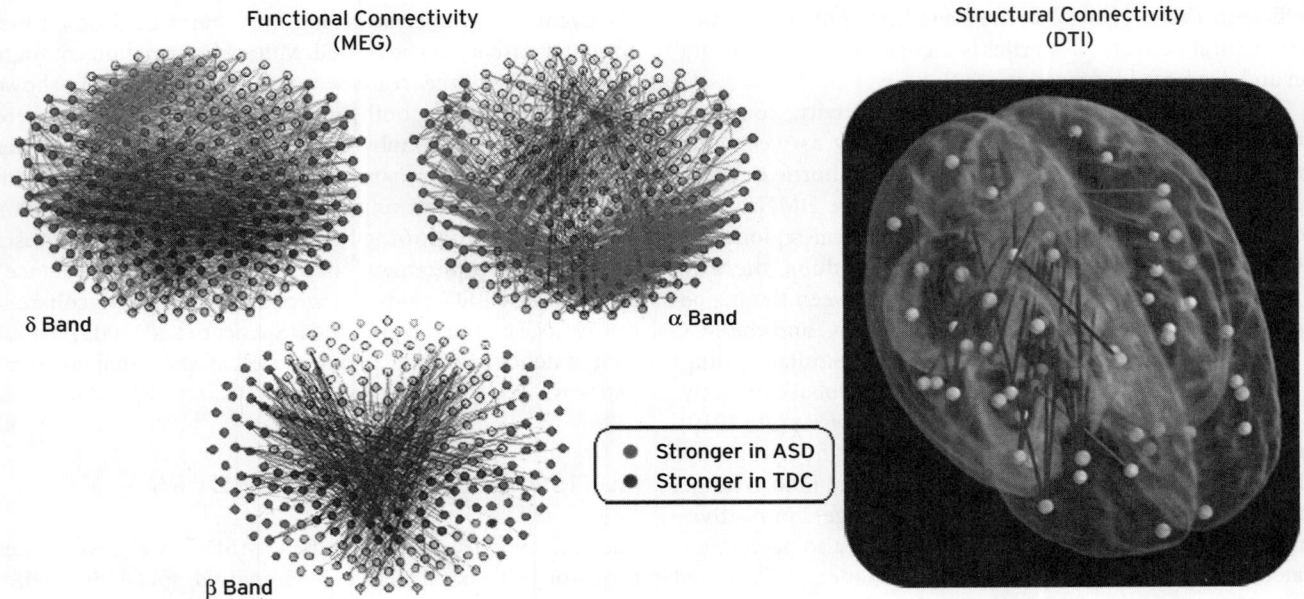

Functional Connectivity (MEG)

δ Band

α Band

β Band

● Stronger in ASD
● Stronger in TDC

Structural Connectivity (DTI)

Figure 75.4 *Structural and functional connectivity differences between ASD subjects and TDCS. Probabilistic tractography was used to compute DTI-based structural connectivity networks for each subject, which were then subjected to statistical analysis. Synchronization likelihood was used to compute functional connectivity networks in five frequency sub-bands of resting state MEG time courses. Shown are the significant different connections in the δ (0.5 to 4 Hz), α (8 to 13 Hz), and β (13 to 30 Hz). Light gray lines indicate connections that are stronger in the ASD population (predominantly shorter range frontal delta-band connections and posterior alpha-band connections), whereas dark gray lines indicated stronger connections in the TDC population (predominantly longer range and interhemispheric connections). (See color insert).*

early diagnosis, prognosis, and stratification for treatment. Differences in the dominant components of MEG-based synchronization likelihood connectivity networks have also been shown (Ghanbari et al., 2012), with ASD subjects lacking a clear interhemispheric connectivity component, but having elevated local frontal delta- and posterior alpha-band connectivity. Figure 75.4 shows representative structural and functional connectivity differences between ASD subjects and typically developing controls (TDCs).

ATTENTION DEFICIT/HYPERACTIVITY DISORDER

One of the most common neurodevelopmental disorders affecting children and adolescents (and, indeed, adults) is attention deficit/hyperactivity disorder (ADHD). Attention deficit/hyperactivity disorder is commonly characterized by impaired attention and concentration, along with increased hyperactivity and impulsivity. Although pharmacological intervention is often successful, the neuronal underpinnings of the disorder remain poorly understood.

A number of rs-fMRI studies (Castellanos and Proal, 2012; Konrad and Eickhoff, 2010) have used ROI-based temporal correlations to examine differences in the connectivity of the default mode network (DMN). Activity in the DMN has been found, driven by decreases in connectivity between the anterior cingulate, the posterior cingulate, and the precuneus. Similarly, ICA analysis of a working memory task (Wolf et al.,

2009) demonstrated decreased connectivity in adults with ADHD, of the anterior cingulate, ventrolateral prefrontal cortex, and superior parietal lobule, as well as increased connectivity in right prefrontal regions, and the left dorsal cingulate, and left cuneus.

Structural connectivity studies of ADHD have shown abnormal structural connectivity in a number of pathways thought to be involved in ADHD symptomatology. Decreases in the FA of the right cingulum and right SLF, both pathways related to executive function, have been demonstrated in ADHD subjects (Makris et al., 2008). Similarly, FA decreases were found in the cortical spinal tract (Hamilton et al., 2008) and the premotor WM regions (Ashtari et al., 2005). Overall, these results support the hypothesis of abnormal structural connectivity in the attention, motor, and executive function networks.

Electrophysiology studies of ADHD have focused primarily on the investigation of differences in local parameters such as spectral power, computed from the time series of each sensor (see Barry et al., 2005 for a comprehensive review). Because source localization techniques have improved, these types of studies have begun to focus on brain regions implicated by other neuroimaging techniques. For instance, Wilson et al. (2011) investigated resting state MEG in the DMN, finding broadband differences in the medial prefrontal cortex activation. More complex connectivity-based analyses are just beginning to be used to study ADHD. Studies using EEG coherence (MSE) to measure connectivity have found differences in intrahemispheric and interhemispheric coherences (Murias et al., 2007a).

OBSESSIVE COMPULSIVE DISORDER

Obsessive compulsive disorder (OCD) is a highly prevalent anxiety disorder that typically presents during childhood or adolescence. Obsessive compulsive disorder is generally characterized by the presence of persistent intrusive thoughts, feelings, and impulses (obsessions), as well as repetitive behaviors (compulsions) such as excessive washing/cleaning, checking, or counting. A growing body of structural and functional neuroimaging research has focused on interactions among the thalamus, striatum, and frontal cortices as being abnormal in subjects with OCD (Del Casale et al., 2011).

More recently, fMRI-based functional connectivity studies have focused on regions participating in the frontal-striatal-thalamic networks in the hopes of better characterizing the nature of their involvement in OCD. Fitzgerald et al. (2011) utilized a seed-based rs-fMRI paradigm to illustrate reduced connectivity among the dorsal striatum, thalamus, and cingulate, while also finding increased connectivity between the dorsal striatum and the medial frontal cortex. Using a task-based fMRI paradigm focused on risk aversion, Admon et al. (2012) found decreased functional connectivity between the amygdala and anterior cingulate, in addition to deceased connectivity between the nucleus accumbens and the orbital frontal areas. Similarly altered interactions between the frontoparietal networks and the DMN have been illustrated using ROI-based rs-fMRI (Stern et al., 2012). Structural connectivity findings based on DW-MRI have been more heterogeneous (Fontenelle et al., 2009), with some studies reporting increased FA in OCD patients (Gruner et al., 2012; Li et al., 2011), whereas others (Admon et al., 2012; Garibotto et al., 2010; Nakamae et al., 2011) report lower FA values.

TOURETTE SYNDROME

Tourette syndrome (TS) is a neuropsychiatric developmental disorder characterized by multiply unwanted physical and vocal tics. Similar to the neuroimaging studies of OCD, many studies of connectivity in TS have focused on the connectivity of frontal regions thought to participate in planning and impulse control.

A number of studies have used rs-fMRI to investigate connectivity in TS. Worbe et al. (2012) used ICA to identify three corticobasal networks (motor, associative, and limbic). ROIs were then placed within these networks and correlation-based connectivity measures were computed. The authors found increased global integration, increased connection strength, and lower characteristic path lengths in all three networks of TS patients. Similarly Church et al. used rs-fMRI to investigate connectivity in task-control networks (Church et al., 2009). They compared these networks with normative data collected on developing adolescents and found that the networks of patients with TS were characterized by *immature* functional connectivity. A task-based fMRI has also been used to investigate connectivity in TS. Wang et al. (2011) used ICA to extract activity that was correlated to both spontaneous and stimulated tics. Using Granger causality, computed between the major ROIs of the ICA networks, the authors showed increases in activity and interregional causality among the regions of the motor pathway. Increased connectivity in the motor system has also been observed using coherence measures computed from MEG data (Franzkowiak et al., 2012). Structural connectivity differences have also been observed in TS. Whole brain analysis of DTI-based scalar metrics have shown decreased FA in the corpus callosum, forceps minor, and internal capsule as well as increase in mean diffusivity in the corticostriatal projections (Govindan et al., 2010; Jackson et al., 2011; Neuner et al., 2010). Probabilistic tractography has also been utilized to quantify connectivity differences in TS, showing decreased connectivity in the fronto-thalamic-striatal networks (Makki et al., 2009).

CONCLUSIONS

Taken together, it can be seen that an emerging body of endeavor and research is focused on advancing our description of brain function to incorporate the dynamics of spatial networks of coordinated regions throughout the brain. In so doing, it is clear that the field is embracing both spatial and spectrotemporal descriptors of brain activity, as well as recognizing the need for increasingly sophisticated mathematical modeling to integrate data, as well as to reduce it to quantifiable metrics of connectivity globally, and of individual connections themselves. As the methodology advances, clinical applications incorporate these analyses providing an increasingly rich description, and ultimately an increasing neurobiological understanding of neuropsychiatric disorders. As with all emerging technologies, the opportunity for erroneous confounds is prevalent, requiring due consideration of both acquisition and analysis steps. Given the multidisciplinary nature of this effort, it seems that "highly connected" teams of clinicians, imagers, and mathematicians are a prerequisite to the successful development of the field.

ACKNOWLEDGMENTS

The authors would like to thank Yasser Ghanbari, Madhura Ingalhalikar, and Alex Smith in creating the synchronization likelihood and ASD-TD group differences figure, and Ted Satterthwaite for his work on default mode networks that made the figure possible. Dr. Roberts would like to thank the Oberkircher family for the Oberkircher Family Chair in Pediatric Radiology.

DISCLOSURES

Dr. Bloy has no conflicts of interest to disclose.

Dr. Verma receives grant support from the NIH (R01 MH092862, R01 MH073174, and R01 MH079938),

Dr. Roberts serves on the Medical Advisory Board of Prism Clinical Imaging for which he has received stock options in that company. He had also received compensation from Elekta for educational presentations. He receives grant support from NIH (R01 DC008871), Simons Foundation, Nancy Lurie Marks Family Foundation, and Seaside Therapeutics.

REFERENCES

Admon, R., Bleich-Cohen, M., et al. (2012). Functional and structural neural indices of risk aversion in obsessive-compulsive disorder (OCD). *Psychiatry Res.* 203(2–3):207–213.

Ameis, S.H., Fan, J., et al. (2011). Impaired structural connectivity of socio-emotional circuits in autism spectrum disorders: a diffusion tensor imaging study. *PLoS One* 6(11):e28044.

Ances, B.M., Leontiev, O., et al. (2008). Regional differences in the coupling of cerebral blood flow and oxygen metabolism changes in response to activation: implications for BOLD-fMRI. *NeuroImage* 39(4):1510–1521.

Ashtari, M., Kumra, S., et al. (2005). Attention-deficit/hyperactivity disorder: a preliminary diffusion tensor imaging study. *Biol. Psychiatry* 57(5):448–455.

Barry, R.J., Clarke, A.R., et al. (2005). Electrophysiology in attention-deficit/hyperactivity disorder. *Int. J. Psychophysiol.* 58(1):1–3.

Barttfeld, P., Wicker, B., et al. (2011). A big-world network in ASD: dynamical connectivity analysis reflects a deficit in long-range connections and an excess of short-range connections. *Neuropsychologia* 49(2):254–263.

Basser, P.J., and Pierpaoli, C. (1996). Microstructural and physiological features of tissues elucidated by quantitative-diffusion-tensor MRI. *J. Magn. Reson. B* 111(3):209–219.

Bassett, D.S., Bullmore, E.T., et al. (2009). Cognitive fitness of cost-efficient brain functional networks. *Proc. Natl. Acad. Sci. USA* 106(28):11747–11752.

Bassett, D.S., Brown, J.A., et al. (2011). Conserved and variable architecture of human white matter connectivity. *NeuroImage* 54(2):1262–1279.

Bastiani, M., Shah, N.J., et al. (2012). Human cortical connectome reconstruction from diffusion weighted MRI: the effect of tractography algorithm. *NeuroImage* 62(3):1732–1749.

Batmanghelich, N.K., Taskar, B., et al. (2012). Generative-discriminative basis learning for medical imaging. *IEEE Trans. Med. Imaging* 31(1):51–69.

Behrens, T.E., Berg, H.J., et al. (2007). Probabilistic diffusion tractography with multiple fibre orientations: what can we gain? *Neuroimage* 34(1):144–155.

Biswal, B., Yetkin, F.Z., et al. (1995). Functional connectivity in the motor cortex of resting human brain using echo-planar MRI. *Magn. Reson. Med.* 34(4):537–541.

Bullmore, E.T., Frangou, S., et al. (1997). The dysplastic net hypothesis: an integration of developmental and dysconnectivity theories of schizophrenia. *Schizophr. Res.* 28(2–3):143–156.

Calhoun, V.D., Kiehl, K.A., et al. (2008). Modulation of temporally coherent brain networks estimated using ICA at rest and during cognitive tasks. *Hum. Brain Mapp.* 29(7):828–838.

Castellanos, F.X., and Proal, E. (2012). Large-scale brain systems in ADHD: beyond the prefrontal-striatal model. *Trends Cogn. Sci.* 16(1):17–26.

Church, J.A., Wenger, K.K., et al. (2009). Task control signals in pediatric tourette syndrome show evidence of immature and anomalous functional activity. *Front. Hum. Neurosci.* 3:38.

Courchesne, E., and Pierce, K. (2005). Why the frontal cortex in autism might be talking only to itself: local over-connectivity but long-distance disconnection. *Curr. Opin. Neurobiol.* 15(2):225–230.

Del Casale, A., Kotzalidis, G.D., et al. (2011). Functional neuroimaging in obsessive-compulsive disorder. *Neuropsychobiology* 64(2):61–85.

Ebisch, S.J., Gallese, V., et al. (2011). Altered intrinsic functional connectivity of anterior and posterior insula regions in high-functioning participants with autism spectrum disorder. *Hum. Brain Mapp.* 32(7):1013–1028.

Fair, D.A., Cohen, A.L., et al. (2009). Functional brain networks develop from a 'local to distributed' organization. *PLoS Comput. Biol.* 5(5):e1000381.

Fitzgerald, K.D., Welsh, R.C., et al. (2011). Developmental alterations of frontal-striatal-thalamic connectivity in obsessive-compulsive disorder. *J. Am. Acad. Child Adolesc. Psychiatry* 50(9):938–948 e933.

Fontenelle, L.F., Harrison, B.J., et al. (2009). Is there evidence of brain white-matter abnormalities in obsessive-compulsive disorder?: a narrative review. *Top. Magn. Reson. Imaging* 20(5):291–298.

Fox, M.D., and Raichle, M.E. (2007). Spontaneous fluctuations in brain activity observed with functional magnetic resonance imaging. *Nat. Rev. Neurosci.* 8(9):700–711.

Franzkowiak, S., Pollok, B., et al. (2012). Motor-cortical interaction in Gilles de la Tourette syndrome. *PLoS One* 7(1):e27850.

Friston, K.J., Frith, C.D., et al. (1993). Functional connectivity: the principal-component analysis of large (PET) data sets. *J. Cereb. Blood Flow. Metab.* 13(1):5–14.

Friston, K.J., Harrison, L., et al. (2003). Dynamic causal modelling. *Neuroimage* 19(4):1273–1302.

Friston, K.J., Ungerleider, L.G., et al. (1994). Characterizing modulatory interactions between areas V1 and V2 in human cortex: a new treatment of functional MRI data. *Hum. Brain Mapp.* 2(4):211–224.

Gandal, M.J., Edgar, J.C., et al. (2012). Gamma synchrony: towards a translational biomarker for the treatment-resistant symptoms of schizophrenia. *Neuropharmacol.* 62(3):1504–1518.

Garibotto, V., Scifo, P., et al. (2010). Disorganization of anatomical connectivity in obsessive compulsive disorder: a multi-parameter diffusion tensor imaging study in a subpopulation of patients. *Neurobiol. Dis.* 37(2):468–476.

Ghanbari, Y., Bloy, L., et al. (2012). Dominant component analysis of electrophysiological connectivity networks. *MICCAI* 15(Pt 3):468–475.

Ghuman, A.S., McDaniel, J.R., et al. (2011). A wavelet-based method for measuring the oscillatory dynamics of resting-state functional connectivity in MEG. *Neuroimage* 56(1):69–77.

Gong, G., Rosa-Neto, P., et al. (2009). Age- and gender-related differences in the cortical anatomical network. *J. Neurosci.* 29(50):15684–15693.

Goodlett, C.B., Fletcher, P.T., et al. (2009). Group analysis of DTI fiber tract statistics with application to neurodevelopment. *Neuroimage* 45(1 Suppl):S133–S142.

Govindan, R.M., Makki, M.I., et al. (2010). Abnormal water diffusivity in corticostriatal projections in children with Tourette syndrome. *Hum. Brain. Mapp.* 31(11):1665–1674.

Gruner, P., Vo, A., et al. (2012). White matter abnormalities in pediatric obsessive-compulsive disorder. *Neuropsychopharmacol.* 37(12):2730–2739.

Hagmann, P., Kurant, M., et al. (2007). Mapping human whole-brain structural networks with diffusion MRI. *PLoS One* 2(7):e597.

Hagmann, P., Sporns, O., et al. (2010). White matter maturation reshapes structural connectivity in the late developing human brain. *Proc. Natl. Acad. Sci. USA* 107(44):19067–19072.

Hamilton, L.S., Levitt, J.G., et al. (2008). Reduced white matter integrity in attention-deficit hyperactivity disorder. *NeuroReport* 19(17):1705–1708.

Hasan, K.M., Sankar, A., et al. (2007). Development and organization of the human brain tissue compartments across the lifespan using diffusion tensor imaging. *Neuroreport* 18(16):1735–1739.

Honey, G.D., Pomarol-Clotet, E., et al. (2005). Functional dysconnectivity in schizophrenia associated with attentional modulation of motor function. *Brain* 128(Pt 11):2597–2611.

Jackson, S.R., Parkinson, A., et al. (2011). Compensatory neural reorganization in Tourette syndrome. *Curr. Biol.* 21(7):580–585.

Jones, D.K. (2010). Challenges and limitations of quantifying brain connectivity *in vivo* with diffusion MRI. *Imaging Med.* 2(3):341–355.

Just, M.A., Keller, T.A., et al. (2012). Autism as a neural systems disorder: a theory of frontal-posterior underconnectivity. *Neurosci. Biobehav. Rev.* 36(4):1292–1313.

Konrad, K., and Eickhoff, S.B. (2010). Is the ADHD brain wired differently? A review on structural and functional connectivity in attention deficit hyperactivity disorder. *Hum. Brain Mapp.* 31(6):904–916.

Kwong, K.K., Belliveau, J.W., et al. (1992). Dynamic magnetic resonance imaging of human brain activity during primary sensory stimulation. *Proc. Natl. Acad. Sci. USA* 89(12):5675–5679.

Lebel, C., Gee, M., et al. (2012). Diffusion tensor imaging of white matter tract evolution over the lifespan. *NeuroImage* 60(1):340–352.

Li, F., Huang, X., et al. (2011). Microstructural brain abnormalities in patients with obsessive-compulsive disorder: diffusion-tensor MR imaging study at 3.0 T. *Radiology* 260(1):216–223.

Lynall, M.E., Bassett, D.S., et al. (2010). Functional connectivity and brain networks in schizophrenia. *J. Neurosci.* 30(28):9477–9487.

Madler, B., Drabycz, S.A., et al. (2008). Is diffusion anisotropy an accurate monitor of myelination? Correlation of multicomponent T2 relaxation and diffusion tensor anisotropy in human brain. *Magn. Reson. Imaging* 26(7):874–888.

Makki, M.I., Govindan, R.M., et al. (2009). Altered fronto-striato-thalamic connectivity in children with Tourette syndrome assessed with diffusion tensor MRI and probabilistic fiber tracking. *J. Child Neurol.* 24(6):669–678.

Makris, N., Buka, S.L., et al. (2008). Attention and executive systems abnormalities in adults with childhood ADHD: a DT-MRI study of connections. *Cereb. Cortex* 18(5):1210–1220.

Markov, N.T., Misery, P., et al. (2011). Weight consistency specifies regularities of macaque cortical networks. *Cereb. Cortex* 21(6):1254–1272.

Montez, T., Linkenkaer-Hansen, K., et al. (2006). Synchronization likelihood with explicit time-frequency priors. *NeuroImage* 33(4):1117–1125.

Murias, M., Swanson, J.M., et al. (2007a). Functional connectivity of frontal cortex in healthy and ADHD children reflected in EEG coherence. *Cereb. Cortex* 17(8):1788–1799.

Murias, M., Webb, S.J., et al. (2007b). Resting state cortical connectivity reflected in EEG coherence in individuals with autism. *Biol. Psychiatry* 62(3):270–273.

Nagae, L.M., Zarnow, D.M., et al. (2012). Elevated mean diffusivity in the left hemisphere superior longitudinal fasciculus in autism spectrum disorders increases with more profound language impairment. *AJNR Am. J. Neuroradiol.* 33:1642–1650.

Nakamae, T., Narumoto, J., et al. (2011). Diffusion tensor imaging and tract-based spatial statistics in obsessive-compulsive disorder. *J. Psychiatr. Res.* 45(5):687–690.

Neuner, I., Kupriyanova, Y., et al. (2010). White-matter abnormalities in Tourette syndrome extend beyond motor pathways. *NeuroImage* 51(3):1184–1193.

Power, J.D., Fair, D.A., et al. (2010). The development of human functional brain networks. *Neuron* 67(5):735–748.

Quian Quiroga, R., Kraskov, A., et al. (2002). Performance of different synchronization measures in real data: a case study on electroencephalographic signals. *Phys. Rev. E. Stat. Nonlin. Soft. Matter Phys.* 65(4 Pt 1):041903.

Roebroeck, A., Formisano, E., et al. (2005). Mapping directed influence over the brain using Granger causality and fMRI. *NeuroImage* 25(1):230–242.

Rosazza, C., and Minati, L. (2011). Resting-state brain networks: literature review and clinical applications. *Neurol. Sci.* 32(5):773–785.

Rubinov, M., and Sporns, O. (2010). Complex network measures of brain connectivity: uses and interpretations. *Neuroimage* 52(3):1059–1069.

Sakkalis, V. (2011). Review of advanced techniques for the estimation of brain connectivity measured with EEG/MEG. *Comput. Biol. Med.* 41(12):1110–1117.

Salmelin, R., and Baillet, S. (2009). Electromagnetic brain imaging. *Hum. Brain. Mapp.* 30(6):1753–1757.

Sameshima, K., and Baccala, L.A. (1999). Using partial directed coherence to describe neuronal ensemble interactions. *J. Neurosci. Methods* 94(1):93–103.

Satterthwaite, T.D., Wolf, D.H., et al. (2012). Impact of in-scanner head motion on multiple measures of functional connectivity: relevance for studies of neurodevelopment in youth. *NeuroImage* 60(1):623–632.

Schoffelen, J.M., and Gross, J. (2009). Source connectivity analysis with MEG and EEG. *Hum Brain Mapp.* 30(6):1857–1865.

Shaw, P., Gogtay, N., et al. (2010). Childhood psychiatric disorders as anomalies in neurodevelopmental trajectories. *Hum. Brain Mapp.* 31(6):917–925.

Smit, D.J., Boersma, M., et al. (2012). The brain matures with stronger functional connectivity and decreased randomness of its network. *PLoS One* 7(5):e36896.

Spencer, K.M., Nestor, P.G., et al. (2003). Abnormal neural synchrony in schizophrenia. *J. Neurosci.* 23(19):7407–7411.

Sporns, O. (2011). The human connectome: a complex network. *Ann. NY Acad. Sci.* 1224:109–125.

Sporns, O., Tononi, G., et al. (2005). The human connectome: a structural description of the human brain. *PLoS Comput. Biol.* 1(4):e42.

Stam, C.J. (2005). Nonlinear dynamical analysis of EEG and MEG: review of an emerging field. *Clin. Neurophysiol.* 116(10):2266–2301.

Stephan, K.E., and Roebroeck, A. (2012). A short history of causal modeling of fMRI data. *Neuroimage* 62(2):856–863.

Stern, E.R., Fitzgerald, K.D., et al. (2012). Resting-state functional connectivity between fronto-parietal and default mode networks in obsessive-compulsive disorder. *PLoS One* 7(5):e36356.

Sundaram, S.K., Kumar, A., et al. (2008). Diffusion tensor imaging of frontal lobe in autism spectrum disorder. *Cereb. Cortex* 18(11):2659–2665.

Supekar, K., Uddin, L.Q., et al. (2010). Development of functional and structural connectivity within the default mode network in young children. *NeuroImage* 52(1):290–301.

Tsiaras, V., Simos, P.G., et al. (2011). Extracting biomarkers of autism from MEG resting-state functional connectivity networks. *Comput. Biol. Med.* 41(12):1166–1177.

Tuch, D.S. (2004). Q-ball imaging. *Magn. Reson. Med.* 52(6):1358–1372.

Van Dijk, K.R., Sabuncu, M.R., et al. (2012). The influence of head motion on intrinsic functional connectivity MRI. *NeuroImage* 59(1):431–438.

Wang, Q., Su, T.P., et al. (2012). Anatomical insights into disrupted small-world networks in schizophrenia. *NeuroImage* 59(2):1085–1093.

Wang, Z., Maia, T.V., et al. (2011). The neural circuits that generate tics in Tourette's syndrome. *Am. J. Psychiatry* 168(12):1326–1337.

Welsh, J.P., Ahn, E.S., et al. (2005). Is autism due to brain desynchronization? *Int. J. Dev. Neurosci.* 23(2–3):253–263.

Weng, S.J., Wiggins, J.L., et al. (2010). Alterations of resting state functional connectivity in the default network in adolescents with autism spectrum disorders. *Brain Res.* 1313: 202–214.

Westin, C.F., Maier, S.E., et al. (2002). Processing and visualization for diffusion tensor MRI. *Med. Image Anal.* 6(2):93–108.

Whitfield-Gabrieli, S., Thermenos, H.W., et al. (2009). Hyperactivity and hyperconnectivity of the default network in schizophrenia and in first-degree relatives of persons with schizophrenia. *Proc. Natl. Acad. Sci. USA* 106(4):1279–1284.

Wilson, T.W., Franzen, J.D., et al. (2011). Broadband neurophysiological abnormalities in the medial prefrontal region of the default-mode network in adults with ADHD. *Hum. Brain Mapp.* 15: 310–320.

Wolf, R.C., Plichta, M.M., et al. (2009). Regional brain activation changes and abnormal functional connectivity of the ventrolateral prefrontal cortex during working memory processing in adults with attention-deficit/hyperactivity disorder. *Hum. Brain Mapp.* 30(7):2252–2266.

Worbe, Y., Malherbe, C., et al. (2012). Functional immaturity of cortico-basal ganglia networks in Gilles de la Tourette syndrome. *Brain* 135(Pt 6):1937–1946.

Yeo, B.T., Krienen, F.M., et al. (2011). The organization of the human cerebral cortex estimated by intrinsic functional connectivity. *J. Neurophysiol.* 106(3):1125–1165.

Zalesky, A., Fornito, A., et al. (2011a). Disrupted axonal fiber connectivity in schizophrenia. *Biol. Psychiatry* 69(1):80–89.

Zalesky, A., Fornito, A., et al. (2010a). Network-based statistic: identifying differences in brain networks. *NeuroImage* 53(4):1197–1207.

Zalesky, A., Fornito, A., et al. (2010b). Whole-brain anatomical networks: does the choice of nodes matter? *NeuroImage* 50(3):970–983.

Zhou, Y., Liang, M., et al. (2007). Functional disintegration in paranoid schizophrenia using resting-state fMRI. *Schizophr. Res.* 97(1–3):194–205.

76 | INTELLECTUAL DISABILITY SYNDROMES

CHARLES E. SCHWARTZ, FIORELLA GURRIERI, AND GIOVANNI NERI

Genetic syndromes that include intellectual disability (ID) as one component manifestation are each individually rare but, taken together, constitute a large group of causally heterogeneous and phenotypically variable conditions. It is difficult, if not impossible, to establish their exact number, given the existence of many "private" conditions, especially those caused by chromosomal imbalances. It is equally hard to provide prevalence estimates, except for some syndromes that are more prevalent and better known, such as Noonan syndrome, Fragile X syndrome, DiGeorge syndrome, Rett syndrome, and Williams syndrome, to mention just a few. Fortunately, significant information can be derived from open access databases (e.g., OMIM—Online Mendelian Inheritance in Man at *http://www.ncbi.nlm.nih.gov/omim*, Orphanet at *http://www.orpha.net*, and DECIPHER at http://decipher.sanger.ac.uk) that collect and store relevant data from the medical literature.

From the point of view of the clinical geneticist, who deals with these rare patients and their families, a useful nosological classification of ID syndromes is by genetic etiology. Knowledge of the genetic cause is the sine qua non for accurate counseling and estimate of recurrence risks. However, even with the help of the most advanced technology, such as chromosome microarray (CMA) and whole exome or other forms of next-generation sequencing, the cause remains unknown probably in one-third or more of the cases seen in genetic clinics. The main etiological classes are listed in Table 76.1, together with tentative prevalence estimates among live born.

Understanding the genes underlying ID is also of great interest for neurobiological studies because they can lead to a molecular and cellular understanding of pathobiology, and gene products represent potential therapeutic targets. One of the most well-known examples of these possibilities arise from Fragile X syndrome, in which animal models with disruptions of the causal gene (*FMR1*) have led to an understanding of synaptic deficits in the disorder, and to novel therapeutics that are beginning to show promise (see, e.g., Berry-Kravis et al., 2012).

The diagnostic approach to the patient who is affected with a syndromic form of ID requires the application of a number of steps. Short of a "gestalt" diagnosis, which may occasionally apply to cases of well-known syndromes, the approach includes the collection of a (at least) three-generation family tree, prenatal and postnatal history, physical examination, relevant imaging data of brain, heart, kidneys, and so on, and functional data, such as EEG. Laboratory tests can be specific for the diagnosis of given syndromes in the presence of a specific clinical suspicion. Otherwise, CMA and analysis of the *FMR1* gene are usually considered first-line tests. Next-generation sequencing is becoming more and more applicable to those cases in which all other approaches failed to reach a causal diagnosis. In the end, it should be made clear to the parents and caregivers alike that lack of a causal diagnosis does not preclude the application of symptomatic, as well as rehabilitating treatments, as deemed appropriate on the basis of the phenotypic manifestations and the patient's needs.

This chapter briefly describes a few selected examples of ID syndromes. The selection was made with the purpose of illustrating various molecular pathways and/or cellular compartments whose disruption as a consequence of genetic mutation cause a disruption of a developmental pathway and, ultimately, an ID syndrome.

This arbitrary selection leaves out numerous syndromic ID conditions even though their causative genes have been identified after incredible research. To get a feel of the genetic burden in ID, some estimates have been attempted: X-linked intellectual disability (XLID) accounts for 5% to 10% of ID in males. More than 150 syndromes, the most common of which is the Fragile X syndrome, have been described. A large number of families with nonsyndromal XLID, 95 of which have been regionally mapped, have been described as well. Mutations in 102 X-linked genes have been associated with 81 of these XLID syndromes and 35 forms of nonsyndromal XLID (Lubs et al., 2012). The distinction between syndromic and non-syndromic ID is not precise, and several genes, initially identified in syndromic conditions, have later been associated with non-syndromic forms (e.g., *ARX, CASK, JARID1C, FGD1,* and *ATRX*).

As for autosomal ID, mutations in approximately 450 genes have been reported, of which 50 genes are associated with non-syndromic ID and 400 genes are associated with syndromic ID (van Bokhoven, 2011). In spite of the rapid progress in disease gene identification, it is difficult to predict how many additional ID genes remain to be identified. Based on the number of approximately 100 known XLID genes (syndromic as well as non-syndromic), a total of 1,500 to 2,000 genes might be a reasonable estimate (van Bokhoven, 2011). The lack of knowledge is even more expansive when it comes to the biological consequences of these mutations on brain functions. Mutant genes encode proteins with a variety of functions including chromatin remodeling, presynaptic and postsynaptic activity, intracellular trafficking, neurogenesis, and neuronal migration. Interestingly, most of the pathways and about half of the genes identified as being involved in ID have also been found

TABLE 76.1. Etiological classification of intellectual disability syndromes

CAUSE	PERCENTAGE
Genomic imbalance (detected cytogenetically or by array-CGH)	20
Mendelian mutations	7
Environmental	23
Unknown but likely of genetic origin	50

(From Curry et al. (1997); Mefford et al. (2012); Ropers (2010); Winnepenninckx et al. (2003).)

to be altered in patients with autism spectrum disorders (ASD) suggesting that these two neurodevelopmental disorders share a common genetic basis (Betancur, 2011).

In the following sections, the selected syndromes are grouped by mode of inheritance: autosomal dominant, autosomal recessive, and X-linked.

AUTOSOMAL DOMINANT

CARDIO-FACIO-CUTANEOUS SYNDROME

Cardio-facio-cutaneous syndrome (CFCS) was first described by Reynolds et al., in 1986. Twenty years later came the demonstration that it is caused by disruption of the RAS-ERK signaling pathway (Narumi et al., 2007; Rodriguez-Viciana et al., 2006), placing it nosologically within the group of RASopathies (Rauen et al., 2010). Although initially it was considered by some authors to be a variant of the Noonan syndrome, the discovery of the causal genes proved it to be a distinct entity, as maintained by Neri et al. (1991).

The incidence of the syndrome is unknown. Since 1986, about 100 cases were reported in the medical literature and more than 100 unpublished cases are known to CFC International, Inc., a family support group operating worldwide (*http://www.cfcsyndrome.org*). This number probably accounts for a fraction of cases because it excludes most mildly affected individuals. All affected subjects to date are sporadic, most likely because of new dominant mutations, as supported by the observation of a paternal age effect (Roberts et al., 2006).

Cardio-facio-cutaneous syndrome has a distinctive clinical presentation starting at pregnancy, which can be uneventful, but is often marked by polyhydramnios. Hypotonia and serious and often longstanding feeding difficulties are hallmarks of the early postnatal period. Feeding problems are especially troublesome, with poor sucking, aspiration, gastroesophageal reflux, oral aversion, hyperemesis, and gastrointestinal dysmotility, leading to serious and long-lasting failure to thrive. These problems are significant enough to require nasogastric tube feeding, or gastrostomy tube placement in some cases. Assisted feeding may be required into middle childhood or beyond. The physical phenotype is characterized by short stature with relative macrocephaly, distinctive facial appearance with high forehead, bitemporal narrowing, downslanting and wide-spaced palpebral

fissures, ptosis, short nose with depressed nasal root, low-set ears with creases on the lobes, sparse curly hair, sparse or absent eyebrows and lashes, ectodermal findings especially follicular keratosis, hyperkeratosis, hyperelastic skin, cutaneous vascular malformations, pigmented nevi, and congenital heart defects, pulmonic stenosis, hypertrophic cardiomyopathy, and atrial septal defects being the most frequent. Intellectual disability, of moderate to severe degree, is almost invariably present. Many children display tactile defensiveness, short attention span, irritability, stubbornness, and obsessive behavior. A minority act aggressively toward others. Nonetheless, parents often comment on a warm and loving personality and an enjoyment of social interactions, particularly music and dance. Epilepsy can be a serious complication in about one-third of cases. It can present as infantile spasms, and absence, generalized, or partial complex seizures. On brain imaging, ventriculomegaly, reduced white matter, and thinning of the corpus callosum are the most common findings. Life expectancy is shortened on average because of the early death of individuals with severe cardiac involvement (Armour and Allanson, 2008).

Noonan syndrome and Costello syndrome, especially the former, are the main differential diagnoses, and there is marked phenotypic overlap among the three conditions. Individuals with Noonan syndrome have normal intelligence or mild psychomotor involvement, less common and less severe failure to thrive, and a history of bleeding disorder. Differences between Costello syndrome and CFCS include skin papillomata, deep palmar and plantar creases, a significant likelihood of chaotic atrial arrhythmia or multifocal atrial tachycardia, and most important, an increased risk of malignant tumors such as rhabdomyosarcoma, transitional cell carcinoma of the bladder, and neuroblastoma.

In 2006, Niihori et al. and Rodriguez-Viciana et al. discovered the genes whose mutations cause CFCS. These are *BRAF*, *KRAS*, *MEK1*, and *MEK2*. Their protein products are components of the RAS-ERK signaling pathway, which is implicated in growth factor-mediated cell proliferation, differentiation, and apoptosis, and plays a crucial role in embryonic development. *RAS* genes encode GTP-binding proteins that function as on-off switches to activate or inhibit downstream molecules. *BRAF* mutations account for the majority of mutation-positive cases (65.8%), followed by *MEK1* and *2* and, more rarely, *KRAS*. Dysregulation of the RAS/ERK pathway is the common underlying mechanism of the phenotypic relatedness of CFCS to Noonan and Costello syndrome, whose genes encode proteins that are also part of the RAS/ERK pathway (Fig. 76.1; Table 76.2).

The role of the RAS/ERK pathway in cellular function is the subject of several recent reviews, including Tidyman and Rauen (2009). In terms of the role of this pathway in the dynamic aspects of CNS function, there is good evidence for a critical role of RAS/ERK signaling in synaptic plasticity and, hence, in learning and memory processes (Mazzucchelli and Brambilla, 2000). This impact on synaptic plasticity is very likely directly related to the impairments in intellectual functioning, and the frequent manifestations of autism spectrum disorder in CFCS.

BRAF and *KRAS* somatic mutations are often reported in human cancers. These are thought to be stronger

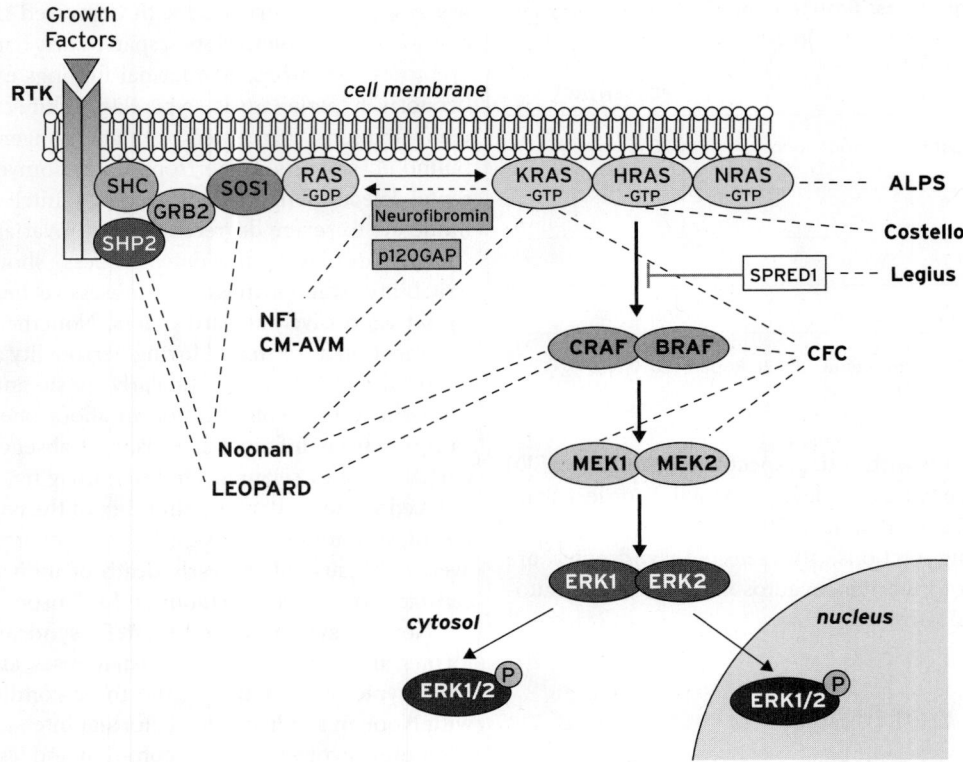

Figure 76.1 The RAS/mitogen-activated protein kinase (MAPK) signaling pathway. This pathway is critical for cell proliferation, differentiation, motility, apoptosis, and senescence. The dashed lines indicate the genes associated with various developmental syndromes. Of interest, some of the syndromes can result from a mutation in more than one of the genes in this pathway. (Adapted from Tidyman, W.E. and Rauen, K.A. (2009). The RASopathies: Developmental syndromes of Ras/MAPK pathway dysregulation. Curr. Opin. Genet. Dev. 19:230–236. Used with permission from Elsevier.)

TABLE 76.2. The RASopathies: syndromes and genes*

SYNDROMES	OMIM	GENES
Noonan	163950	PTPN11, KRAS, RAF1, SOS1, NRAS
Noonan-multiple lentigines	151100	PTPN11, BRAF, RAF1
Costello	218040*	HRAS
Cardio-facio-cutaneous (CFC)	115150	BRAF, MEK1, MEK2, KRAS
Noonan-like with anagen hair	607721	SHOC2
Noonan-like, with or without juvenile myelomonocytic leukemia	613563	CBL
Neurofibromatosis 1	162200	NF1
Legius (neurofibromatosis type1-like syndrome)	611431	SPRED1

*Costello syndrome is autosomal dominant. OMIM number needs updating.

gain-of-function mutations that would be embryo-lethal if present in the zygote. In CFCS, mutations are milder, compatible with (abnormal) development. The same is thought to be true for Noonan and Costello syndrome mutations. Yet, one would expect that patients affected with these syndromes would be more prone to cancer. This is true for Costello syndrome, but not for Noonan and CFCS, with some exceptions. However, it must be noted that all RASopathies patients may one day benefit from the intensive search of new cancer drugs acting as inhibitors of the RAS/ERK pathway, such as lonafarnib, sorafenib, statins, and so on. If and when an effective pharmacological treatment will become available based on these premises, it will be an example of successful translational medicine.

KABUKI SYNDROME

Kabuki syndrome (KS, OMIM #147920), first described in 1981 with the designation of Kabuki make-up syndrome, is characterized by ID, unusual face, large and protruding ears, and postnatal growth delay (Niikawa et al., 1981). The prevalence was estimated at 1:32,000 in the Japanese population (Niikawa et al., 1988), a figure likely to apply also to other ethnicities. Based on the observation of a large number of patients, Niikawa et al. (1988) established the following diagnostic criteria: (1) typical face with long palpebral fissures and eversion of the lateral third of the lower eyelid; arched eyebrows, sparse or notched in their lateral third; depressed nasal tip; large, protruding ears; (2) skeletal anomalies, including cleft and butterfly vertebrae, narrow intervertebral spaces, scoliosis, brachymesophalangy of hands and fifth finger clinodactyly;

(3) persistence of fetal pads on fingertips; (4) mild-to-moderate ID; (5) postnatal growth delay. The neonatal period is characterized by feeding difficulties, which may require tube feeding or gastrostomy, and consequent failure to thrive (Adam, et al., 2011).

A host of different physical anomalies can be present, adding to the complexity of the phenotype (Adam et al., 2011). Nearly half of the individuals with KS have a congenital heart defect, especially coarctation of the aorta (Kawame et al., 1999). Almost three-fourths have a highly arched palate, and one-third have a cleft lip and/or palate. Hypodontia is common, with missing lateral and central incisors. Hearing loss is also common, usually caused by chronic otitis media, but a few patients with true sensorineural hearing loss have been observed. Gastrointestinal anomalies are rare, whereas the genitourinary system is affected in about 25% of individuals with KS. Reported anomalies include fused and/or misplaced kidneys, duplication of collecting system, hypospadias, and cryptorchidism in males (Adam et al., 2011). In females, premature thelarche is fairly common. Brain structural anomalies seem to be rare, with the possible exception of Chiari I malformation, that has been reported in several patients. Immune dysfunction with hypogammaglobulinemia has been reported in a significant proportion of patients (Hoffman et al., 2005).

Most patients with KS have hypotonia, joint laxity, and delay of motoric development. The neuropsychiatric manifestations of KS are interesting. Although mild to moderate ID is reported in more than 90% of patients, the personality of KS children is usually described as pleasant and easy. Verbal and nonverbal reasoning, as well as receptive language seem to represent an area of relative strength, as opposed to expressive language and visuospatial orientation, which show considerable impairment (Mervis et al., 2005). In contrast with many other ID syndromes, autism or autistic spectrum disorders have been reported only rarely. Epilepsy is not a major concern, affecting less than one-third of patients with KS, who tend to respond well to antiepileptic medication.

Kabuki syndrome is an autosomal dominant disorder, with most cases caused by new mutations of the *MLL2* gene, a gene of 54 exons, encoding MLL2, a large protein of 5,262 amino acid residues, which belongs to the SET family of proteins. MLL2 is a histone 3 lysine 4 (H3-K4) methyltransferase, a regulator of gene transcription through epigenetic modulation. H3-K4 methylation is an epigenetic mark of euchromatin, favoring gene transcription. H3-K4 demethylation signals a transition from euchromatin to heterochromatin, inhibiting gene transcription. Loss of *Mll2* in mice causes cellular apoptosis and growth retardation, resulting in embryo lethality. The causative role of *MLL2* in KS was discovered in 2010 by Ng et al., who reported mutations in 10 unrelated patients utilizing whole exome sequencing. Mutations are found in about three-fourths of tested patients. The majority are nonsense or frameshift mutations, predicting a truncated protein and suggesting that haploinsufficiency is the underlying pathogenic mechanism. Mutations are distributed over the entire length of the gene, but are more prevalent in the 3' exons, leading to loss of the SET domain. Some canonical cases of KS without

MLL2 mutation suggest possible genetic heterogeneity of the syndrome.

There are more than 25 known histone methyltransferases in the human genome and several (including *NSD1*, discussed in the following section) have been implicated as genes involved in developmental delay syndromes. There are a similar number of histone demethylase genes, and some of these have also been implicated in developmental delay syndromes.

SOTOS SYNDROME

Sotos syndrome (SoS OMIM #117550) is characterized by overgrowth of prenatal onset persisting during the first years of life, advanced bone age, and characteristic facial features (Baujat and Cormier-Daire, 2007). Birth weight averages 4,200 g in males and 4,000 g in females, whereas mean birth length is 55.6 cm in males and 57.3 cm in females. The newborn period is affected by poor feeding and congenital hypotonia, the latter persisting into adult life. Occipitofrontal head circumference (OFC) tends to exceed the 97th centile by the age of one year. Final height is usually within normal range because of the advanced bone age, present in 84% of patients with SoS. Advanced bone age is common to many overgrowth syndromes, including Weaver and Beckwith-Wiedemann syndrome. However, SoS can be distinguished for the presence of a peculiar (disharmonic) metacarpophalangeal profile. Hand and foot length is often above the 97th centile; dental eruption can occur early; puberty can be precocious. Facial characteristics consist of marked frontal bossing (in 97.5% of patients), high frontal hairline (97.5%), frontoparietal balding, downslanting palpebral fissures (90%), narrow bitemporal diameter, full cheeks, and high palate (70%). The face gradually lengthens with age and the jaw becomes more prominent, with a pointed chin. Pes planus is frequent, and strabismus is found in nearly 40% of patients. The IQ is below average (mean of 78, ranging from 40 to 129), with delay in expressive language. Autistic behavior or other psychological problems, including abnormal social behavior and anxiety, may also be noted (Baujat and Cormier-Daire, 2007; Sarimski, 2003). Seizures have been reported to occur in 50% of cases. Brain magnetic resonance imaging can show a typical pattern of anomalies, including prominence of the trigonus (90%) and the occipital horns (75%), as well as ventriculomegaly (63%). The supratentorial extracerebral fluid spaces and those of the posterior fossa are increased for age in 70% of patients (Schaefer et al., 1997). Heart defects (i.e., septal defects and patent ductus arteriosus) are observed in 8% of patients with SoS, but seem to be as frequent as 35%–41% in patients of Japanese ethnicity. Gastrointestinal and urogenital anomalies have also been reported. Upper respiratory tract infections, especially otitis media, are frequent and may lead to conductive hearing loss. As in most overgrowth syndromes, increased risk of cancer is a concern. Cohen critically reviewed neoplasms reported to occur with SoS (Cohen, 2003). One-third of patients with neoplasia, all males, developed lympho-hematological malignancies (lymphoma or leukemia), which seem to represent the most frequent neoplasias in SoS. Many cases occurred after the age of five (10/22; 45%) or 10 years (4/22; 18%). Thus, it is not easy to give an overall recommendation for cancer surveillance in SoS.

The most frequent cause of SoS was discovered by Kurotaki and colleagues in 2002, who found rearrangements of the *NSD1* gene in SoS patients harboring a chromosomal translocation, encompassing band 5q35. They also identified one nonsense, three frameshift, and 20 submicroscopic deletions of the same gene among 42 sporadic cases (77%). This initial observation was followed by many other reports, confirming that haploinsufficiency of *NSD1* is the major cause of SoS (Niikawa, 2004). A recurrent 2.2-Mb microdeletion at 5q35, including *NSD1* and adjacent genes, is the primary cause of SoS in Japan, accounting for more than 50% of cases. In Europe and United States intragenic mutations cause 60% to 80% of SoS cases, whereas microdeletions are responsible for no more than 10% of cases. Partial *NSD1* deletions, encompassing one or more exons, were detected in SoS cases (6%) without *NSD1* mutation or 5q35 microdeletion (Douglas et al., 2005). In general, children carrying an *NSD1* deletion have severe ID, with no language, major delay in motor milestones, and autistic features. By contrast, in patients carrying *NSD1* point mutations, ID is usually mild to moderate with verbal skills being more affected. There have been suggestions that *NSD1* mutations may also cause the Weaver syndrome, a view that is hard to maintain after the discovery that the original cases of Weaver syndrome are caused by mutation of the *EZH2* gene (Gibson et al., 2012).

The function of the *NSD1* gene (nuclear-receptor-binding SET-domain-containing protein 1) is not entirely clear. Its protein product is likely to act as transcriptional regulator of other genes by various mechanisms, including methylation of histone lysines H3-K36 and H4-K20 (see the preceding), as well as interaction with the transcriptional repressor Nizp1. One may hypothesize that haploinsufficiency of *NSD1* could result in silencing of putative growth regulating genes, the final consequence being accelerated growth. A growth-related role of *NSD1* is further supported by its expression in fetal tissues (Kurotaki et al., 2001).

AUTOSOMAL RECESSIVE

BARDET–BIEDL SYNDROME

This condition was first described in 1866 by Laurence and Moon as an entity characterized by ID, hypogenitalism, retinopathy, and late onset paraplegia. The same clinical phenotype was independently described by Bardet in 1920 and Biedl in 1922. Because of this, the syndrome has been often named with two different eponyms: Laurence–Moon syndrome and Bardet–Biedl syndrome (BBS). Because of the considerable phenotypic overlap, it has been suggested that the two conditions are allelic. Bardet–Biedl syndrome is now the overall used term. Bardet–Biedl syndrome is a pleiotropic genetic disorder with significant clinical variability.

Inheritance is mostly autosomal recessive, although in some instances BBS may be an oligogenic disorder. The prevalence of BBS varies markedly between populations: from 1:160,000 in northern European populations to 1:13,500 in isolated Arabic populations in which a higher level of consanguinity exists.

Bardet–Biedl syndrome is genetically heterogeneous: 16 BBS genes accounting for approximately 80% of clinically diagnosed BBS have been identified so far. The majority of pathogenic mutations are found in BBS1 and BBS10 (23.2% and 20%, respectively). Genotype–phenotype correlations are poor. Some genes seem to have ethnic specific frequency but no mutated genes are detected exclusively in a single ethnic population (Hjortshoj et al., 2010). Whereas most patients show regular autosomal recessive inheritance, in several instances (about 10%) a triallelic pattern of inheritance (three mutations in BBS genes are required for the phenotype to be manifest, or alternatively a third disease locus acts as a modifier) is observed (Beales et al., 2003; Eichers et al., 2004). This irregular pattern of inheritance may raise problems in counseling the parents of affected BBS children for recurrence risk. It has been suggested to counsel anyway according to the autosomal recessive recurrence risk (Abu-Safieh et al., 2012). All the BBS genes encode proteins that are part of the BBsome, localized at the base of the primary cilium and involved in the organization of ciliogenesis and maintenance of the cilium. Overall, BBS can be considered a disease of immotile cilia. Defects in immotile cilia are characterized clinically by retinitis pigmentosa, polydactyly, situs inversus, learning difficulties, and cystic kidneys, liver, and pancreas (Gerdes et al., 2009) (Table 76.3).

The BBS phenotype evolves with age and therefore the diagnosis is not usually suspected until late childhood. The only typical feature at birth may be postaxial polydactyly, rarely associated with brachydactyly or syndactyly. The most common diagnostic finding, which should prompt investigation for BBS, is the development of rod-cone dystrophy. This usually manifests around five years of age but may be present at two. Clinically, patients with BBS experience a gradual onset of night blindness, followed by photophobia and loss of central and color vision. Obesity is another major clinical finding (72%–86% of patients with BBS) mostly developing after the first year. Type 2 diabetes and other signs of metabolic syndrome are frequently observed. Hypogonadism, delayed puberty, hypogenitalism, and infertility are other issues. Speech problems and developmental delay (that can involve specific areas) are common in BBS. Behavior is an issue, as BBS patients may show obsessive-compulsive behavior, difficulties in socialization, autistic features, or psychosis. Renal abnormalities can be a major cause of morbidity and mortality. The renal abnormalities are variable but classically manifest with cystic tubular disease and anatomical malformations. Conductive hearing loss secondary to chronic otitis media is frequent and may worsen the speech defect. Other manifestations include heart malformations and cardiomyopathies, gastrointestinal issues (Hirschsprung disease), hypodontia and enamel hypoplasia, anosmia, ataxia, and poor coordination (Forsythe and Beales, 2012).

It has been suggested that some phenotypic manifestations also occur in mutation heterozygotes, specifically, obesity, increased risk for renal cancers and malformations, as well as retinal dysfunction (Beales et al., 2000; Kim et al., 2007).

TABLE 76.3. The ciliopathies: syndromes and genes

SYNDROMES	OMIM	GENES
Short rib polydactyly type II-III-V	263530, 263520, 263510, 26986	*IFT80, DYNC2H1, WDR35, NEK1*
Asphyxiating thoracic dystrophy	611263, 613091, 613819, 614376	*IFT80, DYNC2H1, TTC21B, WDR19*
Ellis Van Creveld, Weyers acrofacial dysostosis	604831, 614376, 193530	*EVC, EVC2*
Sensenbrenner	613610, 614099, 614378	*WDR19, IFT122, WDR35, IFT43*
Bardet–Biedl, McKusick–Kauffman	209900, 236700	*BBS1–12, BBS15, CEP290, TMEM67, MGC1203, MKS1*
Joubert syndrome	213300	*CEP290, RPGRIPL1, NPHP1, TMEM67, ARL13B, TMEM216, OFD1, AHI1*
Leber congenital amaurosis	204000	*CEP290, RPGRIPL1,*
Senior–Løken syndrome	266900	*CEP290, NPHP1, INVS, NPHP3, NPHP4, NPHP5*
Orofaciodigital syndrome	311200	*TMEM216, OFD1*
Meckel–Gruber syndrome	249000, 267010	*CEP290, NPHP3, TMEM67, RPGRIPL1,*
Nephronophthisis	256100	*CEP290, NPHP1, INVS, NPHP3, NPHP4, NPHP5, TMEM67, RPGRIPL1*

(From Waters, A.M., Beales, P.L., 2011. Ciliopathies: An expanding disease spectrum. *Pediatr Nephrol.* 26(7):1039–1056; Huber, C., Cormier-Daire, V., 2012. Ciliary disorder of the skeleton. *Am. J. Med. Genet. C. Semin. Med. Genet.* 160(3):165–174.)

Because of the many issues in BBS, a multidisciplinary approach is required to manage this pleiotropic condition. Because there is not yet a targeted treatment, the clinical intervention should be focused on symptoms as they arise. In particular, the renal function needs to be monitored and the risk for diabetes insipidus (which is frequent in BBS) should be taken into account. Ophthalmological follow-up is also recommended.

The clinical features of BBS significantly overlap with the manifestations of other ciliopathies. Among those, Alstrom and McKusick–Kauffman syndromes manifest significant overlap with BBS. However, hearing loss and absence of polydactyly differentiate Alstrom syndrome from BBS, and the high prevalence of urogenital anomalies in McKusick–Kauffman syndrome that normally lacks obesity, rod-cone dystrophy, and learning difficulties differentiate this latter condition from BBS.

It is interesting to consider how ciliopathies may contribute to mental illness; several genes in this group have been associated with developmental delay syndromes, including ID and ASD. The means by which cilia are involved in neurodevelopmental processes and by which ciliopathies lead to neurodevelopmental disorders are areas of active research. In addition to the role of motile cilia in mobilizing cerebrospinal fluid, primary cilia, found on most neurons and astrocytes, play roles as modulators of signal transduction during both brain development and homeostasis (Lee and Gleeson, 2011).

COHEN SYNDROME

Cohen syndrome (CS) is a rare autosomal-recessive disorder, first described in 1973, characterized by hypotonia, obesity, ID, characteristic facial appearance, and narrow hands and feet. There is consistent clinical heterogeneity, particularly evident when comparing patients of different ethnic backgrounds, especially when evaluating specific system phenotypes separately, such as the ophthalmic and central nervous systems (Douzgou and Petersen, 2011). The incidence of CS is unknown; however, this condition is overrepresented in Finland owing to the peculiar population structure in genetic isolates. The Finnish CS phenotype is remarkably homogeneous, whereas clinical variability is the rule in non-Finnish patients with CS. Some ethnic group shows peculiarities; for instance, the Amish CS neonatal phenotype is characterized in 50% of cases by respiratory distress syndrome, jaundice, and acidosis, whereas a high-pitched voice and an age-related loss of the left ventricular function have been recurrently reported only in the Finnish CS cohort.

The inheritance is autosomal-recessive and the causative gene, named *VPS13B* or *COH1*, encodes a Golgi-associated matrix protein required for Golgi integrity (Kolehmainen et al., 2003; Seifert et al., 2011). The mutational spectrum is wide and mutations can be present in different portions of the gene; missense, non-sense, and frameshift mutations as well as intragenic deletions have been found in CS patients. Non-Finnish patients are almost always compound heterozygotes (Katzaki et al., 2007). Not much is known of the pathogenesis of CS, but because high levels of urinary hyaluronic acid have been reported, it has been suggested that CS is a connective tissue disorder.

Typical craniofacial features include down-slanting palpebral fissures, thick eyebrows, convex profile of nose, and short philtrum with open mouth and prominent lips exposing the upper central incisors. These features become more evident as the child gets older. In addition, patients with CS exhibit short stature, generalized hypotonia, truncal obesity (evident after five years), delayed puberty, and cryptorchidism. Related to hypotonia is the frequent finding of kyphoscoliosis. Microcephaly can be of prenatal onset and ID, moderate to severe, is usually observed. Seizures are rare and a happy affectionate predisposition is typical.

The hands and feet are narrow, with slender fingers and joint hyperextensibility. Ophthalmological involvement is quite constant. Myopia can develop in up to 90% of patients, and retinal pigmentary degeneration can occur in late childhood in about 80% of cases. However, these lesions only rarely lead to blindness. Neutropenia is also a recurrent, although not constant, laboratory finding. Among these clinical features, some can be considered good indicators for the presence of a mutation in the causative gene: postnatal microcephaly, chorioretinal dystrophy, and neutropenia. It has been suggested that, given the large size of the gene, the mutational analysis should not be indicated in the absence of these features. The follow-up of young patients could be a satisfactory alternative unless there are reproductive issues (El Chehadeh et al., 2010).

The phenotype in CS is quite distinctive, although large-scale mutational analysis has documented the existence of atypical cases. In any case, the diagnosis may be not evident until late childhood when the cardinal features of the condition manifest. A group of ID conditions to be considered as those of syndromes with hypotonia, obesity, and mental retardation, including Prader-Willi syndrome, which clearly has a completely different natural history and clinical appearance. If the phenotypic appearance is not straightforward, quantitative genomic alterations should be ruled out by CMA before considering the diagnosis of non-typical CS.

SMITH–LEMLI–OPITZ SYNDROME

Smith–Lemli–Opitz syndrome (SLOS, #OMIM 270400) was first described in 1964, as a multiple congenital anomalies-mental retardation (MCA-MR) syndrome characterized by microcephaly, peculiar face, developmental delay, syndactyly between the second and third toe, and genital anomalies (Smith et al., 1964). The clinical presentation may be variable in severity, ranging from neonatal death to survival into childhood and adolescence with severe ID and behavioral impairment.

Smith–Lemli–Opitz syndrome is a rare disorder (estimated incidence is between 1:20,000 and 1:60,000 in different populations), but it is not possible to rule out a higher incidence because of mildly affected individuals in whom the condition is difficult to recognize. In any case, it is considered among the most frequent autosomal recessive disorders, with an estimated carrier frequency of 1% to 2% in the general population.

The inheritance is autosomal recessive and the causative gene, named *DHCR7*, encodes the 3-beta-hydroxysterol-delta-7-reductase, an enzyme converting 7-dehydrocholesterol into cholesterol. This defects leads to high plasma levels of 7-dehydrocholesterol and low cholesterol (Irons et al., 1993).

Therefore, the clinical manifestations of SLOS are caused by a defect in cholesterol biosynthesis, a metabolic pathway that is crucial during embryonic development from early on (Porter and Herman, 2011). Because cholesterol is also required for the proper function of the sonic hedgehog (SHH) pathway, some clinical manifestations commonly related to SHH dysfunction, such as holoprosencephaly, can be observed in SLOS. The mutational spectrum of the SLOS gene is wide and mutations in the transmembrane domain or the C-terminal region have been associated with milder phenotypes.

Prenatally, growth retardation, oligohydramnios, and decreased fetal movements can be observed as well as breech presentation and perinatal asphyxia. Increased nucal translucency can be detected by ultrasound (Quelin et al., 2012). Low birth weight is almost always present and failure to thrive is experienced in a high percentage of patients. Death in the neonatal period may occur because of severe feeding difficulties and hepatic dysfunction. Those who survive into childhood usually have short stature and severe intellectual impairment associated with behavioral issues, including autism, aggressiveness, sleep disturbances, and hyperactivity.

Physical anomalies in SLOS can be present in almost any part of the body (DeBarber et al., 2011; Nowaczyk et al., 2012). The brain is often underdeveloped with microcephaly and a constellation of anomalies, including holoprosencephaly, agenesis of the corpus callosum, ventricular dilatation, and cerebellar vermis hypoplasia. Reduced myelination in the cerebral hemispheres, cranial nerves, and peripheral nerves also occur. The face appears round-shaped with hypertelorism, down-slanting palpebral fissures and ptosis, upturned and wide nose, and micrognathia. The mouth shows broad alveolar ridges, small tongue, and rarely lingual cysts. Strabismus and cataract can also be observed. The extremities are also commonly affected, showing most frequently second to third toe syndactyly, postaxial polydactyly, and shortness of the first metacarpals and metatarsals. Positional foot abnormalities are often present as well as hip dislocation. Abnormalities of the external genitalia, mostly reflecting a failure of masculinization, are frequently observed, including cryptorchidism, hypospadias, micropenis, bifid scrotum, ambiguous genitalia, and even sex reversal. The urinary tract can be obstructed or hypoplastic and renal dysplasia (cysts or hypoplasia) can be present. Cardiovascular malformations occur in about 50% of the patients, mostly PDA, VSD, ASD, or tetralogy of Fallot. Other findings include pancreatic islet cells hyperplasia, unilobate lungs, and photosensitivity.

The clinical diagnosis can be confirmed with a biochemical test measuring plasma concentrations of cholesterol (that are usually very low in SLOS) and 7-dehydrocholesterol (increased in SLOS). High levels of 7-dehydrocholesterol can be detected in the amniotic fluid and chorionic villus specimens as well (Kratz and Kelley, 1999).

Supplementary cholesterol is rationally expected to supply the tissues and also reduce the toxic levels of 7-dehydrocholesterol. Simvastatin, aimed at further decreased sterol synthesis, has been also used as potential therapy. Although reported in the literature, the beneficial effects on behavior of dietary cholesterol supplementation have not been formally documented through a randomized clinical trial. Larger studies are still needed to clearly demonstrate the utility of treatment of this metabolic disorder (Tierney et al., 2010).

Chromosomal disorders should be ruled out in newborns with features compatible with the SLOS phenotype. Also, some clinical overlapping exists with Meckel syndrome (in which the cystic kidney dysplasia is typical) and Pallister-Hall syndrome (in which the finding of a hypothalamic hamartoblastoma is quite unique).

X-LINKED

ALLAN–HERNDON–DUDLEY SYNDROME

Allan–Herndon–Dudley syndrome (AHDS, OMIM #300523) was first described in 1944 and was the second X-linked ID syndrome to appear in the literature (Allan et al., 1944). The authors described a large North Carolina (USA) family with 24 affected males over multiple generations. The major clinical findings were hypotonia, muscle hypoplasia, general muscle weakness, which resulted in a "limber neck" (noted by family members), dysarthria, and ataxia. Speech was also limited and there was significant developmental retardation.

The incidence of AHDS is unknown. It is considered one of the more prominent X-linked conditions with more than 25 families having been described, most from the United States and Western Europe. A review of most of the families found that in half of them, there was only one affected male (Schwartz and Stevenson 2007). This same review allowed for a good clinical description of AHDS and an idea of the natural history of the syndrome.

Initially, males with AHDS have birth measurements within the normal range. Most maintain normal postnatal growth. However, muscle hypoplasia was evident early in life and persisted into adulthood.

Facial features appear to be consistent across families. A myopathic face or hypotonic facial appearance with an open mouth and tented upper lip is usually present. There is bitemporal narrowing in most males and the face becomes tall and narrow in adulthood. The ears appear to be simple and cupped.

Neurologically, males with ADHS are hypotonic at birth. The postnatal weakness persists and progresses to spasticity with age. Dystonia and athetoid movements are present. Hyperreflexia becomes evident in adulthood.

Cognitive function is delayed from early in life. There is significant delay in acquiring language and all males with AHDS have severe ID.

The gene for AHDS was mapped to the Xq13-q21 region of the X chromosome when Schwartz and colleagues re-studied the original family (Schwartz et al., 1990). In 2004, both Dumitrescu and colleagues (2004) and Friesema and colleagues (2004) reported families and unrelated males who presented with neurological findings similar to those observed in AHDS. Additionally, the affected individuals had decreased serum T4 levels and significantly elevated serum levels of T3. However, TSH levels in serum were in the high normal range. Both groups identified mutations in the monocarboxylate transporter 8 gene (MCT8, SLC16A2) in their patients. Subsequently, Schwartz and colleagues (2005) showed that mutations in MCT8 were also present in their collection of families with AHDS.

MCT8 is critical for the metabolism of thyroid hormone in the brain. The protein functions as a transporter of T3 into neurons. Without T3, many genes within the neuron are not properly regulated. Thus, the presence of severe cognitive impairment in AHDS patients is not unexpected. However, other aspects of the clinical phenotype observed in AHDS patients do not reflect a defect in thyroid function. Additional studies are needed to explain this disconnect.

The presence of elevated serum T3 levels provides a convenient method for testing for AHDS in at-risk individuals such as males with hypotonia and developmental delay. The prevalence of MCT8 is not known, but with a reliable and rapid test, many AHDS families have been identified. Thus, the prevalence of AHDS may be high relative to other X-linked intellectual disability syndromes.

ALPHA-THALASSEMIA INTELLECTUAL DISABILITY SYNDROME

Alpha-thalassemia intellectual disability or ATRX syndrome (OMIM #301040) is an X-linked recessive condition first noted clinically by Weatherall and colleagues in 1981 when they reported an association of hemoglobin H inclusion bodies in patients with ID. The possibility that this represented an X-linked syndrome was evident by 1990 when Wilkie and colleagues (1991) reported additional patients who did not have any abnormality of the alpha-globin genes located at 16p. The patients were all males and presented with a common phenotype of microcephaly, a hypotonic face (hypotelorism, small triangular nose, tented upper lip, open mouth) and severe ID with mild hemoglobin H disease.

Since the initial descriptions by Weatherall et al. (1981) and Wilkie et al. (1991), many additional patients and families with ATRX have been characterized and a fairly comprehensive review was compiled by Gibbons and Higgs (2000). The clinical spectrum of ATRX consists of hypotonia present in infancy, distinctive facial features of an open mouth with a tented upper lip and prominent lower lip, small upturned triangular nose, and hypertelorism. These facial features become "coarser" with age. Some patients have skeletal anomalies and urogenital anomalies such as cryptorchidism and hypospadias. Speech is severely delayed and maybe absent. There is growth delay and microcephaly is present. One feature noted in the original patients, hemoglobin H inclusion bodies, is not consistently present. Thus, although this was thought to be a useful test for ATRX, many proven cases are not positive for this finding and the test is no longer routinely done in males suspected of having ATRX.

Once ATRX was considered to be an XLID syndrome, Gibbons and colleagues mapped the gene to Xq12-q21.3 by linkage analysis in 1992 (Gibbons et al., 1992). They identified the candidate gene, XNP (X-linked nuclear protein) in 1995 (Gibbons et al., 1995). The availability of a gene test allowed screening of XLID syndromes linked to the Xq13-q21 region as well as some syndromes whose clinical phenotype overlapped with ATRX. As a result, other XLID syndromes were shown to also result from mutations in *XNP*: Carpenter–Waziri, Holmes–Gang, and Chudley–Lowry. Two families with the diagnoses of Juberg–Marsidi and Smith–Fineman–Myers syndromes were found to have mutations in *XNP* (Villard et al., 1996, 2000). However, the families first described with these syndromes (Juberg and Marsidi, 1980; Smith et al., 1980) have not been tested for *XNP* mutations. In fact, the original Juberg-Marsidi family was recently found to have a mutation in the *HUWE1* gene, whereas XNP testing was negative (Abidi and colleagues, unpublished data).

The prevalence of ATRX is unknown in the general population. However, close to 200 males with ATRX syndrome have been reported; thus, it is reasonable to expect the prevalence to be relatively high, about 1% to 2% in males with ID.

One clinical feature that is now considered a hallmark of ATRX is that female carriers of an *XNP* mutation have highly skewed X-inactivation, which probably explains the lack of a clinical phenotype in these females. This distinction, skewed X-inactivation and lack of clinical findings in carriers, allows one to clinically differentiated ATRX from another XLID syndrome, Coffin–Lowry (OMIM #303600). This is critical since both can be confused in early childhood.

Some attempt has been made to construct a genotype/phenotype correlation because of the clinical spectrum of the syndrome and the number of patients with mutations. Unfortunately, this correlation has proved to be less than successful. There does appear to be some association between the loss of the C-terminal end of the protein and the presence of severe urogenital abnormalities (Gibbons and Higgs, 2000). Also, Badens and colleagues (2006) did observe that mutations in the PHD-like domains tended to result in more severe psychomotor delay and more severe urogenital abnormalities. However, overall, no clear genotype/phenotype association has been observed.

One recent observation has been made that may be significant. A fairly common R37X mutation has been found in families who present with a milder form of ATRX (Abidi et al., 2005; Guerrini et al., 2000). This may result from the presence of a small amount of full-length protein as detected by Western blotting and the utilization of an initiation site downstream from the mutation (Abidi et al., 2005; Howard et al., 2004). The *XNP/ATRX* gene was initially cloned and partially characterized by Stayton and colleagues in 1994 (Stayton et al., 1994). They determined it was homologous to members of the helicase II superfamily. Picketts and colleagues (1996) characterized the XNP/ATRX protein further establishing it was a member of the SNF2-like subgroup of proteins, contained helicase domains, a nuclear localization signal, and a C-terminal glutamine-rich region characteristic of a transcription factor. Villard and colleagues (1997) further determined the protein has three zinc finger motifs in the 5′ end of the gene. Last, Gibbons and colleagues (1997) identified a cystine-rich motif, similar to a putative PHD zinc finger domain, in the N-terminal region. With the presence of these various domains, it is not surprising that the XNP/ATRX protein has chromatin remodeling and DNA translocase activities (Gibbons et al., 2003) and with its widespread expression in during embryogenesis (Stayton et al., 1994)

mutations in XNP give rise to a multisystem syndrome. This places *ATRX* into a class of ID and ASD genes that affect regulation of gene expression.

OPITZ–KAVEGGIA SYNDROME (FG SYNDROME)

Opitz–Kaveggia syndrome, better known as FG syndrome (FGS, OMIM #305450) is an X-linked recessive syndrome first reported in 1974 (Opitz and Kaveggia, 1974). The report was based on a single family with macrocephaly, ID, distinctive facial features, hypotonia, broad thumbs, and imperforate anus. The facial features were comprised of hypertelorism, small ears, frontal upsweep of the hair, broad forehead, and down-slanted palpebral fissures. Additionally, partial agenesis of the corpus callosum was found in one of the affected males, but this analysis was not conducted in all affected individuals.

Since the initial FGS description, many other families have been reported to have clinical features of FG syndrome. These publications had expanded the FGS phenotype and led to the identification of multiple FG syndromic loci on the X-chromosome. Genetic heterogeneity as well as clinical variability made the clinical diagnosis difficult and at the same time rather common among males with ID, macrocephaly, and constipation. This was the situation until 2007 when Risheg and colleagues identified the same mutation (c.2881C>T, p.R961W) in the *MED12* gene in six families with an FGS diagnosis (Risheg et al., 2007). The six families included a male from the original family of Opitz and Kaveggia.

After the identification of the *MED12* mutation, many males with a diagnosis of FGS were screened for mutations in *MED12*. This did lead to the identification of other males with the same R961W mutation, but it became evident that it was difficult to confirm the FGS diagnosis in males with a rather non-specific phenotype (Lyons et al., 2009). Based on these results and the fact that the original family had the R961W *MED12* mutation, it was proposed that only males with this alteration be designated as having Opitz–Kaveggia syndrome. To simplify the diagnosis, Clark and colleagues (2009) developed a clinical algorithm for diagnosis based on a clinical evaluation of 23 patients with the R961W mutation as compared with 48 patients who had a clinical diagnosis of FGS but were mutation negative.

The clinical features of Opitz-Kaveggia syndrome are defined as a male with intellectual disability, developmental disability, small ears, a characteristic face (long narrow face with a tall forehead, upsweep of the frontal hairline, open mouth), congenital anomalies of the corpus callosum, anus, heart or skeleton, macrocephaly, early hypotonia, constipation, and an affable, eager-to-please personality (Clark et al., 2009; Graham et al., 2008; Lyons et al., 2009).

The utilization of the clinical diagnosis algorithm developed by Clark and colleagues (2009) has already proved to be useful. Rump and colleagues (2011) screened *MED12* in a Dutch family with three affected male cousins based on the males fitting the clinical criteria for Opitz-Kaveggia syndrome. They found a novel *MED12* mutation, C.2873G>A (p.G958E) in the family. This mutation is three amino acids away from the R961W mutation and is in the same stretch of the highly conserved Leu-Ser rich domain of the MED12 protein.

The prevalence of FGS is unknown. Before the identification of *MED12* as a causative gene, the FGS diagnosis was not uncommon in males with ID, macrocephaly, and constipation; thus, it was thought to be a significant contributor to X-linked ID. Now, it is likely to be a relatively rare XLID entity, probably not exceeding 0.5% of males with ID. Gene testing over the next few years will better address this point. However, it needs to be noted that another syndrome, Lujan syndrome (OMIM #309520) also has a mutation (p.N1007S) in *MED12* (Schwartz et al. 2007) and at least two other *MED12* mutations have been identified in FGS patients (Schwartz et al., unpublished data). Thus, although the FGS associated *MED12* mutation may be rare, other mutations in the gene may be responsible for ID in the male population.

The MED12 protein is a member of the large mediator complex that plays an important regulatory role in the activity of RNA polymerase II (Knuesel, Meyer, Donner, et al., 2009). Mediator also acts as to regulate transcription initiation (Knuesel, Meyer, Bernecky, et al., 2009). Recently, it was shown that Mediator is part of a protein interaction network comprised of G9a histone methyltransferase and REST (RE1 silencing transcription factor) (Ding et al., 2008). This network suppresses neuronal gene expression in non-neuronal cells. Of interest, Ding et al., (2008) have shown the R961W *MED12* mutation disrupts the REST corepressor function of Mediator, suggesting a pathologic basis for the *MED12* mutation.

CONCLUSIONS

There seems to be a common denominator to the pathophysiology of the ID syndromes described in this chapter, expandable to many other conditions, all being disorders of development. All causative genes are in essence "master" genes affecting the expression of other genes either by disrupting signaling pathways, affecting chromatin structure, or altering structures (e.g., the cilium) that are essential for the normal functioning of the cell. The knowledge gained points investigators to other gene defects to explore in patients who do not harbor mutations in the presumptive candidate gene based on the phenotype. In spite of the complexity of the mechanisms involved, the knowledge of the molecular details and protein interactions promises to open the way to pharmacological interventions aimed at specifically correcting or at least ameliorating the basic defect or its metabolic consequences in ID syndromes.

ACKNOWLEDGMENTS

We thank Debra Marler for assisting with the preparation of the manuscript. Dedicated to the memory of Ethan Francis Schwartz, 1996–1998.

DISCLOSURES

Dr. Schwartz: To my knowledge, all of my possible conflicts of interest and those of my coauthors, financial or otherwise, including direct or indirect financial or personal relationships, interests, and affiliations, whether or not directly related to the subject of the chapter, are as follows. I am funded by NICHD and SCDDSN (South Carolina Department of Disabilities and Special Needs). This work was supported in part by a grant from the National Institutes of Health (NICHD) [HD26202 to C.E.S.].

Dr. Gurrieri: No conflicts of interest to disclose.

Dr. Neri: No conflicts of interest to disclose.

REFERENCES

Abidi, F.E., Cardoso, C., et al. (2005). Mutation in the 5′ alternatively spliced region of the XNP/ATR-X gene causes Chudley-Lowry syndrome. *Eur. J. Hum. Genet.* 13(2):176–183.

Abu-Safieh, L., Al-Anazi, S., et al. (2012). In search of triallelism in Bardet-Biedl syndrome. *Eur. J. Hum. Genet.* 20(4):420–427.

Adam, M.P., Hudgins, L., et al. (2011). Kabuki Syndrome. In: Pagon, R.A., et al., eds., *GeneReviewsTM [Internet].* Seattle: University of Washington.

Allan, W., Herndon, C.N., et al. (1944). Some examples of the inheritance of mental deficiency: apparently sex-linked idiocy and microcephaly. *Am. J. Ment. Defic.* 48:325–334.

Armour, C.M., and Allanson, J.E. (2008). Further delineation of cardio-facio-cutaneous syndrome: clinical features of 38 individuals with proven mutations. *J. Med. Genet.* 45(4):249–254.

Badens, C., Lacoste, C., et al. (2006). Mutations in PHD-like domain of the ATRX gene correlate with severe psychomotor impairment and severe urogenital abnormalities in patients with ATRX syndrome. *Clin. Genet.* 70(1):57–62.

Baujat, G., and Cormier-Daire, V. (2007). Sotos syndrome. *Orphanet. J. Rare Dis.* 2:36.

Beales, P.L., Reid, H.A., et al. (2000). Renal cancer and malformations in relatives of patients with Bardet-Biedl syndrome. *Nephrol. Dial. Transplant.* 15(12):1977–1985.

Beales, P.L., Badano, J.L., et al. (2003). Genetic interaction of BBS1 mutations with alleles at other BBS loci can result in non-Mendelian Bardet-Biedl syndrome. *Am. J. Hum. Genet.* 72(5):1187–1199.

Berry-Kravis, E.M., Hessl, D., et al. (2012). Effects of STX209 (Arbaclofen) on neurobehavioral function in children and adults with fragile X syndrome: a randomized, controlled, Phase 2 trial. *Sci. Transl. Med.* 4:152ra127

Betancur, C. (2011). Etiological heterogeneity in autism spectrum disorders: more than 100 genetic and genomic disorders and still counting. *Brain Res.* 1380:42–77.

Clark, R.D., Graham, J.M., Jr., et al. (2009). FG syndrome, an X-linked multiple congenital anomaly syndrome: the clinical phenotype and an algorithm for diagnostic testing. *Genet. Med.* 11(11):769–775.

Cohen, M.M., Jr. (2003). Mental deficiency, alterations in performance, and CNS abnormalities in overgrowth syndromes. *Am. J. Med. Genet. C Semin. Med. Genet.* 117C(1):49–56.

Curry, C.J., Stevenson, R.E., et al. (1997). Evaluation of mental retardation: recommendations of a Consensus Conference: American College of Medical Genetics. *Am. J. Med. Genet.* 72(4):468–477.

DeBarber, A.E., Eroglu, Y., et al. (2011). Smith-Lemli-Opitz syndrome. *Expert Rev. Mol. Med.* 13:e24.

Ding, N., Zhou, H., et al. (2008). Mediator links epigenetic silencing of neuronal gene expression with x-linked mental retardation. *Mol. Cell* 31 (3):347–359.

Douglas, J., Tatton-Brown, K., et al. (2005). Partial NSD1 deletions cause 5% of Sotos syndrome and are readily identifiable by multiplex ligation dependent probe amplification. *J. Med. Genet.* 42(9):e56.

Douzgou, S., and Petersen, M.B. (2011). Clinical variability of genetic isolates of Cohen syndrome. *Clin. Genet.* 79(6):501–506.

Dumitrescu, A.M., Liao, X.H., et al. (2004). A novel syndrome combining thyroid and neurological abnormalities is associated with mutations in a monocarboxylate transporter gene. *Am. J. Hum. Genet.* 74(1):168–175.

Eichers, E.R., Lewis, R.A., et al. (2004). Triallelic inheritance: a bridge between Mendelian and multifactorial traits. *Ann. Med.* 36(4):262–272.

El Chehadeh, S., Aral, B., et al. (2010). Search for the best indicators for the presence of a VPS13B gene mutation and confirmation of diagnostic criteria in a series of 34 patients genotyped for suspected Cohen syndrome. *J. Med. Genet.* 47(8):549–553.

Forsythe, E., and Beales, P.L. (2013). Bardet-Biedl syndrome. *Eur. J. Hum. Genet.* 1:8–13.

Friesema, E.C., Grueters, A., et al. (2004). Association between mutations in a thyroid hormone transporter and severe X-linked psychomotor retardation. *Lancet* 364(9443):1435–1437.

Gerdes, J.M., Davis, E.E., et al. (2009). The vertebrate primary cilium in development, homeostasis, and disease. *Cell* 137(1):32–45.

Gibbons, R.J., Bachoo, S., et al. (1997). Mutations in transcriptional regulator ATRX establish the functional significance of a PHD-like domain. *Nat. Genet.* 17(2):146–148.

Gibbons, R.J., Pellagatti, A., et al. (2003). Identification of acquired somatic mutations in the gene encoding chromatin-remodeling factor ATRX in the alpha-thalassemia myelodysplasia syndrome (ATMDS). *Nat. Genet.* 34(4):446–449.

Gibbons, R.J., and Higgs, D.R. (2000). Molecular-clinical spectrum of the ATR-X syndrome. *Am. J. Med. Genet.* 97(3):204–212.

Gibbons, R.J., Picketts, D.J., et al. (1995). Mutations in a putative global transcriptional regulator cause X-linked mental retardation with alpha-thalassemia (ATR-X syndrome). *Cell* 80(6):837–845.

Gibbons, R.J., Suthers, G.K., et al. (1992). X-linked alpha-thalassemia/mental retardation (ATR-X) syndrome: localization to Xq12-q21.31 by X inactivation and linkage analysis. *Am. J. Hum. Genet.* 51(5):1136–1149.

Gibson, W.T., Hood, R.L., et al. (2012). Mutations in EZH2 cause Weaver syndrome. *Am. J. Hum. Genet.* 90(1):110–118.

Graham, J.M., Jr., Visootsak, J., et al. (2008). Behavior of 10 patients with FG syndrome (Opitz-Kaveggia syndrome) and the p.R961W mutation in the MED12 gene. *Am. J. Med. Genet. A* 146A(23):3011–3017.

Guerrini, R., Shanahan, J.L., et al. (2000). A nonsense mutation of the ATRX gene causing mild mental retardation and epilepsy. *Ann. Neurol.* 47(1):117–121.

Hjortshoj, T.D., Gronskov, K., et al. (2010). Bardet-Biedl syndrome in Denmark—report of 13 novel sequence variations in six genes. *Hum. Mutat.* 31(4):429–436.

Hoffman, J.D., Ciprero, K.L., et al. (2005). Immune abnormalities are a frequent manifestation of Kabuki syndrome. *Am. J. Med. Genet. A* 135(3):278–281.

Howard, M.T., Malik, N., et al. (2004). Attenuation of an amino-terminal premature stop codon mutation in the ATRX gene by an alternative mode of translational initiation. *J. Med. Genet.* 41(12):951–956.

Huber, C., and Cormier-Daire, V. (2012). Ciliary disorder of the skeleton. *Am. J. Med. Genet. C Semin. Med. Genet.* 160(3):165–174.

Irons, M., Elias, E.R., et al. (1993). Defective cholesterol biosynthesis in Smith-Lemli-Opitz syndrome. *Lancet* 341(8857):1414.

Juberg, R.C., and Marsidi, I. (1980). A new form of X-linked mental retardation with growth retardation, deafness, and microgenitalism. *Am. J. Hum. Genet.* 32(5):714–722.

Katzaki, E., Pescucci, C., et al. (2007). Clinical and molecular characterization of Italian patients affected by Cohen syndrome. *J. Hum. Genet.* 52(12):1011–1017.

Kawame, H., Hannibal, M.C., et al. (1999). Phenotypic spectrum and management issues in Kabuki syndrome. *J. Pediatr.* 134(4):480–485.

Kim, L.S., Fishman, G.A., et al. (2007). Retinal dysfunction in carriers of bardet-biedl syndrome. *Ophthalmic. Genet.* 28(3):163–168.

Knuesel, M.T., Meyer, K.D., et al. (2009). The human CDK8 subcomplex is a molecular switch that controls Mediator coactivator function. *Genes Dev.* 23(4):439–451.

Knuesel, M.T., Meyer, K.D., et al. (2009). The human CDK8 subcomplex is a histone kinase that requires Med12 for activity and can function independently of mediator. *Mol. Cell Biol.* 29(3):650–661.

Kolehmainen, J., Black, G.C., et al. (2003). Cohen syndrome is caused by mutations in a novel gene, COH1, encoding a transmembrane protein with a presumed role in vesicle-mediated sorting and intracellular protein transport. *Am. J. Hum. Genet.* 72(6):1359–1369.

Kratz, L.E., and Kelley, R.I. (1999). Prenatal diagnosis of the RSH/Smith-Lemli-Opitz syndrome. *Am. J. Med. Genet.* 82(5):376–381.

Kurotaki, N., Harada, N., et al. (2001). Molecular characterization of NSD1, a human homologue of the mouse Nsd1 gene. *Gene* 279(2):197–204.

Kurotaki, N., Imaizumi, K., et al. (2002). Haploinsufficiency of NSD1 causes Sotos syndrome. *Nat. Genet.* 30(4):365–366.

Lee, J.E., and Gleeson, J.G. (2011). Cilia in the nervous system: linking cilia function and neurodevelopmental disorders. *Curr. Opin. Neurol.* 24:98–105.

Lubs, H.A., Stevenson, R.E., et al. (2012). Fragile X and X-linked intellectual disability: four decades of discovery. *Am. J. Hum. Genet.* 90(4):579–590.

Lyons, M.J., Graham, J.M., Jr., et al. (2009). Clinical experience in the evaluation of 30 patients with a prior diagnosis of FG syndrome. *J. Med. Genet.* 46(1):9–13.

Mazzucchelli, C., and Brambilla, R. (2000). Ras-related and MAPK signalling in neuronaplasticity and memory formation. *Cell. Mol. Life Sci.* 57:604–611.

Mefford, H.C., Batshaw, M.L., et al. (2012). Genomics, intellectual disability, and autism. *N. Engl. J. Med.* 366(8):733–743.

Mervis, C.B., Becerra, A.M., et al. (2005). Intellectual abilities and adaptive behavior of children and adolescents with Kabuki syndrome: a preliminary study. *Am. J. Med. Genet. A* 132A(3):248–255.

Narumi, Y., Aoki, Y., et al. (2007). Molecular and clinical characterization of cardio-facio-cutaneous (CFC) syndrome: overlapping clinical manifestations with Costello syndrome. *Am. J. Med. Genet. A* 143A(8):799–807.

Neri, G., Zollino, M., et al. (1991). The Noonan-CFC controversy. *Am. J. Med. Genet.* 39(3):367–370.

Ng, S.B., Bigham, A.W., et al. (2010). Exome sequencing identifies MLL2 mutations as a cause of Kabuki syndrome. *Nat. Genet.* 42(9):790–793.

Niihori, T., Aoki, Y., et al. (2006). Germline KRAS and BRAF mutations in cardio-facio-cutaneous syndrome. *Nat. Genet.* 38(3):294–296.

Niikawa, N. (2004). Molecular basis of Sotos syndrome. *Horm. Res.* 62(Suppl 3):60–65.

Niikawa, N., Kuroki, Y., et al. (1988). Kabuki make-up (Niikawa-Kuroki) syndrome: a study of 62 patients. *Am. J. Med. Genet.* 31(3):565–589.

Niikawa, N., Matsuura, N., et al. (1981). Kabuki make-up syndrome: a syndrome of mental retardation, unusual facies, large and protruding ears, and postnatal growth deficiency. *J. Pediatr.* 99(4):565–569.

Nowaczyk, M.J., Tan, M., et al. (2012). Smith-Lemli-Opitz syndrome: Objective assessment of facial phenotype. *Am. J. Med. Genet. A* 158A(5):1020–1028.

Opitz, J.M., and Kaveggia, E.G. (1974). Studies of malformation syndromes of man 33: the FG syndrome. An X-linked recessive syndrome of multiple congenital anomalies and mental retardation. *Z. Kinderheilkd.* 117(1):1–18.

Picketts, D.J., Higgs, D.R., et al. (1996). ATRX encodes a novel member of the SNF2 family of proteins: mutations point to a common mechanism underlying the ATR-X syndrome. *Hum. Mol. Genet.* 5(12):1899–1907.

Porter, F.D., and Herman, G.E. (2011). Malformation syndromes caused by disorders of cholesterol synthesis. *J. Lipid Res.* 52(1):6–34.

Quelin, C., Loget, P., et al. (2012). Phenotypic spectrum of fetal Smith-Lemli-Opitz syndrome. *Eur. J. Med. Genet.* 55(2):81–90.

Rauen, K.A., Schoyer, L., et al. (2010). Proceedings from the 2009 genetic syndromes of the Ras/MAPK pathway: From bedside to bench and back. *Am. J. Med. Genet. A* 152A(1):4–24.

Reynolds, J.F., Neri, G., et al. (1986). New multiple congenital anomalies/mental retardation syndrome with cardio-facio-cutaneous involvement—the CFC syndrome. *Am. J. Med. Genet.* 25(3):413–427.

Risheg, H., Graham, J.M., Jr., et al. (2007). A recurrent mutation in MED12 leading to R961W causes Opitz-Kaveggia syndrome. *Nat. Genet.* 39(4):451–453.

Roberts, A., Allanson, J., et al. (2006). The cardiofaciocutaneous syndrome. *J. Med. Genet.* 43(11):833–842.

Rodriguez-Viciana, P., Tetsu, O., et al. (2006). Germline mutations in genes within the MAPK pathway cause cardio-facio-cutaneous syndrome. *Science* 311(5765):1287–1290.

Ropers, H.H. (2010). Genetics of early onset cognitive impairment. *Annu. Rev. Genomics Hum. Genet.* 11:161–187.

Rump, P., Niessen, R.C., et al. (2011). A novel mutation in MED12 causes FG syndrome (Opitz-Kaveggia syndrome). *Clin. Genet.* 79(2):183–188.

Sarimski, K. (2003). Behavioural and emotional characteristics in children with Sotos syndrome and learning disabilities. *Dev. Med. Child Neurol.* 45(3):172–178.

Schaefer, G.B., Bodensteiner, J.B., et al. (1997). The neuroimaging findings in Sotos syndrome. *Am. J. Med. Genet.* 68(4):462–465.

Schwartz, C.E., May, M.M., et al. (2005). Allan-Herndon-Dudley syndrome and the monocarboxylate transporter 8 (MCT8) gene. *Am. J. Hum. Genet.* 77(1):41–53.

Schwartz, C.E., and Stevenson, R.E. (2007). The MCT8 thyroid hormone transporter and Allan-Herndon-Dudley syndrome. *Best Pract. Res. Clin. Endocrinol. Metab.* 21(2):307–321.

Schwartz, C.E., Tarpey, P.S., et al. (2007). The original Lujan syndrome family has a novel missense mutation (p.N1007S) in the MED12 gene. *J. Med. Genet.* 44(7):472–477.

Schwartz, C.E., Ulmer, J., et al. (1990). Allan-Herndon syndrome. II. Linkage to DNA markers in Xq21. *Am. J. Hum. Genet.* 47(3):454–458.

Seifert, W., Kuhnisch, J., et al. (2011). Cohen syndrome-associated protein, COH1, is a novel, giant Golgi matrix protein required for Golgi integrity. *J. Biol. Chem.* 286(43):37665–37675.

Smith, D.W., Lemli, L., et al. (1964). A newly recognized syndrome of multiple congenital anomalies. *J. Pediatr.* 64:210–217.

Smith, R.D., Fineman, R.M., et al. (1980). Short stature, psychomotor retardation, and unusual facial appearance in two brothers. *Am. J. Med. Genet.* 7(1):5–9.

Stayton, C.L., Dabovic, B., et al. (1994). Cloning and characterization of a new human Xq13 gene, encoding a putative helicase. *Hum. Mol. Genet.* 3(11):1957–1964.

Tidyman, W.E., and Rauen, K.A. (2009). The RASopathies: developmental syndromes of Ras/MAPK pathway dysregulation. *Curr. Opin. Genet. Dev.* 19:230–236.

Tierney, E., Conley, S.K., et al. (2010). Analysis of short-term behavioral effects of dietary cholesterol supplementation in Smith-Lemli-Opitz syndrome. *Am. J. Med. Genet. A* 152A(1):91–95.

van Bokhoven, H. (2011). Genetic and epigenetic networks in intellectual disabilities. *Annu. Rev. Genet.* 45:81–104.

Villard, L., Fontes, M., et al. (2000). Identification of a mutation in the XNP/ATR-X gene in a family reported as Smith-Fineman-Myers syndrome. *Am. J. Med. Genet.* 91(1):83–85.

Villard, L., Gecz, J., et al. (1996). XNP mutation in a large family with Juberg-Marsidi syndrome. *Nat. Genet.* 12(4):359–360.

Villard, L., Lossi, A.M., et al. (1997). Determination of the genomic structure of the XNP/ATRX gene encoding a potential zinc finger helicase. *Genomics* 43(2):149–155.

Waters, A.M., and Beales, P.L. (2011). Ciliopathies: an expanding disease spectrum. *Pediatr. Nephrol.* 26(7):1039–1056.

Weatherall, D.J., Higgs, D.R., et al. (1981). Hemoglobin H disease and mental retardation: a new syndrome or a remarkable coincidence? *N. Engl. J. Med.* 305(11):607–612.

Wilkie, A.O., Pembrey, M.E., et al. (1991). The non-deletion type of alpha thalassaemia/mental retardation: a recognisable dysmorphic syndrome with X linked inheritance. *J. Med. Genet.* 28(10):724.

Winnepenninckx, B., Rooms, L., et al. (2003). Mental retardation: a review of the genetic causes. *Br. J. Dev. Disabil.* 49:29–44.

77 | AUTISM SPECTRUM DISORDERS

ALEXANDER KOLEVZON, A. TING WANG, DAVID GRODBERG,
AND JOSEPH D. BUXBAUM

The understanding of autism has evolved dramatically since Kanner and Asperger's original description of the disorder in 1943–44. Autism is characterized by social and language impairments, and restricted and repetitive behaviors and interests. The autism spectrum was historically defined to encompass autistic disorder, Asperger syndrome, and pervasive developmental disorder not otherwise specified (PDD-NOS) and is referred to collectively as autism spectrum disorder (ASD) in this chapter. In the next iteration of the Diagnostic and Statistical Manual for Mental Disorders Fifth Edition (DSM-5) due to be released in May 2013, the nomenclature will shift to Autism Spectrum Disorder to define pervasive developmental disorders currently described in DSM-IV. The first section on phenotype in this chapter describes the clinical features in detail.

The diagnosis of ASD is based on clinical observations of language and behavior, and important shifts in the standard of care have occurred to allow for younger age of diagnosis and earlier intervention. Evidence from studies of behavioral therapy is emerging to support its efficacy in facilitating gains in cognitive functioning, adaptive behavior, and reducing symptom severity. In addition, our knowledge of the neurobiology of ASD has improved in recent years, and much of this gain has been derived from neuroimaging studies, reviewed in the neuroimaging section.

Twin studies in ASD carried out since the 1970s and more recent genetic analyses have come to demonstrate autism as primarily a genetic disorder. Today, most scientists recognize that rare variations in the genetic code account for a significant proportion of cases. Rare variants have been discovered through high-resolution genetic techniques like chromosome microarray (CMA) and next generation or massively parallel sequencing (MPS) and the field is currently in a phase of exponential discovery that is expected to explain a larger proportion of causes of autism in the near future. The section on genetics that follows describes current advances in genetic discovery in ASD.

Understanding the etiological cause of autism is extremely significant for families for several reasons. First, it can provide a medical diagnosis, and in each case, depending on the cause, these genetic aberrations may be associated with other medical comorbidity that will be important to treat and monitor. Second, it can provide families with estimates of recurrence risk for the purpose of family planning. Finally, identifying the cause of autism provides opportunities to develop cellular and animal model systems to better understand the neurobiology

of the disorder and develop targeted novel therapeutics. The final section on therapeutics in this chapter reviews the current state of the evidence in the behavioral and pharmacological treatment of ASD and endeavors to suggest future directions.

PHENOTYPE

The phenomenology of ASD includes the behavioral signs and symptoms described in the current DSM as well as a broadening array of medical and underlying genetic abnormalities. Autism spectrum disorders have traditionally been characterized as having three symptom domains, including communication deficits, social interaction deficits, and repetitive patterns of behavior (American Psychiatric Association, 2000). However, recent evidence suggests that impairments in communication and social interaction are inseparable and may be more accurately conceptualized as one domain (Frazier et al., 2012; Gotham et al., 2007). Accordingly, the proposed DSM-5 revisions combine delays or deviation in social and communicative functioning into a single category (A), alongside a category for repetitive restricted behaviors (B). To explore the phenomenology of ASD, this section first outlines the core features common to those individuals who meet ASD diagnostic criteria, and then describes additional features that contribute to the heterogeneity of the disorder, finishing with a description of medical comorbidities.

CORE FEATURES

Deficits in social communication represent the cardinal features of ASD and manifest as impairments in social–emotional reciprocity, deficits in nonverbal communication, and compromised capacity to develop and maintain age-appropriate relationships with peers. An individual's language skills, which are not contained in the new diagnostic criteria, must be considered *alongside* the social and communicative impairments. For example, a child with delayed language skills may have minimal social impairments, whereas a highly verbal child may only interact by using stereotyped speech or delayed echolalia.

The term joint attention refers to a cluster of behaviors that share the common goal of communicating with another person about a third entity nonverbally. This typically involves eye gaze, gesturing, and showing (Volkmar, 2011). From as early as 12 months, infants with ASD show a lack of interest in the human face and a proclivity to attend to non-social stimuli as opposed to those with social salience (Klin et al., 2009). This gravitation toward non-social stimuli is thought to complicate the interdependent development of joint attention and communication skills. Subsequent early signs of ASD typically involve delays in social communication skills, such as delayed pointing, failure to respond to name, and lack of cooing, babbling, and word production. Over the course of development, these social and communicative deficits typically persist and lead to reduced or total lack of sharing and social interaction as well as impairments in the use and perception of non-verbal social cues.

The repetitive or restricted patterns of behavior of ASD, grouped together into Category B of the proposed DSM-5 criteria, comprise stereotypic or repetitive movements and/or use of speech, insistence on routines, unusual or encompassing preoccupations, and abnormal sensory responses to the environment.

Stereotyped and repetitive motor mannerisms are highly heterogeneous and can be subdivided across multiple dimensions, including fine or gross motor, simple or complex, and with or without objects. Examples are hand flapping, finger flicking, whole-body rocking, and walking on tip-toe. Motor mannerisms are reported in 37% to 95% of individuals with ASD (Filipek et al., 2000). A significant body of research provides evidence for a sensory function of stereotypies (Cunningham and Schreibman, 2008), and repetitive self-injurious behaviors such as head banging, self-biting, or self-pinching are more common in individuals with intellectual impairment. Repetitive speech can take the form of delayed or immediate echolalia, as well as stereotyped speech, which is often characterized by overly formal or idiosyncratic expressions.

Unusual or encompassing preoccupations typically involve interest in the nonfunctional and physical aspects of objects. Such preoccupations may result in stimulation of various sensory modalities such as visual, tactile, vestibular, taste, and smell. Higher functioning individuals may exhibit unusual preoccupations with things such as metal objects, street signs, and toilets. Encompassing preoccupations with areas of circumscribed interests may take over one's life, supplant all other interests or hobbies, and affect functioning in other domains. In addition, individuals may exhibit unusual interests and develop expertise in arcane topics; alternatively, they may exhibit isolated splinter skills, and demonstrate exceptional abilities in areas such as music, drawing, and memory.

A significant proportion of people with ASD exhibit sensory symptoms, which can include heightened or reduced sensitivities to noise, light, or touch as well as paradoxical responses to stimuli such as high and low thresholds for pain. Clinical studies examining rates of sensory symptoms in school-age children with autism report a range from 42% to 88%; scores on the Sensory Profile in young children with autism were significantly higher than in children with other developmental disorders, and high scores were correlated with stereotyped interests and behaviors (Wiggins et al., 2009).

PATTERNS OF ONSET

Children may present in the first year of life with delays in all core domains, whereas some children develop typically and then plateau, and approximately 25% to 30% exhibit frank regression between 12 and 36 months (Ozonoff et al., 2011). The loss of skills observed in regression can occur in the setting of previously typical development or superimposed on an already aberrant developmental trajectory (Ozonoff et al., 2005). Early identification of children at risk for developing ASD is first accomplished through the use of screening tools with high sensitivity and confirmed using the DSM with semi-structured observational tools and parent interviews.

COGNITIVE DEFICITS

A range of cognitive deficits characterize children with ASD. Recent surveillance studies indicate lower rates of intellectual disability—between 45% and 60%—compared with those reported in the 1990s (CDC, 2012; Johnson and Myers, 2007). Lower IQ scores are relatively stable and are associated with worse outcome as well as with a greater risk of developing a seizure disorder in adolescence (Johnson and Myers, 2007; Volkmar et al., 2007). Regardless of the level of general intellectual functioning, the cognitive profile of individuals with ASD is uneven, with marked "scatter" and pockets of skill across cognitive domains (Volkmar et al., 2007). Individuals typically perform better on tasks that require rote, visuospatial, or stimulus-bound perceptual processes as opposed to tasks that require more abstract thinking or higher-order, language-based conceptual processes (Dawson et al., 1998; Minshew et al., 1994; Ozonoff et al., 1991). Accordingly, nonverbal performance (PIQ) is usually stronger than verbally mediated performance (VIQ).

INATTENTION, HYPERACTIVITY, AND IMPULSIVITY

Symptoms of inattention, hyperactivity, and impulsivity are common in individuals with ASD, and may be the primary reason for referral among less impaired patients. In a survey of 487 children and adolescents with ASD, greater than 50% had moderate to severe symptoms of inattention and hyperactivity. In another sample of 101 children with ASD, 95% exhibited attention deficit, 50% demonstrated impulsive behavior, and 75% were found to manifest symptoms consistent with attention deficit hyperactivity disorder (ADHD) (Goldstein and Schwebach, 2004; Lecavalier, 2006). The presence of ADHD symptoms in children with ASD is particularly important to clarify because comorbidity may predict greater impairment in activities of daily life and higher rates of hospitalization than otherwise exist for children with ASD alone.

MEDICAL COMORBIDITY

In approximately 10% to 25% of patients, there is an identifiable medical condition or recognized syndrome associated with the ASD phenotype. Such conditions are typically associated with more severe comorbid global developmental delay and are in some cases considered to be the cause of the ASD symptomatology.

Perhaps the best known association is that of epilepsy. The occurrence of epilepsy in autism is higher than in the general population and there is growing recognition that a subset of ASD patients have epileptiform EEG abnormalities in the absence of clinical seizures (Spence and Schneider, 2009). Depending on the study, 5% to 44% of individuals with ASD have seizure activity. Individuals with more severe intellectual disability are more likely to have epilepsy than those with greater language and cognitive skills (Tuchman and Rapin, 2002). Conversely, behaviors characteristic of autism have also been reported in pediatric patients with different epileptic syndromes. The complex relationship between seizure activity and ASD symptomatology can be seen in children with Landau Kleffner syndrome (LKS). Landau Kleffner syndrome presents with normal development until school age, when children typically develop acquired epileptic aphasia. The loss of previously acquired language milestones and loss of verbal comprehension can take the form of ASD-like symptomatology.

There are many medical genetic conditions associated with ASD. For a comprehensive review, see Betancur (2011) with a few examples noted here. Fragile X syndrome is the most commonly known genetic cause of ASD and intellectual disability in males. The phenotype includes cognitive delays, macrocephaly, large pinnae, hyperorchidism, hypotonia, and joint hyperextensibility. As many as 30% to 50% of individuals with genetically confirmed Fragile X syndrome demonstrate some characteristics of ASD (Rogers et al., 2001).

Additional common causes of ASD are Phelan–McDermid syndrome, Angelman syndrome and 15q duplications, and Rett syndrome. Phelan–McDermid syndrome (PMS) involves a deletion or mutation of the terminal region of chromosome 22 and there is very good evidence for a central role for the loss of SHANK3 as a major determinant for the neurobiological phenotypes in PMS (Buxbaum, 2009). Loss of a functional copy of SHANK3 appears to be second only to Fragile X syndrome in frequency as a monogenic cause of ASD, with estimates of 0.5% to 1% of ASD (Betancur, 2011).

Children with Angelman syndrome, which involves either a 15q deletion or imprinting error, are often nonverbal and present with global developmental delay, hypotonia, wide-based ataxic gait, seizures, and progressive spasticity (Veltman et al., 2005). Many meet criteria for ASD, as do individuals with a duplication of this region (Betancur, 2011).

Females with a mutation of the *MECP2* gene (Rett syndrome) can present with an ASD-like regression; individuals typically exhibit a phenotype characterized by microcephaly, seizures, and hand-wringing stereotypies (Johnson and Myers, 2007). Duplication of this region can also present with an ASD phenotype (Betancur, 2011).

Tuberous sclerosis (TSC) is a neurocutaneous disorder characterized by hypopigmented macules, fibroangioma, kidney lesions, central nervous system hamartomas, seizures, intellectual disability, and autistic and/or ADHD-like behaviors. An estimated 17% to 60% of patients with TSC have ASD (Numis et al., 2011). However, although it is often reported that the rate of TSC in ASD approaches 1%, this is not supported by recent data and the rates of TSC in patients ascertained for ASD are likely to be very low.

Phenylketonuria, often associated with the ASD phenotype in the past, is now considered a rare cause of ASD and ID in the United States because it is preventable through newborn screening and dietary intervention. This serves as an important reminder that there are possibly additional genetic alterations underlying ASD that might be amenable to disease-modifying interventions.

NEUROIMAGING

Although a diagnosis of ASD is made based purely on behavioral symptoms, it is widely accepted that these symptoms have a neurodevelopmental origin. Over the last 20 years, neuroimaging studies have made great contributions to our understanding of the neurobiological underpinnings of the disorder (see Fig. 77.1). There is considerable heterogeneity in the brain phenotype of individuals with ASD, but structural and functional imaging studies have begun to elucidate brain–behavior relationships and move toward developing plausible neural biomarkers of ASD. Here, we summarize emerging themes, recent developments, and promising approaches within the structural and functional neuroimaging literature.

STRUCTURAL NEUROIMAGING

The structural brain imaging field has been plagued by contradictory findings owing in part to variability in both methodology and sample characteristics. However, in recent years, efforts to better understand the effects of age and development on brain structure in ASD have yielded some consistent patterns. The most replicated finding so far is that of increased brain volume in early childhood. Cross-sectional studies across the lifespan suggest that the brain is enlarged by two years of age, but normal or reduced in size by adolescence and adulthood. Taken together with research indicating that head circumference is normal or smaller at birth, these data suggest a period of rapid brain overgrowth in infancy and toddlerhood that is likely followed by a period of arrested growth and perhaps an accelerated rate of decline from adolescence to adulthood (Courchesne et al., 2011). Longitudinal studies have confirmed the findings in young children (e.g., Hazlett et al., 2011), but more work is needed that follows the same individuals through adulthood to confirm the later part of the proposed growth curve.

An important part of understanding brain enlargement in ASD is examining whether there are specific regions that are disproportionately affected. Evidence suggests that there is a gradient, such that the frontal and temporal cortices are most affected and occipital the least (see Courchesne et al., 2007 for a review). With respect to specific brain structures, the *amygdala* has received much recent attention. Although earlier studies yielded highly inconsistent findings, including enlarged size, reduced size, and no difference relative to controls, a metaanalysis revealed that age is an important factor to consider, with enlargement occurring in younger, but not older individuals with ASD (Stanfield et al., 2008). A recent longitudinal study found that the amygdala was enlarged by about 6% by three years of age and, moreover, the magnitude of enlargement was even greater one year later (9%) (Nordahl et al., 2012). Together with earlier evidence from the same

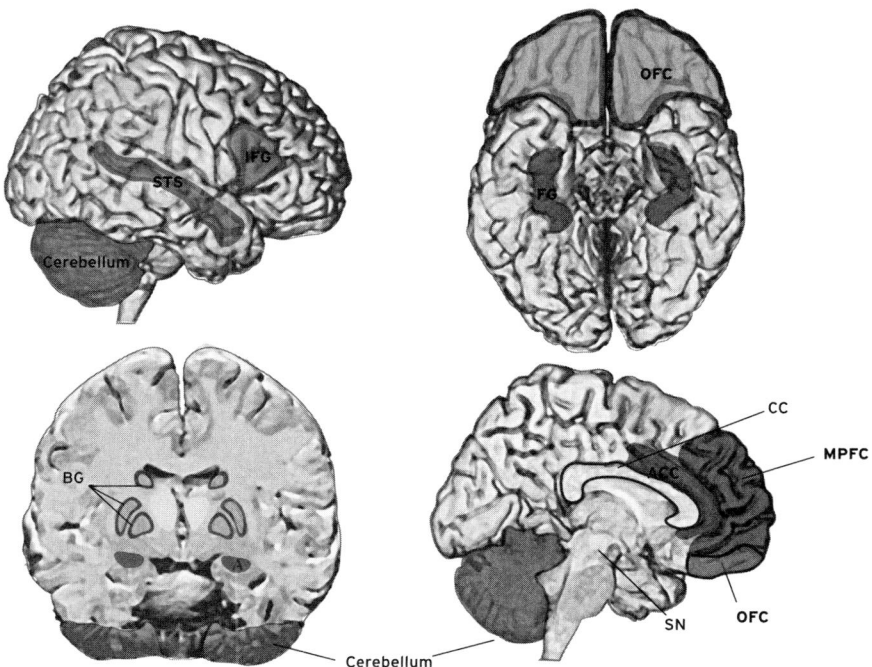

Figure 77.1 Brain areas commonly found to be structurally or functionally abnormal in autism. Regions in bold are considered to be part of the social brain. Structural Differences: A, amygdala; BG, basal ganglia; Cerebellum. CC, corpus callosum. Functional Impairment: ACC, anterior cingulate cortex; A, amygdala; FG, fusiform gyrus; IFG, inferior frontal gyrus; STS, superior temporal sulcus; MPFC, medial prefrontal cortex; OFC, orbitofrontal cortex. (Adapted from Amaral et al. (2008) used with permission from Elsevier.)

group that the amygdala is enlarged by approximately 14% in middle childhood, this suggests that overgrowth of the amygdala begins before age three and continues to accelerate over the next several years. Importantly, abnormal enlargement of the amygdala has been correlated with both the severity of autism symptoms (Schumann et al., 2009) and joint attention abilities (Mosconi et al., 2009), considered to be a pivotal deficit in ASD. Developing such links is critical for understanding brain–behavior relationships and the role of structural abnormalities in the etiology of autism.

Another region that is reportedly enlarged in autism is the *caudate nucleus*, which has been associated with the severity of repetitive behaviors (e.g., Hollander et al., 2005). The *cerebellum* has been widely studied, but findings have been inconsistent. Although a metaanalysis confirmed earlier reports of reduction in cerebellar vermis volumes, there was significant heterogeneity in the data, with age and IQ found to be important factors (Stanfield et al., 2008). Metaanalyses have also revealed that the *corpus callosum* is reduced in autism (Frazier and Hardan, 2009; Stanfield et al., 2008), suggesting that interhemispheric connectivity is impaired. Finally, it is noteworthy that regions thought to play a key role in social cognition and found to be functionally aberrant, such as the fusiform gyrus, the superior temporal sulcus, and the pars opercularis of the inferior frontal gyrus, have also been observed to have structural abnormalities (see Stigler et al., 2011 for a review).

The finding of enlarged brain volume also leads to the question of whether the increase reflects changes in cortical thickness or cortical surface area. These measures are important because they are likely related to distinct biological mechanisms. Cortical thickness is hypothesized to reflect dendritic pruning and arborization or myelination, whereas cortical surface area varies with cortical folding and is thought to depend on the division of progenitor cells in the embryological periventricular area; cortical volume is the product of these two measures. Although newer technology allows for the automated measurement of cortical volume, thickness, and surface area simultaneously, applications to ASD are still in their infancy. In the largest cross-sectional study of this nature to date, Raznahan and colleagues (2010) examined the relationship between age, cortical volume, thickness, and surface area in males with ASD and healthy controls ages 10 to 65 years. They found that within frontal, temporal, and inferior parietal cortices, cortical volume, and thickness decreased significantly with age in healthy controls, but not in the ASD group, such that these measures were reduced relative to controls in childhood, but larger by adolescence and adulthood. However, no such abnormal trajectories were noted in cortical surface area. In contrast, a recent longitudinal study in young children ages two to five years did not find differences in cortical thickness, but did note increases in cortical volume and an estimate of surface area relative to controls at both time points, suggesting that cortical surface area was enlarged before two years of age in the ASD group (Hazlett et al., 2011). Given their potential to shed light on the distinct biological processes underlying brain overgrowth, studies that clarify the relative contributions of cortical thickness and surface area have great potential.

DIFFUSION TENSOR IMAGING

Diffusion tensor imaging (DTI) is a technique that probes the integrity of white matter fibers in the brain. The organization of axons in parallel bundles and the myelination of their sheaths restricts the diffusion of water, producing anisotropic diffusion. Most DTI studies in children and adults with ASD have found reduced fractional anisotropy, usually interpreted as lower coherence and organization of fiber tracts, in a variety of regions (e.g., medial prefrontal, orbitoprefrontal, anterior cingulate, external and internal capsule, corpus callosum, temporal lobe, among others) (see Anagnostou and Taylor, 2011, for a review). However, increased fractional anisotropy has also been observed in young children with ASD, ages 1.8 to 3.3 years (Ben Bashat et al., 2007), which is consistent with the data on early brain overgrowth and further illustrates the need to consider age and developmental trajectory, when designing and parsing neuroimaging studies.

There is a dearth of prospective data on autism from the first year of life, owing to the difficulty in detecting clinical symptoms before 12 months of age (Ozonoff et al., 2010). Recent efforts focused on following infants with high familial risk for ASD are beginning to enable the detection of brain abnormalities before the emergence of behavioral symptoms. For example, Wolff and colleagues (Wolff et al., 2012) used DTI to examine the development of white matter fibers in infants who have an older sibling with autism. Infants were scanned at 6, 12, and 24 months and evaluated for ASD symptoms at 24 months. Trajectories of white matter development, as indexed by fractional anisotropy values, differed significantly in infants who went on to develop ASD compared to infants who did not. Specifically, in most of the fiber tracts evaluated, infants later diagnosed with ASD showed higher fractional anisotropy at six months compared with infants determined to have typical development, but lower values by 24 months, suggesting that a slowed rate of white matter development is associated with an eventual ASD diagnosis among infants with high familial risk. The finding that white matter abnormalities are present and identifiable before the onset of clinical symptoms is exciting because it raises the possibility of developing structural imaging biomarkers for ASD.

FUNCTIONAL NEUROIMAGING

Functional magnetic resonance imaging (fMRI) studies have had a powerful effect on our understanding of autism as a neurobiological disorder. Early fMRI studies attempted to delineate brain–behavior relationships in ASD by designing tasks that tap core symptom domains, including social cognition (e.g., face processing, theory of mind, imitation, joint attention), language (e.g., semantic sentence comprehension, pragmatic/nonliteral language, gesture), and repetitive behaviors (via executive function tasks). A recent metaanalysis revealed that abnormalities in the function of regions considered to be part of the "social brain," such as the *medial prefrontal cortex, orbitofrontal cortex, amygdala, fusiform gyrus,* and *superior temporal sulcus,* are among the most well-replicated findings in the literature (Philip et al., 2012). These studies suggest that ASD is associated with a lack of specialization in systems evolved for social attunement

that are normally automatically engaged. However, so far fMRI studies cannot differentiate whether aberrant brain activity is a cause or consequence of ASD. In fact, there is some evidence indicating that individuals with ASD can show typical levels of activity in key brain regions under certain circumstances—e.g., if the task is personally relevant, allows for cognitive or explicit processing, or draws attention to key social features (see Wang et al., 2007). This suggests the possibility that reduced activity in the social brain may be a result of a lack of social attention or motivation rather than a primary dysfunction in specific brain regions. A better understanding of the circumstances in which normative neural systems are engaged could inform novel treatment approaches.

An abundance of studies have examined the functional connectivity among brain regions that participate in neural networks in ASD. The majority of studies taking this approach have found support for the underconnectivity theory of autism, as coined by Just and colleagues (2004) when they observed decreased synchronization between the time series of activation among regions involved in a sentence comprehension task. Researchers have found underconnectivity in individuals with ASD using task-based approaches, resting-state approaches, and intrinsic approaches that attempt to remove activation effects. However, the findings are not all consistent with the underconnectivity theory and methodology appears to be an important consideration in interpreting the literature; a recent survey of functional connectivity studies found that task-based approaches looking within regions of interest are most likely to support underconnectivity (Muller et al., 2011). Some studies have found increased connectivity between close-range "nonessential" regions, but these findings have been interpreted as increased noise and, therefore, contributing to aberrant connectivity by decreasing signal-to-noise ratio (see Anagnostou and Taylor, 2011, for a review). The underconnectivity theory is appealing in that it offers a unifying, systems-level model of brain dysfunction while accounting for the considerable heterogeneity of ASD (Geschwind and Levitt, 2007). However, reduced functional connectivity between long-range connections has also been observed in a variety of other disorders, including Alzheimer's disease, schizophrenia, chronic heroin use, posttraumatic stress disorder, and dyslexia, so it is not yet clear how underconnectivity accounts for what is common and specific to ASD (see Pelphrey et al., 2011).

One limitation of the extant fMRI literature is that, traditionally, MRI studies of ASD have been restricted to high-functioning older children, adolescents, and adults owing to the fact that obtaining high quality data necessitates that the participant remain still for the duration of a scan. Recently, investigators have extended their samples to infants and toddlers by scanning during natural sleep. Although fMRI signal can be somewhat dampened during sleep, the overall pattern of activation is very similar to that obtained during the awake state. Eyler and colleagues examined brain activity in response to a bedtime story during natural sleep and found that toddlers with ASDs between 12 and 48 months showed abnormalities in lateralization of temporal activity (Eyler et al., 2012). Whereas typically developing toddlers showed the expected left-hemisphere dominant pattern of activity in response to language, children who were later diagnosed with ASD showed reduced activity in the left temporal cortex, a deficit that became more severe with age. This finding is consistent with numerous observations of a similar lack of left-hemisphere language specialization in older children and adults, and extends this work by suggesting that such a lack of specialization emerges early and may be a fundamental aspect of ASD. Scanning during natural sleep should prove to be a useful technique for extending fMRI to even younger ages as well as lower functioning populations.

Similar to the discussion in the structural imaging section, little is known about behavior and brain activation patterns associated with autism in the first year of life, which can lead to delays in diagnosis and treatment. Several research groups are currently trying to remedy this by focusing on prospective longitudinal studies of infants at high risk for autism by virtue of having an older sibling with ASD. A recent study following this approach recorded infants' event-related potentials (ERPs) in response to gaze shifts toward and away from the infant (Elsabbagh et al., 2012). Brain responses to these dynamic gaze shifts at six to 10 months distinguished between at-risk infants who were diagnosed with ASD at 24 or 36 months from both at-risk infants who did not later develop ASD as well as low-risk controls. Significantly, these early differences in brain function were not driven by differences in attention or looking behavior, as eye-tracking data revealed similar visual fixation times on the eyes across risk groups and diagnostic outcomes. The finding that ERP responses to gaze shifts predicted clinical outcomes raises the possibility of developing brain-based screening methods that could lead to early detection and treatment, with the caveat that such a biomarker would need to be established as sensitive and specific to ASD in a population-based sample.

GENETICS

We note in the preceding some medical genetic causes of ASD. More broadly, genetic epidemiological studies have consistently supported a strong role for genetics in ASD. In the nine twin studies conducted over the past 40 years, there has consistently been clear evidence for significantly increased concordance for ASD between monozygotic twins as compared to dizygotic twins (Hallmayer et al., 2011; Lichtenstein et al., 2010; Rosenberg et al., 2009; Taniai et al., 2008). These results indicate that the closer individuals are genetically, controlling for other factors (in this case prenatal, perinatal, and postnatal environment), the more likely they are to share the trait of ASD, which is the sine qua non for a genetic disorder. A strong role for genetics is supported by family studies as well, and most estimates of heritability in ASD are placed at 80% or higher. Clarifying the precise nature of the genetic liability to ASD has remained a challenge, but recent studies have made it clear that a significant proportion of risk resides in rare genetic variants of major effect and in recent genetic variation.

COMMON GENETIC VARIATION

It is informative to consider genetic risk in two dimensions, varying from low to high effect and from rare to common variation (Sullivan et al., 2012). Very few examples of common variants with significant deleterious effect have been described, for the simple reason that if such variants exist, any impact on reproductive fitness would lead to strong purifying selection. One well-known example of such a variant, *APOE4* as a risk allele for Alzheimer's disease, is able to persist in the population because onset of the disorder is late in life. It is therefore likely that for an early onset disorder such as ASD, *common variation* will be associated with only very small effects, and this assertion is supported by both theoretical and empirical data. With several genome-wide association studies having been completed, single nucleotide polymorphism (SNP) variation with odds ratios of above 1.2 have effectively been excluded (Devlin et al., 2011). For SNP associated with smaller odds ratios, there are insufficient sample sizes to be adequately powered to make any conclusions. Based on studies in other psychiatric disorders, most notably schizophrenia, it is likely that there will be SNP association with ASD, but without 15,000 or more samples, we are not likely to identify many of them. One important conclusion from the empirical and theoretical data is that many, and even most, of the candidate gene association studies published in ASD are very likely false-positive findings.

RARE GENETIC VARIATION

When considering rare genetic variation, one can again consider the effect size dimension (Sullivan *et al.*, 2012). Clearly, it would be enormously difficult to reliably identify rare variation associated with very weak effects, so from a practical perspective, we are restricted to a focus on rare variation with higher effect sizes. Here, the field has made enormous progress, with more loci and genes being discovered all the time.

Discovery of rare genetic variation has tracked with technology. From the early days of karyotyping, through high-resolution karyotyping, FISH (fluorescent in situ hybridization), CMA, and now MPS, discovery of ASD loci and genes has been facilitated by the emergent technology (Ledbetter, 2008). Aneuploidies were identified in patients with an ASD using karyotyping, and include Down syndrome, Turner syndrome, Klinefelter syndrome, and additional sex chromosome abnormalities (Betancur, 2011). With the advent of FISH and then CMA, some 40 recurrent microdeletions or microduplications have been associated with ASD (Betancur, 2011; Cooper et al., 2011). Some more common variants include deletions and duplications at 7q11.23 (Williams syndrome), 15q11-q13 (the Prader–Willi/Angelman region), 17p11.2 (Smith–Magenis syndrome), 22q11 (DiGeorge syndrome), and 22q13 (Phelan–McDermid syndrome) and some of these are described briefly in the preceding.

These gene dosage abnormalities, frequently referred to as copy number variation (CNV), are recurrent either because they are subtelomeric or because they are flanked by segmental duplications (also called low copy repeats or LCR) and undergo non-allelic homologous recombination. However, there are many non-recurrent CNVs that have been associated with ASD and there are emerging algorithms to reliably relate a particular CNV to an ASD, taking into account the CNV size, gene content, and *de novo*, inherited, or X-linked inheritance of the CNV. Finally, with traditional and now massively parallel sequencing (MPS), there have been over 100 genes associated with high risk for ASD (Betancur, 2011).

Four recent studies using MPS and focusing on *de novo* single nucleotide variation (SNV) identified at least six new ASD genes (*CHD8, DYRK1A, KATNAL2, NTNG1, POGZ,* and *SCN2A*), highlighting the importance of *de novo* variation in ASD and showing how important MPS approaches will be for further gene discovery (Iossifov et al., 2012; Neale et al., 2012; O'Roak et al., 2012; Sanders et al., 2012). These studies also provided estimates for the total number of dominant ASD genes that can be identified through MPS, now placed at about 800–1000, which suggests that we have identified something in the order of 10% to 20% of ASD genes. As MPS studies accelerate on available samples, it is fairly straightforward to predict that we can readily double the number of confirmed ASD risk genes within just three years. As such genes are identified, cell and animal models can be developed to better understand pathophysiology, which can in turn lead to novel therapeutics (see the following).

MODEL SYSTEMS

Identifying genes for ASD provides an opportunity for cellular and animal models to better understand pathobiology. The high risk associated with genes identified to date means that disruption of these genes in model systems will have strong *construct validity*. A model system of choice has been the genetically modified mouse, and dozens of ASD genes have been disrupted in mouse models (Buxbaum et al., 2012). These models have shown molecular, cellular, and behavioral deficits, which can then be used to dissect out pathobiological mechanisms of ASD that in turn can aid in identifying and assessing novel therapeutics. One recent success is that of fragile X syndrome, where studies in model systems implicate glutamate signaling abnormalities in the phenotype; recent clinical trials indirectly or directly modulating glutamate signaling are showing some very exciting results (Berry-Kravis et al., 2012; Jacquemont et al., 2011). Our work with *SHANK3* (see the preceding) has led to a mouse model where we observed deficits in neuronal glutamate signaling, and evidence for less mature synapses in the hippocampus (Bozdagi et al., 2010). Recently, we have shown that clinical doses of recombinant human insulin-like growth factor 1 (IGF-1) reversed these deficits in mice, and we have recently initiated clinical trials of IGF-1 in *SHANK3* haploinsufficiency (Phelan–McDermid syndrome).

SYSTEMS GENETICS

It should be apparent that with such a complex genetic and genomic architecture for ASD, it will not be straightforward to readily identify targets for drug development. However, systems-level analyses of genes and loci providing high risk for ASD can help identify pathways that underlie an appreciable proportion of ASD risk and can also identify driver genes for such pathways. These driver genes would then represent the high-value targets for drug development. The reader is referred to recent studies on systems-level analyses in ASD, including

evidence for highly connected gene models in ASD (Kou et al., 2012; Neale et al., 2012), a broad role for targets of FMRP (the proteins coded by the fragile X gene) in ASD (Iossifov et al., 2012), and disruption of neuronal gene expression modules in ASD (Voineagu et al., 2011).

THERAPEUTICS

Behavioral interventions are the first-line treatment in ASD. A few commonly used interventions, such as those based in the principles of applied behavioral analysis (ABA), have recently developed the evidence base to be considered empirically supported treatments for ASD (Seida et al., 2009; Warren et al., 2011). There has also been a significant amount of research into pharmacological treatments in ASD, although most medicines have targeted associated features as opposed to core symptom domains (Doyle and McDougle, 2012). This strategy was effective for treatment development, in part, and led to U.S. Food and Drug Administration (FDA) indications for "irritability associated with autism" for risperidone and aripiprazole.

BEHAVIORAL THERAPY

Behavioral interventions can widely be divided into comprehensive programs, including educational models such as TEACCH (Treatment and Education of Autistic and related Communication-handicapped Children), and skill building interventions designed to target specific core or associated symptoms. In general, comprehensive programs deliver behavioral interventions early, intensively, and address several domains of functioning (e.g., language, daily living, behavior, socialization). Comprehensive programs typically enroll children for at least one year and involve parents in the training models. The most studied is Applied Behavioral Analysis (ABA; Lovaas, 1987), which utilizes basic principles of learning and conditioning to systematically teach skills and reduce problematic behaviors. Applied Behavioral Analysis breaks down skills into smaller components and applies positive reinforcement to facilitate incremental improvements in skill performance. In recent years, additional comprehensive treatment models, such as the Early Start Denver Model, have been developed using ABA principles (ESDM; Dawson et al., 2010). Early Start Denver Model integrates ABA with developmental and relationship-based approaches and has shown similar gains in cognitive development seen in traditional ABA models. In a randomized controlled trial, two years of intervention led to an average gain of 17.6 standard IQ points in the ESDM group as compared with seven points in the community treatment controls. In addition, children in the ESDM group showed greater improvements in adaptive functioning and symptom severity (Dawson et al., 2010).

In contrast to comprehensive programs, skill-building programs are focused on one domain or skill and are generally short-term treatments. For example, several skill building treatments are available for language development. One approach for non-verbal children with oral–motor praxis impairments is PROMPT (Prompts for Restructuring Oral

Muscular Phonetic Targets), in which a speech therapist uses modeling and physical manipulation of the mouth and jaw to help the child form speech sounds and awards behavioral reinforcers for successful approximations (Rogers et al., 2006). Picture Exchange Communication Systems (PECS) is an augmentative and alternative communication (AAC) intervention that involves teaching children with ASD to utilize picture symbols to communicate. Metaanalyses suggest that PECS is associated with improved communication skills and behavior (Ganz et al., 2012). Other approaches to teach functional communication in non-verbal children rely on devices using digital voice output, or adapted signs from American Sign Language. With the advent of portable electronic devices, the iPad and other tablets have recently become popular training tools, although the multitude of available applications have not been well studied.

Skill-building interventions are also used to improve socialization impairments in children with ASD. Although several models of social skills intervention exist, commonly used approaches include social skills training groups, Relationship Development Intervention (RDI), peer-mediated interventions, and Social Stories™. Social skills training groups focus on improving ASD-specific impairments through various orientations, including cognitive behavioral therapy (CBT) or play. Relationship Development Intervention is parent-directed and facilitates social learning opportunities for children in naturalistic settings. Peer-mediated interventions train typically developing peers as social interaction facilitators for children with ASD, and Social Stories™ teaches skills through detailed descriptions of social situations that embed direct statements about appropriate behavior expected from a child in a given situation.

Targeted interventions can also be applied to reduce disruptive and repetitive behaviors, such as positive behavioral support (PBS). Positive behavioral support adopts ABA principles to understand environmental triggers for behavioral problems and utilizes systematic observations and data collection known as functional behavioral assessments (FBAs). This approach assumes that disruptive behaviors can be predicted to occur based on antecedent or consequences commonly associated with that behavior. Maladaptive behaviors are believed to be maintained/reinforced because they often allow the child to avoid demands or gain access to a desired object. Once the elements of the setting and specific triggers are understood, the environment is manipulated to replace the disruptive behavior with more adaptive behavior using appropriate reinforcement.

In summary, although widely utilized, only a few behavioral interventions have been rigorously studied and the evidence base for most interventions used in practice is still emerging. Several early, intensive behavioral interventions such as ABA and ESDM are supported by encouraging data in randomized controlled trials. Other models, including social skills interventions and many language interventions, require additional rigorous evaluation. The literature to date does not address several important treatment needs, such as interventions for older individuals with ASD. In addition, moderators and mediators of treatment effects have yet to be identified.

Several collaborative projects, including the Toddler Treatment Network funded by Autism Speaks, are poised to provide valuable data to potentially fill significant gaps in the literature and improve the evidence base in guiding future behavioral treatment in ASD.

PHARMACOTHERAPY

The development of pharmacological treatments in ASD has mainly taken a symptom domain approach to broadly target associated psychiatric features, such as aggression, attention deficit and hyperactivity, and anxiety. This strategy has been only loosely related to what is known about the neurobiology of the disorders and met with mixed success. Several recent papers (Anagnostou and Hansen, 2011; Doyle and McDougle, 2012; Warren et al., 2011) have reviewed the current state of the pharmacological evidence and are cited throughout this section rather than providing individual references to the studies (and see Table 77.1). The section will also be divided into symptom domains in order to be consistent with clinical practice.

AGGRESSION

Aggression and self-injury are among the most distressing associated symptoms in ASD and are treated with a broad range of pharmacological approaches. Various mechanisms have been proposed to explain their prevalence in ASD and biochemical targets include the dopaminergic, serotonergic, adrenergic, and opioid systems, among others. In controlled clinical trials to specifically target aggression, several medications have produced significant improvement as compared with placebo, including risperidone, aripiprazole, methylphenidate, clonidine, tianeptine, and naltrexone. However, only risperidone, aripiprazole, and methylphenidate demonstrate results that have been replicated across at least two well-controlled studies (Anagnostou and Hansen, 2011; Doyle and McDougle, 2012; Warren et al., 2011).

Dopamine dysregulation has specifically been implicated in self-injurious patients with autism and dopaminergic antagonists are most commonly used to prevent the onset and maintenance of aggression and self-injury. Risperidone has the most evidence to support its use for aggression in ASD, and results are consistent across several studies. However, the risks of risperidone include significant weight gain and increased vulnerability to diabetes and cardiovascular disease later in life. At least two controlled trials support the use of aripiprazole for irritability in ASD. As with risperidone, risks of weight gain and metabolic disturbance persist with aripiprazole, although levels of serum prolactin do not appear to increase as they may with risperidone. Other neuroleptics have been studied in ASD. Small open label or retrospective studies of clozapine, quetiapine, ziprasidone, olanzapine, and at least one controlled trial with olanzapine all provide preliminary evidence to support their use to treat disruptive behaviors associated with ASD. Older studies with haloperidol have also demonstrated benefit.

Psychostimulant medications are potent dopaminergic agonists and may act to reduce aggression by increasing the availability of dopamine in the prefrontal cortex and enhancing impulse control though striatal-frontal pathways. At least two controlled

TABLE 77.1. Selected positive controlled trials of medications in ASD

MEDICATION	AUTHORS	DESIGN	SAMPLE	OUTCOME
Risperidone	RUPP (2002)	Placebo Parallel	101 children and adolescents	↓ aggression ↓ hyperactivity
Risperidone	Shea et al. (2004)	Placebo Parallel	80 children	↓ aggression ↓ hyperactivity
Aripiprazole	Owen et al. (2009)	Placebo Parallel	98 children and adolescents	↓ aggression
Aripiprazole	Marcus et al. (2009)	Placebo Parallel	218 children and adolescents	↓ aggression
Valproate	Hollander et al. (2010)	Placebo Parallel	27 children and adolescents	↓ aggression
Clonidine	Jaselkis et al. (1992)	Placebo Crossover	8 children and adolescents	↓ aggression ↓ hyperactivity
Methylphenidate	RUPP (2005)	Placebo Crossover	72 children and adolescents	↓ hyperactivity
Atomoxetine	Hafterkamp et al. (2012)	Placebo Parallel	97 children and adolescents	↓ hyperactivity
Atromoxetine	Arnold et al. (2006)	Placebo Crossover	16 children and adolescents	↓ hyperactivity
Haloperidol	Anderson et al. (1989)	Placebo Crossover	45 children	↓ hyperactivity
Fluvoxamine	McDougle et al. (1996)	Placebo Parallel	30 adults	↓ Repetitive behavior
Fluoxetine	Hollander et al. (2005)	Placebo Crossover	39 children and adolescents	↓ Repetitive behavior

trials found methylphenidate effective for symptoms of aggression and self-injury in ASD, although its effect on aggression is less reliable than on symptoms of attention deficit and hyperactivity in ASD. Notably, the largest study of methylphenidate in ASD to date did not find significant differences on irritability and aggression as compared with placebo, although benefits on hyperactivity were significant (RUPP, 2005).

ATTENTION DEFICIT AND HYPERACTIVITY

Symptoms of attention deficit, hyperactivity, and impulsivity are common in ASD (Lecavalier, 2006). Methylphenidate and atomoxetine effectively treat symptoms of ADHD in ASD, but response rates are lower than what is reported in typically developing children with ADHD alone (Harfterkamp, 2012; RUPP, 2005). Further, in ASD, symptoms of inattention may be less likely to respond than symptoms of hyperactivity and impulsivity. Treatment success may also be limited by tolerability; 18% of subjects with ASD discontinued the RUPP methylphenidate trial, and the most common side effect was irritability.

Many studies have also demonstrated efficacy for antipsychotic medications, and risperidone in particular has consistently shown benefit for hyperactivity in ASD. However, significant concerns about the tolerability of antipsychotics remain and suggest that benefits of these medications must be carefully weighed against the risks, especially in the absence of significant aggression.

Evidence from controlled studies of alpha-two agonists for ADHD-related symptoms in ASD is inconsistent and response rates are relatively low. Open label studies of guanfacine appear promising but additional controlled studies are needed. Alpha-two agonists may nevertheless be a reasonable alternative or augmentation strategy to stimulants and have the advantage of being well tolerated.

Based on evidence of glutamatergic dysregulation in ASD derived from genetic discovery and model systems, amantadine and other NMDA antagonists are of significant interest for the treatment of ASD symptoms. One controlled trial has been published to date with amantadine, and controlled trials are underway with memantine based on positive results from open label and retrospective reports. Despite multiple controlled trials, results with naltrexone are inconsistent and isolated positive findings should be interpreted with caution.

ANXIETY AND REPETITIVE BEHAVIORS

Restrictive, repetitive, and stereotyped behaviors are a core symptom of ASD, and targeting this domain can improve overall outcomes for affected children. Among the various pharmacological options, serotonergic medications are widely used in part because serotonergic dysregulation in ASD is a consistently replicated finding from biochemical, pharmacological challenge, and genetic studies. Fluoxetine is the most rigorously studied serotonergic medication in ASD; numerous case reports, open-label studies, retrospective chart reviews, and small placebo-controlled trials have been published with promising results (Doyle, 2012). However, the Studies of Fluoxetine in Autism (SOFIA) enrolled 158 children and adolescents for a 14-week treatment of placebo or orally disintegrating fluoxetine, but fluoxetine was not more efficacious than placebo for reducing repetitive behaviors.

King and colleagues also published results from a 12-week, multicentered, placebo-controlled trial of liquid citalopram for the treatment of repetitive behaviors in 149 children and adolescents with ASD. No significant differences in response rates were found between the citalopram and placebo group; approximately one-third of participants were rated as responders in both groups. These results were in contrast to two previous retrospective chart reviews of citalopram in ASD, which suggested effectiveness for treating anxiety in ASD (see Doyle and McDougle, 2012).

Other serotonergic medications have also been studied for repetitive behaviors in ASD (Doyle and McDougle, 2012). Fluvoxamine may be effective for adults, but not in children. Open-label studies and case reports suggest improvement with escitalopram, sertraline, and paroxetine and results from one retrospective review of venlafaxine have been positive. Clomipramine has also been used with some success in small studies in children and adults, and several investigators have published case reports documenting improvement with mirtazapine for anxiety and compulsive behaviors in ASD. Among two small trials with buspirone, one did not find improvement in obsessive thinking, while the second found that 76% of 21 children were designated responders on the Clinical Global Impression Scale.

Children with ASD are likely more sensitive to serotonin-associated adverse effects as compared to adults and the appropriate dosing of SSRIs in children with ASD is still in question. A mean dose of only 16.5 mg/day of liquid citalopram caused considerable side effects including behavioral activation, increased energy level, impulsivity, decreased concentration, hyperactivity, and stereotypies in a large randomized controlled trial (Doyle and McDougle, 2012).

Risperidone and other atypical antipsychotics with strong affinity for serotonin receptors, particularly the 5-HT2A receptor, are also used frequently to treat the repetitive behavior domain. Although atypical antipsychotics appear to be effective for reducing repetitive behaviors in ASD, their use is compromised by side effects such as sedation, weight gain, and extrapyramidal symptoms. However, in some cases, repetitive behaviors may reach levels of severity that warrant consideration of antipsychotics when safer options have been unsuccessful.

FUTURE DIRECTIONS

When examined broadly, the field of pharmacological treatment research in ASD has grown in recent years, and significant evidence now exists to support the use of a number of different medications across several symptom domains. However, there has been little progress in targeting core symptoms of social and language impairment. Studying genetic subtypes with single gene causes of ASD, such as Fragile X syndrome, may be necessary to better understand medication efficacy in ASD more broadly. Incorporating biological markers to further characterize ASD phenotypes may also prove useful in predicting treatment response and side effects. Novel measurement instruments also need to be validated to objectively assess core symptoms in ASD. In addition, clinical trials should be designed to examine moderators of treatment response, such as age, developmental level, gender, and intellectual ability. In general, medication treatment of children and adolescents with ASD should be initiated with low starting dosages and slow titrations because these individuals are often very sensitive to side effects. Future studies will improve understanding of medication side effects in ASD and may help identify risk factors to predict which individuals are most vulnerable.

CONCLUSIONS

Autism spectrum disorders involve specific and well-defined deficits in social communication with the presence of repetitive behaviors and restricted interests. However, ASD are clinically and etiologically very heterogeneous. Neuroimaging studies are still evolving but already implicate specific brain regions and brain networks in ASD. Behavioral interventions are important first-line treatments in ASD and there is much progress needed in pharmacological treatments that target core symptoms of ASD. The research community has made great progress in identifying etiological genetic loci for ASD and it is very likely that such findings will explode over the next three to five years with the emergence of MPS. Already, small studies with MPS have identified several new genes. Understanding how the multiple, diverse ASD interact in specific molecular networks is an important means by which high-value therapeutic targets can be identified.

It is important to note that recent genetic discovery and the development of animal model systems have elucidated the neurobiology of several genes implicated in monogenic forms of ASD, including Rett syndrome, tuberous sclerosis, Fragile X syndrome and, in our center, Phelan–McDermid syndrome. These discoveries have in turn led to important opportunities for developing novel treatments. Several large- and small-scale clinical trials are underway in the United States and Europe with potentially disease-modifying medications that target core symptom domains in ASD, arising from neurobiological studies in model systems, and there is even suggestion of positive effects with compounds indirectly or directly modulating glutamate signaling in individuals with fragile X mutation (for example [Berry-Kravis et al., 2012; Jacquemont et al., 2011]). Although the state of the evidence is preliminary, these studies are the basis for enormous optimism in ASD and underscore how neurobiological approaches are likely to lead to novel therapeutics in ASD.

ACKNOWLEDGMENTS

Dr. Kolevzon would like to acknowledge the help of Dr. Latha Soorya for her contribution in researching and writing about behavioral therapy in ASD.

DISCLOSURES

Dr. Kolevzon receives grant support from Seaside Therapeutics and Hoffmann La-Roche.

Drs. Wang and Grodberg have no conflicts of interest to disclose.

Dr. Joseph D. Buxbaum has submitted a patent on therapeutics in SHANK3.

REFERENCES

Anagnostou, E., and Hansen, R. (2011). Medical treatment overview: traditional and novel psycho-pharmacological and complementary and alternative medications. *Curr. Opin. Pediatr.* 23:621–627.

Anagnostou, E., and Taylor, M.J. (2011). Review of neuroimaging in autism spectrum disorders: what have we learned and where we go from here. *Mol. Autism* 2:4.

Anderson, L.T., Campbell, M., et al. (1984). Haloperidol in the treatment of infantile autism: effects on learning and behavioral symptoms. *Am. J. Psychiatry* 141(10):1195–1202.

Arnold, L.E., Aman, M.G., et al. (2006). Atomoxetine for hyperactivity in autism spectrum disorders: placebo-controlled crossover pilot trial. *J. Am. Acad. Child Adolesc. Psychiatry* 45(10):1196–1205.

American Psychiatric Association. (2000). Diagnostic and Statistical Manual of Mental Disorders, 4th Edition, Text Revision. Washington, DC: Author.

Ben Bashat, D., Kronfeld-Duenias, V., et al. (2007). Accelerated maturation of white matter in young children with autism: a high b value DWI study. *NeuroImage* 37:40–47.

Berry-Kravis, E.M., Hessl, D., et al. (2012). Effects of STX209 (Arbaclofen) on neurobehavioral function in children and adults with fragile x syndrome: a randomized, controlled, phase 2 trial. *Sci. Transl. Med.* 4:152ra127.

Betancur, C. (2011). Etiological heterogeneity in autism spectrum disorders: more than 100 genetic and genomic disorders and still counting. *Brain Res.* 1380:42–77.

Bozdagi, O., Sakurai, T., et al. (2010). Haploinsufficiency of the autism-associated Shank3 gene leads to deficits in synaptic function, social interaction, and social communication. *Mol. Autism* 1:15.

Buxbaum, J.D. (2009). Multiple rare variants in the etiology of autism spectrum disorders. *Dialogues Clin. Neurosci.* 11:35–43.

Buxbaum, J.D., Betancur, C., et al. (2012). Optimizing the phenotyping of rodent ASD models: enrichment analysis of mouse and human neurobiological phenotypes associated with high-risk autism genes identifies morphological, electrophysiological, neurological, and behavioral features. *Mol. Autism* 3:1.

Centers for Disease Control (CDC). (2012). Prevalence of autism spectrum disorders: Autism and Developmental Disabilities Monitoring Network, 14 sites, United States, 2008. *MMWR Surveill. Summ.* 61:1–19.

Cooper, G.M., Coe, B.P., et al. (2011). A copy number variation morbidity map of developmental delay. *Nat. Genet.* 43:838–846.

Courchesne, E., Campbell, K., et al. (2011). Brain growth across the life span in autism: age-specific changes in anatomical pathology. *Brain Res.* 1380:138–145.

Courchesne, E., Pierce, K., et al. (2007). Mapping early brain development in autism. *Neuron* 56:399–413.

Cunningham, A.B., and Schreibman, L. (2008). Stereotypy in autism: the importance of function. *Res. Autism Spectr. Disord.* 2:469–479.

Dawson, G., Meltzoff, A.N., et al. (1998). Neuropsychological correlates of early symptoms of autism. *Child. Dev.* 69:1276–1285.

Dawson, G., Rogers, S., et al. (2010). Randomized, controlled trial of an intervention for toddlers with autism: the Early Start Denver Model. *Pediatrics* 125:e17–23.

Devlin, B., Melhem, N., et al. (2011). Do common variants play a role in risk for autism? Evidence and theoretical musings. *Brain Res.* 1380:78–84.

Doyle, C.A., and McDougle, C.J. (2012). Pharmacotherapy to control behavioral symptoms in children with autism. *Exp. Opin. Pharmacother.* 13:1615–1629.

Elsabbagh, M., Mercure, E., et al. (2012). Infant neural sensitivity to dynamic eye gaze is associated with later emerging autism. *Curr. Biol.* 22:338–342.

Eyler, L.T., Pierce, K., et al. (2012). A failure of left temporal cortex to specialize for language is an early emerging and fundamental property of autism. *Brain* 135:949–960.

Filipek, P.A., Accardo, P.J., et al. (2000). Practice parameter: screening and diagnosis of autism: report of the Quality Standards Subcommittee of the American Academy of Neurology and the Child Neurology Society. *Neurology* 55:468–479.

Frazier, T.W., and Hardan, A.Y. (2009). A meta-analysis of the corpus callosum in autism. *Biol. Psychiatry* 66:935–941.

Frazier, T.W., Youngstrom, E.A., et al. (2012). Validation of proposed DSM-5 criteria for autism spectrum disorder. *J. Am. Acad. Child Adolesc. Psychiatry* 51:28–40.e3.

Ganz, J.B., Davis, J.L., et al. (2012). Meta-analysis of PECS with individuals with ASD: investigation of targeted versus non-targeted outcomes, participant characteristics, and implementation phase. *Res. Dev. Disabil.* 33:406–418.

Geschwind, D.H., and Levitt, P. (2007). Autism spectrum disorders: developmental disconnection syndromes. *Curr. Opin. Neurobiol.* 17:103–111.

Goldstein, S., and Schwebach, A.J. (2004). The comorbidity of pervasive developmental disorder and attention deficit hyperactivity disorder: results of a retrospective chart review. *J. Autism Dev. Disord.* 34:329–339.

Gotham, K., Risi, S., et al. (2007). The Autism Diagnostic Observation Schedule: revised algorithms for improved diagnostic validity. *J. Autism Dev. Disord.* 37:613–627.

Hallmayer, J., Cleveland, S., et al. (2011). Genetic heritability and shared environmental factors among twin pairs with autism. *Arch. Gen. Psychiatry* 68:1095–1102.

Harfterkamp, M., van de Loo-Neus, G., et al. (2012). A randomized double-blind study of atomoxetine versus placebo for attention-deficit/hyperactivity disorder symptoms in children with autism spectrum disorder. *J. Am. Acad. Child Adolesc. Psychiatry* 51(7):733–741.

Hazlett, H.C., Poe, M.D., et al. (2011). Early brain overgrowth in autism associated with an increase in cortical surface area before age 2 years. *Arch. Gen. Psychiatry* 68:467–476.

Hollander, E., Anagnostou, E., et al. (2005). Striatal volume on magnetic resonance imaging and repetitive behaviors in autism. *Biol. Psychiatry* 58:226–232.

Hollander, E., Phillips, A., et al. (2005). A placebo controlled crossover trial of liquid fluoxetine on repetitive behaviors in childhood and adolescent autism. *Neuropsychopharmacol.* 30:582–589.

Hollander, E., Chaplin, W., et al. (2010). Divalproex sodium vs placebo for the treatment of irritability in children and adolescents with autism spectrum disorders. *Neuropsychopharmacol.* 35(4):990–998.

Iossifov, I., Ronemus, M., et al. (2012). *De novo* gene disruptions in children on the autistic spectrum. *Neuron* 74:285–299.

Jacquemont, S., Curie, A., et al. (2011). Epigenetic modification of the FMR1 gene in fragile X syndrome is associated with differential response to the mGluR5 antagonist AFQ056. *Sci. Transl. Med.* 3:64ra61.

Jaselskis, C.A., Cook, E.H., et al. (1992). Clonidine treatment of hyperactive and impulsive children with autistic disorder. *J. Clin. Psychopharm.* 12(5):322–327.

Johnson, C.P., and Myers, S.M. (2007). Identification and evaluation of children with autism spectrum disorders. *Pediatrics* 120:1183–1215.

Just, M.A., Cherkassky, V.L., et al. (2004). Cortical activation and synchronization during sentence comprehension in high-functioning autism: evidence of underconnectivity. *Brain* 127:1811–1821.

Klin, A., Lin, D.J., et al. (2009). Two-year-olds with autism orient to non-social contingencies rather than biological motion. *Nature* 459:257–261.

Kou, Y., Betancur, C., et al. (2012). Network- and attribute-based classifiers can prioritize genes and pathways for autism spectrum disorders and intellectual disability. *Am. J. Med. Genet. C Semin. Med. Genet.* 160C:130–142.

Lecavalier, L. (2006). Behavioral and emotional problems in young people with pervasive developmental disorders: relative prevalence, effects of subject characteristics, and empirical classification. *J. Autism Dev. Disord.* 36:1101–1114.

Ledbetter, D.H. (2008). Cytogenetic technology: genotype and phenotype. *N. Engl. J. Med.* 359:1728–1730.

Lichtenstein, P., Carlstrom, E., et al. (2010). The genetics of autism spectrum disorders and related neuropsychiatric disorders in childhood. *Am. J. Psychiatry* 167:1357–1363.

Lovaas, O.I. (1987). Behavioral treatment and normal educational and intellectual functioning in young autistic children. *J. Consult. Clin. Psych.* 55:3–9.

Marcus, R.N., Owen, R., et al. (2009). A placebo-controlled, fixed-dose study of aripiprazole in children and adolescents with irritability associated with autistic disorder. *J. Am. Acad. Child Adolesc. Psychiatry* 48(11):1110–1119.

McDougle, C.J., Naylor, S.T., et al. (1996). A double-blind, placebo-controlled study of fluvoxamine in adults with autistic disorder. *Arch. Gen. Psychiatry* 53(11):1001–1008.

Minshew, N.J., Goldstein, G., et al. (1994). Academic achievement in high functioning autistic individuals. *J. Clin. Exp. Neuropsychol.* 16:261–270.

Mosconi, M.W., Cody-Hazlett, H., et al. (2009). Longitudinal study of amygdala volume and joint attention in 2- to 4-year-old children with autism. *Arch. Gen. Psychiatry* 66:509–516.

Muller, R.A., Shih, P., et al. (2011). Underconnected, but how? A survey of functional connectivity MRI studies in autism spectrum disorders. *Cereb. Cortex* 21:2233–2243.

Neale, B.M., Kou, Y., et al. (2012). Patterns and rates of exonic de novo mutations in autism spectrum disorders. *Nature* 485:242–245.

Nordahl, C.W., Scholz, R., et al. (2012). Increased rate of amygdala growth in children aged 2 to 4 years with autism spectrum disorders: a longitudinal study. *Arch. Gen. Psychiatry* 69:53–61.

Numis, A.L., Major, P., et al. (2011). Identification of risk factors for autism spectrum disorders in tuberous sclerosis complex. *Neurology* 76:981–987.

O'Roak, B.J., Vives, L., et al. (2012). Sporadic autism exomes reveal a highly interconnected protein network of *de novo* mutations. *Nature* 485:246–250.

Owen, R., Sikich, L., et al. (2009). Aripiprazole in the treatment of irritability in children and adolescents with autistic disorder. *Pediatrics* 124(6):1533–1540.

Ozonoff, S., Iosif, A.M., et al. (2010). A prospective study of the emergence of early behavioral signs of autism. *J. Am. Acad. Child Adolesc. Psychiatry* 49:256–266.e1–2.

Ozonoff, S., Iosif, A.M., et al. (2011). Onset patterns in autism: correspondence between home video and parent report. *J. Am. Acad. Child Adolesc. Psychiatry* 50:796–806.e791.

Ozonoff, S., Pennington, B.F., et al. (1991). Executive function deficits in high-functioning autistic individuals: relationship to theory of mind. *J. Child Psychol. Psychiatry* 32:1081–1105.

Ozonoff, S., Williams, B.J., et al. (2005). Parental report of the early development of children with regressive autism: the delays-plus-regression phenotype. *Autism* 9:461–486.

Pelphrey, K.A., Shultz, S., et al. (2011). Research review: Constraining heterogeneity: the social brain and its development in autism spectrum disorder. *J. Child Psychol. Psychiatry* 52:631–644.

Philip, R.C., Dauvermann, M.R., et al. (2012). A systematic review and meta-analysis of the fMRI investigation of autism spectrum disorders. *Neurosci. Biobehav. Rev.* 36:901–942.

Raznahan, A., Toro, R., et al. (2010). Cortical anatomy in autism spectrum disorder: an *in vivo* MRI study on the effect of age. *Cereb. Cortex* 20:1332–1340.

Research Units on Pediatric Psychopharmacology (RUPP). (2002). Risperidone in children with autism and serious behavioral problems. *N. Engl. J. Med.* 347:314–321.

Research Units on Pediatric Psychopharmacology Autism Network (RUPP). (2005). Randomized, controlled, crossover trial of methylphenidate in pervasive developmental disorders with hyperactivity. *Arch. Gen. Psychiatry* 62(11):1266–1274.

Rogers, S.J., Hayden, D., et al. (2006). Teaching young nonverbal children with autism useful speech: a pilot study of the Denver Model and PROMPT interventions. *J. Autism Dev. Disord.* 36:1007–1024.

Rogers, S.J., Wehner, D.E., et al. (2001). The behavioral phenotype in fragile X: symptoms of autism in very young children with fragile X syndrome, idiopathic autism, and other developmental disorders. *J. Dev. Behav. Pediatr.* 22:409–417.

Rosenberg, R.E., Law, J.K., et al. (2009). Characteristics and concordance of autism spectrum disorders among 277 twin pairs. *Arch. Pediat. Adol. Med.* 163:907–914.

Sanders, S.J., Murtha, M.T., et al. (2012). *De novo* mutations revealed by whole-exome sequencing are strongly associated with autism. *Nature* 485:237–241.

Schumann, C.M., Barnes, C.C., et al. (2009). Amygdala enlargement in toddlers with autism related to severity of social and communication impairments. *Biol. Psychiatry* 66:942–949.

Seida, J.K., Ospina, M.B., et al. (2009). Systematic reviews of psychosocial interventions for autism: an umbrella review. *Dev. Med. Child Neurol.* 51:95–104.

Shea, S., Turgay, A., et al. (2004). Risperidone in the treatment of disruptive behavioral symptoms in children with autistic and other pervasive developmental disorders. *Pediatrics* 114:e634–e641.

Spence, S.J., and Schneider, M.T. (2009). The role of epilepsy and epileptiform EEGs in autism spectrum disorders. *Pediatr. Res.* 65:599–606.

Stanfield, A.C., McIntosh, A.M., et al. (2008). Towards a neuroanatomy of autism: a systematic review and meta-analysis of structural magnetic resonance imaging studies. *Eur. Psychiatry* 23:289–299.

Stigler, K.A., McDonald, B.C., et al. (2011). Structural and functional magnetic resonance imaging of autism spectrum disorders. *Brain Res.* 1380:146–161.

Sullivan, P.F., Daly, M.J., et al. (2012). Genetic architectures of psychiatric disorders: the emerging picture and its implications. *Nat. Rev. Genet.* 13:537–551.

Taniai, H., Nishiyama, T., et al. (2008). Genetic influences on the broad spectrum of autism: study of proband-ascertained twins. *Am. J. Med. Genet. B Neuropsychiatr. Genet.* 147B:844–849.

Tuchman, R., and Cuccaro, M. (2011). Epilepsy and autism: neurodevelopmental perspective. *Curr. Neurol. Neurosci. Rep.* 11:428–434.

Tuchman, R., and Rapin, I. (2002). Epilepsy in autism. *Lancet Neurol.* 1:352–358.

Veltman, M.W., Craig, E.E., et al. (2005). Autism spectrum disorders in Prader-Willi and Angelman syndromes: a systematic review. *Psychiatric Genet.* 15:243–254.

Voineagu, I., Wang, X., et al. (2011). Transcriptomic analysis of autistic brain reveals convergent molecular pathology. *Nature* 474:380–384.

Volkmar, F.R. (2011). Understanding the social brain in autism. *Dev. Psychobiol.* 53:428–434.

Volkmar, F.R., Lord, C. (2007). Diagnosis and definition of autism and other pervasive developmental disorders. In: Volkmar, F.R., ed. Autism and the Pervasive Developmental Disorders. Philadelphia: Lippincott Williams & Wilkins, pp. 388–392.

Wang, A.T., Lee, S.S., et al. (2007). Reading affect in the face and voice: neural correlates of interpreting communicative intent in children and adolescents with autism spectrum disorders. *Arch. Gen. Psychiatry* 64:698–708.

Warren, Z., Veenstra-VanderWeele, J., et al. (2011). Therapies for Children with Autism Spectrum Disorders. Rockville, MD: Agency for Healthcare Research and Quality.

Wiggins, L.D., Robins, D.L., et al. (2009). Brief report: sensory abnormalities as distinguishing symptoms of autism spectrum disorders in young children. *J. Autism. Dev. Disord.* 39:1087–1091.

Wolff, J.J., Gu, H., et al. (2012). Differences in white matter fiber tract development present from 6 to 24 months in infants with autism. *Am. J. Psychiatry* 169:589–600.

78 | NEUROBIOLOGY OF ATTENTION DEFICIT/HYPERACTIVITY DISORDER

STEPHEN V. FARAONE AND JOSEPH BIEDERMAN

Attention deficit/hyperactivity disorder (ADHD) is a highly prevalent, early onset, clinically heterogeneous disorder of inattention, hyperactivity, and impulsivity. Its impact on individuals, families, and society is enormous in terms of its financial cost, stress to families, adverse academic and vocational outcomes, and negative effects on self-esteem. Children with ADHD are easily recognized in clinics, schools, and the home. Their inattention leads to daydreaming, distractibility, and difficulties sustaining effort on a single task for a prolonged period of time. As their attention wanders from one stimulus to the next, they often leave parents and teachers with the impression that they are not listening. Their impulsivity makes them accident prone, creates problems with peers, and disrupts classrooms as they blurt out answers, interrupt others, or shift from schoolwork to inappropriate activities. Their hyperactivity, often manifest as fidgeting and excessive talking, is poorly tolerated in schools and is frustrating to parents, who can easily lose them in crowds and cannot get them to sleep at a reasonable hour.

In their teenage years, symptoms of hyperactivity and impulsivity tend to diminish, but—in the majority of cases—the symptoms and impairments of ADHD persist. The teen with ADHD is at high risk for low self-esteem, poor peer relationships, conflict with parents, delinquency, smoking, and substance abuse. A metaanalysis of longitudinal studies found that two-thirds of children with ADHD have impairing ADHD symptoms as adults (Faraone et al., 2006). Studies of clinically referred adults with retrospectively defined childhood-onset ADHD show them to have a pattern of psychosocial disability, psychiatric comorbidity, neuropsychological dysfunction, familial illness, and school failure that resemble the well-known features of children with ADHD, supporting the syndromic continuity between pediatric and adult patients with ADHD.

Throughout the life cycle, an essential clinical feature observed in patients with ADHD is comorbidity with mood, anxiety, and disruptive behavior disorders. Although spurious comorbidity can occur because of referral and screening artifacts, these artifacts cannot explain the high levels of psychiatric comorbidity observed for ADHD. Notably, epidemiological investigators find comorbidity in unselected general population samples—a fact that cannot be caused by the biases inherent in clinical samples (Scahill and Schwab-Stone, 2000).

NEUROTRANSMITTER SYSTEMS AND ATTENTION DEFICIT/HYPERACTIVITY DISORDER

Metaanalyses of pharmacotherapy for ADHD clearly document that three classes of medications reduce the overactivity, impulsivity, and inattentiveness of patients with ADHD: dopamine reuptake inhibitors (the stimulants methylphenidate and amphetamine), norepinephrine reuptake inhibitors (atomoxetine), and alpha2a receptor agonists (clonidine and guanfacine) (Faraone and Glatt, 2010). In addition to improving the core symptoms of ADHD, stimulants also improve associated behaviors, including on-task behavior, academic performance, and social functioning. These effects are dose dependent and are evident in home, school, and occupational settings. Metaanalyses and some direct comparisons suggest that amphetamine is a little more effective than methylphenidate and that both stimulants are more efficacious than non-stimulants (Faraone and Glatt, 2010).

Both stimulant drugs block the dopamine transporter and, by doing so, increase the concentration of dopamine in the synaptic cleft. Because of the distribution of dopamine transporters, these effects are most pronounced in the nucleus accumbens and dorsal striatum (e.g., Kuczenski and Segal, 2002). Although these were initially demonstrated *in vitro* and in animal studies, positron emission tomography (PET) studies in humans show that both methylphenidate and amphetamine administration increase dopamine levels in striatum. Single photon emission tomography (SPECT) and PET studies also show that methylphenidate treatment blocks the dopamine transporter. This suggests that the ultimate effect of methylphenidate's dopamine transporter blockade is to increase the rate of dopamine release.

Rat studies show that low, oral doses of stimulants increase dopamine release in striatum but not in nucleus accumbens, which suggests that oral stimulant administration should not have addictive effects on the brain (Kuczenski and Segal, 2002). Stimulant administration also increased norepinephrine in the hippocampus (important for learning and memory) and dopamine and norepinephrine in the prefrontal cortex (important for maintain executive control) (Kuczenski and Segal, 2002). Both amphetamine and methylphenidate reduce the expression of the norepinephrine transporter. Thus, the efficacy of stimulant medications for treating ADHD suggests that dysfunction of both dopaminergic and noradrenergic systems may underlie the pathophysiology of the disorder.

Further evidence for the relevance of catecholaminergic systems comes from the efficacy of atomoxetine for treating ADHD. Atomoxetine blocks the norepinephrine transporter. Tricyclic antidepressants also block the norepinephrine transporter, but unlike atomoxetine, they also affect other neurotransmitter systems. Neuroimaging studies of primates show that clinical doses of atomoxetine would occupy the norepinephrine transporter almost completely and rat studies show that atomoxetine administration increases norepinephrine and dopamine release in the prefrontal cortex.

Guanfacine and clonidine are alpha2a receptor agonists. They enhance noradrenergic transmission by stimulating postsynaptic alpha2a receptors in prefrontal cortex (Arnsten, 2009). Like the stimulants (Chase et al., 2005), guanfacine also increases the expression of FOS mRNA (Savchenko and Boughter, 2011), suggesting that transcription regulation pathways could be a final common pathway for the activity of ADHD medications. Clonidine also decreases the activity of insulin, which would be expected to decrease the expression of both the dopamine and norepinephrine transporters, suggesting another mechanism of action for this medication.

Because the pharmacological treatment of ADHD implicates dysregulated catecholamine systems, many studies have examined catecholamine metabolites and enzymes in serum and cerebrospinal fluid. Scassellati et al. (2012) completed a metaanalysis of studies comparing ADHD and non-ADHD people on peripheral biochemical markers. They found 71 studies relevant to monoaminergic neurotransmission. After Bonferroni correction, four of these markers significantly discriminated ADHD and non-ADHD samples: increased norepinephrine, decreased 3-methoxy-4-hydroxyphenylethylene glycol (MHPG), decreased monoamine oxidase (MAO), and decreased phenylethylamine. For these significant findings, they found no evidence of publication bias or heterogeneity of effect sizes across studies. They concluded that reduced MAO activity impairs the degradation of norepinephrine and lead to lower levels of MHPG in ADHD patients and that dysregulation of the "MAO-NE-MHPG" pathway may be a compensatory response to hypo-noradrenergic synaptic activity in ADHD. Of note, phenylethylamine, which has a chemical structure that is similar to amphetamine, increases the release of dopamine, which is consistent with the idea that low levels could lead to ADHD.

Animal model studies also support the idea that catecholaminergic systems are impaired in ADHD. One approach has been the use of 6-hydroxydopamine to lesion dopamine pathways in developing rats. Because these lesions created hyperactivity, they were thought to provide an animal model of ADHD. Disruption of catecholaminergic transmission with chronic low-dose N-methyl-4-phenyl-1,2,3,6-tetrahydropyridine (MPTP), a neurotoxin, creates an animal model of ADHD in monkeys. Administration of MPTP to monkeys caused cognitive impairments on tasks thought to require efficient frontal-striatal neural networks, the same networks implicated in ADHD. These cognitive impairments mirrored those seen in monkeys with frontal lesions. Like ADHD

children, MPTP-treated monkeys show attentional deficits and task impersistence. Methylphenidate reversed the behavioral deficits but not the cognitive dysfunction.

Several investigators have used the spontaneously hypertensive rat (SHR) as an animal model of ADHD because of the SHR's locomotor hyperactivity and impaired discriminative performance. Studies using SHR have implicated dopaminergic and noradrenergic systems. The dopamine D2 receptor agonist, quinpirole, caused significantly greater inhibition of DA release from caudate-putamen in SHR compared with control mice. These findings were attributed to increased autoreceptor-mediated inhibition of dopamine release in caudate-putamen slices but not in the prefrontal cortex. Another study showed that the altered presynaptic regulation of dopamine in SHR led to the down-regulation of the dopamine system. The authors hypothesized this may have occurred early in development as a compensatory response to abnormally high DA concentrations.

Other SHR studies implicated an interaction between the noradrenergic and dopaminergic system in the nucleus accumbens, but have ruled out the idea that a dysfunctional locus coeruleus and A2 nucleus impairs dopaminergic transmission in the nucleus accumbens via alpha 2-adrenoceptor mediated inhibition of dopamine release. Papa et al. (1998) used molecular imaging techniques to assess the neural substrates of ADHD-like behaviors in the SHR rat. Their data showed the cortico-striato-pallidal system to mediate these behaviors. Exposure to excess androgen levels early in development led to decreased catecholamine innervation in frontal cortex and enhanced expression of ADHD-like behaviors. Carey et al. (1998) used quantitative receptor autoradiography and computer-assisted image analysis to show a higher density of low-affinity D1 and D5 dopamine receptors in the caudate-putamen, nucleus accumbens, and olfactory tubercle of SHR. Stimulant treatment normalized these receptors by decreasing the number of binding sites and increasing affinity to the control level. Gene expression studies of the SHR brain have implicated genes involved in neural development, immunity, transcription factor, monoamine neurotransmitter, metabolism, signal transduction, and apoptosis as well as genes implicated in human association studies of ADHD (e.g., Dasbanerjee et al., 2008). The SHR has also been shown to have elevated dopamine transporter density in the brain that is normalized by methylphenidate treatment (Roessner et al., 2011).

GENETICS

FAMILY STUDIES

As reviewed in detail elsewhere, family studies consistently support the assertion that ADHD runs in families (Faraone and Doyle, 2001). Table 78.1 presents eight studies providing information about rates of ADHD among the parents of ADHD probands. Table 78.2 shows rates of ADHD and hyperactivity among the siblings of hyperactive probands. There is agreement between early studies of hyperactivity and subsequent studies of ADD and ADHD. These studies find the parents and

TABLE 78.1. Prevalence of attention deficit/hyperactivity disorder (ADHD) in the parents of ADHD and control probands

STUDY	ADHD PROBANDS		CONTROL PROBANDS		RELATIVE RISK	
	FATHERS	MOTHERS	FATHERS	MOTHERS	FATHERS	MOTHERS
Morrison and Stewart (1971)	15	5	2	2	7.5	3.5
Cantwell (1972)	16	4	2	0	8	**
Reeves et al. (1987)	0	1	0	0	0	**
Biederman et al. (1990)	44	18	8	0	5.5	**
Schachar and Wachsmuth (1990)	37	38	19	5	1.9	7.6
Frick et al. (1991)	44	27	18	13	2.4	2.1
Faraone et al. (1992)	17	11	3	2	5.7	5.5
Klein and Mannuzza (1990)	Parents of 219 ADHD probands				No elevated risk	No elevated risk

**Undefined because relative risk has zero denominator.
(From Faraone, S.V. and Doyle, A.E. (2001). The nature and heritability of attention-deficit/hyperactivity disorder. *Child and Adolescent Psychiatric Clinics of North America* 10, 299–316, viii–ix.)

siblings of children with ADHD to have a two- to eightfold increase in the risk for ADHD.

Attention to other psychiatric disorders in family studies of ADHD provided evidence for the genetic heterogeneity of ADHD. Results of analyses from independent samples of children with DSM-III ADD and DSM-III-R ADHD suggested that: (*1*) ADHD and major depression share common familial vulnerabilities; (*2*) ADHD children with conduct and bipolar disorders might be a distinct familial subtype of ADHD; and (*3*) ADHD is familially independent from anxiety disorders and learning disabilities. Thus, stratification by conduct and bipolar disorders may cleave the universe of children with ADHD into more familially homogeneous subgroups. In contrast, major depression may be a nonspecific manifestation of different ADHD subforms.

TWIN STUDIES

The occurrence of twinning creates a natural experiment in psychiatric genetics. If a disorder is strongly influenced by genetic factors, then the risk to co-twins of ill probands should

TABLE 78.2. Prevalence of attention deficit/hyperactivity disorder (ADHD) in the siblings of ADHD and control probands

STUDY	PROBAND DIAGNOSIS		
	ADHD	CONTROL	RELATIVE RISK
Welner et al. (1977)	17	8	2.1
Manshadi et al. (1983)	41	0	**
Pauls et al. (1983)	25	—	—
Biederman et al. (1990)	21	6	3.5
Faraone et al. (1992)	15	5	3

**Undefined because relative risk has zero denominator.

be greatest when the twins are monozygotic. The risk to dizygotic twins should exceed the risk to controls but should not be greater than the risk to siblings.

Twin data are used to estimate heritability, which measures the degree to which a disorder is influenced by genetic factors. Heritability ranges from zero to one, with higher levels indicating a greater degree of genetic determination. Figure 78.1 presents heritability data from 15 twin studies of ADHD. These data attribute about 80% of the etiology of ADHD to genetic factors.

Freitag et al.'s (2010) review of twin studies generated several useful conclusions. They found that studies that used short rating scales with a limited amount of answer categories showed strong rater effects. Parent ratings of ADHD symptoms were more heritable than both teacher ratings and objective measures as hyperactive behaviors by Actigraph. Twin studies also showed that inattentive and hyperactive/impulsive symptoms share susceptibility genes, but each symptom domain also has a unique genetic component. Twin studies of comorbidity suggest that reading disability and inattentive symptoms share risk genes. In contrast, both classes of ADHD symptoms are strongly associated with conduct disorder.

A metaanalysis of twin studies showed that ADHD's heritability remains constant through adolescence (Bergen et al., 2007), which suggests that changes in the mix of genetic and environmental risk factors cannot account for the age-dependent decline of the disorder (Faraone et al., 2006). However, in contrast to the constancy of heritability through adolescence, twin studies have found a lower heritability of ADHD in adult samples. In contrast to the 76% heritability of ADHD in youth, four studies have estimated the heritability of adult ADHD to range from 30% to 40% (Franke et al., 2011). These findings were unexpected given the constancy of heritability during adolescence and data from family studies showing that persistent ADHD was *more* familial than ADHD assessed in childhood. After reviewing the adult ADHD twin data, Franke et al. (2011) concluded that these discrepant findings

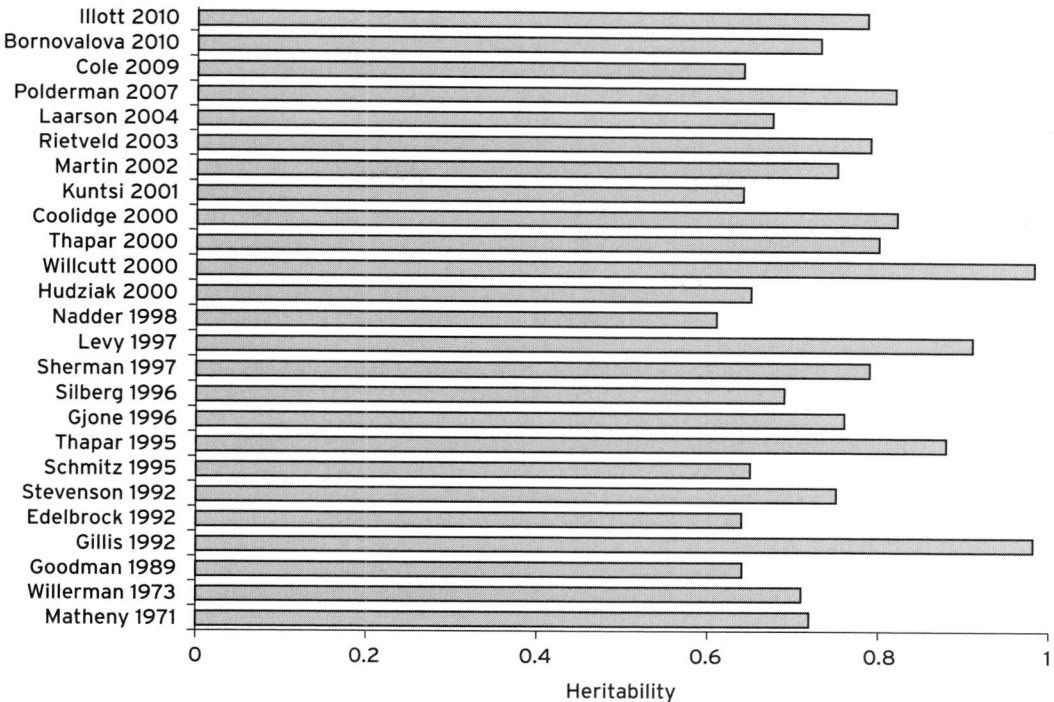

Figure 78.1 *Heritability computed from twin studies of youth with attention deficit/hyperactivity disorder. (See Freitag, C.M., Rohde, L.A., Lempp, T. and Romanos, M. (2010). Phenotypic and measurement influences on heritability estimates in childhood ADHD. Eur. Child Adolesc Psychiatry 19, 311–323; Faraone, S.V. and Mick, E. (2010). Molecular genetics of attention deficit hyperactivity disorder. Psychiatr. Clin. North Am. 33, 159–180.)*

could be caused by methodological issues. Most important, all the twin studies of adult ADHD used self-ratings of ADHD, whereas studies of ADHD youth typically relied on either parent or teacher reports. Notably, twin studies also show that self-ratings of ADHD by adolescents are less heritable than parent or teacher ratings of ADHD symptoms in adolescents. This led Franke et al. (2011) to conclude that self-ratings may be a poorer measure of the genetic liability to ADHD. This could occur simply because of lower reliability, which in a twin study would lower estimates of heritability.

ADOPTION STUDIES

Like twinning, the occurrence of adoption provides another useful experiment for psychiatric genetics. Whereas parents can confer a disease risk to their biological children via both biological and environmental pathways, to adoptive children they can only confer risk via an environmental pathway. Thus, by examining both the adoptive and the biological relatives of ill probands, we can disentangle genetic and environmental sources of familial transmission.

Adoption studies of ADHD also implicate genes in its etiology. Early studies showed that the adoptive relatives of hyperactive children are less likely to have hyperactivity or associated disorders than are the biological relatives of hyperactive children. The adoptive relatives of adopted ADHD probands had rates of ADHD and other associated disorders that were lower than those observed in the biological relatives of non-adopted ADHD probands and similar to those found in relatives of control probands (for details, see Faraone and Mick, 2010).

MOLECULAR GENETIC STUDIES

Molecular genetic studies use two main approaches. The candidate gene approach examines one or more genes based upon some theory (hopefully backed by empirical evidence) about the nature of the disorder. In contrast, the genome scan examines all chromosomal locations without any a priori guesses as to what genes underlie susceptibility to ADHD. In discussing these results, we will differentiate between common and rare DNA variants, using a population prevalence of less than 5% to define a variant as rare. We use the term DNA variant to refer to any piece of DNA sequence including microsatellite polymorphisms, variable number of tandem repeat (VNTR) polymorphisms, single nucleotide polymorphisms (SNPs), and copy number variants (CNVs).

Elsewhere, we have extensively reviewed the hundreds of candidate gene studies of ADHD that are now available (Faraone and Mick, 2010; Franke et al., 2011). These studies have searched for common DNA variants that increase susceptibility to ADHD. A useful summary of these studies can be found in the metaanalysis of Gizer et al. (2009). Among the many DNA variants assessed for association with ADHD, eight showed a statistically significant association with the disorder across multiple studies. These variants implicated six genes: the serotonin transporter gene (*5HTT*), the dopamine transporter gene (*DAT1*), the D4 dopamine receptor gene (*DRD4*), the D5 dopamine receptor gene (*DRD5*), the serotonin 1B receptor gene (*HTR1B*), and a gene coding for a synaptic vesicle regulating protein known as *SNAP25*. As Figure 78.2 shows, the strength of association for each of these DNA variants, as measured by the odds ratio, is fairly small, less than 1.5, which

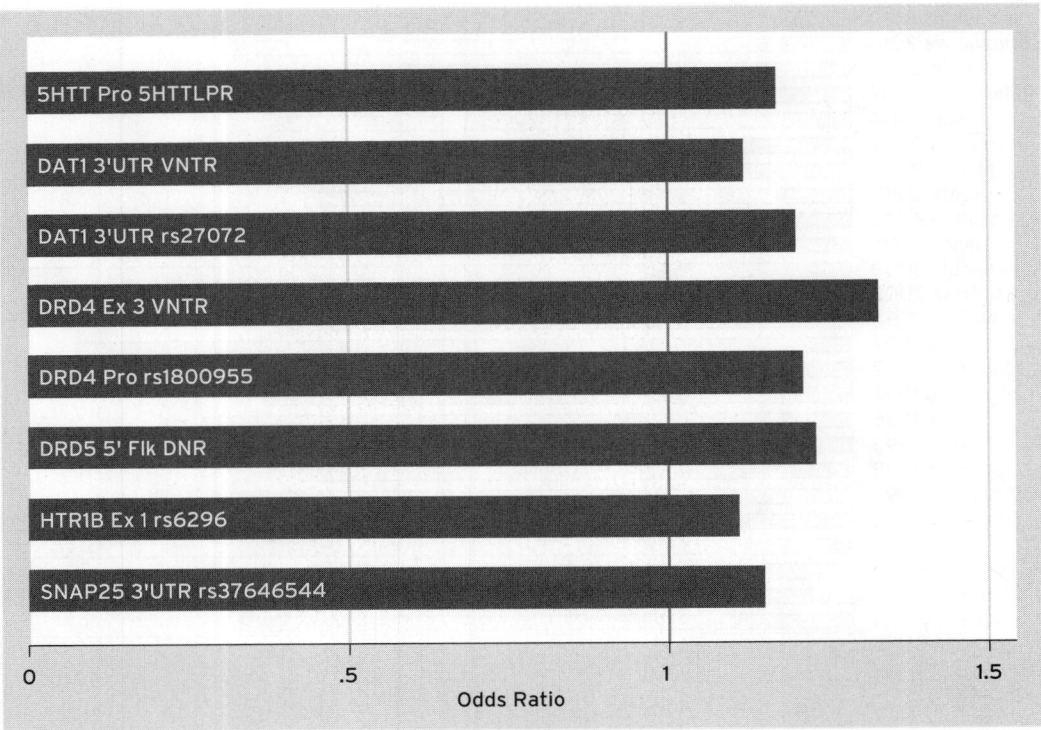

Figure 78.2 *Each bar gives the name of the gene followed by the name of the variant tested for association with attention deficit/hyperactivity disorder. (Based on metaanalysis of Gizer, I.R., Ficks, C. and Waldman, I.D. (2009). Candidate gene studies of ADHD: a meta-analytic review. Hum. Genet. 126, 51–90.)*

means that carrying one of these variants increases one's risk for ADHD by less than 50%.

GENETIC LINKAGE STUDIES

Genome-wide linkage scans examine many DNA markers across the genome to determine if any chromosomal regions are shared more often than expected among family members with ADHD. Because this methodology had been very successful for detecting disease genes for many single gene non-psychiatric disorders, it had been hoped that it would also detect genes for psychiatric disorders. To detect a disease gene, the method requires families having at least two ill family members and a gene that has a very large effect on disease manifestation. Although there is some overlap in nominally significant linkage peaks among linkage studies of ADHD, there is no evidence for the replication of a genome-wide significant finding using strict criteria. However, Zhou et al. (2008) searched for common linkage signals among these studies using Genome Scan Meta-Analysis. They reported genome-wide significant linkage for a region on chromosome 16 between 64 and 83 Mb. Although this finding is intriguing and worthy of follow-up, the lack of significant findings for other loci suggests that common DNA variants having a large effect on ADHD are unlikely to exist.

GENOME-WIDE ASSOCIATION STUDIES

In contrast with the linkage approach, the method of genome-wide association is able to detect common DNA variants having a very small effect on disease etiology. There have been several genome-wide association studies (GWAS) of ADHD. None of these studies reported any DNA variants that achieved current guidelines for asserting genome-wide statistical significance, which require a p-value less than .00000005. This stringent p-value is needed because many SNPs must be examined to fully cover the human genome.

Given the lack of significance of these individual studies, the investigators combined their data and conducted a metaanalysis of the combined sample (Neale et al., 2010). The final sample size consisted of 2,064 trios, 896 cases, and 2,455 controls. No single SNP showed evidence for genome-wide significance, but an analysis of candidate genes suggested that they may be involved in the disorder.

THE SEARCH FOR RARE GENETIC VARIANTS

Rare variants causing ADHD were initially described in scattered, serendipitous, reports of gross chromosomal anomalies cosegregating with ADHD in only a few samples. Examples include the Fragile X syndrome, duplication of the Y-chromosome in boys, velo-cardio facial syndrome, loss of an X-chromosome in girls, and a peri-centric inversion of chromosome 3 co-segregating with ADHD symptoms. One study demonstrated that a rare familial form of ADHD is associated with generalized resistance to thyroid hormone (GRTH), a disease caused by mutations in the thyroid receptor-b gene. The thyroid receptor-b gene cannot account for many cases of ADHD because the prevalence of GRTH is very low among ADHD patients (1 in 2,500) and, among GRTH pedigrees, the

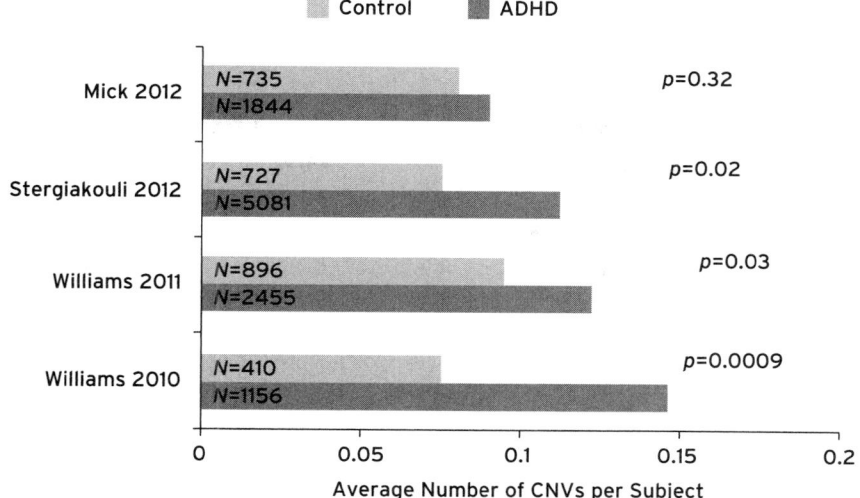

Control ADHD

Mick 2012 — N=735 / N=1844 — p=0.32
Stergiakouli 2012 — N=727 / N=5081 — p=0.02
Williams 2011 — N=896 / N=2455 — p=0.03
Williams 2010 — N=410 / N=1156 — p=0.0009

Average Number of CNVs per Subject

Figure 78.3 *Burden of large (>500 kb) Rare copy number variations.*

association between ADHD and the thyroid receptor-b gene has not been consistently found.

Most of the genotyping technologies used for GWAS can also be used to detect copy number variants (CNVs). Copy number variants are deletions and duplications of DNA segments, which typically are found in genomic regions having repetitive DNA sequences. In addition to being rare, many CNVs have clear implications for gene functioning. Because CNVs delete or duplicate a large portion of a gene, they either completely stop the production of the gene's protein or they lead to a greatly modified protein. This is likely to lead to functional consequences.

Several studies of CNVs in ADHD have now been reported (e.g., Elia et al., 2012; Williams et al., 2012). Four of these used a common method to define CNV burden, which they defined as the average number of large, rare CNVs for ADHD cases and controls. For these analyses, "large" was defined as the CNV being larger than 500 kb, and "rare" was defined as occurring in less than 1% of controls. As Figure 78.3 shows, each study found a greater burden of large, rare CNVs among ADHD patients compared with controls. This finding was significant in three of the four samples and in the combined sample. Another study using a different definition of burden found no difference between ADHD and control subjects. The burden finding suggests that one genetic cause of ADHD is the accumulation of rare deleterious genetic events across the genome.

The CNV studies have also provided insights into which biological systems are affected by rare deletions and duplications to increase the risk for ADHD. In the study by Williams et al. (2012), duplications spanning the *CHRNA7* gene at chromosome 15q13.3 were associated with ADHD in a single-locus analysis. This finding was consistently replicated in an additional 2,242 ADHD case subjects and 8,552 comparison subjects from four independent cohorts from the United Kingdom, the United States, and Canada.

Elia et al. (2012) assayed genome-wide CNVs in 1,013 ADHD cases and 4,105 controls of European ancestry. Positive

findings were evaluated in 2,493 ADHD cases and 9,222 controls of European ancestry. Copy number variants affecting metabotropic glutamate receptor genes were significantly enriched across all cohorts. Their results suggest that variations involving glutamatergic gene networks of the brain contribute to the genetic susceptibility to ADHD.

Other evidence supports a role for glutamate networks in the etiology of ADHD. In a pharmacogenomics GWAS, a SNP in GRM7 was one of the most significant findings (Mick et al., 2008). Defects in the glutamate-stimulated release of dopamine and the functioning of glutamate receptors have been observed in a rat model of ADHD (Russell, 2003). Magnetic resonance spectroscopy in humans shows dysregulation of striatal, and anterior cingulate glutamate and glutamate/glutamine concentrations were greater in the ADHD subjects compared with controls (Dramsdahl et al., 2011).

ENVIRONMENTAL RISK AND PROTECTIVE FACTORS

BIOLOGICAL ADVERSITY

The Feingold hypothesis posits that ADHD symptoms are caused by an allergic reaction to food additives. By eliminating these additives, the Feingold diet was proposed as a treatment for ADHD. Although most studies of the Feingold diet concluded it was not effective for treating ADHD, a metaanalysis concluded that the diet had a very small effect in improving ADHD symptoms (Kavale and Forness, 1983). To put these results into context, the effect of stimulant medication for treating ADHD is about nine times greater than the effect of the Feingold diet. Another series of studies examined the effect of restricted elimination diets on ADHD symptoms. The goal of restricted elimination diets is to eliminate any food to which a child might have a hypersensitivity reaction. Based on metaanalyses of randomized, placebo-controlled studies, Benton (2007) and Nigg et al. (2012) concluded that restricted elimination diets were effective for reducing ADHD symptoms.

However, in some studies, lack of fully blinded assessments may have compromised the results. Another popular theory posited that excessive sugar intake would lead to ADHD symptoms. Although some positive studies supported this idea, the bulk of systematic, controlled research did not (Wolraich et al., 1995).

Iron and zinc have been studied in ADHD because both are required for the production of norepinephrine and dopamine. In a metaanalysis, Scassellati et al. (in press) found nominally significant evidence for low serum ferritin levels (a marker of iron status) to be associated with ADHD. There was substantial heterogeneity in effect sizes across studies, but no evidence of publication bias. The same group also reported highly significant metaanalytical evidence for an association between ADHD and low peripheral zinc levels along with significant heterogeneity and no evidence of publication bias.

Some toxins have been implicated in the etiology of ADHD. Several groups have shown that lead contamination leads to distractibility, hyperactivity, restlessness, and lower intellectual functioning (e.g., Nigg et al., 2008). In a metaanalysis, Scassellati et al. (2012) found that compared with controls, patients with ADHD were more likely to have been exposed to lead. There was substantial heterogeneity across studies but no evidence of publication bias.

The literature examining the association of ADHD with pregnancy and delivery complications (PDCs) presents conflicting results, but tends to support the idea that PDCs can predispose children to ADHD. Specific PDCs implicated in ADHD include toxemia or eclampsia, poor maternal health, maternal age, fetal postmaturity, duration of labor, fetal distress, low birth weight, and antepartum hemorrhage. Notably, the PDCs implicated in ADHD frequently lead to hypoxia and tend to involve *chronic* exposures to the fetus, such as toxemia, rather than *acute*, traumatic events, such as delivery complications. Whether the chronic exposures reflect a larger cumulative "dose" or a higher probability of exposure during a critical period in gestation is unknown.

Animal studies in pregnant mice and rats have shown a positive association between chronic exposure to nicotine and hyperactive offspring. These animal studies show that chronic exposure to nicotine results in tolerance to the drug and an increase in brain nicotinic receptors. Because nicotinic receptors modulate dopaminergic activity and dopaminergic dysregulation may be involved in the pathophysiology of ADHD, it is theoretically compelling to consider maternal smoking as a risk factor for ADHD.

The smoking mother has been shown to be at increased risk for antepartum hemorrhage, low maternal weight, and abruptio placenta. Her fetus is at risk for low birth weight, which has been associated with ADHD. Because smoking increases carboxyhemoglobin levels in both maternal and fetal blood, it places the fetus at risk for a hypoxia, which also has been implicated in ADHD. Thus, it is not surprising that Langley et al.'s (2005) metaanalysis showed that children whose mothers' smoked during pregnancy had a 2.4-fold increased risk for ADHD.

Notably, nicotine amplifies dopamine signals in striatum, interacts with dopamine receptors to cause hyperactivity in rats, and decreases the activity of the dopamine transporter in human striatum. Moreover, ADHD is associated with an increased risk and earlier age of onset of cigarette smoking. Nicotine administration improved both ADHD symptoms and neuropsychological functioning and a nicotine analogue (ABT-418) improved ADHD symptoms. ABT-418 is a selective cholinergic channel activator that is a selective agonist for alpha4beta2 subtype nicotinic receptors. Despite these intriguing findings, studies that question the link between maternal smoking during pregnancy and ADHD suggest that more work is needed to clarify this issue (e.g., Obel et al., 2011).

PSYCHOSOCIAL ADVERSITY

Rutter et al. (1975) examined the prevalence of mental disorders in children living in two very different geographical areas. This research revealed six risk factors within the family environment that correlated significantly with childhood mental disturbances: (1) severe marital discord; (2) low social class; (3) large family size; (4) paternal criminality; (5) maternal mental disorder; and (6) foster placement. This work found that it was the aggregate of adversity factors, rather than the presence of any single one, that impaired development. Other studies also find that as the number of adverse conditions accumulates, the risk of impaired outcome in the child increases proportionally. Biederman et al. (1995a) found a positive association among Rutter's index of adversity and ADHD, measures of ADHD-associated psychopathology, impaired cognition, and psychosocial dysfunction.

Other cross-sectional and longitudinal studies have identified variables such as marital distress, family dysfunction, and low social class as risk factors for psychopathology and dysfunction in children. For example, the Ontario Child Health Study showed that family dysfunction and low income predicted persistence and onset of one or more psychiatric disorders over a four-year follow-up period. Other work implicates low maternal education, low social class, and single parenthood as important adversity factors for ADHD. These studies suggest that the mothers of ADHD children have more negative communication patterns, more conflict with their child, and a greater intensity of anger than do control mothers.

Biederman et al. (1995b) showed that chronic conflict, decreased family cohesion, and exposure to parental psychopathology, particularly maternal psychopathology, were more common in ADHD families compared with control families. The differences between ADHD and control children were not accounted for by social class or parental history of major psychopathology. Moreover, increased levels of family–environment adversity predicted impaired psychosocial functioning. Measures indexing chronic family conflict had a more pernicious impact on the exposed child than those indexing exposure to parental psychopathology. Indeed, researchers have consistently found marital discord to predict disruptive behaviors in boys. This research shows that it is the extent of discord and overt conflict, regardless of whether the parents are separated, that predicts the child's risks for psychopathology and dysfunction.

Thus, dysfunctional family environments appear to be a non-specific risk factor for psychiatric disorders and psychological distress. It is, however, possible that the same risk factors that cause ADHD also contribute to family dysfunction. Reid and Crisafulli (1990) reported a metaanalysis of the impact of marital discord on the psychological adjustment of children and found that parental conflict significantly predicted a variety of child behavior problems. The Ontario Child Health Study provided a prospective example of the impact of parental conflict on children's mental health: family dysfunction (and low income) predicted persistence and onset of one or more psychiatric disorders over a four-year period.

Low maternal warmth and high maternal malaise and criticism have been previously associated with ADHD in children and an epidemiological study examining family attributes in children who had undergone stressful experiences found that children's perceptions of mothers, but not fathers, differentiated stress-resilient and stress-affected children.

An extensive literature documents maternal depression as a risk factor for psychological maladjustment and psychiatric disorder in children (Gelfand and Teti, 1990). This is consistent with the known familial link between ADHD and depression. Moreover, some have suggested that depressed mood may lead mothers to perceive their children as more deviant than warranted by the child's behavior. Richters (1992), however, reviewed 22 studies of this issue and concluded that, because of methodological problems with research in the area, there was no empirical foundation for this claim.

NEUROPSYCHOLOGICAL STUDIES

Satterfield and Dawson (1971) were among the first to propose that ADHD symptoms were caused by fronto-limbic dysfunction. They suggested that weak frontal cortical inhibitory control over limbic functions might lead to ADHD. The success of stimulant medications, and animal models implicating dopamine pathways were taken as support for this model. A review of the neurological literature (Mattes, 1980) articulating the similarities between adult patients with frontal lobe damage and children with ADHD stimulated further research in this area.

Neuropsychological tests measure features of human perception, cognition, or behavior that have been clinically or experimentally linked to specific brain functions. Although useful in developing hypotheses about brain–behavior relationships, these tests are limited in their ability to localize brain dysfunction. Nevertheless, they have several advantages. Many of these tests have been standardized on large normative populations, making it straightforward to define levels of impairment. Because of their extensive use in brain-damaged populations, performance on many of these tests can lead to hypotheses about the locus of brain dysfunction. Thus, they provide a relatively non-invasive and inexpensive means of generating hypotheses about brain pathophysiology that can be tested using the more direct neuroimaging measures of brain structure and function.

In a review of neuropsychological studies, Nigg (2005) showed that ADHD was most consistently associated with deficits in vigilance-attention, cognitive control (i.e., executive functioning), and motivation (as assessed by the processing of reinforcement and incentives). Another metaanalysis of neuropsychological studies concluded that patients with ADHD had deficits in several domains of executive functioning: response inhibition, vigilance, working memory, and planning (Willcutt et al., 2005). From these studies, we can safely conclude that patients with ADHD are at risk for a wide range of neuropsychological dysfunction. However, the differences between ADHD and non-ADHD subjects were not large, which suggests that such deficits are not uniformly seen in patients with ADHD and are not specific to the disorder. The executive function deficits of patients with ADHD lead to difficulties with planning, organization, and time management, which impair their ability to accomplish tasks and function effectively in school and occupational settings (Biederman et al., 2006).

The motivational deficits identified by metaanalysis are often conceptualized as an altered response to reinforcement (Luman et al., 2010). In practical terms, this means that children with ADHD are less able to delay gratification. For example, compared with non-ADHD children, they are more likely to choose small immediate rewards rather than large reward for which they must wait. In experimental paradigms using partial reinforcement, children with ADHD do not function as well normal children. Attention deficit/hyperactivity disorder is also associated with impaired reinforcement–learning and deficits in the extinction of non-rewarded responses (e.g., Luman et al., 2010). Functional magnetic resonance imaging studies and event-related potential studies have reported altered brain activation in experimental paradigms involving the anticipation, receipt, or loss of rewards (Luman et al., 2010).

The wide range of neuropsychological deficits observed in patients with ADHD has motivated the development of several overarching theories that attempt to parsimoniously explain these deficits and ADHD symptoms. These include the Sergeant's Cognitive-Energetic model (Sergeant, 2005), Sonuga-Barke et al.'s (2010) triple pathway model, Tripp and Wickens' (2009) dopamine transfer deficit model, Sagvolden et al.'s (2005) Dynamic Developmental Theory, and Barkley's (1997) model of ADHD as a disorder of deficient self-regulation. We refer readers to the cited articles for further information.

Given that inattention is a hallmark of ADHD, neuropsychological studies of the disorder have focused on the assessment of attention. This led to many vigilance studies finding impaired continuous performance test (CPT) performance in children with ADHD. In these studies, subjects must sustain their attention to subtle sensory signals, avoid being distracted by irrelevant stimuli, and maintain alertness for the duration of the session.

Children with ADHD also perform poorly on tasks requiring inhibition of motor responses, organization of cognitive information, planning, complex problem solving, and the learning and recall of verbal material. Examples of tests that measure these functions are the Stroop test, the Wisconsin Card Sorting Test, the Rey–Osterrieth test, the Freedom from Distractibility factor from Wechsler's tests of intelligence, and the California Verbal Learning Test.

Some studies suggest that the impairments found in children with ADHD cannot be accounted for by psychiatric comorbidity and that the deficits continue through adolescence into adulthood. Moreover, having a family history of ADHD may predict a greater degree of neuropsychological impairment. This latter finding suggests that familial ADHD and neuropsychological impairment identify a more biologically based type of ADHD. In contrast, non-familial cases of ADHD with lesser neuropsychological impairments may be caused by other etiological factors such as psychosocial adversity.

Our description of neuropsychological dysfunction in ADHD describes trends that have emerged in the research literature, not findings that have been consistently replicated. Although there are inconsistencies among studies, it is notable that the pattern of deficits that has emerged is similar to what has been found among adults with frontal lobe damage. Thus, the neuropsychological data tend to support the hypothesis that the frontal cortex or regions projecting to the frontal cortex are dysfunctional in at least some children with ADHD.

Because neuropsychological tests are only indirect measures of brain function, we must be cautious in using them to make inferences about the locus of brain impairment in ADHD. Nevertheless, many of these tests have been standardized on normative populations and administered extensively to brain-damaged populations. Hence, performance on many of these tests can lead to hypotheses about the functional integrity of certain brain regions.

With this caveat in mind, we view the pattern of neuropsychological impairment in children with ADHD as consistent with Satterfield and Dawson's (1971) idea that ADHD is associated with abnormalities of prefrontal cortex and/or its projections to subcortical structures. This inference derives from the clinical and behavioral features that have been linked to regions of the prefrontal cortex. Orbital frontal lesions predict social disinhibition and impulsivity and dorsolateral lesions affect organizational abilities, planning, working memory, and attention. Thus, the neuropsychological test data—along with the clinical features of the disorder—implicate both orbitofrontal and dorsolateral prefrontal dysfunction in ADHD. In contrast, the mesial prefrontal region, in which lesions predict dysfluency and the slowing of spontaneous behavior, is not implicated in ADHD.

Because of the complexity of prefrontal circuitry along with the limitations of neuropsychological inference, whether the "prefrontal" abnormalities in ADHD are owing to "lesions" of prefrontal cortex or to brain areas with prefrontal projections is not yet clear. Thus, the term fronto-subcortical, which denotes a behavioral or cognitive dysfunction that looks "frontal" but may be influenced by subcortical projections, provides a suitable neuropsychological description of ADHD.

It is likely that a network of interrelated brain areas is involved in the attentional-executive impairments of children with ADHD. The cingulate cortex plays a role in motivational aspects of attention and response selection and inhibition. A system mainly involving right prefrontal and parietal cortex is activated during sustained and directed attention across sensory modalities. The inferior parietal lobule and superior temporal sulcus are polymodal sensory convergence areas that provide a representation of extrapersonal space that play an important role in focusing on and selecting a target stimulus. The brainstem reticular activating system and reticular thalamic nuclei, regulate attentional tone and filter interference, respectively. Working memory deficits implicate a distributed network, including anterior hippocampus, ventral anterior and dorsolateral thalamus, anterior cingulate, parietal cortex, and dorsolateral prefrontal cortex.

NEUROIMAGING STUDIES

To overcome the limitations of neuropsychological inference, researchers have turned to brain imaging studies. Because neuroimaging studies provide direct assessments of brain structure and function, they are ideal for testing hypotheses about the locus of brain dysfunction. We discuss three types of ADHD imaging studies. Structural studies ask if patients with ADHD show anomalies of brain structure as evidenced by increases or decreases on the volumes of brain regions. Functional studies ask if the brains of patients with ADHD function differently from the brains of non-ADHD people. Last, functional connectivity studies ask if ADHD is associated with abnormal neural connections among brain regions.

STRUCTURAL IMAGING STUDIES

A comprehensive view of structural brain anomalies in ADHD has been reported in two metaanalyses of studies that examined patients with ADHD with either computed tomography (CT) or magnetic resonance imaging (MRI). Valera et al. (2007) applied metaanalysis to 21 structural imaging studies. Their analysis including all brain regions found globally reduced brain volumes for ADHD subjects compared with controls. They found the largest differences between ADHD and control subjects for cerebellum (especially the posterior inferior region of the vermis) followed by the splenium, right and total cerebral volume, and the right caudate. For these regions, there was no evidence for publication bias, and influence analysis tests indicated that no single study accounted for the significant differences between ADHD and control subjects. Bilateral prefrontal gray matter and right globus pallidus were nominally significant but did not meet criteria for significance after correcting for multiple comparisons.

In another metaanalysis of structural imaging studies, Ellison-Wright et al. (2008) examined seven studies that used MRI, voxel-based morphometry to assess differences in gray matter density and reported the three-dimensional coordinates of brain changes in stereotactic space. This metaanalysis found a single cluster of gray matter decrease associated with ADHD located in the right putamen/globus pallidus region. There was no evidence for gray matter increases in any region to be associated with ADHD. A third metaanalysis of structural imaging data was provided by Nakao et al. (2011). They examined 14 data sets comprising 378 ADHD patients and 344 non-ADHD subjects. Patients with ADHD had significantly decreased global gray matter volumes. Regional analyses showed ADHD to be associated with smaller gray matter volumes in a large cluster in the right lentiform nucleus, which included the caudate nucleus. Attention deficit/hyperactivity disorder was also associated with larger gray matter volumes in the left posterior cingulate cortex/precuneus. In a fourth metaanalysis of brain volumes, Frodl and Skokauskas (2012) examined eleven studies comprising 320 ADHD patients and 288 controls. Consistent with prior structural imaging metaanalyses, these authors reported that ADHD was associated with reduced volumes of the right globus pallidus and putamen as well as the bilateral caudate.

FUNCTIONAL IMAGING STUDIES

Functional imaging studies of ADHD are consistent with the structural studies in implicating fronto-subcortical systems in the pathophysiology of the disorder (Cubillo and Rubia, 2010). The most consistent findings from the functional studies suggest that ADHD is associated with reduced activation of inferior frontostriatal, temporoparietal, and cerebellar brain regions during tasks that require attention and inhibitory control. Dickstein et al. (2006) reported a metaanalysis of 16 fMRI studies, containing 134 foci of activation for patients with ADHD and 180 foci for controls. The authors concluded that ADHD is associated with widely distributed frontal hypoactivity affecting anterior cingulate, dorsolateral prefrontal, inferior prefrontal, and orbitofrontal cortices. They also implicated hypoactivity of the basal ganglia and parietal cortices.

Fassbender and Schweitzer (2006) have interpreted functional imaging studies of ADHD in a developmental context. They point out that patterns of functional brain activity become less diffuse and more focal with maturation. Likewise, for many functional imaging tasks, patients with ADHD activate a more diffuse set of brain regions compared with non-ADHD people. Their review suggested that, for functional imaging tasks requiring higher cognitive functions, ADHD patients activated regions typically associated with motor, visual, and spatial processing whereas, non-ADHD people were more likely to activate brain regions typically associated with executive functioning. Thus, it appears that ADHD brains attempt to solve functional tasks in a manner that is less efficient and less developmentally mature than non-ADHD people. Longitudinal structural MRI studies are also consistent with a developmental delay interpretation of neuroimaging data. Shaw et al. (2007) examined 223 children with ADHD and 223 controls. They indexed cortical maturation with the age of achieving peak cortical thickness. They reported a significant difference in the median age at which 50% of the cortical points achieved their peak thickness: 10.5 years for ADHD patients and 7.5 years for controls. This delay in cortical maturation was greatest for prefrontal regions. These developmental perspectives on ADHD brain imaging data are consistent with the hypothesis that the ADHD brain develops at a slower rate than the non-ADHD brain, which is also consistent with a metaanalysis of longitudinal studies, which reported that about one-third of patients with ADHD remit most signs of the disorder by young adulthood (Faraone et al., 2006). In another study, Shaw et al. (2011) compared 193 typically developing children with 389 longitudinal neuroanatomic magnetic resonance images with 197 children with ADHD having 337 longitudinal scans. This study found a quantitative effect of ADHD symptoms on cortical thinning. Subjects with higher levels of hyperactivity/impulsivity had a slower rate of cortical thinning, with the slowest rate seen for the ADHD sample. For each increase of one point in the hyperactivity/impulsivity score (even among controls), the rate of cortical thinning decreased 0.0054 mm/year. The authors concluded that their data supported a dimensional view of ADHD because cortical thinning was associated with both the diagnosis of ADHD and with the number of ADHD symptoms among non-ADHD children.

Proton magnetic resonance spectroscopy (MRS) is an imaging method that detects neurometabolites in the brain. Perlov et al. (2009) presented a metaanalysis of 16 controlled MRS studies of patients with ADHD. The reviewed studies examined anterior cingulate cortex, prefrontal cortex, the basal ganglia (mostly striatum) and the fronto-striato-thalamo-frontal circuits. The authors concluded that choline compounds (N-acetyl-aspartate and glutamate/glutamine to creatine ratios) were abnormal in ADHD. These results differed somewhat for studies of children and adults. The studies of children provided evidence for increased choline signals in left striatum and right frontal lobe. For adults, increased choline signals were found in the right and left anterior cingulate cortex. The authors noted that these choline signals could implicate abnormal turnover of cell membranes, effects of energy metabolism, or anomalies of cholinergic neurotransmission.

Several studies have measured dopamine transporter (DAT) density in striatum by single photon emission computed tomography (SPECT) or PET. Based on a metaanalysis of nine SPECT and PET studies, Fusar-Poli et al. (2012) concluded that DAT density was 14% higher in patients with ADHD compared with controls. This finding is consistent with the mechanism of action of stimulants, which block the DAT.

Another line of neuroimaging research has examined the functional interregional connectivity between brain regions. These studies ask if ADHD is associated with aberrant neural connectivity. Studies that examine the brain at rest (i.e., while not engaged in a task) find that ADHD is associated with reduced functional connectivity in frontostriatal, frontoparietal, and frontocerebellar regions (Cubillo and Rubia, 2010).

One limitation of brain imaging studies is that many of the patients in these studies had been pharmacologically treated with ADHD, which makes it difficult to disentangle disorder effects from treatment effects. This issue was examined comprehensively in a metaanalysis by Frodl et al. (2012). This metaanalysis examined eleven studies comprising 320 ADHD patients and 288 controls. These authors showed that ADHD associated brain volume reductions in the right globus pallidus and putamen were greatest for those patients that had not received pharmacotherapy, which led them to conclude that pharmacotherapy tended to normalize brain structures. A similar conclusion was reached by the metaanalysis of Nakao et al. (2011), which included 14 data sets comprising 378 ADHD patients and 344 non-ADHD subjects. In that study, use of stimulant medication was associated stimulant medication increased gray matter volume in the right basal ganglia and the right caudate. The authors concluded that treatment with stimulants may be associated with more normal striatal brain structure.

Paloyelis et al.'s (2007) review of fMRI studies concluded that the altered brain activation patterns in children with ADHD are not owing to the effects of long-term pharmacological treatment because many studies of treatment-naïve patients have demonstrated these effects. In the one study that directly compared stimulant treated and non-treated patients, few differences were found. When differences were found, the ADHD group that had received long-term treatment was more similar to the non-ADHD controls than to the untreated ADHD group, which led Paloyelis et al. to conclude that stimulant treatment may normalize neural functioning. This conclusion finds some support in fMRI studies of the acute effects of stimulant treatment. Clinical doses of stimulants boost brain activations in ADHD patients in regions that are typically underactivated in ADHD (i.e., caudate, prefrontal cortex, cingulate, cerebellum), with some studies suggesting normalization of functioning (e.g., Shafritz et al., 2004).

DIFFUSION TENSOR IMAGING STUDIES

Diffusion tensor imaging (DTI) examines the white matter tracts that connect cortical and subcortical structures. Fractional anisotropy assesses cumulative axonal membrane circumference, axonal density, and the thickness of the myelin sheath and is used as an indicator of axonal integrity and organization (Van Ewijk et al., 2012).

Van Ewijk et al. (2012) reported a metaanalysis of 15 DTI studies. They concluded that white matter integrity was reduced in children, adolescents, and adults with ADHD. Their work implicated several white matter regions and tracts: the inferior and superior longitudinal fasciculus, anterior corona radiata, corticospinal tract, cingulum, corpus callosum, internal capsule, caudate nucleus, cerebellum, uncinate fasciculus, forceps minor, areas within the basal ganglia, and widespread differences in the frontal, temporal, parietal, and occipital lobes.

Five clusters were reliably reported across studies of children: the right anterior corona radiate, forceps minor close to the genu of the corpus callosum, right and left internal capsule, and left cerebellar white matter. Studies investigating adolescents or adults did not find group differences in these areas, which led van Ewijk et al. (2012) to speculate that the myelination of these areas had been delayed in children with ADHD. Longitudinal studies are needed to better address this point. Studies focusing on white matter tracts in focused brain regions of interest found decreased fractional anisotropy to be associated with ADHD. In contrast, whole-brain studies identified increased fractional anisotropy. According to van Ewijk et al. (2012), the fact that whole-brain studies have identified increased as well as decreased fractional anisotropy might be owing to including those regions with much fiber crossing.

MODEL OF PATHOGENESIS

History shows that grand theories of psychopathology have short half-lives, but the facts of empirical research endure. Naturally, this leads us to emphasize the empirical generalizations that emerge from the work we have reviewed. All ADHD researchers will agree that the disorder is clinically heterogeneous and most would interpret the variability of findings from neurobiological studies as support for the etiological and pathophysiological heterogeneity of the disorder. It is equally clear that aberrant genes create a vulnerability to the disorder that is not expressed in all environments. We do not know if environmental insults are necessary for the disorder to emerge, but we do know that many environmental agents have been implicated. These run the gamut from psychosocial stressors to toxic and physical assaults on the brain.

The genetic and environmental causes of ADHD most assuredly modify the developing brain, leading to a heterogeneous profile of neuropsychological, structural, and functional abnormalities. Although there is no single pathophysiological profile of ADHD, numerous data implicate dysfunction in the fronto-subcortical-cerebellar pathways that control attention and motor behavior. Moreover, the effectiveness of stimulants, along with animal models of hyperactivity, point to catecholamine dysregulation as at least one source of ADHD brain dysfunction.

Any model of pathogenesis must consider two key points: etiological heterogeneity and multifactorial causation.

ETIOLOGICAL HETEROGENEITY

To ground our work in the empirical realities of ADHD, our heuristic model begins with a nosological theory based on the conceptual framework developed by Robins and Guze, which has guided much empirical psychiatry during the past quarter century. That framework asks if an identified syndrome shows a characteristic course, outcome, family history, and pattern of clinical correlates. This approach has led us to the first proposition of our theory: Rather than being a unitary condition, ADHD is a heterogeneous disorder and its clinical heterogeneity is, in part, an expression of genetic heterogeneity.

To confirm etiological heterogeneity requires that patients with ADHD be separated into at least two classes having different known etiologies and, perhaps, different pathophysiological signatures. In contrast, the homogeneity hypothesis asserts that there is a single necessary and sufficient cause or configuration of causes of ADHD.

To assert either etiological heterogeneity or homogeneity implies that we can fully describe one or more mechanisms of etiology. Although there are many clues to the etiological puzzle, they do not allow a full description because the etiological mechanisms for ADHD have not been worked out in sufficient detail. This tempts researchers to examine descriptive, phenotypical data and infer the presence of one or more etiologies.

Unfortunately, the correspondence between etiology and clinical expression is not isomorphic. Differing etiologies may lead to similar clinical features. For example, Alzheimer's disease can arise from either genetic or non-genetic factors and genetic studies show that there are several genetic subforms. Although the observation of dissimilar phenotypes (clinical heterogeneity) may suggest etiological heterogeneity, such inferences are also limited because a single disease entity, with a homogeneous etiology can have variable expression owing to moderating factors. In genetics the term pleiotropy describes the situation in which a pathogenic genotype can express more than one phenotype. Pleiotropy is not unusual for human genetic diseases and may be the rule rather than the exception for psychiatric disorders.

MULTIFACTORIAL CAUSATION

A simple multifactorial model posits all cases of ADHD to arise from a single pool of genetic and environmental variables—each of small effect—that act in an additive fashion to produce a vulnerability to ADHD. If an individual's cumulative vulnerability exceeds a certain threshold, he or she will manifest the signs and symptoms of ADHD. At lower thresholds, other disorders may be expressed (e.g., neuropsychological disorders). According to the multifactorial model, no single factor is a necessary or sufficient cause for ADHD and each of the etiological factors are interchangeable (i.e., it does not matter which factors one has; only the total number is important).

Multifactorial causation is sometimes viewed as an alternative to etiological heterogeneity, but we argue that both are relevant for the study of ADHD. As we have seen, the etiology of ADHD may involve at least four causal agents: genes, pregnancy and delivery complications, psychosocial adversity, and exposure to toxins. Notably, each of these putative causes is actually a class of potential causes.

The multifactorial model is usually considered a homogeneity model because it assumes that etiological factors are interchangeable. This makes sense for some multifactorial models but not others. For example, if there are 12 causes of ADHD and 11 are needed to develop ADHD, then there would be considerable etiological homogeneity among ADHD patients (i.e., most patients would share the same etiological factors). In contrast, if there were 35 etiological factors (e.g., 10 mutations, eight types of obstetric complications, seven environmental toxins and psychosocial stressors) and five were required to develop ADHD, then there would be considerable etiological heterogeneity. Some cases would be exclusively genetic, others exclusively owing to birth related complications, others would have a toxic etiology, some would be caused solely by psychosocial stress, and many would be caused by the simultaneous action of causes from more than one domain.

Because of these considerations, the second proposition of our theory is that etiologically homogenous subtypes will exist, but will be relatively rare. Most cases of ADHD share some sources of etiological variance with other cases.

IMPLICATIONS FOR PATHOGENESIS

The data we have reviewed provide some evidence for this modified multifactorial model. The genetic studies show that some relatively homogeneous subtypes do exist: Some cases of ADHD—albeit rare—are caused by gross abnormalities of chromosomes. We do not know if the smaller deletions and duplications known as CNVs are necessary and sufficient causes for rare cases of ADHD. As for the large majority of patients with ADHD, the available data reject the most parsimonious version of the hypothesis of etiological homogeneity, that all these cases are caused by the exact same pattern of genetic mutations and adverse environmental exposures.

Instead, there are likely to be several etiological profiles of ADHD. For example, the neuroimaging studies clearly show that there is no single brain lesion that causes ADHD. Instead, and articulated by Makris et al. (2009), ADHD can be viewed as a disorder of the neural networks that mediate attention, executive functions, motor regulation, and emotional regulation. Their model attributes the clinical manifestations of ADHD to four neuroanatomical networks. The first network mediates hyperactivity. It comprises connections among dorsolateral prefrontal cortex, caudate, dorsal anterior cingulate cortex, cerebellum, and the supplementary motor area. The second network mediates inattention and executive dysfunction. It comprises connections among the cerebellar hemisphere, dorsal anterior cingulate cortex, dorsolateral prefrontal cortex, thalamus, and inferior parietal lobule. The third network mediates impulsivity. It comprises connections among cerebellar vermis, perigenual anterior cingulate cortex, orbital frontal cortex, and nucleus accumbens. The fourth network mediates deficient emotional self-regulation. It comprises cerebellar vermis, perigenual anterior cingulate cortex, frontoorbital cortex, and amygdala. Although we cannot say for certain why these brain networks are affected in ADHD, given that the risk factors identified to date are primarily genetic or environmental exposures during fetal development, it is reasonable to speculate that the brains of patients with ADHD are mis-wired during development as opposed to having been subjected to an environmental insult subsequent to the neurodevelopment that occurs *in utero* and early childhood. This suggests a strategy for clarifying the pathophysiology of ADHD. Instead of studying heterogeneous samples of patients with ADHD, neurobiological studies should focus on subgroups that are putatively more homogeneous.

Unraveling these complexities will be a difficult task for ADHD researchers. Technological developments in neuroscience and molecular genetics are moving at a rapid pace. The next decade of work should provide us with more accurate assessments of the brain along with a complete sequence of the human genome. These advances should set the stage for breakthroughs in our understanding of the neurobiology of ADHD and our ability to treat affected individuals.

DISCLOSURES

In the past year, Dr. Faraone received consulting income and/or research support from Shire, Otsuka, Akili, and Alcobra, and research support from the National Institutes of Health (NIH). In previous years, he received consulting fees or was on advisory boards or participated in continuing medical education programs sponsored by Shire, McNeil, Janssen, Novartis, Pfizer, and Eli Lilly. Dr. Faraone receives royalties from books published by Guilford Press: *Straight Talk about Your Child's Mental Health,* and Oxford University Press: *Schizophrenia: The Facts.*

Dr. Joseph Biederman is currently receiving research support from the following sources: Elminda, Janssen, McNeil, and Shire. In 2012, Dr. Joseph Biederman received an honorarium from the MGH Psychiatry Academy and the Children's Hospital of Southwest Florida/Lee Memorial Health System for tuition-funded CME courses. In 2011, Dr. Biederman gave a single unpaid talk for Juste Pharmaceutical Spain, received honoraria from the MGH Psychiatry Academy for a tuition-funded CME course, and received honoraria for presenting at international scientific conference on ADHD. He also received an honorarium from Cambridge University Press for a chapter publication. Dr. Biederman received departmental royalties from a copyrighted rating scale used for ADHD diagnoses, paid by Eli Lilly, Shire, and AstraZeneca; these royalties are paid to the Department of Psychiatry at MGH. In 2010, Dr. Biederman received a speaker's fee from a single talk given at Fundación Dr. Manuel Camelo A.C. in Monterrey Mexico. Dr. Biederman provided single consultations for Shionogi Pharma, Inc. and Cipher Pharmaceuticals, Inc.; the honoraria for these consultations were paid to the Department of Psychiatry at the MGH. Dr. Biederman received honoraria from the MGH Psychiatry Academy for a tuition-funded CME course. In previous years, Dr. Biederman received research support, consultation fees, or speaker's fees from the following additional sources: Abbott, Alza, AstraZeneca, Boston University, Bristol Myers Squibb, Celltech, Cephalon, Eli Lilly and Co., Esai, Fundacion Areces (Spain), Forest, Glaxo, Gliatech, Hastings Center, Janssen, McNeil, Medice Pharmaceuticals (Germany), Merck, MMC Pediatric, NARSAD, NIDA, New River, NICHD, NIMH, Novartis, Noven, Neurosearch, Organon, Otsuka, Pfizer, Pharmacia, Phase V Communications, Physicians Academy, the Prechter Foundation, Quantia Communications, Reed Exhibitions, Shire, the Spanish Child Psychiatry Association, the Stanley Foundation, UCB Pharma Inc., Veritas, and Wyeth.

REFERENCES

Arnsten, A.F. (2009). Toward a new understanding of attention-deficit hyperactivity disorder pathophysiology: an important role for prefrontal cortex dysfunction. *CNS Drugs* 23 (Suppl 1):33–41.

Barkley, R.A. (1997). Attention-deficit/hyperactivity disorder, self-regulation, and time: toward a more comprehensive theory. *J. Dev. Behav. Pediatr.* 18:271–279.

Benton, D. (2007). The impact of diet on anti-social, violent and criminal behaviour. *Neurosci. Biobehav. Rev.* 31:752–774.

Bergen, S.E., Gardner, C.O., et al. (2007). Age-related changes in heritability of behavioral phenotypes over adolescence and young adulthood: a meta-analysis. *Twin Res. Hum. Genet.* 10:423–433.

Biederman, J., Faraone, S.V., et al. (1990). Family-genetic and psychosocial risk factors in DSM-III attention deficit disorder. *J. Am. Acad. Child Adol. Psychiatry* 29:526–533.

Biederman, J., Milberger, S.V., et al. (1995b). Impact of adversity on functioning and comorbidity in children with attention- deficit hyperactivity disorder. *J. Am. Acad. Child Adol. Psychiatry.* 34:1495–1503.

Biederman, J., Milberger, S., et al. (1995a). Family–environment risk factors for attention deficit hyperactivity disorder: A test of Rutter's indicators of adversity. *Arch. Gen. Psychiatry* 52:464–470.

Biederman, J., Petty, C., et al. (2006). Impact of psychometrically defined deficits of executive functioning in adults with attention deficit hyperactivity disorder. *Am. J. Psychiatry* 163:1730–1738.

Cantwell, D.P. (1972). Psychiatric illness in the families of hyperactive children. *Arch. Gen. Psychiatry* 27:414–417.

Carey, M.P., Diewald, L.M., et al. (1998). Differential distribution, affinity and plasticity of dopamine D-1 and D-2 receptors in the target sites of the mesolimbic system in an animal model of ADHD. *Behav. Brain Res.* 94:173–185.

Chase, T.D., Carrey, N., et al. (2005). Methylphenidate regulates c-fos and fosB expression in multiple regions of the immature rat brain. *Brain Res. Dev. Brain Res.* 156:1–12.

Cubillo, A., and Rubia, K. (2010). Structural and functional brain imaging in adult attention-deficit/hyperactivity disorder. *Expert Rev. Neurother.* 10:603–620.

Dasbanerjee, T., Middleton, F.A., et al. (2008). A comparison of molecular alterations in environmental and genetic rat models of ADHD: a pilot study. *Am. J. Med. Genet. B Neuropsychiatr. Genet.* 147B, 1554–1563.

Dickstein, S.G., Bannon, K., et al. (2006). The neural correlates of attention deficit hyperactivity disorder: an ALE meta-analysis. *J. Child Psychol. Psychiatry* 47:1051–1062.

Dramsdahl, M., Ersland, L., et al. (2011). Adults with attention-deficit/hyperactivity disorder—a brain magnetic resonance spectroscopy study. *Front. Psychiatry* 2:65.

Elia, J., Glessner, J.T., et al. (2012). Genome-wide copy number variation study associates metabotropic glutamate receptor gene networks with attention deficit hyperactivity disorder. *Nat. Genet.* 44:78–84.

Ellison-Wright, I., Ellison-Wright, Z., et al. (2008). Structural brain change in attention deficit hyperactivity disorder identified by meta-analysis. *BMC Psychiatry* 8:51.

Faraone, S., Biederman, J., et al. (1992). Segregation analysis of attention deficit hyperactivity disorder: Evidence for single gene transmission. *Psychiatr. Genet.* 2:257–275.

Faraone, S., Biederman, J. et al. (2006). The age dependent decline of attention-deficit/hyperactivity disorder: a meta-analysis of follow-up studies. *Psychol. Med.* 36:159–165.

Faraone, S.V., and Doyle, A.E. (2001). The nature and heritability of attention-deficit/hyperactivity disorder. *Child Adol. Psychiatr. Clin. North Am.* 10:299–316, viii–ix.

Faraone, S.V., and Glatt, S.J. (2010). A comparison of the efficacy of medications for adult attention-deficit/hyperactivity disorder using meta-analysis of effect sizes. *J. Clin. Psychiatry* 71:754–763.

Faraone, S.V., and Mick, E. (2010). Molecular genetics of attention deficit hyperactivity disorder. *Psychiatr. Clin. North Am.* 33:159–180.

Fassbender, C., and Schweitzer, J.B. (2006). Is there evidence for neural compensation in attention deficit hyperactivity disorder? A review of the functional neuroimaging literature. *Clin. Psychol. Rev.* 26(4), 445–465.

Franke, B., Faraone, S.V., et al. (2011). The genetics of attention deficit/hyperactivity disorder in adults, a review. *Mol. Psychiatry* 42:1203–1211.

Freitag, C.M., Rohde, L.A., et al. (2010). Phenotypic and measurement influences on heritability estimates in childhood ADHD. *Eur. Child Adolesc. Psychiatry* 19:311–323.

Frick, P.J., Lahey, B.B., et al. (1991). History of childhood behavior problems in biological relatives of boys with attention deficit hyperactivity disorder and conduct disorder. *J. Clin. Child Psychol.* 20:445–451.

Frodl, T., and Skokauskas, N. (2012). Meta-analysis of structural MRI studies in children and adults with attention deficit hyperactivity disorder indicates treatment effects. *Acta Psychiatr. Scand.* 125:114–126.

Fusar-Poli, P., Rubia, K., et al. (2012). Striatal dopamine transporter alterations in ADHD: pathophysiology or adaptation to psychostimulants? A Meta-Analysis. *Am. J. Psychiatry* 169:264–272.

Gelfand, D.M., and Teti, D.M. (1990). The effects of maternal depression on children. *Clin. Psychol. Rev.* 10:329–353.

Gizer, I.R., Ficks, C., et al. (2009). Candidate gene studies of ADHD: a meta-analytic review. *Hum. Genet.* 126:51–90.

Kavale, K.A., and Forness, S.R. (1983). Hyperactivity and diet treatment: a meta-analysis of the Feingold hypothesis. *J. Learn. Disabil.* 16:324–330.

Klein, R., and Mannuzza, S. (1990). Family history of psychiatric disorders in ADHD. In Presented at the Annual Meeting of the American Academy of Child and Adolescent Psychiatry. American Academy of Child and Adolescent Psychiatry: Chicago.

Kuczenski, R., and Segal, D.S. (2002). Exposure of adolescent rats to oral methylphenidate: preferential effects on extracellular norepinephrine and absence of sensitization and cross-sensitization to methamphetamine. *J. Neurosci.* 22:7264–7271.

Langley, K., Rice, F., et al. (2005). Maternal smoking during pregnancy as an environmental risk factor for attention deficit hyperactivity disorder behaviour. A review. *Minerva Pediatr.* 57:359–371.

Luman, M., Tripp, G., et al. (2010). Identifying the neurobiology of altered reinforcement sensitivity in ADHD: a review and research agenda. *Neurosci. Biobehav. Rev.* 34:744–754.

Makris, N., Biederman, J., et al. (2009). Towards conceptualizing a neural systems-based anatomy of attention-deficit/hyperactivity disorder. *Dev. Neurosci.* 31:36–49.

Manshadi, M., Lippmann, S., et al. (1983). Alcohol abuse and attention deficit disorder. *J. Clin. Psychiatry* 44:379–380.

Mattes, J.A. (1980). The role of frontal lobe dysfunction in childhood hyperkinesis. *Comp. Psychiatry* 21:358–369.

Mick, E., Neale, B., et al. (2008). Genome-wide association study of response to methylphenidate in 187 children with attention-deficit/hyperactivity disorder. *Am. J. Med. Genet. B Neuropsychiatr. Genet.* 147B:1412–1418.

Morrison, J.R., and Stewart, M.A. (1971). A family study of the hyperactive child syndrome. *Biol. Psychiatry* 3:189–195.

Nakao, T., Radua, J., et al. (2011). Gray matter volume abnormalities in ADHD: voxel-based meta-analysis exploring the effects of age and stimulant medication. *Am. J. Psychiatry* 168:1154–1163.

Neale, B.M., Medland, S.E., et al. (2010). Meta-analysis of genome-wide association studies of attention-deficit/hyperactivity disorder. *J. Am. Acad. Child Adolesc. Psychiatry* 49:884–897.

Nigg, J.T. (2005). Neuropsychologic theory and findings in attention-deficit/hyperactivity disorder: the state of the field and salient challenges for the coming decade. *Biol. Psychiatry* 57:1424–1435.

Nigg, J.T., Knottnerus, G.M., et al. (2008). Low blood lead levels associated with clinically diagnosed attention-deficit/hyperactivity disorder and mediated by weak cognitive control. *Biol. Psychiatry* 63:325–331.

Nigg, J.T., Lewis, K., et al. (2012). Meta-analysis of attention-deficit/hyperactivity disorder or attention-deficit/hyperactivity disorder symptoms, restriction diet, and synthetic food color additives. *J. Am. Acad. Child Adolesc. Psychiatry* 51:86–97 e8.

Obel, C., Olsen, J., et al. (2011). Is maternal smoking during pregnancy a risk factor for hyperkinetic disorder? Findings from a sibling design. *Int. J. Epidemiol.* 40:338–345.

Paloyelis, Y., Mehta, M.A., et al. (2007). Functional MRI in ADHD: a systematic literature review. *Expert Rev. Neurother.* 7:1337–1356.

Papa, M., Berger, D.F., et al. (1998). A quantitative cytochrome oxidase mapping study, cross-regional and neurobehavioural correlations in the anterior forebrain of an animal model of attention deficit hyperactivity disorder. *Behav. Brain Res.* 94:197–211.

Perlov, E., Philipsen, A., et al. (2009). Spectroscopic findings in attention-deficit/hyperactivity disorder: review and meta-analysis. *World J. Biol. Psychiatry* 10:355–365.

Reid, W.J., and Crisafulli, A. (1990). Marital discord and child behavior problems: a meta-analysis. *J. Abnormal. Child Psychol.* 18:105–117.

Richters, J.E. (1992). Depressed mothers as informants about their children: a critical review of the evidence for distortion. *Psychol. Bull.* 112:485–499.

Roessner, V., Sagvolden, T., et al. (2011). Methylphenidate normalizes elevated dopamine transporter densities in an animal model of the attention-deficit/hyperactivity disorder combined type, but not to the same extent in one of the attention-deficit/hyperactivity disorder inattentive type. *Neuroscience* 167:1183–1191.

Russell, V.A. (2003). Dopamine hypofunction possibly results from a defect in glutamate-stimulated release of dopamine in the nucleus accumbens shell of a rat model for attention deficit hyperactivity disorder—the spontaneously hypertensive rat. *Neurosci. Biobehav. Rev.* 27:671–682.

Rutter, M., Cox, A., et al. (1975). Attainment and adjustment in two geographical areas: Vol. 1. The prevalence of psychiatric disorders. *Br. J. of Psychiatry* 126:493–509.

Sagvolden, T., Johansen, E.B., et al. (2005). A dynamic developmental theory of attention-deficit/hyperactivity disorder (ADHD) predominantly hyperactive/impulsive and combined subtypes. *Behav. Brain Sci.* 28:397–419; discussion 419–468.

Satterfield, J.H., and Dawson, M.E. (1971). Electrodermal correlates of hyperactivity in children. *Psychophysiology* 8:191–197.

Savchenko, V.L., and Boughter, J.D. (2011). Regulation of neuronal activation by Alpha2A adrenergic receptor agonist. *Neurotox. Res.* 20:226–239.

Scahill, L., and Schwab-Stone, M. (2000). Epidemiology of ADHD in school-age children. *Child Adolesc. Psychiatr. Clin. North Am.* 9:541–555.

Scassellati, C., Bonvicini, C., et al. (2012). Biomarkers and ADHD: a systematic review and meta-analyses. *J. Am. Acad. Child Adol. Psychiatry* 51:1003–1019 e20.

Schachar, R., and Wachsmuth, R. (1990). Hyperactivity and parental psychopathology. *J. Child Psychol. Psychiatry* 31:381–392.

Sergeant, J.A. (2005). Modeling attention-deficit/hyperactivity disorder: a critical appraisal of the cognitive-energetic model. *Biol. Psychiatry* 57:1248–1255.

Shafritz, K.M., Marchione, K.E., et al. (2004). The effects of methylphenidate on neural systems of attention in attention deficit hyperactivity disorder. *Am. J. Psychiatry* 161:1990–1997.

Shaw, P., Eckstrand, K., et al. (2007). Attention-deficit/hyperactivity disorder is characterized by a delay in cortical maturation. *Proc. Natl. Acad. Sci. USA* 104:19649–19654.

Shaw, P., Gilliam, M., et al. (2011). Cortical development in typically developing children with symptoms of hyperactivity and impulsivity: support for a dimensional view of attention deficit hyperactivity disorder. *Am. J. Psychiatry* 168:143–151.

Sonuga-Barke, E., Bitsakou, P., et al. (2010). Beyond the dual pathway model: evidence for the dissociation of timing, inhibitory, and delay-related impairments in attention-deficit/hyperactivity disorder. *J. Am. Acad. Child Adolesc. Psychiatry* 49:345–355.

Tripp, G., and Wickens, J.R. (2009). Neurobiology of ADHD. *Neuropharmacology* 57:579–589.

Valera, E., Faraone, S.V., et al. (2007). Meta-analysis of structural imaging findings in attention-deficit/hyperactivity disorder. *Biol. Psychiatry* 61:1361–1369.

van Ewijk, H., Heslenfeld, D.J., et al. (2012). Diffusion tensor imaging in attention deficit/hyperactivity disorder: a systematic review and meta-analysis. *Neurosci. Biobehav. Rev.* 36:1093–1106.

Welner, Z., Welner, A., et al. (1977). A controlled study of siblings of hyperactive children. *J. Nerv. Ment. Dis.* 165:110–117.

Willcutt, E.G., Doyle, A.E., et al. (2005). Validity of the executive function theory of attention-deficit/hyperactivity disorder: a meta-analytic review. *Biol. Psychiatry* 57:1336–1346.

Williams, N.M., Franke, B., et al. (2012). Genome-wide analysis of copy number variants in attention deficit/hyperactivity disorder confirms the role of rare variants and implicates duplications at 15q13.3 *Am. J. Psychiatry* 169:195–204.

Wolraich, M., Wilson, D., et al. (1995). The effect of sugar on behavior or cognition in children. *JAMA* 274:1617–1621.

Zhou, K., Dempfle, A., et al. (2008). Meta-analysis of genome-wide linkage scans of attention deficit hyperactivity disorder. *Am. J. Med. Genet. B Neuropsychiatr. Genet.* 147B:1392–1398.

79 | TOURETTE SYNDROME AND TIC DISORDERS

KYLE WILLIAMS, MICHAEL H. BLOCH, MATTHEW W. STATE,
AND CHRISTOPHER PITTENGER

Tourette syndrome (TS) was first characterized as a disorder of episodic tics, distinguished from dystonic movements by their spasmodic nature, by the French neurologist Gilles de la Tourette in 1885. Tourette syndrome was long thought to be rare, with a prevalence estimated, as recently as the 1960s, at one case per 2,500 individuals. In recent decades, however, it has been recognized as a far more common condition, affecting between 0.3% and 1% of the population (Robertson et al., 2009). Moreover, it has now been well established that TS is characterized by symptomatology that extends well beyond the pathognomonic motor and vocal tics.

The last 10 years have witnessed striking advances in TS research, with the discovery of rare genetic variants contributing to risk, the emergence of novel insights into the functional and structural neuroanatomy of the syndrome, the identification of specific neuropathological abnormalities in postmortem brains, and the development of new synthetic pathophysiological hypotheses. This chapter presents a summary of these recent advances, addresses current models of TS pathogenesis, reviews available treatments and their putative mechanisms of action, and describes the challenges that lie ahead in developing a deeper understanding of the etiology, natural history, and treatment of TS and related conditions.

PHENOMENOLOGY AND DESCRIPTION OF TIC DISORDERS

Tourette syndrome is a chronic, sometimes disabling disorder, beginning in childhood, that is characterized by stereotyped motor movements and vocalizations termed tics. Tics are discrete, repetitive, involuntary (or semivoluntary) movements or vocalizations. For both diagnostic and treatment purposes tics are described as either motor or phonic. Motor tics may be further classified as either simple, involving a single muscle group (e.g., blinking, sniffing), or complex, involving multiple muscle groups simultaneously with coordinated movement (e.g., head turning, kicking). Phonic tics are similarly classified into simple (e.g., grunting, throat clearing) or complex (e.g., yelling, swearing), based largely on whether or not they result in the production of language.

Tourette syndrome is the most severe end of a spectrum of tic disorders that are hierarchically classified according to both chronicity and tic symptomology. As outlined in the DSM-IV-TR, and in the proposed classification for the forthcoming DSM-5, a diagnosis of Tourette syndrome requires the presence of both a motor and a phonic tic for at least one year, in the absence of any identifiable medical condition responsible for the tics (e.g., stroke, medication). Individuals who display motor tics, phonic tics, or both for less than one year meet criteria for transient tic disorder. Patients who display either motor or phonic tics, but not both, for one year are diagnosed with chronic tic disorder. Finally, individuals with tics who do not meet criteria for a specific tic disorder but do suffer impairment are given the diagnosis of tic disorder not otherwise specified.

Although the specific characteristics of tics differ substantially among individuals, certain trends are broadly recognizable. For example, motor tics manifest more frequently in the muscles of the face and upper limbs than the torso or legs, and, overall, the frequency of simple phonic tics greatly exceeds that of complex phonic tics. One example of a complex phonic tic is coprolalia, or the involuntary yelling of obscenities; this is widely recognized and sometimes described in the lay press as synonymous with TS, but such tics are estimated to occur at some point during the course of the syndrome in only 15% to 20% of patients with TS (Freeman et al., 2009). Recent investigations have outlined the complexity of sensory and motoric processes that are hypothesized to underlie tic symptomology. Ninety percent of adult patients with TS report premonitory "urges" before a tic (Du et al., 2010), and although tics are ultimately involuntary, many patients report an ability to transiently suppress them. Moreover, sensory processing appears to be more generally disrupted in at least some cases of TS. For example, patients often describe either difficulty screening out minor, distracting stimuli and/or the presence of "sensations without sources."

EPIDEMIOLOGY, NATURAL HISTORY, AND COMORBIDITY

Tic disorders are the most common form of movement disorders among children, with an estimated prevalence of 5% (Dooley, 2006). Estimates of the frequency of specific tic disorders vary considerably, and large-scale, well-controlled epidemiological studies are sorely needed; TS itself has an estimated prevalence of 0.6% to 1% of school-aged children (Cavanna and Termine, 2012). Tic disorders in aggregate display a marked gender bias, with boys outnumbering girls 4:1, although this ratio approaches equality when a broader phenotype encompassing both TS and OCD is considered (State, 2011).

By definition, TS onset occurs before adulthood; most patients have an onset of tics between the ages of three and eight, with the highest rate of TS diagnoses occurring from age six to ten (Cavanna and Termine, 2012). Simple motor tics such as eye-blinking or grimacing are generally observed before other tic symptoms, with phonic tics emerging several years following the onset of motor tics. Similarly, simple tics typically precede the onset of complex tics by a number of years (Du et al., 2010).

The clinical course of tic disorders is variable. Tic severity and frequency typically peak at 10 years of age (Jankovic and Kurlan, 2011). Symptoms are dynamic, such that new tics frequently develop or disappear over the course of illness, and their severity and frequency waxes and wanes over weeks to months. Tics are influenced by external factors; they may be exacerbated during periods of stress or fatigue and mitigated during concentration (Du et al., 2010). Most patients experience a significant reduction in tic symptoms with age, with roughly 75% of patients with TS demonstrating improvement by adolescence and as many as one-third displaying complete remission by adulthood (Bloch and Leckman, 2009).

Any description of the clinical phenomenology of tic disorders is incomplete without a discussion of the frequent psychiatric comorbidities observed in affected individuals. Comorbid psychopathology, which Gilles de la Tourette first described as "mental tics," is now appreciated to be the rule rather than the exception, with 60% to 90% of children presenting for evaluation and/or treatment of TS meeting criteria for at least one additional psychiatric disorder. The most frequent comorbidity in clinical populations with tic disorders is attention deficit/hyperactivity disorder (ADHD), with an estimated prevalence of 50% in patients with transient or chronic tic disorders and between 60% and 75% in patients with TS (Du et al., 2010). Similarly high rates of comorbidity are found for obsessive-compulsive disorder (OCD), with an estimated 30% to 50% of patients with TS meeting lifetime diagnostic criteria (Bloch and Leckman, 2009). Finally, the majority of patients with TS also suffer from mood and impulse-control disorders. A recent longitudinal study of TS found 61% of patients to meet criteria for depression by 18 years of age, along with high rates of learning disorders (41%), conduct disorder (23%), and non-OCD anxiety disorders (40%) (Gorman et al., 2010).

Comorbidity can influence the presentation and complicate treatment. Selective serotonin reuptake inhibitor (SSRI) treatment of OCD symptoms is less effective in individuals with a comorbid tic disorder than in those without (March et al., 2007). Psychostimulants, a first-line treatment for ADHD, are no longer contraindicated in patients with tic disorders, as they once were, but are nonetheless thought by many clinicians to exacerbate symptoms in some individuals. A recent metaanalysis failed to support an association, however (Bloch et al., 2009). Comorbid OCD and ADHD diagnoses have been shown to negatively affect quality of life, psychosocial stress, and global functioning in those with TS (Lebowitz et al., 2012). Indeed, comorbid diagnoses may often have a greater impact on quality of life than tics themselves (Bernard et al., 2009), further complicating the long-term treatment of tic disorders and TS.

The frequent comorbidity among OCD, ADHD, and TS has led to the hypothesis that in some individuals these disorders share a common genetic etiology. This hypothesis is indirectly supported by the observation that rates of OCD (or obsessive-compulsive behaviors) and ADHD are higher in relatives of patients with TS than in the general population (O'Rourke et al., 2011). A study using latent-class analysis, a type of structural equation modeling, has reported a highly heritable subclass of comorbid TS + OCD + ADHD in a familial study of TS probands (Grados and Mathews, 2008), although additional studies suggest the shared genetic risk may be related to independent associations between TS + OCD and OCD + ADHD, rather than all three conditions together (Mathews and Grados, 2011). These three disorders all are thought to involve dysfunction of the same basal ganglia circuitry, described in detail in the following, making shared causality quite plausible.

GENETICS

Family studies dating back to the 1970s provide consistent, if indirect, evidence for a genetic contribution to TS. The rate at which first-degree relatives of probands with TS are affected has been found to be on the order of 5% for females and 10% for males, representing an approximately 10-fold increase compared with the general population. Moreover, although relatively small in scale, twin studies have demonstrated that monozygotic twins share a diagnosis of TS much more frequently than do dizygotic twins (State, 2011), suggesting that the observed familial clustering is owing largely to genetic factors.

The earliest studies of TS pedigrees in the mid-1980s were interpreted to suggest that this genetic risk was transmitted as a Mendelian single-gene autosomal-dominant trait with partial and sex-limited penetrance (State, 2011). However, over the subsequent decade, despite intensive efforts, no single genomic locus or gene was identified carrying risk. Given the increasing yield of gene discovery efforts in Mendelian disorders through the 1990s, the continued difficulties in mapping a TS gene, and the completion of additional segregation analyses, it became clear that, like other psychiatric conditions, TS was likely transmitted as a complex trait (Deng et al., 2012) involving multiple genes and their interactions with environmental factors.

This reevaluation led to a series of case control studies focusing on common polymorphisms (typically defined as ≥5% allele frequency in the population) in and around biologically plausible candidate genes. This approach was based on the widely held hypothesis that common genetic variation would underlie common complex disorders. With regard to TS, specific genes interrogated included those encoding dopamine receptors (*DRD2, DRD3, DRD4*), the dopamine transporter (*DAT*), dopamine beta hydroxylase (*DBH*), catechol-*O*-methyltransferase (*COMT*), noradrenergic receptors (*ADRA1C, ADRA2A, ADRA2C*), monoamine oxidase A (*MAO-A*), tyrosine hydroxylase, and several molecules involved in serotonergic neurotransmission (*TPH2, 5HT3, 5HTTLR*) (Deng et al., 2012; Du et al., 2010).

Although this candidate gene approach was popular and relatively easy to implement, such studies generally failed to yield reproducible results in any area of medicine (Hirschhorn and Altshuler, 2002); TS was no exception. More recently, insights into methodological confounds attending hypothesis-driven common variant approaches, combined with key technological advances, have resulted in a shift toward genome-wide association studies (GWAS). This unbiased, genome-wide interrogation of alleles has proved to be a highly reliable means of identifying common variants contributing to common disease. Very recently, the Tourette Syndrome Association International Consortium for Genetics completed a GWAS involving 1496 TS cases and 5249 controls (Scharf et al., 2012). Unfortunately, no locus reached accepted genome-wide thresholds for statistical significance. A likely explanation is that common polymorphisms contributing to TS, like other neuropsychiatric conditions, individually carry very small effects (State, 2011). Consequently, although large relative to other TS genetic efforts, this study was still most likely underpowered to detect common variants influencing risk. Samples on order of magnitude larger than this have played an essential role in identifying common variation contributing to schizophrenia and bipolar disorder (Bergen and Petryshen, 2012).

Although analyses of common variations have generally predominated the field, studies aimed at identifying the contribution of rare mutations have provided important insights. In contrast to the earliest efforts in TS genetics, these more recent rare variant investigations conceptualize the disorder as genetically complex and highly heterogeneous, presupposing that multiple rare mutations, in multiple different genes, may converge on a final common clinical phenotype. Pursuit of this "rare variant, common disease" model has been highly productive in other neurodevelopmental disorders, including autism and schizophrenia (Malhotra and Sebat, 2012).

As early as the mid-1990s, rare chromosomal abnormalities were reported in TS probands or families mapped using traditional and molecular cytogenetic methods, identifying several candidate genes and regions, including 2p12, 3p21.3, 7q35-36, 8q21.4, 9pter, 13q31, and 18q22.3 (Deng et al., 2012). Three results from this work stand out. Verkerk and colleagues reported a complex rearrangement in a father with TS as well as his affected children, disrupting the gene encoding *Contactin-Associated Protein-like 2* (*CNTNAP2*), which is also associated with a rare recessive form of autism and epilepsy and is thought to contribute to common forms of social disability, language delay, and possibly schizophrenia. Lawson-Yuen et al. reported a family with tics and TS transmitting an exonic deletion of the *Neuroligin 4, X-linked* (*NLGN4X*), in which rare mutations also cause autism (State, 2011). These studies point to the now well-established phenomenon of rare variants in a single gene or region leading to highly divergent developmental and neuropsychiatric phenotypes, as has been demonstrated for autism, schizophrenia, epilepsy, and intellectual disability (Malhotra and Sebat, 2012). As discussed in the following, recent studies of structural variation in TS lead to the same conclusion, that variants in the same genes or genomic regions can lead both to TS and other neuropsychiatric conditions.

A third cytogenetic finding has garnered attention because it was the first to lead to the identification of a protein-disrupting rare mutation in a nearby gene. A *de novo* chromosome 13 inversion was identified in a simplex family with TS to a region upstream of the gene *SLITRK1* (*Slit and Trk-like Family Member 1*). Sequencing of a cohort of 179 unrelated affected individuals revealed a frame-shift deletion in the gene in a small pedigree segregating TS and trichotillomania. In addition, two independent instances of a single, very rare single base mutation (var321) were identified in the 3′ untranslated region (UTR) corresponding a micro-RNA (miR-189) binding site. Additional screening for this mutation turned up no additional observations in 4,296 control chromosomes, leading to a significant association with TS ($p = 0.0056$) (State, 2011).

Follow-up studies have yielded mixed results. Sequencing of more than 300 TS subjects has not identified any clearly pathogenic coding mutations in *SLITRK1*, but several putatively disruptive variants were found in a small sample of individuals with trichotillomania. Two candidate gene studies of common variation at the SLITRK1 locus have supported association, but as noted, neither this locus nor any others reached genome-wide significance in GWAS studies of TS. Two studies specifically focused on the 3′ UTR var321 and raised the possibility that this finding may have been the result of occult differences in ancestry among cases and controls (i.e., population stratification). However, the authors of the original paper provided further data and analysis arguing against this interpretation (State, 2011).

A mouse knockout of *SLITRK1* has been described (Aruga et al, 2010). Knockout mice show an anxiety phenotype and increased levels of noradrenaline and its metabolites, mirroring earlier finding in human studies of cerebrospinal fluid in TS (Leckman et al., 1995). Biochemical analyses have demonstrated that SLITRK1 binds to 14-3-3 molecules and regulates neurite outgrowth (Deng et al., 2012), and a mouse knockout of a closely related molecule, *SLITRK5*, shows abnormal corticostriatal dendritic morphology and a rare repetitive grooming/obsessive compulsive phenotype (Shmelkov et al., 2010). Collectively these studies have yielded provocative data; however, the role of *SLITRK1* in TS remains an open question. Given the experience with similarly early rare mutation findings in other areas of psychiatric genetics, such as autism, it is likely that this will only be clarified as larger-scale studies are completed.

The emergence of microarray technology in the early 2000s led to the systematic detection of submicroscopic variations in chromosomal structure called copy number variants (CNVs). These have now been widely studied in a range of disorders, including autism, schizophrenia, bipolar disorder, and others (Malhotra and Sebat, 2012). Two CNV analyses in TS have been reported to date. The first included 111 affected subjects and 73 controls and highlighted the overlap of risks with schizophrenia and autism based on the observation of CNVs in the genes *Neurexin 1* (*NRXN1)* and *Catenin, alpha 3* (*CTNNA3*) (Sundaram et al., 2010). There was no detectable increase in the overall rate of CNVs in cases versus controls, although the power to detect an increase of plausible scale was limited by the small sample size. A later study of 460 TS subjects and 1131 controls similarly found no significant difference in the number of rare CNVs in cases versus controls, though the burden of *de novo* rare exonic variants among 148 TS trios (2.7%) versus 436 control trios (0.7%) approached significance (*p* = .07) (Fernandez et al., 2012). Extrapolating from recent evidence from other disorders, it is likely that a markedly larger sample of affected trios will be required to confirm or refute a significant contribution of *de novo* CNVs to TS. Interestingly, this CNV study provided statistical support for the reported overlap of genes mapping within rare CNVs in TS and ASD. In addition, three large, likely pathogenic *de novo* CNVs were identified, including one disrupting multiple gamma-aminobutyric acid (GABA) receptor genes (Fernandez et al., 2012).

Finally, a recent report of a two-generation family with nine affected members (Ercan-Sencicek et al, 2010) was the first genetic study to suggest a link between TS and histaminergic neurotransmission. The pedigree was found to segregate a rare nonsense mutation in the *HDC* (L-*histidine decarboxylase*) gene, the rate-limiting enzyme in histamine (HA) biosynthesis. In combination with the results of a pathway analysis in the aforementioned CNV study (Fernandez et al., 2012), which found enrichment in CNVs affecting histamine signaling, the finding highlighted a potential role for striatal HA in the genesis or modulation of tics.

Overall, the accumulated evidence demonstrates a critical role for genetic contributors in the etiology of TS, and a series of recent findings have generated intriguing hypotheses regarding molecular pathophysiological mechanisms and the possible overlap of TS risks with other complex neuropsychiatric conditions. Although gene discovery efforts have been less revealing than in other disorders, such as autism and schizophrenia, the prospects for the future are nonetheless extremely bright. Recent studies in autism, schizophrenia, ADHD, and bipolar disorder have all demonstrated that the key to progress is the consolidation of very large samples and the pursuit of studies that address, in an unbiased fashion, the potential contribution of the entire range of allele frequencies, from rare and *de novo* mutations to common polymorphisms (Fig. 79.1). The rapid maturation of genomic technologies, the development of highly reliable analytical methods and the dramatic progress in other complex neuropsychiatric disorders resulting from samples approaching this size point to a clear path forward for TS genetics, one that promises new insights into molecular and cellular mechanisms, and the development of novel and more effective therapeutics.

CORTICOBASAL GANGLIA CONNECTIONS: CORE CIRCUITRY AND CELLULAR COMPONENTS

Dysregulation of the basal ganglia loops connecting the cerebral cortex, striatum (caudate and putamen), globus pallidus, and thalamus—collectively termed the cortico-striato-thalamo-cortical (CSTC) circuitry (Fig. 79.2)—is hypothesized to be

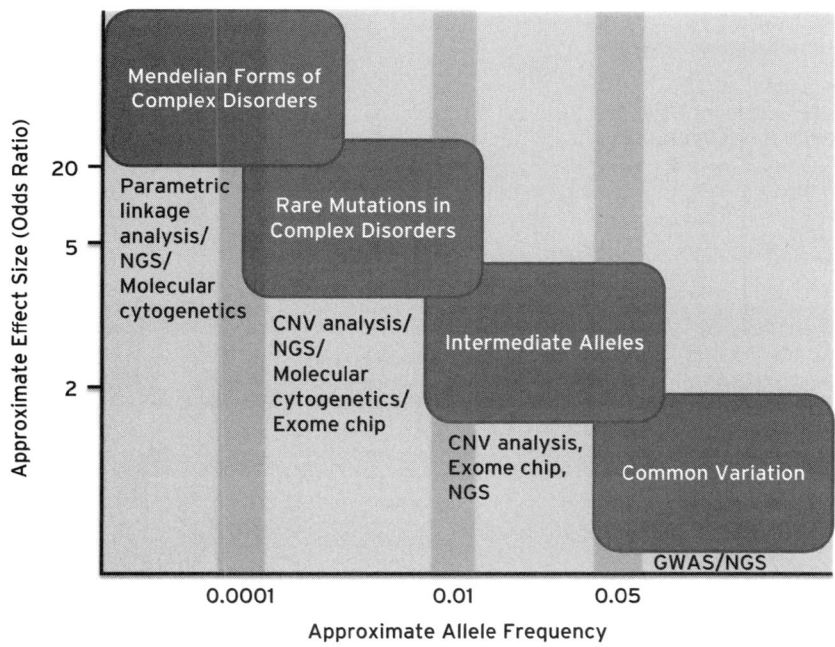

Figure 79.1 *Methodological tools for the discovery of disease-associated alleles of different frequency and effect size. Genetic variation that contributes to disease extends on a continuum of allele frequency and the effect size of disease-associated mutations. These tend to be inversely correlated, as disease alleles of large effect size, particularly for developmental disorders, are subject to purifying selection. Different technologies and analytic approaches are appropriate to characterize alleles at different points along this continuum (as described in the text below the boxes). There is strong evidence for the contribution to TS risk of rare Mendelian forms of TS (e.g., HDC mutations), rare, non-Mendelian mutations (e.g., copy number variation), and common variation. It is very likely that mutations spanning this frequency and effect size spectrum will be found to contribute to both risk and resilience in TS. With the application of the methods noted in the figure, investigations of sufficiently large populations should reveal the genetic architecture of TS in dramatically increased detail over the coming years. Exome-chip, a microarray enriched for probes of recurrent alleles represented at low frequency in the population; NGS, next generation sequencing including whole genome and whole exome analysis. Allele frequencies and effect sizes are approximate and are intended for illustrative purposes.*

central to the pathogenesis of TS. This circuitry is implicated in movement disorders such as Parkinson disease, Huntington disease, and dystonia (Albin et al., 1989). Several lines of evidence suggest that abnormalities in this circuitry also contribute to TS. For example, focal insults to the striatum can produce tics and tic-like phenomenology, as in patients with discrete striatal strokes who may present with motor or phonic tics (Kwak and Jankovic, 2002). Similarly, monkeys develop focal motor tics after local disinhibition of the striatum through injection of the GABA$_A$ antagonist bicuculine (McCairn et al., 2009).

The basal ganglia have been described, to a first approximation, as a series of loops from the cortex, through the striatum and globus pallidus, to the anterior thalamus, and back to the cortex (Alexander et al., 1986). Loops connecting to different cortical regions are hypothesized to quasi-independently process different types of information, although connections between different circuits allow for interactions between domains (Haber et al., 2000). The basal ganglia are unusual in that most of their long-range projections are inhibitory, rather than excitatory. GABAergic medium spiny neurons (MSNs) of the striatum receive excitatory input from the cortex and project through several synapses to the thalamus following two parallel routes, the *direct* (or *striatonigral*) *pathway* and the *indirect* (or *striatopallidal*) *pathway* (see Fig. 79.1). A more recently described third route, the *hyperdirect pathway* constituted by direct cortical projections to the subthalamic nucleus, serves as a reminder that the focus on these two pathways is a convenient simplification.

Activity of MSNs of the direct pathway leads, via two inhibitory synapses, to disinhibition of the thalamus and thus an increase in positive feedback excitation to the cortex. D1 dopamine receptors found on these direct pathway MSNs increase their excitability and firing, thus enhancing excitatory feedback to the cortex. Medium spiny neurons of the indirect pathway, in contrast, produce a net inhibitory effect on the thalamus. D2 dopamine receptors are found on these MSNs and decrease their activity; thus, activation of D2 receptors *also* increases net excitatory feedback to the cortex. This contrasting regulation of direct and indirect pathways by dopamine provides an explanation for the ability of dopamine-enhancing drugs, such as cocaine and amphetamine, to accelerate both behavior and cognition, and for dopamine deficiency in Parkinson disease to produce slowing and deficits in both domains.

This model of the dynamic relationships between nuclei of the basal ganglia neglects their intrinsic microcircuitry; dysregulation of this microcircuitry is likely to have a central role in the pathophysiology of TS. The inhibitory MSNs make up a large majority of striatal neurons, but critical minority populations of interneurons coordinate, sculpt, and integrate MSN firing and thus critically regulate information flow through

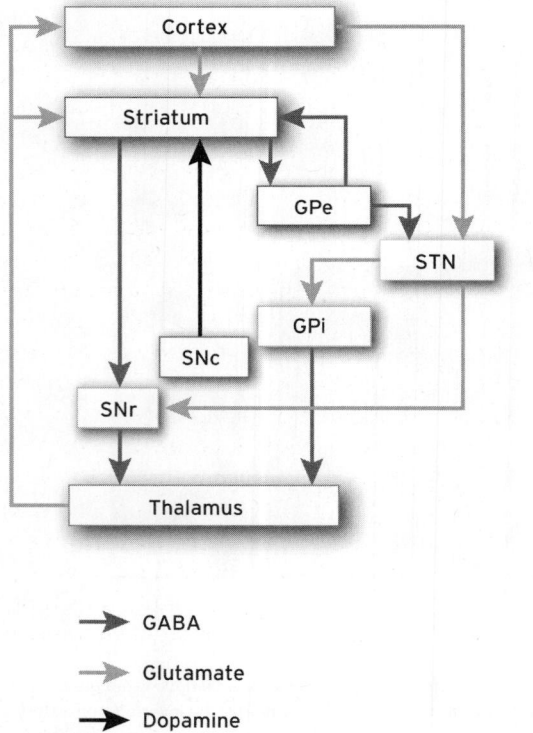

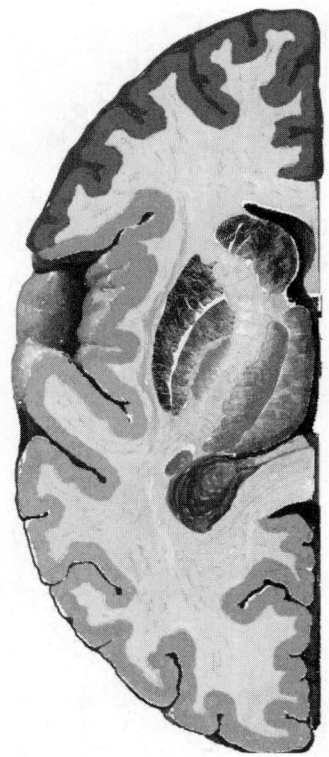

Figure 79.2 *Schematic organization of the cortico-striato-thalamo-cortical circuitry. Major structures and connections of the basal ganglia circuitry are shown. GPe, globus pallidus externa; GPi, globus pallidus interna; STN, subthalamic nucleus; SNc, substantia nigra, pars compacta; SNr, substantia nigra, pars reticulata. D1-expressing MSNs in the striatum (the caudate and putamen) project to the SNr; this constitutes the direct pathway. D2-expressing MSNs project to the GPe, constituting the indirect pathway. (Adapted from Pittenger et al., 2001. Glutamate abnormalities in obsessive compulsive disorder: neurobiology, pathophysiology, and treatment. Pharmaco. The. 132, 314–332.)*

the basal ganglia (Kreitzer, 2009). Prominent among these are the large cholinergic interneurons, hypothesized to be identical to the electrophysiologically identified tonically active neurons (TANs). These intrinsic interneurons provide the only source of modulatory cholinergic tone in the striatum. As their name suggests, the TANs show rhythmic intrinsic activity in the 5-Hz range; this contrasts with the MSNs, which are rather quiet at baseline. Acetylcholine from the TANs acts on both muscarinic and nicotinic receptors, modulating corticostriatal synaptic plasticity (Shen et al., 2008) and interacting with dopamine to gait behavioral reinforcement (Aosaki et al., 2010). Interestingly, the TANs have also recently been shown to release synaptic glutamate (Higley et al., 2011); the implications of this co-release for striatal information processing remain to be clarified.

There are also several populations of GABAergic interneurons in the striatum. The parvalbumin-expressing fast-spiking interneurons (FSIs) have electrophysiological properties similar to those of parvalbumin-expressing interneurons elsewhere in the brain and are capable of firing bursts in excess of 100 Hz. They are thought to mediate feed-forward inhibition from the cortex and may have a role in the synchronization of MSN output (Berke et al., 2004). This suggests that alterations in FSI firing may lead to disorganized striatal information processing. Consistent with this model, pharmacological inhibition of FSI firing produces dyskinetic movements reminiscent of tics (Gittis et al., 2011).

Modulatory neurotransmitters also play a key role in regulating information flow through the basal ganglia, as they do elsewhere in the brain. The roles of dopamine and acetylcholine have been briefly described in the preceding. Certain serotonin receptors, especially the 5-HT1B receptor, are also densely expressed in the basal ganglia. Histaminergic modulation of the basal ganglia has received relatively little attention until recently. However, as summarized previously, the identification of a rare but highly penetrant mutation in the *Hdc* gene that segregates with TS in a dense pedigree creates new interest in the potential role of abnormalities in histaminergic neurotransmission in the pathophysiology of TS. Histamine receptors are prominent in the basal ganglia. Their specific role is an area of active research.

NEUROIMAGING: SUBCORTICAL STRUCTURES

Neuroimaging studies in patients with TS support the presence of anatomical and functional abnormalities in the basal ganglia circuitry. Neuroimaging in patients with TS can be particularly challenging, as tics can generate problematic movement artifacts. Nevertheless, substantial imaging data have been described over the years. The most robust and replicated findings involve volumetric changes in subcortical nuclei, particularly the caudate nucleus. Three volumetric MRI studies, including one with more than 150 subjects, have reported decreases in the volume of the caudate in TS subjects compared with controls. Moreover, reduced caudate volumes are associated with increased tic and OCD symptoms severity in adulthood (Leckman et al., 2010). Changes in the putamen are less well established. One early study suggested a reduction in the size of the lenticular nuclei,

consisting of putamen and globus pallidus (Peterson et al., 2003), whereas subsequent reports have found increased putamenal volumes (Kassubek et al., 2006; Roessner et al., 2011). Two additional large-scale (>100 TS subjects and controls) MRI studies have reported volumetric changes in the hippocampus, amygdala, and thalamic nuclei (Leckman et al., 2010), although the specific findings have yet to be replicated.

With regard to neurotransmitter systems in these brain regions, three PET studies have reported increased dopamine release in response to amphetamine challenge in striatum, although one study failed to find evidence of abnormal dopaminergic transmission (Rickards, 2009). A SPECT study found increased expression of the striatal dopamine transporter compared with controls, consistent with increased dopamine release and turnover. Finally, significant decreases in GABA$_A$ receptor binding throughout subcortical structures (chiefly the basal ganglia, substantia nigra, thalamus, and amygdala) have recently been reported in TS (Lerner et al., 2012). Viewed as a whole, these studies provide evidence for increased dopaminergic activity in TS and altered neurotransmission in CSTC circuitry.

It is worth noting that the majority of these PET and SPECT studies were performed in symptomatic adults. A majority of children with TS experience a significant decrease in their tic symptoms during adolescence. Therefore, adults with clinically significant tics may represent a specific subset of those diagnosed with TS during childhood. It is possible that the pathophysiology of tics in these adult patients differs from that in individuals whose tics remit or substantially improve during adolescence.

Functional imaging studies convey a similar theme. Four PET studies of regional metabolic activity have found decreased basal activity in the striatum and caudate nuclei in subjects with TS compared with controls. Functional MRI (fMRI), which allows better time resolution, has yielded largely consistent results. Functional fMRI studies of brain activation during voluntary tic suppression have revealed increased activation of the caudate nucleus but decreased activation of the putamen and thalamus. Increased striatal activation has been reported in patients with TS during performance of cognitive control tasks. This increase positively correlates with tic severity (Rickards, 2009). Similarly, two studies of inhibitory control, using the Stroop and Simons tasks, showed greater activation of the putamen and globus pallidus, and poorer performance, in children with TS compared with controls (Raz et al., 2009; Rickards, 2009). An fMRI analysis of a simple, non-tic motor task (finger tapping) in medication-free boys with TS found similar increased activation of the caudate nucleus compared to controls, suggesting a generalized inefficiency of this circuitry in both tic-associated and non–tic-associated contexts (Roessner et al., 2012).

Techniques that probe the integrity of neurons and neuronal connections also indicate the presence of abnormalities in the CSTC circuitry in TS. Magnetic resonance spectroscopy (MRS) measurements of *N*-acetylaspartate (NAA), which is thought to reflect neuronal integrity, revealed reductions in the striatum of TS subjects compared with controls (DeVito et al., 2005). Diffusion tensor imaging (DTI), which measures the anisotropic diffusion of water molecules to probe the integrity of white matter tracts, has revealed abnormalities in the organization of the internal capsule, basal ganglia, thalamus, and frontostriatal networks (Felling and Singer, 2011; Govindan et al., 2010).

A consistent theme among these studies is the abnormal structure and function throughout the subcortical components of the CSTC circuitry. The details and functional consequences of these abnormalities remain to be elucidated, and it remains unclear which abnormalities are essential components of the pathophysiology of tic symptomology, as opposed to epiphenomena or compensatory changes. However, the consistency of these findings strongly suggests a role for abnormal CSTC circuit function in the pathophysiology of TS.

NEUROIMAGING: CORTICAL PATHOLOGY IN TOURETTE SYNDROME

Afferent projections to the basal ganglia originate primarily in the cortex and thalamus, and numerous studies have revealed cortical abnormalities in patients with TS. Whether these cortical abnormalities are a primary cause of the subcortical abnormalities described in the preceding or are a consequence of basal ganglia dysregulation is a difficult question to answer. It may be that primary pathology in either region can lead to similar dysregulation of the circuit as a whole and thus to similar symptomatology.

Early postmortem studies identified increased second-messenger enzyme levels in frontal and occipital cortices (Singer et al., 1995), with subsequent findings of increased D_1, D_2, and α_2-adrenergic receptors in the prefrontal cortex of patients with TS compared with controls (Leckman et al., 2010). This later finding is of particular interest because pharmacological treatments for tic disorders are centered upon either dopaminergic or adrenergic modulation.

Neuroimaging provides additional evidence of altered cortical physiology in tic disorders. The most widely replicated findings involve volumetric abnormalities throughout multiple regions of cortex, with cortical thinning in the frontal and parietal cortices, particularly in the sensorimotor regions (Leckman et al., 2010), in adults with TS. These cortical abnormalities appear to follow a specific developmental trajectory, with an *increase* in dorsal prefrontal cortical thickness in children with TS (Peterson et al., 2001), evolving into cortical thinning in adults (Leckman et al., 2010). A similar developmental trajectory of cortical thickness abnormalities has been reported for pre-motor and parieto-occipital cortex, with tic severity inversely correlated to the volume of these structures (Peterson et al., 2001). These findings have been interpreted as suggesting hypertrophied CSTC input in children with TS, with subsequent atrophy of these regions in adulthood. In contrast, the corpus callosum, which interconnects the hemispheres, shows reduced cross-sectional area in children but increased area in adults (Felling and Singer, 2011). An important caveat is that these findings are from cross-sectional studies; no longitudinal studies of cortical thickness or connectivity over time in TS have been reported.

Functional imaging and PET studies complement these structural findings. Studies of resting state connectivity and DTI have identified increased and disorganized connectivity between frontostriatal networks (Felling and Singer, 2011), which has been interpreted as a sign of immature functional connectivity of these neuronal circuits. This finding is congruent with results from task-related fMRI studies, which have repeatedly shown increased recruitment of the frontal cortices during cognitive tasks (Raz et al., 2009; Rickards, 2009), and blink-suppression (Mazzone et al., 2010), in TS subjects compared with controls. Functional imaging during motor tasks has revealed both increased and decreased activation in the sensorimotor and supplementary motor regions during movement when compared with controls (Rickards, 2009; Roessner et al., 2012). However, PET studies have consistently found increased metabolic activity in the premotor and supplementary motor areas in TS subjects, which have positively correlated with tic severity (Felling and Singer, 2011).

In sum, the TS neuroimaging literature—both of cortical and subcortical structures—contains substantial heterogeneity and important open questions, but certain generalizations emerge in which we can have confidence. Multiple cortical areas, especially sensorimotor cortices, are thicker in children but thin over time and are thinner in adults than in matched controls. These same cortical regions appear to be hyperactive at rest and to be more readily recruited during a variety of tasks. The striatum, in contrast, is hypoactive at rest, and the caudate nucleus has a small but significant reduction in volume that correlates with long-term clinical course. In aggregate, these volumetric abnormalities support the hypothesized dysregulation of the CSTC circuitry, although many details remain to be elucidated.

NEUROPATHOLOGY: EVIDENCE FOR BASAL GANGLIA DYSREGULATION IN TOURETTE SYNDROME

Recently, postmortem analysis has provided direct evidence for alterations in striatal interneuron populations in TS (Kataoka et al., 2010). Rigorous quantification of the density of specific populations of interneurons has revealed a significant, approximately 50% decrease in the density of parvalbumin-expressing FSIs throughout the striatum and globus pallidus externa (GPe) of TS subjects when compared with controls (Fig. 79.3). Strikingly, PV+ neurons, although decreased in the GPe, were *increased* by 68% in the adjacent globus pallidus *interna* (GPi) in patients with TS compared with controls. The cholinergic interneurons—the presumptive TANs—were similarly decreased by approximately 50%. These deficits appear specific to the PV+ and ChAT+ interneuron populations, as no differences in total neuronal number or in the density of other, calretinin-expressing interneurons were appreciated. ChAT+ interneurons displayed greater deficits in the sensorimotor and associative regions of the striatum (compared with more ventral limbic regions). There is normally a gradient of TAN density from dorsal to ventral striatum; this regionalized deficit had the effect of abolishing this density gradient seen in control postmortem brains (Kataoka et al., 2010).

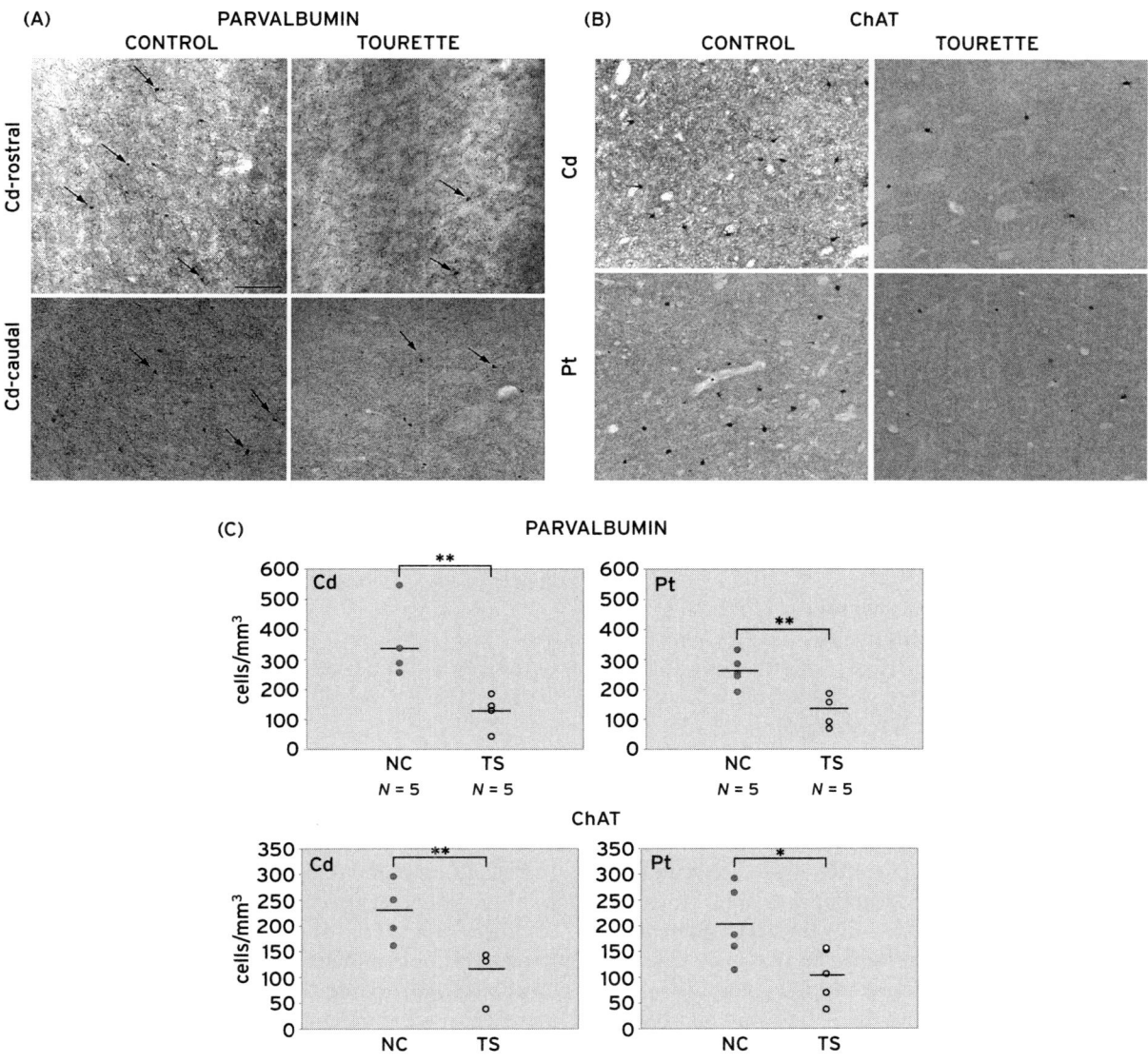

Figure 79.3 Interneuron deficits in postmortem samples from the Tourette syndrome brain. (A) Immunostaining for parvalbumin identifies putative FSI interneurons in postmortem tissue from TS and control brains. (B) Immunostaining for ChAT identifies putatitve TANs. (C) Both categories of interneuron are reduced in number by approximately 50% in the TS brain throughout the caudate and putamen. (Adapted from Kataoka et al., 2010, with thanks to F. Vaccarino and Y. Kataoka. Decreased number of parvalbumin and cholinergic interneurons in the striatum of individuals with Tourette syndrome. The J. Comparat. Neuro. 518, 277–291.)

These important postmortem findings come with some caveats. The total number of TS brains examined remains small (five TS brains and five controls). The subjects were not typical patients with TS. They were adults with lifelong, treatment-refractory disease and had had multiple pharmacotherapy trials. Therefore, it is important to guard against overgeneralizing from these results. Nevertheless, the suggestion that specific interneuron deficits may underlie TS has importantly reoriented the field.

The genesis of the observed deficits in cholinergic interneurons and in PV-expressing interneurons in these postmortem studies remains unclear. In particular, it remains to be established whether these deficits are causal, compensatory, related to the treatment-refractory nature of the particular patients studied, or an epiphenomenon. It is also unclear whether the reduced interneuronal number is caused by a developmental failure or represents a remarkably specific pattern of degeneration. Two arguments support the former possibility. First, the fact that PV-expressing interneurons are not simply missing but rather are maldistributed, with a decreased density in striatum and GPe but an *increased* density in GPi, suggests dysregulated migration during development. Second, recent studies have revealed that these two interneronal populations have a shared developmental origin, and their ontogenesis is regulated by an overlapping set of transcriptional regulators (Fragkouli et al., 2009). This suggests the possibility that disruption in a specific developmental program could produce the remarkably specific observed pattern of interneuron deficits. However, any such proposal remains highly speculative, and many details remain to be worked out.

How might these interneuronal deficits lead to the circuit dysregulation and symptomatology of TS? PV+ interneurons are highly responsive to stimulation from motor and somatosensory cortices (Parthasarathy and Graybiel, 1997) and densely innervate adjacent MSNs (Leckman et al., 2010). They are electrically coupled to one another through gap junctions. *In vivo* recordings in rats suggest that they play a role in synchronizing the firing of MSNs, at least during some behavioral states (Berke et al., 2004); their disruption may lead to dysynchrony of CSTC circuitry. Targeted pharmacological inhibition of PV+ interneurons in the striatum of freely moving mice produces dystonic symptoms, consistent with this prediction (Gittis et al., 2011). Administration of amphetamine has also been shown to increase the firing rates of PV+ interneurons, whereas blockade of the D_2 dopamine receptor decreases firing rates (Wiltschko et al., 2010), suggesting modulation of these neurons from compounds capable of both exacerbating and alleviating tics.

As noted, cholinergic interneurons, identified by their expression of choline acetyltransferase (ChAT), are widely thought to correspond to the sparse tonically active neurons (TANs) found in *in vivo* electrophysiological recordings. These TANs express both D2 and D5 receptors and are also highly responsive to afferent dopaminergic projections, as well as to glutamatergic afferents from both cortex and thalamus. Tonically active neurons synapse richly on MSNs and FSIs, as well as on other TANs and on the terminals of both glutamatergic and dopaminergic afferents (Kreitzer, 2009). Tonically active neuron firing and the burst firing of dopaminergic projections have a complex relationship. When dopaminergic afferents fire in response to an unexpected reward, the TANs coincidentally pause their tonic firing (Goldberg and Reynolds, 2011), possibly through the direct action of these dopaminergic afferents on D2 receptors on the TANs. Recent work suggests activation of ChAT+ interneurons by thalamic afferents may transiently enhance activity of the indirect pathway, inhibiting movement (Ding et al., 2010). It is plausible that dysregulation of this regulatory mechanism leads to impaired indirect pathway activity. However, such interpretations remain highly speculative. The potential consequences of interneuronal dysregulation in TS remain to be clearly elucidated.

ANIMAL MODELS: SUBCORTICAL DYSFUNCTION AND TOURETTE SYNDROME

Both TS and OCD have been associated with dysregulatoin of the CSTC circuitry. An early mouse model of comorbid TS and OCD sought to recapitulate this hyperactivity by expressing the cholera toxin A1 subunit, which potentiates neuronal activity, under the control of the D_1 dopamine receptor promoter. These animals have chronic activation of D_1-containing neurons throughout the cortex and amygdala (Felling and Singer, 2011). They display repetitive behaviors, with bursts of tic-like movements of the head and limbs, and demonstrate

improvement with both α2-agonists and D_2 receptor antagonists. However, these mice also display symptoms outside the scope of TS, such as a reduced seizure threshold, leading to questions regarding the validity of this model.

Another animal model of substantial interest derives from a spontaneous mutation in the Syrian golden hamster: the dystonic or dtsz hamster. These animals display stress-induced facial contortions, hyperextension of limbs, and dystonic posturing; these behaviors are arguably analogous to the symptoms observed in patients with tic disorders. Immunohistochemical analysis revealed a 26% reduction of the PV+ interneuron population in the striatum of mutant hamsters when compared with controls, paralleling what has been described in postmortem human brain, with resultant abnormal burst-firing patterns of globus pallidal neurons recorded using *in vivo* electrophysiology. Remarkably, these mutant hamsters show an age-related decrease in stress-induced dystonias, again analogous to the clinical course of TS, and this improvement of symptoms correlates with an age-related normalization of striatal PV+ interneurons (Leckman et al., 2010).

IMMUNE DYSFUNCTION IN TIC DISORDERS AND TOURETTE SYNDROME

One intriguing hypothesis developed in recent years is that some cases of TS and OCD may derive from autoimmune mechanisms. Proposals along this line have been met with both interest and controversy. One proposed syndrome, termed Pediatric Autoimmune Neuropsychiatric Disorder Associated with Streptococcal infections (PANDAS), hypothesizes that tic disorders in a subset of patients are the result of an autoimmune syndrome initiated by a group A beta-hemolytic streptococcal (GABHS) infection. A more general hypothesis is that more nonspecific inflammatory activity and/or immune dysfunction in the CNS contributes to the pathophysiology of tic disorders more broadly.

PANDAS is characterized by the rapid onset of OCD and/or tic symptoms in a previously healthy child following a recent GABHS infection. This syndrome is conceptualized as a variant of Sydenham chorea, a well-characterized hyperkinetic movement disorder that follows a recent GABHS infection, and shows both radiological evidence of basal ganglia abnormalities and autoimmune antibodies directed against neuronal proteins (Murphy et al., 2010). The clinical scope and diagnostic criteria for PANDAS are defined by an abrupt onset and waxing and waning symptoms associated with GABHS infections.

A thorough discussion of the controversy surrounding the PANDAS diagnosis is beyond the scope of this chapter. Briefly, owing to the lack of biomarkers or diagnostic tools to identify those with PANDAS from children with childhood onset OCD or tic disorder, many investigators have argued that PANDAS represents a spurious association between a ubiquitous infection of childhood (GABHS) and the onset of a common neuropsychiatric disorder (Singer et al., 2011). Cross-sectional studies investigating new-onset diagnoses of TS and GABHS infections, as well as longitudinal studies investigating symptom exacerbations following GABHS infections, have produced conflicting results (Singer et al., 2011).

However, clinical trials using immunomodulatory therapies for children with PANDAS have shown striking reductions in OCD and tic symptoms, as well as normalization of basal ganglia abnormalities on serial MRI exams (Murphy et al., 2010). Furthermore, antibodies against the D_1 and D_2 receptors have been isolated from children with PANDAS (Brimberg et al., 2012), providing a plausible mechanism for an autoimmune etiology in these patients. Additional support comes from two recent animal studies using immunization with GABHS proteins in mice, demonstrating the generation of perseverative behaviors and motor stereotypies, as well as deposition of autoimmune antibodies throughout the CNS, including the basal ganglia (Hoffman et al., 2004; Yaddanapudi et al., 2010). Continued investigation is needed to clarify the validity of this diagnostic entity. A replication trial of immunomodulatory therapy in the treatment of PANDAS is underway at the National Institute of Mental Health.

Multiple investigations suggest individuals with tic disorders display altered immune function, irrespective of any etiopathological link to specific infections. For example, a recent postmortem analysis of RNA transcripts in the basal ganglia of four patients with TS (and four controls) found a 6.5-fold increase in MCP-1, a marker of chronic inflammation and immune cell activation. An additional 2.9-fold increase was observed in IL-2, an inflammatory cytokine involved in immune cell proliferation, replicating a similar finding from a previous study of postmortem putamen in TS subjects. Elevations of inflammatory cytokines in patients with TS compared with controls have been documented in small-scale studies, as have abnormalities in immunoglobulin levels (Murphy et al., 2010). Further research is necessary to discern whether these changes are pathophysiologically related to TS or are an epiphenomenon.

INTEGRATIVE MODELS OF TOURETTE SYNDROME PATHOPHYSIOLOGY

Several themes emerge from this summary of recent advances in our understanding of the pathophysiology of TS. Our insight into the pathophysiology of the disorder remains incomplete; but some integration can be attempted and may guide future investigations.

The initial proposal of the direct and indirect pathways (see Fig. 79.2) suggested that a dynamic balance between them regulates relative levels of activation (Albin et al., 1989). A refinement of the direct/indirect pathway concept, focusing on the concept of *action selection*, has cast further light on how dysregulation of this circuitry may produce tics. In any given context, an organism must select from among different possible actions or responses. The direct pathway is hypothesized to be responsible for selecting an action from among different cortical representations. The indirect pathway, in contrast, suppresses other "off-target" actions (Mink, 2001). In this model, reduced activity in the indirect pathway would be predicted to disinhibit off-target movements, a plausible explanation for tics. D2 blockade, which is an efficacious pharmacotherapy for

TS, would disinhibit the indirect pathway and thereby reduce these off-target movements.

How might such a relative hypoactivity of the indirect pathway develop? We can only speculate. The D2 receptor has a higher affinity for dopamine than the D1 receptor and is thought to be more responsive to tonic, rather than phasic, dopamine stimulation. A chronic, mild elevation of striatal dopamine could thus lead to preferential activation of the D2 receptor and suppression of the indirect pathway, with little or no impact on the direct pathway. Interestingly, H3 histamine receptors are found presynaptically on dopaminergic terminals and are thought to suppress dopamine release; it is plausible, therefore, that reduced histamine (e.g., in patients carrying the rare HDC mutation described in the preceding) could lead to disinhibited dopamine release and produce just such an effect. Amphetamine use, which has been clinically reported to worsen tic severity in some cases, could likewise produce a chronic elevation of striatal dopamine and thus reduced indirect pathway tone. The mechanisms whereby autoimmunity may influence this circuitry in PANDAS are not well understood. However, the observation of antibodies against dopamine receptors in some individuals leads to a plausible explanation for an effect on the flow of information through the system.

How might interneuronal pathology fit into this hypothesis? One possibility is that an interneuronal deficit can differentially affect the medium spiny neurons of the direct and indirect pathways. For example, burst-pause firing of the cholinergic interneurons has recently been shown, in brain slice, to produce a differential silencing of the D2-expressing MSNs of the indirect pathway (Ding et al., 2010). A TAN deficit could plausibly impair this mechanism, producing an indirect pathway-specific deficit (at least phasically). An alternative possibility is that interneuronal deficits lead to a disorganization of striatal information processing. For example, parvalbumin-expressing FSIs are thought to play a role in synchronizing MSN firing, at least during some behavioral states (Berke et al., 2004). Disruption of such a coordinating role could plausibly produce local imbalances of direct and indirect pathway tone, thus disinhibiting fragmentary off-target movements.

These speculations address regulation throughout the basal ganglia (the striatum in particular). But individual tics are typically focal and presumably derive from dysregulated firing of a small domain of the basal ganglia circuitry, not the entirety of the striatum. In support of this supposition, small, localized strokes can produce tics (Kwak and Jankovic, 2002), and local disinhibition of the monkey striatum by infusion of a GABA antagonist produces tic-like movements (McCairn et al., 2009). There are three ways such a local effect may arise. First, there may be a truly local pathology, as occurs after a stroke. Second, there may be a disorganization of striatal network activity such that local areas of dysregulation spontaneously emerge through self-organization of a maladaptive network architecture. Finally, neurochemical or interneuronal abnormalities throughout the basal ganglia circuitry may render it susceptible to aberrant responses to particular patterns of cortical input. This last possibility would potentially provide an explanation for the clinical observation that tics can sometimes be triggered by a particular sensory stimulus, such as a cough, but then appear to become autonomous.

TREATMENT

In many cases, TS and other tic disorders do not require intervention. Because the natural history of the disease is waxing and waning and improvement with age is common, tics can often simply be monitored. Treatment is warranted when tics cause significant distress or impact social or occupational functioning. When tics become self-injurious or damaging, aggressive treatment is critical. We end our discussion of the neurobiology of TS with a brief summary of evidence-based pharmacological and neurosurgical treatments, in the context of the previous discussion of TS pathophysiology.

To date, the only medications approved by the Food and Drug Administration (FDA) for the treatment of TS in children are the neuroleptics haloperidol and pimozide, both potent antagonists of the D_2 receptor. Both haloperidol and pimozide have demonstrated efficacy, compared with placebo, in randomized controlled trials, with one trial suggesting a superior effect of pimozide over haloperidol. Risperidone, a second-generation antipsychotic, has also demonstrated effectiveness in the treatment of tics in randomized, double-blinded controlled trials, with a reported 32% reduction in tic severity at eight weeks. Treatment with these agents is often limited by side effects, with extrapyramidal motor side effects and cardiac effects being of greatest concern for the older agents and weight gain for risperidone.

D2 receptors are particularly concentrated in the caudate and putamen, and D2 blockade has marked effects on basal ganglia function and information processing. In particular, D2 blockade will reduce the normal inhibitory effect of dopamine on activity in the indirect (striatopallidal) pathway through the basal ganglia (see Fig. 79.2). It was speculated in the preceding that tics may represent fragmented off-target movements that are insufficiently inhibited by the indirect pathway. Increasing activity in this pathway may therefore represent the mechanism whereby D2 antagonism mitigates symptoms. D2 receptors are also found on striatal cholinergic interneurons. Blockade of these receptors may disinhibit these interneurons, mitigating some consequences of any deficiency in neuronal number or function. However, these proposed mechanisms remain speculative.

The side effect profile of antipsychotic medications decreases the long-term viability of these treatments for many patients. Agonists of the α_2-adrenergic receptor, clonidine, and guanfacine have shown efficacy in the treatment of tics in double-blind, treatment-controlled studies (Bloch et al., 2011). These medications have a much smaller treatment effect size than the D2 antagonists, but have the benefit of far fewer side effects than the antipsychotics. α_2-adrenergic agonists are also effective therapies for the management of ADHD, making them attractive candidates for those with tic disorders and comorbid ADHD. One barrier to treatment among α_2-adrenergic agonists is their short duration of action. A long-acting preparation has recently been approved by the FDA, although to date no trials in TS have been published. Adrenergic innervation of the basal ganglia is sparse; however, modulation of the frontal cortex is substantial. It is therefore likely that the α_2-adrenergic agonists affect the symptoms of TS by modulating cortical function. Details of this effect remain to be worked out.

We have described the evidence that TS is associated with dysregulation of the CSTC circuitry. This leads to the idea that direct manipulation of activity in this circuit using deep brain stimulation (DBS) may mitigate symptoms in particularly severe, refractory cases. DBS has long been used for Parkinson disease, dystonia, and other movement disorders. In TS, a number of cases and case series of DBS have been described. Targets have included thalamus, globus pallidus, and nucleus accumbens. Reports from these early trials have been promising, with an approximately 60% reduction in tic symptoms across reported studies (Neuner et al., 2009). However, no well-powered placebo-controlled studies have been described to date; therefore, these results must be considered tentative. No consensus exists regarding the optimal structure for stimulation to alleviate tics, and no careful comparison studies have been conducted to date. Further research is needed to identify which targets within the CSTC circuitry give the greatest effect in the DBS treatment of tic symptoms.

CONCLUSIONS

Our understanding of the pathophysiology of TS has advanced remarkably over the past decade, to the point that several specific pathophysiological themes are beginning to coalesce. Multiple strands of evidence from neuroimaging, postmortem, and preclinical studies suggest that abnormalities in the CSTC circuitry are a central component of the neurobiology of TS. Dysregulation of dopaminergic modulation within this circuitry has long been thought to be of central importance. More recent work has focused attention on interneuron abnormalities and potential dysregulation of histaminergic neurotransmission. The genetics of the disorder, long opaque, are now beginning to come into clearer focus, although larger studies are clearly necessary to characterize the contribution of both rare and common genetic variation. Most important, the tools and methodologies necessary to exploit these large samples and clarify the genomic landscape of TS are already in place. Finally, the complex interplay between immunological dysregulation and pathophysiology suggested by the controversial syndrome of PANDAS is a fertile area for ongoing investigation.

Neuropsychiatric diseases are, as a rule, pathophysiologically and genetically complex and heterogeneous. Tourette syndrome is no exception to this generalization, and much work remains to be done before a clear understanding of the genetic and developmental origins, neurobiological correlates, and systems-level abnormalities underlying this fascinating condition can emerge. However, the accelerating pace of discovery in recent years engenders real optimism that the new insights into pathophysiology that emerge will, before long, lead to novel strategies of treatment and prevention.

DISCLOSURES

Dr. Williams is supported by the NIMH (T32MH018268) and the Massachusetts General Hospital Research Fund. He has no real or potential conflicts of interest.

Dr. Bloch is supported by the NIMH (K23MH09124), the Brain and Behavior Research Foundation, the Yale Center for Clinical Investigation (UL1TR000142), and the State of Connecticut through its support of the Abraham Ribicoff Research Facilities at the Connecticut Mental Health Center. He has no real or potential conflicts of interest.

Dr. State is supported by the NIMH and NINDS. He has no conflicts of interest pertaining to the content of this chapter.

Dr. Pittenger's work on this chapter has been supported by the NIMH (K08MH081190; R01MH091861), the Tourette Syndrome Association of America, the Brain and Behavior Research Foundation, and the State of Connecticut through its support of the Abraham Ribicoff Research Facilities at the Connecticut Mental Health Center. He receives research support from Roche Pharmaceuticals for an unrelated project.

REFERENCES

Albin, R.L., Young, A.B., et al. (1989). The functional anatomy of basal ganglia disorders. *Trends Neurosci.* 12:366–375.

Alexander, G.E., DeLong, M.R., et al. (1986). Parallel organization of functionally segregated circuits linking basal ganglia and cortex. *Ann. Rev. Neurosci.* 9:357–381.

Aosaki, T., Miura, M., et al. (2010). Acetylcholine-dopamine balance hypothesis in the striatum: an update. *Geriatr. Gerontol. Int.* 10 (Suppl 1):S148–S157.

Bergen, S.E., and Petryshen, T.L. (2012). Genome-wide association studies of schizophrenia: does bigger lead to better results? *Curr. Opin. Psychiatry* 25:76–82.

Berke, J.D., Okatan, M., et al. (2004). Oscillatory entrainment of striatal neurons in freely moving rats. *Neuron* 43:883–896.

Bernard, B.A., Stebbins, G.T., et al. (2009). Determinants of quality of life in children with Gilles de la Tourette syndrome. *Mov. Disord.* 24:1070–1073.

Bloch, M.H., and Leckman, J.F. (2009). Clinical course of Tourette syndrome. *J. Psychosom. Res.* 67:497–501.

Bloch, M.H., Panza, K.E., et al. (2009). Meta-analysis: treatment of attention-deficit/hyperactivity disorder in children with comorbid tic disorders. *J. Acad. Child Adolesc. Psychiatry* 48:884–893.

Bloch, M., State, M., et al. (2011). Recent advances in Tourette syndrome. *Curr. Opin. Neurol.* 24:119–125.

Brimberg, L., Benhar, I., et al. (2012). Behavioral, pharmacological, and immunological abnormalities after streptococcal exposure: a novel rat model of Sydenham chorea and related neuropsychiatric disorders. *Neuropsychopharmacol.* 37:2076–2087.

Cavanna, A.E., and Termine, C. (2012). Tourette syndrome. *Adv. Exp. Med. Biol.* 724:375–383.

Deng, H., Gao, K., et al. (2012). The genetics of Tourette syndrome. *Nat. Rev. Neurol.* 8:203–213.

DeVito, T.J., Drost, D.J., et al. (2005). Brain magnetic resonance spectroscopy in Tourette's disorder. *J. Am. Acad. Child Adolesc. Psychiatry* 44:1301–1308.

Ding, J.B., Guzman, J.N., et al. (2010). Thalamic gating of corticostriatal signaling by cholinergic interneurons. *Neuron* 67:294–307.

Dooley, J.M. (2006). Tic disorders in childhood. *Seminars in pediatric neurology* 13:231–242.

Du, J.C., Chiu, T.F., et al. (2010). Tourette syndrome in children: an updated review. *Pediatr. Neonatol.* 51:255–264.

Ercan-Sencicek, A., Stillman, A., et al. (2010). L-histidine Decarboxylase and Tourette's Syndrome. *N. Engl. J. Med.* 362:1901–1908.

Felling, R.J., and Singer, H.S. (2011). Neurobiology of Tourette syndrome: current status and need for further investigation. *J. Neurosci.* 31:12387–12395.

Fernandez, T.V., Sanders, S.J., et al. (2012). Rare copy number variants in tourette syndrome disrupt genes in histaminergic pathways and overlap with autism. *Biol. Psychiatry* 71:392–402.

Fragkouli, A., van Wijk, N.V., et al. (2009). LIM homeodomain transcription factor-dependent specification of bipotential MGE progenitors into cholinergic and GABAergic striatal interneurons. *Development* 136:3841–3851.

Freeman, R.D., Zinner, S.H., et al. (2009). Coprophenomena in Tourette syndrome. *Dev. Med. Child Neurol.* 51:218–227.

Gittis, A.H., Leventhal, D.K., et al. (2011). Selective inhibition of striatal fast-spiking interneurons causes dyskinesias. *J. Neurosci.* 31:15727–15731.

Gittis, A.H., Leventhal, D.K., et al. (2011b). Selective inhibition of striatal fast-spiking interneurons causes dyskinesias. *J. Neurosci.* 31:15727–15731.

Goldberg, J.A., and Reynolds, J.N. (2011). Spontaneous firing and evoked pauses in the tonically active cholinergic interneurons of the striatum. *Neuroscience* 198:27–43.

Gorman, D.A., Thompson, N., et al. (2010). Psychosocial outcome and psychiatric comorbidity in older adolescents with Tourette syndrome: controlled study. *Br. J. Psychiatry* 197:36–44.

Govindan, R.M., Makki, M.I., et al. (2010). Abnormal water diffusivity in corticostriatal projections in children with Tourette syndrome. *Hum. Brain. Mapp.* 31:1665–1674.

Grados, M.A., and Mathews, C.A. (2008). Latent class analysis of Gilles de la Tourette syndrome using comorbidities: clinical and genetic implications. *Biol. Psychiatry* 64:219–225.

Haber, S.N., Fudge, J.L., et al. (2000). Striatonigrostriatal pathways in primates form an ascending spiral from the shell to the dorsolateral striatum. *J. Neurosci.* 20:2369–2382.

Higley, M.J., Gittis, A.H., et al. (2011). Cholinergic interneurons mediate fast VGluT3-dependent glutamatergic transmission in the striatum. *PloS One* 6:e19155.

Hirschhorn, J.N., and Altshuler, D. (2002). Once and again-issues surrounding replication in genetic association studies. *J. Clin. Endocr. Metab.* 87:4438–4441.

Hoffman, K.L., Hornig, M., et al. (2004). A murine model for neuropsychiatric disorders associated with group A beta-hemolytic streptococcal infection. *J. Neurosci.* 24:1780–1791.

Jankovic, J., and Kurlan, R. (2011). Tourette syndrome: evolving concepts. *Mov. Disord.* 26:1149–1156.

Kassubek, J., Juengling, F.D., et al. (2006). Heterogeneity of voxel-based morphometry findings in Tourette's syndrome: an effect of age? *Ann. Neurol.* 59:872–873.

Kataoka, Y., Kalanithi, P.S.A., et al. (2010). Decreased number of parvalbumin and cholinergic interneurons in the striatum of individuals with Tourette syndrome. *J. Comp. Neurol.* 518:277–291.

Kreitzer, A.C. (2009). Physiology and pharmacology of striatal neurons. *Ann. Rev. Neurosci.* 32:127–147.

Kwak, C.H., and Jankovic, J. (2002). Tourettism and dystonia after subcortical stroke. *Mov. Disord.* 17:821–825.

Lebowitz, E.R., Motlagh, M.G., et al. (2012). Tourette syndrome in youth with and without obsessive compulsive disorder and attention deficit hyperactivity disorder. *Eur. Child Adoles. Psychiatry* 21(8), 451–457.

Leckman, J.F., Bloch, M.H., et al. (2010). Neurobiological substrates of Tourette's disorder. *J. Child Adol. Psychop.* 20:237–247.

Leckman, J.F., Goodman, W.K., et al. (1995). Cerebrospinal fluid biogenic amines in obsessive compulsive disorder, Tourette's syndrome, and healthy controls. *Neuropsychopharmacol.* 12:73–86.

Lerner, A., Bagic, A., et al. (2012). Widespread abnormality of the gamma-aminobutyric acid-ergic system in Tourette syndrome. *Brain* 135:1926–1936.

Malhotra, D., and Sebat, J. (2012). CNVs: harbingers of a rare variant revolution in psychiatric genetics. *Cell* 148:1223–1241.

March, J.S., Franklin, M.E., et al. (2007). Tics moderate treatment outcome with sertraline but not cognitive-behavior therapy in pediatric obsessive-compulsive disorder. *Biol. Psychiatry* 61:344–347.

Mathews, C.A., and Grados, M.A. (2011). Familiality of Tourette syndrome, obsessive-compulsive disorder, and attention-deficit/hyperactivity disorder: heritability analysis in a large sib-pair sample. *JAAC* 50:46–54.

Mazzone, L., Yu, S., et al. (2010). An fMRI study of frontostriatal circuits during the inhibition of eye blinking in persons with Tourette syndrome. *Am. J. Psychiatry* 167:341–349.

McCairn, K.W., Bronfeld, M., et al. (2009). The neurophysiological correlates of motor tics following focal striatal disinhibition. *Brain* 132:2125–2138.

Mink, J.W. (2001). Basal ganglia dysfunction in Tourette's syndrome: a new hypothesis. *Pediatr. Neurol.* 25:190–198.

Murphy, T.K., Kurlan, R., et al. (2010). The immunobiology of Tourette's disorder, pediatric autoimmune neuropsychiatric disorders associated with streptococcus, and related disorders: a way forward. *J. Child Adol. Psychop.* 20:317–331.

Neuner, I., Podoll, K., et al. (2009). From psychosurgery to neuromodulation: deep brain stimulation for intractable Tourette syndrome. *World J. Biol. Psychiatry* 10:366–376.

O'Rourke, J.A., Scharf, J.M., et al. (2011). The familial association of Tourette's disorder and ADHD: the impact of OCD symptoms. *Am. J. Med. Genet. B Neuropsychiatr. Genet.* 156B:553–560.

Parthasarathy, H.B., and Graybiel, A.M. (1997). Cortically driven immediate-early gene expression reflects modular influence of sensorimotor cortex on identified striatal neurons in the squirrel monkey. *J. Neurosci.* 17:2477–2491.

Peterson, B.S., Staib, L., et al. (2001). Regional brain and ventricular volumes in Tourette syndrome. *Arch. Gen. Psychiatry* 58:427–440.

Peterson, B.S., Thomas, P., et al. (2003). Basal ganglia volumes in patients with Gilles de la Tourette syndrome. *Arch. Gen. Psychiatry* 60:415–424.

Pittenger, C., Bloch, M.H., et al. (2011). Glutamate abnormalities in obsessive compulsive disorder: neurobiology, pathophysiology, and treatment. *Pharmacol. Ther.* 132:314–332.

Raz, A., Zhu, H., et al. (2009). Neural substrates of self-regulatory control in children and adults with Tourette syndrome. *Can. J. Psychiat.* 54:579–588.

Rickards, H. (2009). Functional neuroimaging in Tourette syndrome. *J. Psychosom. Res.* 67:575–584.

Robertson, M.M., Eapen, V., et al. (2009). The international prevalence, epidemiology, and clinical phenomenology of Tourette syndrome: a cross-cultural perspective. *J. Psychosom. Res.* 67:475–483.

Roessner, V., Overlack, S., et al. (2011). Increased putamen and callosal motor subregion in treatment-naive boys with Tourette syndrome indicates changes in the bihemispheric motor network. *J. Child Psychol. Psychiatry* 52:306–314.

Roessner, V., Wittfoth, M., et al. (2012). Altered motor network recruitment during finger tapping in boys with Tourette syndrome. *Hum. Brain Mapp.* 33:666–675.

Scharf, J.M., Yu, D., et al. (2012). Genome-wide association study of Tourette's syndrome. *Mol. Psychiatry.*

Shen, W., Flajolet, M., et al. (2008). Dichotomous dopaminergic control of striatal synaptic plasticity. *Science* 321:848–851.

Shmelkov, S.V., Hormigo, A., et al. (2010). Slitrk5 deficiency impairs corticostriatal circuitry and leads to obsessive-compulsive-like behaviors in mice. *Nat. Med.* 16:598–602, 591

Singer, H.S., Dickson, J., et al. (1995). Second messenger systems in Tourette's syndrome. *J. Neurol. Sci.* 128:78–83.

Singer, H.S., Gilbert, D.L., et al. (2011). Moving from PANDAS to CANS. *J. Pediatr.* 160(5):725–731.

State, M.W. (2011). The genetics of Tourette disorder. *Curr. Opin. Genet. Dev.* 21:302–309.

Sundaram, S., Huq, A., et al. (2010). Tourette syndrome is associated with recurrent exonic copy number variants. *Neurology* 74:1583–1590.

Wiltschko, A.B., Pettibone, J.R., et al. (2010). Opposite effects of stimulant and antipsychotic drugs on striatal fast-spiking interneurons. *Neuropsychopharmacol.* 35:1261–1270.

Yaddanapudi, K., Hornig, M., et al. (2010). Passive transfer of streptococcus-induced antibodies reproduces behavioral disturbances in a mouse model of pediatric autoimmune neuropsychiatric disorders associated with streptococcal infection. *Mol. Psychiatry* 15:712–726.

80 | NOVEL THERAPEUTICS IN CHILDHOOD ONSET PSYCHIATRIC DISORDERS

DOROTHY E. GRICE, ALEXANDER KOLEVZON, WALTER E. KAUFMANN, AND JOSEPH D. BUXBAUM

ntellectual disability (ID) and autism spectrum disorder (ASD) are among the more severe and prevalent neurodevelopmental disorders. It is estimated that the majority (>50 %) of ID cases are traceable to specific genetic causes, and estimates of heritability in ASD are higher, and among the highest in psychiatric disorders (Devlin and Scherer, 2012; van Bokhoven, 2011). Estimates based on gene discovery efforts place the number of genes involved in ID and ASD at 500 or more, with perhaps 20% of ID genes and 10% of ASD genes identified to date (Betancur, 2011; Neale et al., 2012; van Bokhoven, 2011). Widespread use of chromosome microarray (CMA) and massively parallel sequencing (MPS) accelerate gene and locus discovery in these disorders. Many of the genes and loci identified to date are associated with intermediate to high risk for disease (relative risk of approximately 20 to 200; see, e.g., Neale et al., 2012), which allows for the development of cell and animal models with construct validity. The use of neurobiological approaches to analyze these models in turn provides a means to understand disease pathogenesis and identify neurobiologically based targets for future therapeutic interventions. Although the enormous etiological complexity of these neurodevelopmental disorders is daunting, each identified gene provides an additional tool for understanding pathogenesis, and an additional target for novel therapeutics. In this sense, the very complexity of neurodevelopmental disorders may be an advantage for treatment development, especially if some of the causal genes converge on common pathways.

DIRECT AND INDIRECT INHIBITION OF mGluR SIGNALING IN FRAGILE X SYNDROME AND AUTISM SPECTRUM DISORDERS

Neurobiologically driven clinical trials in fragile X syndrome (FXS) are some of the most advanced in the field (Hagerman et al., 2012; Krueger and Bear, 2011). Mice, flies, and worms with disruptions in *FMR1*, the gene mutated in FXS, show alterations in synaptic function. These studies have shown that the *FMR1* gene product (called the FX mental retardation protein, or Fmrp) regulates translation at the synapse, and loss of Fmrp leads to excess translation. Parallel studies have shown that glutamate signaling through group 1 metabotropic glutamate receptors (mGluR) activate translation at the synapse, a

process linked to long-term depression, with Fmrp providing negative feedback for this process. These findings in turn suggest that the mGluR pathway is a therapeutic target in FXS that could be manipulated either by antagonizing these receptors or using reverse agonists to mGluR. More broadly, reducing glutamate transmission through the use of presynaptic GABA$_B$ agonists might represent another mechanism to counter the molecular deficits in FXS. Both of these approaches have been successful in model systems.

Two randomized controlled trials (RCTs) based on these neurobiological approaches have been reported to date. In the first, AFQ056, an mGluR5 antagonist, was studied in 30 males with FXS (Jacquemont et al., 2011). There were no significant effects of treatment on the primary outcome measure, the Aberrant Behavior Checklist-Community Edition (ABC-C). However, exploratory analyses indicated that those individuals with full methylation of the *FMR1* promoter showed significant improvements in total ABC-C and two subscale scores (ABC-Hyperactivity and ABC-Inappropriate speech). This finding is being pursued in independent studies (Table 80.1).

In the second RCT, STX209, which is a GABA$_B$ agonist also known as arbaclofen, was studied in 63 patients with a full *FMR1* mutation (Berry-Kravis et al., 2012). Once again, there was no significant finding in the primary outcome measure, in this case the ABC-Irritability (ABC-I) subscale. In exploratory analyses, there was a positive effect of treatment in the ABC-Social Avoidance scale, a scale derived from ABC-C factor analyses in FXS (Sansone et al., 2012), both in the entire study population and a subgroup of subjects with more severe social impairment. Convergent evidence was provided as they also observed improvements in complementary measures such as the Vineland II-Socialization raw score. Arbaclofen is currently being further assessed as a clinical treatment in both FXS and idiopathic ASD (see Table 80.1). Because mouse models of FXS also display GABAergic deficiency, particularly in the amygdala (Olmos-Serrano et al., 2010), a region implicated in avoidant behaviors, the effects of arbaclofen may be mediated by a combination of GABA agonism and indirect glutamate antagonism.

The Fmrp-binding protein CYFIP1 (cytoplasmic Fmrp-interacting protein 1) is coded by one of five genes found between breakpoints 1 and 2 in the 15q11 region. Loss of one copy of this chromosome interval is associated with increased risk for, or increased severity of, a number of neurodevelopmental and psychiatric disorders, including ID, ASD,

TABLE 80.1. Examples of compounds in clinical trials for pervasive developmental disorders

COMPOUND	TARGET	DISORDER
PHASE I		
Carbetocin	Oxytocin receptor agonist	ASD
RG1662	Gamma-aminobutyric acid receptor A (GABA$_A$) reverse agonist	DS
RG7314	Arginine vasopressin receptor 1A (AVPR1A) antagonist	ASD
STX107	Metabotropic glutamate receptor 5 (mGluR5) antagonist	FXS
PHASE II		
Mecasermin	Insulin like growth factor receptor (IGF1R) agonist	RTT, 22q13DS
STX209 (arbaclofen)	Gamma-aminobutyric acid receptor B (GABA$_B$) agonist	ASD
RO4917523	Metabotropic glutamate receptor 5 (mGluR5) antagonist	FXS
PHASE III		
AFQ056	Metabotropic glutamate receptor 5 (mGluR5) antagonist	FXS
STX209 (arbaclofen)	Gamma-aminobutyric acid receptor B (GABA$_B$) agonist	FXS

22q13DS, 22q13 deletion syndrome; ASD, autism spectrum disorder; DS, Down syndrome; FXS, Fragile X syndrome; RTT, Rett syndrome.

epilepsy, and schizophrenia (reviewed in Bozdagi et al., 2012). Interestingly, mice with a loss of *Cyfip1* show many of the same features of mice with a loss of *Fmr1*, including enhanced long-term depression that is insensitive to protein synthesis inhibitors, and accelerated extinction of inhibitory avoidance. Furthermore, group 1 mGluR antagonists reverse the deficits in synaptic plasticity observed in these mice (Bozdagi et al., 2012). This suggests that the Fmr1/Cyfip1 pathway may be disrupted in multiple neurodevelopmental disorders with the potential for common therapeutic approaches.

IGF-1 IN RETT SYNDROME AND 22q13 DELETION SYNDROME

Rett syndrome is a pervasive developmental disorder almost exclusively found in girls that is characterized by regression, cognitive impairment, deficits in communication, and stereotypic movements and is, in most cases, caused by mutations in the methyl CpG binding protein 2 (*MECP2*) gene (Calfa et al., 2011; Neul et al., 2010). MeCP2 binds to methylated DNA and thereby regulates gene expression. Studies in mouse models of Rett syndrome and human brain tissue have shown that MeCP2 regulates the expression of insulin-like growth factor binding protein 3 (IGFBP3) and that loss of MeCP2 leads to enhanced levels of IGFBP3 (Itoh et al., 2007). Because IGFBP3 functions

to sequester insulin-like growth factor 1 (IGF-1), increased levels of IGFBP3 would lead to reduced IGF-1 signaling.

In one study of *Mecp2*-deficient mice, a peptide derivative of IGF-1 including the first three amino acids of the full-length protein, (1-3)IGF-1, was found to reverse many neurological deficits in the mice (Tropea et al., 2009). One caveat with this study is that the mechanism of action of (1-3)IGF-1 is not fully clear. It does not seem to bind directly to IGF-1 receptors, although it does appear to activate some of the same downstream cascades that are activated by the full-length protein (Corvin et al., 2012). More recently, full-length IGF-1 was shown to reverse deficits in neurons prepared from patients with Rett syndrome (Marchetto et al., 2010). Full-length IGF-1 crosses the blood-brain barrier via its interaction with lipoprotein-related receptor 1 (LRP1), and can be selectively targeted to the brain through local neuronal activity (Nishijima et al., 2010); therefore, peripheral administration of full-length IGF-1, already approved for use in children with Laron-type dwarfism, could be useful in neurodevelopmental disorders.

Two phase I trials with full-length IGF-1 have been completed at the time of this writing. In the first, carried out in six girls with Rett syndrome, six months of twice-daily subcutaneous injection of IGF-1 proved to be safe and showed some positive effects on respiration (Pini et al., 2012). In the second, 12 girls with *MECP2* mutations, most of them with Rett syndrome, have been followed to collect pharmacokinetic and safety data and identify potential biomarkers for phase II trials (Kaufmann et al., unpublished). In addition to showing safety of IGF-1 in this vulnerable population, one important finding of this study is that peripherally administered IGF-1 is found in cerebrospinal fluid.

Loss of one copy of the *SHANK3* gene, either through deletion (termed 22q13 deletion syndrome or Phelan–McDermid syndrome) or point mutation, leads to ID, absent or severely delayed language, and ASD (Grabrucker et al., 2011). A mouse model with a heterozygous loss of the *Shank3* gene shows deficits in synaptic development and plasticity, as well as deficits in motor and social behaviors (e.g., Bozdagi et al., 2010; Yang et al., 2012). The mice show evidence for delayed maturation of glutamatergic synapses via several measures, in addition to reduced levels of postsynaptic density protein 95 (PSD-95), a neuronal protein important for synaptic development and plasticity. Synaptic development and function can be enhanced by IGF-1, and PSD-95 expression increased by IGF-1. Two-week treatment of these mice with full-length IGF-1 reversed the deficits in synaptic signaling, synaptic plasticity, and motor performance (Buxbaum et al., unpublished). A randomized controlled trial is currently underway using IGF-1 in patients with 22q13 deletion syndrome or *SHANK3* mutation (Kolevzon, NCT01525901).

The parallel preclinical findings showing beneficial effects of IGF-1 in two very different disorders (Rett syndrome or loss of *SHANK3*) is a basis for some optimism that even in the face of profound etiological heterogeneity there may be therapeutic approaches effective across neurodevelopmental disorders. Increasing evidence demonstrating mammalian target of rapamycin (mTOR) abnormalities in a variety of disorders associated with ID and ASD (Hoeffer and Klann, 2010) supports this approach to common targets.

GABA$_A$ ANTAGONISTS IN DOWN SYNDROME

Although it is relatively easy to conceptualize treating a monogenic disorder, it is more difficult to consider specific interventions for contiguous gene syndromes. There are dozens of recurrent copy number variants (CNV) associated with neurodevelopmental disorders (Betancur, 2011; Cooper et al., 2011), and many of these likely represent contiguous gene syndromes. In addition, there are larger chromosomal abnormalities associated with ID, including trisomy and monosomy of entire chromosomes. One of the most common trisomies is that affecting chromosome 21, called Down syndrome. Murine chromosome 16 contains large regions syntenic to human chromosome 21, and a mouse with a translocation of a large portion of chromosome 16 has been generated (Ts65DN) that is trisomic for about two-thirds of the human chromosome 21 genes. These mice show excess inhibition in the dentate gyrus and systemic dosing with a GABA$_A$ antagonist has demonstrated beneficial effects on synaptic plasticity (reversing deficits in the induction of long-term potentiation) and cognition (reversing deficits in working memory and in object recognition memory) (Fernandez et al., 2007). A phase I clinical trial with an inverse agonist of the GABA$_A$ receptor 5, a subtype of GABA$_A$ receptor relatively abundant in the hippocampus (Rudolph and Knoflach, 2011), is currently being carried out in young adults with Down syndrome by Hoffmann-La Roche (NCT01436955).

CONCLUSIONS

This chapter summarizes several clinical trials in neurodevelopmental disorders. In each case, the clinical trial was based on preclinical, neurobiological studies in model systems. Although it is premature to assess the clinical success of these approaches, we chose these trials to make several points. First, with a given neurobiological finding, such as dysregulation of translation in FXS, there may be several avenues by which it can be remedied, and we highlight the paths of direct and indirect modulation of glutamate signaling. Second, preclinical studies with IGF-1 in the etiologically distinct conditions of Rett syndrome and *SHANK3*-deficiency syndromes raise the hope that multiple disorders may be treatable with the same or similar therapeutics. Third, even in very complex disorders with multi-gene involvement (e.g., Down syndrome), there may be dominant neurobiological abnormalities that have more profound impact on pathobiology and in turn provide optimal targets for therapeutic intervention. Altogether, the increase in novel therapies in neurodevelopmental disorders represents an important and exciting potential advance in the treatment of mental illness.

DISCLOSURES

Dr. Grice has not reported any conflicts of interest to disclose.

Dr. Kolevzon receives research support from Hoffmann-La Roche and Seaside Therapeutics.

Dr. Kaufmann receives research support from Novartis and Ipsen.

Dr. Buxbaum has filed a patent on the use of IGF-1 in 22q13 deletion syndrome and mGluR antagonists in CYFIP1 deletion.

REFERENCES

Berry-Kravis, E.M., Hessl, D., et al. (2012). Effects of STX209 (arbaclofen) on neurobehavioral function in children and adults with fragile X syndrome: a randomized, controlled, phase 2 trial. *Sci. Transl. Med.* 4:152ra127.

Betancur, C. (2011). Etiological heterogeneity in autism spectrum disorders: more than 100 genetic and genomic disorders and still counting. *Brain Res.* 1380:42–77.

Bozdagi, O., Sakurai, T., et al. (2012). Haploinsufficiency of Cyfip1 produces fragile X-like phenotypes in mice. *PloS One* 7:e42422.

Bozdagi, O., Sakurai, T., et al. (2010). Haploinsufficiency of the autism-associated Shank3 gene leads to deficits in synaptic function, social interaction, and social communication. *Mol. Autism* 1:15.

Calfa, G., Percy, A.K., et al. (2011). Experimental models of Rett syndrome based on Mecp2 dysfunction. *Exp. Biol. Med. (Maywood)* 236:3–19.

Cooper, G.M., Coe, B.P., et al. (2011). A copy number variation morbidity map of developmental delay. *Nat. Genet.* 43:838–846.

Corvin, A. P., Molinos, I., Little, G., Donohoe, G., Gill, M., Morris, D. W., and Tropea, D. (2012). Insulin-like growth factor 1 (IGF1) and its active peptide (1-3)IGF1 enhance the expression of synaptic markers in neuronal circuits through different cellular mechanisms. *Neurosci. Lett.* 520:51–56.

Devlin, B., and Scherer, S. W. (2012). Genetic architecture in autism spectrum disorder. *Curr. Opin. Genet. Dev.* 22:229–237.

Fernandez, F., Morishita, W., et al. (2007). Pharmacotherapy for cognitive impairment in a mouse model of Down syndrome. *Nat. Neurosci.* 10:411–413.

Grabrucker, A.M., Schmeisser, M.J., et al. (2011). Postsynaptic ProSAP/Shank scaffolds in the cross-hair of synaptopathies. *Trends Cell Biol.* 21:594–603.

Hagerman, R., Lauterborn, J., et al. (2012). Fragile X syndrome and targeted treatment trials. *Results Probl. Cell. Differ.* 54:297–335.

Hoeffer, C.A., and Klann, E. (2010). mTOR signaling: at the crossroads of plasticity, memory, and disease. *Trends Neurosci.* 33:67–75.

Itoh, M., Ide, S., et al. (2007). Methyl CpG-binding protein 2 (a mutation of which causes Rett syndrome) directly regulates insulin-like growth factor binding protein 3 in mouse and human brains. *J. Neuropath. Exp. Neur.* 66:117–123.

Jacquemont, S., Curie, A., et al. (2011). Epigenetic modification of the FMR1 gene in fragile X syndrome is associated with differential response to the mGluR5 antagonist AFQ056. *Sci. Transl. Med.* 3:64ra61.

Krueger, D.D., and Bear, M.F. (2011). Toward fulfilling the promise of molecular medicine in fragile X syndrome. *Annu. Rev. Med.* 62:411–429.

Marchetto, M.C., Carromeu, C., et al. (2010). A model for neural development and treatment of Rett syndrome using human induced pluripotent stem cells. *Cell* 143:527–539.

Neale, B.M., Kou, Y., et al. (2012). Patterns and rates of exonic *de novo* mutations in autism spectrum disorders. *Nature* 485:242–245.

Neul, J.L., Kaufmann, W.E., et al. (2010). Rett syndrome: revised diagnostic criteria and nomenclature. *Ann. Neurol.* 68:944–950.

Nishijima, T., Piriz, J., et al. (2010). Neuronal activity drives localized blood-brain-barrier transport of serum insulin-like growth factor-I into the CNS. *Neuron* 67:834–846.

Olmos-Serrano, J.L., Paluszkiewicz, S.M., et al. (2010). Defective GABAergic neurotransmission and pharmacological rescue of neuronal hyperexcitability in the amygdala in a mouse model of fragile X syndrome. *J. Neurosci.* 30:9929–9938.

Pini, G., Scusa, M.F., et al. (2012). IGF1 as a Potential treatment for Rett syndrome: safety assessment in six Rett patients. *Autism Res. Treat.* 2012:679801.

Rudolph, U., and Knoflach, F. (2011). Beyond classical benzodiazepines: novel therapeutic potential of GABA$_A$ receptor subtypes. *Nat. Rev. Drug Discov.* 10:685–697.

Sansone, S.M., Widaman, K.F., et al. (2012). Psychometric study of the Aberrant Behavior Checklist in Fragile X Syndrome and implications for targeted treatment. *J. Autism Dev. Disord.* 42:1377–1392.

Tropea, D., Giacometti, E., et al. (2009). Partial reversal of Rett syndrome-like symptoms in MeCP2 mutant mice. *Proc. Natl. Acad. Sci. USA* 106:2029–2034.

van Bokhoven, H. (2011). Genetic and epigenetic networks in intellectual disabilities. *Annu. Rev. Genet.* 45:81–104.

Yang, M., Bozdagi, O., et al. (2012). Reduced excitatory neurotransmission and mild autism-relevant phenotypes in adolescent Shank3 null mutant mice. *J. Neurosci.* 32:6525–6541.

SECTION IX | SPECIAL TOPIC AREAS

DENNIS S. CHARNEY

81| DSM-5 OVERVIEW AND GOALS

DAVID J. KUPFER AND SUSAN K. SCHULTZ

This chapter reviews the stages of development of the Fifth Edition of the Diagnostic and Statistical Manual (DSM-5) and addresses the present and future goals of the manual regarding its function in informing both diagnostic decision making and serving as a template for integrating neurobiologic information as the field evolves over time. Specifically we review how the last few decades of research have yielded remarkable findings from genetics, neuroimaging, cognitive science, and pathophysiology that significantly affect the way the field conceptualizes many of the major psychiatric disorders. However, our ability to use these findings to draw diagnostic thresholds and inform diagnostic decision making has not yet been fully realized. Indeed, it was one of the main subjects of extensive discussion at a series of international research planning conferences for DSM-5. Furthermore, the task of harmonizing the manual with the International Classification of Disease (ICD) has been another major focus of attention in the DSM development process, including facilitating the adoption of parallel chapter headings that are consistent between the two classifications. Finally, we look ahead to the nosology that will be informed by the NIMH RDoC research agenda and the ability of a neuroscience-based diagnostic framework to ultimately influence the evolution of DSM-5. We have chosen the Arabic numeral five for the express purpose of permitting a DSM-5.1, DSM-5.2, and so on. In sum, DSM-5 does not by any means reduce the value of DSM-IV and in fact DSM-5 is more similar to DSM-IV than dissimilar, but the overarching goal is to combine the tradition of diagnostic reliability while building in new information from the neurosciences that helps refine the nosology through an understanding of the pathophysiology that may help meaningfully separate disorders to optimally convey prognosis and inform treatment decisions.

THE RESEARCH AGENDAS FOR DSM-5

During the DSM planning process, it was anticipated that the emerging scientific advances of the last several decades would affect the assessment and management of mental disorders. To stimulate international discourse and move closer to the objective of rebuilding DSM-5's scientific base, the American Psychiatric Association (APA) convened three research conferences from 1999 to 2002. From these conferences came a series of six white papers, which were published as two monographs, entitled "A Research Agenda for DSM-V" (*A Research Agenda for DSM-V*, 2002) and "Age and Gender Considerations in

Psychiatric Diagnosis: A Research Agenda for DSM-V" (*Age, Gender Considerations in Psychiatric Diagnosis: A Research Agenda for DSM-V*, 2007). These addressed topic discussions in nomenclature, disability and impairment, developmental approaches, advances in neuroscience, cross-cultural issues, and current gaps in the classification system. During the course of this process, the concern was raised that over the last few decades, researchers who have dogmatically adhered to DSM-IV definitions could have been constrained in a way that may have hindered progress in understanding the pathophysiology of mental disorders. Although no one would question the value of having a well-operationalized and universally accepted diagnostic system to facilitate comparisons across studies, the reification of DSM-IV entities such that they are considered equivalent to diseases may be more likely to obscure than elucidate research findings. Research exclusively focused on refining the DSM-defined syndromes may never be successful in uncovering their underlying etiologies. Consequently another important goal of DSM-5 is to transcend the limitations of the current DSM paradigm and encourage a research agenda that goes beyond current ways of thinking to attempt to integrate information from a wide variety of sources and technologies (*A Research Agenda for DSM-V*, 2002).

FINE TUNING THE CONCEPTUAL FRAMEWORK

Following the initial discussions addressing the overall conceptualization of the DSM-5 disorders and the need for new approaches, a series of international research planning conferences were conducted between 2003 and 2008 to solidify the framework of the DSM-5 research agenda. This international research planning conference series, jointly supported by the American Psychiatric Association, the World Health Organization (WHO), and the National Institute of Health (NIH), was began in 2003 and spanned five years. The resulting series of 13 conferences was titled, "The Future of Psychiatric Diagnosis: Refining the Research Agenda for DSM-5." These conferences featured nearly 400 international experts in psychiatry and neuroscience from 39 countries. The experts conducted a multiphase global review of psychiatric diagnosis and classification, and formed the foundation for initial recommendations to the DSM-5 Task Force and Work Groups. The purposes of these conferences were several-fold. First, the conferences sought to examine research evidence for phenomena that cut across traditional diagnostic groups.

For example, such phenomena include the construct of psychosis; hence a conference titled "Deconstructing Psychosis" was convened to examine the current evidence regarding the diagnosis and pathophysiology of common syndromes with psychosis, including: schizophrenia, bipolar disorder, major depressive psychosis, and substance-induced psychosis to address broad issues relating to ways in which psychosis cuts across multiple diagnostic categories (Tamminga et al., 2010). Another conference provided a detailed examination of the heterogeneity and overlap among disorders characterized by fear and avoidance, including posttraumatic stress disorder, panic/agoraphobia, social phobia/social anxiety disorder, and specific phobias. Although these disorders are phenotypically heterogeneous, neuroimaging and neuroanatomy data from human and animal model studies suggest a shared membership in a stress-induced and fear circuitry spectrum, which is conceptually and clinically distinct from other anxiety disorders, such as generalized anxiety disorder, obsessive compulsive disorder, and impulse-control disorders (*Stress-Induced and Fear Circuitry Disorders: Refining the Research Agenda for DSM-V*, 2009). These new conceptualizations could provide useful and novel insights for assessment, treatment, and research.

PURSUING HARMONIZATION ACROSS CLASSIFICATIONS

Another goal for the initial DSM-5 research agenda conferences was to move aggressively toward harmonization with the ICD-11 process. One of the international conferences was dedicated specifically to public health aspects of psychiatric diagnosis and uncovered strategies for using DSM-5 to better address global mental health needs (*Public Health Aspects of Diagnosis and Classification of Mental and Behavioral Disorders: Refining the Research Agenda for DSM-V and ICD-11*, 2012). This conference also served as a springboard for the formation of a DSM-5 Study Group on the interface of general medical disorders with psychiatric disorders. The Psychiatric/General Medical Interface Study Group has sought to specifically examine the link between general medical disorders and psychiatric disorders. Given that most patients with mental illnesses are seen by primary care physicians, the study group was formed to ensure that DSM-5 meets the needs of general medical practitioners as opposed to only specialty mental health clinicians. The study group is also developing revision strategies for the forthcoming DSM-5 for Primary Care, or DSM-5PC, which is intended to be used in primary care settings.

ANTICIPATING THE FUTURE OF NEUROBIOLOGICAL CLASSIFICATIONS

Much of the underlying rationale and discussion associated with the DSM-5 development has been articulated in the research agenda for DSM-5 (*A Research Agenda for DSM-V*, 2002). At the time this volume was published in 2002, it was anticipated that the great gains across the neurosciences addressing pathophysiology and genetics of mental illnesses would affect to a significant degree the diagnosis and classification of mental disorders. However, the anticipation that these research advances would inform psychiatric diagnosis has not evolved to a clinically applicable state as quickly as was expected. It is now clear that findings from genetic, neuroimaging, cognitive science, and pathophysiology will *eventually* be appropriate for DSM documentation, and in fact in some disorders to be discussed later, there is utility to specific biomarker data and validators in diagnostic decision making, but by and large across the manual most disorders await a classification that is fully informed by underlying pathophysiological mechanisms. Consequently, the DSM-5 research planning conferences generated research strategies to identify groups of validators (Andrews, Goldberg et al., 2009; Andrews, Pine et al., 2009; Carpenter et al., 2009; Goldberg et al., 2009; Kendler, 2009; Krueger and South, 2009; Sachdev et al., 2009). As the DSM-5 process has continued, a new research effort, the Research Domain Criteria (RDoC) has been implemented by the NIMH and seeks to classify psychopathology based on dimensions of observable behavior and neurobiological measures (Insel et al., 2010). The NIMH RDoC objective is consistent with the conclusions of the research planning conferences; as described further here, the information that will emerge over time from the RDoC development will likely merge quite well with the template provided by the DSM-5 text structure.

ORGANIZATION OF DIAGNOSTIC CATEGORIES ACROSS DSM-5

The research conferences in the DSM-5 process facilitated an invaluable review of scientific evidence for establishing groups of disorders with shared criteria, and possibly shared etiologies. The dialogue from these conferences prompted a reconceptualization of the process for validating nosologic categories to update the standard originally delineated by Robins and Guze (1970). The new validation process builds on the original concepts to include the following: building a behavioral phenotype of clinical description and course, creating a neurobiological profile, identifying genetic and familial patterns, considering the interaction between biology and environment, and emphasizing treatment response and follow-up studies (Kupfer et al., 2008). Whenever appropriate thresholds for replication have been met, these validators for diagnostic classification have been included.

In addition to a new approach to the assessment of validity, it also became clear during the DSM-5 development process that there was a need for better integration of cross-cutting factors, such as age-related and cultural considerations, which had not been fully addressed in DSM-IV and may have contributed to intradiagnostic variability. One strategy used in the DSM-5 process is actively focusing on overarching themes that may play an essential role in the conceptualization of disease presentation and classification. Such themes include the ways in which diagnoses and symptoms vary across the developmental lifespan and how gender and cultural diversity affect symptomatology. To this end, additional topic-specific study groups were formed, in addition to the Psychiatric/General Medical Interface described in the preceding. These Study Groups included the following: (*1*) Diagnostic Spectra, (*2*) Lifespan and Developmental Approaches, (*3*) Gender and Cross-Cultural Issues, (*4*) Impairment Assessment, and (*5*) Diagnostic Assessment Instruments. Each of these study groups was charged with reviewing the literature on cross-cutting and dimensional issues in their respective areas and disseminating their findings through collaborative interaction with the individual DSM-5 workgroups. This approach may be useful in developing more precise clinical phenotypes to match the neurobiological profiles. Attention to specific cross-cutting issues such as lifespan and development provided an important opportunity to impart key information relevant to age of onset and symptom presentation. Related to this is the concept of how diagnoses change across the lifespan, such as using a developmental approach to elucidate the onset and characterization of pediatric bipolar disorder (Leibenluft and Rich, 2008). The text structure for the individual disorder descriptions in DSM-5 was revised from the DSM-IV format to permit the relevant information such as developmental perspectives to be presented in relevant chapter headings and subheadings. To ensure that these new facets developed within DSM-5 were harmonized with other classifications, discussions with the WHO facilitated the planned adoption of parallel chapter headings that would be consistent across DSM-5 and ICD.

INTEGRATION OF DISORDERS USUALLY FIRST DIAGNOSED IN INFANCY, CHILDHOOD, OR ADOLESCENCE

DSM-5 has implemented a new feature in support of the view that many mental disorders can be viewed as developmental conditions with their roots in childhood or adolescence. DSM-5 does not contain a separate category titled *Disorders Usually First Diagnosed in Infancy, Childhood, or Adolescence* because this category was viewed as creating an artificial distinction among many conditions with strong developmental features. These disorders are now integrated across the manual, some into existing categories and others into new categories. By presenting an overarching lifespan perspective rather than isolating childhood disorders, DSM-5 now aggregates disorders based on similar pathology and emphasizes the salience of development for a broad array of disorders. The reorganization of the childhood disorders permits proximal placement of disorders with the same putative neural substrates in the same section. For example, the separation anxiety disorders are now placed with the anxiety disorders; which optimally reflects their evidence of shared pathophysiology with the anxiety disorders and discordance from other "childhood" disorders, such as attention deficit hyperactivity disorder. This attention to possible shared pathogenesis of disorders may help facilitate future research on diagnostic biomarkers. This approach in DSM-5 provides a template for the role of developmental biology and how it impinges on the manifestation of disease, suggesting that the concept of "developmental validators" may be a useful tool for future use. Data on anxiety disorders and

other mental syndromes emphasize the importance of probabilistic perspectives and a focus on prevention and potential reduction in later morbidity. For example, early problems with anxiety in childhood may constrain patterns of function during adulthood and predict a statistically increased risk for later problems, but they do not invariably predict a chronic, unrelenting pattern of illness from childhood into adulthood (Pine et al., 1998). By facilitating early recognition of risk factors, DSM-5 is positioned to facilitate a focus on early detection and prevention. It is anticipated that the future will hold opportunities for adding relevant developmental biomarkers to the "living" DSM-5 that will be poised to receive ongoing updates as diagnostically useful measures begin to emerge in future research.

THE DEVELOPMENTAL PERSPECTIVE IN DSM-5

Integration of developmental themes for each disorder across the text also provides an opportunity to focus attention on the developmental features of many adult conditions not typically considered to be developmental in nature. For example, major depression did not appear among DSM-IV disorders *Usually First Diagnosed in Infancy, Childhood, or Adolescence*, yet research is increasingly demonstrating that the initial signs of major depression typically arise in adolescence. A complete discussion of these issues has been provided in substantial detail by Pine et al. (2010). The rationale for integrating the childhood disorders across the manual is also supported by the observation that they are more likely to be similar than different in their characteristic features and pathogenesis, and in many cases they likely represent a continuum of the same disorder, as noted by Rutter et al. (2011). It follows intuitively that the end of childhood or adolescence at the age of 18 years does not coincide with resolution of all effects of an illness, and many developmental disorders not only remain persistent into middle and late life but increase in severity as they interact with changing social demands such as parenting, maintaining employment, or entering retirement. In view of this new arrangement, all diagnoses now provide a lifetime perspective with instructions for the ways in which manifestations vary with age.

INTEGRATION OF NEUROBIOLOGICAL, PATHOPHYSIOLOGICAL, AND LABORATORY DATA INTO DSM-5

The text structure of DSM-5 was designed to provide templates for integration of neurobiological information when the data support their diagnostic use. The new text structure DSM-5 includes subheadings that are designed to serve as placeholders or "receptors" for additional subheadings that may not be populated for all disorders in DSM-5, but may be expanded over time as DSM-5.1, DSM-5.2, and so on, evolve. The specific subheadings that may serve as such "receptors" for emerging neurobiological measures and biomarkers may be found within the DSM-5 text in the *Risk and Prognostic Features* section as well as the *Diagnostic Markers* section. The *Risk and Prognostic Features* heading is further subdivided to include: (*1*) temperamental, (*2*) environmental, and (*3*) genetic and physiological factors. The *Risk and Prognostic Factors* section includes a discussion of features thought to portend the development of a disorder, including temperamental or personality features; environmental risks, including toxicities, traumatic exposures, environmental precipitants, and substance use; genetic and physiological factors (e.g., APOE4 for neurocognitive disorders, and other known, replicated familial genetic risks); as well as familial pattern.

In preparation for DSM-5, the use of neurocognitive measures was also extensively considered. For example, the aggregate literature on cognition and schizophrenia was carefully reviewed and a variety of views were carefully considered (Barch et al., 2003; Daban et al., 2006; Keefe and Fenton, 2007). The possibility of adding cognitive impairment as a characteristic symptom was considered, but the Psychotic Disorders Work Group recommended against doing so because of its lack of diagnostic specificity and limited information about the effect of such a change. However, cognition was still considered an essential aspect of schizophrenic psychopathology, and is recommended as one vital dimension to be measured across patients with a psychotic disorder. Continued research in this area, potentially in combination with other biomarkers, may facilitate an increase in diagnostic certainty via multidimensional measures such that the DSM-5 text may ultimately include specific neurocognitive "biomarkers" that have diagnostic significance for schizophrenia and other disorders.

Integration of diagnostic markers based on pathophysiology is already occurring in DSM-5 in the context of neurocognitive disorder due to Alzheimer's disease. For example, in the diagnosis of mild neurocognitive disorder, the Alzheimer's disease (AD) subtype is not commonly diagnosed, however, such a diagnosis is possible if there is evidence of a causative Alzheimer's disease genetic mutation from either genetic testing or family history. This advance in DSM-5 represents one of the first examples of integration of neurobiological information into clinical diagnostic decision making. Along these lines, the sleep-wake disorders represent another group of conditions that have increasingly well-established pathophysiological markers. In the case of the parasomnias, previously sleepwalking and sleep terror disorder were listed as individual parasomnias, yet they represent variations of a single underlying pathophysiology of wake/NREM sleep admixture; consequently, they were proposed to have a single parasomnia heading of "Non-Rapid Eye Movement Sleep Arousal Disorders" in DSM-5, with subtypes including sleepwalking and sleep terrors. This permits an aggregation of the disorders of arousal owing to their shared NREM features as well as expanded explanation of their shared pathoetiology in the DSM-5 text. In sum, the DSM-5 has begun to move toward a manual based in common pathogenic sources as opposed to simply syndromic coherence.

PUBLIC HEALTH IMPLICATIONS AND THE STRUCTURE OF DSM-5

Beyond keeping pace with the science of psychiatry, many of DSM-5's proposed changes represent an opportunity to improve the field from a clinical and public health perspective. This includes the new conceptualization of the neurodevelopmental disorders that has led to a proposed a singular Autism Spectrum Disorder category that would include current DSM-IV autistic disorder (autism), Asperger's disorder, childhood disintegrative disorder, and pervasive developmental disorder not otherwise specified. This decision emerged from data suggesting that these disorders share a pathophysiological substrate. The sharing of neurobiological features can clearly lead to new nosology of disorders, but it will happen in an iterative fashion affecting specific clusters of disorders, rather than the entire nomenclature. As the field continues to grow and the RDoC initiative provides increasing evidence for the pathological substrates that may ideally inform a diagnostic classification, the DSM-5 text template is geared to accommodate additional text that may be presented in future iterations of the "living" DSM.

CONCLUSIONS

It is important to emphasize that DSM-5 does not represent a radical departure from the past, nor does it represent a divergence from the long-term goals of the RDoC. As we gradually build on our knowledge of mental disorders, we begin bridging the gap between what lies behind us (presumed etiologies based on phenomenology) and what hopefully lies ahead (identifiable pathophysiologic etiologies).

DISCLOSURES

Dr. David Kupfer serves as a consultant for the American Psychiatric Association (in his capacity as Chair of the American Psychiatric Association's DSM-5 Task Force).

Dr. Schultz has received support from the National Institute of Health (MH086482, CA122934, AG024904, AG021488), Health Resources and Services Administration (HP19054), Agency for Healthcare Research and Quality (HS019355), the Nellie Ball Trust Fund Foundation, and the Alzheimer's Disease Cooperative Study in partnership with Baxter Healthcare (NCT00818662). She has also received support from the American Psychiatric Association for editorial duties.

REFERENCES

Age, Gender Considerations in Psychiatric Diagnosis: A Research Agenda for DSM-V. (2007). Washington, DC: American Psychiatric Publishing.

Andrews, G., Charney, D.S., et al. (2009a). Stress-Induced and Fear Circuitry Disorders: Refining the Research Agenda for DSM-V. Arlington, VA: American Psychiatric.

Andrews, G., Goldberg, D.P., et al. (2009b). Exploring the feasibility of a meta-structure for DSM-V and ICD-11: could it improve utility and validity? *Psychol. Med.* 39(12):1993–2000.

Andrews, G., Pine, D.S., et al. (2009c). Neurodevelopmental disorders: cluster 2 of the proposed meta-structure for DSM-V and ICD-11. *Psychol. Med.* 39(12):2013–2023.

Barch, D.M., Carter, C.S., et al. (2003). Context-processing deficits in schizophrenia: diagnostic specificity, 4-week course, and relationships to clinical symptoms. *J. Abnorm. Psychol.* 112(1):132–143.

Carpenter, W.T., Bustillo, J.R., et al. (2009). The psychoses: cluster 3 of the proposed meta-structure for DSM-V and ICD-11. *Psychol. Med.* 39(12):2025–2042.

Daban, C., Martinez-Aran, A., et al. (2006). Specificity of cognitive deficits in bipolar disorder versus schizophrenia. A systematic review. *Psychother. Psychosom.* 75(2):72–84.

Goldberg, D.P., Krueger, R.F., et al. (2009). Emotional disorders: cluster 4 of the proposed meta-structure for DSM-V and ICD-11. *Psychol. Med.* 39(12):2043–2059.

Insel, T., Cuthbert, B., et al. (2010). Research domain criteria (RDoC): toward a new classification framework for research on mental disorders. *Am. J. Psychiatry.* 167(7):748–751.

Keefe, R.S., and Fenton, W.S. (2007). How should DSM-V criteria for schizophrenia include cognitive impairment? *Schizophr. Bull.* 33(4):912–920.

Kendler, K.S. (2009). Introduction to a proposal for a meta-structure for DSM-V and ICD-11. *Psychol. Med.* 39:1991–1993.

Krueger, R.F., and South, S.C. (2009). Externalizing disorders: cluster 5 of the proposed meta-structure for DSM-V and ICD-11. *Psychol. Med.* 39(12):2061–2070.

Kupfer, D.J., Regier, D.A., et al. (2008). On the road to DSM-V and ICD-11. *Eur. Arch. Psychiatry Clin. Neurosci.* 258(Suppl 5):2–6.

Leibenluft, E., and Rich, B.A. (2008). Pediatric bipolar disorder. *Annu. Rev. Clin. Psychol.* 4:163–187.

Pine, D.S., Cohen, P., et al. (1998). The risk for early-adulthood anxiety and depressive disorders in adolescents with anxiety and depressive disorders. *Arch. Gen. Psychiatry* 55(1):56–64.

Pine, D.S., Costello, E.J., et al. (2010). Increasing the developmental focus in DSM-V: broad issues and specific potential applications in anxiety. In: Regier, D.A., Narrow, W.E., Kuhl, E.A., and Kupfer, D.J., eds. The Conceptual Evolution of DSM-V. Washington, DC: American Psychiatric, pp. 305–321.

Public Health Aspects of Diagnosis and Classification of Mental and Behavioral Disorders: Refining the Research Agenda for DSM-V and ICD-11. (2012). Arlington, VA: American Psychiatric Publishing.

A Research Agenda for DSM-V. (2002). Washington, D.C.: American Psychiatric Publishing.

Robins, E., and Guze, S.B. (1970). Establishment of diagnostic validity in psychiatric illness: its application to schizophrenia. *Am. J. Psychiatry* 126(7):983–987.

Rutter, M. (2011). Research review: child psychiatric diagnosis and classification: concepts, findings, challenges and potential. *J. Child Psychol. Psychiatry* 52(6):647–660.

Sachdev, P., Andrews, G., et al. (2009). Neurocognitive disorders: cluster 1 of the proposed meta-structure for DSM-V and ICD-11. *Psychol. Med.* 39(12):2001–2012.

Stress-Induced and Fear Circuitry Disorders: Refining the Research Agenda for DSM-V. (2009). Arlington, VA: American Psychiatric Publishing.

Tamminga, C.A., Paul, J., et al. (2010). Deconstructing Psychosis: Refining the Research Agenda for DSM-V. Washington, DC: American Psychiatric.

82 | THE INFIRMITIES OF PSYCHIATRIC DIAGNOSIS

STEVEN E. HYMAN

The major diagnostic systems in psychiatry, the Diagnostic and Statistical Manual of Mental Disorders, 4th edition (American Psychiatric Association [APA], 1994) and the closely related International Classification of Diseases, 10th edition (World Health Organization, 1992), chapter on mental and behavioral disorders are currently undergoing revision. Both the general scientific press (Miller and Holden, 2010) and the lay press have focused a great deal of attention on these revisions because the resulting manuals will exert significant influence on the putative boundaries between health and mental illness, the treatments that patients will receive, reimbursement for services, determinations of disability, and even the sentencing of some individuals convicted of crimes. To the credit of the American Psychiatric Association, each subsequent recent edition of the DSM system has included a disclaimer in the front matter. For example, the current DSM-IV-TR (APA, 2000), states that the diagnostic criteria are "offered as guidelines" because "use of such criteria enhances agreement among clinicians and investigators." The authors of the manual make no truth claims for the classification overall or for any disorder within it. Yet in practice it would be hard to imagine any caveat or disclaimer more widely ignored than this one.

Like any disease classification, the DSM is a cognitive structure imposed on scientific data to make it useful for clinical applications and research. Even the most scientifically useful theoretical frameworks or classification systems eventually outlive their beneficial role. Like Ptolemaic astronomy, a broadly accepted theoretical schema that has outlived its ability to explain emerging data can produce intellectual stagnation by excessively narrowing the focus and even the imagination of investigators (Kuhn, 1962). The DSM system is a central organizer of psychiatric research because it provides a shared language, and more than that, it delineates those specific disorders that can generally be studied within the mainstream psychiatric community. The profound influence of the DSM system grew directly from the success of applying the DSM-III (APA, 1980) to enhance comparability across studies, in marked contrast with the diagnostic free for all (Pope and Lipinski, 1978) that existed before its publication in 1980. Without comparability of subject populations in translational or clinical research, it is simply not possible to replicate results or falsify specific hypotheses with any rigor. The obverse of this benefit is that the DSM system came to dominate thinking about psychiatric disorders at a time when the relevant science was embryonic. Thus the DSM system enhanced the ability of researchers, clinicians, patients, and families to communicate with each other, but also

produced premature intellectual closure—despite the American Psychiatric Association's disclaimer (Hyman, 2007, 2010).

The DSM-III remains—even with the impending publication of DSM-5—the fundamental current prototype for psychiatric disease classification and diagnosis. The DSM approach has been to delineate a large number of distinct diagnostic categories and to define them based on operationalized diagnostic criteria. Given the early state of psychiatric science, all of the current sets of criteria are perforce comprised of clinical descriptions (i.e., phenomenology). It would be possible to imagine that objective tests and biomarkers could be discovered for the existing categories, and their careful incorporation into current sets of criteria would ultimately lead to a modern descendent of the DSM-III. This chapter argues that in contrast to this hopeful view, much clinical and laboratory evidence suggests that there are fundamental structural problems with the DSM system and that the current diagnostic structure may be impeding progress (Hyman, 2007, 2010). For example, essentially all disease-focused grant applications, if they are to be awarded, must select patient populations based on DSM criteria. Similarly, manuscripts submitted for publication must also categorize patients according to the DSM system. Patients entered in clinical trials almost invariably must meet criteria for specific DSM disorders. Indeed, with respect to development of new treatments, DSM-based diagnoses, which are taken to represent the psychiatric community's consensus, strongly influence regulators. Thus, for example, the US Food and Drug Administration takes the DSM system into account in deciding what constellation of symptoms represents a valid indication in psychiatry. Deviations from DSM nomenclature may require special efforts before development of a new drug treatment commences (Buchanan et al., 2005). In addition, psychiatry residents and clinical psychology interns often find themselves memorizing the most recent version of the DSM for certification examinations. It is no wonder that, despite the American Psychiatric Association's disclaimers, the lay press often describes the DSM as psychiatry's bible.

DSM-III ANTEDATED IMPORTANT DEVELOPMENTS IN THE LIFE SCIENCES

Even today we do not understand the etiology or pathophysiology of depression, bipolar disorder, schizophrenia, autism, or any other major disorder under the purview of psychiatry. There are still no objective medical tests that are sensitive or specific enough to use for diagnoses, and there are no validated biomarkers for monitoring treatment. Despite this seemingly dismal picture, which contrasts with significant progress in many other areas of medicine, there is good reason to believe that the science of psychiatry is maturing in ways that will prove highly fruitful. The section that follows, illustrating the potential of newer technological and scientific approaches to psychiatric research is not meant to understate the challenges that remain, but to provide examples of major developments in science relevant to psychiatric disorders, and to underscore that all of these emerged in the decades *after* the publication of DSM-III (APA, 1980).

Much has happened in the life sciences since the gestation of descriptive psychiatry in the 1960s and 1970s and its apotheosis with the publication of DSM-III (APA, 1980) in 1980. Molecular biology, perhaps the dominant force in modern biology and medicine only emerged in the mid-1980s following a moratorium on recombinant DNA technology that ended in 1975 (Wade, 1975). Important discoveries about the nervous system date back to the nineteenth century, but modern neuroscience as an interdisciplinary field is relatively new. The first department of Neuroscience was only founded in 1970, and the field only began to involve clinical disciplines effectively in the ensuing decades. One recent subfield emerging from within neuroscience that is highly relevant to the goals of psychiatry is called "connectomics." This field represents an attempt to provide full descriptions of the brain "wiring diagrams" of both model organisms and humans based on detailed mapping of cells, synapses, and circuits. Beyond a static map, connectomics is also attempting to overlay a dynamic picture of the functional connectivity of the human brain. Because neural circuit function directly underlies thought, emotion, and behavior, in short, the substrate of psychiatric symptoms, the data and understandings that emerge will be critical to understanding psychopathology and ultimately disease classification. Connectomics has become a feasible goal for neuroscientists because of advances in such technologies as microscopy, neuroimaging, computation, and new technologies that utilize molecular tools to study specific neural circuits and their relationship to behavior (Fenno et al., 2011). Noninvasive neuroimaging is giving us important structural and functional views of the human brain. Structural magnetic resonance imaging (MRI) permits the detailed characterization of diverse neural structures; for example, measurements of cerebral cortical thickness or hippocampal volume. Diffusion tensor imaging (DTI) permits the accurate tracing of white matter tracts in the brain. Functional MRI (fMRI) and various modalities of positron emission tomography (PET) make it possible to observe the activation of brain circuits in response to specific tasks and to observe patterns of brain connectivity at rest. PET also permits the labeling and visualization of specific proteins, such as neurotransmitter receptors. To give some historical context, the first published papers using fMRI, now a major contributor to psychiatric neuroscience, only appeared in the mid-1990s.

Genetics is also an important approach to understanding the etiology of mental disorders given that many disorders are highly heritable. Using still-developing technologies motivated by the human genome project (Shendure and Ji, 2008), it has been possible only since 2007 to make significant progress in discovering specific genetic risk factors involved in the pathogenesis of autism (Neale et al., 2012) schizophrenia (Lee et al., 2012), and bipolar disorder. Also in 2007, induced pluripotent cell technology was developed that has made it possible to transform fibroblasts obtained from small skin biopsies of psychiatric patients and healthy comparison subjects into human neurons that can be studied *in vitro* (Takahashi et al., 2007). This technology is already permitting molecular and cellular investigations into the pathogenesis of psychiatric disorders. The intellectual roots of the DSM system lay in the descriptive psychiatry of the 1960s and 1970s (Robins and Guze, 1970), which in turn dates back to the pioneering nineteenth century work of Kraepelin (1899/1991). Descriptive psychiatry was a critically important intellectual movement that helped free the field from the dominant psychoanalytic approaches of the mid-twentieth century that had little place for biology. It should not be surprising, however, that the institutionalization of descriptive psychiatry mediated by the DSM system has provided a poor lens through which to view modern science.

DESCRIPTIVE PSYCHIATRY

Scientifically mature diagnostic systems are generally based on pathophysiology or etiology rather than clinical description in recognition of the fact that multiple factors related to disease processes, patient adaptations, and environmental context may influence the nature and severity of symptoms, functional impairments, and disability. Beginning in the 1950s, new pharmacological treatments had emerged, including antipsychotic drugs, antidepressants, lithium, and benzodiazepines, creating a significant need for a diagnostic system that would permit the selection of homogeneous groups of patients for clinical trials and facilitate the appropriate matching of patients with treatments. One important hurdle was diagnostic reliability, the ability of different observers to reach the same diagnosis for a given patient. Absent understandings of pathophysiology, lacking empirical knowledge of etiology, and even without objective medical tests, careful clinical description would prove to be the best approach available to psychiatry in the mid-twentieth century. In 1970 Robins and Guze (1970) two investigators at Washington University, argued that it would be possible to achieve reliable and valid psychiatric diagnoses based on clinical description, laboratory studies, exclusion of other disorders, follow-up observations, and family studies. They and their colleagues were inspired by the careful phenomenology of Emil Kraepelin (1899/1991), who had argued that psychiatry could identify specific disorders based on careful description of symptoms, signs, and course of illness. Kraepelin used such methods to distinguish what he called dementia praecox (schizophrenia) from manic-depressive illness (bipolar disorder) in the nineteenth century. Following the lead of Robins and Guze, the St. Louis school produced two sets of diagnostic criteria, the Research Diagnostic Criteria (RDC) and the Feighner criteria (Feighner et al., 1972; Spitzer et al., 1975), which were direct forerunners of the DSM-III (APA, 1980). To enhance inter-rater reliability these diagnostic systems employed operationalized criteria (i.e., criteria that specified well defined clinical observations). Validation (i.e., providing evidence that a diagnosis identified a verifiable entity in nature) represented an insurmountable problem given the state of the science in the 1970s. Robins and Guze (1970) argued that validity of diagnoses could be established using multiple forms of evidence, such as the stability of a person's diagnosis over the life course, and the transmission of a disorder within families (Robins and Guze, 1970). As will be seen, however, familial transmission would not prove to be a validator as Robins and Guze had hoped: Disorders defined by purely phenomenological criteria do not breed true (Lichtenstein et al., 2009).

One of the original validating criteria listed by Robins and Guze (1970) was delineation of disorders from each other. Across the RDC, Feighner criteria, and the DSM system, psychiatric disorders are conceptualized as bounded categories that are qualitatively different from each other and from health. All of these diagnostic systems treat psychiatric disorders as discontinuous categories in analogy with infectious diseases such as pneumococcal pneumonia or tuberculosis. The mid-century descriptive psychiatrists eschewed an alternative conceptual schema that has turned out to be more consistent with the accumulated data, which would describe psychiatric disorders in terms of quantitative dimensions that are continuous with normal in analogy with hypertension or diabetes mellitus. In dimensional diagnoses, thresholds for illness are determined empirically based on studies of impairment, disability, or longer-term health outcomes (such as risk of stroke given current blood pressure). Evidence that dimensional approaches better capture psychopathology than categories include the inability to discover discontinuities in the distribution of symptoms from healthy to ill people (e.g., in depression; Lichtenstein et al., 2009) and epidemiological studies that find normal distributions of symptoms in the population (e.g., for attention deficit hyperactivity disorder, autism [Kendler and Gardner, 1998], and schizophrenia) with illness representing extremes of the distribution on multiple dimensions.

An important goal of the early Washington University diagnostic systems (Feighner et al., 1972; Spitzer et al., 1975) and the DSM-III (APA, 1980) was to identify homogeneous populations for research and treatment. The DSM-III attempted to achieve this goal by subdividing psychopathology into a large number of narrowly defined categorical diagnoses. This approach goes to the heart of the deep structural problems of the DSM system: It is based on narrow, highly specified (and therefore, it was thought, reliable), discontinuous categories. Far from producing homogeneity, the DSM approach has resulted in a highly infelicitous combination of overlapping categories that are yet, internally heterogeneous. By slicing psychopathology into many narrow silos, the DSM manuals have produced a situation in which a large number of patients receive more than one diagnosis (so-called co-occurrence or comorbidity.). For example, an individual who receives a single DSM-IV diagnosis often meets criteria for multiple additional disorders, and the pattern of often changes over the lifespan (Kessler et al., 1996, 2005). Thus, for example, children and adolescents with one (and often more than one anxiety disorder diagnosis) may receive a diagnosis of major depression in their teens or twenties. Individuals with autism spectrum disorders have high rates of attention

deficit hyperactivity disorder, obsessive-compulsive disorder, and others (Lichtenstein et al., 2010). Of course, disorders could co-occur at random based on their prevalence or, co-occurrence at a higher rate than predicted by prevalence alone could signify that one disorder is a risk factor for another, just as diabetes mellitus is a risk factor for peripheral vascular disease. Within the DSM system, however, many diagnoses co-occur at frequencies far higher than predicted by their population prevalence, and both emerging understandings of pathogenesis (Kendler et al., 2011; Krueger and Markon, 2006; Krueger and South, 2009) and temporal relationships (Kessler et al., 2005) make it unlikely that one disorder is a risk factor for later onset disorders. The most parsimonious explanation for the plague of comorbidity is that it is largely an artifact of the DSM system, resulting from its having divided shared pathological processes into excessively narrow slices (Krueger and Markon, 2006; Krueger and South, 2009).

The excessively narrow diagnostic silos of the DSM system (which produce comorbidity) do not, unfortunately, generate homogeneity within each category Thus, for example, well-diagnosed schizophrenia does not "breed true"; instead, single families may exhibit schizophrenia schizoaffective disorder, bipolar disorder, and unipolar mood disorders (Craddock et al., 2006; Lichtenstein et al., 2009) even when the etiology of psychopathology appears to rest largely in a single large chromosomal rearrangement (Millar et al., 2000).

Even though, as early as 1967, Gottesman and Shields (1967) recognized that schizophrenia might be polygenic, the Washington University School and the authors of the DSM-III (APA, 1980) understandably did not take this complicating view into account. Had they done so in a sophisticated manner they might have given greater credence to dimensional constructions and might have created a system more tolerant of heterogeneity. What has emerged from family and genetic studies in recent years is that autism (Neale et al., 2012; Sullivan et al., 2012), schizophrenia (Gejman et al., 2011; Lee et al., 2012; Sullivan et al., 2012), bipolar disorder, and indeed all common psychiatric disorders that have been examined (Sullivan et al., 2012), are polygenic. Large numbers of genes contribute to risk of mental disorders in different combinations in different families, where they produce disease phenotypes in combination with stochastic, epigenetic, and environmental factors. In some families genetic risk for mental disorders seems to be caused by many, perhaps hundreds of small variations in DNA sequence (often single nucleotide bases), each causing a very small increment in risk. In other families a copy number variation (CNV), whether a duplication, deletion, or rearrangement of DNA sequence, may play a large role, but still acts against a background of polygenic risk. In some individuals with sporadic autism, rare mutations may occur *de novo*. In others, rare mutations are inherited. In sum, no gene is either necessary or sufficient for risk of a common mental disorder, and genes may produce different symptoms depending on broad genetic background, early developmental influences, life stage, or diverse environmental factors. The DSM myth of narrow homogeneous diagnostic categories seems ready for burial once we recognize the full implications of polygenicity and the variable penetrance and expressivity of many risk genes (Cross-Disorder Group, 2013). Rather than tightly constrained disorder categories, it might be better, for the near term, to rely on broader clinical diagnoses that likely capture etiologically heterogeneous conditions but that might share essential features of pathophysiology and thus produce related (but not identical) symptoms and course.

The DSM-III was based of necessity on clinical phenomenology, and had many important strengths that must be kept in historical context. What went most wrong with the DSM-III were fairly arbitrary decisions to conceptualize psychopathology as discontinuous categories, as if they were infectious diseases, and then to promulgate a very large number of them. A short-term alternative to the use of individual DSM disorders might be the use of disorder clusters that will be embedded in the organization of the DSM-5 (Hyman, 2010), whereas longer term improvements will require substantially new thinking (e.g., National Institutes of Mental Health, Research Domain Criteria). In the meantime, students who use this textbook should recognize that DSM categories are heuristics based on half-century-old science, and are not to be reified, but rather used pragmatically until better approximations of nature arrive.

EPILOGUE: CLASSIFICATION ACCORDING TO BORGES

These ambiguities, redundancies, and deficiencies recall those attributed by Dr. Franz Kuhn to a certain Chinese encyclopedia called the *Heavenly Emporium of Benevolent Knowledge*. In its distant pages it is written that animals are divided into (a) those that belong to the emperor; (b) embalmed ones; (c) those that are trained; (d) suckling pigs; (e) mermaids; (f) fabulous ones; (g) stray dogs; (h) those that are included in this classification; (i) those that tremble as if they were mad; (j) innumerable ones; (k) those drawn with a very fine camel's-hair brush; (l) etcetera; (m) those that have just broken the flower vase; (n) those that at a distance resemble flies.

"John Wilkins' Analytical Language", translator Eliot Weinberger; included in *Selected Non-Fictions: Jorge Luis Borges*", ed. Eliot Weinberger; 1999, New York: Penguin Books, p. 231. The essay was originally published as "El idioma analítico de John Wilkins," *La Nación, February 8, 1942*.

DISCLOSURE

Dr. Steven Hyman serves on the Novartis Science Board and has advised AstraZeneca within the last year. Both advisory roles focus on early stage drug discovery. His research is funded by the Stanley Foundation.

REFERENCES

American Psychiatric Association. (1980). Diagnostic and Statistical Manual of Mental Disorders (3rd edition). Washington, DC: Author.

American Psychiatric Association. (1994). Diagnostic and Statistical Manual of Mental Disorders (4th edition). Washington, DC: Author.

American Psychiatric Association. (2000). Diagnostic and Statistical Manual of Mental Disorders (4th edition, Text Revision). Washington, DC: Author.

Buchanan, R.W., Davis, M., et al. (2005). A summary of the FDA-NIMH-MATRICS workshop on clinical trial design for neurocognitive drugs for schizophrenia. *Schizophr. Bull.* 31:5–19.

Craddock, N., O'Donovan, M.C., et al. (2006). Genes for schizophrenia and bipolar disorder? Implications for psychiatric nosology. *Schizophr. Bull.* 32:9–16.

Cross-Disorder Group of the Psychiatric Genome Consortium (2013). Identification of risk loci with shared effects on five major psychiatric disorders: A genome-wide analysis. *Lancet.* February 28, 2013. Epub ahead of print.

Feighner, J.P., Robins, E., et al. (1972). Diagnostic criteria for use in psychiatric research. *Arch. Gen. Psychiatry* 26:57–63.

Fenno, L., Yizhar, O., et al. (2011). The development and application of optogenetics. *Annu. Rev. Neurosci.* 34:389–412.

Gejman, P.V., Sanders, A.R., et al. (2011). Genetics of schizophrenia: new findings and challenges. *Annu. Rev. Genomics Hum. Genet.* 12:121–144.

Gottesman, I.I., and Shields, J. (1967). A polygenic theory of schizophrenia. *Proc. Natl. Acad. Sci. USA* 58:199–205.

Hyman, S.E. (2007). Can neuroscience be integrated into the DSM-V? *Nat. Rev. Neurosci.* 8:725–732.

Hyman, S.E. (2010). The diagnosis of mental disorders: the problem of reification. *Ann. Rev. Clin. Psychol.* 6:155–179.

Kendler, K.S., Aggen, S.H., et al. (2011). The structure of genetic and environmental risk factors for syndromal and subsyndromal common DSM-IV axis I and all axis II disorders. *Am. J. Psychiatry* 168:29–39.

Kendler, K.S., and Gardner, C.O., Jr. (1998). Boundaries of major depression: an evaluation of DSM-IV criteria. *Am. J. Psychiatry* 155:172–177.

Kessler, R.C., Chiu, W.T., et al. (2005). Prevalence, severity, and comorbidity of 12-month DSM-IV disorders in the National Comorbidity Survey Replication. *Arch. Gen. Psychiatry* 62:617–627.

Kessler, R.C., Nelson, C.B., et al. (1996). Comorbidity of DSM-III-R major depressive disorder in the general population: results from the US National Comorbidity Survey. *Br. J. Psychiatry* 168(Suppl. 30):17–30.

Kraepelin, E. (1899/1991). Psychiatry: A Textbook for Students and Physicians. Transl. ed. H. Metoui, S. Ayed. Canton, MA: Watson Publishers.

Krueger, R.F., and Markon, K.E. (2006). Reinterpreting comorbidity: a model-based approach to understanding and classifying psychopathology. *Annu. Rev. Clin. Psychol.* 2:111–113.

Krueger, R.F., and South, S.C. (2009). Externalizing disorders: cluster 5 of the proposed meta-structure for DSM-V and ICD-11. *Psychol. Med.* 3:2061–2070.

Kuhn, T.S. (1962). The Structure of Scientific Revolutions, 2nd edition. Chicago: University of Chicago Press.

Lee, S.H., DeCandia, T.R., et al. (2012). Estimating the proportion of variation in susceptibility to schizophrenia captured by common SNPs. *Nat. Genet.* 44:247–250.

Lichtenstein, P., Carlstrom, E., et al. (2010). The genetics of autism spectrum disorders and related neuropsychiatric disorders in childhood. *Am. J. Psychiatry* 167:1357–1363.

Lichtenstein, P., Yip, B.H., et al. (2009). Common genetic determinants of schizophrenia and bipolar disorder in Swedish families: a population-based study. *Lancet* 373:234–239.

Millar, J.K., Wilson-Annan, J.C., et al. (2000). Disruption of two novel genes by a translocation cosegregating with schizophrenia. *Hum. Mol. Genet.* 9:1415–1423.

Miller, G., and Holden, C. (2010). Proposed revisions to psychiatry's canon unveiled. *Science* 327:770–771.

National Institutes of Mental Health. *Research Domain Criteria (RDoC)*. http://www.nimh.nih.gov/research-funding/rdoc/index.shtml Accessed December 1, 2012.

Neale, B.M., Kou, Y., et al. (2012). Patterns and rates of exonic *de novo* mutations in autism spectrum disorders. *Nature* 485:242–245.

Pope, H.G., Jr., and Lipinski, J.F., Jr. (1978). Diagnosis in schizophrenia and manic-depressive illness: a reassessment of the specificity of "schizophrenic" symptoms in the light of current research. *Arch. Gen. Psychiatry* 35:811–828.

Robins, E., and Guze, S.B. (1970). Establishment of diagnostic validity in psychiatric illness: its application to schizophrenia. *Am. J. Psychiatry* 126:983–987.

Shendure, J., and Ji, H. (2008). Next-generation DNA sequencing. *Nat. Biotechnol.* 26:1135–1145.

Spitzer, R.L., Endicott, J., et al. (1975). Research diagnostic criteria. *Psychopharmacol. Bull.* 11:22–25.

Sullivan, P.F., Daly, M.J., et al. (2012). Genetic architecture of psychiatric disorders: the emerging picture and its implications. *Nat. Rev. Genet.* 13:537–551.

Takahashi, K., Tanabe, K., et al. (2007). Induction of pluripotent stem cells from adult human fibroblasts by defined factors. *Cell* 131:861–872.

Wade, N. (1975). Conference sets strict controls to replace moratorium. *Science* 187:931–935.

World Health Organization. (1992). The ICD-10 Classification of Mental and Behavioural Disorders. Geneva: Author.

83 | TOWARD PRECISION MEDICINE IN PSYCHIATRY: THE NIMH RESEARCH DOMAIN CRITERIA PROJECT

BRUCE N. CUTHBERT AND THOMAS R. INSEL

Three events transpired between August 2011 and January 2012 that heralded the future of medicine over the next several decades. In August 2011, the FDA issued the first formal approval of a new drug whose use was contingent upon an authorized companion diagnosis: Vemurafenib (trade name Zelboraf) was shown to be effective in extending survival time for late-stage melanoma patients with the BRAF V600E mutation (FDA, 2011). In January 2012, the FDA issued an approval for ivacaftor (trade name Kalydeco), the first non-cancer compound requiring a companion diagnosis. This agent is highly effective in managing cystic fibrosis for the small minority of patients (approximately 4%) who have the G551D mutation of the cystic fibrosis transmembrane regulator gene (FDA, 2012).

These two events bracketed the release in November 2011 of a major report by the Institute of Medicine (IOM) entitled, *Toward Precision Medicine: Building a Knowledge Network for Biomedical Research and a New Taxonomy of Disease* (Committee on a Framework for Developing a New Taxonomy of Disease, 2011; henceforth referred to as the IOM Committee). This report comprised a major proposal for the development of an Information Commons that can incorporate multiple sets of data (genomics, microbiomics, symptoms, environmental influences) to characterize focal groups of patients. Essentially, the report lays out the roadmap for a network of information that could provide an entirely new structure for the integration of research and personalized health care in the United States. Precision medicine is officially, and indubitably, here.

The ability to identify small groups of patients who can benefit from targeted treatments is necessarily built upon two major factors. First, diagnostic tests are required to identify relevant genetic polymorphisms, biomarkers, and other specific aspects of disorders. Second, new interventions must be developed that are targeted directly to the disease mechanisms identified by the diagnostics. Although companion diagnostics—required tests whose use is mandated in tandem with the new therapeutic—may not always be formally necessary, they represent the epitome of the new approach.

Precision medicine thus far is heavily represented by cancer biology, which is well suited for the identification of genetically related abnormalities that directly mediate the disease process. It is not coincidental that two of the first three therapy/companion diagnostic approvals were issued for particular indications in cancer. In other areas of medicine, disease risk is often characterized by multiple genes of small effect, and by substantially greater environmental risk factors. Mental disorders clearly fall in this latter category. Even within this group, however, psychiatry has almost no track record so far, even though research on genetics and neural circuits in the central nervous system has accelerated dramatically over the past two decades.

Comparisons with other comparable disorders illustrate this point. Mortality from heart disease in 2007 was only one-fourth the number projected a decade earlier; 1.1 million fewer deaths occurred in 2007 alone than predictions based on earlier trends (National Heart, Lung, and Blood Institute, 2011). In another area of medicine, a recent report indicated that current survival rates for children with acute lymphoblastic leukemia are greater than 90%, compared with a rate of less than 10% in the 1960s (Hunger et al., 2012). The comparable figures for mental illness present a stark contrast. Prevalence rates for common mental disorders have not declined to any degree over the last several years (Kessler et al., 2005). Diagnosis is typically not made until well after the generally accepted time that symptoms and impairment begin. Mortality resulting from suicide, side effects of medications, and medical comorbidities have not decreased. Very few preventive interventions are available. Finally, and most telling, there are virtually no biomarkers or genetic tests that can help point the way toward the kinds of targeted treatments that precision medicine entails.

There are many, varied reasons for this situation. The brain is easily the most difficult organ in the body to access directly for direct examination or tissue samples. The blood-brain barrier frustrates attempts to introduce many new compounds, and only recently have positron emission tomography scans become available to help indicate whether new chemical entities have reached their intended targets. In another domain, the hopelessness and isolation of mental illness discourage people from seeking treatment quickly or accepting the utility of screening and indicated prevention.

In addition to these difficulties, it has been increasingly clear that standard diagnostic systems in psychiatry—for all their advantages in enhancing reliability in an age when the field retreated from the sway of psychodynamic theory—represent a liability at this point in time regarding the urgent need to link diagnostics with cutting-edge brain science in psychiatric research. This chapter describes a new experimental classification system for research developed by the National

Institute of Mental Health (NIMH) that is intended to inform new versions of nosologies that foster precision medicine for psychiatry. The basic rationale for this initiative can be stated as follows: Psychiatry will never have an empirically derived classification system for precision medicine that is based upon neuroscience until a suitable database is available to inform its development; and obviously, such a database will never become available until research is funded that can generate the relevant literature.

The following sections review the development and organization of this initiative, termed the Research Domain Criteria (RDoC) project, with a particular emphasis upon some of the conceptual foundations and the ways that RDoC could apply to current research issues. Although the latter are illustrated with examples drawn particularly from mood/anxiety disorders and psychotic spectrum disorders, the principles pertain to all areas of mental disorders and mental health.

ORIGINS OF THE RDoC PROJECT

The need to consider an experimental system for classification arose during discussions held in 2007–2008 as the Institute considered topics for its then-new strategic plan. Investigators had noted issues in using the DSM (Diagnostic and Statistical Manual for Mental Disorders; American Psychiatric Association, 2000) in research for some time; these include, for example, comorbidity rates well above chance, heterogeneity, and an inconsistent scientific treatment (e.g., Clark et al., 1995). However, another set of problems emerged with the rise of sophisticated new technologies for studying the neurobiology of disorders. Increasingly, genetics and neuroimaging data failed to map onto standard diagnostic categories, frustrating attempts to develop cohesive theories of etiology or biomarkers (e.g., Hyman, 2007). Thus, although the DSM retained its familiar advantages in clinical utility, the diagnostic system was impeding progress toward research on neuroscience-based conceptions of etiology and pathophysiology.

Such problems were readily apparent to the organizers of the DSM-5 (née DSM-V) revision process. The first volume in an extensive series of reports from the research planning conferences for DSM-5 contained a thoughtful review of the issues for neuroscience-based classification (Charney et al., 2002). The participants were keenly aware of the problems, as well as potential solutions:

…there has been too strong a reliance on the DSM-defined symptom clusters and too little on biologically based symptoms that may cut across the DSM-IV-defined disorders. This over-reification of the DSM categories has led to a form of closed-mindedness on the part of researchers and funding sources. For example, researchers involved in new drug development tend to focus their efforts on treatment of DSM-IV-defined categories, despite widespread evidence that pharmacologic treatments tend to be effective in treating a relatively wide range of DSM

disorders. Furthermore, the erroneous notion that the DSM categories can double as phenotypes may be partly responsible for the lack of success in discovering robust genetic markers. Although a move to an etiologically and pathophysiologically based diagnostic system for psychiatry will be extraordinarily difficult, it is nevertheless essential, based on the increasing belief that many, and perhaps most, of the current symptom clusters of DSM will ultimately not map onto distinct disease states. (p. 34)

It should be emphasized that the DSM has become the standard for regulatory approval of new treatments from the Food and Drug Administration, for pathophysiology research conducted with a view to its eventual translation to new drug targets, and thus for research grant applications and editorial guidelines for publishing. Given the centrality of the DSM throughout the entire mental health system of practice and research, dramatic changes are simply not possible until a clear alternative is evident (see Kupfer and Regier, 2011, for a thoughtful discussion of this point). These facts influenced the NIMH in considering an effort that could provide the data that would be needed for future, neuroscience-based revisions.

Another factor contributing to the momentum for a new initiative was the emergent trend in the literature favoring dimensional approaches both in terms of translational research from non-clinical samples (e.g., Clark, 2005) and from psychopathology, with one of the volumes from the DSM-5 conference series exclusively devoted to dimensional approaches (Helzer et al., 2008). Thus, the NIMH included in its strategic plan Strategy 1.4, to "Develop, for research purposes, new ways of classifying mental disorders based on dimensions of observable behavior and neurobiological measures." (See Table 83.1 for a listing of this aim and the accompanying four-point implementation plan.)

TABLE 83.1. NIMH strategic aim 1.4

Strategy 1.4: Develop, for research purposes, new ways of classifying mental disorders based on dimensions of observable behavior and neurobiological measures.

- Initiate a process for bringing together experts in clinical and basic sciences to jointly identify the fundamental behavioral components that may span multiple disorders (e.g., executive functioning, affect regulation, person perception) and that are more amenable to neuroscience approaches.

- Determine the full range of variation, from normal to abnormal, among the fundamental components to improve understanding of what is typical versus pathological.

- Integrate the fundamental genetic, neurobiological, behavioral, environmental, and experiential components that comprise these mental disorders.

- Develop reliable and valid measures of these fundamental components of mental disorders for use in basic studies and more clinical settings.

RDoC ORGANIZATION AND PROCESS

A workgroup of NIMH staff, supplemented subsequently with a small group of external experts, started the implementation process for Strategy 1.4 in early 2009 and completed an organizational framework and process by March.[1] In July 2009 a meeting was convened that included representatives of the ICD and DSM revision efforts, NIMH staff, and external scientists presenting data that illustrated RDoC goals. The meeting, chaired by former NIMH Director Dr. Steven Hyman, facilitated a discussion that served to highlight the respective areas of emphasis among the three projects, and to prompt an ongoing series of collegial meetings among members of the three agencies that has contributed in multiple ways to efforts both for research purposes and for the clinical utility of classification.

The NIMH workgroup crafted the scientific framework for the new scheme on the basis of multiple areas of research. Five major domains (i.e., the Research Domain Criteria) were designated on the basis of both basic science and clinical research into structural models of disorders: Negative Valence Systems (i.e., those for processing aversive situations), Positive Valence Systems, Cognitive Systems, Systems for Social Processes, and Arousal/Modulatory Systems. The specific dimensions were then nested within each of these domains. As discussed in the following, the dimensions that appear in RDoC are formally denoted as constructs. This follows the traditional definition of the term construct in psychology and similar disciplines, indicating its status as a hypothetical entity that is not necessarily observable and not formally computable, but which serves to organize a set of data that accord with its putative function (Cronbach and Meehl, 1955).

To create a visual framework, the domains and their subordinate constructs were placed in the rows of a two-dimensional matrix. The columns of the matrix contained the various "components" (see the third bullet of Table 83.1) that were to be used to measure the various dimensions, and were termed units of analysis.

Three other important, integral parts of the overall RDoC organization could not be represented in the two-dimensional matrix. One very salient aspect concerns developmental processes, seen as critical for multiple reasons. First, events that occur during childhood affect the trajectories of subsequent development throughout the lifespan. Second, the area of childhood nosology has been particularly fraught with confusion and controversy, because of such factors as the difficulty of assessing behavioral and biological variables and the uncertainty as to whether adult-onset disorders can simply be scaled down to childhood. Third, mental illness is increasingly viewed as a set of neurodevelopmental disorders, with its origins partially stemming from epigenetic programs laid down as a result of such early life effects as maternal diet, maternal stress, and exposure to various infectious agents and toxins (Bale et al., 2010). The exploration of all these effects is best orchestrated by an approach such as RDoC that considers their sequelae in terms of neural circuit development and its associated behavioral activity, given that the most likely outcomes are best represented as dimensions of change in particular areas of functioning.

Environmental influences are a second topic area that could also be represented as another dimension in the matrix. Taken together, development and environmental influences represent one of the most important potential foci of the RDoC effort. Too often, using an infectious-disease model, patients are simply evaluated in terms of their presenting phenomenology so as to provide a diagnosis. Knowledge of past developmental history is sure to be an important step for precision medicine diagnostics.

Third, communicating the dimensionality of a construct ("determine the full range of variation") is difficult in the two-dimensional matrix structure. For symptoms, of course, this would represent severity. One of the important goals that the continuous-dimension framework fosters is the search for nonlinearities, in which sudden change (particularly in symptoms) may result from a relatively small increment in other systems such as behavior or circuit activity—particularly important as the thresholds for diagnosis in the familiar binary, "disease absent/present" format of the DSM and ICD were determined by clinical judgment rather than quantitative modeling. In sum, it would thus require at least a five-dimensional matrix to represent all the aspects that are important for the overall RDoC scheme.

The RDoC project utilized a series of consensus scientific workshops in which experienced scientists met to decide upon a list of constructs for which sufficient evidence existed. Five major workshops were convened, one for each of the five domains (preceded by a "test run" meeting with a single construct, Working Memory, in July 2010). The workshops were planned on an accelerated timetable to hasten the availability of the entire system, with one workshop scheduled every four months between March 2011 and June 2012.

The workshop process was modeled after the NIMH-sponsored CNTRICS initiative (Cognitive Neuroscience for Translational Research in Cognition in Schizophrenia; Barch et al., 2009), which has been successful in generating constructs in cognition that are relevant to schizophrenia (and in fact, formed most constructs of the Cognitive Processes domain).[2] The reader is referred to other RDoC papers for details on the workshop process (e.g., Sanislow et al., 2010). Briefly, participants were charged with producing three products: (1) a listing of constructs for the domain; (2) definitions for each construct; and (3) a set of empirically based elements for each construct at each of the several units of analysis. Participants were instructed that new or altered constructs had to meet the same two criteria that the workgroup used in compiling its draft list: (1) there had to be strong evidence for the validity of the suggested construct as a functional entity (see the following); (2) there had to be strong evidence that the suggested construct maps onto a specific biological system, such as a brain or hormonal circuit.

---

1. The members of the NIMH RDoC workgroup are Bruce Cuthbert (chair), Marjorie Garvey, Robert Heinssen, Michael Kozak, Sarah Morris, Kevin Quinn, Daniel Pine, Rebecca Steiner, Janine Simmons, Rebecca Steiner, and Philip Wang. External consultants are: Deanna Barch, Michael First, and Will Carpenter.

---

2. Grateful thanks are expressed to Drs. Deanna Barch and Cameron Carter for their time and expertise in consulting about the CNTRICS model and the format of the first RDoC conference.

RESEARCH DOMAIN CRITERIA MATRIX

DOMAINS/CONSTRUCTS		Genes	Molecules	Cells	Circuits	Physiology	Behavior	Self-Reports	Paradigms
				— UNITS OF ANALYSIS —					
Negative Valence Systems									
Acute threat ("fear")									
Potential threat ("anxiety")									
Sustained threat									
Loss									
Frustrative nonreward									
Positive Valence Systems									
Approach motivation									
Initial responsiveness to reward									
Sustained responsiveness to reward									
Reward learning									
Habit									
Cognitive Systems									
Attention									
Perception									
Working memory									
Declarative memory									
Language behavior									
Cognitive (effortful) control									
Systems for Social Processes									
Affiliation/attachment									
Social Communication									
Perception/Understanding of Self									
Perception/Understanding of Others									
Arousal/Modulatory Systems									
Arousal									
Biological rhythms									
Sleep-wake									

Figure 83.1 Research domain criteria matrix. The left-hand column shows constructs nested with in domains; the remaining columns show the units of analysis and paradigms.

These twin criteria were one aspect of the workgroup's goal of constructing an integrative approach to the characterization of the various dimensional constructs. Proceedings of the workshops were drafted by members of the RDoC working group with input from the moderators of the breakout groups, and vetted by the workshop participants before being posted on the RDoC website (http://www.nimh.nih.gov/research-funding/rdoc/index.shtml). See Figure 83.1 for a listing of the matrix as of July, 2012 (following the final workshop).

DISTINGUISHING FEATURES OF THE RDoC APPROACH

The basic features of the RDoC initiative are summarized here see Morris and Cuthbert, 2012; Sanislow et al., 2010, for additional details. These points have guided the RDoC project since its inception, and serve to distinguish the RDoC approach from other current nosologies:

1. RDoC takes a strongly translational perspective to mental illness, in which symptoms and disorders are viewed in terms of basic functions (e.g., fear, working memory) and the mechanisms by which their operations become dysregulated in such a way as to eventuate in psychopathology. A keystone of this approach is that these functional dimensions have been found to be implicated in many different disorder categories as currently defined, so that conducting research on the functions themselves, as they cut across multiple disorders (and often in interaction with other dimensions), is the optimal way to analyze how their operations become abnormal.

2. The RDoC approach to psychopathology is strongly dimensional, not only within the range of psychopathology but in the entire range of functioning that runs the gamut from "normal" to extreme pathology.

3. Related to the prior point, one of the goals of RDoC is to support the developmental of appropriate scales and tasks that can provide valid measurement of the entire range for each construct.

4. To foster research designs that address key questions of interest, investigators are free to use measures from any of the units of analysis as the independent variable (IV) in the design (e.g., circuit activation, cognitive performance, targeted symptoms) and dependent variables (DV) from other units of analysis. To put it another way, circuit activation could be an IV in one study and a DV in another, depending on the study aims. This necessitates a two-stage strategy for ascertaining subjects. The first stage is to determine the "sampling frame" for the study; that is, that set of individuals who will comprise the study sample and whose data will generate a reasonable amount of variance regarding the study question. For instance, a specialized facility might not generate sufficient range to

address questions about relationships of genetic variance to different kinds of task deficits, so a clinic seeing a broader range of patients might be more appropriate for this aim. The second stage of the study is then to determine the values of the independent variable(s) through whatever measurement is necessary. In some situations, the value of the independent variable may not be determined until after the subject has been run (e.g., for neuroimaging studies that require extensive data processing).

5. The RDoC model is intended to be integrative across the various units of analysis. Behavioral or cognitive functioning, and the activity of neural circuits and their component elements, are all considered important in characterizing a construct.

6. Particularly at the outset, the project will concentrate on circuits that have strong evidence for their validity and appear especially promising for clinical research. This approach was taken deliberately to gain experience with the overall system and provide a solid platform for future additions. There is no claim at this point to cover the entire range of symptoms or pathology included in the DSM or the ICD.

7. As an experimental classification project, RDoC is committed to incorporating updates on a regular basis. At the same time, it is recognized that overly facile change can prompt instability in the system and confusion among investigators. The RDoC workgroup is developing a process for evaluating proposed changes to the matrix (which will involve criteria similar to those employed originally) so as to foster the continued growth of the literature in this area.

RDoC: CONCEPTUAL STRUCTURE

As a "clean sheet of paper" design, RDoC is unique in many aspects. Accordingly, the considerations and assumptions that went into the overall scheme must be discussed before turning to an examination of how the system will actually work in practice and the kinds of classification issues that might be addressed. The constructs in RDoC are the heart of the system, representing the functional dimensions that are to be explicated, so some elaboration of the way these are treated is necessary.

CONSTRUCTS

In many areas of medicine, symptoms as such are not impairing (lumps under the skin, high blood pressure levels, elevated cholesterol levels), and serve to call attention to palpable (if occult) underlying pathological processes. The DSM generally follows this medical model. Because any combination of X out of Y possible symptoms (e.g., five out of nine for major depressive episode) can define a disorder, any given symptom per se is not seen as critical in and of itself, but merely as a marker of the underlying disorder (granted that impairment is often part of the overall disorder definition). However, the realization

that relatively specific behaviors, cognitive operations, and affective processes are primarily implemented by particular neural circuits suggests a very different view of symptoms. The impairment/disability represented by symptoms and associated dysfunction in relevant neural circuitry are in fact the primary and proper focus of study—the things that ought to be the targets of assessment and treatment—rather than being simply markers. It is for this reason that Strategy 1.4 refers to "dimensions of observable behavior." Such a view is in fact the norm in treatment settings, in that practicing clinicians emphasize treatment of particular symptoms rather than disorders. To restate this critical point, a strong implication of precision medicine for mental disorders is to diagnose and treat specific dysregulated functions that are implemented by particular neural circuits (along with their constituent genes, molecules, and cells), rather than broad syndromes. From this perspective, accordingly, it now becomes a high priority to determine precisely what the functions *are,* and what forms their dysfunction may take.

The precise construal and definition of fundamental dimensions of behavior—and brain-behavior relationships—remains a complex issue, starting with common sense and face validity but heavily dependent upon continual revision and refinement through ongoing empirical studies. For instance, the classic conception by Olds and Milner of a "brain reward system" on the basis of self-stimulation studies (1954) was superseded by a more differentiated and anatomically detailed account that accommodated both the consummatory aspects of pleasure and other brain circuits that implement reward-seeking activity (Berridge, 1995); and subsequently by yet more refined parsing of reward-related processes (Treadway and Zald, 2011). Accordingly, the use of the term construct to denote the primary dimensions in RDoC follows the usual denotation of this term in psychology and areas of biomedical science; that is, a hypothetical entity that is inferred on the basis of a set of measurements that converge on its putative characteristics but do not much overlap with characteristics of other potential functions (Cronbach and Meehl, 1955; MacCorquodale and Meehl, 1948).

The term construct validity was first introduced in the late 1940s and early 1950s to establish standards and procedures for psychological testing, and the principles have been extended to other forms of measurement (e.g., neurophysiological measures). In the current context, constructs are further denoted as functional to indicate their significance to the goals, behaviors, and mental operations of the individual. Although characterizing any particular function may seem to be simply a matter of common sense, it is worth recalling that archaic psychodynamic concepts such as id and superego were once regarded as perfectly acceptable constructs. Thus, it is necessary to consider what the criteria might be for deciding that a construct could be posited, and what its function would comprise. Miller and Kozak (1993), in one of the few systematic analyses of functional constructs in emotional states, relate the question to other areas of science: "...this problem of criteria for judging a proposed function may be approached the way one evaluates any theoretical proposal once made. Does it fit the available data? Does the fit survive various means of convergent validation of the construct?" (p. 41). In other words, various measures that putatively seem to index the hypothesized function should correlate with each other, what Cronbach and Meehl (1955) referred to as the nomological net. These provisions may seem somewhat arcane, but are outlined here because they are directly relevant to the development of the RDoC matrix. One of the two major criteria for including any potential construct in the RDoC matrix held that there must be an adequate body of empirical research validating the construct as a functional entity. As implied by the reward system example in the preceding, the definition and measurement of constructs are subject to continual refinement (or, as for the id, retrenchment) as new data emerge.

"Grain size" for the constructs was a critical parameter that concerned the workgroup from the earliest meetings. As Goldilocks discovered, things needed to be not too big and not too small, but just right. Constructs that were overly large might be vague and ambiguous, and would likely subsume multiple circuits and behavioral functions, resulting in prohibitive theoretical and analytical complexity. Constructs that were overly narrow might suffer from insufficient relevance to clinical issues, have dubious ecological validity, represent undervalidated circuits or functions, and render the system unwieldy as a practical classification tool (even for experimental use). Thus, for instance, fear behavior in animal models can include active avoidance and passive avoidance, which may be somewhat recherché to translate to the clinic. Similarly, a growing number of subcircuits in the amygdala are being elaborated, but it is not yet feasible to measure them in humans and the clinical significance awaits translation. Both these systems, although finding support in the literature, were not included as constructs.

A critical point concerns the initially privileged status of the constructs that emerged from the rigorous workshop and vetting process. Clearly, as an experimental system, a high priority is placed on the ability of RDoC to update the matrix frequently to reflect advancing science. Critics have already pointed out informally the danger that RDoC constructs could suffer the same fate as their DSM/ICD cousins in becoming reified and resistant to constructive change. More to the point, it is obvious that strong consideration for funding must be given to projects that present well-justified (and well-reviewed) proposals for new or altered constructs, else the system will not obtain the data needed for continual improvement of the matrix. The same point holds for research evaluating the various units of analysis.

What, then, is the status of the constructs and elements in the units of analysis in the current version of the matrix? These comprise areas that a large number of scientists have judged as being of particularly high priority for investigations that can revamp our understanding of mental disorders, and that appear most likely to provide traction in building the database for future nosologies; it is anticipated that a substantial proportion of pressing issues can be addressed with these constructs. A clinical researcher could select a construct (or multiple constructs) that match her or his area of interest and then construct the application using the extant constructs and units of analysis, with the assurance that this will be a priority area of study. However, a researcher with a strong background in basic or translational research may well generate hypotheses that fall outside the current matrix. Both have the potential for equally strong contributions.

SYMPTOMS

It has been repeatedly pointed out that one weakness of current psychiatric nosologies is reliance upon presenting signs and symptoms (as opposed to clinical tests) to make a diagnosis (e.g., Hyman, 2010). However, in keeping with the different perspective on symptoms and constructs presented in the preceding, the RDoC workgroup maintained a strong emphasis upon symptoms in formulating the list of constructs to be initially nominated in the matrix. Obviously, symptoms are what prompt patients and families to seek out a clinical facility, and what they wish to see ameliorated by treatment. It is not so much the reliance upon symptoms as such, but the inability to connect them to any systematic bodies of neuroscience or behavioral science that poses a critical problem. A shared consensus among the workgroup members was that the DSM/ICD systems contain virtually all the significant symptoms that have been associated with mental disorders; the concern was thus not so much with the symptoms per se, but rather the ways in which they are clustered to create disorder definitions—with the familiar problems of heterogeneity, overspecification, and comorbidity (Hyman, 2010; Insel et al., 2010).

That said, a number of problems arise in adapting symptoms into the RDoC framework. A first issue is that the symptoms listed in the DSM vary widely in their specificity—another type of "grain size." Thus, one of the criteria for major depressive episode is explicitly quantitative, that is, a gain or loss of weight of more than 5% of body weight in a month. With suitable baseline measurement, there is little uncertainty or subjective judgment about this specific criterion. On the other hand, "depressed mood" is a much broader and more vaguely defined entity that invites serious scientific scrutiny in and of itself. Exactly what is meant by "mood" in any sort of scientific sense, and how would it be measured? Experienced clinicians will typically have a "feel" for the clinical sense of this construct. However, operationalizing and quantifying a construct such as mood is much more challenging from an integrative perspective, and in fact "mood" per se is not included in the matrix. A similar point can be made for the second criterion of major depression (i.e., markedly diminished pleasure) and for many of the symptoms throughout the DSM.

A second and related difficulty in creating a translational framework for psychopathology is that many symptoms are conceived and couched in terms of everyday language constructs that do not have a demonstrated relationship to specific behavioral or neural systems as derived from empirical research. As discussed, the criteria were derived in an era when such a research literature was not available, so the DSM-III can hardly be criticized for the omission; however, the problems has become increasingly obvious as relevant data continue to accumulate three decades later. An example of this problem is given by the "diminished interest or pleasure" criterion for MDE. As has now been noted repeatedly, studies have shown that reward-seeking, the experience of reward, and other processes with respect to appetitive functions can be dissociated on the basis of behavioral and neural systems studies (e.g., see the Positive Valence systems proceedings at the RDoC website: http://www.nimh.nih.gov/research-funding/rdoc/index.shtml). The realization that these functions are distinct to varying degrees has prompted an increasing number of experiments to explore their clinical ramifications and significance (e.g., Treadway and Zald, 2011).

The obvious implication of such considerations is that the nature of a "symptom" must be altered for the RDoC framework, from "a problem that the patient reports or exhibits with respect to traditional feeling-state notions of disorders" to "an abnormality of some degree that can be expressed quantitatively with respect to its deviation from the usual operation of the function(s) attributed to the construct." In some cases, this may be quite close to a DSM symptom (sleep problems), and in others (low mood) not. In some cases, the nature of such an abnormality and its clinical significance will be quite salient. In others, it may be somewhat ambiguous in the early going as to exactly how particular circuit-based dysfunctions relate to an overall clinical picture. (For instance, some investigators have commented that psychosis "looks like a black box" in RDoC, an instance of an invigorating translational question; but see Gold, 2011, for a good example of how relating neural system activity and behavior to reported hedonic states can shed light on an important clinical problem in schizophrenia.) Another way of putting this is that the workgroup members envision a grain size for symptoms that unequivocally reflects clinical level dysfunction, but is sufficiently specific to bear a reasonably strong relationship to the relevant construct both in terms of its function and its neural circuitry. Thus, rather than "low mood," the RDoC symptoms for a particular patient (i.e., in an individuated assessment) might be different combinations of, for example, approach motivation, reward learning, and working memory.

The RDoC workgroup members were mindful of clinical relevance in nominating constructs, and this task will represent one of the challenges facing the enterprise as RDoC moves forward. It may appear in this context that such a shift is unnecessary and needlessly confusing to clinical researchers, accustomed as they are to the current lists of symptoms. The rejoinder is that such change is imperative to fulfill the promise of RDoC; that is, to delineate more sharply the relevance of genetics, neural systems, and behavioral science to an understanding of patients' psychopathology, and in particular, the individual differences in the operation of these systems that can accommodate assessment and intervention in a precision medicine environment. Thus, although it remains unclear as to how well these more empirically derived constructs will relate to the familiar symptoms in the DSM, the long-range goal is that clinicians and researchers alike will perceive the advantage of viewing disorders in terms of fundamental biobehavioral systems.

Yet a third problem involves the lack of tasks and scales to measure "the full range of variation" in dimensions of interest; that is, a range from one extreme to the other. Most scales of characteristics or performance in behavioral science and psychiatry are designed either for normal range traits or clinical symptoms. The result is that either type of assessment lacks sensitivity at the other end. Such scales are now starting to appear with the growing interest in translational research for psychopathology. An excellent example is provided by a scale for the measurement of externalizing spectrum behavior developed by Krueger et al., 2007. These investigators used item-response theory modeling and diverse non-clinical and forensic samples to create an inventory that assesses externalizing behavior along a spectrum ranging from "normal" out to prisoners incarcerated for serious crimes. It is pertinent to quote the authors' conclusions about this dimensional approach.

> Comorbidity among mental disorders has been an impediment to progress because researchers are forced to make a number of confusing choices regarding fundamental issues in research design. For example, in work on the etiology of alcohol use and problems, should persons with antisocial features be included or excluded? The Externalizing Spectrum Model resolves these problems by reconceptualizing the targets for clinical inquiry in a manner derived directly from data on the empirical organization of externalizing phenotypes. (Krueger et al., 2007: p. 661)

Such research will gain increasing priority as the RDoC project advances.

RDoC AND CURRENT DISORDER SPECTRA
MOOD AND ANXIETY DISORDERS

Marked progress has occurred in the science of anxiety disorders (e.g., Ressler and Mayberg, 2007) and mood disorders (e.g., Berton et al., 2012) over the past several years. In spite of this scientific progress, diagnostic and treatment approaches have not changed fundamentally. The essential structure defined by the DSM-III in 1980 remains static, and cognitive-behavioral therapies and drugs acting on monoaminergic systems remain the standard treatments. It has become increasingly clear that the current categorical system poses a variety of obstacles to developing more precise diagnoses and treatments for the anxiety disorders (e.g., Fyer and Brown, 2009) and mood disorders (e.g., Berton et al., 2012). A brief overview of these problems provides a basis for discussing an approach that might be taken from an RDoC perspective.

Extensive co-morbidity represents one of the most substantial problems in investigating the so-called internalizing disorders (Nemeroff, 2002). This is true at both conceptual and practical levels. At the practical level, analyzing co-morbidity in experimental designs is daunting. Although patterns of co-morbidity vary across disorders—e.g., GAD is often observed in conjunction with other diagnoses, but specific phobia much less—myriad combinations are observed. If one were to take the eight major adult anxiety disorders, it would require 246 distinct combinations to account for all possible co-morbidities among these disorders (ranging from two to seven co-morbid conditions). With major depressive episode and dysthymia added to the mix, an investigator would need more than 1,000 categories to account for all potential co-morbidities.

The conceptual problems of co-morbidity are perhaps more knotty, suggesting fundamental mechanisms that are obscured by the lens of categories. The relationships among different internalizing disorders are not random. For more than a decade, structural analyses of disorder co-morbidity in epidemiological and other large samples have revealed two broad classes of so-called internalizing disorders, "fear" versus "distress" or "anxious-misery" (e.g., Krueger, 1999). Such studies have resulted in proposals for a re-alignment of the disorders to reflect this hierarchical arrangement (e.g., Watson, 2005). However, for the most part, the general acknowledgment of this structure has not led to widespread changes in how research grants are funded, or in journal articles, or therapeutic development.

A further complicating factor is the assumption that all patients with a given diagnosis have exactly the same disorder in terms of abnormal psychological or biological functioning. Thus, there are innumerable papers regarding "the" pathophysiology of posttraumatic stress disorder (PTSD), major depression, and so forth. However, as Fyer and Brown conclude regarding heterogeneity in anxiety disorders:

> …categorizing [the anxiety disorder categories] by genetic data creates one set of groupings; using age at onset creates a second set; and latent-class analysis creates a third. There is also considerable within-disorder heterogeneity. These observations suggest that the DSM anxiety categories do not map neatly onto simple, consistent, and distinct etiological pathways. (2009: p. 132)

For example, a recent review of neuroimaging data during symptom provocation in PTSD reported two distinct patterns of response. One pattern was the anticipated hyperarousal but the other was a blunted response that the authors interpreted as dissociative, leading the authors to conclude that "grouping all PTSD subjects, regardless of their different symptom patterns, in the same diagnostic category may interfere with our understanding of posttrauma psychopathology" (Lanius et al., 2006).

Similarly, McTeague and Lang (2012) reported that PTSD patients with a single traumatic event responded with the largest fear-potentiated startle responses (i.e., the difference between fear and neutral images) of several anxiety disorders groups in a symptom-provocation emotional imagery paradigm, whereas patients with PTSD experiencing numerous traumatic events and/or a chronic course showed the smallest startle potentiation of all the groups, with responses during fear not significantly different from those during neutral images. Over the entire sample, patient groups with greater distress and longer chronicity showed consistently smaller startle potentiation. Moreover, startle responses were further attenuated in patients with co-morbid depression. ("Baseline" startles evoked during rest periods did not differ among the groups.) In spite of the marked difference in startle response across groups, patients in all groups reported high subjective arousal during imagery with virtually identical mean scores, an instance of the desynchrony among response systems often noted in emotion research (e.g., Miller and Kozak, 1993).

These results from Lanius et al. (2006) and McTeague and Lang (2012) indicate that a consideration of the "fear circuit dimension" in psychopathology must address not only the canonical notion of hyperreactivity, but also developmental histories that eventuate in a failure to engage appropriate motivational circuits—an important condition both clinically and mechanistically. Beyond anxiety per se, the data further suggest diminished affective responding in patients with overall greater distress (including those with co-morbid depression). Although many recent studies have reported enhanced amygdala activity in depressed patients (e.g., Suslow et al., 2010), others have found various forms of blunted responding during depression (e.g., Vizueta et al., 2012).

A recent intriguing study of monozygotic twins examined those who were discordant for depression (on the basis of epidemiological survey test scores), as well as those who were high- or low-risk concordant (Wolfensberger et al., 2008). For the discordant pairs, high-risk twins showed increased amygdala responses to anxious/angry faces compared to their low-risk sibling. In contrast, concordant high-risk pairs showed blunted amygdala reactivity compared with low-risk pairs. The results indicate that very complex combinations of genetic and environmental risks may affect amygdala reactivity, including interactions with such factors as baseline amygdala activity (as the authors suggest) and with ventromedial prefrontal cortical structures known to modulate amygdala efferents dynamically.

Even such a very brief review serves to indicate that there is significant variability in the types and degrees of dysregulation observed within and across disorders. Integrating the findings across experiments in this area is extremely difficult for several reasons. First, patients are virtually always studied in a particular paradigm with single DSM groups, so that it is impossible to assess the extent to which the same patterns might be present in other groups. Second, reported conclusions for a single diagnosis may differ depending on whether a relatively larger proportion of hyperreactive versus hyporeactive patients happen to be included in the sample (e.g., for PTSD, as discussed). Third, the single-group experimental approach precludes the necessary studies that examine the interactions of the various motivational circuits directly (e.g., the amygdala, vmPFC, areas of the cingulate cortex, nucleus accumbens, HPA axis) across a range of disorders so as to provide a comprehensive accounting of the activity within and among these various systems. To put it more directly, it is only by studying the activity of the neural circuits and relevant behaviors themselves, rather than their variation as a function of one or another diagnosis, that a complete explanation can be sought. A thorough analysis at the systems level also needs to explore carefully the nature of responding as a function of the intensity and temporal characteristics of the stimuli. Many studies of depression have employed very brief and affectively mild face stimuli, whereas other studies employ symptom provocations or other challenges of high intensity. Finally, a developmental perspective

		– – – – – – – – – –		UNITS OF ANALYSIS	– – – – –	– – – – – – – – – – –		
DOMAINS/CONSTRUCTS	Genes	Molecules	Cells	Circuits	Physiology	Behavior	Self-Reports	Paradigms
Negative Valence Systems								
Acute threat ("fear")	IV				IV	DV	DV	
Potential threat ("anxiety")								
Sustained threat								
Loss								
Frustrative nonreward								
Cognitive Systems								
Attention								
Perception								
Working memory	DV			DV	IV			
Declarative memory								
Language behavior								
Cognitive (effortful) control								

Figure 83.2 *Draft research domain criteria matrix. Subsets of the RDoC matrix illustrating examples of independent variables (IV) and dependent variables (DV) in experimental designs.* **Top,** *Example of anxiety disorders study (see text).* **Bottom,** *example psychotic disorders study (see text).*

is absolutely essential to study the trajectories of the systems as maturation interacts with various kinds of life events.

How might an RDoC paradigm be designed to sort out these various considerations? A simple example is given in the top half of Figure 83.2, following roughly the McTeague and Lang (2012) paradigm studied in the preceding. The sampling frame for the study would be all patients seeking treatment at an anxiety disorders clinic, most of whom would receive a primary anxiety disorders diagnosis but with small numbers of patients with depression or personality disorders. The hypothesis of the study would be that magnitude of fear-potentiated startle (or, alternatively, amygdala activation) would predict (inversely) overall symptomatic distress and chronicity, confirming the relationship observed using diagnostic group means. A second aim would predict that patients with elevated startle reactivity would respond well to exposure-based therapies (owing to the presence of a robust response that can be habituated), whereas patients with blunted reactivity would largely fail to profit from exposure. In addition, the independent variable of startle response might be stratified by a genetic factor, for example, the BDNF polymorphism that has been shown to affect extinction learning in normal subjects (Soliman et al., 2010).

Extending the simple example, a longitudinal component might be added to determine the kinds of trajectories that lead to disorder. For example, the Wolfensberger et al. (2008) data (with exaggerated versus blunted amygdalar response in discordant and in concordant high-risk twins, respectively) clearly raise the possibility that some individuals have blunted affective reactivity from an early age, whereas others may be highly reactive initially but then transition to a nonreactive pattern owing to stress-related neuroplastic changes occurring over time. The genetic and epigenetic factors involved with these two patterns would likely be very different, and characteristics that may promote resilience would no doubt modulate these trajectories as well (Southwick and Charney, 2012; Tsankova et al., 2007).

Although an actual study of this type would of course be considerably more complex, the example is deliberately simple to emphasize the point that the main focus of the research is the neural circuits themselves, as modulated by genetic factors and as their activity relates to specific symptoms and behaviors reflecting stress, distress, avoidance, and so forth, but divorced from the procrustean categories that can distort the actual relationships and mechanisms. The reader may readily infer the implications of such work for generating more precise new assessments and intervention tactics.

PSYCHOTIC SPECTRUM DISORDERS

An exciting step forward in biotechnology as applied to mental disorders occurred in May 2011 with the first publication involving the use of human induced pluripotent stem cells (hiPSCs) to study schizophrenia (Brennand et al., 2011). The authors reprogrammed fibroblasts from four patients into hiPSCs, and then differentiated them into neurons. The results revealed nearly 600 genes that showed up- or down-regulated expression compared with control neurons, many of them in areas that had previously been implicated in schizophrenia, such as glutamate, cAMP, and WNT signaling.

This study was justifiably hailed as a first step showing the promise of the still-evolving hiPSC technology to provide information about disorders. The eminent psychiatric geneticist Michael Owen, however, cautioned that it was premature to conclude that the observed differences necessarily underlie schizophrenia: "These disorders are not really disorders. There's no such thing as schizophrenia. It's a syndrome. It's a collection of things psychiatrists have grouped together" (quoted in Callaway, 2011). This viewpoint represents perhaps the extreme of a wide range of opinions as to how psychotic-spectrum disorders should be conceptualized in the current age of genetics and neurobiology. Although the classical Kraepelinian dichotomy between schizophrenia and bipolar disorder has increasingly been questioned since the advent of DSM-III, the issue has risen to the forefront with genetics studies showing a common risk for both disorders, and accumulating findings about the heterogeneity within both disorders.

In spite of the extensive discussion and awareness in the field about such data, the large majority of etiological studies and trials continue to treat both schizophrenia and bipolar disorder as though they are each unitary diseases, each with a common etiology and pathophysiology. Even allowing for the fact that current publications reflect studies initiated seven to ten years ago or more, this seems a remarkable disjunction.

What might a different model look like, and how might it be tested? In an audacious theoretical integration, Craddock and Owen (2010) first reviewed the literature on genetic risks that are shared in common between schizophrenia and bipolar disorder and then considered the comparably large number of copy number variants (CNVs) and familial co-morbidity that are observed in schizophrenia, intellectual disability, and autism. This leads to a model positing an extended gradient of serious mental illness reflecting the extent of neurodevelopmental pathology, ordered as follows (from most to least severe): mental retardation, autism, schizophrenia, schizoaffective disorder, and bipolar/unipolar mood disorders. A second gradient of affective pathology is proposed that is inversely related to the neurodevelopmental gradient (i.e., increasing in intensity toward the bipolar/unipolar end), although the authors acknowledge that this is an oversimplification for presentation purposes. The model roughly resembles the RDoC matrix rotated 90 degrees to the left, with genetic variation underlying the entire gradient; DNA structural variants range from mental retardation through schizoaffective disorder, and SNPs are seen throughout, consistent with the recent literature. Genetic variation contributes to low-level biological systems that, in turn, feed in various ways into neural modules that interact with environmental influences and stochastic variation to eventuate in various forms of cognitive and affective psychopathology across the two gradients.

The implications of this model are far reaching. Rather than discrete entities, the various disorders are seen as differing ranges along an extended spectrum of severe neurodevelopmental pathology. The current interest in exploring relationships between schizophrenia and bipolar disorder, in this model, is constrained to only one segment of the entire spectrum. The challenges of testing such a model are daunting, but even a partially successful explication would go a very long way toward fulfilling the goal of precision medicine in mental illness.

How would one set about testing this model? From an RDoC perspective, the first principle is to examine the data as a function of particular dimensions of interest, rather than as a function of DSM diagnosis. The speculations that Craddock and Owen (2010) offer are quoted at length here, as one could hardly improve upon their statements in framing an RDoC approach to unpacking their complex theories:

...we need to prepare ourselves to move towards more complex and biologically plausible models of illness rather than clinging on to the biology-free models based on clinical empiricism that have been the

tradition of psychiatry....There is a pressing need to characterise the neurocognitive disturbances that underlie the major domains of psychopathology if we wish to develop a more refined taxonomy of mental disorders as well as better entities for genetic and other aetiological studies. It is to be hoped that more fundamental phenotypes might emerge from studies of the biological systems implicated by genetic and other biological findings. A combination of these top-down and bottom-up approaches might ultimately allow us to trace the links between genotype and phenotype. These efforts will require greater integration between different research modalities, including genetics, psychopathology, and cognitive and affective neuroscience, together with insights from systems biology. This should be complemented by consideration of social and other relevant environmental variables, and include a developmental perspective.

Keshavan et al. sound a similar note in discussing the schizophrenia spectrum (2011):

One way ahead is to replace categorical thinking by a continuum model. In such a model, each patient may be placed on a unique location in the multi-dimensional "disease space" along the tripartite coordinates of the patient's genomic and environmental risk/ resilience factors and disease expression (at molecular, physiological and behavioral levels). Doing so is the central tenet of personalized medicine; charting person- specific hallmarks of a complex disorder will not only offer novel targets for future pathophysiological and therapeutic research, but will also help optimize diagnosis and treatment for each individual patient.

Fortunately, good examples of this approach are becoming available in the literature, albeit still within single DSM disorders. For example, Wessman et al. (2009) conducted an unsupervised cluster analysis on the basis of clinical and neuropsychological data, examining a large number of patients diagnosed with schizophrenia as well as affected and unaffected family members. The cluster analysis revealed (aside from a group of unaffected family members) one cluster whose symptoms appeared to be "core schizophrenia" and who showed severe impairment, and a second cluster with a more "psychosis spectrum" pattern (including affective symptoms, although the modal diagnosis was schizophrenia) that showed only mild neurocognitive impairment. A subsequent association study of candidate genes revealed a significant association with the DTNBP1 gene for the former and with DISC1 for the latter. The RDoC sample design in the lower half of Figure 83.2 is somewhat similar to this study, except that the sampling frame would include a broader range of pathology. The IV comprises a neurocognitive task (working memory), and an association study would be conducted on candidate genes (i.e., as a DV). The additional DV in the example might represent, for example, fMRI analyses of dorsolateral prefrontal cortex to examine how circuit activation varies as a function of task performance.

More recently, investigators created sets of genes according to their shared synaptic function (e.g., cell adhesion) and then conducted association studies on the sets of "functional gene groups" rather than individual genes (Lips et al., 2012). The total group of genes encoding synapse-relevant proteins was highly associated with risk for schizophrenia, as compared with a set of matched control genes. Three subgroups of synaptic functioning genes accounted for the most variance: intracellular signal transduction, excitability, and cell adhesion and trans-synaptic signaling. The implications for an RDoC approach are clear, with obvious promise for exploring a greater span of the neurodevelopmental gradient. An obvious hypothesis would predict that different points along the spectrum would be associated with differing total amounts, and/or different types of synaptic group abnormalities. Confirmation would offer systematic inroads toward a mechanistic approach to drug development (e.g., Insel, 2012). Similarly, Brennand et al. conclude from their hiPSC results that "Our data support the "watershed model" of SCZD [schizophrenia] whereby many different combinations of gene malfunction may disrupt the key pathways affected in SCZD. We predict that, as the number of SCZD cases studied using hiPSC neurons increases, a diminishing number of genes will be consistently affected across the growing patient cohort. Instead, evidence will accumulate that a handful of essential pathways can be disrupted in diverse ways to result in SCZD" (Brennand et al., 2011: p. 223). Obviously, as with the Lips et al. study, the results of the Brennand et al. approach could readily be applied to a study of patients across the neurodevelopmental gradient of pathology.

With such powerful tools emerging to make overarching new theories possible, the hope of the NIMH is that RDoC can provide a framework for investigators to use as they explore the daunting new terrain of etiology and precision diagnosis. It is, as yet, somewhat difficult to envision how the diagnostic system of the future will handle these complexities, but direct explorations of the relevant neural systems will provide the kind of database than can inform these future decisions.

RDoC IN TREATMENT

The time frame for the RDoC startup was paralleled by the beginning of a marked withdrawal from central nervous system drug development by pharmaceutical companies (e.g., Miller, 2010). As with any such trend, the reasons are complex; fundamentally, however, the companies regarded central nervous system drug development as an economic liability given recent failures in this area and the lack of good targets for development.

The problems, as well as the opportunities, for precision medicine are outlined by a group of industry scientists: "On average, a marketed psychiatric drug is efficacious in approximately half of the patients who take it. One reason for this low response rate is the artificial grouping of heterogeneous syndromes with different pathophysiological mechanisms into one disorder." However, the potential is that "... by increasing the mechanistic understanding of disease and matching the right treatments to the right patients, one could move from one-size-fits-all to targeted therapy and increase the benefit-risk ratio for patients." They conclude that multi-target, trial-and-error development will be necessary "... until clinical trial design and patient segmentation can improve to the point of matching disease phenotype to circuit-based deficits..." (Wong et al., 2010).

In response to these exigencies, the NIMH has moved to develop a new policy for treatment development that emphasizes an experimental medicine paradigm. New candidate treatments are moved into humans more quickly than in the past, with an emphasis on early trials to demonstrate that the treatment engages its intended target successfully. In the case of compounds, this would ideally involve a PET ligand, but failing that, another measure such as electroencephalography or neurocognitive performance to show that the drug has reached the brain and exerted some effect. Signals of the latter type are also essential for new interventions involving devices or behavioral/psychological treatments. In other words, these very early trials are seen more as probes of target engagement, so that candidate interventions that fail at this step can be shelved quickly ("fast-fail"; see Paul et al., 2010). When target engagement is demonstrated, then the goal is than to move quickly toward early signs of efficacy.

The NIMH has moved forward to implement this new strategy with a slate of contracts for drug development. Termed FAST (for fast-fail), three nearly identical contracts for mood-anxiety spectrum, psychotic disorders spectrum, and autism spectrum disorders were awarded in September 2012 (see the summary at Fedbizopps, 2011). Although still very early in development, RDoC constructs have been integrated into these new trials to provide clinical targets in the form of validated intermediate phenotypes that are closer to the relevant mechanisms (see Meyer-Lindenberg and Weinberger, 2006). The idea is to foster more efficient treatment development by testing a new intervention specifically against the mechanism for which it was developed, rather than a heterogeneous grouping for which the mechanism might be relevant in half or less of the patients. The other function of RDoC would be to provide the measures, in the form of new scale development, that can serve as measures of clinical target engagement and possibly as end points in trials. As yet, the availability of such assessments varies across the domains and constructs, but prior projects have already provided some validated examples and set a model for further developments (e.g., Gold et al., 2012).

In addition to evaluating studies incorporating a fast-fail, experimental medicine approach, these trials will provide the Institute with an opportunity to gain experience with the RDoC dimensional constructs in clinical trials. In addition, this program will no doubt inform the larger RDoC development effort in developing the matrix and the experimental classification scheme.

CONCLUSIONS

This chapter has attempted to provide the reader with a fuller understanding of the conceptual and scientific background for the RDoC project. Such a radical departure from traditional ways of conferring diagnosis in psychiatry necessarily involves many changes, some of them obvious but others more nuanced and subtle. All are equally important to how the system was designed, and to its prospects for generating successful translational research. We have included extensive quotations from scientists with differing areas of expertise to demonstrate the consensus that has grown for developing an experimental system that can inform a nosology for precision medicine in psychiatry.

It is noteworthy that the DSM-5 is moving toward the same goals, albeit from a milieu in which clinical utility and stability are necessarily high priorities. As the leaders of the DSM-5 recently stated:

> It is important to emphasize that DSM-5 does not represent a radical departure from the past, nor does it represent a radical separation from the goals of RDoC. As we gradually build on our knowledge of mental disorders, we begin bridging the gap between what lies behind us (presumed etiologies built on phenomenology) and what we hope lies ahead (identifiable pathophysiologic etiologies). (Kupfer and Regier, 2011: p. 673)

Although the leaders of the ICD-11 revision process must place an even higher priority on clinical utility owing to their international mandate, they also reiterate that clinical practice is ultimately dependent upon validity (e.g., International Advisory Group for the Revision of ICD-10 Mental and Behavioural Disorders, 2011).

It is thus apparent that all the current efforts in psychiatric nosology are converging around a shared direction for precision medicine in psychiatry—toward classifications organized around empirically based conceptions of neural systems that implement particular behavioral functions. Specifying and integrating the various elements of these systems will be an extraordinarily difficult task, as many commentators have noted. However, an emerging consensus indicates that this direction is indeed the way forward for precision diagnoses that lead to tailored treatments. As Craddock and Owen concluded in their review, "At the end of the 19th century, it was logical to use a simple diagnostic approach that offered reasonable prognostic validity. At the beginning of the 21st century, we must set our sights higher" (Craddock and Owen, 2010: p. 95).

DISCLOSURES

Drs. Insel and Cuthbert report no biomedical financial interests or potential conflicts of interest.

ACKNOWLEDGMENTS

Grateful thanks are expressed to Dr. Michael Kozak for his insightful comments on an earlier draft of this paper.

REFERENCES

American Psychiatric Association. (2000). Diagnostic and Statistical Manual of Mental Disorders, 4th Edition, Text Revision. Washington, DC: Author.

Bale, T.L., Baram, T.Z., et al. (2010). Early life programming and neurodevelopmental disorders. *Biol. Psychiatry* 68:314–319.

Barch, D.M., Carter, C.S., et al. (2009). Selecting paradigms from cognitive neuroscience for translation into use in clinical trials: proceedings of the third CNTRICS meeting. *Schizophr. Bull.* 35:109–114.

Berridge, K.C. (1995). Food reward: brain substrates of wanting and liking. *Neurosci. Biobehav. Rev.* 20:1–25.

Berton, O., Hahn, C.-G., et al. (2012). Are we getting closer to valid translational models for major depression? *Science* 338:75–79.

Biomarkers Definitions Working Group. (2001). Biomarkers and surrogate endpoints: preferred definitions and conceptual framework. *Clin. Pharmacol. Ther.* 69:89–95.

Brennand, K.J., Simone, A., et al. (2011). Modelling schizophrenia using human induced pluripotent stem cells. *Nature* 473:221–225.

Callaway, E. (2011). Schizophrenia "in a dish." *Nature.*

Charney, D.S., Barlow, D.H., et al. (2002). Neuroscience research agenda to guide development of a pathophysiologically based classification system. In: Kupfer, D.J., First, M.B., and Regier, D.A., eds. A Research Agenda for DSM-V. Washington, DC: American Psychiatric Association, pp. 31–84.

Clark, L.A. (2005) Temperament as a unifying basis for personality and psychopathology. *J. Abnorm. Psychol.* 114:505–521.

Clark, L.A., Watson, D., et al. (1995). Diagnosis and classification of psychopathology: challenges to the current system and future directions. *Annu. Rev. Psychol.* 46:121–153.

Committee on a Framework for Developing a New Taxonomy of Disease. (2011). Toward Precision Medicine: Building a Knowledge Network for Biomedical Research and a New Taxonomy of Disease. Washington, DC: National Academies Press.

Craddock, N., and Owen, M.J. (2010). The Kraepelinian dichotomy: going, going…but still not gone. *Br. J. Psychiatry* 196:92–95.

Cronbach, L.J., and Meehl, P.E. (1955). Construct validity in psychological tests. *Psychol. Bull.* 52:281–302.

Fedbizopps. (2011). New Experimental Medicine Studies: Fast-Fail Trials in Mood and Anxiety Spectrum Disorders (FAST-MAS). Solicitation notice, published online. https://www.fbo.gov/index?s=opportunity&mode=form&id=01bd3a635f06482ea47a21736b857132&tab=core&_cview=1.

Food and Drug Administration. (2011, August 17). FDA Approves Zelboraf and Companion Diagnostic Test for Late-Stage Skin Cancer. FDA news release. http://www.fda.gov/NewsEvents/Newsroom/PressAnnouncements/ucm268241.htm.

Food and Drug Administration. (2012, January 31). FDA Approves Kalydeco to Treat Rare Form of Cystic Fibrosis. FDA news release. http://www.fda.gov/NewsEvents/Newsroom/PressAnnouncements/ucm289633.htm.

Fyer, A.J., and Brown, T.A. (2009). Stress-induced and fear circuitry disorders: are they a distinct group? In: Andrews, G., Charney, D.S., Sirovatka, P.J., and Regier, D.A., eds. Stress-Induced and Fear Circuitry Disorders: Refining the Research Agenda for DSM-V. Washington, DC: American Psychiatric Association, pp. 125–135.

Gold, J.M. (2011). Imaging emotion in schizophrenia: not finding feelings in all the right places. *Am. J. Psychiatry* 168:237–239.

Gold, J.M., Barch, D.M., et al. (2012). Clinical, functional, and intertask correlations of measures developed by the Cognitive Neuroscience Test Reliability and Clinical Applications for Schizophrenia Consortium. *Schizophr. Bull.* 38:144–152.

Helzer, J.E., Kraemer, H.C., et al., eds. (2008). Dimensional Approaches in Diagnostic Classification: Refining the Research Agenda for DSM-V. Washington, DC: American Psychiatric Association Press.

Hunger, S.P., Lu, X., et al. (2012). Improved survival for children and adolescents with acute lymphoblastic leukemia between 1990 and 2005: a report from the children's oncology group. *J. Clin. Oncol.* 30:1663–1669.

Hyman, S. (2007). Can neuroscience be integrated into the DSM-V? *Nat. Rev. Neurosci.* 8:725–732.

Hyman, S.H. (2010). The diagnosis of mental disorders: the problem of reification. *Annu. Rev. Clin. Psychol.* 6:12.1–12.25.

Insel, T.R. (2012). Next-generation treatments for mental disorders. *Sci. Transl. Med.* 4:155ps19.

Insel, T.R., Cuthbert, B.N., et al. (2010). Research Domain Criteria (RDoC): toward a new classification framework for research on mental disorders. *Am. J. Psychiatry* 167:748–751.

International Advisory Group for the Revision of ICD-10 Mental and Behavioural Disorders. (2011). A conceptual framework for the revision of the ICD-10 classification of mental and behavioural disorders. *World Psychiatry* 10:86–92.

Keshavan, M.S., Nasrallah, H.A., et al. (2011). Schizophrenia, "Just the Facts" 6. Moving ahead with the schizophrenia concept: from the elephant to the mouse. *Schizophr. Res.* 127:3–13.

Kessler, R.C., Demler, R.G., et al. (2005). Prevalence and treatment of mental disorders, 1990 to 2003. *N. Engl. J. Med.* 352:2515–2523.

Krueger, R.F. (1999). The structure of common mental disorders. *Arch. Gen. Psychiatry* 56:921–926.

Krueger, R.F., Markon, K.E., et al. (2007). Linking antisocial behavior, substance use, and personality: an integrative quantitative model of the adult externalizing spectrum. *J. Abnorm. Psychol.* 116:645–666.

Kupfer, D.J., and Regier, D.A. (2011). Neuroscience, clinical evidence, and the future of psychiatric classification in DSM-5. *Am. J. Psychiatry* 168:672–674.

Lanius, R., Bluhm, R., et al. (2006). A review of neuroimaging studies in PTSD: Heterogeneity of response to symptom provocation. *J. Psychiat. Res.* 40:709–729.

Lips, E.S., Cornelisse, L.N., et al. (2012). Functional gene group analysis identifies synaptic gene groups as risk factor for schizophrenia. *Mol. Psychiatry* 17:996–1006.

MacCorquodale, K., and Meehl, P. E. (1948). On a distinction between intervening variables and hypothetical constructs. *Psychol. Rev.* 55:95–107.

McTeague, L.M., and Lang, P.J. (2012). The anxiety spectrum and the reflex physiology of defense: from circumscribed fear to broad distress. *Depress. Anxiety* 29:264–281.

Meyer-Lindenberg, A., and Weinberger, D.R. (2006). Intermediate phenotypes and genetic mechanisms of psychiatric disorders. *Nat. Rev. Neurosci.* 7:818–827.

Miller, G. (2010). Is pharma running out of brainy ideas? *Science* 329:481–482.

Miller, G.A., and Kozak, M.J. (1993). Three-systems assessment and the construct of emotion. In: Birbaumer, N., and Öhman, A., eds. The Structure of Emotion: Physiological, Cognitive and Clinical Aspects. Seattle, WA: Hogrefe & Huber, pp. 31–47.

Morris S.E., and Cuthbert, B.N. (2012). Research domain criteria: cognitive systems, neural circuits, and dimensions of behavior. *Dialogues Clin. Neurosci.* 14:29–37.

National Heart, Lung, and Blood Institute. (2011). NHLBI Fact Book, Fiscal Year 2011. http://www.nhlbi.nih.gov/about/factpdf.htm.

National Institute of Mental Health. (2008). The National Institute of Mental Health Strategic Plan. NIH Publication 08-6368. Bethesda, MD: National Institute of Mental Health. http://www.nimh.nih.gov/about/strategic-planning-reports/index.shtml.

Nemeroff, C.B. (2002). Comorbidity of mood and anxiety disorders: the rule, not the exception? *Am. J. Psychiatry* 159:3–4.

Olds, J., and Milner, P. (1954). Positive reinforcement produced by electrical stimulation of septal area and other regions of rat brain. *J. Comp. Physiol. Psych.* 47:419–427.

Paul, S.M., Mytelka, D.S., et al. (2010). How to improve R&D productivity: the pharmaceutical industry's grand challenge. *Nat. Rev. Drug Discov.* 9:203–214.

Ressler, K.J., and Mayberg, H.S. (2007). Targeting abnormal circuits in mood and anxiety disorders: from the laboratory to the clinic. *Nat. Neurosci.* 10:1116–1124.

Sanislow, C.A., Pine, D.S., et al. (2010). Developing constructs for psychopathology research: research domain criteria. *J. Abnorm. Psychol.* 119:631–639.

Soliman, F., Glatt, C.E., et al. (2010). A genetic variant BDNF polymorphism alters extinction learning in both mouse and human. *Science* 327:863–866.

Southwick, S.M., and Charney, D.S. (2012). The science of resilience: implications for the treatment of depression. *Science* 338:79–82.

Suslow, T., Konrad, C., et al. (2010). Automatic mood-congruent amygdala responses to masked facial expressions in major depression. *Biol. Psychiatry* 15:155–160.

Treadway, M.T., and Zald, D.H. (2011). Reconsidering anhedonia in depression: lessons from translational neuroscience. *Neurosci. Biobehav. Rev.* 35:537–555.

Tsankova, N., Renthal, W., et al. (2007). Epigenetic regulation in psychiatric disorders. *Nat. Rev. Neurosci.* 8:355–367.

Vizueta, N., Rudie, J.D., et al. (2012). Regional fMRI hypoactivation and altered functional connectivity during emotion processing in non-medicated depressed patients with bipolar II disorder. *Am. J. Psychiatry* 169:831–840.

Watson, D. (2005). Rethinking the mood and anxiety disorders: a quantitative hierarchical model for DSM-V. *J. Abnorm. Psychol.* 114:522–536.

Wessman, J., Paunio, T., et al. (2009). Mixture model clustering of phenotype features reveals evidence for association of DTNBP1 to a specific subtype of schizophrenia. *Biol. Psychiatry* 66:990–996.

Wolfensberger, S.P.A., Veltman, D.J., et al. (2008). Amygdala responses to emotional faces in twins discordant or concordant for the risk for anxiety and depression. *NeuroImage* 41:544–552.

Wong, E.H., Yocca, F., et al. (2010). Challenges and opportunities for drug discovery in psychiatric disorders: the drug hunters' perspective. *Int. J. Neuropsychopharmacol.* 13:1269–1284.

World Health Organization. (2010). International Classification of Diseases, vol. 10. Geneva: Author. http://www.nimh.nih.gov/about/strategic-planning-reports/index.shtml.

84 | THE NEUROBIOLOGY OF PERSONALITY DISORDERS: THE SHIFT TO DSM-5

M. MERCEDES PEREZ-RODRIGUEZ, ANTONIA S. NEW, AND LARRY J. SIEVER

nvestigations into the neurobiology of psychiatric disorder increasingly focus on dimensions or domains of psychopathology across diagnoses (as exemplified by the Research Domain Criteria initiative [RDoC]; Insel et al., 2010) and their underlying circuitry problems. Neuropeptides and neurotransmitters then modulate these critical circuits. Gene by environment interactions are a focus for investigating these domains.

Although the study of personality disorder had traditionally been the province of psychoanalytic or behavioral models, there is an emerging neurobiology of personality disorders grounded in altered neurocircuitry associated with individual differences and dimensions such as affective dysregulation (affective instability and negative affectivity), disinhibited aggression, anxiety/avoidance, cognitive/perceptual dysregulation, and social detachment/isolation. Thus, these new directions in psychiatry neurobiological research converge with efforts to identify the neural basis of stable traits in the personality disorders. The Five Factor Model of personality has identified core traits, such as neuroticism, which are stable and quite heritable. Extremes of these traits, expressed in the symptom dimensions, crystallize to the prototypic personality disorders as, for example, borderline personality disorder with affective instability, disinhibition/aggression, and social cognitive/interpersonal impairment. Schizotypal personality disorder is comprised of social isolation/detachment and cognitive/perceptual disorganization. Avoidant personality disorder is characterized by detachment and negative affectivity, whereas obsessive compulsive personality disorder is characterized by negative affectivity and conscientiousness. The cluster of traits that place an individual at risk for the development of a personality disorder also places him or her at risk for other psychiatric illnesses, such as depression and anxiety disorders particularly, accounting for the high rate of co-morbidity with personality disorders. Neurocircuits implicated in the affective instability (negative affectivity) and disinhibition of borderline personality disorder are related to limbic structures such as amygdala and insula as regulated by prefrontal regions including the orbitofrontal cortex (OFC). The cognitive disorganization of schizotypal personality disorder may be related to alterations in the dorsal lateral prefrontal cortex and temporal cortex, whereas deficiencies in ventral striatum dopamine systems may be related to the detachment/anhedonia. The biological underpinnings of avoidant and obsessive compulsive personality disorders are less well understood and because there is not a substantial body of research on these disorders, they are not reviewed in detail in this chapter.

The study of the neurobiology of personality disorders provides a gateway to understanding relationships between brain and behavior building on individual variation in anxiety threshold, affective regulation, social cognition, and inhibition/aggression, and thereby can help us understand the circuitry underlying these critical domains. These specific circuits are modulated by neurotransmitters such as serotonin or norepinephrine for prefrontal cortex, neuropeptides particularly for limbic regions, and these modulators tune the sensitivity and response characteristics of these circuits. The study of the genetics of personality disorders can identify critical genes that regulate the structure of these circuits and their connectivity as well as the modulators that regulate them. Because personality disorders evolve from the interaction of genetics and environment throughout the course of development, understanding the neurobiology of these disorders allows for the characterization of gene by environment interactions as well as the mechanisms by which these interactions unfold in the course of development. Environmental influences also may influence the expression of the genome through epigenetic factors and these are beginning to be investigated in the personality disorders. Finally, through identifying genetic variation and their epigenetic regulation as well as functional aspects of specific neurocircuitry, the molecular mechanisms underlying these differences in personality disorders can be characterized.

CATEGORIES VERSUS DIMENSIONS IN PERSONALITY DISORDERS

Both dimensional and categorical approaches can be used to assess and diagnose personality disorders. There has been controversy about which approach is more valid and a hybrid system utilizing both was proposed for the fifth edition of the Diagnostic and Statistical Manual of Mental Disorders (DSM-5) (Rationale for the Proposed Changes to the Personality Disorders Classification in DSM-5: http://www.dsm5.org/ProposedRevision/Pages/proposedrevision.aspx?rid=17#). The final approved version of DSM-5 will maintain the categorical model and criteria for the 10 DSM-IV personality disorders, and will include the newly proposed trait-specific classification system in a separate area of Section 3.

There has been skepticism about the categorical nature of personality disorders (Eaton et al., 2011; Widiger et al., 2009) based in part on the high levels of co-morbidity among personality disorders and between personality disorders and psychiatric diagnoses categorized in DSM-IV on Axis I. This has led a number of investigators to favor a dimensional model based on elements of the Five Factor Model scales (Costa and Widiger, 2002). Other approaches incorporating a dimensional model include large-scale twin studies, which have supported a different model for personality disorders, suggesting four factors: internalizing, externalizing, anhedonic/introversion, and cognitive/relational disturbance (Kendler et al., 2011a; Roysamb et al., 2011); however, according to this model, the division between Axis I and II in DSM IV is called into question. For example, antisocial personality disorder is more closely linked to Axis I substance abuse disorders, and dysthymia is more closely linked to such disorders as avoidant and dependent personality disorders.

Some have argued that the best way to address the dimensions versus categories controversy for personality disorders classification is to adopt a hybrid dimensional-categorical model (Trull et al., 2011).

Borderline personality disorder (New et al., 2008b), ASPD (Patrick et al., 2009), and STPD (Siever and Davis, 2004) have been studied most comprehensively from a neurobiological vantage point and have the largest empirical evidence of clinical utility and validity among PDs (Skodol et al., 2011). In this chapter, rather than reviewing all of the DSM-IV PDs, we review findings in these three PDs.

Research on the metastructure of comorbidity among common mental disorders suggests that mental disorders can be considered indicators of latent dimensional propensities to two types of psychopathology: internalizing or externalizing (Hasin and Kilcoyne, 2012; Krueger, 1999; Krueger et al., 2002). The externalizing dimension is characterized by antisocial personality disorder and alcohol, nicotine, and drug dependence. The internalizing dimension includes two subdimensions, one involving distress (major depression, dysthymia, generalized anxiety) and the other involving fear (panic, social phobia, specific phobia) (Hasin and Kilcoyne, 2012).

BORDERLINE PERSONALITY DISORDER

The DSM-IV characterizes BPD as a pervasive pattern of instability of interpersonal relationships, self-image, and affects, and marked impulsivity beginning by early adulthood and present in a variety of contexts, as indicated by at least five of nine criteria: (1) frantic efforts to avoid real or imagined abandonment; (2) a pattern of unstable and intense interpersonal relationships characterized by alternating between extremes of idealization and devaluation; (3) identity disturbance: markedly and persistently unstable self-image or sense of self; (4) impulsivity in at least two areas that are potentially self-damaging (e.g., spending, sex, substance abuse, reckless driving, binge eating); (5) recurrent suicidal behavior, gestures, or threats, or self-mutilating behavior; (6) affective instability resulting from a marked reactivity of mood (e.g., intense episodic dysphoria, irritability, or anxiety usually lasting a few hours and only rarely more than a few days); (7) chronic feelings of emptiness; (8) inappropriate, intense anger or difficulty controlling anger (e.g., frequent displays of temper, constant anger, recurrent physical fights); and (9) transient, stress-related paranoid ideation or severe dissociative symptoms (APA, 2000). DSM-5 will maintain the same diagnostic criteria, and will include the newly proposed trait-specific classification system in a separate area of Section 3. In Section 3 of the DSM-5, the diagnosis of BPD is characterized by impairments in personality (self and interpersonal) functioning and the presence of pathological personality traits, including negative affectivity (characterized by emotional lability, anxiousness, separation insecurity, and depressivity), disinhibition (characterized by impulsivity and risk-taking), and antagonism (characterized by hostility).

The proposed traits included in Section 3 of the DSM-5 are based on the Five Factor Model (FFM) of personality (Costa and Widiger, 2002), and arise from the psychology literature. The relation between FFM traits and DSM-IV PDs is supported by considerable data (Samuel and Widiger, 2008). The traits that characterize BPD according to Section 3 of the DSM-5 (negative affectivity, disinhibition, and antagonism) are closely related to the core BPD traits of impulsive aggression and affective dysregulation, which are supported by validating data (Siever and Weinstein, 2009).

EPIDEMIOLOGY

The prevalence of BPD as defined in DSM-IV ranges between 0.5% and 5.9% in epidemiological studies of adults in the general US population (Grant et al., 2008; Leichsenring et al., 2011), making it as prevalent as schizophrenia and bipolar I disorder. This represents a wide range of prevalence, which may reflect the different approaches employed in the studies, although the largest sample of subjects interviewed directly from a community sample reports a lifetime prevalence of 5.9% (Grant et al., 2008). Torgersen et al. (2001) calculated a median prevalence of 1.35%, pooling results from 10 studies. Although earlier research supported a higher prevalence of BPD among women, as reflected in the 3:1 female to male ratio reported in the DSM-IV-TR (APA, 2000), more recent data suggest that there are no sex differences in the prevalence of BPD (Grant et al., 2008).

Borderline personality disorder seems to be less stable over time than expected for personality disorders, with high rates of remission reported in follow-up studies (Skodol et al., 2005; Zanarini et al., 2006) and an inverse relationship between age and prevalence of BPD in the general population (Grant et al., 2008).

COMORBIDITY, ILLNESS BURDEN, AND TREATMENT UTILIZATION

Borderline personality disorder is highly comorbid with both Axis I and II disorders (Grant et al., 2008; Lenzenweger et al., 2007; Skodol et al., 2005): 84.5% of patients with BPD met criteria for one or more 12-month Axis I disorders, most frequently mood disorders, anxiety disorders, and substance use disorders (Grant et al., 2008; Lenzenweger et al., 2007; Skodol et al., 2005). There appear to be gender differences with regard to Axis I comorbidity, with men having higher rates of substance abuse, whereas women are more likely to suffer eating, mood, anxiety, and posttraumatic stress disorders (Grant et al., 2008; Sansone and Sansone, 2011). About one-third of patients with BPD meet criteria for posttraumatic stress disorder (PTSD) during their lifetime (Grant et al., 2008): 73.9% patients with BPD meet criteria for another lifetime Axis II disorder, most frequently schizotypal, narcissistic, and obsessive compulsive PDs (Grant et al., 2008). Men with BPD are more likely than women to have antisocial personality traits (Grant et al., 2008; Sansone and Sansone, 2011). This high comorbidity rates may reflect a common vulnerability for Axis I and II disorders within the externalizing spectrum (Kendler, Aggen et al., 2011).

Individuals with BPD are higher users of mental health resources than patients with major depression (Bender et al., 2006), and they are overrepresented in clinical populations, with a prevalence of greater than 9% of all psychiatric outpatients (Zimmerman et al., 2005).

Borderline personality disorder is associated with severe and persistent functional impairment (Grant et al., 2008; Lenzenweger et al., 2007; Skodol et al., 2005; Skodol et al., 2005). Most—but not all—subjects with BPD have worsening levels of functioning over time, and never regain their initial level of functioning (Zanarini et al., 2006). They also have a high risk of suicide, with a mortality rate around 8% to 10% (Oldham, 2006).

THE ROLE OF TRAUMA

Patients with BPD report many childhood adverse events (e.g., trauma, neglect) and more negative life events than patients with other personality disorders (Bierer et al., 2003; Golier et al., 2003; Yen et al., 2002). However, no strong association between these experiences and the development of psychopathological changes in adulthood has been found (Fossati et al., 1999; Leichsenring et al., 2011). It appears that the interaction between biological (e.g., temperamental) and psychosocial factors (e.g., adverse childhood events) is likely what underlies the development of BPD (Wagner et al., 2009; Wagner et al., 2010).

PATHOPHYSIOLOGY

The neurobiological factors contributing to the genesis of BPD may be conceptualized in relation to core traits of the disorder (affective instability and impulsive aggression).

THE AFFECTIVE DYSREGULATION AND IMPULSIVE AGGRESSION DIMENSIONS

There is considerable support for the model of reduced medial prefrontal modulation of limbic structures (especially the amygdala), which appear to be hyperactive in patients with BPD, and results in dysregulation of emotions and aggression (Bohus et al., 2004; Mauchnik and Schmahl, 2010; New et al., 2012; New et al., 2008a).

One of the most consistent findings in patients with BPD compared with healthy individuals is a decrease in volume (especially gray matter volume) particularly in the anterior cingulate gyrus (ACG) (Hazlett et al., 2005; Minzenberg et al., 2008; Soloff et al., 2008; Tebartz van Elst et al., 2003), which may be especially pronounced in men with BPD (Soloff et al., 2008; Vollm et al., 2009). Other structural abnormalities in BPD include volume reduction in hippocampus (Brambilla et al., 2004; Irle et al., 2005; Nunes et al., 2009; Ruocco et al., 2012; Tebartz van Elst et al., 2003; Zetzsche et al., 2007), orbitofrontal cortex (OFC) (Tebartz van Elst et al., 2003), and amygdala (Nunes et al., 2009; Ruocco et al., 2012; Tebartz van Elst et al., 2007). However, some, but not all studies (de-Almeida et al., 2012) have raised the possibility that the smaller volumes in BPD may relate to comorbidity with PTSD or history of serious trauma for hippocampal volume (Nunes et al., 2009; Schmahl et al., 2009; Weniger et al., 2009) and the effect of comorbid MDD for amygdala volume remains unclear (Zetzsche et al., 2006).

Diffusion tensor imaging (DTI) studies examining white matter tract integrity suggest that there may be decreased fractional anisotropy (a measure of tract coherence) in the OFC in BPD (Grant et al., 2007) and diminished interhemispheric structural connectivity between both dorsal ACGs in BPD (Rusch et al., 2010).

In adolescent BPD, like adult BPD patients, ACG (Goodman et al., 2010; Whittle et al., 2009) and OFC gray matter volumes (Brunner et al., 2010; Chanen et al., 2008) are reduced compared with age-matched controls. One study showed that ACG volume correlated negatively with number of suicide attempts and BPD symptom severity, but not depressive symptoms (Goodman et al., 2010), suggesting that this volume reduction in ACG is related specifically to BPD pathology. This evidence of structural changes in ACG and nearby OFC is consistent with a model of a disruption in frontolimbic circuitry in BPD. This circuit has been studied with functional neuroimaging.

Multiple studies have reported decreased activation of prefrontal areas involved in emotion control in BPD. Early PET imaging studies showed decreased activity of OFC and ACG in BPD compared with controls (Goyer et al., 1994; Leyton et al., 2001; New et al., 2002; Siever et al., 1999; Soloff et al., 2000). A more recent PET study of laboratory-induced aggression using the Point Subtraction Aggression Paradigm found that BPD patients with impulsive aggression showed increased relative glucose metabolic rate in OFC and amygdala in response to provocation, but not in more dorsal brain regions associated with cognitive control of aggression (New et al., 2009). In contrast, during aggression provocation, healthy individuals showed increased relative glucose metabolic response in dorsal regions of prefrontal cortex, involved in top-down cognitive control of aggression, and, more broadly, of emotion (New et al., 2009). Poor connectivity between OFC and amygdala has also been reported in association with aggression (New et al., 2007).

Most functional magnetic resonance imaging (fMRI) studies using emotional stimuli have shown similar results of decreased prefrontal activation in BPD, with some exceptions

(Minzenberg et al., 2007; Schmahl et al., 2006; Schnell et al., 2007). Most studies in BPD have shown less activation (or more deactivation) of frontal areas involved in top-down control of emotions, including OFC and ACG, in BPD compared to healthy controls in response to emotional probes (Koenigsberg et al., 2009b; Minzenberg et al., 2007; Schmahl et al., 2003; Silbersweig et al., 2007; Wingenfeld et al., 2009), although some studies showed heightened prefrontal activation to emotional pictures in BPD (Minzenberg et al., 2007; Schnell et al., 2007) and to unresolved conflicts (Beblo et al., 2006).

Because of its role in emotion encoding and regulation, the amygdala is another region of interest for the study of affective dysregulation in BPD. Several but not all structural studies of BPD have shown volume reduction in the amygdala (Nunes et al., 2009; Tebartz van Elst et al., 2007).

Functional neuroimaging studies also point to abnormalities in the amygdala in BPD patients. Several studies have shown increased amygdala activation to emotional probes (e.g., emotional pictures and faces) (Beblo et al., 2006; Donegan et al., 2003; Koenigsberg et al., 2009b; Schulze et al., 2011). However, the amygdala appears to become deactivated in response to painful stimuli in BPD (Kraus et al., 2009; Niedtfeld et al., 2010; Schmahl et al., 2006), although one study suggests that this finding may be specific to BPD patients with comorbid PTSD (Kraus et al., 2009).

In summary, it seems that in BPD patients, prefrontal brain regions that normally put the brakes on expressions of emotions and more broadly of aggression (e.g., the OFC and ACG) may fail to become activated during emotional provocation, whereas the amygdala appears to hyperrespond to emotional probes.

However, it is important to note that many of the circuits implicated in BPD (including a model of decreased ACG/OFC response with an associated hyperresponse of amygdala) appear to be implicated in other psychiatric disorders, including MDD (Davidson et al., 2003), bipolar disorder (Blumberg et al., 2003), and PTSD (Shin et al., 1999), indicating potential lack of specificity.

Several laboratory psychophysiological tasks also point to abnormal emotional processing in BPD. A study by Hazlett et al. (2007) showed that patients with BPD exhibited larger startle eye blink during unpleasant but not neutral words, interpreted as an abnormality in the processing of unpleasant stimuli.

Studies on the serotonergic system suggest that the putative imbalance between prefrontal regulatory control and limbic responsivity described in the preceding may relate to impaired serotonergic facilitation of "top-down" control. Early cerebrospinal fluid studies on serotonin metabolites found low cerebrospinal fluid 5-hydroxyindolacetic acid in individuals with a history of suicide attempts (Asberg and Traskman, 1981; Asberg et al., 1976) or impulsive aggressive behavior (Coccaro, 1989). Since then, numerous studies have investigated the role of serotonin in BPD. Studies employing a wide variety of methods have replicated decreases in serotonergic responsiveness in disorders characterized by impulsive aggression, such as BPD (Coccaro et al., 1989; Dougherty et al., 1999;

O'Keane et al., 1992), including neuroimaging using pharmacological probes of serotonin (Leyton et al., 2001; New et al., 2002; New et al., 2004; Siever et al., 1999; Soloff et al., 2000). Recently, patients with personality disorders and impulsive aggression showed reduced serotonin transporter availability, as measured by the PET ligand, [11C]McN 5652, in the ACG compared with healthy subjects (Frankle et al., 2005). Moreover, metabolic activity in OFC and ACG in impulsive aggressive individuals is enhanced with fluoxetine treatment (New et al., 2004).

In summary, abnormalities in the serotonergic system may underlie the putative imbalance between prefrontal regulatory influences and limbic responsivity.

Genetics of Impulsive Aggression and Affective Dysregulation

Twin studies of BPD show substantial heritability scores of 0.65 to 0.76 (Distel et al., 2008; New et al., 2008a; Torgersen et al., 2000). A moderate heritability has been reported for dimensional BPD traits (Torgersen et al., 2008). However, there is considerable disagreement about what specific underlying trait or traits predispose to BPD. Some studies have suggested that one highly heritable factor underlies the symptom domains in BPD (Kendler et al., 2011a) and this factor is closely related to affective instability. This same study also describes strong genetic correlations between BPD traits and elements of the five factor personality components, especially neuroticism, and inversely with conscientiousness and agreeableness. Other studies have suggested that the Five Factor Model has more convergent and discriminant validity than the DSM-IV diagnostic criteria for BPD (Samuel and Widiger, 2010) based largely on the superior convergence between self-report and other assessment modalities (e.g., interview, informant interview). The particularly poor ability of BPD patients to describe their own symptoms based on poor ability to mentalize may underlie some of the confusion in the field. The proper approach to describing the underlying neurobiology of BPD symptoms is an active area of investigation and is among the goals of the RDoC's effort through the NIMH. This is important not only for elucidating what underlies BPD and whether new therapeutics might be developed with better neurobiological understanding of this illness, but it also is important because BPD features predispose individuals to other serious disorders, especially treatment-refractory depression (Kornstein and Schneider, 2001).

Candidate genes for impulsive aggression and emotional dysregulation include those that regulate the activity of neuromodulators, such as serotonin and catecholamines, as well as neuropeptides (Siever, 2008; Siever and Weinstein, 2009).

NEUROPEPTIDE MODEL

Neuropeptides are another recent area of interest in BPD. oxytocin has anxiolytic and prosocial effects (Macdonald and Macdonald, 2010), and it reduces amygdala activation in response to a variety of emotional stimuli in healthy individuals (Meyer-Lindenberg, 2008). However, there have been very few studies in BPD and none involving brain imaging. The two empirical studies of oxytocin administration in BPD have shown that oxytocin modestly decreased the subjective anxiety resulting from the Trier Social Stress Test in BPD (Simeon et al., 2011), but it decreased the level of cooperative behavior in BPD (Bartz et al., 2011). We have found that a polymorphism of oxytocin is associated with anger dyscontrol in BPD patients (Siever et al., unpublished data). This association is increased by trauma.

Opioids are also involved in social attachment. One recent imaging study measured μ-opioid receptor binding, by using the μ-opiate ligand [^{11}C] carfentanil, in patients with BPD during induction of neutral and sad sustained emotional states (Prossin et al., 2010). They found greater baseline μ-opioid receptor availability in BPD, interpreted as a deficit in endogenous circulating opioids. Their results also suggest that BPD patients enhance endogenous opiate availability more than controls during sad mood induction, which might reflect a compensatory response and is consistent with lower levels of endogenous opioids in self-injurers (Stanley and Siever, 2010; Stanley et al., 2009). We have found that polymorphisms of the μ-opioid receptor may be associated with affective instability and BPD (Siever et al., unpublished data). These associations also seem exacerbated by trauma, underscoring the interactive effects of genetics and environment.

One theory about self-cutting, a behavior common in BPD, is that it represents a method of releasing endogenous opioids, to compensate for an intrinsic opioid deficit (New and Stanley, 2010; Stanley and Siever, 2010). The interpersonal difficulty that is central to borderline pathology might also be linked to a deficit in endogenous opiates.

A FOCUS ON FUNCTIONAL NEUROIMAGING OF INTERPERSONAL PROCESSES

Very little empirical work has been done on factors underlying interpersonal disruptions in BPD. Several studies have focused on recognition of facial emotional expression in BPD. Borderline personality disorder patients appear to have a heightened ability to identify emotional expressions correctly compared with healthy controls; however, they tend to interpret neutral faces as more angry than controls do (Donegan et al., 2003; Lynch et al., 2006; Wagner and Linehan, 1999). The data suggest that ambiguous stimuli or contexts including time constraints particularly trigger dysfunctional emotional processing in BPD (Dyck et al., 2009). Difficulties in interpreting social affective stimuli also seem to arise when BPD patients are presented stimuli from multiple sensory modalities (Minzenberg et al., 2006).

Even fewer studies have examined more complex social tasks in BPD. One study using a Theory of Mind task during brain imaging found that BPD patients had less activity in superior temporal areas than controls during a task that involved inferring what someone in a picture was feeling, and they had increased activation of anterior insula during a task probing their own responses to emotional pictures (Dziobek et al., 2011). This supports the disturbances of "self" and "other" described in BPD psychopathology (Bender and Skodol, 2007).

A seminal study of complex social interactions showed that BPD patients had difficulty maintaining cooperation in a version of the Trust game (King-Casas et al., 2008). Behaviorally, BPD patients were unable to maintain cooperation, and were impaired in their ability to "repair broken cooperation" when their partner offered a "coaxing" bid. Neurally, healthy individuals activated anterior insula in relation to cooperative "offers" from their partner, whereas BPD patients activated the insula (a brain region predominantly involved in interoception and to a degree social cognition) in relationship to how much the patient him- or herself offered to the other. In a similar version of the Trust game, BPD subjects responded with greater *self*-criticism when given adverse monetary offers from a putative partner (Franzen et al., 2010).

BRAIN IMAGING OF DELIBERATE EMOTION REGULATION IN BORDERLINE PERSONALITY DISORDER

Because psychotherapeutic strategies that enhance emotion regulation skills have proven effective in BPD, another area of growing interest involves the investigation of regional brain activity in response to deliberate emotion regulation (Koenigsberg et al., 2009a; Lang et al., 2012; Schulze et al., 2011). There has also been interest in whether changes in neurocircuitry in response to successful psychotherapeutic treatment can be detected in BPD (Lai et al., 2007). One very small study showed that in dialectical behavior therapy responders, there was a decrease in amygdala activation measured with fMRI in response to emotional stimuli (Goodman et al., unpublished data).

ANTISOCIAL PERSONALITY DISORDER

The DSM-IV characterizes antisocial personality disorder (ASPD) as a pervasive pattern of disregard for and violation of the rights of others that has been occurring since the age of 15 years, as indicated by at least three of seven criteria: (*1*) failure to conform to social norms with respect to lawful behaviors as indicated by repeatedly performing acts that are grounds for arrest; (*2*) deceitfulness, as indicated by repeated lying, use of aliases, or conning others for personal profit or pleasure; (*3*) impulsivity or failure to plan ahead; (*4*) irritability and aggressiveness, as indicated by repeated physical fights or assaults; (*5*) reckless disregard for safety of self or others; (*6*) consistent irresponsibility, as indicated by repeated failure to sustain consistent work behavior or honor financial obligations; (*7*) lack of remorse, as indicated by being indifferent to or rationalizing having hurt, mistreated, or stolen from another (APA, 2000). DSM-5 will maintain the same diagnostic criteria, and will include the newly proposed trait-specific classification system in a separate area of Section 3. In Section 3 of the DSM-5, the diagnosis of ASPD is characterized by impairments in personality (self and interpersonal) functioning and the presence of pathological personality traits, including disinhibition (characterized by irresponsibility, impulsivity, and risk-taking) and antagonism (characterized by manipulativeness, deceitfulness, callousness, and hostility).

Antisocial personality disorder is distinct from psychopathy, a construct characterized by pronounced problems in emotional processing (reduced guilt, empathy, and attachment to significant others; callous and unemotional traits) and increased risk for displaying antisocial behavior (Cleckley, 1941; Hare, 2003). The DSM-IV definition of ASPD has been criticized for focusing on the behavioral outcome such as criminality, and ignoring the core personality features such as affective deficits. Despite its association with ASPD, psychopathy is a distinct disorder: Whereas most of those who are diagnosed with psychopathy will also meet criteria for antisocial personality disorder, only about 10% of those with antisocial personality disorder meet criteria for psychopathy (NCCM) 2010; Table 84.1).

Another essential difference between ASPD and psychopathy is the type of aggression characteristic of each disorder. Two types of aggression have been described, which are given various names in the literature (e.g., proactive or instrumental vs. reactive; premeditated vs. impulsive; predatory vs. defensive). These two types differentiate aggressive behavior that is controlled/planned and serves an instrumental, goal-directed end (i.e., a planned robbery to obtain the victim's money) versus aggressive behavior that is more retaliatory/impulsive (i.e., road rage), occurs in response to a threat or perceived threat and is associated with negative affect (i.e., hostility or anger; Dolan, 2010; Ostrov and Houston, 2008). Reactive aggression has been associated with a lack of impulse control (e.g., in

ASPD, intermittent explosive disorder and BPD), whereas instrumental aggression has been uniquely linked to psychopathic features (Blair, 2010; Dolan, 2010; Ostrov and Houston, 2008).

EPIDEMIOLOGY

The 12-month prevalence of antisocial personality disorder (ASPD) was recently estimated to be 3.6% in a nationally representative general population survey (Grant et al., 2004). Antisocial personality disorder is more common in men, who are also more likely to have a persistent course of antisocial behavior when compared with women (NCCM, 2010).

Antisocial personality disorder is associated with a high risk of disorders within the externalizing spectrum, mainly alcohol, nicotine, and drug dependence (Hasin and Kilcoyne, 2012; Hasin et al., 2011). It has been postulated that this high comorbidity suggests common underlying biological contributors (Krueger et al., 2002).

Antisocial personality disorder is also frequently comorbid with other cluster B PDs. This is thought to result from both common genetic and environmental influences. Research suggests that, etiologically, ASPD and BPD are more closely related to each other than to the other cluster B disorders, with both ASPD and BPD showing a second genetic and non-shared environmental factor above and beyond the genetic factor influencing all cluster B disorders (Torgersen et al., 2008).

DEVELOPMENT AND CHILDHOOD ANTECEDENTS

Longitudinal, epidemiological studies have identified several risk factors for antisocial behavior, including maltreatment, harsh and coercive discipline, smoking during pregnancy, divorce, teen parenthood, peer deviance, parental psychopathology (including depression, antisocial behavior, and alcohol use problems), and social disadvantage (including poverty and neighborhood disadvantage; Jaffee et al., 2012), with varying support for causal effects.

Antisocial symptoms with onset in childhood often persist into adulthood and are associated with decreased functioning in educational, employment, interpersonal, and physical health domains (Jaffee et al., 2012).

THE DIMENSION OF IMPULSIVE AGGRESSION IN ANTISOCIAL PERSONALITY DISORDER AND PSYCHOPATHY

Impulsive aggression is believed to be the core dimension underlying ASPD, and is also seen in all the Axis II cluster B PDs, most typically in BPD. The present review will focus on the pathophysiology of impulsive aggression.

REACTIVE AGGRESSION

Reactive aggression is common in ASPD (Blair, 2010; Dolan, 2010; Ostrov and Houston, 2008).

TABLE 84.1. Items in the Hare Psychopathy Checklist-Revised

FACTOR 1: INTERPERSONAL/AFFECTIVE	FACTOR 2: SOCIAL DEVIANCE
1. Glibness/superficial charm	3. Need for stimulation/ proneness to boredom
2. Grandiose sense of self-worth	9. Parasitic lifestyle
4. Pathological lying	10. Poor behavioral controls
5. Conning/manipulative	12. Early behavioral problems
6. Lack of remorse or guilt	13. Lack of realistic long-term goals
7. Shallow affect	14. Impulsivity
8. Callous/lack of empathy	15. Irresponsibility
16. Failure to accept responsibility for own actions	18. Juvenile delinquency
Additional items	19. Revocation of conditional release
11. Promiscuous sexual behaviour	20. Criminal versatility
17. Many short-term marital relationships	

(Hare, R.D. (2003). *Hare Psychopathy Checklist-Revised*, edn 2. Toronto, Multi-Health Systems.)

Animal research suggests that reactive aggression is part of a gradated response to threat: Distant threats induce freezing, closer threats induce flight, and very close threats in which escape is impossible induce reactive aggression. This progressive response to threat is mediated by a threat system that involves the amygdala, the hypothalamus, and the periaqueductal gray. It is believed that this system is regulated by medial, orbital, and inferior frontal cortices (Blair, 2007, 2010). According to this threat system, those individuals at increased risk of showing reactive aggression should show heightened amygdala responses to emotionally provocative stimuli and reduced frontal emotional regulatory activity (Blair, 2010).

INSTRUMENTAL AGGRESSION

Instrumental aggression is characteristic of psychopathy (Blair, 2010; Dolan, 2010; Ostrov and Houston, 2008). Instrumental aggression is hypothesized to be mediated by the motor cortex and the caudate, like any other form of motor response (Blair, 2007). An individual can choose among several available choices of motor response (e.g., instrumental aggression vs. more prosocial behaviors) based on the costs and benefits associated with each choice. For most individuals, the costs of instrumental aggression (e.g., harm to the victim or oneself, risk of punishment) outweigh the benefits, and more prosocial behaviors are chosen instead of instrumental aggression. However, it is believed that individuals with psychopathy initiate instrumental aggression because of dysfunctional representation of the costs of the behavior, related to amygdala and orbitofrontal cortex (OFC) dysfunction (Blair, 2010).

The amygdala is critical for stimulus reinforcement learning and feeding reinforcement expectancy information forward to the OFC to allow good decision making. Because of the hypothesized dysfunction in amygdala and OFC, individuals with psychopathic traits have difficulty socializing (related to dysfunction in stimulus reinforcement learning) and make poor decisions (because of the OFC dysfunction). According to this model, individuals with psychopathic traits should show reduced amygdala and OFC responses to emotional provocation and during emotion-based decision-making tasks (Blair, 2007, 2010).

Research suggests that healthy individuals are predisposed to find distress cues from others aversive and that we learn to avoid behaviors associated with distress cues (i.e., acts that harm others), which is critical for the development of morality. Distress cues from the victim are believed to act as an inhibitor of aggression (Blair, 1995), but this inhibitory mechanism appears to be defective in psychopathy (Blair, 2007).

NEUROIMAGING OF AGGRESSION IN ANTISOCIAL PERSONALITY DISORDER AND PSYCHOPATHY

Although the data strongly support a disruption of amygdala and prefrontal cortex functioning—specifically, in the OFC, ACG, and dorsolateral prefrontal cortex—in individuals with psychopathic traits and/or antisocial behavior, the data for ASPD itself is less conclusive (Nordstrom et al., 2011; Yang and Raine, 2009). This may be because of the heterogeneity of the ASPD diagnosis itself and of the samples and control groups analyzed (e.g., different demographic groups, psychiatric comorbidities). The majority of the studies and metaanalyses focus on broadly defined antisocial constructs, including individuals with ASPD with or without psychopathy, psychopathy with or without ASPD, antisocial behavior, conduct disorder, oppositional defiant disorder, disruptive behavior disorder, criminals, violent offenders, or aggressive individuals (Yang and Raine, 2009). There is a paucity of studies focusing on ASPD specifically, and even fewer studies assessing the effect of comorbid psychopathy on neuroimaging findings in ASPD subjects (Boccardi et al., 2010; Gregory et al., 2012; Tiihonen et al., 2008).

Structural Findings in Antisocial Personality Disorder

Prefrontal abnormalities

Laakso et al. (2002) observed reductions in volume of the dorsolateral, medial frontal, and orbitofrontal cortices in subjects with ASPD. However, after controlling for substance use and education, they concluded that the observed volume deficits were related more to alcoholism or differences in education rather than the diagnosis of ASPD.

Other authors did find reduced prefrontal volumes in ASPD, even after controlling for the effects of substance use (Dolan, 2010; Raine et al., 2000, 2003; Tiihonen et al., 2008). Raine et al. (2010) observed that individuals with cavum septum pellucidum (CSP), a marker of limbic neural maldevelopment, had significantly higher levels of antisocial personality, psychopathy, arrests, and convictions compared with controls, even after controlling for the effects of potential confounders including prior trauma exposure, head injury, demographic factors, or comorbid psychiatric conditions.

Other abnormalities

Antisocial personality disorder subjects have been reported to have smaller temporal lobes (Barkataki et al., 2006; Dolan et al., 2002), smaller whole brain volumes (Barkataki et al., 2006), larger putamen volumes (Barkataki et al., 2006), larger occipital (Tiihonen et al., 2008) and parietal lobes (Tiihonen et al., 2008), larger cerebellum volumes (Tiihonen et al., 2008), decreased volumes in specific areas of the cingulate cortex, insula, and postcentral gyri (Tiihonen et al., 2008), and cortical thinning in medial frontal cortices (Narayan et al., 2007). Raine et al. (2003) found that psychopathic, antisocial subjects had a longer, thinner corpus callosum with overall increased volume compared with healthy controls.

However, other studies (Gregory et al., 2012) found no differences in gray matter volumes between offenders with ASPD without psychopathy and healthy controls.

Functional Neuroimaging in Antisocial Personality Disorder

Most of the few functional neuroimaging studies with subjects diagnosed with ASPD suggest a dysfunction in brain regions involved in emotional processing and learning (Dolan, 2010). The first functional neuroimaging study in ASPD showed that, compared with healthy controls, subjects with BPD or ASPD activated different neural networks during response inhibition in a go/no-go task (Vollm et al., 2004). Although controls mainly activated the prefrontal cortex—specifically the right dorsolateral and the left OFC—during response inhibition, BPD and ASPD patients showed a more bilateral and extended pattern of activation across the medial, superior and inferior frontal gyri extending to the ACG (Vollm et al., 2004).

Some of the studies suggest that at least part of the neural abnormalities found in ASPD subjects may not be specific to this disorder, but rather associated with aggressive traits that are associated with a tendency to violent behavior. For example, Barkataki et al. (2008) found that both violent ASPD subjects and violent schizophrenia patients, but not nonviolent schizophrenia patients showed reduced thalamic activity, in association with modulation of inhibition in a go/no-go task. However, another study by the same group suggests that, although there are neural alterations related to violence found both in violent schizophrenic and violent ASPD patients in occipital and temporal regions, there are interesting differences specific to ASPD and schizophrenia, respectively. Specifically, they found that the violent ASPD subjects showed attenuated thalamic–striatal activity during later periods in a "threat of electric shock" task—whereas in the violent schizophrenic subjects there was hyperactivation in the same areas (Kumari et al., 2009). This suggests that, although there is a shared biological deficit, violent behaviors may arise from different mechanisms according to the specific disorder.

NEUROCOGNITIVE FUNCTION AND AGGRESSION IN ANTISOCIAL PERSONALITY DISORDER AND PSYCHOPATHY

Previous research investigating whether subjects with ASPD have impaired cognitive functioning has yielded inconsistent findings (Crowell et al., 2003; Morgan and Lilienfeld, 2000). Although some authors have found a broad range of deficits in planning ability and set shifting, response inhibition and visual memory, likely mediated by dorsolateral prefrontal cortex and ventromedial prefrontal cortex function in subjects with ASPD (Dolan and Park, 2002), others have only found circumscribed deficits in processing speed (Barkataki et al., 2005) or response inhibition (Barkataki et al., 2008) in ASPD subjects. Moreover, a metaanalysis of 39 studies including 4,589 participants found that, although antisocial behaviors in general were significantly associated with a large effect size for executive dysfunction, the effect size for executive function deficits among subjects with ASPD was statistically significant but negligible (Morgan and Lilienfeld, 2000), and others could find no differences in executive function between ASPD and healthy or psychiatric controls (Crowell et al., 2003). It should be noted that some authors have studied ASPD samples with high rates of psychopathy. Therefore, it is impossible to tease apart the contributions of psychopathy and ASPD respectively to the deficits reported. For example, Dinn et al. (2000) studied 12 ASPD patients, 11 of whom fulfilled criteria for psychopathy. They found that ASPD subjects showed greater deficits on measures of orbitofrontal dysfunction, but not on classical measures of executive function, in comparison with controls (Dinn and Harris, 2000).

Psychopathy has also been associated with executive function deficits as reported in the metaanalysis described in the preceding (Morgan and Lilienfeld, 2000). However, a more recent study found that among offenders with ASPD there was no significant association between executive function impairment and scores on a measure of psychopathy (Dolan, 2011).

GENETIC VULNERABILITY OF AGGRESSION AND ANTISOCIAL PERSONALITY DISORDER

Family, twin, and adoption studies suggest that antisocial spectrum disorders and psychopathy are heritable, with heritability ranging from 0% to 80% in individual studies, and estimated at around half of the variance in most studies and a metaanalysis of antisocial behavior (Rhee and Waldman, 2002; Viding et al., 2008), and even higher when studying externalizing disorders more broadly (Gunter et al., 2010; Krueger et al., 2002) or for certain subtypes, such as those with callous/unemotional traits (Viding et al., 2008).

In the last decade, considerable scientific energy has been focused on identifying specific genetic factors involved in the development of aggressive behavior, as a trait observed in antisocial spectrum disorders and psychopathy. However, despite the great advances in the field, behavioral genetics has yet to elucidate specific genetic pathways that lead to the genesis of the disorders, or develop molecular genetic tests that may inform diagnosis or treatment (Gunter et al., 2010). Association studies on single candidate genes have not yielded any loci with a major effect size. It has been suggested that examining gene by environmental interactions, performing detailed whole genome association studies, functional imaging studies of genetic variants, and examining the role of epigenetics may provide valuable new targets for research (Craig and Halton, 2009).

One of the challenges of the existing research is the heterogeneity of the phenotypes analyzed in different studies, including individuals with ASPD with or without psychopathy, psychopathy with or without ASPD, antisocial behavior, conduct disorder, oppositional defiant disorder, disruptive behavior disorder, criminals, violent offenders, or aggressive individuals, with only a handful of studies focusing on ASPD specifically (Gunter et al., 2010).

Genome-Wide Linkage and Association Studies

Several genome-wide linkage and association studies have suggested possible genomic locations in chromosomes 1, 2, 3, 4, 9, 11, 12, 13, 14, 17, 19, and 20 for antisocial spectrum disorders, but must be interpreted with caution because very few findings reach genome-wide significance, and even fewer have been replicated (Gunter et al., 2010). These studies have focused on diverse phenotypes, including conduct disorder with or without substance use disorders or attention deficit hyperactivity disorder (ADHD), suicidal behavior as a marker of impulsive aggression, or personality traits of psychoticism and neuroticism (Gunter et al., 2010). Of note, only one of these studies specifically included subjects with a diagnosis of ASPD, and found several regions of interest in the genome

(Ehlers et al., 2008). An interesting question for future studies would be to assess whether other constructs (including dimensional personality approaches) may be closer correlates of the underlying genetic factors than the construct of ASPD itself as currently described in the DSM-IV (APA, 2000).

Candidate Genes

The most widely studied genes in antisocial spectrum disorders have been those related to serotonergic and dopaminergic systems, including catechol-O-methyl transferase (COMT), monoamine oxidase A (MAOA), dopamine beta hydroxylase (DBH), tryptophan hydroxylase 1 and 2 (TPH 1 and 2), dopamine receptor D2 (DRD2), dopamine receptor D4 (DRD4), serotonin receptor 1B (5HTR1B), serotonin receptor 2A (5HTR2A), serotonin transporter (5HTT), and dopamine transporter (DAT). Other targets include androgen receptors (AR), based on the gender differences in frequencies of antisocial spectrum disorders, and novel sites such as SNAP25, which was identified as a region of interest in genome-wide studies (Gunter et al., 2010). Currently, the strongest evidence available points to the MAOA and 5HTT genes in antisocial spectrum disorders (Gunter et al., 2010).

In the decade since the seminal study by Caspi et al. (2002) suggesting that MAO genotypes can moderate children's sensitivity to environmental insults, the analysis of gene–environment interaction has received much attention. Some but not all studies have replicated gene–environment interactions in antisocial spectrum disorders (Gunter et al., 2010).

Other interesting avenues of research are those of analysis of gene expression and epigenetic modification of gene expression via methylation and histone modification, but data on the antisocial spectrum are still very scarce (Gunter et al., 2010). Only one study so far has analyzed the impact of epigenetic mechanisms on the development of ASPD symptoms. Beach et al. observed that the degree of methylation at 5HTT mediated the impact of childhood sex abuse on symptoms of ASPD (Beach et al., 2011).

In summary, there is compelling evidence that genes involved in the serotonergic system are implicated in impulsive aggression.

SUMMARY AND FUTURE DIRECTIONS

The ASPD diagnosis comprises a heterogeneous population, limiting neurobiological research efforts. However, considerable progress has been made in the understanding of impulsive aggression, a core dimension of antisocial spectrum disorders and psychopathy, including the roles of the prefrontal cortex, the amygdala, and neurocognitive deficits. The strongest genetic evidence points to the MAOA and 5HTT genes, and promising new approaches include genome wide analyses, epigenetics, gene expression, and neuroimaging genetics.

Using an interdisciplinary research team and a systems approach to the biology of complex illnesses such as antisocial spectrum disorders and psychopathy may help to shed light on the interplay among genetic factors, neural networks, and behavior (Gunter et al., 2010).

SCHIZOTYPAL PERSONALITY DISORDER

Schizotypal personality disorder (STPD), the prototypic schizophrenia personality disorder, is part of the schizophrenia spectrum disorders, characterized by the presence of attenuated symptoms typically present in chronic schizophrenia. The investigation of STPD offers an opportunity to elucidate the pathophysiological mechanisms giving rise to schizophrenia, in a less impaired and less heavily medicated population.

Schizotypal personality disorder is defined by DSM-IV-TR as "a pervasive pattern of social and interpersonal deficits marked by acute discomfort with, and reduced capacity for, close relationships, as well as by cognitive or perceptual distortions and eccentricities of behavior, beginning by early adulthood and present in a variety of contexts," and requires five or more of the following criteria: (1) ideas of reference (excluding delusions of reference); (2) odd beliefs or magical thinking that influences behavior and is inconsistent with subcultural norms (e.g., superstitiousness, belief in clairvoyance, telepathy, or "sixth sense"; in children and adolescents, bizarre fantasies or preoccupations); (3) unusual perceptual experiences, including bodily illusions; (4) odd thinking and speech (e.g., vague, circumstantial, metaphorical, overelaborate, or stereotyped); (5) suspiciousness or paranoid ideation; (6) Inappropriate or constricted affect; (7) behavior or appearance that is odd, eccentric, or peculiar; (8) lack of close friends or confidants other than first-degree relatives; and (9) excessive social anxiety that does not diminish with familiarity and tends to be associated with paranoid fears rather than negative judgments about self (APA, 2000). DSM-5 will maintain the same diagnostic criteria, and will include the newly proposed trait-specific classification system in a separate area of Section 3. In Section 3 of DSM-5, STPD is characterized by impairments in personality (self and interpersonal) functioning and the presence of pathological personality traits, including psychoticism, detachment, and negative affectivity (http://www.dsm5.org/proposedrevision/Pages/proposedrevision.aspx?rid=15#).

EPIDEMIOLOGY

The median prevalence of STPD had been estimated at 0.7% in the general population (Torgersen et al., 2001); however, recently a lifetime prevalence of 3.9% was reported in a large, nationally representative US community sample (Pulay et al., 2009). Schizotypal personality disorder is more frequent among males than females (Pulay et al., 2009).

More than 80% of those with STPD also suffer other comorbid personality disorders, especially BPD (Pulay et al., 2009) and narcissistic PD (Pulay et al., 2009). Lifetime comorbidity with Axis I disorders is high as well: 67% of individuals with STPD have at least one mood disorder, greater than 70% have at least one anxiety disorder, and greater than 65% have a substance use disorder (Pulay et al., 2009).

Schizotypal personality disorder is one of the DSM-IV PDs most strongly associated with reduced functioning (Pulay et al., 2009) with significantly worse levels of impairment than among patients with other PDs or major depressive disorder (Skodol et al., 2002).

PUTATIVE ETIOLOGIC FACTORS AND PATHOPHYSIOLOGY

The neurobiological factors underlying the genesis of STPD may be conceptualized in relation to each of the core traits of the disorder (psychotic-like symptoms and cognitive organization disturbances). In this way, disturbances in cognitive organization and information processing may contribute to the detachment, desynchrony with the environment, and cognitive/perceptual distortions of STPD and other schizophrenia spectrum personality disorders (Siever and Weinstein, 2009).

PSYCHOTICISM DIMENSION

Psychotic-like symptomatology is characteristic of STPD patients. Like in schizophrenia, increased dopaminergic neurotransmission is associated with more prominent psychotic symptoms, and the dimension of psychotic-like perceptual distortions has been correlated with measures of dopaminergic activity. The fact that STPD patients have less prominent psychotic symptoms than patients with schizophrenia is believed to be caused by better buffered subcortical dopaminergic activity (Siever and Davis, 2004; Siever and Weinstein, 2009). The results of functional and structural imaging and neuroendocrine challenge studies support this hypothesis. This better buffering system may result in less responsiveness to stress by subcortical dopaminergic systems, which may protect against psychosis (Mitropoulou et al., 2004; Siever and Davis, 2004; Siever and Weinstein, 2009).

It has been suggested that dopaminergic activity can be relatively increased or decreased, depending on the predominance of psychosis-like (hypervigilance and stereotypic cognitions/behaviors) or deficit-like (deficits in working memory, cognitive processing, and hedonic tone) symptoms (Siever and Davis, 2004).

Dopaminergic candidate genes including the dopamine D4 receptor and the dopamine β-hydroxylase gene have been found to be associated with psychosis-like symptomatology (Siever and Davis, 2004; Siever and Weinstein, 2009).

In summary, STPD patients share some of the dopaminergic abnormalities underlying psychotic-like symptoms found in schizophrenia, but in a more attenuated form, likely because of better buffered subcortical dopaminergic activity.

COGNITIVE IMPAIRMENT DIMENSION/ DEFICIT SYMPTOMS

Research data suggest that patients with STPD suffer cognitive impairment, likely related to structural brain abnormalities, especially in the temporal cortex, similar to those seen in patients with schizophrenia. Despite these similarities, STPD patients differ from schizophrenia patients in that they have less impaired executive function—likely owing to greater reserves in prefrontal function (Siever and Davis, 2004; Siever and Weinstein, 2009).

Specifically, patients with STPD have increased ventricular volumes, and frontotemporal volume reductions similar but milder than those seen in schizophrenic patients, with sparing of some key regions (Hazlett et al., 2008).

Specific cognitive dimensions found to be impaired in STPD include attention, visual and auditory working memory, verbal learning and memory, and STPD individuals perform poorly on executive function tasks. However, the more generalized intellectual deficits found in schizophrenia are not observed in STPD (McClure et al., 2007; Siever and Weinstein, 2009).

These cognitive deficits may contribute to the impairments in social rapport and inability to read social cues seen in STPD patients. Actually, deficits in working memory have been correlated with interpersonal impairment (Mitropoulou et al., 2005).

Decreased dopaminergic and noradrenergic activity in the prefrontal cortex may contribute to the cognitive impairment in STPD. This is consistent with functional studies showing decreases in frontal activation during executive functioning tasks in STPD subjects. However, unlike schizophrenic patients and normal subjects, STPD subjects appear to activate other compensatory regions during executive function tasks (Koenigsberg et al., 2005).

Working memory has been shown to improve after pharmacological interventions with guanfacine, an alpha2 adrenergic agonist, and pergolide, a D1/D2 agonist (McClure et al., 2007, 2010).

Schizotypal personality disorder subjects also suffer deficits in information processing, reflected in physiological impairments seen in the schizophrenia spectrum. These include deficits in prepulse inhibition (PPI) of the acoustic startle response, the startle blink paradigm, the P50 evoked potential paradigm, or smooth pursuit eye movement among others (see Siever and Davis, 2004, for a review).

In summary, STPD subjects show cognitive and physiological impairments that seem to be partially caused by reduced prefrontal dopaminergic function and that can be partly reversed with dopamine agonists and partially compensated by activation in other brain areas not used by healthy controls.

GENETIC VULNERABILITY

Schizotypal personality disorder is partly heritable (Kendler et al., 2006), and its genetic factors overlap with those for schizophrenia and other schizophrenia spectrum disorders (Fanous et al., 2007; Siever, 2005). It has been suggested that positive and negative symptoms of STPD represent two distinct heritable dimensions. Thus, in disorders of the schizophrenia spectrum, a set of genetic factors expressed as social and cognitive deficits (spectrum phenotype) might be transmitted independently from a second genetic factor set related to psychosis (psychotic phenotype) (Siever and Davis, 2004).

A polymorphism of catechol-o-methyl-transferase (COMT), which metabolizes dopamine and regulates its activity in the frontal cortex, has been associated with working memory deficits and other cognitive deficits both in schizophrenic and schizotypal subjects (Ma et al., 2007; Smyrnis et al., 2007).

A recent study on a risk for psychosis haplotype of the proline dehydrogenase gene found that, in healthy controls, the psychosis variant was associated with PPI and verbal memory deficits as well as higher anxiety and schizotypal personality traits (Roussos et al., 2009).

In a large cohort of young healthy individuals, Stefanis et al. showed an association between common variants in G-protein signaling 4 (RGS4) and D-amino acid oxidase (DAAO) genes with negative schizotypal personality traits; dysbindin (DTNBP1) variants were associated with positive and paranoid schizotypy measures (Stefanis et al., 2007, 2008).

Finally, preliminary results from our group using the custom Consortium on the Genetics of Schizophrenia (COGS) 1,536-SNP chip found a strong association between polymorphisms in ERBB4, NRG1 and genes involved in glutamate, dopamine, GABA and serotonin receptors signaling, as well as cell signal transduction, with categorical clinical diagnosis (STPD vs. healthy controls) and dimensional quantitative phenotypes of STPD, including cognitive impairment, interpersonal deficits, and paranoia (Siever and Roussos, unpublished data).

In summary, several genetic variants have been associated with STPD traits and/or dimensional quantitative phenotypes of STPD, including cognitive impairment symptoms, opening promising avenues for research and pharmacological targets.

CONCLUSIONS

Increasing evidence suggests that several of the personality disorders that have been most studied including BPD, STPD, and ASPD have distinct neurobiological substrates that emerge from genetic susceptibilities, that are beginning to be identified, interacting with the environment. These categorical personality disorders can also be mapped into dimensions that extend across personality disorders and may even extend into normal personality.

A better understanding of the neurocircuitry underlying the personality disorders and their modulation by neuropeptides and neurotransmitters may help us intervene pharmacologically and even provide a base for predictors of outcome and a mechanism of action in the brain for psychosocial treatments for these disorders.

DISCLOSURES

Dr. Perez has no conflicts of interests to disclose. She is funded by the Department of Veterans Affairs (VISN3) Mental Illness Research, Education, and Clinical Center (MIRECC).

Dr. Siever has no conflicts of interest to disclose. His salary comes from the Peters VA and Mt. Sinai Medical school.

Dr. New has no conflicts of interest to disclose. Her salary comes from the James J Peters VA and Mount Sinai School of Medicine.

REFERENCES

American Psychiatric Association (APA). (2000). Diagnostic and Statistical Manual of Mental Disorders, 4th Edition, Text Revision. Washington, DC: Author.

Asberg, M., and Traskman, L. (1981). Studies of CSF 5-HIAA in depression and suicidal behaviour. Adv. Exp. Med. Biol. 133:739–752.

Asberg, M., Traskman-Benz, L., et al. (1976). 5-HIAA in the cerebrospinal fluid a biochemical suicide predictor. Arch. Gen. Psychiatry 33:1193–1197.

Barkataki, I., Kumari, V., et al. (2005). A neuropsychological investigation into violence and mental illness. Schizophr. Res. 74(1):1–13.

Barkataki, I., Kumari, V., et al. (2006). Volumetric structural brain abnormalities in men with schizophrenia or antisocial personality disorder. Behav. Brain Res. 169(2):239–247.

Barkataki, I., Kumari, V., et al. (2008). Neural correlates of deficient response inhibition in mentally disordered violent individuals. Behav. Sci. Law 26(1):51–64.

Bartz, J., Simeon, D., et al. (2011). Oxytocin can hinder trust and cooperation in borderline personality disorder. Soc. Cogn. Affect. Neurosci. 6(5):556–563.

Beach, S.R., Brody, G.H., et al. (2011). Methylation at 5HTT mediates the impact of child sex abuse on women's antisocial behavior: an examination of the Iowa adoptee sample. Psychosom. Med. 73(1):83–87.

Beblo, T., Driessen, M., et al. (2006). Functional MRI correlates of the recall of unresolved life events in borderline personality disorder. Psychol. Med. 36(6):845–856.

Bender, D.S., and Skodol, A.E. (2007). Borderline personality as a self-other representational disturbance. J. Personal. Disord. 21(5):500–517.

Bender, D.S., Skodol, A.E., et al. (2006). Prospective assessment of treatment use by patients with personality disorders. Psychiatr. Serv. 57(2):254–257.

Bierer, L.M., Yehuda, R., et al. (2003). Abuse and neglect in childhood: relationship to personality disorder diagnoses. CNS Spectr. 8(10):737–754.

Blair, R.J. (1995). A cognitive developmental approach to mortality: investigating the psychopath. Cognition 57(1):1–29.

Blair, R.J. (2007). The amygdala and ventromedial prefrontal cortex in morality and psychopathy. Trends Cogn. Sci. 11(9):387–392.

Blair, R.J. (2010). Neuroimaging of psychopathy and antisocial behavior: a targeted review. Curr. Psychiatry Rep. 12(1):76–82.

Blumberg, H.P., Leung, H.C., et al. (2003). A functional magnetic resonance imaging study of bipolar disorder: state- and trait-related dysfunction in ventral prefrontal cortices. Arch. Gen. Psychiatry 60(6):601–609.

Boccardi, M., Ganzola, R., et al. (2010). Abnormal hippocampal shape in offenders with psychopathy. Hum. Brain Mapp. 31(3):438–447.

Bohus, M., Schmahl, C., et al. (2004). New developments in the neurobiology of borderline personality disorder. Curr. Psychiatry Rep. 6(1):43–50.

Brambilla, P., Soloff, P.H., et al. (2004). Anatomical MRI study of borderline personality disorder patients. Psychiatry Res. 131(2):125–133.

Brunner, R., Henze, R., et al. (2010). Reduced prefrontal and orbitofrontal gray matter in female adolescents with borderline personality disorder: is it disorder specific? NeuroImage 49(1):114–120.

Caspi, A., McClay, J., et al. (2002). Role of genotype in the cycle of violence in maltreated children. Science 297(5582):851–854.

Chanen, A.M., Velakoulis, D., et al. (2008). Orbitofrontal, amygdala and hippocampal volumes in teenagers with first-presentation borderline personality disorder. Psychiatry Res. 131(2):125–133.

Cleckley, H. (1941). The Mask of Sanity: An Attempt to Reinterpret the So-Called Psychopathic Personality. St. Louis, MO: Mosby.

Coccaro, E. (1989). Central serotonin and impulsive aggression. Br. J. Psychiatry 155(Suppl. 8):52–62.

Coccaro, E.F., Siever, L.J., et al. (1989). Serotonergic studies in patients with affective and personality disorders: correlates with suicidal and impulsive aggressive behavior. Arch. Gen. Psychiatry 46:587–599.

Costa, P., Jr., and Widiger, T. (2002). Personality Disorders and the Five-Factor Model of Personality, 2nd Edition. Washington, DC: American Psychological Association.

Craig, I.W., and Halton, K.E. (2009). Genetics of human aggressive behaviour. Hum. Genet. 126(1):101–113.

Crowell, T.A., Kieffer, K.M., et al. (2003). Executive and nonexecutive neuropsychological functioning in antisocial personality disorder. Cogn. Behav. Neurol. 16(2):100–109.

Davidson, R.J., Irwin, W., et al. (2003). The neural substrates of affective processing in depressed patients treated with venlafaxine. Am. J. Psychiatry 160(1):64–75.

de-Almeida, C.P., Wenzel, A., et al. (2012). Amygdalar volume in borderline personality disorder with and without comorbid post-traumatic stress disorder: a meta-analysis. CNS Spectr. 17(2):70–75.

Dinn, W.M., and Harris, C.L. (2000). Neurocognitive function in antisocial personality disorder. Psychiatry Res. 97(2–3):173–190.

Distel, M.A., Trull, T.J., et al. (2008). Heritability of borderline personality disorder features is similar across three countries. Psychol. Med. 38(9):1219–1229.

Dolan, M. (2011). The neuropsychology of prefrontal function in antisocial personality disordered offenders with varying degrees of psychopathy. Psychol. Med. 31:1–11.

Dolan, M., and Park, I. (2002). The neuropsychology of antisocial personality disorder. *Psychol. Med.* 32(3):417–427.

Dolan, M.C. (2010). What imaging tells us about violence in anti-social men. *Crim. Behav. Ment. Health.* 20(3):199–214.

Dolan, M.C., Deakin, J.F., et al. (2002). Quantitative frontal and temporal structural MRI studies in personality-disordered offenders and control subjects. *Psychiatry Res.* 116(3):133–149.

Donegan, N.H., Sanislow, C.A., et al. (2003). Amygdala hyperreactivity in borderline personality disorder: implications for emotional dysregulation. *Biol. Psychiatry* 54(11):1284–1293.

Dougherty, D.M., Bjork, J.M., et al. (1999). Laboratory measures of aggression and impulsivity in women with borderline personality disorder. *Psychiatry Res.* 85(3):315–326.

Dyck, M., Habel, U., et al. (2009). Negative bias in fast emotion discrimination in borderline personality disorder. *Psychol. Med.* 39(5):855–864.

Dziobek, I., Preissler, S., et al. (2011). Neuronal correlates of altered empathy and social cognition in borderline personality disorder. *NeuroImage* 57(2):539–548.

Eaton, N.R., Krueger, R.F., et al. (2011). Borderline personality disorder co-morbidity: relationship to the internalizing-externalizing structure of common mental disorders. *Psychol. Med.* 41(5):1041–1050.

Ehlers, C.L., Gilder, D.A., et al. (2008). Externalizing disorders in American Indians: comorbidity and a genome wide linkage analysis. *Am. J. Med. Genet. B Neuropsychiatr. Genet.* 147B(6):690–698.

Fanous, A.H., Neale, M.C., et al. (2007). Significant correlation in linkage signals from genome-wide scans of schizophrenia and schizotypy. *Mol. Psychiatry* 12(10):958–965.

Fossati, A., Madeddu, F., et al. (1999). Borderline personality disorder and childhood sexual abuse: a meta-analytic study. *J. Pers. Disord.* 13(3):268–280.

Frankle, W.G., Lombardo, I., et al. (2005). Brain serotonin transporter distribution in subjects with impulsive aggressivity: a positron emission study with [11C]McN 5652. *Am. J. Psychiatry* 162(5):915–923.

Franzen, N., Hagenhoff, M., et al. (2010). Superior "theory of mind" in borderline personality disorder: an analysis of interaction behavior in a virtual trust game. *Psychiatry Res.* 187(1–2):224–233.

Golier, J.A., Yehuda, R., et al. (2003). The relationship of borderline personality disorder to posttraumatic stress disorder and traumatic events. *Am. J. Psychiatry* 160(11):2018–2024.

Goodman, M., Hazlett, E.A., et al. (2010). Anterior cingulate volume reduction in adolescents with borderline personality disorder and co-morbid major depression. *J. Psychiatr. Res.* 45(6):803–807.

Goyer, P.F., Andreason, P.J., et al. (1994). Positron-emission tomography and personality disorders. *Neuropsychopharmacology* 10(1):21–28.

Grant, B.F., Chou, S.P., et al. (2008). Prevalence, correlates, disability, and comorbidity of DSM-IV borderline personality disorder: results from the Wave 2 National Epidemiologic Survey on Alcohol and Related Conditions. *J. Clin. Psychiatry* 69(4):533–545.

Grant, B.F., Stinson, F.S., et al. (2004). Co-occurrence of 12-month alcohol and drug use disorders and personality disorders in the United States: results from the National Epidemiologic Survey on Alcohol and Related Conditions. *Arch. Gen. Psychiatry* 61(4):361–368.

Grant, J.E., Correia, S., et al. (2007). Frontal white matter integrity in borderline personality disorder with self-injurious behavior. *J. Neuropsychiatry Clin. Neurosci.* 19(4):383–390.

Gregory, S., Ffytche, D., et al. (2012). The antisocial brain: psychopathy matters: a structural MRI investigation of antisocial male violent offenders. *Arch. Gen. Psychiatry* 69(9):962–972.

Gunter, T.D., Vaughn, M.G., et al. (2010). Behavioral genetics in antisocial spectrum disorders and psychopathy: a review of the recent literature. *Behav. Sci. Law* 28(2):148–173.

Hare, R.D. (2003). Hare Psychopathy Checklist-Revised, 2nd Edition. Toronto: Multi-Health Systems.

Hasin, D., Fenton, M.C., et al. (2011). Personality disorders and the 3-year course of alcohol, drug, and nicotine use disorders. *Arch. Gen. Psychiatry* 68(11):1158–1167.

Hasin, D., and Kilcoyne, B. (2012). Comorbidity of psychiatric and substance use disorders in the United States: current issues and findings from the NESARC. *Curr. Opin. Psychiatry* 25(3):165–171.

Hazlett, E.A., Buchsbaum, M.S., et al. (2008). Cortical gray and white matter volume in unmedicated schizotypal and schizophrenia patients. *Schizophr. Res.* 101(1–3):111–123.

Hazlett, E.A., New, A.S., et al. (2005). Reduced anterior and posterior cingulate gray matter in borderline personality disorder. *Biol. Psychiatry* 58(8):614–623.

Hazlett, E.A., Speiser, L.J., et al. (2007). Exaggerated affect-modulated startle during unpleasant stimuli in borderline personality disorder. *Biol. Psychiatry* 62(3):250–255.

Insel, T., Cuthbert, B., et al. (2010). Research domain criteria (RDoC): toward a new classification framework for research on mental disorders. *Am. J. Psychiatry* 167(7):748–751.

Irle, E., Lange, C., et al. (2005). Reduced size and abnormal asymmetry of parietal cortex in women with borderline personality disorder. *Biol. Psychiatry* 57(2):173–182.

Jaffee, S.R., Strait, L.B., et al. (2012). From correlates to causes: can quasi-experimental studies and statistical innovations bring us closer to identifying the causes of antisocial behavior? *Psychol. Bull.* 138(2):272–295.

Kendler, K.S., Aggen, S.H., et al. (2011a). The structure of genetic and environmental risk factors for syndromal and subsyndromal common DSM-IV axis I and all axis II disorders. *Am. J. Psychiatry* 168(1):29–39.

Kendler, K.S., Czajkowski, N., et al. (2006). Dimensional representations of DSM-IV cluster A personality disorders in a population-based sample of Norwegian twins: a multivariate study. *Psychol. Med.* 36(11):1583–1591.

Kendler, K.S., Myers, J., et al. (2011b). Borderline personality disorder traits and their relationship with dimensions of normative personality: a web-based cohort and twin study. *Acta Psychiatr. Scand.* 123(5):349–359.

King-Casas, B., Sharp, C., et al. (2008). The rupture and repair of cooperation in borderline personality disorder. *Science* 321(5890):806–810.

Koenigsberg, H.W., Buchsbaum, M.S., et al. (2005). Functional MRI of visuospatial working memory in schizotypal personality disorder: a region-of-interest analysis. *Psychol. Med.* 35(7):1019–1030.

Koenigsberg, H.W., Fan, J., et al. (2009a). Neural correlates of the use of psychological distancing to regulate responses to negative social cues: a study of patients with borderline personality disorder. *Biol. Psychiatry* 66(9):854–863.

Koenigsberg, H.W., Siever, L.J., et al. (2009b). Neural correlates of emotion processing in borderline personality disorder. *Psychiatry Res.* 172(3):192–199.

Kornstein, S.G., and Schneider, R.K. (2001). Clinical features of treatment-resistant depression. *J. Clin. Psychiatry* 62(16):18–25.

Kraus, A., Esposito, F., et al. (2009). Amygdala deactivation as a neural correlate of pain processing in patients with borderline personality disorder and co-occurrent posttraumatic stress disorder. *Biol. Psychiatry* 65(9):819–822.

Krueger, R.F. (1999). The structure of common mental disorders. *Arch. Gen. Psychiatry* 56(10):921–926.

Krueger, R.F., Hicks, B.M., et al. (2002). Etiologic connections among substance dependence, antisocial behavior, and personality: modeling the externalizing spectrum. *J. Abnorm. Psychol.* 111(3):411–424.

Kumari, V., Das, M., et al. (2009). Neural and behavioural responses to threat in men with a history of serious violence and schizophrenia or antisocial personality disorder. *Schizophr. Res.* 110(1–3):47–58.

Laakso, M.P., Gunning-Dixon, F., et al. (2002). Prefrontal volumes in habitually violent subjects with antisocial personality disorder and type 2 alcoholism. *Psychiatry Res.* 114(2):95–102.

Lai, C., Daini, S., et al. (2007). Neural correlates of psychodynamic psychotherapy in borderline disorders: a pilot investigation. *Psychother. Psychosom.* 76(6):403–405.

Lang, S., Kotchoubey, B., et al. (2012). Cognitive reappraisal in trauma-exposed women with borderline personality disorder. *NeuroImage* 59(2):1727–1734.

Leichsenring, F., Leibing, E., et al. (2011). Borderline personality disorder. *Lancet* 377(9759):74–84.

Lenzenweger, M.F., Lane, M.C., et al. (2007). DSM-IV personality disorders in the National Comorbidity Survey Replication. *Biol. Psychiatry* 62(6):553–564.

Leyton, M., Okazawa, H., et al. (2001). Brain Regional alpha-[11C] methyl-L-tryptophan trapping in impulsive subjects with borderline personality disorder. *Am. J. Psychiatry* 158(5):775–782.

Lynch, T., Rosenthal, M.Z., et al. (2006). Heightened sensitivity to facial expressions of emotion in borderline personality disorder. *Emotion* 6(4):647–655.

Ma, X., Sun, J., et al. (2007). A quantitative association study between schizotypal traits and COMT, PRODH and BDNF genes in a healthy Chinese population. *Psychiatry Res.* 153(1):7–15.

Macdonald, K., and Macdonald, T.M. (2010). The peptide that binds: a systematic review of oxytocin and its prosocial effects in humans. *Harv. Rev. Psychiatry* 18(1):1–21.

Mauchnik, J., and Schmahl, C. (2010). The latest neuroimaging findings in borderline personality disorder. *Curr. Psychiatry Rep.* 12(1):46–55.

McClure, M.M., Barch, D.M., et al. (2007). The effects of guanfacine on context processing abnormalities in schizotypal personality disorder. *Biol. Psychiatry* 61(10):1157–1160.

McClure, M.M., Harvey, P.D., et al. (2010). Pergolide treatment of cognitive deficits associated with schizotypal personality disorder: continued evidence of the importance of the dopamine system in the schizophrenia spectrum. *Neuropsychopharmacology* 35(6):1356–1362.

McClure, M.M., Romero, M.J., et al. (2007). Visual-spatial learning and memory in schizotypal personality disorder: continued evidence for the importance of working memory in the schizophrenia spectrum. *Arch. Clin. Neuropsychol.* 22(1):109–116.

Meyer-Lindenberg, A. (2008). Impact of prosocial neuropeptides on human brain function. *Prog. Brain Res.* 170:463–470.

Minzenberg, M.J., Fan, J., et al. (2007). Fronto-limbic dysfunction in response to facial emotion in borderline personality disorder: an event-related fMRI study. *Psychiatry Res.* 155(3):231–243.

Minzenberg, M.J., Fan, J., et al. (2008). Frontolimbic structural changes in borderline personality disorder. *J. Psychiatr. Res.* 42(9):727–733

Minzenberg, M.J., Poole, J.H., et al. (2006). Social-emotion recognition in borderline personality disorder. *Compr. Psychiatry* 47(6):468–474.

Mitropoulou, V., Goodman, M., et al. (2004). Effects of acute metabolic stress on the dopaminergic and pituitary-adrenal axis activity in patients with schizotypal personality disorder. *Schizophr. Res.* 70(1):27–31.

Mitropoulou, V., Harvey, P.D., et al. (2005). Neuropsychological performance in schizotypal personality disorder: importance of working memory. *Am. J. Psychiatry* 162(10):1896–1903.

Morgan, A.B., and Lilienfeld, S.O. (2000). A meta-analytic review of the relation between antisocial behavior and neuropsychological measures of executive function. *Clin. Psychol. Rev.* 20(1):113–136.

Narayan, V.M., Narr, K.L., et al. (2007). Regional cortical thinning in subjects with violent antisocial personality disorder or schizophrenia. *Am. J. Psychiatry* 164(9):1418–1427.

National Collaborating Centre For Mental Health (2010). Antisocial Personality Disorder: Treatment, Management and Prevention. (NICE Clinical Guidelines, No. 77). Leicester, UK: British Psychological Society.

New, A.S., Buchsbaum, M.S., et al. (2004). Fluoxetine increases relative metabolic rate in prefrontal cortex in impulsive aggression. *Psychopharmacol. (Berl.)* 176(3–4):451–458.

New, A.S., Goodman, M., et al. (2008a). Recent advances in the biological study of personality disorders. *Psychiatr. Clin. North Am.* 31(3):441–461, vii.

New, A.S., Hazlett, E., et al. (2002). Blunted prefrontal cortical 18fluorodeoxyglucose positron emission tomography response to meta-chloropiperazine in impulsive aggression. *Arch. Gen. Psychiatry* 59(7):621–629.

New, A.S., Hazlett, E.A., et al. (2007). Amygdala-prefrontal disconnection in borderline personality disorder. *Neuropsychopharmacology* 32(7):1629–1640.

New, A.S., Hazlett, E.A., et al. (2009). Laboratory induced aggression: a positron emission tomography study of aggressive individuals with borderline personality disorder. *Biol. Psychiatry* 66(12):1107–1114.

New, A.S., Perez-Rodriguez, M.M., et al. (2012). Neuroimaging and borderline personality disorder. *Psychiatr. Ann.* 42(2):65–71.

New, A.S., and Stanley, B. (2010). An opioid deficit in borderline personality disorder: self-cutting, substance abuse, and social dysfunction. *Am. J. Psychiatry* 167(8):882–885.

New, A.S., Triebwasser, J., et al. (2008b). The case for shifting borderline personality disorder to Axis I. *Biol. Psychiatry* 64(8):653–659.

Niedtfeld, I., Schulze, L., et al. (2010). Affect regulation and pain in borderline personality disorder: a possible link to the understanding of self-injury. *Biol. Psychiatry* 68(4):383–391.

Nordstrom, B.R., Gao, Y., et al. (2011). Neurocriminology. *Adv. Genet.* 75:255–283.

Nunes, P.M., Wenzel, A., et al. (2009). Volumes of the hippocampus and amygdala in patients with borderline personality disorder: a meta-analysis. *J. Pers. Disord.* 23(4):333–345.

O'Keane, V., Maloney, E., et al. (1992). Blunted prolactin response to D-fenfluramine in sociopathy: evidence for subsensitivity of central serotonergic function. *Br. J. Psychiatry* 160:643–646.

Oldham, J.M. (2006). Borderline personality disorder and suicidality. *Am. J. Psychiatry* 163(1):20–26.

Ostrov, J.M., and Houston, R.J. (2008). The utility of forms and functions of aggression in emerging adulthood: association with personality disorder symptomatology. *J. Youth Adolescence* 37(9):1147–1158.

Patrick, C.J., Fowles, D.C., et al. (2009). Triarchic conceptualization of psychopathy: developmental origins of disinhibition, boldness, and meanness. *Dev. Psychopathol.* 21(3):913–938.

Prossin, A.R., Love, T.M., et al. (2010). Dysregulation of regional endogenous opioid function in borderline personality disorder. *Am. J. Psychiatry* 167(8):925–933.

Pulay, A.J., Stinson, F.S., et al. (2009). Prevalence, correlates, disability, and comorbidity of DSM-IV schizotypal personality disorder: results from the wave 2 national epidemiologic survey on alcohol and related conditions. *Prim. Care Companion J. Clin. Psychiatry* 11(2):53–67.

Raine, A., Lee, L., et al. (2010). Neurodevelopmental marker for limbic maldevelopment in antisocial personality disorder and psychopathy. *Br. J. Psychiatry* 197(3):186–192.

Raine, A., Lencz, T., et al. (2000). Reduced prefrontal gray matter volume and reduced autonomic activity in antisocial personality disorder. *Arch. Gen. Psychiatry* 57(2):119–127; discussion 128–119.

Raine, A., Lencz, T., et al. (2003). Corpus callosum abnormalities in psychopathic antisocial individuals. *Arch. Gen. Psychiatry* 60(11):1134–1142.

Rhee, S.H., and Waldman, I.D. (2002). Genetic and environmental influences on antisocial behavior: a meta-analysis of twin and adoption studies. *Psychol. Bull.* 128(3):490–529.

Roussos, P., Giakoumaki, S.G., et al. (2009). A risk PRODH haplotype affects sensorimotor gating, memory, schizotypy, and anxiety in healthy male subjects. *Biol. Psychiatry* 65(12):1063–1070.

Roysamb, E., Kendler, K.S., et al. (2011). The joint structure of DSM-IV Axis I and Axis II disorders. *J. Abnorm. Psychol.* 120(1):198–209.

Ruocco, A.C., Amirthavasagam, S., et al. (2012). Amygdala and hippocampal volume reductions as candidate endophenotypes for borderline personality disorder: a meta-analysis of magnetic resonance imaging studies. *Psychiatry Res.* 201(3):245–252.

Rusch, N., Bracht, T., et al. (2010). Reduced interhemispheric structural connectivity between anterior cingulate cortices in borderline personality disorder. *Psychiatry Res.* 181(2):151–154.

Samuel, D.B., and Widiger, T.A. (2008). A meta-analytic review of the relationships between the five-factor model and DSM-IV-TR personality disorders: a facet level analysis. *Clin. Psychol. Rev.* 28(8):1326–1342.

Samuel, D.B., and Widiger, T.W. (2010). Comparing personality disorder models: cross-method assessment of the FFM and DSM-IV-TR. *J. Pers. Disord.* 24(6):721–745.

Sansone, R.A., and Sansone, L.A. (2011). Gender patterns in borderline personality disorder. *Innov. Clin. Neurosci.* 8(5):16–20.

Schmahl, C., Berne, K., et al. (2009). Hippocampus and amygdala volumes in patients with borderline personality disorder with or without posttraumatic stress disorder. *J. Psychiatry Neurosci.* 34(4):289–295.

Schmahl, C., Bohus, M., et al. (2006). Neural correlates of antinociception in borderline personality disorder. *Arch. Gen. Psychiatry* 63(6):659–667.

Schmahl, C.G., Elzinga, B.M., et al. (2003). Neural correlates of memories of abandonment in women with and without borderline personality disorder. *Biol. Psychiatry* 54(2):142–151.

Schnell, K., Dietrich, T., et al. (2007). Processing of autobiographical memory retrieval cues in borderline personality disorder. *J. Affect. Disord.* 97(1–3):253–259.

Schulze, L., Domes, G., et al. (2011). Neuronal correlates of cognitive reappraisal in borderline patients with affective instability. *Biol. Psychiatry* 69(6):564–573.

Shin, L.M., McNally, R.J., et al. (1999). Regional cerebral blood flow during script-driven imagery in childhood sexual abuse-related PTSD: a PET investigation. *Am. J. Psychiatry* 156(4):575–584.

Siever, L.J. (2005). Endophenotypes in the personality disorders. *Dialogues Clin. Neurosci.* 7(2):139–151.

Siever, L.J. (2008). Neurobiology of aggression and violence. *Am. J. Psychiatry* 165(4):429–442.

Siever, L.J., Buchsbaum, M.S., et al. (1999). D,L-fenfluramine response in impulsive personality disorder assessed with [18F]fluorodeoxyglucose positron emission tomography. *Neuropsychopharmacology* 20(5):413–423.

Siever, L.J., and Davis, K.L. (2004). The pathophysiology of schizophrenia disorders: perspectives from the spectrum. *Am. J. Psychiatry* 161(3):398–413.

Siever, L.J., and Weinstein, L.N. (2009). The neurobiology of personality disorders: implications for psychoanalysis. *J. Am. Psychoanal. Assoc.* 57(2):361–398.

Silbersweig, D., Clarkin, J.F., et al. (2007). Failure of frontolimbic inhibitory function in the context of negative emotion in borderline personality disorder. *Am. J. Psychiatry* 164(12):1832–1841.

Simeon, D., Bartz, J., et al. (2011). Oxytocin administration attenuates stress reactivity in borderline personality disorder: a pilot study. *Psychoneuroendocrinology* 36(9):1418–1421.

Skodol, A.E., Bender, D.S., et al. (2011). Personality disorder types proposed for DSM-5. *J. Pers. Disord.* 25(2):136–169.

Skodol, A.E., Gunderson, J.G., et al. (2002). Functional impairment in patients with schizotypal, borderline, avoidant, or obsessive-compulsive personality disorder. *Am. J. Psychiatry* 159(2):276–283.

Skodol, A.E., Gunderson, J.G., et al. (2005). The Collaborative Longitudinal Personality Disorders Study (CLPS): overview and implications. *J. Pers. Disord.* 19(5):487–504.

Skodol, A.E., Pagano, M.E., et al. (2005). Stability of functional impairment in patients with schizotypal, borderline, avoidant, or obsessive-compulsive personality disorder over two years. *Psychol. Med.* 35(3):443–451.

Smyrnis, N., Avramopoulos, D., et al. (2007). Effect of schizotypy on cognitive performance and its tuning by COMT val158 met genotype variations in a large population of young men. *Biol. Psychiatry* 61(7): 845–853.

Soloff, P., Nutche, J., et al. (2008). Structural brain abnormalities in borderline personality disorder: a voxel-based morphometry study. *Psychiatry Res.* 164(3):223–236.

Soloff, P.H., Meltzer, C.C., et al. (2000). A fenfluramine-activated FDG-PET study of borderline personality disorder. *Biol. Psychiatry* 47:540–547.

Stanley, B., Sher, L., et al. (2009). Non-suicidal self-injurious behavior, endogenous opioids and monoamine neurotransmitters. *J. Affect. Disord.* 167(8):925–933.

Stanley, B., and Siever, L.J. (2010). The interpersonal dimension of borderline personality disorder: toward a neuropeptide model. *Am. J. Psychiatry* 167(1):24–39.

Stefanis, N.C., Trikalinos, T.A., et al. (2008). Association of RGS4 variants with schizotypy and cognitive endophenotypes at the population level. *Behav. Brain. Funct.* 4:46.

Stefanis, N.C., Trikalinos, T.A., et al. (2007). Impact of schizophrenia candidate genes on schizotypy and cognitive endophenotypes at the population level. *Biol. Psychiatry* 62(7):784–792.

Tebartz van Elst, L., Hesslinger, B., et al. (2003). Frontolimbic brain abnormalities in patients with borderline personality disorder: a volumetric magnetic resonance imaging study. *Biol. Psychiatry* 54(2):163–171.

Tebartz van Elst, L., Ludaescher, P., et al. (2007). Evidence of disturbed amygdalar energy metabolism in patients with borderline personality disorder. *Neurosci. Lett.* 417(1):36–41.

Tiihonen, J., Rossi, R., et al. (2008). Brain anatomy of persistent violent offenders: more rather than less. *Psychiatry Res.* 163(3):201–212.

Torgersen, S., Czajkowski, N., et al. (2008). Dimensional representations of DSM-IV cluster B personality disorders in a population-based sample of Norwegian twins: a multivariate study. *Psychol. Med.* 38(11):1617–1625.

Torgersen, S., Kringlen, E., et al. (2001). The prevalence of personality disorders in a community sample. *Arch. Gen. Psychiatry* 58(6):590–596.

Torgersen, S., Lygren, S., et al. (2000). A twin study of personality disorders. *Compr. Psychiatry* 41(6):416–425.

Trull, T.J., Distel, M.A., et al. (2011). DSM-5 Borderline personality disorder: at the border between a dimensional and a categorical view. *Curr. Psychiatry Rep.* 13(1):43–49.

Viding, E., Larsson, H., et al. (2008). Quantitative genetic studies of antisocial behaviour. *Philos. Trans. R. Soc. Lond. B Biol. Sci.* 363(1503):2519–2527.

Vollm, B., Richardson, P., et al. (2004). Neurobiological substrates of antisocial and borderline personality disorder: preliminary results of a functional fMRI study. *Crim. Behav. Ment. Health.* 14(1):39–54.

Vollm, B.A., Zhao, L., et al. (2009). A voxel-based morphometric MRI study in men with borderline personality disorder: preliminary findings. *Crim. Behav. Ment. Health* 19(1):64–72.

Wagner, A.W., and Linehan, M.M. (1999). Facial expression recognition ability among women with borderline personality disorder: implications for emotion regulation? *J. Personal. Disord.* 13(4):329–344.

Wagner, S., Baskaya, O., et al. (2010). Modulatory role of the brain-derived neurotrophic factor Val66Met polymorphism on the effects of serious life events on impulsive aggression in borderline personality disorder. *Genes Brain Behav.* 9(1):97–102.

Wagner, S., Baskaya, O., et al. (2009). The 5-HTTLPR polymorphism modulates the association of serious life events (SLE) and impulsivity in patients with Borderline Personality Disorder. *J. Psychiatr. Res.* 43(13):1067–1072.

Weniger, G., Lange, C., et al. (2009). Reduced amygdala and hippocampus size in trauma-exposed women with borderline personality disorder and without posttraumatic stress disorder. *J. Psychiatry Neurosci.* 34(5):383–388.

Whittle, S., Chanen, A.M., et al. (2009). Anterior cingulate volume in adolescents with first-presentation borderline personality disorder. *Psychiatry Res.* 172(2):155–160.

Widiger, T.A., Livesley, W.J., et al. (2009). An integrative dimensional classification of personality disorder. *Psychol. Assess.* 21(3):243–255.

Wingenfeld, K., Rullkoetter, N., et al. (2009). Neural correlates of the individual emotional Stroop in borderline personality disorder. *Psychoneuroendocrinology* 34(4):571–586.

Yang, Y., and Raine, A. (2009). Prefrontal structural and functional brain imaging findings in antisocial, violent, and psychopathic individuals: a meta-analysis. *Psychiatry Res.* 174(2):81–88.

Yen, S., Shea, M.T., et al. (2002). Traumatic exposure and posttraumatic stress disorder in borderline, schizotypal, avoidant, and obsessive-compulsive personality disorders: findings from the collaborative longitudinal personality disorders study. *J. Nerv. Ment. Dis.* 190(8):510–518.

Zanarini, M.C., Frankenburg, F.R., et al. (2006). Prediction of the 10-year course of borderline personality disorder. *Am. J. Psychiatry* 163(5):827–832.

Zetzsche, T., Frodl, T., et al. (2006). Amygdala volume and depressive symptoms in patients with borderline personality disorder. *Biol. Psychiatry* 60(3):302–310.

Zetzsche, T., Preuss, U.W., et al. (2007). Hippocampal volume reduction and history of aggressive behaviour in patients with borderline personality disorder. *Psychiatry Res.* 154(2):157–170.

Zimmerman, M., Rothschild, L., et al. (2005). The prevalence of DSM-IV personality disorders in psychiatric outpatients. *Am. J. Psychiatry* 162(10): 1911–1918.

85 | THE NEUROBIOLOGY OF AGGRESSION

R. JAMES R. BLAIR

ggression, here defined as any form of behavior directed toward the goal of harming or injuring another living being who is motivated to avoid such treatment, is a natural and adaptive phenomenon. However, it can become maladaptive if it is exaggerated, persistent, or expressed out of context (Nelson and Trainor, 2007). As such it is a serious social concern as well as a considerable economic burden on society. Indeed, aggressive and antisocial behaviors are the leading cause of all child and adolescent referrals to mental health clinicians (Berkowitz, 1993). Moreover, each antisocial individual costs society up to ten times more than their healthy counterparts in aggregate health care and social service expenditures (Nelson and Trainor, 2007). An increased risk for aggression can be seen in a variety of psychiatric disorders, including but not limited to mood and personality disorders. Understanding the neurobiology of aggression is thus of considerable importance.

TAXONOMIES OF AGGRESSION

Work with animals has distinguished several forms of aggression (Gregg and Siegel, 2001). We briefly consider the two that, according to the current literature, might be most directly applied to understanding human aggression. These are predatory and reactive aggression.

PREDATORY AGGRESSION

Predatory aggression occurs during food seeking in certain omnivorous and carnivorous species. It involves methodological stalking, well-directed pouncing, and quiet biting attack. If predatory aggression is induced through stimulation of the brain, there will be attacks on live prey but also bites of dead prey. However, attacks on conspecifics will not be initiated. Electrical stimulation of a circuit including dorsolateral hypothalamus and the ventral half of the periaqueductal gray (PAG) has been shown to initiate predatory aggression in both rats and cats (Panksepp, 1998).

REACTIVE AGGRESSION

Animals demonstrate a gradated and instinctual response to threat. Distant threats induce freezing, and then, as the threats draw closer, they induce flight, and finally reactive aggression when they are very close and escape is impossible (Blanchard et al., 1977). As such, reactive aggression involves unplanned,

enraged attacks on the object perceived to be the source of the threat or frustration. The animal exhibits piloerection, autonomic arousal, hissing, and growling during their attack. Reactive aggression appears to be mediated via a circuit that runs from the medial amygdala downward, largely via the stria terminalis to the medial hypothalamus and from there to the dorsal half of the PAG (Gregg and Siegel, 2001; Lin et al., 2011; Nelson and Trainor, 2007; Panksepp, 1998;). There have been suggestions that this is a social behavior network from which aggressive behavior is an emergent property (Nelson and Trainor, 2007). However, more recent data suggest rather that overlapping but distinct neuronal subpopulations are involved in different social behaviors such as fighting and mating (Lin et al., 2011). It has also been argued that orbitofrontal cortex (OFC) has an inhibitory impact on this network (Nelson and Trainor, 2007), a claim that will be considered in greater detail in the following.

HUMAN AGGRESSION

In work on human aggression, a fundamental distinction is drawn between instrumental (proactive/planned) and reactive (affective/defensive/impulsive) aggression. This distinction has been made for some time (Crick and Dodge, 1996) even if consideration of the implications of this distinction for the neurobiology of human aggression is only more recent (Blair, 2001).

Instrumental aggression involves the planned execution of aggression. It can involve both overt and covert actions executed with forethought and a degree of planning. The anticipated outcome is positive as seen from the viewpoint of the aggressor: acquisition of territory or goods, improvement of social status, gratification of a perceived need. Typically, there is a relative absence of intense emotion.

In humans, reactive aggression is unplanned aggression that can be most often characterized as impulsive. These acts are often overt, explosive, and involve the active confrontation of the victim. Accompanying emotions are almost always negative (fear of retaliation, anger, sadness, frustration, and irritation). One notable feature distinguishing human reactive aggression from that studied in animals is that it has been associated with frustration (Berkowitz, 1993). Frustration occurs when an individual continues to do an action in the expectation of a reward but does not actually receive that reward (Berkowitz, 1993).

Instrumental and reactive aggression cluster differentially in confirmatory factor analyses with moderate correlations between the two dimensions (Crick and Dodge, 1996). Studies indicate that approximately 10% of children show elevated levels of instrumental *and* reactive aggression, 3% show elevated instrumental aggression only, and 6% show elevated reactive aggression only (Dodge et al., 1997). Instrumental and reactive aggression have distinct trajectories. (Those with both forms followed a pattern similar to those with instrumental aggression only.) Thus, Dodge and colleagues (1997) observed that children with reactive aggression had an earlier onset (4.5 years vs. 6.5 years for proactive), were more likely (21%) to have experienced physical abuse or aversive parenting, had poorer peer relations, and inadequate problem-solving patterns. The instrumentally aggressive children were more likely to have had aggressive role models in the family and to view aggression positively (Dodge et al., 1997). Similarly, different psychiatric conditions are associated with risks for different forms of aggression. Thus, patients with mood and anxiety conditions (e.g., bipolar disorder and posttraumatic stress disorder, as well as patients with intermittent explosive disorder and borderline personality disorder [BPD]) are at risk for increased reactive aggression. In contrast, individuals with the personality disorder psychopathy show an increased risk for instrumental aggression coupled with an increased risk for reactive aggression (Frick et al., 2005).

It should be noted that the instrumental–reactive dichotomy of aggression has received significant criticism (Bushman and Anderson, 2001). Specifically, whether individual aggressive acts can be reliably classified as reactive or instrumental has been questioned. This criticism may be overstated. Most would agree that the aggression of an individual punching a person who has startled him or her is different from that of an individual pointing a gun at another person and demanding his or her wallet. Moreover, there are identifiable differences in the neural circuitry mediating reactive and instrumental aggression, as detailed in the following. But the criticism of the dichotomy was not without merit. How should one classify the aggression of the person who shoots someone five days after discovering the victim had been having an affair with the shooter's spouse? There is a clear reactive component (anger, frustration, and confrontation), and yet the action is planned and, by using a gun, definitively instrumental. In short, it may be necessary to consider forms of aggression beyond the instrumental–reactive dichotomy such as aggression in which the functional contributions of the neural systems engaged in instrumental and those engaged in reactive aggression are both involved.

INSTRUMENTAL AGGRESSION

There have been suggestions that the animal work on the neurobiology of predatory aggression may provide information on human instrumental aggression (Gregg and Siegel, 2001). However, this appears unlikely. Instrumental aggression is a flexible way of achieving an individual's goals rather than an instinctual response to the presence of a prey animal. It is flexible and highly influenced by the individual's learning environment; for example, environmental factors play a

large role in determining the choice of weapons from fists to pistols. In contrast, whereas predatory aggression in animals may serve the goal of providing the animal with food, it is an instinctual motor program initiated by the presence of prey in the environment that occurs in a relatively fixed fashion; that is, ending with a bite to the neck. Moreover, predatory aggression in animals is not displayed to conspecifics. In contrast, instrumental aggression in humans is almost always displayed to conspecifics. As such, it appears unlikely that most instrumental aggression in humans recruits the subcortical circuits identified in animal work that mediate predatory aggression. Instead, when considering the neurobiology of instrumental aggression in humans, we are considering the neurobiology of instrumental motor responding generally (regions implicated include, e.g., premotor cortex, striatum, and the cerebellum) and, critically, the emotional learning and representational systems that allow the selection of one action over another.

There is only one *clinical* condition associated with an increased risk for *instrumental* aggression: conduct disorder (CD) in childhood and antisocial personality disorder (ASPD) in adulthood. However, it is important to remember that youth with CD and adults with ASPD are not considered to be homogeneous groups (Blair, 2001). Specifically, individuals differ according to their level of callous–unemotional (CU) traits (i.e., the degree to which they show reduced guilt and empathy). Level of CU traits in individuals with CD/ASPD have been shown to modulate BOLD responses within the amygdala to social cues (Marsh et al., 2008; White et al., in press) and within the amygdala and ventromedial frontal cortex (vmPFC) during moral reasoning (Marsh et al., 2011). Callous–unemotional traits are inversely related to mood and anxiety symptoms (Patrick, 1994) and it is individuals with elevated CU traits who are at particular risk for instrumental aggression (Frick et al., 2005).

Instrumental aggression can be adaptive. A starving individual who pushes someone over and takes his or her money is not making a poor decision from that person's own perspective (whatever its value from a societal perspective). The benefit of the soon-to-be purchased food will significantly outweigh the costs of causing (minor) injury to the victim/risking jail. However, an individual who stabs another to death for $80 to purchase a mobile phone is going to be considered, by most individuals, to be making a poor decision. The aggression is maladaptive. The benefits should be represented as significantly less than the costs. An increased risk for (maladaptive) instrumental aggression can emerge *following the specific forms of decision-making impairment seen in individuals with elevated CU traits.*

There are three clear components necessary to make a good decision. The individual must: (*1*) learn the value of the options to be chosen among; (*2*) successfully represent this value information so the options *can* be chosen among; and (*3*) successfully choose among the options. Individuals with elevated CU traits appear to have particular difficulties with at least the first two of these components.

Learning the value of options to be chosen among requires stimulus–reinforcement learning. The individual must associate a reinforcement value with the stimulus. A classic measure of stimulus-reinforcement learning is aversive conditioning—the individual learns that a particular stimulus is associated with threat. Individuals with elevated CU traits show marked impairment in stimulus-reinforcement learning. Indeed, an individual's ability to perform aversive conditioning at 15 years has predictive power regarding whether that individual will display antisocial behavior 14 years later (Raine et al., 1996). Considerable animal and human work shows that the amygdala is critical for aversive conditioning (LeDoux, 2007). Individuals with elevated CU traits show reduced amygdala responses during aversive conditioning (Birbaumer et al., 2005).

A critical cue for reinforcement based learning is the prediction error; that is, the difference between the reinforcement the individual expects to receive and that which he or she does receive. According to learning theory, the greater the prediction error, the faster the learning should occur (Rescorla and Wagner, 1972). Regions implicated in prediction error signaling include the caudate and vmPFC (O'Doherty et al., 2003). Youth with CD and elevated CU traits (requisite studies in adult samples have not been conducted) show indications of impaired prediction error signaling within both the caudate and vmPFC (Finger et al., 2008, 2011).

As the individual learns to associate reinforcement with an object or action, it acquires an expected value. Good decision making by definition involves the selection of an action/stimulus with the highest expected value. VmPFC is critically involved in the representation of expected value (Glascher et al., 2009). Youth with CD show disrupted representation of expected value within vmPFC (Finger et al., 2011).

A critical form of reinforcement for human social interactions involves emotional expressions (Blair, 2003). An individual can show distress by displaying pain, fear, or sadness.

To learn to avoid actions that harm others, one must appropriately represent the distress of others. Youth and adults with elevated CU traits show: (1) reduced autonomic responses to the pain of others (Aniskiewicz, 1979); (2) reduced recognition of fearful and sad expressions (for a metaanalysis, see Marsh and Blair, 2008); and (3) reduced amygdala responses to these expressions (Marsh et al., 2008). The amygdala is thought to allow the individual to associate the distress of others with actions/objects that have caused that distress—this is considered the basis for human socialization (Blair, 2007). Indeed, recent animal work has confirmed that the amygdala is critical for this form of learning (Jeon et al., 2010). In line with their expression processing impairments, the presence of CU traits has been shown to interfere with the child's ability to be socialized using standard parenting techniques (Wootton et al., 1997).

In summary, Figure 85.1 depicts the integrated systems that are dysfunctional in individuals with elevated CU traits and that, through their dysfunction, increase the risk for instrumental aggression. The caudate and vmPFC are involved in prediction error signaling; detecting when a reward or punishment is greater or lesser than expected. Prediction error signals trigger reinforcement learning—they signal to the system that the current reinforcement expectancies are inadequate. If prediction error signaling is disrupted, as data suggest it is in individuals with elevated CU traits, learning about the value of actions and objects will be impaired. The amygdala is involved in stimulus-reinforcement learning allowing the individual to associate reinforcement expectancy values with objects and actions. Again if stimulus-reinforcement learning is disrupted, as data suggest it is in individuals with elevated CU traits, learning about the value of actions and objects will be impaired. A critical type of reinforcement for human social

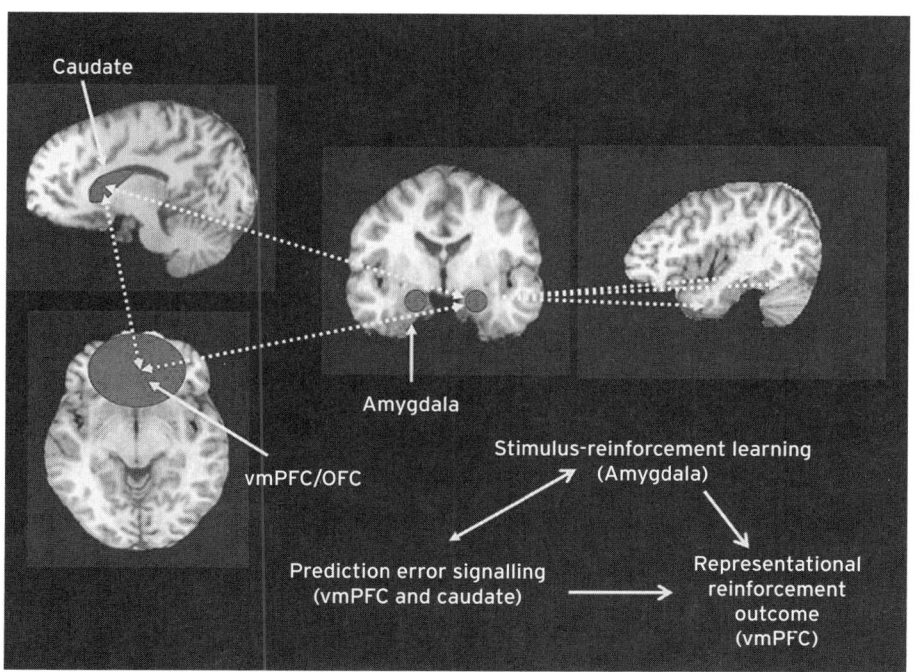

Figure 85.1 The neurobiology of callous–unemotional traits.

interaction is provided by emotional expressions. To learn to avoid actions that harm others one must associate the aversive qualities of the other individual's distress with the object/action that caused this distress. The amygdala is critical for this form of stimulus-reinforcement learning, which again appears disrupted in individuals with elevated CU traits. This learning process is critical for socialization; if disrupted, it will interfere with socialization. Individuals with elevated CU traits show significantly less impact of standard socialization practices than typically developing youth. Poorer stimulus-reinforcement learning and responsiveness to the distress of others lead to an individual who represents more poorly the expected value of objects and actions (including the aversiveness of harmful consequences for others). The VmPFC is critical for the representation of expected value. This representation is also disrupted in individuals with elevated CU traits, further contributing to their decision-making impairment. One manifestation of this decision-making impairment is the selection of maladaptive instrumental aggression/antisocial behavior; that is, choosing antisocial behaviors with inadequate representation of both their potential rewards and their potential aversive consequences.

REACTIVE AGGRESSION

As noted, reactive aggression is considered to be an automatic response to extreme threat that animal work shows is mediated via a circuit that runs from the medial amygdala downward, largely via the stria terminalis to the medial hypothalamus, and from there to the dorsal half of the PAG (Gregg and Siegel, 2001; Panksepp 1998). This circuitry is assumed to mediate reactive aggression in humans also (Blair, 2001) and to be regulated via frontal cortical regions, particularly vmPFC and potentially regions of anterior cingulate cortex (ACC).

There are two main ways that reactive aggression has been investigated in work with humans, by: (1) examining the pathophysiology of patients at increased risk for reactive aggression; and (2) conducting studies with healthy adults performing putative analogues of reactive aggression.

Several psychiatric conditions show a particularly marked increase in the risk for reactive aggression; for example, intermittent explosive disorder, BPD, and severe mood dysregulation in childhood (Coccaro et al., 2009). In addition, Raine and colleagues have done some work with a population of spouse abusers whose aggression was carefully characterized as reactive rather than instrumental (Lee et al., 2008).

Given the animal literature on reactive aggression, it can be predicted that individuals with a heightened risk for the display of reactive aggression will show heightened responsiveness of regions implicated in reactive aggression to emotional provocation (Blair, 2001); that is, the amygdala, hypothalamus, and PAG (Gregg and Siegel, 2001; Lin et al., 2011; Nelson and Trainor, 2007; Panksepp 1998). In line with this suggestion, patients with intermittent explosive disorder and BPD and reactively aggressive spouse abusers all show increased amygdala responsiveness to threatening stimuli relative to comparison individuals (Coccaro et al., 2007; Lee et al., 2008; New et al., 2009). Patients with BPD have also been found to show an increased amygdala response to interpersonal provocation (New et al., 2009). However, none of these studies reported either increased responsiveness of the hypothalamus or the PAG—although this lack likely reflects methodology, neither region is typically investigated in current functional magnetic resonance imaging work.

What about the regulatory role of frontal cortex? Certainly at least some patients with OFC lesions are at increased risk for reactive aggression (Grafman et al., 1996). This is in line with animal work that shows that lesions of the OFC can increase aggression (Izquierdo et al., 2005).

But what is the nature of this regulatory role? The dominant view is that the OFC inhibits ("puts the brakes on") the aggressive responses mediated by the amygdala, hypothalamus, and PAG (Heinz et al., 2011; Nelson and Trainor, 2007), but this view is probably wrong. If the OFC was having an inhibitory effect on systems engaged in threat behavior, one might assume that all threat related behavior would be increased following OFC lesions. In contrast, macaques while showing an increase in mild aggression following OFC lesions showed a significantly *decreased* fear reaction to novel threat stimuli (Izquierdo et al., 2005). Moreover, there are data showing that OFC lesions lead to a reduction in amygdala activity in the context of decision-making paradigms (Schoenbaum and Roesch, 2005).

Work with psychiatric patients at increased risk for reactive aggression is often assumed to support the frontal inhibitory position. It is assumed that patients at risk for reactive aggression will show disruption in the ability to recruit OFC in response to emotional provocation. However, data supporting this hypothesis are notably sparse.

There was a report of reduced activation in spouse abusers proximal to the right ACC and left middle frontal gyrus during the emotional Stroop test (Lee et al., 2008). However, it should be noted that these indications of hypofrontality were not seen in a second study by the same group on this population. Moreover, those from the first study involved a region that was white rather than gray matter and thus must be considered with caution. Similarly, data on patients with BPD have been mixed. For example, although some studies report reduced ACC activity during emotional provocation (New et al., 2009), others do not (Herpertz et al., 2001).

In short, it appears probable that the relationship of vmPFC to the amygdala is not simply suppressive. Animal work clearly demonstrates that lesions of vmPFC do not lead to disinhibited/increased amygdala responding as the "brakes type" regulatory view predicts. Lesions of vmPFC/OFC *decrease* amygdala responding (Schoenbaum and Roesch, 2005) and decrease fear reactions to novel threat stimuli (Izquierdo et al., 2005). Work with patients does not consistently support the view of decreased vmPFC/OFC activity in response to emotional provocation in patients at risk for heightened levels of aggression.

It is perhaps important to consider a core function of vmPFC/OFC outlined in the preceding section (i.e., its role in the representation of the value of an object or action) and the integrated nature of the role with the functioning of the amygdala and caudate. According to this view of integrated functioning, vmPFC/OFC dysfunction should reduce, not increase, amygdala responsiveness (cf., Schoenbaum and Roesch, 2005) and should consequently lead to a reduction, not an increase, in fear reactions to novel threat stimuli (cf., Izquierdo et al., 2005). Within this view, lesions of vmPFC/OFC will increase reactive aggression not because the aggressive response is dis inhibited but rather because the costs and benefits of engaging in reactive aggression are not properly represented. Of course, this view places an instrumental slant on many occasions of reactive aggression; that is, although reactive aggression may be an automatic response to an extreme threat, it may also be a selected response (as fear reactions to novel threat stimuli are too; Izquierdo et al., 2005). In this regard, it is notable that the aggression shown by primates following OFC lesions correlates highly with the aggression shown *to the* primate by other primates (Bachevalier et al., 2011). As such, the increased aggression may be just one reflection of poorer behavioral choices in the primate following the OFC lesion. This point is returned to in the following.

The second main ways that reactive aggression has been investigated in humans involves subjects performing putative analogues of reactive aggression; for example, the Taylor Aggression Paradigm (TAP; Taylor, 1967) and the Point Subtraction Aggression Paradigm (PSAP; Cherek et al., 1997). In the TAP, subjects are instructed that they are playing successive competitive reaction time trials against opponents. They are told that whoever lost a trial would be punished by the opponent with aversive thermal stimulation. Opponents can be predetermined, for example, to differ in provocation (i.e., the amount that they punish the subject). The subject's aggressive responses (retaliatory punishments of the opponent) are a function of provocation level. The similar PSAP examines the subject's responses to the subtraction of points worth money that he or she is accumulating during a testing session in which losses are attributed to the responding of another person. At each moment, the subject can choose to press button A (pressing 100 times earns money), button B (that will take points away from the fictitious person), or button C (that will protect the subject's point total for a set number of trials). Work has demonstrated that increases in provocation by the fictitious player increase retaliatory "aggressive" B responses in the subject (Cherek et al., 1997; New et al., 2009).

Relatively little functional imaging studies have been conducted with these paradigms. There have been reports of increased responding within dorsomedial prefrontal cortex, anterior insula cortex (AIC), and caudate to highly provoking confederates relative to less provoking confederates (Kramer et al., 2008). However, in none of this work was amygdala, hypothalamus, or PAG implicated, with the exception of a study investigating the response of individuals with psychopathy (there was no comparison group; Veit et al., 2010). This study reported that inflicting high relative to low punishments to the competitor was associated with increased activity within the AIC, amygdala, and hypothalamus (extending proximal to the PAG).

The literature on the TAP and PSAP shares interesting similarities with the more extensive literature on social exchange paradigms. In social exchange paradigms, a proposer suggests an allocation of resources and typically the subject decides whether or not to accept this allocation and/or punish the proposer for the unfairness of his offer. As such, social exchange paradigms can be considered social provocation paradigms like the TAP and PSAP. Notably unfair offers are associated with anger, and likely aggression, in the receiving party (Sanfey et al., 2003).

Unfair offers by proposers during social exchange paradigms have been found to elicit activity in subjects within both AIC/inferior frontal cortex (IFC), dorsomedial frontal cortex (dmFC), and striatum (Sanfey et al., 2003; King-Casas et al., 2008; White et al., in press). There have been suggestions that activity within these regions reflects anger elicited by unfairness to the self (Sanfey et al., 2003) or that they play a critical role in detecting and reacting to social norm violations (King-Casas et al., 2008). Indeed, it has been argued AIC/IFC responds to anger/expectations of anger (including in response to norm violations) and organize a behavioral response (Blair and Cipolotti, 2000). In this regard, it appears that part of this organization involves the recruitment of the PAG (e.g., White et al., in press). Decisions to reject the proposer's unfair offers, like decisions to punish another's provocation on the TAP (Veit et al., 2010), are associated with increased activity within dmFC, AIC/IFC, and striatum as well as the PAG (White et al., 2013).

It is interesting in this regard that dmFC and AIC/IFC also show increased activation following unexpected punishments during, for example, reversal learning tasks (e.g., Budhani et al., 2007). Again the assumption is that dmFC responds to the expectation violation (Alexander and Brown, 2011)—in this case the unexpected punishment—and that AIC/IFC organizes a behavioral response. This might involve a change in behavior but it also, as a definitively frustrating event, might involve the initiation of a frustration based reactive aggression episode.

It was argued in the preceding that reactive aggression can be a selected response and that vmPFC lesions increase reactive aggression because the costs and benefits of engaging in reactive aggression are not properly represented. This is important to remember when considering the literature on the PSAP, TAP, or social exchange literature. These paradigms are not modeling an instinctual response to threat or intruders but rather a planned response to another individual's provocative behavior. As successful as these models have been of "reactive aggression," they would appear to be rather more applicable to cases of "instrumental reactive aggression" mentioned in the preceding.

In summary, Figure 85.2 depicts the neural systems involved in the expression of reactive aggression (amygdala, hypothalamus, and PAG) as well as systems implicated in modifying the probability that reactive aggression will be expressed (vmPFC, aIC, and dmFC). Increasing emotional provocation by threat will increase activity in amygdala, hypothalamus, and PAG until, at sufficient strength, reactive aggression will be displayed. Anxiety and mood disorders are associated with an increased

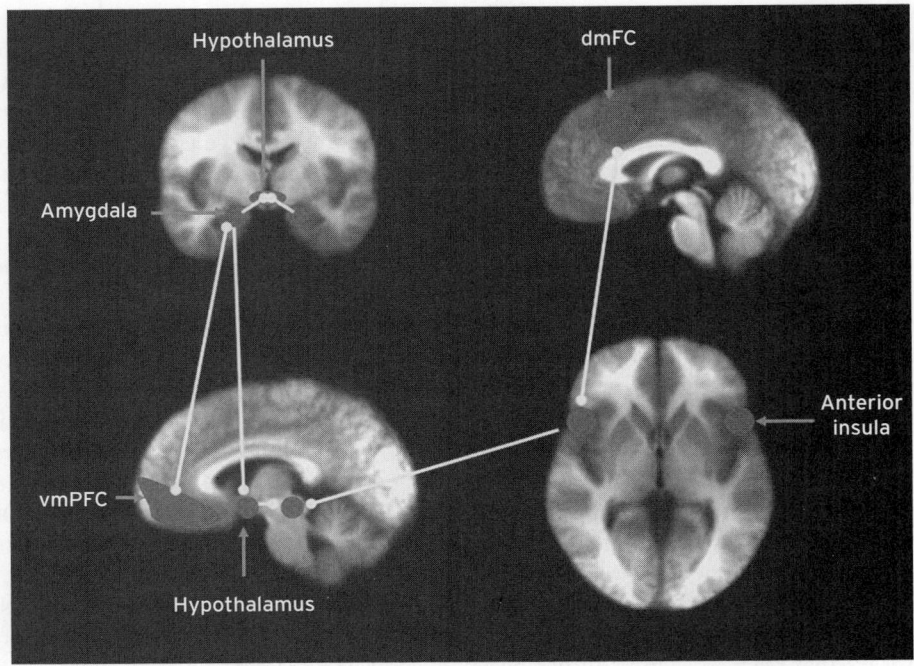

Figure 85.2 *The neural systems involved in the expression of reactive aggression.*

risk for reactive aggression because they involve an increase in the underlying responsiveness of at least parts of this circuit. Emotional regulation, even if it does not involve vmPFC placing the brakes on the amygdala, will reduce responsiveness and thus decrease the probability that reactive aggression will be displayed.

The dmFC and AIC show increased responses to provocation in the context of reactive aggression paradigms (Kramer et al., 2008) and in response to unfair offers in social exchange paradigms (King-Casas et al., 2008; Sanfey et al., 2003; White et al., 2013). They also show increased responses to frustration as initiated by an unexpected punishment for an action expected to result in reward (e.g., Budhani et al., 2007). Retaliatory responses are also associated with dmFC and AIC activity as well as the PAG (White et al., 2013). The suggestion is that the anger initiated by the expectation violation of the other's inappropriate behavior (delivering shocks or making unfair offers) corresponds to expectation violation signaling and behavioral control mediated by dmFC and AIC. The suggestion would be that this activity could be maintained, or at least reinitiated, whenever the individual considers the provocation and this could potentially lead to an angry aggressive response that will have instrumental components (in that it may be planned; e.g., the person goes home to obtain a weapon before attacking the victim).

The vmPFC allows the representation of the value of an object or an action. The suggestion is that vmPFC's role in reactive aggression corresponds to its role in action selection. If it is impaired, reactive aggression may be more likely to be expressed. (The individual may have generated anger following provocation but did not represent the aversive consequences of the expression of this anger to themselves or others.)

MOLECULAR MECHANISMS

Some work has indicated that antisocial personality disorder and aggression are heritable. Reviews have suggested that a genetic effect could account for up to 50% of the variance in aggression (Miles and Carey, 1997). Unfortunately, almost all of the literature has failed to consider the heterogeneity within aggressive individuals. There have been indications that CU traits are highly heritable and that aggression only appears to be highly heritable in those with elevated CU traits (the suggestion has been made the aggression of aggressive individuals with low CU traits is more environmentally determined; Viding et al., 2005). However, it is perhaps unlikely that only CU traits, and not the emotional lability underlying the selectively increased risk for reactive aggression, are under genetic influence. Indeed there is molecular evidence that genetic polymorphisms associated with increased emotional reactivity are associated with an increased risk for reactive aggression (Brunner et al., 1993; Heinz et al., 2011). Given this, an attempt will be made here to filter the existing genetic literature though what is known about the neurocognitive architectures mediating different forms of aggression.

SEROTONIN

Serotonin has long been implicated in the regulation of aggression, particularly reactive aggression. Generally, experimental manipulations that increase 5-HT receptor activation have been found to decrease aggression, whereas those that decrease receptor activation have been found to increase aggression (Heinz et al., 2011).

Some of the most dramatic work indicating a relationship between serotonin and aggression has been molecular genetic work. Prominent among this work are studies examining the gene that encodes monoamine oxidase A (MAOA, a catabolic enzyme that breaks down biogenic amines including serotonin). In a seminal study, a single mutation in this gene was associated with criminal/antisocial behavior (Brunner et al., 1993). Although the human functional knockout is rare, there are common polymorphisms in MAOA. The most studied of these is a variable-number tandem repeat (VNTR) polymorphism in the upstream region of the gene, known as the MAOA uVNTR. Certain alleles in this region are associated with higher MAOA expression (MAOA-H alleles), whereas others are associated with lower expression (MAOA-L alleles) (Heinz et al., 2011). MAOA-L subjects (compared with MAOA-H subjects), like other individuals at increased risk for reactive aggression (see the preceding), show heightened amygdala responsiveness to threat stimuli such as angry and fearful faces (Heinz et al., 2011). Moreover, MAOA-L variant subjects are at increased risk for the display of reactive aggression particularly if the individual has been exposed to abuse (Caspi et al., 2002).

Polymorphisms of the 5-HTT gene (*5-HTTLPR*) also appear to increase risk for reactive aggression particularly if the individual has been exposed to abuse (Reif et al., 2007). Similarly, the common polymorphism of the 5-HTT gene (the *5-HTTLPR* S allele) is associated with increased amygdala activation in response to aversive pictures and with a higher risk of experiencing negative mood states when exposed to traumatic life events (Heinz et al., 2011). The suggestion would be that both these MAOA and 5-HTTLPR polymorphisms and abuse increase responsiveness of the basic threat circuitry (amygdala-hypothalamus-PAG). It appears that the effects of these stressors are interactive rather than simply cumulative; genetic load predisposes the individual to be considerably more impacted by stressful events, considerably increasing the risk for reactive aggression.

DOPAMINE

Considerable animal work has shown that dopamine decreases the threshold for aggressive reaction in response to external stimuli, although an excess of these hormones increases the vulnerability and the risk of uncontrolled responses against stress (Volavka et al., 2004). Much of the human work has considered the involvement of the dopaminergic system in impulsivity rather than aggression. However, there has been some particularly interesting work examining the relationship of the catechol-*O*-methyl transferase (COMT) gene in aggression.

Many studies evaluating the impact of COMT to the genetics of aggression focused on the characterization of the Val158-Met polymorphism. This polymorphism is interesting functionally as there is almost a two fold decrease in the enzymatic activity of the Met158 variant compared to the Val158-encoding allele. In line with animal work showing that heterozygous COMT-deficient male mice exhibited increased aggressive behavior (Heinz et al., 2011), the allele Met158 of COMT has been found to be associated with aggressive personality traits and a propensity for aggression in humans (Rujescu et al., 2003). Importantly, the data again,

for the most part, indicate that individuals with the Met allele show increased amygdala responsiveness to emotional provocation (e.g., Smolka et al., 2005).

γ-AMINOBUTYRIC ACID

Alcohol and benzodiazepines have been consistently shown to increase aggression (Fish et al., 2001). Both have an inhibitory effect on cortical activation, by inducing GABA release and stimulating GABA type A (GABAA) and GABAB receptors and their aggression-heightening effects can be potentiated by their co-administration (Fish et al., 2001).

Acute alcohol use is implicated in approximately one-half of all violent crimes and sexual assaults, and also confers risk for intimate partner violence. Treatment with benzodiazepines has been shown to increase the risk of aggression (Gardner and Cowdry, 1985).

It has been suggested that aggression may result from acute alcohol effects that impair prefrontal cortex mediated executive functions and disinhibit limbic processing of threatening stimuli, and elicit reactive aggression (Heinz et al., 2011). However, current data are rather inconsistent with this view—at least with respect to the disinhibition of limbic responsiveness. Thus, administration of alcohol leads to a *reduction*, rather than an increase, in the amygdala's response to threatening stimuli (Gilman and Hommer, 2008) as does administration of diazepam (Del-Ben et al., 2012). In other words, acute administration of both alcohol and diazepam *inhibits* rather than disinhibits limbic responsiveness.

Alcohol is thought to disrupt decision making in that it increases the probability of maladaptive risk-taking behavior, including risky sexual activity, unsafe driving, and aggression (for a review, see Hommer et al., 2011). However, relatively little work has formally demonstrated decision-making deficits following alcohol ingestion. Somewhat more work has examined reward sensitivity in alcoholics, in which there does appear to be reduced reward sensitivity (Hommer et al., 2011).

In summary, there is a growing literature on the molecular mechanisms underpinning aggression, with some of the most provocative data being provided by molecular genetics. Serotonin decreases the risk for reactive aggression, whereas dopamine increases it. Both alter the sensitivity of the basic threat circuitry (particularly the amygdala). Polymorphisms of serotonin (e.g., MAOA and 5-HTTLPR) and dopamine (e.g., COMT) genes that are associated with an increased risk for aggression are also those polymorphisms associated with increased amygdala responsiveness.

The relationship between alcohol (and probably the benzodiazepines) and aggression appears rather different though. Ingestion of either reduces, rather than increases, amygdala responsiveness to emotional stimuli. Moreover, ingestion of alcohol appears to lead to decision-making impairments (although the precise computational basis of these impairments has not yet been well specified). As such, ingestion of alcohol appears to induce a state of increased CU (although the similarities can only be really determined when the details on the decision-making impairment are specified).

CONCLUSIONS

Considerable progress is continuing to be made in understanding the neurobiological basis of human aggression. The neurobiological circuits distinguishing instrumental from reactive aggression continue to be further specified. However, it is becoming clearer that these circuits can overlap in function. Thus, for example, the expression of rage- and frustration-induced reactive aggressive episodes can come under the control of systems involved in the representation of reinforcement value (vmPFC) that are critical for understanding instrumental aggression.

Instrumental aggression is mediated by the same cortical circuits that mediate other forms of instrumental behavior (e.g., premotor cortex and the cerebellum). Individuals may choose to engage in instrumental aggression if their representations of the benefits of the action outweigh their representations of the costs of the action (particularly if no other more beneficial action is available). Instrumental aggression can be considered maladaptive if the individuals have failed to learn the appropriate reinforcements associated with the action; that is, they have an inadequate representation of the distress of the victim, show impairment in stimulus-reinforcement learning, and show impairment in the representation of reinforcement expectancies. These capacities are reliant on the functional integrity of the amygdala, caudate, and vmPFC. Impairments in these capacities are seen in individuals who show elevated CU traits, individuals who are at risk for increased levels of instrumental aggression.

Reactive aggression involves a motor response driven by the amygdala, hypothalamus, and PAG that is modulated by the vmPFC's role in the representation of reinforcement value. It represents an ultimate response to threat and is displayed to high level threats and (in humans) also to frustration. If the threat or frustration is sufficiently intense the reactive aggression may be relative automatic. However, it is becoming clearer that in humans and other primates that reactive aggression is under considerable modulation by vmPFC. The individual, anticipating displaying reactive aggression, will represent likely future expected reinforcement values of this action; for example, the value associated with the satisfaction of retaliating to the provoker versus that associated with potential jail time.

Although various neurochemical systems are implicated in the expression and modulation of reactive aggression, the roles of serotonin, dopamine, and GABA are perhaps the best understood. Polymorphisms of serotonin (e.g., MAOA and 5-HTTLPR) and dopamine (e.g., COMT) genes that are associated with an increased risk for aggression are also those polymorphisms associated with increased amygdala responsiveness to threat; that is, they increase the responsiveness of systems involved in the expression of reactive aggression. The ingestion of alcohol, in contrast, reduces amygdala responsiveness to distress and leads to decision-making impairments; that is, it proximally induces a state of increased CU.

These are the neural systems that are dysfunctional in individuals with elevated CU traits and that, through their dysfunction, increase the risk for instrumental aggression. The caudate and vmPFC are involved in prediction error signaling,; detecting when a reward or punishment is greater or lesser than expected. Prediction error signals trigger reinforcement learning—they signal to the system that the current reinforcement expectancies are inadequate. If prediction error signaling is disrupted, as data suggest it is in individuals with elevated CU traits, learning about the value of actions and objects will be impaired. The amygdala is involved in stimulus-reinforcement learning allowing the individual to associate reinforcement expectancy values with objects and actions. Again if stimulus-reinforcement learning is disrupted, as data suggest it is in individuals with elevated CU traits, learning about the value of actions and objects will be impaired. A critical type of reinforcement for human social interaction is provided by emotional expressions. To learn to avoid actions that harm others one must associate the aversive qualities of the other individual's distress with the object or action that caused this distress. The amygdala is critical for this form of stimulus-reinforcement learning, which again appears disrupted in individuals with elevated CU traits. This learning process is critical for socialization and if disrupted will interfere with socialization. Individuals with elevated CU traits show significantly less impact of standard socialization practices than typically developing youth. Poorer stimulus-reinforcement learning and responsiveness to the distress of others will lead to an individual who represents more poorly the expected value of objects and actions, including the aversiveness of harmful consequences for others. The VmPFC is critical for the representation of expected value. This representation is also disrupted in individuals with elevated CU traits, further contributing to their decision-making impairment. One manifestation of this decision-making impairment is the selection of maladaptive instrumental aggression/antisocial behavior; that is, choosing antisocial behaviors with inadequate representation of both their potential rewards and their potential aversive consequences.

These neural systems include those responsible for the basic response to threat (amygdala, hypothalamus, and PAG), which when sufficiently activated by sufficient threat will initiate reactive aggression. In addition, they include the dmFC and AIC. The DmFC responds to expectation violations, whether the expectation violation involves another's provocative behavior or the failure to receive an expected reward following task completion. The suggestion is that it organizes potential behavioral responses through AIC, including reactive aggression expressed through the PAG. Finally, they also include vmPFC. The VmPFC allows the representation of the value of an object or an action. The suggestion is that the vmPFC's role in reactive aggression corresponds to its role in action selection. If it is impaired, reactive aggression may be more likely to be expressed. The individual may have generated anger following provocation or experiencing a frustrating event but not represent the aversive consequences of the expression of this anger to him- or herself or others.

DISCLOSURE

Dr. Blair is supported by the Intramural Research Program of the National Institute of Mental Health, National Institutes of Health under grant number 1-ZIA-MH002860-08. He has no financial relationships to disclose.

REFERENCES

Alexander, W.H., and Brown, J.W. (2011). Medial prefrontal cortex as an action-outcome predictor. *Nat. Neurosci.* 14(10):1338–1344.

Aniskiewicz, A.S. (1979). Autonomic components of vicarious conditioning and psychopathy. *J. Clin. Psychol.* 35:60–67.

Bachevalier, J., Machado, C.J., et al. (2011). Behavioral outcomes of late-onset or early-onset orbital frontal cortex (areas 11/13) lesions in rhesus monkeys. *Ann. NY Acad. Sci.* 1239:71–86.

Berkowitz, L. (1993). Aggression: Its Causes, Consequences, and Control. Philadelphia, PA: Temple University Press.

Birbaumer, N., Veit, R., et al. (2005). Deficient fear conditioning in psychopathy: a functional magnetic resonance imaging study. *Arch. Gen. Psychiatry* 62(7):799–805.

Blair, R.J.R. (2001). Neuro-cognitive models of aggression: the antisocial personality disorders and psychopathy. *J. Neurol. Neurosurg. Psychiatry* 71:727–731.

Blair, R.J.R. (2003). Facial expressions, their communicatory functions and neuro-cognitive substrates. *Philos. Trans. R. Soc. Lond. B Biol. Sci.* 358(1431):561–572.

Blair, R.J.R. (2007). The amygdala and ventromedial prefrontal cortex in morality and psychopathy. *Trends Cogn. Sci.* 11(9):387–392.

Blair, R.J.R., and Cipolotti, L. (2000). Impaired social response reversal: a case of "acquired sociopathy." *Brain* 123:1122–1141.

Blanchard, R.J., Blanchard, D.C., et al. (1977). Attack and defensive behaviour in the albino rat. *Anim. Behav.* 25:197–224.

Brunner, H.G., Nelen, M., et al. (1993). Abnormal behavior associated with a point mutation in the structural gene for monoamine oxidase A. *Science* 262(5133):578–580.

Budhani, S., Marsh, A.A., et al. (2007). Neural correlates of response reversal: considering acquisition. *NeuroImage* 34(4):1754–1765.

Bushman, B.J., and Anderson, C.A. (2001). Is it time to pull the plug on the hostile versus instrumental aggression dichotomy? *Psychol. Rev.* 108(1):273–279.

Caspi, A., McClay, J., et al. (2002). Role of genotype in the cycle of violence in maltreated children. *Science* 297(5582):851–854.

Cherek, D.R., Moeller, F.G., et al. (1997). Studies of violent and nonviolent male parolees: I. Laboratory and psychometric measurements of aggression. *Biol. Psychiatry* 41:514–522.

Coccaro, E.F., McCloskey, M.S., et al. (2007). Amygdala and orbitofrontal reactivity to social threat in individuals with impulsive aggression. *Biol. Psychiatry* 62(2):168–178.

Crick, N.R., and Dodge, K.A. (1996). Social information-processing mechanisms on reactive and proactive aggression. *Child Dev.* 67(3):993–1002.

Del-Ben, C.M., Ferreira, C.A., et al. (2012). Effects of diazepam on BOLD activation during the processing of aversive faces. *J. Psychopharmacol.* 26(4):443–451.

Dodge, K.A., Lochman, J.E., et al. (1997). Reactive and proactive aggression in school children and psychiatrically impaired chronically assaultive youth. *J. Abnorm. Psychol.* 106(1):37–51.

Finger, E.C., Marsh, A.A., et al. (2008). Abnormal ventromedial prefrontal cortex function in children with psychopathic traits during reversal learning. *Arch. Gen. Psychiatry* 65(5):586–594.

Finger, E.C., Marsh, A.A., et al. (2011). Disrupted reinforcement signaling in the orbital frontal cortex and caudate in youths with conduct disorder or oppositional defiant disorder and a high level of psychopathic traits. *Am. J. Psychiatry* 168(2):834–841.

Fish, E.W., Faccidomo, S., et al. (2001). Alcohol, allopregnanolone and aggression in mice. *Psychopharmacol. (Berl.)* 153(4):473–483.

Frick, P.J., Stickle, T.R., et al. (2005). Callous-unemotional traits in predicting the severity and stability of conduct problems and delinquency. *J. Abnorm. Child Psychology* 33:471–487.

Gardner, D.L., and Cowdry, R.W. (1985). Alprazolam-induced dyscontrol in borderline personality disorder. *Am. J. Psychiatry* 146:98–100.

Gilman, J.M., and Hommer, D. (2008). Modulation of brain response to emotional images by alcohol cues in alcohol-dependent patients. *Addict. Biol.* 13:423–434.

Glascher, J., Hampton, A.N., et al. (2009). Determining a role for ventromedial prefrontal cortex in encoding action-based value signals during reward related decision making. *Cerebral Cortex* 19:483–495.

Grafman, J., Schwab, K., et al. (1996). Frontal lobe injuries, violence, and aggression: a report of the Vietnam head injury study. *Neurology* 46:1231–1238.

Gregg, T.R., and Siegel, A. (2001). Brain structures and neurotransmitters regulating aggression in cats: implications for human aggression. *Prog. Neuropsychopharmacol. Biol. Psychiatry* 25(1):91–140.

Heinz, A.J., Beck, A., et al. (2011). Cognitive and neurobiological mechanisms of alcohol-related aggression. *Nat. Rev. Neurosci.* 12(7):400–413.

Herpertz, S.C., Dietrich, T.M., et al. (2001). Evidence of abnormal amygdala functioning in borderline personality disorder: a functional MRI study. *Biol. Psychiatry* 50(4):292–298.

Hommer, D.W., Bjork, J.M., et al. (2011). Imaging brain response to reward in addictive disorders. *Ann. NY Acad. Sci.* 1216:50–61.

Izquierdo, A., Suda, R.K., et al. (2005). Comparison of the effects of bilateral orbital prefrontal cortex lesions and amygdala lesions on emotional responses in rhesus monkeys. *J. Neurosci.* 25(37):8534–8542.

Jeon, D., Kim, S., et al. (2010). Observational fear learning involves affective pain system and Cav1.2 Ca2+ channels in ACC. *Nat. Neurosci.* 13(4):482–488.

King-Casas, B., Sharp, C., et al. (2008). The rupture and repair of cooperation in borderline personality disorder. *Science* 321(5890):806–810.

Kramer, U.M., Buttner, S., et al. (2008). Trait aggressiveness modulates neurophysiological correlates of laboratory-induced reactive aggression in humans. *J. Cogn. Neurosci.* 20(8):1464–1477.

LeDoux, J.E. (2007). The amygdala. *Curr. Biol.* 17(20):R868–R874.

Lee, T.M.C., Chan, S.-C., et al. (2008). Strong limbic and weak frontal activation to aggressive stimuli in spouse abusers. *Mol. Psychiatry* 13(7):655–656.

Lin, D., Boyle, M.P., et al. (2011). Functional identification of an aggression locus in the mouse hypothalamus. *Nature* 470(7333):221–226.

Marsh, A.A., and Blair, R.J.R. (2008). Deficits in facial affect recognition among antisocial populations: a meta-analysis. *Neurosci. Behav. Rev.* 32(3):454–465.

Marsh, A.A., Finger, E.C., et al. (2008). Reduced amygdala response to fearful expressions in children and adolescents with callous-unemotional traits and disruptive behavior disorders. *Am J Psychiatry* 165(6):712–720.

Marsh, A.A., Finger, E.C., et al. (2011). Reduced amygdala-orbitofrontal connectivity during moral judgments in youths with disruptive behavior disorders and psychopathic traits. *Psychiatry Res.* 194(3):279–286.

Miles, D.R., and Carey, G. (1997). Genetic and environmental architecture of human aggression. *J. Pers. Soc. Psychol.* 72(1):207–217.

Nelson, R.J., and Trainor, B.C. (2007). Neural mechanisms of aggression. *Nat. Rev. Neurosci.* 8:536–546.

New, A.S., Hazlett, E.A., et al. (2009). Laboratory induced aggression: a positron emission tomograpy study of aggressive individuals with borderline personality disorder. *Biol. Psychiatry* 66:1107–1114.

O'Doherty, J.P., Dayan, P., et al. (2003). Temporal difference models and reward-related learning in the human brain. *Neuron* 38(2):329–337.

Panksepp, J. (1998). Affective Neuroscience: The Foundations of Human and Animal Emotions. New York: Oxford University Press.

Patrick, C.J. (1994). Emotion and psychopathy: startling new insights. *Psychophysiology* 31:319–330.

Raine, A., Venables, P.H., et al. (1996). Better autonomic conditioning and faster electrodermal half-recovery time at age 15 years as possible protective factors against crime at age 29 years. *Dev. Psychol.* 32:624–630.

Reif, A., Rosler, M., et al. (2007). Nature and nurture predispose to violent behavior: serotonergic genes and adverse childhood environment. *Neuropsychopharmacology* 32(11):2375–2383.

Rescorla, R.A., and Wagner, A.R. (1972). A theory of Pavlovian conditioning: variations in the effectiveness of reinforcement and nonreinforcement. In: Black, A.H., and Prokasym, W.F., eds. Classical Conditioning II. New York: Appleton-Century-Crofts, pp. 64–99.

Rujescu, D., Giegling, I., et al. (2003). A functional single nucleotide polymorphism (V158M) in the COMT gene is associated with aggressive personality traits. *Biol. Psychiatry* 54(1):34–39.

Sanfey, A.G., Rilling, J.K., et al. (2003). The neural basis of economic decision-making in the ultimatum game. *Science* 300(5626):1755–1758.

Schoenbaum, G., and Roesch, M. (2005). Orbitofrontal cortex, associative learning, and expectancies. *Neuron* 47(5):633–636.

Smolka, M.N., Schumann, G., et al. (2005). Catechol-O-methyltransferase val158met genotype affects processing of emotional stimuli in the amygdala and prefrontal cortex. *J. Neurosci.* 25(4):836–842.

Taylor, S.P. (1967). Aggressive behavior and physiological arousal as a function of provocation and the tendency to inhibit aggression. *J. Personality* 35:297–310.

Veit, R., Lotze, M., et al. (2010). Aberrant social and cerebral responding in a competitive reaction time paradigm in criminal psychopaths. *NeuroImage* 49(4):3365–3372.

Viding, E., Blair, R.J.R., et al. (2005). Evidence for substantial genetic risk for psychopathy in 7-year-olds. *J. Child Psychol. Psychiatry* 46:592–597.

Volavka, J., Bilder, R., et al. (2004). Catecholamines and aggression: the role of COMT and MAO polymorphisms. *Ann. NY Acad. Sci.* 1036:393–398.

White, S.F., Brislin, S.J., et al. (2012). Callous-unemotional traits modulate the neural response associated with punishing another individual during social exchange: a preliminary investigation. *J. Pers. Disord.* 27(1):99–112.

White, S.F., Marsh, A.A., et al. (2013). Reduced amygdala responding in youth with disruptive behavior disorder and psychopathic traits reflects a reduced emotional response not increased top-down attention to non-emotional features. *Am. J. Psychiatry* 169(7):750–758.

White, S.F., Pope, K., et al. (2013). Disrupted expected value and prediction error signaling in youths with disruptive behavior disorders during a passive avoidance task. *Am. J. Psychiatry* 170(3):315–23.

Wootton, J.M., Frick, P.J., et al. (1997). Ineffective parenting and childhood conduct problems: the moderating role of callous-unemotional traits. *J. Consult. Clin. Psychol.* 65:301–308.

86 | THE NEUROBIOLOGY OF SOCIAL ATTACHMENT

ADAM S. SMITH, KELLY LEI, AND ZUOXIN WANG

Social attachment is a dynamic process, involving multimodal socially relevant sensory information as well as neural systems for attraction, motivation, social recognition, and other cognitive processes to act discriminately in select social environments. Attachments are not simply the absence of social neglect, but these two constructs are not mutually exclusive. Thus, understanding the neurobiological mechanisms underlying social attachment improves knowledge of the neural substrates that govern bond-related behavior, and would provide insight into the etiology of socially related mental disorders. Surprisingly, although social attachments are imperative to survival and success in human and most mammalian societies, the neurobiology behind various bond-dependent behaviors and social attachment itself is only recently coming to light.

The behavioral components of social attachments are highly complex. However, these behaviors that engender infants to bond to their caregivers or two people to fall in love are not beyond appraisal by neurobiological evaluation. In fact, the newly emerged field of social neuroscience (Decety and Cacioppo, 2011) has identified relevantly simple and robust molecular and cellular mechanisms that regulate certain social interactions that propagate social bonding, such as reproductive behavior or parental care (Insel and Fernald, 2004). The form and importance of social attachment depend on the social system. For mammals, mothers are the most vital, if not the only caregiver; thus, reciprocal infant–mother attachments are often crucial to the infant's survival. In monogamous species, two additional attachments emerge, paternal–infant bonds in bi-parental species and pair bonding between committed partners, to dictate the successful navigation of the social environment. These bonds are coupled to species perpetuation and, therefore, have biological function with decisive evolutionary importance. Several observations have highlighted the role of various monoamines and neuropeptides in regulating bond-dependent behaviors, but there is a larger discussion to be had to understand how various neural systems function in congress to govern social attachments. It is the goal of this chapter to describe the current knowledge of the neurobiology behind each of these social attachments by uncoupling the neurochemistry and neuroanatomy of individual bond-related behaviors, reconstructing uniformed neural systems, and correlating these findings to our understanding of human analogues.

PERSPECTIVES ON A SOCIAL BRAIN

Most mammalian species, especially humans, live in highly complex social systems. Integrating social information to develop proper behavioral responses is vital to the survival and success of an individual as well as the ability to successfully form social bonds. In understanding the neurobiology of social attachments, it is first worth determining whether there are governing modules in the brain—neural systems dedicated to categorical information—for social behavior.

The social brain hypothesis suggests that behavioral adaption to ever-increasing complex social society has contributed to the development of neural systems, brain mass, cognitive abilities, processing social information, social communication, and emotionality (Dunbar, 1998). Appropriate behavior during interactions with a conspecific depends on a number of variables associated with the nature of the relationship with the conspecific. For example, the dominant male gorilla (genus *Gorilla*), or silverback, is aggressive toward males intruding into his troop's territory, a display of mate and resource guarding. However, when confronted with an unfamiliar female, the silverback should display more tolerance as to gain new mating opportunities. One cognitive process that is an essential skill for social life in most gregarious species is social recognition, or the ability to distinguish familiar conspecifics from strangers and to remember previous encounters. Without this skill, an animal could not distinguish between lower- or higher-ranking group members or mates from intruders. Indeed, humans have brain regions adept to recognizing faces and facial emotion. Functional neuroimaging and lesion studies have implicated the fusiform area in the inferior temporal lobe and amygdala as two regions in the human brain that are important for face recognition and determining facial expressions (Adolphs, 2003). In addition, non-human primates also have select brain regions that respond to various aspects of faces, such as expression and gaze direction (Perrett et al., 1992). Similar to humans, regions of the temporal lobe such as the superior temporal sulcus are activated when non-human primates look at conspecific faces. Furthermore, facial information from these temporal regions appears to integrate activity of the amygdala. In other mammalian species that rely more on olfactory cues to obtain social information, such as rodents, there are olfactory and vomeronasal neural systems dedicated to processing olfactory and pheromonal signals that provide relevant information about reproductive and social status.

Genetic studies conducted within the last decade have yielded several new insights about the neuroendocrine regulation of social recognition. Social recognition deficits have been observed in individual lines of genetic knockout mice for norepinephrine, oxytocin, and vasopressin and their receptors. Several studies have demonstrated that targeted injections of these neurochemicals into the brain of knockout mice can restore social memory and recognition. Many brain regions have been implicated as sites of action for these neurochemicals in rat social recognition, including the olfactory bulb (OB), amygdala, hippocampus, lateral septum (LS), and medial preoptic area (mPOA). For example, the socially relevant olfactory cues in rodents from the main and accessory olfactory systems converge in the medial subnucleus of the amygdala (MeA). In a series of experiments from Dluzen and colleagues, it was observed that the influence of this pathway on social recognition is mediated by an oxytocin-norepinephrine interaction (reviewed recently in Hammock and Young, 2007). Administration of oxytocin receptor antagonists or antisense DNA into the MeA impaired social recognition in wild-type mice. Similarly, oxytocin-knockout and complete oxytocin receptor-knockout mice have impaired social recognition, but infusion of oxytocin into the MeA of oxytocin-knockout mice reinstates social recognition. Oxytocin infused into the OB minutes before behavioral testing prolongs the social recognition response in rats. Still, oxytocin seems to only enhance regulation of social recognition via norepinephrine action. Blocking oxytocin receptors alone via administration of a selective receptor antagonist does not impede social recognition in rats, but chemical lesions of norepinephrine cells in the OB eliminates the oxytocin-induced enhancements to social recognition in rats. In addition, oxytocin treatments can increase the release of norepinephrine in the OB. Currently, it is suggested that oxytocin promotes norepinephrine action via activation of alpha-2 noradrenergic receptors in the OB, which subsequently suppress local inhibitory granule cells—cells that inhibit output from the OB that is germane to social recognition. This norepinephrine-induced disinhibition of output cells of the OB allows for enhanced signaling from the OB projections to various brain regions to promote social recognition memory. In addition, in a line of forebrain oxytocin receptor-knockout mice, oxytocin receptor expression is reduced in the LS, hippocampus, and ventral pallidum (VP) but remains normal in the MeA, OB, olfactory nucleus, and neocortex compared with wild-type mice. Interestingly, these forebrain oxytocin receptor-knockout mice display only limited social recognition deficits, suggesting a greater role for oxytocin action in non-forebrain structures, such as the OB and MeA, in social recognition.

From the field of social neuroscience (Decety and Cacioppo, 2011) and related fields, there has been evidence to suggest that the social brain has evolved to promote select adaptive social behaviors. These behaviors are associated with and, in a sense, are reinforced by the activation of reward centers in the brain by social cues, ensuring that close social interactions promote positive emotionality, and the negative impact of social stress and loss on mental health and well-being. There has been a major effort to better understand the neurobiological mechanisms governing these behaviors to further appreciate the basis of social bonding. Information gleaned from these studies also has the potential to identify underlying mechanisms of many human mental disorders—such as autism, social anxiety, and schizophrenia—as a major diagnostic component of these disorders includes the inability to properly form social bonds.

PARENT–OFFSPRING BONDING

Proper parenting and formation of parent–infant attachments are considered the cornerstone of an individual's well-being and adaptation throughout life. Discovering the neurobiological basis of the parent–infant bonding process may be invaluable for understanding the natural consequences of disruption to bonds and the etiology of associated pathologies. In accordance to Bowlby's (1958) attachment theory, parent–infant attachments must require neural circuitry that regulates social recognition, motivation and reward, and affiliation and emotional processing pathways. Research has been conducted to outline a number of neural substrates that regulate infant–parent, mother–infant, and, when appropriate and to a lesser extent, father–infant attachment spanning over a number of mammalian species. This section reviews such literature.

INFANT–PARENT ATTACHMENT

Infants form an attachment, or affectional bond or tie, with their caregivers, and this attachment is the main source of safety and security for the child. The bond associated with infant attachment is defined by selective preference, approach, and interaction with their caregivers as well as distress during periods of separation from these individuals. Infant attachments may serve to ensure infant–caregiver proximity and elicit infant care from parents, ultimately increasing the probability of survival until maturity and reproduction in offspring. The characterization of imprinting in birds (Bateson, 1966), early social olfactory learning in rabbits (Hudson, 1993) and rats (Raineki et al., 2010), social behavior development in infant non-human primates (Harlow and Suomi, 1971), and bonding in young children (Bowlby, 1958) have produced a foundation for understanding the inception of infant attachment. Bowlby characterized this attachment in four components: (1) infants rapidly form attachments to their caregivers, (2) infants seek close proximity to their caregivers, (3) caregivers reflect safety and security, and (4) infants will endure considerable abuse to remain with their caregivers. These components reflect a secure infant attachment—providing pleasure, safety, and security for the infant—and are germane for infant attachment observed in humans and throughout the animal kingdom.

Infant attachment to caregivers appears to form during a critical period. For infant–mother attachment, the critical period begins before birth when the infant is exposed to and learns different mother-associated cues (e.g., the mother's voice and odor). After birth, the infant learns the mother's face and continues to form an attachment to the mother when the infant pairs the mother's voice and odor learned in the intrauterine environment to the postnatal environment. Infants can also begin forming attachments in early life to other caregivers, such as the father, in the same manner. These caregiver-associated cues induce innate infant behavior (e.g., proximity-seeking and orienting, caregiver–infant skin-to-skin contact, and nipple attachment and milk suckling). From a neurobiological perspective, more knowledge has been gleaned from separation than attachment, but there are three neurochemical systems that have sufficient evidence to be included into a neural circuit of infant attachment (Fig. 86.1A).

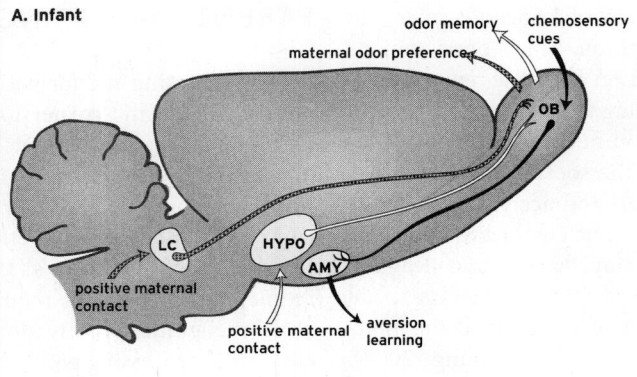

A. Infant

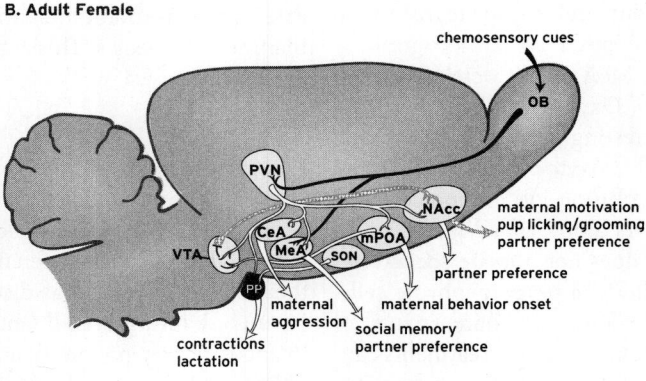

B. Adult Female

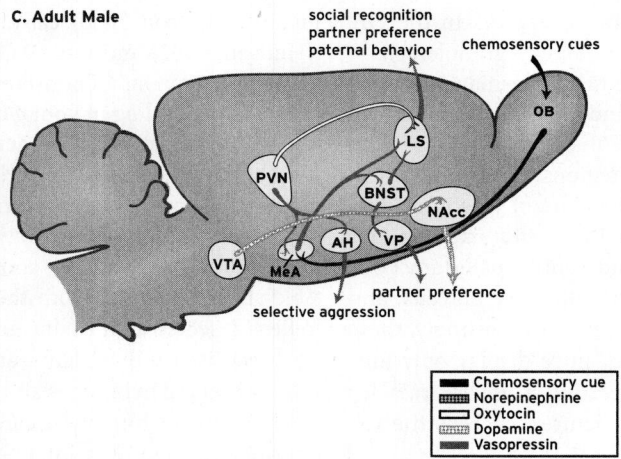

C. Adult Male

Legend:
- Chemosensory cue
- Norepinephrine
- Oxytocin
- Dopamine
- Vasopressin

Figure 86.1 *Schematic representations of the neurocircuitry required for social bonding in infants, adult females, and adult males. (A) In the infant bonding model, neonatal learning of caregiver-associated odor and odor preference occurs during a sensitive period through olfactory bulb activation, facilitated by norepinephrine from the locus coeruleus (LC) and oxytocin from the hypothalamus (HYPO). Odor aversion learning occurs via amygdala (AMY) signaling, but this pathway is inhibited during the sensitive period that leads to infant attachment. (B) In the adult female bonding model, olfactory signals from the mate or infant are transmitted via the OB to the medial subnucleus of the amygdala (MeA) or paraventricular nucleus of the hypothalamus (PVN). Oxytocin from the PVN or supraoptic nucleus of the hypothalamus (SON) acts in the central subnucleus of the amygdala (CeA), MeA, medial preoptic area (mPOA), nucleus accumbens (NAcc), or posterior lobe of the pituitary gland (PP) to facilitate social memory, childbirth, lactation, and various bond-dependent behaviors, including partner preference and maternal behavior onset and aggression. In addition, oxytocin acts in the ventral tegmental area (VTA) to stimulate dopamine release in the NAcc to promote maternal motivation, infant-directed behaviors, and partner preference formation. (C) In the male bonding model, olfactory signals from the mate or infant transmitted to the MeA from the OB. Vasopressin from the PVN is released in the anterior hypothalamus (AH) to induce selective aggression. In addition, vasopressin from the PVN, MeA, and bed nucleus of the stria terminalis (BNST) acts in the MeA, lateral septum (LS), and ventral pallidum (VP) to promote social recognition, partner preference, and paternal behavior. Oxytocin from the PVN and dopamine from the VTA act in the LS and NAcc, respectively, to facilitate partner preference formation.*

NEUROANATOMY AND CHEMICAL SUBSTRATES

In general, altricial species rely, to some degree, on learning about their caregivers to form attachments. This is embodied in the avian imprinting model, occurring at sensitive periods which are limited and restricted to early life (Bateson, 1966). Mammalian infants also display attachment toward their caregivers. For example, the sound and site of their mothers can be strong cues to promote social recognition and attachment for infants, as demonstrated in human infants (DeCasper and Spence, 1986). Mother-associated olfactory cues are also particularly critical for many mammalian species to recognize and preferentially affiliate with the mother, including humans (e.g., Porter and Winberg, 1999). Considering the requisite for infants to display a maternal preference for survival (i.e., orientation, nipple attachment, and huddling), it is advantageous for infants to rapidly form a maternal odor preference and hinder learning that would be aversive to an infant–mother attachment. Olfactory imprinting is particularly important for altricial mammals, like rabbits and rats, as offspring need to remain in the nest while the mother is gone foraging and to orient toward the mother in her presence to procure milk, warmth, and protection. Therefore, infant survival may depend upon the capacity for offspring to learn to approach and remain in close proximity to the mother or other primary caregivers. Sullivan and colleagues have conducted a series of studies noting that during a sensitive period, olfactory discrimination tests show rat pups prefer the odor of the mother (for a recent review, see Raineki et al., 2010). In addition, norepinephrine neurons deriving from the locus coeruleus (LC) regulate function in the OB to promote this maternal odor preference, whereas OB neurons projecting to the amygdala modulate aversion learning. Thus, blocking norepinephrine action in the OB by chemically lesioning the LC or administering a norepinephrine receptor inhibitor hinders learning the mother's odor, or maternal-associated odors, in rat pups. Moreover, odor preferences can be promoted by infusing norepinephrine into the OB, either by exogenous administration or stimulating the LC.

Furthermore, the oxytocin system may promote infant recognition by promoting maternal-associated odor preferences and infant affection by inducing feelings of calmness and stress reduction associated with the mother. Oxytocin facilitates learning of social cues in rat pups, a process inhibited by administration of an oxytocin receptor antagonist (Nelson and Panksepp, 1998). During suckling, the nipple area is a natural source of attraction for the infant, providing significant mother-associated odor and an obvious source of sustenance, and it is during this behavior that oxytocin seems to function in enhancing odor learning. Specifically, this neuropeptide is released in the infant brain during suckling and can act on the OB. In the OB, oxytocin can promote odor memory by augmenting long-term potentiation of neural activation associated with memory (Fang et al., 2008). This provides a significant mechanism in which oxytocin action regulates infant recognition, and ultimately attachment, for the mother. The natural occurrence of skin-to-skin contact between the mother and infant during sucking can also lead to enhanced filial huddling preference in rat pups. Interestingly, release of oxytocin in the hypothalamus is associated with skin-to-skin contact with the mother (Kojima et al., 2012), and oxytocin administration can promote filial huddling preference in rat pups (Kojima and Alberts, 2011). These data coincide with the volume of research indicating that prosocial mother–infant contact induces release of oxytocin, evaluated in the mother during parturition and nursing. Furthermore, it suggests that hypothalamic oxytocin may be released during maternal contact, a source of cutaneous warmth and tactile stimulation, and subsequently regulates the formation of filial huddling preferences and preference for maternal odor.

Infant–mother interactions also require social approach and motivation circuits. There are a few studies to implicate oxytocinergic and dopaminergic pathways in the formation of maternal-associated olfactory cues. However, more research in humans, non-human primates, sheep, and rats have been conducted to indicate that the endogenous opioid systems can attenuate aversion learning induced by stress from maternal separation and are involved in the motivation of an infant to seek maternal contact, perhaps through natural reward neural circuits. First, maternal separation leads to distress vocalizations in infants, but opioid agonists diminish this behavioral response in a number of mammalian species, including rhesus monkeys, dogs, pigs, sheep, and rats (Nelson and Panksepp, 1998). Interestingly, maternal contact can also lead to diminished distress vocalizations in infants, but this maternal buffering effect is ablated by opioid antagonist administration. In addition, endogenous opioids are involved in the attribution of positive value to maternal contact. Maternal contact and milk transferring are natural sources of endogenous opioid release in infants (Weller and Feldman, 2003). Thus, these mother-associated cues may signal the rewarding effects of maternal contact and motivate infants to maintain proximity and establish an affiliative bond with the mother.

CLINICAL CORRELATES: AUTISM

Children with autism often fail to develop, or display limited, recognition of and attachment to their primary caregivers. Thus, much effort has recently been committed to correlate the neurobiology of normally developed infant attachment to those disrupted by autism to better understand this neuropsychological disorder. The positive relationship between oxytocin transmission in the brain and normal infant–mother bonding has led many to speculate on the function of abnormalities in the oxytocin system in the etiology of autism (for a recent review, see Green and Hollander, 2010). Certainly, several studies indicate that variation in the DNA sequences, known as single nucleotide polymorphisms, which encode for the oxytocin and oxytocin receptor genes, are associated with the propensity of autism in children. Furthermore, infusion of oxytocin in adults with autism and other related disorders, such as Asperger disorder, can alter the display of symptoms such as increasing comprehension and memory of word affect as well as reducing repetitive behaviors (e.g., repeating, self-injuring, and touching). In addition, many studies report a number of prosocial effects from intranasal application of oxytocin, including increased trust, generosity, emotional empathy, and salience of social information as well as socially reinforced learning

(Striepens et al., 2011). Despite these correlative data, abnormal function of the brain oxytocin system of children with autism remains to be demonstrated. Furthermore, the neurotransmitter system serotonin has also been associated with autism; nearly 30% of children with autism have increased blood serotonin levels (Cook and Leventhal, 1996). Serotonin acts as a developmental signal in the brain—promoting neural organization and differentiation, neurite outgrowth, synaptogenesis, dendritic branching, and neurogenesis—before assuming its role as a neurotransmitter (Whitaker-Azmitia, 2001). The serotonin system autoregulates its own development via a negative feedback loop and regulates development of other systems such as the oxytocin system (Martin et al., 2012). Therefore, serotonin may also modulate the effects that other neurochemical systems have on the etiology of autism.

MOTHER–INFANT ATTACHMENT

From birth, mammalian infants rely heavily on the care and protection provided by the mother to reassure survival and proper development. Because the mother is the primary, or sole, caregiver for most mammalian species, the onus of maternal investment is great and tethered to infant survival. It seems that mother–infant interactions (e.g., childbirth, infant-related sensory cues, maternal care, and nursing) and the mother's own physiology are skewed to foster maternal attachment and a desire to give warmth, comfort, food, and protection. Mother–infant attachment also manifests via increased intrinsically rewarding properties of contact with offspring, increased protective behavior (i.e., maternal defense or aggression), and reduced stress via mother–infant interaction (i.e., infant buffering). Furthermore, some evidence suggests associations among these effects (e.g., maternal aggression and stress: Bosch and Neumann, 2012; Gammie et al., 2008). Development and maturation of a mother–infant attachment are regulated by a variety of neurochemical systems including, but not limited to, the oxytocin, dopamine, and corticotrophin-releasing hormone (CRH) systems, as well as the interaction between these neural systems (see Fig. 86.1B).

NEUROANATOMY AND CHEMICAL SUBSTRATES

In the peripartum period, the mother's physiology and infant behavior seem to facilitate mother–infant attachments, and oxytocin, a reproductive neuropeptide, may explain these effects. Oxytocin is mainly synthesized in the hypothalamic paraventricular (PVN) and supraoptic (SON) nuclei and is released peripherally via the posterior pituitary in response to distension of the cervix and uterus during labor, leading to contractions of the uterine smooth muscles and succoring birth. After birth, skin-to-skin contact with the newborn, infant pre-feeding behavior (e.g., touching and licking mother's nipples), and breastfeeding also stimulate increased pulsatile release of oxytocin to promote milk ejection (Matthiesen et al., 2001; Nissen et al., 1995). The fact that oxytocin is pivotal in these behaviors and reproductive functions in which maternal bonding occurs initially led to the suggestion that oxytocin may be involved in the bonding process as well (Nelson and

Panksepp, 1998). In fact, the hypothalamic cells that synthesize oxytocin project to various brain regions throughout cortical areas, the olfactory system, the basal ganglia, the limbic system, the thalamus, the hypothalamus, the brainstem, and the spinal cord that express oxytocin receptors, and many of these brain areas are sensitive to social cues and regulate social affiliation (Gimpl and Fahrenholz, 2001). Furthermore, stimulation of neurons in the PVN can lead to release of oxytocin in the brain, acting on neurons expressing oxytocin receptors. Thus, in addition to female reproductive tissue, the central nervous system is sensitive to oxytocin action.

The release of oxytocin in response to childbirth, lactation, and innate infant behavior act on the maternal brain, changing oxytocinergic neuronal morphology and affecting other neural systems that promote maternal behaviors (Insel, 1992). For instance, oxytocin levels during pregnancy and the peripartum period are related to establishing contact with or checking on the infant, attachment-related thoughts, and infant-directed gazing, vocalizations, touching, and positive affect in women (Feldman et al., 2007), maternal olfactory-based recognition in sheep (Kendrick et al., 1997), and grooming and contact of mother rhesus monkeys with their young (Maestripieri et al., 2009). Thus, the hormonal milieu associated with childbirth, breastfeeding, and innate infant behavior (e.g., mother–infant skin contact and milk suckling) leads to oxytocin release, which reinforces maternal behavior. Ultimately, maternal oxytocin levels have also been associated with higher maternal–infant attachment in women (Galbally et al., 2011).

The laboratory rat has been extensively utilized for studying the effect of oxytocin on maternal care as, unlike most mammalian species, female rats show little interest in infants of their own species, even aversions, until just before parturition when they begin to display maternal care (Fig. 86.2A). This shift in behavior is associated with changes to oxytocinergic neuronal morphology during pregnancy and peripartum that promotes onset of maternal care behaviors, including increased oxytocin gene expression and oxytocin receptor binding in the mPOA (Fig. 86.2A,B). Furthermore, in estrogen-primed nulliparous female rats, central administration of oxytocin facilitates the onset of maternal behavior. These effects were first observed when Pedersen and Prange (1979) noted that intracerebroventricular (ICV) administration of oxytocin will induce full maternal response (i.e., nest-building and grouping, licking, crouching, and retrieval of pups) in estrogen-primed nulliparous female rats. Moreover, blockade of oxytocin action in the brain—chemically via oxytocin receptor antagonist or antiserum or by lesioning oxytocinergic neurons in the hypothalamus—significantly impairs onset of rat maternal behavior. These behavioral effects have also been observed when oxytocin action was manipulation in the mPOA or ventral tegmental area (VTA) in rats and the nucleus accumbens (NAcc) in prairie voles (*Microtus ochrogaster*), indicating selective brain regions for oxytocin-induced maternal care (Pedersen, 2004). For instance, oxytocin injections into the mPOA induce a maternal response in most virgin female rats in which chemical blockade of oxytocin receptors in this brain area prevent the onset of maternal behaviors in lactating rats (Fig. 86.2C,D). Interestingly, postpartum rats displaying

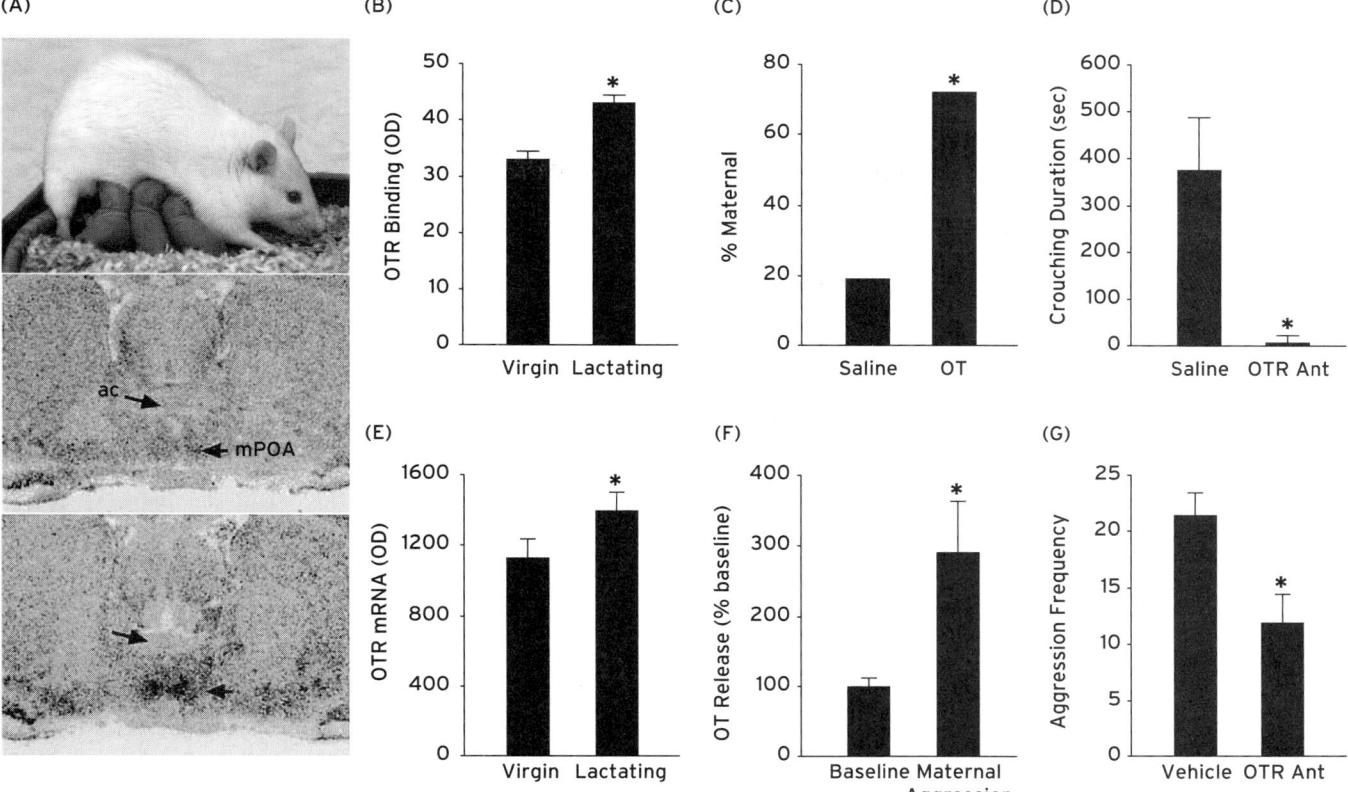

Figure 86.2 Oxytocin (OT) acts in the medial preoptic area (mPOA) to facilitate the onset of maternal behavior and central subnucleus of the amygdala (CeA) to promote maternal aggression in rats. (A) Photo depicts maternal behavior (i.e., arched-back nursing) in female rats (top) as well as differences in oxytocin receptor (OTR) mRNA expression in the mPOA between virgin (middle) and lactating (bottom) female rats. (B) Lactating rats have higher optical densities (OD) of OTR binding in the mPOA than virgin female rats. (C) OT injected in the mPOA induces a higher percentage of virgin female rats to display a full maternal response during a pup interaction test than saline injections. (D) The onset of maternal behavior (e.g., crouching over pups) is inhibited in lactating rats receiving an injection of an OTR antagonist in the mPOA. (E) OTR mRNA expression in the CeA is higher in lactating rats than virgin female rats. (F) OT release in the CeA increases during aggressive interactions with an intruding conspecific during a maternal defense test compared to a period immediately before the onset of the test in which the female rats are undisturbed. (G) Maternal aggression can be reduced via an injection of an OTR antagonist in the CeA. Bars indicate means ± standard error of the mean. *p < 0.05. (Adapted from Bosch et al. (2005); Bosch et al. (2010); Neumann (2008); Pedersen et al. (1982, 1994); Young et al. (1997).)

maternal care are not affected by blocking the central oxytocin system signaling. This suggests that oxytocin is required for the onset of rat maternal behavior but is not involved in the maintenance of these behaviors.

In the brain, oxytocin seems to provide an incentive for the mother to appraise infants as rewarding attachment objects, motivating maternal care and attention. In fact, mothers consider their infants to be intensely rewarding, particularly in the early postpartum months (Swain, 2011). There is also good evidence that the mesocorticolimbic dopamine system promotes the onset of maternal behavior and that hypothalamic oxytocin, particularly from the mPOA, regulates this pathway. For example, intense mother–offspring interactions during suckling result in activation of the dopamine reward system in mothers (Febo et al., 2005). Blockade of local dopamine signaling in the NAcc via lesioning of the VTA, a brain region projecting dopaminergic fibers that innervate the NAcc, reduces maternal behavior as well as the salience of the rewarding properties of pups (for a recent review, see Numan and Stolzenberg, 2009). The oxytocin system seems to innervate dopamine regulation of maternal care in the VTA. Specifically, oxytocin receptors

are expressed in the VTA in rats, and in tract-tracing studies, oxytocin-positive cells and neurons responsive to maternal care in the mPOA have been observed to project to the VTA (Numan and Stolzenberg, 2009; Shahrokh et al., 2010), modulating subsequent VTA-mediated dopamine release in the NAcc. Recent data have also shown that oxytocin action in the VTA can regulate dopamine release in the NAcc associated with pup licking/grooming in female rats. In rats, high licking/grooming mothers have more oxytocinergic neurons in the mPOA and PVN that project into the VTA compared with low licking/grooming mothers. Furthermore, inhibition of oxytocin action in the VTA can impair pup licking/grooming and the amount of dopamine release in the NAcc induced by these behaviors (Shahrokh et al., 2010). Thus, hypothalamic oxytocin seems to interact with the mesocorticolimbic dopamine system in motivating the initial maternal responsiveness toward infants. After a critical period of interaction, it is proposed that the mPOA is reorganized in such a way that pup stimuli alone are sufficient to induce the motivation of maternal behavior and rewarding properties of the infant without the needed regulation of the oxytocin system.

In addition to inducing direct maternal care, oxytocin reduces aggression directed toward neonates and aversion associated with infant cues (Kendrick et al., 1997; Pedersen, 2004). This may be enhanced by the role that oxytocin has in producing the calming and antistress effect associated with infant contact and breastfeeding. In lactating females, oxytocin release during nipple stimulation and breastfeeding reduces basal and stress-induced rises in stress hormones and suppresses heart rates, blood pressure, and stress-related behaviors (Carter and Altemus, 1997). Thus, infant contact during breastfeeding and subsequent oxytocin release could buffer a mother's stress response. This could provide a mechanism through which mother–infant contact ameliorates stress associated with the infant and limits anxiety-induced aggression. Also, there are some data suggesting that maternal stress is associated with maternal defense, and oxytocin mediates this relationship. First, maternal care is associated with increased aggression toward potential threats near the infant. Bosch and Neumann (2012) recently reviewed an emerging body of literature indicating oxytocin may promote intruder-directed maternal aggression. Several brain regions have been identified as sites for oxytocin-mediated maternal aggression, including the central subnucleus of the amygdala (CeA) and PVN and to a lesser extent the bed nucleus of the stria terminalis (BNST) and LS. In the CeA, oxytocin gene expression is increased in this brain area during the peripartum period in rats (Fig. 86.2E). Furthermore, in lactating rats, oxytocin is released in the CeA and PVN during displays of maternal defense, but not during interactions with an unfamiliar conspecific with little or no aggression (Fig. 86.2F). The amount of maternal aggressive behavior displayed by lactating rats during these encounters correlates with the amount of oxytocin released in these brain areas. Administration of oxytocin in the CeA and PVN can also promote maternal aggression. In addition, retrodialysis of an oxytocin receptor antagonist into the CeA or PVN can hinder maternal aggression in lactating rats during a maternal defense test (Fig. 86.2G). Second, maternal stress physiology—such as the release of CRH, a stress hormone regulating one of the major biological stress pathways known as the hypothalamic-pituitary-adrenal (HPA) axis—is negatively associated with the display of maternal aggression. It has been noted that stress and CRH injections can reduce maternal aggression in lactating mice and rats (Gammie et al., 2008). For that reason, inhibition of CRHergic neurons may be a prerequisite for the expression of maternal defensive behavior. The inhibitory action of oxytocin on CRHergic activity, particularly in the PVN, may achieve this requirement (reviewed by Gammie et al., 2008; Smith and Wang, 2012). Therefore, infant-induced activation of central oxytocin—which can be promoted by childbirth, lactation, and innate infant behavior—may minimize negative associations toward infant cues, reducing maternal anxiety and promoting infant proximity and contact, while increasing perceived threats from unfamiliar conspecifics and subsequent maternal protective behaviors. This mechanism could explain the reduced aversion toward infants and enhanced selective aggression toward intruders in mothers.

CLINICAL CORRELATES: MATERNAL NEGLECT

For parental bonding, similar neurochemistry has been observed between humans and other mammalian species, with a focus on oxytocin, dopamine, and vasopressin. However, neural circuitry has primarily been studied in rodent species that only display maternal behavior. Because humans display bi-parental care and have a more complex cortical systems, in comparison with rodents, it will be beneficial to understand how these factors influence the neurobiological regulation of parental bonding in both mothers and fathers. Still, comparing normal variation in the patterns of parental care has led to insights into how different parental brain responses may contribute to aberrant parental bonding, as observed in maternal neglect. Strathearn (2011) noted that insecure attachment—allied with emotional neglect—is associated with the same neural substrates that govern rodent maternal behavior, specifically the oxytocin and mesocorticolimbic dopamine reward systems. Mothers displaying such a dismissive nature have reduced activation of the limbic system as well as decreased peripheral oxytocin response to infant contact. Because oxytocin is released during childbirth and lactation peripherally as well as centrally, as observed in animal literature, one hypothetical mechanism for maternal neglect could include a deficit in brain oxytocin transmission. Women with such a deficit would still be able to have successful deliveries and nurse; however, they would not experience the same reinforcements associated with infant contact or display the same type of responsiveness to infant distress.

FATHER–INFANT ATTACHMENT

A widely accepted benefit of pair bonding in humans, as in other species, is the physical and psychological well-being of children, an effect likely caused by the co-occurrence of pair bonding with the bi-parental care of young. Indeed, paternal involvement in child care has become increasingly recognized as equally important as maternal influences on successful child development in humans, and even more so in some monogamous, bi-parental non-human primate species (for examples, see Solomon and French, 1997). After conception, direct paternal investment in mammals does not manifest until childbirth because males do not gestate. However, during early infancy, the care that fathers provide to their offspring can be equal to that provided by mothers, with the exception of lactation, in many bi-parental species—including humans, prairie voles, degus (Octodon degus) California mice (Peromyscus californicus), marmoset and tamarin monkeys (family Callitrichidae), and titi monkeys (Callicebus moloch). Specifically, fathers from bi-parental mammalian species display a broad range of paternal behaviors, some direct (e.g., carrying, grooming, playing, and eventually feeding) and others indirect (e.g., nest building, paternal defense, and support of the female during pregnancy). Yet, the display of infant care is not always apparent in males that are not pair-bonded or breeding with a female partner. In fact, virgin male California mice are infanticidal rather than paternal, a behavior that persists after mating and through the gestation of their female partner and does not subside until their female partner gives birth. Thus, father–infant attachment may manifest in part by suppressing negative associations to infant stimuli (e.g., progeny of a successful rival male and thus a threat to one's own reproductive success) and promoting care and protective behaviors that are reinforced by stimulating the brain reward centers. In fact, fathers consider their newborns as intensely rewarding (Swain, 2011). However, we know little about the neurobiology of paternal attachment.

NEUROANATOMY AND CHEMICAL SUBSTRATES

One mechanism that has provided some data is the vasopressin system (Fig. 86.1C). Only a few studies have evaluated the effects of pharmacological manipulations of vasopressin signaling on paternal behavior. These studies have been conducted in two closely related *Microtus* rodents, the bi-parental prairie vole (*M. ochrogaster*) and the non-paternal meadow vole (*Microtus pennsylvanicus*). Blockade of vasopressin receptors reduced paternal behavior and increased occurrence of pup attacks in male prairie voles, but this required concurrent inhibition of oxytocin receptors (Bales et al., 2004). In naturally non-paternal meadow voles, vasopressin injections promoted parental behaviors and reduced pup-directed aggression, an effect reversed by a vasopressin receptor antagonist (Parker and Lee, 2001). Thus, *Microtus* paternal behavior seems to be enhanced by the vasopressin system. In addition, Wang et al. (1998) noted that vasopressin injections directly into the LS increased the amount of time male prairie voles engaged in paternal behavior (e.g., contacting and crouching over the pup), whereas pretreatment with a vasopressin 1-alpha receptor (V1aR) antagonist abolished these effects. It is worth mentioning that male prairie voles display high levels of spontaneous paternal behavior, including pup huddling, licking/grooming, and retrieving, which can be augmented further by social experiences, including parental experience and adult male–female bonding. Wang and colleagues noted that parental experience also alters the vasopressin neural system in male prairie voles. Specifically, after parturition of their female partner and parental experience, male prairie voles have less vasopressin-immunoreactive fibers in the LS, which is accompanied by significantly more vasopressin gene expression in the BNST—a brain region that projects to the LS. This reduction in vasopressin immunoreactivity may reflect increased septal vasopressin release because of paternal experience that is not immediately restored. Still, in prairie voles, like many bi-parental species, male infant care is spontaneous. Thus, it may not need hormonal regulation to elicit onset. However, it seems that social experience associated with childbirth and infant contact can enhance neural circuitry that augments the display of male parental behavior while reducing infant-directed aggression. Therefore, father–infant attachment may be associated with altering the perception of an infant from an unfamiliar conspecific or progeny of a rival male, and thus a threat, to an affiliative object that requisites care and protection.

ADULT BONDING

Mammalian societies are often complex and can contain adult relationships fostered by reproduction or kinship (i.e., breeding mates and extended families) or facilitated by environmental pressures such as territorial or predatory defense as well as resource allocation (i.e., group mates, allies, and friendships). In many species, adult relationships include same-sex dyads or coalitions that are required for survival and longevity and sustained by kinship, social tolerance, and even social affiliation. About 3% to 5% of mammalian species, primarily rodents and New World primates, display monogamy as the dominant mating system (Solomon and French, 1997). The dominant relationship in these social groups is defined between the breeding male–female partner, which often includes a stable and enduring social attachment (i.e., pair bond). The formation and maintenance of these bonds are integral to the fabric of human social behavior and implicated in an individual's mental and physical health and well-being. Yet little is known about the underlying neurobiology, potentially because of its inherent complexity and relative rarity in mammals.

Nevertheless, research evaluating the neurobiological basis of pair bonding has provided insight into the regulatory mechanisms of behavioral cornerstones of this bond, including selective social preference and affiliation behavior, mate guarding, bi-parental care, and separation distress. Further, much of this research has focused on *Microtus* rodents or voles because this genus includes closely related species that are either monogamous (e.g., the prairie vole) or non-monogamous (e.g., the meadow vole), and includes similar neurochemical systems involved in parent–infant bonding; namely, oxytocin, vasopressin, and dopamine. From these comparative studies, the differences in social behavior and distribution patterns of central vasopressin and oxytocin systems observed between prairie and meadow voles have been suggested to be related to the divergent life strategies in these species (an example of these results are illustrated in Fig. 86.3A). Instead of delving further into these comparative studies, this section highlights vole research by focusing on the monogamous prairie vole to better understand the neurobiological mechanisms that govern the formation and maintenance of pair bonding in adulthood for females and males (see Fig. 86.1B,C).

PAIR BONDING

Prairie vole pair bonding behaviors have been documented in field research, using radiotelemetry combined with repeated trapping. Sexually naïve prairie voles are highly gregarious and socially tolerant, displaying nonselective affiliative behaviors and low levels of aggression toward conspecifics. However, following extensive mating or cohabitation with the opposite sex, male and female prairie voles remain in close proximity to their breeding partner reinforced by limiting roaming patterns to a defined nest and home range that is shared and protected by the breeding pair, and even traveling together. Bonded adult male and female prairie voles maintain this spatial and social proximity usually until one partner dies, and even then, the survivor rarely forms a new pair bond (Pizzuto and Getz, 1998). Furthermore, male–female breeding partners display behavioral hallmarks of a monogamous pairing such as selective social preferences for their familiar partner (Aragona and Wang, 2004), aggression toward

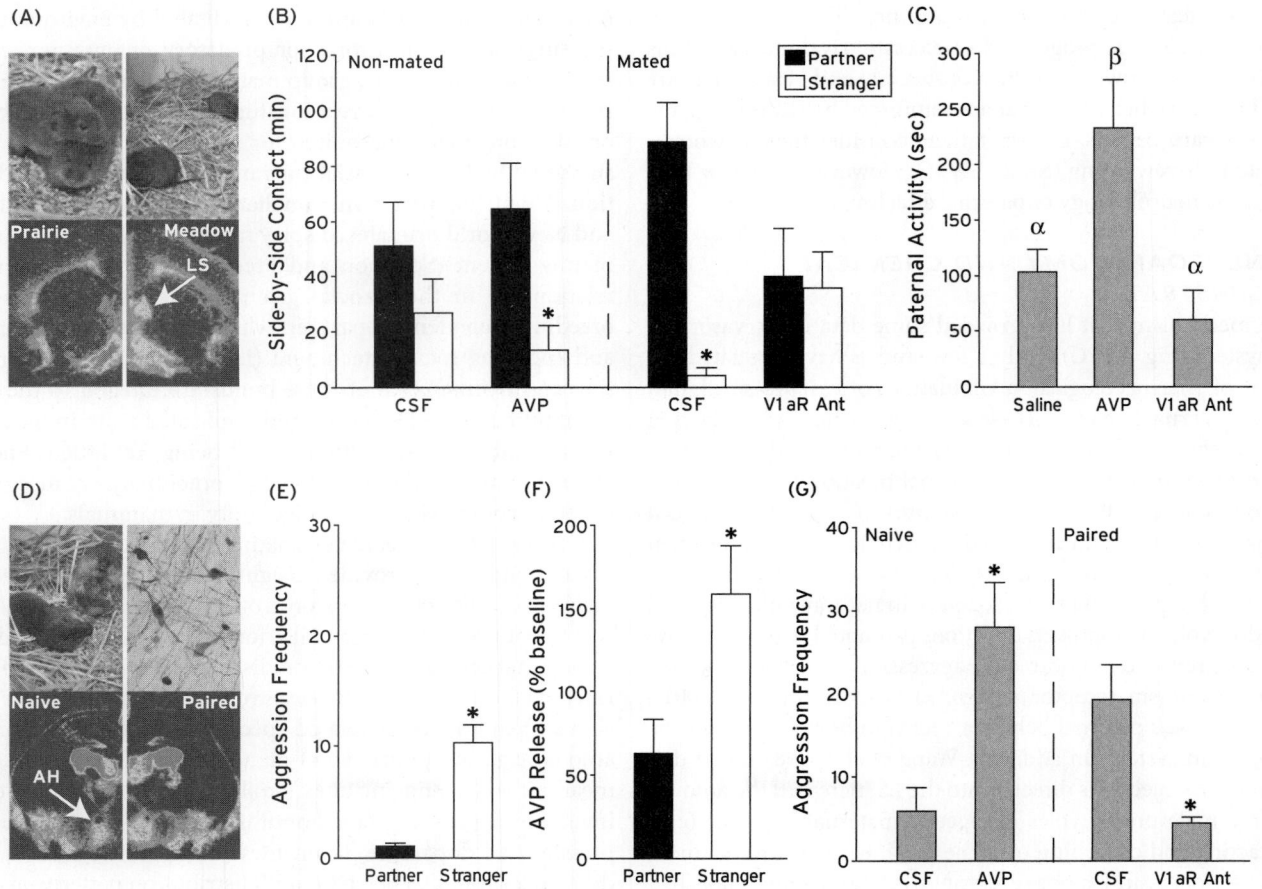

Figure 86.3 *Vasopressin (AVP) regulates partner preference formation and paternal behavior via signaling in the lateral septum (LS) and selective aggression via action in the anterior hypothalamus (AH) in male prairie voles. (A) Photos and photo images illustrating species-specific differences in social affiliation (top) and density of vasopressin 1-alpha receptor (V1aR) binding in the LS (bottom) between the monogamous prairie vole (left) and polygamous, solitary meadow vole (right). (B) AVP injected in the LS facilitates partner preference formation in non-mated male prairie voles, whereas an intra-LS injection of a V1aR antagonist blocks such behavior. (C) An intra-LS injection of AVP, not a V1aR antagonist, can also promote paternal behavior in male prairie voles. (D) Photo and photomicrographs depict selective aggression (top left) and aggression-induced neuronal activity (Fos-immunoreactive cells with dark nuclear staining) in AVP-immunoreactive cells (Dark gray cytoplasmic staining) in the AH (top right) in paired male prairie voles as well as the differences in V1aR binding in the AH between sexually naïve (bottom left) and paired (bottom right) male prairie voles. (E) Paired male prairie voles display significantly more aggression toward an intruding conspecific (stranger) compared with a familiar female partner. (F) AVP release in the AH increases during aggressive interactions, with an intruding conspecific during a resident intruder test compared with a period immediately before the onset of the test in which the male prairie vole is undisturbed. (G) AVP injected in the AH induces intruder-directed aggression in sexually naïve males, whereas an intra-AH injection of a V1aR antagonist blunts such aggression in paired males. Bars indicate means ± standard error of the mean. Bars with different Greek letters differ significantly from each other. *p < 0.05. (Adapted from Gobrogge et al. (2009); Liu et al. (2001); Wang et al. (1994).)*

intruding conspecifics (Gobrogge and Wang, 2011), remaining together through gestation and displaying bi-parental care throughout lactation (Wang et al., 1998), and reducing the stress response and distress associated with social separation or bond loss via social contact and consolatory behaviors (Smith and Wang, 2012). Therefore, these aspects of prairie vole social behavior facilitate and aid in the retention of a pair-bond. Behavioral paradigms have been developed in the laboratory to quantify these behaviors and study the governing neurobiological systems (e.g., oxytocin, vasopressin, and dopamine).

NEUROANATOMY AND CHEMICAL SUBSTRATES

A selective social preference, or partner preference, reflects the extent to which prairie voles seek out social contact with

their partner over other conspecifics, and is a reliable laboratory index of the formation of a pair bond in prairie voles. This selective affiliation can be assessed using a partner preference test first developed in the laboratory of Dr. Sue Carter (Williams et al., 1992). The partner preference test is a three-hour test in which the subject is placed in a three-chamber choice apparatus and allowed to freely roam among the three chambers—an empty cage, which acts as a non-social control environment, and two adjoining cages that house either the subject's social partner or an unfamiliar, opposite-sex conspecific. After 24 hours of cohabitation and mating, male and female prairie voles consistently display a selective preference to spend the majority of time in their partner's cage and affiliating more with their partner compared with the opposite-sex conspecific, indicating a partner preference. The inaugural evidence that two closely related neuropeptidergic systems, namely, oxytocin and vasopressin, regulated partner preference behavior came in the effects of bond-inducing social and sexual behaviors on these systems in the brain. Notably, mating, although not required, can facilitate pair bonding in prairie voles (Williams et al., 1992), and sexually naïve female prairie voles exposed to male chemosensory cues or housed with a male have altered oxytocin receptor density in the anterior olfactory nucleus and release oxytocin in the NAcc from oxytocin-immunoreactive cells originating in the PVN and SON (Ross et al., 2009; Witt et al., 1991). In addition, mating also induces dopamine release in the NAcc in prairie voles. Like maternal attachment, hypothalamic oxytocin can promote dopamine release in the NAcc and, subsequently, promote female pair bonding. In male prairie voles, mating during cohabitation decreases the number of vasopressin-immunoreactive fibers in the LS and increases vasopressin gene expression in the BNST—a brain region that projects to the LS (Wang et al., 1998). Like the paternal experience-induced effects in male prairie voles, these data suggest that sociosexual experience with a female may promote vasopressin release in the LS derived from vasopressinergic cells in the BNST, potentially promoting male pair bonding. Like females, mating induces dopamine release in the NAcc in male prairie voles, providing one behavioral mechanism for partner preference, and thus, motivation to maintain selective social proximity in prairie voles.

More direct evidence for the involvement of oxytocin and vasopressin in prairie vole pair bonding has manifested by use of ICV and site-specific injections of oxytocin, vasopressin, selective antagonists, and viral vectors (reviewed in Aragona and Wang, 2004). Intracerebroventricular administration of oxytocin can facilitate partner preference formation in female prairie voles, and males to a certain degree, diminishing the period of cohabitation required for this behavioral preference to manifest. A selective oxytocin receptor antagonist administered centrally can inhibit the effects of oxytocin release in the brain on partner preference, induced endogenously via mating or cohabitation or administered exogenously. Furthermore, ICV injections of vasopressin can facilitate, whereas a concurrent injection of a selective vasopressin receptor antagonist can inhibit, the display of a partner preference in male prairie voles. In fact, oxytocin and vasopressin both can facilitate partner preference formation in males and females; however, site-specific manipulates indicate sex-specific circuitry. In females, the NAcc and prelimbic cortex (PLC) have been implicated in the oxytocin regulation of partner preferences. Oxytocin injected directly into the NAcc induces partner preferences, whereas an oxytocin receptor antagonist injected into either the NAcc or PLC can inhibit mating-induced female partner preferences. By contrast, oxytocin receptor antagonist administration into the LS can inhibit a partner preference in male prairie voles. Furthermore, vasopressin administration directly into the LS induces male partner preferences in the absence of mating (Fig. 86.3B). Blockade of vasopressin action in the LS by a V1aR antagonist can abolish mating-induced effects on male partner preferences. Vasopressin-immunoreactive fibers are found in dense networks in the LS and extend ventrally into the VP in male prairie vole. Interestingly, overexpression of the V1aR via an adeno-associated viral vector in the VP also facilitates a partner preference in males. As mentioned, an injection

of vasopressin in the LS can also promote paternal behavior in male prairie voles (Fig. 86.3C). Thus, vasopressinergic signaling in the LS seems to promote social bonding in male prairie voles, both as a pair-bonded partner and a father.

Data from a series of experiments have indicated that mesolimbic dopamine activity, particularly in the NAcc, can also promote partner preferences in voles in a receptor-specific manner (Aragona and Wang, 2009; Fig. 86.4A–D). The vole VTA synthesizes dopamine that projects axon fibers that terminate in the NAcc where two families of dopamine receptors are expressed, D1-like (D1R) and D2-like (D2R) receptors (see Fig. 86.4A). They each have opposite intracellular signaling and behavioral effects. Specifically, partner preference formation and expression is stimulated by an injection of a D2R agonist, but blocked by an injection of a D1R agonist, into the NAcc in male prairie voles (see Fig. 86.4B). D1R and D2R have the opposite effects over cyclic adenosine monophosphate (cAMP) signaling (see Fig. 86.4C). D1R signaling activates stimulatory G-proteins that increase conversion of adenosine triphosphate (ATP) to cAMP via adenylyl cyclase activation. This increases cAMP production activates protein kinase A (PKA), leading to activation of transcription factors and gene expression. In contrast, activation of D2R activates inhibitory G-proteins that prevent adenylyl cyclase from converting ATP to cAMP, leaving PKA in an inactive state. Given that when dopamine receptor signaling promotes partner preference formation in prairie voles cAMP signaling-induced PKA activity in the NAcc is decreased, it was hypothesized that blockade of this intracellular signaling pathway was required for partner preference formation. Consistent with the effects of D2R signaling, when PKA activity in the NAcc was pharmacologically depressed in male prairie voles during a short-term cohabitation with a female conspecific, males formed partner preferences, whereas untreated males did not display such preferences (see Fig. 86.4D). Like D1R activation, when PKA activity in the NAcc was chemically increased during a long-term cohabitation, males did not form partner preferences. Thus, dopamine mediates partner preference formation in a receptor-specific manner through intracellular cAMP signaling and PKA activity in the NAcc. In addition, pair-bonded males also have increased D1R expression levels in the NAcc compared to sexually naïve male prairie voles. Because D1R activity inhibits partner preference formation, this may be a neural mechanism that prevents the formation of new pair bonds by attenuating the salience of the rewarding effects of interacting with other conspecifics. Together, these data highlight the functional role and site-specificity of oxytocin, vasopressin, and dopamine in the regulation of partner preference formation in females and males. Nevertheless, although partner preferences persist throughout the adult relationship, even potentially enduring well beyond as prairie voles seldom establish a new pairing after their partner dies, no data have been collected to document the effects of these neurochemicals on the maintenance of this bond-related behavior.

Although selective preference for a partner may facilitate bonding, selective aggression in the form of intruder-directed aggression is one behavior that aids in the maintenance of such a bond. Mating-induced aggression is common in many species. However, this usually takes form as temporary mate guarding,

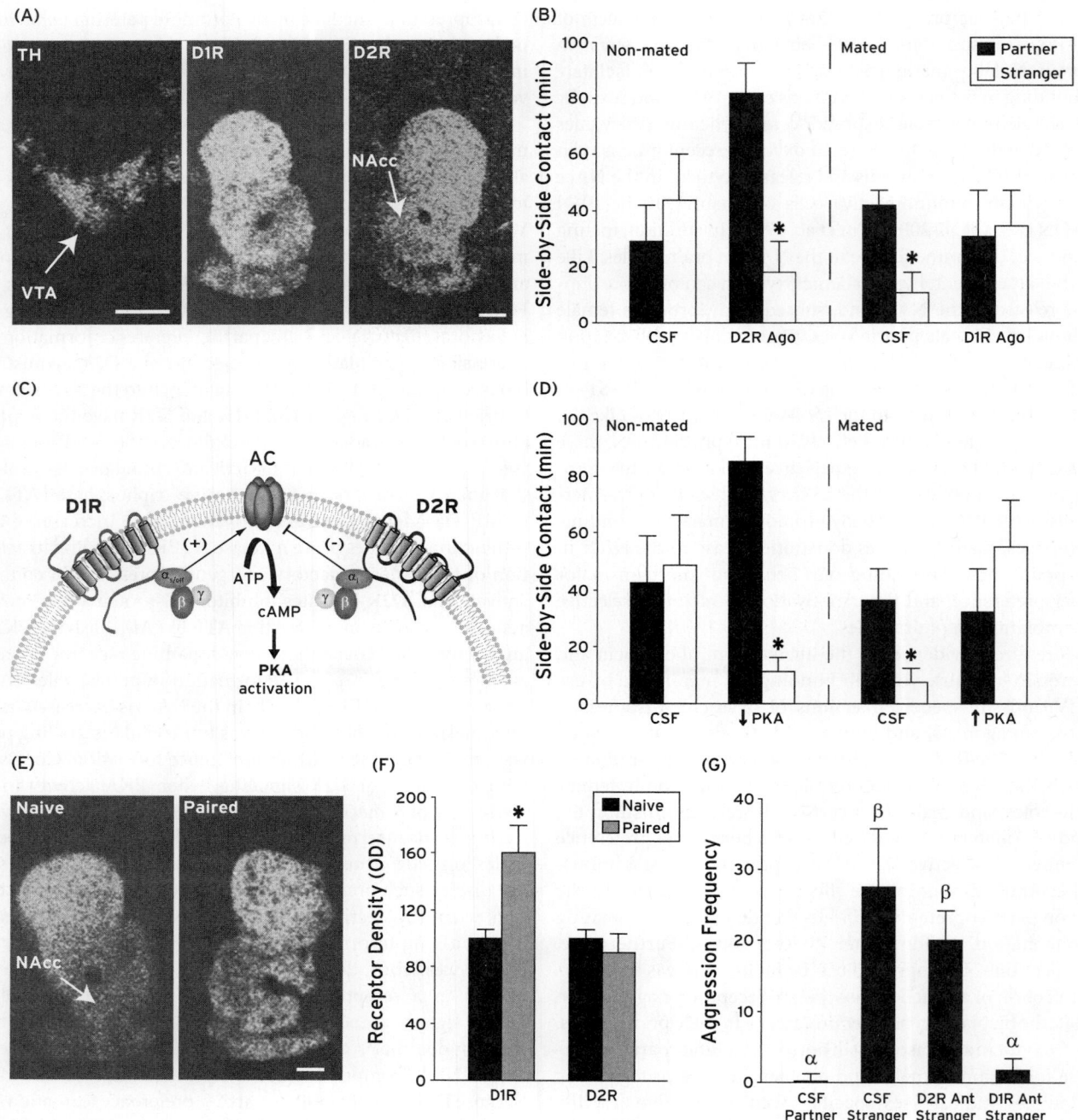

Figure 86.4 *Nucleus accumbens (NAcc) dopamine involvement in partner preference formation, selective aggression, and intracellular signaling pathways in a receptor-specific manner in male prairie voles. (A) Photomicrographs showing immunoreactive staining for tyrosine hydroxylase (TH) mRNA in the ventral tegmental area (left) and receptor binding for D1R (middle) and D2R (right) in the NAcc. (B) D2R agonist (D2R ago) injected in the NAcc induces a partner preference in non-mated males, whereas a D1R agonist (D1R ago) injection blocks partner preference formation in mated males. (C) Illustration representing receptor-specific effects of D1R and D2R on cAMP intracellular signaling. D1R signaling excites stimulatory G-proteins, which promotes ATP conversion to cAMP via adenylyl cyclase (AC) and cAMP-induced PKA activation. In contrast, D2R signaling excites inhibitory G-proteins blocking AC-induced cAMP production and PKA activation via cAMP. (D) Partner preference formation is facilitated in non-mated males via pharmacological inactivation of PKA in the NAcc and blocked in mated males via pharmacological activation of PKA in the NAcc. (E) Photo images portray differences in D1R binding density between sexually naïve and paired male prairie voles. (F) D1R production is increased in paired males compared with sexually naïve males, but D2R production is not. (G) Selective aggression toward strangers can be eliminated by an intra-NAcc injection of a D1R antagonist, but no effect is observed with a D2R antagonist injection. Bars indicate means ± standard error of the mean. Bars with different Greek letters differ significantly from each other. *p < 0.05. (Adapted from Aragona et al., 2006; Aragona and Wang, 2007; Aragona, B.J., Liu, Y., Yu, Y.J., 2006. Nucleus accumbens dopamine differentially mediates the formation and maintenance of monogamous pair bonds. Nat. Neurosci. 9:133–139; Aragona, B.J., Wang, Z. 2007. Opposing regulation of pair bond formation by cAMP signaling within the nucleus accumbens shell. J. Neurosci. 27:13352–13356).*

to improve reproductive success via paternal certainty, leading to intrasexual aggression toward conspecifics. In monogamous species such as prairie voles, mating-induced aggression often facilitates both intra- and intersexual aggression toward unfamiliar conspecifics (see Fig. 86.3D,E), thus thwarting competitors and forgoing potential extra-pair mating opportunities. This is one behavioral mechanism of pair bond maintenance. Interestingly, although vasopressin is involved with promoting selective partner-directed affiliation, there are data to outline its regulatory role in mating-induced intruder-directed aggression in male prairie voles (for a recent review, see Gobrogge and Wang, 2011). Initial experiments indicate that V1aR binding in the anterior hypothalamus (AH) increases after male prairie voles are paired with a female, and neuronal activity, particularly in vasopressin-expressing neurons, increases in the AH and MeA following aggressive interactions with an unfamiliar conspecific compared with non-aggressive interactions or contact with a familiar partner (see Fig. 86.3 D). In addition, aggressive interactions with an unfamiliar conspecific induce increased vasopressin release in the AH (see Fig. 86.3 F). Furthermore, vasopressin injections directly into the AH can promote intruder-directed aggression in male prairie voles, an effect mediated by V1aR as a concurrent injection of a V1aR antagonist can abolish intruder aggression (see Fig. 86.3G). Thus, AH vasopressin is both necessary and sufficient to regulate mating-induced selective aggression in male prairie voles. Given that D1R expression and binding are increased in the NAcc after pairing with a female (see Fig. 86.4E,F), which induces male prairie voles to display selective aggression toward intruders, efforts have been made to also explore the effects of dopamine on this behavior (Aragona and Wang, 2009). Sure enough, when D1R activation was inhibited in the NAcc via an injection of a D1R-specific antagonist, pair-bonded male prairie voles were affiliative, not aggressive, toward intruding, unfamiliar females. However, pair-bonded males receiving a vehicle treatment or a selective D2R antagonist were highly aggressive and displayed little affiliative behavior toward the female intruders (see Fig. 86.4G). Therefore, the plasticity of the vasopressin and mesolimbic dopamine systems underlie the behavioral mechanism of pair bonding that leads to aggressively rejecting new potential mates, ensuring the maintenance of the existing pair bond.

In addition to selective aggression, bi-parental care and separation distress seem to be contributing social factors that promote bond maintenance. First, considerable evidence suggests that the neural processes necessary for parental behavior and pair bonding may be shared in prairie voles. Recent evidence even indicates that prior parental experience can promote activity of the oxytocin and vasopressin systems in the brain and facilitate partner preference in male prairie voles (Kenkel et al., 2012). However, female prairie vole mate choice is dictated by the amount of partner-directed affiliative behavior, not paternal care, that a male displays, and male prairie vole partner-directed affiliation and parental care are not correlated (Ophir et al., 2008). Bi-parental care provides advantages to parental reproductive fitness and the offspring in terms of supporting development and improving mental and physical health and well-being. Nevertheless, although neurobiological substrates have been identified to promote parent–infant bonding in prairie voles and other monogamous species, more research is needed to determine if parental behavior is required to retain a monogamous bond. Second, in a recent review, Smith and Wang (2012) noted that the HPA axis and oxytocin activity may mediate the aversive effects of partner separation, and thus regulate the preservation and maintenance of existing pair bonds. Social separation from a pair-bonded partner during periods of psychological distress can intensify the HPA axis and stress-related behavioral response in prairie voles. However, the response to social separation from familiar conspecifics may depend upon the intensity of existing affiliative bonds because separation from a same-sex conspecific—an adult relationship that is not associated with social bonding in prairie voles—does not affect stress physiology. Social contact with a pair-bonded partner can disrupt the behavioral and physiological stress response in female prairie voles; this is known as social buffering. Interestingly, contact with a pair-bonded partner following a stressful event can induce the release of oxytocin in the PVN in female prairie voles. This release may have functional effects because oxytocin injected into the PVN can also reduce the stress response. Further, the stress-reducing effect of a bonded-partner on the HPA axis response and stress-related behavior in females is marginalized when a selective oxytocin receptor antagonist is injected into the PVN before social contact. Thus, social buffering in prairie voles seems to be regulated by oxytocin action in the PVN that limits the HPA response to stress. Furthermore, disruption of CRH action, and thus HPA axis function, by induction of a CRH receptor antagonist can eliminate behavioral distress associated with social loss in prairie voles (i.e., permanent separation from a pair-bonded partner). Thus, pair bonding maintenance may be enhanced by the benefits of social contact, via oxytocin, and consequences of pair bond disruption, via CRH and the HPA axis. The function of a pair bond on the regulation of the biobehavioral stress response may be one reason why individuals attempt to maintain established bonds, and oxytocin and CRH may be governing neuropeptide systems.

CLINICAL CORRELATE: HUMAN BONDING

Humans develop long-lasting and selective social bonds in adulthood, but the neurobiology of human pair bonding remains unresolved. Certainly, human love and pair bonding in non-human primates are regulated by higher-level cortical structures to a greater degree than social attachments in rodents. But it could be conceived that the same neural substrates that regulate rodent pair bonding such as in prairie voles; namely, oxytocin, vasopressin, and dopamine systems, may also be involved in humans. This would require similarities in the neuroanatomy between prairie voles and humans. The pattern of receptor expression in oxytocin and vasopressin has been examined in humans, and although there is some overlap between human and prairie vole receptor expression, there are brain regions in the human brain analogous to the prairie vole brain that lack these receptors (Gimpl and Fahrenholz, 2001). This may suggest that human pair bonding is mediated by different mechanisms or that these neural systems affect bonding behavior by alternative neural circuitry. Still, there is evidence that human pair bonding is governed, at least in part, by these same neurochemical systems. For example, intranasal application of oxytocin has been reported in a number of studies to promote prosocial effects that would facilitate human bonding, including increased trust, generosity, emotional empathy, conflict resolution, and salience of social information as well as socially reinforced learning (Striepens et al., 2011). In addition, vasopressin is associated with human aggression; the life history of aggression in men and women are positively correlated with the concentration of vasopressin in cerebrospinal fluid (reviewed in Gobrogge and Wang, 2011). Sex could also influence the formation of human pair bonds as it does in monogamous rodents. Although sex is not required for human pair bonding, features of human sexuality such as sexual arousal and organism, even nipple stimulation, may induce the release of oxytocin and vasopressin (Carmichael et al., 1987; Murphy et al., 1987). Furthermore, mesocorticolimbic dopamine activity may propagate romantic love. People had significantly more activity in this pathway while viewing pictures of their romantic partner compared with images of non-romantic friends in a neuroimaging study (Bartels and Zeki, 2000).

CONCLUSIONS

NEUROBIOLOGY OF PARENT–INFANT BONDING

The neurobiological data on the three forms of parent–infant bonding (i.e., infant–parent, mother–infant, and father–infant) focus on neural substrates that regulate social recognition, motivation and reward, and affiliation and emotional processing pathways (see Fig. 86.1). Infant–parent attachment, specifically infant–mother attachment, has centered on the critical capacity for infants to recognize the mother—highlighting olfactory learning—and be motivated to establish close proximity to the mother. From this literature, it seems that norepinephrine projections from the LC and oxytocin from the PVN terminating in the OB are mediating recognition of the mother's odor, beginning from amniotic fluid *in utero* to odors associated with the nipples and milk. In addition, motivation to seek contact with a caregiver is promoted by the endogenous opioid system, although specific opioid centers in the brain have not been clearly identified. Nevertheless, some prognostication may be learned from the neuroanatomical substrates of the infant distress response during maternal separation. Neurophysiological recording and functional brain imaging studies point to the anterior cingulated cortex as a hub for the generation of separation calls and infant crying that can be influenced by decreasing opioid action in this brain region (Newman, 2007). Because maternal buffering of separation distress is promoted by increased opioid activity in the infant brain, the anterior cingulated cortex may be a brain region involved in this regulation. For mother–infant attachment, the onset of maternal behavior is associated with increased neuronal activity, particularly of the oxytocin system, in the mPOA—a brain region that receives projections from the amygdala and BNST. In addition, oxytocinergic fibers from the mPOA innervating the VTA can mediate the activity of the mesocorticolimbic dopamine system, particularly release of NAcc DA, subsequently affecting the regulation of maternal incentive to establish contact with her infant. Maternal aggression and stress are influenced by the social environment and are regulated by oxytocin action in the CeA and PVN, CRH action in the PVN associated with regulation of the HPA axis, and oxytocin–CRH interaction in these brain areas. Finally, father–infant attachment has not been as comprehensively studied. However, there are data to suggest that the vasopressinergic fibers from the BNST project to the LS, and stimulation of the LS can enhance paternal behavior while reducing infant-directed aggression.

NEUROBIOLOGY OF PAIR BONDING

The neurobiological basis of pair bonding focuses on neural substrates that regulate partner preference, selective aggression, bi-parental care, and separation distress (see Fig. 86.1). Partner preference behavior is reinforced by several neurochemical systems—oxytocin, vasopressin, and dopamine. For female prairie voles, male chemosensory cues or cohabitation is required to induce estrus as well as altering oxytocin receptor density in the anterior olfactory nucleus and release oxytocin in the NAcc from oxytocin-immunoreactive cells originating from the PVN and SON (Ross et al., 2009; Witt et al., 1991). Like in mothers, hypothalamic oxytocin may regulate NAcc dopamine release in pair-bonded females, which can itself facilitate the formation and expression of female partner preferences. For male prairie voles, partner preference behavior is enhanced by mating, which can increase BNST vasopressin gene expression and decrease vasopressin fiber density in the LS—a brain region in addition to the VP that vasopressin-expressing neurons from the BNST send axonal projections to. Specific activation of V1aR in the LS and VP can subsequently enhance male partner preferences. Together, vasopressinergic neurons located in the BNST regulate partner preference formation through the release of vasopressin in the LS and VP, promoting vasopressin signaling through V1aR activation. In addition, dopamine release in the NAcc can modulate male partner preference behavior in a receptor-specific manner (i.e., increased via D2R signaling and decreased via D1R signaling). Beyond partner preference formation, the vasopressin system seems to also regulate pair bonding long-term by enhancing selective aggression toward unfamiliar conspecifics. However, it seems that vasopressin action occurs in the MeA and AH to promote intruder aggression rather than the LS and VP as in partner preference formation. Finally, social reinforcement or retention of the pair bond is enhanced via distress associated with bond loss and stress buffering effects associated with social contact and consolatory behaviors. During social loss, the CRH action in the PVN, and subsequent HPA axis function, seems to lead to distress behavior, whereas oxytocin also in the PVN can reduce these stress effects and is necessary for the beneficial effects of social buffering.

EXPLORING A "BONDING BRAIN" AND FUTURE DIRECTIONS

Across all relationships reviewed, the bonding process seems similar: (*1*) initiate contact with potential attachment object (e.g., infant, parent, or partner); (*2*) process socially salient information and learn specific identity of this individual; (3) invest to maintain relationship and develop motivational association to attachment object; and (4) reject other conspecifics. These steps may be achieved by different behaviors, but there seems to be some conservation in the neural processes involved (see Fig. 86.1). Some exceptions include the lack of involvement in different brain regions (e.g., amygdala) in infant attachment, but this may be explained by immature neural circuitry. Also, many of the monoamines and neuropeptides involved in infant, mother, and father attachments as well as adult pair bonding are preserved. Such socially aroused neurochemicals include oxytocin, vasopressin, and dopamine. For example, oxytocin release in the brain of peripartum female rats during pup contact or sexually naïve female prairie voles during contact with a male conspecific can facilitate activation of the mesocorticolimbic dopamine systems, inducing a neural incentive to maintain social proximity. Further, pair bonding and paternal behavior in male prairie voles are associated with increased vasopressin action in the LS, which is innervated by the BNST. Therefore, oxytocin, vasopressin, and dopamine neural circuits may propagate female and male social behavior selectively to promote and protect a social bond. These neural substrates seem generally excitable by social stimuli until a bond manifests and then activation is discriminate to stimulation from a bonded individual. For example, in male prairie voles, NAcc dopamine signaling via D2R activation promotes partner preference formation, whereas D1R activity prevents such behavior. Once males are pair-bonded, D1R expression increases in the NAcc, potentially as a neural mechanism to prevent new bonds from forming. Thus, the rewarding aspects of social interaction with an attachment object may selectively propagate that bond while preventing new bonds from forming.

In the field of social neuroscience, the focus will, in part, be to continue to understand how the oxytocin and vasopressin systems regulate bond-related social behaviors and modulate the mesocorticolimbic dopamine reward center to regulate motivation for social attachments. Nevertheless, in bonded individuals, social behavior is reinforced by stimulation of the brain reward centers by bond-salient stimuli, ensuring attachment objects elicit positive emotionality and consequences to mental health and well-being associated with social stress and loss. From this perspective, the incentive to form new bonds should be similar to the reluctance to break social bonds, providing a need to better understand the neurobiology of bond retention. In addition, research examining sociability in humans is on the rise with new pharmacology, genetic, and neuroimaging techniques. These tools should be implemented in studying human bonding to allow for more substantial comparisons to animal models. Moreover, information derived from studying the neurobiology of social attachment in animal models and humans has the potential to provide insight into the underlying mechanism of many human mental disorders—such as autism, social anxiety, and schizophrenia—as a major diagnostic component of these disorders includes the inability to properly form social bonds.

ACKNOWLEDGMENTS

We would like to thank Y. Liu for her assistance in capturing photo images for several figures. We gratefully acknowledge C. Badland for his photographic contributions for vole images and assistance with the figures. Special thanks to O. Bosch and D. Bayerl also for their photographic contributions for the rat image and to O. Bosch for providing additional data that appear in the figures.

DISCLOSURES

The authors declare there are no conflicts of interest to disclose. Authors are funded by NIMH and NIDA only. Grant support was provided by the National Institutes of Health grants MHF31-095464 to AS and MHR01-58616, MHR01-89852, and DAK02-23048 to ZW.

REFERENCES

Adolphs, R. (2003). Cognitive neuroscience of human social behaviour. *Nat. Rev. Neurosci.* 4:165–178.

Aragona, B.J., Liu, Y., et al. (2006). Nucleus accumbens dopamine differentially mediates the formation and maintenance of monogamous pair bonds. *Nat. Neurosci.* 9:133–139.

Aragona, B.J., and Wang, Z. (2004). The prairie vole (*Microtus ochrogaster*): an animal model for behavioral neuroendocrine research on pair bonding. *ILAR J.* 45:35–45.

Aragona, B.J., and Wang, Z. (2007). Opposing regulation of pair bond formation by cAMP signaling within the nucleus accumbens shell. *J. Neurosci.* 27:13352–13356.

Aragona, B.J., and Wang, Z. (2009). Dopamine regulation of social choice in a monogamous rodent species. *Front. Behav. Neurosci.* 3:15.

Bales, K.L., Kim, A.J., et al. (2004). Both oxytocin and vasopressin may influence alloparental behavior in male prairie voles. *Horm. Behav.* 45:354–361.

Bartels, A., and Zeki, S. (2000). The neural basis of romantic love. *Neuroreport* 11:3829–3834.

Bateson, P.P. (1966). The characteristics and context of imprinting. *Biol. Rev. Camb. Philos. Soc.* 41:177–211.

Bosch, O.J., Meddle, S.L., et al. (2005). Brain oxytocin correlates with maternal aggression: link to anxiety. *J. Neurosci.* 25:6807–6815.

Bosch, O.J., and Neumann, I.D. (2012). Both oxytocin and vasopressin are mediators of maternal care and aggression in rodents: from central release to sites of action. *Horm. Behav.* 61:293–303.

Bosch, O.J., Pfortsch, J., et al. (2010). Maternal behaviour is associated with vasopressin release in the medial preoptic area and bed nucleus of the stria terminalis in the rat. *J. Neuroendocrinol.* 22:420–429.

Bowlby, J. (1958). The nature of the child's tie to his mother. *Int. J. Psychoanal.* 39:350–373.

Carmichael, M.S., Humbert, R., et al. (1987). Plasma oxytocin increases in the human sexual response. *J. Clin. Endocrinol. Metab.* 64:27–31.

Carter, C.S., and Altemus, M. (1997). Integrative functions of lactational hormones in social behavior and stress management. *Ann. NY Acad. Sci.* 807:164–174.

Cook, E.H., and Leventhal, B.L. (1996). The serotonin system in autism. *Curr. Opin. Pediatr.* 8:348–354.

DeCasper, A.J., and Spence, M.J. (1986). Prenatal maternal speech influences newborns' perception of speech sounds. *Infant Behav. Dev.* 9:133–150.

Decety, J., and Cacioppo, J.T. (2011). Handbook of Social Neuroscience. New York: Oxford University Press.

Dunbar, R.I.M. (1998). The social brain hypothesis. *Evol. Anthropol.* 6:178–190.

Fang, L.Y., Quan, R.D., et al. (2008). Oxytocin facilitates the induction of long-term potentiation in the accessory olfactory bulb. *Neurosci. Lett.* 438:133–137.

Febo, M., Numan, M., et al. (2005). Functional magnetic resonance imaging shows oxytocin activates brain regions associated with mother-pup bonding during suckling. *J. Neurosci.* 25:11637–11644.

Feldman, R., Weller, A., et al. (2007). Evidence for a neuroendocrinological foundation of human affiliation: plasma oxytocin levels across pregnancy and the postpartum period predict mother-infant bonding. *Psychol. Sci.* 18:965–970.

Galbally, M., Lewis, A.J., et al. (2011). The role of oxytocin in mother-infant relations: a systematic review of human studies. *Harv. Rev. Psychiatry* 19:1–14.

Gammie, S.C., D'Anna, K.L.L., et al. (2008). Role of corticotropin releasing factor-related peptides in the neural regulation of maternal defense. In: Bridges, R.S., ed. Neurobiology of the Parental Brain. San Diego, CA: Elsevier.

Gimpl, G., and Fahrenholz, F. (2001). The oxytocin receptor system: structure, function, and regulation. *Physiol. Rev.* 81:630–668.

Gobrogge, K.L., Liu, Y., et al. (2009). Anterior hypothalamic vasopressin regulates pair-bonding and drug-induced aggression in a monogamous rodent. *Proc. Natl. Acad. Sci. USA* 106:19144–19149.

Gobrogge, K.L., and Wang, Z. (2011). Genetics of aggression in voles. In: Huber, R., Bannasch, D.L., Brennan, P., eds. Aggression. San Diego, CA: Academic Press, pp. 121–150.

Green, J.J., and Hollander, E. (2010). Autism and oxytocin: new developments in translational approaches to therapeutics. *Neurotherapeutics* 7:250–257.

Hammock, E.A.D., and Young, L.J. (2007). Neuroendocrinology, neurochemistry, and molecular neurobiology of affiliative behavior. In: Lajtha, A., and Blaustein, J.D., eds. Handbook of Neurochemistry and Molecular Neurobiology. New York: Springer, pp. 247–284.

Harlow, H.F., and Suomi, S.J. (1971). Social recovery by isolation-reared monkeys. *Proc. Natl. Acad. Sci. USA* 68:1534–1538.

Hudson, R. (1993). Olfactory imprinting. *Curr. Opin. Neurobiol.* 3:548–552.

Insel, T.R. (1992). Oxytocin: a neuropeptide for affiliation: evidence from behavioral, receptor autoradiographic, and comparative studies. *Psychoneuroendocrinology* 17:3–35.

Insel, T.R., and Fernald, R.D. (2004). How the brain processes social information: searching for the social brain. *Annu. Rev. Neurosci.* 27:697–722.

Kendrick, K.M., Da Costa, A.P., et al. (1997). Neural control of maternal behaviour and olfactory recognition of offspring. *Brain Res. Bull.* 44:383–395.

Kenkel, W.M., Paredes, J., et al. (2012). Neuroendocrine and behavioural responses to exposure to an infant in male prairie voles. *J. Neuroendocrinol.* 24:874–886.

Kojima, S., and Alberts, J.R. (2011). Oxytocin mediates the acquisition of filial, odor-guided huddling for maternally-associated odor in preweanling rats. *Horm. Behav.* 60:549–558.

Kojima, S., Stewart, R.A., et al. (2012). Maternal contact differentially modulates central and peripheral oxytocin in rat pups during a brief regime of mother-pup interaction that induces a filial huddling preference. *J. Neuroendocrinol.* 24:831–840.

Liu, Y., Curtis, J.T., et al. (2001). Differential expression of vasopressin, oxytocin and corticotrophin-releasing hormone messenger RNA in the paraventricular nucleus of the prairie vole brain following stress. *J. Neuroendocrinol.* 13:1059–1065.

Maestripieri, D., Hoffman, C.L., et al. (2009). Mother-infant interactions in free-ranging rhesus macaques: relationships between physiological and behavioral variables. *Physiol. Behav.* 96:613–619.

Martin, M.M., Liu, Y., et al. (2012). Developmental exposure to a serotonin agonist produces subsequent behavioral and neurochemical changes in the adult male prairie vole. *Physiol. Behav.* 105:529–535.

Matthiesen, A.S., Ransjo-Arvidson, A.B., et al. (2001). Postpartum maternal oxytocin release by newborns: effects of infant hand massage and sucking. *Birth* 28:13–19.

Murphy, M.R., Seckl, J.R., et al. (1987). Changes in oxytocin and vasopressin secretion during sexual activity in men. *J. Clin. Endocrinol. Metab.* 65:738–741.

Nelson, E.E., and Panksepp, J. (1998). Brain substrates of infant-mother attachment: contributions of opioids, oxytocin, and norepinephrine. *Neurosci. Biobehav. Rev.* 22:437–452.

Neumann, I.D. (2008). Brain oxytocin: a key regulator of emotional and social behaviours in both females and males. *J. Neuroendocrinol.* 20:858–865.

Newman, J.D. (2007). Neural circuits underlying crying and cry responding in mammals. *Behav. Brain Res.* 182:155–165.

Nissen, E., Lilja, G., et al. (1995). Elevation of oxytocin levels early post partum in women. *Acta Obstet. Gynecol. Scand.* 74:530–533.

Numan, M., and Stolzenberg, D.S. (2009). Medial preoptic area interactions with dopamine neural systems in the control of the onset and maintenance of maternal behavior in rats. *Front. Neuroendocrinol.* 30:46–64.

Ophir, A.G., Crino, O.L., et al. (2008). Female-directed aggression predicts paternal behavior, but female prairie voles prefer affiliative males to paternal males. *Brain Behav. Evol.* 71:32–40.

Parker, K.J., and Lee, T.M. (2001). Central vasopressin administration regulates the onset of facultative paternal behavior in *Microtus pennsylvanicus* (meadow voles). *Horm. Behav.* 39:285–294.

Pedersen, C.A. (2004). Biological aspects of social bonding and the roots of human violence. *Ann. NY Acad. Sci.* 1036:106–127.

Pedersen, C.A., Ascher, J.A., et al. (1982). Oxytocin induces maternal behavior in virgin female rats. *Science* 216:648–650.

Pedersen, C.A., Caldwell, J.D., et al. (1994). Oxytocin activates the postpartum onset of rat maternal behavior in the ventral tegmental and medial preoptic areas. *Behav. Neurosci.* 108:1163–1171.

Pedersen, C.A., and Prange, A.J., Jr. (1979). Induction of maternal behavior in virgin rats after intracerebroventricular administration of oxytocin. *Proc. Natl. Acad. Sci. USA* 76:6661–6665.

Perrett, D.I., Hietanen, J.K., et al. (1992). Organization and functions of cells responsive to faces in the temporal cortex. *Philos. Trans. R. Soc. Lond. B Biol. Sci.* 335:23–30.

Pizzuto, T., and Getz, L.L. (1998). Female prairie voles (*Microtus ochrogaster*) fail to form a new pair after loss of mate. *Behav. Proc.* 43:79–86.

Porter, R.H., and Winberg, J. (1999). Unique salience of maternal breast odors for newborn infants. *Neurosci. Biobehav. Rev.* 23:439–449.

Raineki, C., Pickenhagen, A., et al. (2010). The neurobiology of infant maternal odor learning. *Braz. J. Med. Biol. Res.* 43:914–919.

Ross, H.E., Cole, C.D., et al. (2009). Characterization of the oxytocin system regulating affiliative behavior in female prairie voles. *Neuroscience* 162:892–903.

Shahrokh, D.K., Zhang, T.-Y., et al. (2010). Oxytocin-dopamine interactions mediate variations in maternal behavior in the rat. *Endocrinology* 151:2276–2286.

Smith, A.S., and Wang, Z. (2012). Salubrious effects of oxytocin on social stress-induced deficits. *Horm. Behav.* 61:320–330.

Solomon, N.G., and French, J.A. (1997). Cooperative Breeding in Mammals. New York: Cambridge University Press.

Strathearn, L. (2011). Maternal neglect: oxytocin, dopamine and the neurobiology of attachment. *J. Neuroendocrinol.* 23:1054–1065.

Striepens, N., Kendrick, K.M., et al. (2011). Prosocial effects of oxytocin and clinical evidence for its therapeutic potential. *Front. Neuroendocrinol.* 32:426–450.

Swain, J.E. (2011). The human parental brain: *in vivo* neuroimaging. *Prog. Neuropsychopharmacol. Biol. Psychiatry* 35:1242–1254.

Wang, Z., Ferris, C.F., et al. (1994). Role of septal vasopressin innervation in paternal behavior in prairie voles (*Microtus ochrogaster*). *Proc. Natl. Acad. Sci. USA* 91:400–404.

Wang, Z., Young, L.J., et al. (1998). Voles and vasopressin: a review of molecular, cellular, and behavioral studies of pair bonding and paternal behaviors. *Prog. Brain Res.* 119:483–499.

Weller, A., and Feldman, R. (2003). Emotion regulation and touch in infants: the role of cholecystokinin and opioids. *Peptides* 24:779–788.

Whitaker-Azmitia, P.M. (2001). Serotonin and brain development: role in human developmental diseases. *Brain Res. Bull.* 56:479–485.

Williams, J.R., Catania, K.C., et al. (1992). Development of partner preferences in female prairie voles (*Microtus Ochrogaster*): the role of social and sexual experience. *Horm. Behav.* 26:339–349.

Witt, D.M., Sue, C., et al. (1991). Oxytocin receptor binding in female prairie voles: endogenous and exogenous oestradiol stimulation. *J. Neuroendocrinol.* 3:155–161.

Young, L.J., Muns, S., et al. (1997). Changes in oxytocin receptor mRNA in rat brain during pregnancy and the effects of estrogen and interleukin-6. *J. Neuroendocrinol.* 9:859–865.

87 | THE NEUROBIOLOGY OF SLEEP

GIULIO TONONI AND CHIARA CIRELLI

leep is a state of reduced responsiveness to environmental stimuli, usually associated with immobility and stereotyped postures. This reduced responsiveness is rapidly reversible—distinguishing sleep from coma—but is still potentially dangerous. Considering that such a state of reduced responsiveness occupies one third of our life, that it is universal, being present in every animal species studied, and that it is tightly regulated, it is likely to serve some essential function. However, what that function is remains uncertain to this day. What is certain is that if we stay awake much longer than the usual 16 hours a day, we are soon overcome by sleepiness, and we become cognitively impaired. The brain is spontaneously active during sleep, so changes in sleep rhythms can be a sensitive indicator of changes in brain function in neuropsychiatric disorders.

This chapter first examines how sleep is traditionally subdivided into different stages that alternate in the course of the night. We then consider the brain centers that determine whether we are asleep or awake and examine the negative consequences of sleep deprivation. We then discuss how brain activity changes between sleep and wakefulness and consider how this leads to the characteristic modifications of consciousness experienced during dreaming and dreamless sleep. Finally, we turn to the paramount but still mysterious question of sleep function.

SLEEP STAGES AND CYCLES

The scientific study of sleep and wakefulness came of age in 1928 when Hans Berger developed an amplifier that could record the electrical activity generated by the brain and discovered that the electroencephalogram (EEG) changes dramatically between wakefulness and sleep, mostly because of the appearance of sleep slow waves and spindles (Jung and Berger, 1979). Another key development occurred in 1953, when Aserinsky and Kleitman discovered a stage of sleep during which the EEG was similar to that of wakefulness (Aserinsky and Kleitman, 1953). Because this stage was associated with bursts of eye movements, it was called rapid eye movement (REM) sleep. By contrast, all other sleep has come to be called non-rapid eye movement (NREM) sleep.

Nowadays, sleep is studied for clinical and research purposes by combining behavioral observations with electrophysiological recordings. The EEG records synchronous synaptic activity from millions of neurons underlying electrodes applied to the scalp (Fig. 87.1). The electrooculogram (EOG), which is

recorded from electrodes attached to the skin near the eyes, detects small electrical fields generated by eye movements. The electromyogram (EMG), which is generally recorded from electrodes attached to the chin, is used to detect sustained (tonic) and episodic (phasic) changes in muscle activity that correlate with changes in behavioral state. In the course of the night, the EEG, EOG, and EMG patterns undergo coordinated changes that are used to distinguish among different sleep stages.

WAKEFULNESS

During wakefulness, the EEG is characterized by waves of low amplitude and high frequency. This kind of EEG pattern is known as low-voltage fast-activity or activated. When eyes close in preparation for sleep, EEG alpha activity (8–13 Hz) becomes prominent, particularly in occipital regions. Such alpha activity is thought to correspond to an "idling" rhythm in visual areas. The waking EOG reveals frequent voluntary eye movements and eye blinks. The EMG reveals tonic muscle activity with additional phasic activity related to voluntary movements.

NREM SLEEP STAGE 1

Falling asleep is a gradual phenomenon of progressive disconnection from the environment. Sleep is usually entered through a transitional state, stage 1 (N1), characterized by loss of alpha activity and the appearance of a low-voltage mixed-frequency EEG pattern with prominent theta activity (3–7 Hz). Eye movements become slow and rolling, and muscle tone relaxes. Although there is decreased awareness of sensory stimuli, a subject in stage 1 may deny that he was asleep. Motor activity may persist for a number of seconds during stage 1. Occasionally participants experience sudden muscle contractions (hypnic jerks), sometimes accompanied by a sense of falling and dreamlike imagery. Participants deprived of sleep often have "microsleep" episodes that consist of brief (5–10 seconds) bouts of stage 1 sleep; these episodes can have serious consequences in situations that demand constant attention, such as driving a car.

NREM SLEEP STAGE 2

After a few minutes in stage 1, people usually progress to stage 2 sleep (N2). This stage is heralded in the EEG by the appearance of K-complexes and sleep spindles, which are especially evident over central regions. K-complexes are made up of a high-amplitude negative sharp wave followed by a positive slow

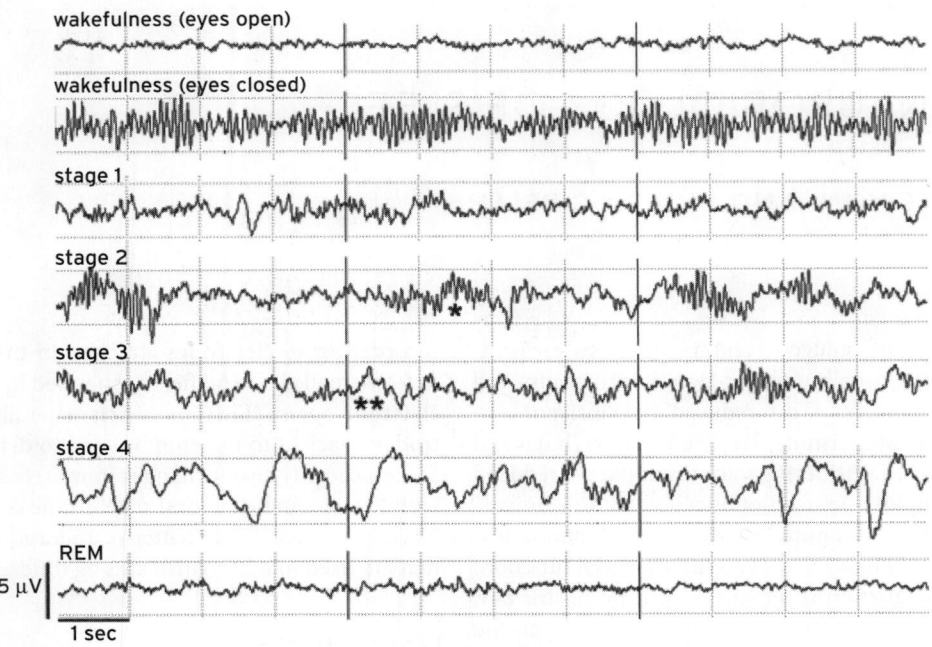

wakefulness (eyes open)

wakefulness (eyes closed)

stage 1

stage 2

stage 3

stage 4

REM

75 µV

1 sec

Figure 87.1 The human electroencephalogram (EEG) during wakefulness and the different stages of sleep (*, sleep spindles; **, slow wave).

wave and are often triggered by external stimuli. Sleep spindles are waxing and waning oscillations at around 12–15 Hz that last about 1 second and occur 5–10 times a minute. Eye movements and muscle tone are much reduced. Stage 2 qualifies fully as sleep because people are partially disconnected from the environment, meaning that they do not respond to the events around them—their arousal threshold is increased. If stimuli are strong enough to wake them up, people in stage 2 will confirm that they were asleep.

NREM SLEEP STAGES 3 AND 4

Particularly at the beginning of the night, stage 2 is generally followed by N3, a period when 20% or more of each sleep epoch consists of slow waves (i.e., waves of 0.5–2 Hz frequencies with peak-to-peak amplitude of >75 µV). N3 is also defined as slow wave sleep, delta sleep, or deep sleep, because arousal threshold increases incrementally from stage N1 to N3. Until recently, slow wave sleep was subdivided according to the proportion of slow waves in the epoch (stage 3, 20–50%; stage 4, >50%), but the validity and biological significance of this subdivision has been called into question and stages 3 and 4 are now together called stage N3 (Silber et al., 2007). Eye movements cease during stages N2 and N3, and EMG activity decreases further. The process of awakening from slow wave sleep is drawn out, and participants often remain confused for some time.

REM SLEEP

After deepening through stage N3, NREM sleep lightens and returns to stage N2, after which the sleeper enters REM sleep. As was mentioned, REM sleep derives its name from the frequent bursts of rapid eye movements (Aserinsky and Kleitman,

1953; Dement and Kleitman, 1957). Rapid-eye-movement (REM) sleep is also referred to as paradoxical sleep (Jouvet, 1962, 1965, 1998) because the EEG during REM sleep is similar to the activated EEG of waking or of stage N1. Indeed, the EEG of REM sleep is characterized by low-voltage fast-activity, often with increased power in the theta band (three–seven Hz). REM sleep is not subdivided into stages but is rather described in terms of tonic and phasic components. Tonic aspects of REM sleep include the activated EEG and a generalized loss of muscle tone, except for the extraocular muscles that drive the REMs, and the diaphragm that keeps us breathing. REM sleep is also accompanied by penile erections (their significance is unknown, but their occurrence can rule out neurological causes of impotence). Phasic features of REM sleep include irregular bursts of REMs and muscle twitches. Behaviorally, REM sleep is deep sleep, with an arousal threshold that is as high as in slow wave sleep.

SLEEP DURING THE LIFE SPAN

Sleep patterns change markedly across the life span (Baker and Colrain, 2011; Carskadon, 2011; Carskadon, 2014; Jenni et al., 2004a, 2004b). Newborn infants spend 16–18 hours per day sleeping, with an early version of REM sleep, called active sleep, occupying about half of their sleep time. At approximately three–four months of age, when sleep starts to become consolidated during the night, the sleep EEG shows more mature waveforms characteristic of NREM and REM sleep. During early childhood, total sleep time decreases, and REM sleep proportion drops to adult levels. The proportion of NREM sleep spent in slow wave sleep increases during the first year of life, reaches a peak, declines during adolescence and adulthood and may disappear entirely by age 60.

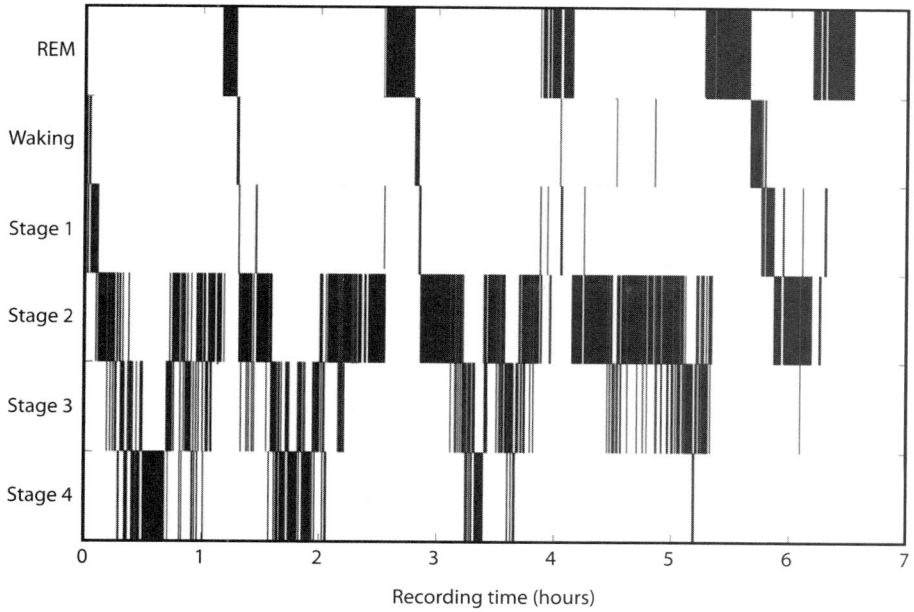

Figure 87.2 *Hypnogram for an all-night recording in a young man. Note the occurrence of five sleep cycles, the predominance of slow wave sleep (stages 3 and 4) early in the night and the increasing length of REM sleep episodes later in the night.*

THE SLEEP CYCLE

The succession of NREM sleep stages followed by an episode of REM sleep is called a *sleep cycle* and lasts approximately 90–110 minutes in humans. As shown in Figure 87.2, there are a total of four to five cycles every night. Slow wave sleep is prominent early in the night, especially during the first sleep cycle, and diminishes as the night progresses. As slow wave sleep wanes, periods of REM sleep lengthen and show greater phasic activity. The proportion of time spent in each stage and the pattern of stages across the night is fairly consistent in normal adults. A healthy young adult will typically spend about 5% of the sleep period in stage N1 sleep, about 50% in stage N2 sleep, 20–25% in slow wave sleep (N3), and 20–25% in REM sleep.

BRAIN CENTERS REGULATING WAKEFULNESS AND SLEEP

Two antagonistic sets of brain structures are responsible for orchestrating the regular alternation between wakefulness and sleep. The neuronal groups that promote wakefulness are located in the basal forebrain, posterior hypothalamus, and in the upper brain stem, whereas those promoting NREM sleep are located in the anterior hypothalamus and basal forebrain (Jones, 2003, 2005; Lin et al., 2011; McGinty, 2008 Saper et al., 2005a; Szymusiak and). Other cellular groups in the dorsal part of the pons and in the medulla constitute the so-called REM sleep generator (Fig. 87.3) (Jouvet, 1962, 1965, 1994; Luppi et al., 2012; McCarley, 2011; Siegel, 2005). The circadian clock, centered on the suprachiasmatic nucleus of the hypothalamus (SCN), exerts an overall control on many of these brain areas, to ensure that sleep occurs at the appropriate time of the 24-hour light–dark cycle (Aston-Jones, 2005; Mistlberger, 2005; Saper et al., 2005b; Zee and Manthena, 2007).

Maintenance of wakefulness is dependent on several heterogeneous cell groups extending from the upper pons and midbrain (the so-called reticular activating system, RAS; Lindsley et al., 1949; Moruzzi and Magoun, 1949) to the posterior hypothalamus and basal forebrain. These cell groups are strategically placed so that they can release, over wide regions of the brain, neuromodulators and neurotransmitters that produce EEG activation, such as acetylcholine, hypocretin, histamine, norepinephrine, and glutamate. The main mechanism by which these neuromodulators and neurotransmitters produce cortical activation is by closing leakage potassium channels on the cell membrane of cortical and thalamic neurons, thus keeping cells depolarized and ready to fire.

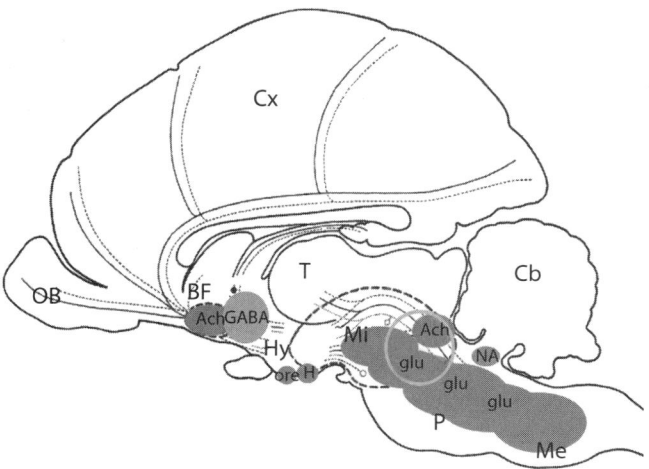

Figure 87.3 *The major brain areas involved in initiating and maintaining wakefulness (glu, glutamate; Ach, acetylcholine; NA, noradrenaline; H, histamine; ore, orexin), NREM sleep (GABA), and REM sleep (Ach).*

ACETYLCHOLINE

Cholinergic cells are located in the basal forebrain and in two small nuclei in the pons: the pedunculopontine tegmental and lateral dorsal tegmental nuclei (PPT/LDT). Basal forebrain and pontine cholinergic cells fire at high rates in wakefulness and REM sleep and decrease or stop firing during NREM sleep (el Mansari et al., 1989; Lee et al., 2005b). Pontine cholinergic cells project to the thalamus, where they help depolarize specific and intralaminar thalamic nuclei. The latter, which are dispersed throughout the thalamus and project diffusely to the cortex, fire at very high frequencies during wakefulness and REM sleep and help to synchronize cortical firing in the gamma (>28 Hz) range (Jones, 2005; McCormick, 1989; Steriade, 2004). They also project to other cholinergic and non-cholinergic (many of them glutamatergic) cells in the basal forebrain, which in turn provide an excitatory input to the entire cortex (Jones, 2003, 2005). Indeed, drugs with anticholinergic activity, including tricyclic antidepressants and atropine, can cause sedation and produce slow waves in the EEG (Domino et al., 1968; Itil and Fink, 1968). On the other hand, cholinergic agonists (e.g., nicotine) usually enhance arousal (Gillin et al., 2005; Metherate et al., 1992). In patients with Alzheimer's disease, loss of cholinergic cells is associated with slowing of the cortical EEG (Dierks et al., 1995; Montplaisir et al., 1998; Prinz et al., 1982; Soininen et al., 1992).

HISTAMINE

Cholinergic neurons in the pons also project to the posterior hypothalamus, where histaminergic neurons are located in the tuberomammillary nucleus (Brown et al., 2001). Histaminergic neurons, which project throughout the cortex, fire at the highest rates during wakefulness and are inhibited during NREM and REM sleep (Takahashi et al., 2006). They have an important wakefulness-promoting function, as shown by the increased sleep and drowsiness when they are experimentally inactivated (Lin et al., 1989, 1996, 2011). Indeed, over-the-counter antihistaminergic drugs are used all over the world to facilitate the induction of sleep (Barbier and Bradbury, 2007).

GLUTAMATE

Probably the largest contingent of the wakefulness-promoting system is made up by cells dispersed throughout the brainstem reticular formation and the basal forebrain that do not release conventional neuromodulators but rather the ubiquitous neurotransmitter glutamate. By binding to metabotropic receptors, glutamate can act as a neuromodulator and influence the excitability of target cells. Most glutamatergic neurons in the basal forebrain discharge at their fastest rates during wakefulness (a subgroup also during REM sleep), although some are most active during slow wave sleep (Hassani et al., 2009). Extracellular glutamate levels in the cortex increase progressively during wakefulness and REM sleep (Dash et al., 2009). The wake-promoting effect of glutamate may also be indirect, via activation of hypothalamic neurons containing hypocretin and histamine (John et al., 2008; Li et al., 2002).

NOREPINEPHRINE

Noradrenergic cells are concentrated in the locus coeruleus in the upper pons, from where they project throughout the brain (Aston-Jones and Cohen, 2005; Berridge and Waterhouse, 2003). They fire tonically during wakefulness and emit short, phasic bursts of activity during behavioral choices or salient events (Aston-Jones and Bloom, 1981a, 1981b; Aston-Jones and Cohen, 2005; Berridge and Abercrombie, 1999; Foote et al., 1980). The release of norepinephrine increases the response of cortical neurons to incoming stimuli, but it is not necessary for EEG activation (noradrenergic lesions induce mild sedation) (Berridge and Espana, 2000; Berridge and Foote, 1991; Cape and Jones, 1998; McCormick, 1989). However, the release of norepinephrine during wakefulness is essential for the induction of genes such as *P-CREB*, *Arc*, and *BDNF*, which are involved in synaptic potentiation and thereby in learning (Cirelli and Tononi, 2000; Cirelli et al., 1996). By contrast, locus coeruleus neurons decrease their firing during NREM sleep and cease firing altogether during REM sleep: in this way, neural activity during sleep does not translate into long-term synaptic potentiation, so we do not end up learning the wrong things and confuse dreams for reality.

SEROTONIN

Serotoninergic cells from the dorsal raphé nucleus also project widely throughout the brain. Serotoninergic neurons, like noradrenergic neurons, fire at higher levels in waking, lower levels in NREM sleep, and fall silent during REM sleep. However, in contrast to noradrenergic neurons, serotoninergic neurons are inactivated when animals make behavioral choices or orient to salient stimuli and are activated instead during repetitive motor activity such as locomoting, grooming, or feeding (Jacobs et al., 2002; McGinty and Harper, 1976). The inactivity of serotonin cells during sleep may contribute to the sensory disconnection from the environment that occurs during sleep. Overall, serotonin has been shown to have a complex, biphasic effect on sleep, first enhancing wakefulness and then facilitating the onset of NREM sleep (Landolt and Wehrle, 2009; Ursin, 2002), at least in part by inhibiting the cholinergic system (Cape and Jones, 1998; Jones, 2005; Jouvet, 1999; Monti and Jantos, 2008).

DOPAMINE

Another aminergic neuromodulator is dopamine (DA). Dopamine-containing neurons located in the substantia nigra and ventral tegmental area innervate the frontal cortex, basal forebrain, and limbic structures (Monti and Monti, 2007). Unlike other aminergic cells, dopaminergic neurons do not appear to change their overall firing rate depending on behavioral state. However, their bursting activity, which is known to induce large synaptic DA release, increases during the consumption of palatable food and during REM sleep relative to NREM sleep (Dahan et al., 2007). Moreover, lesions of areas containing dopaminergic cell bodies in the ventral midbrain or their ascending pathways can lead to loss of behavioral arousal while maintaining cortical activation. Finally, psychostimulants such as amphetamines and cocaine that block reuptake of monoamines including norepinephrine, DA, and serotonin, promote prolonged wakefulness and increase cortical activation and behavioral arousal (Monti and Jantos, 2008). Thus, the evidence for a role of dopamine as a wake-promoting neurotransmitter is substantial.

HYPOCRETIN

The peptide hypocretin (also known as orexin) is produced by cells in the dorsolateral hypothalamus that provide excitatory input to all components of the waking system (Kilduff and Peyron, 2000; Sakurai, 2007). These cells, too, are most active during waking, especially in relation to motor activity and exploratory behavior, and almost stop firing during NREM and REM sleep (Lee et al., 2005a; Mileykovskiy et al., 2005). Specific activation of hypocretin cells, via optogenetic or pharmacogenetic stimulation, facilitates arousal and increases time spent awake (Adamantidis et al., 2007; Sasaki et al., 2011) Most patients with narcolepsy, a disorder characterized by excessive somnolence and cataplectic attacks, have low or undetectable levels of hypocretin in the cerebrospinal fluid (Dauvilliers et al., 2007).

HYPOTHALAMUS, BASAL FOREBRAIN, AND SLEEP

As we seek a quiet, dark, and silent place to fall asleep and close our eyes, the activity of the waking-promoting neuronal groups is decreased because of reduced sensory input. In addition, several of these brain areas are actively inhibited by antagonistic neuronal populations located in the hypothalamic and basal forebrain, and which become active at sleep onset. When the waking-promoting neuronal groups become nearly silent, the decreasing levels of acetylcholine and other waking-promoting neuromodulators and neurotransmitters lead to the opening of leak potassium channels in cortical and thalamic neurons, which become hyperpolarized and begin oscillating at low frequencies.

The importance of hypothalamic structures for sleep induction was recognized at the beginning of the twentieth century during an epidemic of a viral infection of the brain called encephalitis lethargica. Von Economo concluded that if the infection destroyed the posterior hypothalamus, patients became indeed lethargic, but if the anterior hypothalamus was lesioned, patients became severely insomniac (von Economo, 1931). Indeed, subsequent studies confirmed that cell groups within the anterior hypothalamus are involved in the initiation and maintenance of sleep. The ventrolateral preoptic area has been suggested as a possible sleep switch (Sherin et al., 1996; Szymusiak et al., 1998). However, many other neurons scattered through the anterior hypothalamus, for instance in the median preoptic nucleus (Suntsova et al., 2002), also play a major role in initiating and maintaining sleep. These neurons tend to fire during sleep and stop firing during wakefulness. When they are active, many of them release γ-aminobutyric acid (GABA) and the peptide galanin, and inhibit most waking-promoting areas, including cholinergic, noradrenergic, histaminergic,

hypocretinergic, and serotonergic cells. In turn, the latter inhibit several sleep-promoting neuronal groups (Jones, 2003, 2005; Lin et al., 2011; Saper et al., 2005a; Szymusiak and McGinty, 2008). Another group of GABAergic neurons is located in the basal forebrain and projects to the cerebral cortex. GABA levels in the cortex are higher during NREM sleep than during wakefulness or REM sleep (Vanini et al., 2012).

THE REM SLEEP GENERATOR

The REM sleep generator consists of pontine cholinergic cell groups (LDT and PPT) that we have already encountered as waking-promoting areas, and of nearby cell groups in the medial pontine reticular formation and in the medulla (Jouvet, 1962, 1965, 1994; Luppi et al., 2012; McCarley, 2011; Siegel, 2005). Lesions in these areas eliminate REM sleep without significantly disrupting NREM sleep. Rapid eye movement sleep can also be eliminated by certain antidepressants, especially monoamine oxidase inhibitors. As we have seen, pontine cholinergic neurons produce EEG activation by releasing acetylcholine to the thalamus and to cholinergic and glutamatergic basal forebrain neurons that in turn activate the limbic system and cortex. However, though during wakefulness other wak-promoting neuronal groups such as noradrenergic, histaminergic, hypocretinergic, and serotonergic neurons are also active, they are inhibited during REM sleep. Other REM active neurons in the dorsal pons are responsible for the tonic inhibition of muscle tone during REM sleep. Finally, neurons in the medial pontine reticular formation fire in bursts and produce phasic events of REM sleep, such as REMs and muscle twitches.

THE CIRCADIAN CLOCK

In mammals, the primary clock that keeps circadian time is the suprachiasmatic nucleus (SCN) of the hypothalamus. The SCN regulates a number of endocrine and behavioral parameters to coordinate the state of the organism with the 24-hour light–dark cycle, including wakefulness and sleep (Aston-Jones, 2005; Deboer et al., 2007; Mistlberger, 2005; Saper et al., 2005a; Zee and Manthena, 2007). In diurnal animals, the SCN activates waking-promoting areas and inhibits sleep-promoting areas during the day, maximally at the end of the day, whereas the converse is true at night. This makes it difficult to sleep in the early evening or to be awake in the early morning. In animals in which the SCN has been lesioned, sleep is no longer concentrated in one main episode but is dispersed across the entire 24-hour cycle (Bergmann et al., 1987; Mistlberger et al., 1983; Tobler et al., 1983). Each of the ~20,000 cells of the SCN contain a molecular clock that changes their excitability according to a near-24-hour rhythm, and which is reset by light. The SCN produces a coherent output because its cells synchronize among themselves (Mohawk and Takahashi, 2011).

HUMORAL FACTORS

For a long time, it was assumed that sleep was mediated by the accumulation of some humoral factor during wakefulness—a kind of hypnotoxin. Despite a long search, only a few humoral factors have any well-defined role in sleep physiology. One of the best-studied substances is adenosine, not surprising given the well-known wake-promoting effect of the A1 antagonist caffeine (Basheer et al., 2004; Porkka-Heiskanen et al., 2002). Extracellular adenosine levels progressively increase in the basal forebrain during wakefulness, inhibiting cholinergic neurons and promoting sleep (Porkka-Heiskanen et al., 1997). During wakefulness adenosine levels also increase (although not progressively) in cortex and hippocampus, and astrocyte-derived adenosine plays a role in sleep homeostasis (Halassa et al., 2009; Porkka-Heiskanen et al., 2000; Schmitt et al., 2012). Prostaglandin D_2, another sleep promoting substance, acting on the prostaglandin D (PGD) receptor, indirectly activates adenosine A2A-dependent pathways in the basal forebrain (Huang et al., 2007). However, neither A1 nor PGD receptor knockout mice have abnormal baseline sleep. Similarly, a number of lymphokines, such as interleukin-1 (IL-1) and tumor necrosis factor (TNF) alpha, modulate sleep. These effects are often species specific and could be most relevant in the context of acute inflammation or infection. However, the TNF and IL-1 type I receptor knockouts have abnormal sleep, suggesting also a role in baseline sleep regulation (Krueger et al., 2001).

The pineal hormone melatonin is strongly regulated by the circadian clock and peaks at night in diurnal and nocturnal animals (it has been called the "darkness hormone"). Melatonin receptors are highly expressed in the SCN, and melatonin can help reset circadian rhythms and thereby influence sleep (Zee and Manthena, 2007). Light and melatonin can be used to alleviate and correct circadian rhythm disorders and conditions such as jet lag and night shift work. Melatonin is also effective in regularizing the sleep–wake schedule of light-blind subjects whose sleep–wake periods tend to free-run, as well as in children and in the elderly with brain disorders, for example in the treatment of the "sundowning" often seen in dementia (Arendt, 2005; Richardson, 2005).

SLEEP REGULATION AND SLEEP DEPRIVATION

If we are not allowed to sleep and are forced to stay awake longer than usual, sleep pressure mounts and soon becomes overwhelming. Thus, sleep is homeostatically regulated: the more we stay awake, the longer and more intensely we sleep afterwards: arousal thresholds increase, there are fewer awakenings, and during NREM sleep the amplitude and prevalence of slow waves becomes much higher (Fig. 87.4) and there can be a rebound of REM sleep. Sleep pressure only diminishes if one is allowed to sleep, and the number and amplitude of sleep slow waves gradually diminishes.

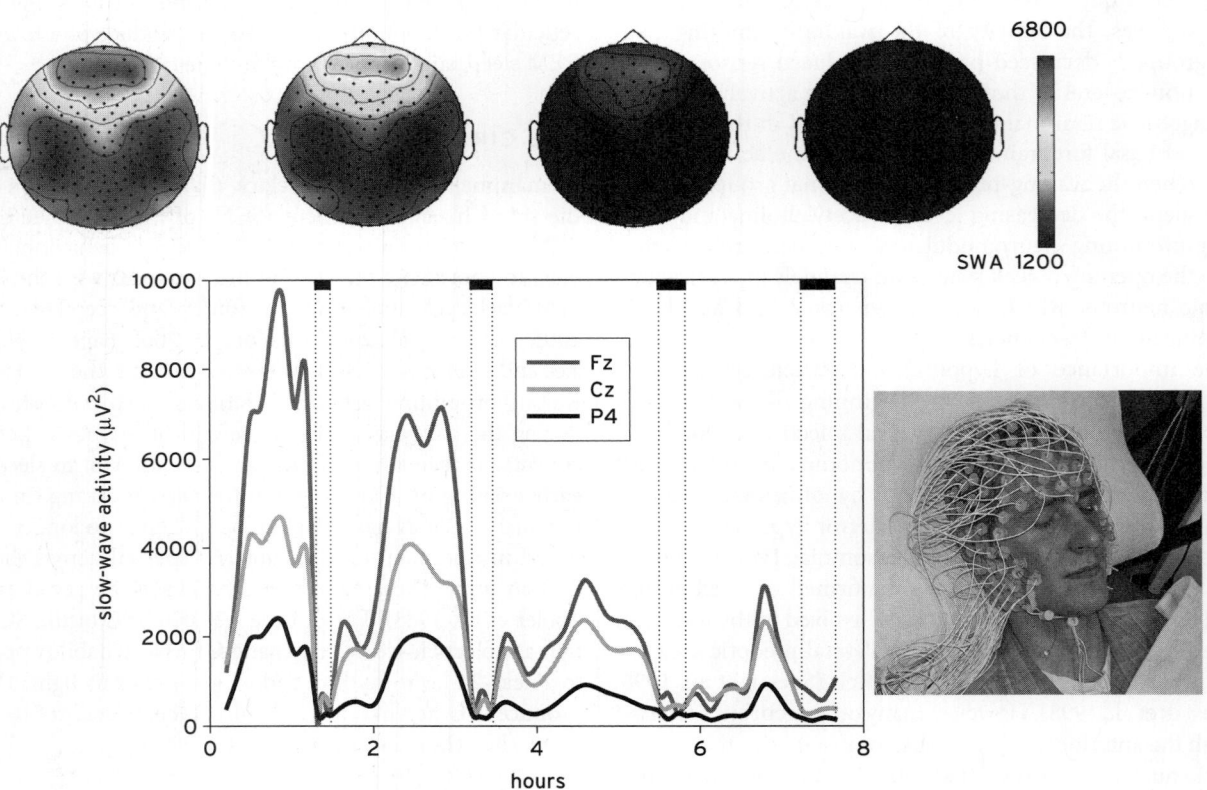

Figure 87.4 *Sleep slow waves as a marker of sleep pressure. Bottom panel: During early sleep, at the end of a day of wakefulness, sleep pressure is maximal. This is reflected in frequent and large sleep slow waves, measured here as slow wave activity (power in the 0.5–4 Hz band, in red for a frontal electroencephalogram (EEG) channel, green for a central channel, and blue for an occipital channel). During sleep slow wave activity decreases exponentially, reflecting a reduction of sleep pressure. The transitory drops in slow-wave activity correspond to episodes of rapid-eye-movement (REM) sleep. Top panel: Topographic display of slow wave activity over the scalp for the four sleep cycles. Notice the frontal predominance and the progressive decline in the course of the night. (See color insert.)*

In humans, the most prominent effect of total sleep deprivation, and even of sleep restriction (for several nights), is cognitive impairment, with striking practical consequences (Banks and Dinges, 2007; Killgore, 2010). A person who is sleep deprived tends to take longer to respond to stimuli, particularly when tasks are monotonous and low in cognitive demands. However, sleep deprivation produces more than just decreased alertness. Tasks emphasizing higher cognitive functions, such as logical reasoning, encoding, decoding, and parsing complex sentences; complex subtraction tasks; and tasks involving a flexible thinking style and the ability to focus on a large number of goals simultaneously, are all significantly affected even after one single night of sleep deprivation. Tasks requiring sustained attention, such as those including goal-directed activities, can be impaired by even a few hours of sleep loss. For example, medical interns make more frequent serious diagnostic errors when they worked frequent shifts of 24 hours or more than when they worked shorter shifts (Barger et al., 2006). Unfortunately, sleep deprived subjects underestimate the severity of their cognitive impairment, often with tragic consequences. Also, lack of sleep does not completely eliminate the capacity to perform but rather makes the performance inconsistent and unreliable (Doran et al., 2001). Thus, a sleepy driver will either respond normally to an emergency or not at all, due to rapid changes in vigilance state and the sudden intrusion of microsleeps during waking. Similarly, people may still be able to transiently perform at baseline levels in short tests even after three–four days of sleep deprivation. However, the same subjects will perform very poorly when engaged in tasks requiring sustained attention. An important issue that remains unresolved is whether the cognitive impairment seen after sleep deprivation and sleep restriction is exclusively caused by sleepiness—the increasing internal pressure to fall asleep presumably mediated by the sleep-promoting areas discussed before—or to progressive cellular dysfunctions in cortical and other circuits that have been awake too long, a veritable form of neuronal tiredness.

It should be mentioned that several well-controlled studies have discredited the once-popular notion that loss of REM sleep might lead to psychosis and suicide. Indeed, REM sleep deprivation, as well as total sleep deprivation or selective slow wave deprivation, improves mood in approximately 50% of people who are depressed (Hemmeter et al., 2010; Landsness et al., 2011).

NEURAL CORRELATES OF WAKEFULNESS AND SLEEP

Wakefulness and NREM and REM sleep are accompanied by distinctive molecular changes, changes in spontaneous neural activity and metabolism, and responsiveness to stimuli.

MOLECULAR CHANGES

It might seem unlikely that the mere change from wakefulness to sleep should lead to changes in the expression of genes in the brain, but this is actually what happens, and on a massive scale. Hundreds of gene transcripts (messenger ribonucleic acids [RNAs]) are expressed at higher levels in the waking brain, and different sets of transcripts are expressed at higher levels in sleep (Cirelli, 2009; Cirelli et al., 2004). Many of these molecular changes are specific to the brain because they do not occur in other tissues such as liver and muscle. Transcripts upregulated during wakefulness code for proteins that help the brain to face high-energy demand, high synaptic excitatory transmission, high transcriptional activity, as well as the cellular stress that may derive from one or more of these processes. Moreover, wakefulness is associated with the increased expression of several genes that are involved in long-term potentiation of synaptic strength, such as *P-CREB, Arc, NGFI-A* and *BDNF* (Cirelli and Tononi, 2000; Cirelli et al., 1996) (Fig. 87.5). As we have seen, one reason these genes are expressed in wakefulness and not in sleep has to do with the release of norepinephrine, which is high during wakefulness, when animals make decisions and learn about the environment, but is low during sleep.

By contrast, the genes that increase their expression during sleep include several that may be involved in long-term depression of synaptic strength and possibly in synaptic consolidation (Cirelli et al., 2004; Cirelli, 2009). Other sleep-related genes appear to favor the rate of protein synthesis, which is

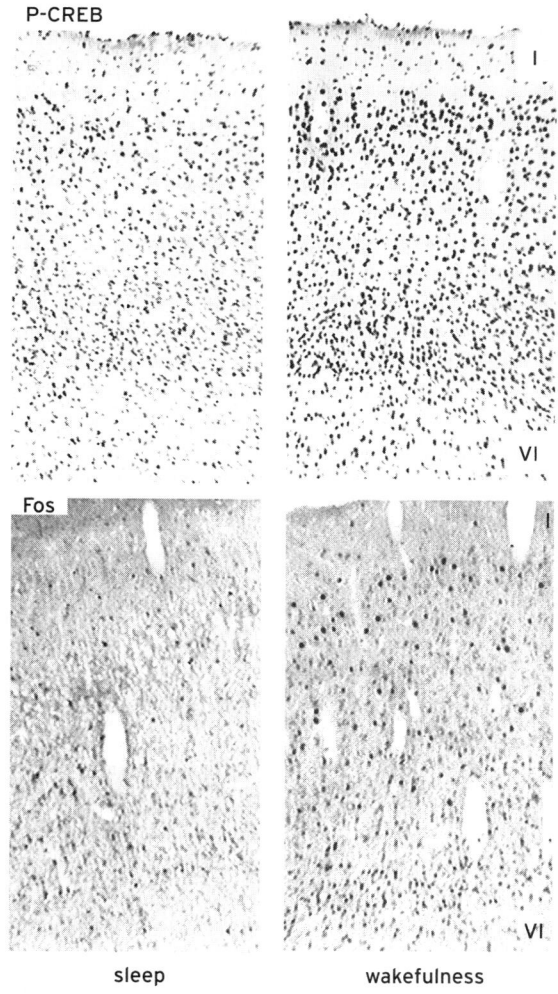

Figure 87.5 *The expression of the transcription factors P-CREB and Fos is high in wakefulness and low in sleep (rat parietal cortex: I, VI, cortical layers I and VI).*

also increased in sleep. Finally, many sleep-related genes play a significant role in membrane trafficking and maintenance. Thus, these findings suggest that although sleep is a state of behavioral inactivity, it is associated not only with intense neural activity, but also with the increased expression of many genes that may favor specific cellular functions.

SPONTANEOUS NEURAL ACTIVITY

WAKEFULNESS

The waking EEG, characterized by the presence of low-voltage fast-activity, is known as activated because most cortical neurons are steadily depolarized close to their firing threshold (Fig. 87.6A), and are thus ready to respond to the slightest change in their inputs. The steady depolarization is caused by the release of acetylcholine and other neurotransmitters and neuromodulators, which close leakage potassium channels on the membrane of cortical neurons. The readiness to respond of cortical and thalamic neurons enables fast and effective interactions among distributed regions of the thalamocortical system, resulting in a continuously changing sequence of specific firing patterns. Because these firing patterns are not globally synchronous across the cortex, the EEG displays rapid fluctuations of low amplitude rather than high-voltage, low-frequency waves. Nevertheless, superimposed on the low-voltage, fast-activity background of wakefulness one frequently observes rhythmic oscillatory episodes within the alpha (8–13 Hz), beta (14–28 Hz), and gamma (>28 Hz) range, which are usually localized to specific cortical areas. These waking rhythms are due to the activation of oscillatory mechanisms intrinsic to each cell as well as to the entrainment of oscillatory circuits among excitatory and inhibitory neurons.

NREM SLEEP

As we have seen, the EEG of NREM sleep is very different from that of wakefulness and is characterized by the occurrence of slow waves (<2 Hz in humans), K-complexes, and sleep spindles. At the beginning of sleep, the release of acetylcholine and other neuromodulators is much reduced, with the consequence that leakage potassium channels on the membrane of cortical and thalamic cells open, positively charged potassium ions leave the cells, and membrane potentials are drawn toward hyperpolarization. This and other neuromodulatory mediated changes trigger a series of membrane currents that lead to an oscillation in cellular membrane potential called the slow oscillation (see Fig. 87.6A) (Steriade et al., 2001). As shown by intracellular recordings, the slow oscillation is made up of a hyperpolarization phase or down-state, which lasts a few hundreds milliseconds, and a slightly longer depolarization phase or up state. The down state is associated with the virtual absence of synaptic activity within cortical networks (OFF periods). During the up state, by contrast, cortical cells fire at rates that are as high or even higher than those seen in waking and may even show periods of fast oscillatory activity in the gamma range.

The slow oscillation is found in virtually every cortical neuron and is synchronized across much of the cortical mantle by corticocortical connections, which is why the EEG records high-voltage, low-frequency waves. Human EEG recordings using 256 channels have revealed that the slow oscillation behaves as a traveling wave that sweeps across a large portion of the cerebral cortex (Massimini et al., 2004). Most of the time, the sweep starts in the very front of the brain and propagates front to back. These sweeps occur very infrequently during stage N1, around 5 times a minute during stage N2, and more than 10–20 times a minute in stage N3. Thus, a wave of depolarization and intense synaptic activity, followed by a wave of hyperpolarization and synaptic silence, sweeps across the brain more and more frequently just as NREM sleep becomes deeper. These waves of activity and inactivity are reminiscent of those of contraction and relaxation that sweep through the cardiac tissue triggered by the electrical activity originating in the sinus pacemaker that travels along the conduction system. It is as if, during NREM sleep, the brain were to unveil its own spontaneous "brain beat."

The various EEG waves that characterize NREM sleep are closely associated with the slow oscillation. Slow oscillations can occur every few seconds at a single cortical source, or can originate at short intervals at multiple cortical sites, in which case they superimpose or interfere, leading to EEG slow waves that are shorter and more fractured (delta waves, 1–2 Hz in humans). Waves in the delta range are also favored by certain intrinsic currents present in cortical and thalamic neurons. Topographically, slow waves are especially prominent over dorsolateral prefrontal cortex. K-complexes are probably nothing more than slow oscillations, usually triggered by external stimuli, which appear particularly prominent because they are not immediately preceded or followed by other slow waves.

Sleep spindles occur during the depolarized phase of the slow oscillation and are generated in thalamic circuits as a consequence of cortical firing. When the cortex enters an up state, strong cortical firing excites GABAergic neurons in the reticular nucleus of the thalamus. These in turn strongly inhibit thalamocortical neurons, triggering intrinsic currents that produce a rebound burst of action potentials. These bursts percolate within local thalamoreticular circuits and produce oscillatory firing at around 12–15 Hz. Thalamic spindle sequences reach back to the cortex and are globally synchronized by corticothalamic circuits, wherein they appear in the EEG as sleep spindles.

Recently, both rodent and human experiments have shown that sleep slow waves and spindles are global at the beginning of sleep, but become mostly local, occurring in some cortical areas and not in others, when sleep pressure has dissipated (Fig. 87.6B) (Nir et al., 2011; Vyazovskiy et al., 2011). Other studies have found that sleep slow waves can be regulated locally, their amplitude and number increasing after experience-dependent plasticity and synaptic potentiation and decreasing after synaptic depression (Faraguna et al., 2008; Hanlon et al., 2009; Huber et al., 2004, 2006, 2008; Hung et al., 2012). Moreover, it was recently found that, the longer a rat stays awake, the more cortical neurons show brief periods of silence in their firing that are essentially indistinguishable from the down states (OFF periods) observed during slow oscillations in a sleeping animal (Vyazovskiy et al., 2011). These OFF periods are local, in that they may

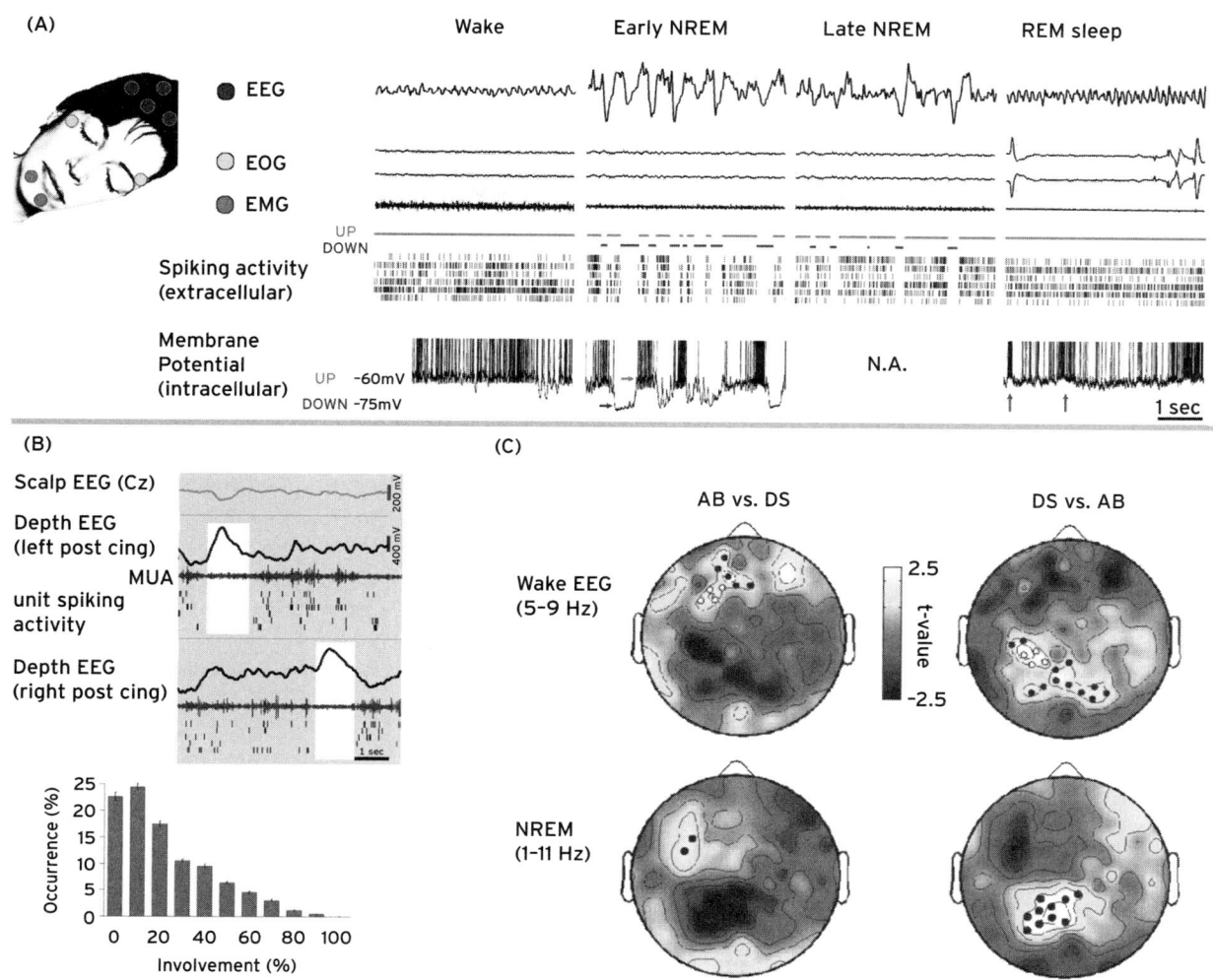

Figure 87.6 (A) Cortical activity in sleep and wake. Intracellular studies have shown that the membrane potential of cortical neurons in both wake and REM sleep is depolarized and fluctuates around −63 mV and −61 mV, respectively. In REM sleep, whenever phasic events such as rapid eye movements occur, neurons increase their firing rates to levels that surpass those found in wake. In early NREM sleep, neurons alternate between two distinct states, each lasting tens to hundreds of milliseconds: UP states (upper arrow) are associated with depolarization and increased firing, whereas in DOWN states (lower arrow) the membrane potential is hyperpolarized around −75 mV, and neuronal firing fades. Extracellular studies found that spiking of individual neurons in REM sleep reaches similar levels as in active wake. In both wake and REM sleep, neurons exhibit tonic irregular asynchronous activity. Sustained activity in wake and REM sleep can be viewed as a continuous UP state. In early NREM sleep, UP states are short and synchronous across neuronal populations, and are frequently interrupted by long DOWN states. In late NREM sleep, UP states are longer and less synchronized. Polysomnography. Waking is characterized by low-amplitude, high-frequency EEG activity, occasional saccadic eye movements, and elevated muscle tone. In early NREM sleep, high-amplitude slow waves (<4 Hz) dominate the EEG. Neuronal UP and DOWN states correspond to positive and negative peaks in the surface EEG, respectively. In late NREM sleep, slow waves are less frequent, whereas spindles (related to UP states and surface EEG positivity) become more common. Eye movements and muscle tone are largely similar to early NREM sleep. In REM sleep, theta activity (4–7 Hz) prevails, rapid eye movements occur and muscle tone is reduced. (B) Top: an example of local sleep slow waves occurring at different times in left and right posterior cingulate cortices. Rows (top to bottom) depict activity in scalp EEG (Cz), left posterior cingulate, and right posterior cingulate. Depth EEG multi-unit activity (MUA); black lines, single-unit spikes. White shadings mark local OFF periods. Bottom: Most slow waves are local. Distribution of slow wave involvement (percentage of monitored brain structures expressing each wave) is shown. (C) Subjects recorded with high-density EEG completed two experiments during which they stayed awake for ≥24 h practicing a language task (AB) or a visuomotor task (DS). Top: topographic distribution of relative power changes from baseline to the last wake session (after 24 h wake) between AB and DS in the theta frequency band (5–9 Hz). Black and white dots show channels with significant increase in spectral power. Bottom: topographic distribution of relative power changes in the low frequencies including slow waves (1–11 Hz) between AB and DS during the recovery night after 24 h wake. Channels showing significant increase in spectral power in AB relative to DS are indicated by black dots. ([A] Modified from Nir and Tononi, 2010; [B] From Nir et al. (2011); [C] Modified from Hung et al. 2012.)

occur at different times in different brain regions, and when they occur in the wrong region at the wrong time they can produce performance deficits. Experience-dependent plasticity extended beyond the normal wake duration also leads to a local slowing of the wake EEG in humans. This slowing is more prominent in the specific brain regions challenged by plasticity, and the subsequent sleep is more intense over the same areas (Fig. 87.6C) (Hung et al., 2012). Thus, it is now clear that the intensity of sleep, as measured by sleep slow waves, can also be regulated at the local level and reflects experience-dependent plasticity occurring during prior wakefulness. Moreover, it appears that the need to sleep is strongly dependent on synaptic plasticity occurring during wake.

REM SLEEP

During REM sleep, the EEG returns to an activated, low-voltage fast-activity pattern that is similar to that of quiet wakefulness or stage 1. As in wakefulness, the tonic depolarization of cortical and thalamic neurons is caused by the closure of leakage potassium channels. In fact, during REM sleep acetylcholine and other neuromodulators are released again at high levels, just as in wakefulness, and neuronal firing rates in several brain areas tend to be even higher.

METABOLISM AND BLOOD FLOW

Recently, the data painstakingly obtained by recording the activity of individual neurons have been complemented by imaging studies that provide a simultaneous picture of synaptic activity over the entire brain, although at much lower resolution (Dang-Vu et al., 2010; Maquet, 2010).

NREM SLEEP

Positron emission tomography (PET) studies show that metabolic activity and blood flow are globally reduced in NREM sleep compared to resting wakefulness. During slow wave sleep, metabolic activity can be reduced by as much as 40%. Metabolic activity is mostly owing to the energetic requirements of synaptic transmission, and its reduction during NREM sleep is thus most likely owing to the hyperpolarized phase of the slow oscillation, during which synaptic activity is essentially abolished. At a regional level, activation is especially reduced in the thalamus, because of its profound hyperpolarization during NREM sleep. In the cerebral cortex, activation is reduced in the dorsolateral prefrontal, orbitofrontal, and anterior cingulate cortex. This deactivation is to be expected given that slow oscillations are especially prominent in these areas. The parietal, precuneus, and posterior cingulate cortex, as well as medial temporal cortex also show relative deactivations. By contrast, primary sensory cortices are not deactivated compared to resting wakefulness. Basal ganglia and cerebellum are also deactivated, probably because of the reduced inflow from cortical areas.

REM SLEEP

During REM sleep absolute levels of blood flow and metabolic activity are high, reaching levels similar to those seen during wakefulness, as would be expected based on the tonic depolarization and high firing rates of neurons. There are, however, interesting regional differences. Some brain areas are more active in REM sleep than in wakefulness. For example, there is a strong activation of limbic areas, including the amygdala and the parahippocampal cortex. Cerebral cortical areas that receive strong inputs from the amygdala, such as the anterior cingulate and the parietal lobule, are also activated, as are extrastriate areas. By contrast, the rest of the parietal cortex, precuneus, and posterior cingulate, and dorsolateral prefrontal cortex are relatively deactivated. As we will see, these regional activations and inactivations are consistent with the differences in mental state between sleep and wakefulness.

Upon awakening, blood flow is rapidly reestablished in brain stem and thalamus, as well as in the anterior cingulate cortex. However, it can take up to 20 minutes for blood flow to be fully reestablished in other brain areas, notably dorsolateral prefrontal cortex. It is likely that this sluggish reactivation is responsible for the phenomenon of sleep inertia—a postawakening deficit in alertness and performance that can last for tens of minutes.

RESPONSIVENESS TO STIMULI

The most striking behavioral consequence of falling asleep is a progressive disconnection from the outside world. We stop responding to stimuli and, to the extent that we remain conscious, our experiences become largely independent of the current environment. This disconnection would appear to be important because we make several behavioral adjustments to bring it about: we seek a quiet environment, find a comfortable position, and close our eyes. However, people (especially small children) can fall asleep in a noisy environment and in uncomfortable positions—in the laboratory people can even sleep with their eyes taped open. Everything else being equal, the threshold for responding to peripheral stimuli gradually increases with the succession of NREM sleep stages 1 to 4 and remains high during REM sleep. Because cortical neurons continue to fire actively during sleep, how does this disconnection come about?

NREM SLEEP

As we have seen, during the transition from wakefulness to NREM sleep, the release of acetylcholine and other neuromodulators is reduced, leading to the progressive hyperpolarization of thalamocortical neurons. As a consequence, sensory stimuli that normally would be relayed to the cortex often fail to do so because they do not manage to fire thalamocortical cells. In addition, the rhythmic hyperpolarization during sleep spindles is especially effective in blocking incoming stimuli because it imposes an intrinsic oscillatory rhythm that effectively decouples inputs from outputs. Thus, the "thalamic gate" to the cerebral cortex is partially closed (Steriade and Timofeev, 2003). However, sensory stimuli in various modalities still elicit evoked potentials from the cerebral cortex, and neuroimaging studies show that primary cortical areas are still being activated (Portas et al., 2000). Studies using transcranial magnetic stimulation (TMS) and high-density EEG have employed direct cortical stimulation to bypass the thalamic gate (Massimini et al., 2005). The results show that during wakefulness TMS induces an initial local response followed for about 300 milliseconds by multiple, fast waves of activity associated with rapidly changing configurations of scalp potentials (Fig. 87.7). With the onset of NREM sleep, however, the brain response to TMS changes markedly. The initial response doubles in amplitude and lasts longer. After this large wave, however, no further TMS-locked activity can be detected, and all TMS-evoked activity ceases by 150 milliseconds. Moreover, this response, which lacks high-frequency components, remains localized and does not propagate to connected brain regions. Apparently, the ability of brain regions to interact causally with each other—their effective connectivity—breaks down during NREM sleep.

REM SLEEP

With the transition from NREM to REM sleep, neurons return to be steadily depolarized much as they are during quiet

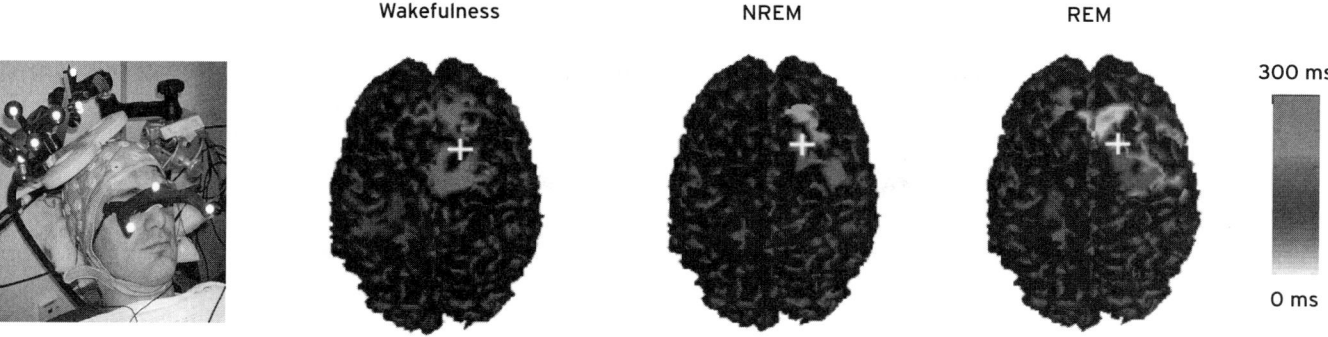

Wakefulness   NREM   REM

300 ms

0 ms

Figure 87.7 *Spatiotemporal cortical current maps of transcranial magnetic stimulation (TMS)-induced activity during wakefulness, non-rapid eye movement (NREM), and REM sleep. On the left is the setup for TMS/EEG. From the electroencephalogram (EEG) data, maximum current sources corresponding to periods of significant activations were plotted and color-coded according to their latency of activation (light blue, 0 ms; red, 300 ms). The yellow cross marks the TMS target on the cortical surface. Note the rapidly changing patterns of activation during wakefulness, lasting up to 300 ms and involving several different areas; the brief activation that remains localized to the area of stimulation during NREM sleep; and an intermediate pattern of activation during REM sleep. (From Massimini M., Ferrarelli F., Huber R., et al., 2005. Breakdown of cortical effective connectivity during sleep. Science 309:2228–2232.) (See color insert.)*

wakefulness, yet we still ignore sensory stimuli. It is as if we are preoccupied with the brain's intrinsic activity rather than with what goes on in the external world (Llinas and Pare, 1991), similar to what happens during states of intense absorption that can occur even when awake, say when one is engrossed in reading a captivating novel. The underlying mechanisms, however, are not clear. As we have seen, prefrontal and parietal cortical areas are deactivated in REM sleep compared to wakefulness. These regions include brain areas important for directing and sustaining attention to what is going on in sensory cortices. Sensory inputs reaching primary cortices would then find themselves to be systematically unattended. It is likely that the reduced activity in these cortical regions is a direct consequence of changes in the neuromodulatory milieu during REM sleep. The reduction of serotonin release during REM sleep may favor a dissociative hallucinogenic state, as seen with certain psychoactive compounds.

Nevertheless, in contrast to a person in a coma or a vegetative state, a sleeping person can always be awakened if stimuli are strong enough, or especially meaningful. For example, it is well known that the sound of one's name, or the wailing of a baby, is among the most effective signals for awakening.

CONSCIOUSNESS DURING SLEEP

Sleep brings about at once the most common and the most dramatic change in consciousness that we are likely to witness—from the near fading of all experience to the bizarre hallucinations of dreams. Indeed, studying mental activity during sleep offers a unique opportunity to find out how changes in brain activity are associated with changes in consciousness (Nir and Tononi, 2010). Typically, subjects are awoken at different times of night and asked to report whatever was going through their mind.

SLEEP ONSET

Reports from sleep onset, that is, stage 1, are very frequent (80–90% of the time), but they are also very short, usually hallucinatory experiences. These are called hypnagogic

hallucinations, from a Greek word meaning "leading into sleep." In contrast to typical dreams, hypnagogic hallucinations are often static, similar to single snapshots or a short sequence of still frames.

NREM SLEEP

Awakenings from NREM sleep yield reports 60–80% of the time. Thus, there is a substantial number of awakenings from NREM sleep that yield no report whatsoever, especially early in the night when stages 3 and 4 are prevalent. The length of NREM reports is widely distributed. However, there are many very short reports early in the night, and much longer reports later in the night, considerably longer than those typically obtained at sleep onset or even during quiet wakefulness. Reports from NREM sleep, especially early in the night, can be thought-like and lack perceptual vividness. However, especially later in the night, they can be much more hallucinatory and, generally speaking, more dreamlike. Indeed, hallucinatory content increases steeply from waking to sleep onset, and then to NREM sleep and REM sleep, whereas thought-like content behaves in the opposite way.

REM SLEEP

Awakenings from REM sleep yield reports 80–90% of the time, a percentage similar to that obtained at sleep onset. Especially in the morning hours, the percentage is close to 100% (the report rate for wakefulness). Remarkably, the median word count of REM sleep reports is even higher than that of wakefulness reports, whether quiet or active. This finding seems to fit with the notion that dreams are single-minded, and thus less frequently interrupted by extraneous thoughts than waking consciousness. The average length of REM reports increases with the duration of the REM sleep episode. By contrast, there is no such relationship for NREM sleep reports.

These observations lead to several conclusions. Contrary to initial claims, some kind of conscious experience during sleep is the rule, rather than the exception. Especially late in the night, several NREM reports must be considered as bona fide dreams, no matter what criteria one uses, although they are on average not as long, vivid, and bizarre as those obtained from REM sleep. Another general conclusion from recent studies is that the length, hallucinatory content, and overall dream-like quality of reports increases from the beginning to the end of the night, irrespective of sleep stage. Thus, the relationship between sleep stages and dream features is probabilistic rather than absolute.

However, we must not forget that a number of NREM reports, especially from the early part of the night, show little evidence of conscious content. Considering that people awakened from stage 3 and 4 NREM sleep, even when they do report something, often take a long time to wake up and confabulate while still half asleep, it seems reasonable to assume that this may be the only time of our regular existence when we are close to losing consciousness altogether. So why does consciousness fade in NREM sleep early in the night, especially considering that spontaneous activity persists? One possibility is that the down state of the slow oscillation, which sweeps the cerebral cortex once a second and produces an intermittent, near-global deactivation, results in the effective disconnection of cortical regions. Indeed, as we have seen above, studies of TMS/EEG have shown a breakdown of cortical effective connectivity during early NREM sleep (Massimini et al., 2005). By contrast, at sleep onset, and in stage 2 NREM sleep toward the morning, there are relatively long periods of activation between slow oscillations that may explain why most participants report dreamlike experiences, although usually short ones. Finally, the long and vivid dreams of REM sleep can occur because brain activation is not interrupted at all by slow oscillations (see Fig. 87.7).

Finally, though the vivid dreams of REM sleep can at times be hard to distinguish from waking experience, usually they share some features that are remarkably consistent with the changes in brain activation revealed by neuroimaging studies. For example, a key feature of dreaming consciousness is the reduced responsiveness to external stimuli, accompanied by vivid hallucinations, especially visual ones. Accordingly, PET studies of REM sleep show reduced activity in primary visual cortex, accompanied by increased activity in higher visual areas. Another relevant difference between dreaming and waking consciousness concerns the ability to reflect on oneself and one's experience, especially the ability to judge the verisimilitude of dreams. As we have seen, dorsolateral prefrontal cortex, which is involved in volitional control and self-monitoring, is especially deactivated during REM sleep. Reduced activation of dorsolateral prefrontal cortex may also contribute to the disorientation, reduction of directed thinking, and working memory observed in dreams, and contributes to dreaming amnesia. Conversely, dreams are characterized by a high degree of emotional involvement, especially fear and anxiety. Correspondingly, imaging studies have revealed a marked activation of limbic and paralimbic structures such as the amygdala, the anterior cingulate cortex, the insula, and medial orbitofrontal cortex during REM sleep. Although we still do not know what is responsible for the changes in brain regional activation that occur during REM sleep, it is likely that neuromodulatory systems may be involved. For example, because monoaminergic systems are silent during REM sleep, acetylcholine is alone in maintaining brain activation. Consistent with imaging results, the cholinergic innervation is especially strong in limbic and paralimbic areas and much weaker in dorsolateral prefrontal cortex.

THE FUNCTIONS OF SLEEP

Why should we periodically abandon daily activities, relinquish the search for food, forgo our reproductive duties, stop monitoring the environment for dangers or opportunities, and slumber for hours into an altered state of consciousness? An appealing idea is that sleep may have evolved from the circadian rest-activity cycle and may thus represent a default state of inactivity that keeps us out of trouble during the dark hours (or the light hours for nocturnal creature) when we have nothing better to do. However, it is likely that sleep serves some more fundamental function. First, why should animals engage in prolonged periods of quiescence during which they are dangerously out of touch? Second, sleep seems to be universal. All animal species carefully studied so far sleep, from invertebrates such as fruit flies and bees to birds and mammals (Cirelli and Tononi, 2008). Nor has evolution found an easy way of getting rid of sleep. Some animals who need continuous vigilance while swimming or flying, for example, certain dolphins and migrating birds, have developed alternating unihemispheric sleep rather than eliminating sleep altogether. Third, sleep need is carefully regulated. If sleep is eliminated or restricted for some time, there is a gradual increase in sleep pressure that rapidly becomes irresistible, and the subsequent sleep is longer and more intense. This suggests that ensuring a certain amount of sleep is as important as preserving appropriate levels of temperature, energy, or electrolytes. Many of the hypotheses that have been put forth over the years fall into two main categories: those that propose a role of sleep in memory, and those that envision a role in brain restitution.

SLEEP AND MEMORY

A connection between sleep and memory was noted a long time ago (Jenkins and Dallenback, 1924). After struggling to learn a new piece of music for much of the day, we often play it better after a night of sleep. Recently, the importance of sleep and even naps occurring after certain types of declarative and non-declarative learning has been documented in well-controlled experiments (Diekelmann and Born, 2010; Stickgold and Walker, 2007). Sleep could indeed offer a favorable context for certain aspects of learning and memory. The sensory disconnection associated with sleep reduces interference between ongoing activities and the consolidation of previously acquired memories. Moreover, sleep permits the repeated reactivation, in an off-line mode, of the neural circuits originally activated during the memorable experience. Studies using multielectrode recordings in animals and PET/ functional magnetic resonance imaging (fMRI) in humans have shown that brain areas or cells activated during waking are preferentially reactivated during subsequent sleep (Buhry et al., 2011; Dang-Vu et al., 2010). A further advantage of sleep is that the relevant neural circuits can be reactivated in a spaced and interleaved fashion. This would favor the integration of new with old memories and would avoid catastrophic interference. The intense, high-frequency bursts of spontaneous neural activity that occur during sleep may be particularly important for triggering molecular mechanisms of synaptic consolidation and to enlarge the network of associations.

Many unknowns remain, however. Whether sleep may favor the consolidation of newly established memories or the maintenance of older ones is not clear. Offline sequential activity also occurs during wakefulness, and in some cases the sequences activated offline correspond to trajectories never experienced by the animal, suggesting that this "reactivation" may be also involved in the maintenance of spatial representation and planning (Buhry et al., 2011). The molecular correlates of such processes are still unclear. Most molecular markers of memory acquisition are turned off during sleep, which may be advantageous given that the intense neural activity of sleep occurs while the animal is disconnected from the environment. Also, much of the early literature connecting sleep and memory was concerned with REM sleep. However, prolonged inhibition of REM sleep in humans through certain antidepressants does not seem to disrupt memory, nor does the complete disappearance of REM sleep after certain brainstem lesions (Siegel, 2001; Vertes, 2004).

SLEEP AND BRAIN RESTITUTION

When we have been awake too long we say we are tired, and after sleep we feel refreshed. Not surprisingly, the most intuitively compelling idea about the function of sleep is that sleep may restore some precious fuel or energy charge that was depleted during wakefulness. It is likely that sleep may indeed reduce energy waste by enforcing body rest in animals with high metabolic rates (this is certainly what hibernation does by drastically reducing body and brain metabolism, shutting off brain activity, and reducing temperature). However, in humans the metabolic savings of spending the night asleep rather than quietly awake are no more than a slice of bread (Horne, 1980). Moreover, we also say we are tired after muscle exertions, yet most bodily organs can recover through quiet wakefulness and do not need sleep. The notable exception is the brain: if we do not sleep, even though we may remain immobile, we rapidly suffer cognitive impairment. Therefore most researchers agree that sleep may be especially important for restoring the brain and provide something not afforded by quiet waking. However, there is great uncertainty when it comes to which chemical or molecular pathway in the brain may be wasted during waking and restored during sleep. For example, it has been suggested that sleep may favor the replenishment of glycogen in glial stores (Benington and Heller, 1995), although recent evidence shows that this may only be true in a few brain regions (Franken et al., 2003, 2006; Gip et al., 2002). The molecular changes that take place between wakefulness and sleep suggest other possibilities as well: sleep could counteract synaptic fatigue by favoring the replenishment of calcium in presynaptic stores, the replenishment of glutamate vesicles, the resting of mitochondria, the synthesis of proteins, or the trafficking and recycling of membranes (Cirelli et al., 2004; Mackiewicz et al., 2007; Mongrain et al., 2010). Unfortunately, most of these possibilities remain unexplored.

SLEEP AND SYNAPTIC HOMEOSTASIS

Memory consolidation and brain restitution are important perspectives on the function of sleep that are not mutually exclusive. A recently hypothesis reconciles these two perspectives by proposing that the main function of sleep is to control the strength of synapses impinging on neurons in the cortex and elsewhere (Tononi and Cirelli, 2003, 2006, 2012). This hypothesis effectively proposes a role for sleep in brain restitution—synaptic strength would increase during wakefulness and return to baseline during sleep. At the same time, the hypothesis claims that sleep is the price we pay because our brains are plastic and is thus related in an important manner to memory.

The hypothesis focuses mostly on NREM sleep, but REM sleep may fulfill a similar role with different mechanisms. The hypothesis says, first, that wakefulness is associated with synaptic potentiation in several cortical circuits (as we have seen, genes involved in synaptic potentiation are indeed unregulated during wakefulness). Although this remarkable plasticity is a good thing, reflecting our ability to learn and adapt, it comes at a cost. Synaptic activity is where the brain spends most of its energy, and increased synaptic strength means increased energy consumption just to keep the brain running (even if we merely sit and do nothing). Increased synaptic strength also means increased housekeeping and space needs. Neural cells have enormous dendritic trees literally covered with synapses, whose maintenance must burden membrane trafficking mechanisms. Moreover, there is very little room inside the brain for adding new synapses or making them bigger. In short, the brain is prone to synaptic overload, and it should have some homeostatic mechanism to save on energy, space, supplies, and to prevent the saturation of its plastic abilities. Therefore, synaptic strength must be regulated and returned to a sustainable level, restoring synaptic homeostasis. In this way, the costs in terms of energy, space, supplies, signal-to-noise ratios, and learning capacity are restored to baseline. The core claim of the hypothesis is that an essential function of sleep is the restoration of synaptic homeostasis, which is best achieved during sleep when there is no demand for learning and neurons can sample most of their inputs in an unbiased manner through off-line spontaneous activity. By contrast, during wake neurons preferentially sample the particular subsets of inputs determined by interactions with the environment, and they are required to learn on-line. Over the last several years much effort has been devoted to evaluating structural, molecular, and physiological indices of synaptic efficacy before and after sleep. So far, evidence obtained using a variety of experimental approaches has been supportive in flies, rodents, and humans: synaptic strength increases during wakefulness and decreases during sleep (Bushey et al., 2011; Donlea et al., 2009, 2011; Gilestro et al., 2009; Huber et al., 2012; Lante et al., 2011; Liu et al., 2010; Maret et al., 2011; Vyazovskiy et al., 2008; Yang and Gan, 2011).

SLEEP AND BRAIN DEVELOPMENT

The ideas and the findings discussed in the preceding usually pertain to adult sleep. However, we have seen that sleep is especially abundant early in development, before birth and during the first year or two. This is a time of intense synaptogenesis as well as remodeling of connections—synaptic density in the cerebral cortex grows exuberantly during the first year of life and then decreases, most prominently during adolescence and then more slowly throughout life (Rakic et al., 1994). The increase in the number of synapses during early development is explosive, and it is bound to pose even greater challenges to neurons (and glia) than the increase in synaptic strength that occurs during wake in adult mammals. It is difficult to imagine how this massive formation of new synapses could be perfectly regulated, with precise titration of the total amount of synaptic weight impinging on each neuron. Instead, most likely during synaptogenesis neurons may undergo a substantial synaptic overload, and for the reasons discussed earlier synaptic rebalancing is best achieved off-line, when a neuron can sample most of its inputs in an unbiased manner. Two recent studies in mice have investigated the occurrence of sleep-dependent synaptic homeostasis during neurodevelopment, and found evidence that during adolescence sleep is associated with a net decrease in the number of synapses (Maret et al., 2011; Yang and Gan, 2011), thus possibly helping to maintain synaptic homeostasis in the face of ongoing synaptogenesis. Many questions remain, however, related to the role of sleep in earlier developmental stages, the role played by different kinds of sleep, and the consequences of sleep deprivation at such critical periods.

CONCLUSIONS

Sleep is characterized behaviorally by immobility and a reduced responsiveness to environmental stimuli that is rapidly reversible. The EEG, EMG, and EOG reveal distinct stages: a transitional stage N1; stage N2 (EEG spindles); stage N3 of NREM sleep (slow waves); and REM sleep (rapid eye movements with wake-like, activated EEG). There are four to five NREM–REM cycles every night. The transitions from wakefulness to sleep and between sleep stages are coordinated by a set of subcortical centers that are neurochemically heterogeneous. Broadly speaking, the reticular activating system in the posterior hypothalamus and upper brain-stem sustains brain activation through the release of neuromodulators such as acetylcholine, glutamate, histamine, and hypocretin; the anterior hypothalamus and basal forebrain coordinate sleep; the upper pons triggers REM sleep; and the suprachiasmatic nucleus is responsible for the circadian modulation of sleep propensity.

Various aspects of brain activity change during sleep, as shown by molecular, unit recordings, and imaging studies, but the brain by no means shuts off. For example, average firing rates in the cerebral cortex are similar to those of quiet wakefulness. However, during NREM sleep cortical cells undergo a characteristic slow oscillation: up to once a second, their membrane potential becomes hyperpolarized and all synaptic activity ceases for a few hundreds of milliseconds. When depolarization returns, it is often accompanied by sleep spindles—faster oscillations generated by interactions between the reticular thalamic nucleus and the thalamus proper. During NREM sleep metabolism in prefrontal and associative areas is reduced, and the brain is relatively disconnected from the environment, due in part to a breakdown of effective connectivity among cortical regions. During REM sleep prefrontal areas are still deactivated, but there is a strong activation of limbic circuits. The interruption of serotonin release during REM sleep may contribute to the persisting disconnection from the environment.

Sleep represents a striking modification of consciousness, which fades early in the night and returns to be vivid later on in the form of dreams. A number of NREM awakenings, especially early in the night, yield little conscious recall. However, more often than not NREM awakenings result in meaningful reports, and in the later part of the night subjects may report full-fledged dreams. Awakenings from REM sleep almost always produce long and vivid dreams. Dreams are usually highly visual, in full color, but do not lack sound, touch, smell and taste, pleasure and pain. Just as in wakefulness, we experience objects, animals, people, faces, places, and so on. We can also have all sorts of thoughts and emotions, especially fear and anxiety. Thus, the dreaming brain is disconnected from the external world, yet it can generate a virtual, imagined world that is fairly similar to the real one. There are, however, some telltale signs of dreaming, including the fading of voluntary control, attention and reflective thought, and an impairment of working memory and episodic memory. By contrast, dreams rely on a network of associations that is less constrained than in waking life.

The periodic and obligatory alteration of consciousness that is forced upon us by sleep is likely to serve an essential function, but what this function might be remains an open issue. Sleep is potentially dangerous, yet it occupies a large fraction of our lives, it is universal in the animal kingdom, and lack of sleep is followed by increasing sleep pressure and cognitive impairment. Various ideas have been put forth, including a role in memory consolidation, in brain restitution, and in brain development. Finally, an intriguing hypothesis is that sleep may be the price we pay for synaptic plasticity during wakefulness.

DISCLOSURES

Dr. Tononi is funded by NIH/NIMH, DARPA, James S. McDonnell Foundation and Philips/Respironics. He is on the Scientific Advisory Board of the Allen Institute for Brain Science with compensation. He is a consultant for Philips/Respironics.

Dr. Cirelli is funded by NIH/NIMH.

REFERENCES

Adamantidis, A.R., Zhang, F., et al. (2007). Neural substrates of awakening probed with optogenetic control of hypocretin neurons. *Nature* 450:420–424.

Arendt, J. (2005). Melatonin: characteristics, concerns, and prospects. *J. Biol. Rhythms* 20:291–303.

Aserinsky, E., and Kleitman, N. (1953). Regularly occurring periods of ocular motility and concomitant phenomena during sleep. *Science* 118:273–274.

Aston-Jones, G. (2005). Brain structures and receptors involved in alertness. *Sleep Med* 6(Suppl. 1):S3–S7.

Aston-Jones, G., and Bloom, F.E. (1981a). Nonrepinephrine-containing locus coeruleus neurons in behaving rats exhibit pronounced responses to non-noxious environmental stimuli. *J Neurosci* 1:887–900.

Aston-Jones, G., and Bloom, F. (1981b). Activity of norepinephrine-containing locus coeruleus neurons in behaving rats anticipates fluctuations in the sleep-waking cycle. *J. Neurosci.* 1:876–886.

Aston-Jones, G., and Cohen, J.D. (2005). An integrative theory of locus coeruleus-norepinephrine function: adaptive gain and optimal performance. *Annu. Rev. Neurosci.* 28:403–450.

Banks, S., and Dinges, D.F. (2007). Behavioral and physiological consequences of sleep restriction. *J. Clin. Sleep Med.* 3:519–528.

Barbier, A.J., and Bradbury, M.J. (2007). Histaminergic control of sleep-wake cycles: recent therapeutic advances for sleep and wake disorders. *CNS Neurol. Disord. Drug Targets* 6:31–43.

Barger, L.K., Ayas, N.T., et al. (2006). Impact of extended-duration shifts on medical errors, adverse events, and attentional failures. *PLoS Med* 3:e487.

Basheer, R., Strecker, R.E., et al. (2004). Adenosine and sleep-wake regulation. *Prog. Neurobiol.* 73:379–396.

Benington, J.H., and Heller, H.C. (1995). Restoration of brain energy metabolism as the function of sleep. *Prog. Neurobiol.* 45:347–360.

Bergmann, B.M., Mistlberger, R.E., et al. (1987). Period-amplitude analysis of rat EEG: stage and diurnal variations and effects of suprachiasmatic nuclei lesions. *Sleep* 10:523–536.

Berridge, C.W., and Abercrombie, E.D. (1999). Relationship between locus coeruleus discharge rates and rates of norepinephrine release within neocortex as assessed by *in vivo* microdialysis. *Neuroscience* 93:1263–1270.

Berridge, C.W., and Espana, R.A. (2000). Synergistic sedative effects of noradrenergic alpha(1)- and beta-receptor blockade on forebrain electroencephalographic and behavioral indices. *Neuroscience* 99:495–505.

Berridge, C.W., and Foote, S.L. (1991). Effects of locus coeruleus activation on electroencephalographic activity in neocortex and hippocampus. *J Neurosci* 11:3135–3145.

Berridge, C.W., and Waterhouse, B.D. (2003). The locus coeruleus-noradrenergic system: modulation of behavioral state and state-dependent cognitive processes. *Brain Res. Brain Res. Rev.* 42:33–84.

Brown, R.E., Stevens, D.R., et al. (2001). The physiology of brain histamine. *Prog. Neurobiol.* 63:637–672.

Buhry, L., Azizi, A.H., et al. (2011). Reactivation, replay, and preplay: how it might all fit together. *Neural. Plast.* 2011:203462.

Bushey, D., Tononi, G., et al. (2011). Sleep and synaptic homeostasis: structural evidence in Drosophila. *Science* 332:1576–1581.

Cape, E.G., and Jones, B.E. (1998). Differential modulation of high-frequency gamma-electroencephalogram activity and sleep-wake state by noradrenaline and serotonin microinjections into the region of cholinergic basalis neurons. *J. Neurosci.* 18:2653–2666.

Carskadon, M.A. (2011). Sleep in adolescents: the perfect storm. *Pediatr. Clin. North Am.* 58:637–647.

Cirelli, C. (2009). The genetic and molecular regulation of sleep: from fruit flies to humans. *Nat. Rev. Neurosci.* 10:549–560.

Cirelli, C., Pompeiano, M., et al. (1996). Neuronal gene expression in the waking state: a role for the locus coeruleus. *Science* 274:1211–1215.

Cirelli, C., Gutierrez, C.M., et al. (2004). Extensive and divergent effects of sleep and wakefulness on brain gene expression. *Neuron* 41:35–43.

Cirelli, C., and Tononi, G. (2000). Differential expression of plasticity-related genes in waking and sleep and their regulation by the noradrenergic system. *J. Neurosci.* 20:9187–9194.

Cirelli, C., and Tononi, G. (2008). Is sleep essential? *PLoS Biol.* 6:e216.

Colrain, I.M., and Baker, F.C. (2011). Changes in sleep as a function of adolescent development. *Neuropsychol. Rev.* 21:5–21.

Dahan, L., Astier, B., et al. (2007). Prominent burst firing of dopaminergic neurons in the ventral tegmental area during paradoxical sleep. *Neuropsychopharmacology* 32:1232–1241.

Dang-Vu, T.T., Schabus, M., et al. (2010). Functional neuroimaging insights into the physiology of human sleep. *Sleep* 33:1589–1603.

Dash, M.B., Douglas, C.L., et al. (2009). Long-term homeostasis of extracellular glutamate in the rat cerebral cortex across sleep and waking states. *J. Neurosci.* 29:620–629.

Dauvilliers, Y., Arnulf, I., et al. (2007). Narcolepsy with cataplexy. *Lancet* 369:499–511.

Deboer, T., Detari, L., et al. (2007). Long term effects of sleep deprivation on the mammalian circadian pacemaker. *Sleep* 30:257–262.

Dement, W., and Kleitman, N. (1957). Cyclic variations in EEG during sleep and their relation to eye movements, body motility, and dreaming. *Electroencephalogr. Clin. Neurophysiol.* 9:673–690.

Diekelmann, S., and Born, J. (2010). The memory function of sleep. *Nat. Rev. Neurosci.* 11:114–126.

Dierks, T., Frolich, L., et al. (1995). Correlation between cognitive brain function and electrical brain activity in dementia of Alzheimer type. *J. Neural. Transm. Gen. Sect.* 99:55–62.

Domino, E.F., Yamamoto, K., et al. (1968). Role of cholinergic mechanisms in states of wakefulness and sleep. *Prog. Brain Res.* 28:113–133.

Donlea, J.M., Ramanan, N., et al. (2009). Use-dependent plasticity in clock neurons regulates sleep need in Drosophila. *Science* 324:105–108.

Donlea, J.M., Thimgan, M.S., et al. (2011). Inducing sleep by remote control facilitates memory consolidation in Drosophila. *Science* 332:1571–1576.

Doran, S.M., Van Dongen, H.P., et al. (2001). Sustained attention performance during sleep deprivation: evidence of state instability. *Arch. Ital. Biol.* 139:253–267.

el Mansari, M., Sakai, K., et al. (1989). Unitary characteristics of presumptive cholinergic tegmental neurons during the sleep-waking cycle in freely moving cats. *Exp. Brain Res.* 76:519–529.

Faraguna, U., Vyazovskiy, V.V., et al. (2008). A causal role for brain-derived neurotrophic factor in the homeostatic regulation of sleep. *J. Neurosci.* 28:4088–4095.

Foote, S.L., Aston-Jones, G., et al. (1980). Impulse activity of locus coeruleus neurons in awake rats and monkeys is a function of sensory stimulation and arousal. *Proc. Natl. Acad. Sci. USA* 77:3033–3037.

Franken, P., Gip, P., et al. (2003). Changes in brain glycogen after sleep deprivation vary with genotype. *Am. J. Physiol. Regul. Integr. Comp. Physiol.* 285:R413–419.

Franken, P., Gip, P., et al. (2006). Glycogen content in the cerebral cortex increases with sleep loss in C57BL/6J mice. *Neurosci. Lett.* 402:176–179.

Gilestro, G.F., Tononi, G., et al. (2009). Widespread changes in synaptic markers as a function of sleep and wakefulness in Drosophila. *Science* 324:109–112.

Gillin, J.C., Drummond, S.P.A., et al. (2005). Medication and substance abuse. In: Kryger, M.H., Roth, T., and Dement, W.C., eds. Principles and Practice of Sleep Medicine, 4th Edition. Philadelphia, PA: Elsevier Saunders, pp. 1345–1358.

Gip, P., Hagiwara, G., et al. (2002). Sleep deprivation decreases glycogen in the cerebellum but not in the cortex of young rats. *Am. J. Physiol. Regul. Integr. Comp. Physiol.* 283:R54–R59.

Halassa, M.M., Florian, C., et al. (2009). Astrocytic modulation of sleep homeostasis and cognitive consequences of sleep loss. *Neuron* 61:213–219.

Hanlon, E.C., Faraguna, U., et al. (2009). Effects of skilled training on sleep slow wave activity and cortical gene expression in the rat. *Sleep* 32:719–729.

Hassani, O.K., Lee, M.G., et al. (2009). Discharge profiles of identified GABAergic in comparison to cholinergic and putative glutamatergic basal forebrain neurons across the sleep-wake cycle. *J. Neurosci.* 29:11828–11840.

Hemmeter, U.M., Hemmeter-Spernal, J., et al. (2010). Sleep deprivation in depression. *Expert Rev. Neurother.* 10:1101–1115.

Horne, J.A. (1980). Sleep and body restitution. *Experientia* 36:11–13.

Huang, Z.L., Urade, Y., et al. (2007). Prostaglandins and adenosine in the regulation of sleep and wakefulness. *Curr. Opin. Pharmacol.* 7:33–38.

Huber, R., Ghilardi, M.F., et al. (2006). Arm immobilization causes cortical plastic changes and locally decreases sleep slow wave activity. *Nat. Neurosci.* 9:1169–1176.

Huber, R., Ghilardi, M.F., et al. (2004). Local sleep and learning. *Nature* 430:78–81.

Huber, R., Maatta, S., et al. (2008). Measures of cortical plasticity after transcranial paired associative stimulation predict changes in electroencephalogram slow-wave activity during subsequent sleep. *J. Neurosci.* 28:7911–7918.

Huber, R., Mäki, H., et al. (2013). Human cortical excitability increases with time awake. *Cereb.Cortex* 23:1–7.

Hung, C.S., Sarasso, S., et al. (2013), Local, experience-dependent changes in the wake EEG after prolonged wakefulness. *Sleep* 36:59–72.

Itil, T., and Fink, M. (1968). EEG and behavioral aspects of the interaction of anticholinergic hallucinogens with centrally active compounds. *Prog. Brain Res.* 28:149–168.

Jacobs, B.L., Martin-Cora, F.J., et al. (2002). Activity of medullary serotonergic neurons in freely moving animals. *Brain Res. Brain Res. Rev.* 40:45–52.

Jenkins, J., and Dallenback, K. (1924). Obliviscence during sleep and waking. *Am. J. Psychol.* 35:605.

Jenni, O.G., Borbely, A.A., et al. (2004a). Development of the nocturnal sleep electroencephalogram in human infants. *Am. J. Physiol. Regul. Integr. Comp. Physiol.* 286:R528–R538.

Jenni, O.G., and Carskadon, M.A. (2004b). Spectral analysis of the sleep electroencephalogram during adolescence. *Sleep* 27:774–783.

John, J., Ramanathan, L., et al. (2008). Rapid changes in glutamate levels in the posterior hypothalamus across sleep-wake states in freely behaving rats. *Am. J. Physiol. Regul. Integr. Comp. Physiol.* 295:R2041–R2049.

Jones, B.E. (2003). Arousal systems. *Front. Biosci.* 8:s438–s451.

Jones, B.E. (2005). Basic mechanisms of sleep-wake states. In: Kryger, M.H., Roth, T., Dement, W.C., eds. 4th Edition. Philadelphia, PA: Elsevier Saunders, pp. 136–153.

Jouvet, M. (1962). Recherches sur les structures nerveuses et les mecanismes responsables des differentes phases du sommeil physiologique. *Archives Italiennes de Biologie* 100:125–206.

Jouvet, M. (1965). Paradoxical sleep: a study of its nature and mechanisms. *Prog. Brain Res.* 18:20–62.

Jouvet, M. (1994). Paradoxical sleep mechanisms. *Sleep* 17:S77–S83.

Jouvet, M. (1998). Paradoxical sleep as a programming system. *J. Sleep Res.* 7(Suppl. 1):1–5.

Jouvet, M. (1999). Sleep and serotonin: an unfinished story. *Neuropsychopharmacology* 21:24S–27S.

Jung, R., and Berger, W. (1979). [Fiftieth anniversary of Hans Berger's publication of the electroencephalogram. His first records in 1924–1931 (author's transl)]. *Arch. Psychiatr. Nervenkr.* 227:279–300.

Kilduff, T.S., and Peyron, C. (2000). The hypocretin/orexin ligand-receptor system: implications for sleep and sleep disorders. *Trends Neurosci.* 23:359–365.

Killgore, W.D. (2010). Effects of sleep deprivation on cognition. *Prog. Brain Res.* 185:105–129.

Krueger, J.M., Obal, F.J., et al. (2001). The role of cytokines in physiological sleep regulation. *Ann. NY Acad. Sci.* 933:211–221.

Landolt, H.P., and Wehrle, R. (2009). Antagonism of serotonergic 5-HT2A/2C receptors: mutual improvement of sleep, cognition and mood? *Eur. J. Neurosci.* 29:1795–1809.

Landsness, E.C., Goldstein, M.R., et al. (2011). Antidepressant effects of selective slow wave sleep deprivation in major depression: a high-density EEG investigation. *J. Psychiatr. Res.* 45:1019–1026.

Lante, F., Toledo-Salas, J.C., et al. (2011). Removal of synaptic Ca(2)+-permeable AMPA receptors during sleep. *J. Neurosci.* 31:3953–3961.

Lee, M.G., Hassani, O.K., et al. (2005b). Cholinergic basal forebrain neurons burst with theta during waking and paradoxical sleep. *J. Neurosci.* 25:4365–4369.

Lee, M.G., Hassani, O.K., et al. (2005a). Discharge of identified orexin/hypocretin neurons across the sleep-waking cycle. *J. Neurosci.* 25:6716–6720.

Li, Y., Gao, X.B., et al. (2002). Hypocretin/orexin excites hypocretin neurons via a local glutamate neuron-A potential mechanism for orchestrating the hypothalamic arousal system. *Neuron* 36:1169–1181.

Lin, J.S., Anaclet, C., et al. (2011). The waking brain: an update. *Cell. Mol. Life Sci.* 68:2499–2512.

Lin, J.S., Hou, Y., et al. (1996). Histaminergic descending inputs to the mesopontine tegmentum and their role in the control of cortical activation and wakefulness in the cat. *J. Neurosci.* 16:1523–1537.

Lin, J.S., Sakai, K., et al. (1989). A critical role of the posterior hypothalamus in the mechanisms of wakefulness determined by microinjection of muscimol in freely moving cats. *Brain Res.* 479:225–240.

Lindsley, D.B., Bowden, J.W., et al. (1949). Effect upon the EEG of acute injury to the brain stem activating system. *Electroencephalogr. Clin. Neurophysiol.* 1:475–486.

Liu, Z.W., Faraguna, U., et al. (2010). Direct evidence for wake-related increases and sleep-related decreases in synaptic strength in rodent cortex. *J. Neurosci.* 30:8671–8675.

Llinas, R.R., and Pare, D. (1991). Of dreaming and wakefulness. *Neuroscience* 44:521–535.

Luppi, P.H., Clement, O., et al. (2012). Brainstem mechanisms of paradoxical (REM) sleep generation. *Pflugers Arch.* 463:43–52.

Mackiewicz, M., Shockley, K.R., et al. (2007). Macromolecule biosynthesis: a key function of sleep. *Physiol. Genomics* 31:441–457.

Maquet, P. (2010). Understanding non rapid eye movement sleep through neuroimaging. *World J. Biol. Psychiatry* 11(Suppl 1):9–15.

Maret, S., Faraguna, U., et al. (2011). Sleep and wake modulate spine turnover in the adolescent mouse cortex. *Nature Neuroscience* 14:1418–1420.

Massimini, M., Ferrarelli, F., et al. (2005). Breakdown of cortical effective connectivity during sleep. *Science* 309:2228–2232.

Massimini, M., Huber, R., et al. (2004). The sleep slow oscillation as a traveling wave. *J. Neurosci.* 24:6862–6870.

McCarley, R.W. (2011). Neurobiology of REM sleep. *Handb. Clin. Neurol.* 98:151–171.

McCormick, D.A. (1989). Cholinergic and noradrenergic modulation of thalamocortical processing. *Trends Neurosci.* 12:215–221.

McGinty, D.J., and Harper, R.M. (1976). Dorsal raphe neurons: depression of firing during sleep in cats. *Brain Research* 101:569–575.

Metherate, R., Cox, C.L., et al. (1992). Cellular bases of neocortical activation: modulation of neural oscillations by the nucleus basalis and endogenous acetylcholine. *J. Neurosci.* 12:4701–4711.

Mileykovskiy, B.Y., Kiyashchenko, L.I., et al. (2005). Behavioral correlates of activity in identified hypocretin/orexin neurons. *Neuron* 46:787–798.

Mistlberger, R.E. (2005). Circadian regulation of sleep in mammals: role of the suprachiasmatic nucleus. *Brain Res. Brain Res. Rev.* 49:429–454.

Mistlberger, R.E., Bergmann, B.M., et al. (1983). Recovery sleep following sleep deprivation in intact and suprachiasmatic nuclei-lesioned rats. *Sleep* 6:217–233.

Mohawk, J.A., and Takahashi, J.S. (2011). Cell autonomy and synchrony of suprachiasmatic nucleus circadian oscillators. *Trends Neurosci.* 34:349–358.

Mongrain, V., Hernandez, S.A., et al. (2010). Separating the contribution of glucocorticoids and wakefulness to the molecular and electrophysiological correlates of sleep homeostasis. *Sleep* 33:1147–1157.

Monti, J.M., and Jantos, H. (2008). The roles of dopamine and serotonin, and of their receptors, in regulating sleep and waking. *Prog. Brain Res.* 172:625–646.

Monti, J.M., and Monti, D. (2007). The involvement of dopamine in the modulation of sleep and waking. *Sleep Med. Rev.* 11:113–133.

Montplaisir, J., Petit, D., et al. (1998). Sleep disturbances and EEG slowing in Alzheimer's disease. *Sleep Res. Online* 1:147–151.

Moruzzi, G., and Magoun, H.W. (1949). Brainstem reticular formation and activation of the EEG. *Electroencephalogr. Clin. Neurophysiol.* 1:455–473.

Nir, Y., Staba, R.J., et al. (2011). Regional slow waves and spindles in human sleep. *Neuron* 70:153–169.

Nir, Y., and Tononi, G. (2010). Dreaming and the brain: from phenomenology to neurophysiology. *Trends Cogn. Sci.* 14:88–100.

Ohayon, M.M., Carskadon, M.A., et al. (2004). Meta-analysis of quantitative sleep parameters from childhood to old age in healthy individuals: developing normative sleep values across the human lifespan. *Sleep* 27:1255–1273.

Porkka-Heiskanen, T., Alanko, L., et al. (2002). Adenosine and sleep. *Sleep Med. Rev.* 6:321–332.

Porkka-Heiskanen, T., Strecker, R.E., et al. (1997). Adenosine: a mediator of the sleep-inducing effects of prolonged wakefulness. *Science* 276:1265–1268.

Porkka-Heiskanen, T., Strecker, R.E., et al. (2000). Brain site-specificity of extracellular adenosine concentration changes during sleep deprivation and spontaneous sleep: an *in vivo* microdialysis study. *Neuroscience* 99:507–517.

Portas, C.M., Krakow, K., et al. (2000). Auditory processing across the sleep-wake cycle: simultaneous EEG and fMRI monitoring in humans. *Neuron* 28:991–999.

Prinz, P.N., Peskind, E.R., et al. (1982). Changes in the sleep and waking EEG's of nondemented and demented elderly subjects. *J. Am. Geriatr. Soc.* 30:86–92.

Rakic, P., Bourgeois, J.P., et al. (1994). Synaptic development of the cerebral cortex: implications for learning, memory, and mental illness. *Prog. Brain Res.* 102:227–243.

Richardson, G.S. (2005). The human circadian system in normal and disordered sleep. *J. Clin. Psychiatry* 66(Suppl 9):3–9; quiz 42–43.

Sakurai, T. (2007). The neural circuit of orexin (hypocretin): maintaining sleep and wakefulness. *Nat. Rev. Neurosci.* 8:171–181.

Saper, C.B., Scammell, T.E., et al. (2005a). Hypothalamic regulation of sleep and circadian rhythms. *Nature* 437:1257–1263.

Saper, C.B., Lu, J., et al. (2005b). The hypothalamic integrator for circadian rhythms. *Trends Neurosci.* 28:152–157.

Sasaki, K., Suzuki, M., et al. (2011). Pharmacogenetic modulation of orexin neurons alters sleep/wakefulness states in mice. *PLoS One* 6:e20360.

Schmitt, L.I., Sims, R.E., et al. (2012). Wakefulness affects synaptic and network activity by increasing extracellular astrocyte-derived adenosine. *J. Neurosci.* 32:4417–4425.

Sherin, J.E., Shiromani, P.J., et al. (1996). Activation of ventrolateral preoptic neurons during sleep. *Science* 271:216–219.

Siegel, J.M. (2001). The REM sleep-memory consolidation hypothesis. *Science* 294:1058–1063.

Siegel, J.M. (2005). REM sleep. In: Kryger, M.H., Roth, T., and Dement, W.C., eds. Principles and Practice of Sleep Medicine, 4th Edition. Philadelphia, PA: Elsevier Saunders, pp. 120–135.

Silber, M.H., Ancoli-Israel, S., et al. (2007). The visual scoring of sleep in adults. *J. Clin. Sleep Med.* 3:121–131.

Soininen, H., Reinikainen, K.J., et al. (1992). Slowing of electroencephalogram and choline acetyltransferase activity in post mortem frontal cortex in definite Alzheimer's disease. *Neuroscience* 49:529–535.

Steriade, M. (2004). Acetylcholine systems and rhythmic activities during the waking: sleep cycle. *Prog. Brain Res.* 145:179–196.

Steriade, M., Timofeev, I., et al. (2001). Natural waking and sleep states: a view from inside neocortical neurons. *J. Neurophysiol.* 85:1969–1985.

Steriade, M., and Timofeev, I. (2003). Neuronal plasticity in thalamocortical networks during sleep and waking oscillations. *Neuron* 37:563–576.

Stickgold, R., and Walker, M.P. (2007). Sleep-dependent memory consolidation and reconsolidation. *Sleep Med.* 8:331–343.

Suntsova, N., Szymusiak, R., et al. (2002). Sleep-waking discharge patterns of median preoptic nucleus neurons in rats. *J. Physiol.* 543:665–677.

Szymusiak, R., Alam, N., et al. (1998). Sleep-waking discharge patterns of ventrolateral preoptic/anterior hypothalamic neurons in rats. *Brain Res.* 803:178–188.

Szymusiak, R., and McGinty, D. (2008). Hypothalamic regulation of sleep and arousal. *Ann. NY Acad. Sci.* 1129:275–286.

Takahashi, K., Lin, J.S., et al. (2006). Neuronal activity of histaminergic tuberomammillary neurons during wake-sleep states in the mouse. *J. Neurosci.* 26:10292–10298.

Tobler, I., Borbely, A.A., et al. (1983). The effect of sleep deprivation on sleep in rats with suprachiasmatic lesions. *Neurosci. Lett.* 42:49–54.

Tononi, G., and Cirelli, C. (2003). Sleep and synaptic homeostasis: a hypothesis. *Brain Res. Bull.* 62:143–150.

Tononi, G., and Cirelli, C. (2006). Sleep function and synaptic homeostasis. *Sleep Med. Rev.* 10:49–62.

Tononi, G., and Cirelli, C. (2012). Time to Be SHY? Some comments on sleep and synaptic homeostasis. *Neural Plast.* 2012:415250.

Ursin, R. (2002). Serotonin and sleep. *Sleep Med. Rev.* 6:55–69.

Vanini, G., Lydic, R., et al. (2012). GABA-to-ACh ratio in basal forebrain and cerebral cortex varies significantly during sleep. *Sleep* 35:1325–1334.

Vertes, R.P. (2004). Memory consolidation in sleep: dream or reality. *Neuron* 44:135–148.

von Economo, C. (1931). Encephalitis Lethargica: Its Sequelae and Treatment. K.O. Newman, Trans. Oxford, UK: Oxford University Press.

Vyazovskiy, V.V., Cirelli, C., et al. (2008). Molecular and electrophysiological evidence for net synaptic potentiation in wake and depression in sleep. *Nat. Neurosci.* 11:200–208.

Vyazovskiy, V.V., Olcese, U., et al. (2011). Local sleep in awake rats. *Nature* 472:443–447.

Yang, G., and Gan, W.B. (2011). Sleep contributes to dendritic spine formation and elimination in the developing mouse somatosensory cortex. *Dev. Neurobiol.* 72:1391–1398.

Zee, P.C., and Manthena, P. (2007). The brain's master circadian clock: implications and opportunities for therapy of sleep disorders. *Sleep Med. Rev.* 11:59–70.

88 | THE NEUROBIOLOGY OF RESILIENCE

ADRIANA FEDER, MARGARET HAGLUND, GANG WU,
STEVEN M. SOUTHWICK, AND DENNIS S. CHARNEY

Resilience is the ability to adapt successfully to severe or chronic stress (Charney, 2004; Rutter, 2006). Resilient individuals are those who are able to demonstrate healthy psychological and physiological stress responses in the face of extreme stress or trauma exposure, thus maintaining "psychobiological allostasis" (Feder et al., 2009; Karatsoreos and McEwen, 2011). Historically, most research on the effects of severe stress focused on its deleterious effects on well-being. The study of resilience began in the 1970s with the study of children exposed to significant adversity during development (Masten, 2001), later extending to the study of trauma-exposed adults (Alim et al., 2008; Bonanno, 2004). More recent epidemiological studies are beginning to look at longitudinal trajectories of posttraumatic stress disorder (PTSD) symptoms and resilience over time, and have begun to distinguish a resistance trajectory, characterized by the absence of symptoms, from a resilience trajectory, characterized by some initial symptom development, followed by prompt recovery (Bonanno et al., 2011; Hobfoll et al., 2009).

In the last decade, there has been a great deal of interest in delineating the neurobiological and psychological profile of resilient individuals. Supplementing studies in humans, animal studies are greatly advancing our understanding of neural and molecular mechanisms underlying resilience to stress (Russo et al., 2012). Identifying the factors that set resilient individuals apart from those who are vulnerable to the effects of stress has clinical significance: understanding the neurobiology and psychology of resilience enables researchers and clinicians to develop new therapies for the prevention and treatment of stress-induced psychopathology in non-resilient individuals. Furthermore, motivated individuals can draw from our increasing understanding of the features of resilience to achieve greater personal resilience to stress (Southwick and Charney, 2012a).

This chapter outlines the current understanding of resilience, from genetic, epigenetic, developmental, psychological, and neurobiological perspectives, and presents promising new therapies for the promotion of resilience to stress.

PREVALENCE OF RESILIENCE

The majority of individuals are exposed to trauma during their lifetime: in the United States, lifetime risk of at least one significant traumatic event, such as sudden unexpected death of a loved one, injury in a motor vehicle accident, or experiencing assault, is estimated at 80–90% (Breslau et al., 1998; Bruce et al., 2001). The prevalence of resilience depends on the particular definition and measure(s) used, on the population studied, and importantly on the severity and chronicity of stress or trauma exposure. In the words of Rutter (2012), "resilience is an inference based on evidence that some individuals have a better outcome than others who have experienced a comparable level of adversity."

Population studies in the United States have estimated the lifetime prevalence of PTSD at 8%, and the conditional probability of PTSD after exposure to trauma at 9% (Breslau et al., 1998; Kessler et al., 1995). Certain types of trauma, however, are significantly more likely to cause PTSD, particularly rape (65%) and combat exposure (38.8%) for men, and rape (45.9%) and physical abuse (48.5%) for women (Kessler et al., 1995). In general, traumatic events that are severe and unpredictable, intentionally caused by other human beings (such as assaultive trauma), and result in loss (of a loved one, property, or physical integrity) are most likely to lead to PTSD (Jordan et al., 1991; Yehuda, 2004). In a study of a high-risk primary care sample, the resilient group had a significantly lower lifetime prevalence of assaultive trauma (46.8% vs. 75.6%), as well as a significantly lower mean number of lifetime experienced trauma types (3.4% vs. 5.1%) than the group with current psychiatric disorders (Alim et al., 2008). Further, studies have shown that the degree of control that an individual has over a stressor or trauma is a key factor in modulating the impact of a stressor (Fleshner et al., 2011).

Recent longitudinal trajectories studies have employed latent growth mixture modeling, a statistical approach that identifies clusters of individuals following distinct courses of longitudinal symptom development without assuming a-priori trajectory types (Nagin and Odgers, 2010; Norris et al., 2009). In these studies, the prevalence of resilience has ranged widely depending on the population studied. For example, the resilience trajectory represented over 80% of the sample in a study of deployed US military service members (Bonanno et al., 2012), whereas it was 35.6% (resistance and resilience trajectories combined) in a sample under ongoing threat of terrorism and rocket attacks (Hobfoll et al., 2009). Of note, the second study used PTSD and depressive symptom measures to define resilience, whereas the first one only measured PTSD symptoms. Despite differences in prevalence across studies, research has shown that a significant percentage of individuals are resilient to the effects of extreme stress.

GENETICS OF RESILIENCE

Studies of gene-by-environment interactions have begun to identify how complex interactions between genetic contributions and an individual's particular history of exposure to environmental stressors yield a unique profile of adaptability of an individual's neurochemical stress responses and neural circuitry function upon exposure to new stressors. Further, as discussed in the following, epigenetic modifications are now understood to modulate stress reactivity by regulating gene expression at the molecular level.

It has long been known that stress-related disorders are at least partially heritable. For example, studies of combat-exposed men enrolled in the Vietnam Twin Registry have found that PTSD, panic disorder, and general anxiety disorder, frequently comorbid conditions, all have significant genetic contributions. It is estimated that up to 40% of the variance in occurrence of these disorders is accounted for by genetic factors, rather than by situation or trauma-related factors (Chantarujikapong et al., 2001; Scherrer et al., 2000; True et al., 1993). Genetic factors are not only important in determining an individual's response to a stressful event, but also influence the likelihood of exposure to that event (Kremen et al., 2012).

A series of studies have identified a range of specific genetic polymorphisms affecting stress reactivity, and thus likely affecting differential vulnerability to stress exposure, of which some examples follow. Regulation of the hypothalamic-pituitary-adrenal (HPA) axis, a key hormonal system involved in adaptation to stress, is affected by genetic factors. Two separate studies have shown that the presence of certain alleles and haplotypes of the gene coding for the corticotropin-releasing hormone (CRH) type 1 receptor moderates the severity of depressive symptoms in adults with a history of childhood abuse (Bradley et al., 2008). Functional polymorphisms of the glucocorticoid receptor (GR) have also been identified: for example, the N363S variant of the GR gene increases cortisol responses to the Trier Social Stress Test, a public speaking and mental arithmetic task (Derijk and de Kloet, 2008). Genetic variation in FKBP5, a gene coding for a protein responsible for regulating GR sensitivity, has been found to affect the efficiency of recovery of HPA axis activation after exposure to the Trier Social Stress Test in healthy individuals (Ising et al., 2008), and to interact with severity of childhood abuse in predicting PTSD symptom severity in adults (Binder et al., 2008). More efficient recovery of HPA axis activation after exposure to environmental stressors is thought to be a key characteristic of resilient individuals. Of note, by combining genetic with gene expression and hormone studies, it is now possible to identify subtypes of PTSD differing, for example, in the nature of HPA axis abnormality (Mehta et al., 2011).

Genetic variations in the serotonergic system have also been found to affect susceptibility to stress-induced psychopathology. The short (S) allele of the serotonin (5-HT) transporter promoter gene (5HTTLPR), which compared with the long (L) allele results in decreased transporter availability and lower uptake of 5-HT from synaptic clefts, has been implicated in a number of studies in a maladaptive response to stress. Although individuals who are carriers for the S allele of 5HTTLPR show elevated risk for depression upon stress exposure in some but not all studies (Caspi et al., 2003; Kendler et al., 2005; Uher and McGuffin, 2010), this finding has been confirmed in a recent large metaanalysis (Karg et al., 2011). S allele carriers also show heightened activation of the amygdala (Hariri et al., 2005) and decreased coupling between the amygdala and the regulatory perigenual cingulate region while viewing fearful or aversive stimuli (Pezawas et al., 2005). Differential neural activation to threat stimuli might represent a biological marker of differential susceptibility to stress. In a recent fMRI study in healthy women, neural systems involved in fear responses and attention to threat showed higher activation during anticipation of a mild shock to the wrist in participants with the SS allele compared with L carriers (Drabant et al., 2012). Further, differential neural activation in medial prefrontal cortex (mPFC) and insula was associated with differential self-reports of anxiety and success at anxiety regulation. Interestingly, recent studies have found that youth homozygous for the short allele of 5HTTLPR were not only more vulnerable to negative parenting, but also more responsive to supportive parenting, showing higher levels of positive affect if parenting was supportive (Hankin et al., 2011). Thus some genetic variations might increase an individual's responsivity to environmental influence, whether good or bad, potentially boosting or decreasing resilience depending on the quality of the environment during development (Homberg and Lesch, 2011). A recent prospective study in female college students found increased acute stress disorder symptoms after a college shooting in students with particular combinations of polymorphisms in the 5-HT transporter gene (Mercer et al., 2012). Variations in other genes affecting serotonin signaling are also being identified. For example, a common functional variation in the gene coding for the serotonin 1A autoreceptor was associated with differential amygdala reactivity to angry and fearful facial expressions in healthy adults, and indirectly with differential trait anxiety (Fakra et al., 2009).

Genetic polymorphisms affecting resilience to stress have been identified in the noradrenergic system as well as in the serotonergic system. Functional polymorphisms in the gene that produces catechol-O-methyltransferase (COMT), an enzyme that degrades dopamine (DA) and norepinephrine (NE), have been identified and found to affect response to stress. Individuals with the low functioning met allele for the enzyme, and hence higher circulating levels of DA and NE, tend to exhibit more anxious behaviors and lower resilience against negative moods (Heinz and Smolka, 2006). They also tend to avoid novelty-seeking behaviors, and while viewing aversive images, show heightened activity in the visuospatial attention system as well as increased reactivity and connectivity in corticolimbic circuits (Drabant et al., 2006), suggesting that they have a heightened awareness for potential threats (Smolka et al., 2005). Another group studying the COMT gene found that carriers of the low functioning met allele exhibited greater plasma endocrine and subjective stress responses in response to psychologically stressful tasks than did carriers of the high-functioning allele (Jabbi et al., 2007).

Polymorphisms in DA receptors and in the DA transporter gene have also been associated with vulnerability to depression and PTSD (Dunlop and Nemeroff, 2007). In a study of combat veterans, for instance, the A1+ allele of the D_2 receptor was associated with more severe PTSD and higher levels of anxiety and depression (Lawford et al., 2006). Polymorphisms in other relevant systems have been identified. A polymorphism (Val66Met) in the gene for brain derived neurotrophic factor (BDNF), a widely expressed protein that stimulates neurogenesis and promotes learning and memory, has been linked with an increased likelihood of suffering stress-induced depression (Kim et al., 2007), and with increased amygdala reactivity in response to emotional stimuli in healthy females (Montag et al., 2008). A single nucleotide polymorphism (rs1617) located in the promoter region of the gene coding for neuropeptide Y (NPY), a peptide released during stress that appears to mitigate the negative effects of the stress response, alters NPY expression and was found to differentially affect stress responses and neural activation to emotional probes (Zhou et al., 2008).

A recent study identified associations between single nucleotide polymorphisms in the genes coding for the pituitary adenylate cyclase-activating polypeptide (PACAP) (involved in regulating the cellular stress response) and its PACAP-PAC1 receptor, and PTSD in females (Ressler et al., 2011). Additional genetic polymorphisms, gene-by-environment, and gene-by-gene-by-environment interactions involved in resilience to stress are currently being identified, the latter exemplified by a study of interactions between a history of childhood trauma and genetic polymorphisms in the CRH type 1 receptor and serotonin transporter genes on depressive symptoms in adults (Ressler et al., 2010). Thus our understanding of the genetics of resilience is likely to increase rapidly in coming years. As more of the genetic factors underlying resilience are uncovered, it may become possible for scientists to design gene or drug therapies specific for individuals with low-resilience genetic profiles.

THE DEVELOPMENT OF RESILIENCE: ROLE OF EARLY LIFE ENVIRONMENT

In addition to genetic makeup, another key contributor to resilience is developmental environment. The study of resilience from a developmental perspective dates back to the early 1970s (Masten and Obradovic, 2006). An important discovery to emerge from this research is that resilience is common, even in children who suffered severe adversity in early life. Studies of adolescents whose development was stunted in childhood due to traumatic experiences such as being orphaned have found that the majority of children rapidly demonstrate "developmental catch-up" when placed in safe and nurturing environments (Masten, 2001). It seems that, under the right circumstances, neural circuits involved in resilience are modifiable for many years after birth, possibly even into adulthood.

Nevertheless, severely traumatic experiences in early life can negatively affect the development of stress response systems, in some cases doing long-lasting damage. Studies of rodents and non-human primates indicate that animals abused by their mothers during the first few weeks after birth have delayed independence and a decreased ability to manage stress later in life, demonstrated by high levels of behavioral anxiety,

a hyperactive HPA axis, and increased basal levels of the anxiogenic CRH in the cerebrospinal fluid (Claes, 2004; McCormack et al., 2006; Strome et al., 2002). Furthermore, non-human primates who suffered damage to their stress response systems as a result of abuse in infancy seem more likely to mistreat their own infants, perpetuating the effects of abuse across generations (Maestripieri et al., 2007).

Studies of human survivors of early life stress and abuse have also found long-lasting alterations in central nervous system circuits and structures involved in psychological well-being. Severe prenatal stress and early childhood abuse have been linked to increased HPA axis activity later in life, putting survivors at risk for the adverse effects of chronic hypercortisolemia (Heim et al., 2000; Janssen et al., 2007 Seckl and Meaney, 2006; Vythilingam et al., 2002). Developmental environment also influences the adult functioning of the locus coeruleus–norepinephrine (LC–NE) system, with severe stress in early life leading to its hyperfunctioning. For instance, one study found that police recruits with a history of childhood trauma had significantly higher levels of a salivary metabolite of NE in response to viewing aversive videos than did healthy controls (Otte et al., 2005). Other research has found that physical or sexual abuse in childhood can lead to smaller-than-average hippocampal volumes; decreased hippocampal volume is commonly seen in individuals with depression or chronic stress disorders (Janssen et al., 2007). Thus, it appears that early abuse can cause long-standing changes in brain structures and circuits associated with resilience.

Although early exposure to unpredictable and uncontrollable stress or trauma commonly leads to later psychopathology, exposure to moderately stressful events that can be mastered to an extent (e.g. family relocation, illness of a parent, or loss of a friendship) seems to enable children to effectively regulate their stress response systems. Children who have experience successfully coping with difficult situations reap benefits when faced with stressors later in life, experiencing less physiological and psychological distress (Boyce and Chesterman, 1990; Khoshaba and Maddi, 1999). It seems that the experience of mastering stress provides a form of immunity against later challenges. This phenomenon is known as stress inoculation, based on the analogy to vaccine-induced inoculation against disease (Rutter, 1993). Just as exposure to a low dose of a pathogen enables the body to mount a long-lasting immune response, exposure to moderate amounts of stress enables organisms to conquer and fight off future stressors.

Research in rodents and primates supports the stress inoculation hypothesis and provides insight into its neurobiological mechanisms. Young monkeys presented with a manageable stressor in the form of periodic short maternal separations from postnatal weeks 17 to 27 experience acute distress during the separation periods, manifested by behavioral agitation and temporarily increased cortisol levels. Later in life, however, the same monkeys demonstrate lower anxiety (e.g. increased exploratory behavior in novel environments) and lower basal stress hormone levels at nine months of age than monkeys who never underwent periods of maternal separation (Parker et al., 2004). Furthermore, these stress-inoculated monkeys demonstrate higher cognitive control assessed at 1.5 years, higher curiosity in a stress-free situation at 2.5 years, and larger ventromedial prefrontal cortex (PFC) volume assessed with neuroimaging at age 3.3 years compared with their non–stress-inoculated peers (Lyons et al., 2009; Parker et al., 2005). Poor control of prefrontal cognition has been associated with depression in humans (Harvey et al., 2005; Murphy et al., 2001). Of note, the size of the ventromedial PFC in humans predicts lower impulsivity, lower harm avoidance, and greater retention of learned fear extinction (Lyons et al., 2009).

Just as in humans, the degree of control that an animal has over a stressor plays a key role in determining whether the event will lead to subsequent vulnerability or resilience to stress. Animals administered unavoidable and unpredictable shocks tend to develop exaggerated fear responses, heightened anxiety states, and deficits in active coping when faced with subsequent stressors: this condition is known as learned helplessness (Overmier and Seligman, 1967). The phenomenon of learned helplessness is a well-known animal model for depression and is thought to lead to dysregulation of the serotonergic neurons in the dorsal raphé nuclei (Greenwood et al., 2003) as well as to reduce hippocampal cell proliferation. Because 5-HT has far-reaching effects in the limbic system, the dysregulations created by learned helplessness likely have serious negative effects on cognition and mood.

In contrast, animals that are administered shocks and given the ability to avoid them by modifying their behavior do not develop learned helplessness. Furthermore, animals that have at one time experienced behavioral control over predictable tail shocks are less likely than naïve animals to develop learned helplessness if they are subsequently exposed to unpredictable and inescapable shocks (Seligman and Maier, 1967). Similarly, human beings that have been "stress inoculated" to one type of stressor by successfully managing the stressor appear to acquire resilience to a broad range of other subsequent stressors (Masten and Obradovic, 2006). As noted by Rutter (2012), limited evidence from human studies suggests that steeling might occur via the acquisition of self-efficacy and mastery.

It is important to note that even among animals administered unpredictable and unavoidable shocks, not all develop learned helplessness. Similarly, in humans exposed to severe, unpredictable, and uncontrollable traumas, not all go on to develop PTSD or other anxiety or panic disorders. Clearly, genetic factors interact with environmental exposures to affect resilience. In some cases, a resilient genetic profile may be enough to overcome even the most adverse developmental circumstances.

EPIGENETICS

Prenatal and early postnatal environments regulate developmental processes at the molecular level via epigenetic mechanisms, affecting gene expression without involving changes in DNA sequence (Dudley et al., 2011). Initial studies in rodents showed that high maternal care early in development can lead to a "permanent increase" in GR expression in the hippocampus, resulting from lower GR promoter DNA methylation, and thereby lowering sensitivity to circulating glucocorticoids (Liu et al., 1997; Weaver et al., 2004). Further epigenetic changes

can occur in response to experiences including drug use, social interactions, and exposure to stress during critical development periods (Dudley et al., 2011).

Stress reactivity in adult animals is partially a result of epigenetic changes stemming from differential early life experience, such as methylation levels of promoter regions in genes of central importance to stress responses (e.g., GR, brain-derived neurotrophic factor), and located in key regions of the brain (e.g., hippocampus, prefrontal cortex) (Roth et al., 2009; Weaver et al., 2004). Similarly, prenatal stress can also result in epigenetic changes, which in turn impact stress reactivity; on the other hand, early evidence suggests that some of these changes are potentially reversible by optimal postnatal experience (Dudley et al., 2011). Studies in humans have begun to identify the role of epigenetic changes, as exemplified by a report of differential methylation of the GR gene in newborn babies of mothers with prenatal depression (Oberlander et al., 2008). There has been a recent surge of animal and human studies investigating the role of epigenetic mechanisms in differential stress reactivity (Mifsud et al., 2011; Radley et al., 2011; Yehuda et al., 2011).

Having reviewed the role of early life environment and recent findings on epigenetic changes, in the following sections we outline what current research holds to be some of the most important factors, psychological and neurobiological, characterizing resilience to extreme stress in the adult.

PSYCHOBIOLOGICAL FEATURES OF RESILIENCE

TRAITS AND BEHAVIORS

POSITIVE EMOTIONS

Positive emotions play an integral role in the capacity to tolerate stress. The broaden-and-build theory holds that positive emotions enable broader psychological and behavioral responses, ultimately building enduring resources (Fredrickson, 2001). Positive affect is associated with health-protecting factors including greater social connectedness and adaptive coping mechanisms (Steptoe et al., 2005). Positive emotions also appear to decrease autonomic arousal (Isen et al., 1987; Folkman and Moskowitz, 2000) and facilitate cardiovascular recovery after negative arousal in response to a stressor (Tugade and Fredrickson, 2004), leading to better physical health. Positive affect has been associated with reduced use of medical services; fewer stress-related illnesses; and decreased neuroendocrine, cardiovascular, and inflammatory reactivity (Carver et al., 1993; Danner et al., 2001; Steptoe et al., 2005; Scheier et al., 1989; Zeidner and Hammer, 1992).

Similarly, optimism has been repeatedly correlated with increased psychological well-being and health (Affleck and Tennen, 1996; Goldman et al., 1996) and with greater life satisfaction (Klohnen, 1996). An optimistic disposition is thought to be in large part inherited; however, motivated individuals can increase their optimism with practice. Optimists maintain positive emotions even in the face of adversity because they tend to view problems as temporary and limited in scope. Pessimists, on the other hand, tend to think of their problems as permanent and pervasive and consequently are more prone to depression (Table 88.1). Optimism has even been correlated with longevity: for example, a study of 180 nuns found that nuns whose diaries from youth reflected optimism lived significantly longer than nuns with more negative diaries (Danner et al., 2001). Optimists are thought to have robust brain reward circuits, which is discussed in further detail later in the chapter.

Dispositional gratitude, another positive emotion related to a generally appreciative outlook toward life, was shown in longitudinal studies to foster social support and protect individuals from stress and depression (Wood et al., 2008).

POSITIVE COGNITIVE REAPPRAISAL

Cognitive reappraisal, or the ability to find the silver lining in every cloud, is closely related to optimism and strongly associated with resilience (Gross, 2002; Southwick et al., 2005; Tugade and Fredrickson, 2004). The technique, also known as cognitive flexibility or cognitive reframing, refers to the purposeful, conscious transformation of emotional experience. Cognitive reframing is the reinterpretation of traumatic events to find their positive meaning, value, or the new opportunity that they provide. It stands in contrast to suppression, which signifies conscious attempts to forget traumatic events. Individuals who use cognitive reappraisal when dealing with trauma have less anger and physiologic arousal than those who use suppression techniques (Gross, 2002). It is thought that cognitive reappraisal works in part by attenuating biological stress responses (Davidson and McEwen, 2012; Disner et al., 2011).

The ability to find personal meaning in tragedy is extraordinarily helpful in successfully overcoming trauma. Viktor Frankl, psychiatrist and Holocaust survivor, attributes his

TABLE 88.1. Selected psychological resilience factors: attitudes and behaviors that can help maintain well-being during stress

1. Positive emotions and positive attitude
   Optimism is strongly related to resilience.
   Optimism is in part inherited but can be learned through therapy.
   Putative neurobiological mechanisms: strengthens reward circuits, decreases autonomic activity
2. Cognitive flexibility and reappraisal
   Finding meaning or value in adversity
   Traumatic experiences can be reevaluated through a more positive lens.
   Trauma can lead to growth: learn to reappraise or reframe adversity, finding its benefits; assimilate the event into personal history; accept its occurrence; and recover.
   Recognize that failure is an essential ingredient for growth.
   Putative neurobiological mechanisms: alters memory reconsolidation, strengthens cognitive control over emotions
3. Moral compass: embrace a set of core beliefs that few things can shatter
   Live by a set of guiding principles.
   For many, moral compass means religious or spiritual faith.
   Altruism strongly associated with resilience: selfless acts increase our own well being.
   Putative neurobiological mechanisms: spirituality/religiosity associated with strong serotonergic systems. Morality has neural basis, likely evolved because adaptive
4. Finding a resilient role model/mentor
   Role models and mentors can help teach resilience: imitation is powerful mode of learning.
   Putative neurobiological mechanisms: oxytocin mediates initial bonding/attachment. "Mirror"/Von Economo neurons involved in neuronal imprinting of human values
5. Facing fears: learning to move through fear
   Fear is normal and can be used as a guide for action.
   Facing and overcoming fears can increase self-esteem and sense of self-efficacy.
   Practice undertaking and completing challenging or anxiety-inducing tasks.
   Putative neurobiological mechanisms: promotes fear extinction, stress inoculation
6. Active coping: seeking solutions, managing emotions
   Resilient individuals use active rather than passive coping skills (dealing with problem and with emotions versus withdrawal, resignation, numbing).
   Can be learned: work on minimizing appraisal of threat, creating positive statements about oneself, focusing on aspects that can be changed
   Putative neurobiological mechanisms: prevents fear conditioning and learned helplessness, promotes fear extinction
7. Establishing and nurturing a supportive social network
   Establish and nurture a supportive social network.
   Very few can "go it alone"; resilient individuals derive strength from close relationships.
   Social support is safety net during stress.
   Putative neurobiological mechanisms: oxytocin mediates bonding/attachment, neural networks subserve automatic emotional responses and voluntary emotion regulation during social interactions
8. Physical exercise and attending to physical well-being
   Physical exercise has positive effects on physical and psychological hardiness.
   Effective at increasing mood and self-esteem
   Putative neurobiological mechanisms: promotes neurogenesis, improves cognition, attenuates HPA activity, aids in regulation of emotion, boosts immune system
9. Other resilience factors
   Training regularly (emotionally and physically), discipline
   Recognizing one's own strengths and fostering them

Modified and reprinted with permission from Cambridge University Press. © 2007, Cambridge University Press. In-depth discussion in Southwick and Charney, 2012a.

survival of concentration camps largely to this process of "meaning making"; in fact, meaning making became the basis for the school of psychotherapy that he founded, known as logotherapy. On a long enforced march, weak from hunger and cold, he wrote, "I forced my thoughts to turn to another subject. Suddenly I saw myself standing on the platform of a well-lit, warm and pleasant lecture room.... I was giving a lecture on the psychology of the concentration camp!" (Frankl, 1959/2006: p. 73). The conscious construction of this narrative and of the meaning he would derive from his experiences provided Dr. Frankl with the psychological endurance to survive his days in concentration camps.

The importance of synthesizing traumatic events into one's personal life narrative was described over a century ago by Pierre Janet, the French neurologist. Janet noted that his patients with posttraumatic pathology had failed to integrate their traumatic memories into a cohesive story. Janet stressed the necessity of cognitive reappraisal in preventing or overcoming posttraumatic stress; traumatic memories "needed to be modified and transformed, that is, placed in their proper context and reconstructed into neutral or meaningful narratives." (van der Kolk and van der Hart, 1989).

PURPOSE IN LIFE

A closely related concept to that of finding meaning is having a sense of purpose in life. Studies are beginning to document an association between higher self-reported purpose in life and resilience or recovery from psychiatric illness in traumatized populations (Alim et al., 2008). Purpose in life was significantly associated with psychological well-being in a study of veterans living with spinal cord injury (deRoon-Cassini et al., 2009). Another study reported greater perceptions of purpose and control in resilient OEF-OIF (Operation Enduring Freedom-Operation Iraqi Freedom) veterans compared with those with PTSD (Pietrzak and Southwick, 2011).

ACTIVE COPING STYLES

Active coping means deploying productive strategies for solving problems, managing stress, and regulating negative emotions that may arise in the aftermath of adverse events. Active coping behaviors include acknowledging and trying to solve problems, accepting that which cannot be changed, facing fears, using humor and physical exercise to alleviate stress, and seeking out social support and role models. Active coping has repeatedly been associated with hardiness and psychological resilience in various populations (Moos and Schaefer, 1993). In contrast, passive coping, including the blunting of emotions through substance use, denial, disengagement, or resignation, is associated with depression and lower levels of hardiness (Maddi, 1999). Several studies have shown an association between avoidance coping and psychopathology (Pietrzak et al., 2011; Thompson et al., 2011).

ACCEPTANCE

Acceptance is an adaptive coping strategy commonly found among people who are able to tolerate extreme and uncontrollable stress (Manne et al., 2003; Siebert, 1996). Acceptance involves recognizing the uncontrollable aspects of certain stressors, changing expectations about outcome based on reality, and focusing on controllable aspects of the stressor. Acceptance is not to be confused with resignation, which is giving up or coping passively. Acceptance has been linked with better physical and psychological health, lower levels of distress, and greater psychological adjustment after trauma exposure (Thompson et al., 2011; Wade et al., 2001). Recent evidence includes the finding that individuals who had an accepting coping style had fewer PTSD symptoms following the terrorist attacks of September 11, 2001 (Silver et al., 2002).

FACING FEARS

Facing fears is a key component of the active coping paradigm. Fear conditioning, which is discussed in greater detail later in the chapter, plays a major role in the development and maintenance of posttraumatic psychopathology. Individuals with PTSD avoid a wide variety of life's opportunities (people, places, events, etc.) that may serve as reminders of the trauma; thus, conditioned fear is maintained rather than extinguished. In contrast, resilient individuals are more adept at managing fear, using it as a guide to critically appraise threat and to select appropriate action.

Active coping at the time of trauma or when exposed to traumatic reminders appears to attenuate fear conditioning, likely by redirecting activity in the lateral and central nuclei of the amygdala away from the brainstem and toward the motor circuits in the ventral striatum. This has the effect of reducing brainstem-mediated responses to fear, such as freezing behavior and autonomic and endocrine responses, and enabling productive action (LeDoux and Gorman, 2002). Resilient individuals have learned to face fears and to actively cope with them; by moving through fear, they avoid fear conditioning and are less likely to develop psychopathology and functional impairments in the aftermath of trauma.

HUMOR

Humor, frequently used by resilient individuals, has been identified as an adaptive coping style and mature defense mechanism (Vaillant, 1977). It appears that humor decreases the probability of developing stress-induced depression (Deaner and McConatha, 1993; Thorson and Powell, 1994). The use of humor has been studied in resilient Vietnam veterans (Haas and Hendin, 1984), surgical patients (Carver et al., 1993), cancer patients (Culver et al., 2002), and at-risk children (Werner and Smith, 1992; Wolin and Wolin, 1993) and has been shown to be protective against distress. Humor is thought to diminish the threatening nature and negative emotional impact of stressful situations (Folkman, 1997), fostering a more positive perspective on challenging circumstances. The use of humor also relieves tension and discomfort (Vaillant, 1992) and attracts social support. Humor is thought to activate a network of subcortical regions that are critically involved in the dopaminergic reward system (Mobbs et al., 2003).

PHYSICAL EXERCISE

Physical exercise has consistently been shown to have positive effects on physical hardiness, mood, and self-esteem. Individuals who exercise regularly report lower depression scores than those who do not exercise (Brosse et al., 2002; Camacho et al., 1991). Physical exercise has effects on a number of neurobiological factors that affect resilience. It attenuates the HPA axis response to stress, increases release of endorphins, and increases levels of plasma monoamines and the 5-HT precursor tryptophan. It is also thought to induce the expression of several genes related to neuroplasticity and neurogenesis, such as hippocampal BDNF (Cotman and Berchtold, 2002). Studies in animals have shown that exercise helps contain the stress response via central sympathetic, serotonergic, and dopaminergic reward pathways, resulting in protection from stress-induced immunosuppression, cytokine elevation, and affective dysregulation (Fleshner et al., 2011). A study of high-impact running in humans suggested that the activity has a beneficial impact on cognitive functioning: high-impact running was associated with improved vocabulary learning and retention as well as a lower likelihood of age-related cognitive diminution (Winter et al., 2006).

SOCIAL SUPPORT

The last active coping strategy we discuss is the seeking out of social support. Higher levels of social support have been associated with better mental and physical health outcomes following a wide variety of stressors (Resick, 2001). Conversely, lower levels of social support have been linked to PTSD and other psychiatric disorders (Tsai et al., 2012). In a study of OEF-OIF veterans, resilience was associated with self-reports of greater family support and understanding (Pietrzak and Southwick, 2011). Social support is thought to decrease appraisals of threat (Fontana et al., 1989), counteract feelings of loneliness (Bisschop et al., 2004), increase sense of self-efficacy, reduce functional impairment (Travis et al., 2004), and increase treatment compliance. Role models and mentors form a valuable part of a strong social support network.

Social isolation and lack of social support are associated with higher rates of mood and anxiety disorders, higher levels of stress, and increased morbidity and mortality from medical illness. Individuals who seek and nurture a supportive social network during times of stress tend to fare better during stress or adversity than individuals who are socially isolated.

MORAL COMPASS: A SET OF GUIDING ETHICAL PRINCIPLES

Moral compass, or an internal framework of belief about right and wrong, is another feature common to resilient individuals (Southwick et al., 2005). This construct may, but does not have to, include adherence to a religious or spiritual system.

Religion and spirituality seem to have a protective effect on physical and psychological well-being. A metaanalysis of 126,000 individuals from 42 independent samples found religious practice or involvement to be associated with lower risk of mortality from all causes (McCullough et al., 2000). In addition, higher levels of religious belief have been correlated with lower incidence of depression and higher rates of remission from depression in a number of populations (Braam et al., 1997, 2002; Kasen et al., 2012; Koenig et al., 1998). Interestingly, one's particular religious affiliation is not implicated in the overall

relationship between religiousness and improved psychological and physical health.

There is some evidence suggesting that spiritual or self-transcendent experiences are associated with increased density of 5-HT_{1A} receptors in the dorsal raphé nuclei, hippocampus, and neocortex (reviewed by Hasler et al., 2004). Chronic stress appears to lead to a down-regulation of 5HT_{1A} receptors; spirituality and religiosity may enhance the functioning of the 5-HT system, fostering resilience and protecting against the development of posttraumatic mental illness.

Religious faith or spirituality is not an essential ingredient in a strong moral compass. In fact, morality appears to have a neural basis and is likely intrinsic to human nature. The idea that morality is inherent to human beings is ancient. Epictetus, a Greek philosopher living in Rome in the first century A.D. wrote: "Every one of us has come into this world with innate conceptions as to good and bad, noble and shameful . . . fitting and inappropriate" (Stockdale, 1991). Moral sense likely developed early in human evolution as our ancestors organized into societies: the successful functioning of society requires cooperation and trust between members. Many studies support the notion that principles of cooperation and reciprocity are ingrained within human nature. Games designed to test participants' morality repeatedly find that human beings act according to the rule that fairness to others should supersede self-interest. For example, in games in which participants are given money to divide between themselves and strangers, most participants choose to divide the money equally among players. Furthermore, participants who play fairly in such games tend to show heightened activation of their dopaminergic reward systems on imaging studies (Fehr and Fischbacher, 2003). These findings provide support for the hypothesis that people know what is right and derive fulfillment from acting accordingly.

ALTRUISM

Altruism, or putting one's moral compass into action, is a powerful contributor to resilience. For example, research on the behavior of citizens after bombing attacks during World War II showed that those who demonstrated altruism by caring for others suffered fewer trauma-related mood and anxiety symptoms than would be expected. Furthermore, individuals who had been symptomatic preattack experienced a meaningful decrease in psychological distress (Rachman, 1979). It appears that, similar to acting fairly, performing acts of altruism activates brain reward circuits. One study found that participants who gave money to charity, whether voluntarily or through taxation, showed heightened activation of the ventral striatum, an important part in reward pathways (Harbaugh et al., 2007).

Some individuals are able to find meaning in personal tragedy by embracing a survivor mission to help others. Rape survivors who go public with their experience to raise social awareness through events such as Take Back the Night, and the mothers who founded Mothers Against Drunk Driving after their children were injured or killed in drunk driving accidents, are examples of this phenomenon.

We now discuss some of the most important neurobiological factors associated with resilience. Individuals with the psychological features of resilience we have discussed likely have a neurobiological profile characterized by optimal levels of these factors.

NEUROBIOLOGICAL PROFILE OF RESILIENCE

A number of neurotransmitters, neuropeptides, and hormones have been implicated in acute and long-term adaptation to stress. A comprehensive review of the many functions and effects of these factors is beyond the scope of this chapter; we focus specifically on the factors' role in mediating the stress response (Table 88.2, Fig. 88.1; see also Color Fig 88.1 in separate insert).

CORTICOTROPIN-RELEASING HORMONE

The hypothalamus releases corticotropin-releasing hormone (CRH) in conditions of stress, activating the pituitary-adrenal axis and triggering the release of cortisol and dehydroepiandrosterone (DHEA). Corticotropin-releasing hormone also has important direct effects in the central nervous system; CRH containing neurons and CRH receptors are distributed widely throughout the brain and gut (Steckler and Holsboer, 1999). Activation of CRH neurons in the amygdala triggers fear-related behaviors, whereas activation of cortical CRH neurons reduces expectation of rewards. It seems that excessive stress in early life can result in abnormally elevated CRH activity in the adult brain (Strome et al., 2002).

Corticotropin-releasing hormone acts via two G-coupled receptors, CRH-1 and CRH-2. These receptors appear to have opposite effects in the response to stress (Bale et al., 2002; Grammatopoulos and Chrousos, 2002); the CRH-1 receptor primarily activates the behavioral, endocrine, and visceral responses to stress. Elevated hippocampal CRH-CRH-1 interaction may contribute to the structural and cognitive impairments associated with early-life stress (Ivy et al., 2010). CRH-1 receptor gene single nucleotide polymorphism rs110402 was found to moderate neural responses to emotional stimuli, thereby potentially increasing vulnerability for the development of psychiatric disorders (Hsu et al., 2012). The CRH-2 receptor generally serves to dampen these effects (Tache and Bonaz, 2007). However, activation of the CRH-2 receptor does produce some anxiogenic effects, for example, enhancing CRH-1 mediated suppression of feeding behavior (Bakshi et al., 2002). A more recent study shows that chronic activation of CRH-2 receptor by overexpressing its specific ligand (urocortin 3) promotes an anxiety-like state, yet with attenuated behavioral and HPA axis response to stress (Neufeld-Cohen et al., 2012). More research is necessary to determine the precise role of both receptors.

Abnormally high CRH levels in the cerebrospinal fluid have been linked to major depression and PTSD (Baker et al., 1999; Bremner et al., 1997; Nemeroff, 2002). Resilient individuals likely have the capacity to effectively regulate CRH levels and/or the relative activity of both receptor subtypes. Gender differences in corticotropin response to CRH challenge may explain differential gender susceptibility to psychopathology following early-life trauma (DeSantis et al., 2011). Although initial studies showed promise for the use of CRH-1 receptor antagonists as potential new pharmacotherapies for anxiety and mood disorders as well as for stress-related gastrointestinal disorders such as irritable bowel syndrome (Tache and Bonaz, 2007; Zoumakis et al., 2006), subsequent clinical trials failed to show a beneficial effect of these compounds in patients with major depression (Binneman et al., 2008) or generalized anxiety disorder (Coric et al., 2010). A randomized controlled trial of a CRH-1 receptor antagonist in patients with PTSD is currently under way.

CORTISOL

Many forms of psychological stress increase the synthesis and release of cortisol, which leads to increased arousal, vigilance, inhibition of growth and reproduction, and containment of the immune response. In resilient individuals, the stress-induced increase in cortisol is effectively constrained via an elaborate negative feedback system involving GR and mineralocorticoid receptors (MR) (de Kloet et al., 2007). Excessive and sustained cortisol secretion can have serious adverse effects, including osteoporosis, immunosuppression, hypertension, metabolic syndrome, depression, and anxiety (Carroll et al., 2007; Whitworth et al., 2005).

Cortisol has important regulatory effects on the hippocampus, amygdala, and PFC. It plays a role in the formation, processing, and retrieval of memories, particularly fearful memories. Cortisol levels appear to be dysregulated in depression and PTSD. Patients with major depressive disorder tend to have higher than normal levels of cortisol and a blunted suppression of cortisol secretion in response to the dexamethasone suppression test (Yehuda, 2001). In contrast, basal circulating cortisol levels are generally lower in individuals with PTSD than in healthy individuals (Bierer et al., 2006; Gill et al., 2008; Griffin et al., 2005; Yang or Brand et al., 2006; Yehuda, 2006). Correspondingly, individuals with PTSD tend to show higher-than-average cortisol suppression during the dexamethasone suppression test, implying that their HPA-axis GRs are hypersensitive. Altered HPA-axis function is associated with impaired fear inhibition in subjects with PTSD (Jovanovic et al., 2010). Women with PTSD having lower basal salivary cortisol levels than men with PTSD may contribute to the gender difference in PTSD prevalence between men and women (Freidenberg et al., 2010).

That patients with PTSD might have lower-than average basal cortisol levels suggests that the disorder may develop in the setting of abnormally low cortisol; this hypothesis is supported by a number of studies showing that steroid administration inhibits traumatic memory formation (Bierer et al., 2006). Patients who are pretreated with stress doses of glucocorticoids before surgery and/or hospitalization in the intensive care unit are less likely to have traumatic memories of their hospital stay after discharge than patients treated with placebo (Brunner et al., 2006; Schelling et al., 2006; Weis et al., 2006). Low activity of 5-alpha reductase, a rate-limiting enzyme for

TABLE 88.2. The neurochemical response patterns to acute stress

NEUROCHEMICAL	ACUTE EFFECTS	BRAIN REGION	KEY FUNCTIONAL INTERACTIONS	ASSOCIATION WITH RESILIENCE	ASSOCIATION WITH PSYCHOPATHOLOGY POTENTIAL FOR TREATMENT?
CRH	Activated fear behaviors, increased arousal, increased motor activity, inhibited neurovegetative function, reduced reward expectations	Prefrontal cortex, cingulated cortex, amygdala, nucleus accumbens, hippocampus, hypothalamus, bed nucleus of the stria terminalis, periaqueductal gray matter, locus coeruleus, dorsal raphe nuclei	CRH-1 receptor anxiogenic, CRH-2 receptor anxiolytic, increases cortisol and DHEA, activates locus coeruleus-norepinephrine system	Reduced CRH release, adaptive changes in CRH-1 and CRH-2 receptors	Persistently increased CRH concentration may predispose to PTSD and mood disorders as well as stress-related gastrointestinal disorders CRH receptor antagonists under investigation as treatments for stress-related disorders
Cortisol	Mobilized energy, increased arousal, focused attention	Prefrontal cortex, hippocampus, amygdala, hypothalamus	Increases amygdala corticotrophin-releasing hormone (CRH), increases hypothalamic CRH	Stress-induced increase rapidly constrained by negative feedback mechanisms	Dysregulated cortisol systems (excessive cortisol release, improperly functioning negative feedback systems) seen in mood disorders and PTSD
Dehydroepi-androsterone (DHEA)	Counteracts deleterious effects of high cortisol Neuroprotective Positive mood effects	Largely unknown; hypothalamus	Antiglucocorticoid actions	High DHEA-cortisol ratios may prevent/lessen severity of PTSD and depression.	Low DHEA response to stress may predispose to PTSD and depression and sensitize to the effects of hypercortisolemia. DHEA supplementation has shown beneficial effects on depressive symptoms.
Locus coeruleus-norepinephrine system	General alarm function activated by extrinsic and intrinsic threat; increased arousal, increased attention, fear memory formation, facilitated motor response	Prefrontal cortex, amygdala, hippocampus, hypothalamus	Activates sympathetic axis, inhibits parasympathetic outflow, stimulates hypothalamic CRH	Reduced responsiveness of locus coeruleus-norepinephrine system	Unrestrained functioning of locus coeruleus-norepinephrine system, seen in some patients with PTSD, leads to chronic anxiety, hyper-vigilance, and intrusive memories. Beta-receptor blockade shortly after trauma exposure has yielded mixed results.
Neuropeptide Y (NPY)	Anxiolytic Improves performance under stress	Amygdala, hippocampus, hypothalamus, septum, periaqueductal gray matter, locus coeruleus	Reduces CRH-related actions at amygdala, reduces rate of firing of locus coeruleus	Adaptive increase in amygdala neuropeptide Y is associated with reduced stress-induced anxiety and depression	Low NPY associated with PTSD Y-1 and Y-2 receptors may be targets for treating mood and anxiety disorders. NPY administration may protect against stress.
Galanin	Involved in anxiety and vulnerability to stress; GAL-1 receptor anxiolytic, GAL-3 anxiogenic	Prefrontal cortex, amygdala, hippocampus, locus coeruleus	Reduces the anxiogenic effects of locus coeruleus-norepinephrine system activation	Adaptive increase in amygdala galanin is associated with reduced stress-induced anxiety and depression.	Low galanin levels likely related to increased vulnerability to PTSD and depression; yet to be studied.
Serotonin (5-HT)	Mixed effects: 5-HT stimulation of 5-HT2 receptors is anxiogenic; 5-HT stimulation of 5-HT$_{1A}$ receptors is anxiolytic	Prefrontal cortex, amygdala, hippocampus, dorsal raphe	High levels of cortisol decrease 5-HT$_{1A}$ receptors	High activity of postsynaptic 5-HT$_{1A}$ receptors may facilitate recovery.	Low activity of postsynaptic 5-HT$_{1A}$ receptors may predispose to anxiety and depression.

Dopamine	High prefrontal cortex and low nucleus accumbens dopamine levels are associated with anhedonic and helpless behaviors	Prefrontal cortex, nucleus accumbens, amygdala	Reciprocal interactions between cortical and subcortical dopamine systems	Within optimal window of activity, preserves functions involving reward and extinction of fear	Excessive mesocortical dopamine release associated with vulnerability to stress Persistently high levels of prefrontal cortical dopamine associated with chronic anxiety and fear Low levels of circulating dopamine linked to depression
Brain-Derived Neurotrophic Factor (BDNF)	Supports neuronal growth, differentiation and survival; involved in fear conditioning, extinction, and inhibitory learning	Hippocampus, cerebral cortex, striatum	Exerts different functions in different brain regions (antidepressant and depression-like effects)	High level of BDNF in hippocampus promotes stress resilience.	Antidepressants can reverse stress-induced decrease in BDNF expression in hippocampus.
Endocannabinoids (eCBs)	Regulate HPA axis activity under basal and stressful conditions	Prefrontal cortex, hypothalamus, amygdala, hippocampus	Actions at CB1 and CB2 receptors; regulation of HPA axis activity	Optimal function of endocannabinoid signaling regulates stress hormone responses.	Enhanced action of endocannabinoids at the CB1 receptor might reduce excessive stress responses.
Glutamate	Excitatory synaptic signaling	Frontal cortex, amygdala, hippocampus, cingulate cortex	Primary receptors NMDA and AMPA; memory formation and learning	Increased AMPA receptor activation may promote antidepressant effects	NMDA receptor antagonism and AMPA receptor activation are novel approaches to depression treatment.

AMPA, alpha-amino-3-hydroxy-5-methyl-4-isoxazole-propionic acid; CRH, corticotrophin-releasing hormone; NMDA, N-methyl-D-aspartate; PTSD, post traumatic stress disorder. (Modified and reprinted with permission from Cambridge Univeristy Press. © 2007, Cambridge University Press)

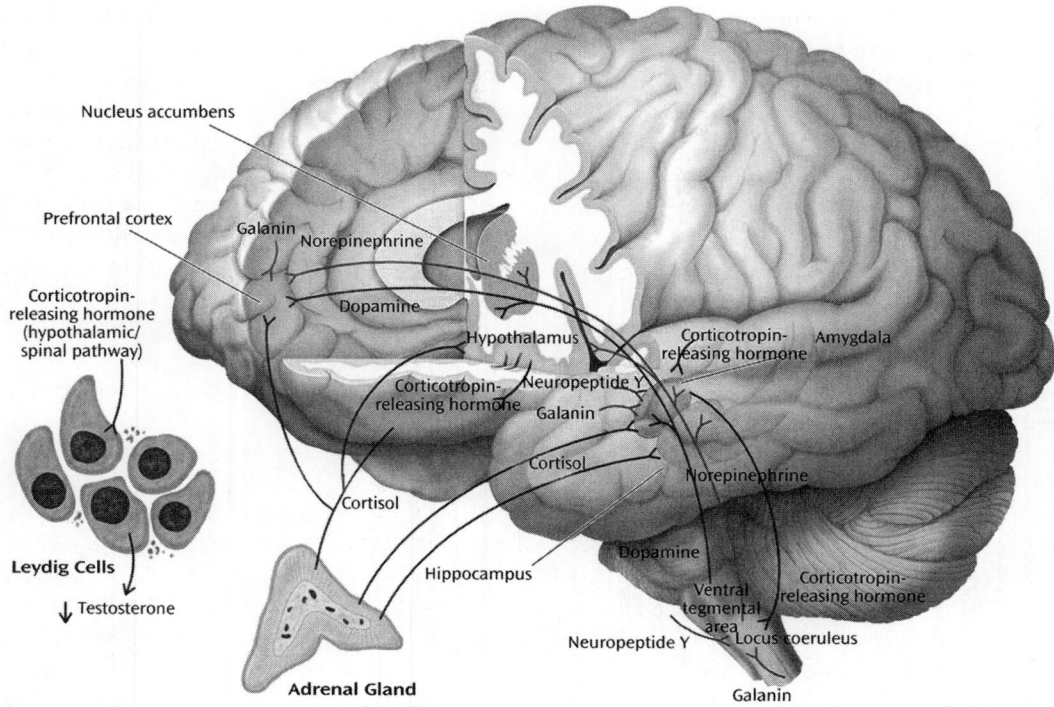

Figure 88.1 *Neurochemical response patterns to acute stress. This figure illustrates some of the key brain structures involved in the neurochemical response patterns following acute psychological stress. The functional interactions among the different neurotransmitters, neuropeptides, and hormones are emphasized. The functional status of brain regions such as the amygdala (neuropeptide Y, galanin, corticotropin-releasing hormone [CRH], cortisol, and norepinephrine), hippocampus (cortisol and norepinephrine), locus coeruleus (neuropeptide Y, galanin, and CRH), and prefrontal cortex (dopamine, norepinephrine, galanin, and cortisol) depends upon the balance among multiple inhibitory and excitatory neurochemical inputs. Functional effects may vary depending on the brain region. For example, cortisol increases CRH concentrations in the amygdala and decreases concentrations in the paraventricular nucleus of the hypothalamus. As described in the text, these neurochemical response patterns may relate to resilience and vulnerability to the effects of extreme psychological stress. (Modified and reprinted with permission from Cambridge University Press, 2007.) (See color insert.)*

cortisol, is associated with avoidance severity and predicts lack of response to psychological treatment for PTSD (Yehuda et al., 2009).

Although there are a great deal of data suggesting that patients with PTSD have lower basal cortisol than healthy controls and that PTSD may develop in the setting of low glucocorticoid levels, there is also conflicting evidence. Some studies have found no difference in cortisol levels between patients with PTSD and healthy controls (Metzger et al., 2008; Wheler et al., 2006); some have even found that patients with PTSD have higher-than-average basal cortisol levels, and that elevated cortisol at the time of trauma may predict subsequent PTSD development (Baker et al., 2005; Inslicht et al., 2006). A significant decrease in salivary cortisol levels has been found in PTSD treatment responders (Gerardi et al., 2010). In summary, though it is clear that cortisol is implicated in the encoding of traumatic memories and in the subsequent development of posttraumatic psychopathology, the exact nature of this effect is still under investigation. Undoubtedly though, dysregulation of cortisol secretion has adverse effects on resilience to stress.

DEHYDROEPIANDROSTERONE

Like cortisol, dehydroepiandrosterone (DHEA) is an adrenal steroid released under stress; in contrast to cortisol, DHEA protects against the negative effects of excessive stress. DHEA is secreted episodically and synchronously with cortisol (Rosenfeld et al., 1971) and has antiglucocorticoid activity in the brain (Browne et al., 1992). DHEA and its metabolites interfere with the normal uptake of GRs in the hippocampus (Bastianetto et al., 1999; Kimonides et al., 1998; Morfin and Starka, 2001), preventing corticosteroid-induced hippocampal neurotoxicity. DHEA derivatives also amplify long-term potentiation of hippocampal neurons, likely by modulating transmission at the N-methylD- aspartate (NMDA) receptor (Chen et al., 2006a). DHEA and fluoxetine were found to have synergistic effects in promoting hippocampal progenitor cell proliferation (Pinnock et al., 2009). The steroid's neuroprotective and potentiating effects in the hippocampus help to facilitate learning and memory.

Studies have shown that DHEA is released under both acute and chronic stress, and that higher levels of DHEA are associated with PTSD and comorbid depression, whereas a higher DHEA-to-cortisol ratio may mitigate symptom severity (Gill et al., 2008; Maninger et al., 2010; Rasmusson et al., 2004). However, one study found no evidence for PTSD-related alterations in cortisol or DHEA secretion in response to stimulation by low doses of ACTH, indicating normal adrenocortical responsiveness in PTSD (Radant et al., 2009).

DHEA appears to enhance cognition and performance under stress. In a study of soldiers undergoing rigorous training as part of military survival school, DHEA-S (dehydroepiandrosterone sulfate) to cortisol ratios were highest in those soldiers who demonstrated the best performance during training. Thus, DHEA-S to cortisol ratios may index the degree to which an individual is buffered against the negative effects of stress (Morgan et al., 2004). In another study, DHEA and DHEA-S levels predicted superior performance in active duty soldiers undergoing an underwater navigation exam (Morgan et al., 2009). Recovery from severe stress in PTSD patients also appears to be facilitated by high levels of DHEA (Rasmusson et al., 2004; Yehuda, 2006; Yang or Brand et al., 2006).

Other studies have also found a negative correlation between plasma DHEA levels and depressive symptoms (Goodyer et al., 1998; Gallagher and Young, 2002; Haren et al., 2007; Young et al., 2002). Studies of DHEA supplementation have shown some beneficial effects on depressive and PTSD symptoms, but further research is needed (Rabkin et al., 2006; Taylor et al., 2012). Animal studies suggest that the antidepressant action of DHEA is mediated via GABA-ergic modulation of the mesolimbic system (Genud et al., 2009). In a recent study, low-dose DHEA supplementation in military men undergoing survival training was found to enhance anabolic balance but did not result in differences in subjective distress (Taylor et al., 2012). More research is needed to determine whether DHEA could enhance resilience if administered prior to trauma exposure.

THE LOCUS COERULEUS–NOREPINEPHRINE SYSTEM

Stress activates the locus coeruleus (LC), which results in increased norepinephrine (NE) release in projection sites of the LC, including the amygdala, PFC, and hippocampus. The LC is activated by a variety of stressors, intrinsic (e.g., hypoglycemia, hypotension) and extrinsic (environmental threats). Such activation serves as a general alarm function and is adaptive in a life-threatening situation. Activation of the LC contributes to the sympathetic nervous system and HPA axis stimulation and inhibits parasympathetic outflow and neurovegetative function, including eating and sleep. A high level of activation of the LC–NE system inhibits function of the PFC, thereby favoring instinctual responses over more complex cognition (Charney, 2004). A recent study in rats showed that during early adolescence, social stress in the form of a resident intruder led to elevated activity of LC neurons, promoting defensive behaviors in this particular age group (Bingham et al., 2011).

The activation of the HPA and LC–NE systems under acute stress facilitates the encoding and relay of aversively charged emotional memories, beginning at the amygdala. Animal studies have shown that injections of NE into the amygdala enhance memory consolidation; on the other hand, blocking NE activity during stress impedes the encoding of fearful memories. In rats, blocking the lateral nucleus of the amygdala to the effects of NE during reactivation of a fearful memory prevents the process of memory reconsolidation and appears to permanently impair that memory (Debiec and LeDoux, 2006).

If unchecked, persistent hyperresponsiveness of the LC-NE system contributes to chronic anxiety, fear, intrusive memories, and an increased risk of cardiovascular disease and hypertension. Findings from an imaging study in humans suggest that disinhibited endogenous NE signaling may contribute to the etiology of PTSD by eliciting exaggerated basolateral amygdala (BLA) responses to fear stimuli (Onur et al., 2009). Noradrenergic activation in the BLA is also involved in the facilitating effects of stress hormones (such as CRH) on the consolidation of emotional memory (Roozendaal et al., 2008). Interestingly, norepinephrine was shown to directly activate multipotent neural precursors in the hippocampus of adult mice via β_3 adrenoreceptors, thus facilitating hippocampal neurogenesis; these findings may pave the way for the development of new types of antidepressants (Jhaveri et al., 2010).

NEUROPEPTIDE Y

Neuropeptide Y (NPY) is an abundant peptide that is widely distributed throughout the brain and acts via at least four G-protein coupled receptors (Y1, Y2, Y4, Y5) (Wu et al., 2011) (Baker and Herkenham, 1995; Karl et al., 2006; Makino et al., 2000 Pieribone et al., 1992; Risold and Swanson, 1997). The Y3 receptor has yet to be cloned and the y6 receptor is a truncated receptor in humans (Sah and Geracioti, 2012; Wu et al., 2011). Neuropeptide Y produces anxiolytic effects and appears to enhance cognitive functioning under stress. There are important functional interactions between NPY and CRH (Britton et al., 2000; Heilig et al., 1994;): NPY counteracts the anxiogenic effects of CRH at various locations within the stress/anxiety circuit, including the amygdala, hippocampus, hypothalamus, and LC (Sajdyk et al., 2006). It may be that the balance between NPY and CRH neurotransmission is critical to maintaining a homeostatic emotional state during stress (Eva et al., 2006; Kask et al., 1997; Sajdyk et al., 2006).

High levels of NPY appear to protect against depression and anxiety, with the Y1 and Y2 receptors playing important roles in the peptide's effects on mood (Heilig et al., 1993; Heilig, 1995, 2004). The Y1 receptor was found to be anxiolytic, whereas the Y2 receptor, a presynaptic autoreceptor, was found to be anxiogenic (reviewed in Wu et al., 2011). Neuropeptide Y activation of the Y1 receptor inhibits several metabolic and behavioral stress responses, including gastrointestinal distress, anxious behavior, and decreased sleep (Eva et al., 2006). Antidepressant drugs and electroconvulsive therapy increase NPY in rodent brains as they decrease depression; this effect is likely mediated by the Y1 receptor (Karl et al., 2006). A variety of antidepressant drugs increase NPY levels in humans as well (Husum and Mathe, 2002).

The potential role of NPY in fear conditioning is under investigation. In one study, central administration of NPY in rats inhibited fear-potentiated startle and enhanced its extinction; the latter effect was counteracted by the Y1 receptor antagonist BIBO3304 (Gutman et al., 2008). In another study, however, whereas fear conditioning was attenuated by exogenous NPY administration, BIBO3304 had no effect on conditioned fear; thus the role of endogenous NPY is more uncertain (Pickens et al., 2009).

Y2 knockout mice exhibit fewer anxious and depressed behaviors and reduced neuronal activation in response to the emotional stressors, and are more adventurous (Carvajal et al., 2006; Nguyen et al., 2009). Site-specific deletion of the Y2 receptor gene in the central and basolateral amygdala, but not in any other amygdaloid nucleus, results in anxiolytic and antidepressant-like effects, suggesting a possible mechanism for Y2 receptor-mediated regulation of anxiety and depression (Tasan et al., 2010). The Y1- and Y2-receptors may therefore be useful targets for treating mood and anxiety disorders in humans.

Elevated NPY levels are associated with better performance under stress (Sah and Geracioti, 2012). NPY treatment after exposure to stress significantly reduced prevalence rates of extreme behavioral responses and trauma-cue freezing responses in animals (Cohen et al., 2012). The Y1 receptor in the basolateral amygdala is implicated in the mediation effects of NPY on stress and may serve as a therapeutic target for the treatment of PTSD (Cui et al., 2008; Hendriksen et al., 2012). Preliminary work with special operations soldiers under extreme training stress indicates that high NPY levels are associated with better performance (Morgan et al., 2000). These findings suggest that the administration of NPY could be an effective intervention for the treatment of depression, anxiety disorders and PTSD, and for enhancing resilience to stress. However, it will first be necessary to design a drug delivery method that enables the peptide to penetrate into the CSF (Born et al., 2002); intranasal administration is currently being investigated.

GALANIN

Galanin, another abundant neuropeptide, has been shown to be involved in a number of physiological and behavioral functions, including anxiety, stress, and alcohol intake (Holmes et al., 2002; Moller et al., 1999). Understanding of galanin's mechanisms of action and effects is still at an early stage; however, overall the peptide appears to mitigate the effects of stress.

Three receptors for galanin have been identified, and two of these (GAL-1 and GAL-3) have been found to affect stress and anxiety (Walton et al., 2006). The GAL-1 receptor, expressed in the amygdala, hypothalamus, and bed nucleus of the stria terminalis, acts as an auto-receptor (Gustafson et al., 1996; Sevcik et al., 1993; Xu et al., 2001) and appears to be involved in anxiolysis: knockout mice for the GAL-1 receptor show increased anxiety-like behaviors (Holmes et al., 2003) and fail to gain stress-resistant responses after galanin injection (Mitsukawa et al., 2009). The GAL-3 receptor, on the other hand, produces anxiogenic effects when activated (Swanson et al., 2005). In humans, certain polymorphisms of the gene for the GAL-3 receptor have been linked with anxiety and alcoholism (Belfer et al., 2006). Few studies have looked at the stress-related effects of the GAL-2 receptor. One study found that it is involved in depressive-like but not anxiety-like behavior (Le Maitre et al., 2011), whereas another study showed that it has both antidepressant-like and anxiolytic effects (Lu et al., 2008).

It has been suggested that galanin recruitment during periods of stress may diminish negative emotions caused by hyperactivity of the noradrenergic system (Karlsson and Holmes, 2006). Galanin appears to inhibit NE, serotonin (5-HT), and DA

neurons from firing, reducing release of these neurotransmitters in forebrain target regions. Enhanced galanin expression in LC from running is associated with suppression of brain norepinephrine in runners and may contribute to the stress-protective effects of exercise (Sciolino and Holmes, 2012). Galanin also prevents toxicity-induced cell death (Counts and Mufson, 2010) and promotes neurogenesis (Abbosh et al., 2011), which may contribute to its antidepressant effect. Galanin was shown to be down-regulated in the CA1 of the hippocampus and the frontal cortex in a PTSD animal model with extreme behavioral response to stressors; immediate postexposure treatment with galnon, a galanin receptor agonist, significantly reduces prevalence rates of extreme responders and trauma-cue freezing responses (Kozlovsky et al., 2009). To our knowledge, galanin function has not been studied in patients exposed to traumatic stress or patients with PTSD or major depression.

SEROTONIN

Serotonin (5-HT) is well known as one of the neurotransmitters most relevant to mood. As a neuromodulator, 5-HT also regulates other neurotransmitter systems involved in mood and anxiety, and dysregulation of the 5-HT system may cause a cascade of changes in brain chemistry. The role of 5-HT as a neuromodulator is demonstrated in tryptophan depletion studies, whereby serotonin levels are lowered by ingestion of a tryptophan-free amino acid mixture. For example, tryptophan depletion led to failure to inhibit appropriate responses to punishing outcomes in healthy females (Robinson et al., 2012), and uncovered a potential vulnerability in never-depressed young adults at high familial risk for depression, who showed increased bias toward negative words while performing an affective go/no-go task in the depletion condition, compared to low-risk controls (Feder et al., 2011).

Acute stress results in increased 5-HT turnover in the PFC, nucleus accumbens, amygdala, and lateral hypothalamus (Kent et al., 2002). Serotonin release may have anxiogenic and anxiolytic effects, depending on the region of the forebrain involved and the receptor subtype activated. 5-HT_{1A} receptors are anxiolytic and may be responsible for adaptive responses to aversive events, whereas anxiogenic effects appear to be mediated by 5-HT_{2A} receptors (Charney and Drevets, 2002). Absence of 5HT_{1A} receptor signaling during early stages of brain maturation predisposes an organism to affective dysfunction later in life (Vinkers et al., 2010). 5HT_{1A} knock-out mice show an increase in anxiety-like behaviors (Heisler et al., 1998; Parks et al., 1998), including behavioral inhibition in ambiguous environments (settings that contain neutral and fear-conditioned cues). This type of behavior represents an inappropriate generalization of fearful behavior, a phenomenon that occurs in some human anxiety disorders, including panic disorder, specific phobias, and PTSD (Klemenhagen et al., 2006). Therefore, lower-than-normal activation of 5HT_{1A} receptors may be involved in the pathophysiology of human anxiety disorders. On the other hand, antagonism of 5HT2A receptor has been shown to prevent the emergence of anxiety behavior and dysregulated stress response following early life stress (Benekareddy et al., 2011).

A scenario has been proposed in which early life stress increases CRH and cortisol levels, which, in turn, downregulate 5-HT$_{1A}$ receptors, resulting in a lower threshold for tolerating stressful life events. Consistent with findings in rodents and non-human primates, a negative association is found between plasma cortisol levels and 5HT$_{1A}$ receptor distribution in humans (Lanzenberger et al., 2010). Alternatively, 5-HT$_{1A}$ receptor density may be partly genetic. Data so far have been mixed. A positron emission tomography (PET) study scanning receptor status in individuals with PTSD found no differences in 5HT$_{1A}$ receptor distribution, binding potential, or tracer delivery (Bonne et al., 2005), whereas a more recent PET study in Rhesus monkeys showed that reduced 5HT$_{1A}$ receptor density during development might be a factor increasing vulnerability to stress-related neuropsychiatric disorders (Sciolino and Holmes, 2012).

DOPAMINE

Dopamine (DA) is released in some areas of the brain and inhibited in others during extreme stress. Stress activates DA release in the mPFC (Cabib et al., 2002) and inhibits DA release in the nucleus accumbens, one of the regions associated with human experience of pleasure and reward (Cabib and Puglisi-Allegra, 1996). Lesions of the amygdala in a conditioned stress model block stress-induced DA activation in the mPFC, implying amygdalar control over stress-induced DA release (Cabib et al., 2002; Goldstein et al., 1996). DA D1 receptors were shown to be responsible for stress-induced deficit of emotional learning and memory (Wang et al., 2012). The degree to which an individual's DA system is activated by stress is in part genetically determined, and individuals whose genetic profile results in excessive mesocortical DA release after stressful events may have a tendency toward vulnerability to stress (Cabib et al., 2002). Variation in the dopamine transporter gene may contribute to one heritable path toward the development of PTSD (Drury et al., 2009). Polymorphisms in the dopamine D2 receptor gene might also contribute to susceptibility to PTSD (Voisey et al., 2009). As mentioned in the earlier discussion on NE, studies of individuals with low-functioning variants of the COMT gene, leading to less DA degradation, display higher anxiety and lower resistance to stress (Heinz and Smolka, 2006).

Although hyperactivity of the dopaminergic system may increase susceptibility to suffering negative effects of stress, it appears that underactivity of dopaminergic neurons in the PFC may be implicated in sustaining posttraumatic stress disorders. Lesions of dopaminergic neurons in the mPFC delay extinction of the conditioned fear response (Morrow et al., 1999), which can sustain PTSD symptoms. Dopamine transporter density is increased in PTSD patients, which may reflect higher dopamine turnover in PTSD (Hoexter et al., 2012).

Reduced levels of circulating DA have also been implicated in depression in a number of studies (Dunlop and Nemeroff, 2007). This link is supported by the fact that individuals with Parkinson's disease (and decreased DA production) have high rates of depression. Postmortem studies of patients who were depressed have found reduced DA metabolites in the cerebrospinal fluid and in brain areas regulating mood and motivation.

Polymorphisms in dopamine transporter and receptor genes in depressed patients appear to be associated with treatment response (Huuhka et al., 2008; Lavretsky et al., 2008).

BRAIN-DERIVED NEUROTROPHIC FACTOR

Brain-derived neurotrophic factor (BDNF) is an important neurotrophic factor that is active in brain regions including the hippocampus, cortex, and basal forebrain (Yamada and Nabeshima, 2003). BDNF helps support neuronal growth, differentiation, and survival (Huang and Reichardt, 2001). BDNF interacts with TrkB and p75 as its two main receptors (Castren and Rantamaki, 2010). The BDNF-TrkB pathway has been implicated in both PTSD in humans and in animal models of fear conditioning, extinction, and inhibitory learning (Mahan and Ressler, 2012). Inhibition of BDNF signaling in the amygdala can lead to impairment of the acquisition and consolidation of fear conditioning (Rattiner et al., 2004), and the consolidation of extinction (Chhatwal et al., 2006).

BDNF exerts different functions in different brain regions. Animal studies showed that, in the hippocampus, stress decreases BDNF expression, which is reversible by antidepressant treatment (Duman and Montaggia, 2006). Hippocampal BDNF expression has been shown to play a critical role in resilience to chronic stress (Taliaz et al., 2011). In the nucleus accumbens, however, stress increases BDNF expression, and this increase is associated with depression-like effects (Berton et al., 2006; Eisch et al., 2003).

There is also increasing evidence for an association between a single nucleotide polymorphism in the BDNF gene (Val66Met) and various psychiatric disorders including depression and PTSD (Mahan and Ressler, 2012). This polymorphism was found to alter BDNF stability and secretion, and might result in activation of the limbic system during memory formation and emotionally-relevant learning (Dennis et al., 2011; Egan et al., 2003; Gonul et al., 2011; Mahan and Ressler, 2012). Studies in Val66Met knock-in mice revealed that mice with the Met/Met genotype exhibited increased anxiety-related behaviors (Chen et al., 2006b).

GLUTAMATE

Glutamate is the most widely distributed excitatory neurotransmitter in the brain. Glutamate functions via activation of its receptors, including ionotropic NMDA, Kainate, and AMPA receptors, as well as metabotropic receptors (Chung, 2012). Glutamate, together with its downstream product GABA, the chief inhibitory neurotransmitter in the nervous system, plays an important role in neuroplasticity, and in modulating cognitive and affective responses to stress (Harvey and Shahid, 2012).

Acute exposure to stress rapidly increases glutamate release in limbic and cortical brain regions, including the hippocampus, amygdala, and prefrontal cortex, areas associated with memory, learning, and affect. The effects of chronic stress on glutamate release are less well understood (Popoli et al., 2011). Numerous studies have found an important role of glutamate in the mediation of stress responsivity, formation of traumatic memories and the pathophysiology of PTSD (Cortese and Phan, 2005; Steckler and Risbrough, 2012). One study in mice found that the induction of DeltaFosB in the nucleus accumbens mediated resilience in response to chronic social defeat stress (Vialou et al., 2010). This effect is produced in part through induction of the GluR2 AMPA subunit of the glutamate receptor, decreasing nucleus accumbens neuron responsiveness to glutamate. In another study, deletion of AMPA receptor subunit GluR-A in mice was associated with increased depression-like symptoms such as learned helplessness, and decreased serotonin and norepinephrine levels (Chourbaji et al., 2008).

Glutamate system dysregulation has been implicated in the pathophysiology of mood disorders, and there is strong interest in drug development targeting the glutamatergic system (Murrough and Charney, 2010; Sanacora et al., 2008; Mathew et al., 2012; Mathews et al., 2012). The NMDA receptor antagonist ketamine has been shown to have antidepressant effects in patients with treatment-resistant depression (aan het Rot et al., 2010, Zarate et al., 2006). It is thought that NMDA receptor antagonist antidepressant effect may be related to a rapid increase in glutamate release, resulting in activation of AMPA receptors and ultimately resulting in changes in synaptic signaling and protein synthesis, and formation of new dendritic spine synapses in the PFC (Autry et al., 2011; Koike et al., 2011; Li et al., 2010). Moreover, antagonism of metabotropic glutamate receptors has also been shown to produce antidepressant-like effects (Belozertseva et al., 2007; Li et al., 2006).

ENDOCANNABINOIDS

Endocannabinoids including anandamide (AEA) and 2-arachidonoyl glycerol (2-AG) are substances naturally produced from within the body that activate cannabinoid receptors such as G protein-coupled CB_1 and CB_2 receptors. The endocannabinoid system is widely distributed throughout neural regions that regulate mood and emotion. The CB_1 receptor and endocannabinoid ligands are found at high densities in regions including the prefrontal cortex, hypothalamus, amygdala, and hippocampus (Herkenham et al., 1991; Hill et al., 2007; Tsou et al., 1998; Moldrich and Wenger, 2000). Activation of CB_1 receptors in these limbic areas can result in both excitatory and inhibitory neurotransmission, as well as the release of monoamines and neuropeptides (Azad et al., 2003; Di et al., 2003; Domenici et al., 2006). The CB_2 receptor is located predominantly in peripheral immune cells and organs (Hillard, 2000; Cota et al., 2003). A growing body of evidence demonstrates that deficits in endocannabinoid signaling may result in depressive and anxiogenic behavioral responses, which could be ameliorated by the pharmacological augmentation of endocannabinoid signaling (Hill and Gorzalka, 2009a).

Preclinical studies showed that CB_1 receptor knockout mice exhibited an increased susceptibility to the anhedonic effects of chronic stress (Martin et al., 2002), as well as increased passive stress coping behaviors in forced swim test and tail suspension test (Aso et al., 2008; Steiner et al., 2008), suggesting that the loss of CB1 receptor signaling promotes a depressive phenotype. CB1 receptor knockout mice also display increased anxiety-like behaviors and impaired extinction of aversive memories (Martin et al., 2002; reviewed in Hill and Gorzalka, 2009a).

Clinical studies in patients with medical conditions showed that the use of CB_1 receptor antagonists rimonabant and taranabant can lead to adverse effects such as developing anxiety and depressive symptoms, suggesting that the disruption of endocannabinoid signaling may promote the emergence of mood and anxiety disorders (Christensen et al., 2007; Hill and Gorzalka, 2009a,b; Nissen et al., 2008). Reduction in circulating endocannabinoid ligands has also been seen in women with major depression (Hill et al., 2008). Little research has investigated the effects of endocannabinoids on symptoms of PTSD, but one study showed that the addition of the synthetic cannabinoid nabilone resulted in reduction of treatment-resistant nightmares in PTSD patients (Fraser, 2009). More research is warranted to elucidate the intricate endocannabinoid signaling in mood and emotion and to explore the therapeutic potential of pharmacological interventions acting on the endocannabinoid system in mood and anxiety disorders.

NEURAL CIRCUITRY OF REWARD: HOW REWARD PATHWAYS IMPACT RESILIENCE TO STRESS

A stable and well-functioning system of reward pathways and response to pleasant stimuli is a prerequisite for dealing successfully with stress and traumatic life experiences. The ability to respond appropriately to positive events and situations is vital to the preservation of reward expectation, optimism, and positive self-concept following stress or trauma. Resilient individuals likely have a robust reward system, which is strongly responsive to reward and/or resistant to change (Table 88.3, Fig. 88.2; see also Color Fig. 88.2 in separate insert).

The dopaminergic system is involved in mediating elements of the reward system, including motivation, incentive, and hedonic tone (Barrot et al., 2002; Wise, 2002). Dopaminergic neurons increase firing when rewards are unexpected or better than expected (Schultz, 2002) and decrease their rate of firing when rewards are absent or less than predicted. Imaging research suggests that the anticipation of reward involves mesolimbic DA pathways through the ventral striatum (Knutson and Cooper, 2005) and other subcortical limbic structures including the dorsal striatum, amygdala, and midbrain ventral tegmental area.

The roles of the orbitofrontal cortex (OFC) and mPFC in reward are somewhat more complex. The OFC, taking input from the nucleus accumbens, assists in discriminating the motivational value of rewarding stimuli (Martin-Soelch et al., 2001; Schultz, 2002). The mPFC appears to be involved in assessing the likelihood of receiving a given reward (as opposed to its magnitude) (Knutson and Cooper, 2005) and providing feedback along glutamatergic projections to the nucleus accumbens and the ventral tegmental area. The anterior insula is involved in producing aversion to risks in the pursuit of reward (Kuhnen and Knutson, 2005). In making decisions about behavior, it appears that a stimulus's potential

TABLE 88.3. Neural mechanisms related to resilience and vulnerability to extreme stress

MECHANISM	NEUROCHEMICAL SYSTEMS	BRAIN REGIONS	ASSOCIATION WITH RESILIENCE	ASSOCIATION WITH PSYCHOPATHOLOGY
Reward	Dopamine, dopamine receptors, glutamate, N-methyl-D-aspartic acid (NMDA) receptors, γ-aminobutyric acid (GABA), opioids, cAMP response element binding protein, ΔFosB	Medial prefrontal cortex, orbital frontal cortex, nucleus accumbens, amygdala, hippocampus, ventral tegmental area, hypothalamus	In resilient individuals, stress does not produce impairment in neurochemical or transcription factor-mediated reward.	Stress-induced reduction in dopamine and increases in cAMP response-element binding protein transcription produces a dysfunction in reward circuitry leading to anhedonia and hopelessness.
Reconsolidation	Glutamate, NMDA receptors, norepinephrine, β-adrenergic receptors, cAMP response-element binding protein	Amygdala, hippocampus	The lability of the memory trace allows a reorganization of original memory that is less traumatic.	Repeated reactivation and reconsolidation may further strengthen the memory trace and lead to persistence of . trauma-related symptoms.
Extinction	Glutamate, NMDA receptors, voltage-gated calcium channels, norepinephrine, dopamine, GABA	Medial prefrontal sensory cortex, amygdala	An ability to quickly attenuate learned fear through a powerful extinction process	Failure in neural mechanisms of extinction may relate to persistent traumatic memories, reexperiencing symptoms, hyperarousal, and phobic behaviors.

cAMP, cyclic adenosine monophosphate; NMDA, N-methyl-D-aspartate.
(Modified and reprinted with permission from Cambridge University Press 2007).

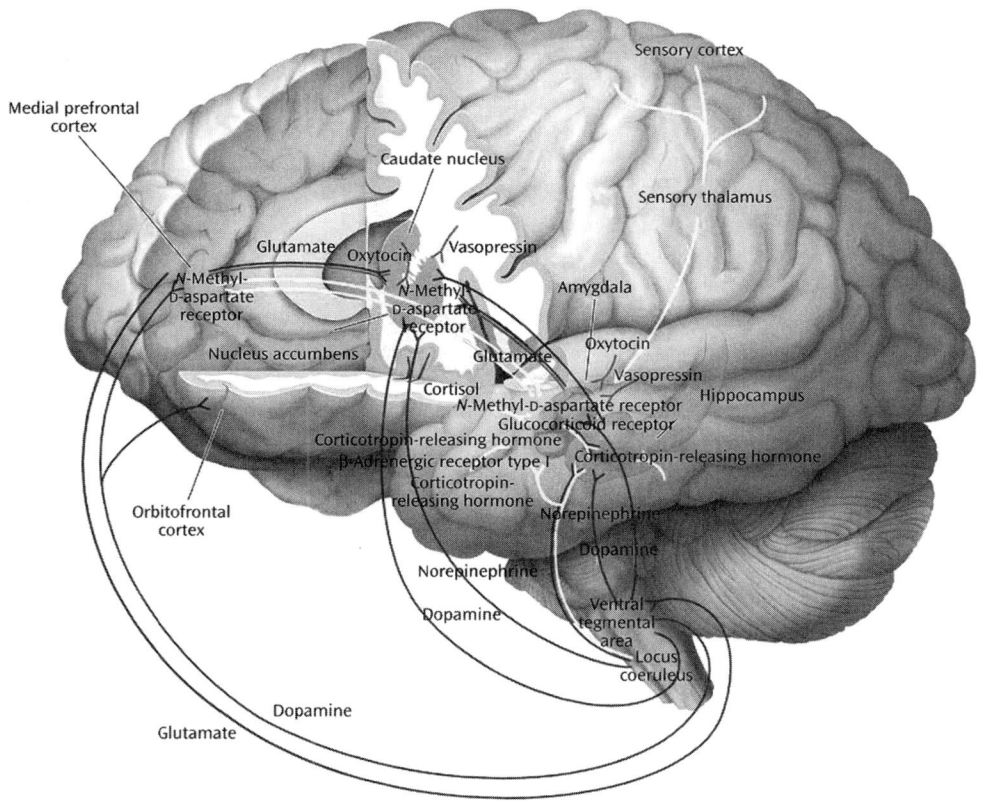

Figure 88.2 Neural circuits associated with reward, fear conditioning, and social behavior. The figure depicts a simplified summary of some of the brain structures and relevant neurochemistry mediating the neural mechanisms of reward (purple paths), fear conditioning and extinction (yellow paths), and social behaviors (blue paths). Only a subset of the many known interconnections among these various regions is shown, and relevant interneurons are not illustrated, yet it can be seen there is considerable overlap in the brain structures associated with these neural mechanisms. This suggests that there may be clinically relevant functional interactions among the circuits. For example, a properly functioning reward circuit may be necessary for the reinforcement of positive social behaviors. An overly responsive fear circuit or impaired extinction process may negatively influence functioning of the reward system. The assessment of these neural mechanisms must be considered in the context of their neurochemical regulation. Alterations in one neurotransmitter, neuropeptide, or hormone system will affect more than one circuit. Several receptors that may be targeted by new anti-anxiety and antidepressant drugs are illustrated. The functional status of these circuits has important influences on stress-related psychopathology and the discovery of novel therapeutics (see text). (Modified and reprinted with permission from Cambridge University Press, 2007) (See color insert).

rewards are assessed in subcortical areas before being analyzed in the mPFC (Knutson and Cooper, 2005).

Strength, persistence, and emotional value of reward memory are modulated by circuits formed by the amygdala, subiculum, bed nucleus of the stria terminalis, nucleus accumbens, and mPFC. Specifically, the cyclic adenosine monophosphate (cAMP) pathway and expression of cAMP response-element binding protein in the amygdala strengthen positive as well as negative associations (Hall et al., 2001; Josselyn et al., 2001). Rodents have been shown to develop persistent anhedonia when increased cAMP response element binding is present in the nucleus accumbens (Barrot et al., 2002).

Stresses, chronic and acute, are correlated with decreased sensitivity to rewarding stimuli and increased sensitivity to aversive stimuli (Bogdan and Pizzagalli, 2006, Pliakas et al., 2001). During performance of a probabilistic reward task, high school student carriers of the S allele of the 5HTTLPR gene showed a larger stress-related reduction in responsiveness to reward as school finals approached, compared with L allele homozygotes (Nikolova et al., 2012). This effect was observed only in males. In a different study, reward learning under a stressful condition was differentially influenced in healthy females depending on their CRH receptor type 1 genotype, and was associated with differential activation to reward in the anterior cingulated cortex (ACC) and OFC (Bogdan et al., 2011). Although exposure to acute stress has the potential to alter reward circuits, decreasing positive response to reward, findings from these studies suggest that some people are more sensitive to the effects of stress, and other, potentially more resilient individuals show reduced stress sensitivity, maintaining highly functional reward systems under adverse conditions. In a recent fMRI study, adolescents and young adults with a parental history of depression showed lower OFC activation to rewarding stimuli and higher lateral OFC and insula activations to aversive stimuli, compared with controls. They also showed blunted ACC activation to both rewarding and aversive stimuli (Mc Cabe et al., 2012). These neural abnormalities suggest a potential mechanism for decreased resilience in individuals at high familial risk for depression.

We thus have a beginning understanding of the neurobiology underlying robust reward systems. There is also some evidence from animal models that provides insight into potential mechanisms. In rodent models, chronic exposure to stressful stimuli will lead to an enduring aversion to social contact. Researchers have found that knocking out *BDNF* in the mesolimbic DA system of the rodents seems to produce a reward system that has lost its plasticity, remaining resistant to change when the rats are subsequently presented with stressors. After undergoing this mesolimbic DA pathway-specific knockdown of *BDNF*, mice become inoculated to the effects of repeated social aggression (Berton et al., 2006). Studies in the social defeat paradigm in mice, whereby mice are exposed to a dominant intruder placed in their cage, have demonstrated that resilient mice, who show appropriate anxiety responses but no defeat, upregulate K+ channels in the VTA, thereby preventing an increase in neuronal excitability and associated BDNF release onto the nucleus accumbens observed by contrast in vulnerable mice (Krishnan et al., 2007).

These findings highlight the major role of the reward system's plasticity in determining resilience and indicate possible mechanisms through which a resistant reward system plays a part in allowing resilient individuals to endure hardships without developing posttraumatic psychopathology.

THE NEURAL CIRCUITRY OF ANXIETY AND FEAR: THE ROLE OF FEAR LEARNING IN RESILIENCE TO STRESS

FEAR CONDITIONING

Individuals with PTSD suffer distress when they encounter traumatic reminders. Over time, patients suffering from PTSD tend to "overgeneralize" fear cues: they begin to associate more and more features in their environment with their past traumas. Often, fear cues are objectively non-threatening and unrelated to trauma. The process through which previously neutral stimuli become fear inducing is known as fear conditioning. In the terminology of fear conditioning, previously neutral stimuli become "conditioned" stimuli by virtue of their association with aversive (unconditioned) stimuli (Blair et al., 2001).

Resilience to the effects of severe stress may be characterized in part by the capacity to avoid overgeneralizing fear-inducing triggers. Resilient individuals are also likely adept at extinguishing of fearful memories; in other words, those who are resistant to stress have an easier time letting go of frightening memories and associations.

Cue-specific conditioned stimuli are transmitted to the thalamus by external and visceral pathways. Afferents reach the lateral amygdala by means of two parallel circuits: a rapid subcortical path directly from the dorsal (sensory) thalamus and a slower regulatory cortical pathway encompassing the primary somatosensory cortices, the insula, and the anterior cingulate/PFC. Contextual conditioned stimuli are projected to the lateral amygdala from the hippocampus and the bed nucleus of the stria terminalis. The lateral nucleus of the amygdala is likely a site of fear memory storage as well as fear acquisition (Schafe et al., 2005). The existence of the long loop pathway (passing through cortical regions) indicates that sensory information relayed to the amygdala undergoes substantial higher-level processing, thereby enabling assignment of significance based on prior exposure to stimuli. This potential for higher-level processing of conditioned stimuli is important because it implies that there is potential for modifying the processing of fear-conditioned stimuli with cognitive therapies.

The lateral amygdala, once engaged, projects to the central and medial nuclei of the amygdala, which project indirectly to the acoustic startle pathway in the brain stem (Davis, 2006). The central nucleus of the amygdala appears to be the primary output nucleus involved in initial memory consolidation; infusions of anisomycin, a protein synthesis inhibitor, into the central nucleus during fear training disrupt consolidation of fear memory (Debiec and LeDoux, 2006). The central nucleus projects to the hypothalamus and brain stem, triggering the cascade of autonomic, endocrine, and behavioral responses associated with fear (Schafe et al., 2001).

The molecular processes underlying fear conditioning is an area of active investigation. Consolidation of fear conditioning is thought to occur via long-term potentiation of synapses in the lateral amygdala. Fear-conditioned rats show increases in an actin polymerization protein, profilin, in dendritic spines in the lateral amygdala; this finding could contribute to a greater understanding of the specific changes underlying synaptic plasticity (Schafe et al., 2005). However, our understanding of the cellular mechanisms underlying the process remains far from complete (Sigurdsson et al., 2007). The currently accepted model to explain how long-term potentiation in the lateral amygdala might lead to the consolidation of fear conditioning was proposed by LeDoux and colleagues (LeDoux, 2000). The model proposes that calcium entry through NMDA receptors and voltage-gated calcium channels initiates the molecular processes to consolidate synaptic changes into long-term memory; short-term memory requires only calcium entry through NMDA receptors (Blair et al., 2001).

Because NMDA receptors are critical in fear learning, which is mediated by glutamate acting in the central nucleus of the amygdala (Davis, 2006), we may be able to impair fear learning by blocking NMDA receptors in the amygdala during stress. This has been demonstrated in rodents (Rodrigues et al., 2001; Walker and Davis, 2000;). Blockade of voltage-gated calcium channels may also prove useful in preventing PTSD in those who are exposed to stress. Of course, because these are mechanisms of initial fear consolidation, it would be necessary to initiate receptor blockade treatment prior to trauma exposure to prevent posttraumatic stress. This might be feasible and useful in populations that are certain to encounter severe stress, for example, soldiers to be deployed in combat, or disaster relief workers.

RECONSOLIDATION AND EXTINCTION

Existing memories, when retrieved or "reactivated" by remembering, become labile and prone to change. Reactivated memories may go down one of two pathways: they may either be strengthened by reconsolidation, or weakened by extinction (Eisenhardt and Menzel, 2007). The processes appear to be mutually exclusive, and may compete for cellular resources (Dudai and Eisenberg, 2004). The processes of memory reactivation, reconsolidation, and extinction involve NMDA and β-adrenergic receptors and require cAMP response element binding protein induction, indicating that nuclear protein synthesis is necessary (Kida et al., 2002). Reconsolidation and extinction are impaired by NMDA and β-adrenergic blockade, and enhanced by the NMDA partial agonist D-cycloserine (Charney and Drevets, 2002; Chhatwal et al., 2006; Debiec and LeDoux, 2006; Przybyslawski et al., 1999; Royer et al., 2000; Sotres-Bayon et al., 2007). Whether the process of reconsolidation or of extinction will be engaged appears to depend on the timing and type of memory retrieval; short memory reactivation sessions tend to lead to reconsolidation, whereas long and intensive extinction training is necessary to achieve extinction (J.L. Lee et al., 2006). Reconsolidation and extinction of a memory are affected by the age of the memory in question (Fulton, 2006). As would be expected, younger memories are more prone to being altered by either process, although intensifying the memory reactivation process helps enhance the lability of older memories (Suzuki et al., 2004).

Similarly, the process of extinction changes over time. Extinction induced immediately after fear acquisition (between 10 minutes and 1 hour later) is thought to occur by "erasing" the learned fear (Myers et al., 2006). However, extinction induced 24–72 hours after initial fear training appears to be a new form of learning altogether (Myers and Davis, 2007). The extinction that is achieved during this later time period may be thought of as the formation of a new, safe association with the original fear cue; this new association is placed, "like a blanket," over the older fear association (Chhatwal et al., 2006). That the original fear association still exists underneath the blanket of safety is suggested by observations that extinguished fears can return spontaneously.

Memory consolidation, reconsolidation, and extinction involve different neural circuits. The central nucleus of the amygdala and hippocampus are involved in initial memory consolidation, the lateral amygdala in reconsolidation, and the basal lateral amygdala in extinction (Bahar et al., 2004; Debiec and LeDoux, 2006). The mPFC is a critical structure in extinction. Since the 1980s, studies have found that lesions of the mPFC result in an impairment of normal extinction (cited in Sotres-Bayon et al., 2006). Failure to achieve an adequate level of activation of the mPFC might lead to persistent fear responses (Herry and Garcia, 2002). Findings from an fMRI study in healthy volunteers suggest that the ability of fear responses to adapt flexibly as threat shifts from one stimulus to another is particularly mediated by the ventromedial PFC (Schiller et al., 2008). Individuals with the capacity to function well after high-stress experiences may have potent mPFC inhibition of amygdala responsiveness. In contrast, patients with PTSD have been shown to exhibit increased left amygdala activation during fear acquisition and decreased activity of the mPFC/anterior cingulate during extinction.

Reconsolidation and extinction of traumatic memories are implicated in vulnerability and resilience to extreme stress. Individuals who are able to attenuate learned fear through extinction are likely highly stress-resilient. Due to our growing understanding of the mechanisms of memory processing, there will likely be ever more possibilities for helping trauma survivors manage their traumatic memories. In particular, recent studies suggest that during reconsolidation, previously stored information becomes labile after retrieval and thus amenable to change as new information is incorporated (Schiller et al., 2010). Recent studies in healthy volunteers, whereby participants underwent extinction during the reconsolidation window, incorporating non-fearful information to the old fear memory, have successfully prevented the expression of fear responses (Schiller et al., 2010; 2012). This effect has been shown to last for at least one year (Schiller et al., 2010) and has been replicated by a different group (Oyarzun et al., 2012). A recent fMRI study in humans demonstrated that suppression of a fear memory by conducting extinction training during the reconsolidation window works by erasing the fear memory representation in the amygdala (Agren et al., 2012). These exciting findings might lead to new interventions for individuals with PTSD. Emerging evidence thus suggests that extinction training during reconsolidation might be a potentially effective treatment approach.

ADDITIONAL NEURAL CIRCUITRY RELEVANT IN RESILIENCE

Stress resilience has been related to a greater capacity for emotion regulation (Johnstone et al., 2007; Masten and Coatsworth, 1998), thought to be mediated by ventral and dorsal neural systems (Phillips et al., 2003a, 2003b). As discussed earlier, studies have linked genetic variation with differential amygdala reactivity to negative stimuli, as well as altered functional coupling between the PFC and the amygdala, a possible mechanism mediating differential vulnerability to stress. In addition, studies of offspring at high and low familial risk for depression have found differences in neural responses to emotional stimuli (Monk et al., 2008) and in attention to negative emotional stimuli during tryptophan depletion (Feder et al., 2011). In a recent study of acutely traumatized individuals, higher trait resilience measured by the Connor-Davidson Resilience Scale was positively correlated with activation in the right thalamus, and the inferior and middle frontal gyri (BA 47), additional areas involved in emotion regulation (Daniels et al., 2012).

The neural basis of a particular form of emotion regulation, cognitive reappraisal, has been examined in several imaging studies. Activation of the lateral PFC, thought to modulate amygdala activation and thus the intensity of emotional responses, has been linked to reappraisal success (Goldin et al., 2008; Ochsner et al., 2004; Wager et al., 2008). Further, greater use of reappraisal in everyday life has been found to correlate with lower amygdala and greater PFC activation to negative stimuli (Drabant et al., 2009).

Other imaging studies have begun to delineate additional neural circuits relevant for social behavior, for example the neural circuitry mediating the capacity for empathy, thought to be comprised of the mirror neuron system in interaction with limbic brain regions (Rizzolatti and Craighero, 2004; Schulte-Rüther et al., 2007). Future studies might uncover possible relationships between the capacity for empathy and resilience. As discussed, social contact and support are known to promote health and well-being (Charuvastra and Cloitre, 2008). Imaging studies are beginning to uncover the neural mechanisms mediating reduced responses to stress in the presence of social support (Coan et al., 2006).

IMPLICATIONS FOR PREVENTION AND TREATMENT OF STRESS-RELATED PSYCHOPATHOLOGY

Our growing understanding of genetic, developmental, psychological, and neurobiological resilience factors continues to lead to the development of therapeutic interventions for enhancing resilience to stress (Southwick and Charney, 2012b).

Cognitive-behavioral therapies emphasize cognitive reappraisal of negatively viewed circumstances into more positive perspectives, and have shown results across a broad range of populations (Beck and Dozois, 2011). Other therapies employing cognitive reappraisal include hardiness training (Maddi, 2008) and well-being therapy (Fava and Tomba, 2009), the latter also showing promising results in school interventions (Ruini and Fava, 2012). Positive psychology-based exercises, including reflecting daily on things that went well that day, were shown to increase positive affect and decrease depression levels in adults (Seligman et al., 2005). Similarly, gratitude interventions, whereby individuals are instructed to identify several things that they are grateful or thankful for in their life, have been associated with increased reports of well-being and positive affect in various populations (Wood et al., 2010).

Meaning-making interventions have been applied to help breast or colorectal cancer patients, resulting in increases in self-esteem, optimism, and self-efficacy, in comparison with a control group (Lee et al., 2006). Mindfulness training for individuals with residual depressive symptoms successfully increased their ability to experience positive emotions and was associated with a reduction in residual depressive symptoms, compared with a waitlist control condition (Geschwind et al., 2011). Research findings on psychological factors associated with resilience have been applied to design a resilience training program for the military (Reivich et al., 2011). Future studies should determine whether these interventions are successful in protecting individuals facing future stressors, thus boosting resilience in general and at-risk populations.

The military, along with first responder groups such as police or firefighters, has a strong tradition of stress inoculation training, in the form of training programs designed to maximize coping self-efficacy and mastery. This training is accomplished by means of exposure to manageable stressors including physical and mental challenges, providing opportunities for mastery by repeated practice and gradual exposure to increasingly challenging situations. A similar approach is applied in outdoor education programs for children and adolescents, such as Outward Bound.

As discussed in the preceding, recent research has made it possible to understand the process of fear extinction further, and current studies are focused on delineating windows of opportunity during memory retrieval when fear memories and responses are more receptive to extinction training, with the goal of developing novel therapeutic interventions (Karatsoreos and McEwen, 2011; Schiller et al., 2012). The principles of fear extinction have already been applied more broadly to the development of exposure therapy, a form of therapy with proven effectiveness in PTSD (Foa, 2011). Extensive investigation is also devoted to potential ways of enhancing stress-resistance and resilience with pharmacologic means, and the combination of pharmacologic and psychotherapy approaches.

Because antagonizing β receptors disrupts the process of consolidation, several trials have investigated the efficacy of β-blockers, in particular propranolol, in disrupting consolidation of traumatic memories shortly after trauma exposure. Although initial trials showed some promise (Pitman et al., 2002; Vaiva et al., 2003), later studies failed to prevent the emergence of PTSD (Hoge et al., 2012; Stein et al., 2007). One possible explanation is that propranolol was administered late in the consolidation window, or after consolidation was already complete (Cain et al., 2012). In a separate series of studies, the N-methyl D-aspartate (NMDA) receptor partial agonist D-cycloserine, which enhances memory reconsolidation and memory extinction, was shown to facilitate the effects of prolonged exposure therapy in humans with anxiety disorders (Hofmann et al., 2006; Ressler et al., 2004). Results in PTSD have been mixed and await further study (Cain et al., 2012).

Animal models are currently being used to investigate the use of other cognitive enhancers that might affect fear extinction, such as agents modulating GABAergic transmission (Kaplan and Moore, 2011). A major area of interest involves the study of the endogenous cannabinoid system, its role in modulating HPA axis activation during stress, and the potential for facilitating fear extinction by targeting endocannabinoid receptors (Hill and Tasker, 2012). Other receptors known to be involved in extinction, such as the BDNF receptor tyrosine kinase b, have been targeted in preclinical trials (Chhatwal et al., 2006).

Additional potential approaches involve targeting the HPA axis. Trials of hydrocortisone, a glucocorticoid receptor agonist, in intensive care unit patients with septic shock or undergoing cardiac surgery resulted in reduced PTSD symptoms and improved health-related quality of life in long-term survivors (Schelling et al., 2006). A pilot study of high-dose hydrocortisone administered immediately after trauma to patients recruited from the emergency department showed promising results (Zohar et al., 2011). Thus, it might be possible to prevent PTSD with treatments administered shortly after trauma exposure or even by pretreating individuals at high risk for trauma exposure. For individuals with chronic PTSD, current trials are investigating the effects of a CRH1 receptor antagonist and the glucocorticoid receptor antagonist mifepristone in separate trials.

Continued progress in understanding the genetic, developmental, biological, and psychological underpinnings of resilience and vulnerability to stress, as well as the interactions between these factors, will aid in moving the field toward the identification, prevention, and treatment of those at risk of developing stress-related psychopathology.

DISCLOSURES

Dr. Feder has no conflicts of interest or disclosures. Her research is funded by CDC/NIOSH and USAMRAA.

Dr. Haglund has no conflicts of interest or disclosures.

Dr. Wu has no conflicts of interest or disclosures.

Dr. Southwick has no conflicts of interest or disclosures. His research is funded by NIH/NIMH, CDC/NIOSH, USAMRAA and the Department of Veterans Affairs.

Dr. Charney and Mount Sinai School of Medicine have been named on a use patent application of Ketamine for the treatment of depression. If Ketamine were shown to be effective in the treatment of depression and received approval from the Food and Drug Administration for this indication, Dr. Charney and Mount Sinai School of Medicine could benefit financially.

Dr. Charney is funded by NIH, NIH/NIMH, NARSAD, USAMRAA.

Dr. Charney is on the following scientific advisory boards with no compensation:

2000	Academic Advisory Board, Pfizer Postdoctoral Fellowship Program
2001	Scientific Advisory Board, Familial Dysautonomia Foundation
2002	National Education Alliance for Borderline Personality Disorder Scientific Advisory Board
2002	National Center for Posttraumatic Stress Disorder
2002	Senior Advisory Board, American Psychiatric Association/American Psychiatric Press Journal: Journal of Lifelong Learning in Psychiatry
2005	Institute of Medicine Committee on Stress of Military Deployment
2006	Institute of Medicine Subcommittee on PTSD
2012	Institute of Medicine Committee on DHS Workforce Resilience

Dr. Charney is also on the following editorial boards with no compensation

1986	Editorial Board, Journal of Affective Disorders
1990	International Editorial Board, Journal of Psychopharmacology
1993	Editorial Board, Journal of Serotonin Research
1994	Editorial Board, Depression and Anxiety
1995	Editorial Board, Seminars in Clinical Neuropsychiatry
1996	Editorial Board, CNS Spectrums
1997	Editorial Board, Human Psychopharmacology
2012	Editorial Board, CNS Spectrums

REFERENCES

Aan het Rot, M., Collins, K.A., et al. (2010). Safety and efficacy of repeated-dose intravenous ketamine for treatment-resistant depression. Biol. Psychiatry 67:139–145.

Abbosh, C., Lawkowski, A., et al. (2011). GalR2/3 mediates proliferative and trophic effects of galanin on postnatal hippocampal precursors. J. Neurochem. 117:425–436.

Affleck, G., and Tennen, H. (1996). Constructing benefits from adversity: adaptational significance and dispositional underpinnings. J. Personality 64:899–922.

Agren, T., Engman, J., et al. (2012). Disruption of reconsolidation erases a fear memory trace in the human amygdala. Science 337:1550–1552.

Alim, T.N., Feder, A., et al. (2008). Trauma, resilience, and recovery in a high-risk African-American population. Am. J. Psychiatry 165:1566–1575.

Aso, E., Ozaita, A., et al. (2008). BDNF impairment in the hippocampus is related to enhanced despair behavior in CB1 knockout mice. J. Neurochem. 105:565–572.

Autry, A.E., Adachi, M., et al. (2011). NMDA receptor blockade at rest triggers rapid behavioural antidepressant responses. *Nature* 475:91–95.

Azad, S.C., Eder, M., et al. (2003). Activation of the cannabinoid receptor type 1 decreases glutamatergic and GABAergic synaptic transmission in the lateral amygdala of the mouse. *Learn Mem.* 10:116–128.

Bahar, A., Dorfman, N., et al. (2004). Amygdalar circuits required for either consolidation or extinction of taste aversion memory are not required for reconsolidation. *Eur. J. Neurosci.* 19:1115–1118.

Baker, D.G., Ekhator, N.N., et al. (2005). Higher levels of basal serial CSF cortisol in combat veterans with posttraumatic stress disorder. *Am. J. Psychiatry* 162:992–994.

Baker, D.G., West, S.A., et al. (1999). Serial CSF corticotropin-releasing hormone levels and adrenocortical activity in combat veterans with posttraumatic stress disorder. *Am. J. Psychiatry* 156:585–588.

Baker, R.A., and Herkenham, M. (1995). Arcuate nucleus neurons that project to the hypothalamic paraventricular nucleus: neuropeptidergic identity and consequences of adrenalectomy on mRNA levels in the rat. *J. Comp. Neurol.* 358:518–530.

Bakshi, V.P., Smith-Roe, S., et al. (2002). Reduction of stress-induced behavior by antagonism of corticotropin-releasing hormone 2 (CRH2) receptors in lateral septum or CRH1 receptors in amygdala. *J. Neurosci.* 22:2926–2935.

Bale, T.L., Picetti, R., et al. (2002). Mice deficient for both corticotropin-releasing factor receptor 1 (CRFR1) and CRFR2 have an impaired stress response and display sexually dichotomous anxiety-like behavior. *J. Neurosci.* 22:193–199.

Barrot, M., Olivier, J.D., et al. (2002). CREB activity in the nucleus accumbens shell controls gating of behavioral responses to emotional stimuli. *Proc. Natl. Acad. Sci. USA* 99:11435–11440.

Bastianetto, S., Ramassamy, C., et al. (1999). Dehydroepiandrosterone (DHEA) protects hippocampal cells from oxidative stress-induced damage. *Brain Res. Mol. Brain Res.* 66:35–41.

Beck, A.T., and Dozois, D.J. (2011). Cognitive therapy: current status and future directions. *Annu. Rev. Med.* 62:397–409.

Belfer, I., Hipp, H., et al. (2006). Association of galanin haplotypes with alcoholism and anxiety in two ethnically distinct populations. *Mol. Psychiatry* 11:301–311.

Belozertseva, I.V., Kos, T., et al. (2007). Antidepressant-like effects of mGluR1 and mGluR5 antagonists in the rat forced swim and the mouse tail suspension tests. *Eur. Neuropsychopharmacol.* 17:172–179.

Benekareddy, M., Vadodaria, K.C., et al. (2011). Postnatal serotonin type 2 receptor blockade prevents the emergence of anxiety behavior, dysregulated stress-induced immediate early gene responses, and specific transcriptional changes that arise following early life stress. *Biol. Psychiatry* 70:1024–1032.

Berton, O., Mcclung, C.A., et al. (2006). Essential role of BDNF in the mesolimbic dopamine pathway in social defeat stress. *Science* 311:864–868.

Bierer, L.M., Tischler, L., et al. (2006). Clinical correlates of 24-h cortisol and norepinephrine excretion among subjects seeking treatment following the World Trade Center attacks on 9/11. *Ann. NY Acad. Sci.* 1071:514–520.

Binder, E.B., Bradley, R.G., et al. (2008). Association of FKBP5 polymorphisms and childhood abuse with risk of posttraumatic stress disorder symptoms in adults. *JAMA* 299:1291–1305.

Bingham, B., Mcfadden, K., et al. (2011). Early adolescence as a critical window during which social stress distinctly alters behavior and brain norepinephrine activity. *Neuropsychopharmacology* 36:896–909.

Binneman, B., Feltner, D., et al. (2008). A 6-week randomized, placebo-controlled trial of CP-316,311 (a selective CRH1 antagonist) in the treatment of major depression. *Am. J. Psychiatry* 165:617–620.

Bisschop, M.I., Knegsman, D.M.W., et al. (2004). Chronic diseases and depression: the modifying role of psychosocial resources. *Soc. Sci. Med.* 59:721–733.

Blair, H.T., Schafe, G.E., et al. (2001). Synaptic plasticity in the lateral amygdala: a cellular hypothesis of fear conditioning. *Learn. Mem.* 8:229–242.

Bogdan, R., and Pizzagalli, D.A. (2006). Acute stress reduces reward responsiveness: implications for depression. *Biol. Psychiatry* 60:1147–1154.

Bogdan, R., Santesso, D.L., et al. (2011). Corticotropin-releasing hormone receptor type 1 (CRHR1) genetic variation and stress interact to influence reward learning. *J. Neurosci.* 31:13246–13254.

Bonanno, G.A. (2004). Loss, trauma, and human resilience: have we underestimated the human capacity to thrive after extremely aversive events? *Am. Psychol.* 59:20–28.

Bonanno, G.A., Mancini, A.D., et al. (2012). Trajectories of trauma symptoms and resilience in deployed U.S. military service members: prospective cohort study. *Br. J. Psychiatry* 200:317–323.

Bonanno, G.A., Westphal, M., et al. (2011). Resilience to loss and potential trauma. *Annu. Rev. Clin. Psychol.* 7:511–535.

Bonne, O., Bain, E., et al. (2005). No change in serotonin type 1A receptor binding in patients with posttraumatic stress disorder. *Am. J. Psychiatry* 162:383–385.

Born, J., Lange, T., et al. (2002). Sniffing neuropeptides: a transnasal approach to the human brain. *Nat. Neurosci.* 5:514–516.

Boyce, W.T., and Chesterman, E. (1990). Life events, social support, and cardiovascular reactivity in adolescence. *J. Dev. Behav. Pediatr.* 11:105–111.

Braam, A.W., Beekman, A.T.F., et al. (1997). Religiosity as a protective or prognostic factor of depression in later life; results from a community survey in The Netherlands. *Acta Psychiatr. Scand.* 96:199–205.

Braam, A.W., Van Den Eeden, P., et al. (2001). Religion as a cross-cultural determinant of depression in elderly Europeans: results from the EURODEP collaboration. *Psychol. Med.* 31:803–814.

Bradley, R.G., Binder, E.B., et al. (2008). Influence of child abuse on adult depression: moderation by the corticotropin-releasing hormone receptor gene. *Arch. Gen. Psychiatry* 65:190–200.

Bremner, J.D., Licinio, J., et al. (1997). Elevated CSF corticotropin-releasing factor concentrations in posttraumatic stress disorder. *Am. J. Psychiatry* 154:624–629.

Breslau, N., Kessler, R.C., et al. (1998). Trauma and posttraumatic stress disorder in the community: the 1996 Detroit Area Survey of Trauma. *Arch. Gen. Psychiatry* 55:626–632.

Britton, K.T., Akwa, Y., et al. (2000). Neuropeptide Y blocks anxiogenic-like behavioral action of corticotropin-releasing factor in an operant conflict test and elevated plus maze. *Peptides* 21:37–44.

Brosse, A.L., Sheets, E.S., et al. (2002). Exercise and the treatment of clinical depression in adults: recent findings and future directions. *Sports Med.* 32:741–760.

Browne, E.S., Wright, B.E., et al. (1992). Dehydroepiandrosterone: antigluco-corticoid action in mice. *Am. J. Med. Sci.* 303:366–371.

Bruce, S.E., Weisberg, R.B., et al. (2001). Trauma and posttraumatic stress disorder in primary care patients. *Prim. Care Companion J. Clin. Psychiatry* 3:211–217.

Brunner, R., Schaefer, D., et al. (2006). Effect of high-dose cortisol on memory functions. *Ann. NY Acad. Sci.* 1071:434–437.

Cabib, S., and Puglisi-Allegra, S. (1996). Different effects of repeated stressful experiences on mesocortical and mesolimbic dopamine metabolism. *Neurosci.* 73:375–380.

Cabib, S., Ventura, R., et al. (2002). Opposite imbalances between mesocortical and mesoaccumbens dopamine responses to stress by the same genotype depending on living conditions. *Behav. Brain Res.* 129:179–185.

Cain, C.K., Maynard, G.D., et al. (2012). Targeting memory processes with drugs to prevent or cure PTSD. *Expert Opin. Investig. Drugs* 21:1323–1350.

Camacho, T.C., Roberts, R.E., et al. (1991). Physical activity and depression—Evidence from the Alameda County Study. *Am. J. Epidem.* 134:220–231.

Carroll, B.J., Cassidy, F., et al. (2007). Pathophysiology of hypercortisolism in depression. *Acta Psychiatr. Scand.* 115 (Suppl. 433):90–103.

Carvajal, C., Dumont, Y., et al. (2006). Emotional behavior in aged neuropeptide Y (NPY) Y2 knockout mice. *J. Mol. Neurosci.* 28:239–245.

Carver, C., Pozo, C., et al. (1993). How coping mediates the effect of optimism on distress: a study of women with early stage breast cancer. *J. Pers. Soc. Psychology* 65:375–390.

Caspi, A., Sugden, K., et al. (2003). Influence of life stress on depression: moderation by a polymorphism in the 5-HTT gene. *Science* 301:386–389.

Castren, E., and Rantamaki, T. (2010). The role of BDNF and its receptors in depression and antidepressant drug action: reactivation of developmental plasticity. *Dev. Neurobiol.* 70:289–297.

Chantarujikapong, S.I., Scherrer, J.F., et al. (2001). A twin study of generalized anxiety disorder symptoms, panic disorder symptoms and post-traumatic stress disorder in men. *Psychiatry Res.* 103:133–145.

Charney, D.S., and Drevets, W.D. (2002). The neurobiological basis of anxiety disorders. In: Davis, K.L., Charney, D.S., Coyle, J.T., and Nemeroff, C., eds. Neuropsychopharmacology: The Fifth Generation of Progress. Philadelphia, PA: Lippincott Williams & Wilkins, pp. 901–930.

Charney, D.S. (2004). Psychobiological mechanisms of resilience and vulnerability: implications for successful adaptation to extreme stress. *Am. J. Psychiatry* 161:195–216.

Charuvastra, A., Cloitre, M. (2008). Social bonds and posttraumatic stress disorder. *Annu. Rev. Psychol.* 59:301–328.

Chen, L., Dai, X.N., et al. (2006a). Chronic administration of dehydroepiandrosterone sulfate (DHEAS) primes for facilitated induction of long-term potentiation via sigma 1 (sigma1) receptor: optical imaging study in rat hippocampal slices. *Neuropharmacology* 50:380–392.

Chen, Z.Y., Jing, D., et al. (2006b). Genetic variant BDNF (Val66Met) polymorphism alters anxiety-related behavior. *Science* 314:140–143.

Chhatwal, J.P., Stanek-Rattiner, L., et al. (2006). Amygdala BDNF signaling is required for consolidation but not encoding of extinction. *Nat. Neurosci.* 9:870–872.

Chourbaji, S., Vogt, M.A., et al. (2008). AMPA receptor subunit 1 (GluR-A) knockout mice model the glutamate hypothesis of depression. *FASEB J.* 22:3129–3134.

Christensen, R., Kristensen, P.K., et al. (2007). Efficacy and safety of the weight-loss drug rimonabant: a meta-analysis of randomised trials. *Lancet* 370:1706–1713.

Chung, C. (2012). New perspectives on glutamate receptor antagonists as antidepressants. *Arch. Pharm. Res.* 35:573–577.

Claes, S.J. (2004). Corticotropin-releasing hormone (CRH) in psychiatry: from stress to psychopathology. *Ann. Med.* 36:50–61.

Coan, J.A., Schaefer, H.S., et al. (2006). Lending a hand: social regulation of the neural response to threat. *Psychol. Sci.* 17:1032–1039.

Cohen, H., Liu, T., et al. (2012). The neuropeptide Y (NPY)-ergic system is associated with behavioral resilience to stress exposure in an animal model of post-traumatic stress disorder. *Neuropsychopharmacology* 37:350–363.

Coric, V., Feldman, H.H., et al. (2010). Multicenter, randomized, double-blind, active comparator and placebo-controlled trial of a corticotropin-releasing factor receptor-1 antagonist in generalized anxiety disorder. *Depress. Anxiety* 27:417–425.

Cortese, B.M., and Phan, K.L. (2005). The role of glutamate in anxiety and related disorders. *CNS Spectr.* 10:820–830.

Cota, D., Marsicano, G., et al. (2003). The endogenous cannabinoid system affects energy balance via central orexigenic drive and peripheral lipogenesis. *J. Clin. Invest.* 112:423–431.

Cotman, C.W., and Berchtold, N.C. (2002). Exercise: a behavioral intervention to enhance brain health and plasticity. *Trends Neurosci.* 25:295–301.

Counts, S.E., and Mufson, E.J. (2010). Noradrenaline activation of neurotrophic pathways protects against neuronal amyloid toxicity. *J. Neurochem.* 113:649–660.

Cui, H., Sakamoto, H., et al. (2008). Effects of single-prolonged stress on neurons and their afferent inputs in the amygdala. *Neuroscience* 152:703–712.

Culver, J.L., Arena, P.L., et al. (2002). Coping and distress among women under treatment for early stage breast cancer: comparing African Americans, Hispanics and non-Hispanic whites. *Psycho-Oncology* 11:495–504.

Daniels, J.K., Hegadoren, K.M., et al. (2012). Neural correlates and predictive power of trait resilience in an acutely traumatized sample: a pilot investigation. *J. Clin. Psychiatry* 73:327–332.

Danner, D.D., Snowdon, D.A., et al. (2001). Positive emotions in early life and longevity: findings from the nun study. *J. Pers. Soc. Psychol.* 80:804–813.

Davidson, R.J., McEwen, B.S. (2012). Social influences on neuroplasticity: stress and interventions to promote well-being. *Nat. Neurosci.* 15:689–695.

Davis, M. (2006). Neural systems involved in fear and anxiety measured with fear-potentiated startle. *Am. Psychol.* 61:741–756.

de Kloet, E.R., Derijk, R.H., et al. (2007). Therapy insight: is there an imbalanced response of mineralocorticoid and glucocorticoid receptors in depression? *Nat. Clin. Prac.* 3:168–179.

Deaner, S.L., and McConatha, J.T. (1993). The relation of humor to depression and personality. *Psychological Rep.* 72:755–763.

Debiec, J., and LeDoux, J.E. (2006). Noradrenergic signaling in the amygdala contributes to the reconsolidation of fear memory: treatment implications for PTSD. *Ann. NY Acad. Sci.* 1071:521–524.

Dennis, N.A., Cabeza, R., et al. (2011). Brain-derived neurotrophic factor val66met polymorphism and hippocampal activation during episodic encoding and retrieval tasks. *Hippocampus* 21:980–989.

Derijk, R.H., and De Kloet, E.R. (2008). Corticosteroid receptor polymorphisms: determinants of vulnerability and resilience. *Eur. J. Pharmacol.* 583:303–311.

deRoon-Cassini, T.A., de St Aubin, E., et al. (2009). Psychological well-being after spinal cord injury: perception of loss and meaning making. *Rehabil. Psychol.* 54:306–314.

Desantis, S.M., Baker, N.L., et al. (2011). Gender differences in the effect of early life trauma on hypothalamic-pituitary-adrenal axis functioning. *Depress. Anxiety* 28:383–392.

Di, S., Malcher-Lopes, R., et al. (2003). Nongenomic glucocorticoid inhibition via endocannabinoid release in the hypothalamus: a fast feedback mechanism. *J. Neurosci.* 23:4850–4857.

Disner, S.G., Beevers, C.G., et al. (2011). Neural mechanisms of the cognitive model of depression. *Nat. Rev.* 12:467–477.

Domenici, M.R., Azad, S.C., et al. (2006). Cannabinoid receptor type 1 located on presynaptic terminals of principal neurons in the forebrain controls glutamatergic synaptic transmission. *J. Neurosci.* 26:5794–5799.

Drabant, E.M., Hariri, A.R., et al. (2006). Catechol O-methyltransferase val158met genotype and neural mechanisms related to affective arousal and regulation. *Arch. Gen. Psychiatry* 63:1396–1406.

Drabant, E.M., McRae, K., et al. (2009). Individual differences in typical reappraisal use predict amygdala and prefrontal responses. *Biol. Psychiatry* 65:367–373.

Drabant, E.M., Ramel, W., et al. (2012). Neural mechanisms underlying 5-HTTLPR-related sensitivity to acute stress. *Am. J. Psychiatry* 169:397–405.

Drury, S.S., Theall, K.P., et al. (2009). The role of the dopamine transporter (DAT) in the development of PTSD in preschool children. *J. Trauma. Stress* 22:534–539.

Dudai, Y., and Eisenberg, M. (2004). Rites of passage of the engram: reconsolidation and the lingering consolidation hypothesis. *Neuron* 44:93–100.

Dudley, K.J., Li, X., et al. (2011). Epigenetic mechanisms mediating vulnerability and resilience to psychiatric disorders. *Neurosci. Biobehav. Rev.* 35:1544–1551.

Duman, R.S., and Monteggia, L.M. (2006). A neurotrophic model for stress-related mood disorders. *Biol. Psychiatry* 59:1116–1127.

Dunlop, B.W., and Nemeroff, C.B. (2007). The role of dopamine in the pathophysiology of depression. *Arch. Gen. Psychiatry* 64:327–337.

Egan, M.F., Kojima, M., et al. (2003). The BDNF val66met polymorphism affects activity-dependent secretion of BDNF and human memory and hippocampal function. *Cell* 112:257–269.

Eisch, A.J., Bolanos, C.A., et al. (2003). Brain-derived neurotrophic factor in the ventral midbrain-nucleus accumbens pathway: a role in depression. *Biol. Psychiatry* 54:994–1005.

Eisenhardt, D., and Menzel, R. (2007). Extinction learning, reconsolidation and the internal reinforcement hypothesis. *Neurobiol. Learn. Mem.* 87:167–173.

Eva, C., Serra, M., et al. (2006). Physiology and gene regulation of the brain NPY Y1 receptor. *Front. Neuroendocrinol.* 27:308–339.

Fakra, E., Hyde, L.W., et al. (2009). Effects of HTR1A C(-1019)G on amygdala reactivity and trait anxiety. *Arch. Gen. Psychiatry* 66:33–40.

Fava, G.A., Tomba, E. (2009). Increasing psychological well-being and resilience by psychotherapeutic methods. *J. Pers.* 77:1903–1934.

Feder, A., Nestler, E.J., et al. (2009). Psychobiology and molecular genetics of resilience. *Nat. Rev. Neurosci.* 10:446–457.

Feder, A., Skipper, J., et al. (2011). Tryptophan depletion and emotional processing in healthy volunteers at high risk for depression. *Biol. Psychiatry* 69:804–807.

Fehr, E., and Fischbacher, U. (2003). The nature of human altruism. *Nature* 425:785–791.

Fleshner, M., Maier, S.F., et al. (2011). The neurobiology of the stress-resistant brain. *Stress* 14:498–502.

Foa, E.B. (2011). Prolonged exposure therapy: past, present, and future. *Depress. Anxiety* 28:1043–1047.

Folkman, S. (1997). Positive psychological states and coping with severe stress. *Soc. Sci. Med.* 45:1207–1221.

Folkman, S., and Moskowitz, J.T. (2000). Positive affect and the other side of coping. *Am. Psychol.* 55:647–654.

Fontana, A.F., Kerns, R.D., et al. (1989). Support, stress, and recovery from coronary heart disease: a longitudinal causal model. *Health Psychol.* 8:175–193.

Frankl, V.E. (2006). Man's Search for Meaning. (I. Lasch, Trans). Boston: Beacon Press. (Original work published 1959).

Fraser, G.A. (2009). The use of a synthetic cannabinoid in the management of treatment-resistant nightmares in posttraumatic stress disorder (PTSD). *CNS Neurosci. Ther.* 15:84–88.

Fredrickson, B.L. (2001). The role of positive emotions in positive psychology. The broaden-and-build theory of positive emotions. *Am. Psychol.* 56:218–226.

Freidenberg, B.M., Gusmano, R., et al. (2010). Women with PTSD have lower basal salivary cortisol levels later in the day than do men with PTSD: a preliminary study. *Physiol. Behav.* 99:234–236.

Fulton, D. (2006). Reconsolidation: does the past linger on? *J. Neuroscience* 26:10935–10936; discussion 10936.

Gallagher, P., and Young, A. (2002). Cortisol/DHEA ratios in depression. *Neuropsychopharmacol.* 26:410.

Genud, R., Merenlender, A., et al. (2009). DHEA lessens depressive-like behavior via GABA-ergic modulation of the mesolimbic system. *Neuropsychopharmacol.* 34:577–584.

Gerardi, M., Rothbaum, B.O., et al. (2010). Cortisol response following exposure treatment for PTSD in rape victims. *J. Aggress. Maltreat. Trauma* 19:349–356.

Geschwind, N., Peeters, F., et al. (2011). Mindfulness training increases momentary positive emotions and reward experience in adults vulnerable to depression: a randomized controlled trial. *J. Consult. Clin. Psychol.* 79:618–628.

Gill, J., Vythilingam, M., et al. (2008). Low cortisol, high DHEA, and high levels of stimulated TNF-alpha, and IL-6 in women with PTSD. *J. Trauma. Stress* 21:530–539.

Goldin, P.R., McRae, K., et al. (2008). The neural bases of emotion regulation: reappraisal and suppression of negative emotion. *Biol. Psychiatry* 63:577–586.

Goldman, S.L., Kraemer, D.T., et al. (1996). Beliefs about mood moderate the relationship of stress to illness and symptom reporting. *J. Psychosom. Res.* 41:115–128.

Goldstein, L.E., Rasmusson, A.M., et al. (1996). Role of the amygdala in the coordination of behavioral, neuroendocrine, and prefrontal cortical monoamine responses to psychological stress in the rat. *J. Neurosci.* 16:4787–4798.

Gonul, A.S., Kitis, O., et al. (2011). Association of the brain-derived neurotrophic factor Val66Met polymorphism with hippocampus volumes in drug-free depressed patients. *World J. Biol. Psychiatry* 12:110–118.

Goodyer, I.M., Herbert, J., et al. (1998). Adrenal steroid secretion and major depression in 8- to 16-year-olds, III. Influence of cortisol/DHEA ratio at presentation on subsequent rates of disappointing life events and persistent major depression. *Psychol. Med.* 28:265–273.

Grammatopoulos, D.K., and Chrousos, G.P. (2002). Functional characteristics of CRH receptors and potential clinical applications of CRH-receptor antagonists. *Trends Endocrin. Metab.* 13:436–444.

Greenwood, B.N., Foley, T.E., et al. (2003). Freewheel running prevents learned helplessness/behavioral depression: Role of dorsal raphe serotonergic neurons. *J. Neurosci.* 23:2889–2898.

Griffin, M.G., Resick, P.A., et al. (2005). Enhanced cortisol suppression following dexamethasone administration in domestic violence survivors. *Am. J. Psychiatry* 162:1192–1199.

Gross, J.J. (2002). Emotion regulation: affective, cognitive, and social consequences. *Psychophysiol.* 39:281–291.

Gustafson, E.L., Smith, K.E., et al. (1996). Distribution of a rat galanin receptor mRNA in rat brain. *Neuroreport.* 7:953–957.

Gutman, A.R., Yang, Y., et al. (2008). The role of neuropeptide Y in the expression and extinction of fear-potentiated startle. *J. Neurosci.* 28:12682–12690.

Haas, A.P., and Hendin, H. (1984). Wounds of War: The Psychological Aftermath of Combat in Vietnam. New York: Basic Books.

Hall, J., Thomas, K.L., et al. (2001). Fear memory retrieval induces CREB phosphorylation and Fos expression within the amygdala. *Eur. J. Neurosci.* 13:1453–1458.

Hankin, B.L., Nederhof, E., et al. (2011). Differential susceptibility in youth: evidence that 5-HTTLPR X positive parenting is associated with positive affect "for better and worse." *Transl. Psychiatry* 1(10):e44.

Harbaugh, W.T., Mayr, U., et al. (2007). Neural responses to taxation and voluntary giving reveal motives for charitable donations. *Science* 316:1622–1625.

Haren, M.T., Malmstrom, T.K., et al. (2007). Lower serum DHEAS levels are associated with a higher degree of physical disability and depressive symptoms in middle-aged to older African American women. *Maturitas* 57:347–360.

Hariri, A.R., Drabant, E.M., et al. (2005). A susceptibility gene for affective disorders and the response of the human amygdala. *Arch. Gen. Psychiatry* 62:146–152.

Harvey, B.H., and Shahid, M. (2012). Metabotropic and ionotropic glutamate receptors as neurobiological targets in anxiety and stress-related disorders: focus on pharmacology and preclinical translational models. *Pharmacol. Biochem. Behav.* 100:775–800.

Harvey, P.O., Fossati, P., et al. (2005). Cognitive control and brain resources in major depression: an fMRI study using the n-back task. *NeuroImage* 26:860–869.

Hasler, G., Drevets, W.C., et al. (2004). Discovering endophenotypes for major depression. *Neuropsychopharmacol.* 29:1765–1781.

Heilig, M. (1995). Antisense inhibition of neuropeptide Y (NPY)-Y1 receptor expression blocks the anxiolytic-like action of NPY in amygdala and paradoxically increases feeding. *Regul. Pept.* 59:201–205.

Heilig, M. (2004). The NPY system in stress, anxiety and depression. *Neuropeptides* 38:213–224.

Heilig, M., Koob, G.F., et al. (1994). Corticotropin-releasing factor and neuropeptide-y: role in emotional integration. *Trends Neurosci.* 17:80–85.

Heilig, M., McLeod, S., et al. (1993). Anxiolytic-like action of neuropeptide Y: mediation by Y1 receptors in amygdala, and dissociation from food intake effects. *Neuropsychopharmacol.* 8:357–363.

Heim, C., Newport, D.J., et al. (2000). Pituitary-adrenal and autonomic responses to stress in women after sexual and physical abuse in childhood. *JAMA* 284:592–597.

Heinz, A., and Smolka, M.N. (2006). The effects of catechol O- methyltransferase genotype on brain activation elicited by affective stimuli and cognitive tasks. *Rev. Neurosci.* 17:359–367.

Heisler, L.K., Chu, H.M., et al. (1998). Elevated anxiety and antidepressant-like responses in serotonin 5-HT1A receptor mutant mice. *Proc. Natl. Acad. Sci. USA* 95:15049–15054.

Hendriksen, H., Bink, D.I., et al. (2012). Re-exposure and environmental enrichment reveal NPY-Y1 as a possible target for post-traumatic stress disorder. *Neuropharmacol.* 63:733–742.

Herkenham, M., Lynn, A.B., et al. (1991). Characterization and localization of cannabinoid receptors in rat brain: a quantitative *in vitro* autoradiographic study. *J. Neurosci.* 11:563–583.

Herry, C., and Garcia, R. (2002). Prefrontal cortex long-term potentiation, but not long-term depression, is associated with the maintenance of extinction of learned fear in mice. *J. Neurosci.* 22:577–583.

Hill, M.N., Barr, A.M., et al. (2007). Electroconvulsive shock treatment differentially modulates cortical and subcortical endocannabinoid activity. *J. Neurochem.* 103:47–56.

Hill, M.N., and Gorzalka, B.B. (2009a). The endocannabinoid system and the treatment of mood and anxiety disorders. *CNS Neurol. Disord. Drug Targets* 8:451–458.

Hill, M.N., and Gorzalka, B.B. (2009b). Impairments in endocannabinoid signaling and depressive illness. *JAMA* 301:1165–1166.

Hill, M.N., Miller, G.E., et al. (2008). Serum endocannabinoid content is altered in females with depressive disorders: a preliminary report. *Pharmacopsychiatry* 41:48–53.

Hill, M.N., and Tasker, J.G. (2012). Endocannabinoid signaling, glucocorticoid-mediated negative feedback, and regulation of the hypothalamic-pituitary-adrenal axis. *Neuroscience* 204:5–16.

Hillard, C.J. (2000). Biochemistry and pharmacology of the endocannabinoids arachidonylethanolamide and 2-arachidonylglycerol. *Prostaglandins Other Lipid Mediat.* 61:3–18.

Hobfoll, S.E., Palmieri, P.A., et al. (2009). Trajectories of resilience, resistance, and distress during ongoing terrorism: the case of Jews and Arabs in Israel. *J. Consult. Clin. Psychol.* 77:138–148.

Hoexter, M.Q., Fadel, G., et al. (2012). Higher striatal dopamine transporter density in PTSD: an *in vivo* SPECT study with [(99m)Tc]TRODAT-1. *Psychopharmacology (Berl.)* 224 (2):337–345.

Hofmann, S.G., Meuret, A.E., et al. (2006). Augmentation of exposure therapy with D-cycloserine for social anxiety disorder. *Arch. Gen. Psychiatry* 63:298–304.

Hoge, E.A., Worthington, J.J., et al. (2012). Effect of acute posttrauma propranolol on PTSD outcome and physiological responses during script-driven imagery. *CNS Neurosci. Ther.* 18:21–27.

Holmes, A., Yang, R.J., et al. (2002). Evaluation of an anxiety-related phenotype in galanin overexpressing transgenic mice. *J. Mol. Neurosci.* 18:151–165.

Holmes, F.E., Bacon, A., et al. (2003). Transgenic overexpression of galanin in the dorsal root ganglia modulates pain related behavior. *Proc. Natl. Acad. Sci. USA* 100:6180–6185.

Homberg, J.R., and Lesch, K.P. (2011). Looking on the bright side of serotonin transporter gene variation. *Biol. Psychiatry* 69:513–519.

Hsu, D.T., Mickey, B.J., et al. (2012). Variation in the corticotropin-releasing hormone receptor 1 (CRHR1) gene influences fMRI signal responses during emotional stimulus processing. *J. Neurosci.* 32:3253–3260.

Huang, E.J., and Reichardt, L.F. (2001). Neurotrophins: roles in neuronal development and function. *Annu. Rev. Neurosci.* 24:677–736.

Husum, H., and Mathe, A.A. (2002). Early life stress changes concentrations of neuropeptide Y and corticotropin-releasing hormone in adult rat brain. Lithium treatment modifies these changes. *Neuropsychopharmacol.* 27:756–764.

Huuhka, K., Anttila, S., et al. (2008). Dopamine 2 receptor C957T and catechol-o-methyltransferase Val158Met polymorphisms are associated with treatment response in electroconvulsive therapy. *Neurosci. Lett.* 448:79–83.

Inslicht, S.S., Marmar, C.R., et al. (2006). Increased cortisol in women with intimate partner violence-related posttraumatic stress disorder. *Ann. NY Acad. Sci.* 1071:428–429.

Isen, A.M., Daubman, K.A., and Nowicki, G.P. (1987). Positive affect facilitates creative problem-solving. *J. Pers. Soc. Psychol.* 52:1122–1131.

Ising, M., Depping, A.M., et al. (2008). Polymorphisms in the FKBP5 gene region modulate recovery from psychosocial stress in healthy controls. *Eur. J. Neurosci.* 28:389–398.

Ivy, A.S., Rex, C.S., et al. (2010). Hippocampal dysfunction and cognitive impairments provoked by chronic early-life stress involve excessive activation of CRH receptors. *J. Neurosci.* 30:13005–13015.

Jabbi, M., Kema, I.P., et al. (2007). Catechol O- methyltransferase polymorphism and susceptibility to major depressive disorder modulates psychological stress response. *Psychiatr. Genet.* 17:183–193.

Janssen, J., Hulshoff Pol, H.E., et al. (2007). Hippocampal volume and subcortical white matter lesions in late-life depression: comparison of early- and late-onset depression. *J. Neurol. Neurosurg. Psychiatry* 78(6):638–640.

Jhaveri, D.J., Mackay, E.W., et al. (2010). Norepinephrine directly activates adult hippocampal precursors via beta3-adrenergic receptors. *J. Neurosci.* 30:2795–2806.

Johnstone, T., van Reekum, C.M., et al. (2007). Failure to regulate: counterproductive recruitment of top-down prefrontal-subcortical circuitry in major depression. *J. Neurosci.* 27:8877–8884.

Jordan, B.K., Schlenger, W.E., et al. (1991). Lifetime and current prevalence of specific psychiatric disorders among Vietnam veterans and controls. *Arch. Gen. Psychiatry* 48:207–215.

Josselyn, S.A., Shi, C., et al. (2001). Long-term memory is facilitated by cAMP response element-binding protein overexpression in the amygdala. *J. Neurosci.* 21:2404–2412.

Jovanovic, T., Norrholm, S.D., et al. (2010). Fear potentiation is associated with hypothalamic-pituitary-adrenal axis function in PTSD. *Psychoneuroendocrinology* 35:846–857.

Kaplan, G.B., and Moore, K.A. (2011). The use of cognitive enhancers in animal models of fear extinction. *Pharmacol. Biochem. Behav.* 99:217–228.

Karatsoreos, I.N., and McEwen, B.S. (2011). Psychobiological allostasis: resistance, resilience and vulnerability. *Trends Cogn. Sci.* 15:576–584.

Karg, K., Burmeister, M., et al. (2011). The serotonin transporter promoter variant (5-HTTLPR): stress, and depression meta-analysis revisited: evidence of genetic moderation. *Arch. Gen. Psychiatry* 68:444–454.

Karl, T., Burne, T.H., et al. (2006). Effect of Y1 receptor deficiency on motor activity, exploration, and anxiety. *Behav. Brain Res.* 167:87–93.

Karlsson, R.M., and Holmes, A. (2006). Galanin as a modulator of anxiety and depression and a therapeutic target for affective disease. *Amino Acids* 31:231–239.

Kasen, S., Wickramaratne, P., et al. (2012). Religiosity and resilience in persons at high risk for major depression. *Psychol. Med.* 42:509–519.

Kask, A., Rago, L., et al. (1997). Alpha-helical CRF(9-41) prevents anxiogenic-like effect of NPY Y1 receptor antagonist BIBP3226 in rats. *Neuroreport* 8:3645–3647.

Kendler, K.S., Kuhn, J.W., et al. (2005). The interaction of stressful life events and a serotonin transporter polymorphism in the prediction of episodes of major depression: a replication. *Arch. Gen. Psychiatry* 62:529–535.

Kent, J.M., Mathew, S.J., et al. (2002). Molecular targets in the treatment of anxiety. *Biol. Psychiatry* 52:1008–1030.

Kessler, R.C., Sonnega, A., et al. (1995). Posttraumatic stress disorder in the National Comorbidity Survey. *Arch. Gen. Psychiatry* 52:1048–1060.

Khoshaba, D.M., and Maddi, S.R. (1999). Early experiences in hardiness development. *Consul. Psychol. J.* 51:106–116.

Kida, S., Josselyn, S.A., et al. (2002). CREB required for the stability of new and reactivated fear memories. *Nat. Neurosci.* 5:348–355.

Kim, J.M., Stewart, R., et al. (2007). Interactions between life stressors and susceptibility genes (5-HTTLPR and BDNF) on depression in Korean elders. *Biol. Psychiatry* 62:423–428.

Kimonides, V.G., Khatibi, N.H., et al. (1998). Dehydroepiandrosterone (DHEA) and DHEA-sulfate (DHEAS) protect hippocampal neurons against excitatory amino acid-induced neurotoxicity. *Proc. Natl. Acad. Sci. USA* 95:1852–1857.

Klemenhagen, K.C., Gordon, J.A., et al. (2006). In HT1A receptor. *Neuropsychopharmacol.* 31:101–111.

Klohnen, E.C. (1996). Conceptual analysis and measurement of the construct of ego-resiliency. *J. Personal Soc. Psychology* 70:1067–1079.

Knutson, B., and Cooper, J.C. (2005). Functional magnetic resonance imaging of reward prediction. *Curr. Opin. Neurol.* 18:411–417.

Koenig, H.G., George, L.K., et al. (1998). Religiosity and remission of depression in medically ill older patients. *Am. J. Psychiatry* 155:536–542.

Koike, H., Iijima, M., et al. (2011). Involvement of AMPA receptor in both the rapid and sustained antidepressant-like effects of ketamine in animal models of depression. *Behav. Brain Res.* 224:107–111.

Kozlovsky, N., Matar, M.A., et al. (2009). The role of the galaninergic system in modulating stress-related responses in an animal model of posttraumatic stress disorder. *Biol. Psychiatry* 65:383–391.

Kremen, W.S., Koenen, K.C., et al. (2012). Twin studies of posttraumatic stress disorder: differentiating vulnerability factors from sequelae. *Neuropharmacol.* 62:647–653.

Krishnan, V., Han, M.H., et al. (2007). Molecular adaptations underlying susceptibility and resistance to social defeat in brain reward regions. *Cell* 131 (2):391–404.

Kuhnen, C.M., and Knutson, B. (2005). The neural basis of financial risk taking. *Neuron* 47:763–770.

Lanzenberger, R., Wadsak, W., et al. (2010). Cortisol plasma levels in social anxiety disorder patients correlate with serotonin-1A receptor binding in limbic brain regions. *Int. J. Neuropsychopharmacol.* 13:1129–1143.

Lavretsky, H., Siddarth, P., et al. (2008). The effects of the dopamine and serotonin transporter polymorphisms on clinical features and treatment response in geriatric depression: a pilot study. *Int. J. Geriatr. Psychiatry* 23:55–59.

Lawford, B.R., Young, R., et al. (2006). The D2 dopamine receptor (DRD2) gene is associated with co-morbid depression, anxiety and social dysfunction in untreated veterans with post-traumatic stress disorder. *Eur. Psychiatry* 21:180–185.

LeDoux, J.E. (2000). Emotion circuits in the brain. *Annu. Rev. Neurosci.* 23:155–184.

LeDoux, J.E., and Gorman, J.M. (2002). A call to action: overcoming anxiety through active coping. *Am. J. Psychiatry* 159:171–171.

Le Maitre, T.W., Xia, S., et al. (2011). Galanin receptor 2 overexpressing mice display an antidepressive-like phenotype: possible involvement of the subiculum. *Neuroscience* 190:270–288.

Lee, J.L., Milton, A.L., et al. (2006). Reconsolidation and extinction of conditioned fear: inhibition and potentiation. *J. Neuroscience* 26:10051–10056.

Lee, V., Robin Cohen, S., et al. (2006). Meaning-making intervention during breast or colorectal cancer treatment improves self-esteem, optimism, and self-efficacy. *Soc. Sci. Med.* 62:3133–3155.

Li, N., Lee, B., et al. (2010). mTOR-dependent synapse formation underlies the rapid antidepressant effects of NMDA antagonists *Science* 329:959–964.

Li, X., Need, A.B., et al. (2006). Metabotropic glutamate 5 receptor antagonism is associated with antidepressant-like effects in mice. *J. Pharmacol. Exp. Ther.* 319:254–259.

Liu, D., Diorio, J., et al. (1997). Maternal care, hippocampal glucocorticoid receptors, and hypothalamic–pituitary–adrenal responses to stress. *Science* 277:1659–1662.

Lu, X., Ross, B., et al. (2008). Phenotypic analysis of GalR2 knockout mice in anxiety- and depression-related behavioral tests. *Neuropeptides* 42:387–397.

Lyons, D.M., Parker, K.J., et al. (2009). Developmental cascades linking stress inoculation, arousal regulation, and resilience. *Front. Behav. Neurosci.* 3:32.

Maddi, S.R. (1999). Hardiness and optimism as expressed in coping patterns. *Consul. Psychology J.* 51:95–105.

Maddi, S.R. (2008). The courage and strategies of hardiness as helpful in growing despite major, disruptive stresses. *Am. Psychol.* 63:563–564.

Maestripieri, D., Lindell, S.G., et al. (2007). Intergenerational transmission of maternal behavior in rhesus macaques and its underlying mechanisms. *Dev. Psychobiol.* 49:165–171.

Mahan, A.L., and Ressler, K.J. (2012). Fear conditioning, synaptic plasticity and the amygdala: implications for posttraumatic stress disorder. *Trends Neurosci.* 35:24–35.

Makino, S., Baker, R.A., et al. (2000). Differential regulation of neuropeptide Y mRNA expression in the arcuate nucleus and locus coeruleus by stress and antidepressants. *J. Neuroendocrinol.* 12:387–395.

Maninger, N., Capitanio, J.P., et al. (2010). Acute and chronic stress increase DHEAS concentrations in rhesus monkeys. *Psychoneuroendocrinology* 35:1055–1062.

Manne, S., Duhamel, K., et al. (2003). Coping and the course of mother's depressive symptoms during and after pediatric bone marrow transplantation. *J. Am. Acad. Child Adol. Psychiatry* 42:1055–1068.

Martin, M., Ledent, C., et al. (2002). Involvement of CB1 cannabinoid receptors in emotional behaviour. *Psychopharmacology (Berl.)* 159:379–387.

Martin-Soelch, C., Leenders, K.L., et al. (2001). Reward mechanisms in the brain and their role in dependence: evidence from neurophysiological and neuroimaging studies. *Brain Res. Brain Res. Rev.* 36:139–149.

Masten, A.S. (2001). Ordinary magic. Resilience processes in development. *Am. Psychol.* 56:227–238.

Masten, A.S., Coatsworth, J.D. (1998). The development of competence in favorable and unfavorable environments. Lessons from research on successful children. *Am. Psychol.* 53:205–220.

Masten, A.S., and Obradovic, J. (2006). Competence and resilience in development. *Ann. NY Acad. Sci.* 1094:13–27.

Mathew, S.J., Shah, A., et al. (2012). Ketamine for treatment-resistant unipolar depression: current evidence. *CNS Drugs* 26:189–204.

Mathews, D.C., Henter, I.D., et al. (2012). Targeting the glutamatergic system to treat major depressive disorder: rationale and progress to date. *Drugs* 72:1313–1333.

McCabe, C., Woffindale, C., et al. (2012). Neural processing of reward and punishment in young people at increased familial risk of depression. *Biol. Psychiatry* 72:588–594.

McCormack, K., Sanchez, M.M., et al. (2006). Maternal care patterns and behavioral development of rhesus macaque abused infants in the first 6 months of life. *Dev. Psychobiol.* 48:537–550.

McCullough, M.E., Hoyt, W.T., et al. (2000). Religious involvement and mortality: a meta-analytic review. *Health Psychology* 19:211–222.

Mehta, D., Gonik, M., et al. (2011). Using polymorphisms in FKBP5 to define biologically distinct subtypes of posttraumatic stress disorder: evidence from endocrine and gene expression studies. *Arch. Gen. Psychiatry* 68:901–910.

Mercer, K.B., Orcutt, H.K., et al. (2012). Acute and posttraumatic stress symptoms in a prospective gene x environment study of a university campus shooting. *Arch. Gen. Psychiatry* 69:89–97.

Metzger, L.J., Carson, M.A., et al. (2008). Basal and suppressed salivary cortisol in female Vietnam nurse veterans with and without PTSD. *Psychiatry Res.* 161:330–335.

Mifsud, K.R., Gutierrez-Mecinas, M., et al. (2011). Epigenetic mechanisms in stress and adaptation. *Brain Behav. Immun.* 25:1305–1315.

Mitsukawa, K., Lu, X., et al. (2009). Bidirectional regulation of stress responses by galanin in mice: involvement of galanin receptor subtype 1. *Neuroscience* 160:837–846.

Mobbs, D., Greicius, M.D., et al. (2003). Humor modulates the mesolimbic reward centers. *Neuron* 40:1041–1048.

Moldrich, G., and Wenger, T. (2000). Localization of the CB1 cannabinoid receptor in the rat brain. An immunohistochemical study. *Peptides* 21:1735–1742.

Moller, C., Sommer, W., et al. (1999). Anxiogenic-like action of galanin after intra-amygdala administration in the rat. *Neuropsychopharmacol.* 21:507–512.

Monk, C.S., Klein, R.G., et al. (2008). Amygdala and nucleus accumbens activation to emotional facial expressions in children and adolescents at risk for major depression. *Am. J. Psychiatry* 165:90–98.

Montag, C., Reuter, M., et al. (2008). The BDNF Val66Met polymorphism affects amygdala activity in response to emotional stimuli: evidence from a genetic imaging study. *NeuroImage* 42:1554–1559.

Moos, R.H., and Schaefer, J.A. (1993). Coping resources and processes: current concepts and measures. In: Goldberger, L., and Breznits, S., eds. Handbook of Stress: Theoretical and Clinical Aspects. New York: Free Press, pp. 234–257.

Morfin, R., and Starka, L. (2001). Neurosteroid 7-hydroxylation products in the brain. *Int. Rev. Neurobiol.* 46:79–95.

Morgan, C.A., III, Rasmusson A., et al. (2009). Relationships among plasma dehydroepiandrosterone and dehydroepiandrosterone sulfate, cortisol, symptoms of dissociation and objective performance in humans exposed to underwater navigation stress. *Biol. Psychiatry* 66:334–340.

Morgan, C.A., III, Southwick, S., et al. (2004). Relationships among plasma dehydroepiandrosterone sulfate and cortisol levels, symptoms of dissociation, and objective performance in humans exposed to acute stress. *Arch. Gen. Psychiatry* 61:819–825.

Morgan, C.A., III, Wang, S., et al. (2000). Hormone profiles in humans experiencing military survival training. *Biol. Psychiatry* 47:891–901.

Morrow, B.A., Elsworth, J.D., et al. (1999). The role of mesoprefrontal dopamine neurons in the acquisition and expression of conditioned fear in the rat. *Neurosci.* 92:553–564.

Murphy, F.C., Rubinsztein, J.S., et al. (2001). Decision making cognition in mania and depression. *Psycholog. Med.* 31:679–693.

Murrough, J.W., Charney, D.S. (2010). Cracking the moody brain: lifting the mood with ketamine. *Nat. Med.* 16:1384–1385.

Myers, K.M., and Davis, M. (2007). Mechanisms of fear extinction. *Mol. Psychiatry* 12:120–150.

Myers, K.M., Ressler, K.J., et al. (2006). Different mechanisms of fear extinction dependent on length of time since fear acquisition. *Learn Mem.* 13:216–223.

Nagin, D.S., and Odgers, C.L. (2010). Group-based trajectory modeling in clinical research. *Annu. Rev. Clin. Psychol.* 6:109–138.

Nemeroff, C.B. (2002). Recent advances in the neurobiology of depression. *Psychopharmacol. Bull.* 36(Suppl 2):6–23.

Neufeld-Cohen, A., Kelly, P.A., et al. (2012). Chronic activation of corticotropin-releasing factor type 2 receptors reveals a key role for 5-HT1A receptor responsiveness in mediating behavioral and serotonergic responses to stressful challenge. *Biol. Psychiatry* 72 (6):437–447.

Nguyen, N.K., Sartori, S.B., et al. (2009). Effect of neuropeptide Y Y2 receptor deletion on emotional stress-induced neuronal activation in mice. *Synapse* 63:236–246.

Nikolova, Y., Bogdan, R., et al. (2012). Perception of a naturalistic stressor interacts with 5-HTTLPR/rs25531 genotype and gender to impact reward responsiveness. *Neuropsychobiology* 65(1):45–54.

Nissen, S.E., Nicholls, S.J., et al. (2008). Effect of rimonabant on progression of atherosclerosis in patients with abdominal obesity and coronary artery disease: the STRADIVARIUS randomized controlled trial. *JAMA* 299:1547–1560.

Norris, F.H., Tracy, M., et al. (2009). Looking for resilience: understanding the longitudinal trajectories of responses to stress. *Soc. Sci. Med.* 68:2190–2198.

Oberlander, T.F., Weinberg, J., et al. (2008). Prenatal exposure to maternal depression, neonatal methylation of human glucocorticoid receptor gene (NR3C1) and infant cortisol stress responses. *Epigenetics* 3:97–106.

Ochsner, K.N., Ray, R.D., et al. (2004). For better or for worse: neural systems supporting the cognitive down- and up-regulation of negative emotion. *NeuroImage* 23:483–499.

Onur, O.A., Walter, H., et al. (2009). Noradrenergic enhancement of amygdala responses to fear. *Soc. Cogn. Affect. Neurosci.* 4:119–126.

Otte, C., Neylan, T.C., et al. (2005). Association between childhood trauma and catecholamine response to psychological stress in police academy recruits. *Biol. Psychiatry* 57:27–32.

Overmier, J.B., and Seligman, M.E. (1967). Effects of inescapable shock upon subsequent escape and avoidance responding. *J. Comp. Physiol. Psychol.* 63:28–33.

Oyarzun, J.P., Lopez-Barroso, D., et al. (2012). Updating fearful memories with extinction training during reconsolidation: a human study using auditory aversive stimuli. *PLoS One* 7:e38849.

Parker, K.J., Buckmaster, C.L., et al. (2005). Mild early life stress enhances prefrontal-dependent response inhibition in monkeys. *Biol. Psychiatry* 57:848–855.

Parker, K.J., Buckmaster, C.L., et al. (2004). Prospective investigation of stress inoculation in young monkeys. *Arch. Gen. Psychiatry* 61:933–941.

Parks, C.L., Robinson, P.S., et al. (1998). Increased anxiety of mice lacking the serotonin1A receptor. *Proc. Natl. Acad. Sci. USA* 95:10734–10739.

Pezawas, L., Meyer-Lindenberg, A., et al. (2005). 5-HTTLPR polymorphism impacts human cingulate-amygdala interactions: a genetic susceptibility mechanism for depression. *Nat. Neurosci.* 8:828–834.

Phillips, M.L., Drevets, W.C., et al. (2003a). Neurobiology of emotion perception I: the neural basis of normal emotion perception. *Biol. Psychiatry* 54:504–514.

Phillips, M.L., Drevets, W.C., et al. (2003b). Neurobiology of emotion perception II: implications for major psychiatric disorders. *Biol. Psychiatry* 54:515–528.

Pickens, C.L., Adams-Deutsch, T., et al. (2009). Effect of pharmacological manipulations of neuropeptide Y and corticotropin-releasing factor neurotransmission on incubation of conditioned fear. *Neuroscience* 164:1398–1406.

Pieribone, V.A., Brodin, L., et al. (1992). Differential expression of mRNAs for neuropeptide Y-related peptides in rat nervous tissues: possible evolutionary conservation. *J. Neurosci.* 12:3361–3371.

Pietrzak, R.H., Harpaz-Rotem, I., et al. (2011). Cognitive-behavioral coping strategies associated with combat-related PTSD in treatment-seeking OEF-OIF Veterans. *Psychiatry Res.* 189:251–258.

Pietrzak, R.H., and Southwick, S.M. (2011). Psychological resilience in OEF-OIF veterans: application of a novel classification approach and examination of demographic and psychosocial correlates. *J. Affect. Disord.* 133:560–568.

Pinnock, S.B., Lazic, S.E., et al. (2009). Synergistic effects of dehydroepiandrosterone and fluoxetine on proliferation of progenitor cells in the dentate gyrus of the adult male rat. *Neuroscience* 158:1644–1651.

Pitman, R.K., Sanders, K.M., et al. (2002). Pilot study of secondary prevention of posttraumatic stress disorder with propranolol. *Biol. Psychiatry* 51:189–192.

Pliakas, A.M., Carlson, R.R., et al. (2001). Altered responsiveness to cocaine and increased immobility in the forced swim test associated with elevated cAMP response element-binding protein expression in nucleus accumbens. *J. Neurosci.* 21:7397–7403.

Popoli, M., Yan, Z., et al. (2011). The stressed synapse: the impact of stress and glucocorticoids on glutamate transmission. *Nat. Rev. Neurosci.* 13:22–37.

Przybyslawski, J., Roullet, P., et al. (1999). Attenuation of emotional and nonemotional memories after their reactivation: role of beta adrenergic receptors. *J. Neurosci.* 19:6623–6628.

Rabkin, J.G., McElhiney, M.C., et al. (2006). Placebo controlled trial of dehydroepiandrosterone (DHEA) for treatment of nonmajor depression in patients with HIV/AIDS. *Am. J. Psychiatry* 163:59–66.

Rachman, S. (1979). Concept of required helpfulness. *Behav. Res. Ther.* 17:1–6.

Radant, A.D., Dobie, D.J., et al. (2009). Adrenocortical responsiveness to infusions of physiological doses of ACTH is not altered in posttraumatic stress disorder. *Front. Behav. Neurosci.* 3:40.

Radley, J.J., Kabbaj, M., et al. (2011). Stress risk factors and stress-related pathology: neuroplasticity, epigenetics and endophenotypes. *Stress* 14:481–497.

Rasmusson, A.M., Vasek, J., et al. (2004). An increased capacity for adrenal DHEA release is associated with decreased avoidance and negative mood symptoms in women with PTSD. *Neuropsychopharmacol.* 29:1546–1557.

Rattiner, L.M., Davis, M., et al. (2004). Brain-derived neurotrophic factor and tyrosine kinase receptor B involvement in amygdala-dependent fear conditioning. *J. Neurosci.* 24:4796–4806.

Reivich, K.J., Seligman, M.E., et al. (2011). Master resilience training in the U.S. Army. *Am. Psychol.* 66:25–34.

Resick, P.A. (2001). Clinical Psychology: A Modular Course. Philadelphia, PA: Taylor & Francis Group.

Ressler, K.J., Bradley, B., et al. (2010). Polymorphisms in CRHR1 and the serotonin transporter loci: gene x gene x environment interactions on depressive symptoms. *Am. J. Med. Genet. B Neuropsychiatr. Genet.* 153B:812–824.

Ressler, K.J., Mercer, K.B., et al. (2011). Post-traumatic stress disorder is associated with PACAP and PAC1 receptor. *Nature* 470:492–497.

Ressler, K.J., Rothbaum, B.O., et al. (2004). Cognitive enhancers as adjuncts to psychotherapy: use of D-cycloserine in phobic individuals to facilitate extinction of fear. *Arch. Gen. Psychiatry* 61:1136–1144.

Risold, P.Y., and Swanson, L.W. (1997). Chemoarchitecture of the rat lateral septal nucleus. *Brain Res. Brain Res. Rev.* 24:91–113.

Rizzolatti, G., Craighero, L. (2004). The mirror-neuron system. *Annu. Rev. Neurosci.* 27:169–192.

Robinson, O.J., Cools, R., et al. (2012). Tryptophan depletion disinhibits punishment but not reward prediction: implications for resilience. *Psychopharmacology (Berl.)* 219:599–605.

Rodrigues, S.M., Schafe, G.E., et al.. (2001). Intraamygdala blockade of the NR2B subunit of the NMDA receptor disrupts the acquisition but not the expression of fear conditioning. *J. Neurosci.* 21:6889–6896.

Roozendaal, B., Schelling, G., et al. (2008). Corticotropin-releasing factor in the basolateral amygdala enhances memory consolidation via an interaction with the beta-adrenoceptor-cAMP pathway: dependence on glucocorticoid receptor activation. *J. Neurosci.* 28:6642–6651.

Rosenfeld, R.S., Hellman, L., et al. (1971). Dehydroisoandrosterone is secreted episodically and synchronously with cortisol by normal man. *J. Clin. Endocrinol. Metab.* 33:87–92.

Roth, T.L., Lubin, F.D., et al. (2009). Lasting epigenetic influence of early-life adversity on the BDNF gene. *Biol. Psychiatry* 65:760–769.

Royer, S., Martina, M., and et al. (2000). Bistable behavior of inhibitory neurons controlling impulse traffic through the amygdala: role of a slowly deinactivating K+ current. *J. Neurosci.* 20:9034–9039.

Ruini, C., Fava, G.A. (2012). Role of well-being therapy in achieving a balanced and individualized path to optimal functioning. *Clin. Psychol. Psychother.* 19:291–304.

Russo, S.J., Murrough, J.W., et al. (2012). Neurobiology of resilience. *Nat. Neurosci.* 15(11):1475–1484.

Rutter, M. (1993). Resilience: some conceptual considerations. *J. Adolesc. Health* 14:626–631.

Rutter, M. (2006). Implications of resilience concepts for scientific understanding. *Ann. NY Acad. Sci.* 1094:1–12.

Rutter, M. (2012). Resilience as a dynamic concept. *Dev. Psychopathol.* 24:335–344.

Sah, R., and Geracioti, T.D. (2012). Neuropeptide Y and posttraumatic stress disorder. *Mol. Psychiatry*:1–10.

Sajdyk, T.J., Fitz, S.D., et al. (2006). The role of neuropeptide Y in the amygdala on corticotropin-releasing factor receptor-mediated behavioral stress responses in the rat. *Stress* 9:21–28.

Sanacora, G., Zarate, C.A., et al. (2008). Targeting the glutamatergic system to develop novel, improved therapeutics for mood disorders. *Nat. Rev. Drug Discov.* 7:426–437.

Schafe, G.E., Doyere, V., et al. (2005). Tracking the fear engram: the lateral amygdala is an essential locus of fear memory storage. *J. Neurosci.* 25:10010–10014.

Schafe, G.E., Nader, K., et al. (2001). Memory consolidation of Pavlovian fear conditioning: a cellular and molecular perspective. *Trends Neurosci.* 24:540–546.

Scheier, M.F., Matthews, K.A., et al. (1989). Dispositional optimism and recovery from coronary artery bypass surgery: the beneficial effects on physical and psychological wellbeing. *J. Pers. Soc. Psychol.* 57:1024–1040.

Schelling, G., Roozendaal, B., et al. (2006). Efficacy of hydrocortisone in preventing posttraumatic stress disorder following critical illness and major surgery. *Ann. NY Acad. Sci.* 1071:46–53.

Scherrer, J.F., True, W.R., et al. (2000). Evidence for genetic influences common and specific to symptoms of generalized anxiety and panic. *J. Affect. Disord.* 57:25–35.

Schiller, D., Levy, I., et al. (2008). From fear to safety and back: reversal of fear in the human brain. *J. Neurosci.* 28:11517–11525.

Schiller, D., Monfils, M.H., et al. (2010). Preventing the return of fear in humans using reconsolidation update mechanisms. *Nature* 463:49–53.

Schiller, D., Raio, C.M., et al. (2012). Extinction training during the reconsolidation window prevents recovery of fear. *J. Vis. Exp.* 66:e3893.

Schulte-Rüther, M., Markowitsch, H.J., et al. (2007). Mirror neuron and theory of mind mechanisms involved in face-to-face interactions: a functional magnetic resonance imaging approach to empathy. *J. Cogn. Neurosci.* 19 (8):1354–1372.

Schultz, W. (2002). Getting formal with dopamine and reward. *Neuron* 36:241–263.

Sciolino, N.R., and Holmes, P.V. (2012). Exercise offers anxiolytic potential: a role for stress and brain noradrenergic-galaninergic mechanisms. *Neurosci. Biobehav. Rev.* 36 (9):1965–1984.

Seckl, J.R., and Meaney, M.J. (2006). Glucocorticoid "programming" and PTSD risk. *Ann. NY Acad. Sci.* 1071:351–378.

Seligman, M.E., and Maier, S.F. (1967). Failure to escape traumatic shock. *J. Exp. Psychol.* 74:1–9.

Seligman, M.E., Steen, T.A., et al. (2005). Positive psychology progress: empirical validation of interventions. *Am. Psychol.* 60:410–421.

Sevcik, J., Finta, E.P., et al. (1993). Galanin receptors inhibit the spontaneous firing of locus coeruleus neurons and interact with mu-opioid receptors. *Eur. J. Pharmacol.* 230:223–230.

Siebert, A. (1996). The Survivor Personality: Why Some People are Stronger, Smarter, and More Skillful at Handling Life's Difficulties...and How You Can Be, Too. New York: Berkely.

Sigurdsson, T., Doyere, V., et al. (2007). Long-term potentiation in the amygdala: a cellular mechanism of fear learning and memory. *Neuropharmacol.* 52:215–227.

Silver, R.-C., Holman, E.A., et al. (2002). Nationwide longitudinal study of psychological responses to September 11. *JAMA* 288:1235–1244.

Smolka, M.N., Schumann, G., et al. (2005). Catechol-Omethyltransferase val158met genotype affects processing of emotional stimuli in the amygdala and prefrontal cortex. *J. Neurosci.* 25:836–842.

Sotres-Bayon, F., Bush, D.E., et al. (2007). Acquisition of fear extinction requires activation of NR2B-containing NMDA receptors in the lateral amygdala. *Neuropsychopharmacol.* 32:1929–1940.

Sotres-Bayon, F., Cain, C.K., et al. (2006). Brain mechanisms of fear extinction: historical perspectives on the contribution of prefrontal cortex. *Biol. Psychiatry* 60:329–336.

Southwick, S.M., and Charney, D.S. (2012a). Resilience: The Science of Mastering Life's Greatest Challenges. New York: Cambridge University Press.

Southwick, S.M. and Charney, D.S. (2012b). The science of resilience: implications for the prevention and treatment of depression. *Science* 338:78–82.

Southwick, S.M., Vythilingam, M., et al. (2005). The psychobiology of depression and resilience to stress: implications for prevention and treatment. *Ann. Rev. Clin. Psychol.* 1:255–291.

Steckler, T., and Holsboer, F. (1999). Corticotropin-releasing hormone receptor subtypes and emotion. *Biol. Psychiatry* 46:1480–1508.

Steckler, T., and Risbrough, V. (2012). Pharmacological treatment of PTSD—established and new approaches. *Neuropharmacol.* 62:617–627.

Stein, M.B., Kerridge, C., et al. (2007). Pharmacotherapy to prevent PTSD: results from a randomized controlled proof-of-concept trial in physically injured patients. *J. Trauma. Stress* 20:923–932.

Steiner, M.A., Wanisch, K., et al. (2008). Impaired cannabinoid receptor type 1 signaling interferes with stress-coping behavior in mice. *Pharmacogenomics. J.* 8:196–208.

Steptoe, A., Wardle, J., et al. (2005). Positive affect and health-related neuroendocrine, cardiovascular, and inflammatory processes. *Proc. Natl. Acad. Sci. USA* 102:6508–6512.

Stockdale, J.B. (1991). Courage Under Fire: Testing Epictetus' Doctrines in a Laboratory of Human Behavior. Stanford, CA: Hoover Institution Press.

Strome, E.M., Wheler, G.H., et al. (2002). Intracerebroventricular corticotropin-releasing factor increases limbic glucose metabolism and has social context-dependent behavioral effects in nonhuman primates. *Proc. Natl. Acad. Sci. USA* 99:15749–15754.

Suzuki, A., Josselyn, S.A., et al. (2004). Memory reconsolidation and extinction have distinct temporal and biochemical signatures. *J. Neurosci.* 24:4787–4795.

Swanson, C.J., Blackburn, T.P., et al. (2005). Anxiolytic- and antidepressant-like profiles of the galanin-3 receptor (Gal3) antagonists SNAP 37889 and SNAP 398299. *Proc. Natl. Acad. Sci. USA* 102:17489–17494.

Tache, Y., and Bonaz, B. (2007). Corticotropin-releasing factor receptors and stress-related alterations of gut motor function. *J. Clin. Invest.* 117:33–40.

Taliaz, D., Loya, A., et al. (2011). Resilience to chronic stress is mediated by hippocampal brain-derived neurotrophic factor. *J. Neurosci.* 31:4475–4483.

Tasan, R.O., Nguyen, N.K., et al. (2010). The central and basolateral amygdala are critical sites of neuropeptide Y/Y2 receptor-mediated regulation of anxiety and depression. *J. Neurosci.* 30:6282–6290.

Taylor, M.K., Padilla, G.A., et al. (2012). Effects of dehydroepiandrosterone supplementation during stressful military training: a randomized, controlled, double-blind field study. *Stress* 15:85–96.

Thompson, R.W., Arnkoff, D.B., et al. (2011). Conceptualizing mindfulness and acceptance as components of psychological resilience to trauma. *Trauma Violence Abus.* 12:220–235.

Thorson, J.A., and Powell, F.C. (1994). Depression and sense of humor. *Psychological. Rep.* 75:1473–1474.

Travis, L.A., Lyness, J.M., et al. (2004). Social support, depression, and functional disability in older adult primary care patients. *Am. J. Geriatr. Psychiatry* 12:265–271.

True, W.R., Rice, J., et al. (1993). A twin study of genetic and environmental contributions to liability for posttraumatic stress symptoms. *Arch. Gen. Psychiatry* 50:257–264.

Tsai, J., Harpaz-Rotem, I., et al. (2012). The role of coping, resilience, and social support in mediating the relation between PTSD and social functioning in veterans returning from Iraq and Afghanistan. *Psychiatry* 75:135–149.

Tsou, K., Brown, S., et al. (1998). Immunohistochemical distribution of cannabinoid CB1 receptors in the rat central nervous system. *Neuroscience* 83:393–411.

Tugade, M.M., and Fredrickson, B.L. (2004). Resilient individuals use positive emotions to bounce back from negative emotional experiences. *J. Pers. Soc. Psychol.* 86:320–333.

Uher, R., and Mcguffin, P. (2010). The moderation by the serotonin transporter gene of environmental adversity in the etiology of depression: 2009 update. *Mol. Psychiatry* 15:18–22.

Vaillant, G. (1977). Adaptation to Life. Boston, MA: Little Brown.

Vaillant, G. (1992). The historical origins and future potential of Sigmund Freud's concept of the mechanisms of defence. *Int. Rev. Psycho Analysis* 19:35–50.

Vaiva, G., Ducrocq, F., et al. (2003). Immediate treatment with propranolol decreases posttraumatic stress disorder two months after trauma. *Biol. Psychiatry* 54:947–949.

van der Kolk, B.A., and van der Hart, O. (1989). Pierre Janet and the breakdown of adaptation in psychological trauma. *Am. J. Psychiatry* 146:1530–1540.

Vialou, V., Robison, A.J., et al. (2010). DeltaFosB in brain reward circuits mediates resilience to stress and antidepressant responses. *Nat. Neurosci.* 13:745–752.

Vinkers, C.H., Oosting, R.S., et al. (2010). Early-life blockade of 5-HT(1A) receptors alters adult anxiety behavior and benzodiazepine sensitivity. *Biol. Psychiatry* 67:309–316.

Voisey, J., Swagell, C.D., et al. (2009). The DRD2 gene 957C>T polymorphism is associated with posttraumatic stress disorder in war veterans. *Depress. Anxiety* 26:28–33.

Vythilingam, M., Heim, C., et al. (2002). Childhood trauma associated with smaller hippocampal volume in women with major depression. *Am. J. Psychiatry* 159:2072–2080.

Wade, S.L., Borawski, E.A., et al. (2001). The relationship of caregiver coping to family outcomes during the initial year following pediatric traumatic injury. *J. Consult. Clin. Psychol.* 69:406–415.

Wager, T.D., Davidson, M.L., et al. (2008). Prefrontal-subcortical pathways mediating successful emotion regulation. *Neuron* 59:1037–1050.

Walker, D.L., and Davis, M. (2000). Involvement of NMDA receptors within the amygdala in short- versus long-term memory for fear conditioning as assessed with fear-potentiated startle. *Behav. Neurosci.* 114:1019–1033.

Walton, K.M., Chin, J.E., et al. (2006). Galanin function in the central nervous system. *Curr. Opin. Drug Discov. Devel.* 9:560–570.

Wang, Y., Wu, J., et al. (2012). Dopamine D1 receptors are responsible for stress-induced emotional memory deficit in mice. *Stress* 15:237–242.

Weaver, I.C., Cervoni, N., et al. (2004). Epigenetic programming by maternal behavior. *Nat. Neurosci.* 7:847–854.

Weis, F., Kilger, E., et al. (2006). Stress doses of hydrocortisone reduce chronic stress symptoms and improve health-related quality of life in high-risk patients after cardiac surgery: a randomized study. *J. Thor. Cardiov. Surg.* 131:277.

Werner, E., and Smith, R. (1992). Overcoming the Odds: High-risk Children from Birth to Adulthood. Ithaca, NY: Cornell University Press.

Wheler, G.H., Brandon, D., et al. (2006). Cortisol production rate in posttraumatic stress disorder. *J. Clin. Endocrinol. Metab.* 91:3486–3489.

Whitworth, J.A., Williamson, P.M., et al. (2005). Cardiovascular consequences of cortisol excess. *Vasc. Health Risk Manag.* 1:291–299.

Wiley, J.L., Beletskaya, I.D., et al. (2002). Resorcinol derivatives: a novel template for the development of cannabinoid CB(1)/CB(2) and CB(2)-selective agonists. *J. Pharmacol. Exp. Ther.* 301:679–689.

Winter, B., Breitenstein, C., et al. (2006). High impact running improves learning. *Neurobiol. Learn Mem.* 87(4):597–609.

Wise, R.A. (2002). Brain reward circuitry: insights from unsensed incentives. *Neuron* 36:229–240.

Wolin, S.J., and Wolin, S. (1993). The Resilient Self: How Survivors of Troubled Families Rise above Adversity. New York: Villard.

Wood, A.M., Froh, J.J., et al. (2010). Gratitude and well-being: a review and theoretical integration. *Clin. Psychol. Rev.* 30:890–905.

Wood, A.M., Maltby, J., et al. (2008). The role of gratitude in the development of social support, stress and depression: two longitudinal studies. *J. Res. Pers.* 42:854–871.

Wu, G., Feder, A., et al. (2011). Central functions of neuropeptide Y in mood and anxiety disorders. *Expert. Opin. Ther. Targets* 15:1317–1331.

Xu, Z.Q., Tong, Y.G., et al. (2001). Galanin enhances noradrenaline-induced outward current on locus coeruleus noradrenergic neurons. *Neuroreport* 12:1779–1782.

Yamada, K., and Nabeshima, T. (2003). Brain-derived neurotrophic factor/ TrkB signaling in memory processes. *J. Pharmacol. Sci.* 91:267–270.

Yehuda, R. (2001). Biology of posttraumatic stress disorder. *J. Clin. Psychiatry* 62(Suppl 17):41–46.

Yehuda, R. (2004). Risk and resilience in posttraumatic stress disorder. *J. Clin. Psychiatry* 65(Suppl 1):29–36.

Yehuda, R., Bierer, L.M., et al. (2009). Cortisol metabolic predictors of response to psychotherapy for symptoms of PTSD in survivors of the World Trade Center attacks on September 11, 2001. *Psychoneuroendocrinology* 34:1304–1313.

Yehuda, R., Brand, S.R., et al. (2006). Clinical correlates of DHEA associated with post-traumatic stress disorder. *Acta Psychiatr. Scand.* 114:187–193.

Yehuda, R., Koenen, K.C., et al. (2011). The role of genes in defining a molecular biology of PTSD. *Dis. Markers* 30:67–76.

Yehuda, R., Yang, R.K., et al. (2006). Alterations in cortisol negative feedback inhibition as examined using the ACTH response to cortisol administration in PTSD. *Psychoneuroendocrinol.* 31:447–451.

Young, A.H., Gallagher, P., et al. (2002). Elevation of the cortisol-dehydroepiandrosterone ratio in drug-free depressed patients. *Am. J. Psychiatry* 159:1237–1239.

Zarate, C.A., Jr., Singh, J.B., et al. (2006). A randomized trial of an N-methyl-D-aspartate antagonist in treatment-resistant major depression *Arch. Gen. Psychiatry* 63:856–864.

Zeidner, M., and Hammer, A.L. (1992). Coping with missile attack—resources, strategies, and outcomes. *J. Personality* 60:709–746.

Zhou, Z., Zhu, G., et al. (2008). Genetic variation in human NPY expression affects stress response and emotion. *Nature* 452:997–1001.

Zohar, J., Yahalom, H., et al. (2011). High dose hydrocortisone immediately after trauma may alter the trajectory of PTSD: interplay between clinical and animal studies. *Eur. Neuropsychopharmacol.* 21:796–809.

Zoumakis, E., Grammatopoulos, D.K., et al. (2006). Corticotropin-releasing hormone receptor antagonists. *Eur. J. Endocrinol.* 155:S85–S91.

89 | THE NEUROBIOLOGY OF EATING DISORDERS

THOMAS B. HILDEBRANDT AND AMANDA DOWNEY

NEUROBIOLOGICAL MODELS OF ANOREXIA NERVOSA

Anorexia nervosa (AN) is an illness that is not homogenous in presentation; rather it is diagnosed upon a range of disturbed behaviors and affective states that constitute the illness. The heterogenic nature of the diagnostic group complicates the process of identifying an underlying neurobiological model for the disease. There are four main factors that make identifying a singular neurobiological model difficult. First, there is more than one source of dysregulation present in the development and maintenance of AN. Predisposing factors that lead to extreme measures to lose weight will most likely be distinct from those that prevent weight restoration and maintenance of adequate caloric intake. Second, it is ethically and scientifically difficult to determine the degree to which systems of dysregulation are a consequence of malnutrition or rather an endophenotype inherent to the individual that predisposes her or him to the illness. Third, sociocultural factors that may play a role in the development of the disorder have often been used to explain the difference in prevalence rates of AN among men and women. No neurobiological basis for this disparity has been elucidated. Finally, the development of AN is correlated with specific temperaments and personality factors. This facet of the disorder makes strict correlation between neurobiology and the disorder complicated because the role of temperament is highly complex and not unique to AN.

NEUROBIOLOGICAL MODELS OF BULIMIA NERVOSA

Bulimia nervosa (BN) is a mental disorder characterized by episodes of binge eating and attempts to compensate for these episodes by self-induced vomiting, abusing laxatives or diet pills, fasting for 24 hours or more, and/or compulsively exercising. They provide positive reinforcement and/or relief from negative symptoms and may be indicative of underlying dysregulation in the serotonergic of dopaminergic systems. A neurobiological model for BN overlaps in many ways with that of AN, although there are several essential differences. First, core behaviors in BN can be studied in the lab, allowing for a more detailed analysis with less confounding factors. Second, most women with BN are within a healthy weight range, which has eliminated the confounding effects of malnutrition on hormonal and neurotransmitter systems. Last, impulsivity is the major temperament associated with BN, as opposed to harm avoidance in AN.

DEVELOPMENT VERSUS MAINTENANCE OF ANOREXIA NERVOSA

The development of AN shows a strong relationship with the onset of puberty, with most patients meeting the full criteria for the disorder before reaching adulthood (Fig. 89.1). Although many recover from symptoms before their mid-twenties, some display behaviors characteristic of other illnesses such as bulimia nervosa. Definitive predictors that can differentiate between the large percentage of patients who remain chronically ill remain elusive, with studies citing highest weight achieved upon weight restoration, time to partial recovery, familial relationships, premorbid asociality, postdischarge weight loss, motivation to recover, and the binge–purge subtype of AN as valuable yet complex predictors (Carter et al., 2012; Strober et al., 1997). Prospective predictors for the development of AN include being female, having feeding problems in infancy, undereating, and having a perfectionist temperament (Tyrka et al., 2002). Furthermore, retrospective studies suggest that perinatal environment may impact an individual's vulnerability to AN. Obstetrical complications (e.g., low birth weight, preterm birth, neonatal cardiac problems, maternal anemia, diabetes mellitus, and preeclampsia) and neonatal dysmaturity may contribute to a dysregulation in prenatal programming of stress response systems and consequently carry some risk for the disorder (Tyrka et al., 2002).

The incidence of AN is approximately eight per 100,000 persons per year. Although considered a rare illness, it is prevalent among young women in Western countries, with a 0.9% lifetime prevalence rate. Anorexia nervosa is highly comorbid with many other DSM-IV disorders, with 56.2% of patients meeting criteria for at least one comorbid psychiatric disorder (Hudson et al., 2007). Incidence rates are highest among females 15 to 19 years old, representing nearly 40% of all cases (Smink et al., 2012). It has the highest rate of mortality among all mental disorders, rendering AN a major public health concern. The incidence of AN in males is significantly less than in females, with estimates of incidence less than one per 100,000 persons per year (Hoek, 2006). Studies have reported conflicting prevalence rates of eating disorders among minority groups, and further population studies are needed. A recent study suggests similar prevalence rates among all ethnic groups in the United States (Smink et al., 2012). Few epidemiological studies have been conducted on AN and BN outside of Western countries. However, it is possible that increased rates of intentional dieting common to

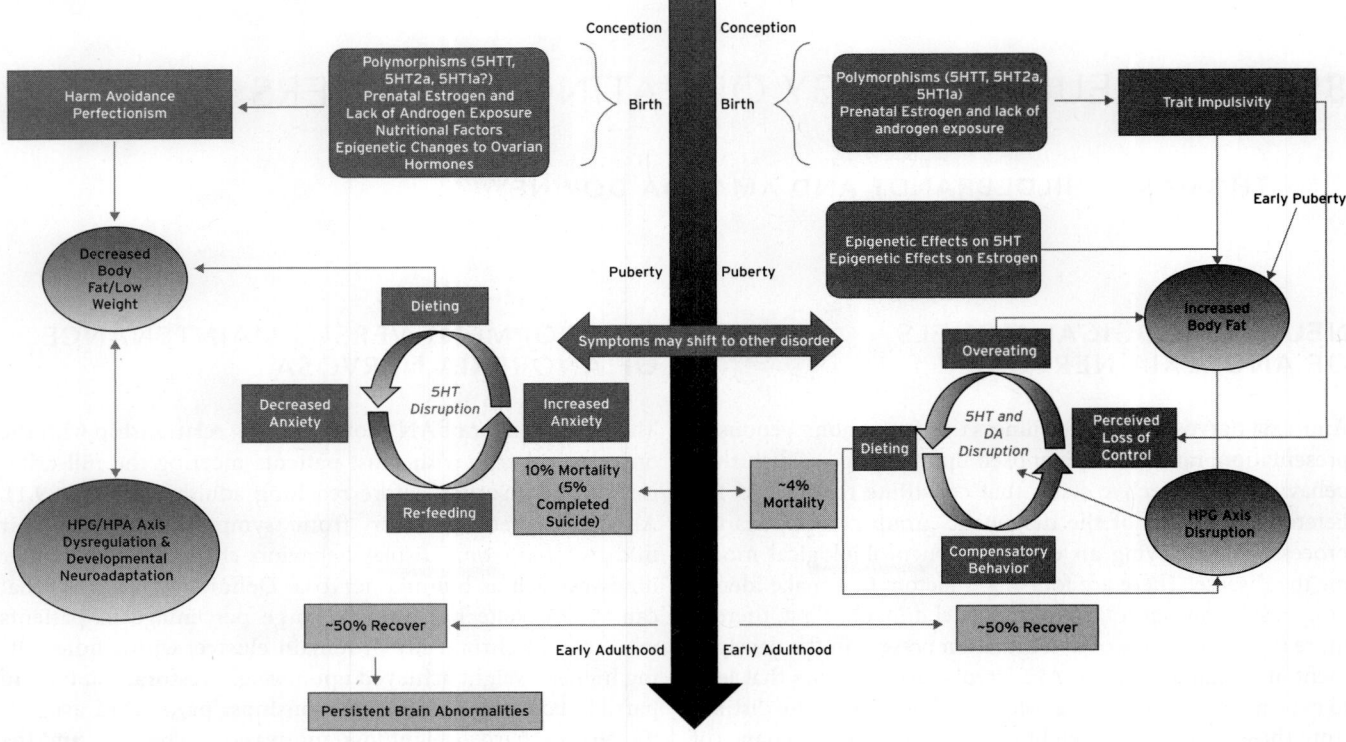

Figure 89.1 *The developmental trajectories for anorexia nervosa (left) and bulimia nervosa (right) indicate periods of accumulating risk which are activated by the environmental and hormonal changes associated with puberty. The hypothalamic pituitary gonadal (HPG) and hypothalamic pituitary adrenal (HPA) axes interact with the dieting-overeating behaviors to support neuronal adaptation to the disease state evidenced by changes in serotonergic (5-HT) and dompaminergic (DA) function that may persist beyond into periods of recovery. For some individuals, the disease state leads to fatal outcomes caused by physical complications of the disease or suicide.*

Western countries may lead to higher incidence rates, particularly in younger individuals.

DEVELOPMENTAL MODEL OF BULIMIA NEROVSA

The onset of bulimia nervosa is characterized by genetic, prenatal, epigenetic, and pubertal conditions (see Fig. 89.1). Vulnerability to BN may be especially influenced by dysregulation in the serotonergic, dopaminergic, and ovarian hormone systems. Furthermore, the emotional and psychosocial impact of an increased propensity for body fat deposition and the propensity for higher BMI among women with BN may contribute to the development of binge episodes and compensatory behaviors. Women with BN tend to undergo pubertal changes earlier than age-matched counterparts. The surge of estrogen accompanying pubertal changes contributes to early visceral fat deposition and weight dissatisfaction for these women (Hildebrandt et al., 2010). This phenomenon leads to both a distancing of the individual from the thin-ideal and activates a range of neurobiological changes that make behavior more difficult to regulate. Additionally, fluctuations in estrogen levels affect mood (e.g., through the serotonin system), appetite, and impulsivity (Rubinow et al., 1998). The combination of these factors within a societal context in which thinness is idealized and dieting is normative leads vulnerable women toward a pattern of dieting in which the binge–purge cycle may begin. Once initiated, the symptoms of BN can have dramatic effects on hypothalamic

regulatory systems that independently of predisposing vulnerabilities can maintain a cycle of overeating and compensatory behavior. Neuroadaptive changes in these hypothalamic hormonal systems make the regulation of mood and stress responses increasingly difficult and are likely partially responsible for alterations in corticolimbic neurocircuitry that characterizes the disorder. Symptoms persist until the individual can achieve some nutritional and affective balance.

The lifetime prevalence of BN remains close to 1%. There is a large gender disparity in the prevalence of the disorder, women being at least three times more likely than men to develop BN (Hudson et al., 2007). This disorder is also highly comorbid with other psychiatric diagnoses, with 94.5% of patients meeting the criteria for at least one disorder. Women with BN are more likely to develop comorbid conditions related to mood, anxiety, impulsecontrol, and substance use, and it is estimated that fewer than half of individuals who meet the criteria for BN seek treatment throughout their lifetime (Hudson et al., 2007).

GENETIC VULNERABILITY TO ANOREXIA NERVOSA

The search for a genetic basis of AN has yet to provide any definitive genetic markers. Family studies have consistently shown significant heritability of AN among first-degree relatives of probands, with a seven- to 12-fold increase in prevalence when compared with control subjects (Strober et al., 2000). Genetic research in AN suggests that a diverse set of genes are potentially

TABLE 89.1. Frequent genetic polymorphisms identified in patients with eating disorders

CATEGORY	GENE	VARIANT	POSSIBLE ASSOCIATION	EPIGENETICS
SEROTONIN				
	Serotonin Transporter (SERT, 5-HTT, SCL6A4)	5-HTTLPR, SLC6A4 44 bp Del/Ins (promoter)	AN/BN	
		5-HTTPLR intron 2 VNTR		
	5-HT$_{1B/1D\beta}$ receptor	821G>C	AN/BN	
		Phe-124-Cys	BN	
	5-HT$_{2A}$ receptor	−1438 G>A		Hypermethylation, increased expression (Polesskaya et al., 2006)
	5-HTR$_{3B}$ receptor	Tyr129Ser	AN	
BRAIN-DERIVED NEUROTROPHIC FACTOR (BDNF)				
		−270C>T, Val-66-Met	AN/BN	
DOPAMINE				
	Catechol-Omethyltransferase gene (COMT)	Val-158-Met		
	D2 receptor	TaqA1	AN/BN	Hypermethylation, decreased expression (Frieling et al., 2010)
		−141 Indel	AN/BN	
	D3 receptor	Ball polymorphism, exon 1	BN	
	D4 receptor	13 bp deletion	BN	
		48 bp deletion	AN/BN	
		Haplotype exon III VNTR, 120 bp repeat, 521 C>T, 809 A>G	AN/BN	
	Neuropeptide Y Y$_1$ receptor	Pst I-polymorphism within the first intron	BN	
	Neuropeptide Y Y$_5$ receptor	1333 G>A (silent)	BN	
LEPTINERGIC-MELANOCORTINERGIC SYSTEM				
	Agouti related protein	526 G>A (silent) in linkage disequilibrium with Ala-67-Thr	AN/BN	
	Melanocortin-4 receptor	Val-103-Ile		
		Ile-251-Thr		
	Endocannabinoid system (CNR1)	rs1049353 rs2180619 rs806379 rs1535255 rs2023239	BN	
		AAT trinucleotide repeat	AN/BN	
	Endocannabinoid system (FAAH)	rs932816 rs324420 rs324419 rs873978 rs2295632	AN/BN	
		rs324420 rs324419 rs873978 rs2295632		

(continued)

TABLE 89.1. (*Continued*)

CATEGORY	GENE	VARIANT	POSSIBLE ASSOCIATION	EPIGENETICS
	Endocannabinoid system (NAAA)	rs2292534 rs4859567 rs10518142 rs6819442	BN	
	Leptin	−1387 G>A (promoter)	BED/BN	
	Glucocorticoids	rs6198	BED	
		rs56149945 (N363S)	AN/BN/BED	
	Pro-opiomelanocortin (POMC)	Insertion of 9 bp between codon 73 and 74	BN	Hypomethylation, increased expression (Ehrlich et al., 2010)
PUBERTY HORMONES				
	Estrogen β receptor (Erβ)	1082 G >A (silent)	AN	
		1730 A >G (silent)		
	β₃—adrenoreceptor	Trp-64-Arg	BN	
OTHER				
	CYP2D6	2 or >2 active genes		
	KCNN3	CAG repeats	AN/BN	
	Uncoupling protein 2, 3	D11S911, flanking microsatellite markers		

(Adapted from Hinney et al. (2000); Monteleone and Maj (2008); Pinheiro et al. (2010).)

involved in the pathogenesis of the disorder. Table 89.1 summarizes the essential genes implicated thus far, although the field is still awaiting completion of ongoing large-scale studies that may provide more clarity in the genetic risks to this disorder.

Candidate gene studies aim to discover consistent genetic polymorphisms that may contribute to the diagnosis of AN, but results have been inconclusive. Strong association between polymorphism and risk of developing an eating disorder could lead to targeted pharmacotherapies and preventive strategies in those at risk. Some association between polymorphism and diagnosis has been found in serotonergic, adrenergic, and dopaminergic genes, genes coding for proteins associated with the melanocortin system, genes for leptin, ghrelin, agouti-related protein, neuropeptide Y, opioids, cannabinoid receptors, potassium channels, brain-derived neurotrophic factor, and reproductive hormones (Pinheiro et al., 2010). Although significant association remains to be found, it is likely that a combination of genetic variants as well as environmental factors contribute to the development of the disorder. Additionally, candidate gene polymorphisms and single nucleotide polymorphisms (SNPs) may be better correlated to endophenotypes and personality traits that correspond to a predisposition to AN rather than finding direct association with the diagnosis itself.

Genome-wide association studies (GWAS) have identified several SNPs associated with the drive for thinness, obsessionality, and other traits associated with AN. Four SNPs on the contactin 5 gene, as well as 1q31.3, 2p11.2, 13q13.3, and rs2048332 are common genetic variations that merit further investigation into possible association with AN (Helder and Collier, 2011).

More recent studies focusing on epigenetic processes may further illuminate the role of genetic processing and expression on the pathology of AN. Epigenetic effects include the breadth of changes to DNA processing within the cell that are not encoded within the genome and therefore reversible, perhaps accounting for the variability in genetically regulated aspects of the disorder. DNA methylation is particularly applicable to eating disorders, having established that methylation patterns in CpG islands at the 5′ end of genes may control long-term regulation of gene expression (Bird, 2002). Diet, genetics, chemical exposure, environment, and other physiological states can influence methylation patterns in humans (Poirier, 2002). Serotonin transporter (5-HTT) mRNA transcription is susceptible to epigenetic modification (Philibert et al., 2008) as is the serotonin receptor 5-HT2a (Polesskaya et al., 2006). Epigenetic modifications support the broad base of evidence for dysregulation in the serotonergic system in AN and likely other systems, including dopaminergic and appetite regulatory systems. Furthermore, epigenetics could account for the sexually dimorphic nature of certain hormones and neurotransmitters, which may shed light on the gender disparity in the prevalence of eating disorders (Gabory et al., 2009). More in-depth study into the mechanism of epigenetic effects on other neurotransmitter systems is warranted.

GENETIC VULNERABILITY TO BULIMIA NERVOSA

Like AN, no definitive genes have been identified that correlate with a diagnosis of BN, although patterns of heritability are evident. Table 89.1 summarizes findings from studies examining this link. Relatives of probands with BN have an approximate four time greater lifetime risk of also developing BN (Strober et al., 2000). Linkage analysis suggests loci with specific genetic polymorphisms and SNPs associated with BN are correlated with age of menarche, body mass index, obsessionality, and concern over mistakes (Bacanu et al., 2005). Polymorphisms in the serotonergic system are particularly evident in patients with BN as compared with control subjects with potential variability residing in the serotonin transporter (5-HTT) and particular serotonin receptors (Monteleone and Maj, 2008). As in AN, epigenetic effects in DNA processing via methylation patterns are being studied both in the serotonergic and dopaminergic systems in women with BN, contributing evidence to the hypothesis that epigenetic dysregulation can affect neurotransmission and play an important role in the pathology of eating disorders (Frieling et al., 2010).

PRENATAL RISK

There is some evidence that the prenatal hormonal environment will affect vulnerability to eating disorders during puberty. Emerging research suggests that exposure to lower levels of testosterone as a fetus in the second trimester may increase sensitivity to fluctuations in estrogen concentrations during puberty, activating a predisposition toward disordered eating (Klump et al., 2006). Androgen hormone exposure in animal models has demonstrated a protective role in the central nervous system, decreasing its sensitivity to estrogens. This genetic influence is hypothesized to originate from a polymorphism within the estrogen receptor beta or in a serotonin receptor (Klump et al., 2006), although there are likely other mechanisms that contribute to this sensitivity. Additionally, higher prenatal androgen exposure may enhance the expression of cytosolic and nuclear androgen receptors, helping to explain the sexually dimorphic nature of some areas of the brain (Resko and Roselli, 1997) and consequently the disparity in prevalence rates of eating disorders between genders.

DYSREGULATION IN HORMONAL SYSTEMS

Figure 89.2 summarizes the changes in hypothalamic hormonal systems that occur during active disease states for those with AN and BN. Acute and chronic starvation produces a unique set of hormonal and neuroendocrine effects that may be involved in the pathophysiology of both AN and BN. Malnutrition induces varying states of adaptation in two hypothalamic regulatory systems—the hypothalamic-pituitary-adrenal (HPA) axis and the hypothalamic-pituitary-gonadal (HPG) axis, resulting in hyper- and hypoactivity of these systems depending on the disease state (e.g., starvation vs. overfeeding) and the associated symptoms (e.g., food avoidance, binge eating). The adaptive hormonal changes included by symptom stress may have implications in a range of cognitive or affective systems, particularly the motivation–reward system (Keating, 2011).

The rapidly changing hormonal environment induced by puberty also contributes to the development of these disorders. The initial surge of ovarian hormones at the onset of puberty may correlate with initial decreased drive to eat, as studies in female rat models have consistently shown a reduction in food intake following the sharpest rise in estrogen levels during the estrous cycle (Butera, 2010). Fluctuations in the menstrual cycle of humans also demonstrate varied caloric intake, notably correlating the luteal phase of the menstrual cycle with highest appetite and lowest levels of estrogen (Buffenstein et al., 1995). The window of vulnerability produced by hormonal fluctuations during puberty provides hormonal mechanisms that may trigger or facilitate existing restrictive or overeating feeding behaviors. The neuroendocrine sequelae of this key developmental window, and the relative impact of malnutrition, have not been completely elucidated. However, morphological changes in the brain caused by the pubertal environment and the steep rise in ovarian hormones may affect the development of several primary neurocircuits involved in motivation, emotional processing, impulsivity, and information processing. It is possible that patients with AN or BN suffer from an impairment in any or all of these pathways (Kaye et al., 2011).

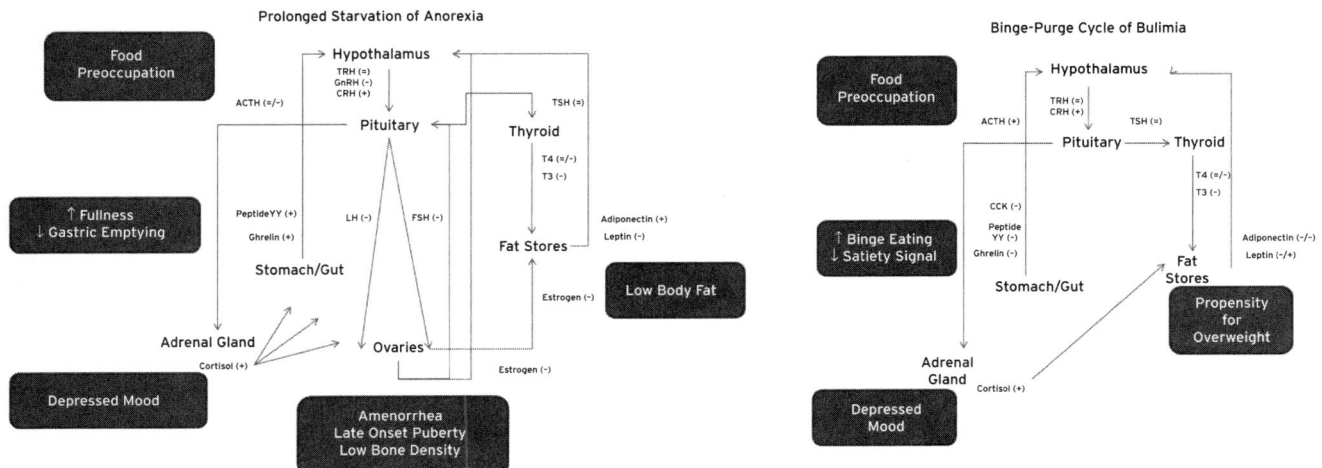

Figure 89.2 The disturbances in gastric, adrenal, and gonadal hormones/peptides are summarized for anorexia nervosa (left) and bulimia nervosa (right) in their relative disease states. TRH =thyrotropin releasing hormone. GnRH = gonadotropin releasing hormone. CRH = corticotropin releasing hormone. TSH = thyroid stimulating hormone. LH = luteinizing hormone. FSH = follicle stimulating hormone. ACTH = Adrenocorticotropic hormone. CCK = Cholecystokinin.

OVARIAN HORMONES

Hyperactivity of the HPA axis that accompanies the malnutrition associated with AN can attenuate the action of the HPG axis, possibly leading to amenorrhea and a reversion in sexual development, including decreased levels of serum estradiol (Stoving et al., 1999). Hyperactivity of the HPA axis leads to increased secretion of cortisol from the adrenal glands, stimulating the release of dopamine from mesolimbic neurons in the brain, thus enhancing the reward system that may reinforce AN (Keating, 2011). Additional studies reinforce this hypothesis and link estrogen levels to the reward–punishment system, correlating lower concentrations of estrogen (hypogonadism secondary to hyperactive HPA axis) with higher levels of dopamine and decreased serotonin secretion, the consequences of which may affect food intake (Keating, 2011). In a state of hypogonadism, it follows that lower rates of estrogen release resulting from HPA axis suppression of the HPG axis would result in increased levels of dopamine and increased sensitivity to the reward system in which eating disordered behaviors are positively reinforced (Barbato et al., 2006).

The ability of estradiol to centrally regulate food intake is dependent upon its interactions with estrogen receptors in the central nervous system, particularly in the hypothalamus and hindbrain (Butera, 2010). The estrogen receptor has two types, alpha and beta, and it remains unclear which of these is primarily responsible for the estrogenic effects on appetite and food intake. Estrogen may centrally modulate the processing of gastrointestinal and hypothalamic neuropeptides, leading to alterations in feeding behavior. There is mounting evidence that serotonergic neurons in the central nervous system are sensitive to and dependent upon exogenous and endogenous estradiol levels (as well as LH, FSH, and GnRH) and are critical to the modulation of affect and mood (Pae et al., 2009).

Recently, the effects of rapid estrogen signaling on AN have come under investigation. Estrogen receptors in the nuclear membrane regulate the transcription of genes in the nucleus and have been extensively studied. New studies show that estrogen receptors in plasma membranes (mERs) may mediate more immediate effects through calcium channels and estrogen-induced protein kinase signaling (Raz et al., 2008). For example, some mERs may increase the excitability of POMC and dopamine neurons (Roepke et al., 2009), whereas others may down-regulate 5-HT1a function (Mize et al., 2001), both having effects on energy homeostasis and food intake. These membranous estrogen receptors may mediate more rapid signaling of estrogen in the brain, and their dysregulation may play a role in AN.

In BN, there is strong evidence for correlation between the frequency of self-induced vomiting and irregular menses (Austin et al., 2008). Frequent vomiting may have a direct effect on hormonal systems. Furthermore, binge eating episodes occur with higher frequency during times in the menstrual cycle when estrogen is the lowest (premenstrual and midluteal phases) (Klump et al., 2008), consistent with aforementioned studies citing the ability of estrogens to centrally inhibit food intake through satiety signals produced by cholecystokinin (CCK) and other regulatory peptides.

APPETITE AND WEIGHT-REGULATING PEPTIDES AND HORMONES

There is evidence that central and peripheral regulatory peptides and hormones function in an altered, dysregulated state in patients with AN and BN. These substances influence feeding motivation for the purposes of weight balance, and the implications of their dysregulation have not yet been fully explored. Substances of interest and ongoing clinical investigation include ghrelin, obestatin, peptide YY, neuropeptide Y, adiponectin, endocannabinoids, IGF-1, cholecystokinin, and insulin.

Cholecystokinin

Cholecystokinin (CCK), an anorexigenic peptide hormone produced in the enteroendocrine cells of the small intestine, functions to inhibit feeding once it has been initiated by enhancing satiation signaling, among other gastrointestinal functions (Chandra and Liddle, 2007). Cholecystokinin-1 receptors relay satiety signals via the vagus nerve to the hindbrain (Chandra and Liddle, 2007). In women with BN, there is evidence that CCK dysregulation may be indicative of gastric dysfunction induced by binge eating episodes. Once CCK has been released in response to a meal, it is released more slowly and in lower concentrations in women with bulimia nervosa as compared with controls (Geracioti and Liddle, 1988). This dysregulation may contribute to the binge–purge cycle, as binge episodes are exacerbated by this dysregulation.

Ghrelin

Ghrelin, a peptide hormone secreted from enteroendocrine cells of the stomach, is unique in its ability to initiate food intake. It reaches sufficiently high circulating levels before a meal and falls drastically a short time afterward. Circulating ghrelin levels are higher in those in acute and chronic starving states secondary to AN as compared with controls and reflect the enteroendocrine system attempting to counteract the state of malnutrition induced by eating-disordered behavior (Monteleone, 2011). Ghrelin is also implicated as a ligand in the secretion of growth hormone (GH) and IGF-1 in maintenance of lean body mass, but has different effects under the catabolic conditions created by malnutrition, implicating further dysregulation in the ghrelin system (Hasan and Hasan, 2011).

Obestatin

Obestatin, another peptide hormone produced from enteroendocrine cells of the gastrointestinal tract, is derived from the same precursor prohormone from which ghrelin is synthesized. Several studies show that obestatin has a complimentary but opposite effect to ghrelin, serving to induce satiety (Monteleone, 2011). Although the functionality of obestatin remains controversial, studies have shown that the ghrelin to obestatin ratio is increased in patients with AN as compared with control subjects, implying further adaptation under conditions of malnutrition to increase the peripheral hunger signal. Altered gene expression of the prohormone from which ghrelin and obestatin originate may also contribute to the apparent dysregulation of ghrelin and obestatin in patients with AN (Monteleone et al., 2008; Zhang et al., 2005).

Neuropeptide Y

Neuropeptide Y (NPY) is a neurotransmitter released in the hypothalamus that serves a role in stimulating appetite and enhances the release of corticotropin-releasing hormone (CRH) (Kaye et al., 1990). Neuropeptide Y in the cerebrospinal fluid of patients with BN is equivalent with that of controls, whereas patients with AN show higher levels of CSF NPY as compared with controls (Kaye et al., 1990). In long-term recovered women with AN and BN, NPY and PYY concentrations return to normal. This suggests that alterations in these systems are secondary to the illness and not traits that may predispose one to the development of an eating disorder (Gendall et al.,1999). Although not a predisposing trait, further study of their influence on metabolic and reproductive systems in the environment of an eating disorder is warranted.

Peptide YY

Peptide YY (PYY) is a peptide hormone secreted by the colon primarily to induce a sensation of satiety following the intake of food. It binds to the receptor of neuropeptide Y, an orexigenic peptide, blocking its ability to signal and functioning as an anorexigenic hormone. Additionally, PYY is able to reduce plasma levels of ghrelin, also contributing to its anorexigenic properties. In several studies of circulating levels of PYY in patients with AN, increased levels of PYY were detected (Misra et al., 2006; Utz et al., 2008). Although earlier studies yielded more inconclusive results, alternate functions of PYY merit investigation (Tong and D'Alessio, 2011). In bulimic patients who had abstained from binging and purging, CSF PYY was significantly increased as compared with controls and patients with AN, perhaps demonstrating dysregulation in this system as contributory to the drive to binge eat in BN (Kaye et al., 1990). Recent functional magnetic resonance imaging (fMRI) studies have shown correlation between elevated PYY concentrations and changes in neural activity in the caudolateral orbitofrontal cortex, allowing researchers to predict feeding behaviors independently of food intake (Batterham et al., 2007). Given that corticolimbic and higher-cortical areas of the brain are influenced by PYY concentration, further research is warranted into the effects of this hormone.

Leptin

Largely synthesized in adipose tissue, leptin is an adipocytokine expressed in various tissues throughout the body. Plasma concentration of leptin is indicative of the adiposity of an individual, especially in females. Levels are low during conditions of starvation, like in AN, and higher in conditions of obesity (Mantzoros et al., 1997). Leptin plays a role in regulating several neuroendocrine functions and promoting energy homeostasis in conditions of starvation, thus it has regulatory properties over the HPA axis. In conditions of starvation, it follows that reproductive and thyroid hormone secretion would be suppressed, to prevent procreation and metabolism, respectively. New approaches to pharmacological therapy in AN under investigation include infusions of leptin as a means of reversing amenorrhea (Chan and Mantzoros, 2005).

Because of the variability in fat percentage and BMI in patients with bulimia nervosa, serum concentrations of leptin have not yielded definitive evidence for dysregulation in these women. In a study of untreated bulimic women, plasma leptin levels were significantly decreased as compared to control subjects which may imply impaired sensitivity to changes in caloric intake or dysregulation in the synthesis of leptin (Monteleone et al., 2000). This dysregulation could play an important role in the pathogenesis of BN.

Adiponectin

Adiponectin is a serum protein synthesized and secreted exclusively by adipocytes. As central and peripheral adiposity increase, adiponectin levels uniformly decrease. Studies have found that acute states of starvation do not significantly affect circulating levels of adiponectin, and adiponectin levels under conditions of chronic starvation remain controversial. Additionally, some studies have demonstrated that adiponectin plays a role in regulating insulin sensitivity, correlating increased adiposity with lower levels of adiponectin and less sensitivity to insulin, but no such studies have been replicated in conditions of starvation (Tagami et al., 2004). There has been some evidence in mouse models of the sexually dimorphic nature of both adiponectin and leptin, making these molecules interesting targets of research into the widely varying rates of prevalence among males and females (Gui et al., 2004).

The Endocannabinoid System

The endocannabinoid system is a lipid signaling system critical to many processes, both physiological and neurological. One emerging role of the endocannabinoid system is in energy balance and lipid metabolism, both within the central nervous system and in peripheral tissues. Two receptors (CB1 and CB2) and two primary endogenous ligands (anandamide and 2-arachidonylglycerol, or 2-AG) comprise the main effectors of the system (Bermudez-Silva et al., 2010). Plasma anandamide concentrations have been found to be significantly elevated in patients with restricting AN as compared with controls, whereas 2-AG has not shown significant fluctuations between patients and controls. The significance of these findings remains under debate. Although higher levels of circulating anandamide should correlate with increased desire for food intake, new hypotheses suggest that the abundance of anandamide may be enhancing the reward system by which pleasure is derived from restrictive behaviors, given the high density of CB1 receptors in areas of the brain associated with the reward system (Kirkham et al., 2002).

Melanocortin

The melanocortin system presents another set of regulators with significant implications in a reward pathway that may serve to reinforce restrictive behaviors in patients with AN in addition to modulating food intake. Agouti related peptide (AGRP) is an orexinergic inverse agonist of melanocortinergic receptors that should encourage food intake. Repeated studies have demonstrated significantly more loss-of-function mutations and polymorhpisms within the gene coding for this peptide in patients with AN as compared with controls, although the significance of this finding warrants further study (Scherag et al., 2010).

HYPOTHALAMIC–PITUITARY–ADRENAL AXIS

Hyperactivation of the HPA axis in response to stress caused by acute and chronic starvation leads to elevated secretion of cortisol. Corticotropin-releasing hormone (CRH) is synthesized in the hypothalamus and transmitted to the pituitary via the portal system, stimulating the synthesis and secretion of substances like adrenocortitropic hormone (ACTH) and beta-endorphin. Adrenocortitropic hormone is transmitted to the adrenal glands, stimulating secretion of cortisol. Hyperactivation of this pathway in patients with AN leads to a state of hypercortisolism through an increased half-life of cortisol and increased pulsatile secretions of cortisol, which enhances gluconeogenesis in the body, helping the body to reestablish glucose stores under conditions of malnutrition (Lo Sauro et al., 2008). Additionally, cortisol stimulates protein breakdown, increases in plasma glucose and insulin, and regulates body adiposity (Licinio et al., 1996). Urine and serum cortisol concentrations have been shown to be positive predictors of truncal adiposity in weight restoration and of the severity of depressive symptoms in patients with AN (Miller, 2011). Hypersecretion of CRH and/or increased sensitivity to CRH at the pituitary may account for increased secretion of cortisol, considering that feedback mechanisms of the HPA axis appear to remain intact (Lo Sauro et al., 2008).

Thyrotropin-Releasing Hormone

Thyrotropin-releasing hormone (TRH) is a hormone synthesized in the hypothalamus and is responsible for the stimulation of secretion of thyroid-stimulating hormone (TSH) from the anterior pituitary. Ultimately, it is responsible for regulation of the thyroid gland. Research has shown that transient hypothyroidism occurs in chronic states of malnutrition, as measured by reduced serum concentrations of T3 and, to a lesser extent, T4 (Swenne et al., 2009). Because hypothyroidism has been linked to feelings of dysphoria, this could account for the symptomatology of dysphoria reported by a subset of patients with AN (Korzekwa et al., 1996).

Endorphins

Beta-endorphin (derived from POMC) and dynorphin are opioid peptides that have recently come under investigation for their role in the regulation of reward-related behaviors and regulation of food intake (Monteleone, 2011). Beta-endorphin levels were detected as reduced in the cerebrospinal fluid of patients with AN and no significant change has been found in the levels of dynorphin (Kaye, 1996). Dysregulation in the opioid system may also contribute to conditions of hypercortisolism in AN (Kaye, 1996). Recent studies show that beta-endorphins have rewarding and reinforcing properties that may be mediated through the mesolimbic dopaminergic system. Additionally, beta-endorphins may play a role in learning and memory (Roth-Deri et al., 2008). These findings further suggest dysregulation in certain opioid peptides may influence the reward system in patients with AN.

Hypothalamic-pituitary-adrenal axis dysregulation in the context of BN has centered around an altered stress response to impulsivity manifesting as self-injury, binge eating, suicidality, depressive symptoms, and so on. Although hyperactivity of the HPA axis is highly prevalent in women with AN, dysregulation of this axis among patients with bulimia nervosa has shown more heterogeneous outcomes. Numerous studies have shown normal, increased, and decreased secretion of cortisol in women with BN, which may imply a dysregulation in the circadian release of cortisol depending on the disease state or the physiological state of the individual. Infusion with exogenous CRH in relapsed and recovered women with BN show stronger ACTH secretory response as compared with control subjects, indicating a hypersensitive HPA response to stress, even after recovery (Birketvedt et al., 2006).

NEUROTRANSMITTER DYSREGULATION

The monoamine neurotransmitters have been extensively studied as part of the attempt to explain a number of traits in AN and BN, including increased anxiety, harm avoidance, perfectionism, impulsivity, mood regulation, and more. Understanding the pathophysiology of these neurotransmitters may help researchers to develop targeted pharmacotherapies in the treatment of eating disorders. Both the dopaminergic and serotonergic systems demonstrate dysregulation in patients with AN, yet there has been no formal integration of the two pathophysiologies to date, only speculation as to their interaction. In BN, serotonergic dysregulation is thought to be the primary factor in the pathology of the illness.

Evidence suggests a severe decrease in serotonergic tone in women with AN. Figure 89.3 demonstrates the cycle by which dysregulation of this system may contribute to the development and maintenance of AN. Those predisposed to developing the disorder might have an imbalance in the ratio between 5-HT1A (inhibitory) and 5-HT2A (excitatory) receptors (Kaye et al., 2005). This imbalance, in conjunction with a predisposition for increased extracellular serotonin (5-HT), may contribute to several traits widely seen in patients with AN, such as harm avoidance, anxiousness, impulse control, and dysregulated feelings of satiety. Positron emission tomography imaging studies suggest that postsynaptic 5-HT1A receptors within mesial temporal and subgenual cingulate regions of the brain are significantly correlated with harm avoidance (Bailer et al., 2005). Extracellular serotonin (and serotonin metabolites in the CSF) are reduced in the starving state because of decreased intake of tryptophan in the diet, an essential amino acid that is a precursor in the synthesis of serotonin, thus reducing anxiety and feelings of dysphoria. This may help to explain why starvation may be reinforced in patients with dysregulated serotonergic systems. In the weight restoration phase of recovery from AN, patients experience surges in serotonin production and excess stimulation of 5-HT1A and 5-HT2A postsynaptic receptors, again increasing dysphoric mood and adding to the challenge of food intake. Although it is logical to assume that selective serotonin reuptake inhibitors (SSRIs) may alleviate symptoms associated with a dysregulated serotonergic system, significant efficacy has not been demonstrated, possibly because of the depleted state of synaptic serotonin caused by severe malnutrition (Kaye et al., 2009). It is important to note that most studies of the serotonergic system and AN are conducted with weight-restored women to avoid the confounding effects of malnutrition on the physiology of the body.

Dysregulation and dysfunction have also been noted in the dopaminergic system of patients with AN. Dopamine is involved in reward pathways, decision-making capabilities, motor movement, and food intake, and thus may have profound effects on the maintenance and development of a disorder like AN. Reduced metabolites in the cerebrospinal fluid of patients both recovered and acutely ill reflect a decrease in dopamine in the extracellular fluid. Additionally, common genetic polymorphisms in dompamine receptors (D2 and D3) are a recurrent finding in patients and PET scans show increased dopamine receptor density in the ventral striatum, a region of the brain heavily involved in reward signaling. These findings correlate with traits of harm avoidance and failure to appropriately respond to salient stimuli (Montague et al., 2004). Recent fMRI studies confirm this theory, showing that patients had difficulty in affective response to salient stimuli but have hyperactive neurocircuits concerned with planning, consequences, and rules (Zastrow et al., 2009).

Modulatory defects in 5-HT function may explain the extremes of mood and binge eating cycles in patients with BN. Although restriction in food intake may lead to reduced synaptic serotonin release and a reduced dysphoric state, less serotonin may lead to unstable mood and a predisposition toward uncontrolled binge episodes (Kaye et al., 1998). Furthermore, serotonergic tone may be dysregulated in patients with BN as evidenced by the genetic polymorphisms associated with serotonergic genes as compared with control subjects. Accumulating PET and fMRI data suggest an imbalance in the expression of specific serotonin receptors and transporters in women with BN that results in functional deficits in impulse control, particularly in response to disease specific stimuli such as food or body evaluation.

The serotonin transporter (5-HTT) is responsible for the reuptake and subsequent conservation of 5-HT from the synaptic cleft (Zhao et al., 2006). Polymorphisms within the allele coding for 5-HTT have been associated with phenotypes associated with patients with bulimia nervosa, like harm avoidance, increased anxiety, and impulsivity. In mice with a mutation in the C-terminus of the 5-HTT resulting in its absence, significantly decreased levels of serotonin were found in the brain. These mice demonstrated anxiety and depression-related behaviors, which confirms that dysfunction in the serotonin transporter correlates with emotional abnormalities (Zhao et al., 2006) that may play a role in the pathogenesis of BN. *In vivo* studies have found decreased hypothalamic and thalamic serotonin transporter availability in patients with BN,

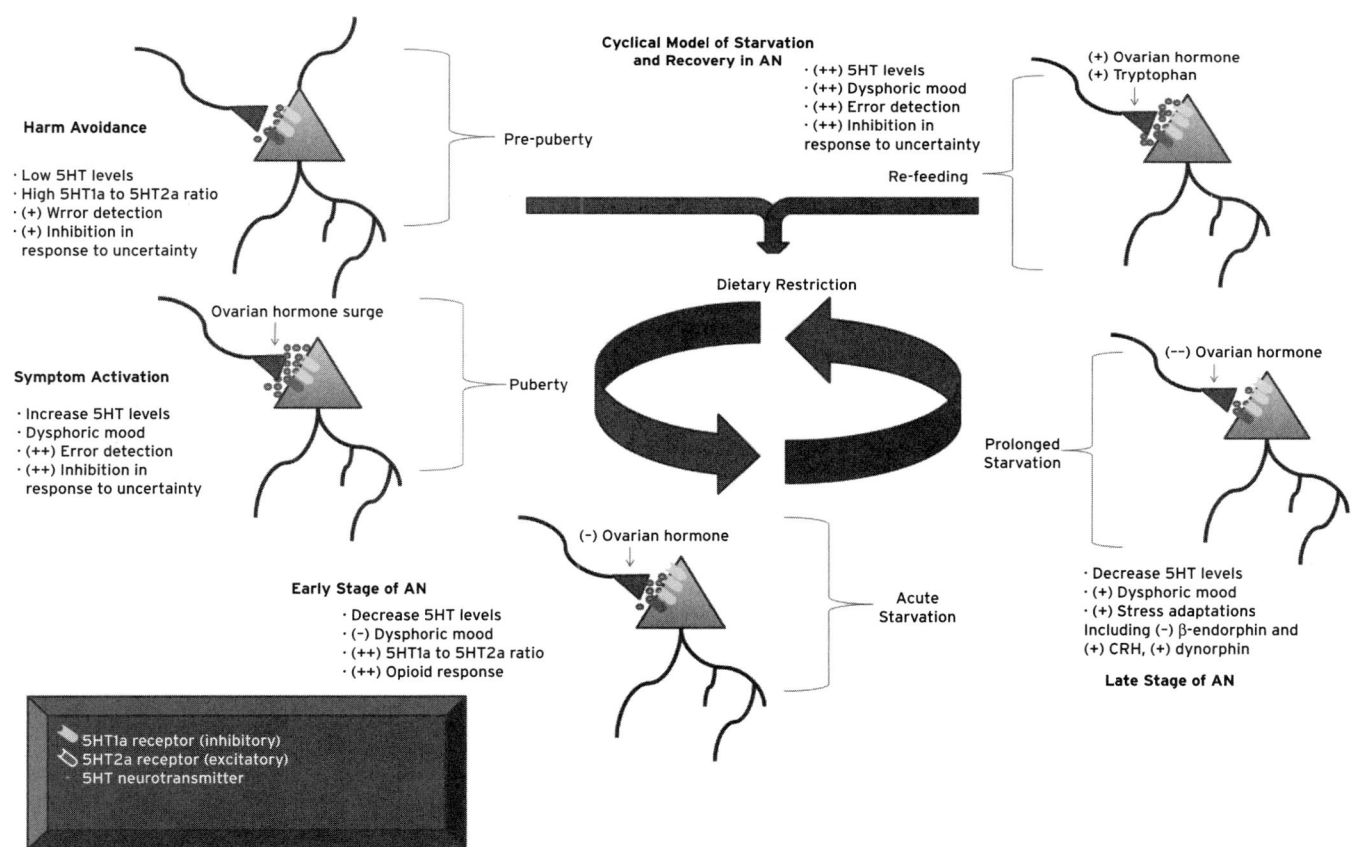

Figure 89.3 The theoretical changes to relevant serotonergic changes that accompany the cycle of starvation and recovery among individuals with anorexia nervosa are thought to be influenced by the increase in ovarian hormones which alter sensitivity to serotonergic signaling. Starvation provides temporary relief which is exacerbated early in recovery by weight gain. The alterations in serotonergic function contribute to cognitive changes in sensitivity to error detection and inhibitory control, particularly in the context of uncertainty.

providing the tangible link between mouse models and the pathology of decreased 5-HTT in patients with bulimia nervosa (Tauscher et al., 2001).

The 5-HT2A receptor is an excitatory postsynaptic serotonin receptor that increases neuronal firing in a number of brain regions involved in the regulation of emotional states within corticolimbic circuits. Studies report conflicting results as to the significance of this receptor in women with bulimia nervosa, but recent PET studies suggest that a decreased receptor density in the acutely ill may result in impaired communication in neurocircuits regulating emotion and impulsivity, which may be a result of a polymorphism in the receptor's gene (Nomura et al., 2006).

The 5-HT1A receptor is an inhibitory postsynaptic serotonin receptor implicated in the termination of signaling between two serotonergic neurons. High densities of this receptor are found in limbic brain areas, like the hippocampus, lateral septum, cortical areas, and the mesencephalic raphe nuclei. Receptors are located both on post- and presynaptic neurons (Barnes and Sharp, 1999). Reduced 5-HT1A binding is implicated in many anxiety disorders, with dysregulation manifesting in enhanced harm avoidance. Both over- and under-expression of the receptor has been shown in relation to a variety of mental illnesses related to anxiety (Akimova et al., 2009). In women with BN, 5-HT1A receptor binding is increased in areas of high receptor density, reflecting dysregulation associated with impulse control as it may relate to impulsive binge eating (Tiihonen et al., 2004). Colocalization and dysregulated ratios of 5-HT1A and 5-HT2A receptors in the medial prefrontal cortex may further illuminate the complexities of behavioral disinhibition in BN (Carli et al., 2006).

The dopaminergic system, like in AN, has also been implicated in the pathogenesis of BN. Positron emission tomography studies have demonstrated that dopamine in the dorsal striatum is involved in food motivation, as well as regulating reward pathways involving food in the nucleus accumbens (Volkow et al., 2002). Recent PET imaging studies have found decreased D2 receptor density in women with BN, indicative of inhibited dopamine response. This blunted response may reflect an adaptation in the motivation–reward system that seeks more potent reinforcers, impairing the ability of women with BN to use alternate reinforcers of behaviors like binge eating and/or purging (Broft et al., 2012). These findings are consistent with findings in individuals with substance abuse illnesses, although the link between the disorders remains complicated by a plethora of hormonal, cerebral, and sociocultural factors.

NEUROCIRCUITRY IMPLICATED IN ANOREXIA NERVOSA

A number of corticolimbic thalamic circuits are dysregulated in AN and they are likely to play a significant role in primary and secondary features of the illness. These complex circuits are involved in the regulation and integration of appetite, energy, emotional processing, and the motivation–reward pathway. Functional neuroimaging has helped to illuminate potential sources of dysregulation among these systems, but the data collected from these imaging studies are increasingly complicated

by a number of factors. First, the wide array of morphological changes to the brain during the acute illness phase of AN make functional imaging of the brain difficult to interpret. Enlarged ventricles, cerebral atrophy, decreased total gray matter volume, and decreased cerebrospinal fluid are observed morphological changes that recover with weight restoration, but at varying rates. The anterior cingulate cortex (ACC) and insular cortex regions of the brain, for example, may be slower to recover as compared with other regions, complicating data comparisons (Muhlau et al., 2007). Second, investigations into neurocircuits tend to compare activity to some baseline, or control, measurement, while failing to study the relationships between neurocircuits in a starved state. Therefore, there is a failure to formally integrate cause and effect relationships that may exist and give insight into the functionality of certain neurocircuits.

With the many brain regions and neurocircuits being investigated in the pathogenesis of AN, the anterior insula stands out as an integrative center incorporating them all. It has been hypothesized that this region is the key to the dysregulation of these neurocircuits (Nunn et al., 2008). The insula has been described as a bridge, facilitating connections between the frontal, temporal and parietal lobes, and the limbic system. This strategic location implicates that the insula is involved in regulation of the autonomic nervous system, the regulation of appetite and eating, taste and visceral memory, monitoring of the body state, integration of thoughts and feelings, the regulation of the experience of pain, the experience of disgust, interoceptive processing and anxiety, and empathy (Nunn et al., 2011). Disease-specific effects of puberty, dieting, genetics, societal pressures, and early developmental are hypothesized to carry some pathogenic effect on the insula (Nunn et al., 2011). Particularly intriguing to this insula hypothesis is the association between feelings of disgust and activation of the anterior insula (Phillips et al., 1997). Enhanced disgust responses to food in patients with AN as compared with control subjects suggest an important impairment in the insula that may play a role in the pathogenesis of the illness (Aharoni and Hertz, 2012).

NEUROCIRCUITRY IMPLICATED IN BULIMIA NERVOSA

Much of the neurocircuitry implicated in BN follows that of AN. Similar patterns of dysregulation are found in both illnesses, which are likely to reflect similarities in trait disturbances found in both disorders. Patients with BN have increased volume in the medial orbitofrontal cortex (mOFC) and enlarged nucleus accumbens (Schafer et al., 2010). Enlarged mOFC may represent altered reward processing because this region has much to do with the processing of rewards and punishments (Kringelbach and Rolls, 2004). The enlarged gray matter of the nucleus accumbens has been positively correlated with frequency of purging, although there is no clear causal link between this region and purging. It may be that chronic use of this area of the brain in the context of negative reinforcement strategies and compensatory behaviors like purging may lead to the increased volume (Schafer et al., 2010).

NEUROCIRCUITS INVOLVED IN APPETITE

Appetite is a complex drive that relies on many psychobiological processes. To understand such processes, a number of studies have focused on imaging to quantify the activity of brain regions involved in the regulation of appetite. Patients undergoing an fMRI scan are administered a sweet-taste perception task mediated by tongue receptors. Signals travel via a number of neural pathways to the primary gustatory cortex and the anterior insula, which is responsible for responding to various physical properties of the food. Food deprivation in controls activates the insula and associated regions, like the amygdala, anterior cingulate cortex (ACC), and the orbitofrontal cortex (OFC). A self-reported rating of the pleasantness of sweet foods also positively correlates with activity of the insula (Schoenfeld et al., 2004). Conversely, weight-restored women with AN show a significantly reduced activation level of the insula and associated regions. Additionally, self-reported rating of the pleasantness of sweet foods provided no correlation with activity of the insula, giving credibility to the argument that perception of taste may be altered in AN (Wagner et al., 2008).

The ability of the central nervous system to integrate physiological sensations and sensory information is a process known as interoceptive processing and primarily occurs in the anterior insula. Because of the strong body of evidence demonstrating the dysregulated neurocircuitry of the anterior insula as well as its crucial role in interoceptive awareness, some believe the pathology of AN is best studied in the context of the anterior insula. Dysregulation in this part of the brain may suggest that women suffering from this disorder have a fundamentally and physiologically altered sense of self (Kaye et al., 2009).

In BN, sweet-taste perception tasks show hypoactivation of the reward system, regulated by hyeractivation of the anterior insula. Patients with BN show reduced responsiveness to taste reward stimuli, as evidenced by hyperactivation of the insula and amygdala, which leads to reduced activation of the ventral putamen, which may correlate to reduced dopaminergic activity via down-regulation of D2 receptors (Frank et al., 2011). This dopaminergic taste reward system functions in much the same way as that seen in substance abuse. Speculation has been made as to an addiction state mediated by dysregulation of the dopaminergic system in women with BN in which episodically the drive for food stimulation leads to binge eating, and the consequent fears of excessive weight gain trigger excessive exercise or purging (Frank et al., 2011).

NEUROCIRCUITS INVOLVED IN EMOTIONAL PROCESSING

The ventral neurocircuit mentioned previously, including regions of the amygdala, insula, ventral striatum, ventral regions of the ACC, and the prefrontal cortex, is important in assigning emotional significance to stimuli as well as regulating affect and response to these stimuli (Kaye et al., 2009). Positron emission tomography imaging studies have demonstrated that this cognitive-limbic neurocircuit contains increased densities of 5-HT1A inhibitory neurons and decreased densities of 5-HT2A excitatory neurons in weight-restored women, thus locating a major source of dysregulation in the serotonergic system (Frank et al., 2002). Although suggestive of a mechanism

for the personality disturbances that may be associated with AN, it does not help to clarify whether the dysregulation is a consequence of starvation or rather a genetic predisposition.

An additional dorsal neurocircuit that includes the hippocampus, dorsal regions of the caudate, and the dorsolateral prefrontal cortex (DLPC) is the cognitive neurocircuit involved in more strategic processes like sequencing, planning, and the modulation of attention. This neurocircuit is also shown to be dysregulated in weight-restored women with AN. The emotional salience of food is further dysregulated as evidenced by fMRI research showing hyperactivity of the ACC and medial PFC (mPFC) in both acutely ill and weight-restored women (Fisher et al., 2009).

During tasks that require behavioral inhibition, women with BN display dysregulation in neurocircuitry implicated in emotional regulation like the ACC (Penas-Lledo et al., 2007). Self-regulatory processes are altered in these women as evidenced by their failure to activate frontostriatal circuitry (left inferolateral prefrontal cortex, lenticular nucleus, inferior frontal gyrus, ACC, putamen, and caudate regions) as compared with control subjects during conflict trials that required self-regulatory control for appropriate responses (Marsh et al., 2009). These activation deficits may correlate with decreased or dysfunctional serotonin metabolism and neurotransmission. Diminished activity within these areas may also explain the loss of control sensation of binge episodes reported by women with BN.

NEUROCIRCUITS INVOLVED IN BODY IMAGE PERCEPTION

The parietal cortex plays a vital role in proprioception and the development and maintenance of one's own body image. When presented with body image stimuli, acutely ill patients show decreased activity in the parietal cortex that is reversed with weight restoration. Positron emission tomography imaging studies suggest that these observations are consistent with the increased density of 5-HT2A receptors and the decreased density of 5-HT1A receptors in this region (Fisher et al., 2009). Additionally, patients with AN have a higher negative affective reaction when looking at images of another's body and reduced activation of relevant brain areas when looking at their own body as measured by fMRI, suggestive of body-related avoidance behaviors (Vocks et al., 2010). They also demonstrate emotionally bound body-size perception deficiencies (Cash and Deagle, 1997). Other studies suggest that dysregulation in body image perception lies in an impaired cognitive ability to mentally rotate objects and dysregulation when reconstructing or manipulating shapes (Skrzypek et al., 2001). Another psychopathology exhibiting this type of dysregulation is body dysmporphic disorder.

Many of the findings from fMRI studies of body image stimuli in patients with AN is applicable to bulimia nervosa as disturbances in neurocircuitry pertaining to body image are similar in both disorders. For BN, the anterior insula plays an especially crucial role in the construct of body image disturbance when estimating body size, which may serve to maintain the illness (Mohr et al., 2011). Women with BN may also demonstrate special perception deficiencies, as evidenced by nonactivation of the middle frontal gyrus during body size estimation tasks as compared with control subjects, reflecting a less functional spatial manipulation capacity (Mohr et al., 2011). Body image disturbance in eating disorders is not yet fully understood.

STARVATION VERSUS PSYCHOPATHOLOGY

Many of the aforementioned morphological, hormonal, and neurotransmitter changes described in the pathology of AN are reversed upon weight restoration, insinuating that they are consequences of starvation rather than predisposing factors to illness. The observed reduction in brain matter in starving individuals is consistent with the hyperactive HPA axis that induces catabolic changes in conditions of stress, leading to other effects such as hypercotisolism and decreased secretion of brain derived neurotrophic factor (BDNF), which is crucial to neuronal outgrowth and differentiation, synaptic connectivity, and neuronal repair (Monteleone, 2011). There is emerging evidence that some changes induced by starvation are not reversed upon weight restoration, including ACC volume and anterior insula volume. There is also evidence of permanently reduced metabolism in the prefrontal, parietal, temporal, and cingulate cortices, manifesting as larger ventricles and wider gaps between sulci as compared with controls (Muhlau et al., 2007). Although most studies investigate pathologies in weight-restored women with AN to avoid the confounding factors associated with starvation, it remains an ethical and practical challenge to differentiate between those pathologies that predispose one to develop AN and those factors that are a result of starvation.

GENDER DIFFERENCES

Females are more commonly affected by AN than are males with a female-to-male ratio of greater than ten to one (Hoek and van Hoeken, 2003). Interestingly, no published data exist as to the neurobiology and psychopathology of the illness specifically in males; therefore, no credible explanation exists for the gender disparity in prevalence rates of AN. Only speculation as to the possible sources of gender differences can be made. Further study into sexually dimorphic regulation systems is warranted (e.g., of the endocannabinoid system) and may implicate that peripheral differences between men and women account the disparity in prevalence. Furthermore, different gonadal hormones and hypothalamic axis differences would be a valid beginning for exploration into the gender-specific neurobiology of AN.

TEMPERAMENT AND ANOREXIA NERVOSA
HARM AVOIDANCE AND PERFECTIONISM

Harm avoidance and perfectionism remain two of the most prevalent traits among patients with AN and as such are considered predisposing factors in the development of the disorder, although they are also common among women with BN. Harm avoidance, a heritable trait, has been correlated with

specific brain regions and neurotransmitter dysregulation, like increased 5-HT1A receptor density (Bailer et al., 2004). More recently, decreased intrasynaptic dopamine and increased dopamine receptor density have also been linked to characteristic harm avoidance (Bailer et al., 2004). Overall perfectionism, when quantified using different analyses, is highly correlated with AN. Several genes associated with predisposition to AN have also been associated with perfectionism and may help to explain the endophenotype (Bachner-Melman et al., 2005).

IMPULSE CONTROL

The inability to inhibit impulsive behaviors is a temperament associated with certain groups of women with AN, although the trait is less pervasive than that of perfectionism and harm avoidance. These patients may exhibit behaviors of self-harm, trauma, binge eating and purging, substance abuse, lack of self-control, and aggression. The neurobiological basis for dysregulation in impulse control may also lie within the serotonergic system. Genetic polymorphisms in the serotonin transporter (5-HTT) have been linked to issues of impulse control (Kaye et al., 1991).

ACTIVITY-BASED ANOREXIA

There are no credible animal models of self-induced starvation and consequently a limit to many of the translational models of eating disorders. One exception is the activity-based anorexia (ABA) model, which capitalizes on the phenomena of increased physical activity found among starved rodents. Inducing hyperactivity, decreasing caloric intake, and enhancing activity of the HPA axis in adolescent rats creates an environment of ABA in which anxiety behaviors can be measured over subsequent weeks into rat adulthood. To date, it has been shown that exposure to ABA in adolescent rats produces symptoms of heightened anxiety into adulthood, paralleling the increased anxiety found in those with adolescent onset AN. Although causality has not been established, human studies have also correlated anxiety symptoms with high levels of exercise (Klein et al., 2004). These studies may have implications for patient care and treatment in the future (Kinzig and Hargrave, 2010).

BINGE EATING DISORDER

Binge eating disorder (BED) is characterized by periods of binge eating in which an abnormally large amount of food is consumed and accompanied by a feeling of being out of control. The disorder is similar to BN except that patients do not engage in compensatory behaviors following a binge episode. Lifetime prevalence rates of BED are 3.5% among women, and 2% among men (Hudson et al., 2007). This disorder remains a public health concern because of its associated comorbidities, including obesity and depression (Mathes et al., 2009). There is, however, opposition to characterizing binge eating as a disorder, questioning the validity of the distinction between BED and other behaviors of overeating. Research shows that

BED individuals and obese control subjects both exhibit high sensitivity to rewards and display enhanced anxiety, impulsivity, and addictive personality traits as compared with control subjects, which complicates the categorization of BED as a psychiatric illness. There is evidence that BED patients differ from obese controls in that binge episodes are significantly more hedonic, which may imply neurobiological dysregulation that merits further investigation (Davis et al., 2008).

FOOD ADDICTION

With the current advances in our knowledge of neurobiological mechanisms and neuroimaging, the link between binge eating and food addiction is being explored and debated. More than half of patients with BED meet self-reported diagnostic criteria for food addiction (Gearhardt et al., 2012). These patients may respond to clinical intervention based on the neurobiological dysregulation associated with their disorder. The heterogeneous nature of overeating and obesity has others questioning the validity of the studies that find significant correlation between food addiction and binge eating, focusing on neuroimaging studies like PET ligand studies and fMRI studies that present inconclusive and conflicting results in the context of a unified neurobiological profile of patients with BED demonstrating food addiction (Ziauddeen et al., 2012). Careful and sound investigation into the mechanism of binge eating and food addiction is warranted to avoid hasty categorization and subsequent clinical practices that could be costly and ineffective.

DISCLOSURE

Dr. Hildebrandt is an advisory board member and minority equity owner of Noom Inc. The content of this chapter is not directly relevant to Dr. Hildebrandt's role or interest in this company.
Ms. Downey has no conflicts or other interests to declare.

REFERENCES

Aharoni, R., and Hertz, M.M. (2012). Disgust sensitivity and anorexia nervosa. *Eur. Eat. Disord. Rev.* 20(2):106–110.
Akimova, E., Lanzenberger, R., et al. (2009). The serotonin-1A receptor in anxiety disorders. [Review]. *Biol. Psychiatry* 66(7):627–635.
Austin, S.B., Ziyadeh, N.J., et al. (2008). Irregular menses linked to vomiting in a nonclinical sample: findings from the National Eating Disorders Screening Program in high schools.. *J. Adolesc. Health* 42(5):450–457.
Bacanu, S.A., Bulik, C.M., et al. (2005). Linkage analysis of anorexia and bulimia nervosa cohorts using selected behavioral phenotypes as quantitative traits or covariates. *Am. J. Med. Genet. B Neuropsychiatr. Genet.* 139B(1):61–68.
Bachner-Melman, R., Gritsenko, I., et al. (2005). Dopaminergic polymorphisms associated with self-report measures of human altruism: a fresh phenotype for the dopamine D4 receptor.. *Mol. Psychiatry* 10(4):333–335.
Bailer, U.F., Frank, G.K., et al. (2005). Altered brain serotonin 5-HT1A receptor binding after recovery from anorexia nervosa measured by positron emission tomography and [carbonyl11C]WAY-100635. *Arch. Gen. Psychiatry* 62(9):1032–1041.
Bailer, U.F., Price, J.C., et al. (2004). Altered 5-HT(2A) receptor binding after recovery from bulimia-type anorexia nervosa: relationships

to harm avoidance and drive for thinness. *Neuropsychopharmacology* 29(6):1143–1155.
Barbato, G., Fichele, M., et al. (2006). Increased dopaminergic activity in restricting-type anorexia nervosa. *Psychiatry Res.* 142(2–3):253–255.
Barnes, N.M., and Sharp, T. (1999). A review of central 5-HT receptors and their function. [Review]. *Neuropharmacology* 38(8):1083–1152.
Batterham, R.L., ffytche, D.H., et al. (2007). PYY modulation of cortical and hypothalamic brain areas predicts feeding behaviour in humans. [Randomized Controlled Trial]. *Nature* 450(7166):106–109.
Bermudez-Silva, F.J., Viveros, M.P., et al. (2010). The endocannabinoid system, eating behavior and energy homeostasis: the end or a new beginning? *Pharmacol. Biochem. Behav.* 95(4):375–382.
Bird, A. (2002). DNA methylation patterns and epigenetic memory. *Genes Dev.* 16(1):6–21.
Birketvedt, G.S., Drivenes, E., et al. (2006). Bulimia nervosa—a primary defect in the hypothalamic-pituitary-adrenal axis? *Appetite* 46(2):164–167.
Broft, A., Shingleton, R., et al. (2012). Striatal dopamine in bulimia nervosa: a pet imaging study. *Int. J. Eat. Disord.* 45(5):648–656.
Buffenstein, R., Poppitt, S.D., et al. (1995). Food intake and the menstrual cycle: a retrospective analysis, with implications for appetite research. *Physiol. Behav.* 58(6):1067–1077.
Butera, P.C. (2010). Estradiol and the control of food intake. *Physiol. Behav.* 99(2):175–180.
Carli, M., Baviera, M., et al. (2006). Dissociable contribution of 5-HT1A and 5-HT2A receptors in the medial prefrontal cortex to different aspects of executive control such as impulsivity and compulsive perseveration in rats. *Neuropsychopharmacology* 31(4):757–767.
Carter, J.C., Mercer-Lynn, K.B., et al. (2012). A prospective study of predictors of relapse in anorexia nervosa: implications for relapse prevention. *Psychiatry Res.*
Cash, T.F., and Deagle, E.A., 3rd. (1997). The nature and extent of body-image disturbances in anorexia nervosa and bulimia nervosa: a meta-analysis. [Meta-Analysis]. *Int. J. Eat. Disord.* 22(2):107–125.
Chan, J.L., and Mantzoros, C.S. (2005). Role of leptin in energy-deprivation states: normal human physiology and clinical implications for hypothalamic amenorrhoea and anorexia nervosa. *Lancet* 366(9479):74–85.
Chandra, R., and Liddle, R.A. (2007). Cholecystokinin. *Curr. Opin. Endocrinol. Diabetes Obes.* 14(1):63–67.
Davis, C., Levitan, R.D., et al. (2008). Personality and eating behaviors: a case-control study of binge eating disorder. *Int. J. Eat. Disord.* 41(3):243–250.
Fisher, P.M., Meltzer, C.C., et al. (2009). Medial prefrontal cortex 5-HT(2A) density is correlated with amygdala reactivity, response habituation, and functional coupling. *Cereb. Cortex* 19(11):2499–2507.
Frank, G.K., Kaye, W.H., et al. (2002). Reduced 5-HT2A receptor binding after recovery from anorexia nervosa. *Biol. Psychiatry* 52(9):896–906.
Frank, G.K., Reynolds, J.R., et al. (2011). Altered temporal difference learning in bulimia nervosa. *Biol. Psychiatry* 70(8):728–735.
Frieling, H., Romer, K.D., et al. (2010). Epigenetic dysregulation of dopaminergic genes in eating disorders. *Int. J. Eat. Disord.* 43(7):577–583.
Gabory, A., Attig, L., et al. (2009). Sexual dimorphism in environmental epigenetic programming. *Mol. Cell Endocrinol.* 304(1–2):8–18.
Gearhardt, A.N., White, M.A., et al. (2012). An examination of the food addiction construct in obese patients with binge eating disorder. *Int. J. Eat. Disord.* 45(5):657–663.
Gendall, K.A., Kaye, W.H., et al. (1999). Leptin, neuropeptide Y, and peptide YY in long-term recovered eating disorder patients. *Biol. Psychiatry* 46(2):292–299.
Geracioti, T.D., Jr., and Liddle, R.A. (1988). Impaired cholecystokinin secretion in bulimia nervosa. *N. Engl. J. Med.* 319(11):683–688.
Gui, Y., Silha, J.V., et al. (2004). Sexual dimorphism and regulation of resistin, adiponectin, and leptin expression in the mouse. *Obes. Res.* 12(9):1481–1491.
Hasan, T.F., and Hasan, H. (2011). Anorexia nervosa: a unified neurological perspective. *Int. J. Med. Sci.* 8(8):679–703.
Helder, S.G., and Collier, D.A. (2011). The genetics of eating disorders. *Curr. Top. Behav. Neurosci.* 6, 157–175.
Hildebrandt, T., Alfano, L., et al. (2010). Conceptualizing the role of estrogens and serotonin in the development and maintenance of bulimia nervosa. *Clin. Psychol. Rev.* 30(6):655–668.
Hoek, H.W. (2006). Incidence, prevalence and mortality of anorexia nervosa and other eating disorders. *Curr. Opin. Psychiatry* 19(4):389–394.
Hoek, H.W., and van Hoeken, D. (2003). Review of the prevalence and incidence of eating disorders. *Int. J. Eat. Disord.* 34(4):383–396.
Hudson, J.I., Hiripi, E., et al. (2007). The prevalence and correlates of eating disorders in the National Comorbidity Survey Replication. *Biol. Psychiatry* 61(3):348–358.

Kaye, W., Gendall, K., et al. (1998). Serotonin neuronal function and selective serotonin reuptake inhibitor treatment in anorexia and bulimia nervosa. *Biol. Psychiatry* 44(9):825–838.

Kaye, W.H. (1996). Neuropeptide abnormalities in anorexia nervosa. *Psychiatry Res.* 62(1):65–74.

Kaye, W.H., Berrettini, W., et al. (1990). Altered cerebrospinal fluid neuropeptide Y and peptide YY immunoreactivity in anorexia and bulimia nervosa. *Arch. Gen. Psychiatry* 47(6):548–556.

Kaye, W.H., Frank, G.K., et al. (2005). Serotonin alterations in anorexia and bulimia nervosa: new insights from imaging studies. *Physiol. Behav.* 85(1):73–81.

Kaye, W.H., Fudge, J.L., et al. (2009). New insights into symptoms and neurocircuit function of anorexia nervosa. *Nat. Rev. Neurosci.* 10(8):573–584.

Kaye, W.H., Gwirtsman, H.E., et al. (1991). Altered serotonin activity in anorexia nervosa after long-term weight restoration. Does elevated cerebrospinal fluid 5-hydroxyindoleacetic acid level correlate with rigid and obsessive behavior? *Arch. Gen. Psychiatry* 48(6):556–562.

Kaye, W.H., Wagner, A., et al. (2011). Neurocircuity of eating disorders. [Review]. *Curr. Top. Behav. Neurosci.* 6, 37–57.

Keating, C. (2011). Sex differences precipitating anorexia nervosa in females: the estrogen paradox and a novel framework for targeting sex-specific neurocircuits and behavior. [Review]. *Curr. Top. Behav. Neurosci.* 8, 189–207.

Kinzig, K.P., and Hargrave, S.L. (2010). Adolescent activity-based anorexia increases anxiety-like behavior in adulthood. *Physiol. Behav.* 101(2):269–276.

Kirkham, T.C., Williams, C.M., et al. (2002). Endocannabinoid levels in rat limbic forebrain and hypothalamus in relation to fasting, feeding and satiation: stimulation of eating by 2-arachidonoyl glycerol. *Br. J. Pharmacol.* 136(4):550–557.

Klein, D.A., Bennett, A.S., et al. (2004). Exercise "addiction" in anorexia nervosa: model development and pilot data. *CNS Spectr.* 9(7):531–537.

Klump, K.L., Gobrogge, K.L., et al. (2006). Preliminary evidence that gonadal hormones organize and activate disordered eating. *Psychol. Med.* 36(4):539–546.

Klump, K.L., Keel, P.K., et al. (2008). Ovarian hormones and binge eating: exploring associations in community samples. *Psychol. Med.* 38(12):1749–1757.

Korzekwa, M.I., Lamont, J.A., et al. (1996). Late luteal phase dysphoric disorder and the thyroid axis revisited. *J. Clin. Endocrinol. Metab.* 81(6):2280–2284.

Kringelbach, M.L., and Rolls, E.T. (2004). The functional neuroanatomy of the human orbitofrontal cortex: evidence from neuroimaging and neuropsychology. *Prog. Neurobiol.* 72(5):341–372.

Licinio, J., Wong, M.L., et al. (1996). The hypothalamic-pituitary-adrenal axis in anorexia nervosa. *Psychiatry Res.* 62(1):75–83.

Lo Sauro, C., Ravaldi, C., et al. (2008). Stress, hypothalamic-pituitary-adrenal axis and eating disorders. *Neuropsychobiology* 57(3):95–115.

Mantzoros, C., Flier, J.S., et al. (1997). Cerebrospinal fluid leptin in anorexia nervosa: correlation with nutritional status and potential role in resistance to weight gain. *J. Clin. Endocrinol. Metab.* 82(6):1845–1851.

Marsh, R., Steinglass, J.E., et al. (2009). Deficient activity in the neural systems that mediate self-regulatory control in bulimia nervosa. *Arch. Gen. Psychiatry* 66(1):51–63.

Mathes, W.F., Brownley, K.A., et al. (2009). The biology of binge eating. *Appetite* 52(3):545–553.

Miller, K.K. (2011). Endocrine dysregulation in anorexia nervosa update. *J. Clin. Endocrinol. Metab.* 96(10):2939–2949.

Misra, M., Miller, K.K., et al. (2006). Elevated peptide YY levels in adolescent girls with anorexia nervosa. *J. Clin. Endocrinol. Metab.* 91(3):1027–1033.

Mize, A.L., Poisner, A.M., et al. (2001). Estrogens act in rat hippocampus and frontal cortex to produce rapid, receptor-mediated decreases in serotonin 5-HT(1A) receptor function. *Neuroendocrinology* 73(3):166–174.

Mohr, H.M., Roder, C., et al. (2011). Body image distortions in bulimia nervosa: investigating body size overestimation and body size satisfaction by fMRI. *NeuroImage* 56(3):1822–1831.

Montague, P.R., Hyman, S.E., et al. (2004). Computational roles for dopamine in behavioural control. [Review]. *Nature* 431(7010):760–767.

Monteleone, P. (2011). New frontiers in endocrinology of eating disorders. *Curr. Top. Behav. Neurosci.* 6, 189–208.

Monteleone, P., Bortolotti, F., et al. (2000). Plamsa leptin response to acute fasting and refeeding in untreated women with bulimia nervosa. *J. Clin. Endocrinol. Metab.* 85(7):2499–2503.

Monteleone, P., and Maj, M. (2008). Genetic susceptibility to eating disorders: associated polymorphisms and pharmacogenetic suggestions. *Pharmacogenomics* 9(10):1487–1520.

Monteleone, P., Serritella, C., et al. (2008). Deranged secretion of ghrelin and obestatin in the cephalic phase of vagal stimulation in women with anorexia nervosa. *Biol. Psychiatry* 64(11):1005–1008.

Muhlau, M., Gaser, C., et al. (2007). Gray matter decrease of the anterior cingulate cortex in anorexia nervosa. *Am. J. Psychiatry* 164(12):1850–1857.

Nomura, M., Kusumi, I., et al. (2006). Involvement of a polymorphism in the 5-HT2A receptor gene in impulsive behavior. *Psychopharmacology (Berl.)*:187(1):30–35.

Nunn, K., Frampton, I., et al. (2011). Anorexia nervosa and the insula. *Med. Hypotheses* 76(3):353–357.

Nunn, K., Frampton, I., et al. (2008). The fault is not in her parents but in her insula—a neurobiological hypothesis of anorexia nervosa. *Eur. Eat. Disord. Rev.* 16(5):355–360.

Pae, C.U., Mandelli, L., et al. (2009). Effectiveness of antidepressant treatments in pre-menopausal versus post-menopausal women: a pilot study on differential effects of sex hormones on antidepressant effects. *Biomed. Pharmacother.* 63(3):228–235.

Penas-Lledo, E.M., Loeb, K.L., et al. (2007). Anterior cingulate activity in bulimia nervosa: a fMRI case study. *Eat. Weight Disord.* 12(4):e78–e82.

Philibert, R.A., Sandhu, H., et al. (2008). The relationship of 5HTT (SLC6A4) methylation and genotype on mRNA expression and liability to major depression and alcohol dependence in subjects from the Iowa Adoption Studies. *Am. J. Med. Genet. B Neuropsychiatr. Genet.* 147B(5):543–549.

Phillips, M.L., Young, A.W., et al. (1997). A specific neural substrate for perceiving facial expressions of disgust. *Nature* 389(6650):495–498.

Pinheiro, A.P., Bulik, C.M., et al. (2010). Association study of 182 candidate genes in anorexia nervosa. *Am. J. Med. Genet. B Neuropsychiatr. Genet.* 153B(5):1070–1080.

Poirier, L.A. (2002). The effects of diet, genetics and chemicals on toxicity and aberrant DNA methylation: an introduction. *J. Nutr.* 132(Suppl 8):2336S–2339S.

Polesskaya, O.O., Aston, C., et al. (2006). Allele C-specific methylation of the 5-HT2A receptor gene: evidence for correlation with its expression and expression of DNA methylase DNMT1. *J. Neurosci. Res.* 83(3):362–373.

Raz, L., Khan, M.M., et al. (2008). Rapid estrogen signaling in the brain. *Neurosignals* 16(2–3):140–153.

Resko, J.A., and Roselli, C.E. (1997). Prenatal hormones organize sex differences of the neuroendocrine reproductive system: observations on guinea pigs and nonhuman primates. *Cell. Mol. Neurobiol.* 17(6):627–648.

Roepke, T.A., Qiu, J., et al. (2009). Cross-talk between membrane-initiated and nuclear-initiated oestrogen signalling in the hypothalamus. *J. Neuroendocrinol.* 21(4):263–270.

Roth-Deri, I., Green-Sadan, T., et al. (2008). Beta-endorphin and drug-induced reward and reinforcement. *Prog. Neurobiol.* 86(1):1–21.

Rubinow, D.R., Schmidt, P.J., et al. (1998). Estrogen-serotonin interactions: implications for affective regulation. *Biol. Psychiatry* 44(9):839–850.

Schafer, A., Vaitl, D., et al. (2010). Regional grey matter volume abnormalities in bulimia nervosa and binge-eating disorder. *NeuroImage* 50(2):639–643.

Scherag, S., Hebebrand, J., et al. (2010). Eating disorders: the current status of molecular genetic research. *Eur. Child Adolesc. Psychiatry* 19(3):211–226.

Schoenfeld, M.A., Neuer, G., et al. (2004). Functional magnetic resonance tomography correlates of taste perception in the human primary taste cortex. *Neuroscience* 127(2):347–353.

Skrzypek, S., Wehmeier, P.M., et al. (2001). Body image assessment using body size estimation in recent studies on anorexia nervosa. A brief review. *Eur. Child. Adolesc. Psychiatry* 10(4):215–221.

Smink, F.R., van Hoeken, D., et al. (2012). Epidemiology of eating disorders: incidence, prevalence and mortality rates. *Curr. Psychiatry Rep.*

Stoving, R.K., Hangaard, J., et al. (1999). A review of endocrine changes in anorexia nervosa. *J. Psychiatr. Res.* 33(2):139–152.

Strober, M., Freeman, R., et al. (2000). Controlled family study of anorexia nervosa and bulimia nervosa: evidence of shared liability and transmission of partial syndromes. *Am. J. Psychiatry* 157(3):393–401.

Strober, M., Freeman, R., et al. (1997). The long-term course of severe anorexia nervosa in adolescents: survival analysis of recovery, relapse, and outcome predictors over 10–15 years in a prospective study. *Int. J. Eat. Disord.* 22(4):339–360.

Swenne, I., Stridsberg, M., et al. (2009). Triiodothyronine is an indicator of nutritional status in adolescent girls with eating disorders. *Horm. Res.* 71(5):268–275.

Tagami, T., Satoh, N., et al. (2004). Adiponectin in anorexia nervosa and bulimia nervosa. *J. Clin. Endocrinol. Metab.* 89(4):1833–1837.

Tauscher, J., Pirker, W., et al. (2001). [123I] beta-CIT and single photon emission computed tomography reveal reduced brain serotonin transporter availability in bulimia nervosa. *Biol. Psychiatry* 49(4):326–332.

Tiihonen, J., Keski-Rahkonen, A., et al. (2004). Brain serotonin 1A receptor binding in bulimia nervosa. *Biol. Psychiatry* 55(8):871–873.

Tong, J., and D'Alessio, D. (2011). Eating disorders and gastrointestinal peptides. *Curr. Opin. Endocrinol. Diabetes Obes.* 18(1):42–49.

Tyrka, A.R., Waldron, I., et al. (2002). Prospective predictors of the onset of anorexic and bulimic syndromes. *Int. J. Eat. Disord.* 32(3):282–290.

Utz, A.L., Lawson, E.A., et al. (2008). Peptide YY (PYY) levels and bone mineral density (BMD) in women with anorexia nervosa. *Bone* 43(1):135–139.

Vocks, S., Busch, M., et al. (2010). Neural correlates of viewing photographs of one's own body and another woman's body in anorexia and bulimia nervosa: an fMRI study. *J. Psychiatry Neurosci.* 35(3):163–176.

Volkow, N.D., Wang, G.J., et al. (2002). "Nonhedonic" food motivation in humans involves dopamine in the dorsal striatum and methylphenidate amplifies this effect. *Synapse* 44(3):175–180.

Wagner, A., Aizenstein, H., et al. (2008). Altered insula response to taste stimuli in individuals recovered from restricting-type anorexia nervosa. *Neuropsychopharmacology* 33(3):513–523.

Zastrow, A., Kaiser, S., et al. (2009). Neural correlates of impaired cognitive-behavioral flexibility in anorexia nervosa. *Am. J. Psychiatry* 166(5):608–616.

Zhang, J.V., Ren, P.G., et al. (2005). Obestatin, a peptide encoded by the ghrelin gene, opposes ghrelin's effects on food intake. *Science* 310(5750):996–999.

Zhao, S., Edwards, J., et al. (2006). Insertion mutation at the C-terminus of the serotonin transporter disrupts brain serotonin function and emotion-related behaviors in mice. *Neuroscience* 140(1):321–334.

Ziauddeen, H., Farooqi, I.S., et al. (2012). Obesity and the brain: how convincing is the addiction model? *Nat. Rev. Neurosci.* 13(4):279–286.

INDEX

autosomal recessive, 1014–1017
BBS and, 1014–1015
  comorbidities with, 1015
  diagnosis of, 1014
  discovery of, 1014
  genetic expression of, 1014
  prevalence of, 1014
  treatment of, 1015
causes of, 972–973
CFCS and, 1011–1012
  clinical indications for, 1011
  Costello syndrome and, 1011
  gene mutations and, 1011–1012
  Noonan syndrome and, 1011
  pregnancy and, 1011
  prevalence rates for, 1011
CNVs in, 939, 946–947
CS and, 1015–1016
  clinical indications for,
    1015–1016
  phenotypes for, 1015
definition of, 933
deletion syndromes in, 946
DGS, 973–974, 982
diagnosis of, 933, 946, 1010
Down syndrome, 939
  animal models of, 972–973
  spine pathology with, 990
  transgenic models, 110
duplication syndromes in, 946
etiological classification of, 1011
exome sequencing for, 947–948
as extreme variant trait, 937
FGS, 1018–1019
  clinical features of, 1018
  diagnosis of, 1018
  gene mutations in, 1018
  prevalence of, 1019
FXS, 940
  animal models of, 971,
    974–975
  clinical trials for, 1062
  epigenetics for, 101
  mGluR5 receptors in, 1061–1062
  phenotypes for, 130
  stem cell modeling for, 130
  treatment therapies for,
    1031–1032
genetic sources of, 933, 1010
  single-gene syndromes, 940
heritability of, 935–936
IQ and, 946
KS and, 101, 1012–1013
  comorbidities with, 1013
  diagnostic criteria for,
    1012–1013
  gene mutations with, 1013
  prevalence rates for, 1012
prevalence rates for, 935–936
rasopathies with, 1012–1015
reproductive disadvantage with,
  939
SLOS and, 1016–1017
  clinical indications for, 1016
  comorbidities with, 1016
  diagnosis of, 1016
  prevalence rates for, 1016
  treatment therapies for,
    1016–1017
SNVs in, 947–948
SoS and, 1013–1014
  causes of, 1014

clinical indications for,
  1013–1014
NSD1 gene and, 1014
trajectory into adulthood, 934
X linked, 975, 1017–1019
intellectual quotient (IQ), 946
interleaved scanning
  DBS, 218
  tDCS, 215
  TMS, 216
interleukin-6 (IL-6), 84
intermittent explosive disorder (IED),
  951
International Classification of Disease
  (ICD)
  development of, 369–370
  DSM-V and, 1067, 1068
  WHO adoption of, 370
International Classification of Disease,
  10th Revision (ICD-10)
  bipolar disorder in, 227–228, 229
  development of, 370
  mood disorder diagnostic systems
    and, 371, 372–385
  schizoaffective disorder in,
    227–229
  schizophrenia in, 226, 227–228
  synaptic disease in, 321–322
Internet and computer-based
  psychotherapy (ICT), 631
  CBT and, 631
  cost effectiveness of, 632
  effectiveness of, 633–634
  mechanisms of action for, 633
interpersonal therapy (IPT), 521
interpretive bias modification (CBM-I)
  therapy, 628
  cost effectiveness of, 632
  empirical evidence for, 628–629
intracranial self-stimulation (ICSS),
  678
intrauterine growth restriction (IUGR)
  phenotypes, 959–960
intrinsic plasticity, of brain, 67–71. *See*
  also ion channels
  AD and, 71
  AHP and, 70
  AIS and, 68–69
  AUD and, 71
  axons and, 69
  at axo-somatic level, 68
  definition of, 67–68
  dendrites and, 68
  drug abuse and, 71
  experience-dependent, 70–71
  features of, 67–68
  in learning, 70–71
  in memory, 70–71
  molecular substrates and, 69–70
  morphine exposure and, 71
  in neurological disorders, 71
  postnatal brain development and,
    988
  rule learning and, 70–71
  in saving, 70
  at subcellular level, 68–69
  SUD and, 675
  after TBI, 71
  voltage-gated ion channels and,
    67–68
in utero electroporation (IUE), 142
in vivo recording, 32–33

in vivo transplantation, 133
IOM. *See* Institute of Medicine
ion channels. *See also* voltage-gated ion
    channels
  ligand-gated, 31
  mental illness and, 34–35
  molecular substrates and, 69–70
  neurons and, 27
  neurotransmitter-gated, 40–42
  in signal transduction pathways,
    40–41
  in synaptic disease, 313
ionotropic receptors, 32
  addiction and, 687–688
ion pumps, 27
Iowa Gambling task, 278
IP₃ receptors. *See* inositol-
    trisphosphate receptors
iproniazid, 508
iPSCs. *See* induced pluripotent stem
    cells
IPSP. *See* inhibitory postsynaptic
    potential
IPT. *See* interpersonal therapy
IQ. *See* intellectual quotient
iron levels, ADHD and, 1040
ischemia, VCI and, 900–901, 909
  SBI, 903
  WMH and, 903
  treatment therapies for, 910–911
isocarboxazid, 511
IUE. *See* in utero electroporation
IUGR phenotypes. *See* intrauterine
    growth restriction
    phenotypes
ivacaftor, 1076

J
Jackson, John Hughlings, 223
Jakob, Alfons, 915
Janet, Pierre, 369
Janus tyrosine kinase-signal transducer
    and activator of transcription
    (JAK-STAT) receptors, 46
Jaspers, Karl, 224
Joubert syndrome, 982
Jun proteins, 83
  as IEG, 83

K
Kabuki syndrome (KS), 101,
    1012–1013
  comorbidities with, 1013
  diagnostic criteria for, 1012–1013
  gene mutations with, 1013
  prevalence rates for, 1012
Kahlbaum, Karl, 368
Kalirin, 335
Kalydeco. *See* ivacaftor
Katzman, Robert, 791
ketamine, 36
  in antidepressants, 433–434
    biomarkers in, 442–444
    molecular mechanisms in, 442
  clinical trials with, 442
  in glutamatergic system, 439–444
  limitations of, 441–442
  for MDD, 425
  side effects of, 442
knockout mouse models, 111–113
  conditional, 116–117

NT-3 factors, 116
RTT, 116
vesicle function, 116–117
disease models, 112
dopaminergic system and, 112, 114
ES cell line modifications, 111
haplo-insufficiency, 112
lethality issues, 113
limitations of, 112–113
Reeler gene, 112
of schizophrenia, 292
TH, 113
transgenic compared to, 111
knockout rat models, 112
Kraepelin, Emil, 232, 223
  mood disorder diagnosis under,
    368
  neuroimaging methodologies
    influenced by, 256
  phenomenology of, 1073
KS. *See* Kabuki syndrome
Kuhn, Franz, 1075
Kuru, neuropathology of, 927

L
Landau Kleffner syndrome (LKS),
    1023–1024
language deficits
  with LBD, 876
  with PDD, 876
large-clone transgenic mouse models
    for disease states, 110
  Down Syndrome, 110
  GFP, 110
large-scale sequencing studies,
    242–245
late life, onset of disease in.
    See also late onset
    Alzheimer's disease
  bipolar disorder, 384
  depression
    AD and, 478
    AGTR genes, 477
    basal ganglia circuits and, 475
    BDNF and, 477
    brain systems in, 471–472
    circuit changes in, 473–475
    degenerative diseases and, 478
    dorsal circuit and, 473–474
    genetics of, 477
    historical recognition of, 470
    5HTTLPR polymorphism, 477
    lesions and, location of,
      470–473
    metabolomic studies for,
      477–478
    MRI for, 470
    neurobiology of, 471–472
    PD and, 478
    subcortical ischemic disease
      and, 476
    in twin studies, 472–473
    vascular, 476–477
    ventral circuit and, 474–475
  MDD, 384
  mood disorders, diagnostic systems
    for, 384
  subcortical ischemic disease,
    475–476
    depression and, 476
latent growth mixture modeling
    (LGMM), 1144

Omniscan, 151
1000 Genomes Project, 164
opioids. *See also* heroine,
        neuroimaging for; morphine,
        intrinsic plasticity of brain
        and
    BPD and, 1093
    for depression, 451
    MRS studies of, 747–751
    neuroimaging for, 727
    self-cutting and, 1093
Opitz-Kaveggia syndrome (FGS),
        1018–1019
    clinical features of, 1018
    diagnosis of, 1018
    gene mutations in, 1018
    prevalence of, 1019
opponent-process models, of
        addiction, 737
opsin genes, 138, 138–140
    optimization of, 139
    rhodopsins and, 138
    SFOs, 139–140
    SSFOs, 139–140
Optison, 148
optogenetic technology, for disease
        research
    action spectrum engineering for,
        145
    for addiction, 690
    biochemical-signaling expansion
        in, 146
    biophysics and, 145–146
    electric-inhibitory channels in, 146
    experimental potential of, 141
    functions of, 138
    genomics in, 145–146
    halorhodopsins, 138
        light-activated, 141
    light-sensors in, 145–146
    mammalian biology issues and, 144
    neuropsychiatric disease models,
        141–144
        for anxiety disorders, 142
        combinatorial optogenetics, 144
        excitation-inhibition imbalance
            in, 142, 144
        fiberoptic neural interface, 142
        IUE, 142
        for memory deficits, 142
        projection targeting in, 142
    neuroscience applications, 141–144
    non-genetically tractable cell types
        in, 145
    opsin genes, 138, 138–140
        optimization of, 139
        rhodopsins and, 138
        SFOs, 139–140
        SSFOs, 139–140
    reverse engineering in, 145
    3D light delivery in, 144–145
    tool functionality, 138–141
    tool mutations in, 146
    versatile strategizing with, 144
    wiring extraction patterns and, 145
orbital prefrontal cortex (OFC),
        474–475
    aggression and, 1106
    in personality disorders, 1089
    in reward, 735
orexin, 22
organotherapy, 483
orofaciodigital syndrome, 982

overconsolidation theory, of PTSD, 561
Owen, Michael, 1084
oxytocin
    in adult bonding animal models,
        1121
    in BPD treatment, 1092–1093
    infant-parental attachment and,
        1115
    mother-infant attachment and,
        1116–1118

P

PACAP. *See* pituitary adenylate cyclase-
        activating polypeptide
pair bonding, 1119–1120
    animal models of, 1120–1123
paliperidone, 351
PANDAS. *See* Pediatric Autoimmune
        Neuropsychiatric Disorder
        Associated with Streptococcal
        infections
panic disorder, 532
    DCS therapy for, 625
    family studies for, 537
    GABA and, 567
    neurobiology of, 615–616
        amygdala and, 615
        insula and, 615–616
        PFC activity and, 616
    symptoms of, 637
    treatment therapy for
        with DCS, 625
        first-line approaches to, 637–640
        second-line approaches to,
            640–641
    twin studies for, 537
paradoxical sleep, 1128. *See also* rapid-
        eye movement sleep
parent-offspring bonding
    father-infant attachment,
        1118–1119
        chemical substrates in, 1119
        display behaviors in, 1118–1119
        neuroanatomy of, 1119
    infant-parental attachment,
        1113–1116
        autism and, 1115–1116
        development of, 1113
        motivation circuits in, 1115
        neurobiology of, 1115
        social approaches to, 1115
    mother-infant attachment,
        1116–1118
        chemical substrates of,
            1116–1118
        development of, 1116
        maternal neglect and, 1118
        neuroanatomy of, 1116–1118
        neurobiology of, 1116–1118
        oxytocin and, 1116–1118
    neurobiology of, 1113–1119, 1124
        for infant-parental attachment,
            1115, 1113–1116
        for mother-infant attachment,
            1116–1118
Parkinson, James, 872
Parkinson's disease (PD)
    animal models of, 810
        MPTP model, 810
    autonomic dysfunction with, 877
    deprenyl and, 16
    dopamines and, 131
    gene editing in, 131

genetic mutations in, 130–131
    late life depression and, 478
    neuropathology of, 878
    PDD
        cognitive impairments in, 872
        depression with, 876
        development of, 872
        diagnostic criteria for, 873
        DLB compared to, 874
        executive function deficits in,
            874–875
        hallucinations with, 876
        language deficits with, 876
        memory deficits with, 876
        neuropathology of, 878
    phenotypes in, 131
    prevalence rates for, 872
    stem cell modeling for, 130–131
    viral-mediated gene transfer and,
        117–118
    ZFN and, 131
Parkinson's disease dementia (PDD)
    cognitive impairments in, 872
    depression with, 876
    development of, 872
    diagnostic criteria for, 873
    DLB compared to, 874
    executive function deficits in,
        874–875
    hallucinations with, 876
    language deficits with, 876
    memory deficits with, 876
    neuropathology of, 878
Parnate. *See* tranylcypromine
paroxetine, 641, 895, 1031
partial directed coherence (PDC), 1003
parvalbumin (PV) neurons,
        304–309
pathological anxiety, 552
    animal models of, 560–564
        avoidance in, 563–564
        coping processes in, 562–564
        developmental manipulations
            in, 561
        for fear extinction, 562–563
        genetic manipulations in, 561–562
        incubation in, 563
        individual differences in, 562
        psychological manipulations
            in, 561
        reconsolidation in, 563
        stress-enhanced fear learning
            in, 561
        treatment processes in, 562–564
    defensive responding and, 552
    neurobiology of, 606
    stress responses to, 552
pathological fear, 552
    animal models of, 560–564
        avoidance in, 563–564
        coping processes in, 562–564
        developmental manipulations
            in, 561
        for fear extinction, 562–563
        genetic manipulations in,
            561–562
        incubation in, 563
        individual differences in, 562
        psychological manipulations
            in, 561
        reconsolidation in, 563
        stress-enhanced fear learning
            in, 561

treatment processes in, 562–564
defensive responding and, 552
neurobiology of, 606
stress responses to, 552
pathways. *See* axon pathways; signal
        transduction pathways
Pavlovian threat conditioning (PTC),
        554–558
    behavioral aspects of, 554
    molecular mechanisms of, 556
    neurocircuitry in, 554–556
    procedure variations for, 556–558
    synaptic plasticity, 556
PBS. *See* positive behavioral support
PcG proteins. *See* Polycomb-Group
        proteins
PCP. *See* phenylcyclidine
PCr. *See* phosphocreatine
PD. *See* Parkinson's disease
PDC. *See* partial directed coherence
PDD. *See* Parkinson's disease
        dementia
pediatric anxiety disorders
    age of onset for, 539
    family studies for, 539
        design of, 539
        OAD, 540
    separation anxiety disorder, 539
    SOC, 539
    twin studies for, 539
Pediatric Autoimmune
        Neuropsychiatric Disorder
        Associated with Streptococcal
        infections (PANDAS),
        1056–1057
Pepeu, Giancarlo, 811
peptide transmitters
    classical compared to, 21
    hypocretin, 22
    inactivation of, 22
    orexin, 22
    release of, 22
    storage of, 21–22
    synthesis of, 21–22
    types of, 1014
peptide YY (PYY), 1177
perfectionism, AN and, 1182
perimenopausal depression, 491–492
    hormones
        in studies, 491–492
        in therapy treatments, 492
    onset triggers for, 492
    risk predictors for, 491
personality
    BPD
        diagnostic criteria for, 1090
        FFM and, 1090
        emotional regulation and, 589
        FFM for, 1089, 1090
        Five Factor Model, 1089, 1090
        LBD and, 876–877
personality disorders. *See also*
        obsessive-compulsive
        disorder
    ASPD, 1093–1097
        aggression and, 1094–1095
        candidate gene studies for, 1097
        childhood antecedents for, 1094
        clinical indications for,
            1093–1094
        cognitive function and, 1096
        comorbidities with, 1094
        development of, 1094

reward prediction
    errors, 733
    wanting and, 275, 277–280
reward sensitivity, 681
rhodopsins
    ChRs, 138
        red-shifting, 140–141
    opsin genes and, 138
    optogenetic technology, 138
ribonucleic acid (RNA), 76–77.
        See also gene expression;
        transcription control, for
        genomes
    base pairing in, 76
    DNA transcription into, 77
    information flow in, to proteins,
        77–78
    miRNAs, 77, 98
    mRNA, 14, 77
    ncRNA, 77, 95–96
    nucleosomes in, 79
    ribosomes in, 77–78
    RNAi, 93–94
    transcription phases, 79
ribosomes, 77–78
riluzole, 445, 657
risperidone, 351, 641–642, 895,
        1029–1030, 1031, 1058
The Rites of Zhou, 368
rivastigmine, 811, 844, 882
RNA. *See* ribonucleic acid
RNA interference (RNAi), 93–94
ROI. *See* region-of-interest
Roth, Martin, 791
RTT. *See* Rett syndrome
Rubinstein-Taybi syndrome (RSTS),
        101
rules, learning of, 70–71
ryanodine receptors, 47

S
Sacks, Elyn, 346
SAD. *See* seasonal affective disorder
S-adenosylmethionine (SAM-e), 522
SADS. *See* Schedule for Affective
        Disorders and
        Schizophrenia
SAM-e. *See* S-adenosylmethionine
satellite DNA, 78
saving, 70
SBI. *See* silent brain ischemia
scanning. *See* interleaved scanning
Schedule for Affective Disorders and
        Schizophrenia (SADS), 230
schizoaffective disorder
    in DSM-IV, 226–228
    in ICD-10, 227–229
    RDoC for, 226, 225
schizophrenia
    academic development of, as
        psychosis, 223
    affect and, 223
    affective deficits and, 280–281
    ambivalence and, 223
    animal models for, 37–38
    antipsychotic drugs for, 329
    ASD and, 252, 223
    associations and, 223
    autism and, 223
    Bleuler and, 223
    CNVs and, 235–237, 248
        deletions, 248–253
        duplications, 250–253

loci review, 248–253, 249
    in mouse models, 289–290
cognitive deficits and, 280–281
context processing in, 269–270
COS, 328, 949–950
    CNVs in, 949–950
    epigenetics in, 955–956
    exome sequencing for, 950
    SNVs in, 950
cost-benefit analysis and, 275–276
DISC1 gene and, 134, 335
    neuronal pathways for, 334
    Wnt pathways and, 332
DNA methylation and, 97
dopamine hypothesis, 347
in DSM-IV, 226
effort computations in, 278
EM and, 273–275
    cognitive deficits and, 274–275
    cognitive neuroscience models,
        273
    hippocampal activity, 273, 274
    impairments, 273–275
    PFC and, 273
epidemiology for, 232–234
    environmental factors, 233–234
    family studies in, 232–233
    genetic overlap with bipolar
        disorder, 233
    incidence rates for, 232, 247
    non-inherited factors, 233–234
    twin studies in, 232–233
epigenetics and, 97–98, 955–956
factor analysis of, 223
family studies for, 161
Feigner Criteria for, 225
four A's of, 223
functional connectivity in, 1005
GABA and, 304–310
    alterations specific to, 307–309
    in alternate brain regions, 307
    calretinin cells in, 307
    CCK cell alterations, 306, 309
    GAD1 genes, 308
    network oscillations and, 309
    neurotransmission of, 304
    NMDA hypofunction in, 308
    PV neurons, 304–309
    reduced excitation consequences
        in, 309
    SST neurons and, 307
    synthesis alterations, 304
    TrkB genes, 308
    uptake alterations, 304
    in vivo measurements, 307
    WM and, 309
gene expression in, 187
    variations in, 329–330
genetic mapping technologies for,
        168
genetic study methods for,
        234–235
    with candidate genes, 235
    future applications for, 245
    linkage analysis, 234–235
genomic syndromes in
    evidence sources for, 247–248
    low-resolution approaches to,
        247
    mutation rates in, 253
    selection coefficients in, 253,
        254
    VCFS, 247

goal-directed action and, 278–279
goal representations in, 275–280
    effort computation and, 276
    outcome achievements and,
        276
groups, 223
GWAS for, 237–240
    as genetic study method, 234
    linkage disequilibrium
        variances, 237–238
    MHC and, 238–240
    overlap with bipolar disorder,
        242
    risks in, 238
hedonics and liking and, 275,
        276–277
hippocampal dysfunction, 263
    EM and, 273, 274
histone protein modifications and,
        97–98
in ICD-10, 226, 227–228
iPSCs and, 132
Jackson and, 223
large-scale sequencing studies for,
        242–245
MDD and, 398–399
    family studies for, 399
    GenRED study, 398–399
microRNA and, 98
miRNA
    expression and, 98
    pathways, 335
motivational deficits in, 275–280
mouse models of
    behavioral tests in, 295–296
    CNV and, 289–290
    DISC1 genes, 291–292,
        292–293
    dysbindin genes, 290
    etiologic models, 287
    future developments for,
        295–296
    genetic, 288
    through GWAS, 289
    knockout, 292
    with linkage study genes,
        290–292
    non-genetic, 288
    NRG1 genes, 290–291
    pathogenic, 288
    pathophysiological, 287
    PCP-induced hyperactivity in,
        288
    pharmacological, 288
    phenotypic, 287
    risk allele, 292
    symptom-oriented, 288
neural mechanisms for
    cortical-subcortical network
        dysfunction, 263–264
    in cortico-striatal models, 264
    hippocampal dysfunction, 263
    network models, 262–263
    PFC alterations in, 263
neurobiology of
    challenges for, 343–344
    electrophysiology for, 343
    neurobehavioral performance,
        338–339
    neurocognition in, 338–339
    neuroimaging for, 339–342
    neurotransmitters in, 342–343
    olfactory identification in, 339

prodromal concept, 338
    social cognition in, 339
neurodevelopmental model of,
        327–329
    antibodies in, 327–328
    brain volume in, 328
    channel pathways in, 335
    environmental effects in,
        327–328
    immigrant status and, 327
    minority status as influence
        in, 327
    myelin in, 328–329
    neonatal influences in, 327
    neurotransmitters in, 329
    oligodendrocytes in, 328–329
    stress factors in, 327
neuroimaging for, 258–259.
        See also neurobiology, of
        schizophrenia
    with DTI, 341–342
    with fMRI, 342
    with MRI, 340–341
neuronal pathways for, 330–334
    DISC1 genes, 334
    early developmental, 330
neuropathology of, 328
onset of
    during adolescence, 328
    during childhood, 328
PFC and, 258
    alterations as influence on, 263
    DLPFC and, 278–279
    EM and, 273
    in proactive control mechanisms,
        270
    WM and, 272
polygenic sources of, 1074
proactive control in, 270
RDoC for, 225–227, 1085–1086
reactive control in, 270
recurrence risks for, 234
reward prediction/wanting and,
        275, 277–280
risk factors, 132
stem cell modeling for, 132
SUD and, 780
symptoms
    core, 269
    FRS, 223
    negative, 223
    positive, 223
    second rank, 223
synaptic disease and, 322
synaptic pathways, 334
synaptic transmission, 335
SZ, 132
WM in, 270–273
    altered default mode processing
        during, 272–273
    behavioral findings on, 271
    cognitive neuroscience models,
        270–271
    deficit expression, 271
    encoding phases of, 271
    maintenance phase of, 271
    PFC recruitment in, 272
    temporal aspects of, 271
Wnt pathways, 330–334
    canonical signaling, 331–332
    cell morphologies, 333–334
    DISC1 genes, 332
    for neuronal development, 332